Williams
Obstetrics
19th Edition

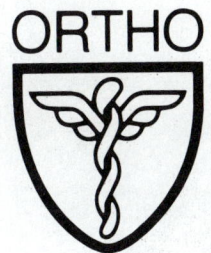

ORTHO

Williams
Obstetrics
—————19ᵗʰ Edition–

F. Gary Cunningham, MD
Professor and Chairman, Department of Obstetrics
  & Gynecology
Jack A. Pritchard Professor of Obstetrics & Gynecology
The University of Texas Southwestern Medical Center
  at Dallas
Chief of Obstetrics & Gynecology, Parkland
  Memorial Hospital

Paul C. MacDonald, MD
Professor, Department of Obstetrics & Gynecology
  and Biochemistry
Cecil H. and Ida Green Distinguished Chair in
  Reproductive Biology
The University of Texas Southwestern Medical Center
  at Dallas
Attending Staff, Parkland Memorial Hospital

Kenneth J. Leveno, MD
Gillette Professor, Department of Obstetrics
  & Gynecology
The University of Texas Southwestern Medical Center
  at Dallas
Chief of Obstetrics, Parkland Memorial Hospital

Norman F. Gant, MD
Professor, Department of Obstetrics & Gynecology
The University of Texas Southwestern Medical Center
  at Dallas
Attending Staff, Parkland Memorial Hospital
Executive Director, American Board of Obstetrics
  & Gynecology

Larry C. Gilstrap III, MD
Professor, Department of Obstetrics & Gynecology
Director of Maternal–Fetal Medicine Fellowship and
  Clinical Genetics
The University of Texas Southwestern Medical Center
  at Dallas
Attending Staff, Parkland Memorial Hospital

ORTHO

APPLETON & LANGE
Norwalk, Connecticut

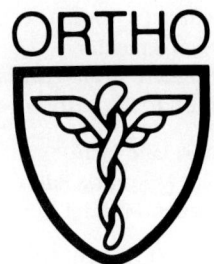

93 94 95 96 97 / 10 9 8 7 6 5 4 3 2 1

Prentice Hall International (UK) Limited, *London*
Prentice Hall of Australia Pty. Limited, *Sydney*
Prentice Hall Canada, Inc., *Toronto*
Prentice Hall Hispanoamericana, S.A., *Mexico*
Prentice Hall of India Private Limited, *New Delhi*
Prentice Hall of Japan, Inc., *Tokyo*
Simon & Schuster Asia Pte. Ltd., *Singapore*
Editora Prentice Hall do Brasil Ltda., *Rio de Janeiro*
Prentice Hall, *Englewood Cliffs, New Jersey*

Library of Congress Cataloging-in-Publication Data

Williams obstetrics. — 19th ed. / F. Gary Cunningham . . . [et al.]
    p. cm.
    Previous ed cataloged under: Williams, J. Whitridge.
    Includes bibliographical references and index.
    ISBN 0-8385-9634-7
    1. Obstetrics. I. Cunningham, F. Gary. II. Williams, J.
Whitridge (John Whitridge), 1866–1931. III. Title: Obstetrics.
    [DNLM: 1. Obstetrics. WQ 100 W7283 1993]
    RG524.W7   1993
    618.2—dc20
    DNLM/DLC
    for Library of Congress   93-6569

Listed here are some recently translated editions of this book and the publishers:

Indonesian (*17th edition*), Airlangga University Press
Italian (*15th edition*), Piccin
Japanese (*15th edition*), Hirokawa
Persian, Franklin
Portuguese (*16th edition*), Ed. Gunabara Koogan
Spanish (*18th edition*), Salvat

Editor: Jane Licht
Senior Managing Editor: John Williams
Designer: Michael Kelly

ISBN 0-8385-9634-7

PRINTED IN THE UNITED STATES OF AMERICA

■ Dedication ■

This book is dedicated to all those medical professionals who provide health care for pregnant women. We especially want to cite the unceasing efforts of the many people who care for underprivileged women and their infants at Parkland Hospital and at community women's clinics throughout Dallas. The hard work of nurses, nurse practitioners, and certified nurse midwives is acknowledged and appreciated. Similarly, we cite the expert care provided by resident physicians, fellows, and faculty of the Departments of Obstetrics & Gynecology, Pediatrics, and Anesthesiology. Importantly, we acknowledge the help of countless unsung heroes who help make such a massive clinical service reach out and touch with dignity the lives of the thousands of mothers and their infants; thus, we thank the ward clerks, orderlies, housekeeping attendants, and others for their dedication and hard work. Without administrative support, both from Parkland and UT Southwestern, such a large clinical service would never operate optimally; we are grateful for help and guidance provided by Parkland's chief executive officer, chief financial officer, and vice president for Women and Children's Services, as well as our president, vice-president for clinical affairs, and dean. Finally, we must include in this dedication the many, many pregnant women who have for almost 40 years entrusted their maternity care to what those aforementioned often affectionately refer to as "Parkland Obstetrics."

Contents

■ Preface ■

Obstetrics is art and science combined, and its practitioners must be concerned simultaneously with the lives of at least two intricately interwoven patients–the mother and her fetus(es). Because the expectation of life with continued good health for these two (or more) persons typically exceed 120 years, it is apparent that the responsibility of the obstetrician is enormous, but then so are the humanitarian rewards of successful pregnancy management.

At first glance, this Nineteenth Edition of *Williams Obstetrics* in some ways suggests a radical change from its predecessor Eighteenth Edition. On closer inspection, however, it becomes apparent that the differences are qualified quantity. For example, for the first time there are five authors, representing an addition of expertness and knowledge to enable us to remain abreast of the myriad developments in normal and abnormal human reproduction. Overall, there are 20 more chapters and the book is 40 percent longer. Fortunately, technology in paper chemistry has allowed a significant increase in bulk without diminished reading quality.

Where is the emphasis with over 400 newly added pages? We again have strived to emphasize the basic principles of sound obstetrical practice based on scientific observations. These principles provide the framework upon which to build an understanding of management of abnormal pregnancy. Therefore, the major changes reflect principally the closer embracing of developments that have been forthcoming since the scientific approach to obstetrics began in earnest in the mid-1960s and which culminated in the development of the relatively new subspecialty of maternal–fetal medicine. Selected sections or chapters of the Eighteenth Edition have been expanded significantly to include more in-depth coverage of topics important to contemporaneous obstetrics. Some examples include the detailed description of the physiological and pathological principles of intrapartum fetal heart and uterine pressure monitoring. Complementing this is an expanded section to include chapters describing various antepartum assessments of fetal health. There now is a chapter devoted to the discussion of pregnancy at the extremes of reproductive life, an important subject for the 1990s. A significant expansion of the application of genetic principles and prenatal diagnosis for obstetricians is included in this edition. There also is a thorough compendium of the effects of drugs and medications that may be taken by the pregnant woman as well as a complete description of the effects of diagnostic radiation during pregnancy. Finally, the section on medical and surgical diseases complicating pregnancy has been doubled compared with that in the previous edition. In addition to a more detailed discussion of diagnosis and management of these conditions, this section now includes a chapter devoted to critical care and trauma.

To accomplish these extensive revisions, the voluminous literature relevant to all aspects of obstetrics and maternal–fetal medicine published since the completion of the Eighteenth Edition was reviewed. More than 3000 references have been added, along with 200 new figures and tables. Continuing the tradition of the past five editions, we cite frequently our cumulative clinical experience provided by the large obstetrical service at Parkland Hospital. We do so to develop unambiguous recommendations for the management of a variety of obstetrical problems and complications. We emphasize, as we have before, that these should not be interpreted as the only acceptable management schemes to obtain a favorable pregnancy outcome. Indeed, the "Parkland way"—as it is referred to, almost (ir)reverently, by our faculty, fellows, housestaff, and nurses—is but one established approach; nonetheless, it is one that certainly has served the women we care for well. Indeed, this approach has been our cornerstone in the development of obstetrical care plans that have proved useful for the successful management of more than a third of a million pregnant women and their fetuses.

The production of a textbook is not possible without the dedication and hard work of many uncited but vitally important people. Certainly an incredible amount of time is necessary for a revision of this magnitude. The contributions and participation of many persons in the Department of Obstetrics & Gynecology were essential to ensure the timely printing of the Nineteenth Edition. To these individuals, we are truly grateful. Once again, Dr. Alvin "Bud" Brekken took on yet a third job and provided strong leadership for the Department when the writing chores took their heaviest toll. Dr. Linette Casey facilitated the incorporation of important basic science principles that underlay clinical obstetrics and in particular parturition. Providing expert advice from their specialized fields were Dr. David Hemsell for ectopic pregnancy, Dr. George Wendel for sexually transmitted diseases, Dr. Tom Lowe for medical and surgical illnesses complicating pregnancy, Drs. Barry Schwarz and Uel Crosby for family planning, Drs. Mark Maberry, Bert Little, Mary Jo Harrod, and Nancy Schneider for genetics and teratology, Drs. Rigoberto Santos and Diane Twickler for ultrasonography, Dr. Donald Wallace for obstetrical anesthesia, and Dr. David Miller for trophoblastic disease. Dr. Gary Hankins from Wilford Hall USAF Hospital provided expert help in the discussions of critical care. Just as important, numerous unmentioned faculty and fellows readily and graciously helped to assume our duties and "took up the slack" at particularly busy times. To name but a few, particular thanks is given to those maternal–fetal medicine faculty members who cheerfully assumed additional clinical burdens: Drs. Charles Brown, Ralph DePalma, Kenneth Goldaber, Michael Lucas, Mark Peters, and Susan Ramin. As before, the inquiring minds of the obstetrical housestaff and maternal–fetal medicine fellows served as a constant stimulus. We are pleased, therefore, to acknowledge that this Nineteenth Edition is the product of the efforts of an entire Department.

From the beginning of the development of this edition, planning, assistance, and encouragement were provided by our colleagues at Appleton & Lange. At the outset, Lin Paterson provided encouragement and advice in developing the new format. We note sadly Lin's death after a lengthy battle with cancer—her courage is an inspiration to everyone that she touched. Subsequently, Jane Licht has resumed editorial responsibilities for us, and she and John Williams have guided us capably through rough waters and provided expertise with more planning and guidance, editorial production, and importantly, attention to details.

In our Department, Rosemary Bell, Laurie Daniels, Julie Jackson, Beverly King, Carol Lewis, Lynne McDonnell, Kimberly McKinney, and Janet Rensmeyer spent many overtime hours preparing manuscript to meet deadlines. New and beautifully revised artwork was provided by the very talented Nancy Marshburn. As with the Eighteenth Edition, the success of such a massive endeavor would be doomed without a project director. Once again, Marsha Congleton provided vast experience and great expertness as production coordinator, as severe taskmaster, and importantly, as mother confessor. To all of these people, and to many more who are unnamed, we are grateful.

During the thousands of hours spent during the year in which the manuscript was produced, we again neglected our families even more so than usual. Despite this neglect, they have been understanding, supportive, and helpful. Clearly, the Nineteenth Edition also is a "family production." To family, as well as to our friends and colleagues, we give our sincerest thanks and deepest affection.

Williams
Obstetrics
—— 19th Edition —

Juan F Posada

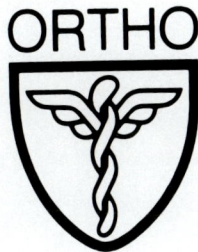

ORTHO

■ SECTION I ■
Human Pregnancy

■

CHAPTER 1
Obstetrics in Broad Perspective

Obstetrics is the branch of medicine that deals with parturition, its antecedents, and its sequels (*Oxford English Dictionary,* 1933). It is principally concerned, therefore, with the phenomena and management of pregnancy, labor, and the puerperium, in both normal and abnormal circumstances.

In a broader sense, obstetrics is concerned with the reproduction of a society. Obstetrical care, when appropriately practiced, should promote health and well-being, both physical and mental, among couples and their offspring, and should help them to develop healthy attitudes toward sex, family life, and the place of the family in society. Obstetrics is concerned with all the physiological, pathological, psychological, and social factors that profoundly influence both the quantity and the quality of human reproduction. The problems of population growth are the natural heritage of obstetrics. The vital statistics of the nation, published monthly by the National Center for Health Statistics, attest to society's concern with the charge of this specialty.

The word *obstetrics* is derived from the Latin term *obstetrix,* meaning "midwife." The etymology of *obstetrix,* however, is obscure. In most dictionaries, it is connected with the verb *obstare,* which means "to stand by" or "in front of." The rationale of this derivation is that the midwife stood by or in front of the parturient. This has long been attacked by some etymologists, who believe that the word was originally *adstetrix* and that the *ad* was changed to *ob.* In that case, *obstetrix* would mean "the woman assisting the parturient." The fact that on certain inscriptions *obstetrix* is also spelled *opstetrix* has led to the conjecture that it was derived from *ops* (*aid*) and *stare,* meaning "the woman rendering aid." According to Temkin,* the most likely interpretation is that *obstetrix* meant "the woman who stood by the parturient." Whether it alluded merely to the midwife's standing in front of or near the parturient, or whether it

carried the additional connotation of rendering aid, is not clear.

The term *obstetrics* is of relatively recent usage. The *Oxford English Dictionary* gives the earliest example from a book published in 1819, and indicates that in 1828 it was necessary to apologize for the use of the word *obstetrician.* Kindred terms, however, are much older. For example, *obstetricate* is found in English works published as early as 1623; *obstetricatory,* in 1640; *obstetricious,* in 1645; and *obstetrical,* in 1775. These terms were often used figuratively. As an example of such usage, the adjective *obstetric* appears in Pope's *Dunciad* (1742) in the famous couplet:

> There all the Learn'd shall at the labour stand, and
> Douglas lend his soft, obstetric hand.

The much older term *midwifery* was used instead of *obstetrics* until the latter part of the 19th century in both the United States and Great Britain. It is derived from the Middle English *mid,* meaning "with," and *wif,* meaning "wife" in the sense of a woman. The term *midwife* was used as early as 1303, and *midwifery* in 1483.

Aims of Obstetrics. The transcendent objective of obstetrics is that every pregnancy be wanted, and that it culminate in a healthy mother and a healthy baby. Obstetrics strives to minimize the number of women and infants who die as a result of the reproductive process or who are left physically, intellectually, or emotionally injured from the process. Obstetrics is further con-

---

* Previous communication. Dr. Owsei Temkin, Associate Professor of the History of Medicine, Johns Hopkins University School of Medicine, graciously devoted time to a study of the etymology of the word *obstetrics,* and the comments cited are entirely his.

cerned with the number and spacing of children so that both mother and offspring, indeed all the family, may enjoy optimal physical and emotional well-being. Finally, obstetrics strives to analyze and influence the social factors that impinge on reproductive efficiency.

Vital Statistics. To aid in the reduction of mothers and infants who die as a consequence of pregnancy and labor, it is important to know how many such deaths there are in this country each year and in what circumstances. To evaluate these data correctly, a variety of events concerned with pregnancy outcomes have been defined by various agencies:

- **Birth.** This is the complete expulsion or extraction from the mother of a fetus irrespective of whether the umbilical cord has been cut or the placenta is attached. Fetuses weighing less than 500 g are usually not considered as births, but rather as *abortuses,* for purposes of perinatal statistics. In the absence of a birthweight, a body length of 25 cm, crown to heel, is usually equated with 500 g. Approximately 20 weeks' gestational age is commonly considered to be equivalent to 500 g fetal weight; however, a 500 g fetus is actually more likely to be 22 (menstrual) weeks' gestational age.
- **Birthrate.** The number of live births per 1000 population is the birthrate, or crude birthrate. The birthrate in the United States for the year ending May 1991 was 16.5 (National Center for Health Statistics, 1991).
- **Fertility rate.** This term refers to the number of live births per 1000 female population aged 15 through 44 years. In 1991 this was 70.9.
- **Live birth.** Whenever the infant at or some time after birth breathes spontaneously, or shows any other sign of life such as heartbeat or definite spontaneous movement of voluntary muscles, a live birth is recorded.
- **Stillbirth.** None of the signs of life are present at or after birth.
- **Neonatal death.** Early neonatal death refers to death of a live-born infant during the first 7 days after birth. Late neonatal death refers to death after 7 but before 29 days.
- **Stillbirth rate (fetal death rate).** The number of stillborn infants per 1000 infants born, including live births and stillbirths.
- **Neonatal mortality rate.** The number of neonatal deaths per 1000 live births.
- **Perinatal mortality rate.** This rate is defined as the number of stillbirths plus neonatal deaths per 1000 total births.
- **Low birthweight.** If the first newborn weight obtained after birth is less than 2500 g, the infant is termed low birthweight.

- **Term infant.** An infant born anytime after 37 completed (menstrual) weeks of gestation through 42 completed weeks of gestation (260 to 294 days) is considered by most to be a term infant. Such a definition implies that birth at any time within this period is optimal, whereas birth before or afterward is not. Such an implication is not warranted. Some infants born between 37 and 38 weeks are at risk of functional prematurity, as with the development of respiratory distress in the newborn infant of a diabetic mother (see Chap. 53, p. 1201). In the past, some considered gestation extending past 41 weeks to be postterm; however, any risk to the fetus that might be imposed by remaining in utero until 42 weeks rather than 41 weeks does not appear to be appreciable (see Chap. 38, p. 871).
- **Preterm infant.** An infant born before 37 completed weeks has been so classified, although born before 38 completed weeks would seem more appropriate for reasons stated above. In the past, *prematurity* was used synonymously with preterm birth.
- **Postterm infant.** An infant born anytime after completion of the 42nd week has been classified by some as postterm.
- **Abortus.** A fetus or embryo removed or expelled from the uterus during the first half of gestation (20 weeks or less), weighing less than 500 g, or measuring less than 25 cm is also referred to as an abortus.
- **Direct maternal death.** Death of the mother resulting from obstetrical complications of pregnancy, labor, or the puerperium, and from interventions, omissions, incorrect treatment, or a chain of events resulting from any of the above is considered a direct maternal death. An example is maternal death from exsanguination resulting from rupture of the uterus.
- **Indirect maternal death.** An obstetrical death not directly due to obstetrical causes but resulting from previously existing disease, or a disease that developed during pregnancy, labor, or the puerperium, but which was aggravated by the maternal physiological adaptation to pregnancy, is classified as an indirect maternal death. An example is maternal death from complications of mitral stenosis.
- **Nonmaternal death.** Death of the mother resulting from accidental or incidental causes in no way related to the pregnancy may be classified as a nonmaternal death. An example is death from an automobile accident.
- **Maternal mortality ratio.** The number of maternal deaths that result from the reproductive process per 100,000 live births. Used more commonly, but less accurately, are the terms *ma-*

ternal mortality rate or *maternal death rate*. The term *ratio* is more accurate because it includes in the numerator the number of deaths regardless of pregnancy outcome (e.g., live births, stillbirths, ectopic pregnancies), while the denominator includes the number of live births (Koonin and colleagues, 1989).

The Birthrate and Fertility Rate. One index of the need for obstetrical personnel and facilities is the number of births each year. Additional indices are the birthrate and the fertility rate. From these data, particularly the fertility rate, the expected number of births in future years can be estimated.

According to the National Center for Health Statistics (1991), there were 4.14 million live births in the United States for the year ending May 1991. This was the largest number of births recorded since 1964. The fertility rate was 70.4 in 1991, while it was 64.9 in 1986. There also was an increase in the number of women in the childbearing years, and thus, the reason for more births in 1991 was an increase in the number of women between 15 and 44 years of age as well as a slight increase in their fertility. According to the center, women born during the post–World War II "baby boom" accounted for much of this increase (see Chap. 30, p. 653).

Maternal Mortality

United States. In the United States, the number of maternal deaths per 100,000 live births has decreased remarkably in the past half century. From 1979 through 1986, according to the Centers for Disease Control (Koonin and colleagues, 1991), a total of 2726 pregnancy-related deaths were reported, for a maternal mortality ratio of 9.1 per 100,000 live births. By way of comparison, there were 12,544 maternal deaths, or 582 per 100,000 live births in 1935! Values for intervening years are presented in Table 1–1.

TABLE 1–1. MATERNAL MORTALITY IN THE UNITED STATES, 1935–1985

Maternal Deaths		Ratio Per 100,000 Live Births			Other/White
Year	Number	Total	White	Other	Ratio
1935	12,544	582.1	530.6	945.7	1.8
1940	8876	376.0	319.8	773.5	2.4
1945	5668	107.2	172.1	454.8	2.6
1950	2960	83.3	61.1	221.6	3.6
1955	1901	47.0	32.8	130.3	4.0
1960	1579	37.1	26.0	97.9	3.8
1965	1189	31.6	21.0	83.7	4.0
1970	803	21.5	14.4	55.9	3.9
1975	403	12.8	9.1	29.0	3.2
1980	334	9.2	6.7	19.8	3.0
1985	295	7.8	5.2	18.1	3.5

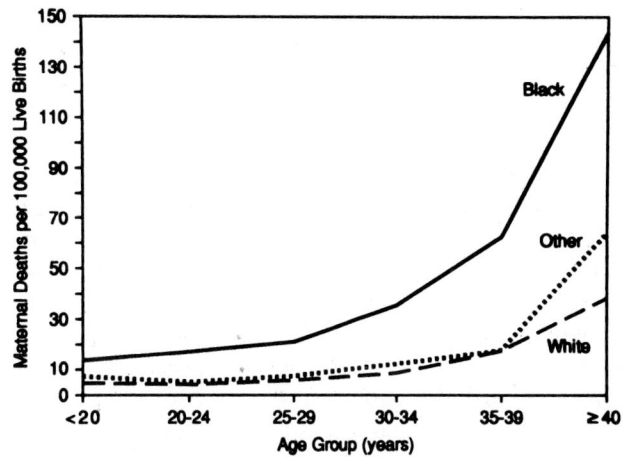

Fig. 1–1. Maternal mortality ratio, by age group and race. Figures for the United States, 1979 through 1986, as reported to the Centers for Disease Control. (From Koonin and colleagues, 1991.)

The maternal mortality ratio for African-American women compared with white women is increased appreciably (Fig. 1–1). The differences in maternal mortality appears to result primarily from social and economical factors, such as a relative lack of skilled personnel and appropriate facilities at delivery, lack of antepartum care, lack of family planning services, faulty health education, and dietary deficiencies. Other conditions commonly cited are higher mortality rates due to induced abortion and ectopic pregnancy. As these unfavorable social and economical conditions are improved, the racial difference in the maternal death rates hopefully will decrease, but a nonwhite woman in the United States still has a threefold greater incidence of death during pregnancy than a white woman (Table 1–1). **This unfortunately has not changed in the richest country in the world!** In fact, the maternal death ratio for nonwhite women in 1985 was approximately the same as that for white women 20 years before.

As shown in Figure 1–1, the maternal mortality ratio also varies with the age of the mother (see Chap. 30, p. 655). In all races, the remarkable increase in mortality with advancing age can be explained only on the basis of an intrinsic maternal factor(s). The increasing frequency of hypertension with advancing years and the greater tendency to uterine hemorrhage contribute significantly to the increased mortality rate. Advanced age and high parity act independently to increase the risk of childbearing, but their effects are usually additive. In the actual analysis of cases, it is difficult to dissociate these two factors.

The World. In 1991, the World Health Organization estimated that nearly 500,000 women die annually from pregnancy-related causes. Tragically, all but 6000 of these are in undeveloped countries. They cited that a woman's likelihood of death from pregnancy in Africa is 1 in 20!

Common Causes of Maternal Mortality. Hemorrhage, hypertension that is either induced or aggravated by pregnancy, and infection still account for half of direct maternal deaths in the United States (Atrash and colleagues, 1990, Kaunitz and associates, 1985). Common causes of maternal mortality are shown in Figure 1–2. The causes of obstetrical hemorrhage are multiple and include postpartum hemorrhage, bleeding in association with abortion, bleeding from ectopic pregnancy, bleeding as the result of abnormal placental location or separation (placenta previa and abruptio placentae), and bleeding from uterine rupture. Hypertension, induced or aggravated by pregnancy, complicates about 5 percent of pregnancies and is commonly accompanied by edema and proteinuria (preeclampsia), and in some severe cases by convulsions and coma (eclampsia). Puerperal infection, or postpartum pelvic infection, usually begins as uterine and parametrial infection, but sometimes it undergoes extension to cause peritonitis, thrombophlebitis, and bacteremia. Trauma accounted for almost one half of maternal deaths in Cook County from 1986 through 1989 (Fildes and associates, 1992). Details of the origin, prevention, and treatment of these conditions form a considerable portion of the subject matter of obstetrics.

Unfortunately, maternal deaths are underreported. The Centers for Disease Control, in conjunction with the American College of Obstetricians and Gynecologists, established the Maternal Mortality Collaborative to determine the accuracy of voluntary reporting (Koonin

and colleagues, 1989, Rochat and associates, 1988). Over the 6-year period from 1980 through 1985, 19 reporting areas, including 16 states, reported a total of 601 maternal deaths. This number was 40 percent more than deaths reported for these areas by the National Center for Health Statistics.

Reasons for Decline in Maternal Mortality. Many factors and agencies are responsible for the dramatic fall in the maternal death rate in this country over the past 50 years. Obviously, there has been a general improvement in medical practice. The widespread use of blood transfusion and antimicrobial drugs, and the maintenance of fluid, electrolyte, and acid-base balance in the serious complications of pregnancy and labor, have materially changed obstetrical practice. Equally important is the development of widespread obstetrical training and continuing educational programs, which have provided more and better qualified specialists. Similarly, training programs in anesthesia, as well as the recognition that obstetrical anesthesia requires special personnel and equipment, have substantially lowered the maternal death rate from its use.

Obstetrics is unique in that no other branch of medicine is subject to such careful public scrutiny. Not only are births a matter of public record, but maternal and perinatal deaths are examined by municipal, state, and national health authorities. In many areas, at least in the past, local medical or obstetrical and gynecological societies also examined such deaths, and mortality conferences were frequently conducted as part of the continuing medical education of the obstetrician. Unfortunately, because these proceedings are subject to

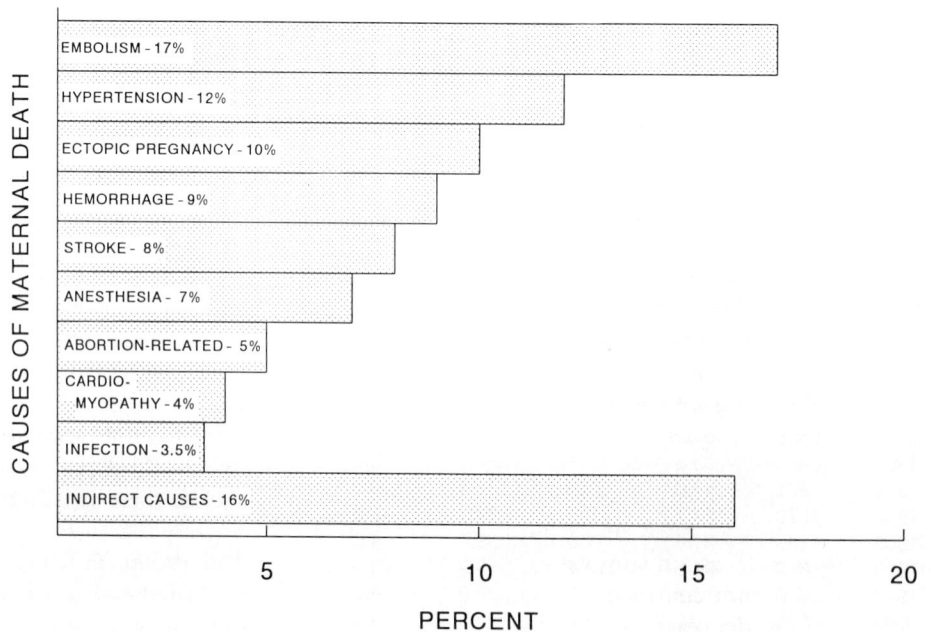

Fig. 1–2. Major causes of 601 maternal deaths in the United States from 1980 through 1985 and evaluated by the Maternal Mortality Collaborative. (From Koonin and colleagues, 1989.)

CAUSES OF MATERNAL DEATH

EMBOLISM - 17%
HYPERTENSION - 12%
ECTOPIC PREGNANCY - 10%
HEMORRHAGE - 9%
STROKE - 8%
ANESTHESIA - 7%
ABORTION-RELATED - 5%
CARDIO-MYOPATHY - 4%
INFECTION - 3.5%
INDIRECT CAUSES - 16%

PERCENT

TABLE 1–2. REPRODUCTIVE MORTALITY IN THE UNITED STATES BY CAUSE—1955, 1976, AND 1982

| | Estimated Number of Deaths | | | | | | | |
| | Pregnancy Related | | | Contraception Related | | | | |
Year	Ectopic Pregnancy	Abortion	Other Deaths	OC[a]	IUD[a]	Sterilization	Total Deaths	Reproductive Mortality Rate[b]
1955	139	485	2065	—	—	14	2703	7.8
1975	50	49	428	452	6	14	999	2.1
1982	—	7	369	327	25	23	751	1.4

[a] OC = oral contraceptives; IUD = intrauterine device (neither used in 1955).
[b] Rate per 100,000 women aged 15 to 44.
Data from Rosenberg and Rosenthal (1987); Sachs and associates (1982).

subpoena to substantiate alleged malpractice claims, their utility has been diminished, and this has detracted greatly from their educational value.

The *sine qua non* of good work in any field is well-trained personnel, but they could not have achieved the excellent results had there not been a great expansion in facilities for good obstetrical care. Despite increased facilities, there remain areas in the United States where obstetrical services woefully are inadequate, particularly in rural areas and in some large inner cities.

From the viewpoint of safer care during labor, the outstanding advance of the past 40 years has been the great increase in the proportion of hospital deliveries. As recently as 1940, only 60 percent of white births took place in hospitals, but this figure now exceeds 99 percent. Hospital births not only mean better facilities but imply care by individuals specially trained in obstetrics and perinatology. More recently, *birthing centers* have become popular as nonhospital facilities to provide maternity care for low-risk women. Although Rooks and colleagues (1989) contend that such birth centers are safe and acceptable alternatives for selected pregnant women, it appears that their use is associated with more intrapartum fetal deaths compared with hospital deliveries (Leveno and Cunningham, 1990). Because about 1 in 10 women who labor in these centers develop complications, a close hospital alliance is mandatory. Indeed, Lieberman and Ryan (1989) suggest that such centers should be located in hospitals.

Reproductive Mortality. In more recent years, as the maternal mortality rate decreased markedly, some deaths were occurring as the consequence of a great increase in the use of various contraceptive techniques. The sum of the mortalities from pregnancy and from the use of these techniques to prevent pregnancy has been termed *reproductive mortality.* As shown in Table 1–2, in spite of the innovation and widespread use of oral contraceptives and intrauterine devices accompanied by a marked increase in surgical sterilization, the number of deaths from contraception was slight compared with the larger decrease in maternal mortality.

Perinatal Mortality. The sum of stillbirths and neonatal deaths is termed *perinatal mortality.* The perinatal death rate has fallen by nearly 50 percent in the past 25 years (Table 1–3). Currently, there are about 180 perinatal deaths for every maternal death. With the current very low incidence of maternal deaths, perinatal loss rates not only are a better index of the level of obstetrical care, but also give a valid indication of an equally important obstetrical indicator, *infant morbidity.* To some extent, the total perinatal loss is correlated with the age and parity of the mother. The rates tend to be highest for the firstborn of very young women and births of the order of six and over.

Factors Affecting the Stillbirth Rate. About half of perinatal deaths are stillbirths. Stillbirths tend to decline as the quality of care during and throughout pregnancy improves. With improvement in prenatal care and proper hospitalization, some of these deaths are preventable. In too large a proportion of fetal deaths, un-

TABLE 1–3. PERINATAL MORTALITY IN THE UNITED STATES, 1950–1989

Year	Perinatal[a] Number	Rate[d]	Fetal[b] Number	Rate[d]	Neonatal[c] Number	Rate[e]
1950	141,117	39.0	68,262	18.8	72,855	20.5
1960	148,213	34.3	68,480	15.8	79,733	18.7
1970	109,240	28.9	52,961	14.0	56,279	15.1
1980	63,971	17.5	33,353	9.1	30,618	8.5
1985	55,840	14.7	29,661	7.8	26,179	7.0
1986	54,184	14.3	28,972	7.7	25,212	6.7
1987	53,976	14.1	29,349	7.6	24,627	6.5
1988	54,132	13.7	29,442	7.5	24,690	6.3
1989	55,637	13.7	30,469	7.5	25,168	6.2

[a] Includes fetal deaths of 20 weeks' gestation or greater and infant deaths of less than 28 days.
[b] Fetal deaths of 20 weeks' gestation or more.
[c] Infant deaths of less than 29 days.
[d] Rate per 1000 live births and fetal deaths.
[e] Rate per 1000 live births.
From National Center for Health Statistics (1985, 1986, 1987, 1988, 1992); unpublished data courtesy of Drs. Donna Hoyert and Harry Rosenberg of the National Center for Health Statistics.

fortunately, there may be no obvious explanation. Fretts and colleagues (1992) reported that deaths due to intrapartum fetal asphyxia almost have disappeared, and there has been a significant decline in unexplained antepartum fetal deaths.

Neonatal Deaths. In 1977, for the first time in the United States, there were fewer neonatal deaths than fetal deaths (stillbirths). Nearly half of the neonatal deaths occur in the first day of life. The number of deaths during those 24 hours exceeds that from the second month to the completion of the first year. The causes of this huge wastage during the neonatal period are numerous, but the most important is low birthweight, usually as the consequence of preterm delivery. The proportion of low-birthweight infants differs among ethnic groups, ranging from about 60 per 1000 for white mothers to approximately 120 per 1000 for African-American women. The interracial difference in the rates of low birthweight accounts for the major difference in neonatal mortality between these two groups. Although social and environmental factors heavily affect this difference, lack of access to medical care is likely a major factor. As well as deaths, low birthweight has contributed appreciably to infant morbidity, and to a large fraction of the neurological and intellectual deficits that are tragic individually and collectively costly to society. Why some women go into labor before term is one of the greatest unsolved problems of obstetrics.

The second most common cause of neonatal death is congenital malformations. These first two causes also contribute significantly to infant mortality, or deaths after 28 days but before 1 year of life (National Center for Health Statistics, 1991). Another common cause is injury to the central nervous system. Here the word *injury* is used in its broadest sense to indicate both cerebral injury resulting from hypoxia in utero and traumatic injury to the brain during labor and delivery. Fortunately, both are becoming very uncommon.

The Birth Certificate. In all 50 states and the District of Columbia, a birth certificate is required by law to be submitted promptly to the local registrar. An extensively revised document was implemented in January 1989. After a birth has been registered, notification is sent to the parents of the child, and a complete report is forwarded to the National Center for Health Statistics in Washington.

There are many reasons why complete and accurate registration of births is essential. Certification of the facts of birth is needed as evidence of age, citizenship, and family relationships. Moreover, the data provided are of immeasurable importance to all agencies (social, public health, demographic, or obstetrical) dealing with human reproduction. For instance, the data presented in the foregoing paragraphs were obtained almost entirely from information published by the National Center for Health Statistics on the basis of birth certificates, and this represents only a small fraction of the information obtainable from that source. A birth certificate provides even more data of direct obstetrical importance. **Hence, the prompt and accurate completion of this certificate after each birth is not only a legal duty but a contribution to the broad field of obstetrical knowledge.**

Obstetrics and Other Branches of Medicine. Obstetrics is a multifaceted discipline with close and numerous relations to other branches of medicine. It is related so intimately to the kindred subject of gynecology that obstetrics and gynecology are generally regarded as one specialty. Gynecology deals with the physiology and the pathology of the female reproductive organs in the nonpregnant state, whereas obstetrics deals with the pregnant state and its sequels. Correct differential diagnosis in either obstetrics or gynecology entails an intimate acquaintance with the clinical syndromes met in both, and the methods of examination and many operative techniques are common to both disciplines. Indeed, Pearse (in press) has rightfully encouraged that obstetrician–gynecologists lead the movement for comprehensive women's health care.

The scope of fetal diagnosis and treatment has broadened remarkably, as discussed especially in Chapter 41. This, as well as the concern of obstetrics with the newborn infant, has brought the subject into close relation with pediatrics and given rise to the concept of perinatology. The boundaries between obstetrics and neonatology are not sharp, but rather overlap to the benefit of the fetus and infant. Even in metropolitan centers, inconvenient hours of birth often impose on the obstetrician the management of a newborn during the most critical hour of life. The obstetrician must be knowledgeable, therefore, in the management of the infant at this time as well as before birth.

Because pregnant and nonpregnant women are subject to the same diseases, the obstetrician commonly encounters and therefore must be knowledgeable about a variety of diseases in pregnant women. As emphasized in Section XIII, the clinical picture presented by some of these disorders may be altered remarkably during pregnancy and the immediate puerperium; likewise, these diseases may affect the course of gestation.

Obstetrics is related closely to most clinical and preclinical sciences. The study of spontaneous abortion, for example, depends on knowledge of anomalies in the development of the early embryo and trophoblast. Abortion may also involve hormonal defects, a condition that would link the subjects of obstetrics and endocrinology; or abortion may result from chromosomal defects, and such a condition forges a link to cytogenetics. The concept of erythrocyte antigen isoimmunization has shown how immunological factors may interfere with the successful outcome of pregnancy, but in turn, by appropriate immunotherapy, how such interference may be successfully prevented. Obstetrics and general pathology meet closely in the rapidly developing field of perinatal pathology. In studies of fetal malformation, clinical genetics is of prime importance. Other important relations of obstetrics to preclinical sciences include microbiology, in the study of maternal and fetal infections; biochemistry and physiology, in relation to myriad events including labor; pharmacology, in the action and metabolism of drugs in the mother and in the fetus and newborn infant; and molecular genetics, from which techniques are used to identify fetuses with an ever-increasing number of inherited disease. The numerous applications of the preclinical sciences to problems of human reproduction are evident in the relatively short but remarkable history of the National Institute of Child Health and Human Development.

Obstetrics is also related to certain fields that are not strictly medical. Because nutritional requirements are altered by pregnancy, obstetrics requires knowledge of the science of nutrition. Because the mother–child relationship is the basis of the family unit, the obstetrician continually is dealing with psychological and sociological problems. Economics play a prominent role in obstetrics because health care may be quite expensive. Additionally, obstetrics has important legal aspects, especially with respect to the increasing number of suits alleging malpractice.

Obstetrics, the Mother, and Her Family. In spite of the remarkable record of safety for the hospitalized expectant mother and her fetus-infant that has been achieved in recent years, there has evolved a small but quite vocal group of dissidents made up of former parturients, their partners, and those who would attempt to provide care during home delivery. Hopefully, those complaints about hospitalization for which there are real bases can be resolved short of sacrificing the safety that hospitalization for delivery can provide the mother and especially her fetus-infant.

There is no question that some individuals who collaborate in the effort to provide optimal in-hospital care for the mother and the fetus-infant have not been as considerate of the pregnant woman and her family as they should have been. The expectant woman has commonly been treated as if she were seriously ill, even when she was quite healthy. All too often she has been forced to conform to a common pathway of care that stripped her of most of her individuality and much of her dignity. Pleasant surroundings have not always been provided; instead, hospital austerity has prevailed. Hospital administrators have tended not to seek her business, claiming they lost money on obstetrics. In recent years, obstetricians, for many good reasons, have worked mostly in groups and as a consequence, about

the time of delivery—the ultimate event in the minds of the woman and her family—there may have either been a "changing of the obstetrical guard" or the obstetrician may have created the appearance of wanting to hurry the labor and delivery because he or she would soon be "going off duty." The same picture has been presented by the nurses and other personnel intimately involved in providing care for the woman and her fetus-infant. Too often the expectant mother has felt that her fate, and the fate of her baby, were dependent not so much on skilled personnel but upon an electronical cabinet that appeared to possess some great power that prevailed above all others. Fortunately, appropriate applications of medical science do not require that excellent care be a dehumanizing ordeal. Excellent obstetrical care and the many benefits that accrue from it can be provided in a hospital setting that, at the same time, is enjoyed by the woman and her family, and is acceptable economically to all parties involved.

The Future. Although the recent decline in maternal mortality rate has been enormous, continuous improvements in maternal health care are needed. If the nonwhite mortality rate were reduced to the level of that of white women by providing equal care, and if the deaths in all women considered preventable by many mortality studies were averted, approximately two thirds of current maternal deaths could be prevented. Maternal mortality most seriously affects the socially and economically deprived. Many of these deaths result from sheer lack of adequate facilities, including lack of properly distributed units for antepartum care, lack of suitable hospital arrangements, and lack of readily available blood for transfusion. Others are caused by errors of management by the obstetrical personnel. Errors of omission include failure to provide antepartum care, failure to follow the woman and fetus carefully throughout labor and the early puerperium, and failure to obtain appropriate consultation.

These several deficiencies in maternity care obviously must be corrected first if maternal and perinatal mortality rates are to be brought to the irreducible minimum. Indeed, the United States Public Health Service (1989) has identified significant maternal and fetal priorities in its *Year 2000 Objectives for the Nation.* Some of these goals include significant lowering of the neonatal and fetal mortality rates. They can and doubtless will be lowered to that level by the same methods that have proved efficacious in the past: more and better trained personnel and well-equipped facilities available to all pregnant women and their fetuses. Davidson (1991) appropriately calls for intense scrutiny of fetal and infant mortality by committees, modeled after maternal mortality committees.

Along with these improvements to better insure pregnancy outcome is the realization that costs for obstetrical care are rising in an unprecedented fashion.

Simply put, technology is expensive, and the addition to routine prenatal care of various screening tests to detect relatively uncommon diseases will continue to increase the costs of prenatal care. For example, maternal serum screening is now used to detect high or low alphafeto-protein concentration that may suggest a neural-tube defect or chromosomally abnormal fetus. Although the yield of such screening techniques is low, the technological and counseling services needed to support such programs are expensive. Along with the availability of easily performed and widely accessible techniques of molecular genetics to diagnose inherited diseases during early pregnancy comes the formidable pricetag for the use of such technology.

Commonly used methods of fetal health assessment include ultrasound to visualize the fetus for anatomical aberrations as well as to measure fetal growth. Electronical assessment of fetal heart rate and its reaction to a variety of stimuli is used to predict fetal well-being. Many times, a combination of fetal heart rate reactivity and ultrasonic evaluation is conducted simultaneously. Such innovations are also expensive, both from the technological as well as personnel standpoints. Thus, obstetrical care has become expensive for consumers, who typically are young couples getting started in life, and who can least afford to bear escalating and sometimes overwhelming medical costs.

The impact of malpractice litigation on obstetrics cannot be ignored. The Institute of Medicine (1989) reviewed the status of professional liability on the practice of obstetrics in the United States. The committee concluded that there indeed is a professional liability crisis in our country. Although the intensive surveillance of perinatal outcome by patients and plaintiff attorneys has served, in some instances, to improve some obstetrical practices, it is unreasonable and unfair to assume automatically that a less than salutary outcome is always caused by neglect or incompetence. An example is cerebral palsy, which, as discussed in Chapter 44, seldom follows recognizable perinatal insults, but whose identification commonly places the health-care providers in a defensive posture, forced to prove that medical mismanagement **did not** cause the injury. In these and similar cases with imperfect outcomes, litigation is instituted too frequently by overzealous and oftentimes self-serving avaricious attorneys in search of huge settlements. Too often, in many of these cases, "expert" witnesses readily provide dogmatic opinions to chronicle alleged obstetrical mismanagement. Such practices have also served to increase the cost of obstetrical care, because malpractice insurance premiums necessarily are passed on to patients. Another adverse effect of the so-called "litigation crisis" is that a large number of skilled clinicians are voluntarily retiring from the practice of obstetrics. Finally, high-cost litigation has also decreased the already marginal availability of obstetrical care for indigent women.

Nevertheless, the concept of the right of every child to be physically, mentally, and emotionally "well-born" is fundamental to human dignity. If obstetrics is to serve a role in the realization of this goal, the specialty must maintain and even extend its role in the control of population growth. The right to be "well-born" in its broadest sense is simply incompatible with unrestricted fertility. Yet our knowledge of the forces operative in the fluctuation and control of population growth is still rudimentary. This concept of obstetrics as a social as well as a biological science impels us to accept a responsibility unprecedented in American medicine. What remains to be done by society is to accept with us the responsibility for these pregnant women and their fetus-infants. This responsibility includes the economical means to provide the same quality and quantity of care for socially and economically disadvantaged women. Finally, medical progress does not "just happen," and progress is based upon laboratory and clinical research. Without research there is no progress; and without this progress women and children will continue to suffer and die needlessly.

References

Atrash HK, Koonin LM, Lawson HW, Franks AL, Smith JC: Maternal mortality in the United States, 1979–1986. Obstet Gynecol 76:1055, 1990

Davidson EC Jr: A strategy to reduce infant mortality. Obstet Gynecol 77:1, 1991

Fildes J, Reed L, Jones N, Martin M, Barrett J: Trauma: The leading cause of maternal death. J Trauma 32:643, 1992

Fretts RC, Boyd ME, Usher RH, Usher HA: The changing pattern of fetal death, 1961–1988. Obstet Gynecol 79:35, 1992

Institute of Medicine: Medical Professional Liability and the Delivery of Obstetrical Care, Vol I. Washington, DC, National Academy Press, 1989

Kaunitz AM, Hughes JM, Grimes DA, Smith JC, Rochat RW, Kafrissen ME: Causes of maternal mortality in the United States. Obstet Gynecol 65:605, 1985

Koonin LM, Atrash HK, Lawson HW, Smith JC: Maternal mortality surveillance, United States, 1979–1986. MMWR 40:1, 1991

Koonin LM, Atrash HK, Rochat RW, Smith JC: Maternal mortality surveillance, United States, 1980–1985. MMWR 37:19, 1989

Leveno KJ, Cunningham FG: Outcome of care in birth centers. N Engl J Med 322:1528, 1990

Lieberman E, Ryan KJ: Birth-day choices. N Engl J Med 321:1824, 1989

National Center for Health Statistics: Births, marriages, divorces, and deaths for May, 1991. Monthly Vital Stat Rep 40:5, 1991

National Center for Health Statistics: *Vital Statistics of the United States*, Vol. II. Mortality. Washington, DC, NCHS, 1985, 1986, 1987, 1988

National Center for Health Statistics: Advance report of final mortality statistics, 1989. Monthly Vital Stat Rep 40(8), 1992

Pearse WH: Bright seashells in the sand. Am J Obstet Gynecol (in press)

Rochat RW, Koonin LM, Atrash HK, Jewett JJ, and the Maternal Mortality Collaborative: Maternal mortality in the United States: Report from the Maternal Mortality Collaborative. Obstet Gynecol 72:91, 1988

Rooks JP, Weatherby NL, Ernst EKM, Stapleton S, Rosen D, Rosenfield A: Outcomes of care in birth centers: The National Birth Center study. N Engl J Med 321:1804, 1989

Rosenberg MJ, Rosenthal SM: Reproductive mortality in the United States: Recent trends and methodologic considerations. Am J Public Health 77:833, 1987

Sachs BP, Layde PM, Rubin GL, Rochat RW: Reproductive mortality in the United States. JAMA 247:2789, 1982

United States Public Health Service: Promoting health/ preventing disease: Year 2000 objectives for the nation. U.S. Department of Health and Human Services, September, 1989

CHAPTER 2
Pregnancy: Overview and Diagnosis; Ovarian Function and Ovulation

Overview of Reproductive Function in Women

The biomedical science and practice of obstetrics is intertwined with all phases of human reproduction: sexual maturation, gonadal function, gamete release and transport, ovum fertilization, zygote cleavage, blastocyst transport and implantation, pregnancy adaptations, fetal development, parturition, puerperal adaptation, breast feeding, and gonadal senescence. And in addition, consideration must be given to all manner of abnormalities that may affect each of these processes. Clinical obstetrics, therefore, must be concerned with all aspects of women's health; and in turn, all physicians must be cognizant of the profound impact of reproductive biological processes on women's health and well-being, both physical and mental.

To this end, it is important to recognize the enormous physiological expenditures, involuntarily obliged, in women to ensure the perpetuation of humankind. Physiologically, women are the limiting resource in human reproduction, as is true of the female of all mammals. In other mammalian species, however, the adult female experiences cyclic episodes of estrus during a defined time of the year (i.e., the breeding season). In women, spontaneous, cyclic ovulation continues throughout the year, from menarche to menopause, for about 38 years in most women. During this time, in the absence of pregnancy or pharmacological intervention, about 10,000 ovarian follicles are recruited and 500 are chosen for ovulation.

On the one hand, for the woman who chooses not to be pregnant, 500 ovarian cycles with massive progesterone secretion and withdrawal and thence menstruation are obliged for no physiological purpose. In consequence, many women choose to use some form of contraception that necessitates continued cyclic menstruation because safe methods for effecting amenorrhea and infertility have not been developed.

On the other hand, for the woman who does not choose to use contraception, there are 500 opportunities for pregnancy, which likely can be achieved by sexual intercourse on any one of 1500 days. In consequence, physicians of all specialities must be constantly vigilant and sensitive to the possibility that women of reproductive age may be pregnant irrespective of their presenting complaint.

Human Reproduction Today. From one vantage point, the success of human reproduction is the cause for one of the greatest problems of humankind—overpopulation of the world, a tragedy in progress because of a population explosion that is worsening. In an expression of worldwide interest and concern for the rapid rate of population increase, and because of apprehension about the consequences of continued rapid growth, The United Nations designated 1974 as World Population Year. Two decades later, this fear of overpopulation of the world is believed by many, and with considerable justification, to continue as the greatest hazard to the health and the environmental and economic future of humankind.

Until about 10,000 years ago, at least 35,000 years were required for the population of the earth to double. In the late 1970s, the doubling time of the world population was estimated to be 35 years. At this rate, 10 doublings (350 years) would produce a population of more than 4 trillion! (Coale, 1974). The population doubling time in some countries today is believed to be less than 20 years, perhaps as low as 12 or 15. The population of the world has already passed the 5 billion mark!

In the United States, one of the momentous social problems of the day is that of the high and increasing number of unwanted pregnancies among teenage girls. The sexually transmitted, acquired immune deficiency syndrome (AIDS) threatens the world with a horrific, deadly epidemic. At this time, more than 120,000 persons in the United States have died of AIDS, and it is believed that 1 in 100 men are infected with HIV. Reports from the International Conference on AIDS held in Amsterdam (1992) are gloomy on all fronts. Therefore, one view of the current status of human reproduction is that of a worldwide sexual orgy that is unencumbered by the use of contraceptive methods or protection against sexually transmitted disease, a dilemma that will soon be reconciled by way of competition between overpopulation-induced starvation and AIDS-induced sure death.

From another vantage point, however, the problem of human reproduction that haunts many women and men and their physicians is that of absolute or relative infertility, which may approach 20 percent for married couples. This major factor in human reproductive failure is coupled with a living newborn pregnancy success rate for in vitro fertilization and embryo transfer that seems to be paralyzed at no more than 25 percent. At the same time, and in concert with this dilemma, pregnancy failure caused by embryonic or fetal wastage seems to occur at every possible step of human reproduction. Commencing with failure of oocyte fertilization, and proceeding through failure of zygote cleavage and blastocyst implantation, losses are high; and high fetal losses from spontaneous abortion, fetal malformations, and preterm birth are major concerns (Chap. 30). From this perspective, it would be easy to reach the judgment that difficulty will be encountered in maintaining the human race, either quantitatively or qualitatively.

Human Reproduction in Biological and Intellectual Evolutionary Perspective.

For physicians, researchers, demographers, and anthropologists—indeed for all those interested in reproductive biology sciences and those entrusted with the health care of women—it is important to be able to envision a theoretical norm: human reproduction uncluttered by social, religious, or pharmacological intervention. To gain such a vision, it would be essential to comprehend the natural history of human reproduction. But such an understanding and such a vision are difficult to attain because of the cunning of women and men. According to Short (1976a, 1980), the reproductive variables that ordinarily would lead to some sort of reproductive equilibrium would include (1) age of puberty, (2) extent of embryonic and fetal death, (3) neonatal (perinatal) mortality, and (4) the duration of lactational amenorrhea (i.e., anovulation or infertility). But in humans, these constraints have been modified, albeit at times unwittingly.

Therefore, the natural history of reproduction in our species has been obscured by social overlay (Short, 1976a). Nonetheless, it is worth remembering, as pointed out by Short, *that genetically speaking we are still primitive hunter-gatherers; it is only 80 generations since the birth of Christ, and at most a few hundred since the dawn of civilization, hardly time for any meaningful genetic change to have occurred.*

Reproduction in Other Primates. One perspective of *"natural human reproduction"* may be gained from an examination of reproduction in closely related primates living in the wild. Among female chimpanzees in the jungle, the birth interval is almost 6 years; but this interval is shortened by infant death, suggesting that the long interval between successive births in the chimpanzee is normally caused by lactation-induced infertility (anovulation and amenorrhea). Chimpanzees in the wild suckle their young several times per hour, secrete a milk similar to humans, and sleep with the infant at their breast during the night (Short, 1984). Therefore, one factor in the social evolution of human reproductive

successes or failures may have evolved about the duration of breast feeding of the newborn. Before modern times, the duration of breast feeding was usually dictated by the availability of soft foods for the infants.

Chimpanzees are one of the few primates that experience menstruation (Chap. 4); but in chimpanzees living in the wild, menstruation is rare because of repeated pregnancy and lactation-induced anovulation and amenorrhea. Is it possible that the same would be true of ovulation and menstruation in women were it not for their advanced intellectual development, which has enabled women to choose infertility and limit the duration of lactation. Women have accepted ovulation and menstruation in place of near continuous pregnancy and lactation.

Reproduction in Primitive Societies. To address this question, it would be necessary to remove some of the social overlay that obscures our view of uncluttered reproduction in the human. To do so, anthropologists from around the world have studied a particular primitive tribe, the !Kung hunter-gatherers of the Kalahari Desert of South Africa. These people provide useful clues as to the impact of demographic changes that have affected reproduction in humans. (The exclamation point in "!Kung" denotes an alveolar-palatal click. The tip of the tongue is pressed against the roof of the mouth and then drawn away sharply, producing a hollow popping sound [Kolata, 1974]). The !Kung have lived as hunter-gatherers for at least 11,000 years; but recently, some have begun to live in agrarian villages near those of the Bantus.

Among nomadic !Kung women, who are hunters as well, the age of menarche is relatively late, 15½ years. This lateness of menarche has been attributed to the leaner body mass of the young nomadic !Kung women compared with that of the more sedentary women who now live in farming-like villages. The !Kung women marry in early puberty; but the nomadic women do not conceive until 19½ years of age on average, presumably because of postmenarchal anovulation (and oligoamenorrhea). The !Kung do not practice any form of contraception, and the time interval between births is about 4.1 years. Because of the nomadic, hunter-gatherer lifestyle of these women, there is very little soft food available for their babies. Probably for this reason, the !Kung women breast feed their small children for 4 to 5 years. And, they choose to breast feed frequently, as many as four times per hour during the daytime, even if only for a minute or so at a time. Additionally, the !Kung women sleep with their infants and small children who suckle the breasts during the night. This may contribute to the long birth interval, because there seems to be a closer relationship between the number of times per day that the infant suckles and the duration of anovulation and amenorrhea, than between the total time of suckling or the amount of milk produced and the duration of lactation-induced infertility. During lactation-induced anovulation and amenorrhea, fertility is low, as reviewed by Kolata (1974) and Short (1976a, 1984). Among nomadic !Kung women, the average completed family size is 4.7 children; and the population doubling time of the nomadic !Kung people is estimated to be 300 years. Because of the duration of pregnancy and breast feeding, menstruation among !Kung women is infrequent. By definition, therefore, the recurrence of premenstrual syndrome-like symptoms among !Kung women also is rare.

In !Kung women who recently have adopted the agrarian life-style, menarche occurs earlier; first pregnancy occurs earlier; and the interval between births is diminished. *"Population explosion among the !Kung!"* (Short, 1980).

Possibly menarche in more sedentary women occurs earlier because of increased body fat. The time of menarche is most closely related to body weight. Lactation-induced amenorrhea intervals are shortened by the availability of soft food and alternate (animal) sources of milk for the babies, permitting a reduction in the duration of breast feeding. In the !Kung, therefore, *"we may be witnessing in microcosm the transformation that occurred in human fertility as we changed from a nomadic to an agrarian way of life"* (Short, 1976b).

Reproduction in the North American Hutterites. The ethnic Hutterites of North America are an example of an agrarian people with an exceptionally high rate of fertility. This group is an anabaptist religious sect that lives in hamlets, which they refer to as colonies. By "anabaptist" is meant that they reject the notion of baptism of infants. Rather, baptism is conducted as a ritual of adulthood and is a prerequisite for marriage; the mean age of marriage for Hutterite women in 1950 was 22.0 years of age (Eaton and Mayer, 1953).

Reproduction among the Hutterites is encouraged; but premarital sex is forbidden, and very rarely practiced. In Hutterite women age 25 to 29, the age-specific nuptial fertility rate is 498—that is, there are 498 births per year for each 1000 married women between the ages of 25 and 29. Stated differently, there is one birth per woman every 2 years. The average completed family size of Hutterite women is 10.6 children.

The average maximum fecundity of the Hutterite population has been estimated assuming an earlier marriage (e.g., 15 years of age). The average maximum fecundity computed was 12 to 14 children, or only about 1 to 3 children more than the actual number in the completed family. The largest number of children (live births) reported for Hutterite women is 16. This is considerably fewer than the 32 infants (all but 4 of them live born) born to the wife of a Viennese linen-weaver (Pearl, 1929, cited by Eaton and Mayer, 1953). The incidence of sterility in Hutterites is very low, 3.4 per-

cent; nonetheless, 33 percent of Hutterite women have 3 children or fewer. Menstruation among Hutterite women is uncommon.

Compared to the nomadic !Kung women, Hutterite women experience earlier puberty and ovulation, breast feed their children on a rigid schedule, and supplement breast feeding with soft foods early in the infant's life. Based on the reproductive history of the Hutterite women, the population doubling time of this group was estimated to be 16 years, as reviewed by Eaton and Mayer (1953) and Short (1976a, 1984).

Reproduction in Modern Women. It seems reasonable to conclude that the sedentary, agrarian way of life of the past few centuries has contributed to a change in body composition and mass that favors earlier menarche and ovulation. Menarche in women in the United States today occurs at about 12½ years of age (Fig. 4–6, p. 95); and whereas anovulation is more common immediately after menarche than later in reproductive life, most young postmenarchal girls today are ovulatory and therefore potentially fertile. And today, of the women who choose to breast feed their newborns, few will continue to do so for more than a few weeks or at most a few months. Most women who do breast feed their infants choose to suckle the baby no more than 8 times per 24 hours compared with 48 times per 12 hours of daylight for !Kung women (Short, 1984).

Therefore, there appear to be two major factors that have affected the natural course of human reproduction: nutrition and woman's intellectual capacity to choose infertility. Nutritional advances have led to (1) earlier menarche (and ovulation); (2) artificial feeding of the newborn, resulting in decreased duration of lactation and associated anovulation and amenorrhea after childbirth; and (3) longer infant survival. Women in the United States today, on average, choose to have two pregnancies and to breast feed for only a few weeks, if at all. In consequence, no more than 20 ovulatory (menstrual) cycles are eliminated by the amenorrhea of pregnancy and lactation. It is for these reasons that in the absence of pharmacological intervention, modern women experience 450 ovulatory cycles with massive progesterone secretion and withdrawal and attendant menstruation because they have chosen infertility.

The Ovary and Human Reproduction

It is important for students of reproductive biology, medicine, and, in particular, obstetrics to recognize these incredible endocrinological, physiological, and anatomical expenditures that are obliged, involuntarily, in reproductive-age women to ensure the recurrent opportunity for pregnancy. The depth of this investment is so great that Short (1984) comes to the view that *"women are physiologically ill-adapted to spend the greater part of their reproductive lives in the nonpregnant state."* There can be no doubt that the physiological animus of the ovarian cycle and its hormones, as well as the accompanying morphological accommodations of the reproductive tract in response to the actions of ovarian sex steroid hormones, is ovulation, fertilization, and implantation—namely, the establishment of pregnancy. There are fail-safe systems that become operative if there is failure of fertilization of the ovum or failure of implantation of the blastocyst; and these culminate in menstruation. Menstruation, therefore, is indisputable evidence of fertility failure, whether purposefully chosen or naturally occurring.

The consequences of the slow (and now absent) natural biological evolution of humans compared with the advanced intellectual development of women on reproductive processes, general health, and well-being are further considered in Chapter 4.

Ovulation: Cardinal Function of the Ovary.

Ordinarily one egg is released by way of ovulation each month; this process is repeated faithfully every 22 to 35 days from menarche to menopause, or for about 35 to 40 years, so long as pregnancy does not intervene and so long as sufficient numbers of follicles remain in the ovary. The endocrine events of the ovarian cycle are optimized to create a hormonal environment that promotes ovulation. The endocrine milieu that evolves during the ovarian cycle is also optimal for the regeneration of endometrium after completion of a failed fertility cycle (menstruation) in preparation of the uterus for the next pregnancy opportunity.

The somatic effects of estrogen—for example, those on bone density—must be considered as coincidental benefits of follicular estrogen that is produced in such a manner as to regulate ovarian–brain–pituitary function and follicular maturation, which eventuates in ovulation. For example, there is no physiological mechanism in place by which somatic tissues can act to regulate the rate of ovarian estrogen secretion. Except for ovary and brain–pituitary, this is true of all estrogen-responsive tissues, including breast, uterus, bone, skin, vagina, and liver. In addition, there is no advantage to the widely fluctuating levels of estrogen during the ovarian cycle for metabolic processes other than those directly involved in reproduction. These considerations are important not only to an understanding of the reproductive biology of women but for developing rational therapeutic practices when the administration of estrogen to hypogonadal women is considered. This issue is also addressed in Chapter 4.

Considering the relatively uncommon occurrence of menstruation among female chimpanzees living in the wild and among nomadic !Kung women and Hutterite women, it seems reasonable to conclude that repetitive, cyclic ovulation and menstruation are not the biological evolutionary norm, however universal this phenomenon may be among most young women today. Rather, recurrent ovulation and menstruation are the consequence of the greater intellectual than biological evolution of humans. Infertility can be chosen; but the physiological futility that results, and the endocrinopathy that may accrue from this choice is appreciable. From this analysis, we do not suggest that there is a metabolic or health advantage to be gained from repeated episodes of pregnancy and lactation. On the contrary, we conclude that we are nowhere near finding a reasonable method for fertility control, one that would provide for optimum benefits from estrogen without the necessity for recurrent progesterone secretion or menstruation.

The Ovary as an Endocrine Organ.

The function and functional regulation of the human ovary during the reproductive years is unlike that known for any other human endocrine gland. Generally, endocrine glands respond to appropriate trophic stimuli by producing the major hormone(s) characteristic of that gland: for example, cortisol is secreted by the adrenal cortex in response to the action of adrenocorticotropin (ACTH) on the adrenal cortex; thyroxine is released in response to the action of TSH (thyroid-stimulating hormone) on the thyroid; testosterone in response to LH (luteinizing hormone) on the testes; but this straightforward response to trophic agents does not obtain for the ovary and gonadotropins. Estrogen formation is largely confined to the granulosa cells of one ovary at a time, and more specifically, to the granulosa cells of a single follicle—the chosen follicle, the dominant follicle, the follicle that is destined for ovulation in that ovarian cycle. And the rate of formation and secretion of estradiol (estradiol-17β, the biologically potent, naturally occurring estrogen), by the granulosa cells of the chosen follicle corresponds to the final stages of the maturation and development of that follicle. Indeed, when the follicular apparatus of the ovaries is depleted, ovarian endocrine function ceases (i.e., the menopause). Thereafter, the ovaries do not secrete estrogen and do not respond to gonadotropins by an increase in estrogen formation (Chap. 4).

During the first and last few days of each menstrual cycle, very little estradiol is synthesized in the ovarian follicle(s) or corpus luteum. Rather, most of the estrogen produced at these times is estrone, which arises by way of the extraglandular aromatization (the rate-limiting enzymatic process in estrogen biosynthesis) of a plasma C_{19}-steroid (namely androstenedione, which is secreted by the adrenal cortex and ovary). This occurs primarily in adipose tissue. The extraglandular pathway of estrogen formation is that by which most estrogen is produced in men, children, and in postmenopausal and anovulatory women.

Therefore, it is readily apparent that the ovary is

not an endocrine gland of the same type as the adrenal cortex, thyroid, or even the testis. The formation of estrogen and thence progesterone in the ovary is closely linked to the ovulatory process. At the midfollicular phase of each ovarian cycle, there is a gradual and thence a sudden increase in the rate of follicular development and estradiol secretion. These momentous endocrine events are parallel to and essential for the development and maturation of the follicle and for the regulation of gonadotropin secretion, including the sudden release, or *surge,* in LH secretion at midcycle, which brings about ovulation of the "chosen" follicle.

After ovulation, the corpus luteum develops in the site of the ruptured follicle and progesterone is produced therein in prodigious amounts. In fact, the rate of progesterone secretion by the corpus luteum is greater than that of any steroid hormone produced in men or nonpregnant women, including cortisol secreted by the adrenal cortex (see Chap. 4 and Fig. 4–8). Progesterone is accepted as the "pro gestation steroid"—that is, it is generally believed that progesterone is essential to the maintenance of pregnancy in most mammalian species (Chap. 12). Progesterone withdrawal, by way of surgical removal of the human corpus luteum, before 8 weeks of pregnancy, results in abortion, as does the pharmacological inhibition of progesterone action (as with a progesterone receptor antagonist such as RU-486). **But apart from pregnancy and pregnancy-related phenomena, there is no known metabolic utility of progesterone.** Rather, the repetitive secretion of progesterone at monthly intervals for long times may be an endocrinopathy that gives rise to distressing, sometimes disabling symptoms in women at the times of progesterone secretion and withdrawal—that is, the premenstrual syndromes (Chap. 4).

Reproductive Function of Women in Physiological Perspective.

Therefore, the reproductive processes in women can also be envisioned as follows: The most intricate and complex function of the ovary is the extrusion of an egg at cyclic intervals; and if this is accomplished, all other aspects of ovarian function, including the hypothalamic–pituitary participation in this event, must be normal. The function of the fallopian tubes evolves singularly about sperm, egg, and zygote transport and the provision of an environment conducive to fertilization of the ovum and early cleavage of the zygote. The endometrium may be the optimal (but not the only) site for blastocyst implantation. The implantation of the blastocyst in the uterine cavity, however, provides for a mechanism by which the fetus can ultimately be delivered, namely, access to the outside world. Thus, reproductive function in women is focused in a highly directed and obligate manner toward the achievement of pregnancy and then nourishment and delivery of the fetus.

Modern Woman's Partner in Reproduction.

From the vantage point of optimal reproductive success, men (compared with most other male mammals) are relatively inefficient contributors to successful reproduction. There are large numbers of abnormal spermatozoa in the ejaculates of men, which is not true of other male mammals. If ejaculation occurs more often than once every 48 to 72 hours in men, semen volume and sperm numbers decline appreciably. There are relatively small reserves of spermatozoa in the testes of men compared with those in some other mammals. For example, the male chimpanzee has very large testes with an enormous sperm reserve and is able to copulate repeatedly with several female chimpanzees who come into estrus on the same day. The ejaculate of the chimpanzee contains 603 million sperm. And the chimpanzee testes produce 2737 million sperm per day, sufficient for at least four ejaculates. By comparison, the ejaculate of men contains 253 million sperm but only 176 million sperm are produced by the testes each day, fewer than the number in one ejaculate (Short, 1980). It has been reasoned that the large sperm reservoirs of the chimpanzee serve to permit genetic competition among the males. The male that deposits the greatest number of sperm in the vaginas of the estrus females is likely to be the male whose genetic material is transmitted by way of the winning sperm (Harcourt and associates, 1981).

The Future.

Optimistically, we are pressing toward the time that the regulation of reproductive function to achieve or not to achieve pregnancy can be the choice of every woman. At that time, women can elect to control the destiny of their own reproductive function. This meritorious goal must be shared by all interested physicians and scientists. Indeed, the topic of the 1988 plenary session of the annual meeting of the Institute of Medicine was "Advances in Reproductive Biology: Implications for Research, Application, and Policy Development." And in 1992, the Institute of Medicine published the findings of a 2-year study entitled *Strengthening Research in Academic OB/GYN Departments.* The time for making great progress in improving the health care of women and promoting the well-being of women through research is now. Presently, the National Institutes of Health and the National Institute of Mental Health, with the urging of the Congress of the United States, are dedicated to the improvement of women's health and well-being.

Given the possibility that we can approach this meritorious plateau in science and civilization, we as obstetricians are challenged as never before to contribute to the goal of guaranteeing that every newborn is well born. We also look forward to the time that women can choose infertility without obliging the endocrinopathy of recurrent progesterone secretion in massive amounts, which also necessitates the associated distress of menstruation that this choice now brings. We submit that each woman should be able to select when to be (or not to be) pregnant as a positive demonstration of her own choice without being obliged to make such a choice from a variety of inadequate options.

Pregnancy Organization: The Fetal–Maternal Communication System

Development of the Communication System. There is no doubt that ovulation is dependent upon brain–pituitary–ovarian interactions; but after conception, the establishment and maintenance of pregnancy is highly dependent upon contributions made by the blastocyst, the trophoblasts, the embryo, and thence the fetus. A biomolecular communication system is established between the zygote/blastocyst/embryo/fetus and mother that is operative from before the time of nidation and persists through the time of parturition and possibly beyond. Indeed, by way of breast feeding, this communication persists after birth; and, through maternal–infant bonding, a communication system, in some form, may be established that is lifelong. This fetal–maternal communication system is essential to the success of blastocyst implantation, maternal recognition of pregnancy, immunological acceptance, fetal contributions to the maintenance of pregnancy, maternal adaptation to pregnancy, fetal nutrition, and probably fetal participation in the initiation of parturition. These physiological processes evolve primarily from fetal-directed modifications of maternal responses.

In the past, we have envisioned this communication system as being operative primarily to provide nutritive supplies from the mother to the fetus. By way of this communication system, it was presumed that the mother serves up nutrients that are effectively taken up by fetal trophoblasts and transferred to the embryo-fetus. But the importance of the contributions of the fetus to this communication system is enormous. The blastocyst is the dynamic force of pregnancy beginning at the time of implantation. Thereafter, the embryo-fetus continues as the moving force throughout pregnancy, delivery, and beyond, including the involvement of the fetus-newborn in creating the hormonal milieu that culminates in lactation and thence in milk let-down during suckling.

There are two major anatomical and functional arms of this fetal–maternal communication system. One is the **placental arm,** in which a variety of functional components are operative, for example, nutritive, endocrine, and immunological components. The other is the **paracrine arm,** the functional components of which include pregnancy maintenance, immunological acceptance, amnionic fluid volume homeostasis, physical protection of the fetus, and perhaps parturition (Fig. 2–1).

The placental arm of the fetal–maternal communication system is in place by way of blood-borne conduits that involve (1) the endometrial/decidual spiral arterial supply of maternal blood to the placental intervillous space; this maternal blood directly bathes the

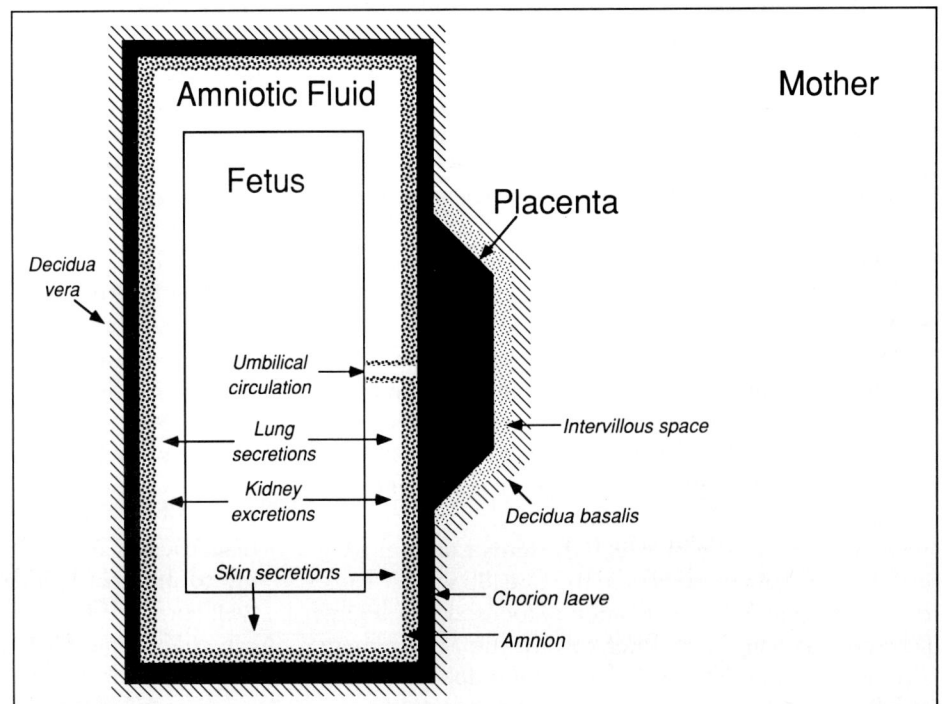

Fig. 2–1. The fetal–maternal communication system. The proximal anatomical parts of the two arms of this system, the placental arm and the paracrine arm, are depicted. Fetal blood perfuses the placenta by way of the fetal villous capillaries. Maternal blood directly bathes the trophoblasts. Amnionic fluid, comprised in large measure of fetal urine, and containing secretions from fetal lung and skin, bathes the avascular amnion, which is contiguous with avascular chorion laeve. The chorion laeve and decidua vera (parietalis) are in direct cell-to-cell contact. A trophoblastic "shell" separates embryo-fetus from maternal cells and blood at all anatomic sites.

villous syncytiotrophoblast; and (2) fetal blood, which is confined within the fetal villous capillaries that traverse within the intravillous space. The paracrine arm of the communication system is established by direct cell-to-cell contact and biomolecular trafficking between fetal membranes (chorion laeve) and maternal decidua parietalis. In turn, the amnion, the innermost avascular fetal membrane, which is contiguous with the chorion laeve on one side and is bathed by the amnionic fluid on the other side, is a component of this paracrine system. And amnionic fluid, which is rich in fetal excretions (kidney) and secretions (lung, skin), provides for a peculiar direct communication system between the fetus and mother. The constituents of amnionic fluid, derived from fetal excretions and secretions, may act via the fetal membranes; and constituents of amnionic fluid arising in maternal tissues enter the fetus because amnionic fluid, in large volumes, is both inspired into the lungs and swallowed by the fetus.

Organization of the Communication System.
At the very commencement of pregnancy (i.e., at the time of blastocyst implantation), there is, anatomically, only one distinguishable communication link between blastocyst and mother. This is established between the trophectoderm of the blastocyst and the uterine endometrium (decidua) and thence maternal blood. But even then, the functional progenitors of the two mature arms of the communication system are developing (Fig. 2–1).

Placental Arm of the Fetal–Maternal Communication System (Nutrient Transfer and Endocrine System).
The placenta (villous trophoblast; syncytium) becomes the principal site of nutrient transfer between mother and fetus and the principal endocrine tissue of pregnancy, albeit one that is highly dependent upon the provision of blood-borne, preformed precursors for placental steroid hormone formation (Chap. 6). **Ultimately, the proximal anatomical parts of the placental arm (nutrient transfer and endocrine function) of the fetal–maternal communication system are the fetal blood, the syncytium, and the maternal blood.** The human placenta is of the hemochorioendothelial type. As stated already, this means that syncytiotrophoblast is bathed directly by maternal blood, but the fetal blood is contained within fetal capillaries in the intravillous space of the placenta; therefore, fetal blood is separated from the syncytiotrophoblast by the wall of the fetal capillaries, the mesenchyme in the intravillous space, and the cytotrophoblasts (Chap. 5); in consequence, fetal and maternal blood do not come into direct contact except in abnormal conditions. It should be noted that the walls of the fetal capillaries and other fetal vessels within the placenta are not comprised of smooth muscle cells or endothelium as are other vessels (Chap. 5).

Paracrine Arm of the Fetal–Maternal Communication System (Fetal Membranes–Decidua).
As the embryo and extraembryonic tissues grow, the amnion and chorion laeve develop as tough, avascular membranous structures that come to lie adjacent to the entire surface of the decidua vera (parietalis) that is not occupied by the placenta (Chap. 5). This anatomical arrangement gives rise to the fetal–decidual paracrine arm of the communication system. We refer to this as a paracrine arm because (1) the fetal membranes are avascular and (2) there are cell-to-cell interactions that take place between the fetal membranes and the maternal decidua. **Therefore, the proximal anatomical parts of the paracrine arm of the fetal–maternal communication system are the amnionic fluid, amnion, chorion laeve, and decidua parietalis.** Communication between fetus and mother by way of this paracrine arm is possible through several mechanisms. After about 16 weeks of gestation, fetal urine becomes an important constituent of amnionic fluid. Fetal lung secretions also enter amnionic fluid by way of fetal thoracic movements (fetal "breathing"). Therefore, the amnionic fluid serves as a conduit for the transmission of fetal signals to maternal tissues in the paracrine arm of this communication system. In the reverse direction, decidual products as well as some maternal blood constituents enter amnionic fluid, and these products enter the fetus by way of the fetal lung and fetal swallowing. In some cases, there is preferential entry of decidual products into amnionic fluid. For example, large amounts of prolactin are formed in decidua; but little or none of decidual prolactin enters maternal blood. Instead, decidual prolactin enters amnionic fluid almost exclusively (Chap. 5). In addition, biologically potent vasoactive peptides and growth factors are synthesized in amnion directly and these agents enter amnionic fluid.

Three other anatomical and functional components that are anatomical extensions of this paracrine communication system must be considered. The amnion also covers the fetal surface of the placenta (i.e., the placental amnion) and the umbilical cord. In addition, amnion is present between fetuses of twin pregnancies with diamnionic–dichorionic and diamnionic–monochorionic types of twin placentae. Chorion laeve does not extend over the surface of the placenta or the cord; rather, only the amnion is present to cover the fetal surface of the placenta and the umbilical cord. Therefore, the entire epithelial surface of the amnion is contiguous with amnionic fluid, but on the basal surface, the placental amnion is directly adjacent to the adventitial surface of the chorionic vessels, which traverse over the fetal surface of the placenta as part of the chorionic plate.

Recently, Casey and co-workers have shown that powerful vasoactive peptides are produced in human amnion, namely endothelin-1 (a vasoconstrictor) and parathyroid hormone-related protein (a vasorelaxant) (Casey and co-workers, 1991, 1992; Germain and associates, 1992; Sunnergren and colleagues, 1990). Thus, it is possible that vasoactive peptides generated in the placental amnion are available to act in a paracrine manner to modulate vascular tone in the chorionic vessels that transfer blood between the fetus and placenta (Chap. 5). These vessels, along the surface of the placenta (before branching into the cotyledons), are comprised of smooth muscle and endothelial cells as are other vessels. These vessels are responsive, therefore, to vasoactive agents. Endothelin-1 and parathyroid hormone-related protein are also present in amnionic fluid. Amnion covering the umbilical cord is contiguous with Wharton jelly, that is, the extracellular matrix of the cord through which the two umbilical arteries and one umbilical vein traverse from the fetus to the placenta (Chap. 5).

The Dynamic Role of the Fetus in Pregnancy

Until relatively recently, the fetus was commonly envisioned as a passive passenger (parasite) of the pregnancy unit; nothing could be further from the truth. To comprehend the magnitude of the fetal contributions to the regulation of human pregnancy, it is important to recognize that whereas the fetus enjoys a position of protection from the external environment that is never to be experienced again in life, at the same time the fetus is the dynamic force in the orchestration of its own destiny.

From the time of conception, a molecular dialogue is established between fetal and maternal tissues; in several mammalian species—the horse for example—there are even clear-cut differences between the transport of fertilized and nonfertilized ova in the fallopian tube.

The chemical impetus for implantation is derived from the trophoblasts and blastocyst products; invasion of the maternal endometrium and blood vessels in the process of implantation and development of the placenta is under the active direction of bioactive products of the trophoblasts; the maternal recognition of pregnancy is brought about by way of signals generated by the trophoblast that act upon the maternal ovary; the immunological acceptance of the semiallogenic tissues of the conceptus is modulated by trophoblasts; the maintenance of pregnancy is orchestrated by fetal contributions to steroid hormone formation in trophoblast; the physiological changes of pregnancy derive from products formed and secreted by the placenta; indeed, it is probable that fetal-induced retreat from the maintenance of pregnancy is the penultimate event in the spontaneous initiation of parturition at term. From these interactions, it is established that there is trafficking, at the biomolecular level, that involves intimate signal transmission and responses between tissues of the fetus and those of its mother.

To understand the organization and the functional components that serve to promote the maintenance of pregnancy and the physiological adaptations of the maternal organism to the developing fetus, it is essential that we understand the anatomical and physiological arrangements provided by this communication system in appreciable detail.

Overview. Fertilization of the human ovum by a spermatozoan occurs in the fallopian tube within a short time (minutes to a few hours) after ovulation; and 6 days after fertilization, the blastocyst begins to implant in the endometrium; pregnancy has begun. Based on the proposition that the fetus is the dynamic force in the orchestration of the physiological events of pregnancy, the concept clearly emerges that the maternal organism is constitutively passive, responding to signals emanating from the fetus or extraembryonic fetal tissues (the placenta and fetal membranes). The biological behavior of the fetus and extraembryonic fetal tissues in pregnancy is not dissimilar to that of a nonmetastasizing, but rapidly growing, neoplasm. The developing embryo-fetus is very demanding; and in general, its demands are met at whatever cost to the maternal organism because of efficient placental mechanisms for nutrient uptake and transfer. But in other respects, the fetus is a benevolent, albeit self-serving, parasite in that it provides for the development of physiological changes that facilitate maternal adaptation to this rapidly growing, semiallogenic, tumorlike graft. These systems include, among many others, those that permit a sizable expansion of the maternal blood volume, an increase in cardiac output, blood vessel refractoriness to pressor agents, increases in renal blood flow, and efficient utilization of energy sources (Chap. 8).

The fetus is also able to "tap in" to maternal systems that provide for protection, as in the transplacental passage of selected antibodies; and in general, the fetus occupies a privileged and protected position during pregnancy. But the fetus is not totally isolated from the maternal environment, being subject to adverse effects of teratogens and some infectious agents and to profound alterations in maternal metabolic function and uteroplacental blood flow.

To illustrate the active role of the blastocyst/embryo/fetus in guaranteeing its own optimum outcome (Fig. 2–2), consider the examples given in the following sections.

Implantation. Clearly, the endometrium is not essential to implantation; ectopic pregnancies occur in the fallopian tube, ovary, peritoneal cavity, and even in the spleen; and in experimental studies, the blastocyst can be implanted successfully into many tissues, including the testis. Thus, it must be surmised that the blastocyst (trophoblasts) is the driving force in implantation.

There are components of both the neoplastic and

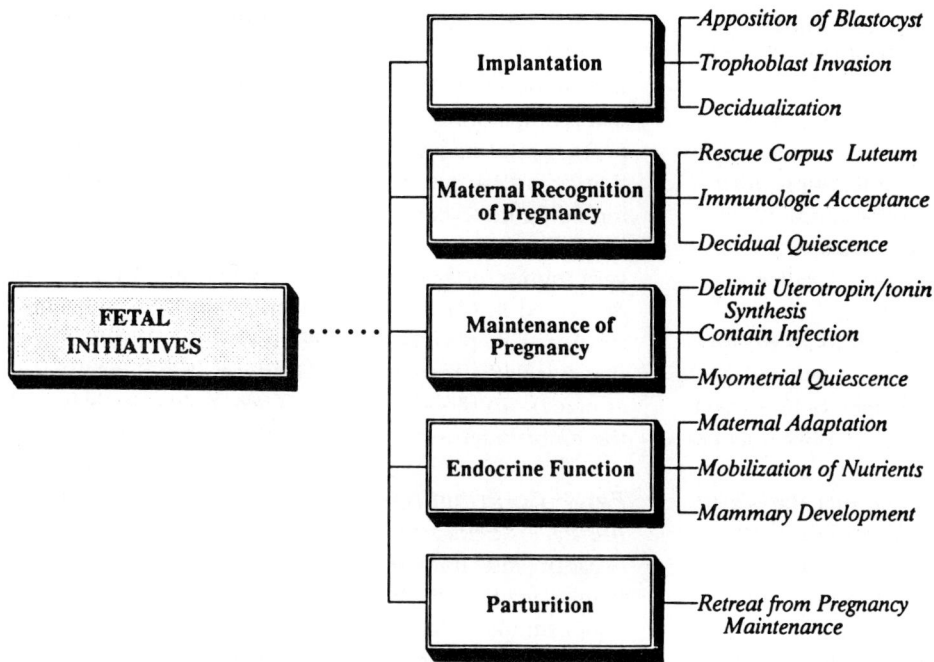

Fig. 2–2. Fetal contributions to the maintenance of pregnancy. The fetus and extraembryonic fetal tissues are the dynamic, driving force in the establishment and maintenance of pregnancy. The contributions of the fetus include processes essential to implantation and maternal recognition of pregnancy; but more than this, the physiological and metabolic accommodations in the maternal organism that contribute to successful pregnancy are orchestrated by fetal-directed biomolecular initiatives.

the inflammatory process involved in blastocyst implantation; the blastocyst produces or else provokes the formation of prostaglandins, platelet-activating factor, and plasminogen activator. In fact, complete decidualization of endometrium in human pregnancy takes place only after blastocyst implantation. It is possible that the blastocyst provides an essential growth factor, such as transforming growth factor-β that serves to foster the completion of decidualization (Chap. 4). There can be no doubt that the blastocyst is an efficient, invasive, aggressive, dynamic force that enables both the commencement and maintenance of successful pregnancy.

Fetal-Induced Maternal Recognition of Pregnancy. Among the early physiological arrangements provided by the fetal–maternal communication system is one referred to by Short (1969) as the **maternal recognition of pregnancy.** This is an extraordinarily important concept in mammalian pregnancy physiology. But we suggest that the arrangement should be redesignated, for an important reason, as the **fetal-induced maternal recognition of pregnancy.** Whereas there is no doubt that there is, physiologically, maternal recognition of pregnancy, this response is effected by *fetal contributions to the early maintenance of pregnancy.* The importance of this distinction is to acknowledge the essential contributions made by fetal tissues to the success of pregnancy. Conceptually, this interpretation also is important in defining the role of the fetus in the initiation of parturition (Chap. 12).

The "maternal recognition" of pregnancy encompasses a series of processes (Bazer and colleagues, 1986) that culminate in prolongation of the life span of the corpus luteum to ensure continued progesterone secretion and trophoblast modification of the expression of major histocompatibility complex (HLA) antigens to ensure maternal tissue acceptance of the fetal graft. Chorionic gonadotropin (hCG) produced by trophoblasts serves to rescue the corpus luteum and to promote progesterone formation by the ovary until such time as the trophoblasts are able to synthesize sufficient amounts of progesterone to maintain pregnancy (Chaps. 6 and 12). Receptors for low-density lipoprotein (the source of cholesterol for placental progesterone production) are discernible in trophoblasts by 6 weeks of gestation, but are very likely present and functional even earlier.

In some mammalian species, involution of the corpus luteum during a nonfertile cycle is induced in response to the luteolytic action of prostaglandin $PGF_{2\alpha}$ produced in endometrium (possibly in response to ovarian oxytocin). In particular, if blastocyst implantation does not occur, $PGF_{2\alpha}$ is produced in the endometrium; the $PGF_{2\alpha}$ enters the uterine venous circulation; in sheep and other species, the uterine vein crosses over the ovarian artery. $PGF_{2\alpha}$ is transferred from the uterine vein to the ovarian artery by a transvascular mechanism, and the $PGF_{2\alpha}$ acts on the corpus luteum as a luteolytic agent, bringing an end to the function of the corpus luteum to produce progesterone. This process has been referred to as the *murder of the corpus luteum.* There are certain analogies between the regulation of corpus luteum function (luteolysis) and the initiation of parturition. For example, progesterone withdrawal occurs before the initiation of parturition in most mammalian species (primates excepted), including those species in which progesterone during pregnancy is produced in the corpus luteum and in those in which progesterone is produced in placenta (Chap. 12). This does not appear to be the case in the human, however. There is no evidence of endometrial production of a luteolytic agent in women, because after hysterectomy normal ovarian function including the development of corpora lutea with normal life spans and progesterone secretion continues. And, there is no evidence of progesterone withdrawal (i.e., a decrease in the plasma progesterone concentrations) before the onset of human parturition. Nonetheless, hCG, produced by human trophoblasts, functions to prolong the life span of the human corpus luteum to provide a source of progesterone early in pregnancy before there is sufficient syncytiotrophoblast to accomplish this essential endocrine function of pregnancy.

There is also appreciable evidence that the blastocyst and embryo produce agents that serve directly to effect decidual quiescence, thus facilitating the maintenance of pregnancy. The most clear-cut example of such an agent is that of ovine trophoblast protein-1 (oTP-1) produced by the sheep embryo. OTP-1 (M_r about 18,000) is the major secretory product of the early (13- to 21-day) sheep blastocyst (Godkin and co-workers, 1984). There is appreciable homology between the amino acid sequence of this protein and that of interferon-α (Imakawa and associates, 1987). Receptors for oTP-1 are present in sheep endometrium. OTP-1 is produced transiently by sheep blastocyst, and serves to prevent luteolysis, possibly by inhibiting $PGF_{2\alpha}$ formation in the endometrium (Hansen and colleagues, 1985). A similar protein is produced by the bovine conceptus (bTP). To illustrate the validity of this concept, the infusion of bovine interferon-α into the uterine lumen of the cow prolongs the life span of the corpus luteum (Plante and co-workers, 1988).

There is no evidence that the human blastocyst produces a protein similar to oTP or bTP, but Hearn and colleagues (1991) propose that an unknown embryonic signal that acts on corpus luteum may be secreted by the human blastocyst even before bioactive hCG can be detected. They present evidence from studies of nonhuman primates (e.g., the marmoset monkey), that increased function of the corpus luteum (e.g., inhibin secretion), commences before hCG is detected. As reviewed by Hearn and associates, mRNA for hCG has been found in 6- to 8-cell human (triploid) zygotes by in situ hybridization techniques. Additionally, mRNA for both α- and β-subunits of hCG are demonstrable in trophoectoderm of preimplantation blastocysts, but the β-subunit mRNA is not found in cytotrophoblasts of the villus. Thus, it is not clear whether intact hCG is produced in the preimplantation trophoblasts. They point out that a number of preimplantation blastocyst signals have been proposed—early pregnancy factor, platelet-activating factor, histamine-releasing factor, and hCG. It is unlikely that the "rescue" of the corpus luteum is as simplistic as the stimulation by hCG.

Fetal Contributions to Maternal Acceptance of Semiallogenic Fetal Graft. Just after, or at about the time of blastocyst implantation, the expression of major histocompatibility complex (HLA) antigens is suppressed in extraembryonic fetal tissues (trophoblasts)—that is, in tissues that directly embrace maternal tissues, including maternal blood. This may be the most critical mechanism by which the blastocyst and embryo-fetus gain immunological acceptance by maternal tissues. As described in Chapter 5, the trophoblasts form an uninterrupted trophoblastic shell around the embryo such that normally, maternal tissues never come into direct contact with blood or other nontrophoblastic tissues of the embryo-fetus.

Fetal Contributions to Endocrinology of Pregnancy. The hormonal changes of human pregnancy (in breadth and amount) are monumental and unprecedented in the annals of mammalian endocrinology and endocrinopathology (Chap. 6). But without exception, the endocrine changes of human pregnancy evolve as the consequence of fetal–placental function, either directly or indirectly—thus, the fetus is also responsible for the endocrine milieu of human pregnancy. The formation of estrogens during pregnancy takes place by way of the placental aromatization of C_{19}-steroids, which in turn are produced primarily in the fetal adrenals. Progesterone is also produced in the syncytium in massive quantities by way of the utilization of maternal plasma LDL cholesterol; indeed, the rate of trophoblast consumption of maternal plasma LDL for progesterone formation at term is so great in some pregnancies as to be equivalent to the total daily turnover of LDL in nonpregnant women (Chap. 6). But even in capturing LDL cholesterol, the fetus is an aggressive and efficient parasite. The hydrolysis of the cholesterol esters yield essential fatty acids and the hydrolysis of the LDL apoprotein gives free amino acids, including essential amino acids.

A fraction of placental progesterone is converted, in extraadrenal maternal and fetal tissues to deoxycorticosterone, a potent mineralocorticosteroid; placental progesterone, secreted into the maternal compartment, serves as the stimulus for increased maternal adrenal aldosterone secretion to a rate 20 times or more than that found in men and nonpregnant women. Increased mineralocorticosteroid formation (aldosterone and deoxycorticosterone) is essential for the expansion of the blood volume in pregnant women. All of these endocrine changes, and many more, are effected by way of fetal tissue-produced or fetal tissue hormone-induced endocrine changes that accompany normal human pregnancy (Chaps. 6 and 8).

Placental Sequestration of Nutrients. Fetal villous syncytiotrophoblast is remarkably efficient in extracting or sequestering essential nutrients from the maternal circulation. For example, in women with profound iron-deficiency anemia during pregnancy, the iron stores of the fetus are normal; in women with severe folic acid deficiency during pregnancy causing severe anemia, the fetal hematocrit is normal (Chaps. 7 and 8). The fetus is a demanding and efficient parasite.

We have long been fascinated by the fact that the amount of calcium assembled into the shell of the egg of the chicken in a period of 18 hours is equivalent to the amount of calcium contained in the entire bony skeleton of the hen. Thus, even in the avian, a species that arguably is never pregnant (absence of implantation), the demands of the embryo are met at whatever cost to the maternal organism.

Fetal Retreat from Participation in Pregnancy Maintenance: Initiation of Parturition. It is probable that the fetus is also in control of its own destiny with respect to the timely onset of parturition. Presumably this comes about by way of fetal-induced suspension of the maintenance of the remarkable uterine quiescence that characterizes 90 to 95 percent of normal pregnancy (phase 0 of parturition; see Chap. 12). A good example of the importance of the fetus in the maintenance of pregnancy and the initiation of parturition is found in cases of fetal death. Even with death of the fetus, labor usually does not immediately ensue. It is common for pregnancies, after the fetus has died, to continue for days, weeks, or even months before the onset of labor. It has been observed that with death of the fetus caused by Rh isoimmunization before 35 weeks gestation, 50 percent of such pregnancies remain undelivered, at least in the absence of intervention, for up to 5 weeks after the death of the fetus (Townsend and Shelton, 1964). Removal of the fetus with the placenta left in situ in rhesus monkey pregnancy, results in spontaneous delivery of the placenta sometime well after the expected time of delivery (Nathanielsz and associates, 1992). It seems that there is no built-in mechanism for emptying the uterus through processes independently initiated within the maternal compartment in response to death or removal of the fetus. The delivery of such pregnancies may come about only after progesterone withdrawal, which may eventuate with degeneration of the placenta after prolonged absence of fetal–placental blood flow.

Fetal-Newborn Contributions to Lactation and Milk Let-Down. During pregnancy, estrogen and progesterone, together with prolactin, act on maternal mammary tissue to induce optimal morphological and biochemical maturational processes that prepare the maternal mammary tissue for lactation or milk production. Progesterone also acts to prevent lactogenesis itself; but with progesterone withdrawal after delivery of the placenta, lactogenesis promptly commences. Thereafter, suckling of the breasts by the newborn induces episodic secretion of oxytocin from the maternal neurohypophysis-posterior pituitary; oxytocin acts on the myoepithelial

cells of the breast ducts to cause milk let down. Obviously, the fetus-infant acts to ensure its own survival.

These are but a few examples to indicate unambiguously that the embryo-fetus, extraembryonic fetal tissues, or both, direct the orchestration of the physiological adaptations of pregnancy. The maternal organism passively responds—even at times to the point of her own detriment. We will refer to this particular arrangement frequently as we consider the physiological adaptations of maternal systems to pregnancy (Chap. 8), acceptance of the fetal semiallogenic graft (Chap. 5), fetal growth and development (Chap. 7), and the initiation of parturition (Chap. 12).

Diagnosis of Pregnancy

Pregnancy is ordinarily a physiological state, but the importance of the correct diagnosis of pregnancy cannot be overstated. In the life of women, few diagnoses are more important than that of pregnancy. For the woman who may be pregnant, there are few diagnoses that can evoke emotions of such absolute joy or else such pains of profound despair. And for all physicians entrusted with the medical management of women of reproductive age, knowledge of the existence of pregnancy is crucial to the proper diagnosis and treatment of all disease processes. For all of these reasons, every physician who assumes the responsibility for the medical care of any woman of reproductive age, irrespective of the nature of the physician's practice or special interest, must always raise the question, *Is she pregnant?* Failure to do so often leads to incorrect diagnoses, inappropriate treatment, and, at times, to medicolegal embroilment.

Many of the normal physiological adaptations of pregnancy are easily recognized and constitute important clues that facilitate the diagnosis of pregnancy and the evaluation of pregnancy progress. Namely, the physiological changes of pregnancy are predictable with sufficient timeliness to constitute important milestones that mark the accommodations of the pregnant woman to the growth, maturation, and function of the fetus.

The diagnosis of pregnancy is ordinarily very easy to establish; but unfortunately, this is not always the case. On occasion, pharmacological or pathophysiological processes may cause endocrine or anatomical changes that mimic those of pregnancy and cause confusion for the woman and sometimes the physician. At times, therefore, the diagnosis of pregnancy is not easy to make; but rarely is it impossible if appropriate clinical and laboratory tests are carefully conducted. Ordinarily, the woman is aware of the likelihood or at least the possibility of pregnancy when she consults a physician, although she may not volunteer this information unless asked specifically. Mistakes in diagnosis of pregnancy are most frequently made in the first several weeks while the uterus is still a pelvic organ. Although it is possible to mistake the enlarged uterus of pregnancy, even at term, for a tumor of some nature, such errors are commonly the result of hasty or incomplete examination.

The endocrinological, physiological, and anatomical alterations that accompany pregnancy give rise to symptoms and signs that provide evidence that pregnancy exists. These symptoms and signs are classified into three groups: presumptive evidence, probable signs, and positive signs of pregnancy.

Presumptive Evidence of Pregnancy

Presumptive evidence of pregnancy is based largely on subjective symptoms and signs that include (1) nausea with or without vomiting, (2) disturbances in urination, (3) fatigue, and (4) the perception of fetal movement. The presumptive signs of pregnancy include (1) cessation of menses, (2) anatomical changes in the breasts, (3) discoloration of the vaginal mucosa, (4) increased skin pigmentation and the development of abdominal striae, and especially important (5) **does the woman believe that she is pregnant?**

Symptoms of Pregnancy

Nausea With or Without Vomiting. Pregnancy is commonly characterized by disturbances of the digestive system, manifested particularly by nausea and vomiting. This so-called *morning sickness of pregnancy* usually commences during the early part of the day but passes off in a few hours, although occasionally it persists longer and may occur at other times. This disturbing symptom usually appears about 6 weeks after the commencement (first day) of the last menstrual period and ordinarily disappears spontaneously 6 to 12 weeks later.

Disturbances in Urination. During the first trimester of pregnancy, the enlarging uterus, by exerting pressure on the urinary bladder, may cause frequent micturition. Gradually, the frequency of urination diminishes as pregnancy progresses and as the uterus rises up into the abdomen. The symptom of frequent urination reappears near the end of pregnancy, however, when the fetal head descends into the maternal pelvis, impinging upon the volume capacity of the bladder.

Fatigue. Easy fatigability is such a frequent characteristic of early pregnancy that it provides a noteworthy diagnostic clue.

Perception of Fetal Movement. Sometime between 16 and 20 weeks (menstrual age) gestation, the pregnant woman becomes conscious of slight fluttering movements in the abdomen, and these movements gradually increase in intensity. These sensations are caused by fetal movements, and the time that these are first rec-

ognized by the pregnant woman is designated as *quickening,* or the perception of life. This sign provides only corroborative evidence of pregnancy, however, and in itself is of little diagnostic value. Quickening is nonetheless a milestone of the progress of pregnancy that, if dated accurately, can provide corroborative evidence in establishing the duration of gestation.

Signs of Pregnancy

Cessation of Menses. In a healthy woman who previously has experienced spontaneous, cyclic, predictable menstruation, the abrupt cessation of menses is highly suggestive of pregnancy. There is appreciable variation in the length of the ovarian (and thus menstrual) cycle among women, and even in the same woman; therefore, it is not until 10 days or more after the time of expected onset of the menstrual period that the absence of menses is a reliable indication of pregnancy. When a second menstrual period is missed, the probability of pregnancy is very much greater.

Although cessation of menstruation is an early and very important indication of pregnancy, gestation may begin without prior menstruation, that is, in a girl in whom menarche has not occurred. In certain Asian countries, where girls marry at a very early age, and in sexually promiscuous groups, pregnancy sometimes commences before menarche. We have provided the medical management of a girl who experienced four normal pregnancies and deliveries without ever having a menstrual period. She delivered her fourth child at age 16, and conceived her first child at age 12 before menarche, presumably with first ovulation. Nursing mothers, who usually do not menstruate during lactation because of lactation-induced anovulation, sometimes ovulate and conceive at that time; and more rarely, women who believe they recently passed the menopause will ovulate again and may become pregnant.

Uterine bleeding, somewhat suggestive of menstruation, occurs occasionally after conception. For example, during the first half of pregnancy, one or two episodes of bloody discharge, reminiscent of and sometimes misinterpreted as menstruation, are not uncommon. Almost always, however, such bleeding is brief and scant. In a series of 225 consecutive pregnant women who did not abort, Speert and Guttmacher (1954) observed that macroscopic vaginal bleeding, which occurred between the time of conception and the 196th day of pregnancy, was reported by 22 percent of these women. In the absence of cervical lesions, the bleeding began on or before the 40th day of pregnancy in 8 percent. They interpreted such bleeding to be physiological, the consequence of implantation. Bleeding during pregnancy was three times more frequent among multiparas than among primigravidas. Of 83 multiparas, 25 percent experienced bleeding.

Alleged instances in which women are said to have

"menstruated" every month throughout pregnancy are incorrect; true uterine bleeding during pregnancy is undoubtedly the result of some abnormality of the reproductive organs. **Bleeding per vagina at any time during pregnancy must be regarded as abnormal and portends a much greater likelihood of serious pregnancy complications.**

Cessation or absence of menstruation can be caused by a number of conditions other than pregnancy. The most common cause of a delay in the time of onset of the expected next menstrual period (other than pregnancy) is anovulation, which in turn may be the consequence of a number of factors that include severe illness and physiological aberrations induced by emotional disorders, including the fear of pregnancy. Environmental changes as well as a variety of chronic disease processes also may suppress ovulation by inducing anestrogenic or estrogenic anovulation. Delays in the onset of menstruation have also been attributed to persistent corpus luteum function (e.g., in association with cystic corpora lutea); but in our view, the evidence for this entity is not convincing. Most, if not all, instances of prolonged function of the corpus luteum are caused by a pregnancy episode, even though the pregnancy may be unrecognized, as in the case of early missed or incomplete abortion or even undiagnosed ectopic pregnancy.

Changes in the Breasts. Generally, the anatomical changes in the breast that accompany pregnancy are quite characteristic in primiparas, but are less obvious in multiparas, whose breasts may contain a small amount of milky material or colostrum for months or even years after the birth of their last child, especially if breast feeding was chosen. Occasionally, changes in the breasts similar to those caused by pregnancy are found in women with prolactin-secreting pituitary tumors and in women taking drugs that induce hyperprolactinemia. Instances also have been reported of similar breast changes in women with spurious or imaginary pregnancy (*pseudocyesis,* p. 31).

Discoloration of the Vaginal Mucosa. During pregnancy, the vaginal mucosa frequently appears dark bluish or purplish-red and congested; this is the so-called *Chadwick sign* (Chadwick, 1886). This appearance of the vagina is taken as presumptive evidence of pregnancy; but it is not conclusive. Similar changes in vaginal appearance may be induced by any condition that causes intense congestion of the pelvic organs.

Increased Skin Pigmentation and Appearance of Abdominal Striae. These cutaneous manifestations are common to, but not diagnostic of, pregnancy. These signs may be absent during pregnancy; conversely, these changes may be associated with the ingestion of estrogen–progestin contraceptives.

Probable Evidence of Pregnancy

The probable signs of pregnancy include (1) enlargement of the abdomen; (2) changes in the shape, size, and consistency of the uterus; (3) anatomical changes in the cervix; (4) Braxton Hicks contractions; (5) ballottement; (6) physical outlining of the fetus; and (7) positive results of endocrine tests for the presence of hCG in urine or serum.

Enlargement of the Abdomen. By 12 weeks of gestation, the uterus can usually be palpated through the abdominal wall just above the symphysis as a tumor; thereafter, the uterus gradually increases in size until the end of pregnancy. In general, any enlargement of the abdomen in women during the childbearing period is strongly suggestive of pregnancy.

The abdominal enlargement in primiparous women is usually less pronounced than in multiparous women, in whom some of the tone of the abdominal musculature was lost in previous pregnancies; indeed, in some multiparous women, the abdominal wall is so flaccid that the uterus sags forward and downward, producing a pendulous abdomen. This difference in abdominal tone between first and subsequent pregnancies is sometimes so obvious that it is not rare for women in the latter part of a second pregnancy to suspect a twin pregnancy because of the apparent greater size of their abdomen, as compared with that in the corresponding month of their previous pregnancy. The abdomen of the pregnant woman also undergoes significant changes in shape depending on the woman's body position. The uterus is, of course, much less prominent when the woman is in the supine position.

Changes in Size, Shape, and Consistency of the Uterus. During the first few weeks of pregnancy, the increase in size of the uterus is limited principally to the anterioposterior diameter, but at a little later time in gestation, the body of the uterus is almost globular; an average uterine diameter of 8 cm is attained by 12 weeks of pregnancy. On bimanual examination, the body of the uterus during pregnancy feels doughy or elastic and sometimes becomes exceedingly soft.

At about 6 to 8 weeks after the onset of the last menstrual period, the *Hegar sign* becomes manifest. With one hand of the examiner on the abdomen and two fingers of the other hand placed in the vagina, the still-firm cervix is felt, with the elastic body of the uterus above the compressible soft isthmus, which is between the two. Occasionally, the softening at the isthmus is so marked that the cervix and the body of the uterus seem to be separate organs. At this time in pregnancy, the inexperienced examiner may mistakenly conclude that the cervix is a small uterus, and that the softened body of the fundus is a tumor of the ovaries or oviducts. This sign of Hegar is not, however, positively diagnostic of pregnancy, because occasionally it may be present when the walls of the nonpregnant uterus are excessively soft for reasons other than pregnancy.

Changes in the Cervix.

By 6 to 8 weeks' gestation, the cervix often becomes considerably softened. In primigravidas, the consistency of the cervical tissue that surrounds the external os is more similar to that of the lips of the mouth than to that of the nasal cartilage, as it is in nonpregnant women. Other conditions, however, may bring about softening of the cervix. Estrogen–progestin contraceptives, for example, commonly act to cause some softening and congestion of the uterine cervix.

As pregnancy progresses, the cervical canal may become sufficiently patulous as to admit the tip of the examiner's finger. In certain inflammatory conditions, as well as with carcinoma, the cervix may remain firm during pregnancy, yielding only with the onset of labor, if at all.

Braxton Hicks Contractions.

During pregnancy, the uterus undergoes palpable but ordinarily painless contractions at irregular intervals from the early stages of gestation. These contractions may increase in number and amplitude when the uterus is massaged. These Braxton Hicks contractions, however, are not positive signs of pregnancy, because similar contractions are sometimes observed in uteri of women with hematometra and occasionally in the uterus in which there are soft myomas, especially those of the pedunculated, submucous variety. The detection of Braxton Hicks contractions, however, may be helpful in excluding the existence of an ectopic abdominal pregnancy.

Ballottement.

Near midpregnancy, the volume of the fetus is small compared with the volume of amnionic fluid; and consequently, sudden pressure exerted on the uterus may cause the fetus to sink in the amnionic fluid and then rebound to its original position; the tap produced (ballottement) is felt by the examining fingers.

Outlining the Fetus.

In the second half of pregnancy, the outlines of the fetal body may be palpated through the maternal abdominal wall, and the outlining of the fetus becomes easier the nearer that term is approached. Occasionally, subserous myomas may be of such a size and shape as to simulate the fetal head, small parts, or both, thus causing serious diagnostic errors. A positive diagnosis of pregnancy cannot be made, therefore, from this sign alone.

Endocrine Tests of Pregnancy.

The presence of (human) chorionic gonadotropin (hCG) in maternal plasma and its excretion in urine provides the basis for the endocrine tests for pregnancy. This hormone can be identified in body fluids by any one of a variety of immunoassay or bioassay techniques.

Detection of Chorionic Gonadotropin

One constituent of the **fetal-induced maternal recognition of pregnancy** system that arises in trophoblast provides for a convenient chemical test of pregnancy: the production of the glycoprotein hormone, hCG. The production of hCG by fetal trophoblast is important for the maternal recognition of pregnancy because hCG acts to rescue the corpus luteum, the principal site of progesterone formation in the first 6 to 8 weeks of pregnancy, by preventing its involution. HCG is a luteinizing hormone (LH)-like agent that acts as an LH surrogate in responsive tissues, such as the ovary (corpus luteum) and testis (Leydig cells). Specifically, hCG acts by way of the LH receptor. The detection of hCG in biological fluids, either urine or serum of the woman that is tested, is by far the most common test of pregnancy used throughout the world. For this reason, it is imperative that the student of obstetrics become familiar with the chemistry, biological action, and detection of this unique hormone.

History of the Discovery of hCG

The evolution of our understanding of the biological, physiological, and chemical nature of hCG occupies an important niche in the history of obstetrics. It is interesting to recall that the species in which a chorionic gonadotropin was first discovered was the human, and that the formation of chorionic gonadotropin is limited to primates. Hirose (1919) is credited with the initial demonstration of a trophic effect of human placental tissue fragments on the ovaries and uteri of the rabbit; and it was the demonstration of the *pregnancy hormone* in urine of pregnant women by Ascheim and Zondek (1927) that formed the basis for the original consideration of the detection of hCG in urine as a test for pregnancy.

Hertz (1980) related the story of an interesting conversation that he had with Bernhard Zondek. In that conversation, Zondek recounted with good humor that he once chastised his technician for the reporting of a positive pregnancy test that was obtained with the urine of a man. Hertz recounts that the matter was complicated further because the man's last name was the same as that of one of the pregnant women whose urine was tested in the same assay. Ultimately, it was found that the man in question was one in whom there was a testicular tumor that was producing hCG. Now we know that a number of human *neoplasias* produce hCG. Zondek made amends and never doubted that technician's findings again.

The discovery of the *pregnancy hormone* led to the development of the first pregnancy test, and even the laity were familiar with the *Ascheim–Zondek*, or *A-Z test* and the *Friedman tests* for pregnancy because, as Hertz points out, these became household terms. These tests were bioassays that took advantage of the biological property of hCG to stimulate the gonads of experimental animals, either sexually immature animals (the rat) or else induced ovulators (the rabbit). Indeed, the A-Z test, or variations on the theme—stimulation of the follicles of the ovaries of experimental animals, as well as the induction of ovulation in induced ovulators (rabbits) by urine of pregnant women—was the standard test for pregnancy in women for more than 40 years.

Zondek believed that there were two pregnancy-related gonadotropin activities because he observed that concentrates of urine of pregnant women evoked both follicular development and ovulation and corpus luteum formation. For these reasons, he believed that there were two separate agents, and he referred to these putative agents as *prolan A* and *prolan B*. Soon there was considerable controversy as to the relationship between the gonadotropin(s) in urine of pregnant women and those extracted from pituitary tissue. Hertz recounts the history of, and the resolution of, this controversy as follows: Zondek (1931) and others emphasized that, by use of the bioassay procedures employed, there was, in the urine of postmenopausal women, follicle-stimulating activity. It was also demonstrated that whereas the avian gonad and the ovary of the immature rhesus monkey were responsive to extracts of the pituitary, there was no such response to concentrates of urine of pregnant women. Convincing evidence that the two preparations, the pituitary extracts and concentrates of urine of pregnant women, were different in gonadotropin properties was obtained by Reichert and co-workers (1932), who demonstrated that the hypophysectomized rat was virtually unresponsive to extracts of urine of pregnant women but readily responsive to extracts of pituitary tissue.

In 1938, the placental source of hCG was solidified further and verified by Gey and co-workers, who demonstrated the production of the hormone by trophoblast cells maintained in tissue culture. Based on the work of these pioneering investigators, we since have come to know (1) the nature as well as structure of hCG; (2) in large measure, the molecular events involved in its mechanism of action; (3) the nature of its biosynthesis and processing; and (4) the utility of this glycoprotein hormone in the evaluation of certain neoplastic processes. Trials have been conducted to ascertain if the hormone could be used as an antigen for the development of antibodies to hCG as a means of immunization against pregnancy in women.

Chemistry of hCG. HCG is a glycoprotein with a high carbohydrate content; the molecule is a heterodimer comprised of two dissimilar subunits, designated α and β, which are noncovalently linked. These subunits have been separated, isolated in pure form, and the primary structure of each has been characterized (Chap. 6).

Levels of hCG in Pregnancy. HCG is produced in placenta exclusively by syncytiotrophoblast and not by cytotrophoblasts (Chap. 6). As the syncytium is derived from cytotrophoblasts (Chap. 5), however, the synthesis of hCG constitutes an important function of the differentiated trophoblast.

The production of hCG in trophoblasts begins very early in pregnancy, almost certainly on the day of implantation. Thereafter, the levels of hCG in maternal plasma and urine rise very rapidly. Certainly with a sensitive test, such as a radioimmunoassay using antibodies directed against the β-subunit of hCG (which are specific for hCG and not cross-reactive with LH), the pregnancy hormone can be demonstrated in maternal plasma or urine by 8 to 9 days after ovulation. It is estimated that, in early pregnancy, the doubling time of the concentration of hCG in plasma is 1.4 to 2.0 days (Chartier and colleagues, 1979). The levels of hCG in blood and urine increase from the day of implantation until about 60 to 70 days of pregnancy. Thereafter, the concentration of hCG declines slowly until a nadir is reached at about 100 to 130 days of pregnancy. The levels of hCG in the urine of pregnant women closely parallel the levels in serum; peak levels are attained between 60 and 70 days of gestation. A good rule of thumb is that the amount of hCG contained in 1 liter of maternal plasma is equivalent to that contained in 24 hours of urine. Thus, if the urine excreted per 24 hours were 1 liter, the concentration of hCG in serum and in urine would be similar.

Although most curves constructed from mean values for hCG in serum or urine, as a function of gestational age, appear to be quite similar, these curves are not reflective of the considerable variations in the levels of this hormone in blood or urine among individual women at the same time of gestation.

Pregnancy Tests

In this time of wide utilization of the principles of immunoassay for the measurement of thousands of compounds, at a time when radioreceptor assays are common, as are radioenzymatic assays and the use of monoclonal antibodies, it seems strange that we used bioassays for the detection (and quantification) of hCG in biological fluids for nearly 4 decades. On the one hand, it was obviously necessary to establish the general principles of immunoassay before these could be applied to the measurement of hCG as a means of sensitive and accurate testing for pregnancy. But on the other hand, it is reasonably impressive to recall that several of the bioassays for hCG, especially those in which the development of ovarian hyperemia in the immature rat was used as the end-point, were, while insensitive, remarkably accurate by 4 to 5 weeks after ovulation or at least by the time of the second missed menses. This attests to the specific bioaction of hCG and to the enormous amount of this glycoprotein produced in human pregnancy.

Today, there are inexpensive kits available commercially that can be used for pregnancy testing that can be completed in 3 to 5 minutes or less, with high accuracy and (with certain precautions) high precision. The chemical detection of pregnancy involves the demonstration of hCG in blood or urine of the woman to be tested. Many different test systems are available in kit form. Each test, however, is dependent upon the same principle: recognition of hCG (or a subunit thereof) by an antibody to the hCG molecule or the β-subunit thereof. Bandi and colleagues (1987) found that there were 39 commercially available kits for urine pregnancy tests in 1986. Cole and Kardana (1992) observed that in 1991 there were more than 50 commercial kits marketed for measuring hCG in serum. The tests for detecting hCG involve the principles of agglutination inhibition, radioimmunoassay, enzyme-linked immunosorbent assay (ELISA), and immunochromatography.

Antibodies to hCG. In the past, some of the immunoassays and all of the bioassays commonly used for pregnancy testing were not absolutely specific for hCG. Antibodies raised against the complete (intact) hCG molecule also recognized LH. The amino acid sequence of the α-subunit of four glycoprotein hormones—FSH, TSH, LH, and hCG—is identical (Chap. 6). Conversely, the β-subunit for each of these hormones is distinct. Antibodies raised against the complete hCG molecule, therefore, will recognize epitopes on the α-subunit of LH as well as hCG. The apparent hCG activity in biological fluids was sometimes found to differ appreciably, depending upon whether immunoassay or bioassay was employed. Wide and Hobson (1967), and also Bridson and associates (1970), demonstrated that hCG synthesized in vitro by cloned choriocarcinoma cells yielded values twice as great by immunoassay as by bioassay. They suggested that the reduction in biologically active material compared with that found by immunoassays was the result of alterations in the hormone molecule after it was secreted by the trophoblast. We now know, however, that such cells secrete the α-subunit, the β-subunit, and complete hCG; the separate subunits are biologically inactive but are recognized by antibodies in varying degrees of reactivities, dependent upon the particular antibody used.

With the recognition that LH and hCG were composed of an α- and a β-subunit, that the two subunits of each molecular species could be separated and purified, and that the β-subunits of each were structurally distinct, at least at the COOH-terminus (Chap. 6), Vaitukaitis and colleagues (1972) set out to develop

antibodies that would recognize epitopes specific to the β-subunit of hCG. Thereby, an antibody could be used that would discriminate between LH and hCG. The development of such antibodies has provided incredibly useful tools for investigations of physiological processes, for early detection of pregnancy, and for monitoring hCG production in persons with neoplastic trophoblastic disease, both before and during treatment.

Therefore, antibodies, with high specificity for the β-subunit of hCG, with little or no discernible cross-reactivity against LH, have been raised by immunization of animals (polyclonal antibodies) or by hybridoma techniques (monoclonal antibodies) against recognition sites on the β-subunit of hCG; and antibodies have been raised against the free α-subunit of hCG and LH (which are identical).

Immunoassays of hCG

Agglutination Inhibition. In many immunoassay procedures, the principle of agglutination inhibition is used, the prevention of flocculation of hCG-coated particles, such as latex particles to which hCG is covalently bound. The kits commercially available to offices and laboratories that employ failure of agglutination of latex particles to detect hCG in urine, contain two reagents. One is a suspension of latex particles coated with or covalently bound to hCG, and the other contains a solution of hCG antibody. To test for hCG, one drop of urine is mixed with one drop of the antibody-containing solution on a black glass slide. If hCG is not present in the urine tested, antibody will remain available to agglutinate the hCG-coated latex particles, which are added subsequently. Agglutination of the latex particles can be easily observed when a bright light source is illuminated against the dark background of the glass slide. If hCG were present in the urine, it would bind to the antibody and thus prevent antibody-induced agglutination of the hCG-coated latex particles. Therefore, the pregnancy test is positive if no agglutination occurs; the pregnancy test is negative when agglutination occurs.

Radioimmunoassays. In radioimmunoassays, [^{125}I] iodohCG is used as the radiolabeled ligand for antibodies raised against hCG and is dependent upon displacement of (or competition with) the radiolabeled ligand by nonradiolabeled hCG in the biological sample to be tested. In radioimmunoassays, "free" and "bound" [^{125}I]iodohCG are separated and radioactivity that is unbound is assayed. From a construction of standard curves, hCG is quantified with great accuracy and sensitivity by this method. In this immunoassay, antibodies against the β-subunit of hCG are also used.

Enzyme-linked Immunosorbent Assay (ELISA). The enzyme-linked immunosorbent assay (ELISA) is useful for the quantification of extremely small amounts of materials in biological samples. In the ELISA for hCG, a monoclonal antibody, bound to a solid phase support (usually plastic), binds the hCG in the test sample; a second antibody is added to "sandwich" the hCG. It is the second antibody to which an enzyme (e.g., alkaline phosphatase) is linked; when substrate for this enzyme is added, a blue color develops, the intensity of which is related directly to the amount of enzyme and thus to the amount of second antibody bound. This in turn is determined by the amount of hCG present in the test sample. The sensitivity of ELISA for hCG in serum is 50 mIU/mL.

Vallejo (1990) evaluated the utility of an hCG ELISA in detecting hCG in blood stains for forensic pregnancy diagnosis. She found that for qualitative purposes, hCG was stable for 3 months but not necessarily for 6 months in cotton clothing stains at room temperature and even at elevated temperatures (56° C).

Accuracy of Pregnancy Tests. In a multicenter collaborative study sponsored by the National Institutes of Health, Jovanovic and associates (1987) concluded that laboratories conducting routine clinical tests could detect hCG accurately at the time of "missed" menses, but not necessarily before this time.

For some purposes, the precise quantification of hCG in biological fluid (e.g., serum) is important to clinical management. Among these indications are the monitoring of pregnancy (to exclude ectopic pregnancy) and to evaluate the course of neoplastic trophoblastic disease or its treatment (e.g., hydatidiform mole, choriocarcinoma, and selected nontrophoblastic malignancies). For this purpose, some of the commercial kits may give discordant results (Cole and Kardana, 1992). This dilemma appears to be primarily attributable to the fact that immunoreactive "hCG" in serum is a mixture of α- and β-subunit-related molecules with varying recognition by the antibodies to hCG used. For example, there is intact (normal) hCG, "nicked" hCG (missing peptide linkage at the β44-45 or β47-48 amino acids), carbohydrate variants of hCG, hCG missing the β-subunit c-terminal segment, hCG β-subunit core fragment, hCG free α-subunit, and possibly others.

"Do-It-Yourself" Pregnancy Test Kits. Today there are a large number of relatively inexpensive over-the-counter pregnancy test kits for use at home. In several of the tests, the principle of hemagglutination inhibition using sheep erythrocytes is employed with antibodies to hCG and the subject's urine.

Valanis and Perlman (1982) evaluated the prevalence of home pregnancy testing among a wide distribution of subjects according to age, race, and socioeconomic status. They also investigated test results. They found that among 144 women interviewed in the settings of a private physician's office, a Planned Parent-

hood clinic, and a public obstetrics–gynecology clinic, almost one third of the subjects had used a home pregnancy-testing kit. They also found that the false-negative test result incidence was nearly 25 percent, and that only one third of the subjects complied with test kit instructions. They also found greater use among white compared with black women and greater use among middle-income women and among women consulting private physicians. These investigators voiced concern about the high false-negative test results even among women who did ultimately seek medical advice. In this study, only women who did initiate medical care were evaluated. Subsequently, Doshi (1986) found that when women conducted their own in-home pregnancy tests, the predictive value of a negative result was 56 percent and the predictive value of a positive result was 83 percent. Jeng and colleagues (1991) also found that 33 percent of 4700 women surveyed, who recently delivered a child, used a home pregnancy test. The women surveyed were from a variety of socioeconomic backgrounds. Lee and Hart (1990) summarized the reports of several investigators. In all cases, the results obtained by laypersons using the home tests were less accurate than results obtained by trained technologists, even though the home test kits were capable of greater than 97 percent accuracy.

Current progress in the development of home pregnancy-testing kits is centered about the creation of one-step tests. The essential features of this type of test are the use of (1) an absorbent wick that is held in contact with a porous membrane that contains three separate zones of antibody and (2) the principles of immunochromatography. The first zone of antibody is deposited so as to be mobilizable; it consists of colored latex particles sensitized with monoclonal antibodies to the β-subunit of hCG, which is immobilized in the membrane. If the urine contains hCG, it will react with the anti-α-hCG on the latex, and this will be trapped by the second, anti-β-subunit hCG zone antibody, causing the formation of a colored line in the large window (May, 1991).

Physician opinion is divided concerning the wisdom of making pregnancy testing available to nonprofessionals. Some argue that such tests will give results that will prompt women to see physicians earlier. We are of the view that the reverse may be more likely in those complicated situations in which early physician consultation is urgently needed.

Pharmacological Endocrine Assay of Pregnancy. Progestin-induced withdrawal uterine bleeding was used in the past in attempts to differentiate pregnancy from other causes of amenorrhea. In the absence of pregnancy, withdrawal bleeding usually occurs 3 to 5 days after a test dose of progestin in estrogen-producing anovulatory women. This response, of course, requires an estrogen-primed endometrium. Withdrawal of the progestin results in uterine bleeding if there is little or no endogenous progesterone production. If there is sufficient production of endogenous progesterone or if the endometrium is not estrogen-primed, withdrawal bleeding does not occur.

In general, this method offers little that cannot be accomplished by a careful evaluation of the woman's history and by ascertaining, at the time of pelvic examination, whether cervical mucus is present and, if so, whether the spread and dried mucus crystallizes to form a fern or a cellular pattern (Chap. 4). If copious thin mucus is present and if a fern pattern develops on drying, early pregnancy is very unlikely and the woman almost certainly will experience uterine bleeding after treatment with and withdrawal of progestin. If little cervical mucus is present and a highly cellular pattern forms, she may or may not be pregnant. If not pregnant, she may or may not sustain uterine bleeding after receiving progestin, depending upon her own supply of endogenous progesterone. Moreover, currently there is fear that progestins are potential teratogens (Chap. 42). Therefore, progestins should not be used in women who are believed to be pregnant except in unusual circumstances (e.g., after removal of the corpus luteum before completion of the 8th week of pregnancy).

Summary and Critique of Pregnancy Tests for hCG. **None of the chemical tests of pregnancy is sufficiently accurate to provide positive proof of pregnancy. Unfortunately, pregnancy tests conducted by women at home may give rise to false security or unnecessary alarm if she cannot evaluate the likely validity of the results of such tests in light of other signs or symptoms.**

Measurement of hCG in Gynecological Disorders

Ectopic pregnancy is a common gynecological disorder that may present a variety of difficulties in diagnosis and management (Chap. 32). Frequently, the routinely used clinical tests for pregnancy, when the embryo is implanted outside the endometrial cavity (ectopic pregnancies), are negative for hCG. This is the case for a variety of reasons, likely the most common being reduction in placentation for the stage of gestation because of the ectopic site of implantation, disruption of trophoblasts by hemorrhage, or embryonic death. Nonetheless, hCG is present in plasma and urine of most (probably all) women with ectopic pregnancies, albeit generally in lower concentrations than in women with normal intrauterine pregnancies at comparable stages of gestations (Barnes and associates, 1985).

In many instances of unruptured ectopic pregnancy, the diagnosis may be difficult. For this reason, the detection of hCG in biological fluids of such women, or the demonstration of declining levels of hCG, may be of considerable assistance in reaching a definitive diagnosis. By use of sensitive radioimmunoassay procedures with antibodies directed toward the β-subunit of the molecule, this goal ordinarily is achieved. If the case under study is not an emergency situation, the demonstration of a decline in hCG levels early in pregnancy, or else a failure of the levels to increase with time, is indicative of impending spontaneous abortion or else ectopic pregnancy. Unfortunately, the reverse does not obtain. Namely, normal levels of hCG are sometimes found in women in whom there is an ectopic pregnancy.

Early in pregnancy, the levels of hCG in plasma double about every 2 days. If this doubling time can be demonstrated, a successful pregnancy outcome can be expected in 90 percent of cases (Pelosi and associates, 1983). This same doubling time in the increase in plasma levels of hCG is found in only 20 percent of women with an ectopic pregnancy. Kadar and colleagues (1981) found that the level of hCG in plasma increased by at least 66 percent in 48 hours early in normal pregnancy but by less than this amount in women with an ectopic pregnancy.

By use of sensitive assays for hCG, positive results have been obtained in 80 to 99 percent of proven cases of ectopic pregnancy by various investigators. It is important to remember, however, that low or falling levels of hCG are not sufficiently distinctive so as to distinguish between ectopic pregnancy and impending spontaneous abortion (Barnes and co-workers, 1985).

Lagrew and colleagues (1983) found that the concentration of hCG in plasma of pregnant women increased in an exponential fashion between 30 and 60 days of pregnancy (dated from first day of last menses). By use of a regression line constructed from measurement of hCG in a large population of pregnant women, these investigators found that the level of hCG at this time in pregnancy was an accurate reflection of the duration of gestation. Thus, in women with infertility and ovulation induction or in other instances in which the last normal menses may not be helpful for pregnancy dating, the levels of hCG in early pregnancy may be informative.

In some cases of elective abortion, postabortion evaluation of hCG may be useful in determining the possibility of persistent trophoblastic function, which could be indicative of the possibilities that abortion was not accomplished (for example, very early in pregnancy—menstrual extraction), that abortion was incomplete, or that the pregnancy was (and is) ectopically implanted. Yet another explanation could be that a twin pregnancy existed, but only one fetus (placenta) was removed. Given the long half-life of hCG, early postabortal testing, however, is of limited utility. Postabortion follow-up testing for hCG, if indicated, is best conducted 2 to 3 weeks after the procedure (Derman and colleagues, 1981).

Positive Signs of Pregnancy

The three positive signs of pregnancy are (1) identification of fetal heart action separately and distinctly from that of the pregnant woman, (2) perception of active fetal movements by the examiner, and (3) recognition of the embryo and fetus at most any time in pregnancy by sonographic techniques or of the more mature fetus radiographically in the latter half of pregnancy.

Identification of Fetal Heart Action. Hearing or observing the pulsations of the fetal heart assures the diagnosis of pregnancy. Contractions of the fetal heart can be identified by auscultation with a special fetoscope, by use of the *Doppler principle* with ultrasound, and by use of sonography.

The heartbeat of the fetus can be detected by auscultation with a stethoscope by 17 weeks' gestation, on average, and by 19 weeks in nearly all pregnancies in nonobese women (Jimenez and co-workers, 1979). Normally, the fetal heart rate at this stage of gestation and beyond ranges from 120 to 160 beats per minute and is heard as a double sound resembling the tick of a watch under a pillow. To establish the diagnosis of pregnancy, it is not sufficient merely to "hear" the "fetal" heart; it must be different from that of the maternal pulse. During much of pregnancy, the fetus moves freely in the amnionic fluid; and consequently, the site on the maternal abdomen where the fetal heart sounds can be heard best will vary as the position of the fetus changes.

Several instruments are available that make use of the *Doppler principle* to detect the action of the fetal heart. By use of these instruments, ultrasound is directed toward the moving blood of the fetus. The sound reflected by the moving blood undergoes a shift in frequency, the echo of which is detected by a receiving crystal immediately adjacent to the transmitting crystal. Because of the difference in heart rates, pulsatile flow in the fetus is easily differentiated from that of the mother unless there is severe fetal bradycardia or else significant maternal tachycardia. Fetal cardiac action can be detected almost always by the 10th week of gestation with appropriate equipment in which the Doppler principle is employed.

Echocardiography can be used to detect fetal heart action as early as 48 days after the first day of the last normal menses (Robinson, 1972). *Real-time sonography* can be used to detect fetal heart action and fetal movement after the second month of pregnancy.

Upon auscultation of the abdomen of the pregnant woman in the later months of pregnancy, the examiner may often hear sounds other than those produced by fetal heart action, the most common of which are (1) the funic (umbilical cord) souffle, (2) the uterine souffle, (3) sounds resulting from movement of the fetus, (4) the maternal pulse, and (5) the gurgling of gas in the intestines of the pregnant woman.

The *funic souffle* is caused by the rush of blood through the umbilical arteries. It is a sharp, whistling sound that is synchronous with the fetal pulse and can be heard in perhaps 15 percent of pregnancies. It is inconstant, sometimes being recognizable distinctly at the time of one examination, but not found in the same pregnancy on other occasions.

The *uterine souffle* is heard as a soft, blowing sound that is synchronous with the maternal pulse; it is usually heard most distinctly during auscultation of the lower portion of the uterus. This sound is produced by the passage of blood through the dilated uterine vessels and is characteristic not only of pregnancy but of any condition in which the blood flow to the uterus is greatly increased. Accordingly, a uterine souffle may be heard in nonpregnant women with large uterine myomas or large tumors of the ovaries.

Frequently, the maternal pulse can be heard distinctly by auscultation of the abdomen; and in some women, the pulsation of the aorta is unusually loud. Occasionally during examination, the pulse of the mother may become so rapid as to simulate the fetal heart sounds.

In addition to the sounds described, it is not unusual to hear certain other sounds that are produced by the passage of gases or liquids through the intestines of the pregnant woman.

Perception of Fetal Movements. The second positive sign of pregnancy is the detection, by the examiner, of movements by the fetus. After about 20 weeks' gestation, active fetal movements can be felt, at indeterminate intervals, by placing the examining hand on the woman's abdomen. These fetal movements vary in intensity from a faint flutter early in pregnancy to brisk motions at a later period; the latter are sometimes visible as well as palpable. Occasionally, somewhat similar sensations may be produced by contractions of the intestines or the muscles of the abdominal wall of the pregnant woman, although these should not deceive an experienced examiner.

Ultrasonic Recognition of Pregnancy. A normal intrauterine pregnancy may be demonstrated by abdominal pulse echo sonography after only 4 to 5 weeks of gestation (menstrual age) (Fig. 2–3). After 6 weeks, the small white gestational ring is so characteristic that failure to identify it raises doubts about pregnancy. Thus, there may be ultrasonic confirmation of pregnancy by the time that some of the common tests for hCG in urine become positive. By careful scanning, distinct echoes from the embryonic poles can be demonstrated within the gestational ring by 7 weeks after commencement of the last normal menstrual period. By 8 weeks, fetal brain is seen and heart action can be detected using Doppler or real-time sonography. By this time, from the length of the embryo, the gestational age can be estimated quite

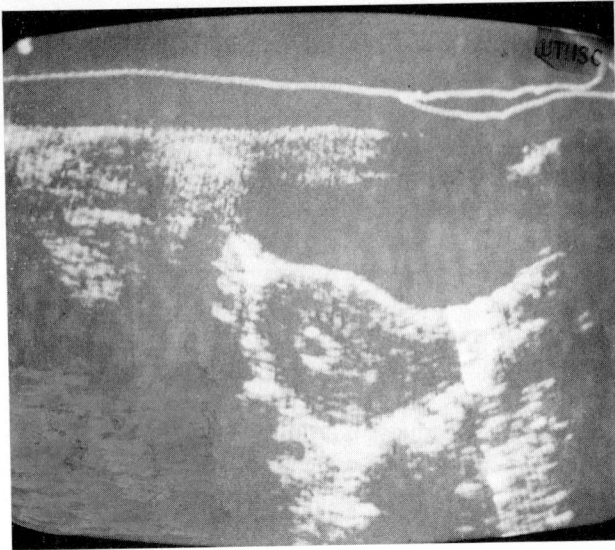

Fig. 2–3. Longitudinal abdominal sonogram in which a gestational sac at 5 to 6 weeks of gestational (menstrual) age is demonstrated.

accurately (Fig. 2–4). Up to 12 weeks, the crown–rump length is predictive of gestational age within 4 days (American College of Obstetricians and Gynecologists, 1988).

In addition to the early identification of normal pregnancy, the findings of sonography may also permit the identification of gestations in which there is a blighted ovum—that is, the embryo is dead and an abortion will ultimately occur. The characteristic features of a blighted ovum are (1) loss of definition of the gestational sac, (2) an unusually small gestational sac, and (3)

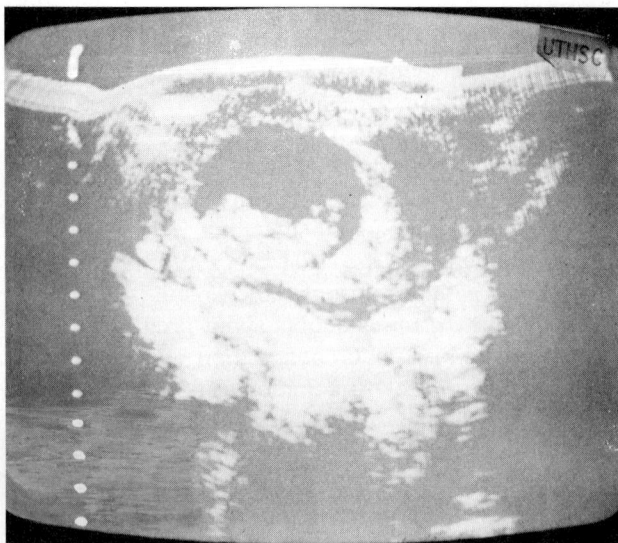

Fig. 2–4. Transverse abdominal sonographic view of amnionic sac in which there is a fetus of 10 to 12 weeks' gestational age.

the absence of echoes emanating from the fetus after 8 weeks' gestation.

By 11 weeks of amenorrhea, the pregnancy ring is normally no longer distinctly identifiable in the uterine cavity by sonography. By the 14th week, the fetal head and thorax can be identified; and soon thereafter, the placental site can be visualized by ultrasound techniques. First-trimester fetal ultrasonic findings were reviewed by Green and Hobbins (1988).

Subsequently, ultrasonography can be used to identify the number of fetuses, the presenting part(s), various fetal anomalies, and hydramnios, and to assess the rate of fetal growth by measuring, serially, the biparietal diameter of the fetal head, the circumference of the fetal abdomen, and other fetal structures.

Vaginal Sonography in Early Pregnancy. Ultrasonic scanning, using a vaginal probe, provides a number of methodological advantages for selected diagnostic purposes in obstetrics and gynecology (Bernaschek and colleagues, 1988). By use of this technique, a gestational sac in the uterine cavity as small as 2 mm in diameter can be identified. This corresponds to a time about 16 days after ovulation or 10 days after implantation. Rempen (1990) found that visualization of the chorionic cavity is possible by 2 weeks after conception, the yolk sac at 3 weeks, and cardiac activity is readily recognized at 4 postconceptional weeks by vaginal sonography. The threshold value (i.e., the earliest) at which fetal heart motion was detected corresponded to 26 days postconception (40 menstrual days), an hCG level of 6770 mIU/mL, and a crown–rump length of 2 mm. This technique, therefore, provides a valuable means for establishing fetal life in complicated cases of early pregnancy.

The findings of sonography almost always provide as much, and usually much more, information than do those of radiography without the potential, albeit undefined, risks of irradiation. To date, no adverse effects on the human embryo or fetus have been identified from exposure to energies comparable to those used for clinical sonographic examinations.

Fetal Recognition by Radiography. Whenever the fetal skeleton is distinguished radiologically, the diagnosis of pregnancy is certain. This method of positive identification of pregnancy is usually not valid, however, until after 16 weeks of gestation, and it is not used today for this purpose. On occasion, however, radiological examination of the abdomen is obliged or is conducted without knowledge of the existence of pregnancy. By x-ray examination, Bartholomew and co-workers (1921) were able to make a positive diagnosis of pregnancy by 20 weeks' gestation in only one third of the women examined who were pregnant and in only one half by 24 weeks. Just how early the fetal skeleton is visible in the radiograph depends, in part, upon the thickness of the abdominal wall of the mother and the radiological technique used. Foci of ossification in the fetus have been demonstrated as early as 14 weeks, although ordinarily the gestation must have reached 16 weeks or more before the fetal skeleton can be visualized.

Differential Diagnosis of Pregnancy

The uterus of pregnancy is sometimes mistaken for other tumors occupying the pelvis or abdomen; less frequently, the opposite error is made. The uterine changes of the early weeks of pregnancy may be simulated through enlargement of the uterus caused by myomas, hematometra, adenomyosis, or by apparent enlargement that actually is due to a contiguous but extrauterine mass or masses. As a rule, the enlarged uterus in these circumstances is firmer than it is in pregnancy and is less elastic and boggy. Except in hematometra, moreover, such conditions are usually not attended by cessation of the menses.

Spurious Pregnancy

Imaginary pregnancy, or *pseudocyesis,* usually occurs in women nearing the menopause or in women with an intense desire to be pregnant. Such women may present all the subjective symptoms of pregnancy in association with a considerable increase in the size of their abdomen, caused either by deposition of fat, by gas in the intestinal tract, or by abdominal fluid. In such women, the menses do not as a rule disappear, but may become unpredictable in time of onset and in amount and duration of bleeding. Changes in the breasts, including enlargement; the appearance of galactorrhea; and increased areolar pigmentation sometimes occur. In a majority of these women, there is morning sickness, probably of psychogenic origin.

The ingestion of a variety of phenothiazines can lead to amenorrhea, hyperprolactinemia, breast enlargement, and galactorrhea. Obviously, the underlying emotional problem may be compounded by these changes.

The supposed fetal movements that are perceived by women with pseudocyesis can usually be ascribed to intestinal peristalsis or to muscular contractions of her abdominal wall, but occasionally these are so marked as to deceive physicians. Careful examination of such women usually leads to a correct diagnosis without great difficulty because the small uterus can be palpated on bimanual examination. The greatest difficulty encountered in the care of such women may be that of convincing them of the correct diagnosis. The delusion of pregnancy may persist for years in emotionally distressed women.

Distinction Between First and Subsequent Pregnancies

Occasionally, it is of practical importance to ascertain whether a woman is pregnant for the first time or has previously borne children. Ordinarily, but not always, there are indelible traces of a former term pregnancy.

In a nullipara, the abdomen is usually tense and firm, and the uterus is felt through it with difficulty. The characteristic old abdominal striae and the distinctive changes in the breasts are absent. The labia majora are usually in close apposition and the frenulum is intact. The vagina is usually narrow and characterized by well-developed rugae. The cervix is softened but usually does not admit the tip of the examiner's finger until the very end of pregnancy.

In multiparas, the abdominal wall is usually lax and, at times, pendulous, and through it the uterus is palpated readily. In addition to the pink abdominal striae associated with the present pregnancy, the silvery cicatrices of past pregnancies also may be present. Usually, the breasts are not so firm as in women during their first pregnancy, and frequently there are striae in the skin over the breast tissue similar to those on the abdomen. The vulva of a woman who previously has delivered vaginally usually gapes open to some extent, the frenulum has disappeared, and the hymen is transformed into the myrtiform caruncles. In multiparas who previously have delivered vaginally, the external os of the cervix, even in the early months of pregnancy, may admit the tip of the examiner's finger, which can be extended up to the internal os. Moreover, the sites of healed lacerations of the cervix can usually be identified.

Identification of Fetal Life or Death

A learned review of the problems of diagnosis and management of fetal death was presented by Pitkin (1987). He observed that all too often the occurrence of fetal death comes *"utterly without warning in a pregnancy that has previously seemed entirely normal."* Regrettably, the cause of this tragic event may go undiscovered; in fact, the "unknown" cause group may constitute 50 percent of the total. The scenario that ensues, Pitkin says, is all too commonly as follows: The woman, with anxiety in her voice, reports that she has not felt fetal movement for hours or for 1 or 2 days. The fetal heart is not heard by auscultation or identified by real-time ultrasound examination. Failure to detect heart wall motion after 10 to 12 weeks gestation by real-time ultrasonography is reliable evidence of fetal death. Ancillary findings of sonography in the case of fetal death include scalp edema and the sequelae of maceration.

In the early months of pregnancy, the diagnosis of

fetal death may present difficulty. Unless ultrasonic techniques are employed, the diagnosis of fetal death can be made with certainty only after it can be shown by repeated examinations that the uterus has remained constant in size or that there has actually been a decrease in size over a number of weeks. Because trophoblasts of the placenta may continue to produce hCG for several weeks after death of the embryo or fetus, a positive endocrine test for pregnancy is not necessarily indicative that the fetus is alive.

In the latter half of pregnancy, the cessation of fetal movements usually alerts the woman to the possibility of fetal death, but if fetal cardiac action can still be identified distinct from that of the mother, the fetus is certainly alive. If, by careful auscultation, the fetal heart tones are not heard, however, the fetus probably is dead. There is a possibility of error, of course, especially in pregnancies in which the fetal heart is remote from the examiner, as when the woman is obese or if hydramnios exists.

Ultrasonic examinations in which the Doppler shift principle is employed, as described, are of considerable value in the evaluation of pregnancies in which the fetal heart cannot be heard by auscultation with a stethoscope. The use of Doppler ultrasound is especially valuable when fetal death is suspected but fetal "heart action" can be identified. If fetal heart action is not demonstrated after careful examination, it can be stated that very likely, but not absolutely, the fetus is dead. Real-time ultrasonic examination, when carefully performed, will serve to accurately identify the presence or absence of fetal heart motion. It has also been observed that, by vaginal ultrasonography, an enlarged amnionic cavity, compared with the crown–rump length, in early gestation is indicative of embryonic death (Horrow, 1992).

If the fetus has been dead for some time, it can usually be shown by careful examination that the uterus does not correspond in size to the estimated duration of pregnancy, or that the uterus has actually become smaller than previously observed. With the death of the fetus, maternal weight gain usually ceases; and not infrequently, there is even a slight decrease in her weight. At the same time, retrogressive changes usually have occurred in the breasts. Sometimes the diagnosis of fetal death cannot be made from the findings of a single examination, but fetal death certainly must be considered when the signs just mentioned are identified and fetal cardiac action cannot be detected.

Occasionally, a positive diagnosis of fetal death can be established by palpating the collapsed fetal skull through the partially dilated cervix; in that event, the loose bones of the fetal head feel as though these are contained in a flabby bag.

Radiographic techniques were used in the past but are rarely indicated today to establish fetal death. There are three principal radiological signs of fetal death:

1. Significant overlap of the skull bones (Spalding sign), caused by liquefaction of the brain, a process that requires several days to develop. A similar sign may develop occasionally with a living fetus, as when the fetal head is compressed in the maternal pelvis.
2. Exaggerated curvature of the fetal spine. Because the development of this sign depends on maceration of the spinous ligaments, its development also requires several days; moreover, mild degrees of curvature of the spine in living fetuses may be misleading.
3. Demonstration of gas in the fetus is an uncommon but reliable sign of fetal death (Fig. 2–5).

In instances in which the fetus has been dead for several days to weeks, the amnionic fluid is red to brown and usually turbid rather than nearly colorless and clear. The finding of such amnionic fluid is not absolutely diagnostic of fetal death, however, because prior hemorrhage into the amnionic sac, as rarely occurs during amniocentesis, may lead to similar discoloration of the amnionic fluid even though the fetus is alive.

Overview of Ovarian Function

Obstetrician as Endocrinologist. The obstetrician, as endocrinologist, enjoys a significant advantage over his internist colleagues who are obliged to deal with endo-

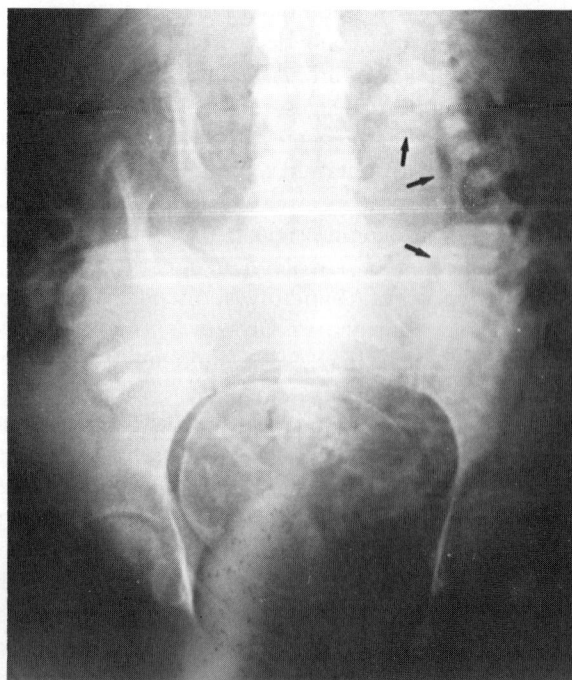

Fig. 2–5. Fetal death is established by the presence of gas in a major vessel. The close proximity to the fetal spine implies that the vessel is the aorta.

crine problems in men. The clinical manifestations of abnormalities of the ovarian cycle are easily detected, informative guides to the endocrine milieu of women. Only a few of us will become students of the molecular events that serve to regulate ovarian endocrine function, ovum maturation, or ovulation, but we all should be knowledgeable of the reproductive physiology and pathophysiology of women.

Despite the likelihood that repetitive cyclic ovulation for long times is an aberration of societal development, the faithful repetition of the ovarian cycle itself—predictable alterations in hormone production and cyclic extrusion of a single ovum at approximately 1-month intervals—is the rule and not the exception. It is true that some women, on occasion, are anovulatory—and a few are permanently so—but this situation is relatively uncommon compared with the reverse: regular, predictable, cyclic ovulation. This fact stands in further testimony to the remarkable physiological expenditures that are obliged involuntarily, but faithfully fulfilled, in reproductive-age women to achieve pregnancy. If it is accepted that the month after month repetition of ovulation is not the biological evolutionary norm, the monotonous success of this process in women who have chosen to be infertile is even more astounding.

The Ovary and Cyclic, Spontaneous, Predictable Menses. We also know that the occurrence of spontaneous, predictable menses at reasonable intervals (21 to 35 days) is strong evidence for recurrent ovulation. Moreover, if such menses are associated with some degree of discomfort, which may vary from only a prodroma of impending menstruation to that of severe dysmenorrhea, the likelihood of cyclic ovulation is even greater. This is probably true because progesterone withdrawal-induced menstruation (i.e., that which is characteristic of ovulation) is associated with the endometrial formation of $PGF_{2\alpha}$ and possibly endothelin-1, which can cause vasoconstriction of the endometrial spiral arteries and myometrial contractions, the pseudoparturition of fertility failure (Chap. 4).

Recurrent Ovulation Equals Normal Sex Hormone Production. We do not accept the proposition that regular, predictable menses occur in anovulatory women (excepting in those who are ingesting sex steroids, such as oral contraceptives). Therefore, the term *"anovulatory cycles"* is a nonsequitur. This being the case, two equations can be derived: (1) cyclic, predictable, spontaneous menses = ovulation; (2) ovulation = normal sex hormone production. In women who are ovulatory, therefore, it can be assumed, with great confidence, that the production of pituitary gonadotropins, both FSH and LH, as well as estrogens, androgens, and progesterone, is appropriate. Very rare exceptions to this general rule can be found, as in women with so-called *luteal phase*

deficiency, and in women with abetalipoproteinemia. But almost always, the history of cyclic, predictable, spontaneous menstruation is more valuable than the results of many hundreds of dollars worth of endocrine tests.

For this reason, a thorough and carefully obtained menstrual history is of real as well as potential value. Consider the woman, for example, who experiences the regular, cyclic, predictable onset of menstruation, but who sustains abnormal bleeding thereafter. Such a woman almost invariably will have some organic disease of the uterus to account for the abnormal uterine bleeding. At the same time, except in women over 40 years of age, the occurrence of unpredictable uterine bleeding—unpredictable in onset, amount, or duration of bleeding—which is usually painless, is most often the result of chronic anovulation or undiagnosed pregnancy rather than organic uterine disease. In women past 40, the possibility of endometrial carcinoma as a cause of abnormal uterine bleeding increases and must be considered. The same is true of women before age 40 who are chronically anovulatory; but in these women, regular, cyclic, spontaneous menses do not occur.

Overview of the Regulation of Ovarian Function.

The history of the study of the physiological regulation of the ovarian cycle and its hormones is not dissimilar to that of the investigations of many other endocrine glands. From a very simplistic, but at the same time quite sophisticated interpretation of events—that the pituitary served as the "master gland"—we have marched through a host of hypotheses. Many of these were meritorious and supported by experimental findings that, while convincing at the time, were obviously incomplete. The prevailing theory of the preceding 2 or 3 decades has been one in which it was envisioned that the brain—and in particular, specialized functions of the hypothalamus—served as the central processing site for receipt of and thence transmittal of signals that regulated the function of the anterior pituitary. The release of small peptides into the hypophyseal–portal blood was, and is now, considered to be of signal importance in the hypothalamic regulation of anterior pituitary release of gonadotropins and prolactin.

In the past decade, however, many investigators have guided our thinking to include a consideration of intraovarian control mechanisms that may constitute fail-safe systems vitally important to the successful maintenance of cyclic ovarian function that eventuates in ovulation.

Intra-Ovarian Fail-Safe Systems to Ensure Ovulation.

We know that the levels of various hormones in blood at any given stage of the ovarian cycle vary widely among women, and even in a given woman from one cycle to the next. Yet, the *sine qua non* of perfection in ovarian function—that is, ovulation—is accomplished.

Likely this is facilitated by intraovarian regulatory factors that serve in a fail-safe manner to ensure ovulation. The nature of the molecular events that are controlled by these fail-safe systems are of such real and potential importance that new, descriptive, and even somewhat romantic terms are used to describe some of the putative agents involved: inhibins and activins, growth factors, cybernins, gonadocrinins and gonadostatins, cytokines, and monokines.

Perhaps one of the most important aspects of the recognition of these intraovarian regulators is that we can set aside the long-standing notion that the hypothalamic–pituitary–ovarian cycle is *"delicately balanced and controlled."* Nonsense! If this were the case, a population explosion would not be the major health, environmental, and economic problem of the world today. Rather, ovulation is the rule even with appreciable fluctuations in sex steroid hormone levels and with considerable differences in gonadotropin levels at various stages of the cycle. And it is probable that the intra-ovarian fail-safe control systems act as the buffer systems that permit ovulation despite the presence of other endocrine disorders, morbid obesity, severe pelvic inflammatory disease, and many other anomalies of physiological function that would upset a "delicate" system much more readily.

The Ovary, the Follicle, and Ovulation

George W. Corner (1943) provided a translation of the observations (written in Latin) of the celebrated Dutch anatomist, Regner de Graaf (1641–1673), for whom the graafian follicle is named, concerning the anatomy and function of the human ovaries, which, de Graaf initially referred to as the female testes.

> The testes of women differ much from those of the male as to position, form, size, substance, integuments, and function.... [They] are located in the interior cavity of the abdomen, in order that they may be nearer the uterus and serve the better and more easily their intended purpose.

We have emphasized that the physiological expenditures involuntarily obliged in women to achieve pregnancy are phenomenal. In the absence of pharmacological intervention, ovarian function is directed by single purpose to the success of ovulation: pregnancy. Indeed, de Graaf long ago espoused a rather similar view:

> Thus, the general function of the female testicles is to generate the ova, to nourish them, and to bring them to maturity so that they serve the same purpose in women as the ovaries of birds. On this account, many have considered these bodies useless, but this is incorrect, because they are indis-

pensable for reproduction. Hence, they should rather be called ovaries than testes because they show no similarity, either in form or contents, with the male testes properly so called.

Embryology of the Ovary. The anatomical, morphological, and physiological parade of events that lead to the development of the mature graafian follicle and release of the mature ovum at ovulation begins early in embryonic development (Chap. 3). Baker (1978) states, with considerable conviction, that *"One of the most important concepts in reproductive physiology is that the definitive germ cells—the eggs and spermatozoa—are derived solely from the primitive sex cells [that are] found early in embryonic development."* He goes on to say that there is *"a continuity of the germ-cell line from embryo to adult."* As Baker again emphasizes, *"there is overwhelming evidence in support of the classical view of the continuity of the germ-cell line,"* but no evidence for *"the transformation of epithelial (somatic) cells into those of the germinal line."*

About 3 weeks after conception, the germ cells in the human embryo are localized in the epithelium of the yolk sac near the developing allantois (Baker, 1978; Fig. 2–6). Thereafter, these germ cells migrate to the connective tissue of the hindgut and thence move progressively to the gonadal primordia or ridges (Fig. 2–6). The number of germ cells increases by mitosis. There may

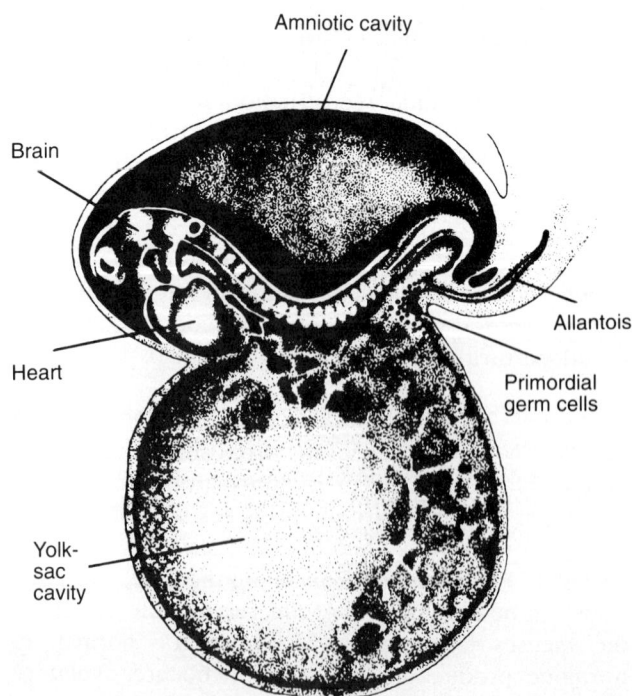

Fig. 2–6. Reconstruction of 24-day human embryo and its amnion. The primordial germ cells (black dots) are grouped at the top of the yolk sac and in the ventral wall of the developing hindgut. (From Baker, 1978.)

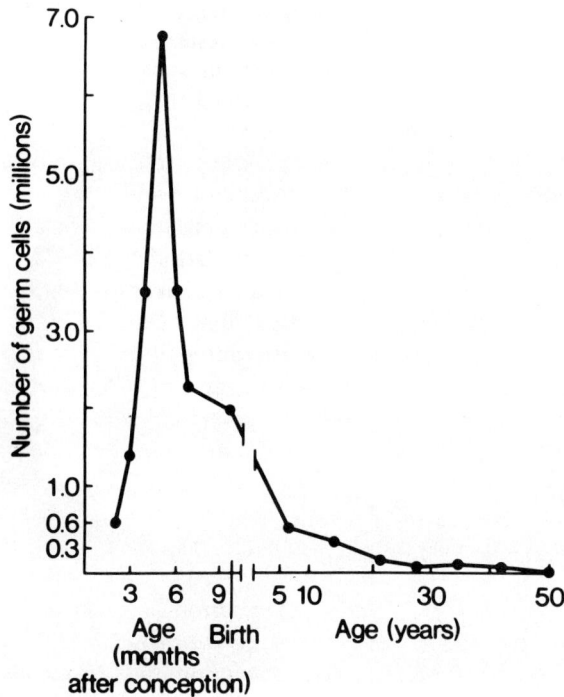

Fig. 2–7. Changes in the total population of germ cells in the human ovary with increasing age. (From Baker, 1971.)

be a substance (telopheron) that directs the anatomical migration of the germ cell to the genital ridge. The exact means by which germ cells migrate is not fully defined; ameboid activity, chemotactic substances, and lytic enzyme activities may all be involved. Generally, the germ cells remain in the cortex if the presumptive gonad is to be an ovary; and the differentiation of the embryonic female gonad is late compared with that of the male.

The number of germ cells in developing ovaries, by mitosis, changes rapidly during gestational development (Fig. 2–7). After a definitive number of mitoses, the oogonia are transformed into oocytes—at this time, prophase is entered, which is the first of two meiotic divisions; thereafter, there are no new oocytes formed. Therefore, as oogonia are eliminated from the ovary—before birth primarily—the population of germ cells can only be reduced in number.

Prodigality, as Baker states, is the *keynote* in the early history of the germ cells—that is, the oogonia. But if this were true of ova, consider the extraordinary extent of prodigality in the case of spermatogonia, when hundreds of millions are ejaculated in a single copulation.

The lifetime history of germ cell maturation, loss, atresia, development, and ovulation is illustrated in Figure 2–7, which is reproduced, in large measure, from data assembled by Baker. As stated, there is no evidence in support of the proposition that ova are formed in the human after birth. Rather, it has been estimated that there are 600,000 oogonia in the ovaries of female fetuses at 2 months and 6,800,000 at 5 months gestation. Degeneration occurs thereafter, and 2 million are found at birth, but only 300,000 to 400,000 remain in the ovaries of prepubertal girls (Baker, 1978; Fig. 2–7).

Ovarian Folliculogenesis. Before puberty, mature graafian follicles are found only in the deeper portions of the cortex. Later, however, mature follicles also develop in the superficial portions of the ovary. During each ovarian cycle, one follicle makes its way to the surface, and appears there as a transparent vesicle that may vary from only a few to 10 or 12 mm in diameter. As the follicle approaches the surface of the ovary, the wall becomes thinner but more abundantly supplied with vessels (Fig. 2–8), except in the very most prominent projecting portion, which appears to be almost bloodless. This small, avascular locus is called the stigma, which is the site on the follicle wall where rupture is to occur with ovulation.

After formation of the oocytes in the early primordial follicles, the ovum is surrounded by flattened epithelial-like cells (Fig. 2–9). As folliculogenesis progresses, these granulosa cells proliferate and become cuboidal (Figs. 2–10 and 2–11) and then commence to secrete a fluid that ultimately accumulates into one large pool—and in this manner, an antrum is formed.

The ovarian stromal cells differentiate and form the theca externa and theca interna (Figs. 2–10 and 2–11). Through this stage of development, follicular growth appears to proceed independently of gonadotropin action. Hereafter, an integrated set of metabolic events is obliged for complete maturation of the follicle—the choosing of the dominant follicle, which is destined to be the one follicle of the ovary that releases its ovum in a given cycle. Thereafter, as folliculogenesis continues, there is an orderly and progressive sequence of hormonally responsive and operative events that permit and facilitate the final stages of maturation of the dominant follicle in preparation for ovulation.

During this time of folliculogenesis, two major functions emerge: (1) a gonadotropin hormone-receptor adenylate cyclase-coupling system develops in the granulosa cells and (2) a cell-contact system for intercellular communication is established. It is recognized that not only do gonadotropins serve to stimulate and to activate the enzymatic processes of the cells of the follicles, but estradiol, synthesized by the granulosa cells, also acts to alter gonadotropin receptor content and to stimulate growth and development of gap junctions in preantral follicles. Thereby, gonadotropins and estradiol formed in the granulosa cells in situ act in a synergistic manner that results in an exponential growth and secretory phase of the cycle.

The great majority of vesicular follicles, including all of those before puberty, undergo degeneration at various stages of formation (Baker, 1978; Fig. 2–7). As

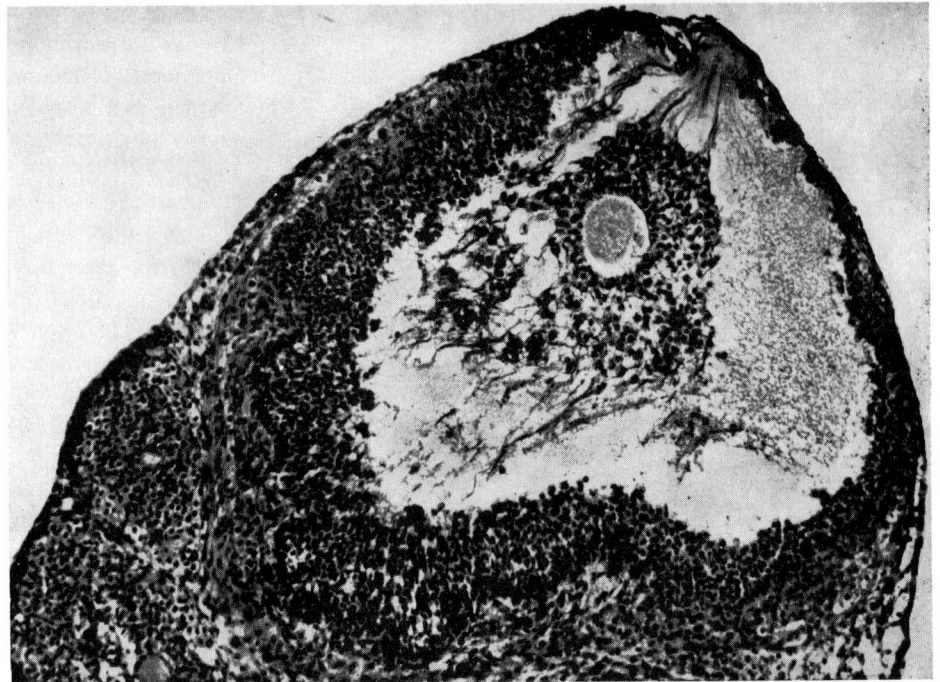

Fig. 2–8. Rat ovary just prior to ovulation. (Courtesy of Dr. Richard J. Blandau.)

Short (1980) puts it, *"only a minute proportion of the total population of oocytes in the ovary present at birth are ever ovulated; the majority perish through atresia."*

During any one ovarian cycle, 20 or more follicles appear to embark on the processes that lead to ovulation. We know little, in fact nothing, of how these few of so many thousand are chosen, let alone how one of these 20 or so follicles becomes the dominant or **chosen one.** As follicular maturation progresses, the order of events is as follows: (1) increase in size of the oocyte; (2) alteration in granulosa cell morphology from flat to cuboidal, followed by granulosa cell replication; and (3) formation of the zona pellucida. The zona pellucida is a clear, mucoid band that envelops the ovum and persists until after the fertilized ovum reaches the uterus (Figs. 2–12 and 2–13).

Thereafter, the theca interna becomes highly vascularized and surrounded by the theca externa (Figs. 2–14 and 2–15). At this time, the increase in follicle size is disproportionately greater than that of the ovum (Fig. 2–16).

Mature Graafian Follicle. The mature follicle is known as a *graafian follicle;* de Graaf described this structure in 1677. Referring to the microscopic structure of the ovary, de Graaf wrote the following.

> From what has just been said, everyone will readily gather that it is the vesicles or their contents solely, which the nerves, arteries, veins, integuments, and the other structures normally observed in the [female] testes are designed to serve. These vesicles have been described under various names by Vesalius, Fallopius, Volcher, Coiter, Laurentius, Castro, Riolan, Bartholin, Wharton, Marchettis, and others. Fallopius says: "I have seen in them indeed certain vesicles, as it were, swollen out with a watery humor, in some yellow, in others transparent." Castro also says: "The [female] testes have within them, besides the vessels, certain cavities full of a thin and watery humor which is like whey or white of egg." But the celebrated Dr. van Horne in his prodromum preferred to call them ova, a term which since it seems to me more convenient than the others, we shall in the future use, and we shall call these vesicles ova.

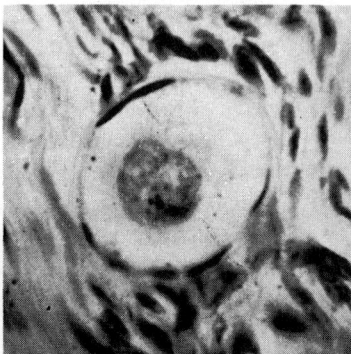

Fig. 2–9. Primordial follicle from ovary of an adult woman.

It seems, therefore, that de Graaf mistook the entire follicle as an ovum, but correctly deduced, nonetheless,

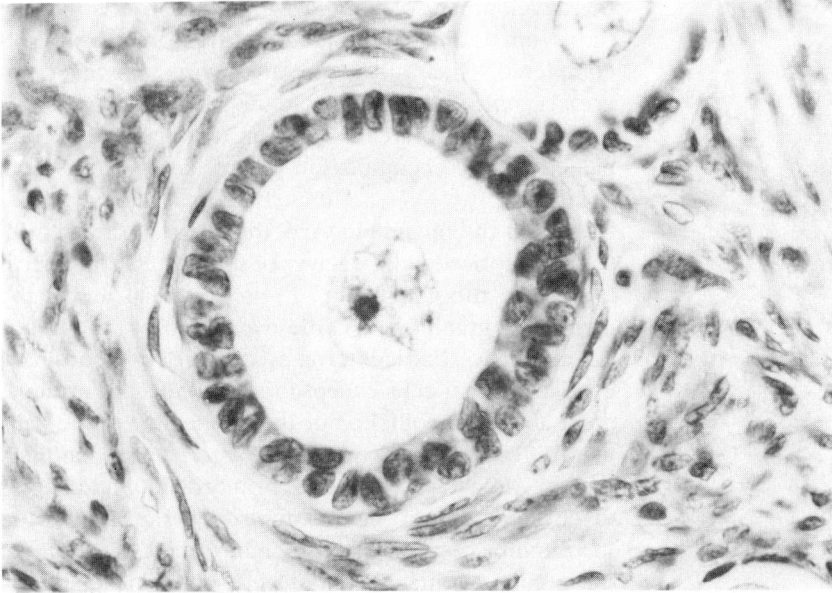

Fig. 2–10. An early growing follicle in an ovary of a 4-year-old girl. A theca layer begins to form. (From Peters, 1979.)

that these were the structures from which the female germ cells were derived.

The follicular cells—the granulosa cells that immediately surround the ovum—constitute the *cumulus oophorus* and *discus proligerus,* a group of granulosa cells that project into the now-abundant follicular fluid in the antrum of the mature follicle. As the graafian follicle grows, the stromal cells that surround the entire follicle enlarge, the capillary net about these cells becomes closer, and the theca interna is formed (Fig. 2–15). The cells of the theca interna are the site of synthesis of C_{19}-steroids, and in particular androstenedione, which serves as the preformed steroid precursor for estradiol formation in the granulosa cells. After ovulation, the cells of the theca interna persist about the collapsed follicle and lie immediately adjacent to the

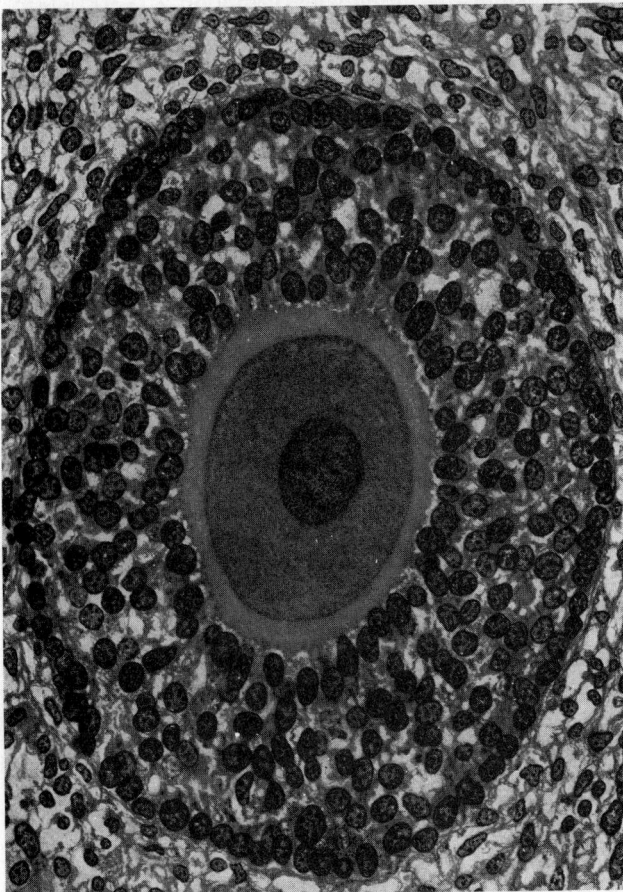

Fig. 2–11. Developing follicle.

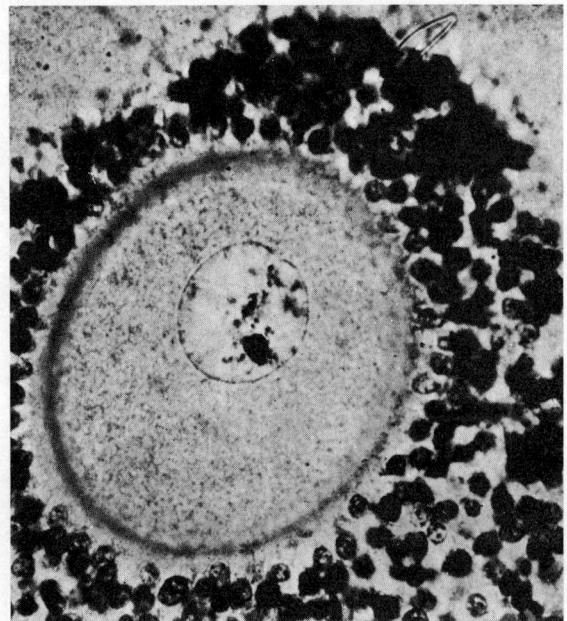

Fig. 2–12. Human oocyte from a large graafian follicle. (Courtesy of Carnegie Institute.)

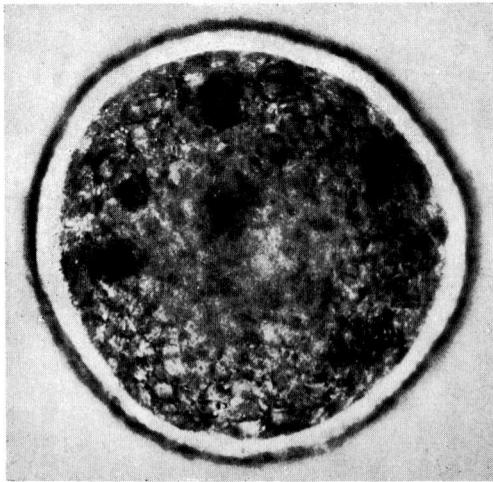

Fig. 2–13. Human ovum washed from fallopian tube. Fresh specimen, surrounded by semitransparent zona pellucida, consists largely of lipoid masses. Ovum measured 0.136 mm in the living state. (Carnegie Collection No. 6289, Dr. W.H. Lewis.)

the development of the graafian follicle, the volume of the ovum increases about 40-fold before maturity is completed. The nucleus of the ovum, however, increases only about threefold in size during this period. The large increase in ovum cytoplasm is accompanied by the accumulation of nutrients such as yolk granules.

From the outside inward, the mature graafian follicle is comprised of (1) a layer of specialized connective tissue, the theca folliculi; (2) an epithelial lining, the membrana granulosa; (3) the ovum; and (4) the liquor folliculi. The theca externa is comprised of ordinary ovarian stromal cells except for the concentric arrangement about the follicle; but the connective tissue cells that differentiate as the theca interna are modified greatly. Almost as soon as the primordial follicle begins to develop, mitotic figures appear in the cells of the surrounding stroma, considerable multiplication of these cells occurs, and these cells become distinctly larger than those of the surrounding connective tissue. As the follicle increases in size, these *theca lutein cells* accumulate lipid and a yellowish pigment, which gives rise to a granular appearance. Simultaneously, there is a striking increase in the vascularity and number of lymphatic spaces of the theca.

Before ovulation, the theca cells are separated from the granulosa cells by a highly polymerized membrane. It is possible that luteinizing hormone acts to depoly-

remaining enlarged granulosa cells, which are then called the granulosa lutein cells, or luteinized granulosa cells.

From the results of measurements of the diameters of ova in sections of well-preserved ovaries, there are indications that although the ovum grows slowly during

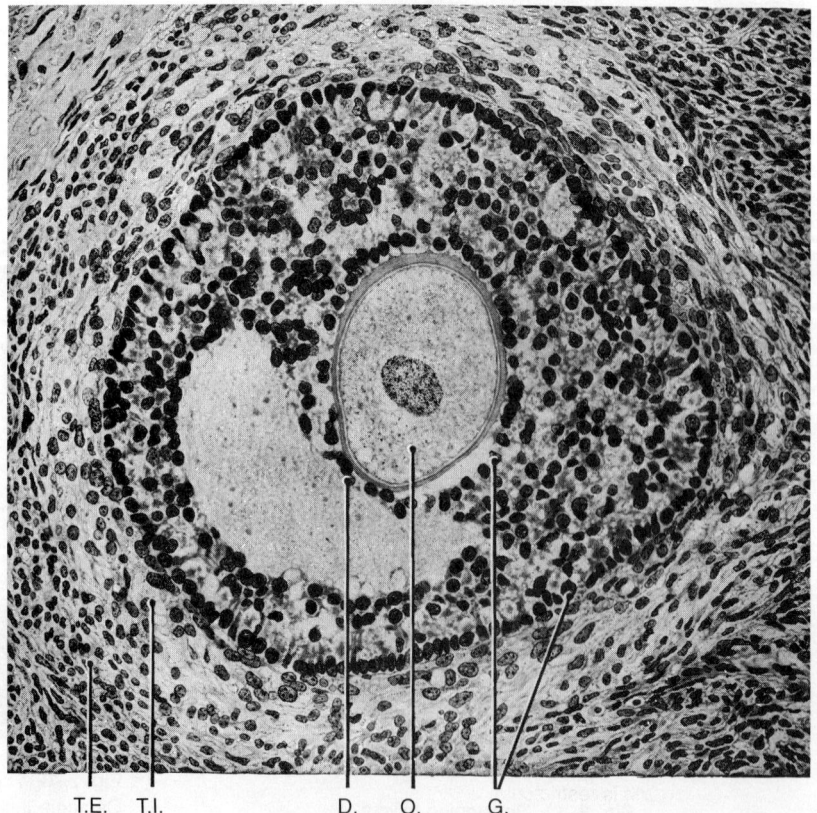

Fig. 2–14. Graafian follicle approaching maturity. (T.E. = theca externa; T.I. = theca interna; D. = discus proligerus [cumulus oophorus]; O. = ovum; G. = granulosa cell layer.)

T.E.   T.I.   D.   O.   G.

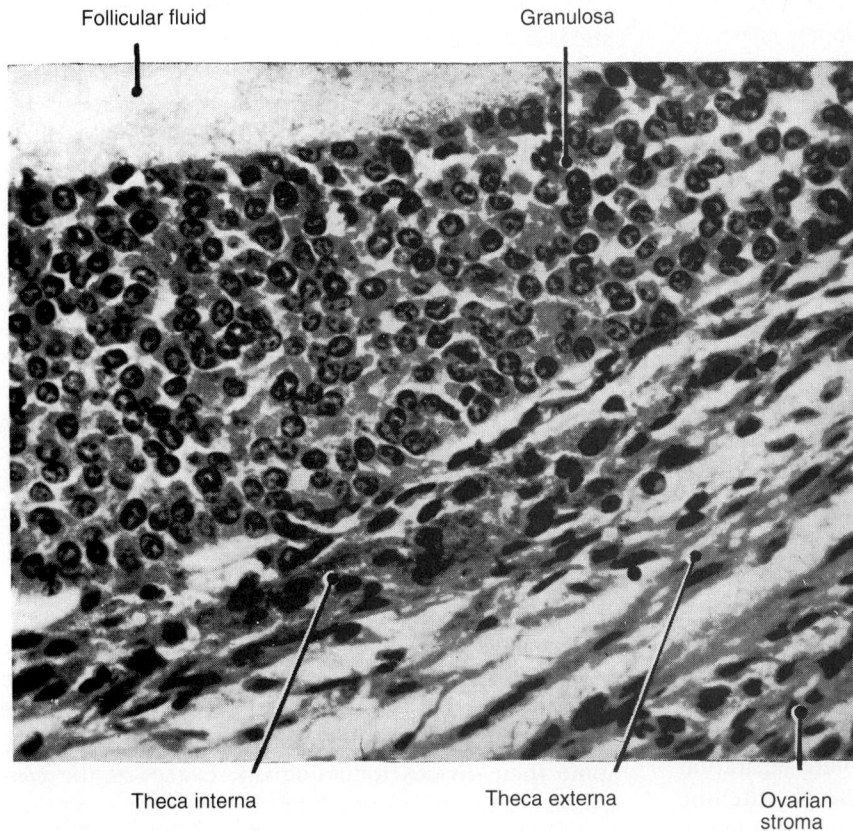

Follicular fluid   Granulosa

Theca interna   Theca externa   Ovarian stroma

Fig. 2–15. Section through the wall of a mature graafian follicle.

merize this membrane at about the time of ovulation. Such an event would facilitate angiogenesis and thereby contribute to the vascularization of the granulosa cells after ovulation in the formation of the corpus luteum. The epithelial lining of the follicle, or membrana granulosa, consists of several layers of small polygonal or cuboid cells in which there are round, darkly staining nuclei; the larger the follicle, the fewer the number of layers. At one time, the membrana granulosa is much

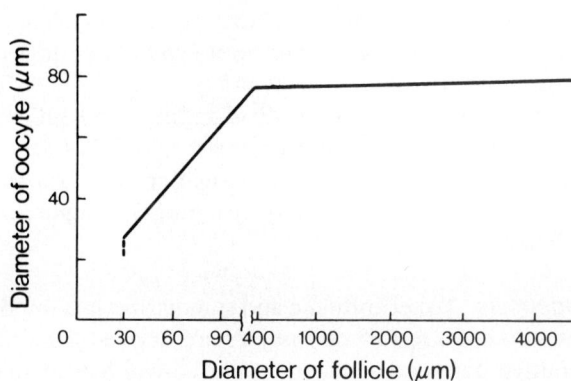

Fig. 2–16. Growth of the oocyte and follicle in the human ovary. First the oocyte alone enlarges, and then both grow at a corresponding pace; finally, growth is restricted almost entirely to the follicle. (From Baker, 1978.)

thicker than elsewhere, and a mound is formed in which the ovum is included—that is, the cumulus oophorus.

The follicle is filled with a clear, proteinaceous fluid, the *liquor folliculi* (the follicular fluid). The usual fat stains are not taken up by the granulosa cells until the stage of preovulatory swelling, a time of rapid growth that commences about 24 hours before ovulation and is apparently related to the onset of, or preparation for, the secretion of progesterone. Before ovulation, the granulosa cells are dependent for steroidogenesis upon precursor substrate that enters the follicular fluid from the theca interna.

Ovarian follicles develop throughout childhood and occasionally attain considerable size, but normally do not rupture at this time. Instead, these follicles undergo atresia in situ. The relative rates of increase in oocyte size and follicular size with maturation are considerably different (Fig. 2–16). Even in adult women, many follicles that reach a diameter of 5 mm or more undergo atresia.

Concerning ovarian development, de Graaf wrote,

Moreover, their size varies not a little with age, for in developing girls and [in women] in the flower of their life they weigh almost one and a half drachms, so that they attain a size about half that of the male testis, although in proportion they are wider and more succulent. In the old and decrepit, they are smaller, firmer, and more dried up, and slowly wither more and more, but never disappear completely; we have observed that the smallest testicles of old women weigh from five grains to half a scruple.

The Mature Ovum. When brightly illuminated on a dark background, the human ovum, as it approaches maturity, is barely visible to the naked eye. According to Hartman (1929) and Allen and co-workers (1930), the average diameter of the mature human ovum is 0.133 mm.

If the nearly mature ovum is examined in the follicular fluid or in physiological saline, the structures that can be distinguished in and about it are as follow: (1) a surrounding corona radiata; (2) a zona pellucida; (3) a perivitelline space; (4) a small clear zone of protoplasm; (5) a broad, finely granulated zone of protoplasm; (6) a central, deutoplasmic zone; (7) the nucleus, or germinal vesicle, within it a germinal spot; and, if appropriately stained, (8) many small spheroidal mitochondria. The ovum is free to rotate within the zona pellucida even though the outer vitelline membrane of the ovum appears to be applied closely to it. After fertilization, shrinkage of the ovum results in its complete separation from the zona pellucida as it floats in the perivitelline fluid. During growth, the oocyte accumulates deutoplasm (yolk granules). Before ovulation, the ovum, in the living state, is transparent with a faint yellowish tinge. There are also larger lipoid granules, which in preserved material appear to surround the nucleus (germinal vesicle). Numerous mitochondria are distributed through the cytoplasm. The spherical nucleus is located near the center of the oocyte; and in it, there is a large nucleolus and sparsely distributed chromatin. Shortly before ovulation, the nucleus migrates toward the periphery, and meiosis is reinitiated. At the completion of the first and second meiotic divisions, the number of chromosomes in the oocyte is halved, and two polar bodies are formed: the first before ovulation and the second after penetration of the oocyte by a spermatozoan. Both polar bodies are extruded into the perivitelline space.

Gametogenesis. Primitive germ cells are present in the human embryo by the end of the third week of development. Both *oogenesis,* in the course of which mature ova are formed from primitive oogonia, and *spermatogenesis,* which results in the production of spermatids, share a basic biological feature of maturation—reduction and division (Fig. 2–17). Such special cellular division, known as *meiosis,* is limited to germ cells. The process of meiosis is characterized by a long and unusual prophase, and involves a process that provides for the exchange of genetic material between homologous chromosomes and the reduction of the *diploid* number of chromosomes to the *haploid* number.

In all primitive germ cells of the human (*oogonia* and *spermatogonia*) there are a diploid number of chromosomes (46). When these stem cells divide to produce primary oocytes and spermatocytes, each chromosome undergoes replication by splitting longitudinally to form a double-stranded structure. During this typical *mitosis,* one strand of each chromosome enters each daughter cell; and in this manner, the identical chromosomal components of the parent cells are obtained.

When the primary oocytes and spermatocytes continue maturation to form secondary oocytes and spermatocytes, respectively, however, the meiotic division that ensues is quite different; this is the case in that each of the newly formed cells receives only 23, or the haploid number of chromosomes. The basic difference between meiosis and mitosis is the prolonged prophase in meiosis, in which there is preliminary pairing of homologous chromosomes before division. During the *leptotene* stage of meiotic prophase, the 46 chromosomes appear as single slender threads; in the next stage, the *zygotene,* the homologous chromosomes are aligned in a parallel manner, one to the other, in *synapsis,* with the formation of 23 bivalent components. Each chromosome then divides longitudinally, except at the *centromere,* and the ensuing *pachytene* stage is comprised of *tetrads* of 4 chromatids, the shape of which is dependent upon the position of the centromere. At this stage, the chromatids break and thence recombine with strands from the homologous chromosome to effect an exchange of genetic material. During the next, *diplotene,* stage, the homologous strands separate. During the metaphase of the first meiotic division, the bivalents (2 chromatids that comprise each chromosome) become oriented on the spindle; and when the cell divides, the members of each pair move toward opposite poles into the daughter cells, which then contain the haploid number of chromosomes, still as chromatid pairs. *The individual chromosomes now are no longer genetically identical with those of the parent cell.* Each secondary oocyte will thus receive 22 autosomes and an X chromosome, and each secondary spermatocyte will receive 22 autosomes and either an X or Y chromosome.

At the second meiotic division, the *diad* splits at the centromere to form two *monads,* one of which becomes associated with each daughter cell, probably having already undergone a typical mitotic longitudinal replication.

Oogenesis. To recapitulate and summarize, it is important to recognize that all oocytes are derived from the primitive germ cells. Blandau and co-workers (1963) recorded, cinematographically, in the mouse, the ameboid-like migration of primitive germ cells from the yolk sac to the germinal ridges. The primitive oogonia, furthermore, continue movements locally within the de-

NORMAL GAMETOGENESIS

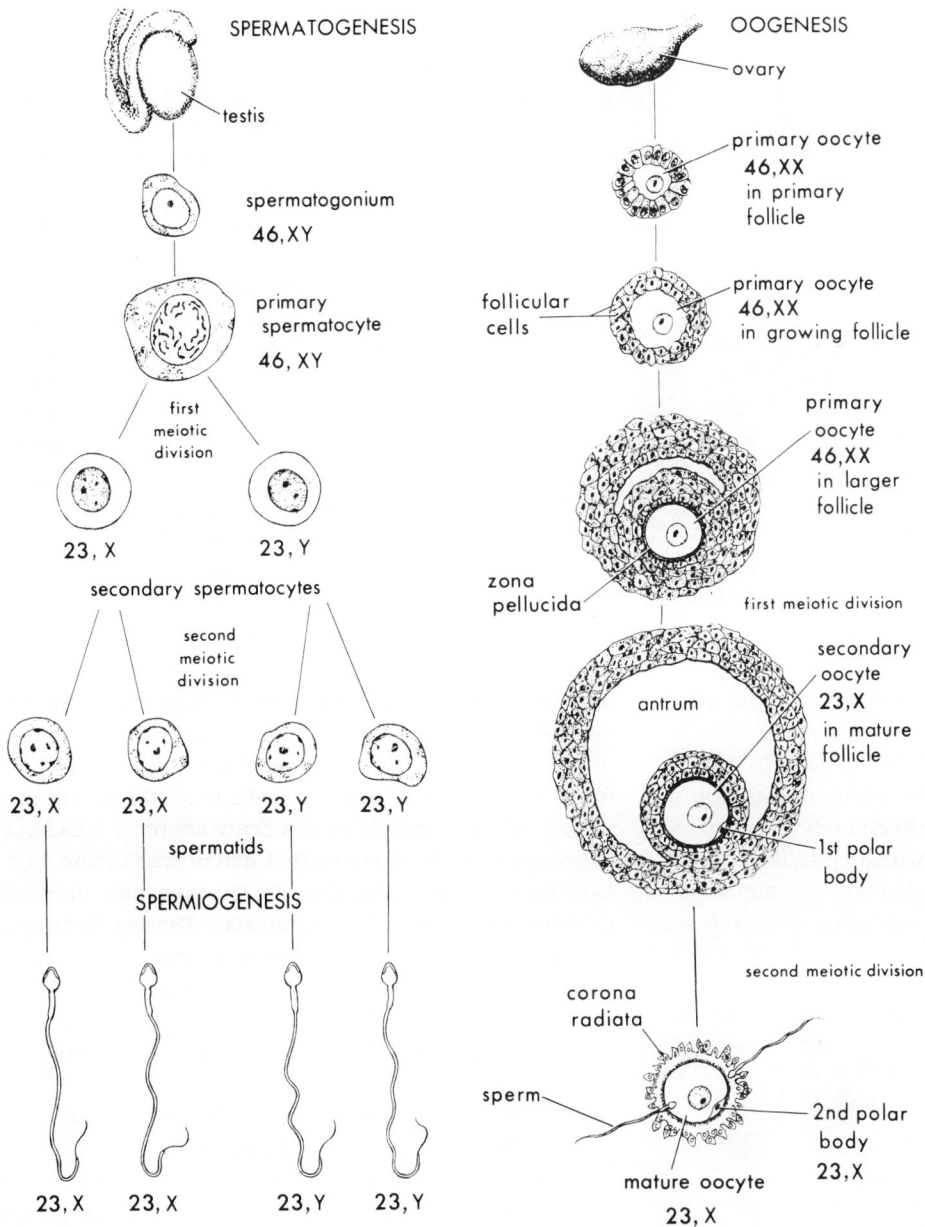

SPERMATOGENESIS

testis

spermatogonium
46,XY

primary
spermatocyte
46, XY

first
meiotic
division

23, X   23, Y

secondary spermatocytes

second
meiotic
division

23, X   23, X   23, Y   23, Y

spermatids

SPERMIOGENESIS

23, X   23, X   23, Y   23, Y

OOGENESIS

ovary

primary oocyte
46,XX
in primary
follicle

follicular
cells

primary oocyte
46,XX
in growing follicle

primary
oocyte
46,XX
in larger
follicle

zona
pellucida

first meiotic division

secondary
oocyte
23,X
in mature
follicle

antrum

1st polar
body

second meiotic division

corona
radiata

sperm

2nd polar
body
23,X

mature oocyte
23, X

Fig. 2–17. Drawings to compare spermatogenesis and oogenesis. The chromosome complement of the germ cells is shown at each stage. The number designates the total number of chromosomes, including the sex chromosome(s) shown after the comma. Note that (1) after the two meiotic divisions, the diploid number of chromosomes, 46, is reduced to the haploid number, 23; (2) four sperm form from one primary spermatocyte, whereas only one mature oocyte (ovum) results from maturation of a primary oocyte; and (3) the cytoplasm is conserved during oogenesis to form one large cell, the mature oocyte (ovum). (From Moore, 1988.)

veloping ovary even after the pachytene stage of meiosis is reached.

The primary oocytes increase in size, and cuboidal granulosa cells proliferate to form increasingly thick coverings around them (Fig. 2–18). The granulosa cells, furthermore, deposit on the surface of the oocyte an *acellular* glycoprotein mantle that thickens gradually to form the *zona pellucida* (Figs. 2–18 and 2–19). Irregular fluid-filled spaces between the granulosa cells then coalesce to form an antrum. The radially elongated granulosa cells that surround the zona pellucida form the corona radiata (Fig. 2–18). A solid mass of granulosa cells, the cumulus oophorus, surrounds the ovum in a developing vesicular ovarian follicle (Figs. 2–18 and

2–19). As the follicle nears maturity, the cumulus projects further into the antrum, and as a consequence, the oocyte appears to be supported by this column of granulosa cells. At this stage, the follicle may vary from 6 to 12 mm in diameter and lies immediately beneath the surface of the ovary. The formation of the oocyte completes the first meiotic division, which was begun before birth, during the final stage of transformation of the primordial follicle into the mature graafian follicle. The important result is the formation of two daughter cells, each with 23 chromosomes but of greatly unequal size. One cell receives almost all of the cytoplasm of the mother cell and becomes a secondary oocyte; the other, the first polar body, receives very little cytoplasm. The

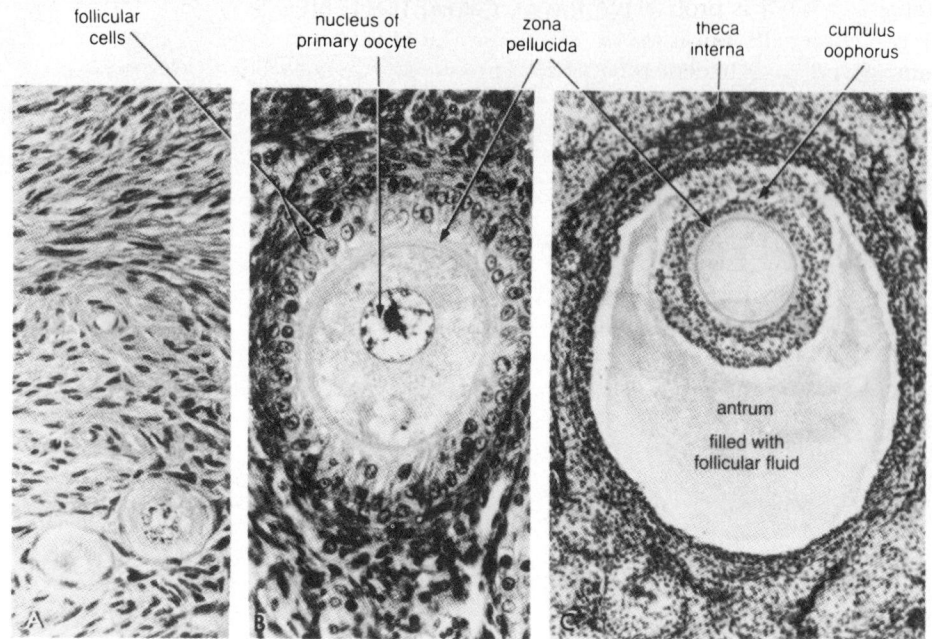

follicular cells   nucleus of primary oocyte   zona pellucida   theca interna   cumulus oophorus

antrum filled with follicular fluid

Fig. 2–18. Photomicrographs of sections from ovaries of adult women. **A.** Ovarian cortex showing two primordial follicles that contain primary oocytes that have completed the prophase of the first meiotic division and have entered the dictyotene stage, a "resting" stage between prophase and metaphase ($\times$ 250). **B.** Growing follicle that contains a primary oocyte, surrounded by the zona pellucida and a stratified layer of follicular cells ($\times$ 250). **C.** An almost mature follicle with a large antrum. The oocyte, embedded in the cumulus oophorus, does not show a nucleus because it has been sectioned tangentially ($\times$ 100). (From Moore, 1988.)

polar body lies between the zona pellucida and the vitelline membrane of the secondary oocyte.

The Chosen Ovum. Not only is there a chosen or dominant follicle; there must be a dominant oocyte, because it is the only oocyte in the preovulatory follicles that matures; all others do not develop beyond the immature dictyotene state (Channing and colleagues, 1982). It is believed that a cybernin called *oocyte maturation inhibitor* (OMI) may serve an important role in regulating oocyte maturation. OMI appears to be present in all follicles except preovulatory ones. From the results of a variety of experiments beginning with those of Chang (1955), and as summarized by Channing and Pomerantz (1981), it is reasonably clear that a substance in follicular fluid that arises from granulosa cells inhibits oocyte

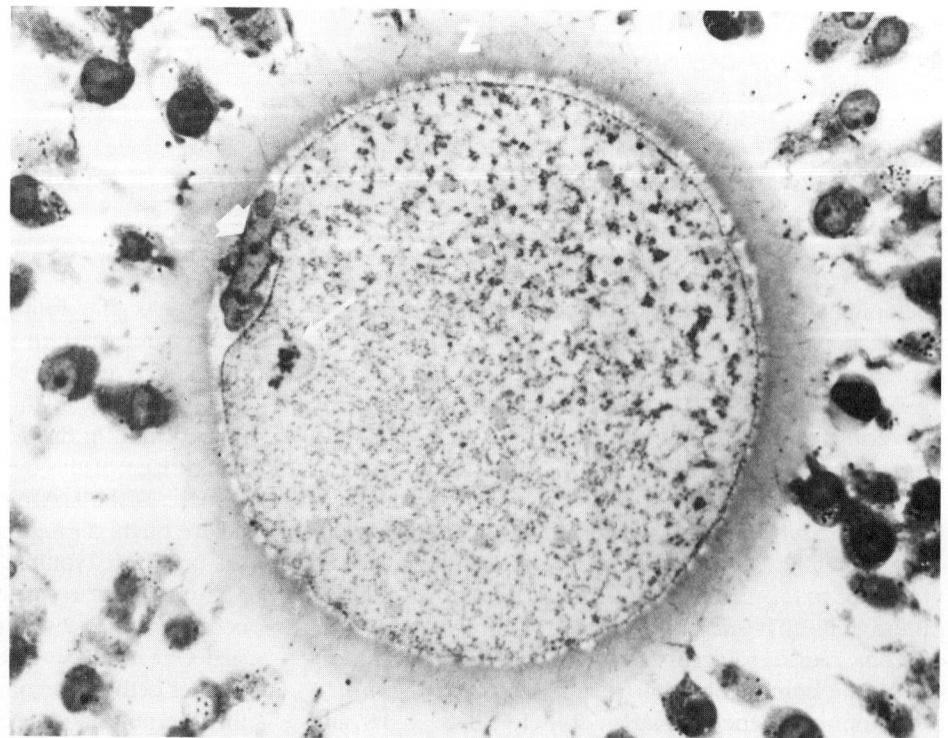

Fig. 2–19. Light micrograph of a human follicular oocyte. The first polar body (*short arrow*) has been liberated and lies in the perivitelline space, which separates the oocyte from the zona pellucida (Z). The oocyte chromosomes are aligned on the equator of the meiotic spindle (*long arrow*). These will remain in this position until penetration of the fertilizing spermatozoan, when the second meiotic division will resume. The cells of the cumulus oophorus are more dispersed than in the previous stages. Some of these cells are undergoing regression, as shown by the presence of numerous fat droplets in the cytoplasm and pyknosis of nuclei. These features represent the onset of the denudation of the oocyte, a process that will be completed in the oviduct ($\times$ 1500). (From Ferenczy and Richart, 1974.)

maturation. OMI is probably a peptide that is secreted by granulosa cells, but it may act by way of cells of the cumulus. LH, in all likelihood, acts on the chosen follicle to block the action of the OMI.

The first polar body is cast off while still in the ovary (Hertig and Rock, 1944). A second division is consummated in the formation of the second polar body at about the moment that the sperm penetrates the egg.

The second maturation division is completed in human ova only if the ovum is fertilized. If penetration by a spermatozoan does not occur within a few hours of ovulation, the ovum begins to degenerate. Although it is not certain that the first polar body always undergoes subsequent division, fertilized ova have been found that were accompanied by three polar bodies. During maturation, the diameter of the human ovum increases from 19 microns in the original oocyte to 135 microns in the fully mature ovum, a sevenfold increase in size.

Transport of Ova and Spermatozoa

Tubal Transport. Eddy and Pauerstein (1980) have presented an excellent review of the anatomy and physiology of the fallopian tube. The ovaries in women normally lie free in the peritoneal cavity except for the supporting mesovarium and ovarian ligament. About the time of ovulation, however, the fimbriae of the oviduct, possibly as the consequence of appropriate hormonal (probable) and neural (doubtful) regulation, are believed to cover the ovary completely at the site of ovulation. Ovulation is not an explosive phenomenon; instead, as the stigma of the follicular wall is digested by proteolytic enzymes, there is a gentle outpouring of the contents of the follicle, which includes the egg still surrounded by the zona pellucida and the cumulus oophorus. The cumulus cells appear to be important for uptake and transport of the ovum by the oviduct. In the oviduct of the monkey, ciliary action is believed to be the prominent force in the movement of the ovum in the tube, whereas peristalsis appears to be so in the rabbit. The relative contribution of each of these mechanisms to sperm and ovum transport in women is not known. Because fertilization in mammals usually occurs in the ampulla, whatever the roles of the tubal cilia and peristalsis may be, an adequate theory must be one to explain movement of ova and spermatozoa in opposite directions.

Migration of Fertilized Ovum. In most mammals, the fertilized ovum migrates through the oviduct and reaches the cavity of the uterus about 3 to 4 days after ovulation. In women, the ovum is believed to be able to wander across the pelvis and then to be taken up by the opposite tube (*external migration*) or else, theoretically, the ovum may cross inside the uterus and migrate up to the opposite tube (*internal migration*). Presumptive clinical evidence of migration of the ovum includes

a successful intrauterine pregnancy in women who have only one tube and only the contralateral ovary. It is likely, however, that the entire subject of migration of the ovum in women has received more attention than it deserves. In consideration of known normal anatomical relationships, as observed at laparotomy, both tubes are usually freely mobile, and the fimbriated extremities lie posterior to the uterus and in rather close approximation. In view of the recognized motility of the fallopian tubes, it is reasonable to presume that the ovum may be taken up directly by the opposite tube, without recourse to complicated explanations that involve mechanisms of internal or external migration.

Transport of Spermatozoa. During human coitus, there is in each ejaculate, on average, a volume of seminal fluid of 2 to 5 mL, in which there are approximately 70 million sperm per mL that are deposited in the vagina. Of these 200 million or more spermatozoa, of which between 80 and 90 percent are presumed to be normal forms, perhaps fewer than 200 actually reach the site of fertilization, the ampulla of the tube. For successful fertilization, Eddy and Pauerstein (1980) asked the important question as to why *"so many sperm are required in the ejaculate when so few arrive at the site of fertilization?"* Only one spermatozoan must meet, in the upper portion of the fallopian tube, the single mature ovum that is released during each ovulatory cycle.

A few sperm sometimes reach the site of fertilization in the ampulla of the oviduct quickly (often only 5 minutes) after ejaculation, a time that is much faster than can be explained by the flagellar action of spermatozoa. Eddy and Pauerstein are of the view that there are reservoirs for spermatozoa (the ejaculate and the uterus may be considered such), whereas *"the cervix, uterotubal junctions, and possibly the oviductal isthmus may be considered as barriers to the passage of sperm."* An unbelievably sharp decrement occurs in the number of sperm between those deposited in the vagina and those that reach the ampulla of the fallopian tube.

It still remains a biological curiosity that a few spermatozoa can reach the ampulla of the fallopian tube with such rapidity from the time of insemination. Indeed as stated, it has been reported that this transit time may be no more than 5 minutes, but on average, a time of 4 to 6 hours seems more reasonable. The loss of sperm in the ejaculate, however, is remarkable. In one study, it was estimated that for every 14 million sperm deposited in the vagina, only one could be recovered from the fallopian tubes within 15 to 45 minutes of insemination. It is clear, however, that there are mechanisms operative in the genital tract of women that provide for accelerated transport of sperm. It is believed that the movement of spermatozoa that is caused by flagellar action is necessary for maintenance of the sperm in suspension and in the facilitation of transport; moreover, such movement is believed to be necessary for transit of the spermatozoan through the cumulus oophorus and zona pellucida of the ovum.

It also is presumed that the spermatozoa must make their own way through the mucus that fills the cervical canal. The first spermatozoa appear to burrow through the mucus by chemical as well as mechanical processes; the leaders among the spermatozoa very likely depolymerize the cervical mucus by releasing proteinases that are contained in the acrosome, and thereby render the mucus more easily penetrable by the spermatozoa that follow and successfully enter the uterine cavity. The uterine cavity in vivo may well be nearly obliterated, except for canals that extend from the internal os of the cervix to the uterotubal junctions; as the consequences of such canals, sperm are directed to the oviduct.

Fertilization of the Ovum. As soon as the sperm penetrates the zona pellucida and comes in contact with the vitelline membrane, a second polar body is formed and the female pronucleus, as well as the male pronucleus, are evident in the ovum. Ordinarily, the penetration of the zona pellucida and vitelline membrane by one sperm acts in a manner to inhibit entry by other sperm; but on rare occasions, more than one sperm does enter.

Zona Pellucida of the Ovum. The role of zona pellucida in fertilization was reviewed by Dean (1992). The zona pellucida is an extracellular matrix that surrounds the ovum and contains the primary and secondary sperm receptors. The plasma membrane of the ovum and the zona, immediately after fertilization, are modified to prevent polyspermy. Motile sperm pass through the cumulus oophorus cells and bind to the zona pellucida. The human zona pellucida is composed of three major glycoproteins, designated ZP1, ZP2, and ZP3.

ZP3 (from unfertilized eggs) inhibits sperm binding to the plasma membrane of the ova. ZP2 may be a secondary sperm receptor that binds sperm only after induction of the sperm acrosome reaction. The acrosome is an organelle that is bound and anteriorly positioned in the head of the sperm. It is believed that the binding of sperm to ZP3 induces the aggregation of a sperm 95-kDa protein with tyrosine kinase activity, which leads to the acrosome reaction, namely release of the acrosome contents. The enzymes of the acrosome facilitate passage of a motile sperm through the zona pellucida.

Immediately after fertilization, polyspermy is prevented by modifications in the plasma membrane of the fertilized ovum and by enzyme modification of the zona pellicuda that inhibits further sperm binding and zona-bound sperm penetration.

Dickman and Noyes (1961) found that the zona pellucida in the rat is shed from the blastocyst during the fifth day after fertilization. The shedding, moreover, appears unrelated to a specific uterine environment, but rather is an intrinsic manifestation of growth and matu-

ration of the blastocyst. The zona clearly is not necessary for implantation; on the contrary, its removal is a prerequisite for implantation. The escape of the fertilized ovum from the zona pellucida has been referred to as the "hatching of the human egg."

Aging of Gametes. The increased incidence of the trisomy 21 variety of Down syndrome late in reproductive life is well-established. It may be related to an increased tendency toward nondisjunction in ova that have remained dormant in the ovary for 40 years or more. Although the incidence of this syndrome in the population as a whole is only 3 per 2000 live births, the incidence increases to about 1 in 100 in women by age 40 (Chap. 40).

Aging also exerts an adverse effect of gametes of males on the embryo and fetus (Tesh and Glover, 1969). They reported that aging of rabbit sperm in the male reproductive tract led to a decrease in the capacity for fertilization. Moreover, if eggs were fertilized by such sperm, an increase in embryonic anomalies resulted. Friedman (1981) found that the risk of new autosomal dominant mutations in children is increased many times among the offspring of fathers who are 40 years of age or older. Indeed, he found that such risk was similar to that of Down syndrome in infants of 35- to 40-year-old mothers. Thus, aging of spermatozoa before or after maturation is potentially harmful.

Vickers (1969) observed that delayed fertilization also led to an increase in chromosomal anomalies of the embryo. In mice, in which fertilization was delayed 7 to 13 hours, triploidy, for example, was increased ninefold. Vickers postulated that the chromosomal aberrations may have resulted from errors in meiosis, fertilization, or cleavage. Thus, the timing of ovum fertilization may be extraordinarily important to the quality of the zygote in human pregnancy. As women do not experience estrus (periodic sexual receptivity), aged sperm or ova may become involved in fertilization. This may lead to pregnancy wastage (Chap. 31).

Theca–Granulosa Cell Cooperativity in Ovarian Steroidogenesis

Final Stages of Follicular Maturation and Ovulation. It now is clear that a variety of molecular events in the theca and granulosa cells of the ovaries of women are subject to regulatory processes that involve the actions of steroids as well as gonadotropins. It is recognized that follicular maturation can proceed to the preantral stage of development and even to replication of granulosa cells to a finite point—four-cell-layer thickness in the absence of pituitary hormone stimulation. Beyond this stage of development, however, gonadotropins and sex steroid hormones produced within the follicle in response to gonadotropin action are required for full expression of follicular maturation and responsiveness.

Two-Cell Hypothesis of Ovarian Steroidogenesis.

The characteristic cyclicity of secretion of estradiol and progesterone, as well as the formation of the C_{19}- steroids, androstenedione, dehydroepiandrosterone, and testosterone by the ovaries of young women, is regulated by mechanisms that are considerably different with respect to C_{18}- and C_{21}-steroids (estrogen and progesterone) as compared with those of the C_{19}-steroids (androgen or androgen-like).

Follicle-stimulating hormone (FSH) acts in granulosa cells to increase the enzyme activity that catalyzes the aromatization of C_{19}-steroids to produce estrogen. Aromatase activity is believed to be modulated by an increase in cyclic AMP, by an increase in adenylate cyclase activity, and by "androgens" that act in an as yet undefined manner to increase aromatization. But more than that, estradiol synthesized by the dominant follicle also appears to act to increase the follicular cell actions of FSH to enhance LH responsiveness. The stimulation of aromatase activity by cAMP is likely mediated by cAMP-dependent phosphorylation of a number of cellular proteins, and by an increase in the rate of transcription of the specific gene that encodes for the aromatase protein. And it is only after FSH priming that cells become competent to LH action. This is believed to be the result of an FSH-induced increase in LH receptors. Thus, FSH acts

to cause an increase in aromatase activity (by way of synthesis of new enzyme) as well as an increase in LH receptors.

More than three decades ago, a "new" or revised hypothesis, *the two-cell hypothesis,* was put forward and championed by Ryan and Smith (1959) to describe the pathways of steroid synthesis in the ovary, and in particular the maturing follicle. This postulate described the potential cooperativity between theca and granulosa cells in estrogen formation. Since that time, considerable support has been added to strengthen this postulate.

LH acts in theca cells to increase cholesterol side-chain cleavage enzyme activity (which is believed to be the rate-limiting step in steroidogenesis in many steroidogenic tissues) and to increase the activities of steroid 17α-hydroxylase/17,20-lyase ($P450_{17\alpha}$), an enzyme that is crucial to the formation of C_{19}-steroids—that is, androgen-like compounds such as dehydroepiandrosterone, androstenedione, and testosterone.

Androstenedione, formed in theca, diffuses into the follicular fluid and becomes available to the granulosa cells for aromatization to form estrone, which is then converted to estradiol (Fig. 2–20). There is little or no de novo synthesis of steroids in granulosa cells because of limited capacity for the de novo synthesis of cholesterol and the absence of $P450_{17\alpha}$ before ovulation. We will return to this latter issue in a consideration of the synthesis of progesterone by the luteinized granulosa cells of the corpus luteum.

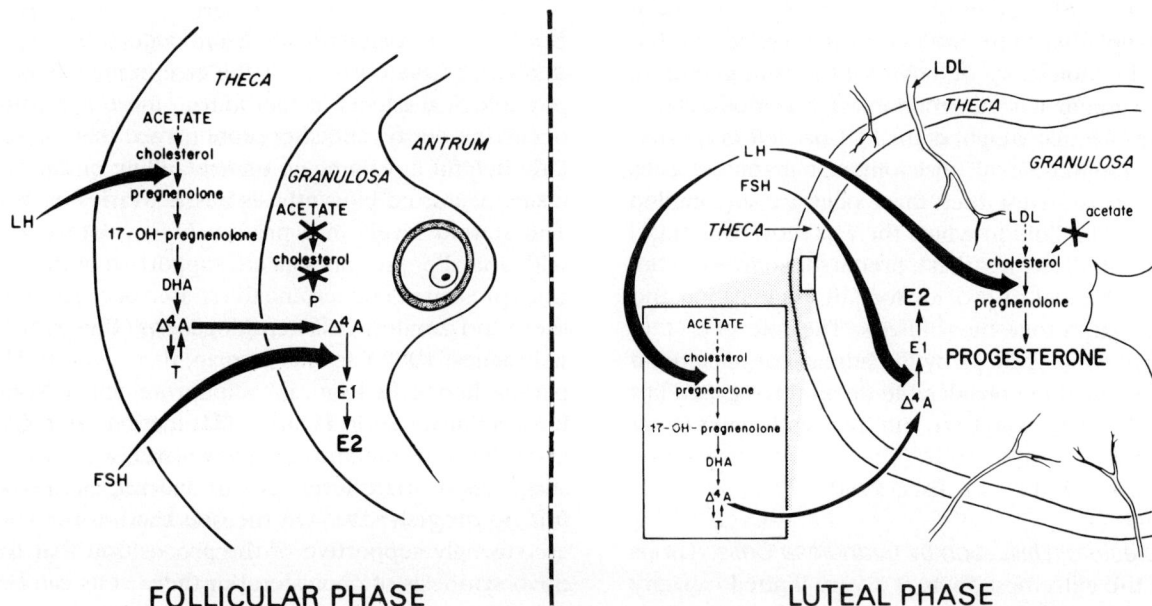

FOLLICULAR PHASE   **LUTEAL PHASE**

Fig. 2–20. Relation between theca and granulosa cells in estradiol-17β (E2) production. Androstenedione (Δ⁴-A) is synthesized by way of pregnenolone and dehydroepiandrosterone (DHA) formation in theca cells. Note that LH stimulates the formation of pregnenolone by increasing side-chain cleavage of cholesterol. Aromatization occurs in granulosa cells to give E2 by way of estrone (E1). The aromatization of androstenedione is stimulated by FSH. Progesterone synthesis from plasma low-density lipoprotein (LDL) cholesterol occurs in luteinized granulosa cells. Testosterone (T) is also synthesized in the ovary.

Source of Cholesterol in the Follicle and Corpus Luteum for Steroidogenesis. We have known for many decades that cholesterol is the ultimate precursor of all steroid hormones. What we did not consider, until relatively recently, was that the source of cholesterol for a given steroidogenic cell may differ. From the pioneering studies of Brown and colleagues (1979), who demonstrated that many extrahepatic tissues assimilate cholesterol by uptake and processing of circulating lipoproteins, it was soon demonstrated that similar processes are applicable to the assimilation of cholesterol for steroidogenesis in human endocrine glands and trophoblast (Chap. 6).

The specific form and source of cholesterol utilized by a given gland, however, varies widely among species and perhaps within a given cell type of a given gland in the same species. By way of example, the source of cholesterol for progesterone biosynthesis by the corpus luteum of various mammals is among the most diverse. In the rabbit, cholesterol is synthesized in the corpus luteum de novo, from 2-carbon fragments such as acetate. In the rat, however, circulating plasma high-density lipoprotein (HDL) is used as the cholesterol source. But in women, there is little de novo synthesis of cholesterol in granulosa cells, including the luteinized granulosa cells of the corpus luteum, and HDL is not assimilated by human granulosa cells.

Rather, low-density lipoprotein (LDL) is the near exclusive form of cholesterol that is used for progesterone biosynthesis. The same is true of progesterone formation in the human syncytiotrophoblast, although the syncytium is capable of limited de novo cholesterol synthesis (Chap. 6). Comparing these two cell types (granulosa and syncytiotrophoblast) to produce progesterone, the impairment in cholesterol de novo synthesis in granulosa cells is severe; in syncytiotrophoblast, it is moderate.

The molecular weight of the LDL particle is approximately 3 million. Recall that follicular granulosa cells are not vascularized; rather, these cells are surrounded by the follicular fluid in which there is little or no LDL. It is apparent, therefore, that a precursor source of cholesterol is essential to provide for full luteinization and optimal progesterone biosynthesis. The role of LDL in progesterone biosynthesis by the human corpus luteum has been defined in considerable detail through studies conducted by Simpson, Carr, and their colleagues (Carr and associates, 1981, 1982; Ohashi and colleagues, 1982; Simpson and co-workers, 1980).

LDL Cholesterol Utilization by Granulosa Cells. Let us consider the extremes. There is a very limited capacity for de novo synthesis of cholesterol in human granulosa cells, and these cells do not utilize HDL as a source of cholesterol. In the follicular fluid that surrounds the avascular granulosa cells, there is little or no LDL; the LDL particle is too large to enter the follicular fluid. Thus, it is obvious that little or no steroidogenesis can proceed in

the granulosa cells by the utilization of LDL cholesterol in this unique environment. Therefore, before ovulation, progesterone is not formed by human granulosa cells. It has been shown that the small amount of progesterone in plasma of women before ovulation arises by secretion from the adrenal cortex (Judd and co-workers, 1992). The principal steroid produced by granulosa cells, estradiol, is synthesized from androstenedione, which is taken up from the follicular fluid. The androstenedione diffuses into the follicular fluid from the theca interna cells in which it is synthesized.

If granulosa cells obtained from the follicles of women are placed in culture, these cells become luteinized and respond to appropriate trophic stimuli by producing progesterone in large amounts. It must be remembered, however, that the culture medium that bathes these cells usually contains serum—and thus LDL. Therefore, the "spontaneous" luteinization of granulosa cells in culture and thence the biosynthesis of progesterone is attributable, in large part, to the addition of a utilizable source of cholesterol (LDL) to these cells. LH acts to increase cholesterol side-chain cleavage, thereby facilitating the conversion of cholesterol (taken up from LDL) to pregnenolone, the immediate precursor of progesterone. This is an important concept in understanding the rate of progesterone synthesis by the corpus luteum in women. The number of granulosa cells remaining in the follicle is a limiting factor in progesterone synthesis as the uptake of LDL is dependent upon the number of LDL receptors, which is largely dependent upon the number of granulosa cells that remain in the ovary after ovulation.

Source of Cholesterol for Steroidogenesis in Theca and Granulosa Cells. As is the case in many studies of physiological events in the human, there is a naturally occurring entity, abetalipoproteinemia, that is particularly helpful in gaining an understanding of the mechanisms of steroid biosynthesis in the ovaries of women. The steroid levels in a presumably ovulatory woman with abetalipoproteinemia are supportive of the deductions presented concerning the source of cholesterol for theca and ganulosa cell steroidogenesis (Illingworth and colleagues, 1982). In this woman, there was no LDL in plasma, hence the term, abetalipoproteinemia. Nonetheless, as illustrated in Figure 2–21, there appeared to be cyclic ovarian function in this woman: a midcycle LH surge, appropriate levels of FSH and LH, and estradiol, *but no progesterone!* On the one hand, these findings are strongly supportive of the proposition that the de novo synthesis of cholesterol in theca cells can be sufficient to support the biosynthesis of C_{19}-steroids that enter follicular fluid and become available to the granulosa cells for estradiol production. On the other hand, there was no post-LH-surge synthesis of progesterone in this woman. We take this as evidence that the granulosa cells are dependent almost exclusively upon LDL as the

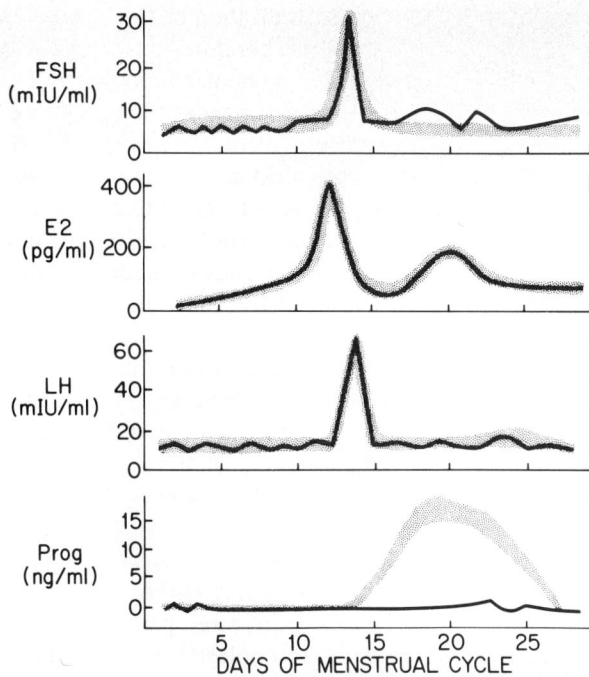

Fig. 2–21. Hormones throughout the menstrual cycle. The shaded areas represent mean values in normal ovulatory women. The solid lines represent those values determined in serum of a woman with abetalipoproteinemia. (Adapted from Illingworth and associates, 1982.)

source of cholesterol precursor for progesterone biosynthesis. This woman was undoubtedly ovulatory, because she became pregnant and delivered a normal child at term (Chap. 12).

Thus, the *two-cell hypothesis* seems to be almost complete. We cannot set aside the possibility that the theca cells utilize LDL-cholesterol; but, from the findings in the case of the woman with abetalipoproteinemia presented, it seems likely that sufficient de novo synthesis of cholesterol can proceed in theca, in the absence of LDL, to provide adequate quantities of androstenedione for granulosa cell estradiol synthesis. At the same time, we cannot conclude that LDL-cholesterol is the only factor required for granulosa cells to produce progesterone. Stimulation of granulosa cells by LH to synthesize the P450 cholesterol side-chain cleavage enzyme also is required. Thus, LDL and LH are the primary regulators of progesterone synthesis in the human corpus luteum, a conclusion also reached in a study conducted by Richardson and colleagues (1992). The mechanism(s) of estradiol formation by the human corpus luteum, however, are not so clear. Nonetheless, it is well established that estradiol is produced by the human corpus luteum.

Ovulation

As the graafian follicle grows to a size of 10 to 12 mm in diameter, it gradually reaches the surface of the ovary and ultimately protrudes above it. Necrobiosis of the overlying tissues, rather than pressure within the follicle, is the principal factor resulting in follicular rupture. The cells at the exposed tip of the follicle float away at the site of the pale stigma on the wall of the ovarian follicle so that the region becomes transparent. The thinnest clear area then ruptures and the follicular liquid and the ovum, surrounded by the zona pellucida and corona radiata and cumulus oophorus, are extruded at the time of ovulation.

The actual rupture of the follicle is not explosive; nonetheless, the discharge of the ovum together with the zona pellucida and attached follicular cells takes no more than a few seconds. Excellent motion pictures of the process of ovulation in the rat have been obtained by Richard Blandau and others. Two frames from these movies are shown in Figures 2–8 and 2–22. The follicle is pictured just before ovulation and the expulsion of the ovum also is shown. In the first (Fig. 2–8), the stigma is clearly visible, whereas in the second (Fig. 2–22), the actual release of the ovum is illustrated. A scanning electron micrograph of an oocyte and the follicle of a mouse at the time of ovulation is presented in Figure 2–23.

Strickland and Beers (1979) demonstrated that granulosa cells produce the plasminogen activator enzyme, and that the extracellular level of this enzyme is correlated closely with ovulation. The activity of the enzyme is modulated by the action of gonadotropins, cyclic nucleotides, and prostaglandins. Further, by the action of this enzyme on plasminogen, which is present in follicular fluid, plasmin, the proteolytic enzyme, is generated, which acts to weaken the wall of the follicle (Beers, 1975).

Day of Ovulation. The exact time of ovulation in the cycle is of the utmost importance for several reasons. First, because the life span of both the spermatozoa and the unfertilized ovum is limited, fertilization must take place within hours (preferably minutes) after ovulation if conception is to occur in that cycle. In some infertile couples, knowledge of the time of ovulation and appropriate adjustment of the time of coitus are important considerations in therapy. Also, for couples who use the "rhythm method" to avoid conception, coitus must be limited to that part of the cycle several days removed from the time of ovulation, or the "safe period." Ovulation usually approximately marks the midpoint of both the ovarian and menstrual cycles. The period from the first day of menstrual bleeding to ovulation is designated as the follicular or proliferative phase of the ovarian/menstrual cycle. The proliferative phase encompasses roughly the first half of the menstrual cycle; the *postovulatory phase* is known as the secretory phase (Chap. 4).

Various methods have been used to determine the time of ovulation in women. Allen and colleagues

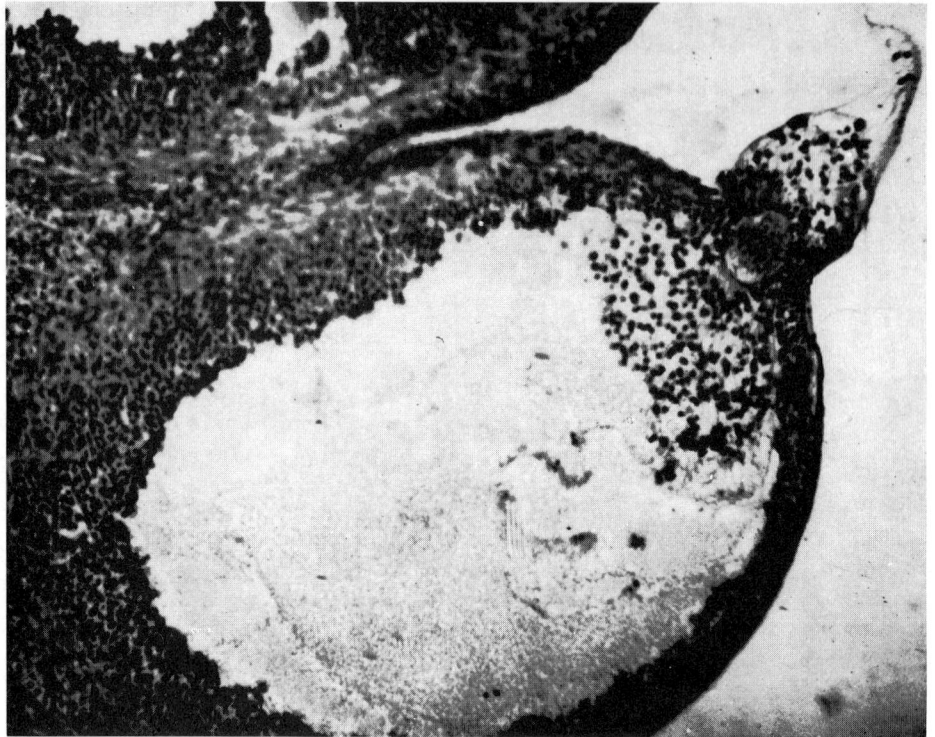

Fig. 2–22. Moment of ovulation in the rat. (Courtesy of Dr. Richard J. Blandau.)

(1930) recovered mature unfertilized ova from the fallopian tube on the 12th, 15th, and 16th days of the cycle and concluded that ovulation occurs approximately on day 14 of an idealized 28-day cycle. Other indirect methods by which to ascertain the time of ovulation are the examination of fertilized ova and evaluation of the changes that have taken place at the site of the ruptured follicle. By use of these approaches, it has been demonstrated that, although ovulation frequently occurs between the 12th and 16th days of the cycle, there is considerable variation in the timing of ovulation. It is not uncommon for ovulation to take place at any time between the 8th and 20th days (Fig. 2–24).

The time of ovulation bears a much closer temporal relation to the onset of the next menstrual period than to the previous menses. Ovulation usually occurs ap-

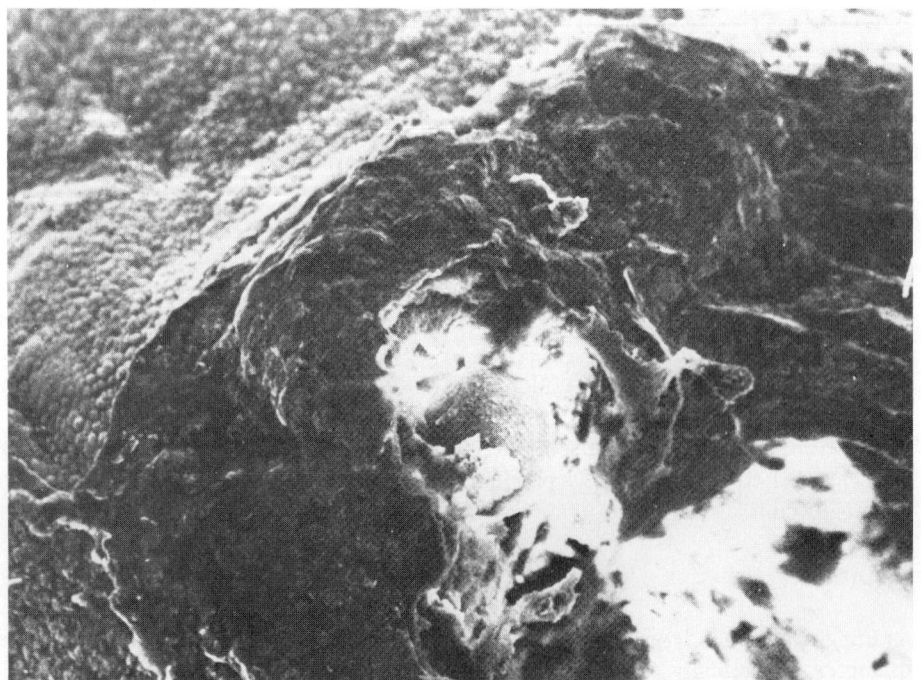

Fig. 2–23. Scanning electron micrograph of an oocyte and the follicle of a mouse at the time of ovulation. (From Motta and Hafez, 1980.)

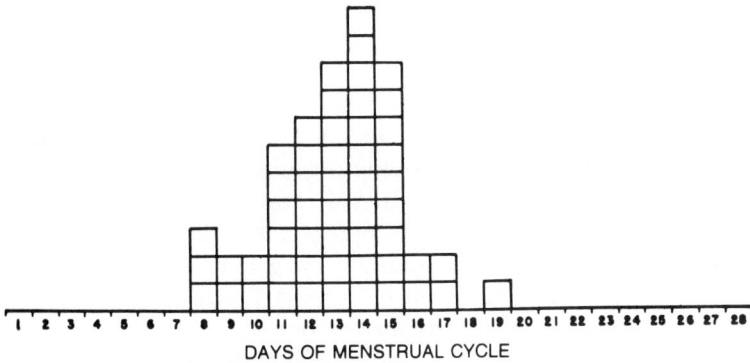

Fig. 2–24. Day of ovulation in 54 women calculated form the apparent age of the corpus luteum. Each block represents an observation of one woman.

proximately 14 days before the first day of the succeeding menstrual bleeding. For purposes of timing ovulation, urinary LH levels can be monitored by use of commercially available test kits similar to those used for home testing of hCG for pregnancy diagnosis. The purpose of such testing is to define the time of the "LH surge," which precedes ovulation by 24 to 36 hours.

Signs and Symptoms of Ovulation. On or about the day of ovulation, as many as 25 percent of women experience lower abdominal discomfort on the involved side. This so-called *Mittelschmerz* is believed to be caused by peritoneal irritation caused by follicular fluid or blood that escapes from the ruptured follicle. The symptoms rarely occur during every cycle.

A useful means of detecting ovulation is by documentation of a shift in basal body temperature from a relatively constant lower level during the follicular or preovulatory phase to a somewhat higher level early in the luteal or postovulatory phase (Fig. 2–25). Most likely, ovulation occurs just before or during the shift in temperature. The increase in the basal body temperature is believed to be caused by the thermogenic action of progesterone in the brain. This phenomenon may be induced by the action of 5β-reduced metabolites of

progesterone, which are known to cause fever, at least when given intramuscularly (for review: MacDonald and colleagues, 1991). A similar thermal response can be induced by the injection of progesterone into a castrated woman. The rise in basal body temperature, therefore, may be evidence for the development of a corpus luteum and the secretion of progesterone. Extensive luteinization of the granulosa cells, however, may occur in a follicle that still contains an ovum (luteinized follicle or entrapped ovum). Such an event is believed to be one cause of a short luteal phase.

Corpus Luteum Formation

De Graaf also provided a clear description of the corpus luteum:

> Those structures, which thought normal, are only at certain times found in the testes of women, are globular bodies in the form of conglomerate glandulae which are composed of many particles, extending from the center to the circumference in straight rows, and are enveloped by a special membrane. We assert that these globules do not exist at

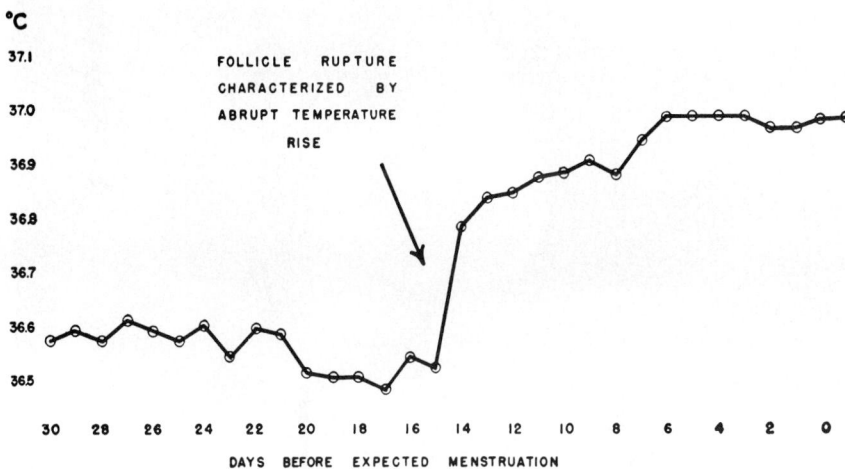

Fig. 2–25. Basal temperature shift characteristic of rupture of follicle. (From Palmer, 1949.)

all times in the testicles of females; on the contrary, they are only detected in them after coitus, [being] one or more in number according as the animal brings forth one or more foetuses from that congress.

Probably, de Graaf concluded that coitus brought about the appearance of the corpus luteum because of comparisons he made with anatomical findings in animals that are induced ovulators, such as the cat and rabbit.

The corpus luteum forms in the ovary at the site of the ruptured follicle immediately after ovulation (Fig. 2–26). It is colored by a golden pigment, from which it derives its name, which means "yellow body." Microscopically, it has been observed that the corpus luteum undergoes four stages of development and demise: proliferation, vascularization, maturity, and regression.

When the mature graafian follicle ruptures, the ovum, follicular liquid, and a considerable portion of the surrounding granulosa cells are discharged from the ruptured follicle. The collapsed walls of the empty follicle form convolutions about the blood-filled cavity (Fig. 2–27). The remaining granulosa cells appear polyhedral, with round, vesicular nuclei and frothy cytoplasm. There are many large lacunae that contain extravasated blood but, initially, no blood vessels. The theca interna is invaginated, and its vascular channels are greatly dilated. Endothelial sprouts from the vessels penetrate the hemorrhagic cavity of the ruptured follicle. Hertig (1964) described the K cells (Fig. 2–28) that can be recognized in the mature graafian follicle as stellate cells in which there is deeply eosinophilic, homogenous cytoplasm. During the proliferative stage, strands of K cells, which migrate from the theca, extend into the membrana granulosa to a position as far as the central coagulum.

In the stage of vascularization (which follows soon after ovulation), the blood-filled cavity of the ruptured follicle undergoes rapid organization. Grossly, the central coagulum appears pale gray with only a few hemorrhagic foci. Microscopically, there are fibroblasts, but no capillaries, within the coagulum. Elsewhere in the granulosa layer, dilated capillaries are conspicuous. As the stage of vascularization of the corpus luteum progresses to maturity, there is vacuolation in the periphery of the luteinized cells that originated from granulosa; this finding is suggestive that the luteinized cells are physiologically active. The theca interna cells are also vacuolated; when stained for lipid, many more coarse droplets are present in the theca interna cells than in the granulosa lutein cells. The K cells continue to constitute a prominent portion of the corpus luteum cell mass at that stage and also contain lipid, as well as alkaline phosphatase activity in great amounts. The mature corpus luteum is usually 1 to 3 cm in diameter but occasionally may occupy one third or more of the entire ovary. At this stage, the corpus luteum characteristically is bright yellow.

In the absence of blastocyst implantation, regressive changes occur in the corpus luteum, occasionally as early as the 23rd day of the menstrual cycle. These changes become progressively more marked, up to the onset of menstruation, until the central coagulum has been obliterated by connective tissue, and blood pigment has been removed by leukocytes. There is no further capillary proliferation; the nuclei of the granu-

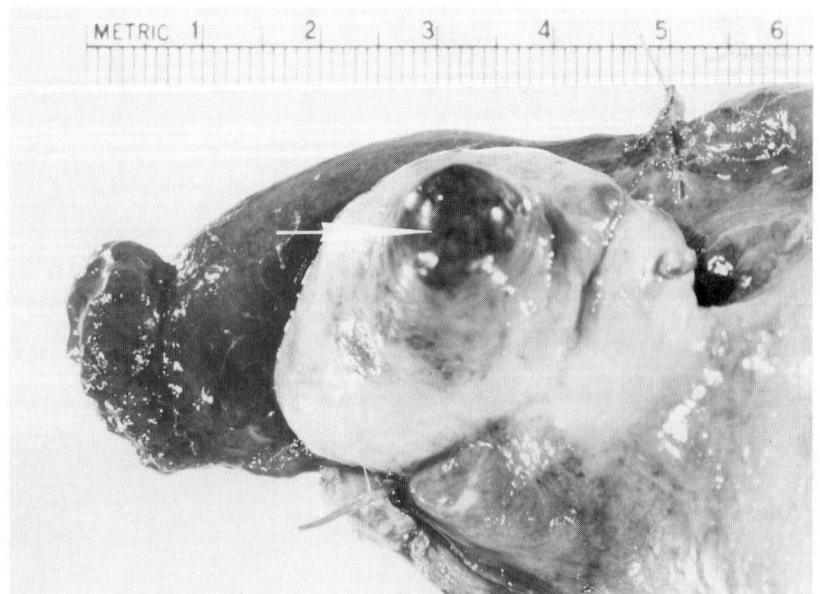

Fig. 2–26. Arrow points to an intact corpus luteum of early pregnancy. (Courtesy of Dr. R. Vogt.)

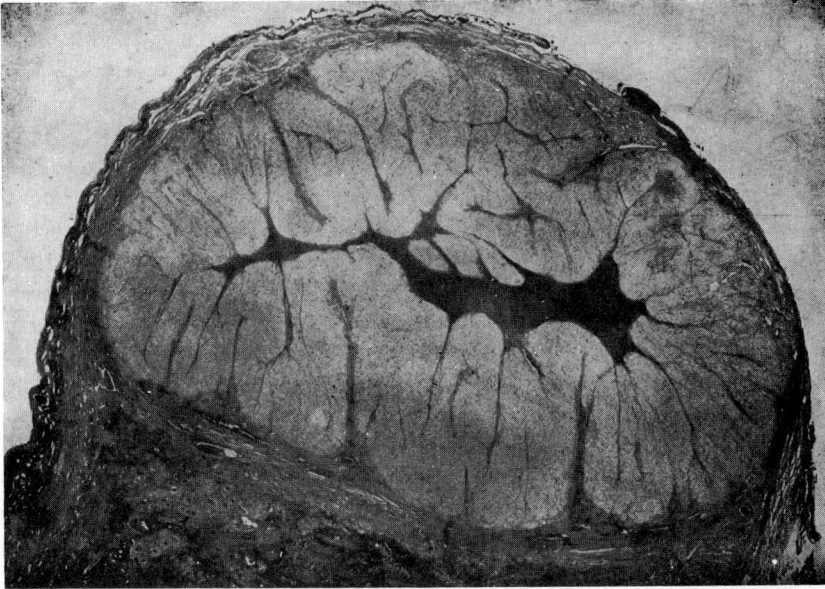

Fig. 2–27. Corpus luteum of pregnancy. (Low power; see also Fig. 2–29.)

losa lutein cells become pale, and vacuolization of the peripheral cytoplasm decreases as coarse lipid droplets accumulate. The theca cells can be seen only in widely separated clumps. The K cells develop hyperchromatic nuclei, and the cellular outlines almost disappear. There is a progressive loss of lipid-staining material throughout the entire corpus luteum. Complete regression of the corpus luteum takes place before menstruation. If implantation does not take place, the corpus luteum is destined to be a short-lived *corpus luteum of menstruation*. If implantation does take place, the corpus luteum is rescued by the action of

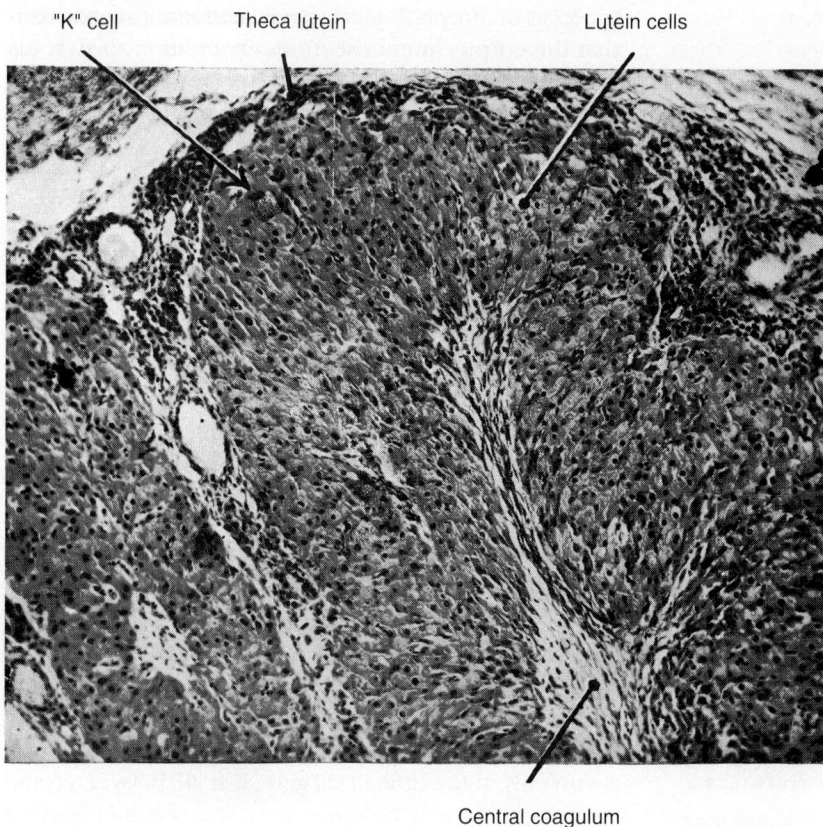

"K" cell   Theca lutein   Lutein cells

Central coagulum

Fig. 2–28. Section through the wall of a mature corpus luteum of menstruation.

trophoblast hCG and a *corpus luteum of pregnancy* is maintained, and there is a temporary postponement of the degenerative changes that otherwise would occur (Fig. 2–29).

Corpus Luteum of Pregnancy. The duration and the function of the corpus luteum of pregnancy are the subjects of much speculation and investigation (Chap. 6). The scientific validity of hormonal therapy in the prevention of early abortion when surgical removal of the corpus luteum is obliged depends on an understanding of the function of this structure.

Hertig (1964) enumerated the morphological criteria of a very early corpus luteum of pregnancy; these include (1) a surge of hyperplasia from the 23rd to 28th day after the last menstrual period, which results presumably, at least in part, from the stimulus of hCG; (2) an increasing number of K cells; and (3) the absence of atrophic, ischemic, or regressive changes similar to those that appear when menstruation is imminent. The degenerative changes in the corpus luteum are delayed for a variable time but take place most frequently at about 6 months of gestation, although corpora lutea that appear to be normal have been found at term. Progesterone secretion by the corpus luteum of pregnancy declines much earlier, however, at about 8 weeks.

Ultrastructure of the Corpus Luteum of Pregnancy. Adams and Hertig (1969) compared the ultrastructure of human corpora lutea obtained during the 6th, 10th, 16th,

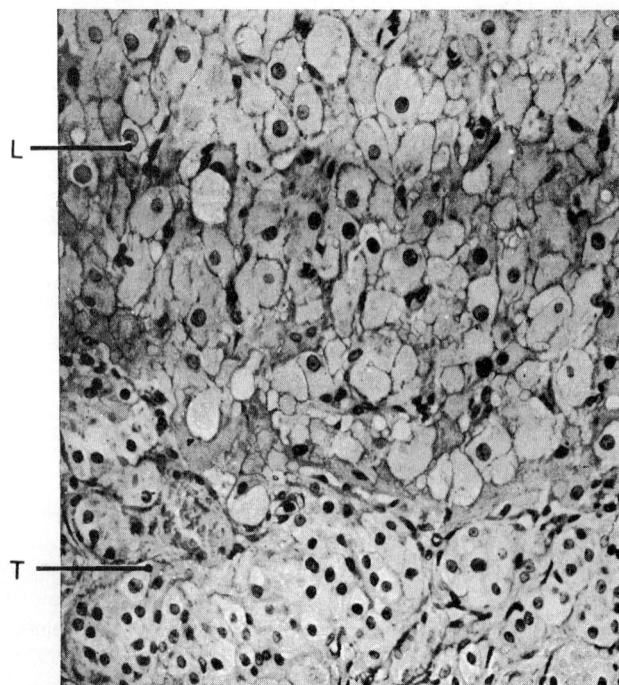

Fig. 2–29. Corpus luteum of pregnancy. (High power; L = granulosa lutein cells; T = theca lutein cells.)

and 35th weeks of pregnancy with that of those obtained during the menstrual cycle. In pregnancy, the luteal cell appears to be more highly compartmentalized, with a peripheral mass of endoplasmic reticulum and a central area in which mitochondria and Golgi complexes are concentrated. The area that is rich in mitochondria and Golgi complexes extends to the cell surface where microvilli are found that face a vascular space. In certain luteal cells with irregular nuclear membranes, there are vesicular aggregates within the peripheral nucleoplasm or the perinuclear cytoplasm. These nuclear vesicular aggregates and certain spherical bodies may be reflective of prolonged endocrine stimulation and thence secretory exhaustion, which ultimately produce electron-dense cells in which there are pyknotic nuclei.

Crisp and co-workers (1970), in an ultrastructure study, compared the granulosa and theca lutein cells of human corpora lutea. In early pregnancy, luteinized granulosa cells may be distinguished from theca lutein cells on the basis of more homogeneous, electronlucent matrix, enlarged pleomorphic mitochondria, abundant endoplasmic reticulum, and several other important ultrastructural features. Furthermore, granulosa lutein cells of early pregnancy may be distinguished from those of the progestational phase of the ovarian cycle by a well-developed endoplasmic reticulum, large spherical mitochondria, more numerous membrane-bound granules, and greater numbers of intercellular canaliculi. These investigators suggested that these differences are a result of the action of hCG during early gestation. On the basis of morphological specializations, it seems likely that the corpus luteum secretes, in addition to steroids, proteinaceous products. In fact, we now know that the corpus luteum secretes relaxin, activins, inhibins, and at times, oxytocin (Chap. 6).

Progesterone Secretion by the Corpus Luteum in Pregnancy. It is generally agreed that progesterone produced by the corpus luteum during the first 8 weeks (menstrual age) of human gestation is important to the maintenance of pregnancy. Thereafter, progesterone synthesis in syncytiotrophoblast becomes dominant.

Sometimes, however, the obstetrician must face certain therapeutic choices when obliged to remove the corpus luteum from the ovary in early pregnancy of a woman who wishes to continue that pregnancy. Our choice is the use of a parenteral progestin, 17α-hydroxyprogesterone caproate (Delalutin, 150 mg) when the corpus luteum is removed prior to 10 weeks' gestation. We choose 17α-hydroxyprogesterone caproate because (1) the duration of action is predictable, (2) rarely if ever does such treatment lead to virilization of a female fetus, and (3) it can be given intramuscularly. Beyond 8 weeks' gestation, we administer the progestin only at the time of surgery, if at all. Between 6 and 8 weeks, there may be some merit in a second injection 1 week after surgery.

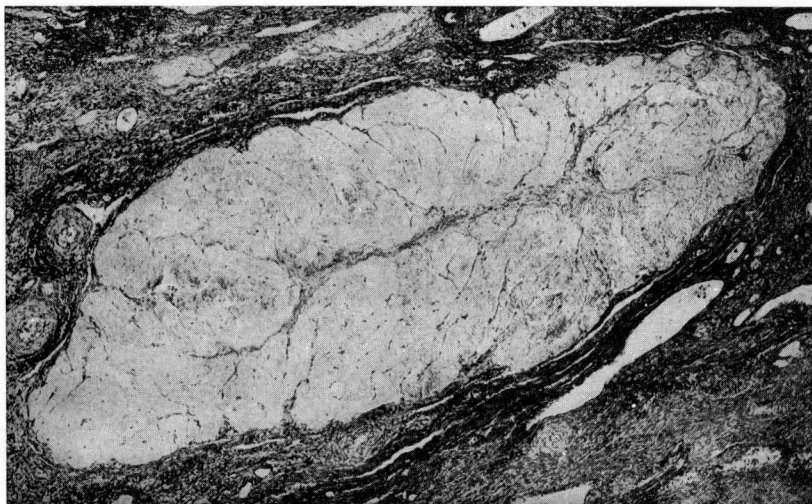

Fig. 2–30. Corpus albicans.

Corpora Albicantia. In the absence of pregnancy, degenerated lutein cells are rapidly resorbed; and in a short time, the corpus luteum is replaced by newly formed connective tissue that closely resembles that of the surrounding ovarian stroma. The structures formed, called corpora albicantia, appear, on cut-section, to be dull and white, somewhat like scar tissue (Fig. 2–30); these are, however, invaded gradually by the surrounding stroma and are broken up into increasingly smaller hyaline masses, which eventually are completely resorbed. Ultimately, the site of the original follicle is indicated only by an area of slightly thickened connective tissue. In older women, this process may be slower and less complete. In women near the age of menopause, it is not uncommon to find that the ovaries are almost filled by scars of various sizes.

Atretic Ovarian Follicles. The theca lutein cells serve a prominent role in the life history of follicles that degenerate without rupture. This process, *follicular atresia,* is particularly pronounced during pregnancy. In this circumstance, after the follicle has attained a certain size, the ovum undergoes cytolysis, while the membrana granulosa degenerates, is cast off into the liquor folliculi, and eventually is resorbed. As these changes are in progress, the theca lutein cells proliferate to form, about the follicle, a tunic many layers thick that frequently becomes yellowish. Eventually, as the follicular fluid disappears, the walls of the follicle collapse and there are fatty and hyaline changes in the theca cells that surround it. Finally, an irregular hyaline body results that cannot be distinguished from a similar structure that was derived from a corpus luteum.

Artesia is the fate of the vast majority of follicles that develop beyond the primordial stage; the process begins during intrauterine life and continues until after the menopause. Corpora lutea, however, always develop only from the comparatively few follicles, usu-ally one each ovarian cycle, that rupture after reaching maturity.

References

Adams EC, Hertig AT: Studies on the human corpus luteum, I. Observations on the ultrastructure of development and regression of the luteal cells during the menstrual cycle. J Cell Biol 41:696, 1969

Allen E, Pratt JP, Newell QU, Bland LJ: Human tubal ova: Related early corpora lutea and uterine tubes. Contrib Embryol 22:45, 1930

American College of Obstetricians and Gynecologists: Ultrasound in pregnancy. Technical Bulletin no. 116, May 1988

Ascheim S, Zondek B: Anterior pituitary hormone and ovarian hormone in the urine of pregnant women. Klin Wochenschr 6:248, 1927

Baker TG: Oogenesis and ovulation. In Austin CR, Short RV (eds): Reproduction in Mammals, I. Germ Cells and Fertilization. Cambridge, Cambridge University Press, 1978

Baker TG: Radiosensitivity of mammalian oocytes with particular reference to the human female. Am J Obstet Gynecol 110:746, 1971

Bandi ZL, Schoen I, DeLara M: Enzyme-linked immunosorbent urine pregnancy tests: Clinical specificity studies. Am J Clin Pathol 87:236, 1987

Barnes RB, Roy S, Yee B, Duda MJ, Mishell DR: Reliability of urinary pregnancy tests in the diagnosis of ectopic pregnancy. J Reprod Med 30:827, 1985

Bartholomew RA, Sale BE, Calloway JT: Diagnosis of pregnancy by the roentgen ray. JAMA 76:912, 1921

Bazer RW, Vallet JL, Roberts RM, Sharp DC, Thatcher WW: Role of conceptus secretory products in establishment of pregnancy. J Reprod Fert 76:841, 1986

Beers WH: Follicular plasminogen and plasminogen activator and the effect of plasmin on ovarian follicle wall. Cell 6:379, 1975

Bernaschek G, Rudelstorfer R, Csaicsich P: Vaginal sonography versus serum human chorionic gonadotropin in early detection of pregnancy. Am J Obstet Gynecol 158:608, 1988

Blandau RJ, White BJ, Rumery RE: Observations on the movements of the living primordial germ cells in the mouse. Fertil Steril 14:482, 1963

Bridson WE, Ross GT, Kohler PO: Immunologic and biologic activity of chorionic gonadotropin synthesized by cloned choriocarcinoma cells in tissue culture. Clin Res 18:356, 1970

Brown MS, Kovanen PT, Goldstein JL: Receptor-mediated uptake of lipoprotein cholesterol and its utilization for steroid synthesis in the adrenal cortex. Recent Prog Horm Res 35:215, 1979

Carr BR, MacDonald PC, Simpson ER: The role of lipoproteins in the regulation of progesterone by the human corpus luteum. Fertil Steril 38:303, 1982

Carr BR, Sadler RK, Rochelle DB, Stalmach MA, MacDonald PC, Simpson ER: Plasma lipoprotein regulation of progesterone biosynthesis by human corpus luteum tissue in organ culture. J Clin Endocrinol Metab 52:875, 1981

Casey ML, Mibe M, Erk A, and MacDonald PC: Transforming growth factor-β_1 stimulation of parathyroid hormone-related protein expression in human uterine cells in culture: mRNA levels and protein secretion. J Clin Endocrinol Metab 74:950, 1992

Casey ML, Word RA, and MacDonald PC: Endothelin-1 gene expression and regulation of endothelin mRNA and protein biosynthesis in avascular human amnion. J Biol Chem 266:5762, 1991

Chadwick JR: Value of the bluish coloration of the vaginal entrance as a sign of pregnancy. Trans Am Gynecol Soc 11:399, 1886

Chang MC: The maturation of rabbit oocytes in culture and their maturation, activation, fertilization and subsequent development in the fallopian tubes. J Exp Zool 128:378, 1955

Channing CP, Anderson LD, Hoover DJ, Kolena J, Osteen KG, Pomerantz SH, Tanabe K: The role of nonsteroidal regulators in control of oocyte and follicular maturation. Recent Prog Horm Res 38:331, 1982

Channing CP, Pomerantz SH: Studies on an oocyte maturation inhibitor partially purified from porcine and human follicular fluids. In Franchimont P, Channing CP (eds): Intragonadal Regulation of Reproduction. New York, Academic Press, 1981, p 81

Chartier M, Roger M, Barrat J, Michelon B: Measurement of plasma chorionic gonadotropin (hCG) and CG activities in the late luteal phase: Evidence of the occurrence of spontaneous menstrual abortions in infertile women. Fertil Steril 31:134, 1979

Coale AJ: The history of the human population. Sci Am 231:41, 1974

Cole LA, Kardana A: Discordant results in human chorionic gonadotropin assays. Clin Chem 38:263, 1992

Corner GW: On the female testes or ovaries, by Regner de Graaf. In Farquar ST, Leake CD, Lyons WR, Simpson ME (eds): Essays in Biology. Los Angeles, University of California Press, 1943, p 123

Crisp TM, Dessouky DA, Denys FR: The fine structure of the human corpus luteum of early pregnancy and during the progestational phase of the menstrual cycle. Am J Anat 127:37, 1970

Dean J: Biology of mammalian fertilization: role of the zona pellucida. J Clin Invest 89:1055, 1992

de Graaf R: De Mulierum organis generationi inservientibus. Lugd, Batav, 1677, p 161

Derman R, Corson LS, Horwitz CA, Lau HD, Solderstrom R: Early diagnosis of pregnancy: A symposium. J Reprod Med 26:149, 1981

Dickman Z, Noyes RW: Zona pellucida at the time of implantation: Fertil Steril 12:310, 1961

Doshi ML: Accuracy of consumer performed in-home tests for early pregnancy detection. Am J Public Health 76:512, 1986

Eaton JW, Mayer AJ: The social biology of very high fertility among the Hutterites: The demography of a unique population. Hum Biol 25:206, 1953

Eddy CA, Pauerstein CJ: Anatomy and physiology of the fallopian tube. Clin Obstet Gynecol 23:1177, 1980

Ferenczy A, Richart RM: The Female Reproductive System. Dynamics of Scan and Electron Microscopy. New York, Wiley, 1974

Friedman JM: Genetic disease in the offspring of older fathers. Obstet Gynecol 57:745, 1981

Germain AM, Attaroglu H, MacDonald PC, Casey ML: Parathyroid hormone-related protein mRNA in avascular human amnion. J Clin Endocrinol Metab 75:1173, 1992

Gey GO, Jones GES, Hellman LM: The production of a gonadotrophic substance (prolan) by placental cells in tissue culture. Science 88:306, 1938

Godkin JD, Bazer FW, Roberts RM: Ovine trophoblast protein-1, an early secreted blastocyst protein, binds specifically to uterine endometrium and affects protein synthesis. Endocrinology 114:120, 1984

Green JJ, Hobbins JC: Abdominal ultrasound examination of the first-trimester fetus. Am J Obstet Gynecol 159:165, 1988

Hansen PJ, Anthony RV, Bazer RW, Baumbach GA, Roberts RM: In vitro synthesis and secretion of ovine trophoblast protein-1 during the period of maternal recognition of pregnancy. Endocrinology 117:1424, 1985

Harcourt AH, Harvey PH, Larson SG, Short RV: Testis weight, body weight and breeding system in primates. Nature 293:55, 1981

Hartman CG: How large is the mammalian egg? Q Rev Biol 4:581, 1929

Hearn JP, Webley GE, Gidley-Baird AA: Chorionic gonadotrophin and embryo-maternal recognition during the peri-implantation period in primates. J Reprod Fert 92:497, 1991

Hertig AT: Gestational hyperplasia of endometrium: A morphologic correlation of ova, endometrium, and corpora lutea during early pregnancy. Lab Invest 13:1153, 1964

Hertig AT, Rock J: On the development of the early human ovum with special reference to the trophoblast of the previllous stage: A description of 7 normal and 5 pathologic human ova. Am J Obstet Gynecol 47:149, 1944

Hertz R: Early studies of chorionic gonadotropin and antihormones. In Segal SJ (ed): Chorionic Gonadotropin. New York, Plenum, 1980

Hirose T: Experimentalle histologische Studie fur genese Corpus luteum. Mitt ad med Fakultd t Univ Z U, Tokyo 23:63, 1919

Horrow MM: Enlarged amniotic cavity: A new sonographic sign of early embryonic death. AJR 158:359, 1992

Illingworth DR, Corbin DK, Kemp ED, Keenan EJ: Hormone changes during the menstrual cycle in abetalipoproteinemia: Reduced luteal phase progesterone in a patient with homozygous hypobetalipoproteinemia. Proc Natl Acad Sci USA 79:6685, 1982

Imakawa K, Anthony RV, Kazemi M, Marotti KR, Polites HG, Roberts RM: Interferon-like sequence of ovine trophoblast protein secreted by embryonic trophectoderm. Nature 330:377, 1987

Jeng LL, Moore Jr RM, Kaczmarek RG, Placek PJ, Bright RA: How frequently are home pregnancy tests used? Results from the 1988 national maternal and infant health survey. Birth 18:11, 1991

Jimenez JM, Tyson JE, Santos-Ramos R, Duenhoelter JH: Comparison of obstetric and pediatric evaluation of gestational age. Pediatr Res 13:498, 1979

Jovanovic L, Singh M, Saxena BB, Mills JL, Tulchinsky D, Holmes LB, Simpson JL, Metzger BE, Labarbera A, Aarons J, Van Allen MI: NICHD-DIEP Study Group: Verification of early pregnancy tests in a multicenter trial. Proc Soc Exp Biol Med 184:201, 1987

Judd S, Terry A, Petrucco M, White G: The source of pulsatile secretion of progesterone during the human follicular phase. J Clin Endocrinol Metab 74:299, 1992

Kadar N, Caldwell BV, Romero R: A method of screening for ectopic pregnancy and its indications. Obstet Gynecol 58:162, 1981

Kolata GB: !Kung hunter-gatherers: Feminism, diet and birth control. Science 185:932, 1974

Lagrew DC, Wilson EA, Jawad MJ: Determination of gestational age by serum concentrations of human chorionic gonadotropin. Obstet Gynecol 62:37, 1983

Lee C, Hart LL: Accuracy of home pregnancy tests. DICP 24:712, 1990

MacDonald PC, Dombroski RA, Casey ML: Recurrent secretion of progesterone in large amounts: An endocrine/metabolic disorder unique to young women? Endocr Rev 12:372, 1991

May K: Home tests to monitor fertility. Am J Obstet Gynecol 165:2000, 1991

Moore KL: The Developing Human: Clinically-Oriented Embryology, 4th ed. Philadelphia, Saunders, 1988

Motta PM, Hafez ES: Biology of the Ovary. The Hague, Martinus Nijhoff, 1980

Nathanielsz PW, Figueroa JP, Honnebier MB: In the rhesus monkey placental retention after fetectomy at 121 to 130 days' gestation outlasts the normal duration of pregnancy. Am J Obstet Gynecol 166:1529, 1992

Ohashi M, Carr BR, Simpson ER: Lipoprotein-binding sites in human corpus luteum membrane fractions. Endocrinology 110:1477, 1982

Palmer A: The diagnostic use of the basal body temperature in gynecology and obstetrics. Obstet Gynecol Surv 4:1, 1949

Pelosi MC, Apuzzi J, Dwyer JW: Early diagnosis of pregnancy, I. Workup and laboratory tests. Female Patient 8:38, 1983

Peters H: In Midgley, Sadler (eds). Aspects of Early Follicular Development, New York, Raven, 1979

Pitkin RM: Fetal death: Diagnosis and management. Am J Obstet Gynecol 157:583, 1987

Plante C, Hansen PJ, Thatcher WW: Prolongation of luteal lifespan in cows by intrauterine infusion of recombinant bovine alpha-interferon. Endocrinology 122:2342, 1988

Reichert FL, Pencharz FI, Simpson ME, Meyer K, Evans HM: Relative ineffectiveness of prolan in hypophysectomized animals. Am J Physiol 100:157, 1932

Rempen A: Diagnosis of viability in early pregnancy with vaginal sonography. J Ultrasound Med 9:711, 1990

Richardson MC, Davies DW, Watson RH, Dunsford ML, Inman CB, Masson GM: Cultured human granulosa cells as a model for corpus luteum function: Relative roles of gonadotrophin and low density lipoprotein studied under defined culture conditions. Hum Reprod 7:12, 1992

Robinson HP: Detection of fetal heart movement in first trimester of pregnancy using pulsed ultrasound. Br Med J 4:66, 1972

Ryan KJ, Smith OW: Biogenesis of estrogens by the human ovary: I. Conversion of acetate-1-C^{14} to estrone and estradiol. J Biol Chem 234:268, 1959

Short RV: Breast feeding. Sci Am 250:35, 1984

Short RV: The origins of human sexuality. In Austin CR, Short RV (eds): Reproduction in Mammals: Human Sexuality. Cambridge, Cambridge University Press, 1980, p 2

Short RV: Definition of the problem: The evolution of human reproduction. In Short RV, Baird DT (eds): Contraceptives of the Future. Cambridge, University Printing House, 1976a, p 3

Short RV: The evolution of human reproduction. Proc Roy Soc Lond 195:3, 1976b

Short RV: Maternal recognition of pregnancy. In Wolstenhome GEW, O'Connor M (eds): Foetal Autonomy. London, Churchill, 1969, p 2

Simpson ER, Rochelle DB, Carr BR, MacDonald PC: Cytochrome plasma lipoprotein in follicular fluid of human ovaries. J Clin Endocrinol Metab 52:1469, 1980

Speert H, Guttmacher AF: Frequency and significance of bleeding in early pregnancy. JAMA 155:172, 1954

Strickland S, Beers WH: Studies of the enzymatic basis and hormonal control of ovulation. In Midgley AR, Sadler WA (eds): Ovarian Follicular Development. New York, Raven, 1979

Sunnergren KP, Word RA, Sambrook JF, MacDonald PC, Casey ML: Expression and regulation of endothelin precursor mRNA in avascular human amnion. Mol Cell Endocrinol 68:R7, 1990

Tesh JM, Glover TD: Aging of rabbit spermatozoa in the male tract and its effect on fertility. J Reprod Fertil 20:287, 1969

Townsend L, Shelton JG: Intrauterine death due to fetal erythroblastosis. Aust NZ J Obstet Gynaecol 4:84, 1964

Vaitukaitis JL, Braunstein GD, Ross GT: A radioimmunoassay which specifically measures chorionic gonadotropin in the presence of human luteinizing hormone. Am J Obstet Gynecol 113:751, 1972

Valanis BG, Perlman CS: Home pregnancy testing kits: Prevalence of use, false-negative rates, and compliance with instructions. Am J Public Health 72:1034, 1982

Vallejo G: Human chorionic gonadotropin detection by means of enzyme immunoassay: A useful method in forensic pregnancy diagnosis in bloodstains. J Forensic Sci 35:293, 1990

Vickers AD: Delayed fertilization and chromosomal anomalies in mouse embryos. J Reprod Fertil 20:69, 1969

Wide L, Hobson B: Immunological and biological activity of human chorionic gonadotropin in urine and serum of pregnant women and women with a hydatidiform mole. Acta Endocrinol 54:105, 1967

Zondek B: Die Hormone des Ovariums und des Hypophysenvordelappens. Berlin, Springer, 1931

CHAPTER 3
Anatomy of the Reproductive Tract of Women

The organs of reproduction of women are classified as either external or internal. The external organs and the vagina serve for copulation; the internal organs provide for ovulation, a site of ovum fertilization and blastocyst transport, implantation, and thence development and birth of the fetus. There may be marked variation in anatomical structures in a given patient, and this is especially true for major blood vessels and nerves.

External Generative Organs

The *pudenda*, or the external organs of generation, are commonly designated the *vulva*, which includes all structures visible externally from the pubis to the perineum, that is, the mons pubis, labia majora and minora, clitoris, hymen, vestibule, urethral opening, and various glandular and vascular structures (Fig. 3–1).

Mons Pubis. The mons pubis, or mons veneris, is the fat-filled cushion that lies over the anterior surface of the symphysis pubis. After puberty, the skin of the mons pubis is covered by curly hair that forms the *escutcheon*. Generally, the distribution of pubic hair differs in the two sexes. In women, it is distributed in a triangular area, the base of which is formed by the upper margin of the symphysis, and a few hairs are distributed downward over the outer surface of the labia majora. In men, the escutcheon is not so well circumscribed; hairs from the pubic area grow in a region that extends upward toward the umbilicus and downward and inward over the inner surface of the thighs.

Labia Majora. There are two rounded folds of adipose tissue that are covered with skin, and that extend downward and backward from the mons pubis; these are the labia majora. Among adult women, these structures vary somewhat in appearance, principally according to the amount of fat that is contained within these tissues. Embryologically, the labia majora are homologous with the male scrotum. The round ligaments terminate at the upper borders of the labia majora. After repeated childbearing, the labia majora are less prominent, and in old age usually begin to shrivel. Ordinarily, these structures are 7 to 8 cm in length, 2 to 3 cm in width, and 1 to 1.5 cm in thickness, and are somewhat tapered at the lower extremities. In children and nulliparous women, the labia majora usually lie in close apposition, and thereby completely conceal the underlying tissues; whereas in multiparous women, the labia majora may gape widely (Fig. 3–2). The labia majora are continuous directly with the mons pubis above and merge into the perineum posteriorly, at a site where these structures are joined medially to form the *posterior commissure*.

Before puberty, the outer surface of the labia is similar to that of the adjacent skin, but after puberty they are covered with hair. In nulliparous women, the inner surface is moist and resembles a mucous membrane; whereas in multiparous women, the inner surface becomes more skinlike, but is not covered with hair. The labia majora are richly supplied with sebaceous glands. Beneath the skin, there is a layer of dense connective tissue that is rich in elastic fibers and adipose tissue, but is nearly void of muscular elements. Unlike the squamous epithelium of the vagina and cervix, there are epithelial appendages in parts of the vulvar skin. Beneath the skin, there is a mass of fat, which provides the bulk of the volume of the labium; this tissue is supplied with a plexus of veins that, as the result of injury, may rupture to create a hematoma.

Labia Minora. Two flat reddish folds of tissue are visible when the labia majora are separated; these structures are the labia minora, or nymphae, structures that join at the upper extremity of the vulva. The labia minora vary greatly in size and shape. In nulliparous women, they usually are not visible behind the nonseparated labia majora, whereas in multiparous women, it is common for the labia minora to project beyond the labia majora.

Each labium minus is a thin fold of tissue that, when projected, is moist and reddish in appearance and is similar to that of a mucous membrane. These structures, however, are covered by stratified squamous epithelium into which numerous papillae project. There are no hair follicles in the labia minora, but there are many sebaceous follicles and, occasionally, a few sweat glands. The interior of the labial folds is comprised of connective tissue with many vessels and some smooth muscular fibers, as is the case in typical erectile structures. These structures are supplied with a variety of nerve endings and are extremely sensitive.

The tissues of the labia minora converge superiorly, where each is divided into two lamellae, the lower pair

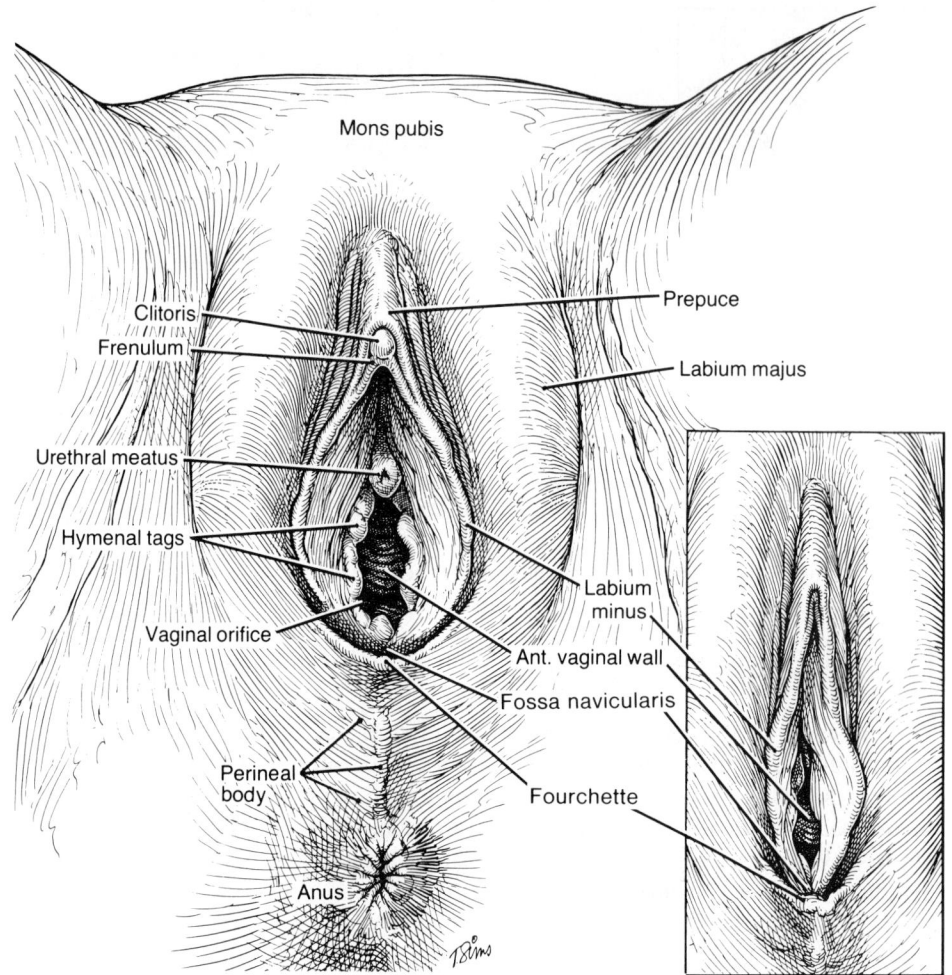

Fig. 3–1. External organs of reproduction of women. The lower anterior vaginal wall is visible through the labia minora. In nulliparous women, the vaginal orifice is not so readily visible (*inset*) because of the close apposition of the labia minora.

of which fuses to form the *frenulum of the clitoris*, and the upper pair of which merges to form the *prepuce* of the clitoris. Inferiorly, the labia minora extend to approach the midline as low ridges of tissue that fuse to form the *fourchette* in nulliparous women; in multiparous women the labia minora usually are imperceptibly contiguous with the labia majora.

Clitoris. The clitoris is the homologue of the penis and is located near the superior extremity of the vulva. This erectile organ projects downward between the branched extremities of the labia minora, which, as stated, converge to form the prepuce and frenulum of the clitoris. The clitoris is comprised of a glans, a body (corpus), and two crura. The glans is made up of spindle-shaped cells, and in the body there are two corpora cavernosa, in the walls of which are smooth muscle fibers. The long, narrow crura arise from the inferior surface of the ischiopubic rami and fuse just below the middle of the pubic arch to form the corpus.

Rarely does the clitoris exceed 2 cm in length, even in a state of erection (Verkauf and associates, 1992), and

it is bent sharply by traction that is exerted by the labia minora. As a result, the free end of the clitoris is pointed downward and inward toward the vaginal opening. The glans, which rarely exceeds 0.5 cm in diameter, is covered by stratified squamous epithelium that is richly supplied with nerve endings and is, therefore, extremely sensitive. The vessels of the erectile clitoris are connected with the vestibular bulbs; the clitoris is believed to be one, if not the principal, erogenous organ of women.

In the labia majora, as well as the labia minora and clitoris, Krantz (1958) reported that there is a delicate network of free nerve endings, the fibers of which terminate in small knoblike thickenings in or adjacent to the cells. These nerve endings are encountered more frequently in the papillae than elsewhere; moreover, tactile discs are also found in abundance in these areas. The number of genital corpuscles, which are considered the main structures that are mediators of erotic sensation, varies considerably. These structures are distributed sparsely and randomly in the labia majora deep in the corium, but are abundant in the labia minora and in the skin that overlies the glans clitoris.

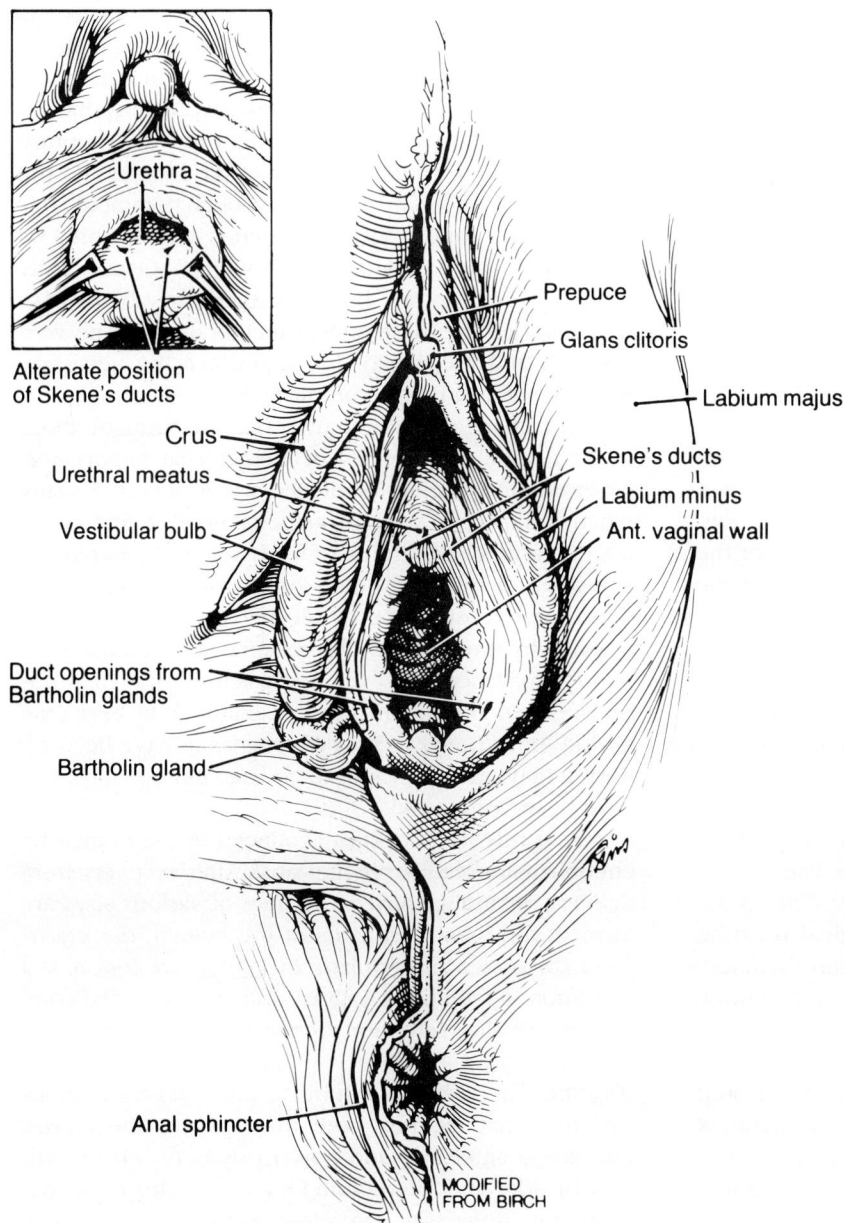

Urethra

Alternate position
of Skene's ducts

Crus

Urethral meatus

Vestibular bulb

Duct openings from
Bartholin glands

Bartholin gland

Anal sphincter

Prepuce

Glans clitoris

Labium majus

Skene's ducts

Labium minus

Ant. vaginal wall

MODIFIED
FROM BIRCH

Fig. 3–2. The external genitalia with the skin and subcutaneous tissue removed from the right side.

Vestibule. The vestibule is an almond-shaped area that is enclosed by the labia minora laterally and extends from the clitoris to the fourchette. The vestibule is the functionally mature female structure of the urogenital sinus of the embryo; in the mature state it usually is perforated by six openings: the urethra, the vagina, the ducts of the Bartholin glands, and, at times, the ducts of the paraurethral glands, also called the Skene ducts and glands (Fig. 3–2). The posterior portion of the vestibule between the fourchette and the vaginal opening is called the *fossa navicularis*, and is usually observed only in nulliparous women.

The *Bartholin glands* (Fig. 3–2) are a pair of small compound structures that are about 0.5 to 1 cm in diameter. Each is situated beneath the vestibule on ei-

ther side of the vaginal opening and they are the *major vestibular glands*. The Bartholin glands lie under the constrictor muscle of the vagina and sometimes are found to be covered partially by the vestibular bulbs. The gland ducts are 1.5 to 2 cm long and open on the sides of the vestibule just outside the lateral margin of the vaginal orifice. The small gland lumen ordinarily admits only the finest of probes. At times of sexual arousal, mucoid material is secreted from these glands. These glands may harbor *Neisseria gonorrhoeae*, or other bacteria, which in turn may cause suppuration and a Bartholin gland abscess.

Urethral Opening. The lower two thirds of the urethra lies immediately above the anterior vaginal wall. The urethral opening or meatus is in the midline of the vestibule, 1 to 1.5 cm below the pubic arch, and a short distance above the vaginal opening. The urethral orifice appears as a vertical slit, which can be distended to 4 or 5 mm in diameter. Ordinarily, the *paraurethral ducts*, also known as the Skene ducts, open onto the vestibule on either side of the urethra; but occasionally they open on the posterior wall of the urethra just inside the meatus (Fig. 3–2). These ducts are about 0.5 mm in diameter, and of variable length.

Vestibular Bulbs. Beneath the mucous membrane of the vestibule on either side are the vestibular bulbs, which are almond-shaped aggregations of veins, 3 to 4 cm long, 1 to 2 cm wide, and 0.5 to 1 cm thick. These bulbs lie in close apposition to the ischiopubic rami and are partially covered by the ischiocavernosus and constrictor vaginae muscles. The lower terminations of the vestibular bulbs usually are at about the middle of the vaginal opening, and anteriorly, the vestibular bulbs extend upward toward the clitoris.

Embryologically, the vestibular bulbs correspond to the anlage of the corpus spongiosum of the penis. The vestibular bulbs of women, during childbirth, usually are pushed up beneath the pubic arch; because the posterior ends partially encircle the vagina, however, these structures are liable to injury and rupture, which may result in a vulvar hematoma or hemorrhage.

Vaginal Opening and Hymen. The vaginal opening varies considerably in size and shape. In virginal women, it most often is hidden by the overlapping labia minora, and when exposed, it usually appears almost completely closed by the membranous hymen.

There also are marked differences in shape and consistency of the hymen, which is comprised mainly of elastic and collagenous connective tissue. Both the outer and inner surfaces are covered by stratified squamous epithelium. Connective tissue papillae are more numerous on the vaginal surface and at the free edge. There are no glandular or muscular elements in the hymen and it is not richly supplied with nerve fibers.

In the newborn, the hymen is very vascular and redundant; in pregnant women, the epithelium is thick and the tissue is rich in glycogen; after menopause, the epithelium of the hymen is thin and focal cornification may develop. In adult virginal women, the hymen is a membrane of various thickness that surrounds the vaginal opening more or less completely; among virginal women, the aperture of the hymen varies in diameter from that of a pinpoint to a caliber that admits the tip of one or even two fingers. The hymenal opening usually is crescentic or circular, but occasionally may be cribriform, septate, or fimbriated. The fimbriated type of hymen in virginal women may be indistinguishable from one that has been penetrated during intercourse; thus, it is not possible to determine virginity by such an examination.

As a rule, the hymen is torn at several sites during first coitus, usually in the posterior portion. The edges of the torn tissue soon cicatrize, and the hymen becomes divided permanently into two or more portions that are separated by narrow sulci. The extent to which rupture occurs varies with the structure of the hymen and the extent to which it is distended. Although commonly it is believed that rupture of the hymen is accompanied by bleeding, this is not evident in all women. Occasionally with hymenal rupture, however, there may be profuse bleeding. Rarely, the hymenal membrane may be very resistant and incision of the tissue may be necessary before coitus can be accomplished.

The changes in the hymen that are brought about by coitus are occasionally of medicolegal importance, especially in instances of alleged sexual assault. Usually when nulliparous women are examined a few hours after an attack, the finding of fresh hymenal lacerations, abrasions, or bleeding points on the hymen constitutes corroborative evidence of recent vaginal penetration, possibly by intercourse. The absence of such findings is of no significance, however, because the hymen may not be lacerated even with repeated coitus in a short time period. In fact, many cases of pregnancy have been reported in women in whom the hymen did not appear to have been "ruptured."

As a rule, the changes produced in the hymen by childbirth are readily recognizable. After recovery from delivery, several cicatrized nodules of various sizes are formed, the tissue remnants of the hymen, the *myrtiform caruncles*. *Imperforate hymen*, a rare lesion, is a condition in which the vaginal orifice is occluded completely, causing retention of the menstrual discharge.

Vagina. The vagina is a tubular, musculomembranous structure that extends from the vulva to the uterus, interposed anteriorly and posteriorly between the urinary bladder and the rectum (Fig. 3–3). This organ has many functions: the excretory canal of the uterus, through which uterine secretions and menstrual flow escape; the female organ of copulation; and part of the birth canal. The upper portion of the vagina arises from the müllerian ducts while the lower portion is formed from the urogenital sinus. Anteriorly, the vagina is in contact with the bladder and urethra, from which it is separated by connective tissue, often referred to as the vesicovaginal septum. Posteriorly, between the lower portion of the vagina and the rectum, there are similar tissues that, together, form the rectovaginal septum. Usually, the upper fourth of the vagina is separated from the rectum by the rectouterine pouch, also called the cul-de-sac of Douglas.

Normally, the anterior and posterior vaginal walls lie in contact with only a slight space that intervenes between the lateral margins. Thus, when not distended, the vaginal canal on transverse section is H-shaped (Fig. 3–4). The vagina can be distended

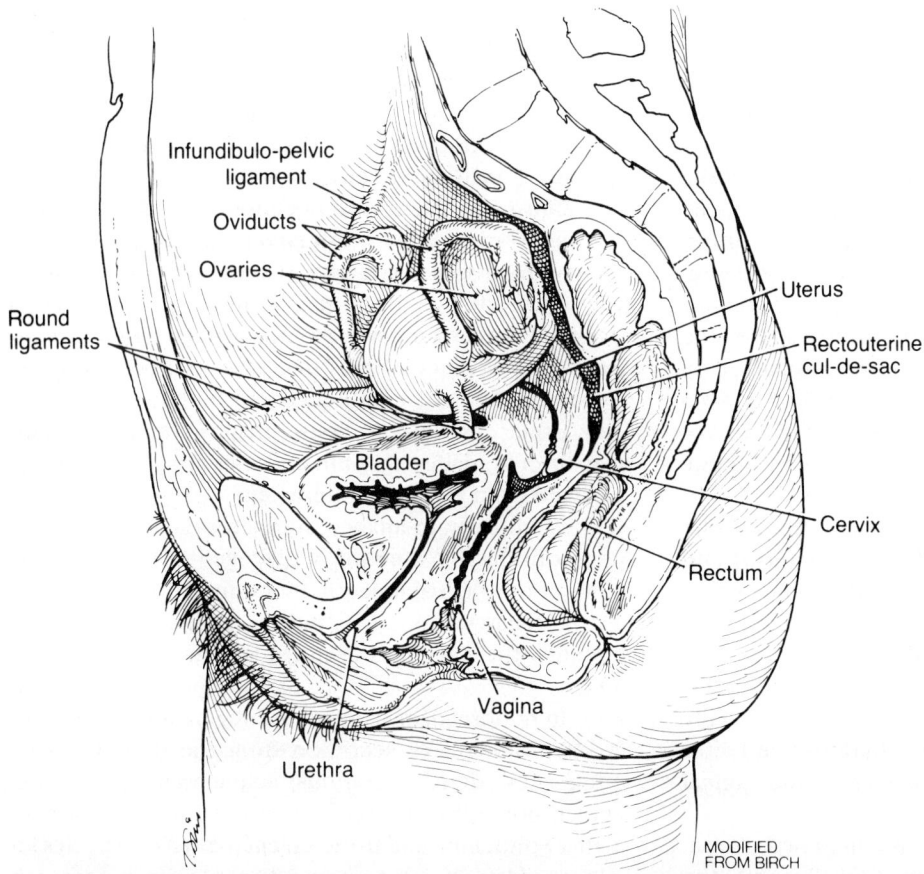

Fig. 3–3. Sagittal section of the pelvis of an adult woman showing relations of pelvic viscera.

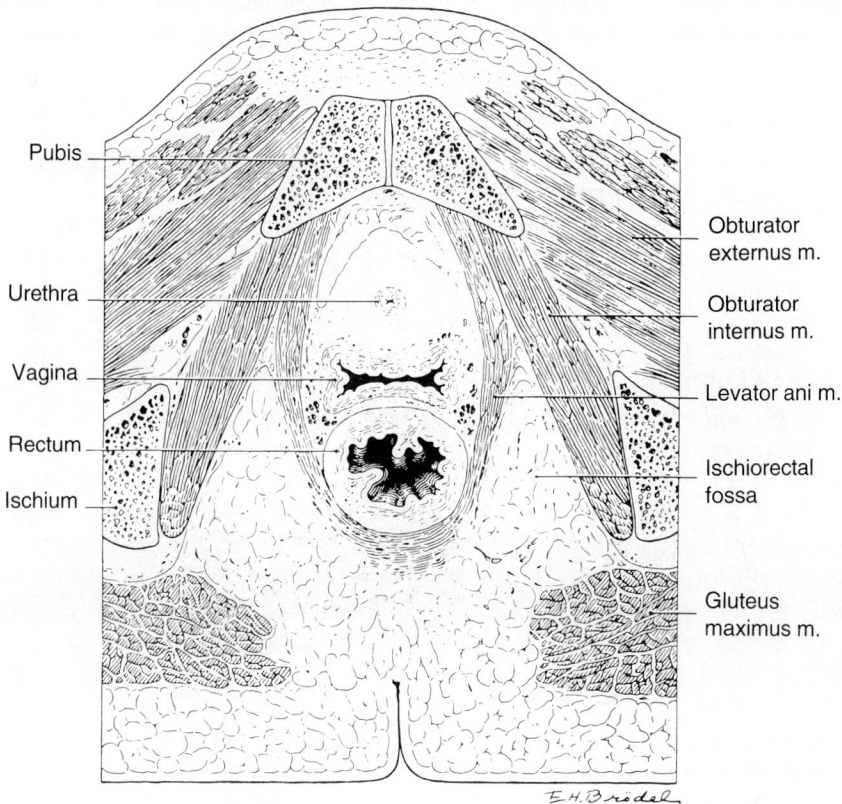

Fig. 3–4. Cross-section of the pelvis of an adult woman; the H-shaped lumen of the vagina is apparent. (m. = muscle.)

markedly, a characteristic that is most evident during childbirth.

The upper end of the vaginal vault is subdivided into the anterior, posterior, and two lateral fornices by the uterine cervix. Because the vagina is attached higher up on the posterior wall than on the anterior wall of the cervix, the depth of the posterior fornix is appreciably greater than the anterior. The lateral fornices are intermediate in depth. The fornices are of considerable clinical importance because the internal pelvic organs usually can be palpated through the thin walls of the fornices. Moreover, the posterior fornix usually provides ready surgical access to the peritoneal cavity. Vaginal length varies considerably; commonly, the anterior and posterior vaginal walls are, respectively, 6 to 8 cm, and 7 to 10 cm in length.

Prominent longitudinal ridges project into the vaginal lumen from the midlines of both the anterior and posterior walls. In nulliparous women, numerous transverse ridges, or *rugae*, extend outward from, and almost at right angles to, the longitudinal vaginal ridges. The rugae are such as to form a corrugated surface, which is not present before menarche and is one that gradually becomes obliterated after repeated childbirth and after menopause. In elderly multiparous women, the vaginal walls often are smooth.

The vaginal mucosa (Fig. 3–5) is comprised of noncornified stratified squamous epithelium. Beneath the epithelium there is a thin fibromuscular coat, usually consisting of an inner circular layer and an outer longitudinal layer of smooth muscle. There is a thin layer of connective tissue that overlies the mucosa and the muscularis, one that is rich in blood vessels, and one in which there are a few small lymphoid nodules. The mucosa and muscularis are attached very loosely to the underlying connective tissue. Some argument remains as to whether this connective tissue, often referred to as perivaginal endopelvic fascia, is a definite fascial plane in the strict anatomical sense.

Normally, glands are not present in the vagina. In parous women, however, fragments of stratified epithelium, which sometimes give rise to cysts, are occasionally embedded in the vaginal connective tissue. These *vaginal inclusion cysts* are not glands, but rather are remnants of mucosal tags that were buried during the repair of vaginal lacerations after childbirth. Occasionally, other cysts may be found that are lined by columnar or cuboidal epithelium and that are believed to be derived from embryonic remnants.

From early in infancy until after menopause, there is a considerable amount of glycogen in the superficial cells of the vaginal mucosa. By examination of cells that are exfoliated from the vaginal epithelium, one can identify the various hormonal events of the ovarian cycle.

In nonpregnant women, the vagina is kept moist by a small amount of secretion from the uterus. During pregnancy, there is copious, acidic vaginal secretion, which normally consists of a curdlike product of exfoliated epithelium and bacteria. *Lactobacillus* species are recovered from most pregnant women in higher concentrations than in nonpregnant women (Larsen and Galask, 1980). These are the predominant bacteria of the vagina during pregnancy. The acidic reaction is attributable to the presence of lactic acid, which arises from the metabolism of glycogen from the mucosal cells

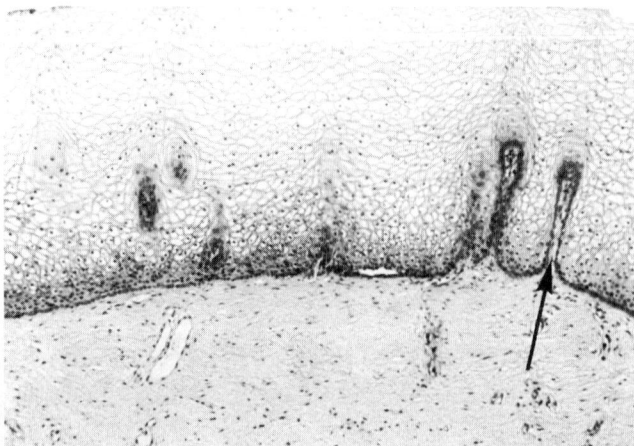

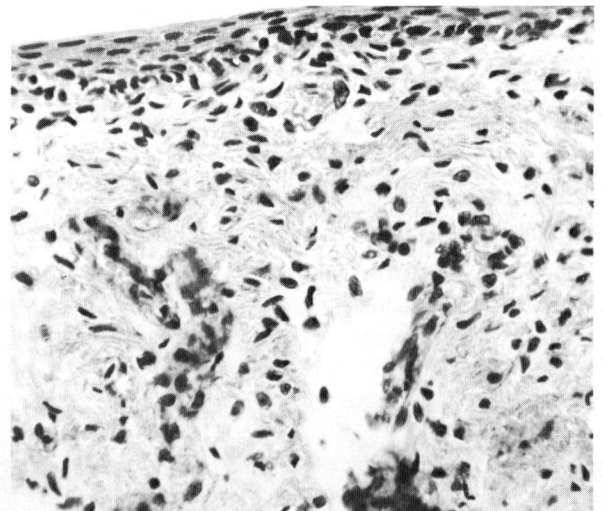

A

B

Fig. 3–5. A. Photomicrograph of the vagina of an adult woman that is characterized by noncornified, thick, stratified squamous epithelium; note that epithelial appendages are not present. Arrow is pointed to a papilla.
B. Photomicrograph of typical thin vaginal epithelium of a prepubertal girl.

by lactobacilli. The pH of the vaginal secretion varies with the nature of the ovarian hormones that are secreted. Before puberty, the pH of the secretions of the vagina varies between 6.8 and 7.2, whereas in adult women it generally ranges from 4.0 to 5.0.

There appear to be both qualitative and quantitative changes in the microbial flora during pregnancy. In 80 percent of women with normal flora before pregnancy, the flora remains normal (Hiller and colleagues, 1992). Most investigators report that *Lactobacillus* species are isolated more commonly during pregnancy, and probably in higher concentrations. There is also evidence that anaerobic organisms commonly isolated from nonpregnant women are not as numerous during pregnancy. However, during the postpartum period, anaerobic bacteria increase dramatically and are the most common isolates causing infection in puerperal women (Larsen and Galask, 1980).

There is an abundant vascular supply to the vagina; the upper third is supplied by the cervicovaginal branches of the uterine arteries, the middle third by the inferior vesical arteries, and the lower third by the middle rectal and internal pudendal arteries. The vaginal artery may branch directly from the internal iliac artery. There is an extensive venous plexus that immediately surrounds the vagina, vessels that follow the course of the arteries; eventually, these veins empty into the internal iliac veins. For the most part, the lymphatics from the lower third of the vagina, along with those of the vulva, drain into the inguinal lymph nodes; those from the middle third drain into the internal iliac nodes; and those from the upper third drain into the iliac nodes. According to Krantz (1958), although the vagina is devoid of any special nerve endings (genital corpuscles), occasionally free nerve endings are found in the papillae.

The Perineum. The many structures that make up the perineum are illustrated in Figure 3–6. Most of the support of the perineum is provided by the pelvic and urogenital diaphragms. The *pelvic diaphragm* consists of the levator ani muscles plus the coccygeus muscles posteriorly and the fascial coverings of these muscles. The levator ani muscles form a broad muscular sling that originates from the posterior surface of the superior rami of the pubis, from the inner surface of the ischial spine, and between these two sites, from the obturator fascia. The muscle fibers are inserted in several locations as follows: around the vagina and rectum to form efficient functional sphincters for each; into a raphe in the midline between the vagina and rectum; into a midline raphe below the rectum; and into the coccyx. The *urogenital diaphragm* is positioned external to the pelvic diaphragm, that is, in the triangular area between the ischial tuberosities and the symphysis pubis. The urogenital diaphragm is comprised of the deep transverse perineal muscles, the constrictor of the urethra, and the internal and external fascial coverings.

The major blood supply to the perineum is via the internal pudendal artery and its branches. Branches of the internal pudendal artery include the inferior rectal artery and posterior labial artery.

The innervation of the perineum is primarily via the pudendal nerve and its branches. The pudendal nerve originates from the S_2, S_3, and S_4 portion of the spinal cord.

Perineal Body. The median raphe of the levator ani, which is positioned between the anus and the vagina, is reinforced by the central tendon of the perineum, on which converge the bulbocavernosus muscles, superficial transverse perineal muscles, and external anal sphincter. These structures, which contribute to the perineal body and provide much of the support for the perineum, often are lacerated during delivery unless an adequate episiotomy is made.

Internal Generative Organs

Uterus. The uterus is a muscular organ that is covered, partially, by peritoneum, or serosa. The cavity of the uterus is lined by the endometrium. During pregnancy, the uterus serves for reception, implantation, retention, and nutrition of the conceptus, which it then expels during labor.

Anatomical Relationships. The uterus of the nonpregnant woman is situated in the pelvic cavity between the bladder anteriorly and the rectum posteriorly. Almost the entire posterior wall of the uterus is covered by serosa, or peritoneum, the lower portion of which forms the anterior boundary of the *recto-uterine cul-de-sac*, or pouch of Douglas. Only the upper portion of the anterior wall of the uterus is so covered (Fig. 3–7). The lower portion is united to the posterior wall of the bladder by a well-defined but normally loose layer of connective tissue (Figs. 3–3 and 3–8).

Size and Shape. The uterus is a structure that resembles a flattened pear in shape (Figs. 3–7 and 3–8) and consists of two major but unequal parts: an upper triangular portion, the *body*, or *corpus*; and a lower, cylindrical, or fusiform portion, the *cervix*, which projects into the vagina. The anterior surface of the body of the uterus is almost flat, whereas the posterior surface is distinctly convex. The oviducts, or fallopian tubes, emerge from the *cornua* of the uterus at the junction of the superior and lateral margins. The convex upper segment between the points of insertion of the fallopian tubes is called the *fundus*. Laterally, the portion of the uterus below the insertion of the fallopian tubes is not covered directly by peritoneum, but is the site of the attachments of the broad ligaments.

The uterus varies widely in size and shape, and the

Colles' fascia

Ischiocavernosus m.

Bulbocavernosus m.

Urogenital diaphragm
Inferior fascia

Sup. transv. perineal m.

Central tendon

Pelvic diaphragm
Inferior fascia

Ext. sphincter ani m.

Gluteus maximus m.

Post. labial a.

Urethral meatus

Labium minus

Hymen

Perineal a.

A. of clitoris

Int. pudendal a.

Iliococcygeus m.

Inf. hemorrhoidal a.

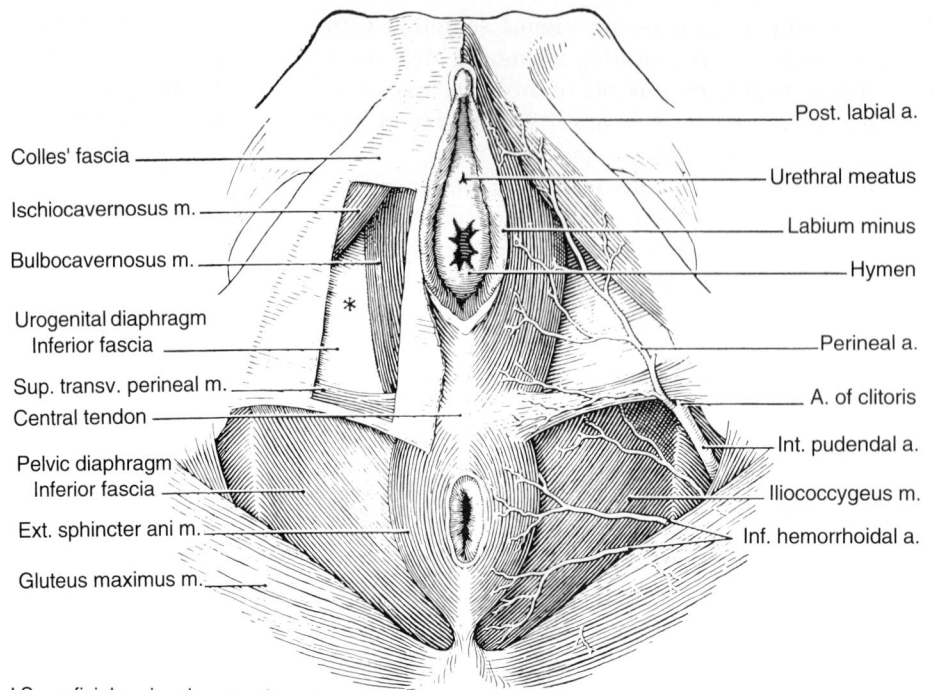

✳Superficial perineal compartment

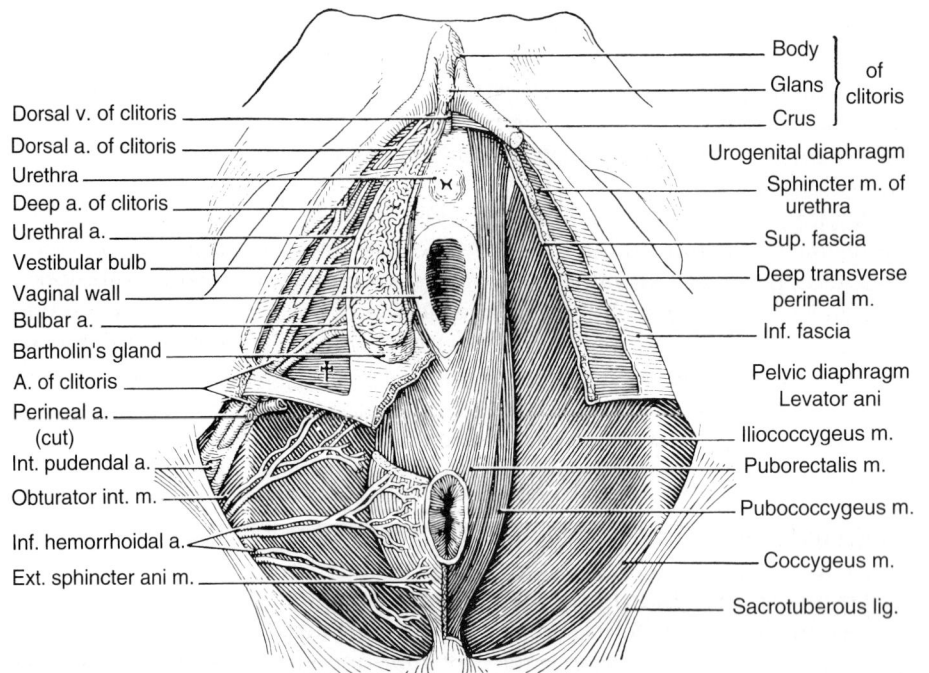

Dorsal v. of clitoris

Dorsal a. of clitoris

Urethra

Deep a. of clitoris

Urethral a.

Vestibular bulb

Vaginal wall

Bulbar a.

Bartholin's gland

A. of clitoris

Perineal a.
(cut)

Int. pudendal a.

Obturator int. m.

Inf. hemorrhoidal a.

Ext. sphincter ani m.

Body
Glans   of
Crus   clitoris

Urogenital diaphragm

Sphincter m. of
urethra

Sup. fascia

Deep transverse
perineal m.

Inf. fascia

Pelvic diaphragm
Levator ani

Iliococcygeus m.

Puborectalis m.

Pubococcygeus m.

Coccygeus m.

Sacrotuberous lig.

E. H. Brödel

Fig. 3–6. The perineum. The more superficial components are illustrated above and the deeper structures below. (m. = muscle; a. = artery; lig. = ligament; Int. = internal; Ext. = external; Inf. = inferior.)

† Deep perineal compartment

age and parity of women influence this tremendously. Before puberty, the organ varies in length from 2.5 to 3.5 cm. The uterus of adult nulliparous women is from 6 to 8 cm in length as compared with 9 to 10 cm in multiparous women (Fig. 3–8). Uteri of nonparous and parous women also differ considerably in weight, averaging from 50 to 70 g for the former, and 80 g or more for the latter (Langlois, 1970). The relationship between the length of the body of the uterus and that of the

cervix likewise varies widely. In the premenarchal girl, the body of the uterus is only half as long as the cervix. In nulliparous women, the two are about equal in length. In multiparous women, the cervix is only a little more than one third of the total length of the organ (Fig. 3–8).

The great bulk of the body of the uterus, but not the cervix, is comprised of muscle. The inner surface of the anterior and posterior walls of the uterus lie almost in contact; the cavity between these walls forms a mere slit

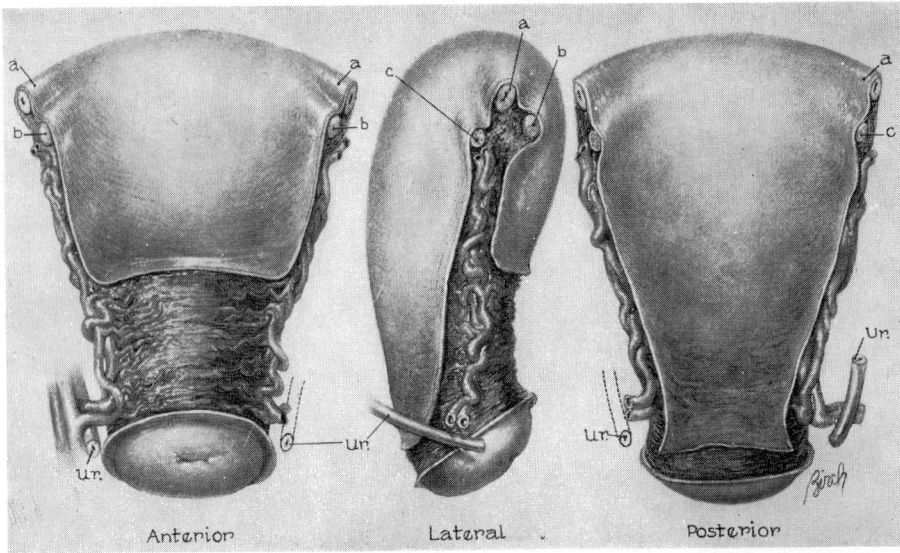

Fig. 3–7. Anterior, right lateral, and posterior views of the uterus on an adult woman. (a, oviduct; b, round ligament; c, ovarian ligament; Ur. = ureter.)

(Fig. 3–8). The cervical canal is fusiform and is open at each end by small apertures, the *internal os* and the *external os.* On frontal section, the cavity of the body of the uterus is triangular, whereas that of the cervix is fusiform in shape. The margins of parous uteri become concave instead of convex, and hence the triangular appearance of the uterine cavity is less pronounced. After menopause, the size of the uterus decreases as a consequence of atrophy of both the myometrium and the endometrium. The *isthmus* (Fig. 3–8) is of special obstetrical significance because, in pregnancy, it is essential to the formation of the lower uterine segment (See Chap. 12, p. 341).

Uterus During Pregnancy. As described in Chapter 8 (p. 209), the uterus during pregnancy undergoes re-

markable growth due to hypertrophy of muscle fibers. Its size increases from 70 g in the nonpregnant state to about 1100 g at term. Its total volume averages about 5 L. As growth proceeds, the uterine fundus, a previously flattened convexity between tubal insertions, now becomes dome-shaped (Fig. 3–9). The round ligaments now appear to insert at the junction of the middle and upper thirds of the organ. The fallopian tubes elongate, but the ovaries grossly appear unchanged.

Uterine Cervix. The cervix is the specialized portion of the uterus that is below the isthmus. Anteriorly, the upper boundary of the cervix, the internal os, corresponds approximately to the level at which the peritoneum is reflected upon the bladder.

The cervix is divided by the attachment of the

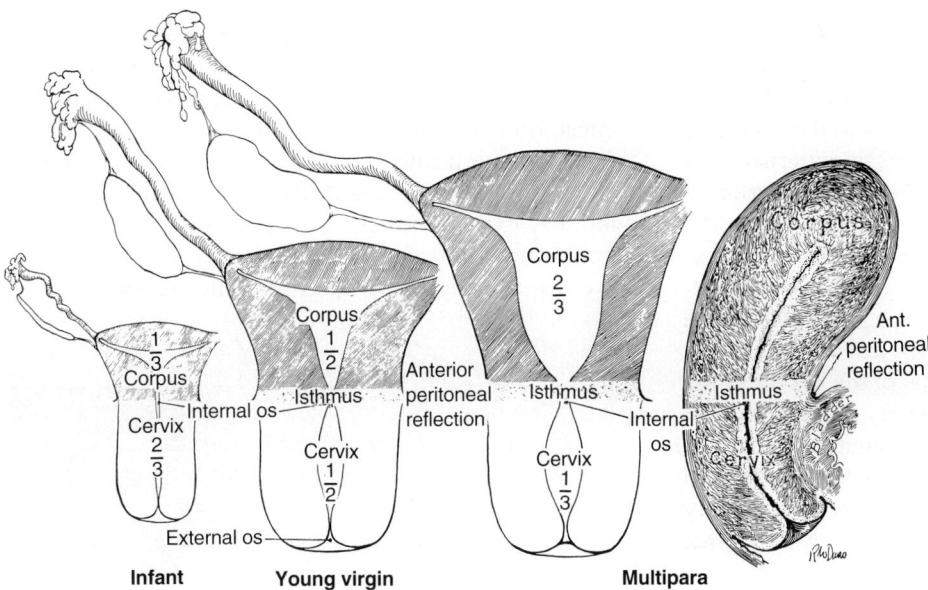

Fig. 3–8. Comparison of the size of uteri of prepubertal girls and adult nonparous and parous women by frontal and sagittal sections.

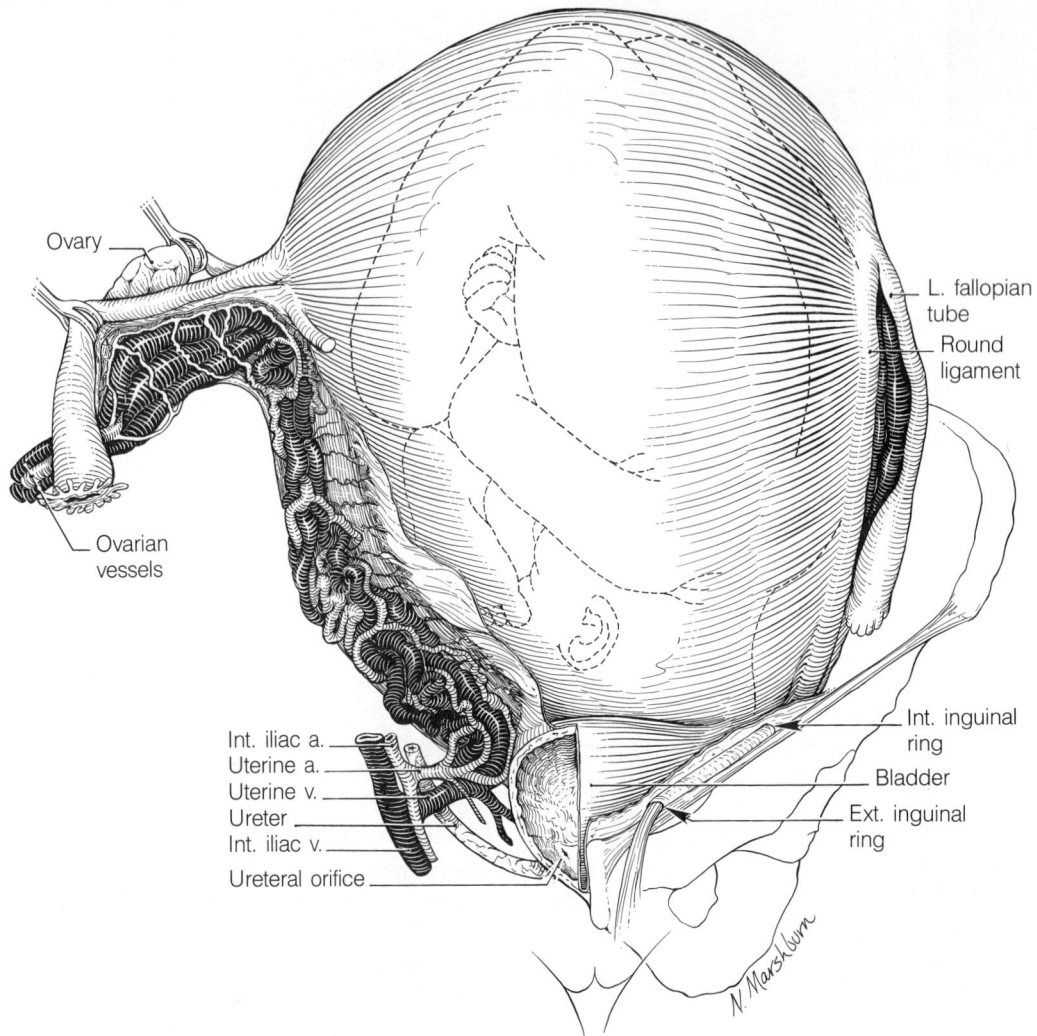

Ovary

L. fallopian
tube

Round
ligament

Ovarian
vessels

Int. iliac a.
Uterine a.
Uterine v.
Ureter
Int. iliac v.
Ureteral orifice

Int. inguinal
ring

Bladder

Ext. inguinal
ring

N. Marshburn

Fig. 3–9. Uterus of near-term pregnancy. The fundus is now dome-shaped and the tubes and round ligaments appear to insert in the upper middle portion of the uterine body. Note the markedly hypertrophied vascular supply.

vagina into vaginal and supravaginal portions. The supravaginal segment on its posterior surface is covered by peritoneum. Laterally, it is attached to the cardinal ligaments; and anteriorly, it is separated from the overlying bladder by loose connective tissue. The external os is located at the lower extremity of the vaginal portion of the cervix, the *portio vaginalis*.

The external cervical os varies greatly in appearance. Before childbirth, it is a small, regular, oval opening; after childbirth, the orifice is converted into a transverse slit that is divided such that there are the so-called anterior and posterior lips of the cervix. If the cervix was torn deeply during delivery, it might heal in such a manner that it appears to be irregular, nodular, or stellate. These changes are sufficiently characteristic to permit an examiner to ascertain with some certainty whether a given woman has borne children by vaginal delivery (Figs. 3–10 and 3–11).

The cervix is composed predominantly of collagenous tissue plus elastic tissue and blood vessels, although it does contain some smooth muscle fibers. The transition from the primarily collagenous tissue of the cervix to the primarily muscular tissue of the body of the uterus, although generally abrupt, may be gradual, and may extend over as much as 10 mm. The results of studies by Danforth and colleagues (1960) are suggestive that the physical properties of the cervix are deter-

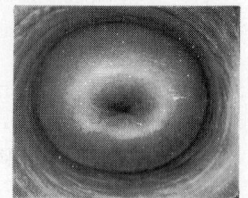

Fig. 3–10. Cervical external os of a nonparous woman.

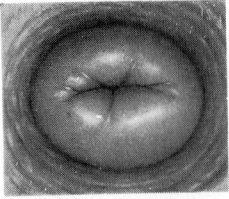

Fig. 3–11. Cervical external os of a parous woman.

mined, in large measure, by the state of the connective tissue, and that during pregnancy and labor the remarkable ability of the cervix to dilate is the result of dissociation of collagen. Buckingham and co-workers (1965) quantified the amount of muscle and collagen in the tissue of the cervix of women. In the normal cervix, the proportion of muscle is, on average, about 10 percent, whereas in women with an *incompetent cervix,* sometimes the proportion of muscle is appreciably greater.

The mucosa of the cervical canal is composed of a single layer of very high, columnar epithelium that rests upon a thin basement membrane. The oval nuclei are situated near the base of the columnar cells, the upper portions of which appear to be rather clear because of content of mucus. These cells are supplied abundantly with cilia.

There are numerous cervical glands that extend from the surface of the endocervical mucosa directly into the subjacent connective tissue; because there is no submucosa as such, these glands furnish the thick, tenacious secretion of the cervical canal. If the ducts of the cervical glands are occluded, retention cysts, known as *Nabothian follicles* or *Nabothian cysts,* are formed.

Normally, the squamous epithelium of the vaginal portion of the cervix and the columnar epithelium of the cervical canal form a sharp line of demarcation very near the external os, that is, the squamo-columnar junction. In response to inflammation or trauma, however, the stratified epithelium may extend gradually up the cervical canal and come to line the lower third, or occasionally even the lower half, of the canal. This change is more marked in multiparous women, in whom the lips of the cervix often are everted. Uncommonly, the two varieties of epithelium abut on the vaginal portion outside the external os, as in *congenital ectropion.*

Body of the Uterus. The wall of the body of the uterus is composed of serosal, muscular, and mucosal layers. The serosal layer is formed by the peritoneum that covers the uterus, and to which it is firmly adherent except at sites just above the bladder and at the lateral margins where the peritoneum is deflected in a manner to form the broad ligaments.

Endometrium. The endometrium is the innermost portion of the uterus, or its mucosal layer that lines the uterine cavity in nonpregnant women. It is a thin, pink, velvet-like membrane, which on close examination is found to be perforated by a large number of minute openings; these are the ostia of the uterine glands. Because of the repetitive cyclical changes during the reproductive years, the endometrium normally varies greatly in thickness, and measures from 0.5 mm to as much as 5 mm. The endometrium is comprised of surface epithelium, glands, and interglandular mesenchymal tissue in which there are numerous blood vessels.

The epithelium of the endometrial surface is comprised of a single layer of closely packed, high columnar, ciliated cells. During much of the endometrial cycle, the oval nuclei are situated in the lower portions of the cells but not so near the base as in the endocervix. Cilia have been demonstrated in endometrial cells of many mammals; the ciliated cells are located in discrete patches, whereas secretory activity appears to be limited to nonciliated cells. The ciliary current in both the fallopian tubes and the uterus is in the same direction and extends downward from the fimbriated end of the tubes toward the external os.

The tubular *uterine glands* are invaginations of the epithelium, which, in the resting state, are reminiscent of the fingers of a glove. The glands extend through the entire thickness of the endometrium to the myometrium, which is occasionally penetrated for a short distance. Histologically, the inner glands resemble the epithelium of the surface and are lined by a single layer of columnar, partially ciliated epithelium that rests upon a thin basement membrane. The glands secrete a thin alkaline fluid that serves to keep the uterine cavity moist.

In the classical monograph of Hitschmann and Adler (1908), the endometrium was described as undergoing constant, hormonally controlled changes during each ovarian cycle. These three fundamental phases—*menstrual, proliferative (follicular), and secretory (luteal)*—are discussed in detail in Chapter 4 in the section on menstruation. After menopause, the endometrium is atrophic and the epithelium flattens. The glands gradually disappear, and the interglandular tissue becomes more fibrous.

The connective tissue of the endometrium, between the surface epithelium and the myometrium, is a mesenchymal stroma. Immediately after menstruation, the stroma is comprised of closely packed cells with oval- and spindle-shaped nuclei, around which there is very little cytoplasm. When separated by edema, the cells appear to be stellate, with cytoplasmic processes that branch to form anastomoses. These cells are packed more closely around the glands and blood vessels than elsewhere. Several days before menstruation, the stromal cells usually become larger and more vesicular, like decidual cells; and at the same time, there is a diffuse leukocytic infiltration.

The vascular architecture of the endometrium is of signal importance in the phenomena of menstruation and pregnancy. Arterial blood is transported to the uterus by way of the uterine and ovarian arteries. As the arterial branches penetrate the uterine wall obliquely inward and reach its middle third, these vessels ramify in a plane that is parallel to the surface; these vessels are therefore named the *arcuate arteries*. Radial branches extend from the arcuate arteries at right angles toward the endometrium. The endometrial arteries are comprised of *coiled* or *spiral arteries*, which are a continuation of the radial arteries, and *basal arteries*, which branch from the radial arteries at a sharp angle, as illustrated in Figures 3–12 and 3–13. The coiled arteries supply most of the midportion and all of the superficial third of the endometrium. The walls of these vessels are responsive, that is, sensitive, to the action of a number of hormones, especially by vasoconstriction, and thus probably serve an important role in the mechanism(s) of menstruation. The straight basal endometrial arteries are smaller in both caliber and length than are the coiled vessels. These vessels extend only into the basal layer of the endometrium, or at most a short distance into the middle layer, and are not responsive to hormonal action.

Myometrium. The myometrium, which makes up the major portion of the uterus, is comprised of bundles of smooth muscle that are united by connective tissue in which there are many elastic fibers. According to Schwalm and Dubrauszky (1966), the number of muscle fibers of the uterus progressively diminishes caudally such that in the cervix, muscle comprises only 10 percent of the tissue mass. In the inner wall of the body of the uterus, there is relatively more muscle than in the outer layers; and in the anterior and posterior walls, there is more muscle than in the lateral walls. During pregnancy, the myometrium increases greatly via hypertrophy with no significant change in the muscle content of the cervix. The anatomical changes that occur in the myometrium during pregnancy are presented in detail in Chapter 8.

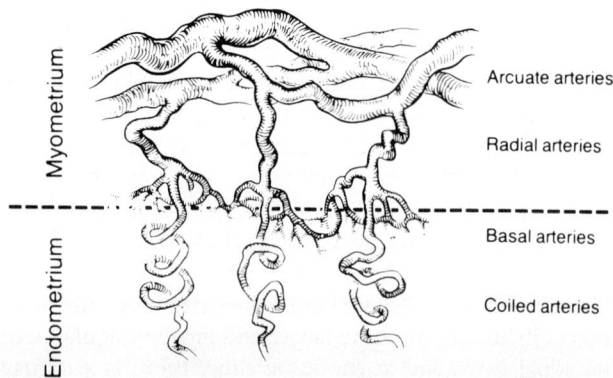

Fig. 3–13. Corrosion cast of the complexly branching endometrial capillary network of the upper compact layer of a Rhesus monkey on the 25th day of the menstrual cycle × 400. (From Ferenczy and Richart, 1974.)

Ligaments of the Uterus. The broad, round, and uterosacral ligaments extend from either side of the uterus. The *broad ligaments* are comprised of two winglike structures that extend from the lateral margins of the uterus to the pelvic walls and thereby divide the pelvic cavity into anterior and posterior compartments. Each broad ligament consists of a fold of peritoneum, and there are superior, lateral, inferior, and medial margins. The inner two thirds of the superior margin form the *mesosalpinx*, to which the fallopian tubes are attached. The outer third of the superior margin of the broad ligament, which extends from the fimbriated end of the oviduct to the pelvic wall, forms the *infundibulopelvic ligament* (suspensory ligament of the ovary), through which the ovarian vessels traverse.

At the lateral margin of each broad ligament, the peritoneum is reflected onto the side of the pelvis. The base of the broad ligament, which is quite thick, is continuous with the connective tissue of the pelvic floor. The most dense portion—referred to as the *cardinal ligament*, transverse cervical ligament, or Mackenrodt ligament—is composed of connective tissue that medially is united firmly to the supravaginal portion of the cervix. In the base of the broad ligament, the uterine vessels and the lower portion of the ureter are enclosed.

A vertical section through the uterine end of the broad ligament is triangular and the uterine vessels are found within its broad base (Fig. 3–14). In its lower part, it is widely attached to the connective tissues that are adjacent to the cervix, that is, the *parametrium*. The upper part is comprised of three folds that nearly cover

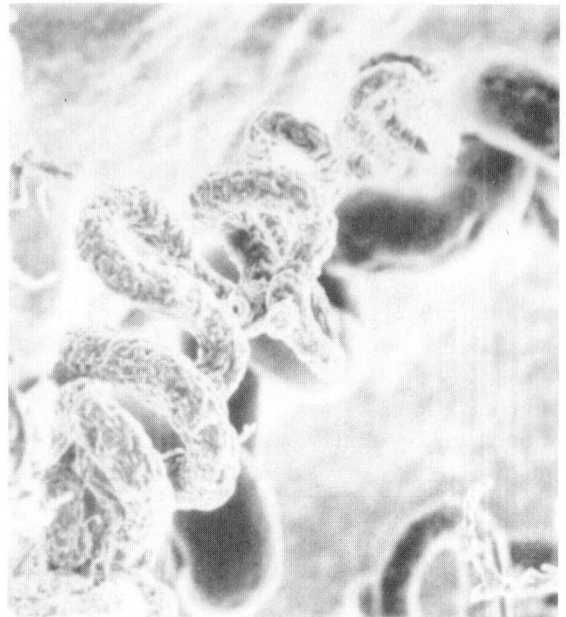

Fig. 3–12. Stereographic representation of myometrial and endometrial arteries in the macaque. Above, parts of myometrial arcuate arteries from which myometrial radial arteries course toward the endometrium. Below, the larger endometrial coiled arteries and the smaller endometrial basal arteries. (From Okkels and Engle, 1938.)

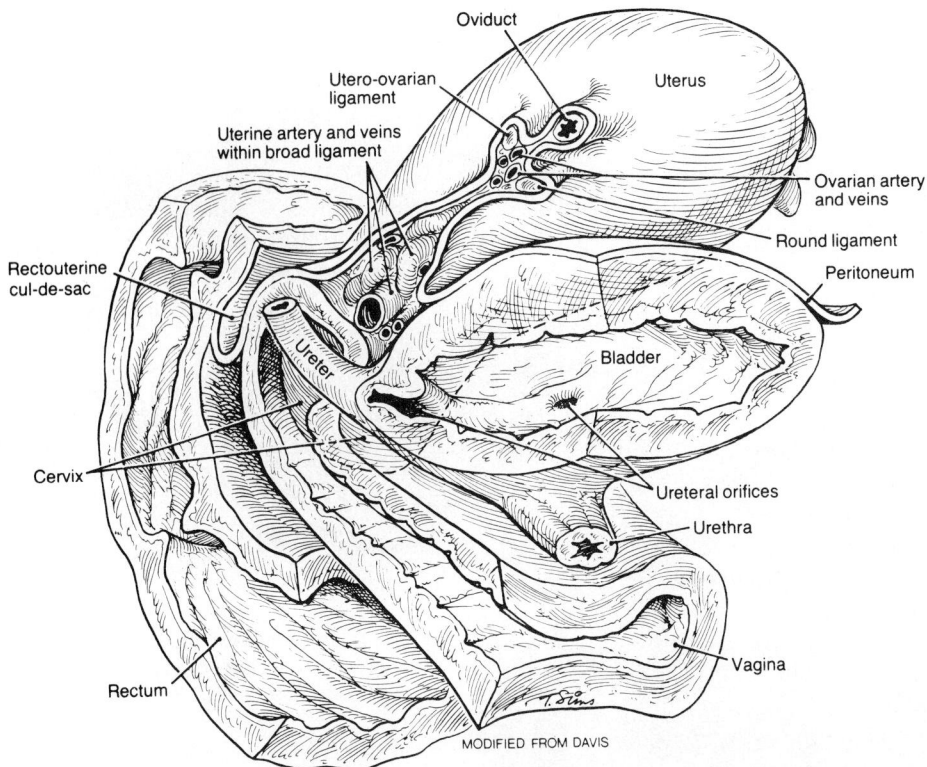

Fig. 3–14. Vertical section through uterine end of right broad ligament.

the oviduct, the utero-ovarian ligament, and the round ligament.

The *round ligaments* extend from the lateral portion of the uterus, arising somewhat below and anterior to that of the origin of the oviducts. Each round ligament is located in a fold of peritoneum that is continuous with the broad ligament and extends outward and downward to the inguinal canal, through which it passes to terminate in the upper portion of the labium majus. In nonpregnant women, the round ligament varies from 3 to 5 mm in diameter, and is comprised of smooth muscle cells that are continuous directly with those of the uterine wall and a certain amount of connective tissue. The round ligament corresponds, embryologically, to the gubernaculum testis of men. During pregnancy, the round ligaments undergo considerable hypertrophy and increase appreciably in both length and diameter.

Each *uterosacral ligament* extends from an attachment posterolaterally to the supravaginal portion of the cervix to encircle the rectum, and thence insert into the fascia over the second and third sacral vertebrae. The uterosacral ligaments are comprised of connective tissue and some smooth muscle and are covered by peritoneum. These ligaments form the lateral boundaries of the rectouterine cul-de-sac, or pouch of Douglas.

Position. When a nonpregnant woman stands upright, the body of the uterus most often is almost horizontal, flexed somewhat anteriorly with the fundus resting upon the bladder, whereas the cervix is directed back-

ward toward the tip of the sacrum with the external os approximately at the level of the ischial spines. The position of the body of the uterus is variable as a function of the degree of distension of the bladder, rectum, or both.

Normally, the uterus is a partially mobile organ; whereas the cervix is anchored, the body of the uterus is free to move in the anteroposterior plane. Therefore, posture and gravity are factors that influence the position of the uterus. The posterior directed, or retroflexed uterus, that is, with the fundus resting on the rectum, is a normal variant and is encountered in many women.

Blood Vessels. The vascular supply of the uterus is derived principally from the uterine and ovarian arteries. The uterine artery, a main branch of the internal iliac (hypogastric) artery (Fig. 3–15), enters the base of the broad ligament, and makes its way medially to the side of the uterus. In so doing, it crosses anterior to the ureter, as described subsequently. Immediately adjacent to the supravaginal portion of the cervix, the uterine artery is divided into two main branches. The smaller cervicovaginal artery supplies blood to the lower portion of the cervix and the upper portion of the vagina. The main branch turns abruptly upward and extends thereafter as a highly convoluted vessel that traverses along the margin of the uterus; a branch of considerable size extends to the upper portion of the cervix and numerous other branches penetrate the body of the uterus. Just before the main branch of the uterine artery

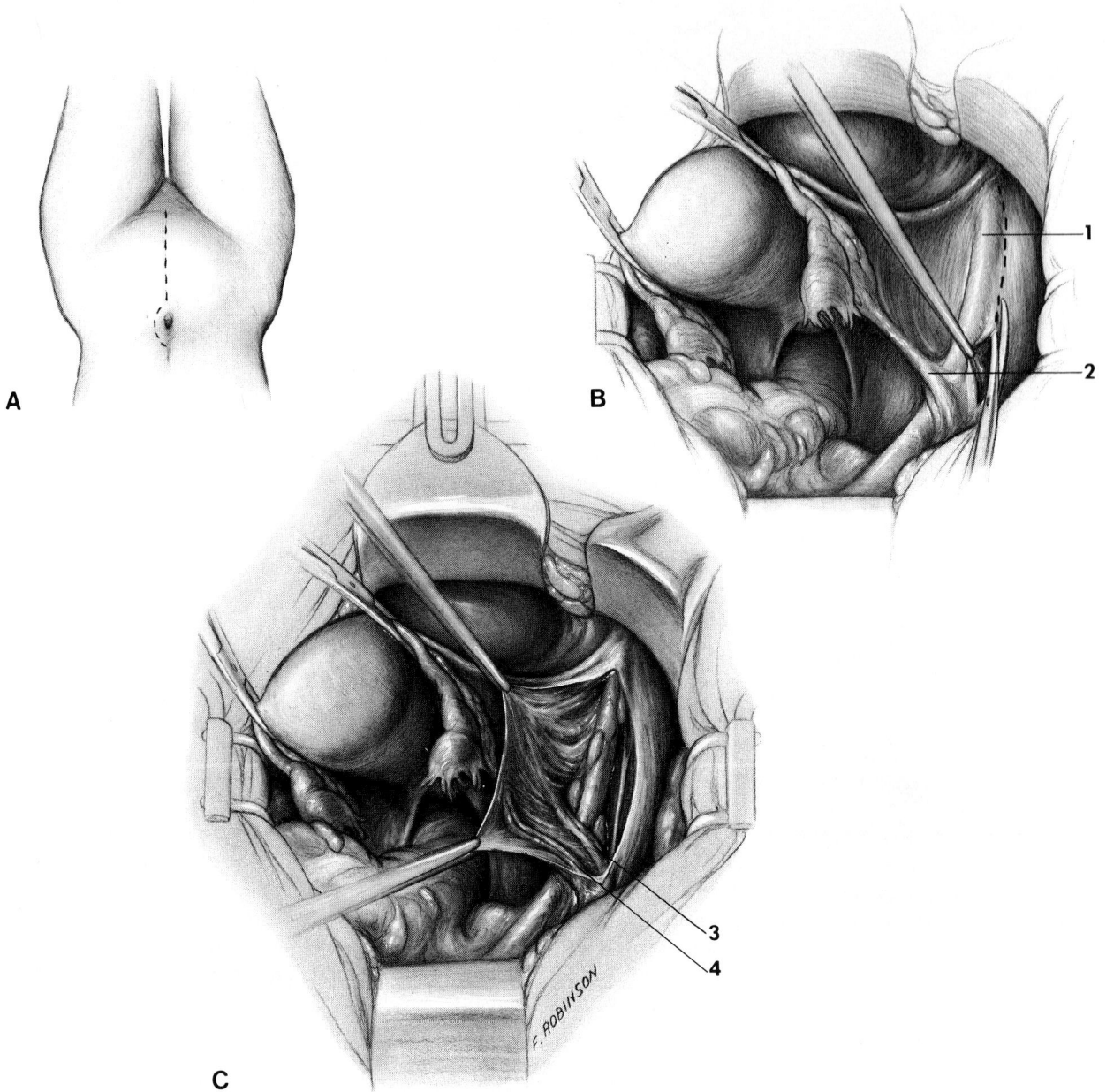

Fig. 3–15. Illustrated are the pelvic viscera as seen through a long midline incision **(A)** made in the lower abdomen. **B.** Retractors have been placed to spread the abdominal incision. The small intestine and omentum that overlie the pelvic contents have been displaced from the operative field. The oviducts, utero-ovarian ligaments, and round ligaments have been clamped bilaterally at their origin immediately adjacent to the uterus. Peritoneum just lateral to the right external iliac artery (1) is incised and the right infundibulopelvic ligament (2) is tensed by pulling the uterus to the left. **C.** The right broad ligament has been opened laterally. The right ureter (3) is now visible as it crosses the iliac vessels at the pelvic brim and courses medially and downward toward the cervix and bladder. The right ovarian artery and vein (4) are visible after dissection of the infundibulopelvic ligament.

reaches the oviduct, it divides into three terminal branches: fundal, tubal, and ovarian. The ovarian branch of the uterine artery anastomoses with the terminal branch of the ovarian artery; the tubal branch makes its way through the mesosalpinx and supplies part of the oviduct; and the fundal branch is distributed to the uppermost portion of the uterus.

About 2 cm lateral to the cervix, the uterine artery crosses over the ureter, as shown in Figures 3–7, 3–15, and 3–16. The proximity of the uterine artery and uterine vein to the ureter at this point is of great surgical significance because, during hysterectomy, the ureter may be injured or ligated in the process of clamping and ligating the uterine vessels.

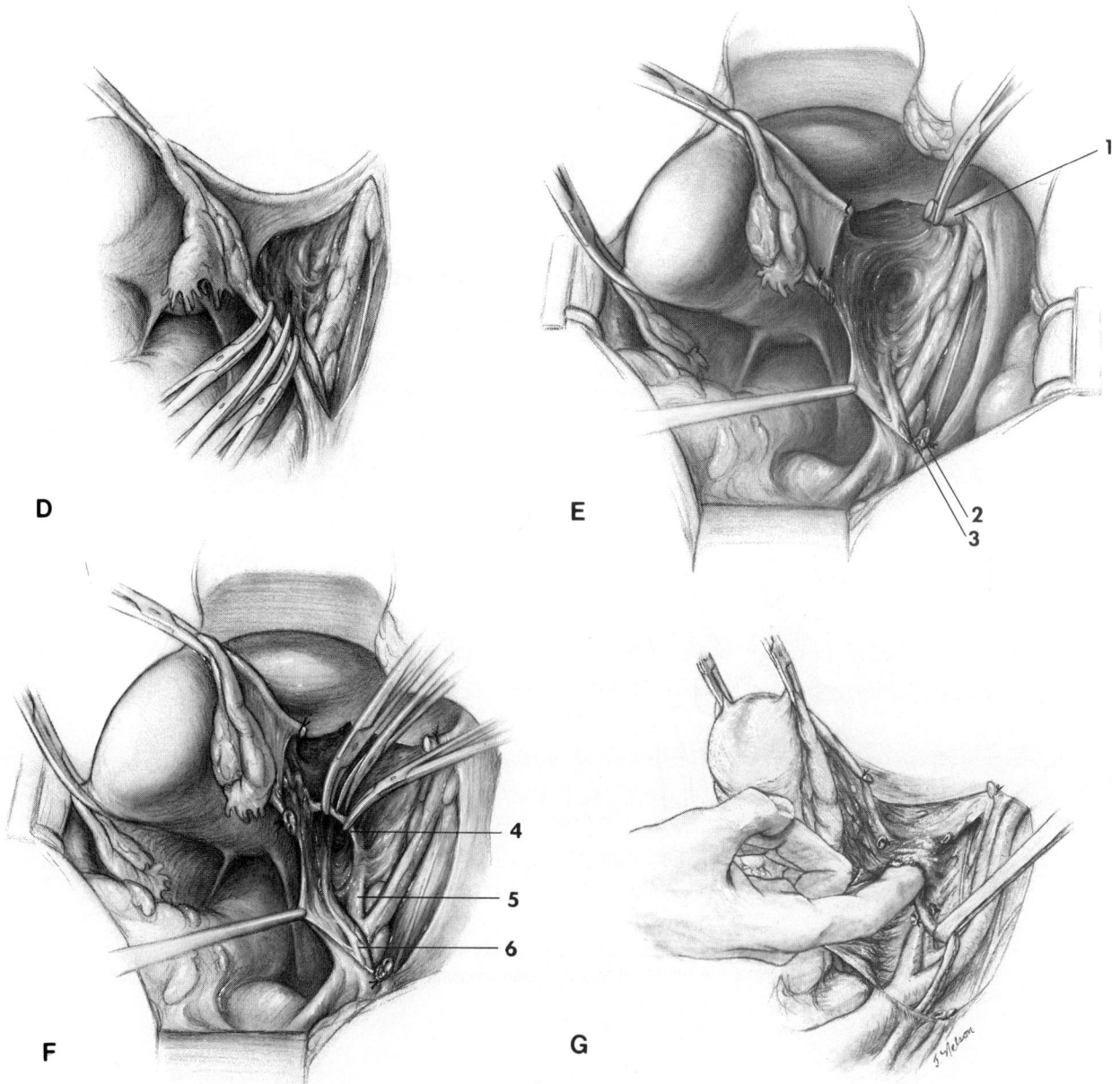

Fig. 3–15 (continued). D. The ovarian vessels have been clamped and are being severed. The uterus is retracted to the left and the external iliac artery is seen to the right. **E.** The round ligament (1) and the ovarian vessels (2) have been ligated and severed. More of the ureter is visible (3). **F.** The origin of the right uterine artery (4) from the internal iliac artery (5) is illustrated. Note the ureter (6) coursing beneath the uterine artery (4) just lateral to the junction of the cervix and body of the uterus. **G.** The operator's finger is in the paracervical ureteral tunnel through the right cardinal ligament just lateral to supravaginal portion of the cervix. The ureter is being retracted laterally. (From Nelson, 1977.)

A major portion of the blood supply to the pelvis is via the branches of the internal iliac artery, as shown in the arteriogram in Figure 3-17. In the past, this commonly was referred to as the hypogastric artery. Other branches of the anterior division of the internal iliac artery besides the uterine artery include the umbilical, middle and inferior vesical, middle rectal, obturator, internal pudendal middle hemorrhoidal, vaginal, and inferior gluteal arteries. The branches of the posterior division of the internal iliac artery include the lateral sacral, superior gluteal, and iliolumbar arteries (Table 3–1).

The *ovarian artery*, a direct branch of the aorta, enters the broad ligament through the infundibulopelvic ligament. At the ovarian hilum, it is divided into a number of smaller branches that enter the ovary; whereas the main stem of the ovarian artery traverses

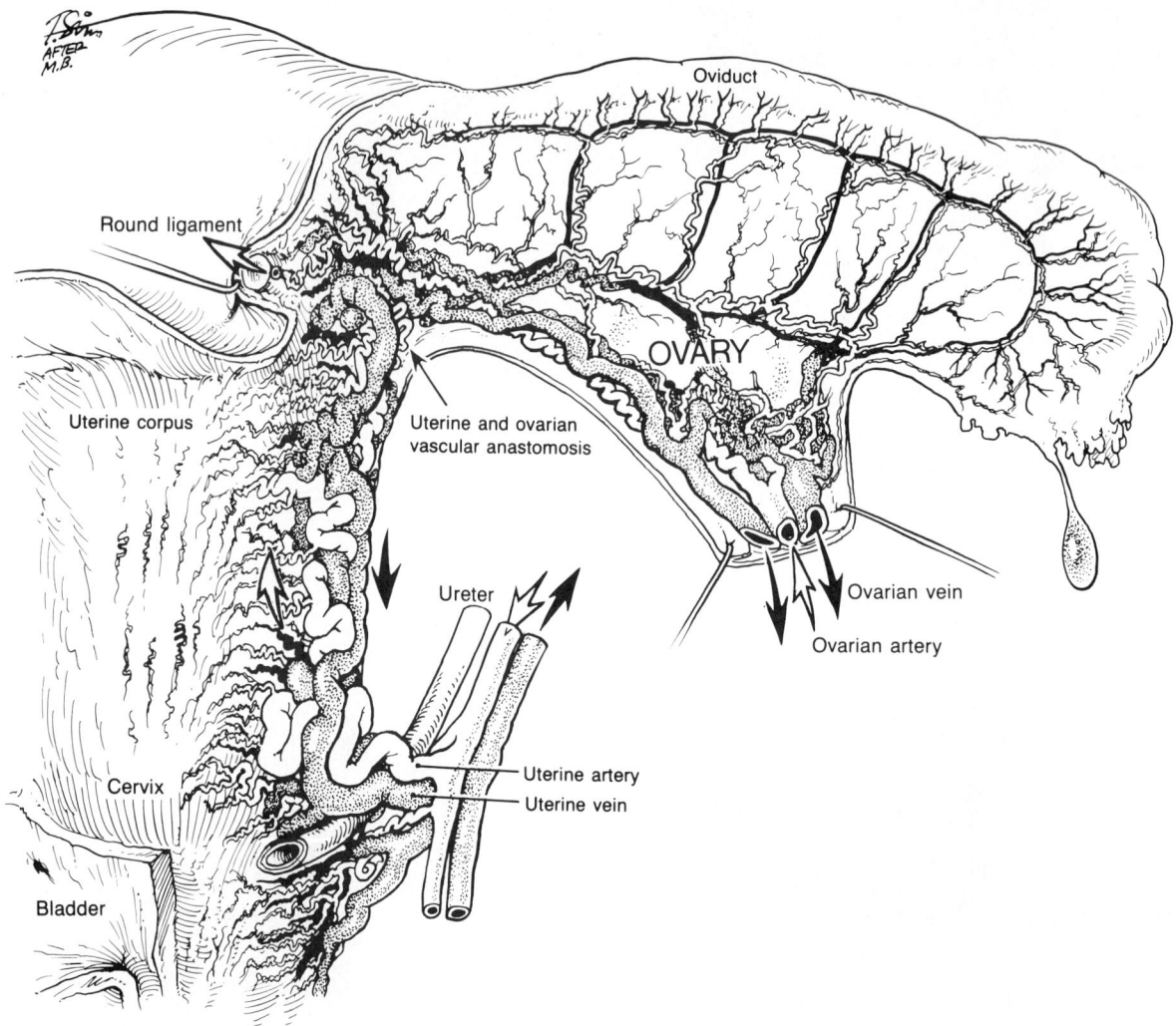

Fig. 3–16. Blood supply to the left ovary, left oviduct, and the left side of the uterus. The ovarian and uterine vessels anastomose freely. Note the uterine artery and vein crossing over the ureter that lies immediately adjacent to the cervix.

the entire length of the broad ligament very near the mesosalpinx and makes its way to the upper portion of the lateral margin of the uterus, where it anastomoses with the ovarian branch of the uterine artery. There are numerous additional communications among the arteries on both sides of the uterus.

When the uterus is in a contracted state, its numerous venous lumens are collapsed; however, in injected specimens the greater part of the uterine wall appears to be occupied by dilated venous sinuses. On either side, the arcuate veins unite to form the *uterine vein*, which empties into the internal iliac vein and thence into the common iliac vein.

Some of the blood from the upper part of the uterus and blood from the ovary and upper part of the broad ligament is collected by several veins that, within the broad ligament, form the large *pampiniform plexus*,

the vessels that terminate in the ovarian vein. The right ovarian vein empties into the vena cava, whereas the left ovarian vein empties into the left renal vein.

During pregnancy, there is marked hypertrophy of the blood supply to the uterus (Fig. 3–9). As discussed in Chapter 8 (p. 210), this accommodates uteroplacental blood flow estimated at 500 to 700 mL per minute.

Lymphatics. The endometrium is abundantly supplied with lymphatics, but true lymphatic vessels are confined largely to the basal layer. The lymphatics of the underlying myometrium are increased in number toward the serosal surface and form an abundant lymphatic plexus just beneath it, especially on the posterior wall of the uterus and, to a lesser extent, on the anterior wall.

The lymphatics from the various segments of the uterus drain into several sets of lymph nodes. Those

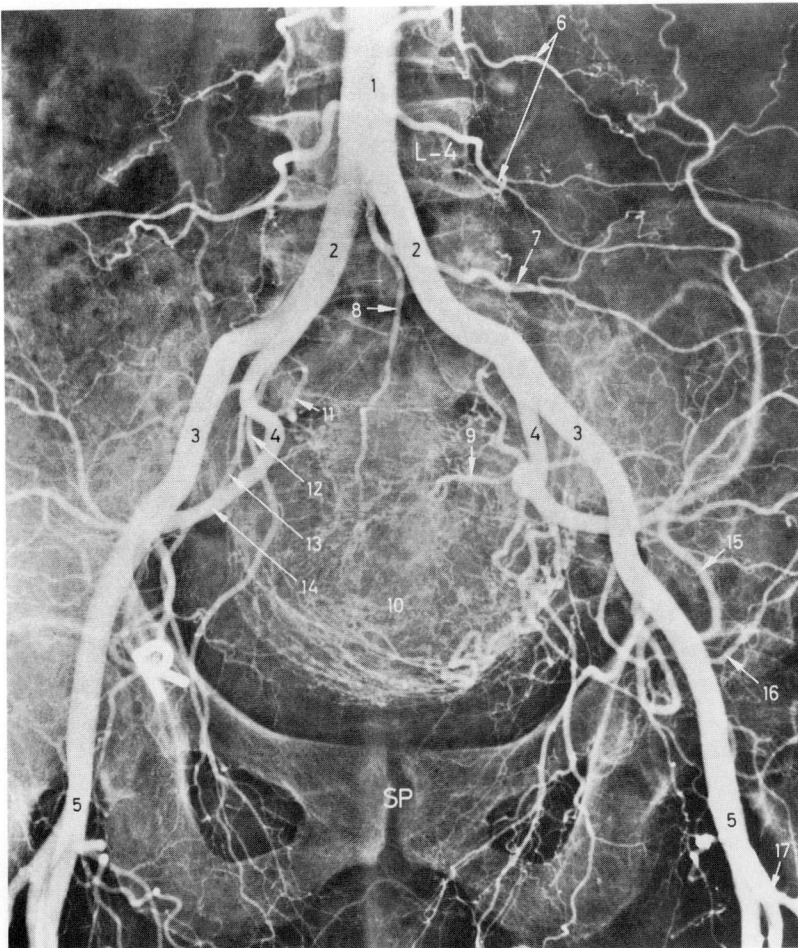

Fig. 3–17. Iliac arteriogram. It can be seen that the bifurcation of the aorta (1) into the two common iliac arteries (2) occurs at the lower border of the body of the L-4 vertebra. The common iliac vessels branch into external (3) and internal (4) iliac arteries. The internal iliac artery (4) on each side serves a number of branches to the pelvis, perineum, and gluteal region, while the external iliac artery (3), after giving off the inferior epigastric (15) and deep circumflex iliac (16) arteries, becomes the femoral artery below the inguinal ligament. (Also shown: 5 = femoral artery; 6 = lumbar arteries; 7 = iliolumbar artery; 8 = median sacral artery; 9 = uterine artery; 10 = uterus; 11 = lateral sacral artery; 12 = obturator artery; 13 = internal pudendal artery; 14 = superior gluteal artery; 17 = deep femoral artery; L4-4 = the lumbar vertebra; SP = symphysis pubis.) (From Wicke, 1982, with permission.)

from the cervix terminate mainly in the hypogastric nodes, which are situated near the bifurcation of the common iliac vessels. The lymphatics from the body of the uterus are distributed to two groups of nodes. One set of vessels drains into the internal iliac nodes; the other set, after joining certain lymphatics from the ovarian region, terminates in the periaortic lymph nodes.

Innervation. The nerve supply is derived principally from the sympathetic nervous system, but also partly from the cerebrospinal and parasympathetic systems.

TABLE 3–1. BRANCHES OF THE INTERNAL ILIAC ARTERY

Anterior Division	Posterior Division
Uterine artery	Superior gluteal artery
Umbilical artery	Inferior gluteal artery
Inferior vesical artery	Iliolumbar artery
Obturator artery	
Internal pudendal artery	
Inferior gluteal artery	
Middle vesical artery	
Middle hemorrhoidal artery	
Vaginal artery	

The parasympathetic system is represented on either side by the pelvic nerve, which is comprised of a few fibers that are derived from the second, third, and fourth sacral nerves; it loses its identity in the cervical ganglion of Frankenhaüser. The sympathetic system enters the pelvis by way of the internal iliac plexus that arises from the aortic plexus just below the promontory of the sacrum. After descending on either side, it also enters the uterovaginal plexus of Frankenhaüser, which is comprised of ganglia of various sizes, but particularly of a large ganglionic plate that is situated on either side of the cervix and just above the posterior fornix in front of the rectum.

Branches from these plexuses supply the uterus, bladder, and upper vagina and are comprised of both myelinated and nonmyelinated fibers. Some of these fibers terminate freely between the muscular fibers, whereas others accompany the arteries into the endometrium.

In the 11th and 12th thoracic nerve roots, there are sensory fibers from the uterus that transmit the painful stimuli of uterine contractions to the central nervous system. The sensory nerves from the cervix and upper part of the birth canal pass through the pelvic nerves to the second, third, and fourth sacral nerves, whereas those from the lower portion of the birth canal pass primarily through the pudendal nerve.

Oviducts. The oviducts or fallopian tubes vary from 8 to 14 cm in length, are covered by peritoneum, and their lumen is lined by mucous membrane. Each fallopian tube is divided into an *interstitial portion, isthmus, ampulla,* and *infundibulum.* The interstitial portion is embodied within the muscular wall of the uterus. Its approximate course is obliquely upward and outward from the uterine cavity. The isthmus, or the narrow portion of the tube that adjoins the uterus, passes gradually into the wider, lateral portion, or *ampulla.* The *infundibulum,* or fimbriated extremity, is the funnel-shaped opening of the distal end of the fallopian tube (Fig. 3–18). The oviduct varies considerably in thickness; the narrowest portion of the isthmus measures from 2 to 3 mm in diameter, and the widest portion of the ampulla measures from 5 to 8 mm. The oviduct is surrounded completely by peritoneum except at the attachment of the mesosalpinx.

The fimbriated end of the infundibulum opens into the abdominal cavity. One projection, the *fimbria ovarica,* which is considerably longer than the other fimbriae, forms a shallow gutter that approaches or reaches the ovary.

The musculature of the fallopian tube is arranged, in general, in two layers, an inner circular and an outer longitudinal layer. In the distal portion of the oviduct, the two layers are less distinct and, near the fimbriated extremity, are replaced by an interlacing network of muscular fibers. The tubal musculature undergoes rhythmic contractions constantly, the rate of which varies with the hormonal changes of the ovarian cycle. The greatest frequency and intensity of contractions is reached during transport of ova. Contractions are slowest and weakest during pregnancy.

The fallopian tube is lined by a single layer of columnar cells, some of them ciliated and others secretory. The ciliated cells are most abundant at the fimbriated extremity; elsewhere, these cells are found in discrete patches. There are differences in the proportions of these two types of cells in different phases of the ovarian cycle. Because there is no submucosa, the epithelium is in close contact with the underlying muscle. In the tubal mucosa, there are cyclical histological changes similar to, but much less striking than, those of the endometrium. The postmenstrual phase is characterized by a low epithelium that rapidly increases in height. During the follicular phase, the cells are taller; the ciliated elements are broad, with nuclei near the margin; and the nonciliated cells are narrow, with nuclei nearer the base. During the luteal phase, the secretory cells enlarge, project beyond the ciliated cells, and the nuclei are extruded. During the menstrual phase, these changes are even more marked. Changes in the fallopian tubes during late pregnancy and in the puerperium include the development of a low mucosa, plugging of the capillaries with leukocytes, and a decidual reaction.

The mucosa of the oviducts is arranged in longitudinal folds that are more complex toward the fimbriated end; consequently, the appearance of the lumen varies from one portion of the tube to another. On cross sections through the uterine portion, four simple folds are

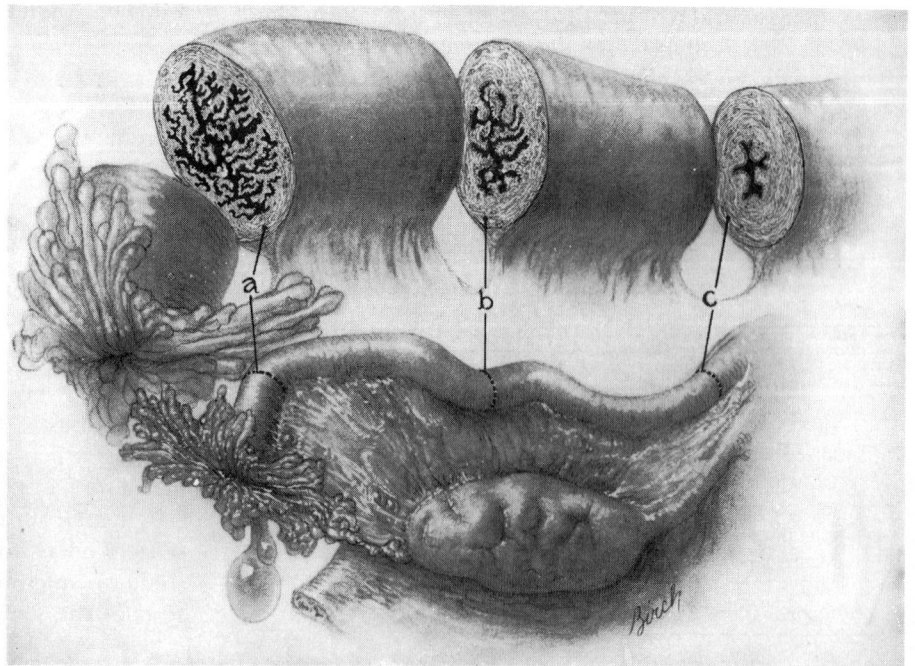

Fig. 3–18. The oviduct of an adult woman with cross-sectioned illustrations of the gross structure of the epithelium in several portions: a, infundibulum; b, ampulla; c, isthmus.

found that form a figure that resembles a Maltese cross. The isthmus is more complex; in the ampulla, the lumen is occupied almost completely by the arborescent mucosa, which consists of very complicated folds (Fig. 3–18).

The current produced by the tubal cilia is such that the direction of flow is toward the uterine cavity; indeed, minute foreign bodies that are introduced into the abdominal cavities of animals may eventually appear in the vagina after these are transported through the tubes and the cavity of the uterus. Tubal peristalsis also is believed to be an extraordinarily important factor in transport of the ovum.

The tubes are supplied richly with elastic tissue, blood vessels, and lymphatics. Sympathetic innervation of the tubes is extensive, in contrast to parasympathetic innervation. The role of these nerves in tubal function is poorly understood (Hodgson and Eddy, 1975).

Diverticula may extend occasionally from the lumen of the tube for a variable distance into the muscular wall and reach almost to the serosa. These diverticula may serve a role in the development of ectopic pregnancy (see Chap. 32, p. 691). Pertinent information concerning the gross anatomical, histological, and ultrastructural aspects of the human oviduct was summarized well by Woodruff and Pauerstein (1969).

Embryological Development of the Uterus and Oviducts. The uterus and fallopian tubes arise from the müllerian ducts, which first appear near the upper pole of the urogenital ridge in the fifth week of embryonic development. This ridge is comprised of the mesonephros, gonad, and associated ducts. The first indication of the development of the müllerian duct is a thickening of the coelomic epithelium at about the level of the fourth thoracic segment. This thickening becomes the fimbriated extremity of the fallopian tube, which invaginates and grows caudally to form a slender tube at the lateral edge of the urogenital ridge. In the sixth week of embryonic life, the growing tips of the two müllerian ducts approach each other in the midline and reach the sinus 1 week later. At that time, a fusion of the two müllerian ducts is begun at the level of the inguinal crest, or gubernaculum (primordium of the round ligament), to form a single canal. Thus, the upper ends of the müllerian ducts produce the oviducts and the fused parts give rise to the uterus. The uterine lumen from the fundus to the vagina is completed during the third month of fetal life. According to Koff (1933), the vaginal canal is not patent throughout its entire length until the sixth month of fetal life.

The Ovaries. The ovaries are almond-shaped organs, the functions of which are the development and extrusion of ova and the synthesis and secretion of steroid hormones. The ovaries vary considerably in size, and during childbearing years, they are 2.5 to 5 cm in length,

1.5 to 3 cm in breadth, and 0.6 to 1.5 cm in thickness. After menopause, ovarian size diminishes remarkably.

Normally, the ovaries are situated in the upper part of the pelvic cavity and rest in a slight depression on the lateral wall of the pelvis between the divergent external and internal iliac vessels—the ovarian fossa of Waldeyer. The position of the ovaries is subject to marked variation, and it is rare to find both ovaries at exactly the same level.

The ovary is attached to the broad ligament by the *mesovarium*. The *utero-ovarian ligament* extends from the lateral and posterior portion of the uterus, just beneath the tubal insertion, to the uterine, or lower pole of the ovary. Usually, it is several centimeters long and 3 to 4 mm in diameter. It is covered by peritoneum and is made up of muscle and connective tissue fibers that are continuous with those of the uterus. The *infundibulopelvic* or *suspensory ligament of the ovary* extends from the upper, or tubal, pole to the pelvic wall (Fig. 3–15B); through it course the ovarian vessels and nerves.

The exterior surface of the ovary varies in appearance with age. In young women, the organ is smooth, with a dull white surface through which glisten several small, clear follicles. As the woman grows older, the ovaries become more corrugated; in elderly women, the exterior surfaces may be convoluted markedly.

The general structure of the ovary can be studied best in cross sections, in which two portions may be distinguished, the *cortex* and *medulla*. The cortex, or outer layer, varies in thickness with age and becomes thinner with advancing years. It is in this layer that the ova and graafian follicles are located. The cortex of the ovary is composed of spindle-shaped connective tissue cells and fibers, among which there are scattered primordial and graafian follicles that are in various stages of development. As the woman grows older, the follicles become less numerous. The outermost portion of the cortex, which is dull and whitish, is designated as the *tunica albuginea*; on its surface, there is a single layer of cuboidal epithelium, the germinal epithelium of Waldeyer.

The medulla, or central portion, of the ovary is composed of loose connective tissue that is continuous with that of the mesovarium. There are a large number of arteries and veins in the medulla and a small number of smooth muscle fibers that are continuous with those in the suspensory ligament; the muscle fibers may be functional in movements of the ovary.

Both sympathetic and parasympathetic nerves are supplied to the ovaries. The sympathetic nerves are derived, in large part, from the ovarian plexus that accompanies the ovarian vessels; a few are derived from the plexus that surrounds the ovarian branch of the uterine artery. The ovary is richly supplied with nonmyelinated nerve fibers, which for the most part accompany the blood vessels. These are merely vascular nerves, whereas others form wreaths around normal and atretic follicles, and these give off many minute branches that have been traced up to, but not through, the membrana granulosa.

Development of the Ovary. The developmental changes in the human urogenital system have been described in ovaries from the third gestational week after conception to maturity. At first, the changes in the gonads are the same in both sexes. The earliest sign of a gonad is one that appears on the ventral surface of the embryonic kidney at a site between the eighth thoracic and fourth lumbar segments at about 4 weeks. As illustrated in Figure 3–19, the coelomic epithelium is thickened, and clumps of cells are seen to bud off into the underlying mesenchyme. This circumscribed area of the coelomic epithelium often is called the *germinal epithelium.* By the fourth to sixth week, however, there are many large ameboid cells in this region that have migrated into the body of the embryo from the yolk sac; these cells have been recognized in this region as early as the third week. These *primordial germ cells* are distinguishable by a large size and certain mor-

phological and cytochemical features. They react strongly in tests for alkaline phosphatase (McKay and associates, 1949), and are recognizable even after repeated divisions.

When the primordial germ cells reach the genital area, some enter the germinal epithelium and others mingle with the groups of cells that proliferate from it or lie in the mesenchyme. By the end of the fifth week, rapid division of all these types of cells results in development of a prominent *genital ridge.* The ridge projects into the body cavity medially to a fold in which there are the mesonephric (wolffian) and the müllerian ducts (Fig. 3–20). Because the growth of the gonad at the surface is more rapid, it enlarges centrifugally. By the seventh week (Figs. 3–19 and 3–20), it is separated from the mesonephros except at the narrow central zone, the future hilum, where the blood vessels enter. At this time, the sexes can be distinguished, because the testes can be recognized by well-defined radiating strands of cells (sex cords). These cords are separated from the germinal epithelium by mesenchyme that is to

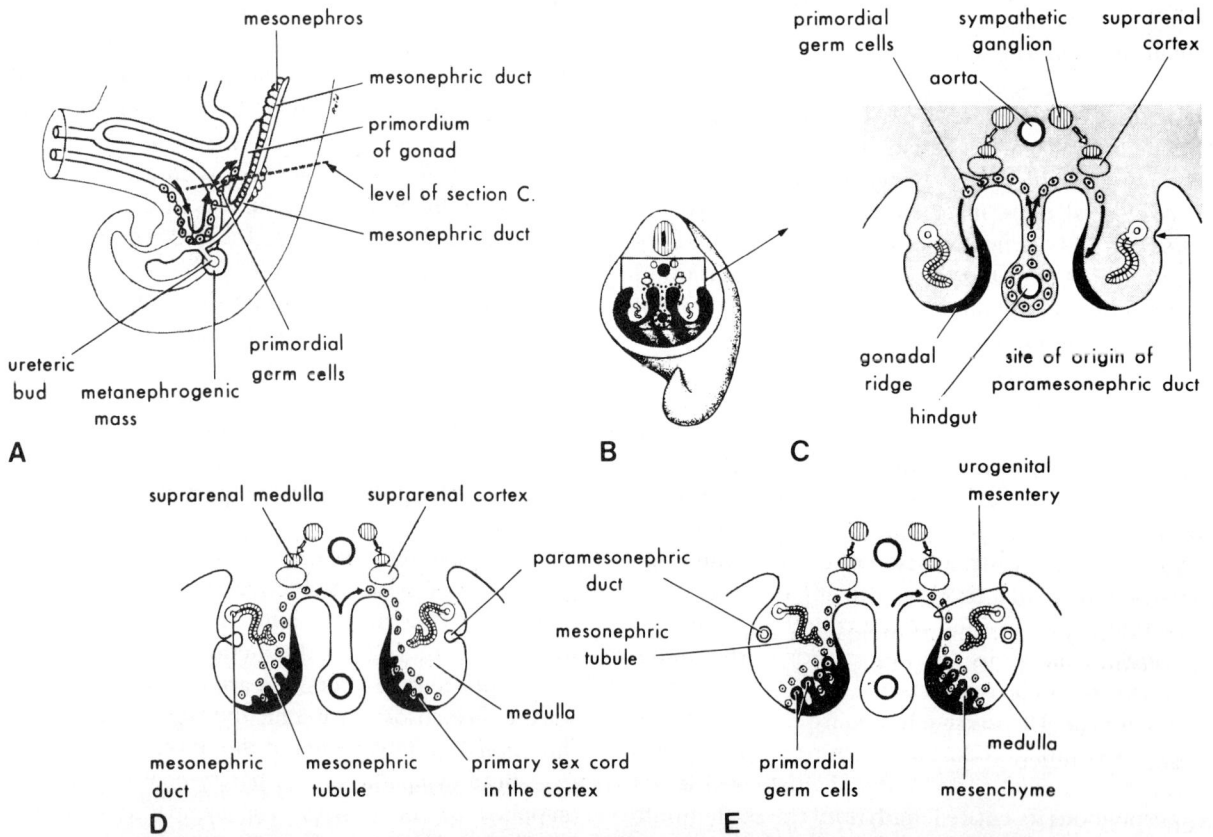

Fig. 3–19. A. Sketch of 5-week embryo illustrating the migration of primordial germ cells. **B.** Three-dimensional sketch of the caudal region of a 5-week embryo showing the location and extent of the gonadal ridges on the medial aspect of the urogenital ridges. **C.** Transverse section showing the primordium of the adrenal glands, gonadal ridges, and migration of primordial germ cells. **D.** Transverse section through a 6-week embryo showing the primary sex cords and developing paramesonephric ducts. **E.** Similar section at later stage showing the indifferent gonads and the mesonephric and paramesonephric ducts. (From Moore, 1983.)

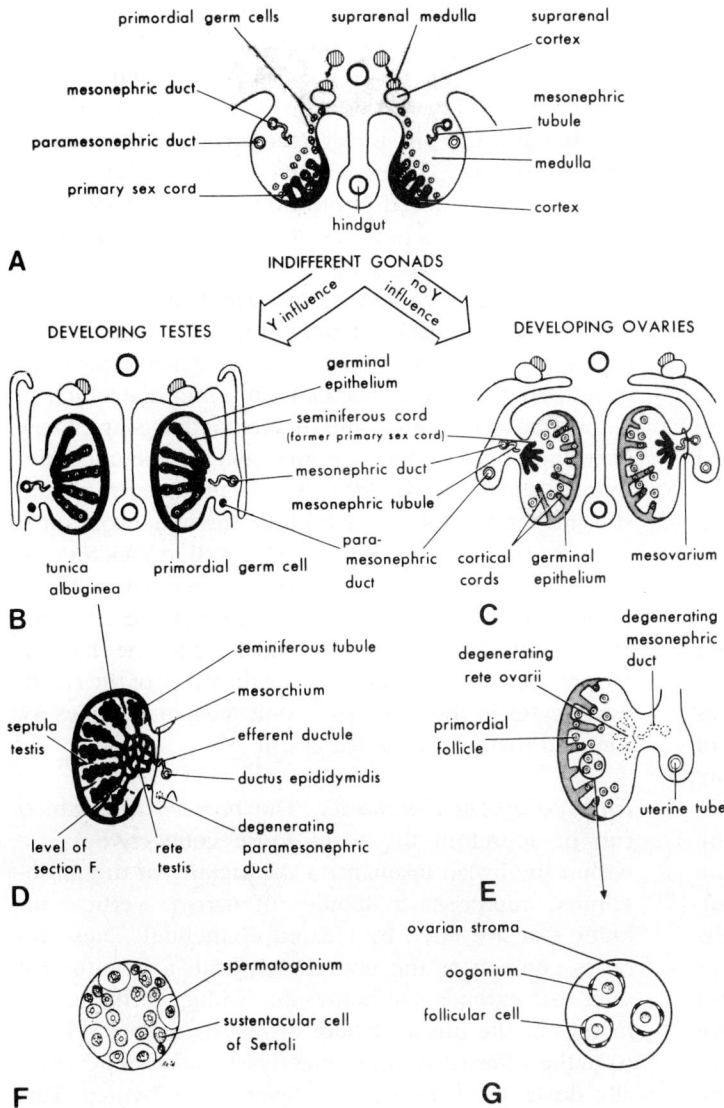

Fig. 3–20. Schematic sections illustrating the differentiation of the indifferent gonads into testes or ovaries. **A.** Six weeks, showing the indifferent gonads that are comprised of an outer cortex and an inner medulla. **B.** Seven weeks, showing testes developing under the influence of a Y chromosome. Note that the primary sex cords have become seminiferous cords and that they are separated from the surface epithelium by the tunica albuginea. **C.** Twelve weeks, showing ovaries beginning to develop in the absence of Y chromosome influence. Cortical cords have extended from the surface epithelium, displacing the primary sex cords centrally into the mesovarium, where they form the rudimentary rete ovarii. **D.** Testis at 20 weeks, showing the rete testis and the seminiferous tubules derived from the seminiferous cords. An efferent ductule has developed from a mesonephric tubule, and the mesonephric tubule and duct are regressing. **F.** Section of a seminiferous tubule from a 20-week fetus. Note that no lumen is present at this stage and that the seminiferous epithelium is comprised of two kinds of cells. **G.** Section from the ovarian cortex of a 20-week fetus showing three primordial follicles. (From Moore, 1983.)

become the tunica albuginea. The sex cords, which consist of large germ cells and smaller epithelioid cells derived from the germinal epithelium, develop into the seminiferous tubules and tubuli rete. The rete, probably derived from mesonephric elements, establishes connection with the mesonephric tubules that develop into the epididymis (Fig. 3–20). The mesonephric ducts become the vas deferens.

In the female, the germinal epithelium continues to proliferate for a much longer time. The groups of cells thus formed lie at first in the region of the hilum. As connective tissue develops between them, these appear as sex cords. These give rise to the medullary cords and persist for variable times (Forbes, 1942). By the third month, medulla and cortex are defined, as illustrated in Figure 3–20. The bulk of the organ is comprised of cortex, a mass of crowded germ and epithelioid cells that show some signs of grouping, but there are no

distinct cords as in the testis. Strands of cells extend from the germinal epithelium into the cortical mass, and mitoses are numerous. The rapid succession of mitoses soon reduces the size of the germ cells to the extent that these no longer are differentiated clearly from the neighboring cells; these cells are now called *oogonia*. Some of the oogonia in the medullary region are soon distinguishable by a series of peculiar nuclear changes. Large masses of nuclear chromatin appear, very different from the chromosomes of the oogonial divisions. This change marks the beginning of *synapsis*, which involves interactions between pairs of chromosomes that are derived originally from father and mother. Various stages of synapsis soon can be seen throughout the cortex; because similar changes occur in adjacent cells, groups (or "nests") appear. During one stage of synapsis, the chromatin is massed at one side of the nucleus, and the cytoplasm becomes highly fluid. Unless the in vitro preservation is prompt and perfect, these cells appear to be degenerating.

By the fourth month, some germ cells, again in the medullary region, having passed through synapsis, begin to enlarge. These are called *primary oocytes* at the beginning of the phase of growth that continues until maturity is reached. During this period of cell growth, many oocytes undergo degeneration, both before and after birth. The primary oocytes soon become surrounded by a single layer of flattened *follicle* cells that were derived originally from the germinal epithelium. These structures are now called *primordial follicles* and are first seen in the medulla and later in the cortex. Some follicles begin to grow even before birth and some are believed to persist in the cortex almost unchanged until menopause.

By 8 months of gestation, the ovary has become a long, narrow, lobulated structure that is attached to the body wall along the line of the hilum by the *mesovarium*, in which lies the *epoophoron*. At that stage of development, the germinal epithelium has been separated for the most part from the cortex by a band of connective tissue (tunica albuginea), which is absent in many small areas where strands of cells, usually referred to as cords of Pflüger, are in contact with the germinal epithelium. Among these cords are cells believed by many investigators to be oogonia that have come to resemble the other epithelial cells as a result of repeated mitoses. In the underlying cortex, there are two distinct zones. Superficially, there are nests of germ cells in synapsis, interspersed with Pflüger cords and strands of connective tissue. In the deeper zone, there are many groups of germ cells in synapsis, as well as primary oocytes, prospective follicular cells, and a few primordial follicles.

At term, the various types of ovarian cells in the human female fetus may still be found. In some cases, there are vesicular follicles in the medulla, which are all doomed to early degeneration.

Microscopical Structure of Ovary. From the first stages of its development until after the menopause, the ovary undergoes constant change. The number of oocytes at the onset of puberty has been estimated variously at 200,000 to 400,000. Because only one ovum ordinarily is cast off during each ovarian cycle, it is evident that a few hundred ova suffice for purposes of reproduction.

Mossman and co-workers (1964), in an attempt to clarify the terminology of glandular elements of ovaries of adult women, distinguished interstitial, thecal, and luteal cells. The interstitial glandular elements are formed from cells of the theca interna of degenerating or atretic follicles; the thecal glandular cells are formed from the theca interna of ripening follicles; and the true luteal cells are derived from the granulosa cells of ovulated follicles and from the undifferentiated stroma that surround them.

The huge store of primordial follicles at birth is exhausted gradually during the time of sexual maturation. Block (1952) found that there is a gradual decline from a mean of 439,000 oocytes in girls under 15 years to a mean of 34,000 in women over the age of 36.

In the young girl, the greater portion of the ovary is comprised of the cortex, which is filled with large numbers of closely packed primordial follicles. Those nearest the central portion of the ovary are at the most advanced stages of development. In young women, the cortex is relatively thinner but still contains a large number of primordial follicles that are separated by bands of connective tissue cells in which there are spindle-shaped or oval nuclei. Each primordial follicle is comprised of an oocyte and its surrounding single layer of epithelial cells, which are small and flattened, spindle-shaped, and somewhat sharply differentiated from the still smaller and spindly cells of the surrounding stroma.

The oocyte is a large, spherical cell in which there is clear cytoplasm and a relatively large nucleus that is located near the center of the ovum. In the nucleus, there is one large and several smaller nucleoli, and numerous masses of chromatin. The diameter of the smallest oocytes in the ovaries of adult women averages 33 μm, and that of the nuclei, 20μm.

Embryological Remnants. The *parovarium*, which can be found in the scant loose connective tissue within the broad ligament in the vicinity of the mesosalpinx, comprises a number of narrow vertical tubules that are lined by ciliated epithelium. These tubules connect at the upper ends with a longitudinal duct that extends just below the oviduct to the lateral margin of the uterus, where ordinarily it ends blindly near the internal os; infrequently, it may extend laterally down the vagina to the level of the hymen. This canal, the remnant of the wolffian (mesonephric) duct in women, is called the *Gartner duct*. The parovarium, also a remnant of the wolffian duct, is homologous, embryologically, with the caput epididymis in men. The cranial portion of the parovarium is the *epoophoron*, or organ of Rosenmüller; the caudal portion, or *paroophoron*, is a group of vestigial mesonephric tubules that lie in or around the broad ligament. It is homologous, embryologically, with the paradidymis of men. Usually the paroophoron in adult women disappears, but on occasion macroscopic cysts are formed from these remnants.

REFERENCES

Block E: Quantitative morphological investigation of the follicular system in women. Acta Anat 14:108, 1952

Buckingham JC, Buethe RA Jr, Danforth DN: Collagen–muscle ratio in clinically normal and clinically incompetent cervices. Am J Obstet Gynecol 91:232, 1965

Danforth DN, Buckingham JC, Roddick JW Jr: Connective tissue changes incident to cervical effacement. Am J Obstet Gynecol 80:939, 1960

Ferenczy A, Richart RM: Female Reproductive System: Dynamics of Scanning and Transmission Electron Microscopy. New York, Wiley, 1974

Forbes TR: On the fate of the medullary cords of the human ovary. Contrib Embryol 30:9, 1942

Hillier SL, Krohn MA, Nugent RP, Gibbs RS, Vaginal Infections and Prematurity Study Group: Characteristics of three vaginal flora patterns assessed by gram stain among pregnant women. Am J Obstet Gynecol 166:938, 1992

Hitschmann F, Adler L: The structure of the endometrium of the sexually mature woman. Monatschr Geburtsh Gynaek 27:1, 1908

Hodgson BJ, Eddy CA: The autonomic nervous system and its relationship to tubal ovum transport—A reappraisal. Gynecol Invest 6:161, 1975

Koff AK: Development of the vagina in the human fetus. Contrib Embryol 24:59, 1933

Krantz KE: Innervation of the human vulva and vagina. Obstet Gynecol 13:382, 1958

Langlois PL: The size of the normal uterus. J Reprod Med 4:220, 1970

Larsen B, Galask RP: Vaginal microbial flora: Practical and theoretic relevance. Obstet Gynecol 55:100S, 1980

McKay DG, Robinson D, Hertig AT: Histochemical observations on granulosa cell tumors, thecomas and fibromas of the ovary. Am J Obstet Gynecol 58:625, 1949

Moore K: The Developing Human, Philadelphia, Saunders, 1983

Mossman HW, Koering MJ, Ferry D Jr: Cyclic changes in interstitial gland tissue of the human ovary. Am J Anat 115:235, 1964

Nelson JH: Atlas of Radical Pelvic Surgery, 2nd ed. New York, Appleton, 1977, p 133

Okkels H, Engle ET: Studies on the finer structure of the uterine blood vessels of the macacus monkey. Acta Pathol Microbiol Scand 15:150, 1938

Schwalm H, Dubrauszky V: The structure of the musculature of the human uterus-muscles and connective tissue. Am J Obstet Gynecol 94:391, 1966

Verkauf BS, Von Thron J, O'Brien WF: Clitoral size in normal women. Obstet Gynecol 80:41, 1992

Wicke L: Atlas of Radiologic Anatomy, 3rd ed. Baltimore, Urban & Schwarzenberg, 1982

Woodruff JD, Pauerstein CJ: The Fallopian Tube. Baltimore, Williams & Wilkins, 1969

Physiology of Pregnancy

■

CHAPTER 4

The Endometrium and Decidua: Menstruation and Pregnancy

Maternal Tissues of the Fetal–Maternal Communication System

The endometrium is the mucosal lining of the uterine cavity; the decidua is the highly modified, specialized endometrium of pregnancy. The single physiological function of the endometrium and decidua is to serve as the maternal tissue interface of pregnancy. This tissue is the anatomical site of blastocyst apposition, implantation, and placental development. From the evolutionary perspective, the human endometrium is the most functionally sophisticated example of this tissue among all mammalian species, being the most highly developed and modified for hemochorioendothelial implantation. Endometrial development of a magnitude anywhere similar to that observed in women, replete with the special spiral (or coiling) arteries, is restricted to only a few primates, the great apes, and Old World monkeys. Indeed, it is only in these few primates that menstruation is obliged with infertile ovarian cycles to shed the highly developed endometrium.

Direct cell-to-cell contact between fetal and maternal tissues is first established about 6 days after fertilization of the ovum; it is then that the blastocyst embraces and becomes adherent to the endometrial surface epithelium. This is the time of blastocyst *apposition*; and for a brief time, the endometrial surface is the only maternal tissue in direct cell-to-cell contact with the blastocyst; but already, dialogue between fetal and maternal tissues is operative. Soon after apposition, the blastocyst begins the process of implantation; and, the fundamental components of implantation, immunological acceptance of the blastocyst, maternal recognition of pregnancy, pregnancy maintenance, and fetal nutrition are established.

In some manner, trophoblast invasion incites further decidualization of the secretory (progesterone-dominated) endometrium. It is likely that the stimuli for advanced decidualization (in addition to estrogen and progesterone) involve essential elements of the inflammatory process, including blastocyst (trophoblast) generation of or induction of endometrial formation of prostaglandins, platelet-activating factor, serine proteases (e.g., plasminogen activator), and possibly histamine release. In addition, it is now suspected that specific growth factors, arising in the blastocyst and possibly from maternal platelets and endometrium, may be operative to finalize stromal cell decidualization. In the experimental animal, appropriately treated with estrogen and progesterone, trauma to the endometrium is a potent artificial stimulus to deciduoma formation. This brings to mind the products of platelets; and, attractive candidates for the promotion of the final stages of decidualization are transforming growth factor-β (TGF-β) and platelet-derived growth factor (PDGF), delivered to the site of endometrial vessel disruption by maternal platelets, generated in trophoblasts of the blastocyst, or both. In addition to its action to promote the formation of extracellular matrix and inhibit the formation of metalloproteinases, TGF-β1 is perhaps the most potent agent in promoting TGF-β1 gene transcription—that is, autoinduction. Indeed, a wavelike propagation of TGF-β1 expression, spreading from blastocyst implantation site across the endometrium, is observed in the decidua during the periimplantation period in the mouse (Tamada and colleagues, 1990).

Functionally, there are two maternal tissues directly involved in the fully developed fetal–maternal communication system: (1) maternal uterine decidua (basalis and parietalis) and (2) maternal blood. As the blastocyst invades the endometrium during implantation, trophoblasts become readily recognizable cells, histologically distinct from the embryo-forming cells; and the two distinct arms of the communication system are created

(Chap. 5). Trophoblasts invade the endometrial blood vessels, and in consequence become surrounded by "lakes" of maternal blood, the lacunae, which later will coalesce to form the intervillous space. At this time, **the placental arm of the communication system** is operative. The portion of the decidua invaded by trophoblasts becomes the decidua basalis; these trophoblasts will create the villous placenta and the extravillous anchoring cytotrophoblasts. And as the embryo and extraembryonic fetal tissues grow, the extraembryonic fetal membranes (amnion and chorion laeve) are formed. Much later in pregnancy (14 to 16 weeks), the chorion laeve comes to lie adjacent to all of the uterine decidua not occupied by villous placenta, namely the decidua parietalis; this completes the establishment of **the paracrine arm of the fetal–maternal communication system** (Chaps. 2 and 5).

From the immunological perspective, it is important to recognize that trophoblasts separate the embryo from direct contact with maternal tissues at all sites and at all stages of pregnancy. Thereby, the embryo-fetus is encased in a "protective" shell, the trophoblastic shell, which constitutes an immunological buffer zone between the embryo-fetus and maternal tissues and blood (Fig. 2–1). And whereas the trophoblasts are of fetal origin, derived from the fertilized ovum, the expression of major histocompatibility complex (HLA) antigens (including paternal antigens) in these extraembryonic cells is modified markedly (Chap. 5).

Pregnancy, the Cardinal Function of the Uterus.
To gain greater insights into the function and functional regulation of the uterus (endometrium, myometrium), it is worthwhile to critically consider the potential contributions of this unique organ to all physiological processes. From the conduct of such an inventory, we have concluded, as have most others before us, that the single salutary metabolic function of the uterus is the accommodation of a conceptus (pregnancy). There is no known hormonal or other physiological function of the endometrium or myometrium, independent of pregnancy, that contributes to metabolic homeostasis or to the physical well-being of women. There is no evidence that removal of the endometrium and myometrium (hysterectomy) serves to affect adversely the life span or health of women, unless of course this results in undesired sterility or complications of the surgical procedure. On the contrary, dysmenorrhea, blood loss with menstruation or from other causes, malignant transformation, infections, or benign tumors of this organ may cause significant disability, disease, and all too often, death. In fact, the association between hormonal treatment and an increased incidence of neoplasia in humans is established most clearly in the case of endometrium (estrogen treatment and endometrial adenocarcinoma).

Ramsey (1977) has reviewed the history of the evolution of knowledge concerning the anatomy of the uterus. She observed that during the Middle Ages (the "Dark Ages"), the popular theory was that the uterus was multicompartmental, the most popular number of compartments was believed to be seven. It was commonly accepted that male embryos developed in the three right-hand cells, females in the three on the left, and hermaphrodites in the one in the middle. An alternative view was that the female reproductive tract was a mirror image of that of the male, the vagina being a penis turned inside out and the uterus an inverted scrotum.

In 1315, Mondino dei Luzzi conducted the first authorized public dissection of a human body; and from his findings, the uterus, cervix, and vagina were described almost as we know these structures today. Leonardo da Vinci correctly depicted the anatomical relationship between the ovaries, tubes, and ligaments. Clearly, he considered the uterus to consist of a single cavity; and at about the same time, Beringario da Carpi stated that *"it is a pure lie—to say that the uterus has seven cavities."*

The Renaissance in anatomy can be focused on Vesalius, whose epic *De Humani Corporis Fabrica* appeared in 1543. The frontispiece of *Fabrica* is a picture of Vesalius presiding over the dissection of a female cadaver; and the presentation of the gross anatomy of the human female reproductive tract presented in this masterpiece was as we know it today (Chap. 3). The term *uterus* was first used in this treatise; since that time, we have come to understand the morphology and, to some extent, the physiological function of this organ in appreciably greater detail.

Overview of Endometrial Function.
There are relatively few cell types in humans that continue to replicate in adult life; among these few, those of the endometrium of reproductive-age women are particularly noteworthy. The growth and functional characteristics of the endometrium of women are unique and astonishing. This obtains not only because the epithelial (glandular) and stromal cells, as well as the blood vessels, of the endometrium replicate at a rapid rate, but because this tissue is regenerated during each endometrial (ovarian–menstrual) cycle. Namely, two thirds of the entire endometrium is shed and regenerated more than 450 times, on average, in the life of most women. There is no other example in humans of the cyclic shedding and regrowth of an entire tissue. With this many endometrial cells formed, it is likely that endometrial carcinoma in all women is prevented only because of the short half-life and thereby the shedding of these cells.

To place menstruation in yet another perspective, the lifetime cumulative menstrual blood loss associated with normal endometrial shedding is 10 to 20 liters or more, an amount of blood that contains at least three times the total body iron content of the average adult woman. The 38-year reproductive lifetime cumulative production of progesterone for the woman who chooses two pregnancies and experiences 450 ovarian cycles is about 150,000 milligrams (150 grams), which is about equal to the cumulative amount of cortisol secreted in most women during the same 38 years. And, as we have observed before (in the seventeenth edition of this book), if the doubling time of endometrial growth experienced from the 5th to 20th day of the ovarian cycle were maintained for 1 year, the weight of endometrium would approach 1 ton!

This incredible investment in tissue growth and thence cyclic shedding is clearly the consequence of infertile ovarian cycles; but at the same time, this process constitutes cyclic renewal of this entire functional tissue of the endometrium in preparation of the uterus for the next pregnancy opportunity. Therefore, for the woman who elects to be infertile, the ovarian–menstrual cycle constitutes anatomical, endocrinological, and physiological futility. We will return to this important theme in a consideration of the disabilities caused as a direct consequence of the ovarian–menstrual cycles of women who are not desirous of pregnancy.

Pregnancy, the Cardinal Function of the Endometrium and Decidua.

The importance of the uterine endometrium (decidua) in the success of pregnancy cannot be underestimated, but at the same time it should not be overstated. It is clear that the endometrium is the optimal site for blastocyst implantation and embryo and fetal development; but it cannot be claimed that this function of the endometrium and decidua is unique because of the success, albeit limited, of ectopic pregnancies (pregnancies in which the blastocyst implants and the fetus develops outside of the uterine cavity). "Decidualization" of tissues in which ectopic pregnancies implant (e.g., the mucosal lining of the fallopian tube, peritoneum, and ovary) is prominent.

There may also be a role for the endometrium in sperm capacitation; but again, it cannot be argued that this function is unique to the endometrium, as evidenced by the success of sperm capacitation and fertilization of the ovum in vitro.

The decidua—the highly specialized endometrium of pregnancy—is largely comprised of decidual cells, which (under the influence of progesterone and other stimuli) develop from the stromal cells (mesenchyme) of the endometrium. In addition, there are normally many bone-marrow-derived cells (a variety of leukocytes) in the decidua. Most of the glandular epithelium and glandular structure of the human endometrium is lost as gestation progresses.

Today, there is appreciable evidence that the maintenance of pregnancy and the initiation of parturition are closely aligned in all mammalian species by way of rigid regulation (prevention) of myometrial contractions throughout 90 to 95 percent of pregnancy (phase 0 of parturition, Chap. 12). Normally, it is only at term, with timely retreat from continued pregnancy maintenance, that parturition begins. For this reason, we suggest that endometrial (decidual) function is coordinately directed

to the success of biomolecular processes that forestall the initiation of labor until the achievement of fetal maturity. But sometime thereafter, once the stronghold on myometrial quiescence is released when retreat from pregnancy maintenance has been sounded, the decidua is a potential site of formation of uterotonins (myometrial smooth muscle contractants) that may support the active labor (phase 2) function of the parturitional process. It is known that a number of potent uterotonins can be synthesized in decidua: prostaglandins, endothelin-1, and oxytocin. Later (Chap. 12), we refer to this special time in pregnancy as the transition from phase 1 to phase 2 of parturition. A *uterotropin* is an agent that acts to promote the synthesis of functional proteins that prepare the uterus for labor. A *uterotonin* is an agent that acts directly to cause myometrial smooth muscle cell contraction (Chap. 12).

Perhaps the most important feature of the decidua that contributes to successful pregnancy outcome resides in the obvious. Namely, the implantation of the blastocyst in the decidua provides a means for the birth of the fetus. The decidua is a tissue that lines the endometrial cavity and thereby is continuous with the birth canal—that is, there is access from the decidual surface to the cervical canal and vagina, channels that enable delivery of the fetus. This anatomical arrangement also provides for a mechanism of expulsion of the fetus by the action of the myometrial contractions of labor that effect the dilatation of the cervix and descent of the fetus.

Any decidual function beyond these anatomical distinctions is a plus; and many such added functions have been proposed. The decidua is an immunologically privileged tissue; the hormonal responsiveness of the endometrium and decidua facilitates apposition and implantation of the blastocyst; the endometrium and decidua and their unique blood vessels provide for early blastocyst nutrition; the decidua may contribute cytokines and growth factors to promote placental growth and function; the decidua may serve first to accept and thence to limit the extent of trophoblast invasion; and the decidua becomes an endocrine tissue, producing prolactin, 1,25-dihydroxy-vitamin-D_3, corticotropin releasing hormone (CRH), parathyroid hormone-related protein (PTH-rP), relaxin, insulin-like growth factor binding protein, and multiple pregnancy-specific proteins.

For these reasons, the functional characteristics of the decidua are important in the acceptance of the semiallogenic fetal graft, the physiology of pregnancy maintenance, fetal nutrition, and in parturition through support of labor. It also is possible that the functional characteristics of the decidua will be profoundly important in devising strategies for the prevention of preterm labor. **Premature perturbation, activation, or stimulation of decidual tissue to produce uterotonins, could be one cause of preterm birth** (Chap. 12).

The role of the decidua in placental growth and function is a topic of great research interest in many laboratories around the world. Many such studies are directed toward a definition of the role of cytokines and growth factors, produced in the decidua, that will cause trophoblast replication and differentiation or modify growth factor receptors in the trophoblasts. Among the agents under intense study are epidermal growth factor; macrophage colony-stimulating factor (M-CSF or CSF-1); insulin-like growth factor; and the cytokines interleukin-6 (IL-6), IL-1β, and IL-2. From the findings of these studies, it seems likely that trophoblasts can incite the decidua to promote further growth and differentiation of the placenta in a handshake, cooperative, paracrine arrangement. The specifics of this coordinated action are not yet defined, but there seems to be little doubt that trophoblasts are capable of enlisting maternal decidual tissue assistance in supporting placental growth, development, and survival. This may be accomplished by the contributions of both decidual and bone-marrow-derived cells (leukocytes) of the decidua to trophoblast growth, differentiation, and functioning. This interrelationship has been reviewed by Casey and MacDonald, 1992a.

Specialized Functions of the Endometrium and Decidua. As stated, the endometrial cavity is patent—anatomically open through the cervical canal, which in turn is open to the vagina, which in turn is open to the external environment. The same is true of the decidua during pregnancy, at least at the lower pole of the interface between the chorion laeve and decidua parietalis. To be sure, there is functional closure of the cervical canal during pregnancy by way of a mucus "plug," and there are antimicrobial properties ascribed to the cervical mucus. Nonetheless, because of the anatomical reality of patency of the female reproductive tract, it is reasonable to presume that the decidua must normally be endowed with unique and extraordinary capacities to effectively respond to microbial and immunological challenges without causing the abortion of the fetus. It is highly likely that, normally, the decidua functions to contain infectious processes at the lower pole of chorion laeve–decidual interface as a means of preventing the onset of preterm labor (Chap. 12). Many of the mediators of the inflammatory process, including the prostaglandins and platelet-activating factor, are known to be uterotonins or else are capable of promoting the formation of uterotonins (IL-1β and TNF-α) and thereby uterine contractions.

The Relationship of Menstruation to Parturition. In Chapter 2, we observed that menstruation is the consequence of failed fertility; it is probable that the biomolecular processes that eventuate in the initiation of menstruation constellate about some of the same fundamental processes for which the function of the endometrium is destined, that is, pregnancy and parturition. Progesterone withdrawal is clearly the endocrinological event that leads to the onset of menstruation; and progesterone withdrawal seems to be the key endocrine event that heralds the initiation of parturition in many (if not all) mammalian species (Chap. 12). Others have referred to the process of parturition as *delayed menstruation* (Gustavii, 1972). We choose another philosophical interpretation: With failed fertility, menstruation is initiated by cellular and biomolecular processes similar to those involved in parturition; therefore, **menstruation is the pseudoparturition of fertility failure.** Indeed, the uterine contractions that occur during menstruation are important in emptying the uterus of blood and cellular debris, thus facilitating preparation of the endometrium for the next pregnancy opportunity.

Hormonal Regulation of the Endometrium

The endometrium has become a model tissue for investigations to define the mechanisms of action of sex steroid hormones and other agents, such as growth factors, polyamines, prostaglandins, oncogenes, peptide hormones, and cytokines. The ready accessibility of human endometrial tissue for study, together with the fact that endometrial glandular epithelium can be easily separated from stroma, have rightfully attracted the interest of endocrinologists, molecular biologists, and immunologists who seek to establish the molecular nature of the action(s) of these agents in target tissues. Moreover, the functional relationships and interactions between endometrial glandular epithelium and stroma may be a model for study of interrelationships between mesenchyme and epithelium of a given tissue.

Estrogen Action. Estradiol, the biologically potent, naturally occurring estrogen secreted by the dominant ovarian follicle, acts to promote responses of the endometrium in a manner that now stands as a model for the mechanism of steroid hormone action. In 1961, Elwood Jensen presented a scintillating lecture, entitled "Basic guides to the mechanism of estrogen action," to the Laurentian Hormone Conference (Jensen and Jacobson, 1962). By use of estrogens of high specific radioactivity, these investigators demonstrated that nonmetabolized (radiolabeled) estradiol is sequestered in estrogen-responsive tissues, notably the uterus. This seems to have been the beginning of the contemporary era of the study of the mechanisms of steroid action through binding to specific steroid receptor proteins. One of us was privileged to be present at this brilliant lecture and will never forget that Jensen ended this dissertation with a limerick:

> *To a tissue that's trying to grow*
> *We hope these experiments show:*
> *With steroids phenolic*
> *Don't get metabolic,*
> *Just grab on, and never let go!*

Indeed, plasma estradiol enters the endometrial cells by simple diffusion; but in estrogen-responsive cells, estradiol, in some manner, is *sequestered* and translocated to the nucleus, where it becomes bound to the estrogen receptor protein. The receptor is a macromolecule that is characterized by high affinity, but low capacity, for estradiol and other biologically active estrogens, including synthetic estrogens. The estradiol–receptor complex, probably after transformational changes, becomes associated with the estrogen response element of specific genes. This brings about estrogen-specific gene transcription that results in synthesis of specific messenger RNAs and, thereafter, the synthesis of specific proteins.

Among the many proteins synthesized in response to estrogen action in the endometrium are macromolecules that are characterized by high affinity for progesterone (*progesterone receptors*) as well as additional estrogen receptors. Thus, the actions of estradiol on the endometrium include those that provide both for the perpetuation of the cellular milieu in which estrogen can act, and those for the initiation of processes that provide for a response to progesterone. In the past, it was believed that cytosolic receptors became bound to steroid hormones and that the cytosolic receptor–steroid complex and thereafter the steroid–receptor complex was translocated to the nucleus. It now seems likely that the finding of receptors in cytosolic preparations was, at least in large part, an artifact of the process of tissue preparation, and that in vivo the receptors for steroid hormones are principally concentrated in the nucleus.

Progesterone Action. Progesterone also enters the endometrial cells by diffusion, and thence becomes associated with nuclear receptors with high affinity, but low capacity, for progesterone. Generally however, the concentration of progesterone receptors is dependent on previous estrogen action. The progesterone–receptor complex is also active in promoting gene transcription, but the attendant response is strikingly different from that evoked by the estradiol–receptor complex. Progesterone acts to bring about specific responses characteristic of progesterone; but in addition, the progesterone–receptor complex acts to cause a decrease in the production of estrogen receptor molecules (Tseng and Gurpide, 1975), an action that serves as one means by which progesterone attenuates the action of estrogen. Progesterone also acts to cause an increase in the enzyme *estradiol dehydrogenase,* which catalyzes the interconversion of estradiol and estrone. Tseng and Gurpide (1974) found that the reaction kinetics of estradiol dehydrogenase in endometrium are such that the net formation of estrone, a biologically weaker estrogen than estradiol, is favored. Progesterone also acts to increase sulfurylation of estrogen (*estrogen sulfotransferase*), another means of estrogen inactivation (Tseng and Liu, 1981). Thus, progesterone serves as an antiestrogen—that is, to attenuate estrogen action in endometrium—in at least three ways: (1) by reducing the rate of synthesis of estrogen receptors, (2) by bringing about a reduction in the intracellular level of estra-

diol (through conversion to estrone), and (3) by effecting estrogen inactivation through sulfurylation.

The findings of important studies such as these have also provided tools for investigators to identify markers of estrogen and progesterone action—markers believed to be important in the identification of and thence in the management of hormone-responsive tumors. For example, one useful marker of estrogen action in a given tissue (or tumor) is the presence of progesterone receptors. Horwitz and colleagues (1975) have pioneered the delineation of estrogen-responsive breast cancers by showing that tumors in which progesterone receptors are demonstrable are likely to be more responsive, therapeutically, to endocrine ablation procedures that lead to reduced endogenous estrogen formation or to the action of antiestrogenic compounds.

The presence of, or an increase of, estradiol dehydrogenase activity in endometrium after progestin treatment is also indicative of estrogen action to promote progesterone receptors and of progesterone responsiveness as well; and an increase in this enzyme activity in endometrial carcinoma tissue may signal responsiveness, therapeutically, of such tumors to progesterone or synthetic progestational agents.

Steroid hormones, however, may be activated by mechanisms other than the classic receptor-mediated, genomic process just described. This may be more evident for progesterone than for any other steroid. Progesterone or its metabolites can exert profound biological actions by way of receptors other than the progesterone receptor and by receptor-independent, nongenomic processes described later in this chapter in a consideration of the potential role of progesterone in the biogenesis of the premenstrual syndromes (PMS).

The Endometrial Cycle

Histology: History. Hitschmann and Adler (1908) were the first to describe cyclical histological changes in the endometrium. And almost 60 years ago, Rock and Bartlett (1937) suggested that the histological features of the endometrium were sufficiently characteristic to permit "dating" the ovarian cycle of the woman from whom the endometrial tissue was obtained. The histological changes that occur in the endometrium during the menstrual cycle are summarized in Figure 4–1; the findings are taken from those of Noyes and associates (1950). This manuscript, in which the day-to-day changes in endometrial histology were described, as noted by Benirschke (1986), was the first paper published in the then-new journal *Fertility and Sterility.*

Hormone-Induced Morphological Changes. In response to the changes that are evoked by the actions of sex steroid hormones produced in the ovary during each ovulatory cycle, there are morphological changes in the endometrium that evolve with such precise regularity

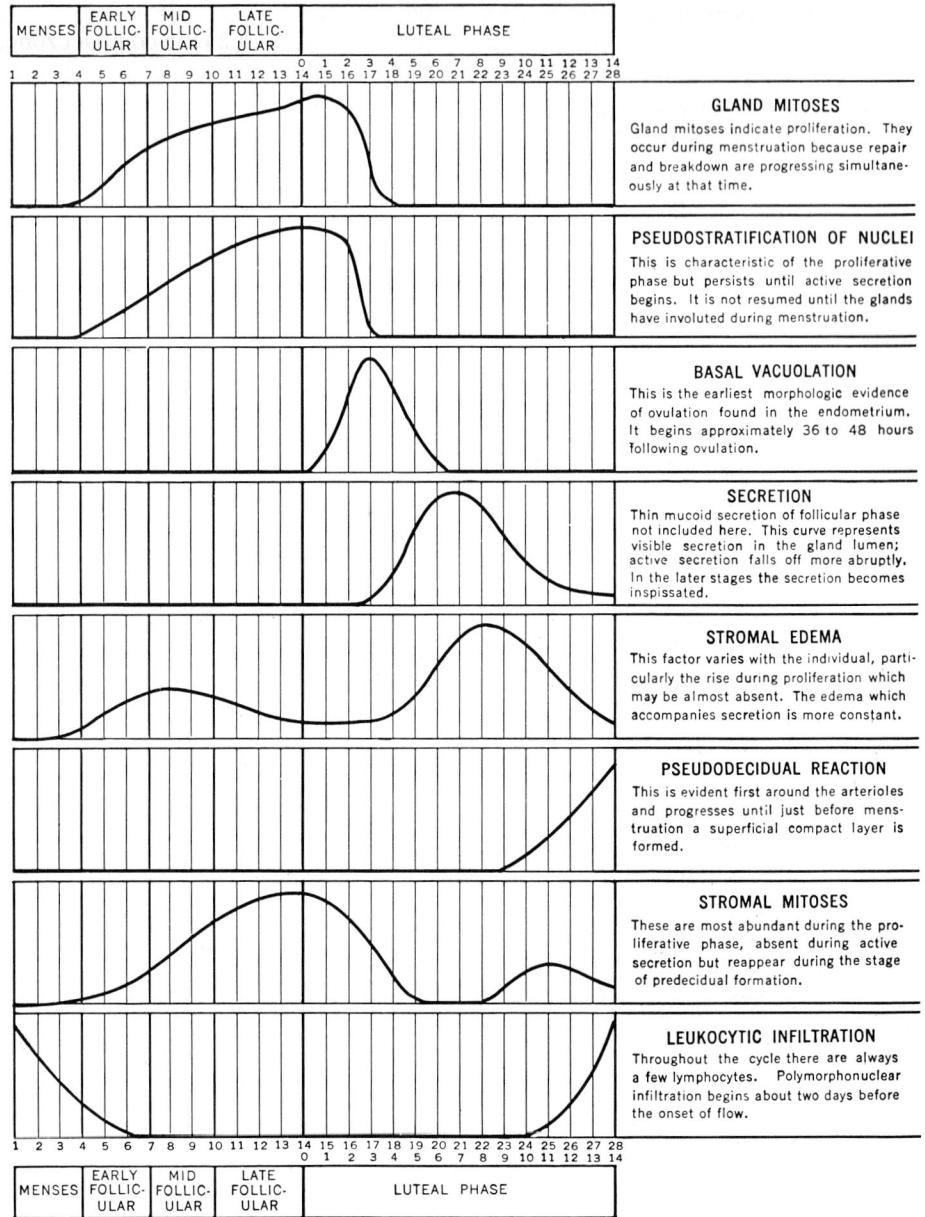

Fig. 4–1. Dating of the endometrium according to the day of the menstrual cycle during a hypothetical 28-day ovarian cycle. Correlation of typical morphological findings. (From Noyes and associates, 1950.)

that the histological features of the endometrium can be used by an experienced morphologist to estimate the day of the ovarian cycle on which the endometrium was removed. The sex steroid hormonal changes during the ovarian cycle can be summarized as follows: (1) During the preovulatory, or follicular, phase of the ovarian cycle, estradiol is secreted (principally by the dominant follicle of the ovary) in increasing quantities until just before ovulation. (2) During the postovulatory, or luteal, phase of the cycle, progesterone is secreted in massive amounts by the corpus luteum. (3) During the premenstrual phase, the corpus luteum regresses and the rates of secretion of both estradiol and progesterone diminish progressively.

In response to these changes in sex steroid hormone secretion during the ovarian cycle, there are five main stages of the endometrial cycle: (1) menstrual/

postmenstrual *reepithelialization*; (2) *endometrial proliferation* in response to stimulation (directly or indirectly) by estradiol; (3) abundant glandular *secretion*, which results from the combined action of estrogen and progesterone; (4) *premenstrual ischemia*, which results from endometrial involution, which causes stasis of blood in the spiral arteries; and (5) *menstruation*, which is preceded and accompanied by vasoconstriction of the endometrial spiral arteries and collapse and desquamation of all but the deepest layer of the endometrium. In the final analysis, menstruation is the consequence of progesterone withdrawal.

The follicular (preovulatory or proliferative) phase, and the postovulatory (luteal or secretory) phase, are customarily divided into early and late stages. The normal secretory phase may be subdivided rather finely (almost day by day), by histological criteria, beginning shortly after ovulation until the onset of menstruation.

Early Proliferative Phase. During menstruation, about two thirds of the functional endometrium is fragmented and shed. Reepithelialization commences, however, even before menstrual bleeding has ceased; and by the fifth day (first day of menses equals day 1), the epithelial surface of the endometrium has been restored. This important event is associated with revascularization of the endometrium. During the early proliferative phase of the cycle, the endometrium is thin, usually less than 2 mm in depth (thickness). Histologically, the glands at this time are narrow, tubular structures that pursue almost a straight and parallel course (one with the other) from the surface toward the basal layer. The glandular epithelium is low columnar, and the nuclei are round and basal. In the deeper part of the endometrium, the cells of the stroma are packed rather densely and the nuclei of these cells are deep-staining and small. In the superficial or reorganizing layer, the stromal cells are packed more loosely and the nuclei are more nearly round, more vesicular, and larger than those in the deeper layers.

Mitotic figures, especially in the glands, are present by the fifth day after the commencement of menstruation, and mitotic activity in both glandular epithelium and stroma persists thereafter until 2 to 3 days after ovulation. Although the blood vessels are numerous and prominent, there is no extravasated blood or lymphocytic infiltration in the endometrium at this stage.

Late Proliferative Phase. The endometrium in the late proliferative phase has become thicker, as a result of both glandular hyperplasia and an increase in stromal ground substance (edema and proteinaceous material). The loose stroma is especially prominent superficially, and the glands are widely separated compared with those of the deeper zone, where the glands are crowded and tortuous and the stroma is more dense. Gradually, the glandular epithelium becomes taller and pseudostratified at about the time of ovulation.

Day-by-day "dating" of the endometrium during the proliferative phase is not possible, however, because of the considerable variation among women in the length of the follicular phase of the ovarian cycle. Whereas the luteal or secretory (i.e., postovulatory) phase of the cycle among women is remarkably constant in duration (12 to 14 days), the length of the proliferative or follicular (i.e., preovulatory) phase varies greatly. In apparently normal, fertile women, the follicular phase may vary from 7 to 21 days.

Early Secretory Phase. After ovulation, the changes in the morphology of the endometrium occur with such regularity that the endometrium can be dated (relative to the day of ovulation) by the histological appearance of the tissue. During the secretory stage, three zones of the endometrium become well defined: (1) the basal zone, which is the layer adjacent to the myometrium; (2) the compact zone, or layer immediately beneath the endometrial surface adjacent to and lining the endometrial cavity; and (3) the spongy zone, or layer between the compact and basal layers. Actually, the basal layer undergoes little if any histological change during the endometrial (menstrual) cycle, except that mitoses are found in the glands. The spongy middle layer is comprised of a lacy labyrinth with little stroma between the tortuous, serrated glands that characterize the luteal phase. In the compact superficial layer, the glands are more nearly straight and narrower, but the glandular lumens are often filled with secretions. Edema of the abundant stroma is an important factor in causing the thickening of the endometrium, but there is also an increase in dry weight.

Mid to Late Secretory Phase. At the time of the midluteal phase of the cycle, the endometrium is extremely vascular, succulent, and rich in glycogen; presumably, it is ideally suited at this time for the implantation and growth of the blastocyst. It is estimated that on average there are about 15,000 endometrial glands that open onto the endometrial surface at this time. The stromal cells, and in particular those stromal cells immediately around the blood vessels, undergo hypertrophic changes similar to, but less extensive than, those of the true decidual cells of pregnancy. This intimate relationship between the arteries and arterioles, and decidualization of the contiguous stromal cells, is important in the process of decidualization and in the initiation of menstruation, as we will describe.

During the late secretory phase of the cycle, the formation of a pericellular basement membrane around stromal cells commences, one that will come to completely surround each stromal cell as decidualization progresses. This very peculiar pericellular basement membrane and the components thereof are considered in greater detail in the analysis of decidual tissue.

Spiral (Coiled) Arteries of the Endometrium and Decidua. Boyd and Hamilton (1970) emphasize the extraordinary importance of the peculiar arteries of the human endometrium, pointing out that William Hunter in 1774 referred to these vessels as the "curling arteries." Ultimately, the endometrial spiral arteries arise from the uterine arteries, namely from the arcuate arteries, which are branches of the uterine vessels. It is worth repeating that the marked spiraling and twisting of the endometrial arteries is characteristic only of those few primates (among all mammals) that sustain menstruation, the apes, Old World monkeys, and women. An important characteristic of the secretory-phase endometrium is the striking growth and development of these *spiral,* or *coiled arteries,* which become much more tortuous at this time. In the compact layer, the arteries branch and the arterioles break up into capillaries within this zone. Superficially, a capillary network forms near the surface of the endometrium, and these are the vessels first invaded by the trophoblasts of the implanting blastocyst. Modifications of the spiral arteries are essential to the initiation of menstruation and in the establishment of the maternal blood supply to the syncytiotrophoblast, namely, the delivery of maternal blood to the intervillous space.

Premenstrual Phase. The premenstrual phase of the endometrial cycle encompasses the 2 to 5 days that precede menstruation, and corresponds in time to the regression of the corpus luteum and, in consequence, to the steady decline in plasma levels of progesterone and estradiol. During this latter stage of the secretory phase, there is regression of the endometrial growth cycle, which is characterized first by loss of tissue fluid in the superficial zone of the endometrium. This causes a striking reduction in the thickness of the endometrium; and as the thickness of the endometrium is reduced, the glands collapse. This obliges the spiral arteries to become even more coiled than before, resulting in increased resistance to arterial blood flow in these vessels. The stasis of blood that results brings about hypoxia of the endometrial tissue.

Another notable histological characteristic of the late premenstrual phase is the infiltration of the stroma by polymorphonuclear and mononuclear leukocytes, by which a pseudoinflammatory appearance is imparted to the tissue. The infiltration of neutrophils occurs primarily on the day or two immediately preceding the onset of menstruation. It has been demonstrated that the endometrial stromal cells produce interleukin-8 (IL-8), a chemotactic/activating factor for neutrophils (Arici and associates, 1992a). IL-8, produced in endometrial stromal cells, may act to recruit neutrophils to the endometrium just prior to the onset of menstruation. Similarly, the endometrial stromal cells are capable of synthesis of monocyte chemotactic peptide-1 (MCP-1) (Arici and associates, 1991, 1992b), a potent chemoattractant for monocytes as is TGF-β. Thus, the stromal cells also may function to recruit bone marrow-derived cells to the endometrium through the in situ formation of leukocyte chemoattractants.

Endometrial Ischemia. In a classic study, Markee (1940) was able to describe the tissue and vascular changes that occur before menstruation from direct observations of these alterations in endometrial tissue explants transplanted to the anterior chamber of the eye of the rhesus monkey. Markee studied, at magnifications of up to 150, 2 to 72 menstrual cycles in pieces of endometrial tissue in each of 41 monkeys. Markee observed 432 cycles during a 9-year study period. Each menstrual cycle of one monkey was studied for 6½ years! It was common practice for Markee to observe these transplants for 15 hours a day during times of menstruation. From these many detailed observations, Markee chose to describe the cyclic changes that occur in endo-

metrium as growth cycles. Menstruation, he concluded, occurred during a phase of regression of endometrial growth. He also emphasized that menstruation occurs only when regression in endometrial growth is sufficiently rapid and extensive. In particular, he found that regression in endometrial size (thickness) always preceded, accompanied, and followed bleeding; and this period of regression in endometrial growth began 2 to 5 days before the onset of menstrual bleeding.

Markee deduced that it was the marked changes in blood flow to the endometrium during the time of growth regression (as estrogen and progesterone withdrawal occurred) that determined whether menstruation eventuates in a given species. He also emphasized that the endometrium is supplied with blood by two types of vessels: (1) "straight" arteries supply the basal one third of endometrium and (2) "coiled" or spiral (curling) arteries supply the superficial two thirds of this tissue. During and preceding menstruation, the "straight" arteries do not contract.

Recall that the spiral arteries, during the time of endometrial growth, lengthen at a rate that is appreciably greater than the rate of increase in endometrial tissue volume (height or thickness); this discordance in growth between the two tissues causes an even greater coiling of these vessels. (Perrot-Applanat and associates, [1988] demonstrated the presence of progesterone and estrogen receptors in the smooth muscle cells of the uterine arteries, including the spiral arteries.) Recall also that with regression in the endometrial growth cycle, which commences concomitantly with the decline in corpus luteum function during an infertile cycle, an even greater coiling of the spiral arteries is obliged. When the coiling of the spiral arteries becomes severe, increased resistance to blood flow is created in these vessels; this becomes so striking that the severe stasis leads to hypoxia of the endometrium; and possibly in response to this hypoxia, vasodilatation at this time was sometimes observed (45 percent of cycles). Somewhat later, at 4 to 24 hours before the onset of bleeding into the endometrium, there was invariably a period of intense vasoconstriction of the spiral arteries. In consequence, the anemic appearance of the functional zone of the endometrium that results during this time of vasoconstriction may be striking.

Markee emphasized that *"the period of vasoconstriction preceding the onset of menstruation is the most striking and constant event of the menstrual cycle."* In his many observations, vasoconstriction preceded every menstrual period, always beginning 4 to 24 hours before the onset of bleeding. Based on this sequence of events, Markee reasoned that the vasoconstriction of these vessels served to limit blood loss at menstruation, whereas the reduction in spiral artery flow and resultant stasis prior to vasoconstriction was the primary mechanism operative to induce endometrial ischemia and thence tissue degeneration.

Markee hypothesized that a *"substance"* from the

hypoxic endometrium acted to induce the vasospasm of the spiral arteries. Thus, Markee's observations led him to surmise that a paracrine mechanism was involved in the induction of the characteristic premenstrual vasospasm of the spiral arteries; namely, a vasoconstrictor was produced by endometrial stromal cells. Casey and associates (Casey and MacDonald, 1992b; Economos and colleagues, 1992) suggest that this stromal cell "vasoconstrictor substance" may be endothelin-1.

Markee also noted that when, after a period of constriction, an individual coiled artery relaxed, hemorrhage occurred from that artery or its branches. Then, in sequence, the arterioles of these constricted arteries relax and bleed; the succession of small hemorrhages from individual arterioles or capillaries continues for a variable but very short time (seconds to a few minutes). Although this sequence of vasoconstriction, relaxation, and hemorrhage appears to be well established, the mechanism(s) that actually brings about the escape of blood from the vessels is not certain. It is possible that the damage to the walls of the vessels, which occurs during the period of intense vasoconstriction, results in the rupture of these vessels when the constricted segment relaxes and then blood flow is resumed.

In summary, Markee observed two (and sometimes three) entirely different vascular phenomena in endometrial transplants during the few days that precede menstrual bleeding. Beginning 1 to 5 days before the onset of menstruation, there is a period of slowed circulation, or relative *stasis*, during which *vasodilatation* sometimes occurs. Thereafter, there is a period of *vasoconstriction* that commences 4 to 24 hours before the extravasation of any blood. The period of stasis is extremely variable, from less than 24 hours to 4 days. It was Markee's opinion that the slowing of the circulation that leads to stasis is caused by the increased resistance to blood flow caused by the intense coiling of the spiral arteries. He observed that as more coils were added, the blood flow became increasingly slower. Another explanation, however, must be invoked for bleeding during anovulatory cycles and for bleeding that follows withdrawal of estrogen, in which circumstances the arteries may be quite simple or relatively uncoiled.

Menstrual Phase. Menstrual bleeding is of both arterial and venous origin, but arterial bleeding is, quantitatively, appreciably greater than venous. Bleeding appears at the outset to result from rhexis of an arteriole of a coiled artery with consequent formation of a hematoma, but occasionally it takes place by leakage through the vessel. When a hematoma forms, the superficial endometrium is distended and then ruptures. Subsequently, fissures develop in the adjacent functional layers, and blood, as well as fragments of tissue of various sizes, are detached. Although some tissue autolysis occurs, as a rule fragments of endometrium can be identified in the menstrual discharge collected from the vagina. Hemorrhage stops when the arterioles are again

constricted. The changes that accompany partial necrosis also serve to seal off the tip of the vessel; and in the superficial portion, often only the endothelium remains. The surface of the endometrium is restored, according to Markee, by growth of the flanges, or collars, that form the everted free ends of the uterine glands. These flanges increase in diameter very rapidly, and the continuity of the epithelium is reestablished by the fusion of the edges of these sheets of thin, migrating cells.

Role of Vasoactive Peptides Produced in the Endometrium in Menstruation. The prostaglandins, a unique class of bioactive tissue autacoids, are commonly synthesized in the cells in which these substances act or else in nearby cells. Thus, prostaglandins usually are autocrine- or paracrine-acting agents rather than endocrine or humoral hormones. In most tissues, prostaglandins are degraded rapidly in the tissues of origin or in nearby tissues, as well as in more remote sites such as the lungs. The prostaglandins are synthesized from an essential fatty acid, arachidonic acid. Arachidonic acid is present in tissues in an esterified form, primarily in the *sn*-2 position of glycerophospholipids. In this esterified form, arachidonic acid *cannot* be converted to prostaglandins. The enzyme, *phospholipase A₂*, catalyzes the hydrolysis of the *sn*-2 fatty acid ester of certain glycerophospholipids (e.g., phosphatidylcholine) to effect the release of free arachidonic acid. Other lipases, such as *phospholipase C*, which commonly act in concert in a series of reactions, catalyze the hydrolysis of arachidonic acid from other lipid stores, notably phosphatidylinositol. The rate of release of free arachidonic acid is commonly the rate-limiting step in the formation of prostaglandins in many tissues. Both endometrium and decidua are richly endowed with prostaglandin synthase activity. It also has been shown that the decidua is enriched with arachidonic acid. The potential role of prostaglandin formation in decidua in the maintenance of labor, after the initiation of parturition by other processes, is discussed in Chapter 12.

A role for prostaglandins in the initiation of menstruation has also been envisioned by many investigators. The administration of prostaglandins to nonpregnant women will cause the onset of menstruation, which is believed to be mediated by the induction of vasoconstriction of the endometrial spiral arteries. Large amounts of prostaglandins are found in menstrual blood, and prostaglandin administration to women gives rise to symptoms that mimic those of dysmenorrhea, which is commonly associated with normal ovulatory menses (menses initiated by progesterone withdrawal).

NAD^+-dependent 15-hydroxyprostaglandin dehydrogenase (PGDH), the enzyme that catalyzes the first reaction in the degradation of prostaglandins, is found in endometrium, principally in the cells of the glandular epithelium (Casey and co-workers, 1980). The specific activity of this enzyme is highest in endometrial tissues obtained during the early midluteal phase of the cycle, whereas it is barely detectable or absent on days 26 to 28, just before the onset of menses, and on days 1 to 5 during menses (Fig. 4–2). Thus, the specific activity of PGDH in endometrium initially appears to follow the levels of progesterone. But as progesterone levels reach a plateau, prostaglandin dehydrogenase activity falls precipitously. The half-life of this enzyme in tissue is very short. It has been hypothesized that the fall in prostaglandin dehydrogenase activity, as the levels of progesterone decline, and, in turn, the reduced rate of degradation of prostaglandins, may serve to permit an increase in the levels of prostaglandins in the endometrium, and thereby spiral artery vasoconstriction. Abel (1985) has provided a review of the role of prostaglandins in the endometrial cycle.

Another possibility, however, must be entertained in establishing the role of prostaglandins in the vascular control of the endometrium (Casey and MacDonald, 1992b). Prostaglandins are known to be produced in response to inflammation, hypoxia, or trauma, and are thereby one of the mediators of the inflammatory process. This comes about because with tissue insult, membrane glycerophospholipid hydrolysis occurs, resulting in arachidonic acid release. The cell must deal with free arachidonic acid; and a major mechanism for metabolizing arachidonic acid is through the formation of prostaglandins. Thus, prostaglandin formation in endometrium may be obliged because of the hypoxia caused by stasis of blood in the spiral arteries during progesterone withdrawal. This may account, in part, for Markee's observation that vasodilatation sometimes accompanied stasis of blood flow in the spiral arteries. PGE_2 and PGI_2 both act to cause vasodilation.

Therefore, a different paracrine system may be operative in the regulation of endometrial blood flow, namely the endothelin/enkephalinase system as proposed by Casey and associates. The endothelins (endothelin-1, -2, and -3) are small (21 amino acids) peptides that are the products of three separate genes. Endothelin-1 is a very potent vasoconstrictor, apparently the most potent ever described of natural origin. The prototype, endothelin-1, was first identified as a product of vascular endothelial cells (Yanagisawa and colleagues, 1988). It is synthesized as a much larger molecule (preproendothelin-1; 212 amino acids) that is processed in cellular sites of synthesis to big endothelin-1 (38 amino acids), which is, intrinsically, biologically inactive. Big endothelin-1 is converted by an unidentified enzyme(s) (endothelin converting enzyme) to mature endothelin-1, which is highly bioactive. The conversion of big endothelin-1 to endothelin-1 can occur in the cellular site of preproendothelin-1 biosynthesis, or in nearby cells, or even in cells distal to the site of synthesis after big endothelin-1 is transported by blood. Mature endothelin-1 acts in responsive cells by way of specific receptors designated A and B. The type A receptor is found in vascular smooth muscle cells, and type B receptors are generally identified in cells other than smooth muscle (Arai and colleagues, 1990; Sakurai and co-workers, 1990).

In considering the potential role of endothelin-1 as the spiral artery vasoconstrictor, it is interesting and potentially important to recognize that endothelin-1 is sometimes more potent as a vasoconstrictor when applied to the adventitial surface of blood vessels than when presented to the luminal surface. This response is likely attributable to the fact that endothelin-1 acts upon the luminal surface of endothelial cells to cause the formation of the vasorelaxants PGI_2 and endothelium-derived relaxing factor. Casey and colleagues proposed that endothelin-1, synthesized in endometrial stromal cells, acts upon the adventitial surface of the contiguous spiral arteries to cause the characteristic premenstrual vasoconstriction of these vessels. In support of this idea, they found that the preproendothelin-1 mRNA is expressed constitutively in human endometrium, and that the level of preproendothelin-1 mRNA is greater in tissues obtained during the premenstrual and menstrual

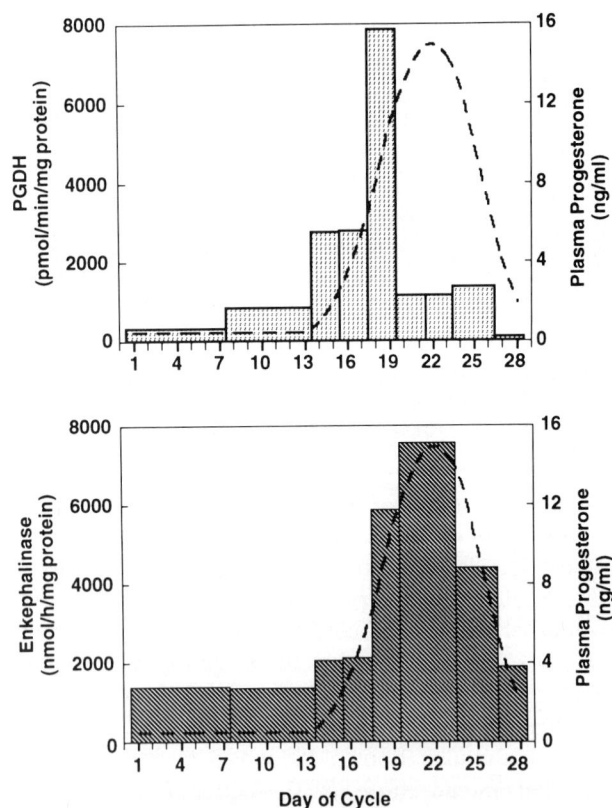

Fig. 4–2. *Top.* Specific activity (mean ± SEM) of PGDH in cytosolic fractions of human endometrial tissues obtained on various days of the menstrual cycle. *Bottom.* Specific activity of enkephalinase in endometrial tissue. Days of the menstrual cycle were idealized to that of a 28-day ovulatory cycle according to menstrual history, histological appearance of the endometrium, and serum progesterone concentrations on the day of endometrial sampling. (From Casey and colleagues, 1980, 1991.)

phases than at other times of the cycle. They also found that preproendothelin-1 mRNA is expressed constitutively in isolated endometrial stromal cells maintained in culture and the level of preproendothelin-1 mRNA in these cells is decreased by progestin treatment but increased by treatment with TGF-β1 and interleukin-1. These cells also secrete immunoreactive endothelin-1 into the culture medium.

They also pointed to the possibility that the net bioaction of endothelin-1 in endometrium can be regulated in a number of ways: (1) the rate of synthesis of big endothelin-1, (2) the conversion of inactive big endothelin-1 to mature endothelin-1, and (3) the degradation of endothelin-1. Endothelin-1 is degraded by the action of the enzyme enkephalinase, membrane metalloendopeptidase (EC 3.4.24.11), a plasma membrane ectoenzyme that is present in many cells. Enkephalinase serves to degrade a number of highly bioactive small (MW < 3000) peptides, including endothelin-1, -2, and -3, the enkephalins, atrial natriuretic peptide, and substance P. This enzyme is found in high specific activity, however, in only a few cells, specifically in cells in which the substrates it degrades are bioactive. For example, in brain cells, enkephalins; in kidney, atrial natriuretic peptide; in bronchial epithelium and intestine, substance P; and in endometrium, endothelin. This enzyme is localized in endometrial stromal cells, and the specific activity of enkephalinase in endometrial tissue increases strikingly as the blood level of progesterone increases. The highest specific activity of enkephalinase is found at the time of the midluteal phase of the ovarian cycle (Casey and associates, 1991). Thereafter, the specific activity of enkephalinase steadily declines as the plasma levels of progesterone decrease with regression of the corpus luteum (Fig. 4–2). By immunocytochemical techniques, enkephalinase is found localized in the stromal cells of the endometrium (Head and colleagues, in press).

The progesterone-induced increase in the specific activity of enkephalinase in endometrial stromal cells may be indicative of a mechanism for maintaining low tissue levels of endothelin-1 at the expected time of blastocyst implantation. By contrast, the decline in enkephalinase activity with regression of the corpus luteum should favor increased tissue levels of endothelin-1 during the premenstrual phase. In addition, increased levels of preproendothelin-1 mRNA and secretion of endothelin-1 should also be favored by progesterone withdrawal. In this reciprocal but coordinated manner, endothelin-1 derived from stromal cells is available to act as the premenstrual vasoconstrictor of the contiguous endometrial spiral arteries.

Very recently, the synthesis of another vasoactive peptide has been demonstrated in these same endometrial stromal cells. Parathyroid hormone-related protein (PTH-rP) and parathyroid hormone (PTH) are potent vasorelaxants. PTH-rP mRNA is expressed constitutively and immunoreactive PTH-rP is secreted by endometrial stromal cells in culture (Casey and associates, 1992). PTH-rP is the humoral hypercalcemia factor of malignancy, being identified in a wide assortment of neoplastic tissues and neoplastic cells in culture. PTH-rP acts in part as a PTH surrogate by way of the PTH plasma membrane receptor; and in this manner, PTH-rP, when secreted in large amounts by malignant tumors of the breast, ovary, lung, and other tissues, gives rise to a syndrome similar to hyperparathyroidism. PTH is an 84-amino acid peptide; PTH-rP is most commonly a 141-amino acid protein (but sometimes 139 or 173 amino acids). There is amino acid sequence homology between PTH and PTH-rP in only 8 or the first 13 N-terminal amino acids. There is no homology in the remaining portion of the PTH and PTH-rP molecules, which are products of separate genes on separate chromosomes.

The action of PTH and PTH-rP at the PTH receptor are accounted for principally (if not exclusively) by the N-terminal 27 amino acids. Acting by way of the PTH receptor, the two peptides are usually indistinguishable in bioaction and potency. Both serve as powerful stimulators of adenylate cyclase in responsive cells; and importantly, as stated, both act as vasorelaxants. Thus, it is possible that there is an endothelin-1/enkephalinase/PTH-rP system in endometrial stromal cells that is operative in modulating endometrial spiral arterial blood flow in a local, but hormonally responsive manner. The multiple potential roles of PTH-rP in other reproductive processes is further discussed in Chapters 6, 7, and 12.

Dating of the Endometrium by Histological Criteria. Benirschke (1986), in an excellent review, summarized the histological features of the endometrium that permit accurate dating of the tissues obtained after ovulation. Immediately after ovulation, days 14 to 16 (assuming ovulation on day 14) of an idealized 28-day menstrual cycle, and in response to the action of progesterone secreted by the developing corpus luteum, characteristic subnuclear, glycogen-rich vacuoles develop in the glandular epithelium. By day 17 to 18, the vacuoles have displaced the nuclei toward the middle of the cells, and mitoses are rare; by day 18, mitosis has ceased. The cellular migration of vacuoles continues past the nuclei toward the luminal surface of the glands, and by day 20, near-maximum secretion into the lumen is evident. At this time, only a few vacuoles remain in the glandular cells. During the early luteal phase of the cycle, mitosis ceases but the glands become more tortuous as the luteal response continues.

Simultaneously, there are hormonally induced changes in the stroma—indeed, by days 20 to 21, there is considerable interstitial edema and abundant ground substance. Predecidualization is underway by days 23 to 24 of the menstrual cycle, a process that consists of an increase in the cytoplasm of stromal cells—commencing first in cells around the spiral arterioles. Thereafter, the predecidual changes extend throughout the stroma. This is an interesting occurrence because progesterone secretion by the corpus luteum has already begun to decline by this time in infertile ovarian cycles, and decidualization is believed to be caused in large measure by the action of progesterone. This is suggestive that other stimuli are necessary to evoke decidualization; in fact, complete decidualization of the human endometrium does not occur until after blastocyst implantation.

The premenstrual phase of the endometrial cycle (days 24 to 28) is characterized by a marked decrease in thickness of the endometrium, extravasation of blood, and disassociation and thence disintegration of stromal cells. In Benirschke's description of these morphological changes, he points out that, "amazingly," at a time when the surface epithelium of the premenstrual endometrium is still intact, there is extensive hemorrhage into and disintegration of the stroma.

Ultrastructure. From the findings of Wynn and associates (1967a,b) and White and Buchsbaum (1973), who studied the ultrastructure of the endometrium, there is secretion of cytoplasmic components of the endometrial cells into the glandular lumens throughout the menstrual cycle (Figs. 4–3 and 4–4). The terms *prolif-*

erative and *secretory* therefore, less accurately reflect the histological pattern of the endometrium than the terms *preovulatory* (follicular) and *postovulatory* (luteal).

The Endometrial Cycle in Retrospect. The correlations of the hormonal events of the ovarian cycle, the morphological changes of the endometrial cycle, and the action of the pituitary gonadotropic hormones are summarized in Table 4–1 and in Figure 4–5. Commonly, we presume (incorrectly) that the ovarian cycle and the endometrial or menstrual cycle are coincident in time. And again, somewhat incorrectly, the follicular phase of the ovarian cycle is presumed to be coincident with the proliferative phase of the endometrial or menstrual cycle. At the same time, the terms *luteal phase* and *secretory phase* have been regarded, in terms of the cycle, to be coincident if not synonymous.

The ovarian cycle as we now understand it, and the menstrual cycle as we define it (the endometrial cycle that begins on the first day of menses), are not coincident. The recruitment of follicles in the ovary, presumably brought about in part by a modest but significant increase in FSH secretion, commences not with menstruation but a few days before the onset of menses, at a time during maximum regression of the corpus luteum;

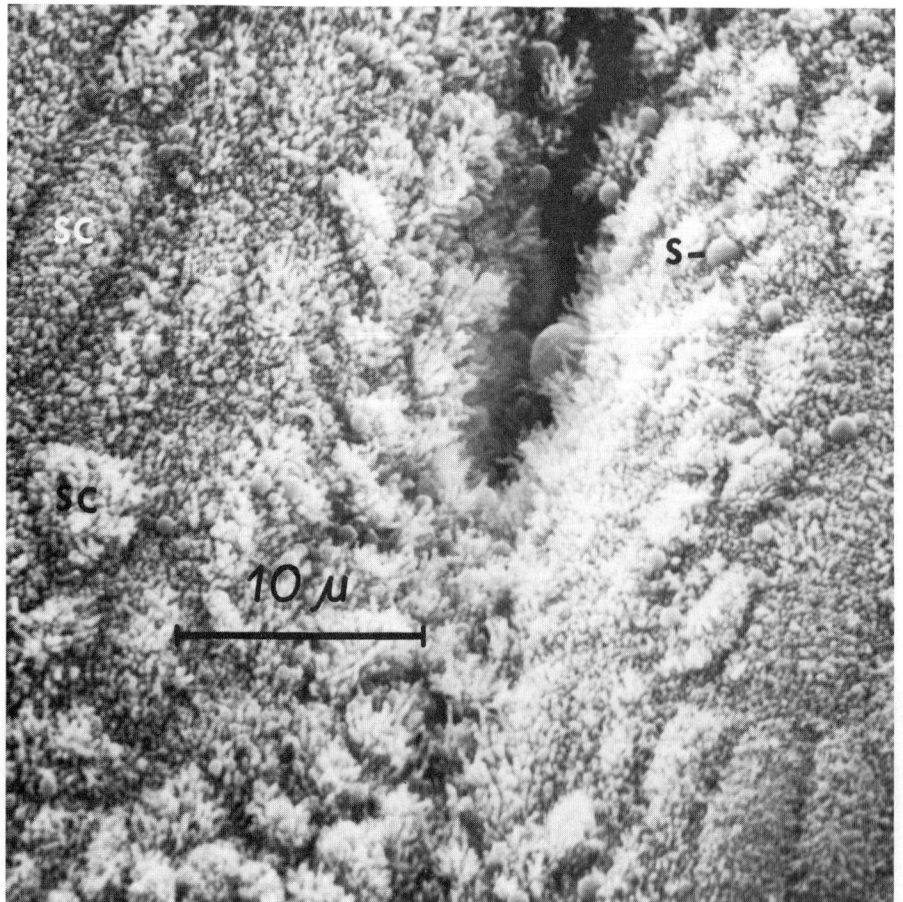

Fig. 4–3. Gland ostium and surrounding endometrium in preovulatory phase by scanning electron microscopy. Many secretory droplets are seen on cell surfaces. Microvilli are prominent on secretory cells (SC) and individual cell margins are identified. (From White and Buchsbaum, 1973.)

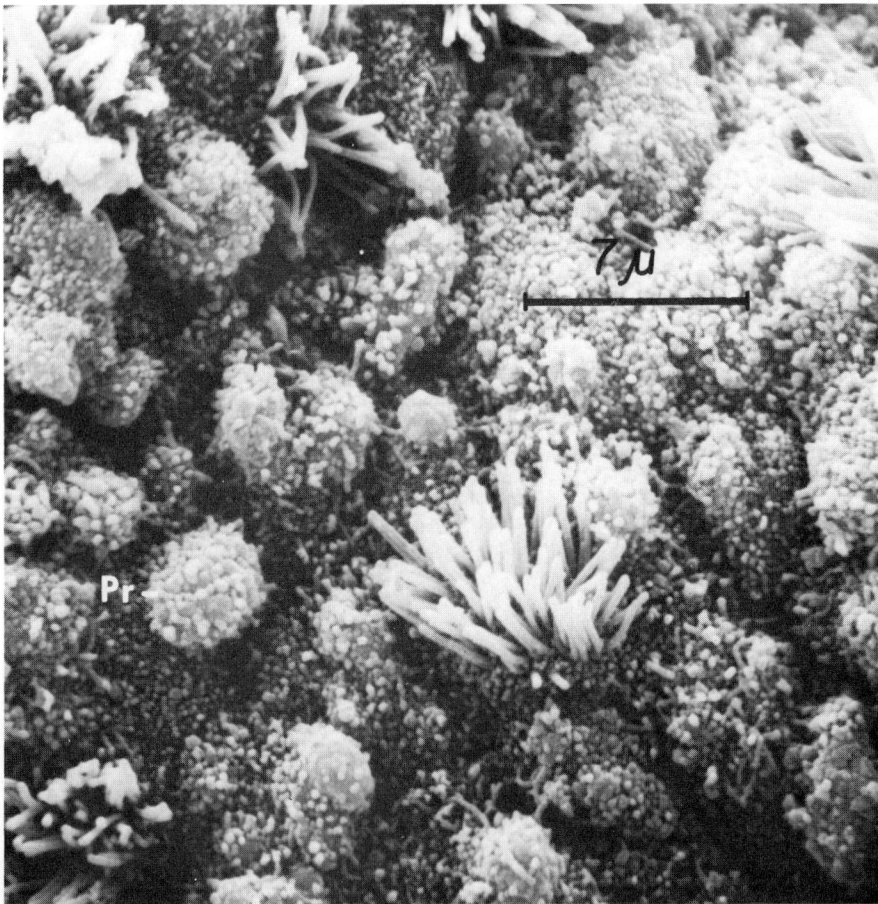

Fig. 4–4. Cellular detail for phase endometrium on day 24 of the menstrual cycle, demonstrated by scanning electron microscopy. Microvilli are prominent and cellular protuberances are evident. (From White and Buchsbaum, 1973.)

indeed, the preceding ovarian cycle terminates before the onset of menstruation as the corpus luteum of the succeeding ovarian cycle regresses.

Although the cycles are divided into phases for descriptive purposes and for convenience of description, the changes are continuous throughout an ovulatory cycle. Furthermore, there is considerable individual variation in both the activity of the endocrine glands and in the response of the target organ, the uterus. Secretory changes that closely resemble those of the luteal phase may occasionally appear before ovulation.

Anovulatory cycles sometimes occur in otherwise apparently normal women, but the incidence is difficult to establish because adequate observations of the ovaries are rarely possible. It appears that in some such cycles, a follicle enlarges but then becomes cystic and degenerates. In others, no follicles grow beyond a few millimeters throughout the entire cycle. Withdrawal of progesterone, therefore, is not absolutely essential for uterine bleeding because uterine bleeding, albeit unpredictable in time of onset, duration, and amount, sometimes occurs in anovulatory women. **In women with persistent anovulation, endometrial bleeding is not cyclic unless the women are ingesting sex steroids that promote bleeding.**

At about 27 to 35 days after the first day of the last menstrual period, there may be bleeding around the site of implantation of the fertilized ovum, an event that results in slight vaginal bleeding that is sometimes mistaken for menses. This "placental sign" of bleeding always occurs during pregnancy in the rhesus monkey (Hartman, 1932).

Clinical Aspects of Menstruation

Menstruation per se is the periodic discharge of blood, mucus, and cellular debris from the uterine mucosa and occurs at more or less regular, cyclic, and predictable intervals from menarche to menopause except during periods of pregnancy, lactation, anovulation, or pharmacological intervention. It is convenient and more accurate to use the word menstruation to refer to the bleeding that accompanies progesterone withdrawal after ovulation, and to refer to other episodes of endometrial hemorrhage as uterine bleeding.

From the biological perspective, menstruation is clear-cut evidence of fertility failure. And from this perspective, the role of repetitive ovulation and the formation of progesterone in massive quantities is brought

TABLE 4–1. IMPORTANT MILESTONES IN THE CORRELATION OF OVARIAN AND ENDOMETRIAL (MENSTRUAL) CYCLES (IDEALIZED 28-DAY CYCLE)

	Phase					
Menstrual (1–5 days)	**Early Follicular (6–8 days)**	**Advanced Follicular (9–13 days)**	**Ovulation (14 days)**	**Early Luteal (15–19 days)**	**Advanced Luteal (20–25 days)**	**Premenstrual (26–28 days)**
Ovary						
Formation of corpus albicans from corpus luteum of preceding cycle. Recruitment of follicles.	Folicular maturation and development of the chosen or dominant follicle.		Ovulation and luteinization of granulosa cells in the ruptured follicle.	Vascularization of granulosa lutein cells and formation of corpus luteum. Follicular atresia.	Mature corpus luteum and continued follicular atresia.	Involution of corpus luteum and initiation of follicular recruitment for the next cycle.
Estrogen						
Low; derived principally from extraglandularly produced estrone; little estradiol-17β secretion by the ovary.	Estradiol-17β secretion, principally by granulosa cells of the dominant follicle, increases strikingly, maximal rates being attained just prior to the LH surge.		Immediately after, or coincident with, ovulation, there is an abrupt, indeed, precipitous decline in estradiol-17β secretion.	Gradual and progressive postovulatory rise in estradiol-17β secretion by the corpus luteum.	Maximal rates of postovulatory estradiol-17β secretion are attained; luteal phase estradiol-17β secretion rates, however, are not nearly as great as those observed in the immediate preovulatory phase.	Estradiol-17β secretion declines precipitously and, as during menstruation, the principal estrogen produced is estrone, which is formed in extraglandular sites.
Progesterone						
Low secretion; there is little secretion of progesterone by the adrenal cortex and the corpus luteum of the preceding ovarian cycle has regressed.	During the follicular phase of the ovarian cycle, progesterone levels remain low. This is due to the fact that human granulosa cells cannot synthesize cholesterol, the obligate precursor of progesterone, but are dependent upon LDL cholesterol that can be obtained only from the blood after vascularization of the granulosa cells after ovulation.		Progesterone secretion increases steadily as the consequence of the availability of LDL and LH action to effect cholesterol side-chain cleavage.	Progesterone secretion remains high until the end of the advanced luteal phase.		Precipitous decline in progesterone secretion.
Endometrium						
Menstrual desquamation and early reorganization of endometrial glandular epithelium.	Proliferation of glandular epithelium with many mitoses.	Pseudostratification of nuclei—no secretion, early stromal changes.	Appearance of subnuclear vacuoles that are rich in glycogen.	Migration of vacuoles to the luminal surface; cessation of mitosis. The endometrial glands become very tortuous.	Vacuoles have been secreted and decidualization commences. Stromal edema and enlargement of stromal cells is prominent.	Disruption and disintegration of stromal cells. Leukocyte infiltration and interstitial hemorrhage.
Pituitary Secretion: FSH						
Continuing decline in FSH levels that had become modestly increased coincident with the decline in steroid secretion by the regressing corpus luteum of the preceding cycle.	FSH secretion is at all times pulsatile in nature, but during the proliferative phase of the ovarian cycle, prior to the time of the LH surge at midcycle, FSH levels remain low.		There is a significant surge of FSH secretion, albeit less prominent than that of LH, that heralds the commencement of the ovulatory process.	After the midcycle gonadotropin surge, FSH levels fall abruptly to levels similar to those found during the preovulatory phase of the cycle.		As steroid secretion by the regressing corpus luteum diminishes, there is a modest but significant increase in FSH.
Pituitary Secretion: LH						
The levels of LH are low and reasonably constant until just prior to ovulation.			Coincident with, or just after, the striking increase in estradiol-17β secretion by the dominant follicle, there is a striking increase in LH secretion—the LH "surge."	The levels of LH are low and reasonably constant until just prior to ovulation.		

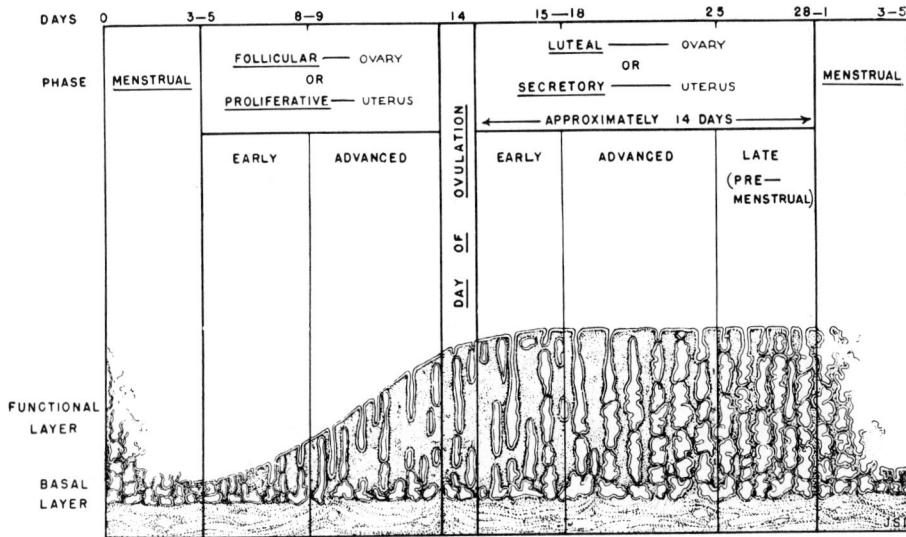

Fig. 4–5. Cyclic changes in thickness and in form of glands and arteries of endometrium and the relation of these changes to those of the ovarian cycle.

into a *pathophysiological* mode rather than an evolutionarily developed physiological process. Namely, we must consider the formation of progesterone by the corpus luteum in nonfertile cycles as an endocrinopathy; this is the case because in the absence of pregnancy, the formation of progesterone is clear-cut physiological futility. This issue is considered further in a discussion of the biogenesis of the premenstrual syndromes.

The Menarche and Puberty. Historically, the age at which menstruation begins, *menarche,* has declined steadily until recent years (Fig. 4–6). This decline in age of menarche has ceased in women living in the United States. The average time at which menstruation begins is now between 12 and 13 years of age, but in

a small number of apparently normal girls, menarche may occur as early as the 10th or as late as the 16th year. The term menarche refers specifically to the first menstruation, whereas puberty is a more general term that encompasses the entire transitional stage between childhood and sexual maturity. The menarche is just one sign of puberty; but if menarche is the consequence of ovulation (and attendant hormonal secretion), it is indicative of the completion of the fundamental physiological events of puberty, namely the release of an ovum.

Interval. Although the *modal interval* at which menstruation recurs is considered to be 28 days, there is considerable variation among women in general, as well as in the cycle lengths of a given woman. Marked variation in the intervals between menstrual cycles does not necessarily mean infertility.

Arey (1939), who analyzed 12 studies comprising about 20,000 calendar records from 1500 women, reached the conclusion that there is no evidence of perfect menstrual cycle regularity. In a study by Gunn and co-workers (1937) of 479 normal British women, the typical difference between the shortest and the longest cycle was 8 or 9 days. In 30 percent of women, it was more than 13 days, but in no woman was it fewer than 2 days. Arey found that in an average adult woman, one third of her cycles departed by more than 2 days from the mean of the lengths of her cycles. Arey's analysis of 5322 cycles in 485 normal women was indicative of an average interval of 28.4 days; his finding for the average cycle length in pubertal girls was longer, 33.9 days. Chiazze and associates (1968) analyzed the intervals between 30,655 menstrual cycles of 2316 women. The mean for all cycles was 29.1 days. For cycles that range from 15 to 45 days, the average length was 28.1 days. The degree of variability was such that only 13

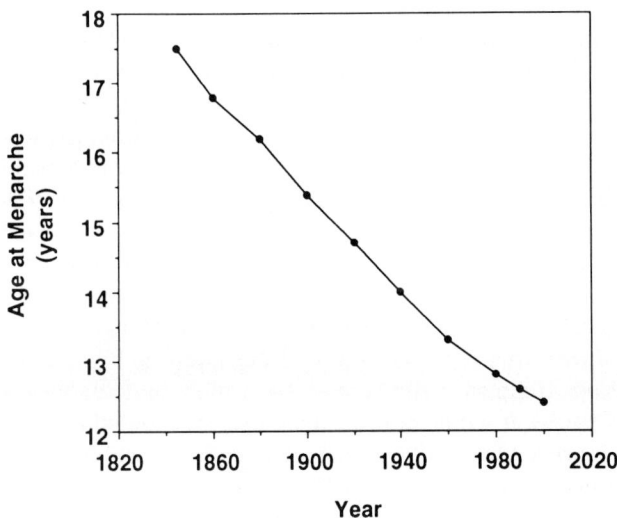

Fig. 4–6. Age of menarche from 1830 to 1990. (From MacDonald and colleagues, 1991, with permission.)

percent of the women experienced cycles that varied in length by less than 6 days. Haman (1942) surveyed 2460 cycles in 150 housewives who attended a clinic where special attention was directed to recording accurately the length of the menstrual cycles. Arey's data and those of Haman, which are similar, and the distribution curves (computed from averages of these data), are shown in Figure 4–7.

Duration and Amount. The duration of menstrual flow is also variable; the usual duration is 4 to 6 days, but bleeding for 2 to 8 days may be considered normal. In any individual woman, however, the duration of the menstrual flow is usually reasonably similar from cycle to cycle.

The menstrual discharge consists of shed fragments of endometrium mixed with a variable quantity of blood. Usually the blood is liquid, but if the rate of hemorrhage is excessive, clots of various sizes may appear. Considerable attention has been directed to the usual state of incoagulability of menstrual blood. The most logical explanation for the incoagulability is that the blood was coagulated as it was shed, but thereafter was liquefied by fibrinolytic activity. There are potent thromboplastic properties of endometrium that promptly initiate clotting, but there are also potent fibrinolytic properties (plasmin) that effect prompt lysis of fibrin clots. Plasmin is formed by way of the action of plasminogen activator (produced in endometrium) on blood-borne plasminogen. It is quite likely that hormonal regulation of plasminogen activator and plasminogen activator inhibitor are important cellular features of the biochemical regulation of menstruation.

The extrusion of clots with uterine bleeding is also suggestive of anovulation (bleeding that occurs without benefit of progesterone action and withdrawal).

The average amount of blood lost by women during a normal menstrual period has been determined by several groups of investigators, who found it to range from about 25 to 60 mL (Baldwin and associates, 1961; Barker and Fowler, 1936; Hallberg and co-workers, 1966; Hytten and associates, 1964; Millis, 1951). With a normal hemoglobin concentration of 14 g/dL and a hemoglobin iron content of 3.4 mg/g, these volumes of blood contain from 12 to 29 mg of iron and represent a blood loss equivalent to 0.4 to 1.0 mg of iron for every day of the cycle, or from 150 to 400 mg/year. Finch (1959) determined the rate of decrease in the specific activity of the miscible iron of the body for a period of years after the injection of [55]Fe to ascertain the rate of loss of iron from the body. In women who menstruated, the iron loss on average was 0.6 mg/day more than the iron loss in men or postmenopausal women. Because the amount of iron that is absorbed from the diet is usually quite limited, this seemingly "negligible" iron loss is quantitatively important, because it contributes further to the low iron stores that are present in the majority of women (Hallberg and co-workers, 1968; Scott and Pritchard, 1967).

Actually, the blood loss at menstruation is relatively small, especially considering that the surface area of the endometrium of normal uteri of nonpregnant women is 10 to 45 cm^2 (Chimbira and colleagues, 1980). Therefore, there must be an effective means of hemostasis in the endometrium during menstruation. The control of blood loss is likely not appreciably effected by myometrial contractions to compress uterine vessels, because inhibitors of prostaglandin synthesis usually serve to reduce blood loss during menstruation. On the other hand, excessive blood loss is common in women with coagulation or platelet disorders. It is likely, therefore, that hemostasis in endometrium is effected by hemostatic plug formation as in other tissues (Christiaens and associates, 1985) and by spiral artery vasoconstriction.

Changes in Body Weight During the Ovarian Cycle. It has been frequently reported that about 30 percent of women gain 1 to 3 pounds shortly before the onset of menstruation, an amount of weight that is promptly lost as menstruation begins. Although only a minority of women manifest weight gains, there has been a tendency to regard the increase in weight as a normal characteristic of the cycle that is reflective of the influence of steroid hormones. Actually, the average weight gain is insignificant, perhaps a quarter of a pound, as shown in a statistical study of this question by Chesley and Hellman (1957) and by Golub and associates (1965). It would appear, therefore, that the concept of appreciable premenstrual weight gain as a physiological phenomenon is not valid. Preece and co-workers (1975) could find no consistent change in total body water during the menstrual cycle.

On the other hand, it is possible that we have not

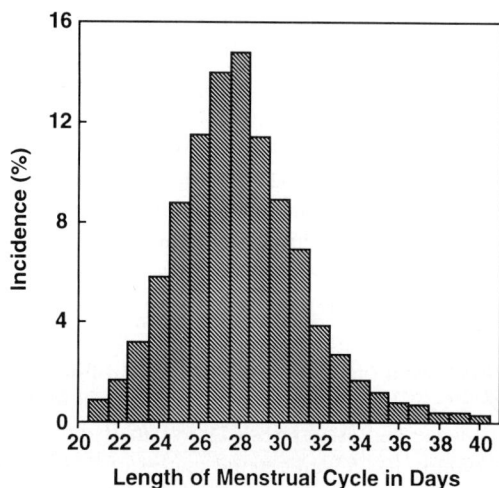

Fig. 4–7. Duration of menstrual cycle based on distribution data of Arey (1939) and Haman (1942).

conducted the proper studies to evaluate weight gain due to increases in body water. Most studies have been performed by carefully weighing women in the morning after first micturition. First, it is possible that the increased glomerular filtration rate of the supine position during sleep leads to a water diuresis and thus eliminates from consideration the excess water loss that occurred during the night. Second, it is likely that significant fluid retention during the luteal phase affects only a portion of ovulatory women.

These are important considerations in future evaluations of the changes in sodium and water homeostasis during the luteal phase of the ovarian cycle and in deciphering the potential causes of the premenstrual syndromes. During the midluteal phase of the ovarian cycle, there is a sizable increase in the rate of secretion of aldosterone by the adrenal cortex. Presumably this increase in aldosterone secretion is in response to the natriuretic effect of progesterone, which is produced in large amounts by the corpus luteum. Increased sodium excretion favors the release of renin from the juxtaglomerular apparatus of kidney, leading to increased angiotensin II formation; and, angiotensin II is the principal stimulus of aldosterone secretion by the adrenal gland. But in addition, there is a striking increase in the production of another mineralocorticosteroid, deoxycorticosterone, during the midluteal phase of the ovarian cycle and during pregnancy. This comes about by way of the extraadrenal conversion of plasma progesterone to deoxycorticosterone through the action of a steroid 21-hydroxylase activity in nonadrenal tissues, including tissues of mineralocorticosteroid action. But there is a wide variation among women (30-fold) in the extent of conversion of plasma progesterone to deoxycorticosterone (Casey and MacDonald, 1982).

The increase in mineralocorticosteroid formation during the luteal phase of the cycle, which persists in fertile cycles and increases as pregnancy progresses, is one of the early adaptations of the maternal organism to pregnancy (Chap. 8), facilitating the expansion of the maternal blood volume.

Premenstrual Syndromes

In Chapter 2, we put forward the notion that the recurrent secretion and withdrawal of progesterone in women who choose to be infertile is clearly physiological futility. There is no doubt that the extraordinary physiological expenditures of the ovarian cycle are invested in ovulation, fertilization, and implantation—that is, in pregnancy.

There is no physiological merit of any sort known for progesterone secretion and action, other than pregnancy. This is a very important concept because it obliges a consideration of the potential undesirable side effects of progesterone when this steroid is produced repetitively in massive amounts and then withdrawn for no physiological purpose, when pregnancy is not desired.

It is reasonable to suspect, therefore, that repetitive ovulation and menstruation in modern women is the result of far greater intellectual than biological evolution. As cited in Chapter 2, in populations of women in whom early marriage was the rule and in whom contraception was not practiced, menstruation was uncommon. Pregnancy occurred with ovulation in early adolescence; and after delivery, anovulation and amenorrhea persisted during lactation; and, breast feeding was continued for 2 or 3 years or more, depending upon the availability of soft food for the infant. Thereafter, pregnancy occurred again and again, and by the time that 6 to 10 pregnancy–lactation episodes were completed, death occurred or ovarian function and ovulation ceased at menopause. Menstruation was rare.

In modern times, the development of safe and effective contraceptive agents, according to Baird (1985), who also referred to the writings of his father, Sir Dugald Baird, *"has relieved [women] from the tyranny of excessive fertility—'the fifth freedom.' Because the social and physical demands of continuous [pregnancy and] breast-feeding are unlikely to be acceptable to women of the 20th century,"* they have chosen menstruation as an alternative, *"in the absence of a simple, safe means of inducing amenorrhea pharmacologically."* Accordingly, menstruation must be viewed, in a physiological sense, as the end-result of fertility failure, whether the infertility was purposefully chosen or naturally occurring.

This perspective on reproductive function in women is appropriate in a treatise on obstetrics for two reasons. First, it emphasizes the natural propensity of humans to reproduce; and, as we will emphasize repeatedly, obliges all physicians involved in the health care of women to be constantly alert to the possibility that pregnancy may exist in any woman in the reproductive age range who seeks medical care.

Second, a variety of maladies, sometimes disabling, beset many ovulatory women in a recurrent manner during the luteal phase of the ovarian cycle. The biological basis for this association is not defined; much evidence, however, points to the involvement of progesterone in the biogenesis of these *premenstrual syndromes* (PMS) (MacDonald and associates, 1991).

Recurrent Progesterone Secretion As an Endocrinopathy. The symptoms of PMS include disorders in mood, behavior, and physical well-being. And commonly, characteristic clusters of such symptoms recur in the same woman month after month. It is important to recognize that the cyclic recurrence of these symptoms of PMS is restricted to women in whom progesterone is produced in large amounts and then withdrawn, and that the symptoms of PMS recur and are limited to the time of progesterone secretion or withdrawal. Specifically, PMS is limited to ovulatory women. These symptoms do not recur in prepubertal, postmenopausal, anovulatory, or castrate women; and PMS-like symptoms do not recur in women treated with estrogen, whether given continuously or cyclically. Moreover, the symptoms of PMS are relieved by treatment with gonadotropin releasing hormone (GnRH) agonists to arrest ovarian function, and by oophorectomy. All of these correlates point directly to an involvement of progesterone in the biogenesis of PMS.

The Biogenesis of PMS.

We suggest that a major impediment to progress in defining the biological basis of PMS is attributable to the view of clinicians, basic scientists, and the general public alike that recurrent ovulation (with massive progesterone secretion) and thence menstruation is the biological evolutionary norm for young women. In consequence, many researchers have presumed that aberrations in well-being should not accrue from processes that are physiologically normal. Therefore, they have searched for a physiological abnormality to explain PMS. With all good intentions, we have reassured our daughters that cyclic menstruation is normal; and from this perspective, it has been assumed by many women that repetitive menstruation is equated with femininity. If this prevalant premise that recurrent ovulation is the biological evolutionary norm were incorrect, it would be easier to accept the likelihood that the recurrent secretion and withdrawal of progesterone is an endocrinopathy that is pivotal in the development of luteal phase disabilities.

The idea that recurrent ovulation with massive progesterone secretion is an endocrinopathy is not a new concept, but it is one that has been difficult to embrace and heretofore not possible to establish. Indeed, the high incidences of PMS frequently reported have puzzled some observers, as it seemed pejorative to identify upwards of 75 percent of women as ill or physically incapacitated. Rather, it has been generally accepted that (aside from pregnancy) cyclic ovulation and menstruation is the pinnacle of endocrinological normality in reproductive-age women. In the past several editions of this book, we have emphasized, with great conviction, that such a history is highly suggestive of recurrent ovulation, corpus luteum formation, and progesterone secretion; and from the perspective of ovarian function, therefore, recurrent, cyclic, spontaneous menstruation is evidence of the potential for fertility. Indisputably, the brain–pituitary–ovarian cycle that culminates in ovulation is one of the most majestic physiological events in biology; and, the sex-hormone–induced biochemical and morphological antecedents of menstruation, eventuating in intense vasospasm of the endometrial spiral arterioles, and culminating in the near-complete shedding of the endometrium, add a unique physiological finale to this remarkable process.

Natural History of Human Reproduction.

But even though ovulation is the penultimate in ovarian physiological achievement, the long-standing repetition of this process at approximately monthly intervals (with attendant menstruation) cannot be considered to be the norm for women. **Therefore, it is misleading to assume that repetitive ovulation/progesterone secretion/menstruation for many years is the evolutionary norm, however universal these phenomena may be among young women.** If the vast majority of women about us were prepubertal, postmenopausal, pregnant, or lactating, then repetitive, cyclic ovulation (and menstruation) would not be viewed as normal. Even the recognition of this predicament is not new; over 75 years ago Whitehouse (1914) observed: *"Periodic uterine hemorrhage is, in fact, one of the sacrifices which women must offer at the altar of evolution and civilization."*

And in recent years, this problem has worsened. It was only 150 years ago that the average age of menarche among European girls was 17½ years (Tanner, 1962). As menarche today occurs, on average, at 12½ years, this difference in age of menarche alone has increased the number of ovulatory cycles for today's woman, who lives until menopause, by 15 percent (or approximately 65 cycles). With menarche at 17½ years of age, and eight pregnancy–lactation episodes of 4 years each, menstruation was eliminated almost completely. This is not an unreasonable number of pregnancies for women who do not practice contraception (Chap. 2).

This formulation of the reproductive status of modern woman is not intended to imply that there is a metabolic advantage to be gained from repeated pregnancy–lactation episodes. On the contrary, we submit that the biological evolution of humans has stood still compared with the intellectual development of women and their biological needs for optimal well-being. It is from this perspective, however, that we do argue in favor of a role for progesterone, and its metabolites, in the pathogenesis of PMS, which occurs commonly but *uniquely* in ovulatory women.

The Case for Progesterone and PMS.

Progesterone is produced in massive amounts during the luteal phase of each ovarian cycle; indeed, the secretory rate of progesterone at these times is greater, by a large margin, than that of any other steroid hormone produced in men or nonpregnant women (Fig. 4–8).

The question is: How does progesterone bring about PMS in some but not all women? Until relatively recently, it was believed that progesterone action was mediated singularly by way of the progesterone receptor (and the progesterone response element in selected genes). Thereby, genomic actions were effected in responsive cells—cells in which the progesterone receptor is expressed. Based on this presumption, there was no known action of progesterone that

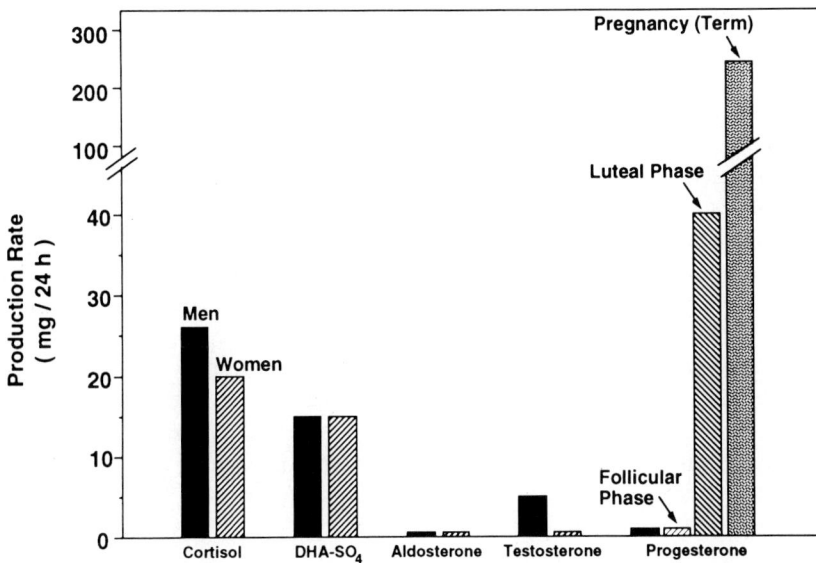

Fig. 4–8. Steroid production rates in men and women. (From MacDonald and colleagues, 1991, with permission.)

would implicate progesterone in the biogenesis of PMS, let alone explain the striking differences among ovulatory women in the spectrum or severity of PMS symptoms that are known to characterize this disorder(s).

During the past decade we have learned that the biological actions of progesterone are mediated not only by the progesterone receptor through classical genomic processes, but in addition, progesterone can exert biological effects by a number of other cellular mechanisms. As examples, progesterone acts at the level of the plasma membrane of selected cells by a nongenomic mechanism to inhibit the activation of adenylate cyclase (e.g., in oocytes and in spermatozoa). Progesterone, after extraadrenal 21-hydroxylation to form deoxycorticosterone, acts by way of the mineralocorticosteroid receptor. And the metabolites of progesterone, formed by reduction at C-5 and C-3, act in brain in a nongenomic manner on the gamma-aminobutyric acid (GABA)$_A$ receptor to modulate the actions of GABA.

Based on these newly discovered actions of progesterone, it has been theorized that PMS may be caused by progesterone and its metabolites. Specifically, it has been proposed that (1) the extrahepatic metabolism of progesterone is strikingly dissimilar among women and (2) that there will be a close correlation between the metabolic fate of progesterone and the recurrence of PMS (MacDonald and associates, 1991). This theory evolved first from the findings that (1) the fractional metabolism of progesterone to deoxycorticosterone varies by 30-fold among women and (2) the 5α-reduced metabolites of progesterone are bioactive in brain to modulate the action of the neuroinhibitory amino acid, GABA.

GABA acts by way of the GABA$_A$ receptor as an anxiolytic-type of neurotransmitter. The GABA$_A$ receptor complex is a chloride channel; GABA acts to maintain this channel in an open state favoring the influx of chloride ions into the cell. GABA producing neurons and GABA$_A$ receptors are widely distributed in brain. Increased chloride entry into brain cells serves to hyperpolarize the cell membrane and thereby to inhibit neural transmission. The benzodiazepine class of drugs act at the GABA$_A$ receptor in a manner analogous to that of the 5α-reduced metabolites of progesterone, namely to modify the affinity of the GABA$_A$ receptor for GABA. The end result is increased GABA action and anxiolysis or anesthesia.

It has been known for more than 50 years that metabolites of progesterone, administered to experimental animals or to humans, causes anesthesia. Based on this information, steroidal anesthetics were produced for use in humans. Many hundreds of cesarean sections have been conducted in Great Britain with the steroid anesthetic, althesin, which is 11-keto-5α-pregnane-3α-ol-20-one. These types of metabolites of progesterone are produced endogenously in women during the luteal phase of the cycle when progesterone levels are high.

The importance of these bioactive metabolites of progesterone in the biogenesis of PMS likely resides in the sterospecificity of their actions and in differences in the rates of formation of these compounds because of variation among women in extrahepatic progesterone metabolism.

It has already been demonstrated that the fractional conversion of plasma progesterone to deoxycorticosterone varies markedly (30-fold) among women, thus accounting for wide variations among women in the production rate of deoxycorticosterone during the luteal phase of the ovarian cycle. Thus, when progesterone is present in plasma, deoxycorticosterone is produced in a manner that is not regulated by ACTH or angiotensin II. Extraadrenal deoxycorticosterone formation is governed by the plasma levels of progesterone, and a given woman's inherent capacity for 21-hydroxylation in nonadrenal tissues (for review: Casey and MacDonald, 1982).

A similar variability among women in the relative rates of formation of anxiolytic steroid metabolites of progesterone may give rise to modifications in mood and behavior during times of progesterone production and withdrawal in the late luteal phase of the ovarian cycle.

In addition, we now know that progesterone acts in the endometrium to induce an increase in enkephalinase activity (Casey and colleagues, 1991). If progesterone also acts in brain to cause an increase in enkephalinase, enkephalin withdrawal will occur; this event will also favor the development of the symptoms of PMS.

Metabolism of Progesterone. It is difficult to believe that before 1990, the metabolic fate of the vast majority of progesterone produced in women was unknown. To be sure, there were well-characterized metabolites of progesterone that had been isolated from urine. But the total urinary and fecal excretion of identifiable progesterone metabolites accounted for only 30 to 40 percent of progesterone produced or of radiolabeled progesterone administered. The majority of identified progesterone metabolites were reduced in the C-5β position, for example, 5β-pregnanolone and 5β-pregnanediol. We now recognize that these metabolites were found because 5β-reduced metabolites are formed in liver, and the hepatocytes are conjugated with glucuronic acid. The 5β-reduced compounds are better substrates for the hepatic glucuronyl transferase enzyme. The highly water soluble glucuronic acid-conjugated metabolites are readily excreted in urine. Recently it has been demonstrated that the majority (50 to 70 percent) of progesterone is metabolized by 5α-reduction, and much of this metabolic pathway is accounted for in extrahepatic tissues. Ultimately, most of the 5α-reduced metabolites are conjugated with sulfuric acid in the liver; the sulfate conjugates are excreted in bile; and in the intestine, these sulfoconjugates are acted upon by intestinal bacterial enzymes to give products that are not readily identifiable (MacDonald and associates, 1991.)

The Metabolic Futility of Progesterone Production. Therefore, the recurrent secretion of progesterone during infertile ovarian cycles not only constitutes physiological futility but may represent an endocrinopathy that causes significant emotional and physical disability in women. It is vitally important that research be directed to find a reasonable means of establishing effective human contraception. As an intermediate goal, women must be able to choose infertility without obliging the endocrinopathy of recurrent progesterone secretion and withdrawal or the pharmacologically substituted and equally futile process of repetitious exogenous hormone-induced menstruation.

The Menopause and Climacteric

Menopause is the cessation of menses. There are wide variations in the age at which menopause occurs. About one half of all women cease menstruating between the ages of 45 and 50, about one quarter stop before the age of 45, and another one quarter continue cyclic menstruation until past 50 years of age. The term *climacteric* is derived from the Greek word that means "rung of a ladder," and bears the same relation to the menopause as the term *puberty* bears to menarche. The climacteric refers to the time in a woman's life known to the laity as the "change of life."

For a variety of clinical reasons, it is important to understand the role of the postmenopausal ovary in sex steroid hormone formation. There have been claims that estrogen is produced by postmenopausal ovaries and that the C_{19}-steroids, androstenedione and testesterone, are secreted by postmenopausal ovaries as well. Nonsense! The old adage, *"a difference, to be a difference, must make a difference,"* was never more appropriate than it is to describe this nondilemma. If ovarian tissue obtained from postmenopausal women is incubated with selected substrates of high specific radioactivity, small conversions to estrone, androstenedione, and testosterone are sometimes found. But this is true of many tissues that contribute little or nothing to net steroid production. Aromatase enzyme activity, for example, is demonstrable in adipose tissue, skin, bone, brain, liver, hair follicles, and muscle of men and women. Moreover, the demonstration of a small arterial–venous difference in the concentration of a steroid across the postmenopausal ovary is meaningless because of the liability of technical error and the very small blood flow to these glands. The important issue is that removal of the postmenopausal ovaries does not result in a significant difference in the daily blood production rates of sex steroid hormones. In the absence of ovarian tumors, the postmenopausal ovaries should not be considered as tissue sites of origin of metabolically meaningful amounts of sex steroid hormone production.

Menstrual Blood

Another issue is worthy of restatement: normal menstruation, that which occurs in ovulatory women (progesterone withdrawal), is characterized by the extrusion of incoagulable blood; and there is indirect evidence in favor of the probability that serine proteases (and inhibitors thereof) are produced in endometrium in a cyclic manner that is suggestive of hormonal regulation.

Among these, plasminogen activator is recognized as an important enzyme in the fibrinolytic system.

Hahn (1980) quoted John Hunter who described this event more than 200 years ago (1774): *"In healthy menstruation, the blood which is discharged does not coagulate; in the irregular or unhealthy it does."* Perhaps a remarkably profound insight into the biomolecular regulation of this event was provided as early as 1914 by Whitehouse, who observed that *"as the blood escapes into the tissues it is brought into contact with cells rich in thrombokinase, and this induces rapid coagulation. The thrombus is then disintegrated by the enzyme contained in the secretion of the endometrial glands. These two processes are normally balanced, but it will be obvious that abnormalities in either may lead to the production of excessive bleeding."*

These several physiological correlates are extraordinarily informative and useful in constructing a reasonable hypothesis to explain the hormonal and cellular control of menstruation; in particular, the hormonal regulation of formation of serine proteases and inhibitors thereof in endometrium may be pivotal not only in the fibrinolytic action of endometrium but also in the processing of other proteins.

The Decidua

The decidua is the specialized, highly modified endometrium of pregnancy, and is formed by prolonged stimulation of the endometrium by estrogen and progesterone and by stimuli provided by the implanting blastocyst or maternal platelets during trophoblast invasion of the endometrium and its vessels. The special relationship that exists between the endometrium or decidua and the invading trophoblast seemingly defies the laws of transplantation immunology. The success of this unique autograft is not only a curiosity but may involve processes that many investigators believe could harbor solutions to the future of successful transplantation surgery and perhaps the control of neoplasia as well. The means by which immunological acceptance of the blastocyst is accomplished are considered in Chapter 5.

Decidual Structure. William Hunter, the 19th-century British gynecologist, wrote the first comprehensive treatise on the uterus of pregnant women. In that book, he provided the first scientific description of the *membrana decidua.* According to Damjanov (1985), the term was coined in the best tradition of formal logic applied to scientific writing—*membrana*, denoting its gross appearance, while the qualifier, *decidua*, was added in analogy with deciduous leaves and deciduous teeth to indicate its ephemeral nature and the fact that it is shed from the rest of the uterus at the time of delivery. Wewer and associates (1985) provided evi-

dence that, in Damjanov's opinion, decidua indeed qualifies to be called a membrane, not only because of its gross appearance but because it contains most, if not all, of the major basement membrane components. But more than this, each mature decidual cell becomes surrounded by a basement membrane, one major component of which is *laminin,* which is produced in decidual cells.

In the development of this pericellular membrane of decidual cells, there is at first what appears to be a gradual development of the extracellular matrix. In proliferative endometrium, laminin cannot be identified in association with the stromal cells. In late secretory endometrium, punctate areas of laminin are identified in extracellular sites. In early pregnancy (8 to 16 weeks), the vast majority of the decidual cells are completely surrounded by the laminin-rich basement membranes (large mature decidual cells). But in addition, there also are intermediate-size decidual cells, and these cells are characterized by pericellular or intracellular basement membrane proteins.

Thus, the human decidual cells clearly build walls around themselves and possibly around the fetus. In addressing this issue, Damjanov was reminded of the verse from Robert Frost, *"Before I build a wall I'd ask to know, what I was walling in or walling out."* Perhaps a partial answer to this poetic question, in the case of the decidual cell may serve to answer unsolved riddles regarding the immunological acceptance of the blastocyst and biomolecular trafficking between decidual cells and trophoblasts.

The Decidual Reaction. The decidual reaction encompasses the changes that begin in response to progesterone produced after ovulation that prepare the endometrium for implantation and nutrition of the blastocyst. Predecidual changes commence first around the spiral arteries and arterioles, spreading in waves throughout the mucosa of the uterus. During development of the decidua, the endometrial stromal cells enlarge and form polygonal or round *decidual cells.* In human pregnancy, the decidual reaction is not completed until several days after nidation. The nuclei become round and vesicular, and the cytoplasm becomes clear, slightly basophilic, and surrounded by a translucent membrane. During pregnancy, the decidua thickens, eventually attaining a depth of 5 to 10 mm. With a magnifying glass, furrows and numerous small openings, representing the mouths of uterine glands, can be detected. Later in pregnancy, as the fetus grows and the amnionic fluid expands, the thickness of the decidua decreases, presumably due to the pressure of the intrauterine contents.

The portion of the decidua directly beneath the site of blastocyst implantation forms the *decidua basalis;* that overlying the enlarging blastocyst and separating it from the rest of the uterine cavity is the *decidua cap-*

sularis (Figs. 4–9 and 4–10). The decidua capsularis is most prominent about the second month of pregnancy, consisting of decidual cells covered by a single layer of flattened epithelial cells without traces of glands; internally, it contacts the chorion laeve. The remainder of the uterus is lined by *decidua parietalis,* sometimes called the *decidua vera* when decidual capsularis and decidua parietalis are ultimately joined. Initially, there is a space between the decidua capsularis and the decidua parietalis because the gestational sac does not fill the entire uterine cavity during the early weeks of pregnancy. By 14 to 16 weeks, the growing sac fills the uterine cavity; and with fusion of the decidua capsularis and parietalis, the uterine cavity is obliterated.

The decidua parietalis and the decidua basalis, like the secretory endometrium, are each composed of three layers: a surface, or compact zone (*zona compacta*); a middle portion, or spongy zone (*zona spongiosa*), with remnants of glands and numerous small blood vessels; and a basal zone (*zona basalis*). The compacta and the spongiosa together form the functional zone (*zona functionalis*). The basal zone remains after delivery and gives rise to new endometrium.

Decidual Blood Supply. The blood supply to the various portions of decidua is fundamentally changed as a consequence of implantation. The blood supply to the decidua capsularis is lost as the embryo-fetus grows into the uterine cavity. The blood supply to the decidua parietalis persists by way of the spiral arteries, as in the endometrium before pregnancy during the luteal phase of the cycle. These spiral arteries in the decidua pari-

etalis, therefore, retain a smooth muscle wall and remain responsive to vasoactive agents that act upon the smooth muscle or endothelial cells of the spiral arteries and arterioles. The arterial system supplying the decidua basalis over the implanting blastocyst, and ultimately the intervillous space surrounding the syncytiotrophoblast, is altered remarkably. The spiral arterioles and arteries are invaded by the implanting trophoblasts, and the spiral artery vessel walls are destroyed, leaving only a shell without smooth muscle or endothelial cells. In consequence, these vascular conduits are not responsive to vasoactive agents (Chap. 5).

Decidual Histology. The compact layer of the decidua consists of large, closely packed, epithelioid, polygonal, lightly staining cells with round vesicular nuclei (Fig. 4–11). Many stroma cells appear stellate, particularly when the decidua is edematous, with long protoplasmic processes that anastomose with those of adjacent cells. Numerous small round cells, which contain very little cytoplasm, are scattered among typical decidual cells, especially early in pregnancy. Variously considered in the past to be lymphocytes or decidual cells, these cells are now established as the uterine large granular lymphocytes, which are bone-marrow-derived cells that enter endometrium from peripheral blood (Chap. 5).

Early in pregnancy, the spongy layer of the decidua consists of large distended glands, often exhibiting marked hyperplasia but separated by minimal stroma. At first, the glands are lined by typical cylindrical uterine epithelium with abundant secretory activity. Presumably, the glandular secretion contributes to the nourish-

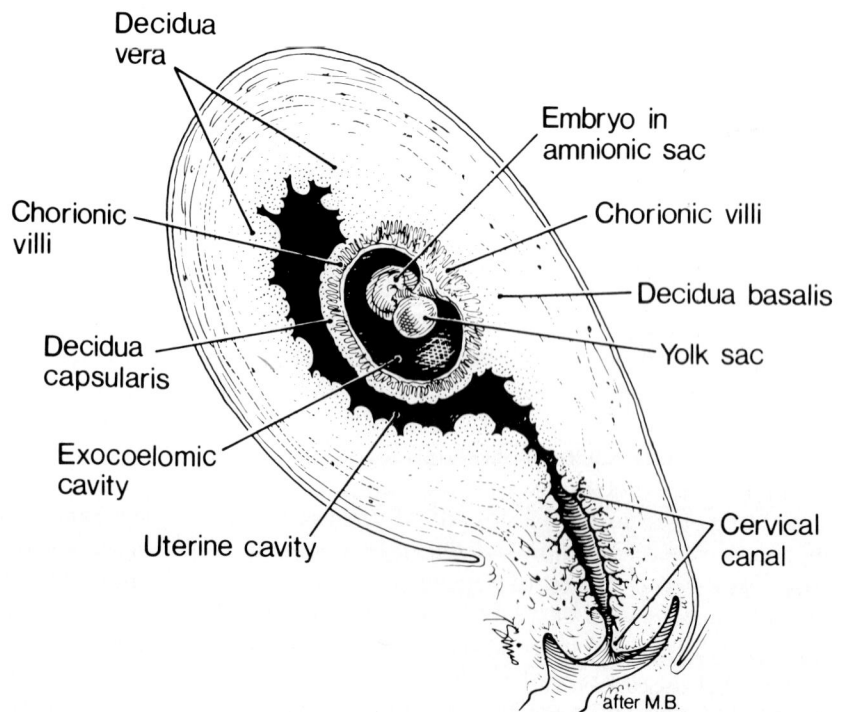

Fig. 4–9. Three portions of the decidua (basalis, capsularis, and parietalis, or vera) of early pregnancy are illustrated.

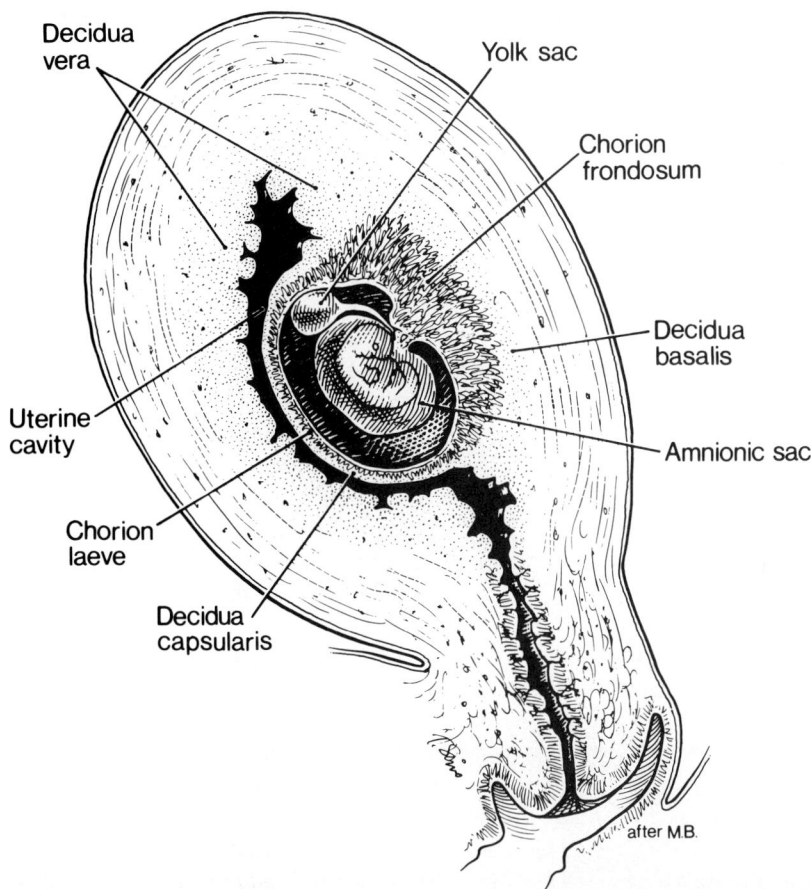

Fig. 4–10. More advanced stage of pregnancy, showing atrophic chorion laeve and chorion frondosum (chorionic villi) proliferating into decidua basalis.

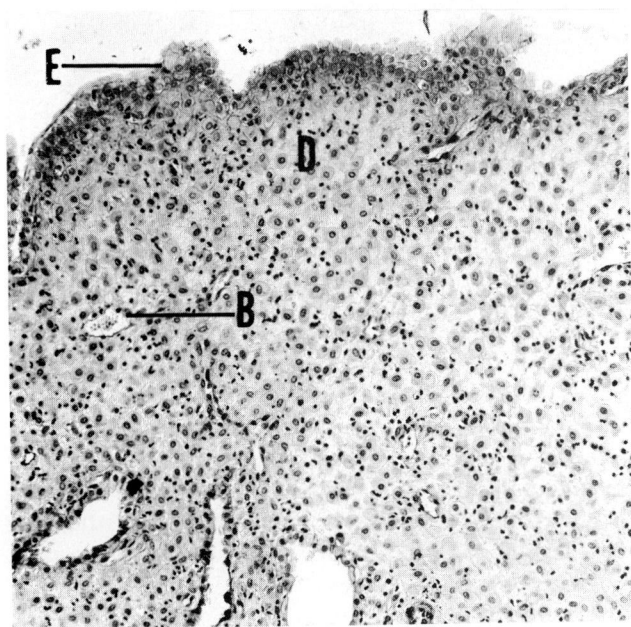

Fig. 4–11. Photomicrograph of decidua vera (parietalis) in which epithelium (E), decidualized stromal cells (D), and blood vessels (B) are shown. (Courtesy of Dr. Ralph M. Wynn.)

ment of the blastocyst during its histotrophic phase, before the establishment of a placental circulation. The epithelium gradually becomes cuboidal or even flattened, later degenerating and sloughing to a greater extent into the lumens of the glands. The stroma of the spongy zone undergoes little change. Later in pregnancy, the glandular elements of the decidua largely disappear.

In comparing the decidua parietalis at 16 weeks gestation with the early proliferative endometrium of the uterus of nonpregnant women, it is clear that during decidual transformation of the endometrial stroma, there is marked hypertrophy but only slight hyperplasia.

The decidua basalis enters into the formation of the *basal plate* of the placenta, and differs histologically from the decidua parietalis in two respects (Fig. 4–12). First, the spongy zone of the decidua basalis consists mainly of arteries and widely dilated veins; by term, as noted, the glands have virtually disappeared. Second, the decidua basalis is invaded extensively by trophoblastic giant cells, which first appear as early as the time of implantation. The number and depth of penetration of the giant cells vary greatly. Although generally confined to the decidua, these cells may penetrate the myometrium. In such circumstances, their number and invasiveness may be so extensive as to be suggestive of choriocarcinoma to the inexperienced observer.

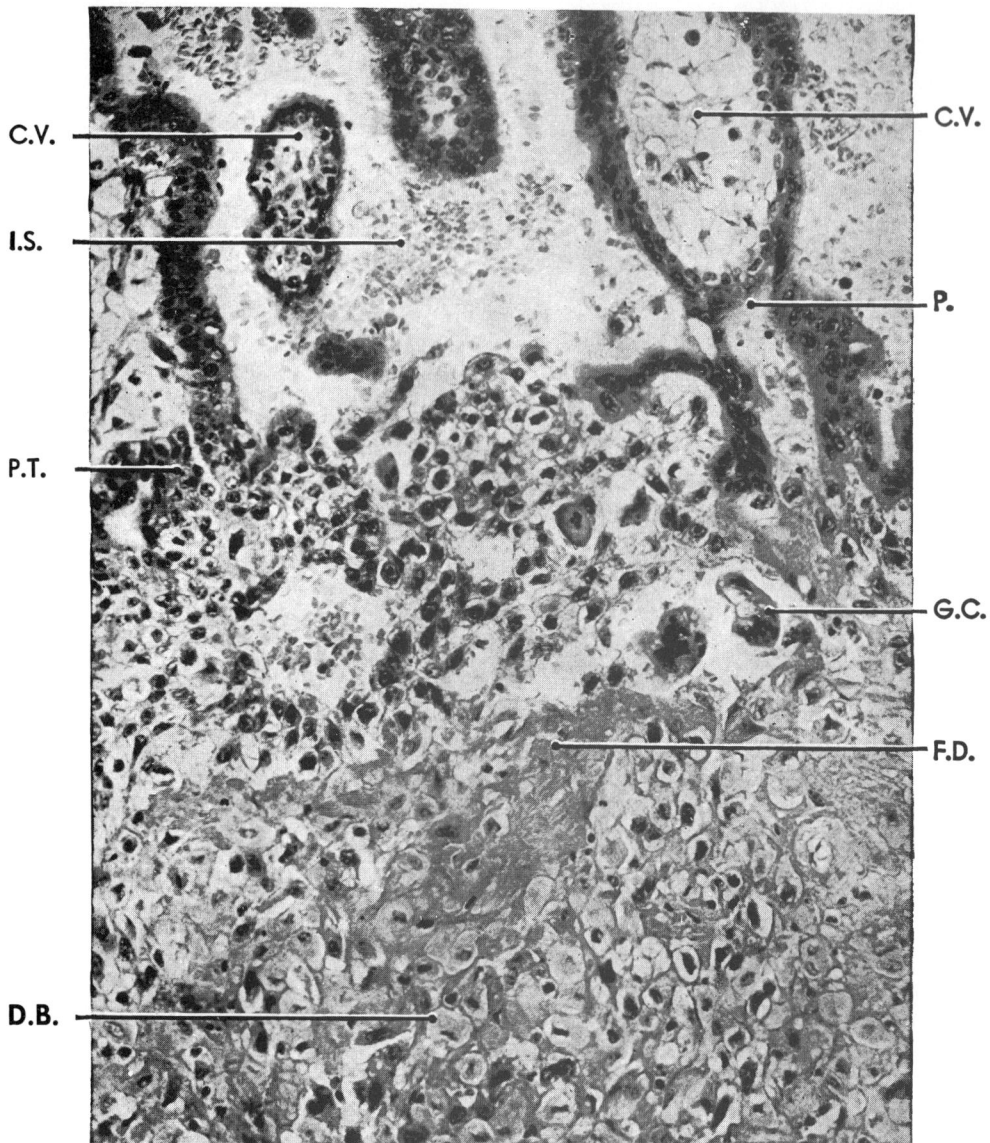

Fig. 4–12. Section through junction of chorion and decidua basalis. Fourth month of gestation. (C.V. = chorionic villi; D.B. = decidua basalis; F.D. = fibrinoid degeneration; G.C. = giant cell; I.S. = intervillous space containing maternal blood; P. = fastening villus; P.T. = proliferating trophoblast.)

Aging of the Decidua. Where invading trophoblast meets the decidua, there is a zone of fibrinoid degeneration, *Nitabuch's layer.* Whenever the decidua is defective, as in placenta accreta (see Chap. 35), Nitabuch layer is usually absent. There is also an inconstant deposition of fibrin, *Rohr stria,* at the bottom of the intervillous space and surrounding the fastening villi. McCombs and Craig (1964) found that decidual necrosis is a normal phenomenon in the first and probably the second trimester. The presence of necrotic decidua obtained through curettage after spontaneous abortion in the first trimester should not, therefore, be interpreted as necessarily either a cause or an effect of the abortion.

Bioactive Substances in the Decidua. The unique nature and histology and endocrine and immunological

function of the decidual cell distinguishes it clearly from "fibroblasts."

Prolactin. Convincing evidence has been presented by Riddick and co-workers (1979) and Golander and associates (1978) that the decidua is the source of prolactin that is present in enormous amounts in the amnionic fluid during human pregnancy. Decidual prolactin is not to be confused with placental lactogen (hPL), which is produced only by the syncytiotrophoblast. Rather, decidual prolactin is a product of the same gene that encodes for pituitary prolactin.

Levels of prolactin of 10,000 ng/mL of amnionic fluid are found during the 20th to 24th week of pregnancy compared with levels of 150 ng/mL in plasma of near-term pregnant women (Tyson and co-workers,

1972). As described in Chapter 8, the concentration of prolactin in amnionic fluid is extraordinarily high compared with the levels in fetal or maternal plasma. Importantly, prolactin produced in decidua preferentially enters amnionic fluid and little or none enters maternal blood. This is a classic example of the peculiar trafficking of molecules between maternal and fetal tissues of the paracrine arm of the fetal–maternal communication system.

There is no doubt that prolactin arises in the decidua (Riddick and co-workers, 1983). There are a number of lines of evidence in favor of this conclusion: (1) prolactin concentrations in decidua are extraordinarily high; (2) the synthesis of prolactin persists in decidual tissue maintained in organ culture; (3) prolactin has been isolated from culture medium of dispersed decidual cells in monolayer culture; (4) pituitary and decidual prolactin are immunologically indistinguishable, as are the biological activities of pituitary and decidual prolactin; (5) cycloheximide treatment of decidual tissue in culture inhibits prolactin secretion; (6) radiolabeled leucine is incorporated into prolactin by decidual tissue; (7) bromocriptine treatment of pregnant women, while causing a striking reduction in the concentration of prolactin in fetal and maternal plasma, does not affect the concentration of prolactin in amnionic fluid; and (8) prolactin formation is demonstrable in secretory endometrium of nonpregnant women and in appropriately treated separated endometrial stromal cells (prepared from endometrium of nonpregnant women) in culture.

The factor(s) that regulates prolactin secretion in decidua is not clearly defined. Those factors known to affect, either negatively or positively, the rate of secretion of prolactin by the anterior pituitary—for example, dopamine and dopamine agonists and thyrotropin-releasing hormone—do not act either in vivo or in vitro to alter the rate of decidual prolactin secretion. It has been reported that arachidonic acid, but not PGE_2 or $PGF_{2\alpha}$, will attenuate the rate of decidual prolactin secretion (Handwerger and colleagues, 1981).

Blithe and co-workers (1991) find that "free alpha" molecules stimulate prolactin synthesis and the secretion of prolactin by human decidual cells. Free alpha is the α-subunit of several glycoprotein hormones including hCG, FSH, LH, and TSH. Free alpha is produced by placenta (Chap. 6). The levels of free α-subunit increase as pregnancy advances; in part, this is the case because the synthesis of the β-subunit of hCG in placenta is limiting in the formation of complete hCG (Chap. 6).

The physiological role of prolactin produced in decidua is not known. Because all or most all of prolactin produced in decidua enters amnionic fluid, it has been speculated that there may be a role for this hormone in solute and water transport across the chorioamnion, and thus in the maintenance of amnionic fluid volume homeostasis.

It has recently been shown that prolactin receptors are present in a number of bone-marrow-derived immune cells, and that prolactin acts on these cells to modify selected immune functions (for recent review: Pellegrini and colleagues, 1992). Recall that many bone-marrow-derived leukocytes are present in endometrium and in decidua throughout pregnancy. And the function of these immune cells is modified appreciably in this tissue site. The question must be addressed, therefore, as to whether the function of these cells is regulated, in part, by the action of prolactin produced in the decidual cells.

Various other roles for decidual prolactin have been suggested, but presently these must be considered as speculative. Excellent reviews of the synthesis of prolactin in decidua have been presented by Tyson and McCoshen (1983) and by Bigazzi (1983).

Other Decidual Bioactive Agents. The mysteries of the human decidua continue to increase. It now is established that *relaxin, β-endorphin,* and *1,25-dihydroxyvitamin D_3* also are produced in human decidua; and, numerous *pregnancy-specific proteins,* and a number of *cytokines* are produced in this macrophage-like tissue. Most recently, the formation of corticotropin-releasing hormone (CRH; Chap. 6) and parathyroid hormone-related protein have been demonstrated in decidua and in endometrial stromal cells in culture (Casey and co-workers, 1992).

Polyamine Synthesis and Metabolism in the Decidua.
Many investigators have established the probability that the accelerated production of the polyamines—putrescine, spermidine, and spermine—is essential in processes that involve both hypertrophy and hyperplasia. Human pregnancy would seem to be a physiological process in which extraordinary rates of polyamine production exist. Not only is there a rapidly growing fetus and placenta but there is extensive hypertrophy of the uterus and other tissues as well. Yet, as discussed in Chapter 8, increased levels of polyamines are demonstrable in the urine of pregnant women only briefly during pregnancy, at about 12 to 14 weeks' gestation. The enzyme that catalyzes the first and rate-limiting step in polyamine formation, *ornithine decarboxylase,* is present in and has been characterized in decidua of women (Garza and co-workers, 1983). Thus, it seems enigmatic and, in view of the growth of the fetus, disappointing that the levels of polyamines in maternal blood and urine are not reflective of the rate of growth of fetus, decidua, and the uterus; if this were the case, it could be that the measurement of polyamines would be useful as an index of fetal growth.

An explanation, however, may be offered for this apparent paradox. The activity of the enzyme *diamine oxidase,* also known as *histaminase,* rises dramatically in blood of pregnant women early in pregnancy at about the time that the levels of polyamines begin to decline, namely at about 14 weeks' gestation. The importance of this observation is that diamine oxidase is the enzyme that catalyzes the metabolism of putrescine. Thus, it may be that the rate of polyamine synthesis is indeed accelerated and increases throughout pregnancy but the rate of catabolism of these compounds is greater than the rate of synthesis. This is easily envisioned when one considers that diamine oxidase activity in plasma of pregnant women may increase a thousandfold by 20 weeks' gestation (Ahlmark, 1944). It is believed that this increased amount of diamine oxidase is principally of decidual origin (Swanberg, 1948), but the direct secretion of diamine oxidase by trophoblasts has been demonstrated.

For this reason and others, many investigators have determined the activity of diamine oxidase in plasma of pregnant women in the hope of using such values as an index of fetal well-being. Although some correlates appear to exist, it is generally accepted that such measurements are not useful in the selection of clinical management plans (Resnik and Levine, 1969).

It is possible that diamine oxidase serves to degrade histamine, which is known to cause uterine contractions. Thus, diamine oxidase may be an example of the many enzymes that act to degrade potential uterotonins. This is one mechanism by which uterine quiescence is maintained during the first 90 to 95 percent of pregnancy (phase 0 of parturition, Chap. 12). Other potential uterotonins are also degraded by enzymes that are increased during pregnancy, such as endothelin-1: enkephalinase; prostaglandins:prostaglandin dehydrogenase; and oxytocin:oxytocinase Chap. 12).

Cervical, Vaginal, and Tubal Cycles

Cervix. Cyclic changes occur in the endocervical glands, especially during the follicular phase of the ovarian cycle. During the early follicular phase, the glands are only slightly tortuous, and the secretory cells are not very tall. Secretion of mucus is meager. The late follicular phase, however, is characterized by pronounced tortuosity of the glands, deep invagination, tumescence of the epithelium, high columnar cells, and abundant secretion. The connective tissue acquires a looser texture and more extensive vascularization. After ovulation, these characteristics regress.

The secretory activity of the endocervical glands is maximal at about the time of ovulation, and is the result of estrogenic stimulation. Only at that time, in most women, is the quality of the cervical mucus such as to permit penetration by the spermatozoa. The property of the cervical mucus that permits it to be drawn out in long strands is termed *spinnbarkeit*, a property of mucus that is maximal at the time of ovulation. The synchronization of the height of secretory activity in the

cervical and endometrial cycles is precise and purposeful. In the cervix, where the mucus facilitates passage of the spermatozoa, it occurs just before the ovum is to be released (i.e., at ovulation), a period probably of not more than about 36 to 48 hours. In the endometrium, where the purpose of the highly developed secretory activity seems to be to provide a site favorable for nidation of the fertilized ovum, the changes are maximum about 6 to 7 days later, when the fertilized ovum is ready to implant.

Cervical Mucus. If cervical mucus is aspirated, spread on a glass slide, allowed to dry for a few minutes, and examined microscopically, characteristic patterns can be discerned that are dependent on the stage of the ovarian cycle and the presence or absence of pregnancy (i.e., progesterone secretion in large amounts). From about the 7th day of the menstrual cycle to about the 18th day, a fern-like pattern of dried cervical mucus is seen (Fig. 4–13); it is sometimes called a process of "arborization" or the "palm leaf pattern." After approximately the 21st day of the menstrual cycle, this fern pattern does not develop, but rather there is a quite different pattern that forms, giving a beaded or cellular appearance (Fig. 4–14). This beaded pattern is usually also encountered in pregnancy. The crystallization of the mucus, which is necessary for the production of the fern, or arborized pattern, is dependent upon the concentration of electrolytes, principally sodium chloride, in the secretion. In general, a concentration of sodium chloride of 1 percent is required for the full develop-

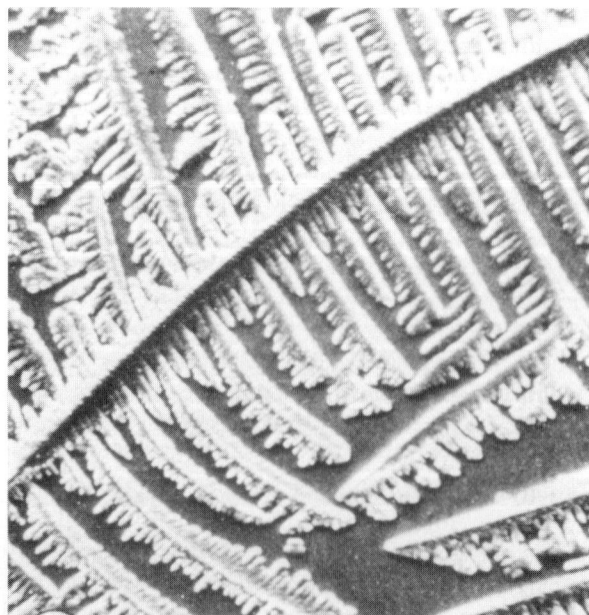

Fig. 4–13. Scanning electron microscopy of cervical mucus obtained on day 11 of the menstrual cycle. (From Zaneveld and colleagues, 1975.)

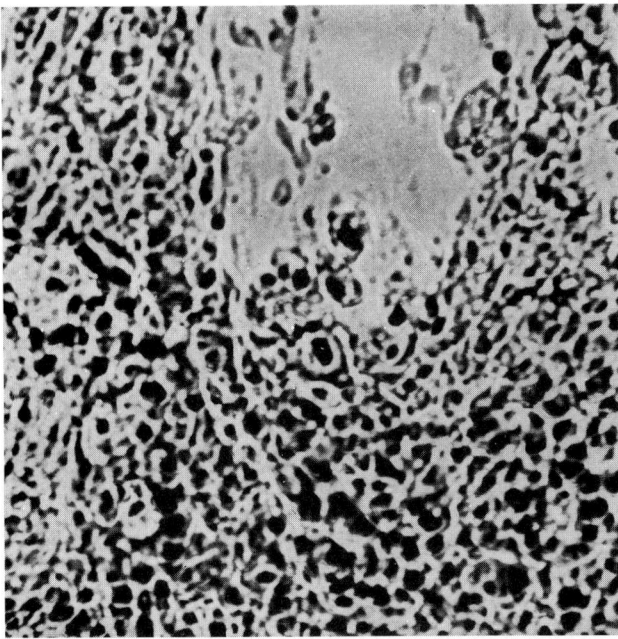

Fig. 4–14. Photomicrograph of dried cervical mucus obtained from the cervical canal of a woman pregnant at 32 to 33 weeks. The beaded pattern is characteristic of progesterone action on the endocervical gland mucus composition. (Courtesy of Dr. J.C. Ullery.)

ment of a fern pattern; below that concentration, either a beaded pattern or an atypical or incomplete arborization is seen.

The concentration of sodium chloride, and in turn the presence or absence of the fern pattern, is determined by the response of the cervix to hormonal action. Whereas the cervical mucus is relatively rich in sodium chloride when estrogen, but not progesterone, is being produced, the secretion of progesterone (even without a reduction in the rate of secretion of estrogen) promptly acts to lower the sodium chloride concentration of the mucus, either cervical or nasal, to levels at which ferning will not occur as the specimen dries. During pregnancy, progesterone usually exerts a similar effect, even though the amount of estrogen produced is enormous compared with that produced during a normal ovarian cycle.

Vagina. There is constant desquamation of the superficial cells of the vaginal epithelium. Consequently, the nature of maturity of the cells in the vaginal fluid is reflective to some degree of the changes in the epithelium of the surface of the vagina that occur in response to hormone action. Vaginal epithelium, under estrogenic stimulation, is characterized by cyclic changes during which the greatest development is reached at the end of the follicular phase. This stage is characterized by enlargement, flattening, and spreading of the superficial cells and by relative leukopenia, whereas in the smear

taken in the luteal phase, there is an increase in the number of basophilic cells and leukocytes, as well as irregular grouping of the cells.

Fallopian Tubes. Fertilization of the ovum occurs in the fallopian tube soon after ovulation. Based on considerable experience assembled by investigators around the world, there is evidence that the milieu of the fallopian tube is optimized for early cleavage and development of the zygote. Recapitulation of this environment has been the goal of many investigators seeking to idealize conditions for in vitro fertilization.

References

Abel MH: Prostanoids and menstruation. In Baird DT, Michie EA (eds): Mechanisms of Menstrual Bleeding. New York, Raven, 1985, p 139

Ahlmark A: Studies on the histominolytic power of plasma with special reference to pregnancy. Acta Physiol Scand 9 (suppl 28):1, 1944

Arai H, Hori S, Aramori I, Ohkubo H, Nakanishi S: Cloning and expression of a cDNA encoding an endothelin receptor. Nature 348:730, 1990

Arey LB: The degree of normal menstrual irregularity: An analysis of 20,000 calendar records from 1,500 individuals. Am J Obstet Gynecol 37:12, 1939

Arici A, Head JR, MacDonald PC, Casey ML: Interleukin-8 gene expression in human endometrium/decidua: Regulation in human endometrial stromal and epithelial cells in culture. Manuscript submitted, 1992a

Arici A, MacDonald PC, Casey ML: Differential expression of transforming growth factor-β1 (TGF-β1) in human endometrial stromal cells. Am Fert Soc, 1992b. Abstract

Arici A, MacDonald PC, Economos K, Casey ML, Head JR: Expression of neutrophil activating peptide/interleukin-8 (NAP/IL-8) and monocyte chemotactic protein (MCP-1) in human endometrial stromal cells. Abstract presented at 38th annual meeting of Society for Gynecological Investigation, San Antonio, March 1991

Baird DT: Preface. In Baird DT, Michie EA (eds): Mechanisms of Menstrual Bleeding. New York, Raven, 1985, p v

Baldwin RM, Whalley PJ, Pritchard JA: Measurements of menstrual blood loss. Am J Obstet Gynecol 81:739, 1961

Barker AP, Fowler WM: The blood loss during normal menstruation. Am J Obstet Gynecol 31:979, 1936

Benirschke K: The endometrium. In Yen SSC, Jaffe RB (eds): Reproductive Endocrinology: Physiology, Pathophysiology and Clinical Management. Philadelphia, Saunders, 1986, p 385

Bigazzi M: Specific endocrine function of human decidua. Semin Reprod Endocrinol 1:343, 1983

Blithe DL, Richards RG, Skarulis MC: Free alpha molecules from pregnancy stimulate secretion of prolactin from human decidual cells: A novel function for free alpha in pregnancy. Endocrinology 129:2257, 1991

Boyd JD, Hamilton WJ: The Human Placenta. Cambridge, England, Heffer, 1970

Casey ML, Hemsell DL, MacDonald PC, Johnston JM: NAD$^+$-dependent 15-hydroxyprostaglandin dehydrogenase activity in human endometrium. Prostaglandins 19:115, 1980

Casey ML, MacDonald PC: Cytokines in the human placenta, fetal membranes, uterine decidua, and amniotic fluid. In Rice G, Brennecke S (eds): Molecular Aspects of Placental and Fetal Membrane Autacoids. CRC Press, 1992a (in press)

Casey ML, MacDonald PC: Modulation of endometrial flood flow: Regulation of endothelin-1 biosynthesis and degradation in human endometrium. In Alexander NJ (ed): Exogenous Hormones and Dysfunctional Bleeding. AAAS Press, 1992b (in press)

Casey ML, MacDonald PC: Extraadrenal formation of a mineralocorticosteroid: Deoxycorticosterone and deoxycorticosterone sulfate biosynthesis and metabolism. Endocrine Rev 3:396, 1982

Casey ML, Mibe M, Erk A, MacDonald PC: Transforming growth-β stimulation of parathyroid hormone-related protein expression in human uterine cells in culture: mRNA levels and protein secretion. J Clin Endocrinol Metab 74:950, 1992

Casey ML, Smith JW, Nagai K, Hersh LB, MacDonald PC: Progesterone-regulated cyclic modulation of membrane metalloendopeptidase (enkephalinase) in human endometrium. J Biol Chem 266:23041, 1991

Chesley LC, Hellman LM: Variations in body weight and salivary sodium in the menstrual cycle. Am J Obstet Gynecol 74:582, 1957

Chiazze L, Brayer FT, Macisco JJ, Parker MP, Duffy BJ: The length and variability of the human menstrual cycle. JAMA 203:377, 1968

Chimbira TH, Anderson ABM, Turnbull AC: Relation between measured menstrual blood loss and patient's subjective assessment of loss, duration of bleeding, number of sanitary towels used, uterine weight and endometrial surface area. Br J Obstet Gynaecol 87:603, 1980

Christiaens GCML, Sixma JJ, Haspels AA: Vascular and haemostatic changes in menstrual endometrium. In Baird DT, Michie EA (eds): Mechanism of Menstrual Bleeding. Serono Symposia, Vol XXV. New York, Raven, 1985, p 27

Damjanov I: Editorial: Vesalius and Hunter were right: Decidua is a membrane. Lab Invest 53:597, 1985

Economos K, MacDonald PC, Casey ML: Endothelin-1 gene expression and protein biosynthesis in human endometrium. Potential modulator of endometrial blood flow. J Clin Endocrinol Metab 74:14, 1992

Finch CA: Body iron exchange in man. J Clin Invest 38:392, 1959

Garza JR, MacDonald PC, Johnston JM, Casey ML: Characterization of ornithine decarboxylase activity in human uterine decidua vera. Am J Obstet Gynecol 145:509, 1983

Golander A, Hurley T, Barret J, Hizi A, Handwerger S: Prolactin synthesis by human chorion decidual tissue: A possible source of prolactin in the amniotic fluid. Science 202:311, 1978

Golub LJ, Menduke H, Conly SS Jr: Weight changes in college women during the menstrual cycle. Am J Obstet Gynecol 91:89, 1965

Gunn DL, Jenkin PM, Gunn AL: Menstrual periodicity: Statistical observations on a large sample of normal cases. J Obstet Gynaecol Br Emp 44:839, 1937

Gustavii B: Labour: A delayed menstruation? Lancet 2:1149, 1972

Hahn L: Composition of menstrual blood. In Diczfalusy E, Fraser IS, Webb FTG (eds): Endometrial Bleeding and Steroidal Contraception. Proceedings of Symposium on Steroid Contraception and Mechanism of Menstrual Bleeding. Bath, England, Pitman Press, 1980, p 107

Hallberg L, Hallgren J, Hollender A, Hogdahl AM, Tibblin G: Occurrence of iron deficiency anemia in Sweden. Symp Swed Nutri Found 6:19, 1968

Hallberg L, Hogdahl AM, Nilsson L, Rybo G: Menstrual blood loss, a population study: Variation at different ages and attempts to define normality. Acta Obstet Gynecol Scand 45:320, 1966

Haman JO: The length of the menstrual cycle: A study of 150 normal women. Am J Obstet Gynecol 43:870, 1942

Handwerger S, Barry S, Barrett J, Markoff E, Zeitler P, Cwikel B, Siegel M: Inhibition of the synthesis and secretion of decidual prolactin by arachidonic acid. Endocrinology 109:2016, 1981

Hartman CG: Studies in the reproduction of the monkey *Macaca (Pithecus) rhesus* with special reference to menstruation and pregnancy. Contrib Embryol 23:1, 1932

Head JR, MacDonald PC, Casey ML: Cellular localization of membrane metalloendopeptidase (enkephalinase) in human endometrium during the ovarian cycle. J Clin Endocrinol Metab, 1992 (in press)

Hitschmann F, Adler L: Der Bau der Uterusschleimhaut des geschlechtsreifen Weives mit besonderer Berücksichtigung der Menstruation. Monatsschr Geburtshilfe Gynaekol 27:1, 1908

Horwitz KB, McGuire WL, Pearson OH, Segaloff A: Predicting response to endocrine therapy in human breast cancer: A hypothesis. Science 189:726, 1975

Hytten FE, Cheyne GA, Klopper AI: Iron loss at menstruation. J Obstet Gynaecol Br Commonw 71:255, 1964

Jensen EV, Jacobson HI: Basic guides to the mechanism of estrogen action. Recent Prog Horm Res 18:387, 1962

MacDonald PC, Dombroski RA, Casey ML: Recurrent secretion of progesterone in large amounts: An endocrine/metabolic disorder unique to young women? Endocrine Rev 12:372, 1991

Markee JE: Menstruation in intraocular endometrial transplants in the rhesus monkey. Contrib Embryol 28:219, 1940

McCombs HL, Craig MJ: Decidual necrosis in normal pregnancy. Obstet Gynecol 24:436, 1964

Millis J: The iron losses of healthy women during consecutive menstrual cycles. Med J Aust 2:874, 1951

Noyes RW, Hertig AT, Rock J: Dating the endometrial biopsy. Fertil Steril 1:3, 1950

Pellegrini I, Lebrun JJ, Ali S, Kelly PA: Expression of prolactin and its receptor in human lymphoid cells. Mol Endocrinol 6:1023, 1992

Perrot-Applanat M, Groyer-Picard MT, Garcia E, Lorenzo F, Milgrom E: Immunocytochemical demonstration of estrogen and progesterone receptors in muscle cells of uterine arteries in rabbits and humans. Endocrinology 123:1511, 1988

Preece PE, Richards AR, Owen GM, Hughes LE: Mastalgia and total body water. Br Med J 4:498, 1975

Ramsey EM: History. In Wynn RM (ed): Biology of the Uterus. New York, Plenum, 1977, p 1

Resnik R, Levine RJ: Plasma diamine oxidase activity in pregnancy: A reappraisal. Am J Obstet Gynecol 104:1061, 1969

Riddick DH, Daly DC, Walters CA: The uterus as an endocrine compartment. Clin Perinatol 10:627, 1983

Riddick DH, Luciano AA, Kusmik WF, Maslar IA: Evidence for a nonpituitary source of amniotic fluid prolactin. Fertil Steril 31:35, 1979

Rock J, Bartlett M: Biopsy studies of human endometrium. JAMA 108:2022, 1937

Sakurai T, Yanagisawa M, Takuwa Y, Miyazaki H, Kimura S, Goto K, Masaki T: Cloning of a cDNA encoding a nonisopeptide-selective subtype of the endothelin receptor. Nature 348:732, 1990

Scott DE, Pritchard JA: Iron deficiency in healthy young college women. JAMA 199:897, 1967

Swanberg H: Source of histaminolytic enzyme in blood of pregnant women. Acta Physiol Scand 16:83, 1948

Tamada H, McMaster MT, Flanders KC, Andrews GK, Dey SK: Cell type-specific periimplantation period. Mol Endocrinol 4:965, 1990

Tanner JM: Growth at Adolescence. Oxford, Blackwell Scientific, 1962, p 325

Tseng L, Gurpide E: Effects of progestins on estradiol receptor levels in human endometrium. J Clin Endocrinol Metab 41:402, 1975

Tseng L, Gurpide E: Estradiol and 20α-dihydroprogesterone dehydrogenase activities in human endometrium during the menstrual cycle. Endocrinology 94:419, 1974

Tseng L, Liu HC: Stimulation of acylsulfotransferase activity by progestins in human endometrium in vitro. J Clin Endocrinol Metab 53:418, 1981

Tyson JE, Hwang P, Guyda H, Friesen HG: Studies of prolactin secretion in human pregnancy. Am J Obstet Gynecol 113:14, 1972

Tyson JE, McCoshen JA: Decidual prolactin: An enigmatic cybernin in human reproduction. Semin Reprod Endocrinol 1:197, 1983

Wewer UM, Faber M, Liotta LA, Albrechtsen R: Immunochemical and ultrastructural assessment of the nature of the pericellular basement membrane of human decidual cells. Lab Invest 53:624, 1985

White AJ, Buchsbaum HJ: Scanning electron microscopy of the human endometrium. Gynecol Oncol 1:330, 1973

Whitehouse HB: Pathological uterine haemorrhage. Lancet 1:951, 1914

Wynn RM, Harris JA: Ultrastructural cyclic changes in the human endometrium, I. Normal preovulatory phase. Fertil Steril 18:632, 1967a

Wynn RM, Woolley RS: Ultrastructural cyclic changes in the human endometrium, II. Normal postovulatory phase. Fertil Steril 18:721, 1967b

Yanagisawa M, Kurihara H, Kimura S, Tomobe Y, Kobayashi M, Mitsui Y, Yazaki Y, Goto K, Masaki T: A novel potent vasoconstrictor peptide produced by vascular endothelial cells. Nature 332:411, 1988

Zaneveld LJ, Tauber PF, Port C, Propping D: Scanning electron microscopy of cervical mucus crystallization. Obstet Gynecol 46:419, 1975

CHAPTER 5
The Placenta and Fetal Membranes

Overview

Benirschke (1981) observed that *"the placenta is the most accurate record of the infant's prenatal experiences."* He went on to suggest that *"physicians generally are uncomfortable with the task of examining the placenta. Yet, it is a task they should willingly undertake. . . . Submitting this organ to a reasonably knowledgeable look and touch can provide much insight into prenatal life; the results are often helpful in caring for the neonate; the findings provide a record pediatricians and obstetricians can use to plan the future care for mother and child; and, most important, much of what can be learned cannot be put into the maternal prenatal history if the information is discarded with the organ."* But despite these strong admonitions, Salafia and Vintzileos (1990) observed that *"it would surprise neither obstetricians nor pathologists if a governmental survey concluded that the single group expressing the most consistent interest in the (human) placenta was the cosmetics industry, which purchases tons of placentas yearly for the extraction of hormones and proteins to be used in hair, face, and skin care treatments."*

Fetal Tissues of the Fetal–Maternal Communication System

The basic organization of the fetal–maternal communication system of human pregnancy, which is comprised of two arms (placental and paracrine), was described in Chapters 2 and 4 (Fig. 2–1). The villous and extravillous trophoblasts are the fetal tissues of the anatomical interface of the placental arm; and the fetal membranes (i.e., the amnion and chorion laeve) are the fetal tissues of the anatomical interface of the paracrine arm of this communication system. Ultimately, a link between mother and fetus is established by way of the placental arm as follows: maternal blood directly bathes the villous trophoblasts; but fetal blood is contained within fetal capillaries that traverse the villi within the intravillous space. Thus, a *hemochorioendothelial* type of placentation develops and is operative throughout human pregnancy. The link established by the paracrine arm of the communication system is through the anatomical and biomolecular juxtaposition of (fetal) chorion laeve and (maternal) decidua parietalis tissues. **Therefore, at all sites of direct contact, maternal tissue (decidua and blood) is juxtaposed to fetal trophoblasts and not to embryonic cells or fetal blood.** This is an important consideration that will be emphasized again in an evaluation of the immunological success of the maternal acceptance of the conceptus.

Interest in the placenta has properly derived primarily from its role in nidation and in the transfer of nutrients from mother to the developing fetus. Scientific interest in the placenta also evolves from its enormous diversity of form and function and from the unique metabolic, endocrine, and immunological properties of its trophoblasts. Today, we recognize that important metabolic functions of the fetal–maternal communication system are also accomplished by way of the fetal avascular membranes and uterine decidua parietalis. In this paracrine arm of the communication system, there is direct cell-to-cell molecular trafficking between extraembryonic fetal (trophoblasts) and maternal tissues.

Evolution of Knowledge of the Placenta

Boyd and Hamilton (1970) presented a marvelous account of the history of placental research. They observe that the term *placenta* is believed to have been introduced by Realdus Columbus in 1559 when he used the Latin word for a *circular cake*. In 1937, Mossman defined *placenta* as that portion of the fetal membranes that was in apposition with or fused to the uterine mucosa. Historically, as pointed out by Boyd and Hamilton, knowledge about the *afterbirth* can be traced far back in human history.

In the Old Testament, the placenta was considered as the external soul and was sometimes described as being tied up in the so-called bundle of life, which probably included the umbilical cord. It is believed that Aristotle (384–322 BC) was the first to use the word *chorion*. Chori means separate, distinct. It was not, however, until the early 16th century, a time of renaissance of anatomy, that opinions were given concerning placental function. But even then, as recounted by Boyd and Hamilton, Leonardo da Vinci (1452–1519) and Vesalius (1514–1564) illustrated the human placenta incorrectly. Vesalius, in 1555, corrected his error in the second edition of his outstanding book.

The concept of the placental circulation apparently was introduced by Harvey in 1628; but it was John Mayow (1643–1679) who more adequately described its nature. Placental endocrine function was not recognized until much later, because the function of hormones in general must necessarily have preceded such an understanding. It was not until 1564 that Arantius, by careful dissections, discounted the concept that there was continuity between maternal and fetal vascular systems. Harvey, in 1651, set forth clearly that there was a fetal arterial and venous circulation to the placenta, but it was Malpighi, in 1660, who established the concept of a capillary network as the anatomical basis for the regional circulation. By the end of the 17th century there was a remarkably accurate concept of the structure and functional significance of the placenta. The basic idea that there was a *placental barrier* was already formulated clearly in the late 17th or early 18th century. John and William Hunter, around 1750, injected liquid wax into the uterine artery; the wax did not appear in the fetal circulation. This finding finally set aside the notion of anastomoses between maternal and fetal vessels (Ramsey, 1985).

William Hunter, in 1774, is credited with the first accurate description of the decidua and, even then, he distinguished a parietal lining (decidua parietalis) from a capsular one (decidua capsularis). In 1821, John Hunter described the decidua basalis. It was probably William and John Hunter, although each claimed credit separately, who accurately described what we now know as the intervillous spaces. It was not until the middle of the 19th century that the true nature of the chorionic villi was appreciated; by 1880, however, the basic knowledge of the nature of blood circulation in the intervillous space was established. In 1882, a notable contribution was made by Langhans, who demonstrated clearly that the villi were covered by two layers of cells. Indeed, it is the inner layer of cells, the cytotrophoblasts (which line the intravillous space), that are referred to as the *Langhans cells*. It was in 1889 that the term *trophoblast* was introduced by Hubrecht to distinguish the portion of blastocyst cells that do not contribute to the cellular portion of the embryo. The superficial layer of the chorionic villi was eventually demonstrated to be syncytial in nature, and is now generally referred to as the syncytiotrophoblast. Syncytium is used as a term to designate a multinucleate condition that results from the fusion of cells that initially were separate.

Development of the Human Placenta

Fertilization. Moore (1973) provides a quote by George W. Corner, who may have described fertilization best: *"The fertilization of an egg by a sperm is one of the greatest wonders of nature, an event in which magnificently small fragments of animal life are driven by cosmic forces toward their appointed end, the growth of a living being. As a spectacle it can be compared only with an eclipse of the sun or the eruption of a volcano. . . . It is, in fact, the most common and the nearest to us of nature's cataclysms, and yet it is very*

seldom observed because it occurs in a realm most people never see, the region of microscopic things."

We also have been captivated by Richard Blandau's pictorial comparison of the ejaculation of seminal fluid with an atomic explosion; and we have realized with him that a population explosion in the world can be as devastating as atomic blasts. Few, if any, naturally occurring phenomena are of greater importance to humankind than the union of egg and sperm. Fertilization of the human egg by a spermatozoan occurs in the fallopian tube within 2 minutes or no more than a few hours after ovulation.

Definitions. The following definitions are taken from Moore (1973).

- **Zygote:** The cell that results from the fertilization of the ovum by a spermatozoan.
- **Blastomeres:** Mitotic division of the zygote (cleavage) gives rise to daughter cells called blastomeres.
- **Morula:** The solid ball of cells formed by 16 or so blastomeres.
- **Blastocyst:** After the morula reaches the uterus, a fluid-filled cavity is formed, converting the morula to a blastocyst.
- **Embryo:** The embryo-forming cells, which are grouped as an inner cell mass, give rise to the embryo, which usually is designated when the bilaminar embryonic disc forms. The *embryonic period* extends until the end of the seventh week, at which time the major structures are present.
- **Fetus:** After the embryonic period, the developing conceptus is referred to as the fetus.
- **Conceptus:** This term is used to refer to all tissue products of conception—embryo (fetus), fetal membranes, and placenta. Specifically, the conceptus includes all tissues that develop from the zygote, both embryonic and extraembryonic.

Human Embryo Development

Cleavage of the Zygote. The mature ovum, after fertilization in the fallopian tube, becomes a zygote—a diploid cell with 46 chromosomes—which then undergoes segmentation, or cleavage, into blastomeres.

The first typical mitotic division of the segmentation nucleus of the zygote results in the formation of two blastomeres. In a photomicrograph of a living, segmenting zygote of the monkey (Fig. 5–1), the suspension of blastomeres and polar bodies in the perivitelline fluid, which is surrounded by the zona pellucida, is shown. In a fertilized human ovum (Fig. 5–2), there are similar changes.

While still within the fallopian tube, the zygote undergoes slow cleavage for 3 days; indeed, fertilized

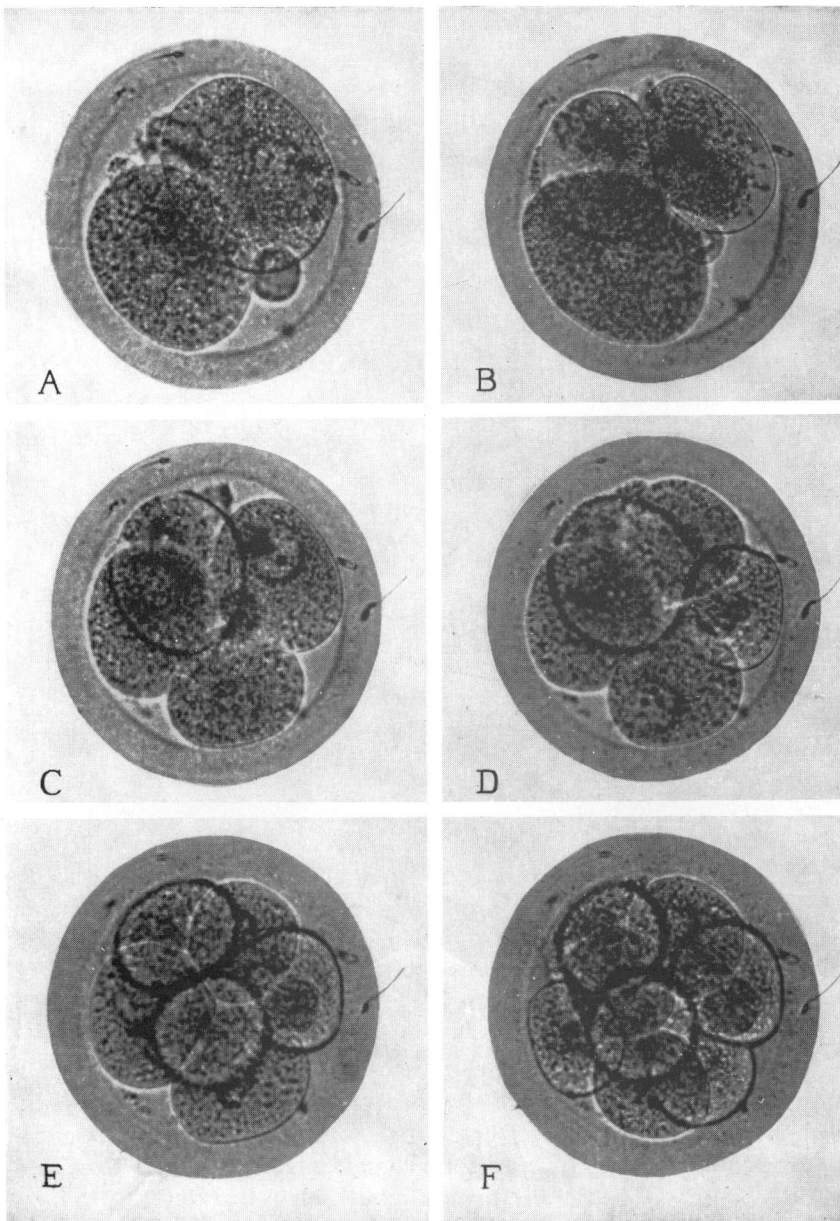

Fig. 5–1. Photomicrographs (× 300) of living monkey fertilized ovum showing its cleavage divisions. The fertilized ovum was washed out of the tube and cultivated in plasma; its growth changes were recorded cinematographically. The illustrations are enlargements from single frames of the film. **A.** 2-cell stage, 29 hours and 30 minutes after ovulation. **B.** 3-cell stage, 36 hours and 4 minutes after ovulation. **C.** 4-cell stage, 37 hours and 35 minutes after ovulation. **D.** 5-cell stage, 48 hours and 39 minutes after ovulation. **E.** 6-cell stage, 48 hours and 48 minutes after ovulation. **F.** 8-cell stage, 49 hours exactly after ovulation. These cleavages normally occur as the ovum passes down the fallopian tube. Note the spermatozoan in the zona pellucida. (After Lewis and Hartman, 1933.)

human ova that are recovered from the uterine cavity may be comprised of only 12 to 16 blastomeres. As the blastomeres continue to divide, a solid mulberry-like ball of cells, the *morula,* is produced. The morula enters the uterine cavity about 3 days after fertilization of the ovum; and the gradual accumulation of fluid between blastomeres within the morula results in the formation of the blastocyst. At one pole of the blastocyst, there is a compact mass of cells, the *inner cell mass,* which is destined to produce the embryo (Fig. 5–3), and an outer mass of cells destined to be the *trophoblasts.*

The Early Human Zygote. In a presumably normal two-cell zygote that was flushed from the oviduct (Fig. 5–2A), Hertig and co-workers (1954) found that the blastomeres (and a polar body, which was free in the

perivitelline fluid) were surrounded by a thick zona pellucida. In a 58-cell blastocyst (Fig. 5–2B), the outer cells (which presumably are destined to produce the trophoblasts) can be distinguished from the inner cells (those that form the embryo). The next stage that was obtained was a 107-cell blastocyst (blastodermic vesicle) that was no larger than the earlier cleavage stages, despite the accumulated fluid (Fig. 5–2C). It measured 0.153 by 0.155 mm in diameter before fixation and after the disappearance of the zona pellucida. The 8 formative (embryo-producing) cells were surrounded by 99 trophoblastic cells. The fertilized "ovum," now a blastocyst, was ready for implantation.

Implantation. Before implantation, the zona pellucida disappears and the blastocyst adheres to the endome-

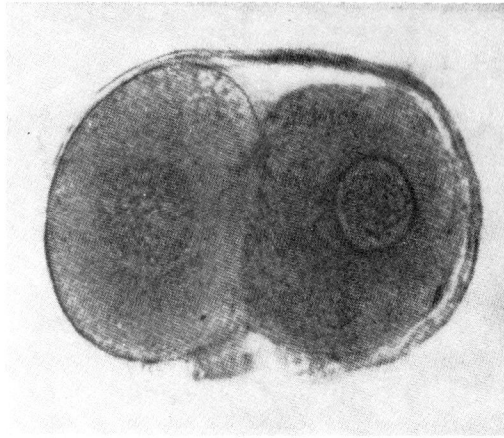

A

Fig. 5–2. Human preimplantation stages. **A.** 2-cell stage. Intact fertilized ovum surrounded by zona pellucida, photographed after fixation. Washed from fallopian tube about 1½ days after conception. Nuclei shimmer through granular cytoplasm. Polar body in perivitelline space. (Carnegie Collection no. 8698; × 500.) **B.** 58-cell blastula with intact zona pellucida found in uterine cavity 3 to 4 days after conception. Thin section showing outer (probably trophoblastic) and inner (embryo-forming) cells and beginning segmentation cavity. (Carnegie Collection no. 8794; × 600.) **C.** 107-cell blastocyst found free in uterine cavity about 5 days after conception. A shell of trophoblastic cells enveloping fluid-filled blastocele and inner cell mass consisting of embryo-forming cells. (Carnegie Collection no. 8663; × 600.) (From Hertig and associates, 1954.)

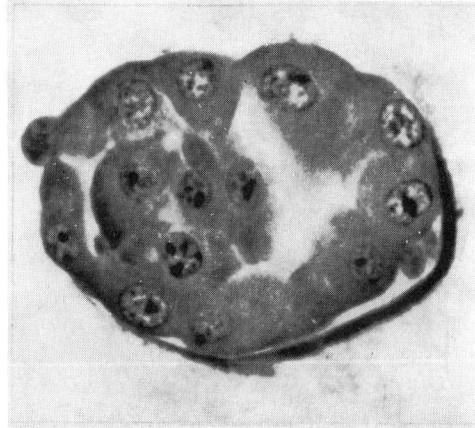

B

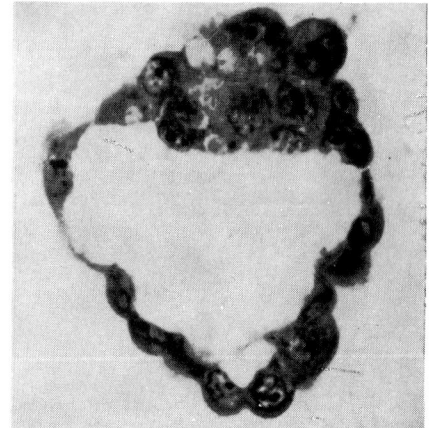

C

trial surface; this is the time of *apposition* and occurs when the blastocyst is composed of 107 to 256 cells. Most commonly, implantation occurs in the upper part and somewhat more often on the posterior wall of the uterus. After erosion between epithelial cells of the surface endometrium, the blastocyst invades deeper in and soon becomes totally encased within the endometrium—that is, **the implanting blastocyst is completely buried in and covered over by the endometrium.**

At the time of blastocyst implantation, the invading conceptus is very analogous to a locally invasive tumor, but a very unusual one because it is theoretically a semiallogenic graft. This graft is qualified as "theoretically" semiallogenic because whereas there is no question that the embryo bears and expresses paternal antigens, it is likely that HLA gene expression is inhibited in trophoblast. At this time, the innermost trophoblasts, i.e., some of the trophoblasts contiguous with and invading the endometrium coalesce to become an amorphous, multinucleated, continuous membrane uninterrupted by intercellular spaces, i.e., the syncytium. Thus, the syncytiotrophoblast is derived from the inner cytotrophoblasts. This is an important concept, so let us

restate it. **The cytotrophoblasts are the cellular progenitors of the syncytiotrophoblast, i.e., the syncytium.** As Benirschke points out, it is incorrect to refer to "syncytiotrophoblasts" as there are no individual cells, only a continuous lining; therefore it is syncytiotrophoblast or the syncytium. At this time, there clearly are two distinguishable layers of trophoblasts. Thus, the syncytiotrophoblast is contiguous with maternal decidua (and later, maternal blood) whereas the cytotrophoblasts are the innermost (embryonic side) layer and ultimately come to be the cells nearest the intravillous space, in which the fetal vessels traverse as one conduit of the placental arm of the fetal–maternal communication system. The extravillous, forward wave of trophoblasts that come to form the anchoring cells remain as single or cytotrophoblast-like cells.

Recall again that the entire blastocyst becomes imbedded in the maternal endometrium. Therefore, as the trophoblasts begin to replicate, the blastocyst is covered by both trophoblasts and endometrium—decidua. As the developing blastocyst and its surrounding trophoblasts and covering decidua grow, one pole of this mass extends toward the cavity of the uterus and one pole remains buried in the endometrium—decidua. The in-

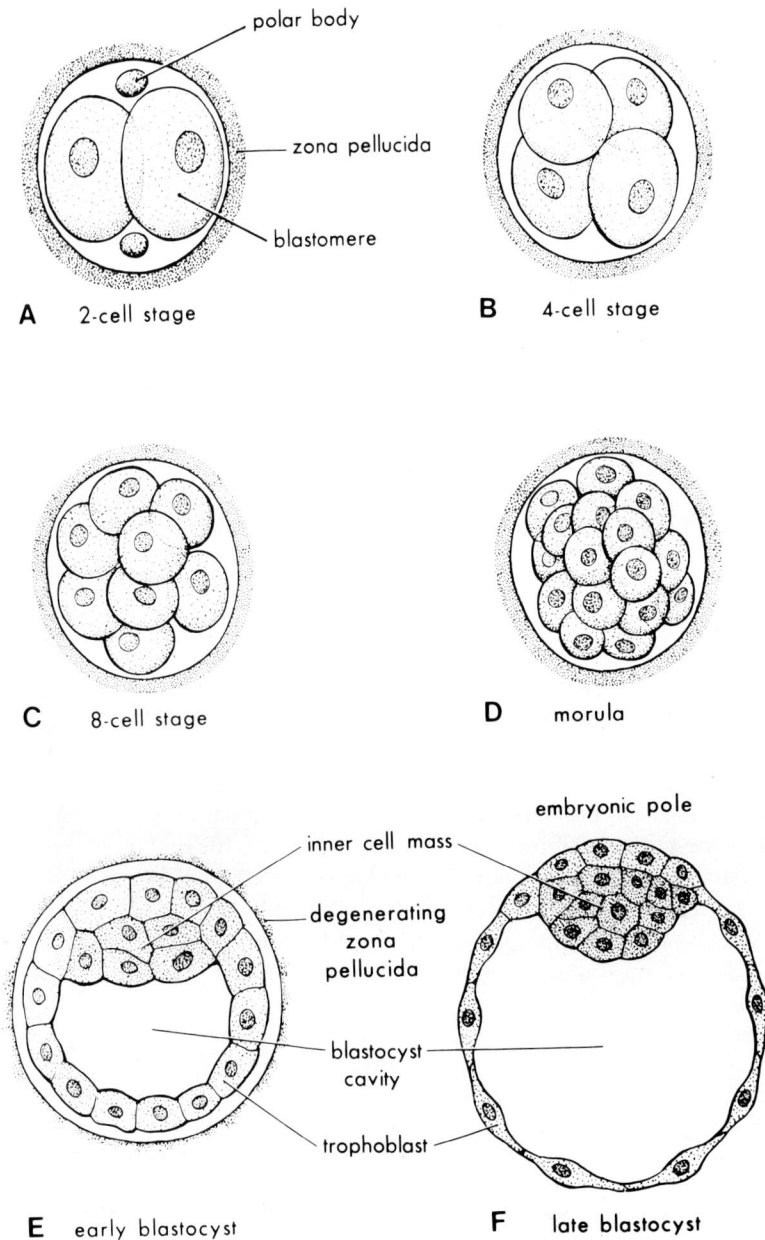

Fig. 5–3. Cleavage of the zygote and formation of the blastocyst. **A** to **D** show various stages of cleavage. The period of the morula begins at the 12- to 16-cell stage and ends when the blastocyst forms, which occurs when there are 50 to 60 blastomeres present. **E** and **F** are sections of blastocysts. The zona pellucida has disappeared by the late blastocyst stage (5 days). The polar bodies shown in **A** are small, nonfunctional cells that soon degenerate. (From Moore, 1988.)

nermost pole ultimately forms the placenta (i.e., the villous trophoblasts), whereas the pole developing toward the endometrial cavity is covered by the chorion frondosum, which at this time is covered by decidua (capsularis). **In this manner, the fetal tissues that will form the two arms (placental and paracrine) of the fetal–maternal communication system are clearly distinguished.**

With continued embryonic growth, the blood supply of the chorion facing the endometrial cavity becomes restricted, and the villous nature of this tissue is lost as is its blood supply; at that time, it becomes an avascular fetal membrane, the chorion laeve (i.e., the smooth chorion). With continued expansion, the chorion laeve will come to lie contiguous with the en-

tire maternal decidua (parietalis) not occupied by the villous and anchoring extravillous trophoblasts. The chorion laeve, therefore, is comprised of cytotrophoblasts and fetal mesodermal cells that survive in a relatively low oxygen atmosphere. As the embryo expands, the decidua capsularis comes to be merged with the decidua parietalis—but probably the decidua capsularis is largely lost by way of pressure and loss of blood supply. This area of the decidua, where decidua capsularis and decidua parietalis merge, is sometimes referred to as the decidua vera.

One of the earliest implanting blastocysts discovered by Hertig and Rock (1944) is shown in Figure 5–4. It measured only 0.36 by 0.31 mm; and it was believed to have been in the process of penetrating the endo-

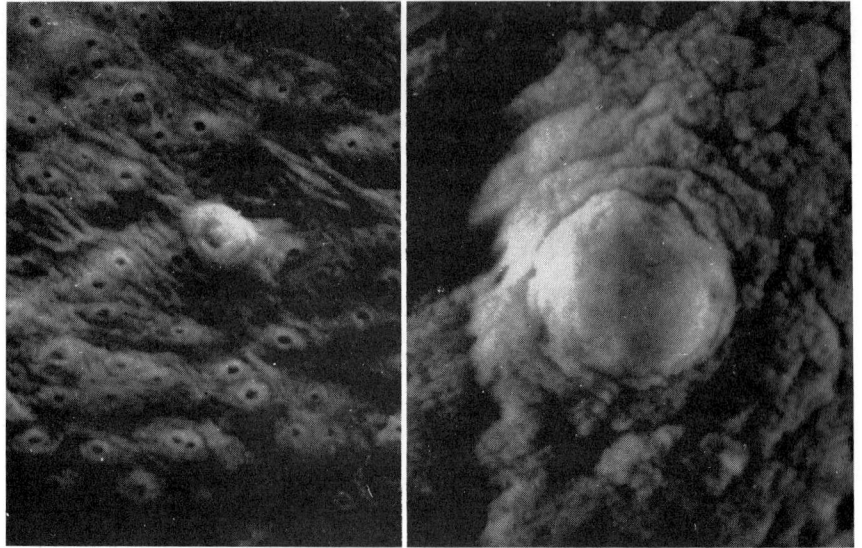

Fig. 5–4. Low- and high-power photomicrographs of surface view of an early human implantation obtained on day 22 of the endometrial cycle, less than 8 days after conception. Site was slightly elevated and measured 0.36 × 0.31 mm. Mouths of uterine glands appear as dark spots surrounded by halos. (Carnegie Collection no. 8225.) (From Hertig and Rock, 1944.)

metrium, with the thin outer wall of the blastocyst still within the uterine cavity. An implanting blastocyst at a similar stage of development, 7½ days after fertilization, is shown in Figure 5–5. It appears to have been flattened in the process of penetrating the uterine epithelium; the enlargement and multiplication of the trophoblastic cells in contact with the endometrium are alone responsible for the increase in size of the implanted blastocyst as compared with the free one. The hole in the uterine epithelium that is created by the blastocyst 9½ days after fertilization (Fig. 5–6), as it implants, is indicative of the size of the blastocyst at the time of penetration of the endometrial surface. The defect is bounded by a zone of maternal endometrial epithelium that shriveled as the trophoblast spread out beneath it. When correction was made for the additional artifactual shrinkage, which results from preparation of the histological sections, the diameter of the fertilized ovum at the moment

of implantation was estimated to be 0.23 mm. We now understand that the human blastocyst penetrates the endometrial surface gently by intrusion between endometrial epithelial cells.

According to Hertig and Rock, implantation of the human blastocyst takes place 6 days after ovum fertilization. As the blastocyst contacts the endometrium, syncytiotrophoblast is differentiated from cytotrophoblast. Development of syncytiotrophoblast is undoubtedly a major goal in successful endometrial invasion. In the human, a full decidual response in endometrium is not elicited until the trophoblast has eroded the superficial uterine epithelium, suggesting that the trophoblasts contribute to the decidualization process.

In the human, the free blastocytic period (fertilization to apposition) is 4 to 6 days; but in some species, there is a *developmental diapause,* or delayed implantation, during which time the blastocysts may remain

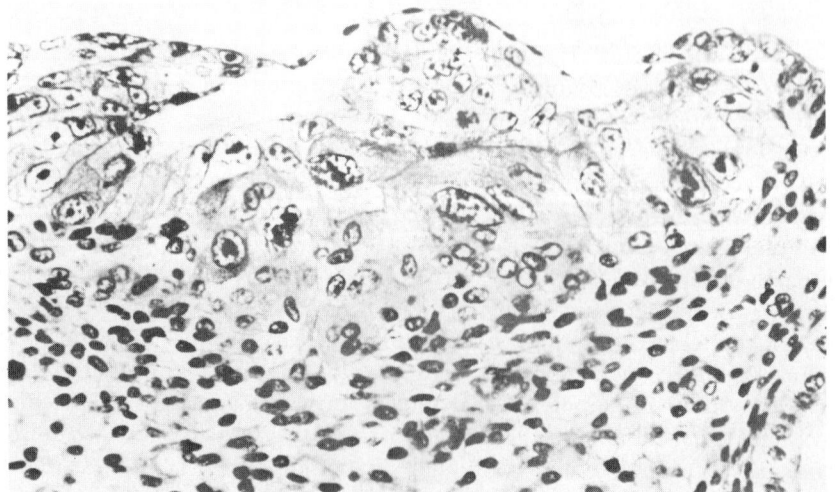

Fig. 5–5. An implanting human blastocyst 7½ days after fertilization. (From Potter and Craig, 1975.)

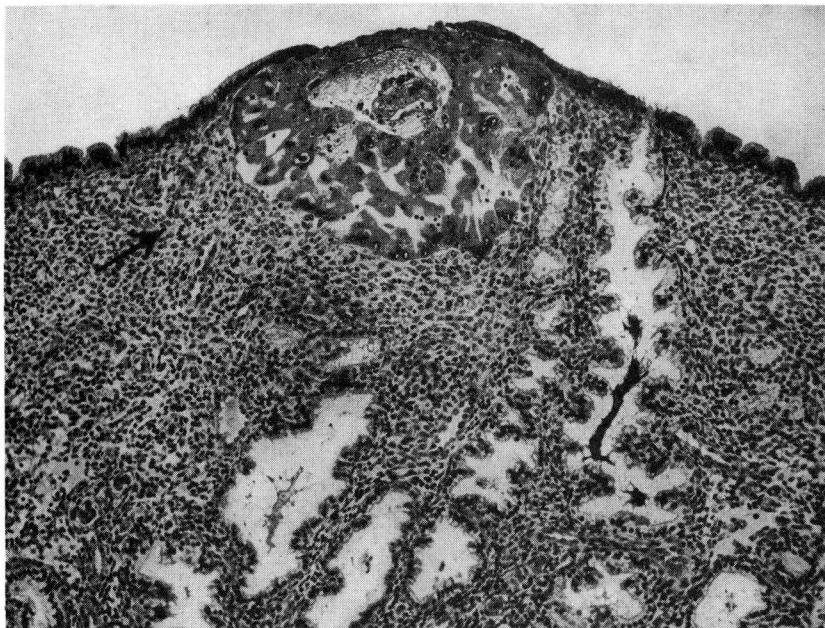

Fig. 5–6. A thin section of fertilized ovum obtained on 25th day of cycle, 9½ days or less after fertilization. Area still exposed to uterine lumen as in Figure 5–9. Syncytiotrophoblast, a complex network fills enlarged implantation site. Within cytotrophoblastic shell, 2-layered embryo and amnion-forming cells. Arrow is pointed to zone of enlarged stromal cells. (Carnegie Collection no. 8004; × 100.) (From Hertig and Rock, 1945.)

unattached for much longer intervals (e.g., 6 months or more in the pine marten).

Early Trophoblasts. In a description of the earliest stages of the human blastocyst, the wall of the primitive blastodermic vesicle was described as consisting of a single layer of ectoderm (Fig. 5–2). As early as 72 hours after fertilization, Hertig (1962) observed that the 58-cell blastula had differentiated into 5 embryo-producing cells and 53 cells destined to form trophoblasts. Although trophoblasts have not been distinguished before blastocyst implantation, both cellular and syncytiotrophoblast are identifiable in the earliest implanted monkey blastocyst. Indeed, evidence has been presented that the expression of chorionic gonadotropin (hCG) by cells of the blastocyst may commence before implantation (Chap. 6).

Soon after implantation, the trophoblasts proliferate rapidly and invade the surrounding decidua. Early trophoblasts resemble choriocarcinoma in their invasive and cytolytic behavior, in histologically characteristic cytoplasmic vacuolization, and in ultrastructure (see Chap. 35). On the one hand, it seems reasonably clear that the impetus for implantation–invasion is provided by products of the blastocyst (trophoblasts). On the other hand, it is speculated that limitation of trophoblast invasion is provided by decidua, and in particular, the large granular lymphocytes of this tissue. This issue is discussed in some detail below.

As endometrial invasion by trophoblasts proceeds, maternal blood vessels are tapped to form lacunae, which are soon filled with maternal blood. To understand the nature of human placentation, it is imperative that we recall again the importance of the human type of placentation—that is, **hemochorioendothelial** placentation. The "hemo" refers to maternal blood, which directly bathes the syncytiotrophoblast ("chorio"), which in turn are separated from fetal blood by the wall of the fetal capillaries ("endothelial") that traverse the intravillous space. This is not true of all species, but it is a consideration of signal importance in human placentation. This arrangement is illustrated in Figures 5–7 and 5–8. As the lacunae join, a complicated labyrinth is formed that is partitioned by solid trophoblastic columns. The trophoblast-lined labyrinthine channels and the solid cellular columns form the intervillous space and primary villous stalks, respectively.

Much of our knowledge of the formation of the intervillous space of both the human and the macaque is based on the findings of the classic studies of Wislocki and Streeter (1938). Initially, the capillary network of the most superficial portion of the endometrium is invaded by trophoblasts. **Ultimately, the arterioles and thence the spiral arteries are invaded, and the walls of these vessels are destroyed.**

Let us consider this proposition in some detail because of its great importance to an understanding of uteroplacental blood flow. Hamilton and Boyd (1966) give credit to Friedlander (1870) for the first description of the striking structural changes of the spiral arteries of the decidua basalis during placentation. They observed that during implantation of the human blastocyst, the spiral arteries acquire a lining of cells within the endothelium that are derived from the invading cytotrophoblasts. During this invasive process, degenerative changes occur in the vessel wall, affecting all layers. The most striking change involves the vascular smooth muscle, which ceases to be recognizable. The

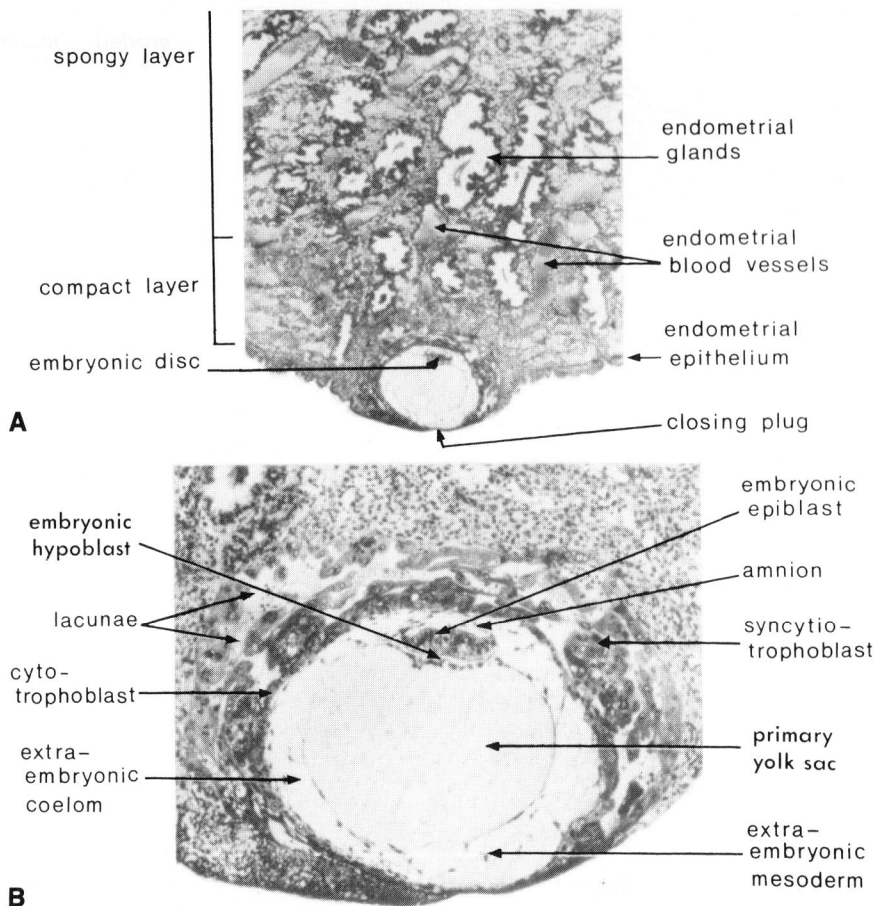

Fig. 5–7. A. Section through the implantation site of a human embryo 12 days after fertilization. The embryo is embedded in the compact layer of endometrium (× 30). **B.** Higher magnification of the conceptus and surrounding endometrium (× 100). (From Hertig and Rock, 1941. Courtesy of Carnegie Institution of Washington, as modified by Moore, 1988.)

cytotrophoblasts that invade the spiral arteries can pass several centimeters along the vessel lumen; indeed, Hamilton and Boyd noted their occurrence in myometrial portions of these vessels. They also emphasize that these vascular changes are not observed in the decidua parietalis—that is, in tissue sites removed from the invading trophoblasts. The intraluminal trophoblastic cells diminish in number near term. But in earlier pregnancy (midtrimester), trophoblasts are present in all of the spiral arteries of the decidua at the placental site. Hamilton and Boyd took special notice of several curious features of their observations: (1) the trophoblasts in the vessels do not appear to replicate; (2) oddly, these cells are not readily dislodged by the flow of blood; (3) in fact, the cells appear to migrate against the arterial flow and pressure; (4) there is no obvious adhesion of these cells one to the other; and (5) the maternal vascular invasion of trophoblasts involves only the arteries, not the veins. Veins do transport trophoblasts, but this process occurs in a completely different manner by a separate mechanism that is referred to as villous deportation.

Maternal blood enters the intervillous space through the spiral arteries in fountain-like bursts; thus, maternal blood (which is totally outside of maternal vessels) sweeps over and bathes the syn-

cytiotrophoblast. The maternal surface of the syncytiotrophoblast consists of a complex microvillous structure; and during the course of pregnancy, there is continual shedding and reformation of these microvilli.

Embryonic Development After Implantation. At 7½ days of development, the stage shown in Figure 5–5, the wall of the blastocyst that faces the uterine lumen consists of a single layer of flattened cells, whereas the thicker opposite wall is comprised of two zones—the trophoblast and the embryo-forming inner cell mass. Among the trophoblasts, two subdivisions of cells are distinguishable, the *cytotrophoblast,* comprised of individual cells with relatively pale-staining cytoplasm, and the *syncytiotrophoblast,* in which dark-staining nuclei are distributed irregularly within a common basophilic cytoplasm. Mitotic figures, however, are confined to the cellular (cytotrophoblast) elements. As early as 7½ days after fertilization, the inner cell mass, now called the *embryonic disc,* is already differentiated into a thick plate of primitive ectoderm and an underlying endoderm layer. Between the embryonic disc and the trophoblast, some small cells appear that soon enclose a space that will become the amnionic cavity.

To illustrate the next stage of development, a thin section of the 9½-day fertilized ovum (Fig. 5–6) is

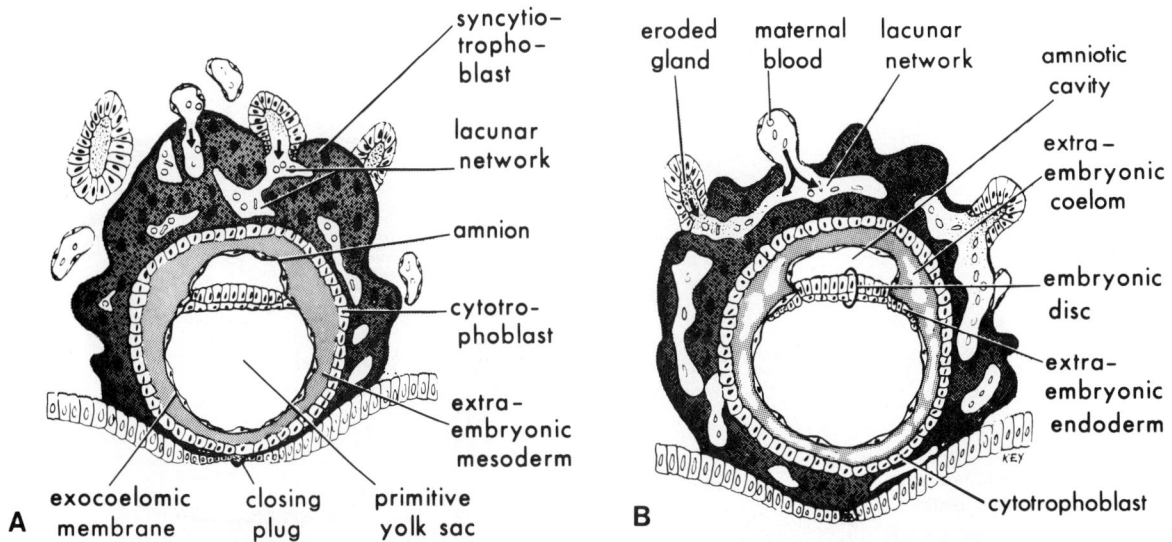

Fig. 5–8. Drawings of sections through implanted blastocysts. **A.** 10 days. **B.** 12 days after fertilization. The stage of development is characterized by the intercommunication of the lacunae filled with maternal blood. Note in **B** that large cavities have appeared in the extraembryonic mesoderm, forming the beginning of the extraembryonic coelom. Also note that extraembryonic endodermal cells have begun to form on the inside of the primary yolk sac. (From Moore, 1988.)

shown; the increase in size is the result primarily of development of the syncytium, which comprises a complex network of protoplasmic strands that enclose irregular fluid-filled spaces, the *lacunae*, which later become confluent. The embryonic disc now consists of a "dorsal" ectoderm, which is made up of tall columnar cells, and a "ventral" endoderm, which is formed of somewhat irregular cells. The remainder of the blastocyst is occupied by a proteinaceous coagulum, which is limited externally by a layer of flattened cells—the *exocoelomic,* or *Heuser membrane*—the origin of which is uncertain. The amnionic cavity dorsal to the embryonic disc is now well defined.

As the embryo enlarges, more maternal (decidua basalis) tissue is invaded and the walls of the superficial endometrial–decidual capillaries are eroded; the result is that maternal blood enters the lacunae. With deeper burrowing and blastocystic invasion into the decidua, the trophoblastic strands branch to form the solid primitive villi that traverse the lacunae. Originally located over the entire blastocyst surface, the villi later disappear except over the most deeply implanted portion, which is the site destined to form the placenta.

The mesenchyme first appears as isolated cells within the cavity of the blastocyst. When the cavity is completely lined with mesoderm, it is termed the *chorionic vesicle,* and its membrane, now called the *chorion,* is composed of trophoblasts and mesenchyme.

The diameter of the 12-day embryo, as shown in Figure 5–7, is almost 1 mm. The mesenchymal cells within the cavity are most numerous about the embryo, where these eventually condense, to form the *body stalk* that serves to join the embryo to the nutrient chorion and later develops into the umbilical cord. Thereafter, the site of entry of the blastocyst into the endometrium is covered by regenerated epithelium. The defect itself is plugged by fibrin and cellular debris.

The syncytiotrophoblast of the chorionic shell is permeated by a system of intercommunicating channels of trophoblastic lacunae that contain maternal blood. At the same time, a decidual reaction intensifies in the surrounding endometrial stroma, which is characterized by enlargement of the endometrial stromal cells and storage of glycogen therein. The amnionic cavity is then lined by ectoderm, which is apparently contiguous with that of the embryonic disc. At this stage, the endoderm probably delaminates from the inferior surface of the embryonic disc and soon spreads peripherally beyond the disc to line the blastocoele; this process results in the formation of the yolk sac. The remainder of the blastocyst is filled with primary mesoderm, which consists of sparse mesenchymal cells in a loose matrix. It is believed that the mesoderm arises from the embryonic cells, but its precise mode of origin in the human is still not clear.

The Germ Layers. The amnion and yolk sac, with both epithelial and mesenchymal components, are illustrated in Figures 5–8 and 5–9. The body stalk, from which the caudal end of the embryo arises, also can be recognized at this stage. Cellular proliferation in the embryonic disc marks the beginning of a thickening in the midline that is clearly indicative of the embryonic axis and is called the *primitive streak.* Cells spread out laterally from the

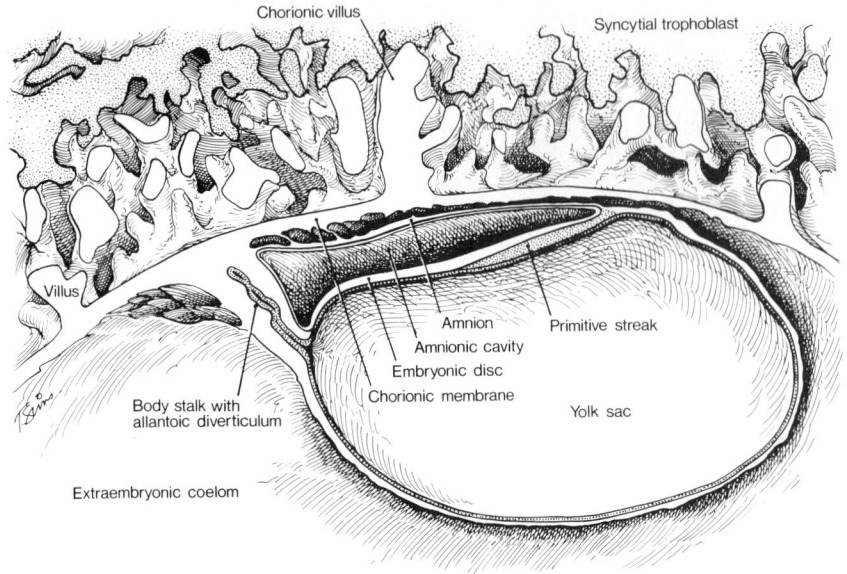

Fig. 5–9. Median view of a drawing of a wax reconstruction of Mateer fertilized ovum, showing the amnionic cavity and its relations to chorionic membrane and yolk sac (× 50). (After Streeter, 1920.)

primitive streak between ectoderm and endoderm to form the mesoderm. These three germ layers give rise to the various organs of the developing embryo. The entire nervous system, central and peripheral, and the epidermis, with such derivatives as the crystalline lens and the hair, are derived from the *ectoderm*. The *endoderm* develops into the lining of the gastrointestinal tract, from pharynx to rectum, and such derivative organs as the liver, pancreas, and thyroid. The dermis, skeleton, connective tissues, vascular and urogenital systems, and most skeletal and smooth muscles arise from the *mesoderm*. The cavity that later divides the somatic and visceral sheets of intraembryonic mesoderm is the *coelom*.

Formation of the Somites. During the third week after fertilization (fifth week of gestation), the primitive streak becomes a prominent structure, and the cephalic and caudal ends of the embryo become distinguishable. As cells proliferate rapidly and spread laterally from the primitive streak, a midline *primitive groove* develops. Simultaneously, the yolk sac enlarges, and hence the embryonic disc is spread out upon it. A well-defined body stalk into which a narrow endodermal diverticulum, the allantois, has extended, is shown in Figure 5–9. In many mammals, the allantois develops into a large sac that vascularizes the chorion. A forward extension of the primitive streak, the *notochord* (Fig. 5–10), constitutes the primordial supporting structure of vertebrates and remains as a continuous column of cells throughout embryonic life. Remnants of the notochord persist in the adult as the nucleus pulposus of the intervertebral discs.

Because differentiation of structures proceeds from cephalic to caudal ends in a sequence characteristic of all vertebrate embryos, most of the substance of the early embryo will enter into formation of the head; the

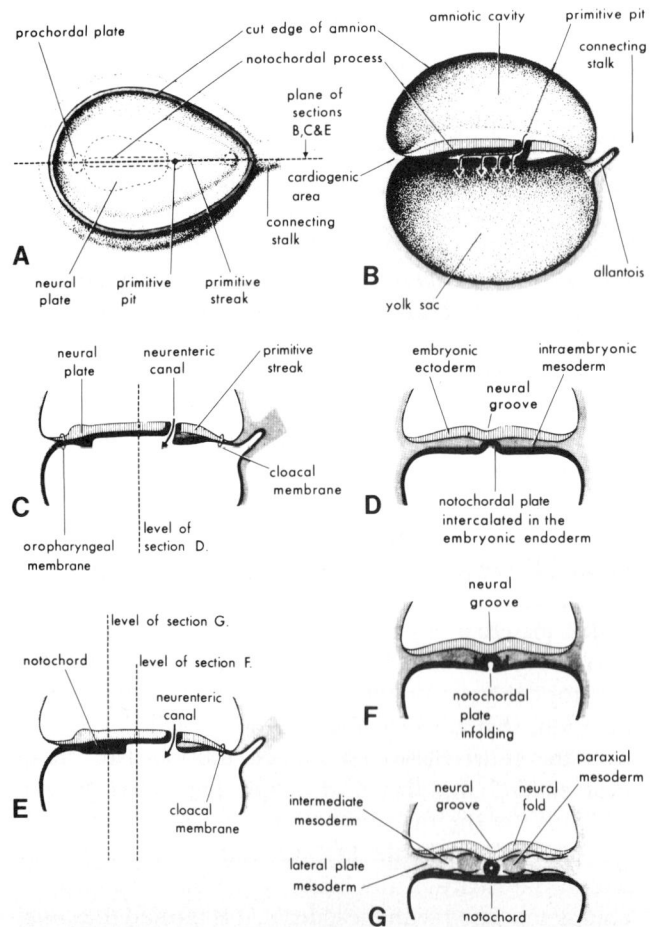

Fig. 5–10. Drawings illustrating final stages of notochord development. **A.** Dorsal view of the embryonic disc at about 18 days, exposed by removing the amnion. **B.** Three-dimensional sagittal section of the embryo. **C** and **E.** Sagittal sections of embryos of about 18 to 19 days. **D, F,** and **G.** Transverse sections of the embryonic disc. (From Moore, 1988.)

subsequent development of the primitive streak provides material for the rest of the body. Soon, a *neural groove* develops as neural folds arise on either side. The cavity of the future neural tube is connected with the future lumen of the gut by the *neurenteric canal.* As the neural folds develop, the underlying lateral mesoderm is divided into discrete blocks, the *somites,* which give rise to the skeletal and connective tissues, the muscles, and the dermis. The first three or four somites enter into formation of the occipital region of the head. The primordium of the heart already has appeared beneath the pharynx and is separated from the yolk sac by a fold that also lifts the cephalic end of the embryo above the level of the yolk sac. In Figure 5–11, the elevation of the neural folds is shown as is the closure of these folds to form a tube, which is wider from the outset in the region of the fourth pair of somites. Although the head remains relatively enormous during the embryonic period, the rest of the body takes form after the fourth week, and the head becomes smaller in proportion. By the seventh week after fertilization, the neck can be recognized, the tail filament has disappeared, and the embryo can be identified as human. From the eighth week after fertilization, changes in the shape of the human fetus are less striking. Some of the principal features are presented in Chapter 7.

Biology of the Trophoblast

Origin of the Syncytiotrophoblast. Of all placental components, the trophoblast is the most variable in

structure, function, and development. Its invasiveness provides for attachment of the blastocyst to the uterus; its role in nutrition of the conceptus is reflected in its name; and its function as an endocrine organ is essential to maternal physiological adaptation to pregnancy. Morphologically, the trophoblast may be cellular or syncytial and it may appear as uninuclear cells or multinuclear giant cells. The true syncytial character of the human syncytiotrophoblast (syncytium) has been confirmed by electron microscopy. Its mechanism of growth, however, was a mystery, in view of the discrepancy between an increase in the number of nuclei in the syncytiotrophoblast and only equivocal evidence of intrinsic nuclear replication. Mitotic figures are completely absent from the syncytium, being confined to the cytotrophoblast.

It now is clear that the cytotrophoblast is the germinal cell, and the syncytium, the secretory cells, are derived from the cytotrophoblasts. Each cytotrophoblast is characterized as a single cell with well-demarcated borders and a single, distinct nucleus, and among the cytotrophoblasts there are frequent mitoses. These characteristics are lacking, however, in the syncytium, in which the cytoplasm is amorphous, lacking cell borders, and the nuclei are multiple and diverse in size and shape (Ramsey, 1985).

Trophoblast Function in Implantation. Ulloa-Aguirre and co-workers (1987), in an elegant series of studies, have demonstrated the in vitro conversion of cytotrophoblasts to a morphologically and functionally characteristic syncytium; and they have shown that at least a

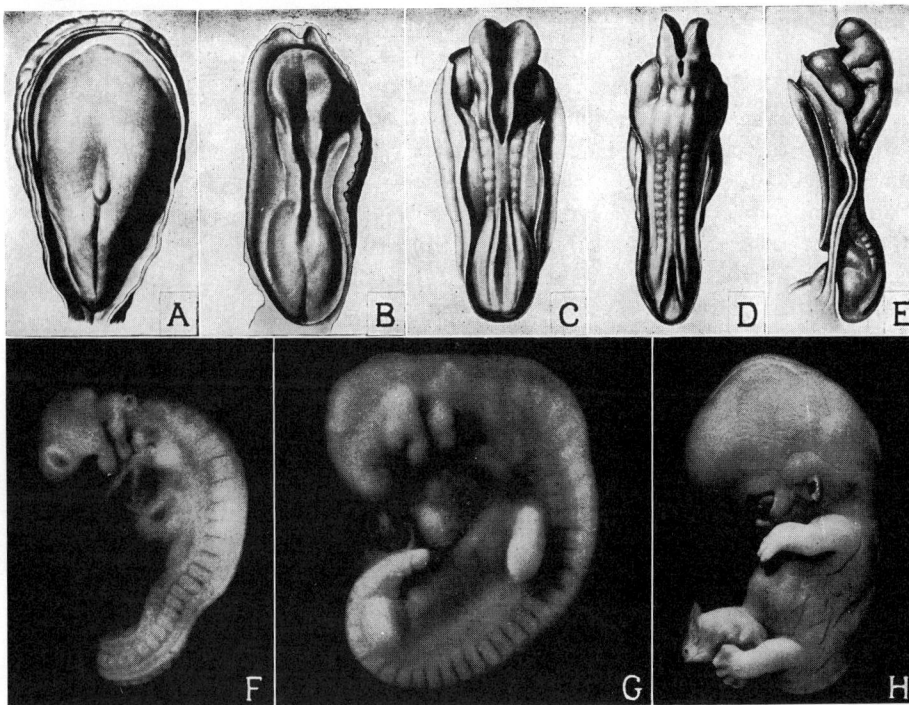

Fig. 5–11. Human embryogenesis. **A.** Heuser, 19 days (× 30). **B.** Ingalls (× 28). **C.** Payne (× 23). **D.** Corner (× 23). **E.** Atwell, 21 to 22 days (× 15.5). **F.** 4th week (× 12). **G.** 5th week (× 8.5). **H.** 8th week (× 2.5). (Carnegie Collection. From Streeter, 1931.)

part of this differentiation process involves the action of cyclic adenosine monophosphate (cAMP). They also present a model for the formation of the syncytiotrophoblast in which it is envisioned that isolated cytotrophoblasts migrate toward each other to form aggregates. The aggregates fuse to form the syncytiotrophoblast (Kliman and colleagues, 1986; Ulloa-Aguirre and co-workers, 1987).

Coutifaris and associates (1991) have provided a succinct and informative review of the process of human trophoblast implantation as well as an overview of in vitro systems useful for the study of this process. They point out that after apposition of the trophectoderm of the blastocyst to the endometrial epithelial cells, implantation commences by intrusion of the trophoblast cells between endometrial epithelial cells. Upon coming into contact with the basement membrane, degradation of this structure occurs, permitting invasion of trophoblasts through the stroma to the endometrial vessels.

Using methods for the isolation and characterization of human cytotrophoblasts that they developed, in vitro systems have been established to evaluate blastocyst implantation (Kliman and associates, 1986; Ringler and Strauss, 1990). These investigators observed that isolated cytotrophoblasts in serum-containing medium migrate towards one another, form aggregates, and finally form a syncytium during a period of 3 to 4 days. They also observed that these phenomena occur in the absence of serum provided that extracellular matrix components are present to serve as a lattice for the movement of the cells. The syncytium produced is covered by microvilli.

The aggregation of cytotrophoblasts is dependent upon protein synthesis and they find evidence that the calcium-dependent cell adhesion molecule (CAM), E-cadherin, is intimately involved in the aggregation process. Desmosomes develop between the cells. As the cells fuse, the expression of E-cadherin disappears. The cytotrophoblasts can bind to various extracellular matrix components and thence produce the proteinases that enable the degradation of the same molecules, possibly describing the process involved in the migration of these cells. Urokinase-type plasminogen activator and metalloproteinases produced by trophoblasts likely are involved in the degradation of the extracellular matrix proteins.

Co-cultures of isolated human endometrial glandular cells with human cytotrophoblasts permit the study of the direct interaction of trophoblasts and endometrium. Interestingly, Coutifaris and co-workers (1991) point out that this trophoblast intrusion appears to be a *"gentle"* process in which the separation of junctions between endometrial cells is gradual, not destroying the endometrial epithelial cells. In this manner, the dislodged epithelial cells will come to be remodeled around the invading trophoblasts, eventually totally encasing the trophoblasts.

Trophoblast Production of Oncofetal Fibronectin. As described by Feinberg and colleagues (1991), oncofetal fibronectin (onfFN) molecules are those with a unique glycopeptide within the type III connecting segment (IIICS) of the fibronectin molecule. They used an antibody with specificity toward an O-linked glycosylated hexapeptide within IIICS, but no reactivity to normal adult fibronectin, to localize onfFN to the junction of trophoblast with extracellular matrix. Specifically, fibronectin was localized to the extracellular matrix connecting extravillous trophoblasts and trophoblastic cell columns to the uterine decidua. They found that isolated cytotrophoblasts in culture synthesize and secrete onfFN, but when treated with cAMP agonists, its synthesis is markedly inhibited.

They refer to onfFN as *"trophouteronectin"* or *"trophoblast glue"* to suggest a critical role for this protein in the migration and attachment of trophoblasts. The glycosylation of onfFN is believed to reduce its binding efficiency for other components of the extracellular matrix. As onfFN is associated with extravillous trophoblasts, including those of chorion laeve, it may facilitate the separation of these tissues from the uterus at delivery. Lockwood and colleagues (1991) have evaluated the appearance of onfFN in cervical and vaginal secretions in association with term and preterm labor. These findings are further discussed in Chapter 12.

Trophoblast Ultrastructure. From the electron microscopic studies of Wislocki and Dempsey (1955), basic data were provided upon which the functional interpretation of the fine structure of the placenta is based. The prominent microvilli of the syncytial surface, corresponding to the so-called brush border of light microscopy, and the associated pinocytotic vacuoles and vesicles, are related to the absorptive and secretory placental functions. The inner layer of cytotrophoblasts, which persists to term although often compressed against the trophoblastic basal lamina, retains its ultrastructural simplicity. There are few specialized organelles in these cells, with abundant free ribosomes but scant ergastoplasm. Desmosomes connect individual cytotrophoblast cells with one another and with the syncytium, from which complete plasma membranes are absent. Ultrastructurally, the syncytium is relatively complex, containing abundant endoplasmic reticulum, Golgi bodies, and mitochondria, as well as numerous secretory droplets, lipid granules, and highly convoluted plasma membranes. As the syncytium matures, the fine structural changes are reflective of functional maturation. The early syncytiotrophoblast often exhibits a microvesicular endoplasmic reticulum; later, at the height of active protein synthesis, flattened ergastoplasmic channels assume prominence; and still later, associated with storage and transport of proteins, dilated cisternae of endoplasmic reticulum appear, the largest of which are visible with the light microscope. Secretory granules, at least those believed to be glycoproteins and osmophilic lipid granules, correspond to PAS-positive and sudanophilic droplets, respectively (Figs. 5–12 to 5–14).

As the human placenta matures, the placental membrane may be reduced anatomically to a thin covering of trophoblast, capillary wall, and trophoblastic and endothelial basement membranes separated by mere wisps of connective tissue.

The term *barrier* as applied to placental physiology should therefore be replaced by the more accurate term *placental membrane.* Furthermore, the number of layers is a poor index of the true approximation of the fetal and maternal circulations.

Organization of Placenta

Chorionic Villi. Villi can first be distinguished easily in the human placenta on about the 12th day after fertilization. When the solid trophoblast column is invaded by

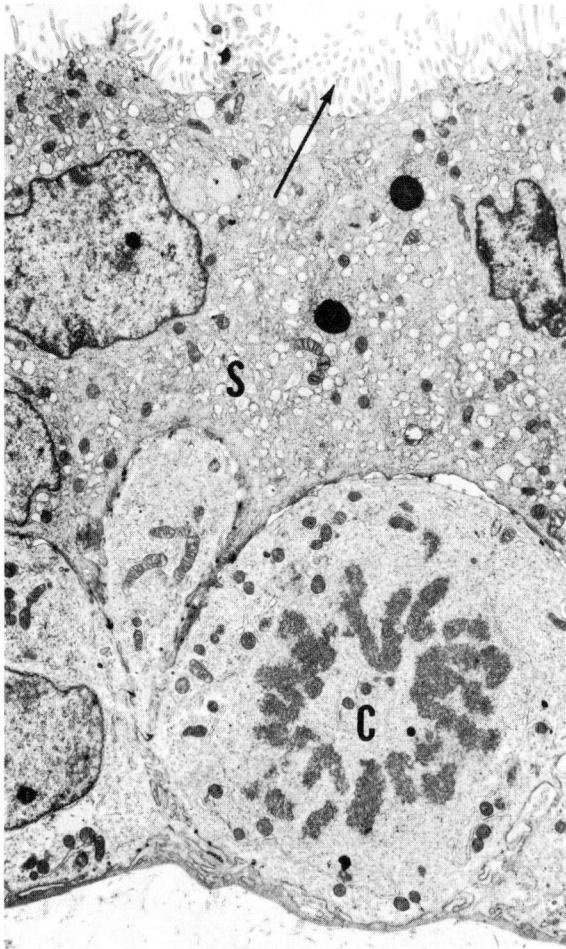

Fig. 5–12. Electron micrograph of human placenta at 6 weeks' gestation. Note prominent border of microvilli (*arrow*), syncytium (S), and mitotic figure in cytotrophoblast (C). (Courtesy of Dr. Ralph M. Wynn.)

a mesenchymal cord, presumably derived from cytotrophoblasts, secondary villi are formed. After angiogenesis occurs in situ from the mesenchymal cores, the resulting villi are termed *tertiary.*

Maternal venous sinuses are tapped early, but until the 14th or 15th day after fertilization, maternal arterial blood does not enter the intervillous space. By about the 17th day, both fetal and maternal blood vessels are functional and a placental circulation is established. The fetal–placental circulation is completed when the blood vessels of the embryo are connected with the chorionic blood vessels, which are likely formed in situ from cytotrophoblasts. Some villi, in which absence of angiogenesis results in a lack of circulation, may distend with fluid and form vesicles. A striking exaggeration of this process is present in the development of hydatidiform mole (see Chap. 35).

Proliferation of cellular trophoblasts at the tips of the villi produces the trophoblastic cell columns, which are not invaded by mesenchyme but are anchored to the decidua at the basal plate. Thus, the floor of the intervillous space (maternal side) consists of cytotrophoblasts from the cell columns, the peripheral syncytium of the trophoblastic shell, and decidua of the basal plate. The floor of the chorionic plate, consisting of the two trophoblasts externally and fibrous mesoderm internally, forms the roof of the intervillous space.

Between the 18th and 19th days of development, the blastocyst (including the chorionic shell) measures 6 by 2.5 mm in diameter. At this time, the embryo is in the primitive-streak stage, with a maximal length of 0.6 to 0.7 mm. The trophoblastic shell is thick, with villi formed of cytotrophoblastic projections, a central core of chorionic mesoderm in which blood vessels are developing, and an external covering of the syncytiotrophoblast, or syncytium. At this time, the blastocyst lies buried in the decidua and is separated from the myometrium by the decidua basalis and from the uterine epithelium by the decidua capsularis. The embryo itself is trilaminar, and its endoderm is continuous with the lining of the yolk sac. An intermediate layer of intraembryonic mesoderm can be traced and found to be contiguous with the extraembryonic mesoderm, which later forms part of the walls of the amnion and yolk sac and connects the embryonic structures to the chorionic mesoderm by the body stalk, or abdominal pedicle, the forerunner of the umbilical cord.

By about 3 weeks after fertilization, the relation of chorion to decidua is clearly evident in the human embryo. The chorionic membrane consists of an inner connective tissue layer and an outer epithelium from which rudimentary villi project. The connective tissue consists of spindly cells with protoplasmic processes within a loose intercellular matrix. The trophoblast differentiates into cuboidal or nearly round cells with clear cytoplasm and light-staining vesicular nuclei (cytotrophoblasts or Langhans cells) and an outer syncytium containing ir-

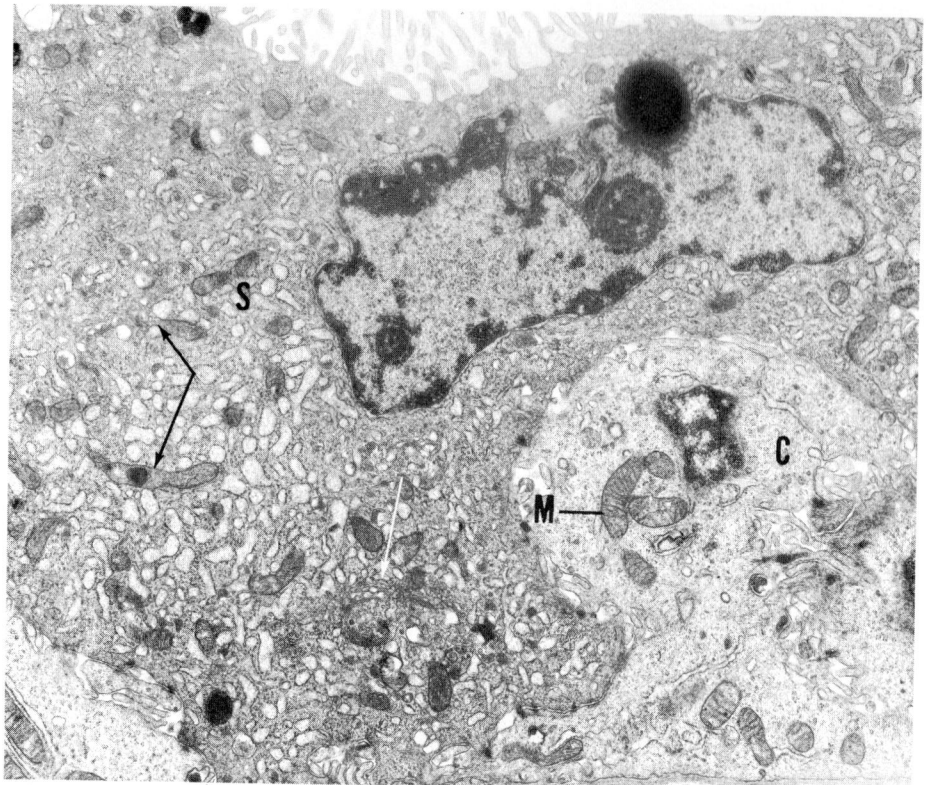

Fig. 5–13. First-trimester human placenta, showing well-differentiated syncytiotrophoblast (S) with numerous mitochondria (*black arrows*) and Golgi complexes (*white arrow*). Cytotrophoblast (C) has large mitochondria (M) but few other organelles. (Courtesy of Dr. Ralph M. Wynn.)

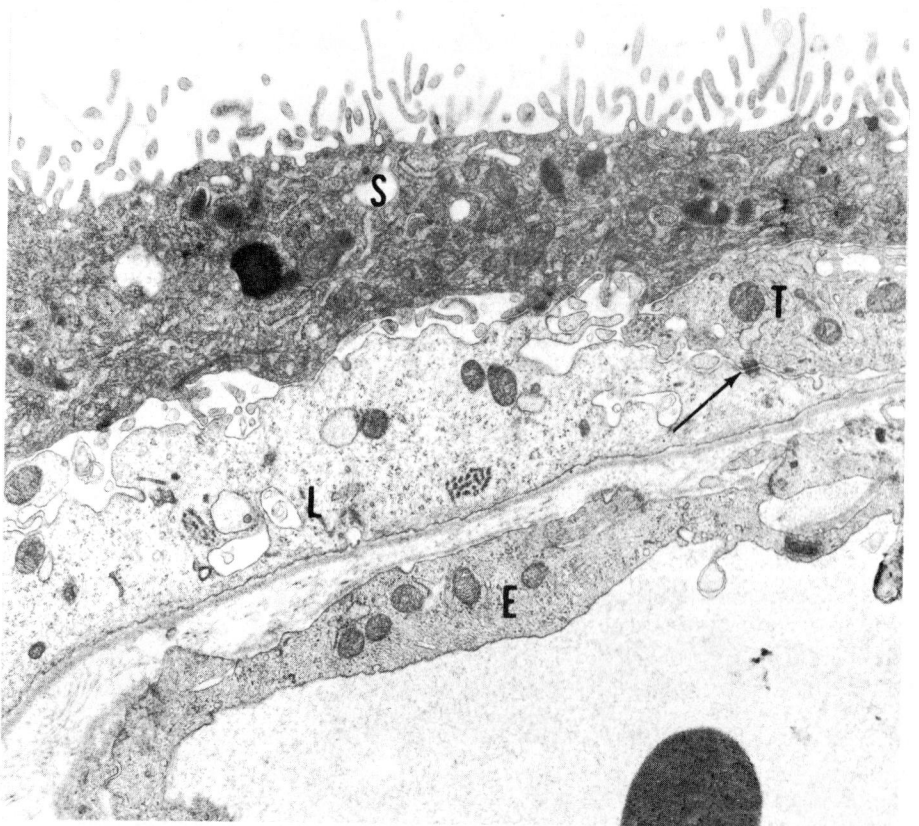

Fig. 5–14. Term human placenta showing electron-dense syncytium (S), Langhans cells (L), transitional cytotrophoblast (T), and capillary endothelium (E). Arrow points to desmosome. (Courtesy of Dr. Ralph M. Wynn.)

regularly scattered, dark-staining nuclei within a coarsely granulated cytoplasm (syncytiotrophoblast).

In early pregnancy, the villi are distributed over the entire periphery of the chorionic membrane; grossly, an ovum dislodged from the endometrium at this stage of development appears shaggy (Fig. 5–15). The villi in contact with the decidua basalis proliferate to form the leafy chorion, or *chorion frondosum,* the fetal component of the placenta; whereas those in contact with the decidua capsularis cease to grow and undergo almost complete degeneration, the *chorion laeve.* The greater part of the chorion, thus denuded of villi, is designated the smooth, or bald, chorion or the chorion laeve. It is formed, according to Hertig (1962), as the result of a combination of direct pressure and interference with its vascular supply. The chorion laeve is generally more nearly translucent than the amnion even though rarely exceeding 1 mm in thickness. The chorion laeve contains ghost villi and, clinging to its surface, shreds of decidua. Until near the end of the third month, the chorion laeve remains separated from the amnion by the exocelomic cavity. Thereafter, the amnion and chorion are in intimate contact (Fig. 5–16). **In the human, the chorion laeve and amnion form an avascular amniochorion, which is an important site of transfer and metabolic activity.** The chorion laeve is the fetal tissue of the interface of the paracrine arm of the fetal–maternal communication system. It is important to recognize that the chorion laeve does not traverse over the surface of the fetal side of the placenta. Only amnion covers the chorionic vessels (the branches of the umbilical vessels) that fan out in the chorionic plate.

Placental Cotyledons. Certain villi of the chorion frondosum extend from the chorionic plate to the decidua and serve as anchoring villi. Most villi, however,

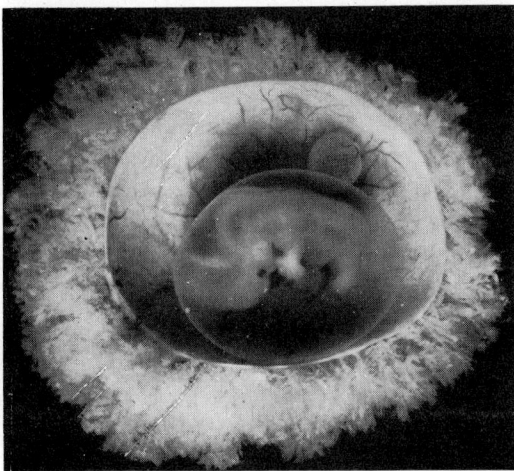

Fig. 5–15. Human chorionic vesicle. Ovulatory age, 40 days. (Carnegie Collection no. 8537.)

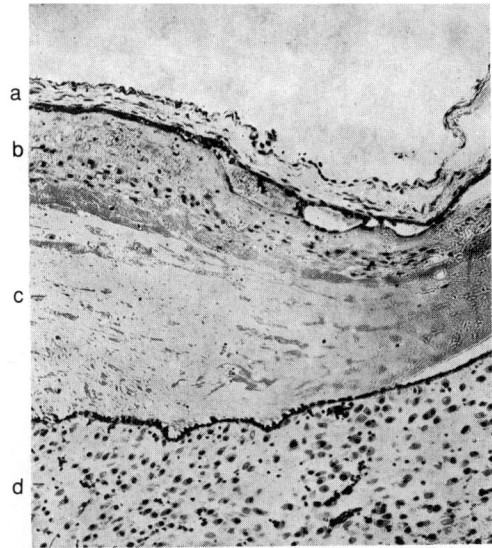

Fig. 5–16. Unfused decidua parietalis and capsularis. Section through uterus at 10 weeks' gestation, showing that the decidua parietalis and capsularis have not yet fused. (a = amnion-chorionic membrane; b = degenerating decidua capsularis; c = uterine cavity; d = decidua parietalis.)

arboresce and end freely in the intervillous space without reaching the decidua (Fig. 5–17). As the placenta matures, the short, thick, early stem villi branch repeatedly, forming progressively finer subdivisions and greater numbers of increasingly small villi (Fig. 5–18). Each of the main stem (truncal) villi and its ramifications (rami) constitute a placental cotyledon (lobe), the fetal tissue interface of the placental arm of the fetal–maternal communication system. Each cotyledon is supplied with a branch (truncal) of the chorionic artery; and for each cotyledon there is a vein, resulting in a 1:1:1 ratio of artery to vein to cotyledon.

Placental Septa. The origin and exact composition of the placental septa continue to stimulate controversy. These appear to consist of decidual tissue in which trophoblastic elements are encased, and are thus very likely of dual fetal and maternal origin. Especially recommended for an elegant pictorial and written description of human placentation is Boyd and Hamilton's extensively illustrated treatise, *The Human Placenta* (1970).

Placental Size and Weight. The data obtained from weighing the placenta vary considerably, depending upon how the placenta is prepared. If membranes and most of the cord are left attached and adherent maternal blood clot is not removed, the weight may be increased by nearly 50 percent (Thomson and co-workers, 1969). Crawford (1959) suggested that the total number of cotyledons remains the same throughout gestation; but

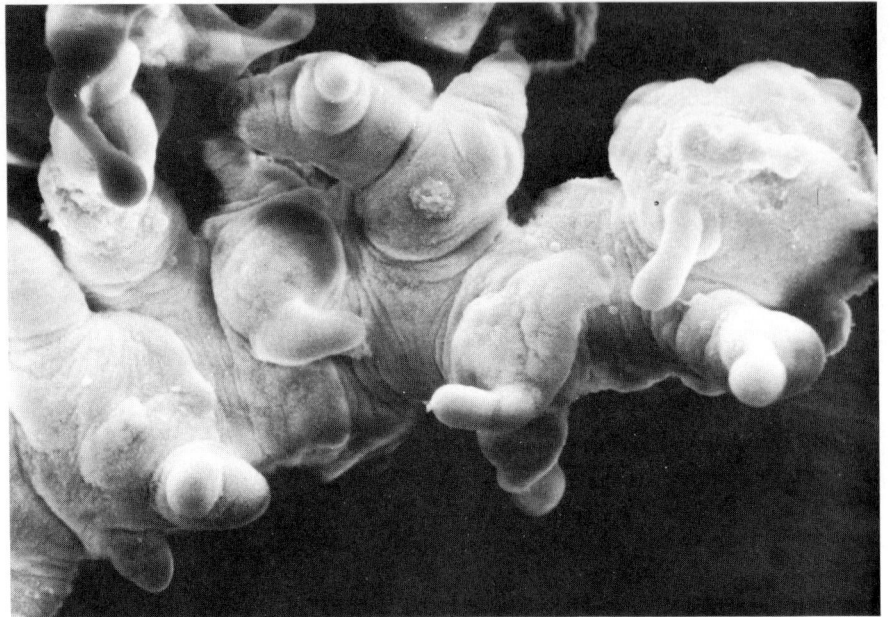

Fig. 5–17. Scanning electron micrograph of placental villi at 10 to 14 weeks' gestation. Note the larger stem villi and the small syncytial sprouts at various stages of formation. Furrows or creases on the surface also are evident, especially at the bases of larger villi (× 289). (From King and Menton, 1975.)

individual cotyledons continue to grow until term, although less actively in the final weeks.

The Placenta at Term. According to Boyd and Hamilton (1970), the placenta at term is, on average, 185 mm in diameter and 23 mm in thickness, with an average volume of 497 mL and weight of 508 g; but these measurements vary widely. There are multiple shapes and forms of the human placenta and a variety of types of umbilical cord insertions (see Chap. 35). Viewed from the maternal surface, there is a variable number (10 to 38) of slightly elevated convex areas called lobes (or if small, lobules). These lobes are separated, incompletely, by grooves of variable depth, which are referred to as placental septa. The lobes are often called cotyledons. Boyd and Hamilton suggest that the smallest macroscopic subdivision of the human placenta is a lobule that corresponds to a single placentome and thus possesses one fetal cotyledon. Thus, the larger lobes are compound placentomes. Each fetal cotyledon is supplied by a primary branch of the chorionic arteries of the chorionic plate; the branch that pierces the chorionic plate is referred to as the truncal artery.

Placental Aging. As the villi continue to branch and the terminal ramifications become more numerous and smaller, the volume and prominence of cytotrophoblasts (Langhans cells) in the villi decrease, although cytotrophoblasts remain obvious in the placental floor. As the syncytium thins and forms knots, the vessels become

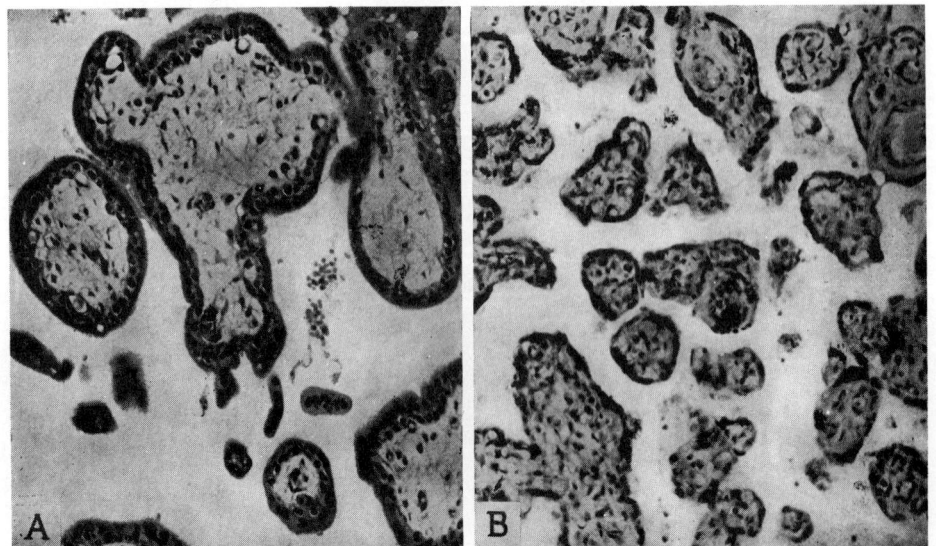

Fig. 5–18. Comparison of chorionic villi in early and late pregnancy. **A.** 2-months' gestation. Note inner Langhans cells (cytotrophoblasts) and outer syncytial layer. **B.** Term placenta. Syncytial layer is obvious, but Langhans cells are difficult to recognize at low magnification in light micrographs.

more prominent and lie closer to the surface. The stroma of the villi also exhibits changes associated with aging. In placentas of early pregnancy, the branching connective tissue cells are separated by an abundant loose intercellular matrix; later, the stroma becomes denser and the cells more spindly and more closely packed. Another change in the stroma involves the so-called *Hofbauer cells,* which are likely fetal macrophages. These are nearly round cells with vesicular, often eccentric nuclei and very granular or vacuolated cytoplasm. These cells are characterized histochemically by intracytoplasmic lipid and are readily distinguished from plasma cells.

As the placenta grows and ages, certain of the accompanying histological changes are suggestive of an increase in the efficiency of transport to meet the growing fetal metabolic requirements. Such changes involve a decrease in thickness of the syncytium, partial disappearance of Langhans cells, decrease in the stroma, and an increase in the number of capillaries and their approximation to the syncytial surface. By 4 months, the apparent continuity of the cytotrophoblasts is broken, and the syncytium forms knots on the more numerous, smaller villi. At term, the covering of the villi may be focally reduced to a thin layer of syncytium with minimal connective tissue; and the fetal capillaries seem to abut the trophoblast. The villous stroma, Hofbauer cells, and Langhans cells are markedly reduced, and the villi appear filled with thin-walled capillaries. Other changes, however, appear to decrease the efficiency for placental exchange; these changes include the thickening of basement membranes of capillaries and trophoblast, obliteration of certain vessels, deposition of fibrin on the surface of the villi, and deposits of fibrin in the basal and chorionic plates and elsewhere in the intervillous space.

Immunological Considerations

The success of the fetal semiallogenic graft appears to defy the laws of transplantation immunology. Today, it still is enigmatic that the mother tolerates the fetal graft; but we have reached a time in the investigation of this issue such that a reasonable explanation seems to be very close.

Immunology of Trophoblasts and Endometrium–Decidua.
Attempts to explain the survival of the semiallogenic fetal graft have occupied the attention of many outstanding biologists. The first explanation based on antigenic immaturity of the fetus must be discarded in light of Billingham's demonstration (1964) that transplantation antigens (in embryonic tissues) appear very early in life. But ordinarily in the fetal–maternal communication system, only extraembryonic fetal tissues are in direct contact with maternal tissues. And more

specifically, trophoblasts are the fetal tissues directly contiguous with maternal blood and decidua. And except for the abnormal passage of fetal blood cellular elements through "breaks" in the placenta, cells of the embryo do not come into direct contact with maternal tissues. Nonetheless, except in parthenogenesis, or in situations in which both parents are genetically identical, the trophoblasts could theoretically confront the mother with foreign paternal antigens.

A second explanation, based on diminished immunological reactivity of the mother during pregnancy, provides at best only an ancillary factor in the prevention of the development of maternal isoimmunization during pregnancy. If the uterus were an immunologically privileged site, as in a third explanation, advanced ectopic pregnancies could never occur. Because transplantation immunity can be evoked and expressed in the uterus as elsewhere, the survival of the homograft must be related to a peculiarity of the conceptus, primarily the trophoblasts, rather than of the uterus.

Ancillary Immunological Considerations.
Siiteri and co-workers (1977) demonstrated that the rejection of grafted hamster skin is delayed by the presence of progesterone in high local concentrations.

Maternal lymphocyte function may be altered during pregnancy, as reflected by a reduction in phytohemagglutinin-induced transformation (Finn and colleagues, 1972; Purtilo and associates, 1972). It has been suggested that both trophoblasts and decidua produce agents that suppress lymphocyte immune responses. Sargent and co-workers (1987) reviewed these associations.

Breaks in the Placental "Barrier."
The failure of the placenta to maintain absolute integrity of the fetal and maternal circulations is documented by numerous findings of the passage of cells between mother and fetus in both directions, and best exemplified clinically by the occurrence of erythroblastosis fetalis (see Chap. 44, p. 1004). Typically, a few fetal blood cells are found in the mother's blood; and, rarely, the fetus may exsanguinate into the maternal circulation. Leukocytes from the fetus may replicate in the mother; leukocytes bearing a Y chromosome have been identified in women for up to 5 years after giving birth to a son (Ciaranfi and colleagues, 1977). Desai and Creger (1963) labeled maternal leukocytes and platelets with atabrine and found that these cells crossed the placenta from mother to fetus. Lymphocytes passing into the fetus create the possibility of chimerism, the subject of a review by Benirschke (1970).

Cells of fetal origin other than constituents of the blood have also been identified in the maternal circulation. Cells morphologically identical with trophoblast have been identified in uterine venous blood (Douglas and associates, 1959), as well as in cord blood (Salvaggio and co-workers, 1960). The immunological significance of continuous release of fetal elements into the maternal circulation is not yet explained.

HLA Antigen Expression in Fetal Trophoblasts.

Head and co-workers (1987) have provided an excellent review of an attractive hypothesis for the unique success of fetal acceptance by its immunocompetent maternal host. They point out that as early as 1932, Witebsky and Reich found that blood group antigens are lacking in human trophoblasts. Subsequently, much research has been focused on the expression of the major histocompatibility complex (MHC) antigens as a function of trophoblast development. (Human leukocyte antigens, or HLA, by international agreement, is the analogue of the human major histocompatibility complex.) Before blastocyst implantation in the mouse, low levels of MHC class I antigens are expressed on the trophectoderm, but these antigens disappear at the time of implantation, not to reappear except later in selected subpopulations of trophoblasts in the mature placenta. **Class II MHC antigens are absent from trophoblasts at all stages of gestation.**

The same generalities of HLA expression are applicable to human trophoblasts. Evidence began to accrue, however, that the class I antigens expressed in human trophoblasts were novel. Moreover, it seemed possible that the expression of these antigens may be modulated (e.g., by the action of interferons). This latter issue is important, because it is clear that increased expression of class I antigens after exposure to interferon leads to better killing of allogenic and virus-infected targets.

The important question finally posed, therefore, was related to the potential immunogenicity of trophoblasts. Expression of class II HLA antigens is believed to be important in the immunogenicity of tissue and organ allografts; the complete absence of class II antigens in human (and other mammalian) trophoblasts is no doubt important in maternal acceptance of the fetus. The elimination of class II antigen-presenting macrophages from kidney permits transplantation of this tissue in experimental animals without immunosuppression (Schreiner and associates, 1988).

Role of HLA Class I Antigens on Trophoblasts.

The absence of class I antigens from trophoblasts during the peri-implantation period and the absence of class II antigens on trophoblasts in contact with maternal blood could provide the "immunological buffer zone" between maternal and embryonic or fetal tissues (Head and colleagues, 1987). Therefore, the most simplistic answer to maternal acceptance of the semiallogenic graft would have been the complete absence of major histocompatibility class antigens. This is not the case for class I antigens, but it is for class II. It therefore seemed possible that selected expression of class I antigens, both in time and type, may be beneficial to pregnancy. As pointed out by Head and co-workers (1987), one

possibility is that such antigen expression may elicit the formation of growth-promoting cytokines. Other possibilities include the participation of class I antigens with the binding of peptide hormones to the cell surface. Such a proposal has been made in the case of insulin and epidermal growth factor.

Uterine Large Granular Lymphocytes. At this time, however, it appears that several recently discovered aspects of trophoblasts and selected lymphocyte functions may provide a provisional explanation. To consider these findings, recall that there are large numbers of granulated cells in the endometrium at the expected time of implantation. The origin of these cells was controversial in the past, but it is now clear that these are lymphoid cells of bone marrow origin. The cells are distinctive, and are referred to as uterine *large granular lymphocytes* (LGL). It is believed that these cells are of the natural killer (NK) cell lineage, but the precise phenotype of these lymphocytes is distinctive. These cells are characterized by a high surface density of CD56, which is identical with neural cell adhesion molecule. The density of CD56 in uterine large granular lymphocytes is more than 20 times that found on circulating natural killer cells (for review: King and Loke, 1991). The uterine LGL account for upwards of 70 percent of bone marrow cells at the time of implantation and in the decidua during the early phases of pregnancy. Importantly, the number of uterine LGL varies during the ovarian cycle, being greatest at the midluteal phase. It is believed that the increase in uterine LGL is the result of replication of these cells in situ in the endometrium and is not the consequence of increased migration (recruitment) from peripheral blood.

Uterine LGL replicate in response to interleukin-2, and such treatment also results in increased NK-like killing properties. Interestingly, the high-affinity interleukin-2 receptor (CD25) is not expressed by uterine large granular lymphocytes. It is presumed that interleukin-2 responsiveness of these cells is mediated by the β-chain (p75) of the interleukin-2 receptor (IL-2Rβ), which is expressed in uterine LGL (King and Loke, 1991). It has been proposed that uterine LGL represent an immature stage of NK cell differentiation or else a distinct NK/LGL subset specific to the uterus. The latter option is consistent with the finding that this LGL phenotype is localized to the uterine mucosal surface and is not found in any other tissue. Moreover, these lymphocytes are confined to endometrium–decidua and are not present in cervix or fallopian tube, excepting in foci of decidualization. The uterine LGL may originate in blood from the small number of these cells found in peripheral blood. Interestingly, there are more of these cells in blood of women than of men.

LGL function has not been established. But as King and Loke (1991) point out, LGL are present in endometrium–decidua in large numbers only during the period of placentation. Therefore, it seems reasonable to suspect that these cells are involved in placentation. King and Loke present an interesting hypothesis that normal pregnancy is dependent upon controlled trophoblast invasion of maternal endometrium–decidua, including the spiral arteries. Specifically, there must be a mechanism in place for permitting and yet limiting trophoblast invasion.

HLA Expression in Human Trophoblasts. As reviewed by Hunt and Orr (1992), it is established that the HLA genes are the products of multiple genetic loci of the major histocompatibility complex (MHC) found within the short arm of chromosome 6 at 6p21.1 to 6p21.3. Seventeen class I genes spanning almost 2000 kb of DNA have been identified. First, there are the three classical genes (HLA-A, -B, and -C) that encode the major class I transplantation antigens. In addition, there are three other class I genes, designated HLA-E, -F, and -G, that encode class I HLA antigens. The remaining DNA sequences are pseudogenes and partial gene fragments. The nonclassical HLA-E, -F, and -G genes are known to be nonpolymorphic, whereas the classical HLA-A, -B, and -C genes are each characterized by a large pool of alleles in the population. Importantly, the HLA-G gene is expressed only in extraembryonic tissues. This is highly suggestive of tissue-specific, that is, selective, expression of the HLA-G gene. The levels of HLA-G messenger RNA (assessed by gene specific RNase protection assays) in placenta decrease as gestation progresses. HLA-G is expressed in cytotrophoblasts, including extravillous cytotrophoblasts in the decidua basalis and those in the chorion laeve.

The regulation of class I HLA genes is as follows: (1) transcription of all class I heavy-chain genes is inhibited in syncytiotrophoblast; (2) translation controls are operative in cytotrophoblasts such that early placentas contain HLA-G mRNA but do not synthesize protein in detectable levels; (3) extravillous cytotrophoblastic cells transcribe the HLA-G class I gene and synthesize HLA-G class I antigen. But in addition, in the 5′-flanking region of HLA-G, there is a 13-bp deletion that is located within the A/IFN (interferon) consensus sequence region characteristic of other class I HLA genes.

They suggest that the permission of, but the limitation to, trophoblast invasion is accomplished by the interaction of uterine LGL with the unusual HLA-G class I gene expressed by cytotrophoblasts. In this theorem, it is important that HLA-G expression is confined to extravillous trophoblasts that invade the decidua and spiral arteries and those that form the chorion laeve. And importantly, HLA-G is nonpolymorphic. The syncytiotrophoblast expresses neither HLA class I nor II antigens.

To extend the theory, King and Loke also emphasize that in many model systems, NK cells preferentially kill target cells with few or no HLA molecules; this phenomenon has given rise to the "missing self" hypothesis. Namely, the absence of self-HLA molecules on target cells is detected by NK cells rather than by the presence of some specific recognition molecule. Through the expression of monomorphic HLA-G, extravillous trophoblast may be regarded by uterine large granular lymphocytes as self, and therefore not killed by these maternal NK-like cells. Cells from the inner cell mass of the blastocyst (i.e., those that form the embryo), gradually develop both class I and II HLA antigens during the progress of gestation, but these tissues are not in direct contact with maternal tissues or blood. Thus the regulation of HLA-G class I antigen expression on extravillous trophoblasts may be crucial to permitting and thence inhibiting the invasion of these cells in the endometrium–decidua.

Circulation in the Mature Placenta

Elizabeth Ramsey (1985), the preeminent researcher of the contemporary era of investigations of placental circulation, states that *"the modern era in the understanding of the placenta could not have commenced while scientists still thought that maternal and fetal vessels were anastomosed end to end."* Because the placenta functionally represents a rather intimate presentation of the fetal capillary bed to maternal blood, its gross anatomy primarily concerns vascular relations. Recall that the human placenta at term is a discoid organ measuring approximately 20 cm in diameter and 2 to 3 cm in thickness. It weighs approximately 500 g and is generally located in the uterus anteriorly or posteriorly near the fundus. The fetal surface is covered by transparent amnion beneath which the fetal chorionic vessels course, with the arteries passing over the veins. A section through the placenta in situ (Figs. 5–19 to 5–21) includes amnion, chorion, chorionic villi and intervillous spaces, decidual plate, and myometrium. It is important to note that the chorion laeve does not extend over the placental surface; the amnion is in direct contact with the adventitial surface of the chorionic vessels and the chorionic plate on the fetal surface of the placenta.

The maternal surface of the placenta (Fig. 5–22) is divided into irregular lobes by furrows produced by septa, which consist of fibrous tissue with sparse vessels confined mainly to their bases. The broad-based septa ordinarily do not reach the chorionic plate, thus providing only incomplete partitions.

Fetal Circulation. Fetal blood flows to the placenta through the two umbilical arteries, which carry deoxygenated, or "venous-like," blood. At the juncture of the umbilical cord with the placenta, the umbilical vessels branch repeatedly beneath the amnion and again within the dividing villi, forming capillary networks in the ter-

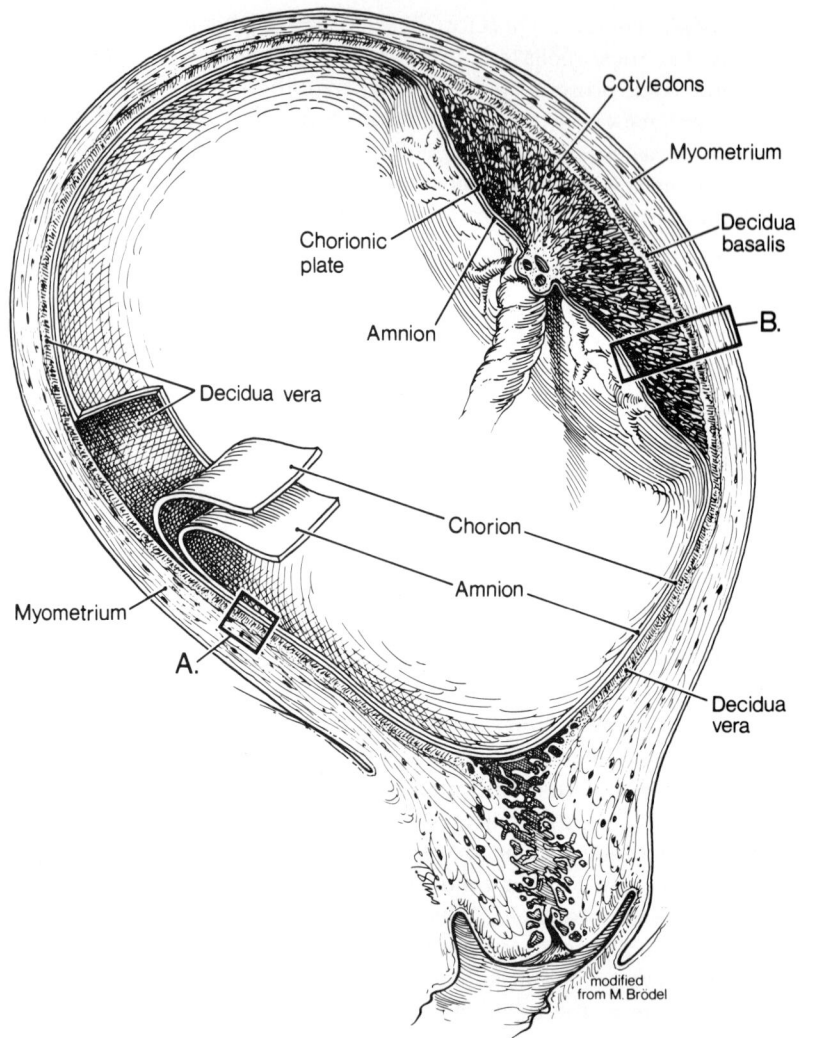

Fig. 5–19. Uterus of pregnant woman showing normal placenta in situ. **A.** Location of section shown in Fig. 5–20. **B.** Location of section shown in Fig. 5–21.

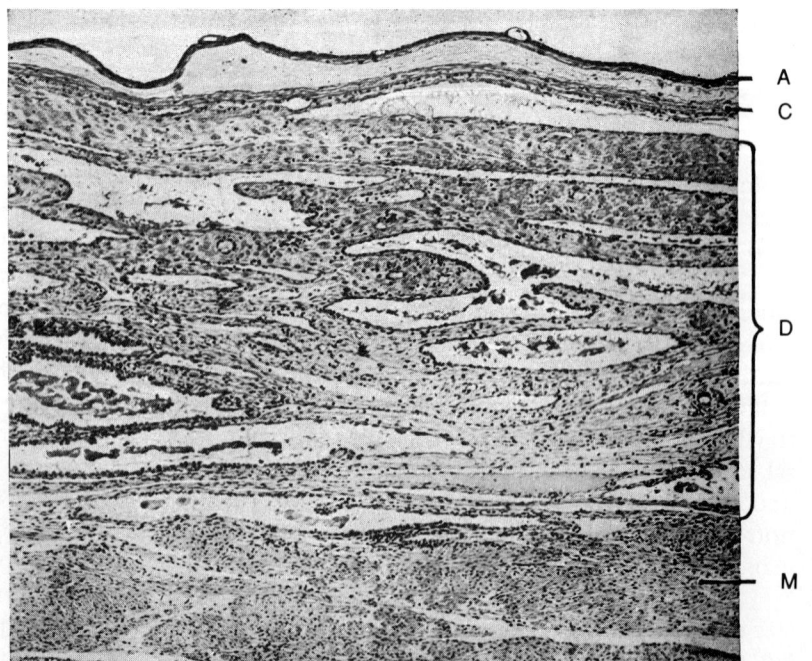

Fig. 5–20. Section of fetal membranes and uterus opposite placental site at A in Fig. 5–19. (A = amnion; C = chorion laeve; D = decidua parietalis; M = myometrium.)

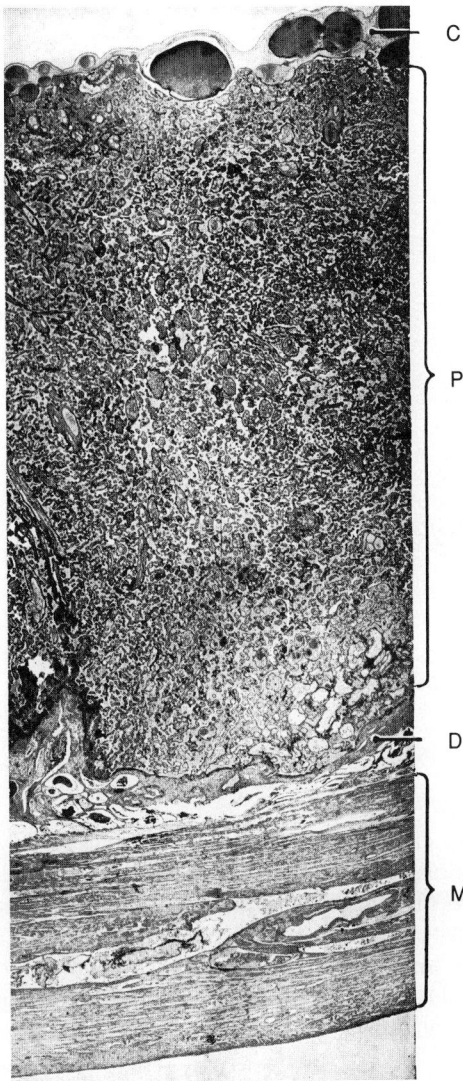

Fig. 5–21. Section of placenta and uterus through B in Fig. 5–19. (C = chorionic plate with fetal blood vessels; P = placental villi; D = decidua basalis; M = myometrium.)

minal divisions (Fig. 5–23). Blood, with a significantly higher oxygen content, returns to the fetus from the placenta through the single umbilical vein (see Chap. 7).

The branches of the umbilical vessels that traverse along the fetal surface of the placenta (the chorionic plate) are referred to as placental surface or chorionic vessels. Anatomically, morphologically, histologically, and functionally, these are curious vessels. Immediately before or just after entering the chorionic plate, the two umbilical arteries are joined by a transverse anastomosis, referred to as the Hyrtl anastomosis. Rarely, this anastomosis is missing.

The two umbilical arteries separate at the chorionic plate and supply branches to the cotyledons. Two different patterns of chorionic artery branching are recognized: *disperse* (63 percent of cases) and *magistral* (37 percent of cases). The chorionic vessels are known to be responsive to a number of vasoactive substances.

In the disperse type, the pattern of distribution is that of a fine network of vessels that traverse from the site of insertion of the umbilical cord to the various cotyledons. The magistral pattern is characterized by arteries that traverse to the edge of the placenta without an appreciable decrease in the diameter of the vessel. The arteries are end arteries. The arteries individually supply one cotyledon as the branch turns downward to pierce the chorionic plate. Importantly, there is a 1:1 relationship between the cotyledenary artery and vein. **The surface or chorionic arteries always cross over the veins.** This is an interesting phenomenon; in fact, identification of chorionic artery and vein is most readily accomplished in this manner because, as Benirschke points out, it is nearly impossible to distinguish the two by histological criteria.

As the perforating branches of the chorionic arteries pass through the chorionic plate, these are called the *truncal arteries*. Each truncal artery supplies one cotyledon. There is a decrease in smooth muscle of the vessel wall and an increase in the caliber of the vessel as it penetrates through the basal plate; and the loss in smooth muscle continues as the truncal arteries branch into the rami; the same is true of the vein walls.

At about 10 postconceptional weeks' gestation, the pattern of umbilical blood velocity waveforms changes abruptly (Fisk and colleagues, 1988; Loquet and associates, 1988). Before this time, there are no "end-diastolic frequencies." Later in gestation, this finding would be considered abnormal. Also at 8 to 10 weeks, the "definitive" chorionic plate is formed as the amnionic and primary chorionic plate mesenchyme fuse with each other. This is accomplished by expansion of the amnionic sac, which also surrounds the connective stalk and the allantois and joins them to form the umbilical cord (Kaufmann and Scheffen, 1992). There is another curious feature of the chorionic vessels; the thickness of the wall of these vessels is asymmetric, being much thinner on the side contiguous with the amnion (the fetal side). It is believed that the thinning, primarily of the arterial wall, also commences after 10 weeks' gestation.

The joining of amnion to the chorionic plate presents not only an interesting anatomical but also an important functional consideration. The "placental" amnion, or the amnion of the chorionic plate, is directly contiguous with the adventitial surface of the chorionic vessels. (Chorion laeve is contiguous only with the reflected amnion.) At least some vasoactive peptides are produced by the amnion, namely endothelin-1 (a vasocontractant) and parathyroid hormone-related protein (a vasorelaxant).

Maternal Circulation. The physiological particulars of the maternal placental circulation have been explained in physiological terms only relatively recently. Insofar as fetal homeostasis is dependent on efficient maternal–

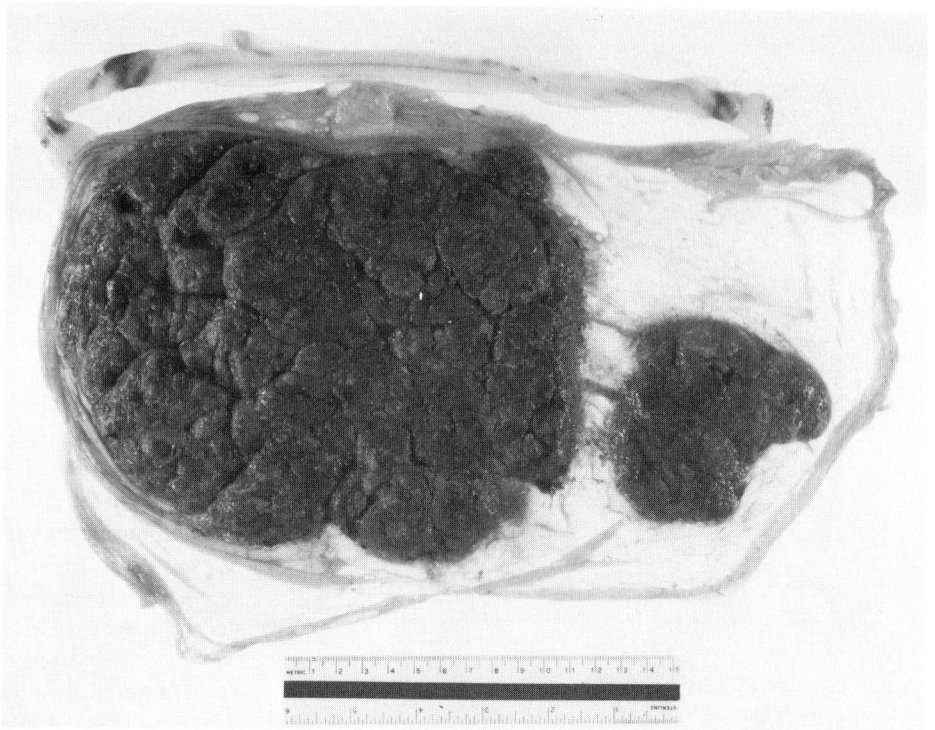

Fig. 5–22. Maternal surface of term placenta. Variably discrete, irregularly shaped adjacent lobes are evident plus a large separate (succenturiate) lobe.

placental circulation, the extensive efforts of investigators to define the factors that regulate the flow of blood into and from the intervillous space have led to important practical applications in obstetrics. An adequate theory must explain how blood actually may leave the maternal circulation, flow into an amorphous space lined by trophoblastic syncytium rather than capillary endothelium, and return through maternal veins without producing arteriovenous-like shunts that would prevent the blood from remaining in contact with the villi long enough for adequate exchange.

It was not until the studies of Ramsey and co-workers (1963, 1966) that a "physiological" mechanism of placental circulation, consistent with both experimental and clinical findings, was available (Fig. 5–23). Discarding the crude corrosion technique of their predecessors, by careful, slow injections of radiocontrast material under low pressure that avoided disruption of the circulation, they proved that the arterial entrances as well as the venous exits are scattered at random over the entire base of the placenta.

The maternal blood entering through the basal plate is driven by the head of maternal arterial pressure high up toward the chorionic plate before lateral dispersion occurs. After bathing the chorionic villi, the blood drains through venous orifices in the basal plate and enters the uterine veins. The maternal blood thus traverses the placenta randomly without preformed channels, propelled by the maternal arterial pressure. The spiral arteries generally are perpendicular and the veins parallel to the uterine wall, an arrangement that

facilitates closure of the veins during a uterine contraction and prevents squeezing of essential maternal blood from the intervillous space. According to Brosens and Dixon (1963), there are about 120 spiral arterial entries into the intervillous space of the human placenta at term, discharging blood in spurts that displace the adjacent villi, as described by Borell and co-workers (1958).

Ramsey and Harris (1966) compared the decidual vasculature and circulation of the rhesus monkey with those of the human. The most significant morphological variation is the greater dilatation of human spiral arteries. In the human, particularly in early pregnancy, there may be multiple openings from a single arterial stem into the intervillous space. The force of the spurts of blood is eventually dissipated with the creation of a small lake of blood roughly 5 mm in diameter about halfway toward the chorionic plate. The closeness of the villi slows the flow of blood, providing adequate time for exchange.

Ramsey's concept is supported by the findings of numerous arteriographic studies. Clearly, the spiral arterial spurts are associated with the "lakes" and the closure of uteroplacental veins is effected by pressure produced at the beginning of uterine contractions. Corroboration has been provided by results of cineradioangiography, in which it was shown how, in the macaque, debouching streams from the spiral arteries connect with and develop into the small lakes, which then disperse in a general effusion of blood throughout the intervillous space (Fig. 5–24).

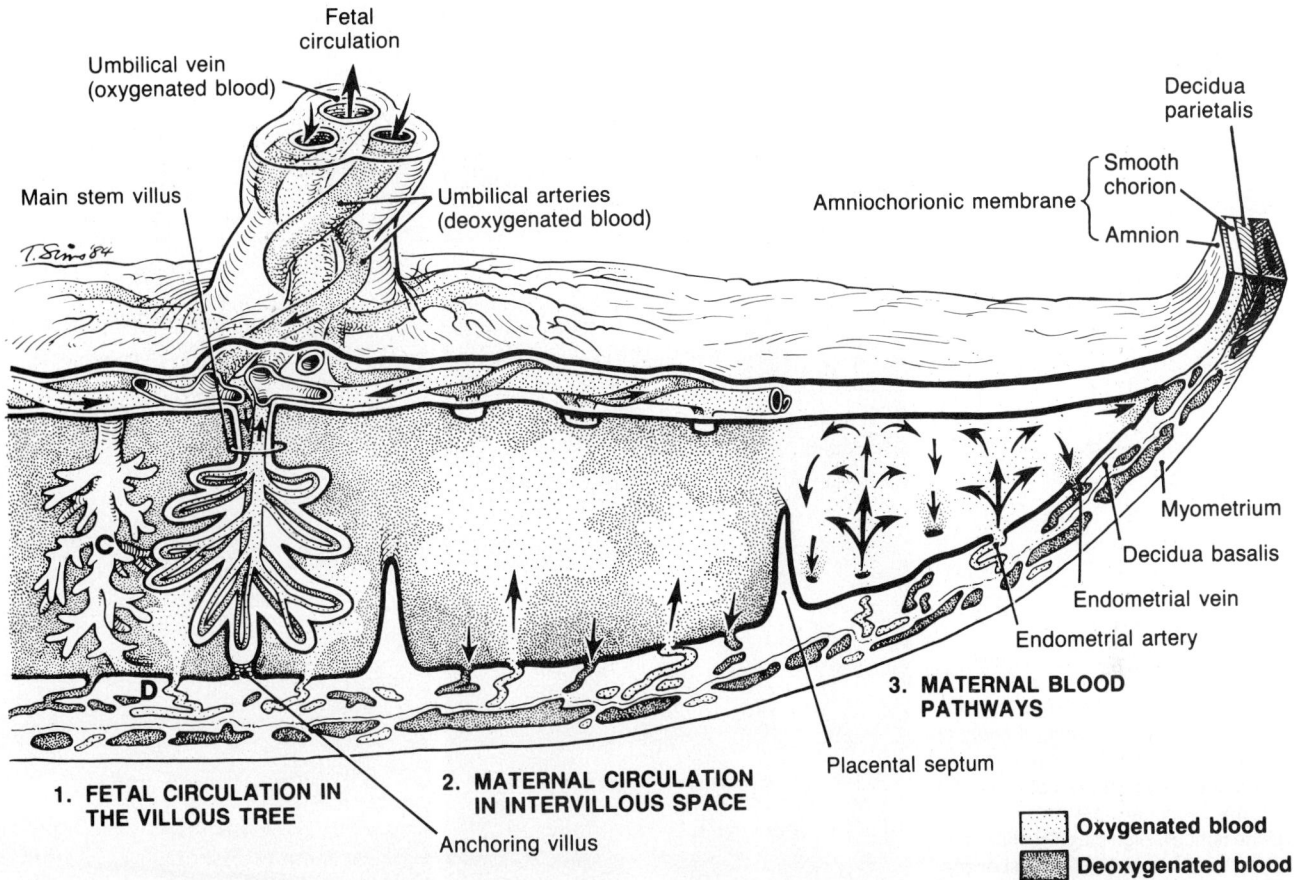

Fig. 5–23. Schematic drawing of a section through a full-term placenta: **1.** The relation of the villous chorion (C) to the decidua basalis (D) and the fetal placental circulation. **2.** The maternal placental circulation. Maternal blood flows into the intervillous spaces in funnel-shaped spurts, and exchanges occur with the fetal blood as the maternal blood flows around the villi. **3.** The inflowing arterial blood pushes venous blood into the endometrial veins, which are scattered over the entire surface of the decidua basalis. Note also that the umbilical arteries carry deoxygenated fetal blood to the placenta and that the umbilical vein carries oxygenated blood to the fetus. Note that the cotyledons are separated from each other by placental (decidual) septa. Each cotyledon consists of two or more mainstem villi and their many branches. (Based on Moore, 1988.)

In Ramsey's motion pictures, the effect of myometrial contractions upon placental circulation is shown unequivocally to involve diminution of arterial inflow and cessation of venous drainage. Continued observation of the contrast medium by televised fluoroscopy was indicative that myometrial contractions cause a slight delay in appearance of the contrast medium in the veins of the uterine wall when injection occurs during a strong contraction. The pressure in the intervillous space may be decreased to the point at which blood cannot be expressed against the prevailing myometrial pressure. Ramsey has provided further evidence of independent activity of the spiral arteries, as indicated by the appearance of spurts in different locations even when injections are performed under conditions of minimal myometrial pressure. Not all endometrial spiral arteries are continuously patent, nor do all spiral arteries necessarily discharge blood into the intervillous space simultaneously.

In summary, Ramsey's concept holds that the maternal blood enters the intervillous space in spurts produced by the maternal blood pressure. The *vis a tergo* forces blood in discrete streams toward the chorionic plate until the head of pressure is reduced. Lateral spread then occurs. Continuing influx of arterial blood exerts pressure on the contents of the intervillous space, pushing the blood toward exits in the basal plate, from which it is drained through uterine veins. During uterine contractions, both inflow and outflow are curtailed, although the volume of blood in the intervillous space is maintained, thus providing for continual, albeit reduced, exchange.

Bleker and associates (1975) used serial sonography to study pregnancies of normally laboring women and found that the length, thickness, and surface of the placenta increased during contractions. They attributed these changes to distension of the intervillous spaces by blood as the consequence of relatively greater impair-

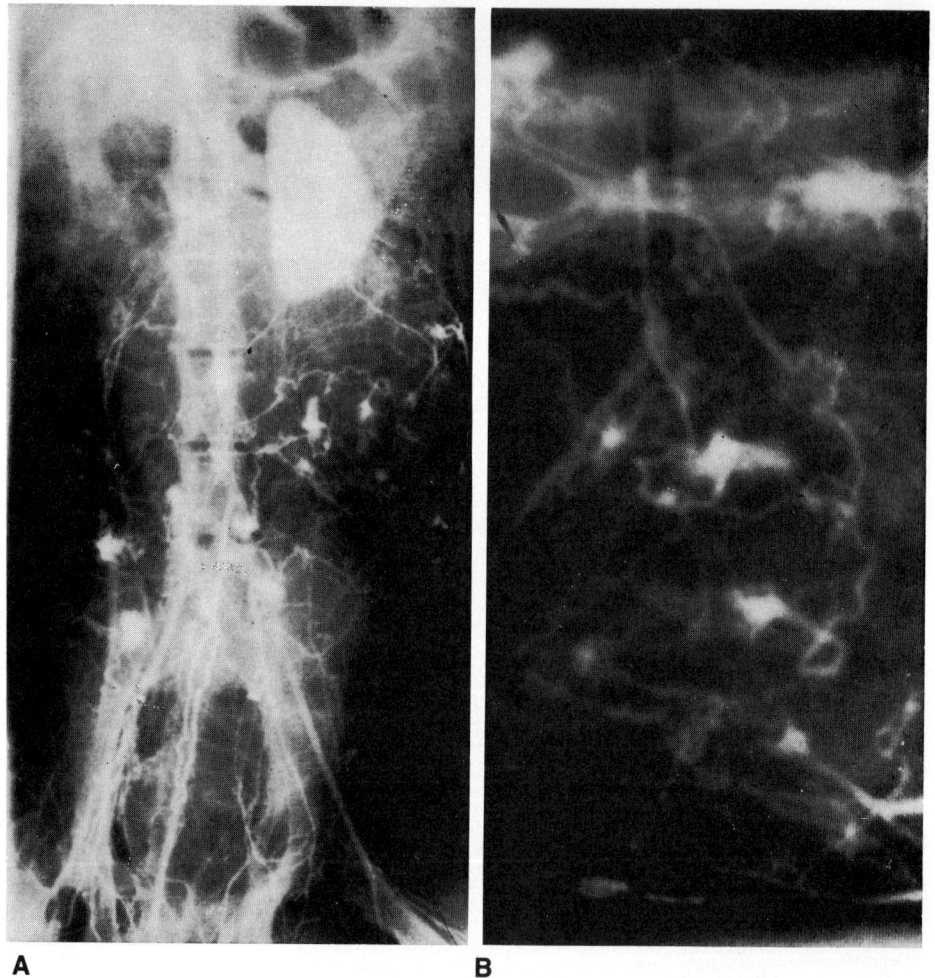

Fig. 5–24. A. Radiogram 6 seconds after injection of a radiopaque contrast medium into the right femoral artery of a monkey on day 111 of pregnancy. The primary placenta is below on the left; the secondary placenta is above on the right. **B.** High magnification of an artery at the center of the secondary placenta in the same monkey. (Courtesy of Dr. Elizabeth M. Ramsey.)

A   **B**

ment of venous outflow compared with arterial inflow. During contractions, therefore, a somewhat larger volume of blood is available for exchange even though the rate of flow is decreased. More recently, by use of Doppler velocimetry, it was shown that diastolic flow velocity in spiral arteries is diminished during uterine contractions.

The principal factors regulating blood flow in the intervillous space, therefore, include arterial blood pressure, intrauterine pressure, the pattern of uterine contraction, including the contour of the individual contraction wave, and factors acting specifically upon the arteriolar walls.

Ramsey and Donner (1980) presented a summary of anatomical studies of the uteroplacental vasculature. They noted that cytotrophoblastic elements are initially confined to the terminal portions of the uteroplacental arteries but later extend proximally. By the 16th week, cytotrophoblasts are found in many of the arteries of the inner layer of myometrium, as noted before from the observations of Hamilton and Boyd. Intraarterial accumulation of trophoblasts may ultimately stop circulation through some of these vessels. The number of arterial

openings into the intervillous space is gradually reduced by cytotrophoblasts and by breaching of the walls of the more proximal parts of the arteries by deeply penetrating trophoblasts. After the 30th week, a prominent venous plexus separates the decidua basalis from the myometrium, thus participating in providing a plane of cleavage for separation of the placenta.

The Amnion

Early in the process of blastocyst implantation, a space develops between the embryonic cell mass and adjacent trophoblasts (Fig. 5–7). Small cells that line this inner surface of trophoblasts have been called amniogenic cells, which are the precursors of the amnionic epithelium. By expansion of the cleft that separates these cells from the embryo, the amnionic cavity develops and slowly comes to surround the embryo (Benirschke and Kaufman, 1990). Heretofore, there has been considerable disagreement concerning the histogenesis of the amnionic epithelium. It is now reasonably clear that the epithelial cells are derived from fetal ectoderm (the embryonic disc), and not by delamination from trophoblasts. This is an important consideration not only from the embryological but from the functional perspective. For example, HLA class I gene expression in amnion is more characteristic of embryo cells than trophoblasts. In addition to the epithelial cells that line the innermost (amnionic fluid) side of the amnion, there is a layer of fibroblast-like cells that may also be derived from the embryo (i.e., from embryonic mesoderm), but this is not certain. The important "missing" elements of human amnion are smooth muscle cells, nerves, lymphatics, and most importantly, blood vessels.

The human amnion likely develops about the seventh or eighth day of development of the normal blastocyst. Initially a minute vesicle (see Fig. 5–8), the amnion develops into a small sac that covers the dorsal surface of the embryo. As the amnion enlarges, it gradually engulfs the growing embryo, which prolapses into its cavity. Distension of the amnionic sac eventually brings it into contact with the interior surface of the chorion laeve; apposition of the mesoblasts of chorion laeve and amnion near the end of the first trimester results in obliteration of the extraembryonic coelom. The amnion and chorion laeve, though slightly adherent, are never intimately connected, and usually can be separated easily, even at term.

The normal amnion is 0.2 to 0.5 mm in thickness. The epithelium normally consists of a single layer of nonciliated, cuboid cells. (Fig. 5–25). According to Bourne (1962), the amnion is comprised of five layers: starting from within, the epithelium, basement membrane, compact layer, fibroblastic layer, and spongy layer. Electron microscopic studies of amnion by Hoyes (1968), however, did not confirm such sharply defined layers.

There are four anatomically distinct portions of the amnion. First, the reflected amnion is that portion that is contiguous with the chorion laeve. Second, the placental amnion overlies the fetal surface of the placenta, being directly contiguous with the adventitial surface of the chorionic vessels. Third, the amnion also covers the umbilical cord, being contiguous with Wharton jelly, the extracellular matrix through which the umbilical vessels traverse. Fourth, in diamnionic–dichorionic twin pregnancies and in diamnionic–monochorionic twin pregnancies, there is "fused" amnion, which in the former is contiguous with "fused" chorion laeve and in the latter amnion is fused with amnion. The amnion is clearly more than a simple membrane to contain amnionic fluid. It is metabolically active, involved in solute and water transport to maintain amnionic fluid homeostasis, and it produces a variety of interesting peptides.

Casey and colleagues have demonstrated the capacity of amnion to produce vasoactive peptides, namely endothelin-1 (a potent vasoconstrictor) and parathyroid hormone-related protein (a vasorelaxant). In addition, the enzyme enkephalinase, which degrades endothelin-1, is present in chorion laeve in high specific activity. Thus, the vasoactive peptides produced in amnion may act directly upon the adventitial surface of the chorionic vessels of the placenta (Casey and associates, 1991, 1992; Germain and co-workers, 1992; Sunnegren and colleagues, 1990). These findings are suggestive that the placental amnion may serve a role in modulating chorionic vessel tone and blood flow.

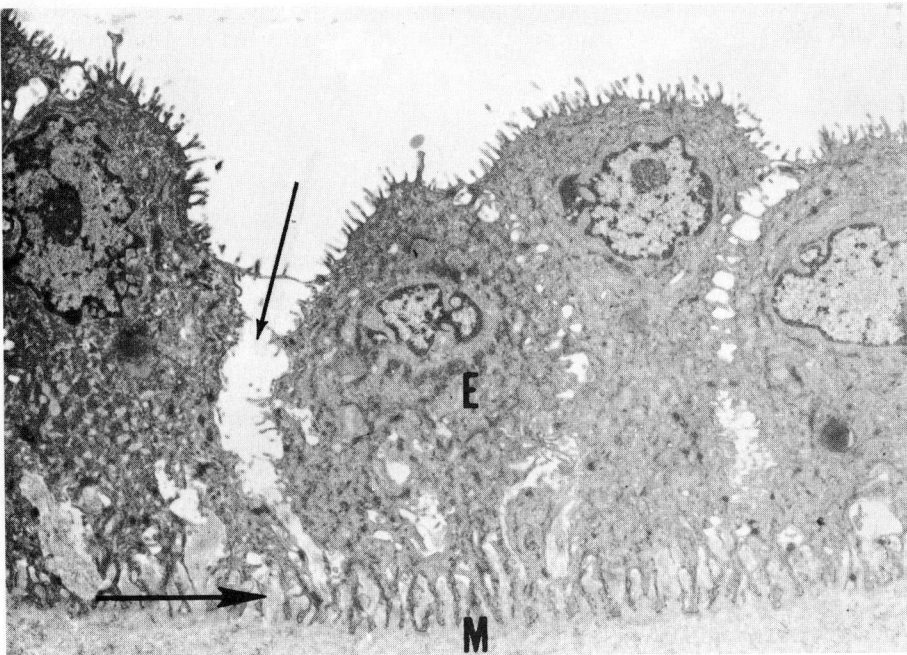

Fig. 5–25. Electron micrograph of human amnion at term. Epithelium (E) and mesenchyme (M) are shown. Thin arrow indicates intercellular space. Thick arrow points to specializations of basal plasma membranes. (Courtesy of Dr. Ralph M. Wynn.)

Amnionic Fluid. The normally clear fluid that collects within the amnionic cavity increases in quantity as pregnancy advances until near term, when it normally decreases. An average volume of about 1000 mL is found at term, although this may vary widely from a few milliliters to many liters in abnormal conditions (oligohydramnios and polyhydramnios, or hydramnios). The origin, composition, and function of the amnionic fluid are further discussed in Chapters 12 and 34.

Umbilical Cord and Related Structures

Development. The yolk sac and the umbilical vesicle into which it develops are quite prominent at the beginning of pregnancy. At first, the embryo is a flattened disc interposed between amnion and yolk sac. Because the dorsal surface grows faster than the ventral surface, in association with the elongation of the neural tube, the embryo bulges into the amnionic sac and the dorsal part of the yolk sac is incorporated into the body of the embryo to form the gut. The allantois projects into the base of the body stalk from the caudal wall of the yolk sac or, later, from the anterior wall of the hindgut. As pregnancy advances, the yolk sac becomes smaller and its pedicle relatively longer. By about the middle of the third month, the expanding amnion obliterates the exocelom, fuses with the chorion laeve, and covers the bulging placental disc and the lateral surface of the body stalk, which is then called the umbilical cord, or funis. Remnants of the exocelom in the anterior portion of the cord may contain loops of intestine, which continue to develop outside the embryo. Although the loops are later withdrawn, the apex of the midgut loop retains its connection with an attenuated vitelline duct that terminates in a crumpled, highly vascular sac 3 to 5 cm in diameter lying on the surface of the placenta between amnion and chorion or in the membranes just beyond the placental margin, where occasionally it may be identified at term.

The cord at term normally has two arteries and one vein. The right umbilical vein usually disappears early during fetal development, leaving only the original left vein. Sections of any portion of the cord frequently reveals, near the center, the small duct of the umbilical vesicle, lined by a single layer of flattened or cuboid epithelial cells. In sections just beyond the umbilicus, but never at the maternal end of the cord, another duct representing the allantoic remnant occasionally is found. The intra-abdominal portion of the duct of the umbilical vesicle, which extends from umbilicus to intestine, usually atrophies and disappears, but occasionally it remains patent, forming the Meckel diverticulum. The most common vascular anomaly in humans is the absence of one umbilical artery. This subject is further discussed in Chapter 35 (p. 745).

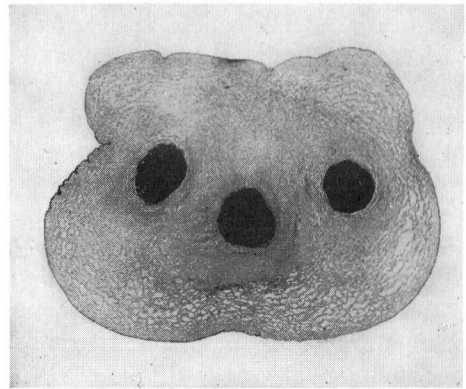

Fig. 5–26. Cross section of umbilical cord fixed after blood vessels had been emptied. The umbilical vein, carrying oxygenated blood to the fetus, is in the center; on either side are the two umbilical arteries carrying deoxygenated blood from the fetus to the placenta. (From Reynolds, 1954.)

Structure and Function of the Umbilical Cord. The umbilical cord, or funis, extends from the fetal umbilicus to the fetal surface of the placenta (the chorionic plate). Its exterior is dull white, moist, and covered by amnion, through which three umbilical vessels may be seen. Its diameter is 0.8 to 2.0 cm, with an average length of 55 cm and a usual range of 30 to 100 cm. Generally, cord length less than 32 cm is considered abnormally short. Folding and tortuosity of the vessels, which are longer than the cord itself, frequently create nodulations on the surface, or *false knots*, which are essentially varices. The extracellular matrix, which is a specialized connective tissue, consists of Wharton jelly (Figs. 5–26 and 5–27). After fixation, the umbilical vessels appear empty, but Figure 5–27 more accurately is representative of the situation in vivo, when the vessels are not emptied of blood. The two arteries are smaller in diameter than the vein. When fixed in its normally dis-

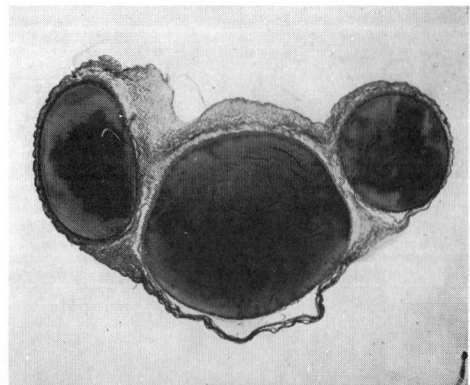

Fig. 5–27. Cross section of the same umbilical cord shown in Fig. 5–26, but through a segment from which the blood vessels had not been emptied. This photograph probably represents more accurately the conditions in utero. (From Reynolds, 1954.)

tended state, the umbilical arteries exhibit transverse intimal *folds (valves) of Hoboken* across part of their lumens (Chacko and Reynolds, 1954). The mesoderm of the cord, which is of allantoic origin, fuses with that of the amnion.

The flow of blood from the umbilical vein is by way of two routes, the ductus venosus, which empties directly into the inferior vena cava, and numerous smaller openings into the fetal hepatic circulation and thence into the inferior vena cava by the hepatic vein. The blood takes the path of least resistance through these alternate routes. Resistance in the ductus venosus is controlled by a sphincter, which is situated at the origin of the ductus at the umbilical recess and innervated by a branch of the vagus nerve.

Ellison and co-workers (1970) studied the innervation of the umbilical cord of the rat by means of localization of acetylcholinesterase and catecholamines. Cholinesterase-positive nerves were confined to periarterial plexus, while adrenergic nerves were entirely absent from the cord. By these techniques, certain nerves could be traced to the placenta but not into it.

Anatomically, the umbilical cord can be regarded as a fetal membrane. The vessels contained in the cord are characterized by spiraling or twisting. The spiraling may occur in a clockwise (dextral) or anticlockwise (sinistral, accounting for 50 to 90 percent of cases) direction. It is believed that the spiraling serves to attenuate "snarling," which occurs in all hollow cylinders subjected to torsion. Boyd and Hamilton note that the *"twists are not really spirals, but cylindrical helices in which a constant curvature is maintained equidistant from a central axis."*

References

Ahlmark A: Studies on the histaminolytic power of plasma with special reference to pregnancy. Acta Physiol Scand 9(suppl 28):1, 1944

Benirschke K: The placenta: How to examine it and what you can learn. Contemp Obstet Gynecol 17:117, 1981

Benirschke K: Spontaneous chimerism in mammals: A critical review. In Current Topics in Pathology. Berlin, Springer-Verlag, 1970, p 1

Benirschke K, Kaufman P: Pathology of the Human Placenta. New York, Springer Verlag, 1990, p 130

Billingham RE: Transplantation immunity and the maternal–fetal relation. N Engl J Med 270:667, 1964

Bleker OP, Kloosterman GJ, Mieras DJ, Oosting J, Salle HJA: Intervillous space during uterine contractions in human subjects: An ultrasonic study. Am J Obstet Gynecol 123:697, 1975

Borell U, Fernstrom I, Westman A: An arteriographic study of the placental circulation. Geburtshilfe Frauenheilkd 18:1, 1958

Bourne GL: The Human Amnion and Chorion. Chicago, Year Book, 1962

Boyd JD, Hamilton WJ: The Human Placenta. Cambridge, England, Heffer, 1970

Brosens I, Dixon HG: The anatomy of the maternal side of the placenta. Br J Obstet Gynaecol 73:357, 1963

Casey ML, Mibe M, Erk A, MacDonald PC: Transforming growth factor-β1 stimulation of parathyroid hormone-related protein expression in human uterine cells in culture: mRNA levels and protein secretion. J Clin Endocrinol Metab 74:950, 1992

Casey ML, Word RA, MacDonald PC: Endothelin-1 gene expression and regulation of endothelin mRNA and protein biosynthesis in avascular human amnion. J Biol Chem 266:5762, 1991

Chacko AW, Reynolds SRM: Architecture of distended and nondistended human umbilical cord tissues, with special references to the arteries and veins. Contrib Embryol 35:135, 1954

Ciaranfi A, Curchod A, Odartchenko N: Survie de lymphocytes foetaux dans de sang maternal post-partum. Schweiz Med Wschr 107:134, 1977

Coutifaris C, Babalola GO, Abisogun AO, Kao LC, Chin U, Vadillo-Ortega F, Osheroff J, Kliman HJ, Strauss III JF: In vitro systems for the study of human trophoblast implantation. Ann NY Acad Sci 622:191, 1991

Crawford JM: A study of human placental growth with observations on the placenta in erythroblastosis foetalis. Br J Obstet Gynaecol 66:855, 1959

Desai RG, Creger WP: Maternofetal passage of leukocytes and platelets in man. Blood 21:665, 1963

Douglas GW, Thomas L, Carr M, Cullen NM, Morris R: Trophoblast in the circulating blood during pregnancy. Am J Obstet Gynecol 78:960, 1959

Ellison JP, Hibbs RG, Ferguson MA, Mahan M, Blasini EJ: The innervation of the umbilical cord. Anat Rec 166:302, 1970

Feinberg RF, Kliman HJ, Lockwood CJ: Is oncofetal fibronectin a trophoblast glue for human implantation? Am J Pathol 138:537, 1991

Finn R, St Hill CA, Govan AJ, Ralfs IG, Gurney FJ, Denye V: Immunological responses in pregnancy and survival of fetal homograft. Br Med J 3:150, 1972

Fisk NM, Maclachlan N, Ellis C, Tannirandorm Y, Tonge HM, Rodeck CH: Absent endodiastolic flow in first trimester umbilical artery. Lancet 2: 1256, 1988

Germain AM, Attaroglu H, MacDonald PC, Casey ML: Parathyroid hormone-related protein mRNA in avascular human amnion. J Clin Endocrinol Metab 75:1173, 1992

Hamilton WJ, Boyd JD: Trophoblast in human utero-placental arteries. Nature 212:906, 1966

Head JR, Drake BL, Zuckermann FA: Major histocompatibility antigens on trophoblast and their regulation: Implications in the maternal–fetal relationship. Am J Reprod Immunol Microbiol 15:12, 1987

Hertig AT: The placenta: Some new knowledge about an old organ. Obstet Gynecol 20:859, 1962

Hertig AT, Rock J: Two human ova of the pre-villous stage, having a developmental age of about seven and nine days respectively. Contrib Embryol 31:65, 1945

Hertig AT, Rock J: On the development of the early human ovum, with special reference to the trophoblast of the pre-villous stage: A description of 7 normal and 5 pathologic human ova. Am J Obstet Gynecol 47:149, 1944

Hertig AT, Rock J: Two human ova of the pre-villous stage, having an ovulation age of about eleven and twelve days respectively. Contrib Embryol 29:127, 1941

Hertig AT, Rock J, Adams EC, Mulligan WJ: On the preimplantation stages of the human ovum. Contrib Embryol 35:199, 1954

Hoyes AD: Fine structure of human amniotic epithelium in early pregnancy. Br J Obstet Gynecol 75:949, 1968

Hunt JS, Orr HT: HLA and maternal–fetal recognition. FASEB J 6:2344, 1992

Kaufmann P, Scheffen I: Placental Development. In Polin RA, Fox WW (eds): Fetal and Neonatal Physiology. Philadelphia, Saunders, 1992, p 47

King A, Loke YW: On the nature and function of human uterine granular lymphocytes. Immunol Today 12:432, 1991

King BF, Menton DN: Scanning electron microscopy of human placental villi from early and late in gestation. Am J Obstet Gynecol 122:824, 1975

Kliman HJ, Nestler JE, Sermasi E, Sanger JM, Strauss JF: Purification, characterization, and in vitro differentiation of cytotrophoblasts from human term placenta. Endocrinology 118:1567, 1986

Lewis WH, Hartman CG: Early cleavage stages of the egg of the monkey (macacus rhesus). Contrib Embryol 24:187, 1933

Lockwood CJ, Senyei AE, Dische MR, Casal D, Shah KD, Thung SN, Jones L, Deligdisch L, Garite TJ: Fetal fibronectin in cervical and vaginal secretions as a predictor of preterm delivery. N Engl J Med 325:669, 1991

Loquet P, Broughton-Pipkin F, Symonds EM, Rubin PC: Blood velocity waveforms and placental vascular formation. Lancet 2:1252, 1988

Moore KL: The Developing Human: Clinically Oriented Embryology, 4th ed. Philadelphia, Saunders, 1988

Moore KL: The Developing Human: Clinically Oriented Embryology, 1st ed. Philadelphia, Saunders, 1973

Mossman HW: Comparative morphogenesis of the fetal membranes and accessory uterine structures. Contrib Embryol 26:129, 1937

Potter EL, Craig JM: Pathology of the fetus and the infant. Chicago, Year Book, 1975

Purtilo DT, Hallgren H, Yunis EJ: Depressed maternal lymphocyte response to phytohaemagglutinin in human pregnancy. Lancet 1:769, 1972

Ramsey EM: What we have learned about placental circulation. J Reprod Med 30:312, 1985

Ramsey EM, Davis RW: A composite drawing of the placenta to show its structure and circulation. Anat Rec 145:366, 1963

Ramsey EM, Donner MW: Placental Vascular and Circulation. Philadelphia, Saunders, 1980

Ramsey EM, Harris JWS: Comparison of uteroplacental vasculature and circulation in the rhesus monkey and man. Contrib Embryol 38:59, 1966

Reynolds SRM: Hemodynamic characteristics of the fetal circulation. Am J Obstet Gynecol 68:69, 1954

Reynolds SRM, Freese UE, Bieniarz J, Caldeyro-Barcia R, Mendez-Bauer C, Escarcena L: Multiple simultaneous intervillous space pressures recorded in several regions of the hemochoroidal placenta in relation to functional anatomy of the fetal cotyledon. Am J Obstet Gynecol 102:1128, 1968

Ringler GE, Strauss III JF: In vitro systems for the study of human placental endocrine function. Endo Rev 11:105, 1990

Salafia CM, Vintzileos AM: Why all placentas should be examined by a patholgist in 1990. Am J Obstet Gynecol 163:1282, 1990.

Salvaggio AT, Nigogosyan G, Mack HC: Detection of trophoblasts in cord blood and fetal circulation. Am J Obstet Gynecol 80:1013, 1960

Sargent IL, Redman CWG: The placenta as a graft. In Lavery JP (ed): The Human Placenta: Clinical Perspectives. Rockville, MD, Aspen, 1987, p 79

Schreiner GF, Flye W, Brunt E, Korber K, Lefkowith JB: Essential fatty acid depletion of renal allografts and prevention of rejection. Science 240:1032, 1988

Siiteri PK, Febres F, Clemens LE, Chang JR, Gondos B, Sites D: Progesterone and maintenance of pregnancy: Is progesterone nature's immunosuppressant? Ann NY Acad Sci 286:384, 1977

Streeter GL: A human embryo (Mateer) of the presomite period. Contrib Embryol 9:389, 1920

Streeter GL: Development of the egg as seen by the embryologist. Sci Monthly 32:495, 1931

Sunnergren KP, Word RA, Sambrook JF, MacDonald PC, Casey ML: Expression and regulation of endothelin precursor mRNA in avascular human amnion. Mol Cell Endocrinol 68:R7, 1990

Thomson AM, Billewicz WZ, Hytten FE: The weight of the placenta in relation to birthweight. Br J Obstet Gynaecol 76:865, 1969

Ulloa-Aguirre A, August AM, Golos TG, Kao LC, Sakuragi N, Kliman HJ, Strauss JF: 8-Bromo-adenosine 3′, 5′-monophosphate regulates expression of chorionic gonadotropin and fibronectin in human cytotrophoblasts. J Clin Endocrinol Metab 64:1002, 1987

Wislocki GB, Dempsey EW: Electron microscopy of the human placenta. Anat Rec 123:133, 1955

Wislocki GB, Streeter GL: On the placentation of the macaque (Macaca mulatta), from the time of implantation until the formation of the definitive placenta. Contrib Embryol 27:1, 1938

Witebsky ES, Reich H: Zur gruppenspezifischen Differenzierung der Placentarorgan. Klin Wochenschr 11:1960, 1932

CHAPTER 6
The Placental Hormones

Overview

The first suggestion that the placenta was an endocrine organ was made by Halban in 1905. Since then, many investigators have contributed to a definition of the endocrine functions of the human placenta, including the formation of steroid and protein hormones. From the demonstration of a unique relationship between the incredible hyperestrogenic state of human pregnancy and the fetal adrenal secretion of massive quantities of C_{19}-steroids (which are used as precursors for estrogen synthesis in placental syncytiotrophoblast), the existence of an interactive fetal–placental hormone production system in human pregnancy was established. Similarly, an interactive system for trophoblast utilization of maternal plasma, low-density lipoprotein (LDL) cholesterol for progesterone biosynthesis has been defined. The rates of estrogen and progesterone production in most pregnant mammals, including subhuman primates, are miniscule compared with those of human pregnancy. A compendium of steroid hormone production rates in near-term pregnant women and in nonpregnant women is presented in Table 6–1. From a perusal of these values, it is evident that the steroid hormone alterations that accompany human pregnancy are the most unique and astounding in both breadth and quantity that are recorded in mammalian physiology or pathophysiology.

In addition to these increases in the formation of sex steroid and mineralocorticosteroid hormones, there are striking increases in the levels of plasma renin, angiotensinogen, and angiotensin II (Chap. 8), together with the daily production of 1 to 3 grams of placental lactogen (hPL), and massive quantities of chorionic gonadotropin (hCG). The placenta also produces chorionic adrenocorticotropin (ACTH), as well as other products of pro-opiomelanocortin (POMC), chorionic thyrotropin (hCT), parathyroid hormone-related protein (PTH-rP), and hypothalamic-like releasing and inhibiting hormones; that is, thyrotropin-releasing hormone (TRH), gonadotropin-releasing hormone (GnRH) or luteinizing hormone-releasing hormone (LHRH), corticotropin-releasing hormone (CRH), somatostatin, and growth hormone-releasing hormones (GHRH). It also produces inhibins, activins, and a variety of proteins that are unique to pregnancy (pregnancy-specific) or neoplastic processes.

It is understandable, therefore, that one of the more remarkable phenomena of human pregnancy is the development of physiological adaptations whereby the gravid woman is able to cope with this unusual endocrine milieu. Maternal adaptations to pregnancy are considered in appreciable detail in Chapter 8.

The proximal anatomical parts of the endocrine component of the placental arm of the fetal–maternal communication system are the fetal pituitary, adrenal glands, and liver, fetal blood, placental trophoblasts (cytotrophoblasts and syncytium), and maternal blood, including maternal plasma LDL cholesterol. Endocrine responsive tissues of both mother and fetus are the end-organs of this remarkable endocrine system (Fig. 6–1).

Protein Hormones of the Placenta

Chorionic Gonadotropin. The early history of the discovery of chorionic gonadotropin (hCG) is recounted in Chapter 2. HCG is a glycoprotein hormone with biological activity like luteinizing hormone (LH), that is produced almost exclusively during pregnancy, namely in the syncytium of the placenta. HCG acts on responsive cells by way of the plasma membrane LH receptor; but the half-life of hCG (24 hours) in plasma is much longer than is that of LH (2 hours). A variety of malignant tumors produce this glycoprotein, sometimes in reasonably large amounts; and possibly, the pituitary of normal men and nonpregnant women produces very small quantities of hCG in an episodic fashion (Odell and Griffin, 1987). Nonetheless, the detection of hCG in blood or urine of reproductive-age women by customary procedures used to identify hCG is almost always indicative of the presence of fetal trophoblasts (i.e., pregnancy), including neoplastic fetal trophoblastic disease (Chaps. 2 and 35).

Incredible amounts of hCG are produced during human pregnancy; but this is not true in all mammalian species. Chorionic gonadotropin has been found only in primates, and no other primate has been identified in which amounts of chorionic gonadotropin are produced as large as those produced by the human placenta.

Chemical Characteristics of hCG. HCG is a glycoprotein (M_r about 36,700) with a high carbohydrate (30 percent) content; indeed, this is the highest carbohydrate content of any human hormone. The carbohydrate component, and especially the terminal sialic acid, protects the molecule from catabolism; the enzymatic removal of the terminal sialic acid greatly accelerates the rate of clearance of hCG from the circulation.

TABLE 6–1. STEROID PRODUCTION RATES IN NONPREGNANT AND NEAR-TERM PREGNANT WOMEN

Steroid[a]	Production Rate (mg/24 hr)	
	Nonpregnant	*Pregnant*
Estradiol-17β	0.1–0.6	15–20
Estriol	0.02–0.1	50–150
Progesterone	0.1–40	250–600
Aldosterone	0.05–0.1	1–2
Deoxycorticosterone	0.05–0.5	1–12
Cortisol	10–30	10–20

[a] Estrogens and progesterone are produced by placenta. Aldosterone is produced by the maternal adrenal in response to the stimulus of angiotensin II. Deoxycorticosterone is produced in extraglandular tissue sites by way of the 21-hydroxylation of plasma progesterone. Cortisol production during pregnancy is not increased, even though the blood levels are elevated because of decreased clearance caused by increased cortisol-binding globulin.

The hCG molecule is comprised of two dissimilar subunits, designated α and β, which are noncovalently linked. The α- and β-subunits are held together by electrostatic and hydrophobic forces that can be separated in vitro by treatment with acidified urea. The two subunits of hCG have been isolated in pure form; and the primary structure of each has been characterized and cDNAs cloned. There is no intrinsic biological activity of either separated subunit (neither subunit binds to the LH receptor); but if the subunits are recombined, near

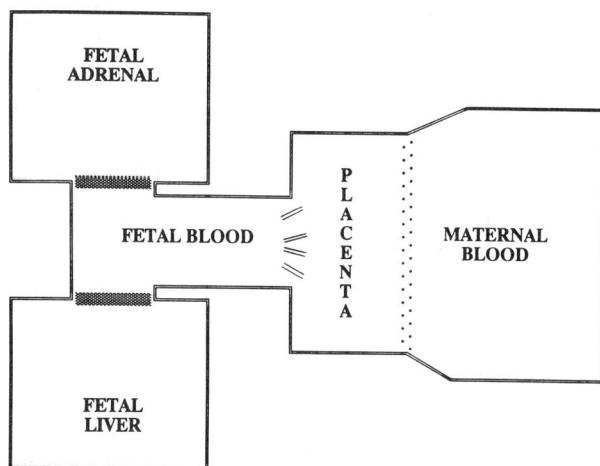

Fig. 6–1. The anatomical parts of the endocrine component of the placental arm of the fetal–maternal communication system. Fetal liver is the principal site of production of low-density lipoprotein (LDL) cholesterol, the principal precursor for fetal adrenal steroidogenesis. Dehydroepiandrosterone sulfate, secreted in prodigious amounts by the fetal adrenal, is converted to 16α-hydroxydehydroepiandrosterone sulfate in fetal liver. These steroids, dehydroepiandrosterone and 16α-hydroxydehydroepiandrosterone, are converted in placenta to estrogens, namely, estradiol and estriol, respectively. Cholesterol derived from LDL in maternal plasma serves as the precursor for progesterone biosynthesis in placenta. The majority (90 percent) of the steroids formed in placenta (both estrogens and progesterone) enters maternal blood; 10 percent enters fetal blood.

100 percent of bioactivity is restored. Talamantes and Ogren (1988) have presented an excellent review of the chemistry of hCG.

The characteristics of the purified subunits are of considerable interest to both clinicians and researchers (Chap. 2). HCG is structurally related to three other glycoprotein hormones—LH, follicle-stimulating hormone (FSH), and thyroid-stimulating hormone (TSH). The amino acid structure of the α-subunits of all four of these human glycoprotein hormones is identical; but in contrast, while sharing certain similarities, there are distinctive differences among the amino acid sequences of the β-subunits of FSH and TSH, as well as those of hCG and LH. The β-subunits of hCG and LH, however, are more similar one to the other; there is 80 percent sequence homology of the first 121 amino acids of β-LH and β-hCG, but there is a 24-amino acid extension at the carboxy-terminus in the hCG β-subunit, which is not present in β-hLH. Recombination of an α- and a β-subunit of the four glycoprotein hormones gives rise to a molecule with biological activity characteristic of the hormone from which the β-subunit was derived.

The carbohydrate moieties of the molecules apparently are not crucial to receptor binding or antibody recognition, but may be important in the coupling of the hormone to adenylate cyclase in responsive cells.

Biosynthesis of hCG. The synthesis of the α- and β-chains of hCG is regulated separately; a single gene codes for the α-subunit of all four glycoprotein hormones; but there are 8 separate genes of the family that codes β-hCG and β-LH. Seven of these genes code for β-hCG and one for β-LH. All eight of the genes for the β-subunit are on chromosome 19. Only 3 of the β-hCG genes are expressed. It is speculated that the 7 β-hCG genes evolved from an ancestral gene for β-LH. This seems likely because chorionic gonadotropin is produced only in trophoblasts of primates. Commonly, trophoblasts are thought of as primitive-type cells; but in an evolutionary sense, this is not the case. As with hCG, a number of genes expressed in human placenta seem to have evolved from genes normally expressed in adult tissues even in lower species. This also is the case for hPL, which is believed to have evolved from the prolactin gene; and in the case of other genes (e.g., aromatase), alternate promoters are used in trophoblast to initiate gene transcription compared with the promoters used to transcribe this gene in nontrophoblastic cells.

The rate of synthesis of the β-subunit is limiting in the formation of the complete hCG molecule. Trophoblasts of normal placenta and those of hydatidiform mole and choriocarcinoma tissues secrete the free α- and β-subunits as well as complete hCG; but there is an excess of hCG α-subunits in placenta and in plasma of pregnant women, whereas the hCG β-subunit is present in plasma in small or undetectable quantities. Interestingly, the same obtains for the synthesis and secretion of the free α- and β-subunits of LH by the pituitary.

Both the α- and β-subunits are synthesized as larger molecular weight precursors; the signal sequences are cleaved by microsomal endopeptidases. Once intact hCG is synthesized, the molecule is rapidly released from the cell; but the regulation of the cellular secretion of hCG is not understood.

Cellular Site of Origin of hCG. The complete hCG molecule is synthesized principally in the syncytiotrophoblast rather than in cytotrophoblasts. It has been demonstrated, however, that mRNA for α-hCG is present in cytotrophoblasts and syncytiotrophoblast, whereas mRNA for β-hCG is primarily restricted to the syncytiotrophoblast.

It is somewhat paradoxical, therefore, that the greatest concentration of hCG in plasma of pregnant women is found at a time in gestation when there are the greatest number of cytotrophoblasts in the placenta, in early pregnancy at 8 to 10 weeks' gestation. As the number of cytotrophoblasts in the placenta declines, the levels of hCG in maternal plasma also decline. Later in gestation, with some pregnancy complications there is a reappearance of cytotrophoblasts, such as in pregnancies with D-antigen isoimmunization and an affected fetus and in pregnancies of some women with severe or poorly regulated diabetes mellitus. In these circumstances, there is also an increase in the plasma concentration of hCG. Indeed, in some such pregnancies, theca lutein cysts develop in the ovaries late in pregnancy, possibly in response to the increase in the concentration of hCG in maternal plasma.

It is possible, as will be subsequently addressed, that GnRH, produced in cytotrophoblasts, acts in a paracrine manner on syncytiotrophoblast to stimulate the secretion of hCG in a manner analogous to the stimulation of pituitary LH release by hypothalamic GnRH. In addition, interleukin-6 (IL-6), if produced in trophoblasts, is believed to stimulate hCG synthesis by way of a GnRH and GnRH receptor-independent mechanism (Li and co-workers, 1992).

Concentrations of hCG in Serum and Urine. The intact (complete) hCG molecule is detectable in the plasma of pregnant women within 8 to 10 days after the midcycle surge of LH that precedes ovulation. Thus, it is likely that hCG enters maternal blood on the day of blastocyst implantation (Chap. 2). Thereafter, the levels of hCG in blood increase rapidly, maximal levels being attained at about 10 weeks of pregnancy. There is no discernible predictable rhythmicity in the secretion of hCG during the day, but appreciable fluctuations in the levels of hCG in plasma are observed from time to time on the same day in the same pregnant woman.

The level of hCG in fetal plasma is about 3 percent of that in maternal plasma. The pattern of appearance of hCG in fetal blood (as a function of gestational age) is similar to that in the mother. HCG is present in amnionic fluid; and early in pregnancy, the concentration of hCG in this biological space is similar to that in maternal plasma. As pregnancy progresses, however, the amnionic fluid concentration of hCG declines to levels that are about one fifth of those in maternal plasma.

Beginning at about 10 to 12 weeks of pregnancy, the level of hCG in maternal plasma begins to decline, a nadir being reached by about 20 weeks' gestation. But this lower plasma level of hCG persists during the remainder of pregnancy. The plasma level of hCG is closely parallel to that in urine, rapidly rising from approximately 1 IU/mL by 6 weeks after the commencement of the last menstrual period to an average value of about 100 IU/mL between the 60th and 80th days after the last menses (Fig. 6–2).

The levels and the gestational pattern of the concentrations of both the free α- and β-subunits in plasma of pregnant women are substantially different from those of the intact molecule. As cited, the levels of the β-subunit in plasma are low or undetectable throughout human pregnancy (Fig. 6–2). On the other hand, the plasma levels of the free α-subunit increase gradually and steadily until about 36 weeks of gestation, when a plateau is attained that is maintained for the remainder of pregnancy. This pattern is similar to that of the plasma hPL levels (Ashitaka and co-workers, 1980; see also Fig. 6–2), as discussed subsequently. Thus, the secretion of α-hCG corresponds to placental mass, whereas the secretion of the complete hCG molecule is maximal at 8 to 10 weeks' gestation. The plasma concentration of

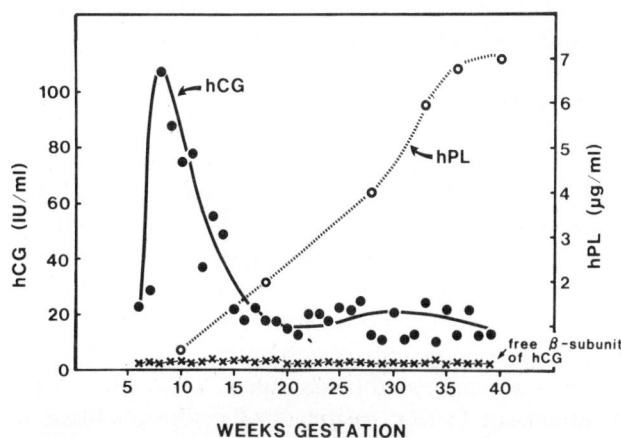

Fig. 6–2. Mean concentration of hCG and hPL in serum of women throughout normal pregnancy. Free β-subunit of hCG is in low concentration or else undetectable throughout pregnancy. The concentration of free α-subunit of hCG in serum increases gradually during pregnancy in a manner similar to that of hPL, albeit in much smaller amounts. (Data from Ashitaka and colleagues, 1980; Selenkow and co-workers, 1971.)

α-hCG, however, is always much less (10 percent or less) than that of intact hCG.

Significantly higher plasma levels of hCG are likely to be found in pregnancies with multiple fetuses, in pregnancies with a single erythroblastotic fetus resulting from maternal isoimmunization, and especially in women with hydatidiform mole and choriocarcinoma. Interestingly, a variety of nontrophoblastic tumors also produce hCG; and, Yoshimoto and co-workers (1979) have demonstrated that many normal tissues also synthesize hCG, albeit in very small amounts. It has been shown that the β-subunit of hCG is produced in fetal kidney (McGregor and co-workers, 1981); moreover, it also has been demonstrated that a number of fetal tissues produce the intact hCG molecule (McGregor and associates, 1983).

Nicks in the hCG Molecule. During the past 5 years, it has been determined that hCG in serum and urine contains nicks, or missing peptide linkages. This is true of purified standard preparations and in individual samples of serum and urine as well. These nicks occur primarily between β-subunit amino acids 44-45 and 47-48. The extent of nicking in standard preparations from pooled urine is 10 to 20 percent, but in individual samples it varies from 0 to 100 percent. The origin of these nicks is likely attributable to enzymatic action on the molecule that occurs near the cellular site of synthesis of the β-subunit (e.g., catalyzed by leukocyte elastase). The biological importance of these nicked molecules is unknown, but the bioactivity of nicked hCG is diminished strikingly, and the immunoreactivity to monoclonal antibodies may be severely attenuated but variable among different antibodies (for review: Cole and associates, 1991). This can be an issue of some concern when monitoring changes in hCG levels as a function of time, treatment, or both, as in the clinical management of persons with trophoblastic disease. With assays conducted with different antibodies, quantitative data may vary appreciably.

Regulation of hCG Biosynthesis. The complete hCG molecule is synthesized in the syncytiotrophoblast. The amount of total mRNA for both the α- and β-subunits of hCG is greater in trophoblast from the first trimester than from trophoblast at term. The finding of mRNA for the α- and β-subunits of hCG in cytotrophoblasts or in intermediate trophoblasts is suggestive that the genes for hCG are expressed before full differentiation of the trophoblasts. In fact, treatment of cytotrophoblasts in culture with cAMP causes hCG secretion without the formation of syncytium.

This conclusion is also supported by the fact that cytotrophoblasts begin to disappear from the placenta at the end of the first trimester; and when there is a reappearance of cytotrophoblasts, hCG levels rise, as with

D-antigen isoimmunization. Alternatively, as stated, GnRH produced in cytotrophoblasts may act on the syncytium to stimulate hCG formation. There are several lines of evidence in favor of a role for placental GnRH in the regulation of hCG formation. Recently, a role for placental inhibin in the regulation of hCG has also been proposed. In fact, it has been demonstrated that a number of agents act to increase hCG secretion by trophoblasts in vitro. Among these are butyrated derivatives of cyclic AMP, GnRH, IL-6, and epidermal growth factor; but dibutyryl cyclic GMP, AMP, insulin, progesterone, epinephrine, and prostaglandin do not cause an increase in hCG secretion.

Metabolic Clearance of hCG. The metabolic clearance rate (MCR) of hCG is about 3 mL/min; that is, about 4 liters of plasma are cleared of hCG each day. The renal clearance of hCG as the native molecule accounts for 30 percent of the total MCR, the remainder being metabolized by pathways other than renal excretion, likely in liver and kidney (Nishula and Wehmann, 1980). The MCR of the β-subunit and of the α-subunit are about 10-fold and 30-fold, respectively, greater than that of intact hCG. By contrast, the renal clearance rates of the subunits are considerably less than that of hCG. Thus, renal clearance is not the means by which the subunits are cleared so rapidly from plasma.

Assay of hCG. The methods for detecting hCG are of considerable importance, because these assays form the basis for the majority of tests for pregnancy in women (Chap. 2).

Biological Functions of hCG. The best known function of hCG in pregnancy is the rescue and maintenance of the function of the corpus luteum during early gestation—that is, continued progesterone production. Bradbury and colleagues (1950) demonstrated that the progesterone-producing life span of the corpus luteum could be prolonged by the administration of hCG to nonpregnant women during the luteal phase of the ovarian cycle. Until recently, however, this action of hCG, while accepted without question, seemed to provide an incomplete explanation for the physiological role of hCG in ovarian function. This obtained because the maximum plasma concentrations of hCG are attained at a time in gestation after the function of the corpus luteum, with respect to progesterone formation, has declined, at 8 to 10 weeks' gestation (Fig. 6–2). Although not rigorously proven, a tentative explanation for this observation may be formulated. HCG, which is present in high concentrations at 8 to 10 weeks' gestation, may cause "down-regulation" of the hCG/LH receptors in corpus luteum; the consequence would be a decrease in the rate of cholesterol side-chain cleavage, and thereby a reduction in the rate of corpus luteum progesterone secretion at a time in gestation when trophoblasts are capable of producing sufficient progesterone for the maintenance of pregnancy.

There seems to be another important role for hCG that is more correspondent in time, physiologically, with the plasma levels of hCG. Fetal testicular testosterone secretion is maximum at the same time in gestation when the rate of placental secretion of hCG is maximum. Thus, at a critical time in sexual differentiation of the male fetus, hCG in fetal plasma acts as an LH surrogate, stimulating Leydig cells of the fetal testes to synthesize testosterone and thereby to promote male sexual differentiation (Chap. 7).

In the ovaries of nonpregnant women, appropriately primed by FSH, hCG induces ovulation and is sometimes used therapeutically, together with FSH, in the treatment of infertility caused by anovulation resulting from hypogonadotropic hypogonadism. For this purpose, it is important to reiterate that the half-life of hCG is quite long (24 hours) compared with that of LH (2 hours), which may account for a longer life span of the corpus luteum after ovulation induction with hCG compared with that when ovulation is induced by LH in hypophysectomized women.

Human Placental Lactogen

History of hPL Discovery. Prolactin-like activity in the human placenta was first described by Ehrhardt in 1936. The protein responsible for this hormone activity was isolated from extracts of human placenta and retroplacental blood and partially purified by Ito and Higashi (1961) and by Josimovich and MacLaren (1962). Because of potent lactogenic and growth hormone-like bioactivity (and an immunochemical resemblance to human growth hormone), it was first called *human placental lactogen* or *chorionic growth hormone.* This hormone has also been referred to as chorionic somatomammotropin. Recently, most authors have used the original name, human placental lactogen (hPL). Grumbach and Kaplan (1964) found, by immunofluorescence studies, that this hormone, like hCG, was concentrated in the syncytiotrophoblast. HPL is detected in the trophoblast as early as the second or third week after fertilization of the ovum.

Chemical Characteristics of hPL. HPL consists of a single polypeptide chain with a molecular weight of 22,279 Da, derived from a precursor of 25,000 Da that has a 26 amino acid signal sequence. The gene for hPL has been cloned, and the nucleotide sequence for DNA complementary to the mRNA encoding for hPL has been determined (Shine and colleagues, 1977). Placental lactogen contains 191 amino acid residues, compared with 188 in human growth hormone; the amino acid sequence in each hormone is strikingly

similar (94 percent homology, including conservative substitutions). HPL also is structurally similar to human prolactin (hPRL), with about 67 percent amino-acid-sequence homology. For these reasons, it has been suggested that the genes for hPL, hPRL, and hGH evolved from a common ancestral gene (probably PRL) by repeated gene duplication (reviewed by Talamantes and Ogren, 1988). Large molecular weight forms of hPL (dimers and higher oligomers) are found in serum and in extracts of the placenta.

HPL Gene Structure and Expression. There are five genes in the growth hormone–placental lactogen gene family; the genes are linked and located on chromosome 17. Two of these genes, hCS-A and hCS-B, both code for hPL, and the amount of mRNA for each (in term placentas) is similar. The gene for hPRL is located on chromosome 6 (Owerbach and co-workers, 1980, 1981).

The mRNA for hPL in placenta is localized exclusively in the syncytiotrophoblast not in cytotrophoblasts, indicating that the genes for hPL are expressed only in the fully differentiated trophoblast. Incredibly, hPL represents 7 to 10 percent of the peptides synthesized by placental ribosomes at term. In fact, 20 percent of the mRNA of term placenta is hPL mRNA. The synthesis of hPL is stimulated by insulin and cAMP. PGE_2 and $PGF_{2\alpha}$ seem to inhibit the secretion of hPL.

HPL Secretion and Metabolism. The MCR of hPL, about 175 L/day, is considerably greater than that of hCG; and the production rate near term, 1 to 3 g/day, is the greatest of any known hormone in the human.

Concentration of hPL in Serum. HPL is demonstrable in syncytiotrophoblast within 5 to 10 days after conception; and hPL can be detected in the serum of pregnant women as early as the fifth week of gestation (3 weeks after fertilization). The concentration of hPL rises steadily until about the 34th to 36th week of pregnancy, and the concentration in maternal blood is approximately proportional to placental mass. The concentration of hPL in maternal serum, as measured by radioimmunoassay, reaches higher levels in late pregnancy (5 to 15 µg/mL) than those of any other known protein hormone (Fig. 6–2). These high hPL plasma levels, coupled with a very short plasma half-life, attest to a rate of production of hPL by the placenta of considerable magnitude. The half-life of hPL in maternal plasma is between 10 and 30 minutes (for review: Walker and associates, 1991).

Very little hPL is found in the circulation of the human fetus or in the urine of the mother or newborn; the concentration of the hPL in amnionic fluid is somewhat lower than that in maternal plasma. Because hPL is secreted primarily into the maternal circulation, with only very small amounts in cord blood, it appears that the role of the hormone in pregnancy, if any, is mediated through action in maternal rather than in fetal tissues. Nonetheless, there has recently been increasing interest in the possibility that hPL in the fetus serves select functions in fetal growth.

Regulation of hPL Biosynthesis. The levels of mRNA for hPL in syncytiotrophoblast remain relatively constant throughout pregnancy. This finding is also supportive of the likelihood that the rate of hPL secretion is proportional to placental mass. As stated, the absence of mRNA for hPL in cytotrophoblasts may be indicative that only the mature, differentiated cell produces hPL; the finding of very high levels of hCG in blood of women with neoplastic trophoblastic disease, together with low levels of plasma hPL of these same women, is also supportive of this view.

Prolonged starvation in the first half of pregnancy leads to an increase in the plasma concentration of hPL. Short-term changes in plasma glucose or insulin, however, have relatively little effect on plasma levels of hPL.

Metabolic Actions of hPL. It has been postulated that hPL participates, directly or indirectly, in a number of important metabolic processes. These putative actions include (1) lipolysis and an increase in the levels of circulating free fatty acids (thereby providing a source of energy for maternal metabolism and fetal nutrition) and (2) an anti-insulin action of hPL, leading to an increase in maternal levels of insulin, which favors protein synthesis; this in turn ensures a mobilizable source of amino acids for transport to the fetus.

HPL, however, does not appear to be required for a successful pregnancy outcome. Nielsen and associates (1979) described a pregnancy in which hPL could not be identified in either maternal serum or in the placenta when analyzed by several techniques in a number of laboratories. Since the account of Nielsen and co-workers, other cases of very low or undetectable plasma levels of hPL in otherwise normal pregnancies have been described. It has been estimated that deficiency in hPL production may occur in about 1 of 12,000 pregnancies. Hubert and associates (1983) found that the level of hPL mRNA in placental tissue of a pregnancy in which plasma hPL was undetectable, was very low compared with that in a normal placenta.

These findings are consistent with the likelihood that hPL functions primarily as a fail-safe mechanism to ensure nutrient supply to the fetus, for example, in times of maternal starvation. As cited in Chapters 2 and 4, there has been little time as yet for significant genetic change in the evolution of humans. Many bodily functions are likely carryovers from the time that humans were hunters-gatherers when periods of sparse food supply were common. HPL may represent such an example; in times of starvation, hPL could function to ensure a nutrient supply to the developing fetus by efficient mobilization of maternal tissue stores.

Spellacy and Buhi (1969) could not detect hPL in the early postpartum period, and also noted a deficient output of pituitary growth hormone at this time. They suggested that this relative lack of insulin antagonism is associated with low fasting levels of blood glucose during this period.

HPL production is not restricted to the trophoblast. The hormone has been detected by direct radioimmunoassay in sera from men and women with various malignancies, other than those originating in trophoblast or gonad, including bronchogenic carcinoma, hepatoma, lymphoma, and pheochromocytoma (Weintraub and Rosen, 1970).

Chorionic Adrenocorticotropin. An ACTH-like protein has been isolated from placental tissue and considerable evidence has accrued to support the proposition that this compound is of placental origin. There are several lines of evidence that are supportive of the likelihood that ACTH is produced in chorionic tissue. Odagiri and colleagues (1979) found that ACTH, lipotropin, and β-endorphin are all found in placental extracts and presumably are derived from the same or a similar 31-kDa precursor molecule, pro-opiomelanocortin (POMC) (Fig. 6–3), as are the pituitary peptides. Liotta and colleagues (1977) also found that ACTH is produced by dispersed placental cells.

Dexamethasone treatment of women does not alter the levels of bioactive or immunoreactive ACTH in placental tissue. To evaluate the biosynthesis of ACTH and ACTH-like compounds in placental tissue, the incorporation of $[^{35}S]$methionine and $[^3H]$leucine into ACTH

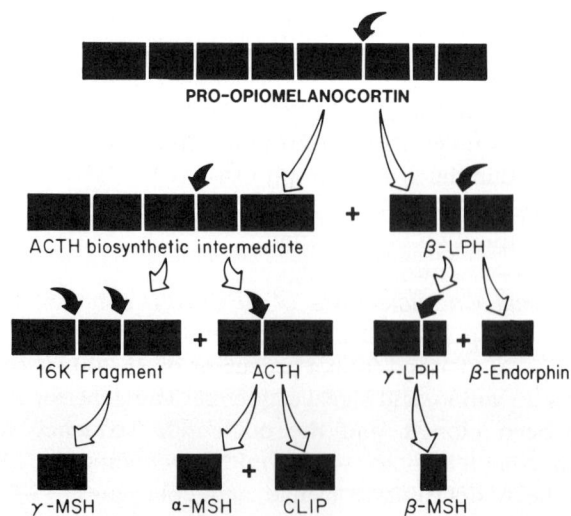

Fig. 6–3. Processing of pituitary pro-opiomelanocortin (31-kDa protein).

and related peptides by dispersed trophoblastic cells was demonstrated. By use of pulse-chase studies, the radiolabel was first incorporated into a high molecular weight (M_r about 34,000) peptide similar to that of the ACTH, β-lipotropin precursor of the pituitary and hypothalamus. With longer incubations, the radiolabel disappeared progressively from the high molecular weight form and began to appear, in increasing amounts, in smaller peptides that corresponded to peptides with antigenic determinants of ACTH and α-MSH, as well as β-lipotropin and β-endorphin. For a review of the placental processing of pro-opiomelanocortin, see Simpson and MacDonald (1981) and Krieger (1982).

Nonetheless, the physiological role of placental ACTH and related compounds is unclear. In pregnant women, the plasma levels of ACTH at all times in pregnancy (before labor) are lower than those in men and nonpregnant women; nonetheless, the concentration of immunoreactive ACTH in maternal plasma increases as pregnancy advances, but the levels of ACTH at all times are less than those in nonpregnant women (Carr and colleagues, 1981). The placenta may produce ACTH that is secreted into the mother or fetus during pregnancy, but it is likely that ACTH does not cross the placenta (i.e., from mother to fetus). The administration of dexamethasone to pregnant women does not cause suppression of urinary free cortisol levels as effectively as it does in men and nonpregnant women. CRH produced in placenta stimulates the synthesis and release of chorionic ACTH, as we will discuss subsequently.

Chorionic Thyrotropin. There is also evidence that the placenta produces a chorionic thyrotropin, but there is as yet no evidence that there is a significant biological role for this substance in normal human pregnancy. The neoplastic trophoblasts of hydatidiform mole and choriocarcinoma may produce a family of chorionic thyrotropins, but the increased thyroid-stimulating activity in women with neoplastic trophoblastic disease is attributed primarily to the thyroid-stimulating properties of hCG, which are low; but, enormous quantities of hCG are produced in women with hydatidiform mole (Chap. 35); and binding of hCG to the TSH receptor in thyroid has been demonstrated (Tomer and associates, 1992).

Parathyroid Hormone-related Protein. The history of the discovery of parathyroid hormone-related protein (PTH-rP) and the chemical relationships between PTH and PTH-rP were described in Chapters 4 and 5. Briefly, PTH-rP was identified, sequenced, and the gene was cloned in 1987. In the short time since those notable observations were made, many potential functions of PTH-rP have been suggested. In particular, the synthesis of PTH-rP has been demonstrated in a number of tissues of the adult, especially in organs of reproduction including the uterus, both myometrium and endometrium in

the human, and in the corpus luteum. Moreover, a number of fetal tissues synthesize PTH-rP, including the fetal parathyroid and the placenta. Recall that PTH-rP is not produced in the normal parathyroid glands of adults.

Because of the production of PTH-rP by fetal tissues and because immunoreactive PTH is not readily detected in fetal blood, it has been proposed that PTH-rP serves as the parathormone of the fetus (Chap. 7). The findings of recently conducted studies are supportive of this view. The adult parathyroid responds to changes in the extracellular concentration (plasma level) of Ca^{2+} by variations in the secretion of PTH. This is not the case for PTH-rP in other tissues. That is to say, the rate of synthesis of PTH-rP is not governed by the plasma concentration of Ca^{2+} in any tissue studied, except the placenta.

In the case of the trophoblast, Hellman and associates (1992) found that this generalization did not hold. They point to the observation that there is active Ca^{2+} transport across trophoblast from mother to fetus, thus accounting for the higher concentration of Ca^{2+} in fetal plasma. It also is established that intact PTH-rP$_{(1-141)}$ infused into the fetal circulation causes increased Ca^{2+} transport in ovine placenta whereas intact PTH$_{(1-84)}$ will not. Therefore, the discovery that cytotrophoblasts express the same unique Ca^{2+} sensing receptor mechanism as the parathyroid cells (Juhlin and associates, 1990) was suggestive that PTH-rP synthesis/secretion by cytotrophoblasts may be responsive to the extracellular Ca^{2+} concentration. This proved to be correct; increases in extracellular levels of Ca^{2+} cause a decrease in cytotrophoblast formation of both PTH-rP and 1,25-dihydroxy-vitamin D_3.

Hypothalamic-like–releasing Hormones of the Placenta. For each of the known hypothalamic-releasing or -inhibiting hormones described, namely GnRH, TRH, CRH, GHRH, and somatostatin, there is an analogous hormone produced in human placenta, as reviewed by Siler-Khodr (1988) and Petraglia and colleagues (1992). The role of these hypothalamic-like releasing or inhibiting hormones in trophoblasts, however, cannot be completely resolved presently. Many investigators have proposed that the finding of these substances in placental tissue is indicative that there may be a hierarchy of control of the synthesis of chorionic trophic agents such as hCG, hCT, and POMC-derived peptides of the placenta; and appreciable evidence has been assembled in support of this view.

Gonadotropin-releasing Hormone. There is a reasonably large amount of immunoreactive gonadotropin-releasing hormone (GnRH) in placenta (Siler-Khodr, 1988; Siler-Khodr and Khodr, 1978). Interestingly, these investigators also found that immunoreactive GnRH was present in cytotrophoblasts, but not in the syncytiotrophoblast. Siler-Khodr (1983) has referred to this substance as hCG-releasing hormone. Gibbons and co-workers (1975) and Khodr and Siler-Khodr (1980) demonstrated that the human placenta can synthesize both GnRH and TRH in vitro.

It has also been shown that GnRH stimulates the secretion of hCG from placental explants and isolated cells in culture; and first-trimester trophoblasts are more responsive to GnRH than are cells from term placentae (Currie and co-workers, 1992). It also seems possible that inhibin and activin, also synthesized in trophoblast, may act in a paracrine manner to regulate GnRH synthesis.

Corticotropin-releasing Hormone. Attempts to isolate and identify hypothalamic corticotropin-releasing hormone (CRH) were in progress for 40 years; sometimes great controversy raged over the existence of this putative factor, presumably of hypothalamic origin. We were privileged to follow this field of neuroendocrinology for most of these 4 decades. Because of this interest, one of our favorite scientific manuscripts was published in *Science* in 1981. Wylie Vale and associates had isolated, purified, sequenced, and synthesized hypothalamic corticotropin-releasing factor (CRF) or hormone (CRH). The scientific accomplishment was most impressive; but the abstract of that publication was a true gem! In its entirety, the abstract reads as follows:

> A peptide with high potency and intrinsic activity for stimulating the secretion of corticotropin-like and β-endorphin-like immunoactivities by cultured anterior pituitary cells has been purified from ovine hypothalamic extracts. The primary structure of this 41-residue corticotropin-and β-endorphin-releasing factor has been determined to be: H-Ser-Gln-Glu-Pro-Pro-Ile-Ser-Leu-Asp-Leu-Thr Phe-His-Leu-Leu-Arg-Glu-Val-Leu-Glu-Met-Thr-Lys-Ala-Asp-Gln-Leu-Ala-Gln-Gln-Ala-His-Ser-Asn-Arg-Lys-Leu-Leu-Asp-Ile-Ala-NH$_2$.

It is now established that CRH also is synthesized in placenta, amnion, chorion laeve, and decidua; and the same gene (long arm of chromosome 8) is expressed in these tissues as that in the formation of CRH in hypothalamic tissues.

In nonpregnant women, the plasma level of CRH is about 15 pg/mL. The levels of CRH in maternal plasma increase to a level of about 250 pg/mL in the early third trimester and to a level of 1 to 2 ng/mL at term (Goland and associates, 1988), levels rising abruptly during the last 5 to 6 weeks of pregnancy. By 24 hours postpartum, CRH in maternal plasma is undetectable, concentrations declining after delivery with a half-life of about 1 hour.

CRH is also found in umbilical venous blood (in about one tenth the concentration as that in maternal plasma), indicative of placental secretion of this peptide into the fetal compartment. Margioris and associates

(1988) demonstrated that placental fragments infused in vitro release immunoreactive CRH.

CRH levels are increased in maternal and umbilical cord plasma in several abnormal states, namely, pregnancy-induced hypertension, preterm labor, fetal asphyxia, and fetal growth retardation. The levels of CRH mRNA in placenta are correlated with the levels of CRH in maternal plasma. The plasma levels of CRH are also elevated in twin pregnancies, being on average about four times greater than those in plasma of women at term with a singleton fetus (Warren and associates, 1990). Also, during the course of labor, the maternal plasma levels of CRH increase by about two- to three-fold (Petraglia and colleagues, 1989, 1990).

Riley and co-workers (1991) found that immunoreactive CRH is localized in syncytium of placenta and also in intermediate trophoblasts, amnion, chorion laeve, and in decidual stromal cells. The biological function of CRH synthesized in these tissues is not so clear.

Several investigators have reported the finding of CRH-binding proteins (BP) in human plasma; and the binding of CRH to these proteins inactivates the CRH. These findings were reviewed by Potter and colleagues (1991), who isolated, cloned, and characterized a cDNA for CRH-BP from human liver and rat brain. They were also able to confirm that this CRH-BP served to inhibit CRH-induced ACTH release by pituitary cells in vitro. The amount of CRH-BP in plasma does not vary appreciably during pregnancy. The affinity constant (Ka) of CRH-BP is about 5×10^9 M^{-1} (Linton and associates, 1990). It has been postulated that this CRH-BP serves to protect against inappropriate maternal pituitary–adrenal stimulation in pregnancy.

It seems unlikely, therefore, that chorionic CRH in the maternal compartment can act to stimulate maternal pituitary ACTH secretion. This is consistent with observations that the levels of ACTH in maternal plasma do not parallel the rise in CRH late in pregnancy. Curiously, CRH-BP is found in plasma only in humans and binds only human CRH (rat CRH is identical to that of the human) (Linton and associates, 1990). The CRH-BP is expressed in human liver, placenta, and brain. This tissue distribution of CRH-BP mRNA in humans is interesting, as pointed out by Potter and associates, because in the rat, for example, a species in which there is very little CRH produced in placenta, CRH-BP mRNA is found only in brain.

Receptors for CRH are present in many tissues: placenta, adrenal, sympathetic ganglia, lymphocytes, gastrointestinal tract, pancreas, and gonads. In most circumstances, CRH acts locally, that is, in a paracrine or neuroendocrine fashion. CRH receptors are coupled to adenylate cyclase. Prostaglandin formation in placenta, amnion, chorion laeve, and decidua is increased by treatment with CRH (Jones and Challis, 1989).

In the hypothalamus, glucocorticosteroids act to inhibit CRH release, but in the trophoblast, glucocorticosteroids stimulate the expression of the CRH gene, with two- to fivefold increases in CRH mRNA and protein after treatment of human trophoblasts in culture with dexamethasone (Robinson and associates, 1988). Therefore, the possibility exists of a positive feedback loop in placenta that involves placental CRH stimulation of placental ACTH formation, placental ACTH stimulation of glucocorticosteroid formation, and finally, glucocorticosteroid stimulation of placental CRH expression (Riley and colleagues, 1991).

There have been a few cases reported of the development of Cushing syndrome during pregnancy with spontaneous resolution after delivery (Aron and coworkers, 1990). It would be interesting to know if the abnormality in such cases resided in a deficiency in the formation of CRH-BP such that placental CRH were effective in such women, when pregnant, to stimulate ACTH formation in the anterior pituitary.

Thyrotropin-releasing Hormone. The synthesis of chorionic thyroid-releasing hormone (TRH) in placenta has been demonstrated, but relatively little is known of the regulation of synthesis or biological role of this chorionic releasing factor.

Neuropeptide-Y. Neuropeptide-Y (NPY) is a small (36 amino acid) peptide that is widely distributed in brain. NPY is also found in the periphery, that is, in sympathetic neurons innervating the cardiovascular, respiratory, gastrointestinal, and genitourinary systems. NPY has been isolated from placenta and localized in cytotrophoblasts (Petraglia and colleagues, 1989). In these studies, it was shown that placental cells released NPY into the medium and that K^+, in high concentrations, increased the release of NPY from trophoblasts. Receptors for NPY have been demonstrated in placenta, and treatment of placental cells with NPY causes the release of CRH.

Growth Hormone-releasing Hormone. Growth hormone-releasing hormone (GHRH), somatocrinin, is expressed in selected human tumors and is implicated in the development of acromegaly in persons with such tumors. The mRNA for GHRH has been identified in human placenta, but the cellular site of GHRH expression is not defined (Berry and co-workers, 1992). In mouse and rat, GHRH has been localized to cytotrophoblasts. The function of placental GHRH is not known.

Inhibin and Activin. Inhibin, a glycoprotein hormone that acts preferentially to inhibit FSH release by the pituitary, is produced by human testis and by the granulosa cells of the human ovary including the corpus luteum. Inhibin is a heterodimer (i.e., composed of dissimilar α- and β-subunits). Activin is closely related to inhibin. The inhibin β-subunit is composed of one of two distinct peptides, βA or βB. The combination

of two β-subunits provides a separate dimer, activin. The placenta produces inhibin α-, βA- and βB-subunits with the greatest levels present at term (Petraglia and colleagues, 1991). Inhibin, produced in placenta, in conjunction with the large amounts of sex steroid hormones produced in human pregnancy, may serve to inhibit FSH secretion and thereby preclude ovulation during pregnancy. Originally it was believed that inhibin was produced in cytotrophoblasts and may serve, in a paracrine fashion, to regulate syncytiotrophoblast function (e.g., the synthesis of hCG). Qu and associates (1992) found that inhibin also is localized in syncytiotrophoblast in vitro. Petraglia and coworkers (1992) suggest that syncytiotrophoblast is a site of storage of inhibin, activin, and GnRH, whereas cytotrophoblasts are the cells in which synthesis occurs. HCG and cyclic AMP analogues stimulate inhibin secretion in isolated cytotrophoblasts, and antibodies to the inhibin α-subunit cause an increase in hCG secretion, suggesting that inhibin may act via GnRH to regulate hCG synthesis/secretion in placenta (Petraglia and associates, 1987). It is possible, perhaps likely, that chorionic activin and inhibin serve functions in placental endocrinology or metabolic processes other than GnRH synthesis as in other tissue sites in nonpregnant women. As yet, these functions have not been established.

Estrogens

Estrogen Production in Pregnancy. Normal human pregnancy, near term, is a hyperestrogenic state of nearly unbelievable proportions, and estrogen is produced almost exclusively by synthesis in syncytiotrophoblast. The amount of estrogen produced each day by syncytiotrophoblast during the last few weeks of pregnancy is similar to that produced in a day, on average, by the ovaries of no fewer than 1000 ovulatory women. By way of another analogy, during the course of one normal human pregnancy, more estrogen is produced by the placenta than is secreted by the ovaries of 200 ovulatory women during the same 40 weeks. This hyperestrogenic state is one of continually increasing magnitude as pregnancy progresses, terminating abruptly after delivery of the fetus and placenta.

The small amount of estrogen produced by the maternal ovaries is limited to the first 2 to 4 postovulatory weeks of pregnancy. There was no reduction in the levels of urinary estrogens after bilateral oophorectomy conducted as early as the 78th day of pregnancy (Diczfalusy and Borell, 1961). Similar results were obtained in several studies of urinary estrogen excretion by pregnant women after surgical removal of the corpus luteum. As early as the seventh week of gestation, more than 50 percent of the estrogens entering the maternal circulation is produced in placenta (MacDonald, 1965; Siiteri and MacDonald, 1963, 1966a).

Estrogen Biosynthesis in Placenta. The biosynthetic pathway of estrogen formation in human pregnancy differ from those in men and nonpregnant women. In the ovary, androstenedione, the immediate precursor of estrone, is produced de novo, from acetate or cholesterol, in theca cells of the developing follicle. Androstenedione is transferred from the theca cells into the follicular fluid and utilized by the granulosa cells for estrogen synthesis. Therefore, it is clear that estradiol synthesized in the granulosa cells is produced from an ovarian theca cell precursor, androstenedione, which in turn is produced de novo from acetate or cholesterol (Chap. 2).

This is not true of placenta. Neither acetate nor cholesterol, nor even progesterone, can serve as precursor for estrogen biosynthesis in the human placenta. Steroid 17α-hydroxylase/17,20-desmolase activity is not expressed in the human placenta; and consequently, the conversion of C_{21}-steroids to C_{19}-steroids, the latter being the immediate precursors of estrogen, is not possible in human syncytium.

Steroid 17α-hydroxylase/17,20-desmolase activity is present in the placenta of several mammalian species, but not in the placenta of most primates. In those species in which steroid 17α-hydroxylase/17,20-desmolase is present in placenta, the induction of this enzyme is usually possible by treatment with glucocorticosteroids (e.g., cortisol of fetal adrenal origin); and increased placental 17α-hydroxylase/17,20-desmolase activity leads to a fall in progesterone secretion and a "surge" in estrogen formation, endocrine antecedents that herald the onset of parturition in many species, but not in the human (Chap. 12).

Placental Aromatase. Estrogen formation from androstenedione is catalyzed by an enzyme complex termed aromatase, which is comprised of a specific cytochrome P-450, aromatase cytochrome P-450 (P-450_{AROM}; P-450_{XIX}, that is, the product of the CYP19 gene), and a flavoprotein, NADPH-cytochrome P-450 reductase (which is ubiquitously distributed among many cells). The principal cellular location of P-450_{AROM} is human syncytiotrophoblast and granulosa cells of the ovary. But in addition, CYP19 is expressed in other cells—adipose tissue (principally stromal cells), neoplastic trophoblasts, Sertoli and Leydig cells of the testis, brain (hypothalamus), and fetal liver. The product estrogen in each of these cells is dependent in part on the substrate available, and in part on the net activity of 17β-hydroxysteroid dehydrogenase (estradiol dehydrogenase) in that tissue. In ovary and testis, estradiol is the product hormone. In particular, androstenedione in these cells is aromatized to estrone, which then is converted (by estradiol dehydrogenase) to estradiol before secretion. In placenta, estradiol is one secretory product; and in addition, 16α-hydroxyandrostenedione is converted to 16α-hydroxyestrone in placenta; this es-

trogen is converted to estriol before secretion by trophoblast. In adipose tissue, however, androstenedione is converted to estrone and the estrone formed (without conversion in situ to estradiol) enters the blood.

Simpson and colleagues have isolated the gene encoding P-450_{AROM} and found it to be unique among all P-450 genes in that (1) it is the largest P-450 gene and (2) the first exon of CYP19 in placenta is untranslated. Moreover, alternate promoters are used in different tissues for initiation of aromatase gene transcription. In trophoblasts, both normal and neoplastic, the primary aromatase transcript is attributable to a different promoter than that used by granulosa cells and adipose tissue stromal cells (Kilgore and colleagues, 1992; Mahendroo and associates, 1991; Means and co-workers, 1991).

This is suggestive that the expression of aromatase is regulated in part by tissue-specific or developmentally regulated promoters. This set of findings, therefore, is consistent with tissue-specific regulation of cis- and trans-regulatory elements for controlling aromatase activity. Furthermore, it seems possible, as Simpson and colleagues point out, that the use of alternate promoters may represent an evolutionary process whereby selected genes in human trophoblasts are expressed.

Precursors for Placental Estrogen Biosynthesis. In classic experiments, Ryan (1959a) found that there is an exceptionally high capacity of placenta to convert certain C_{19}-steroids to estrone and estradiol. He found that dehydroepiandrosterone, androstenedione, and testosterone were efficiently converted to estrone, estradiol, or both by preparations of human placental tissue. These findings were crucial in investigations conducted later to define the role of preformed C_{19}-steroids delivered to placenta in maternal or fetal plasma as precursors for the biosynthesis of estrogen.

Plasma-borne Precursors for Placental Estrogen Formation. Prophetically, Amoroso (1960) suggested that the placenta might, through its abundant enzymatic activity, bring about the formation of active agents by way of the conversion of inactive materials derived from elsewhere in the body. Support for this deduction was provided by Frandsen and Stakemann (1961), who discovered that the level of urinary estrogen in women pregnant with an anencephalic fetus was approximately one tenth that found in women pregnant with a normal fetus at the same stage of gestation. Pointing to the characteristic absence of the fetal zone of the adrenal cortex in anencephalic human fetuses, Frandsen and Stakemann deduced that the fetal adrenal may be the site of origin of a substance(s) that serves to promote placental estrogen formation.

The first proof that the placenta uses plasma-borne precursors as substrates for estrogen biosynthesis was provided by the demonstration that radiolabeled dehydroepiandrosterone sulfate, introduced into the maternal circulation, was converted extensively to radioactive estrogens by the placenta (Baulieu and Dray, 1963; Siiteri and MacDonald, 1963). It was also shown that other C_{19}-steroids, namely, nonconjugated dehydroepiandrosterone, androstenedione, and testosterone, when introduced into the maternal circulation, were also converted to estrogens.

The abundance of dehydroepiandrosterone sulfate in the plasma and the much longer half-life of this sulfate ester, however, uniquely qualified this steroid as the principal circulating precursor of placental estrone and estradiol. The presentation of dehydroepiandrosterone to the placenta as a sulfate conjugate does not preclude its use in the synthesis of estrogen; this obtains because the placenta is normally a rich source of sulfatase activity (Pulkkinen, 1961; Warren and Timberlake, 1962). By the 30th week of pregnancy, 25 percent or more of dehydroepiandrosterone sulfate secreted by the maternal adrenals is converted to estradiol in the placenta (Siiteri and MacDonald, 1963, 1966a).

Metabolism of Maternal Plasma Dehydroepiandrosterone Sulfate.

The extensive utilization of maternal plasma dehydroepiandrosterone sulfate for placental estradiol biosynthesis accounts, in part, for the progressive decrease in the concentration of dehydroepiandrosterone sulfate in the plasma of pregnant women as pregnancy progresses, as well as the decrease in the amount of 11-deoxy-17-ketosteroids excreted in the urine of pregnant women (Migeon and associates, 1955; Milewich and colleagues, 1978; Siiteri and MacDonald, 1966b).

Gant and co-workers (1971) found that there is a striking increase in the MCR of plasma dehydroepiandrosterone sulfate in normally pregnant women at term compared with the MCR of this steroid in men and nonpregnant women. The MCR of dehydroepiandrosterone sulfate in men and nonpregnant women is small, 6 to 8 liters per 24 hours; but the rate of clearance of this steroid sulfoconjugate from plasma of pregnant women at term is increased 10- to 20-fold. Because the production rate of dehydroepiandrosterone sulfate in the maternal adrenals is not changed significantly during human pregnancy, the plasma concentration must decrease as the rate of clearance increases.

The increase in the MCR of plasma dehydroepiandrosterone sulfate in pregnancy appears to be attributable to two processes: (1) removal through conversion to estradiol in the syncytium and (2) increased 16α-hydroxylation of dehydroepiandrosterone sulfate in the maternal compartment (probably in maternal liver). Approximately 30 percent of plasma dehydroepiandrosterone sulfate in pregnant women is converted to 16α-hydroxydehydroepiandrosterone sulfate (Madden and associates, 1976, 1978). The extent of these conversions is high; nonetheless, because the maternal adrenal does not produce large amounts of dehydroepiandros-

terone sulfate during pregnancy, **the fetal adrenal is the quantitatively important source of placental estrogen precursors in the human.**

Fetal Adrenal Glands

Fetal Adrenal Function and Estrogen Formation in Placenta.

As pregnancy progresses, the placental utilization of maternal plasma dehydroepiandrosterone sulfate accounts for only a small fraction of total placental estrogen formation. The observation by Frandsen and Stakemann (1961) of lower urinary excretion of estrogens in women pregnant with an anencephalic fetus, in whom the fetal zone of the adrenal cortex characteristically is absent, together with the finding of high levels of dehydroepiandrosterone sulfate in the cord blood of normal infants (Colas and co-workers, 1964), were suggestive that the fetal adrenal cortex was the principal source of placental estrogen precursors, especially estriol.

Confirmation for part of this hypothesis was provided by Bolté and co-workers (1964a,b) who demonstrated that dehydroepiandrosterone sulfate, introduced into the umbilical artery and perfused through the placenta in situ, was converted to estrone and estradiol. Ultimately it was established that, near term, about 50 percent of estradiol produced in placenta arises from the utilization of maternal plasma dehydroepiandrosterone sulfate and 50 percent arises from fetal plasma dehydroepiandrosterone sulfate (Siiteri and MacDonald, 1966a).

Fetal Adrenal Contribution to Estriol Formation in Placenta.

Therefore, dehydroepiandrosterone sulfate, circulating in both fetal and maternal plasma, is converted to estrone and estradiol by the placenta. Nonetheless, these findings did not provide an explanation for the inordinately large amount of estriol produced in human pregnancy.

In nonpregnant women, the estrogen secreted by the granulosa cells of the "chosen" follicle is estradiol; the estrogen formed from plasma androstenedione in extraglandular tissues is estrone; and from these two primary estrogens, the multiple estrogenic urinary metabolites (including estriol) are derived. The ratio of the concentration of urinary estriol to that of estrone plus estradiol in nonpregnant women is approximately one. But during pregnancy, this ratio increases to ten or even much more near term; thus there is a disproportionate increase in estriol formation during pregnancy.

The greater estriol excretion during human pregnancy could not be accounted for by a change in metabolism of estrone or estradiol with pregnancy. Brown (1956) demonstrated that the metabolism of estradiol in pregnant women was not significantly different from that in nonpregnant women. Moreover, it has not been possible to show the conversion of more than trace amounts of estradiol to estriol in the placenta, indicating that the critical step of 16α-hydroxylation necessary for the biosynthesis of estriol from estrone/estradiol is not possible in human syncytium.

Ryan (1959b) had demonstrated that 16α-hydroxylated C_{19}-steroids such as 16α-hydroxydehydroepiandrosterone, 16α-hydroxy-Δ^4-androstenedione, and 16α-hydroxytestosterone were converted to estriol by preparations of human placental tissue. In addition, large amounts of 16α-hydroxydehydroepiandrosterone sulfate are found in umbilical cord blood (Colas and coworkers, 1964). Finally, the conversion of radiolabeled 16α-hydroxydehydroepiandrosterone and 16α-hydroxydehydroepiandrosterone sulfate, introduced into the maternal circulation, to radiolabeled estriol was demonstrated (MacDonald and Siiteri, 1965a; Madden and associates, 1978).

The disproportionate increase in estriol formation during human pregnancy, therefore, results from the direct placental synthesis of estriol from 16α-hydroxy-C_{19}-steroids, principally 16α-hydroxydehydroepiandrosterone sulfate, rather than from an alteration in the metabolism of estrone or estradiol to estriol in mother or fetus or from 16α-hydroxylation in placenta. 16α-Hydroxydehydroepiandrosterone sulfate arises by synthesis in the fetal adrenal and by 16α-hydroxylation of fetal plasma dehydroepiandrosterone sulfate in the fetal liver (Fig. 6–4). **The fetus is the source of 90 percent of the precursor of estriol formed in placenta in near-term normal human pregnancy** (Siiteri and MacDonald, 1966a).

Maternal plasma dehydroepiandrosterone sulfate is also converted to estriol by way of an estrone/estradiol-independent pathway; namely, plasma dehydroepiandrosterone sulfate is converted in maternal liver to 16α-hydroxydehydroepiandrosterone sulfate, which in placenta is converted to estriol (MacDonald and Siiteri, 1965a,b; Madden and colleagues, 1976, 1978).

Fetal Adrenal Function: An Overview. Because of the importance of the fetal adrenal in the synthesis of placental estrogen precursors and based on the potential importance of fetal adrenal secretions in lung maturation (Chap. 8) and in the initiation of labor (Chap. 12), much effort has been expended to define the factors that regulate the growth and steroidogenic activity of this remarkable gland.

The fetal adrenal cortex is unique. Compared with organs of the adult, it is the largest organ of the fetus; but it is an unusual structure in other ways. At term, the weight of the fetal adrenals approximates the weight of the adult adrenals; but more than 85 percent of the fetal adrenal gland is normally composed of the peculiar fetal zone, which is not found in the adult adrenals.

Direct measurements of fetal adrenal steroid secretory rates are not possible; nonetheless, it can be esti-

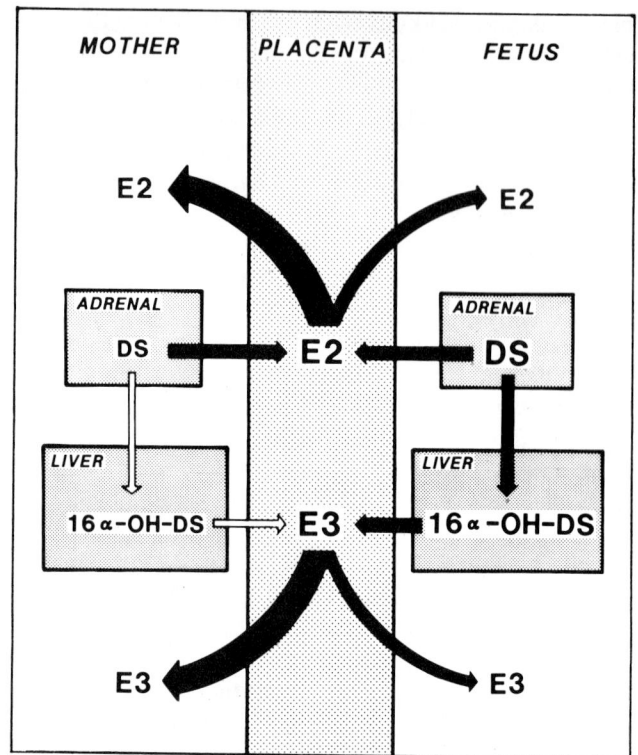

Fig. 6–4. Schematic presentation of the biosynthesis of estrogen in human placenta. Near term, half of estradiol is derived from fetal adrenal dehydroepiandrosterone sulfate (DS) and half from maternal DS. On the other hand, 90 percent of estriol in placenta arises from fetal 16α-OH-dehydroepiandrosterone sulfate (16α-OH-DS) and only 10 percent from all other sources. Most (80 to 90 percent) of steroids produced in placenta are secreted into the maternal blood.

mated that near term, the daily fetal adrenal steroid production is 100 to 200 mg or more steroids per day. The normal rate of steroid secretion by the adrenals of nonstressed, resting adults rarely exceeds 20 to 30 mg per day; from this comparison, it is apparent that the human fetal adrenal is a truly remarkable steroidogenic tissue.

During the neonatal period, the adrenal cortex undergoes rapid involution immediately after birth; and the weight of the adrenals decreases strikingly during the first few weeks of life. The size attained by the fetal adrenals just before birth is not achieved again until late in adolescent or early adult life (Fig. 6–5).

Early Fetal Adrenal Development. Early in embryonic life, the adrenal cortex is composed of cells that resemble those that later in development comprise the fetal zone; these cells appear early in the embryonic period and proliferate rapidly prior to the time that vascularization of the pituitary by the hypothalamus is complete. This is suggestive that the early development of the fetal adrenal is under trophic influences that do not conform to those of the adult (Mulchahey and colleagues, 1987). ACTH does not cross the placenta. Pos-

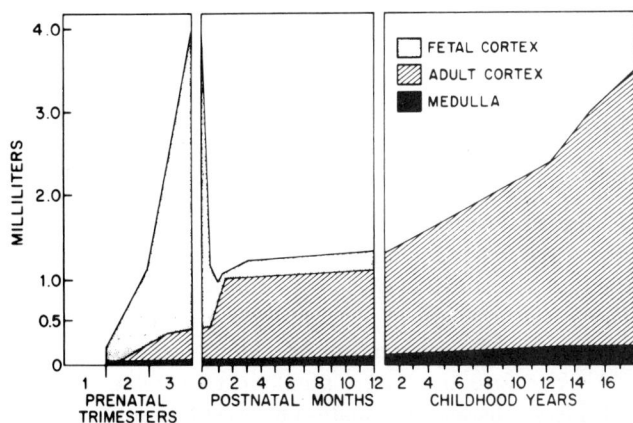

Fig. 6–5. Size of the adrenal gland and its component parts in utero, during infancy, and during childhood. (Adapted from Bethune, 1974.)

sibly, ACTH is secreted by the fetal pituitary in the absence of hypothalamic CRH, or else ACTH (or CRH) arises from a source(s) other than the fetal pituitary, such as chorionic ACTH (or CRH), that is synthesized by trophoblasts. But there are other possibilities, including the likelihood that there is an agent(s) other than ACTH that promotes the growth of the fetal zone of the adrenal glands.

The normal fetal adrenal cortex continues to grow throughout gestation; and during the last 5 to 6 weeks of pregnancy, there is a rapid increase in size of the fetal adrenal. It is quite clear that the rate of fetal adrenal growth and steroid secretion are not controlled by a single trophic stimulus (ACTH), but rather must be regulated by more than one growth-promoting substance. The peculiar development, growth rate, and steroid synthetic pattern that are characteristic of the human fetal adrenals can seemingly be explained in only this way.

Enzymatic Considerations. There is a severe deficiency in the expression of the microsomal enzyme 3β-hydroxysteroid dehydrogenase,$\Delta^{5,4}$-isomerase in the fetal zone cells. The absence of this enzyme activity limits the conversion of pregnenolone to progesterone, an obligatory step in cortisol biosynthesis. In the past few years, it has become clear the absence of 3β-hydroxysteroid dehydrogenase is because of lack of synthesis of this enzyme in fetal zone cells (Doody and associates, 1990). The failure of expression of 3β-hydroxysteroid dehydrogenase causes a relative inefficiency in cortisol biosynthesis. By contrast, there is very active steroid sulfotransferase activity in the fetal adrenal. In consequence, the principal secretory products of the fetal adrenals are pregnenolone sulfate and dehydroepiandrosterone sulfate. Comparatively, cortisol, which likely arises primarily in the neocortex and not in the fetal zone, is a minor secretory product of the human fetal adrenal.

Fetal Adrenal Size and Steroidogenesis. Relative to body weight, the adrenals of the human fetus at term are 25 times larger than those of the adult. Because of the enormous size of the fetal adrenals and the equally enormous capacity for steroid production, many investigators have deduced that there must be more than one growth stimulus for this gland. That is, it is probable that ACTH alone does not bring about the total growth and steroid secretory capacity characteristic of the human fetal adrenals; in fact, there is a continual decrease in the concentration of immunoreactive ACTH in human fetal plasma as pregnancy progresses (Winters and associates, 1974). But during this time, the fetal adrenal is growing most rapidly. And generally, ACTH acts to evoke hypertrophy but not replication of adrenal cells.

For all of these reasons, many investigators have searched for a second growth-promoting agent that acts cooperatively with ACTH to stimulate the fetal adrenal cortex. In this quest, every compound known to be secreted by the pituitary (Fig. 6–3) and each of the peptide hormones of the placenta have been evaluated as potential candidates for this role. By way of brief summary, none of these agents acts on fetal adrenal tissues acutely to cause significant increases in steroid production.

It is likely, however, that the rate of growth of the fetal adrenal is determined by growth factors that may not affect directly the rate of steroidogenesis. There appears to be sufficient ACTH in the fetal circulation at all stages of gestation to ensure adequate activity of the cholesterol side-chain cleavage enzyme, the rate-limiting step in adrenal steroidogenesis. If this were correct, it follows that stimulation of fetal adrenal growth leading to an increased mass of functional cells would result in a striking increase in the capacity of the gland for steroid formation even if the putative growth factor did not act directly to increase steroidogenesis. Therefore, growth of the human fetal adrenal cortex may be determined, in part, by factors that affect cell replication without necessarily altering the rate of synthesis or activities of steroidogenic enzymes.

The unique pattern of fetal adrenal steroid synthesis, that is, the secretion of large amounts of pregnenolone sulfate and dehydroepiandrosterone sulfate and small amounts of cortisol, is reminiscent of the adrenal steroid secretory patterns sometimes observed with adrenal adenomas that cause virilization in women.

In yet another pathophysiological state, hyperprolactinemia caused by microadenomas of the anterior pituitary, high plasma levels of dehydroepiandrosterone sulfate and normal levels of cortisol are sometimes observed. Importantly, when such women were treated with dopamine agonists, which lower the plasma levels of prolactin, the plasma levels of dehydroepiandrosterone sulfate also decreased appreciably. Thus, a second hormone that may serve a role in fetal adrenal steroidogenesis is fetal pituitary prolactin. In support of this view, it has been demonstrated that whereas the levels of immunoreactive ACTH in fetal plasma decline throughout the course of gestation, the prolactin levels increase. Indeed, the fetal plasma levels of prolactin are very high during the time of maximum fetal adrenal growth (Winters and associates, 1975).

Most investigators, including ourselves, however, have been unable to show a direct stimulatory effect of prolactin on fetal adrenal steroidogenesis. Therefore, it appears that if there is a role for prolactin in fetal adrenal steroidogenesis, it must be indirect, perhaps by way of an effect on the growth of the fetal adrenal without necessarily increasing steroidogenesis in a given cell.

It is likely that the third trophic agent for the human fetal adrenal (ACTH and LDL being the first two established) will be one that acts as a growth-promoting factor, perhaps a growth factor itself, and possibly one produced in placenta. This would account for continued growth of the fetal adrenal throughout gestation but rapid involution immediately after birth.

The Source of Precursor for Fetal Adrenal Steroidogenesis.
Because of the very high rate of steroid biosynthesis in the fetal adrenal, yet another consideration becomes pivotal. Namely, **what is the precursor used for steroid biosynthesis in the fetal adrenals?**

In the past, it was proposed that progesterone and pregnenolone produced by the placenta may serve as precursors for fetal adrenal cortisol and dehydroepiandrosterone sulfate biosynthesis, respectively. The conversion of radiolabeled progesterone, introduced into the fetal circulation, to radiolabeled cortisol has been demonstrated. The quantitative importance, however, of this pathway of cortisol formation in the fetal adrenal is small compared with the synthesis of cortisol from cholesterol. It is also clear that the fetal adrenal utilization of plasma pregnenolone cannot account for more than a tiny fraction of the enormous quantity of dehydroepiandrosterone sulfate secreted by the fetal adrenals near term. Therefore, it was reasonable to assume that the precursor for fetal adrenal steroidogenesis must be cholesterol.

The rate of steroid biosynthesis in the fetal adrenal, however, is so great that fetal adrenal steroid hormone production alone requires the utilization of an amount of cholesterol equivalent to one fourth to one fifth of the total daily LDL cholesterol turnover in the adult. If the size of the fetus relative to that of the adult is taken into account, it can be computed that the rate of turnover of the fetal cholesterol pool must be six times that of the total cholesterol turnover in the adult just to accommodate the needs of the fetal adrenal for steroidogenesis, not taking into account the utilization of cholesterol for fetal adrenal cell membrane synthesis in this rapidly growing tissue.

LDL Cholesterol and Fetal Adrenal Steroidogenesis.
This brings us to another important question concerning the regulation of fetal adrenal steroidogenesis; namely, what is the source of cholesterol that is used for fetal adrenal steroidogenesis? Several investigators have demonstrated that fetal adrenal tissue in serum-free medium in vitro synthesizes steroid hormones. Therefore, it is clear that the fetal adrenal can synthesize cholesterol from two carbon fragments, that is, acetate. Nonetheless, the rate of de novo cholesterol synthesis by fetal adrenal tissue is insufficient to account for more than a fraction of the steroids produced by the fetal adrenals at term.

Therefore, the fetal adrenal must assimilate cholesterol from the fetal circulation to meet the demands for optimal steroidogenesis. Cholesterol and cholesterol esters in plasma are present principally in the form of lipoproteins. Lipoproteins are designated according to density as determined by ultracentrifugation; very-low-density lipoprotein (VLDL), low-density lipoprotein (LDL), and high-density lipoprotein (HDL). In studies of human fibroblasts in culture, Goldstein and Brown (1974) demonstrated the presence of specific plasma membrane receptors with high affinity for LDL. After binding of LDL to the plasma membrane receptor, LDL is internalized by an adsorptive endocytotic process. The internalized endocytotic vesicles fuse with lysosomes and the hydrolytic enzymes of the lysosomes catalyze the hydrolysis of the protein component of LDL, which gives rise to amino acids, and the hydrolysis of the cholesterol esters of LDL, which gives rise to cholesterol and free fatty acids.

Simpson, Carr and co-workers conducted important experiments to ascertain if human fetal adrenals take up circulating lipoproteins as a source of cholesterol for steroidogenesis. Using explants of human fetal adrenal tissue maintained in organ culture, they found that when LDL was present in the culture medium, steroidogenesis by ACTH-treated fetal adrenal tissue was markedly stimulated. HDL was much less effective than LDL, and VLDL was devoid of stimulatory activity. These investigators also evaluated the relative contribution of cholesterol synthesized de novo and that of cholesterol derived from the uptake of LDL for fetal adrenal steroidogenesis. First, they found that the activity of the rate-limiting enzyme in the de novo cholesterol synthesis in the fetal adrenal, that is, 3-hydroxy-3-methylglutaryl coenzyme A (HMG CoA) reductase, could account for only a fraction of the cholesterol required for fetal adrenal steroidogenesis. Second, they demonstrated that if LDL were removed from the medium of fetal adrenal explants in organ culture, the rate of steroidogenesis decreased, even in the presence of ACTH. Thus, the fetal adrenal is highly dependent upon circulating LDL as a source of cholesterol for optimum rates of steroidogenesis (Carr and colleagues, 1980, 1982; Carr and Simpson, 1981b; Ohashi and co-workers, 1981, 1982; Simpson and associates, 1979).

A model of cholesterol metabolism in the fetal adrenal as described by Carr and Simpson is shown in Figure 6–6.

Regulation of Cholesterol Levels in the Human Fetus.

The next important question addressed was the source of cholesterol in human fetal plasma. Pitkin and co-workers (1972), from the results obtained in studies of subhuman primates, and in the study of one human pregnancy, concluded that no more than 20 percent of cholesterol in fetal plasma could be accounted for by transfer from the mother.

Carr and Simpson (1984) demonstrated that most of the LDL in fetal plasma arises by de novo synthesis in the fetal liver. The low level of LDL-cholesterol in the plasma of the fetus is not the consequence of limited LDL production in the fetus but rather is the result of rapid clearance of LDL by the fetal adrenal for steroidogenesis. Early in human pregnancy, the fetal plasma levels of LDL-cholesterol are similar to those of the adult. But as pregnancy progresses, the levels of LDL-cholesterol in fetal plasma decline as the fetal adrenal grows. In the normal newborn delivered at term, the concentration of LDL-cholesterol is only about 30 mg/dL (Parker and associates, 1980, 1983a). In the anencephalic newborn in whom the adrenal is atrophic, the levels of LDL cholesterol in umbilical cord plasma are high. Moreover, the level of LDL in cord blood of newborn infants of women with hypertension (in whom estriol levels are low) is also high; thus there is an inverse correlation between the cord plasma levels of LDL and dehydroepiandrosterone sulfate (Parker and associates, 1983b, 1986a).

Secretion of Steroids Produced in Syncytium into the Maternal and Fetal Blood.

Estrogens synthesized in syncytium preferentially enter the maternal circulation. Gurpide and co-workers (1966) have shown that more than 90 percent of estradiol and estriol formed in syncytiotrophoblast enters maternal plasma. The same is true of progesterone formed in the syncytium. Gurpide and co-workers (1972) also found that 85 percent or more of placental progesterone enters maternal plasma; and very little maternal plasma progesterone crosses the placenta to the fetus.

The primary placental estrogen that enters the maternal compartment is estradiol; but somewhat surprisingly, estrone as well as estradiol enter the fetus—there is preferential entry of estrone rather than estradiol into the fetal plasma (Gurpide and co-workers, 1982; Walsh and McCarthy, 1981). This finding, however, as Gurpide and colleagues point out, may be attributed to extratrophoblastic conversion of secreted estradiol to estrone in fetal tissues or erythrocytes. Estriol synthesized in trophoblasts enters both fetal and maternal plasma, but most (90 percent) enters the mother.

Fetal Adrenal Function and Fetal "Stress."

In the past, it was commonly assumed that the fetus would respond physiologically to adverse conditions, such as hypoxia, as the adult responds to stress. This is not always the case. Much of the adult response to stress involves the "fight or flight" phenomenon, which includes fear. So far as we know, the fetus does not experience fear. Fight, flight, and fear in the adult are preludes to increased ACTH secretion and, in consequence, an increase in cortisol secretion by the adrenal cortex.

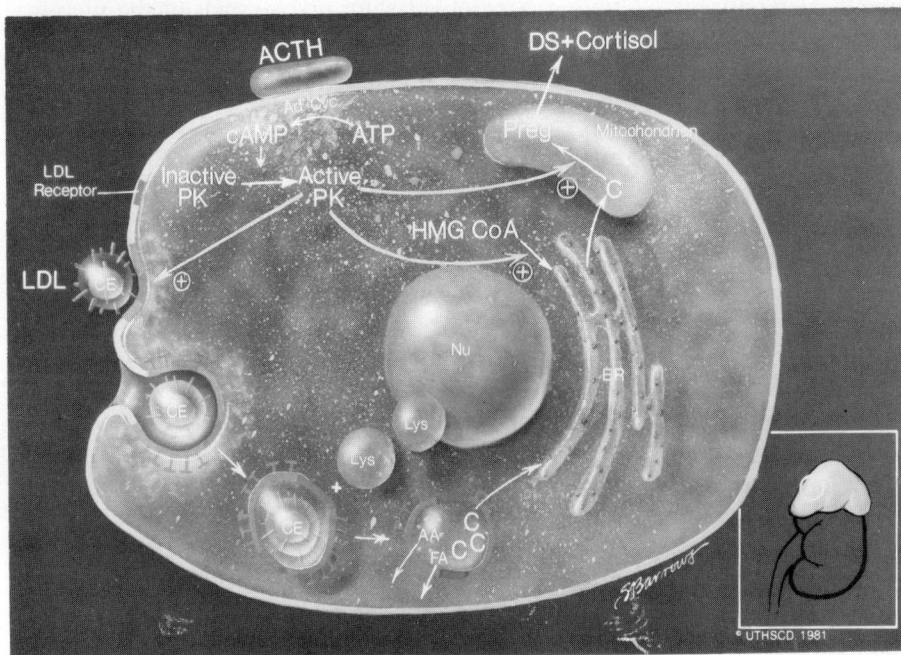

Fig. 6–6. A model proposed for the regulation of fetal adrenal steroidogenesis, lipoprotein utilization, and cholesterol metabolism in the human fetal gland. (Lys = lysosome; Nu = nucleus; ER = endoplasmic reticulum; Ad. Cyc. = adenylate cyclase; Preg = pregnenolone; CE = cholesterol esters; AA = amino acids; C = cholesterol; FA = fatty acids; PK = protein kinase; + = stimulation.) (From Carr and Simpson, 1981b, with permission.)

The importance of this issue is related to the response of the fetus during times of hypoxia or asphyxia insofar as maturation of key fetal tissues is concerned. For example, it has been observed that "stressed" fetuses sometimes experience more rapid lung maturation than is the case in nonstressed fetuses. Commonly, it has been assumed that this circumstance may be related to increased secretion of glucocorticosteroids by the adrenal cortex of the "stressed" fetus. There is probably an additional, if not alternative explanation, however, for these observations.

In pregnancies complicated by a presumed decrease in uteroplacental blood flow, as with maternal hypertension, the levels of maternal plasma and urinary estrogens sometimes are reduced. The decrease in estrogen levels is the result of reduced placental estrogen formation because of inadequate supply of fetal adrenal precursor, dehydroepiandrosterone sulfate (and 16α-hydroxydehydroepiandrosterone sulfate) for estrogen synthesis. Thus, in times of moderate or chronic fetal "stress," fetal adrenal function, at least with respect to the secretion of dehydroepiandrosterone sulfate, may be suppressed. Because of decreased adrenal steroidogenesis, the utilization of fetal plasma LDL cholesterol by the fetal adrenal is reduced; thereby, LDL cholesterol levels in fetal blood of affected fetuses are increased. Indeed, alterations in LDL cholesterol levels in cord plasma appear to be highly dependent, inversely, upon the rate of fetal adrenal steroid biosynthesis before birth (Parker and colleagues, 1980, 1983a, 1983b).

On the other hand, several groups of investigators have found increased levels of arginine vasopressin (AVP) in blood of newborns who are more severely or acutely "stressed" in utero (Chap. 7). AVP acts to increase ACTH secretion. Nonetheless, it has been difficult to establish increased cortisol secretion in such fetuses. Higher blood levels of cortisol in these newborns may be accounted for by transfer of cortisol from the mother to the fetus. During labor, for example, the levels of cortisol in maternal plasma are appreciably increased.

Alterations in Net Transfer of Steroids from Trophoblasts into Maternal and Fetal Blood. Recall that the placental arm of the fetal–maternal communication system of human pregnancy is established by way of hemochorioendothelial placentation. Therefore, steroids secreted from the syncytiotrophoblast enter directly into maternal blood in the intervillous space. There is no evidence of specific estrogen binding within the trophoblast; therefore, net transfer between trophoblast and intervillous space favors entry into maternal blood, which rapidly enters the general circulation of the mother.

Steroids that leave the syncytium toward the fetal compartment, however, do not enter fetal blood directly. First, steroids traveling toward the fetus must traverse the cytotrophoblasts and then enter the intravillous space.

Steroids in this space can reenter the syncytium. Second, steroids that escape the intravillous space toward the fetus must then traverse the wall of the fetal capillaries to reach fetal blood. And steroids in the fetal capillaries of the intravillous space can reenter the intravillous space and thence the syncytium.

The net result of this hemochorioendothelial arrangement is that there is substantially greater release of steroids formed in syncytium into the maternal circulation compared with the amount of steroids that enter the fetal blood.

An interesting phenomenon exists with respect to the distribution of steroids formed in syncytium to the maternal and fetal compartments in pregnancies in which there is decreased uteroplacental blood flow. In newborn infants of women with pregnancy-induced hypertension, chronic hypertension, and severe forms of diabetes mellitus, the umbilical cord plasma levels of estrogens and progesterone are significantly greater than in newborn infants of normal women. Initially, this was a surprise, because with decreased uteroplacental blood flow, estrogen production in placenta is decreased, as are the levels of estrogen in the maternal compartment.

These seemingly discordant findings can be interpreted as follows: as uteroplacental blood flow is reduced, there is relative stasis of maternal blood in the intervillous space. This results in a redistribution of steroids formed in syncytium in favor of the fetal compartment. In particular, there is a decrease in the net exit of steroids into the maternal circulation, probably because of stasis of intervillous blood and thereby greater reentry of steroids from the intervillous space into the syncytium. This favors a relative increase in the transfer of steroids from the syncytiotrophoblast into the fetal compartment. Thereby, there is an increase in the concentration of trophoblast-formed steroids in the umbilical vein. This occurs even in the face of a decrease in total placental estrogen formation and, in consequence, a decrease in estrogen levels in the maternal compartment. This is an important concept that may be important in evaluations of the role(s) of steroids produced in the placenta in fetal development, as with lung maturation, which may be accelerated in fetuses of pregnancies in which uteroplacental blood flow is believed to be reduced (Parker and associates, 1987; see also Chap. 7).

Estrogen Production in Pregnancy: Clinical Correlations. A schematic representation of the pathways of estrogen formation in the placenta is presented in Figure 6–4.

Fetal Anencephaly. In the absence of the fetal zone of the adrenal cortex, as in anencephaly, the rate of formation of placental estrogens (especially estriol) is limited severely because of the lack of C_{19}-steroid precursor formation in the fetus. Verification of the diminished levels of precursors in anencephalic fetuses was provided by the finding of low levels of dehydroepiandrosterone sulfate in cord blood of such newborns (Nichols and co-workers, 1958). Therefore, almost all of the estrogens produced in women pregnant with an anencephalic fetus can be accounted for by the placental utilization of maternal plasma dehydroepiandrosterone sulfate. Furthermore, in such pregnancies the production of estrogens can be increased by the administration (to the mother) of ACTH, which stimulates the rate of dehydroepiandrosterone sulfate secretion by the maternal adrenal (ACTH does not cross the placenta). Finally, placental production of estrogens is decreased in women pregnant with an anencephalic fetus during the administration of a potent glucocorticosteroid, which suppresses ACTH secretion and thus decreases the rate of secretion of dehydroepiandrosterone sulfate from the maternal adrenal cortex (MacDonald and Siiteri, 1965a,b).

Maternal Adrenal Dysfunction. In pregnant women with Addison disease, the maternal urinary estrogen is reduced (Baulieu and co-workers, 1956); but the decrease principally affects estrone and estradiol because the fetal contribution to the synthesis of estriol, particularly in the latter part of pregnancy, is quantitatively much more important.

Maternal Ovarian Androgen-producing Tumors. The extraordinary efficiency of the placenta in the aromatization of C_{19}-steroids may be exemplified by two considerations. First, Edman and associates (1981) found that the placental clearance of maternal plasma androstenedione to estradiol was very similar (when corrected to total blood cleared) to the estimated blood flow to the placenta. This means that virtually all of the androstenedione entering the intervillous space is converted to estradiol and none of this C_{19}-steroid escaped into the fetus. Second, it is rare that a female fetus is virilized in a pregnant woman who is known to have an androgen-secreting ovarian tumor. This finding also indicates that the placenta efficiently converts aromatizable C_{19}-steroids (including bioactive testosterone) to estrogens, thereby precluding transplacental passage of bioactive aromatizable androgen from the mother to the fetus. Indeed, it may be that virilized female fetuses of women with an androgen-producing tumor are cases in which a nonaromatizable C_{19}-steroid androgen is produced by the tumor (e.g., 5α-dihydrotestosterone).

Placental Sulfatase Deficiency. Generally, estrogen formation in placenta is regulated by the availability of C_{19}-steroid prohormones in fetal and maternal plasma. Specifically, there is no rate-limiting enzymatic reaction in placenta in the sequence leading to estrogen biosynthesis. And aside from minor alterations in placental aromatase induced by xenobiotics, the excess of the placental enzymatic machinery for estrogen formation is

large. An exception to this generality was found by France and Liggins (1969), who were the first to establish placental sulfatase deficiency as the cause of very low estrogen levels in otherwise normal (except possibly for dysfunctional labor) pregnancies. Sulfatase deficiency precludes the hydrolysis of C_{19}-steroid sulfate precursors of estrogen, the first enzymatic step in the placental use of these circulating prehormones for estrogen biosynthesis. This is an X-linked disorder (all affected fetuses are male) that is associated with the development of icthyosis later in life (for review: Bradshaw and Carr, 1986).

Placental Aromatase Deficiency. A second exception has been reported, namely, a case of placental aromatase deficiency that resulted in virilization of the pregnant woman and the female fetus of the affected pregnancy. This is the only well-documented example of aromatase deficiency reported. Before this well-studied case was described (Shozu and colleagues, 1991), it was commonly believed that such an enzyme deficiency in the fetilized ovum was incompatible with pregnancy. This view was based on the presumption that the blastocyst production of estrogen seems to be required to promote blastocyst implantation in some species. In the case described, fetal adrenal dehydroepiandrosterone sulfate, which is produced in large quantities, was converted in placenta to androstenedione. Because of the aromatase deficiency, the androstenedione could not be metabolized to estradiol. Rather, C_{19}-steroids, including testosterone, produced in placenta were secreted into the maternal and fetal circulations. Subsequently, the aromatase gene defect in this placenta was defined and found to be caused by *an insert* of 87 base pairs *in frame*, giving rise to a modified gene that encodes an abnormal protein that contains an additional 29 amino acids. In consequence, the aromatase activity of this protein was about 6 percent of normal (Harada and colleagues, 1992). The pregnancy was further complicated by frequent episodes of uterine contractions before term, but ultimately the fetus was born alive, and early in life has grown normally.

Glucocorticosteroid Treatment. The administration of glucocorticosteroids, in moderate to high doses, to pregnant women causes a striking reduction in placental estrogen formation. Glucocorticosteroids act to inhibit ACTH secretion by the maternal and fetal pituitary, resulting in decreased maternal and fetal adrenal secretion of placental estrogen precursor, dehydroepiandrosterone sulfate.

Neoplastic Trophoblastic Disease. In the case of neoplastic trophoblastic disease—namely, hydatidiform mole or choriocarcinoma—there is no fetal adrenal source of C_{19}-steroid precursor for trophoblast estrogen biosynthesis. Thereby, estrogen formation is limited to the utilization of C_{19}-steroids in the maternal plasma, and therefore the estrogen produced is principally estradiol (MacDonald and Siiteri, 1964, 1966). Great variation is observed in the rates of both estradiol and progesterone formation in such cases that is not necessarily related to the volume of neoplastic trophoblastic tissue. This is due to variable disruption of large masses of molar tissue from the uterine wall by blood clots. In this manner, variable amounts of tissue are separated from the maternal blood supply of precursors for estradiol and progesterone formation (MacDonald and Siiteri, 1964, 1966).

Deficiency in Fetal LDL-Cholesterol Biosynthesis. A successful pregnancy in a woman with abetalipoproteinemia has been described (Parker and colleagues, 1986b). This pregnancy is extraordinarily interesting for many endocrinological reasons. The absence of LDL in the maternal plasma led to little or no progesterone formation in the corpus luteum and restricted the amount of progesterone formation in the placenta; in addition, the levels of estriol were also lower than normal (Chap. 12). Presumably, the depressed estrogen production was the result of decreased LDL formation in the fetus, who was heterozygous for the LDL deficiency. Decreased fetal LDL formation could limit fetal adrenal production of dehydroepiandrosterone sulfate and thereby reduce the availability of precursor for placental estrogen synthesis. The fetal adrenal glands are dependent upon plasma LDL as well as the de novo synthesis of cholesterol as precursor for steroidogenesis (Carr and Simpson, 1981a; Mason and Rainey, 1987).

Decreased Fetal Adrenal Utilization of LDL. The most common cause of decreased placental estrogen formation (aside from fetal death) is an acquired reduction in fetal adrenal utilization of plasma LDL. This leads to a reduction in the rate of formation of dehydroepiandrosterone sulfate and thereby a reduction in placental estrogen precursor availability. This sequence of events is observed most commonly in pregnancies complicated by hypertension or more severe forms of diabetes mellitus (Parker and associates, 1984, 1987). As noted before, the final consequence may be as follows: Estrogen formation in placenta is decreased and estrogen levels in maternal blood and urine are decreased. The levels of dehydroepiandrosterone sulfate in umbilical venous blood are decreased, but the levels of LDL are increased. At the same time, because of a redistribution of placental estrogens, the levels of estriol in umbilical venous blood may be increased.

Estriol as a Test of Fetal Well-Being

Rationale. With the discovery that there are large amounts of estrogens in the urine of pregnant women and that these originate in the placenta, measurements of these urinary metabolites were conducted to provide an index of *placental function* or *fetal well-being.* Because the principal estrogen in the urine of pregnant women is estriol, most investigators concentrated on developing reliable methods for the measurement of this estrogen metabolite. With the discovery that the fetus serves an important role in contributing precursors for the synthesis of estriol, there was added impetus provided for the postulate that fetal well-being may be recognized or monitored by the evaluation of urinary or plasma levels of estriol.

Urinary Estriol. It has been known for many decades that death of the human fetus is followed by a striking reduction in the levels of urinary estrogens. Moreover, it was demonstrated that after ligation of the umbilical cord with the fetus and placenta left in situ, there was an abrupt and striking decrease in the production of placental estrogens (Cassmer, 1959). The findings of Cassmer's classic study were subject to at least two interpretations. The first explanation was that maintenance of the fetal placental circulation is essential to the functional integrity of the placenta. This explanation was unlikely to be correct, however, because in Cassmer's study, the placental production of progesterone was maintained after occlusion of the umbilical cord. A second explanation for the marked decrease in urinary estrogens was that after umbilical cord ligation, an important source of precursors of placental estrogen (but not progesterone) biosynthesis was eliminated—that is, the fetus.

In the past, there was clinical usefulness for the measurements of estriol as corroborative evidence of fetal death. But the critical question always has been whether measurements of estrogens provide a clinically useful index of placental function or useful insights into the condition of the living fetus. The clinical value of such tests can be established only by proof of increased infant salvage that is the direct result of therapeutic regimens predicated upon the results of estriol measurements.

Thirty years ago, the development of this aspect of obstetrical endocrinology was extensively discussed by Frandsen and Stakemann (1963). They reviewed the development of methods for measuring urinary estriol and described reliable procedures for the estimation of urinary estriol levels throughout normal human pregnancy. The range of variation in the amount of urinary estriol excreted among different normal pregnant women is great, as illustrated in Figure 6–7. With reliable urine collections and accurate chemical methods, however, they found that the day-to-day variation of estriol excretion by the same pregnant woman was relatively small; in four fifths of the women in this study, there was less than 20 percent day-to-day variation in estriol levels during the last 30 weeks of pregnancy.

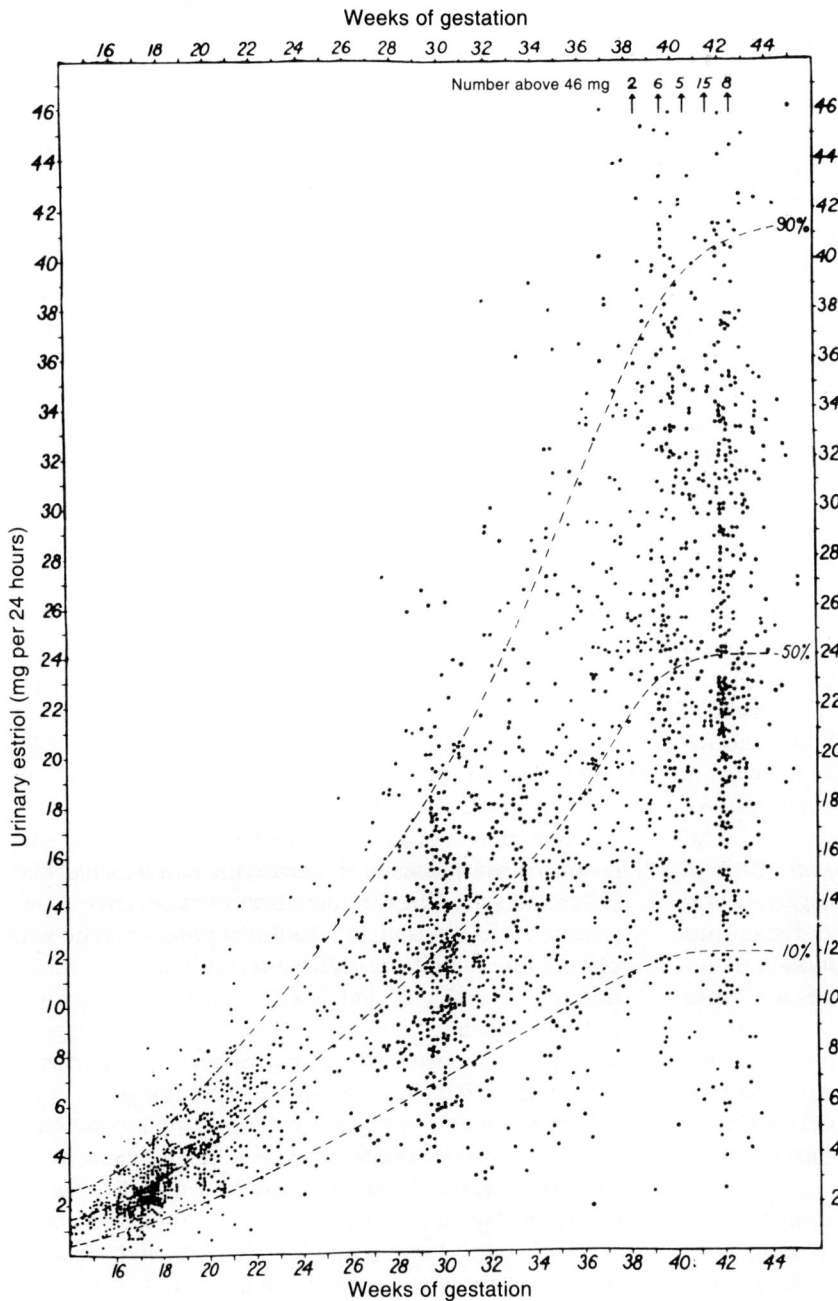

Fig. 6–7. Urinary estriol values from 14 weeks of gestation showing 10th, 50th, and 90th percentiles. (From Beischer and associates, 1969.)

Clinical Utility. The greatest problem in obstetrical management is the proper timing of delivery when complications of a given pregnancy threaten the life or well-being of the fetus. The difficult but common problem is to make the choice between prematurity on the one hand and high risk for the fetus (if intrauterine existence in a deteriorating environment is continued) on the other. In such situations, notably including diabetes mellitus, pregnancy-induced or chronic hypertension, poor previous obstetrical history, fetal growth retardation, and suspected postmaturity, the need for an accurate index of fetal well-being is urgent.

It has been emphasized by several investigators, however, that there is little evidence that obstetrical management plans based on levels of urinary or plasma estriol increased the rate of infant salvage beyond that accomplished by sound clinical judgment alone (Barnes, 1965). Moreover, the results of the only prospective, controlled study reported to date are suggestive that the measurement of estriol has little or no clinical utility in reducing perinatal mortality or morbidity (Duenhoelter and co-workers, 1976). Specifically, the results of this study were supportive of the conclusion that expert clinical management offers greater potential for reduction of perinatal mortality and morbidity, and that the measurement of hormones produced by the placenta offers no unique insight into a complicated pregnancy in which the fetus is at high risk. In a study of pregnancies complicated by mild chronic hypertension, it was found that estriol measurements were of no utility in the management of such complicated pregnancies (Arias and Zamora, 1979). Similarly, it was concluded that 24-hour urinary estriol excretion, measured three times per week, was of no value in the management of postterm pregnancies (Schneider and colleagues, 1978); and Dooley and associates (1984) found such measurements of no value—in fact, misleading—in the management of pregnant women with diabetes. Regrettably, there is no evidence of clinical utility for the measurement of urinary or plasma estriol in the selection of management options for the pregnancy believed to be at high risk for the fetus.

Progesterone

Tissue Site of Production. After the first 6 to 8 weeks of human pregnancy, the biosynthesis of progesterone is accomplished by the utilization of maternal plasma LDL cholesterol in syncytiotrophoblast. Recall that the capacity for de novo synthesis of progesterone in placenta is limited; this is because of low rates of cholesterol formation in trophoblasts.

After the first few weeks of gestation, very little of the progesterone produced arises in the ovary (Diczfalusy and Troen, 1961). Surgical removal of the corpus luteum or even bilateral oophorectomy conducted during the 7th to 10th weeks of pregnancy does not cause a decrease in the rate of excretion of urinary pregnanediol, the principal urinary metabolite of progesterone. There is a gradual increase in the levels of plasma progesterone as well as those of estradiol and estriol in normal human pregnancy, as shown in Figure 6–8.

Progesterone Production Rate. Isotope dilution techniques for the measurement of the rates of endogenous hormone production in humans were first applied to the study of progesterone in pregnancy. The results of these studies, conducted by Pearlman in 1957, were that the daily production of progesterone in late normal, singleton pregnancies was about 250 mg. The findings of studies in which other methods have been employed since then are in agreement with this value. In some pregnancies with multiple fetuses, however, the daily progesterone production rate may exceed 600 mg/day.

Source of Cholesterol Precursor for Progesterone Biosynthesis. Progesterone is formed from cholesterol in all steroidogenic tissues in a two-step enzymatic reaction. First, cholesterol is converted, in mitochondria, to the steroid intermediate pregnenolone, in a reaction catalyzed by cytochrome P-450 cholesterol side-chain cleavage enzyme. In turn, pregnenolone is

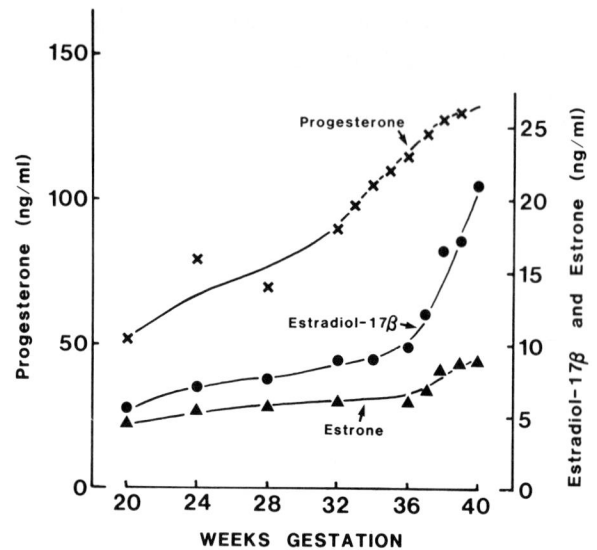

Fig. 6–8. Mean plasma levels (± SEM) of progesterone, unconjugated estradiol, and unconjugated estriol in 33 normal women during the last 9 weeks before delivery. (Adapted from Tungsubutra and France, 1978.)

converted to progesterone, in microsomes, by 3β-hydroxysteroid dehydrogenase,Δ^{5-4}-isomerase.

Solomon and colleagues (1954) found that perfusion of the placenta in vitro with radiolabeled cholesterol resulted in the formation of radiolabeled progesterone. In addition, incubation of pregnenolone with placental tissue preparations also resulted in the formation of progesterone; and an exceedingly great capacity of the placenta to convert pregnenolone to progesterone was demonstrated by in situ placental perfusion studies conducted in Diczfalusy's laboratories.

But whereas the placenta produces a prodigious amount of progesterone, there is a limited capacity for the biosynthesis of cholesterol in this organ. The rate of incorporation of radiolabeled acetate into cholesterol by placental tissue proceeds very slowly, and the activity of the rate-limiting enzyme in cholesterol biosynthesis, 3-hydroxy-3-methylglutaryl coenzyme A (HMG CoA) reductase, in placental tissue microsomes is small. This raised the question as to the source of cholesterol for placental progesterone formation.

Bloch (1945) and Werbin and co-workers (1957) demonstrated that after the intravenous administration of radiolabeled cholesterol to pregnant women, the specific activity of urinary pregnanediol was similar to that of plasma cholesterol. Hellig and associates (1970) also found that maternal plasma cholesterol was the principal precursor (up to 90 percent) of progesterone biosynthesis in human pregnancy. These findings are consistent with the conclusion that in vivo the de novo synthesis of cholesterol in trophoblast is minimal. But in part, this is due to the inhibition of HMG CoA reductase by the high levels of LDL in blood, causing inhibition of synthesis of this enzyme. With LDL deficiency, de novo cholesterol synthesis in trophoblast is appreciable, albeit less than optimum to meet the needs of placenta for both membrane synthesis and normal progesterone synthesis.

Placental Utilization of Maternal Plasma LDL Cholesterol. In studies similar to those described by use of fetal adrenal tissue, Simpson and associates demonstrated that the trophoblast preferentially uses LDL-cholesterol for progesterone biosynthesis. Thus, the formation of placental progesterone, like that of placental estrogens, occurs through the uptake and utilization of circulating precursors; but unlike estrogens, which are formed principally from fetal adrenal precursors, placental progesterone biosynthesis proceeds by way of the utilization of a maternal precursor, LDL cholesterol. This subject was reviewed recently by Casey and colleagues (1992).

These findings provide insights not only into the biochemical mechanisms of placental progesterone formation, but also may provide insights into other aspects of maternal–placental–fetal physiology. The rate of progesterone biosynthesis is largely dependent on the number of LDL receptors on the plasma membrane of the trophoblasts, and thereby, primarily independent of uteroplacental blood flow. This obtains for several reasons:

1. Cholesterol side-chain cleavage activity in placental mitochondria is continually in a highly activated state.
2. De novo synthesis of cholesterol by the placenta is limited but not absent, and is increased in the absence of maternal plasma LDL. Reduced placental progesterone formation was observed in a successful pregnancy of a woman with abetalipoproteinemia (i.e., a homozygous deficiency in LDL formation) (Parker and co-workers, 1986b; see also Chap. 12).
3. The fetus contributes little or no precursors for placental progesterone biosynthesis in normal human pregnancy.
4. Maternal levels of LDL cholesterol are normally not rate limiting in the placental assimilation of cholesterol from the maternal circulation.

The metabolism of LDL by the trophoblasts results in the hydrolysis of the apoprotein and the cholesterol esters of the LDL particle. This may represent a significant source of essential fatty acid and amino acids because such a prodigious amount of LDL is processed each day by the near-term placenta. It can be computed that the placenta alone may process an amount of LDL cholesterol equal to the total daily LDL turnover in nonpregnant women. The hydrolysis of the protein component of LDL gives rise to amino acids, many of which are essential amino acids. The hydrolysis of the cholesterol esters of LDL gives rise to cholesterol, which is used for progesterone biosynthesis, and to fatty acids. The principal fatty acid of LDL cholesterol esters is linoleic acid, an essential fatty acid. It seems reasonable to speculate, therefore, that the metabolism of LDL by trophoblast constitutes a means of obtaining cholesterol for placental progesterone biosynthesis and a mechanism for sequestering essential fatty acids and amino acids for transport to the fetus.

Simpson and Burkhart (1980) also found that progesterone, in concentrations similar to those found in placental tissue, inhibits the activity of the enzyme that catalyzes cholesterol esterification. It can be envisioned that this physiological event serves to ensure a supply of cholesterol for progesterone biosynthesis by preventing the sequestration of cholesterol into a nonusable storage form, cholesterol esters, and will protect liberated essential fatty acids from reesterification with cholesterol.

The intimate relationships that exist between fetal well-being and the placental production of estrogen cannot be demonstrated in the case of progesterone. Fetal death, ligation of the umbilical cord with the fetus and placenta remaining in situ, and anencephaly, are all conditions associated with very low maternal plasma levels and urinary excretion of estrogens. In these circumstances, however, there is no concomitant decrease in the plasma levels of progesterone to anywhere near the same extent as those of estrogen until some indeterminate time after fetal death. Thus, placental endocrine function, including the formation of protein hormones such as hCG, and progesterone biosynthesis, may persist for long periods (weeks) after death of the fetus.

Trophoblast LDL Receptor. The LDL receptors are localized in coated pits on the microvillous membranes of syncytium and are demonstrable as early as 4 weeks after conception. The affinity of these receptors for LDL remains constant throughout human pregnancy and similar to that in other tissues. The trophoblast is unique in that two mRNA species for the LDL receptor are found in human trophoblast, the usual 5.3-kb mRNA and an additional 3.7-kb mRNA. Furuhashi and colleagues (1989) have proposed that the differential utilization of splicing sites may give rise to the smaller LDL receptor mRNA. The expression of LDL receptor gene in trophoblast is highest in the first trimester of pregnancy; this high level of expression may be important in trophoblast growth at this time of pregnancy as well as in provision of progesterone precursor. There is a decrease in the 5.3-kb mRNA for the LDL receptor as pregnancy progresses.

Progesterone Metabolism During Pregnancy. The MCR of progesterone in pregnant women is similar to that found in men and nonpregnant women. This is an

cells of human placenta. Arch Biochem Biophys 293:174, 1992

Hubert C, Descombey D, Mondon F, Daffos F: Plasma human chorionic somatomammotropin deficiency in a normal pregnancy is the consequence of low concentration of messenger RNA coding for human chorionic somatomammotropin. Am J Obstet Gynecol 147:676, 1983

Ito Y, Higashi K: Studies on prolactin-like substance in human placenta, II. Endocrinol Jpn 8:279, 1961

Jones SA, Challis JRG: Steroid, corticotropin-releasing hormone, ACTH and prostaglandin interactions in the amnion and placenta of early pregnancy in man. J Endocrinol 125:153, 1990

Jones SA, Challis JRG: Local stimulation of prostaglandin production by corticotropin-releasing hormone in human fetal membranes and placenta. Biochem Biophys Res Commun 159:192, 1989

Josimovich JB, MacLaren JA: Presence in human placenta and term serum of highly lactogenic substance immunologically related in pituitary growth hormone. Endocrinology 71:209, 1962

Juhlin C, Lundgren S, Johansson H, Lorentzen J, Rask L, Larsson E, Rastad J, Akerstrom G, Klareskog L: 500-Kilodalton calcium sensor regulating cytoplasmic Ca^{2+} in cytotrophoblast cells of human placenta. J Biol Chem 265:8275, 1990

Khodr GS, Siler-Khodr TM: Placental luteinizing hormone-releasing factor and its synthesis. Science 207:315, 1980

Kilgore MW, Means GD, Mendelson CR, Simpson ER: Alternative promotion of aromatase P-450 expression in the human placenta. Mol Cell Endocrinol 83:R9, 1992

Krieger DT: Placenta as a source of "brain" and "pituitary hormones." Biol Reprod 26:55, 1982

Li Y, Matsuzaki N, Masuhiro K, Kameda T, Taniguchi T, Saji F, Yone K, Tanizawa O: Trophoblast-derived tumor necrosis factor-α induces release of human chorionic gonadotropin using interleukin-6 (IL-6) and IL-6-receptor-dependent system in the normal human trophoblasts. J Clin Endocrinol Metab 74:184, 1992

Linton EA, Behan DP, Saphier PW, Lowry PJ: Corticotropin-releasing hormone (CRH)-binding protein: Reduction in the adrenocorticotropin-releasing activity of placental but not hypothalamic CRH. J Clin Endocrinol Metab 70:1574, 1990

Liotta A, Osathanondh R, Ryan KJ, Krieger DT: Presence of corticotropin in human placenta: Demonstration of in vitro synthesis. Endocrinology 101:1552, 1977

MacDonald PC: Placental steroidogenesis. In Wynn RM (ed): Fetal Homeostasis, Vol I. New York, New York Academy of Sciences, 1965, p 265

MacDonald PC, Dombroski RA, Casey ML: Recurrent secretion of progesterone in large amounts: An endocrine/metabolic disorder unique to young women? Endocr Rev 12:372, 1991

MacDonald PC, Siiteri PK: The in vivo mechanisms of origin of estrogen in subjects with trophoblastic tumors. Steroids 8:589, 1966

MacDonald PC, Siiteri PK: Origin of estrogen in women pregnant with an anencephalic fetus. J Clin Invest 44:465, 1965a

MacDonald PC, Siiteri PK: The conversion of isotope-labeled dehydroisoandrosterone and dehydroisoandrosterone sulfate to estrogen in normal and abnormal pregnancy. In Paulsen CA (ed): Estrogen Assays in Clinical Medicine. Seattle, University of Washington Press, 1965b, p 251

MacDonald PC, Siiteri PK: Study of estrogen production in women with hydatiform mole. J Clin Endocrinol Metab 24:685, 1964

Madden JD, Gant NF, MacDonald PC: Studies of the kinetics of conversion of maternal plasma dehydroisoandrosterone sulfate to 16α-hydroxydehydroisoandrosterone sulfate, estradiol and estriol. Am J Obstet Gynecol 132:392, 1978

Madden JD, Siiteri PK, MacDonald PC, Gant NF: The pattern and rates of metabolism of maternal plasma dehydroisoandrosterone sulfate in human pregnancy. Am J Obstet Gynecol 125:915, 1976

Mahendroo MS, Means GD, Mendelson CR, Simpson ER: Tissue-specific expression of human P-450AROM. The promoter responsible for expression in adipose tissue is different from that utilized in placenta. J Biol Chem 266:11276, 1991

Majewska MD, Ford-Rice F, Falkay G: Pregnancy-induced alterations of GABA_A receptor sensitivity in maternal brain: An antecedent of post-partum "blues?" Brain Res 482:397, 1989

Margioris AN, Grino M, Protos P, Gold PW, Chrousos GP: Corticotropin-releasing hormone and oxytocin stimulate the release of placental proopiomelanocortin peptides. J Clin Endocrinol Metab 66:922, 1988

Mason JI, Rainey WE: Steroidogenesis in the human fetal adrenal: A role for cholesterol synthesized de novo. J Clin Endocrinol Metab 64:140, 1987

McGregor WG, Kuhn RW, Jaffe RB: Biologically active chorionic gonadotropin: Synthesis by the human fetus. Science 220:306, 1983

McGregor WG, Raymoure WJ, Kuhn RW, Jaffe RB: Fetal tissue can synthesize a placental hormone: Evidence for chorionic gonadotropin β-subunit synthesis by human fetal kidney. J Clin Invest 68:306, 1981

Means GD, Kilgore MW, Mahendroo MS, Mendelson CR, Simpson ER: Tissue-specific promoters regulate aromatase cytochrome P450 gene expression in human ovary and fetal tissues. Mol Endocrinol 5:2005, 1991

Migeon CJ, Keller AT, Holmstrom EG: Dehydroisoandrosterone, androsterone and 17-hydroxycorticosteroid levels in maternal and cord plasma in cases of vaginal delivery. Bull Johns Hopkins Hosp 97:415, 1955

Milewich L, Gomez-Sanchez CE, Madden JD, Bradfield DJ, Parker PM, Smith SL, Carr BR, Edman CD, MacDonald PC: Dehydroisoandrosterone sulfate in peripheral blood of premenopausal, pregnant, and postmenopausal women and men. J Steroid Biochem 9:1159, 1978

Milewich L, Gomez-Sanchez CE, Madden JD, MacDonald PC: Isolation and characterization of 5α-pregnane-3,20-dione and progesterone in peripheral blood of pregnant women: Measurement throughout pregnancy. Gynecol Invest 6:291, 1975

Mulchahey JJ, DiBlasio AM, Martin MC, Blumenfeld A, Jaffe RB: Hormone production and peptide regulation of the human fetal pituitary gland. Endocr Rev 8:406, 1987

Nichols J, Lescure OL, Migeon CJ: Levels of 17-hydroxycorticosteroids and 17-ketosteroids in maternal and cord plasma in term anencephaly. J Clin Endocrinol 18:444, 1958

Nielsen PV, Pedersen J, Kampmann EM: Absence of human placental lactogen in an otherwise uneventful pregnancy. Am J Obstet Gynecol 135:322, 1979

Nishula BC, Wehmann R: Distribution, metabolism, and excretion of human chorionic gonadotropin and its subunits in man. In Segal S (ed): Chorionic Gonadotropin. New York, Plenum, 1980, p 199

Odagiri E, Sherrill BJ, Mount CD, Nicholson WE, Orth DN: Human placental immunoreactive corticotropin, lipotropin, and β-endorphin: Evidence for a common precursor. Proc Natl Acad Sci USA 16:2027, 1979

Odell WD, Griffin J: Pulsatile secretion of human chorionic gonadotropin in normal adults. N Engl J Med 317:1688, 1987

Ohashi M, Carr BR, Simpson ER: Low density lipoprotein receptors in adrenal tissue of a human anencephalic fetus. Early Hum Dev 7:149, 1982

Ohashi M, Carr BR, Simpson ER: Effects of adrenocorticotropic hormone on low density lipoprotein receptors of human fetal adrenal tissue. Endocrinology 108:1237, 1981

Owerbach D, Martial JA, Baxter JD, Rutter WJ, Shows TB: Genes for growth hormone, chorionic somatomammotropin, and growth hormone–like gene on chromosome 17 in humans. Science 209:289, 1980

Owerbach D, Rutter WJ, Cooke NE, Martial JA, Shows TB: The prolactin gene is located on chromosome 6 in humans. Science 212:815, 1981

Parker CR Jr, Carr BR, Simpson ER, MacDonald PC: Decline in the concentration of low-density lipoprotein-cholesterol in human fetal plasma near term. Metabolism 32:919, 1983a

Parker CR Jr, Carr BR, Winkel CA, Casey ML, Simpson ER, MacDonald PC: Hypercholesterolemia due to elevated low-density lipoprotein-cholesterol in newborns with anencephaly and adrenal atrophy. J Clin Endocrinol Metab 57:37, 1983b

Parker CR Jr, Hankins GDV, Carr BR, Gant NF, MacDonald PC, Porter JC: Prolactin levels in umbilical cord serum and its relation to fetal adrenal activity in newborns of women with pregnancy-induced hypertension. Pediatr Res 20:876, 1986a

Parker CR Jr, Hankins GDV, Carr BR, Leveno KJ, Gant NF, MacDonald PC: The effect of hypertension in pregnant women on fetal adrenal function and fetal plasma lipoprotein-cholesterol metabolism. Am J Obstet Gynecol 150:263, 1984

Parker CR Jr, Hankins GDV, Guzick DS, Rosenfeld CR, MacDonald PC: Ontogeny of unconjugated estriol in fetal blood and the relation of estriol levels at birth to the development of respiratory distress syndrome. Pediatr Res 21:386, 1987

Parker CR Jr, Illingworth DR, Bissonnette J, Carr BR: Endocrinology of pregnancy in abetalipoproteinemia: Studies in a patient with homozygous familial hypobetalipoproteinemia. N Engl J Med 314:557, 1986b

Parker CR Jr, Simpson ER, Bilheimer DW, Leveno KJ, Carr BR, MacDonald PC: Inverse relation between low-density lipoprotein-cholesterol and dehydroisoandrosterone sulfate in human fetal plasma. Science 208:512, 1980

Pearlman WH: [16-³H]Progesterone metabolism in advanced pregnancy and in oophorectomized-hysterectomized women. Biochem J 67:1, 1957

Petraglia F, Calza L, Giardino L, Sutton S, Marrama P, Rivier J, Genazzani AR, Vale W: Identification of immunoreactive neuropeptide-(gamma) in human placenta: Localization, secretion, and binding sites. Endocrinology 124:2016, 1989

Petraglia F, Garuti GC, Calza L, Roberts V, Giardino L, Genazzani AR, Vale W, Meunier H: Inhibin subunits in human placenta: Localization and messenger ribonucleic acid levels during pregnancy. Am J Obstet Gynecol 165:750, 1991

Petraglia F, Giardino L, Coukos G, Calza L, Vale W, Genazzani AR: Corticotropin-releasing factor and parturition: plasma and amniotic fluid levels and placental binding sites. Obstet Gynecol 75:784, 1990

Petraglia F, Sawchenko P, Lim AT, Rivier J, Vale W: Localization, secretion, and action of inhibin in human placenta. Science 237:187, 1987

Petraglia F, Woodruff TK, Botticelli G, Botticelli A, Genazzani AR, Mayo KE, Vale W: Gonadotropin-releasing hormone, inhibin, and activin in human placenta: Evidence for a common cellular localization. J Clin Endocrinol Metab 74:1184, 1992

Pitkin RM, Connor WE, Lin DS: Cholesterol metabolism and placental transfer in the pregnant rhesus monkey. J Clin Invest 51:2584, 1972

Potter E, Behan DP, Fischer WH, Linton EA, Lowry PJ, Vale WW: Cloning and characterization of the cDNAs for human and rat corticotropin-releasing factor-binding proteins. Nature 349:423, 1991

Pulkkinen MO: Arylsulphatase and the hydrolysis of some steroid sulphates in developing organism and placenta. Acta Physiol Scand 180(suppl):52, 1961

Qu J, Ying SY, Thomas K: Inhibin production and secretion in human placental cells cultured in vitro. Obstet Gynecol 79:705, 1992

Riley SC, Walton JC, Herlick JM, Challis JRG: The localization and distribution of corticotropin-releasing hormone in the human placenta and fetal membranes throughout gestation. J Clin Endocrinol Metab 72:1001, 1991

Robinson BG, Emanuel RL, Frim DM, Majzoub JA: Glucocorticoid stimulates expression of corticotropin-releasing hormone gene in human placenta. Proc Natl Acad Sci USA 85:5244, 1988

Ryan KJ: Biological aromatization of steroids. J Biol Chem 234:268, 1959a

Ryan KJ: Metabolism of C-16-oxygenated steroids by human placenta: The formation of estriol. J Biol Chem 234:2006, 1959b

Schneider JM, Olson RW, Curet LB: Screening for fetal and neonatal risk in the postdate pregnancy. Am J Obstet Gynecol 131:473, 1978

Selenkow HA, Varina K, Younger D, White P, Emerson K Jr: Patterns of serum immunoreactive human placental lactogen (IR-HPL) and chorionic gonadotropin (IR-HCG) in diabetic pregnancy. Diabetes 20:696, 1971

Shine J, Seeburg PH, Marial JA, Baxter JD, Goodman HM: Construction and analysis of recombinant DNA for human chorionic somatomammotropin. Nature 270:494, 1977

Shozu M, Akasofu K, Harada T, Kubota Y: A new cause of female pseudohermaphroditism: Placental aromatase deficiency. J Clin Endocrinol Metab 72:560, 1991

Siiteri PK, MacDonald PC: Placental estrogen biosynthesis during human pregnancy. J Clin Endocrinol Metab 26:751, 1966a

Siiteri PK, MacDonald PC: The origin of placental estrogen precursor: During human pregnancy. Excerpta Medica Int Cong Ser 132:726, 1966b

Siiteri PK, MacDonald PC: The utilization of circulating dehydroisoandrosterone sulfate for estrogen synthesis during human pregnancy. Steroids 2:713, 1963

Siler-Khodr TM: Chorionic peptides. In McNellis D, Challis JRG, MacDonald PC, Nathanielsz PW, Roberts JM (eds): The Onset of Labor: Cellular and Integrative Mechanisms. An NICHD Workshop. Ithaca, Perinatology Press, 1988, p 213

Siler-Khodr TM: Hypothalamic-like peptides of the placenta. Semin Reprod Endocrinol 1:321, 1983

Siler-Khodr TM, Khodr GS: Content of luteinizing hormone-releasing factor in the human placenta. Am J Obstet Gynecol 130:216, 1978

Simpson ER, Burkhart M: Acyl CoA: Cholesterol acyl transferase activity in human placental microsomes: Inhibition by progesterone. Arch Biochem Biophys 200:79, 1980

Simpson ER, Carr BR, Parker CR, Milewich L, Porter JC, MacDonald PC: The role of serum lipoproteins in steroidogenesis by the human fetal adrenal cortex. J Clin Endocrinol Metab 49:146, 1979

Simpson ER, MacDonald PC: Endocrine physiology of the placenta. Annu Rev Physiol 43:163, 1981

Solomon S, Lentz AL, VandeWiele RL, Lieberman S: Pregnenolone as intermediate in the biogenesis of progesterone and the adrenal hormones. Proc Am Chem Soc Abstract 29C, 1954

Spellacy WN, Buhi WC: Pituitary growth hormone and placental lactogen levels measured in normal term pregnancy and at the early and late postpartum periods. Am J Obstet Gynecol 105:888, 1969

Talamantes F, Ogren L: The placenta as an endocrine organ: Polypeptides. In Knobil E, Neill J (eds): The Physiology of Reproduction. New York, Raven, 1988, p 2093

Tomer Y, Huber GK, Davies TF: Human chorionic gonadotropin (hCG) interacts directly with recombinant human TSH receptors. J Clin Endocrinol Metab 74:1477, 1992

Tungsbutra GV, France JT: Steroid levels in pregnancy. Aust NZ J Obstet Gynaecol 18:97, 1978

Vale W, Spiess J, Rivier C, Rivier J: Characterization of a 41-residue ovine hypothalamic peptide that stimulates secretion of corticotropin and β-endorphin. Science 213:1394, 1981

Walker WH, Fitzpatrick SL, Barrera-Saldana HA, Resendez-Perez D, Saunders GF: The human placental lactogen genes: structure, function, evolution and transcriptional regulation. Endocr Rev 12:316, 1991

Walsh SW, McCarthy MS: Selective placental secretion of estrogens into fetal and maternal circulations. Endocrinology 109:2152, 1981

Warren JC, Timberlake CE: Steroid sulfatase in the human placenta. J Clin Endocrinol 22:1148, 1962

Warren WB, Goland RS, Wardlaw SL, Stark RI, Fox HE, Conwell IM: Elevated maternal plasma corticotropin releasing hormone levels in twin gestation. J Perinat Med 18:39, 1990

Weintraub D, Rosen SW: Ectopic production of human chorionic somatomammotropin (HCS) in patients with cancer. Clin Res 18:375, 1970

Werbin H, Plotz EJ, LeRoy GV, David ME: Cholesterol: A precursor of estrone in vivo. J Am Chem Soc 79:1012, 1957

Winters AJ, Colston C, MacDonald PC, Porter JC: Fetal plasma prolactin levels. J Clin Endocrinol Metab 41:626, 1975

Winters AJ, Oliver C, Colston C, MacDonald PC, Porter JC: Plasma ACTH levels in the human fetus and neonate as related to age and parturition. J Clin Endocrinol Metab 39:269, 1974

Yoshimoto Y, Wolfsen AR, Hirose F, Odell WD: Human chorionic gonadotropin-like material: Presence in normal human tissues. Am J Obstet Gynecol 134:729, 1979

CHAPTER 7
The Morphological and Functional Development of the Fetus

Fetal Development

Contemporary Obstetrics and the Fetus. The high purposes of obstetrics are to maintain the health and well-being of each pregnant woman and to ensure that every newborn is physically invested, *mens sana in corpore sano,* sound in mind and body, for the lifelong pursuit of the quintessence of earthly existence. To this end, investigations of the nature of human life in utero have been, and will continue to be, among the most fascinating and rewarding in all of biomedical research. This obtains, in large measure, because the findings of these inquiries are of momentous import to all humankind.

It is for this reason that the contemporary era of obstetrics, arbitrarily defined as that period encompassed by the past quarter of a century, has found much of obstetrical research focused on the physiology and pathophysiology of the fetus, its development, and its environment. As an important consequence, the status of the fetus has been elevated to that of a patient who, in large measure, can be given the same meticulous care that obstetricians have long given the pregnant woman.

During this same time, we have come to understand that the conceptus is the dynamic force in the pregnancy unit; the maternal organism, in general, responds passively to signals generated in embryonic/fetal or extraembryonic fetal tissues. Therefore, research directed toward an understanding of embryonic and fetal development and maturation must necessarily take cognizance of the fetal contributions to implantation, maternal recognition of pregnancy, immunological acceptance, endocrine function, nutrition, and parturition (Fig. 2–1).

In this chapter, we consider the development of the normal fetus. In Chapters 41, 45, and 46, the techniques currently used for identifying fetal well-being, or fetal health, are considered in greater detail; and in Chapters 41 and 44, anomalies, injuries, and diseases that affect the fetus and newborn infant are addressed.

Dating of Pregnancy. Several different terms are commonly used to indicate the duration of pregnancy, and thus fetal age; and these are somewhat confusing. *Menstrual age or gestational age* is estimated by computing from the first day of the last menstrual period, a time that precedes conception; this usually is about 2 weeks before ovulation and fertilization and nearly 3 weeks before implantation of the blastocyst. About 280 days, or 40 weeks, elapse, on average, between the first day of the last menstrual period and delivery of the infant; 280 days corresponds to 9⅓ calendar months, or 10 units of 28 days each. The unit of 28 days has been referred to, commonly but imprecisely, as a lunar month of pregnancy; actually, the time from one new moon to the next is 29½ days.

Obstetricians customarily calculate *gestational age* as the menstrual age of a given pregnancy. Embryologists, however, cite events in days or weeks from the time of ovulation (*ovulation age*) or conception (*post-conception age*), these latter two being nearly identical. Occasionally, it is of some value to divide the period of gestation into 3 units of 3 calendar months each, or 3 *trimesters,* because some important obstetrical milestones may be designated conveniently by trimesters. The possibility of spontaneous abortion, for example, is limited principally to the first trimester of pregnancy, whereas the likelihood of survival of the infant born preterm is increased greatly in pregnancies that reach the third trimester.

A short description of various periods of development of the fertilized ovum and embryo is presented. For a more detailed description, based on Streeter's (1920) timetables of human development, *"Horizons,"* the reader is referred to the text by Hamilton and Mossman (1972).

The Ovum, Zygote, and Blastocyst. During the first 2 weeks after ovulation, there are several successive phases of development: (1) ovulation; (2) fertilization of the ovum; (3) formation of free blastocyst (the events of the first week after ovulation are illustrated in Fig. 7–1); and (4) implantation of the blastocyst, a process that begins at the end of the first week after conception. Primitive chorionic villi begin to form soon after implantation. It is conventional to refer to the products of conception after the development of chorionic villi not as a fertilized ovum, or zygote, but as an embryo. The early stages of preplacental development, and the formation of the placenta, are described in Chapter 5.

165

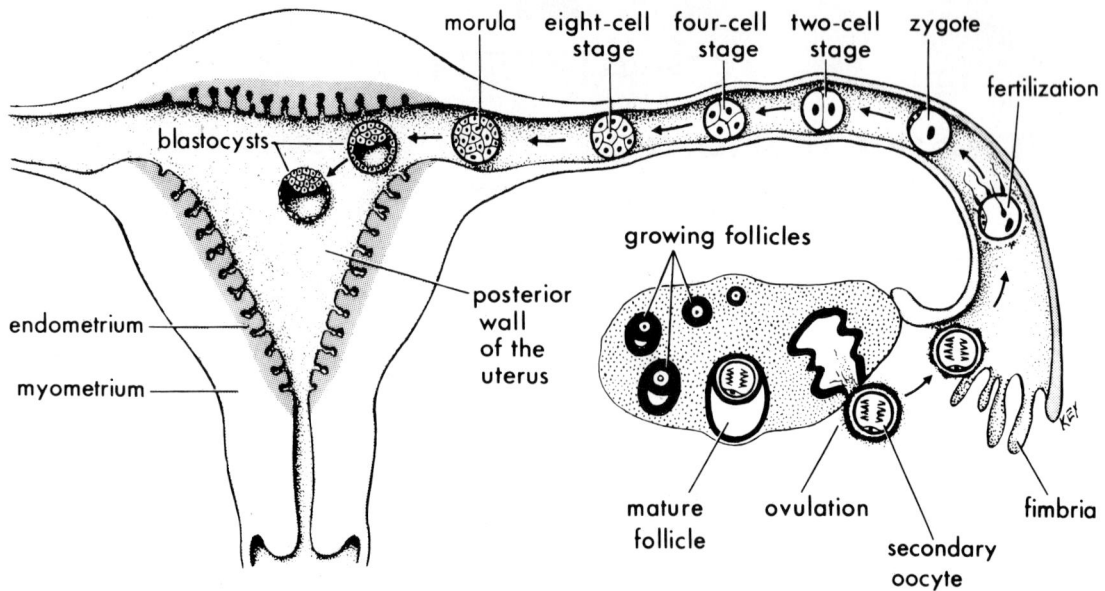

Fig. 7–1. Diagrammatic summary of the ovarian cycle, fertilization, and human development during the first week. Developmental stage 1 begins with fertilization and ends when the zygote forms. Stage 2 (days 2 to 3) comprises the early stages of cleavage (from 2 to about 16 cells, or the morula). Stage 3 (days 4 to 5) consists of the free unattached blastocyst. Stage 4 (days 5 to 6) is represented by the blastocyst attaching to the center of the posterior wall of the uterus, the usual site of implantation. (From Moore, 1988.)

The Embryo. The commencement of the embryonic period is taken as the beginning of the third week after ovulation (fertilization), and coincides in time with the expected time of the next menstruation. Most pregnancy tests (for hCG) in clinical use are positive by this time (Chap. 2). At this stage, the embryonic disc is well defined and the body stalk is differentiated; the chorionic sac measures approximately 1 cm in diameter (Figs. 7–2 and 7–3). There is a true intervillous space that contains maternal blood and villous cores in which there is angioblastic chorionic mesoderm.

By the end of the fourth week after ovulation, the chorionic sac measures 2 to 3 cm in diameter, and the embryo about 4 to 5 mm in length (Fig. 7–4). The heart and pericardium are very prominent because of the dilatation of the chambers of the heart. Arm and leg

buds are present, and the amnion is beginning to ensheath the body stalk, which thereafter becomes the umbilical cord.

At the end of the sixth week after fertilization, the embryo is 22 to 24 mm in length, and the head is quite large compared with the trunk. Fingers and toes are present, and the external ears form definitive elevations on either side of the head.

The Fetus. The end of the embryonic period and the beginning of the fetal period are arbitrarily designated by most embryologists to occur 8 weeks after fertilization, or 10 weeks after the onset of the last menstrual period. At this time, the embryo is nearly 4 cm long. Few, if any, new major structures are formed thereafter; development during the fetal period of gestation con-

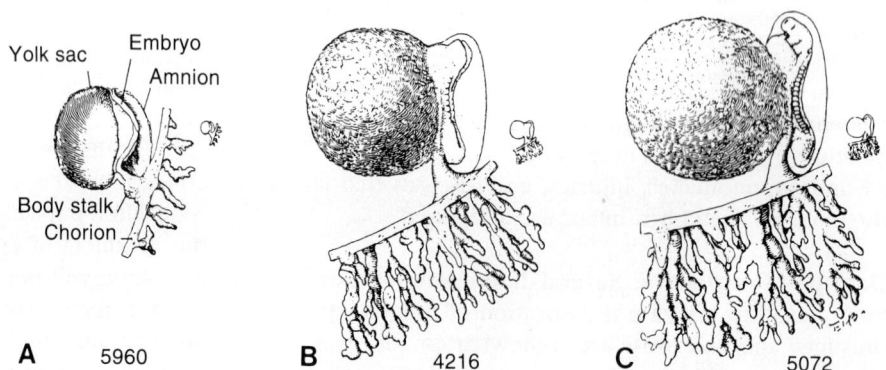

Fig. 7–2. Early human embryos. Only the chorion adjacent to the body stalk is shown. Small outline to right of each embryo gives its actual size. Ovulation ages: **A.** 19 days (presomite). **B.** 21 days (7 somites). **C.** 22 days (17 somites). (After drawings and models in the Carnegie Institute.)

A   5960   B   4216   C   5072

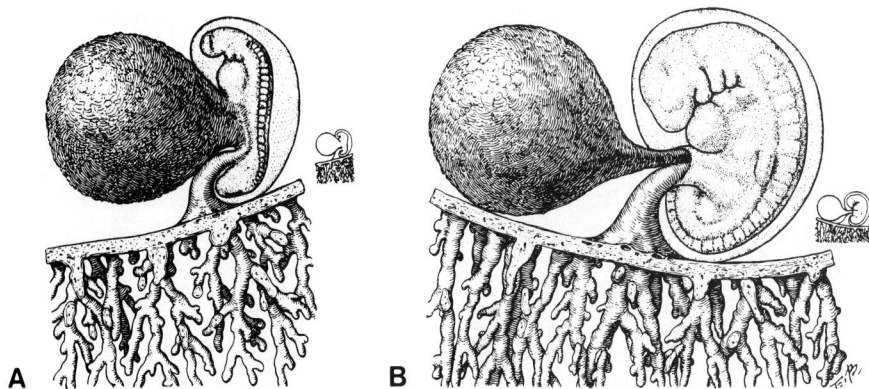

Fig. 7–3. Early human embryos. Small outline to right of each embryo gives its actual size. Ovulation ages: **A.** 22 days. **B.** 23 days. (After drawings and models in the Carnegie Institute.)

sists of growth and maturation of structures that were formed during the embryonic period.

Twelve Gestational Weeks. By the end of the 12th week of pregnancy, the crown–rump length of the fetus is 6 to 7 cm (Figs. 7–5 and 7–6); and by this time, the uterus is usually palpable just above the symphysis pubis. Centers of ossification have appeared in most of the fetal bones; the fingers and toes have become differentiated and are provided with nails; scattered rudiments

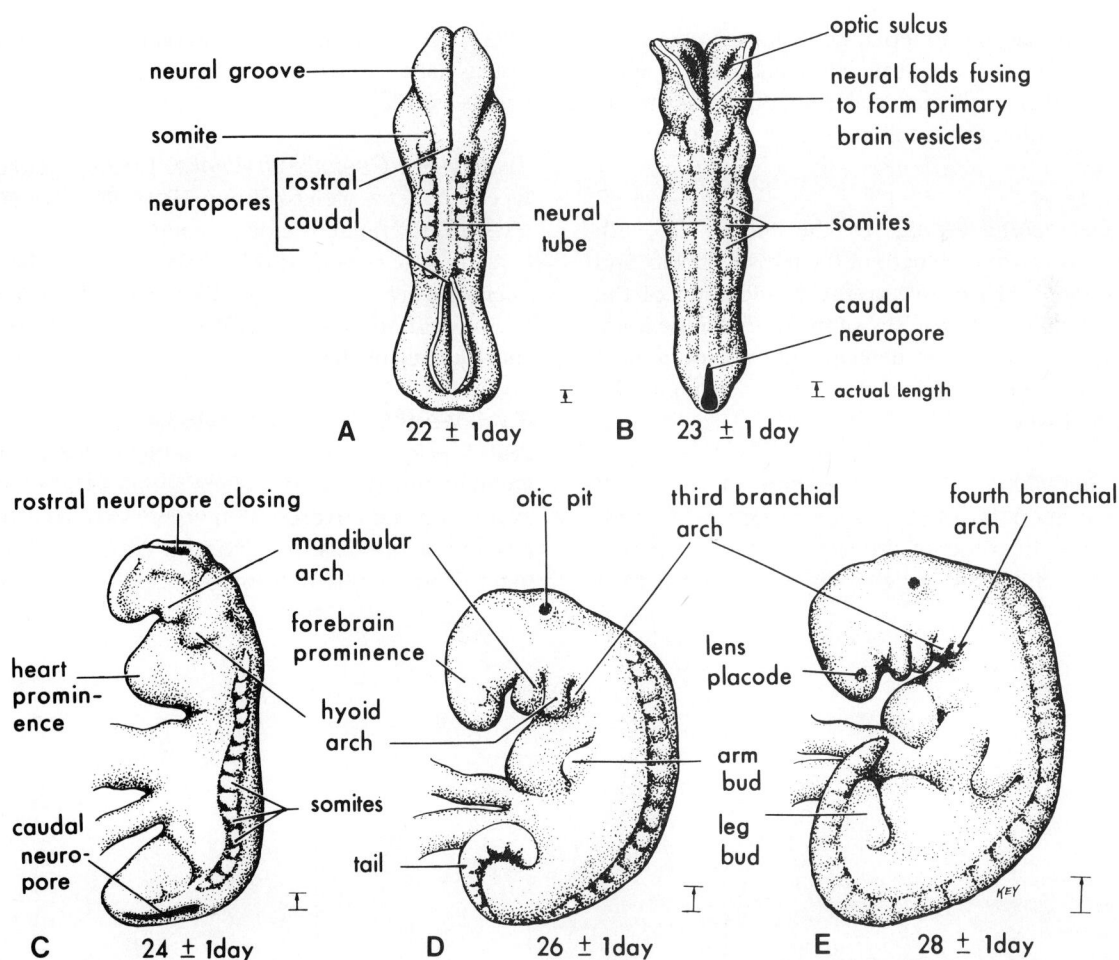

Fig. 7–4. Three- to four-week-old embryos. **A, B.** Dorsal views of embryos during stage 10 of development (about 22 to 23 days) showing 8 and 12 somites, respectively. **C–E.** Lateral views of embryos during stages 11, 12, and 13 of development (24 to 28 days), showing 16, 27, and 33 somites, respectively. (From Moore, 1988.)

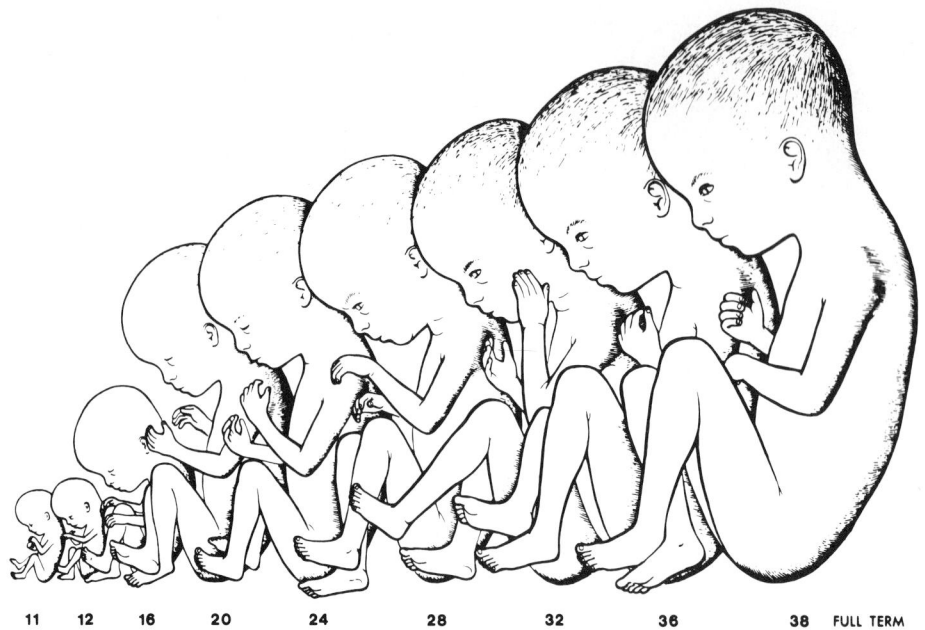

Fig. 7–5. The embryonic period ends at the point of the eighth week after fertilization; by this time, the beginnings of all essential structures are present. The fetal period, extending from the ninth week until birth, is characterized by growth and elaboration of structures. Sex is clearly distinguishable by 12 weeks. (From Moore, 1988.)

of hair appear; and the external genitalia are beginning to show definite signs of male or female sex. A fetus delivered at this time may make spontaneous movements if still within the amnionic sac or if immersed in warm saline.

Sixteen Gestational Weeks. By the end of the 16th week, the crown–rump length of the fetus is 12 cm, and it weighs about 110 g. By careful examination of the external genital organs, the sex of the fetus can be identified. Sex can be correctly determined by experienced observers from inspection of the external genitalia by 14 menstrual weeks.

Twenty Gestational Weeks. The end of the 20th week is the midpoint of pregnancy or gestation as estimated from the time of the last normal menstrual period. The fetus now weighs somewhat more than

300 g. The fetal skin has become less transparent, a downy lanugo covers its entire body, and some scalp hair is visible.

Twenty-four Gestational Weeks. By the end of the 24th week, the fetus weighs about 630 g. The skin is characteristically wrinkled, and fat is deposited beneath it. The head is still comparatively quite large; eyebrows and eyelashes are usually recognizable. A fetus born at this period will attempt to breathe, but almost always dies shortly after birth.

Twenty-eight Gestational Weeks. By the end of the 28th week, a crown–rump length of about 25 cm is attained and the fetus weighs about 1100 g. The thin skin is red and covered with vernix caseosa. The pupillary membrane has just disappeared from the eyes. An infant born at this time in gestation moves his or her

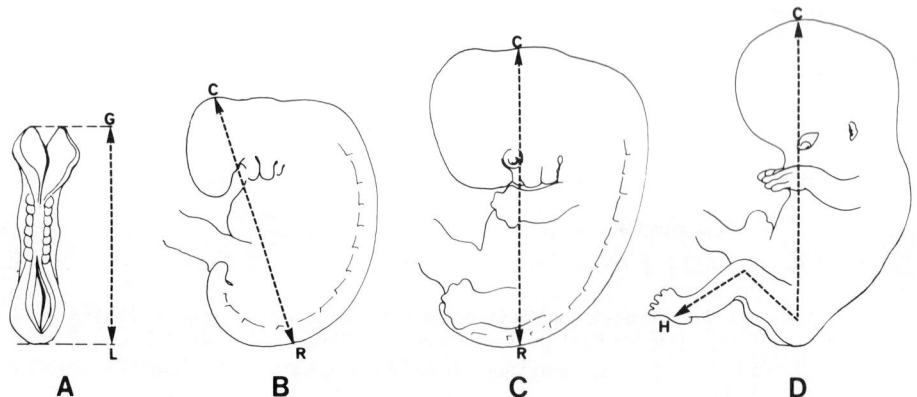

Fig. 7–6. Sketches showing methods of measuring the length of embryos. **A.** Greatest length. **B,C.** Crown–rump length. **D.** Crown–heel length. (From Moore, 1988.)

limbs quite energetically and cries weakly. The infant of this gestational age, with expert care, most often will survive.

Thirty-two Gestational Weeks. At the end of 32 gestational weeks, the fetus has attained a crown–rump length of about 28 cm and a weight of about 1800 g. The surface of the skin is still red and wrinkled. Infants born at this period, with proper care, usually survive.

Thirty-six Gestational Weeks. At the end of 36 weeks gestation, the average crown–rump length of the fetus is about 32 cm and the weight is about 2500 g. Because of the deposition of subcutaneous fat, the body has become more rotund, and the previous wrinkled appearance of the face is lost. Infants born at this time have an excellent chance of survival with proper care.

Forty Gestational Weeks. Term is reached at 40 weeks after the onset of the last menstrual period. At this time, the fetus is fully developed, with the characteristic features of the newborn infant to be described here. The average crown–rump length of the fetus at term is about 36 cm, and the weight is approximately 3400 g, with variations to be discussed subsequently.

Length of Fetus. Because of the variability in the length of the legs and the difficulty of maintaining them in extension, measurements corresponding to the sitting height (crown to rump) are more accurate than are those corresponding to the standing height (Fig. 7–6). The average sitting height and weight of the fetus at the end of each lunar month were determined by Streeter (1920) from 704 specimens; and these values are similar to those found more recently, as shown in Table 7–1. Such values are approximate, but generally, the length is a more accurate criterion of the gestational age of a fetus than is the weight.

Haase (1875) suggested that, for clinical purposes, the length in centimeters of the fetus measured from crown to heel may be approximated during the first 5 months by squaring the number of the lunar month to which the pregnancy has advanced; and in the second half of pregnancy, by multiplying the month by 5.

Weight of the Newborn. The average term infant at birth weighs about 3000 to 3600 g, depending upon race, parental economic status, size of the parents, and parity of the mother, with boys about 100 g (3 oz) heavier than girls. During the second half of pregnancy, the fetal weight increases in a linear manner with time until about the 37th week of gestation, and then the rate slows variably. The principal determinants of fetal growth late in pregnancy are related, in large part, to the socioeconomic status of the mother. In general, the greater the socioeconomic deprivation, the slower the rate of late fetal growth.

Birthweights over 5000 g occur occasionally, but

TABLE 7–1. CRITERIA FOR ESTIMATING AGE DURING THE FETAL PERIOD

Age (wk) Menstrual	Fertilization	CR Length (mm)[a]	Foot Length (mm)[a]	Fetal Weight (g)[b]	Main External Characteristics
11	9	50	7	8	Eyes closing or closed. Head more rounded. External genitalia still not distinguishable as male or female. Intestines are in the umbilical cord.
12	10	61	9	14	Intestines in abdomen. Early fingernail development.
14	12	87	14	45	Sex distinguishable externally. Well-defined neck.
16	14	120	20	110	Head erect. Lower limbs well developed.
18	16	140	27	200	Ears stand out from head.
20	18	160	33	320	Vernix caseosa present. Early toenail development.
22	20	190	39	460	Head and body (lanugo) hair visible.
24	22	210	45	630	Skin wrinkled and red.
26	24	230	50	820	Fingernails present. Lean body.
28	26	250	55	1000	Eyes partially open. Eyelashes present.
30	28	270	59	1300	Eyes open. Good head of hair. Skin slightly wrinkled.
32	30	280	63	1700	Toenails present. Body filling out. Testes descending.
34	32	300	68	2100	Fingernails reach fingertips. Skin pink and smooth.
38	36	340	79	2900	Body usually plump. Lanugo hairs almost absent. Toenails reach toe tips.
40	38	360	83	3400	Prominent chest; breasts protrude. Testes in scrotum or palpable in inguinal canals. Fingernails extend beyond fingertips.

[a] These measurements are averages and so may not apply to specific cases; dimensional variations increase with age. The method for taking CR (crown–rump) measurements is illustrated in Fig. 7–6.
[b] These weights refer to fetuses that have been fixed for about two weeks in 10 percent formalin. Fresh specimens usually weigh about 5 percent less.
From Moore (1977).

most tales of huge babies vastly exceeding this figure were based on hearsay or inaccurate measurements at best. Presumably, the largest baby recorded in the medical literature is that described by Belcher (1916), a stillborn female weighing 11,340 g (25 lb). Term infants, however, frequently weigh less than 3200 g, and sometimes as little as 2250 g (5 lb) or even less. In the past, it was customary when the birthweight was 2500 g or less, to classify the infant as preterm, even though in some cases the low birthweight was not the consequence of preterm birth but rather was caused by retardation in growth during intrauterine development.

Fetal Head. Obstetrically, the head of the fetus is a most important body part, because an essential feature of labor is the adaptation between the fetal head and the maternal bony pelvis. Only a comparatively small part of the head of the fetus at term is represented by the face; the rest is composed of the firm skull, which is made up of two frontal, two parietal, and two temporal bones, along with the upper portion of the occipital bone and the wings of the sphenoid.

These bones are not united rigidly, but rather are separated by membranous spaces, the *sutures* (Fig. 7–7). The most important sutures are the *frontal*, between the two frontal bones; the *sagittal*, between the two parietal bones; the two *coronal*, between the frontal and parietal bones; and the two *lambdoid*, between the posterior margins of the parietal bones and upper margin of the occipital bone. With vertex presentation, all of the sutures are palpable during labor, except the *temporal* sutures, which are situated on either side between the inferior margin of the parietal and upper margin of the temporal bones, covered by soft parts, and cannot be felt in the living fetus.

Where several sutures meet, an irregular space forms, which is enclosed by a membrane and designated as a *fontanel* (Fig. 7–7). Three such structures are usually distinguished, namely the greater, the lesser, and the temporal fontanels. The *greater*, or *anterior fontanel* is a lozenge-shaped space that is situated at the junction of the sagittal and the coronal sutures. The *lesser*, or *posterior fontanel*, is represented by a small triangular area at the intersection of the sagittal and lambdoid sutures. Both can be palpated readily during labor, and the localization of these fontanels gives important information concerning the presentation and position of the fetus. The *temporal*, or *casserian* fontanels, situated at the junction of the lambdoid and temporal sutures, have no diagnostic significance. It is customary to measure certain critical *diameters* (Fig. 7–8) and *circumferences* of the infant's head. The diameters most frequently used, and the average lengths thereof, are as follows:

1. The *occipitofrontal* (11.5 cm), which follows a line extending from a point just above the root of the nose to the most prominent portion of the occipital bone.
2. The *biparietal* (9.5 cm), the greatest transverse diameter of the head, which extends from one parietal boss to the other.
3. The *bitemporal* (8.0 cm), the greatest distance between the two temporal sutures.
4. The *occipitomental* (12.5 cm), from the chin to the most prominent portion of the occiput.
5. The *suboccipitobregmatic* (9.5 cm), which follows a line drawn from the middle of the large fontanel to the undersurface of the occipital bone just where it joins the neck (Figs. 7–7 and 7–8).

The greatest circumference of the head, which corresponds to the plane of the occipitofrontal diameter, averages 34.5 cm; and the smallest circumference, corresponding to the plane of the suboccipitobregmatic diameter, is 32 cm. As a rule, white infants have larger heads than do nonwhite infants; boys, somewhat larger than girls; and the infants of multiparas, larger heads than those of nulliparas. Because of the widely varying

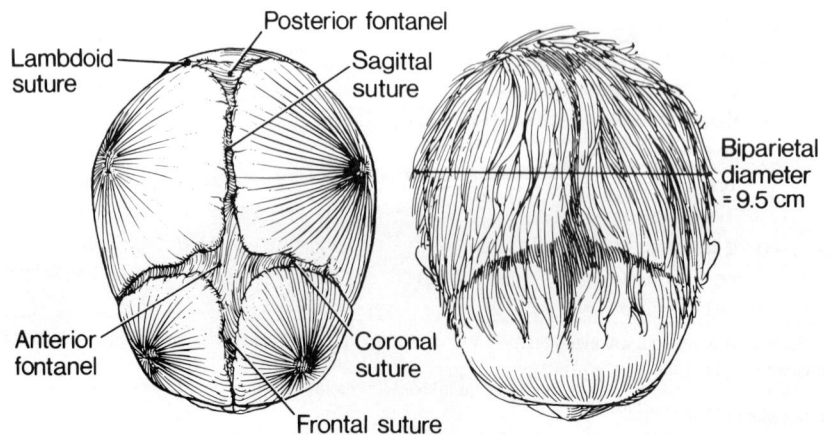

Fig. 7–7. Fetal head at term showing various fontanels, sutures, and the biparietal diameter.

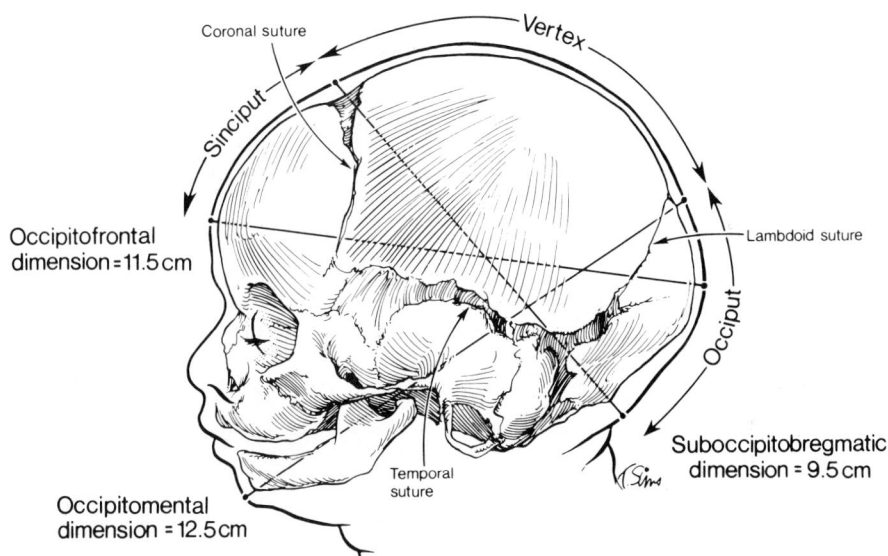

Fig. 7–8. Diameters of the fetal head at term.

mobility between the bones of the skull at the sutures, fetal heads differ appreciably in adaptation to the maternal pelvis by *molding*. The bones of one fetus may be soft and readily molded, whereas those of another are firmly ossified, only slightly mobile, and therefore incapable of significant reduction in size. This variation undoubtedly contributes to fetopelvic disproportion, a leading indication for cesarean delivery (Chaps. 20 and 21).

Fetal Brain. As pregnancy advances, the fetal brain changes remarkably in appearance as well as function (Fig. 7–9). Therefore, it is possible to identify fetal age rather precisely from the external appearance of the brain (Dolman, 1977).

The Fetal–Maternal Communication System: Placental Arm

The transfer of oxygen and a great variety of nutrients from the mother to the fetus, and conversely the transfer of carbon dioxide and other metabolic wastes from fetus to mother, is accomplished by way of the nutritive component of the placental arm of the fetal–maternal communication system. Thus, the placenta is the organ of transfer between mother and fetus. The placenta, and to a limited extent the attached membranes, supply all material for fetal growth and energy production while removing all products of fetal catabolism.

There are no direct communications between the fetal blood (contained in the fetal capillaries in the intravillous space of the chorionic villi) and the maternal blood (in the intervillous space). The one exception to this generalization regarding the independence of the circulations is the development of occasional breaks in the chorionic villi, permitting the escape of fetal erythrocytes (and leukocytes), in various numbers, into the maternal circulation. This leakage is the mechanism by which some D-negative women become sensitized by the erythrocytes of their D-positive fetus (see Chap. 44). These occasional leaks, however, do not controvert the basic principle that there is no gross intermingling of the macromolecular constituents of the two circulations. The transfer of substances from mother to fetus and from fetus to mother, therefore, depends primarily on the mechanisms that permit or facilitate the transport of such substances through the syncytiotrophoblast of the intact chorionic villi.

The Intervillous Space: Maternal Blood. The intervillous space is the maternal biological compartment of transfer; the maternal blood in this extravascular compartment directly bathes the trophoblasts. Transfer of substances from mother to fetus is accomplished first by transfer from the intervillous space into the syncytiotrophoblast. This also is the biological space into which substances from the fetus are transported by way of the syncytium. Because this process of transfer supplies the fetus with oxygen as well as nutrients and provides for elimination of metabolic waste products, the chorionic villi and the intervillous space, together, function for the fetus as lung, gastrointestinal tract, and kidney. Fetal urination commences early in pregnancy, and the fetal urine enters amnionic fluid, especially after 16 weeks' gestation. But fetal kidney function develops slowly as pregnancy progresses, as is true of other fetal organs.

The circulation of maternal blood within the intervillous space is described in Chapter 5. The residual volume of the intervillous space of the delivered term

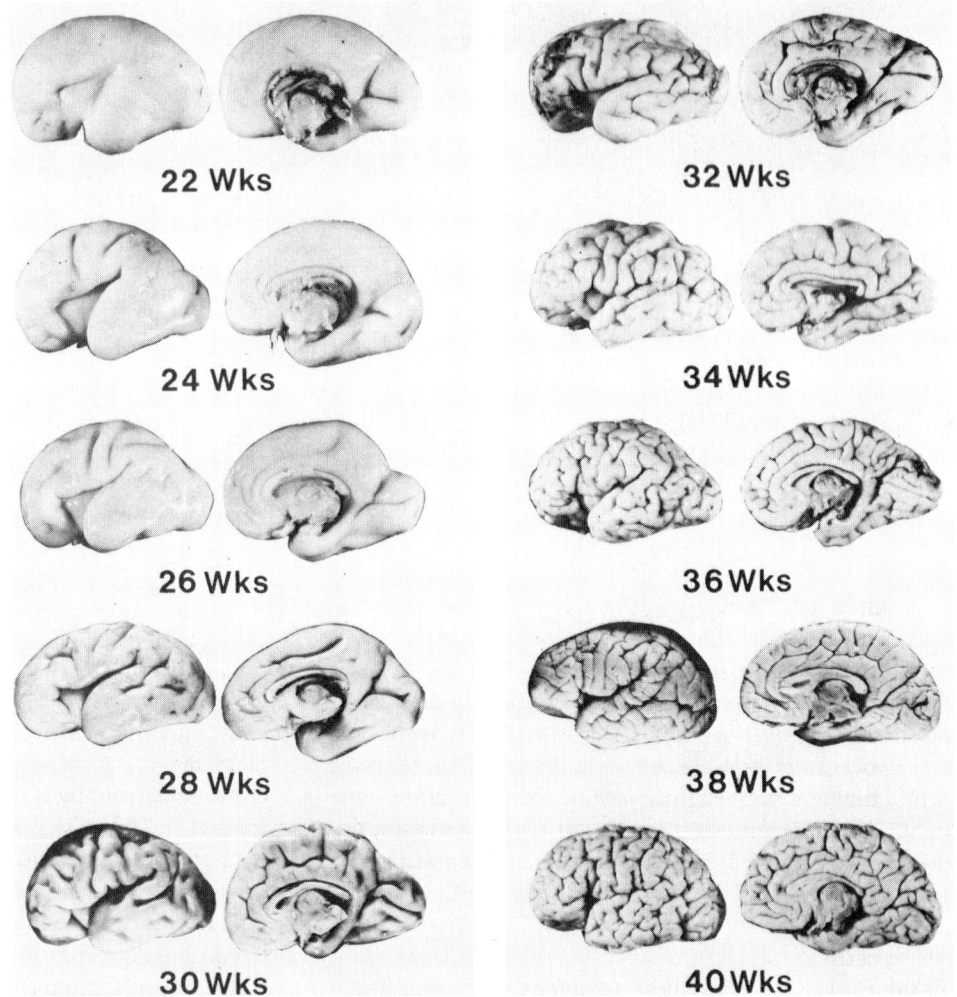

Fig. 7–9. Characteristic configuration of fetal brains from 22 to 40 weeks of gestation at 2-week intervals. (From Dolman, 1977.)

placenta measures about 140 mL; the normal volume of the intervillous space before delivery, however, may be twice this value (Aherne and Dunnill, 1966). Uteroplacental blood flow near term has been estimated to be about 700 to 900 mL/min, with most of the blood apparently going to the intervillous space.

Uterine contractions cause a reduction in the flow of blood into the intervillous space, the degree of reduction depending in large measure upon the intensity of the contraction. Blood pressure within the intervillous space is significantly less than the uterine arterial pressure, but somewhat greater than uterine venous pressure. Uterine venous pressure, in turn, varies depending upon several factors, including the body position of the pregnant woman. When she is supine, for example, pressure in the lower part of the inferior vena cava is elevated; consequently, in this position, pressure in the uterine and ovarian veins, and in turn the intervillous space, is increased. An even greater increase in intervillous pressure is likely when she is standing.

Fetal Capillaries of the Intravillous Space: Fetal Blood. The hydrostatic pressure in the fetal capillaries that traverse the chorionic villi is probably not appreciably different from that in the intervillous space. During normal labor, the rise in fetal blood pressure must be parallel to the pressure in the amnionic fluid and the intervillous space. Otherwise, the capillaries in the chorionic villi would collapse and fetal blood flow through the placenta would cease.

Placental Transfer

Chorionic Villus. Substances that pass from the maternal blood to the fetal blood must traverse (1) trophoblast, (2) stroma of the intravillous space, and (3) fetal capillary wall. Although this histological "barrier" separates the blood in the maternal and fetal circulations, it does not behave uniformly like a simple physical barrier. Throughout pregnancy, syncytiotrophoblast either actively or passively permits, facilitates, and adjusts the amount and rate of transfer of a wide range of substances to the fetus. After midpregnancy, the number of Langhans cells, or cytotrophoblasts, decreases, and the villous epithelium then consists predominantly of syncytiotrophoblast. The walls of the villous capillaries likewise become thinner, and the relative number of fetal vessels increases in relation to the villous connective tissue. It is important to recall that the fetal placental surface vessels after branching from the truncal arteries of the chorionic vessels do not contain smooth muscle cells in the walls of these vessels (Chap. 5).

Several attempts have been made to estimate the total surface area of chorionic villi in the human placenta at term. The planimetric measurements made by Aherne and Dunnill (1966) of the villous surface area of the placenta indicate that there is a close correlation with fetal weight. They calculated that the total surface area at term was approximately 10 m^2.

Regulation of Placental Transfer.

The syncytiotrophoblast is the fetal tissue interface of the placental arm of the transport system. The maternal-facing surface of this tissue is characterized by a complex microvillous structure. The fetal-facing (basal) cell membrane of the trophoblast is the site of transfer to the intravillous space through which the fetal capillaries traverse. In the case of transport from the intravillous space into fetal blood, or vice versa, the fetal capillaries pose an additional transport site.

At least 10 variables are important in determining the effectiveness of the human placenta as an organ of transfer:

1. The concentration of the substance under consideration in the maternal plasma, and in some instances the extent to which it is bound to another compound, such as a carrier protein.
2. The rate of maternal blood flow through the intervillous space.
3. The area available for exchange across the villous trophoblast epithelium.
4. If the substance is transferred by diffusion, the physical properties of the tissue barrier interposed between blood in the intervillous space and in the fetal capillaries.
5. For any substance actively transported, the capacity of the biochemical machinery of the placenta for effecting active transfer (e.g., specific receptors on the plasma membrane of the trophoblast).
6. The amount of the substance metabolized by the placenta during transfer.
7. The area for exchange across the fetal capillaries in the placenta.
8. The concentration of the substance in the fetal blood, exclusive of any that is bound.
9. Specific binding or carrier proteins in the fetal or maternal circulation.
10. The rate of fetal blood flow through the villous capillaries.

Transfer by Diffusion.

Most substances with a molecular mass less than 500 d diffuse readily through the placental tissue interposed between the maternal and fetal circulations. Molecular weight clearly is important in determining the rate of transfer by diffusion; all other things equal, the smaller the molecule, the more rapid the transfer rate. Simple diffusion, however, is by no means the only mechanism of transfer of low molecular weight compounds. The syncytiotrophoblast actually facilitates the transfer of a variety of small compounds, especially those that are in low concentration in maternal plasma but are essential for the normal growth and development of the fetus.

Simple diffusion appears to be the mechanism involved in the transfer of oxygen, carbon dioxide, water, and most (but not all) electrolytes. Anesthetic gases also pass through the placenta rapidly by simple diffusion.

Insulin, steroid hormones, and thyroid hormones cross the placenta but at very slow rates. The hormones synthesized in situ in the trophoblasts enter both the maternal and fetal circulations but not to the same degree (Chap. 6). For example, the concentrations of hCG and hPL are very much lower in fetal plasma than in maternal plasma. Substances of very high molecular weight usually do not traverse the placenta, but there are important exceptions, such as immune gamma globulin G (IgG; its M_r is about 160,000), which is transferred by way of a specific trophoblast receptor-mediated mechanism.

Transfer of Oxygen and Carbon Dioxide.

Morriss and Boyd (1988), in an excellent account of placental transport, provide an interesting observation. They recall that Mayow, in 1674, suggested that the placenta served as the fetal lung. Moreover, Erasmus Darwin, in 1796, only 22 years after the discovery of oxygen, reasoned that the function of the placenta was comparable with that of lungs and gills. Inasmuch as Darwin observed that the color of blood passing through each organ became bright red, he deduced that *"from the structure as well as the use of the placenta, it appears to be a respiratory organ, like the gills of the fish, by which the fetus becomes oxygenated."*

The transfer of carbon dioxide across the placenta is diffusion limited; but the transfer of oxygen is blood-flow limited. As shown in Figure 7–10, there are other limitations. The placenta supplies about 8 mL O_2 per min/per kg weight of fetus; and because the fetal blood oxygen stores are sufficient for only 1 to 2 minutes, this supply must be continuous (Longo, 1991). Normal values for oxygen, carbon dioxide, and pH in maternal and

Fig. 7–10. Changes in umbilical vein blood PO_2 during progressively increasing maternal blood PO_2 in the sheep. Note that when the maternal blood PO_2 was raised to about 300 mm Hg by ventilating the maternal lungs with 100 percent oxygen (black dots), umbilical vein blood PO_2 remained below 60 mm Hg. This illustrates the boundary imposed on fetal oxygenation. Only when maternal blood PO_2 was increased by hyperbaric oxygenation (open circles) did the fetal blood PO_2 increase to high levels. (From Assali, 1974.)

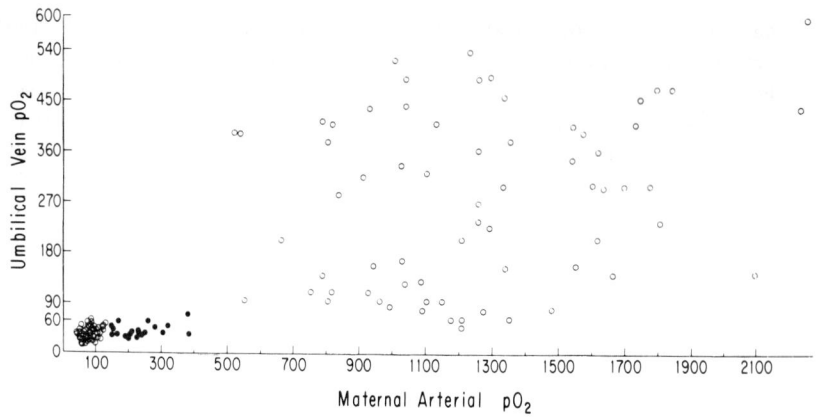

fetal blood, as compiled by Longo (1987), are presented in Table 7–2. Because of the continuous passage of oxygen from the maternal blood in the intervillous space to the fetus, the oxygen saturation of this blood resembles that in the maternal capillaries; namely, it is somewhat less than that of the mother's arterial blood. The average oxygen saturation of intervillous space blood is estimated to be 65 to 75 percent, with a partial pressure (PO_2) of about 30 to 35 mm Hg. The oxygen saturation of umbilical vein blood is similar, but with an oxygen partial pressure somewhat lower.

Despite the relatively low PO_2, the fetus normally does not suffer from lack of oxygen. The human fetus probably behaves like the lamb fetus, and therefore has a cardiac output considerably greater per unit of body weight than does the adult. The high cardiac output and, late in pregnancy, the increased oxygen-carrying capacity of fetal blood (attributable to fetal hemoglobin), and a higher hemoglobin concentration than in adults, compensate effectively for the low oxygen tension. Both of these mechanisms are considered further in this chapter under "Fetal Circulation" and "Fetal Blood." Additional evidence that the fetus normally does not experience lack of oxygen is provided by measurements of the

lactic acid content of fetal blood, which is only slightly higher than that of the mother.

In general, the transfer of carbon dioxide from the fetus to the mother is accomplished by diffusion, the placenta being highly permeable to carbon dioxide, which traverses the chorionic villus more rapidly than does oxygen. Near term, the partial pressure of carbon dioxide in the umbilical arteries is estimated to average about 48 mm Hg, or about 5 mm or so more than in the maternal blood in the intervillous space. Fetal blood has somewhat less affinity for carbon dioxide than does the blood of the mother, thereby favoring the transfer of carbon dioxide from the fetus to the mother. Also, mild hyperventilation by the pregnant woman results in a fall in PCO_2 favoring a transfer of CO_2 from the fetal compartment into maternal blood.

Selective Transfer and Facilitated Diffusion. Although diffusion is an important method of placental transfer, the trophoblasts and the chorionic villus unit exhibit enormous selectivity in transfer, maintaining different concentrations of a variety of metabolites on the two sides of the villus.

The concentrations of a number of substances, which are not synthesized by the fetus, are several times higher in fetal than in maternal blood. Ascorbic acid is a good example of this phenomenon. This relatively low molecular weight substance resembles the pentose and hexose sugars and might be expected to traverse the placenta by simple diffusion. The concentration of ascorbic acid, however, is two to four times higher in fetal plasma than in maternal plasma (Morriss and Boyd, 1988). The unidirectional transfer of iron across the placenta provides another example of the unique capabilities of the human placenta for transport. Typically, iron is present in the plasma at a lower concentration in the pregnant women than in her fetus; and at the same time, the iron-binding capacity of the plasma is much greater in the pregnant woman than in the fetus. Nonetheless, iron is transported actively from maternal to fetal

TABLE 7–2. NORMAL VALUES FOR OXYGEN, CARBON DIOXIDE, AND pH IN HUMAN MATERNAL AND FETAL BLOOD

	Uterine		Umbilical	
	Artery	*Vein*	*Vein*	*Artery*
PO_2 (mm Hg)	95	40	27	15
O_2Hb (percent saturation)	98	76	68	30
O_2 content (mL/dL)	15.8	12.2	14.5	6.4
Hemoglobin (g/dL)	12.0	12.0	16.0	16.0
O_2 capacity (mL O_2/dL)	16.1	16.1	21.4	21.4
PCO_2 (mm Hg)	32	40	43	48
CO_2 content (mM/L)	19.6	21.8	25.2	26.3
HCO_3 (mM/L)	18.8	20.7	24.0	25.0
pH	7.40	7.34	7.38	7.35

From Longo (1987).

plasma; and in the human fetus, the amount transferred appears to be independent of maternal iron status.

Fetal infections caused by viruses, bacteria, and protozoa are occasionally encountered (Chap. 44). Many viruses, including those responsible for rubella, chickenpox, measles, mumps, smallpox, vaccinia, poliomyelitis, cytomegalic inclusion disease, coxsackie virus disease, and western equine encephalitis, may cross the placenta and infect the fetus. *Treponema pallidum, Toxoplasma, Plasmodium* species, and *Mycobacterium tuberculosis* may also produce fetal infection. With protozoal and bacterial, but not necessarily viral, infections, there is almost always histological evidence of involvement of the placenta.

Rarely, malignant cells arising in neoplasias in the pregnant woman can be transferred to the placenta, fetus, or both. According to Read and Platzer (1981), approximately 50 percent of these are malignant melanomas or else are hematopoietic in origin (see Chap. 44).

Nutrition of the Fetus

During the first 2 months of pregnancy, the embryo consists almost entirely of water; in later months, relatively more solids are added. The amounts of water, fat, nitrogen, and certain minerals in the fetus at successive weeks of pregnancy are given in Table 7–3. Because of the small amount of yolk in the human ovum, growth of the fetus from the very early stage of development depends on nutrients obtained from the mother. During the first few days after implantation, the nutrition of the blastocyst arises directly from the interstitial fluid of the endometrium and from the surrounding maternal tissue. Within the next week, the forerunners of the intervillous space are formed; in the beginning, there are simply lacunae filled with maternal blood. During the third week after fertilization, fetal blood vessels appear in the chorionic villi. During the fourth week after ovulation, a cardiovascular system has formed, and thereby a true circulation, both within the embryo and between the embryo and the chorionic villi.

Ultimately, the maternal diet is the source of the nutrients supplied to the fetus; but ingested foodstuff is translated into storage forms that are then made available continuously, in an orderly way, to meet the demands for energy, tissue repair, and new growth, including those related to pregnancy. Three major storage depots—the liver, muscle, and adipose tissue—and the storage hormone insulin, are intimately involved in the metabolism of the nutrients absorbed from the maternal gut. Insulin is released from the maternal islands of Langerhans in response to various materials liberated from food during digestion and absorption. The secretion of insulin is sustained by rising levels of blood glucose and amino acids. The net effect is to store glucose as glycogen primarily in the liver and muscle, to retain some amino acids as protein, and to store the excess as fat. This storage of maternal fat peaks in the second trimester, and then declines as fetal demands increase in late pregnancy (Pipe and colleagues, 1979).

During the fasting state, glucose is released from glycogen, but glycogen stores in the mother are not large and these cannot provide an adequate amount of glucose to meet the requirements of the mother and fetus for energy and growth. The cleavage of triacylglycerols, stored in adipose tissue, however, provides the mother with energy in the form of free fatty acids. The process of lipolysis is activated, directly or indirectly, by a number of hormones, including glucagon, norepinephrine, human placental lactogen (hPL), glucocorticosteroids, and thyroxine.

Glucose. The transfer of D-glucose across the placenta is accomplished by a carrier-mediated, stereospecific, nonconcentrating process that can be saturated—*facilitated diffusion.* Transporter proteins for D-glucose have been isolated from the plasma membrane of the

TABLE 7–3. TOTAL AMOUNTS OF FAT, NITROGEN, AND MINERALS IN THE BODY OF THE DEVELOPING FETUS

Body Weight (g)	Approx. Fetal Age (wk)	Water (g)	Fat (g)	N (g)	Ca (g)	P (g)	Mg (g)	Na (mEq)	K (mEq)	Cl (mEq)	Fe (mg)	Cu (mg)	Zn (mg)
30	13	27	0.2	0.4	0.09	0.09	0.003	3.6	1.4	2.4	—	—	—
100	15	89	0.5	1.0	0.3	0.2	0.01	9	2.6	7	5.1	—	—
200	17	177	1.0	2.8	0.7	0.6	0.03	20	7.9	14	10	0.7	2.6
500	23	440	3.0	7.0	2.2	1.5	0.10	49	22	33	28	2.4	9.4
1000	26	860	10	14	6.0	3.4	0.22	90	41	66	64	3.5	16
1500	31	1270	35	25	10	5.6	0.35	125	60	96	100	5.6	25
2000	33	1620	100	37	15	8.2	0.46	160	84	120	160	8.0	35
2500	35	1940	185	49	20	11	0.58	200	110	130	220	10	43
3000	38	2180	360	55	25	14	0.70	240	130	150	260	12	50
3500	40	2400	560	62	30	17	0.78	280	150	160	280	14	53

From Widdowson (1968).

microvilli of human trophoblasts (Morriss and Boyd, 1988).

Because glucose is a major nutrient for growth and energy in the fetus, it would seem advantageous during pregnancy for the operational mechanisms to be those that minimize glucose utilization by the mother and thereby make the limited maternal supply available to the fetus. One metabolic action of hPL, a hormone normally present in abundance in the mother but not the fetus, is believed to be the blocking of the peripheral uptake and utilization of glucose by maternal tissues while promoting the mobilization and utilization of free fatty acids. HPL does not appear to be absolutely required for a normal pregnancy outcome (Chap. 6). The fetus is not exposed to a constant supply of glucose; even in normal pregnant women, the plasma levels may vary by up to 75 percent. Whereas the fetus is quite dependent on the mother for nutrition, the fetus is not a passive parasite; it actively participates in providing for its own nutrition. At midpregnancy, fetal glucose concentration is independent of and may exceed maternal levels (Bozzetti and colleagues, 1988).

Lactate. Lactate also is transported across the placenta by facilitated diffusion. By way of co-transport with hydrogen ions, lactate is probably transported as lactic acid. Among mammalian neonates, the newborn human infant has a large proportion of fat, 16 percent of body weight on average (Kimura, 1991). This is indicative that late in pregnancy, a greater part of substrate transferred to the human fetus is stored as fat.

Free Fatty Acids and Triglycerides. Neutral fat (triacylglycerols) does not cross the placenta, but glycerol does. The extent of transport of free fatty acids is not known, although the transfer of palmitic acid from the maternal to the fetal side of the human placenta perfused in vitro has been demonstrated (Szabo and associates, 1969). Lipoprotein lipase is present on the maternal but not on the fetal surface of the placenta. This arrangement should favor hydrolysis of triacylglycerols in the maternal intervillous space while preserving these neutral lipids in the fetal blood.

In Chapter 6, we pointed to the likelihood that the placental uptake and use of low-density lipoprotein (LDL) by the placenta may account for an additional mechanism for the assimilation of essential fatty acids and essential amino acids. The LDL particle of maternal plasma becomes bound to specific LDL receptors in the coated-pit region of the microvilli on the maternal-facing side of the trophoblasts. The LDL particle is taken up by a process of endocytosis. The apoprotein and cholesterol esters of LDL are hydrolyzed by lysosomal enzymes in trophoblasts to give (1) cholesterol for progesterone synthesis; (2) free amino acids (including essential amino acids); and (3) an essential fatty acid, linoleic acid, from the hydrolysis of the cholesterol es-

ters of LDL. Indeed, the concentration of arachidonic acid in fetal plasma is greater than that in maternal plasma; most of the arachidonic acid arises from linoleic acid assimilated from the diet.

Amino Acids. In addition to the use of LDL, the placenta is known to concentrate a large number of amino acids intracellularly (Lemons, 1979). Neutral amino acids from maternal plasma are taken up by trophoblasts by at least three specific processes. Presumably, the amino acids, concentrated in trophoblasts, are thence transferred to the fetal side by diffusion.

Proteins and Other Large Molecules. Generally, the transfer of larger proteins across the placenta is very limited. There are important exceptions. A major one is immunoglobulin G (IgG). In the human, IgG crosses the placenta in major amounts.

Near term, IgG is present in approximately the same concentrations in cord and maternal sera, but IgA and IgM are considerably lower in cord serum. Although IgA and IgM of maternal origin are effectively excluded from the fetus, IgG crosses the placenta with considerable efficiency (Gitlin and colleagues, 1972). Fc receptors are present on trophoblasts; and the transport of IgG is accomplished by way of these receptors through a classic process of endocytosis. *Increased amounts of IgM are found in the fetus only after the fetal immune system has been provoked into antibody response by an infection in the fetus.*

Ions and Trace Metals. Iodide transport across the placenta is clearly carrier mediated by an active process; indeed the placenta concentrates iodide. Iron is accumulated in placenta by an active, energy-requiring process. The concentrations of zinc in the fetal plasma are also greater than those in maternal plasma.

Calcium. Calcium and phosphorus are also actively transported across the placenta from mother to fetus. A calcium-binding protein is present in placenta. Parathyroid hormone-related protein (PTHrP), as the name implies, acts as does PTH in many systems, including the activation of adenylate cyclase and the movement of Ca^{2+}. The history and special proposed actions of PTH-rP in endometrium are described in Chapter 4. The production of PTH-rP in placenta is addressed in Chapter 6 and the potential role of this agent in myometrium is cited in Chapter 12. PTH-rP is not produced in normal adult parathyroid, but is produced in the fetal parathyroid and in the placenta and other fetal tissues. Indeed, PTH is not demonstrable in fetal plasma, but PTH-rP is found in fetal blood. Some investigators refer to PTH-rP as the fetal parathormone (Abbas and associates, 1990). An interesting feature of PTH-rP is that the intact (141 amino acid) molecule stimulates Ca^{2+} transport across the sheep placenta. Another interesting feature is that a

Ca^{2+}-sensing receptor is present in trophoblast, as in parathyroid glands (Juhlin and colleagues, 1990). And unlike any other cell studied, the extracellular concentration of Ca^{2+} modulates the formation of PTH-rP in cytotrophoblasts (Hellman and co-workers, 1992).

Vitamins

Vitamin A (Retinol). The concentration of vitamin A is greater in fetal than in maternal plasma. Vitamin A in fetal plasma is bound to retinol-binding protein and to prealbumin.

Vitamin C (Ascorbic Acid). The transport of vitamin C across the placenta from mother to fetus is accomplished by an energy-dependent carrier-mediated process.

Vitamin D (Cholecalciferol). The levels of the principal vitamin D metabolites, including 1,25-dihydroxycholecalciferol, are greater in maternal plasma than are those in fetal plasma. The 1α-hydroxylation of 25-hydroxyvitamin D_3 is known to take place in placenta and in decidua.

Maternal Nutrition. For obvious reasons, a great deal of investigative effort continues to be focused on maternal nutrition and its effect on the growth and development of the fetus. Fetal size is not just a function of fetal age. For example, in some forms of maternal diabetes mellitus (i.e., those without significant maternal vascular disease), the fetus may be larger than normal; but if severe maternal vascular disease further complicates the diabetes, the fetus may be appreciably smaller than normal (see Chap. 38). Fetal macrosomia usually complicates the pregnancy when maternal diabetes is not well controlled.

Physiology of the Fetus

The fetus swallows amnionic fluid; and late in gestation, large volumes are ingested. Nonetheless, it is unlikely that this represents a major source of nutrients to the fetus. On the other hand, there may be an important function of amnionic fluid in fetal development other than physical protection of the fetus. In fetal conditions in which amnionic fluid is not taken into the lungs by fetal thoracic excursions (fetal breathing), lung hypoplasia invariably results. Heretofore, this phenomenon was attributed to failure of lung expansion by amnionic fluid, and no doubt this is a partial explanation. But on the other hand, we also know that epidermal growth factor (EGF)-like growth factors may serve an important role in fetal lung development. Thus, the ingestion of amnionic fluid into the lung and gastrointestinal tract of the fetus may promote growth and differentiation by way of growth factors in amnionic fluid.

Fetal Circulation. Because almost all nutrient materials required for fetal growth and maturation are delivered to the fetus from the placenta by the umbilical vein, the fetal circulation must differ fundamentally from that of the adult (Fig. 7–11). The single umbilical vein in the umbilical cord carries oxygenated, nutrient-bearing blood from the placenta to the fetus. The *umbilical vein* enters the fetus through the umbilical ring and ascends along the anterior abdominal wall toward the liver. The vein then divides into the portal sinus and the ductus venosus, the former carrying blood to the hepatic veins primarily on the left side of the liver, and the latter or major "branch" of the umbilical vein traversing the liver to enter directly the *inferior vena cava.* The blood flowing to the fetal heart from the inferior vena cava, therefore, consists of an admixture of "arterial-like" blood that passes through the ductus venosus and less well-oxygenated blood that collects from most of the veins below the level of the diaphragm. As a consequence, the oxygen content of blood delivered to the heart from the inferior vena cava is less than that which leaves the placenta, but it is greater than that from the superior vena cava.

The *foramen ovale* opens directly off the inferior vena cava, so that blood from the inferior vena cava is, for the most part, immediately deflected by the *crista dividens* through the foramen ovale into the left atrium (Dawes, 1962). Little or none of the less-well oxygenated blood from the *superior vena cava* normally passes through the foramen ovale. The preferential flow of blood from the inferior vena cava through the foramen ovale to the left atrium bypasses the right ventricle and pulmonary circulation and permits delivery to the left ventricle of more highly oxygenated blood than if complete admixture had occurred in the right atrium. The more highly oxygenated blood that passes through the foramen ovale and is ejected from the left ventricle perfuses two vital organs, the heart and the brain. The blood that is typically venous in character, coming from the superior vena cava and ejected from the right ventricle into the pulmonary trunk, is for the most part shunted through the *ductus arteriosus* into the descending aorta.

The lamb fetus has been studied intensively by several groups of investigators who take the view that the circulatory function of the mature lamb fetus is similar in many respects to that of the mature human fetus. Before birth, in human and in sheep, both ventricles of the fetal heart, as the consequence of the shunts just described, work in parallel rather than in series. Attempts to measure cardiac output in the lamb fetus have yielded somewhat variable results. Assali and associates (1968, 1974) found a mean value of about 225 mL/kg per minute, but with considerable individual variation; Paton and co-workers (1973) found very similar values in baboon fetuses. Such a high fetal cardiac output, which per unit of weight is

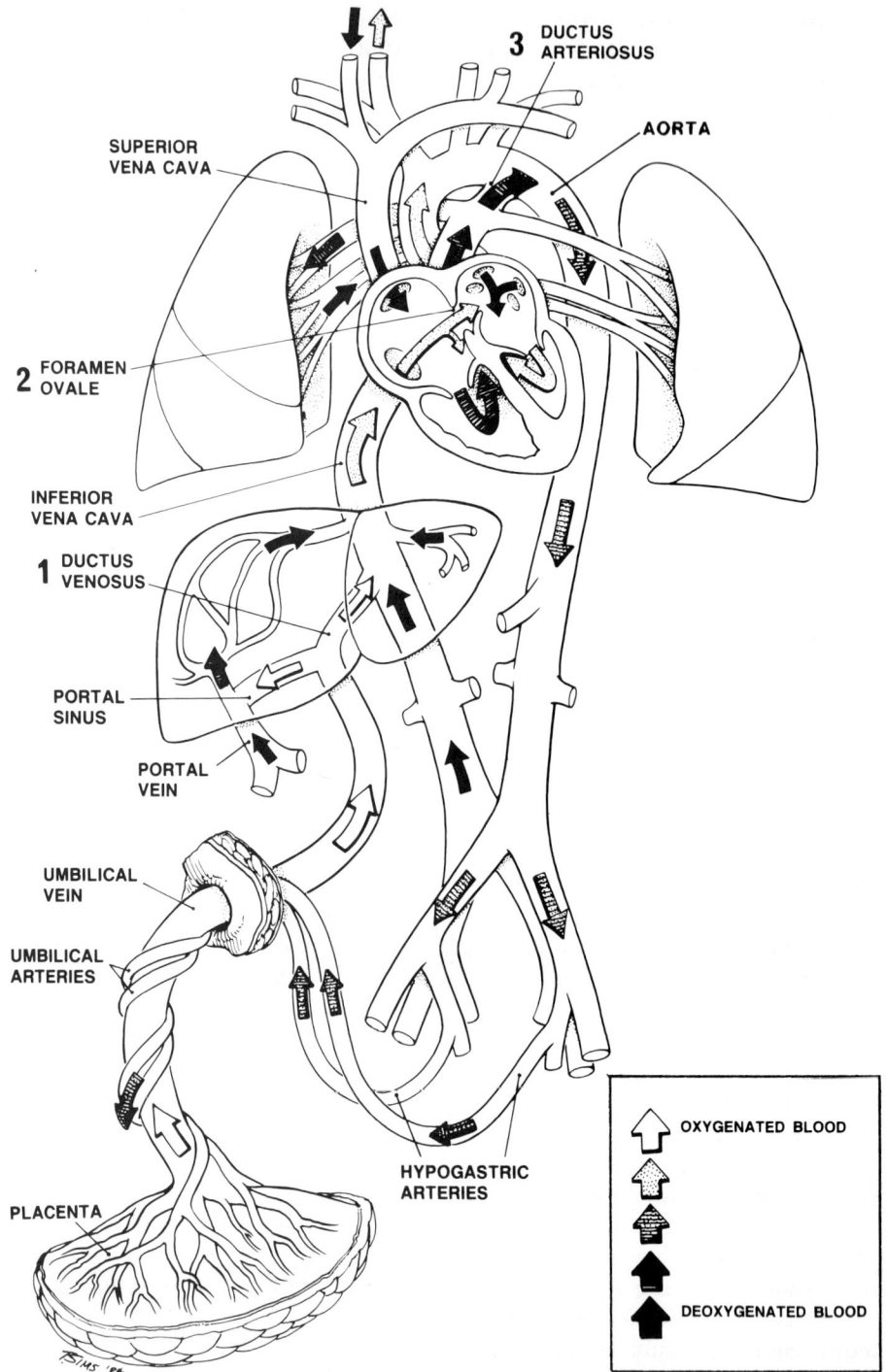

Fig. 7–11. The intricate nature of the fetal circulation is evident. The degree of oxygenation of blood in various vessels differs appreciably from that in the postnatal state as the consequence of oxygenation being provided by the placenta rather than the lungs and the presence of three major vascular shunts: **1.** Ductus venosus. **2.** Foramen ovale. **3.** Ductus arteriosus.

about three times that of an adult at rest, would serve to compensate for the low oxygen content of fetal blood. The high cardiac output is accomplished, in part, by the fast heart rate of the fetus and a low systemic (peripheral) resistance.

Before birth and expansion of the lungs, the high pulmonary vascular resistance accounts for the high pressure and the low blood flow in the fetal pulmo-

nary circuit. At the same time, resistance to flow through the ductus arteriosus and the umbilicoplacental circulation is low, probably accounting for the overall low fetal systemic vascular resistance. It is estimated that in the fetal lamb, about one half the combined output of the two ventricles goes to the placenta. Injecting isotopically labeled plastic microspheres into the fetal lamb circulation at various sites, the distribution of cardiac output during the last third of gestation was determined to be approximately as follows: placenta, 40 percent; carcass, 35 percent; brain, 5 percent; heart, 5 percent; gastrointestinal tract, 5 percent; lungs, 4 percent; kidneys, 2 percent; spleen, 2 percent; and liver (hepatic artery only), 2 percent (Rudolph and Heymann, 1968).

Blood is returned to the placenta through the two *hypogastric arteries,* which distally become the *umbilical arteries.*

After birth, the umbilical vessels, ductus arteriosus, foramen ovale, and ductus venosus normally constrict or collapse, and consequently the hemodynamics of the fetal circulation undergo pronounced changes. Clamping of the umbilical cord and expansion of the fetal lungs, either through spontaneous breathing or artificial respiration, promptly induce a variety of hemodynamic changes in sheep (Assali, 1974; Assali and associates, 1968). The systemic arterial pressure initially falls slightly, apparently the result of the reversal in the direction of blood flow in the ductus arteriosus, but it soon recovers and then rises above the control value. These investigators concluded that several factors served to regulate the flow of blood through the ductus arteriosus, including the difference in pressure between the pulmonary artery and aorta, and especially the oxygen tension of the blood passing through the ductus arteriosus. They were able to influence flow through the ductus arteriosus by altering the Po_2 of the blood. When the lungs were ventilated with oxygen and the Po_2 rose above 55 mm Hg, ductus flow dropped, but ventilation with nitrogen, initially at least, returned the ductus flow to the original pattern. The ductus is functionally closed by 10 to 96 hours after birth, and anatomically closed by 2 to 3 weeks (Clymann and Heymann, 1981).

The effects from variations in oxygen tension of blood flowing through the ductus arteriosus are believed to be mediated through the actions of prostaglandins on the ductus. Prostaglandin E_2 dilates the constricted ductus arteriosus and is intimately involved in maintaining normal patency in utero. Inhibitors of prostaglandin synthase, when given to the mother, may lead to premature closure of the ductus arteriosus (see Chap. 38), but can be used pharmacologically to close a symptomatic patent ductus arteriosus postnatally (Brash and associates, 1981).

The more distal portions of the hypogastric arteries, which course from the level of the bladder along the abdominal wall to the umbilical ring and into the cord as the umbilical arteries, undergo atrophy and obliteration within 3 to 4 days after birth, to become the *umbilical ligaments;* intra-abdominal remnants of the umbilical vein form the *ligamentum teres.* The ductus venosus constricts and its lumen closes, resulting in the formation of the *ligamentum venosum.*

Fetal Blood

Hematopoiesis. Hematopoiesis, in the very early embryo, is demonstrable first in the yolk sac. The next major site of erythropoiesis is the liver and finally the bone marrow. The contributions made by each site throughout the growth and development of the embryo and fetus are graphically demonstrated in Figure 7–12.

The first erythrocytes formed in the fetus are nucleated and macrocytic, but as fetal development progresses, more and more of the circulating erythrocytes are nonnucleated. As the fetus grows, not only does the volume of blood in the common circulation of the fetus and placenta increase, but the hemoglobin concentration rises as well. The hemoglobin of fetal blood rises to the adult male level of about 15 g/dL at midpregnancy, and at term it is somewhat higher, about 18 g/dL. Fetal blood at or near term is characterized, therefore, by a hemoglobin concentration that is high by maternal standards (Walker and Turnbull, 1953).

The reticulocyte count falls from a very high level in the very young fetus to about 5 percent at term. Pearson (1966), using a variety of techniques, found the life span of erythrocytes from more mature fetuses to be approximately two thirds that of erythrocytes of normal adults; but erythrocytes of less mature fetuses have an even shorter life span. This is related undoubtedly to their large volume, and these data are supportive of the concept that fetal erythrocytes are "stress erythrocytes." The erythrocytes of the fetus differ structurally and metabolically from those of the adult. Fetal erythrocytes are more deformable, which serves to offset their higher viscosity, and they contain several enzymes that have appreciably different activities (Smith and co-workers, 1981).

Erythropoiesis. The fetus is capable of making erythropoietin in increased amounts when severely anemic,

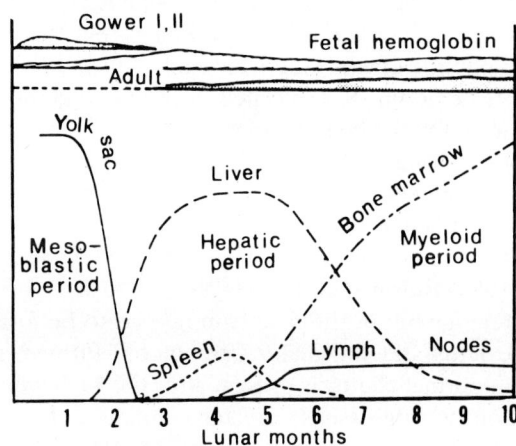

Fig. 7–12. Sites of hematopoiesis and kinds of hemoglobin synthesized at various stages of fetal development. (From Brown, 1968.)

and of excreting it into the amnionic fluid (Finne, 1966; Zivny and co-workers, 1982). Evidence of a physiological role for erythropoietin in fetal erythropoiesis has been provided by Zanjani and co-workers (1974). The injection of antierythropoietin into the sheep fetoplacental circulation was followed by a decrease in reticulocytes and decreased incorporation of radioiron into erythrocytes; moreover, induction of anemia in the fetus resulted in elevated levels of erythropoietin-like material. In utero, the fetal liver, rather than the kidney, appears to be an important source of erythropoietin. After birth, erythropoietin normally may not be detectable for up to 3 months.

Fetal Blood Volume. Precise measurements of the volume of blood contained in the human fetoplacental circulation are lacking. Usher and associates (1963), however, have measured the volume of blood of term normal infants very soon after birth and found an average of 78 mL/kg when immediate cord-clamping was conducted. Gruenwald (1967) found the volume of blood of fetal origin contained in the placenta after prompt cord-clamping to average 45 mL per kg of fetus. Thus, fetoplacental blood volume at term is approximately 125 mL per kg of fetus. Pritchard and co-workers (unpublished observations) measured the volumes of blood in infants with erythroblastosis fetalis as well as their placentas and cords immediately after delivery. The "fetoplacental" blood volume in these circumstances was very close to 120 mL per kg of infant weight.

Fetal Hemoglobin. In the embryo and fetus, the globin moiety of much of the hemoglobin differs from that of the normal adult. In the embryo, three major forms of hemoglobin may be found. The most primitive forms are Gower-1 and Gower-2 (Pearson, 1966). The third form is hemoglobin Portland. The globin moiety of Gower-1 consists of two ξ-peptide chains and two γ-chains per molecule of protein, whereas in Gower-2 there are two α- and two ε-chains. All normal hemoglobins elaborated after Gower-1 contain a pair of α-chains, but the other pair of peptide chains differs for each kind of hemoglobin. Hemoglobin F (so-called fetal hemoglobin or alkaline-resistant hemoglobin) contains a pair of α-peptide chains and a pair of γ-chains per molecule of hemoglobin. Actually, two varieties of γ-chains have been identified in hemoglobin F, the ratios changing steadily as the fetus and infant mature (Fadel and Abraham, 1981; Huisman and colleagues, 1970).

Hemoglobin A, the final hemoglobin to be formed by the fetus and the major hemoglobin formed after birth in normal adults, is present after the 11th week of gestation in progressively greater amounts as the fetus matures (Pataryas and Stamatoyannopoulos, 1972).

Evidence has been presented that the switch from hemoglobin F to hemoglobin A that begins at 32 to 34 weeks' gestation is associated with methylation of the γ-globin genes. In newborns of women with diabetes mellitus, there is commonly a persistence of the hemoglobin F and there is hypomethylation of the γ-globin genes (Perrine and associates, 1988). The globin of hemoglobin A is made up of a pair of α-chains and a pair of β-chains. Hemoglobin A_2, the globin of which contains a pair of α-chains and a pair of δ-chains, is present in very small concentrations in the mature fetus but increases after birth. Thus, as growth proceeds, there is a shift not only in the amounts but also in the kinds of globin synthesized by the embryo and fetus.

As illustrated in Figure 7–13, at any given oxygen tension and at identical pH, fetal erythrocytes that contain mostly hemoglobin F bind more oxygen than do erythrocytes that contain nearly all hemoglobin A. The major reason for this difference is that hemoglobin A binds 2,3-diphosphoglycerate more avidly than does hemoglobin F (De Verdier and Garby, 1969), and 2,3-diphosphoglycerate so bound lowers the affinity of the hemoglobin molecule for oxygen. The increased oxygen affinity of the fetal erythrocyte results from a lower concentration of 2,3-diphosphoglycerate compared with that of the maternal erythrocyte, in which the 2,3-diphosphoglycerate level is increased compared with the nonpregnant state. Gilbert and associates (1983) found that, at higher temperatures, the affinity of fetal blood for oxygen decreases. They concluded that increases in fetal temperature as a consequence of ma-

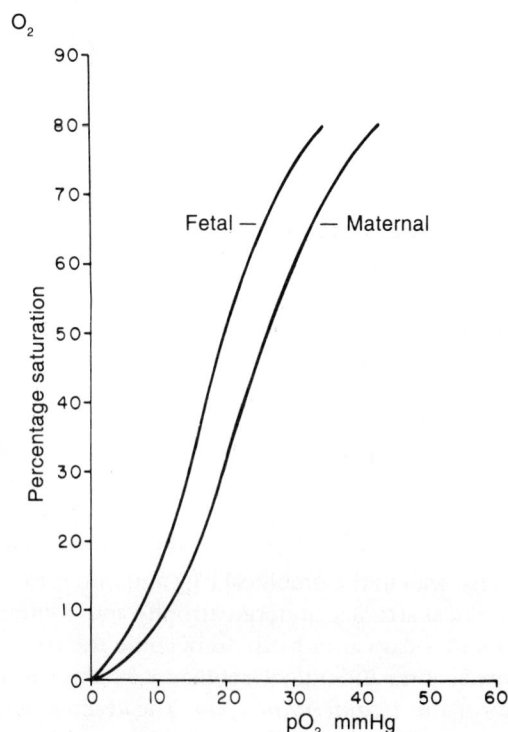

Fig. 7–13. Oxygen dissociation curves of fetal and maternal human bloods prepared at pH 7.40. (Courtesy of Dr. Andre Hellergers.)

ternal hyperthermia could significantly compound fetal hypoxia.

Because fetal erythrocytes that are formed late in pregnancy contain less hemoglobin F and more hemoglobin A than do the cells formed earlier, the content of hemoglobin F of the fetal erythrocytes falls somewhat during the latter weeks of pregnancy. At term, about three fourths of the total hemoglobin normally is hemoglobin F. During the first 6 to 12 months of life, the proportion of hemoglobin F continues to decrease, eventually to reach the low level found in erythrocytes of normal adults (Schulman and Smith, 1953).

Coagulation Factors in the Fetus. The concentrations of several coagulation factors at birth are appreciably below the levels that develop within a few weeks after birth (Sell and Corrigan, 1973). The factors that are low in cord blood are II, VII, IX, X, XI, XII, XIII, and fibrinogen. Without prophylactic vitamin K, vitamin K-dependent coagulation factors usually decrease even further during the first few days after birth, especially in breast-fed infants, and may lead to hemorrhage in the newborn infant. Platelet counts in cord blood are in the normal range for nonpregnant adults, while fibrinogen levels are somewhat less than in nonpregnant adults. For reasons unknown, the time for conversion of fibrinogen in plasma to fibrin clot when thrombin is added (thrombin time) is somewhat prolonged compared with that of older children and adults. The measurement of factor VIII coagulant activity in the cord is of value in accurately making or excluding the diagnosis of hemophilia in male infants (Kasper and colleagues, 1964). Functional factor XIII (fibrin-stabilizing factor) levels in plasma are significantly reduced compared with those in normal adults (Henriksson and co-workers, 1974), but the clinical diagnosis of factor XIII deficiency is usually made by observing a continuous "ooze" from the umbilical stump. Nielsen (1969) described the finding of low levels of plasminogen and somewhat increased fibrinolytic activity in cord plasma compared with that in maternal plasma. This may be due to a structurally and functionally different fetal plasminogen (Estelles and co-workers, 1980).

Fetal Plasma Proteins. The mean total plasma protein and plasma albumin concentrations in maternal and cord blood are similar. For example, Foley and associates (1978) identified maternal and cord total plasma proteins to average 6.5 and 5.9 g/dL, respectively, with maternal and cord plasma albumin levels of 3.6 and 3.7 g/dL, respectively.

Immunocompetence of the Fetus. In the absence of a direct antigenic stimulus in the fetus, such as infection, the immunoglobulins in the fetus consist almost totally of immune globulin G (IgG) synthesized by the mother

and subsequently transferred across the placenta by receptor-mediated processes in trophoblast, as described later in this chapter. Therefore, the antibodies in the fetus and the newborn infant most often reflect the immunological experiences of the mother.

Immunoglobulin G. IgG transport from mother to fetus begins at about 16 weeks' gestation and increases as gestation proceeds. But the bulk of IgG is acquired by the fetus (from the mother) during the last 4 weeks of pregnancy (Gitlin, 1971). Accordingly, preterm infants are endowed relatively poorly with maternal antibodies. Newborns begin to produce IgG, but slowly; adult values are not attained until 3 years of age.

Immunoglobulin M. IgM is not transported from mother to fetus; therefore, any IgM in the fetus or newborn is that which was produced in the fetus. Very little IgM is produced by normal, healthy fetuses; that which is produced may include antibody to maternal T lymphocytes (Hayward, 1983). Increased levels of IgM are found in newborns with congenital infection (rubella, cytomegalovirus, toxoplasmosis). Adult levels of IgM are normally attained by 9 months of age.

Lymphocytes. The immune system begins to mature early in fetal life. B lymphocytes appear in liver by 9 weeks and are present in blood and spleen by 12 weeks' gestation. T lymphocytes begin to leave the thymus at about 14 weeks (Hayward, 1983).

Monocytes. Monocytes of newborns are able to process and present antigen when tested with maternal antigen-specific T cells.

Ontogeny of the Immune Response. The transfer of some IgG antibodies from mother to fetus is harmful rather than protective to the fetus. The classic clinical example of antibodies of maternal origin that are dangerous to the fetus is hemolytic disease of the fetus and newborn resulting from D-antigen isoimmunization. In this disease, maternal antibody to fetal erythrocyte antigen crosses the placenta to destroy the fetal erythrocytes.

Infections in utero have provided an opportunity to examine some of the mechanisms for immune response by the human fetus. The opinion that the fetus is immunologically incompetent is no longer tenable. Indeed, morphological evidence of immunological competence in the human fetus has been reported as early as 13 weeks' gestational age by Altshuler (1974), who described infection of the placenta and fetus by cytomegalovirus with characteristic severe inflammatory cell proliferation as well as virus inclusions. Moreover, synthesis of complement late in the first trimester by fetal organs has been demonstrated by Kohler (1973) and confirmed by Stabile and co-workers (1988). All components of human complement are produced at an early stage of fetal development. In cord blood at or near term, the average level for most components of complement are about one half the values for adults (Adinolfi, 1977).

The newborn responds poorly to immunization, and especially poorly to bacterial capsular polysaccharides. This immaturity of response may be due to (1) deficient response of newborn B cells to polyclonal activators or (2) lack of T cells that proliferate in response to specific stimuli (Hayward, 1983).

Differing from many animals, the human newborn infant does not acquire much in the way of passive immunity from the absorption of humoral antibodies ingested in the colostrum. Nevertheless, IgA ingested in colostrum may provide protection against enteric infections, because the antibody resists digestion and is effective on mucosal surfaces. The same is possibly true for IgA ingested with amnionic fluid before delivery.

In the adult, production of immune globulin M (IgM) in response to antigen is superseded in a week or so predominantly by production of IgG. In contrast, the IgM response is dominant in the fetus and remains so for weeks to months in the newborn. IgM serum levels in umbilical cord blood and identification of specific antibodies may be of aid in the diagnosis of intrauterine infection.

Nervous System and Sensory Organs

Synaptic function is sufficiently developed by the eighth week of gestation to demonstrate flexion of neck and trunk (Temiras and co-workers, 1968). If the fetus is removed from the uterus during the 10th week, spontaneous movements may be observed, although movements in utero are usually not felt by the mother until several weeks later. At 10 weeks, local stimuli may evoke squinting, opening the mouth, incomplete finger closure, and plantar flexion of the toes. Complete finger closure is achieved during the fourth lunar month. Swallowing and respiration are also evident at 14 to 16 weeks, but the ability to suck is not present until 24 weeks or even later (Lebenthal and Lee, 1983).

During the third trimester of pregnancy, integration of nervous and muscular function proceeds rapidly, so that the majority of fetuses delivered after the 32nd week of gestation survive.

By 28 weeks, the eye is sensitive to light, but perception of form and color is not complete until long after birth.

The internal, middle, and external components of the ear are well developed by midpregnancy. The fetus apparently hears some sounds in utero as early as the 24th to 26th week of gestation.

Taste buds are evident histologically in the third

lunar month; and by 28 weeks of gestation, the fetus is responsive to variations in the taste of ingested substances.

Digestive System

Gastrointestinal Tract

Development. By the 11th week of gestation, the small intestine undergoes peristalsis and is capable of transporting glucose actively (Koldovsky and colleagues, 1965). Gastrointestinal function is sufficiently developed at 16 weeks to allow the fetus to swallow amnionic fluid, absorb much of the water from it, and propel unabsorbed matter as far as the lower colon (Fig. 7–14). Hydrochloric acid and some adult digestive enzymes are present in very small amounts in the early fetus; therefore, in the premature infant, transient deficiencies of these enzymes are often present depending upon the gestational age of the infant when born (Lebenthal and Lee, 1983).

Fetal Swallowing. Fetal swallowing at various stages of pregnancy has been measured by introducing a small

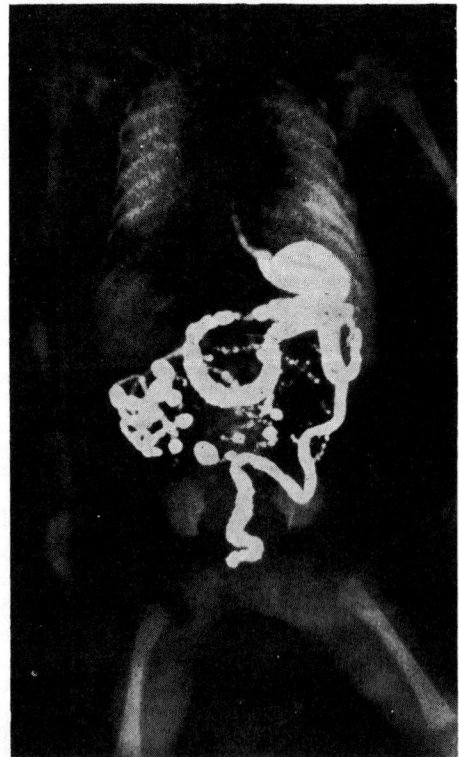

Fig. 7–14. X-ray of 115-g fetus in which Thorotrast is present in the lungs, esophagus, stomach, and entire intestinal tract following injection into the amnionic cavity 26 hours before delivery. This demonstrates not only intrauterine respiration of the fetus but also active swallowing of amnionic fluid. (From Davis and Potter, 1946.)

volume of maternal erythrocytes labeled with isotopic chromium into the amnionic sac and subsequently measuring the chromium that accumulated in the gastrointestinal tract either directly in fetuses that succumbed from immaturity after delivery or in the meconium and feces passed after birth by more mature fetuses (Pritchard, 1965, 1966). Term-size fetuses are believed to swallow relatively large volumes of amnionic fluid; in one study, the amount appeared to average nearly 450 mL per 24 hours. Gitlin and associates (1972) found that the rate of clearing of radiolabeled albumin from amnionic fluid, presumably by swallowing, was very similar to this value. It is likely, however, that the volumes of amnionic fluid swallowed directly by the fetus are less than what has been reported. Probably some of the label in the amnionic fluid was removed by inhalation; and the inspired radiolabeled material, in turn, was either absorbed across the lung or was propelled from the lung by ciliary movement into the pharynx from which it was swallowed.

Fetal swallowing appears to have little effect on the amnionic fluid volume early in pregnancy, because the volume swallowed is small compared with the total volume of amnionic fluid present. Late in pregnancy, however, the volume of amnionic fluid appears to be regulated substantially by fetal swallowing, for when swallowing is inhibited, hydramnios is common (see Chap. 44).

The act of swallowing may enhance growth and development of the alimentary canal and condition the fetus for alimentation after birth, although anencephalic fetuses, which usually swallow little amnionic fluid, have gastrointestinal tracts that appear normal. In late pregnancy, swallowing serves to remove some of the insoluble debris that is normally shed into the amnionic sac and sometimes abnormally excreted into it. The undigested portions of the swallowed debris can be identified in meconium collected at birth. The amnionic fluid swallowed probably contributes little to the caloric requirements of the fetus but may contribute essential nutrients. Gitlin (1974) demonstrated that late in pregnancy about 0.8 g of soluble protein, approximately one-half albumin, appears to be ingested by the fetus each day.

Meconium. *Meconium* consists not only of undigested debris from swallowed amnionic fluid, but to a larger degree, of various products of secretion, excretion, and desquamation by the gastrointestinal tract. The dark greenish-black appearance is caused by pigments, especially biliverdin. Hypoxia has been implicated in the evacuation of meconium from the large bowel into the amnionic fluid. This mechanism may result from the release of arginine vasopressin (AVP) from the fetal pituitary secondary to hypoxia. The AVP thus released stimulates the smooth muscle of the colon to contract,

resulting in intraamnionic defecation (DeVane and coworkers, 1982; Rosenfeld and Porter, 1985).

Small-bowel obstruction may lead to vomiting in utero (Shrand, 1972). Fetuses who suffer from congenital chloride diarrhea may have diarrhea in utero, which leads to hydramnios and preterm delivery (Holmberg and associates, 1977).

Liver and Pancreas

Liver. Hepatic function in the fetus differs, in several ways, from that of the adult. Many enzymes of the fetal liver are present in considerably reduced amounts compared with those in later life. The liver has a very limited capacity for converting free *bilirubin* to bilirubin diglucuronoside (see Chap. 44). The more immature the fetus, the more deficient the system for conjugating bilirubin.

Because the life span of the fetal erythrocyte is shorter than that of normal adult erythrocytes, relatively more bilirubin is produced. Only a small fraction of the bilirubin is conjugated by the fetal liver and excreted through the biliary tract into the intestine and ultimately oxidized to biliverdin. Bashore and associates (1969) demonstrated that radiolabeled unconjugated bilirubin is cleared promptly from the monkey fetal circulation by the placenta to the maternal liver where it is conjugated and excreted through maternal bile. The transfer of the unconjugated bilirubin across the placenta, however, is bidirectional. This observation is supported by the rarely encountered case of high levels of unconjugated bilirubin in maternal plasma. Conjugated bilirubin is not exchanged to any significant degree between mother and fetus.

Most of the cholesterol in the fetus is produced in fetal liver. Indeed, the large demand for LDL cholesterol by the fetal adrenal is met primarily by fetal hepatic synthesis.

Glycogen appears in low concentration in fetal liver during the second trimester of pregnancy, but near term there is a rapid and marked increase in normal fetuses to levels two to three times those in adult liver. After delivery, the glycogen content falls precipitously.

Pancreas. It is interesting to remember that the discovery of insulin by Banting and Best (1922) came from its extraction from the pancreas of the fetal calf. Insulin-containing granules can be identified in the human fetal pancreas by 9 to 10 weeks' gestation, and insulin in fetal plasma is detectable at 12 weeks (Adam and associates, 1969). The fetal pancreas responds to hyperglycemia by increasing plasma insulin (Obenshain and colleagues, 1970). Although the precise role of insulin of fetal origin is not clear, fetal growth must be determined to a considerable extent by the amounts of basic nutrients from the mother and, through the action of insulin, the anabolism of these materials by the fetus. Insulin levels are high in serum from newborn infants of diabetic mothers and in other large-for-gestational-age infants, but insulin levels are low in infants who are small for gestational age (Brinsmead and Liggins, 1979).

Glucagon has been identified in the fetal pancreas at 8 weeks' gestation. Induced hypoglycemia and infused alanine cause an increase in glucagon levels in the rhesus mother, yet similar stimuli to the fetus do not. Within 12 hours of birth, however, the infant is capable of responding (Chez and co-workers, 1975). Moreover, fetal alpha cells of the pancreas are capable of responding to L-dopa (Epstein and associates, 1977). Therefore, alpha cell nonresponsiveness to hypoglycemia and infused alanine is likely the consequence of failure of glucagon release rather than inadequate production of the hormone.

The exocrine function of the fetal pancreas appears to be limited but not necessarily absent. For example, radioiodine-labeled human albumin injected into the amnionic sac and swallowed by the fetus is absorbed from the fetal intestine. It is not absorbed as undigested protein, however, because the iodine is excreted promptly in the maternal urine when pretreatment with iodide has been provided to enhance the clearance of the digested radiolabeled iodine (Pritchard, 1965).

Urinary System

Two primitive urinary systems, the pronephros and the mesonephros, precede the development of the metanephros. Embryological failure of either of the first two may result in anomalous development of the definitive urinary system.

By the end of the first trimester, the nephrons have some capacity for excretion through glomerular filtration, although the kidneys are functionally immature throughout fetal life. The ability to concentrate and modify the pH of urine is quite limited even in the mature fetus. Fetal urine is hypotonic with respect to fetal plasma because of low concentrations of electrolytes. In the lamb fetus, and most likely in the human fetus, the fraction of the cardiac output perfusing the kidneys is low and renal vascular resistance is high, compared with these values later in life (Assali and colleagues, 1968; Rudolph and Heymann, 1968). In the lamb fetus, urine flow varies considerably in response to stress. Transient marked fetal polyuria postoperatively that apparently dissipates with recovery of fetal well-being has been noted by Gresham and co-workers (1972).

Urine is usually found in the bladder even in small fetuses. Wladimiroff and Campbell (1974) estimated urine production for human fetuses using an ultrasonic method to determine bladder volumes. They found a mean production of 10 mL/hr at 30 weeks, with an increase at term to 27 mL/hr, or 650 mL/day. Maternally administered diuretic (furosemide) increases fetal urine formation. Kurjak and associates (1981) confirmed the findings of Wladimiroff and Campbell and measured fetal glomerular filtration rates and fetal tubular water reabsorption. All three measurements were decreased in 33 percent of growth-retarded infants and in 17 percent of infants of diabetic mothers. All values were normal in anencephalic infants and in cases of polyhydramnios.

After obstruction of the urethra, the bladder, ureters, and renal pelves may become quite dilated; the bladder may become sufficiently distended that dystocia results. The kidneys in these circumstances seem capable of excreting urine until back pressure ultimately destroys the renal parenchyma. Kidneys are not essential for survival in utero, but are important in the control of the composition and volume of amnionic fluid (see Chap. 44). Abnormalities that cause chronic anuria are most often accompanied by oligohydramnios and hypoplasia of the lungs.

Amnionic Fluid

The fluid filling the amnionic sac serves several important functions. It provides a medium in which the fetus can readily move, cushions the fetus against possible injury, helps maintain an even temperature, and provides, when appropriately tested, useful information concerning the health and maturity of the fetus (see Chap. 41). If the presenting part of the fetus is not closely applied to the lower uterine segment during labor, the hydrostatic action of the amnionic fluid also may be important in dilating the cervix.

By the 12th day after fertilization of the ovum, a cleft enclosed by primitive amnion has formed adjacent to the embryonic plate. Rapid enlargement of the cleft and fusion of the surrounding amnion first with the body stalk, and later with the chorion, create the amnionic sac, which fills with an essentially colorless fluid. The amnionic fluid increases rapidly to an average volume of 50 mL at 12 weeks' gestation and 400 mL at midpregnancy; it reaches a maximum of about 1000 mL at 36 to 38 weeks' gestation. The volume then decreases as term approaches, and if the pregnancy is prolonged, amnionic fluid may become relatively scant (see Chap. 38). There are rather marked individual differences in amnionic fluid volume, however, as reported by Fuchs (1966). Similar data reported by Gillibrand (1969a) are shown in Figure 7–15. The physician performing amniocentesis for diagnostic purposes soon appreciates the considerable variability in the volume of amnionic fluid present at the same time in different pregnancies as well as at different times in the same pregnancy.

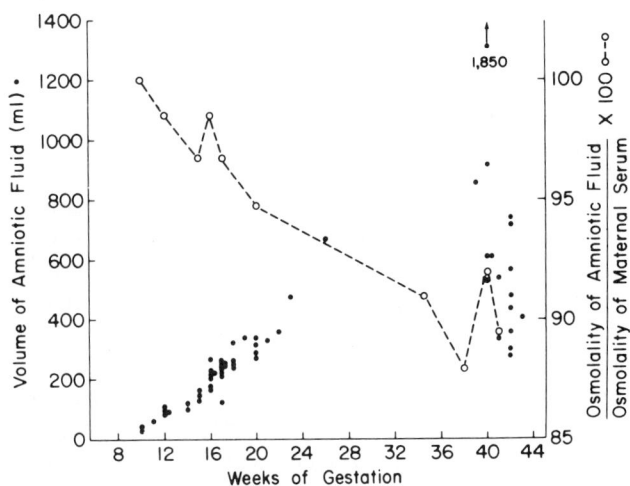

Fig. 7-15. Amnionic fluid volume (black dots) and osmolality (open circles). The first and second trimesters are characterized by a rather orderly increase in volume, but at term the volume is quite variable. The osmolality decreases in approximately linear fashion as pregnancy advances. (From Gillibrand, 1969a, 1969b.)

The composition and volume of amnionic fluid change as pregnancy advances. In the first half of pregnancy, the fluid is the same as the extracellular fluid of the fetus, and it is nearly devoid of particulate matter.

Ions and small molecules move rapidly into and out of amnionic fluid but at rates that are specific for each substance. In contradistinction to bulk movement of amnionic fluid, as with swallowing, this process simply involves molecular or ionic trade across a membrane without necessarily inducing changes in volume or concentration (Plentl, 1968).

There is no single mechanism that will account for all the variations in composition and volume of amnionic fluid that have been observed during the course of a normal pregnancy. One relatively simple explanation is that amnionic fluid in early pregnancy is a product primarily of the amnionic membrane covering the placenta and cord. It is likely that fluid also passes across the fetal skin at this time (Lind and colleagues, 1972). As pregnancy advances, the surface of the amnion expands and the volume of fluid increases, but from about the fourth month, the fetus is capable of modifying amnionic fluid composition and volume by urinating and swallowing progressively larger amounts of fluid. At the same time, movement of fluid into and out of the respiratory tract is likely to modify further the volume and composition of amnionic fluid.

As gestation advances, fetal urine makes an increasingly important contribution to the amnionic fluid. Fetal urine is quite hypotonic compared with maternal or fetal plasma, because of the lower electrolyte concentration in the urine, but it contains more urea, creatinine, and uric acid than does plasma. The net effect is

that the osmolality of fluid decreases with increasing length of gestation. These observations have been shown to exist in utero as early as the 24th week of pregnancy. Mandelbaum and Evans (1969) examined urine obtained inadvertently from the fetal bladder at the time of attempted transfusion and compared the concentrations of several of the constituents of the urine with those of amnionic fluid. Even at 24 weeks' gestation, the urea and creatinine concentrations were two to three times higher in the urine, whereas the concentrations of sodium, potassium, and chloride were only about one third to one fifth as great as those in the amnionic fluid. The admixture of sizable volumes of fetal urine with the amnionic fluid, therefore, would logically be expected to lower the osmolality, as shown in Figure 7–15, and at the same time to raise the concentration of urea, creatinine, and uric acid. Indeed, late in pregnancy, amnionic fluid normally differs from plasma in precisely these ways.

As pregnancy progresses, glycerophospholipids, primarily from the lung, accumulate in the fluid, and variable amounts of particulate matter in the form of desquamated fetal cells, lanugo and scalp hair, and vernix caseosa are shed into the fluid. The concentrations of various solutes also change significantly, and as a consequence the osmolality decreases on the average about 20 to 30 mOsm, or about 10 percent (Fig. 7–15).

The fetus swallows amnionic fluid during much of pregnancy. Often, but not always, a great excess of amnionic fluid (hydramnios) develops whenever fetal swallowing is greatly impaired. A classic example of a lesion in which fetal swallowing cannot take place and thereby leads to hydramnios is fetal esophageal atresia. Conversely, when urination in utero cannot take place, as in instances of renal agenesis or atresia of the urethra, the volume of amnionic fluid surrounding the fetus typically is extremely limited (oligohydramnios).

Although lack of fetal swallowing with continuous production of normal amounts of fluid by the amnion and by the fetal kidneys may lead to hydramnios, this mechanism is certainly not the sole cause of hydramnios. Progressive hydramnios has been observed in instances in which a normal fetus was known to ingest relatively large amounts of amnionic fluid, and in which maternal diseases known to predispose to hydramnios, such as diabetes, were not identified (Pritchard, 1966). Presumably, in these instances, increased production by the amnion or, unlikely, intense fetal polyuria, or even both, cause the increase in amnionic fluid volume. Whether the respiratory tract is involved at times in the development of hydramnios is not clear. What is clear, however, is that if the volume of amnionic fluid is reduced to abnormal levels, as may occur in anephric fetuses or in instances of early and prolonged rupture of the fetal membranes, fetal pulmonary hypoplasia may result to such a severe degree that extrauterine life is impossible (Fliegner and co-workers, 1981; Wigglesworth and Desai, 1982).

Respiratory System

Fetal Lung. The timetable of lung maturation and the identification of biochemical indices of lung functional maturity in the fetus are of considerable importance and concern to the obstetrician. This obtains because functional immaturity of the lung at birth leads to the development of the respiratory distress syndrome.

Respiratory Distress Syndrome

History. Keidel and Gluck (1975), as well as Farrell and Avery (1975), have succinctly recounted the history of the clinical identification of the respiratory distress syndrome. The signs and symptoms of this disorder were first described in 1903 by Hocheim, who observed a nebulous lining in the lungs of two infants who died shortly after birth. His observation led to the use of the descriptive phrase *hyaline membrane disease,* which is used to describe the pathological features of the respiratory distress syndrome. In 1929, von Neergard compared the pressure–volume curves of lungs distended with air with those of lungs distended with a gum arabic solution; and from the results of these studies, he concluded that the forces that promote deflation or collapse of the air-containing lung are those that result principally from surface tension at the air–tissue interface of the alveolus. Clements (1957) found that a surface tension-lowering material was present in saline extracts of lung lavage material. Subsequently, it was demonstrated that the surface-active properties of the alveoli are attributable to the components of a complex lipoprotein known as *surfactant.*

Surfactant. Klaus and associates (1961) determined that the principal surface-active component of surfactant was attributable to a specific *lecithin, dipalmitoylphosphatidylcholine,* a unique phosphatidylcholine moiety in which palmitate is present in both the *sn*-1 and *sn*-2 positions of this glycerophospholipid. This is a peculiar species of phosphatidylcholine; this is true because it is rare to find a saturated fatty acid in both the *sn*-1 and -2 positions of a glycerophospholipid. Ordinarily there is a saturated fatty acid in the *sn*-1 position but a polyunsaturated fatty acid in the *sn*-2 position.

Avery and Mead (1959) were the first to point out that the respiratory distress syndrome is caused by a deficiency in surfactant biosynthesis in fetal and neonatal lung. Subsequently, several investigators have shown that augmented surfactant synthesis normally appears in fetal lungs according to a developmental timetable; and it is known that of the 40 cell types of the lung, surfactant is formed specifically in the type II pneumonocytes that line the alveoli (Fig. 7–16). The type II cells are characterized by multivesicular bodies (Fig. 7–16), the cellular progenitors of the lamellar bodies (Figs. 7–17 and 7–18) in which surfactant is assembled. Ultimately, the lamellar bodies are secreted from the lung. During late fetal life, at a time when the alveolus is characterized by a water-to-tissue interface, the intact lamellar

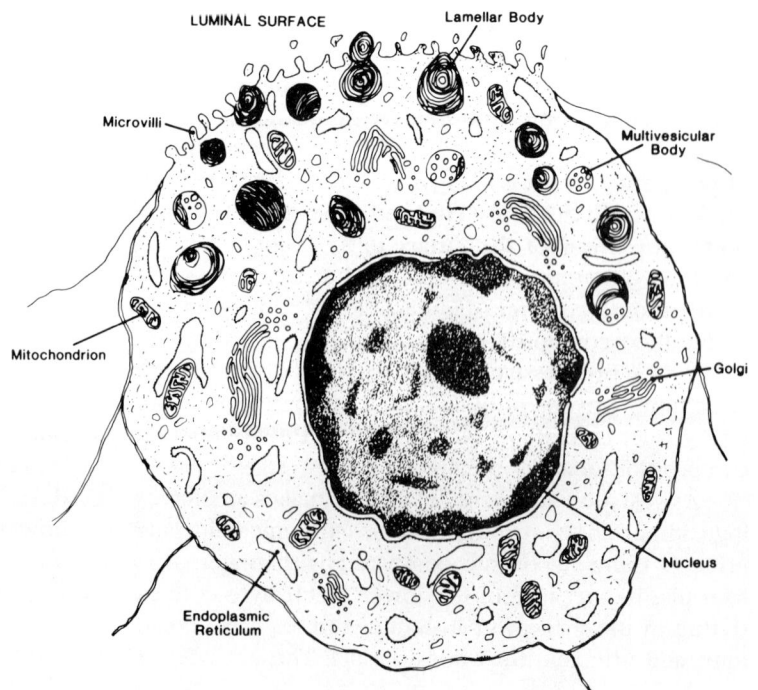

Fig. 7–16. Type II pneumonocyte. There are prominent microvilli identifiable on the apical surface. Many multivesicular bodies, the precursor of lamellar bodies, and many lamellar bodies (rich in surfactant) that are migrating toward the luminal surface prior to extrusion into the alveolar space are illustrated.

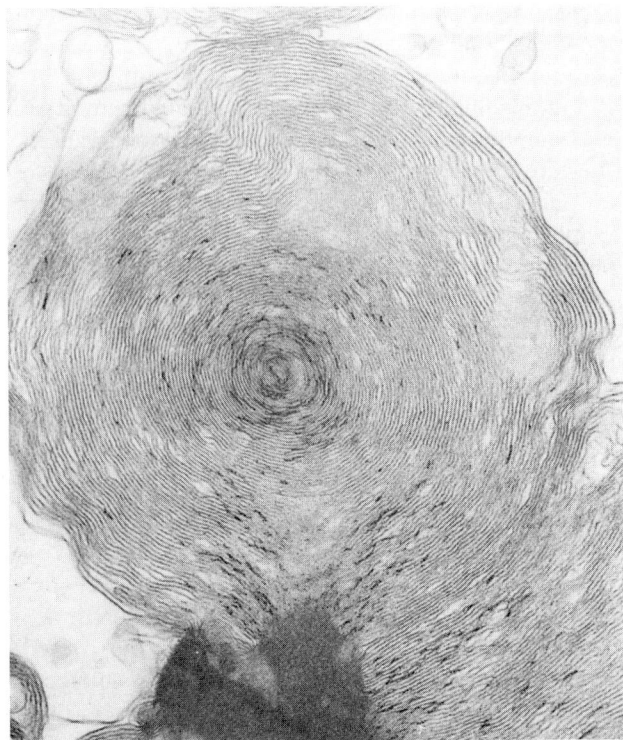

Fig. 7–17. Transmission electron micrograph of fused human fetal lung lamellar bodies. (Courtesy of Drs. J. Snyder and J. M. Johnston.)

bodies are swept into the amnionic fluid during fetal respiratory-like movements (i.e., fetal breathing).

This is a particularly important feature of human pregnancy because the appearance of surfactant in amnionic fluid heralds the commencement of functional maturation of the fetal lungs. In other species, lung secretions do not necessarily enter amnionic fluid; for example, in the sheep fetus, the lung secretions are swallowed.

After birth, with the first breath, an air-to-tissue interface is produced in the lung alveolus of the newborn. This permits the "uncoiling" of surfactant from the lamellar bodies, and this surface tension-lowering material then spreads to line the alveolus and thereby prevent alveolar collapse during expiration. Therefore, it is the capacity for fetal lungs to produce surfactant, and not the actual laying down of this material in utero, that characterizes lung maturity before birth.

Surfactant Composition. The recognition of the important role of surfactant in the prevention of respiratory distress syndrome prompted many investigators to study the composition of this lipoprotein (Fig. 7–19). About 90 percent of surfactant (dry weight) is lipid; and approximately 80 percent of the glycerophospholipids are comprised of phosphatidylcholines (lecithins); but importantly, a single phosphatidylcholine, *dipalmitoylphosphatidylcholine* (*disaturated phosphatidylcholine* or *disaturated lecithin*), accounts for nearly 50 percent of the glycerophospholipids of surfactant. There also is an unusually high content of *phosphatidylglycerol* in surfactant, 9 to 15 percent, an amount that is much greater than that found in any other mammalian tissue (Keidel and Gluck, 1975).

Phosphatidylglycerol is the second most surface-active glycerophospholipid component of surfactant; but more importantly, phosphatidylglycerol appears to confer a certain unique feature to the surfactant moiety,

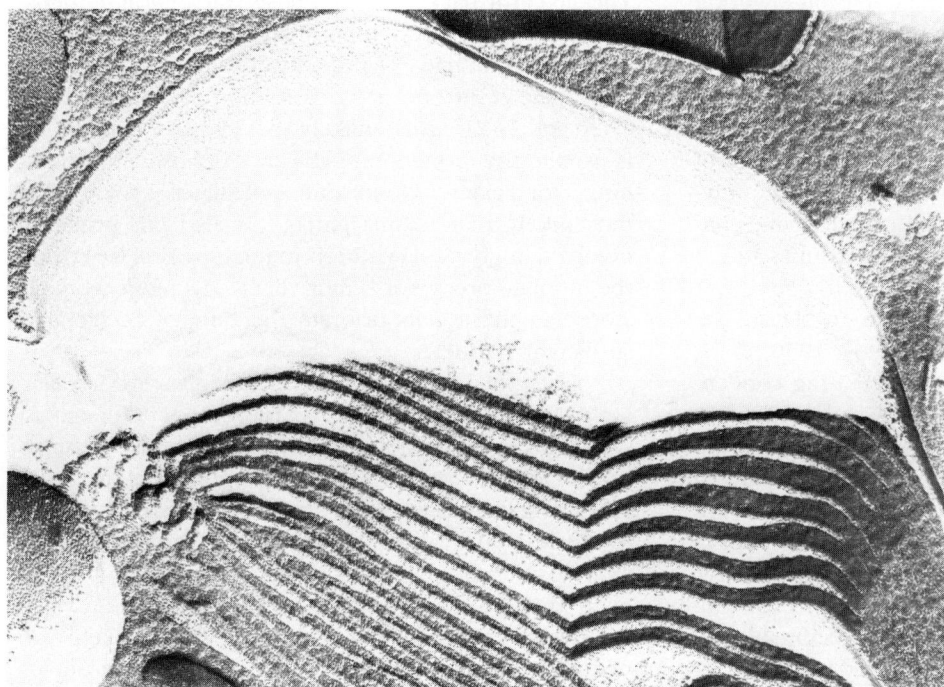

Fig. 7–18. Freeze-fracture scanning electron micrograph of a lamellar body. (Courtesy of Drs. R. C. Reynolds and J. M. Johnston.)

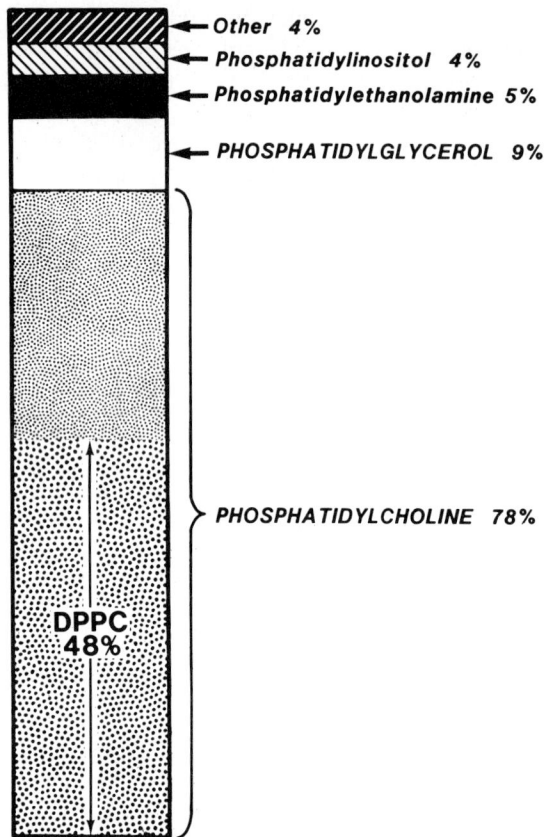

← Other 4%

← Phosphatidylinositol 4%

← Phosphatidylethanolamine 5%

← PHOSPHATIDYLGLYCEROL 9%

PHOSPHATIDYLCHOLINE 78%

DPPC 48%

Fig. 7–19. Glycerophospholipid composition of "mature" surfactant. Surfactant is especially enriched in lecithin (phosphatidylcholine) and, in particular, the surface-active dipalmitoylphosphatidylcholine (DPPC, 48 percent). The phosphatidylglycerol content of surfactant (8 to 15 percent) is also very high.

a surface-active property that is over and above that which can be attributed to its surface tension-lowering properties alone. This as-yet ill-defined action of phosphatidylglycerol is believed to be important in the prevention of the respiratory distress syndrome, because infants born before the appearance of phosphatidylglycerol in surfactant are at increased risk of development of the respiratory distress syndrome even in those newborns in whom the dipalmitoylphosphatidylcholine content of the surfactant is normal for mature lungs.

Regulation of Surfactant Synthesis. In an elegant series of studies, Gluck and associates (1967, 1970, 1971, 1972, 1974) demonstrated that an increasing concentration of dipalmitoylphosphatidylcholine (lecithin) in amnionic fluid, relative to that of sphingomyelin (the lecithin to sphingomyelin, or L/S, ratio), constitutes a marker of fetal lung maturation. These studies were successful because of the ingenious idea of determining the concentration of sphingomyelin as a reference for glycerophospholipid synthesis by the lung in general, whereas the measurement of acetone-precipitable dipalmitoylphosphatidylcholine (disaturated lecithin) is a

specific index of surfactant synthesis in type II pneumonocytes. Hallman and co-workers (1976) later demonstrated that the identification of phosphatidylglycerol in amnionic fluid is also an indicator of lung maturation.

From these many and complementary observations, it became apparent that augmented synthesis of surfactant, and specifically that which is enriched with dipalmitoylphosphatidylcholine and phosphatidylglycerol, is essential for the successful preparation of the fetal lung for the transition from a water–alveolar interface to an air–alveolar interface, events that must take place if alveolar collapse on expiration after birth is to be prevented. Thus, the regulation of the rate of synthesis of dipalmitoylphosphatidylcholine and phosphatidylglycerol in fetal lung is of signal importance. The biosynthetic pathways involved in the formation of the glycerophospholipids of surfactant are illustrated in Figures 7–20 through 7–22.

In the past few years, we also have come to appreciate and understand the nature and regulation of synthesis of the apoproteins of surfactant. The protein moiety is essential not only to the synthesis of surfactant but also to the function and recycling of the lipoprotein in the alveolus of the lung.

Regulation of Surfactant Formation

GLYCEROPHOSPHOLIPIDS. Surfactant biosynthesis is confined to the type II cells of the lung. The apoproteins are produced in the endoplasmic reticulum. The surface-active components of surfactant, the glycerophospholipids, are synthesized by way of cooperative interactions of several cellular organelles. Common reactions are involved in the initial steps in the biosynthesis of phosphatidylcholine and phosphatidylglycerol. The glycerol backbone for phosphatidylcholine, phosphatidylinositol, and phosphatidylglycerol synthesis (phosphatidic acid) is provided by dihydroxyacetone phosphate from one or two reaction sequences (Figs. 7–20 and 7–21). It is unlikely that glycerol from blood is used in the formation of glycerol-3-phosphate in fetal lung (for review: Odom and colleagues, 1986). It is most likely that plasma glucose is also not primarily involved in glycerol synthesis in the type II cells; rather, the ultimate precursor is more likely glycogen, which is stored in these cells prior to the time of accelerated surfactant synthesis.

Glycerol-3-phosphate is acylated in a stepwise fashion in a process that gives rise to phosphatidic acid, in which there are two of a variety of fatty acids. Phosphatidic acid is the precursor of all the glycerophospholipids of surfactant. Generally, there is a saturated fatty acid in the *sn*-1 position and an unsaturated fatty acid in the *sn*-2 position of phosphatidic acid. In lung tissue, however, there is considerable capacity for the de novo synthesis of palmitic acid, and thus a greater likelihood of finding palmitate in the *sn*-2 position of glycerolipids

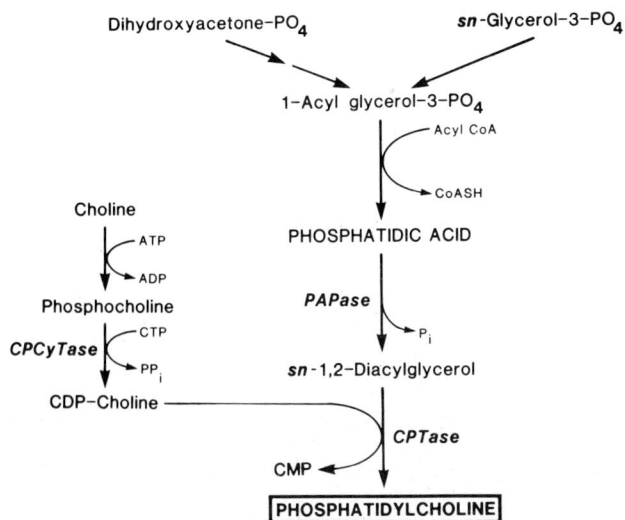

Fig. 7–20. Biosynthetic pathway for phosphatidylcholine (lecithin) synthesis in type II pneumonocytes. (PAPase = phosphatidate phosphohydrolase; CPTase = choline phosphotransferase; CPCyTase = choline phosphate cytidylyltransferase; CDP = choline diphosphate; CMP = cytidine monophosphate.)

in lung tissue compared with that in other tissues. In the biosynthesis of phosphatidic acid by lung tissue, however, there is no evidence for preferential incorporation of palmitoyl-CoA in the *sn*-2 position.

It is important to emphasize that phosphatidic acid is a substrate common to the formation of the two

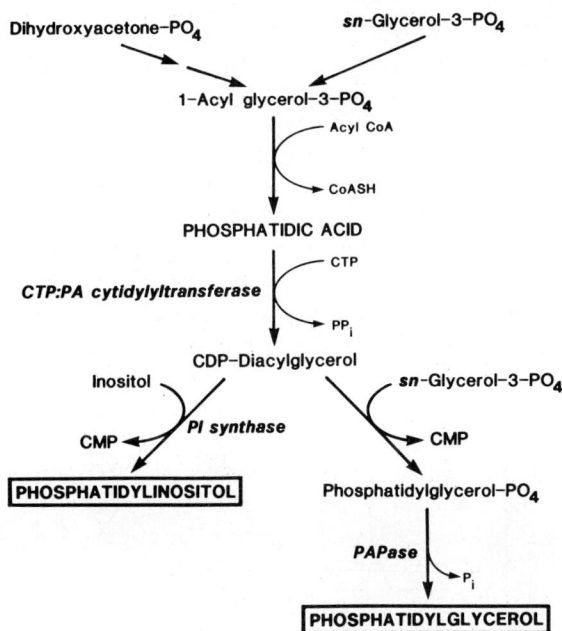

Fig. 7–21. Biosynthetic pathway for the synthesis of phosphatidylinositol and phosphatidylglycerol in type II pneumonocytes. (CTP:PA = cytidine triphosphate:phosphatidic acid. For other abbreviations, see Fig. 7–20.)

principal surface-active glycerophospholipids, dipalmitoylphosphatidylcholine and phosphatidylglycerol (Figs. 7–20 through 7–22). Thus, the metabolism of phosphatidic acid constitutes a critical branch point in the regulation of the biosynthesis of the principal surface-active glycerophospholipids of surfactant.

LECITHIN (DIPALMITOYLPHOSPHATIDYLCHOLINE). Dipalmitoylphosphatidylcholine is the major glycerophospholipid of surfactant. In the synthesis of lecithin, phosphatidic acid is hydrolyzed, through the action of the enzyme phosphatidate phosphohydrolase (PAPase), to give *sn*-1,2-diacylglycerols (Fig. 7–20). The *sn*-1,2-diacylglycerols serve as co-substrate with cytidine diphosphate (CDP)-choline in the formation of phosphatidylcholines. This latter reaction is catalyzed by the enzyme choline phosphotransferase (CPTase). The co-substrate, CDP-choline, is formed in a sequence of reactions; through the action of choline kinase, phosphorylcholine is formed. Phosphorylcholine, in turn, is converted to CDP-choline in a reaction that is catalyzed by cytidine triphosphate (CTP)-phosphocholine cytidylyltransferase (CTP-CyT; Fig. 7–20). In the resultant phosphatidylcholines, there may be a saturated fatty acid, commonly palmitic acid, in the *sn*-1 position, whereas an unsaturated fatty acid may be present in the *sn*-2 position.

Obviously, some molecular rearrangement of such phosphatidylcholines must occur to produce dipalmitoylphosphatidylcholine, the surface-active lecithin. Two separate mechanisms have been proposed to account for the enrichment of phosphatidylcholines with palmitic acid in the *sn*-2 position. In both mechanisms, the action of the enzyme phospholipase A_2 is required. The action of phospholipase A_2 results in the deacylation of glycerophospholipids at the *sn*-2 position. One product of this reaction is *sn*-1-palmitoyllysophosphatidylcholine. This lysophosphatidylcholine product may be acylated with palmitoyl-CoA through the action of acyltransferase, resulting in the product dipalmitoylphosphatidylcholine (Lands, 1958). It is interesting that this pathway was first demonstrated in lung tissue. Alternatively, the remodeling of phosphatidylcholine can come about as the result of the transfer of the acyl moiety from the *sn*-1 position of an *sn*-1-palmitoyllysophosphatidylcholine to the *sn*-2 position of a second *sn*-1-palmitoyllysophosphatidylcholine. Dipalmitoylphosphatidylcholine can also be formed by way of this pathway.

PHOSPHATIDYLGLYCEROL. The regulation of phosphatidylglycerol synthesis is especially important because Hallman and co-workers (1976) have shown that increased concentrations of phosphatidylglycerol, together with decreased concentrations of phosphatidylinositol, in surfactant also herald lung maturation. Some infants who are born of diabetic mothers develop the respiratory distress syndrome despite high concentrations of di-

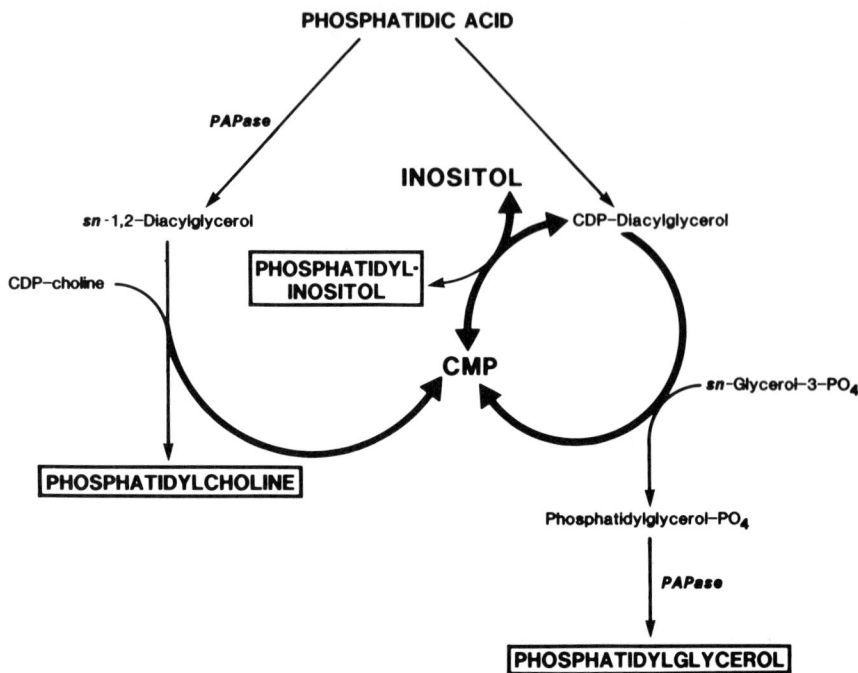

Fig. 7–22. The proposed CMP cycle for the regulation of the relative rates of synthesis of phosphatidylcholine, phosphatidylinositol, and phosphatidylglycerol.

palmitoylphosphatidylcholine in their amnionic fluid. The surfactant in lung and amnionic fluid of affected fetuses and neonates is characterized by low levels of phosphatidylglycerol and high levels of phosphatidylinositol. Furthermore, it has been shown that phosphatidylglycerol also acts to increase the activity of the lung tissue enzyme CTP:phosphocholine cytidylyltransferase, an enzyme necessary for phosphatidylcholine biosynthesis.

The regulation of phosphatidylinositol and phosphatidylglycerol biosynthesis is incompletely understood. It seems likely that the decrease in concentration of phosphatidylinositol that is associated with a concomitant increase in phosphatidylglycerol in surfactant with lung maturation is brought about by a change in the flux of CDP-diacylglycerol through the pathways involved in the synthesis of these acidic glycerophospholipids (Bleasdale and colleagues, 1979) (Figs. 7–21 and 7–22). In any event, it is known that with fetal lung maturation there is first a "surge" in phosphatidylcholine synthesis that is followed, in time, by an increase in phosphatidylglycerol together with a concomitant decrease in phosphatidylinositol in surfactant (Fig. 7–23).

From an evaluation of the metabolic pathways involved in the biosynthesis of phosphatidylglycerol and phosphatidylinositol, it was difficult to envision a mechanism that could account for (1) the increase in phosphatidylcholine synthesis for surfactant formation with lung maturation, which thereafter is followed in time by (2) an increase in phosphatidylglycerol content, and (3) a concomitant decrease in phosphatidylinositol concentration in surfactant. The difficulty in resolving the mechanisms involved was related to the proposition

that each of these glycerophospholipids is ultimately derived from a common precursor, phosphatidic acid; but more than that, phosphatidylinositol and phosphatidylglycerol are both derived from a common precursor that is a product of phosphatidic acid, namely CDP-diacylglycerol.

Batenburg and co-workers (1982) reviewed the three mechanisms by which the switchover from phosphatidylinositol to phosphatidylglycerol synthesis for surfactant could come about:

1. An increase in enzymatic activity for glycerol-phosphate phosphatidyltransferase.

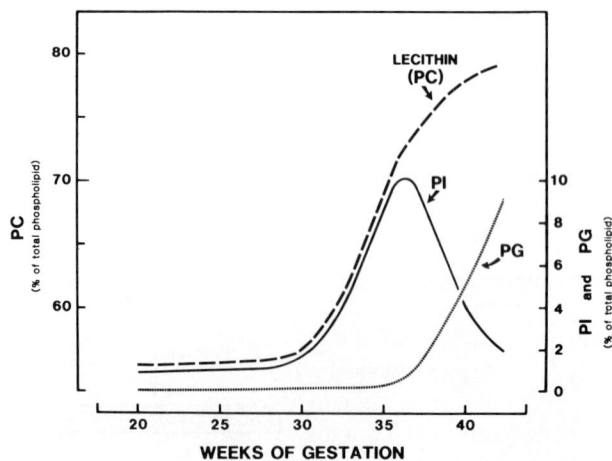

Fig. 7–23. Relation between the levels of lecithin (dipalmitoylphosphatidylcholine, PC), phosphatidylinositol (PI), and phosphatidylglycerol (PG) in amnionic fluid as a function of gestational age.

2. A decrease in fetal plasma inositol.
3. Increased levels of cytidine monophosphate (CMP), resulting from increased phosphatidylcholine (lecithin) synthesis.

Based on findings of studies conducted in isolated type II cells of the adult rat lung, Batenburg and co-workers (1982) concluded that mechanism 2 was most important. Bleasdale and associates (1979) presented convincing evidence in favor of mechanism 3. There is little support for mechanism 1. Possibly the solution is to be found through a combination of mechanisms 2 and 3.

APOPROTEINS. Surfactant is primarily composed of glycerophospholipids; but in the past 10 years, the functional importance of the unique apoproteins of surfactant has been defined. Three surfactant-associated proteins are known: surfactant protein A, B, and C (for review: Whitsett, 1992). The major apoprotein is surfactant A (SP-A), a glycoprotein (M_r about 28,000 to 35,000). The SP-A is synthesized in the type II cells, and increased synthesis is related temporally to increased surfactant formation in maturing fetal lungs. The amnionic fluid content of SP-A also increases as does the L/S ratio as a function of gestational age and fetal lung maturity. Synthesis of SP-A is known to be increased by treatment of fetal lung tissue with cyclic AMP (analogues) and by epidermal growth factor and triiodothyronine. On the other hand, glucocorticosteroids may inhibit SP-A synthesis (Whitsett and associates, 1987), and insulin definitely inhibits its synthesis (Snyder and Mendelson, 1987).

SP-A seems to be important in the structural transformation of the secreted lamellar body into tubular myelin within the lumen of the alveolus. SP-A also may be involved in the endocytosis and recycling of secreted surfactant by the type II cells. In addition to SP-A, there are a number of smaller molecular weight proteins of surfactant (M_r about 5000 to 18,000). These lower molecular weight surfactant proteins (SP-B and SP-C) are believed to be important in optimizing the surface-active properties of surfactant. In addition, SP-A, after being taken back into the type II cells by receptor-mediated endocytosis, acts to inhibit surfactant glycerophospholipid synthesis and secretion.

Increases in surfactant apoprotein synthesis precede the increase in surfactant glycerophospholipid synthesis (Mendelson and associates, 1986). SP-A gene expression is not detectable at 16 to 20 weeks' gestation (Snyder and colleagues, 1988).

In studies of surfactant replacement therapy, natural surfactants that contain the surfactant proteins are more effective than are synthetic lipid mixtures. And surfactant therapy, using natural surfactants, is meritorious in preventing or treating respiratory distress syndrome in newborns.

Alterations in the Timetable of "Mature" Surfactant Formation. If this were a correct formulation of the means by which the relative amounts of glycerophospholipids and apoproteins in surfactant are regulated, it can be envisioned that certain physiological or pathophysiological events may cause a delay in the timetable of fetal lung maturation. By way of example, if the levels of plasma *myo*-inositol were elevated, phosphatidylinositol formation, at the expense of phosphatidylglycerol, would be favored (Fig. 7–22). This pattern of surfactant formation—one rich in phosphatidylcholine and phosphatidylinositol and deficient in phosphatidylglycerol—is characteristic of that found in some newborn infants of diabetic mothers. Such infants are at greater risk of respiratory distress syndrome in spite of high levels of lecithin in amnionic fluid. Inositolemia and inositol intolerance are common in persons with diabetes mellitus. Quirk and Bleasdale (1984) and Odom and colleagues (1986) have presented in-depth reviews of the maturation of the fetal lung in pregnancies complicated by maternal diabetes mellitus. At the same time, hyperinsulinemia of the fetus may serve to inhibit the synthesis of the apoprotein of surfactant.

Hormonal Regulation of Surfactant Formation in Human Fetal Lung. Although it is of signal importance to define the biochemical events involved in the synthesis and release of surfactant, it is equally important to define the mechanisms involved in the control of the synthesis and release (secretion) of surfactant. Many substances (generally hormones) have been proposed as potentially important modulators of these processes. Ballard (1986) has presented a comprehensive review of this subject. The interest of most investigators who have directed their attention to this question, however, has been centered on only a few agents. Of these, the most intensively investigated compounds are hormones, in particular cortisol and other glucocorticosteroids and thyroxine.

Cortisol and Fetal Lung Maturation. The basis for suspecting that glucocorticosteroids promote lung maturation was first provided by Liggins (1969). In studies designed to induce preterm labor in the sheep (Chap. 12), he observed that there appeared to be accelerated lung maturation in prematurely delivered lambs that had been treated with glucocorticosteroids prior to birth. Since that time, many investigators have suggested that cortisol produced in the fetal adrenal is the natural stimulus for augmented surfactant synthesis.

There is appreciable evidence in support of the view that glucocorticosteroids, when administered in large amounts to the mother at certain critical times during gestation, effect an increase in the rate of maturation of the human fetal lung as indicated by a reduced incidence of respiratory distress syndrome in newborn infants of such glucocorticosteroid-treated mothers compared with that in those whose mothers were not so treated (Liggins and Howie, 1972).

The precise role of glucocorticosteroids in fetal lung maturation has not been fully defined, however; and from the evidence available, it cannot be concluded that cortisol is the single physiological regulator of the activities of enzymes involved in surfactant formation in most species, including humans.

There is little doubt that the administration of glucocorticosteroids to pregnant women during the 29th to 33rd weeks of gestation is associated with a reduced incidence of respiratory distress in their prematurely born infants; but various conclusions have been reached regarding the mechanism(s) by which such treatment is effective. Some investigators have found that the lecithin (phosphatidylcholine)-to-sphingomyelin ratio in amnionic fluid increases after glucocorticosteroid treatment of the mother (Spellacy and colleagues, 1973; Zuspan and associates, 1977); yet Liggins and Howie (1972) found no consistent increase.

Johnson and colleagues (1978) found that the administration of glucocorticosteroids to pregnant subhuman primates was not associated with an increase in surfactant content in the fetal lungs. Rather, they found that the principal alteration in the fetal lungs of corticosteroid-treated pregnant monkeys was a decrease in the content of collagenous tissue.

Most investigators have concluded that cortisol is not the single stimulus for augmented surfactant formation in the maturing human fetal lung (Hauth and co-workers, 1978). This conclusion is strengthened by the well-known clinical observation that the respiratory distress syndrome is not necessarily observed in many human neonates in whom the capacity to secrete cortisol is limited. Such infants include those with anencephaly, adrenal hypoplasia, and congenital adrenal hyperplasia. It may be that cortisol is one of several hormones that act cooperatively to effect fetal lung maturation. For example, cortisol is believed to stabilize the ribosomal–endoplasmic reticulum complex of mammary tissue such that this organ can respond to prolactin and insulin and thereby secrete milk (Oka and Topper, 1971).

Fibroblast Pneumocyte Factor. Smith (1978) observed that a factor produced in stromal cells of lung (fibroblast pneumocyte factor, or FPF) may serve as an intermediate modulator for type II cell maturation. Purified type II cells responded poorly to glucocorticosteroids; but in the presence of fibroblasts or partially purified FPF, the cells do respond. Post and co-workers (1984) demonstrated that antibodies raised against partially purified FPF inhibited cortisol-stimulated surfactant formation.

Snyder and colleagues (1981) have developed an elegant system for the study of human fetal lung maturation in vivo. They find that there is a striking morphological and biochemical maturation in explants of fetal lung tissue (16 to 20 weeks' gestational age abortuses)

that are maintained in organ culture. In such tissues, there is a remarkable increase in phosphatidylcholine formation and a rapid (4 to 5 days of culture) appearance of multivesicular bodies and lamellar bodies in type II pneumonocytes in these tissues. In such preparations, Mendelson and co-workers (1981) found that cortisol plus prolactin (but neither hormone alone) caused an acceleration in the rate of increase in phosphatidylcholine synthesis by human fetal lung tissue in organ culture. Thus, cortisol and prolactin, acting in concert, may be the lead hormones in the orchestration of a multihormonal stimulation of surfactant biosynthesis in fetal lung.

If the account presented were an accurate description of the events that transpire in vivo, it easily can be envisioned that other hormones may serve a supportive role in this orchestration of fetal lung maturation. Estrogens affect phospholipid turnover in many tissues, act to promote prolactin release from the anterior pituitary, and may be involved in the synthesis of prolactin receptors. Quirk and colleagues (1982) have reviewed the role of prolactin in fetal lung maturation.

Estrogens and Fetal Lung Maturation. It is of interest that in many of the tissues in which there are prolactin receptors, there also are receptors for estrogens. In fact, it appears that estrogens, directly or indirectly, act to regulate the number of prolactin receptors in the liver and mammary gland (Gelato and co-workers, 1975; Kelly and associates, 1975; Posner and Kelly, 1975). Many of the actions of prolactin and estrogens appear to be interrelated, especially with regard to lipid metabolism and growth. Estrogens are anabolic steroids that are known to regulate lipoprotein synthesis in the liver (Luskey and co-workers, 1974) and lipid metabolism in the rat uterus (Chan and colleagues, 1976). Increased lipid synthesis is one of the earliest and most dramatic responses of the rat uterus to estrogenic hormones (Aizawa and Mueller, 1961). Spooner and Gorski (1972) showed that estrogens caused enhanced fatty acid synthesis and an increase in rate of the incorporation of choline into glycerophospholipids of the rat uterus. Dickey and Robertson (1969) found that maternal and neonatal urinary estrogens in infants in whom respiratory distress subsequently developed were decreased. Pasqualini and associates (1976), studying guinea pig fetuses, demonstrated a high concentration of estradiol receptors in lung tissue cytosol as well as nuclear binding of the steroid. The number of estrogen receptors in the lung of the guinea pig fetus increased with gestational age (Sumida and colleagues, 1977). Mendelson and associates (1980) have demonstrated high-affinity estrogen binding in cytosolic fractions prepared from rat and human fetal lung tissues. Moreover, Khosla and Rooney (1979) found that when pregnant rabbits were injected with estradiol, fetal lung surfactant content was increased. Rooney and Brehier (1982) suggested that the estrogen-induced increase in the incorporation of choline into phosphatidylcholine is mediated by changes in CTP:phosphocholine cytidylyltransferase activity.

Nonetheless, the human fetus appears to be relatively estrogen-insensitive, at least in many tissues other than brain. Therefore, a role for estrogen in human fetal lung maturation may be indirect—for example, by way of the modulation of pituitary prolactin secretion.

Thyroxine and Fetal Lung Maturation. A role for thyroxine in the rate of surfactant synthesis has been proposed by a number of investigators. Thyroxine administration to rabbit fetuses at 24 to 25 days of gestation is associated with accelerated maturation of the fetal lung and an early appearance of osmophilic lamellar inclusions within the type II pneumonocytes (Rooney and colleagues, 1974; Wu and associates, 1971, 1973). Smith and Torday (1974) found that thyroxine treatment was associated with an increased incorporation of choline into phosphatidylcholine in cultured cells prepared from rabbit fetuses of 28 days' gestation. On the other hand, Rooney and co-workers (1974) found no effect of thyroxine treatment on the activities of lysophosphatidic acid acyltransferase, CPTase, CDP-diglyceride:inositol phosphatidyltransferase, glycerolphosphate phosphatidyltransferase, acyltransferase, or fatty acid biosynthesis. Mason (1973), in a study of the effect of thyroxine treatment on the concentration of dipalmitoylphosphatidylcholine in lungs of hyperthyroid and in euthyroid rats, found that thyroxine had little effect on the concentration of dipalmitoylphosphatidylcholine. Thus, the role of thyroxine, if any, in the biochemical maturation of the fetal lung type II pneumonocyte is unclear.

Growth Factors and Fetal Lung Maturation. Epidermal growth factor (EGF) acts to promote surfactant secretion and specifically to increase the synthesis of SP-A, the major apoprotein of surfactant (Whitsett and colleagues, 1987).

Platelet-Activating Factor (PAF). There is an increase in PAF concentration in fetal lung that is concomitant with the decrease in glycogen content. And PAF treatment of lung tissue causes a decrease in glycogen (Hoffman and colleagues, 1986, 1988). PAF is found in amnionic fluid in association with surfactant; and it has been proposed that lung is one source of amnionic fluid PAF (Chap. 12).

Conclusion. Presently, it seems reasonable to conclude that the hormonal stimulation of surfactant synthesis in the type II pneumonocytes of developing fetal lung is brought about by a complex interaction of several hormones. It is well established that pretreatment of breast tissue with estrogens, followed by cortisol, prolactin,

and insulin treatment, is essential for lactation. Perhaps a similar sequence of events leads to accelerated surfactant formation in maturing fetal lungs.

On the other hand, it now seems most reasonable to conclude that the regulation of fetal lung maturation (1) does not evolve singularly about the maturation of the type II pneumonocyte and (2) does not necessarily involve similar stimuli for the synthesis of both the glycerophospholipids and the apoproteins of surfactant. Moreover, it is clear that lung growth and maturation are not synonymous—perhaps the two events are not even complementary; for example, lung growth may involve processes that inhibit functional maturation. If this were true, considerable initial confusion would be presented to investigators seeking to define the regulation of fetal lung growth, maturation, and function.

Several curious features of human fetal lung development are supportive of this proposition. For example, glucocorticosteroid treatment of pregnant women to effect fetal lung maturation is generally effective only during one brief window in gestation, from 29 to 33 weeks. This may be indicative that the therapeutic benefits of glucocorticosteroids at this time are derived from processes largely independent of accelerated surfactant formation. Possibly, the benefits are the consequence of alterations in extracellular matrix that facilitate lung expandability, a proposition suggested before from studies of the rhesus fetus (Johnson and associates, 1978).

Respiration. Within a very few minutes after birth, the respiratory system must be able to provide oxygen as well as eliminate carbon dioxide if the neonate is to survive. Development of air ducts and alveoli, pulmonary vasculature, muscles of respiration, and coordination of their activities through the central nervous system to a degree that allows fetal survival, at least for a time, can be demonstrated by the end of the second trimester of pregnancy. The majority of fetuses born before this time succumb immediately or during the next few days from respiratory insufficiency, as pointed out in Chapters 38 and 44.

Movements of the fetal chest wall have been detected by ultrasonic techniques as early as 11 weeks' gestation (Boddy and Dawes, 1975). From the beginning of the fourth month, the fetus is capable of respiratory movement sufficiently intense to move amnionic fluid in and out of the respiratory tract. In the radiograph in Figure 7–14, obtained 26 hours after injection of Thorotrast into the amnionic sac, the contrast medium is present in fetal lung. Davis and Potter (1946) reported that the longer the exposure in utero after a single injection of Thorotrast, the greater the apparent concentration in the lungs.

Duenhoelter and Pritchard (1976, 1977) demonstrated in both the human and the rhesus fetus that chromium-labeled erythrocytes and other labeled parti-

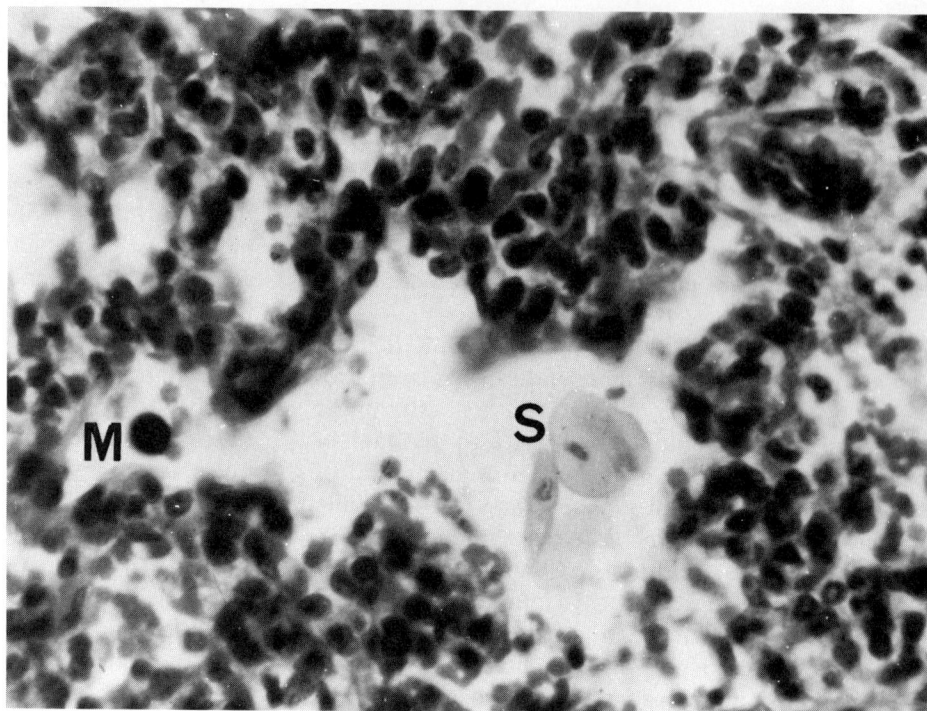

Fig. 7–24. Photomicrograph of lung of a near-term rhesus fetus delivered 24 hours after labeling the amnionic fluid with radio-strontium-labeled microspheres as well as chromium-labeled erythrocytes. Contained in the alveolus immediately adjacent to the dense microsphere (M) are labeled erythrocytes that were also inhaled, as were fetal squamous cells, or squames (S). From the amount of chromium within the lungs, it was calculated that at least 62 mL of amnionic fluid was inhaled in 24 hours by a fetus that weighed 281 g. (From Duenhoelter and Pritchard, 1976.)

cles injected into the amnionic sac accumulated in the lungs as well as the gastrointestinal tract (Fig. 7–24). They concluded that throughout the last two trimesters progressively larger volumes of amnionic fluid are normally inspired and presumably expired by the fetus. The pressure changes with some inspirations are sufficient to account for such movement in the rhesus fetus (Martin and co-workers, 1974).

Boddy and Dawes (1975) identified fetal breathing movements in the normal human fetus that are episodic and irregular, their frequency typically ranging from 30 to 70 per minute. Asphyxia was followed by cessation of normal breathing movements and the initiation of gasping respiratory efforts. Such cessation of normal respiratory movements may be the consequence of increased levels of fetal β-endorphin (Browning and co-workers, 1983).

Vagitus Uteri. Crying in utero is a rare phenomenon. After rupture of the membranes, air may gain access to the amnionic cavity and be inspired by the fetus. Thiery and associates (1973) described three cases in which fetal crying was heard during vaginal examination, amnioscopy, or application of a clip electrode to the fetus. Fetal hiccuping is a more common phenomenon, and frequently the movement produced by the fetus is appreciated by the mother.

Endocrine Glands

Anterior Pituitary. Mulchahey and associates (1987), in an elegant review of the ontogenesis of fetal pituitary

gland function and regulation, put forward an interesting and plausible view. First, they discounted the validity of the concept that the control of fetal anterior pituitary secretion was dependent upon maturation of the central nervous system. Second, they pointed out that the fetal endocrine system is functional for some time before "*the central nervous system completes its synaptogenesis and other integrative systems have reached a state of maturity competent to perform many of the tasks associated with homeostasis.*" Third, they go on to suggest that the endocrine system of the fetus does not necessarily mimic that of the adult but nonetheless may be one of the first homeostatic systems to develop.

Ultimately, the fetal anterior pituitary differentiates into five cell types, which secrete six protein hormones: (1) lactotropes, producing prolactin (PRL); (2) somatotropes, producing growth hormone (GH); (3) corticotropes, producing corticotropin (ACTH); (4) thyrotropes, producing thyroid-stimulating hormone (TSH); and (5) gonadotropes, producing luteinizing hormone (LH) and follicle-stimulating hormone (FSH). ACTH is first detected in the fetal pituitary at 7 weeks' gestation; and before the end of the 17th week, the fetal pituitary is able to synthesize and store all pituitary hormones. GH, ACTH, and LH have been identified in the pituitary of the human fetus by 13 weeks' gestation. Moreover, the fetal pituitary is responsive to hypophysiotropic hormones and is capable of secreting these hormones from early in gestation (Grumbach and Kaplan, 1974).

The levels of pituitary *growth hormone* are rather high in cord blood, although the role for the hormone in fetal growth and development is not clear. Decapitation in utero does not appreciably impair the growth of the rest of the animal fetus, as shown by Bearn (1967) as well as others. Furthermore, human anencephalic fetuses, with little pituitary tissue, are not remarkably different in weight from normal fetuses.

The fetal pituitary produces and releases β-endorphin in a manner separate from maternal plasma levels (Browning and colleagues, 1983). Furthermore, cord blood levels of β-endorphin and β-lipotrophin were found to decrease with declining fetal pH but correlate in a positive manner with fetal P_{CO_2}.

Neurohypophysis. The fetal neurohypophysis is well developed by 10 to 12 weeks' gestation and oxytocin and arginine vasopressin (AVP) are demonstrable. In addition, the neurohypophyseal hormone of submammalian vertebrates, arginine vasotocin (AVT), is present in fetal pituitary and pineal glands. AVT is present only in fetal life in the human (Fisher, 1986). In adult animals, the infusion of AVT promotes sleep and stimulates prolactin release.

It is probable that oxytocin as well as AVP are functional in the fetus to conserve water; but these actions may be largely at the level of lung and placenta rather than kidney. PGE_2 formation in fetal kidney may serve to attenuate AVP action in this organ.

Several investigators have found that the levels of AVP in umbilical cord plasma are increased strikingly compared with the levels found in maternal plasma (Chard and associates, 1971; Polin and co-workers, 1977). Additionally, AVP in cord and fetal blood appears to be elevated by fetal stress (DeVane and Porter, 1980; DeVane and co-workers, 1982).

Fetal Intermediate Pituitary. There is a well-developed intermediate lobe of the pituitary in the human fetus. The cells of this structure begin to disappear before term and are absent from the pituitary of adults. The principal secretory products of the intermediate lobe cells are α-melanocyte-stimulating hormone (α-MSH) and β-endorphin. The levels of fetal α-MSH decrease progressively with gestation.

Thyroid. The pituitary–thyroid system is capable of function by the end of the first trimester (Table 7–4). Until midpregnancy, however, secretion of thyroid-stimulating hormone and thyroid hormones is low. There is a considerable increase after this time (Fisher, 1975, 1985; Fisher and Klein, 1981). Probably very little *thyrotropin* crosses the placenta from mother to fetus, whereas the long-acting thyroid stimulators LATS and LATS-protector do so when present in high concentrations in the mother (see Chap. 8, p. 237). Also, maternal IgG antibodies against thyroid-stimulating hormone (TSH) also may cross the placenta, resulting in falsely high TSH levels in the neonate (Lazarus and associates, 1983).

TABLE 7–4. PHASES OF THYROID MATURATION IN THE HUMAN FETUS AND NEWBORN INFANT

Phase	Events	Gestational Age
I	Embryogenesis of pituitary–thyroid axis	2 to 12 weeks
II	Hypothalamic maturation	10 to 35 weeks
III	Development of neuroendocrine control	20 weeks to 4 weeks after birth
IV	Maturation of peripheral monodeiodination systems	30 weeks to 4 weeks after birth

From Fisher (1979).

The human placenta actively concentrates iodide on the fetal side; and throughout the second and third trimesters of pregnancy, the fetal thyroid concentrates iodide more avidly than does the maternal thyroid. Therefore, the hazard to the fetus of administering either radioiodide or appreciable amounts of ordinary iodide to the mother is obvious.

Thyroid hormones of maternal origin cross the placenta to a very *limited* degree, with triiodothyronine crossing more readily than thyroxine. There is limited action of thyroid hormones during fetal life. The athyroid human fetus is normally grown at birth. Only selected fetal tissues may be responsive to thyroid hormone (e.g., brain and lung).

Immediately after birth there are major changes in thyroid function and metabolism. Atmospheric cooling evokes sudden and marked increase in thyrotropin secretion, which in turn causes a progressive increase in serum thyroxine levels maximal 24 to 36 hours after birth. There are nearly simultaneous elevations of serum triiodothyronine levels.

Adrenal Glands. The *adrenal* of the human fetus is very much larger in relation to total body size than is that of the adult; the bulk of the enlargement is made up of the inner or so-called fetal zone of the adrenal cortex. The normally hypertrophied fetal zone involutes rapidly after birth. The fetal zone is scant to absent in rare instances where the fetal pituitary is congenitally absent. The function of the fetal adrenal and the control of fetal adrenal steroidogenesis (dehydroepiandrosterone sulfate and cortisol) are discussed in detail in Chapter 6.

The fetal adrenal also synthesizes *aldosterone*. In one study, aldosterone levels in cord plasma near term exceeded those in maternal plasma, as did renin and renin substrate (Katz and colleagues, 1974). The renal tubules of the newborn, and presumably the fetus, appear relatively insensitive to aldosterone (Kaplan, 1972).

Gonads. Siiteri and Wilson (1974) demonstrated the synthesis of testosterone by the fetal testis from progesterone and pregnenolone by 10 weeks' gestation. Moreover, Leinonen and Jaffe (1985) found that fetal testicular Leydig cells escape desensitization characteristic of adult testes subjected to repeated hCG challenges. This phenomenon in fetal testis may be due to (1) absence of estrogen receptors in the fetal testes and (2) prolactin stimulation of hCG/LH receptors in fetal testes. Therefore, there is a close relationship between (1) the appearance of development of Leydig cells in fetal testes and levels of hCG, (2) fetal testicular testosterone formation and levels of hCG, (3) receptor concentration for LH/hCG and hCG levels, and (4) the absence of down-regulation of LH/hCG receptors and continued fetal testicular testosterone secretion during the time that hCG levels are high. The formation of estrogen in fetal ovaries has been demonstrated, but estrogen formation in the ovaries is not required for female phenotypic development.

Sex of the Fetus

Sex Ratio. The accepted secondary sex ratio—that is, the sex ratio of human fetuses that reach viability—is approximately 106 males to 100 females. This figure has been obtained by the examination of term and preterm infants. Many attempts have been made to establish a sex ratio for fetuses of earlier gestational age. In general, such studies have been misleading, for as Wilson (1926) showed, the appearance of external genitals is an unreliable index of sex before the 50-mm stage.

Because, theoretically, there should be as many Y-bearing as X-bearing sperm, the primary sex ratio, or the ratio at the time of fertilization, should be one to one. If so, the secondary sex ratio of 106 to 100 is suggestive that more females than males are lost during the early months of pregnancy. Establishment of the primary sex ratio in humans is at present impracticable, for it requires the recovery and assignment of zygotes that fail to cleave and blastocysts that fail to implant. The results of Carr's studies (1963), nevertheless, are suggestive that the primary sex ratio in the human may be unity.

Sexual Differentiation. One of the greatest responsibilities of the obstetrician is the assignment of sex to the newborn. But if the external genitalia of the newborn are ambiguous (with respect to complete male or female development), a profound dilemma is faced.

Griffin and Wilson (1986) have stated that *"it is no exaggeration to say that the detection of sexual ambiguity in the newborn constitutes a true medical emergency."* An incorrect assignment of sex portends grave psychological and social problems for the baby and family. Yet, we are of the view that the proper functional sex assignment for the newborn can almost always be made at the time of delivery, even in newborns with ambiguity of the external genitalia. To address this issue, and to address the issue of establishing a definitive di-

agnosis as to the cause of development of ambiguous external genitalia, the mechanisms of normal and abnormal sexual differentiation must be understood.

It is clear that male phenotypic sexual differentiation is directed by the function of the fetal testis. **In the absence of the testis, female differentiation ensues irrespective of the genetic sex.**

Chromosomal Sex. Genetic sex, XX or XY, is established at the time of fertilization of the ovum. Thereafter, however, for the first 8 weeks, the development of male and female embryos is identical. It is the differentiation of the primordial gonad into testis or ovary that heralds the establishment of gonadal sex (Fig. 7–25).

Gonadal Sex. In the process of gonadal differentiation, it is known that the Y-chromosome is of paramount importance in the direction of gonadal differentiation into testes. It is reasonably clear that the testis-determining gene is located near the centromere on the short arm of the Y-chromosome. This subject was reviewed in an in-depth analysis by George and Wilson (1988). Nonetheless, it is still not clear how the Y-chromosome directs testicular differentiation. It is known that there are male-specific, cell-surface proteins, such as the H-Y antigen(s), that are correlated with testicular development in many species. Indeed, evidence has been presented that H-Y antigen actually induces testicular differentiation (Ohno and associates, 1978). It may be, however, that the structural gene that specifies H-Y antigen is located on an autosome with positive regulation caused by a locus on the Y-chromosome and a negative regulatory control caused by a locus on the X-chromosome (Wolf, 1981). As pointed out by Silvers and colleagues (1982), however, there are likely a number of male-specific antigens; and at present, no invariable relation can be defined between the presence of a given antigen and the development of a testis.

The contribution of chromosomal sex to gonadal sex may be best deciphered from an understanding of the apparent paradox presented by the XX male. The incidence of 46,XX phenotypic human males is estimated to be about 1 in 20,000 to 24,000 male births. Most cases in the human seem to result from interchange of a Y-chromosome fragment with the X-chromosome. Translocation of a testis-determining region of the Y-chromosome to the X-chromosome during meiosis of male germ cells gives rise to this possibility (George and Wilson, 1988).

Nonetheless, with establishment of the gonadal sex, there is the very rapid development of the phenotypic sex. It should be emphasized, however, that there is an appreciable difference in the *determination* of sex and in *sexual differentiation,* the latter being determined by fetal testicular secretory products.

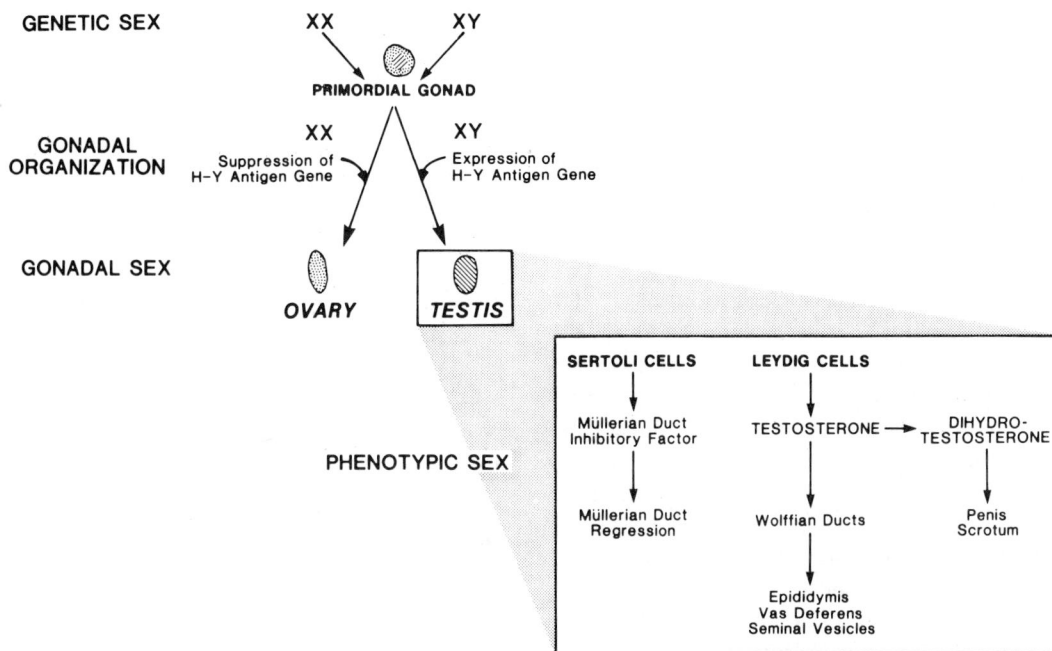

Fig. 7–25. Sexual differentiation. Genetic sex is established at the time of fertilization of the ovum. At a time thereafter, the primordial gonad is acted upon by male-specific substances (e.g., H-Y antigen) that effect the organization of the gonad as a testis, the secretions of which effect male phenotypic sex differentiation.

Phenotypic Sex. The urogenital tract of the human fetus is identical in the two sexes before the eighth week of gestation. Thereafter, development (differentiation) of the internal and external genitalia of the male phenotype is dependent upon testicular function.

The fundamental experiments to determine the role of the testis in male sexual differentiation were conducted by a French anatomist, Alfred Jost. Ultimately, he established that the induced-phenotype is male and that secretions from the gonad, including the ovary, are not necessary for female differentiation.

Fetal Castration. Jost and associates (1973) found that if castration of the rabbit fetus were conducted before differentiation of the genital anlagen, all newborns were phenotypic females with female external genitalia; and the müllerian ducts had developed into uterus, fallopian tubes, and upper vagina.

Fetal Castration Plus Testis Implant. If castration of the fetus were conducted before differentiation of the genital anlagen and this was followed by implantation of a testis on one side, the phenotype of all fetuses was male; the external genitalia of such fetuses was masculinized; and on the side of the testicular implant, there was wolffian duct development in that a vas deferens, epididymis, and seminal vesicle were formed. On the side of the testicular implant, müllerian structures—the uterine horn and fallopian tube—were not present. On the other hand, the müllerian duct did develop on the side of castration in which there was no testis graft.

Fetal Castration Plus Androgen Pellet Implant. Jost also found that if after castration of the fetus, at the sexually indifferent stage, a testosterone pellet were implanted on one side (in the site of a removed gonad), the external genitalia masculinized, as did the wolffian duct; but the müllerian duct did not regress, that is, the uterine horn and fallopian tubes did develop in spite of the "androgen" implant.

These fundamental observations, together with those of Wilson and collaborators (Wilson and Gloyna, 1970; Wilson and Lasnitzki, 1971), form the basic framework of our understanding of the mechanisms of sexual differentiation.

Testosterone Conversion to 5α-Dihydrotestosterone. Wilson and Gloyna (1970) demonstrated convincingly that in most androgen-responsive tissues, the androgen testosterone is converted to 5α-dihydrotestosterone in a reaction catalyzed by the enzyme 5α-reductase. In these tissues, androgen action is amplified by way of this 5α-reduced metabolite. The 5α-dihydrotestosterone is bound to the androgen-binding protein (the androgen receptor) and the steroid-receptor protein complex in the nucleus becomes associated with chromatin. Thus, in the genital tubercle and urogenital sinus, testosterone acts only after conversion to 5α-dihydrotestosterone.

There is a notable and important exception, however, to this generalization for testosterone action in genital tissues. Namely, Wilson and Lasnitzki (1971) also demonstrated that testosterone, as testosterone, acts on the wolffian duct of the embryo to cause development of the male ductal system; indeed, this action of testosterone is expressed before 5α-reductase activity is detectable in this tissue.

Physiological and Biomolecular Basis of Sexual Differentiation. Based on these observations, the biochemical basis of sexual differentiation can be formulated as illustrated diagrammatically in Figure 7–25 and summarized as follows:

1. Genetic sex is established at the time of fertilization of the ovum.
2. Gonadal sex is determined by organizing factor(s) that may arise on autosomes, but by way of genic action that is affected positively by factors encoded on loci on the Y-chromosome or negatively by factors encoded on loci on the X-chromosome. By way of these coordinated processes, differentiation of the primitive gonad as a testis is accomplished.
3. The fetal testis secretes a proteinaceous substance called *müllerian-inhibiting substance,* a dimeric glycoprotein (M_r about 140,000) that acts locally (i.e., not as a hormone) to cause regression of the müllerian duct—that is, it prevents the development of uterus, fallopian tube, and upper vagina. Müllerian-inhibiting substance is produced by the Sertoli cells of the seminiferous tubules; importantly, the seminiferous tubules appear in fetal gonads before the Leydig cells, the cellular site of origin of testosterone. And müllerian-inhibiting substance is produced by Sertoli cells even before differentiation of the seminiferous tubules. Therefore, regression of the müllerian ducts is initiated at a time in fetal development before testosterone secretion commences. Müllerian-inhibiting substance acts locally, near its site of formation; therefore, if a testis were absent on one side, the müllerian duct on that side would persist and the uterus and fallopian tubes would develop from it. It also may be that müllerian-inhibiting substance is important in testicular descent, because the testes of newborn boys with cryptorchidism contain less müllerian-inhibiting substance than those of normal newborns.
4. The fetal testis, initially under the influence of the action of chorionic gonadotropin (hCG) and later fetal pituitary LH, secretes testosterone that acts directly on the wolffian duct to effect the development of the vas deferens, epididymides, and seminal vesicles. Testosterone, of fetal testicular origin, enters the blood, reaches the genital tubercle and urogenital sinus, and in these tissues, testosterone is converted to 5α-dihydrotestosterone, the active androgen that brings about the virilization of the external genitalia.

Genital Ambiguity of the Newborn. **The development of ambiguous genitalia is brought about, invariably, by abnormal androgenic representation in utero.** This means, simply, excessive androgen expression for an embryo that was destined to be female or too little androgenic representation for an embryo or a fetus that was destined to be male.

In the case of the fetus destined to be male, inadequate androgenic representation may be caused by deficient fetal testicular secretion of testosterone or else by a tissue deficiency in responsiveness to testosterone or 5α-dihydrotestosterone in tissues that nominally respond to androgen.

Based on these premises, we believe that all abnormalities of sexual differentiation can be assigned to one of three general categories:

1. Female pseudohermaphroditism
2. Male pseudohermaphroditism
3. Dysgenetic gonads and true hermaphroditism

Category 1. Female pseudohermaphroditism. In this category, abnormalities are found that conform to several guidelines as follow: (1) müllerian-inhibiting substance is *not* produced; (2) androgen exposure of the embryo and fetus is variable; (3) karyotype is 46,XX; and (4) ovaries are present. Therefore, all subjects in this category were destined to be female by virtue of genetic and gonadal sex.

Thus, the only abnormality that can occur is androgenic excess. Because müllerian-inhibiting substance was not produced (ovaries, not testes, are present), the uterus, fallopian tubes, and upper vagina are present in each subject of this category. If such embryos were exposed to a small androgenic excess reasonably late in fetal development, the only abnormality would be slight clitoral hypertrophy, with an otherwise normal female phenotype. With somewhat greater androgenic excess, clitoral hypertrophy and posterior labial fusion may develop. With progressively increasing androgenic excess, somewhat earlier in embryonic development, there is greater virilization. This process of virilization can proceed through the formation of labioscrotal folds, the development of a urogenital sinus (in which the vagina empties into the posterior urethra), and even to the development of a penile urethra with scrotal formation, the "empty scrotum" syndrome.

The cause of female pseudohermaphroditism is excessive androgen for a fetus that was destined to be female. The androgenic excess most commonly arises by androgen secretion from the fetal adrenal because of increased secretion of androgen or androgen prehormones as a result of enzymatic defects in the pathway to cortisol formation in the adrenal cortex, that is, congenital adrenal hyperplasia. With inadequate cortisol synthesis, it is presumed that ACTH secretion is elevated.

Excessive stimulation of the adrenals leads to excessive secretion of precursors of cortisol and metabolites thereof, which include androgens or androgenic prehormones that can be converted, principally by way of androstenedione to testosterone, in extraglandular tissues. The enzyme deficiency may involve any of the five enzymatic reactions in the pathway to cortisol biosynthesis: cholesterol side-chain cleavage, 3β-hydroxysteroid dehydrogenase, 17α-hydroxylase/17,20-lyase, 21-hydroxylase, or 11β-hydroxylase.

Another cause of female pseudohermaphroditism is androgen excess in the fetus that is caused by increased androgen formation in the maternal compartment. Excess androgen in the mother may arise by secretion from maternal ovaries (i.e., hyperreactio lutealis), or from tumors of the maternal ovary (e.g., luteomas, arrhenoblastomas [Sertoli/Leydig cell tumor], or hilar cell tumors).

Most commonly, however, the female fetus of a pregnant woman with an androgen-secreting tumor is not virilized. During most, and perhaps all, of pregnancy, the female fetus is protected from excess androgen in the maternal circulation because of the extraordinary capacity of the trophoblast to convert aromatizable C_{19} steroids (androgens) to estrogens. The only exception to this generality was the one case report of placental aromatase deficiency, causing maternal and fetal virilization, as described in Chapters 6 and 12.

In addition, if certain drugs are given to pregnant women, virilization of their female fetuses may occur. Most commonly, such drugs are synthetic progestins. It is not altogether clear how progestins cause virilization of the female fetus. On the one hand, some of these compounds, especially those of the 19-nortestosterone configuration, may act on fetal tissues as androgens. On the other hand, these agents may act to inhibit aromatization in the placenta and thus allow the transfer to the fetus of androgens that escape aromatization.

Importantly, all subjects of category 1 (except the subject with aromatase deficiency) can be normal, fertile women if the proper diagnosis is made and appropriate therapy is initiated.

Category 2. Male pseudohermaphroditism. In this category, we find abnormalities that conform to several guidelines as follow: (1) müllerian-inhibiting substance is produced; (2) androgenic representation is variable; (3) karyotype is 46,XY; and (4) testes, or else no gonads, are present. All subjects in this category were destined to be male by virtue of genetic sex. Thus, the abnormalities in sexual differentiation are the result of incomplete virilization, that is, inadequate androgenic representation.

Incomplete masculinization of the fetus can be caused by inadequate production of testosterone by the fetal testis or else by diminished responsiveness of the genital anlagen to normal quantities of androgen, including failure of in situ formation of 5α-dihydrotestosterone in tissues destined to form the external genitalia.

Because müllerian-inhibiting substance was produced during embryonic life in these subjects (testes present, at least at some time in embryonic life), the uterus, fallopian tubes, and upper vagina did not develop.

DIMINISHED FETAL TESTICULAR TESTOSTERONE SECRETION. *Deficient fetal testicular testosterone production* may occur if there is an enzymatic defect in the testis that involves any one of the four enzymes (which catalyze five enzymatic reactions) in the biosynthetic pathway to testosterone formation (Fig. 7–26). Defects in each of these enzymatic reactions, as a cause of abnormal sex

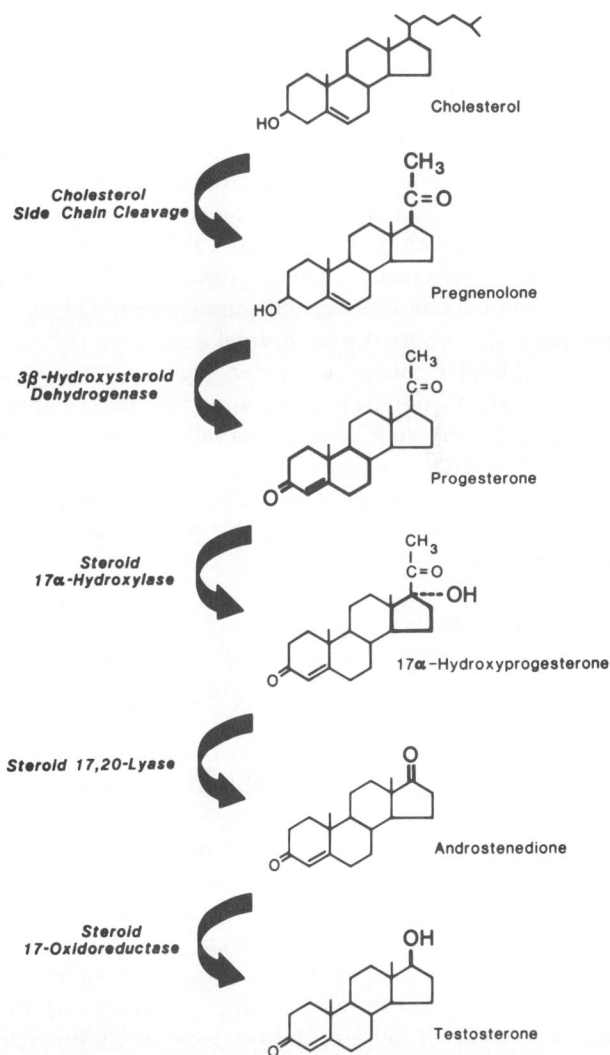

Fig. 7–26. Biosynthetic pathway of testosterone formation in the testis. There are five enzymatic reactions involved in the conversion of cholesterol to testosterone. A defect in each of these enzymes has been identified as the cause of inadequate fetal testicular testosterone production.

differentiation, have been described. Enzymatic defects in testicular testosterone biosynthesis give rise to decreased rates of fetal testosterone secretion, and incomplete masculinization of the external genitalia is the consequence. The phenotype of such newborns is variable in the degree of ambiguity, because the degree of enzyme deficiency varies, and thereby the deficiency in fetal testosterone production also varies.

EMBRYONIC TESTICULAR REGRESSION. Embryonic or fetal loss of testes gives rise to a phenotype that is dependent upon the time in embryonic life that the testes regressed. If the testes regress during embryonic or fetal life, there will be, thereafter, deficient testosterone production. Such an occurrence has been referred to as embryonic testicular regression (Edman and associates, 1977).

The time course of gonadal development and sexual differentiation is illustrated in Figure 7–27. Edman and associates (1977) analyzed the phenotypes of reported cases of agonadism in 46,XY persons, and in 3 cases of their own. They compared these findings with those that would be expected to occur if the testes regressed at various stages of development according to embryological findings of the time course of human sexual differentiation (Jirasek, 1967, 1970, 1971). They found that a spectrum of phenotypes (cases *a* to *i*, Fig. 7–27) had been described, and among affected persons the phenotypes varied from normal female with absent uterus, fallopian tubes, and upper vagina, to that of a normal male phenotype but with anorchia. Because müllerian duct regression commences before virilization is initiated in embryonic life, such a spectrum of phenotypes was to be expected if testicular regression were to occur at various times during the process of sexual differentiation.

ANDROGEN RESISTANCE. Deficiencies in androgen responsiveness are caused by an abnormal androgen receptor protein in androgen-responsive tissues, or else may be due to failure of conversion of testosterone to 5α-dihydrotestosterone in such tissues because of deficient 5α-reductase enzyme activity (Wilson and MacDonald, 1978).

The most extreme form of the disorders of androgen resistance is that of *testicular feminization*. In this entity, there appears to be little or no tissue responsiveness to androgen. In affected subjects, there is a female phenotype and a short, blind-ending vagina, no uterus or fallopian tubes, and no wolffian duct structures. At the expected time of puberty, testosterone levels in such women rise to values similar to or greater than those found in normal adult men. Nonetheless, virilization does not occur, and even sexual hair (pubic and axillary hair) does not develop because of end-organ resistance to androgen action. Presumably, because of androgen resistance at the level of the brain and pituitary, LH

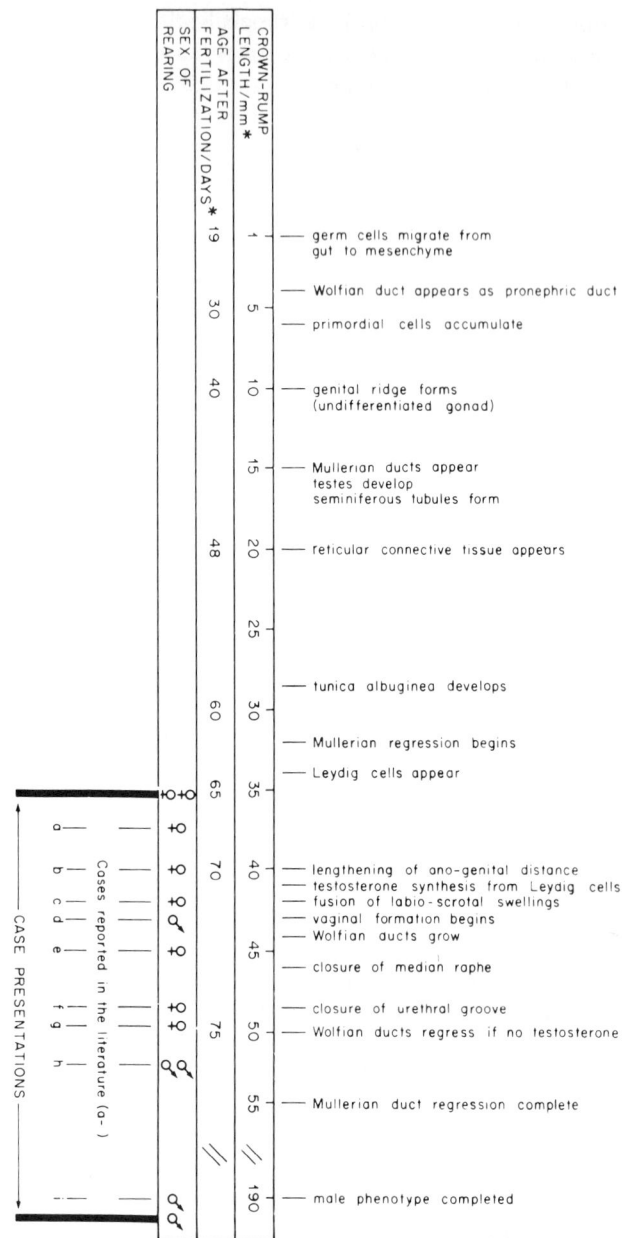

Fig. 7–27. The temporal relations of the sequence or morphological changes that occur during male embryogenesis, and a comparison of this sequence to the phenotypes reported in subjects with embryonic testicular regression.

levels are elevated in these women. In response to LH, in high concentrations there is also increased testicular secretion of estrogen compared with that found in normal men (MacDonald and colleagues, 1979). The increased estrogen, together with the absence of androgen responsiveness, may act in concert to cause feminization (breast development).

In the disorder referred to as *incomplete testicular feminization,* there appears to be slight androgen responsiveness. In such subjects, there is ordinarily modest clitoral hypertrophy at birth; but at the expected time of puberty, virilization does not occur, although pubic and axillary hair do develop. These women also develop feminine breasts, presumably through the same endocrine mechanisms as in women with the complete form of testicular feminization (Madden and co-workers, 1975).

A third syndrome of androgen resistance has been referred to as *familial male pseudohermaphroditism,* type I (Walsh and colleagues, 1974). This entity is also commonly referred to as *Reifenstein syndrome,* but constitutes a spectrum of abnormalities of genital virilization varying from a phenotype similar to that of women with incomplete testicular feminization to that of a male phenotype with only a bifid scrotum, infertility, and gynecomastia. In these subjects, androgen resistance was also established by the demonstration of diminished 5α-dihydrotestosterone-binding capacity in fibroblasts grown in culture from genital skin biopsies.

A fourth form of androgen resistance is caused by 5α-*reductase deficiency* in androgen-responsive tissues. Because androgen action in the genital tubercle and urogenital sinus is mediated by the action of 5α-dihydrotestosterone, in persons with 5α-reductase deficiency there are female external genitalia (modest clitoral hypertrophy). But because androgen action in the wolffian duct of the embryo is mediated by testosterone itself, in such persons there are well-developed epididymides, seminal vesicles, and vas deferens, and the male ejaculatory ducts empty into the vagina (Walsh and associates, 1974).

Causes of Androgen Resistance

5α-Reductase Deficiency. Andersson and co-workers (1989, 1991) have demonstrated that there are two genes that encode for steroid 5α-reductase, genes 1 and 2. The 5α-reductase gene 1 is expressed in many tissues. The 5α-reductase gene 2 is primarily expressed in androgen-responsive tissues. It is this gene that is abnormally expressed in persons with 5α-reductase deficiency. In persons with abnormalities in sexual differentiation, the high level of 5α-reductase gene 2 expression that is present in androgen-responsive tissues of nonaffected persons is missing.

Deficiency in Androgen Receptor. Many different abnormalities of the gene encoding for the androgen receptor have been demonstrated. This accounts for the wide variability in androgen responsiveness among persons in whom the androgen receptor protein is abnormal (McPhaul and associates, 1991).

A composite photograph of the genitalia of subjects with each of the four types of androgen resistance is shown in Figure 7–28.

Category 3. In this category of our classification, we find subjects with abnormalities of sexual differentiation that conform to several guidelines as follows: (1) müllerian-inhibiting substance was not produced; (2) fetal androgen exposure among subjects was variable; (3) karyotype varies among subjects and is commonly abnormal; and (4) neither ovaries nor testes are present (but rarely, both are). In all of the subjects of this category, there is a uterus, fallopian tubes, and upper vagina.

In the majority of subjects in category 3, dysgenetic gonads are found. With the typical case of gonadal dysgenesis (e.g., those with Turner syndrome) there is a female phenotype; but at the time of expected puberty, sexual infantilism persists. In some persons with gonadal dysgenesis, there are ambiguous genitalia, a finding that is indicative that an abnormal gonad produced androgen, albeit in small amounts, during embryonic development. Generally, in such subjects, we find mixed gonadal dysgenesis (such as, a dysgenetic gonad on one side and an abnormal testis or dysontogenetic tumor on the other side). In most subjects with true hermaphroditism, the guidelines for category 3 are met. True hermaphrodites are those persons in whom both ovarian and testicular tissues are present; and in particular, the germ cells (ova and sperm) of both sexes are found in the abnormal gonads.

Preliminary Diagnosis of the Cause of Genital Ambiguity. A preliminary diagnosis of the etiology and pathogenesis of genital ambiguity can be made at the time of birth of an affected child. By physical and ultrasonic examination of the newborn, the experienced examiner can ascertain whether the child has a uterus. If the uterus is present, the diagnosis must be female pseudohermaphroditism, testicular or gonadal dysgenesis, or true hermaphroditism. A family history of congenital adrenal hyperplasia is helpful. If the uterus is not present, the diagnosis is male pseudohermaphroditism. Androgen resistance and enzymatic defects in testicular testosterone biosynthesis are familial.

Sex Assignment. The critical decision of sex assignment by the obstetrician, in our view, is usually easy, although sometimes a painful decision to make. In our judgment, any newborn with ambiguity of the genitalia so severe as to represent more than hypospadias should be designated as female. This conclusion is reached on the basis of several considerations: (1) all persons in category 1 of our classification (i.e., female pseudohermaphroditism) can be normal, fertile women; (2) the subjects of category 2 of this classification either cannot produce testosterone or else are refractory to its action, and all subjects of category 2 will be infertile; and (3) currently, reconstruction of the penis in persons with androgen resistance is possible, but the achievement of male sexual function, let alone fertility, is not.

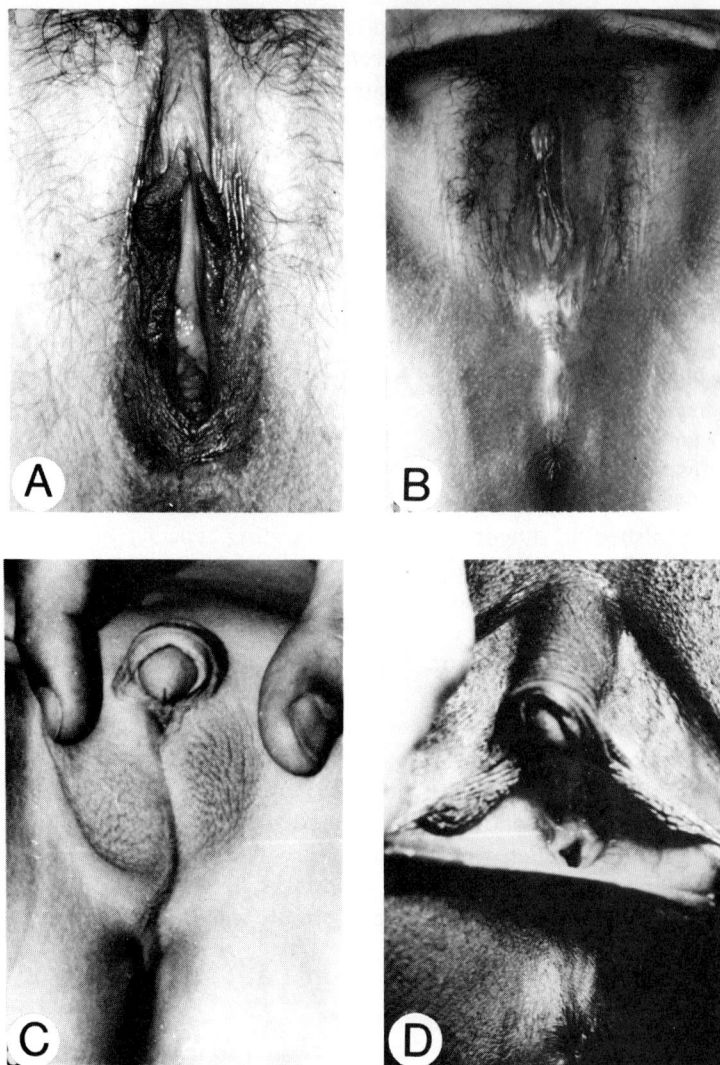

Fig. 7–28. External genitalia of representative patients with male pseudohermaphroditism due to androgen resistance. **A.** Testicular feminization. **B.** Incomplete testicular feminization. **C.** Familial male pseudohermaphroditism, type I (Reifenstein syndrome). **D.** 5α-reductase deficiency. (From Wilson and MacDonald, 1978.)

References

Abbas SK, Pickard DW, Illingworth D, Storer J, Purdie DW, Moniz C, Dixit M, Caple IW, Ebeling PR, Rodda CP, Martin TJ, Care AD: Measurement of PTH-rP protein in extracts of fetal parathyroid glands and placental membranes. J Endocrinol 124:319, 1990

Adam PAJ, Teramo K, Raiha N, Gitlin D, Schwartz R: Human fetal insulin metabolism early in gestation: Response to acute elevation of the fetal glucose concentration and placental transfer of human insulin-I-131. Diabetes 18:409, 1969

Adinolfi M: Human complement: Onset and site of synthesis during fetal life. Am J Dis Child 131:1015, 1977

Aherne W, Dunnill MS: Morphometry of the human placenta. Br Med Bull 22:1, 1966

Aizawa Y, Mueller GC: The effect in vivo and in vitro of estrogens on lipid synthesis in the rat uterus. J Biol Chem 236:381, 1961

Altshuler G: Immunologic competence of the immature human fetus. Obstet Gynecol 43:811, 1974

Andersson S, Berman DM, Jenkins EP, Russell DW: Deletion of steroid 5 alpha-reductase 2 gene in male pseudohermaphroditism. Nature 354:159, 1991

Andersson S, Bishop RW, Russell DW: Expression cloning and regulation of steroid 5 alpha-reductase, an enzyme essential for male sexual differentiation. J Biol Chem 264:16249, 1989

Assali NS: In Gluck L (ed): Modern Perinatal Medicine. Chicago, Year Book, 1974

Assali NS, Bekey GA, Morrison LW: Fetal and neonatal circulation. In Assali NS (ed): Biology of Gestation, Vol II. The Fetus and Neonate. New York, Academic Press, 1968

Avery ME, Mead J: Surface properties in relation to atelectasis and hyaline membrane disease. Am J Dis Child 97:517, 1959

Ballard PL: Hormones and lung maturation. Monographs in Endocrinology, Vol XXVIII. New York. Springer-Verlag, 1986

Banting FG, Best CH: Pancreatic extracts. J Lab Clin Med 1:464, 1922

Bashore RA, Smith F, Schenker S: Placental transfer and disposition of bilirubin in the pregnant monkey. Am J Obstet Gynecol 103:950, 1969

Batenburg JJ, Klazinga W, Van Golde LMG: Regulation of phosphatidylglycerol and phosphatidylinositol synthesis in alveolar type II cells isolated from adult rat lung. FEBS Lett 147:171, 1982

Bearn JG: Role of fetal pituitary and adrenal glands in the development of the fetal thymus of the rabbit. Endocrinology 80:979, 1967

Belcher DP: A child weighing 25 pounds at birth. JAMA 67:950, 1916

Bleasdale JE, Wallis P, MacDonald PC, Johnston JM: Characterization of the forward and reverse reactions catalyzed by CDP-diacylglycerol: Inositol transferase in rabbit lung tissue. Biochem Biophys Acta 575:135, 1979

Boddy K, Dawes GS: Fetal breathing. Br Med Bull 31:3, 1975

Bozzetti P, Ferrari MM, Marconi AM, Ferrazzi E, Pardi G, Makowski EL, Battaglia FC: The relationship of maternal and fetal glucose concentrations in the human from midgestation until term. Metabolism 37:358, 1988

Brash AR, Hickey DE, Graham TP, Stahlman MT, Oates JA, Cotton RB: Pharmacokinetics of indomethacin in the neonate: Relation of plasma indomethacin levels to response of the ductus arteriosus. N Engl J Med 305:67, 1981

Brinsmead MW, Liggins, GC: Somadomedin-like activity, prolactin, growth hormone and insulin in human cord blood. Aust NZ J Obstet Gynecol 19:129, 1979

Brown AR: In Assali NS (ed): Biology of Gestation, Vol II, The Fetus and Neonate. New York, Academic Press, 1968, p 361

Browning AJF, Butt WR, Lynch SS, Shakespear RA: Maternal plasma concentrations of β-lipotropin, β-endorphin and γ-lipotrophin throughout pregnancy. Br J Obstet Gynaecol 90:1147, 1983

Carr D: Chromosome studies in abortuses and stillborn infants. Lancet 2:603, 1963

Chan L, Jackson RL, O'Malley BW: Synthesis of very low density lipoproteins in the cockerel: Effects of estrogen. J Clin Invest 58:368, 1976

Chard T, Hudson CN, Edwards CRW, Boyd NRH: Release of oxytocin and vasopressin by the human foetus during labour. Nature 234:352, 1971

Chez RA, Mintz DH, Reynolds WA, Hutchinson DL: Maternal–fetal plasma glucose relationships in late monkey pregnancy. Am J Obstet Gynecol 121:938, 1975

Clements JA: Surface tension of lung extracts. Proc Soc Exp Biol Med 95:170, 1957

Clymann RI, Heymann MA: Pharmacology of the ductus arteriosus. Pediatr Clin North Am 28:77, 1981

Davis ME, Potter EL: Intrauterine respiration of the human fetus. JAMA 131:1194, 1946

Dawes GS: The umbilical circulation. Am J Obstet Gynecol 84:1634, 1962

DeVane GW, Naden RP, Porter JC, Rosenfeld CR: Mechanism of arginine vasopressin release in the sheep fetus. Pediatr Res 16:504, 1982

DeVane GW, Porter JC: An apparent stress-induced release of arginine vasopressin by human neonates. J Clin Endocrinol Metab 51:1412, 1980

De Verdier CH, Garby L: Low binding of 2,3-diphosphoglycerate to hemoglobin F. Scand J Clin Lab Invest 23:149, 1969

Dickey RP, Robertson AF: Newborn estrogen excretion. Am J Obstet Gynecol 104:551, 1969

Dolman CL: Characteristic configuration of fetal brains from 22 to 40 weeks gestation at two week intervals. Arch Pathol Lab Med 101:193, 1977

Duenhoelter JH, Pritchard JA: Fetal respiration. A review. Am J Obstet Gynecol 129:326, 1977

Duenhoelter JH, Pritchard JA: Fetal respiration: Quantitative measurements of amnionic fluid inspired near term by human and rhesus fetuses. Am J Obstet Gynecol 125:306, 1976

Edman CD, Winters AJ, Porter JC, Wilson J, MacDonald PC: Embryonic testicular regression. A clinical spectrum of XY agonadal individual. Obstet Gynecol 49:208, 1977

Epstein M, Chez RA, Oakes GK, Mintz DH: Fetal pancreatic glucagon responses in glucose-intolerant nonhuman primate pregnancy. Am J Obstet Gynecol 127:268, 1977

Estelles A, Aznar J, Gilabert J, Parrilla JJ: Dysfunctional plasminogen in full-term newborn. Pediatr Res 14:1180, 1980

Fadel HE, Abraham EC: Minor fetal hemoglobins in relation to gestational age. Am J Obstet Gynecol 141:704, 1981

Farrell PM, Avery ME: Hyaline membrane disease. Am Rev Respir Dis 111:657, 1975

Finne PH: Antenatal diagnosis of the anemia in erythroblastosis. Acta Paediatr Scand 55:609, 1966

Fisher DA: The unique endocrine milieu of the fetus. J Clin Invest 78:603, 1986

Fisher DA: Control of thyroid hormone production in the fetus. In Albrecht ED, Pepe GJ (eds): Research in Perinatal Medicine, Vol IV: Perinatal Endocrinology. Ithaca, NY, Perinatology Press, 1985, p 55

Fisher DA: Ross Conference on Obstetrical Decisions and Neonatal Outcome, San Diego, 1979

Fisher DA: Fetal thyroid hormone metabolism. Contemp Ob/Gyn 3:47, 1975

Fisher DA, Klein AH: Thyroid development and disorders of thyroid function in the newborn. N Engl J Med 304:702, 1981

Fliegner JR, Fortune DW, Eggers TR: Premature rupture of the membranes, oligohydramnios and pulmonary hypoplasia. Aust NZ J Obstet Gynaecol 21:77, 1981

Foley ME, Isherwood DM, McNicol GP: Viscosity, haematocrit, fibrinogen and plasma proteins in maternal and cord blood. Br J Obstet Gynaecol 85:500, 1978

Fuchs F: Volume of amniotic fluid at various states of pregnancy. Clin Obstet Gynecol 9:449, 1966

Gelato M, Marshall S, Boudreau M, Bruni J, Campbell GA, Meit J: Effects of thyroid and ovaries on prolactin binding activity in rat liver. Endocrinology 96:1292, 1975

George FW, Wilson JD: Sex determination and differentiation. In Knobil E, Neill J (eds): The Physiology of Reproduction. New York, Raven Press, 1988, p 3

Gilbert RD, Lis L, Longo LD: Temperature effects on O_2 affinity of fetal blood. Paper presented at the 30th annual meeting of the Society for Gynecologic Investigation, Washington, DC, March 17–20, 1983

Gillibrand PN: Changes in amniotic fluid volume with advancing pregnancy. J Obstet Gynaecol Br Commonw 76:527, 1969a

Gillibrand PN: Changes in the electrolytes, urea, and osmolality of the amniotic fluid with advancing pregnancy. J Obstet Gynaecol Br Commonw 76:898, 1969b

Gitlin D: Protein transport across the placenta and protein turnover between amnionic fluid, maternal and fetal circulation. In Moghissi KS and Hafez ESE (eds): The Placenta. Springfield, IL, Thomas, 1974

Gitlin D: Development and metabolism of the immune globulins. In Kaga BM, Stiehm ER (eds): Immunologic Incompetence. Chicago, Year Book, 1971

Gitlin D, Kumate J, Morales C, Noriega L, Arevalo N: The turnover of amniotic fluid protein in the human conceptus. Am J Obstet Gynecol 113:632, 1972

Gluck L, Kulovich MV, Borer RC: The interpretation and significance of the lecithin–sphingomyelin ratio in amniotic fluid. Am J Obstet Gynecol 120:142, 1974

Gluck L, Kulovich MV, Borer RC, Brenner PH, Anderson GG, Spellacy WN: Diagnosis of the respiratory distress syndrome by amniocentesis. Am J Obstet Gynecol 109:440, 1971

Gluck L, Kulovich MV, Eidelman AI, Cordero L, Khazin AF: Biochemical development of surface activity in mammalian lung, IV. Pulmonary lecithin synthesis in the human fetus and newborn and etiology of the respiratory distress syndrome. Pediatr Res 6:81, 1972

Gluck L, Landowne RA, Kulovich MV: Biochemical development of surface activity in mammalian lung, III. Structural changes in lung lecithin during development of the rabbit fetus and newborn. Pediatr Res 4:352, 1970

Gluck L, Motoyama EK, Smits HL, Kulovich MV: The biochemical development of surface activity in mammalian lung, I. The surface-active phospholipids; the separation and distribution of surface-active lecithin in the lung of the developing rabbit fetus. Pediatr Res 1:237, 1967

Gresham EL, Rankin JHG, Makowski EL, Meschia G, Battaglia FC: An evaluation of fetal renal function in unstressed pregnancies. J Clin Invest 51:149, 1972

Griffin JE, Wilson JD: Disorders of sexual differentiation. In Walsh PC, Gittes RF, Perlmutter AD, Stamey RA (eds): Campbell's Urology. Philadelphia, Saunders, 1986, p 1819

Gruenwald P: Growth of the human foetus. In McLaren A (ed): Advances in Reproductive Physiology. New York, Academic Press, 1967

Grumbach MM, Kaplan SL: Fetal pituitary hormones and the maturation of central nervous system regulation of anterior pituitary function. In Gluck L (ed): Modern Perinatal Medicine. Chicago, Year Book, 1974

Haase W: Maternity annual report for 1875. Charite Annalen 2:669, 1875

Hallman M, Kulovich MV, Kirkpatrick E, Sugarman RG, Gluck L: Phosphatidylinositol and phosphatidylglycerol in amniotic fluid: Indices of lung maturity. Am J Obstet Gynecol 125:613, 1976

Hamilton WJ, Mossman HW: Human Embryology, 4th ed. Baltimore, Williams & Wilkins, 1972

Hauth JC, Parker CR Jr, MacDonald PC, Porter JC, Johnston JM: A role of fetal prolactin in lung maturation. Obstet Gynecol 51:81, 1978

Hayward AR: The human fetus and newborn: Development of the immune response. Birth Defects 19:289, 1983

Hellman P, Ridefelt P, Juhlin C, Akerstrom G, Rastad J, Gylfe E: Parathyroid-like regulation of parathyroid hormone-related protein release and cytoplasmic calcium in cytotrophoblast cells of human placenta. Arch Biochem Biophys 293:174, 1992

Henriksson P, Hedner V, Nilsson IM, Boehm J, Robertson B, Lorand L: Fibrin-stabilization factor XIII in the fetus and the newborn infant. Pediatr Res 8:789, 1974

Hocheim H: Cited by Kiedel W and Gluck L in Scarpelli (ed): Pulmonary Physiology of the Fetus, Newborn, and Child. Philadelphia, Lea & Febiger, 1975

Hoffman DR, Truong CT, Johnston JM: The role of platelet-activating factor in human fetal lung maturation. Am J Obstet Gynecol 155:70, 1986

Hoffman DR, White RG, Angle MJ, Maki N, Johnston JM: Platelet-activating factor induces glycogen degradation in fetal rabbit lung in utero. J Biol Chem 263:9316, 1988

Holmberg C, Perheentupa J, Launiala K, Hallman N: Congenital chloride diarrhoea. Arch Dis Child 52:255, 1977

Huisman THJ, Schroder WA, Brown AK: Changes in the nature of human fetal hemoglobin during the first year of life. Paper presented at Meeting of Society for Pediatric Research, Atlantic City, NJ, May 1, 1970

Jirasek JE: Development of the genital system in human embryos and fetuses. Development of the Genital System and Male Pseudohermaphroditism. Baltimore, Johns Hopkins Press, 1971

Jirasek JE: The relationship between differentiation of the testicle, genital ducts and external genitalia in fetal and postnatal life. In Rosenberg E, Paulsen CA (eds): The Human Testis: Advances in Experimental Medicine and Biology, Vol X. New York, Plenum, 1970

Jirasek JE: The relationship between the structure of the testis and differentiation of the external genitalia and phenotype in man. In Wolstenholme GEW, O'Connor M (eds): Ciba Foundation Colloquia on Endocrinology: Endocrinology of the Testis. Boston, Little, Brown, 1967

Johnson JWC, Mitzner W, Lindon WJ, Palmer AE, Scott R, Kearney K: Glucocorticoids and the rhesus fetal lung. Am J Obstet Gynecol 130:905, 1978

Jost A, Vigier B, Prepin J: Studies on sex differentiation in mammals. Recent Prog Horm Res 29:1, 1973

Juhlin C, Lundgren S, Johansson H, Lorentzen J, Rask L, Larsson E, Rastad J, Akerstrom G, Klareskog L: 500-Kilodalton calcium sensor regulating cytoplasmic Ca^{2+} in cytotrophoblast cells of human placenta. J Biol Chem 265:8275, 1990

Kaplan S: Disorders of the endocrine system. In Assali NS (ed): Pathophysiology of Gestation, Vol III. Fetal and Neonatal Disorders. New York, Academic Press, 1972

Kasper CK, Hoag MS, Aggeler PM, Stone S: Blood clotting factors in pregnancy: Factor VIII concentrations in normal and AHF-deficient women. Obstet Gynecol 24:242, 1964

Katz FH, Beck P, Makowski EL: The renin–aldosterone system in mother and fetus at term. Am J Obstet Gynecol 118:51, 1974

Keidel W, Gluck L: Lipid biochemistry and biochemical development of the lung. In Scarpelli E (ed): Pulmonary Physiology of the Fetus, Newborn, and Child. Philadelphia, Lea & Febiger, 1975, p 96

Kelly PA, Posner BI, Friesen HG: Effects of hypophysectomy, ovariectomy, and cycloheximide on specific binding sites for lactogenic hormones in rat liver. Endocrinology 97:1408, 1975

Khosla SS, Rooney SA: Stimulation of fetal lung surfactant production by administration of 17β-estradiol to the maternal rabbit. Am J Obstet Gynecol 133:213, 1979

Kimura RE: Lipid metabolism in the fetal–placental unit. In Cowett RM (ed): Principles of Perinatal–Neonatal Metabolism. New York, Springer-Verlag, 1991, p 291

Klaus MH, Clements JA, Havel RJ: Composition of surface-active material isolated from beef lung. Proc Natl Acad Sci USA 47:185, 1961

Kohler PF: Maturation of the human complement system. J Clin Invest 52:671, 1973

Koldovsky O, Heringova A, Jirsova U, Jirasek JE, Uher J: Transport of glucose against a concentration gradient in everted sacs of jejunum and ileum of human fetuses. Gastroenterology 48:185, 1965

Kurjak A, Kirkinen P, Latin V, Ivankovic D: Ultrasonic assessment of fetal kidney function in normal and complicated pregnancies. Am J Obstet Gynecol 141:266, 1981

Lands WE: Metabolism of glycerolipids: A comparison of lecithin and triglyceride synthesis. J Biol Chem 231:883, 1958

Lazarus JH, John R, Ginsberg J, Hughes IA, Shewring G, Smith BR, Woodhead JS, Hall R: Transient neonatal hyperthyrotrophinaemia: A serum abnormality due to transplacentally acquired antibody to thyroid stimulating hormone. Br Med J 286:592, 1983

Lebenthal E, Lee PC: Interactions of determinants of the ontogeny of the gastrointestinal tract: A unified concept. Pediatr Res 1:19, 1983

Leinonen PK, Jaffe RB: Leydig cell desensitization by human chorionic gonadotropin does not occur in the human fetal testis. J Clin Endocrinol Metab 61:234, 1985

Lemons JA: Fetal placental nitrogen metabolism. Semin Perinatol 3:177, 1979

Liggins GC: Premature delivery of foetal lambs infused with glucocorticoids. J Endocrinol 45:515, 1969

Liggins GC, Howie MB: A controlled trial of antepartum glucocorticoid treatment of prevention of the respiratory distress syndrome in premature infants. Pediatrics 50:515, 1972

Lind R, Kendall A, Hytten FE: The role of the fetus in the formation of amniotic fluid. J Obstet Gynaecol Br Commonw 79:289, 1972

Longo LD: Respiration in the fetal–placental unit. In Cowett RM (ed): Principles of Perinatal–Neonatal Metabolism. New York, Springer-Verlag, 1991, p 304

Longo LD: Respiratory gas exchange in the placenta. In Fishman AP, Farhi LE, Tenney SM (eds): Handbook of Physiology, Sec. 3. The Respiratory System, Vol IV. Gas Exchange. Washington, DC, American Physiological Society, 1987, p 351

Longo L: Disorders of placental transfer. In Assali NS (ed): Pathophysiology of Gestation, Vol II. New York, Academic Press, 1972

Luskey KL, Brown MS, Goldstein JL: Stimulation of the synthesis of very low density lipoproteins in rooster liver by estradiol. J Biol Chem 249:5939, 1974

MacDonald PC, Madden JD, Brenner PF, Wilson JD, Siiteri PK: Origin of estrogen in normal men and in women with testicular feminization. J Clin Endocrinol Metab 49:905, 1979

Madden JD, Walsh PC, MacDonald PC, Wilson JD: Clinical and endocrinological characterization of a patient with syndrome of incomplete testicular feminization. J Clin Endocrinol 41:751, 1975

Mandelbaum B, Evans TN: Life in the amniotic fluid. Am J Obstet Gynecol 104:365, 1969

Martin CB, Murata Y, Petrie RH: Respiratory movements in fetal rhesus monkeys. Am J Obstet Gynecol 119:934, 1974

Mason RJ: Disaturated lecithin concentration of rabbit tissues. Am Rev Respir Dis 107:678, 1973

McPhaul MJ, Marcelli M, Tilley WD, Griffin JE, Wilson JD: Androgen resistance caused by mutations in the androgen receptor gene. FASEB J 5:2910, 1991

Mendelson CR, Chen C, Boggaram V, Zacharias C, Snyder JM: Regulation of the synthesis of the major surfactant apoprotein in fetal rabbit lung tissue. J Biol Chem 261:9938, 1986

Mendelson CR, Johnston JM, MacDonald PC, Snyder JM: Multihormonal regulation of surfactant synthesis by human fetal lung *in vitro*. J Clin Endocrinol Metab 53:307, 1981

Mendelson CR, MacDonald PC, Johnston JM: Estrogen binding in human fetal lung cytosol. Endocrinology 106:368, 1980

Moore KL: The Developing Human: Clinically Oriented Embryology, 4th ed. Philadelphia, Saunders, 1988

Moore KL: The Developing Human, 2nd ed. Philadelphia, Saunders, 1977

Morriss FH Jr, Boyd RDH: Placental transport. In Knobil E, Neill J (eds): The Physiology of Reproduction. New York, Raven, 1988, p 2043

Mulchahey JJ, DiBlasio AM, Martin MC, Blumenfeld Z, Jaffe RB: Hormone production and peptide regulation of the human fetal pituitary gland. Endocr Rev 8:406, 1987

Nielsen NC: Coagulation and fibrinolysin in normal women immediately postpartum and in newborn infants. Acta Obstet Gynecol Scand 48:371, 1969

Obenshain SS, Adam PAJ, King KC, Teramo K, Raivio KO, Raiha N, Schwartz R: Human fetal insulin response to sustained maternal hyperglycemia. N Engl J Med 283:566, 1970

Odom MJ, MacDonald PC, Bleasdale JE: Diabetes and fetal lung maturation. Williams Obstetrics, 17th ed (suppl 7). Norwalk, CT, Appleton & Lange, July/August, 1986

Ohno S, Najai Y, Cicares S: Testicular cells lyso-stripped by H-Y antigen organize ovarian follicle-like aggregates. Cytogenet Cell Genet 20:351, 1978

Oka T, Topper YJ: Hormone-dependent accumulation of rough endoplasmic reticulum in mouse mammary epithelial cells *in vitro*. J Biol Chem 246:7701, 1971

Pasqualini JR, Sumida C, Gelly C: Cytosol and nuclear [^{3}H]oestradiol binding in the foetal tissues of guinea pig. Acta Endocrinol 83:811, 1976

Pataryas HA, Stamatoyannopoulos G: Hemoglobins in human fetuses: Evidence for adult hemoglobin production after the 11th gestational week. Blood 39:688, 1972

Paton JB, Fisher DE, DeLannoy CW, Behram RE: Umbilical blood flow, cardiac output, and organ blood flow in the immature baboon fetus. Am J Obstet Gynecol 117:560, 1973

Pearson HA: Recent advances in hematology. J Pediatr 69:466, 1966

Perrine SP, Greene MF, Cohen RA, Faller DV: A physiological delay in human fetal hemoglobin switching is associated with specific globin DNA hypomethylation. FEBS Lett 228:139, 1988

Pipe NGJ, Smith T, Halliday D, Edmonds CJ, Williams C, Coltart TM: Changes in fat, fat-free mass and body water in human normal pregnancy. Br J Obstet Gynaecol 86:929, 1979

Plentl AA: Physiology of the placenta: III. Dynamics of amniotic fluid. In Assali NS (ed): Biology of Gestation, Vol I. The Maternal Organism. New York, Academic Press, 1968

Polin RA, Husain MK, James LS, Frantz AG: High vasopressin concentrations in human umbilical cord blood—lack of correlation with stress. J Perinat Med 5:114, 1977

Posner BI, Kelly PA: Prolactin receptors in rat liver: Possible induction by prolactin. Science 188:57, 1975

Post M, Foros J, Smith BT: Inhibition of lung maturation by monoclonal antibodies against fibroblast-pneumocyte factor. Nature 308:284, 1984

Pritchard JA: Fetal swallowing and amniotic fluid volume. Obstet Gynecol 28:606, 1966

Pritchard JA: Deglutition by normal and anencephalic fetuses. Obstet Gynecol 25:289, 1965

Quirk JG, Bleasdale JE: Fetal lung maturation in the pregnancy complicated by diabetes mellitus. In DiRenzo GC, Hawkins PF (eds): Perinatal Medicine: Updates and Controversies. London, Wiley, 1984

Quirk JG, MacDonald PC, Johnston JM: Role of fetal pituitary prolactin in fetal lung maturation. Semin Perinatol 6:328, 1982

Read EJ Jr, Platzer PB: Placental metastasis from maternal carcinoma of the lung. Obstet Gynecol 58:387, 1981

Rooney SA, Brehier A: The CDP-choline pathway: Cholinephosphate cytidylyl-transferase. In Farrell PM (ed): Lung Development: Biological and Clinical Perspectives, Vol I. New York, Academic Press, 1982, p 317

Rooney SA, Gross I, Motoyama EK, Warshaw JB: Effects of cortisol and thyroxine on fatty acid and phospholipid biosynthesis in fetal rabbit lung. Physiologist 17:323, 1974

Rosenfeld CR, Porter JC: Arginine vasopressin in the developing fetus. In Albrecht ED, Pepe GJ (eds): Research in Perinatal Medicine, IV. Perinatal Endocrinology. Ithaca, NY, Perinatology Press, 1985, p 91

Rudolph AM, Heymann MA: The fetal circulation. Annu Rev Med 19:195, 1968

Schulman I, Smith CH: Fetal and adult hemoglobins in premature infants. Am J Dis Child 86:354, 1953

Sell EJ, Corrigan JJ Jr: Platelet counts, fibrinogen concentrations, and factor V and factor VIII levels in healthy infants according to gestational age. J Pediatr 82:1028, 1973

Shrand II: Vomiting in utero with intestinal atresia. Pediatrics 49:767, 1972

Siiteri PK, Wilson JD: Testosterone formation and metabolism during male sex differentiation in human embryo. J Clin Endocrinol 38:113, 1974

Silvers WK, Glasser DL, Eicher EM: H-Y antigen, serologically detectable male antigen and sex determination. Cell 28:439, 1982

Smith BT: Fibroblast-pneumocyte factor: Intercellular mediator of glucocorticoid effect on fetal lung. In Stern L (ed): Intensive Care in the Newborn. New York, Masson, 1978, p 25

Smith BT, Torday JS: Factors affecting lecithin synthesis by fetal lung cells in culture. Pediatr Res 8:848, 1974

Smith CM II, Tukey DP, Krivit W, White JG: Fetal red cells (FC) differ in elasticity, viscosity, and adhesion from adult red cells (AC). Pediatr Res 15:588, 1981

Snyder JM, Johnston JM, Mendelson CR: Differentiation of type II cells of human fetal lung in vitro. Cell Tissue Res 220:17, 1981

Snyder JM, Kwun JE, O'Brien JA, Rosenfeld CR, Odom MJ: The concentration of the 35 kDa surfactant apoprotein in amniotic fluid from normal and diabetic pregnancies. Pediatr Res 24:728, 1988.

Snyder JM, Mendelson CR: Insulin inhibits the accumulation of the major lung surfactant apoprotein in human fetal lung explants maintained *in vitro.* Endocrinology 120:1250, 1987

Spellacy WN, Buhi WC, Riggall FC, Holsinger KL: Human amniotic fluid lecithin/sphingomyelin ratio changes with estrogen or glucocorticoid treatment. Am J Obstet Gynecol 115:216, 1973

Spooner PM, Gorski J: Early estrogen effects on lipid metabolism in the rat uterus. Endocrinology 91:1273, 1972

Stabile I, Nicolaides KH, Bach A, Teisner B, Rodeck C, Westergaard JG, Grudzinskas JG: Complement factors in fetal and maternal blood and amniotic fluid during the second trimester of normal pregnancy. Br J Obstet Gynaecol 95:281, 1988

Streeter GL: Weight, sitting height, head size, foot length, and menstrual age of the human embryo. Contrib Embryol 11:143, 1920

Sumida C, Gelly C, Nguyen BL, Pasqualini JR: Cytosol and nuclear ^{3}H-estradiol receptors in fetal guinea pig kidney, lung, and uterus during fetal development. Acta Endocrinol 85(suppl 212):36, 1977

Szabo AJ, Grimaldi RCD, Jung WF: Palmitate transport across perfused human placenta. Metabolism 18:406, 1969

Temiras PS, Vernadakis A, Sherwood NM: Development and plasticity of the nervous system. In Assali NS (ed): Biology of Gestation, Vol. VII. The Fetus and Neonate. New York, Academic Press, 1968

Thiery M, Yo Le Sian A, Vrijens M, Janssens D: Vagitus uterinus. J Obstet Gynaecol Brit Commonw 80:183, 1973

Usher R, Shephard M, Lind J: The blood volume of the newborn infant and placental transfusion. Acta Paediatr 52:497, 1963

Von Neergard K: Neue Auffassungen über einen Grundbegriff der Atemmechanik die Retrakionskraft der Lunge abhangig von der Oberflach enspannung in den Alveolen. Z Ges Exp Med 66:373, 1929

Walker J, Turnbull EPN: Haemoglobin and red cells in the human foetus and their relation to the oxygen content of the blood in the vessels of the umbilical cord. Lancet 2:312, 1953

Walsh PC, Madden JD, Harrod MJ, Goldstein JL, MacDonald PC, Wilson JD: Familial incomplete male pseudohermaphroditism, type 2: Decreased dihydrotestosterone formation in pseudovaginal perineoscrotal hypospades. N Engl J Med 291:944, 1974

Whitsett JA: Composition of Pulmonary Surfactant Lipids and Proteins. In Polin RA, Fox WW (eds): Fetal and Neonatal Physiology. Philadelphia, Saunders, 1992, p 941

Whitsett JA, Weaver TE, Lieberman MA, Clark JC, Daugherty C: Differential effects of epidermal growth factor and transforming growth factor-β on synthesis of $M_r = 35,000$ surfactant-associated protein in fetal lung. J Biol Chem 262:7908, 1987

Widdowson EM: Growth and composition of the fetus and newborn. In Assali NS (ed): Biology of Gestation, Vol II. The Fetus and Neonate. New York, Academic Press, 1968

Wigglesworth JS, Desai R: Is fetal respiratory function a major determinant of perinatal survival? Lancet 1:264, 1982

Wilson JD, Gloyna RE: The intranuclear metabolism of testosterone in the accessory organs of reproduction. Recent Prog Horm Res 26:309, 1970

Wilson JD, Lasnitzki I: Dihydrotestosterone formation in fetal tissues of the rabbit and rat. Endocrinology 89:659, 1971

Wilson JD, MacDonald PC: Male pseudohermaphroditism due to androgen resistance: Testicular feminization and related syndromes. In Stanbury JB, Wyngaarden JD, Frederickson DS (eds): The Metabolic Basis of Inherited Disease. New York, McGraw-Hill, 1978

Wilson KM: Correlation of external genitalia and sex-glands in the human embryo period. Contrib Embryol 18:23, 1926

Wladimiroff JW, Campbell S: Fetal urine-production rates in normal and complicated pregnancy. Lancet 1:151, 1974

Wolf U: Genetic aspects of H-Y antigen. Hum Genet 58:25, 1981

Wu B, Kikkawa Y, Orzalesi MM, Motoyama EK, Kaibara M, Zigas CJ, Cook CD: The effect of thyroxine on the maturation of fetal rabbit lungs. Biol Neonate 22:161, 1973

Wu B, Kikkawa Y, Orzalesi MM, Motoyama EK, Kaibara M, Zigas CJ, Cook CD: Accelerated maturation of fetal rabbit lungs by thyroxine. Physiologist 14:253, 1971

Zanjani ED, Peterson EN, Gordon AS, Wasserman LR: Erythropoietin production in the fetus: Role of the kidney and maternal anemia. J Lab Clin Med 83:281, 1974

Zivny J, Kobilkova J, Neuwirt J, Andrasova V: Regulation of erythropoiesis in fetus and mother during normal pregnancy. Obstet Gynecol 60:77, 1982

Zuspan FR, Cordero L, Semchyshyn S: Effects of hydrocortisone on lecithin–sphingomyelin ratio. Am J Obstet Gynecol 128:571, 1977

CHAPTER 8
Maternal Adaptations to Pregnancy

The anatomical, physiological, and biochemical adaptations that take place in women during the short span of human pregnancy are profound. Many of these changes begin soon after fertilization and continue throughout gestation, and as noted already (Chaps. 2 and 5 through 7), most of these remarkable adaptations occur in response to physiological stimuli provided by the fetus or fetal tissues. Equally astounding is that the woman who was pregnant is returned almost completely to her prepregnancy state after delivery and cessation of lactation. The understanding of these adaptations to pregnancy remains a major goal of obstetrics, and without such knowledge, it is almost impossible to understand the disease processes—pregnancy induced or coincidental—that can threaten women during pregnancy and the puerperium.

Uterus

Hypertrophy and Dilatation. The capacity of the uterus to increase rapidly in size during pregnancy, and then to return almost to its original state within a few weeks, is remarkable. In the nonpregnant woman, the uterus is an almost-solid structure weighing 70 g or so and with a cavity of 10 mL or less. During pregnancy, the uterus is transformed into a relatively thin-walled muscular organ of sufficient capacity to accommodate the fetus, placenta, and amnionic fluid. The total volume of the contents of the uterus at term averages about 5 L but may be as much as 20 L or more, so that by the end of pregnancy the uterus has achieved a 500 to 1000 times greater capacity than in the nonpregnant state. There is a corresponding increase in uterine weight, and the body of the uterus at term weighs approximately 1100 g.

During pregnancy, uterine enlargement involves stretching and marked hypertrophy of existing muscle cells, whereas the appearance of new muscle cells is limited. At the time of parturition, a single myometrial cell is about 500 μm in length, and the nucleus is eccentrically placed in the thickest part of the cell. The myometrial smooth muscle cell is surrounded by an irregular array of collagen fibrils. The force of contraction is transmitted from the contractile proteins of the muscle cell to the surrounding connective tissue through the reticulum of collagen.

Accompanying the increase in size of the uterine muscle cells during pregnancy, there is an accumulation of fibrous tissue, particularly in the external muscle layer, together with a considerable increase in elastic tissue. The network that is formed adds materially to the strength of the uterine wall. Concomitantly, there is a great increase in size and number of blood vessels and lymphatics. The veins that drain the placental site are transformed into large uterine sinuses, and there is hypertrophy of the nerves exemplified by the increase in size of the Frankenhäuser cervical ganglion.

During the first few months of pregnancy, uterine hypertrophy is probably stimulated chiefly by the action of estrogen and perhaps that of progesterone. It is apparent that early hypertrophy is not entirely in response to mechanical distension by the products of conception because similar uterine changes are observed when the embryo is implanted ectopically. But after about 12 weeks, the increase in uterine size is in large part related in some manner to the effect of pressure exerted by the expanding products of conception.

Rapid growth of most, and perhaps all, tissues is correlated with increased synthesis of *polyamines*, which include *spermidine* and *spermine* and their immediate precursor, *putrescine*. These polyamines are believed to occupy crucial roles in tissue growth and cell hypertrophy. Russell and colleagues (1978) found that polyamine levels in the urine of normally pregnant women are strikingly elevated, and that the highest levels are attained at 13 to 14 weeks' gestation. But equally important, at 13 to 14 weeks there is a 1000-fold increase in *diamine oxidase* activity in blood. This enzyme is probably produced in decidua but is released into blood in large amounts. It catalyzes the metabolism of polyamines. Thus, it is likely that the rate of polyamine formation is increased strikingly throughout pregnancy, but the rate of metabolism of these growth-promoting agents increases so remarkably, due to the action of diamine oxidase, that the levels of polyamines decline after 12 to 14 weeks.

During the first few months of pregnancy, the uterine walls become considerably thicker, but as gestation advances the walls gradually thin. At term, the walls of the corpus are only about 1.5 cm or less in thickness. Early in pregnancy, the uterus loses the firmness and resistance characteristic of the nonpregnant organ. In the later months, the uterus is changed into a muscular sac with thin, soft, readily indentable walls, demonstrable by the ease with which the fetus usually can be palpated through the abdominal wall and by the readiness with which the uterine walls yield to the movements of the fetal extremities.

Uterine enlargement is not symmetrical and it is most marked in the fundus. The differential growth is readily apparent by observing the relative positions of the attachments of the fallopian tubes and ovarian and round ligaments. In the early months of pregnancy, these structures insert only slightly below the apex of the fundus, whereas in the later months, they are inserted slightly above the middle of the uterus. The position of the placenta also influences the extent of uterine hypertrophy, because the portion of the uterus surrounding the placental site enlarges more rapidly than does the myometrium distal to the site of placental implantation.

Arrangement of the Muscle Cells

Uterine musculature during pregnancy is arranged in three strata: (1) an external hoodlike layer, which arches over the fundus and extends into the various ligaments; (2) an internal layer, consisting of sphincter-like fibers around the orifices of the tubes and the internal os; and (3) lying between these two, a dense network of muscle fibers perforated in all directions by blood vessels. The main portion of the uterine wall is formed by the middle layer, which consists of an interlacing network of muscle fibers between which extend the blood vessels. Each cell in this layer has a double curve, so that the interlacing of any two gives approximately the form of the figure eight. As a result of this arrangement, when the cells contract after delivery they constrict the penetrating blood vessels and thus act as ligatures.

The muscle cells composing the uterine wall in pregnancy, especially in its lower portion, overlap one another like shingles on a roof. One end of each fiber arises beneath the serosa of the uterus and extends obliquely downward and inward toward the decidua, forming a large number of muscular lamellae that are interconnected by short muscular processes. When the tissue is slightly spread apart, it appears sieve-like and, on closer examination, is found to comprise innumerable rhomboidal spaces.

Changes in Uterine Size, Shape, and Position. As the uterus increases in size, it also undergoes important modifications in shape. For the first few weeks, its original pear shape is maintained, but as pregnancy advances the corpus and fundus soon assume a more globular form, becoming almost spherical by the third lunar month. Subsequently, the organ increases more rapidly in length than in width and assumes an ovoid shape (Fig. 3–9).

By the end of 12 weeks, the uterus has become too large to remain totally within the pelvis. Thereafter, as the uterus continues to enlarge, it contacts the anterior abdominal wall, displaces the intestines laterally and superiorly, and continues to rise, ultimately reaching almost to the liver. As the uterus rises, tension is exerted upon the broad ligaments, which partly unfold their median and lower portions, and upon the round ligaments.

During pregnancy, the uterus is movable. With the pregnant woman standing, the longitudinal axis of the uterus corresponds to an extension of the axis of the pelvic inlet. The abdominal wall supports the uterus and, unless it is quite relaxed, maintains this relation between the long axis of the uterus and the axis of the pelvic inlet. When the pregnant woman is supine, the uterus falls back to rest upon the vertebral column and the adjacent great vessels, especially the inferior vena cava and the aorta.

With ascent of the uterus from the pelvis, it usually undergoes rotation to the right, resulting in the left margin facing anteriorly. This *dextrorotation* likely results in large measure from the presence of the rectosigmoid on the left side of the pelvis.

Changes in Contractility. From the first trimester of pregnancy onward, the uterus undergoes irregular contractions, which are normally painless. In the second trimester, these contractions may be detected by bimanual examination. The relaxed uterus transiently becomes firm and then returns to its original relaxed state. Since attention was first called to this phenomenon in 1872 by J. Braxton Hicks, the contractions have been known by his name. Such contractions appear unpredictably and sporadically, are usually nonrhythmic, and their intensity varies between approximately 5 and 25 mm Hg (Alvarez and Caldeyro-Barcia, 1950). Until the last month of gestation, *Braxton Hicks contractions* are infrequent, but increase in frequency during the last week or two. At this time, the contractions may occur as often as every 10 to 20 minutes and may also assume some degree of rhythmicity. Late in pregnancy, these contractions may cause some discomfort and account for so-called *false labor*. Unfortunately, normalizing patient reports of uterine activity as "Braxton Hicks" contractions without performing cervical examinations has often negated early diagnosis of preterm labor (Hill and Lambertz, 1990).

Uteroplacental Blood Flow. The delivery of most substances essential for the growth and metabolism of the fetus and placenta, as well as the removal of most metabolic wastes, is dependent upon adequate perfusion of the placental intervillous space (Chap. 5). There is little experimental evidence available concerning the mechanics of blood flow in the human uterus during pregnancy, and most of what is known is from the elegant primate experiments by Ramsey and colleagues (1959), who observed:

Arterial blood enters the placenta (intervillous space) from the myometrial arteries under a head of maternal pressure sufficiently higher than that prevailing in the vast, amorphous lake of the intervillous space so that the incoming stream is driven high up toward the chorionic plate. Gradually this force is spent and lateral dispersion occurs aided by the villi which acting as baffles, promote mixing and slowing and, by their own pulsation, effect a mild stirring. Eventually the blood in the intervillous space falls back upon the orifices in the basal plate which connect with maternal veins, and, since there is an additional fall in blood pressure between the intervillous space and the myometrial veins, drainage is accomplished.

Placental perfusion by maternal blood is dependent in turn upon blood flow to the uterus through the uterine and ovarian arteries. There is no question that there is a progressive increase in uteroplacental blood flow during pregnancy. The reported values, which average about 500 mL/min late in pregnancy, must be viewed as approximations because of inherent errors in the methods of measurement as well as the undoubtedly appreciable changes in uterine blood flow that are likely induced by changes in body positions (Kauppila and associates, 1980).

Assali and co-workers (1953, 1960) and Metcalfe and colleagues (1955), using the nitrous oxide method to estimate uteroplacental blood flow in human pregnancy, found that the total flow averages about 500 mL/min at term. Rekonen and co-workers (1976) attempted measurement of intervillous and myometrial blood flow in pregnant women in the supine position using intravenously injected ^{133}Xe. For a placenta of 500 g and a uterus of 1000 g, uteroplacental blood flow estimated by this technique average 650 mL/min. Edman and colleagues (1981) calculated minimal placental intervillous blood flow from the placental clearance rate of maternal plasma Δ^4-androstenedione through placental estradiol-17β formation. They reported values of approximately 450 mL/min for intervillous flow at or near term.

Assali and co-workers (1968), using electromagnetic flow meters, studied the effects of spontaneous and oxytocin-induced labor on uteroplacental blood flow in sheep and dogs at term. They found that uterine contractions, either spontaneous or induced, caused a decrease in uterine blood flow that was approximately proportional to the intensity of the contraction and that a tetanic contraction caused a precipitous fall in uterine blood flow. Harbert and associates (1969) made similar observations in gravid monkeys, and the same pattern of change undoubtedly follows the myometrial contractions of human parturition.

Janbu and Nesheim (1987) measured uterine artery velocities during labor using pulsed Doppler spectrum analysis. They studied normal women in labor and correlated these Doppler waveforms with intrauterine pressure readings. They found an almost linear correlation between pressure and decreased velocity. With contractions generating 50 mm Hg pressure, velocity was decreased by 60 percent. However, Brar and colleagues (1988) reported no adverse effects on umbilical artery flow.

Control of Uteroplacental Blood Flow.

Factors that serve to regulate uteroplacental perfusion remain largely unknown. By the use of animal models and indirect methods of assessing human uteroplacental perfusion, however, a partial understanding is evolving.

Increases in total uterine blood flow occur progressively throughout gestation in both the human and sheep. In sheep, however, there is a definite redistribution of blood flow within the gravid uterus (Makowski and co-workers, 1968). Before pregnancy, uterine blood flow is divided equally between myometrium, endometrium, and future placental implantation sites (caruncles). By the end of the first third of ovine pregnancy, endometrial blood flow is 50 percent of the total. By term, blood flow to the placental cotyledons accounts for approximately 90 percent of total uterine blood flow (Rosenfeld and associates, 1974).

What actually induces the increase in uterine blood flow during the first two thirds of ovine pregnancy is not clearly understood. There is, however, no doubt that it is in part the consequence of increasing placental size and number of blood vessels (Teasdale, 1976). The increase in maternal–placental blood flow principally occurs by means of vasodilation, whereas fetal–placental blood flow is increased by a continuing increase in placental vessels (Teasdale, 1976). This appears to result in an optimal match of maternal and fetal placental blood flows such that maternal–fetal transfer should be maximal. It appears likely that this late-pregnancy vasodilation is at least in part the consequence of estrogen stimulation (Rosenfeld and co-workers, 1976). Naden and Rosenfeld (1985) showed that estradiol-17β administration to nonpregnant sheep induced cardiovascular changes similar to those observed in pregnant animals.

Catecholamines

Both epinephrine and norepinephrine cause significant decreases in placental perfusion in sheep even in the absence of any change in arterial blood pressure (Rosenfeld and co-workers, 1976; Rosenfeld and West, 1977). Such a response is likely the consequence of a greater sensitivity to catecholamines of the uteroplacental vascular beds when compared with the systemic vasculature.

Angiotensin II

Vascular refractoriness to the pressor effects of angiotensin II appears to be a normal response of both human (Chesley and associates, 1965; Gant and co-workers, 1973) and ovine pregnancy (Rosenfeld and Gant, 1981). Despite a marked refractoriness of the systemic vasculature to angiotensin II, the uterine vasculature in sheep is even more refractory. This is clearly illustrated in Figure 8–1, where greater changes in mean arterial blood pressure and systemic vascular resistance are found at lower doses of infused angiotensin II compared with changes in uterine vascular resistance.

The physiological implications of uterine vascular refractoriness to angiotensin II are not immediately apparent but may be of signal importance. For example, this response may result in a potential advantage to the fetus when there is a decreased refractoriness of the systemic vasculature to pressor agents (increased sensitivity to pressor agents). This is likely in women destined to develop pregnancy-induced hypertension and where uterine vascular refractoriness to pressor agents is maintained, at least initially. This would be expected to result in an increased uteroplacental perfusion in such pregnancies prior to the development of actual hypertension. Such a situation is known to occur in women destined to develop pregnancy-induced hypertension (Gant and associates, 1976). In these women, uteroplacental blood flow, as reflected by the metabolic clearance rate of dehydroisoandrosterone sulfate, is initially increased, and then falls as pregnancy advances and hypertension develops or worsens. The initial increase in uteroplacental blood flow likely results as a consequence of a blunted uterine vascular resistance to angiotensin II, and possibly other pressor agents as well, compared with systemic vascular resistance (Fig. 8–1). Uteroplacental perfusion then decreases as uterine vascular resistance increases compared with systemic vascular resistance. This is analogous to the effect observed on the uteroplacental vasculature that occurs at higher doses of infused angiotensin II, when uterine vascular resistance exceeds mean arterial pressure, resulting in decreased uterine blood flow.

These observations have additional clinical significance as to whether mild to moderate blood pressure increases, such as in women with chronic hypertension, should be treated with antihypertensive drugs during pregnancy. Antihypertensive drugs may cause a greater decrease in vascular resistance than in uterine vascular resistance, thereby resulting in a greater fall in uterine blood flow.

Changes in the Cervix. During pregnancy, there is pronounced softening and cyanosis of the cervix, often demonstrable as early as a month after conception. These changes comprise two of the very earliest physical signs of pregnancy (Chap. 2, p. 23). The factors responsible for these changes are increased vascularity and edema of the entire cervix, together with hypertrophy and hyperplasia of the cervical glands.

As shown in Figure 8–2, the glands of the cervical mucosa undergo such marked proliferation that by the end of pregnancy, they occupy approximately one half of the entire cervical mass, rather than a small fraction as in the nonpregnant state. Moreover, the septa separating the glandular spaces become progressively thinner, resulting in the formation of a structure resembling a honeycomb, the meshes of which are filled with tenacious mucus. Soon after conception a clot of very thick mucus obstructs the cervical canal. At the onset of labor, if not before, this so-called *mucus plug* is expelled, resulting in a *bloody show.* The glands near the external os proliferate beneath the stratified squamous epithelium of the portio vaginalis, giving the cervix the velvety consistency characteristic of pregnancy.

So-called cervical *erosions* are common during pregnancy. These lesions are customarily red and velvety in appearance and are covered by columnar epithelium, spreading from the external os to involve the portio vaginalis of the cervix to various degrees. The high frequency of these normal pregnancy-induced changes is best explained in that they represent an extension, or *eversion,* of the proliferating endocervical glands and the columnar endocervical epithelium. Although the term *erosion* implies an "eating out" or ulceration of the covering epithelium, the cause in pregnancy is rarely inflammatory.

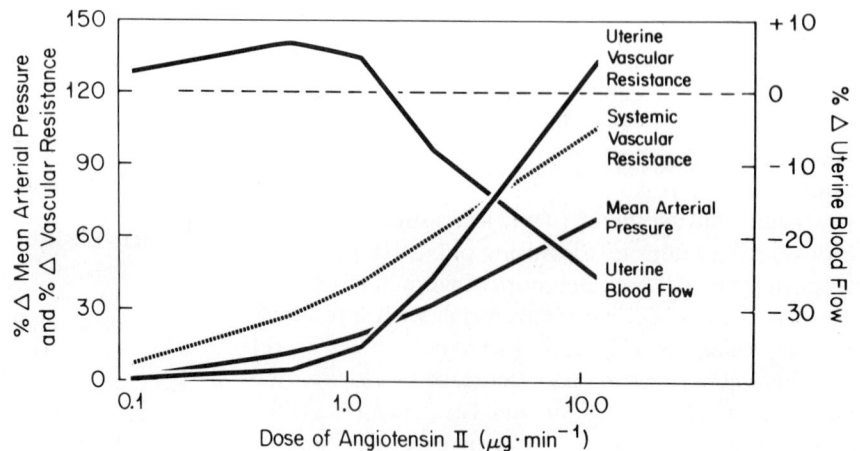

Fig. 8–1. The relative changes in uterine blood flow, mean arterial pressure, systemic vascular resistance, and uterine vascular resistance during the systemic infusion of angiotensin II in term pregnant ewes. Responses were recorded after 4 to 5 minutes of stabilization at each dose of angiotensin II. (From Rosenfeld, 1984, with permission.)

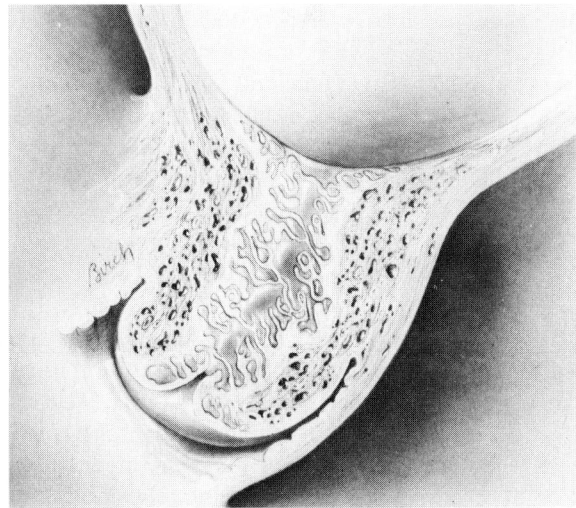

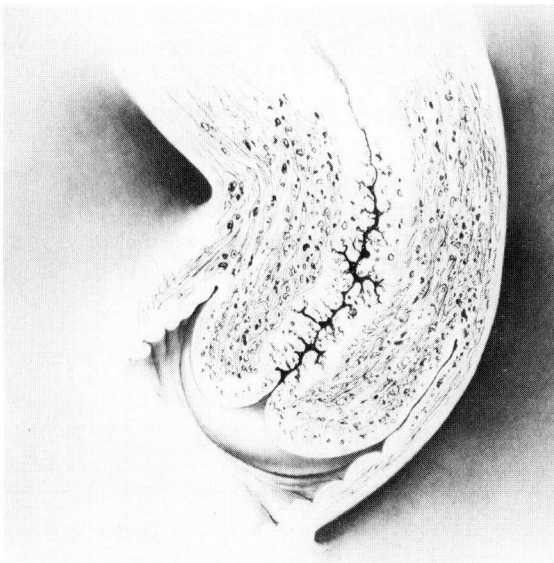

A

B

Fig. 8–2. Changes in the cervix induced by pregnancy. **A.** Cervix in the nonpregnant woman. **B.** Cervix in pregnancy. Note the elaboration of the mucosa into a honeycomb-like structure, the meshes of which are filled with a tenacious mucus plug.

During pregnancy, there is a change in the consistency of the cervical mucus. In the great majority of pregnant women, cervical mucus, spread and dried on a glass slide, is characterized by fragmentary crystallization, or *beading,* typical of the effect of progesterone (see Chap. 4, p. 106). In some women, arborization of the crystals, or *ferning,* is observed.

During pregnancy, basal cells near the squamocolumnar junction histologically are likely to be prominent in size, shape, and staining qualities. These changes are considered to be estrogen induced (Hellman and colleagues, 1954). Although the cervix contains a small amount of smooth muscle, its major component is connective tissue. The cervix undergoes profound changes during pregnancy, including a rearrangement of collagen-rich connective tissue to produce a 12-fold reduction in mechanical strength (Rechberger and colleagues, 1988).

Ovaries and Fallopian Tubes

Ovarian Function. Ovulation ceases during pregnancy and the maturation of new follicles is suspended. Ordinarily, only a single corpus luteum of pregnancy can be found in the ovaries of pregnant women (Chap. 2). In gonadotropin-induced pregnancies, Yoshima and associates (1969) found that the level of plasma progesterone, after having risen during the luteal phase of the ovarian cycle, reached a nadir by the eighth week of pregnancy (sixth week post-ovulation) and then rose again. Such a nadir was not observed by Tulchinsky and Hobel (1973) in spontaneous ovulatory cycles, but in-

stead a less rapid increase or plateau in plasma progesterone levels was found. By contrast, maternal plasma 17α-hydroxyprogesterone levels continued to decline in early pregnancy to a level only somewhat greater than those found during the luteal phase. Thus, the corpus luteum of pregnancy most likely functions maximally during the first 6 to 7 weeks of pregnancy (4 to 5 weeks post-ovulation), and thereafter, the corpus luteum contributes relatively little to progesterone production. This has been confirmed in vivo by the surgical removal of the corpus luteum before 7 weeks' gestation (5 weeks post-ovulation), which results in a rapid fall in maternal serum progesterone and abortion (Csapo and co-workers, 1973). After this time in pregnancy, however, corpus luteum removal ordinarily does not cause abortion or labor.

Relaxin. Human relaxin (M_r about 6000) is a protein hormone composed of nonidentical A and B chains of similar length. There are structural features of relaxin that are similar to insulin and insulin-like growth factors I and II. As in the case for insulin, relaxin is synthesized initially as a single-chain preprohormone that includes the signal peptide (B chain) and connecting peptide (A chain). Although the gene for human insulin is located on the short arm of chromosome 11 and the two genes for relaxin on the short arm of chromosome 9, Crawford and associates (1984) concluded that the insulin and relaxin genes separated during a chromosomal translocation involving a breakpoint between the two genes. Relaxin gene 2 appears to be the functional member of the two.

Human relaxin is secreted by the corpus luteum of

pregnancy and possibly by uterine decidua during pregnancy. The pattern of secretion is similar to human chorionic gonadotropin (Eddie and co-workers, 1986). Therefore, secretion of relaxin differs from that of ovarian steroid hormones. Whereas 17α-hydroxyprogesterone and likely progesterone secretion by the corpus luteum declines to negligible rates by the seventh to eighth gestational week, appreciable relaxin secretion continues throughout pregnancy (Eddie and associates, 1986).

The role of relaxin during human pregnancy is not defined. Although it is a major myometrial inhibitory substance in the pregnant guinea pig uterus (Porter, 1972), it is not essential to the maintenance of human pregnancy (Bryant-Greenwood, 1982). The mechanism of action of relaxin in producing uterine relaxation during rat pregnancy is very similar to the action of β-mimetic drugs. Specifically, relaxin appears to react or combine with a β-adrenergic receptor on the cell membrane to stimulate an increase in adenylate cyclase, which in turn increases cyclic AMP and protein kinase. The result is uterine muscle relaxation (Sanborn, 1986). Whether such a mechanism occurs in the human as either a primary or secondary modulating system for maintaining uterine relaxation is not known.

The role of human relaxin in producing softening and effacement of the uterine cervix is also unknown. The topical administration of pharmacological doses of a highly purified porcine relaxin to the human cervix, however, results in cervical softening and effacement, as well as a more successful rate of labor inductions in treated versus untreated women (Evans and colleagues, 1983; Porter, 1980).

A variety of other actions of relaxin have been reported in animals including changes in blood pressure, changes in symphysis mobility, regulation of lactation, and remodeling of connective tissues. For example, Kakouris and associates (1992) reported that relaxin has powerful chronotropic and inotropic effects on the rat heart. Such effects vary from animal species to species, but there is a little evidence to support such actions in the human (Sherwood, 1988).

Pregnancy Luteoma. In 1963, Sternberg described a solid ovarian tumor that developed during pregnancy that was composed of large acidophilic luteinized cells. The observations of Krause and Stembridge (1966) and Garcia-Bunuel and co-workers (1975) are consistent with the view that a luteoma of pregnancy represents an exaggeration of the luteinization reaction of the ovary of normal pregnancy and is not a true neoplasm. The luteoma regresses after delivery, and normal ovarian function returns even in those instances in which the luteoma is responsible transiently for maternal virilization. In the immediate puerperal state, the luteoma may be responsive to exogenously administered chorionic gonadotropin (hCG) (Cohen and associates, 1982). Luteomas may recur in subsequent pregnancies (Shortle and associates, 1987).

Even though maternal virilization may be prominent, the female fetus is usually not affected, presumably because of the protective role of the placenta through its high capacity to convert androgens and androgen-like steroids to estrogens (Edman and co-workers, 1979). There is no question, however, that a female fetus can in some cases be virilized (Cohen and associates, 1982).

Hyperreactio Luteinalis. Hyperreactio luteinalis is a second benign lesion of the ovary that causes maternal virilization during pregnancy. Although the cellular pattern is similar to that of a luteoma of pregnancy, the two tumors are different grossly. The luteoma is solid and hyperreactio luteinalis is a cystic tumor. Additionally, hyperreactio luteinalis is commonly associated with extremely high hCG values (Muechler and colleagues, 1987).

A case of hyperreactio luteinalis managed at Parkland Hospital highlights many of the features of this clinical entity (Bradshaw and co-workers, 1986). The primigravida developed temporal balding, hirsutism, and clitoromegaly during the third trimester. Levels of androstenedione and testosterone were elevated massively in maternal serum but normal in umbilical cord blood. Maternal serum levels of hCG were twice the mean for normal late pregnancy. Bilateral multicystic ovarian masses obstructed fetal descent during labor and necessitated cesarean delivery. Increased ovarian responsiveness to hCG was confirmed 8 weeks postpartum.

Other Changes. A *decidual* reaction on and beneath the surface of the ovaries, similar to that found in the endometrial stroma, is common in pregnancy and may be observed at cesarean section. These elevated patches of tissue bleed easily and may, on first glance, resemble freshly torn adhesions. Similar decidual reactions are occasionally seen on the posterior uterine serosa and upon or within other pelvic or even extrapelvic abdominal organs.

The enormous caliber of the ovarian veins viewed at cesarean section is startling. Through actual measurement, Hodgkinson (1953) found that the diameter of the ovarian vascular pedicle increased during pregnancy from 0.9 cm to approximately 2.6 cm at term.

Fallopian Tubes. The musculature of the fallopian tubes undergoes little hypertrophy during pregnancy. The epithelium of the tubal mucosa is flattened during gestation, compared with that of the nonpregnant state. Decidual cells may develop in the stroma of the endosalpinx, but a continuous decidual membrane is not formed.

Vagina and Perineum

During pregnancy, increased vascularity and hyperemia develop in the skin and muscles of the perineum and vulva, and there is softening of the normally abundant connective tissue of these structures.

Increased vascularity prominently affects the vagina. The copious secretion and the characteristic violet color of the vagina during pregnancy (*Chadwick sign*), similar to the cervical changes during pregnancy, probably result chiefly from hyperemia. The vaginal walls undergo striking changes seemingly in preparation for the distension that occurs during labor, with a considerable increase in thickness of the mucosa, loosening of the connective tissue, and hypertrophy of the smooth-muscle cells to nearly the same extent as in the uterus. These changes effect such an increase in length of the vaginal walls that sometimes, in parous women, the lower portion of the anterior vaginal wall protrudes slightly through the vulvar opening. The papillae of the vaginal mucosa also undergo considerable hypertrophy, creating a fine hobnailed appearance.

Vaginal Secretions. The considerably increased cervical and vaginal secretions during pregnancy consists of a somewhat thick, white discharge. Its pH is acidic, varying from 3.5 to 6, the result of increased production of lactic acid from glycogen in the vaginal epithelium by the action of *Lactobacillus acidophilus*. The acidic pH probably serves to control the rate of multiplication of pathogenic bacteria in the vagina.

Vaginal Cytology. Early in pregnancy the vaginal epithelial cells are similar to those found during the luteal phase of the menstrual cycle (see Chap. 4, p. 107), but as pregnancy advances, two patterns of response may be seen: (1) Small intermediate cells, called navicular cells by Papanicolaou, are found in abundance in small, dense clusters. These ovoid cells contain a vesicular, somewhat elongated nucleus. (2) Vesicular nuclei without cytoplasm, or so-called naked nuclei, are evident along with an abundance of *Lactobacillus*.

Abdominal Wall and Skin

Striae Gravidarum. In the later months of pregnancy, reddish, slightly depressed streaks commonly develop in the skin of the abdomen and sometimes in the skin over the breasts and thighs. These striae gravidarum occur in about half of pregnant women. In multiparous women, in addition to the reddish striae of the present pregnancy, glistening, silvery lines that represent the cicatrices of previous striae frequently are seen.

Diastasis Recti. Occasionally the muscles of the abdominal walls do not withstand the tension to which they are subjected, and the rectus muscles separate in the midline, creating a diastasis recti of varying extent. If severe, a considerable portion of the anterior uterine wall is covered by only a layer of skin, attenuated fascia, and peritoneum. In extreme instances, herniation of the gravid uterus through the diastasis may be so great that the fundus of the uterus drops below the level of the pelvic inlet when the woman is standing.

Pigmentation. In many women, the midline of the abdominal skin becomes markedly pigmented, assuming a brownish-black color to form the *linea nigra*. Occasionally, irregular brownish patches of varying size appear on the face and neck, giving rise to *chloasma* or *melasma gravidarum* (*mask of pregnancy*), which, fortunately, usually disappears, or at least regresses considerably, after delivery. Oral contraceptives may cause similar pigmentation in these same women. There is very little known of the nature of these pigmentary changes, although melanocyte-stimulating hormone, a polypeptide similar to corticotropin, has been shown to be elevated remarkably from the end of the second month of pregnancy until term. Estrogen and progesterone are reported to have melanocyte-stimulating effects. These changes also are discussed in Chapter 56 (p. 1259).

Pro-opinomelanocorticotropin is metabolized in the intermediate lobe of the pituitary to β-endorphin and to α-melanotropin (α-MSH). This activity is under the inhibitory influence of dopamine control, which when blocked results in a marked increase in β-endorphin plasma levels in pregnant *but not in nonpregnant women* (Abou-Samra and co-workers, 1984). The response in pregnant women is likely due to hypertrophy of the intermediate lobe of the pituitary gland. Thus, it may be that estrogen and progesterone stimulation during pregnancy results in hypertrophy of the intermediate lobe with an increased release of β-endorphin and *possibly* α-MSH.

Cutaneous Vascular Changes. Angiomas, called *vascular spiders*, develop in about two thirds of white women and approximately 10 percent of African American women during pregnancy. These are minute, red elevations on the skin, particularly common on the face, neck, upper chest, and arms, with radicles branching out from a central body. The condition is often designated as nevus, angioma, or telangiectasis. *Palmar erythema* is encountered in pregnancy in about two thirds of white women and one third of black women. The two conditions are frequently seen together, but are of no clinical significance and disappear in most women shortly after pregnancy. The high incidence of vascular spiders and palmar erythema in pregnancy is most likely the consequence of the hyperestrogenemia of pregnancy.

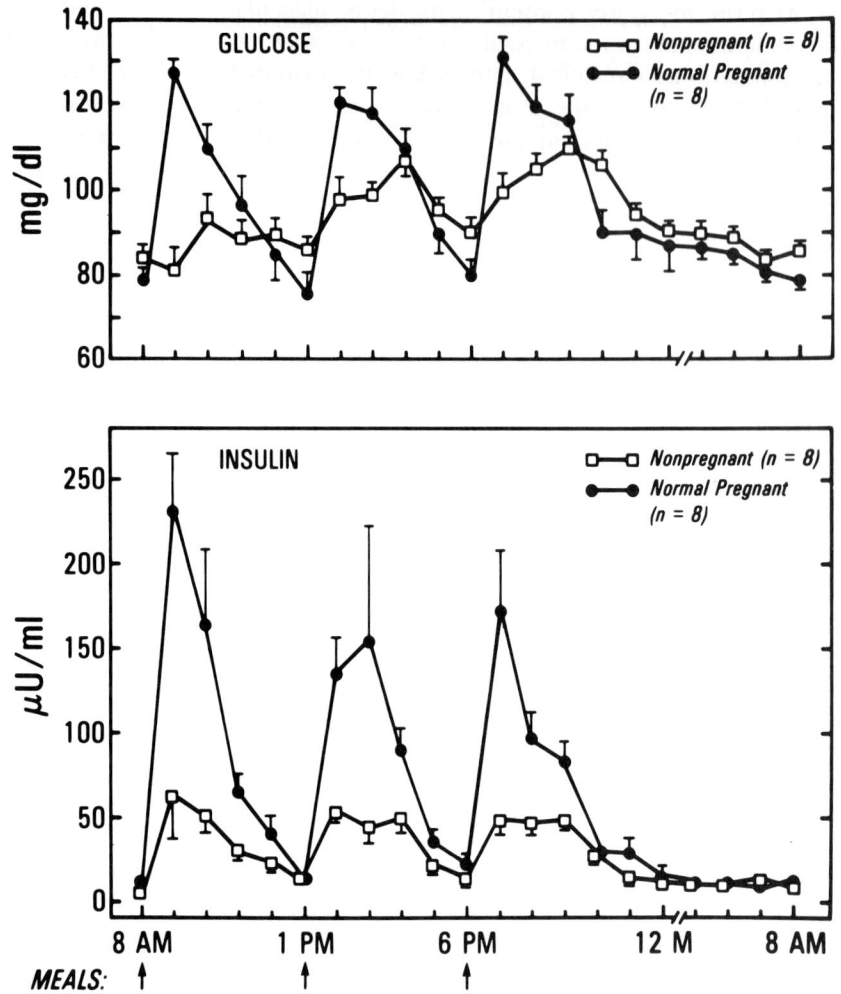

Fig. 8–4. The effect of normal late pregnancy on the diurnal changes in plasma glucose and insulin. Asterisks indicate values during pregnancy that are significantly elevated. (From Phelps and colleagues, 1981, with permission.)

tance to insulin (Freinkel and colleagues, 1985; Lind, 1979).

Tissue resistance to insulin during pregnancy is suggested by three observations: (1) increased insulin response to glucose (increased plasma level and duration); (2) reduced peripheral uptake of glucose (increased plasma level and duration); and (3) suppressed glucagon response (Lind, 1979). The mechanism(s) responsible for insulin tissue resistance is not completely understood. Progesterone and estrogen may act, directly or indirectly to mediate this resistance (Baumann and colleagues, 1981; Tsibris and co-workers, 1980). Plasma levels of human placental lactogen increase with gestation, and this protein hormone is characterized by growth hormone-like action that may result in increased lipolysis and increased liberation of free fatty acids (Freinkel, 1980). The increased concentration of circulating free fatty acids also may facilitate increased tissue resistance to insulin.

The mechanisms cited ensure that a continuous supply of glucose is available for transfer to the fetus. The pregnant woman, however, changes rapidly from a postprandial state characterized by elevated and sustained glucose levels to a fasting state characterized by decreased plasma glucose and amino acids such as alanine. There also are higher plasma concentrations of free fatty acids, triglycerides, and cholesterol in the pregnant woman during fasting (Fig. 8–5). Freinkel and colleagues (1985) have referred to this pregnancy-induced switch in fuels from glucose to lipids as **accelerated starvation.** Certainly, when fasting is prolonged in the pregnant woman, these alterations are exaggerated and ketonemia rapidly appears (Bender and Chickering, 1985).

There is *insulinase* activity in the human placenta. It seems unlikely, however, that accelerated insulin degradation contributes appreciably to the diabetogenic state induced by pregnancy, because the rate of degra-

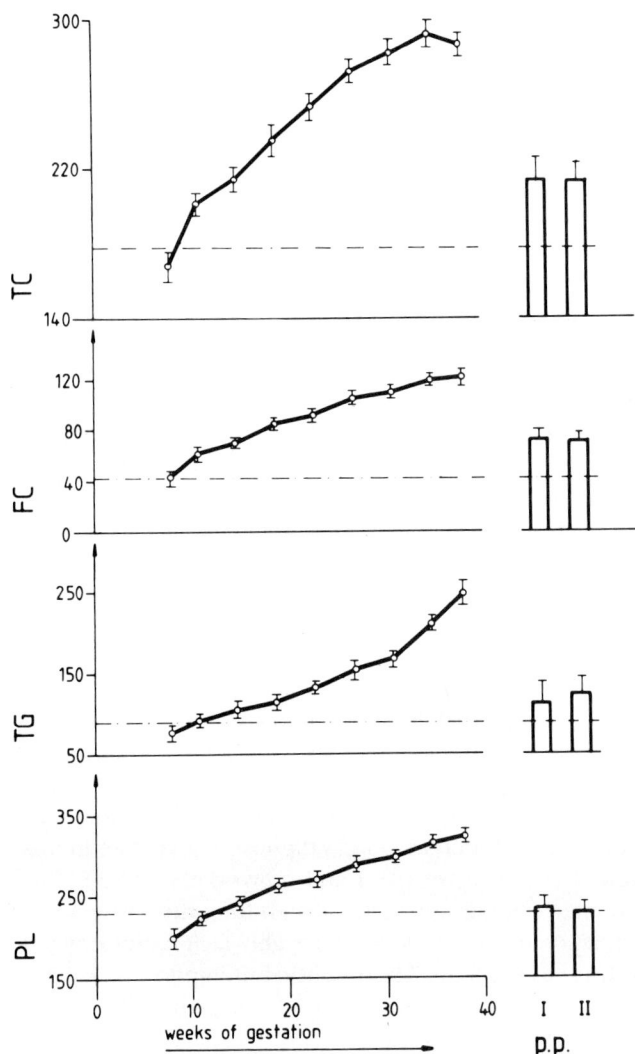

Fig. 8–5. Mean (± SEM) plasma lipid concentrations (mg/dL) throughout gestation (n = 42) and during the luteal (I) and follicular (II) phases postpartum (p.p.; n = 23). The dashed lines represent the mean values of the control group (n = 24). (TC = total cholesterol; FC = free cholesterol; TG = triglycerides; PL = phospholipids.) (From Desoye and associates, 1987, with permission.)

dation of radiolabeled insulin in vivo does not appear to differ among pregnant and nonpregnant women (Burt and Davidson, 1974).

The role of glucagon during pregnancy is not totally defined. Hornnes and Kuhl (1980) measured glucagon and insulin responses to a standard glucose stimulus in the same women late in normal pregnancy and again postpartum. The insulin response to glucose infusion was increased about four times in late pregnancy. In contrast, plasma glucagon concentrations were suppressed, and the degree of suppression was similar in late pregnancy and the puerperium. These results are consistent with the view that β-cell sensitivity to a glucose challenge is increased significantly in normal pregnant women, but that the α-cell sensitivity to a glucose stimulus is unaltered.

Fat Metabolism. The concentrations of lipids and lipoproteins and apolipoproteins in plasma increase appreciably during pregnancy. Plasma lipid levels increase continuously throughout gestation, and Desoye and co-workers (1987) found by time-series analysis that there were positive correlations between the concentrations of lipids shown in Figure 8–5 and those of estradiol, progesterone, and human placental lactogen.

Apolipoproteins AI, AII, and B concentrations increase until weeks 25, 28, and 28, respectively, and then usually remain unchanged until delivery. The concentration changes in apolipoprotein B are similar to those of estradiol after a 2-week time shift, and this effect may be related causally (Desoye and associates, 1987).

Plasma lipoprotein cholesterol levels also change significantly during pregnancy. Low-density lipoprotein cholesterol (LDL-C) levels peak at approximately week 36. High-density lipoprotein cholesterol (HDL-C) peaks at week 25, decreases until week 32, and remains constant for the remainder of pregnancy. High-density lipoprotein-2 and -3 cholesterol levels peak at approximately 28 weeks and remain unchanged throughout the remainder of pregnancy.

The increase in LDL-C is likely the consequence of the hepatic effects of estradiol and progesterone (Desoye and associates, 1987). The decrease in LDL-C before term was paralleled by a fall in the estradiol to progesterone ratio. This in fact might be the consequence of increased utilization of LDL-C for placental progesterone production, because the estradiol to progesterone ratio change was principally due to an increase in progesterone relative to estradiol.

The increase in HDL-C levels in the first half of gestation is believed to be caused by estrogen. Interestingly, the decrease after weeks 22 to 24 coincides with the onset of increasing resistance to insulin and the increase in concentration of plasma insulin. Therefore, the HDL-C concentration may be controlled, in part, by insulin.

After approximately 30 weeks, HDL-C levels plateau. One possible explanation for this is that human placental lactogen, through its lipolytic activity, causes an increase in plasma concentrations of free fatty acids. The free fatty acids then may be incorporated into triglycerides and very low-density lipoproteins in the liver. The increased specific activity of hepatic lipase induced by progesterone in turn likely results in increased concentrations of high-density lipoproteins (Desoye and co-workers, 1987). Maternal lipoprotein lipase activity favors hypertriglyceridemia (Herrera and colleagues, 1988).

Handwerger and colleagues (1987) found that high-density lipoproteins stimulate, in a dose-dependent manner, the release of human placental lactogen from placental tissue explants. The stimulation also was observed after dilipidation of apolipoproteins AI, AII, and

CI. Furthermore, dilipidation of high-density lipoprotein did not prevent its activity but tryptic digestion did. It is likely, therefore, that the high-density lipoprotein effect is due to its apoprotein components. Finally, placental cells have specific high-density lipoprotein receptors. These results are consistent with the view that high-density lipoproteins are involved in the regulation of human placental lactogen release during pregnancy in a manner possibly independent from the usual role of the lipoprotein as a plasma lipid carrier.

After delivery, the concentrations of these lipids, lipoproteins, and apolipoproteins decrease at different rates (Desoye and co-workers, 1987). Lactation increases the rate of decrease of many of these compounds (Darmady and Postle, 1982).

In pregnant women, starvation induces a more intense ketonemia (see p. 218) than occurs in nonpregnant women. For example, remarkably increased levels of plasma-free fatty acids, glycerol, and ketones were observed in women at midpregnancy who were starved experimentally for up to 4 days prior to abortion (Bender and Chickering, 1985).

Hytten and Thomson (1968) and Pipe and co-workers (1979) concluded that storage of fat occurs primarily during midpregnancy, the fat being deposited mostly in central rather than peripheral sites. Later in pregnancy, as fetal nutritional demands increase remarkably, fat storage decreases. Hytten and Thomson (1968) cited some evidence that progesterone may act to reset a "lipostat" in the hypothalamus, and at the end of pregnancy the lipostat returns to its previous nonpregnant level and the added fat is lost. Such a mechanism for energy storage, theoretically at least, might protect the mother and fetus during times of prolonged starvation or hard physical exertion.

Mineral Metabolism. The requirements for iron during pregnancy are considerable and often exceed the amounts available (p. 222). With respect to most other minerals, pregnancy induces little change in their metabolism other than their retention in amounts equivalent to those used for growth of fetal and, to a lesser extent, maternal tissues (see Chap. 7, p. 176 and Chap. 9, p. 257).

Copper and ceruloplasmin in the plasma increase considerably early in pregnancy because of the increases in estrogens, which will produce the same changes when administered to nonpregnant subjects (Russ and Raymunt, 1956). Vir and co-workers (1981) reported that copper levels in hair were similar in nonpregnant and pregnant women, but plasma values in pregnancy decreased from the first through third trimesters.

During pregnancy, calcium and magnesium levels are reduced very slightly, the reduction probably reflecting for the most part the lowered plasma protein concentration and, in turn, the consequent decrease in the amount of each electrolyte that is bound to protein.

However, Fogh-Andersen and Schultz-Larsen (1981) demonstrated a small but significant increase in free calcium ion concentration in late pregnancy by correcting for blood pH changes. Serum phosphorus levels are within the nonpregnant range. Cole and co-workers (1987) reported that bone turnover was reduced during early pregnancy, returned toward normal during the third trimester, and increased in postpartum lactating women.

Acid-Base Equilibrium and Plasma Electrolytes. Normally, the pregnant woman hyperventilates, compared with the nonpregnant subject, and this causes a respiratory alkalosis by lowering the P_{CO_2} of the blood. A moderate reduction in plasma bicarbonate from about 26 to about 22 mmol/L *partially* compensates for the respiratory alkalosis. As a result, there is only a minimal increase in blood pH. The increase in blood pH shifts the oxygen dissociation curve to the left and increases the affinity of maternal hemoglobin for oxygen (*Bohr effect*), thereby decreasing the oxygen-releasing capacity of maternal blood. Thus, the hyperventilation that results in a reduced maternal P_{CO_2} facilitates transport of carbon dioxide from the fetus to the mother but *appears to impair* release of oxygen from maternal blood to the fetus. The increase in blood pH, however, while minimal, stimulates an increase in 2,3-diphosphoglycerate in maternal erythrocytes (Tsai and co-workers, 1982). This counteracts the Bohr effect by shifting the oxygen dissociation curve back to the right, facilitating oxygen release to the fetus. These subtle but important changes insure that the fetus has every advantage from blood gas exchange.

Despite large accumulations during pregnancy of sodium and potassium, the serum concentration of these electrolytes decreases. During normal pregnancy, nearly 1000 mEq of sodium and 300 mEq of potassium are retained (Lindheimer and colleagues, 1987b). Brown and colleagues (1986, 1988) showed that sodium and potassium excretion are unchanged during pregnancy despite the fact that their glomerular filtration is increased. Fractional excretion of these electrolytes is decreased, and it has been postulated that progesterone counteracts the natriuretic and kaliuretic effects of aldosterone (see p. 238).

Hematological Changes of Normal Pregnancy

Blood Volume. The maternal blood volume increases markedly during pregnancy. In a study of 50 normal women, the blood volumes at or very near term averaged about 45 percent above their nonpregnant levels (Pritchard, 1965). The degree of expansion varies considerably; in some women there is only a modest increase, while in others the blood volume nearly doubles.

A fetus is not essential for the development of hypervolemia during pregnancy, for increases in blood volume identical with those found during normal pregnancy have been demonstrated in some women with hydatidiform mole (Pritchard, 1965). The degree of expansion varies considerably; in some women there is only a modest increase, while in others the blood volume doubles.

The pregnancy-induced hypervolemia serves to meet the demands of the enlarged uterus with its greatly hypertrophied vascular system; to protect the mother, and in turn the fetus, against the deleterious effects of impaired venous return in the supine and erect positions; and very importantly, to safeguard the mother against the adverse effects of blood loss associated with parturition. As shown in Figure 8–6, maternal blood volume starts to increase during the first trimester, expands most rapidly during the second trimester, and then rises at a much slower rate during the third trimester to plateau during the last several weeks of pregnancy.

Increased blood volume results from an increase in both plasma and erythrocytes. The usual pattern is that of an initial rise in the plasma volume, followed by an increase in the volume of erythrocytes. Although more plasma than erythrocytes is usually added to the maternal circulation, the increase in the volume of circulating erythrocytes is considerable, averaging about 450 mL, or an increase of about 33 percent. The importance of this increase in creating a demand for iron is discussed below. The increase in the volume of erythrocytes in pregnancy is accomplished by accelerated production rather than by prolongation of the life span of the erythrocyte (Pritchard and Adams, 1960).

The mean age of circulating maternal red cells is lower during the latter half of pregnancy because the rate of red cell production exceeds that of destruction. The *mean cell volume* is increased with the red blood cells becoming more spherical due to a decreased diameter and an increased thickness (Bolton and colleagues, 1982).

Moderate erythroid hyperplasia is present in the bone marrow, and the reticulocyte count is elevated slightly during normal pregnancy. This is almost certainly due to increased maternal plasma erythropoietin levels which increase two to threefold. This is seen only after 20 weeks' gestation, thus corresponding to the time in gestation when erythrocyte production is most marked (Widness and co-workers, 1984).

Jepson and Friesen (1968) reported that administration of purified human placental lactogen to polycythemic mice accelerated the incorporation of iron into their erythrocytes, an effect that was abolished by its incubation with antibody to placental lactogen but not with antisheep erythropoietin. Cotes and co-workers (1983) reported that serum erythropoietin levels and placental lactogen were related significantly. Apparently quite normal pregnancies, however, develop with no detectable levels of placental lactogen.

Atrial Natriuretic Peptide and Plasma Volume. Another group of hormones recently implicated in normal plasma volume homeostasis is the atrial natriuretic peptide system. This group of biologically active peptides is synthesized and secreted by atrial myocytes. Three separate forms (α, β, Δ) have been isolated from human atrial cells (Kangawa and Matsu, 1984; Kangawa and co-workers, 1985). The biologically active form of the peptide is not definitely known, but indirect evidence has accrued that the 28-amino-acid α-atrial natriuretic peptide is the active form (Sagnella and associates, 1985).

Atrial natriuretic peptide has been reported to produce significant natriuresis and diuresis in humans. The peptide induces an increase in renal blood flow and glomerular filtration rate and decreased renin secretion (Burnett, 1984). However, the actual mechanism(s) responsible for the natriuresis remains unclear, with evidence consistent for both a hemodynamically induced natriuresis (Wakitani and colleagues, 1985) and an inhibitory effect upon tubular sodium reabsorption (Borenstein, 1983).

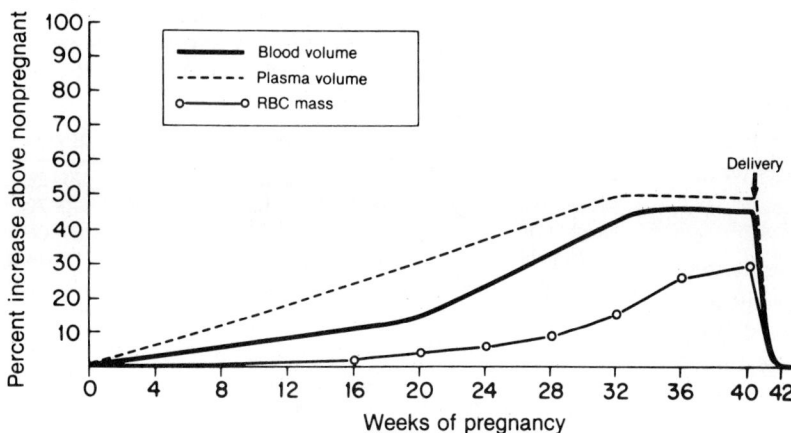

Fig. 8–6. Blood volume changes during pregnancy. (From Scott, 1972, with permission.)

The atrial natriuretic peptides also have been shown to reduce basal release of aldosterone from cultured zona glomerulosa cells and to blunt corticotropin and angiotensin II-stimulated release of aldosterone as well (Atarashi and associates, 1984). As mentioned, renin secretion is also inhibited by this peptide. Finally, atrial natriuretic peptides also have a direct vasorelaxant action upon vascular smooth muscle stimulated by angiotensin II or norepinephrine. Thus, the peptide appears to behave as a functional antagonist to endogenous vasoconstrictors (Kleinert and co-workers, 1984).

Increased secretion of atrial natriuretic peptides follows volume expansion and atrial stretch, and also occurs in response to a high-sodium diet (Sagnella and co-workers, 1985). Conversely, a low-sodium diet results in a decrease in peptide concentration.

Milson and co-workers (1988) measured immunoreactive plasma atrial natriuretic peptide in 12 normal pregnancies and correlated the results to maternal hemodynamics during each trimester and the puerperium. Plasma atrial natriuretic peptide increased throughout pregnancy concomitant with the expected increase in cardiac output, stroke volume, and heart rate. They concluded that increased atrial natriuretic peptide release probably represented one of the several mechanisms that maintain circulatory and volume homeostasis during normal pregnancy. In contrast, this observation was not confirmed by Rutherford (1987), Grace (1987), Hirai (1988), or Steegers (1987) and their co-workers, who found no increase in atrial natriuretic peptide. The reason for this discrepancy is not apparent but may be the result of different assay techniques. Interestingly, Rutherford and Steegers (1987) found that the peptide rapidly increased in concentration during the first few days postpartum with a resulting prompt natriuresis likely due to a puerperal shift of fluid from the extravascular space into the vascular compartment.

The actual effect of this peptide on plasma volume in the normally pregnant woman remains to be defined. However, most available data indicate that plasma levels are inappropriately low in pregnancy compared with nonpregnant volume-expanded states (Hatjis and colleagues, 1990). In other words, the volume sensors that control atrial natriuretic peptide release are apparently reset to sense the expanded plasma volume of pregnancy as near normal. Despite this, the peptide has a rapid and effective action upon plasma volume during the early puerperium. It seems unlikely that such a potent mediator of volume and sodium hemostasis would not have an effect during pregnancy as well.

Changes in Hematocrit.
In spite of an augmented erythropoiesis, the concentrations of hemoglobin and erythrocytes, as well as the hematocrit, decrease slightly during normal pregnancy. Consequently, whole blood viscosity decreases (Huisman and colleagues, 1987). In a careful study in which iron was readily available to the

mother for erythropoiesis, Pritchard and Hunt (1958) found that the hemoglobin concentration at term averaged 12.5 g/dL; in only 6 percent was this below 11.0 g/dL. Thus in most women, a hemoglobin concentration below 11.0 g/dL, especially late in pregnancy, should be considered abnormal and usually due to iron deficiency, rather than to hypervolemia of pregnancy (see Chap. 9, p. 257).

Iron Metabolism

Iron Stores. While the total body iron content averages about 4 g in men, in healthy young women of average size, it is probably half that amount (Table 8–2). Commonly, iron stores of normal young women are only about 300 mg (Pritchard and Mason, 1964; Scott and Pritchard, 1967). As in men, heme iron in myoglobin and enzymes and transferrin-bound circulating iron together total only a few hundred milligrams. The total iron content of normal adult women ranges from 2.0 to 2.5 g.

Iron Requirements. The iron requirements of normal pregnancy total about 1 g. About 300 mg are actively transferred to the fetus and placenta and about 200 mg are lost through various normal routes of excretion (Widdowson and Spray, 1951). These are obligatory losses and occur even when the mother is iron deficient. The average increase in the total volume of circulating erythrocytes of about 450 mL during pregnancy, when iron is available, uses another 500 mg of iron because 1 mL of normal erythrocytes contains 1.1 mg of iron. Practically all the iron for these purposes is used during the latter half of pregnancy. Therefore, the iron requirement becomes quite large during the second half of pregnancy, averaging 6 to 7 mg/day (Pritchard and Scott, 1970). Because this amount is not available from body stores in most women, the desired increase in maternal erythrocyte volume and hemoglobin mass will not develop unless exogenous iron is made available in ade-

TABLE 8–2. MEASUREMENT OF HEMOGLOBIN IRON AND IRON STORES IN HEALTHY NULLIGRAVID WOMEN WHO NEVER EXPERIENCED ABNORMAL BLOOD LOSS

	Average	Range
Age	23	21–26
Weight (kg)	60	49–72
Height (in)	65	60–68
Hemoglobin (g/dL)	14.1	13–15.6
Serum iron (μg/dL)	105	76–132
Hemoglobin mass (g)	443	358–492
Hemoglobin iron (mg)	1505	1210–1670
Iron stores[a] (mg)	347	150–629

[a] Iron converted to hemoglobin following repeated phlebotomies.
From Pritchard and Mason (1964).

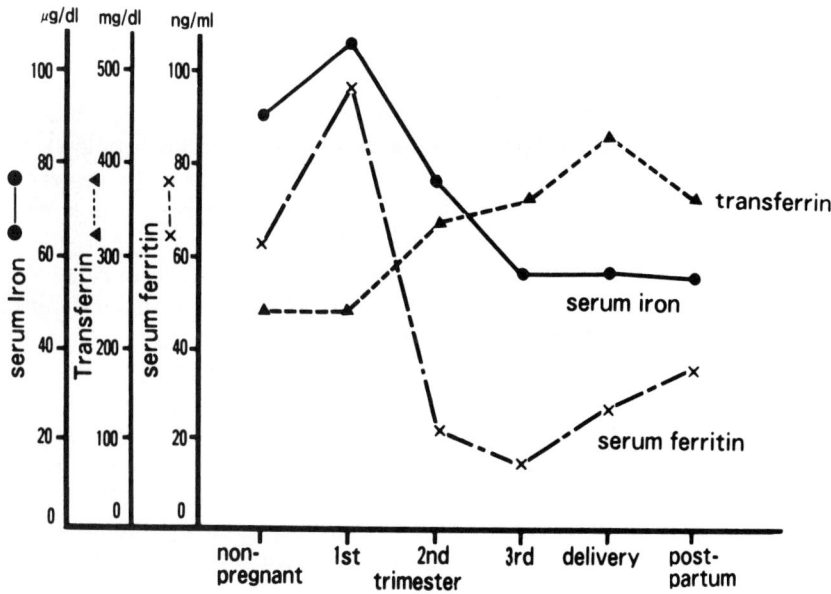

Fig. 8–7. Indices of iron turnover during pregnancy in women without overt anemia but who were not given iron supplementation. (From Kaneshige and colleagues, 1981, with permission.)

quate amounts. In the absence of added exogenous iron, the hemoglobin concentration and hematocrit fall appreciably as the maternal blood volume increases. Hemoglobin production in the fetus, however, will not be impaired, because the placenta obtains iron from the mother in amounts sufficient for the fetus to establish normal hemoglobin levels even when the mother has severe iron-deficiency anemia.

The amount of iron absorbed from diet, together with that mobilized from stores, is usually insufficient to meet the demands imposed by pregnancy. This is true even though gastrointestinal tract iron absorption appears to be moderately increased during pregnancy (Hahn and associates, 1951). If the pregnant woman who is not anemic is not given supplemental iron, serum iron and ferritin concentrations decline during the second half of pregnancy (Fig. 8–7). The somewhat unexpected early pregnancy increases in serum iron and ferritin are thought to be due to minimal iron demands during the first trimester as well as to a positive iron balance because of amenor-

rhea. These values, summarized in Table 8–3, show that standard deviations for a given mean value are quite large. For example, in pregnant women without overt anemia and not given supplemental iron, serum ferritin levels can vary from 7.0 to 22.4 ng/mL during the third trimester. Also shown in Figure 8–7 is the increase in iron-binding capacity (transferrin) that occurs even when iron deficiency has been eliminated by oral iron supplementation.

Blood Loss. Not all the iron added to the maternal circulation in the form of hemoglobin is necessarily lost from the mother. During normal vaginal delivery and through the next few days, only about one half of the erythrocytes added to the maternal circulation during pregnancy are lost from the majority of women by way of the placental implantation site, the placenta itself, the episiotomy wound and lacerations, and in the lochia. On the average, an amount of maternal erythrocytes corresponding to about 500 to 600 mL of predelivery blood is lost during and after vaginal de-

TABLE 8–3. CONCENTRATIONS OF HEMOGLOBIN, SERUM IRON, TRANSFERRIN, AND SERUM FERRITIN DURING PREGNANCY IN WOMEN WITHOUT OVERT ANEMIA AND NOT GIVEN DIETARY IRON SUPPLEMENTATION

Concentration	Nonpregnant (n = 10)	1st Trimester (n = 17)	2nd Trimester (n = 26)	3rd Trimester (n = 17)	At Delivery (n = 33)	Postpartum (n = 27)
Hemoglobin (g/dL)	13.0± 0.6	12.2± 1.3	10.9± 0.8	11.0± 0.9	12.4± 1.0	11.5± 1.0
Serum iron (µg/dL)	90.0±32.9	106.5±24.5	75.3±37.8	56.0±31.0[a]	57.1±31.2[a]	56.0±21.8[a]
Transferrin (mg/dL)	242.1±52.7	244.6±52.7	336.2±72.6[a]	362.8±55.4[a]	438.2±80.0[a]	363.4±40.5[a]
Serum ferritin (ng/mL)	63.0±34.7	97.4±39.4[a]	22.2±14.6[b]	14.7± 7.7[b]	27.6±15.6[b]	36.0±23.0[b]

Each value represents the mean ± standard deviation.
Significantly different from nonpregnant value:
[a] P < .05,
[b] P < .005.
From Kaneshige (1981), with permission.

livery of a single fetus (Pritchard, 1965; Ueland, 1976). The average blood loss associated with cesarean delivery or with the vaginal delivery of twins is about 1000 mL, or nearly twice that lost with the delivery of a single fetus. It is not rare for the quantity of erythrocytes lost to equal or exceed the added volume accumulated during pregnancy.

Generally, the pattern of change in maternal blood volume during labor, vaginal delivery, and puerperium is as follows: (1) there is some hemoconcentration during labor, which varies with the degree of muscular activity and dehydration; (2) during and soon after delivery there is a further reduction in volume, which closely parallels the amount of blood lost; (3) during the first few days of the puerperium there is little change in blood volume; and (4) by 1 week after delivery there is a further reduction in plasma volume to the extent that the maternal blood volume is only slightly greater than several months later (Pritchard, 1965).

After delivery, any excess circulating hemoglobin above the amount normally present in the nonpregnant state ultimately yields iron for storage. The mechanism by which this occurs is most likely not accelerated erythrocyte destruction during the late puerperium, but rather normal destruction with reduced production of new erythrocytes. A similar process occurs after a normal nonanemic person receives transfused cells, or when a normal person with polycythemia, induced by high altitude, returns to sea level.

Immunological and Leukocyte Functions.

Pregnancy has been assumed to be associated with suppression of a variety of humoral and cellularly mediated immunological functions in order to accommodate the "foreign" semiallogeneic fetal graft. In fact, humoral antibody titers against several viruses—for example, herpes simplex, measles, and influenza A—decrease during pregnancy. The decrease in titers, however, is accounted for by the hemodilutional effect of pregnancy (Baboonnian and Griffiths, 1983). The prevalence of a variety of autoantibodies is unchanged (Patton and colleagues, 1987). Furthermore, α-interferon, which is present in almost all fetal tissues and fluids, is most often absent in normally pregnant women (Chard and co-workers, 1986). There is evidence, as yet unexplained, that polymorphonuclear leukocyte chemotaxis and adherence functions are depressed beginning in the second trimester and continuing throughout pregnancy (Krause and associates, 1987). It is possible that these depressed leukocyte functions of pregnant women account in part for the improvement observed in some with autoimmune diseases and the possibly increased susceptibility to certain infections. Thus, both function and absolute numbers of leukocytes appear to be important factors when considering the leukocytosis of normal pregnancy.

The blood leukocyte count varies considerably during normal pregnancy. Usually it ranges from 5000 to 12,000 per mL. During labor and the early puerperium it may become markedly elevated, attaining levels of 25,000 or even more; however, the concentration averages 14,000 to 16,000 per mL (Taylor and co-workers, 1981). The cause for the marked increase is not known, but the same response occurs during and after strenuous exercise. It probably represents the reappearance in the circulation of leukocytes previously shunted out of the active circulation.

C-reactive protein is an acute-phase serum reactant originally named because it precipitates with the C-polysaccharide extract of *Streptococcus pneumoniae.* Serum concentrations rise rapidly to 1000-fold in response to tissue trauma or inflammation. Watts and colleagues (1991) measured C-reactive protein sequentially during 81 normal pregnancies to establish normal values. Median C-reactive protein values during pregnancy were higher than values for nonpregnant individuals, and these values were elevated further in labor. In women not in labor, 95 percent of values were 1.5 mg/dL or less, and gestational age did not affect maternal serum levels.

Beginning quite early in pregnancy, the activity of **leukocyte alkaline phosphatase** is increased. Such elevated activity is not peculiar to pregnancy but occurs in a wide variety of conditions, including most inflammatory states. During pregnancy there is a neutrophilia that consists predominantly of mature forms; however, an occasional myelocyte is found.

Basic immunology, the immunology of implantation and placentation, and maternal immune responses were recently reviewed elegantly by Stirrat (1991).

Blood Coagulation.

The levels of several blood coagulation factors are increased during pregnancy. Plasma fibrinogen (factor I) in normal nonpregnant women averages about 300 mg/dL and ranges from about 200 to 400. During normal pregnancy, fibrinogen concentration increases about 50 percent to average about 450 mg/dL late in pregnancy, with a range from 300 to 600. The increase in the concentration of fibrinogen undoubtedly contributes greatly to the striking increase in the *erythrocyte sedimentation rate* in normal pregnancy (Ozanne and co-workers, 1983). Increased sedimentation in pregnancy, therefore, has no diagnostic or prognostic value when employed for usual clinical purposes, such as the assessment of the activity of lupus erythematosus.

Other clotting factor activities that are increased appreciably during normal pregnancy are factor VII (proconvertin), factor VIII (antihemophilic globulin), factor IX (plasma thromboplastin component or Christmas factor), and factor X (Stuart factor). Usually the level of factor II (prothrombin) is increased only slightly, whereas activities of factors XI (plasma thromboplastin antecedent) and XIII (fibrin-stabilizing factors) are decreased somewhat (Coopland and associates, 1969; Kasper and colleagues, 1964; Talbert and Langdell, 1964). The Quick one-stage prothrombin time and the partial thromboplastin time both are shortened slightly as pregnancy progresses.

There is a moderate decrease in the number of platelets per unit volume as pregnancy progresses (Pitkin and Witte, 1980). This may be the consequence of increased platelet consumption throughout normal pregnancy (Fay and co-workers, 1983). The clotting times of whole blood in either plain glass tubes (wettable surface) or silicone-coated or plastic tubes (nonwettable surface) do not significantly differ in normal pregnant and nonpregnant women. Some, but not all, of the pregnancy-induced changes in the levels of coagulation factors can be duplicated by the administration of estrogen plus progestin contraceptive tablets.

High-molecular-weight soluble fibrin–fibrinogen complexes circulate in normal pregnancy. Also, an increased capacity for neutralizing heparin has been described, but plasma antithrombin III does not appear to be reduced during pregnancy (Weiner and Brandt, 1980). Some of these alterations in coagulation factors during normal pregnancy may be equated with continuing low-grade intravascular coagulation. In support of this concept, Tygart and associates (1986) observed a mildly elevated mean platelet volume and a significant increase in platelet distribution width as pregnancy advanced. They interpreted these observations to represent an increased level of thrombocytopoiesis as a consequence of both dilutional and consumptive stimuli of normal pregnancy. Rakoczi and co-workers (1979) reported a shorter half-life for platelets in pregnant compared with nonpregnant women. Beta-thromboglobulin, a platelet-specific protein, also is increased during the second half of pregnancy in normally pregnant women (Douglas and associates, 1982). Bonnar (1978) used electron microscopy and identified fibrin deposited in the intervillous space of the placenta and in the walls of the spiral arteries that supply blood to the intervillous space.

During normal pregnancy, the level of maternal plasminogen (profibrinolysin) in plasma increases considerably, a phenomenon that can be induced by estrogen treatment. Even so, fibrinolytic, or plasmin, activity, measured either as the time for clotted plasma to dissolve or as the time for the clotted euglobulin fraction from plasma to undergo lysis, is distinctly prolonged compared with that of the normal nonpregnant state. Astedt (1972) implicated the placenta in the reduced fibrinolytic activity that characterizes normal pregnancy, because delivery is normally followed by a prompt increase in plasma fibrinolytic activity (Ratnoff and co-workers, 1954). At the same time, fibrin degradation

products usually rise slightly after delivery (Woodfield and associates, 1968).

Cardiovascular System

During pregnancy and the puerperium there are remarkable changes involving the heart and the circulation. These changes are graphically summarized in Figure 8–8, which also shows the important effects of maternal posture on hemodynamic events during pregnancy. The effects of those profound changes in pregnant women with heart disease is discussed in Chapter 48.

Heart. The resting pulse rate increases about 10 to 15 beats per minute during pregnancy. As the diaphragm becomes progressively elevated, the heart is displaced to the left and upward, while at the same time it is rotated somewhat on its long axis. As a result, the apex of the heart is moved somewhat laterally from its position in the normal nonpregnant state, and an increase in the size of the cardiac silhouette is found in radiographs

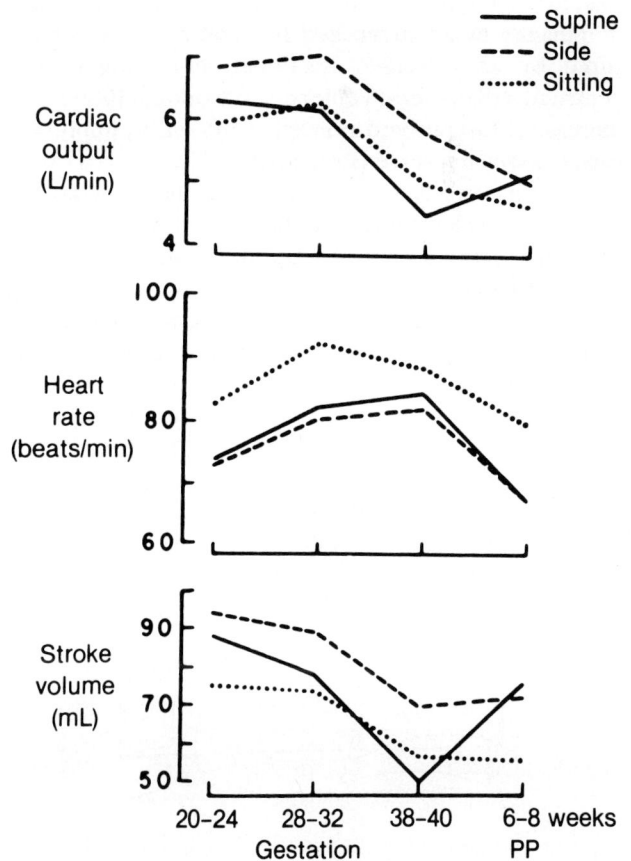

Fig. 8–8. Effect of maternal posture on hemodynamics. (From Ueland and Metcalfe, 1975, with permission.)

(Fig. 8–9). The extent of these changes is influenced by the size and position of the uterus, the strength of the abdominal muscles, and the configurations of the abdomen and thorax. Furthermore, normally pregnant women apparently have some degree of benign pericardial effusion, which may increase the cardiac silhouette on x-ray (Enein and colleagues, 1987). Variability of these factors makes it difficult to identify precisely moderate degrees of cardiomegaly by physical examination or by simple x-ray studies. Therefore, a diagnosis of pathological cardiomegaly during pregnancy should be made cautiously.

In several studies using frontal and sagittal x-rays, the cardiac volume was found to increase normally by about 75 mL, or a little more than 10 percent, between early and late pregnancy (Ihrman, 1960). Katz and co-workers (1978) studied left ventricular performance during pregnancy and the puerperium using echocardiography. Both left ventricular wall mass and end-diastolic dimensions increased during pregnancy, as did heart rate, calculated stroke volume, and cardiac output. The changes in stroke volume were directly proportional to end-diastolic volume, implying, at least, that there is little change in the inotropic state of the myocardium during normal singleton pregnancy and the puerperium. In multifetal pregnancies, however, cardiac output is increased even more than in singleton pregnancies. This is accomplished predominantly by an **increased inotropic effect** as measured by an increased fractional shortening of the ventricular diameters (Veille and co-workers, 1985). The increased heart rate and inotropic contractility imply that cardiovascular reserve is reduced.

During pregnancy, some of the cardiac sounds may be altered to the extent that they would be considered abnormal in the absence of pregnancy. Cutforth and Mac-Donald (1966) obtained phonocardiograms at varying stages of pregnancy in 50 normal women and documented the following changes: (1) an exaggerated split-ting of the first heart sound with increased loudness of both components; no definite changes in the aortic and pulmonary elements of the second sound; and a loud, easily heard third sound; and (2) a systolic murmur in 90 percent of pregnant women, intensified during inspiration in some or expiration in others, and disappearing very shortly after delivery; a soft diastolic murmur transiently in 20 percent; and continuous murmurs arising apparently in the breast vasculature in 10 percent. Thus, the significance of murmurs during pregnancy must be assessed carefully, especially systolic murmurs.

Normal pregnancy induces no characteristic changes in the *electrocardiogram* other than slight deviation of the electrical axis to the left as a result of the altered position of the heart.

Cardiac Output. During normal pregnancy, arterial blood pressure and vascular resistance decrease while blood volume, maternal weight, and basal metabolic rate increase. Each of these events would be expected to affect cardiac output with some leading to decreased output but others causing an increase. It is now evident that cardiac output *at rest*, when measured in the lateral recumbent position, increases appreciably beginning in early pregnancy, and continues to increase and remains elevated during the remainder of pregnancy (Fig. 8–10). Typically, cardiac output in late pregnancy is appreciably higher when the woman is in the lateral recumbent position than when she is supine, because in the supine position the large uterus often impedes cardiac venous return. Ueland and Hansen (1969), for example, found

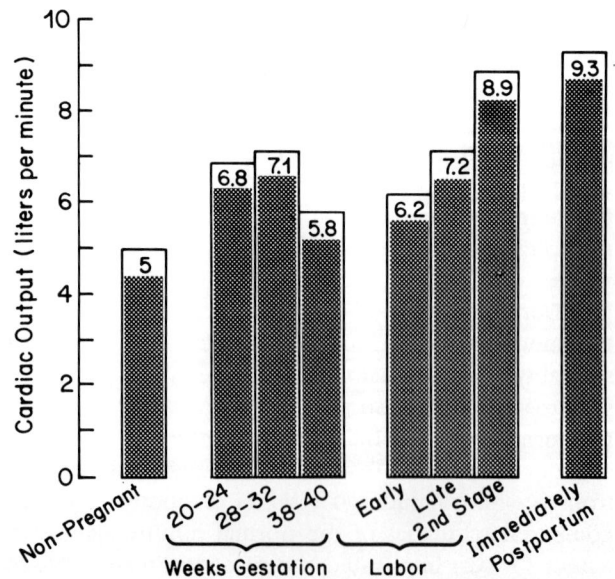

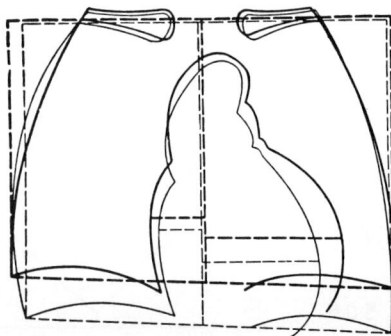

Fig. 8–9. Change in cardiac outline that occurs in pregnancy. The light lines represent the relations between the heart and thorax in the nonpregnant woman, and the heavy lines represent the conditions existing in pregnancy. These findings are based on x-ray findings in 33 women. (From Klafen and Palugyay, 1927.)

Fig. 8–10. Cardiac outputs during three stages of gestation, labor, and immediately postpartum are compared with values of nonpregnant women. All values were determined with women in the lateral recumbent position. (Adapted from Ueland and Metcalfe, 1975, with permission.)

cardiac output to increase 1100 mL (22 percent) when the pregnant woman was moved from her back onto her side. When she assumes the standing position after sitting, cardiac output in the pregnant woman falls to the same degree as in the nonpregnant woman (Easterling and associates, 1988).

Cardiac output in response to physical activity by the ambulatory woman must be greater late in pregnancy than it would be if she were not pregnant. Increase in mass alone demands such a response. During the first stage of labor, cardiac output increases moderately, and during the second stage, with vigorous expulsive efforts, it is appreciably greater (Fig. 8–10). Most of the increase in cardiac output induced by pregnancy is lost very soon after delivery (Ueland and Metcalfe, 1975).

Antepartum Hemodynamic Values for Late Pregnancy.

Clark and colleagues (1989) have conducted important studies of maternal cardiovascular hemodynamics that serve to define normal antepartum hemodynamic values late in pregnancy (Table 8–4). Right heart catheterization was performed in 10 healthy nulliparous women at 35 to 38 weeks' gestation, and again at 11 to 13 weeks postpartum. Late pregnancy was associated with the expected increases in heart rate, stroke volume, and cardiac output. Systemic vascular and pulmonary vascular resistance both decreased significantly, as did colloid osmotic pressure. Pulmonary capillary wedge pressure and central venous pressure did not change appreciably between late pregnancy and the puerperium. These investigators concluded that normal late pregnancy is not associated with hyperdynamic left ventricular function as determined by Starling function curves.

Factors Controlling Vascular Reactivity in Pregnancy.

Gant and associates (1973) conducted a prospective study of vascular reactivity to angiotensin II throughout pregnancy to ascertain when vascular refractoriness to angiotensin II was lost in women who later became hypertensive. The results of these studies are given in Figure 36–1 (p. 770). Briefly, 192 young primigravid women were studied sequentially, and at each clinic visit they were infused with angiotensin II in doses sufficient to increase baseline diastolic blood pressure by 20 mm Hg. The dose of angiotensin II in ng/kg per minute required to elevate diastolic blood pressure 20 mm Hg was recorded as the *effective pressor dose.* Women destined to develop pregnancy-induced hypertension became progressively more sensitive to the pressor effects of infused angiotensin II after 18 weeks. In a retrospective analysis of the data obtained between 28 and 32 weeks, it was ascertained that more than 90 percent of women in whom the effective pressor dose of angiotensin II was less than 8 ng/kg per minute developed hypertension 10 to 14 weeks later. Conversely, hypertension did not develop in over 90 percent of those women who remained refractory to angiotensin II infusion at doses greater than this.

The early and clear divergence the effective pressor dose of angiotensin II observed in normal and subsequently preeclamptic women was likely the result of significant alterations in a variety of physiological processes that serve to control vascular reactivity to angiotensin II. Gant and associates (1974b) speculated that possible factors included alterations in circulating plasma levels of renin, angiotensin II, aldosterone, and possibly prostaglandins. Certainly, in pregnancies complicated by pregnancy-induced hypertension, plasma renin concentration, renin activity, angiotensin II, and aldosterone levels are lower than in normotensive women (Chesley, 1978).

Renin, Angiotensin II, and Plasma Volume.

Pressor responsiveness to angiotensin II and the renin–angiotensin–aldosterone system is altered remarkably in pregnancy. In normotensive pregnant women, there are marked increases in the concentrations of plasma renin, renin activity, renin substrate, angiotensin II, and aldos-

TABLE 8–4. CENTRAL HEMODYNAMIC CHANGES IN 10 NORMAL NULLIPAROUS WOMEN BETWEEN 35 AND 38 WEEKS' GESTATION AND AGAIN WHEN 11 TO 13 WEEKS POSTPARTUM

	Pregnant[a]	Postpartum	Change
Mean arterial pressure (mm Hg)	90 ± 6	86 ± 8	No change
Pulmonary capillary wedge pressure (mm Hg)	8 ± 2	6 ± 2	No change
Central venous pressure (mm Hg)	4 ± 3	4 ± 3	No change
Heart rate (beats/min)	83 ± 10	71 ± 10	+ 17%
Cardiac output (L/min)	6.2 ± 1.0	4.3 ± 0.9	+ 43%
Systemic vascular resistance (dyne/sec/cm^{-5})	1210 ± 266	1530 ± 520	− 21%
Pulmonary vascular resistance (dyne/sec/cm^{-5})	78 ± 22	119 ± 47	− 34%
Serum colloid osmotic pressure (mm Hg)	18.0 ± 1.5	20.8 ± 1.0	− 14%
COP-PCWP gradient (mm Hg)	10.5 ± 2.7	14.5 ± 2.5	− 28%
Left ventricular stroke work index (g/m/m^2)	48 ± 6	41 ± 8	No change

COP = colloid osmotic pressure; PCWP = pulmonary capillary wedge pressure.
[a] Made in lateral recumbent position.
Adapted from Clark and colleagues (1989), with permission.

terone, as well as a blunted pressor response to infused angiotensin II (Chesley, 1978). Gant and co-workers (1974b) and Cunningham and associates (1975) found that various volume loads, including normal saline (1000 mL), dextran (500 mL), and packed red blood cells (950 mL), did not alter pressor responsiveness to angiotensin II in normotensive pregnant women despite significant increases in blood volume and decreases in renin plasma levels. Therefore, the increased refractoriness to angiotensin II characteristic of normal pregnancy is likely the consequence of individual vessel refractoriness to angiotensin II. That is, in the woman destined to develop preeclampsia, or in the woman already acutely ill with preeclampsia, the increased sensitivity to angiotensin II was the result of an alteration in vessel wall refractoriness *rather* than the consequence of changes in blood volume or circulating renin-angiotensin levels.

Prostaglandins. Prostaglandins are potent mediators of vascular reactivity in several organs under a variety of conditions. Terragno and colleagues (1974) reported that late in canine pregnancy, uterine blood flow was related to the concentration of prostaglandin E in uterine venous blood. They also observed that the intravenous infusion of angiotensin II into pregnant dogs led to an increase in uterine blood flow and a rise in the level of prostaglandin E in uterine blood.

Everett and co-workers (1978c) evaluated the effect of prostaglandin synthase inhibitors on the effective pressor dose of angiotensin II in normally pregnant women after 28 weeks. They found that indomethacin and aspirin resulted in a significant reduction in the amount of infused angiotensin II required to evoke an increase in diastolic blood pressure of 20 mm Hg. Thus, the refractoriness to angiotensin II usually observed during normal human pregnancy may be mediated in part by the action of prostaglandin-related substances that are produced in situ by arteriolar endothelium. Decreases in the rate of prostaglandin synthesis, or increases in the rate of prostaglandin catabolism, might therefore result in increased vascular responsiveness to infused angiotensin II, a characteristic of the pregnant woman who has developed or is destined to develop pregnancy-induced hypertension.

The likelihood of prostaglandin involvement in the regulation of vascular reactivity in pregnancy was confirmed by Broughton-Pipkin and Meirelles (1982). They infused prostaglandin E_2 intravenously into pregnant women and found that the amount of angiotensin II required to raise diastolic blood pressure by 20 mm Hg was increased.

Progesterone and Progesterone Metabolites. Other factors appear to participate in modulating vascular responsiveness to angiotensin II during pregnancy. Gant and associates (1977) observed that normally pregnant

women lose pregnancy-acquired vascular refractoriness to angiotensin II within 15 to 30 minutes after the placenta is delivered. Moreover, large amounts of intramuscular progesterone given during late labor delayed this loss. On the other hand, intravenously administered progesterone does not restore angiotensin II refractoriness to women with pregnancy-induced hypertension; however, the infusion of a major progesterone metabolite—5α-pregnane-3, 20-dione (5α-dihydroprogesterone)—does. Although the mechanism by which 5α-dihydroprogesterone restores vascular refractoriness to women with pregnancy-induced hypertension is not known, infusion of this steroid into five normally pregnant women who had been rendered angiotensin II-sensitive by the administration of indomethacin also restored vascular refractoriness (Everett and associates, 1978a).

Thus, a progestin-induced mechanism may modulate the prostaglandin-mediated vascular responsiveness to the pressor effects of angiotensin II that is characteristic of normal human pregnancy. Alternatively, the steroid may act independently of prostaglandin action(s).

Alterations in Cyclic AMP. Administration of theophylline to angiotensin II-sensitive pregnant women with early-onset pregnancy-induced hypertension more than doubled the mean effective pressor dose of angiotensin II, restoring the vascular refractoriness characteristic of normal pregnancy (Everett and co-workers, 1978b). This effect of theophylline likely results from its inhibition of the enzyme phosphodiesterase, a principal regulator of intracellular cyclic nucleotide accumulation. Phosphodiesterase activity inhibition would promote the accumulation of cyclic adenosine monophosphate (cAMP) within vascular smooth muscle and should lead to the promotion of vascular smooth muscle relaxation.

Alterations in Calcium Entry to Vascular Smooth Muscle. Reductions in vascular refractoriness to infused angiotensin II have been reported in normal women and several different animals after the administration of various agents that act as calcium-channel blockers (Anderson, 1987; Hof, 1984, 1985; Pasanisi, 1985; Vierhapper, 1982; and their co-workers).

Endothelin. Decreased vascular tone in pregnancy may be attributed in part to changes in the synthesis of endothelial-derived vasoactive substances. It is likely that vascular endothelium generates vasodilators and vasoconstrictor substances that may be crucial to the adaptive changes of pregnancy. It was recently shown that the vascular endothelium produces endothelin[-1], a 21-amino-acid residue peptide with potent vasoconstrictor properties (Yanagisawa and colleagues, 1988). This discovery has prompted interest in the role of endothelin in the control of vascular responsiveness during pregnancy. It is thought to act at its site of production as a local regulator of tissue blood supply. Moreover, endothelin^{-1} is a potent stimulator of arachidonic acid metabolism (Zoja and colleagues, 1990), and therefore is a hormone capable theoretically of mediating both prostacyclin and prostaglandin E_2 synthesis. In one of the early studies of endothelin during human pregnancy, Benigni and co-workers (1991) found significantly increased renal synthesis of endothelin^{-1} after the second trimester (see also Chaps. 4 and 12).

Summary: Control of Vascular Reactivity. It appears likely that vascular reactivity in human pregnancy is controlled at least in part by (1) the action of a prostaglandin(s) or prostaglandin-related substance(s) on vascular smooth muscle, (2) progestin action that may modify the prostaglandin effect, (3) alterations in the cyclic nucleotide system of vascular smooth muscle, (4) changes in intracellular calcium concentration, and (5) endothelium-derived factors that cause vasodilation or vasoconstriction.

Circulation. The posture of the pregnant woman affects *arterial blood pressure.* Typically, blood pressure in the brachial artery is highest when sitting, lowest when lying in the lateral recumbent position, and intermediate when supine, except for some women who become quite hypotensive in the supine position. Usually, arterial blood pressure decreases to a nadir during the second trimester or early third trimester and rises thereafter. A sustained rise of 30 mm Hg systolic or 15 mm Hg diastolic pressure under basal conditions may be indicative of an abnormality, most likely pregnancy-induced hypertension (see Chap. 36, p. 763).

The antecubital *venous pressure* remains unchanged during pregnancy, but in the supine position the femoral venous pressure rises steadily, from 8 cm H_2O early in pregnancy to 24 cm H_2O at term (Fig. 8–11). Employing radiolabeled tracers, Wright and co-workers (1950) and others have demonstrated that blood flow in the legs is retarded during pregnancy except when the lateral recumbent position is assumed. This tendency toward stagnation of blood in the lower extremities during the latter part of pregnancy is attributable to the occlusion of the pelvic veins and inferior vena cava by pressure of the enlarged uterus. The elevated venous pressure returns to normal if the pregnant woman lies on her side and immediately after delivery (McLennan, 1943). From a clinical viewpoint, the retarded blood flow and increased lower extremity venous pressure are of great importance. These alterations contribute to the dependent edema frequently experienced by women as they approach term, and to the development of varicose veins in the legs and vulva, as well as hemorrhoids.

Supine Hypotension. In the supine position, the large pregnant uterus rather consistently compresses the

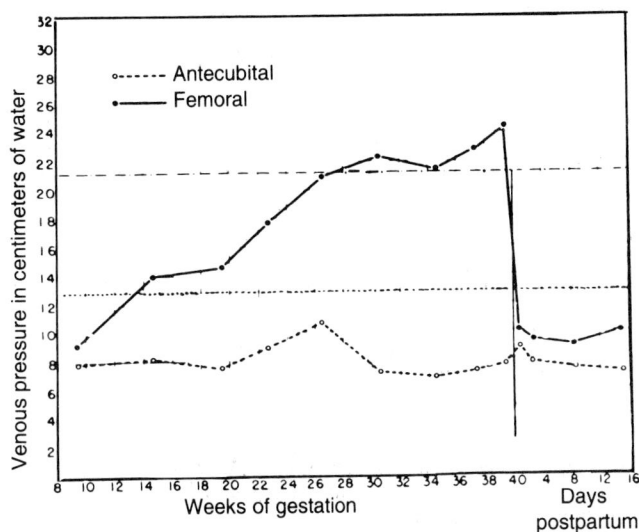

Fig. 8–11. Serial changes in antecubital and femoral venous blood pressure throughout normal pregnancy and early puerperium. These measurements were made on women in the supine position. (From McLennan, 1943.)

venous system that returns blood from the lower half of the body to the extent that cardiac filling may be reduced and cardiac output decreased. Infrequently, this causes significant arterial hypotension, sometimes referred to as the *supine hypotensive syndrome* (Howard and colleagues, 1953). Bieniarz and associates (1968) observed that in the supine position, the large pregnant uterus may compress the aorta sufficiently to lower arterial blood pressure below the level of compression. They demonstrated that the usual measurement of blood pressures in the brachial artery does not provide a reliable estimate of the pressure in the uterine or other arteries that lie distal to aortic compression. When the pregnant woman is supine, uterine arterial pressure is significantly lower than that in the brachial artery. In the presence of systemic hypotension, as occurs with spinal analgesia, the decrease in uterine arterial pressure is even more marked than in arteries above the level of aortic compression.

Gant and associates (1974a) reported that an appreciable number of women destined to develop pregnancy-induced hypertension exhibited more than a 20 mm Hg increase in diastolic blood pressure when they were turned from the lateral to the supine position. They called this a *supine pressor test,* but its exact mechanism remains to be defined.

Blood Flow to Skin. Increased cutaneous blood flow in pregnancy is thought to serve to dissipate excess heat generated by increased metabolism (Spetz, 1964).

Respiratory Tract

Anatomical Changes. The diaphragm rises about 4 cm during pregnancy. The subcostal angle widens appreciably as the transverse diameter of the thoracic cage increases about 2 cm. The thoracic circumference increases about 6 cm, but not sufficiently to prevent a reduction in the residual volume of air in the lungs created by the elevated diaphragm. The idea that the elevated diaphragm was "splinted" during normal pregnancy has been disproved using fluoroscopic studies (Möbius, 1961). Diaphragmatic excursion is actually greater during pregnancy than when nonpregnant. As a result, the tidal volume increases.

Pulmonary Function. At any stage of normal pregnancy, the amount of oxygen delivered by the increase in tidal volume clearly exceeds the oxygen need imposed by the pregnancy. Moreover, the amount of hemoglobin in the circulation, and in turn the total oxygen-carrying capacity, increases appreciably during normal pregnancy, as does cardiac output. As the consequence, *maternal arteriovenous oxygen* difference is decreased.

The respiratory rate is little changed during pregnancy but the *tidal volume, minute ventilatory volume,* and *minute oxygen uptake* increase appreciably as pregnancy advances (Table 8–5). The *maximum breathing capacity* and *forced or timed vital capacity* are not altered appreciably. The *functional residual capacity* and the *residual volume* of air are decreased as the consequence of the elevated diaphragm. *Lung compliance* is unaffected by pregnancy while *airway conductance* is increased and *total pulmonary resistance* is reduced, possibly effected by progesterone action.

The *closing volume,* or the lung volume at which airways in the dependent parts of the lung begin to close during expiration, has been considered to be higher in pregnancy by some investigators but not by others (DeSwiet, 1991). If indeed it was increased, this would suggest that the caliber of the small airways is decreased.

An increased awareness of a desire to breathe is common even early in pregnancy (Milne and colleagues,

1978). This may be interpreted as dyspnea, which in turn suggests pulmonary or cardiac abnormalities when none exists. The mechanism of physiological dyspnea is thought to be increased tidal volume that lowers the blood P_{CO_2} slightly, which paradoxically causes dyspnea.

The increased respiratory effort and in turn the reduction in P_{CO_2} during pregnancy is most likely induced in large part by progesterone and to a lesser degree estrogen. Medroxyprogesterone has been administered to stimulate an increased respiratory drive in obese nonpregnant subjects who hypoventilate. Their site of action appears to be central through a direct stimulatory effect on the respiratory center.

Although pulmonary function is not impaired by pregnancy, disease of the respiratory tract may be more serious during gestation (see Chap. 49). Important factors are undoubtedly the increased oxygen requirements imposed by pregnancy and perhaps an increase in closing volume, especially when supine.

Urinary System

Remarkable changes in both structure and function take place in the urinary tract during normal pregnancy.

Kidney. The kidney increases slightly in size during pregnancy. Bailey and Rolleston (1971), for example, found that the kidney was 1.5 cm longer during the early puerperium than when measured 6 months later.

The glomerular filtration rate (GFR) and renal plasma flow (RPF) increase early in pregnancy, the former as much as 50 percent by the beginning of the second trimester, and the latter not quite so much (Chesley, 1963; Dunlop, 1981). The precise mechanism by which these are increased in pregnancy has not been identified. Elevated glomerular filtration has been found by most investigators to persist to term (Fig. 8–12), whereas renal plasma flow decreases during late pregnancy.

Most studies of renal function conducted during pregnancy have been performed while the subjects were supine, a position that late in pregnancy may produce marked systemic hemodynamic changes (see p. 229) that lead to alterations in several aspects of renal function. Late in pregnancy, for instance, urinary flow and sodium excretion are significantly affected by posture, averaging less than half the rate of excretion in the supine position, compared with the lateral recumbent position.

Whereas posture clearly affects sodium and water excretion in late pregnancy, its impact on glomerular filtration and renal plasma flow seems to be much more variable. For example, Chesley and Sloan (1964) found both to be reduced when the pregnant woman was in the supine position, whereas Dunlop (1976) identified little or no reduction. Pritchard (1955) detected de-

TABLE 8–5. VENTILATORY FUNCTION IN PREGNANT WOMEN COMPARED WITH NONPREGNANT WOMEN

Function	Non-pregnant	Pregnant	Change (%)
Respiratory rate	15	16	—
Tidal volume (mL)	485	680	+39[a]
Minute ventilation (mL)	7270	10,340	+42[a]
Minute O₂ uptake	201	265	+32[a]
Vital capacity (mL)	3260	3310	+ 1
Maximum breathing capacity (%) of predicted)	102	97	− 5
Inspiratory capacity (mL)	2625	2745	+ 5
Residual volume (mL)	965	770	−20[a]

[a] Significant differences.
From Cugell and associates (1953).

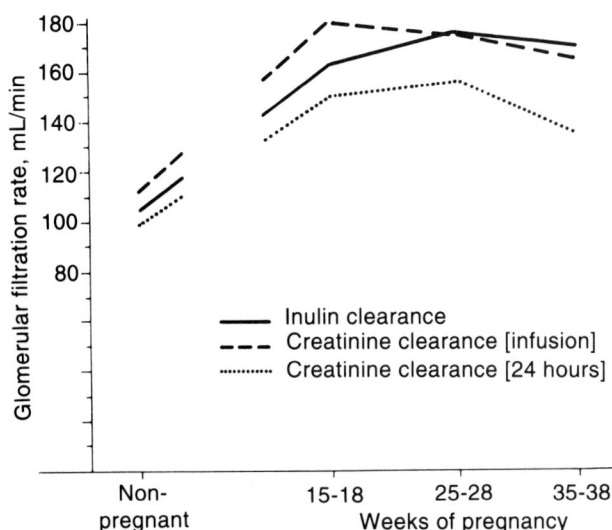

Fig. 8–12. Mean glomerular filtration rate in healthy women over a short period with infused inulin (*solid line*), simultaneously as creatinine clearance during the inulin infusion (*broken line*), and over 24 hours as endogenous creatinine clearance (*dotted line*). (From Davison and Hytten, 1974.)

creases in these while supine compared with lateral recumbent in some, but not most, of the late pregnant woman studied. Ezimokhai and associates (1981) presented evidence that the late pregnancy decrease in renal plasma flow is not due simply to a positional effect. Davison and Hytten (1974) rightfully pointed out that an estimate of glomerular filtration rate is only valid for the conditions under which it is measured and that changes with posture represent the real-life situation rather than artifact.

Loss of Nutrients. One unusual feature of the pregnancy-induced changes in renal excretion is the remarkably increased amounts of various nutrients in the urine. Amino acids and water-soluble vitamins are lost in the urine of pregnant women in much greater amounts than in the urine of nonpregnant women (Hytten and Leitch, 1971).

Tests of Renal Function. The results of several tests of renal function in general clinical use may be altered during normal pregnancy and therefore may be quite misleading. During pregnancy the plasma concentrations of creatinine and urea normally decrease as a consequence of their increased glomerular filtration. At times, the urea concentration may be so low as to suggest impaired hepatic synthesis, which sometimes occurs with severe liver disease.

Creatinine clearance is a useful test to estimate renal function in pregnancy provided that complete urine collection is made over an accurately timed period, preferably several hours at least. *Urine concentration tests* may give results that are misleading (Davison

and colleagues, 1981). During the day, pregnant women tend to accumulate water in the form of dependent edema (see p. 229); and at night, while recumbent, they mobilize this fluid and excrete it via the kidneys. This reversal of the usual nonpregnant diurnal pattern of urinary flow causes nocturia, and the urine is more dilute than in the nonpregnant state. The failure of a pregnant woman to excrete a concentrated urine after withholding fluids for approximately 18 hours does not signify renal damage. In fact, the kidney in these circumstances functions perfectly normally by excreting mobilized extracellular fluid of relatively low osmolality.

Urinalysis. *Glucosuria* during pregnancy is not necessarily abnormal. The appreciable increase in glomerular filtration, together with impaired tubular reabsorptive capacity for filtered glucose, accounts in most cases for the glucosuria (Davison and Hytten, 1975). Chesley (1963) calculated that for these reasons alone about one sixth of all pregnant women should spill glucose in the urine. Even though glucosuria is common during pregnancy, the possibility of diabetes mellitus cannot be ignored. *Proteinuria* normally does not occur during pregnancy except occasionally in slight amounts during or soon after vigorous labor. Lopez-Espinoza and colleagues (1986) measured serial urinary albumin excretion using a sensitive radioimmunoassay in 14 healthy pregnant women. There was a slight but significant rise from a median of 7 to 18 mg per 24 hours from early to late pregnancy; however, albuminuria was not detected using conventional testing methods. If not the result of contamination during collection, blood cells in the urine during pregnancy are compatible with a diagnosis of urinary tract disease. Difficult labor and delivery, of course, can cause hematuria because of trauma to the lower urinary tract.

Hydronephrosis and Hydroureter. In pregnant women, after the uterus rises completely out of the pelvis, it rests upon the ureters, compressing them at the pelvic brim. Increased intraureteral tonus above the level of the pelvic brim compared with that of the pelvic portion of the ureter has been identified (Rubi and Sala, 1968). No such differences were demonstrable in nonpregnant women.

Schulman and Herlinger (1975) found ureteral dilatation to be greater on the right side in 86 percent of pregnant women studied (Fig. 8–13). A similar result has been reported by Peake and co-workers (1983) using ultrasonic techniques. The unequal degrees of dilatation may result from a cushioning provided the left ureter by the sigmoid colon and perhaps from greater compression of the right ureter as the consequence of dextrorotation of the uterus. Bellina and co-workers (1970) emphasized that the right ovarian vein complex, which is remarkably dilated during pregnancy, lies

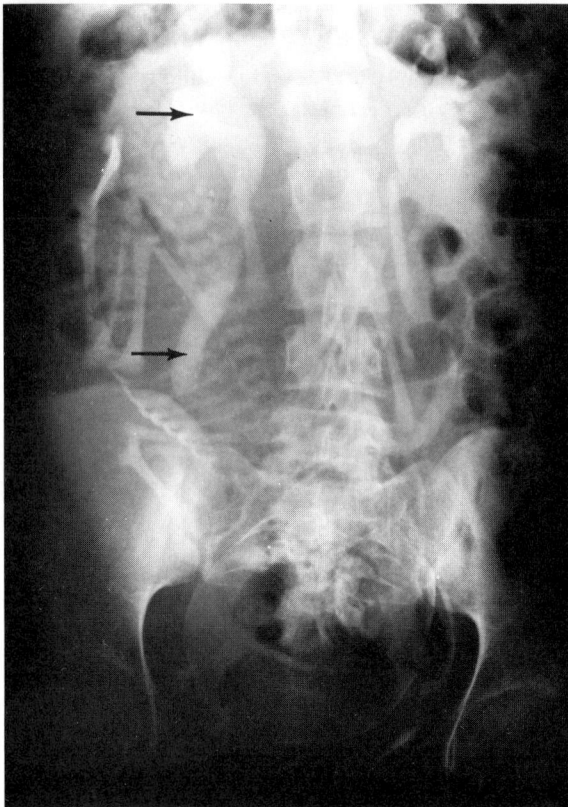

Fig. 8–13. Normal intravenous pyelogram at 36 weeks' gestation. Pregnancy-induced hydronephrosis (*upper arrow*) and hydroureter (*lower arrow*) are more marked on the right. Elongation, dilation, and peristalsis of the ureter create the appearance of ureteral discontinuity.

obliquely over the right ureter and may contribute significantly to right ureteral dilatation.

Another possible mechanism causing hydronephrosis and hydroureter is hormonal, presumably an effect of progesterone. Major support for this concept was provided by Van Wagenen and Jenkins (1939), who described in the monkey further dilatation of the ureters after removal of the fetus if the placenta remained in situ. The relatively abrupt onset of dilatation in women at midpregnancy is more consistent with ureteral compression from a translocated enlarging uterus than a hormonal effect.

Elongation accompanies distension of the ureter, which is frequently thrown into curves of varying size, the smaller of which may be sharply angulated, producing (at least theoretically) partial or complete obstruction. These so-called kinks are poorly named, because the term connotes obstruction. They are usually single or double curves, which when viewed in the radiograph taken in the same plane as the curve, appear as more or less acute angulations of the ureter (Fig. 8–13). Another exposure at right angles nearly always identifies them to be more gentle curves rather than kinks. The ureter, in both its abdominal and pelvic portions, undergoes not

only elongation but frequently lateral displacement by the pressure of the enlarged uterus.

Urinary Bladder. There are few significant anatomical changes in the bladder before the fourth month of pregnancy. From that time onward, however, the increased size of the uterus, together with the hyperemia that affects all pelvic organs and the hyperplasia of the muscle and connective tissues, elevates the bladder trigone and causes thickening of its posterior, or intraureteric, margin. Continuation of this process to the end of pregnancy produces marked deepening and widening of the trigone. The bladder mucosa undergoes no change other than an increase in the size and tortuosity of its blood vessels.

Using urethrocystometry, Iosif and colleagues (1980) found that bladder pressure doubled from 8 cm H_2O early in primigravid pregnancy to 20 cm H_2O at term. To compensate for reduced bladder capacity, absolute and functional urethral lengths increased by 6.7 and 4.8 mm, respectively. Finally, to preserve continence, maximal intraurethral pressure increased from 70 to 93 cm H_2O.

Toward the end of pregnancy, particularly in nulliparas in whom the presenting part often engages before the onset of labor, the entire base of the bladder is pushed forward and upward, converting the normal convex surface into a concavity. As a result, difficulties in diagnostic and therapeutic procedures are greatly increased. In addition, the pressure of the presenting part impairs the drainage of blood and lymph from the base of the bladder, often rendering the area edematous, easily traumatized, and probably more susceptible to infection. Both urethral pressure and length have been shown to be decreased in women following vaginal but not abdominal delivery (Van Geelen and co-workers, 1982). These investigators suggest that a weakness of the urethral sphincter mechanism due to pregnancy or delivery may play a role in the pathogenesis of urinary stress incontinence.

Normally there is little residual urine in nulliparas, but occasionally it develops in the multipara with relaxed vaginal walls and a cystocele. Incompetence of the ureterovesical valve may supervene, with the consequent probability of vesicoureteral reflux of urine.

Gastrointestinal Tract

As pregnancy progresses, the stomach and intestines are displaced by the enlarging uterus. As the result of the positional changes in these viscera, the physical findings in certain diseases are altered. The appendix, for instance, is usually displaced upward and somewhat laterally as the uterus enlarges, and at times it may reach the right flank (Chap. 51, p. 1151).

It is widely accepted that gastric emptying and intestinal transit times are delayed in pregnancy on the basis of hormonal or mechanical factors. For example, this may be the result of progesterone or decreased levels of *motilin,* a hormonal peptide known to have smooth-muscle stimulating effects (Christofides and associates, 1982). Macfie and colleagues (1991) studied gastric emptying times using paracetoneal absorption in nonpregnant women compared to antepartum women in each trimester of pregnancy and found gastric emptying times to be unchanged. However, during labor, especially after administration of analgesic agents, *gastric-emptying time* is typically prolonged appreciably. A major danger of general anesthesia for delivery is regurgitation and aspiration of either food-laden or highly acidic gastric contents (see Chap. 16, p. 427).

Pyrosis (heartburn), common during pregnancy, is most likely caused by reflux of acidic secretions into the lower esophagus (see Chap. 51, p. 1147). The altered position of the stomach probably contributes to its frequent occurrence; however, lower esophageal sphincter tone is also decreased. Intraesophageal pressures are lower and intragastric pressures higher in pregnant women. At the same time, esophageal peristalsis has lower wave speed and lower amplitude (Ulmsten and Sundström, 1978).

The gums may become hyperemic and softened during pregnancy and may bleed when mildly traumatized, as with a toothbrush. A focal, highly vascular swelling of the gums, the so-called *epulis* of pregnancy, develops occasionally but typically regresses spontaneously after delivery. Most evidence indicates that pregnancy does not incite tooth decay.

Hemorrhoids are fairly common during pregnancy. They are caused in large measure by constipation and the elevated pressure in veins below the level of the enlarged uterus.

Liver and Gallbladder

Liver. Although the liver in some animals increases remarkably in size during pregnancy, there is no evidence for such an increase during human pregnancy (Combes and Adams, 1971). Histological evaluation of liver biopsies, including examination with the electron microscope, have shown no distinct changes in liver morphology in normal pregnant women (Ingerslev and Teilum, 1946). The results of the very few measurements of hepatic blood flow during pregnancy are conflicting, and there is perhaps a slight increase.

Some of the laboratory tests commonly used to evaluate hepatic function yield appreciably different results during normal pregnancy. Moreover, the changes induced by pregnancy often occur in the same direction as those found in patients with hepatic disease. Total *alkaline phosphatase* activity in serum almost doubles during

normal pregnancy and commonly reaches levels that would be considered abnormal in the nonpregnant woman. Much of the increase is attributable to placental alkaline phosphatase isozymes, which are heat-stable up to 65° C. Whether all of the increase is caused by placental enzymes is not clear, because nonpregnant women given estrogen in amounts comparable with those found in pregnancy frequently have increased serum alkaline phosphatase activity (Song and Kappas, 1968).

Mendenhall (1970) reconfirmed the presence of a decrease in *plasma albumin* concentration, showing it to average 3.0 g/dL late in pregnancy compared with 4.3 g/dL in nonpregnant women. The reduction in albumin concentrations, combined with a normal slight increase in plasma globulins, results in a decrease in the albumin to globulin ratio similar to that seen in certain hepatic diseases. Plasma *cholinesterase* activity is reduced during normal pregnancy. The magnitude of the decrease is about the same as the decrease in the concentration of albumin (Kambam and associates, 1988; Pritchard, 1955).

Leucine aminopeptidase activity is markedly elevated in serum from pregnant women and at term it reaches a level approximately three times the nonpregnant value. The increase in total serum leucine aminopeptidase activity during pregnancy results from the appearance of a pregnancy-specific enzyme (or enzymes) with distinct substrate specificities (Song and Kappas, 1968). Pregnancy-induced aminopeptidase has oxytocinase activity.

Combes and associates (1963) demonstrated that the capacity of the liver for excreting sulfobromophthalein into bile is somewhat decreased during normal pregnancy, while at the same time the ability of the liver to extract and store sulfobromophthalein is increased. The administration of estrogens to nonpregnant women induces comparable changes. *Spider nevi* and *palmar erythema*, both of which occur in patients with liver disease, are commonly found in normal pregnant women, most likely as a result of the increased circulating estrogens during pregnancy, but they disappear soon after delivery.

Gallbladder. Gallbladder function is altered during pregnancy. Braverman and co-workers (1980), using ultrasonography, have shown the gallbladder to be sluggish during pregnancy. Specifically, there is impaired contraction and high residual volume. It has been suggested that the female hormones, especially progesterone, impair gallbladder contraction by inhibiting cholecystokinin-mediated smooth muscle stimulation, which is the primary regulator of gallbladder contraction. Such impaired gallbladder smooth muscle contraction leads to stasis, and this, associated with the increased cholesterol saturation of pregnancy, may serve to explain the increased prevalence of cholesterol stones in women who have been pregnant (Cohen, 1980).

The effects of pregnancy on bile acids in the maternal circulation have been incompletely characterized despite the long acknowledged propensity for pregnancy to cause intrahepatic cholestasis and pruritus gravidarum (see Chap. 51, p. 1153) due to retained bile salts. Cholestasis has been linked to high circulating levels of estrogen, which inhibit intraductal transport of bile acids. The primary bile acids include cholic and chenodeoxycholic acid, and 90 percent of these go through the enterohepatic circulation, which results in secondary bile acids, deoxycholic and chenodeoxycholic, formed by bacterial degradation in the gut. Carter (1991) measured postprandial venous plasma levels of total bile acids and found small but progressively increased levels during pregnancy. Specifically, mean levels were 5.3 μmol/L at 16 weeks compared with 6.5 μmol/L at term.

Endocrine Glands

Some of the most important endocrine changes of pregnancy have been discussed elsewhere, especially in Chapter 6.

Pituitary Gland. The pituitary enlarges during pregnancy by approximately 135 percent compared with nonpregnant controls (Gonzalez and colleagues, 1988). An example of this increase in size caused by hyperplasia of lactotrophs is shown in Figure 8–14. Although there have been suggestions that it may increase sufficiently to compress the optic chiasma and reduce visual fields, such visual changes during normal pregnancy are either absent or minimal. Scheithauer and colleagues (1990) have provided evidence that the incidence of pituitary prolactinomas is not increased during pregnancy. However, in some cases, enlargement of such adenomas does occur (see Chap. 53, p. 1221).

The maternal pituitary gland is not essential for maintenance of pregnancy. A number of women have undergone hypophysectomy, completed pregnancy successfully, and have undergone spontaneous labor while receiving glucocorticoids along with thyroid hormone and vasopressin. Extensive destruction of both the maternal and the fetal pituitary glands in monkeys during the second trimester does not interrupt gestation (Hutchinson and co-workers, 1962). In these hypophysectomized primates, marked adrenal atrophy did not occur; thus the placenta may be a source of an adrenal corticotropin in this species.

Growth Hormone. Although placental lactogen (hPL) is abundant in the blood of pregnant women, the level of pituitary growth hormone is increased only slightly. During the first trimester, serum and amnionic fluid growth hormone concentrations are within nonpregnant values of 0.5 to 7.5 ng/mL (Kletzky and associates, 1985). Serum values increase slowly from approximately 3.5 ng/mL at 10 weeks to plateau after 28 weeks at approximately 14 ng/mL. Growth hormone in amnionic fluid peaks at 14 to 15 weeks and slowly declines thereafter to reach baseline values after 36 weeks. After delivery, placental lactogen rapidly disappears, but growth hormone is elevated for some time but at levels lower than late pregnancy values (Spellacy and Buhi, 1969). The relative lack of these hormones, with the loss of their diabetogenic effect, may account in part for the usually abrupt and rather marked reduction in insulin requirements of women with diabetes mellitus during the early puerperium.

Prolactin. During the course of human pregnancy, there is a marked increase in the maternal plasma levels of prolactin. In fact, as shown in Figure 8–15, the levels increase to such an extent that mean concentrations of 150 ng/mL, values 10 times greater than those in normal nonpregnant women, are observed at term (Kletzky and associates, 1985). Paradoxically, after delivery, there is a decrease in plasma prolactin concentration even in women who are breastfeeding. During early lactation,

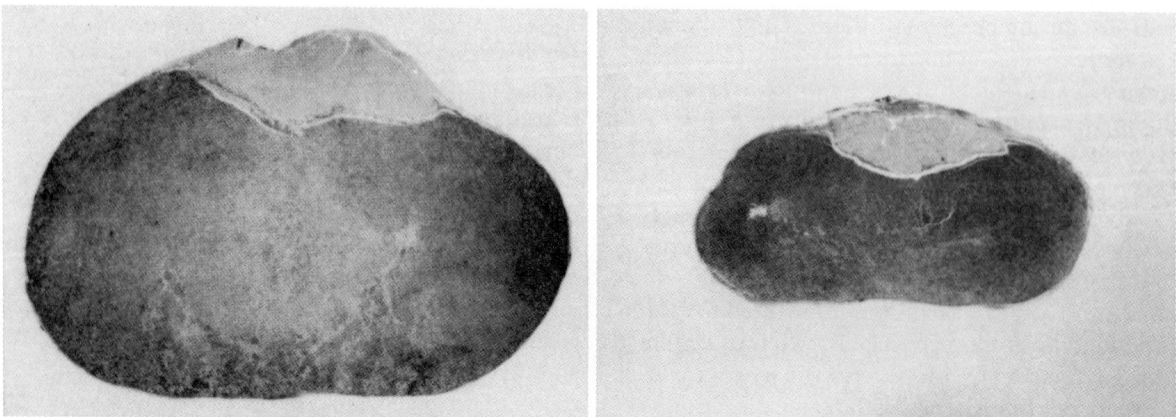

Fig. 8–14. Photographs of pituitary glands showing normal hypertrophy during pregnancy on the left compared to normal gland size in a nonpregnant woman. Both pituitary glands magnified times 6. (From Scheithauer and colleagues, 1990.)

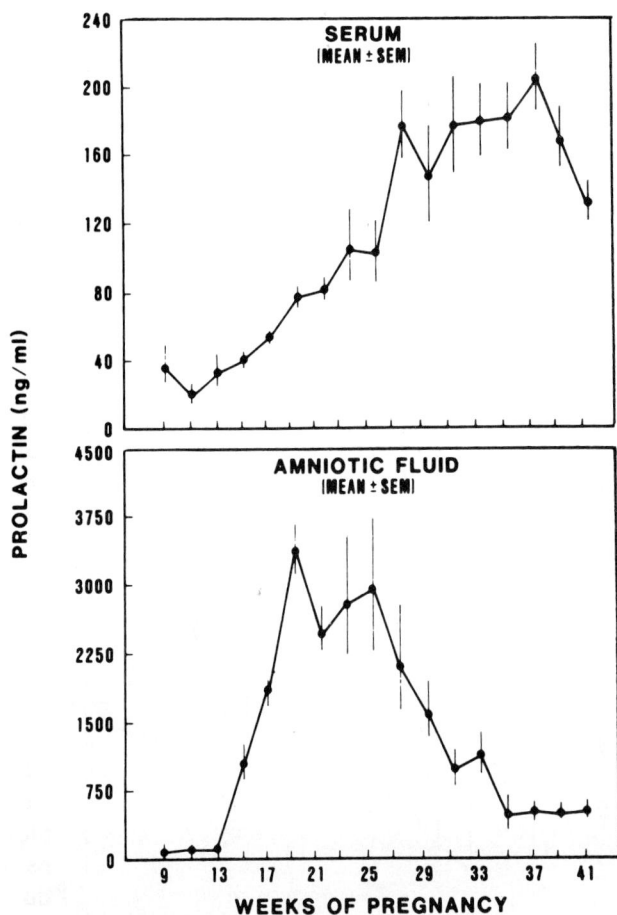

Fig. 8–15. Mean (± SEM) concentrations of human prolactin in maternal serum and in amnionic fluid throughout pregnancy. (From Kletzky and associates, 1985, with permission.)

there are pulsatile bursts of prolactin secretion apparently in response to suckling. The physiological cause of the marked increase in prolactin prior to parturition is not entirely certain; however, estrogen stimulation increases the number of anterior pituitary lactotrophs and may stimulate the release of prolactin from these cells (Andersen, 1982). Thyroid-releasing hormone acts to cause an increased prolactin level in pregnant compared with nonpregnant women but the response decreases in each trimester as pregnancy advances (Andersen, 1982; Miyamoto, 1984). Serotonin also is believed to increase prolactin but prolactin-inhibiting factor (probably identical to dopamine) is believed to inhibit its secretion (Andersen, 1982).

The principal function of maternal serum prolactin is believed to ensure lactation. Early in pregnancy, prolactin acts to initiate DNA synthesis and mitosis of glandular epithelial cells and the presecretory alveolar cells of the breast. Prolactin also increases the number of estrogen and prolactin receptors in these same cells. Finally, prolactin promotes mammary alveolar cell RNA synthesis, galactopoiesis, and production of casein and lactalbumin, lactose, and lipids (Andersen, 1982). Kaup-

pila and co-workers (1987) found that a woman with an isolated prolactin deficiency failed to lactate after two pregnancies, establishing the absolute necessity of prolactin for lactation but *not* for successful pregnancy outcome.

Prolactin also is found, throughout the course of gestation, in high concentration in the fetal plasma, attaining highest concentrations during the last 5 weeks of pregnancy (Winters and associates, 1975). Considerable evidence has accrued that is supportive of the view that prolactin in fetal plasma is of fetal pituitary origin and not of maternal pituitary origin.

Prolactin is present in amnionic fluid in high concentrations, and indeed, levels of up to 10,000 ng/mL are found in the amnionic fluid at 20 to 26 weeks' gestation (Fig. 8–15). Several groups of investigators have presented convincing evidence that the uterine decidua is the site of prolactin synthesis in amnionic fluid (Chap. 4). The levels of prolactin in amnionic fluid decrease after about 26 weeks and reach a nadir after 34 weeks at approximately 500 ng/mL.

The function of amnionic fluid prolactin is not known. Some investigators have suggested that it impairs the transfer of water from the fetal into the maternal compartment, thus preserving fetal extracellular fluid and preventing fetal dehydration during late pregnancy, when amnionic fluid is normally hypotonic (Andersen, 1982).

β-Lipotrophin. The major precursor for a number of pituitary and likely chorionic peptide hormones is proopiomelanocortin, a large peptide chain that is processed at a variety of sites by specific proteolytic enzymes (see Chap. 6, p. 144, and Fig. 6–3). One of the major fragments from this process is a 91-amino-acid chain, β-lipotrophin. This compound may then be cleaved again to give two additional fragments, one a 51-amino-acid peptide called γ-lipotrophin and the other a 31-amino-acid chain called β-endorphin, which is a potent endogenous opioid that is elevated in a variety of stressful situations, including labor, in parallel with pituitary corticotropin (Fletcher and associates, 1980; Genazzani and colleagues, 1981; Goland and associates, 1981).

Maternal plasma concentrations of β-lipotrophin, β-endorphin, and γ-lipotrophin are increased steadily throughout pregnancy (Browning and co-workers, 1983a and 1983b; Newnham and associates, 1983). Their levels are lower in women delivered vaginally who have epidural analgesia than in women receiving either a narcotic or no analgesics. The specific physiological function for these opioid agents in maternal plasma during pregnancy and labor has not been established. However, such agents obviously could serve to blunt the pain of childbirth.

Thyroid Gland. There are important changes in thyroidal economy during pregnancy that are due to three modifications in the regulation of thyroid hormones. First, pregnancy induces a marked increase in circulating levels of the major thyroxine transport protein, thyroxine-binding globulin, in response to high estrogen levels. Second, several thyroidal stimulatory factors of placental origin are produced in excess. Although it is well recognized that hyperthyroidism may develop in women with elevated chorionic gonadotropin due to trophoblastic disease, the role of this hormone in normal pregnancy still is debated. However, there is mounting evidence that the thyroid is under dual control of both thyrotropin and chorionic gonadotropin during normal and abnormal pregnancy (Kennedy and Darn, 1991). Third, pregnancy is accompanied by a decreased availability of iodide for the maternal thyroid. This is due to increased renal clearance and losses to the fetoplacental unit during late gestation, and it results in a relative iodine-deficiency state.

Glinoer and co-workers (1990) recently reported a landmark investigation of normal thyroid physiology during pregnancy. Their prospective investigation included a cohort of 606 healthy women, and they provided cross-sectional and longitudinal data of maternal thyroid functions throughout pregnancy. As shown in Figure 8–16, thyroxine-binding globulin (TBG) increased beginning early in the first trimester, reached its zenith at about 20 weeks, and stabilized at approximately double baseline values for the remainder of pregnancy. Total (free and bound thyroxine) serum thyroxine (T_4) increased sharply between 6 and 9 weeks, and thereafter only slowly, eventually reaching a plateau value of 152 nmol/L (approximately 11.5 mg/dL) at 18 weeks' gestation. In contrast to thyroxine, the rise in total triiodothyronine (T_3) was more pronounced up to 18 weeks; thereafter, it plateaued at an average value of 3.6 nmol/L (approximately 240 mg/dL). An important finding was that after 10 weeks' gestation, serum T_4 and, to a lesser extent, serum T_3, did not rise as quickly as levels of thyroxine-binding globulin observed during the first half of gestation.

The modifications in serum free T_4 and T_3 concentrations and thyroxine-binding globulin saturation as a function of gestational age are shown in Figure 8–17. There was a progressive decrease in thyroxine-binding globulin saturation, from 40 percent at 6 to 9 weeks, to an average plateau level of 30 percent saturation after 20 weeks. Similarly, free T_4 and T_3 levels decreased. The decrease in free hormones was a logical consequence of TBG desaturation, although free T_4 concentrations remained within the reference range for nonpregnant women.

Glinoer and colleagues (1990) further observed that the adjustment of thyroidal output of T_4 and T_3 was not similar for all pregnant women. Specifically, in about one third of women, there was relative hypothyroxinemia, preferential T_3 secretion, and higher (albeit normal) serum thyrotropin levels. These results suggest

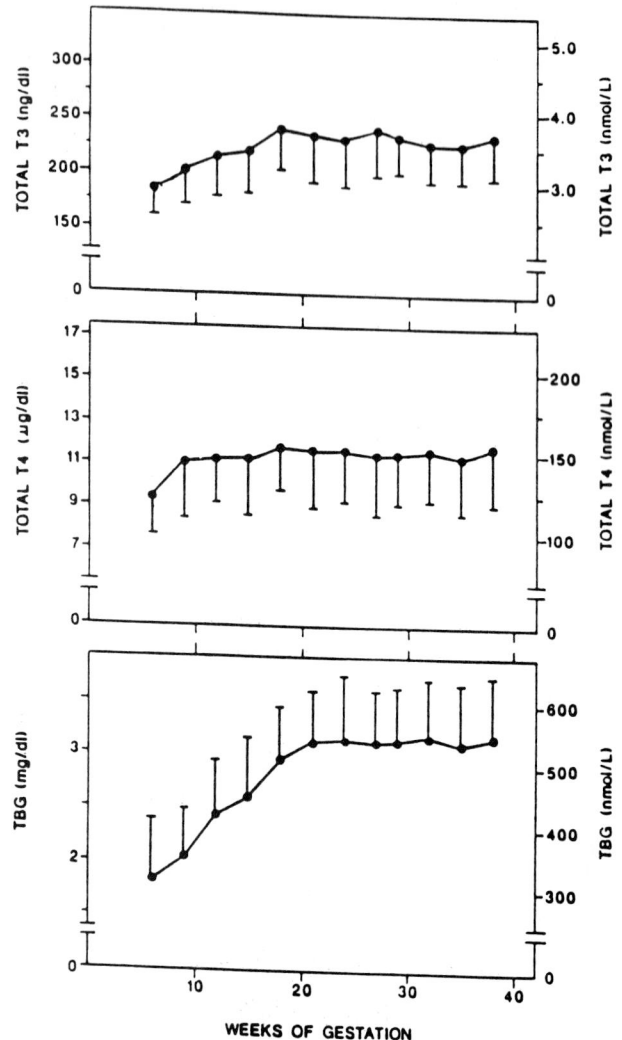

Fig. 8–16. Maternal serum triiodothyronine (T_3), thyroxine (T_4), and thyroxine-binding globulin (TBG) as a function of gestational age. Each point gives the mean value (± SD). (Adapted from Glinoer and co-workers, 1990, with permission.)

considerable variability in thyroidal adjustments during normal pregnancy.

The modifications in serum thyroid stimulating hormone and chorionic gonadotropin as a function of gestational age are illustrated in Figure 8–18. There was an inverse relationship between the rise in chorionic gonadotropin and diminishing thyrotropin concentrations. Indeed, thyrotropin levels increased in more than 80 percent of the women, even though levels remained in the normal range for nonpregnant individuals. Thus, high serum chorionic gonadotropin levels are associated with thyroid stimulation, and these data are consistent with a thyrotropin-like effect of chorionic gonadotropin on the thyroid gland.

During pregnancy there is a moderate enlargement of the thyroid caused by hyperplasia of the glandular tissue and increased vascularity. Glinoer and colleagues (1990) assessed thyroid gland volume from 552 ultra-

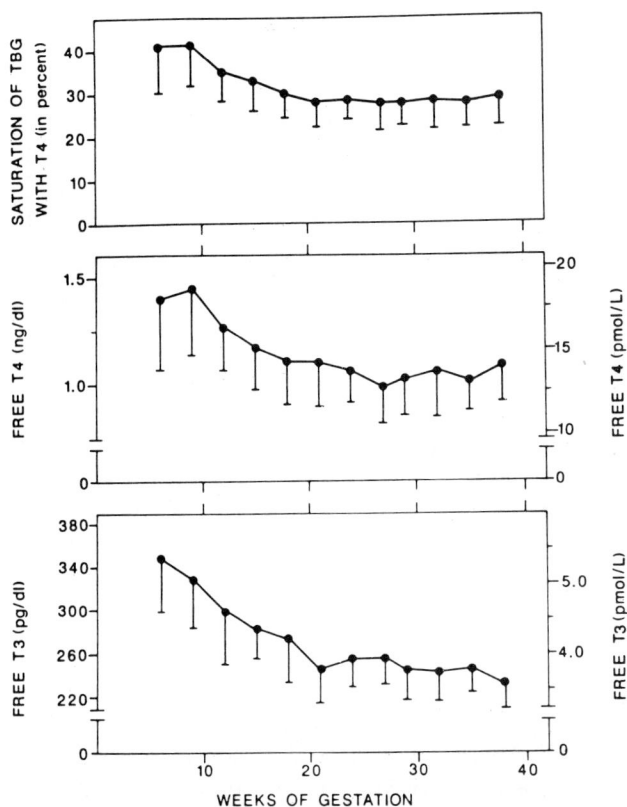

Fig. 8–17. Maternal serum free thyroxine (T_4) and triiodothyronine (T_3) concentrations and thyroxine-binding globulin (TBG) saturation related to gestational age. Thyroxine-binding globulin saturation by T_4 corresponds to the molar T_4/TBG ratio expressed as a percentage. Each point gives the mean value ($\pm$ SD). (From Glinoer and co-workers, 1990, with permission.)

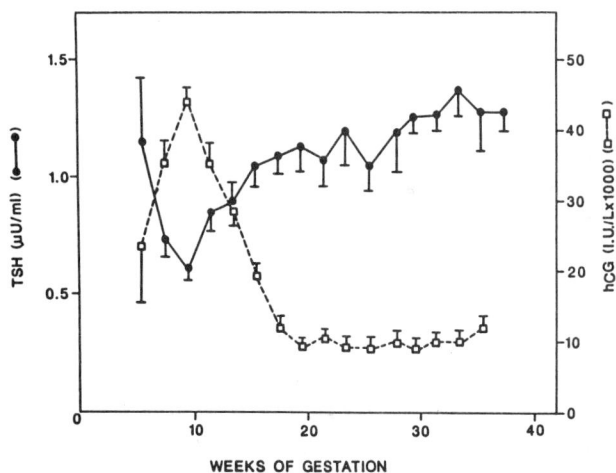

Fig. 8–18. Serum thyrotropin (TSH) and chorionic gonadotropin (hCG) levels related to gestational age. The symbols depict the mean value ($\pm$ SE). Each point corresponds to the average of 33 determinations for gonadotropin and 49 for thyrotropin. (From Glinoer and co-workers, 1990, with permission.)

sound examinations. Total gland volume increased from 12.1 mL $\pm$ 4.5 (SD) in the first trimester to 15.0 mL $\pm$ 6.8 at delivery. This increase was observed in the majority of women. Total volume also was found to be inversely proportional to thyrotropin serum concentrations. As emphasized by Levy and co-workers (1980), normal pregnancy does not typically cause significant thyromegaly, and any goiter in pregnancy should be investigated.

These many complex alterations in thyroid regulation during pregnancy do not alter maternal thyroid status as measured by using metabolic studies. Although basal metabolic rate increases progressively during normal pregnancy by as much as 25 percent, most of this increase in oxygen consumption is the result of fetal metabolic activity. If fetal body surface area is considered along with that of the mother, the predicted and observed basal metabolic rates are quite similar.

Reverse Triiodothyronine. Reverse triiodothyronine (rT_3) is formed from the inner ring (5-deiodinase) monodeiodination of thyroxine. Its level in maternal blood is three to five times less than in fetal blood and amnionic fluid (Roti and associates, 1983). This is likely because the conversion of thyroxine to reverse triiodothyronine takes place in fetal membranes and in the placenta.

There is almost no transfer of thyroxine, triiodothyronine, or reverse triiodothyronine from the maternal into the fetal compartment. Therefore, fetal thyroid function appears to be independent of maternal thyroid status. This protection of the fetus is likely the consequence of placental inner ring thyroxine deiodination.

Long-acting Thyroid Stimulator. The usually protected status of the fetal thyroid is overcome in some cases of Graves disease. Long-acting thyroid stimulator (LATS) may cross the placenta in women with Graves disease and stimulate the fetal thyroid to produce neonatal thyrotoxicosis. LATS is now recognized to be only one of a variety of thyroid-stimulating immunoglobulins that may be detected in women with Graves disease (Roti and co-workers, 1983).

Thyroid-releasing Hormone. Thyroid-releasing hormone (TRH) is a neurotransmitter present throughout the brain but in highest concentrations in the hypothalamus. It stimulates synthesis and release of thyrotropin from the anterior pituitary. It is not increased during normal pregnancy, but it does cross the placenta and may stimulate the fetal pituitary to secrete thyrotropin (Thorpe-Beeston and associates, 1991). The role, if any, served by maternal TRH in fetal homeostasis is not clear at this time.

Parathyroid and Calcium Metabolism. The regulation of calcium concentration is closely interrelated to magnesium, phosphate, parathyroid hormone, vitamin

D, and calcitonin physiology. Any alteration of one of these factors is likely to change the others.

Parathyroid Hormone and Calcium Interrelationships. Acute or chronic decreases in plasma calcium or acute decreases in magnesium stimulate the release of parathyroid hormone, whereas increases in calcium and magnesium suppress parathyroid hormone levels. The net effect of the action of this hormone on bone resorption, intestinal absorption, and kidney reabsorption is to increase extracellular fluid calcium and decrease phosphate.

Parathyroid hormone concentrations in plasma decrease during the first trimester, and then increase progressively throughout the remainder of pregnancy (Pitkin, 1985). Increased parathyroid hormone levels likely result from increased plasma volume, increased glomerular filtration rate, and increased fetal transfer of calcium, all resulting in a chronic suppression of calcium concentration in the pregnant woman. Despite the well-observed decrease in total calcium concentration during pregnancy, ionized calcium, which is the major feedback mechanism regulating secretion of parathyroid hormone, is decreased only slightly during pregnancy (Pitkin, 1985). Reitz and co-workers (1977) suggest that during pregnancy a new "set point" exists between ionized calcium and parathyroid hormone. Estrogens also appear to block the action of parathyroid hormone on bone resorption resulting in another mechanism to increase parathyroid hormone during pregnancy. The net result of these actions is a "physiological hyperparathyroidism" of pregnancy, likely in order to supply the fetus with adequate calcium.

The potential roles of parathyroid hormone-related peptide production in the fetus, placenta, and maternal tissues are discussed in Chapters 4 through 7.

Calcitonin and Calcium Interrelationships. The calcitonin-secreting C cells are derived embryologically from the neural crest and are located predominantly in the perifollicular areas of the thyroid gland. Calcium and magnesium increase the biosynthesis and secretion of calcitonin. Various gastric hormones (gastrin, pentagastrin, glucagon, and pancreoxymin) and food ingestion also increase calcitonin plasma levels.

The known actions of calcitonin are generally considered to oppose those of parathyroid hormone and vitamin D to protect skeletal calcification during times of calcium stress. Pregnancy and lactation are two examples of profound calcium stress; and during these times, calcitonin levels are appreciably higher than in nonpregnant women (Whitehead and associates, 1981).

Vitamin D and Calcium Interrelationships. Vitamin D is synthesized in the skin or ingested and is converted into 25-hydroxyvitamin D_3 by the liver. This product is then converted in the kidney, decidua, and placenta to 1,25-dihydroxyvitamin D_3 (Weisman and co-workers, 1979).

This most likely is the biologically active compound, and it stimulates resorption of calcium from bone and absorption in the intestines.

The actual control of 1,25-dihydroxyvitamin D_3 production and release is unknown, but the conversion of 25-hydroxyvitamin D_3 to 1,25-dihydroxyvitamin D_3 is facilitated by parathyroid hormone and by low calcium and phosphate plasma levels and opposed by calcitonin (Tsang and associates, 1976). A possible role of prolactin has been suggested by Robinson and colleagues (1982). They found that in the lactating rat, prolactin increased the plasma levels of 1,25-dihydroxyvitamin D_3, and this in turn increased intestinal absorption of calcium. As yet, this effect has not been reported in the human, but 1,25-dihydroxyvitamin D_3 levels are increased during normal pregnancy (Whitehead and associates, 1981).

Adrenal Glands. In normal pregnancy, there is probably very little morphological change in the maternal adrenal glands. There are, however, profound changes in secretion of some of its cortical hormones.

Cortisol. There is a considerable increase in the serum concentration of circulating cortisol, but much of it is bound by cortisol-binding globulin, *transcortin.* The rate of cortisol secretion by the maternal adrenal is not increased, and probably it is decreased compared with the nonpregnant state. The metabolic clearance rate of cortisol, however, is lower during pregnancy; in a pregnant woman, the half-life of intravenously injected radiolabeled cortisol is nearly twice as long as it is in nonpregnant women (Migeon and associates, 1957). Administration of estrogen, including most oral contraceptives, causes changes in levels of cortisol and transcortin similar to those of pregnancy.

In early pregnancy, the levels of circulating corticotropin (ACTH) are reduced strikingly. As pregnancy progresses, the levels of corticotropin and free cortisol rise. This apparent paradox is not understood completely. Nolten and Rueckert (1981) have presented evidence that the higher free cortisol levels observed in pregnancy are the result of a "resetting" of the maternal feedback mechanism to higher levels. They further propose that the "resetting" might result from *tissue refractoriness* to cortisol. Thus an elevated free cortisol would be needed during pregnancy to maintain homeostasis.

Aldosterone. As early as 15 weeks of normal pregnancy, the maternal adrenal glands secrete considerably increased amounts of aldosterone. By the third trimester, about 1 mg per day is secreted. If sodium intake is restricted, aldosterone secretion is elevated even further (Watanabe and co-workers, 1963). At the same time, levels of renin and angiotensin II substrate are normally increased, especially during the latter half of pregnancy (Geelhoed and Vander, 1968; Massani and associates, 1967). This gives rise to increased plasma levels of angiotensin II, which by acting on the zona glomerulosa of the maternal adrenal glands, likely accounts for the markedly elevated secretion of aldosterone. It has been suggested that the increased aldosterone secretion during normal pregnancy affords protection against the natriuretic effect of progesterone. Progesterone administered to nonpregnant women is associated with a prompt increase in aldosterone excretion (Laidlaw and colleagues, 1962).

Deoxycorticosterone. There is a striking increase in the maternal plasma levels of deoxycorticosterone (DOC) during pregnancy. Brown and co-workers (1972) and Nolten and associates (1978) found that in nonpregnant women and during the first two trimesters of pregnancy, the levels of plasma deoxycorticosterone are less than 100 pg/mL. During the last few weeks of pregnancy, these levels rise to 1500 pg/mL or more. Interestingly, Nolten and associates (1978) found that the administration of the potent glucocorticoid, dexamethasone, to pregnant women to reduce corticotropin secretion is not accompanied by a reduction in plasma deoxycorticosterone levels. Moreover, ACTH administration to pregnant women is not accompanied by an increase in plasma deoxycorticosterone concentration. This was highly suggestive that deoxycorticosterone and its sulfate (DOC-SO$_4$) in plasma of pregnant women do not arise principally by maternal adrenal secretion. The levels of deoxycorticosterone and DOC-SO$_4$ in fetal blood are appreciably higher than those in maternal blood, and this suggests transfer of fetal deoxycorticosterone into the maternal compartment.

Most of the deoxycorticosterone in maternal plasma, however, arises from maternal extraadrenal 21-hydroxylation of plasma progesterone (Winkel and associates, 1980). The product of the fractional conversion of plasma progesterone to deoxycorticosterone, and the plasma production rate of progesterone, is nearly equal to the total production rate of deoxycorticosterone in the maternal compartment. This is a very interesting and potentially important phenomenon for several reasons. First, the extraadrenal conversion of plasma progesterone to deoxycorticosterone is known to occur in tissue sites of mineralocorticosteroid action (kidney, skin, and blood vessels). Thus, there is in situ formation of a potent mineralocorticosteroid in its potential site of action. Second, there is great individual variation, up to 30-fold, in the fractional conversion of plasma progesterone to deoxycorticosterone (Casey and MacDonald, 1982). This is very unusual for steroid conversions or interconversions. For these two reasons, it is quite possible that much more deoxycorticosterone is produced during pregnancy in one woman compared with another, and the hormone may be formed largely in tissues that are mineralocorticosteroid responsive. Obviously, adaptation to pregnancy includes accommodations for marked increases in the formation of both aldosterone and deoxycorticosterone without the development in most of pregnancy-induced hypertension. It is probable that the increased formation of mineralocorticosteroids is important in the plasma volume expansion that accompanies pregnancy.

The mechanisms of origin of DOC-SO$_4$ during pregnancy are equally or more provocative than are those of deoxycorticosterone. It is clearly established that plasma deoxycorticosterone is not converted to plasma DOC-SO$_4$. Plasma progesterone is not converted to DOC-SO$_4$. Recently, however, evidence was obtained that DOC-SO$_4$ in the blood of pregnant women probably arises by way of a fetal–placental interaction. It has been known for some time that the fetal plasma concentration of pregnenolone-3,21-disulfate is elevated strikingly, with fetal plasma levels to 1000 ng/mL. Yet it is believed that pregnenolone and pregnenolone sulfate are not good substrates for steroid 21-hydroxylase activity in the fetal adrenal glands. On the other hand, large amounts of pregnenolone sulfate are known to be secreted by the fetal adrenal glands. From the work of Casey and associates (1987), it is likely that pregnenolone sulfate is converted in fetal liver to pregnenolone-3,21-disulfate; and in the placenta, the latter is converted to DOC-SO$_4$, which is secreted into the maternal compartment.

Dehydroepiandrosterone Sulfate. As discussed in Chapter 6 (p. 149), the levels of *dehydroepiandrosterone sulfate* circulating in maternal blood and excreted in the urine are not increased during normal pregnancy, but rather decreased as a consequence of an increased rate of removal, through extensive 16α-hydroxylation in the maternal liver and estrogen formation in the placenta.

Androstenedione and Testosterone. Maternal plasma levels of *androstenedione* and *testosterone* are increased during pregnancy. This finding is not totally explained by alterations in the metabolic clearance rates of these steroids. Maternal plasma androstenedione and testosterone are converted to estradiol in the placenta, which increases the rate of clearance. Conversely, there is an increased amount of sex hormone-binding globulin in plasma of pregnant women, which retards the rate of testosterone clearance. Thus, there is an increased plasma production rate of maternal testosterone and androstenedione during human pregnancy. The source of this increased C$_{19}$-steroid production is unknown but it likely originates in the ovary. Interestingly, little or no testosterone in maternal plasma enters the fetal circulation as testosterone. Even when massive testosterone levels are found in the circulation of pregnant women with androgen-secreting tumors, the testosterone level in umbilical cord venous plasma is likely to be too low to be detected. This finding is the result of the near complete conversion of testosterone to 17β-estradiol by the trophoblast (Edman and associates, 1979).

Musculoskeletal System

Progressive *lordosis* is a characteristic feature of normal pregnancy. Compensating for the anterior position of the enlarging uterus, the lordosis shifts the center of gravity back over the lower extremities. There is increased mobility of the sacroiliac, sacrococcygeal, and pubic joints during pregnancy, presumably as a result of hormonal changes. Their mobility may contribute to the alteration of maternal posture, and in turn cause discomfort in the lower portion of the back, especially late in pregnancy. During late pregnancy, aching, numbness, and weakness are occasionally experienced in the upper extremities, possibly as a result of the marked lordosis with anterior flexion of the neck and slumping of the shoulder girdle, which in turn produces traction on the ulnar and median nerves (Crisp and DeFrancesco, 1964).

Eyes

Pregnancy causes changes in the eyes, which have been reviewed by Sunness (1988). Intraocular pressure decreases during pregnancy, and this has been attributed in part to increased vitreous outflow. Corneal sensitivity is also decreased, with the greatest changes late in gestation. Most pregnant women demonstrate a measurable but slight increase in corneal thickness thought to be due to edema. Consequently, pregnant women may have difficulty with previously comfortable contact lenses. Brownish-red opacities on the posterior surface of the cornea (*Krukenberg spindles*) have also been observed with a higher than expected frequency during pregnancy. Hormonal effects are postulated as the cause of this increased pigmentation.

Other than transient loss of accommodation reported with both pregnancy and lactation, visual function is unaffected by pregnancy. Historically, the normal increase in pituitary size associated with pregnancy was implicated by some investigators as the cause for their reported changes in visual fields. However, methodological problems in objectively measuring visual fields, and the realization that pregnant women do not complain subjectively of visual field change, has prompted most investigators to conclude that visual fields are not affected.

References

Aboul-Khair SA, Crooks J, Turnbull AC, Hytten FE: The physiological changes in thyroid function during pregnancy. Clin Sci 27:195, 1964

Abou-Samra AB, Pugeat M, Dechaud H, Nachury L, Tourniaire J: Acute dopaminergic blockage by sulpiride stimulates β-endorphin secretion in pregnant woman. Clin Endocrinol 21:583, 1984

Alvarez H, Caldeyro-Barcia R: Contractility of the human uterus recorded by new methods. Surg Gynecol Obstet 91:1, 1950

Anderson GH, Howland T, Domascek P, Streeten DHP: Effect of sodium balance and calcium channel blocking drugs on blood pressure responses. Hypertension 10:239, 1987

Andersen JR: Prolactin in amniotic fluid and maternal serum during uncomplicated human pregnancy. Dan Med Bull 29:266, 1982

Assali NS, Dilts PV, Pentl AA, Kirschbaum TH, Gross SJ: Physiology of the placenta. In Assali NS (ed): Biology of Gestation, Vol I. The Maternal Organism. New York, Academic Press, 1968

Assali NS, Douglass RA, Baird WW, Nicholson DB, Suyemoto R: Measurement of uterine blood flow and uterine metabolism, IV. Results in normal pregnancy. Am J Obstet Gynecol 66:248, 1953

Assali NS, Rauramo L, Peltonen T: Measurement of uterine blood flow and uterine metabolism, VIII. Uterine and fetal blood flow and oxygen consumption in early human pregnancy. Am J Obstet Gynecol 79:86, 1960

Astedt B: Significance of placenta in depression of fibrinolytic activity during pregnancy. J Obstet Gynaecol Br Commonw 79:205, 1972

Atarashi K, Mulrow PJ, Franco-Saenz R, Snajdar R, Rapp J: Inhibition of aldosterone production by an atrial extract. Science 224:992, 1984

Baboonian C, Griffiths P: Is pregnancy immunosuppressive? Humoral immunity against viruses. Br J Obstet Gynaecol 90:1168, 1983

Bailey RR, Rolleston GL: Kidney length and ureteric dilatation in the puerperium. J Obstet Gynaecol Br Commonw 78:55, 1971

Baumann G, Puavilai G, Freinkel N, Domont LA, Metzger BE, Levene HB: Hepatic insulin and glucagon receptors in pregnancy: Their role in the enhanced catabolism during fasting. Endocrinology 108:1979, 1981

Bellina JH, Dougherty CM, Mickal A: Pyeloureteral dilation and pregnancy. Am J Obstet Gynecol 108:356, 1970

Bender HS, Chickering WR: Minireview: Pregnancy and diabetes: The maternal response. Life Sci 37:1, 1985

Benigni A, Gaspari F, Orisio S, Bellizzi L, Amuzo G, Frusca T, Remuzzi G: Human placenta expresses endothelin gene and corresponding protein is executed in increasing amounts during normal pregnancy. Am J Obstet Gynecol 164:844, 1991

Bieniarz J, Branda LA, Maqueda E, Morozovsky J, Caldeyro-Barcia R: Aortocaval compression by the uterus in late pregnancy, III. Unreliability of the sphygmomanometric method in estimating uterine artery pressure. Am J Obstet Gynecol 102:1106, 1968

Bolton FG, Street MJ, Pace AJ: Changes in erythrocyte volume and shape in pregnancy. Br J Obstet Gynecol 89:1018, 1982

Bonnar J: Hemostatic function and coagulopathy during pregnancy. In Wynn R (ed): Obstetrics and Gynecology Annual. New York, Appleton-Century-Crofts, 1978, p 195

Borenstein AB: The effect of natriuretic atrial extract on renal hemodynamics and urinary excretion in anesthetized rats. J Physiol 334:133, 1983

Bradshaw KD, Santos-Ramos R, Rawlins SC, MacDonald PC, Parker CR: Endocrine studies in a pregnancy complicated by ovarian thecalutein cysts and hyperreaction luteinalis. Obstet Gynecol 67:665, 1986

Brar HS, Platt LD, DeVore GR, Horenstein J, Medearis AL: Qualitative assessment of maternal uterine and fetal umbilical artery blood flow and resistance in laboring patients by Doppler velocimetry. Am J Obstet Gynecol 158:95, 1988

Braverman DZ, Johnson ML, Kern Jr F: Effects of pregnancy and contraceptive steroids on gallbladder function. N Engl J Med 302:362, 1980

Broughton-Pipkin F, Meirelles RS: Prostaglandin E_2 attenuates the pressor response to angiotensin II in pregnant subjects but not in nonpregnant subjects. Am J Obstet Gynecol 142:168, 1982

Brown MA, Gallery EDM, Ross MR, Esber RP: Sodium excretion in normal and hypertensive pregnancy: A prospective study. Am J Obstet Gynecol 159:297, 1988

Brown MA, Sinosich MJ, Saunders DM, Gallery EDM: Potassium regulation and progesterone–aldosterone interrelationships in human pregnancy: A prospective study. Am J Obstet Gynecol 155:349, 1986

Brown RD, Strott CA, Liddle GW: Plasma desoxycorticosterone in normal and abnormal human pregnancy. J Clin Endocrinol Metab 35:736, 1972

Browning AJF, Butt WR, Lynch SS, Shakespear RA: Maternal plasma concentrations of β-endorphin and γ-lipotrophin throughout pregnancy. Br J Obstet Gynaecol 90:1147, 1983a

Browning AJF, Butt WR, Lynch SS, Shakespear RA, Crawford JS: Maternal and cord plasma concentrations of β-lipotrophin, β-endorphin, and Δ-lipotrophin at delivery: Effect of analgesia. Br J Obstet Gynaecol 90:1152, 1983b

Bryant-Greenwood GD: Relaxin as a new hormone. Endocrinol Rev 3:62, 1982

Burnett JC: Effects of synthetic ANF on renal function and renin release. Am J Physiol F863, 1984

Burt RL, Davidson IWF: Insulin half-life and utilization in normal pregnancy. Obstet Gynecol 43:161, 1974

Calloway DH: Nitrogen balance during pregnancy. In Winick M (ed): Nutrition and Fetal Development, Vol II. New York, Wiley, 1974

Carter J: Serum bile acids in normal pregnancy. Br J Obstet Gynecol 98:540, 1991

Casey ML, MacDonald PC: Metabolism of deoxycorticosterone and deoxycorticosterone sulfate in men and women. J Clin Invest 70:312, 1982

Casey ML, Winkel CA, Guerami A, MacDonald PC: Mineralocorticosteroids and pregnancy: Regulation of extraadrenal deoxycorticosterone production by estrogen. J Steroid Biochem 27:1013, 1987

Chard T, Craig PH, Menabawey M, Lee C: Alpha interferon in human pregnancy. Br J Obstet Gynaecol 93:1145, 1986

Chesley LC: Renal function during pregnancy. In Carey HM (ed): Modern Trends in Human Reproductive Physiology. London, Butterworth, 1963

Chesley LC: Renin, angiotensin, and aldosterone in pregnancy. In Chesley LC (ed): Hypertensive Disorders in Pregnancy. New York, Appleton-Century-Crofts, 1978, p 236

Chesley LC: Weight changes and water balance in normal and toxic pregnancy. Am J Obstet Gynecol 48:565, 1944

Chesley LC, Sloan DM: The effect of posture on renal function in late pregnancy. Am J Obstet Gynecol 89:754, 1964

Chesley LC, Talledo OE, Bohler CS, Zuspan FP: Vascular reactivity to angiotensin II and norepinephrine in pregnant and

nonpregnant women. Am J Obstet Gynecol 91:837, 1965

Christofides ND, Ghatei MA, Bloom SR, Borberg C, Gillmer MDG: Decreased plasma motilin concentrations in pregnancy. Br Med J 285:1453, 1982

Clark SL, Cotton DB, Lee W, Bishop C, Hill T: Central hemodynamic assessment of normal term pregnancy. Am J Obstet Gynecol 161:1439, 1989

Cohen DA, Daughaday WH, Weldon VV: Fetal and maternal virilization associated with pregnancy. Am J Dis Child 136:353, 1982

Cohen S: The sluggish gallbladder of pregnancy. N Engl J Med 302:397, 1980

Cole DEC, Gundberg CM, Stirk LJ, Atkinson SA, Hanley DA, Ayer LM, Baldwin LS: Changing osteocalcin concentrations during pregnancy and lactation: Implications for maternal mineral metabolism. J Clin Endocrinol Metab 65:290, 1987

Combes B, Adams RH: Pathophysiology of the liver in pregnancy. In Assali NS (ed): Pathophysiology of Gestation, Vol I. New York, Academic Press, 1971

Combes B, Shibata H, Adams R, Mitchell BD, Trammell V: Alterations in sulfobromophthalein sodium-removal mechanisms from blood during normal pregnancy. J Clin Invest 42:1431, 1963

Coopland A, Alkjaersig N, Fletcher AP: Reduction in plasma factor XIII (fibrin stabilization factor) concentration during pregnancy. J Lab Clin Med 73:144, 1969

Cotes PM, Canning CE, Lind T: Changes in serum immunoreactive erythropoietin during the menstrual cycle and normal pregnancy. Br J Obstet Gynecol 90:304, 1983

Crawford RJ, Hudson P, Shine J, Niall HD, Eddy RL, Shows TB: Two human relaxin genes are on chromosome 9. EMBO J 3:2341, 1984

Crisp WE, DeFrancesco A: The hand syndrome of pregnancy. Obstet Gynecol 23:433, 1964

Csapo AI, Pulkkinen MO, Wiest WG: Effects of hysterectomy and progesterone replacement in early pregnant patients. Am J Obstet Gynecol 115:759, 1973

Cugell DW, Frank NR, Gaensler ER, Badger TL: Pulmonary function in pregnancy, I. Serial observations in normal women. Am Rev Tuberc 67:568, 1953

Cunningham FG, Cox K, Gant NF: Further observations on the nature of pressor responsivity to angiotensin II in human pregnancy. Obstet Gynecol 46:581, 1975

Cusson JR, Gutkowska J, Rey E, Michon N, Boucher M, Larochelle P: Plasma concentration of atrial natriuretic factor in normal pregnancy. N Engl J Med 313:1230, 1985

Cutforth R, MacDonald CB: Heart sounds and murmurs in pregnancy. Am Heart J 71:741, 1966

Darmady JM, Postle AD: Lipid metabolism in pregnancy. Br J Obstet Gynaecol 89:211, 1982

Davison JM, Hytten FE: The effect of pregnancy on the renal handling of glucose. Br J Obstet Gynaecol 82:374, 1975

Davison JM, Hytten FE: Glomerular filtration during and after pregnancy. J Obstet Gynaecol Br Commonw 81:588, 1974

Davison JM, Vallotton MB, Lindheimer MD: Plasma osmolality and urinary concentration and dilution during and after pregnancy: Evidence that lateral recumbency inhibits maximal urinary concentrating ability. Br J Obstet Gynaecol 88:472, 1981

Dennis KJ, Bytheway WR: Changes in the body weight after delivery. J Obstet Gynaecol Br Commonw 72:94, 1965

Desoye G, Schweditsch MO, Preiffer KP, Zechner R, Kostner

GM: Correlation of hormones with lipid and lipoprotein levels during normal pregnancy and postpartum. J Clin Endocrinol Metab 64:704, 1987

DeSwiet M: The respiratory system. In Hytten FE, Chamberlain G (eds): Clinical Physiology in Obstetrics, 2nd ed. Oxford, Blackwell, 1991, p 83

Douglas JT, Shah M, Lowe GDO, Betch JF, Forbes CD, Prentice CRM: Plasma fibrinopeptide A and beta-thromboglobulin in pre-eclampsia and pregnancy hypertension. Thromb Haemost 47:54, 1982

Dunlop W: Serial changes in renal haemodynamics during normal human pregnancy. Br J Obstet Gynaecol 88:1, 1981

Dunlop W: Investigations into influence of posture on renal plasma flow and glomerular filtration rate during late pregnancy. Br J Obstet Gynaecol 83:17, 1976

Easterling TR, Schmucker BC, Benedetti TJ: The hemodynamic effects of orthostatic stress during pregnancy. Obstet Gynecol 72:550, 1988

Eddie LW, Bell RJ, Lester A, Geier M, Bennett G, Johnston PD, Niall HD: Radioimmunoassay of relaxin in pregnancy with an analogue of human relaxin. Lancet 1:1344, 1986

Edman CD, Devereux WP, Parker CR, MacDonald PC: Placental clearance of maternal androgens: A protective mechanism against fetal virilization. Abstract 112 presented at the 26th annual meeting of the Society for Gynecologic Investigation, San Diego, 1979. Gynecol Invest 67:68, 1979

Edman CD, Toofanian A, MacDonald PC, Gant NF: Placental clearance rate of maternal plasma androstenedione through placental estradiol formation: An indirect method of assessing uteroplacental blood flow. Am J Obstet Gynecol 131:1029, 1981

Enein M, Zina AAA, Kassem M, El-Tabbakh G: Echocardiography of the pericardium in pregnancy. Obstet Gynecol 69:851, 1987

Evans MI, Dougan MB, Moawad AH, Evans WJ, Bryant-Greenwood GD, Greenwood FC: Ripening of the human cervix with porcine ovarian relaxin. Am J Obstet Gynecol 147:410, 1983

Everett RB, Worley RJ, MacDonald PC, Gant NF: Modification of vascular responsiveness to angiotensin II in pregnant women by intravenously infused 5α-dihydroprogesterone. Am J Obstet Gynecol 131:352, 1978a

Everett RB, Worley RJ, MacDonald PC, Gant NF: Oral administration of theophylline to modify pressor responsiveness to angiotensin II in women with pregnancy-induced hypertension. Am J Obstet Gynecol 132:359, 1978b

Everett RB, Worley RJ, MacDonald PC, Gant NF: Effect of prostaglandin synthetase inhibitors on pressor response to angiotensin II in human pregnancy. J Clin Endocrinol Metab 46:1007, 1978c

Ezimokhai M, Davison JM, Philips PR, Dunlop W: Non-postural serial changes in renal function during the third trimester of normal human pregnancy. Br J Obstet Gynaecol 88:465, 1981

Faure A, Sutter-Dub MT, Sutter BCJ, Assan R: Ovarian–adrenal interactions in regulation of endocrine pancreatic function in the rat. Diabetologia 24:122, 1983

Fay RA, Hughes AO, Farron NT: Platelets in pregnancy: Hyperdestruction in pregnancy. Obstet Gynecol 61:238, 1983

Fletcher JE, Thomas TA, Hill RG: β-Endorphin and parturition. Lancet 1:310, 1980

Fogh-Andersen N, Schultz-Larsen P: Free calcium ion concentration in pregnancy. Acta Obstet Gynecol Scand 60:309, 1981

Freinkel N: Banting lecture 1980: Of pregnancy and progeny. Diabetes 29:1023, 1980

Freinkel N, Dooley SL, Metzger BE: Care of the pregnant woman with insulin-dependent diabetes mellitus. N Engl J Med 313:96, 1985

Gallery EDM, Brown MA: Control of sodium excretion in human pregnancy. Am J Kidney Dis 9:290, 1987

Gant NF, Chand S, Worley RJ, Andersen GD: Unpublished observations, 1977

Gant NF, Chand S, Worley RJ, Whalley PJ, Crosby UD, MacDonald PC: A clinical test for predicting the development of acute hypertension in pregnancy. Am J Obstet Gynecol 120:1, 1974a

Gant NF, Daley GL, Chand S, Whalley PJ, MacDonald PC: The nature of pressor responsiveness to angiotensin II in human pregnancy. Obstet Gynecol 43:854, 1974b

Gant NF, Daley GL, Chand S, Whalley PJ, MacDonald PC: A study of angiotensin II pressor response throughout primigravid pregnancy. J Clin Invest 52:2682, 1973

Gant NF, Madden JD, Chand S, Worley RJ, Strong JS, MacDonald PC: Metabolic clearance rate of dehydroisoandrosterone sulfate, V. Studies of essential hypertension complicating pregnancy. Obstet Gynecol 47:319, 1976

Garcia-Bunuel R, Berek JS, Woodruff JD: Luteomas of pregnancy. Obstet Gynecol 45:407, 1975

Geelhoed GW, Vander AJ: Plasma renin activities during pregnancy and parturition. J Clin Endocrinol 28:412, 1968

Genazzani AR, Facchinetti F, Parrini D: β-Lipotrophin and β-endorphin plasma levels during pregnancy. Clin Endocrinol 141:409, 1981

Glinoer D, DeNayer P, Bourdoux P, Lemone M, Robyn C, Van Steirteghem A, Kinthaert J, Lejeune B: Regulation of maternal thyroid during pregnancy. J Clin Endocrinol Metab 71:276, 1990

Goland RS, Wardlaw SL, Stark RI, Frantz AG: Human plasma β-endorphin during pregnancy, labour and delivery. J Clin Endocrinol Metab 52:74, 1981

Gonzalez JG, Elizondo G, Saldivar D, Nanez H, Todd LE, Villarreal JZ: Pituitary gland growth during normal pregnancy: An in vivo study using magnetic resonance imaging. Am J Med 85:217, 1988

Grace AA, D'Souza V, Menon RK, O'Brien S, Dandona P: Atrial natriuretic peptide concentrations during pregnancy. Lancet 1:1267, 1987

Habicht J, Yarbrough C, Lechtig A, Klein RE: Relationships of birthweight, maternal nutrition and infant mortality. Nutr Rep Int 7:533, 1973

Hahn PF, Carothers EL, Darby WJ, Martin M, Sheppard CW, Cannon RO, Beam AS, Densen PM, Peterson JC, McClellan GS: Iron metabolism in human pregnancy as studied with the radioactive isotope Fe[59]. Am J Obstet Gynecol 61:477, 1951

Handwerger S, Quarfordt S, Barrett J, Harman I: Apolipoproteins AI, AII, and CI stimulate placental lactogen release from human placental tissue. J Clin Invest 79:625, 1987

Harbert GM, Cornell GW, Littlefield JB, Kayan JB, Thornton WN: Maternal hemodynamics associated with uterine contraction in gravid monkeys. Am J Obstet Gynecol 104:24, 1969

Hatjis CG, Kofinas AD, Greelish JP, Swain M, Rose JC: Interrelationships between atrial natriuretic factor concentrations and acute volume expansion in pregnant and nonpregnant women. Am J Obstet Gynecol 63:45, 1990

Hellman LM, Rosenthal AH, Kistner RW, Gordon R: Some factors influencing the proliferation of the reserve cells in the human cervix. Am J Obstet Gynecol 67:899, 1954

Herrera E, Lasunción MA, Gomez-Coronado D, Aranda P, López-Luna P, Maier I: Role of lipoprotein lipase activity on lipoprotein metabolism and the fate of circulating triglycerides in pregnancy. Am J Obstet Gynecol 158:1575, 1988

Hill WC, Lambertz EL: Let's get rid of the term "Braxton Hicks Contractions." Obstet Gynecol 75:709, 1990

Hirai N, Yanaihara T, Nakayama T, Ishibashi M, Yamaji T: Plasma levels of atrial natriuretic peptide during normal pregnancy and in pregnancy complicated by hypertension. Am J Obstet Gynecol 159:27, 1988

Hodgkinson CP: Physiology of the ovarian veins in pregnancy. Obstet Gynecol 1:26, 1953

Hof RP: Modification of vasopressin- and angiotensin II-induced changes by calcium antagonists in the peripheral circulation of anaesthetized rabbits. Br J Pharmacol 85:75, 1985

Hof RP: The calcium antagonists PY 108-068 and verapamil diminish the effects of angiotensin II: Sites of interaction in the peripheral circulation of anaesthetized cats. Br J Pharmacol 82:51, 1984

Hornnes PJ, Kuhl C: Plasma insulin and glucagon responses to isoglycemic stimulation in normal pregnancy and post partum. Obstet Gynecol 55:425, 1980

Howard BK, Goodson JH, Mengert WF: Supine hypotensive syndrome in late pregnancy. Obstet Gynecol 1:371, 1953

Hubinont CJ, Balasse H, Dufrane SP, Leclercq-Meyer V, Sugar J, Schwers J, Malaisse WJ: Changes in pancreatic B cell function during late pregnancy, early lactation and postlactation. Gynecol Obstet Invest 25:89, 1988

Hudson P, Haley J, John M, Cronk M, Crawford R, Haralambidis J, Gregear G, Shine J, Niall H: Structure of a genomic clone encoding biologically active human relaxin. Nature 301:628, 1983

Huisman A, Aarnoudse JG, Heuvelmans JHA, Goslinga H, Fidler V, Huisjes HJ, Zijlstra WJ: Whole blood viscosity during normal pregnancy. Br J Obstet Gynaecol 94:1143, 1987

Hutchinson DL, Westoner JL, Well DW: The destruction of the maternal and fetal pituitary glands in subhuman primates. Am J Obstet Gynecol 83:857, 1962

Hytten FE: Weight gain in pregnancy. In Hytten FE, Chamberlain G (eds): Clinical Physiology in Obstetrics, 2nd ed. Oxford, Blackwell, 1991, p 173

Hytten FE, Leitch I: The Physiology of Human Pregnancy, 2nd ed. Philadelphia, Davis, 1971

Hytten FE, Thomson AM: Maternal physiological adjustments. In Assali NS (ed): Biology of Gestation, Vol I. The Maternal Organism. New York, Academic Press, 1968

Ihrman K: A clinical and physiological study of pregnancy in material from northern Sweden, VII. The heart volume during and after pregnancy. Acta Soc Med Upsal 65:326, 1960

Illingworth PJ, Jung RG, Howie PW, Tsles TE: Reduction in postprandial energy expenditure during pregnancy. Br Med J 294:1573, 1987

Ingerslev M, Teilum G: Biopsy studies on the liver in pregnancy, II. Liver biopsy on normal pregnant women. Acta Obstet Gynecol Scand 25:352, 1946

Iosif S, Ingemarsson I, Ulmsten U: Urodynamic studies in normal pregnancy and the puerperium. Am J Obstet Gynecol 137:696, 1980

Janbu T, Nesheim BI: Uterine artery blood velocities during contractions in pregnancy and labour related to intrauterine pressure. Br J Obstet Gynaecol 94:1150, 1987

Jepson JH, Friesen HG: The mechanism of action of human placental lactogen on erythropoiesis. Br J Haematol 15:465, 1968

Kakouris H, Eddie LW, Summers RJ: Cardiac effects of relaxin in rats. Lancet 339:1076, 1992

Kambam JR, Perry SM, Entman S, Smith BE: Effect of magnesium on plasma cholinesterase activity. Am J Obstet Gynecol 159:309, 1988

Kaneshige E: Serum ferritin as an assessment of iron stores and other hematologic parameters during pregnancy. Obstet Gynecol 57:238, 1981

Kangawa K, Fukuda A, Matsuo H: Structural identification of β- and Δ-human atrial natriuretic polypeptides. Nature 313:397, 1985

Kangawa K, Matsu H: Purification and complete amino acid sequence of a human atrial natriuretic polypeptide (α-hANP). Biochem Biophys Res Commun 111:131, 1984

Kasper CK, Hoag MS, Aggelar PM, Stone S: Blood clotting factors in pregnancy: Factor VIII concentrations in normal and AHF-deficient women. Obstet Gynecol 24:242, 1964

Katz R, Karliner JS, Resnik R: Effects of a natural volume overload state (pregnancy) on left ventricular performance in normal human subjects. Circulation 58:434, 1978

Kauppila A, Chatelain P, Kirkinen P, Kivinen S, Ruokonen A: Isolated prolactin deficiency in a woman with puerperal alactogenesis. J Clin Endocrinol Metab 64:309, 1987

Kauppila A, Koskinen M, Puolakka J, Tuimala R, Kuikka J: Decreased intervillous and unchanged myometrial blood flow in supine recumbency. Obstet Gynecol 55:203, 1980

Kennedy RL, Darne J: The role of hCG in regulation of the thyroid gland in normal and abnormal pregnancy. Obstet Gynecol 78:298, 1991

Killingsworth LM: Plasma protein patterns in health and disease. CRC Crit Rev Clin Lab Sci 11:1, 1979

King JC: Protein metabolism during pregnancy: Symposium on nutrition. Clin Perinatol 2:243, 1975

Klafen, Palugyay: Vergleichende Uutersuchungen über lage und ausdehrung von Herz und Lunge in der Scherangerschaft und im Wochenbatt. Arch Gynaekol 131:347, 1927

Kleinert HD, Maack T, Atlas SA, Januszewicz A, Sealy JE, Laragh JH: ANF inhibits angiotensin-, norepinephrine-, and potassium-induced vascular contractility. Hypertension 6:143, 1984

Kletzky OA, Rossman F, Bertolli SI, Platt LD, Mischell DR: Dynamics of human chorionic gonadotropin, prolactin, and growth hormone in serum and amniotic fluid throughout normal human pregnancy. Am J Obstet Gynecol 151:878, 1985

Krause DE, Stembridge VA: Luteomas of pregnancy. Am J Obstet Gynecol 95:192, 1966

Krause PJ, Ingardia CJ, Pontius LT, Malech HL, LoBello TM, Maderazo EG: Host defense during pregnancy: Neutrophil chemotaxis and adherence. Am J Obstet Gynecol 157:274, 1987

Laidlaw JC, Ruse JL, Gornall AG: The influence of estrogen and progesterone on aldosterone excretion. J Clin Endocrinol 22:161, 1962

Levy RP, Newman DM, Rejali LS, Barford DAG: The myth of goiter in pregnancy. Am J Obstet Gynecol 137:701, 1980

Lind T: Metabolic changes in pregnancy relevant to diabetes mellitus. Postgrad Med J 55:353, 1979

Lind T, Bell S, Gilmore E, Huisjes HJ, Schally AV: Insulin disappearance rate in pregnant and non-pregnant women, and in non-pregnant women given GHRIH. Eur J Clin Invest 7:47, 1977

Lindheimer MD, Barron WM, Dürr J, Davison JM: Water homeostasis and vasopressin release during rodent and human gestation. Am J Kidney Dis 9:270, 1987a

Lindheimer MD, Richardson DA, Ehrlich EN, Katz AI: Potassium homeostasis in pregnancy. J Repro Med 32:517, 1987b

Lopez-Espinoza I, Dhar H, Humphreys S, Redman CWG: Urinary albumin excretion in pregnancy. Br J Obstet Gynaecol 93:176, 1986

Macfie AG, Magides AP, Richmond MN, Reilly CS: Gastric emptying in pregnancy. Br J Anaesth 67:54, 1991

Makowski EL, Meschia G, Droegemueller W, Battaglia FC: Distribution of uterine blood flow in the pregnant sheep. Am J Obstet Gynecol 101:409, 1968

Massani ZM, Sanguinetti R, Gallegos R, Raimondi D: Angiotensin blood levels in normal and toxemic pregnancies. Am J Obstet Gynecol 99:313, 1967

McLennan CE: Antecubital and femoral venous pressure in normal and toxemic pregnancy. Am J Obstet Gynecol 45:568, 1943

Mendenhall HW: Serum protein concentrations in pregnancy, I. Concentrations in maternal serum. Am J Obstet Gynecol 106:388, 1970

Metcalfe J, Romney SL, Ramsey LH, Reid DE, Burwell CS: Estimation of uterine blood flow in normal human pregnancy at term. J Clin Invest 34:1632, 1955

Migeon CJ, Bertrand J, Wall PE: Physiological disposition of 4-C^{14} cortisol during late pregnancy. J Clin Invest 36:1350, 1957

Milne JS, Howie AD, Pack AI: Dyspnoea during normal pregnancy. Br J Obstet Gynaecol 85:260, 1978

Milsom J, Hedner J, Hedner T: Plasma atrial natriuretic peptide (ANP) and maternal hemodynamic changes during normal pregnancy. Acta Obstet Gynecol Scand 67:717, 1988

Miyamoto J: Prolactin and thyrotropin responses to thyrotropin-releasing hormone during the periportal period. Obstet Gynecol 63:639, 1984

Möbius W von: Atmung und Schwangerschaft. Munch Med Wochenschr 103:1389, 1961

Muechler EK, Fichter J, Zongrone J: Human chorionic gonadotropin, estriol, and testosterone changes in two pregnancies with hyperreactio luteinalis. Am J Obstet Gynecol 157:1126, 1987

Naden RP, Rosenfeld CR: Systemic and uterine responsiveness to angiotensin II and norepinephrine in estrogen-treated nonpregnant sheep. Am J Obstet Gynecol 153:417, 1985

Newnham JP, Tomlin S, Ratter SJ, Bourne GL, Rees LH: Endogenous opiod peptides in pregnancy. Br J Obstet Gynaecol 90:535, 1983

Nielsen JH: Effects of growth hormone, prolactin, and placental lactogen on insulin content and release, and deoxyribonucleic acid synthesis in cultured pancreatic islets. Endocrinology 110:600, 1982

Nolten WE, Lindheimer MD, Oparil S, Ehrlich EN: Desoxycorticosterone in pregnancy, I. Sequential studies of the secretory patterns of desoxycorticosterone, aldosterone and cortisol. Am J Obstet Gynecol 132:414, 1978

Nolten WE, Rueckert PA: Elevated free cortisol index in pregnancy: Possible regulatory mechanisms. Am J Obstet Gynecol 139:492, 1981

Oian P, Maltau JM, Noddeland H, Fadnes HO: Oedema-preventing mechanisms in subcutaneous tissue of normal pregnant women. Br J Obstet Gynaecol 92:1113, 1985

Ozanne P, Linderkamp O, Miller FC, Meiselman HJ: Erythrocyte aggregation during normal pregnancy. Am J Obstet Gynecol 147:576, 1983

Pasanisi F, Elliott HL, Reid JL: Vascular and aldosterone responses to angiotensin II in normal humans: Effects of nicardipine. J Cardiovasc Pharmacol 7:1171, 1985

Patton PE, Coulam CB, Bergstralh E: The prevalence of autoantibodies in pregnant and nonpregnant women. Am J Obstet Gynecol 157:1345, 1987

Peake SL, Roxburgh HB, Langlois SLP: Ultrasonic assessment of hydronephrosis of pregnancy. Radiology 146:167, 1983

Phelps RL, Metzger BE, Freinkel N: Carbohydrate metabolism in pregnancy, XVII. Diurnal profiles of plasma glucose, insulin, free fatty acids, triglycerides, cholesterol, and individual amino acids in late normal pregnancy. Am J Obstet Gynecol 140:730, 1981

Pipe NGJ, Smith T, Halliday D, Edmonds CJ, Williams C, Coltart TM: Changes in fat, fat free mass and body water in human normal pregnancy. Br J Obstet Gynaecol 86:929, 1979

Pitkin RM, Reynolds WA, Williams GA, Hargis GK: Calcium metabolism in pregnancy: A longitudinal study. Am J Obstet Gynecol 151:99, 1985

Pitkin RM, Witte DL: Platelet and leukocyte counts in pregnancy. JAMA 242:2696, 1980

Porter DG: Myometrium of the pregnant guinea pig: The probable importance of relaxin. Biol Reprod 7:458, 1972

Porter DG: Relaxin and cervical softening. In Anderson AM, Ellwood DA (eds): The Cervix in Pregnancy and Labour. Edinburgh, Churchill Livingstone, 1980

Pritchard JA: Changes in the blood volume during pregnancy and delivery. Anesthesiology 26:393, 1965

Pritchard JA: Plasma cholinesterase activity in normal pregnancy and in eclamptogenic toxemias. Am J Obstet Gynecol 70:1083, 1955

Pritchard JA, Adams RH: Erythrocyte production and destruction during pregnancy. Am J Obstet Gynecol 79:750, 1960

Pritchard JA, Hunt CF: A comparison of the hematologic responses following the routine prenatal administration of intramuscular and oral iron. Surg Gynecol Obstet 106:516, 1958

Pritchard JA, Mason RA: Iron stores of normal adults and their replenishment with oral iron therapy. JAMA 190:897, 1964

Pritchard JA, Scott DE: Iron demands during pregnancy. In Iron Deficiency-Pathogenesis: Clinical Aspects and Therapy. London, Academic Press, 1970, p 173

Rakoczi F, Tallian F, Bagdany S, Gati I: Platelet life-span in normal pregnancy and pre-eclampsia as determined by a non-radioisotope technique. Thromb Res 15:553, 1979

Ramsey EM, Corner GW, Long WN, Stran NM: Studies of amniotic fluid and intervillous space pressures in the rhesus monkey. Am J Obstet Gynecol 77:1016, 1959

Ratnoff OD, Colopy JE, Pritchard JA: The blood-clotting mechanism during normal parturition. J Lab Clin Med 44:408, 1954

Rechberger T, Uldbjerg N, Oxlund H: Connective tissue changes in the cervix during normal pregnancy and pregnancy complicated by cervical incompetence. Obstet Gynecol 71:563, 1988

Reitz RE, Thomas AD, Woods JR, Weinstein RL: Calcium, magnesium, phosphorus, and parathyroid hormone interrelationships in pregnancy and newborn infants. Obstet Gynecol 50:701, 1977

Rekonen A, Luotola H, Pitkänen M, Kuikka J, Pyörälä M: Measurement of intervillous and myometrial blood flow by an intravenous ^{133}Xe method. Br J Obstet Gynaecol 83:723, 1976

Robinson CJ, Spanos E, James MF, Pike JW, Haussler MR, Makeen AM, Hillyard CJ, MacIntyre I: Role of prolactin in vitamin D metabolism and calcium absorption during lactation in the rat. J Endocrinol 94:443, 1982

Rosenfeld CR: Consideration of the uteroplacental circulation in intrauterine growth. Semin Perinatol 8:42, 1984

Rosenfeld CR, Barton MD, Meschia G: Effects of epinephrine on distribution of blood flow in the pregnant ewe. Am J Obstet Gynecol 124:156, 1976

Rosenfeld CR, Gant NF Jr: The chronically instrumented ewe. A model for studying vascular reactivity to angiotensin II in pregnancy. J Clin Invest 67:486, 1981

Rosenfeld CR, Morriss FH Jr, Makowski EL, Meschia G, Battaglia FC: Circulatory changes in the reproductive tissues of ewes during pregnancy. Gynecol Invest 5:252, 1974

Rosenfeld CR, West J: Circulatory response to systemic infusion of norepinephrine in the pregnant ewe. Am J Obstet Gynecol 127:376, 1977

Roti E, Gnudi A, Braverman LE: The placental transport, synthesis and metabolism of hormones and drugs which affect thyroid function. Endocrinol Rev 4:131, 1983

Rubi RA, Sala NL: Ureteral function in pregnant women, III. Effect of different positions and of fetal delivery upon ureteral tonus. Am J Obstet Gynecol 101:230, 1968

Russ EM, Raymunt J: Influence of estrogens on total serum copper and ceruloplasmin. Proc Soc Exp Biol Med 92:465, 1956

Russell DH, Giles HR, Christian CD, Campbell JL: Polyamines in amniotic fluid, plasma, and urine during normal pregnancy. Am J Obstet Gynecol 132:649, 1978

Rutherford AJ, Anderson JV, Elder MG, Bloom SR: Release of atrial natriuretic peptide during pregnancy and immediate puerperium. Lancet 1:928, 1987

Sagnella GA, Markandu ND, Shore AC, MacGregor GA: Effects of changes in dietary sodium intake and saline infusion on immunoreactive atrial natriuretic peptide in human plasma. Lancet 1:1208, 1985

Sanborn BM: The role of relaxin in uterine function. In Huszar G (ed): Physiology and Biochemistry of the Uterus in Pregnancy and Labor. Boca Raton, CRC Press, 1986, p 225

Scheithauer BW, Sano T, Kovacs KT, Young WF Jr, Ryan N, Randah RV: The pituitary gland in pregnancy: A clinicopathologic and immunohistochemical study of 69 cases. Mayo Clin Proc 65:461, 1990

Scott DE: Anemia during pregnancy. Obstet Gynecol Annu 1:219, 1972

Scott DE, Pritchard JA: Iron deficiency in healthy young college women. JAMA 199:897, 1967

Schulman A, Herlinger H: Urinary tract dilatation in pregnancy. Br J Radiol 48:638, 1975

Sherwood OD: Relaxin. In Knobil E, Neil J (eds): The Physiology of Reproduction. New York, Raven, 1988, p 585

Shortle BE, Warren MP, Tsin D: Recurrent androgenicity in pregnancy: A case report and literature review. Obstet Gynecol 70:462, 1987

Song CS, Kappas A: The influence of estrogens, progestins and pregnancy on the liver. Vitam Horm 26:147, 1968

Spellacy WN, Buhi WC: Pituitary growth hormone and placental lactogen levels measured in normal term pregnancy and at the early and late postpartum periods. Am J Obstet Gynecol 105:888, 1969

Spetz S: Peripheral circulation during normal pregnancy. Acta Obstet Gynecol Scand 43:309, 1964

Steegers EAP, Hein PR, Groeneveld EAM, Jongsma HW, Tan ACITL, Benraad TJ: Atrial natriuretic peptide concentrations during pregnancy. Lancet 1:1267, 1987

Sternberg WH: Non-functioning ovarian neoplasms. In Grady HG, Smith DE (eds): International Academy of Pathology Monograph, no. 3. The Ovary. Baltimore, Williams & Wilkins, 1963

Stirrat G: The immune system. In Hytten F, Chamberlain C (eds): Clinical Physiology in Obstetrics, 2nd ed. Oxford, Blackwell, 1991

Sunness JS: The pregnant woman's eye. Surv Ophthalmol 32:219, 1988

Talbert LM, Langdell RD: Normal values of certain factors in the blood clotting mechanism in pregnancy. Am J Obstet Gynecol 90:44, 1964

Taylor DJ, Phillips P, Lind T: Puerperal haematological indices. Br J Obstet Gynaecol 88:601, 1981

Teasdale F: Numerical density of nuclei in the sheep placenta. Anat Rec 185:186, 1976

Terragno NA, Terragno DA, Pacholczyk D, McGiff JC: Prostaglandins and the regulation of uterine blood flow in pregnancy. Nature 249:57, 1974

Thorpe-Beeston JG, Nicolaides KH, Snijders RJM, Butler J, McGregor AM: Fetal thyroid-stimulating hormone response to maternal administration of thyrotropin-releasing hormone. Am J Obstet Gynecol 164:1244, 1991

Tsai CH, deLeeuw NKM: Changes in 2,3-diphosphoglycerate during pregnancy and puerperium in normal women and in β-thalassemia heterozygous women. Am J Obstet Gynecol 142:520, 1982

Tsang RC, Donovan EF, Steichen JJ: Calcium physiology and pathology in the neonate. Pediatr Clin North Am 23:611, 1976

Tsibris JCM, Raynor LO, Buhi WC, Buggie J, Spellacy WN: Insulin receptors in circulating erythrocytes and monocytes from women on oral contraceptives or pregnant women near term. J Clin Endocrinol Metab 51:711, 1980

Tulchinsky D, Hobel CJ: Plasma human chorionic gonadotropin, estrone, estradiol, estriol, progesterone, and 17α-hydroxyprogesterone in human pregnancy, III. Early normal pregnancy. Am J Obstet Gynecol 117:884, 1973

Tygart SG, McRoyan DK, Spinnato JA, McRoyan CJ, Kitay DZ: Longitudinal study of platelet indices during normal pregnancy. Am J Obstet Gynecol 154:883, 1986

Ueland K: Maternal cardiovascular dynamics, VII. Intrapartum blood volume changes. Am J Obstet Gynecol 126:671, 1976

Ueland K, Hansen JM: Maternal cardiovascular dynamics, II. Posture and uterine contractions. Am J Obstet Gynecol 103:1, 1969

Ueland K, Metcalfe J: Circulatory changes in pregnancy. Clin Obstet Gynecol 18:41, 1975

Ulmsten U, Sundström G: Esophageal manometry in pregnant and nonpregnant women. Am J Obstet Gynecol 132:260, 1978

Van Geelen JM, Lemmens WAJG, Eskes TKAB, Martin CB Jr: The urethral pressure profile in pregnancy and after delivery in healthy nulliparous women. Am J Obstet Gynecol 144:636, 1982

Van Wagenen G, Jenkins RH: An experimental examination of factors causing ureteral dilatation of pregnancy. J Urol 42:1010, 1939

Veille JC, Morton MJ, Burry KJ: Maternal cardiovascular adaptations to twin pregnancy. Am J Obstet Gynecol 153:261, 1985

Vierhapper H, Waldhäusl W: Reduced pressor effect of angiotensin II and of noradrenaline in normal man following the oral administration of the calcium-antagonist nifedipine. Eur J Clin Med 12:263, 1982

Vir SC, Love AHG, Thompson W: Serum and hair concentrations of copper during pregnancy. Am J Clin Nutr 34:2382, 1981

Vulsma T, Gons MH, de Vijlder JJM: Maternal-fetal transfer of thyroxine in congenital hypothyroidism due to a total organification defect or thyroid agenesis. N Engl J Med 321:13, 1989

Wakitani K, Cole BR, Geller DM, Currie MG, Adams SP, Fok KF, Needleman P: Atriopeptins: Correlation between renal vasodilatation and natriuresis. Am J Physiol 249:F49, 1985

Watanabe M, Meeker CI, Gray MJ, Sims EAH, Solomon S: Secretion rate of aldosterone in normal pregnancy. J Clin Invest 42:1619, 1963

Watts DH, Krohn MA, Wener M, Escheubach DA: C-reactive protein in normal pregnancy. Obstet Gynecol 77:176, 1991

Weiner CP, Brandt J: Plasma antithrombin III activity in normal pregnancy. Obstet Gynecol 56:601, 1980

Weisman Y, Harell A, Edelstein S, David M, Spirer Z, Golander A: 1,25-Dihydroxyvitamin D_3 and 24,25-dihydroxyvitamin D in vitro synthesis by human decidua and placenta. Nature 281:317, 1979

Whitehead M, Lane G, Young O, Campbell S, Abeyasekera G, Hillyard CJ, MacIntyre I, Phang KG, Stevenson JC: Interrelations of calcium-regulating hormones during normal pregnancy. Br Med J 283:10, 1981

Widdowson EM, Spray CM: Chemical development in utero. Arch Dis Child 26:205, 1951

Widness JA, Clemons GK, Garcia JF, Schwartz R: Plasma immunoreactive erythropoietin in normal women studied sequentially during and after pregnancy. Am J Obstet Gynecol 149:646, 1984

Winkel CA, Parker CR Jr, Milewich L, Simpson ER, Gant NF, MacDonald PC: The conversion of plasma progesterone to desoxycorticosterone (DOC) in men, nonpregnant and pregnant women, and adrenalectomized subjects: Evidence for steroid 21-hydroxylase activity in non-adrenal tissues. J Clin Invest 66:803, 1980

Winters AJ, Colston C, MacDonald PC, Porter JC: Fetal plasma prolactin levels. J Clin Endocrinol Metab 41:626, 1975

Woodfield DG, Cole SK, Allan AGE, Cash JD: Serum fibrin degradation products throughout normal pregnancy. Br Med J 4:665, 1968

Wright HP, Osborn SB, Edmonds DG: Changes in rate of flow of venous blood in the leg during pregnancy, measured with radioactive sodium. Surg Gynecol Obstet 90:481, 1950

Yanagisawa M, Kurihara H, Kimura S, Tomobe Y, Kobayashi M, Mitsui Y, Yazaki Y, Goto K, Masaki T: A novel potent vasoconstrictor peptide produced by vascular endothelial cells. Nature 332:411, 1988

Yoshima T, Strott CA, Marshall JR, Lipsett MD: Corpus luteum function early in pregnancy. J Clin Endocrinol Metab 29:225, 1969

Zoja C, Benigui A, Reuzi D, Piccinelli A, Perico N, Remuzzi G: Endothelin and eicosanoid synthesis in cultured mesangial cells. Kidney Int 37:927, 1990

■ SECTION III ■
Antepartum: Management of Normal Pregnancy

■

CHAPTER 9
Prenatal Care

The objective of prenatal care is to assure that every wanted pregnancy culminates in the delivery of a healthy baby without impairing the health of the mother.

Overview. Before the evolution of modern obstetrics, the pregnant woman usually had but a single antepartum interview with a physician. At that time not much more was accomplished than an attempt to anticipate the date of delivery. When next seen, she might be in the throes of an eclamptic convulsion, or suffering severe chills and high fever from pyelonephritis, or struggling to expel a very large but dead fetus.

Organized prenatal care in the United States was introduced largely by social reformers and nurses (Merkatz and colleagues, 1990). In 1901, Mrs. William Lowell Putnam of the Boston Infant Social Service Department began a program of nurse visits to women enrolled in the home delivery service of the Boston Lying-in Hospital. This work was so successful that an outpatient prenatal clinic was established in 1911, and women were urged to enroll as early in pregnancy as possible. Mrs. Putnam subsequently convinced Dr. J. Whitridge Williams to support systematic prenatal care at the Johns Hopkins Hospital. In a 1914 study, Williams estimated that organized prenatal care could have reduced fetal mortality by 40 percent. Dr. Nicholas J. Eastman credited the movement to organized prenatal care with having "done more to save mothers' lives in our time than any other single factor."

Since 1979, approximately 75 percent of American women have begun prenatal care during the first trimester, with no change in this proportion in the ensuing decade (National Center for Health Statistics, 1991). The median number of visits made in 1989 by women who had any prenatal care was 12. The proportion of women who received late prenatal care, beginning in the third trimester, or no care at all, has remained 6 percent since 1983. The United States Public Health Service (1992) goal for the year 2000 is for at least 90 percent of American women to commence prenatal care in the first trimester.

Recent Developments. In 1986, the Department of Health and Human Services convened an expert panel to review the content of prenatal care (Rosen, 1991). This was in response to a report by the Institute of Medicine and National Institutes of Health on the importance of prenatal care in reducing the incidence of low-birthweight infants as a national agenda. The panel was made up of obstetricians, pediatricians, and nurse midwives, and there also were economists, consumer advocates, ethicists, social workers, psychologists, nutritionists, statisticians, and epidemiologists. The panel concluded that many medical conditions (e.g., diabetes mellitus) and personal behaviors (e.g., alcohol abuse) associated with bad pregnancy outcomes could be identified and modified *prior to conception*. Because health during pregnancy depends on health before pregnancy, it is logical that preconception care should be an integral part of prenatal care.

Moreover, the panel emphasized that prenatal care should provide an opportunity to focus on the total health and well-being of the family to include medical, psychological, social, and environmental variables affecting health. Systematic health care beginning long before pregnancy undoubtedly proves quite beneficial to the physical and emotional well-being of the prospective mother and, in turn, her child-to-be. As the consequence of such a program, many acquired diseases and developmental abnormalities will be recognized before pregnancy. Thus, appropriate steps can be taken to eradicate these, or at least to minimize deleterious effects. A striking example is that diabetic women can be advised of probable benefits for the embryo-fetus to be achieved from near normalization of blood glucose levels before conception (see Chap. 53, p. 1207).

Detailed recommendations were provided for preconceptional care beginning within a year of a planned pregnancy, the first pregnancy visit at 6 to 8 weeks, and visits throughout pregnancy. These were summarized by Rosen and colleagues (1991). The most controversial recommendation made by the expert panel was their proposal to reduce the number of prenatal visits in women at no apparent risk. They suggested that such women would best be served by return visits targeted at specific times (e.g., alphafetoprotein screening at 16 weeks) and therefore with a meaningful purpose for the visit. We have used such an approach for all pregnancies at Parkland Hospital since late 1988. Parous women with normal obstetrical histories are seen even less frequently than has been the traditional practice. The approach has been to limit visits in the first 6 months to specific purposes. Tyson and co-workers (1990), in an analysis of almost 29,000 deliveries at Parkland Hospital from 1977 to 1980, observed that there were substantial perinatal outcome benefits from prenatal care after 30 weeks' gestation, but not from early prenatal care.

The intervals for routine tests and those indicated for selected patients during pregnancy, as recommended by the American College of Obstetricians and Gynecologists Committee on Obstetrics (1992), are summarized in Table 9–1.

Perhaps somewhat paradoxically, it must be emphasized that prenatal care should do no harm, because at times it has been a two-edged sword. Instead of improving pregnancy outcome, on occasion the opposite was brought about in a variety of ways, including inappropriate dietary advice to achieve rigid weight restriction, the unnecessary prescription of potentially dangerous drugs such as powerful diuretics, and failure to encourage immediate reporting of an abnormal event, allowing the woman to wait to do so at the next scheduled visit.

A priori pregnancy should be considered a normal physiological state. Unfortunately, the complexity of the functional and anatomical changes that accompany gestation tends in the minds of some to stigmatize normal pregnancy as a disease process. For example, a hemoglobin concentration of 10.5 g/dL is abnormally low for the woman who is not pregnant, but not for one who is in the late second trimester; a plasma thyroxine level of 16 μg/dL is normal during pregnancy but is very strongly suggestive of hyperthyroidism in nonpregnant women. At times pregnancy imposes other changes that when modest in degree are normal, but when more intense

TABLE 9–1. RECOMMENDED INTERVALS FOR ROUTINE AND INDICATED TESTS AND PROCEDURES DURING PRENATAL CARE

Time (wk)	Assessment
Initial (as early as possible)	Hemoglobin or hematocrit
	Urinalysis, including microscopic examination and infection screen
	Blood group and Rh type
	Antibody screen
	Rubella antibody titer
	Syphilis screen
	Cervical cytology
	Hepatitis B virus screen
8–18	Ultrasound
	Amniocentesis
	Chorionic villus sampling
16–18	Maternal serum alphafetoprotein
26–28	Diabetes screening
	Repeat hemoglobin or hematocrit
28	Repeat antibody test for unsensitized Rh-negative patients
	Prophylactic administration of Rho(D) immune globulin
32–36	Ultrasound
	Testing for sexually transmitted disease
	Repeat hemoglobin or hematocrit

From the American College of Obstetrics and Gynecologists (1992), with permission.

decidedly are abnormal. For example, edema of the feet and ankles after ambulation is the normal consequence of regional physical forces imposed by the large pregnant uterus and by gravity. Generalized edema obvious in the face, hands, and abdomen, however, is definitely abnormal. **It is essential for the physician who assumes responsibility for prenatal care to be familiar with the normal physiological changes, as well as the pathological changes, that may develop during pregnancy.**

Good prenatal care is vital for the accomplishment of the objective stated at the outset, namely, the delivery of a healthy baby from a healthy mother. An attempt has been made in this chapter to delineate many of the ingredients essential to good prenatal care. **Bad prenatal care may be worse than none.** All too often, inappropriate prenatal care provides the expectant mother with an unwarranted sense of security that allows her to ignore signs and symptoms for which, if left to her own instincts, she might have urgently sought advice.

Terminology

Definitions

- A **primipara** is a woman who has been delivered only once of a fetus or fetuses who reached viability. Therefore, completion of any pregnancy beyond the stage of abortion (see Chap. 31, p. 665) bestows parity upon the mother.

- A **multipara** is a woman who has completed two or more pregnancies to viability. It is the number of pregnancies reaching viability, and not the number of fetuses delivered, that determines *parity*. Parity is not greater if a single fetus, twins, or quintuplets were delivered, nor lower if the fetus or fetuses were stillborn.
- A **nulligravida** is a woman who is not now and never has been pregnant.
- A **gravida** is a woman who is or has been pregnant, irrespective of the pregnancy outcome. With the establishment of the first pregnancy, she becomes a primigravida, and with successive pregnancies a multigravida. A **nullipara** is a woman who has never completed a pregnancy beyond an abortion. She may or may not have had a spontaneous or elective abortion(s).
- A **parturient** is a woman in labor.
- A **puerpera** is a woman who has just given birth.

In certain clinics it is customary to summarize past obstetrical history by a series of digits connected by dashes as follows: 6–1–2–6. The first digit refers to the number of term infants, the second to the number of preterm infants, the third to the number of abortions, and the fourth to the number of children currently alive. For the example given, 6–1–2–6, the woman has had 6 term deliveries, 1 preterm delivery, 2 abortions, and she currently has 6 children alive. This series of digits serves to summarize the obstetrical history somewhat better than the designation *gravida* 9, *para* 7, *abortus* 2, only when the recipient of the information understands the code.

Normal Duration of Pregnancy. The mean duration of pregnancy calculated from the first day of the last normal menstrual period for a large number of healthy women has been identified to be very close to 280 days, or 40 weeks. Three studies are cited: Kortenoever (1950), in an analysis of 7504 pregnancies, found the average duration to be 282 days. A mean value of 281 days was calculated from the data of the Obstetrical Statistical Cooperative for 77,300 women who underwent spontaneous labor and whose infants weighed at least 2500 g. Nakano (1972) identified the mean duration for 5596 pregnancies in Osaka, Japan to be 279 days from the first day of the last menstrual period, with two standard deviations of + 17 days.

It is customary to estimate the expected date of delivery by adding 7 days to the date of the first day of the last normal menstrual period and counting back 3 months (Naegele's rule). For example, if the last menstrual period began on September 10, the expected date of delivery would be June 17. It is apparent that pregnancy is erroneously considered to have begun about 2 weeks before ovulation if the duration is so calculated. Nonetheless, clinicians persist in using *gestational age* or *menstrual age*, calculated from the first day of the last menstrual period, to identify temporal events in pregnancy. Embryologists and other reproductive biologists more often employ *ovulatory age* or *fertilization age*, both of which are typically 2 weeks shorter. It currently is usually the practice to calculate delivery dates from the last menses with the aid of "pregnancy wheels" provided by several pharmaceutical companies. Bracken and Belanger (1989) tested the accuracy of such devices provided by three companies and found that the wheels were remarkably prone to error. Specifically, incorrect delivery dates were predicted in 40 to 60 percent of estimates, with a 5-day error being typical.

It has become customary to divide pregnancy into three equal parts, or *trimesters,* of approximately 3 calendar months each. Historically, the first trimester extended through the completion of 14 weeks, the second through 28 weeks, and the third trimester included the 29th through 42nd weeks of pregnancy. Put another way, trimesters can be obtained by division of 42 into three periods of 14 weeks each. There are certain major obstetrical problems that cluster in each of these time periods. For example, most spontaneous abortions occur during the first trimester, whereas practically all cases of pregnancy-induced hypertension become clinically evident during the third trimester. However, it is no longer true that no infant will survive if born earlier than the third trimester.

The clinical use of trimesters to describe the duration of a specific pregnancy fosters imprecision and should be abandoned. For example, it is inappropriate in case of uterine hemorrhage to categorize the problem temporally as "third-trimester bleeding." Appropriate management for the mother and her fetus will vary remarkably, depending upon whether the bleeding is encountered early or late in the third trimester. **Precise knowledge of the age of the fetus is imperative for ideal obstetrical management!** Therefore, expert attention must be given to this important measurement. The clinically appropriate unit of measure is *weeks of gestation completed.*

General Procedures

Every word and every act by all who come in contact with the pregnant woman should impress upon her both the importance and the availability of prenatal care. All too often, especially in public clinics, the strong impression has been propagated that such care is really not available without great expenditure of physical and emotional effort by her, and too often, of money beyond her ability to pay. It is tragic when women and their fetuses are denied adequate prenatal care simply because of lack of funds. Humanitarian aspects notwithstanding, the cost for good prenatal care is modest compared with the expense of caring subsequently for serious, but preventable, complications in the mother, her fetus-infant, or both. For example, at Parkland Hospital not only is the frequency of low-birthweight infants much higher for pregnancies without prenatal care, but the cost is nearly doubled for newborn care (Leveno and colleagues, 1985).

Initial Care. Prenatal care should be initiated as soon as there is reasonable likelihood of pregnancy. This may be as early as a few days after a missed menstrual period, especially for the woman who desires an abortion, but it should be no later than the second missed period for anyone.

In order to initiate antepartum care early, a system was developed at Parkland Hospital that has, in general, proved effective. The woman is seen for initial screening any day of the week without an appointment. At this initial visit nurses familiar with obstetrical care identify the following: (1) the probability of pregnancy (including urine testing for chorionic gonadotropin when indicated); (2) the woman's desire for the pregnancy to continue; (3) any current health problems; (4) any previous major illnesses, including those in previous pregnancies; (5) the outcomes of previous pregnancies; and (6) all medications being taken. The woman is instructed to bring with her at the next visit a few days later all drugs that she has been taking.

Physical evaluation initiated at the initial screening visit by the nurse includes determination of blood pressure, height, and weight.

The following laboratory tests are initiated at the first visit:

- *Blood*: Hemoglobin, hematocrit, red cell indices, white blood cell and platelet count, sickle cell screening for black women, glucose and creatinine concentration, serological test for syphilis, identification of blood type and abnormal red cell antibodies, presence of antibody to rubella, and screening for hepatitis B antigen. Voluntary human immunodeficiency virus (HIV) antibody testing with appropriate counseling and consent is offered to all women and encouraged for those at risk (American College of Obstetricians and Gynecologists, 1991e).
- *Urine*: Glucose, protein, and quantitative culture of clean-catch midstream sample to identify significant bacteriuria.

Physicians are continually available in the clinic and are consulted by the nurse whenever a problem is suspected that might require immediate attention. Any woman who is considering abortion is offered counseling. Moreover, every woman is specifically asked if she wishes to see a physician at this screening visit. Finally, she is given explicit instructions on how to get help promptly in case of a problem.

It is difficult to convince the pregnant woman of the importance of prenatal care if, when she seeks it, the physician delays for many weeks her initial care! Even in the absence of identified pregnancy problems, all women are given appointments within 14 days for the completion by a physician, or nurse practitioner with expertise in prenatal care, of a comprehensive general health evaluation. Previous health records and laboratory data are reviewed at that time.

Initial Comprehensive Evaluation

Goals. The major goals are (1) to define the health status of the mother and fetus, (2) to determine the gestational age of the fetus, and (3) to initiate a plan for continuing obstetrical care. Once the health status of the mother and fetus have been defined, the initial plan for subsequent care may range from relatively infrequent routine visits to that of prompt hospitalization because of serious maternal or fetal disease.

History. For the most part, the same essentials go into appropriate history-taking from the pregnant woman as elsewhere in medicine. The history is obtained unhurriedly in a private setting to establish the good rapport so necessary for a successful outcome. Although it is undesirable for the woman to wait for protracted periods of time before interview, it is worse for her to be hurriedly and indifferently interrogated. **It is mandatory that all data important to the care of the mother and fetus be clearly recorded so that all members of the health care team can interpret them correctly.**

The *menstrual history* is extremely important. The woman who spontaneously menstruates regularly every 28 days or so is most likely to ovulate at midcycle. Thus, the gestational age (menstrual age) becomes simply the number of weeks since the onset of the last menstrual period. If her menstrual cycles were significantly longer than 28 to 30 days, ovulation more likely occurred well beyond 14 days; or if the intervals were much longer and irregular, chronic anovulation is likely to have preceded some of the episodes of vaginal bleeding identified as menses. In the latter instance, menstrual data are unreliable for calculating duration of the gestation. **Without regular, predictable, cyclic, spontaneous menses that suggest ovulatory cycles, accurate dating of pregnancy by physical examination is difficult.**

It is important to ascertain whether or not *steroidal contraceptives* were used before the pregnancy and, if so, when. It is now common, but not necessarily recommended, for women who sustain regularly recurring withdrawal bleeding while using oral contraceptives to cyclically stop their use and to conceive without any further menstrual-like bleeding. Ovulation, however, may not have resumed 2 weeks after the onset of the last withdrawal bleeding, but instead at an appreciably later but highly variable date. The difficult problem of predicting the time of ovulation in this circumstance is similar to that in which pregnancy follows delivery or abortion prior to the reestablishment of normal menstrual periods.

The possibility of the presence of an *intrauterine device* should be ascertained, because certain pregnancy complications are increased by its presence in utero (see Chap. 61, p. 1341). If present, its fate also must be clearly recorded.

Obstetrical Examination. The cervix is visualized employing a speculum lubricated with warm water. Next, in order to identify cytological abnormalities, a gentle swabbing from the lower half of the endocervical canal, and then a scraping from the squamocolumnar junction, are obtained, spread on slides, and fixed immediately in ether-alcohol or by an appropriate aerosol spray. The outer half of the cervical canal is again swabbed slowly to obtain material to culture and identify *Neisseria gonorrhoeae.* The applicator stick is rolled over the transport medium while the container is held vertically to prevent loss of the carbon dioxide–enriched air in the culture bottle. The specimens are labeled immediately and accurately.

Bluish-red passive hyperemia of the cervix is characteristic, but not of itself diagnostic, of pregnancy. Dilated, occluded cervical glands bulging beneath the exocervical mucosa, so-called *Nabothian cysts,* may be prominent. If the cervix is dilated appreciably, fetal membranes may be visualized through the cervical canal, implying at least that expulsion of the products of conception may be imminent.

The character of vaginal secretions is noted. A moderate amount of white mucoid discharge is normal. The presence of foamy yellow liquid in the vagina is strongly suggestive of *Trichomonas,* whereas the presence of a curd-like discharge is consistent with *Candida* infection (p. 268). Material may be swabbed from the vagina for microscopical examination and culture.

The speculum is removed and the digital pelvic examination is completed by palpation, with special attention given to the consistency, length, and dilatation of the cervix; to the fetal presenting part, especially if late in pregnancy; to the bony architecture of the pelvis; and to any anomalies of the vagina and perineum, including cystocele, rectocele, and relaxed or torn perineum. The vulva and contiguous structures are also carefully inspected. (The pelvic examination is described in more detail in Chapter 14, p. 372.) All cervi-

cal, vaginal, and vulvar lesions are evaluated further by appropriate use of colposcopy, biopsy, culture, or dark-field examination. The perianal region should be visualized and digital rectal examination done to identify hemorrhoids or other lesions.

Between 18 and 32 weeks' gestation, there is good correlation between the gestational age of the fetus in weeks and the height of the uterine fundus in centimeters, when measured as the distance over the abdominal wall from the top of the symphysis pubis to the top of the fundus, with the bladder empty. During this time period, the height in centimeters approximates the gestational age in weeks. Therefore, it is important for the examiner to carefully document the height of the fundus.

Physical Examination. The general physical examination should be thorough. It includes evaluation of the teeth and repair of carious teeth should be undertaken promptly. When varicose veins are identified, frequent postural drainage should be urged and elastic support stockings provided.

Further Instructions. After the history and physical examination have been completed, the woman is instructed about diet, relaxation and sleep, bowel habits, exercise, bathing, clothing, recreation, sexual intercourse, smoking, drug and alcohol ingestion, and follow-up visits, including steps to take if an appointment is missed. Usually it is possible to assure her that she may anticipate an uneventful pregnancy followed by an uncomplicated delivery. **At the same time, she is tactfully instructed about the following danger signals, which must be reported immediately, day or night:**

1. Any vaginal bleeding
2. Swelling of the face or fingers
3. Severe or continuous headache
4. Dimness or blurring of vision
5. Abdominal pain
6. Persistent vomiting
7. Chills or fever
8. Dysuria
9. Escape of fluid from the vagina
10. Marked change in frequency or intensity of fetal movements

Prognosis. All information obtained should be employed to accurately identify the gestational age of the fetus and to anticipate the kinds and the magnitude of morbidity, both maternal and fetal, that may subsequently develop. Often, when morbidity is anticipated, its intensity can be minimized by appropriate care.

High-Risk Pregnancies. Considerable attention has been directed toward identifying complicated or "high-risk" pregnancies, and indeed, risk-assessment programs have been demonstrated to be effective for identifying most pregnancies at increased risk (Hobel and associates, 1979; Sokol and co-workers, 1977). Creasy and colleagues (1980) have used a risk-scoring system modified after Papiernik and Kaminski (1974) in an attempt to identify women at risk for preterm labor (see Chap. 38, p. 857). In this system scores of 1 to 10 are given to a variety of pregnancy factors, including socioeconomic status, reproductive history, daily habits, and current pregnancy complications. Women with scores of 10 or more are considered at high risk for preterm delivery. In practice, one problem inherent in such attempts to identify the high-risk pregnancy has been a tendency to subsequently ignore the pregnancy that early on had been categorized as low risk yet proved later to be high risk. Nonetheless, there are major categories for increased risk that should be identified antepartum and given appropriate consideration in subsequent pregnancy management. These include (1) preexisting medical illness; (2) previous poor pregnancy performance, such as perinatal mortality, preterm delivery, fetal growth retardation, malformations, placental accidents, and maternal hemorrhage; and (3) evidence of maternal undernutrition.

Subsequent Prenatal Care

Return Visits. Traditionally the timing of subsequent prenatal examinations has been scheduled at intervals of 4 weeks until 28 weeks, then every 2 weeks until 36 weeks, and weekly thereafter. Rather often, however, important information can be gained from a more flexible appointment schedule. For example, at midpregnancy, certain clinically discernible events characteristically occur that, when precisely identified, enhance the reliability of the estimate of gestational age.

Audible Fetal Heart Sounds. In essentially all pregnancies, the fetal heart can first be heard between 16 and 19 weeks when carefully listened for with a DeLee fetal stethoscope (see Chap. 2, p. 28). Obviously, the ability of an examiner to hear unamplified fetal heart sounds will depend upon several factors, including, among others, patient size and the examiner's hearing acuity. Herbert and co-workers (1987) reported that the fetal heart was audible by 20 weeks in 80 percent of women with regular menses. By 21 weeks audible fetal heart sounds were present in 95 percent, and by 22 weeks in all.

Fundal Height. Measurement of the height of the uterine fundus above the symphysis can provide useful information. For example, Jimenez and co-workers (1983)

demonstrated that between 20 and 31 weeks the fundal height in centimeters equaled the gestational age in weeks. Utilizing a tape calibrated in centimeters and applied over the abdominal curvature, they measured the distance from the top of the fundus to the top of the symphysis pubis. The top of the fundus was identified by percussion and by palpation, and the tape was placed there and extended to the top of the symphysis. Quaranta and associates (1981) and Calvert and colleagues (1982) reported essentially identical observations up to 34 weeks' gestation. *The bladder must be emptied before making the measurement.* Worthen and Bustillo (1980), for example, demonstrated that at 17 to 20 weeks' gestation the fundal height was 3 cm higher with a full bladder.

Gestational Age. **For the great majority of pregnancies, the most important question to be answered through prenatal examination is "How old is the fetus?"** Fortunately, it is possible to identify gestational age with considerable precision through an appropriately timed, carefully performed clinical examination, coupled with knowledge of the time of onset of the last menstrual period. When the date of onset of the last menstrual period and the fundal height are repeatedly in temporal agreement, the duration of gestation can be firmly established. When gestational age cannot be clearly identified, sonography may be of considerable value (see Chap. 46, p. 1045).

Later in pregnancy, previously acquired precise knowledge of gestational age is of considerable importance, because a number of pregnancy complications may develop, for which the optimal treatment will depend on fetal age. For example, with the development of preeclampsia at 38 weeks, very often delivery is the treatment most beneficial to both mother and fetus. However, if the duration of gestation is only 28 weeks when preeclampsia develops, attempts at conservative management and delay of delivery may be more beneficial.

Prenatal Surveillance. At each return visit steps are taken to identify the well-being of both the expectant mother and her fetus. Certain information, obtained by oral history and by examination, is especially important:

Fetal

1. Fetal heart rate(s).
2. Size of fetus(es), actual and rate of change.
3. Amount of amnionic fluid.
4. Presenting part and station (late in pregnancy).
5. Fetal activity.

Maternal

1. Blood pressure, actual and extent of change.
2. Weight, actual and amount of change.
3. Symptoms, including headache, altered vision,

abdominal pain, nausea and vomiting, bleeding, fluid from vagina, and dysuria.

4. Distance to uterine fundus from symphysis.
5. A carefully performed vaginal examination late in pregnancy often provides valuable information as follows:
   a. Confirmation of the presenting part.
   b. Station (depth in the pelvis) of the presenting part (see Chap. 14, p. 372).
   c. Clinical mensuration of the pelvis and an appreciation of its general configuration (see Chap. 11, p. 288–290).
   d. The consistency, effacement, and dilatation of the cervix. Digital exploration must be conducted with care lest membranes be ruptured or an undiagnosed low-lying placenta be separated, causing severe hemorrhage.

Subsequent Laboratory Tests. If the initial results were quite normal, most of the procedures need not be repeated. Hematocrit determination and the serological test for syphilis, if syphilis prevails in the population cared for, should be repeated at about 28 to 32 weeks. A cervical culture for gonorrhea may be repeated at this time if gonorrhea is common.

Determination of maternal serum alphafetoprotein concentration at 16 to 18 weeks is recommended to screen for open neural-tube defects and some chromosomal anomalies (American College of Obstetricians and Gynecologists, 1991a). Precise knowledge of gestational age is paramount for accuracy of this screening test (see Chap. 41, p. 942).

Screening for cystic fibrosis, the most common serious autosomal recessive disease in North American caucasians of European ancestry, is now possible (American College of Obstetricians and Gynecologists, 1991c). However, current recommendations limit such testing to couples with a family history of cystic fibrosis, including a parent, sibling, uncle, aunt, niece, nephew, or cousin. It is emphasized that under current circumstances, population-based screening is not recommended for individuals and couples with a negative family history (see Chap. 41, p. 944).

For women at risk for gestational diabetes, screening for glucose intolerance between 24 and 28 weeks is recommended by the American College of Obstetricians and Gynecologists (1986a). Following a 50-g oral glucose challenge, if plasma glucose at 1 hour exceeds 140 mg/dL, then a 3-hour 100-g test is recommended (see Chap. 53, p. 1205). Some recommend that all women be tested with a 1-hour 50-g glucose challenge. For women without risk factors for gestational diabetes we prefer to obtain a random plasma glucose level to rule out overt diabetes.

For pregnant women at high risk for sexually transmitted diseases the American College of Obstetricians and Gynecologists (1985) recommends that diagnostic testing for *Chlamydia trachomatis* be performed, if possible at the first prenatal visit and then again in the third trimester (see Chap. 59, p. 1304).

Other screening tests may be applied selectively to populations at high risk for the condition sought. For example, serological testing for HIV should be considered for women who take illicit intravenous drugs or who may be at risk for other reasons (see Chap. 59, p. 1310).

Routine urinalysis at every clinic visit is rarely warranted. Practically all women who develop preeclampsia develop a significant rise in blood pressure, and many have a sudden gain in weight before overt proteinuria develops. Therefore, in general, after the initial examination, proteinuria need only be looked for selectively in women who develop an increase in blood pressure or marked increase in weight. Fasting and postprandial plasma glucose levels are much more informative than are tests for glucosuria, especially in the case of the woman at risk for diabetes. Nonetheless, glucosuria, if detected, should not be ignored.

All pertinent information obtained at each visit must be recorded legibly and be sufficiently descriptive that anyone who uses the pregnancy record at any time can appreciate the significance of the information.

Nutrition During Pregnancy

Throughout most of this century, the diets of pregnant women have been the subject of endless discussions that often resulted in considerable contradiction and confusion. Various enthusiasts have urged pregnant women to adhere to a wide variety of diets, ranging from those that emphasized rigid caloric restriction to those that provided unusually large amounts of protein as well as calories. Faulty reasoning led some obstetricians to advise rigid caloric restriction, a recommendation that stemmed primarily from the observation that a prominent feature of preeclampsia and eclampsia was excessive weight gain. It was not generally appreciated that the abnormal weight gain in preeclampsia and eclampsia resulted from fluid retention rather than excessive caloric intake.

Meaningful studies of nutrition in human pregnancy are exceedingly difficult to design. For ethical reasons, experimental dietary deficiency must not be produced deliberately. In those instances in which severe nutritional deficiencies have been induced as a consequence of social, economic, or political disaster, coincidental events often have created many variables, the effects of which are not amenable to quantification. Some past experiences suggest, however, that in otherwise healthy women a state of near starvation is required to establish clear differences in pregnancy outcome. Such an example is the acute starvation imposed on pregnant women during the German occupation of the Netherlands late in World War II.

During the winter of 1944–1945 nutritional deprivation of known intensity prevailed in a well-circumscribed area of the Netherlands. As pointed out by Stein and associates (1972), the type and the degree of nutritional deprivation during the famine was identified with a precision unequaled in any large population before or since. At the lowest point, rations reached 450 kcal per day, with generalized undernutrition rather than selective malnutrition. Shortly after the end of the war, Smith (1947) analyzed the outcomes of pregnancies that were in progress during this 6-month period of famine. The median birthweights of infants were decreased about 250 g. The birthweights rose again after food became available in a way that indicated that birthweight can be significantly influenced by starvation during the latter half of pregnancy. The perinatal mortality rate, however, was not altered, nor was the incidence of malformations significantly increased. Smith also identified the frequency of pregnancy toxemia (preeclampsia–eclampsia), defined by three different sets of criteria, to have declined during this "hunger-winter." Subsequent analysis by Ribeiro and associates (1982) identified an overall decline in maternal blood pressure near delivery during the famine.

Evidence of impaired brain development has been obtained in some animal fetuses whose mothers during pregnancy had been subjected to intense dietary deprivation. These animal studies in turn stimulated interest in the subsequent intellectual development of the young adults in the Netherlands whose mothers had been starved during pregnancy. The comprehensive study by Stein and co-workers (1972) was made possible by the fact that practically all males at age 19 undergo compulsory examination for military service. They concluded that the severe dietary deprivation during pregnancy caused no detectable effects on the mental performance of the surviving male offspring.

More recently, Nilsen and colleagues (1984) reported no adverse effects of low birthweight on intelligence in Norwegian men who weighed less than 2500 g at birth from a variety of causes. These young men were evaluated for physical fitness and intelligence at compulsory military induction, and when compared with other 18 year olds, they were indistinguishable except for somewhat smaller size and increased frequency of minor visual defects. The results of intelligence tests were the same for both groups.

Caution must be exercised in extrapolating from one species to another. For example, severe protein deprivation of a few days' duration in the pregnant rat, in which gestation is only 21 days and in which total fetal weight represents one fourth of maternal weight, may lead to serious reproductive casualties. In human pregnancy, which lasts 13 times longer and in which fetal weight is only about one twentieth of that of the mother, failure to ingest protein for the same number of days hardly could be expected to produce an insult of the same intensity.

Weight Gain During Pregnancy. According to Hytten (1991), the London physiologist widely considered the preeminent authority on weight gain during pregnancy,

> The range of weight change in pregnancy is wide, from a loss to a gain of 23 kg or more. The incidence of clinical complications rises at the extremes of the range, but a normal outcome is possible throughout, and there is no simple figure for weight change in pregnancy that can be regarded as "normal," with the implication that different figures are abnormal.

Hytten has reviewed available literature regarding weight gain during pregnancy for at least the past 2 decades and has found only two reports methodologically acceptable. One is by Humphreys (1954), who weighed 1000 healthy, normal women sequentially from the 12th week during pregnancy. The other report is by Thomson and Billewicz (1957), who calculated the weight gain of 2868 normotensive primigravidas from the 13th week. In these reports, total maternal weight gain in British women averaged 11.5 kg (about 25 lb), excluding the first trimester. Very little information exists on weight gain during early pregnancy, but most estimates have indicated approximately 1 kg weight gain during the first trimester. Using these estimates, Hytten observed that total weight gain throughout pregnancy in healthy primigravidas eating without restrictions is approximately 12.5 kg (27.5 lb). Normal physiological events cumulatively account for about 9 kg as fetus, placenta, amnionic fluid, uterine hypertrophy, increase in maternal blood volume, breast enlargement, and maternal extracellular and extravascular fluid (see Table 8–1, p. 216). The remainder of the 12.5 kg appears to be mostly maternal storage fat. Hytten and Leitch (1971) had earlier examined the rate of weight gain during the second half of pregnancy in primigravidas of at least 5 ft 3 in (160 cm) who delivered between the 39th and 41st weeks of a normal pregnancy. The rate of weight gain between 20 weeks' gestation and delivery was about 1 lb per week, with a wide range of weight gain (Fig. 9–1).

Remarkably similar results were obtained by Petitti and co-workers (1991) in their analysis of weight gain by gestational age in both African-American and white women who delivered infants with birthweights of 3000 g or more. Specifically, weight gain from 8 to 20 weeks was about 0.7 lb/wk and about 1 lb/wk from 20 weeks to delivery. Weight gains were nearly identical for white and black women with prenatal care and delivery of infants weighing 3000 g or more. Perhaps the most remarkable findings about weight gain in pregnancy are that a wide range is compatible with good clinical outcomes, and that departures from "normality" are very nonspecific for any adverse outcome in a given individual. Indeed, some have questioned the necessity of routinely weighing women during antenatal care (Dawes and co-authors, 1992).

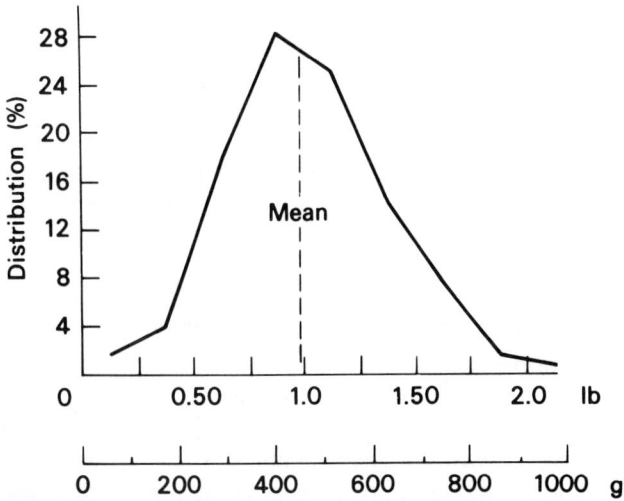

Fig. 9–1. Distribution of weekly weight gain from 20 weeks' gestation to delivery in healthy young primigravidas. (From Hytten, 1991, with permission.)

For the past 2 decades at least, the American College of Obstetricians and Gynecologists (1989) and others have recommended that pregnant women gain around 10 to 12 kg (22 to 27 lb) during pregnancy. In 1990, a committee of the National Academy of Science, through the Institute of Medicine, summarized and published studies on weight gain during pregnancy and concluded that weight gain in U.S. women was higher at every gestational age compared with the British study populations that Hytten used to formulate his conclusions cited above. The Institute recommended weight gains of 12.5 to 18 kg (28 to 40 lb) for underweight women, 11.5 to 16 kg (25 to 35 lb) for normal weight women, and 7 to 11.5 kg (15 to 25 lb) for overweight women. These categories were based on *body mass index* (*BMI*) defined as prepregnant weight divided by height^2. Underweight women had an index less than 19.8 kg/m^2 and overweight women exceeded 26 kg/m^2. They further suggested that young girls and African-American women gain toward the upper limit within their pregravid weight ranges. It was also observed that fetal growth effects of maternal weight gain during pregnancy were greatest in thin women and least in overweight women.

Several possible disadvantages as a consequence of the fetus-infant being heavier must be considered. For example, it seems likely that larger fetuses will cause an increased incidence of dystocia with an increased incidence of cesarean delivery. Parker and Abrams (1992) examined the associations between maternal weight gains outside the recommendations of the Institute of Medicine and three pregnancy outcomes (small-for-gestational age, large-for-gestational age, and cesarean delivery) in 6690 singleton live births in San Francisco. The average prepregnancy weight was 57 kg (125 lb), and the average maternal weight gain was 15.2 ± 5.2 kg

(33.4 ± 11.4 lb) in these predominantly white and Asian women. Less than half of the women studied gained weight within the Institute's recommendations for their habitus. Maternal weight gains within the recommendations reduced the risk of the outcomes studied. Specifically, low weight gains for a given habitus was associated with small-for-gestational age infants. Conversely, excessive weight gains were linked to large-for-gestational age infants and increased cesarean delivery rates (16 versus 21.5 percent, respectively).

Not all the weight put on during pregnancy is lost during and immediately after parturition (Hytten, 1991). The normal woman who gains 12.5 kg (27.5 lb) in pregnancy is about 4.4 kg (9 lb) above her prepregnant weight when she leaves the hospital postpartum. Schauberger and co-workers (1992) studied prenatal and postpartum weights in 795 women delivered in La Crosse, Wisconsin. Average weight gain was 13.0 ± 4.8 kg (28.6 ± 10.6 lb). As shown in Figure 9–2, the majority of maternal weight loss (about 5.5 kg or 12.1 lb) occurred at delivery and in the ensuing 2 postpartum weeks (about 4 kg or 8.8 lb). An additional 2.5 kg (5.5 lb) was lost between 2 weeks and 6 months postpartum. The average total weight loss was 12.2 ± 4.6 kg (26.8 ± 10.1 lb), resulting in an average retained weight of 1.4 ± 4.8 kg (3 ± 10.5 lb) due to pregnancy. Overall, the more weight gained during pregnancy, the more that was lost postpartum. Parous women retained more of their pregnancy weight, but the interval between pregnancies was not linked to long-term obesity. The effects of breast feeding on maternal weight loss was negligible.

Recommended Dietary Allowances

Periodically the Food and Nutrition Board of the National Research Council recommends dietary allow-

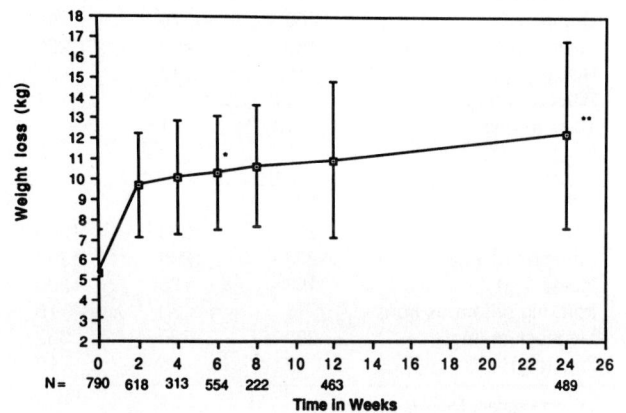

Fig. 9–2. Cumulative weight loss from last antepartum visit to 6 months postpartum. (From Schauberger and co-workers, 1992, with permission.)

ances for women, including those who are pregnant or lactating. Their latest recommendations are summarized in Table 9–2. Recommended daily allowances are not intended for application to individuals, but as guides to the needs of populations and groups, because individuals undoubtedly vary widely in their requirements. Directions on the labels of certain prenatal vitamin-mineral supplements may lead to intakes well in excess of the 1989 *Recommended Dietary Allowances.* This is not readily apparent to either the consumer or physician issuing the prescription, because label information is expressed in terms of the Food and Drug Administration's *U.S. Recommended Daily Allowances,* which are substantially different for several nutrients (Institute of Medicine, 1990). Moreover, the use of excessive supplements—for example, 10 times the Recommended Daily Allowances—which often are self-prescribed, by a substantial portion of the general public has lead to concern about nutrient toxicities during pregnancy. Nutrients that can potentially exert toxic effects include iron, zinc, selenium, and vitamins A, B_6, C, and D.

The Institute of Medicine (1990) made significant recommendations concerning nutrient supplementation during pregnancy, concluding that iron was the only known nutrient for which requirements could not be

met by diet alone. The Institute did not recommend routine multivitamin supplementation. For women who do not consume an adequate diet, the Institute recommended beginning in the second trimester with a daily multivitamin-mineral supplement containing 30 mg of iron, 15 mg of zinc, 2 mg of copper, 250 mg of calcium, 2 mg of vitamin B_6, 300 μg of folate, 50 mg of vitamin C, and 5 μg of vitamin D.

Calories. A daily caloric increase of 300 kcal throughout pregnancy has been recommended by the Food and Nutrition Board. Calories are necessary for energy, and whenever caloric intake is inadequate, protein is metabolized for energy rather than being spared for its vital role in growth and development. Total physiological requirements during pregnancy are not necessarily the sum of ordinary nonpregnant requirements plus those specific to pregnancy. For example, the additional energy required during pregnancy may be compensated in whole or in part by reduced physical activity (Hytten, 1991).

The importance of adequate caloric intake was emphasized by a nutrition intervention study in Guatemala that identified infant birthweights to be larger when the at most marginal maternal diets were supplemented (Delgado and associates, 1977). In two of four villages, a high-protein plus calorie supplement was made available; in the other two villages a drink that provided calories without protein was offered. Birthweights were influenced by the number of calories ingested rather than by the protein content. For those pregnancies in which less than 10,000 supplemental kcal were ingested, birthweight averaged 2986 g, and 18.3 percent of the infants weighed less than 2500 g. For those pregnancies in which more than 20,000 kcal were consumed in the form of supplements, the mean birthweight was 3120 g, and only 9.4 percent of the infants weighed less than 2500 g at birth.

In a more recent investigation of the impact of caloric supplementation on birthweights of infants of Gambian women, a threshold effect was apparent (Prentice and co-workers, 1983, 1987). Food supplementation that provided throughout much of pregnancy somewhat more than 400 kcal per day on average improved birthweights for infants whose mothers were in marked negative energy balance as the consequence of both food shortage and heavy workload. For example, the frequency of low-birthweight infants decreased threefold with maternal calorie supplementation. However, for women who were in positive energy balance, even though they were consuming only 60 percent of the recommended dietary allowance, supplementation had no demonstrable beneficial effect on birth outcome. These studies serve especially to emphasize the deleterious effect on fetal growth imposed by severe restriction of caloric intake.

TABLE 9–2. NATIONAL RESEARCH COUNCIL RECOMMENDED DAILY DIETARY ALLOWANCES FOR WOMEN BEFORE AND DURING PREGNANCY AND LACTATION

Nutrient	Non-pregnant[a]	Pregnant	Lactating
Kilocalories	2200	2500	2600
Protein (g)	55	60	65
Fat-soluble vitamins			
A (μg RE)[b]	800	800	1300
D (μg)	10	10	12
E (mg TE)[c]	8	10	12
K (μg)	55	65	65
Water-soluble vitamins			
C (mg)	60	70	95
Folate (μg)	180	400	280
Niacin (mg)	15	17	20
Riboflavin (mg)	1.3	1.6	1.8
Thiamin (mg)	1.1	1.5	1.6
Pyridoxine B_6 (mg)	1.6	2.2	2.1
Cobalamin B_{12} (μg)	2.0	2.2	2.6
Minerals			
Calcium (mg)	1200	1200	1200
Phosphorus (mg)	1200	1200	1200
Iodine (μg)	150	175	200
Iron (mg of ferrous iron)	15	30	15
Magnesium (mg)	280	320	355
Zinc (mg)	12	15	19

[a] For nonpregnant females age 15–18.
[b] 1 μg retinol = 1 retinol equivalent (RE).
[c] TE = tocopherol equivalent.
From the National Research Council (1989).

Protein. To the basic protein needs of the nonpregnant woman for repair of her tissues are added the demands for growth and repair of the fetus, placenta, uterus, and breasts, and increased maternal blood volume. During the last 6 months of pregnancy about 1 kg of protein is deposited, amounting to 5 to 6 g per day on average (Hytten and Leitch, 1971). Amino acids in maternal plasma have been incompletely studied other than to observe a marked fall in the concentrations of ornithine, glycine, taurine, and proline (Hytten, 1991). Exceptions during pregnancy are glutamic acid and alanine, which rise in concentration.

It is desirable that the majority of the protein be supplied from animal sources, such as meat, milk, eggs, cheese, poultry, and fish, because they furnish amino acids in optimal combinations. Milk and milk products have long been considered nearly ideal sources of nutrients, especially protein and calcium, for pregnant or lactating women. Nonetheless, milk (lactose) intolerance in the form of gastrointestinal disturbances that include bloating, flatulence, and cramps is a problem in some adults. For example, some degree of lactose intolerance was found in 81 percent of African-American adults, compared with 12 percent of whites (Bayless and co-workers, 1975). As little as 240 mL of milk caused the unpleasant symptoms. Villar and co-workers (1988) studied lactose digestion during pregnancy and found improvement in intestinal handling of milk lactose.

Minerals. The intakes recommended by the Food and Nutrition Board for a variety of minerals are presented in Table 9–2 and are discussed below. There is good evidence that only one mineral—iron—provides any demonstrated benefit when provided as a supplement to pregnant women. Practically all diets that supply sufficient calories for appropriate weight gain will contain enough of the other minerals to prevent a mineral deficiency if iodized salt is used.

Iron. The reasons for increased iron requirements during pregnancy are discussed in Chapter 8 (p. 222). Of the approximately 300 mg of iron transferred to the fetus and placenta and the 500 mg incorporated, if available, into the expanding maternal hemoglobin mass, nearly all is utilized during the latter half of pregnancy. During that time, the average iron requirements imposed by pregnancy are about 6 mg a day, and in addition there is the need for nearly 1 mg to compensate for maternal excretion, a total of about 7 mg of iron per day (Pritchard and Scott, 1970). Very few women have sufficient iron stores to supply this amount of iron. Moreover, the diet seldom contains enough iron to meet this demand. The recommendation by the Food and Nutrition Board (Table 9–2) of 15 mg of dietary iron per day for nonpregnant women represents the ceiling imposed by caloric requirements. To ingest any more iron from dietary sources would simultaneously provide an undesirable excess of calories. The board has acknowledged that because of small iron stores, the pregnant woman will often be unable to meet the iron requirements, and therefore supplementation is recommended.

Supplementation with medicinal iron is practiced commonly in the United States and elsewhere, although the merits of this practice continue to be questioned by a minority of investigators, cited below. Scott and co-workers (1970) established that as little as 30 mg of iron supplied in the form of a simple iron salt such as ferrous gluconate, sulfate, or fumarate, taken regularly once each day throughout the latter half of pregnancy, provided sufficient iron to meet the requirements of pregnancy and to protect any preexisting iron stores. This amount should also provide for the iron requirements of lactation. The pregnant woman may benefit from 60 to 100 mg of iron per day if she is large, has twin fetuses, is late in pregnancy, takes iron irregularly, or if her hemoglobin level is somewhat depressed. The woman who is overtly anemic from iron deficiency responds well to 200 mg of iron per day in divided doses (see Chap. 52, p. 1173).

The availability for absorption of iron contained in at least some prenatal vitamin-mineral supplements has been questioned (Seligman and associates, 1983). Undoubtedly, calcium and magnesium compounds included in such mixtures can inhibit iron absorption, as they do when taken as antacids. **A very effective and inexpensive way to avoid impairment of iron absorption by such agents is to prescribe simple iron salts alone!**

Because iron requirements are slight during the first 4 months of pregnancy, it is *not* necessary to provide supplemental iron during this time. Withholding iron supplementation during the first trimester of pregnancy avoids the risk of aggravating nausea and vomiting. Ingestion of iron at bedtime also appears to minimize the possibility of an adverse gastrointestinal reaction. Moreover, keeping the container of iron tablets in proximity to toothpaste enhances the ability of the expectant mother to remember to ingest the supplement regularly. Iron-containing medication must be kept out of the reach of small children lest they ingest a large number of the usually quite attractive tablets or capsules.

In some circumstances, compromised fetal well-being may be associated with an above-average maternal hemoglobin concentration. Murphy and co-workers (1986) reported findings from the Cardiff Births Survey of 54,382 singleton pregnancies and observed that women with hemoglobin values greater than 13.2 g/dL at 13 to 18 weeks had excessive perinatal mortality, low birthweight, and preterm delivery. Importantly, pregnancy-induced hypertension was substantively increased in nulliparas with higher hemoglobin levels. Unfortunately, findings such as these have led to the supposition by some that iron ingested prenatally, by stimulating an abnormally high hemoglobin concentration, is actually detrimental and therefore should not be used (Goodlin, 1982). Even vigorous iron administration does not raise the hemoglobin concentration of iron-sufficient women (Taylor and associates, 1982). Almost certainly, reduced blood volume from failure of expansion of plasma volume is the important culprit in the genesis of impaired fetal well-being. Failure of the hemoglobin concentration to fall is but one consequence of inadequate expansion. (If hemoglobin concentration in itself were an important factor, phlebotomy or even leeches might again come into vogue!)

Calcium. The pregnant woman retains about 30 g of calcium, most of which is deposited in the fetus late in pregnancy (Pitkin, 1985). This amount of calcium represents only about 2.5 percent of total maternal calcium, most of which is in bone, and which can readily be mobilized for fetal growth. Moreover, Heaney and Skillman (1971) demonstrated increased calcium absorption by the intestine and progressive retention throughout pregnancy. In a few places in the world, *osteomalacia* is still recognized in women who are reproducing, but only under the very unusual circumstances of almost total avoidance of sunlight coupled with low vitamin D and calcium intake for very long periods. According to Pitkin (1985), bound calcium levels, but not ionized calcium, fall slightly in maternal plasma as the concentration of albumin decreases (Chap. 8, p. 238).

Belizán and colleagues (1988) reviewed the relationship between calcium intake and pregnancy-induced hypertension and found no firm evidence that calcium supplementation was protective. Although widely practiced in the United States, supplementation is unlikely to be of any benefit. One quart of cow's milk provides approximately 1 g of calcium.

Phosphorus. The ubiquitous distribution of phosphorus ensures an adequate intake during pregnancy. Plasma levels of inorganic phosphorus do not differ appreciably from nonpregnant levels.

Zinc. Severe zinc deficiency may lead to poor appetite, suboptimal growth, and impaired wound healing. Profound zinc deficiency may cause dwarfism and hypogonadism. It may also lead to a specific skin disorder, *acrodermatitis enteropathica*, which is a rare, severe congenital zinc deficiency.

Zinc in plasma is only about 1 percent of total body zinc. Moreover, plasma zinc is almost entirely bound to several plasma proteins and amino acids. Therefore, low plasma concentrations are generally the consequence of changes in concentration of the various binders in plasma rather than true zinc depletion (Swanson and King, 1983). Even though the concentration is reduced, the total zinc plasma pool of normally pregnant women is actually increased as the consequence of the large increase in pregnancy-induced plasma volume. There is no strong evidence that dietary supplementation with zinc is of any benefit to the mother or fetus. Moreover, the level of zinc supplementation that is safe for pregnant women has not been clearly established. The rationale for slightly increasing the recommended zinc intake during pregnancy (Table 9–2) is not altogether clear.

Iodine. The use of iodized salt by all pregnant women is recommended to offset the increased need for fetal requirements and increased maternal renal losses. Severe maternal iodine deficiency predisposes offspring to endemic cretinism, characterized by multiple severe neurological defects (see Chap. 53, p. 1215). In parts of New Guinea where this condition was endemic, the intramuscular injection of iodized oil very early in pregnancy successfully prevented cretinism (Pharoah and associates, 1971). Iodine ingestion in pharmacological amounts during pregnancy may depress thyroid function and induce a sizable fetal goiter. The consumption of large amounts of seaweed by food faddists may do the same.

Magnesium. Magnesium deficiency as the consequence of pregnancy has not been recognized. Undoubtedly, during prolonged illness with no magnesium intake, the plasma level might become critically low, as it would in the absence of pregnancy. We have observed magnesium deficiency during pregnancy complicated by the consequences of previous intestinal bypass surgery. Sibai and co-workers (1989) randomized 400 normotensive primigravid women to placebo tablets or 365 mg elemental magnesium supplementation from 13 to 24 weeks' gestation. Supplementation did not improve any measures of pregnancy outcome.

Copper. Copper-containing enzymes such as cytochrome oxidase play key roles in many oxidative processes, and hence in the production of most of the energy required for metabolism. Pregnancy has a major effect on maternal copper metabolism, with marked increases in serum ceruloplasmin and plasma copper. Copper deficiency has not been documented in humans during pregnancy. No studies of copper supplementation of pregnant women have been reported, although several prenatal multivitamin-mineral preparations currently marketed provide 2 mg of copper per tablet.

Selenium. Selenium is an essential component of the enzyme glutathione peroxidase, which catalyzes the conversion of hydrogen peroxide to water; thus, selenium is an important defensive component against free radical damage. Selenium deficiency has been identified in a large area of the People's Republic of China, where there is a severe geochemical deficiency of this micronutrient. The deficiency is manifested by a frequently fatal cardiomyopathy in young children and women of childbearing age. Conversely, selenium toxicity due to oversupplementation has also been observed. There is no reported need to supplement selenium in American women during pregnancy.

Chromium. Chromium is believed to play a physiological role as a cofactor for insulin, facilitating the initial attachment of the hormone to its peripheral receptors. The extent to which chromium is important in human nutrition remains uncertain, and there are no data suggesting that chromium supplementation is advisable during pregnancy.

Manganese. Manganese-activated enzymes include the glycosyltransferases, which are necessary for the synthesis of polysaccharides and glycoproteins. Manganese deficiency has not been observed in human adults, including pregnant women, and manganese supplements are not indicated during pregnancy.

Potassium. The concentration of potassium in maternal plasma decreases by about 0.5 mEq/L by midpregnancy (Brown and colleagues, 1986). Potassium deficiency develops in the same circumstances as when the patient is not pregnant. Prolonged nausea and vomiting may lead to hypokalemia and metabolic alkalosis. A previously rather common cause—the use of diuretics—has nearly disappeared.

Sodium. Sodium deficiency during pregnancy is most unlikely unless diuretics are prescribed or dietary sodium intake is reduced drastically. In general, salting food to taste will provide an abundance of sodium. Plasma sodium concentration normally decreases a few mEq during pregnancy; however, sodium excretion is unchanged, and averages 100 to 110 mEq/day (Brown and colleagues, 1986).

> In the not too distant past much was said about the dangers of inciting preeclampsia–eclampsia through sodium ingestion during pregnancy and, by implication at least, of the benefits to be achieved from rigid restriction of sodium intake. Next, sodium restriction by pregnant women was cited as being detrimental, undoubtedly because rigid sodium restriction in pregnant rats caused abnormalities in the dams' adrenals. About this time it was claimed that extra salt in the maternal diet, especially rock salt, prevented preeclampsia–eclampsia (Robinson, 1958). Nonetheless, the ingestion of exorbitant amounts of sodium may prove harmful. However, there is no good evidence that rigorous sodium restriction is beneficial. Indeed, it too may be harmful.

Fluoride. The value of supplemental fluoride during pregnancy has been questioned. Horowitz and Heifetz (1967) investigated the prevalence of caries in temporary and permanent teeth of children with the same postnatal exposure to optimally fluoridated water but different patterns of prenatal exposure. They concluded that there were no meaningful additional benefits from maternal ingestion of fluoridated water if the offspring ingested such water from birth.

Glenn and associates (1982) reported a remarkably lower incidence (99 percent) of caries in children whose mothers ingested 2.2 mg of sodium fluoride daily during pregnancy, compared with those whose mothers used only fluoridated water. They strongly recommended that for structurally superior and caries-free teeth, 2.2 mg of sodium fluoride daily be ingested during pregnancy. Obviously, further investigations are needed to confirm these benefits and at the same time to detect deleterious effects, if any, from the fluoride. Fluoride supplementation during pregnancy has not been endorsed by the American Dental Association (Institute of Medicine, 1990).

Supplemental fluoride ingested by the lactating woman does not increase the fluoride concentration in her milk (Ekstrand, 1981).

Vitamins. Most evidence concerning the importance of vitamins for successful reproduction has been obtained from animal experiments. Typically, severe deficiency has been produced in the animal either by withholding the vitamin completely, beginning long before the time of pregnancy, or by giving a very potent vitamin antagonist. The administration of some vitamins in great excess to pregnant animals has been shown to exert deleterious effects on the fetus and newborn.

The increased requirements for vitamins during pregnancy (Table 9–2) in practically all circumstances can be supplied by any general diet that provides adequate amounts of calories and protein. The possible exception is folic acid during times of unusual requirements, such as pregnancy complicated by protracted vomiting, hemolytic anemia, or multiple fetuses.

Folic Acid. Maternal benefits to be derived from folic acid supplementation are not distinct. In the 1960s, several investigators implicated maternal folate deficiency in a variety of reproductive casualties, including placental abruption, pregnancy-induced hypertension, and fetal anomalies. For the most part, these reports have not been confirmed (Emery, 1977; Hall, 1977; Pritchard and coworkers, 1969; Whalley and associates, 1969).

There is abundant evidence that maternal folate requirements are increased somewhat during pregnancy. In the United States, this increase frequently leads to lowered plasma folate levels, less often to hypersegmentation of neutrophils, infrequently to megaloblastic erythropoiesis, but only rarely to megaloblastic anemia.

The amount of folic acid supplement that will prevent these changes varies considerably, depending primarily on the diet consumed. Because 1 mg of folic acid per day produces a vigorous hematological response in pregnant women with severe megaloblastic anemia, this amount would almost certainly provide very effective prophylaxis (Pritchard and co-workers, 1969). Chanarin and associates (1977) found that as little as 100 μg of folic acid per day raises the blood folate levels to the normal nonpregnant range.

The possibility of increased frequency of fetal malformations as the consequence of maternal folate deficiency has long been discussed, especially neural-tube defects (Smithells and colleagues, 1983). Recognition that aminopterin, a folic acid antagonist, was a human teratogen, and that such agents caused neural-tube defects in animals, focused attention on the possible etiological role of folic acid.

Mills and co-workers (1989), in a case-control study in which history of periconceptional multivitamin use was obtained 1 month after delivery, concluded that folate-containing supplements did not decrease the risk of having an infant with a neural-tube defect. Milunsky and colleagues (1989) reached different conclusions. Specifically, they examined the relation of multivitamin intake in general, and folic acid in particular, to the risk of neural-tube defects in a cohort of 23,491 women undergoing maternal serum alpha-fetoprotein screening or amniocentesis around 16 weeks' gestation. The prevalence of neural-tube defects in women who used multivitamins containing folic acid during the first 6 weeks of pregnancy was 0.9 per 1000 compared with 3.3 per 1000 when folic acid was not taken. The British Medical Research Council (1991) reported a randomized double-blind study of folic acid use before conception and during early pregnancy. This 8-year study, which involved 33 centers, included women who had a previous pregnancy complicated by an infant or fetus with a neural-tube defect. A total of 1817 such women were randomized to be given either folic acid (4 mg per day), other vitamins, both, or neither. Folic acid supplementation *before* conception significantly reduced the incidence of recurrent neural-tube defects. This report prompted the Centers for Disease Control (1991) to recommend folic acid supplementation for women who previously had an infant or fetus with spina bifida, anencephaly, or encephalocele. The guideline called for the consumption of a 4.0 mg daily dose of folic acid, from at least one month before conception through the first 3 months of pregnancy. Subsequently, the Centers for Disease Control (1992) recommended that all fertile American women consume 0.4 mg of folic on a regular continuous basis as a public health measure. Folate intake of 0.4 mg per day can be obtained from diet through careful selection of foods or from use of supplement pills.

Vitamin B_{12}. The level of vitamin B_{12} in maternal plasma decreases variably in otherwise normal pregnancies (Sauberlich, 1978). The decrease is thought to result mostly from a reduction in plasma binders and is prevented only in part by supplementation. However, maternal vitamin B_{12} deficiency develops in special circumstances. Vitamin B_{12} occurs naturally only in foods of animal origin. It is now established that *strict vegetarians* may give birth to infants whose vitamin B_{12} stores are low. Moreover, because breast milk of a vegetarian mother most likely contains little vitamin B_{12}, the deficiency may become profound in the breast-fed infant (Higginbottom and associates, 1978). Excessive ingestion of vitamin C can also lead to a functional deficiency of vitamin B_{12}.

Vitamin B_6. A variety of biochemical changes induced by vitamin B_6 deficiency, including excessive excretion of xanthurenic acid after the ingestion of tryptophan, have been summarized by Sauberlich (1978). Several of the changes accompany otherwise normal pregnancy and have been identified in women who use estrogen-containing contraceptives.

Some investigators have related impaired glucose tolerance during pregnancy to altered metabolic pathways induced by low vitamin B_6 levels and, in turn, a lowering of the biological activity of endogenous insulin. However, neither the observations of Perkins (1977) nor those of Gillmer and Mazibuko (1979) provide support for this premise. Gillmer and Mazibuko investigated 13 pregnant women who had abnormal glucose tolerance tests and who excreted elevated amounts of xanthurenic acid after a tryptophan load. Treatment with pyridoxine, 100 mg daily for 2 to 3 weeks, restored the urinary excretion of xanthurenic acid to levels normal for nonpregnant individuals, but improvement in the glucose tolerance test was observed in only 2 women, with no change in 5, and deterioration in 6.

As the consequence of these observations, an increase in the recommended daily dietary allowance for pyridoxine intake during pregnancy has been urged by some. However, to modify some of the biochemical changes that imply a deficiency of vitamin B_6 during pregnancy requires more of the vitamin than is now recommended and would likely necessitate specific supplementation. For example, Cleary and associates (1975) emphasized that to raise pyridoxal phosphate levels in maternal plasma to those characteristic of normal nonpregnant women required a daily supplement of pyridoxine of more than 2.5 mg. The benefits that might accrue from larger supplements do not appear at this time to warrant so vigorous an undertaking.

Vitamin C. The recommended dietary allowance for vitamin C during pregnancy is 70 mg per day, or about 20 percent more than when nonpregnant (Table 9–2). A reasonable diet should readily provide this amount. The maternal plasma level declines during pregnancy while the cord level is higher, a phenomenon observed with most water-soluble vitamins. The ingestion of 1 g or more of vitamin C for prophylaxis against the common cold has become commonplace, even though there is no good evidence that it is of any benefit. Conversely, there is evidence that it may prove harmful during pregnancy. Scurvy has been identified in normally fed infants whose mothers had ingested large doses of vitamin C during pregnancy (Cochrane, 1965). Large doses of vitamin C also can interfere with vitamin B_{12} absorption and metabolism, and this may not be overcome by vitamin B_{12} supplementation (Herbert and Jacob, 1974).

Pragmatic Nutritional Surveillance

While the science of nutrition continues in its perpetual struggle to identify the ideal amounts of protein, calories, vitamins, and minerals for the pregnant woman and her fetus, those directly responsible for their care may best discharge their duties as follows:

1. In general, advise the pregnant woman to eat what she wants in amounts she desires and salted to taste.
2. Make sure that there is ample food to eat, especially in the case of the socioeconomically deprived woman.
3. Make sure, by serially weighing every expectant mother, that she is gaining weight, with a goal of about 22 to 27 pounds.
4. Periodically, explore the food intake by dietary recall to uncover the ingestion of any bizarre diet. In this way the occasional nutritionally absurd diet will be discovered—for example, the ingestion of a peck of grapes per day or a pound of Argo Gloss Starch.
5. Give tablets of simple iron salts that provide 30 to 60 mg of iron daily.
6. Recheck the hematocrit or hemoglobin concentration at 28 to 32 weeks, so as to detect any significant decrease.

General Hygiene

Exercise. In general, it is not necessary for the pregnant woman to limit exercise, provided she does not become excessively fatigued or risk injury to herself or her fetus. The current enthusiasm for jogging also has attracted a number of pregnant women. In fact, several women, even late in pregnancy, have run safely in marathons.

Hauth and co-workers (1982) studied fetal heart rate reactivity throughout the third trimester of pregnancy in 7 women who jogged at least 1.5 miles three times a week before and during pregnancy. Upon completion of a run the women immediately climbed three flights of stairs to undergo evaluation. Fetal heart reactivity was evident in spite of the vigorous, very recent maternal exercise, and appreciable fetal tachycardia so induced persisted for up to one half hour. Carpenter and colleagues (1988) observed that submaximal exercise (maternal heart rate 148 beats per min or less) was not followed by fetal bradycardia; however, it was common after maximal exercise. Fetal heart rate responses to maximal maternal exercise with a treadmill or swimming was investigated by Watson and colleagues (1991). They documented fetal bradycardia during 15 percent of the exercise sessions when maternal heart rate averaged about 180 beats per min.

Clapp (1989a) studied 18 women with clinically normal singleton gestations to determine the amount of oxygen required to complete a specific treadmill exercise before, during, and after pregnancy. Those women who maintained a regular exercise regimen during pregnancy actually improved their metabolic efficiency. Specifically, the amount of oxygen required to complete a treadmill exercise actually *decreased* during pregnancy! Pivarnik and co-workers (1990) compared cardiovascular responses of 7 healthy women to aerobic exercise (cycle or treadmill) using pulmonary and radial artery catheters during late pregnancy with 3 months postpartum. Oxygen consumption ($\dot{V}O_2$), heart rate, stroke volume, and cardiac output all increased appropriately in response to exercise during pregnancy.

The effects of maternal exercise on pregnancy outcomes, including spontaneous abortion (Clapp, 1989b), the course of labor (Clapp, 1990a), and birthweight (Clapp and Capeless, 1990b), have been recently described. Continuation of aerobic exercise at intensities between 50 and 85 percent of their maximum capacity in 47 recreational runners and 40 aerobic dancers during the periconceptional period had no affect on the incidence of spontaneous abortion. Well-conditioned women who perform aerobics or run regularly were found to have shorter active labors and fewer cesarean deliveries, less meconium-stained amnionic fluid, and less fetal distress in labor. However, continuation of regular aerobic or running exercise programs did result in reduced birthweight (average 310 g) due to fetal growth restriction that primarily affected neonatal fat mass.

With some pregnancy complications, the mother and her fetus may benefit from a very sedentary existence; for example, women with pregnancy-induced hypertension appear to benefit (see Chap. 36, p. 789), as do women pregnant with two or more fetuses (see Chap. 39, p. 908), women suspected of having a growth-retarded fetus (see Chap. 38, p. 880), or those with severe heart disease (see Chap. 48, p. 1086).

The American College of Obstetricians and Gynecologists (1986b) recommends that women who are accustomed to aerobic exercise before pregnancy should be allowed to continue this during pregnancy. It cautions against starting new aerobic exercise programs or intensifying training efforts. For example, in women who were previously sedentary, aerobic activity more strenuous than walking is not recommended.

Employment. The legal and social movements in the United States to provide equality of opportunity in the workplace have reached women who are or might become pregnant. Annas (1991) has thoroughly reviewed the legal issues involved with employment during pregnancy. Importantly, the United States Supreme Court has buttressed the Pregnancy Discrimination Act of 1978 by ruling in 1991 that federal law prohibits employers from excluding women from job categories on the basis that they are or might become pregnant.

It is estimated that nearly one half of women of childbearing-age in the United States are in the labor force. Even larger proportions of socioeconomically less fortunate women are working. According to the report of Naeye and Peters (1982), working during pregnancy can be deleterious to pregnancy outcome. They identified birthweights of infants whose mothers worked during the third trimester to be 150 to 400 g less than those of newborns whose mothers did not work, even though the length of gestation was the same for both groups. Reduction in birthweight was greatest for mothers who were underweight before pregnancy and whose weight gain during pregnancy was low, for mothers who were hypertensive, and for mothers whose work required standing. The data were collected between 1959 and 1966, and therefore the results were possibly influenced by the widespread practice of dietary restrictions and use of drugs then in vogue to try to control weight gain and dependent edema.

Manshande and colleagues (1987) reported a sevenfold increased incidence of low-birthweight infants in women from Zaire who worked hard in the fields. Teitelman and co-workers (1990) evaluated maternal work activity and pregnancy outcome in 4186 women delivered at Yale–New Haven Hospital. Women were classified according to the type of jobs they held. *Standing* jobs, such as those of a cashier, bank teller, or dentist, required standing in the same position for more than 3 hours per day. *Active* jobs, such as physicians, waitresses, and real estate agents, involved continuous or intermittent walking. *Sedentary* jobs, such as librarian, bookkeeper, or bus driver, required less than an hour of standing per day. They found that pregnant women who work at jobs that require prolonged standing are at greater risk for preterm delivery, but this was not observed to have any effect on intrauterine growth. Klebanoff and colleagues (1990) also found that prolonged periods of standing (8 hours or longer per day) were

associated with a small increased risk of preterm delivery in a prospective study of over 7100 women. However, heavy work, defined as sufficient to cause sweating, was not found to be deleterious.

Common sense dictates that any occupation that subjects the pregnant woman to severe physical strain should be avoided. Ideally, no work or play should be continued to the extent that undue fatigue develops. Adequate periods of rest should be provided during the working day. Women with previous pregnancy complications that are likely to be repetitive, such as, low-birthweight infants, probably should minimize physical work.

Travel. The restriction of travel to short trips had been a rule for obstetrical patients until World War II, when many women found it necessary to follow their husbands regardless of distance or mode of travel. The data compiled during that era are consistent with the conclusion that travel by the healthy woman has no harmful effect on pregnancy. Travel in properly pressurized aircraft offers no unusual risk. For example, American Airlines permits unrestricted travel as long as the pregnant woman feels well and is not within 7 days of her expected delivery date. Delta Airlines has no travel restrictions, but does recommend that the pregnant woman check with her physician if travel is scheduled after the eighth month of pregnancy. At least every 2 hours, the pregnant woman should walk about. Perhaps the greatest risk with travel, especially international travel, is the development of a complication remote from facilities adequate to manage the complication.

The American College of Obstetricians and Gynecologists (1991b) has formulated guidelines for use of automobile passenger restraints during pregnancy. There is no evidence that safety restraints increase the chance of fetal injury. Indeed, the leading cause of fetal death in a motor accident is the death of the mother. Therefore, pregnant women should be encouraged to wear properly positioned 3-point restraints throughout pregnancy while riding in automobiles. The lap belt portion of the restraining belt should be placed under her abdomen and across her upper thighs. The belt should be as snug as comfortably possible. The shoulder belt also should be snugly applied and positioned between the breasts, although no serious harm appears to occur if the breast is compressed during a collision.

Bathing. There is no objection to bathing during pregnancy or the puerperium. During the last trimester, the heavy uterus usually upsets the balance of the pregnant woman and increases the likelihood of her slipping and falling in the bathtub. For that reason, tub baths at the end of pregnancy may be inadvisable.

Clothing. The clothing worn during pregnancy should be practical and nonconstricting. Supporting girdles are no longer routinely used. The increasing mass of the breasts may make them pendulous and painful, and well-fitting supporting brassieres may be indicated. Constricting garters should be avoided during pregnancy because of the interference with venous return and the aggravation of varicosities. Backache and pressure associated with lordotic posture and a pendulous abdomen may be relieved by a properly fitted maternity girdle. There is no reason for insisting that the pregnant woman wear only low-heeled shoes, unless she develops backache from the increased lordosis that results from shoes with high heels, or if she is unable to maintain balance.

Bowel Habits. During pregnancy, bowel habits tend to become more irregular, presumably because of generalized relaxation of smooth muscle and compression of the lower bowel by the enlarging uterus early in pregnancy or by the presenting part of the fetus late in pregnancy (see Chap. 51, p. 1150). In addition to the discomfort caused by the passage of hard fecal material, bleeding and painful fissures may develop in the edematous and hyperemic rectal mucosa. There is also greater frequency of *hemorrhoids* and, much less commonly, of prolapse of the rectal mucosa.

Women whose bowel habits are reasonably normal in the nonpregnant state may prevent constipation during pregnancy by close attention to bowel habits, sufficient quantities of fluid, and reasonable amounts of daily exercise, supplemented when necessary by a mild laxative, such as prune juice, milk of magnesia, bulk-producing substances, or stool-softening agents. Nonabsorbable oil preparations are discouraged because of their possible interference with the absorption of lipid-soluble vitamins. The use of harsh laxatives and enemas is not recommended.

Coitus. Whenever abortion or preterm labor threatens, coitus should be avoided. Otherwise it has been generally accepted that in healthy pregnant women, sexual intercourse usually does no harm before the last 4 weeks or so of pregnancy. It has long been the custom of many obstetricians to recommend abstinence from intercourse during the last 4 weeks of pregnancy, a recommendation undoubtedly not followed in many instances.

The risks versus possible benefits from intercourse late in pregnancy have not been clearly delineated. Pugh and Fernandez (1953), for example, did not find that intercourse caused preterm labor, rupture of the membranes, bleeding, or infection. They concluded that it is not necessary to abstain from coitus during the final weeks of gestation.

Goodlin and associates (1972) were more concerned about possible injurious effects from intercourse late in pregnancy. They identified transient fetal bradycardia with increased uterine tension during maternal orgasms induced by vulvar and vaginal manipulation at 39 weeks' gestation. The painful uterine contractions ceased within 15 minutes after the last orgasm. Whether such changes commonly accompany orgasm and whether they are harmful to the fetus is not known. They also reported the incidence of orgasm after 32 weeks to have been significantly higher for women who subsequently delivered prematurely. Grudzinkas and co-workers (1979) found no association between gestational age at delivery and the frequency of coitus during the last 4 weeks of pregnancy. However, women who were sexually active in the last 4 weeks showed a higher incidence of fetal distress.

Naeye (1979), using data from the Collaborative Perinatal Project, investigated the impact of coitus during the month before delivery, and reported that amnionic fluid infections and perinatal mortality were significantly increased if mothers reported intercourse once or more weekly. Nielson and Mutambira (1989) studied the effects of coitus in 126 Zimbabwean women with increased risk for preterm delivery due to twin gestation. It was uncommon for study participants to report coital frequency more than once per week. Coital frequency decreased with advancing gestation and was not linked with preterm delivery.

On occasion, the couple's sexual drive in the face of admonishment against intercourse late in pregnancy has led to sexual practices with disastrous consequences. Aronson and Nelson (1967), for instance, describe fatal cases of air embolism late in pregnancy as a result of air blown into the vagina during cunnilingus. Other near-fatal cases have been described (Bernhardt and associates, 1988).

Douches. If douching in pregnancy is desirable because of excessive cervical and vaginal secretions, the following precautions should be observed:

1. Hand bulb syringes must be absolutely forbidden, because several deaths in pregnancy from air embolism have followed their use (Forbes, 1944).
2. The douche bag should be placed not more than 2 feet above the level of the hips to prevent high fluid pressure.
3. The nozzle should not be inserted more than 3 inches through the vulva.

Care of Breasts and Abdomen. Special breast care during pregnancy is often advised to increase the ability to nurse by toughening the nipples and thereby reducing the incidence of cracking, and by effecting enlargement and eversion of the nipples. From the available data it is concluded that ointments, massage, and traction on the nipples do not always improve these functions, but such practices are usually harmless. Massages and ointments do not significantly alter the incidence of striae on the breasts or abdomen. In general, the extent of striation is proportional to the size of the uterus and maternal weight gain.

Care of the Teeth. Examination of the teeth should be included in the prenatal general physical examination. Pregnancy is rarely a contraindication to needed dental treatment. The concept that dental caries are aggravated by pregnancy is unfounded.

Immunization. There has been some concern over the safety of various immunization techniques during pregnancy. The recommendations of the American College of Obstetricians and Gynecologists (1991d), with appropriate updating for specific immunizations during pregnancy, are summarized in Table 9–3.

Smoking. Mothers who smoke during pregnancy have infants whose birthweight average less than nonsmokers. There is also evidence that smoking mothers have a significantly greater incidence of perinatal deaths. Goldstein (1977) estimated that about 4600 infants die in the United States every year because their mothers smoke. Many of the data to support these statements were presented in the publication, *Smoking and Health, Report to the Surgeon General of the Public Health Service* (1979). Since 1984 the Surgeon General's warning labels on cigarette packages have carried messages specifically aimed at pregnant women. One warning reads, "Smoking by pregnant women may result in fetal injury, premature birth, and low birthweight."

To explain these adverse effects from smoking, various investigators have implicated the following: (1) carbon monoxide and its functional inactivation of fetal and maternal hemoglobin; (2) vasoconstrictor action of nicotine, causing reduced placental perfusion; (3) reduced appetite and, in turn, reduced caloric intake; (4) decreased maternal plasma volume; and (5) an unexplained predisposition in certain women that persists even when they quit smoking.

Astrup and associates (1972), Socol and co-workers (1982), and Bureau and colleagues (1982) implicated carbon monoxide in the genesis of low birthweight on the basis of their studies on women, monkeys, and rabbits. D'Souza and co-workers (1978) identified the hemoglobin level in cord blood to average 17.8 g/dL if the mother smoked during pregnancy, compared with 16.3 g/dL if she did not smoke. A plausible explanation to account for these differences is bone marrow stimulation from chronic fetal hypoxia. Low birthweight has been described, however, for infants whose mothers did not smoke but rather chewed tobacco (Krushna, 1978).

Rush (1974) and Davies and co-workers (1976) have contended that lower birthweight of infants whose mothers smoke is primarily the consequence of lower pregnancy weight gain by smoking mothers. However, Haworth and co-workers (1980) identified birthweights to be lower for infants whose mothers smoked than for those whose mothers did not, even though maternal weight gain and dietary intake were the same for both groups.

Boomer and Christensen (1982) identified evidence for increased high maternal hematocrits and low-birthweight infants in pregnancies of women who smoked. They considered these events to most likely reflect the decrease in plasma volume among pregnant women who smoked described by Pirani and MacGillivray (1978). Brown and colleagues (1988) found that extensive placental calcification at 37 weeks was doubled (36 versus 14 percent) in smokers. Wen and co-workers (1990) analyzed the effects of smoking on birthweight, fetal growth retardation, and prematurity in over 17,000 pregnancies. Smoking lowered birthweight both by decreasing fetal growth and by decreasing gestational age at delivery.

Doppler velicometry has recently been used to evaluate maternal–fetal blood flow effects of smoking, and in particular, nicotine and carbon monoxide. Lindblad and colleagues (1988) observed

---

TABLE 9–3. SUMMARY OF RECOMMENDATIONS FOR IMMUNIZATION DURING PREGNANCY

Live Virus Vaccines	**Inactivated Bacterial Vaccines**	**Hyperimmune Globulins**
Measles—contraindicated	Cholera—to meet international travel requirements	Hepatitis B—postexposure prophylaxis: give along with hepatitis B vaccine initially, then vaccine alone at 1 and 6 months
Mumps—contraindicated		
Poliomyelitis—not routine; increased risk exposure	Pneumococcus—same as nonpregnant	
Rubella—contraindicated	Plague—selective vaccination of exposed persons	Rabies—postexposure prophylaxis
Yellow fever—travel to high-risk areas only	Typhoid—travel to endemic areas	Tetanus—postexposure prophylaxis
		Varicella—consider for postexposure (within 96 hours)
Inactive Virus Vaccines	**Toxoids**	**Pooled Immune Serum Globulins**
Influenza—serious underlying diseases	Tetanus-Diphtheria—same as nonpregnant	Hepatitis A—postexposure prophylaxis
Rabies—same as nonpregnant		Measles—postexposure prophylaxis
Hepatitis B—at high risk and negative for B antigen		

Modified with permission from the American College of Obstetricians and Gynecologists (1991d).

immediate increases in maternal heart rate, blood pressure, fetal heart rate, and fetal aortic and umbilical vein blood flow due to nicotine but not carbon monoxide. Monrow and co-workers (1988) observed that maternal smoking caused a direct increase in placental vascular resistance from the placental side because uterine artery vascular resistance, as measured by the systolic/diastolic velocity ratio, was unaffected by smoking.

In view of the obvious dangers to people who smoke, cigarettes should be avoided completely by women, irrespective of any deleterious effects on pregnancy. Benowitz (1991) has reviewed use of nicotine chewing gum or transdermal patches during pregnancy.

Alcohol. Because alcohol use during pregnancy can be harmful to the fetus (see Chap. 42, p. 973), the Surgeon General recommends that women who are pregnant or considering pregnancy abstain from using any alcoholic beverages (U.S. Department of Health and Human Services, 1981). During the past decade, many state and national organizations have instituted educational programs to discourage alcohol use during pregnancy (U.S. Department of Health and Human Services, 1986). Serdula and co-workers (1991) surveyed alcohol consumption in American women and found a decline in the prevalence of alcohol consumption during pregnancy from 32 percent in 1985 to 20 percent in 1988. However, there was no decline observed among those less educated or under the age of 25 years. From the evidence available, the best advice to the woman pregnant or about to become pregnant would seem to be **don't consume alcohol**. Hopefully, the adverse effects of alcohol on pregnancy do not linger after the woman stops drinking.

Caffeine. In 1980 the Food and Drug Administration advised pregnant women to limit caffeine intake. The Fourth International Caffeine Workshop concluded shortly thereafter that there was no evidence that caffeine increased teratogenic or reproductive risk (Dews and colleagues, 1984). In small laboratory animals, caffeine is not a teratogen, but it does potentiate mutagenic effects of radiation and some chemicals if given in massive doses. When infused intravenously into sheep, it decreases uterine blood flow by 5 to 10 percent (Conover and colleagues, 1983).

Most studies of human pregnancy report no association between caffeine consumption and birth defects or low birthweight (Kurppa and co-workers, 1983; Leviton, 1988; Linn and colleagues, 1982). Narod and associates (1991) have reviewed the reproductive effects of coffee.

Illicit Drugs. Chronic use during pregnancy of illicit drugs, including opium derivatives, barbiturates, and amphetamines, in large doses, is harmful to the fetus.

Intrauterine distress, low birthweight, and serious compromise as the consequence of drug withdrawal soon after birth are well documented. Often the mother who uses hard drugs does not seek prenatal care, and even if she does, she may not admit to the use of such substances. Detection of scars from venipunctures may be the first clue. The management of pregnancy and delivery and successful care of the newborn infant may be extremely difficult (Edelin and associates, 1988). Early abortion should be considered for the addicted pregnant woman who wants to try to "kick the habit."

The effects of a number of illicit drugs are considered in detail in Chapter 42 (p. 973).

Medications. With rare exception, any drug that exerts a systemic effect in the mother will cross the placenta to reach the embryo and fetus. Some drugs commonly ingested during pregnancy, and their possible adverse fetal effects, are considered in detail in Chapter 42 (p. 961). All physicians should develop the habit of ascertaining the likelihood of pregnancy before prescribing drugs for any woman, because a number of medications in common use can be injurious to the embryo and the fetus. Package inserts provided by pharmaceutical companies and approved by the Food and Drug Administration should be consulted before drugs are prescribed for pregnant women. If a drug is administered during pregnancy, the advantages to be gained must clearly outweigh any risks inherent in its use.

Common Complaints

Nausea and Vomiting. Nausea and vomiting are common complaints during the first half of pregnancy. Typically they commence between the first and second missed menstrual period and continue until about the time of the fourth missed period. Nausea and vomiting are usually worse in the morning, but may continue throughout the day.

The genesis of pregnancy-induced nausea and vomiting is not clear. Possibly the hormonal changes of pregnancy are responsible. Chorionic gonadotropin, for instance, has been implicated on the basis that its levels are rather high at the same time that nausea and vomiting are most common. Moreover, in women with hydatidiform mole, in which levels of chorionic gonadotropin typically are very much higher than in normal pregnancy, nausea and vomiting are often prominent clinical features. However, Soules and co-workers (1980), as well as Depue and colleagues (1987), found no relationship between the serum levels of chorionic gonadotropin and the incidence and severity of nausea and vomiting in pregnant women, including those with a hydatidiform mole.

Emotional factors undoubtedly can contribute to

the severity of the nausea and vomiting of pregnancy. Very infrequently vomiting may be so severe that dehydration, electrolyte and acid-base disturbances, and starvation become serious problems.

Seldom is the treatment of nausea and vomiting of pregnancy so successful that the affected expectant mother is afforded complete relief. However, the unpleasantness and discomfort can usually be minimized. Eating small feedings at more frequent intervals but stopping short of satiation is of value. Because the smell of certain foods often precipitates or aggravates the symptoms, such foods should be avoided as much as possible. Management of hyperemesis gravidarum is described in Chapter 51 (p. 1146).

Backache. Backache occurs to some extent in most pregnant women. Minor degrees follow excessive strain or fatigue and excessive bending, lifting, or walking. Mild backache usually requires little more than elimination of the strain and occasionally a lightweight maternity girdle. Severe backaches should not be attributed simply to pregnancy until a thorough orthopedic examination has been conducted. Muscular spasm and tenderness, which often are classified clinically as acute strain or fibrositis, respond well to analgesics, heat, and rest.

In some women, motion of the symphysis pubis and lumbosacral joints, and general relaxation of pelvic ligaments, may be demonstrated. In severe cases the pregnant woman may be unable to walk or even remain comfortable without support furnished by a heavy girdle and prolonged periods of rest. Occasionally, anatomical, congenital, or traumatic defects are found. Pain caused by herniation of an intervertebral disc occurs during pregnancy with about the same frequency as at other times.

Varicosities. Varicosities, generally resulting from congenital predisposition, are exaggerated by prolonged standing, pregnancy, and advancing age. Usually varicosities become more prominent as pregnancy advances, as weight increases, and as the length of time spent upright is prolonged. As discussed in Chapter 8 (p. 229), femoral venous pressure increases appreciably as pregnancy advances. The symptoms produced by varicosities vary from cosmetic blemishes on the lower extremities and mild discomfort at the end of the day to severe discomfort that requires prolonged rest with the feet elevated.

The treatment of varicosities of the lower extremities is generally limited to periodic rest with elevation of the legs, elastic stockings, or both. Surgical correction of the condition during pregnancy is generally not advised, although occasionally the symptoms may be so severe that injection, ligation, or even stripping of the veins is necessary in order to allow the pregnant woman to remain ambulatory. In general, these operations

should be postponed until after delivery. Vulvar varicosities may be aided by application of a foam rubber pad suspended across the vulva by a belt of the type used with a perineal pad. Rarely, large varicosities may rupture, resulting in profuse hemorrhage.

A severe case of massive varicosities that involved both legs and the vulva of a woman of high parity is demonstrated in Figure 9–3. Treatment during pregnancy consisted of elastic stockings, frequent elevation of the legs throughout the day to provide drainage, and avoidance of injury to the affected parts. Delivery was accomplished spontaneously without laceration. Aggressive ambulation with elastic support stockings was initiated soon after delivery and after tubal sterilization. Surgical intervention with extensive vein stripping was performed late in the puerperium.

Occasionally, *superficial thrombophlebitis* complicates preexisting varicose veins.

Hemorrhoids. Varicosities of the rectal veins occasionally first appear during pregnancy. More often, pregnancy causes an exacerbation or recurrence of previous hemorrhoids. Their development or aggravation during

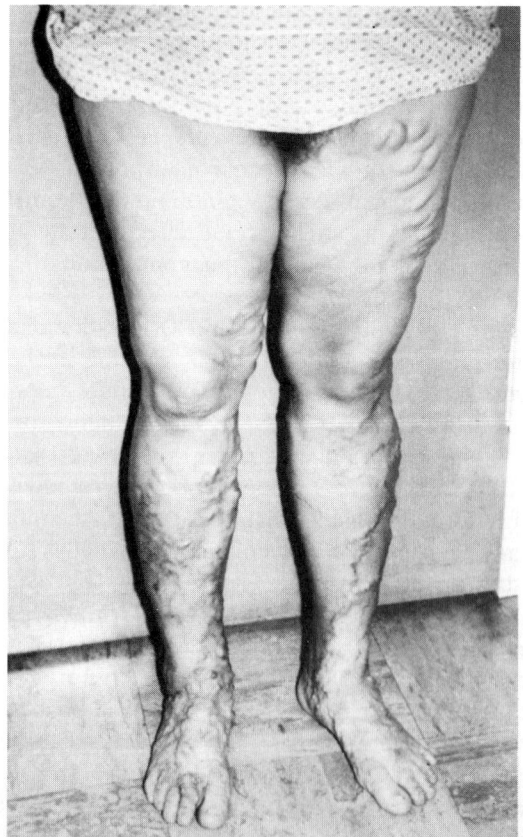

Fig. 9–3. In a multiparous woman, before this pregnancy a leg varix had ruptured with severe hemorrhage necessitating transfusion. During this pregnancy, massive varices developed. Well-fitting support hose provided considerable relief until surgical correction was performed late in the puerperium.

pregnancy is undoubtedly related to increased pressure in the rectal veins caused by obstruction of venous return by the large uterus, and to the tendency toward constipation during pregnancy. Usually pain and swelling are relieved by topically applied anesthetics, warm soaks, and agents that soften the stool. Thrombosis of a rectal vein can cause considerable pain, but the clot can usually be evacuated by incising the wall of the involved vein with a scalpel under topical anesthesia.

Bleeding from rectal veins occasionally may result in loss of sufficient blood to cause iron-deficiency anemia. The loss of only 15 mL of blood results in the loss of 6 to 7 mg of iron, an amount equal to the daily requirements during latter pregnancy. If bleeding is persistent, hemorrhoidectomy may be required. In general, however, hemorrhoidectomy is not desirable during pregnancy, because most often hemorrhoids become asymptomatic soon after delivery.

Heartburn. Heartburn, one of the most common complaints of pregnant women, is caused by reflux of gastric contents into the lower esophagus. The increased frequency of regurgitation during pregnancy most likely results from the upward displacement and compression of the stomach by the uterus combined with decreased gastrointestinal motility. In most pregnant women, symptoms are mild and relieved by a regimen of more frequent but smaller meals and avoidance of bending over or lying flat. Antacid preparations may provide considerable relief. Aluminum hydroxide, magnesium trisilcate, or magnesium hydroxide, alone or in combination (for example, Amphojel, Gelusil, Maalox, or milk of magnesia), should be used in preference to sodium bicarbonate. The pregnant woman who tends to retain sodium can become edematous as the result of ingestion of excessive amounts of sodium bicarbonate. Management for symptoms that do not respond to these simple measures is discussed in Chapter 51 (p. 1147).

Pica. Occasionally during pregnancy, bizarre cravings for strange foods develop, and at times for materials hardly considered edible, such as laundry starch, clay, and even dirt. For example, at Parkland Hospital, interrogation of recently delivered mothers has disclosed that the following items were craved and consumed by them during the current pregnancy: Argo Gloss Starch, flour, baking powder, baking soda, clay, baked dirt, powdered bricks, and frost scraped from the refrigerator (pagophagia).

The ingestion of starch (amylophagia) or clay (geophagia) or related items is practiced more often by socioeconomically less privileged pregnant women. The desire for dry lump starch, clay, chopped ice, or even refrigerator frost has been considered by some to be triggered by severe iron deficiency. Although women with severe iron deficiency sometimes crave these items, and although the craving is usually ameliorated

after correction of the iron deficiency, not all pregnant women with pica are necessarily iron-deficient.

The consumption of starch in sufficient quantities to provide a significant portion of the calories ingested or to cause ptyalism is not healthful, nor is the ingestion of clay to the extent that the intestine is sufficiently filled to cause obstruction of labor or fecal impaction. Nonetheless, it is quite unlikely that either laundry starch or clay free of parasites is distinctly harmful to the pregnancy if consumed in moderation and if the diet is nutritionally adequate.

Ptyalism. Women during pregnancy are occasionally distressed by profuse salivation. The cause of the ptyalism sometimes appears to be stimulation of the salivary glands by the ingestion of starch. This cause should be looked for and eradicated if found.

Fatigue. Early in pregnancy, most women complain of fatigue and desire for excessive periods of sleep. The condition usually remits spontaneously by the fourth month of pregnancy and has no special significance.

Headache. Headache early in pregnancy is a frequent complaint. A few cases may result from sinusitis or ocular strain caused by refractive errors. In the vast majority, however, no cause can be demonstrated. Treatment is largely symptomatic. By midpregnancy, most of these headaches decrease in severity or disappear. The pathological significance of headaches as the consequence of pregnancy-induced hypertension that develops later in pregnancy is considered in Chapter 36 (p. 784).

Leukorrhea. Pregnant women commonly develop increased vaginal discharge, which in many instances has no pathological cause. Increased mucus formation by cervical glands in response to hyperestrogenemia is undoubtedly a contributing factor. If the secretion is troublesome, the woman may be advised to douche with water mildly acidified with vinegar. The precautions for douching listed on page 263 should be stressed.

Occasionally, troublesome leukorrhea is the result of an infection caused by *Trichomonas vaginalis* or *Candida albicans*.

Trichomonas vaginalis. In as many as 20 percent of women *Trichomonas vaginalis* can be identified during prenatal examination; however, symptomatic infection is much less prevalent. It has been suggested that trichomonal infestation is a cause of preterm labor (see Chap. 59, p. 1314). Trichomonal vaginitis is characterized by foamy leukorrhea with pruritus and irritation. Trichomonads are demonstrated readily in fresh vaginal secretions as flagellated, pear-shaped, motile organisms that are somewhat larger than leukocytes.

Metronidazole has proved effective in eradicating

Trichomonas vaginalis. The drug may be administered orally or vaginally. When ingested by the mother, metronidazole crosses the placenta and enters the fetal circulation. The possibility of teratogenicity from first-trimester exposure has been raised: however, the earlier described chromosomal abnormalities following metronidazole therapy for Crohn disease now are thought to have been the consequence of sulfasalazine (Mitelman and associates, 1980). As discussed in Chapter 42 (p. 963), Rosa and colleagues (1987) found no increased frequency of birth defects in over 1000 women given metronidazole during early pregnancy.

Candida albicans. Candida can be cultured from the vagina in about 25 percent of women approaching term. Asymptomatic vaginal candidiasis requires no treatment. However, it sometimes may cause an extremely profuse irritating discharge. Miconazole, clotrimazole, and nystatin are effective for the treatment of candidiasis during pregnancy. Infection is likely to recur, thereby requiring repeated treatment during pregnancy; but usually it subsides at the end of gestation.

References

American College of Obstetricians and Gynecologists: Guidelines for perinatal care, 3rd ed. Committee on Obstetrics, 1992

American College of Obstetricians and Gynecologists: Alphafetoprotein. Technical bulletin no. 154, April 1991a

American College of Obstetricians and Gynecologists: Automobile passenger restraints for children and pregnant women. Technical bulletin no. 151, January 1991b

American College of Obstetricians and Gynecologists: Current status of cystic fibrosis carrier screening. Committee opinion no. 101, November 1991c

American College of Obstetricians and Gynecologists: Immunization during pregnancy. Technical bulletin no. 160, October 1991d

American College of Obstetricians and Gynecologists: Voluntary testing for human immunodeficiency virus. Committee opinion no. 97, September 1991e

American College of Obstetricians and Gynecologists: Standards for obstetric–gynecologic services. Washington, DC, American College of Obstetricians and Gynecologists, 1989

American College of Obstetricians and Gynecologists: Management of diabetes mellitus in pregnancy. Technical bulletin no. 92, March 1986a

American College of Obstetricians and Gynecologists: Women and exercise. Technical bulletin no. 87, September 1986b

American College of Obstetricians and Gynecologists: Gonorrhea and chlamydial infections. Technical bulletin no. 89, November 1985

Annas GJ: Fetal protection and employment discrimination—The Johnson controls case. N Engl J Med 325:740, 1991

Aronson ME, Nelson PK: Fatal air embolism in pregnancy resulting from an unusual sex act. Obstet Gynecol 30:127, 1967

Astrup P, Olsen HM, Trolle D, Kjeldsen K: Effect of moderate carbon-monoxide-exposure on fetal development. Lancet 2:1220, 1972

Bayless TM, Rothfeld B, Massa C, Wise L, Paige D, Bedine M: Lactose and milk intolerance: Clinical implications. N Engl J Med 292:1156, 1975

Belizán JM, Villar J, Repke J: The relationship between calcium intake and pregnancy-induced hypertension: Up-to-date evidence. Am J Obstet Gynecol 158:898, 1988

Benowitz NL: Nicotine replacement therapy during pregnancy. JAMA 266:3174, 1991

Bernhardt TL, Goldmann RW, Thombs PA, Kindwall EP: Hyperbaric oxygen treatment of cerebral air embolism from urogenital sex during pregnancy. Crit Care Med 16:729, 1988

Boomer AL, Christensen BL: Antepartum hematocrit, maternal smoking and birth weight. J Reprod Med 27:387, 1982

Bracken MB, Belanger K: Calculation of delivery dates. N Engl J Med 321:1483, 1989

British Medical Research Council Vitamin Study Research Group: Prevention of neural tube defects: Results of the medical research council vitamin-study. Lancet 338:131, 1991

Brown HL, Miller JM, Khawli O, Gabert HA: Premature placental calcification in maternal cigarette smokers. Obstet Gynecol 71:914, 1988

Brown MA, Sinosich MJ, Saunders DM, Gallery ED: Potassium regulation and progesterone–aldosterone interrelationships in human pregnancy: A prospective study. Am J Obstet Gynecol 155:349, 1986

Bureau MA, Monette J, Shapcott D, Paré C, Mathieu JL, Lippé J, Blovin D, Berthiaume Y, Begin R: Carboxyhemoglobin concentration in fetal cord blood and in blood of mothers who smoked during labor. Pediatrics 69:371, 1982.

Calvert JP, Crean EE, Newcombe RG, Pearson JF: Antenatal screening of measurement of symphysis-fundus height. Br Med J 285:846, 1982

Carpenter MW, Sady SP, Hoegsberg B, Sady MA, Haydon B, Cullinane EM, Coustan DR, Thompson PD: Fetal heart rate response to maternal exertion. JAMA 259:2006, 1988

Centers for Disease Control: Recommendations for the use of folic acid to reduce the number of cases of spina bifida and other neural tube defects. MMWR 41:1, 1992

Centers for Disease Control: Use of folic acid for prevention of spina bifida and other neural tube defects. MMWR 40:513, 1991

Centers for Disease Control: Prevention of perinatal transmission of hepatitis B virus: Prenatal screening of all pregnant women for hepatitis B surface antigen. MMWR 37:341, 1988

Centers for Disease Control: Influenza vaccine: Preliminary statement. Ann Intern Med 89:373, 1978

Chanarin I, McFayden IR, Kyle R: The physiological macrocytosis of pregnancy. Br J Obstet Gynaecol 84:504, 1977

Clapp JC: The course of labor after endurance exercise during pregnancy. Am J Obstet Gynecol 163:1799, 1990a

Clapp JC, Capeless EL: Neonatal morphometrics after endurance exercise during pregnancy. Am J Obstet Gynecol 163:1805, 1990b

Clapp JC: Oxygen consumption during treadmill exercise before, during, and after pregnancy. Am J Obstet Gynecol 161:1458, 1989a

Clapp JC: The effects of maternal exercise on early pregnancy outcome. Am J Obstet Gynecol 161:1453, 1989b

Cleary RE, Lumeng L, Li YK: Maternal and fetal plasma levels of pyridoxal phosphate at term: Adequacy of vitamin B_6 supplementation during pregnancy. Am J Obstet Gynecol 121:25, 1975

Cochrane WA: Overnutrition in prenatal and neonatal life: A problem? Can Med Assoc J 93:893, 1965

Conover WB, Key TC, Resnik R: Maternal cardiovascular response to caffeine infusion in the pregnant ewe. Am J Obstet Gynecol 145:534, 1983

Creasy RK, Gummer BA, Liggins GC: System for predicting spontaneous preterm birth. Obstet Gynecol 55:692, 1980

Davies DP, Gray OP, Ellwood PC, Abernathy M: Cigarette smoking in pregnancy: Associations with maternal weight gain and fetal growth. Lancet 1:385, 1976

Dawes MC, Green J, Ashurst H: Routine weighing in pregnancy. Br Med J 304:487, 1992

Delgado H, Lechug A, Yarbrough C, Martorell R, Klein RE, Irwin M: Maternal nutrition—Its effects on infant growth and development and birthspacing. In Moghissi KS, Evans TN (eds): Nutritional Impacts on Women. Hagerstown, MD, Harper & Row, 1977, p 133

Depue RH, Bernstein L, Ross RK, Judd HL, Henderson BE: Hyperemesis gravidarum in relation to estradiol levels, pregnancy outcome, and other maternal factors: A seroepidemiologic study. Am J Obstet Gynecol 156:1137, 1987

Dews P, Grice HC, Neims A, Wilson J, Wurtman R: Report of Fourth International Caffeine Workshop, Athens, 1982. Food Chem Toxicol 22:163, 1984

D'Souza SW, Black PM, Williams N, Jennison RF: Effect of smoking during pregnancy upon the haematological values of cord blood. Br J Obstet Gynaecol 85:495, 1978

Edelin KC, Gurganious L, Golar K, Oellerich D, Kyei-Aboagye K, Hamid MA: Methadone maintenance in pregnancy: Consequences to care and outcome. Obstet Gynecol 71:399, 1988

Ekstrand J: No evidence of transfer of fluoride from plasma to breast milk. Br Med J 283:761, 1981

Emery AEH: Folates and fetal central-nervous-system malformations. Lancet 1:703, 1977

Food and Drug Adminstration: Clinical implications of Surgeon General's report on smoking and health. FDA Drug Bull 9:4, 1979

Forbes G: Air embolism as complication of vaginal douching in pregnancy. Br Med J 2:529, 1944

Gillmer MDG, Mazibuko D: Pyridoxine treatment of chemical diabetes in pregnancy. Am J Obstet Gynecol 133:499, 1979

Glenn FB, Glenn WD III, Duncan RC: Fluoride tablet supplementation during pregnancy for caries immunity: A study of the offspring produced. Am J Obstet Gynecol 143:560, 1982

Goldstein H: Smoking in pregnancy: Some notes on the statistical controversy. Br J Prevent Soc Med 31:13, 1977

Goodlin RC: Why treat "physiologic" anemias of pregnancy? J Reprod Med 27:639, 1982

Goodlin RC, Keller DW, Raffin M: Orgasm during late pregnancy: Possible deleterious effects. Obstet Gynecol 38:916, 1971

Goodlin RC, Schmidt W, Creevy DC: Uterine tension and fetal heart rate during maternal orgasm. Obstet Gynecol 39:125, 1972

Grudzinkas JG, Watson C, Chard T: Does sexual intercourse cause fetal distress? Lancet 2:692, 1979

Hall MH: Folates and the fetus. Lancet 1:648, 1977

Hauth JC, Gilstrap LC III, Widmer K: Fetal heart rate reactivity before and after maternal jogging during the third trimester. Am J Obstet Gynecol 142:545, 1982

Haworth JC, Ellestad-Sayed JJ, King J, Dilling LA: Fetal growth retardation in cigarette-smoking mothers is not due to decreased maternal food intake. Am J Obstet Gynecol 137:719, 1980

Heaney RP, Skillman TG: Calcium metabolism in normal human pregnancy. J Clin Endocrinol 33:661, 1971

Herbert V, Jacob E: Destruction of vitamin B_{12} by ascorbic acid. JAMA 230:241, 1974

Herbert WNP, Bruninghaus HM, Barefoot AB, Bright TG: Clinical aspects of fetal heart auscultation. Obstet Gynecol 69:574, 1987

Higginbottom MC, Sweetman L, Nyhan WL: A syndrome of methylmalonic aciduria, homocystinuria, megaloblastic anemia and neurologic abnormalities in a vitamin B_{12}-deficient breast-fed infant of a strict vegetarian. N Engl J Med 299:317, 1978

Hobel CJ, Youkeles L, Forsythe A: Prenatal and intrapartum high-risk screening: II. Risk factors reassessed. Am J Obstet Gynecol 135:1051, 1979

Horowitz HS, Heifetz SB: Effects of prenatal exposure to fluoridation on dental caries. Public Health Rep 82:297, 1967

Humphreys RC: An analysis of the maternal and foetal weight factors in normal pregnancy. J Obstet Gynaecol Br Commonw 61:764, 1954

Hytten FE: Weight gain in pregnancy. In Hytten FE, Chamberlain G (eds): Clinical Physiology in Obstetrics, 2nd ed. Oxford, Blackwell, 1991, p 173

Hytten FE, Leitch I: The Physiology of Human Pregnancy, 2nd ed. Oxford, Blackwell, 1971

Institute of Medicine: Nutrition During Pregnancy: I, Weight Gain; II, Nutrient Supplements. National Academy Press, Washington, DC, 1990

Jimenez JM, Tyson JE, Reisch JS: Clinical measures of gestational age in normal pregnancies. Obstet Gynecol 61:438, 1983

Klebanoff MA, Shiono PH, Carey JC: The effect of physical activity during pregnancy on preterm delivery and birthweight. Am J Obstet Gynecol 163:1450, 1990

Kortenoever ME: Pathology of pregnancy: Pregnancy of long duration and postmature infant. Obstet Gynecol Surv 5:812, 1950

Krushna K: Tobacco chewing in pregnancy. Br J Obstet Gynaecol 85:726, 1978

Kurppa K, Holmberg PC, Kuosma E, Saxen L: Coffee consumption during pregnancy and selected congenital malformations: A nationwide case-control study. Am J Public Health 73:1397, 1983

Leveno KJ, Cunningham FG, Roark ML, Nelson SD, Williams ML: Prenatal care and the low birth weight infant. Obstet Gynecol 66:599, 1985

Leviton A: Caffeine consumption and the risk of reproductive hazards. J Reprod Med 33:175, 1988

Lindblad A, Marsal K, Andersson KE: The effect of nicotine on human fetal blood flow. Obstet Gynecol 72:371, 1988

Linn S, Schoenbaum SC, Monson RR, Rosner B, Stubblefield PG, Ryan KJ: No association between coffee consumption and adverse outcomes of pregnancy. N Engl J Med 306:141, 1982

Manshande JP, Eeckels R, Manshande-Desmet V, Vlietinck R:

Rest versus heavy work during the last weeks of pregnancy: Influence on fetal growth. Br J Obstet Gynaecol 94:1059, 1987

Merkatz IR, Thompson JE, Walsh LV: History of prenatal care. In Merkatz IR, Thompson JE (eds): New Perspectives on Prenatal Care. New York, Elsevier, 1990, p 14

Mills JL, Rhoads GG, Simpson JL, Cunningham GC, Conley MR, Lassman MR, Walden ME, Depp OR, Hoffman HJ: The absence of a relation between the periconceptual use of vitamins and neural tube defects. N Engl J Med 321:430, 1989

Milunsky A, Jick H, Jick SS, Bruell CL, MacLaughlin DS, Rothman KJ, Willett W: Multivitamin/folic acid supplementation in early pregnancy reduces the prevalence of neural tube defects. JAMA 262:2847, 1989

Mitelman F, Strombeck B, Ursing B: No cytogenic effect of metronidazole. Lancet 1:1249, 1980

Monrow RJ, Ritchie JW, Bull SB: Maternal cigarette smoking: The effects on umbilical and uterine blood flow velocity. Am J Obstet Gynecol 159:1069, 1988

Murphy JF, Newcomb RG, O'Riodan J, Coles EC, Pearson JF: Relation of haemoglobin levels in first and second trimesters of outcome of pregnancy. Lancet 1:993, 1986

Naeye RL: Coitus and associated amniotic-fluid infections. N Engl J Med 301:1198, 1979

Naeye RL, Peters EC: Working during pregnancy: Effects on the fetus. Pediatrics 69:724, 1982

Nakano R: Post-term pregnancy. Acta Obstet Gynecol Scand 51:217, 1972

Narod SA, de Sanjose S, Victora C: Coffee during pregnancy: A reproductive hazard? Am J Obstet Gynecol 164:1109, 1991

National Center for Health Statistics: Advance report of final mortality statistics, 1989. Monthly Vital Statistics Report 40:11, 1991

National Research Council: Recommended Dietary Allowances, 10th ed. Washington, National Academy Press, 1989, p 240

Nilsen ST, Finne PH, Bergs JO, Stamnes O: Males with low birthweight examined at 18 years of age. Acta Paediatr Scand 73:168, 1984

Nilson JP, Mutambira M: Coitus, twin pregnancy, and preterm labor. Am J Obstet Gynecol 160:416, 1989

Papiernik E, Kaminski M: Multifactorial study of the risk of prematurity at 32 weeks of gestation: A study for the frequency of 30 predictive characteristics. J Perinat Med 2:30, 1974

Parker JD, Abrams B: Prenatal weight gain advice: An examination of the recent prenatal weight gain recommendations of the Institute of Medicine. Obstet Gynecol 79:664, 1992

Perkins RP: Failure of pyridoxine to improve glucose tolerance in gestational diabetes mellitus. Obstet Gynecol 50:370, 1977

Petitti DB, Croughan-Minihane MS, Hiatt RA: Weight gain by gestational age in both black and white women delivered of normal-birth-weight and low-birth-weight infants. Am J Obstet Gynecol 164:801, 1991

Pharoah POD, Buttfield IH, Hetzel BS: Neurological damage to the fetus resulting from severe iodine deficiency during pregnancy. Lancet 1:308, 1971

Pirani BBK, MacGillivray I: Smoking during pregnancy: Its effects on maternal metabolism and fetoplacental function. Br J Obstet Gynaecol 52:257, 1978

Pitkin RM: Calcium metabolism in pregnancy and the perinatal period: A review. Am J Obstet Gynecol 151:99, 1985

Pivarnik JM, Lee W, Clark SL, Cotton DB, Spillman HT, Miller JF: Cardiac output responses to primigravid women during exercise determined by the direct Fick technique. Obstet Gynecol 75:954, 1990

Prentice AM, Cole TJ, Foord FA, Lamb WH, Whitehead RG: Increased birthweight after prenatal dietary supplementation of rural women. Am J Clin Nutr 46:912, 1987

Prentice AM, Whitehead RG, Watkinson M, Lamb WH, Cole TJ: Prenatal dietary supplementation of African women and birth-weight. Lancet 1:489, 1983

Pritchard JA, Scott DE: Iron demands during pregnancy. In Hallberg L, Harwerth HG, Vannotti A (eds): Iron Deficiency: Pathogenesis, Clinical Aspects, Therapy. New York, Academic Press, 1970

Pritchard JA, Scott DE, Whalley PJ: Folic acid requirements in pregnancy induced megaloblastic anemia. JAMA 208:1163, 1969

Pugh WE, Fernandez FL: Coitus late in pregnancy. Obstet Gynecol 2:636, 1953

Quaranta P, Currell R, Redman CWG, Robinson JS: Prediction of small-for-date infants by measurements of symphysial-fundal height. Br J Obstet Gynaecol 88:115, 1981

Ribeiro MD, Stein Z, Susser M, Cohen P, Neugut R: Prenatal starvation and maternal blood pressure. Am J Clin Nutr 35:535, 1982

Robinson M: Salt in pregnancy. Lancet 1:178, 1958

Rosa FW, Baum C, Shaw M: Pregnancy outcomes after first trimester vaginitis drug therapy. Obstet Gynecol 69:751, 1987

Rosen MG, Merkatz IR, Hill JG: Caring for our future: A report by the expert panel on the content of prenatal care. Obstet Gynecol 77:782, 1991

Rush D: Lower weight gain among smokers explains most of the effect of smoking on birthweight. Pediatr Res 8:450, 1974

Sauberlich HE: Vitamin indices. In: Laboratory Indices of Nutritional Status in Pregnancy. Washington, DC, National Research Council Committee on Nutrition of the Mother and Preschool Child, National Academy of Sciences, 1978, p 109

Schauberger CW, Rooney BL, Brimer LM: Factors that influence weight loss in the puerperium. Obstet Gynecol 79:424, 1992

Scott DE, Pritchard JA, Saltin A-S, Humphreyes SM: Iron deficiency during pregnancy. In Hallberg L, Harwerth HG, Vannotti A (eds): Iron Deficiency: Pathogenesis, Clinical Aspects, Therapy. New York, Academic Press, 1970

Seligman PA, Caskey JH, Frazier JL, Zucker RM, Podell ER, Allen RH: Measurements of iron absorption from prenatal multivitamin-mineral supplements. Obstet Gynecol 61:356, 1983

Serdula M, Williamson DF, Kendrick JS, Anda RF, Byers T: Trends in alcohol consumption by pregnant women: 1985 through 1989. JAMA 265:876, 1991

Sibai BM, Villar MA, Brau E: Magnesium supplementation during pregnancy; A double-blind randomized controlled clinical trial. Am J Obstet Gynecol 161:115, 1989

Smith CA: Effects of maternal undernutrition upon the newborn infant in Holland (1944–1945). Am J Obstet Gynecol 30:229, 1947

Smithells RW, Sellar MJ, Harris R, Fielding DW, Schorah CJ,

Nevin NC, Sheppard S, Read AP, Walker S, Wild J: Further experience of vitamin supplementation for prevention of neural tube defect recurrences. Lancet 1:1027, 1983

Socol ML, Manning FA, Murata Y, Druzin ML: Maternal smoking causes fetal hypoxia: Experimental evidence. Am J Obstet Gynecol 142:214, 1982

Sokol RJ, Rosen MG, Stojkov J, Chik J: Clinical application of high-risk scoring on an obstetric service. Am J Obstet Gynecol 128:652, 1977

Soules MR, Hughes CL Jr, Garcia JA, Livengood CH, Prystowski MR, Alexander E III: Nausea and vomiting of pregnancy: Role of human chorionic gonadotropin and 17-hydroxyprogesterone. Obstet Gynecol 55:696, 1980

Stein Z, Susser M, Saenger G, Marolla F: Nutrition and mental performance. Science 178:708, 1972

Swanson CA, King JC: Reduced serum zinc concentration during pregnancy. Obstet Gynecol 62:313, 1983

Taylor DJ, Mallen C, McDougall N, Lind T: Effect of iron supplementation on serum ferritin levels during and after pregnancy. Br J Obstet Gynaecol 89:1011, 1982

Teitelman AM, Welch LS, Hellenbrand KG, Bracken MB: Effect of maternal work activity on preterm birth and low birthweight. Am J Epidemiol 131:104, 1990

Thomson AM, Billewicz WZ: Clinical significance of weight trends during pregnancy. Br Med J 1:243, 1957

Tyson J, Guzick D, Rosenfeld CR, Lasky R, Gant N, Jiminez J, Heartwell S: Prenatal care evaluation and cohort analyses. Pediatrics 85:195, 1990

United States Department of Health and Human Services, Public Health Service: The 1990 health objectives for the nation: A midcourse review. Washington, DC, 1986, p 49

United States Department of Health and Human Services: Surgeon General's advisory on alcohol and pregnancy. FDA Drug Bull 11:9, 1981

US Public Health Service: Healthy People 2000, National Health Promotion and Disease Preventing Objectives. US Department of Health and Human Services, Public Health Service, 1992, p 381

Villar J, Kestler E, Castillo P, Juarez A, Menendez R, Solowons NW: Improved lactose digestion during pregnancy: A case of physiologic adaptation? Obstet Gynecol 71:697, 1988

Watson MJ, Katz VL, Hackney AC, Gall MM, McMurray RG: Fetal responses to maximal swimming and cycling exercise during pregnancy. Obstet Gynecol 77:382, 1991

Wen SW, Goldenberg RL, Cutter GC, Hoffman HJ, Cliver JP, Davis RO, DuBaid MB: Smoking, maternal age, fetal growth and gestational age at delivery. Am J Obstet Gynecol 162:53, 1990

Whalley PJ, Scott DE, Pritchard JA: Maternal folate deficiency and pregnancy wastage: I. Placental abruption. Am J Obstet Gynecol 105:670, 1969

Worthen N, Bustillo M: Effect of urinary bladder fullness on fundal height measurements. Am J Obstet Gynecol 138:759, 1980

CHAPTER 10

Lie, Presentation, Attitude, and Position of the Fetus

At the onset of labor, the position of the fetus, with respect to the birth canal, is critical to the route of delivery. For example, if at the time of labor, the fetus is transverse to the birth canal, cesarean delivery is the only option for a viable infant. Therefore, it is of paramount importance to know the position of the fetus within the uterine cavity at the onset of labor.

By convention, the fetal position within the uterine cavity is described with respect to fetal lie, presentation, attitude, and position. These can be established clinically by abdominal palpation, vaginal examination, and auscultation, or by technical means using x-ray or sonography. Clinical assessment is less accurate, or even sometimes impossible to perform and interpret in obese patients.

Lie of the Fetus. The lie is the relation of the long axis of the fetus to that of the mother, and is either *longitudinal* or *transverse*. Occasionally, the fetal and the maternal axes may cross at a 45-degree angle, forming an *oblique* lie, which is unstable and always becomes longitudinal or transverse during the course of labor. Longitudinal lies are present in over 99 percent of labors at term.

Presentation and Presenting Part. The presenting part is that portion of the body of the fetus that is either foremost within the birth canal or in closest proximity to it. The presenting part is that portion of the fetus that is felt through the cervix on vaginal examination. The presenting part determines the presentation. Accordingly, in longitudinal lies, the presenting part is either the fetal head or the breech, creating cephalic and breech presentations, respectively. When the fetus lies with the long axis transversely, the shoulder is the presenting part. Thus, a shoulder presentation is felt through the cervix on vaginal examination.

Cephalic Presentation. Cephalic presentations are classified according to the relation of the head to the body of the fetus (Fig. 10–1). Ordinarily the head is flexed sharply so that the chin is in contact with the thorax. In this circumstance the occipital fontanel is the presenting part, and such a presentation is usually referred to as a *vertex* or *occiput presentation.* (The vertex´ actually lies just in front of the occipital fontanel, and the occiput just behind the fontanel, as il-

lustrated in Fig. 7–7, p. 170). Much less commonly, the fetal neck may be sharply extended so that the occiput and back come in contact and the face is foremost in the birth canal (*face presentation*). The fetal head may assume a position between these extremes, partially flexed in some cases, with the anterior (large) fontanel, or bregma, presenting (*sinciput presentation*), or partially extended in other cases, with the brow presenting (*brow presentation*). These latter two presentations are usually transient. As labor progresses, sinciput and brow presentations are almost always converted into vertex or face presentations by flexion or extension, respectively.

Breech Presentation. When the fetus presents as a breech, the thighs may be flexed and the legs extended over the anterior surfaces of the body (*frank breech presentation;* Fig. 10–2); or the thighs may be flexed on the abdomen and the legs upon the thighs (*complete breech presentation*) (Fig. 10–3), and one or both feet, or one or both knees, may be lowermost (*incomplete, or footling, breech presentation*) (Fig. 10–4).

Fetal Attitude or Posture. In the later months of pregnancy the fetus assumes a characteristic posture described as *attitude* or *habitus* (Fig. 10–1). As a rule, the fetus forms an ovoid mass that corresponds roughly to the shape of the uterine cavity. The fetus becomes folded or bent upon itself in such a manner that the back becomes markedly convex; the head is sharply flexed so that the chin is almost in contact with the chest; the thighs are flexed over the abdomen; the legs are bent at the knees; and the arches of the feet rest upon the anterior surfaces of the legs. In all cephalic presentations, the arms are usually crossed over the thorax or become parallel to the sides, and the umbilical cord lies in the space between them and the lower extremities. This characteristic posture results partly from the mode of growth of the fetus and partly from a process of accommodation to the uterine cavity.

Abnormal exceptions to this attitude occur as the fetal head becomes progressively more extended from the vertex to the face presentation (Fig. 10–1). This results in a progressive change in fetal attitude from a convex (flexed) to a concave (extended) contour of the vertebral column.

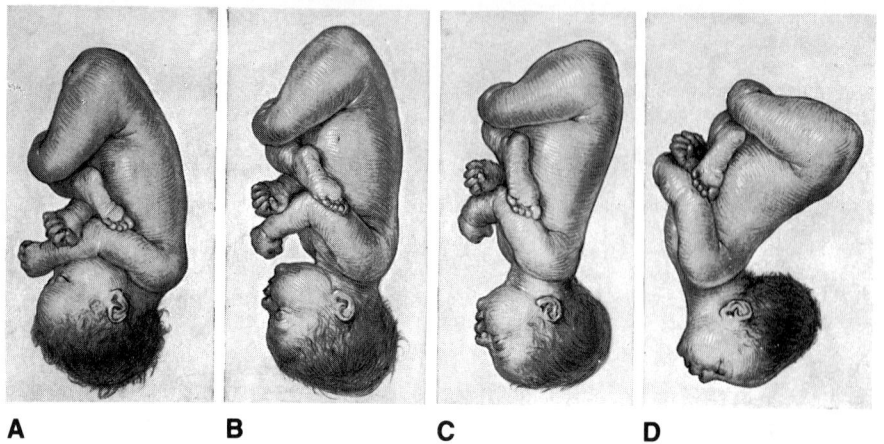

Fig. 10–1. Longitudinal lie. Cephalic presentation. Differences in attitude of fetal body in (**A**) vertex, (**B**) sinciput, (**C**) brow, and (**D**) face presentations. Note changes in fetal attitude in relation to fetal vertex as the fetal head becomes less flexed.

A   B   C   D

Position. Position refers to the relation of an arbitrarily chosen portion of the fetal presenting part to the right or left side of the maternal birth canal. Accordingly, with each presentation there may be two positions, right or left. The fetal occiput, chin (mentum), and sacrum are the determining points in vertex, face, and breech presentations, respectively (Figs. 10–5 to 10–8).

Variety. For still more accurate orientation, the relation of a given portion of the presenting part to the anterior, transverse, or posterior portion of the mother's pelvis is considered. Because there are two positions, it follows

that there must be three varieties for each position (either right or left) and six varieties for each presentation (three right and three left) (Figs. 10–5 to 10–8).

Nomenclature. Because the presenting part in any presentation may be in either the left or right position, there are left and right occipital, left and right mental, and left and right sacral presentations, abbreviated as LO and RO, LM and RM, and LS and RS, respectively. Because the presenting part in each of the two positions may be directed anteriorly (A), transversely (T), or posteriorly (P), there are six varieties of each of these three

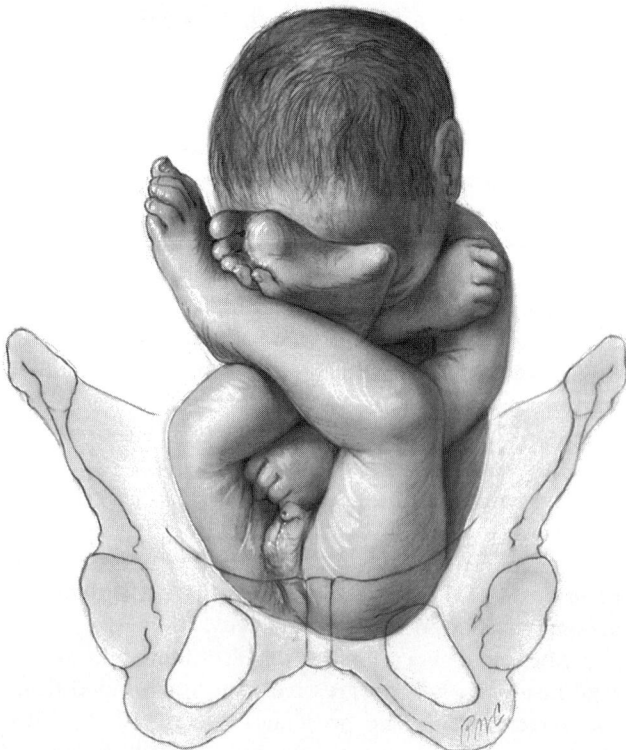

Fig. 10–2. Longitudinal lie. Frank breech presentation.

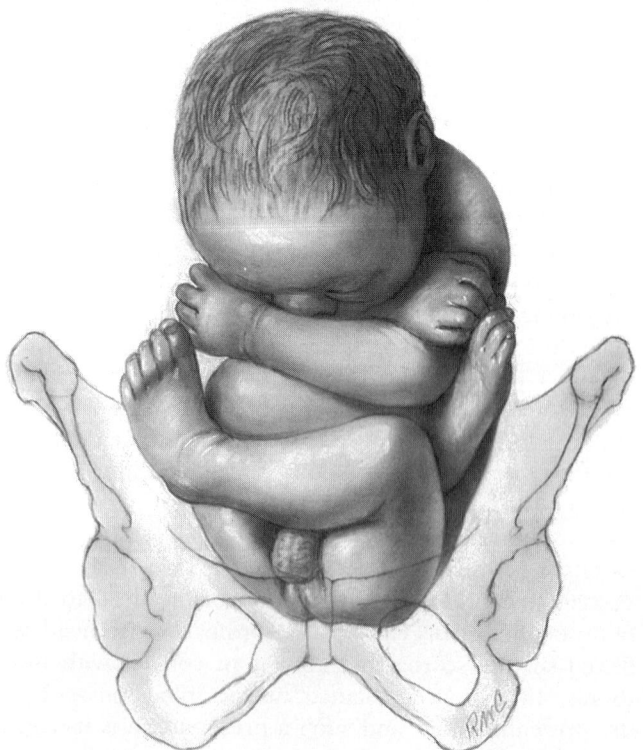

Fig. 10–3. Longitudinal lie. Complete breech presentation.

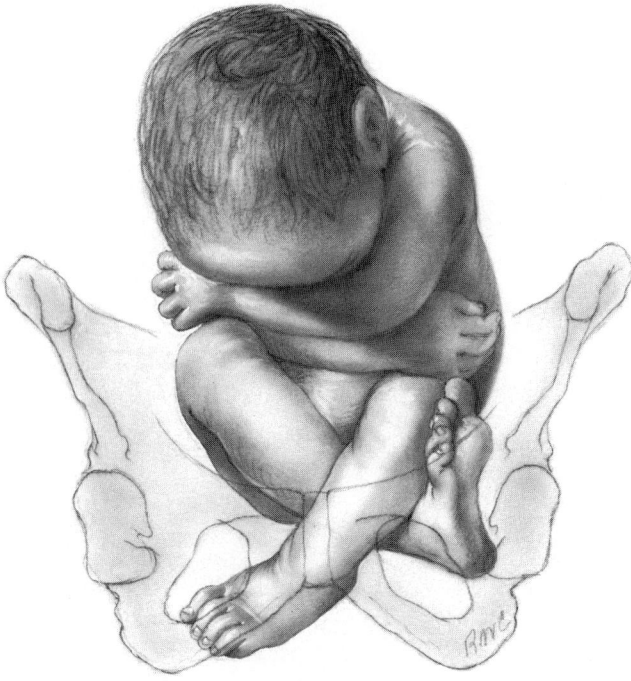

Fig. 10–4. Longitudinal lie. Incomplete, or footling, breech presentation.

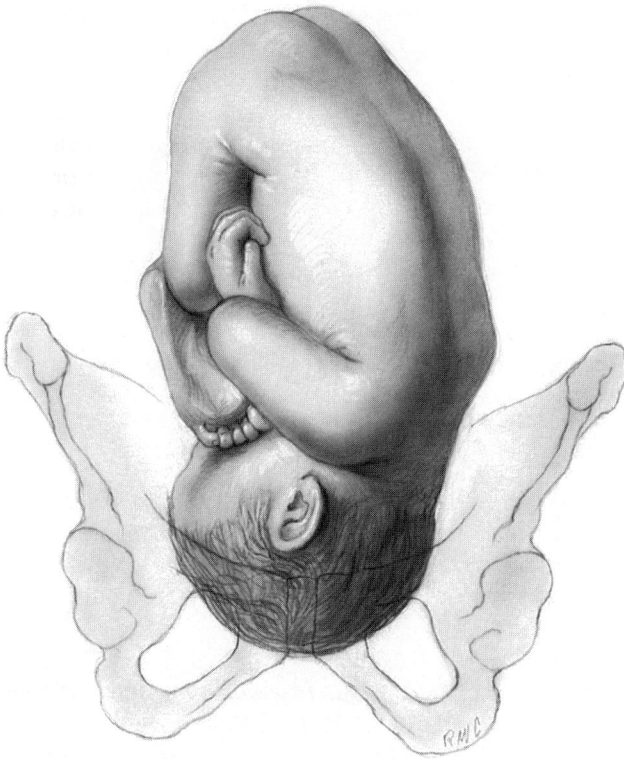

A

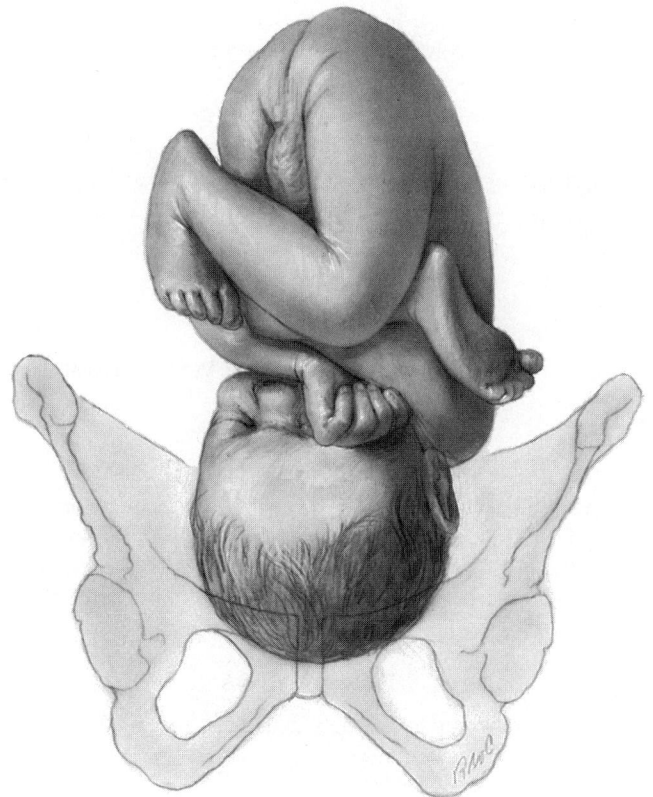

B

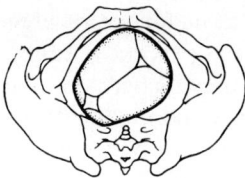

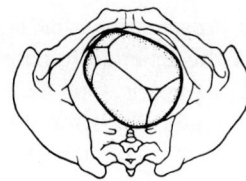

Fig. 10–5. Longitudinal lie. Vertex presentation. **A.** Left occiput anterior (LOA). **B.** Left occiput posterior (LOP).

A   B

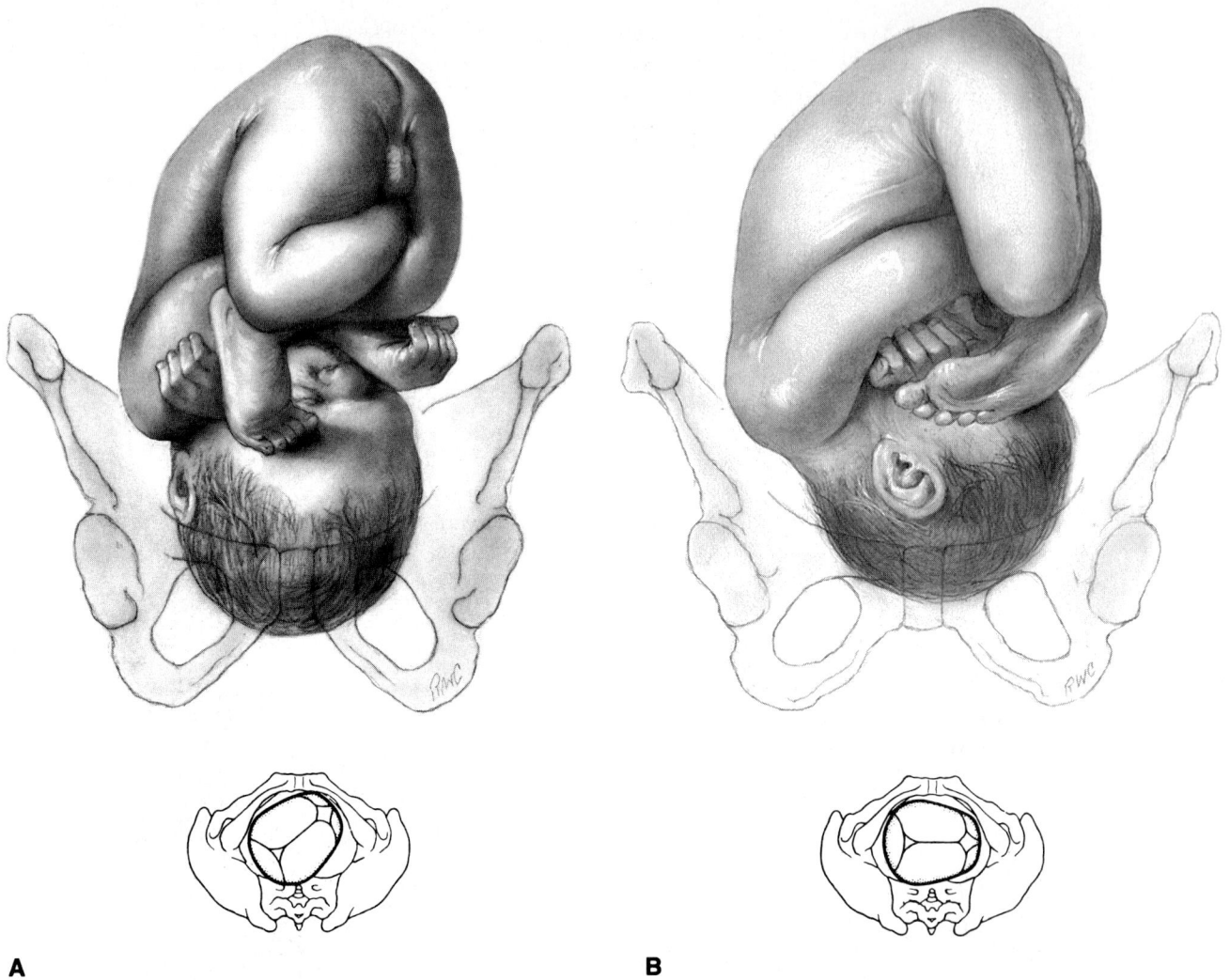

Fig. 10–6. Longitudinal lie. Vertex presentation. **A.** Right occiput posterior (ROP). **B.** Right occiput transverse (ROT).

presentations (Figs. 10–5 to 10–8). Thus, in an occiput presentation, the presentation, position and variety may be abbreviated in clockwise fashion as

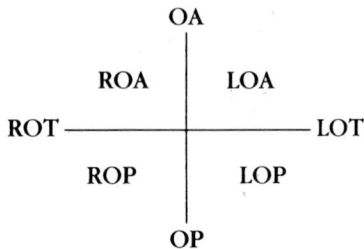

```
                        OA

            ROA    |    LOA

   ROT ─────────────┼───────────── LOT

            ROP    |    LOP

                        OP
```

In shoulder presentations the acromion (scapula) is the portion of the fetus arbitrarily chosen to orient it with the maternal pelvis. One example of the terminology sometimes employed for the purpose is illustrated in Figure 10–9. The acromion or back of the fetus may be directed either posteriorly or anteriorly and superiorly or inferiorly (see Chap. 20, p. 503). However, because it is impossible to differentiate ex-

actly the several varieties of shoulder presentation by clinical examination, and because such differentiation serves no practical purpose, it is customary to refer to all transverse lies of the fetus simply as shoulder presentations.

Frequency of the Various Presentations and Positions. At or near term the incidence of the various presentations is approximately as follows: vertex, 96 percent; breech, 3.5 percent; face, 0.3 percent; and shoulder, 0.4 percent. About two thirds of all vertex presentations are in the left occiput position, and one third in the right.

Although the incidence of breech presentation is only a little over 3 percent at term, it is much greater earlier in pregnancy. Scheer and Nubar (1976), using ultrasonography, found the incidence of breech presentation to be 14 percent between 29 and 32 weeks gestation (see Table 20–1). Subsequently, the breech converted spontaneously to vertex in increasingly higher percentages as term approached.

C

Fig. 10–6 (continued). C. Right occiput anterior (ROA).

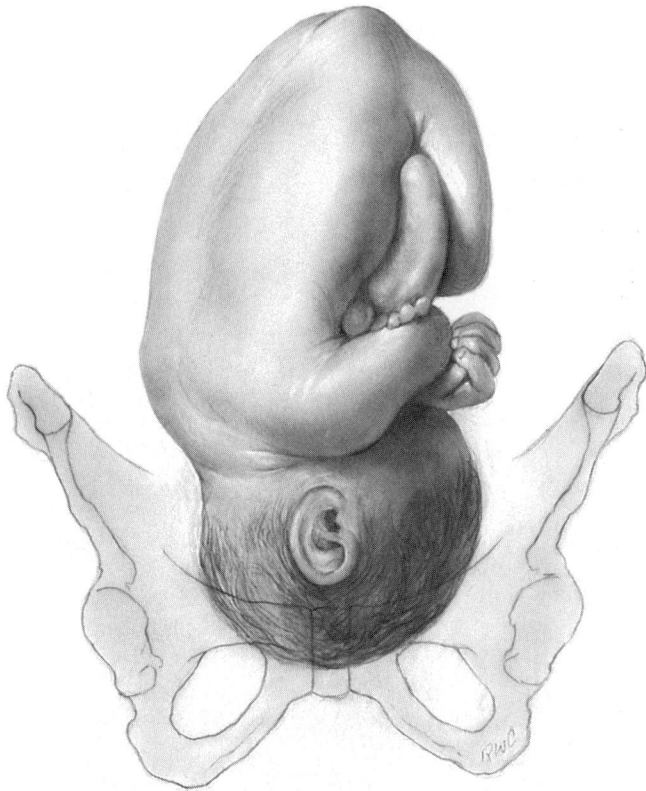

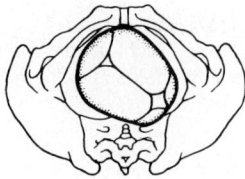

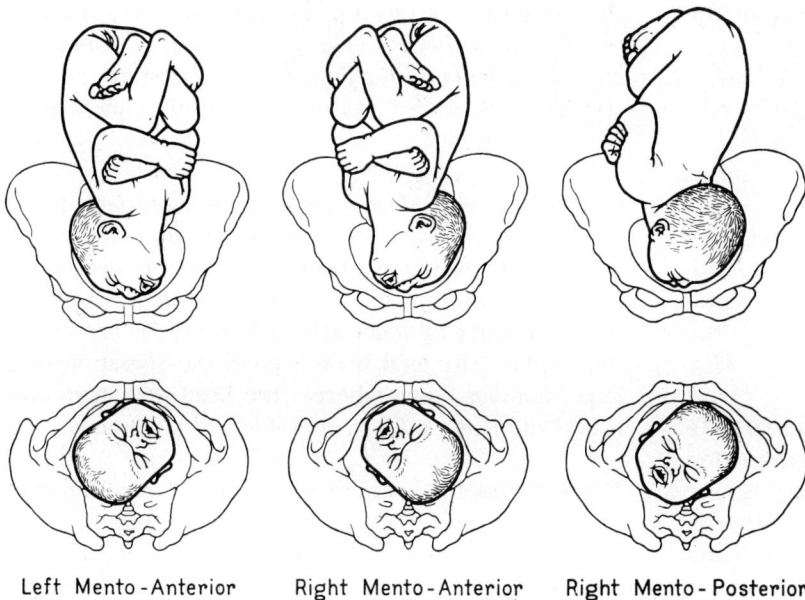

Reasons for the Predominance of Cephalic Presentations and Clinical Significance. Of the several reasons that have been advanced to explain why the fetus at term usually presents by the vertex, the most logical explanation seems to be that this is because the uterus is piriform shaped. Although the fetal head at term is slightly larger than the breech, the entire podalic pole of the fetus—that is, the breech and its flexed extremities—is bulkier than the cephalic pole and more movable. The cephalic pole is comprised of the fetal head only, because the upper extremities are removed some distance, are small, and are less protruding than the buttocks and lower extremities combined. Until about the 32nd week, the amnionic cavity is large compared to the fetal mass, and there is no crowding of the fetus by the uterine walls. At approximately this time, however, the ratio of amnionic fluid volume to fetal mass becomes altered by relative diminution of amnionic fluid and by increasing fetal size. As a result, the uterine walls are apposed more closely to the fetal parts, and then the fetal lie is more nearly dependent upon the piriform shape of the uterus. The fetus, if presenting by the breech, often changes polarity in order to make use of the roomier fundus for its bulkier and more movable podalic pole. The high incidence of breech presentation in hydrocephalic fetuses (see Chap. 20, p. 493) is in accord with this theory, because in this circumstance the cephalic pole of the fetus is definitely larger than the podalic pole.

The cause of breech presentation may be some circumstance that prevents the normal version from taking place, for example, a septum that protrudes into the uterine cavity (Chap. 33, p. 724). A peculiarity of

Left Mento-Anterior   Right Mento-Anterior   Right Mento-Posterior

Fig. 10–7. Longitudinal lie. Face presentation. Left and right anterior and right posterior positions.

Fig. 10–9. Transverse lie. Right acromiodorsoposterior position (RADP). The shoulder of the fetus is to the mother's right, and the back is posterior.

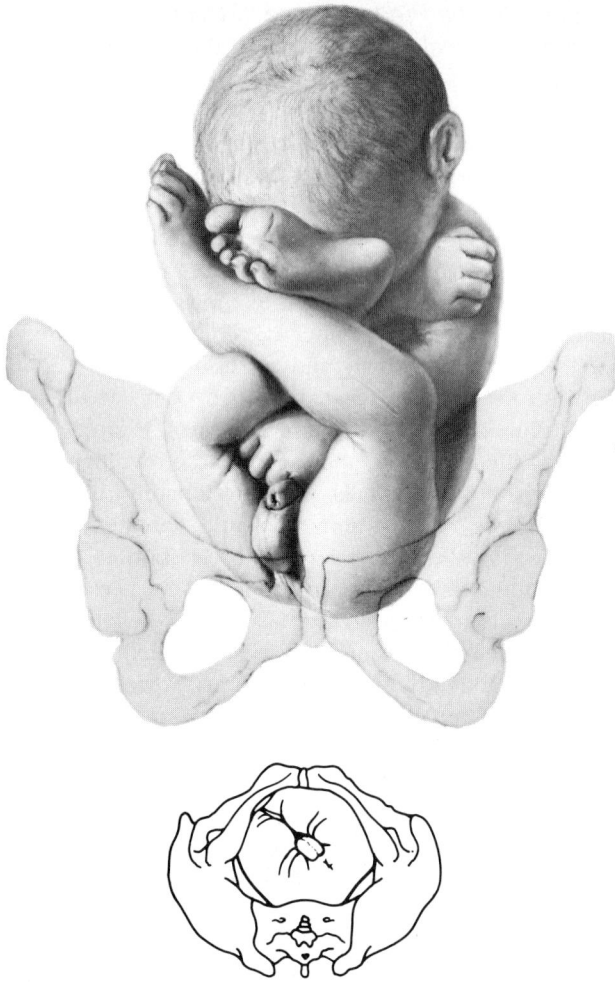

Fig. 10–8. Longitudinal lie. Breech presentation. Left sacrum posterior position (LSP).

fetal attitude, particularly extension of the vertebral column as seen in frank breeches, also may prevent the fetus from turning.

Diagnosis of Presentation and Position of the Fetus

There are several methods that can be used to diagnose fetal presentation and position. These include abdominal palpation, vaginal examination, combined examination, auscultation, and in certain doubtful cases, ultrasonography or radiography.

Abdominal Palpation—Leopold's Maneuvers. In order to obtain satisfactory results, the examination should be conducted systematically employing the four maneuvers suggested by Leopold and Sporlin (1894). The mother should be on a firm bed or examining table, with her abdomen bared. During the first three maneuvers, the examiner stands at the side of

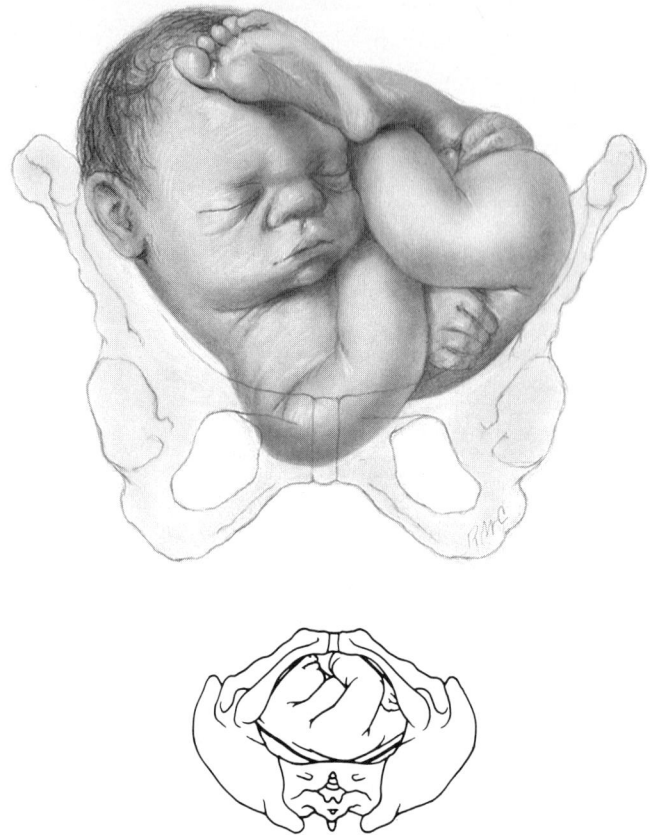

the bed that is most convenient and faces the patient; the examiner reverses this position and faces her feet for the last maneuver (Fig. 10–10). These maneuvers may be difficult, if not impossible, to perform and interpret in the obese patient or if the placenta is anteriorly implanted.

First Maneuver. After outlining the contour of the uterus and ascertaining how nearly the fundus approaches the xiphoid cartilage, the examiner gently palpates the fundus with the tips of the fingers of both hands in order to define which fetal pole is present in the fundus. The fetal breech gives the sensation of a large, nodular body, whereas the head feels hard and round and is more freely movable and ballottable.

Second Maneuver. After the determination of the pole of the fetus that lies in the fundus, the palms of the examiner's hands are placed on either side of the abdomen, and gentle but deep pressure is exerted. On one side, a hard, resistant structure is felt, the back; and on

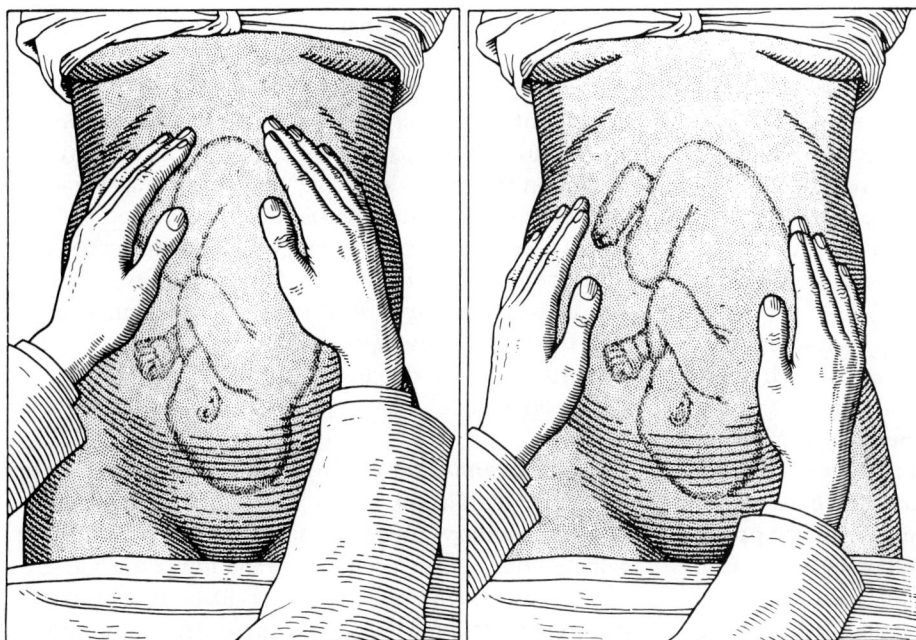

First maneuver

Second maneuver

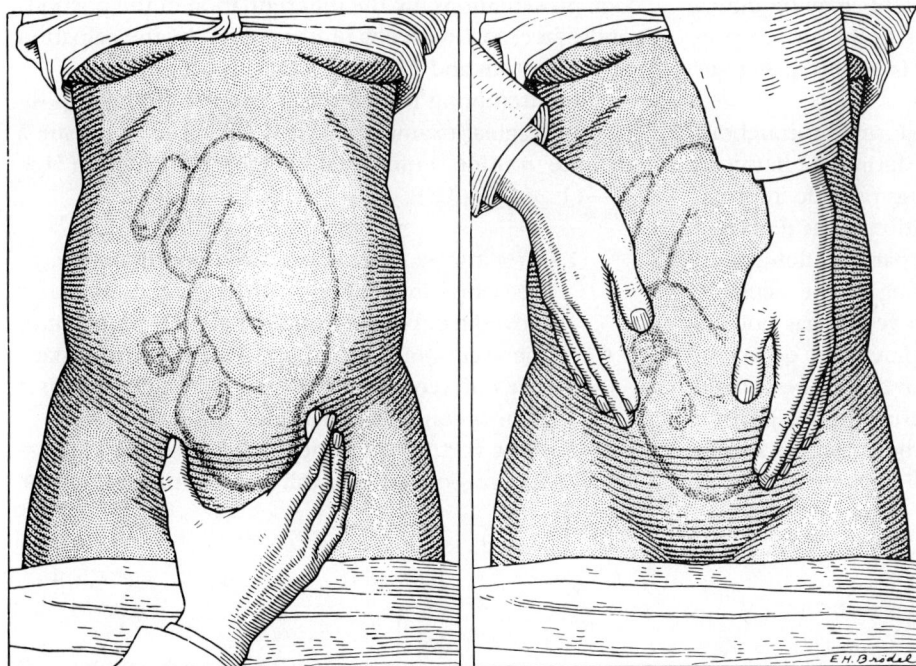

Third maneuver

Fourth maneuver

Fig. 10–10. Longitudinal lie. Palpation in left occiput anterior position (LOP) (maneuvers of Leopold). See also Figure 11–5A.

the other, numerous nodulations, the small parts. In pregnant women with thin abdominal walls, the fetal extremities can be differentiated readily, but in heavier women only irregular nodulations may be felt. In the presence of obesity or considerable amnionic fluid, the back is felt more easily by exerting deep pressure with one hand while palpating with the other. By next noting whether the back is directed anteriorly, transversely, or posteriorly, a more accurate picture of the orientation of the fetus is obtained.

Third Maneuver. Employing the thumb and fingers of one hand, the examiner grasps the lower portion of the maternal abdomen, just above the symphysis pubis. If the presenting part is not engaged, a movable body will be felt, usually the fetal head. The differentiation between head and breech is made as in the first maneuver. If the presenting part is not engaged, the examination is almost complete; with the location of the fetal head, breech, back, and extremities known, all that remains to be defined is the attitude of the head. If by careful palpation it can be shown that the cephalic prominence is on the same side as the small parts, the head must be flexed, and therefore the vertex is the presenting part. When the cephalic prominence of the fetus is on the same side as the back, the head must be extended. If the presenting part is deeply engaged, however, the findings from this maneuver are simply indicative of the fact that the lower pole of the fetus is fixed in the pelvis; the details are then defined by the last (fourth) maneuver.

Fourth Maneuver. The examiner faces the mother's feet and, with the tips of the first three fingers of each hand, exerts deep pressure in the direction of the axis of the pelvic inlet. If the head presents, one hand is arrested sooner than the other by a rounded body, the cephalic prominence, while the other hand descends more deeply into the pelvis. In vertex presentations, the prominence is on the same side as the small parts; and in face presentations, on the same side as the back. The ease with which the prominence is felt is indicative of the extent to which descent has occurred. In many instances, when the fetal head has descended into the pelvis, the anterior shoulder of the fetus may be differentiated readily by the third maneuver. In breech presentations, the information obtained from this maneuver is less precise.

Abdominal palpation can be performed throughout the latter months of pregnancy and during the between the contractions of labor. The findings provide information about the presentation and position of the fetus and the extent to which the presenting part has descended into the pelvis. For example, so long as the cephalic prominence is readily palpable, the vertex has not descended to the level of the ischial spines. The degree of cephalopelvic disproportion, moreover, can be gauged by evaluating the extent to which the anterior portion of the fetal head overrides the mother's symphysis pubis. With experience, it is possible to estimate the size of the fetus and even to map out the presentation of the second fetus in a twin gestation.

During labor, palpation also may provide information about the lower uterine segment. When there is obstruction to the passage of the fetus, a pathological retraction ring sometimes may be felt as a transverse or oblique ridge extending across the lower portion of the uterus (see Chap. 19, p. 489). Even in normal cases, the contracting body of the uterus and the passive lower uterine segment may be distinguished by palpation. During a contraction, the upper portion of the uterus is firm or hard, whereas the lower segment feels elastic or almost fluctuant.

Vaginal Examination. Before labor, the diagnosis of fetal presentation and position by vaginal examination is often inconclusive, because the presenting part must be palpated through a closed cervix and lower uterine segment. During labor, however, after dilatation of the cervix, important information may be obtained. In vertex presentations, the position and variety are recognized by differentiation of the various sutures and fontanels; in face presentations, by the differentiation of the portions of the face; and in breech presentations, by the palpation of the sacrum and maternal ischial tuberosities.

In attempting to determine presentation and position by vaginal examination, it is advisable to pursue a definite routine, comprised of four maneuvers (Figs. 10–11 and 10–12):

1. After the woman is prepared appropriately, as described in Chapter 14, two fingers of either gloved hand of the examiner are introduced into the vagina and carried up to the presenting part. The differentiation of vertex, face, and breech is then accomplished readily.
2. If the vertex is presenting, the examiner's fingers are introduced into the posterior aspect of the

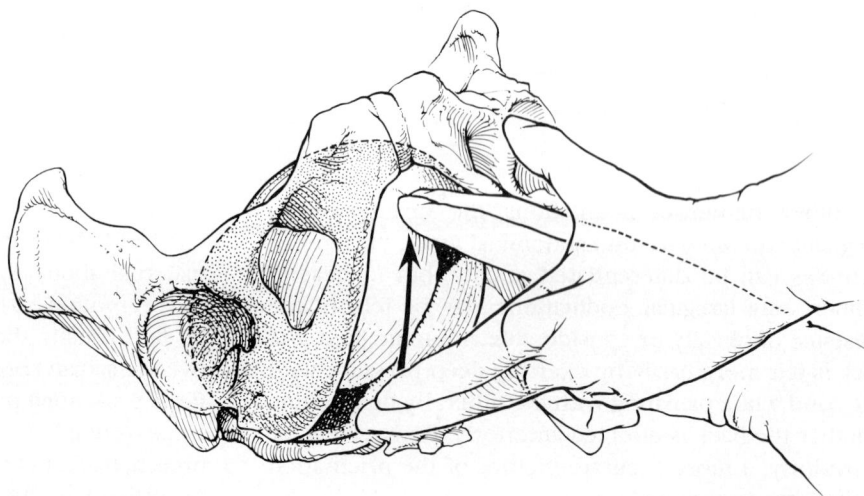

Fig. 10–11. Locating the sagittal suture by vaginal examination.

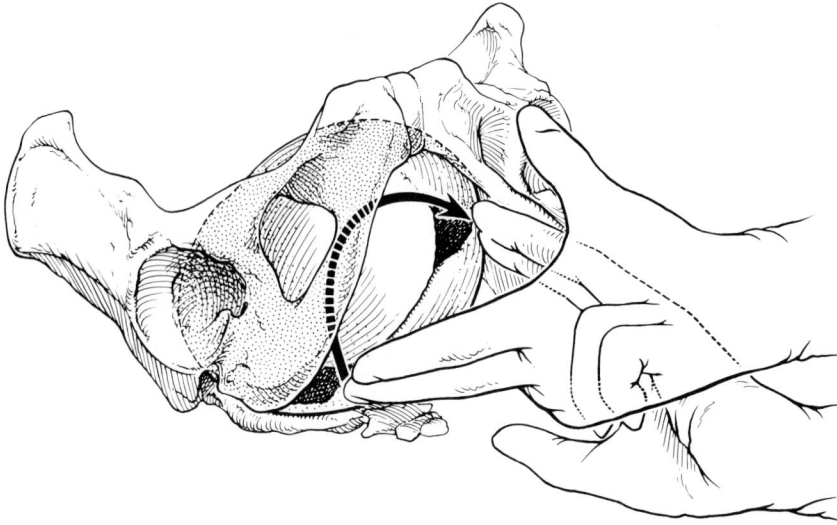

Fig. 10–12. Differentiating the fontanels by vaginal examination.

vagina. The fingers are then swept forward over the fetal head toward the maternal symphysis (Fig. 10–11). During the performance of this movement, the examiner's fingers necessarily cross the fetal sagittal suture. When it is felt, its course is outlined, with small and large fontanels at the opposite ends.

3. The positions of the two fontanels then are ascertained. The examiner's fingers are passed to the anterior extremity of the sagittal suture, and the fontanel encountered there is examined carefully and identified; then by a circular motion, the fingers are passed around the side of the head until the other fontanel is felt and differentiated (Fig. 10–12).

4. The station (extent to which the presenting part has descended into the pelvis) can also be established at this time (see Chap. 11, p. 290).

Using these three maneuvers, the various sutures and fontanels (Chap. 7, p. 170) are located readily, and the possibility of error is lessened considerably. In face and breech presentations, errors are minimized, because the various parts are distinguished more readily.

Auscultation. Auscultation alone does not provide reliable information concerning the presentation and position of the fetus, but auscultory findings sometimes reinforce results obtained by palpation. Ordinarily, fetal heart sounds are transmitted through the convex portion of the fetus that lies in intimate contact with the uterine wall. Therefore, fetal heart sounds are heard best through the fetal back in vertex and breech presentations, and through the fetal thorax in face presen-

tations. The region of the abdomen in which fetal heart sounds are heard most clearly varies according to the presentation and the extent to which the presenting part has descended. In cephalic presentations, fetal heart sounds are best heard midway between the maternal umbilicus and the anterior superior spine of her ilium, whereas in breech presentations it is usually at or slightly above the level of the umbilicus. In occipitoanterior positions, heart sounds usually are heard best a short distance from the midline; in the transverse varieties, they are heard more laterally; and in the posterior varieties, they are best heard well back in the mother's flank.

Sonography. Improvements in ultrasonic technique have provided another diagnostic aid of particular value in doubtful cases. In obese women or in women whose abdominal walls are rigid, a sonographic examination may provide information to solve many diagnostic problems and lead to early recognition of a breech or shoulder presentation that might otherwise have escaped detection until late in labor. Employing ultrasonography, the fetal head and body can be located without the *potential* hazards of radiation (see Chap. 43, p. 981). On infrequent occasions, however, the information obtained radiographically far exceeds the minimal risk from a single diagnostic x-ray exposure.

References

Leopold, Sporlin: Conduct of normal births through external examination alone. Arch Gynaekol 45:337, 1894

Scheer K, Nubar J: Variation of fetal presentation with gestational age. Am J Obstet Gynecol 125:269, 1976

CHAPTER 11
The Normal Pelvis

The mechanisms of labor are essentially processes of accommodation of the fetus to the bony passage through which the fetus must pass. Accordingly, the size and shape of the pelvis are extremely important in obstetrics. In both women and men the pelvis forms the bony ring through which body weight is transmitted to the lower extremities, but in women it has a special form that adapts it to childbearing (Fig. 11–1). The pelvis is composed of four bones: the sacrum, coccyx, and two innominate bones. Each innominate bone is formed by the fusion of the ilium, ischium, and pubis. The innominate bones are joined to the sacrum at the sacroiliac synchondroses and to one another at the symphysis pubis. Consideration of the pelvis will be limited to those features of importance in childbearing.

Pelvic Anatomy: Obstetrical Considerations

The false pelvis lies above the linea terminalis and the true pelvis below this anatomical boundary (Fig. 11–1). The false pelvis is bounded posteriorly by the lumbar vertebrae and laterally by the iliac fossae, and in front the boundary is formed by the lower portion of the anterior abdominal wall. The false pelvis varies considerably in size according to the flare of the iliac bones, but this has no obstetrical significance.

The true pelvis is the portion important in childbearing. It is bounded above by the promontory and alae of the sacrum, the linea terminalis, and the upper margins of the pubic bones, and below by the pelvic outlet. The cavity of the true pelvis can be described as an obliquely truncated, bent cylinder with its greatest height posteriorly, because its anterior wall at the symphysis pubis measures about 5 cm and its posterior wall about 10 cm (Figs. 11–2 and 11–3). With the woman upright, the upper portion of the pelvic canal is directed downward and backward, and its lower course curves and becomes directed downward and forward.

The walls of the true pelvis are partly bony and partly ligamentous. The posterior boundary is the anterior surface of the sacrum, and the lateral limits are formed by the inner surface of the ischial bones and the sacrosciatic notches and ligaments. In front the true pelvis is bounded by the pubic bones, the ascending superior rami of the ischial bones, and the obturator foramina.

The sidewalls of the true pelvis of the normal adult woman converge somewhat; therefore, if the

planes of the ischial bones were extended downward, they would meet near the knee. Extending from the middle of the posterior margin of each ischium are the ischial spines. The ischial spines are of great obstetrical importance because the distance between them usually represents the shortest diameter of the pelvic cavity. Moreover, because the ischial spines can be felt readily by vaginal or rectal examination, they serve as valuable landmarks in assessing the level to which the presenting part of the fetus has descended into the true pelvis (p. 289).

The sacrum forms the posterior wall of the pelvic cavity. Its upper anterior margin corresponds to the body of the first sacral vertebra and is designated as the promontory. The promontory may be felt on vaginal examination in small pelves and can provide a landmark for clinical pelvimetry. Normally the sacrum has a marked vertical and a less pronounced horizontal concavity, which in abnormal pelves may undergo important variations. A straight line drawn from the promontory to the tip of the sacrum usually measures 10 cm, whereas the distance along the concavity averages 12 cm.

The appearance of the pubic arch is characteristic. The descending inferior rami of the pubic bones unite at an angle of 90 to 100 degrees to form a rounded arch under which the fetal head must pass.

Pelvic Inclination. The normal position of the pelvis, in the standing woman, can be reproduced by holding a skeletal specimen with the incisures of the acetabula pointing directly downward. The same result is achieved when the anterior superior spines of the ilium and the pubic tubercles are placed in the same vertical plane.

Pelvic Joints

Symphysis Pubis. Anteriorly, the pelvic bones are joined together by the symphysis pubis. This structure consists of fibrocartilage and the superior and inferior pubic ligaments; the latter is frequently designated the *arcuate ligament of the pubis* (Fig. 11–4). The symphysis has a certain degree of mobility, which increases during pregnancy, particularly in multiparas. This fact was demonstrated by Budin (1897), who reported that if a finger was inserted into the vagina of a pregnant woman and she then walked, the ends of the pubic bones could be felt moving up and down with each step.

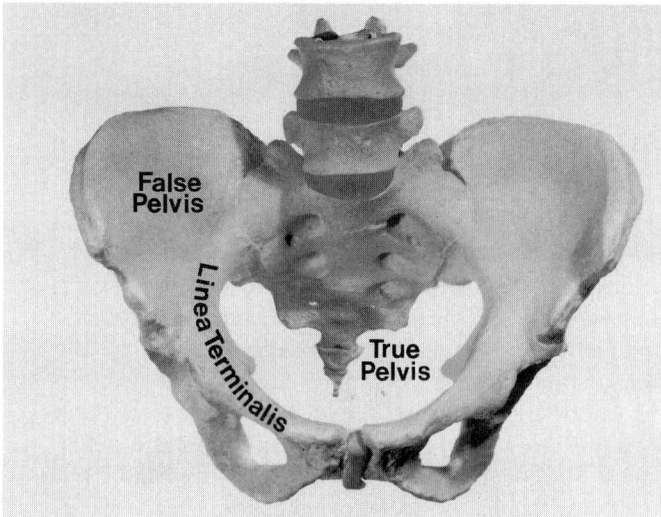

Fig. 11–1. Normal female pelvis with the false and true pelvis identified.

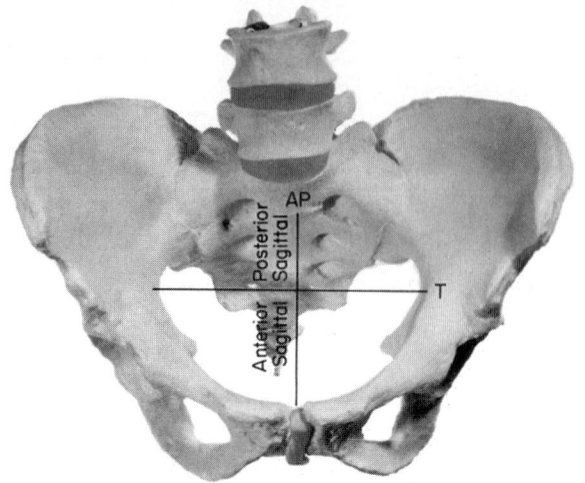

Fig. 11–3. Adult female pelvis. Anteroposterior (AP) and transverse (T) diameters of the pelvic inlet are illustrated, as well as the posterior sagittal of the inlet.

Sacroiliac Joints. Posteriorly the pelvic bones are joined by the articulations between the sacrum and the iliac portion of the innominate bones (sacroiliac joints). These joints also have a certain degree of mobility.

Relaxation of the Pelvic Joints. During pregnancy, relaxation of these joints likely results from hormonal changes. Abramson and co-workers (1934) observed that relaxation of the symphysis pubis commenced in women in the first half of pregnancy and increased during the last 3 months. These investigators reported that regression of relaxation began immediately after parturition and was completed within 3 to 5 months. The

symphysis pubis also increases in width during pregnancy (more in multiparas than in primigravidas), and returns to normal soon after delivery. By careful radiographic studies, Borell and Fernstrom (1957) demonstrated that the rather marked mobility of the pelvis of women at term was caused by an upward gliding movement of the sacroiliac joint. The displacement, which is greatest in the dorsal lithotomy position, may increase the diameter of the outlet by 1.5 to 2.0 cm. **This is the main justification for placing a woman in this position for a vaginal delivery.** It should be noted, however, that the increase in the diameter of the pelvic outlet occurs *only* if the sacrum is allowed to rotate

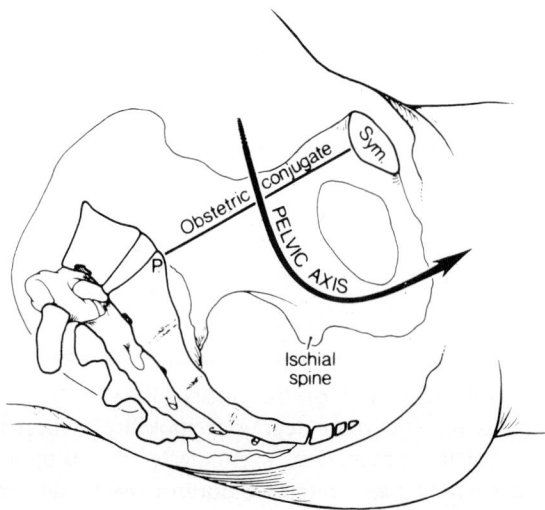

Fig. 11–2. The cavity of the true pelvis is comparable to an obliquely truncated, bent cylinder with its greatest height posteriorly. Note the curvature of the pelvic axis.

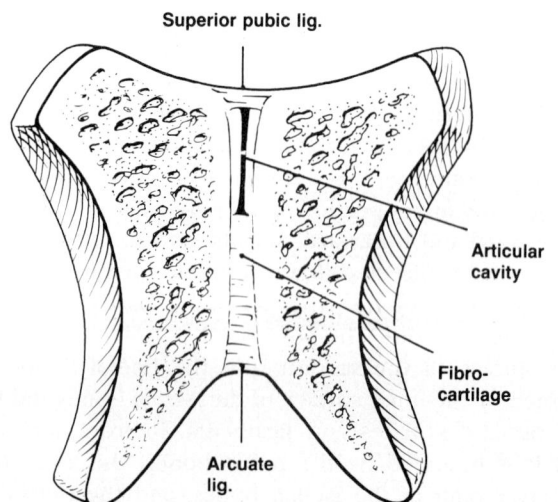

Fig. 11–4. Frontal section through symphysis pubis. (Redrawn from Spalteholz, 1933.)

posteriorly, that is, only if the sacrum is not forced anteriorly by the weight of the maternal pelvis against the delivery table or bed (Russell, 1969, 1982). This is likely the reason the McRoberts maneuver often is successful in releasing an obstructed shoulder in a case of shoulder dystocia (see also Chap. 20, p. 511). Gardosi and co-workers (1989) reported in a randomized controlled trial that a modified squatting position in the second stage of labor resulted in a shorter second stage of labor and fewer perineal lacerations. There was an increase in labial lacerations, however. In this trial conducted during the second stage of labor, women used a modified squatting position on a specialized pillow. The authors attributed the "success" of the method to increasing the interspinous diameter and the diameter of the pelvic outlet (Russell, 1969, 1982) as well as to improving the "pushing efforts" of the laboring woman. Although these observations are unconfirmed, such a squatting position is assumed by many primitive women as the "normal" position for birth (Gardosi and associates, 1989; Russell, 1982).

Planes and Diameters of the Pelvis

Because of its complex shape, it is difficult to describe the exact location of an object within the pelvis. For convenience, therefore, the pelvis is described as having four imaginary planes: (1) the plane of the pelvic inlet (superior strait), (2) the plane of the pelvic outlet (inferior strait), (3) the plane of the midpelvis (least pelvic dimensions), and (4) the plane of greatest pelvic dimensions. Because this last plane has no obstetrical significance, it is not considered further.

Pelvic Inlet. The pelvic inlet (superior strait) is bounded posteriorly by the promontory and alae of the sacrum, laterally by the linea terminalis, and anteriorly by the horizontal rami of the pubic bones and symphysis pubis (Figs. 11–2, 11–3, 11–5, and 11–6). The configuration of the inlet of the human female pelvis typically is more nearly round than ovoid. Caldwell and co-workers (1934) identified radiographically a nearly round or *gynecoid* pelvic inlet in approximately 50 percent of the pelves of white women.

Four diameters of the pelvic inlet are usually described: anteroposterior, transverse, and two obliques. The obstetrically important anteroposterior diameter is the shortest distance between the promontory of the sacrum and the symphysis pubis, and is designated the *obstetrical conjugate* (Figs. 11–2, 11–3, and 11–5). Normally, the obstetrical conjugate measures 10 cm or more, but it may be considerably shortened in abnormal pelves.

The transverse diameter is constructed at right angles to the obstetrical conjugate and represents the greatest distance between the linea terminalis on either side. It usually intersects the obstetrical conjugate at a point

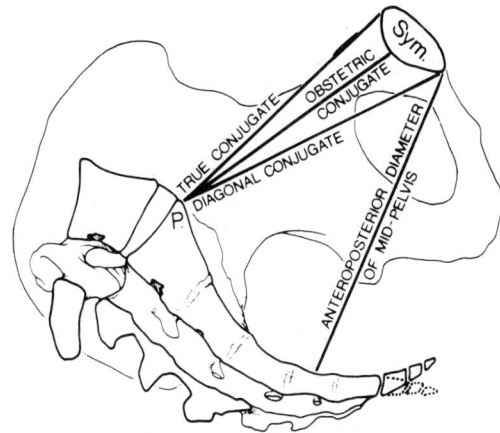

Fig. 11–5. Three anteroposterior diameters of the pelvic inlet are illustrated: the true conjugate, the more important obstetrical conjugate, and the clinically measurable diagonal conjugate. The anteroposterior diameter of the midpelvis is also shown. (P = sacral promontory; Sym = symphysis pubis.)

about 4 cm in front of the promontory (Fig. 11–3). The segment of the obstetrical conjugate from the intersection of these two lines to the promontory is designated the *posterior sagittal* diameter of the inlet.

Each of the oblique diameters extends from one of the sacroiliac synchondroses to the iliopectineal eminence on the opposite side of the pelvis. They average just under 13 cm and are designated right and left, according to whether they originate at the right or left sacroiliac synchondrosis.

The anteroposterior diameter of the pelvic inlet that has been identified as the *true conjugate* does not represent the shortest distance between the promontory of the sacrum and symphysis pubis (Fig. 11–5). The shortest distance is the *obstetrical conjugate,* which is the shortest anteroposterior diameter through which

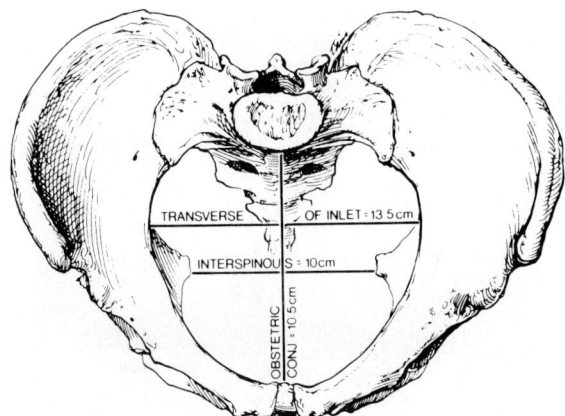

Fig. 11–6. Adult female pelvis demonstrating anteroposterior and transverse diameters of the pelvic inlet and transverse (interspinous) diameter of the midpelvis. The obstetrical conjugate is normally greater than 10 cm.

the head must pass in descending through the pelvic inlet (Figs. 11–2, 11–3, and 11–5).

The obstetrical conjugate cannot be measured directly with the examining fingers; therefore, various instruments have been designed in an effort to obtain such a measurement. Unfortunately, none of these instruments has proven to be reliable. For clinical purposes, it is sufficient to estimate the length of the obstetrical conjugate indirectly. This is accomplished by measuring the distance from the lower margin of the symphysis to promontory of the sacrum, that is, the *diagonal conjugate* (Fig. 11–5), and subtracting 1.5 to 2 cm from the result, according to the height and inclination of the symphysis pubis (see "Pelvic Size and Its Clinical Estimation" later in the chapter).

Midpelvis. The midpelvis at the level of the ischial spines (midplane, or plane of least pelvic dimensions) is of particular importance following engagement of the fetal head in obstructed labor. The interspinous diameter, 10 cm or somewhat more, is usually the smallest diameter of the pelvis (Fig. 11–6). The anteroposterior diameter, through the level of the ischial spines, normally measures at least 11.5 cm (Fig. 11–5). The posterior component (posterior sagittal diameter), between the sacrum and the line created by the interspinous diameter, is usually at least 4.5 cm.

Pelvic Outlet. The outlet of the pelvis consists of two approximately triangular areas not in the same plane but having a common base, which is a line drawn between the two ischial tuberosities (Fig. 11–7). The apex of the posterior triangle is at the tip of the sacrum, and the lateral boundaries are the sacrosciatic ligaments and the ischial tuberosities. The anterior triangle is formed by the area under the pubic arch. Three diameters of the pelvic outlet usually are described: the anteroposterior,

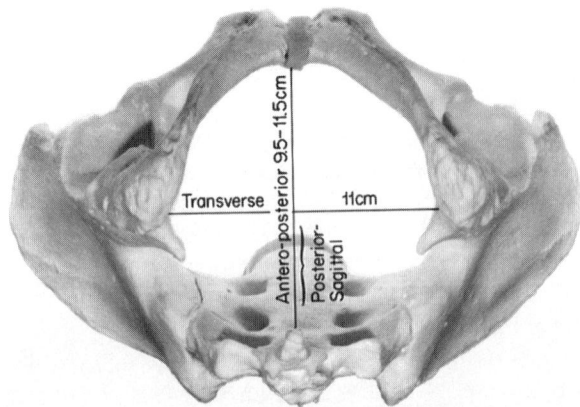

Fig. 11–7. Pelvic outlet with diameters marked. Note that the anteroposterior diameter may be divided into anterior and posterior sagittal diameters.

transverse, and posterior sagittal. The anteroposterior diameter (9.5 to 11.5 cm) extends from the lower margin of the symphysis pubis to the tip of the sacrum (Fig. 11–7). The transverse diameter (11 cm) is the distance between the inner edges of the ischial tuberosities. The posterior sagittal diameter extends from the tip of the sacrum to a right-angle intersection with a line between the ischial tuberosities. The normal *posterior sagittal diameter* of the outlet usually exceeds 7.5 cm (Fig. 11–7).

In obstructed labors caused by a narrowing of the midpelvis and/or pelvic outlet, the prognosis for vaginal delivery often depends on the length of the posterior sagittal diameter of the pelvic outlet (Figs. 21–4 and 21–5).

Pelvic Shapes

In the years before the *potential* hazards of diagnostic x-rays were appreciated, but before antimicrobial drugs and blood transfusions were generally available, the real and immediate risks of cesarean delivery were formidable. At this time, x-ray pelvimetry was used with greater frequency in women with suspected cephalopelvic disproportion or fetal malpresentation. Pelvic radiography also was used as an aid in understanding the general architecture and configuration of the pelvis, as well as its size. Caldwell and Moloy (1933, 1934) developed a classification of the pelvis that is still used. The classification is based upon the shape of the pelvis, and familiarity with the classification helps the physician to understand the mechanisms of labor in normally and abnormally shaped pelves. This information is useful in helping the physician to manage abnormal labors due to various types of pelvic contractions.

Caldwell–Moloy Classification. A line drawn through the greatest transverse diameter of the inlet divides it into anterior and posterior segments. The shapes of these segments are important determinants in this method of classification (Fig. 11–8). The character of the posterior segment determines the type of pelvis, and the character of the anterior segment determines the tendency. Many pelves are not pure but mixed types, for example, a gynecoid pelvis with android "tendency," means that the posterior pelvis is gynecoid and the anterior pelvis is android in shape.

Gynecoid Pelvis. The gynecoid pelvis has the anatomical characteristics ordinarily associated with the female pelvis. The posterior sagittal diameter of the inlet is only slightly shorter than the anterior sagittal. The sides of the posterior segment are well rounded and wide. Because the transverse diameter of the inlet is either slightly greater than or about the same as the antero-

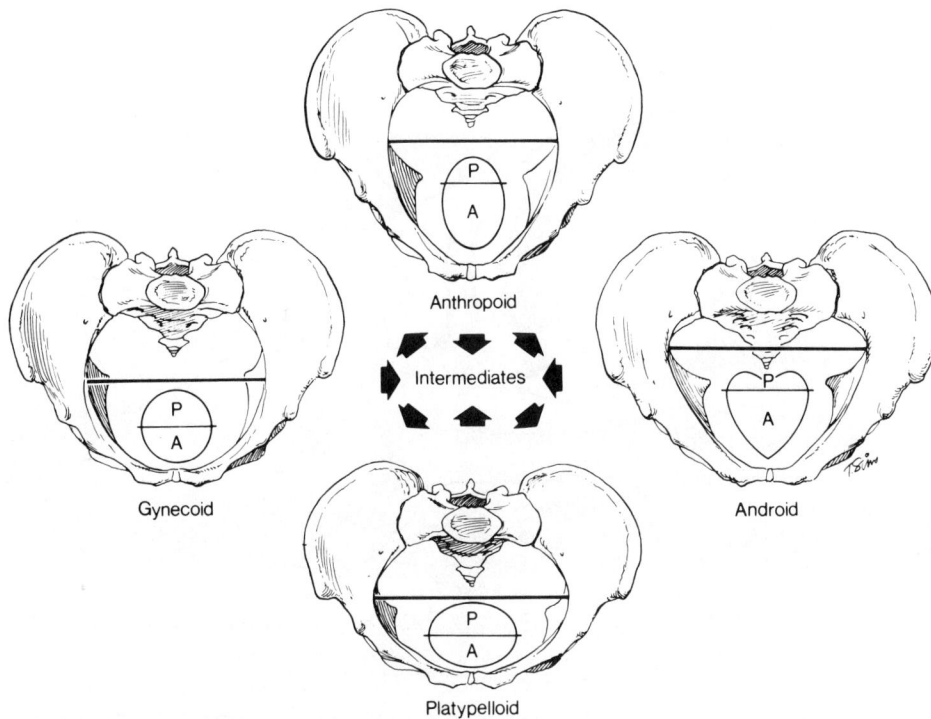

Fig. 11–8. The four parent pelvic types of the Caldwell–Moloy classification. A line passing through the widest transverse diameter divides the inlet into posterior (P) and anterior (A) segments.

posterior diameter, the inlet is either slightly oval or round. The sidewalls of the pelvis are straight, the spines are not prominent, the pubic arch is wide, and the transverse diameter at the ischial spines is 10 cm or more. The sacrum is inclined neither anteriorly nor posteriorly. The sacrosciatic notch is well rounded and never narrow. Caldwell and co-workers (1939) ascertained the frequency of the four parent pelvic types by study of Todd's collection, and they reported the gynecoid pelvis was found in almost 50 percent of women.

Android Pelvis. With the android pelvis, the posterior sagittal diameter at the inlet is much shorter than the anterior sagittal, limiting the use of the posterior space by the fetal head. The sides of the posterior segment are not rounded but tend to form, with the corresponding sides of the anterior segment, a wedge at their point of junction. The anterior pelvis is narrow and triangular. The sidewalls are usually convergent, the ischial spines are prominent, and the subpubic arch is narrowed. The bones are characteristically heavy, and the sacrosciatic notches are narrow and highly arched. The sacrum is set forward in the pelvis and usually is straight, with little or no curvature, and the posterior sagittal diameter is decreased from inlet to outlet by the forward inclination of the sacrum. Not infrequently there is considerable forward inclination of the sacral tip.

The extreme android pelvis presages a poor prognosis for vaginal delivery. The frequency of difficult forceps operations and stillbirths increases substantively

when there is a *small* android pelvis. Android-type pelves made up one third of pure-type pelves encountered in white women and one sixth in nonwhite women in the Todd collection.

Anthropoid Pelvis. The anthropoid pelvis is characterized by an anteroposterior diameter of the inlet greater than the transverse. This results in an oval anteroposteriorly, with the anterior segment somewhat narrow and pointed. The sacrosciatic notches are large, and the sidewalls often are convergent. The sacrum usually has six segments and is straight, making the anthropoid pelvis deeper than the other types.

The ischial spines are likely to be prominent. The subpubic arch frequently is narrowed but well shaped. The anthropoid pelvis is more common in nonwhite women, whereas the android form is more frequent in white women. Anthropoid-type pelves make up one fourth of pure-type pelves in white women and nearly one half of those in nonwhite women.

Platypelloid Pelvis. The platypelloid pelvis has a flattened gynecoid shape, with a short anteroposterior and a wide transverse diameter. The latter is set well in front of the sacrum, as in the typical gynecoid pelvis. The angle of the anterior pelvis is very wide, and the anterior puboiliac and posterior iliac portions of the iliopectineal lines are well curved. The sacrum usually is well curved and rotated backward. Thus, the sacrum is short and the pelvis shallow, creating wide sacrosciatic notches. The

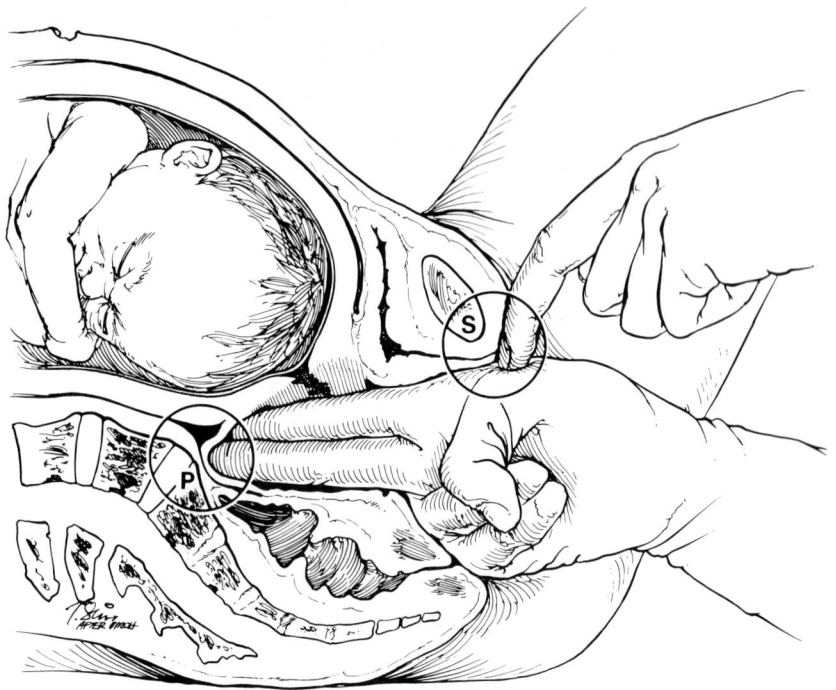

Fig. 11–9. Vaginal examination to determine the diagonal conjugate. (P = sacral promontory; S = symphysis pubis.)

platypelloid pelvis is the rarest of the pure varieties and is found in less than 3 percent of women.

Intermediate-type Pelves. Intermediate or mixed types of pelves are much more frequent than pure types.

Pelvic Size and Its Clinical Estimation

Pelvic Inlet Measurements

Diagonal Conjugate. In many abnormal pelves, the anteroposterior diameter of the pelvic inlet (the obstetrical conjugate) is considerably shortened. It is important therefore to determine its length, but this measurement can be obtained only by radiographic techniques. The distance from the sacral promontory to the lower margin of the symphysis pubis (the diagonal conjugate), however, can be measured clinically (Figs. 11–9 to 11–11). **The diagonal conjugate measurement is most important. Every practitioner of obstetrics should be thoroughly familiar with the technique of its measurement and the interpretation of the information gained from its use.**

To obtain this measurement, the patient is placed upon an examining table with her knees drawn up and her feet supported by suitable stirrups. If such an examination cannot be arranged conveniently, she should be brought to the edge of the bed, where a firm pillow should be placed beneath her buttocks. The examiner introduces two fingers into the vagina; and before measuring the diagonal conjugate, the mobility of the coc-

cyx is evaluated and the anterior surface of the sacrum is palpated. The mobility of the coccyx is tested by palpating it with the fingers in the vagina and attempting to move it to and fro. The anterior surface of the sacrum is then palpated from below upward, and its vertical and lateral curvatures are noted. In normal pelves only the last three sacral vertebrae can be felt without indenting the perineum, whereas in markedly contracted pelves the entire anterior surface of the sacrum usually is readily accessible. Occasionally, the mobility of the coccyx and the anatomical features of the lower sacrum may be defined more easily by rectal examination.

Except in extreme degrees of pelvic contraction, in order to reach the promontory of the sacrum, the examiner's elbow must be depressed and, unless the ex-

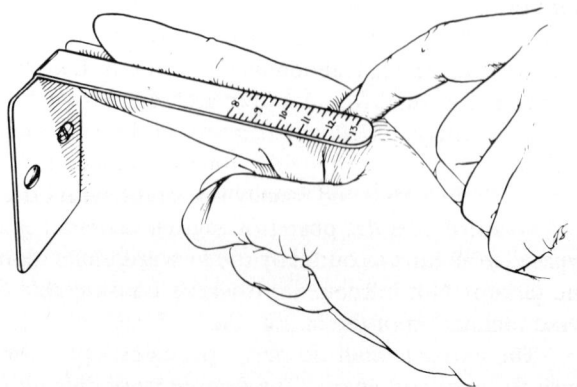

Fig. 11–10. Metal scale fastened to wall for measuring the diagonal conjugate diameter as ascertained manually.

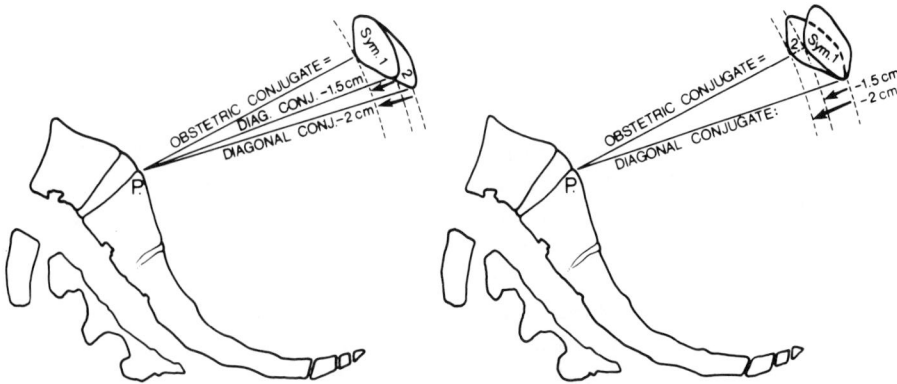

Fig. 11–11. Variations in length of diagonal conjugate dependent on height and inclination of the symphysis pubis. (P = sacral promontory; Sym = symphysis pubis.)

aminer's fingers are unusually long, the perineum forcibly indented by the knuckles of the examiner's third and fourth fingers. The index and the second fingers, held firmly together, are carried up and over the anterior surface of the sacrum. By sharply depressing the wrist, the promontory may be felt by the tip of the second finger as a projecting bony margin. With the finger closely applied to the most prominent portion of the upper sacrum, the vaginal hand is elevated until it contacts the pubic arch; and the immediately adjacent point on the index finger is marked, as shown in Figure 11–9. The hand is withdrawn, and the distance between the mark and the tip of the second finger is measured. Because measurement using a pelvimeter often introduces an error of 0.5 to 1 cm, it is better to employ a rigid measuring scale attached to the wall, as shown in Figure 11–10. The diagonal conjugate is determined, and the obstetrical conjugate is computed by subtracting 1.5 to 2.0 cm, depending upon the height and inclination of the symphysis pubis, as illustrated in Figure 11–11. If the diagonal conjugate is greater than 11.5 cm, it is justifiable to assume that the pelvic inlet is of adequate size for vaginal delivery of a normal-sized fetus.

Objection to measurement of the diagonal conjugate is sometimes raised on the basis that it is painful to the patient. This discomfort can be minimized if the examination is properly performed and if it is deferred until the latter half of pregnancy, when the vagina and perineum are more distensible.

Transverse contraction of the inlet can be measured only by imaging pelvimetry (discussed later in the chapter). Such a contraction is possible even in the presence of an adequate anteroposterior diameter.

Engagement. Engagement refers to the descent of the biparietal plane of the fetal head to a level below that of the pelvic inlet (Figs. 11–12 and 11–13). When the biparietal, or largest, diameter of the normally flexed fetal head has passed through the inlet, the head is engaged. Although engagement of the fetal head usually is regarded as a phenomenon of labor (and is discussed later in that connection), in nulliparas it commonly oc-

curs during the last few weeks of pregnancy. When it does so, it is confirmatory evidence that the pelvic inlet is adequate for that fetal head. **With engagement, the fetal head serves as an internal pelvimeter to demonstrate that the pelvic inlet is ample for that fetus.**

Whether the head is engaged may be ascertained by rectal or vaginal examination or by abdominal palpation. After gaining experience with vaginal examination, it becomes relatively easy to locate the station of the lowermost part of the fetal head in relation to the level of the ischial spines. If the lowest part of the occiput is at or below the level of the spines, the head usually, but not always, is engaged, because the distance from the plane of the pelvic inlet to the level of the ischial spines is approximately 5 cm in most pelves, and the distance from the biparietal plane of the unmolded fetal head to the vertex is about 3 to 4 cm. Under these circumstances, the vertex cannot possibly reach the level of the spines unless the biparietal diameter has passed the inlet, or unless there has been considerable elongation of

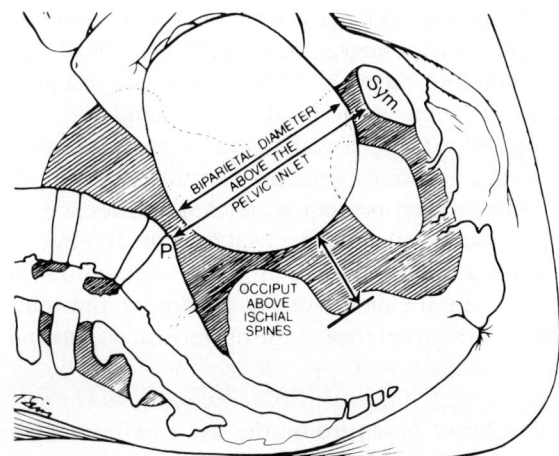

After Schlossberg

Fig. 11–12. When the lowermost portion of the fetal head is above the ischial spines, the biparietal diameter of the head is not likely to have passed through the pelvic inlet and therefore is not engaged. (P = sacral promontory; Sym = symphysis pubis.)

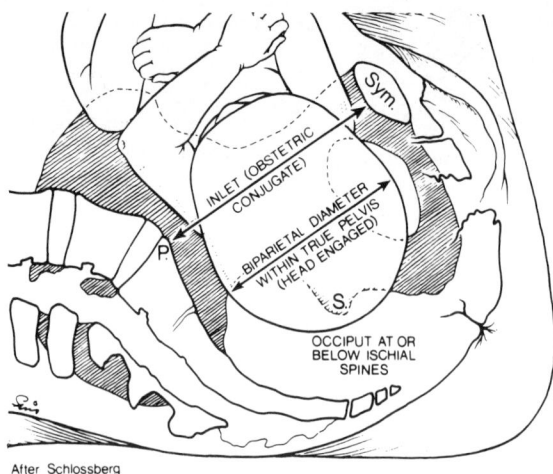

After Schlossberg

Fig. 11–13. When the lowermost portion of the fetal head is at or below the ischial spines, it is usually engaged. Exceptions occur when there is considerable molding, caput formation, or both. (P = sacral promontory; S = ischial spine; Sym = symphysis pubis.)

the fetal head because of molding and formation of a caput succedaneum (see Chap. 13, p. 368).

Engagement may be ascertained less satisfactorily by abdominal examination. If the biparietal plane of a term-sized infant has descended through the inlet, the examining fingers cannot reach the lowermost part of the head. Thus, when pushed downward over the lower abdomen, the examining fingers will slide over that portion of the head proximal to the biparietal plane (nape of the neck) and diverge. Conversely, if the head is not engaged, the examining fingers can easily palpate the lower part of the head and will converge (the fourth Leopold maneuver, Chap. 10, p. 277).

Fixation of the fetal head is its descent through the pelvic inlet to a depth that prevents its free movement in any direction when pushed by both hands placed over the lower abdomen. Fixation is not necessarily synonymous with engagement. Although a head that is freely movable on abdominal examination cannot be engaged, fixation of the head is sometimes seen when the biparietal plane is still 1 cm or more above the pelvic inlet, especially if the head is molded appreciably.

Although engagement is conclusive evidence of an adequate pelvic inlet for that fetal head, its absence is by no means always indicative of pelvic contraction. Nevertheless, the incidence of contraction of the inlet is higher in this group than in the obstetrical population at large.

Pelvic Outlet Measurements. An important dimension of the pelvic outlet that is accessible for clinical measurement is the diameter between the ischial tuberosities, variously called the *biischial diameter, intertuberous diameter,* and *transverse diameter of the outlet.* A measurement of over 8 cm is considered normal. The

measurement of the transverse diameter of the outlet can be estimated by placing a closed fist against the perineum between the ischial tuberosities, after first measuring the width of the closed fist (Fig. 11–14). Usually the closed fist is wider than 8 cm. The shape of the subpubic arch also can be evaluated at the same time by palpating the pubic rami from the subpubic region toward the ischial tuberosities.

Midpelvis Estimation. Clinical estimation of midpelvis capacity by any direct form of measurement is not possible. If the ischial spines are quite prominent, the sidewalls are felt to converge, and the concavity of the sacrum is very shallow; if the biischial diameter of the outlet is less than 8 cm (Chap. 21, p. 525), suspicion is aroused about a contraction in this region. Unfortunately, the midpelvis can be measured precisely only by using imaging studies.

Imaging Pelvimetry: X-ray, Computed Tomography, Ultrasound, and Magnetic Resonance

X-ray Pelvimetry

Status of X-ray Pelvimetry. The prognosis for successful vaginal delivery in any given pregnancy cannot be established on the basis of x-ray pelvimetry alone because the pelvic capacity is but one of several factors that determine the outcome. As enumerated by Mengert (1948), there are at least five factors concerned: (1) size and shape of the bony pelvis, (2) size of the fetal head, (3) force of the uterine contractions, (4) moldability of the fetal head, and (5) presentation and position of the

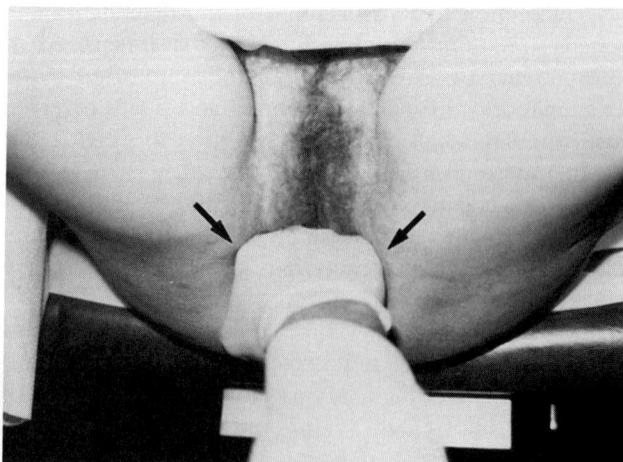

Fig. 11–14. Measurement of the biischial diameter. The distance across the top of a closed fist can be measured, and this can be used as a frame of reference to estimate the distance between the ischial tuberosities (*arrows*).

fetus. Only the first of these factors is amenable to reasonably precise radiographic measurement, and it is possible to eliminate only this one factor from the category of the unknown. Today x-ray pelvimetry no longer is considered necessary in the management of a labor with a cephalic fetal presentation in which the mother is suspected of having a contracted pelvis. If vaginal delivery is anticipated for a fetus presenting as a breech, however, x-ray pelvimetry still is used in many medical centers, including our own (see Chap. 20, p. 494 and Chap. 25, p. 578).

X-ray pelvimetry has the following advantages over manual estimation of pelvic size:

1. It can provide mensuration to a degree of precision unobtainable clinically. The clinical importance of such precision becomes evident when the shortcomings of the diagonal conjugate measurement are considered. When the diagonal conjugate exceeds 11.5 cm, the anteroposterior dimension of the inlet (the obstetrical conjugate) very rarely is contracted. When the diagonal conjugate is under 11.5, however, it is not always a reliable index of the obstetrical conjugate because the difference between these two diameters, usually about 1.5 cm, may range from less than 1 to more than 2 cm. For example, two women may have diagonal conjugates of 10.5 cm, but in one the obstetrical conjugate may be 10.2 cm, whereas in the other it may be 8.2 cm. Such information may prove critical during a breech delivery.
2. It can provide exact mensuration of two important diameters not otherwise obtainable, namely, the transverse diameter of the inlet and the interischial spinous diameter (transverse diameter of the midpelvis).

Indications for X-ray Pelvimetry. Because of the expense involved, as well as *potential* radiation hazards (Table 11–1), radiographic pelvic measurement is not necessary in the great majority of cases (Barton and co-workers, 1982; Laube and associates, 1981; Parsons and Spellacy, 1985). There are, however, certain clinical circumstances in which x-ray pelvimetry is a part of good obstetrical practice. One is the woman with a previous injury or disease likely to affect the bony pelvis. Another is in the case of a breech presentation when vaginal delivery is anticipated.

Before obtaining x-ray or other types of imaging pelvimetry, it is essential to ask two important questions. First, is the information to be obtained likely to affect the subsequent management of labor and delivery? If cesarean delivery almost certainly is going to be performed regardless of the radiographic information, the use of x-ray pelvimetry is difficult to justify. Second, are other types of imaging techniques available for pelvimetry measurements that can give similar results with lower or no radiation exposure?

TABLE 11–1. CHILDHOOD LEUKEMIA FOLLOWING ANTEPARTUM X-RAYS

Year	Author	Relative Risk	P Value
1958	Kaplan	1.37	NS
1958	Stewart and associates	2.00	< 0.05
1959	Murray and co-workers	1.00	NS
1959	Ford and colleagues	1.66	< 0.05
1959	Polhemus and Koch	1.34	< 0.05
1960	Court-Brown and cohorts	0.86	NS
1960	Lewis	0.42	NS
1961	Wells and Steer	0.72	NS
1962	MacMahon	1.52	< 0.05
1964	Gunz and Atkinson	1.13	NS
1965	Ager and associates	1.21	NS
1972	Bross and Natarajan	1.40	< 0.05
1973	Diamond and colleagues	2.81	< 0.05
1975	Bithell and Stewart	1.41	< 0.05
1975	Oppenheim and co-authors	1.73	NS
1985	Harvey and co-workers	2.40	< 0.05
1990	Magnani and associates	1.10 and 2.40	NS

NS = not statistically significant.
Adapted from Klapholz (1983).

Hazards of Diagnostic Radiation. An increasing awareness of the potential hazards of radiation has focused attention on the true value of diagnostic x-rays in obstetrics, as compared with the potential damage to the mother, her fetus, and future generations (see also Chap. 43). The recognized dangers to the fetus from diagnostic radiation are death, mental retardation, microcephaly, germ cell mutations, and increased risk of malignancy later in life. There is no proof that any diagnostic radiation before 8 weeks and after 25 weeks' gestation will result in fetal death, mental retardation, or central nervous system damage (Committee on Biological Effects, 1990). There is, however, an increased risk of microcephaly and severe mental retardation associated with high-dose radiation exposure between 8 and 25 weeks' gestation. The risk appears to be greatest between 8 to 15 weeks' gestation and likely is a nonthreshold linear function of the dose absorbed by the fetus. For example, the incidence of severe mental retardation between 8 and 15 weeks increases with radiation exposure as follows: 4 percent at 0.1 Gy, 20 percent at 0.5 Gy, 40 percent at 1 Gy, and 60 percent at 1.5 Gy (Committee on Biological Effects, 1990; Hall, 1991). Between 8 and 15 weeks' gestation, because of the nonthreshold relationship, even very small doses of radiation may increase the risk of mental retardation compared with the general population (Hall, 1991). Larger doses are necessary between 16 to 25 weeks to cause the same degree of mental retardation. Still many, but not all, geneticists and radiobiologists believe, on the basis of animal experimentation, that the only entirely safe dose of irradiation is zero (Gaulden, 1974).

The possibility of childhood malignancy was raised by Stewart and associates (1956), who identified an increased incidence of leukemia in children of women x-rayed during pregnancy. Since then, there have been several other reports supportive of the thesis that diagnostic radiation absorbed by the fetus increases the risk of subsequent development of leukemia and other malignancies (Table 11–1). A comparison made by Brent (1974) of the apparent risk of leukemia developing in various risk groups is presented in Table 11–2. He showed a relative risk of 1.5 for leukemia developing in children exposed to x-ray pelvimetry. Oppenheim and associates (1975) emphasized, however, that increased morbidity and mortality have not been identified uniformly among children exposed prenatally to diagnostic x-rays. If the mother underwent examination because of a medical indication, there was increased morbidity and mortality in the offspring, compared to that found in offspring of healthy women in whom irradiation was for pelvimetry. Finally, the risk of childhood malignancy may also be the consequence of other antenatal factors, such as maternal cigarette smoking or narcotic analgesics, and postnatal factors such as viral infections (Magnani and associates, 1990; McKinney and associates, 1987; Stjernfeldt and co-workers, 1986).

Certainly not all investigators have reported a risk of leukemia developing in children whose mothers were x-rayed antepartum (Table 11–1). **The slight risk from x-ray pelvimetry, however, seems justifiable whenever information critical to the welfare of the fetus or mother is likely to be obtained.**

The concept that x-ray pelvimetry should be limited has been endorsed by the American College of Radiology (1979) and the American College of Obstetricians and Gynecologists (1979). The Bureau of Radiological Health of the Food and Drug Administration (U.S. Department of Health and Human Resources, 1980) convened a panel composed of radiologists and obstetricians to examine available information on x-ray pelvimetry. A statement concerning the uses of such x-rays was developed and unanimously endorsed by the panel. The statement adopted by the American College of Radiology (1979) is:

Pelvimetry is not usually necessary or helpful in making the decision to perform a cesarean section. Therefore, pelvimetry should be performed only when the physician caring for the patient feels that pelvimetry will contribute to the decisions concerning diagnosis or treatment. In those few instances, the reason for requesting the pelvimetry should be written on the patient's chart. This statement does not apply to x-ray examinations for purposes other than measurement of the pelvis.

The following statement by the American College of Obstetricians and Gynecologists (1979) was published in the *ACOG Newsletter:*

X-ray pelvimetry provides limited additional information to physicians involved in the management of labor and delivery. It should not be a prerequisite to clinical decisions concerning obstetrical management. Reasons for requesting x-ray pelvimetry should be individually established.

Other X-ray Examinations. Not only have recommendations been made to limit x-ray pelvimetry exposure, but similar advice has been given to limit diagnostic radiation exposure to the pelvis of any woman at any time in the childbearing years. As emphasized by Brent (1987, 1989), radiation exposure of less than 0.5 Gy, except for carcinogenesis, likely represents no measurable risk to the conceptus, especially late in pregnancy (see Chap. 43).

Computed Tomographic Scanning

Status of Computed Tomography. Because of the small but *potential* risk of childhood malignancy discussed above, digital radiographs obtained with computed tomographic scanners have been used to measure pelvic diameters in attempts to reduce radiation exposure. The International Commission on Radiological Protection recommended that the radiation dose to the fetus not exceed 0.01 Gy during pregnancy (Reekie and colleagues, 1967). With conventional x-ray pelvimetry, the mean gonadal exposure is estimated to be 0.00885 ± 0.00111 Gy by the Committee on Radiological Hazards to Patients (Osborn, 1963). Thus, even without additional x-ray views, the average radiation dose approaches the 0.01 Gy value. These doses likely are lower today utilizing newer machines and shorter exposure times (Twickler and associates, 1992).

Federle and associates (1982) reported that adequate images of the bony pelvis could be obtained utilizing anteroposterior and lateral digital radiographs in a tomogram machine with an average absorbed dose of 0.00022 Gy each, and a single computed tomograph at the level of the ischial spines with an average absorbed dose of 0.0038 Gy. This has since been confirmed by others (Claussen and co-workers, 1985; Gimovsky and

TABLE 11–2. RISK OF CHILDHOOD LEUKEMIA AFTER IN UTERO RADIATION EXPOSURE BY PELVIMETRY

Risk Category	Approximate Risk, First 10 Years	Relative Risk
White children, United States (control)	1 : 2800	1
Exposure in utero to x-ray pelvimetry	1 : 2000	1.5
Siblings of leukemic children	1 : 710	4
Identical twin of leukemic child	1 : 3	1000

Adapted from Brent (1974).

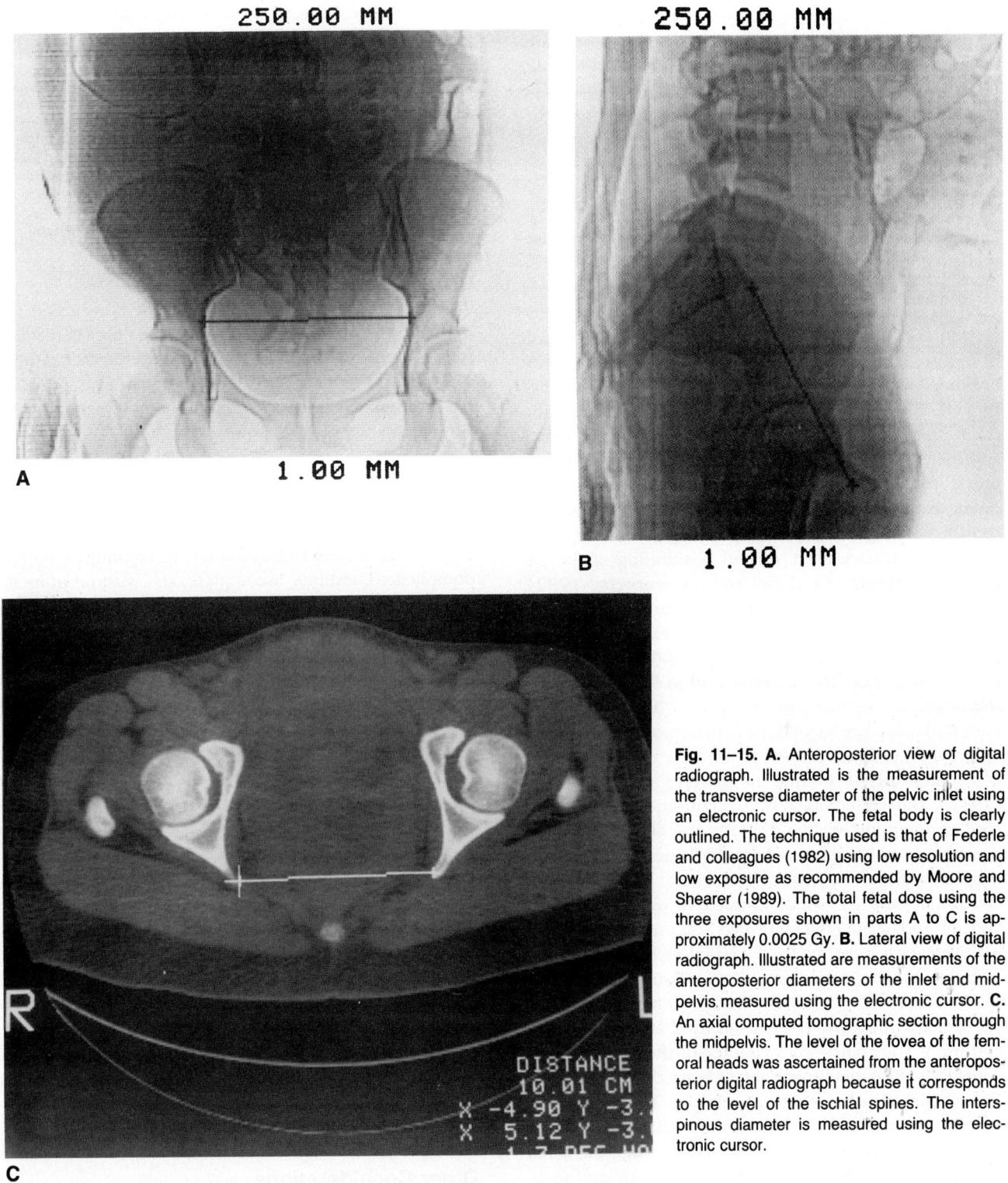

Fig. 11–15. A. Anteroposterior view of digital radiograph. Illustrated is the measurement of the transverse diameter of the pelvic inlet using an electronic cursor. The fetal body is clearly outlined. The technique used is that of Federle and colleagues (1982) using low resolution and low exposure as recommended by Moore and Shearer (1989). The total fetal dose using the three exposures shown in parts A to C is approximately 0.0025 Gy. **B.** Lateral view of digital radiograph. Illustrated are measurements of the anteroposterior diameters of the inlet and midpelvis measured using the electronic cursor. **C.** An axial computed tomographic section through the midpelvis. The level of the fovea of the femoral heads was ascertained from the anteroposterior digital radiograph because it corresponds to the level of the ischial spines. The interspinous diameter is measured using the electronic cursor.

associates, 1985; Kopelman and co-workers, 1986; Lenke and Shuman, 1986). Adam and associates (1985) reported that two digital radiographs (anteroposterior and lateral views) usually are sufficient to measure the necessary pelvic diameters, including the interspinous, provided appropriate corrections are made. Moore and Shearer (1989) maintain that adequate pelvimetry can be obtained with a fetal dose of only 0.0025 Gy.

Despite these claims of low-dose exposures, newer tomography equipment often emits higher doses of ionizing radiation for an equivalent study (Twickler and associates, 1992). Additionally, exposure of the fetus is dependent upon maternal thickness, fetal size and position, distance from the radiation source, and time of exposure to name but a few factors (Twickler and colleagues, 1992). Thus, fetal exposure can vary from

0.0025 to 0.015 Gy with computed tomography pelvimetry, depending upon the method used (Moore and Shearer, 1989). Each radiology department likely should calculate expected fetal exposure based upon their type machine and the technique used. Based upon this information, the obstetrician then can make an informed decision concerning the use the service offered.

Technique for Computed Tomographic Pelvimetry. Digital views are obtained for anteroposterior and lateral projections, and a single axial tomogram also is obtained at the level of the fovea of the femoral heads, a level accurately selected from the anteroposterior projection (Federle and associates, 1982). In this projection, the fetus presenting as a breech also can be evaluated for hyperextension of the head and the type of breech. Electronic calipers are used to measure the transverse diameter of the inlet (anteroposterior view) and the anteroposterior diameters of the inlet and midpelvis from the lateral view (Fig. 11–15). There is little or no distortion or magnification as long as the patient remains at the center of the table. Thus, when the electronic calipers are used, careful positioning of the patient is essential (Federle and co-workers, 1982). Maternal movement is kept at a minimum because maternal or fetal movement may cause artifacts (Brody and associates, 1986). The digital radiograph at the level of the ischial spines can be eliminated in some cases and the interspinous diameter measured when appropriate compensations are made for distortion, as described by Adam and colleagues (1985).

Using the technique of Federle and associates (1982), and employing low resolution and low exposure as recommended by Moore and Shearer (1989), computed tomographic pelvimetry is performed in our hospital with a fetal exposure of approximately 0.0025 Gy. Briefly, the technique consists of obtaining lateral and anterior scout (digital) views and one axial section. All three views are made at 120 kilovolts (peak). The lateral scout film is made at 70 mA, 75 mm per sec, and the anteroposterior view is made at 40 mA, 75 mm per sec. Finally, the axial view is obtained at 20 mA, 2 sec (40 mA). The transverse diameter of the inlet and the anteroposterior diameters are measured directly from the images with electronic calipers (Fig. 11–15A and B). In order to measure the interspinous diameter (Figure 11–15C), an axial section is obtained through the fovea of the femoral heads as described by Federle and associates (1982).

Advantages of Computed Tomographic Pelvimetry. The obvious advantage of this technique is a reduction in radiation exposure, with a range of 0.00044 Gy (Adam and associates, 1985) to 0.00425 Gy (Federle and co-workers, 1982). The accuracy is greater than conventional x-ray pelvimetry, and it is easier to perform (Adam and associates, 1985; Gimovsky and co-workers, 1985;

TABLE 11–3. NORMAL MEASUREMENTS FOR COMPUTED TOMOGRAPHIC PELVIMETRY

Plane	Diameters (cm)[a]	
	Anterior–Posterior	Transverse
Inlet	10.5	11.5
Midpelvis	11.5	10.0

[a] All normal values are equal to or exceed these measurements.
Modified from Collea and associates (1980).

Twickler and colleagues, 1992). Depending upon the machine and technique employed, fetal doses may range from 0.0025 to 0.015 Gy (Moore and Shearer, 1989). The cost is comparable to conventional x-ray pelvimetry. Normal values for inlet and midpelvis diameters are listed in Table 11–3.

Ultrasound. Despite the significant advances in obstetrics achieved with the use of diagnostic ultrasound, accurate measurement of maternal pelvic diameters has not been achieved. Unfortunately, all techniques remain complicated, tedious, incomplete, and without immediate clinical utility (Nakano, 1981; Nakano and co-workers, 1977). Morgan and Thurnau (1988) described a *fetal-pelvic index* calculated from x-ray and ultrasonically derived measurements. Although they reported that the use of this index was helpful in predicting cephalopelvic disproportion with fetuses weighing more than 4000 g, their observations remain to be confirmed, as does their report that the index is useful in women attempting vaginal birth after a previous cesarean delivery (Thurnau and colleagues, 1991).

Magnetic Resonance Imaging. The advantages of magnetic resonance imaging include the lack of ionizing radiation, accurate pelvic measurements, and complete imaging of the fetus, as well as providing the potential for evaluating reasons for soft tissue dystocia (McCarthy, 1986; Stark and co-workers, 1985). Currently this methodology is limited because of expense, time involved for adequate imaging studies, and availability of equipment. At least for now, this new and promising technology is experimental.

Other Considerations

Because of their limited clinical applicability, previously presented discussions of the pelvis of the newborn, sexual differences in the adult pelvis, and transformation of the fetal into the adult pelvis are not included in the 19th edition of Williams Obstetrics. These topics have been covered extensively in previous editions, and the interested reader is referred to the 17th edition, Chapter 11, page 231.

References

Abramson D, Roberts SM, Wilson PD: Relaxation of the pelvic joints in pregnancy. Surg Obstet Gynecol 58:595, 1934

Adam PH, Alberge AY, Castellano S, Kassab M, Escude B: Pelvimetry by digital radiography. Clin Radiol 36:327, 1985

Ager EA, Schuman LM, Wallace HM, Rosenfeld AB, Gullen WH: An epidemiological study of childhood leukemia. J Chronic Dis 18:113, 1965

American College of Obstetricians and Gynecologists: ACOG Bull 23:10, 1979

American College of Radiology: ACR Bull 35:2, 1979

Barton JJ, Garbaciak JA Jr, Ryan GM: The efficacy of x-ray pelvimetry. Am J Obstet Gynecol 143:304, 1982

Bithell J, Stewart A: Prenatal irradiation and childhood malignancy: A review of British data from the Oxford Survey. Br J Cancer 31:271, 1975

Borell U, Fernstrom I: Movements at the sacroiliac joints and their importance to changes in pelvic dimensions during parturition. Acta Obstet Gynecol Scand 36:42, 1957

Brent RL: Comment on editorial. J Reprod Med 12:6, 1974

Brent RL: Ionizing radiation. Contemp Obstet Gynecol 30:20, 1987

Brent RL: The effect of embryonic and fetal exposure to x-ray, microwaves, and ultrasound: Counseling the pregnant and nonpregnant patient about these risks. Semin Oncol 16:347, 1989

Brody AS, Saks BJ, Field DR, Skinner SR, Capra RE: Artifacts seen during CT pelvimetry: Implications for digital systems with scanning beams. Radiology 160:269, 1986

Bross IDJ, Natarajan N: Leukemia from low level radiation. N Engl J Med 287:107, 1972

Budin RC: X-radiography of a Naegele pelvis. Obstetrique Par 2:499, 1897

Caldwell WE, Moloy HC: Anatomical variations in the female pelvis and their effect in labor with a suggested classification. Am J Obstet Gynecol 26:479, 1933

Caldwell WE, Moloy HC, D'Esopo DA: Further studies on the pelvic architecture. Am J Obstet Gynecol 28:482, 1934

Caldwell WE, Moloy HC, Swenson PC: The use of the roentgen ray in obstetrics, I. Roentgen pelvimetry and cephalometry; technic of pelviroentgenography. Am J Roentgenol 41:305, 1939

Claussen C, Köhler D, Christ F, Golde G, Lochner B: Pelvimetry by digital radiography and its dosimetry. J Perinat Med 13:287, 1985

Collea JV, Chein C, Quilligan EJ: The randomized management of term frank breech presentation: A study of 208 cases. Am J Obstet Gynecol 137:235, 1980

Committee on Biological Effects of Ionizing Radiation, National Research Council: Other somatic and fetal effects. In Beir V (ed): Effects of Exposure to Low Levels of Ionizing Radiation. Washington, DC, National Academy Press, 1990

Court-Brown WM, Doll R, Hill AB: Incidence of leukaemia after exposure to diagnostic x-ray in utero. Br Med J 2:1539, 1960

Diamond EL, Schmerler H, Lilienfeld AM: The relationship of intrauterine radiation to subsequent mortality and development of leukemia in children (a prospective study). Am J Epidemiol 97:283, 1973

Federle MP, Cohen HA, Rosenwein MF, Brant-Zawadzki MN,

Cann CE: Pelvimetry by digital radiography: A low-dose examination. Radiology 143:733, 1982

Ford DD, Paterson JCS, Treuting WL: Fetal exposure to diagnostic x-rays and leukemia and other malignant disease in childhood. JNCI 22:1903, 1959

Gardosi J, Hutson N, Lynch CB: Randomised, controlled trial of squatting in the second stage of labour. Lancet 2:74, 1989

Gaulden ME: Possible effects of diagnostic x-rays on the human embryo and fetus. J Arkansas Med Soc 70:424, 1974

Gimovsky ML, Willard K, Neglio M, Howard T, Zerne S: X-ray pelvimetry in a breech protocol: A comparison of digital radiography and conventional methods. Am J Obstet Gynecol 153:887, 1985

Gunz FW, Atkinson HR: Medical radiations and leukaemia: A retrospective survey. Br Med J 1:389, 1964

Hall EJ: Scientific view of low-level radiation risks. Radiographics 11:509, 1991

Harvey EB, Boice JD, Honeyman M, Flannery JT: Prenatal x-ray exposure and childhood cancer in twins. N Engl J Med 312:541, 1985

Kaplan HS: An evaluation of the somatic and genetic hazards of the medical uses of radiation. Am J Roentgenol Radium Ther Nucl 80:696, 1958

Klapholz H: Evaluation of fetopelvic relationships. In Cohen WR, Friedman EA (eds): Management of Labor. Baltimore, University Park Press, 1983, p 33

Kopelman JN, Duff P, Karl RT, Schipul AH, Read JA: Computed tomographic pelvimetry in the evaluation of breech presentation. Obstet Gynecol 68:455, 1986

Laube DW, Varner MW, Cruikshank DP: A prospective evaluation of x-ray pelvimetry. JAMA 246:2187, 1981

Lenke RR, Shuman WP: Computed tomographic pelvimetry. J Reprod Med 31:958, 1986

Lewis TLT: Leukaemia in childhood after antenatal exposure to x-rays (a survey at Queen Charlotte's Hospital). Br Med J 2:1551, 1960

MacMahon B: Prenatal x-ray exposure and childhood cancer. JNCI 28:1173, 1962

McCarthy S: Magnetic resonance imaging in obstetrics and gynecology. Magn Reson Imaging 4:59, 1986

McKinney PA, Cartwright RA, Saiu JMT, Mann JR, Stiller CA, Draper GJ, Harley AL, Hopton PA, Birch JM, Waterhouse JAH, Johnston HE: The interregional epidemiological study of childhood cancer (IRESCC): A case control study of aetiological factors in leukaemia and lymphoma. Arch Dis Child 62:279, 1987

Magnani C, Pastor G, Luzzatto L, Terracini B: Parental occupation and other environmental factors in the etiology of leukemias and non-Hodgkin's lymphomas in childhood: A case-control study. Tumori 76:413, 1990

Mengert WF: Estimation of pelvic capacity. JAMA 138:169, 1948

Moore MM, Shearer DR: Fetal dose estimates for CT pelvimetry. Radiology 171:265, 1989

Morgan MA, Thurneau GR: Efficacy of the fetal-pelvic index for delivery of neonates weighing 4000 grams or greater: A preliminary report. Am J Obstet Gynecol 158:1133, 1988

Murray R, Heckel P, Hempelmann LH: Leukemia in children exposed to ionizing radiation. N Engl J Med 261:585, 1959

Nakano H: Assessment of dystocia pelvis by ultrasound pelvimetry. Acta Obstet Gynaecol Jpn 7:1077, 1981

Nakano H, Koyanagi T, Nii F, Kumano Y, Kubota S, Sakamoto C,

Taki I: Study on the female pelvis by ultrasonic tomography. Acta Obstet Gynaecol Jpn 29:431, 1977

Oppenheim BE, Briem ML, Meier P: The effects of diagnostic x-ray exposure on the human fetus: An examination of the evidence. Radiology 114:529, 1975

Osborn SB: The implications of the Committee on Radiological Hazards to Patients (Adrian Committee), I. Variations in the radiation dose received by the patient in diagnostic radiology. Br J Radiol 36:230, 1963

Parsons MT, Spellacy WN: Prospective randomized study of x-ray pelvimetry in the primigravida. Obstet Gynecol 66:76, 1985

Polhemus DW, Koch R: Leukemia and medical radiation. Pediatrics 23:453, 1959

Reekie D, Davison M, Davidson JK: The radiation hazard in radiography of the female abdomen and pelvis. Br J Radiol 40:849, 1967

Russell JGB: Moulding of the pelvic outlet. J Obstet Gynaecol Br Commonw 76:817, 1969

Russell JGB: The rationale of primitive delivery positions. Br J Obstet Gynaecol 89:712, 1982

Spalteholz: Hand Atlas of Human Anatomy, Vol I. Philadelphia, Lippincott, 1933

Stark DD, McCarthy SM, Filly RA, Parer JT, Hricak H, Callen PW: Pelvimetry by magnetic resonance imaging. Am J Radiol 144:947, 1985

Stewart A, Webb J, Giles D, Hewitt D: Malignant disease in childhood and diagnostic irradiation in utero. Lancet 2:447, 1956

Stewart A, Webb J, Hewitt D: A survey of childhood malignancies. Br Med J 1:1495, 1958

Stjernfeldt M, Berglund K, Lindsten J, Ludvigsson J: Maternal smoking during pregnancy and risk of childhood cancer. Lancet 1:1350, 1986

Thurnau GR, Scates DH, Morgan MA: The fetal–pelvic index: A method of identifying fetal–pelvic disproportion in women attempting vaginal birth after previous cesarean delivery. Am J Obstet Gynecol 165:353, 1991

Twickler DM, Clarke G, Cunningham FG: Diagnostic imaging in pregnancy. Williams Obstetrics, 18 ed (suppl 18). Norwalk, CT, Appleton & Lange, June/July 1992

US Department of Health and Human Resources: The selection of patients for x-ray examinations: The pelvimetry examination. HHS pub (FDA) 80:8128, July 1980

Wells J, Steer CM: Relationship of leukemia in children to abdominal radiation of mothers during pregnancy. Am J Obstet Gynecol 81:1059, 1961

◼ SECTION IV ◼

Normal Labor and Delivery and the Puerperium

◼

CHAPTER 12

Parturition: Biomolecular and Physiologic Processes

PHYSIOLOGICAL AND BIOCHEMICAL PROCESSES

Overview and Definitions

Parturition: the act of bringing forth or being delivered of young; the act of giving birth; childbirth.
—*Webster's New Twentieth Century Dictionary, 1979*

Parturition, the bringing forth of young, encompasses all physiological processes involved in birthing: the prelude to, the preparation for, the process of, and the parturient's recovery from childbirth. This physiological description of the factors involved in parturition, however comprehensive, does not provide an answer to a fundamentally important question: **When does parturition begin?**

The mechanism(s) by which human parturition is initiated spontaneously, either at term or preterm, is not known. It is understandable, therefore, that a reasonable and lucid answer to this question is crucial to (1) the development of a logical parturition research agenda, (2) the selection of optimal clinical management strategies for preventing preterm birth, and (3) expediting communication among researchers and clinicians.

This query could be treated philosophically by proposing that parturition is initiated at the time of conception. And notwithstanding our wish to be reasonable and practical, there is merit in this position, even though it appears to be without discernible usefulness in deciphering the cause of spontaneous parturition at term or

that of preterm birth. Obviously, migration of the fertilized ovum to the uterine cavity and implantation of the blastocyst in the endometrium, rather than in some ectopic site, is essential for successful parturition. Hypertrophy of uterine smooth muscle cells is necessary for the generation of forceful contractions required to propel the fetus through the cervix and birth canal during labor and delivery. Even the proper orientation of the long axis of the fetus with the maternal pelvis is crucial for delivery. Nonetheless, we reject the notion that parturition begins at conception, because such a definition lacks clinical or research applicability in gaining a better understanding of parturition initiation.

At the same time, however, it must be emphasized that from the time of conception until late in gestation, successful parturition is dependent upon the systems that cause near-absolute myometrial contractile unresponsiveness. The uterus is inherently a contractile tissue. The uterine tranquility of pregnancy does not exist by default; rather this state is dependent upon highly activated biochemical processes. The contractile function of the uterus must be rendered unresponsive until fetal organs attain sufficient physiological maturity to enable the fetus to survive the transition to extrauterine life.

The question "When does parturition begin?" also could be addressed in a pragmatic fashion by proposing that parturition begins when labor begins. But this is a very narrow-sighted view. Clearly, the usefulness of this definition of the initiation of parturition is diminished by several realities. First, it is not possible to determine when labor begins. There is no objective method available to ascertain when, in the course of human pregnancy, effective myometrial contractions commence. In consequence, we are obliged to rely upon each woman's recollection of the time that labor "pains" were first perceived. Obviously, this approach is severely flawed. Second, the commencement of forceful labor is a continuum that involves a change from uterine contractures to painless contractions to the forceful contractions that cause labor "pains" (Nathanielsz, 1989). Third, selected modifications in uterine function must be effected before the coordinated myometrial contractions of successful labor are possible. At parturition, uterine preparedness precedes active labor in all pregnant mammals examined. Fourth, some of the biological and chemical findings at parturition are the consequences, indeed the sequelae, of labor. This causes confusion for the researcher; oftentimes cause-and-effect relationships cannot be distinguished. Parturition research has been plagued by this dilemma when the ill-defined onset of labor was taken as the initiation of parturition.

After pondering this question as to when parturition begins for many years, we regrettably conclude that there is no precise manner to establish a point in time when parturition is initiated in a given pregnancy. Nonetheless, we suggest that the initiation of parturition can be defined in an understandable way that is useful for clinical, research, and pharmacological purposes. The several sequential modifications of uterine function, which are obliged during pregnancy for successful parturition, must be recognized.

Beginning before implantation, a protracted period of incredible uterine quiescence follows; this prelude to parturition normally persists for the first 90 to 95 percent of gestation. There are multiple maternal physiological adaptations during this time, and key fetal organs mature. Many of the maternal physiological adaptations are crucial to successful parturition; and the maturation of key organ systems is mandated for the successful transition from fetal to extrauterine life.

At the end of this parturitional diapause, the uterus that was rendered highly unresponsive for the preceding 36 to 38 weeks must be awakened. The myometrium must be prepared for the generation of coordinated contractions of sufficient force to cause cervical dilatation and fetal descent that eventuates in childbirth. For this to happen, the cervix must be softened, ripened. The myometrial cells' capacity to regulate cytoplasmic Ca^{2+} concentrations must be restored; myometrial cell responsivity and intercellular communicability must be reinstituted. Then, labor can begin. For a time immediately after delivery, the myometrium must be held in a state of persistent contraction and retraction. This causes compression and thrombosis of the large uterine vessels, limiting uterine bleeding and preventing fatal postpartum hemorrhage. In the puerperium, the production of milk in maternal mammary glands, in an evolutionary sense, is crucial to the bringing forth of young; and finally, involution of the uterus, which restores this organ to the nonpregnant state, must be accomplished in preparation for the next pregnancy.

Uterine Phases of Parturition. As indicated above, an ordered sequence of diverse demands must be met by the myometrium and cervix for successful childbirth. Accordingly, the uterine parturitional process is divided into four functional states: phases 0, 1, 2, and 3. The divisions are made in recognition of the major uterine accommodations that characterize each parturitional phase and to define the morphological and functional transitions that must be made to progress in an orderly and timely manner from one phase to the next (Fig. 12–1).

Phase 0. Phase 0 is the prelude to parturition, the time of uterine smooth muscle contractile tranquility and cervical rigidity; this phase is normally maintained from before implantation until late in gestation. Phase 0 is established by harnessing the potential power of the uterus, by rendering this organ unresponsive to natural stimuli, and by imposing contractile paralysis against enormous mechanical and chemical challenges to empty its contents.

Phase 1. Phase 1 is the interval of uterine preparedness for labor when functional changes in myometrium and cervix, which are required for labor, are implemented. This phase is commonly identifiable clinically during the last days of pregnancy by distinctive signs: ripening of the cervix, increasing frequency of reasonably painless

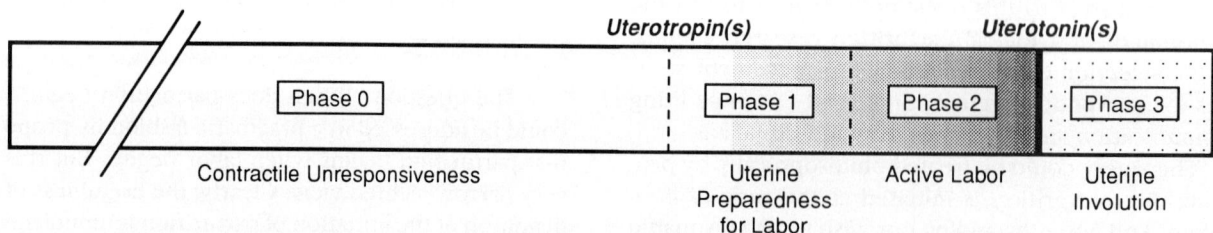

Fig. 12–1. The uterine phases of parturition. Phase 0: the prelude to parturition. Phase 1: uterine preparedness for labor. Phase 2: the process of active labor. Phase 3: parturient recovery from parturition.

uterine contractions, development of the lower uterine segment, and myometrial irritability. Phase 1 is dependent upon suspension of phase 0. Indeed, phase 1 may be the outcome of suspending phase 0. Similarly, phase 2 is dependent upon the completion of phase 1; phase 2 may be the outcome of phase 1 implementation.

Phase 2. Phase 2 is the period of *active labor,* that is, the uterine contractions that bring about progressive cervical dilatation, fetal descent, and delivery of the conceptus. This phase of parturition is customarily further divided into *the three stages of labor.*

Phase 3. During phase 3 parturient recovery takes place, which culminates in uterine involution and restored fertility. Four to 6 weeks are required to complete uterine recovery (involution); but the duration of phase 3 is dependent on the duration of breast feeding. Generally, so long as breast feeding is continued, infertility persists because of lactation-induced anovulation and amenorrhea.

The Initiation of Parturition: Definition. We choose to reject both the philosophical and the pragmatic approaches to defining the initiation of parturition in favor of a practical option:

The initiation of parturition is the transition from uterine phase 0 to phase 1 of parturition. This is the time late in pregnancy when uterine quiescence is suspended, enabling the recovery of the contractile competency of the uterus preparatory to labor.

According to this definition, the initiation of parturition and retreat from continued maintenance of uterine tranquility are synonymous (Fig. 12–2) (Casey and MacDonald, 1988a,c). But more than this, the suspension of uterine phase 0 may be the only impetus required to proceed through phase 1 into phase 2.

It is important to recognize, however, that by this definition, the initiation of parturition and the *"onset of labor,"* as the latter is customarily defined, are not synonymous and in fact are functionally distinct and separated in time. The commencement of phase 2 of parturition and the "onset of labor" are theoretically synonymous, but ill-defined in time, both clinically and physiologically. By defining the initiation of parturition as the transition from uterine phase 0 to phase 1, important physiological questions can be formulated more easily, and the sequence of the parturitional processes more clearly envisioned (Fig. 12–2).

Establishment of the Parturition Phases: Clinical and Biochemical Considerations. Whereas the "time" of the onset of labor cannot be identified, the absence of labor can be established. The absence of forceful contractions and the absence of cervical dilatation are easily determined. This permits the conclusion that uterine phase 2 of parturition has not begun. By fulfilling these criteria, the pregnancy must be either in uterine phase 1 or 0 of parturition. By clinical criteria alone, the transition from phase 0 to phase 1 can be suspected, but not conclusively established by current standards of clinical assessment. For research purposes, however, this may be an achievable goal. The functional changes of uterine phase 1 can be identified by morphological and biochemical criteria; thus, the precise sequence of the uterine changes of phase 1 can be ascertained. Moreover, it is reasonable to suspect that there may be an "early marker" and "later markers" of the uterine modifications that bring about the awakening of the uterus. At the very least, a specific research agenda for defining the processes involved the transition from phase 0 to phase 1—that is, in the initiation of parturition—can be set forth.

Is Labor Irreversible? By defining the initiation of parturition as the transition from uterine phase 0 to phase 1, we must consider the possibility that parturition, once initiated, may be a reversible process. We do not subscribe to the long-standing dictum that labor (phase 2 of parturition), once begun, inevitably proceeds to delivery. Perhaps this postulate was useful 40 or 50 years ago for support in clinical decision making, but not today. Clearly there are large numbers of pregnancies in which

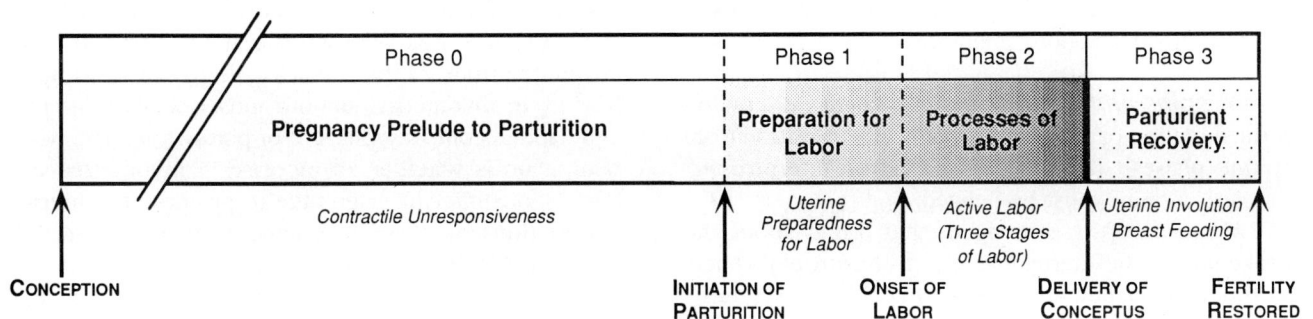

Fig. 12–2. The initiation of parturition and the "onset of labor."

uterine contractions (of sufficient force to cause cervical effacement and dilatation) begin and then cease. This is a relatively common occurrence preterm; and many of these pregnancies go undelivered with no specific pharmacological intervention. To argue that such pregnancies were not in labor, that is, not in uterine phase 2 of parturition, because delivery did not occur, is to define the parturitional process by default. This is a defensive posture that serves only to hide, not overcome, our ignorance. It cannot be ascertained as yet whether such pregnancies were complicated by some aberrant, unidentified process that caused the uterus to contract or whether the normal sequence of parturitional processes was initiated too early but ceased. Nonetheless, and for whatever reason that such episodes occur, this problem must not be ignored.

This issue is highly relevant to the processes involved in preterm labor. Many investigators find that upwards of two thirds of pregnancies believed to be complicated by preterm labor do not deliver when treated only with placebos. In these complicated pregnancies, many possibilities must be considered. The most common answer given is that such pregnancies were misdiagnosed and that preterm labor did not in fact exist. This analysis, however, provides an incomplete and unsatisfactory explanation for the myometrial contractions and cervical changes observed in such pregnancies.

Potential Cessation of Labor. It may be that parturition, when initiated by way of the ordered sequence normally involved in the spontaneous initiation of parturition, is an irreversible process both at term and preterm. If uterine phase 0 processes are suspended and set aside, labor and delivery may be the inevitable consequence. If, however, in response to extraneous factors, uterine phase 0 was only partly interrupted, the myometrial contractions that result may or may not be irreversible. For example, if Ca^{2+} extrusion mechanisms were critical for the maintenance of phase 0 and this capacity was temporarily impaired, but gap junctions did not develop and oxytocin receptors did not appear, myometrial contractions of sufficient force to cause cervical effacement and some dilatation may ensue. If the factor that precipitated this condition were removed and the myometrial cell Ca^{2+} extrusion system(s) were reactivated, contractions might cease.

Uterotropins and Uterotonins. To begin a discussion of the initiation of parturition, that is, the transition from uterine phase 0 to phase 1—the terms "uterotropin" and "uterotonin" must be defined.

A **uterotropin** is an agent that brings about the awakening of the uterus; namely, a uterotropin(s) acts on the myometrium and cervix to enable the synthesis of functional elements that prepare the uterine tissues for labor (Casey and MacDonald, 1988a). Phase 1 functional elements are those that facilitate myometrial contractile effectiveness (e.g., gap junctions and oxytocin receptors) and cervical softening. The transition from phase 0 to phase 1 necessitates the action of a uterotropin(s) that can effect the suspension of phase 0. Theoretically, a uterotropin can be produced in the myometrium or delivered by paracrine or endocrine mechanisms. A uterotropin may act by disabling phase 0 in a manner that is tantamount to the withdrawal of progesterone. The term "uterotropin" is not used to describe an agent that causes uterine growth, but neither is it intended to exclude substances that otherwise may be important in myometrial cell hypertrophy, such as sex steroid hormones or growth factors.

A **uterotonin** is a uterine smooth muscle contractant, such as oxytocin, prostaglandins, and endothelin-1. Uterotonins act directly on responsive myometrial smooth muscle cells to cause myometrial cell contraction. It is possible that a particular uterotonin, such as a prostaglandin, may also be a uterotropin. Some uterotonins can be formed in tissues within the uterus and act in an autocrine or paracrine manner; other uterotonins could be produced in extrauterine sites and act in an endocrine manner after delivery to the uterus through the maternal circulation (Casey and MacDonald, 1988b,c). Several uterotonins are produced as sequelae of labor; these uterotonins probably never reach the myometrium and are produced only coincidentally, that is, in tissue sites in which inflammation is a normal byproduct of labor.

Are Uterotonins Required for Parturition? The uterus is a smooth muscle tissue with an enormous inherent propensity to contract; therefore if the contractile unresponsiveness of phase 0 were suspended, does it follow that spontaneous contractions will commence? Is it possible that the discontinuation of uterine tranquility, in and of itself, is sufficient to effect not only uterine preparedness for labor, but also the commencement of myometrial contractions? Is phase 2 of parturition the inevitable outcome of the completion of phase 1?

Ca^{2+} Movement and Myometrial Cell Contraction. Perhaps this line of questioning is begging the obvious, but we think not. Clearly, an increase in the intracellular (cytoplasmic, free) Ca^{2+} concentration (abbreviated as $[Ca^{2+}]_i$) is essential for the generation of smooth muscle contractions. At the very least, therefore, a change in $[Ca^{2+}]_i$ in myometrial smooth muscle cells must precede and accompany phase 2 of parturition. The pertinent issue is whether an increase in myometrial cell $[Ca^{2+}]_i$ of sufficient magnitude to promote the uterine contractions of phase 2 is effected when phase 0 is suspended. It is possible that uterotonins are not required to induce myometrial contractions in the face of increased myometrial contractile responsiveness together with the development of contractile synchrony

through the formation of gap junctions. Alternatively, maximal contractile force may be dependent upon an increase in myometrial cell $[Ca^{2+}]_i$ achievable only by the action of uterotonins such as oxytocin, prostaglandins, or endothelin-1, even after phase 0 is discontinued.

Uterotonins and Ca^{2+} Movement. The uterotonins act to cause an increase in myometrial cell $[Ca^{2+}]_i$ by one or more of several signal transduction systems, presumably acting through the membrane receptor for that uterotonin.

OXYTOCIN. Oxytocin acts through a specific plasma membrane receptor(s) to stimulate phosphatidylinositol hydrolysis and thereby the formation of inositol phosphates. In turn, inositol phosphates cause the release of Ca^{2+} from intracellular stores. There is some evidence from in vitro studies that oxytocin acts to inhibit the plasma membrane Ca^{2+}-adenosinetriphosphatase (Ca^{2+}-ATPase) pump, which should allow entry of extracellular Ca^{2+} into the cell; but such an increase has not been demonstrable with intact cells. The synthesis of oxytocin receptors, which are required for oxytocin action, may be inhibited by the action of progesterone during phase 0 of parturition. The number of these receptors in the myometrium is increased during phase 1.

PROSTAGLANDINS. In strips of myometrial tissues obtained from the uteri of pregnant women, prostaglandin (PG)E_2 and $PGF_{2\alpha}$ are relatively ineffective in promoting an increase in myometrial cell $[Ca^{2+}]_i$ and in causing a contractile response (Word and co-workers, 1992). The uterotonic action of administered prostaglandins may be mediated indirectly. Extraordinary amounts of these agents are required to induce abortion or labor when administered intraamnionically.

ENDOTHELIN-1. Endothelin-1 acts to increase markedly the frequency of contractions in myometrial tissue strips obtained from the uteri of nonpregnant women. This action is mediated through an increase in $[Ca^{2+}]_i$ by the release of Ca^{2+} from intracellular stores and an influx of extracellular Ca^{2+} (Word and colleagues, 1990). Endothelin-1 is less effective in myometrial muscle tissue of pregnant women (Word and colleagues, 1992).

Myometrial Cell Ca^{2+} and Phase 0 of Parturition. The myometrium, during phase 0 of parturition, is generally less responsive to a variety of contractile stimuli, suggesting that the myometrial cell $[Ca^{2+}]_i$ is held more rigidly constant during this phase of parturition. The extracellular Ca^{2+} concentration (1 to 2 mM) is far greater (10,000-fold) than $[Ca^{2+}]_i$ ($\sim$100 to 120 nM). It is obvious, therefore that myometrial (and other) cells must be extraordinarily efficient in regulating Ca^{2+} entry into and extrusion from the cytoplasm of the cell. An increase in myometrial cell $[Ca^{2+}]_i$ from 100 to only about 500 nM will cause a maximal contractile response.

There are several potential mechanisms whereby $[Ca^{2+}]_i$ could be held constant at low levels during uterine phase 0 to prevent activation of contractile responses. One of the major means of regulating myometrial cell $[Ca^{2+}]_i$ is through the plasma membrane and sarcoplasmic reticulum calcium pumps, which are ATPase-dependent Ca^{2+}-extrusion systems. The plasma membrane Ca^{2+}-pump extrudes Ca^{2+} from the cell to the extracellular fluid; the sarcoplasmic reticulum Ca^{2+}-ATPase pump transports cytoplasmic Ca^{2+} to the sarcoplasmic reticulum wherein Ca^{2+} is sequestered, perhaps by a calcium-binding protein (e.g., calsequestrin) (reviewed by Broderick and Broderick, 1990). Increases in $[Ca^{2+}]_i$ can be effected by the mobilization of Ca^{2+} into the cytoplasm from the extracellular fluid or from sequestered stores in the sarcoplasmic reticulum. The concentration of Ca^{2+} in sarcoplasmic reticulum is similar to that in the extracellular space; and if released into the cytoplasm, there is sufficient Ca^{2+} to cause a maximal contractile response in some smooth muscle cells (reviewed by Carsten and Miller, 1990).

Other means of maintaining myometrial cell $[Ca^{2+}]_i$ at lower levels may involve putative intracellular Ca^{2+}-binding proteins (other than calmodulin, which is required for Ca^{2+} activation of myosin light chain kinase). Ca^{2+}-binding proteins could be localized in either the cytoplasm or sarcoplasmic reticulum of the myometrial cells.

It seems likely that the activities (capacities) of the Ca^{2+} pumps or the concentration of Ca^{2+}-sequestering proteins, or both, in myometrial cells are increased during uterine phase 0, possibly in response to the action of the sex steroid hormones (estrogen and progesterone), acting directly or indirectly.

Role of Uterotonins in Parturition

Ca^{2+} Movement and Phase 1 of Parturition. If the Ca^{2+}-ATPase pumps of the plasma membrane and sarcoplasmic reticulum are activated during uterine phase 0, it is possible that this increased Ca^{2+}-extrusion capability is abolished during the suspension of phase 0. Alternatively, if active sequestration of Ca^{2+} (e.g., by way of binding proteins) is effected during phase 0, the interruption of phase 0 may involve a decrease in the myometrial cell levels of such binders.

The importance of these possibilities is as follows: If uterine phase 1 of parturition includes increased myometrial cell contractile responsiveness because of relief from whatever mechanism(s) may be in place to reduce $[Ca^{2+}]_i$, then phase 2 of parturition is automatically instituted. On the other hand, if phase 1 of parturition does not include such a modification in contractile response, a uterotonin may be obliged to effect an increase in $[Ca^{2+}]_i$ of sufficient magnitude to cause the optimal myometrial force generation of uterine phase 2 of parturition.

But it also may be that both a decrease in Ca^{2+} extrusion and sequestration capacity and the action of a uterotonin are necessary to achieve the necessary $[Ca^{2+}]_i$. Teleologically, it seems that the most effective biological scheme for successful parturition would involve a system that promotes uterotonin formation as phase 1 is completed. The formation of uterotonins before the uterus is functionally prepared for labor is physiologically counterproductive unless these uterotonins masquerade as uterotropins in the face of an effective Ca^{2+} extrusion, sequestration, and binding system.

Increased Uterotonin Formation During Labor. There is no doubt that there is increased uterotonin formation during active labor. Presently, it is not possible to know the physiological meaning, if any, of the increase in uterotonins at labor for two reasons. First, there is no evidence that an increase in the formation of any uterotonin precedes the onset of phase 2 (even as active labor is customarily defined), let alone precedes or accompanies the initiation of parturition, the transition from phase 0 to phase 1. Second, a number of uterotonins are produced as sequelae of labor. Inflammatory responses obliged by anatomical changes in fetal membranes and decidua (in the formation of the forebag compartment of the amnionic fluid) result in uterotonin formation; but these uterotonins are produced coincidental to labor and are not available to the myometrium. This coincidental production of uterotonins is so great, however, as to mask the putative synthesis of uterotonins functionally available to the myometrium.

Heretofore evidence for increased uterotonin formation during labor has come from measurements of known uterotonins in amnionic fluid, blood, or urine. These include prostaglandins, oxytocin, platelet-activating factor (PAF), and endothelin-1. As we will describe, the uterotonins in these biological fluids may have arisen primarily as the consequence of sequelae of the labor process and were never accessible to the myometrium.

Induction of Uterotonin Formation by Myometrial Contractions. The formation of uterotonins directly in myometrium or decidua is an attractive alternative whereby uterotonins may participate in phase 2 of parturition. Uterotonins produced in these tissue sites may not enter amnionic fluid and may constitute a very small fraction of the total uterotonin pool in blood. As stated, changes in myometrial cell contractile responsiveness during phase 1 may lead to an increase in $[Ca^{2+}]_i$ of sufficient magnitude to permit the commencement of uterine contractions. The increase in $[Ca^{2+}]_i$ and the contractions of the myometrium could then promote uterotonin formation. This, in turn, would support the attainment of optimal $[Ca^{2+}]_i$ and, thence, the forceful

contractions of phase 2 of parturition. For this to be an effective fail-safe system—which seems likely for such a momentous event—the increased formation of several uterotonins could be expected.

Increases in $[Ca^{2+}]_i$ favor increased prostaglandin formation by activating Ca^{2+}-dependent phospholipases that serve to mobilize arachidonic acid from storage forms, the glycerophospholipids. Hypoxia caused by uterine contractions also favors prostaglandin production by acceleration of glycerophospholipid hydrolysis, as does the action of oxytocin by way of the oxytocin receptor-mediated hydrolysis of phosphatidylinositol. Shear stress and hypoxia stimulate the production of endothelin-1. Thereby, if uterine contractions are induced by an increase in $[Ca^{2+}]_i$ in myometrial cells as uterine phase 0 processes are suspended, a cascade would automatically follow that vaults the uterus into phase 2 of parturition.

Uterine Phase 0 of Parturition

Uterine phase 0 is the prelude to the initiation of parturition, characterizing the normal state of the uterus during the first 36 to 38 weeks of human pregnancy. All systems that permit, facilitate, favor, or promote myometrial contractility or cervical softening are rendered inoperative during uterine phase 0 of parturition. The myometrium is maintained in a state of remarkable quiescence as the cervix remains rigid. For the purpose of sorting out and thence aligning the uterine modifications of parturition in the proper sequence, the most remarkable phenomenon of uterine phase 0 is the completeness and success of the systems that act to immobilize the intrinsic contractile properties of the uterus.

Myometrium: Inherent Propensity to Contract. The phasic smooth muscle of the myometrium of nonpregnant women contracts readily. Strips of human myometrial tissue placed in an isotonic bath contract in a rhythmical fashion without added stimuli. Uterine contractions facilitate the transport of spermatozoa along the uterine cavity to the fallopian tubes. The dysmenorrhea of menstruation is caused in large measure by painful uterine contractions that function to empty the uterus of blood and endometrial tissue debris. Small intrauterine devices, inserted for contraception, commonly provoke such painful uterine contractions that removal is necessitated. Not infrequently, intense and painful uterine contractions cause the delivery of pedunculated submucous leiomyomata or endometrial polyps through the cervical canal into the vagina in nonpregnant women. Indeed, the uterus enlarged by leiomyomata is often mistaken for the uterus of pregnancy; and the extrusion of a large submucous myoma through a dilated cervix has been misinterpreted as delivery of a fetal head. Stretching, cell replication, inflammation, trauma, and foreign tissue grafts are stimuli of uterotonin formation; and each of these processes is involved in the establishment and progress of mammalian pregnancy. The human uterus increases in size during pregnancy from an organ of about 50 to 70 g to one that at term weighs more than 1 kg. This comes about primarily by cellular hypertrophy, with a 10-fold increase in myometrial cell size; during this same time, the volume capacity of the uterus increases by several orders of magnitude.

Collectively, the authors have managed hundreds of pregnancies with multiple fetuses; but recently, one of us became the grandfather-to-be of twins. This obstetrician-researcher was placed in a professionally disembodied, but profoundly concerned and philosophical posture. During the last 20 weeks of this pregnancy, we marveled, most every minute of each passing day (and in great appreciation), at the tranquility of the uterus of this young woman. Ultimately, at 39 weeks' gestation, when the myometrium was still absolutely tranquil, the uterus was emptied by cesarean delivery of healthy, happy grandbabies, 6 pound Melissa and 8 pound Ryan, together with 3 pounds of placenta and fetal membranes and 4 pounds of amnionic fluid. Having observed similar pregnancies for years as the obstetrician, we were still prompted to ask ourselves how indeed is it possible to expand the cavity of a 50 g smooth muscle organ sufficiently to accommodate 21 pounds, which includes vigorously kicking twins, without provoking violent uterine contractions. This and similar, and even much more exaggerated experiences, are the more puzzling knowing the inherent tendency of the uterus to contract, and knowing that the capacity for the formation of a number of powerful uterotonins in intrauterine tissues of human pregnancy is substantial. Recognizing the great force that will be generated by the contracting myometrium during labor, we, like others before us for thousands of years, are continually reminded of the ancient, but still highly relevant (somewhat paraphrased) cliché: **It is amazing that the burden of human pregnancy is tolerated with such functional myometrial equanimity.**

Progesterone and Uterine Phase 0 of Parturition.
For most of this century, it has been presumed that the biological action of progesterone is obliged for the successful maintenance of pregnancy. Yet neither the biomolecular particulars of this presumed progesterone-mediated stronghold on myometrial contractile responsiveness, nor the role of other putative agents in the promotion of this tolerant uterine state, are clearly defined.

Notwithstanding this large gap in our knowledge, it is clear that, unlike the human, there is an unequivocal and precipitous decline in the maternal plasma levels of progesterone that precedes and is temporally related to the initiation of parturition in most mammalian species (Challis and Olson, 1988). In these species, progester-

one withdrawal is the invariable antecedent event that heralds the initiation of parturition. And this is true irrespective of whether, during pregnancy in a given species, progesterone arises in the corpus luteum or in the placenta.

Therefore, in most mammals, the suspension of uterine phase 0, permitting the implementation of phase 1 of parturition, occurs as progesterone is withdrawn. This is highly suggestive that progesterone acts directly, or indirectly, to establish and maintain uterine phase 0 of parturition. In support of this contention, phase 0 of parturition is suspended irrespective of whether the withdrawal of progesterone is naturally occurring or pharmacologically or surgically induced. As defined herein, this is the initiation of parturition.

But in a few mammalian species, including humans (and some other primates and the guinea pig), progesterone withdrawal does not take place at the end of pregnancy; that is, there is no decrease in the concentration of plasma progesterone in these species before (or even during) labor (Challis and Olson, 1988). In these species, progesterone withdrawal occurs only after delivery of the placenta. Nonetheless, the biochemical and morphological adaptations of the uterus that prepare this organ for labor (i.e., uterine phase 1 of parturition) are seemingly the same in type and timing in species in which progesterone withdrawal does not occur as in those in which progesterone withdrawal is well defined.

It is important, therefore, to examine the particulars of the processes that are operative to establish uterine phase 0 for clues as to the mechanisms whereby uterine phase 0 in human pregnancy can be suspended. So far as is known, progesterone is also the principal mediator of phase 0 phenomena in human pregnancy. The question remains, therefore, as to how uterine phase 0 can be interrupted during human parturition without the removal of progesterone.

Phase 0 of Parturition: Myometrium.
There is no doubt that uterine phase 0 of parturition is implemented by active, cooperative, highly effective, coordinated processes that cause (1) inhibition of myometrial cell contractile responsiveness, (2) limited availability of uterotonins to the myometrium, and (3) severe limitations to the propagation of myometrial contractile signals. The paralytic effectiveness of phase 0 on uterine contractility is normally very complete. It is understandable, therefore, that the uterus placed into this unresponsive mode must be awakened and rejuvenated before the forceful contractions of labor can begin.

Depressed Myometrial Contractile Responsiveness.
There are substantial changes in the myometrial cell contractile responsiveness that operate in a very efficient manner during uterine phase 0. Very little is known of the processes that cause this contractile refractoriness. It seems likely, however, that this phenom-

enon must be accomplished by multiple processes that prevent an increase in the effective myometrial cell $[Ca^{2+}]_i$; or stated differently, the capacity of cellular processes that promote the extrusion of Ca^{2+} from the cell, the sequestration of Ca^{2+} in sarcoplasmic reticulum, or the intracellular binding of Ca^{2+}, must be increased or activated to establish uterine phase 0.

Uterotonin Degradation. In addition to the pregnancy-induced myometrial cell contractile refractoriness, there are striking increases in the activities of enzymes (in uterine tissues and plasma, or erythrocytes) that degrade endogenously produced uterotonins, e.g., prostaglandins: prostaglandin dehydrogenase (PGDH); endothelin:enkephalinase; oxytocin:oxytocinase; histamine:diamine oxidase; catecholamines:catechol-O-methyl transferase (COMT); angiotensin-II:angiotensinase(s); and, PAF:PAF-acetylhydrolase. The activities of several of these enzymes are known to be increased by progesterone action. Examples include enkephalinase in endometrium (Casey and associates, 1991a), diamine oxidase in decidua, PAF-acetylhydrolase in plasma (Yasuda and Johnston, 1992), PGDH in many tissues including endometrium (Casey and colleagues, 1980), and possibly COMT in erythrocytes (reticulocytes) (Bates and co-workers, 1979).

Thus, one action of progesterone in promoting phase 0 of parturition seems to be mediated through an increased capacity for the enzymatic degradation of uterotonins.

Inhibition of Myometrial Cell Contractile Signal Propagation. Propagation of contractile signals in myometrium during uterine phase 0 is severely limited. Gap junctions between myometrial cells are rare and oxytocin receptors are few; and this is true of the myometrial tissues of all mammals that have been examined during uterine phase 0. No doubt other myometrial cell signal propagation systems, not yet clearly identified, are also disabled during this time. The formation of gap junctions and the synthesis of oxytocin receptors also seems to be prevented by the action of progesterone.

Phase 0 of Parturition: Cervix.
During phase 0 of parturition, as the myometrium is quiescent and reasonably flaccid, the cervix must remain rigid and unyielding. The maintenance of cervical anatomical and structural integrity is essential to phase 0 of parturition. Premature cervical dilatation, structural incompetence, or both, portend an unfavorable pregnancy outcome that commonly ends in preterm delivery.

Uterine Phase 0 of Parturition: Summary.
Before the initiation of parturition, pregnancy is a physiological state in which a biomolecular stronghold is placed on uterine tissues to prevent coordinated, forceful myometrial contractions. Obviously, the biomolecular systems that establish uterine phase 0 are effective and unrelenting. The only clue to the mechanism by which this stronghold on myometrial contractile responsiveness is effected is the action of progesterone.

Uterine Phase 1 of Parturition

During uterine phase 1 of parturition, the uterus must be made ready for action so violent as never to be revisited—except at the next time of active labor. But during phase 0 of parturition, the uterus was deprived of all means of emptying its contents; all processes that support coordinated, forceful uterine contractions were suspended. Before labor can begin, the uterus must be awakened: Cooperative myometrial cell arrangements must be restored, myometrial cell responsiveness must be rekindled, and the rigidity of the cervix must be discarded in favor of softening.

This transition from uterine phase 0 to phase 1 is the initiation of parturition (Fig. 12–2).

Role of the Fetus in the Transition from Phase 0 to Phase 1.
It is satisfying to believe that the fetus, after sufficient maturation of vital organs, provides a signal that parturition should commence. Teleologically, it seems that this is the most logical manner by which parturition could begin in a timely fashion.

Fetal Contributions to Suspension of Phase 0. Many investigators, including ourselves, have searched for a *fetal signal* that will lead to the suspension of uterine phase 0. Regrettably, such a fetal signal has not been discovered in human pregnancy. Signals from the human fetus could be transmitted in one of several ways; but however this is accomplished, the end-result must be the suspension of uterine phase 0. In sheep, the parturition signal seems to arise in the fetal brain; the suspension of phase 0 in sheep pregnancy is accomplished by the withdrawal of progesterone. The signal transmission system in the sheep fetus proceeds via the brain, pituitary, adrenal, fetal blood, and trophoblasts. The sheep fetus promotes the interruption of uterine phase 0 through a fetal adrenal cortisol-induced increase in the transcription of a gene that encodes a steroidogenic enzyme in trophoblast. The sheep fetus provides a signal that results in the transition from uterine phase 0 to phase 1.

Similarly, the human fetus may act to cause the suspension of uterine phase 0 through a fetal blood-borne agent that acts upon the placenta. Alternatively, a signal could be transmitted from the fetal lungs or kidneys by secretions or excretions of these organs, which enter the amnionic fluid (the paracrine arm of the fetal–maternal communication system).

It seems unlikely, however, that the initial signal for the commencement of parturition is a uterotonin, such as oxytocin, prostaglandins, or endothelin-1. It is rather more likely that uterine phase 0 of parturition must first be rendered inoperative. Until this is accomplished, increased production of a uterotonin would be ineffective and counterproductive.

The termination of phase 0, however, could be caused by the action of a uterotropin. If a uterotropin (produced in the fetus, or in the placenta in response to a fetal signal) acts on myometrium to suspend the processes promoting phase 0, the transition to uterine phase 1 would result. An experimental example of the interruption of phase 0 and the inauguration of phase 1 has been provided by the inhibition of progesterone action at the level of the progesterone receptor (e.g., the administration of the synthetic antiprogestin steroid, RU-486).

Fetal Contributions to Initiation of Parturition. The bovine, ovine, and human fetus each appear to negotiate the timely onset of parturition. Anomalies of the brain of the fetal calf, fetal lamb, and human fetus interfere with the normal timing of parturition. When there is congenital absence of the pituitary in the bovine fetus, the gestation period of the cow is prolonged by several weeks. Adrenal hypoplasia in the bovine fetus also causes a delay in the onset of parturition.

If the pregnant ewe, early in pregnancy, grazes on the foliage of a *Veratrum californicum* (a vetch called skunk cabbage), which grows wild in the northwestern United States, the sheep embryo develops a teratogen-induced, characteristic cyclopean deformity. The anomalies of such a fetus include abnormal vascularization of the fetal pituitary from the hypothalamus. In such a fetus, there is adrenal hypoplasia and the pregnancy is prolonged. Such a pregnancy goes far beyond term, and the cyclopean sheep fetus continues to grow and ultimately dies in utero without the ewe ever going into labor. These naturally occurring parturitional phenomena have been reviewed by Thorburn (1983) and by Challis and Olson (1988).

Speigelberg, in 1882 (cited by Thorburn), put forward the idea that the signal for the initiation of human parturition also originated in the fetus. In 1898, Rea observed an association between anencephaly in the human fetus and prolonged gestation. In 1933, Malpas extended these observations and described a well-documented human pregnancy with an anencephalic fetus that went far beyond term, to 374 days (53 weeks). He concluded that the association between fetal anencephaly and prolonged gestation seemed to be attributable to the anomalous brain–pituitary–adrenal function of the anencephalic fetus. The adrenal glands of the anencephalic fetus are very small, and at term may be only 5 to 10 percent as large as those of a normal fetus. The smallness of the adrenal glands is caused by failure of development of the fetal zone—the structure that accounts for most of the adrenal mass and C_{19}-steroid

biosynthesis in the human fetal adrenal glands (Chap. 6). These findings were suggestive that in humans, as in sheep, the fetal adrenal glands serve an important role in the timely onset of parturition. There is another corollary between prolonged gestation and a fetal adrenal anomaly in human pregnancy. In pregnancies in which there is a fetus with adrenal hypoplasia (Anderson and Turnbull, 1973), as in sheep in which the fetal adrenal glands have been rendered inactive either by hypophysectomy or adrenalectomy (Liggins, 1973), the onset of labor may be delayed.

Most investigators have reasoned that the relationship between fetal adrenal dysfunction and prolongation of human pregnancy or delayed parturition is likely more related to deficient placental estrogen formation than to defective fetal adrenal cortisol production. In support of this deduction, delays in the onset of parturition (or else dysfunctional labor) are sometimes encountered in pregnancies with placental sulfatase deficiency and low estrogen formation, but with normal fetal adrenal cortisol production. At this juncture in the development of analogies between the sheep and human models of parturition initiation, however, there is a divergence between the preparturitional endocrinology of the two species of considerable magnitude, as we will describe in detail later. In brief, there is no clear-cut increase in the fetal plasma concentration of cortisol before the onset of human parturition—and there is no evidence of a decline in the concentration of progesterone in maternal or fetal plasma before or during labor in human pregnancy.

The Human Fetus and Parturition: Summary. Today there is fragmentary, and inconsistent, evidence that pregnancies with relative hypoestrogenism (fetal anencephaly, fetal adrenal hypoplasia, and placental sulfatase deficiency) are associated with prolonged gestation or dysfunctional labor. With each of these conditions, prolonged gestation is sometimes but not invariably observed. Normal amounts of estrogen for human pregnancy may facilitate the development of optimal and timely parturitional processes, but the rate of estrogen formation is not the critical functional key to the timing of the initiation of human parturition. In all of these conditions, estrogen formation is much less than that in normal pregnancy but much, much more than that in nonpregnant women. In the only well-documented case of placental aromatase deficiency, causing even more severe hypoestrogenism, the pregnancy was plagued by inappropriate preterm uterine contractions beginning in the late midtrimester of pregnancy; but at 38 weeks, spontaneous labor began, but was dysfunctional, requiring uterotonin administration to effect delivery (Shozu and associates, 1991). Perhaps in this pregnancy, estrogen formation was impaired so severely as to preclude adequate synthesis of progesterone receptors in uterine tissues. Other fetal abnormalities that prevent or severely reduce the entry of fetal urine (absence of fetal kidneys) or lung secretions (pulmonary hypoplasia) into amnionic fluid do not cause prolongation of human pregnancy. Thus, a signal from the fetus (e.g., from the fetal lungs or kidneys) through the paracrine arm of the fetal–maternal communication system is not mandated for the initiation of human parturition.

The Human Fetus and Parturition: Speculations. Teleologically it seems reasonable to expect that maturation of some fetal tissue(s) or system(s) is central to the fetal-induced suspension of uterine phase 0. Intuitively, it seems less likely that such a profound responsibility rests with the maturation of a single fetal organ. There are too many examples of human fetal organ abnormalities that are not associated obligatorily with aberrations in the timing of parturition for this to be tenable. Yet, brain (or adrenal or both) maturation in the sheep fetus (and other mammalian fetuses) seems to be the means of initiating a parturition signaling system. This brain–pituitary–adrenal response may represent one maturational event that is part of a more generalized developmental milestone of the fetus—one as yet not identified, but one that possibly is common to all mammalian fetuses in generating the signal necessary for the suspension of uterine phase 0. McDonald and Nathanielsz (1991) presented a similar view, citing the probability that the signal from the fetal sheep brain is transmitted in response to the brain's interpretation of *"a multitude of sensory inputs in determining maturational status of the fetus to initiate parturition when a critical level of maturity has been achieved."* They suggest that the fetal brain receives and interprets signals that are indicative of fetal organ maturity. Once the fetal brain interprets these multiple signals as representing sufficient organ maturity, the fetal pituitary is called upon to be the messenger.

Phase 1 of Parturition: Functional Elements and Uterotropins. The functional modifications of uterine tissues known to take place during phase 1 of parturition are: (1) cervical softening and ripening, (2) an increase in the population of oxytocin receptors in myometrial cells, (3) an increase in gap junctions (number and size) between myometrial cells, (4) increased myometrial contractile responsiveness to uterotonins, and (5) transition of the uterus from a state in which contractures occur to one in which more frequent mild contractions develop. There is no doubt that many other modifications of the uterus take place late in pregnancy. Some of these almost certainly are integral components of the preparation of the uterus for labor, acting either as functional elements or regulatory agents in the transition to and establishment of uterine phase 1.

We suggest, therefore, that the institution of uterine phase 1 processes must include two types of agents acting on the uterus: regulatory agents (uterotropins)

and functional elements. A given agent not directly involved in establishing the functional uterine changes of phase 1 itself, that is, a uterotropin, may act to initiate the synthesis of the functional components. Alternatively, a given process of phase 1, once initiated (e.g., a given protein once synthesized), may promote the next uterine modification of phase 1. Yet another possibility exists, one that we favor. A uterotropin or a uterotropin-stimulating agent may be delivered to the uterus in the maternal circulation. In this case, the plasma-borne uterotropin (or its agent) may promote further uterotropin formation directly in the myometrium.

If only a single uterotropin were involved in the promotion of phase 1 processes, at least one function of this uterotropin must be to negate or somehow interrupt selected actions of progesterone, either directly or indirectly. Stated differently, a uterotropin must act to suspend the continuation of uterine phase 0. A major milestone would be reached in deciphering the physiological sequence of human parturitional processes if the "regulatory" uterotropin(s) that serves to suspend phase 0 were identified. The regulation of the transition from uterine quiescence to phase 1 of parturition with or without progesterone withdrawal should become more understandable. Perhaps a particular biochemical modification of myometrium will be identified as an early marker of phase 1 processes and thereby provide the long-awaited major clue to the identity of the primary uterotropin(s).

In species in which progesterone withdrawal signals the onset of parturition, the uterine modifications of phase 1 commence as progesterone levels decline. Lest we forget, however, phase 1 preparatory processes also take place faithfully, and in a timely manner, in uterine tissues of women during the initiation of parturition despite the absence of progesterone withdrawal or definitive evidence of progesterone deprivation.

Phase 1 of Parturition: Myometrium

Oxytocin Receptors. The uterus is refractory to the induction of labor during phase 0 of parturition even when oxytocin is infused intravenously in large amounts. This is because the population of oxytocin receptors in myometrial cells during uterine phase 0 is sparse. Late in pregnancy, before commencement of uterine phase 2 of parturition, there is a striking increase in the number of oxytocin receptors in myometrium (Fuchs and associates, 1982). The increase in oxytocin receptors coincides with an increase in uterine contractile responsiveness to oxytocin in all mammalian species studied, including the human (Riemer and colleagues, 1986; Soloff and co-workers, 1979). Moreover, prolonged gestation in humans and rats is associated with a delay in the increase in oxytocin receptors in myometrium (Bercu and colleagues, 1980; Fuchs and collaborators, 1984). Most studies conducted to evaluate the regulation of myometrial oxytocin receptor synthesis have been performed in the rat in vivo or with rat uterine tissues in vitro. Estrogen and progesterone are produced by the corpus luteum in rat pregnancy, and progesterone withdrawal commences 2 to 3 days before parturition. Estradiol treatment of ovariectomized rats causes an increase in myometrial oxytocin receptors; this action of estradiol is prevented by simultaneous treatment with progesterone (Fuchs and colleagues, 1983). Similarly, estradiol treatment of rat uterine tissue explants in vitro leads to increased oxytocin receptors, whereas progesterone treatment causes a sharp reduction. Progesterone may act to increase oxytocin receptor degradation (Soloff and colleagues, 1983).

The physiological increase in oxytocin receptors in myometrium of the pregnant rat during phase 1 of parturition occurs abruptly, within 24 hours of the onset of labor. The number of uterine oxytocin receptors is greatest during labor, but falls to a low level by 1 to 2 days postpartum. These changes in the oxytocin receptor population in vivo are correlated with alterations in the plasma levels of estrogen and progesterone (Alexandrova and Soloff, 1980a).

Oxytocin receptors are also present in endometrium of nonpregnant women and in decidua at term; and it is likely that oxytocin receptor protein synthesis in endometrium or decidua is also regulated by estrogen and progesterone as in the myometrium (Fuchs and colleagues, 1985). Oxytocin acts in decidual tissue in vitro to stimulate prostaglandin production (Fuchs and associates, 1981); and, oxytocin receptors are also present in amnion and chorion–decidual tissues (Benedetto, 1990). Human myometrial smooth muscle cells in culture are responsive to oxytocin, which stimulates prostaglandin formation and a small increase in myometrial cell $[Ca^{2+}]_i$ and the phosphorylation of myosin light chains (MacKenzie and associates, 1990). The human oxytocin receptor has been isolated and a cDNA cloned (Kimura and colleagues, 1992). The level of oxytocin receptor mRNA in human uterine tissues obtained at term is far greater than that in uterine tissues of nonpregnant women. Thus, the increase in oxytocin receptor number in myometrium at term (Fuchs and associates, 1982) is probably attributable to increased oxytocin gene transcription. Collectively, these data are suggestive that progesterone acts on estrogen-stimulated myometrial cells to inhibit oxytocin receptor synthesis, to increase oxytocin receptor protein degradation, or both. With the availability of cDNAs for the oxytocin receptor, this issue should be resolved expeditiously. It should be possible to define the role of progesterone in the regulation of oxytocin receptor number and to place the time of appearance of oxytocin receptors in the correct order in the sequence of phase 1 processes.

Gap Junction Protein (Connexin43). The physiological importance of optimal numbers (area) of functional, permeable gap junctions between myometrial cells at parturition is believed to be the provision of improved electrical synchrony in the myometrium to effect coordination of contractions and thereby greater force. Gap junctions are transcellular membrane channels comprised of connexons; a connexon is a hexameric assemblage of a specific connexin (the gap junction protein), which is joined in mirror symmetry with a connexon in the membrane of an adjacent cell (Fig. 12–3). These pairs of connexons are a conduit for the exchange of small molecules (M_r <1000) and ions between cells. Thereby, communication is established between coupled cells for the passage of current (electrical or ionic coupling) or metabolites (metabolite coupling). In heart and myometrium, connexin43 (a 43-kDa protein) is the principal gap junction protein (Beyer and associates, 1989).

In the human and in the rat, the number and size of gap junctions between myometrial cells increase before the onset of labor (i.e., during phase 1 of parturition), and then decrease quickly after delivery. This is true whether parturition occurs at term or preterm (Garfield and associates, 1977; Garfield and Hayashi, 1981). In the rat, estrogen treatment promotes gap junction formation in the myometrium (by increasing connexin43 synthesis). The simultaneous administration of antiestrogens prevents the estrogen-induced increase in gap junctions (Burghardt and colleagues, 1984). Progesterone treatment negates the stimulatory effect of estrogen on the development of gap junctions in the rat and sheep uterus; and the administration of an antiprogestin, such as RU-486, leads to premature development of gap junctions, preterm labor, and delivery in pregnant rats. Chwalisz and colleagues (1991) found that a progesterone antagonist (ZK 98 299) administered to pregnant guinea pigs late in gestation increased uterine sensitivity to oxytocin with no change in oxytocin receptor number. They obtained evidence that this increase in sensitivity to oxytocin is due to an increase in the number of gap junctions.

Considerably less is known about the regulation of connexin43 biosynthesis and gap junction formation in human myometrium. In myometrial tissue obtained from pregnant rats or pregnant women before labor (when the number of gap junctions is small), a spontaneous increase in the number of gap junctions occurs in vitro (Hayashi and collaborators, 1985). This is suggestive that the excised tissue was relieved from a pregnancy endocrine milieu that prevents gap junction development in vivo. As in the case of the oxytocin receptor, it appears that progesterone acts to inhibit gap junction protein synthesis. In the case of human uterine phase 1 development, therefore, the question again must be asked, does a uterotropin act to antagonize or override the action of progesterone that prevents gap junction formation?

Modifications in gap junctional permeability have been demonstrated in a variety of systems in response to

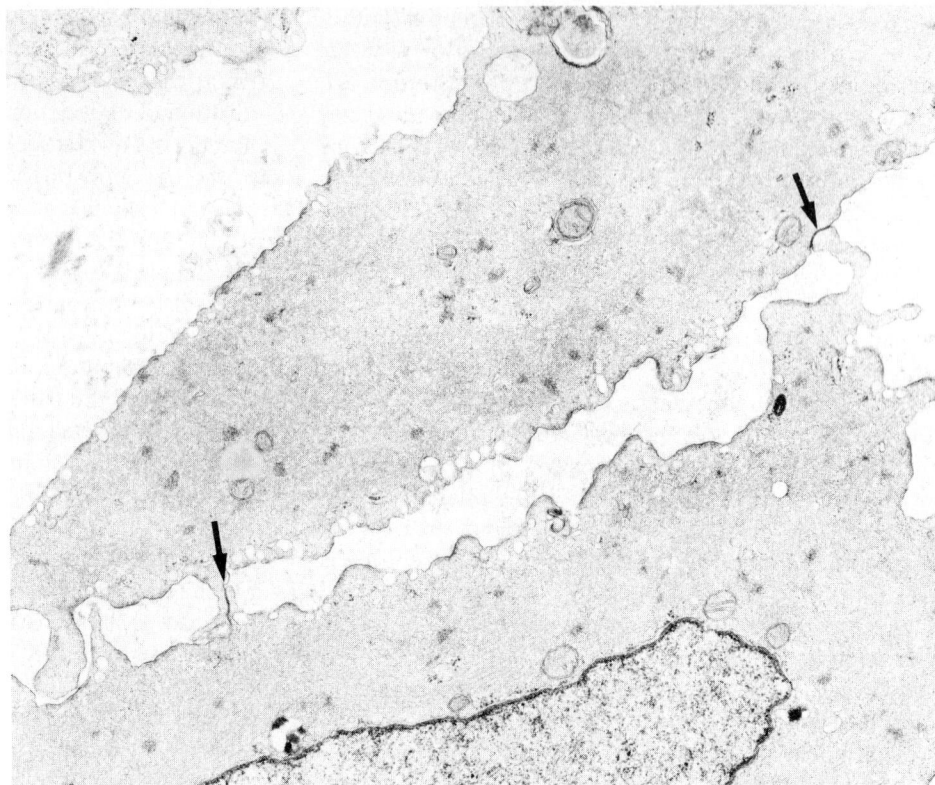

Fig. 12–3. Electron photomicrograph of gap junctions in human myometrial cells. Tissue obtained after labor commenced. (Courtesy of Dr. R. Garfield.)

various hormones, neurotransmitters, Ca^{2+}, cAMP, and phorbol esters. Using strips of rat myometrial tissue, Cole and Garfield (1986) found that cAMP analogs (or activators of adenylate cyclase) caused a decrease in gap junction permeability. In studies of strips of human myometrial tissues, similar findings were obtained by Sakai and co-workers (1992). Collectively, these findings are suggestive that intercellular myometrial communication via gap junctions may be regulated by the level (synthesis/degradation) of connexin43, the assembly of connexons, and the permeability of the gap junctions. Opportunities for researchers to define the regulation of gap junction protein biosynthesis and degradation have been advanced greatly by the development of antibodies specific for the connexin proteins and by the cloning of cDNAs for the gap junction mRNAs, including connexin43 (Beyer and co-workers, 1987).

Potential Phase 1 Proteins. As stated, there is no doubt that agents not presently recognized as uterotropins or uterine phase 1 functional elements will be discovered. As these compounds are identified, the prospects for solving the cause of the initiation of human parturition puzzle will be enhanced appreciably.

Parathyroid Hormone-related Protein. Parathyroid hormone-related protein (PTH-rP) is expressed in myometrium during phase 1 of parturition; PTH-rP may therefore be a participant in phase 1 processes. It is not clear, however, whether PTH-rP is a phase 1 functional element, uterotropin, or both. PTH-rP was identified in a search for the parathormone-like agent responsible for the "humoral hypercalcemia of malignancy syndrome," a complication of cancer with malignant tumors of a wide assortment. PTH-rP was isolated and characterized, and cDNAs were cloned from human malignant cells in culture (Martin and colleagues, 1989). Parathyroid hormone (PTH), an 84-amino acid protein, is secreted exclusively by the parathyroid gland. PTH-rP, most commonly a 141-amino acid protein, is not secreted by the normal adult parathyroids (Chaps. 6 and 7). The amino acid homology between PTH and PTH-rP is limited to 8 of the first 13 amino acids of the N-terminus of the two proteins. PTH-rP is secreted by a host of malignant cells and by a number of normal tissues. PTH-rP expression is especially prominent in several tissues of reproduction and fetal development. PTH-rP, produced in the fetus (by the fetal parathyroid, placenta, and other tissues), is believed to substitute for PTH, acting as the "parathormone of the fetus" (Chaps. 5 to 7; Abbas and colleagues, 1990). All of the *known* actions of PTH can be accounted for by the N-terminal 27 amino acids and a single type of plasma membrane PTH receptor. Generally, it has been presumed that PTH-rP acts via the plasma membrane receptor for PTH because the actions of $PTH_{(1-34)}$ and $PTH\text{-}rP_{(1-34)}$ are usually indistinguishable. There is evidence, however, that intact $PTH\text{-}rP_{(1-141)}$, or segments longer than 1 to

34, act to promote processes not effected by intact $PTH_{(1-84)}$. For example, PTH-$rP_{(1-141)}$, but not $PTH_{(1-84)}$, will increase Ca^{2+} transport in ovine placenta; PTH-rP, but not PTH, mediates selected transforming growth factor-β (TGF-β)-like actions; and PTH-rP is more potent in stimulating adenylate cyclase in some cells than is PTH (for review: Mallette, 1991).

Thiede and associates (1990, 1991a, 1991b) have made a number of important observations suggestive of a role for PTH-rP in myometrium during late pregnancy and parturition. They found that PTH-rP is expressed in the rat uterus (myometrium) during pregnancy and that the highest levels of PTH-rP mRNA in myometrium are in uterine horns (occupied by fetuses) just before and during labor. Estrogen treatment of nonpregnant animals caused an increase in myometrial PTH-rP mRNA levels, but the levels were not nearly as great as those in myometrial tissues in fetus-occupied uterine horns at term. Casey and associates (1992) demonstrated that PTH-rP mRNA is present constitutively in human myometrial cells in culture and that immunoreactive PTH-rP is secreted into the medium of these cells. They also demonstrated that TGF-β treatment of human myometrial cells causes an increase in the levels of PTH-rP mRNA and the secretion of immunoreactive PTH-rP into the medium.

Thiede and colleagues also found PTH-rP mRNA and protein in the avian oviduct, especially in the serosal (vascular-enriched) tissues. In laying hens, a temporal relationship was discovered between the specific anatomical site of increase in PTH-rP mRNA in the oviduct and egg transport. Whereas the function of PTH-rP in uterine physiology is not established, Thiede and co-workers (from studies of avian oviduct) suggest that PTH-rP may act, by way of the promotion of vasodilatation, to increase blood flow in the avian oviduct during egg transport and oviposition. Indeed, it is known that both PTH and PTH-rP are effective vasorelaxants (Mok and colleagues, 1989). Thus, PTH-rP, acting as a vasorelaxant, may serve to maximize uterine blood flow during myometrial contractions. In addition, through activation of adenylate cyclase, PTH-rP may also act as a uterotropin to promote the development of other phase 1 processes.

Calbindin D-9K. As is true for oxytocin receptors, gap junctions, and PTH-rP, there is also an increase in the level of calbindin D-9K in rat myometrium late in gestation (Mathieu and associates, 1989). This protein (~9 kDa) binds Ca^{2+} with high affinity and is believed to be important in the transport of Ca^{2+} across epithelial cells of the intestine, kidney, yolk sac, and possibly the uterus of mouse and rat. In the rat and mouse, Bruns and colleagues (1985, 1988) found that calbindin D-9K is present in myometrial cells and in uterine stromal cells. The expression of calbindin D-9K is increased in rat myometrium late in gestation, leading these investiga-

tors to postulate that this protein is involved in the regulation of uterine contractions. Calbindin D-9K levels in myometrium are not regulated by 1,25-dihydroxyvitamin D_3 as in the intestine; but L'Horset and colleagues (1990) demonstrated that estrogen treatment of ovariectomized rats causes an increase in myometrial calbindin D-9K gene expression. Estrogen acts (1) to increase the rate of calbindin D-9K gene transcription (via estrogen response elements in this gene) and (2) to increase calbindin D-9K mRNA stability as well (Darwish and colleagues, 1991). Thus, calbindin D-9K is a potential candidate for a role in the biogenesis of uterine phase 1 processes. The status of calbindin D-9K in uterine tissues of women, however, is not defined.

Transforming Growth Factor-βs. Casey and associates (1992) found that transforming growth factor-βs (TGF-β) acts on human myometrial smooth cells in culture to cause an increase in the levels of PTH-rP mRNA and immunoreactive PTH-rP protein secretion into the medium. In addition, they found that TGF-β1 acts to increase prepro-endothelin-1 mRNA and protein (Casey and associates, 1991b), and that TGF-β1 and TGF-β3 mRNAs are present in myometrium of pregnant women at term before and after the onset of spontaneous labor (Casey and MacDonald, unpublished). Therefore, it may be that both PTH-rP and TGF-β are expressed in myometrium in greater amounts during phase 1 of parturition. Possibly TGF-β is one of the regulatory agents (uterotropins) that promote the synthesis of the functional elements of uterine phase 1.

Other Potential Uterine Phase 1 Proteins. Other myometrial components of phase 1 processes will no doubt be identified. Among those that are under investigation are myometrial endothelin-1 and the endothelin receptors (A and B). The specific activity of enkephalinase (the enzyme that degrades endothelin) is high in rat myometrium during uterine phase 0 but falls precipitously during phase 1 of parturition (Ottlexa and associates, 1991). The mRNA for oxytocin has been identified in rat myometrium (Fantoni and co-workers, 1992) and placenta (Lefebvre and colleagues, 1992b) and in human placenta (Chibbar and colleagues, 1991).

Phase 1 of Parturition: Cervix. The body of the uterus (the fundus) and the cervix, although parts of the same organ, must respond to the uterotropins–uterotonins of parturition in quite different ways. On the one hand, it is essential that during most of pregnancy, the myometrium be dilatable but remain quiescent. On the other hand, the cervix must remain unyielding and rigid. Coincident with the initiation of parturition, however, the cervix must soften, yield, and become more readily dilatable. The fundus must be transformed from the relatively relaxed, unresponsive organ characteristic of most of pregnancy to one capable of thunderous contractions that drive the fetus through the yielding cervix and on through the birth canal. Failure of a coordinated interaction between the functions of cervix and fundus portends an unfavorable pregnancy outcome. But despite the apparent reversal of roles between cervix and fundus from before to during labor, it is likely that both processes are regulated by common agents.

Composition of the Cervix. There are three principal structural components of the cervix: smooth muscle, collagen, and the connective tissue or ground substance (extracellular matrix). Constituents of the cervix important in cervical modifications at parturition are those in the extracellular matrix or ground substance, the glycosaminoglycans dermatan sulfate and hyaluronic acid. The smooth muscle content of cervix is much less than that of the fundus and varies, anatomically, from 25 to only 6 percent. The role for smooth muscle in the cervical "ripening" process is not clear; but it is probably more important than previously believed. The cervical ripening process principally involves changes that occur in collagen, connective tissue, and its ground substance.

Cervical Ripening. Cervical ripening is associated with two complementary changes: (1) collagen breakdown and rearrangement of the collagen fibers and (2) alterations in the relative amounts of the various glycosaminoglycans. Hyaluronic acid is associated with the capacity of a tissue to retain water. Near term, there is a striking increase in the relative amount of hyaluronic acid in cervix, with a concomitant decrease in dermatan sulfate.

PGE$_2$ and PGF$_{2\alpha}$, applied directly to the cervix, induce the maturational changes of cervical ripening, that is, modification of collagen and alterations in the relative concentration of the glycosaminoglycans. Prostaglandin suppositories, placed intravaginally adjacent to the cervix, are used clinically to effect cervical softening and ripening to facilitate the induction of labor. In some species, these same events can be recapitulated in response to an alteration in the "effective" endogenous estrogen-to-progesterone ratio by manipulations that favor estrogen. Yet other compounds may serve as active participants in the activation or orchestration of these coordinated events. Relaxin, for example, acts to effect cervical ripening while maintaining the uterus in a quiescent state. If this relaxin-mediated process were operative in human pregnancy, it would represent a very early phase 1 functional modification, and thereby relaxin could be regarded as a uterotropin, that is, a regulatory agent of phase 1. But despite the enormous importance of cervical ripening to the success of parturition in all species, relatively little is known of the precise sequence or the regulation of the biochemical processes involved.

Phase 1 of Parturition: Summary. In summary, phase 1 of parturition normally commences during the final days of gestation, marking the time in pregnancy when the stronghold on myometrium to prevent contractions is abolished. *Accordingly, retreat from pregnancy maintenance* and *the initiation of parturition are synonymous as we define these processes.* During uterine phase 1, the functional modifications of this organ for the efficient, powerful uterine contractions of active labor are set in place. But from the analyses presented, we are still left with the presumption that progesterone is the most likely mediator of the biochemical processes that sustain uterine phase 0 of parturition. It follows, therefore, that progesterone must be withdrawn or else its actions selectively inhibited to permit the momentous transition of the uterus to phase 1 of parturition. It has been established that progesterone treatment of women will not prolong uterine phase 0. Therefore, we deduce that at the time of human parturition, the actions of progesterone are inhibited. If this were the case, it is possible that only selected actions of progesterone are abolished. Possibly only selected progesterone-responsive genes are affected, establishing an evolutionary hierarchy in human parturition for the modulation of progesterone action.

Uterine Phase 2 of Parturition

Uterine phase 2 of parturition is the period of active labor—the forceful uterine contractions that cause cervical dilatation, fetal descent, and delivery of the conceptus.

Myometrial Smooth Muscle

Anatomical Features. There are unique anatomical features of myometrial muscle (and other smooth muscles) compared with skeletal muscle. Huszar and Walsh (1989) and Huszar and Roberts (1982) point out that these differences create a peculiar advantage for myometrial smooth muscle in the development of uterine contractions and the delivery of the fetus. First, the degree of shortening in smooth muscle cells with contraction may be one order of magnitude greater than that attained in striated muscle cells. Second, forces can be exerted in smooth muscle cells in any direction, whereas the contraction force generated by skeletal muscle is always aligned with the axis of the muscle fibers. Third, smooth muscle is not organized in the same manner as skeletal muscle; in myometrium, the thick and thin filaments are found in long, random bundles throughout the cells. This arrangement facilitates the greater shortening and force-generating capacity of smooth muscle. Fourth, there is the advantage that multidirectional force generation in myometrial smooth muscle permits versatility in expulsive force directionality that can be brought to bear irrespective of the lie or presentation of the fetus.

Regulation of Smooth Muscle Contractions. The interaction of myosin and actin is essential to muscle contraction. Myosin (M_r ~500,000) is comprised of multiple light and heavy chains and is laid down in thick myofilaments. The interaction of myosin and actin, which causes activation of ATPase, ATP hydrolysis, and force generation, is effected by enzymatic phosphorylation of the 20-kDa light chain of myosin (reviewed by Stull and colleagues, 1988). This phosphorylation reaction is catalyzed by the enzyme *myosin light chain kinase,* which is activated by Ca^{2+} (Fig. 12–4). Ca^{2+} binds to calmodulin, a calcium-binding regulatory protein, which in turn binds to and activates myosin light chain kinase. Thereby, agents that act on myometrial smooth muscle cells to cause an increase in $[Ca^{2+}]_i$ promote contraction. Conditions that cause a decrease in $[Ca^{2+}]_i$ favor relaxation. Agents that cause an increase in the intracellular concentration of cyclic adenosine monophosphate (cAMP) promote uterine relaxation; an example is β-adrenergic agonists (reviewed by Diamond, 1990). It is believed that cAMP acts to cause a decrease in $[Ca^{2+}]_i$, although the exact mechanism is not defined. One possibility is that cAMP promotes the sequestration of Ca^{2+} in the sarcoplasmic reticulum (for review: Roberts and associates, 1988). Alternatively, it has been proposed that phosphorylation of myosin light chain kinase, by cAMP-dependent protein kinase(s), causes inactivation of this enzyme, and thereby the phosphorylation of myosin light chain is inhibited. The decrease in activity of the phosphorylated enzyme is attributable to a decrease in the affinity for Ca^{2+}-calmodulin. Dephosphorylation of the myosin light chain by the action of phosphatase also causes muscle relaxation (Fig. 12–4). The biochemistry and physiology of smooth muscle contractility has been reviewed by Stull and associates (1988) and Barany and Barany (1990). Roberts and colleagues have studied the regulation of rabbit uterine contractile responsiveness by sex steroids. They find that estrogen treatment promotes α_1-adrenergic-mediated contractile responsiveness whereas progesterone treatment promotes β-adrenergic-mediated relaxation by relieving α_2-adrenergic-mediated inhibition of adenylate cyclase (Roberts and associates, 1989).

Phase 2 of Parturition: Three Stages of Labor. Customarily, and for good clinical reasons, active labor (phase 2 of parturition) is divided into three separate stages.

The *first stage of labor,* by custom, is said to com-

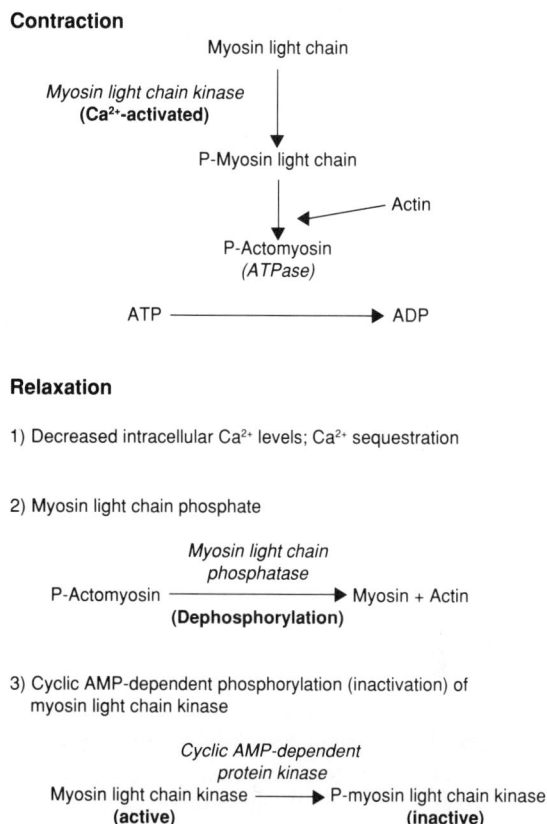

Contraction

Relaxation

1) Decreased intracellular Ca^{2+} levels; Ca^{2+} sequestration

2) Myosin light chain phosphate

3) Cyclic AMP-dependent phosphorylation (inactivation) of myosin light chain kinase

Fig. 12–4. Metabolic regulation of myometrial smooth muscle contraction and relaxation. An increase in intracellular, cytoplasmic, free Ca^{2+} activates myosin light chain kinase, which catalyzes the phosphorylation of the 20-kd light chain of myosin. Phosphorylated myosin interacts with actin and thereby activates ATPase; with the hydrolysis of ATP, force is generated and the muscle shortens. Relaxation is promoted by sequestration of Ca^{2+} in the sarcoplasmic reticulum, dephosphorylation of phosphorylated myosin by the action of phosphatase, and possibly phosphorylation (inactivation) of myosin light chain kinase by a cAMP-dependent protein kinase. (Illustration courtesy of Dr. L. Casey.)

mence when uterine contractions of sufficient *frequency, intensity,* and *duration* are attained to bring about readily demonstrable effacement and dilatation of the cervix. The first stage of labor ends when the cervix is fully dilated, that is, when the cervix is sufficiently dilated (about 10 cm) to allow passage of the fetal head. The first stage of labor, therefore, is that stage in which *cervical effacement and dilatation* occur. There is no increase in oxytocin levels in plasma during this stage of labor. Prostaglandin levels in amnionic fluid and maternal blood increase after the first stage of labor is in progress, but not before.

The *second stage of labor* begins when dilatation of the cervix is complete and ends with delivery of the fetus. The second stage of labor is the stage of *expulsion of the fetus.* During this stage of labor, maternal plasma oxytocin levels are increased.

The third stage of labor begins immediately after delivery of the fetus and ends with the delivery of the placenta and fetal membranes. The third stage of labor is the stage of *separation and expulsion of the placenta.*

Delivery of the Placenta and Fetal Membranes. We must not overlook the fact that successful parturition includes not only the delivery of the fetus but also the delivery of the placenta and fetal membranes. Before the time of readily available blood for transfusion and antibiotics to combat infection, retention of the placenta and/or fetal membranes was sometimes a major obstetrical complication. On some occasions, maternal death occurred because of hemorrhage, shock, and infection, which are complications of retained placental fragments and membranes.

It seems reasonable to presume, therefore, that there are active chemical processes that serve together with mechanical forces to effect delivery of these tissues. We must acknowledge this possibility so as not to confuse whatever these processes may encompass as part of a more global involvement of these tissues in parturition. The trophoblasts directly contiguous with maternal decidua produce a modified fibronectin, oncofetal fibronectin. As emphasized by Feinberg and colleagues (1991), oncofetal fibronectin (*trophoblast glue*) is less avidly bound to extracellular matrix. For this reason, oncofetal fibronectin may facilitate the separation of chorion laeve from decidua parietalis at delivery. Increases in the levels of oncofetal fibronectin in cervical and vaginal fluids are observed in women during labor, both at term and preterm (Lockwood and associates, 1991). This is supportive of the view that fetal membrane separation is in progress during labor, before delivery. Other products of amnion, chorion laeve, and decidua may also facilitate the separation and delivery of the fetal membranes. These may include the prostaglandins and other mediators of the inflammatory process. Some cytokines, for example, act to increase the degradation of extracellular matrix proteins by stimulating the formation of metalloproteinases. The involvement of amnion and chorion laeve as tissue participants in metabolic processes of parturition is discussed further later in this chapter.

Uterine Phase 3 of Parturition

Uterine phase 3 is the time of parturient recovery, which encompasses important postpartum events: (1) uterine contraction and retraction to prevent puerperal hemorrhage, (2) initiation of lactation and milk ejection to facilitate breast feeding, (3) involution of the uterus, and (4) restoration of fertility. The uterotonins, oxytocin and endothelin-1, are likely important in regulating several processes of phase 3 of parturition. Endothelin-1,

acts, as does oxytocin, to contract smooth muscle cells (i.e., the myometrium and myoepithelium of the breasts). The increase in the plasma concentration of oxytocin during the second stage of labor is suggestive that oxytocin supports the expulsive phase of labor. Suckling of the maternal breasts by the newborn also elicits oxytocin release from the maternal neurohypophysis-posterior pituitary. The practice of placing the newborn infant to the mother's breast immediately after delivery may have evolved in part from the observations of midwives that uterine hemorrhage may be lessened by such a practice.

Parturition Research

Overview. The contemporary era of parturition research began almost 30 years ago. At that time, reproductive biologists began to define the processes involved in the fetal–maternal communication system of human pregnancy. During these 3 decades, important discoveries have been made and new concepts have been formulated. Some parturition theorems have been discarded and others revisited. As recently as the 18th edition of *Williams Obstetrics* (1989) the possibility was reviewed that the cause of preterm labor (at least some forms thereof) might be discovered before the mechanisms were understood by which parturition is normally initiated at term.

There was optimism then that the biomolecular processes that cause preterm labor in a sizable fraction of human pregnancies would be defined. This hopeful notion was based on the belief that preterm labor commonly was caused by the actions of products of microorganisms, that is, bacterial toxins. If this proposition had proven to be correct, great insights might have been gained into the biomolecular processes of parturition, whether occurring normally at term or preterm. Today, it seems more likely that infection, as a cause of preterm labor in pregnancies with intact fetal membranes, is a rare occurrence. Notwithstanding this disappointment, investigations of the processes involved in the initiation of human parturition are strengthened by numerous new findings.

Over these 3 decades, parturition researchers have been struggling with two general theorems. Simplistically stated, these can be referred to as the retreat from pregnancy maintenance hypothesis and the uterotonin theory.

There are many combinations of selected tenets of each of these two postulates in the theorems of most investigators. It is commonly presumed, for example, that the mature fetus, in some manner, provides a signal that initiates the procession of parturitional processes. Namely, the fetus is believed to be in charge of its own destiny with respect to the timing of birth. There-

fore, fetal-induced retreat from pregnancy maintenance is a satisfying consideration. An obligatory role
for increased uterotonin formation has also been included in the parturition theories of most investigators,
either as a primary or a secondary phenomenon in the
physiological sequence of parturition processes proposed.

***Experimental Basis for Modern Parturition Re-
search.*** Two independent observations made almost
30 years ago have influenced the direction of parturition research up until now. One of these was the discovery of the mechanism by which estrogen is produced in human pregnancy. At that time, it was known
that human pregnancy was a hyperestrogenic state of
incredible proportions (Chap. 6) in which the placenta was virtually the sole tissue site of estrogen synthesis. But it also was known that the human placenta
could not synthesize estrogen de novo from acetate or
cholesterol, or even from C_{21}-steroid precursors such
as pregnenolone or progesterone. These potential in-
consistencies were reconciled by the discovery that
the human adrenal glands produce a prodigious
amount of C_{19}-steroids, which is transported by way of
the fetal circulation to the placenta; and in syncytiotrophoblast, the fetal adrenal steroid precursors are
metabolized with great efficiency to estrogens. Thus,
the human placenta, with respect to estrogen biosynthesis, is an incomplete endocrine organ. This finding
permitted an expansion of the fetal–maternal communication system concept; namely, by way of an interactive organ system, steroid prehormones synthesized
in the fetal adrenal glands serve as substrates in the
syncytium for the synthesis of estrogens that enter the
maternal and fetal circulation. The estrogens produced
in this manner totally account for the hyperestrogenic
state of human pregnancy (Siiteri and MacDonald,
1963).

Liggins and associates (1967, 1968) established that
the sheep fetus provides the initial signal that culminates in the timely onset of parturition. They conducted
elegant experiments to define the physiological processes involved in the initiation of parturition in sheep.
In clever and technically demanding investigations, they
demonstrated on the one hand that adrenalectomy or
hypophysectomy of the sheep fetus (but not the ewe)
caused a delay in the time of delivery. On the other
hand, infusion of ACTH or cortisol (or a synthetic glucocorticosteroid) into the sheep fetus caused the premature onset of parturition. From these findings, Liggins
and colleagues deduced that fetal sheep brain–pituitary–
adrenal function gives rise to a signal that leads to the
initiation of parturition (Challis and Olson, 1988; Liggins, 1973; Liggins and associates, 1973). Therefore, it
seemed possible that in some way the fetal adrenal
glands or brain–pituitary–adrenal function might be

central to the regulation of the initiation of parturition
in all mammalian species, if only we could discover the
specifics of the regulation and contribution of these fetal
organs among species.

The Sheep Model of Parturition. The most complete
scheme for the physiological sequence of events of parturition among all mammalian species has been established in sheep. Liggins and colleagues (1967, 1973)
and other investigators from around the world have
discovered many of the physiological particulars for
sheep parturition (see Challis and Olson, 1988 for an
excellent review). The sheep model is presently the
"gold standard" of mammalian parturition research despite the probability that greater progress has been made
during the past 30 years in defining the endocrinology
of human pregnancy than in any other species. The
specific components of the fetal–maternal communication system are defined most clearly in the human; and
in many specific areas, there is more knowledge of the
biomolecular processes involved in selected phenomena of human parturition than in other animals. Nonetheless, a plausible sequence of physiological events
involved in human parturition has not been developed
as it has in the sheep.

A profound conundrum has been faced by investigators attempting to define the cause of the initiation of
parturition in human pregnancy, because an endocrinological or metabolic alteration that precedes the initiation of human parturition has not been identified. Many
investigators have struggled to understand the biological meaning of the differences in the endocrine physiology of parturition in primates and other mammalian
species. Most students of parturition subscribe to the
premise that the fundamental biomolecular events of
the parturitional process must be similar in all mammals
irrespective of apparent differences in endocrine physiology that precedes or follows the commencement of
parturition. Even as we are overcome by ignorance, and
no doubt shrouded in misconceptions, we still cling to
this belief.

The Fetal Sheep Signal for Parturition. Near the end of
sheep pregnancy, a signal arising in the fetal sheep brain
initiates retreat from the continued maintenance of
phase 0 of parturition (McDonald and Nathanielsz,
1991). Ultimately, this signal results in the suspension of
uterine phase 0. This fetal signal promotes the beginning
of a coordinated sequence of events that brings about
progesterone withdrawal and thereafter increased formation of a uterotonin, $PGF_{2\alpha}$, in uterine decidua. The
parturition signal from fetal brain is transmitted to the
fetal pituitary to effect increased ACTH release. In consequence of the increased release of and adrenal responsiveness to ACTH, fetal adrenal cortisol secretion
increases (Myers and colleagues, 1992).

Fetal Cortisol Alters Placental Steroid Production in the Sheep. It is presumed that fetal cortisol acts (directly or indirectly) to increase the expression of trophoblast cytochrome P-450 17α-hydroxylase/17,20-lyase (P-450$_{17\alpha}$). As P-450$_{17\alpha}$ activity in trophoblast increases, placental pregnenolone is diverted away from the synthesis of progesterone into 17α-hydroxypregnenolone; the increase in activity of this single steroidogenic enzyme causes two dramatic modifications in the hormonal milieu of sheep pregnancy (Fig. 12–5). Namely, progesterone "withdrawal" is effected (a precipitous decline in progesterone secretion) and, concomitantly, estrogen synthesis is increased. The latter is the result of increased availability of substrate for placental P-450-aromatase through the pathway: 17α-OH-pregnenolone → dehydroepiandrosterone → androstenedione → estrone → estradiol (Fig. 12–6).

Compared with 17α-hydroxypregnenolone, 17α-hydroxyprogesterone is a poor substrate for the steroid-17,20 desmolase reaction; thus, androstenedione, the immediate precursor of estrogen in sheep placenta, arises primarily from 17α-OH-pregnenolone via dehydroepiandrosterone and not from 17α-hydroxyprogesterone (France and associates, 1988). Fetal cortisol also acts, directly or indirectly, to cause a modest increase in aromatase activity in sheep trophoblast; but aromatase is not rate-limiting in estrogen formation in the sheep placenta; rather, the supply of C$_{19}$-steroid precursors (dehydroepiandrosterone → androstenedione) formed de novo in sheep placenta is rate-limiting (France and colleagues, 1987) (Fig. 12–6).

Progesterone Withdrawal and Sheep Parturition. A single signal emanating from fetal brain triggers a sequence of processes that brings about an increase in the expression of a single gene in trophoblast. In some manner related to progesterone withdrawal, but otherwise not defined, this change in sex steroid hormone production leads to the suspension of uterine phase 0, which enables the development of phase 1 of parturition, uterine preparedness for labor. It is also believed that the withdrawal of progesterone ultimately causes (again in some undefined manner) increased uterotonin (PGF$_{2\alpha}$) formation in decidua and thereby the onset of phase 2 of parturition (Fig. 12–7).

Human Parturition: Divergence from the Sheep Model. As stated, it has always seemed reasonable to presume that the fundamental biomolecular processes of parturition are similar among all mammalian species, even though the particulars of the antecedent event(s) (endocrine or otherwise) may differ in some specific details. But crucial differences in key endocrine events that seem to be pivotal in the initiation of parturition in sheep and humans have so far obstructed the realization of this expectation. Among the important differences in the endocrinology of human and sheep pregnancy before the initiation of parturition are the following: (1) there is no appreciable increase in cortisol formation by the human fetal adrenals as there is in the sheep fetus before the onset of parturition; (2) the infusion of ACTH or cortisol into the human fetus does not initiate parturition as it does in the sheep; (3) glucocorticosteroid treatment in human pregnancy causes a pronounced decrease in estrogen formation (by inhibiting fetal adrenal C$_{19}$-steroid formation) and no change in the levels of progesterone; in contrast, glucocorticosteroid treatment of the sheep fetus causes an increase in placental estrogen synthesis and a decrease in progesterone formation; (4) in human pregnancy, there is no decrease in the rate of secretion or the plasma levels of progesterone before the onset of labor; in the sheep model there

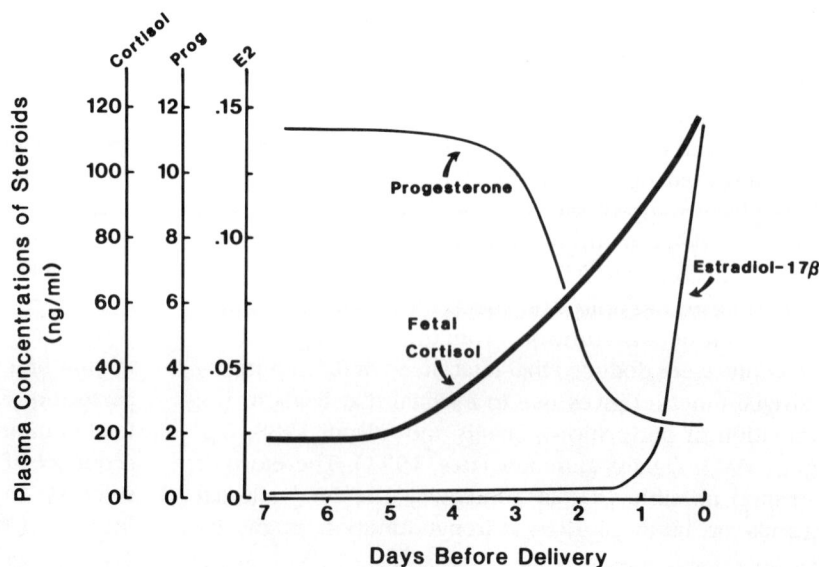

Fig. 12–5. Endocrine antecedents of parturition in the sheep. As the levels of fetal plasma cortisol increase, the levels of maternal plasma progesterone decline. Thereafter, there is an increase in estradiol production by the placenta.

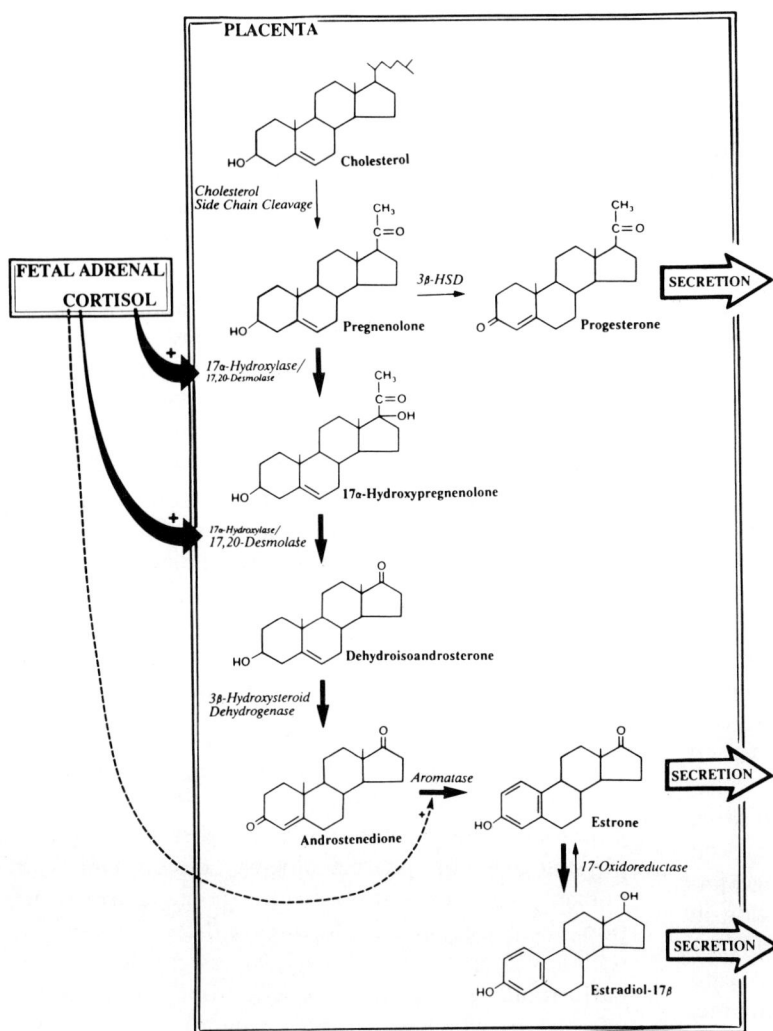

Fig. 12–6. Fetal cortisol action to increase the expression of placental steroid 17α-hydroxylase/17,20-lyase to modify progesterone and estrogen biosynthesis prior to the initiation of parturition in the sheep.

is a precipitous decline in the plasma levels of progesterone in the ewe before the onset of phase 1 of parturition; (5) placental progesterone production in sheep pregnancy is small compared with that in the human; (6) the sheep fetal adrenal glands are not the source of placental estrogen precursors as are the fetal adrenal glands in humans, and estrogen production in sheep pregnancy is small compared with that in the human; (7) steroid 17α-hydroxylase/17,20-desmolase is expressed in sheep (but not in human) placenta; and (8) intrauterine prostaglandin formation during labor in sheep (Liggins, in discssion of Flower, 1977) is at least 20 times that produced in uterine tissues during human labor (Casey and MacDonald, 1988c).

Human Parturition: Progesterone Synthesis and Progesterone Withdrawal.

There is no reduction in the plasma level or production rate of progesterone before the initiation of human parturition. Little and colleagues (1966) found that the metabolic clearance rate of plasma progesterone during human pregnancy is the same as that found in men and nonpregnant women

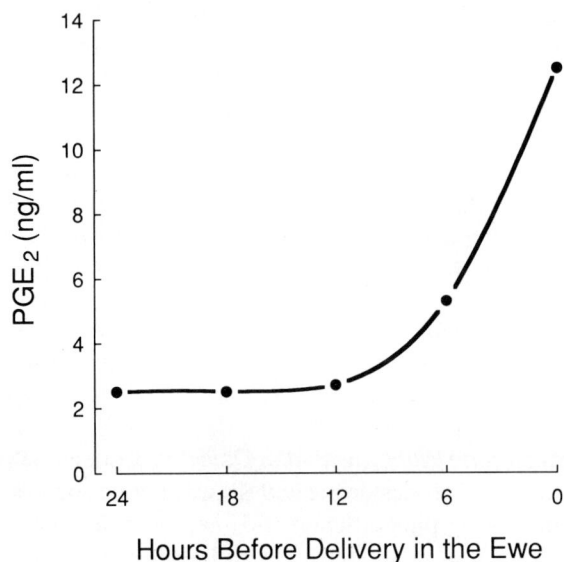

Fig. 12–7. Concentration of PGE_2 in amnionic fluid of the sheep during labor, as a function of hours before delivery. (Data from Mitchell, 1976.)

(Billiar and associates, 1974; Lin and co-workers, 1972). Therefore, the plasma level of progesterone is directly proportional to its production rate. Progesterone production declines in human pregnancy only after delivery of the placenta, that is, after phase 2 of parturition.

Nonetheless, it still is not possible to abandon the notion that progesterone action is crucial to the success of uterine phase 0 of human parturition. But by clinging to this belief, there is no explanation for the suspension of uterine phase 0 in human pregnancy. Many investigators, including ourselves, have searched for some kind of "loophole" to explain this conundrum: (1) the absence of progesterone withdrawal before the onset of human parturition; (2) the observation that progesterone withdrawal, if experimentally or surgically induced in human pregnancy, usually causes the initiation of parturition; but (3) the fact that progesterone treatment of women will not prevent spontaneous parturition or arrest preterm labor. Researchers have asked whether there could be some alternate form of progesterone withdrawal, sequestration, inhibition, or whatever, to explain the initiation of human parturition. In particular, can there be some sort of hidden form of progesterone deprivation during human pregnancy, even in selected tissues, that leads to the onset of parturition?

Many possibilities have been considered, and some subjected to intense scrutiny, but all have come up short of a convincing explanation whereby progesterone action can be interrupted without a reduction in plasma levels of progesterone. To summarize the findings of the studies of many investigators, there is no substantive evidence for alterations in progesterone metabolism, compartmentalization (sequestration) of progesterone, or for alterations in progesterone-binding proteins or receptor numbers to account for some hidden form of progesterone deprivation near the end of human pregnancy. For these reasons, we have concluded in the past, however reluctantly, that progesterone withdrawal is not a fundamental component of the initiation of parturition in human pregnancy (Casey and MacDonald, 1988a).

It is time to search again! It is time to evaluate the possibility that some unusual form of progesterone deprivation might take place late in human pregnancy to bring about the transition from uterine phase 0 to phase 1. One largely unexplored means by which progesterone action could be abolished is by the action of a naturally occurring, endogenously produced antiprogestin.

Progesterone Withdrawal After Delivery. Conceptually, the timing of progesterone withdrawal among species is an interesting phenomenon and may provide clues to the absence of progesterone withdrawal enigma of human pregnancy. Progesterone inhibits lactogenesis. The initiation of lactogenesis is a well-established biological end-point of progesterone withdrawal in all mammalian pregnancies. This is true in species in which progesterone withdrawal occurs before the onset of parturition (e.g., sheep, goats, rats, mice, rabbits) and in those in which progesterone withdrawal occurs after delivery (e.g., humans, some other primates, and the guinea pig). In some newborn species (e.g., the sheep) the ingestion of liquids very soon after birth is essential to survival; in these species, progesterone withdrawal occurs well before delivery, enabling the early elaboration of milk. In other species, liquids are not required by the newborn for several days after birth; in the human, progesterone withdrawal is postponed until after delivery and lactation begins 2 to 3 days after birth. The human fetus requires little, if any, fluid for the first 48 to 72 hours of life. In the guinea pig, in which progesterone withdrawal also occurs after delivery, the newborn is mature enough to munch on lettuce! These findings are suggestive that if progesterone action were interrupted to initiate human parturition, it is only selected actions of progesterone that are affected—not, for example, the inhibition of lactogenesis, which occurs only with progesterone withdrawal.

Surgical, Pathological, or Pharmacological Induction of Progesterone Withdrawal in Human Pregnancy. Progesterone withdrawal is sometimes observed in pathophysiological or pharmacological circumstances in human pregnancy, but not before spontaneous parturition. There are important features of these progesterone withdrawal episodes that may give insights into human parturitional processes. If progesterone withdrawal is effected, by whatever means, during human pregnancy, abortion, labor, or increased myometrial sensitivity ensues. Removal of the corpus luteum in early human pregnancy (before 8 weeks' gestation) results in abortion. In ectopic pregnancies or with fetal demise, a decrease in progesterone formation may precede the onset of spontaneous uterine contractions and the delivery of a decidual cast (ectopic pregnancy, Chap. 32) or a dead fetus. Progesterone withdrawal is not an immediate accompaniment of fetal demise. Trophoblasts commonly survive the fetus and trophoblast utilization of maternal plasma LDL for progesterone synthesis continues sometimes for weeks after fetal death (Chap. 6).

Pharmacologically induced inhibition of progesterone formation (inhibition of 3β-hydroxysteroid dehydrogenase) or progesterone action (receptor antagonist, RU-486) also causes abortion, increased sensitivity of the myometrium to uterotonins, or both. Therefore, if progesterone withdrawal is effected in human pregnancy, parturition is favored, as in other mammalian species.

Progesterone Administration to Prevent Parturition. The administration of progesterone will, in many mammalian species, prevent the initiation of parturition. This is true in species in which progesterone withdrawal precedes the initiation of parturition. The administration of progesterone to women, however, does not prevent or arrest labor at term or preterm (for review: Casey and MacDonald, 1988a). These findings are supportive of the absence of progesterone withdrawal in the initiation of human parturition.

Is an Antiprogestin Produced in Human Pregnancy? The commencement of uterine phase 1 processes at the end of pregnancy might properly be referred to as the awakening of the uterus. We suggest again that the identity of the signal(s) that sounds this alarm in uterine tissues is critical to a solution of the puzzle of the initiation of human parturition. If this piece of the puzzle were in place, we should be able to design experimental protocols to define the role of the human fetus in determining the timing of its own birth. It also seems reasonable to surmise that a means for modifying the time of the initiation of parturition will be accomplished by resetting the alarm for this awakening process.

Based on the findings in most experimental animals, it also seems probable that the endocrine physiology of human pregnancy must somehow be involved in the timing and regulation of the processes that govern the transition from uterine phase 0 to phase 1 of parturition. Therefore, progesterone withdrawal is difficult to dismiss as the phase 1 alarm system, because progesterone action is the only viable clue to an understanding of the mechanisms by which uterine phase 0 of parturition is established and maintained. The attractiveness of the progesterone withdrawal theory is so compelling that all possible mechanisms for instituting progesterone deprivation—both genomic and nongenomic—are worthy of evaluation.

An Evolutionary Hierarchy of Progesterone Withdrawal Systems. Perhaps the very pinnacle of evolutionary development of systems for the withdrawal of progesterone would be the attenuation of progesterone action on specific genes. If some actions of progesterone could be subjugated to permit the disabling of phase 0 of parturition, while other salutary actions of progesterone (not essential to parturition, such as inhibition of lactogenesis), were preserved until delivery of the placenta, a more sophisticated system of parturition initiation has evolved.

Inhibition of Progesterone Action. It seems that the only remaining viable option for the suspension of uterine phase 0 in human parturition is that an endogenous antiprogestin is produced and acts in a tissue-specific or gene-specific manner before the initiation of human parturition.

If an endogenous antiprogestin were targeted so as to alter the expression of specific genes, this could be accomplished by modifying progesterone-regulated gene transcriptional activity, mRNA stability, or protein function and stability. The specificity of progesterone antagonism could be modulated at the molecular level (utilization of specific promoters, specificity of *trans*-acting factors); at the biochemical level (protein function, enzyme activity); or at the cellular level (antiprogestin receptor synthesis and function). A gene-specific block of progesterone action could account for the interruption of selected functions of progesterone in a manner that would not be overcome by exogenous progesterone. This possibility is both reasonable and attractive: (1) The opposing effects of two or more substances on the expression of a single gene are well-established as common; (2) such a gene-specific antiprogesterone system would provide for highly selective progesterone "withdrawal" consistent with the evolutionary hierarchy of humans in reproductive processes, allowing other important progesterone functions to be maintained even during labor (e.g., inhibition of lactogenesis, refractoriness to vasopressors); (3) such a process would explain the absence of effectiveness of administered progesterone to delay or prevent the onset of human parturition at term or preterm; and (4) similar systems may be involved in physiological and pathophysiological phenomena that seemingly are unique to human pregnancy.

The expression of the genes or proteins of the functional elements of phase 1 of parturition in human pregnancy are consistent with such a gene-specific form of disabling progesterone action. Possibly, the biosynthesis of oxytocin receptors, connexin43 gene or protein expression, PTH-rP gene expression, endothelin-1 gene expression, enkephalinase enzyme activity, and others are subject to the action of a gene-specific antiprogestin, likely a protein rather than a steroid.

The Missing Piece of the Human Parturition Puzzle. There is a very important missing piece for the solution of the human parturition puzzle. This piece must fit between those of progesterone-induced uterine unresponsiveness of phase 0 of parturition and the suspension of these processes to permit the implementation of phase 1 of parturition. There must be an intermediate step, one not yet defined. There must be a uterotropin or intermediate modulator that acts in a manner that is analogous to, or serves to cause a condition tantamount to progesterone withdrawal. Heretofore, we guessed that this intermediate modulator might be a cytokine, interleukin-1β (Casey and MacDonald, 1990). Later, this possibility was rejected (MacDonald and co-workers, 1991) in favor of a more likely alternative: this protein should be a uterotropin that acts as an antiprogestin in a gene-specific manner rather than as a mediator of the inflammatory process (Fig. 12–8).

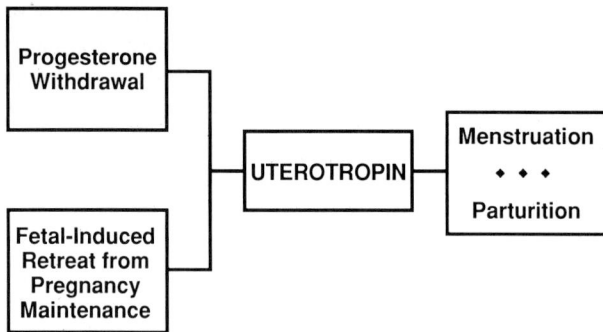

Fig. 12–8. A uterotropin as the intermediate modulator of parturition. (Illustration courtesy of Dr. L. Casey.)

AMNION, CHORION LAEVE, DECIDUA PARIETALIS, AND PARTURITION

Paracrine Systems and Parturition

The amnion, chorion laeve, and decidua parietalis comprise a tissue unit that constitutes a paracrine system, the paracrine arm of the fetal–maternal communication system (Chap. 2). Many investigators have theorized that selected regulatory phenomena of parturition are invested in these tissues.

Contributions of the placenta are considered separately because products of the villous trophoblasts (syncytium) enter maternal blood (the intervillous space) (Chap. 6). Oxytocin, delivered to the myometrium in the maternal circulation from the maternal neurohypophysis–posterior pituitary, also constitutes an endocrine mechanism and is considered separately.

There are many potential advantages of a paracrine system in parturitional processes. For example, if uterotonins were required for the success of labor after parturition has been initiated, it is metabolically expedient to deliver these agents in a paracrine manner. Some uterotonins, if present in the circulation in appreciable amounts, cause devastating effects: hypertension, hypotension, platelet aggregation, intravascular coagulation, pulmonary dysfunction, bronchospasm, nausea and vomiting, and diarrhea.

These tissues (amnion, chorion laeve, and decidua parietalis) have been studied most often to define the role of each in promoting parturition. But another possibility must be considered for each of these tissues: It may be more likely that the fetal membranes and decidua contribute to protection against the initiation of parturition, acting to ensure the success of uterine phase 0 of parturition.

Anatomical Changes in Amnion, Chorion Laeve, and Decidua Parietalis During Labor

The anatomical changes in the fetal membrane–decidual tissues obliged during labor must be taken into account

in analyses of the putative contributions of these tissues to parturition. Beginning very early in phase 2 of parturition, these tissues of the paracrine system are subjected to intense trauma and inflammatory challenges. This process is described in detail in "The Forebag of the Amnionic Fluid and Parturition" later in the chapter. It is imperative that the fundamentals of this process be understood before interpreting the contributions of these tissues to parturitional processes.

Briefly, the forebag is formed by a traumatic process that involves tearing part of the decidua parietalis tissue away from the lower uterine segment and then exposing these tissues to the vaginal fluids that contain microorganisms, bacterial toxins, and cytokines. The surface area of these tissues that is exposed increases as labor progresses, the result of the opening of the cervix (i.e., cervical dilatation). This is a normal process and consequence of normal labor. The trauma to and exposure of these tissues to bioactive agents, however, provokes an inflammatory response in these tissues. Some of the mediators of the inflammatory response are uterotonins and others induce uterotonin formation. The uterotonins produced in these tissues as sequelae of the labor process, however, do not gain access to the myometrium, but accumulate in the forebag amnionic fluid and in the vagina. Heretofore, this process has caused confusion about the role of these tissues and the agents produced in the parturitional process. In the formation of the forebag, two compartments of amnionic fluid are created that are anatomically and functionally separated. As a result, products formed in the forebag tissues accumulate in the amnionic fluid of the forebag. If amnionic fluid is obtained during labor by amniotomy, it is forebag amnionic fluid. The fluid of the upper compartment is more representative of the paracrine system of amnion, chorion laeve, and decidua parietalis.

The Amnion and Parturition

Amnion: Uterine Phase 0 of Parturition. There are several reasons to conclude that the amnion is as crucial to pregnancy maintenance as is uterine phase 0 of parturition. Oftentimes the more obvious contributions of amnion to pregnancy go unnoticed. Unlike other mammalian species, human amnion is avascular, providing a uniquely tough shield that precludes fetal hemorrhage by rupture of fetal amnion vessels with trauma to the mother. The amnionic fluid contained by the amnion provides physical protection for the fetus against trauma and maintains a constant environmental temperature. The amnion is very resistant to penetration by leukocytes, microorganisms, and neoplastic cells. Amnion is contiguous with the chorion laeve and covers the placenta and umbilical cord. In partnership, these fetal membranes act as a physical, metabolic, and immunological shield. Maternal tissues are protected from constituents of the amnionic fluid that may adversely affect decidual or myometrial function and thereby fetal well-being. Bioactive products of the amnion, as well as the constituents of the amnionic fluid, are selectively transported and oftentimes degraded before gaining access to contiguous maternal tissues. Many bioactive products, such as prostaglandins and endothelin-1, accumulate in amnionic fluid because of decreased metabolism and lack of transport to vascularized uterine decidua. Prostaglandin formation in amnion in vivo is limited severely, not by low enzymatic capacity for prostaglandin synthesis but by lack of extracellular arachidonic acid. Because amnionic fluid is contained in a specific space bounded by the microvillar apical surface of the amnion epithelial cells, the amnionic fluid is an extension of the extracellular fluid of amnion cells. Essential nutrients (those that cannot be synthesized de novo) for amnion cells must come from the amnionic fluid. Among these is arachidonic acid, the precursor of prostaglandins, which is present in very low concentrations in amnionic fluid. Moreover, unique inhibitors of amnion phospholipase A_2 are present in amnionic fluid (Wilson and collaborators, 1989).

The amnion serves as a selective filter to prevent fetal squames as well as lung and skin secretions in amnionic fluid from entering the maternal compartment. The amniochorion is an immunological barrier, constituting a protective shell around the fetus because of the absence of HLA class I and II gene expression (except for monomeric HLA-G) in the cytotrophoblasts of the chorion laeve (Chap. 5).

The fetus near term swallows large volumes of amnionic fluid (~500 mL/24 hr); and by fetal thoracic movements, there is a large exchange of fluids between amnionic fluid and fetal lung secretions. Thus, a number of agents in amnionic fluid are available to the fetus in sizeable quantities by swallowing or inspiratory movements: prolactin, epidermal growth factor (EGF), PTH-rP, endothelin-1, IL-6, and IL-8. The precise role(s) of these agents in fetal development, if any, is not known. But the expansion of the fetal lungs by inspired amnionic fluid is essential to fetal lung development. Selected constituents of amnionic fluid, such as EGF and prolactin, are believed to be involved in fetal lung maturation and accelerated surfactant formation.

Thus, many functions of the amnion appear to protect the fetus, to protect the decidua, to protect against interruption of fetal well-being, and to protect against interruption of the uterine tranquility of uterine phase 0 of parturition.

Amnion: Contributions to Parturition. In contradistinction to the theorem that amnion protects against premature parturition, investigations were begun almost 20 years ago to define the metabolic functions of the amnion that might contribute to the initiation of parturition (MacDonald and associates, 1974). The majority of studies of amnion tissue (or of epithelial cells derived therefrom) since then have been conducted to evaluate prostaglandin biosynthesis in amnion. More recently, the biosynthesis of other uterotonins (e.g., endothelin-1, PAF, and oxytocin) in amnion has been investigated. More human parturition research (as judged by the number of published manuscripts) has been devoted to basic studies of amnion than to all other tissues of the uterus and fetus combined.

In retrospect, it is difficult to understand the enormous interest in this tissue in the biological affairs of parturition. One reason for this incredible focus on amnion may simply be the large amounts of tissue available together with the ease of separating this fetal membrane from other tissues. A second reason is that this tissue can be obtained under a variety of pregnancy and parturition circumstances. A third reason was that a role for amnion in the initiation of parturition was envisioned from clinical experiences and correlations. For example, rupture or infection of the membranes as well as exposure of the membranes to hypertonic solutions, and stripping of the membranes away from the uterine wall, sometimes cause the onset of labor or abortion. A fourth reason, albeit a very unfortunate one, is the assumption that uterotonins and other bioactive agents found in amnionic fluid at parturition may have arisen in amnion and may be involved in the initiation of uterine contractions. To establish a role for amnion in metabolic processes that contribute to the initiation of parturition, however, it seems that the many functions of the amnion to maintain pregnancy would have to be set aside.

Amnion: Histology and Anatomy. The surface of the amnion that is bathed by amnionic fluid is composed of a single layer of epithelial cells. These cells line a thick, membranous, extracellular matrix in which there are other (mesenchymal-type) cells, presumably of embryonic mesodermal origin. Sometimes these mesenchymal cells seem to be aligned in a plane parallel to the surface of amnion. The histogenesis of these cells is not clear, but some functions presently ascribed to amnion epithelium may rather be accounted for by these mesenchymal cells.

The amnion is a most unusual tissue. Not only is it void of blood vessels, lymphatics, and nerves, but it lies contiguous with avascular chorion laeve on one side and on the other side is bathed by a large volume of amnionic fluid in which the O_2 saturation is very low. In addition to its pivotal anatomical location, the amnion is capable of complicated metabolic functions that belie its avascular, oxygen-deprived status.

Fetus, Amnionic Fluid, and Amnion. The fetus exists in the aqueous environment of the amnionic fluid, which is contained within the fetal amnion-chorion laeve; these tissues are contiguous with the entire surface of the uterine cavity (about 0.6 m^2) not occupied by placenta.

Direct chemical communication between the fetus and amnion is possible through the amnionic fluid, which is enriched in fetal excretions and secretions from kidney, lung, umbilical cord, and skin (Fig. 2–1). During the last two thirds of pregnancy, the amnionic fluid is comprised principally of fetal urine. The fetus is free to move in this space, but at the same time is cushioned from external trauma.

The amnionic fluid has been used extensively to evaluate the concentrations of substances believed to be involved in the initiation of parturition, such as uterotonins. The findings of PGE_2 and $PGF_{2\alpha}$ in amnionic fluids in high concentrations during labor focused attention on the amnion as one potential tissue site of origin of these autacoids. More recently, other uterotonins have been identified in amnion tissue or in the culture medium of amnion cells and in the amnionic fluid (e.g., endothelin-1 and PAF).

Amnion: Endothelin-1. The history of the discovery of endothelin-1 as well as the biosynthesis and processing of this extraordinarily potent smooth muscle contractant is given in Chapter 4. Soon after its discovery (Yanagisawa and colleagues, 1988), research was commenced to ascertain if endothelin-1 may be involved in the parturitional process. In addition to its action on vascular smooth muscle as a powerful vasoconstrictor, endothelin-1 was shown to be a powerful uterotonin that acts on human myometrial smooth muscle cells to cause contraction by a rapid increase in myometrial cell $[Ca^{2+}]_i$ (Word and colleagues, 1990).

Endothelin-1 Synthesis in Amnion. At the beginning of endothelin-1 research, it was generally believed that this vasoactive peptide was produced exclusively by vascular endothelial cells. Because of its great potency in causing myometrial cell contraction, however, Casey and colleagues set out to determine if endothelin-1 was synthesized in uterine or extraembryonic fetal tissues. In the conduct of these initial studies, amnion was used as a suspected negative control tissue for endothelin-1 expression because of the absence of vascular endothelial cells in this tissue. As it turned out, however, the level of prepro-endothelin-1 mRNA in amnion tissue was decidedly greater than that in chorion laeve, decidua, or myometrial tissues (Casey and associates, 1991b; Casey and MacDonald, 1992; Sunnergren and co-workers, 1990). Since the finding of prepro-endothelin-1 gene expression in amnion, it has been discovered that endothelins are produced in a number of cell types other than the vascular endothelium.

REGULATION OF AMNION ENDOTHELIN-1 SYNTHESIS. Endothelin-1 is synthesized in the epithelial cells of both the reflected and placental amnion (Casey and associates, 1991b; Germain and colleagues, 1992); and endothelin-1 immunoreactivity is found in the amnion

epithelial cells that cover the umbilical cord (Salamonsen and colleagues, 1992). The levels of prepro-endothelin-1 mRNA and the rate of immunoreactive endothelin-1 secretion by human amnion epithelial cells in culture is increased by treatment with EGF, IL-1β, or TGF-β. These amnion epithelial cells may be the principal source of immunoreactive endothelin-1 that is present in amnionic fluids from all gestational ages studied, midtrimester to term. There are some reports that the levels of endothelin-1 in amnionic fluid obtained during labor are increased (Casey and colleagues, 1991b; Usuki and associates, 1990). The levels of endothelin-1 are greater in the forebag compartment than in the upper compartment of amnionic fluid (Casey and MacDonald, 1992). Thus, it may be that mediators of the inflammatory response, such as IL-1β, which accumulate in forebag amnionic fluid, stimulate endothelin-1 biosynthesis in amnion cells. We will return to this issue in "The Forebag of the Amnionic Fluid and Parturition" section later in the chapter.

In addition to amnion, chorion laeve, decidual cells, monocytes, and macrophages all are potential sites of synthesis of endothelin-1 that enters amnionic fluid (Casey and MacDonald, 1992; Ehrenreich and colleagues, 1990).

METABOLIC FATE OF AMNION ENDOTHELIN-1. With respect to parturition, another question is whether endothelin-1 can be transported from its site of synthesis in reflected amnion (or from amnionic fluid), without degradation, to the myometrium. To do so, the peptide must traverse the underlying layer of amnion extracellular matrix proteins and the mesenchymal cells that are contained therein, the chorion laeve, and then the decidua parietalis. The transport of bioactive endothelin-1 across these tissues in a nonmetabolized (i.e., intact) bioactive form is unlikely. Using "full thickness membranes"— that is, fetal membranes plus attached decidua in vitro— Eis and colleagues (1992) found that endothelin-1 placed in the culture medium that bathed the amnion epithelial cells of these preparations did not traverse the full-thickness membranes and decidual tissues to enter the medium bathing the decidua. One obstacle to endothelin-1 transport across the fetal membranes is the enzyme enkephalinase (more properly called membrane metalloendopeptidase), which is present in the mesenchymal cells of amnion and in the cytotrophoblasts of chorion laeve with high specific activity (Casey and MacDonald, 1992; Head and colleagues, unpublished). As described in Chapter 4, enkephalinase catalyzes the degradation of endothelin-1 as well as a number of other small, bioactive peptides (e.g., the enkephalins, substance P, and atrial natriuretic peptide). Thus, the myometrium is protected from endothelin-1 produced in amnion as well as that which accumulates, in relatively high levels, in amnionic fluid. **The fetal membranes protect against parturition.**

POTENTIAL FUNCTIONS OF AMNION ENDOTHELIN-1. Endothelin-1 also is formed in the placental amnion. Recall that the placental amnion is in direct contact with the adventitial surface of the chorionic vessels (branches of the umbilical vessels) that traverse the chorionic plate prior to branching into the placental cotyledons (Chap. 5). One possibility is that endothelin-1 is released from the basal surface of the placental amnion cell (Wagner and colleagues, 1992) and acts via the adventitial surface of these vessels to modulate vascular tone (Germain and associates, 1992; see also Chap. 5). This is one of many examples of potential amnion functions that sometimes appear to be related to parturition, but which may in fact be more relevant to the many other biological functions of this unique tissue.

Amnion: Oxytocin.

There is preliminary evidence that the oxytocin gene is expressed in human amnion; Chibbar and co-workers (1991) identified oxytocin mRNA (in relatively low levels) in human amnion tissues obtained after delivery at term. In their studies, the synthesis of oxytocin protein was not demonstrated, however. The transfer of oxytocin synthesized in amnion (or from amnionic fluid) across the fetal membranes and decidua to myometrium is also highly unlikely for reasons similar to those cited for amnion-derived endothelin-1; namely, the activity of oxytocinase in intervening tissues is high and should protect the myometrium from oxytocin transferred in this manner. But again, there are possibilities for amnion oxytocin action independent of parturition. Oxytocin receptors have been identified in amnion and chorion–decidual tissue (Benedetto and associates, 1990), suggesting that oxytocin may serve a non-uterotonic function in fetal membranes and decidua. For example, oxytocin may act on amnion in the regulation of amnionic fluid volume homeostasis in a manner more analogous to the action of oxytocin in kidney.

Amnion: Prostaglandins.

From the demonstration of PGE_2 in amnionic fluid before and during labor and PGE_2 biosynthesis in amnion tissue in vitro, it commonly has been assumed that the increase in PGE_2 levels in amnionic fluid at parturition are attributable, at least in part, to increased PGE_2 formation in amnion. Based on these unfounded assumptions, however, yet more severe extrapolations have been made more recently, so that it is now commonplace for research reports to begin by stating that: *"amnion prostaglandins are 'known' to be involved in the initiation of parturition."* There are no data to substantiate this assumption. Rather, there is appreciable evidence, direct as well as indirect, that PGE_2 formation in amnion in vivo is very limited and that the transfer of PGE_2 from amnion (or amnionic fluid) to myometrium is severely if not completely precluded.

Anatomical, Metabolic, and Functional Peculiarities of Amnion.

Compared with all other human tissues, the metabolic posture of the amnion is absolutely unique. Possibly for this reason, the functional potential of amnion is sometimes misinterpreted.

The extracellular fluid of amnion epithelial cells is enormous and composed of unique substances that enter amnionic fluid. The conditions of the amnion tissue in vivo are, in some ways, difficult to recapitulate in vitro. And commonly, studies with amnion cells have been conducted in vitro under conditions that never exist for amnion tissue in vivo. These conditions have given rise to findings that are unlikely to be relevant to amnion function in vivo.

Potential for PGE₂ Formation in Amnion In Vivo.

This dilemma is best illustrated, perhaps, by a consideration of the potential for prostaglandin synthesis in amnion. Prostaglandins of the 2-series (e.g., PGE_2 and $PGF_{2\alpha}$) are metabolites of arachidonic acid. This polyunsaturated fatty acid cannot by synthesized de novo but must be ingested or synthesized from the essential fatty acid, linoleic acid. Yet, amnion tissue is relatively well-stocked in arachidonic acid. Approximately 20 percent of the fatty acids of amnion is arachidonic acid, which is found in the *sn*-2 position of the majority of the phosphatidylinositol and phosphatidylethanolamine molecules of human amnion (Okita and co-workers, 1982a). This is an interesting situation.

Fetal plasma-borne arachidonic acid cannot be the source of arachidonic acid in amnion (or chorion laeve) because these tissues are avascular. How is it possible for the avascular fetal amnion positioned between avascular fetal chorion laeve and amnionic fluid to be so well supplied with an essential fatty acid that must have arisen in the maternal diet? There are two possibilities: arachidonic acid in fetal membranes is acquired either from the decidua or the amnionic fluid; that is, from maternal albumin (to which arachidonic acid is bound) in amnionic fluid or in maternal plasma (decidua).

Source of Arachidonic Acid in Amnion Tissue.

This dilemma was solved in a study of the content and distribution of arachidonic acid among lipids in the amnion and chorion laeve of diamnionic–dichorionic human twin pregnancies when Okita and colleagues (1983a) discovered that arachidonic acid in the human amnion is acquired from the amnionic fluid. The content and distribution of arachidonic acid in the fused portion of the amnion of twin pregnancies was the same as that in the nonfused, reflected portion of the same amnion and the same as that in amnions of singleton pregnancies. The arachidonic acid in the fused portion of amnion must have arisen from the amnionic fluid. The arachidonic acid content of fused chorion laeve was appreciably less (about 50 percent) than that of nonfused (reflected) chorion laeve and less than that of fused or nonfused amnion. Thus, arachidonic acid in reflected chorion laeve of singleton fetus pregnancies is acquired both from amnionic fluid and contiguous maternal decidua parietalis.

The knowledge that human amnion assimilates arachidonic acid singularly from amnionic fluid is critical for the interpretation of studies on arachidonic acid accumulation in the fetal membranes and utilization for PGE_2 formation in vivo.

AMNION: ARACHIDONIC ACID IN EARLY DEVELOPMENT. Expansion of the amnion proceeds for the first 12 to 14 weeks of gestation before the volume of the amnionic cavity (by the accumulation of amnionic fluid and fetal growth) causes fusion of the amnion and chorion laeve with the decidua parietalis. At this time, the uterine cavity is obliterated. Up until this time, there can be no fetal-independent maternal arachidonic acid contribution to the amnionic fluid. The fetus must assimilate arachidonic (or linoleic) acid from the maternal circulation. Prior to fusion of amniochorion with the decidua parietalis, the amnionic fluid is more similar to fetal extracellular fluid than to fetal urine. Thus, arachidonic acid may enter amnionic fluid early in pregnancy as a transudate with plasma albumin through the thin integument of fetal skin.

AMNION: ARACHIDONIC ACID CONTENT BEFORE AND DURING LABOR. The arachidonic acid content of amnion tissues decreases significantly sometime during the earlier part of phase 2 of parturition (active labor) (equal to or less than 4 cm cervical dilatation). There is a specific decrease in the arachidonic acid content of phosphatidylinositol and (diacyl)phosphatidylethanolamine in amnion before approximately 4 cm dilatation of the cervix (Okita and colleagues, 1982a). In these studies, the entire reflected amnion was used for analysis and therefore it is not possible to know if there were specific reductions in amnion arachidonic acid content in a particular anatomic portion of this tissue (e.g., in amnion of the forebag) during early labor.

Heretofore, the decrease in arachidonic acid content of amnion during early labor was interpreted by some to mean that arachidonic acid from amnion was converted to PGE_2. This is not necessarily the case either before or during early labor, and may not ever obtain for the amnion of the upper compartment.

Later in labor (at or more than 5 cm cervical dilatation), the arachidonic acid content of the fetal membranes is restored and remains as great for the remainder of labor as that which existed before labor commenced. The free arachidonic acid content of forebag amnionic fluid increases appreciably during labor. Therefore, there is a net gain in the arachidonic acid content of the amnion cellular and extracellular compartment during labor. Accordingly there is no identifiable loss in arachidonic acid in the amnion–amnionic fluid compartment.

AMNION GLYCEROPHOSPHOLIPID REMODELING. All of these findings point to the likelihood of continuous glycerophospholipid turnover in amnion throughout pregnancy, which is accelerated during labor. In support of this view, (1) there is an increase in the content of palmitic acid in the glycerophospholipids of amnion during labor; (2) diacylglycerols accumulate in the amnion during labor; and (3) the fatty acid content of the diacylglycerols is the same as that of the phosphatidylinositol of this tissue, suggestive of increased hydrolysis of phosphatidylinositol (Okita, 1981; Okita and associates, 1982b). Thus, during early labor there is an exchange of arachidonic acid with palmitate in amnion. The relative increase in palmitic acid in the amnion is reflective of the utilization of fatty acids in amnionic fluid for remodeling these lipids. There is a striking increase in the palmitic acid content of fetal lung secretions late in pregnancy, accounting for increased levels of palmitate in amnionic fluid (Chap. 7).

AMNIONIC FLUID ARACHIDONIC ACID. Two studies have been conducted to quantify free arachidonic acid in amnionic fluid before and during labor. In one, the amnionic fluid was sampled by needle aspiration of the forebag during labor (MacDonald and colleagues, 1974); in the other, amnionic fluid was collected during labor by amniotomy, thus also representing forebag amnionic fluid (Keirse and co-workers, 1977). In the first study, a disproportionate increase in the concentration of arachidonic acid compared with that of all other free fatty acids in amnionic fluid during labor also was found. The importance of the concentration of free arachidonic acid in amnionic fluid evolves about the question of whether amnion produces PGE_2 in vivo. Before labor, arachidonic acid concentration of the extracellular fluid of the amnion cells in vivo (amnionic fluid) is low (~ 0.2 μM). During labor, there is a 5- to 10-fold increase in the concentration of free arachidonic acid in the "amnionic fluid" (1 to 2 μM). The findings of studies conducted in vitro are helpful in evaluating this proposition further.

AMNION: CELL REQUIREMENT FOR EXTRACELLULAR ARACHIDONIC ACID FOR PROSTAGLANDIN SYNTHESIS. Amnion cells, maintained in monolayer culture, produce very little PGE_2; but these cells are stimulated to produce PGE_2 by a variety of agents, including EGF, IL-1, tumor necrosis factor-α (TNF-α), tumor-promoting phorbol esters, vanadate, and calcium ionophores. In the absence of arachidonic acid in the medium, however, the rate of PGE_2 formation in amnion cells in response to these stimuli is restricted (Casey and associates, 1987, 1988a).

These findings are relevant to the in vivo situation of human pregnancy because of the very low concentration of arachidonic acid in amnionic fluid before the onset of labor. It is not known, but highly probable, that the arachidonic acid content of upper-compartment amnionic fluid during labor is less than that in forebag amnionic fluid, a value intermediate between that in the amnionic fluid before labor and that in the forebag during labor.

In amnion cells in culture, the concentration of arachidonic acid (bound to albumin) must be raised to about 2.5 to 3 μM to effect an increase in amnion cell PGE_2 formation. So long as the concentration of arachidonic acid in the extracellular space of amnion cells in culture is low, PGE_2 formation is curtailed even with stimuli (EGF, IL-1) that cause an increase in amnion PGH_2-synthase. We interpret this to mean that the release of arachidonic acid from amnion cells does not lead to PGE_2 formation until the concentration of free arachidonic acid in the extracellular space is increased to a critical level. Before this concentration is achieved, liberated arachidonic acid is preferentially utilized for reacylation of lipids. Thus, prior to labor, when the level of arachidonic acid in amnionic fluid is low, PGE_2 production by amnion should be severely restricted. But even after labor is well in progress, the concentration of arachidonic acid in amnionic fluid is likely too low to support appreciable PGE_2 formation.

AMNION: NET GAIN IN AMNION–AMNIONIC FLUID ARACHIDONIC ACID DURING LABOR. The net increase in arachidonic acid in this avascular compartment most likely arises by way of the release of arachidonic acid from decidua parietalis during labor. Stimulation of macrophages also causes the release of 50 percent of the arachidonic acid of these cells. In this regard, therefore, the inflammation-induced activation of decidua and the stimulation of macrophages are similar, as reviewed by Casey and Mac-Donald (1988a, 1988c, 1990). Exposure of the forebag compartment tissues by processes that involve trauma, hypoxia, and inflammation during normal labor likely accounts for the release of arachidonic acid from cells in the decidual tissue of the forebag and transfer of the free arachidonic acid into the amnionic fluid of the forebag (MacDonald and associates, 1991).

Source of Amnionic Fluid PGE₂ During Early Labor. There is little opportunity for amnion to produce PGE_2 before labor commences. After labor is in progress, there is an increase in the concentration of PGE_2 and $PGF_{2\alpha}$ in the amnionic fluid (Fig. 12–9). As this occurs, there is initially a greater increase in PGE_2 than in $PGF_{2\alpha}$ and 13,14-dihydro-15-keto-$PGF_{2\alpha}$ (PGFM). Previously, the greater rate of increase of PGE_2 compared with $PGF_{2\alpha}$ and PGFM in amnionic fluid during early labor was interpreted to be indicative that amnion (or chorion laeve or both) was the source of this PGE_2, because $PGF_{2\alpha}$ and also PGE_2 are produced in decidua (Fig. 12–10). But, because of the severe restrictions on amnion PGE_2 formation due to low amnionic fluid concentration of arachidonic acid, there is a more plausible explanation. The exposure of the forebag tissues in the vagina obliges stimulation of the macrophages of the decidua and an influx of leukocytes to this site of inflammation. These cells produce primarily PGE_2 and are a likely source of PGE_2 that enters forebag amnionic fluid early after cervical dilatation.

As labor progresses, there is a considerably greater increase in the amnionic fluid concentrations of $PGF_{2\alpha}$ and PGFM; and the levels of PGF ultimately exceed that of PGE_2 (Dray and Frydman, 1976; Reddi and collaborators, 1984); (Fig. 12–9). Decidua produces $PGF_{2\alpha}$ preferentially (compared with PGE_2).

The Metabolic Fate of Amnion (or Amnionic Fluid) PGE₂. But even if PGE_2 were produced in amnion, it is unlikely to be available to the myometrium to serve as a uterotonin. The fate of amnion (or amnionic fluid) PGE_2 that diffuses toward maternal tissues is that of rapid inactivation by prostaglandin dehydrogenase in chorion

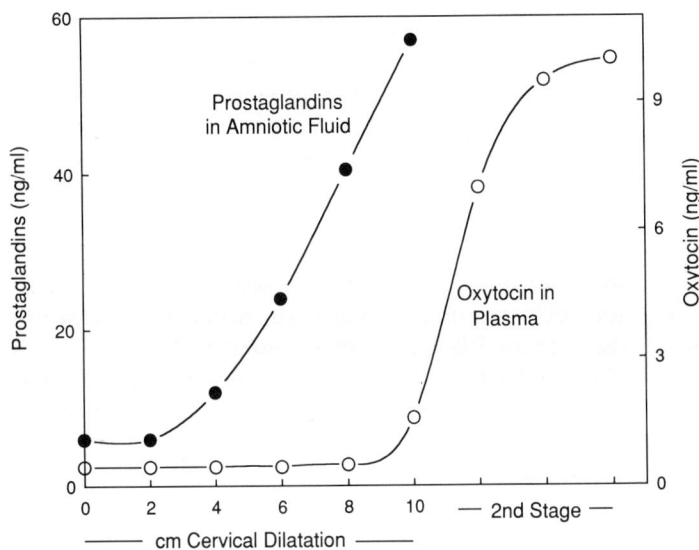

Fig. 12–9. Prostaglandins in amnionic fluid during human labor. (Data from MacDonald and Casey, 1993; Leake, 1990.)

AMNION	CHORION	DECIDUA
PGE_2	PGE_2	$PGE_2 + PGF_{2\alpha}$
✖ ↓	↓ PGDH	↓ PGDH
	inactive metabolites	inactive metabolites

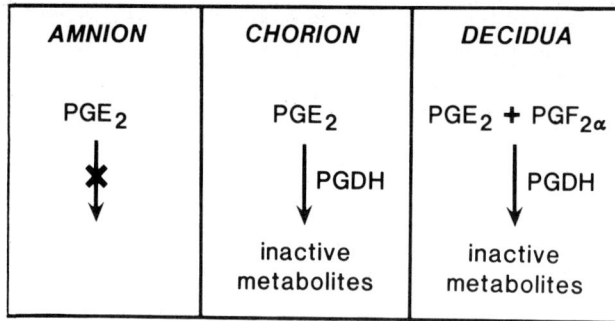

Fig. 12–10. Prostaglandin biosynthesis and metabolism in amnion, chorion laeve, and decidua. The greatest prostaglandin synthase activity is in amnion, in which only PGE_2 is formed; in amnion PGE_2 is not metabolized. In chorion laeve, PGE_2 is the principal prostanoid produced, yet there is considerable NAD^+-dependent PGDH activity. In decidua, PGE_2 and $PGF_{2\alpha}$ are formed; PGDH is active in decidua.

laeve, decidua, or both. The specific activity of prostaglandin dehydrogenase in chorion laeve is very high (Keirse and Turnbull, 1975; Okazaki and associates, 1981). Using experimental models in vitro, McCoshen and co-workers (1987, 1990) found that all of the PGE_2 transferred across the membranes from amnion to decidua was metabolized enzymatically to an inactive form(s), first by prostaglandin dehydrogenase and then by other enzymes.

Amnion: Platelet-Activating Factor Formation.

Platelet-activating factor (PAF) is a potent uterotonin, acting, as do other uterotonins, on myometrial cells to increase $[Ca^{2+}]_i$. PAF receptors have been demonstrated in myometrial cells (Zhu and associates, 1992). The capacity of amnion to produce PAF in vitro (Johnston and Maki, 1989) by a process referred to as the "remodeling pathway" is appreciable (Uemura and colleagues, 1991). By this mechanism, the lysophospholipid product of phospholipase A_2 action on selected lipids of amnion cells is utilized for the formation of PAF. The other product of phospholipase A_2 action is arachidonic acid. PAF is also produced in increased amounts as a part of the inflammatory response (which involves the activation of phospholipase A_2).

It has been proposed that PAF may act to cause the myometrial contractions of labor. PAF is present in amnionic fluid and the levels are increased in forebag amnionic fluid obtained during labor (Billah and colleagues, 1983; Nishihara and associates, 1984).

But it is likely that PAF is produced, like prostaglandins, cytokines, and endothelin-1, as a result of the inflammation that is obliged with cervical dilation and exposure of the traumatized forebag tissues to the vaginal fluids. Whereas PAF is synthesized in amnion tissue, it is not released from amnion cells. PAF produced in mononuclear phagocytes is released. Thus, it is likely

that decidua (including the leukocytes therein) produces PAF, prostaglandins, a number of cytokines, and endothelin-1 during phase 2 of parturition, as described in the section "Decidua Parietalis and Parturition" later in the chapter).

The accessibility of PAF from amnionic fluid to myometrium is uncertain but highly unlikely. PAF is inactivated enzymatically by PAF-acetylhydrolase; this enzyme is present in high amounts in macrophages (Prescott and associates, 1990), which are present in large numbers in decidua. Thus, the myometrium may be protected from PAF action by PAF-acetylhydrolase. This protective mechanism is analogous to that suggested for other uterotonins: oxytocin and oxytocinase, endothelin-1 and enkephalinase, and (as presented) prostaglandins and prostaglandin dehydrogenase.

Amnion and Parturition in Perspective.

There is little doubt that the amnion, at least that portion of the amnion of the forebag, is activated to new levels of metabolic activity during human parturition; but these processes may not include the formation of appreciable amounts of PGE_2. There are several reasons to conclude that amnion is not a source of uterotonins that can reach the myometrium, even if uterotonins were involved in the initiation of parturition. But more than that, it is unlikely that PGE_2 in amnionic fluid (or if produced by amnion in vivo) can be involved in inducing myometrial contractions at any phase of parturition.

The instillation of PGE_2 or free arachidonic acid into the amnionic fluid in the human causes abortion or labor (MacDonald and associates, 1974). But it has always been curious that the amounts of these agents required to cause labor were extraordinarily large. In fact, the amount required is several orders of magnitude more than is produced during spontaneous parturition. And the extraovular instillation of arachidonic acid in the rhesus monkey does not cause labor (Robinson and colleagues, 1979). The obvious explanation for these findings is that amnion (or amnionic fluid) PGE_2 is not a uterotonin of human parturition. Moreover, neither PGE_2 nor $PGF_{2\alpha}$ are effective uterotonins when applied directly to tissue strips of myometrium of pregnant women in vitro (Word and associates, 1992). And the prostaglandins produced in the forebag tissues are formed after labor begins, and are functionally isolated to the forebag compartment.

Amnion and Parturition: Summary.

There is no direct evidence for amnion PGE_2 production before or during early labor. PGE_2 in amnionic fluid does not cross chorion laeve and decidua without degradation. The same applies to endothelin-1 produced in amnion. Indeed, PGE_2 formation in amnion in vivo is likely to be restricted even during labor because of the low concentration of free arachidonic acid in the extracellular fluid of these cells, namely the amnionic fluid. It is more likely that the PGE_2 that accumulates in amnionic fluid in early labor arises in mononuclear phagocytes in the decidua parietalis of the forebag or in these cells after entry into amnionic fluid. PAF is not secreted from amnion. We suggest that all evidence taken together is supportive of a role for amnion in protecting the fetus from many different types of onslaughts, including parturition. We deduce that the amnion and chorion laeve (as discussed in the next section) are more important contributors to the prevention of parturition than to its initiation.

Chorion Laeve and Parturition

The chorion laeve is composed of cytotrophoblasts derived from the chorion frondosum that extended toward the endometrial cavity with growth of the embryo after blastocyst implantation (Chap. 5). These cytotrophoblasts are highly modified, however, and are functionally distinct from villous cytotrophoblasts and syncytium and from anchoring cytotrophoblasts in the decidua basalis. The villous structure of this tissue was lost as was its blood supply during expansion of the embryo-fetus and the amnionic fluid. Throughout most of pregnancy, these cells survive in a highly reduced O_2 atmosphere. Therefore, chorion laeve is an avascular, membranous tissue that is sandwiched between the avascular amnion and the maternal decidua parietalis. There also are mesenchymal cells in the chorion laeve tissue, presumably of fetal mesodermal cell origin; but the precise histogenesis of these cells is not certain.

Chorion Laeve: Parturition Research. Much less research has been conducted to evaluate the role of the chorion laeve in parturition than has been conducted with the amnion or decidua parietalis. In large part, this has been because it is appreciably more difficult to work with isolated chorion laeve and its cytotrophoblastic cells than with isolated amnion and its epithelial cells or with decidua and isolated decidual cells. It is very difficult to separate chorion laeve tissue completely from tightly adherent fragments of decidua parietalis, and vice versa. Sometimes, the fused chorion laeve tissues of diamnionic–dichorionic twin placentae are used to avoid decidual tissue contamination. In doing so, however, the influence of decidual tissue on chorion laeve function, if any, is not present.

Clearly, the potential contributions of chorion laeve in parturitional processes are deserving of greater scrutiny. The chorion laeve is the central fetal tissue of the anatomical core of the paracrine arm of the fetal–maternal communication system. As in the case of amnion, however, the chorion laeve may make a contribution primarily as a protective tissue—physical protection, immunological acceptance, and in the prevention of parturition.

Chorion Laeve: Endothelin-1. Prepro-endothelin-1 mRNA is present in chorion laeve at midtrimester and at term. The expression of prepro-endothelin-1, however, as judged by the level of mRNA in chorion laeve tissue, is decidedly less than that in amnion (Casey and MacDonald, 1992).

Chorion Laeve: Prostaglandins. In vitro, the chorion laeve, like the amnion, produces PGE_2 almost exclusively and little or no $PGF_{2\alpha}$. There is no evidence that PGE_2 is produced by chorion laeve in vivo.

Chorion Laeve: Arachidonic Acid Metabolism. As in the case of amnion, the chorion laeve is likely stimulated to new levels of metabolic activity at parturition.

Okita and colleagues (1982a) found that during early labor (before 5 cm cervical dilatation) there is significantly less arachidonic acid in two glycerophospholipids of chorion laeve tissue, (diacyl)phosphatidylethanolamine and phosphatidylinositol. But as in the case of amnion, the arachidonic acid content of the chorion laeve is restored later in labor. During labor, there is also fatty acid remodeling of glycerophospholipids of chorion laeve as in amnion (Okita, 1981).

As chorion laeve also is avascular, the arachidonic acid incorporated into lipids must be derived from a source other than fetal blood. From a comparison of the arachidonic acid composition of chorion laeve tissues of diamnionic–dichorionic twin pregnancies with that of singleton pregnancies, Okita and colleagues (1983a) demonstrated that chorion laeve tissue assimilates arachidonic acid from both the amnionic fluid (possibly by way of the amnion) and from maternal decidua (blood). The arachidonic acid content of fused chorion laeve in diamnionic–dichorionic twin pregnancies was about one half that found in reflected chorion laeve tissue of both twin and singleton pregnancies. The fatty acid pattern of glycerophospholipid remodeling in chorion laeve during labor is suggestive that a part of the fatty acids utilized in this process were assimilated from amnionic fluid.

Chorion Laeve: Oncofetal Fibronectin. Fetal chorion laeve is juxtaposed to maternal decidual tissue. One function of chorion laeve in parturition may be related to its production of oncofetal fibronectin, which provides less tightly adherent junctions (than would fibronectin) to the extracellular matrix of decidual cells (Feinberg and colleagues, 1991). This may facilitate separation and thence delivery of the fetal membranes (Chap. 5). Oncofetal fibronectin is present in large amounts in vaginal and cervical fluids during labor (both at term and preterm)(Lockwood and associates, 1991), likely because of partial and traumatic separation of chorion laeve and lower uterine segment decidua during labor. This traumatic process is obliged in the formation of the forebag as the decidua parietalis is torn away from the uterus. As described in "The Forebag of the Amnionic Fluid and Parturition" later in the chapter, the chorion laeve, especially in the lower uterine segment, is pulled away from the uterus during cervical effacement and dilatation. In this process, fragments of decidua parietalis are torn away from the remainder of the decidua.

Chorion Laeve: Uterotonin Degradation. Evidence is accumulating that chorion laeve is a tissue that, like amnion, protects against rather than contributes to the initiation of parturition. In the case of chorion laeve, however, this function is subserved in part by highly efficient enzyme systems that degrade uterotonins. The chorion laeve forms a protective metabolic wall around the amnionic fluid that precludes the transfer of amnion (or amnionic fluid) uterotonins to decidua or myometrium.

Prostaglandin Dehydrogenase. In contrast to the amnion, the chorion laeve is extraordinarily rich in prostaglandin dehydrogenase activity, the initial and rate-limiting enzyme in prostaglandin inactivation (Fig. 12–10). Even if PGE_2 were produced in amnion and transferred toward chorion laeve, it is evident that no more than a small fraction could escape metabolism in chorion laeve tissue. PGE_2 is an appreciably better substrate for this enzyme than is $PGF_{2\alpha}$.

Enkephalinase. The chorion laeve is very rich in enkephalinase. The specific activity of enkephalinase in homogenates of this tissue is very high (Casey and MacDonald, 1992), and enkephalinase protein is readily apparent in chorion laeve by immunohistochemical analysis (Head and colleagues, unpublished). Because enkephalinase is present in such high amounts in chorion laeve, it is unlikely that endothelin-1 formed in amnion or chorion laeve could escape metabolism by this enzyme.

Chorion Laeve and Parturition in Perspective. Because of the very high specific activities of prostaglandin dehydrogenase and enkephalinase in chorion laeve, it seems virtually indisputable that this tissue is a metabolic barrier protecting decidua and myometrium from the potent uterotonic or vasoconstrictor action of PGE_2 and endothelin-1 synthesized in amnion or chorion laeve (or that from amnionic fluid that might otherwise traverse the membranes). Thus, with respect to functions related to parturition, it is most likely that chorion laeve, like amnion, serves principally to forestall the initiation of parturition.

Decidua Parietalis and Parturition

The highly modified endometrium of pregnancy is an extraordinarily versatile tissue, producing a number of protein hormones (hPRL, relaxin, PTH-rP, CRH), vari-

ous cytokines, 1,25-dihydroxy-vitamin D_3, growth factors, endothelin-1, and unique binding proteins. The decidual cells also are richly supported by bone-marrow-derived leukocytes, which include uterine large granular lymphocytes and resident tissue macrophages in large numbers (Chap. 4).

Decidua: Anatomical and Functional Considerations. The decidua parietalis is contiguous on the fetal side with the chorion laeve, and on the other side with the myometrium. A metabolic contribution of decidua parietalis to parturition has been an appealing possibility to many investigators for a number of reasons, both anatomical and functional. Being situated contiguous with the myometrium, the generation of paracrine-acting uterotropins or uterotonins in this multifunctional tissue is an interesting option. There are several lines of evidence that *"decidual activation"* is an accompaniment of human parturition (for review: Casey and MacDonald, 1988a, 1988c, 1990; MacDonald and colleagues, 1991).

The Bioactive Agent Set. In a reasonably large number of normal pregnancies, a set of bioactive agents accumulates in amnionic fluid during labor. This group of compounds is referred to as a *bioactive agent set* because the compounds are commonly produced simultaneously in increased amounts during inflammation. These agents (PGE_2, PGF_α, PGFM, PAF, free arachidonic acid, IL-1β, IL-6, IL-8, TNF-α, and endothelin-1) are mediators of the inflammatory response. Several of these compounds are not produced (or secreted) by amnion or chorion laeve: $PGF_{2\alpha}$, PGFM, and IL-1β. Therefore, decidual cells and mononuclear phagocytes in or recruited to the forebag decidua are the likely sources of these agents that accumulate in amnionic fluid.

Decidual Activation. The finding of the bioactive agent set in amnionic fluid during labor, and other supportive data, form the basis of the *"decidual activation"* concept. An important consideration for the decidual activation theorem is that this tissue is supplied, albeit poorly, with maternal blood, and is highly enriched with mononuclear phagocytes (macrophages and, during labor, stimulated monocytes). The activation of decidua and the particular portion of the decidua parietalis activated is important to understanding the origin and significance of the accumulation of bioactive agents in the amnionic fluid and the vagina during labor.

Decidual Activation: Lipid Metabolites in Amnionic Fluid

$PGF_{2\alpha}$ and PGFM. There is an increase in the concentration of PGE_2, $PGF_{2\alpha}$, and PGFM in amnionic fluid after labor is in progress; and thereafter, the concentrations of these prostaglandins continue to increase as labor

progresses (Fig. 12–9). The $PGF_{2\alpha}$ and PGFM in amnionic fluid are particularly important to an analysis of the origin of prostaglandins in amnionic fluid, because amnion and chorion laeve cannot synthesize $PGF_{2\alpha}$; rather, the fetal membranes are capable only of PGE_2 synthesis. Mononuclear phagocytes produce PGE_2 almost exclusively. The decidua, on the other hand, produces both $PGF_{2\alpha}$ and PGE_2.

$PGF_{2\alpha}$ FORMATION AND CERVICAL DILATATION. It is probable that the continuing increase in the concentration of prostaglandins in amnionic fluid (as labor progresses) is attributable to two factors: First, it is the result of accumulation of prostaglandins in amnionic fluid and not the consequence of a continually increasing rate of prostaglandin synthesis per unit tissue mass. The level of PGFM in maternal blood is also increased during labor. Second, as the surface area of the forebag increases with cervical dilatation, more decidual tissue is exposed, providing a new tissue source of $PGF_{2\alpha}$ substrate, arachidonic acid. Because the decidual tissue of the forebag is largely devascularized during the formation of the forebag, arachidonic acid is limiting. The concentrations of prostaglandins in forebag amnionic fluid during labor are much greater (10-fold) than those in the upper compartment (MacDonald and Casey, in press).

OTHER POTENTIAL SOURCES OF $PGF_{2\alpha}$ IN AMNIONIC FLUID: FETAL URINE. The amount of $PGF_{2\alpha}$ in fetal urine during labor is much too low to account for the $PGF_{2\alpha}$ in amnionic fluid (Casey and colleagues, 1983).

OTHER POTENTIAL SOURCES OF $PGF_{2\alpha}$ IN AMNIONIC FLUID: MYOMETRIUM. The myometrium also produces $PGF_{2\alpha}$; it is unlikely to represent a quantitatively important source of amnionic fluid $PGF_{2\alpha}$, however, because of (1) the ready accessibility of myometrial prostaglandins to maternal blood and (2) the likelihood of reduced myometrial prostaglandin production in response to the action of cortisol, the levels of which are increased in the blood of pregnant women during labor (Casey and colleagues, 1985; Richardson and associates, 1986). Therefore, increased $PGF_{2\alpha}$ entry into amnionic fluid is both a marker of decidual activation and a marker of active labor.

OTHER POTENTIAL SOURCES OF $PGF_{2\alpha}$ IN AMNIONIC FLUID: PGE_2 9-KETOREDUCTASE IN DECIDUA. The possibility was considered that PGE_2, originating in amnion, chorion laeve, or both, is converted to $PGF_{2\alpha}$ in decidua. The activity of the enzyme that catalyzes the conversion of PGE_2 to $PGF_{2\alpha}$ (PGE_2 9-ketoreductase) is demonstrable in decidual tissue (Niesert and associates, 1986; Schlegel and co-workers, 1984). There are, however, at least four findings that mitigate against the possibility that decidual $PGF_{2\alpha}$ arises from PGE_2 produced in the fetal membranes. (1) The specific activity of PGE_2 9-ketoreductase

in decidual tissue and in subcellular fractions of decidual tissue is low. (2) The specific activity of this enzyme is appreciably less than that of 15-hydroxyprostaglandin dehydrogenase, the enzyme that catalyzes the first step in the inactivation of both PGE_2 and $PGF_{2\alpha}$. (3) Prostaglandin dehydrogenase in decidua preferentially catalyzes the metabolism of PGE_2, compared with $PGF_{2\alpha}$ (Casey and associates, 1989b). (4) In incubations conducted with intact decidual cells, there is little or no conversion of PGE_2 to $PGF_{2\alpha}$, reflective of the low activity of PGE_2 9-ketoreductase, limited entry of PGE_2 into decidual cells, or both. Therefore, $PGF_{2\alpha}$ and PGFM in amnionic fluid during labor are almost certainly synthesized in decidua, most likely in the exposed decidua of the forebag of the amnionic fluid.

Prostaglandin Dehydrogenase in Decidua. As stated, prostaglandin dehydrogenase is present in high activity in decidua and preferentially inactivates PGE_2. Prostaglandin dehydrogenase in decidua can therefore serve, with chorion laeve, to prevent the transport of PGE_2 (from amnionic fluid, amnion, chorion laeve, or decidua itself) to myometrium.

Decidual Activation: Arachidonic Acid in Amnionic Fluid. During labor there is a net gain in the arachidonic acid content of amnion and its extracellular fluid, the amnionic fluid. As fetal breathing is diminished during labor, precluding an arachidonic acid source from fetal lung, the arachidonic acid almost certainly was released from decidual tissue. Arachidonic acid release (phospholipase A_2 action) is a component of the inflammatory response. Hypoxia and trauma, also stimuli of inflammation, cause arachidonic acid release even in the absence of infection. Therefore, as described on p. 323, the increase in arachidonic acid concentration in the forebag amnionic fluid during labor is likely attributable to the release of arachidonic acid from forebag decidual tissues.

Decidual Activation: Platelet-activating Factor in Amnionic Fluid. Platelet-activating factor (PAF) accumulates in amnionic fluid during labor (Billah and Johnston, 1983; Nishihara and associates, 1984), and PAF can be synthesized in amnion and decidua (Ban and associates, 1986). The tissue site(s) of origin of PAF in amnionic fluid during human labor, however, is not established. Whereas PAF can be synthesized in amnion, it is not released from this tissue (which is true of PAF synthesized in most cells other than leukocytes). Several suggestions have been made as to the origin of amnionic fluid PAF; among these are fetal urine, fetal lung secretions, and decidua (Angle and associates, 1988; Johnston and colleagues, 1987). Stimulation of macrophages causes a marked increase in glycerophospholipid hydrolysis, arachidonic acid release, prostaglandin formation (Kunkel and Chensue,

1986), and the production of PAF (Albert and Snyder, 1983). PAF release by mononuclear phagocytes is a characteristic of the inflammatory response; and PAF is a mediator of this response. The release of arachidonic acid from 1-alkyl-2-arachidonoyl phosphatidylcholine favors the formation of PAF because the other product of this reaction, 1-alkyl-lysophosphatidylcholine, is the cosubstrate for PAF biosynthesis. The potential role of PAF in parturition was reviewed by Johnston and associates (1987). Because of the likelihood of increased glycerophospholipid hydrolysis in decidua during labor, together with activation and recruitment of mononuclear phagocytes, it is reasonable to suspect that the PAF that accumulates in amnionic fluid during labor arises in decidua, possibly in mononuclear phagocytes in this tissue. Thus, activation of forebag decidua parietalis tissue by an inflammatory reaction will give free arachidonic acid, PGE_2, $PGF_{2\alpha}$, PGFM, and PAF. All of these products are indicative of increased glycerophospholipid turnover.

Decidual Activation: Cytokines in Amnionic Fluid.

Cytokines—the interleukins, tumor necrosis factors, and colony-stimulating factors—are produced by leukocytes, especially mononuclear phagocytes, in rapid response to inflammatory or immunological challenges. Some of these cytokines (e.g., IL-6, IL-8, and CSFs) are found as normal constituents of amnionic fluid obtained before labor at various stages of pregnancy from midtrimester to term. Other cytokines (IL-1β, TNF-α) are found in some (25 to 40 percent) amnionic fluid samples collected during labor. Because of the multiple biological functions of these agents, including the stimulation of uterotonin formation, many studies have been conducted to quantify various cytokines in amnionic fluid and to explore the action of these cytokines in fetal membranes, decidua, and myometrium. Among the cytokines that have been identified in amnionic fluid are IL-1β, IL-1α, IL-6, IL-8, TNF-α, and M-CSF.

Interleukin-1 in Amnionic Fluid.

Two forms of IL-1 are synthesized, IL-1α and IL-1β (reviewed by Dinarello, 1986). Originally, these two cytokines were distinguished by differences in isoelectric point. The two IL-1s, however, are the products of two separate genes, the organizational structures of which are quite similar. There is relatively little amino acid sequence homology (26 percent) between the two proteins. In most systems, the biological actions of IL-1α and IL-1β are indistinguishable, and the mature forms of the cytokines (M_r about 17,000) act by way of a common receptor. The IL-1β gene probably evolved more recently; and in most cells, IL-1β formation exceeds that of IL-1α by at least an order of magnitude. The transcription of the two genes for IL-1 seems to be regulated similarly by stimuli that eventuate in increased IL-1 formation. Pro-IL-1α/β is synthesized principally in mononuclear phagocytes but

also in other tissues in response to specific stimuli. But the processing of pro-IL-1β is requisite for secretion of bioactive IL-1β and is limited to a few cell types, principally monocytes and macrophages. This issue is addressed in a subsequent section.

Before the onset of labor, IL-1β is not present in amnionic fluid in quantities detectable by sensitive immunoassay techniques (ELISA). In some normal pregnancies with intact fetal membranes, however, the concentration of IL-1β in amnionic fluid during labor is very high. In about 25 to 40 percent of pregnancies during spontaneous labor at term, there is readily measurable IL-1β in concentrations of about 100 to 5000 pg/mL (Cox and associates, 1988a; Romero and colleagues, 1990).

The most extensive studies of amnionic fluid IL-1β were first conducted with amnionic fluid samples obtained during preterm labor. The finding of IL-1β in amnionic fluid in these earlier studies was believed to constitute corroborative evidence of infection-induced preterm labor. At the time of this interpretation, however, it was not realized that IL-1β was found with about equal frequency (25 to 40 percent) in amnionic fluid samples obtained from pregnancies at term during spontaneous labor. This latter finding obliged a consideration of the likelihood that IL-1β might be just another mediator or marker of inflammation that accumulates in amnionic fluid as a normal sequela of labor. But in this case, it was a protein rather than a lipid derivative that entered amnionic fluid.

Origin of IL-1β in Amnionic Fluid.

As in the case of lipid derivatives that enter amnionic fluid during labor, IL-1β almost certainly is produced as a consequence of activation of the decidual tissues of the forebag during labor. The entry of IL-1β from forebag decidua into amnionic fluid, however, cannot be compared directly with the entry of prostaglandins. First, IL-1β is a protein (M_r ~17,000). It is probable that the transfer of IL-1β from decidua across the fetal membranes of the forebag is severely limited. IL-1β is secreted from forebag decidua into the vagina, but IL-1β is not found in 60 to 75 percent of the amnionic fluids collected during labor. The secretion of IL-1β in decidua is probably limited to mononuclear phagocytes in this tissue and governed by the bioactive agents in vaginal fluids, that is, endotoxin, microorganisms, and IL-1β per se. IL-1β is a strong autoinducer of IL-1β expression. Very specific features of IL-1β synthesis, processing, and secretion are important to an evaluation of the cellular origin of IL-1β that enters amnionic fluid.

IL-1β SYNTHESIS, PROCESSING, AND SECRETION. IL-1β is synthesized as pro-IL-1β, a (34-kDa) precursor form in which there is no leader sequence and which, at least at the plasma membrane receptor level, is biologically inactive. If pro-IL-1β is not converted to mature, bioactive

(17-kd) IL-1β, the pro-IL-1β accumulates in the cytosol, (that is, is not secreted from the cell) (Auron and colleagues, 1987).

Many divergent types of cells (e.g., decidual cells) express the pro-IL-1β gene; and upon appropriate stimulation, pro-IL-1β mRNA as well as pro-IL-1β protein accumulates in these cells. But, these cells do not secrete mature IL-1β. The function of intracellular pro-IL-1β is not known; pro-IL-1β is not incorporated into the cell membrane; and as stated, pro-IL-1β is not active by way of the plasma membrane receptor for IL-1β (for review: Mosley and collaborators, 1987). Mature IL-1β (17 kDa) is synthesized and secreted almost exclusively by mononuclear phagocytes, that is, stimulated monocytes or activated macrophages, in a very precise manner that is critically important to an understanding of decidual activation during parturition. Specifically, the processing of pro-IL-1β to mature IL-1β in vivo is believed to be (1) confined to mononuclear phagocytes (and possibly neutrophils); (2) catalyzed by a specific intracellular pro-IL-1β converting enzyme, which is present in mononuclear phagocytes and neutrophils; (3) co-linked to the release of mature, 17-kDa, bioactive IL-1β; (4) absent in extracellular sites; and (5) increased in compromised or injured monocytes and macrophages (Hogquist and colleagues, 1991; Howard and associates, 1991; Webb and co-workers, 1987). IL-1β is not found in fetal urine either before or after the onset of labor.

Therefore, IL-1β, when present in amnionic fluid, must have arisen in mononuclear phagocytes (from activated resident tissue macrophages in the decidua of the forebag or else from maternal blood-borne monocytes, or from neutrophils recruited to this inflammatory reaction in decidual tissue of the forebag and into the amnionic fluid).

IL-1β mRNA IN FOREBAG DECIDUA. The levels of IL-1β mRNA in the decidual tissues of the forebag of term spontaneous labor pregnancies are appreciably greater than those in decidual tissues attached to chorion laeve in the upper amnionic fluid compartment of the same tissues (MacDonald and colleagues, 1991).

CELLULAR ORIGIN OF AMNIONIC FLUID IL-1β. Based on all data available, the most likely option for the origin of mature IL-1β in amnionic fluid is that it is produced in the amnionic fluid space directly. Namely, IL-1β, when present in amnionic fluid, likely arises in this space in situ by secretion from mononuclear phagocytes (probably maternal monocytes) recruited into the amnionic fluid.

There are very few macrophages in the amnionic fluid of normal pregnancies before the onset of labor. In response to the inflammatory reaction in the forebag decidua during labor, however, leukocytes are recruited to the amnionic fluid. There is a highly significant correlation between the presence of stimulated monocytes

and the concentration of IL-1β in amnionic fluid (Head and colleagues, personal communication). The amount of IL-1β in amnionic fluid may be determined by the number of monocytes recruited, the activational status of these cells, or the effect of constituents of amnionic fluid on the rate of secretion of IL-1β by mononuclear phagocytes.

MONONUCLEAR PHAGOCYTES IN AMNIONIC FLUID. The number of monocytes recruited to the amnionic fluid may be dependent upon several factors, including the vascular integrity of the exposed decidua of the forebag, the capacity of monocyte chemoattractant formation in decidua, the amount of decidual tissue separated from the uterus during the formation of the forebag, and the microorganisms of the vaginal fluid of a given pregnancy.

The activational status of the monocytes may be partly dependent upon the toxins elaborated by the microorganisms prevalent in the vagina of a given woman at the time labor begins. Modifications in monocyte IL-1β secretory capacity by constituents of amnionic fluid may be gestational age-dependent and related to the amnionic fluid concentration of agents known to modify monocyte IL-1β synthesis (e.g., TGF-β). We have observed, albeit in a relatively small number of pregnancies, that very high levels of IL-1β in amnionic fluid during preterm labor are found principally in the earlier gestational age group, 24 to 28 weeks. At this stage of gestation, the decidua is still a thick, lush tissue; the amount (volume) of decidua decreases rapidly thereafter as pregnancy progresses to term.

Decidual Activation: Other Cytokines in Amnionic Fluid.

IL-1β is the primary cytokine that promotes the synthesis of other cytokines. The processing and secretion of cytokines such as IL-6 and IL-8 are not as complex as those of IL-1β. A cell that is stimulated to synthesize IL-6 or IL-8, secretes IL-6 and IL-8. IL-1β stimulates the synthesis of IL-6, IL-8, TNF-α, prostaglandins, M-CSF, and endothelin-1—that is, the bioactive agent set that accumulates in some amnionic fluids during labor. Thus, the accumulation of these agents in amnionic fluid may be principally a response to IL-1β action. IL-1β stimulates amnion cells to secrete IL-6, IL-8, and endothelin-1.

INTERLEUKIN-6. Interleukin-6 (IL-6) is a multifunctional cytokine that is produced in many tissues, especially in response to IL-1β action. IL-6 stimulates the synthesis of acute phase proteins by hepatocytes, stimulates immunoglobulin synthesis by B cells, and seems to be involved in a host of other immunological responses. IL-6 is present in amnionic fluid in reasonably large amounts at term and at midtrimester of pregnancy, irrespective of the presence or absence of labor. Thus, IL-6 is a normal constituent of amnionic fluid. The levels of IL-6 in forebag amnionic fluid are greater than those in the upper compartment during labor. IL-6 mRNA is demonstrable in decidual tissue, and the levels of IL-6 mRNA are increased in response to treatment with IL-1 and TNF-α (as well as bacterial toxins, which may act primarily to increase IL-1 production). Amnion and chorion laeve also are potential sites of IL-6 production; both amnion cells and cytotrophoblasts from chorion laeve express IL-6 mRNA and secrete IL-6 into the culture medium. Moreover, IL-1β stimulates IL-6 formation and secretion by amnion. Therefore, an increase in IL-6 levels in amnionic fluid during labor is likely to occur in response to IL-1β action whenever IL-1β gains access to the amnionic fluid.

INTERLEUKIN-8. Interleukin-8 (IL-8) is a cytokine polypeptide with neutrophil chemotactic/activating and T-cell chemotactic activity. IL-8 is produced by a number of cell types including peripheral blood monocytes, endothelial cells, fibroblasts, keratinocytes, synovial cells, pulmonary epithelial cells, and neutrophils. The major secreted form of IL-8 is a 72-amino-acid protein that is formed by successive removal of amino-terminal residues from a 99-amino-acid precursor. IL-8 is also present in considerable amounts in amnionic fluid at midtrimester and at term, irrespective of labor status. Thus, IL-8 is also a normal constituent of amnionic fluid. The levels of IL-8 in amnionic fluid increase during labor and are greater in fluids in which there is other direct evidence of inflammation or infection (increased numbers of monocytes, fever, chorioamnionitis, and IL-1β). It has been suggested that IL-8 may be responsible for recruitment of leukocytes to the endometrium or decidua.

Arici and associates (1992) find that IL-8 mRNA is present in varying amounts in human endometrium and decidua at midtrimester and at term. In addition, IL-8 mRNA is present and IL-8 protein is produced by endometrial stromal cells in culture (Arici and colleagues, 1991, 1992). In these cells, IL-1α, TNF-α, and serum act to increase the levels of IL-8 mRNA and immunoreactive IL-8 protein secreted into the culture medium as is known to occur in other cell types. Based on the results of studies conducted in endometrial stromal cells, Arici and associates suggested that IL-8 mRNA stability can be modified by cytokines in a manner that effectively leads to increased gene expression (i.e., increased IL-8 production).

As in the case of IL-6, increases in IL-8 levels in amnionic fluid are likely the result of IL-1β action whenever this primary cytokine is present in amnionic fluid. IL-8 also is produced by amnion cells, and IL-1β stimulates amnion cell IL-8 secretion.

TUMOR NECROSIS FACTOR-α. Tumor necrosis factor-α (TNF-α), also known as cachectin, is another cytokine produced by macrophages in response to a variety of challenges, in particular bacterial endotoxin and IL-1β. TNF-α is not found in amnionic fluid of normal pregnan-

cies at any stage of gestation before the onset of labor. But TNF-α is sometimes found in amnionic fluid of normal, term pregnancies during labor and in pregnancies complicated by preterm labor (Casey and associates, 1989a; Romero and colleagues, 1989b). These findings also are indicative of the inflammation of decidua of the forebag that is exposed to vaginal fluids after cervical dilatation.

COLONY-STIMULATING FACTORS. The colony-stimulating factors (CSFs) are glycoproteins that regulate the formation of mature macrophages and granulocytes from immature progenitor cells (Stanley, 1986). Selected CSFs are produced by stimulated macrophages; and in turn, one particular CSF, *macrophage CSF* (M-CSF), usually produced in mesenchymal (stromal) cells of tissues, acts on macrophages and their precursors to promote replication and differentiation of these cells. Uniquely, the receptor for M-CSF, which is the product of the c-*fms* proto-oncogene, is present in decidual and trophoblastic tissue (Visvader and Verma, 1989). Heretofore c-*fms* was believed to be present only in monocytes and macrophages.

The concentration of M-CSF in mouse uterine tissue during pregnancy is increased strikingly (1000-fold), compared with that present in the uterus of nonpregnant animals (Bartocci and colleagues, 1986; Rosendaal, 1975). It has been suggested that M-CSF produced in decidua acts on trophoblasts as a growth or differentiating factor (Rettenmier and associates, 1986).

Presently it is not possible to deduce the exact role of CSFs in the regulation of decidual and placental function or in parturition. There is, however, suspicion that such a role exists, because CSF concentrations of a type not yet defined are increased during labor in amnionic fluid (Ringler and colleagues, 1989). And it is known that there is a marked increase in the number of neutrophils in the blood of women during labor and in the puerperium, possibly indicating an increase in granulocyte-macrophage (GM)-CSF formation during labor. The finding of increased concentrations of colony stimulating factors in amnionic fluid during labor may be another indication of activation of the mononuclear phagocytes and decidual cells in the forebag decidua.

Decidual Activation: Endothelin-1 in Amnionic Fluid. Endothelin-1 mRNA is present in decidual tissues at midtrimester of human pregnancy and at term, irrespective of the presence or absence of labor. Immunoreactive endothelin-1 is secreted into the culture medium of decidual tissue explants. The cell(s) in decidual tissue that produces endothelin-1, however, has not been identified, but both decidual cells themselves and macrophages are potentially involved, as well as the vascular endothelial cells of this tissue. As discussed in Chapter 4, endometrial stromal cells (the progenitor of the decidual cell) synthesize and secrete endothelin-1. In these cells, the levels of endothelin-1 mRNA are increased by TGF-β treatment and decreased by progestin treatment. Macrophages are also known to synthesize endothelin-1, and the production of endothelin-1 by both of these cell types is increased in response to treatment with IL-1β and TNF-α. As stated previously, the levels of endothelin-1 are increased in the forebag amnionic fluid compartment, together with those of cytokines such as IL-1β, IL-6, IL-8, and TNF-α. As IL-1β and TNF-α are effective stimulators of endothelin-1 biosynthesis (mRNA levels and protein production) in amnion cells, endometrial stromal cells, and other cell types, it is possible that all of these tissues contribute to the endothelin-1 that accumulates in the forebag amnionic fluid during the inflammatory response in forebag tissues that is obliged with cervical dilatation.

Decidual Activation and Parturition: Summary.

As the cervix dilates, the decidual tissue of the forebag is traumatized and exposed to vaginal fluids. Specifically, the outer lining of the forebag consists of partially devascularized decidua that has been torn away from the lower uterine segment. Trauma, hypoxia, and exposure to LPS, microorganisms, and IL-1β in the vaginal fluids provokes an inflammatory reaction. In response to this reaction, mediators of inflammation are released (arachidonic acid) or synthesized: prostaglandins, PAF, IL-1β, IL-6, IL-8, TNF-α, CSF-1 and endothelin-1. The fatty acids and PAF can cross the membranes into the amnionic fluid. The inflammatory reaction incites leukocytic infiltration. The leukocytes, which include activated monocytes, can penetrate the inflamed tissues of the forebag into the amnionic fluid space. Mononuclear phagocytes in the amnionic fluid synthesize and process IL-1β. IL-1β acts on the mononuclear phagocytes and amnion to stimulate the synthesis of IL-6, IL-8, and endothelin-1. Thus, the accumulation of mediators of the inflammatory response in amnionic fluid is a consequence of labor. The inflammatory reaction induced in the forebag is an inevitable and consistent sequela of labor. Therefore, the accumulation of these agents in amnionic fluid cannot be taken as evidence of the involvement of these mediators of inflammation in processes that initiate parturition.

The Forebag of the Amnionic Fluid and Parturition

An understanding of the tissue sites of origin of the *bioactive agent set* that sometimes accumulates in amnionic fluid during labor, and of the cellular mechanisms involved in the generation of these agents, is crucial to an interpretation of the role of these compounds in parturition. It is likely that these agents are produced in *activated decidua* or in response to decidual products.

During labor, the lowermost pole of the fetal membranes, with attached fragments of decidua parietalis, is involved in a very important structural modification, namely, the formation of the forebag of the amnionic sac. In the active phase of labor, the forebag serves as the leading wedge that promotes cervical dilatation (provided the membranes are intact) prior to the time when the fetal presenting part descends sufficiently to fulfill this role. The forebag is important to parturition not only because of its mechanical role in promoting cervical dilatation, but also because the forebag tissues are major sites of synthesis of substances that accumulate in the amnionic fluid during labor. The forebag is formed during the process of cervical effacement and dilatation.

Mechanism of Cervical Effacement.

Effacement ("obliteration" or "taking up") of the cervix is the shortening of the cervical canal from a length of about 2 cm so that the canal is replaced by a mere circular orifice with almost paper-thin edges. This process takes place from above downward; it occurs as the muscular fibers in the vicinity of the internal os are pulled upward, or "taken up," into the lower uterine segment, while the condition of the external os remains temporarily unchanged. As illustrated in Figures 12–11 through 12–14, the edges of the internal os are drawn upward several centimeters to become a functional part of the lower uterine segment. Effacement may be compared with a funneling process in which the whole length of a narrow cylinder is converted into a very obtuse, flaring funnel with only a small circular orifice for an outlet. As the result of increased myometrial activity during phase 1 of parturition, appreciable effacement of the ripened cer-

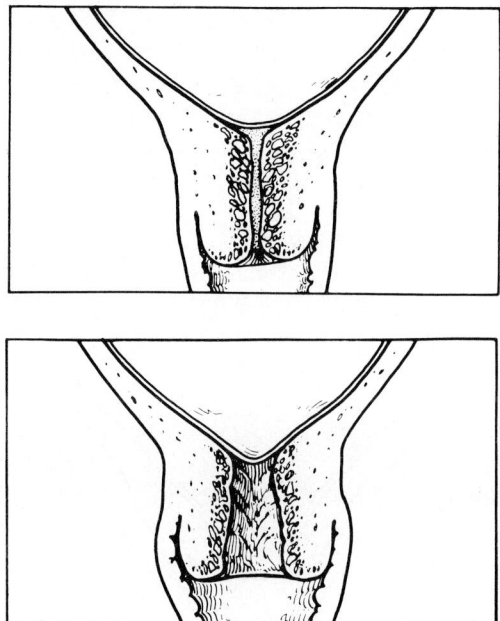

Fig. 12–11. Cervix near the end of pregnancy but before labor. Top, primigravida; bottom, multipara.

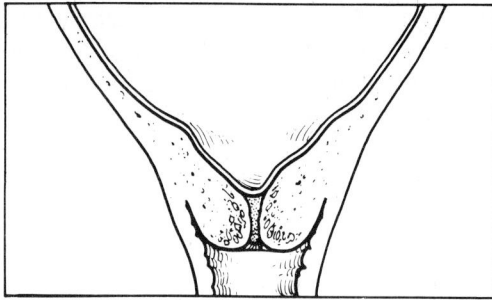

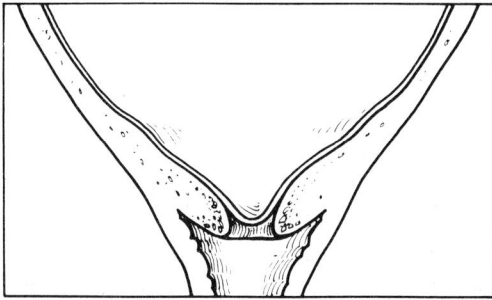

Fig. 12–12. Beginning effacement of cervix. Note dilatation of internal os and funnel-shaped cervical canal. Top, primigravida; bottom, multipara.

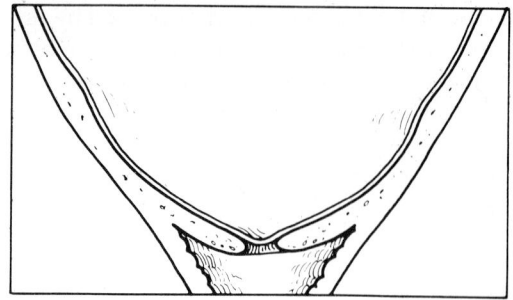

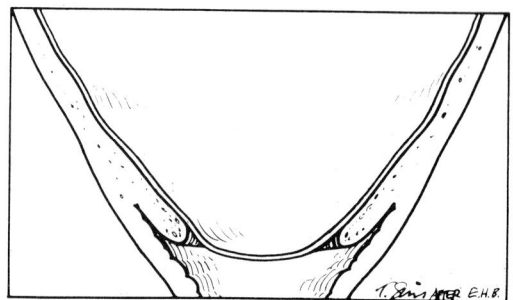

Fig. 12–14. Cervical canal obliterated—that is, the cervix is completely effaced. Top, primigravida; bottom, multipara.

vix is sometimes attained even before active labor begins. Such effacement usually facilitates expulsion of the mucus plug from the cervical canal as it is shortened.

Mechanism of Cervical Dilatation. Compared with the body of the uterus, the lower uterine segment and cervix are regions of lesser resistance. Therefore, dur-

Fig. 12–13. Further effacement of cervix. Top, primigravida; bottom, multipara.

ing a contraction, these structures are subjected to distension, in the course of which a centrifugal pull is exerted on the cervix (Figs. 12–15 to 12–17). As the uterine contractions cause pressure on the membranes, the hydrostatic action of the amnionic sac, in turn, dilates the cervical canal like a wedge. In the absence of intact membranes, the pressure of the presenting part against the cervix and lower uterine segment is similarly effective. Early rupture of the membranes ("dry birth") does not retard cervical dilatation so long as the presenting part of the fetus is positioned to exert pressure against the cervix and lower uterine segment.

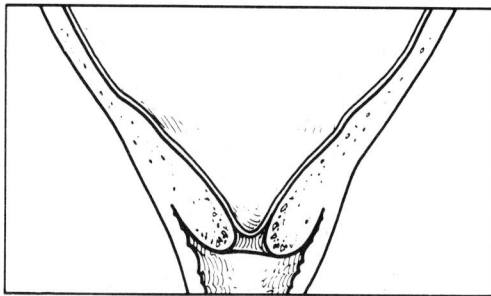

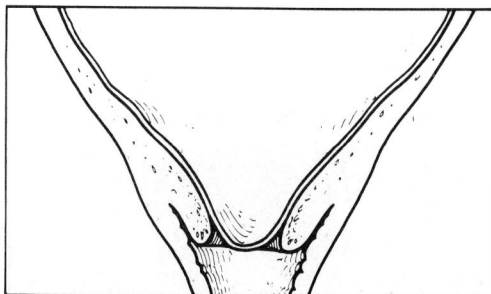

Decidua Parietalis of the Forebag. The decidua parietalis of the lower uterine segment is thin and poorly developed. The slightest movement of the underlying muscle, therefore, allows the fetal membranes with attached decidua parietalis to pull away and slip back and forth over fragments of decidua parietalis that remain attached to the myometrium. This loosening of the membranes and tearing decidua away from the lower segment is a normal feature of early labor and a prerequisite to successful cervical dilatation. Membranes that slide readily over the lower segment and partly through the cervix are much more efficacious dilators than if more firmly attached. This process serves to expose the decidua attached to the forebag to fluids and secretions in the vagina.

Anatomy of the Forebag. Recall that the fetal membranes, during the final 24 to 28 weeks of pregnancy, are

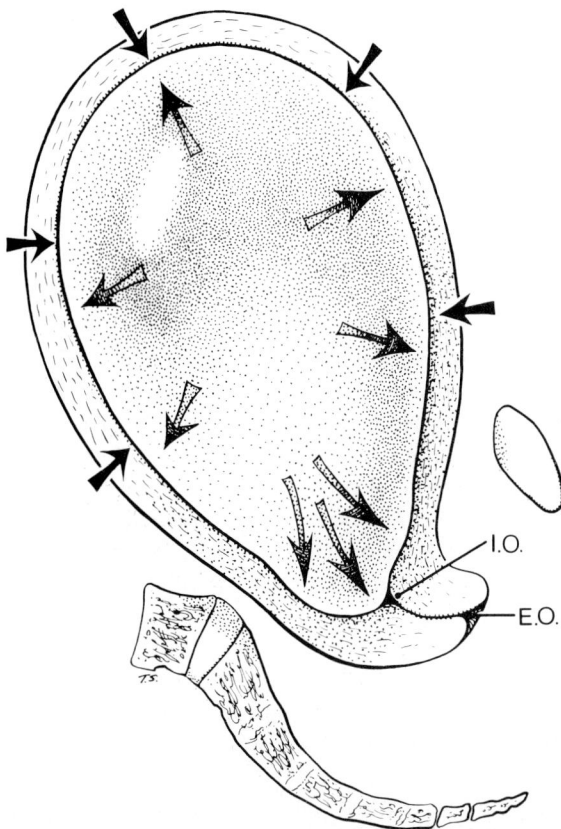

Fig. 12–15. Hydrostatic action of membranes in effecting cervical effacement and dilatation. In the absence of intact membranes, the presenting part, applied to the cervix and forming the lower uterine segments, acts similarly. In this and Figs. 12–16 and 12–17, note changing relations of the external os (E.O.) and internal os (I.O.).

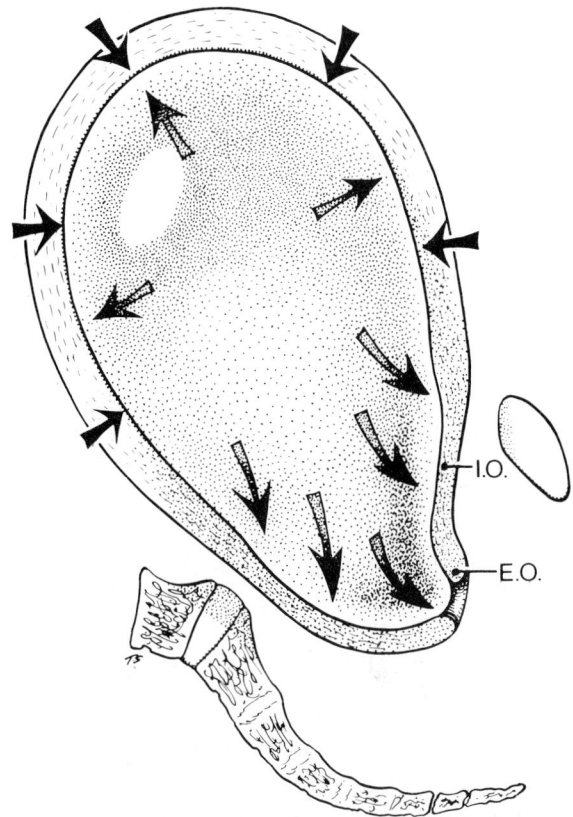

Fig. 12–16. Hydrostatic action of membranes at completion of effacement.

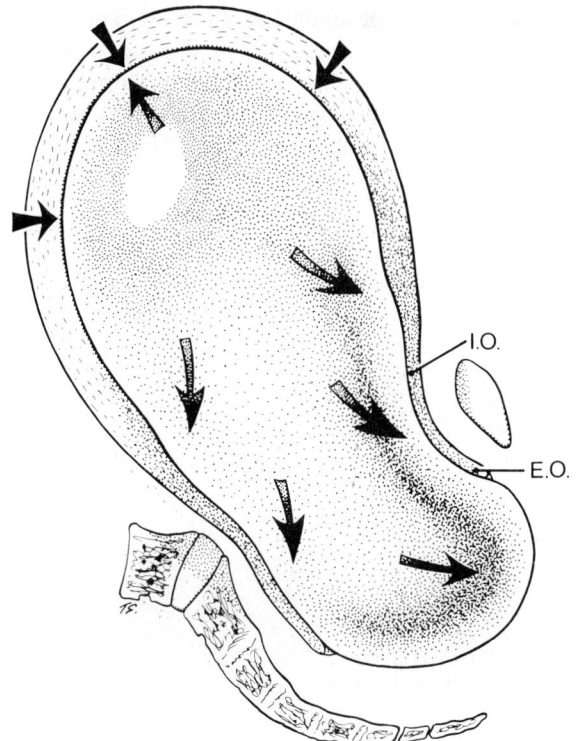

Fig. 12–17. Hydrostatic action of membranes at full cervical dilatation.

contiguous with and attached to the uterine decidua parietalis; the cells of the chorion laeve are interdigitated with those of the decidua by way of extracellular matrix proteins, in part accounted for by oncofetal fibronectin, synthesized by the extravillous cytotrophoblasts (Chap. 5). As the cervix dilates, more and more of the decidua parietalis from the lower uterine segment is torn away from the uterus.

Once the cervix is opened in this manner, the lowermost pole of the amnionic sac is exposed, like the tip of a fluid-filled balloon under pressure being pushed through an enlarging diameter of a hollow cylinder. The surface area of the exposed tissues increases as cervical dilatation progresses during phase 2 of parturition.

The inner surface of the wall of the forebag is the amnion, which on its apical epithelial surface is still bathed by the amnionic fluid. The traumatized, hypoxic decidual tissue torn away from the uterus lines the outer surface of the forebag. This outer surface is exposed to and bathed by the secretions and fluids present in the vagina. These fluids contain a large number and variety of microorganisms, bacterial toxins in large amounts, as well as IL-1β even before labor commences. The tissue trauma involved in the exposure of the forebag tissues and the action of the constituents of the vaginal fluids on these tissues produce an inflammatory response therein (Fig. 12–18). This is an unavoidable, natural accompaniment of labor. It must occur in all pregnancies. In consequence, mediators of the inflammatory process, including prostaglandins and cytokines, are produced in the decidual lining of the forebag in large amounts. The magnitude of the inflammatory response, as judged by the amounts of bioactive agents produced, may be highly dependent on the amount of decidual tissue that remains attached to the forebag chorion laeve. This inflammatory reaction is a consequence of labor; and the inflammatory products formed are sequelae of the inflammatory process that the events of normal labor oblige (MacDonald and associates, 1991).

Amnionic Fluid at Parturition

Constituents. The intact sac of amnionic fluid constitutes a remarkable repository. Measurements conducted of constituents of this fluid, if correctly interpreted, are useful for deciphering some of the biomolecular processes of parturition, including labor and its accompanying events (cervical dilatation). This biological fluid is not only contiguous with tissues that are intimately involved in the labor process, but also seems to be a medium in which important bioactive products are temporarily stored. We choose the term "stored" because the half-life of selected compounds in amnionic fluid is much longer than those of the same compounds in blood. For example, the half-life of $PGF_{2\alpha}$ and PGE_2 in blood is only 6 to 8 minutes; but the half-life of PGE_2 and $PGF_{2\alpha}$ in amnionic fluid is 4 to 6 hours. Therefore, during times of rapid intrauterine physiological or inflammatory or traumatic change, as during labor, substances

accumulate in amnionic fluid so long as the fetal membranes are intact. This provides an opportunity to identify and quantify these compounds in a relatively accessible and uniquely positioned biological fluid of pregnancy.

Anatomical Separation of Amnionic Fluid Compartments. The formation of the forebag is finalized as the forceful myometrial contractions of labor cause the long axis of the fetus to be pushed downward so that the fetal head is wedged into the maternal pelvis. In consequence, amnionic fluid, in variable amounts, in front of the fetal head is trapped between the leading surface of the presenting fetal part and the inner surface of the lower pole of the amnionic sac, that is, the forebag (Fig. 12–18). As the fetal presenting part is engaged in the maternal pelvis, this *forebag compartment* of amnionic fluid is isolated anatomically from the remainder of the amnionic fluid, which is the *upper compartment.* This results in the formation of two anatomically and functionally distinct compartments of amnionic fluid. The surface area of the forebag exposed in the vaginal vault at full cervical dilatation (10 cm) constitutes a large surface area of tissue, 78.5 cm^2.

Functional Separation of Amnionic Fluid Compartments. The two compartments of amnionic fluid become functionally separated because of the following factors. (1) Fetal swallowing, urination, and thoracic movements (effecting exchange between fetal lungs) continues in the upper compartment, but not in the isolated forebag compartment. (2) The upper compartment of the amnionic fluid persists as a component of the paracrine arm of the fetal–placental communication system, and the blood supply to the decidua parietalis of the upper compartment is not compromised. (3) The blood supply to the decidua parietalis that is torn away from the forebag membranes is compromised. (4) The amnion epithelial surface lining of the forebag is contiguous with the amnionic fluid on one side, but the chorion laeve and decidual surface on the other side is bathed by the vaginal secretions. Because of this anatomical arrangement, products of the forebag tissues enter both the amnionic fluid (of the forebag) and the vagina. (5) Compounds produced in forebag tissues that enter the forebag amnionic fluid after the isolation of this compartment do not equilibrate with amnionic fluid in the upper compartment. (6) Therefore, agents formed in the tissues of the forebag accumulate in this space or else are secreted into the vagina.

Inflammation of the Forebag Tissues. The tissue trauma and compromise in the blood supply of the decidua parietalis that are obliged in creation of the forebag, together with the exposure of the decidual fragments to the vaginal contents result in the development of an inflammatory response in these tissues.

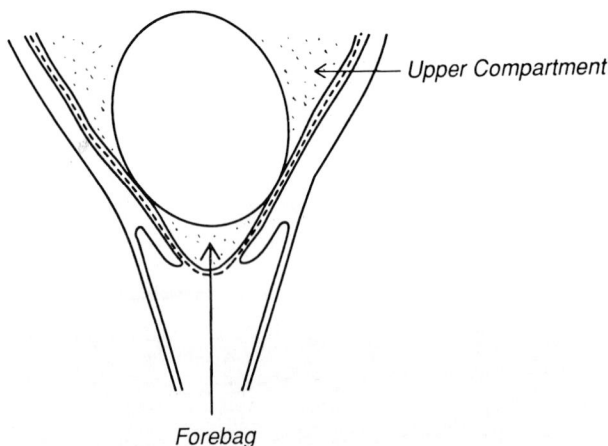

Fig. 12–18. Development of two compartments of the amnionic fluid. As the fetal head engages the maternal pelvis, two amnionic fluid compartments are formed and the forebag is isolated.

The entry into amnionic fluid of prostaglandins (formed in forebag tissues), which are arachidonic acid derivatives ($M_r \sim 300$), is accomplished readily as is the secretion of prostaglandins into the vaginal fluids.

It also is likely that prostaglandins from these tissues enter the maternal circulation after these compounds are secreted from the forebag into the vagina. This also may explain the findings that surgical rupture of the membranes and manipulation of the cervix give rise to increased levels of PGFM in maternal plasma. For example, it has been demonstrated that rupture of the forebag (amniotomy) and manipulations of these tissues (cervical examination) cause an increase in the concentration of PGFM in maternal plasma (Mitchell and colleagues, 1977).

A major line of evidence presented in support of a role for prostaglandins in the initiation of parturition was the finding of high levels of prostaglandins in amnionic fluid during labor. The same is true of platelet-activating factor (PAF). More recently, the accumulation of prostaglandins, PAF, and cytokines in amnionic fluid has been cited as evidence of infection as a cause of preterm labor.

We suggest that most of the prostaglandins, PAF, and cytokines that accumulate in the forebag amnionic fluid during labor arise because of inflammation of the forebag tissues that is obliged during labor (MacDonald and Casey, in press).

Distribution of Bioactive Agents in Amnionic Fluid Compartments. Because of the anatomical and functional separation of the amnionic fluid compartments, there are enormous differences in the concentrations of bioactive agents in the two compartments. The differences are attributable to (1) differences in the amounts of the bioactive agents produced with access to a given compartment, (2) differences in clearance (rate or method) of the bioactive agents from a given compartment, and (3) differences in the amnionic fluid volumes of the two compartments. For example, the levels of prostaglandins in forebag amnionic fluid are much greater than in the upper compartment (10-fold), and the same is true for endothelin-1 concentrations in the two compartments (MacDonald and Casey, in press).

Amnionic Fluid Sampling. Amnionic fluid has been the biological fluid used most commonly to evaluate increases in prostaglandin formation at parturition. Unfortunately, the methods used to collect amnionic fluid and sites of sampling during labor have probably contributed to artifactual results. In most studies, amnionic fluids obtained during labor were collected by amniotomy, surgical rupture of the fetal membranes per vagina. These samples are, by definition, forebag amnionic fluids. Generally, amniotomy is performed electively only with fetal cephalic presentations and only after there is reasonably complete formation of two amnionic fluid

compartments. If the forebag tissues were the principal or only site of production of prostaglandins that enter amnionic fluid during labor, the isolated fluid of this functionally separated space is not representative of the formation of prostaglandins that could be involved in parturition. Additional artifactual results are introduced, however, when these amniotomy-collected fluids contact, and thence are "contaminated" by, vaginal secretions as the fluid flows through the vagina. The vaginal secretions contain PGE_2 and $PGF_{2\alpha}$ in variable, but large, amounts compared with those in amnionic fluid before or during labor (MacDonald and colleagues, unpublished data). These fluids, therefore, are useless for the evaluation of amnionic fluid levels of prostaglandins.

In other studies, amnionic fluids were collected during labor by way of catheters placed into the amnionic sac after rupture of the fetal membranes. The catheters are placed for the purpose of monitoring uterine contractions. These fluids are also useless for the determination of prostaglandin levels. This obtains because immediately after rupture of the membranes, an inflammatory reaction commences in the amnionic sac that includes an influx of mononuclear phagocytes, cytokine formation, and prostaglandin synthesis. Thereby prostaglandin generation independent of the parturitional process gives artifactual results for these fluids.

Amnionic fluids obtained before labor are collected by amniocentesis. Generally, such fluids are obtained by transabdominal amniocentesis conducted for diagnostic purposes. Alternatively, some such fluids are collected by transuterine amniocentesis at the time of cesarean delivery conducted electively before the onset of labor. Fluids sometimes can be collected during labor by sampling the upper compartment by transuterine amniocentesis at cesarean section; and forebag fluid can be sampled during labor by direct needle aspiration per vagina (MacDonald and Casey, in press).

PROSTAGLANDINS AND PARTURITION

The most popular parturition research topic during the past 25 years has been an evaluation of the role of prostaglandins in the initiation of parturition. There has been persuasive evidence that an increase in the rate of prostaglandin formation in one or more uterine or extraembryonic fetal tissues is intimately involved in some obligatory manner in human parturition. This also has been true for all other mammalian species studied. Moreover, Hertelendy (1983) demonstrated that prostaglandins are produced during oviposition (the laying of hard-shelled eggs by birds).

Based upon several lines of evidence, many researchers elected to study the tissue sites of origin and the regulation of prostaglandin synthesis as the most promising clue to the initiation of the parturitional process in human pregnancy. In retrospect, it is clear that this choice was made in part because of the obstacle presented by the absence of progesterone withdrawal before the onset of human parturition. As a result, investigations of human parturition were often conducted after uterine phase 2 of parturition was already in progress. The findings of these studies were compared with those obtained during uterine phase 0 (i.e., before the initiation of parturition). In the conduct of biomedical research, this approach has always been hazardous because it is ultimately necessary to sort out cause-and-effect relationships. Commonly, a particular phenomenon that once was believed to be involved in the biogenesis of a physiological or pathophysiological process may be studied only to discover later that the phenomenon was an aftermath of the process. This predicament has plagued obstetrical research to determine the cause of pregnancy-induced hypertension. For 50 years or more, these investigations have been sidetracked repeatedly by uncertainty as to which processes are causative and which are simply sequelae of preeclampsia.

We and many other investigators conducting parturition research accepted and fostered the view (which, unfortunately, has achieved a status tantamount to pragmatic sanction) that prostaglandins, particularly $PGF_{2\alpha}$ and PGE_2, are somehow obligatorily involved in the biomolecular processes of spontaneous parturition at term. In defense of these studies, there were several lines of evidence in support of a role for prostaglandins in human parturition.

Evidence for Prostaglandin Involvement in Human Parturition.
First, the treatment of pregnant women with prostaglandins, by any of several routes of administration, will cause abortion or labor at all stages of gestation (reviewed by Novy and Liggins, 1980). Second, the levels of prostaglandins (or metabolites thereof) in amnionic fluid, maternal plasma, and maternal urine are increased during labor (Keirse, 1979). Third, it is commonly believed, although not rigorously proven (Keirse, 1990), that the administration of PGH_2 synthase inhibitors to pregnant women will delay the time of onset of induced abortion or spontaneous parturition and sometimes arrest preterm labor (Besinger and Neibyl, 1990). Fourth, prostaglandins cause the contraction of many smooth muscle tissues in vitro.

Collectively, these findings were sufficiently convincing to prompt us and others to search for the tissue site(s) of increased prostaglandin production at parturition and to identify the mechanisms governing prostaglandin formation in that tissue(s). Let there be no doubt: The evidence in favor of the involvement of prostaglandins in parturition is persuasive; but we now suggest that this evidence is deceptive.

Obstacles to the Prostaglandin Theory of Parturition.
In contradistinction to the evidence in favor of a pivotal role for prostaglandins in the initiation of parturition, other considerations that impinge upon the validity of this postulate have been disturbing.

Increased Prostaglandin Formation at Parturition.
There is no evidence to show that there is an increase in prostaglandin formation before the onset of phase 2 of parturition. Contrarily, there is appreciable evidence that this is not the case. On the one hand, it may be that the interval between increased prostaglandin formation and the commencement of forceful uterine contractions is too short to permit realistically the sampling of fluids necessary to obtain such evidence; but on the other hand, the striking increase in the levels of prostaglandins in biological fluids after labor is in progress could be caused by one or more labor-associated processes (e.g., the formation of the forebag and the obligatory involvement of the forebag tissues in an inflammatory reaction).

Importantly, there is no evidence for an increase in prostaglandin formation during the time of transition from uterine phase 0 to phase 1, that is, during the initiation of parturition.

Prostaglandin Induction of Labor or Abortion.
The administration of $PGF_{2\alpha}$ or PGE_2 to pregnant women will cause abortion or labor; but it cannot be concluded from this finding alone that prostaglandins are physiologically involved in the initiation of parturition. Many agents, which almost certainly are not involved physiologically in the initiation of parturition, will cause myometrial smooth muscle to contract; consequently, the success of prostaglandin administration to induce myometrial contractions and thence labor or abortion may reside in pharmacological properties of these agents, which are unrelated to the physiological processes of parturition initiation. This possibility is supported by the finding that with muscle strips prepared from myometrial tissues of pregnant women, prostaglandins are ineffective in inducing contractions (Word and associates, 1992).

Moreover, the amounts of prostaglandins required to cause abortion or labor are enormous, far greater than those generated in vivo. For example, the maximum total amount of PGE_2 that accumulates in the amnionic fluid during term labor is no more than 30 μg; yet the intraamnionic administration of 40 mg of PGE_2 does not always induce abortion.

Inhibition of Prostaglandin H_2 Synthase to Prevent or Arrest Labor.
Rigorous testing of the proposition that inhibitors of prostaglandin synthesis will prevent or arrest labor has not been conducted in human pregnancy (Keirse, 1990). Fear of adverse effects on the fetus caused by pharmacological inhibition of prostaglandin synthesis has prevented most investigators from conducting such studies. If prostaglandins were produced only after the initiation of parturition, the temporary arrest or delay of labor by inhibitors of prostaglandin

synthesis could cause confusion as to the sequence of events involved in parturition. This type of response is not unprecedented. Ritodrine administration may cause a temporary diminution in myometrial contractions (for 24 to 28 hours) without decreasing the incidence of preterm delivery (Canadian Preterm Labor Investigators Group, 1992; Leveno and Cunningham, 1992).

But, there is another important problem in evaluating studies of the inhibition of PGH$_2$ synthesis. Most investigators find that the majority of pregnancies that initially are believed to be complicated by preterm labor do not continue in labor to delivery—that is, with no treatment at all, labor ceases. About two thirds of suspected preterm labor pregnancies remain undelivered without pharmacological intervention. This obstacle alone presents severe limitations in the interpretation of findings of studies to evaluate prostaglandin synthesis inhibition to arrest preterm labor. Few such studies have been conducted that included placebo-treated pregnancies.

Inflammation and Prostaglandin Formation. It is important to emphasize that prostaglandins are mediators of the inflammatory response. With tissue damage, prostaglandins are produced rapidly in large amounts. This is true of blunt and sharp trauma, hypoxia, thermal injury, infection, menstruation, immunological challenge, and others (including labor, we suggest). This rapid response to tissue damage is caused by hydrolysis of cellular membrane glycerophospholipids, which causes the release of arachidonic acid. This obliges prostaglandin formation as a normal metabolic function of the cell in the metabolism of free arachidonic acid.

Inflammation of the Forebag and Prostaglandin Formation. Clearly, the formation of the forebag is a traumatic event that involves hypoxia of the decidua and exposure to multiple prostaglandin synthesis stimulatory agents in vaginal secretions. Therefore, prostaglandin formation in forebag tissues is obliged, but this metabolic obligation is clearly a sequela of labor and cannot be taken as evidence for the involvement of prostaglandins in the spontaneous initiation of human parturition. The concentration of prostaglandins in forebag amnionic fluid is much greater (10-fold) than that in amnionic fluid of the upper compartment during labor.

Yet in attempts to define the sequence of parturitional processes, prostaglandins have been looked upon primarily as physiological modulators of uterine function rather than as sequelae of labor. The fundamental importance of this problematic issue cannot be overstated! Regrettably, it seems that a state of confusion presently exists in our understanding of the sequence of human parturitional processes. The question that must be raised is as follows:

Does inflammation cause the onset of parturition, or does labor normally, indeed inevitably, **bring about an inflammatory process (at term and preterm)?**

Pregnancy, Prostaglandins, and Parturition: A Perspective. There is no doubt that a variety of prostaglandins are produced in large amounts during human parturition. There also is no doubt that prostaglandin formation is a sequela of the trauma and inflammation of the normal processes of labor. Prostaglandin production at parturition can be attributed, in a large part, directly to the inflammatory processes involving the forebag tissues of the amnionic fluid. Absorption of prostaglandin metabolites from the vagina probably accounts for much of the PGFM in plasma during labor.

Prostaglandins and Phase 2 of Parturition. Nonetheless, these findings do not answer the question as to whether prostaglandins are involved in physiological processes of parturition. Presently there are no data to support or to refute this possibility. It is quite possible that at the end of uterine phase 1 processes, there is increased prostaglandin formation in tissues (cells) in close proximity to the myometrium, perhaps including the myometrial cells themselves. Prostaglandins produced in this putative tissue site may not enter amnionic fluid. Moreover, the contribution of this source of prostaglandin to the plasma pool of prostaglandin metabolites may be small compared with the amount contributed by extraneous inflammatory processes of labor. The same analysis may describe the formation of other uterotonins, such as endothelin-1, oxytocin, PAF, and possibly others.

Prostaglandins and Other Uterotonins During Phase 2 of Parturition. As discussed previously, it is reasonable to assume that relief from continued maintenance of uterine phase 0 is tantamount to the initiation of parturition and causes the cascade of the parturitional process. To optimize force generation of the contractions of labor sufficiently to effect cervical dilatation and delivery, uterotonins may be required. Because an increase in $[Ca^{2+}]_i$ is required for myometrial contractions and stimulates uterotonin formation, a synergistic, physiological handshake arrangement may be instituted such that the progression from uterine phase 1 to phase 2 of human parturition is facilitated, sustained, and supported.

THE OXYTOCIN THEORY OF PARTURITION

A variety of uterotonins have been proposed as agents that cause the initiation of parturition. Among these are the prostaglandins, platelet-activating factor, endothelin-1 and others. But the classical example of a uterotonin is oxytocin.

Because of the success of oxytocin administration in causing the safe induction of labor in near-term pregnant women, it was natural to consider the possibility that oxytocin or a similar agent was involved in the spontaneous initiation of parturition. Herein, perhaps, lies the basis for the great research interest in uterotonins in the parturitional process. The history of oxytocin research is a caricature of the history of parturition research. On the one hand, oxytocin administration to near-term pregnant women recapitulates very precisely the parturition process. But on the other hand, the administration of oxytocin will not cause the commencement of labor in pregnancies not yet at term.

These two observations are consistent with the proposition that there are distinctive uterine parturitional phases. Oxytocin is ineffective as a uterotonin before the uterus is "ripe" or "sensitized." This sensitization of the myometrium to oxytocin is caused by the appearance of oxytocin receptors during uterine phase 1 of parturition.

The logical interpretation of this observation is that parturition must be initiated before oxytocin can act. Namely, the myometrium must undergo transition from uterine phase 0 to phase 1 of parturition before oxytocin is effective. Therefore, oxytocin cannot be the agent that initiates parturition. This points to the necessity for the suspension of phase 0 of parturition in favor of phase 1 in the initiation of parturition.

This is a very important physiological distinction. Therapeutic schemes to prevent preterm labor will be successful only if the initiation of parturition is prevented. After the transition of the uterus to phase 1 of parturition, it is far more difficult to arrest the parturitional process.

These propositions are also presented as a global argument against the possibility that a uterotonin is the agent involved in parturition initiation unless, as stated before, a particular uterotonin is able to masquerade as a uterotropin. Rather, uterotonins are effective only after the myometrium is awakened and prepared for labor, that is, after the initiation of parturition.

To illustrate this point, the oxytocin theory of parturition is reviewed as the classical example of a theorem in which a role for a uterotonin in the initiation of parturition has been postulated.

Oxytocin: Overview

Oxytocin means *"quick birth"*; and oxytocin was the first uterotonin to be implicated in the initiation of parturition. In 1906, Sir Henry Dale discovered uterotonic bioactivity in extracts of the posterior pituitary. By 1909, the uterotonic property of these extracts was demonstrated after the administration of these crude preparations to women; and by 1911, these same preparations were in use in clinical obstetrics. In 1950, Pierce and Du Vigneaud determined the structure of oxytocin, the uterotonic agent of the posterior pituitary; Du Vigneaud was awarded the Nobel Prize for his pioneering work in the elucidation of peptide structure.

Oxytocin is a nonapeptide synthesized in the magnocellular neurons of the supraoptic and paraventricular neurons. The oxytocin prohormone is transported with a carrier protein, neurophysin, along the axons to the neural lobe of the posterior pituitary in membrane-bound vesicles for storage and later release. Oxytocin prohormone is converted enzymatically to oxytocin during transport. Gainer and colleagues (1988) and Leake (1990) have presented learned reviews of the synthesis and secretion of oxytocin.

A Role for Oxytocin in the Initiation of Parturition

A role for oxytocin in the initiation of parturition was supported by several lines of evidence. Oxytocin is known to be a very potent uterotonin, causing (in very low concentrations) uterine contractions in a sensitized uterus. And we have known for more than three quarters of a century that the administration of this potent uterotonic agent will bring about orderly labor in near-term pregnant women in a manner that recapitulates uterine phase 2 of normal spontaneous parturition at term. The key issue, however, is that oxytocin is effective only in a sensitized uterus. This means that oxytocin receptors must be present in myometrium for oxytocin to act; and in turn, this means that uterine phase 0 of parturition must have been suspended and uterine phase 1 processes instituted before oxytocin is a functionally competent uterotonin.

Nonetheless, the effectiveness of oxytocin in inducing labor at term, the very great potency of this uterotonin, and its natural occurrence in humans were considered sufficient reasons for investigating a physiological role for oxytocin in the initiation of spontaneous parturition at term. Other discoveries provided additional support for a role for oxytocin in parturition: (1) there is a striking increase in the number of oxytocin receptors in myometrial tissue near the end of gestation; (2) oxytocin acts upon endometrial (decidual) tissue to promote the release of prostaglandins; and (3) most recently, it was discovered that oxytocin may be synthesized in uterine tissues themselves (Lefebvre and colleagues, 1992a) or in the placenta (Chibbar and colleagues, 1991; Lefebvre and associates, 1992b).

Arguments Against Oxytocin in the Initiation of Parturition

Notwithstanding the importance of these findings in the physiology and biochemistry of oxytocin action, we conclude that all of the evidence, examined critically, does not favor a primary role for oxytocin in the initiation of parturition. Later in the parturitional process, perhaps primarily at the end of uterine phase 2 (second stage of labor) and during phase 3 of parturition, oxytocin is a very important uterotonin. It also is possible that oxytocin serves, together with other uterotonins produced within the uterus, to facilitate optimal increases in myometrial cell $[Ca^{2+}]_i$ after the transition from phase 0 to phase 1 of parturition is already accomplished. In addition, oxytocin may act on amnion to facilitate the maintenance of amnionic fluid homeostasis as described.

Oxytocin Action. There are several reasons for rejecting a physiological role for oxytocin in the initiation of spontaneous parturition: Oxytocin does not act as an antiprogestin; there is no evidence that oxytocin is involved in the development of phase 1 of parturition (preparation of the uterus for labor); oxytocin does not induce gap junction formation between myometrial cells; and oxytocin does not act to induce oxytocin receptors. Most commonly, failures of labor induction with oxytocin are encountered when there has been no antecedent cervical softening or ripening. Indeed, the infusion of oxytocin in relatively large amounts is ineffective in inducing labor in human pregnancy except near term; oxytocin seems to be an effective uterotonin only in those pregnancies in which uterine phase 0 has been suspended and the transition to phase 1 of parturition, preparation of the uterus for active labor, is underway.

Oxytocin Plasma Production Rates

Plasma Levels of Oxytocin. Another important factor that mitigates against a role for oxytocin in the initiation of parturition is that the levels of oxytocin in maternal blood do not increase before or during labor, at least not until late, that is, during the second stage of labor (Fig. 12–9). It has been argued that the increase in concentration of oxytocin receptors in myometrium (or decidua or both) late in pregnancy is so great that oxytocin action can be effected with only subtle or perhaps no change in the level of circulating oxytocin. An increase in oxytocin receptor levels in these tissues immediately before the onset of labor, however, has not been demonstrated; rather, the level of oxytocin receptors is increased strikingly in human myometrium for some time (several days at least) before active labor begins. But if oxytocin does not induce oxytocin receptor synthesis and oxytocin receptors are required for oxytocin action, the issue is moot. Oxytocin does not act to initiate parturition.

Metabolic Clearance Rate of Oxytocin. It has also been suggested that the metabolic clearance rate of oxytocin (MCR-oxy) from plasma is so great that increases in the rate of secretion of oxytocin from the neurohypophysis–

posterior pituitary could occur without detectable increases in the plasma concentration of oxytocin. This argument is untenable. Oxytocin secreted or released from the posterior pituitary is a hormone, transported from its site of storage to tissue sites of action by way of the circulation. The accuracy of measurements of oxytocin in plasma and the plasma clearance rate of oxytocin are, therefore, crucial in analyses of the role of posterior pituitary-derived oxytocin in the initiation of parturition (Leake, 1983, 1990).

The MCR-oxy concentration in the human, determined by several investigators, is about 1700 to 2000 L plasma per 24 hours in pregnant women, men, and nonpregnant women (Leake and associates, 1980, 1990). This rate of clearance of plasma oxytocin is somewhat less than that of many steroids, including progesterone, androstenedione, dehydroepiandrosterone, and aldosterone.

Secretion Rate of Oxytocin. The secretion rate (SR) of oxytocin from brain in pregnant women before and during labor is computed as follows: SR-oxy = MCR-oxy $\times$ $[oxy]_p$, where $[oxy]_p$ is the concentration of oxytocin in plasma. Most investigators find that the plasma concentration of oxytocin in pregnant women is 2 to 10 pg/mL (Leake and colleagues, 1981). Taking a value of 5 pg/mL as representative (and an MCR-oxy as 2000 L per 24 hours), the SR-oxy in pregnant women is 10 μg/day, or about 7 ng/min. The plasma concentrations of oxytocin do not change during phase 1 or 2 of parturition, at least not until the very end of active labor (the second stage of labor).

Oxytocin Infusion. The infusion of oxytocin at a rate of 20 ng/min will cause labor in most women at term (1 μU oxytocin equals 2 pg). This rate of infusion will effect an increase in blood levels of about three- to sevenfold. In fact, the infusion of oxytocin at a constant rate less than that required to induce labor causes a predictable increase in the plasma concentrations of oxytocin.

A number of investigators have also been successful in monitoring increases in the levels of oxytocin in blood during breast suckling. The rates of oxytocin secretion during breast feeding are similar to the rates of oxytocin infusion that often will induce labor. For all of these reasons, it is difficult to believe that increases in oxytocin secretion from the neurohypophysis–posterior pituitary or placenta of sufficient magnitude to induce labor can go undetected. But even if oxytocin secretion were increased, but not detected because of woefully inadequate oxytocin assays, the absence of oxytocin action without oxytocin receptors negates the possibility of oxytocin initiating parturition.

Oxytocin Formation in the Uterus. Recently, evidence was presented for the expression of the oxytocin gene in the uterus of pregnant rats near term (Lefebvre and co-workers, 1992a). If it were established that oxytocin is produced in uterine or intrauterine tissues, new possibilities for oxytocin in parturition might emerge: uterine oxytocin, acting in a paracrine or autocrine manner, would diminish the obligation for an increase in the blood level of this uterotonin to establish an increased level of oxytocin in the myometrium. But even then, it is likely that oxytocin of myometrial or fetal membrane or decidual origin would facilitate the success of phase 2 of parturition only after the initiation of parturition, as defined by the transition of the uterus from phase 0 to phase 1 of parturition. Specifically, the prior formation of oxytocin receptors (uterine phase 1) seems to be essential for oxytocin action, irrespective of the tissue site of oxytocin biosynthesis.

Fetal Oxytocin. In several mammalian species (e.g., rats and guinea pigs), the fetal pituitary content of oxytocin decreases during birth. There is also evidence of increased fetal oxytocin secretion during human parturition. Oxytocin levels are higher in umbilical arterial than venous plasma and higher after spontaneous labor than before parturition begins. There is no evidence, however, that oxytocin can escape placental degradation and enter the maternal circulation (Leake, 1990).

Oxytocin and Parturition in Perspective. The increase in oxytocin receptors in the uterus before the onset of labor is an important marker of the preparatory events of parturition (phase 1). Oxytocin may act as a uterotonin to maximize the myometrial forces involved in the expulsive phase (second stage of phase 2) of labor; oxytocin likely acts to promote uterine contraction and retraction after delivery to limit uterine blood loss; oxytocin may act synergistically with other uterotonins produced within the uterus to facilitate the success of uterine phase 2 of parturition; and oxytocin is important in causing milk ejection during lactation. But there is no evidence that oxytocin is involved in the initiation of human parturition (i.e., promoting the transition from phase 0 to phase 1).

CLINICAL COURSE OF LABOR: PHASE 2 OF PARTURITION

Spontaneous Parturition at Term

Early Signs

"Lightening." A few weeks before the onset of active labor, it is common for the abdomen of the pregnant woman to undergo a change in shape. The fundal height decreases somewhat; at times this event is described by the mother as "The baby dropped." This is a clinical manifestation of phase 1 of parturition. With the development of a well-formed lower uterine segment, the fetal head descends to or even through the pelvic inlet. Additionally, there is a small reduction in the volume of amnionic fluid.

"Show." A rather dependable sign of the impending onset of active labor (provided no rectal or vaginal examination has been performed in the preceding 48 hours) is "show" or "bloody show," which consists of the discharge of a small amount of blood-tinged mucus from the vagina, representing the extrusion of the plug of mucus that was filling the cervical canal during pregnancy. "Show" is a late sign, because labor usually ensues during the next several hours to few days (or has already begun). Normally, only a few drops of blood escape with the mucus plug; more substantial bleeding is suggestive of an abnormal condition.

False Labor. For a variable time before the establishment of true or effective labor (phase 2 of parturition), women may experience so-called *false labor.* The uterine contractions of false labor are characterized by irregularity in occurrence and by brevity of duration; most often, the discomfort produced is confined to the lower abdomen and groin. In contrast, the discomfort produced by the uterine contractions that are characteristic of true labor begins first in the fundal region and then radiates over the uterus and through to the lower back.

Uterine irritability that causes discomfort but that does not represent phase 2 of parturition (in that cervical dilatation does not occur) may develop at any time during pregnancy. False labor is observed most commonly late in pregnancy and in parous women. It often stops spontaneously but may proceed rapidly to the effective contractions of true labor. Therefore, the report of relatively infrequent and short-lived, but uncomfortable, uterine contractions cannot be summarily dismissed. All too frequently when this is done, delivery takes place without benefit of the assistance of professional personnel or facilities essential for optimal care of the mother and fetus-infant.

Characteristics of Uterine Contractions of Labor. Unique among physiological muscular contractions, those of uterine smooth muscle of labor are painful. Therefore, the common designation, in many languages, for such a contraction is "pain." The cause of the pain is not known definitely, but several have been suggested: (1) hypoxia of the contracted myometrium (as in angina pectoris), (2) compression of nerve ganglia in the cervix and lower uterus by the tightly interlocking muscle bundles, (3) stretching of the cervix during dilatation, and (4) stretching of the peritoneum overlying the fundus. Compression of nerve ganglia in the cervix and lower uterine segment by the contracting myometrium is an especially attractive hypothesis. Paracervical infiltration with a local anesthetic drug typically produces appreciable relief of pain during subsequent uterine contractions (see Chap. 16).

Uterine contractions are involuntary and for the most part independent of extrauterine control. Neural blockage from caudal or epidural analgesia, if initiated quite early in labor, is sometimes associated with a reduction in the frequency and intensity of uterine contractions; but this is not the case after labor is well established. Moreover, in paraplegic women there are normal, though painless, contractions as in women after bilateral lumbar sympathectomy.

Mechanical stretching of the cervix enhances uterine activity in several species, including the human. This phenomenon has been referred to as the *Ferguson reflex.* The exact mechanism by which mechanical dilatation of the cervix causes increased myometrial contractility is not clear. Release of oxytocin was suggested as the cause by Ferguson (1941), but this is not proven. Manipulation of the cervix and "stripping" the fetal membranes causes an increase in prostaglandin $F_{2\alpha}$ metabolites in blood (Mitchell, 1976). Likely, this is attributable to additional trauma to the decidua of the forebag or lower uterine segment and the uptake of PGFM from the vaginal fluid.

The interval between contractions diminishes gradually from about 10 minutes at the onset of the first stage of labor to as little as 1 minute or less in the second stage. Periods of relaxation between contractions, however, are essential to the welfare of the fetus, because unremitting contraction of the uterus compromises uteroplacental blood flow and ultimately fetal–placental flow, sufficiently to cause fetal hypoxia. In the active phase of labor, the duration of each contraction ranges from 30 to 90 seconds, averaging about 1 minute. There is appreciable variability in the intensity of uterine contractions during apparently normal labor, as emphasized by Schulman and Romney (1970). They recorded the amnionic fluid pressures generated by uterine contractions in women during spontaneous labor; the pressures averaged about 40 mm Hg, but varied from 20 to 60 mm Hg.

Differentiation of Uterine Activity. During uterine phase 2 of parturition, the uterus differentiates into two distinct parts. The actively contracting upper segment becomes thicker as labor advances; the lower portion, comprising the lower segment of the uterus and the cervix, is relatively passive compared with the upper segment, and it develops into a much more thinly walled passage for the fetus. The lower uterine segment is analogous to a greatly expanded and thinned-out isthmus of the uterus of nonpregnant women, the formation of which is not solely a phenomenon of labor. The lower segment develops gradually as pregnancy progresses and then thins remarkably during labor (Figs. 12–19 and 12–20). By abdominal palpation, even before rupture of the membranes, the two segments can be differentiated during a contraction. The upper uterine segment is quite firm or hard, whereas the consistency of the lower uterine segment is much less firm. The former represents the actively contracting part of the uterus; the latter is the distended, normally much more passive, portion.

If the entire sac of uterine musculature, including the lower uterine segment and cervix, were to contract simultaneously and with equal intensity, the net expulsive force would be decreased markedly. Herein lies the importance of the division of the uterus into an actively contracting upper segment and a more passive lower

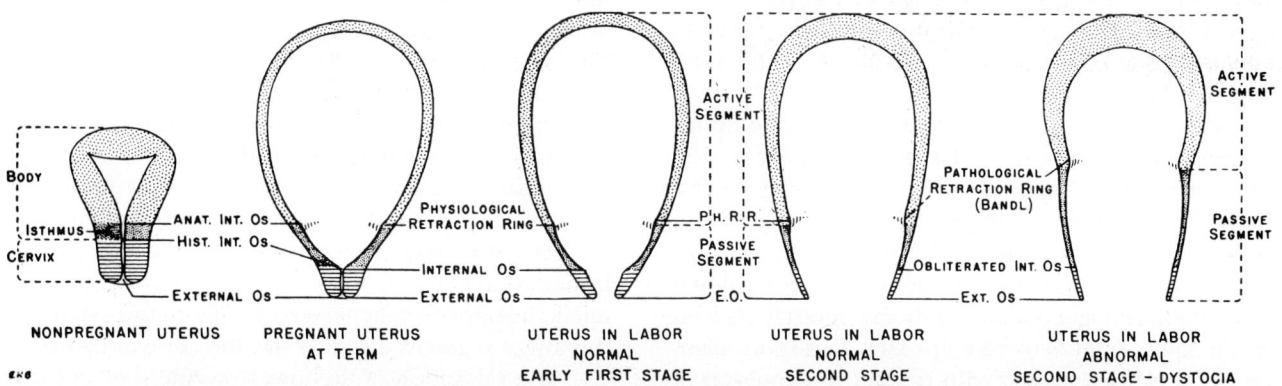

Fig. 12–19. Sequence of development of the segments and rings in the uterus in pregnant women at term and in labor. Note comparison between the uterus of a nonpregnant woman, the uterus at term, and the uterus during labor. The passive lower segment of the uterine body is derived from the isthmus; the physiological retraction ring develops at the junction of the upper and lower uterine segments. The pathological retraction ring develops from the physiological ring. (Anat. Int. Os = anatomical internal os; Hist. Int. Os = histological internal os; Ph.R.R. = physiological retraction ring; E.O. = external os.)

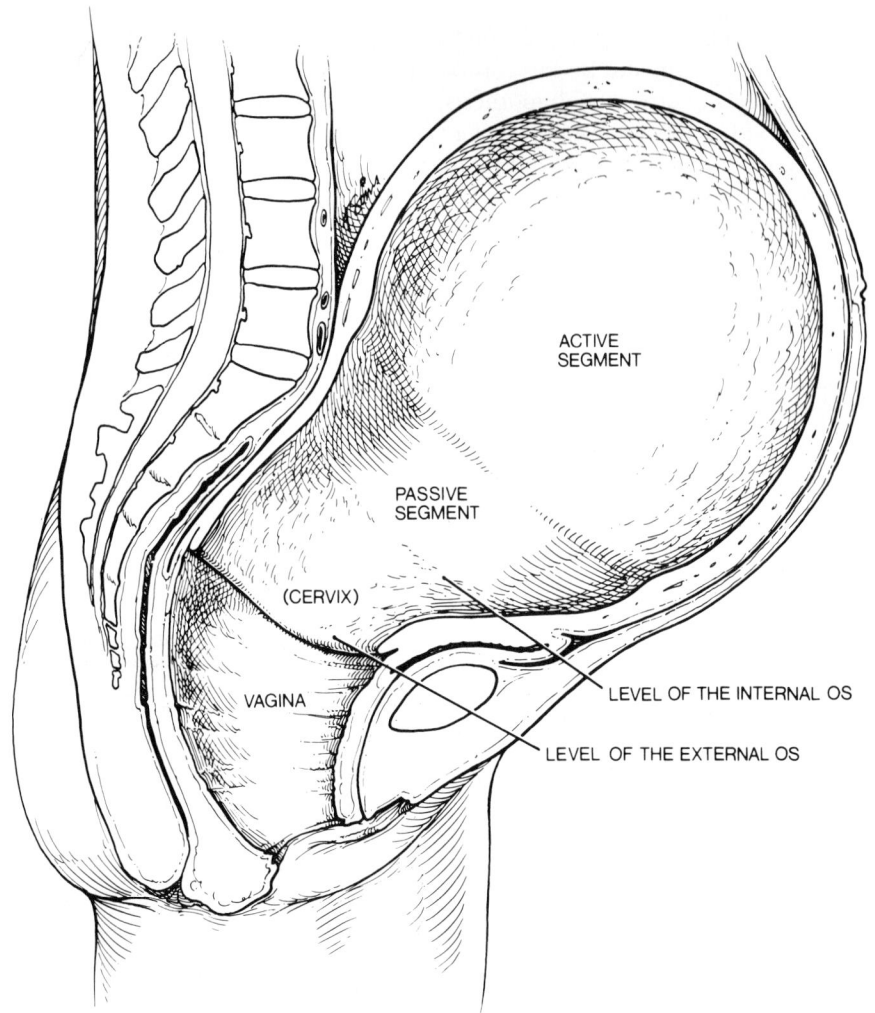

Fig. 12–20. The uterus at the time of vaginal delivery. The active upper segment of the uterus retracts about the fetus as the fetus descends through the birth canal. In the passive lower segment, there is considerably less myometrial tone.

segment that differ not only anatomically but also physiologically. The upper segment contracts, retracts, and expels the fetus; in response to the force of the contractions of the upper segment, the ripened lower uterine segment and cervix dilate and thereby form a greatly expanded, thinned-out muscular and fibromuscular tube through which the fetus can be extruded.

After contractions, the myometrium of the upper uterine segment does not relax to its original length; rather, it becomes relatively fixed at a shorter length. The tension, however, remains the same as before the contraction. The effect of the ability of the upper portion of the uterus, or active segment, to contract down on its diminishing contents with myometrial tension remaining constant is to take up slack, that is, to maintain the advantage gained with respect to expulsion of the fetus, and to maintain the uterine musculature in firm contact with the intrauterine contents. As the consequence of retraction, each successive contraction commences where its predecessor left off, so that the upper part of the uterine cavity becomes slightly smaller with each successive contraction. Because of the suc-

cessive shortening of its muscular fibers with each contraction, the upper uterine segment (active segment, Fig. 12–19) becomes progressively thickened throughout the first and second stages of labor and tremendously thickened immediately after delivery of the fetus. The phenomenon of retraction of the upper uterine segment is contingent upon a decrease in the volume of its contents. For its contents to be diminished, particularly early in labor when the entire uterus is virtually a closed sac with only a minute opening at the cervix, there is a requirement that the musculature of the lower segment stretch, permitting increasingly more of the intrauterine contents to occupy the lower segment. Indeed, the upper segment retracts only to the extent that the lower segment distends and the cervix dilates.

The relaxation of the lower uterine segment is by no means complete relaxation, but rather the opposite of retraction. The fibers of the lower segment become stretched with each contraction of the upper segment, after which these are not returned to the previous length but rather remain relatively fixed at the longer length; the tension, however, remains essentially the same as before. The musculature still manifests tone, still resists stretch, and still contracts somewhat on stimulation.

The successive lengthening of the muscular fibers in the lower uterine segment, as labor progresses, is accompanied by thinning, normally to only a few millimeters in the thinnest part. As a result of the thinning of the lower uterine segment and the concomitant thickening of the upper, the boundary between the two is marked by a ridge on the inner uterine surface, the *physiological retraction ring.* When the thinning of the lower uterine segment is extreme, as in obstructed labor, the ring is very prominent, forming a *pathological retraction ring* (the ring of Bandl), an abnormal condition illustrated in Figure 12–19 and one further discussed in Chapter 19. From quantitative measurements of the difference in behavior of the upper and lower parts of the uterus during normal labor it was found that there is normally a gradient of diminishing physiological activity from the fundus to the cervix. Several ingenious devices have been used to evaluate uterine forces, including the tocodynamometer, intrauterine receptors, and intramyometrial catheters.

In the tocodynamometer, three strain gauges set in heavy brass ring mountings are employed; the gauges may be placed anywhere on the abdomen. When the uterus contracts, the increased convexity of the local arc of the uterus underlying the ring pushes upward on the gauge and applies a strain to its elements proportional to the local force of the uterine contraction. A record is obtained electrometrically, an example of which is shown in Figure 12–21. It is evident from these tracings that the intensity of each contraction is greater in the fundal zone than in the midzone, and greater in the midzone than lower down. Equally noteworthy is the differential in the duration of the contractions; those in the midzone are much briefer than those above, whereas the contractions in the lower zone are extremely brief and sometimes absent. This subsidence of contractions in the midzone, at a time when the upper zone is still contracting, is indicative that the upper part of the corpus, throughout a substantial portion of each contraction, comes to exert pressure caudally on the more relaxed parts of the uterus. Occasionally, when labor is not progressing, this gradient is absent, and both the intensity and the duration of the contractions may be the same in all three zones.

These findings of Reynolds (1949) were confirmed by Karlson (1949) through the use of an entirely different apparatus. By his technique, the internal pressure in the uterus at any point was measured by means of so-called receptors (metal capsules about 12 mm long with a diameter of 4.5 mm), in the middle of which is a small aperture. On the inner side of this aperture there is a membrane that is sensitive to pressure. Pressure exerted against the window is carried and registered electrometrically; an example of one of Karlson's tracings is shown in Figure 12–22. Here again, there is a gradient of di-

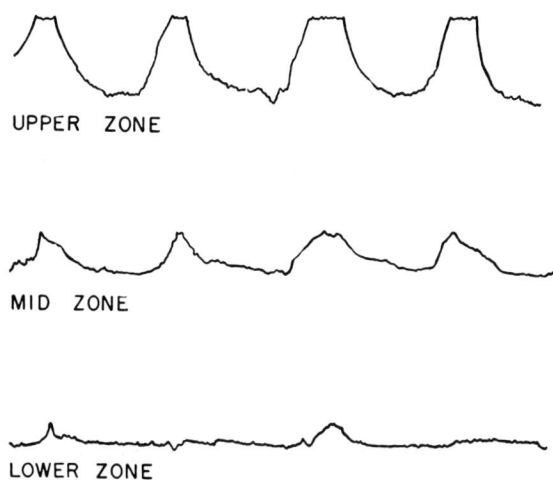

Fig. 12–21. Uterine contractions in various parts of the uterus recorded by Reynolds tocodynamometer. The lower zone probably corresponds to the lower uterine segment. The woman studied was a primigravida in active labor; the cervix was 5 cm dilated, and contractions were occurring at about 3-minute intervals. The original tracings have been inked over for clearer reproduction. (From Reynolds and co-workers, 1948.)

minishing activity from the fundus to the lower uterine segment. Karlson's other tracings, like those of Reynolds, are indicative that in the absence of this gradient—that is, when the intensity of contraction of the lower segment equals or exceeds that of the fundus—cervical dilatation may cease. Similar results were obtained by Caldeyro-Barcia and associates (1950), who inserted small intramyometrial balloons or open-ended catheters at various levels and recorded the pressures during contractions.

Change in Uterine Shape. Each contraction produces an elongation of the uterine ovoid with a concomitant decrease in horizontal diameters. By virtue of this

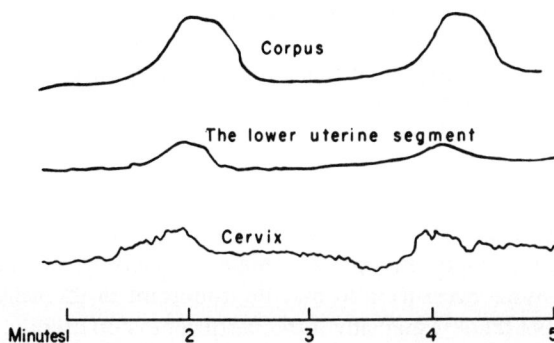

Fig. 12–22. Uterine contractions in various parts of the uterus recorded by Karlson by means of intrauterine receptors. The woman studied was in early labor, but from the time this tracing was made, progress of labor was rapid. To permit clearer reproduction the background of the original record has been eliminated and the tracings have been inked over. (Modified from Karlson, 1949.)

change in shape, there are important effects on the process of labor:

1. The decrease in horizontal diameter produces a straightening of the fetal vertebral column, pressing its upper pole firmly against the fundus of the uterus, whereas the lower pole is thrust farther downward and into the pelvis. The lengthening of the fetal ovoid thus produced has been estimated as between 5 and 10 cm. The pressure so exerted is known as fetal axis pressure.

2. With lengthening of the uterus, the longitudinal fibers are drawn taut; because the lower segment and cervix are the only parts of the uterus that are flexible, these are pulled upward over the lower pole of the fetus. This effect on the musculature of the lower segment and on the cervix is an important factor in cervical dilatation. The round ligaments also contain smooth muscle, which can contract and pull the uterus forward. These actions, however, are not essential for successful labor and delivery.

Other Forces Concerned in Labor

Intra-abdominal Pressure. After the cervix is dilated fully, the force that is principally important in the expulsion of the fetus is that produced by increased intra-abdominal pressure created by contraction of the abdominal muscles simultaneously with forced respiratory efforts with the glottis closed. In obstetrical jargon this is usually referred to as pushing. The nature of the force produced is similar to that involved in defecation, but usually the intensity is much greater. The important role that is served by intra-abdominal pressure in fetal expulsion is most clearly attested to by the labors of women who are paraplegic. Such women suffer no pain, although the uterus may contract vigorously. Cervical dilatation, in large measure the result of uterine contractions acting on a ripened cervix, proceeds normally, but expulsion of the infant is rarely possible except when the woman is instructed to bear down and can do so at the time that the obstetrician identifies uterine contractions. Although increased intra-abdominal pressure is required for the spontaneous completion of labor, it is futile until the cervix is fully dilated. In other words, it is a necessary auxiliary to uterine contractions in the second stage of labor, but pushing accomplishes little in the first stage, except to fatigue the mother. Intra-abdominal pressure also may be important in the third stage of labor, especially if the parturient is unattended. After the placenta has separated, its spontaneous expulsion is aided by the mother's bearing down, that is, by an increase in intra-abdominal pressure.

Resistance. Mechanically, work is the generation of motion against resistance. Labor is work. The forces involved in labor are those of the uterus and the abdomen, which act to expel the fetus, and those that must overcome the resistance offered by the cervix to dilatation and the friction created by the tissues of the birth canal during passage of the presenting part. In addition, forces of resistance may be exerted by the muscles of the pelvic floor. The work involved in labor, according to Gemzell and colleagues (1957), is only a fraction of the maximal functional capacity of the normal woman.

Changes Induced in the Cervix. The effective force of the first stage of labor is the uterine contraction, which in turn exerts hydrostatic pressure through the membranes against the cervix and lower uterine segment. In the absence of intact membranes, the presenting part is forced directly against the cervix and lower uterine segment. As the result of the action of these forces, two fundamental changes—effacement and dilatation—take place in the previously ripened cervix.

Cervical Effacement and Dilatation. For the head of the average fetus at term to pass through the cervix, the cervical canal must dilate to a diameter of about 10 cm. When sufficient dilatation is attained for the fetal head to pass through, the cervix is said to be completely dilated or fully dilated. There may be no fetal descent during cervical effacement, but as a rule the presenting part descends somewhat as the cervix dilates. During the second stage of labor, descent of the fetal presenting part typically occurs rather slowly but steadily in nulliparas. In multiparas, however, particularly those of high parity, descent may be very rapid.

Pattern of Cervical Dilatation. Friedman, in his treatise on labor (1978), stated, *"The clinical features of uterine contractions—namely, frequency, intensity, and duration—cannot be relied upon as measures of progression in labor nor as indices of normality.... Except for cervical dilatation and fetal descent, none of the clinical features of the parturient ... appears to be useful in assessing labor progression."* The pattern of cervical dilatation that takes place during the course of normal labor takes on the shape of a sigmoid curve. As depicted in Figure 12–23, two phases of cervical dilatation can be defined: the latent phase and the active phase.

The active phase has been subdivided further as the acceleration phase, phase of maximum slope, and the deceleration phase (Friedman, 1978). The duration of the latent phase is more variable and subject to sensitive changes by extraneous factors and by sedation (prolongation of latent phase) and myometrial stimulation (shortening of latent phase). The duration of the latent phase has little bearing on the subsequent course of labor, whereas the characteristics of the accelerated phase are usually predictive of the outcome of a partic-

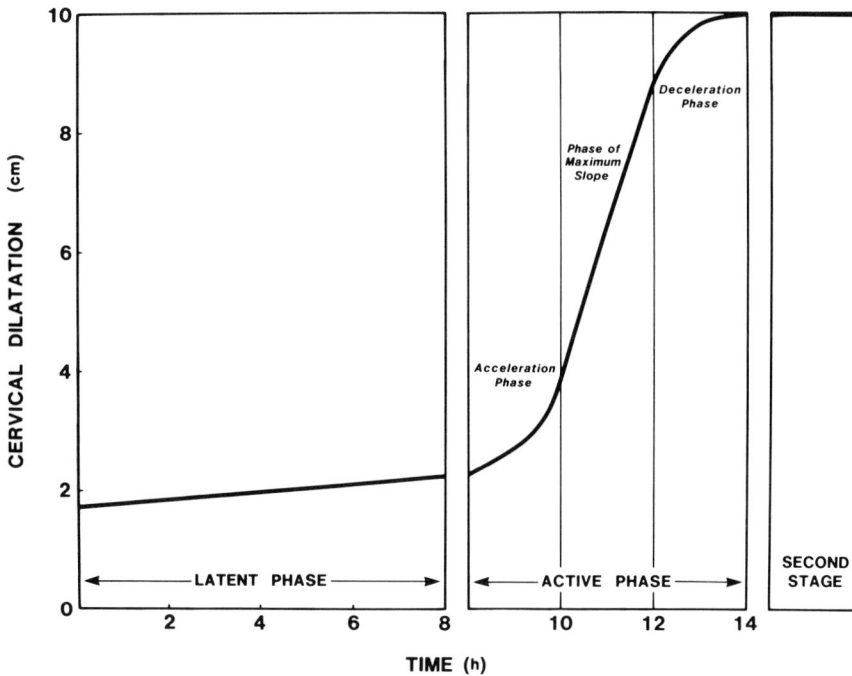

Fig. 12–23. Composite of the average dilatation curve for nulliparous labor based on analysis of the data derived from the patterns traced by a large, nearly consecutive, series of gravidas. The first stage is divided into a relatively flat latent phase and a rapidly progressive active phase. In the active phase, there are three identifiable component parts: an acceleration phase, a linear phase of maximum slope, and a deceleration phase. (Illustration courtesy of Dr. L. Casey, redrawn from Friedman, 1978.)

ular labor. Friedman considers the maximum slope as a *"good measure of the overall efficiency of the machine,"* whereas the nature of the deceleration phase is more reflective of fetopelvic relationships. The completion of cervical dilatation during the active phase of labor is accomplished by cervical retraction about the presenting part of the fetus. After complete cervical dilatation, the second stage of labor commences; thereafter, only progressive descent of the presenting fetal part is available to assess the progress of labor.

Pattern of Descent. In many nulliparas, engagement of the fetal head is accomplished prior to the onset of labor, and further descent does not occur until late in labor. In others in whom engagement of the fetal head is initially not so complete, further descent occurs during the first stage of labor. In the descent pattern of normal labor, a typical hyperbolic curve is formed when the station of the fetal head is plotted as a function of the duration of labor. Active descent usually takes place after cervical dilatation has progressed for some time. In nulliparas, increased rates of descent are observed ordinarily during the phase of maximum slope of cervical dilatation. At this time, the speed of descent increases to a maximum, and this maximal rate of descent is maintained until the presenting fetal part reaches the perineal floor (Friedman, 1978).

First and Second Stages of Labor. Friedman also sought to select criteria that would delimit normal labor and thus enable identification of significant abnormalities in labor. The limits, admittedly arbitrary, appear to be logical and clinically useful. The group of women

studied were nulliparas and multiparas with no fetopelvic disproportion, no fetal malposition or malpresentation, no multiple pregnancy, and none were treated with heavy sedation or conduction analgesia, oxytocin, or operative intervention. All had a normal pelvis and were at term with a vertex presentation and delivered average-sized infants. From these studies, Friedman developed the concept of three functional divisions of labor—preparatory, dilatational, and pelvic—to describe the physiological objectives of each division (Fig. 12–24). He found that the preparatory division of labor may be sensitive to sedation and conduction analgesia. Although little cervical dilatation occurs during this time, considerable changes take place in the ground substance (collagen and other connective tissue components) of the cervix (Danforth and colleagues, 1960). The dilatational division of labor, during which time dilatation is occurring at the most rapid rate, is principally unaffected by sedation or conduction analgesia. The pelvic division of labor commences with the deceleration phase of cervical dilatation. The classic mechanisms of labor that involve the cardinal movements of the fetus take place principally during the pelvic division of labor. The time of onset of the pelvic division of labor is seldom clinically identifiable separate from the dilatational division of labor. Moreover, the rate of cervical dilatation does not always decelerate as full dilatation is approached; in fact, it may accelerate.

Rupture of Membranes. Spontaneous rupture of the fetal membranes most often occurs sometime during the course of active labor. Typically, **rupture of the membranes is evident by a sudden gush of a variable**

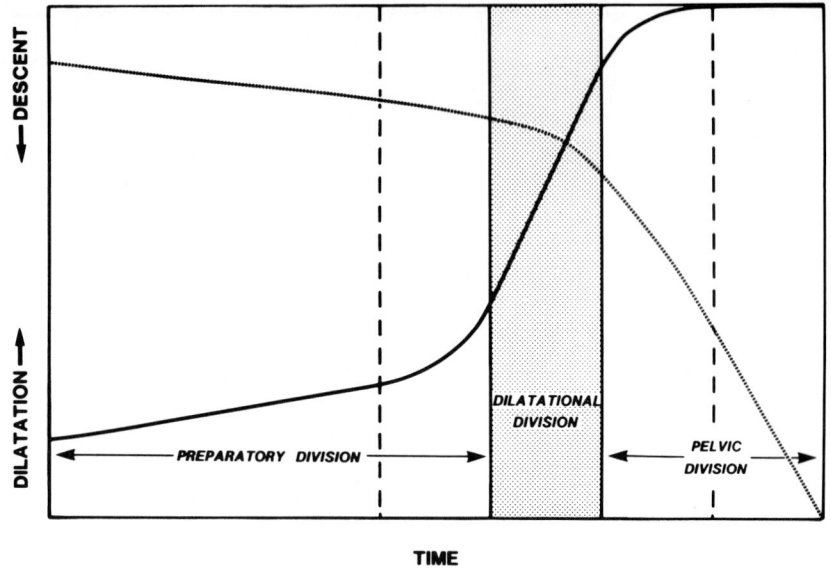

Fig. 12–24. Labor course divided functionally on the basis of expected evolution of the dilatation and descent curves into (1) a preparatory division, including latent and acceleration phases; (2) a dilatational division, occupying the phase of maximum slope of dilatation; and (3) a pelvic division, encompassing both deceleration phase and second stage while concurrent with the phase of maximum slope of descent. (Illustration courtesy Dr. L. Casey, redrawn from Friedman, 1978.)

quantity of normally clear or slightly turbid, nearly colorless fluid. Less frequently, the membranes remain intact until the time of delivery of the infant. If by chance the membranes remain intact until completion of delivery, the fetus is born surrounded by them, and the portion covering the head of the newborn infant is sometimes referred to as the *caul.*

Changes in the Vagina and Pelvic Floor. The birth canal is supported and is closed functionally by a number of layers of tissues that together form the pelvic floor. From within outward these tissues are (1) peritoneum, (2) subperitoneal connective tissue, (3) internal pelvic fascia, (4) levator ani and coccygeus muscles, (5) external pelvic fascia, (6) superficial muscles and fascia, (7) subcutaneous tissue, and (8) skin.

Anatomy of the Pelvic Floor. The most important of these structures of the pelvic floor are the levator ani muscle and the fascia covering its upper and lower surfaces, which for practical purposes may be considered as the pelvic floor (see Chap. 3). This muscle (or group of muscles) closes the lower end of the pelvic cavity as a diaphragm and thereby a concave upper and a convex lower surface is presented, as illustrated in Figures 12–25 and 12–26. On either side, the levator ani consists of a pubic and iliac portion. The former is a band 2 to 2.5 cm in width arising from the horizontal ramus of the pubis, 3 to 4 cm below its upper margin, and 1 to 1.5 cm from the symphysis pubis. Its fibers pass backward to encircle the rectum and possibly give off a few fibers that pass behind the vagina. The greater, or iliac, portion of the muscle arises on either side of the pelvis from the white line (the tendinous arch of the pelvic fascia) and from the ischial spine at a distance of about 5 cm below

the margin of the pelvic inlet. The greater part of the muscle passes backward and unites with that from the other side of the rectum; the posterior portions meet in the tendinous raphe in front of the coccyx, with the most posterior fibers attached to the bone itself. The posterior and lateral portions of the pelvic floor, which are not filled out by the levator ani, are occupied by the piriformis and coccygeus muscles on either side. The levator ani varies in thickness from 3 to 5 mm, though its margins encircling the rectum and vagina are somewhat thicker. During pregnancy, the levator ani usually undergoes hypertrophy. By vaginal examination, the internal margin of this muscle can be felt as a thick band that extends backward from the pubis and encircles the vagina about 2 cm above the hymen. On contraction, the levator ani draws both the rectum and vagina forward and upward in the direction of the symphysis pubis and thereby acts to close the vagina. The more superficial muscles of the perineum are too delicate to serve more than an accessory function.

The internal pelvic fascia, which forms the upper covering of the levator ani, is attached to the margin of the pelvic inlet, where it is joined by the fascia of the iliac fossa and by the transverse fascia of the obturator internus and is attached firmly to the periosteum covering the lateral wall of the pelvis. The white line is indicative of its point of deflection from the periosteum. From there the internal pelvic fascia spreads out over the upper surface of the levator ani and coccygeus muscles. The inferior fascial covering of the pelvic diaphragm is divided into two parts by a line drawn between the ischial tuberosities. The posterior portion consists of a single layer, which, taking its origin from the sacrosciatic ligament and the ischial tuberosity, passes up over the inner surface of the ischial bones and

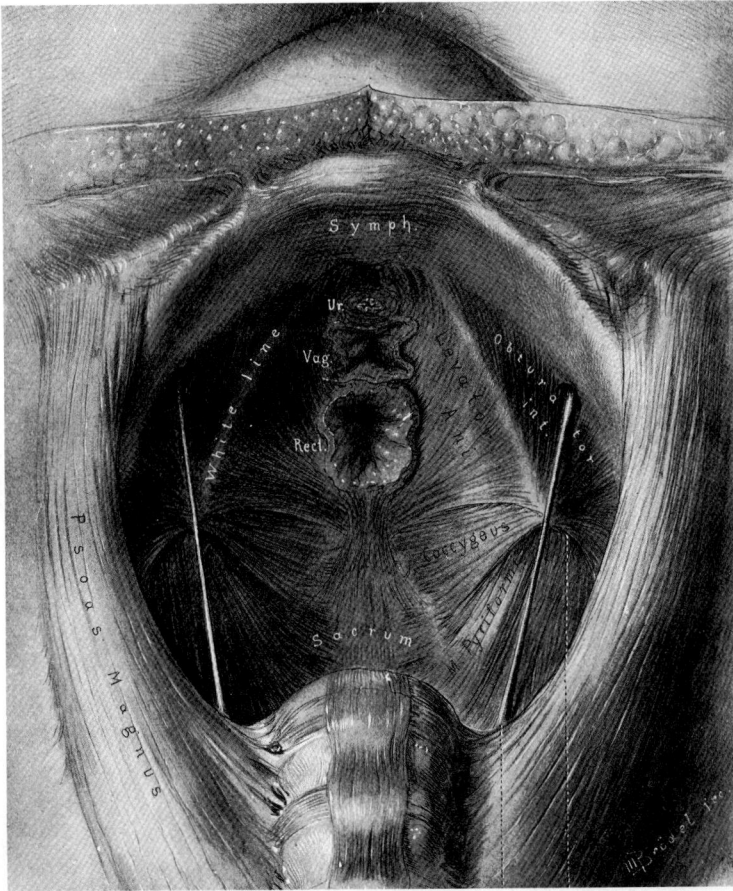

Fig. 12–25. The pelvic floor seen from above. Uterus, tubes, ovaries, peritoneum, supporting ligaments, and internal fascial coverings have been removed. (Symph. = symphysis; Ur. = urethra; Vag. = vagina; Rect. = rectum). (From Kelly, 1906.)

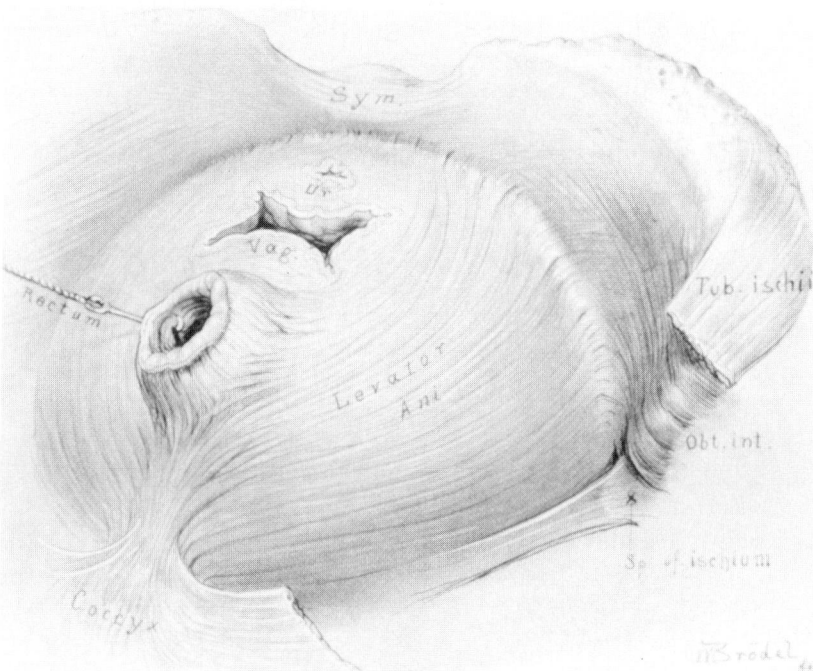

Fig. 12–26. The deep muscles of the pelvic floor seen from below. (Sym. = symphysis; Ur. = urethra; Vag. = vagina; Sp. of Ischium = ischial spine; Obt. int. = obturator internus muscle; Tub. ischii = ischial tuberosity.)

the obturator internus to the white line, in the formation of which it takes part. From this tendinous structure it is reflected at an acute angle over the inferior surface of the levator ani; the space induced between the latter and the lateral pelvic wall forms the *ischiorectal fossa.* The structure filling out the triangular space between the pubic arch and a line joining the ischial tuberosities is known as the *urogenital diaphragm,* which, exclusive of skin and subcutaneous fat, principally consists of three layers of fascia: (1) the deep perineal fascia, which covers the anterior portion of the inferior surface of the levator ani muscle and is continuous with the fascia just described; (2) the middle perineal fascia, which is separated from the former by a narrow space in which are situated the pubic vessels and nerves; and (3) the superficial perineal fascia, which together with the layer just described, forms a compartment in which the superficial perineal muscles lie, with the exception of the sphincter ani, the rami of the clitoris, the vestibular bulbs, and the vulvovaginal glands (see Chap. 3).

The superficial perineal muscles are comprised of the bulbocavernosus, ischiocavernosus, and superficial transverse perineal muscles. These muscles are delicately formed and are of no major obstetrical importance except that the superficial transverse perineal muscles are always torn in the case of perineal lacerations.

In the first stage of labor, the membranes and presenting part of the fetus serve a role in dilating the upper portion of the vagina. After the membranes have ruptured, however, the changes in the pelvic floor are caused entirely by pressure that is exerted by the presenting part of the fetus. The most marked change consists of the stretching of the fibers of the levator ani muscles and the thinning of the central portion of the perineum, which becomes transformed from a wedge-shaped mass of tissue 5 cm in thickness to (in the absence of an episiotomy) a thin, almost transparent membranous structure that is less than 1 cm in thickness. When the perineum is distended maximally, the

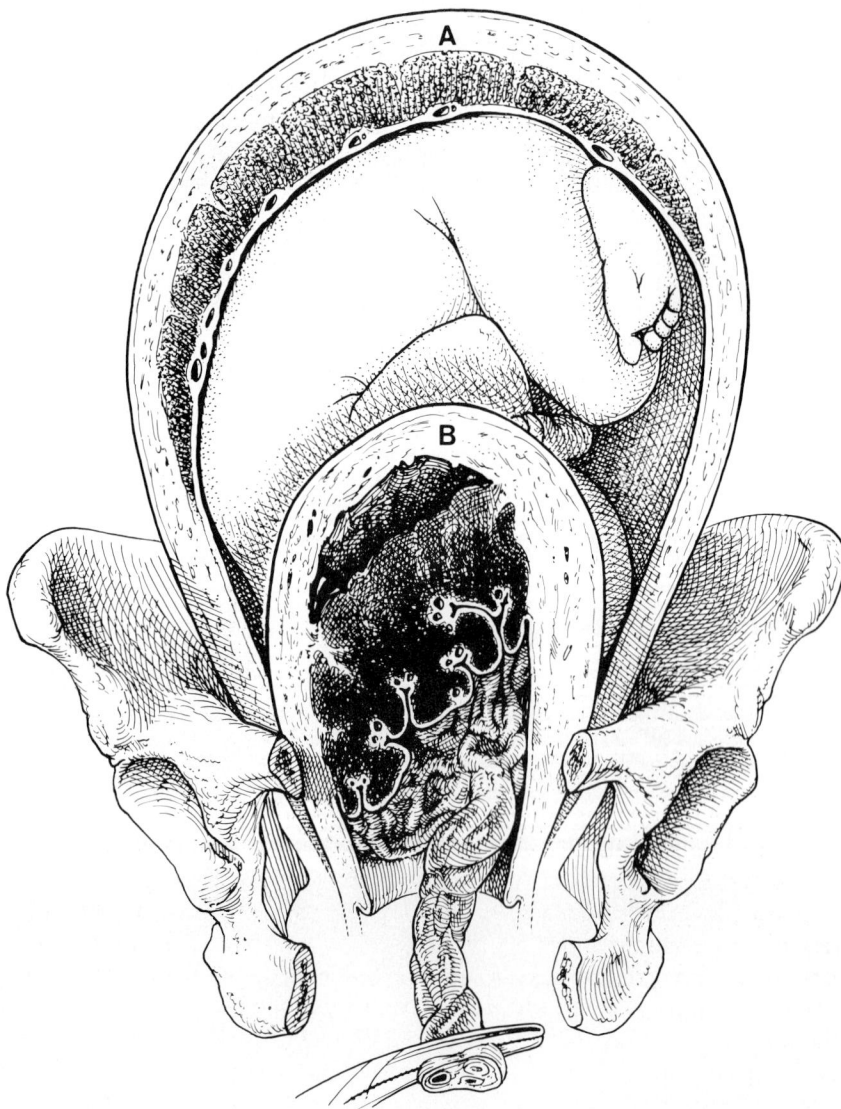

Fig. 12–27. Diminution in size of placental site after birth of baby. **A.** Spatial relations before birth of the infant. **B.** Placental spatial relations after birth of the infant.

anus becomes markedly dilated and presents an opening that varies from 2 to 3 cm in diameter and through which the anterior wall of the rectum bulges. The extraordinary number and size of the blood vessels that supply the vagina and pelvic floor is such as to cause a great increase in the amount of blood loss when these tissues are torn.

Third Stage of Labor. The third stage of labor, which begins immediately after delivery of the fetus, involves the separation and expulsion of the placenta. After delivery of the placenta and fetal membranes, phase 2 of parturition is completed.

The Phase of Placental Separation. As the baby is born, the uterus spontaneously contracts down on its diminishing contents. Normally, by the time the infant is completely delivered, the uterine cavity is nearly obliterated and the organ consists of an almost solid mass of muscle, the walls of which are several centimeters thick above the lower segment, and the fundus of which lies just below the level of the umbilicus. This sudden diminution in uterine size is inevitably accompanied by a decrease in the area of the placental implantation site (Fig. 12–27). For the placenta to accommodate itself to this reduced area, it increases in thickness, but because of limited placental elasticity, it is forced to buckle. The resulting tension causes the weakest layer of the decidua—the spongy layer, or decidua spongiosa—to give way, and cleavage takes place at that site. Therefore, separation of the placenta results primarily from a disproportion created between the unchanged size of the placenta and the reduced size of the underlying implantation site. During cesarean section, this phenomenon may be directly observed when the placenta is implanted posteriorly. Cleavage of the placenta is greatly facilitated by the nature of the loose structure of the spongy decidua, which may be likened to the row of perforations between postage stamps. As separation proceeds, a hematoma forms between the separating placenta and the remaining decidua. Formation of the hematoma is usually the result, rather than the cause, of the separation, because in some cases bleeding is negligible. The hematoma may, however, accelerate the process of cleavage. Because the separation of the placenta is through the spongy layer of the decidua (see Chap. 4), part of the decidua is cast off with the placenta, whereas the rest remains attached to the myometrium (Fig. 12–28). The amount of decidual tissue retained at the placental site varies.

Most investigators have found that placental separation occurs within a very few minutes after delivery. Brandt (1933) and others, based on results obtained in combined clinical and radiographic studies, supported the idea that because the periphery of the placenta is probably the most adherent portion, separation usually begins elsewhere. Occasionally some degree of separa-

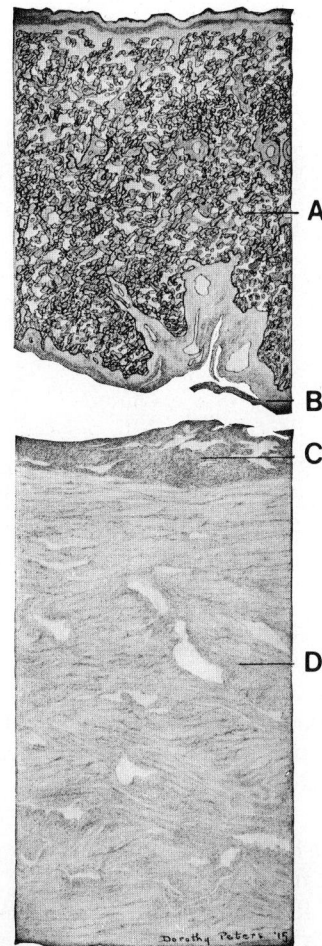

Fig. 12–28. Separation of placenta with cleavage of the decidua. **A.** Placenta. **B.** Decidua cast off with placenta. **C.** Decidua retained in utero. **D.** Myometrium.

tion begins even before the third stage of labor commences, probably accounting for certain cases of fetal distress that occur just before expulsion of the infant.

Separation of Amniochorion. The great decrease in the surface area of the cavity of the uterus simultaneously causes the fetal membranes (amniochorion) and the parietal decidua to be thrown into innumerable folds that increase the thickness of the layer from less than 1 mm to 3 to 4 mm. The lining of the uterus (Fig. 12–29) early in the third stage indicates that much of the parietal layer of decidua parietalis is included between the folds of the festooned amnion and chorion laeve. The membranes usually remain in situ until the separation of the placenta is nearly completed. These are then peeled off the uterine wall, partly by the further contraction of the myometrium and partly by traction that is exerted by the separated placenta, which lies in the flabby lower uterine segment or in the upper portion of the vagina. The body of the uterus at that time normally forms an almost solid mass of muscle, the anterior and posterior

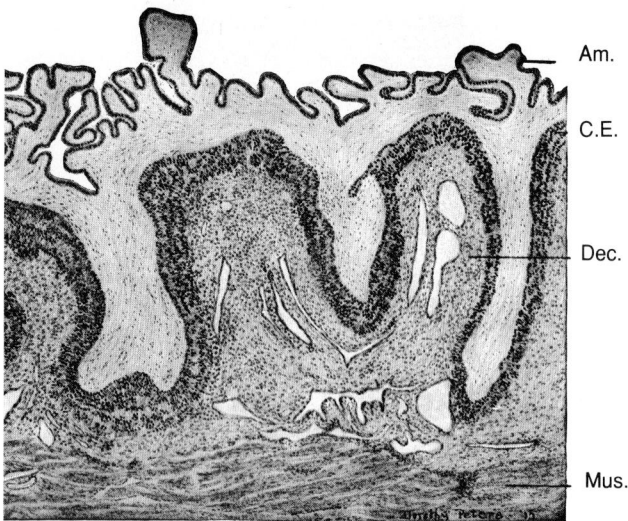

Fig. 12–29. Folding of membranes as uterine cavity decreases in size. (Am. = amnion; C.E. = epithelium of chorion laeve; Dec. = decidua vera; Mus. = myometrium.)

walls of which, each measuring 4 to 5 cm in thickness, lie in close apposition such that the uterine cavity is almost obliterated.

The Phase of Placental Extrusion. After the placenta has separated from its implantation site, the pressure exerted upon it by the uterine walls causes it to slide downward into the flaccid lower uterine segment or the upper part of the vagina. In some cases the placenta may be expelled from those locations by an increase in abdominal pressure, but women in the recumbent position frequently cannot expel the placenta spontaneously. An artificial means of completing the third stage is therefore generally required. The usual method employed is alternately to compress and elevate the fundus, while exerting minimal traction on the umbilical cord (see Chap. 14, p. 384)

Mechanisms of Placental Extrusion. When the central, or usual, type of placental separation occurs, the retroplacental hematoma is believed to push the placenta toward the uterine cavity, first the central portion and then the rest. The placenta, thus inverted and weighted with the hematoma, then descends. Because the surrounding membranes are still attached to the decidua, the placenta can descend only by dragging the membranes along; the membranes then peel off its periphery. Consequently, the sac formed by the membranes is inverted, with the glistening amnion over the placental surface presenting at the vulva. The retroplacental hematoma either follows the placenta or is found within the inverted sac. In this process, known as *the Schultze mechanism* of placental expulsion, blood from the placental site pours into the inverted sac, not escaping externally until after extrusion of the

placenta. The other method of placental extrusion is known as *the Duncan mechanism,* in which separation of the placenta occurs first at the periphery, with the result that blood collects between the membranes and the uterine wall and escapes from the vagina. In this circumstance, the placenta descends to the vagina sideways, and the maternal surface is the first to appear at the vulva.

Preterm Labor

An untimely birth is one of the major health hazards of humans. Preterm birth is the greatest cause of neonatal morbidity and mortality; but more than this, the sequelae of an untimely birth, for those infants who survive, oftentimes causes lifelong disabilities. A large number of permanently institutionalized persons are mentally or physically impaired because of an untimely birth. To suffer the agony of lifelong mental and physical impairment is surely one of the greatest tragedies that can beset a person, his or her family, society, and even the economies of the world. An untimely birth may portend grave and horrendous impositions on the most innocent and vulnerable of our society: the newborn. Guaranteeing the optimal quality of life for newborns, who should expect to enjoy 70 to 80 years or more of good health, must be a major goal of scientists, physicians, and economists concerned with the health care needs of all humans.

The Clinical Problem. A survey of chairpersons of departments of obstetrics and gynecology in the United States and Canada was conducted recently by the Institute of Medicine to define a research agenda for clinician-investigators in this discipline. By an overwhelming majority, preterm birth was identified as the most pressing problem (Townsend, 1992).

Notwithstanding our ignorance of the precise biomolecular processes involved in birthing, there is no doubt that the timeliness of this momentous happening is among the most important biological determinants in establishing the quality of human life. Delivery of the fetus nominally occurs about 260 days after implantation of the blastocyst; but all too commonly, parturition is initiated far in advance of the achievement of full fetal maturation; some 6 to 8 percent of newborns are delivered preterm, that is, before the completion of 37 weeks of gestation.

Today, however, this is not as meaningful a statistic as before. It is true that there has been no reduction in the rate of preterm births for decades; and this is true despite the extensive use of tocolytic agents. Fortuitously, most infants born after 34 completed weeks of gestation now survive; this happy outcome, however, is attributable to the extraordinary advances in neonatal care provided to preterm infants by our neonatology colleagues. Therefore, mortality and morbidity from preterm birth today is primarily a problem for those newborns delivered before the end of 34 weeks' gestation; and it is during the 24- to 34-week gestational period that a reduction in preterm births must be established as a major worldwide clinical and research health objective of highest priority.

Causes of Preterm Birth. Preterm birth, however, is not singularly the consequence of preterm parturition. There are three major sets of problems that affect human pregnancy that culminate in premature delivery: (1) preterm, premature rupture of the fetal membranes; (2) spontaneous preterm labor in pregnancies with intact fetal membranes; and (3) complications of pregnancy that severely jeopardize fetal or maternal health (or both) and mandate delivery for reasons independent of labor or rupture of the membranes. In many hospitals, preterm delivery (before completion of 34 weeks of gestation) occurs most commonly (sometimes 40 percent of the total) in association with preterm premature rupture of the fetal membranes. And in some institutions with a large high-risk pregnancy population, mandated preterm delivery because of deteriorating fetal or maternal health may account for 25 percent of births before 34 weeks of gestation.

Preterm Birth: Premature Rupture of the Membranes. The term "premature rupture of the membranes" is to denote rupture of the membranes before the onset of labor, whether at term or preterm. In some institutions, including Parkland Memorial Hospital, as many or more preterm deliveries are associated with premature rupture of the membranes as with spontaneous preterm labor (Chap. 38).

It has not been possible, however, to study these pregnancies in the same manner as those in which preterm labor begins while the fetal membranes are intact, for two reasons. First, colonization of the fetal membranes by microorganisms commonly occurs very rapidly after rupture and thus causes confusion about the role of infection as a causative agent in preterm rupture of the membranes. Second, after rupture of the membranes, the repository, traplike nature of the amnionic fluid compartment and thereby evaluations of this fluid for etiological clues is lost. Both of these factors render the evaluation of bioactive agents in residual amnionic fluid problematic.

Many investigators suspect that infection may lead to the induction of metalloproteinases that act upon extracellular matrix proteins of the membranes to weaken and thence cause rupture. Whereas this is an attractive hypothesis, the supportive evidence so far is highly circumstantial. An alternative theory being addressed experimentally is that apoplexy of a spiral artery in the decidua parietalis is the basis for membrane rupture. The extracellular matrix of the fetal membranes in

vitro is exquisitely sensitive to a variety of metalloproteinases. The generation of collagenase(s) or stromelysin, or both, in a segment of hypoxic decidua and the action of these metalloproteinases on amniochorion could result in rupture of the membranes at any anatomical site.

The expression of collagenase and stromelysin genes has been demonstrated by the presence of mRNA for both of these metalloproteinases in human decidua and in endometrial stromal cells in culture (Nagai and colleagues, 1991). In addition, tissue inhibitor of metalloproteinase I is expressed in amnion and the levels of mRNA can be regulated in amnion cells in culture.

Nonetheless, the pathogenesis of premature rupture of the membranes is obscure; and unfortunately, new insights into the prevention of this devastating disorder have not emerged. The management of pregnancies complicated by this problem is considered in Chapter 38.

Preterm Delivery: Compromised Fetal and Maternal Health. A host of pregnancy disorders may oblige preterm delivery. Most commonly, these situations cause deteriorating fetal health so that the life or well-being of the fetus is severely compromised. All too often, this unfortunate occurrence obliges a decision between preterm delivery and a worsening intrauterine existence for the fetus. Many examples may be cited, but the most common complications are centered about maternal hypertension, severe diabetes mellitus, fetal growth retardation, and abruptio placenta. Each of these conditions is considered separately in great detail.

Less often, maternal health and survival are also threatened severely by continued pregnancy, and the decision must be made to deliver the pregnancy preterm to preserve the health or life of the mother. And not uncommonly, the health of both fetus and mother are of concern in preterm delivery decisions.

Preterm Delivery: Spontaneous Preterm Labor. The preterm onset of labor in pregnancies in which the fetal membranes are intact is the group of pregnancies most commonly referred to in discussions of preterm labor. Clearly, these pregnancies (for clinical as well as research purposes) must be distinguished from those in which there is preterm, premature rupture of the membranes.

Preterm labor pregnancies, however, do not constitute a homogenous group that is characterized singularly by the onset of parturition too early in pregnancy. Among the more common associated problems are preterm cervical dilatation, anatomical incompetence of the cervix, uterine (fundal) abnormalities, fetal anomalies, multifetal pregnancies, extrauterine infection (appendicitis, peritonitis, pyelonephritis, pneumonia, and others), maternal thermal injury (body burns), autoimmune diseases, pregnancy-induced hypertension, severe

IL-1β IN AMNIONIC FLUID. In our experience, IL-1β is not detected in amnionic fluid at any stage of gestation before the onset of labor. The results of studies of amnionic fluids collected during preterm labor, from all laboratories reporting, have been virtually identical. Namely, in a reasonably large number of preterm labor pregnancies (25 to 40 percent), the primary cytokine, IL-1β, and often microorganisms and LPS, are present in the amnionic fluid (Cox and colleagues, 1988b; Romero and associates, 1987). Based on these initial findings, it was hoped that one cause of preterm labor had been established, confirming what many obstetricians had suspected for decades, that "silent" infection is a relatively common cause of preterm labor.

It was soon discovered, however, that IL-1β is also present in upwards of 25 to 40 percent of amnionic fluids obtained during spontaneous labor at term. Importantly, these amnionic fluids were collected by transabdominal amniocentesis or by direct needle aspiration of fluid from the forebag. These findings of IL-1β in amnionic fluids during spontaneous labor at term in a similar fraction of pregnancies as in preterm labor necessitated a reevaluation of the original hypothesis.

MICROORGANISMS IN AMNIONIC FLUID. The penetrability of tissues by microorganisms varies appreciably among bacteria and among tissues. The microbial penetrability through the tissues exposed in the vagina is likely dependent upon the vaginal flora of a given woman, the duration of exposure of the tissues in the vagina, the numbers of specific microorganisms, the integrity of the fetal membranes exposed, the pH of the vaginal fluids, cooperative actions among microorganisms, and no doubt other unknown factors. Some microorganisms are found in amnionic fluid more commonly than others (e.g., *Fusobacterium sp*). Heretofore, some researchers interpreted these findings as presumptive evidence that certain microorganisms are more commonly involved as pathogens in causing preterm labor. Another view, however, is that given access to the membranes (after cervical dilatation), these microorganisms are better suited to penetrate them.

Fusobacteria, for example, is not an organism that is commonly found in the vagina; but it is the one microorganism most commonly isolated from amnionic fluid during preterm labor. Altshuler and Hyde (1988) found that fusobacteria burrow through the amnion and may be present in large numbers in amnion tissues as if penetrating between the amnion epithelial cells. They also identified (with intrauterine infections) large numbers of fusobacteria in the Wharton jelly of the umbilical cord, suggesting a peculiar propensity for these microorganisms to penetrate amnion, which also covers the umbilical cord. Fusobacteria produce a variety of toxins, some of which are extraordinarily potent in stimulating cytokine forma-

tion in mononuclear phagocytes. We interpret these data, and Hyde and Altshuler concur (personal communication, 1992), to mean that fusobacteria and possibly other microorganisms penetrate the fetal membranes after the tissues are exposed to these microorganisms in the vagina. This would provide an explanation for the low incidence of fusobacteria in vaginal fluids but the high incidence in positive cultures of amnionic fluids.

LEUKOCYTES IN AMNIONIC FLUID. Macrophages are present in amnionic fluid in very small numbers before the onset of labor, except with fetal anomalies, such as open-tube neural defects (anencephaly), when fetal macrophages enter amnionic fluid from the tissue wound of the fetus. Indeed, leukocytes do not readily penetrate normal fetal membranes either in vivo or in vitro. With inflammation of the exposed decidua of the tissues that form the forebag during preterm labor, however, maternal leukocytes are recruited into the amnionic fluid (presumably in response to chemoattractants produced at the site of inflammation in the decidua of the forebag). The same phenomenon is noted at term. Leukocyte activation is accelerated in sites of inflammation, and the activated leukocytes are able to penetrate the fetal membranes.

OTHER CYTOKINES IN AMNIONIC FLUID DURING PRETERM LABOR. Other cytokines in amnionic fluid samples of preterm labor pregnancies have been quantified. Among these are IL-6, IL-8, TNF-α, and M-CSF. There is a strong correlation between the concentration of these cytokines and that of IL-1β, as should be expected. IL-1β stimulates the secretion of IL-6 and IL-8 from a number of cells, of both immune and nonimmune origin. Thus, the finding of increased levels of cytokines other than IL-1β is most likely indicative of the stimulation of cells that produce these other cytokines (e.g., amnion) by the primary cytokine IL-1β. The same is true of endothelin-1 and PTH-rP. IL-1β acts on amnion to increase the synthesis of both endothelin-1 and PTH-rP, and these two vasoactive proteins are found in increased amounts in amnionic fluid of the forebag.

Preterm Labor and High Levels of Amnionic Fluid Cytokines. In a fraction (probably about 10 to 15 percent) of preterm labor pregnancies, the levels of cytokines in amnionic fluid are strikingly increased, that is, much greater than the highest levels in amnionic fluid found during labor at term. Indeed, the levels of IL-1β may be 10 to 100 times the maximum values encountered at term. As yet there is no satisfactory explanation for this finding, but there are several viable possibilities.

If it were correct that most of IL-1β in amnionic fluid arises in mononuclear phagocytes recruited to this space, then the variables of IL-1β formation in amnionic fluid must somehow evolve about these cells: cell number, extent of stimulation, and modifying factors in the amnionic fluid that affect mononuclear cell IL-1β synthesis and processing. It is also possible that the rate of IL-1β degradation or IL-1β binding to another macromolecule in amnionic fluid may be involved.

It is possible, but unlikely in our view, that the very high levels of IL-1β sometimes found in amnionic fluid during preterm labor are somehow indicative that infection was present in these particular pregnancies before labor began. A more likely option, however, may be that processes related to gestational age, preterm cervical dilatation, or occult rupture of the membranes are the cause of high numbers of mononuclear cells in the amnionic fluid, and that these cells give rise to larger amounts of IL-1β in some preterm labor pregnancies.

Sometimes there is a crucial difference in the management of labor in pregnancies at term compared with the management of preterm labor. In the former, management is directed toward effecting delivery in a safe and expedient manner. In the latter, management is commonly directed toward delaying delivery. In consequence, it is rare for recognized labor to extend beyond 18 hours in term pregnancies. It is common for the cervix to be dilated for days, sometimes weeks, when the pregnancy is preterm.

The finding of very high levels of IL-6, IL-8, or TNF-α are probably less relevant to the issue, because these cytokines are produced in response to IL-1β. And as stated, the amnion produces IL-6 and IL-8 and the rate of synthesis of these cytokines in amnion is increased by IL-1β treatment.

Therefore, the entry of IL-1β into or else the in situ formation of IL-1β in cells recruited to the amnionic fluid is the central issue in determining cytokine concentration in amnionic fluid.

Inflammatory Mediators in Amnionic Fluid: Interpretation. Thus, the bioactive agents that accumulate in some amnionic fluids during labor are typical of the compounds produced in an inflammatory response. And these are the same as the bioactive agent set that accumulates in a similar percent of pregnancies at term. The only unique feature of this response to intrauterine tissues is that several of the agents produced could serve as uterotonins: PGE_2, $PGE_{2\alpha}$, PAF, the leukotrienes, and endothelin-1. But these agents, produced in the tissues exposed in the vagina, are formed after (not before) parturition begins and are largely unavailable to the myometrium.

Inflammation and Preterm Labor: Critique. The important question that must be asked is the following:

Does inflammation cause the onset of parturition; or rather, does labor beget inflammation?

To address this question, it is useful to consider the following: There are no substantive differences in the data obtained by all investigators despite the fact that these studies were conducted with socioeconomically divergent obstetrical populations. Therefore, the question is one of data interpretation:

1. Does the inflammatory response and accompanying accumulation of bioactive agents in amnionic fluid precede the initiation of parturition, or does the inflammation develop as a normal sequelae of processes essential for labor, both at term and preterm?
2. Do the uterotonins produced during this inflammatory response gain access to the myometrium or simply accumulate in the amnionic fluid and vagina?
3. Is a uterotropin produced as a part of the inflammatory response to cause the initiation of parturition prematurely, or was a uterotropin produced that caused the preterm initiation of parturition before the inflammatory response existed?
4. Perhaps, most importantly, would antibiotic treatment have prevented the onset of preterm labor in those pregnancies in which evidence of an inflammatory response is found by evaluations of the amnionic fluid for mediators of inflammation?

We are of the view that the answers to these questions, for the overwhelming majority of preterm labor pregnancies, can be summarized as follows: Infection is rarely the cause of preterm labor; but progressive labor, both at term and preterm, always results in inflammation of the tissues exposed by cervical dilatation. Therefore, antibiotic treatment of women can be expected to prevent so few cases of preterm labor that a cause-and-effect relationship cannot be established by statistical comparisons of antibiotic treatment with placebo treatment.

This view is based upon the same lines of reasoning that were applied to an analysis of the finding of inflammatory response mediators in forebag amnionic fluids obtained during spontaneous labor at term. Therefore, it is worth repeating that **it is not possible to traumatize and devascularize the tissues of the forebag and then expose these tissues to the constituents of the vaginal fluid without eliciting an inflammatory response, either at term or preterm.**

It is important to recognize that evidence for infection as a cause of preterm labor has been obtained only by examinations of amnionic fluid (or other biological fluids or tissues) that were collected after labor began.

Preterm Labor: Summary. Preterm labor is not a single etiology disorder. There are clearly uterine abnormalities of both the cervix and fundus that favor preterm labor. A large number of fetal anomalies as well as multifetal pregnancies favor preterm parturition. The most important current question to resolve is whether preterm labor is caused by infection in pregnancies in which the fetal membranes are intact. We conclude that the evidence in favor of this proposition is largely circumstantial and somewhat artifactual. An inflammatory process involving the tissues exposed in the vagina by cervical dilatation is a normal accompaniment of labor, both at term and preterm. The accumulation of mediators of the inflammatory response in amnionic fluid is representative of this natural event of labor and cannot be taken as evidence of infection as the cause of preterm birth.

References

Abbas SK, Pickard DW, Illingworth D, Storer J, Purdie DW, Moniz C, Dixit M, Caple IW, Ebeling PR, Rodda CP, Martin TJ, Care AD: Measurement of PTH-rP protein in extracts of fetal parathyroid glands and placental membranes. J Endocrinol 124:319, 1990

Albert DH, Snyder F: Biosynthesis of 1-alkyl-2-acetyl-sn-glycero-3-phosphocholine (platelet activating factor) from 1-alkyl-2-acyl-sn-glycero-3-phosphocholine by rat alveolar macrophages. Phospholipase A_2 and acetyl transferase activities during phagocytosis and ionophore stimulation. J Biol Chem 258:97, 1983

Alexandrova M, Soloff MS: Oxytocin receptors and parturition, I. Control of oxytocin receptor concentration in the rat myometrium at term. Endocrinology 106:730, 1980a

Altshuler G, Hyde S: Clinicopathologic considerations of fusobacteria chorioamnionitis. Acta Obstet Gynecol Scand 67:513, 1988

Anderson ABM, Turnbull AC: Comparative aspects of factors involved in the onset of labor in ovine and human pregnancy. In Klopper A, Gardner J (eds): Endocrine Factors in Labour. London, Cambridge University Press, 1973, p 141

Angle M, Maki N, Johnston JM: Bioactive metabolites of glycerophospholipid metabolism in relation to parturition. In McNellis D, Challis JRG, MacDonald PC, Nathanielsz P, Roberts J (eds): Cellular and Integrative Mechanisms in the Onset of Labor. An NICHD workshop. Ithaca, NY, Perinatology Press, 1988, p 125

Arici A, MacDonald PC, Casey ML: Transforming growth factor-β1 (TGF-β1) modulates interleukin-8(IL-8) expression in endometrial stromal cells by affecting the mRNA stability. Abstract presented at 39th annual meeting of Society for Gynecological Investigation, San Antonio, March 1992

Arici A, MacDonald PC, Economos K, Casey ML, Head J: Expression of neutrophil activating peptide/interleukin-8 (NAP/IL-8) and monocyte chemotactic protein (MCP-1) in human endometrial stromal cells. Abstract presented at 38th annual meeting of Society for Gynecological Investigation, San Antonio, March, 1991

Auron PE, Warner SJ, Webb DA, Cannon JG, Bernheim HA, McAda KJ, Rossenwasser LJ, LoPreste G, Mucci SJ, Dinarello CA: Studies on IL-1. J Immunol 138:1447, 1987

Ban C, Billah MM, Truong CT, Johnston JM: Metabolism of platelet-activating factor (1-0-alkyl-2-acetyl-sn-glycero-3-phosphocholine) in human fetal membranes and decidua vera. Arch Biochem Biophys 246:9, 1986

Barany K, Barany M: Myosin light chain phosphorylation in uterine smooth muscle. In Carsten ME, Miller JD (eds): Uterine Function: Molecular and Cellular Aspects. Plenum, New York, 1990, p 71

Bartocci A, Pollard JW, Stanley ER: Regulation of colony-stimulating factor 1 during pregnancy. J Exp Med 164:956, 1986

Bates GW, Edman CD, Porter JC, MacDonald PC: Catechol-O-methyltransferase activity in erythrocytes of women taking oral contraceptive steroids. Am J Obstet Gynecol 133:691, 1979

Benedetto MT, DeCicco F, Rossiello F, Nicosia AL, Lupi G, Dell'Acqua S: Oxytocin receptor in human fetal membranes at term and during labor. J Steroid Biochem 35:205, 1990

Bercu BB, Hyashi A, Poth M, Alexandrova M, Soloff MS, Donahoe PK: LHRH induced delay of parturition. Endocrinology 107:504, 1980

Besinger RE, Neibyl JR: The safety and efficacy of tocolytic agents for the treatment of preterm labor. Obstet Gynecol Surv 415, 1990

Beutler B, Cerami A: Cachectin and tumor necrosis factor as two sides of the same biological coin. Nature 320:584, 1986

Beyer EC, Kistler J, Paul DL, Goodenough DA: Antisera directed against connexin43 peptides react with a 43-kD protein localized to gap junctions in myocardium and other tissues. J Cell Biol 108:595, 1989

Beyer EC, Paul DL, Goodenough DA: Connexin43: A protein from rat heart homologous to a gap junction protein from liver. J Cell Biol 105:2621, 1987

Billah MM, Johnston JM: Identification of phospholipid platelet-activating factor (1-0-alkyl-2-acetyl-sn-glycero-3-phosphocholine) in human amnionic fluid and urine. Biochem Biophys Res Commun 113:51, 1983

Billiar RB, Jassani M, Little B: The metabolic clearance rate and uterine extraction of progesterone at midgestation. Endocr Res Commun 1:339, 1974

Brandt ML: Mechanism and management of the third stage of labor. Am J Obstet Gynecol 25:662, 1933

Broderick R, Broderick KA: Ultrastructure and calcium stores in the myometrium. In Carsten ME, Miller JD (eds): Uterine Function. Molecular and Cellular Aspects. New York, Plenum, 1990, p 1

Bruns ME, Kleeman E, Mills SE, Bruns DE, Herr JC: Immunochemical localization of vitamin D-dependent calcium-binding protein in mouse placenta. Anat Rec 231:514, 1985

Bruns ME, Overpeck JG, Smith GC, Hirsch GN, Mills SE, Bruns DE: Vitamin D-dependent calcium binding protein in rat uterus: Differential effects of estrogen, tamoxifen, progesterone and pregnancy on accumulation and cellular localization. Endocrinology 122:2371, 1988

Burghardt RC, Mitchell PA, Kurten RC: Gap junction modulation in rat uterus, II. Effects of antiestrogens on myometrial and serosal cells. Biol Reprod 30:249, 1984

Caldeyro-Barcia R, Alvarez H, Reynolds SRM: A better understanding of uterine contractility through simultaneous recording with an internal and a seven channel external method. Surg Gynecol Obstet 91:641, 1950

Canadian Preterm Labor Investigators Group: Treatment of

preterm labor with the beta-adrenergic agonist ritodrine. N Engl J Med 327:308, 1992

Carsten ME, Miller JD: Calcium control mechanisms in the myometrial cell and the role of the phosphoinositide cycle. In Carsten ME, Miller JD (eds): Uterine Function. Molecular and Cellular Aspects. New York, Plenum, 1990, p 121

Casey ML, Cox SM, Beutler B, Milewich L, MacDonald PC: Cachectin (tumor necrosis factor-α) production in human decidua: Potential role of cytokines in infection-induced preterm labor. J Clin Invest 83:430, 1989a

Casey ML, Cutrer SI, Mitchell MD: Origin of prostanoids in human amniotic fluid: The fetal kidney as a source of amniotic fluid prostanoids. Am J Obstet Gynecol 147:547, 1983

Casey ML, Delgadillo M, Cox KA, Niesert S, MacDonald PC: Inactivation of prostaglandins in human decidua vera (parietalis) tissue: Substrate specificity of prostaglandin dehydrogenase. Am J Obstet Gynecol 160:3, 1989b

Casey ML, Hemsell DL, MacDonald PC, Johnston JM: NAD$^+$-dependent 15-hydroxyprostaglandin dehydrogenase activity in human endometrium. Prostaglandins 19:115, 1980

Casey ML, Korte K, MacDonald PC: Epidermal growth factor-stimulation of prostaglandin E_2 biosynthesis in amnion cells: Induction of PGH$_2$ synthase. J Biol Chem 263:7846, 1988a

Casey ML, MacDonald PC: The endothelin/enkephalinase system of human fetal membranes and chorionic vessels. Abstract presented at 39th annual meeting of Society for Gynecological Investigation, San Antonio, March, 1992

Casey ML, MacDonald PC: Biomolecular mechanisms in human parturition: Activation of uterine decidua. In d'Arcangues C, Fraser IS, Newton JR, Odlind V (eds): Contraception and Mechanisms of Endometrial Bleeding, Cambridge, UK, Cambridge University Press, 1990, p 501

Casey ML, MacDonald PC: Biomolecular processes in the initiation of parturition: Decidual activation. Clin Obstet Gynecol 31:533, 1988a

Casey ML, MacDonald PC: The role of a fetal–maternal paracrine system in the maintenance of pregnancy and the initiation of parturition. In Jones CT (ed): Fetal and Neonatal Development. Ithaca, NY, Perinatology Press, 1988b, p 521

Casey ML, MacDonald PC: Decidual activation: The role of prostaglandins in labor. In McNellis D, Challis JRG, MacDonald PC, Nathanielsz P, Roberts J (eds): Cellular and Integrative Mechanisms in the Onset of Labor. An NICHD workshop. Ithaca, NY, Perinatology Press, 1988c, p 141

Casey ML, MacDonald PC, Mitchell MD: Despite a massive increase in cortisol secretion in women during parturition, there is an equally massive increase in prostaglandin synthesis: A paradox? J Clin Invest 75:1852, 1985

Casey ML, Mibe M, Erk A, MacDonald PC: Transforming growth factor-β1 stimulation of parathyroid hormone-related protein expression in human uterine cells in culture: mRNA levels and protein secretion. J Clin Endocrinol Metab 74:950, 1992

Casey ML, Mitchell MD, MacDonald PC: Epidermal growth factor-stimulated prostaglandin E_2 production in human amnion cells: Specificity and nonesterified arachidonic acid dependency. Mol Cell Endocrinol 53:169, 1987

Casey ML, Smith JW, Nagai K, Hersh LB, MacDonald PC: Progesterone-regulated cyclic modulation of membrane metalloendopeptidase (enkephalinase) in human endometrium. J Biol Chem 266:23041, 1991a

Casey ML, Word RA, MacDonald PC: Endothelin-1 gene ex-

pression and regulation of endothelin mRNA and protein biosynthesis in avascular human amnion: Potential source of amniotic fluid endothelin. J Biol Chem 266:5762, 1991b

Challis JRG, Olson DM: Parturition. In Knobil E, Neill JD (eds): The Physiology of Reproduction, Vol II. New York, Raven, 1988, p 2177

Chibbar R, Miller FD, Mitchell BF: Oxytocin is synthesized in human fetal membranes. Abstract presented at 38th annual meeting of Society for Gynecological Investigation, San Antonio, March, 1991

Chwalisz K, Fahrenholz F, Hackenberg M, Garfield R, Elger W: The progesterone antagonist onapristone increases the effectiveness of oxytocin to produce delivery without changing the myometrial oxytocin receptor concentrations. Am J Obstet Gynecol 165:1760, 1991

Cole WC, Garfield RE: Evidence for the physiological regulation of myometrial gap junction permeability. Am J Physiol 251:C411, 1986

Cox SM, MacDonald PC, Casey ML: Decidual activation is synchronous with spontaneous parturition and with bacterial endotoxin [lipopolysaccharide (LPS)]-induced preterm labor. Proc Soc Gynecol Invest 35:89, 1988a. Abstract

Cox SM, MacDonald PC, Casey ML: Assay of bacterial endotoxin (lipopolysaccharide) in human amniotic fluid: Potential usefulness in diagnosis and management of preterm labor. Am J Obstet Gynecol 159:99, 1988b

Dale HH: On some physiologic actions of ergot. J Physiol (Lond) 34:163, 1906

Danforth DN, Buckingham JC, Roddick JW: Connective tissue changes incident to cervical effacement. Am J Obstet Gynecol 80:939, 1960

Darwish H, Krisinger J, Furlow JD, Smith C, Murdoch FE, DeLuca HF: An estrogen-responsive element mediates the transcriptional regulation of calbindin D-9K gene in rat uterus. J Biol Chem 266:551, 1991

Diamond J: β-Adrenoceptors, cyclic AMP, and cyclic GMP in control of uterine motility. In Carsten ME, Miller JD (eds): Uterine Function: Molecular and Cellular Aspects. New York, Plenum, 1990, p 249

Dinarello CA: Interleukin-1: Amino acid sequences, multiple biological activities, and comparison with tumor necrosis factor (cachectin). Year Immunol 2:69, 1986

Ehrenreich H, Anderson RW, Fox CH, Rieckmann P, Hoffman GS, Travis WD, Coligan JE, Kehrl JH, Fauci AS: Endothelins, peptides with potent vasoactive properties, are produced by human macrophages. J Exp Med 172:1741, 1990

Eis AW, Mitchell MD, Myatt L: Endothelin transfer and endothelin effects on water transfer in human fetal membranes. Obstet Gynecol 79:411, 1992

Fantoni G, Casparis D, Magini A, Del Carlo P, Giannini S, Gloria L, Barni T, Vannelli GB, Maggi M: Endothelin in human uterus during pregnancy. Abstract presented at 74th annual meeting of the Endocrine Society, San Antonio, June, 1992

Feinberg RF, Kliman HJ, Lockwood CJ: Is oncofetal fibronectin a trophoblast glue for human implantation? Am J Pathol 138:537, 1991

Ferguson JKW: A study of the motility of the intact uterus at term. Surg Gynecol Obstet 73:359, 1941

Flower RJ: The role of prostaglandins in parturition, with special reference to the rat. In Knight J, O'Connor M (eds): The Fetus and Birth. Ciba Foundation Symposium 47. Amsterdam, Elsevier, 1977, p 297

France JT, Magness RR, Murry BA, Rosenfeld CR, Mason JI: The regulation of ovine placental steroid 17α-hydroxylase and aromatase by glucocorticoid. Mol Endocrinol 2:193, 1988

France JT, Mason JI, Magness RR, Murry BA, Rosenfeld CR: Ovine placental aromatase: Studies of activity level, kinetic characteristics and effects of aromatase inhibitors. J Steroid Biochem 28:155, 1987

Friedman EA: Labor: Clinical Evaluation and Management, 2nd ed. New York, Appleton-Century-Crofts, 1978

Fuchs AR, Fuchs F, Husslein P, Soloff MS: Oxytocin receptors in the human uterus during pregnancy and parturition. Am J Obstet Gynecol 150:734, 1984

Fuchs AR, Fuchs F, Husslein P, Soloff MS, Fernström MJ: Oxytocin receptors and human parturition. A dual role for oxytocin in the initiation of labor. Science 215:1396, 1982

Fuchs AR, Fuchs F, Soloff MS: Oxytocin receptors in nonpregnant human uterus. J Clin Endocrinol Metab 60:37, 1985

Fuchs AR, Husslein P, Fuchs F: Oxytocin and the initiation of human parturition, II. Stimulation of prostaglandin production in human decidua by oxytocin. Am J Obstet Gynecol 141:694, 1981

Fuchs AR, Periyasamy S, Alexandrova M, Soloff MS: Correlation between oxytocin receptor concentration and responsiveness to oxytocin in pregnant rat myometrium: Effect of ovarian steroids. Endocrinology 113:742, 1983

Gainer H, Alstein M, Whitnall MH, Wray S: The biosynthesis and secretion of oxytocin and vasopressin. In Knobil E, Neill J (eds): The Physiology of Reproduction, Vol II, New York, Raven, 1988, p 2265

Garfield RE, Hayashi RH: Appearance of gap junctions in the myometrium of women during labor. Am J Obstet Gynecol 140:254, 1981

Garfield RE, Sims SM, Daniel EE: Gap junctions: Their presence and necessity in myometrium during parturition. Science 198:958, 1977

Gemzell CA, Robbe H, Stern B, Strom G: Observation on circulatory changes and muscular work in normal labor. Acta Obstet Gynecol Scand 36:75, 1957

Germain AM, Attaroglu H, MacDonald PC, Casey ML: Parathyroid hormone-related protein mRNA in avascular human amnion. J Clin Endocrinol Metab 75:1173, 1992

Hayashi RH, Garfield RE, Harper MJK: Regulation of human myometrial gap junctions: In vitro studies. In (ed): The Physiological Development of the Fetus and Newborn. London, Academic Press, 1985, p 411

Hertelendy F: Regulation of oviposition. In MacDonald PC, Porter JC (eds): Initiation of Parturition: Prevention of Prematurity. Fourth Ross Conference on Obstetric Research. Columbus, OH, Ross Laboratories, 1983, p 79

Hogquist KA, Unanue ER, Chaplin DD: Release of IL-1 from mononuclear phagocytes. J Immunol 147:2181, 1991

Howard AD, Kostura MJ, Thornberry N, Ding GJF, Limjuco G, Weidner J, Salley JP, Hogquist KA, Chaplin DD, Mumford RA, Schmidt JA, Tocci MJ: IL-1-converting enzyme requires aspartic acid residues for processing IL-1β precursor. J Immunol 147:2964, 1991

Huszar G, Roberts JB: Biochemistry and pharmacology of the myometrium and labor: Regulation at the cellular and molecular levels. Am J Obstet Gynecol 142:225, 1982

Huszar G, Walsh MP: Biochemistry of the myometrium and

cervix. In Wynn RM, Jollie WP (eds): Biology of the Uterus, 2nd ed. New York, Plenum, 1989, p 355

Iams JD, Clapp DH, Contox DA, Whitehurst R, Ayers LW, O'Shaughnessy RW: Does extraamniotic infection cause preterm labor: Gas-liquid chromatography studies of amniotic fluid in amnionitis, preterm labor, and normal controls. Obstet Gynecol 70:365, 1987

Johnston JM, Bleasdale JE, Hoffman DR: Functions of PAF in reproduction and development: Involvement of PAF in fetal lung maturation and parturition. In Snyder F (ed): Platelet-Activating Factor and Related Lipid Mediators. New York, Plenum, 1987

Johnston JM, Maki N: PAF and fetal development. In Barnes PJ, Page CP, Henson PM (eds): PAF in Health and Disease. Oxford, Blackwell, 1989, p 297

Karlson S: On the motility of the uterus during labour and the influence of the motility pattern on the duration of the labour. Acta Obstet Gynecol Scand 28:209, 1949

Keirse MJNC: Eicosanoids in human pregnancy and parturition. In M Mitchell (ed): Eicosanoids in Reproduction. Boca Raton, FL, CRC Press, 1990, p 199

Keirse MJNC: PGs in parturition. In Keirse M, Anderson A, Gravenhorst J (eds): Human Parturition. The Hague, Netherlands, Martinus Nijhoff, 1979, p 101

Keirse MJNC, Hicks BR, Mitchell MD, Turnbull AC: Increase in the prostaglandin precursor, arachidonic acid, in amniotic fluid during spontaneous labour. Br J Obstet Gynaecol 84:937, 1977

Keirse MJNC, Turnbull AC: Metabolism of prostaglandins within the human pregnant uterus. Br J Obstet Gynaecol 82:887, 1975

Kelly HA: Operative Gynecology, 2nd ed. New York, Appleton, 1906

Kimura T, Tanizawa O, Mori K, Brownstein M, Okayama H: Structure and expression of a human oxytocin receptor. Nature 356:526, 1992

Kunkel SL, Chensue SW: The role of arachidonic acid metabolites in mononuclear phagocytic cell interaction. Int J Dermatol 25:83, 1986

Leake RD: Oxytocin in the initiation of labor. In Carsten ME, Miller JD (eds): Uterine Function. Molecular and Cellular Aspects. New York, Plenum, 1990, p 361

Leake RD: Oxytocin. In MacDonald PC, Porter JC (eds): Initiation of Parturition: Prevention of Prematurity. Fourth Ross Conference on Obstetric Research. Columbus, OH, Ross Laboratories. 1983, p 43

Leake RD, Weitzman RE, Fisher DA: Pharmacokinetics of oxytocin in the human subject. Obstet Gynecol 56:701, 1980

Leake RD, Weitzman RE, Glatz TH, Fisher DA: Plasma oxytocin concentrations in men, nonpregnant women, and pregnant women before and during labor. J Clin Endocrinol Metab 53:730, 1981

Lefebvre DL, Giaid A, Bennett H, Lariviere R, Zingg HH: Oxytocin gene expression in rat uterus. Science 256:1553, 1992a

Lefebvre DL, Giaid A, Zingg HH: Expression of the oxytocin gene in rat placenta. Endocrinology 130:1185, 1992b

Leveno KJ, Cunningham FG: β-adrenergic agonists for preterm labor. N Engl J Med 327:349, 1992

L'Horset F, Perret C, Brehier A, Thomasset M: 17β-Estradiol stimulates the calbindin-D9K (CaBP9K) gene expression at the transcriptional and post transcriptional levels in the rat uterus. Endocrinology 127:2891, 1990

Liggins GC: Fetal influences on myometrial contractility. Clin Obstet Gynecol 16:148, 1973

Liggins GC: Premature parturition after infusion of corticotrophin or cortisol into foetal lambs. J Endocrinol 42:323, 1968

Liggins GC, Fairclough RJ, Grieves SA, Kendall JZ, Knox BS: The mechanism of initiation of parturition in the ewe. Recent Prog Horm Res 29:111, 1973

Liggins GC, Kennedy PC, Holm LW: Failure of initiation of parturition after electrocoagulation of the pituitary of the fetal lamb. Am J Obstet Gynecol 98:1080, 1967

Lin TJ, Billiar RB, Little B: Metabolic clearance of progesterone in the menstrual cycle. J Clin Endocrinol Metab 35:879, 1972

Little B, Tait JF, Tait SA, Erlenmeyer F: The metabolic clearance rate of progesterone in males and ovariectomized females. J Clin Invest 45:901, 1966

Lockwood CJ, Senyei AE, Dische MR, Casal D, Shah KD, Thung SN, Jones L, Deligdisch L, Garite TJ: Fetal fibronectin in cervical and vaginal secretions as a predictor of preterm delivery. N Engl J Med 325:669, 1991

MacDonald PC, Casey ML: The accumulation of prostaglandins (PG) in amniotic fluid is an aftereffect of labor and not indicative of a role for PGE_2 or $PGE_{2\alpha}$ in the initiation of human parturition. J Clin Endocrinol Metab (in press)

MacDonald PC, Cox SM, Casey ML: Infection-associated preterm labor as a model for parturition. In Genazzani AR, Petraglia F, Volpe A, Facchinetti F (eds): Advances in Gynecological Endocrinology, Vol I. Carnforth, UK, Parthenon, 1988, p 487

MacDonald PC, Koga S, Casey ML: Decidual activation in parturition: Examination of amniotic fluid for mediators of the imflammatory response. Ann NY Acad Sci 622:315, 1991

MacDonald PC, Schultz FM, Duenhoelter JH, Gant NF, Jimenez JM, Pritchard JA, Porter JC, Johnston JM: Initiation of human parturition, I. Mechanism of action of arachidonic acid. Obstet Gynecol 44:629, 1974

MacKenzie LM, Word RA, Casey ML, Stull JT: Myosin light chain phosphorylation in human myometrial smooth muscle cells. Am J Physiol 258:C92, 1990

Mallette LE: Parathyroid polyhormone actions: New concepts. Endocr Rev 12:110-117, 1991

Malpas P: Postmaturity and malformation of the fetus. J Obstet Gynaecol Br Emp 40:1046, 1933

Martin TJ, Allan EH, Caple IW, Care AD, Danks JA, Diefenbach-Jagger H, Edeling PR, Gillespie MT, Hammonds G, Heath JA, Hudson PJ, Kemp BE, Kubota M, Kukreja SC, Moseley JM, Ng KW, Raisz LG, Rodda CP, Simmons HA, Suva LJ, Wettenhall REH, Wood WI: Parathyroid hormone-related protein. Recent Prog Horm Res 45:467, 1989

Mathieu CL, Burnett SH, Mills SE, Overpeck JG, Bruns DE, Bruns ME: Gestational changes in calbindin-D_{9K} in rat uterus, yolk sac, and placenta: Implications for maternal–fetal calcium transport and uterine muscle function. Proc Natl Acad Sci USA 86:3433, 1989

McCoshen JA, Hoffman DR, Kredentser JV, Araneda C, Johnston JM: Fetal membranes regulating production, transport of PGE_2. Am J Obstet Gynecol 163:1632, 1990

McCoshen JA, Johnson KA, Dubin NH, Ghodgaonkar RB: PGE_2 release on the fetal and maternal sides of the amnion chorion–decidua. Am J Obstet Gynecol 156:173, 1987

McDonald TJ, Nathanielsz PW: Bilateral destruction of the fetal paraventricular nuclei prolongs gestation in sheep. Am J Obstet Gynecol 165:764, 1991

Mitchell MD: Studies on prostaglandins in relation to parturition in the sheep. D. Phil. thesis, Oxford University, 1976

Mitchell MD, Flint AP, Bibby J, Brunt J, Arnold JM, Anderson AB, Turnbull AC: Rapid increases in plasma prostaglandin concentrations after vaginal examination and amniotomy. Br Med J 2:1183, 1977

Mok LL, Nickols GA, Thompson JC, Cooper CW: Parathyroid hormone as a smooth muscle relaxant. Endocr Rev 10:420, 1989

Mosley B, Urdal DL, Prickett KS, Larsen A, Cosman D, Conlon PJ, Gillis S, Dower SK: The IL-1 receptor binds the IL-1α precursor but not the IL-1β precursor. J Biol Chem 262:2941, 1987

Myers DA, McDonald TJ, Nathanielsz PW: Effect of bilateral lesions of the ovine fetal hypothalamic paraventricular nuclei at 118–122 days of gestation on subsequent adrenocortical steroidogenic enzyme gene expression. Endocrinology 131:305, 1992

Nagai K, MacDonald PC, Casey ML: Gene expression of collagenase, stromelysin, and tissue inhibitor of metalloproteinase in human fetal membranes and decidua. Proc Soc Gynecol Invest 38:208, 1991. Abstract

Nathanielsz PW: The regulation of the switch from myometrial contractures to contractions in late pregnancy. In Gluckman PD, Johnston BM, Nathanielsz PW (eds): Advances in Fetal Physiology. Ithaca, NY, Perinatology Press, 1989, p 409

Niesert S, Christopherson WA, Korte K, Mitchell MD, MacDonald PC, Casey ML: Prostaglandin E_2 9-keto-reductase activity in human decidua vera tissue. Am J Obstet Gynecol 155:1348, 1986

Nishihara J, Ishibashi T, Mai Y, Muramatsu T: Mass spectrometric evidence for the presence of platelet-activating factor (1-0-alkyl-2-sn-glycero-3-phosphocholine) in human amniotic fluid during labor. Lipids 19:907, 1984

Novy MJ, Liggins GC: Role of prostaglandin, prostacyclin, and thromboxanes in the physiologic control of the uterus and in parturition. Semin Perinatol 4:45, 1980

Okazaki T, Casey ML, Okita JR, MacDonald PC, Johnston JM: Initiation of human parturition, XII. Biosynthesis and metabolism of prostaglandins in human fetal membranes and uterine decidua vera. Am J Obstet Gynecol 139:373, 1981

Okita JR: Alternations in arachidonic acid content of specific glycerophospholipids of amnion and chorion laeve during human parturition. Doctoral dissertation, University of Texas Southwestern Medical School, Dallas, 1981

Okita JR, Johnston JM, MacDonald PC: Source of prostaglandin precursor in human fetal membranes: Arachidonic acid content of amnion and chorion laeve of diamnionic–dichorionic twin placentae. Am J Obstet Gynecol 147:477, 1983a

Okita JR, MacDonald PC, Johnston JM: Mobilization of arachidonic acid from specific glycerophospholipids of human fetal membranes during early labor. J Biol Chem 247:14029, 1982a

Okita JR, MacDonald PC, Johnston JM: Initiation of human parturition, XIV. Increase in the diacylglycerol content of amnion during parturition. Am J Obstet Gynecol 142:432, 1982b

Ottlexa A, Walker S, Conrad M, Starcher B: Neutural metalloendopeptidase associated with the smooth muscle cells of pregnant rat uterus. J Cell Biochem 45:401, 1991

Pierce JG, du Vigneaud V: Studies on high potency oxytotic materials from beef posterior pituitary lobes. J Biol Chem 186:77, 1950

Prescott SM, Zimmerman GA, McIntyre TM: PAF. J Biol Chem 265:17381, 1990

Rea C: Prolonged gestation, acrania, monstrosity and apparent placenta praevia in one obstetrical case. JAMA 30:1166, 1898

Reddi K, Kambaran SR, Norman RJ, Joubert SM, Philpott RH: Abnormal concentrations of prostaglandins in amniotic fluid during delayed labour in multigravid patients. Br J Obstet Gynaecol 91:781, 1984

Rettenmier CW, Sacca R, Furman WL, Roussel MF, Holt JT, Neinhuis AW, Stanley ER, Sherr CJ: Expression of the human c-fms proto-oncogene product (colony-stimulating factor-1 receptor) on peripheral blood mononuclear cells and choriocarcinoma cell lines. J Clin Invest 77:1740, 1986

Reynolds SR: Physiology of the Uterus with Clinical Correlations, 2nd ed. New York, Hoeber, 1949

Reynolds SR, Hellman LM, Bruns P: Pattern of uterine contractility in women during pregnancy. Obstet Gynecol Surv 3:629, 1948

Richardson MR, Mitchell MD, MacDonald PC, Casey ML: Glucocorticosteroid regulation of prostaglandin biosynthesis in human myometrial smooth muscle cells in monolayer culture. J Steroid Biochem 25:521, 1986

Riemer RK, Goldfien AC, Goldfien A, Roberts JM: Rabbit uterine oxytocin receptors and in vitro contractile response: Abrupt changes at term and the role of eicosanoids. Endocrinology 119:669, 1986

Ringler GE, Coutifaris C, Strauss JF, Allen JI, Geier M: Accumulation of colony stimulating factor 1 in amniotic fluid during human pregnancy. Am J Obstet Gynecol 160:655, 1989

Roberts JM, Riemer RK, Bottari SP, Wu YY, Goldfien A: Hormonal regulation myometrial adrenergic responses: The receptor and beyond. J Dev Physiol 11:125, 1989

Roberts JM, Riemer RK, Bottari SP, Wu YY, Goldfien A: Myometrial postreceptor responses: Targets for steroidal regulation. In McNellis D, Challis JRG, MacDonald PC, Nathanielsz P, Roberts J (eds): Cellular and Integrative Mechanisms in the Onset of Labor. An NICHD workshop. Ithaca, NY, Perinatology Press, 1988, p 37

Robinson JS, Chapman RL, Challis JR, Mitchell MD: Administration of extra-amniotic arachidonic acid and the suppression of uterine prostaglandin synthesis during pregnancy in the rhesus monkey. J Reprod Fertil 54:369, 1979

Romero R, Durum S, Dinarello CA, Oyarzun E, Hobbins JC, Mitchell MD: Interleukin-1 stimulates prostaglandin biosynthesis by human amnion. Prostaglandins 37:13, 1989a

Romero R, Kadar N, Hobbins JC, Duff GW: Infection and labor: The detection of endotoxin in amniotic fluid. Am J Obstet Gynecol 157:815, 1987

Romero R, Manogue KR, Mitchell MD, Wu YK, Oyarzun E, Hobbins JC, Cerami A: Infection and labor, IV. Cachectin-tumor necrosis factor in the amniotic fluid of women with intraamniotic infection and preterm labor. Am J Obstet Gynecol 161:336, 1989b.

Romero R, Mazor M, Wu YK, Sirtori M, Oyarzun E, Mitchell MD, Hobbins JC: Infection in the pathogenesis of preterm labor. Semin Perinatol 12:262, 1988

Romero R, Parvizi ST, Oyarzun E, Mazor M, Wu YK, Avila C,

Athanassiadis AP, Mitchell MD: Amniotic fluid IL-1 in spontaneous labor at term. J Reprod Med 35:235, 1990

Rosendaal M: Colony-stimulating factor (CSF) in the uterus of the pregnant mouse. J Cell Sci 19:411, 1975

Sakai N, Tabb T, Garfield RE: Modulation of cell-to-cell coupling between myometrial cells of the human uterus during pregnancy. Am J Obstet Gynecol 167:472, 1992

Salamonsen LA, Butt AR, Macpherson AM, Rogers PAW, Findlay JK: Immunolocalization of the vasoconstrictor endothelin in human endometrium during the menstrual cycle and in umbilical cord at birth. Am J Obstet Gynecol 167:163, 1992

Schlegel W, Kruger S, Korte K: Purification of prostaglandin E_2-9-oxoreductase from human decidua vera. FEBS Lett 171:141, 1984

Schulman H, Romney SL: Variability of uterine contractions in normal human parturition. Obstet Gynecol 36:215, 1970

Semer D, Reisler K, MacDonald PC, Casey ML: Responsiveness of human endometrial stromal cells to cytokines, Ann NY Acad Sci 622:99, 1991

Shozu M, Akasofu K, Harada T, Kubota Y: A new cause of female pseudohermaphroditism: Placental aromatase deficiency. J Clin Endocrinol Metab 72:560, 1991

Siiteri PK, MacDonald PC: The utilization of circulating dehydroisoandrosterone sulfate for estrogen synthesis during human pregnancy. Steroids 2:713, 1963

Soloff MS, Alexandrova M, Fernström MJ: Oxytocin receptors: Triggers for parturition and lactation? Science 204:1313, 1979

Soloff MS, Fernström MA, Periyasamy S, Soloff S, Baldwin S, Wieder M: Regulation of oxytocin receptor concentration in rat uterine explants by estrogen and progesterone. Can J Biochem Cell Biol 61:625, 1983

Stanley ER: Action of the colony-stimulating factor, CSF-1. In Evered D, Nugent J, O'Connor M (eds): Biochemistry of Machrophages. Ciba Foundation Symposium 118. New York, Wiley, 1986, p 29

Stull JT, Taylor DA, MacKenzie LW, Casey ML: Biochemistry and physiology of smooth muscle contractility. In McNellis D, Challis JRG, MacDonald PC, Nathanielsz P, Roberts J (eds): Cellular and Integrative Mechanisms in the Onset of Labor. An NICHD Workshop. Ithaca, NY, Perinatology Press, 1988, p 17

Sunnergren KP, Word RA, Sambrook JF, MacDonald PC, Casey ML: Expression and regulation of endothelin precursor mRNA in avascular human amnion. Mol Cell Endocrinol 68:R7, 1990

Thiede MA, Daifotis AG, Weir EC, Brines ML, Burtis WJ, Ikeda K, Dreyer BE, Garfield RE, Broadus AE: Intrauterine occupancy controls expression of the parathyroid hormone-related peptide gene in preterm rat myometrium. Proc Natl Acad Sci USA 87:6969, 1990

Thiede MA, Harm SC, Hasson DM, Gardner RM: In vivo regulation of PTH-rP messenger ribonucleic acid in the rat uterus by 17β-estradiol. Endocrinology 128:2317, 1991a

Thiede MA, Harm SC, McKee RL, Grasser WA, Duong LT, Leach Jr RM: Expression of the PTH-rP gene in the avian oviduct. Endocrinology 129:1958, 1991b

Thorburn GD: Past and present concepts on the initiation of parturition. In MacDonald PC, Porter JC (eds): Initiation of

Parturition: Prevention of Prematurity. Fourth Ross conference on obstetric research. Columbus, OH, Ross Laboratories, 1983, p 2

Townsend J, ed. Strengthening Research in Academic Ob/Gyn Departments. Washington, DC, Institute of Medicine, National Academy Press, 1992

Uemura Y, Lee TC, Snyder F: A coenzyme A-independent transacylase is linked to the formation of platelet-activating factor (PAF) by generating the lyso-PAF intermediate in the remodeling pathway. J Biol Chem 266:8268, 1991

Usuki S, Saitoh T, Sawamura T, Suzuki N, Shigemitsu S, Yanagisawa M, Goto K, Onda H, Fujino M, Masaki T. Increased maternal plasma concentration of endothelin-1 during labor pain or on delivery and the existence of a large amount of endothelin-1 in amniotic fluid. Gynecol Endocrinol 4:85, 1990

Visvader J, Verma IM: Differential transcription of exon 1 of the human c-*fms* gene in placental trophoblasts and monocytes. Mol Cell Biol 9:1336, 1989

Wagner OF, Christ G, Wojta J, Vierharpper H, Parzer S, Nowotny PJ, Schneider B, Waldhäusal W, Binder BR: Polar secretion of endothelin-1 by cultured endothelial cells. J Biol Chem 267:16066, 1992

Webb AC, Rosenwasser LJ, Auron PE: Molecular organization and expression of the prointerleukin-1β gene. In Gillis S (ed): Recombinant Lymphokines and Their Receptors. New York, Marcel Dekker, 1987, p 139

Wilson T, Liggins GC, Joe L: Purification and characterization of a uterine phospholipase inhibitor that loses activity after labor onset. Am J Obstet Gynecol 35:602, 1989

Word RA, Kamm KE, Casey ML: Contractile effects of prostaglandins, oxytocin, and endothelin in human myometrium in vitro. Refractoriness of myometrial tissue of pregnant women to prostaglandin E_2 and $F_{2\alpha}$. J Clin Endocrinol Metab 75:1027, 1992

Word RA, Kamm KE, Stull JT, Casey ML: Endothelin increases cytoplasmic calcium and myosin phosphorylation in human myometrium. Am J Obstet Gynecol 162:1103, 1990

Yanagisawa M, Kurihara H, Kimura S, Tomobe Y, Kobayashi M, Mitsui Y, Yazaki Y, Goto K, Masaki T: A novel potent vasoconstrictor peptide produced by vascular endothelial cells. Nature 332:411, 1988

Yasuda K, Johnston JM: The hormonal regulation of PAF-acetylhydrolase in the rat. Endocrinology 130:708, 1992

Zahl PA, Bjerknes C: Induction of decidua-placental hemorrhage in mice by the endotoxins of certain gram-negative bacteria. Proc Soc Exp Biol Med 54:329, 1943

Zhu YP, Word RA, Johnston JM: The presence of PAF binding sites in human myometrium and its role in uterine contraction. Am J Obstet Gynecol 166:1222, 1992

CHAPTER 13
Mechanism of Normal Labor in Occiput Presentation

The fetus is in the occiput or vertex presentation in approximately 95 percent of all labors. The fetal presentation is most commonly ascertained by abdominal palpation and confirmed by vaginal examination sometime before or at the onset of labor. In the majority of cases, the vertex enters the pelvis with the sagittal suture in the transverse pelvic diameter (Caldwell and associates, 1934).

Diagnosis of Occiput Presentation

Occiput Transverse Positions. For diagnosis by abdominal examination, the four maneuvers of Leopold are employed (see Fig. 10–10). The fetus enters the pelvis in the left occiput transverse (LOT) position in 40 percent of all labors, compared with 20 percent in the right occiput transverse (ROT) position (Caldwell and associates, 1934). The following findings are obtained for the LOT position by abdominal examination (Fig. 10–10):

- *First maneuver:* Fundus occupied by the breech.
- *Second maneuver:* Resistant plane of the back felt directly to the examiner's right, readily palpated through the mother's left flank.
- *Third maneuver:* Negative if the head is engaged (biparietal diameter through the pelvic inlet); otherwise, the movable head is detected at or above the pelvic inlet.
- *Fourth maneuver:* Negative if head is engaged; otherwise, cephalic prominence on the maternal right side.

In the ROT position, palpation yields similar information (see Fig. 10–6B), except that the fetal back is in the mother's right flank and the small parts and cephalic prominence are on the left. On vaginal examination the sagittal suture occupies the transverse diameter of the pelvis more or less midway between the sacrum and the symphysis. In LOT positions, the smaller posterior fontanel is to the left in the maternal pelvis and the larger anterior fontanel is directed to the opposite side. In ROT positions, the reverse holds true. The fetal heart in right and left positions is usually heard in the right and left flank, respectively, at or slightly below the level of the umbilicus.

Occiput Anterior Positions. In occiput anterior positions (LOA or ROA), the head either enters the pelvis with the occiput rotated 45 degrees anteriorly from the transverse position, or subsequently does so. *This degree of anterior rotation produces only slight differences on abdominal examination* (see Figs. 10–5A and 10–6C). The mechanism of labor usually is very similar to that in occiput transverse positions.

Occiput Posterior Positions. The incidence of occiput posterior positions when the fetus first enters the pelvis is approximately 20 percent. The right occiput posterior (ROP) is slightly more common than the left (LOP) (Caldwell and associates, 1934). It appears likely from evidence obtained from radiographic studies that posterior positions are more often associated with a narrow forepelvis.

On vaginal or rectal examination in the ROP position, the sagittal suture occupies the right oblique diameter, the small fontanel is felt opposite the right maternal sacroiliac synchondrosis, and the large fontanel is directed toward the left iliopectineal eminence (see Fig. 10–6A). In the LOP position the reverse is true (see Fig. 10-5B). In many cases, particularly in the early part of labor, because of imperfect flexion of the head, the larger anterior fontanel lies at a lower level than in anterior positions and is felt more readily.

Cardinal Movements of a Labor in Occiput Presentation

Because of the irregular shape of the pelvic canal and the relatively large dimensions of the mature fetal head, it is evident that not all diameters of the head necessarily can pass through all diameters of the pelvis. It follows that a process of adaptation or accommodation of suitable portions of the head to the various segments of the pelvis is required for completion of childbirth. These positional changes in the presenting part constitute the mechanisms of labor. *The cardinal movements of labor are engagement, descent, flexion, internal rotation, extension, external rotation, and expulsion.* These movements are illustrated in Figure 13–1.

For purposes of instruction, the various movements often are described as though they occurred separately and independently. In reality the mechanism of labor

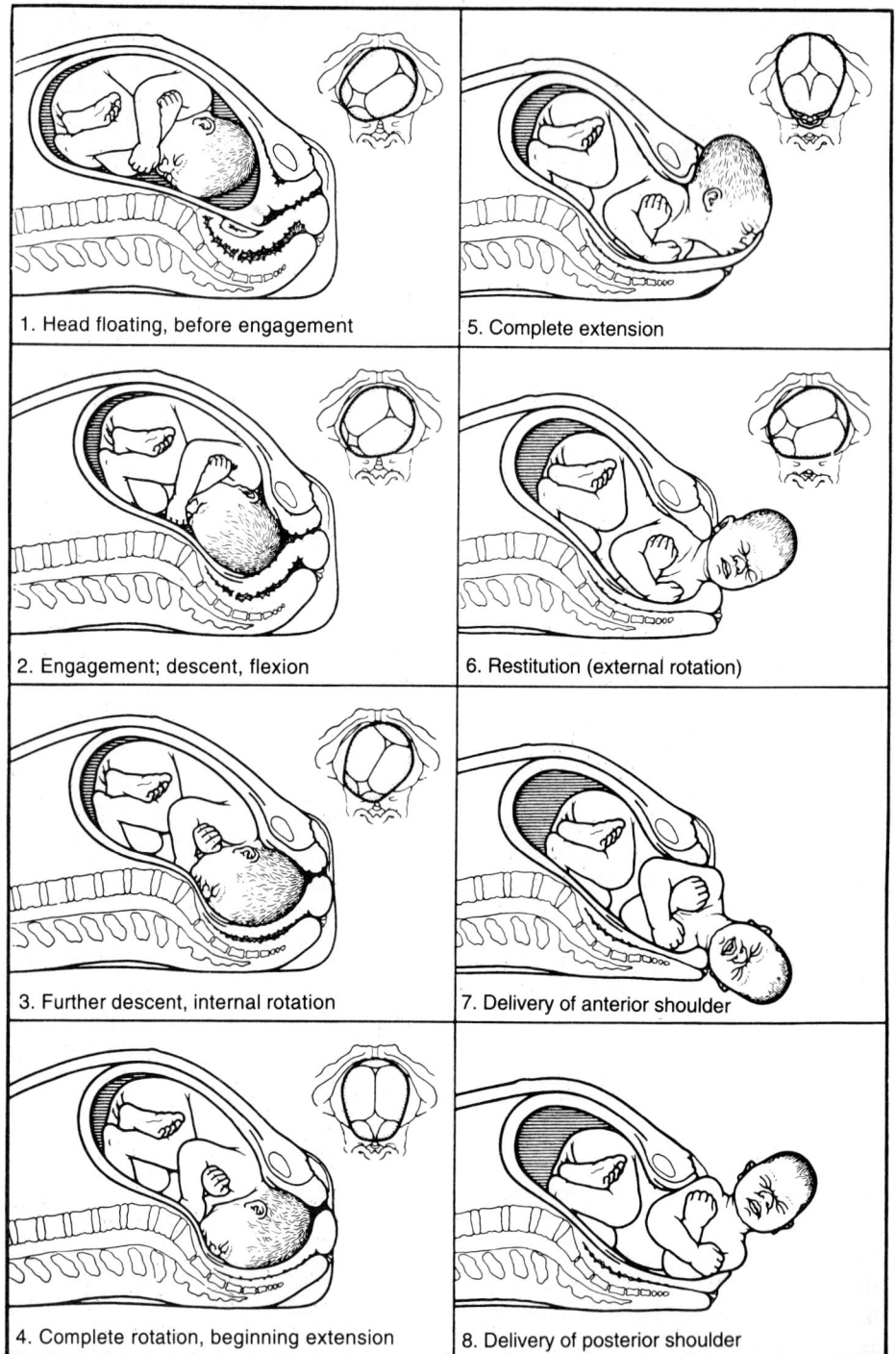

Fig. 13–1. Movements in the mechanism of labor and delivery, left occiput anterior position.

1. Head floating, before engagement

2. Engagement; descent, flexion

3. Further descent, internal rotation

4. Complete rotation, beginning extension

5. Complete extension

6. Restitution (external rotation)

7. Delivery of anterior shoulder

8. Delivery of posterior shoulder

consists of a combination of movements that are ongoing simultaneously. For example, as part of the process of engagement there is both flexion and descent of the head. It is impossible for the movements to be completed unless the presenting part descends simultaneously. Concomitantly, the uterine contractions effect important modifications in the fetal attitude, or habitus, especially after the head has descended into the pelvis. These changes consist principally of a straightening of the fetus, with loss of dorsal convexity and closer application of the extremities to the body. As a result, the fetal ovoid is transformed into a cylinder, with normally the smallest possible cross section passing through the birth canal.

Engagement. As discussed in Chapter 11 (p. 289), the mechanism by which the biparietal diameter, the greatest transverse diameter of the fetal head in occiput pre-

Anterior asynclitism
Naegele's obliquity

Normal synclitism

Posterior asynclitism
Litzmann's obliquity
Ear presentation

Anterior
parietal

Sagittal
suture

Occipito-
frontal plane
Pelvic inlet
plane

Posterior
parietal

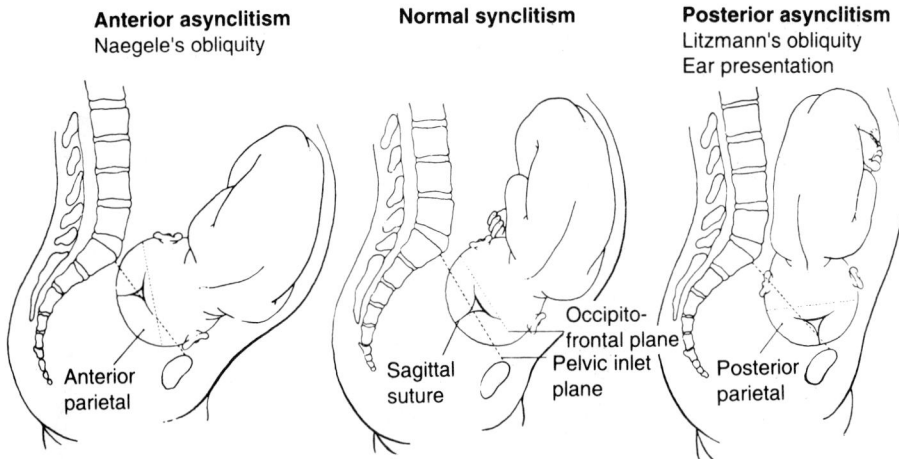

Fig. 13–2. Synclitism and asynclitism.

sentations, passes through the pelvic inlet is designated *engagement*. This phenomenon may take place during the last few weeks of pregnancy, or it may not occur until after the commencement of labor. In many multiparous and some nulliparous women, at the onset of labor the fetal head is freely movable above the pelvic inlet. In this circumstance, the head is sometimes referred to as "floating." A normal-sized head usually does not engage with its sagittal suture directed anteroposteriorly. Instead, the fetal head usually enters the pelvic inlet either in the transverse diameter or in one of the oblique diameters (Caldwell and colleagues, 1934).

Asynclitism. Although the fetal head tends to accommodate to the transverse axis of the pelvic inlet, the sagittal suture, while remaining parallel to that axis, may not lie exactly midway between the symphysis and sacral promontory. The sagittal suture frequently is deflected either posteriorly toward the promontory or anteriorly toward the symphysis (Fig. 13–2). Such lateral deflection of the head to a more anterior or posterior position in the pelvis is called *asynclitism*. If the sagittal suture approaches the sacral promontory, more of the anterior parietal bone presents itself to the examining fingers, and the condition is called *anterior asynclitism*. If, however, the sagittal suture lies close to the symphysis, more of the posterior parietal bone will present, and the condition is called *posterior asynclitism*. Moderate degrees of asynclitism are the rule in normal labor, but if severe, the asynclitism may lead to cephalopelvic disproportion even with an otherwise normal-sized pelvis. Successive changes from posterior to anterior asynclitism facilitate descent by allowing the fetal head to take advantage of the roomiest areas of the pelvic cavity.

Descent. The first requisite for birth of the infant is descent. With the nulliparous woman, engagement may occur before the onset of labor, and further descent may occur before the onset of labor, and further descent may

not follow necessarily until the onset of the second stage of labor. In multiparous women descent usually begins with engagement. Descent is brought about by one or more of four forces: (1) pressure of the amnionic fluid, (2) direct pressure of the fundus upon the breech, (3) contraction of the abdominal muscles, and (4) extension and straightening of the fetal body.

Flexion. As soon as the descending head meets resistance, whether from the cervix, walls of the pelvis, or pelvic floor, flexion of the head normally results. In this movement, the chin is brought into more intimate contact with the fetal thorax, and the appreciably shorter suboccipitobregmatic diameter is substituted for the longer occipitofrontal diameter (Figs. 13–3 and 13–4).

Internal Rotation. Internal rotation is a turning of the head in such a manner that the occiput gradually moves

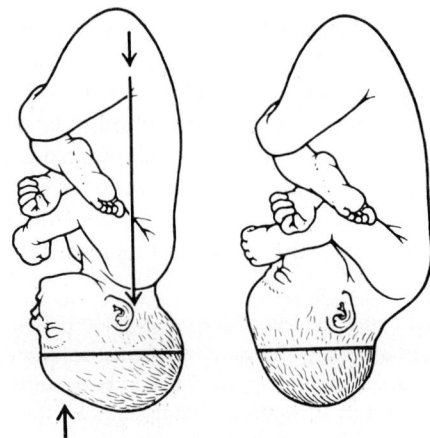

Fig. 13–3. Lever action producing flexion of the head; conversion from occipitofrontal to suboccipitobregmatic diameter typically reduces the anteroposterior diameter from nearly 12 to 9.5 cm.

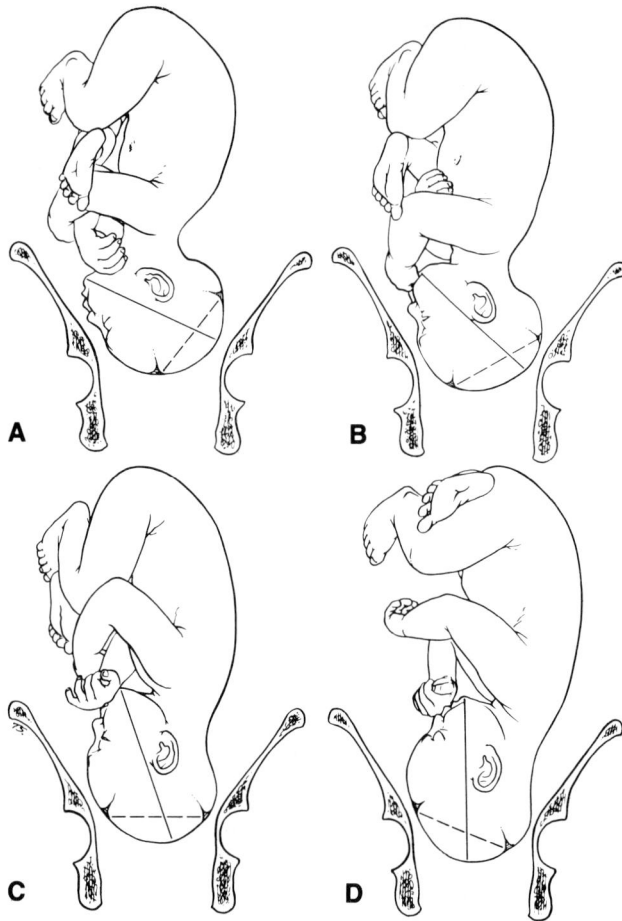

Fig. 13–4. Four degrees of head flexion. Indicated by the solid line is the occipitomental diameter; the broken line connects the center of the anterior fontanel with the posterior fontanel: **A.** Flexion poor. **B.** Flexion moderate. **C.** Flexion advanced. **D.** Flexion complete. Note that with flexion complete, the chin is on the chest and the suboccipitobregmatic diameter, the shortest anteroposterior diameter of the fetal head, is passing through the pelvic inlet. (Modified from Rydberg, 1954.)

from its original position anteriorly toward the symphysis pubis or, less commonly, posteriorly toward the hollow of the sacrum (Figs. 13–5 to 13–7). Internal rotation is essential for the completion of labor, except when the fetus is unusually small. Internal rotation, which always is associated with descent of the presenting part, is usually not accomplished until the head has reached the level of the spines and therefore is engaged.

Calkins (1939) studied more than 5000 patients in labor to ascertain the time of internal rotation. He concluded that in approximately two thirds of women, internal rotation is completed by the time the head reaches the pelvic floor; in about one fourth, internal rotation is completed very shortly after the head reaches the pelvic floor; and in about

5 percent, anterior rotation does not take place. When rotation fails to occur until the head reaches the pelvic floor, it takes place during the next one or two contractions in multiparas, and in nulliparas during the next three to five. Rotation before the head reaches the pelvic floor is more frequent in multiparas than in nulliparas, according to Calkins.

Extension. When, after internal rotation, the sharply flexed head reaches the vulva, it undergoes another movement that is essential to its birth, namely, extension, which brings the base of the occiput into direct contact with the inferior margin of the symphysis pubis (Fig. 13–6). Because the vulvar outlet is directed upward and forward, extension must occur before the head can pass through it. If the sharply flexed head, on reaching the pelvic floor, did not extend but was driven farther downward, it would impinge upon the posterior portion of the perineum and, if the force from behind were sufficiently strong, would eventually be forced through the tissues of the perineum. When the head presses upon the pelvic gutter, however, two forces come into play. The first, exerted by the uterus, acts more posteriorly, and the second, supplied by the resistant pelvic floor and the symphysis, acts more anteriorly. The resultant force is in the direction of the vulvar opening, thereby causing extension.

With increasing distension of the perineum and vaginal opening, an increasingly larger portion of the occiput gradually appears. The head is born by further extension as the occiput, bregma, forehead, nose, mouth, and finally the chin pass successively over the anterior margin of the perineum. Immediately after its birth, the head drops downward so that the chin lies over the maternal anal region.

External Rotation. The delivered head next undergoes restitution. If the occiput was originally directed toward the left, it rotates toward the left ischial tuberosity; if it was originally directed toward the right, the occiput rotates to the right. The return of the head to the oblique position (restitution) is followed by completion of external rotation to the transverse position, a movement that corresponds to rotation of the fetal body, serving to bring its bisacromial diameter into relation with the anteroposterior diameter of the pelvic outlet. Thus, one shoulder is anterior behind the symphysis and the other is posterior. This movement is apparently brought about by the same pelvic factors that produced internal rotation of the head.

Expulsion. Almost immediately after external rotation, the anterior shoulder appears under the symphysis pubis, and the perineum soon becomes distended by the posterior shoulder. After delivery of the shoulders, the rest of the body is quickly extruded.

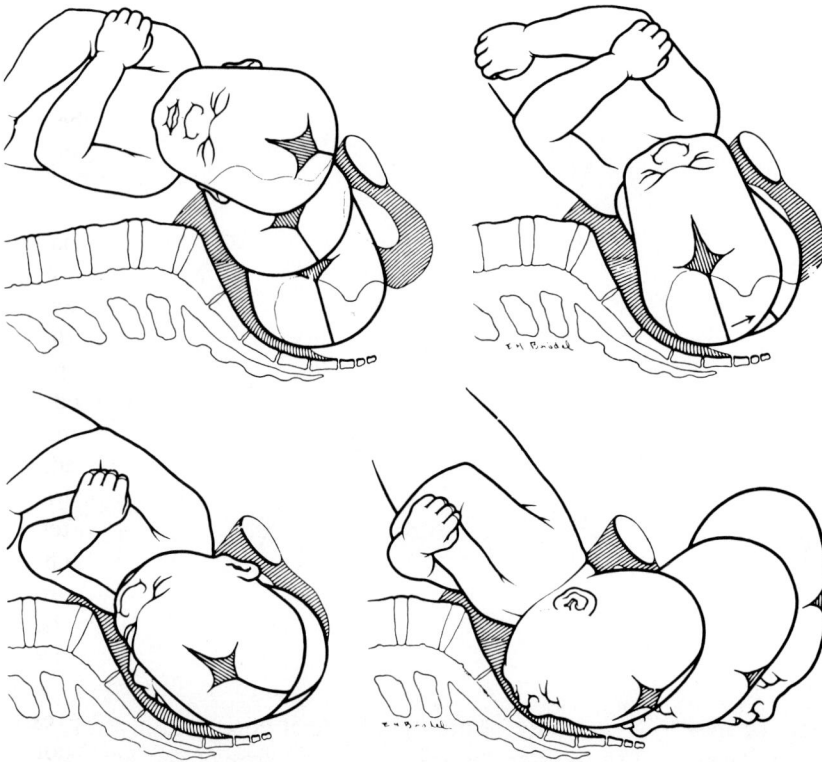

Fig. 13–5. Mechanism of labor for the left occiput transverse position, lateral view. Anterior asynclitism at the pelvic brim followed by lateral flexion, resulting in posterior asynclitism after engagement, further descent, rotation, and extension. (From Steele and Javert, 1942.)

Labor in Occiput Posterior Positions. In the great majority of labors in the occiput posterior positions, the mechanism of labor is identical to that observed in the transverse and anterior varieties, except that the occiput has to rotate to the symphysis pubis through 135 degrees, instead of 90 and 45 degrees, respectively (Fig. 13–7).

With effective contractions, adequate flexion of the head, and a fetus of average size, the great majority of posteriorly positioned occiputs rotate promptly as soon as they reach the pelvic floor, and labor is not lengthened appreciably. In perhaps 5 to 10 percent of cases, however, these favorable circumstances do not occur. For example, with poor contractions, faulty flexion of

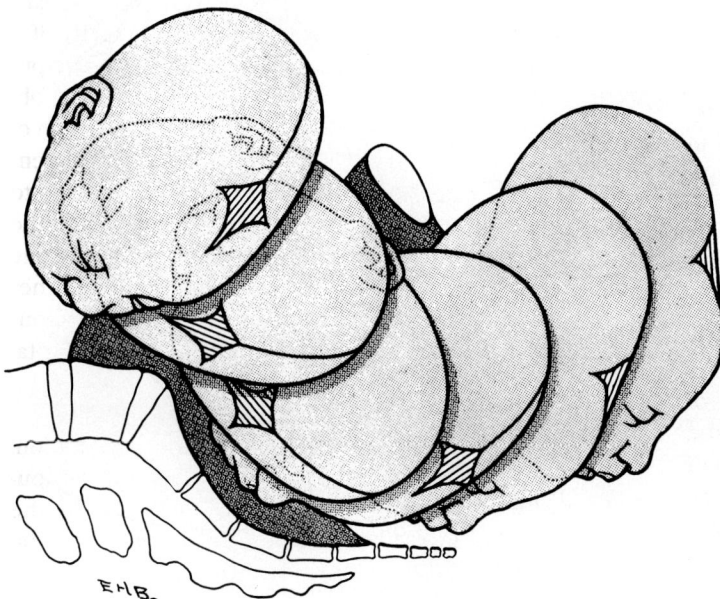

Fig. 13–6. Mechanism of labor for left occiput anterior position.

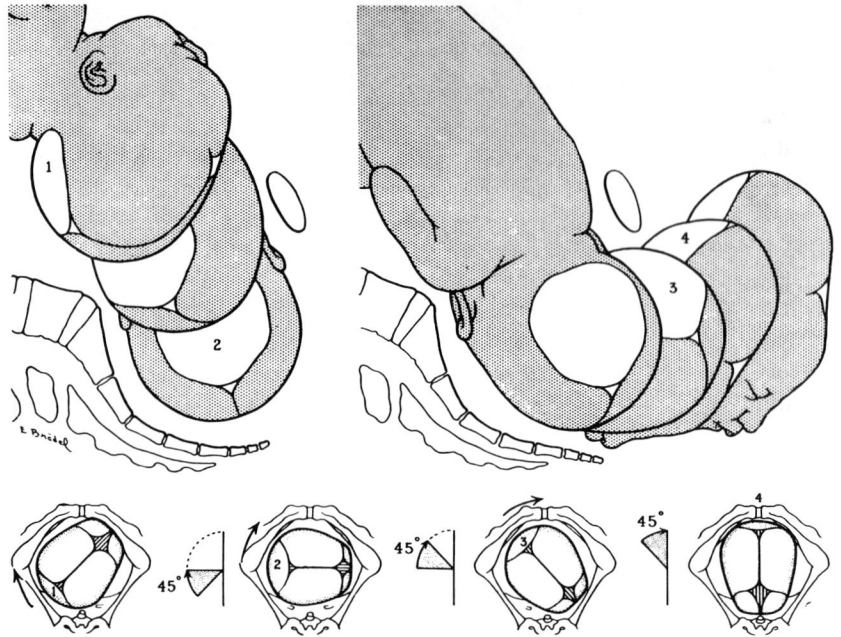

Fig. 13–7. Mechanism of labor for right occiput posterior position, anterior rotation.

the head, or both, rotation may be incomplete or may not take place at all, especially if the fetus is large. Epidural analgesia, which diminishes abdominal muscular pushing as well as relaxing the muscles of the pelvic floor, also predisposes to incomplete rotation (see Chap. 16, p. 438). If rotation is incomplete, *transverse arrest* results. If rotation toward the symphysis does not take place, the occiput usually rotates to the direct occiput posterior position, a condition known as *persistent occiput posterior*. Both transverse arrest and persistent occiput posterior represent deviations from the normal mechanisms of labor and are considered further in Chapter 20.

Changes in the Shape of the Fetal Head

Caput Succedaneum. In vertex presentations the fetal head undergoes important characteristic changes in shape as the result of the pressures to which it is subjected during labor. In prolonged labors before complete dilatation of the cervix, the portion of the fetal scalp immediately over the cervical os becomes edematous, forming a swelling known as the *caput succedaneum* (Fig. 13–8). It usually attains a thickness of only a few millimeters, but in prolonged labors it may be sufficiently extensive to prevent the differentiation of the various sutures and fontanels. More commonly the caput is formed when the head is in the lower portion of the birth canal and frequently only after the resistance of a rigid vaginal outlet is encountered. Because it occurs over the most dependent portion of the head, in LOT position it is found over the upper and posterior

extremity of the right parietal bone, and in ROT positions over the corresponding area of the left parietal bone. It follows that after labor the original position often may be ascertained by noting the location of the caput succedaneum.

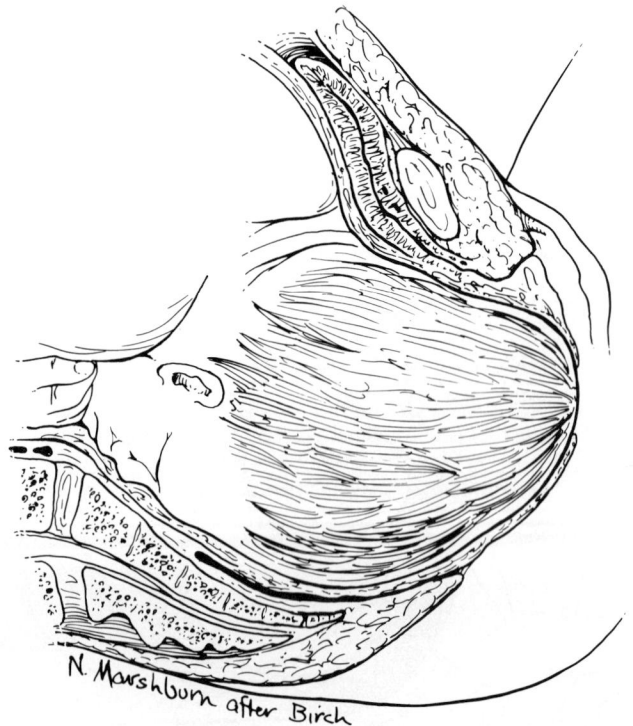

Fig. 13–8. Formation of caput succedaneum.

Molding. Of considerable importance is the degree of molding that the head undergoes. Because the various bones of the skull are not firmly united, movement may occur at the sutures. Ordinarily the margins of the occipital bone, and more rarely those of the frontal bone, are pushed under those of the parietal bones. In many cases one parietal bone may overlap the other, the anterior parietal usually overlapping the posterior. These changes are of greatest importance in contracted pelves, when the degree to which the head is capable of molding may make the difference between successful vaginal delivery and a major obstetrical operation. Molding may account for a diminution in biparietal and suboccipito-bregmatic diameters of 0.5 to 1.0 cm, or even more in prolonged labors.

References

Caldwell WE, Moloy HC, D'Esopo DA: A roentgenologic study of the mechanism of engagement of the fetal head. Am J Obstet Gynecol 28:824, 1934

Calkins LA: The etiology of occiput presentations. Am J Obstet Gynecol 37:618, 1939

Rydberg S: The Mechanism of Labour. Springfield, IL: Thomas, 1954

Steele KB, Javert CT: The mechanism of labor for transverse positions of the vertex. Surg Gynecol Obstet 75:477, 1942

CHAPTER 14
Conduct of Normal Labor and Delivery

Psychological Considerations

Most pregnant women have two major fears: "Will my baby be all right?" and "Will labor and delivery be extremely painful?" These concerns should also be uppermost in the minds of everyone who participates in caring for the mother and her fetus. All things possible should be done to make "yes" the answer to the first question, and "no" to the second.

Is labor easy because a woman is calm, or is she calm because her labor is easy? Is a woman in pain and frightened because her labor is difficult, or is her labor difficult and painful because she is frightened? After scrutinizing many cases, the late British obstetrician Read concluded: *"Fear is in some way the chief pain-producing agent in otherwise normal labor."*

It is not an easy task to dispel the age-old fear of pain during labor and delivery; but from the first prenatal visit, a conscious effort should be made on the part of all persons involved to emphasize that labor and delivery are normal physiological processes. These professionals must demonstrate competence and also instill confidence that they are the woman and her baby's friend and advocate, sincerely desirous of sparing her all possible pain within the limits of safety. Physicians, nurses, and students should note especially that the morale of a woman in labor may sometimes be destroyed by careless remarks or actions. Casual comments outside the labor room are often overheard by her and misinterpreted. Laughter is frequently interpreted as directed toward her.

Physiological Childbirth. To eliminate the harmful influence of fear in labor, there has developed a school of thought that emphasizes the advantages of "natural childbirth" or "physiological childbirth." This concept entails antepartum education that emphasizes elimination of fear, exercises to promote relaxation, muscle and breathing control, and adroit management throughout labor by constant attendance of a professional skilled in reassurance of the mother.

Cook (1982), in his monograph on natural childbirth, emphasized that the natural order results in very high maternal, fetal, and neonatal death rates and uncounted forms of morbidity. He stressed that it was medical intervention in this *natural process* that resulted in the dramatic drop in maternal and perinatal mortality. He supported many of the natural childbirth movement's goals of education, husbands in the delivery room, breast feeding, and limitation of unnecessary sedation and analgesia; but he also frankly discussed the risks to both gravida and fetus of placing the desire for a *meaningful experience* before the needs of the fetus-infant. He concluded that as long as the *outcome* of childbirth is not subjugated to the *experience*, these features should be incorporated into patient care.

Most proponents of physiological childbirth have never claimed that labor can be made devoid of pain or that delivery should be conducted without anesthetic aids. With natural childbirth, most women experience some pain, and analgesics and anesthetics are not withheld when they are indicated. Physiological, or psychoprophylactic, childbirth also is considered in Chapter 16, p. 426.

Admittance Procedures

The woman should be urged to report early in labor rather than to procrastinate until delivery is imminent for fear that she might be experiencing false labor. Early admittance to the labor and delivery unit is important, but especially so if during antepartum care the woman, her fetus, or both have been identified as being at risk.

Identification of Labor. **One of the most critical diagnoses in obstetrics is the accurate diagnosis of labor.** If labor is falsely diagnosed, inappropriate interventions to augment labor may be made. Conversely, if labor is not diagnosed, the fetus-infant may be damaged by unexpected complications occurring in sites remote from medical personnel and adequate medical facilities. Although the differential diagnosis between false and true labor is difficult at times, it usually can be made on the basis of the following features.

Contractions of True Labor

- Contractions occur at regular intervals.
- Intervals gradually shorten.
- Intensity gradually increases.
- Discomfort is in back and abdomen.
- Cervix dilates.
- Discomfort is not stopped by sedation.

Contractions of False Labor

- Contractions occur at irregular intervals.
- Intervals remain long.

- Intensity remains unchanged.
- Discomfort is chiefly in lower abdomen.
- Cervix does not dilate.
- Discomfort is usually relieved by sedation.

In those instances when a diagnosis of labor cannot be established with certainty, it often is wise to observe the woman over a longer period of time. The general condition of mother and fetus should be ascertained accurately by history and physical examination, including blood pressure, temperature, and pulse. The frequency, duration, and intensity of the uterine contractions should be documented and the time established when they first become uncomfortable. The degree of discomfort that the mother displays is noted. The heart rate, presentation, and size of the fetus should be determined and documented on admission. **The fetal heart rate should be checked, especially at the end of a contraction and immediately thereafter, to identify pathological slowing of the heart rate** (Chap. 15, p. 375). Inquiries are made about the status of the fetal membranes and whether there has been any vaginal bleeding. The questions of whether fluid has leaked from the vagina and, if so, how much and when the leakage first commenced, are also addressed (American College of Obstetricians and Gynecologists, 1992).

Electronic Admission Testing. Some authorities recommend that a nonstress test (NST) or contraction stress test (CST) be performed on all patients admitted to the labor and delivery unit, the so-called "admission test" (Ingemarsson and associates, 1986). Such fetal surveillance is in reality an assessment of fetal heart rate accelerations or lack of the same with fetal movement (NST); or an assessment of fetal heart rate before, during, and following a uterine contraction if the patient is in labor (CST) (Freeman and colleagues, 1991) (also see Chap. 15). Fetal heart rate variability and variable decelerations also are used in these evaluations (Ingemarsson and colleagues, 1986, 1988). It is alleged that such tests of fetal well-being, alone or in combination with fetal acoustic stimulation, will identify unsuspected cases of fetal jeopardy (Ingemarsson and associates, 1988; Sarno and co-workers, 1990). This assertion remains to be proven, but the added costs of such procedures are self-evident. If the woman is to be discharged from the labor unit undelivered, however, this practice may be justified to ensure, as nearly as possible, that fetal compromise could not be identified at this time.

Admittance Vaginal Examination. Most often, *unless there has been bleeding in excess of bloody show,* a vaginal examination under aseptic conditions is performed as described below. Careful attention to the following items is essential in order to obtain the greatest amount of information and to minimize bacterial contamination from multiple examinations.

1. *Amnionic fluid.* If there is a question of membrane rupture, the vulva and vaginal introitus are cleansed, a sterile speculum is carefully inserted, and fluid is sought in the posterior vaginal fornix. Any fluid is observed for vernix or meconium; if the source of the fluid remains in doubt, it is collected on a swab for further study, as described below.
2. *Cervix.* Softness, degree of effacement (length), extent of dilatation, and location of the cervix with respect to the presenting part and vagina are ascertained, as described below. The presence of membranes with or without amnionic fluid below the presenting part often can be felt by careful palpation. The fetal membranes often can be visualized if they are intact and the cervix is dilated somewhat.
3. *Presenting part.* The nature of the presenting part should be positively determined and, ideally, its position as well, as described in Chapter 10 (p. 278).
4. *Station.* The degree of descent of the presenting part into the birth canal is identified as described below; and if the fetal head is high in the pelvis (above the level of the ischial spines), the effect of firm fundal pressure on descent of the fetal head is tested.
5. *Pelvic architecture.* The diagonal conjugate, ischial spines, pelvic sidewalls, and sacrum are reevaluated for adequacy (see Chapt. 11, p. 288).

Cervical Effacement. The degree of cervical effacement is usually expressed in terms of the length of the cervical canal compared to that of an uneffaced cervix (see Chap. 12, p. 344). When the length of the cervix is reduced by one half, it is 50 percent effaced; when the cervix becomes as thin as the adjacent lower uterine segment, it is completely, or 100 percent, effaced.

Cervical Dilatation. The amount of cervical dilatation is ascertained by estimating the average diameter of the cervical opening. The examining finger is swept from the margin of the cervix on one side to the opposite side, and the diameter traversed is expressed in centimeters. The cervix is said to be dilated fully when the diameter measures 10 cm, because the presenting part of a term-size infant usually can pass through a cervix this widely dilated (see Chap. 12, p. 344).

Position of the Cervix. The relationship of the cervical os to the fetal head is categorized as posterior, midposition, or anterior. A posterior position is suggestive of preterm labor.

Station. The level of the presenting fetal part in the birth canal is described in relationship to the ischial spines, which are halfway between the pelvic inlet and the pelvic outlet. When the lowermost portion of the presenting fetal part is at the level of the ischial spines, it is designated as being at zero (0) station. In the past, the long axis of the birth canal above the ischial spines has been arbitrarily divided into thirds. That is, if the presenting part is at the level of the pelvic inlet, it is at −3 station; if it has descended one third the distance from the pelvic inlet to the ischial spines, it is at −2 station; if it has reached a level two thirds the distance from the inlet to the spines, it is at −1 station.

The long axis of the birth canal between the level of the ischial spines and the outlet of the pelvis has been similarly divided into thirds. If the level of the presenting part in the birth canal is one third or two thirds the distance between the ischial spines and the pelvic outlet, it is at +1 or +2 station, respectively. When the presenting fetal part reaches the perineum, its station is +3.

Friedman (1978) recommended that the stations above and below the ischial spines be divided into fifths, supposedly to more accurately represent the centimeters above and below the spines. Thus, as the presenting fetal part descends from the inlet toward the ischial spines, the designation is −5, −4, −3, −2, −1, then 0 station. Below the ischial spines, the presenting fetal part passes +1, +2, +3, +4, and +5 stations to delivery.

This degree of accuracy (in centimeters) is likely impossible to achieve clinically. Nevertheless, in view of its increasing use and in order to avoid confusion between the "thirds" and "fifths" systems, it seems reasonable for the practitioner to identify their preferred system using the following designations. The system used should be the denominator and the station the numerator. Thus for the "fifths" system, the stations would be designated −5/5, −4/5, −3/5, −2/5, −1/5, 0, +1/5, +2/5, +3/5, +4/5, +5/5. For, the "thirds" system the stations would be −3/3, −2/3, −1/3, 0, +1/3, +2/3, +3/3.

If the vertex is at 0 station or below, most often engagement of the head has occurred; that is, the biparietal plane of the fetal head has passed through the pelvic inlet. **If the head is unusually molded, or if there is an extensive caput formation, or both, engagement might not have taken place even though the vertex is at 0 station or even lower.** Progressive cervical dilatation with no change in the station of the presenting part, in a woman of low parity, implies fetopelvic disproportion.

Detection of Ruptured Membranes. The pregnant woman should be instructed during the antepartum period to be aware of leakage of fluid from the vagina and to report such an occurrence promptly. Rupture of the membranes is significant for three reasons. First, if the presenting part is not fixed in the pelvis, the possibility

of prolapse of the umbilical cord and cord compression is greatly increased. Second, labor is likely to occur soon if the pregnancy is at or near term. Third, if delivery is delayed for 24 hours or more after membrane rupture, there is likelihood of serious intrauterine infection.

A firm diagnosis of rupture of the membranes is not always easy to make unless amnionic fluid is seen or felt escaping from the cervical os by the examiner. Although several diagnostic tests for the detection of ruptured membranes have been recommended, none is completely reliable. Perhaps the most widely employed procedure involves testing the acidity or alkalinity of the vaginal fluid. The basis for this test is the fact that the pH of vaginal secretions normally ranges between 4.5 and 5.5, whereas that of the amnionic fluid is usually 7.0 to 7.5.

Nitrazine Test. The use of the indicator nitrazine for the diagnosis of ruptured membranes, first suggested by Baptisi (1938), is a simple and fairly reliable method. Test papers are impregnated with the dye, and the color of the reaction is interpreted by comparison with a standard color chart. The pH of the vaginal secretion is estimated by inserting a sterile cotton-tipped applicator deeply into the vagina and then touching it to a strip of the nitrazine paper and comparing the color of the paper with the chart supplied with the paper. A pH above 6.5 is consistent with ruptured membranes.

Baptisi (1938) emphasized that a false reading is likely to be encountered in women with intact membranes who have an unusually large amount of bloody show, because blood, like amnionic fluid, is not acidic. A more extended study of the nitrazine test by a slightly different technique was made by Abe (1940), who reported the nitrazine test to be correct in 98.9 percent of women with known membrane rupture, and in 96.2 percent of women with intact membranes. In clinical practice, however, these tests will not yield such accurate results, because they are used in questionable cases in which the amount of fluid is small and therefore more susceptible to a change in pH by admixed blood and vaginal secretions.

Other tests have been used as markers for rupture of the membranes. Several have achieved transient popularity, including (1) cervical mucus ferning due to the high estrogen content in the amnionic fluid bathing the cervical mucus (Gorodeski and associates, 1979); (2) nile blue sulfate staining of fetal squamous cells in the suspected amnionic fluid (Gorodeski and co-workers, 1979); (3) identification of high values of glucose, fructose, prolactin, alphafetoprotein, or diamine oxidase in the suspected amnionic fluid (Friedman, 1969; Gorodeski, 1979; Hjertberg, 1987; Smith, 1976; Wishart, 1979; and all their colleagues); and (4) injection of various dyes, including Evans blue, methylene blue, and flouorescan, into the amnionic sac via abdominal amniocentesis when the diagnosis is uncertain (Atlay and

Sutherst, 1970; Cowett and associates, 1976; Smith, 1976). It must be noted that these invasive procedures are not without the risk of rupture of the membranes, fetal trauma, infection, and possibly even adverse effects from the dyes. Finally, there may be extra-ovular injection or leakage of the dye, which may result in false-positive or false-negative tests depending upon when and if the dye reaches the cervical os. Unfortunately, none of these tests or procedures has proven to be more practical then the nitrazine test.

Other Admittance Procedures

Vital Signs and Review of Pregnancy Record. The maternal blood pressure, temperature, pulse, and respiratory rate are checked for any abnormality, and these are recorded. The pregnancy record is promptly reviewed to identify complications. Any problems identified during the antepartum period, as well as any that were anticipated, should be displayed prominently in the pregnancy record.

Preparation of Vulva and Perineum. The woman is placed on a bedpan with her legs widely separated. While washing the region, the attendant holds a sponge to the woman's introitus to prevent wash water from running into the vagina. Scrubbing is directed from above downward and away from the introitus. Attention should be paid to careful cleansing of the vulvar folds during this procedure. As the scrub sponge passes over

the anal region, it is discarded. In many hospitals the hair on the lower half of the vulva and the perineum is removed either by shaving or clipping.

Vaginal Versus Rectal Examinations. Ideally, after the vulvar and perineal regions have been properly prepared, and the examiner has donned sterile gloves, the thumb and forefinger of one hand are used to separate the labia widely to expose the vaginal opening and prevent the examining fingers from coming in contact with the inner surfaces of the labia. The index and second fingers of the other hand are then introduced into the vagina (Fig. 14-1). During vaginal examination, a precise routine of evaluation, as described under "Admittance Vaginal Examination" earlier in the chapter, should be followed. It is important to avoid the anal region and be sure not to withdraw the fingers from the vagina until the examination is completed.

A vaginal examination, *properly performed with appropriate preparation and care,* is probably not much more likely than a rectal examination to carry pathogenic bacteria through the dilating cervix into the uterus. The number of vaginal examinations during labor, however, do correlate with morbidity, especially in cases of early membrane rupture.

Enema. Early in labor, a cleansing enema usually is given to minimize subsequent contamination by feces, which otherwise may be a problem, especially during delivery. A ready-to-use enema solution of sodium phos-

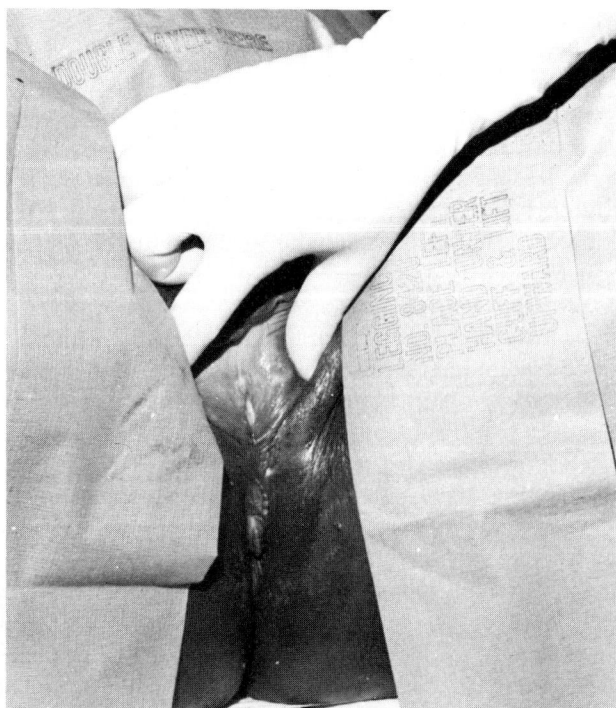 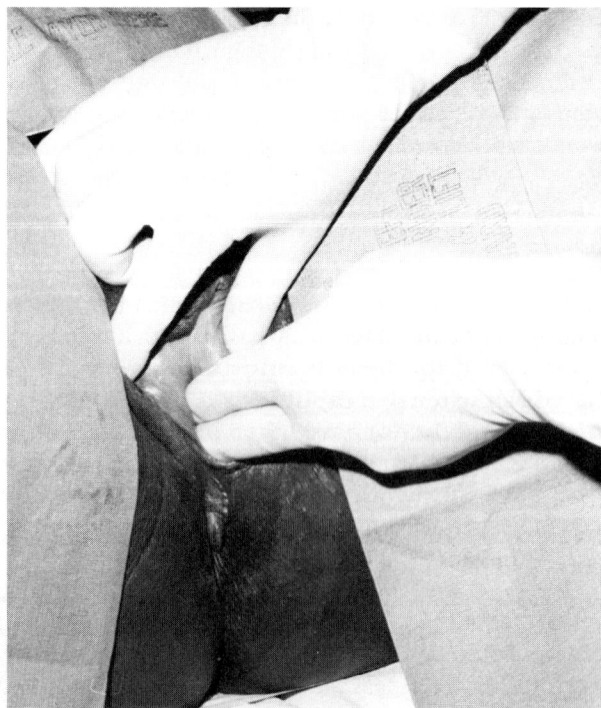

A   **B**

Fig. 14–1. A. Vaginal examination. The labia are separated with a sterile gloved hand. **B.** Vaginal examination. The first and second fingers of the other sterile gloved hand are carefully inserted through the introitus.

phates in a disposable container (Fleet enema) has proven satisfactory in many hospitals.

Laboratory. When the woman is admitted in labor, most often the hematocrit, or hemoglobin concentration, should be rechecked. The hematocrit can be measured easily and quickly. Blood may be collected in a plain tube from which a heparinized capillary tube is filled immediately. By employing a small microhematocrit centrifuge in the labor-delivery unit, the value can be obtained in 3 minutes. A labeled tube of blood is allowed to clot and is kept on hand for blood group and screen, if needed, and another is used for routine serology. In some units, a voided urine specimen, as free as possible of debris, is examined for protein and glucose. We obtain a urine specimen for protein analysis only in hypertensive women. Patients who have had no prenatal care should be considered to be at risk for syphilis, hepatitis B, and human immunodeficiency virus (HIV) (American College of Obstetricians and Gynecologists, 1992). In unregistered patients, these laboratory studies as well as a blood type, Rh, and antibody screen for atypical antibodies should be performed, remembering that various restrictions apply to testing for immunodeficiency virus in different states.

Management of First Stage of Labor

As soon as possible after admittance, the remainder of the general physical examination is completed. The physician can reach a conclusion about the normalcy of the pregnancy only when all examinations, including record and laboratory review, are completed. A rational plan for monitoring labor then can be established based on the needs of the fetus and the mother. If no abnormality is identified or suspected, the mother should be reassured. Although the average duration of the first stage of labor in nulliparous women is about 8 hours and in parous women about 5 hours, there are marked individual variations. Any precise statement as to the duration of labor, therefore, is unwise (See Chap. 19, p. 476).

Monitoring Fetal Well-being During Labor. The word *monitor* is currently equated in the minds of some only with continuous electronic recording of the fetal heart rate and intrauterine pressure. The desirability, let alone the necessity, of electronic monitoring for *all* labors certainly has not been established, as will be discussed subsequently. It is mandatory, however, that for a good pregnancy outcome, a well-defined program be established that provides careful surveillance of the well-being of both mother and fetus. All observations must be appropriately recorded. The frequency, intensity, and duration of uterine contractions, and the response of the fetal heart rate to the contractions, are of considerable concern. These features can be promptly evaluated in logical sequence.

Fetal Heart Rate. The fetal heart rate may be identified with a suitable stethoscope or any of a variety of Doppler ultrasonic devices. Changes in the fetal heart rate that most likely are ominous almost always are detectable immediately after a uterine contraction. Therefore, it is imperative that the fetal heart be monitored by auscultation immediately after a contraction. To avoid confusing maternal and fetal heart rates, the maternal pulse should be counted as the fetal heart rate is counted. Otherwise, maternal tachycardia may be misinterpreted as a normal fetal heart rate.

Fetal jeopardy, compromise or distress—that is, loss of fetal well-being—is suspected if the fetal heart rate immediately after a contraction is repeatedly below 120 beats per minute. Fetal jeopardy very likely exists if the rate is heard to be less than 100 per minute, even though there is recovery to a rate in the 120 to 160 range before the next contraction. When decelerations of this magnitude are found after a contraction, the fetus may be in jeopardy, and further labor, if allowed, is best monitored electronically, as described in Chapter 15.

The appropriate frequency of fetal heart rate auscultation is not known. Leveno and associates (1986) reported that in low-risk pregnancies, auscultation at least every 30 minutes resulted in perinatal outcomes similar to those obtained with continuous electronic fetal monitoring. Accordingly, the American College of Obstetricians and Gynecologists (1992) recommends that during the first stage of labor, in the absence of any abnormalities, the fetal heart should be checked immediately after a contraction at least every 30 minutes and then every 15 minutes during the second stage. For women with pregnancies at risk, continuous electronic monitoring may be used with evaluation of the tracing every 15 minutes during the first stage of labor, and every 5 minutes during the second stage. Alternatively, intermittent auscultation may be every 15 minutes during the first stage of labor and every 5 minutes during the second stage. The latter technique is equivalent to continuous electronic fetal heart rate monitoring as long as there is a 1 : 1 nurse to patient ratio (American College of Obstetricians and Gynecologists, 1992).

Uterine Contractions. With the palm of the hand lightly on the uterus, the examiner determines the time of onset of the contraction. The intensity of the contraction is gauged from the degree of firmness the uterus achieves. At the acme of effective contractions, the finger or thumb cannot readily indent the uterus. Next, the time that the contraction disappears is noted. This sequence is repeated in order to evaluate the frequency, duration, and intensity of uterine contractions. It is inappropriate to simply describe ongoing uterine contractions, or labor, as "good." "Good" uterine contractions can be identified only retrospectively—that is, if the contractions produced orderly effacement and dilatation of the cervix with descent of the presenting part followed by uncomplicated delivery of an uncompromised infant.

Attendance in Labor. Ideally, the person who performs these measurements is able to remain with the woman throughout labor to provide psychological support as well as to discern promptly any fetal or maternal abnormalities. Haverkamp and co-workers (1976, 1979) demonstrated that an equally satisfactory outcome for the fetus can be achieved without continuous electronic monitoring of the fetal heart rate, continuous intrauterine pressure recording, and fetal scalp blood pH measurement *if the mother and fetus are closely attended by appropriately trained labor room personnel.*

The concept that universal electronic fetal monitoring will not improve pregnancy outcome was confirmed by Leveno and co-workers (1986) in a prospective comparison of selective versus universal electronic fetal monitoring in 34,995 pregnancies. Pregnancy outcomes in which universal electronic fetal monitoring was used (13,956 of 17,586 women, or 79 percent) were compared to those in which selective electronic monitoring was used when the fetus was judged to be at high risk (6420 of 17,409 women, or 37 percent). Major risk factors included oxytocin stimulation of labor, dysfunctional labor, abnormalities of the fetal heart rate, and meconium-stained amnionic fluid. Perinatal outcomes, as reflected by intrapartum fetal deaths, low Apgar scores, assisted ventilation of the neonates, admissions to the neonatal intensive care unit, and incidence of neonatal seizures, were not significantly different between the two groups (Table 14–1). There was, however, a small but significantly increased incidence of cesarean delivery for fetal distress in low-risk women who were universally monitored (Table 14–2). These authors stressed that many women judged to be at low risk at the onset of labor subsequently were assigned to a high-risk category and thus were electronically monitored. They concluded that clinical monitoring is mandatory for all laboring women, and that this

TABLE 14–1. COMPARISON OF OUTCOMES THAT SUGGESTED FETAL ASPHYXIA IN SELECTIVE VERSUS UNIVERSAL MONITORING

Outcome[a]	Selective Monitoring	Universal Monitoring
Fetuses alive upon admission to labor and delivery	17,410	17,641
Fetal deaths in labor and delivery (≥ 500 g)	25 (1.4/1000)	30 (1.7/1000)
Assisted ventilation of neonate	1259 (7.2%)	1315 (7.5%)
5-minute Apgar score ≤ 5	293 (1.7%)	296 (1.7%)
Neonates admitted to intensive care nursery	428 (2.5%)	460 (2.6%)
Neonates with seizures	45 (2.6/1000)	53 (3.0/1000)

[a] Any differences in outcome between groups is not significant.
Modified from Leveno and co-workers (1986).

TABLE 14–2. MATERNAL AND NEONATAL OUTCOMES WITH SELECTIVE VERSUS UNIVERSAL MONITORING IN 14,618 LOW-RISK PREGNANCIES[a]

Outcome	Selective Monitoring (n = 7330) No. (%)	Universal Monitoring (n = 7288) No. (%)	P Value[b]
Abnormal fetal heart rate	196 (2.7)	551 (7.6)	< 0.01
Cesarean section for fetal distress	28 (0.4)	64 (0.9)	< 0.01
Intrapartum fetal deaths	None	None	NS
Neonatal deaths	5 (0.1)	4 (0.1)	NS
Assisted ventilation of newborn	102 (1.4)	119 (1.6)	NS
5-minute Apgar score ≤ 5	14 (0.2)	18 (0.2)	NS
Admission to intensive care nursery	17 (0.2)	25 (0.3)	NS
Neonates with seizures	3 (0.04)	1 (0.01)	NS

[a] Low risk defined as single fetus in cephalic presentation; spontaneous, uncomplicated labor; and birthweight more than 2500 g.
[b] NS = not significant.
Modified from Leveno and co-workers (1986).

type of "screening" procedure for fetuses considered to be at low risk was as efficacious as universal electronic fetal monitoring.

Given a choice, most women probably would prefer the reassurance of the nearly continuous presence of the obstetrician or a compassionate well-trained obstetrical associate to that of a metal cabinet with its wires and tubes that invade her and her fetus. Because of the ease of operation, the constant threat of legal action, and simply because the trend to continuous electronic fetal monitoring has become almost an accepted reality, it seems highly unlikely that there will be less continuous electronic fetal monitoring. It is important to note that the monitor itself is not a mystical talisman. Electronic monitors are merely extensions of doctors' and nurses' eyes and hands. All information obtained from these electrical devices is of no value unless processed through the human brain in a timely and appropriate fashion. For example, an isolated, ominous-appearing fetal heart rate tracing may have no clinical significance. Alternatively, subsequent contractions may be associated with a picture consistent with a worsening fetal condition. **Simply stated, the physician or nurse must be present to interpret the information gathered from electronic monitors. It is the interpretation and action taken that is the important feature of fetal surveillance during labor, not merely the collection of reams of monitor tracings.** As mentioned above, if continuous electronic fetal heart rate monitoring is used, with or without external or internal uterine contraction monitoring, the tracing should be evaluated at least every 15 minutes during the first stage and every 5 minutes during the second stage of labor in which the fetus is at risk (American College of Obstetricians and Gynecologists, 1992). There is no reason, in most instances, why the machine and health care providers cannot be combined to provide a safe and a compassionate environment for the laboring woman.

Maternal Monitoring and Management During Labor

Maternal Position During Labor. The normal laboring woman need not be confined to bed early in labor prior to use of analgesia. A comfortable chair may be beneficial psychologically and perhaps physiologically. In bed, the laboring woman should be allowed to assume the position she finds most comfortable, which will be lateral recumbency most of the time. She must not be restricted to lying supine.

Subsequent Vaginal Examinations. During the first stage of labor, the need for subsequent vaginal examinations to identify the status of the cervix and the station and position of the presenting part will vary considerably. When the membranes rupture, an examination should be repeated immediately if the fetal head was not definitely engaged at the previous vaginal examination. In any event, the fetal heart rate should be checked immediately and during the next uterine contraction in order to detect an occult umbilical cord compression.

Analgesia. Most often, analgesia is initiated on the basis of the woman's discomfort, a uterine contraction pattern of established labor, and cervical dilatation of at least 2 cm. The kinds of analgesia, amounts, and frequency of administration should be based on the need to allay pain on the one hand and the likelihood of delivering a depressed infant on the other (see Chap. 16, p. 426).

The timing, method of administration, and size of initial and subsequent doses of systemically acting analgesic agents are based to a considerable degree on the anticipated interval of time until delivery. A repeat vaginal examination is often appropriate before administering more analgesia. With the onset of symptoms characteristic of the second stage of labor, that is, an urge to bear down or "push," the status of the cervix and the presenting part should be reevaluated.

Maternal Vital Signs. In our delivery unit, maternal temperature and pulse are evaluated every 1 to 2 hours. If fetal membranes have been ruptured for many hours before the onset of labor, or if there is a borderline temperature elevation, the temperature should be checked hourly. Moreover, with prolonged membrane rupture, the pregnancy should be considered to be at high risk. Blood pressure usually is taken more fre-

quently and is obtained between contractions, because it normally rises during a contraction (Kjeldsen, 1979).

Amniotomy. If the membranes are intact, there is a great temptation even during normal labor to perform amniotomy. The presumed benefits are more rapid labor, earlier detection of instances of meconium staining of amnionic fluid, and the opportunity to apply an electrode to the fetus and insert a pressure catheter into the uterine cavity. Rosen and Peisner (1987) reported that *spontaneous* rupture of the membranes during labor was followed by a shorter duration of labor when compared with *artificial* rupture or no rupture. When membranes were artificially ruptured, there was a slightly shorter labor than recorded with intact membranes. Amniotomy may shorten the length of labor slightly, but there is no evidence that shorter labor is necessarily beneficial to the fetus or to the mother. Indeed, the reverse may be true (Caldeyro-Barcia and associates, 1974). If amniotomy is performed, an aseptic technique should be used. Importantly, the fetal head must not be dislodged from the pelvis to hasten the escape of amnionic fluid; such an action invites prolapse of the umbilical cord.

Oral Intake. In essentially all circumstances, food and oral fluids should be withheld during active labor and delivery. Gastric emptying time is remarkably prolonged once labor is established and analgesics are administered. As a consequence, ingested food and most medications remain in the stomach and are not absorbed; instead, they may be vomited and aspirated (see Chap. 16, p. 429).

Intravenous Fluids. Although it has become customary in many hospitals to establish an intravenous infusion system routinely early in labor, there is seldom any real need for such in the normally pregnant woman at least until analgesia is administered. An intravenous infusion system is advantageous during the immediate puerperium in order to administer oxytocin prophylactically, and at times therapeutically when uterine atony persists. Moreover, with longer labors, the administration of glucose, some sodium, and water to the otherwise fasting woman at the rate of 60 to 120 mL per hour is efficacious to combat dehydration and acidosis.

Urinary Bladder Function. Bladder distension must be avoided, because it can possibly lead to obstructed labor and to subsequent bladder hypotonia and infection. During each abdominal examination, the suprapubic region should be palpated in order to detect a filling bladder. If the bladder is readily palpated above the symphysis, the woman should be encouraged to void. At times she can ambulate with assistance to a toilet and successfully void, even though she could not void on a bedpan. If the bladder is distended and she cannot void, **catheterization** is indicated.

Active Management of Labor. As the cesarean delivery rate began to increase during the 1970s, the Dublin group proposed that their active labor management scheme described as early as 1969 would decrease this trend (O'Driscoll and colleagues, 1984, 1988). Active management, as defined by the Irish investigators, includes artificial amniotomy upon detection of painful uterine contractions accompanied by passage of blood-stained mucus or complete cervical effacement, regardless of dilatation. Afterwards, frequent cervical examinations are made, and oxytocin is given if cervical dilatation does not progress at least 1 cm per hour. Oxytocin is commenced at 6 mU per minute. If necessary, this is increased by 6 mU per minute every 15 minutes, not to exceed 40 mU per minute. Although this plan was associated with a very low cesarean delivery rate in nulliparas (5 percent), the incidence of intrapartum fetal death was increased sevenfold and the incidence of neonatal seizures was increased twofold when compared with contemporaneous obstetrical data from Parkland Hospital (Leveno and colleagues, 1985, 1988).

Iffy and co-workers (1990) also compared American obstetrical practices and results with those described from the National Maternity Hospital. Specifically, they compared the use of cesarean delivery and perinatal outcomes from their Newark hospital for 1983 through 1987 with data from the Dublin hospital. Their analysis included 12,164 Newark deliveries and 37,428 Dublin deliveries. Iffy and colleagues (1990) confirmed results discussed above for Parkland Hospital. Thorp and associates (1988), however, reported no adverse perinatal outcomes with so-called active management using high-dose oxytocin in 612 nulliparas.

More recently, Cahill and colleagues (1992) from the National Maternity Hospital disputed that active management increased perinatal risk. For example, they observed that the incidence of neonatal asphyxial seizures was 2.2 per 1000 with active management compared with 1.3 per 1000 without such management. Although they reported the significance of data was 0.06, reanalysis using the Mantel–Haenszel chi-square test gives a probability of 0.03, thus indicating that active management definitely may have adverse consequences.

Although Turner (1988), Akoury (1988), and their co-workers were able to decrease the primary cesarean delivery rate with similar, but not identical management, Cohen and associates (1987) reported no differences in two populations randomly assigned to routine versus active management. Certainly, if the primary cesarean rate is 30 percent, then we agree with Boylan and Frankowski (1986) that active intervention may be successful in lowering it. Indeed, any *obstetrical* management might be expected to lower such a rate.

The difficulty in trying to access the impact of "active management" on labor is that no single group, including the group at the National Maternity Hospital in Dublin, has consistently used the same methods to effect "active management." For example, the reports by O'Driscoll and colleagues over a 15-year period from 1970 through 1984, are modified by changing factors in each report such as induction versus augmentation of labor. Also, the time to ensure delivery changed from 24 to 12 hours. Nevertheless, the reports from Dublin have been provocative and useful in directing attention to this critically needed area of labor management. This has resulted not only as a consequence of O'Driscoll's reports, but also as a result of investigations cited below.

Boylan and co-workers (Boylan, 1989; Boylan and Parisi, 1990; Boylan and co-workers, 1987; Thorpe and associates, 1988) reported success similar to the Dublin group in employing "active management" of labor. They, however, used different doses of oxytocin and have used and not used oxytocin infusion pumps and electronic fetal heart rate monitoring. Regardless, perinatal outcomes have been similar in all studies, and cord blood gases (Thorpe and associates, 1988) have not been different in actively managed pregnancies versus controls. Unfortunately, the incidence of uterine hyperstimulation was not mentioned in any of the reports by Boylan, O'Driscoll, or Cahill and their associates.

Turner and associates (1988), using a similar approach to the Dublin group, reported a progressive decrease in cesarean deliveries in nulliparas from 14.5 percent in 1981 to 10.8 percent in 1985 using a modified "active management" program that included the use of electronic fetal monitors and prostaglandin gel. They reported no significant increase in perinatal mortality or morbidity during this 5-year period. Lopez-Zeno and co-workers (1992) also reported that using their method of active management reduced cesarean deliveries from 14.1 to 10.5 percent.

Cohen and associates (1987), in a randomized prospective study, used "aggressive management of early labor" versus a control group, and found no differences in mode of delivery, perinatal outcome, or course and duration of labor. The authors noted that their study was *not* designed to replicate the Dublin protocol.

Akoury and co-workers (1988) reduced their cesarean delivery rate from 13 to 4.3 percent ($P < 0.005$) and forceps deliveries from 29 to 19 percent ($P < 0.005$) in actively managed women compared with controls. Perinatal outcome variables were not different between the two groups, and the authors noted no uterine hyperstimulation causing fetal distress. In 1991, however, they reported that oxytocin augmentation of "nonprogressive labor," using the same regimen as reported in 1988, resulted in "uterine hyperstimulation" in 18 percent of "actively managed" women compared with 14 percent hyperstimulation for control patients. The difference was not significant.

Active management of labor is a concept, not merely an oxytocin dose (see Chap. 19, p. 484). At Parkland Hospital, Satin and associates (1992) compared low-dose with high-dose oxytocin to augment or induce labor. No other tenets of active management were employed. The low-dose regimen used in 1251 pregnancies consisted of 1 mU per min with incremental increases at 20-minute intervals up to 8 mU per min, and then incremental increases of 2 mU per min up to 20 mU per min. The high-dose regimen used in 1537 women consisted of 6 mU per min in 20-minute intervals to a maximum dose of 42 mU per min. The high-dose regimen shortened labor by more than 3 hours ($P < 0.0001$), decreased neonatal sepsis from 1.3 to 0.2 percent ($P < 0.01$), and decreased cesarean deliveries for dystocia from 12 to 9 percent ($P < 0.04$). The hyperstimulation rate with high-dose oxytocin was 55 percent compared with 42 percent ($P < 0.0001$) for the low-dose regimen. No adverse fetal effects were observed, but the incidence of cesarean delivery for fetal distress (6 versus 3 percent, $P = 0.05$) was increased in women given the high-dose regimen compared with low-dose oxytocin.

Conclusions. The following conclusions can be drawn. (1) The rate of cesarean delivery in the United States for "failure to progress" or "cephalopelvic disproportion" *probably* is too high. (2) The rate of cesarean delivery for the same reasons at the National Maternity Hospital in Dublin probably is too low to be entirely safe for the fetus. (3) The term "active management of labor" is imprecise even when used by O'Driscoll and colleagues. Indeed, reports of so-called "active management" have excluded and included electronic fetal monitoring, infusion pumps, prostaglandin gel, scalp pH determinations, different doses of oxytocin, and the reporting or nonreporting of the incidence of uterine hyperstimulation using different definitions. Controls have been used in only a few series. Thus, it is *impossible to compare methods and outcomes* between these different reports. (4) The use of higher doses of oxytocin is associated with uterine hyperstimulation in about half of cases, probably resulting in increased cesarean deliveries for fetal distress. (5) The rate of cesarean delivery probably can be lowered in the United States and elsewhere for "failure to progress" and "cephalopelvic disproportion" by accurately diagnosing the onset of labor and by augmenting labor appropriately when necessary.

Management of Second Stage of Labor

Identification. With full dilatation of the cervix, which signifies the onset of the second stage of labor, the woman typically begins to bear down, and with descent of the presenting part she develops the urge to defecate. Uterine contractions and the accompanying expulsive forces may last 1½ minutes and recur at times after a myometrial resting phase of no more than a minute.

Duration. The median duration of the second stage is 50 minutes in nulliparas and 20 minutes in multiparas,

but it can be highly variable. In a woman of higher parity with a stretched vagina and perineum, two or three expulsive efforts after the cervix is fully dilated may suffice to complete the delivery of the infant. Conversely, in a woman with a contracted pelvis or a large fetus, or with impaired expulsive efforts from conduction analgesia or intense sedation, the second stage may become abnormally long.

Fetal Heart Rate. For the low-risk fetus, the heart rate should be auscultated during the second stage of labor at least every 15 minutes, whereas in those at high risk, 5-minute intervals are recommended (American College of Obstetricians and Gynecologists, 1992). Slowing of the fetal heart rate induced by head compression is common during a contraction and the accompanying maternal expulsive efforts. If recovery of the fetal heart rate is prompt after the contraction and expulsive efforts cease, labor is allowed to continue. Not all instances of fetal heart rate slowing during second-stage labor are the consequence of head compression. The vigorous force generated within the uterus by its contraction and by maternal expulsive efforts may reduce placental perfusion appreciably. Descent of the fetus through the birth canal and the consequent reduction in uterine volume may trigger some degree of premature separation of the placenta, with further compromise of fetal well-being. Descent is more likely to tighten a loop or loops of umbilical cord around the fetus, especially the neck, sufficiently to obstruct umbilical blood flow. Prolonged, uninterrupted maternal expulsive efforts can be dangerous to the fetus in these circumstances. Maternal tachycardia, which is common during the second stage, must not be mistaken for a normal fetal heart rate.

Maternal Expulsive Efforts. In most cases, bearing down is reflex and spontaneous during second-stage labor, but occasionally the woman does not employ her expulsive forces to good advantage and coaching is desirable. Her legs should be half-flexed so that she can push with them against the mattress. Instructions should be to take a deep breath as soon as the next uterine contraction begins and, with her breath held, to exert downward pressure exactly as though she were straining at stool. She should not be encouraged to "push" beyond the time of completion of each uterine contraction. Instead, she and her fetus should be allowed to rest and recover from the combined effects of the uterine contraction, breath holding, and considerable physical effort. Gardosi and associates (1989) have recommended a squatting or semi-squatting position using a specialized pillow. They claim that this shortens second-stage labor by increasing expulsive forces and by increasing the diameter of the pelvic outlet.

Usually, bearing down efforts are rewarded by increasing bulging of the perineum—that is, by further descent of the fetal head. The woman should be in-

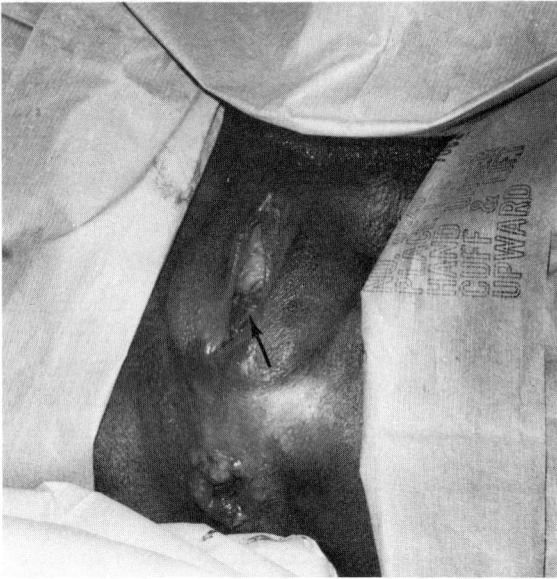

Fig. 14–2. Scalp (*arrow*) appearing at vulva during a contraction.

formed of such progress, for encouragement at this stage is very important. During this period of active bearing down, the fetal heart rate auscultated immediately after the contraction is likely to be slow, but should recover to normal range before the next expulsive effort.

As the head descends through the pelvis, small particles of feces are frequently expelled. As they appear at the anus, they should be sponged downward, away from the vagina, with large pledgets soaked in diluted soap solution. As the head descends still farther, the perineum begins to bulge and the overlying skin becomes tense and glistening. Now the scalp of the fetus may be visible through the vulvar opening (Fig. 14–2). At this time, or before in instances where little perineal resis-

tance to expulsion is anticipated, the woman and her fetus are prepared for delivery.

Preparation for Delivery. Actual delivery of the fetus can be accomplished with the mother in a variety of positions. The most widely used and often the most satisfactory one is the dorsal lithotomy position in order to increase the diameter of the pelvic outlet (Chap. 11, p. 284). In placing the legs in leg-holders, care should be taken not to separate the legs too widely or place one leg higher than the other. The popliteal region should rest comfortably in the proximal portion and the heel in the distal portion of the leg-holder. Too often the leg is forced to conform to the existing setting. Cramps in the legs may develop during the second stage, in part, because of pressure by the fetal head on nerves in the pelvis. Such cramps may be relieved by changing the position of the leg or by brief massage, but leg cramps should never be ignored.

No one should be permitted in the delivery room without a scrub suit, a mask covering both nose and mouth, and a cap that completely covers the hair. Preparation for actual delivery entails thorough vulvar and perineal scrubbing and usually covering with sterile drapes in such a way that only the immediate area about the vulva is exposed (Fig. 14–3).

Scrubbing and Gloving. Because sterile gloves are punctured easily and occasionally tear, the necessity for meticulously cleaning the hands before putting on gloves is apparent. Even with these precautions, the possibility of disseminating bacteria within the genital tract is not eliminated entirely because the organisms may be carried up from the vaginal outlet by the gloved finger. In the past, the major reason for care in scrubbing, gowning, and gloving was to protect the laboring woman from the introduction of infectious agents. Al-

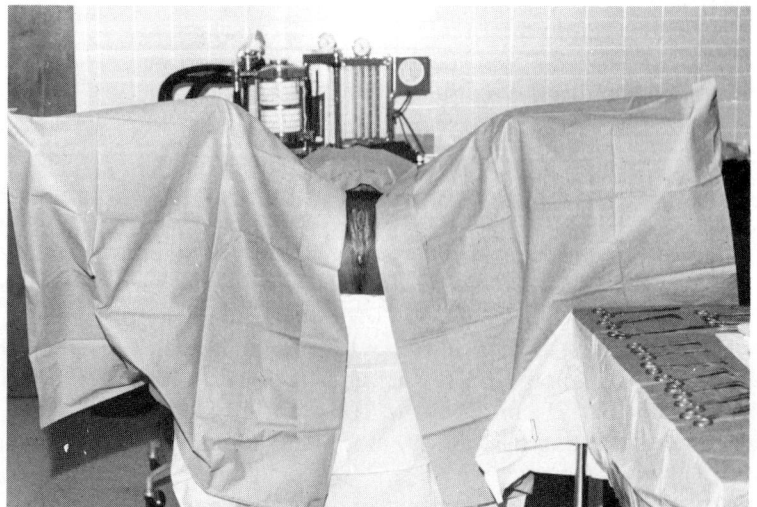

Fig. 14–3. Following thorough scrubbing of the vulva, perineum, and adjacent regions, the field is sterile-draped in preparation for delivery.

though this reason remains valid, concern today also must be extended to the health care providers, because of the threat of exposure to human immunodeficiency virus. Recommendations for protection of those who care for women during labor and delivery are summarized in Chapter 59 (p. 1312).

Spontaneous Delivery

Delivery of the Head. With each contraction, the perineum bulges increasingly and the vulvovaginal opening becomes more dilated by the fetal head (Fig. 14–4), gradually forming an ovoid and finally an almost circular opening. With the cessation of each contraction, the opening becomes smaller as the head recedes. As the head becomes increasingly visible, the vaginal outlet and vulva are stretched further until they ultimately encircle the largest diameter of the baby's head (Fig. 14–5). This encirclement of the largest diameter of the fetal head by the vulvar ring is known as *crowning*.

Unless an episiotomy has been made, as described later in the chapter, the perineum by now is extremely thin and, especially in the case of the nulliparous woman, almost at the point of rupture with each contraction. At the same time, the anus becomes greatly stretched and protuberant, and the anterior wall of the rectum may be easily seen through it. Failure to perform an episiotomy by this time likely invites perineal lacerations.

Ritgen Maneuver. By the time the head distends the vulva and perineum (during a contraction) enough to open the vaginal introitus to a diameter of 5 cm or more, a towel-draped, gloved hand should be used to exert forward pressure on the chin of the fetus through the perineum just in front of the coccyx. At the same time, the other hand exerts pressure superiorly against the occiput (Fig. 14–6). Although this maneuver is simpler than that originally described by Ritgen (1855), it is customarily designated the Ritgen maneuver, or the modified Ritgen maneuver. It allows the physician to control the delivery of the head. It also favors extension, so that the head is delivered with its smallest diameters passing through the introitus and over the perineum (Fig. 14–7). The head is delivered slowly with the base of the occiput rotating around the lower margin of the symphysis pubis as a fulcrum, while the bregma (anterior fontanel), brow, and face pass successively over the perineum (Fig. 14–8).

Clearing the Nasopharynx. To minimize the likelihood of aspiration of amnionic fluid debris and blood that might occur once the thorax is delivered and the infant can inspire, the face is quickly wiped and the nares and mouth are aspirated as demonstrated in Figure 14–9.

Nuchal Cord. Next the finger should be passed to the neck of the fetus to ascertain whether it is encircled by one or more coils of the umbilical cord (Fig. 14–10). Nuchal cords occur in about 25 percent of cases and ordinarily do no harm. If a coil of umbilical cord is felt, it should be drawn down between the fingers and, if loose enough, slipped over the infant's head. If it is applied too tightly to the neck to be slipped over the

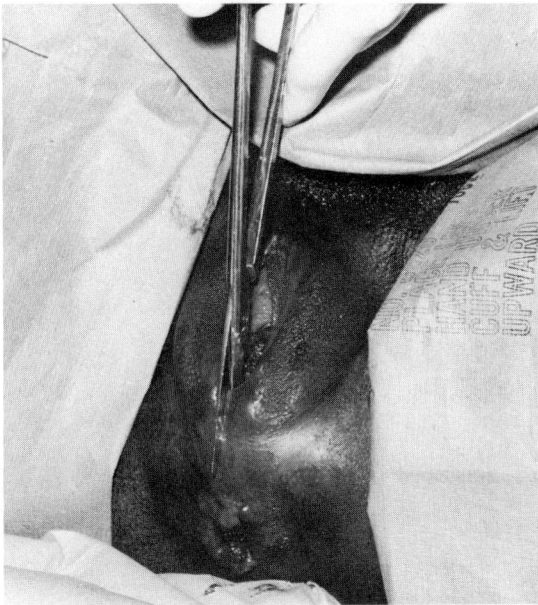

Fig. 14–4. Vulva partially distended by fetal head. Midline episiotomy being made.

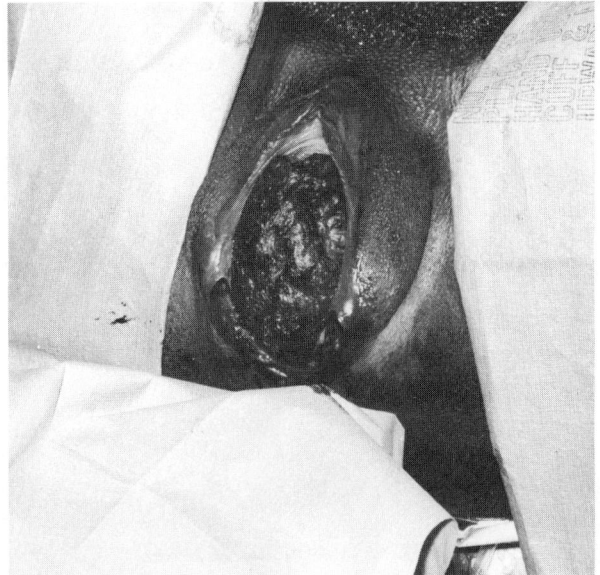

Fig. 14–5. Birth of head. The occiput is being kept close to the symphysis by moderate pressure to the fetal chin at the tip of the maternal coccyx.

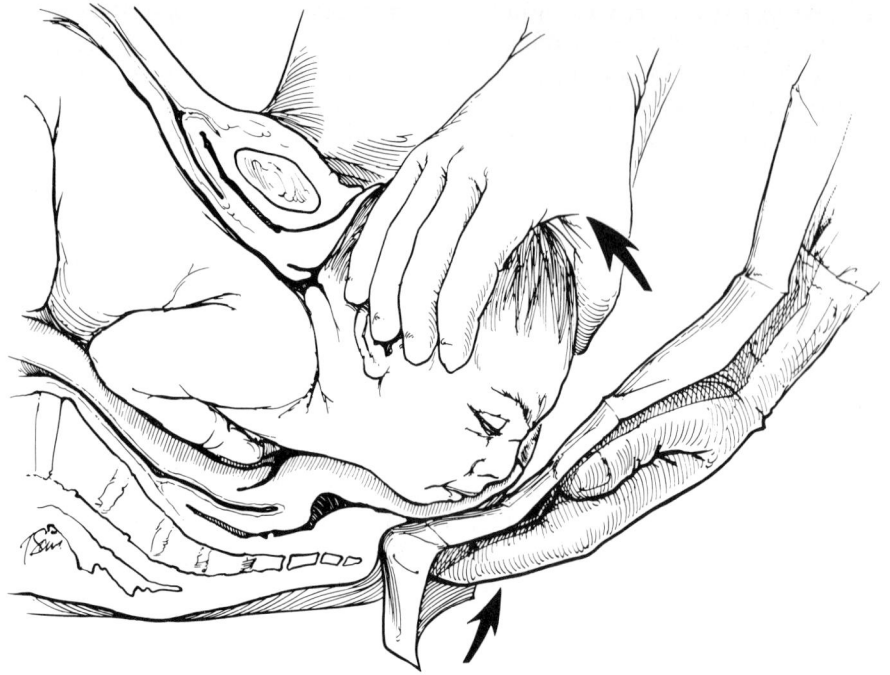

Fig. 14–6. Near completion of the delivery of the fetal head by the modified Ritgen maneuver. Moderate upward pressure is applied to the fetal chin by the posterior hand covered with a sterile towel while the suboccipital region of the fetal head is held against the symphysis.

head, it should be cut between two clamps and the infant promptly delivered.

Delivery of Shoulders. After its birth, the head falls posteriorly, bringing the face almost into contact with the anus. As described in Chapter 13, the occiput promptly turns toward one of the maternal thighs so that the head assumes a transverse position (Fig. 14–9). The movement of restitution (external rotation) indicates that the bisacromial diameter (transverse diameter of the thorax) has rotated into the anterioposterior diameter of the pelvis.

Most often, the shoulders appear at the vulva just after external rotation and are born spontaneously. Oc-

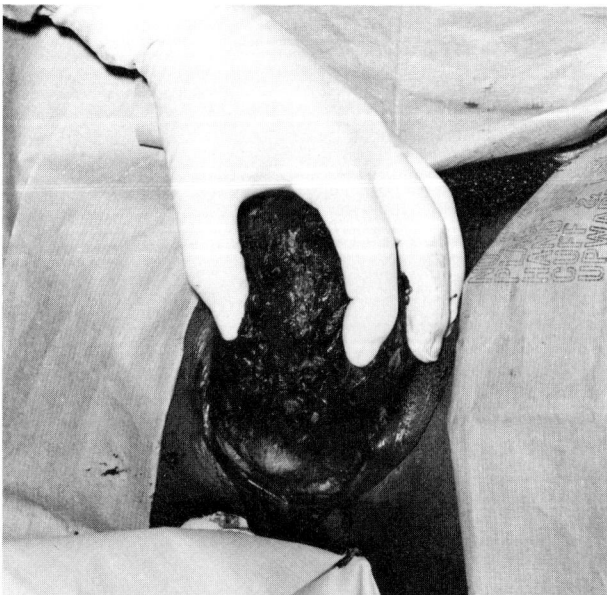

Fig. 14–7. Pressure is applied through the towel covering the hand to the underside of the chin of the infant as soon as the occiput is beyond the symphysis. This extends the head. At the same time, the fingers of the other hand simultaneously elevate the scalp to help extend the head.

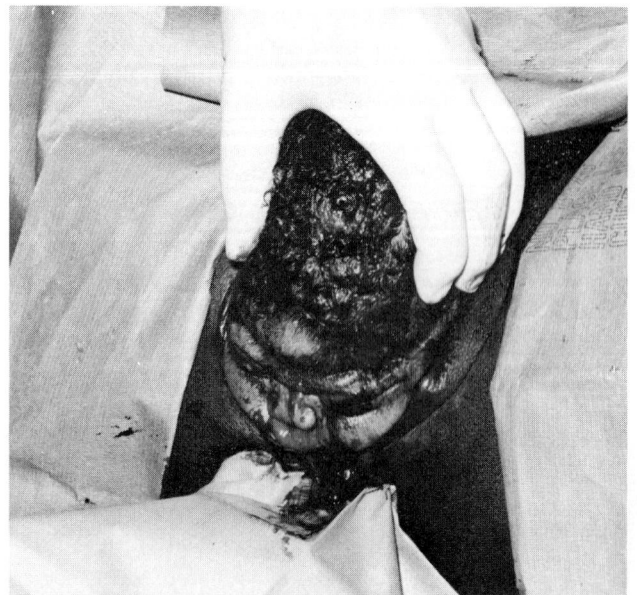

Fig. 14–8. Birth of head; the mouth appears over perineum.

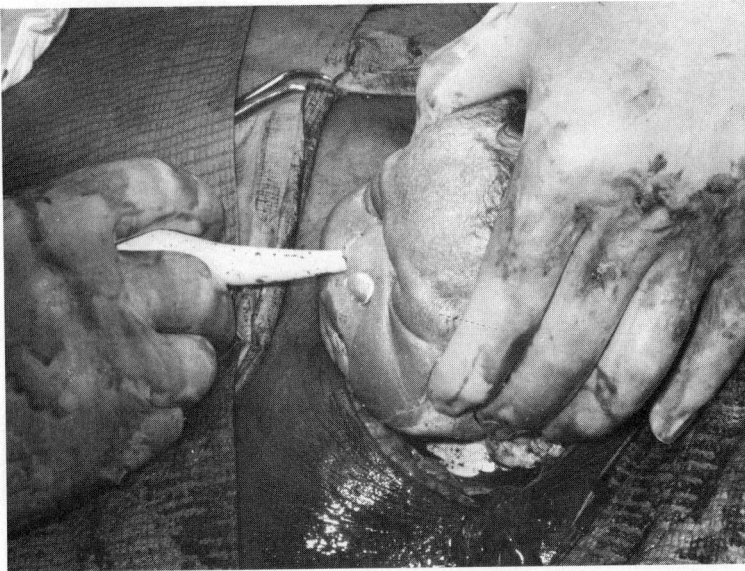

Fig. 14–9. Aspirating the nose and mouth immediately after delivery of the head.

casionally, a delay occurs and immediate extraction may appear advisable. In this event, the sides of the head are grasped with the two hands and *gentle* downward traction applied until the anterior shoulder appears under the pubic arch. Then, by an upward movement, the posterior shoulder is delivered (Fig. 14–11).

The rest of the body almost always follows the shoulders without difficulty; but in case of prolonged delay, its birth may be hastened by *moderate* traction on the head and moderate pressure on the uterine fundus. Hooking the fingers in the axillae should be avoided because this may injure the nerves of the upper extremity, producing a transient or possibly even a permanent

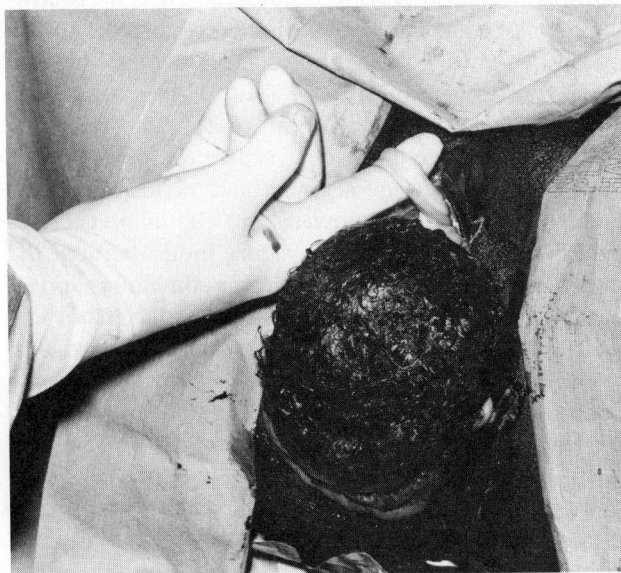

Fig. 14–10. Cord identified around the neck. It readily slipped over the head.

paralysis. Traction, furthermore, should be exerted only in the direction of the long axis of the infant, for if applied obliquely it causes bending of the neck and excessive stretching of the brachial plexus.

Immediately after delivery of the infant, there is usually a gush of amnionic fluid, often tinged with blood but not grossly bloody.

Clamping the Cord. The umbilical cord is cut between two clamps placed 4 or 5 cm from the fetal abdomen, and later an umbilical cord clamp is applied 2 or 3 cm from the fetal abdomen. A plastic clamp (Hollister, Double Grip Umbilical Clamp) that is safe, efficient, easy to sterilize, and fairly inexpensive is shown in Figure 14–12.

Timing of Cord Clamping. If, after delivery, the infant is placed at or below the level of the vaginal introitus for 3 minutes and the fetoplacental circulation is not immediately occluded by clamping the cord, an average of 80 mL of blood may be shifted from the placenta to the infant (Yao and Lind, 1974). One benefit to be derived from placental transfusion is that the hemoglobin in 80 mL of placental blood that shifts to the fetus eventually provides about 50 mg of iron, which reduces the frequency of iron-deficiency anemia later in infancy. In the presence of accelerated destruction of erythrocytes, as occurs with maternal alloimmunization, the bilirubin formed from the added erythrocytes contributes further to the danger of hyperbilirubinemia (see Chap. 44, p. 1007). Although the theoretical risk of circulatory overloading from gross hypervolemia is formidable, especially in preterm and growth-retarded infants, addition of placental blood to the infant's circulation ordinarily does not cause difficulty.

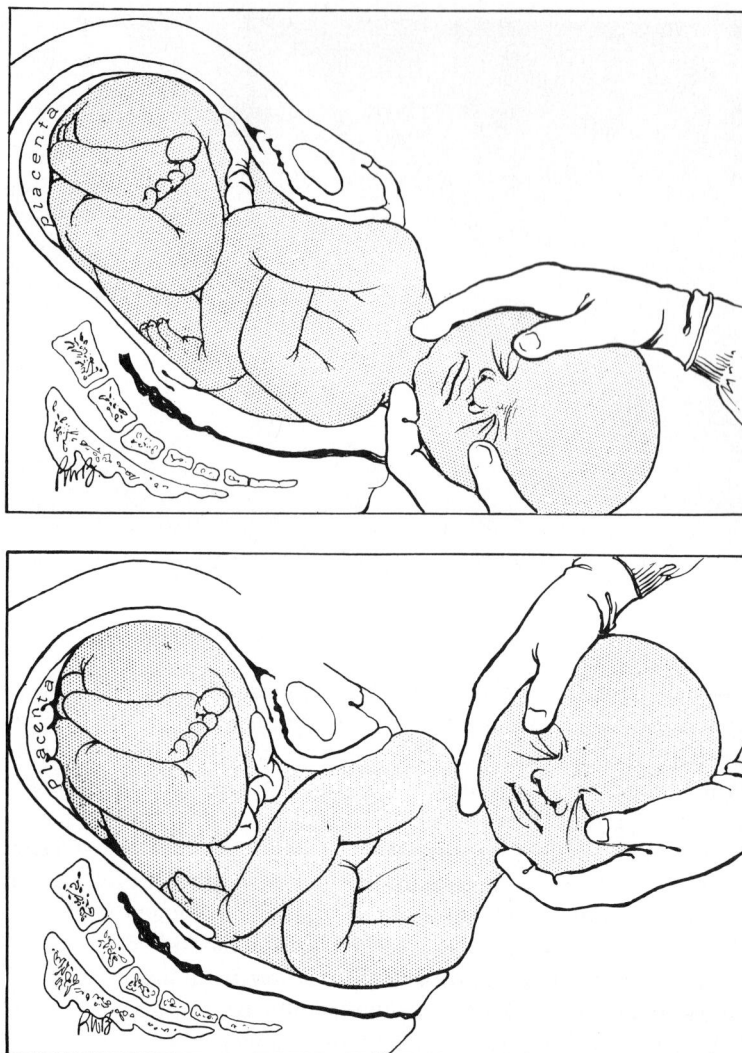

Fig. 14–11. *Gentle* downward traction to bring about descent of anterior shoulder (*top*). Delivery of anterior shoulder completed; *gentle* upward traction to deliver the posterior shoulder (*bottom*).

Our policy is to clamp the cord after first thoroughly clearing the infant's airway, all of which usually takes about 30 seconds. The infant is not elevated above the introitus at vaginal delivery or much above the maternal abdominal wall at the time of cesarean delivery. The cord is then clamped.

Management of Third Stage of Labor

Immediately after delivery of the infant, the height of the uterine fundus and its consistency are ascertained. As long as the uterus remains firm and there is no unusual bleeding, watchful waiting until the placenta is separated is the usual practice. No massage is practiced; the hand is simply rested on the fundus frequently, to make certain that the organ does not become atonic and filled with blood behind a separated placenta.

Signs of Placental Separation. Because attempts to express the placenta prior to its separation are futile and possibly dangerous, it is most important that the following signs of placental separation be recognized: (1) The uterus becomes globular and, as a rule, firmer. This sign is the earliest to appear. (2) There is often a sudden gush of blood. (3) The uterus rises in the abdomen because the placenta, having separated, passes down into the lower uterine segment and vagina, where its bulk pushes the uterus upward. (4) The umbilical cord protrudes farther out of the vagina, indicating that the placenta has descended. These signs sometimes appear within about a minute after delivery of the infant and usually within 5 minutes. When the placenta has separated, it should be ascertained that the uterus is firmly contracted. The mother may be asked to bear down, and the intraabdominal pressure so produced may be adequate to expel the placenta. If these efforts fail, or if spontaneous expulsion is not possible because of anesthesia, and after ensuring that the uterus is contracted firmly, pressure is exerted with the hand on the fundus to propel the detached placenta into the vagina, as depicted and described in Figure 14–13.

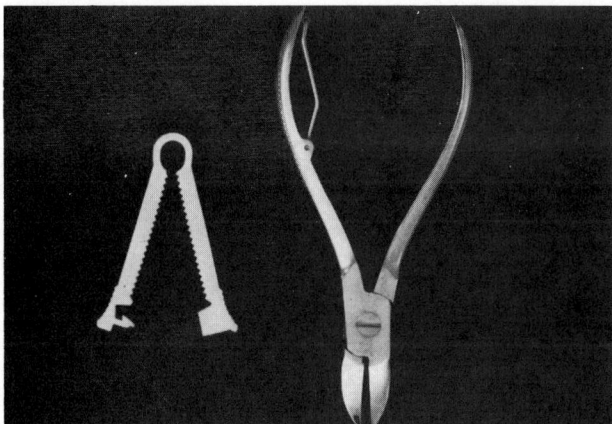

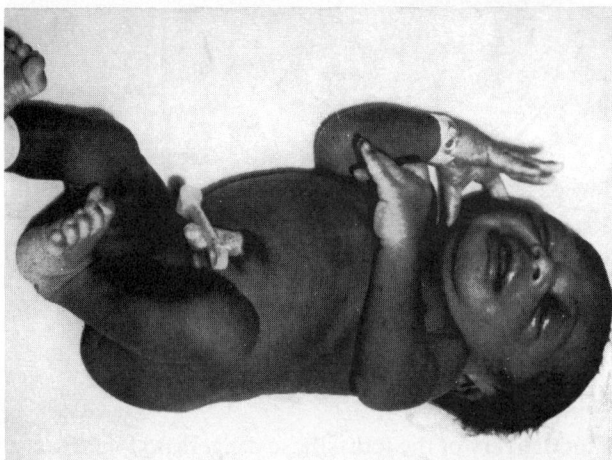

Fig. 14–12. Plastic cord clamp. These clamps lock in place and cannot slip. They are removed on the second or third day simply by cutting the plastic at the loop, or they can be allowed to drop off with the cord.

Delivery of the Placenta. Placental expression should never be forced before placental separation lest the uterus be turned inside out. *Inversion of the uterus* is one of the grave complications associated with delivery (see Chap. 27, p. 622). As pressure is applied to the body of the uterus (Fig. 14–13), the umbilical cord is kept slightly taut. The uterus is lifted cephalad with the abdominal hand. This maneuver is repeated until the placenta reaches the introitus (Prendiville and associates, 1988b). Draining the umbilical cord and placenta do not hasten placental separation and delivery (Thomas and associates, 1990).

Traction on the umbilical cord must not be used to pull the placenta out of the uterus. As the placenta passes through the introitus, pressure on the uterus is stopped. The placenta is then gently lifted away from the introitus (Fig. 14–14). Care is taken to prevent the membranes from being torn off and left behind. If the membranes start to tear, they are grasped with a clamp and removed by gentle traction (Fig. 14–15). The maternal surface of the placenta should be examined carefully to insure that no placental fragments are left in the uterus.

Manual Removal of Placenta. Occasionally, the placenta will not separate promptly. If at any time there is brisk bleeding and the placenta cannot be delivered by these techniques, manual removal of the placenta is indicated, using the safeguards described in Chapter 27 (p. 618). A question to which there is no definite answer concerns the length of time that should elapse in the absence of bleeding before the placenta is manually removed. Manual removal of the placenta is rightfully practiced much sooner and more often than in the past. In fact, some obstetricians practice routine manual removal of any placenta that has not separated spontaneously by the time they have completed delivery of the infant and care of the cord. Proof of the efficacy of this practice, however, has not been established, and most await spontaneous placental separation unless bleeding is excessive.

"Fourth Stage" of Labor. The placenta, membranes, and umbilical cord should be examined for completeness and for anomalies, as described in Chapters 34 and 35. The hour immediately following delivery is a critical period and has been designated by some as the "fourth stage of labor." Even though oxytocics are administered, as described below, postpartum hemorrhage as the result of uterine relaxation is more likely at this time. As emphasized in Chapter 18 (p. 468), it is mandatory that the uterus be frequently evaluated throughout this period by a competent attendant, who frequently places a hand on the fundus and massages it at the slightest sign of uterine relaxation. At the same time, the perineal region is also inspected frequently to allow prompt identification of any excessive bleeding.

Oxytocic Agents

After the uterus has been emptied and the placenta has been delivered, the primary mechanism by which hemostasis is achieved at the placental site is vasoconstriction produced by a well-contracted myometrium (see Chap. 37, p. 820). Oxytocin (Pitocin, Syntocinon), ergonovine maleate (Ergotrate), and methylergonovine maleate (Methergine) are employed in various ways in the conduct of the third stage of labor, principally to reduce blood loss by stimulating myometrial contractions. (Prendiville and associates, 1988a; Thornton and colleagues, 1988).

Oxytocin. The synthetic form of the octapeptide oxytocin is commercially available in the United States as Syntocinon and Pitocin; 1 mg of oxytocin is equal to about 500 USP units. Each mL of injectable oxytocin contains 10 USP units of oxytocin, which is not effective

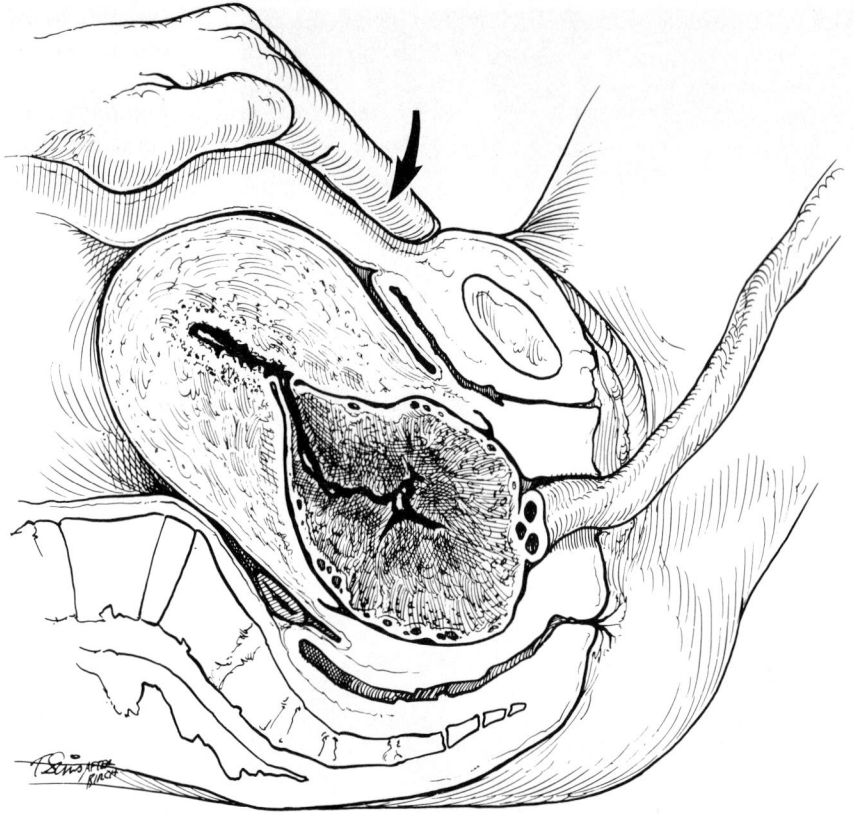

Fig. 14–13. Expression of placenta. Note that the hand is *not* trying to push the fundus of the uterus through the birth canal! As the placenta leaves the uterus and enters the vagina, the uterus is elevated by the hand on the abdomen (arrow) while the cord is held in position. The mother can aid in the delivery of the placenta by bearing down. As the placenta reaches the perineum the cord is lifted, which, in turn, lifts the placenta out of the vagina. Adherent membranes are eased away from thin attachments so as to prevent their being torn off and retained in the birth canal.

by mouth. The half-life of intravenously infused oxytocin is very short, perhaps 3 minutes.

Before delivery, the spontaneously laboring uterus is very likely to be exquisitely sensitive to oxytocin. Even with an intravenous dose of a few mU per minute, the pregnant uterus may contract so violently as to kill the fetus, rupture itself, or both (see Chap. 19, p. 487).

After delivery of the fetus, these dangers no longer exist. Nonetheless, at this time, there are other potentially grave dangers from inappropriate use of oxytocin.

Cardiovascular Effects. Deleterious effects may on occasion follow the intravenous injection of a bolus of oxytocin. Hendricks and Brenner (1970) demonstrated

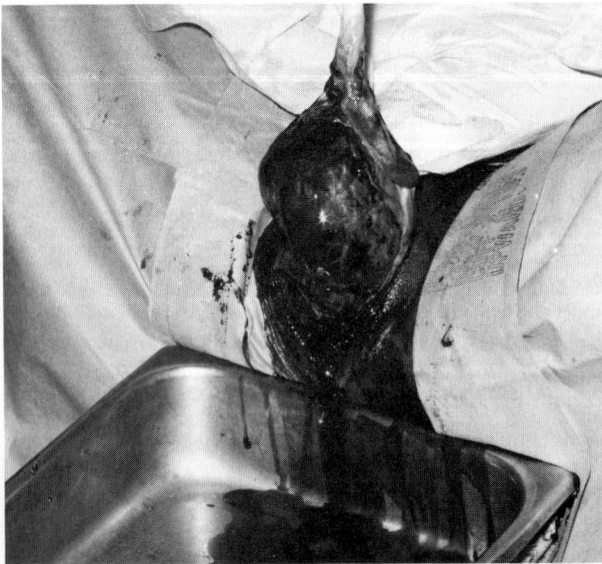

Fig. 14–14. The placenta is removed from the vagina by lifting the cord.

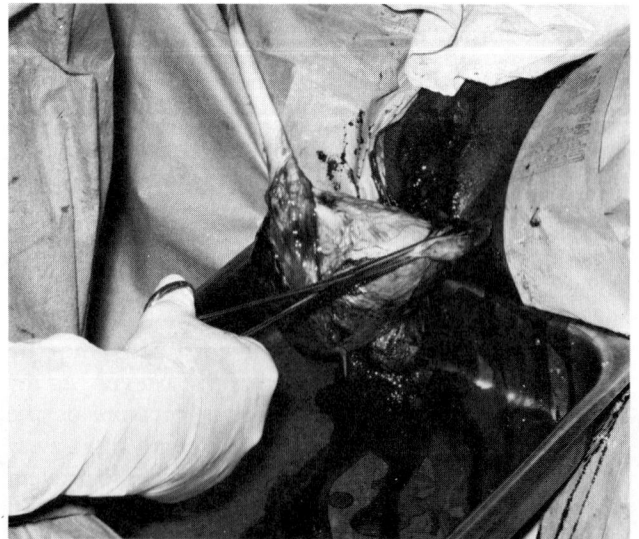

Fig. 14–15. Membranes that were somewhat adherent to the uterine lining are separated by gentle traction with a ring forceps.

with the rapid intravenous injection of 5 units (0.5 mL) of oxytocin that the uterus contracted tetanically for several minutes and maternal blood pressure decreased simultaneously. In one dramatic instance of hypotension from uterine bleeding following delivery of twins, they noted that a bolus injection of 5 units of oxytocin intravenously was promptly followed by a further decrease in blood pressure from 70/42 to 44/26 mm Hg (Fig. 14–16). After rapid administration of 500 mL of saline, the blood pressure increased and the mother again became responsive.

Secher and co-workers (1978) consistently observed that, even in healthy women, an intravenous bolus of 10 units of oxytocin caused a transient but marked fall in arterial blood pressure that was followed by an abrupt increase in cardiac output. They too concluded that these hemodynamic changes could be dangerous to women already hypovolemic from hemorrhage, or who had cardiac disease that limited cardiac output. The same danger is present for women with right-to-left cardiac shunts. **Oxytocin should not be given intravenously as a large bolus,** but rather as a much more dilute solution by continuous intravenous infusion (p. 388), or be injected intramuscularly in a dose of 10 USP units.

Antidiuresis. Another important adverse effect of oxytocin is antidiuresis, caused primarily by reabsorption of free water. Abdul-Karim and Assali (1961) demonstrated clearly that in both pregnant and nonpregnant women oxytocin has considerable antidiuretic activity. In women who are undergoing diuresis in response to the administration of water, the continuous intravenous infusion of 20 mU of oxytocin per minute usually produces a demonstrable decrease in urine flow. When the rate of infusion is raised to 40 mU per minute, urinary flow is strikingly reduced. With doses of this magnitude, it is possible to produce water intoxication if the oxytocin is administered in a large volume of electrolyte-free aqueous dextrose solution (Eggers and Fliegner, 1979; Whalley and Pritchard, 1963).

The hyponatremic, hypoosmotic state is not limited to just the mother. Schwartz and Jones (1978), for example, described convulsions in both the mother and her newborn following the administration of 6.5 liters of 5 percent dextrose solution and 36 units of oxytocin predelivery. The concentration of sodium in cord plasma was 114 mEq/L. In general, if oxytocin is to be administered in high doses for a considerable period of time, its concentration should be increased rather than increasing the rate of flow of a more dilute solution. The antidiuretic effect of intravenously administered oxytocin disappears within a few minutes after the infusion is stopped. Oxytocin injected intramuscularly in doses of 5 to 10 units (0.5 to 1 mL) every 15 to 30 minutes also causes antidiuresis, but the possibility of water intoxication is not nearly so great because large volumes of electrolyte-free aqueous solution are not required as a vehicle (Whalley and Pritchard, 1963).

Ergonovine and Methylergonovine. Ergonovine is an alkaloid obtained from ergot, a fungus that grows on rye and some other grains, or it is synthesized in part from lysergic acid. Methylergonovine is a very similar alkaloid made from lysergic acid. The alkaloids are dispensed as the maleate (Ergotrate and Methergine, respectively) either in solution for parenteral use or in tablets for oral use.

Effects. There is no convincing evidence of any appreciable difference in the actions of ergonovine and methylergonovine. Whether given intravenously, intramuscularly, or orally, ergonovine and methylergonovine are powerful stimulants of myometrial contraction, exerting an effect that may persist for hours. The sensitivity of the pregnant uterus to ergonovine and methylergonovine is very great. In pregnant women, an intravenous dose of as little as 0.1 mg, or an oral dose of only 0.25 mg, results in a tetanic uterine contraction that occurs almost immediately after intravenous injection of the drug and within a few minutes after intra-

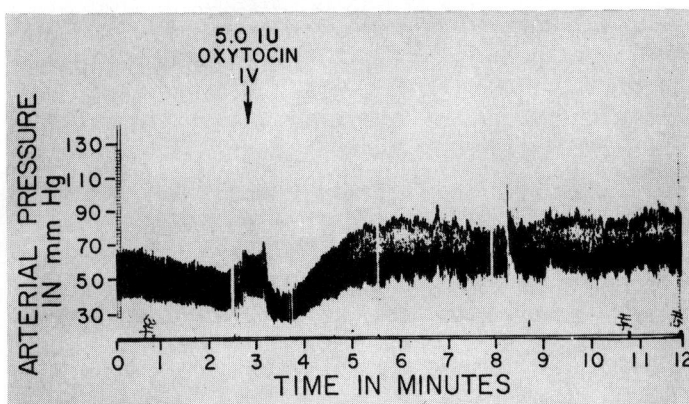

Fig. 14–16. Adverse effect of the intravenous bolus of 5 units of oxytocin in a case of postpartum hemorrhage 18 minutes postdelivery. The hypotension worsened to a level of 44/26 mm Hg until saline was infused rapidly. (From Hendricks and Brenner, 1970.)

muscular or oral administration. Moreover, the response is sustained with little tendency toward relaxation. The tetanic effect of ergonovine and methylergonovine is effective for the prevention and control of postpartum hemorrhage but is very dangerous for the fetus and the mother prior to delivery.

The parenteral administration of these alkaloids, especially by the intravenous route, sometimes initiates transient but severe hypertension. Such a reaction is most likely when conduction analgesia is used for delivery and in women who are prone to develop hypertension. Browning (1974) described four instances of serious postdelivery side effects attributable to 0.5 mg of ergonovine administered intramuscularly. Two women promptly became severely hypertensive, the third became hypertensive and convulsed, and the fourth suffered a cardiac arrest. Because of the frequency of hypertension among our obstetrical population, we do not use these alkaloids routinely.

Prostaglandins. Prostaglandin compounds are not used routinely for management of the third stage of labor. Their use is restricted to the management of postpartum hemorrhage due to uterine atony, which is discussed in Chapter 27 (p. 618).

Oxytocics During and After Delivery. Oxytocin, ergonovine, and methylergonovine are all employed widely in the conduct of the normal third stage of labor, but the timing of their administration differs in various institutions. Oxytocin, and especially ergonovine, given before delivery of the placenta will decrease blood loss somewhat (Prendiville and associates, 1988a). There is, however, a significant danger associated with this practice. The use of oxytocin, and especially ergonovine or methylergonovine, before delivery of the placenta may entrap an undiagnosed, undelivered second twin. This may prove injurious, if not fatal, to the entrapped fetus. In most cases following uncomplicated vaginal delivery, the third stage of labor can be conducted with reasonably small blood loss without using these agents before delivery of the placenta.

If an intravenous infusion is in place, our standard practice has been to add 20 units (2 mL) of oxytocin per liter. This solution is administered after delivery of the placenta at a rate of 10 mL per minute for a few minutes until the uterus remains firmly contracted and bleeding is controlled. The infusion rate then is reduced to 1 to 2 mL per minute until the mother is ready for transfer from the recovery suite to the postpartum unit. At this time, the infusion usually is discontinued.

Lacerations of the Birth Canal. Lacerations of the vagina and perineum are classified as first, second, third, or fourth degree. Such lacerations most often are pre-ventable with an appropriate episiotomy and avoidance of midforceps deliveries.

First-degree lacerations involve the fourchet, perineal skin, and vaginal mucous membrane but not the underlying fascia and muscle.

Second-degree lacerations involve, in addition to skin and mucous membrane, the fascia and muscles of the perineal body but not the rectal sphincter (Fig. 14–17). These tears usually extend upward on one or both sides of the vagina, forming an irregular triangular injury.

Third-degree lacerations extend through the skin, mucous membrane, and perineal body, and involve the anal sphincter.

A *fourth-degree laceration* is distinguished by a third-degree tear that extends through the rectal mucosa to expose the lumen of the rectum. Tears in the region of the urethra are also likely to occur with this type of laceration unless an adequate episiotomy is performed. These periurethal tears may bleed profusely.

Because the repair of perineal tears is virtually the same as that of episiotomy incisions, albeit often less satisfactory because of irregular lines of tissue cleavage, the technique of repairing lacerations is discussed in the following section.

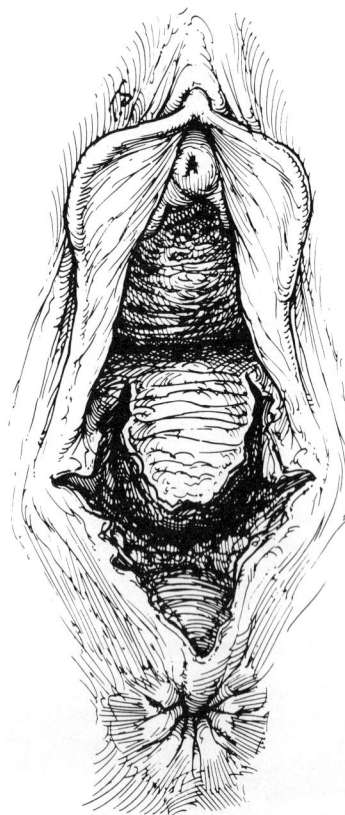

Fig. 14–17. Deep second-degree laceration of perineum and vagina.

Episiotomy and Repair

Episiotomy, in a strict sense, is incision of the pudenda. Perineotomy is incision of the perineum. In common parlance, however, episiotomy is often used synonymously with perineotomy, a practice that will be followed here. The incision may be made in the midline (median or midline episiotomy), or it may begin in the midline but be directed laterally and downward away from the rectum (mediolateral episiotomy).

Purposes of Episiotomy. Episiotomy is the most common operation in obstetrics. The reasons for its popularity among obstetricians are clear. It substitutes a straight, neat surgical incision for the ragged laceration that otherwise frequently results. It is easier to repair, but the long-held beliefs that postoperative pain is less and healing improved with an episiotomy compared to a tear appear *not* to be true (Larsson and colleagues, 1991). With a mediolateral episiotomy, the likelihood of a laceration into the rectum is reduced but not eliminated.

The advantages provided by an episiotomy have been questioned by some individuals (Borgatta, 1989; Larsson, 1991; Sleep, 1984; Thacker, 1983; Thorp, 1987, 1989; Viktrup, 1992; Wilcox, 1989; and all their co-workers). One commonly cited but unproven benefit of routine episiotomy is that it prevents pelvic relaxation, that is, cystocele, rectocele, and urinary incontinence. Obviously, if the perineal incision is made at the time of maximal distension, then this benefit might be limited. Borgatta (1989), Gass (1986), Thorp (1987, 1989), Wilcox (1989), and their co-workers maintain that routine episiotomy is associated with an increased incidence of anal sphincter and rectal tears. Reynolds and Yudkin (1987) studied nearly 25,000 deliveries at the John Radcliffe Hospital at Oxford, and they reported that the episiotomy rate in nulliparas decreased from 73 percent in 1980 to 45 percent in 1984. During this same time, the incidence of second-degree tears increased from 7 to 20 per 1000; but the incidence of third-degree lacerations was unchanged at about 5 per 1000.

In summary, episiotomy should not be performed routinely. The procedure should be applied selectively for appropriate indications, some of which include fetal indications (preterm delivery, shoulder dystocia, breech delivery), forceps or vacuum extractor operations, occiput posterior positions, and in instances where it is obvious that failure to perform an episiotomy will result in perineal rupture. The final rule is that there is no substitute for surgical judgment and common sense.

The important questions if an episiotomy is to be utilized are:

1. How long before delivery should it be performed?
2. Should a midline or mediolateral incision be made?
3. Should the incision be sutured before or after expulsion of the placenta?
4. What are the best techniques and suture materials to employ?

Timing of Episiotomy. If episiotomy is performed unnecessarily early, bleeding from the incision may be considerable during the interim between the episiotomy and the delivery. If episiotomy is performed too late, the muscles of the perineal floor already will have undergone excessive stretching, and one of the objectives of the operation is defeated. It is common practice to perform episiotomy when the head is visible during a contraction to a diameter of 3 to 4 cm (Fig. 14–4).

In this connection, the question arises whether episiotomy should be performed before or after the application of forceps. Application and articulation of forceps with widely separated shanks, as with Simpson forceps, may cause tearing of the introitus (see Chap. 24, p. 556). The application of those with narrow overlapping shanks, such as Tucker–McLane forceps, before episiotomy is not as likely to be so traumatic. Although it is slightly more awkward to perform an episiotomy with the forceps in place, blood loss from the episiotomy is somewhat less with this technique, because immediate traction on the forceps can be exerted; and the resultant tamponade of the perineal floor by the fetal head is effected earlier than could otherwise be achieved.

Midline Versus Mediolateral Episiotomy. The advantages and disadvantages of the two types of episiotomies are summarized in Table 14–3. Except for the important issue of third- and fourth-degree extensions, midline episiotomy is superior. With proper selection of cases, it is possible to secure the advantages of midline episiotomy and at the same time reduce to a minimum this one disadvantage. In addition to a midline episiotomy, Combs and associates (1990) reported the following factors to be associated with an increased risk for third- and fourth-degree lacerations: nulliparity, second-stage

TABLE 14–3. MIDLINE VERSUS MEDIOLATERAL EPISIOTOMY

Characteristic	Episiotomy	
	Midline	**Mediolateral**
Surgical repair	Easy	More difficult
Faulty healing	Rare	More common
Postoperative pain	Minimal	Common
Anatomical results	Excellent	Occasionally faulty
Blood loss	Less	More
Dyspareunia	Rare	Occasional
Extensions	Common	Uncommon

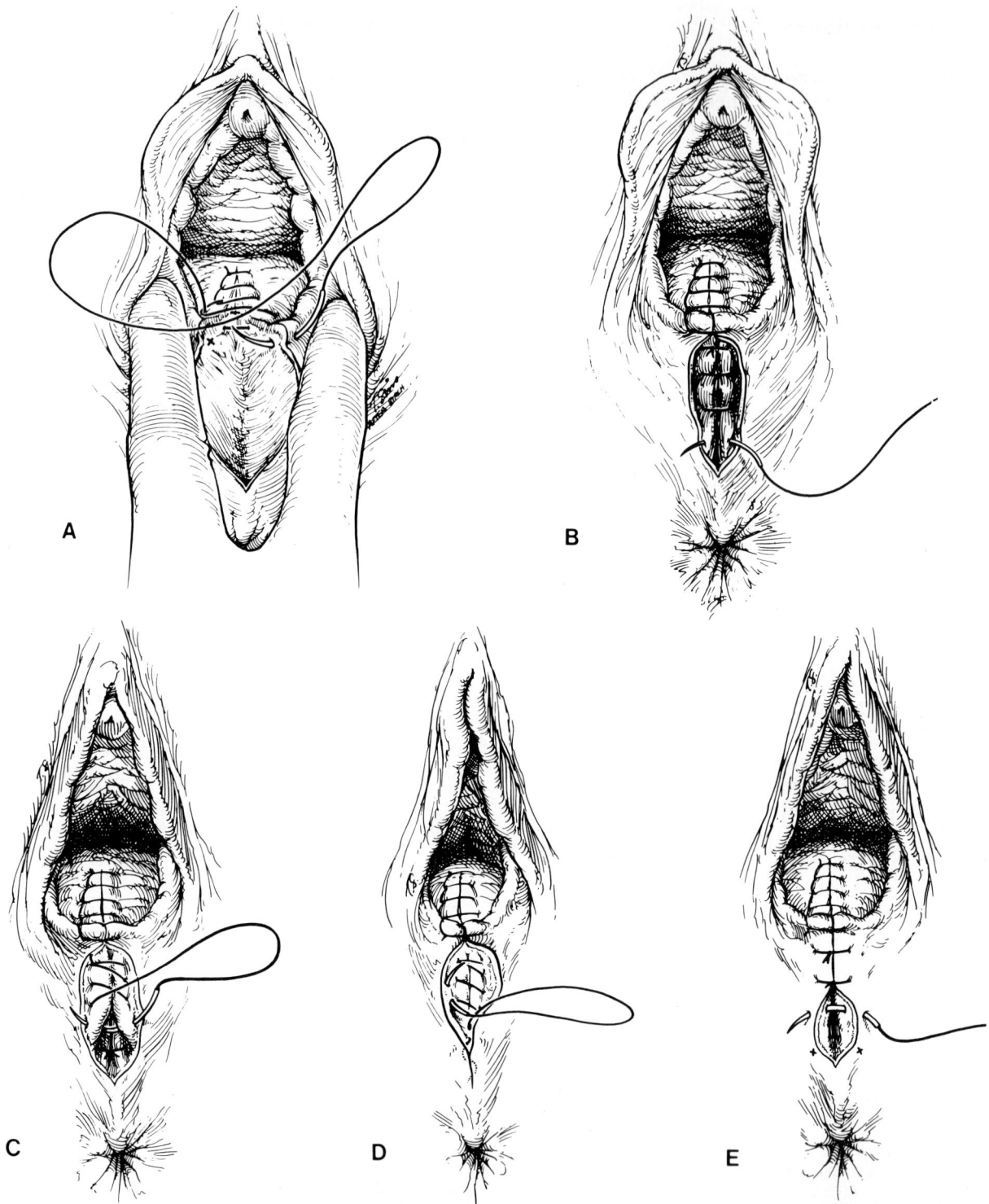

Fig. 14–18. Repair of median episiotomy. **A.** Chromic catgut 00, or preferably 000, is used as a continuous suture to close the vaginal mucosa and submucosa. **B.** After closing the vaginal incision and reapproximating the cut margins of the hymenal ring, the suture is tied and cut. Next, 3 or 4 interrupted sutures of 00 or 000 catgut are placed in the fascia and muscle of the incised perineum. **C.** A continuous suture is carried downward to unite the superficial fascia. **D.** Completion of repair. The continuous suture is carried upward as a subcuticular stitch. (An alternative method of closure of skin and subcutaneous fascia is illustrated in E.) **E.** Completion of repair of median episiotomy. A few interrupted sutures of 000 chromic catgut are placed through the skin and subcutaneous fascia and loosely tied. This closure avoids burying two layers of catgut in the more superficial layers of the perineum.

arrest of labor, persistent occiput posterior position, mid- or low-forceps instead of a vacuum extractor, use of local anesthetics, and Asian race.

It is good practice, in general, to use a mediolateral episiotomy when a third- or fourth-degree extension is likely, but to employ the midline incision otherwise. Even with careful selection, however, the total number of third- and fourth-degree lacerations sustained with this policy is probably greater than with routine mediolateral episiotomy. In any case, sharply pointed scissors should not be used lest they inadvertently penetrate the rectum.

Benyon (1974) described her experiences with a policy of mandatory midline episiotomy. Of 1166 nulliparas who underwent a midline episiotomy, there was extension through the anal sphincter with involvement of *the rectum in 8 percent*. The technique of repair was similar to that described below. She emphasized that the episiotomies and repairs were performed primarily by house officers in training. Following repair, there was no special emphasis on bowel action. Suppositories, rectal tubes, and enemas were not allowed and rectal examinations were avoided. Only one woman developed a rectovaginal fistula. Therefore, a third-degree laceration as the consequence of a midline episiotomy need not be a major catastrophe. Such benign outcomes, however, are not always observed. Venkatesh and colleagues (1989) reported a 5 percent incidence of third- and fourth-degree perineal tears in 20,500 vaginal deliveries. Ten percent of these 1040 primary repairs had a wound disruption and 67 of the 101 required surgical correction. Goldaber and associates (1993) discussed our experiences. They reported that 21 of 390 (5.4 percent) women with fourth-degree lacerations experienced significant morbidity. There were 7 (1.8 percent) dehiscences, 11 (2.8 percent) infections with dehiscences, and 3 (0.8 percent) infections alone. While administration of perioperative antibiotics (cefazolin sodium, 2 g intravenously) appeared to reduce this morbidity, it did not totally eliminate it (Goldaber and associates, unpublished observations).

Timing of the Repair of Episiotomy. The most common practice is to defer episiotomy repair until the placenta has been delivered. This policy permits undivided attention to the signs of placental separation and delivery. Early delivery of the placenta is believed to decrease blood loss from the implantation site because it prevents the development of extensive retroplacental bleeding. A further advantage is that episiotomy repair is not interrupted or disrupted by the obvious necessity of delivering the placenta, especially if manual removal must be performed.

Technique. There are many ways to close an episiotomy incision, but *hemostasis and anatomical restoration without excessive suturing are essential* for

success with any method. A technique that commonly is employed is shown in Figure 14–18. The suture material ordinarily used is 000 chromic catgut, but Grant (1989) recommends suture composed of derivatives of polyglycolic acid. A decrease in postsurgical pain is cited as the major advantage of the newer materials despite the occasional need to remove some of the suture from the site of repair.

Fourth-Degree Laceration. The technique of repairing a fourth-degree laceration is shown in Figure 14–19. Various techniques have been recommended; but in all instances, it is essential to approximate the torn edges of the rectal mucosa with muscularis sutures placed approximately 0.5 cm apart. This muscular layer then is covered with a layer of fascia. Finally, the cut ends of the anal sphincter are isolated, approximated, and sutured together with two or three interrupted stitches. The remainder of the repair is the same as for an episiotomy. Stool softeners should be prescribed for a week, and enemas should be avoided. Prophylactic antibiotics probably should be administered, as described by Goldaber and Wendall (unpublished observations). Unfortunately, normal function is not always assured even with

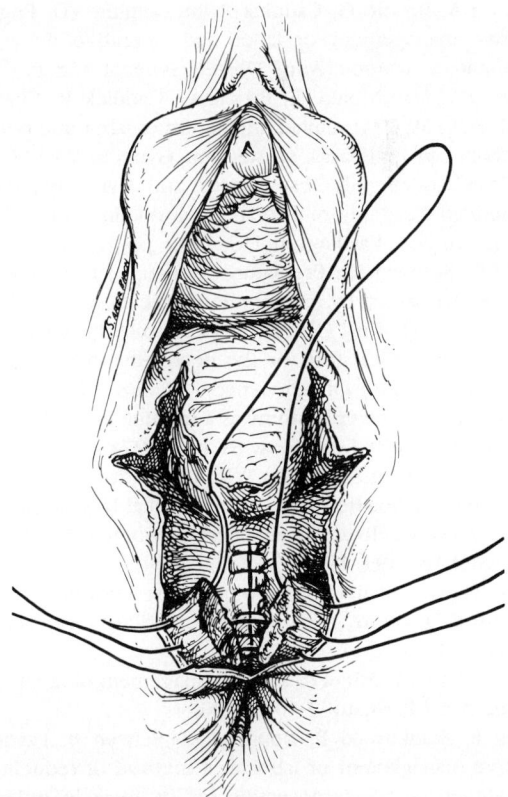

Fig. 14–19. Repair of complete perineal tear. The rectal mucosa has been repaired with interrupted, fine chromic catgut sutures. The torn ends of the sphincter ani are next approximated with 2 or 3 interrupted chromic catgut sutures. The wound is then repaired, as in a second-degree laceration or an episiotomy.

correct and complete surgical repair. Some women may experience continuing fecal incontinence due to injury to the innervation of the pelvic floor musculature (Roberts and co-workers, 1990).

Pain After Episiotomy. For the relief of episiotomy pain, a heat lamp has been a standard remedy; but during warm weather especially, it may produce more discomfort than relief. An ice collar applied early tends to reduce swelling and allay discomfort. Aerosol sprays containing a local anesthetic are helpful at times. Analgesics such as codeine give considerable relief. **Because pain may be a signal of a large vulvar, paravaginal, or ischiorectal hematoma or perineal cellulitis, it is essential to examine these sites carefully if pain is severe or persistent.** Management of these complications is discussed in Chapter 29 (p. 644).

References

Abdul-Karim R, Assali NS: Renal function in human pregnancy: V. Effects of oxytocin on renal hemodynamics and water and electrolyte excretion. J Lab Clin Med 57:522, 1961

Abe T: The detection of the rupture of fetal membranes with the nitrazine indicator. Am J Obstet Gynecol 39:400, 1940

Akoury HA, Brodie G, Caddick R, McLaughin VD, Pugh PA: Active management of labor and operative delivery in nulliparous women. Am J Obstet Gynecol 158:255, 1988

Akoury HA, MacDonald FJ, Brodie G, Caddick R, Chaudhry NM, Frize M: Oxytocin augmentation of labor and perinatal outcome in nulliparas. Obstet and Gynecol 78:227, 1991

American College of Obstetricians and Gynecologists and American Academy of Pediatrics: Guidelines for Perinatal Care, 3rd ed., Washington, DC, 1992, pp 72, 76

Atlay RD, Sutherst JR: Premature rupture of the fetal membranes confirmed by intra-amniotic injection of dye (Evans blue T-1824). Am J Obstet Gynecol 108:993, 1970

Baptisti A: Chemical test for the determination of ruptured membranes. Am J Obstet Gynecol 35:688, 1938

Benyon CL: Midline episiotomy as a midline procedure. J Obstet Gynaecol Br Commonw 81:126, 1974

Borgatta L, Piening SL, Cohen WR: Association of episiotomy and delivery position with deep perineal laceration during spontaneous delivery in nulliparous women. Am J Obstet Gynecol 160:294, 1989

Boylan P: Active management of labor: Results in Dublin, Houston, London, New Brunswick, Singapore, and Valparaiso. Birth 16:114, 1989

Boylan P, Parisi V: Effect of active management of latent phase labor. Am J Perinatol 7:363, 1990

Boylan P, Frankowski R, Rountree R, Selwyn B, Parrish K: Active management of labor as a method of reducing the incidence of cesarean section for dystocia in nulliparas. Trans Am Gynecol Obstet Soc 5:122,1987.

Boylan P, Frankowski R: Dystocia, parity, and the cesarean problem. Am J Obstet Gynecol 155:455, 1986

Browning DJ: Serious side effects of ergometrine and its use in routine obstetric practice. Med J Austral 1:957, 1974

Cahill DJ, Boylan PC, O'Herlihy C: Does oxytocin augmentation increase perinatal risk in primigravid labor? Am J Obstet Gynecol 166:847, 1992

Caldeyro-Barcia R, Schwarcz R, Belizan JM, Martell M, Nieto F, Sabatino H, Tenzer SM: Adverse perinatal effects of early amniotomy during labor. In Gluck L (ed): Modern Perinatal Medicine. Chicago, Year Book, 1974

Cohen CR, O'Brien WF, Lewis L, Knuppel RA: A prospective randomized study of the aggressive management of early labor. Am J Obstet Gynecol 157:1174, 1987

Combs CA, Robertson PA, Laros RK: Risk factors for third-degree and fourth-degree perineal lacerations in forceps and vacuum deliveries. Am J Obstet Gynecol 163:100, 1990

Cook WA: Natural Childbirth: Fact and Fallacy. Chicago, Nelson-Hall, 1982

Cowett RM, Hakason DO, Kocon RW, Oh W: Untoward neonatal effect of intra-amnionitic administration of methylene blue. Obstet Gynecol 48(suppl):74, 1976

Eggers TR, Fliegner JR: Water intoxication and syntocinon intoxication. Aust NZ J Obstet Gynaecol 19:59, 1979

Freeman K, Garite Tj, Nageotte MP: Pitfalls in intrapartum fetal monitoring. In Freeman K, Garite TJ, Nageotte MP (eds): Fetal Heart Rate Monitoring, 2nd ed. Baltimore, Williams & Wilkins, 1991, p 206

Freidman EA: Labor, Clinical Evaluation and Management, 2nd ed. New York, Appleton, 1978

Friedman ML, McElin TW: Diagnosis of ruptured fetal membranes. Clinical study and review of the literature. Am J Obstet Gynecol 104:544, 1969

Gardosi J, Hutson N, Lynch CB: Randomised, Controlled trial of squatting in the second stage of labour. Lancet 2:74, 1989

Gass MS, Dunn C, Styes SJ: Effect of episiotomy on the frequency of vaginal outlet lacerations. J Reprod Med 31:240, 1986

Goldaber KG, Wendel PJ, McIntire DD, Wendel GD: Postpartum morbidity after fourth-degree perineal repair. Am J Obstet Gynecol, (in press)

Gorodeski IG, Paz M, Insler V, Fishel J: Diagnosis of rupture of the fetal membranes by glucose and fructose measurements. Obstet Gynecol 53:611, 1979

Grant A: The choice of suture materials and techniques for repair of perineal trauma: An overview of the evidence from controlled trials. Br J Obstet Gynaecol 96:1281, 1989

Haverkamp AD, Orleans M, Langendoerfer S, McFee J, Murphy J, Thompson HE: A controlled trial of the differential effects of intrapartum fetal monitoring. Am J Obstet Gynecol 134:399, 1979

Haverkamp AD, Thompson HE, McFee JG, Cetrulo C: The evaluation of continuous fetal heart rate monitoring in high risk pregnancy. Am J Obstet Gynecol 125:310, 1976

Hendricks CH, Brenner WE: Cardiovascular effects of oxytocic drugs used postpartum. Am J Obstet Gynecol 108:751, 1970

Hjertberg R, Belfrage P, Eneroth P: Latex agglutination test for α-fetoprotein in the diagnosis of premature rupture of the amniotic membranes (PROM). Acta Obstet Gynecol Scand 66:437, 1987

Iffy L, Apuzzio JJ, Castillo M, Ganesh V, Hopp L, Tiger M: Rates of cesarean section and perinatal mortality: An intercontinental dispute. Isr J Obstet Gynecol 1:5, 1990

Ingemarsson I, Arulkumaran S, Ingemarsson E, Tambyraja RL,

Ratnam SS: Admission Test: A screening test for fetal distress in labor. Obstet Gynecol 68:800, 1986

Ingemarsson I, Arulkumaran S, Paul RH, Ingemarsson E, Tambyraja RL, Ratnam SS: Fetal acoustic stimulation in early labor in patients screened with the admission test. Am J Obstet Gynecol 158:70, 1988

Kjeldsen J: Hemodynamic investigations during labour and delivery. Acta Obstet Gynecol Scand 89(suppl):1, 1979

Larsson P, Platz-Christensen J, Bergman B, Wallstersson G: Advantage or disadvantage of episiotomy compared with spontaneous perineal laceration. Gynecol Obstet Invest 31:213, 1991

Leveno KJ, Cunningham FG, Nelson S, Roark M, Williams ML, Guzick D, Dowling S, Rosenfeld CR, Buckley A: A prospective comparison of selective and universal electronic fetal monitoring in 34,995 pregnancies. N Engl J Med 315:615, 1986

Leveno KJ, Cunningham FG, Pritchard JA: Cesarean section: The House of Horne revisited. Am J Obstet Gynecol 160:78, 1989

Leveno KJ, Cunningham FG, Pritchard JA: Cesarean section: An answer to the House of Horne. Am J Obstet Gynecol 153:838, 1985

Lopez-Seno JA, Peaceman AM, Adashek JA, Socol ML: A controlled trial of a program for the active management of labor. N Engl J Med 326:450, 1992

O'Driscoll K, Foley M, MacDonald D: Active management of labor as an alternative to cesarean section for dystocia. Obstet Gynecol 63:485, 1984

O'Driscoll K, Foley M, MacDonald D, Stronge J: Cesarean section and perinatal outcome: Response from the House of Horne. Am J Obstet Gynecol 158:449, 1988

O'Driscoll K, Jackson RJA, Gallagher JT: Prevention of prolonged labour. Br Med J 2:477, 1969

Prendiville W, Elbourne D, Chalmers I: The effects of routine oxytocic administration in the management of the third stage of labour: An overview of the evidence from controlled trials. Br J Obstet Gynaecol 95:3, 1988a

Prendiville WJ, Harding JE, Elbourne DR, Stirrat GM: The Bristol third stage trial: Active versus physiological management of third stage of labour. Br Med J 297:1295, 1988b

Reynolds JL, Yudkin PL: Changes in the management of labour: II. Perineal management. Can Med Assoc J 136:1045, 1987

Ritgen G: Concerning his method for protection of the perineum. Monatschrift für Geburtskunde 6:21, 1855. See English translation, Wynn RM: Am J Obstet Gynecol 93:421, 1965

Roberts PL, Coller JA, Schoetz DJ, Veidenheimer MC: Manometric assessment of patients with obstetric injuries and fecal incontinence. Dis Colon Rectum 33:16, 1990

Rosen MG, Peisner DB: Effect of amniotic membrane rupture on length of labor. Obstet Gynecol 70:604, 1987

Sarno AP, Ahn MO, Phelan JP, Paul RH: Fetal acoustic stimulation in the early intrapartum period as a predictor of subsequent fetal condition. Am J Obstet Gynecol 162:762, 1990

Satin AJ, Leveno KJ, Sherman ML, Brewster DS, Cunningham FG: High versus low-dose oxytocin for labor stimulation. Obstet Gynecol 80:111, 1992

Schwartz RH, Jones RWA: Transplacental hyponatremia due to oxytocin. Br Med J 1:152, 1978

Secher NJ, Arnso P, Wallin L: Haemodynamic effects of oxytocin (Syntocinon) and methylergometrine (Methergin) on the systemic and pulmonary circulations of pregnant anaesthetized women. Acta Obstet Gynecol Scand 57:97, 1978

Sleep J, Grant A, Garcia J, Elbourne D, Spencer J, Chalmers I: West Berkshire perineal management trial. Br Med J 289:587, 1984

Smith RP: A technique for the detection of rupture of the membranes: Review and preliminary report. Obstet Gynecol 48:172, 1976

Thacker SB, Banta HD: Benefits and risks of episiotomy: An interpretive review of the English language literature, 1860–1980. Obstet Gynecol Surv 38:232, 1983

Thomas IL, Jeffers TM, Brazier JM, Burt CL, Barr KE: Does cord drainage of placental blood facilitate delivery of the placenta? Aust NZ J Obstet Gynaecol 30:314, 1990

Thornton S, Davison JM, Baylis PH: Plasma oxytocin during third stage of labour: comparison of natural and active management. Br Med J 297:167, 1988

Thorp JA, Boylan PC, Parisi VM, Heslin EP: Effects of high-dose oxytocin augmentation on umbilical cord blood gas values in primigravid women. Am J Obstet Gynecol 159:670, 1988

Thorp JM, Bowes WA Jr: Episiotomy: Can its routine use be defended? Am J Obstet Gynecol 160:1027, 1989

Thorp JM Jr, Bowes WA Jr, Brame RG, Cefalo R: Selected use of midline episiotomy: Effect of perineal trauma. Obstet Gynecol 70:260, 1987

Turner MJ, Brassil M, Gordon H: Active management of labor associated with a decrease in the cesarean section rate in nulliparas. Obstet Gynecol 71:150, 1988

Venkatesh KS, Ramanujam PS, Larson DM, Haywood MA: Anorectal complications of vaginal delivery. Dis Colon Rectum 32:1039, 1989

Viktrup L, Lose G, Rolff M, Barfoed K: The symptom of stress incontinence caused by pregnancy or delivery in primiparas. Obstet Gynecol 79:945, 1992

Whalley PJ, Pritchard JA: Oxytocin and water intoxication. JAMA 186:601, 1963

Wilcox LS, Strobino DM, Baruffi G, Dellinger WS: Episiotomy and its role in the incidence of perineal lacerations in a maternity center and a tertiary hospital obstetric service. Am J Obstet Gynecol 160:1047, 1989

Wishart MM, Jenkins DT, Knott ML: Measurement of diamine oxidase activity in vaginal fluid—an aid to diagnosis of ruptured fetal membranes. Aust NZ J Obstet Gynaecol 19:23, 1979

Yao AC, Lind J: Placental transfusion. Am J Dis Child 127:128, 1974

CHAPTER 15
Intrapartum Assessment

Intrapartum Fetal Surveillance. A goal to be pursued constantly during labor is preservation of fetal well-being by early detection and relief of fetal distress. To monitor means simply to watch or check on a person or thing. In the minds of many in obstetrics, however, the word *monitor* has come specifically to mean surveillance of fetal heart and uterine activity by an electronic device. It is sometimes forgotten that clinical monitoring has produced meritorious results when applied conscientiously by appropriately trained individuals.

Continuous electronic fetal heart rate monitoring is a marvelous invention introduced into obstetrical practice during the late 1960s. No longer was the perception of fetal distress limited to heart sounds; the continuous graph paper portrayal of the fetal heart rate was potentially diagnostic in assessing pathophysiological events affecting the fetus. There were great expectations for certain assumptions: (1) that electronic fetal heart rate monitoring provided accurate information; (2) that this information was of value in diagnosing fetal distress; (3) that it would be possible to intervene to prevent fetal death or morbidity; and (4) that continuous electronic fetal heart rate monitoring was superior to intermittent methods.

Early Experiences with Electronic Fetal Heart Rate Monitoring. A major impetus for the use of continuous electronic fetal heart rate monitoring rather than intermittent surveillance was a study from the American Collaborative Perinatal Study (Benson and co-workers, 1968). They analyzed perinatal outcomes in nearly 25,000 singleton pregnancies delivered between 1959 and 1965 at 15 institutions. Their purpose was to determine if auscultated fetal heart rate accurately defined perinatal risk. The auscultation protocol included measurement of fetal heart rate every 15 minutes during the first stage of labor and every 5 minutes during the second stage. Fetal heart rate was not measured during contractions or for 30 seconds thereafter. Only one to five fetal heart rate measurements were made in one third of pregnancies, and "variable periods of observation" (i.e., the protocol was not always followed) were described.

These investigators found that auscultated abnormal fetal heart rate was linked, albeit poorly, to low 5-minute Apgar scores (3 or less) and fetal and neonatal deaths. Abnormal fetal heart rate was not linked to abnormal neurological outcomes. The major difficulty with interpretation of auscultated fetal heart rate was the nonspecificity of an abnormal rate. Thus, this study did not prove auscultation ineffective in identifying compromised fetuses; rather, it showed that abnormal fetal heart rate was nonspecific because most infants were born in good condition. The group concluded: "Naivete and wishful thinking inspired our hope for a single rule-of-thumb estimate of fetal distress. Obviously, the problem is much too complex for such an easy appraisal." It was in this setting that the first commercial electronic fetal heart rate monitors became available in the United States in the late 1960s.

The first report to describe clinical application of electronic fetal monitoring in the United States was from Paul and Hon (1970). They described their experiences with electronic monitoring in 6 percent of 4561 deliveries at Yale–New Haven Hospital. Indications for monitoring included: abnormal fetal heart rate by auscultation, meconium, inadequate labor, ruptured membranes, and other complications such as hypertension or prolonged pregnancy. They compared these results with those from the Collaborative Perinatal Study and found no difference in the incidence of various Apgar scores. However, they concluded that electronic monitoring was beneficial in complicated pregnancies because of finding "a lesser number of depressed babies in the monitored group than might be expected."

By 1978 it was estimated that nearly two thirds of American women were being monitored electronically during labor (Banta and Thacker, 1979). Indeed, a 1976 survey of obstetricians showed that 77 percent believed all women in labor should receive such monitoring (Heldfond and co-workers, 1976). Thus when first introduced, electronic fetal heart rate monitoring was used primarily in complicated pregnancies, but gradually it came to be used in most pregnancies.

Internal Electronic Fetal Heart Rate Monitoring

The fetal heart rate may be measured by attaching a bipolar spiral electrode directly to the fetus (Fig. 15–1). The wire spiral electrode penetrates the fetal scalp and the second pole is the metal wing on the electrode panel. Vaginal body fluids create a saline electrical bridge that completes the circuit and permits measurement of the voltage differences between the two poles. The electrical fetal cardiac signal (P wave, QRS complex, and T wave) is amplified and fed into a cardio-

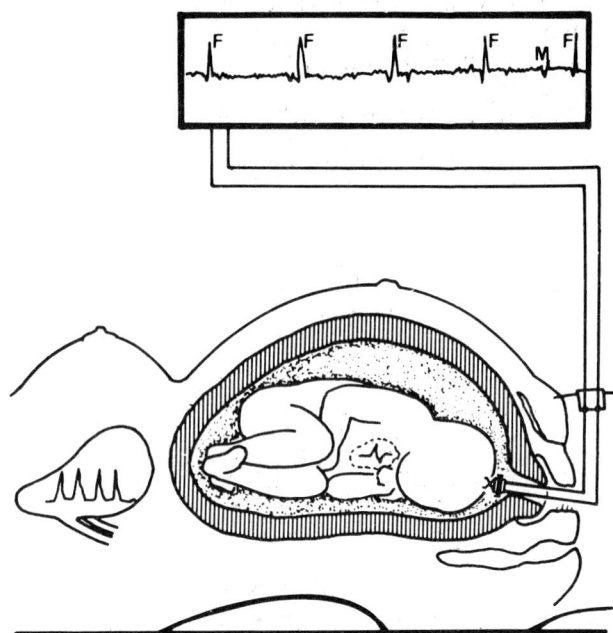

Fig. 15–1. Schematic representation of bipolar electrode attached to fetal scalp for detection of fetal QRS complexes (F). Also shown is the maternal heart and corresponding electrical complexes (M). (From Klavan and co-authors, 1977).

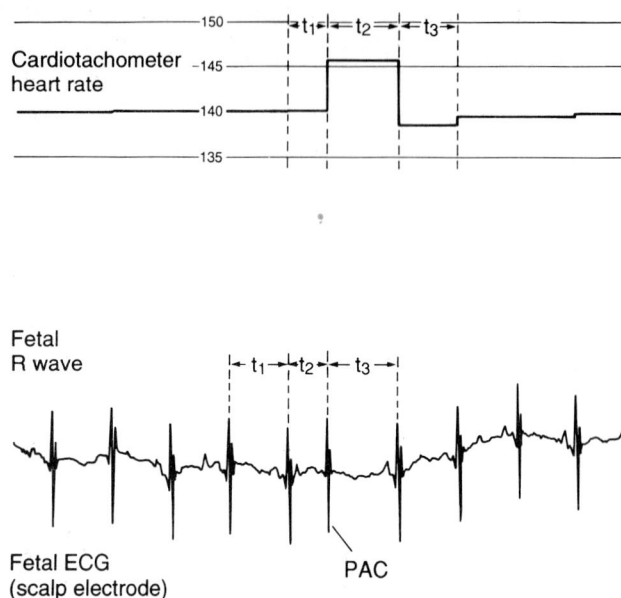

Fig. 15–2. Schematic representation of fetal electrocardiographic signals used to compute continuing beat-to-beat heart rate with scalp electrodes. Time intervals (t_1, t_2, t_3) in seconds between successive fetal R waves are used by cardiotachometer to compute instantaneous fetal heart rate. (PAC = premature atrial contraction.)

tachometer for heart rate calculation. The peak R-wave voltage is the portion of the fetal electrocardiogram most reliably detected. The two wires of the bipolar electrode are attached to a reference electrode on the maternal thigh to eliminate electrical interference. Shown in Figure 15–2 is an example of the method of fetal heart rate processing employed when a scalp electrode is used. Time (t) in milliseconds between fetal R waves is fed into a cardiotachometer where a new fetal heart rate is set with the arrival of each new R wave. As shown in Figure 15–2, a premature atrial contraction is computed as a heart rate acceleration because the interval (t_2) is shorter than the preceding one (t_1). The phenomena of continuous R wave to R wave fetal heart rate computation is known as "beat to beat" variability. However, the physiological event being counted is not a mechanical event corresponding to a heartbeat but rather an electrical event.

Electrical cardiac complexes detected by the fetal scalp electrode include those generated by the mother. The relative amplitude of maternal R waves is approximately one fifth those of the fetus, which vary between 50 and 100 microvolts (Freeman and co-authors, 1991). However, spontaneous variations in fetal R-wave amplitude are not rare during labor (Lee and Hon, 1965). These are likely due to frequent changes in fetal position, thus changing the fetal cardiac axis and corresponding electrical vectors (Roche and Hon, 1965). Although the maternal electrocardiogram (ECG) signal is approximately five times stronger than the fetal ECG,

its amplitude is diminished when it is recorded through the fetal scalp electrode. In a live fetus, this low maternal ECG signal is detected but masked by the "noise" of the fetal ECG. If the fetus is dead, the smaller maternal signal will be amplified by the automatic gain control circuitry in the fetal monitor and displayed as "fetal" heart rate (Freeman and co-authors, 1991).

Shown in Figure 15–3 are simultaneous recordings of maternal chest wall ECG signals and fetal scalp electrode ECG signals. This fetus is experiencing premature atrial contractions, which cause the cardiotachometer to rapidly and erratically seek new heart rates, resulting in the "spiking" of rate shown in the standard fetal monitor tracing. Occasionally, a similar fetal monitor tracing with spiking will occur due to voltage equality of maternal and fetal R-wave amplitude. In this circumstance maternal R waves are counted rather than the intended fetal complexes, and the cardiotachometer constantly seeks new rates of considerably different values.

Importantly, and as shown in Figure 15–4, when the fetus is dead, the maternal R waves are still detected by the scalp electrode and are counted by the cardiotachometer as the next best signal.

External (Indirect) Electronic Fetal Heart Rate Monitoring

The necessity for membrane rupture and uterine invasion may be avoided by use of external detectors to

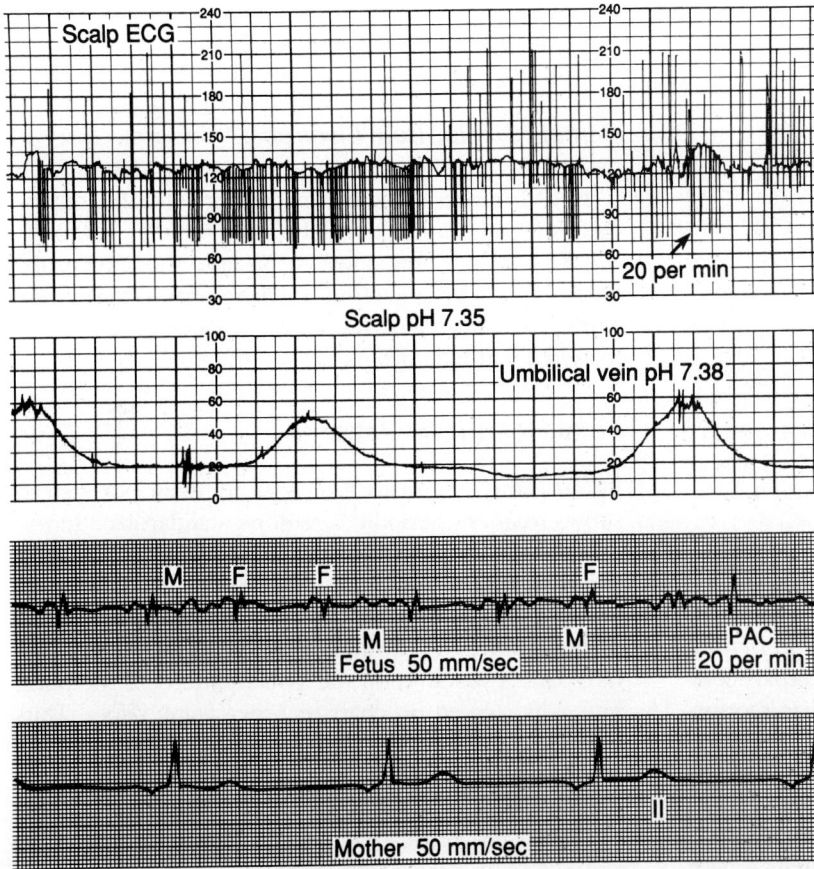

Fig. 15–3. Standard fetal monitor tracing of heart rate using fetal scalp electrode shown at top. Bottom two tracings represent cardiac electrical complexes detected from fetal scalp and maternal chest wall electrodes. Spiking of the fetal rate in the monitor tracing is due to the premature atrial contractions. (F = fetus; M = mother; PAC = fetal premature atrial contraction.)

monitor fetal heart action and uterine activity. External monitoring does not provide the precision of fetal heart measurement or the quantification of uterine pressure afforded by internal monitoring.

The fetal heart rate may be detected in a number of ways through the maternal abdominal wall. The easiest technique employs the *ultrasound Doppler principle*

(Fig. 15–5). Ultrasonic waves undergo a shift in frequency as they are reflected from moving fetal heart valves and from blood ejected in pulsatile fashion during systole. The unit consists of a transducer that emits ultrasound and a sensor to detect a shift in frequency of the reflected sound. The transducer is placed on the maternal abdomen at a site where fetal heart action is best

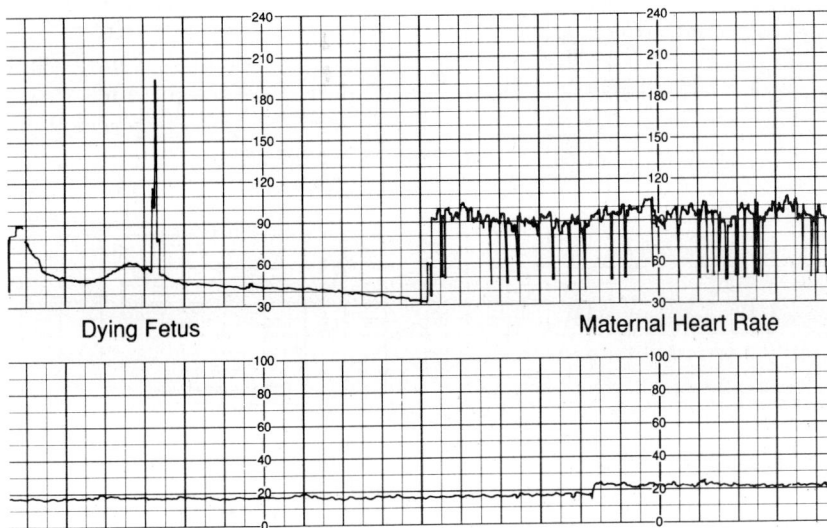

Fig. 15–4. Placental abruption: The fetal scalp electrode detected heart rate first of the dying fetus. After fetal death, maternal ECG complex is detected and recorded.

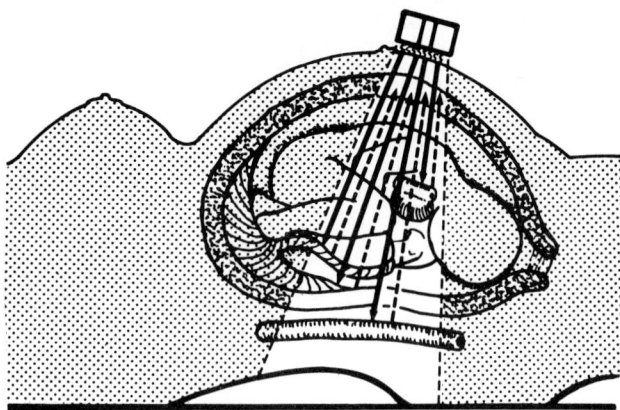

Fig. 15–5. Ultrasound Doppler principle used externally to measure fetal heart motions. Pulsations of the maternal aorta may also be detected and counted. (From Klavan and co-authors, 1977).

detected. A coupling gel must be applied because air conducts ultrasound poorly. The device is held in position by a belt. Care should be taken that maternal aortic pulsations are not confused with fetal cardiac motion.

Ultrasound Doppler signals are edited electronically before fetal heart rate data are printed onto the bedside monitor tracing paper. Reflected ultrasound signals from moving fetal heart valves are put through a microprocessor that compares incoming signals with the most recent previous signal. This process is called *autocorrelation* and is based on the premise that the fetal heart rate has regularity whereas "noise" is random and without regularity. Essentially, several fetal heart motions must be deemed electronically acceptable by

the microprocessor before the fetal heart rate is printed. Such electronic manipulation has greatly improved the tracing quality of externally recorded fetal heart rate.

Remote Display from Electronic Monitors. Observation of the fetal heart rate and uterine contraction patterns of laboring women by means of centrally located electronic display units has become popular. Although this enables one individual to observe these recorded functions at a distance from the laboring women, attendants must still regularly visit the bedside to determine maternal and fetal progress.

Fetal Heart Rate Patterns

Because the fetal heart rate is rarely fixed but instead shows frequent periodic variations, standardized terminology was proposed to more precisely describe both baseline activity and periodic variations from the baseline (Freeman and co-authors, 1991). It is important to recognize that interpretation of electronic fetal heart rate data is based upon the visual pattern of the heart rate as portrayed on chart recorder graph paper. Thus the choice of vertical and horizontal scaling directly affects the appearance of the fetal heart rate. Typical scaling factors employed in the United States are 30 beats/min per vertical cm (range 30 to 240 beats/min) and 3 cm/min chart recorder paper speed. For example (Figure 15–6), fetal heart rate variation is falsely displayed at the slower 1 cm/min paper speed when compared with the smoother baseline recorded at 3 cm/min. Thus, pattern recognition can be considerably distorted depending on the scaling factors used.

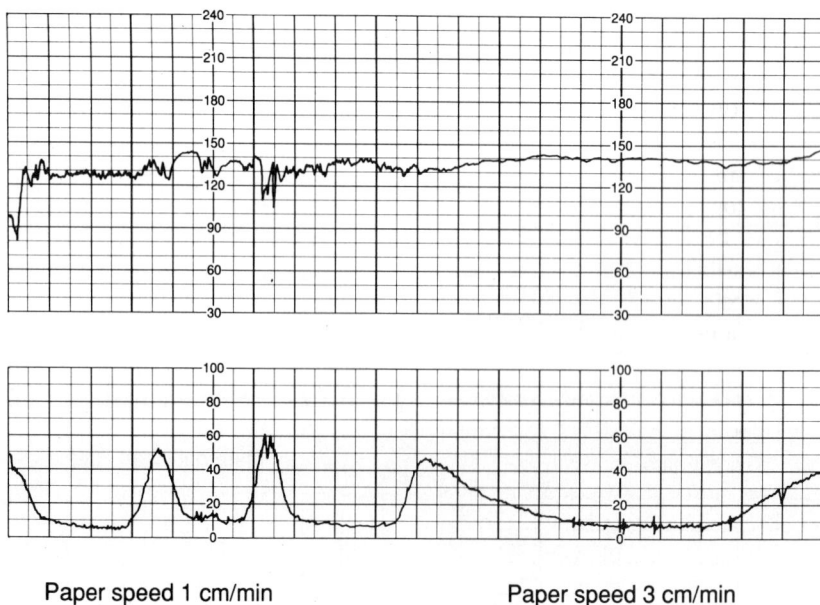

Fig. 15–6. Fetal heart rate obtained by a scalp electrode and recorded at 1 cm/min compared with 3 cm/min chart recorder paper speed.

Paper speed 1 cm/min   Paper speed 3 cm/min

Baseline Fetal Heart Activity. Baseline fetal heart activity refers to the modal characteristics that prevail apart from periodic accelerations or decelerations associated with uterine contractions. Descriptive characteristics of baseline fetal heart activity include *rate, beat-to-beat variability, fetal arrythmia,* and distinct patterns such as *sinusoidal* or *saltatory* fetal heart rates.

RATE. With increasing fetal maturation, the mean heart rate decreases. This continues postnatally such that the average rate is 90 beats/min by age 8 (Behrman, 1992). Pillai and James (1990) longitudinally studied fetal heart rate characteristics in 43 normal human pregnancies from 16 to 40 weeks' gestation. The baseline fetal heart rate decreased an average of 24 beats/min between 16 weeks and term, or approximately 1 beat/min per week. At 16 weeks the average baseline rate was about 160 beats/min, which decreased to 140 at 40 weeks. It is postulated that this normal gradual slowing of the fetal heart rate corresponds to maturation of parasympathetic (vagal) heart control (Renou and co-workers, 1969).

During the third trimester, the normal average baseline fetal heart rate is generally accepted to be between 120 and 160 beats/min. The average fetal heart rate is considered to be the result of tonic balance between *accelerator* and *decelerator* influences on pacemaker cells. In this concept, the sympathetic system is the accelerator influence, and the parasympathetic is the decelerator factor mediated via vagal slowing of heart rate (Dawes, 1985). Heart rate is also under the control of arterial chemoreceptors such that both hypoxia and hypercapnia can modulate rate. More severe and prolonged hypoxia with a rising blood lactate and severe metabolic acidemia, induces a prolonged fall of heart rate due to direct effects on the myocardium.

BRADYCARDIA. Bradycardia is a baseline fetal heart rate under 120 beats/min that lasts 15 minutes or longer (Freeman and co-authors, 1991). However, a rate between 100 and 119 beats/min, in the absence of other changes, is usually not considered to represent fetal compromise (American College of Obstetricians and Gynecologists, 1989). Such low but potentially normal baseline heart rates have also been attributed to head compression from occiput posterior or occiput transverse positions, particularly during second-stage labor (Young and Weinstein, 1976). Such mild bradycardias were observed in 2 percent of monitored pregnancies and averaged about 50 minutes in duration. Moderate bradycardias are defined as 80 to 100 beats/min, and severe bradycardias are less than 80 beats/min, for 3 minutes or longer (American College of Obstetricians and Gynecologists, 1989).

Mild bradycardia without deceleration or acceleration is not necessarily evidence for fetal compromise. Umbilical arterial blood acidemia (pH less than 7.2) was

identified by Gilstrap and co-workers (1987) in one third of 53 neonates with mild bradycardia of 90 to 119 beats/min during second-stage labor. None of these acidemic neonates required resuscitation. They also found umbilical arterial blood acidemia in 40 percent of 63 neonates with moderate to severe bradycardia defined as less than 90 beats/min.

Other causes of fetal bradycardia include congenital heart block and serious fetal compromise. Figure 15–7 depicts bradycardia in a fetus dying from placental abruption. Maternal hypothermia under general anesthesia for repair of a cerebral aneurysm or during maternal cardiopulmonary bypass for open-heart surgery can also cause fetal bradycardia (see Chap. 48, p. 1089). These infants are apparently not harmed by several hours of such bradycardia.

Other nonperiodic but sudden slowings of the fetal heart rate often are termed fetal "bradycardias." Instead, these are probably best considered *prolonged decelerations*, which are subsequently discussed. Some causes include uterine hyperactivity; paracervical or conduction analgesia; pelvic examination, presumably due to manual fetal head compression; cord prolapse; uterine rupture; placental abruption; maternal hypoperfusion (e.g., supine hypotension syndrome or hemorrhage due to trauma); and maternal hypoxia (e.g., eclampsia).

TACHYCARDIA. Tachycardia is considered *mild* if the baseline rate is between 161 and 180 beats/min and *severe* if 181 or more (American College of Obstetricians and Gynecologists, 1989). The most common explanation for fetal tachycardia is maternal fever from amnionitis, although fever from any source can increase baseline fetal heart rate. Such infections have also been observed

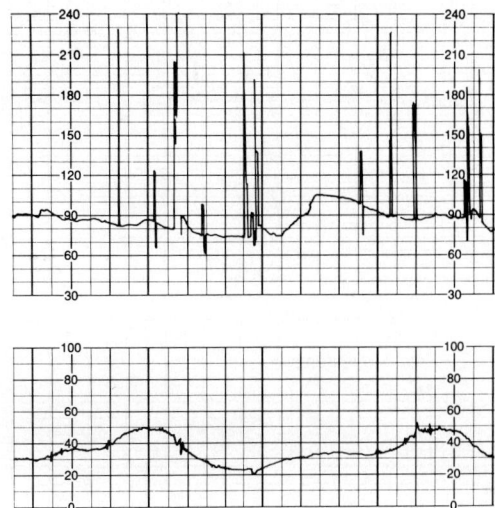

Fig. 15–7. Fetal bradycardia measured with a scalp electrode in a pregnancy complicated by placental abruption and subsequent fetal death.

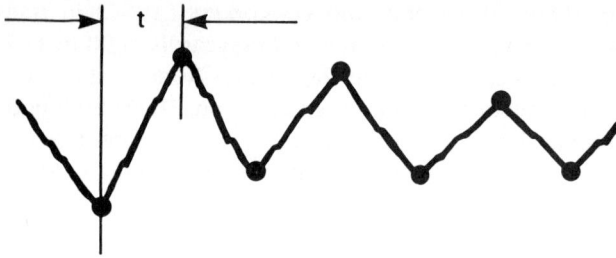

Fig. 15–8. Schematic representation of short-term beat-to-beat variability measured by a fetal scalp electrode. (t = time interval between successive fetal R waves.) (From Klavan and co-authors, 1977.)

to induce fetal tachycardia before overt maternal fever is diagnosed (Gilstrap and associates, 1987). Fetal tachycardia caused by maternal infection is typically not associated with fetal compromise unless there are associated periodic heart rate changes or fetal sepsis.

Other causes of fetal tachycardia include fetal compromise, cardiac arrhythmias, and administration of parasympathetic (e.g., atropine) or sympathomimetic (e.g., ritodrine hydrochloride) drugs to the mother. The key to fetal compromise in association with tachycardia seems to be concomitant heart rate decelerations. However, prompt relief of the compromising event, such as correction of maternal hypotension caused by epidural analgesia, can result in fetal recovery.

BEAT-TO-BEAT VARIABILITY. Baseline fetal heart rate variability is an important index of cardiovascular function and appears to be regulated largely by the autonomic

nervous system. The baseline rate normally exhibits an oscillating form, reflective of beat-to-beat changes in rate, which gives it varying degrees of irregularity or variability when printed on graph paper. Such deviations in heart rate are defined as baseline variability. Variability is further divided into *short term* and *long term*.

Short-term variability reflects the instantaneous change in fetal heart rate from one beat (or R wave) to the next. This variability is a measure of the time interval between cardiac systoles (Fig. 15–8). *It can most reliably be determined to be normally present only when electrocardiac cycles are measured directly with a scalp electrode.* External Doppler ultrasound recording methods can create artifactual "normal" variability. However, *absence* of variability (Fig. 15–9) during external Doppler fetal heart recording can suggest loss of beat-to-beat variability.

Long-term variability is used to describe the oscillatory changes that occur during the course of 1 minute and result in the waviness of the baseline (Fig. 15–10). The normal frequency of such waves is three to five cycles per min (Freeman and co-authors, 1991).

Decreased beat-to-beat variability is diagnosed when the fetal heart rate baseline is flat or nearly flat with absent short-term variability and fewer than two cyclic changes per minute of long-term variability (American College of Obstetricians and Gynecologists, 1989). It should be recognized, however, that precise quantitative analysis of both short- and long-term variability presents a number of frustrating problems due to technical and scaling factors. For example, Parer and co-workers (1985) evaluated 22 mathematical formulas designed to quantify heart rate variability and most were unsatisfactory. Consequently, most clinical interpretation is based on visual analysis with subjective judgement of the "smoothness" or "flatness" of the baseline.

Several physiological and pathological processes can affect or interfere with beat-to-beat variability. Dawes and co-workers (1981) described increased beat-to-beat variability during **fetal breathing.** In healthy infants, short-term variability is attributable to respiratory sinus arrhythmia (Divon and co-workers, 1986). Moreover, this respiratory variability can be reduced by asphyxia. **Fetal body movements** affect variability.

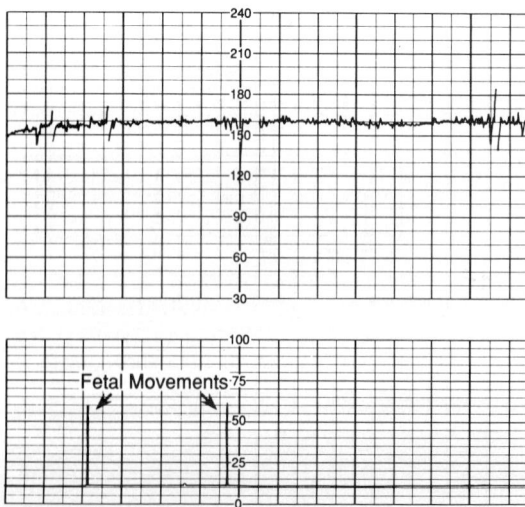

Fig. 15–9. External fetal heart rate recording obtained using Doppler technique and showing a "flat" baseline suggesting loss of beat-to-beat variability. No response to infrequent fetal movements was observed. This fetus was acidemic due to chronic placental insufficiency.

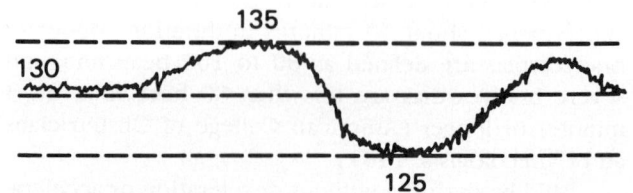

Fig. 15–10. Schematic representation of long-term beat-to-beat variability of the fetal heart rate ranging between 125 and 135 beats/min. (From Klavan and co-authors, 1977.)

Granat and co-investigators (1979) observed that fetuses exhibited 40- to 80-minute cycles of movements thought to correspond to fetal "wakefulness." Van Geijn and co-workers (1980) analyzed electroencephalographic data in healthy term infants and observed 30- to 70-minute sleep cycles corresponding to fetal physical inactivity. Pillai and James (1990) reported increased baseline variability with **advancing gestation.** Up to 30 weeks, baseline characteristics were similar during both fetal rest and activity. After 30 weeks, fetal inactivity was associated with diminished baseline variability and, conversely, variability was increased during fetal activity.

It is important to recognize that the baseline fetal heart rate becomes more physiologically "fixed" (i.e., less variable) as the rate increases. Conversely, there is more instability or variability of the baseline at lower heart rates. This phenomena presumably reflects less cardiovascular physiological wandering as beat-to-beat intervals shorten due to increasing heart rate. It is generally believed that all of these physiological processes modulate variability via the autonomic nervous system (Renou and co-workers, 1969). That is, sympathetic and parasympathetic control of the sinoatrial node mediates moment-to-moment or beat-to-beat oscillation of the baseline heart rate.

Diminished beat-to-beat variability can be an ominous sign indicating a seriously compromised fetus. Paul and co-workers (1975) reported that loss of variability in combination with decelerations was associated with fetal acidemia. They analyzed variability in the 20 minutes preceding delivery in 194 pregnancies. They defined decreased variability as 5 or fewer beats/min excursion of the baseline (Fig. 15–11), whereas acceptable variability exceeded this range. This definition apparently prevailed for both short- and long-term variability, because these two features were not distinguished. Fetal scalp pH was measured 1119 times in these pregnancies, and mean values were progressively more acidemic when decreased variability was added to progressively intense heart rate decelerations. For example, mean fetal scalp pH was about 7.10 when severe decelerations were combined with 5 beats/min or less variability, compared with a pH about 7.20 when greater variability was associated with similarly severe decelerations. Analysis of beat-to-beat variability independent of decelerations revealed slightly lower Apgar scores when variability was 5 or fewer beats/min. Indeed, diminished variability can be associated with severe fetal acidemia (Figure 15–12).

Severe **maternal acidemia** can also cause de-

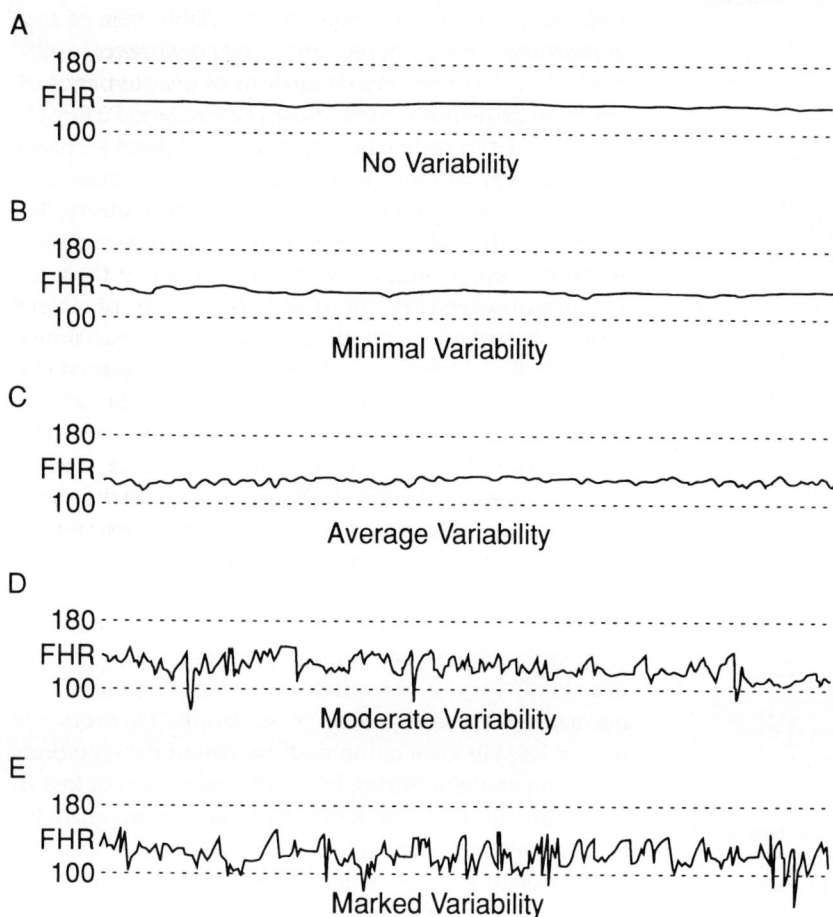

Fig. 15–11. Examples of baseline fetal heart rate variability. Panels A and B indicate *decreased* variability (5 beats/min or less), whereas average or acceptable variability is shown in panels C through D. (Redrawn from Paul and co-workers, 1975, with permission.)

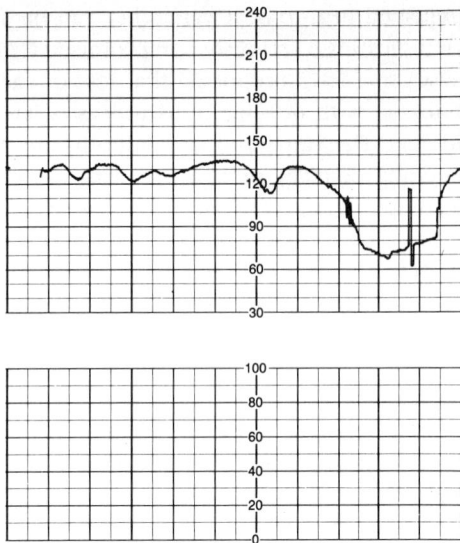

Fig. 15–12. Diminished short- and long-term variability (2 waves or less per minute) due to uterine rupture caused by a motor vehicle accident. Umbilical artery blood pH was 6.7 and the 1735-g infant succumbed despite emergency cesarean delivery.

creased fetal heart rate beat-to-beat variability, as shown in Figure 15–13 in a mother with diabetic ketoacidosis. The precise pathological mechanisms by which fetal hypoxemia results in diminished beat-to-beat variability is not understood totally.

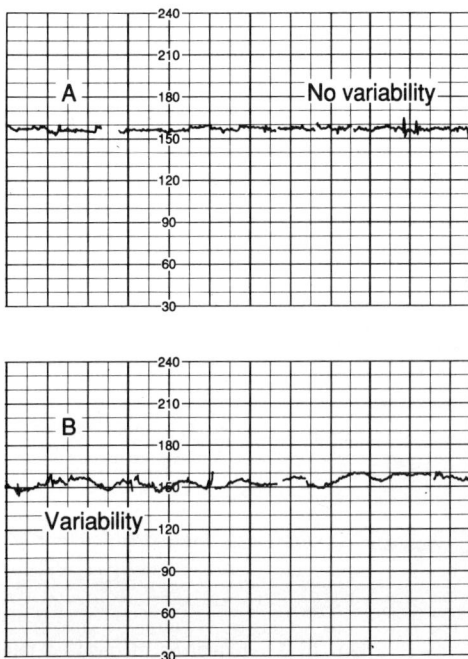

Fig. 15–13. A. External fetal heart recording showing diminished long-term variability at 31 weeks during maternal diabetic ketoacidosis (pH 7.09). **B.** Recovery of fetal long-term variability after correction of maternal acidemia.

Although loss of variability and its ominous significance, such as shown in Figure 15–12, are familiar to most obstetricians, mild degrees of fetal hypoxemia during human labor have been reported to *increase* variability, at least at the outset of the hypoxic episode (Huck and co-workers, 1977). According to Dawes (1985) it seems probable that the loss of variability (as shown in Fig. 15–12) is a result of metabolic acidemia that causes depression of the fetal brainstem or the heart itself. Thus, diminished beat-to-beat variability, when a reflection of compromised fetal condition, likely reflects acidemia rather than "hypoxia" per se.

A common cause of diminished beat-to-beat variability is analgesic drugs given during labor. A large variety of central nervous system depressant drugs can cause transient diminished beat-to-beat variability. Included are narcotics, barbiturates, phenothiazines (e.g., promethazine), tranquilizers (e.g., diazepam) and general anesthetics. Diminished beat-to-beat variability occurs regularly following meperidine administration, and the effects may last 30 to 45 minutes or longer depending on the route given. Reduced fetal heart rate variability has been reported when fentanyl was administered epidurally for labor analgesia (Viscomi and co-workers, 1990). Obviously, such drug-induced effects can greatly confuse interpretation of the fetal significance of diminished variability.

It is generally believed that reduced baseline heart rate variability is the single most reliable sign of fetal compromise. For example, Smith and co-workers (1988) performed a computerized analysis of beat-to-beat variability in growth-retarded fetuses before labor. They observed that diminished beat-to-beat variability (4.2 beats/min or less) that was maintained for 1 hour is diagnostic of developing acidemia and imminent fetal death. We have reported similar experiences (Leveno and co-workers, 1983). Snijders and colleagues (1992) more recently observed a relationship between significant fetal growth retardation and diminished baseline variability. They studied 13 fetuses over 25 days and observed that long-term fetal heart rate variation decreased gradually with time and fell below normal at about the same time decelerations due to placental insufficiency appeared.

In summary, beat-to-beat variability and its short- and long-term components are affected by a variety of physiological mechanisms. Fetal heart rate variability has considerably different meaning depending on the clinical setting. Prolonged loss of both short- and long-term variability before labor in growth-retarded fetuses can signify serious placental insufficiency. Similarly, abnormally decreased baseline oscillations (5 beats per min or less) in association with persistent decelerations is also meaningful during labor. Interpretation of loss of variability during labor in otherwise normal pregnancies is, however, seriously confused by a variety of fetal behavioral states, all of which are depressed by administration of many different drugs to the mother.

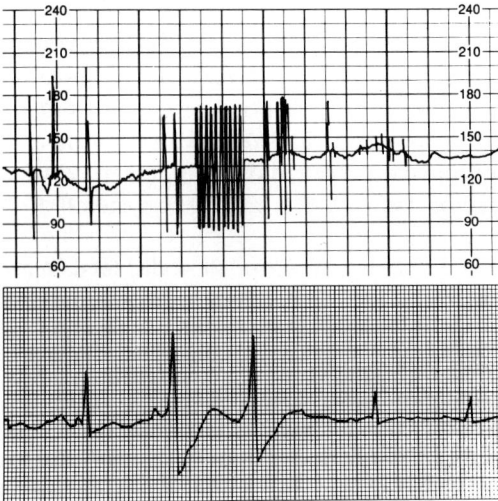

Fig. 15–14. Internal fetal monitoring at term showed occasional abrupt beat-to-beat fetal heart rate spiking due to erratic extrasystoles shown in the superimposed fetal electrocardiogram. The normal infant was delivered spontaneously and had a normal cardiac rhythm in the nursery.

CARDIAC ARRHYTHMIA. Young and co-workers (1979) reported the incidence of fetal cardiac arrhythmias to be 1 percent during electronically monitored labors. Of 15 cases diagnosed during 2 years, 13 were supraventricular and two were ventricular in origin. Southall and co-authors (1980) studied antepartum fetal cardiac rate and rhythm disturbances in 934 normal pregnancies between 30 and 40 weeks. Cardiac arrhythmias and episodes of bradycardia less than 100 beats/min, or tachycardia greater than 180 beats/min, occurred in 3 percent.

When fetal cardiac arrhythmias are first suspected using electronic monitoring, findings can include baseline bradycardia, tachycardia, or most commonly in our experience, abrupt baseline **spiking** (Fig. 15–14). Intermittent baseline bradycardia is frequently due to congenital heart block.

Documentation of an arrhythmia during electronic monitoring can only be accomplished, practically speaking, when scalp electrodes are used. Most fetal monitors can be adapted to output the scalp electrode signals into an electrocardiographic recorder. However, only a single ECG lead is obtained, thus severely restricting interpretation to analysis of rhythm and rate disturbances.

Gleicher and Elkayam (1990) reviewed the many supraventricular, nodal, and ventricular arrhythmias reported in fetuses. Most supraventricular arrhythmias are of little fetal significance during labor unless there is coexistent heart failure as evidenced by hydrops. Not uncommonly, most supraventricular arrhythmias disappear in the immediate neonatal period, although some are associated with structural cardiac defects. Maxwell and associates (1988) reported 23 fetuses with su-

praventricular arrhythmias diagnosed before labor; 12 had supraventricular tachycardia, 8 atrial flutter, and 3 a mixture of these two. No relation was found between the rate or type of arrythmia and fetal heart failure. Outcome for hydropic fetuses was dependent on maturity at delivery and in utero cardioversion by maternal administration of digoxin, verapamil, or both. Spontaneous delivery was not injurious to nonhydropic fetuses; most hydropic fetuses were either delivered electively by cesarean delivery or required abdominal delivery for fetal distress.

Other than ectopic systoles, which are as common in fetuses as in adults, ventricular arrhythmias are unusual in utero. As discussed in Chapter 54 (p. 1232), conduction defects, most commonly complete AV block, are usually found in association with connective-tissue diseases.

The clinical significance of intrapartum fetal arrhythmias continues to be a complex problem. Most arrhythmias are of little consequence during labor when there is no evidence for fetal hydrops. However, such arrhythmias impair interpretation of intrapartum heart rate tracings. Ultrasonic survey of fetal anatomy as well as echocardiography may be useful, particularly when the arrythmia is suspected antepartum. Some clinicians use fetal scalp sampling as an adjunct. Generally, in the absence of fetal hydrops, neonatal outcome is not measurably improved by pregnancy intervention. At Parkland Hospital, intrapartum fetal cardiac arrhythmias, especially in the presence of clear amnionic fluid, are managed conservatively.

SINUSOIDAL HEART RATES. The discovery of sinusoidal fetal heart rate is attributed to Kubli and co-workers (1972) and Manseau and colleagues (1972). A sinusoidal pattern is frequently observed in conjunction with serious fetal anemia (Fig. 15–15). Insignificant sinusoidal patterns have been reported following administration of meperidine, morphine, alphaprodine, and butorphanol

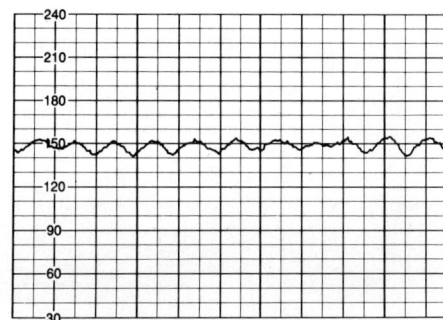

Fig. 15–15. Antepartum fetal heart tracing obtained using a Doppler transducer and showing a sinusoidal pattern that was intermittent. The fetus was severely anemic due to fetal–maternal hemorrhage as a consequence of maternal blunt abdominal trauma. Sine waves are occurring at a rate of 3 cycles/min.

(Angel, 1984; Egley, 1991; Epstein, 1982; Gray, 1978; and their associates). The pattern also has been described with fetal distress (Gal and co-workers, 1978), umbilical cord occlusion (Ayromlooi and co-workers, 1978–1979), and with amnionitis (Gleicher and co-workers, 1980).

Young and co-workers (1980c) and Johnson and colleagues (1981) concluded that intrapartum sinusoidal fetal heart patterns were not associated with fetal compromise. Modanlou and Freeman (1982), based on extensive review of the literature, proposed adoption of a strict definition: (1) stable baseline heart rate of 120 to 160 beats/min with regular oscillations, (2) amplitude of 5 to 15 beats/min (rarely greater), (3) frequency of 2 to 5 cycles/min long-term variability, (4) fixed or flat short-term variability, (5) oscillation of the sinusoidal waveform above or below a baseline, and (6) absence of accelerations. Although these criteria were selected to define a sinusoidal pattern that is most likely ominous, they observed that the pattern associated with alphaprodine is indistinguishable. Some have defined intrapartum sine-wavelike baseline variation with periods of acceleration as *pseudo-sinusoidal*. Murphy and co-workers (1991) reported that such patterns were identified in 15 percent of fetuses electronically monitored. Even using the stricter definition proposed above, Egley and associates (1991) observed a sinusoidal pattern in 4 percent of fetuses monitored during labor.

The case shown in Figure 15–15 is a sinusoidal pattern observed with fetal–maternal hemorrhage. Shown in Figure 15–16 is a sinusoidal pattern seen with maternal meperidine administration. An important difference between the two patterns is the frequency of sine waves. The frequency is 3 cycles/min with fetal anemia and 6 cycles/min when due to narcotics.

The pathophysiology of sinusoidal patterns is unclear. This is in part due to the various definitions. There seems to be general agreement that antepartum sine wave baseline undulation portends severe fetal anemia; however, few D-isoimmunized fetuses develop this pattern (Nicolaides, 1989). Moreover, the sinusoidal pattern has been reported to develop or disappear after fetal transfusion (Del Valle and associates, 1992; Lowe and co-workers, 1984). Murata and co-investigators (1985) found that interruption of the vagus nerve was required to produce sinusoidal patterns in fetal lambs. The sinusoidal heart rate did not appear to be under the influence of the α- or β-sympathetic systems.

Periodic Fetal Heart Rate. Periodic fetal heart rate refers to deviations from baseline that are related to uterine contractions. **Acceleration** refers to an increase in fetal heart rate above baseline and **deceleration** to a decrease below baseline rate. The most commonly used system in the United States is based on the *timing* of the deceleration in relation to contractions—thus, **early, late,** or **variable** in onset compared with the corresponding uterine contraction. The waveform of these decelerations is also significant for pattern recognition. In early and late decelerations, the slope of fetal heart rate change is gradual, resulting in a curvilinear and uniform or symmetrical waveform. With variable decelerations, the slope of fetal heart rate change is abrupt and erratic, giving the waveform a jagged appearance.

Another system now used less often for description of decelerations is based on the pathophysiological events considered most likely to cause the pattern. In this system, early decelerations are termed *head compression,* late decelerations are termed *uteroplacental insufficiency,* and variable decelerations become *cord compression patterns.* The nomenclature of type I (early), type II (late), and type III (variable) "dips" proposed by Caldeyro-Barcia and co-workers (1973) is not used as often in the United States.

ACCELERATIONS. An acceleration is an increase in the fetal heart rate of at least 15 beats/min, usually of 15 to 20 seconds duration (American College of Obstetricians and Gynecologists, 1989). According to Freeman and co-authors (1991), accelerations occur most commonly antepartum, in early labor, and in association with variable decelerations. Proposed explanations for intrapartum acceleration include fetal movement, stimulation by uterine contractions, umbilical cord occlusion, and fetal stimulation during pelvic examination. Fetal scalp blood sampling and acoustic stimulation both incite fetal heart rate acceleration (Clark and co-workers, 1982; Read and Miller, 1977). Finally, acceleration can also occur during labor without any apparent stimulus.

Accelerations seem to have the same physiological explanations as beat-to-beat variability in that they represent intact neurohormonal cardiovascular control mechanisms linked to fetal behavioral states. Krebs and co-workers (1982a) analyzed electronic heart rate tracings in nearly 2000 fetuses and found sporadic accelerations during labor in 99.8 percent. Accelerations during the first and/or last 30 minutes was a favorable sign for fetal well-being. However, the absence of fetal

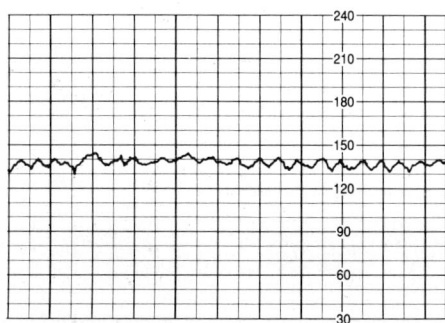

Fig. 15–16. Sinusoidal fetal heart rate pattern associated with maternal intravenous meperidine administration. Sine waves are occurring at a rate of 6 cycles/min.

heart accelerations during labor cannot be construed an unfavorable sign.

EARLY DECELERATION. *Early* deceleration of the fetal heart rate was first described by Hon (1958). He observed that there was a "drop" in heart rate with uterine contractions, and that this was related to cervical dilatation. He considered these physiological. Compressing the fetal head produced *variable* type decelerations in 18 of 19 attempts (Ball and Parer, 1992). Similar decelerations were elicited by locking of forceps and initiation of traction.

Freeman and co-authors (1991) defined early decelerations as those generally seen in active labor between 4 and 7 cm dilatation. In their definition, the degree of deceleration is generally proportional to the contraction strength and rarely falls below 100 to 110 beats/min or 20 to 30 beats/min below baseline. An example consistent with this definition is shown in Figure 15–17. Such decelerations are not typical of active labor and they are quite uncommon. They are not associated with baseline fetal heart rate changes. Importantly, early decelerations, as shown in Figure 15–17, are not associated with fetal hypoxia, acidemia, or low Apgar scores.

Ball and Parer (1992) provided an excellent review of the mechanisms responsible for fetal heart rate changes due to head compression. Head compression probably causes vagal nerve activation due to dural stimulation that mediates heart rate deceleration (Paul and co-workers, 1964). Ball and Parer (1992) concluded that fetal head compression is a likely cause not only for the decelerations shown in Figure 15–17, but also for those shown in Figure 15–18, which typically

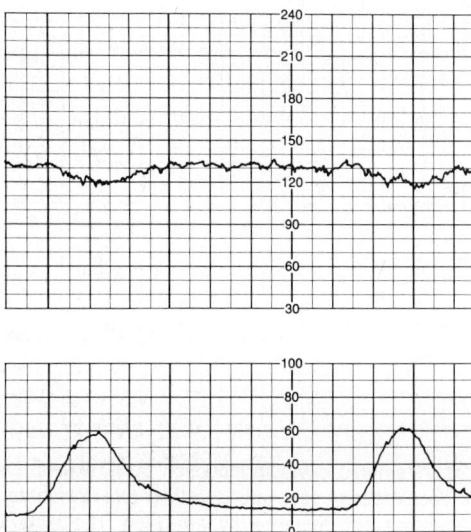

Fig. 15–18. Two different fetal heart rate patterns during second-stage labor that are likely both due to head compression. Maternal bearing down efforts correspond to the spikes with uterine contractions. Fetal heart rate deceleration C is consistent with the pattern of head compression shown in Figure 15–17. Deceleration B, however, is "variable" in appearance because of its jagged configuration, and may also represent cord occlusion.

occur during second-stage labor. Indeed, they observed that head compression is the likely cause of many variable decelerations (see subsequent discussion) classically attributed to cord occlusion. Sufficiently intense vagal stimulation-mediated fetal heart rate deceleration may result in decreased fetal cardiac output and umbilical blood flow leading to "variable" type patterns commonly seen just before delivery.

LATE DECELERATION. The fetal heart rate response to uterine contractions can be an index of either uterine perfusion or placental function. Because even normal uterine contractions interdict uteroplacental perfusion, it was anticipated very early in the history of electronic fetal monitoring that the stress of uterine contractions could become the basis for a clinical test for placental respiratory function. A late deceleration is a symmetrical decrease in fetal heart rate beginning at or after the peak of the contraction and returning to baseline only after the contraction has ended (American College of Obstetrics and Gynecologists, 1989). According to Freeman and co-authors (1991), late decelerations are uniform in shape and typically begin 30 seconds or more after the onset of the contraction. As shown in Figure 15–19, the nadir of deceleration is after the contraction acme, and the return to baseline is well after the contraction is over. **Descent and return of the fetal heart rate are gradual and smooth.** The magnitude of late decelerations reportedly is rarely more than 30 to 40 beats/min below baseline, and typically not more than

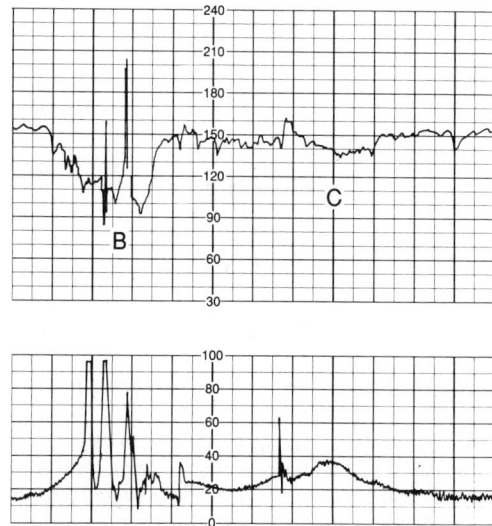

Fig. 15–17. Early fetal heart rate deceleration coinciding with spontaneous uterine contractions at 4 cm cervical dilatation. (Tracing courtesy of Scottie Brewster, RN.)

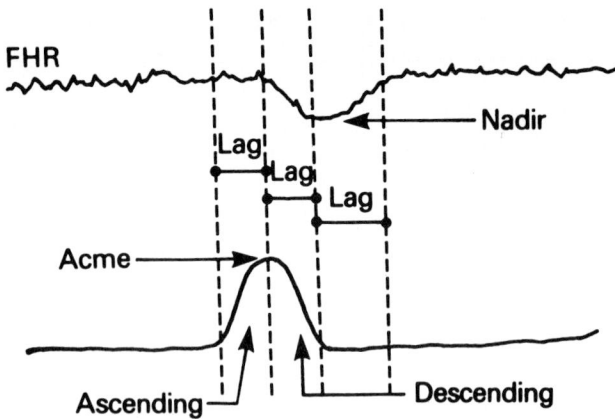

Fig. 15–19. Schematic representation of a late fetal heart rate deceleration related to a uterine contraction. Three different lag (or latency) periods that have been linked to fetal oxygenation are also shown. (From Klavan and co-authors, 1977.)

10 to 20 beats/min in intensity. Late decelerations are usually not accompanied by accelerations.

Myers and associates (1973) studied monkeys in which they compromised uteroplacental perfusion by lowering blood pressure in the maternal aorta. They showed that the time interval, or lag periods (Fig. 15–19), from the onset of a contraction to the onset of a late deceleration is directly related to basal fetal oxygenation. They demonstrated that the length of the lag phase was predictive of the fetal P_{O_2}, but not fetal pH. Both the slope and amplitude of deceleration correlated with fetal oxygen tension. Thus, late decelerations are dependent on fetal hypoxia already present prior to the stress of contractions. The lower the fetal P_{O_2} prior to contractions, the shorter the lag phase to onset of late decelerations. This lag period reflected the time necessary for the fetal P_{O_2} to fall below a critical level necessary to stimulate arterial chemoreceptors which mediated decelerations.

Murata and co-workers (1982) also showed that late deceleration was the first fetal heart rate consequence of uteroplacental induced hypoxia. During the course of progressive hypoxia that led to fetal death over 2 to 13 days, the fetuses invariably exhibited late decelerations before the development of acidemia. Variability of the baseline heart rate disappeared as acidemia developed.

The precise pathophysiological mechanisms whereby fetal hypoxia is translated into fetal heart rate effects is unclear. Harris and colleagues (1982) studied mechanisms of late decelerations in fetal lambs and concluded that there are two pathophysiological pathways: (1) chemoreceptor mediated vagal reflex and (2) hypoxic myocardial depression. They observed that it often is noticed clinically that sudden maternal hypotension or uterine hyperstimulation with oxytocin in a previously normal fetus results in late decelerations with retention

of beat-to-beat variability. They postulated that the chemoreceptor–vagal nerve reflex mechanism is involved in such circumstances. In contrast, with prolonged fetal hypoxia, late deceleration is mediated via direct myocardial depression. In the latter circumstance, baseline variability is absent.

The method for inducing uteroplacental insufficiency and late decelerations in animal experiments cited above was interference with maternal aortic blood flow. A similar mechanism of maternal hypoperfusion frequently leads to late decelerations when conduction analgesia is used during labor. Thomas (1975) observed late deceleration patterns in one fourth of normal laboring women given epidural analgesia. Such late decelerations are typically transient and are not considered harmful.

A large number of clinical circumstances can result in late decelerations. Generally, any process that causes maternal hypotension, excessive uterine activity, or placental dysfunction can induce late decelerations. The most common etiology is uterine hyperactivity due to oxytocin stimulation of labor. Maternal diseases such as hypertension (Fig. 15–20), diabetes, and collagen–vascular disorders can cause chronic placental dysfunction. A rare cause is severe chronic maternal anemia without hypovolemia. Placental abruption can cause acute and severe late decelerations (Fig. 15–21).

VARIABLE DECELERATIONS. The most common deceleration patterns encountered during labor are variable decelerations attributed to umbilical cord occlusion. Release of

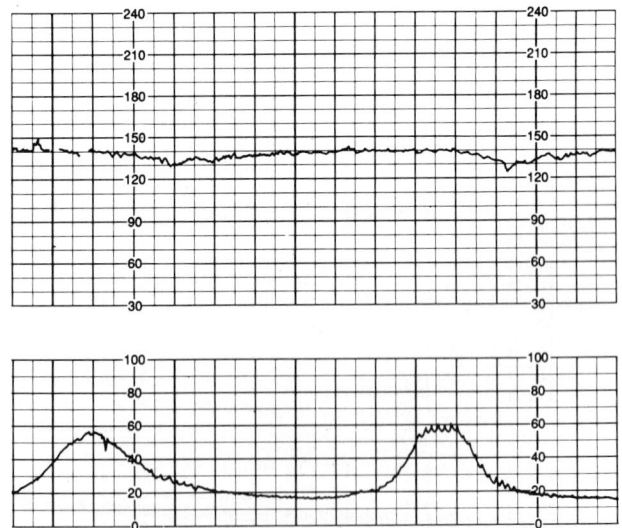

Fig. 15–20. Attempted oxytocin induction at 38 weeks. Late fetal heart rate decelerations seen are due to chronic placental insufficiency associated with maternal hypertension. The fetus was severely growth retarded. Milder contractions did not elicit late decelerations compared with more intense contractions. The fetus was delivered by cesarean section and was hypoxic and acidemic at birth.

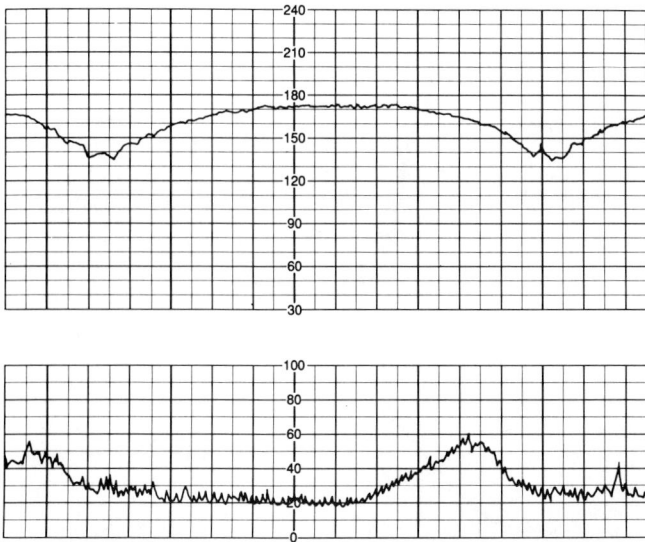

Fig. 15–21. Late decelerations due to uteroplacental insufficiency resulting from placental abruption. Immediate cesarean delivery was performed. Umbilical artery pH was 7.05 and the PO_2 was 11 mm Hg.

amnionic fluid and fetal descent during parturition are conducive to umbilical cord entrapment. A third of fetuses have one or more loops of cord wound around the neck. Similarly, short—less than 35 cm—and long—more than 80 cm—cords are found in 6 percent of

births and are associated with variable decelerations (Rayburn and associates, 1981). Melchior and Bernard (1985) identified variable decelerations in 40 percent of over 7000 monitor tracings when labor had progressed to 5 cm dilatation and in 83 percent by the end of the first stage.

Very early in the development of electronic monitoring, Hon (1959) tested the effects of umbilical cord compression on fetal heart rate (Fig. 15–22). Similar complete occlusion of the umbilical cord in experimental animals produces abrupt, jagged-appearing deceleration of the fetal heart rate (Fig. 15–23). Concomitantly, fetal aortic pressure increases. Itskovitz and co-workers (1983) observed that variable decelerations in fetal lambs occurred only after umbilical blood flow was reduced by at least 50 percent.

Two types of variable decelerations are shown in Figure 15–24. The deceleration denoted by "A" is very much like that seen with complete umbilical cord occlusion in experimental animals (Fig. 15–23). However, deceleration "B" has a different configuration because of the "shoulders" of acceleration before and after the deceleration component. Lee and co-workers (1975) pro-

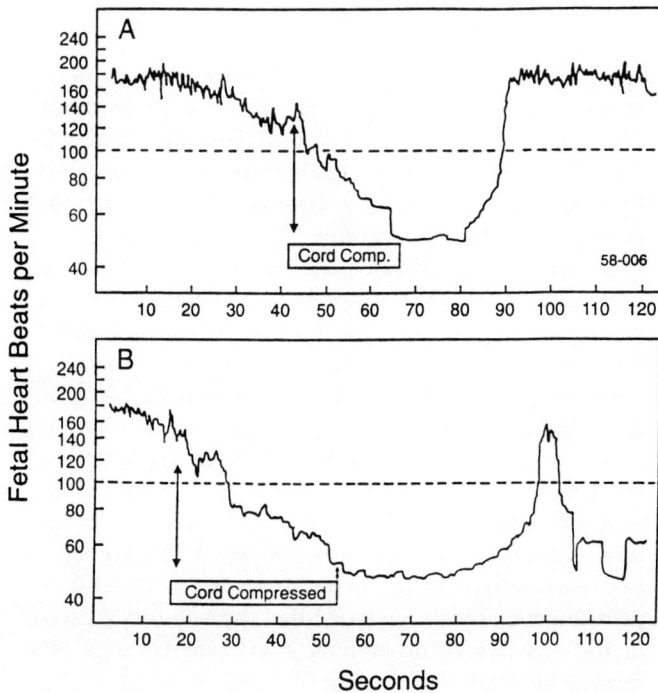

Fig. 15–22. Fetal heart rate effects of manual compression of a prolapsed umbilical cord in a 25-week footling breech. **A** shows the effects of 25-sec compression compared with 40 sec in **B**. (Redrawn from Hon, 1959, with permission.)

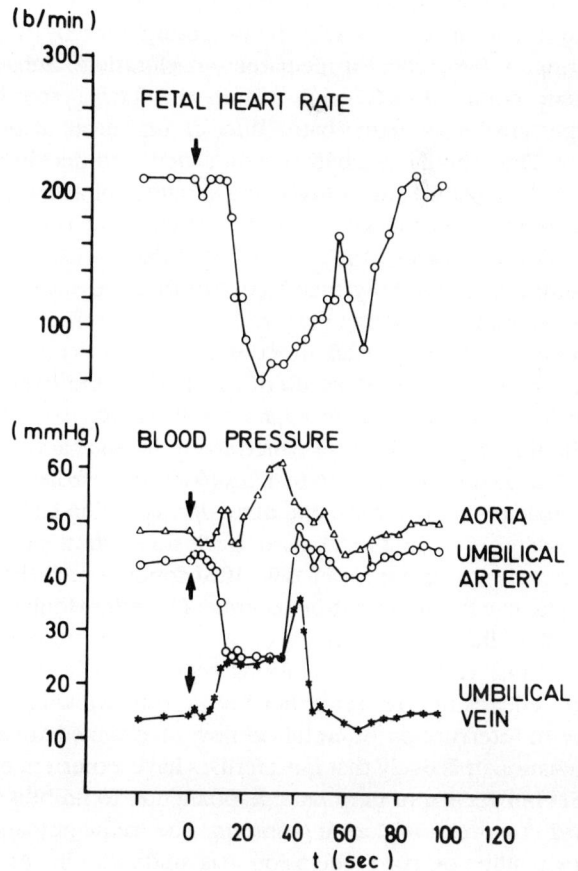

Fig. 15–23. Total umbilical cord occlusion (*arrow*) in the sheep fetus is accompanied by increase in fetal aortic blood pressure. Blood pressure changes in the umbilical vessels are also shown. (From Kunzel, 1985, with permission.)

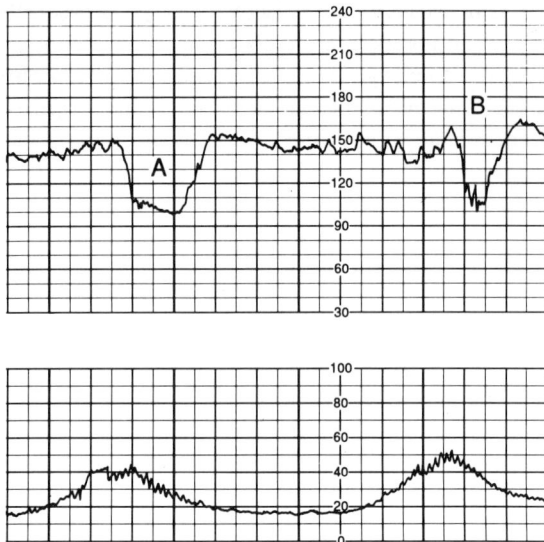

Fig. 15–24. Varying (variable) fetal heart rate decelerations. Deceleration **B** exhibits "shoulders" of acceleration compared with deceleration **A.**

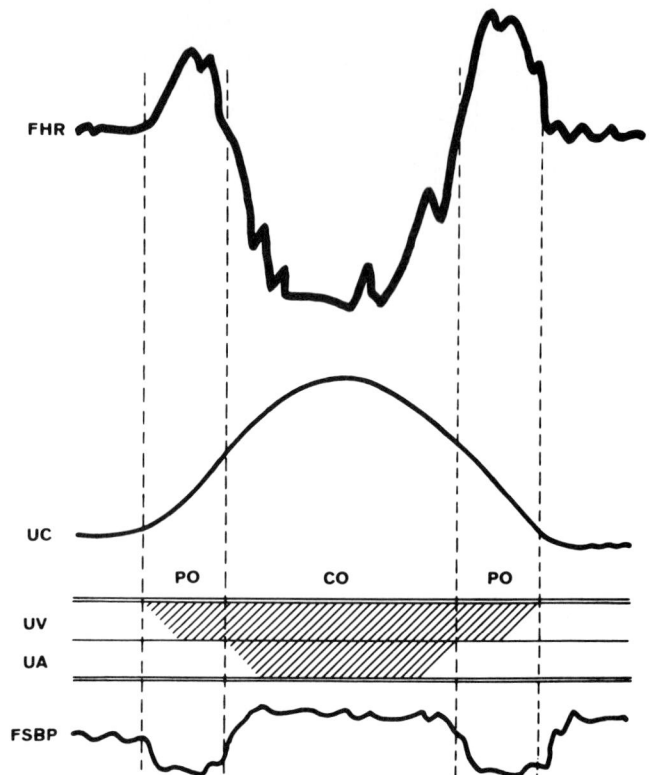

Fig. 15–25. Schematic representation of the fetal heart rate (FHR) effects of partial occlusion (PO) and complete occlusion (CO) of the umbilical cord. (UC = uterine contraction; UV = umbilical vein; UA = umbilical artery; FSBP = fetal systemic blood pressure.) (From Lee and co-authors, 1975.)

posed that the variation of variable decelerations was caused by differing degrees of partial cord occlusion. In this physiological scheme (Figure 15–25), occlusion of only the vein reduces fetal blood return thereby triggering a baroreceptor-mediated acceleration. Subsequent complete occlusion results in fetal systemic hypertension due to obstruction of umbilical artery flow. This stimulates a baroreceptor-mediated deceleration. Presumably, the aftercoming shoulder of acceleration represents the same events occurring in reverse.

Ball and Parer (1992) concluded that variable decelerations are vagally mediated and that the vagal response may be due to chemoreceptor or baroreceptor activity or both. Partial or complete cord occlusion (baroreceptor) produces afterload increase and hypertension and decreases in fetal arterial oxygen content (chemoreceptor), both of which result in vagal activity leading to deceleration. In fetal monkeys the baroreceptor reflexes appear to be operative during the first 15 to 20 seconds of umbilical cord occlusion followed by decline in Po_2 at approximately 30 seconds, which then serves as a chemoreceptor stimulus (Mueller-Heubach and Battelli, 1982).

Thus, variable decelerations represent fetal heart rate reflexes that reflect either blood pressure changes due to interruption of umbilical flow or changes in oxygenation. It is likely that most fetuses have experienced brief but recurrent periods of hypoxia due to umbilical cord compression during gestation. The frequency and inevitability of cord occlusion has undoubtedly provided the fetus with these physiological mechanisms as a means of coping. Hence, we have elected to term these reflexes "physiological" rather than pathophysiological. The great dilemma for the obstetrician in man-

aging variable fetal heart rate decelerations is determining when variable decelerations are pathological. The American College of Obstetricians and Gynecologists (1989) has defined **significant** variable decelerations as those decreasing to less than 70 beats/min and lasting more than 60 seconds.

Other fetal heart rate patterns have been associated with umbilical cord compression. **Saltatory** baseline heart rate (Fig. 15–26) was first described by Hammacher and co-workers (1968) and linked to umbilical cord complications during labor. The pattern is considered due to rapidly recurring couplets of acceleration and deceleration causing relatively large oscillations of the baseline fetal heart rate. We also observed a relationship between cord occlusion and the saltatory pattern (Leveno and associates, 1984). Although Cibils (1978) reported these to be associated with fetal depression, we are unconvinced that the saltatory pattern, in the absence of other fetal heart rate findings, is a marker for fetal compromise.

Goldkrand and Speichinger (1975) described a **mixed cord compression** pattern consisting of an acceleration immediately followed by a deceleration associated with abnormal cord positions at delivery. Aladjem

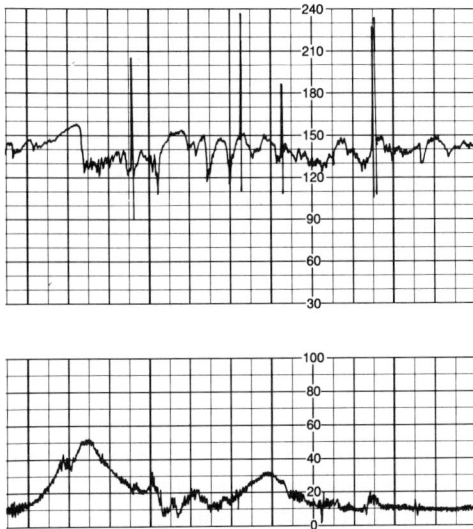

Fig. 15–26. Saltatory fetal heart rate baseline showing rapidly recurring couplets of acceleration combined with deceleration.

and associates (1977) subsequently termed this acceleration–deceleration combination the **lambda** pattern and attributed it to fetal movement (Fig. 15–27). Brubaker and Garite (1988) identified the lambda pattern in 4 percent of labors and concluded that it was not associated with adverse outcomes. The pattern shown in Figure 15–27 also could be interpreted to represent slow or delayed return of a variable deceleration to baseline. Some investigators have concluded such slow recovery is indicative of fetal compromise (Cibils, 1978; Young and associates, 1980b).

PROLONGED DECELERATION. Prolonged decelerations (Fig. 15–28) are defined as isolated decelerations lasting more than 60 to 90 seconds (Freeman and co-authors, 1991). However, this description does not define the maximum duration. Put another way, when does a prolonged deceleration cease being a periodic heart rate change and become a rate bradycardia? Because baseline rate refers to a baseline lasting 15 minutes or longer (see page 399), then prolonged decelerations, would be those lasting more than 60 and 90 seconds and less than 15 minutes. Their incidence during first-stage labor is unclear; however, Melchior and Bernard (1985) described them in approximately one third of second-stage labors. The significance of the amplitude of prolonged decelerations is also unclear; presumably, guidelines for interpretation of baseline bradycardias should prevail.

Prolonged decelerations are difficult to interpret because they are seen in many different clinical situations. Tejani and associates (1975) reported that some of the more common causes included cervical examination, uterine hyperactivity, cord entanglement, and maternal supine hypotension. The longest prolonged deceleration in this study was 12 minutes. Only one of the fetuses was mildly acidemic (pH 7.18) measured by scalp sampling 20 minutes following recovery from the prolonged deceleration. They concluded that prolonged decelerations are temporary and are typically followed by fetal recovery.

Other causes of prolonged deceleration include epidural, spinal, or paracervical analgesia; maternal hypoperfusion or hypoxia due to any cause; placental abruption; umbilical cord knots or prolapse; maternal

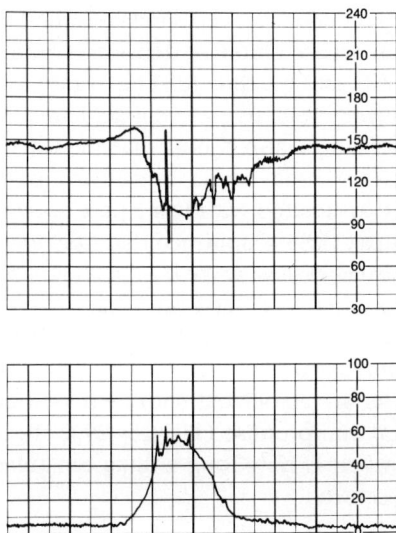

Fig. 15–27. Cord occlusion causing "lambda" fetal heart rate pattern of acceleration immediately followed by deceleration with slow recovery.

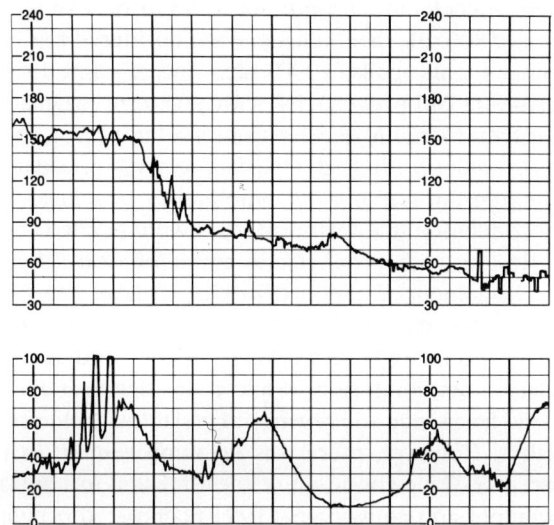

Fig. 15–28. Prolonged fetal heart rate deceleration due to uterine hyperactivity. Approximately 3 minutes are shown, but the fetal heart rate returned to normal after uterine hypertonus resolved. Vaginal delivery later ensued.

seizures including eclampsia and epilepsy; application of a fetal scalp electrode; impending birth; or even maternal valsalva maneuver.

Freeman and co-authors (1991) have observed that the placenta is very effective in resuscitating the fetus if the original insult does not recur immediately. Occasionally, such self-limited prolonged decelerations are followed by loss of beat-to-beat variability, baseline tachycardia, and even a period of late decelerations; all which resolve as the fetus recovers. Freeman and co-authors (1991) emphasize rightfully that the fetus may die during prolonged decelerations. Thus, management of prolonged decelerations can be extremely tenuous. Management of isolated prolonged decelerations is based on bedside clinical judgment, which will inevitably be imperfect given the unpredictability of these decelerations. Similarly, harsh "morning after" criticisms of such clinical judgments are frequently inappropriate.

Amnioinfusion. Gabbe and co-workers (1976) showed in monkeys that removal of amnionic fluid produced variable decelerations and that replenishment of fluid with saline relieved the decelerations. Miyazaki and Taylor (1983) infused saline through the intrauterine pressure catheter in laboring women who had either variable decelerations or prolonged decelerations attributed to cord entrapment. They found that such therapy improved the heart rate pattern in half. Miyazaki and Nevarez (1985) subsequently randomized 96 pregnancies and found that nulliparous women in labor with cord compression patterns who were treated with amnioinfusion less often required cesarean delivery for fetal distress. One infant was born depressed after cord prolapse 2 hours after successful amnioinfusion. Room temperature saline was infused by gravity at 15 to 20 mL/min. If variable decelerations were not relieved by a single infusion of 800 mL, then infusion was considered a failure. Owen and colleagues (1990) randomized saline amnioinfusion in 100 pregnancies with postterm pregnancy, intrapartum variable decelerations, preterm labor, or oligohydramnios with suspected fetal growth retardation. Amnioinfusion was not overwhelmingly beneficial, and they concluded that further studies were needed.

Results with prophylactic amnioinfusion—that is, for management of oligohydramnios without heart rate patterns due to umbilical cord occlusion—have been mixed. Nageotte and co-workers (1991) found that prophylactic amnioinfusion resulted in significantly decreased frequency and severity of variable decelerations in labor. However, there was no improvement in the cesarean rate or condition of term infants. In contrast, Schrimmer and co-workers (1991) compared pregnancies with oligohydramnios treated with about 500 mL of saline amnioinfusion with untreated controls. Sonography was used to estimate amnionic fluid volume after amnioinfusion. In 175 treated women, amnioinfusion was associated with a reduction in the rate of cesarean

delivery for fetal distress from 19 percent to 4 percent compared with 130 untreated women. Infant outcome, measured by umbilical artery blood pH and Apgar scores, likewise was improved significantly.

Amnioinfusion may produce uterine overdistension with adverse fetal effects. Tabor and Maier (1987) and Posner and co-workers (1990) described elevated intrauterine pressures leading to abnormal heart rate patterns. In one instance, baseline uterine pressure increased from about 5 mm Hg to almost 35 mm Hg during amnioinfusion; the fetus responded with a sustained heart rate deceleration.

Second-stage Labor Fetal Heart Rate Patterns. Melchior and Bernard (1985) reported that only 1.4 percent of over 7000 deliveries *did not* have fetal heart rate decelerations during second-stage labor. Both cord compression and fetal head compression have been implicated to cause decelerations and baseline bradycardia during second-stage labor. The high incidence of such patterns minimized their potential significance during early development of electronic monitoring. For example, Boehm (1975) described profound, prolonged fetal heart rate deceleration in the 10 minutes preceding vaginal delivery of 18 healthy infants. Subsequently, Herbert and Boehm (1981) reported another 18 pregnancies with similar prolonged decelerations during second-stage labor, but now associated with one stillbirth and one neonatal death. These experiences attest to the unpredictability of second-stage labor fetal heart rate.

Picquard and co-workers (1988) analyzed heart rate patterns during second-stage labor in 234 women in an attempt to identify specific patterns to diagnose fetal compromise. Fetal scalp blood was obtained for pH, lactic acid, and PCO_2 determinations at the beginning of the second stage, and similar studies were done on umbilical artery blood at delivery. Loss of beat-to-beat variability and baseline fetal heart rate less than 90 beats/min were predictive of fetal acidemia. Krebs and co-workers (1981) also found that persistent or progressive baseline bradycardia, as well as baseline tachycardia, were associated with low Apgar scores. Gilstrap and associates (1984) confirmed that baseline bradycardia, tachycardia, or absent beat-to-beat variability were somewhat predictive of fetal acidemia.

Thus, abnormal baseline heart rate, absent beat-to-beat variability, or both, in the presence of second-stage decelerations, are associated with increased but not inevitable fetal compromise (Fig. 15–29). The unknown factor, however, is how long a fetus can tolerate such heart rate patterns.

Fetal Scalp Blood Sampling

Measurements of the pH of appropriately collected capillary blood may help to identify the fetus in serious

Second Stage

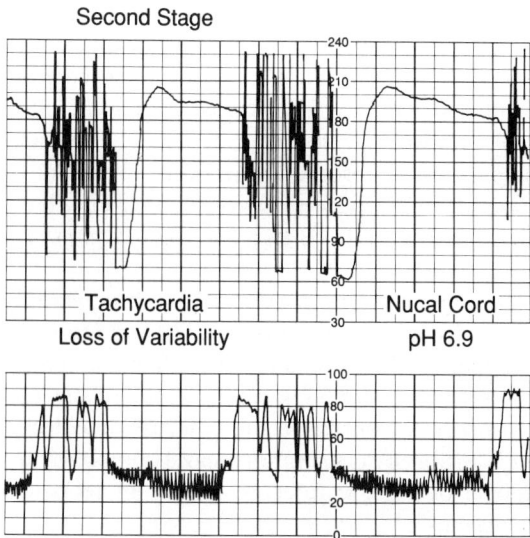

Fig. 15–29. Cord compression fetal heart rate decelerations in second-stage labor associated with tachycardia and loss of variability. The umbilical cord arterial pH was 6.9.

distress. A suitably illuminated endoscope is inserted through the sufficiently dilated cervix and ruptured membranes so as to press firmly against fetal skin, usually the scalp (Fig. 15–30). The skin is wiped clean with a cotton swab and coated with a silicone gel to cause the blood to accumulate as discrete globules. An incision is made through the skin to a 2 mm depth with a special blade on an appropriately long handle. As a drop of blood forms on the surface, it is immediately collected into a heparinized glass capillary tube and the pH of the blood is promptly measured.

The pH of fetal capillary blood is usually lower than arterial blood and approaches that of venous blood. Saling (1964) initially proposed a pH of 7.2 as the critical value for identification of serious fetal distress, while Mann (1978) and some others recommended immediate delivery whenever scalp blood pH was 7.25 or less. Zalar and Quilligan (1979) recommended the following protocol to try to confirm fetal distress: If the pH is greater than 7.25, labor is observed. If the pH is between 7.20 and 7.25, the pH measurement is repeated within 30 minutes. If the pH is less than 7.20, another scalp blood sample is collected immediately and the mother is taken to an operating room and prepared for surgery. Delivery is performed promptly if the low pH is confirmed. Otherwise, labor is allowed to continue and scalp blood samples are repeated periodically. The only benefits reported for scalp pH testing were estimates of fewer cesarean deliveries for fetal distress (Young and co-workers, 1980a).

Adhering too closely to a critical pH value in actual practice may prove disadvantageous, because it will tend to allay suspicion of early hypoxic acidosis. A fall in pH is a relatively late effect of hypoxia, and when samples of fetal blood are obtained intermittently, detection of hypoxia of rapid onset may be unduly delayed. It must also be kept in mind that the pH of fetal capillary blood need not accurately reflect the degree of fetal hypoxia, because the pH will be appreciably influenced by that of the mother. The severely hypoxic fetus becomes overtly acidotic, which is reflected by a low blood pH except when the mother is alkalotic—for example, from hyperventilation. Conversely, the fetus may have a low blood pH without being remarkably hypoxic if the mother is acidotic—for example, following a seizure. Bowen and co-authors (1986) have reviewed maternal-fetal pH interrelationships.

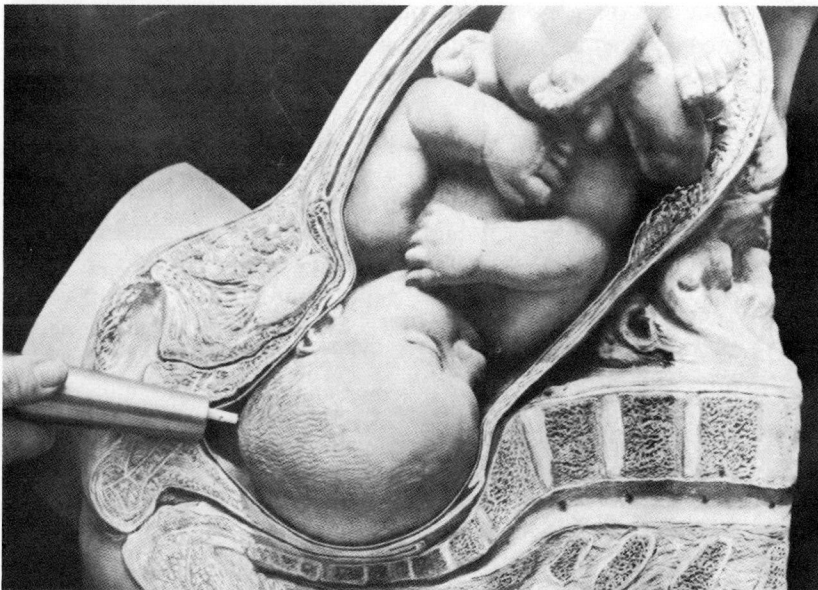

Fig. 15–30. The technique of fetal scalp sampling utilizing an amnioscope. The end of the endoscope is displaced from the fetal vertex approximately 2 cm to show disposable blade against the fetal scalp before incision. (From Hamilton and McKeown, 1974.)

Clark and Paul (1985) maintain that although fetal scalp sampling remains a valuable clinical tool in select cases, the technique should be deemphasized in clinical practice. They believe that the clinician can detect fetal distress without scalp blood sampling.

Scalp Stimulation. Clark and associates (1984) have suggested that scalp stimulation is an alternative to scalp blood sampling. An Allis clamp was used to pinch the fetal scalp just prior to obtaining scalp blood for pH measurement. Acceleration of the heart rate in response to pinching was invariably associated with a normal scalp blood pH. Conversely, failure to provoke acceleration was not uniformly predictive of fetal acidemia. Fetal heart rate acceleration in response to vibroacoustic stimulation has also been recommended as a substitute for scalp sampling by some (Edersheim and colleagues, 1987). Richards and associates (1988), however, reported that the vibroacoustic startle stimulus provoked variable fetal heart rate decelerations in 19 pregnancies and prolonged decelerations in 2 cases.

Complications from Electronic and Physicochemical Monitoring

There are potential dangers inherent in monitoring the fetal heart rate by direct application of a fetal electrode, measuring uterine pressure by an indwelling uterine catheter, or incising the fetal scalp to measure blood pH. A strong orientation toward universal use of internal monitoring is likely to predispose to *early amniotomy* and its potential dangers, including cord prolapse, infection, and possibly more cord compression because of less amnionic fluid. Studies performed in late gestation in monkeys by Gabbe and associates (1976), and similar studies in sheep, serve to reemphasize the protective cushion against cord compression provided by amnionic fluid. Acute reduction of amnionic fluid volume led to variable decelerations and fluid restoration eliminated the abnormal pattern.

Injury to the fetal scalp by the electrode is rarely a major problem, although application at some other site (for example, the eye in case of a face presentation), can prove serious. A fetal vessel in the placenta may be ruptured by catheter placement. Trudinger and Pryse-Davies (1978) observed four such accidents, two of which led to perinatal death from exsanguination. They also identified one instance of severe cord compression from entanglement with the catheter. Penetration of the placenta causing hemorrhage and uterine perforation during catheter insertion has led to serious morbidity, as well as spurious recordings that resulted in inappropriate management.

Both the fetus and the mother may be at increased risk of *infection* as the consequence of internal monitoring. Scalp wounds from the electrode may become infected by organisms of the vaginal flora. McGregor and McFarren (1989) have reviewed scalp electrode site infections and described a case of cranial osteomyelitis. A modest increase in maternal infections following internal monitoring has been reported. Faro and associates (1990) observed puerperal infection to be increased from 12 percent in women externally monitored compared with 18 percent when an internal apparatus was used.

Although external monitoring techniques obviate the necessity of ruptured membranes and uterine invasion, as well as direct fetal trauma, their use commonly results in the mother lying supine much of the time so as to protect placement of the external detectors. The supine position, by causing aortocaval compression, may be deleterious if the fetus is already in jeopardy for other reasons.

Three troublesome complications resulting from fetal scalp blood sampling are infection, blade breakage, and bleeding. If vaginal bleeding is encountered at any time following scalp blood sampling, fetal bleeding must be ruled out. Marked deficiencies of vitamin K-dependent coagulation factors have been implicated in the genesis of such hemorrhage in some infants, and hemophilia has subsequently been diagnosed in a few others (Hull, 1972). Negative pressure from use of a vacuum extractor to effect delivery after scalp blood sampling may incite troublesome hemorrhage.

Fetal Heart Rate Patterns and Brain Damage. Despite more than 30 years of research into electronic fetal monitoring, there have been remarkably few claims in the medical literature linking fetal heart rate patterns to brain damage. Clark and Paul (1986) cited a report by Painter and co-workers (1978) as the only extensive investigation that showed a correlation between fetal heart rate patterns and neurological performance at 1 year. They identified 38 term infants with the "most ominous" intrapartum fetal heart patterns and compared neurological outcomes with those of 12 normal births. Severe variable and late deceleration patterns were present in 60 percent of these ominous tracings. The remainder were less intense variable decelerations. At 1 year, hypotonia of the lower extremities was observed in 23 infants with ominous intrapartum fetal heart rate patterns. The authors concluded that such hypotonia was consistent with prolonged partial asphyxia. Subsequent follow-up of these same infants at 6 to 9 years, indicated that they "outgrew" their neurological deficits and now were normal functioning children (Painter and associates, 1988). Remarkably, one of the fetuses with normal childhood outcome apparently sustained 975 minutes of severe fetal heart rate decelerations (Painter, 1989).

Shields and Schifrin (1988) described what they considered a unique fetal heart rate pattern characteristic of impaired fetal neurological development. This pattern consisted of a normal baseline rate with persistently absent variability and mild variable decelerations with "overshoot." This pattern was frequently found in association with postmaturity, meconium staining, fetal growth retardation, and neonatal seizures. There was no acidemia at birth, and they concluded that such patterns represented chronic, antenatal intermittent cord compression from oligohydramnios that resulted in repetitive central nervous system ischemia.

Experimental Evidence. Fetal heart rate patterns necessary for perinatal brain damage have been studied in experimental animals. Myers (1972) described the effects of complete and partial asphyxia in rhesus monkeys in studies of brain damage due to perinatal asphyxia. Complete asphyxia was produced by total occlusion of umbilical blood flow which led to a prolonged deceleration (Fig. 15–31). Fetal arterial pH did not reach 7.0 until about 8 minutes after complete cessation of oxygenation and umbilical flow. At least 10 minutes of such prolonged deceleration was required before there was evidence of brain damage in successfully resuscitated fetuses.

Partial asphyxia was produced in these monkeys by impeding maternal aortic blood flow. This resulted in late decelerations due to uterine and placental hypoperfusion. Myers (1972) observed that several hours of these late decelerations did not damage the fetal brain unless the pH fell below 7.0. Indeed, Adamsons and Myers (1977) reported subsequently that late decelerations were a marker of partial asphyxia long *before* brain damage occurred. Put another way, late decelerations were a marker for the absence of fetal brain damage!

Human Evidence. The contribution of intrapartum events to subsequent neurological handicaps has, until fairly recently, been greatly overestimated (Nelson and Ellenberg, 1986). Low and co-workers (1989) examined temporal relationships of neuropathological conditions caused by perinatal asphyxia severe enough to kill the infant. They divided perinatal brain damage into the three categories based on microscopical findings: (1) 18 to 48 hours, neuronal necrosis with pyknosis or lysis of the nucleus in shriveled eosinophilic cells; (2) 48 to 72 hours, more intense neuronal necrosis with macrophage response; and (3) more than 3 days, all the preceding plus astrocyte response with gliosis and, in some, early cavitation. Abnormal brain histopathology was not observed with acute, lethal asphyxia. Moreover, 43 percent of brain damage episodes occurred prior to labor and 25 percent were in the neonatal period. Infants with brain damage during labor (25 percent) were in pregnancies complicated by placental hemorrhage, severe preeclampsia, and meconium aspiration.

In another investigation, Low and co-workers (1984) estimated that more than 1 hour of fetal hypoxia associated with profound metabolic acidemia (pH less than 7.0) was required before neurological abnormalities could be diagnosed at 6 to 12 months of age. Low and co-workers (1988) followed 37 term infants with profound metabolic acidemia at birth to 1 year and found major neurological deficits in 13 percent of the infants. Minor deficits were diagnosed in 10 infants, and the remaining 60 percent were normal.

Clearly, for brain damage to occur, the fetus must be exposed to much more than a brief period of hypoxia. Moreover, the hypoxia must cause profound, just barely sublethal metabolic acidemia. Fetal heart rate patterns consistent with these sublethal conditions are fortunately rare. Conversely, it seems prudent that lesser and pervasive fetal heart rate patterns should not be overinterpreted in attributing fetal brain damage to intrapartum events. Brain damage, manifest as cerebral palsy, first received medical recognition approximately 150 years ago, at which time this affliction was attributed to birthing (see Chap. 44, p. 997). This belief has continued to dominate societal concepts concerning the etiology of fetal brain damage, despite the fact that the obstetrical management prevailing 150 years ago

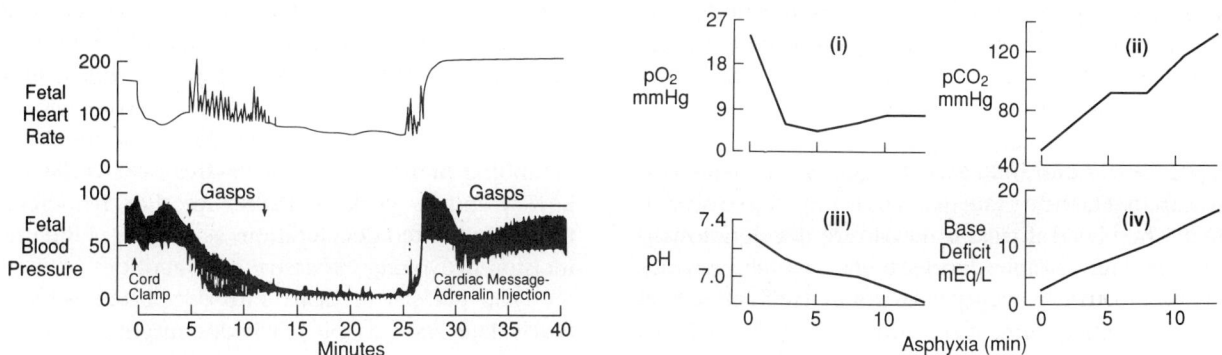

Fig. 15–31. Prolonged deceleration in a rhesus monkey shown with blood pressure and biochemical changes during total occlusion of umbilical cord blood flow. (Redrawn from Myers and colleagues, 1972, with permission.)

cannot conceivably be equated with modern intrapartum care.

Fetal Distress and Fetal Damage

Definition of "Fetal Distress." Use of the word *distress* conjures up any number of synonyms that include *danger, calamity, suffering, wretchedness, oppression,* or even *harassment.* The words **fetal distress** are too broad and vague to be applied with any precision to clinical situations. For example, some element of fetal distress (danger) is almost universal at some time during normal human parturition. Uncertainty about the diagnosis of "fetal distress" based upon interpretation of fetal heart rate patterns has given rise to use of descriptions such as *reassuring* or *nonreassuring.* "Reassuring" suggests a restoration of confidence by a particular pattern, whereas "nonreassuring" suggests inability to remove doubt. These patterns during labor are dynamic such that they can rapidly change from reassuring to nonreassuring and vice versa. In this situation, obstetricians are essentially experiencing surges of both confidence and doubt. Put another way, most diagnoses of fetal distress using heart rate patterns occur when obstetricians lose confidence or cannot assuage doubts about the condition of a fetus. *These fetal assessments are entirely subjective clinical judgments inevitably subject to imperfection and must be recognized as such.*

Why is diagnosis of fetal distress based on heart rate patterns so tenuous? One explanation is that heart rate patterns are more a reflection of fetal physiology than pathology. Physiological control of heart rate includes a variety of interconnected mechanisms that depend on blood flow as well as oxygenation. Moreover, the activity of these control mechanisms is influenced by the preexisting state of fetal oxygenation, as seen, for example, with chronic placental insufficiency. Importantly, the fetus is tethered by an umbilical cord, where blood flow is constantly in jeopardy, which demands that the fetus have a strategy for survival. Moreover, normal labor is a process of increasing acidemia (Modanlou and co-workers, 1973). Thus, normal parturition is a process of repeated fetal hypoxia resulting in acidemia. Put another way, and assuming that "asphyxia" can be defined as hypoxia leading to acidemia, then normal parturition is an asphyxiating event for the fetus.

Diagnosis of Fetal Distress. Diagnosis of fetal distress based upon fetal heart rate patterns is too often oversimplified. The classical triad of heart rate decelerations—early, late, and variable decelerations—which provides clues about in utero events, does not in itself define fetal damage. A critical dimension—duration of the in utero event—is essentially ignored in deliberations on fetal distress. There have been several research efforts aimed at quantifying the duration of abnormal heart rate patterns necessary to portend significant fetal effects. The most common, due to umbilical cord occlusion, requires considerable time to significantly affect the fetus in experimental animals. Watanabe and associates (1992) showed that sequential complete occlusion of the umbilical cord for 40 seconds followed by 80 seconds of release for 30 minutes in sheep resulted in only moderate fetal acidemia. Similarly, Clapp and colleagues (1988) partially occluded the umbilical cord for 1 minute every 3 minutes in fetal sheep and observed brain damage after 2 hours.

Myers and co-workers (1972) observed that more than 20 late decelerations were necessary in humans for a depressed Apgar score. Low and co-workers (1977), using profound fetal metabolic acidemia as an endpoint, reported that heart rate patterns could only be correlated with outcome during the last *2 hours* of labor, and moreover, only in those 2-hour segments showing decelerations with more than 35 percent of uterine contractions. Fleischer and co-workers (1982) also observed that abnormal heart rate patterns had to persist for 120 to 140 minutes before the incidence of fetal acidemia increased significantly.

Severely abnormal fetal heart rate deceleration patterns cannot be attributed to have significant fetal impact when these patterns are intermittent and of short duration. There is also evidence that the prognostic significance of heart rate changes is increased by combining several patterns. For example, Gaziano (1979) observed that variable decelerations in conjunction with abnormal baseline rate (either tachycardia or bradycardia) and loss of variability more often predicted poor fetal condition compared with variable decelerations without baseline changes.

Inevitably, the timing and route of delivery are scrutinized in deliberations about "fetal distress." It is generally assumed that cesarean delivery would have improved the infant outcome. Keegan and associates (1985) emphasized that prompt intervention, within 30 minutes of diagnosis of fetal distress, did not prevent newborn seizures. Moreover, Krebs and colleagues (1982b) observed that fetuses with abnormal heart rate patterns in the last portion of labor were in worse metabolic condition when delivered by cesarean delivery compared with those delivered vaginally. Interestingly, cesarean delivery itself, as well as the choice of anesthetic, can affect the fetal heart rate. Prolonged decelerations have been reported during abdominal wall scrubbing in 10 percent of cesarean deliveries (Petrikovsky and co-workers, 1988). Another 10 percent of fetuses exhibited decelerations as a result of the uterine incision provoking excessive contractility.

The pattern of heart rate decelerations in labor (early, late, and variable) provides insight into the physiological in utero event affecting the fetus. Baseline heart rate and beat-to-beat variability provide important clues about the fetal impact of these events. The most frequent cause of worrisome patterns during human labor is umbilical cord compression. Management of variable fetal heart decelerations, in the absence of baseline changes, is difficult because of the unpredictability of cord occlusion.

Management. Management of significant fetal heart rate patterns consists of correcting the potential fetal insult, if possible (American College of Obstetricians and Gynecologists, 1989). Measures may include discontinuing oxytocin, moving the mother to a lateral position, increasing fluid infusions to improve intervillous perfusion, giving oxygen by mask at 8 to 10 L/min, and correcting hypotension associated with regional analgesia. If these measures are not effective, preparations should be made for prompt delivery by the most expeditious route. Most evidence indicates that even such ideal management of abnormal fetal heart patterns will not always prevent fetal death or brain damage in the infant.

Benefits of Electronic Fetal Heart Rate Monitoring

By the end of the 1970s questions about the efficacy, safety, and costs of electronic monitoring were being voiced from the Office of Technology Assessment, Congress of the United States, and Centers for Disease Control. Banta and Thacker (1979) examined the evidence and after analysis of 158 reports, they concluded that "the technical advances required in the demonstration that reliable recording could be done seems to have blinded most observers to the fact that this additional information will not necessarily produce better outcomes." They attributed the apparent lack of benefit to the imprecision of electronic monitoring for the diagnosis of fetal distress. Moreover, increased usage was linked to more frequent cesarean delivery. They also estimated that additional costs of childbirth in the United States, if 50 percent of labors had electronic monitoring, was approximately $400 million per year.

The National Institute of Child Health and Human Development appointed a task force that published its consensus in 1979. This group included research scientists, obstetricians, pediatricians, economists, ethicists, lawyers, and consumers. After an exhaustive review of electronic monitoring literature, the group concluded that the evidence only suggested a trend toward improved infant outcome in complicated pregnancies. No evidence demonstrated improved outcome in uncomplicated pregnancies. They emphasized that few scientifically conducted investigations had been done to address the perinatal benefits of such monitoring. Importantly, and largely ignored in the current obstetrical litigation crisis, the task force concluded that "Courts of law should recognize intrapartum hypoxia as only one

of the many potential factors involved in the development of handicaps and perinatal death, and current research and clinical data do not allow comprehensive definition of antepartum or intrapartum risk, nor means to reduce risk of adverse outcome."

Randomized Electronic Fetal Heart Rate Monitoring Studies. The first five randomized, prospective studies of electronic monitoring involved 3100 pregnancies (Haverkamp, 1976, 1979; Kelso, 1978; Renou, 1976; Wood, 1981; and their many colleagues). Only complicated pregnancies were studied in three of these. In four studies, no perinatal benefits of electronic monitoring were found.

The National Maternity Hospital, Dublin, between 1981 and 1983, was the site of the largest randomized study of electronic monitoring (MacDonald and co-workers, 1985). Nearly 13,000 pregnancies were entered. Most were uncomplicated pregnancies; however, about one fourth had the following complications: diabetes, preeclampsia, chronic hypertension, renal and cardiac disease, prior perinatal death, prior neurological abnormality, prior low birthweight, prolonged pregnancy, multiple gestation, breech presentation, or gestational age less than 34 weeks. The incidence of forceps delivery was more frequent in the electronically monitored group, but cesarean delivery rates did not differ. No differences were found in the incidence of intrapartum stillbirths or neonatal deaths. Although the number of infants suffering seizures in the auscultation group was increased, there was an equal number of neurologically damaged infants in either group at follow-up.

Luthy and co-workers (1987) studied the effects of electronic monitoring on neurobehavioral development of low-birthweight infants. They studied the neurological outcomes of 212 live-born infants weighing 700 to 1750 g whose intrapartum management had been randomly assigned to either electronic monitoring or periodic fetal heart rate auscultation. Electronic monitoring was not associated with significantly improved neurological outcomes. Cerebral palsy was diagnosed in 13 percent of infants with electronic monitoring compared with 8 percent in those in whom auscultation had been used.

The Parkland Hospital Electronic Fetal Heart Rate Monitoring Study. Continuous electronic monitoring was first used at Parkland Hospital in 1974. Pregnancies complicated by meconium, those requiring oxytocin stimulation of labor, and those with auscultated fetal heart rate abnormalities were transferred for electronic monitoring to a centralized unit with nursing staff in constant attendance. Regular labor rooms were equipped with Doppler ultrasound transducers and the fetal heart rate was measured at 30-minute intervals during first-stage labor. By 1982, approximately one third of pregnancies were being selected for continuous nursing supervision and electronic monitoring.

In July 1982, an investigation was designed to ascertain whether all women in labor should undergo electronic monitoring (Leveno and co-workers, 1986). In alternating months, universal electronic monitoring was rotated with selective heart rate monitoring, which was the existing practice. During the 3-year investigation, 17,410 fetuses were managed with selective monitoring practices. These were compared with 17,641 fetuses managed using universal electronic monitoring (Table 15–1). No significant differences were found in any perinatal outcomes; however, there was a statistically significant small increase in the frequency of primary cesarean delivery for fetal distress associated with universal electronic monitoring. Thus, increased application of electronic monitoring at Parkland Hospital did not improve perinatal results, but it increased the frequency of cesarean delivery for fetal distress.

Why Unfulfilled Expectations? There are several fallacious assumptions behind expectations of improved perinatal outcome with electronic monitoring. One assumption is that fetal distress is a slowly developing phenomenon and that electronic monitoring makes possible early detection of the compromised fetus. This assumption is illogical; how can all fetuses die slowly? Another presumption is that all fetal damage develops in the hospital. Only recently has attention focused on the reality that many damaged fetuses have suffered insults before their arrival to labor units (see Chap. 44, p. 997). The very term implies that this inanimate technology in some fashion "monitors." The assumption is made that if a dead or damaged infant is delivered, the tracing strip must provide some clue, because this device was "monitoring" fetal condition. Last, and despite contrary evidence, many have hypothesized that fetal distress cannot be detected reliably without electronic instrumentation. All of these assumptions led to great expectations and fostered the belief that all dead or damaged neonates are preventable. These unwarranted expectations have greatly fueled the current litigation crisis in obstetrics.

Too many fetuses demonstrate fetal heart rate abnormalities during labor to permit accurate detection of those who are actually compromised. Indeed, most "fetal distress" does not represent an overtly compromised fetus. As discussed, fetal heart rate abnormalities are quite common in labor. In one study of electronic monitoring in over 900 uncomplicated pregnancies, more than two thirds demonstrated decelerations during labor, 25 percent had poor beat-to-beat variability, and 20 percent had an abnormal baseline rate (Krebs and co-workers, 1980). Importantly, debate continues about interpretation of many heart rate patterns. Ironically, this state of affairs for electronic monitoring does not differ from that of Benson and co-workers (1968) in their report on auscultation: "Naivete and wishful thinking inspired our hope for a simple rule-of-thumb estimate of fetal distress. Obviously, the problem is much too complex for such an easy appraisal."

Current Recommendations. The methods most commonly used for intrapartum fetal heart rate monitoring include auscultation with a fetal stethoscope or a Doppler ultrasound device or continuous electronic monitoring of the heart rate and uterine contractions. There is no scientific evidence that has identified the most effective method, including frequency or duration of fetal surveillance, that ensures optimum results. Shown in Table 15–2 are the current recommendations of the American College of Obstetricians and Gynecologists (1989). Intermittent auscultation or continuous electronic monitoring are considered acceptable methods of intrapartum surveillance in both low- and high-risk pregnancies. However, the recommended interval for checking the heart rate is longer in the uncomplicated pregnancy. When auscultation is used, it is recommended that it be performed during a contraction and for 30 seconds thereafter. It is also recommended that a 1:1 nurse–patient ratio be used if auscultation is employed. Thus, the number of nurses available in a labor and delivery may preclude use of intermittent auscultation.

TABLE 15–1. THE PARKLAND HOSPITAL ELECTRONIC MONITORING STUDY

Perinatal Outcomes	Monitoring Method[a]			
	Selective		Universal	
Singleton pregnancies		17,410		17,641
Fetal deaths in labor and delivery (≥ 500 g)	25	(1.4/1000)	30	(1.7/1000)
Assisted ventilation	1259	(7.2%)	1315	(7.5%)
5-minute Apgar score ≤ 5	293	(1.7%)	296	(1.7%)
Admission to intensive care nursery	428	(2.5%)	460	(2.6%)
Neonatal seizures	45	(2.6/1000)	53	(3/1000)

[a] All comparisons statistically insignificant.
From Leveno and co-workers (1986).

TABLE 15–2. GUIDELINES FOR INTRAPARTUM FETAL HEART RATE SURVEILLANCE

Surveillance	Low-risk Pregnancies	High-risk Pregnancies
Acceptable methods		
Intermittent auscultation	Yes	Yes
Continuous electronic monitoring	Yes	Yes
Evaluation intervals		
First-stage labor (active)	30 min	15 min[a]
Second-stage labor	15 min	5 min[a]

[a] Includes tracing evaluation and charting with continuous electronic monitoring.
From American College of Obstetricians and Gynecologists (1989), with permission.

Intrapartum Surveillance of Uterine Activity

A new dimension in the analysis of labor was afforded by the development of electronic monitoring. Although uterine contractions are also depicted, most interest has been focused on the fetal heart rate. Analysis of electronically measured uterine activity permits some generalities concerning the relationship of certain patterns of uterine contractions to labor outcome. There is considerable normal variation, however, and caution must be exercised before judging true labor or its absence solely from study of a monitor tracing. Uterine muscle efficiency to effect delivery varies greatly. To use an analogy, 100-meter sprinters all have the same muscle groups yet cross the finish line at different times.

Internal Uterine Pressure Monitoring. Measurements of intrauterine pressure—that is, the pressure of amnionic fluid, between and during contractions—are made in clinical practice by a fluid-filled plastic catheter positioned in utero so that the distal tip is located in amnionic fluid above the presenting fetal part. First, a plastic catheter guide that contains the distal portion of the catheter is inserted just through the cervical os, and the fluid-filled catheter is then gently pushed beyond the guide into the uterine cavity. To minimize risk to the placenta from the catheter tip, when the site of placental implantation is known, the tip of the catheter inserter should be positioned so that the catheter is likely to be inserted away from the placental site. The opposite end of the catheter, filled with saline, is connected to a strain-gauge pressure sensor adjusted to the same level as the catheter tip in the uterus. The amplified electrical signal produced in the strain gauge by variations in pressure within the fluid system is recorded on a calibrated moving paper strip, simultaneously with the recording of the fetal heart rate. Free communication between amnionic fluid and fluid in the catheter is essential. If the catheter tip becomes obstructed, it can usually be relieved by injecting a small volume of sterile saline from a syringe through the catheter.

External Uterine Contraction Monitoring. Uterine contractions can be measured by a displacement transducer placed on the abdomen close to the fundus. The transducer button ("plunger") is held against the abdominal wall and, as the uterus contracts, the button moves in proportion to the strength of the contraction. This movement is converted into a measurable electrical signal that indicates the *relative* intensity of the contraction—it does not give an accurate measure of contraction intensity. However, if carefully supervised, external monitoring can give a good indication of the onset, acme, and end of the contraction, and it is an easy-to-use, noninvasive technique.

Patterns of Uterine Activity. Caldeyro-Barcia and Poseiro (1960) from Montevideo, Uruguay, were pioneers who have done much to elucidate the patterns of spontaneous uterine activity throughout pregnancy. Their investigations were made possible by the development of electronic means of recording and quantifying in situ uterine contractions of the pregnant woman before and during labor. Contractile waves of uterine activity were usually measured using intraamnionic pressure catheters, but early in their studies as many as four simultaneous intramyometrial microballoons were also used to record uterine pressure. They also introduced the concept of **Montevideo units** to define uterine activity. By this definition, uterine performance is the product of the intensity—that is, increased uterine pressure above baseline tone—of a contraction in mm Hg multiplied by contraction frequency per 10 minutes. For example, 3 contractions in 10 minutes, each of 50 mm Hg intensity, would equal 150 Montevideo units. These studies during the 1960s were unique and provided useful insights for understanding normal labor. Similarly, Hendricks (1968) has also provided useful information concerning the characteristics of normal human uterine activity during prelabor, labor, and in the immediate puerperium.

During the first 30 weeks, uterine activity measured in Montevideo units is comparatively quiescent (Fig. 15–32). Uterine contractions are seldom greater than 20 mm Hg, and these have been equated with those first

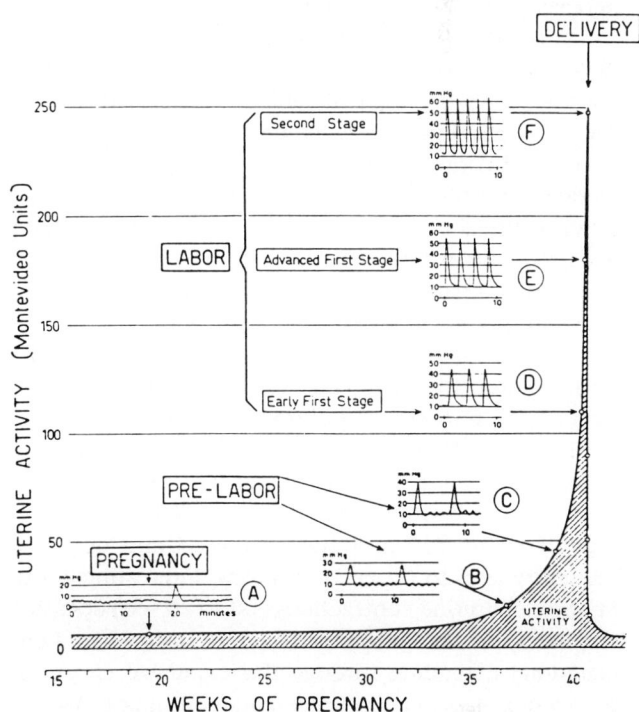

Fig. 15–32. The development of spontaneous uterine activity (*striped area*) throughout pregnancy and labor. Typical schematic tracings of uterine contractility are shown for each stage of labor. (From Caldeyro-Barcia and Poseiro, 1960.)

Prelabor   First stage   Second stage

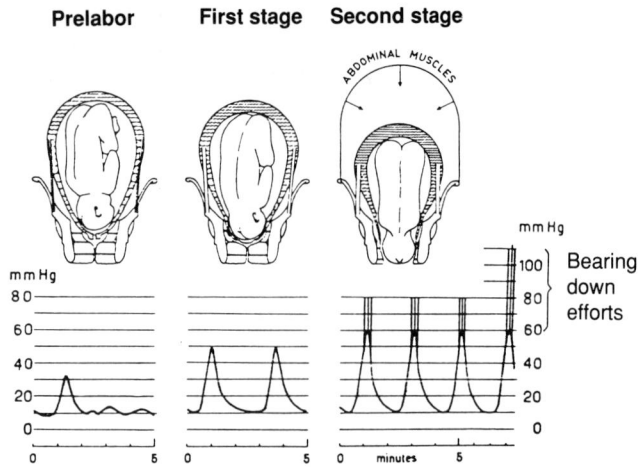

Fig. 15–33. Intrauterine pressures in normal labor. In the upper part are shown three schematic frontal sections of the uterus, fetus, and pelvis. In the lower part are three schematic tracings of amnionic fluid pressure corresponding to stages of labor. (From Caldeyro-Barcia and Poseiro, 1960.)

described in 1872 by John Braxton Hicks. Uterine activity increases gradually after 30 weeks, and it is noteworthy that those contractions—commonly referred to as Braxton Hicks contractions—also increase in intensity and frequency. Further increases in uterine activity are typical of the last weeks of pregnancy, termed **prelabor** by Caldeyro-Barcia and colleagues. During prelabor, the cervix ripens, presumably as a consequence of increasing uterine contractions (see Chap. 12).

According to Caldeyro-Barcia and Poseiro (1960), clinical labor usually commences when uterine activity reaches values between 80 and 120 Montevideo units (Fig. 15–33). This translates into approximately three 40 mm Hg contractions per 10 minutes, or 120 Montevideo units. Importantly, there is no clear-cut division between prelabor and labor, but rather a gradual and progressive transition.

During first-stage labor, uterine contractions increase progressively in intensity from about 25 mm Hg at commencement of labor to 50 mm Hg at the end. At the same time, frequency increases from 3 to 5 contractions per 10 minutes, and uterine baseline tone from 8 to 12 mm Hg. Uterine activity further increases during second-stage labor, aided by maternal abdominal muscles during bearing down (Fig. 15–33). Indeed, contractions of 80 to 100 mm Hg are typical and occur as frequently as 5 to 6 per 10 minutes. Interestingly, the duration of uterine contractions (60 to 80 sec) does not increase appreciably from early active labor (3 to 4 cm dilatation) extending through the expulsive efforts of the second-stage (Pontonnier and colleagues, 1975). Presumably, this constancy of duration serves a fetal respiratory gas-exchange function. That is, functional fetal "breath holding" during a uterine contraction,

which results in isolation of the intervillous space where respiratory gas exchange occurs, has a 60- to 80-second limit that remains relatively constant.

Caldeyro-Barcia and Poseiro (1960) also observed empirically that uterine contractions are clinically palpable only after their intensity exceeds 10 mm Hg. Moreover, until the intensity of the contractions reaches 40 mm Hg, the uterine wall can readily be depressed by the finger, but at greater intensity, it then becomes so hard that it resists easy depression. Uterine contractions are usually not associated with pain until their intensity exceeds 15 mm Hg, presumably because this is the minimum pressure required for distending the lower segment and cervix. It follows that Braxton Hicks contractions exceeding 15 mm Hg may be perceived as uncomfortable because distension of the uterus, cervix, and birth canal is generally thought to elicit discomfort, the uterine contraction otherwise being relatively painless.

Hendricks (1968) observed that "the clinician makes great demands upon the uterus. He expects it to remain well relaxed during pregnancy, to contract effectively but intermittently during labor, and then to remain in a state of almost constant contraction for several hours postpartum." Figure 15–34 demonstrates an example of normal uterine activity during one labor, measured through a catheter similar to that used today. As also described by Caldeyro-Barcia and Poseiro

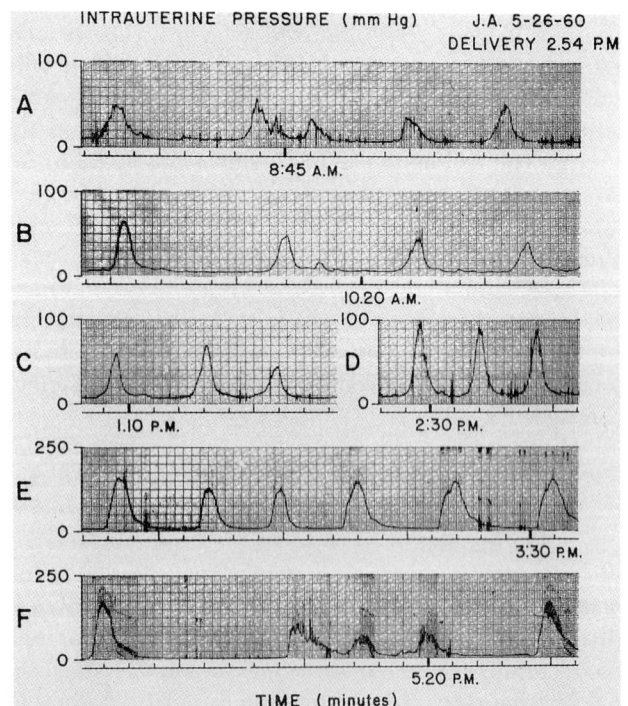

Fig. 15–34. Intrauterine pressure recorded through a single catheter. **A.** Prelabor. **B.** Early labor. **C.** Active labor. **D.** Late labor. **E.** Spontaneous activity ½ hour postpartum. **F.** Spontaneous activity 2½ hours postpartum. (From Hendricks, 1968.)

(1960), uterine activity progressively and gradually increases from prelabor through late labor. Interestingly, and as shown in Figure 15–34, uterine contractions after birth are identical to those resulting in delivery of the infant. Indeed, the pattern of uterine activity is one of gradual subsidence or reverse of that leading up to delivery. It is therefore not surprising that the uterus that performs poorly before delivery is also prone to atony and puerperal hemorrhage.

Origin and Propagation of Uterine Contractions. The uterus, unlike the heart, has not been extensively studied in terms of its nonhormonal physiological mechanisms of function. The normal contractile wave of labor originates near the uterine end of one of the fallopian tubes; thus these areas act as "pacemakers" (Fig. 15–35). The right pacemaker usually predominates over the left and starts the great majority of contractile waves. The contraction spreads from the pacemaker area throughout the uterus at 2 cm/sec, depolarizing the whole organ within 15 seconds. This depolarization wave propagates downward toward the cervix; the intensity is greatest in the fundus and it diminishes in the lower uterus. This phenomenon is thought to reflect reductions of myometrial thickness from the fundus to the cervix. Presumably, this descending gradient of uter-

ine pressure serves to direct fetal descent toward the cervix and efface the cervix. That is, the lower parts of the uterus are distended and yield as a result of the propagation of fundal dominant contractions. Importantly, all parts of the uterus are synchronized and reach their peak pressure almost simultaneously, giving rise to the curvilinear waveform shown in Figure 15–35.

The pacemaker theory also serves to explain the varying intensity of adjacent coupled contractions shown in Lines A and B of Figure 15–34. Such coupling is termed **incoordination** by Caldeyro-Barcia and Poseiro (1960). A contractile wave begins in one cornual-region pacemaker, but does not synchronously depolarize the entire uterus. As a result, another contraction begins in the contralateral pacemaker and produces the second contractile wave of the couplet. These small contractions alternating with larger ones appear to be typical of early labor, and indeed, labor may progress with such uterine activity but at a slower pace. They also observed that labor would progress slowly if regular contractions were hypotonic—that is, contraction intensity less than 25 mm Hg or frequency less than 2 contractions per 10 minutes. Similar observations were made by Seitchik (1981) in a computer-aided analysis comparing women in active labor with those with arrested labor. Normal labor was characterized by a minimum of 3 contractions that averaged greater than 25 mm Hg and less than 4-minute intervals between contractions. Less than this amount of uterine activity was associated with arrest of active labor. He cautioned that the prospective diagnosis of hypotonic labor based simply on a few uterine pressures cannot be accomplished reliably. He did report, however, that modest dosages of oxytocin (usually 8 mU/min or less) restored uterine contractions in women with hypocontractile patterns.

Caldeyro-Barcia and Poseiro (1960) attempted to quantify uterine work necessary to dilate the cervix from 2 cm to complete dilatation. Labor was induced by infusing oxytocin in parous women, and the total uterine contraction pressure in mm Hg necessary to accomplish complete dilatation was summed. They found that between 4000 and 8000 mm Hg of total contraction pressure was required. If the contractions had an average intensity of 50 mm Hg, then 80 to 160 contractions were necessary. Moreover, if the contraction frequency ranged from 4 to 5 per 10 minutes, then the duration of the first stage of labor would be between 3 and 6 hours. Calculations such as these apply to many normal labors and, although applicable to some pregnancies, the extreme biological variation of normal labor defies efforts to mathematically describe it for the purpose of determining departure from normal.

Hauth and co-workers (1986) quantified uterine contraction pressures in 109 women at term who received oxytocin for labor induction or augmentation. Most of these women with successfully stimulated labor

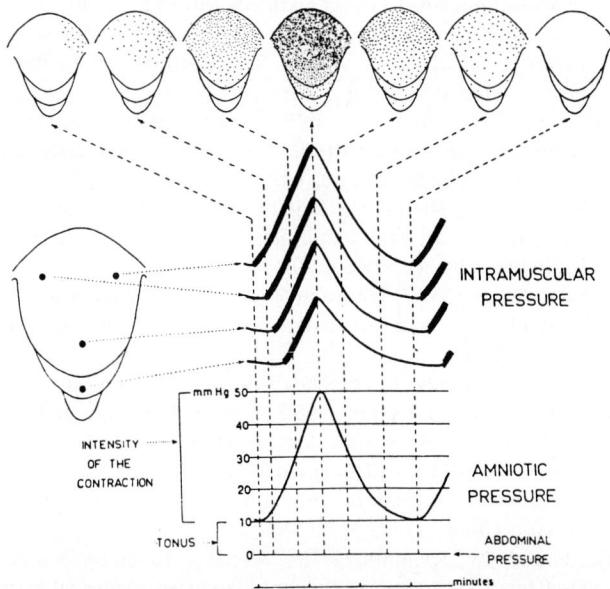

Fig. 15–35. Schematic representation of the normal contractile wave of labor. Large uterus on the left shows the four points at which intramyometrial pressure was recorded with microballoons. Four corresponding pressure tracings are shown in relation to each other by shading on the small uteri. (From Caldeyro-Barcia and Poseiro, 1960.)

achieved 200 to 225 Montevideo units, and 40 percent up to 300 Montevideo units to effect spontaneous delivery. They suggested that these levels of uterine activity should be sought before consideration of cesarean delivery for presumed dystocia.

References

Adamsons K, Myers RE: Late decelerations and brain tolerance of the fetal monkey to intrapartum asphyxia. Am J Obstet Gynecol 128:893, 1977

Aladjem S, Feria A, Stojanovic J: Fetal heart rate responses to fetal movements. Br J Obstet Gynaecol 84:487, 1977

American College of Obstetricians and Gynecologists: Intrapartum fetal heart rate monitoring. Technical bulletin no. 132, September 1989

Angel J, Knuppel R, Lake M: Sinusoidal fetal heart rate patterns associated with intravenous butorphanol administration. Am J Obstet Gynecol 149:465, 1984

Ayromlooi J, Berg P, Tobias M: The significance of sinusoidal fetal heart rate patterns during labor and its relation to fetal status and neonatal outcome. Int J Gynaecol Obstet 16:341, 1978–1979

Ball RH, Parer JT: The physiologic mechanisms of variable decelerations. Am J Obstet Gynecol 166:1683, 1992

Banta HD, Thacker SB: Assessing the costs and benefits of electronic fetal monitoring. Obstet Gynecol Surv 34:627, 1979

Behrman RE: The cardiovascular system. In Behrman RE, Kliegman RM, Nelson WE, Vaughn VC (eds): Nelson Textbook of Pediatrics, 14th ed. Philadelphia, Saunders, 1992, p 1127

Benson RC, Shubeck F, Deutschberger J, Weiss W, Berendes H: Fetal heart rate as a predictor of fetal distress. A report from the collaborative project. Obstet Gynecol 32:259, 1968

Boehm FH: Prolonged end stage fetal heart rate deceleration. Obstet Gynecol 45:579, 1975

Bowen LW, Kochenour NK, Rehm NE, Woolley FR: Maternal–fetal pH difference and fetal scalp pH as predictors of neonatal outcome. Obstet Gynecol 67:487, 1986

Brubaker K, Garite TJ: The lambda fetal heart rate pattern: An assessment of its significance in the intrapartum period. Obstet Gynecol 72:881, 1988

Caldeyro-Barcia R, Mendez-Bauer C, Poseiro JJ, Pose S: Fetal monitoring in labor. In Walloch HJ, Gold EM, Lis EF (eds): Maternal and Child Health Practices. Springfield, IL, Thomas, 1973, p 332

Caldeyro-Barcia R, Poseiro JJ: Physiology of the uterine contraction. Clin Obstet Gynecol 3:386, 1960

Cibils LA: Clinical significance of fetal heart rate patterns during labor, V. Variable decelerations. Am J Obstet Gynecol 132:791, 1978

Clapp JF, Peress NS, Wesley M, Mann LI: Brain damage after intermittent partial cord occlusion in the chronically instrumented fetal lamb. Am J Obstet Gynecol 159:504, 1988

Clark SL, Gimovsky ML, Miller FC: The scalp stimulation test: A clinical alternative to fetal scalp blood sampling. Am J Obstet Gynecol 148:274, 1984

Clark SL, Gimovsky ML, Miller FC: Fetal heart rate response to scalp blood sampling. Am J Obstet Gynecol 14:706, 1982

Clark SL, Paul RH: Fetal heart rate monitoring patterns. Am J Obstet Gynecol 155:914, 1986. Letter to the editor

Clark SL, Paul RH: Intrapartum fetal surveillance. The role of fetal scalp sampling. Am J Obstet Gynecol 153:717, 1985

Dawes GS: The control of fetal heart rate and its variability in counts. In Kunzel W (ed): Fetal Heart Rate Monitoring. Berlin, Springer-Verlag, 1985, p 188

Dawes GS, Visser GHA, Goodman JDS, Levine DH: Numerical analysis of the human fetal heart rate: Modulation by breathing and movement. Am J Obstet Gynecol 140:535, 1981

Del Valle GO, Joffe GM, Izquierdo LA, Smith JF, Kasnic T, Gilson GJ, Chatterjee MS, Curet LB: Acute post traumatic fetal anemia treated with fetal intravascular transfusion. Am J Obstet Gynecol 166:127, 1992

Divon MY, Winkler H, Yeh SY, Platt LD, Langer O, Merkatz IR: Diminished respiratory sinus arrhythmia in asphyxiated term infants. Am J Obstet Gynecol 155:1263, 1986

Edersheim TG, Hutson JM, Druzin ML, Kogut EA: Fetal heart rate response to vibratory acoustic stimulation predicts fetal pH in labor. Am J Obstet Gynecol 157:1557, 1987

Egley CC, Bowes WA, Wagner D: Sinusoidal fetal heart rate pattern during labor. Am J Perinatol 8:197, 1991

Epstein H, Waxman A, Gleicher N, Lauersen NH: Meperidine induced sinusoidal fetal heart rate pattern and reversal with naloxone. Obstet Gynecol 59:225, 1982

Faro S, Martens MG, Hammill HA, Riddle G, Tortolero G: Antibiotic prophylaxis: Is there a difference? Am J Obstet Gynecol 162:900, 1990

Fleischer A, Schulman H, Jagani N, Mitchell J, Randolph G: The development of fetal acidosis in the presence of an abnormal fetal heart rate tracing, I. The average for gestational age fetus. Am J Obstet Gynecol 144:55, 1982

Freeman RK, Garite TH, Nageotte MP: Fetal Heart Rate Monitoring, 2nd ed. Baltimore, Williams & Wilkins, 1991

Gabbe SG, Ettinger BB, Freeman RK, Martin CB: Umbilical cord compression associated with amniotomy: laboratory observations. Am J Obstet Gynecol 126:353, 1976

Gal D, Jacobson LM, Ser H, Park SA, Taucer ML: Sinusoidal patterns: An alarming sign of fetal distress. Am J Obstet Gynecol 125:903, 1978

Gaziano EP: A study of variable decelerations in association with other heart rate patterns during monitored labor. Am J Obstet Gynecol 135:360, 1979

Gilstrap III LC, Hauth JC, Hankins GDV, Beck AW: Second-stage fetal heart rate abnormalities and type of neonatal acidemia. Obstet Gynecol 70:191, 1987

Gilstrap LC, Hauth JC, Toussaint S: Second stage fetal heart rate abnormalities and neonatal acidosis. Obstet Gynecol 63:209, 1984

Gleicher N, Elkayam U: Fetal heart rate and rhythm disorders. In Elkayam U, Gleicher (eds): Cardiac Problems in Pregnancy, 2nd ed. New York, Liss, 1990, p 723

Gleicher N, Runowicz CD, Brown B: Sinusoidal fetal heart rate patterns in association with amnionitis. Obstet Gynecol 56:109, 1980

Goldkrand JW, Speichinger JP: "Mixed cord compression," fetal heart rate pattern and its relation to abnormal cord position. Am J Obstet Gynecol 122:144, 1975

Granat M, Lavie P, Cedar D, Sharf M: Short-term cycles in human fetal activity. Am J Obstet Gynecol 134:696, 1979

Gray JH, Cudmore DW, Luther ER, Martin TR, Gardner AJ: Sinusoidal fetal heart rate pattern associated with alphaprodine administration. Obstet Gynecol 52:678, 1978

Hamilton LA Jr, McKeown MJ: Biochemical and electronic

monitoring of the fetus. In Wynn RM (ed): Obstetrics and Gynecology Annual, 1973. New York, Appleton-Century-Crofts, 1974

Hammacher K, Huter K, Bokelmann J, Werners PH: Foetal heart frequency and perinatal conditions of the fetus and newborn. Gynaecologia 166:349, 1968

Harris JL, Krueger TR, Parer JT: Mechanisms of late deceleration of the fetal heart rate during hypoxia. Am J Obstet Gynecol 144:491, 1982

Hauth JC, Hankins GV, Gilstrap LC, Strickland DM, Vance P: Uterine contraction pressures with oxytocin induction/augmentation. Obstet Gynecol 68:305, 1986

Haverkamp AD, Orleans M, Langendoerfer S, McFee J, Murphy J, Thompson HE: A controlled trial of the differential effects of intrapartum fetal monitoring. Am J Obstet Gynecol 134:399, 1979

Haverkamp AD, Thompson HE, McFee JG, Cetrulo C. The evaluation of continuous fetal heart rate monitoring in high-risk pregnancy. Am J Obstet Gynecol 125:310, 1976

Heldfond AJ, Walker CN, Wade ME: Do we need fetal monitoring in a community hospital? Trans Pac Coast Obstet Gynecol Soc 43:25, 1976

Hendricks CH: Uterine contractility changes in the early puerperium. In Anderson GV, Quilligan EJ (eds): Clinical Obstetrics and Gynecology, Thromboembolic Disorders, Physiology of Labor. New York, Harper & Row, 1968, p 125

Herbert CM, Boehm FH: Prolonged end-stage fetal heart deceleration: A reanalysis. Obstet Gynecol 57:589, 1981

Hicks JB: On the contractions of the uterus throughout pregnancy. Trans Obstet Soc Lond 13, 1872

Hon EH: The fetal heart rate patterns preceding death in utero. Am J Obstet Gynecol 78:47, 1959

Hon EH: The electronic evaluation of the fetal heart rate. Am J Obstet Gynecol 75:1215, 1958

Huck A, Huck R, Schneider H, Rooth G: Continuous transcutaneous monitoring of fetal oxygen torsion during labour. Br J Obstet Gynaecol 84 (supp 1):1, 1977

Hull MGR: Perinatal coagulopathies complicating fetal blood sampling. Br Med J 3:319, 1972

Itskovitz J, LaGamma EF, Rudoloph AM: Heart rate and blood pressure response to umbilical cord compression in fetal lambs with special reference to the mechanisms of variable deceleration. Am J Obstet Gynecol 147:451, 1983

Johnson TR Jr, Compton AA, Rotmeusch J, Work BA, Johnson JC: Significance of the sinusoidal fetal heart rate pattern. Am J Obstet Gynecol 139:446, 1981

Keegan KA, Waffarn F, Quilligan EJ: Obstetric characteristics and fetal heart rate patterns of infants who convulse during the newborn period. Am J Obstet Gynecol 153:732, 1985

Kelso IM, Parsons RJ, Lawrence GF, Arora SS, Edmonds DK, Cooke ID: An assessment of continuous fetal heart rate monitoring in labor. Am J Obstet Gynecol 131:526, 1978

Klavan M, Laver AT, Boscola MA: Clinical concepts of fetal heart rate monitoring. Waltham MA, Hewlett-Packard Co, 1977

Krebs HB, Petres RE, Dunn LJ: Intrapartum fetal heart rate monitoring, V. Fetal heart rate patterns in the second stage of labor. Am J Obstet Gynecol 140:435, 1981

Krebs HB, Petres RE, Dunn LJ, Segreti A: Intrapartum fetal heart rate monitoring, IV. Observations on elective and nonelective fetal heart rate monitoring. Am J Obstet Gynecol 138:213, 1980

Krebs HB, Petres RE, Dunn LJ, Smith PJ: Intrapartum fetal heart rate monitoring, VI. Prognostic significance of accelerations. Am J Obstet Gynecol 142:297, 1982a

Krebs HB, Petres RE, Dunn LJ, Smith PJ: Intrapartum fetal heart rate monitoring, VII: The impact of mode of delivery on fetal outcome. Am J Obstet Gynecol 143:190, 1982b

Kubli F, Ruttgers H, Haller U, Bogdan C, Ramzin M: Die antepartale fetal Herzfrequenz, II. Baseline levels, baseline irregularity and decelerations with antepartum fetal death. Z Gerburtshilfe Perinatol 176:309, 1972

Kunzel W: Fetal heart rate alterations in partial and total cord occlusion. In Kunzel W (ed): Fetal Heart Rate Monitoring: Clinical Practice and Pathophysiology. Berlin, Springer-Verlag, 1985, p 114

Lee CV, DiLaretto PC, Lane JM: A study of fetal heart rate acceleration patterns. Obstet Gynecol 45:142, 1975

Lee ST, Hon EH: The fetal electrocardiogram, IV. Unusual variations in the QRS complex during labor. Am J Obstet Gynecol 92:1140, 1965

Leveno KJ, Cunningham FG, Nelson S: Prospective comparison of selective and universal electronic fetal monitoring in 34,995 pregnancies. N Engl Med 315:615, 1986

Leveno KJ, Quirk JG, Cunningham FG, Nelson SD, Santos R, Toufanian A, DePalma RT: Prolonged pregnancy: Observations concerning the causes of fetal distress. Am J Obstet Gynecol 150:465, 1984

Leveno K, Williams L, DePalma R, Whalley P: Perinatal outcome in the absence of antepartum fetal heart rate accelerations. Obstet Gynecol 61:347, 1983

Low JA, Galbraith RS, Muir DW, Killen HL, Pater EA, Karchmar EJ: Motor and cognitive deficits after intrapartum asphyxia in the mature fetus. Am J Obstet Gynecol 158:356, 1988

Low JA, Galbraith RS, Muir DW, Killen HL, Pater EA, Karchmar EJ: Factors associated with motor and cognitive deficits in children after intrapartum fetal hypoxia. Am J Obstet Gynecol 148:533, 1984

Low JA, Pancham SR, Worthington DN: Intrapartum fetal heart rate profiles with and without fetal asphyxia. Am J Obstet Gynecol 127:729, 1977

Low JA, Robertson DR, Simpson LL: Temporal relationships of neuropathologic conditions caused by perinatal asphyxia. Am J Obstet Gynecol 160:608, 1989

Lowe TW, Leveno KJ, Quirk JG, Santos-Ramos R, Williams ML: Sinusoidal fetal heart rate patterns after intrauterine transfusion. Obstet Gynecol 64:215, 1984

Luthy DA, Shy KK, van Belle G, Larson EB, Hughes JP, Benedetti TJ, Brown ZA, Effer S, King JF, Stenchever MA: A randomized trial of electronic fetal monitoring in preterm labor. Obstet Gynecol 69:687, 1987

MacDonald D, Grant A, Sheridan-Pereira M, Boylan P, Chalmers I: The Dublin randomized controlled trial of intrapartum fetal heart rate monitoring. Am J Obstet Gynecol 152:524, 1985

Mann L: Intrapartum fetal monitoring: Scalp blood pH is a useful tool. Contemp Obstet Gynecol 11:25, 1978

Manseau P, Vaquier J, Chavinie J, Sureau C: Sinusoidal fetal cardiac rhythm. An aspect evocative of fetal distress during pregnancy. J Gynecol Obstet Biol Reprod (Paris) 1:343, 1972

Maxwell DJ, Crawford DC, Curry PV, Tynan MJ, Allan LD: Obstetric importance, diagnosis, and management of fetal tachycardias. Br Med J 297:107, 1988

McGregor JA, McFarren T: Neonatal cranial osteomyelitis: A complication of fetal monitoring. Obstet Gynecol 73:490, 1989

Melchior J, Bernard N: Incidence and pattern of fetal heart rate alterations during labor. In Kunzel W (ed): Fetal Heart Rate Monitoring: Clinical Practice and Pathophysiology. Berlin, Springer-Verlag, 1985, p 73

Miyazaki FS, Nevarez F: Saline amnioinfusion for relief of repetitive variable decelerations: A prospective randomized study. Am J Obstet Gynecol 153:301, 1985

Miyazaki FS, Taylor NA: Saline amnioinfusion for relief of variable or prolonged decelerations. Am J Obstet Gynecol 146:670, 1983

Modanlou H, Freeman RK: Sinusoidal fetal heart rate pattern: Its definition and clinical significance. Am J Obstet Gynecol 142:1033, 1982

Modanlou H, Yeh SY, Hon EH, Forsythe A: Fetal and neonatal biochemistry and Apgar score. Am J Obstet Gynecol 117:942, 1973

Mueller-Heubach E, Battelli AF: Variable heart rate decelerations and transcutaneous pO_2 (tc pO_2) during umbilical cord occlusion in the fetal monkey. Am J Obstet Gynecol 144:796, 1982

Murata Y, Martin CB, Ikenoue T, Hasimoto T, Taira S, Saqawa T, Sakata H: Fetal heart rate accelerations and late decelerations during the course of intrauterine death in chronically catheterized rhesus monkeys. Am J Obstet Gynecol 144:218, 1982

Murata Y, Miyake U, Yamamoto T, Higuchi M, Hesser J, Ibara S, Bessho T: Experimentally produced sinusoidal fetal heart rate patterns in the chronically instrumented fetal lamb. Am J Obstet Gynecol 153:693, 1985

Murphy KW, Russell V, Collins A, Johnson P: The prevalence, aetiology and clinical significance of pseudo-sinusoidal fetal heart rate patterns in labour. Br J Obstet Gynaecol 98:1093, 1991

Myers GG, Krapohl AJ, Peterson RD, Caldyro-Barcia R: New method for measuring lag time between human uterine contraction and the effect on fetal heart rate. Am J Obstet Gynecol 112:39, 1972

Myers RE: Two patterns of perinatal brain damage and their conditions of occurrence. Am J Obstet Gynecol 112:246, 1972

Myers RE, Mueller-Heubach E, Adamsons K: Predictability of the state of fetal oxygenation from a quantitative analysis of the components of late deceleration. Am J Obstet Gynecol 115:1083, 1973

Nageotte MP, Bertucci L, Towers CV, Lagrew DL, Modanlou H: Prophylactic amnioinfusion in pregnancies complicated by oligohydramnios: A prospective study. Obstet Gynecol 77:677, 1991

National Institute of Child Health and Human Development. Consensus Development Conference, III. Predictors of intrapartum fetal distress. In: Antenatal Diagnosis. Bethesda, US Department of Health, Education and Welfare, Public Health Service, National Institutes of Health, 1979

Nelson KB, Ellenberg JH: Antecedents of cerebral palsy. N Engl J Med 315:81, 1986

Nicolaides KH, Sadovsky G, Cetin E: Fetal heart rate patterns in red blood cell isoimmunized pregnancies. Am J Obstet Gynecol 161:351, 1989

Owen J, Hanson BV, Hauth JC: A prospective randomized study of saline solution amnioinfusion. Am J Obstet Gynecol 162:1146, 1990

Painter MJ: Fetal heart rate patterns, perinatal asphyxia, and brain injury. Pediatr Neurol 5:137, 1989

Painter MJ, Depp R, O'Donoghue PD: Fetal heart rate patterns and development in the first year of life. Am J Obstet Gynecol 132:271, 1978

Painter MJ, Scott M, Hirsch R, O'Donoghue P, Depp R: Fetal heart rate patterns during labor: Neurologic and cognitive development at 6–9 years of age. Am J Obstet Gynecol 159:854, 1988

Parer WJ, Parer JT, Holbrook RH, Block BSB: Validity of mathematical models of quantitating fetal heart rate variability. Am J Obstet Gynecol 153:402, 1985

Paul RH, Hon EH: A clinical fetal monitor. Obstet Gynecol 35:161, 1970

Paul RH, Snidon AK, Yeh SY: Clinical fetal monitoring, VII. The evaluation and significance of intrapartum baseline FHR variability. Am J Obstet Gynecol 123:206, 1975

Paul WM, Quilligan EJ, MacLachlan T: Cardiovascular phenomena associated with fetal head compression. Am J Obstet Gynecol 90:824, 1964

Petrikovsky B, Cohen M, Fastman D, Tancer ML: Electronic fetal heart rate monitoring during cesarean section. Int J Gynecol Obstet 26:203, 1988

Picquard F, Hsiung R, Mattauer M, Schaefer A, Haberey P: The validity of fetal heart rate monitoring during the second stage of labor. Obstet Gynecol 72:746, 1988

Pillai M, James D: The development of fetal heart rate patterns during normal pregnancy. Obstet Gynecol 76:812, 1990

Pontonnier G, Puech F, Grandjean H, Rolland M: Some physical and biochemical parameters during normal labour. Fetal and maternal study. Biol Neonate 26:159, 1975

Posner MD, Ballagh SA, Paul RH: The effect of amnioinfusion on uterine pressure and activity: A preliminary report. Am J Obstet Gynecol 163:813, 1990

Rayburn WF, Beynen A, Brinkman DL: Umbilical cord length and intrapartum complications. Obstet Gynecol 57:450, 1981

Read LR, Miller FC: Fetal heart rate acceleration in response to acoustic stimulation as a measure of fetal well-being. Am J Obstet Gynecol 129:512, 1977

Renou P, Chang A, Anderson I, Wood C: Controlled trial of fetal intensive care. Am J Obstet Gynecol 126:470, 1976

Renou P, Warwick N, Wood C: Autonomic control of fetal heart rate. Am J Obstet Gynecol 105:949, 1969

Richards DS, Cefalo RC, Thorpe JM, Salley M, Rose D: Determinants of fetal heart rate response to vibroacoustic stimulation in labor. Obstet Gynecol 71:535, 1988

Roche JB, Hon EH: The fetal electrocardiogram, V. Comparison of lead systems. Am J Obstet Gynecol 92:1149, 1965

Saling EZ: Die Blutgasverhaltnisse und der saure Basen-Haushalt der Feten bei ungerstörtem Geburtsablauf. Z Geburtsh Gynaekol 161:262, 1964

Schrimmer DB, Macri CJ, Paul RD: Prophylactic amnioinfusion as a treatment for oligohydramnios in laboring patients: A prospective, randomized trial. Am J Obstet Gynecol 165:972, 1991

Seitchik J: Quantitating uterine contractility in a clinical context. Obstet Gynecol 57:453, 1981

Shields JR, Schifrin BS: Perinatal antecedents of cerebral palsy. Obstet Gynecol 71:899, 1988

Smith JH, Anand KJ, Cotes PM, Dawes GD, Harkness RA, Howlett TA, Rees LH, Redman CW: Antenatal fetal heart rate variation in relation to the respiratory and metabolic status of the compromised human fetus. Br J Obstet Gynaecol 95:980, 1988

Snijders RJ, Ribbert LS, Visser GH, Mulder EJ: Numeric analysis of heart rate variation in intrauterine growth-retarded fetuses: A longitudinal study. Am J Obstet Gynecol 166:22, 1992

Southall DP, Richards J, Hardwick RA, Shinebourne EA, Gibbens GL, Jones HT, DeSwiet M, Johnston PG: Prospective study of fetal heart rate and rhythm patterns. Arch Dis Child 55:506, 1980

Tabor BL, Maier JA: Polyhydramnios and elevated intrauterine pressure during amnioinfusion. Am J Obstet Gynecol 156:130, 1987

Tejani N, Mann LI, Bhakthavathsalan A, Weiss RR: Prolonged fetal bradycardia with recovery—its significance and outcome. Am J Obstet Gynecol 122:975, 1975

Thomas G: The aetiology, characteristics and diagnostic relevance of late deceleration patterns in routine obstetric practice. Br J Obstet Gynaecol 82:121, 1975

Trudinger BJ, Pryse-Davies J: Fetal hazards of the intrauterine pressure catheter: Five case reports. Br J Obstet Gynaecol 85:567, 1978

van Geijn HP, Jongsma HN, deHaan J, Eskes TK, Prechtl HF: Heart rate as an indicator of the behavioral state. Am J Obstet Gynecol 136:1061, 1980

Viscomi CM, Hood DD, Melone PJ, Eisenach JC: Fetal heart rate variability after epidural fentanyl during labor. Anesth Analg 71:679, 1990

Watanabe T, Okamura K, Tanigawara S, Shintaku Y, Akagi K, Endo H, Yajima A: Changes in electrocardiogram T-wave amplitude during umbilical cord compress is predictive of fetal condition in sheep. Am J Obstet Gynecol 166:246, 1992

Wood C, Renou R, Oats J, Farrell E, Beischer N, Anderson I: A controlled trial of fetal heart rate monitoring in a low-risk obstetric population. Am J Obstet Gynecol 141:527, 1981

Young DC, Gray JH, Luther ER, Peddle LJ: Fetal scalp blood pH sampling: Its value in an active obstetric unit. Am J Obstet Gynecol 136:276, 1980a

Young BK, Katz M, Klein SA: Intrapartum fetal cardiac arrythmia. Obstet Gynecol 54:427, 1979

Young BK, Katz M, Wilson SJ: Fetal blood and tissue pH with variable deceleration patterns. Obstet Gynecol 56:169, 1980b

Young BK, Katz M, Wilson SJ: Sinusoidal fetal heart rate, I. Clinical significance. Am J Obstet Gynecol 136:587, 1980c

Young BK, Weinstein HM: Moderate fetal bradycardia. Am J Obstet Gynecol 126:271, 1976

Zalar RW, Quilligan EJ: The influence of scalp sampling on the cesarean section rate for fetal distress. Am J Obstet Gynecol 135:239, 1979

CHAPTER 16
Analgesia and Anesthesia

Pain relief in labor presents unique problems. These may be best appreciated by comparing several important differences between obstetrical and surgical (nonobstetrical) analgesia and anesthesia:

1. **Infant.** In surgical procedures, there is but one patient to consider, whereas during labor there are two patients—mother and fetus. Sedative and anesthetic drugs, when given to the laboring woman, rapidly traverse the placenta and may cause respiratory depression in the newborn.

2. **Indications.** Anesthesia is essential to the safe, satisfactory, and humane performance of surgical procedures, and it also is essential for many abnormal deliveries. Although neither anesthesia nor analgesia is absolutely necessary for all spontaneous vaginal deliveries, it may relieve unnecessary suffering.

3. **Duration.** In most surgical cases, analgesia is required for only a few hours. Obstetrical analgesia may be required for 12 hours or even longer.

4. **Effects on Labor.** Analgesic agents should exert little or no deleterious effect on uterine contractions and voluntary expulsive efforts. If they do, labor may be prolonged and postpartum hemorrhage may be an added risk.

5. **Timing.** Labor begins without warning, and obstetrical anesthesia may be required within a few hours of a full meal. Moreover, gastric emptying is delayed during pregnancy and prolonged even more during labor, especially after analgesics are given. Vomiting with aspiration of gastric contents, therefore, is a constant threat and often a major cause of serious maternal morbidity and mortality.

Because of these inherent difficulties, as yet no completely safe and satisfactory method of pain relief has been developed for obstetrics. Analgesia and anesthesia, when employed by skilled personnel, may be beneficial rather than detrimental to both fetus and mother. For example, adequate pain relief often forestalls inappropriate operative interventions. The importance of recognizing obstetrical anesthesia as a subspecialty will allow analgesia and anesthesia provided for the parturient by the obstetrician and anesthesiologist working in concert.

Pain relief during labor and delivery is a benefit-versus-risk issue. According to the Maternal Mortality Collaborative (Rochat and colleagues, 1988), 8 percent of direct maternal deaths in 19 reporting areas from 1980 to 1985 were caused by anesthesia complications. With the introduction of obstetrical anesthesia as a special priority, however, the maternal mortality rate from anesthetic-related accidents in Massachusetts decreased significantly over 3 decades—with only 3 deaths over the last decade (Sachs and associates, 1989). In a recent review of 2644 maternal deaths from 1979 through 1986, Atrash and associates (1990) reported that 3.3 percent were anesthesia-related. The rate of death from anesthetic complication was less than 0.4 per 100,000 live births.

In 1986, Gibbs and colleagues reported that less than half of the hospitals with fewer than 500 deliveries per year had general anesthesia for cesarean delivery provided by an anesthesiologist. According to McGrady (1992), the paucity of anesthesiologists continues to be a major problem for hospitals providing obstetrical care. Other major problems that he cites include poor communication between the obstetrician and the anesthesiologist and inadequate supervision of junior personnel.

General Principles

Obstetrical Anesthesia Services. The American College of Obstetricians and Gynecologists and the American Academy of Pediatrics (1992) recently reaffirmed guidelines concerning anesthesia care for obstetrics. They recommend that a qualified person readily be available to administer an appropriate anesthetic and to maintain support of vital functions in an obstetrical emergency. In larger facilities with complicated patients, 24-hour in-house anesthesia is recommended. Moreover, hospitals providing obstetrical care should be capable of starting a cesarean delivery within 30 minutes from the time the decision is made. They also stressed the importance of properly trained individuals capable of managing anesthetic complications. In a recent committee opinion (American College of Obstetricians and Gynecologists, 1992), the importance of assessing the obstetrical patient for various anesthetic risk factors was emphasized. Some of these risk factors are as follows:

1. Marked obesity.
2. Severe edema or anatomical anomalies of the face and neck.

3. Protuberant teeth or difficulty in opening the mouth.
4. Short stature or short neck.
5. Asthma or other serious medical or obstetrical complications.
6. Previous history of anesthetic complications.

Meaningful interpersonal relationships and communication between obstetricians and anesthesiologists cannot be stressed enough!

Principles of Pain Relief. The three essentials of obstetrical pain relief are simplicity, safety, and preservation of fetal homeostasis. With respect to the latter, the most important factor is the transfer of oxygen, which is dependent on the concentration of inhaled oxygen, uterine blood flow, oxygen gradient across the placenta, and umbilical blood flow. Impaired fetal oxygenation most often is the consequence of either compression of the umbilical cord or prolonged or repeated decreases in placental perfusion. Prominent causes of reduced placental perfusion include hypertonic uterine contractions, severe preeclampsia, hemorrhage, premature separation of the placenta, and hypotension from spinal or epidural analgesia.

The woman who is given any form of analgesia should be supervised closely. Without close supervision, she may fall out of bed or vomit and aspirate gastric contents. Similarly, assiduous attention is directed to blood pressure and anesthetic levels after administration of spinal or epidural analgesia.

The obstetrician should become proficient in local, pudendal, and low spinal ("saddle block") analgesia. Continuous lumbar epidural analgesia also may be administered by the obstetrician when he or she has been properly trained and in appropriately selected circumstances. In general, however, it is preferable for an anesthesiologist or anesthetist to provide this care so that the obstetrician can focus attention on the delivery (American Academy of Pediatrics and American College of Obstetricians and Gynecologists, 1992). General anesthesia such as that produced by the combination of thiopental (Pentothal), nitrous oxide, succinylcholine, and a halogenated agent should be available immediately for laparotomy, but also should be administered only by those with special training.

Nonpharmacological Methods of Pain Control. The proper psychological management of the pregnant woman throughout pregnancy and labor is a valuable basic "tranquilizer." **Fear potentiates pain.** A woman who is free from fear, and who has confidence in the obstetrical staff that cares for her, usually requires smaller amounts of analgesia.

Great benefits can be obtained by women and their spouses or "significant others" who attend childbirth-preparation classes. Pregnant women who are taught what to expect regarding pain with labor generally have less fear regarding childbirth. Conversely, women who attempt natural childbirth, but who eventually request intrapartum analgesia, should never be allowed to feel as if they have failed.

Continuous emotional support during labor may also prove of great benefit. In a study by Kennell and associates (1991), 412 nulliparous women in labor were randomized to two groups; one received continuous emotional support from an experienced companion or "doula," and the other was monitored only by an inconspicuous observer who did not interact with the laboring women. The cesarean delivery rate was significantly lower in the continuous support group (8 versus 13 percent) as was the frequency of epidural analgesia for vaginal delivery (7.8 versus 22.6 percent). The use of oxytocin and duration of labor also were less in this group.

Read (1944) emphasized that the intensity of pain during labor is related in large measure to emotional tension. He urged that women be well informed about the physiology of parturition and the various hospital procedures to which they will be subjected during labor and delivery. Lamaze (1970) subsequently described his psychoprophylactic method, which emphasized childbirth as a natural physiological process. Both taught that pain can be minimized by appropriate training in breathing and appropriate psychological support. These concepts have had a considerable impact on the reduction of potent analgesic, sedative, and amnestic drugs used during labor, as well as the reduced use of general anesthesia for delivery. The presence of a supportive spouse or other family member, of conscientious labor attendants, and of a considerate obstetrician who instills confidence, contributes greatly to accomplishing this goal.

Although psychoprophylaxis will not be successful universally, it should be available for those who desire it and are willing to make the effort. At the same time, women who attempt psychoprophylaxis but find the discomforts of labor too great should not be denied the relief provided by appropriate analgesics. It is not unusual for Lamaze-prepared women in the United States to be given a narcotic during labor and conduction analgesia for delivery (Hughey and colleagues, 1978).

Analgesia and Sedation During Labor

When uterine contractions and cervical dilatation cause discomfort, pain relief with a narcotic such as meperidine, plus one of the tranquilizer drugs such as promethazine, usually is indicated. The mother should rest quietly between contractions with a successful program of analgesia and sedation. In this circumstance, discomfort usually is felt at the acme of an effective uterine contraction, but the pain generally is not unbearable. Appropriate drug selection and administration should accomplish these objectives for the great majority of women in labor, without risk to them or their infants.

Meperidine and Promethazine. Meperidine, 50 to 100 mg, with promethazine, 25 mg, may be administered intramuscularly at intervals of 3 to 4 hours. In general, a small dose given more frequently is preferable to a large one administered less often. Then, if delivery follows during the next hour or so after the injection, the neonate is less likely to be depressed by the medication. The size of the mother must be taken into account in determining the size of the dose.

A more rapid effect is achieved by giving these drugs intravenously, but in general, not more than 50 mg of meperidine or more than 25 mg of promethazine should be given at one time by this route. Whereas analgesia is maximal about 45 minutes after an intramuscular injection, it develops almost immediately following intravenous administration. The depressant effect in the fetus follows closely behind the peak analgesic effect in the mother.

Effect of Meperidine on Labor. There is no convincing evidence that meperidine prolongs labor. In fact, Riffel and co-workers (1973) evaluated the effects of meperidine alone and meperidine plus promethazine on labor; they observed not a decrease but a slight increase in uterine activity following injection of these drugs. DeVoe and co-workers (1969) reported similar observations. It seems reasonable to postulate that this increase in uterine activity may be related to a decrease in epinephrine or other catecholamines.

Other Drugs. Other narcotic analgesics such as alphaprodine (Nisentil), butorphanol (Stadol), and nalbuphine (Nubain) have been used to provide pain relief during labor. A great variety of sedative agents and tranquilizers has been administered with such narcotics or, at times, alone. It is important to recognize that all narcotics and tranquilizers rapidly cross the placenta and may produce significant neonatal respiratory depression.

The synthetic narcotic butorphanol, given in 1- to 2-mg doses, compares favorably with 40 to 60 mg of meperidine (Quilligan and colleagues, 1980). Neonatal respiratory depression is reported to be less than with meperidine, but care must be taken that the two drugs are not given contiguously because butorphanol antagonizes the narcotic effects of meperidine. Angel and colleagues (1984) and Hatjis and Meis (1986) described a sinusoidal fetal heart rate pattern following butorphanol administration.

Nalbuphine also is a synthetic narcotic. When given in a dose of 15 to 20 mg intravenously, it does not cause neonatal depression (Wilson and associates, 1986).

Narcotic Antagonists. Meperidine or other narcotics used during labor may cause newborn respiratory depression. Naloxone hydrochloride (Narcan) is a narcotic antagonist capable of reversing respiratory depression induced by opioid narcotics by displacing the narcotic from specific receptors in the central nervous system. Withdrawal symptoms may be precipitated in recipients who are physically dependent on narcotics. The recently revised suggested dose for the newborn infant is 0.1 mg per kg of body weight injected into the umbilical vein (American Academy of Pediatrics and American College of Obstetricians and Gynecologists, 1992). This usually acts within 2 minutes with an effective duration of at least 30 minutes. The naloxone injection may have to be repeated.

In the absence of narcotics, naloxone exhibits little, if any, adverse activity and is the drug of choice for treating narcotic depression in the newborn.

GENERAL ANESTHESIA

Without exception, all anesthetic agents that depress the maternal central nervous system cross the placenta and depress the fetal central nervous system. Another constant hazard with any general anesthetic is aspiration of gastric contents and particulate matter that will obstruct airways and ultimately may lead to pneumonitis, pulmonary edema, and death. Fasting before the time of anesthesia is not always an effective safeguard, because fasting gastric juice, even if free of particulate matter, is likely to be strongly acidic and thus can produce fatal aspiration pneumonitis. At the same time, tracheal intubation is valuable to ensure a satisfactory airway and minimize the risk of aspiration. **Failed tracheal intubation** fortunately is uncommon, but is a major cause of anesthesia-related maternal deaths (Endler and colleagues, 1988; King and Adams, 1990).

With inhalation, the concentration of the anesthetic agent increases in the lungs of the pregnant woman somewhat more rapidly because the functional residual capacity and residual volume of the lungs are reduced. For the same reason, residual oxygen in the lung after expiration is appreciably less, a factor of importance when there is delay in intubation and oxygenation after injection of a muscle relaxant. **Trained personnel and specialized equipment are mandatory for the safe use of general anesthesia.**

Inhalation Anesthesia

Gas Anesthetics. Nitrous oxide (N_2O) is the only anesthetic gas in current use for obstetrical analgesia in the United States. It may be used to provide pain relief during labor as well as at delivery. This agent produces analgesia and altered consciousness, but by itself does not provide true anesthesia. Nitrous oxide does not prolong labor or interfere with uterine contractions. Satisfactory analgesia often is obtained with a concentration of 50 percent nitrous oxide and 50 percent oxygen. During the second stage of labor, when a uterine contraction begins, a well-fitting clear mask is placed on the woman's face and she is encouraged to take three deep breaths and then to bear down.

Nitrous oxide commonly is used as part of a **balanced general anesthesia** that is popular for cesarean delivery and some forceps deliveries. It is given along with oxygen in a 50 : 50 mixture, and a short-acting barbiturate (usually thiopental) is given intravenously along with a muscle relaxant (usually succinylcholine) just prior to tracheal intubation. With this technique, high concentrations of potent inhalational anesthetics are avoided.

Volatile Anesthetics. Halothane (Fluothane), enflurane (Ethrane), and isoflurane (Forane) are used to supplement nitrous oxide during maintenance of general anesthesia. These halogenated hydrocarbons cross the placenta readily and are capable of producing narcosis in the fetus.

Halothane is a potent, nonexplosive agent that produces remarkable uterine relaxation when given in high inhaled concentrations. Its use should be restricted to those very uncommon situations in which uterine relaxation is a requisite rather than a hazard. It is one of the anesthetic agents of choice for the now very uncommon procedures of internal podalic version of the second twin, breech decomposition, and replacement of the acutely inverted uterus. As soon as the maneuver has been completed, halothane administration should be stopped and immediate efforts made to promote myometrial contraction to minimize hemorrhage from the placental implantation site. Because of its cardiodepressant and hypotensive effects, halothane may intensify the adverse effects of maternal hypovolemia. Halothane has occasionally been associated with *hepatitis* and *massive hepatic necrosis.*

Enflurane and *isoflurane* are used by some because of possible halothane hepatotoxicity. In doses that provide analgesia, they are likely to cause unconsciousness. Also, like halothane, they may cause myometrial relaxation. We now use isoflurane preferentially to induce uterine relaxation for version and extraction of the second twin. Enflurane should not be given to anyone suspected of impaired renal function.

Methoxyflurane is pleasant to take and may be self-administered in low concentration to provide analgesia during the first and second stages of labor and during delivery. Overdose may be a major complication when methoxyflurane is self-administered for analgesia. This agent is rarely used today.

Balanced General Anesthesia. Nitrous oxide and oxygen given for balanced general anesthesia have been

associated with some degree of maternal awareness when these women were interviewed postpartum (Hodgkinson and colleagues, 1978; Warren and associates, 1983). For this reason, as well as to be able to increase the inspired concentration of oxygen, many anesthesiologists recommend the addition of one of the halogenated agents in concentrations of less than 1 percent (Warren and colleagues, 1983). Piggott and co-workers (1990) studied 200 women undergoing cesarean delivery and randomized them to either nitrous oxide (50 percent) and oxygen (50 percent) or oxygen (100 percent), both supplemented with isoflurane. There were no instances of awareness in either group, and babies of mothers who received 100 percent oxygen required less resuscitation and had higher Apgar scores.

The major concern regarding halogenated agents has been their possible association with increased blood loss (Gilstrap and associates, 1987). Andrews and colleagues (1992) reported a significantly greater decrease in the postpartum hematocrit when general anesthesia with a halogenated agent was compared with regional techniques for women undergoing elective repeat cesarean delivery. Others also have reported an increased risk of hemorrhage associated with their use (Combs and associates, 1991). Conversely, other studies have not reported such associations, especially if women at high risk for bleeding are excluded (Abboud and co-workers, 1985; Camann and Datta, 1991; Lamont and associates, 1988; Warren and colleagues, 1983). Volatile agents such as halothane, enflurane, and isoflurane are of paramount importance in general anesthetic techniques, and their possible association with increased blood loss is not viewed as a general condemnation of their use during cesarean delivery (Camann and Datta, 1991).

Anesthetic Gas Exposure and Pregnancy Outcome. Sufficient data have accrued to cause concerns for the welfare of the embryo and fetus of pregnant women who work in operating rooms where they are chronically exposed to anesthetic gases. In some reports, but not all, the spontaneous abortion rate of female workers exposed was about twice that for unexposed personnel, and the minor malformation rate in children of exposed male workers was slightly greater (Knill-Jones and colleagues, 1975). In England and Wales, a comparison has been made between pregnancy outcomes of women doctors exposed to anesthetic gases during pregnancy and those not so exposed (Pharah and colleagues, 1977). Conception while the woman was actively engaged in practicing anesthesiology resulted in slightly smaller babies (3350 versus 3390 g), an increased frequency of cardiovascular malformations (1.4 versus 0.4 percent), and more stillbirths (1.7 versus 0.8 percent). Spontaneous abortions were the same for both groups (14 percent). However, Ericson and Källen (1979) found no differences in pregnancies of operating-room workers in Sweden. From Denmark, Husum and co-workers (1983) detected no effects from long-term exposure to trace concentrations of waste anesthetic gases. Sister chromatid exchanges and structural chromosomal aberrations in lymphocytes were no more common in operating-room personnel than in unexposed control subjects. Thus, although the exact fetal risk of chronic maternal exposure of waste anesthetic gas is unknown, available data would suggest that there is not a substantial risk for either pregnancy loss or congenital anomalies (Friedman, 1988).

Intravenous Drugs During Anesthesia

Thiopental. Intravenous thiopental (Pentothal) is used widely in conjunction with other agents for general anesthesia in obstetrics. The drug offers the advantages of ease and extreme rapidity of induction, ready controllability, and prompt recovery with minimal risk of vomiting. Thiopental and similar compounds are poor analgesic agents, and the administration of sufficient drug given alone to maintain anesthesia may cause appreciable newborn depression. Thus, thiopental is not used as the sole anesthetic agent, but in a dose that induces sleep, it is given along with a muscle relaxant, usually succinylcholine, and nitrous oxide plus oxygen.

General anesthesia should not be induced until all steps preparatory to actual delivery have been completed, so as to minimize transfer of the anesthetic agent to the fetus and, in turn, avoid respiratory depression in the newborn. General anesthesia, however, need not cause appreciable neonatal depression. Zagorzycki and Brinkman (1982) compared the status of infants immediately after cesarean delivery whose mothers received either epidural analgesia or general anesthesia, the technique for which consisted of preoxygenation, thiopental (4 mg per kg), muscle relaxant, nitrous oxide (50 percent), and halothane (0.5 percent). No difference was found in Apgar scores at 1 and 5 minutes. No appreciable differences in mean scores or in the frequency of scores below 7 were evident.

When the time from induction of anesthesia to delivery is prolonged appreciably, there is an increased likelihood of neonatal depression. Often the delay is the consequence of obstetrical difficulties necessitating manipulation of the uterus and the fetus, leading to fetal depression.

Ketamine. Occasionally ketamine is utilized in obstetrics to produce analgesia and sedation (0.5 mg per kg). Larger doses (1 to 2 mg per kg) are often sufficient to induce general anesthesia. It may prove useful in women with acute hemorrhage because it is not associated with hypotension like thiopental. In fact, it usually causes a rise in blood pressure and thus it generally should be avoided in women already hypertensive. Unpleasant delirium and hallucinations commonly are induced by this agent. When given in high doses, ketamine may cause respiratory depression and hypertonus sufficient to impair efforts at newborn ventilation.

Aspiration During General Anesthesia

Pneumonitis from inhalation of gastric contents has been the most common cause of anesthetic death in obstetrics. In its survey of over 2700 maternal deaths between 1979 and 1986, the Centers for Disease Control (Atrash and colleagues, 1990) identified inhalation of gastric contents to be associated with at least one fourth of all anesthetic deaths. The aspirated material from the stomach may contain undigested food and thereby cause airway obstruction and tissue damage that, unless promptly relieved, may prove rapidly fatal. Although gastric juice is likely to contain less particulate matter during fasting, it is extremely acidic and capable of inducing a lethal chemical pneumonitis.

Prophylaxis. Important to effective prophylaxis are (1) fasting for at least 6 and preferably 12 hours before anesthesia; (2) use of agents to reduce gastric acidity during the induction and maintenance of general anesthesia; (3) skillful tracheal intubation accompanied by pressure on the cricoid cartilage to occlude the esophagus; (4) at completion of the operation, extubation with the mother awake and lying on her side with head lowered; and (5) utilization of regional anesthetic techniques when appropriate.

Fasting. Steps should be taken to lessen the likelihood of danger from aspiration of both particulate matter and acidic gastric secretions. These measures should be included also for women for whom conduction analgesia is planned. For elective obstetrical procedures, fasting for 12 hours usually rids the stomach of undigested food but not necessarily of acidic liquid. Sutherland and colleagues (1986) studied women undergoing early pregnancy termination or minor gynecological surgery, and they showed that despite overnight fasting, the mean stomach juice volume was 20 mL, with a pH of 1.6. In women at term undergoing elective cesarean delivery, Lewis and Crawford (1987) showed that women given a light meal of only tea and toast had twice the volume of gastric contents as fasted controls at 4 hours, and particulate matter was identified in 20 percent. Gastric emptying in labor is even more retarded, and women in early labor should be advised to fast before coming to the hospital, and certainly thereafter. **Despite these precautions, it should be assumed that any woman in labor has both gastric particulate matter as well as acidic contents.**

Antacids. **The practice of administering antacids shortly before induction of anesthesia probably has done more to decrease mortality from obstetrical anesthesia than any other single practice.** It is essential that the antacid disperse promptly throughout all of the gastric contents to neutralize the hydrogen ion effectively. It is equally important that the antacid, if aspirated, not incite comparably serious pulmonary problems.

Gibbs and colleagues (1984) reported that 30 mL of 0.3 M sodium citrate with citric acid (Bicitra), given about 45 minutes before surgery, neutralized gastric contents (mean volume 70 mL) in nearly 90 percent of women undergoing cesarean delivery. For several years now at Parkland Hospital, we have routinely administered 30 mL of Bicitra within a few minutes of the anticipated time of anesthesia induction, either general or by major regional block. If more than 1 hour has passed since the first dose was given and anesthesia induction, then a second dose is given.

Magnesium hydroxide, or milk of magnesia, also effectively neutralizes gastric acid (Wheatley and colleagues, 1979), and its favorable effects last long enough for cesarean delivery to be completed. Gibbs and associates (1979) demonstrated in dogs that pulmonary instillation of a suspension of milk of magnesia and aluminum hydroxide can induce pneumonitis; however, we have observed no long-term effects on the respiratory tract in those instances in which women aspirated the compound.

Cimetidine, given sometime before general anesthesia for delivery, also has been recommended (Hodgkinson and colleagues, 1983). At least 60 minutes are required after parenteral administration to decrease gastric acidity to relatively safe levels. Therefore, in emergency situations, either an antacid or antacid plus cimetidine should be used (Moir, 1983). Thorburn and Moir (1987) studied 100 women undergoing emergency cesarean delivery who were given cimetidine, 200 mg intravenously, along with 30 mL of sodium citrate orally. The time interval from cimetidine administration to induction of general anesthesia was 5 to 208 minutes. None of the women had a gastric pH of less than 2.7 and all but one had a pH of 3.0 or higher.

Another histamine H_2-antagonist, ranitidine, can be given the night before surgery and will result in decreased gastric section through the next morning. This agent might prove useful when given along with a second dose on the morning of surgery for scheduled elective cesarean deliveries (Burchman, 1992). Yau and associates (1992), in a study of 49 women undergoing cesarean delivery who received ranitidine and sodium citrate, reported that only one patient (2 percent) had an intragastric pH of less than 2.5 and a volume greater than 25 mL.

Intubation. Various positions have been tried to minimize aspiration before and during tracheal intubation and cuff inflation, but the disadvantages from positions other than supine outweigh any advantage. Cricoid pressure from the time of induction of anesthesia until intubation should be performed by a trained associate. In special instances, intubation may be performed with the mother awake. In these cases, local anesthesia usually is applied. Appropriately applied topical spray generally will not significantly depress the laryngeal reflex.

Extubation. At the completion of the surgical procedure, the tracheal tube may be safely removed only if the woman is conscious to a degree to follow commands and is capable of maintaining oxygen saturation with spontaneous respiration.

Pathology. Aspiration pneumonitis associated with obstetrical anesthesia was described by Mendelson in 1946. Teabeaut (1952) demonstrated experimentally that if the pH of aspirated fluid was below 2.5, severe chemical pneumonitis developed. In one study the pH of gastric juice of nearly half of women tested intrapartum without treatment was below 2.5 (Taylor and Pryse-Davies, 1966). The right mainstem bronchus usually offers the simplest pathway for aspirated material to reach the lung parenchyma, and therefore the right lower lobe most often is involved. In severe cases, there is bilateral widespread involvement.

The woman who aspirates may develop evidence for respiratory distress immediately or as long as several hours after aspiration, depending in part upon the material aspirated, the severity of the process, and the acuity of the attendants. Aspiration of a large amount of solid material causes obvious signs of airway obstruction. Smaller particles without acidic liquid may lead to patchy atelectasis and later to bronchopneumonia.

When highly acidic liquid is inspired, decreased oxygen saturation along with tachypnea, bronchospasm, rhonchi, rales, atelectasis, cyanosis, tachycardia, and hypotension likely are to develop. At the sites of injury, protein-rich fluid containing numerous erythrocytes exudes from capillaries into the lung interstitium and alveoli to cause decreased pulmonary compliance, shunting of blood, and severe hypoxemia. Radiographic changes may not appear immediately and they may be quite variable, although the right lobe most often is affected. Therefore, a chest x-ray alone should not be used to exclude aspiration.

Treatment. In recent years, the methods recommended for treatment of aspiration have changed appreciably, indicating that previous therapy was not very successful. Suspicion of aspiration of gastric contents demands very close monitoring for evidence of any pulmonary damage.

Suction and Bronchoscopy. As much as possible of the inhaled fluid should be immediately wiped out of the mouth and removed from the pharynx and trachea by suction. Saline lavage may further disseminate the acid throughout the lung. If large particulate matter is inspired, prompt bronchoscopy may be indicated to relieve airway obstruction. Otherwise, bronchoscopy not only is unnecessary but may contribute to morbidity and mortality.

Corticosteroids. There is no clinical evidence that corticosteroid therapy is unequivocally beneficial (Bynum and Pierce, 1976). Furthermore, experimental evidence is not consistent with the conclusion that appreciable benefits accrue from the use of corticosteroids. Nonetheless, the clinical impression of some has been that the immediate intravenous administration of 500 mg of methylprednisolone sodium succinate (Solu-Medrol), with repeated doses of 250 mg every 8 hours for 24 hours, is beneficial. It has not been our practice to utilize steroids.

Oxygen and Ventilation. Oxygen delivered through a tracheal tube in increased concentration by intermittent positive pressure may be required to raise and maintain the arterial Po_2 at 60 mm Hg or higher. Frequent suctioning is necessary to remove secretions including edema fluid. Mechanical ventilation that produces positive end-expiratory pressure may prove lifesaving by preventing the complete collapse of the now surfactant-poor lung on expiration. Treatment for the adult respiratory distress syndrome is described in Chapter 47 (p. 1069).

Antimicrobials. Although the likelihood of bacterial contamination and infection from aspiration is appreciable, the use of antimicrobials prophylactically is controversial (Bynum and Pierce, 1976). Bartlett and associates (1974) identified anaerobic bacteria in 50 of 54 cases of pneumonia caused by aspiration. They concluded that anaerobes play a key role in most cases of infection after aspiration, and they suggested the use of clindamycin or chloramphenicol for those anaerobes not sensitive to penicillin. We do not give antimicrobials unless there is clinical evidence of infection.

Failed Intubation

As mentioned previously, failed intubation remains a significant cause of anesthetic-related maternal mortality. According to Morgan (1987) and King and Adams (1990), the incidence of failed intubation actually is higher in the obstetrical patient compared with the general surgery patient. Although its exact incidence is unknown, it has been estimated to occur in approximately 1 in 300 obstetrical patients in whom intubation is attempted (Lyons, 1985; Morgan, 1987).

Prevention. A detailed history to elicit previous difficulties with intubation as well as a careful assessment of anatomical features of the neck, maxillo-facial, pharyngeal, and laryngeal structures may help predict a difficult intubation (King and Adams, 1990). Unfortunately, this

serious complication may be encountered unexpectedly in women without such a history, or in women with normal-appearing anatomical features (King and Adams, 1990).

Morbid obesity also is a risk factor for failed or difficult intubation. Of paramount importance in these women is appropriate preoperative preparation to include the immediate availability of a short-hand laryngoscope, fiber-optic laryngoscope, and the liberal use of awake nasal or oral intubation techniques (Blass, 1991).

Management. An important principle is to start the operative procedure only after it has been ascertained that tracheal intubation has been successful and that adequate ventilation can be accomplished. Although the surgeon is eager to begin surgery as soon as the tube appears to be in place, especially in the presence of an abnormal fetal heart rate pattern, initiation of cesarean delivery will serve only to complicate matters if there is difficulty or failure in tracheal intubation. Most often these women must be allowed to awaken and a different technique utilized such as an awake intubation or a regional analgesic. On occasion, fetal bradycardia may occur as a manifestation of failed or difficult intubation. Again, it is better to allow the mother to awaken and the fetus to recover *in utero* than to proceed with an emergency cesarean delivery in the presence of inadequate maternal ventilation.

Following failed intubation, the patient should be ventilated by mask and cricoid pressure applied to reduce the chance of aspiration (Malan and Johnson, 1992). Again it is usually more prudent to allow the patient to awaken in this scenario.

REGIONAL ANALGESIA

A variety of nerve blocks have been developed over the years to provide pain relief for the woman in labor and at delivery. Because they are designed to be implemented without loss of consciousness (anesthesia), they are correctly referred to as regional analgesics.

Sensory Innervation of Genital Tract

Uterine Innervation. Pain in the first stage of labor is generated largely from the uterus. Visceral sensory fibers from the uterus, cervix, and upper vagina traverse through the *Frankenhäuser ganglion,* which lies just lateral to the cervix, into the pelvic plexus, and then to the middle and superior internal iliac plexuses. From there, the fibers travel in the lumbar and lower thoracic sympathetic chains to enter the spinal cord through the white rami communicantes associated with the 10th, 11th, and 12th thoracic and first lumbar nerves. Early in the first stage of labor, the pain of uterine contractions is transmitted predominantly through the 11th and 12th thoracic nerves.

The motor pathways to the uterus leave the spinal cord at the level of the seventh and eighth thoracic vertebrae. Theoretically, any method of sensory block that does not also block the motor pathways to the uterus can be used for analgesia during labor.

Lower Genital Tract Innervation. Although painful uterine contractions continue during the second stage of labor, much of the pain of vaginal delivery arises from the lower genital tract. Painful stimuli from the lower genital tract are transmitted primarily through the *pudendal nerve*, the peripheral branches of which provide sensory innervation to the perineum, anus, and the more medial and inferior parts of the vulva and clitoris. The pudendal nerve passes across the posterior surface of the sacrospinous ligament just as the ligament attaches to the ischial spine (Fig. 16–1). The sensory nerve fibers of the pudendal nerve are derived from the ventral branches of the 2nd, 3rd, and 4th sacral nerves.

Anesthetic Agents

A variety of compounds currently are used in obstetrics to induce local or regional analgesia. Some of the more commonly used local anesthetics, along with their usual concentration, doses, and duration of actions, are shown in Table 16–1. **The physician is cautioned to carefully study the package insert for each product before use.** Some preparations suitable for epidural analgesia are not suitable for subarachnoid injection because the preservative may cause inflammation. Some preparations contain a dilute solution of epinephrine to prolong the action of the anesthetic or to produce symptoms when a test dose is inadvertently given intravenously. We find that there is sufficient flexibility in the choice of plain solutions, and thus we avoid the potential hazard of severe hypertension from epinephrine. The dose of each agent varies widely, and is dependent upon the indicated nerve block and physical status of the woman. When the dose is increased, onset, duration, and quality of analgesia are enhanced, but only incremental dosage of small-volume boluses allows safety through careful monitoring for early warning signs of toxicity. **Administration of these agents must be followed by appropriate monitoring for adverse reactions, and equipment and personnel to manage these reactions must be immediately available.**

Most often, serious toxicity follows injection of an anesthetic into a vessel, but it may also be induced by administration of excessive amounts. Because many of these agents are manufactured in more than one concentration and ampule size to be used for specific local or regional blocks, a thorough knowledge of the ones selected for use is essential for safety. Two manifestations of systemic toxicity from local anesthetics are

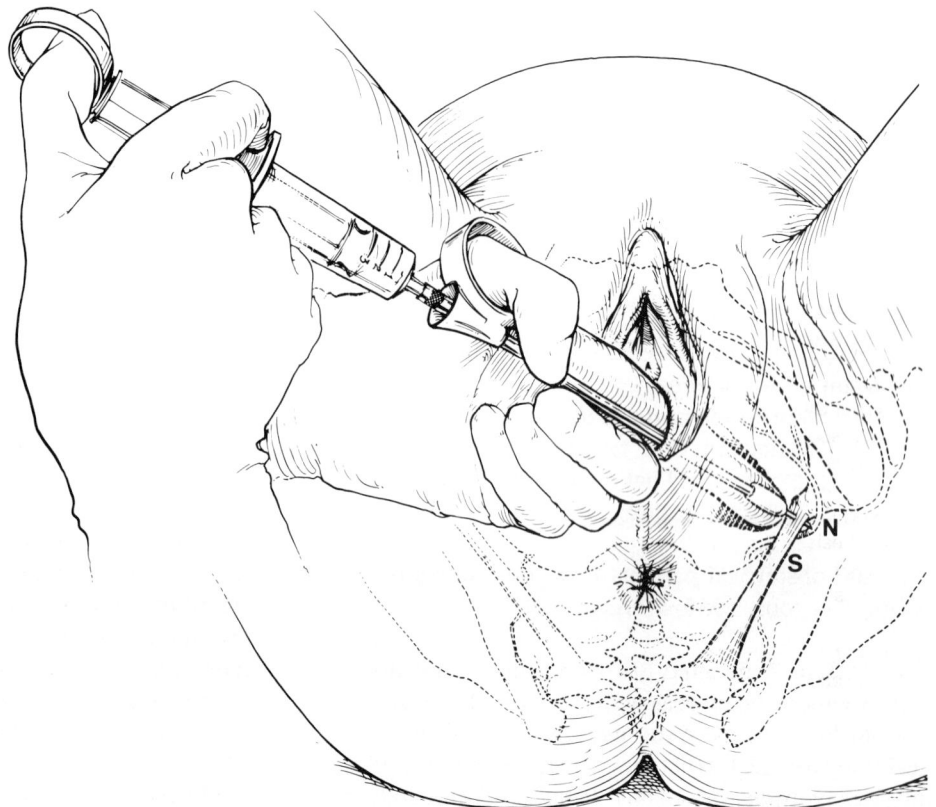

Fig. 16–1. Local infiltration of the pudendal nerve. Transvaginal technique showing the needle extended beyond the needle guard and passing through the sacrospinous ligament (S) to reach the pudendal nerve (N).

TABLE 16–1. SOME LOCAL ANESTHETIC AGENTS USED IN OBSTETRICS

| Anesthetic Agent | Plain Solutions | | | | Clinical Use |
	Usual Concentration (%)	Usual Volume (mL)	Usual Dose (mg)	Average Duration (min)	
Amino-esters					
2-Chloroprocaine	1–2	20–30	400–600	15–30	Local infiltration and pudendal block
	2–3	15–25	300–750	30–60	Epidural for cesarean delivery
	2	8–10	160–200	30–60	Epidural for labor analgesia
Tetracaine	0.2	2	4	75–150	Low spinal block with 6% glucose
	0.5	—	7–10	75–150	Spinal for cesarean delivery with 5% glucose
Amino-amides					
Lidocaine	1	20–30	200–300	30–60	Infiltration and pudendal block
	1.5	8–10	120–150	60–90	Epidural for labor analgesia
	1.5–2	15–30	300–450	60–90	Epidural for cesarean delivery
	5	1–2	50–75	45–60	Spinal for cesarean delivery with 7.5% glucose
Bupivacaine	0.5	10–20	50–100	90–150	Epidural for cesarean delivery
	0.25	8–10	20–25	60–90	Epidural for labor analgesia

those of the central nervous and cardiovascular systems. Both are life threatening and may follow any route of administration.

Central Nervous System Toxicity. Characteristically there is excitation followed by depression. Symptoms include lightheadedness, dizziness, tinnitus, bizarre behavior, slurred speech, metallic taste, numbness of the tongue and mouth, muscle fasciculation and excitation, generalized convulsions, and loss of consciousness (Table 16–2). The convulsions should be controlled, an airway established, and oxygen delivered. Succinylcholine abolishes the peripheral manifestations of the convulsions and allows tracheal intubation. Thiopental or diazepam acts centrally to inhibit convulsions. In the few instances in which it has been tried at Parkland Hospital, magnesium sulfate administered according to the regimen for eclampsia also has controlled effectively

TABLE 16–2. CLINICAL MANIFESTATIONS AND TREATMENT OF CENTRAL NERVOUS SYSTEM TOXICITY FROM LOCAL ANESTHETIC AGENTS

Signs and Symptoms
Slurred speech
Dizziness
Metallic taste
Tinnitus
Paresthesia of the mouth
Syncope
Seizures
Coma

Treatment
Oxygenation
Ventilation (consider intubation)
Thiopental or diazepam for seizures
Correction of hypotension—uterine displacement, fluids, ephedrine

Adapted from Gilstrap and Hankins (1988).

the convulsions. Fetal distress, manifested by either late heart rate decelerations or persistent bradycardia, may develop as the consequences of maternal hypoxia and lactic acidosis induced by convulsions. With arrest of the convulsions, administration of oxygen, and application of other supportive measures, the fetus likely will recover more quickly in utero than following immediate cesarean delivery. Moreover, maternal well-being usually is better served by waiting until the intensity of the hypoxia and the metabolic acidosis have diminished.

Cardiovascular Toxicity. Cardiovascular manifestations from local anesthetic toxicity do not always follow central nervous system involvement. Generally, they develop later than those from cerebral toxicity, because they are induced by higher blood levels of drug. They also are characterized first by stimulation and then depression. Accordingly, there is hypertension and tachycardia, which soon is followed by hypotension and cardiac arrhythmias. The hypotension and arrhythmias contribute appreciably to impaired uteroplacental perfusion and fetal distress. Hypotension initially is managed by turning the woman onto her side to avoid aortocaval compression. A crystalloid solution is infused rapidly along with intravenously administered ephedrine. **The temptation to perform emergency cesarean delivery for fetal distress must be resisted, because this may prove fatal for the mother if done before she is resuscitated.** As with convulsions, the fetus is likely to recover more quickly in utero once maternal cardiac output is reestablished.

Inadvertent intravenous injection of local anesthetic is likely to cause these adverse effects. Another mechanism is repeated injections of the drug at multiple sites, resulting in an increase in total dose. Such an example is the administration of an ineffective epidural, followed by pudendal block that was not satisfactory for repairing an episiotomy or lacerations, followed by local infiltration.

Local Infiltration

Local infiltration is of no value for analgesia during labor, but is employed for delivery. Local infiltration is of especial value in the following circumstances: (1) before episiotomy and delivery, (2) after delivery into the site of lacerations to be repaired, and (3) around the episiotomy wound if there is inadequate analgesia. From the standpoint of safety, local infiltration analgesia is preeminent.

Pudendal Block

A tubular director that allows 1.0 to 1.5 cm of a 15 cm-long 22-gauge needle to protrude beyond its tip is used to guide the needle into position over the pudendal nerve (Fig. 16–1). The end of the director is placed against the vaginal mucosa just beneath the tip of the ischial spine. The needle is pushed beyond the tip of the director into the mucosa and a mucosal wheal is made with 1 mL of 1 percent lidocaine solution or an equivalent dose of another local anesthetic with similarly high tissue penetration and rapid action. **Aspiration is attempted before this and all subsequent injections to guard against intravascular infusion.** The needle is then advanced until it touches the sacrospinous ligament, which is infiltrated with 3 mL of lidocaine. The needle is advanced farther through the ligament, and as it pierces the loose areolar tissue behind the ligament, the resistance of the plunger decreases. Another 3 mL of the anesthetic solution is injected into this region. Next, the needle is withdrawn into the guide, the tip of the guide is moved to just above the ischial spine, and the needle is inserted through the mucosa. After again aspirating to avoid intravascular injection, the rest of 10 mL of solution is deposited.

Within 3 to 4 minutes of the time of injection, the successful pudendal block will allow pinching of the lower vagina and posterior vulva bilaterally without pain. It is often of benefit before pudendal block to infiltrate the fourchette, perineum, and adjacent vagina directly at the site where the episiotomy is to be made with 5 to 10 mL of 1 percent lidocaine solution. Then, if delivery occurs before pudendal block becomes effective, an episiotomy can be made without pain. By the time of the repair, the pudendal block usually has become effective.

Pudendal block usually works well and is an extremely safe and relatively simple method of providing analgesia for spontaneous delivery. From 1988 to 1991

at Parkland Hospital, 25 percent of over 48,000 women delivered vaginally were managed effectively with bilateral pudendal block and local analgesia. Some of these women had been given epidural analgesia during labor.

Pudendal block, however, may not provide adequate analgesia for forceps delivery or when delivery requires manipulation. Moreover, analgesia limited to pudendal block usually is inadequate for women in whom complete visualization of the cervix and upper vagina, or manual exploration of the uterine cavity, are indicated. Under these circumstances, the addition of an intravenously administered narcotic analgesic such as 50 mg of meperidine may provide appreciable, although not total, relief from the pain of examination.

Complications. Intravascular injection of a local anesthetic agent may cause serious systemic toxicity characterized by stimulation of the cerebral cortex leading to convulsions (Table 16–2). A troublesome hematoma, the consequence of perforation of a blood vessel, is most likely to occur when there is defective coagulation such as that induced by heparin or by severe placental abruption. Rarely, severe infection may originate at the injection site. The infection may spread to the region posterior to the hip joint, into the gluteal musculature, or into the retropsoal space (Svancarek and associates, 1977). Death or severe permanent impairment in some survivors has been recorded (Wenger and Gitchell, 1973).

Paracervical Block

Paracervical block serves to relieve the pain of uterine contractions, but because the pudendal nerves are not blocked, additional analgesia is required for delivery. Usually lidocaine or chloroprocaine, 5 to 10 mL of a 1 percent solution, is injected at 3 and 9 o'clock. Because these anesthetics are relatively short acting, paracervical block may have to be repeated during labor.

Complications. Although good to excellent pain relief usually is achieved from paracervical block during the first stage of labor, *fetal bradycardia* is a worrisome complication that has been reported in 10 to 70 percent of such blocks. Bradycardia usually develops within 10 minutes and may last up to 30 minutes. Several investigators stress that bradycardia is not a sign of fetal asphyxia, because it usually is transient and the newborns are in most instances vigorous at birth. There are reports, however, in which fetal scalp blood pH and Apgar scores were sometimes found to be low, and a few fetuses have died. The effect may be the consequence of transplacental transfer of the anesthetic agent or its metabolites and, in turn, a depressant effect on the heart. However, Greiss (1976) and Fishburne (1979) and their associates, based on studies in pregnant ewes, believe that fetal bradycardia results from decreased placental perfusion as the consequence of drug-induced uterine artery vasoconstriction and myometrial hypertonus. For these reasons, paracervical block should not be used in situations of potential fetal compromise (Carlsson and colleagues, 1987).

Spinal (Subarachnoid) Block

Introduction of a local anesthetic into the subarachnoid space to effect spinal block long has been used for uncomplicated cesarean delivery and for vaginal delivery of normal women of low parity. Because of the smaller subarachnoid space during pregnancy, the same amount of anesthetic agent in the same volume of solution produces much higher blockade in parturients than in nonpregnant women. The smaller space is the consequence most likely of engorgement of the internal vertebral venous plexus.

Vaginal Delivery. Low spinal block is a popular form of analgesia for delivery. The level of analgesia extends to the 10th thoracic dermatome, which corresponds to the level of the umbilicus. Blockade to this level provides excellent relief from the pain of uterine contractions. The term *saddle block* has been incorrectly applied to this level of analgesia, because the area of skin anesthetized is appreciably greater than that which would be in contact with a saddle.

Nearly all local anesthetic agents have been used for spinal analgesia, but for many years one that has proved quite satisfactory for vaginal delivery is tetracaine in a dose of 4 mg already dissolved in 2 mL of a 6 percent solution of dextrose in water (Table 16–1). With 4 mg of tetracaine, satisfactory anesthetic in the lower vagina and the perineum persists for about an hour. Lidocaine given in a hyperbaric solution also produces excellent spinal analgesia and has the advantage of a shorter duration. Neither is administered for vaginal delivery until the cervix is fully dilated and all other criteria for safe forceps delivery have been fulfilled (see Chap. 24, p. 560). Spinal analgesia is not recommended before this time because of the frequency of disruption of orderly labor by the anesthetic. Preanalgesic intravenous hydration with a liter of crystalloid solution will prevent hypotension in many cases.

Cesarean Delivery. For cesarean delivery, a higher level of spinal sensory blockade is essential to at least the level of the eighth thoracic dermatome, which is just below the xiphoid process of the sternum. **Because a larger area is to be anesthetized, a larger dose of anesthetic agent is necessary, and this increases the frequency and intensity of toxic reactions.** Depending upon maternal size, 8 to 10 mg of tetracaine or 50 to 75 mg of lidocaine are adminis-

tered. The addition of 0.2 mg of morphine improves pain control during delivery and postoperatively (Abouleish and colleagues, 1988). Undue delay between intrathecal injection of anesthetic agent and delivery of the infant should be avoided if a safe dose of the anesthetic drug is to be used, yet have spinal analgesia of sufficient intensity and duration to allow completion of abdominal delivery without serious discomfort. Therefore, catheterization of the bladder and shaving of the operative field should be done before the anesthetic is administered.

Complications with Spinal Analgesia. A number of complications may follow induction of spinal analgesia. Close clinical monitoring of vital signs is imperative, and this includes assessment of the level of analgesia, which should stabilize by 10 to 20 minutes.

Hypotension. Maternal hypotension may develop very soon after injection of the analgesic agent. This is the consequence of vasodilatation from sympathetic blockade compounded by obstructed venous return caused by uterine compression of the vena cava and adjacent large veins. Importantly, in the supine position, even in the absence of maternal hypotension measured in the brachial artery, placental blood flow still may be reduced significantly. Important to prophylaxis and to treatment of spinal hypotension are (1) uterine elevation and displacement to the left of the abdomen; (2) acute hydration with a balanced salt solution; and (3) at the first sign of a decrease in blood pressure after hydration, the intravenous injection of 10 to 15 mg of ephedrine (Table 16–3).

Total Spinal Blockade. Complete spinal blockade with respiratory paralysis may complicate spinal analgesia. Most often, total spinal blockade is the consequence of administration of a dose of analgesic agent far in excess of that tolerated by pregnant women. Hypotension and apnea promptly develop and must be immediately treated to prevent cardiac arrest. In the undelivered woman, the uterus is displaced laterally to minimize aortovenal compression. Effective ventilation is established, through a tracheal tube when possible, to protect

TABLE 16–3. PROPHYLAXIS AND TREATMENT FOR COMPLICATIONS ASSOCIATED WITH SUBARACHNOID BLOCK

Hypotension
   Uterine displacement
   Hydration with 500 to 1000 mL of a balanced salt solution
   Ephedrine 10 to 15 mg intravenously if hypotension develops
Total Spinal Block
   Treat associated hypotension
   Tracheal intubation
   Ventilatory support

against aspiration. When the woman is hypotensive, intravenous fluids are given and ephedrine may be helpful to increase cardiac output.

Anxiety and Discomfort. Everyone in the operating room must remember that the woman under regional analgesia is awake. The mother should not misinterpret remarks or actions as an indication that she or her fetus may be in jeopardy. She usually is aware of surgical manipulation, identifying each maneuver as a feeling of pressure. She may painfully be aware of any manipulation above the level of the spinal sensory blockade. At times, the degree of pain relief from spinal analgesia is inadequate. In this circumstance, a significant measure of relief can be provided before delivery by administering 50 to 70 percent nitrous oxide with oxygen. Immediately after clamping the cord, a variety of techniques can be employed to provide effective analgesia. Morphine, meperidine, or fentanyl given intravenously at this time often provide excellent analgesia and euphoria as the operation is completed.

Spinal (Postpuncture) Headache. Leakage of cerebrospinal fluid from the site of puncture of the meninges is thought to be the major factor in the genesis of spinal headache. Presumably, when the woman sits or stands, the diminished volume of cerebrospinal fluid allows traction on pain-sensitive central nervous system structures. The likelihood of this unpleasant complication can be reduced by using a small-gauge spinal needle and avoiding multiple punctures of the meninges. There is no good evidence that placing the woman absolutely flat on her back for several hours is very effective in preventing headache. Vigorous hydration has been claimed to be of value, but also without compelling evidence to support its use. Abdominal support with a girdle or abdominal binder does seem to afford relief, and is worth trying. Typically, the headache is remarkably improved by the third day and absent by the fifth. Application of a blood patch is effective; a few mL of the woman's blood obtained aseptically without anticoagulant is injected into the epidural space at the site of the dural puncture. Relief is immediate. Saline similarly injected in larger volumes also has been claimed to provide relief.

Convulsions. In rare instances, post-dural puncture cephalgia is associated with blindness and convulsions. We have observed 8 cases associated with 19,000 regional analgesics, and presume that they too are caused by cerebrospinal fluid hypotension (Shearer and colleagues, 1991).

Bladder Dysfunction. With spinal analgesia, bladder sensation is likely to be obtunded and bladder emptying impaired for the first few hours after delivery. As a consequence, bladder distension is a frequent complication of the puerperium, especially if appreciable volumes of intravenous fluid have been or are being administered. Combinations of (1) infusion of a liter or more of fluid, (2) neural blockade from epidural or spinal analgesia, (3) antidiuretic effect of oxytocin infused for a time after delivery and then stopped, (4) discomfort from a sizable episiotomy, (5) failure to observe the woman very closely for bladder distension, and (6) failure to relieve bladder distension promptly by catheterization, are very likely to lead to quite troublesome bladder dysfunction and possibly urinary tract infection.

Oxytocics and Hypertension. Paradoxically, hypertension from ergonovine (Ergotrate) or methylergonovine (Methergine) injected following delivery is most common in women who have received a spinal or epidural block.

Arachnoiditis and Meningitis. No longer are the ampules of local anesthetic stored in alcohol, formalin, or other highly toxic preservatives or solutes. Needles and catheters now are rarely subjected to cleaning by chemical treatment so that they can be reused. Instead, disposable equipment is used, and these current practices, coupled with strict aseptic technique, have made meningitis and arachnoiditis rarities.

Contraindications to Spinal Analgesia. The common serious complication from spinal block is hypotension. The supine position late in pregnancy commonly predisposes to a reduction in return of blood from veins below the level of the large pregnant uterus and, in turn, a reduction in cardiac output. Moreover, sympathetic blockade from spinal analgesia usually is extensive, and it leads to further pooling of blood in dilated blood vessels below the blockade. Obstetrical complications that in themselves predispose to maternal hypovolemia and hypotension are contraindications to the use of spinal block. Thus, severe decrease in blood pressure can be predicted when subarachnoid analgesia is used in the presence of hemorrhage or severe pregnancy-induced or aggravated hypertension. **The woman with preeclampsia is exquisitely sensitive to the hypotensive effects caused by subarachnoid block.** Thus, spinal block is contraindicated in severe preeclampsia (Malinow and Ostheimer, 1987).

The cardiovascular effects of spinal block in the presence of acute blood loss but in the absence of the hemodynamic effects of pregnancy have been investigated by Kennedy and co-workers (1968). In 15 nonpregnant volunteers, spinal analgesia to the 5th thoracic sensory level was induced twice, the second time after a phlebotomy of 10 mL per kg. In the case of subarachnoid block without hemorrhage, the mean arterial blood pressure fell 10 percent while cardiac output rose slightly. In the case of hemorrhage without subarachnoid block, the mean blood pressure fell to the same degree and again the cardiac output rose slightly. However, when there was subarachnoid block after the modest hemorrhage, the mean arterial pressure fell nearly 30 percent and cardiac output fell 15 percent. Undoubtedly, the presence of a large pregnant uterus serves in the supine position to magnify appreciably these deleterious changes from spinal analgesia after overt hemorrhage.

Disorders of coagulation and defective hemostasis preclude the use of spinal analgesia. Subarachnoid puncture is contraindicated when the skin or underlying tissue at the site of needle entry is infected. Neurological disorders are considered by many to be a contraindication, if for no other reason than exacerbation of the neurological disease might be attributed to the anesthetic agent. Conversely, as discussed in Chapter 55, epidural analgesia is recommended by many for a number of neurological disorders complicating pregnancy.

Epidural Analgesia

Relief from the pain of uterine contractions and delivery, vaginal or abdominal, can be accomplished by injecting a suitable local anesthetic agent into the epidural or peridural space. The epidural space, in effect, is a potential area that contains areolar tissue, fat, lymphatics, and the internal venous plexus, which becomes engorged during pregnancy so that it appreciably reduces the volume of the space. It is limited peripherally by the ligamentum flavum and centrally by the dura matter, and it extends from the base of the skull almost to the end of the sacrum. The portal of entry into the epidural space for obstetrical analgesia is through either a lumbar intervertebral space *(lumbar epidural analgesia)* or through the sacral hiatus and sacral canal *(caudal epidural analgesia)*. Although one injection may be used, much more often these are repeated through an indwelling plastic catheter, or they are given by continuous infusion using a volumetric pump.

Continuous Lumbar Epidural Block. Complete analgesia for the pain of labor and vaginal delivery necessitates a block from the 10th thoracic to 5th sacral dermatomes. For abdominal delivery, the block is essential beginning at the 8th thoracic level and extending to the 1st sacral dermatome. The spread of the epidurally injected anesthetic agent will depend upon the location of the catheter tip as well as the dose, concentration, and volume of anesthetic agent used (Table 16–1), and whether the woman is placed in the head-down, horizontal, or head-up position.

Before any injection of the local anesthetic agent, a *test dose* is given and the woman observed for features of toxicity from intravascular injection and signs of spinal blockade from subarachnoid injection. If there is no evidence for these, then a full dose is given carefully and

analgesia is maintained by intermittent boluses of similar volume, or small volumes of the drug are delivered continuously by infusion pump. The addition of small doses of a short-acting narcotic, either fentanyl or sufentanil, has been shown to improve analgesic efficacy for labor or cesarean delivery (Chestnut and colleagues, 1988; Phillips, 1988; Preston and associates, 1988).

When vaginal delivery is anticipated in 10 to 15 minutes, a rapidly acting agent is given through the epidural catheter to effect perineal analgesia.

Caudal Analgesia

At the lower end of the sacrum, on its posterior surface, there is a foramen resulting from the nonclosure of the laminae of the last sacral vertebra. It is screened by a thin layer of fibrous tissue. This foramen, called the sacral hiatus, leads to the caudal canal or space, which is actually the lowest extent of the epidural, or peridural space. Through the caudal space, a rich network of sacral nerve passes downward after having emerged from the dural sac several centimeters cephalad. The dural sac separates the caudal canal from the spinal cord and its surrounding fluid. A suitable anesthetic solution that fills the caudal canal may abolish the sensation of pain carried via the sacral nerves and anesthetize the pelvis, producing analgesia suitable for vaginal delivery. Higher levels with continuous caudal technique provide analgesia both in the first and second stages and for delivery. Caudal analgesia is infrequently used today.

Complications. Both lumbar and caudal epidural analgesia for labor and delivery may provide most pleasant relief from the pain of labor. There are certain problems inherent in their use and, as with spinal blockade, it is imperative that close monitoring, including the level of analgesia, be performed by trained personnel.

Inadvertent Spinal Blockade. Dural puncture, along with inadvertent subarachnoid injection, is always a potential complication; personnel and facilities must be immediately available to manage the complications of high spinal block (see p. 435). Postspinal headache is a less serious but troublesome complication of inadvertent entry.

Ineffective Analgesia. The extent to which pain relief during labor can be obtained with lumbar epidural analgesia varies. In the best of circumstances, according to Crawford (1979), about 85 percent of laboring women are free of pain, 12 percent experience partial relief, and 3 percent have no relief. Nonetheless, establishment of effective pain relief with maximum safety takes time. Epidural analgesia for women of higher parity in rapid active labor is likely to prove not worth the risk and expense. If the epidural analgesia is allowed to dissipate before another injection of anesthetic drug, subsequent pain relief may be delayed, incomplete, or both.

At times, perineal analgesia for delivery is difficult to obtain, especially with the lumbar epidural technique. When this condition is encountered, a low spinal or pudendal block, or systemic analgesia, is added.

Hypotension. By blocking sympathetic tracts, epidurally injected analgesic agents may cause hypotension. In the nonhypertensive and normally hypervolemic pregnant women, hypotension induced by epidural analgesia can usually be prevented by rapid infusion of a balanced salt solution, or treated successfully as described for spinal analgesia. Despite these precautions, hypotension is the most common side effect. Brizgys and colleagues (1987) studied 583 women given epidural analgesia for cesarean delivery and reported that hypotension developed in 32 percent, even after volume expansion with 1 L of lactated Ringer's solution. In another group of women, similarly prehydrated but also given 25 mg of intramuscular ephedrine prophylactically, the incidence was 25 percent (Fig. 16–2). Although there were no differences in umbilical arterial and venous Po_2 and Pco_2, neonates born to women with hypotension had a lower mean pH.

It is important that with each injection of analgesic the blood pressure be measured every 2 minutes for the next 20 minutes. Brizgys and colleagues (1987) showed that rapid correction of hypotension with crystalloid infusion, left uterine displacement, and intravenous ephedrine resulted in delivery of healthy infants.

Central Nervous Stimulation. Convulsions are an uncommon but serious complication, the immediate management of which was described previously (Table 16–2).

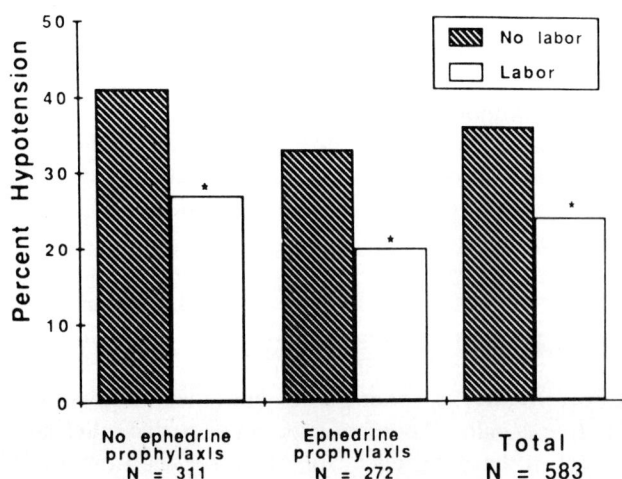

Fig. 16–2. The incidence of hypotension following epidural analgesia given for cesarean delivery. Asterisk indicates significant difference between women with and without labor. (From Brizgys and colleagues, 1987.)

Effect on Labor. Epidural block induced prior to well-established labor may be followed by desultory labor. The precise role played by epidural analgesia in this phenomenon is not clear, because this sequence of events also is seen in its absence. Lowensohn and co-workers (1974) reported significant depression of uterine activity for about 30 minutes following the epidural injection of lidocaine. Akamatsu and Bonica (1974) suggested that epinephrine injected with the anesthetic agent may impair labor. During the second stage of labor, epidural analgesia that provides effective pain relief likely is to reduce appreciably maternal expulsive efforts. As a consequence, an epidural block may lead to delay or, less frequently, failure of descent of the presenting part and spontaneous rotation to the occiput anterior position, and hence an increased incidence of operative vaginal delivery as well as cesarean delivery (Chap. 24, p. 557).

Maternal Pyrexia. Epidural analgesia in labor may be associated with maternal pyrexia. Fusi and associates (1989) compared temperature in laboring women who were given meperidine versus epidural for analgesia. The mean temperature in the epidural group was significantly higher after 6 hours of labor, and this was not attributed to infection. These investigators concluded that this rise in temperature may be secondary to both vascular and thermoregulatory modifications induced by epidural analgesia.

Safety. The relative safety of epidural analgesia is attested to by the extraordinary experiences reported by Crawford (1985) from the Birmingham Maternity Hospital in England. From 1968 through 1985, nearly 26,000 women were given epidural analgesia for labor, and there were no maternal deaths. Crawford outlined the significant complications encountered, and divided these into the categories shown in Table 16–4. As expected, the nine potentially life-threatening complications followed either inadvertent intravenous or intrathecal injections of lidocaine, bupivacaine, or both.

Contraindications. As with spinal analgesia, the contraindications include actual or anticipated serious maternal hemorrhage, infection at or near the sites for puncture, and suspicion of neurological disease. Rolbin and colleagues (1988) advise against epidural analgesia if the platelet count is below 100,000 per µL. Conversely, Rasmus and associates (1989) found no cases in which bleeding was caused by regional analgesia in thrombocytopenic women. They recommended consideration for this method if the patient may be difficult to intubate or ventilate.

Severe Preeclampsia–Eclampsia. Disagreements persist over the use of epidural analgesia in the presence of preeclampsia (Cunningham and Lindheimer, 1992; Ma-

TABLE 16–4. COMPLICATIONS WITH LUMBAR EPIDURAL ANALGESIA GIVEN DURING LABOR TO 26,490 WOMEN AT BIRMINGHAM MATERNITY HOSPITAL, ENGLAND

Complication Category	Example (n)	Outcome
Potentially life-threatening (1 : 3000)	Intravenous injection (3)	Loss of consciousness
	Intrathecal injection (6)	1 cardiac arrest (recovered)
Serious, not life-threatening (1 : 13,000)	Epidural space fibrosis (1)	Laminectomy (improved)
	Epidural abscess (1)	Laminectomy (improved)
Moderately serious	Prolonged hypotension (2)	Recovered
During labor (1 : 2000)	Severe hypertension, headache (1)	Recovered
	Failed analgesia, paresis (1)	Recovered
After delivery (1 : 2000)	Backache, leg pain (1)	Recovered
	Numbness and weakness (2)	Recovered

Data from Crawford (1985).

linow and Ostheimer, 1987). Some obstetrical anesthesiologists urge regional analgesia for women with overt hypertension (Gutsche and Cheek, 1987; Moir, 1986). Proponents contend that regional blockade diminishes responses to painful uterine contractions, thus minimizing hazards of hypertensive crisis. Another reason given for the use of regional analgesia in preeclamptic women undoubtedly stems from the fact that the blood pressure is very often lowered by regional analgesia. As emphasized by Shnider and Levinson (1979) *"Sudden falls in blood pressure can rapidly produce fetal distress and demise as the uteroplacental circulation becomes further compromised."* Because of these earlier experiences, in over 400 consecutive cases of antepartum or intrapartum eclampsia at Parkland Hospital, spinal and epidural blockade have been avoided deliberately. Instead, local or pudendal block plus nitrous oxide–oxygen analgesia have been used for vaginal deliveries; and general analgesia with thiopental, succinylcholine, and nitrous oxide–oxygen is used for the occasional difficult vaginal delivery and for cesarean deliveries. Perinatal and maternal mortality rates have been very low in these pregnancies complicated by eclampsia (Pritchard and co-workers, 1984).

In most medical centers, a more liberal view of epidural analgesia has been taken. This undoubtedly stems from the availability of continuous anesthesia coverage by physicians with expertise in obstetrical analgesia and anesthesia. As discussed in Chapter 36, epidural analgesia for women with severe preeclampsia-eclampsia can be safely used when specially trained anesthesiologists and obstetricians are responsible for the woman and her fetus (American College of Obste-

tricians and Gynecologists, 1988; Cunningham and Lindheimer, 1992; Moore and colleagues, 1985). In a more recent evaluation of regional analgesia for cesarean delivery in women with severe preeclampsia at Parkland Hospital, Wallace and colleagues (1992) randomized 66 such women to receive general anesthesia, epidural analgesia, or a combined spinal–epidural analgesia. Importantly, maternal hypotension developed in 30 percent of the women given epidural analgesics and 22 percent of those given spinal–epidural analgesia. Despite this, there were no significant differences in neonatal acid-base studies or the frequency of 5-minute Apgar scores of less than 4 among the three groups.

Epidural Opiate Analgesia. Injection of opiates into the epidural space to relieve pain was described in 1979 by Wang and colleagues. This method of relieving pain from labor is now quite popular, especially because complications with this technique are less worrisome than those seen with epidural injections of local anesthetics alone. The mechanism of action of opiates given epidurally is from their interaction with specific receptors in the dorsal horn and dorsal roots. Apparently both cerebral and spinal opioid receptors are stimulated by these narcotics (Ackerman and colleagues, 1992; Yeung and Rudy, 1980).

In general, opiates alone will not provide adequate analgesia and they most often are given with a local anesthetic agent such as bupivacaine (Chestnut and associates, 1988; Phillips, 1988; Preston and co-workers, 1988). The major advantages of utilizing a combination of opiates and local anesthetics is the rapid onset of pain relief, a decrease in shivering, and the absence of motor blockade from the smaller doses of bupivacaine required (Ackerman and colleagues, 1992). Steinberg and associates (1989) reported that sufentanil may provide adequate epidural analgesia when utilized alone.

Some of the epidural opioids utilized in obstetrical patients for labor, cesarean delivery, or postoperative pain relief are summarized in Table 16–5. The few sys-

TABLE 16–5. EPIDURAL OPIOIDS THAT HAVE BEEN UTILIZED IN OBSTETRICAL PATIENTS.

Alfentanil
Buprenorphine
Butorphanol
Fentanyl
Hydromorphone
Meperidine
Methadone
Morphine
Nalbuphine
Pentazocine
Sufentanil

Adapted from Ackerman and colleagues (1992).

temic symptoms encountered are from low levels of the drug following vascular absorption. Side effects include pruritus, nausea and vomiting, urinary retention, and either immediate or delayed respiratory depression (Ackerman and colleagues, 1992). Naloxone, given intravenously, will abolish these systems without affecting the analgesic action.

Recently, Cohen and colleagues (1992), in a randomized study of epidural buprenorphine plus bupivacaine versus fentanyl plus bupivacaine, reported that both epidural opioids were equally efficacious.

Huntoon and co-workers (1992) have also reported that clonidine administered epidurally may be effective in providing postoperative pain relief without the side effects associated with opioids.

The risk of adverse fetal effects such as respiratory depression associated with epidural opiates in combination with local anesthetic agents appears to be very low (Ackerman and associates, 1992). Hunt and colleagues (1989) have reported a fetal sinusoidal heart rate pattern associated with maternal administration of epidural butorphanol and bupivacaine.

References

Abboud TK, Kim SH, Henriksen EH, Chen T, Eisenman R, Levinson G, Shnider SM: Comparative maternal and neonatal effects of halothane and enflurane for cesarean section. Acta Anesthesiol Scand 29:663, 1985

Abouleish E, Rawal N, Fallow K, Hernandez D: Combined intrathecal morphine and bupivacaine for cesarean section: Anesth Analg 67:370, 1988

Ackerman WE, Juneja M, Spinnato JA: Epidural opioids' OB advantages. Contemp Obstet Gynecol 37:68, 1992

Akamatsu TJ, Bonica JJ: Spinal and extradural analgesia-anesthesia for parturition. Clin Obstet Gynecol 17:183, 1974

American College of Obstetricians and Gynecologists: Anesthesia for emergency deliveries. ACOG Committee Opinion, no. 104, March 1992

American Academy of Pediatrics and American College of Obstetricians and Gynecologists: Guidelines for Perinatal Care, 3rd ed, 1992

American College of Obstetricians and Gynecologists: Obstetric anesthesia and analgesia. Technical Bulletin, no. 112, January 1988

Andrews WW, Ramin SM, Wallace DH, Shearer V, Black S, Maberry MC, Dax JS: Effect of type of anesthesia on blood loss at elective repeat cesarean section. Am J Perinatol 9:197, 1992

Angel JL, Knuppel RA, Lake M: Sinusoidal fetal heart rate pattern associated with intravenous butorphanol administration: A case report. Am J Obstet Gynecol 149:465, 1984

Atrash HK, Koonin LM, Lawson HW, Franks AL, Smith JC: Maternal mortality in the United States, 1979–1986. Obstet Gynecol 76:1055, 1990

Bartlett JG, Gorbach SL, Finegold SM: The bacteriology of aspiration pneumonia. Am J Med 56:202, 1974

Blass NH: The morbidly obese pregnant patient. In Datta S (ed): Anesthetic and Obstetric Management of High-risk Pregnancy. St. Louis, Mosby, 1991, p 59

Brizgys RV, Dailey PA, Shnider SM, Kotelko DM, Levinson G: The incidence and neonatal effects of maternal hypotension during epidural anesthesia for cesarean section. Anesthesiology 67:782, 1987

Burchman CA: Maternal aspiration. In Ostheimer GW (ed): Manual of Obstetric Anesthesia, 2nd ed. New York, Churchill Livingstone, 1992, p 161

Bynum LJ, Pierce AK: Pulmonary aspiration of gastric contents. Am Rev Respir Dis 114:1129, 1976

Camann WR, Datta S: Red cell use during cesarean delivery. Transfusion 31:12, 1991

Carlsson BM, Johansson M, Westin B: Fetal heart rate pattern before and after paracervical anesthesia. A prospective study. Acta Obstet Gynecol Scand 66:391, 1987

Chestnut DH, Owen CL, Bates JN, Ostman LG, Choi WW, Geiger MW: Continuous infusion epidural analgesia during labor: A randomized, double-blind comparison of 0.625% bupivacaine/0.0002% fentanyl versus 0.125% bupivacaine. Anesthesiology 68:754, 1988

Cohen S, Amar D, Pantuck CB, Pantuck EJ, Weissman AM, Landa S, Singer N: Epidural patient-controlled analgesia after cesarean section: Buprenorphine–0.015% bupivacaine with epinephrine versus fentanyl–0.015% bupivacaine with and without epinephrine. Anesth Analg 74:226, 1992

Combs CA, Murphy EL, Laros RK Jr: Factors associated with hemorrhage in cesarean deliveries. Obstet Gynecol 77:77, 1991

Crawford JS: Continuous lumbar epidural analgesia for labour and delivery. Br Med J 1:72, 1979

Crawford JS: Some maternal complications of epidural analgesia for labour. Anesthesia 40:1219, 1985

Cunningham FG, Lindheimer M: Hypertension in pregnancy. N Engl J Med 326:927, 1992

DeVoe SJ, DeVoe K Jr, Rigsby WC, McDaniels BA: Effects of meperidine on uterine contractility. Am J Obstet Gynecol 105:1004, 1969

Endler GC, Mariona FG, Sokol RJ, Stevenson LB: Anesthesia-related maternal mortality in Michigan, 1972 to 1984. Am J Obstet Gynecol 159:187, 1988

Ericson A, Källen B: Survey of infants born in 1973 or 1975 to Swedish women working in operating rooms during their pregnancies. Anesth Analg 58:302, 1979

Fishburne JI Jr, Greiss FC Jr, Hopkinson R, Rhyne AL: Response of the gravid uterine vasculature to arterial levels of local anesthetic agents. Am J Obstet Gynecol 133:753, 1979

Friedman JM: Teratogen update: Anesthetic agents. Teratology 37:69, 1988

Fusi L, Steer PJ, Maresh MJA, Beard RW: Maternal pyrexia associated with the use of epidural analgesia in labour. Lancet 1:1250, 1989

Gibbs CP, Banner TC: Effectiveness of Bicitra/Pr as a preoperative antacid. Anesthesiology 61:97, 1984

Gibbs CP, Schwartz DJ, Wynne JW, Hood CI, Kuck EJ: Antacid pulmonary aspiration in the dog. Anesthesiology 51:380, 1979

Gilstrap LC, Hankins GDV: The uncomplicated patient. In Phelan JP, Clark SL (eds): Cesarean Delivery. New York, Elsevier, 1988, p 140

Gilstrap LC, Hauth JC, Hankins DG, Patterson AR: Effect of type of anesthesia on blood loss at cesarean section. Obstet Gynecol 69:328, 1987

Greiss FC Jr, Still JG, Anderson SG: Effects of local anesthetic agents on the uterine vasculatures and myometrium. Am J Obstet Gynecol 124:889, 1976

Gutsche BB, Cheek TG: Anesthetic considerations in pre-eclampsia-eclampsia. In Shnider SM, Levinson G (eds): Anesthesia for Obstetrics, 2nd ed. Baltimore, Williams & Wilkins, 1987, p 225

Hatjis CG, Meis PJ: Sinusoidal fetal heart rate pattern associated with butorphanol administration. Obstet Gynecol 67:377, 1986

Hodgkinson R, Bhatt M, Kim SS, Grewal G, Marx GF: Neonatal neurobehavioral tests following cesarean section under general and spinal anesthesia. Am J Obstet Gynecol 132:670, 1978

Hodgkinson R, Glassenberg R, Joyce TH, Coombs DW, Ostheimer GW, Gibbs CP: Comparison of cimetidine (Tagamet) with antacid for safety and effectiveness in reducing gastric acidity before elective cesarean section. Anesthesiology 59:86, 1983

Hughey MJ, McElin TW, Young T: Maternal and fetal outcome of Lamaze prepared patients. Obstet Gynecol 51:643, 1978

Hunt CO, Naulty JS, Malinow AM, Datta S, Ostheimer GW: Epidural butorphanol–bupivacaine for analgesia during labor and delivery. Anesth Analge 68:323, 1989

Huntoon M, Eisenach JC, Boese P: Epidural clonidine after cesarean section. Appropriate dose and effect of prior local anesthetic. Anesthesiology 76:187, 1992

Husum B, Wulf HC, Norgaard I: Sister chromatid exchanges and structural chromosome aberrations in lymphocytes in operating room personnel. Acta Anaesthesiol Scand 27:262, 1983

Kennedy WF Jr, Bonica JJ, Akamatsu TJ, Ward RJ, Martin WE, Grinstein A: Cardiovascular and respiratory effects of subarachnoid block in the presence of acute blood loss. Anesthesiology 29:29, 1968

Kennell J, Klaus M, McGrath S, Robertson S, Hinkley C: Continuous emotional support during labor in a US hospital: A randomized controlled trial. JAMA 265:2197, 1991

King TA, Adams AP: Failed tracheal intubation. Br J Anaesth 65:400, 1990

Knill-Jones RP, Newman BJ, Spence AA: Anaesthetic practice and pregnancy. Lancet 2:807, 1975

Lamaze F: Painless Childbirth: Psychoprophylactic Method. Chicago, Henry Regnery, 1970

Lamont BJ, Pennant JH, Wallace DH, Jennings LW, Giesecke AH: Directly measured uterine tone and blood loss during anesthesia for cesarean section. Anesth Analg 67S:126, 1988. Abstract

Lewis M, Crawford JS: Can one risk fasting the obstetric patient for less than 4 hours? Br J Anaesth 59:312, 1987

Lowensohn RI, Paul RH, Fales S, Yeh SY, Hon EH: Intrapartum epidural anesthesia: An evaluation of effects on uterine activity. Obstet Gynecol 44:388, 1974

Lyons G: Failed intubation. Six years' experience in a teaching maternity unit. Anaesthesia 40:759, 1985

Malan TP, Johnson MD: Failed intubation. In Ostheimer GW (ed): Manual of Obstetric Anesthesia, 2nd ed. New York, Churchill Livingstone, 1992, p 161

Malinow AM, Ostheimer GW: Anesthesia for the high-risk parturient. Obstet Gynecol 69:951, 1987

McGrady EM: Maternal mortality. In Ostheimer GW (ed): Manual of Obstetric Anesthesia, 2nd ed. New York, Churchill Livingstone, 1992, p 402

Mendelson CL: The aspiration of stomach contents into the lungs during obstetric anesthesia. Am J Obstet Gynecol 52:191, 1946

Moir DD: Cimetidine, antacids, and pulmonary aspiration. J Anesthesiol 59:81, 1983

Moir DD: Local anaesthetic techniques in obstetrics. Br J Anaesth 58:747, 1986

Moore TR, Key TC, Reisner LS, Resnick R: Evaluation of the use of continuous lumbar epidural anesthesia for hypertensive pregnant women in labor. Am J Obstet Gynecol 152:104, 1985

Morgan M: Anaesthetic contribution to maternal mortality. Br J Anaesth 59:842, 1987

Pharah POD, Alberman E, Doyle P: Outcome of pregnancy among women in anesthetic practice. Lancet 1:34, 1977

Phillips G: Continuous infusion epidural analgesia in labor: The effect of adding sufentanil to 0.125% bupivacaine. Anesth Analg 67:462, 1988

Piggott SWE, Bogod DG, Rosen M, Rees GA, Harmer M: Isoflurane with either 100% oxygen or 50% nitrous oxide in oxygen for cesarean section. Br J Anaesth 65:325, 1990

Preston PG, Rosen MA, Hughes SC, Glosten B, Ross BK, Daniels D, Shnider SM, Dailey PA: Epidural anesthesia with fentanyl and lidocaine for cesarean section: Maternal effects and neonatal outcome. Anesthesiology 68:938, 1988

Pritchard JA, Cunningham FG, Pritchard SA: The Parkland Memorial Hospital protocol for treatment of eclampsia: Evaluation of 245 cases. Am J Obstet Gynecol 148:951, 1984

Quilligan EJ, Keegan KA, Donahue MJ: Double-blind comparison of intravenously injected butorphanol and meperidine in parturients. Int J Gynaecol Obstet 18:363, 1980

Rasmus KT, Rottman RL, Kotelko DM, Wright WC, Stone JJ, Rosenblatt RM: Unrecognized thrombocytopenia and regional anesthesia in parturients: A restrospective review. Obstet Gynecol 72:943, 1989

Read GD: Childbirth Without Fear. New York, Harper, 1944, p 192

Riffel HD, Nochimson DJ, Paul RH, Hon EHG: Effects of meperidine and promethazine during labor. Obstet Gynecol 42:738, 1973

Rochat RW, Koonin LM, Atrash HK, Jewett JF, and The Maternal Mortality Collaborative: Maternal Mortality in the United States: Report from the Maternal Mortality Collaborative. Obstet Gynecol 72:91, 1988

Rolbin SH, Abbott D, Musclow E, Papsin F, Lie LM, Freedman J: Epidural anesthesia in pregnant patients with low platelet counts. Obstet Gynecol 71:918, 1988

Sachs BP, Oriol NE, Ostheimer GW, Weiss JB, Driscoll S, Acker D, Brown DA, Jewett JF: Anesthetic related maternal mortality, 1954 to 1985. J Clin Anesth 1:333, 1989

Shearer VE, Cunningham G, Wallace DH, Giesecke AH: Seizures following post dural puncture headache in postpartum women. A series with suggested etiology. Anesthesiology 75:A852, 1991

Shnider SM, Levinson G: Anesthesia for Obstetrics. Baltimore, Williams & Wilkins, 1979

Steinberg RB, Powell G, Hu XH, Dunn SM: Epidural sufentanil for analgesia for labor and delivery. Reg Anesth 14:225, 1989

Sutherland AD, Stock JG, Davies JM: Effects of preoperative fasting on morbidity and gastric contents in patients undergoing day-stay surgery. Br J Anaesth 58:876, 1986

Svancarek W, Chirino O, Schaefer G Jr, Blythe JG: Retropsoas and subgluteal abscesses following paracervical and pudendal anesthesia. JAMA 237:892, 1977

Taylor G, Pryse-Davies J: The prophylactic use of antacids in the prevention of the acid pulmonary aspiration syndrome. Lancet 1:288, 1966

Teabeaut JR II: Aspiration of gastric contents: An experimental study. Am J Pathol 28:51, 1952

Thornburn J, Moir DD: Antacid therapy for emergency cesarean sections. Anaesthesia 42:352, 1987

Wallace DH, Leveno KJ, Cunningham FG, Shearer V, Black S, Holloway J: Randomized study of generalized anesthesia versus epidural or spinal-epidural analgesia complicated by severe preeclampsia. Am J Obstet Gynecol 166:302, 1992. Society of Perinatal Obstetricians abstract 77

Wang JK, Nauss LE, Thomas JE: Pain relieved by intrathecally applied morphine in man. Anesthesiology 50:149, 1979

Warren TM, Datta S, Ostheimer GW, Naulty JS, Weiss JB, Morrison JA: Comparison of the maternal and neonatal effects of halothane, enflurane, and isoflurane for cesarean delivery. Anesth Analg 62:516, 1983

Wenger DR, Gitchell RG: Severe infections following pudendal block anesthesia: Need for orthopaedic awareness. J Bone Joint Surg (Am) 55:202, 1973

Wheatley RG, Kallus FT, Reynolds RC, Giesecke AH: Milk of magnesia is an effective pre-induction antacid in obstetrical anesthesia. Anesthesiology 50:514, 1979

Wilson SJ, Errick JK, Balkon J: Pharmacokinetics of nalbuphine during parturition. Am J Obstet Gynecol 155:340, 1986

Yau G, Kan AF, Gin T, Oh TE: A comparison of omeprazole and ranitidine for prophylaxis against aspiration pneumonitis in emergency cesarean section. Anesthesia 47:2, 1992

Yeung JC, Rudy TA: Multiplicative interaction between narcotic agonisms expressed at spinal and supraspinal sites of antinociceptive action as revealed by concurrent intrathecal and intracerebroventricular injections or morphine. J Pharm Exp Ther 215:633, 1980

Zagorzycki MT, Brinkman CR III: The effect of general and epidural anesthesia upon neonatal Apgar scores in repeat cesarean section. Surg Gynecol Obstet 155:641, 1982

CHAPTER 17
The Newborn Infant

Adaptation of the Newborn to Air Breathing

The First Breath of Air. As the infant is born and the fetoplacental circulation ceases to function, the infant is subjected to rapid and profound physiological changes (Chap. 7, p. 179). Survival depends upon a prompt and orderly interchange of oxygen and carbon dioxide between the new environment and the pulmonary circulation. For efficient interchange, the fluid-filled alveoli of the lungs must fill with air, the air must be exchanged by appropriate respiratory motion, and a vigorous microcirculation must be established in close proximity to the alveoli.

Intrauterine Respiration. It was once believed that the fetus breathed only at times of hypoxic stress. In recent years, however, conclusive evidence of episodic respiratory movements in utero has been obtained during normal human pregnancy. Breathing movements are commonly observed when the fetus is evaluated by ultrasound. Pressure changes during inspiration appear sufficiently intense to induce movement of amnionic fluid into and out of the fetal lungs, as demonstrated in both monkey and human fetuses (Duenhoelter and Pritchard, 1976; Martin and co-workers, 1974).

Initiation of Air Breathing. Very soon after birth, the breathing pattern shifts from one of shallow episodic inspirations, which characterizes fetal breathing, to that of regular deeper inhalations. Aeration of the newborn lung is not the inflation of a collapsed structure, but instead, the rapid replacement of bronchial and alveolar fluid by air. In the lamb, and presumably in the human infant, residual alveolar fluid after delivery is cleared through the pulmonary circulation and, to a lesser degree, through pulmonary lymphatics (Chernick, 1978). Delay in the removal of fluid from the alveoli probably contributes to the syndrome of **transient tachypnea of the newborn**. As fluid is replaced by air, there is considerable reduction in pulmonary vascular compression and, in turn, lowered resistance to blood flow. With the fall in pulmonary arterial blood pressure, the ductus arteriosus normally closes. Closure of the foramen ovale is more variable.

High negative intrathoracic pressures are required to bring about the initial entry of air into fluid-filled alveoli. Normally, from the first breath after birth, progressively more residual air accumulates in the lung, and with each successive breath, lower pulmonary opening pressure is required. In the mature normal infant, by about the fifth breath of air, the pressure–volume changes achieved with each respiration are very similar to those of the normal adult.

Alveolar Surface Tension and Lung Surfactant. The successful filling of the lungs with air and the rapid establishment of a physiological pattern of pressure–volume changes on inspiration and expiration require the presence of surface-active material that will lower surface tension in the alveoli and thereby prevent the collapse of the lung with each expiration (Chap. 7, p. 186). Lack of sufficient surfactant, common in preterm infants, leads to the prompt development of the respiratory distress syndrome (Chap. 44, p. 991).

The Stimuli to Breathe Air. Normally, the newborn begins to breathe and cry almost immediately after birth, indicating the establishment of active respiration. All the factors involved in the first breath of air have been difficult to elucidate, undoubtedly because many individually subtle stimuli contribute simultaneously. For example, *physical stimulation*, such as handling the infant during delivery and contact with various relatively rough surfaces, is believed to provoke respiration through stimuli reaching the respiratory center reflexly from the skin.

Compression of the thorax during the second stage of labor forces some fluid from the respiratory tract. Saunders (1978) found that considerable pressure often is produced by chest compression during vaginal delivery. He estimated that lung fluid is expelled equivalent to one fourth to one third of ultimate functional residual capacity. Although babies born by cesarean usually cry satisfactorily and sometimes just as quickly as babies born vaginally, they are likely to have more fluid and less gas in their lungs throughout the first 6 hours of life (Milner and colleagues, 1978). Thoracic compression incidental to vaginal delivery and the expansion that follows delivery may, nevertheless, be an auxiliary factor in the initiation of respiration.

Deprivation of oxygen and accumulation of carbon dioxide may stimulate respiration. Blood samples obtained from catheters implanted into vessels of experimental animal fetuses for prolonged periods of time, as well as funipuncture in humans, have revealed that P_{O_2} is low by adult standards. In animals, a further decrease in P_{O_2} diminishes or abolishes fetal respiratory motion, whereas an elevation of P_{CO_2} increases the frequency and magnitude of fetal breathing movements (Dawes, 1974). For the foregoing reasons, it seems that the fetus-infant most likely responds to hypoxia and to hypercapnea the same way in utero and after birth. This likely explains, in part, why hypercapnia (increase in P_{CO_2}) is the initiating event resulting in fetal meconium aspiration.

Management of Delivery

Immediate Care. As the head of the infant is delivered, either vaginally or by cesarean delivery, the face is immediately wiped and the mouth and nares suctioned, as discussed in Chapter 14 (p. 383) (Fig. 14–9). A soft rubber ear syringe or its equivalent inserted with care is quite suitable for the purpose. Before clamping and severing the cord, while the infant is still being held head down, it may be beneficial to aspirate the mouth and pharynx again. Once the cord has been divided, the infant is immediately placed supine with the head lowered and turned to the side in a heated unit that has appropriate thermal regulation and is equipped for immediate intensive care (Fig. 17–1). To minimize heat loss, the baby is wiped dry.

Evaluation of the Infant. Before and during delivery, careful considerations must be given to the following determinants of neonatal well-being: (1) health status of the mother; (2) prenatal complications; (3) labor complications; (4) gestational age; (5) duration of labor; (6) duration of ruptured membranes; (7) kinds, amounts, times, and routes of administration of analgesics; (8) kind and duration of anesthesia; and (9) any difficulty with delivery. The obstetrician inspects the infant for any visible abnormalities during delivery and until the cord is severed, and then the infant is handed to a trained associate for further care.

The person immediately in charge of caring for the neonate should observe respirations closely and identify the heart rate. The heart rate can be determined by auscultation over the chest or by palpating the base of the umbilical cord. A readily discernible heartbeat of 100 or more is acceptable. Persistent bradycardia requires prompt resuscitation. Next, the mouth, nares, and pharynx are suctioned carefully.

Most normal infants take a breath within a few seconds of birth and cry within half a minute. If respirations are infrequent, suction of the mouth and pharynx, followed by light slapping of the soles of the feet and rubbing of the back, usually together serve to stimulate breathing. Prolongation of these intervals beyond 1 and 2 minutes, respectively, indicates an abnormality. Continued lack of breathing indicates either marked central depression or mechanical obstruction and demands active resuscitation.

Lack of Effective Respirations. Important causes of failure to establish effective respirations include the following: (1) fetal hypoxemia or acidosis from any cause; (2) drugs administered to the mother; (3) gross fetal immaturity, (4) upper airway obstruction; (5) pneumothorax; (6) other lung abnormalities, either intrinsic (e.g., hypoplasia) or extrinsic (e.g., diaphragmatic hernia); (7) aspiration of amnionic fluid grossly contaminated with meconium; (8) central nervous system injury; and (9) septicemia.

Methods Used to Evaluate the Newborn's Condition

Apgar Score. A useful aid in evaluation of the infant is the Apgar scoring system applied at 1 minute and again at 5 minutes after birth (Table 17–1). In general, the higher the score, up to a maximum of 10, the better is the condition of the infant. The 1-minute Apgar score determines the need for immediate resuscitation. Most

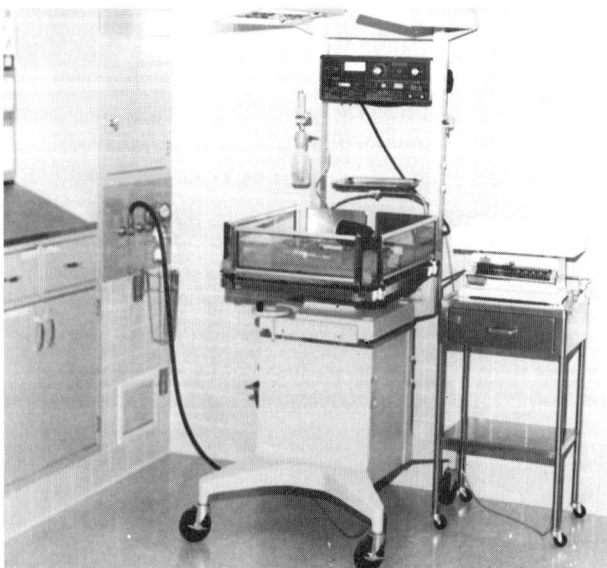

Fig. 17–1. Thermostatically controlled infant care unit in delivery room.

TABLE 17–1. APGAR SCORING SYSTEM

Sign	0	1	2
Heart rate	Absent	Below 100	Over 100
Respiratory effort	Absent	Slow, irregular	Good, crying
Muscle tone	Flaccid	Some flexion of extremities	Active motion
Reflex irritability	No response	Grimace	Vigorous cry
Color	Blue, pale	Body pink, extremities blue	Completely pink

infants at birth are in excellent condition, as indicated by Apgar scores of 7 to 10, and require no aid other than perhaps simple nasopharyngeal suction. *Mildly to moderately depressed infants* score 4 to 6 at 1 minute, demonstrating depressed respirations, flaccidity, and pale to blue color. Heart rate and reflex irritability, however, are good. *Severely depressed infants* score 0 to 3, with heart rate slow to inaudible and reflex response depressed or absent. Resuscitation, including artificial ventilation, should be started immediately. Often, babies who need immediate active intervention are obvious. They are flaccid, apneic, and often covered with meconium, and the heart rate is below 100. Pharyngeal suction, tracheal intubation and suction, and positive pressure oxygenation should be instituted as soon as possible.

For many years, the Apgar score as described above was used to assess the newborn condition immediately after birth. The score has been a useful clinical tool to help identify those neonates who might require resuscitation, as well as the effectiveness of any resuscitative measures. Unfortunately, attempts have been made to relate the score to ultimate long-term outcomes. Additionally, for reasons that are not entirely clear, erroneous definitions of asphyxia have been established, based upon the Apgar score alone. Because of these misconceptions, the Committee on Maternal and Fetal Medicine of the American College of Obstetricians and Gynecologists (1986) and the Committee on Fetus and Newborn of the American Academy of Pediatrics (1986) issued a joint statement on the use and misuse of the Apgar score. This statement was reaffirmed in 1991. Because of its importance, and with permission from the American College of Obstetricians and Gynecologists, it is reprinted here in its entirety.

Use and Misuse of the Apgar Score

The Apgar score, devised in 1952 by Dr. Virginia Apgar, is a quick method of assessing the state of the newborn (Apgar, 1953; Apgar and co-workers, 1958). The ease of scoring by this method has led to its use in many studies of neonatal outcome. Its misuse, however, as appears in the ninth revision of the International Classification of Disease (ICD-9-CM) Coding, has led to an erroneous definition of asphyxia. Intrapartum asphyxia implies fetal hypercarbia and hypoxemia, which if prolonged will result in metabolic acidemia. Since the intrapartum disruption of uterine or fetal blood flow is rarely, if ever, absolute, asphyxia is an imprecise, general term. Terms such as hypercarbia, hypoxia, metabolic, respiratory, or lactic acidemia are more precise, both for immediate assessment of the newborn and for retrospective assessment of intrapartum management.

Although the Apgar score continues to provide a convenient shorthand for reporting the state of the newborn and the effectiveness of resuscitation, the purpose of this statement is to place the Apgar score in its proper perspective as a tool for assessing asphyxia and predicting future neurological deficit.

Factors That May Affect Apgar Scores

The Apgar score comprises five components: heart rate, respiratory effort, tone, reflex irritability, and color, each of which can be given a score of 0, 1, or 2 (Table 17–1). Although rarely stated, it is important to recognize that elements of the score such as tone, color, and reflex irritability are partially dependent on the physiologic maturity of the infant. The normal premature infant may thus receive a low score purely because of immaturity, with no evidence of anoxic insult or cerebral depression.

Maternal sedation or analgesia may decrease tone and responsiveness. Neurologic conditions such as muscle disease and cerebral malformations may decrease tone and interfere with respiration. Cardiorespiratory conditions may interfere with heart rate, respiration, and tone. Thus, to equate the presence of a low Apgar score solely with asphyxia or with future neurologic outcome represents a misuse of the score.

Apgar Score and Subsequent Disability

The 1-minute Apgar score may be used to indicate the infant who requires special attention. A low 1-minute score, however, does not correlate with future outcome (Fields and associates, 1983).

The 5-minute Apgar score, particularly the change in the score between 1 and 5 minutes, is a useful index of the effectiveness of resuscitation efforts. However, even a 5-minute score of 0 to 3, although possibly due to hypoxia, is limited in indicating the severity of the problem and correlates poorly with future neurologic outcome (Nelson and Ellenberg, 1981). An Apgar score of 0 to 3 at 5 minutes is associated with an increased risk of cerebral palsy, but this risk increases only from 0.3 percent to 1 percent. A 5-minute Apgar score of 7 to 10 is considered normal. Scores of 4, 5, and 6 are intermediate and are not markers of high risk of later neurologic dysfunction. As mentioned, such scores are affected by physiologic immaturity, sedation, the presence of congenital malformations, and other factors.

Because Apgar scores at 1 and 5 minutes correlate poorly with either cause or outcome, these scores alone should not be considered either evidence of or consequent to substantial asphyxia. Therefore, a low 5-minute Apgar score alone does not prove that later cerebral palsy was caused by perinatal asphyxia.

Later Scores

Correlation of the Apgar score with future neurologic outcome increases when the score is 0 to 3 at 10, 15, and 20 minutes (Nelson and Ellenberg, 1981). Although cerebral asphyxia may be brief or transient and may be manifested as a low Apgar score at 5 minutes, substantial cerebral hypoxia leading to cerebral palsy can be presumed only when three criteria are met:

1. Apgar score is 0 to 3 at 10 minutes (in the absence of other cause)
2. Infant remains hypotonic for at least several hours (Finer and associates, 1983; Sarnat and Sarnat, 1976)
3. Infant has seizures (Mellits and colleagues, 1982)

Confirmation of suspected hypoxia (asphyxia) may be obtained by demonstrating metabolic acidemia in umbilical cord blood. The absence of metabolic acidemia in umbilical cord blood makes intrapartum asphyxia unlikely.

Cerebral palsy is the only neurologic deficit clearly linked to perinatal asphyxia. Although mental retardation and epilepsy may accompany cerebral palsy, there is no evidence that these conditions are caused by perinatal asphyxia unless cerebral palsy is also present (U.S. Department of Health and Human Services, 1985). The Apgar score alone cannot establish the occurrence of sufficient hypoxia to cause cerebral palsy. An infant with an Apgar score of 0 to 3 at 5 minutes whose 10-minute score improves to 4 or better has a 99 percent chance of not having cerebral palsy at 7 years of age. It should also be noted that 75 percent of children in whom cerebral palsy has developed had normal Apgar scores at birth (Nelson and Ellenberg, 1981).

In an infant with a low Apgar score, the presence of umbilical cord acidemia in the absence of maternal acidemia, large base deficit, and nucleated erythrocytes in the peripheral blood may provide supporting evidence of asphyxia; liver, renal, and cardiac dysfunction may also provide evidence of asphyxia. To date, however, none of these indications has been convincingly correlated with central nervous system outcome.

Summary

Low Apgar scores at 1 and 5 minutes are excellent indicators for identification of infants needing resuscitation. Although low scores may be evidence of hypoxia, they are influenced by other factors affecting tone, responsiveness, and respiration. Apgar scores alone are not evidence of sufficient hypoxia to result in neurologic damage. In a child who later is found to have cerebral palsy, low 1- or 5-minute Apgar scores provide insufficient evidence that the damage was due to hypoxia. To substantiate that hypoxia led to adverse neurologic outcome, additional perinatal evidence, such as Apgar scores of 0 to 3 at 10 minutes, early perinatal seizures, and prolonged hypotonia, is required. One of these elements alone is insufficient evidence that prolonged or severe asphyxia has occurred. In the absence of such evidence, subsequent neurologic deficits cannot be ascribed to perinatal asphyxia (Brann and Dykes, 1977).

Umbilical Cord Blood Acid-base and Blood Gas Measurements.

Umbilical cord blood pH and acid-base status are objective measures of neonatal well-being and can be utilized retrospectively, in most cases, to assess the effects of labor on the fetus. Furthermore, because the absence of metabolic acidemia in umbilical cord blood makes intrapartum asphyxia unlikely, it is critical to distinguish clearly between the commonly used terms *acidemia, acidosis,* and *asphyxia* and to define the types of acidemia.

Acidemia has been defined as an increase in hydron ion concentration in umbilical arterial blood resulting in a pH of less than 7.2 (Gilstrap and co-workers, 1984b, 1987; Wible and associates, 1982; Yeomans and colleagues, 1985). Yeomans and associates (1989) subsequently reported that a pH between 7.10 and 7.19 was associated with a vigorous neonate in 83 percent of cases. Gilstrap and associates (1989) and Freeman and Nelson (1988) suggested that clinically significant acidemia actually begins below a pH of 7.00. The American College of Obstetricians and Gynecologists (1989a) also supports this latter view, which was further strengthened by the observations of Goldaber and associates (1991) that there were significantly more neonatal deaths and neurological dysfunction if a pH cutoff value of less than 7.00 was used (Table 17–2).

A possible reason for the earlier reported normal values of pH greater than 7.20 has been provided by Vintzileos and colleagues (1992), who reported that umbilical arterial acidemia for *laboring women* should be defined as less than pH 7.15 and for *nonlaboring women* as less than pH 7.2. Thus in earlier reports, the mixing of values from fetuses delivered of laboring and nonlaboring women likely resulted in a higher estimation of "normal" arterial pH than was clinically relevant.

Acidosis ideally should be defined as an increase in hydrogen ion concentration in tissues. Although an abnormal value is likely a tissue pH of less than 7.00, most authors agree on a pH value of less than 7.20.

Asphyxia is best defined as hypoxia with or without hypercarbia of sufficient *severity and duration* to produce *metabolic acidosis.* The clinical diagnosis of

TABLE 17–2. UMBILICAL ARTERIAL BLOOD pH RELATED TO NEONATAL MORBIDITY, MORTALITY, AND APGAR SCORES IN TERM INFANTS

	Umbilical Artery pH			
	< 7.00 (n = 85)	7.00–7.04 (n = 95)	7.05–7.09 (n = 290)	7.10–7.14 (n = 798)
Seizure	9 (10.6)	3 (3.2)	0	2 (0.3)
Neonatal deaths	7 (8.2)	2 (2.1)	0	3 (0.4)
Intensive care nursery	17 (20.5)	5 (5.3)	4 (1.4)	7 (0.9)
Intubated	32 (37.6)	3 (3.2)	9 (3.1)	10 (1.3)
Apgar scores ≤ 3				
1 minute	23 (27.1)	6 (6.3)	12 (4.1)	19 (2.4)
5 minutes	9 (10.6)	0	5 (1.7)	0

From Goldaber and associates (1991).

TABLE 17–3. UMBILICAL ARTERIAL AND VENOUS pH AND BLOOD GAS DETERMINATIONS AT BIRTH IN 146 NORMAL NEONATES

	Arterial Values				Venous Values			
	Mean	*SD[a]*	*Range*	*SEM[b]*	*Mean*	*SD[a]*	*Range*	*SEM[b]*
pH	7.28	0.05	7.15–7.43	0.004	7.35	0.05	7.24–7.49	0.0004
PCO_2 (mm Hg)	49.2	8.4	31.1–74.3	0.68	38.2	5.6	23.2–49.2	0.46
PO_2 (mm Hg)	18.0	6.2	3.8–33.8	0.50	29.2	5.9	15.4–48.2	0.48
Bicarbonate (mEq/L)	22.3	2.5	13.3–27.5	0.20	20.4	2.1	15.9–24.7	0.17

[a] SD = standard deviation.
[b] SEM = standard error of the mean.
Modified from Yeomans and associates (1985).

asphyxia remains simple to establish, but strict criteria are required (see below) based not only upon an assignment of clinical criteria (see "Use and Misuse of the Apgar Score" earlier in the chapter) and acidemia (pH) but also upon the type of acidemia—that is, metabolic, respiratory, or mixed respiratory–metabolic. Also, an interpretation of base deficit or excess may be critical in assessing cases of mixed respiratory–metabolic acidemia. Therefore, a brief discussion on the analysis of umbilical cord blood acid-base status is presented.

Analysis of Umbilical Cord Blood Acid-base Status: Types of Acidemia. Umbilical cord blood gas and acid-base analysis can be informative and reassuring, but sometimes misleading. For example, an umbilical cord arterial pH above 7.2 is convincing evidence that obstetrical management of labor did not result in fetal asphyxia. The detection of an umbilical cord pH of less than 7.2, or even 7.0, however, may be the result of a respiratory, metabolic, or mixed acidemia. Most often, such a low pH is not due to metabolic acidemia, and **it is only a metabolic acidosis of severe magnitude and long duration or a mixed respiratory–metabolic acidosis with a marked base deficit** that results in serious fetal damage (Gilstrap and Cunningham, 1989). Therefore, it is important to ascertain in the acidemic fetus the type of acidemia present and the likely etiology. If such information is not available, an arterial cord blood pH of less than 7.2 can be misleading.

Normal values for acid-base and blood gas measurements were reported by Yeomans and associates (1985) and are listed in Table 17–3. It is important to note that these values were obtained in neonates who had normal fetal heart rate tracings, and who were delivered at term from women without complications. Ruth and Raivio (1988) reported similar values. Finally, these values are not different in preterm neonates when compared with term infants (Ramin and associates, 1989; Vintzileos and co-workers, 1992).

Ramin and colleagues (1989) reported observations from 77 preterm and 1292 term neonates and found no significant difference in the frequency of aci-

demia based on gestational age. They also observed that preterm neonates had significantly lower Apgar scores than had been reported by other investigators (Catlin and associates, 1986; Goldenberg and colleagues, 1984). The lack of correlation between low Apgar scores and the frequency of acidemia in preterm neonates is illustrated in Table 17–4. Using the erroneous International Classification of Disease (ICD-9-CM, 1980) coding of asphyxia based merely on a 1-minute Apgar score of less than 7 (see "Use and Misuse of the Apgar Score," earlier in the chapter), 36 percent of preterm infants would have been labeled as having mild birth asphyxia (Apgar 6 or less) and 12 percent as having severe birth asphyxia (1-minute Apgar score 3 or less); however, only 8 percent had acidemia based on a high cut-off pH value of 7.20 or less. Thus, in the study by Ramin and associates (1989), it is apparent that a most important factor influencing the Apgar score is gestational age. Dickinson and colleagues (1992), in a larger study of the effect of preterm birth on umbilical cord blood gases, arrived at the same conclusion. **This, again, emphasizes that an Apgar score of 7 in a preterm neonate should be considered the upper normal value. More importantly, umbilical cord gas indices may be of more value than Apgar scores in preterm infants.**

Two other variables also may alter umbilical cord

TABLE 17–4. FREQUENCY OF ACIDEMIA AND LOW APGAR SCORES IN PRETERM INFANTS COMPARED WITH TERM INFANTS

	Preterm Infants (n = 77) No. (%)	Term Infants (n = 1292) No. (%)
Acidemia (pH < 7.20)	6 (8)	129 (10)
Apgar score ≤ 3		
1 minute	9 (12)[a]	13 (1)
5 minute	2 (2.3)	0
Apgar score ≤ 6		
1 minute	28 (36)[a]	31 (2.4)
5 minute	11 (14)	0

[a] $P < 0.05$ when compared with 5-minute score.
Adapted from Gilstrap and Cunningham (1989) and Ramin and colleagues (1989).

blood gases; altitude and sepsis. Yancey and associates (1992) noted that mean arterial umbilical cord blood pH was increased and mean P_{CO_2} decreased in infants born above 6000 feet. Birthweights were lower and hematocrits higher in these same neonates compared with those born near sea level. Sepsis has been reported to decrease mean arterial umbilical cord blood pH in term but not preterm infants (Meyer and colleagues, 1992). The decrease was correlated significantly with a longer duration of labor.

Fetal Acid-base Physiology. The fetus produces carbonic and organic acids. Carbonic acid (H_2CO_3) is formed by oxidative metabolism of CO_2. The fetus can rapidly clear CO_2 through the placental circulation; but when H_2CO_3 accumulates in fetal blood without an increase in organic acids, this is known as a respiratory acidemia. Organic acids primarily are formed by anaerobic metabolism and include lactic and β-hydroxybutyric acids. These organic acids are cleared slowly from fetal blood, and when they accumulate without an increase in H_2CO_3, this results in a metabolic acidemia, and bicarbonate (HCO_3) *decreases* as it is used to buffer the organic acid. An increase in H_2CO_3 and an increase in organic acid (seen as a decrease in HCO_3) is known as a mixed respiratory–metabolic acidemia.

The actual pH of blood is dependent upon the proportion of carbonic acid and organic acids as well as the amount of bicarbonate that is the major buffer in blood. This can best be illustrated by the Henderson–Hasselbalch equation.

$$pH = pK + \log \frac{[base]}{[acid]} \text{ or } pH = pK + \log \frac{HCO_3}{H_2CO_3}$$

For clinical purposes, HCO_3 represents the metabolic component and is reported as HCO_3 in mEq per L. The H_2CO_3 concentration represents the respiratory component and is reported as the P_{CO_2} in mm Hg. Thus:

$$pH = pK + \log \frac{\text{metabolic } (HCO_3 \text{ mEq/L})}{\text{respiratory } P_{CO_2} \text{ mm Hg})}$$

In summary,

1. Metabolic acidemia = pH < 7.20 with decreased HCO_3 (mEq/L) accompanied by a normal P_{CO_2}.
2. Respiratory acidemia = pH < 7.20 with increased P_{CO_2} (mm Hg) accompanied by a normal HCO_3.
3. Mixed respiratory–metabolic acidemia = pH < 7.20 with increased P_{CO_2} and decreased HCO_3.

Delta base is a calculated number used as a measure of the change in buffering capacity of bicarbonate (HCO_3). For example, bicarbonate will be decreased in concentration with a metabolic acidemia as it is consumed in order to maintain a normal pH. A **base deficit** occurs

when HCO_3 concentration decreases to below normal levels, and a **base excess** occurs when HCO_3 values are above normal. It must be emphasized again that a large base deficit and a low HCO_3 (less than 12 mEq/L) associated with mixed respiratory–metabolic acidemia is more often associated with a depressed neonate than is a mixed acidemia with a minimal base deficit and a more nearly normal HCO_3 (Gilstrap and Cunningham, 1989).

All of the above considerations are based upon the assumption that maternal pH and blood gases are normal. Any major change in maternal values will result in similar fetal changes. The values used to define types of fetal acidemia are listed in Table 17–5.

Clinical Diagnosis of Asphyxia. As emphasized by the Maternal–Fetal Medicine Committee of the American College of Obstetricians and Gynecologists (1991), the term **birth asphyxia** is imprecise and should not be used. Furthermore, acidemia is not sufficient evidence to establish that there has been hypoxic injury. In order to establish that hypoxia near delivery was severe enough to cause hypoxic ischemic encephalopathy, all of the following must be present:

1. Umbilical artery metabolic or mixed respiratory–metabolic acidemia with pH < 7.00.
2. A persistent Apgar score of 0 to 3 for more than 5 minutes.
3. Neonatal neurological sequelae, such as seizures, coma, or hypotonia.
4. Multiorgan system dysfunction (see "Use and Misuse of the Apgar Score," earlier in the chapter).

Umbilical Cord Blood Collection. A 10- to 20-cm segment of umbilical cord is clamped **immediately** following delivery with two clamps near the neonate and two clamps nearer the placenta (Lievaart and deJong, 1984). The cord is then cut between the two proximal and two distal clamps. *Arterial blood* is drawn from the isolated segment of cord into a 1- to 2-mL plastic syringe that has been flushed with a heparin solution containing 1000 units/mL. The needle is then capped, and the capped syringe is placed into a plastic sack containing crushed

TABLE 17–5. CRITERIA USED TO DEFINE TYPES OF ACIDEMIA IN NEWBORNS WITH UMBILICAL ARTERIAL BLOOD pH LESS THAN 7.20

Classification	P_{CO_2} (mm Hg)	HCO_3 (mEq/L)	Base Deficit (mEq/L)
Respiratory	> 65	≥ 22	− 6.4 ± 1.9
Metabolic	< 65	≤ 17	− 15.9 ± 2.8
Mixed	≥ 65	≤ 17	− 9.6 ± 2.5

Adapted from American College of Obstetricians and Gynecologists (1989a), Gilstrap and colleagues (1987).

ice and immediately transported to the laboratory. Although there is little change in Pco_2 or pH in uniced blood for up to 60 minutes (Duerbeck and associates, 1992; Strickland and colleagues, 1984), most clinical laboratories will not accept blood gas samples that are not immediately placed and transported in ice.

Recommendations for Blood Gas Determinations.

A cost-effectiveness analysis for universal cord blood gas measurements has not been conducted. The American College of Obstetricians and Gynecologists (1991) recommended that cord blood gas and pH analyses be used in neonates with low Apgar scores to distinguish metabolic acidemia from hypoxia or other causes that might result in a low Apgar score. We have concluded that although umbilical cord acid-base blood determinations have a low predictability for either immediate or long-term adverse neurological outcome, they are helpful to exclude intrapartum or birth events that cause acidosis (Gilstrap and Cunningham, 1989). Since 1988, we have performed universal umbilical arterial blood gas and acid-base analysis on all neonates, regardless of the clinical circumstances. A similar approach has been adopted at the University of Florida (Johnson and colleagues, 1990).

Active Resuscitation

Although resuscitative measures beyond the stimulation provided by suctioning the mouth and nares, patting the feet, and rubbing the back are needed by only a small percentage of infants, more active measures, skillfully performed, are lifesaving for that small group. It must be mentioned that the first rule of resuscitation is to recognize rapidly the neonate who requires these measures. Also, it should be remembered that suctioning of the mouth, nares, and trachea can result in significant vagal stimulation and reflex slowing of the neonate's heart rate, *unnecessary* or *overvigorous* suctioning of these areas should be avoided.

Successful active resuscitation requires (1) skilled personnel who are immediately available; (2) a suitably heated, well-lighted, appropriately large work area (Fig. 17–1); (3) equipment to deliver oxygen by intermittent positive pressure through a face mask and to carry out tracheal intubation with suction and positive-pressure oxygenation; and (4) drugs, syringes, needles, and catheters for possible intravenous administration of naloxone (Narcan), sodium bicarbonate, and epinephrine. The site of every delivery, vaginal or abdominal, must be so equipped for resuscitation, and the equipment should be thoroughly checked before each delivery. An extremely useful method to ensure that such supplies are available is a wall clipboard system arranged so that any missing equipment or drug is immediately apparent (Fig. 17–2).

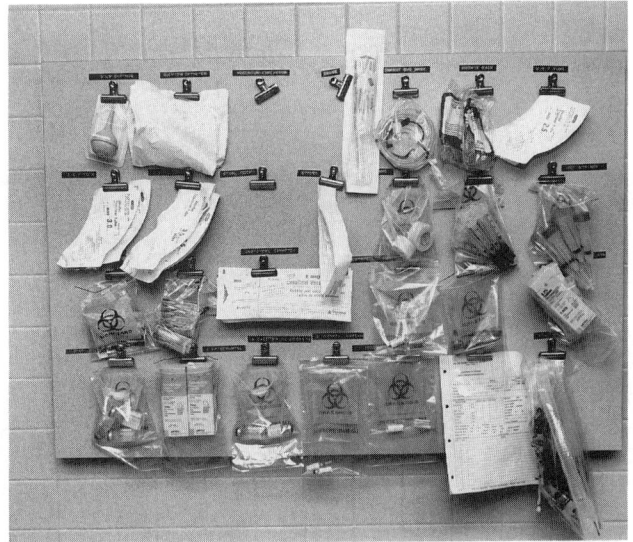

Fig. 17–2. Wall clipboard system used to display equipment and drugs needed for neonatal resuscitation. As shown, a missing item can be identified at a glance and replaced between deliveries.

Ventilation by Mask. Inadequate respirations that persist much beyond a minute lead to a falling heart rate and decreased muscle tone, and call for a quick but careful examination, especially of the mouth, nose, pharynx, neck, and chest, and the administration of oxygen. If the mouth and pharynx are free of liquid and foreign material and no physical obstruction to breathing is identified, oxygen may be delivered through a well-fitting mask at a pressure of about 20 cm H_2O in 1- to 2-second bursts. If this maneuver does not *promptly* stimulate breathing and correct the evidence of hypoxemia, tracheal intubation is necessary under direct visualization with an appropriate laryngoscope.

Tracheal Intubation. The head of the supine infant is kept level. The laryngoscope is introduced into the right side of the mouth and then directed posteriorly toward the oropharynx (Fig. 17–3). The laryngoscope is next gently moved into the space between the base of the tongue and the epiglottis. Gentle elevation of the tip of the laryngoscope will pick up the epiglottis and expose the glottis and the vocal cords. The tracheal tube is introduced through the right side of the mouth and is inserted through the vocal cords until the shoulder of the tube reaches the glottis. Care must be exercised to ensure that the tube is in the trachea and not in the esophagus. The laryngoscope is then removed. Any foreign material encountered in the tracheal tube is immediately removed by suction. Meconium, blood, mucus, and particulate debris in amnionic fluid or in the birth canal may have been inhaled in utero or while passing through the birth canal. The resuscitator using an appropriate ventilation bag attached to the tracheal tube should deliver puffs of oxygen-rich air into the tube at 1-

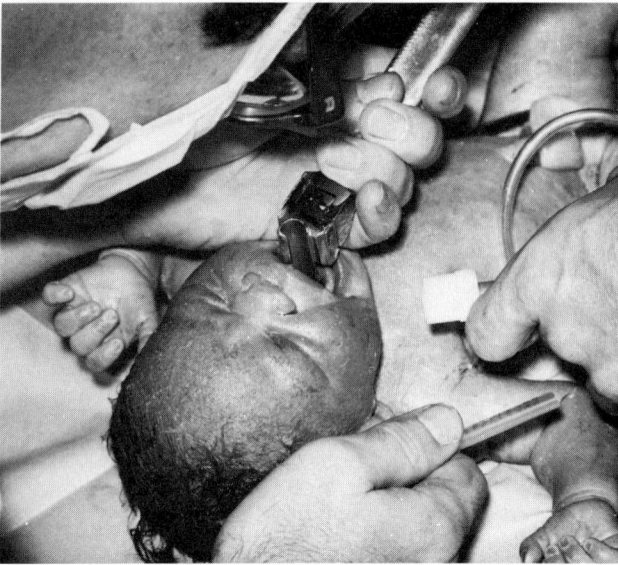

Fig. 17–3. Use of laryngoscope to insert tracheal tube under direct vision. Oxygen is being delivered from curved tube held by an assistant.

to 2-second intervals with a force adequate to lift the chest wall gently. Pressures of 25 to 35 cm H_2O are desired to expand the alveoli yet not cause pneumothorax or pneumomediastinum. If the stomach expands, the tube is almost certainly in the esophagus rather than in the trachea. Once adequate spontaneous respirations have been established, the tube can usually be removed safely.

Causes of Persistent Depression of the Newborn

Acidosis. The treatment of acidosis is correction of the cause. Sodium bicarbonate may be useful in prolonged resuscitation to help correct documented acidosis, but it is not recommended for brief episodes of bradycardia or cardiac arrest. Thus, 1 mEq/kg is injected through the umbilical vein of the severely depressed, hypoxemic newborn who does not respond promptly to establishment of an airway and positive-pressure oxygen administration. This dose may be repeated if a favorable clinical response is not achieved. It is essential that the infant be ventilated effectively so that carbon dioxide can be dissipated. Otherwise, respiratory acidosis will develop, as well as a metabolic acidosis. Further administration of sodium bicarbonate is dependent upon results of measurements of blood gases and pH.

Opioid Drugs. Meperidine (Demerol) and similar drugs given to the mother an hour or less before delivery may cause respiratory depression in the newborn infant. In such cases, naloxone (Narcan) may be given in a dose of 0.1 mg/kg (see Chap. 16, p. 427). This dose may be repeated in 3 to 5 minutes if there is no immediate

response. If there is no response after 2 or 3 doses, the neonatal depression most likely is not due to narcotic effect (American College of Obstetricians and Gynecologists, 1989b). If narcotics have not been given within 4 hours, naloxone at 10 times the usual dose provides no benefit in the resuscitation of depressed newborns (Chernick and colleagues, 1988).

Hypovolemia. Some severely depressed newborn infants are hypovolemic. The infant may be hypovolemic without evidence for fetal hemorrhage. Some causes are sepsis, fetal-to-maternal hemorrhage, trauma to the placenta, cord compression with obstruction of the umbilical vein and pooling of blood in the placenta, and twin-to-twin transfusion. At least partial restoration of intravascular volume and correction of severe anemia are essential for improvement in the volume-depleted infant.

Cardiac Massage. If fetal heart action was present just before delivery but cannot be demonstrated after birth, or if the heart stops after birth, external cardiac massage may be initiated. Immediately, the airway must be cleared, the trachea intubated, and adequate pulmonary ventilation established. External cardiac massage is effected with pressure from two fingers applied to the anterior chest wall in the lower midline at a rate of about 120 per minute. Four compressions of the chest are alternated with each inflation of the lung. Epinephrine may be of value in resuscitating the arrested heart. Epinephrine, 0.1 mL/kg of a 1 : 10,000 dilution, is injected through the tracheal tube or into the umbilical venous line. A delay of several minutes in cardiac massage will most likely result in an unfortunate outcome, either death or permanent marked impairment of central nervous system function.

Common Errors in Resuscitation of the Newborn. If resuscitation efforts are not rapidly successful, the apparent failure may be the consequence of an easily correctable technical error. Even the most skilled and experienced operator can experience difficulties, and the possibility of technical errors should always be kept in mind when an infant fails to respond to resuscitation. These common errors include the following:

1. Failure to check resuscitation equipment beforehand:
   a. Damaged resuscitation bag
   b. Laryngoscope with dull or flickering light
2. Use of a cold resuscitation table
3. Unsuccessful intubation:
   a. Hyperextension of neck
   b. Inadequate suctioning
   c. Excessive force
4. Inadequate ventilation:
   a. Improper head position
   b. Improper application of mask

    c. Placement of tracheal tube into esophagus or right mainstem bronchus

    d. Failure to secure the tracheal tube

5. Failure to detect and determine cause of poor chest movement or persistent bradycardia
6. Failure to detect and treat hypovolemia
7. Failure to perform cardiac massage

Routine Newborn Care

Estimation of Gestational Age. A rapid yet rather precise estimate of gestational age of the newborn may be made very soon after delivery by examining (1) sole creases, (2) breast nodules, (3) scalp hair, (4) ear lobes, and (5) in the case of the male, testes and scrotum (Table 17–6). A more definitive estimate can be made in a few days with the help of neurological examination (see Chap. 38, p. 856). Unfortunately, estimates of gestational age based upon physical and neurological examination frequently are unacceptably inaccurate in preterm and growth-retarded infants (Spinnato and co-workers, 1984). It is unwise to rely on these evaluations alone in such neonates.

Care of the Eyes. Because of the possibility of neonatal eye infection during passage through the vagina of a mother with gonorrhea, Credé, in 1884, introduced the practice of instilling into each eye immediately after birth one drop of a 1 percent solution of silver nitrate, which was later washed out with saline. This procedure led to a marked decrease in the frequency but not the elimination of *gonococcal ophthalmia* and resulting blindness. In most states, the use of an efficacious regimen is required by law.

Technique for Silver Nitrate Prophylaxis

As a preliminary precaution, the region about each eye should be irrigated with sterile water applied to the nasal side of the eye and allowed to run off the opposite side. The lower lid should then be drawn down and the 1 percent silver nitrate solution dropped into the lower cul-de-sac. The silver nitrate produces a discernible chemical conjunctivitis in over half the cases, manifested by redness, edema, or discharge, which develops in 24 hours and lasts 2 to 3 days.

Neonatal Eye Prophylaxis

Gonococcal Ophthalmia Neonatorum

Fortunately, since the introduction of 1 percent silver nitrate solution, blindness due to neonatal infection from *Neisseria gonorrhoeae* has been largely eliminated. More recently a variety of antibiotics have also proven to be extremely effective in preventing gonococcal ophthalmia (Table 17–7). Penicillin ointment in the strength of 100,000 U/g as an ophthalmic ointment has proven to be extremely effective, as has aqueous penicillin G, 50,000 units administered intramuscularly (Siegel and associates, 1982). Tetracycline ophthalmic ointment (1 percent) and erythromycin ointment (0.5 percent) both afford effective prophylaxis (Dillon, 1986; Laga and colleagues, 1988).

Unfortunately, with the emergence of penicillinase-producing *Neisseria gonorrhoeae* (PPNG) strains, penicillin may no longer be effective prophylaxis. A switch to prophylaxis using cefotaxime 100 mg/kg as a single intramuscular injection (Lepage and associates, 1988, 1990), or a single 125 mg intramuscular injection of ceftriaxone, will likely be effective, because these agents have proven to be effective therapy for ophthalmia neonatorum caused by penicillinase-producing strains (Fransen and Klauss, 1988).

Chlamydial Conjunctivitis/Ophthalmia Neonatorum

The problem of providing adequate neonatal prophylaxis against chlamydial infection is much more complex. Although it is reasonable to expect that tetracycline and erythromycin ophthalmic ointments applied at birth should reduce the incidence of chlamydial conjunctivitis/ophthalmia, results with these agents and silver nitrate solution have been disappointing (Table 17–7). Buisman and associates (1988) reported that silver nitrate eye prophylaxis was ineffective against chlamydia. Hammerschlag and co-workers (1989) reported the same for silver nitrate as well as tetracycline and erythromycin ophthalmic ointments. Observations of Laga and colleagues (1988) support this conclusion (Table 17–7). Therefore, truly effective prophylaxis against

---

TABLE 17–6. RAPID ESTIMATION OF GESTATIONAL AGE OF THE NEWBORN

Sites	Gestational Age		
	36 Weeks or Less	*37 to 38 Weeks*	*39 Weeks or More*
Sole creases	Anterior transverse crease only	Occasional creases anterior two-thirds	Sole covered with creases
Breast nodule diameter	2 mm	4 mm	7 mm
Scalp hair	Fine and fuzzy	Fine and fuzzy	Coarse and silky
Ear lobe	Pliable, no cartilage	Some cartilage	Stiffened by thick cartilage
Testes and scrotum	Testes in lower canal, scrotum small, few rugae	Intermediate	Testes pendulous, scrotum full, extensive rugae

TABLE 17–7. EFFECTIVENESS OF NEONATAL EYE PROPHYLAXIS

	Silver Nitrate (1%) Ophthalmic Solution			Tetracycline (1%) Ophthalmic Ointment			Erythromycin (0.5%) Ophthalmic Ointment		
	GC[a]	Chlam[b]	Non[c]	GC[a]	Chlam[b]	Non[c]	GC[a]	Chlam[b]	Non[c]
Incidence (%)									
Laga and associates (1988)	0.4	0.7	8.9	0.1	0.5	4.5	—	—	—
Buisman and colleagues (1988)	0.9	1.8	2.9	—	—	—	—	—	—
Hammerschlag and co-workers (1989)	0.008	—	—	0.02	—	—	0.03	—	—
Attack Rates (%)									
Laga and associates (1988)	7.0	10.1	—	3.0	7.2	—	—	—	—
Hammerschlag and co-workers (1989)	—	20.0	—	—	11.0	—	—	14.0	—

[a] Gonococcal ophthalmia neonatorum.
[b] Chlamydial conjunctivitis/ophthalmia neonatorum.
[c] Nongonococcal, nonchlamydial conjunctivitis/ophthalmia neonatorum.

chlamydial conjunctivitis/ophthalmia neonatorum is not available currently (Chandler, 1989; Isenberg, 1990; Schachter, 1989; Whitcher, 1990).

Several new approaches to the problem of chlamydial ophthalmia have been reported but remain to be proven. A new diagnostic technique, the immune dot-blot test (IDBT), detects chlamydial lipopolysaccharide (LPS) antigen. Bishop and associates (1991) evaluated this test over a 2-year period in both adult and infant eye infections. They found the test more than twice as sensitive as culture. Its use may identify the neonate who should receive prophylaxis or therapy. The new erythromycin analogue, azithromycin, has proven to be effective in treating genital and ocular *Chlamydia trachomatis* in adults using a single 1-g oral dose (Birsum and associates, 1990; Jones, 1991; Stamm, 1991). Prophylactic treatment of the pregnant woman prior to delivery and/or the prophylactic treatment of her infant might result in better outcomes than those using ocular tetracycline or erythromycin. The use of a systemically administered agent such as azithromycin for eye prophylaxis against *Chlamydia trachomatis* might also prevent chlamydial pneumonia, which occurs in 10 to 20 percent of exposed infants.

Other Causes of Neonatal Conjunctivities

In addition to gonorrhea and chlamydia, other organisms such as *Staphylococcus aureus, Streptococcus pneumoniae, Neisseria meningitidis, Pseudomonas aeruginosa, Hemophilus influenzae, Escherichia coli* and other coliform organisms may cause neonatal conjunctivitis. Other streptococci as well as herpesvirus also may cause neonatal conjunctivitis. Fortunately, these pathogens are unusual causes of neonatal conjunctivitis (Repoza and co-workers, 1986), but they should not be forgotten in persistent or refractory cases.

Permanent Infant Identification. Proper identification of each infant is of prime importance. A foolproof system must be operative at all hours. Mother and infant should not be separated until identification is complete.

The system should provide a record easily recognized by the mother, such as an identification band or row of beads that spell the infant's name. A permanent record, often including footprints, should be kept on file at the hospital.

Definitive ridges on the palms, fingers, and feet begin to form several months before birth and remain throughout life. Most hospitals today use footprints rather than fingerprints or palmprints in identifying infants, because the ridges in the feet are more pronounced and it is easier to obtain prints from them in newborn infants. For the footprint to be satisfactory, close attention must be paid to technique. Too often the ridges are not discrete and, therefore, the print is of no value (Clark and associates, 1981). After we found that such identification was not considered valid by the Federal Bureau of Investigation for investigating kidnapping cases, we discontinued footprinting procedures at Parkland Hospital in 1985.

Subsequent Care

Temperature. The temperature of the infant drops rapidly immediately after birth. If the naked newborn is left exposed in the usual cool delivery room or nursery, chilling incites shivering and increases oxygen requirements. Consequently, the infant must be cared for in a warm crib in which temperature control is regulated closely. During the first few days of life, the infant's temperature is unstable, responding to slight stimuli with considerable fluctuations above or below the normal level.

Vitamin K. Routine administration of vitamin K is urged, as described in Chapter 44 (p. 1017).

Hepatitis B Immunization. Routine immunization of all newborns against hepatitis B should be initiated prior to hospital discharge (American Academy of Pediatrics and American College of Obstetricians and Gynecologists, 1992). If the mother is hepatitis B surface antigen positive, the neonate should also be passively immunized with hepatitis B immune globulin (see also Chap. 44). This is only the start of the immunization process, not only for hepatitis, but also for all other immunizations. The mother should understand this fact and the importance of keeping all well-baby appointments.

Umbilical Cord. Loss of water from Wharton jelly leads to mummification of the cord shortly after birth. Within 24 hours it loses its characteristic bluish white, moist appearance and soon becomes dry and black. Gradually the line of demarcation appears just beyond the skin of the abdomen, and in a few days the stump sloughs, leaving a small, granulating wound, which after healing forms the umbilicus. Separation usually takes place within the first 2 weeks, with a range of 3 to 45 days (Novack and colleagues, 1988). The umbilical cord dries more quickly and separates more readily when exposed to the air, and therefore a dressing is not recommended.

Formerly, disregard for asepsis in cord management frequently resulted in serious infection transmitted through the umbilical vessels. Even today serious umbilical infections are sometimes encountered, usually but not always indicating a lack of care. The offending organisms are often *Staphylococcus aureus, Escherichia coli,* or group B *Streptococcus.* Because the umbilical stump in such cases may present no outward sign of infection, the diagnosis cannot be made with certainty except by autopsy. Strict aseptic precautions should therefore be observed in the immediate care of the cord. Most apply triple dye or bacitracin ointment (American College of Obstetricians and Gynecologists, 1992). Gladstone and colleagues (1988) found that povidone–iodine applied daily was effective and acceptable.

Neonatal *tetanus* continues to kill infants in developing countries. Hygienic practices applied to the cutting and subsequent management of the umbilical cord will serve to eliminate this serious complication. In addition, active immunization of the mother against tetanus with passage of antibody to the fetus can serve to reduce the risk to the neonate.

Skin Care. Infants should be promptly patted dry to minimize heat loss caused by evaporation. In most hospitals, not all the vernix caseosa is removed, but the excess, as well as blood and meconium, is gently wiped off. The vernix is readily absorbed by the baby's skin and disappears entirely within 24 hours. It is unwise to wash newborns until their temperature has stabilized, and handling of babies during this time should be minimized.

Stools and Urine. For the first 2 or 3 days after birth, the contents of the colon are composed of soft, brownish-green *meconium,* which is composed of desquamated epithelial cells from the intestinal tract, mucus, and epidermal cells and lanugo (fetal hair) that have been swallowed with amnionic fluid. The characteristic color results from bile pigments. During intrauterine life and for a few hours after birth, the intestinal contents are sterile, but bacteria soon gain access. The passage of meconium and urine in the minutes immediately after birth or during the next few hours indicates patency of the gastrointestinal and urinary tracts. Of all newborns, 90 percent pass meconium within the first 24 hours; most of the rest do so within 36 hours. Voiding, although usually occurring shortly after birth, may not occur until the second day of life. Failure of the infant to eliminate meconium or urine after these times suggests a congenital defect, such as imperforate anus or a urethral valve. These events should be recorded as they occur.

After the third or fourth day, as the consequence of ingesting milk, meconium is replaced by light yellow homogeneous feces with a characteristic odor. For the first few days the stools are unformed, but soon thereafter they assume a cylindrical shape.

Icterus Neonatorum. About one third of all babies, between the second and fifth day of life, develop so-called ***physiological jaundice of the newborn.*** Serum bilirubin levels at birth are 1.8 to 2.8 mg/dL. These levels increase during the next few days but with wide individual variation. Between the third and fourth day, the bilirubin in mature infants commonly reaches somewhat more than 5 mg/dL, the concentration at which jaundice usually becomes noticeable. Most of the bilirubin is free, or unconjugated. One cause, but not the sole cause, is immaturity of the hepatic cells, resulting in less conjugation of bilirubin with glucuronic acid and reduced excretion in bile (Chap. 44, p. 1014). Reabsorption of free bilirubin as the consequence of the enzymatic splitting of bilirubin glucuronide by intestinal conjugase activity in the newborn intestine also appears to contribute significantly to the transient hyperbilirubinemia. In preterm infants, jaundice is more common and usually more severe and prolonged than in term infants, because of less hepatic enzymatic maturity. Term, but small-for-gestational-age infants, however, metabolize bilirubin in a manner similar to term infants. Increased erythrocyte destruction from any cause contributes to hyperbilirubinemia.

Initial Weight Loss. Because most infants receive little nutriment for the first 3 or 4 days of life, and at the same time produce a considerable amount of urine, feces, and sweat, they progressively lose weight until the flow of maternal milk or other feeding has been established. Preterm infants lose relatively more weight and regain their birthweight more slowly than do term infants. Infants that are small for gestational age but otherwise healthy regain their initial weight more quickly when fed than do preterm infants.

If the normal infant is nourished properly, birthweight usually is regained by the end of the 10th day. Subsequently, the weight typically increases steadily at the rate of about 25 g/day for the first few months, to double the birthweight by 5 months of age and to triple it by the end of the first year.

Feeding. It is advisable, because of the stimulating effect of nursing on mother and baby, to commence regular nursing within the first 12 hours postpartum. Most term infants thrive best when fed at intervals of about 4 hours. Preterm or growth-retarded infants require feedings at shorter intervals. In most instances a 3-hour interval is satisfactory. The proper length of each feeding depends on several factors, such as the quantity of breast milk, the readiness with which it can be obtained from the breast, and the avidity with which the infant nurses. It is generally advisable to allow the baby to remain at the breast for 10 minutes at first; 4 to 5 minutes are sufficient for some infants, however, and 15 to 20 minutes are required by others. It is satisfactory for the baby to nurse for 5 minutes at each breast for the first 4 days, or until the mother has a supply of milk. After the fourth day, the baby nurses up to 10 minutes on each breast. A baby receiving proper nourishment should increase steadily in weight. Breast feeding and formula choices also are discussed in Chapter 18 (p. 464).

Circumcision. The Committee on the Fetus and Newborn of the American Academy of Pediatrics in 1971 and 1975 recommended that routine circumcision of newborn males not be performed. The same position was reconfirmed by the Academy along with the American College of Obstetricians and Gynecologists in their 1983 publication *Guidelines for Perinatal Care.* We adopted these recommendations at Parkland Memorial Hospital, and they were apparently also adopted throughout other parts of the United States, because by 1987 only 61 percent of newborn males were circumcised (Poland, 1990).

In the 1992 *Guidelines for Perinatal Care* (American Academy of Pediatrics and American College of Obstetricians and Gynecologists), circumcision was no longer condemned, but it also was not recommended. This change likely resulted from the American Academy of Pediatrics Report of the Task Force on Circumcision (1989). The task force concluded that properly performed newborn circumcision prevented phimosis, paraphimosis, and balanoposthitis, and it decreased the incidence of penile cancer. The committee could not agree that circumcision resulted in a decreased incidence of urinary infections in babies because of the lack of well-designed prospective studies. They also agreed that an increased incidence of cancer of the cervix had been reported in sexual partners of uncircumcised men infected with human papillomavirus. Finally, the task force could not agree on whether circumcision resulted in a decreased incidence of sexually transmitted diseases.

They concluded (without a recommendation) that newborn circumcision was generally a safe procedure when performed by an experienced operator, and circumcision should be an elective procedure performed in a healthy stable neonate. Local anesthesic (dorsal penile nerve block) appeared to reduce the pain of the procedure, but the anesthestic was not without its own complications. In a noncommital last paragraph, the Task Force stated "Newborn circumcision has potential medical benefits and advantages as well as disadvantages and risks. When circumcision is being considered, the benefits and risks should be explained to the parents and informed consent obtained."

We have not changed our policy at Parkland Hospital.

Anesthesia for Circumcision

Stang and colleagues (1988) reported that dorsal penile nerve block reduced behavioral distress and modified adrenocortical stress response in neonates undergoing circumcision. This observation now has been confirmed in several other clinical studies (Arnett and co-workers, 1990; Fontaine and Toffler, 1991; Toffler and associates, 1990). Masciello (1990) reported that local anesthesia is better than a single dorsal penile nerve block, but Blass and Hoffmeyer (1991) maintain that even a sucrose-flavored pacifier proves adequate anesthesia for the procedure.

Complications of Circumcision

As with any surgical procedure, there is a risk of bleeding, infection, and hematoma formation. These risks, however, are low (Braun, 1990; Moreno and Realini, 1989; Wiswell and associates, 1991). More unusual complications have been reported as isolated cases, including denudation of the penis (Orozco-Sanchez and Neri-Vela, 1991), penile destruction with electrocautery (Gearhart and Rock, 1989), and finally ischemia following the **inappropriate use of lidocaine with epinephrine** (Berens and Pontus, 1990). Schoen and Fischell (1991) advise caution before local anesthesia is used widely because of local and systemic side effects of lidocaine.

Rooming-in. Rooming-in involves keeping the infant in a crib at the mother's bedside rather than in the nursery, thus permitting the mother to take care of the baby. This practice stems, in part, from a trend to make all phases of childbearing as natural as possible and to foster proper mother–child relationships at an early date. By the end of 24 hours, the mother is generally fully ambulatory; thereafter, with rooming-in, she can conduct for herself and for the infant practically all routine care. An obvious advantage is the mother's increased ability to assume full care of the baby when she arrives home.

Abnormalities of the Newborn. These are considered throughout the text, and especially in Chapters 38 and 44.

References

American Academy of Pediatrics: Report of the Task Force on Circumcision. Errata Pediatrics 84:761, 1989

American Academy of Pediatrics: Report of the Task Force on Circumcision. Pediatrics 84:388, 1989

American Academy of Pediatrics: Report of the ad hoc Task Force on Circumcision. Pediatrics 56:610, 1975

American Academy of Pediatrics, Committee on Fetus and Newborn: Use and abuse of the Apgar score. Pediatrics 78:1148, 1986

American Academy of Pediatrics, Committee on the Fetus and Newborn. Standards and recommendations for hospital care of newborn infants, 5th ed. Evanston, American Academy of Pediatrics, 1971, p 110

American Academy of Pediatrics and the American College of Obstetricians and Gynecologists: Guidelines for perinatal care. 3rd ed. Washington, DC, 1992, pp 103, 109, 155

American Academy of Pediatrics and the American College of Obstetricians and Gynecologists: Guidelines for perinatal care, 2nd ed. Washington, DC, 1983.

American College of Obstetricians and Gynecologists: Utility of umbilical cord blood acid-base assessment. ACOG MFM Committee Opinion no. 91, February 1991

American College of Obstetricians and Gynecologists: Assessment of newborn acid-base status. Technical Bulletin no. 127, 1989a

American College of Obstetricians and Gynecologists: Naloxone use in newborns. ACOG Committee Opinion no. 70, August 1989b

American College of Obstetricians and Gynecologists, Committee on Maternal and Fetal Medicine: Use and misuse of the Apgar score. November 1986; reaffirmed 1991

Apgar V: A proposal for a new method of evaluation of the newborn infant. Curr Res Anesth Analg 32:260, 1953

Apgar V, Holaday DA, James LS, Weisbrot IM, Berrien C: Evaluation of the newborn infant—second report. JAMA 168:1985, 1958

Arnett RM, Jones JS, Horger EO III: Effectiveness of 1% lidocaine dorsal penile nerve block in infant circumcision. Am J Obstet Gynecol 163:1074, 1990

Berens R, Pontus SP Jr: A complication associated with dorsal penile nerve block. Reg Anaesth 15:309, 1990

Birsum T, Dannevig L, Strvold G, Melby K: Chlamydia trachomatis: In vitro susceptibility of genital and ocular isolates to some quinolones, amoxicillin and azithromycin. J Chemother 36:407, 1990

Bishop PN, Tullo AB, Killough R, Richmond SJ: An immune dot-blot test for the diagnosis of ocular infection with Chlamydia trachomatis. Eye 5:305, 1991

Blass E, Hoffmeyer LB: Sucrose as an analgesic for newborn infants. Pediatrics 87:215, 1991

Brann AW Jr, Dykes FD: The effects of intrauterine asphyxia on the full-term neonate. Clin Perinatol 4:149, 1977

Braun D: Neonatal bacteremia and circumcision. Pediatrics 85:135, 1990

Buisman NJ, Abong Mwemba T, Garrigue G, Durand JP, Stilma JS, van Balen TM: Chlamydial ophthalmia neonatorum in Cameroon. Doc Ophthalmol 70:257, 1988

Catlin EA, Carpenter MW, Brann BS, Mayfield SR, Shaul PW, Goldstein M, Oh W: The Apgar score revisited: Influence of gestational age. J Pediatr 109:865, 1986

Chandler JW: Controversies in ocular prophylaxis of newborns. Arch Ophthalmol 107:814, 1989

Chernick V: Fetal breathing movements and the onset of breathing at birth. Clin Perinatol 5:257, 1978

Chernick V, Manfreda J, DeBooy V, Davi M, Rigatto H, Seshia M: Clinical trial of naloxone in birth asphyxia. J Pediatr 113:519, 1988

Clark DA, Thompson J, Cahill J, Salisbury B: Footprinting the newborn—cost effective? Pediatr Res 15:552, 1981

Credé CSF: Die Verhütung der Augenenzündung der Neugeborenen. Berlin, Hirschwald, 1884

Dawes GS: Breathing before birth in animals or man. N Engl J Med 290:557, 1974

Dickinson JE, Eriksen NL, Meyer BA, Parisi VM: The effect of preterm birth on umbilical cord blood gases. Obstet Gynecol 79:575, 1992

Dillon HC Jr: Prevention of gonococcal ophthalmia neonatorum. N Engl J Med 315:1414, 1986

Duenhoelter JH, Pritchard JA: Fetal respiration: Quantitative measurements of amnionic fluid inspired near term by human and rhesus fetuses. Am J Obstet Gynecol 125:306,1976

Duerbeck NB, Chaffin DG, Seeds JW: A practical approach to umbilical artery pH and blood gas determinations. Obstet Gynecol 79:959, 1992

Fields LM, Entman SS, Boehm FH: Correlation of the one-minute Apgar score and the pH value of the umbilical arterial blood. South Med J 76:1477, 1983

Finer NN, Robertson CM, Peters KL, Coward JH: Factors affecting outcome in hypoxic–ischemic encephalopathy in term infants. Am J Dis Child 137:21, 1983

Fontaine P, Toffler WL: Dorsal penile nerve block for newborn circumcision. Am Fam Physician 43:1327, 1991

Fransen L, Klauss V: Neonatal ophthalmia in the developing world. Epidemiology, etiology, management and control. Int Ophthalmol 11:189, 1988

Freeman JM, Nelson KB: Intrapartum asphyxia and cerebral palsy. Pediatrics 82:240, 1988

Gearhart JP, Rock JA: Total ablation of the penis after circumcision with electrocautery: A method of management and long-term followup. J Urol 142:799, 1989

Gilstrap LC, Cunningham FG: Cord blood acid-base analysis. Cunningham FG, MacDonald PC, Gant NF (eds): Williams Obstetrics, 18th ed, supplement 1. Norwalk, CT, Appleton & Lange, 1989

Gilstrap LC, Hauth JC, Hankins GDV, Beck AW: Second-stage fetal heart rate abnormalities and type of neonatal acidemia. Obstet Gynecol 70:191, 1987

Gilstrap LC, Hauth JC, Schiano S, Connor KD: Neonatal acidosis and method of delivery. Obstet Gynecol 63:681, 1984a

Gilstrap LC, Hauth JC, Toussaint S: Second-stage fetal heart rate abnormalities and neonatal acidosis. Obstet Gynecol 62:209, 1984b

Gilstrap LC, Leveno KJ, Burris J, Williams ML, Little BB: Diagnosis of birth asphyxia based on fetal pH, Apgar score, and newborn cerebral dysfunction. Am J Obstet Gynecol 161: 825, 1989

Gladstone IM, Clapper L, Thorp JW, Wright DI: Randomized study of six umbilical cord care regimens. Comparing length of attachment, microbial control, and satisfaction. Clin Pediatr 27:127, 1988

Goldaber KG, Gilstrap LG, Leveno KJ, Dax JS: Pathologic fetal acidemia. Obstet Gynecol 78:1103, 1991

Goldenberg RL, Huddleston JF, Nelson KG: Apgar scores and umbilical arterial pH in preterm newborn infants. Am J Obstet Gynecol 149:651, 1984

Hammerschlag MR, Cummings C, Roblin PM, Williams TH, Delke I: Efficacy of neonatal ocular prophylaxis for the prevention of chlamydial and gonococcal conjunctivitis. N Engl J Med 320:769, 1989

Isenberg SJ: The dilemma of neonatal ophthalmic prophylaxis. West J Med 153:190, 1990

Johnson JWC, Richards DS, Wagaman RA: The case for routine umbilical blood acid-base studies at delivery. Am J Obstet Gynecol 162:621, 1990

Jones RB: New treatments for chlamydia trachomatis. Am J Obstet Gynecol 164:1789, 1991

Josten BE, Johnson TRB, Nelson JP: Umbilical cord blood pH and Apgar scores as an index of neonatal health. Am J Obstet Gynecol 157:843, 1987

Laga M, Plummer FA, Piot P, Datta P, Namaara W, Ndinya-Achola JO, Nzanze H, Maitha G, Ronald AR, Pamba HO, Brunham RC: Prophylaxis of gonococcal and chlamydial ophthalmia neonatorum: A comparison of silver nitrate and tetracycline. N Engl J Med 318:653, 1988

Lepage P, Bogaerts J, Kestelyn P, Meheus A: Single-dose cefotaxime intramuscularly cures gonococcal ophthalmia neonatorum. Br J Ophthalmol 72:518, 1988

Lepage P, Kestelyn P, Bogaerts J: Treatment of gonococcal conjunctivitis with a single intramuscular injection of cefotaxime. J Antimicrob Chemother 26(suppl A):23, 1990

Lievaart M, deJong PA: Acid-base equilibrium in umbilical cord blood and time of cord clamping. Obstet Gynecol 63:44, 1984

Martin CB Jr, Murata Y, Petrie RH, Parer JT: Respiratory movements in fetal rhesus monkeys. Am J Obstet Gynecol 119:939, 1974

Masciello AL: Anesthesia for neonatal circumcision: Local anesthesia is better than dorsal penile nerve block. Obstet Gynecol 75:834, 1990

Mellits ED, Holden KR, Freeman JM: Neonatal seizures: II. A multivariate analysis of factors associated with outcome. Pediatrics 70:177, 1982

Meyer BA, Dickinson JE, Chambers C, Parisi VM: The effect of fetal sepsis on umbilical cord blood gases. Am J Obstet Gynecol 166:612, 1992

Milner AD, Saunders RA, Hopkins IE: The effect of delivery by caesarean section on lung mechanics and lung volume in the human neonate. Arch Dis Child 53:545, 1978

Moreno CA, Realini JP: Infant circumcision in an outpatient setting. Texas Med J 85:37, 1989

Nelson KB, Ellenberg JH: Apgar scores as predictors of chronic neurologic disability. Pediatrics 68:36, 1981

Novack AH, Mueller B, Ochs H: Umbilical cord separation in the normal newborn. Am J Dis Child 142:220, 1988

Orozco-Sanchez J, Neri-Vela R: Total denudation of the penis in circumcision. Description of a plastic technique for repair of the penis. Bol Med Hosp Infant Mex 48:565, 1991

Poland RL: The question of routine neonatal circumcision. N Engl J Med 322:1312, 1990

Ramin SM, Gilstrap LC, Leveno KJ, Burris JC, Little BB: Umbilical artery acid-base status in the preterm infant. Obstet Gynecol 74:256, 1989

Repoza P, Quinn T, Kiessling L, Taylor H: Epidemiology of neonatal conjunctivitis. Ophthalmology 93:456, 1986

Ruth VJ, Raivio KO: Perinatal brain damage: Predictive value of metabolic acidosis and the Apgar score. Br Med J 297:24, 1988

Sarnet HB, Sarnet MS: Neonatal encephalopathy following fetal distress: A clinical and electroencephalographic study. Arch Neurol 33:696, 1976

Saunders RA: Pulmonary/volume relationships during the last phase of delivery and the first postnatal breaths in human subjects. J Pediatr 93:667, 1978

Schachter J: Why we need a program for the control of *Chlamydia trachomatis*. N Engl J Med 320:802, 1989

Schoen EJ, Fischell AA: Pain in neonatal circumcision. Clin Pediatr 30:429, 1991

Siegel JD, McCracken GH Jr, Threlkeld N, DePasse BM, Rosenfeld CR: Single-dose penicillin prophylaxis of neonatal group B streptococcal disease. Lancet 2:1426, 1982

Spinnato JA, Sibai BM, Shaver DC, Anderson GD: Inaccuracy of Dubowitz gestational age in low birth weight infants. Obstet Gynecol 63:491, 1984

Stamm WE: Azithromycin in the treatment of uncomplicated genital chlamydial infections. Am J Med 91:19S, 1991

Stang JH, Gunnar MR, Snellman L, Condon LM, Kestenbaum R: Local anesthesia for neonatal circumcision. Effects on distress and cortisol response. JAMA 259:1507, 1988

Strickland DM, Gilstrap LC, Hauth JC, Widmer K: Umbilical cord pH and P_{CO_2}: Effects of interval from delivery to determination. Am J Obstet Gynecol 148:191, 1984

Toffler WL, Sinclair AE, White KA: Dorsal penile nerve block during newborn circumcision: Underutilization of a proven technique? J Am Board Fam Pract 3:171, 1990

US Department of Health and Human Services: The International Classification of Diseases ICD-9-CM, DHHS pub. no. (PHS) 80-1260. Washington, DC, Government Printing Office, 1980

US Department of Health and Human Services, Public Health Service, National Institutes of Health, National Institute of Child Health and Human Development; Freeman JM (ed): Prenatal and Perinatal Factors Associated with Brain Disorders, NIH pub. no. 85-1149. Washington, DC, Government Printing Office, 1985

Vintzileos AM, Egan J, Campbell WA, Rodis JF, Scorza WE, Fleming AD, McLean DA: Asphyxia at birth as determined by cord blood pH measurements in preterm and term gestations: Correlation with neonatal outcome. J Matern Fetal Med 1:7, 1992

Whitcher JP: Neonatal ophthalmia: Have we advanced in the last 20 years? Int Ophthalmol Clin 30:39, 1990

Wible JL, Petrie RH, Koons A, Perez A: The clinical use of umbilical cord acid-base determinations in perinatal surveillance and management. Clin Perinatol 9:387, 1982

Wiswell TE, Curtis J, Dobek AS, Zierdt CH: Staphylococcus aureus colonization after neonatal circumcision in relation to device used. J Pediatr 119:302, 1991

Yancey MK, Moore J, Brady K, Milligan D, Strampel W: The effect of altitude on umbilical cord blood gases. Obstet Gynecol 79:571, 1992

Yeomans ER, Gilstrap LC, Leveno KJ, Burris JS: Meconium in the amniotic fluid and fetal acid-base status. Obstet Gynecol 73:175, 1989

Yeomans ER, Hauth JC, Gilstrap LC III, Strickland DM: Umbilical cord pH, P_{CO_2} and bicarbonate following uncomplicated term vaginal deliveries. Am J Obstet Gynecol 151:798, 1985

CHAPTER 18
The Puerperium

Definition. Puerperium is defined literally as the period of confinement during and just after birth. By popular use, however, the meaning includes the subsequent weeks during which normal pregnancy involution occurs. Most consider the first 6 weeks postpartum to be the puerperium. During this time, the reproductive tract returns anatomically to a normal nonpregnant state, and in most women who are not breast feeding, ovulation is reestablished.

Involution of the Genital and Urinary Tracts

Involution of the Body of the Uterus. Immediately after placental expulsion, the fundus of the contracted uterus is slightly below the umbilicus. The uterine body then consists mostly of myometrium covered by serosa and lined by basal decidua. The anterior and posterior walls, in close apposition, each measure 4 to 5 cm in thickness. Because its vessels are compressed by the contracted myometrium, the puerperal uterus on section appears ischemic when compared to the reddish-purple hyperemic pregnant organ. After the first 2 days, the uterus begins to shrink, so that within 2 weeks, it has descended into the cavity of the true pelvis and can no longer be felt above the symphysis. It regains its previous nonpregnant size within about 4 weeks. The rapidity of the process is remarkable. The immediately postpartum uterus weighs approximately 1 kg. As the consequence of *involution*, 1 week later it weighs about 500 g, decreasing at the end of the second week to about 300 g, and soon thereafter to 100 g or less. The total number of muscle cells does not decrease appreciably; instead, the individual cells decrease markedly in size. The mechanism by which the individual muscle cell divests itself of excess cytoplasm, including contractile protein, remains to be elucidated. The involution of the connective tissue framework occurs equally rapidly.

Because separation of the placenta and membranes involves the spongy layer of the decidua, basal decidua remains in the uterus. The decidua that remains has striking variations in thickness, an irregular jagged appearance, and is infiltrated with blood, especially at the placental site.

Regeneration of Endometrium. Within 2 or 3 days after delivery, the remaining decidua becomes differentiated into two layers. The superficial layer becomes necrotic, and it is sloughed in the lochia. The basal layer adjacent to the myometrium, which contains the fundi of endometrial glands, remains intact and is the source of new endometrium. The endometrium arises from proliferation of the endometrial glandular remnants and the stroma of the interglandular connective tissue.

Endometrial regeneration is rapid, except at the placental site. Within a week or 10 days, the free surface becomes covered by epithelium, and the entire endometrium is restored during the third week. Sharman (1953) identified fully restored endometrium in all biopsy specimens obtained from the 16th postpartum day onward. Endometrium was normal except for occasional hyalinized decidual remnants and leukocytes. The so-called endometritis identified histologically during the reparative days of the puerperium is only part of the normal process of repair. Similarly, in almost half of postpartum women, fallopian tubes, between 5 and 15 days, demonstrate microscopical inflammatory changes characteristic of acute salpingitis; however, this is not infection, but only part of the normal involutional process (Andrews, 1951).

Involution of the Placental Site. According to Williams (1931), complete extrusion of the placental site takes up to 6 weeks. This process is of great clinical importance, for when it is defective, late puerperal hemorrhage may ensue. Immediately after delivery, the placental site is about the size of the palm of the hand, but it rapidly decreases thereafter. By the end of the second week, it is 3 to 4 cm in diameter. Within hours of delivery, the placental site normally consists of many thrombosed vessels that ultimately undergo the typical organization of a thrombus (Fig. 18–1).

If involution of the placental site comprised only these events, each pregnancy would leave a fibrous scar in the endometrium and subjacent myometrium, thus eventually limiting the number of future pregnancies. Williams (1931) explained involution of the placental site as follows:

> Involution is not effected by absorption in situ, but rather by a process of exfoliation which is in great part brought about by the undermining of the placental implantation site by the growth of endometrial tissue. This is affected partly by extension and downgrowth of endometrium from the margins of the placental site and partly by the development of endometrial tissue from the glands and stroma left in the depths of the decidua basalis after the sepa-

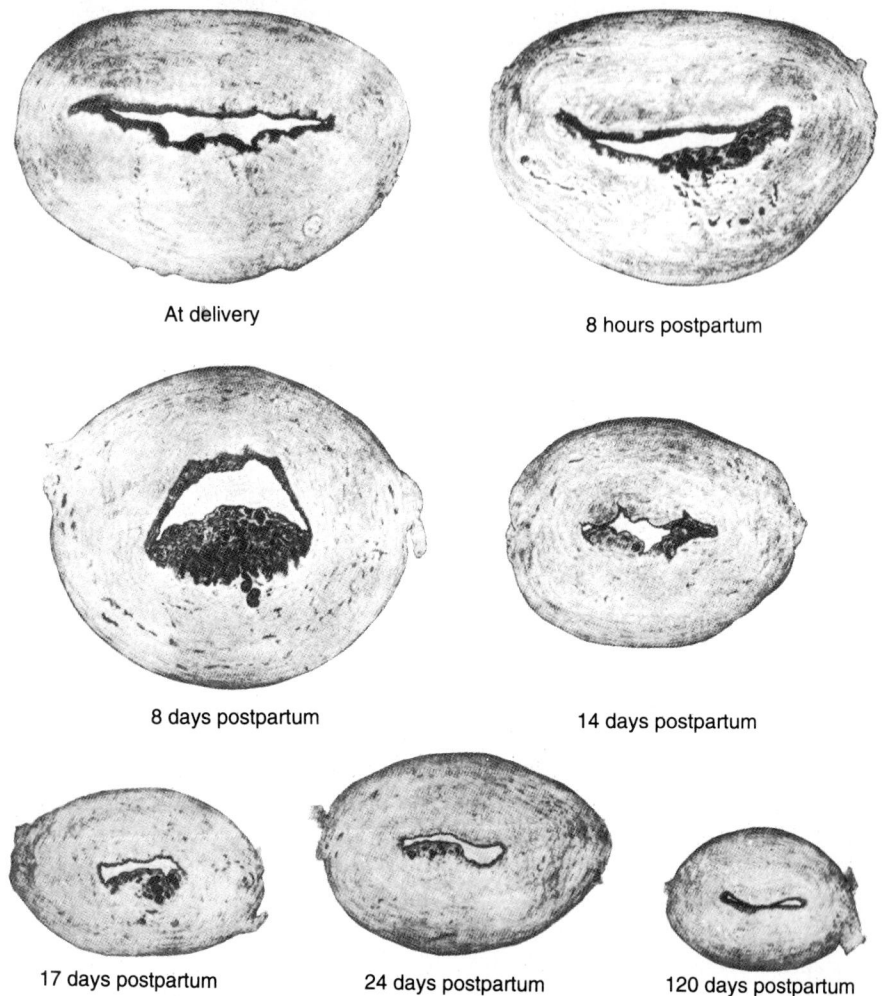

At delivery

8 hours postpartum

8 days postpartum

14 days postpartum

Fig. 18–1. Cross sections of uteri made at the level of the involuting placental site at varying times after delivery. (From Williams, 1931.)

17 days postpartum

24 days postpartum

120 days postpartum

ration of the placenta.... Such a process of exfoliation should be regarded as very conservative, and as a wise provision on the part of nature; otherwise great difficulty might be experienced in getting rid of the obliterated arteries and organized thrombi which, if they remained in situ, would soon convert a considerable part of the uterine mucosa and subjacent myometrium into a mass of scar tissue with the result that after a few pregnancies it would unlikely be possible for it to go through its usual cycle of changes, and the reproductive career would come to an end.

Anderson and Davis (1968) concluded that placental site exfoliation is brought about as the consequence of a necrotic slough of infarcted superficial tissues followed by a reparative process not unlike that which takes place on any denuded epithelium-covered structure.

Changes in the Uterine Vessels. Successful pregnancy requires a great increase in uterine blood flow. To provide for this, arteries and veins within the uterus, and especially to the placental site, enlarge remarkably, as do transport vessels to and from the uterus (Chap. 8, p.

211). Within the uterus, growth of new vessels also provides for the marked increase in blood flow. After delivery, the caliber of extrauterine vessels decreases to equal, or at least closely approximate, that of the prepregnant state.

Within the puerperal uterus, blood vessels are obliterated by hyaline changes, and vessels that are smaller replace them. Resorption of the hyalinized residue is accomplished by processes similar to those observed in the ovaries following ovulation and corpus luteum formation. Minor vestiges, however, may persist for years, thus affording a microscopical means of differentiating between the uteri of parous and nulliparous women.

Changes in the Cervix and Lower Uterine Segment. Immediately after the third stage of labor, the cervix and lower uterine segment are thin, collapsed, flabby structures. The outer margin of the cervix, which corresponds to the external os, is usually lacerated, especially laterally. The cervical opening contracts slowly, and for a few days immediately after labor, it readily admits two fingers. By the end of the first week, it has narrowed to a one-finger diameter. As the cervical opening narrows, the cervix thickens, and a canal is reformed. At the completion of involution, however, the external os does not resume its pregravid appearance completely. It remains somewhat wider, and typically, bilateral depressions at the site of lacerations remain as permanent changes that characterize the parous cervix (Fig. 3–11, p. 67).

After delivery, the markedly thinned-out lower uterine segment contracts and retracts but not as forcefully as the body of the uterus. Over the course of a few weeks, the lower segment is converted from a clearly evident structure, large enough to contain most of the head of the term fetus, into a barely discernible uterine isthmus located between the body of the uterus above and the internal os of the cervix below (Fig. 3–8, p. 65).

Vagina and Vaginal Outlet. Early in the puerperium, the vagina and vaginal outlet form a capacious, smooth-walled passage that gradually diminishes in size but rarely returns to nulliparous dimensions. Rugae reappear by the third week. The hymen is represented by several small tags of tissue, which during cicatrization are converted into the *myrtiform caruncles* characteristic of parous women.

Changes in the Peritoneum and Abdominal Wall.

As the myometrium contracts and retracts after delivery, the peritoneum covering much of the uterus is formed into folds and wrinkles. The broad and round ligaments are much more lax than in the nonpregnant condition, and they require considerable time to recover from the stretching and loosening that occurred during pregnancy.

As a result of the rupture of elastic fibers in the skin and the prolonged distention caused by the enlarged pregnant uterus, the abdominal walls remain soft and flabby. Return to normal for these structures requires several weeks, but recovery is aided by exercise. Except for silvery striae, the abdominal wall usually resumes its prepregnancy appearance; but when muscles remain atonic, the abdominal wall also remains lax. There may be a marked separation, or diastasis, of the rectus muscles. In this condition, the abdominal wall in the vicinity of the midline is formed only by peritoneum, attenuated fascia, subcutaneous fat, and skin.

Changes in the Urinary Tract.

Postpartum cystoscopic examination discloses not only edema and hyperemia of the bladder wall, but also submucous extravasation of blood. In addition, the puerperal bladder has an increased capacity and a relative insensitivity to intravesical fluid pressure. Therefore, overdistention, incomplete emptying, and excessive residual urine must be watched for closely. The paralyzing effect of anesthesia, especially conduction analgesic, and the temporarily disturbed neural function of the bladder, are undoubt-

edly contributory factors. Residual urine and bacteriuria in a traumatized bladder, coupled with the dilated renal pelves and ureters, create optimal conditions for the development of urinary tract infection (Chap. 50, p. 1128). Dilated ureters and renal pelves return to their prepregnant state from 2 to 8 weeks after delivery (Chap. 8, p. 231).

Kerr-Wilson and colleagues (1984) studied the effect of labor on postpartum bladder function using urodynamic techniques. They concluded that, as long as prolonged labors were avoided and if catheterization was done promptly for bladder distention, there was no evidence for bladder hypotonia. Although they reported that epidural analgesia did not predispose to bladder hypotonia postpartum, Weil and colleagues (1983) found that 35 percent of women who had epidural analgesia had asymptomatic urinary retention. Careful attention to all postpartum women, with prompt catheterization for those who cannot void, will prevent most urinary problems.

Viktrup and colleagues (1992) followed 305 nulliparous women during pregnancy and then postpartum; 7 percent developed stress incontinence after delivery. The stretching and dilatation during pregnancy do not cause permanent changes in the renal pelves and ureters. Obstetrical factors such as length of second-stage labor, infant head circumference, birthweight, and episiotomy were associated with the development of stress incontinence after delivery. Conversely, cesarean delivery seemed to protect against its development. Impaired muscle function in or around the urethra during vaginal delivery was proposed as the pathophysiology underlying puerperal incontinence. Most women returned to normal micturition by 3 months postpartum.

Changes in Mammary Glands

Anatomy of the Breasts. Anlagen of mammary glands are contained in ectodermal ridges that form on the ventral surface of the embryo and extend laterally from forelimb to hindlimb. The multiple pairs of buds normally disappear from the embryo except for one pair in the pectoral region that eventually develops into the two mammary glands (Fig. 18–2). At times, however, the buds elsewhere may not completely disappear, but instead they may participate to an amazing degree in the pattern of growth that characterizes the two normal mammary glands (Fig. 29–5).

At midpregnancy, each of the two fetal mammary buds destined to form the breasts begins to grow and divide; this results in the formation of 15 to 25 secondary buds that provide the basis for the duct system in the mature breast. Each secondary bud elongates into a cord, bifurcates, and differentiates into two concentric layers of cuboidal cells and a central lumen. The inner layer of cells eventually gives rise to the secretory epi-

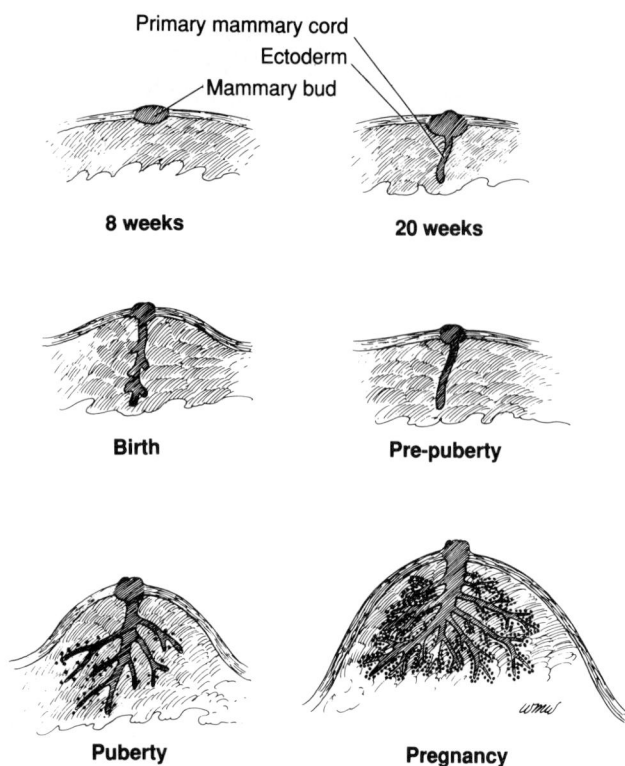

Fig. 18–2. Sequential growth of the mammary gland is illustrated from 8 weeks embryonic age through puberty and during pregnancy. (Courtesy of Dr. John C. Porter.)

thelium, which synthesizes the milk, while the outer layer becomes myoepithelium, which provides the mechanism for milk ejection (Fig. 18–3A, B).

Thelarche is the onset of rapid breast growth that begins about the time of puberty when estrogen production rises. The previously infantile mammary glands respond to estrogen with growth and development of mammary ducts and fat deposition. With the onset of ovulation, progesterone stimulates development of the alveoli and sets the stage for future lactation.

Anatomically, each mature mammary gland is composed of 15 to 25 lobes that arose from the secondary mammary buds described above. The lobes are arranged radially and are separated from one another by varying amounts of fat. Each lobe consists of several lobules, which in turn are made up of large numbers of alveoli (Fig. 18–3A, B). Every alveolus is provided with a small duct that joins others to form a single larger duct for each lobe (Fig. 18–3B). These lactiferous ducts open separately upon the nipple, where they may be distinguished as minute but distinct orifices. The alveolar secretory epithelium synthesizes the various milk constituents (Fig. 18–3C).

Lactation. Colostrum is the deep lemon-yellow colored liquid secreted by the breasts for the first 5 postpartum days. It usually can be expressed from the

nipples by the second postpartum day, but actual milk production usually is not established until puerperal day 5.

Colostrum. Compared with mature milk, colostrum contains more minerals and protein, much of which is globulin, but less sugar and fat. Colostrum nevertheless contains large fat globules in so-called colostrum corpuscles; these are thought by some to be epithelial cells that have undergone fatty degeneration and by others to be mononuclear phagocytes containing fat. Colostrum secretion persists for about 5 days, with gradual conversion to mature milk during the ensuing 4 weeks. Antibodies are demonstrable in the colostrum, and its content of immunoglobulin A may offer protection for the newborn against enteric pathogens, as described below. Other host resistance factors, as well as immunoglobulins, are found in human colostrum and milk. These include complement, macrophages, lymphocytes, lactoferrin, lactoperoxidase, and lysozymes.

Milk. The major components of milk are proteins, lactose, water, and fat. Milk is isotonic with plasma, with lactose accounting for half of the osmotic pressure. Major proteins, including α-lactalbumin, β-lactoglobulin, and casein, are synthesized in the rough endoplasmic reticulum of the alveolar secretory cell. Essential amino acids are derived from blood, and nonessential amino acids are derived in part from blood or synthesized in the mammary gland. Most milk proteins are unique and not found elsewhere. Whey from human milk has been shown to contain large amounts of interleukin-6 (Saito and co-workers, 1991). Peak levels of this cytokine were found in colostrum, and there was a positive correlation between its concentration and the number of mononuclear cells in human milk. Additionally, interleukin-6 was associated closely with local immunoglobulin A production by the breast. Prolactin appears to be actively secreted into breast milk (Yuen, 1988), and epidermal growth factor (EGF) has been identified in human milk (Koldovsky and associates, 1991; McCleary, 1991). Because epidermal growth factor is not destroyed by gastric proteolytic enzymes, it may be absorbed and promote growth and maturation of the infant's intestinal mucosa. Somatostatin and vasoactive intestinal peptide are concentrated in rat milk, but not produced by the breast (Koch and associates, 1991). Furthermore, somatostatin is absorbed intact and biologically active from the gut of neonatal rats. If this is found in humans, it will allow a new understanding of glucose metabolism and fat deposition in neonates.

Major changes in milk composition occur 30 to 40 hours postpartum, including a sudden increase of lactose concentration. The synthesis of lactose from glucose in alveolar secretory cells is catalyzed by lactose synthetase (Fig. 18–4). Some lactose enters the maternal circulation and is excreted by the kidney. This may

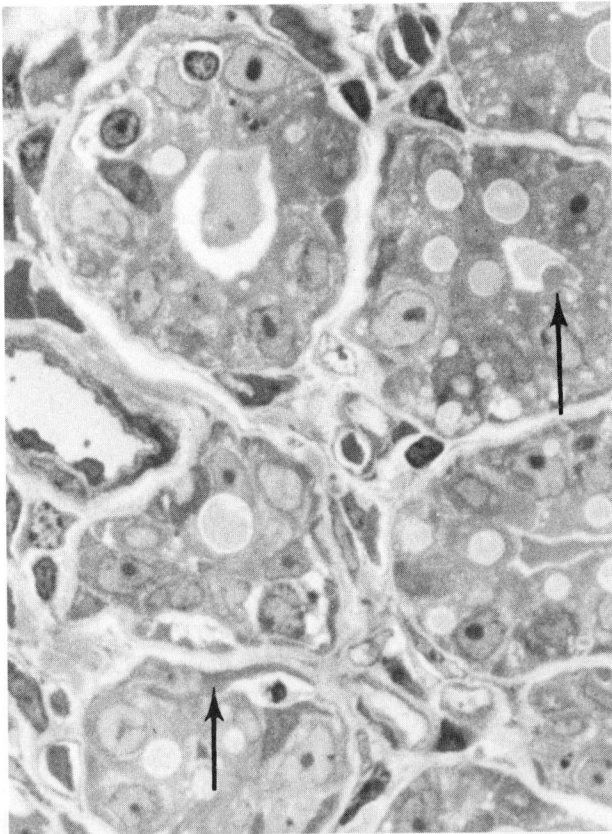

A

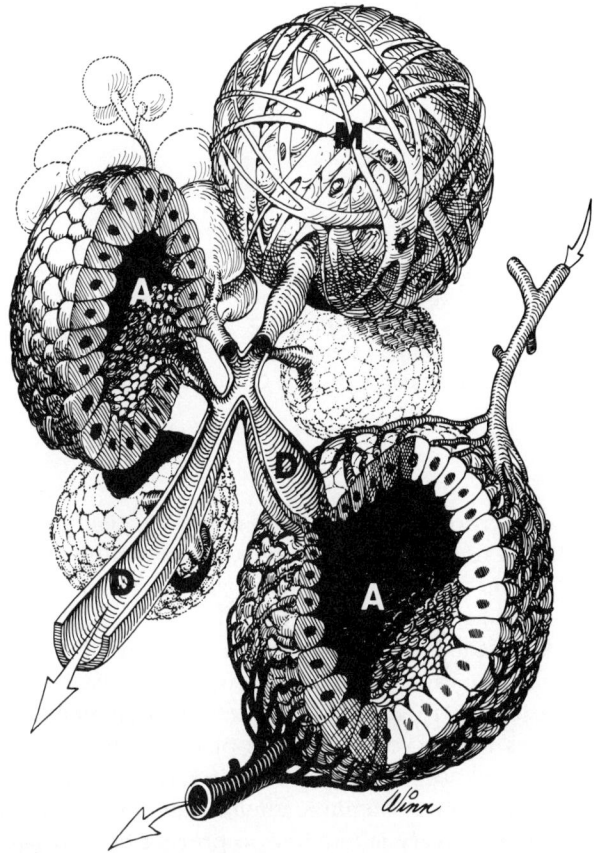

B

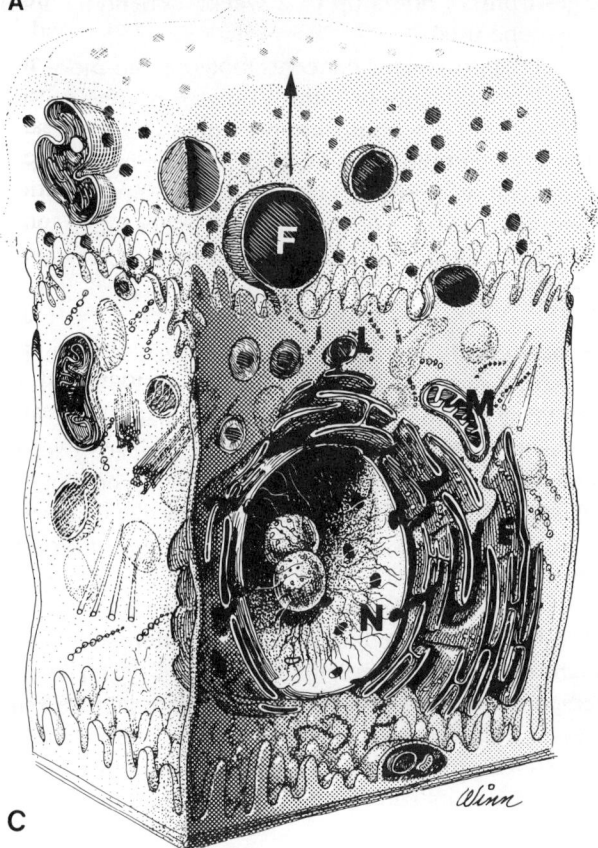

C

Fig. 18–3. A. Histology of maternal breast at 32 weeks' gestation in preparation for lactation. Secretions are evident in the lumen of each alveolus. Myoepithelial cells are evident around alveoli (*lower left arrow*). Secretions are being delivered by exocytosis into the lumen of one alveolus (*upper right arrow*). **B.** Graphic demonstration of alveolar and ductal system shown in **A.** Note the myoepithelial fibers (M) that surround the outside of the uppermost alveolus. The secretions from the glandular elements are extruded into the lumen of the alveoli (A) and ejected by the myoepithelial cells into the ductal system (D), which empties through the nipple. Arterial blood supply to the alveolus is identified by the upper right arrow and venous drainage by arrow beneath. **C.** Individual secretory cell. Two nucleoli are located within the nucleus (N). The endoplasmic reticulum (E) surrounds the nucleus. Mitochondria (M) are evident. Lactose granules (L) and fat droplets (F) migrate to the luminal margin of the cell and there are secreted by exocytosis into an alveolus (*arrow*). (Courtesy of Dr. John C. Porter.)

Uridine diphosphate (UDP) + glucose galactose → Lactose + UDP → Water osmotically drawn into Golgi vesicle → Discharge by exocytosis of contents of Golgi vesicle into lumen

Lactose synthetase

Galactosyl transferase ("A" protein)   α-Lactalbumin ("B" protein)   β-Lactoglobulin caseinogen

Protein aggregated within Golgi vesicles

Proteins synthesized in rough endoplasmic reticulum

Prolactin stimulates
Progesterone inhibits

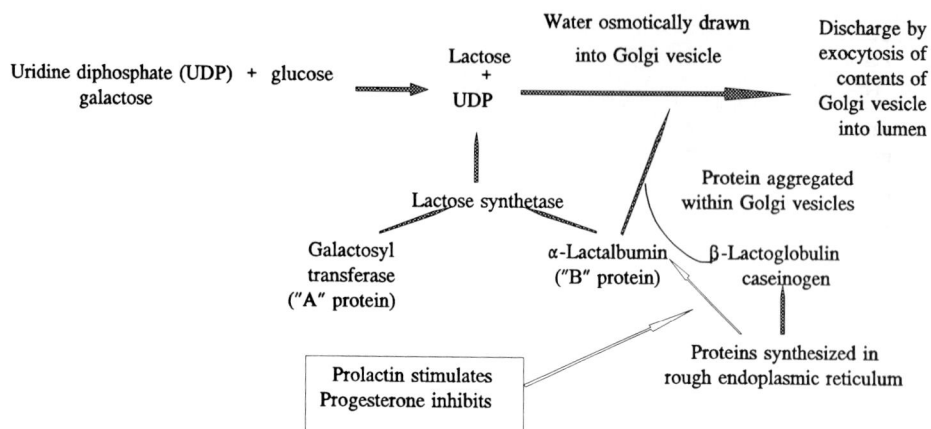

Fig. 18–4. Relation of protein, lactose, and water secretion on lactation. Note that progesterone inhibits production of α-lactalbumin and prolactin stimulates its production. (Courtesy of Dr. John C. Porter.)

be misinterpreted as glucosuria unless specific glucose oxidase is used in testing. Fatty acids are synthesized in the alveoli from glucose and are secreted by an apocrine-like process (Fig. 18–3A).

All vitamins except vitamin K are found in human milk, but in variable amounts (American Academy of Pediatrics, 1981), and maternal dietary supplementation increases the secretion of most of these. Because the mother does not provide the vitamin K requirements for breast-fed infants, vitamin K administration to the infant soon after delivery is required to prevent hemorrhagic disease of the newborn (Chap. 44, p. 1017).

Human milk contains a low iron concentration, but iron is better absorbed from human milk than it is from cow's milk. Maternal iron stores do not seem to influence the amount of iron in breast milk. Therefore, the use of supplemental iron-fortified infant formulas, or a weaning formula also fortified with iron (American Academy of Pediatrics, 1989b), is recommended. The use of such iron-fortified formulas apparently has eliminated iron-deficiency anemia during childhood (Hertrampf and co-workers, 1986; Vazquez-Seoane and colleagues, 1985; Yip and associates, 1987). Such iron-containing formulas are well tolerated by most infants (Nelson and associates, 1988), and there is no evidence that these formulas impair absorption of zinc or copper (Yip and colleagues, 1985).

Mennella and Beauchamp (1991) have recently documented what experienced nursing mothers have long known: breast-fed infants are aware of what their mothers eat and drink. They studied the infant effects of maternal ingestion of the ethanol equivalent of one can of beer prior to nursing. Such consumption caused the infants to suck more frequently during the first minute of feeding, but ultimately they consumed significantly less milk.

The mammary gland, like the thyroid gland, concentrates iodine and several other minerals including gallium, technetium, indium, and possibly sodium. Therefore, these radioactive minerals should not be

given to nursing women because they rapidly appear in breast milk. The American Academy of Pediatrics, Committee on Drugs (1989a) recommends consultation with a nuclear medicine physician before performing a diagnostic study, so that a radionuclide with the shortest excretion time in breast milk can be used. They further recommend that the mother pump her breasts before the study and store enough milk in a freezer for feeding the infant. After the study, she should pump her breasts to maintain milk production, but discard all milk produced during the time that radioactivity is present. This ranges from 15 hours up to 2 weeks, depending upon the isotope used.

The approximate concentrations of the more important components of human colostrum, mature human milk, and cow's milk are presented in Table 18–1. These concentrations may vary depending upon maternal diet and when studied in the puerperium (Brasil and co-workers, 1991; Giovannini and colleagues, 1991; Karra and colleagues, 1988; Ogunleye and associates, 1991).

Endocrinology of Lactation. The precise humoral and neural mechanisms involved in lactation are complex. Progesterone, estrogen, and placental lactogen, as well as prolactin, cortisol, and insulin, appear to act in concert to stimulate the growth and development of the milk-secreting apparatus of the mammary gland (Porter, 1974). With delivery, there is an abrupt and profound decrease in the levels of progesterone and estrogen, which removes the subcellular inhibitory influence of progesterone on production of α-lactalbumin by the rough endoplasmic reticulum (Fig. 18–4). The increased α-lactalbumin serves to stimulate lactose synthetase and ultimately an increase in milk lactose. Progesterone withdrawal also allows prolactin to act unopposed in its stimulation of α-lactalbumin production.

In otherwise normal circumstances, the intensity and duration of subsequent lactation are controlled, in

TABLE 18–1. COMPOSITION OF MATURE HUMAN MILK, COW'S MILK, AND A TYPICAL FORMULA USED FOR TERM INFANTS

Composition per 100 mL	Mature Breast Milk	Cow's Milk	Formula with Iron
Calories	75	69	67
Protein (g)	1.1	3.5	1.5
Lactalbumin (%)	80	18	60
Casein (%)	20	82	40
Water (mL)	87.1	87.3	90
Fat (g)	4.5	3.5	3.8
Carbohydrates	7.1	4.9	6.9
Ash (g)	0.21	0.72	0.34
Minerals (mg)			
Na	16	50	21
K	53	144	69
Ca	33	118	46
P	14	93	32
Mg	4	13	5.3
Fe	0.05	Trace	1.3
Zn	0.15	0.4	0.42
Vitamins			
A (IU)	182	140	210
C (mg)	5	1	5.3
D (IU)	2.2	42	42
E (IU)	0.18	0.04	0.83
Thiamine (mg)	0.01	0.03	0.04
Riboflavin (mg)	0.04	0.17	0.06
Niacin (mg)	0.2	0.1	0.7
pH	Alkaline	Acid	Acid
Bacterial content	Sterile	Nonsterile	Sterile

Modified from Avery and Fletcher (1987).

large part, by the repetitive stimulus of nursing. Prolactin is essential for lactation; women with extensive pituitary necrosis, as in Sheehan syndrome, do not lactate (Chap. 27, p. 617). Although plasma prolactin falls after delivery to lower levels than during pregnancy, each act of suckling triggers a rise in prolactin levels (McNeilly and associates, 1983). Presumably a stimulus from the breast curtails the release of prolactin-inhibiting factor from the hypothalamus; this, in turn, transiently induces increased prolactin secretion.

The neurohypophysis, in pulsatile fashion, secretes oxytocin, which stimulates milk expression from a lactating breast by causing contraction of myoepithelial cells in the alveoli and small milk ducts. In fact, this mechanism has been utilized to assay oxytocin activity in biological fluids. Milk ejection, or "letting down," is a reflex initiated especially by suckling, which stimulates the neurohypophysis to liberate oxytocin (McNeilly and associates, 1983). Milk ejection may be provoked even by the cry of the infant or inhibited by fright or stress.

In women who continue lactating but who resume ovulation, there are acute alterations in breast milk composition 5 to 6 days before and 6 to 7 days following ovulation (Hartmann and Prosser, 1984). These changes are abrupt and characterized by increased concentra-

tions of sodium and chloride, along with decreased potassium, lactose, and glucose concentrations. In women who become pregnant but who continue to breast feed, milk composition undergoes progressive alterations suggesting gradual loss of metabolic and secretory breast activity (Hartmann and Prosser, 1984).

Immunological Consequences of Breast Feeding.
Antibodies are present in human colostrum and milk but are poorly absorbed, if at all, from the infant's gut. Indeed, no anti-D antibodies have been detected in the sera of infants fed milk containing a high titer of anti-D antibodies. This circumstance, however, does not lessen the importance of at least some of the antibodies in breast milk. The predominant immunoglobulin in milk is secretory IgA, a macromolecule that is important in antimicrobial processes in mucous membranes across which it is secreted. In this context, it is envisioned that secretory IgA contained in breast milk may act locally within the infant's gastrointestinal tract. For example, milk contains secretory IgA antibodies against *Escherichia coli* (Cravioto and associates, 1991), and it is known that breast-fed babies are less prone to enteric infections than are bottle-fed babies. It has been suggested that IgA exerts its action by preventing bacterial adherence to epithelial cells surfaces, thus preventing tissue invasion (Cravioto and colleagues, 1991; Samra and associates, 1991).

Much attention has been directed to an elucidation of the role of maternal breast milk lymphocytes in fetal immunological processes. Human milk contains both T and B lymphocytes, but milk T lymphocytes appear to differ from those found in blood. Specifically, milk T lymphocytes are almost exclusively composed of cells that exhibit specific membrane antigens including the LFA-1 high memory T-cell phenotype. These memory T cells appear to be another mechanism by which the neonate benefits from maternal immunological experience (Bertotto and associates, 1990). Lymphocytes in colostrum undergo blastoid transformation in vitro following exposure to specific antigens. In experimental animals, Beer and Billingham (1976) observed a transmission of viable lymphocytes from mother to infant through breast milk. As mentioned above, interleukin-6 is present in colostrum and appears to stimulate an increase in mononuclear cells in breast milk (Saito and co-workers, 1991). The amounts of protective factors in human milk appear to vary appreciably, being much richer in the milk of young women compared to that of older women (Whitehead, 1983), and present in higher quantities in colostrum.

Nursing.
The ideal food for neonates is mother's milk. Human lactation has an average efficiency of 95 percent (Frigerio and associates, 1991). Moreover, breast-fed preterm infants evaluated at 1½ and 7½ years of age

compared with similar preterm infants not given breast milk had higher intelligence quotient (IQ) scores (Lucas and colleagues, 1992). Appropriately, the frequency of breast feeding has increased considerably in recent years. In one recent survey in the United States, nearly two thirds of women were breast feeding their 1-week-old infants, compared with less than one third 25 years before.

In most instances, even though the supply of milk at first appears insufficient, it becomes adequate if suckling is continued. Nursing also accelerates uterine involution because repeated stimulation of the nipples releases oxytocin, which contracts uterine muscle. There are known lactation inhibitors. For example, oral contraceptives decrease the volume of milk production. They are not contraindicated in lactating women, but they should not be started until lactation is well established (American Academy of Pediatrics and American College of Obstetricians and Gynecologists, 1992). The progestin-only contraceptive ("minipill") may be the agent of choice, because there is evidence that it has minimal effects on milk production, neonatal growth, and early development (Fraser, 1991). It must be noted that while progesterone in high doses will suppress lactation (see p. 464), progestins have less of an effect. Newer contraceptive progestin-only compounds include the time-release levonorgestrel implant (Norplant) and the vaginal ring, which releases 10 mg of progesterone per 24 hours. Neither device appears to impair successful lactation (Shaaban, 1991). Smoking significantly reduces breast milk volume and decreases infant growth rates (Vio and associates, 1991).

Nursing is contraindicated in women with known cytomegalovirus, chronic hepatitis B, and human immunodeficiency virus infection (American Academy of Pediatrics and American College of Obstetricians and Gynecologists, 1992). Cytomegalovirus and hepatitis B virus are excreted in milk, and even with passive and active neonatal immunization against hepatitis B, breast feeding is unjustifiable. The actual risk of human immunodeficiency virus transmission through breast milk is unknown, but for now, infected women are advised against breast feeding. Women with active herpes simplex virus may suckle their infants if there are no breast lesions, and particular care is directed to hand washing before nursing.

Care of the Breasts and Nipples. Decisions about breast feeding determine appropriate breast care. In addition to promoting maternal–infant interaction, breast feeding alone can satisfy the infant's nutritional needs for the first 4 to 6 months of life. As noted earlier, in a recent survey in the United States carried out by a manufacturer of infant formula, nearly two thirds of women were breast feeding their 1-week-old infants, compared with less than one third 25 years before.

The nipples require little attention in the puerperium other than cleanliness and attention to fissures. Because dried milk is likely to accumulate and irritate the nipples, cleaning of the areola with water and mild soap is helpful before and after nursing. Occasionally, with irritated nipples, it is necessary to use a nipple shield for 24 hours or longer. Inverted or retracted nipples may be troublesome; however, these can usually be teased out by gently pulling with the finger and thumb. This is best done during pregnancy to prepare the nipples for subsequent nursing.

The woman who does not desire to breast feed should be reassured that stopping milk production is not a major problem. During the stage of engorgement, the breasts become painful and should be supported with a well-fitting brassiere. Ice packs and oral analgesics for 12 to 24 hours may be required to relieve discomfort. Breast binders, rather than hormonal suppression of lactation, are routinely used at Parkland Hospital in women not desiring to nurse their infant. Indeed, the Food and Drug Administration has removed painful postpartum breast engorgement as an indication for the use of bromocriptine and sex hormones (American College of Obstetricians and Gynecologists, 1990).

Drugs Secreted in Milk. Most drugs given to the mother are secreted in breast milk. Many factors influence their excretion, including the concentration of drugs in plasma, degree of protein binding of the drug, plasma and milk pH, degree of ionization, lipid solubility, and molecular weight. Drugs are usually secreted into milk in concentrations no higher than in maternal plasma. Consequently, the amount of drug ingested by the infant is typically small.

The Committee on Drugs of the American Academy of Pediatrics (1989a) has provided an extensive list of drugs and other chemicals that are transferred into breast milk. The committee acknowledges that only those drugs that have been reported to have, or possibly to have, adverse effects on lactation or the infant are included in the report. Contraindicated drugs are listed in Table 18–2. Drugs are further divided into (1) drugs of abuse that are contraindicated—amphetamines, cocaine, heroin, marijuana, nicotine, and phencyclidine; (2) radiopharmaceuticals that require temporary cessation of breast feeding—[67]gallium, [111]indium, [125]iodine, [131]iodine, radioactive sodium, and [99]technetium; (3) drugs whose effect on nursing infants is unknown but may be of concern—psychotropic drugs, antianxiety drugs, antidepressants, antipsychotics, chloramphenicol, metoclopramide, metronidazole, and tinidazole; and (4) drugs that have caused significant effects on some nursing infants and should be given to nursing mothers with caution (too numerous to list). If drugs in this last category are prescribed, the committee recommended that, if possible, blood concentrations of the drug be measured in the infant.

TABLE 18–2. DRUGS AND CHEMICALS CONTRAINDICATED DURING BREAST FEEDING

Drug		Sign or Symptom in Infant
Generic Name	Trade Name	or Effect on Lactation
Bromocriptine	Parlodel	Suppresses lactation
Cocaine	—	Cocaine intoxication
Cyclophosphamide	Cytoxan or Neosar	Possible immune suppression; unknown effect on growth or association with carcinogenesis
Doxorubicin[a]	Adriamycin	Same as cyclophosphamide
Ergotamine	Cafergot (ergotamine tartrate with caffeine)	Vomiting, diarrhea, convulsions (doses used in migraine medications)
Lithium	Lithobid or Cibalith	⅓ to ½ therapeutic blood concentration in infants
Methotrexate	Folex or Mexate	Possible immune suppression; unknown effect on growth or association with carincogenesis; neutropenia
Phencyclidine (PCP)	—	Patient hallucinogen
Phenidione (not available in USA)	Hedulin or Eridione	Anticoagulant; increased prothrombin and partial thromboplastin time in one infant

[a] Drug concentrated in human milk.
Modified from the American Academy of Pediatrics: Committee on Drugs (1989a).

Clinical and Physiological Aspects of the Puerperium

Temperature. Engorgement of the breasts with milk, which is common on the third or fourth day of the puerperium, was once thought to cause a rise in temperature. This so-called *milk fever* was regarded as physiological. Extreme vascular and lymphatic engorgement may result in fever, but it does not last more than 24 hours (see Chap. 29, p. 646). **Any fever in the puerperium implies an infection—most likely somewhere in the genitourinary tract—until otherwise proven.**

Afterpains. In primiparas the puerperal uterus tends to remain tonically contracted. If blood clots, placental fragments, or other foreign bodies are retained, hypertonic contractions may result as the uterus contracts in an effort to expel them. Particularly in multiparas, the uterus often contracts vigorously at intervals, giving rise to "afterpains." Occasionally these pains are severe enough to require an analgesic; and in some women, they may last for several days. Afterpains are noticeable particularly when the infant suckles, likely because of oxytocin release. Usually, they decrease in intensity and become mild by the third postpartum day.

Lochia. Early in the puerperium, sloughing of decidual tissue results in a vaginal discharge of variable quantity; this is termed *lochia*. Microscopically, lochia consists of erythrocytes, shreds of decidua, epithelial cells, and bacteria. Microorganisms are found in lochia pooled in the vagina and are present in most cases even when the discharge has been obtained from the uterine cavity.

For the first few days after delivery, blood in the lochia is sufficient to color it red, or *lochia rubra*. After 3 or 4 days, lochia becomes progressively paler, or *lo-chia serosa*. After the 10th day, because of an admixture of leukocytes and a reduced fluid content, lochia assumes a white or yellowish-white color, or *lochia alba*. Foul-smelling lochia is suggestive of infection, but such an odor is not diagnostic.

In some centers, it is routine to prescribe an oxytocic agent to hasten uterine involution by promoting uterine contractility. This also presumably diminishes bleeding complications. Adams and Flowers (1960) reported, however, that routine use of oral methylergonovine (Methergine) was unwarranted. Newton and Bradford (1961) similarly concluded that after the period immediately following delivery, routine administration of intramuscular oxytocin to normal women was of no value in decreasing blood loss or hastening uterine involution.

A reddish color in lochia may be maintained for a longer period. When this persists for more than 2 weeks, however, it is indicative of retention of small portions of placenta, imperfect involution of the placental site, or both.

Urine. Diuresis regularly occurs between the second and fifth days, even when intravenous fluids were not infused vigorously during labor and delivery. Normal pregnancy is associated with an appreciable increase in extracellular water, and puerperal diuresis is a physiological reversal of this process. The fluid-retaining stimuli of pregnancy-induced hyperestrogenism and elevated venous pressure in the lower half of the body dissipate after delivery, and residual hypervolemia is lost. In preeclampsia, both retention of fluid antepartum and diuresis postpartum may be greatly increased (Chap. 36, p. 798).

Occasionally, substantial amounts of sugar may be found in urine during the first week of the puerperium. The sugar most likely is lactose, which is not detected by test systems using glucose oxidase. After a long labor, acetonuria also may be identified as a consequence of starvation.

Blood. Rather marked leukocytosis occurs during and after labor, the leukocyte count sometimes reaching 30,000 per μL (see Chap. 8, p. 224). The increase is predominantly granulocytes. There also is a relative lymphopenia and an absolute eosinopenia.

Normally, during the first few postpartum days, hemoglobin, hematocrit, and erythrocyte counts fluctuate moderately. If they fall much below the levels present just prior to labor, a considerable amount of blood has been lost (Chap. 37, p. 819). By 1 week after delivery, the blood volume has returned to near its nonpregnant level. Robson and colleagues (1987) showed that cardiac output remains elevated for at least 48 hours postpartum. Most likely, this is due to increased stroke volume from venous return, because the heart rate falls at the same time. By 2 weeks, these changes have returned to normal nonpregnant values.

Pregnancy-induced changes in blood coagulation factors persist for variable periods during the puerperium. Elevation of plasma fibrinogen is maintained at least through the first week, and as a consequence, the elevated sedimentation rate normally found during pregnancy remains high.

Weight Loss. In addition to the loss of about 5 to 6 kg due to uterine evacuation and normal blood loss, there is usually a further decrease of 2 to 3 kg through diuresis. Chesley and co-workers (1959) demonstrated a decrease in sodium space of about 2 L, or 2 kg during the first week postpartum.

According to Schauberger and co-investigators (1992), an almost universal desire expressed by postpartum women is to lose weight and to get back into shape. They found that most women approach their self-reported prepregnancy weight 6 months after delivery but still retain an average surplus of 1.4 kg (3 lbs). Factors that increased puerperal weight loss included weight gain during the pregnancy, primiparity, early return to work outside the home, and smoking. Breast feeding, age, or marital status did not affect weight loss. Greene and colleagues (1988) analyzed data from the collaborative perinatal study, and found that prenatal weight gain in excess of 20 lbs was associated with postpartum weight retention.

Care of the Mother During the Puerperium

Attention Immediately After Labor. For the first hour after delivery, maternal blood pressure and pulse should be taken every 15 minutes, or more frequently if indicated. The amount of vaginal bleeding should be noted, and the uterine fundus should be palpated to ensure that it is well contracted. After delivery of the placenta, the uterus should be firm, with its upper margin just below the umbilicus. As long as it remains in this condition, there is little danger of postpartum hemorrhage from *uterine atony*. If relaxation is detected, the uterus should be massaged through the abdominal wall until it remains contracted. Blood may accumulate within the uterus without external evidence of bleeding. This condition may be detected early by identifying uterine enlargement through frequent fundal palpation during the first few hours postpartum. Because the likelihood of significant hemorrhage is greatest immediately postpartum, even in normal cases, a trained attendant should remain with the mother for at least 1 hour after completion of the third stage of labor.

Following regional analgesia or general anesthesia, the mother should be observed in an appropriately equipped and staffed recovery area (see Chap. 16, p. 425). This area should include complete cardiopulmonary resuscitation equipment and a staff trained to operate it.

Early Ambulation. Immediately after World War II, early ambulation became an accepted puerperal practice. Women are now out of bed within a few hours after delivery. The many advantages of early ambulation are confirmed by numerous well-controlled studies. Women state that they feel better and stronger after early ambulation. Bladder complications and constipation are less frequent. Importantly, early ambulation has also reduced the frequency of puerperal venous thrombosis and pulmonary embolism (see Chap. 49, p. 1111). For the first ambulation at least, an attendant should be present to help prevent injury if the woman should become syncopal.

Care of the Vulva. The patient should be taught to cleanse the vulva from anterior to posterior (vulva toward anus). An ice bag applied to the perineum may help reduce edema and discomfort during the first several hours after episiotomy repair. Beginning about 24 hours after delivery, moist heat as provided with warm sitz baths can be used to reduce local discomfort. The interdiction of tub bathing after uncomplicated delivery is without foundation.

Bladder Function. Bladder filling after delivery may be quite variable. In most hospitals, intravenous fluids are infused during labor and for an hour after delivery. Oxytocin, in doses that have an antidiuretic effect, is commonly infused after the third stage of labor. As a consequence of infused fluid and the sudden withdrawal of the antidiuretic effect of oxytocin, rapid bladder filling is common. Moreover, both bladder sensation and the capability of the bladder to empty spontaneously may be diminished by anesthesia, especially conduction analgesia, as well as by painful lesions in the genital tract, such as extensive episiotomy, lacerations, or hematomas. It is not surprising, therefore, that urinary retention with bladder overdistention is a common complication of the early puerperium. Once overdistention occurs, bladder function becomes further impaired, and ascending infection of the urinary tract is a likely consequence.

Prevention of overdistention demands close observation after delivery to ensure that the bladder does not overfill and that with each voiding it empties adequately. The bladder may be palpated as a cystic mass suprapubically, or the enlarged bladder may be evident abdominally only indirectly as a consequence of elevating the uterine fundus above the umbilicus.

If the woman has not voided within 4 hours after delivery, it is likely she cannot. Ambulation to a toilet usually should be tried before resorting to catheterization. The woman who has trouble voiding initially is likely to have further trouble. At times, an indwelling catheter is necessary, as described in Chapter 29 (p. 645). The likelihood of hematomas of the genital tract must be considered when the woman cannot void postpartum. Whenever the bladder becomes overdistended, an indwelling catheter should be left in place until the factors causing the retention have abated. Harris and colleagues (1977) reported that 40 percent of such women will develop bacteriuria; thus, a short course of antimicrobial therapy seems reasonable after catheter removal.

Bowel Function. At times, the lack of a bowel movement is no more than the expected consequence of an efficient cleansing enema administered before delivery. With both early ambulation and early feeding of a general diet, constipation has become much less of a problem in the puerperium. Routine prescription of a stool softener is a common practice.

Subsequent Discomfort. The discomfort from cesarean delivery, its causes, and its management are considered in Chapter 26 (p. 607). During the first few days after vaginal delivery, the mother may be uncomfortable for a variety of reasons, including afterpains, episiotomy and lacerations, breast engorgement, and at times, postspinal puncture headache. It is prudent to provide codeine, 60 mg; aspirin, 600 mg; or acetaminophen, 500 mg; at intervals as frequent as every 3 hours during the first few days after delivery. Uterine contractions are commonly accentuated during nursing, giving rise at times to troublesome afterpains.

An episiotomy or lacerations may be uncomfortable, as discussed in Chapter 14 (p. 389). Early application of an ice bag to the perineum may minimize swelling and discomfort. The majority of women also appear to obtain a measure of relief from the periodic application of a local anesthetic spray on the site of episiotomy or laceration. Severe discomfort may mean that a sizable hematoma has formed in the genital tract. Therefore, careful examination is warranted, especially whenever ordinary orally ingested analgesics do not provide relief. The episiotomy incision normally is firmly healed and nearly asymptomatic by the third week after delivery.

Mild Depression. There is strong tradition in the psychiatric literature to consider *postpartum depression* a distinct diagnosis. However, and according to Whiffen (1991), the empirical evidence indicates that, in terms of etiology and relapse rates, postpartum depression is indistinguishable from depression at any other time. Symptomatically, postpartum "depression" seems to involve a milder disturbance suggesting that it is best seen as an adjustment disorder. The concept that depression surfaces only during the puerperium is likely incorrect. Gotlib and co-workers (1989) examined the prevalence of depression in a heterogenous sample of 360 pregnant women. Approximately 10 percent of the women met diagnostic criteria for depression during pregnancy and 7 percent were depressed postpartum. However, only half of the cases of postpartum depression were new onset, indicating that many women who were depressed during the puerperium also were depressed during pregnancy.

It is fairly common for a mother to exhibit some degree of depression a few days after delivery. The transient depression, or *postpartum blues*, most likely is the consequence of a number of factors. Prominent in its genesis are (1) the emotional letdown that follows the excitement and fears that most women experience during pregnancy and delivery, (2) the discomforts of the early puerperium that have been described above, (3) fatigue from loss of sleep during labor and postpartum in most hospital settings, (4) anxiety over her capabilities for caring for her infant after leaving the hospital, and (5) fears that she has become less attractive to her husband. In the great majority of cases, effective treatment need be nothing more than anticipation, recognition, and reassurance.

As stressed by Robinson and Stewart (1986), this mild disorder is self-limited and usually remits after 2 to 3 days, although it sometimes persists for up to 10 days. Should postpartum blues persist, or worsen, then careful attention is given to searching for symptoms of psychotic depression, which requires prompt consultation (Chap. 55, p. 1254). Women particularly susceptible to more severe depression are those with unwanted pregnancies or those with major marital difficulties. Watson and co-workers (1984) reported that 12 percent of women developed clinically relevant depressive disorders by 6 weeks after delivery; however, in 90 percent of these individuals, situational aspects or long-standing problems had important etiological roles.

Abdominal Wall Relaxation. An abdominal binder is unnecessary. It does not help restore the mother's figure. If the abdomen is unusually flabby or pendulous, an ordinary girdle is often more satisfactory than an abdominal binder. Exercises to restore abdominal wall tone may be started any time after vaginal delivery and as soon as abdominal soreness diminishes after cesarean delivery.

Diet. There are no dietary restrictions for women who have been delivered vaginally. An appetizing general diet is recommended. Two hours after a normal vaginal delivery, if there are no complications likely to necessitate an anesthetic, the woman should be given something to drink and eat if she desires. The diet of lactating women, compared with that consumed during pregnancy, should be increased in calories and protein, as recommended by the Food and Nutrition Board of the National Research Council (Table 9–2, p. 256). If the mother does not breast feed her infant, her dietary requirements are the same as for a normal nonpregnant woman.

It is standard practice in our hospital to continue iron supplementation for at least 3 months after delivery. The hematocrit also is checked at the first postpartum visit, which is scheduled during the third week of the puerperium.

Immunizations. The D-negative woman who is not isoimmunized and whose baby is D-positive is given 300 μg of anti-D immune globulin shortly after delivery (see Chap. 44, p. 1008). Women who are not already immune to rubella are excellent candidates for vaccination before discharge (Chap. 9, p. 250). Unless it is contraindicated, we administer a diphtheria-tetanus toxoid booster injection at this time. Beginning in 1991, women delivered at Parkland Hospital have been given measles (rubeola) immunization prior to postpartum discharge. This recommendation is based upon (1) the failure of previously immunized persons to develop protective immunity (Centers for Disease Control, 1989), (2) significant outbreaks of measles in the community, and (3) maternal morbidity and mortality due to measles pneumonitis.

Time of Discharge. Following vaginal delivery, if there are no puerperal complications, hospitalization is seldom warranted for more than 48 hours, excluding the day of delivery. Following an uncomplicated postoperative cesarean delivery, women usually are ready for discharge on the third or fourth day.

Before discharge, the woman should receive instructions concerning the anticipated normal physiological changes of the puerperium, including changes in lochia patterns, weight loss due to diuresis, and when to expect milk let down. She also should receive instructions concerning what to do if she becomes febrile, has excessive vaginal bleeding, or develops leg pain, swelling, or tenderness. Any shortness of breath or chest pains should warrant her immediate concern and prompt contact with her health-care provider.

Early Discharge. Because of prohibitive hospital costs, many women request discharge after a 1-day stay. This is acceptable as long as the mother has had an uncomplicated antepartum course and a normal vaginal delivery. All laboratory values must be checked and appropriately managed. Other procedures, education, and immunization are handled as outlined above.

Contraception. During the postpartum hospital stay, a concerted effort should be made to provide family planning education. Steroidal contraception and its effects on lactation are discussed on p. 466. Other forms of contraception are discussed in Section XIV.

Coitus. There is no definite time after delivery when coitus should be resumed; however, hemorrhage and infection are less likely 14 to 21 days postpartum. Resumption of intercourse this soon may prove to be unpleasant, if not frankly painful, due to incomplete uterine involution and incomplete healing of the episiotomy and lacerations.

The best rule to follow is one of common sense. Specifically, coitus should not be resumed prior to 2 weeks postpartum for the reasons listed above. After 2 weeks, coitus may be resumed *based upon the patient's desire and comfort.* Robson and Kumar (1981) longitudinally interviewed 119 nulliparous women throughout pregnancy and for 1 year postpartum to determine aspects of sexuality. They reported that the diminished sexual activity and enjoyment from intercourse seen in late pregnancy may persist for at least a year after delivery. Only 35 percent of women resumed intercourse by 6 weeks, and at 3 months, 40 percent of those having intercourse reported pain and discomfort. The patient should be advised that breast feeding will cause a prolonged period of suppressed estrogen production with a resulting vaginal atrophy and dryness. Such a physiological state results in decreased vaginal lubrication during sexual arousal. Therefore, a vaginal lubricant likely should be used by lactating women prior to coitus.

Infant Follow-up. Special arrangements must be made to insure that the neonate receives appropriate follow-up care. The neonate discharged early should be term, normal, and have stable vital signs. All laboratory studies should be normal including direct Coombs test, bilirubin, hemoglobin and hematocrit, and blood glucose. The maternal serological test for syphilis and hepatitis B surface antigen should be nonreactive. Initial hepatitis B vaccine should be administered, and all screening tests required by law should be performed. These always include testing for phenylketonuria (PKU) and hypothyroidism. If subsequent phenylketonuria retesting is required after the neonate has consumed milk, the mother must be so instructed. Finally, the importance of subsequent neonatal and well-baby care should be stressed and an emphasis placed on infant immunizations.

Return of Menstruation and Ovulation. If the woman does not nurse her child, menses usually return within 6 to 8 weeks. At times, however, it is difficult clinically to assign a specific date to the first menstrual period after delivery. A minority of women bleed small to moderate amounts intermittently, starting soon after delivery. Menses may not appear so long as the infant is nursed, but great variations are observed; in lactating women the first period may occur as early as the second or as late as the 18th month after delivery.

Sharman (1966), by means of histological dating of the endometrium, identified ovulation as early as 42 days after delivery; Perez and associates (1972) did so as early as 36 days. Moreover, a corpus luteum has been observed 6 weeks after delivery at the time of sterilization. Thus, the necessity for avoiding delay in instituting contraceptive techniques for sexually active women is obvious.

Ovulation is much less frequent in women who breast feed compared to those who do not. Nonetheless, pregnancy can occur with lactation. Hefnawi and Badraoui (1977) studied 340 lactating Egyptian women who used no contraception after delivery; one fourth had conceived again within 12 months. Of those who became pregnant, one fourth had not menstruated since delivery. Onset of menses increased from 8 percent the first month after delivery to 61 percent by 12 months. Among those who menstruated, ovulation—identified by examinations of cervical mucus and endometrial biopsies—increased from 3 percent at 1 month to 60 percent at 12 months.

It is generally believed that amenorrhea during lactation is due to a lack of appropriate ovarian stimulation by pituitary gonadotropins. This concept is consistent with the data illustrated in Figure 18–5. The levels of luteinizing hormone (LH) and follicle-stimulating hormone (FSH) in this carefully studied lactating woman were appreciably lower during the time of amenorrhea than they were after resumption of menstruation. Bonnar and co-workers (1975) reported that in some breast-feeding women, plasma estrogens did not increase despite a rise in FSH. The lack of response was attributed to an inhibitory effect of the increased prolactin levels on follicular development.

Follow-up Care. By the time of discharge, women who had a normal delivery and puerperium can resume most

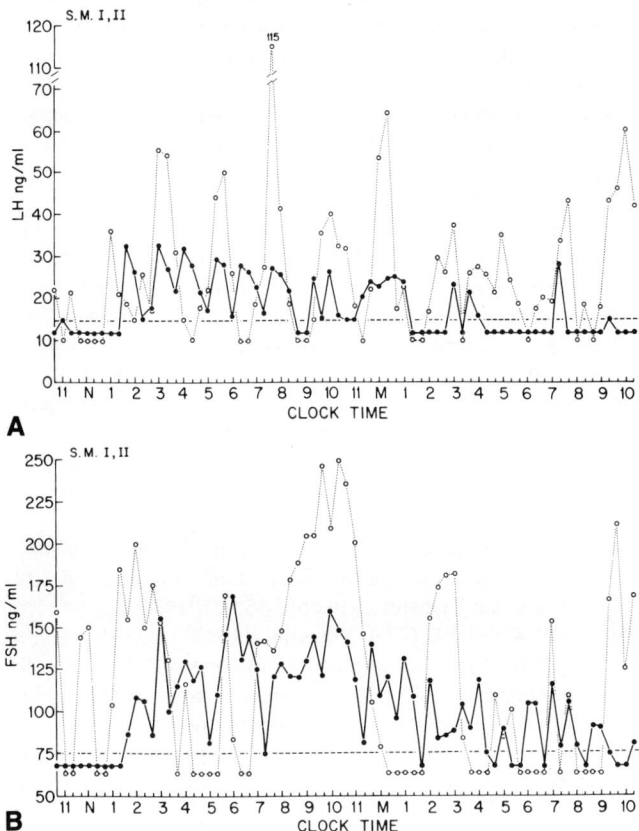

Fig. 18–5. A. Comparison of the 24-hour secretory patterns of LH in the lactating woman. The closed circles denote plasma LH levels during the period of amenorrhea. The open circles correspond to the plasma LH concentrations after menses had resumed. B. Comparison of the 24-hour secretory patterns of FSH in the lactating woman. The closed circles denote plasma FSH levels during the period of amenorrhea. The open circles correspond to the plasma FSH concentrations after menses had resumed. (From Madden and co-workers, 1978.)

activities, including bathing, driving, and household functions. Although it has been customary for some obstetricians to recommend that patients not resume employment or return to school for several weeks, there is no evidence that to do so earlier causes any physical harm. Jimenez and Newton (1979) tabulated cross-cultural information on 202 societies from different geographic regions of the world. Postnatally, most societies did not restrict maternal work activity, and about half expected a return to full duties within 2 weeks. Tulman and Fawcett (1988) reported, however, that only half of women had regained their usual level of energy by 6 weeks postpartum. Women who delivered vaginally were twice as likely to have normal energy levels at this time compared with those who had cesarean deliveries. Ideally, the care and nurturing received by the neonate should be provided by the mother with ample help from the father. For the mother to provide this care, her presence at home with the infant precludes her early return to full-time work or school.

Since 1969, puerperal women at our hospital have been given appointments for follow-up examination during the third postpartum week. This has proven quite satisfactory both to identify any abnormalities of the later puerperium as well as to initiate contraceptive practices. Estrogen plus progestin oral contraceptives started at this time have proven to be effective without increased morbidity. Moreover, the frequencies of uterine perforation, expulsions, and pregnancies when intrauterine devices were inserted during the third week postpartum were no greater than when the devices were inserted 3 months or more postpartum. Family planning techniques and follow-up care are further discussed in Section XIV (Chaps. 60 to 62).

References

Adams H, Flowers CE: Oral oxytocic drugs in the puerperium. Obstet Gynecol 15:280, 1960

American Academy of Pediatrics, Committee on drugs: Transfer of drugs and other chemicals into human milk. Pediatrics 84:924, 1989a

American Academy of Pediatrics, Committee on nutrition: Follow-up or weaning formulas. Pediatrics 83:1067, 1989b

American Academy of Pediatrics, Committee on nutrition: Nutrition and lactation. Pediatrics 68:435, 1981

American Academy of Pediatrics and American College of Obstetricians and Gynecologists: Guidelines for perinatal care, 3rd ed. 1992, p 183

American College of Obstetricians and Gynecologists, Newsletter, April 1990, p 8

Anderson WR, Davis J: Placental site involution. Am J Obstet Gynecol 102:23, 1968

Andrews MC: Epithelial changes in the puerperal fallopian tube. Am J Obstet Gynecol 62:28, 1951

Avery GB, Fletcher AB: Nutrition. In Avery GB (ed): Neonatology, Pathophysiology and Management of the Newborn, 3rd ed. Philadelphia, Lippincott, 1987, p 1192

Beer AE, Billingham RE: The immunobiology of mammalian reproduction. Englewood Cliffs, NJ, Prentice-Hall, 1976, p 198

Bertotto A, Gerli R, Gabietti G, Crupi S, Arcangeli C, Scalis F, Vaccaro R: Human breast milk T lymphocytes display the phenotype and functional characteristics of memory T cells. Eur J Immunol 20:1877, 1990

Bonnar J, Franklin M, Nott PN, McNeilly AS: Effect of breast-feeding on pituitary–ovarian function after childbirth. Br Med J 4:82, 1975

Brasil AL, Vitolo MR, Lopez FA, De Nobrega FJ: Fat and protein composition of mature milk in adolescents. J Adolesc Health 12:365, 1991

Centers for Disease Control: Measles prevention: Recommendations of the Immunization Practice Advisory Committee. MMWR 38(suppl 9):1, 1989

Chesley LC, Valenti C, Uichano L: Alterations in body fluid compartments and exchangeable sodium in early puerperium. Am J Obstet Gynecol 77:1054, 1959

Cravioto A, Tello A, Villafan H, Ruiz J, del Vedovo S, Neeser JR: Inhibition of localized adhesion of enteropathogenic Escherichia coli to HEp-2 cells by immunoglobulin and oligosaccharide fractions of human colostrum and breast milk. J Infect Dis 163:1247, 1991

Fraser IS: A review of the use of progestogen-only minipills for contraception during lactation. Reprod Fertil Dev 3:245, 1991

Frigerio C, Schutz Y, Prentice A, Whitehead R, Jequier E: Is human lactation a particularly efficient process? Eur J Clin Nutr 45:459, 1991

Giovannini M, Agostoni C, Salari PC: The role of lipids in nutrition during the first months of life. J Int Med Res 19:351, 1991

Gotlib IH, Whiffen VE, Mount JH, Milne K, Cordy NI: Prevalence rates and demographic characteristics associated with depression in pregnancy and the postpartum. J Consult Clin Psychol 57:269, 1989

Greene GW, Smiciklas-Wright H, Scholl TO, Karp RJ: Postpartum weight change: How much of the weight gained in pregnancy will be lost after delivery? Obstet Gynecol 71:701, 1988

Harris RE, Thomas VL, Jui GW: Postpartum surveillance for urinary tract infection: Patients at risk of developing pyelonephritis after catheterization. South Med J 70:1273, 1977

Hartmann PE, Prosser CG: Physiological basis of longitudinal changes in human milk yield and composition. Fed Proc 43:2448, 1984

Hefnawi F, Badraoui MHH: The benefits of lactation amenorrhea as a contraceptive. Fertil Steril 28:320, 1977

Hertrampf E, Cayazzo M, Pizarro F, Stekel A: Bioavailability of iron in soy-based formula and its effect on iron nutriture in infancy. Pediatrics 78:640, 1986

Jimenez MH, Newton N: Activity and work during pregnancy and the postpartum period: A cross-cultural study of 202 societies. Am J Obstet Gynecol 135:171, 1979

Karra MV, Kirksey A, Galal O, Bassily NS, Harrison GG, Jerome NW: Zinc, calcium, and magnesium concentrations in milk from American and Egyptian women throughout the first 6 months of lactation. Am J Clin Nutr 47:642, 1988

Kerr-Wilson RJH, Thompson SW, Orr JW, Davis RO, Cloud GA: Effect of labor on the postpartum bladder. Obstet Gynecol 64:115, 1984

Koch Y, Werner H, Fridkin M: Hypothalamic hormones in milk, Endocr Regul 25:128, 1991

Koldovsky O, Britton J, Grimes J, Schaudies P: Milk-borne epidermal growth factor (EGF) and its processing in developing gastrointestinal tract. Endocr Regul 25:58, 1991

Lucas A, Morley R, Cole TJ, Lister G, Leeson-Payne C: Breast milk and subsequent intelligence quotient in children born preterm. Lancet 339:261, 1992

Madden JD, Boyar R, MacDonald PC, Porter JC: Analysis of secretory patterns of prolactin and gonadotropins during twenty-four hours in a lactating woman before and after resumption of menses. Am J Obstet Gynecol 132:436, 1978

McCleary MJ: Epidermal growth factor: An important constituent of human milk. J Human Lactation 7:123, 1991

McNeilly AS, Robinson ICA, Houston MJ, Howie PW: Release of oxytocin and prolactin in response to suckling. Br Med J 286:257, 1983

Mennella JA, Beauchamp GK: The transfer of alcohol to human milk. N Engl J Med 325:981, 1991

Nelson SE, Ziegler EE, Copeland AM, Edwards BB, Fomon SJ: Lack of adverse reactions to iron-fortified formula. Pediatrics 81:360, 1988

Newton M, Bradford WM: Postpartal blood loss. Obstet Gynecol 17:229, 1961

Ogunleye A, Fakoya AT, Niizeki S, Tojo H, Sasajima I, Kobayashi M, Tateishi S, Yamaguchi K: Fatty acid composition of breast milk from Nigerian and Japanese women. J Nutr Sci Vitaminol 37:435, 1991

Perez A, Vela P, Masnic GS, Potter RG: First ovulation after childbirth: The effect of breastfeeding. Am J Obstet Gynecol 114:1041, 1972

Porter JC: Hormonal regulation of breast development and activity. J Invest Dermatol 63:85, 1974

Robinson GE, Stewart DE: Postpartum psychiatric disorders. Can Med Assoc J 134:31, 1986

Robson KM, Kumar R: Maternal sexuality during first pregnancy and after childbirth. Br J Obstet Gynecol 88:882, 1981

Robson SC, Dunlop W, Hunter S: Haemodynamic changes during the early puerperium. Br Med J 294:1065, 1987

Saito S, Maruyama M, Kato Y, Moriyama I, Ichijo M: Detection of IL-6 in human milk and its involvement in IgA production. J Reprod Immunol 20:267, 1991

Samra HK, Ganguly NK, Mahajan RC: Human milk containing specific secretory IgA inhibits binding of *Giardia lamblia* to nylon and glass surfaces. J Diarrhoeal Dis Res 9:100, 1991

Schauberger CW, Rooney BL, Brimer LM: Factors that influence weight loss in the puerperium. Obstet Gynecol 79:424, 1992

Shaaban MM: Contraception with progestogens and progesterone during lactation. J Steroid Biochem Mol Biol 40:705, 1991

Sharman A: Ovulation in the post-partum period. Excerpta Medica International Congress Series, no. 133, 1966, p 158

Sharman A: Postpartum regeneration of the human endometrium. J Anat 87:1, 1953

Tulman L, Fawcett J: Return of functional ability after childbirth. Nurs Res 37:77, 1988

Vazquez-Seoane P, Windom R, Pearson HA: Disappearance of iron deficiency anemia in a high-risk infant population given supplemental iron. N Engl J Med 313:1239, 1985

Viktrup L, Lose G, Rolff M, Barfoed K: The symptoms of stress incontinence caused by pregnancy or delivery in primipara. Obstet Gynecol 79:945, 1992

Vio F, Salazar G, Infante C: Smoking during pregnancy and lactation and its effects on breast-milk volume. Am J Clin Nutr 54:1011, 1991

Watson JP, Elliott SA, Rugg AJ, Brough DI: Psychiatric disorders in pregnancy and the first postnatal year. Br J Psychol 144:453, 1984

Weil A, Reyes H, Rottenberg RD, Begiun F, Herrmann WL: Effect of lumbar epidural analgesia on lower urinary tract function in the immediate postpartum period. Br J Obstet Gynaecol 90:428, 1983

Whiffen VE: The comparison of postpartum with non-postpartum depression: A rose by any other name. J Psychiatry Neurosci 16:160, 1991

Whitehead RG: Nutritional aspects of human lactation. Lancet 1:167, 1983

Williams JW: Regeneration of the uterine mucosa after delivery with especial reference to the placental site. Am J Obstet Gynecol 22:664, 1931

Yip R, Binkin NJ, Fleshood L, Trowbridge FL: Declining prevalence of anemia among low-income children in the United States. JAMA 258:1619, 1987

Yip R, Reeves JD, Lönnerdal B, Keen CL, Dallman PR: Does iron supplementation compromise zinc nutrition in healthy infants? Am J Clin Nutr 42:683, 1985

Yuen BH: Prolactin in human milk: The influence of nursing and the duration of postpartum lactation. Am J Obstet Gynecol 158:583, 1988

■ SECTION V ■
Abnormal Labor

■

CHAPTER 19

Dystocia Due to Abnormalities of the Expulsive Forces

Dystocia—literally, difficult labor—is characterized by abnormally slow progress of labor. It is the consequence of four distinct abnormalities that may exist singly or in combination:

1. Abnormalities of the expulsive forces, either uterine forces insufficiently strong or appropriately coordinated to efface and dilate the cervix (uterine dysfunction), or inadequate voluntary muscle effort during the second stage of labor (Chap. 19).
2. Abnormalities of presentation, position, or development of the fetus (see Chap. 20).
3. Abnormalities of the maternal bony pelvis—that is, pelvic contraction (see Chap. 21).
4. Abnormalities of the birth canal other than those of the bony pelvis that form an obstacle to fetal descent (see Chap. 22).

Pelvic contraction is often accompanied by uterine dysfunction, and the two together constitute the most common cause of dystocia. Similarly, faulty presentation or unusual fetal size or shape may be accompanied by uterine dysfunction. *As a generalization, uterine dysfunction is common whenever there is disproportion between the presenting part of the fetus and the birth canal.*

Dystocia is the most common contemporary indication for primary cesarean delivery. Shiono and colleagues (1987) found that 43 percent of primary cesarean deliveries were done for dystocia, whereas the next leading category was fetal distress, which accounted for only 14 percent of primary operations. Inevitably, methods of labor management, including oxytocin induction and augmentation, are receiving renewed interest as obstetricians grapple with means of controlling escalating cesarean delivery rates. Dystocia

is very complex, and although its definition (abnormal progress in labor) seems simple, there is no consensus as to what "abnormal progress" means. Given this difficulty, it seems prudent to attempt a better understanding of normal labor in order to determine departure(s) from normal.

Labor Diagnosis

The greatest impediment to understanding normal labor is recognizing its commencement. The strict definition of labor—*uterine contractions that bring about demonstrable effacement and dilatation of the cervix*—does not easily aid the clinician in determining when labor has actually commenced, because this diagnosis is confirmed only after the event. Several options may be used to deal with this dilemma. One is to instruct the woman to quantify uterine contractions for some specified period, and then define labor onset as the clock time when painful contractions become regular. Obviously, this is very subjective and frequently is a source of considerable frustration for both the obstetrician and the patient. Indeed, uterine irritability that causes discomfort, but that does not represent true labor, may develop at any time during pregnancy. False labor is most commonly observed late in pregnancy and in parous women. Although it often stops spontaneously, it may proceed rapidly into the effective contractions of true labor. Thus, the report of relatively infrequent and short-lived, albeit uncomfortable, uterine contractions, cannot be summarily dismissed. All too frequently when this is done, delivery takes place without benefit of professional assistance or facilities essential for optimal care.

A second option is to define the onset of labor to begin at the time of admission to the labor unit. This simplistic definition also suffers because it depends on somewhat subjective admission criteria. At the National Maternity Hospital in Dublin (O'Driscoll and Meagher, 1980), efforts have been made to codify admission criteria, following which labor management is disciplined carefully. Criteria for admission at term require painful uterine contractions accompanied by any one of the following: (1) ruptured membranes, (2) bloody "show," or (3) complete effacement of the cervix. These admission criteria are not used in Dublin to equate with true labor, which is still defined as cervical dilatation accompanied by painful uterine contractions; these are only useful indices for deciding admission. In the Irish scheme, the duration of labor is determined based on the elapsed time from admission to delivery, thus implying that "labor" commences upon admission.

In the United States, admission for the diagnosis of labor is frequently based on the extent of cervical dilatation accompanied by painful uterine contractions. When the woman presents for examination with intact membranes, cervical dilatation of 3 to 4 cm or greater is presumed to be a reasonably reliable threshold for the diagnosis of active labor. In this case, onset of labor commences with the time of the admission examination. This presumptive method of diagnosing true labor obviates many of the uncertainties in diagnosing labor during earlier stages of cervical dilatation.

To summarize, labor may be presumed to have begun either at home when the woman had the onset of regular, painful uterine contractions, or after presentation to a maternity unit and when certain admission criteria have been met. In either case, it must be admitted that the woman's perceptions of what is or is not labor largely influence the diagnosis of true labor. O'Driscoll and Meagher (1980) observed that "this procedure, which leaves the initiative in the hands of patients, has no parallel in other branches of medicine."

First Stage of Labor. Assuming that the diagnosis of labor has been confirmed, then what are the expectations for the progress of normal labor? Historically, normal progress was usually described in terms of simple elapsed time, with the realization that the diagnosis of normal labor could be made only after the fact. Indeed, for many years, labor was not considered prolonged unless 24 to 48 hours had elapsed, and hence the maxim: "Never let the sun set twice on a laboring woman." A scientific approach to the study of labor was begun by Friedman in 1954, who began to describe pioneering studies that demonstrated a characteristic sigmoid pattern for labor when analyzed by graphing cervical dilatation against time. This graphic approach, based on statistical observations, eventually resulted in a change in the management of labor. This graphic, and thus visual, description helped to dispel many of the myths about labor and placed the treatment of dysfunctional labor on a more logical basis.

Based on more than two decades of scholarly analysis of the labor patterns of a large number of women, Friedman also sought to select criteria that would delimit normal labor and thus enable us to identify its significant abnormalities. From these studies, Friedman developed the concept of three functional divisions of labor—preparatory, dilatational, and pelvic—to describe the physiological objectives of each division. (Fig. 19–1). Although little cervical dilatation occurs during the **preparatory division,** considerable changes take place in the ground substance (collagen) and other connective tissue components of the cervix. Friedman found that this division of labor may be sensitive to sedation and conduction analgesia. The **dilatational division** of labor, during which time dilatation proceeds at its most rapid rate, is unaffected by sedation or conduction analgesia. The **pelvic division** of labor commences with the deceleration phase of cervical dilatation. The classical mechanisms of labor that involve the cardinal movements of the fetus in the cephalic presentation—engagement, flexion, descent, internal rotation, extension, and external rotation—take place principally during the pelvic division. In actual practice, however, the time of onset of the pelvic division is seldom clearly identifiably separate from the dilatational division.

As shown in Figure 19–2, the pattern of cervical dilatation during the preparatory and dilatational divisions of normal labor takes on the shape of a sigmoid curve. As also depicted in Figure 19–2, two phases of cervical dilatation are defined: the **latent phase** corresponds to the preparatory division and the **active phase** to the dilatational division. Friedman subdivided the active phase into the *acceleration phase, phase of maximum slope,* and the *deceleration phase.*

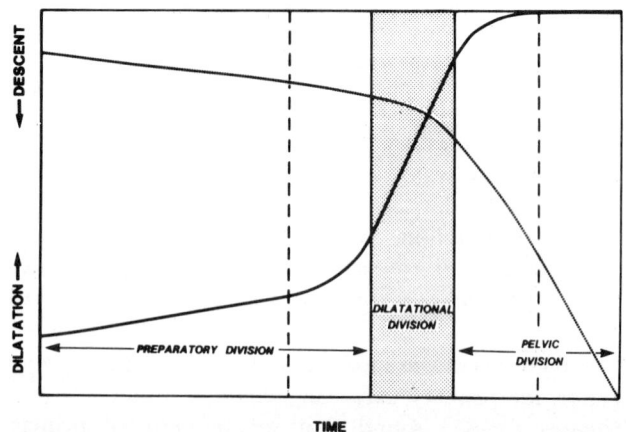

Fig. 19–1. Labor course divided functionally on the basis of expected evolution of the dilatation and descent curves into (1) a preparatory division, including latent and acceleration phases; (2) a dilatational division, occupying the phase of maximum slope of dilatation; and (3) a pelvic division, encompassing both deceleration phase and second stage while concurrent with the phase of maximum slope of descent. (Illustration courtesy of Dr. L. Casey; redrawn from Friedman, 1978.)

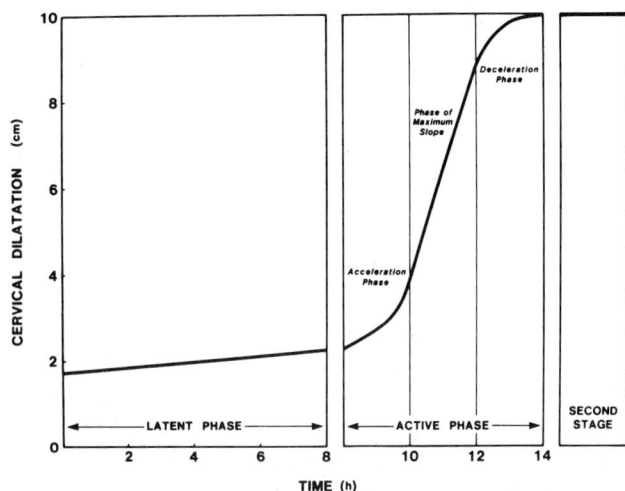

Fig. 19–2. Composite of the average dilatation curve for nulliparous labor based on analysis of the data derived from the patterns traced by a large, nearly consecutive series of gravidas. The first stage is divided into a relatively flat latent phase and a rapidly progressive active phase. In the active phase, there are three identifiable component parts: an acceleration phase, a linear phase of maximum slope, and a deceleration phase. (Illustration courtesy of Dr. L. Casey; redrawn from Friedman, 1978.)

Latent Phase. Latent labor onset is defined according to Friedman (1972) as the point at which the mother perceives regular contractions. He described the latent phase as an interval during which orientation of uterine contractions takes place along with cervical softening and effacement in preparation for active dilatation. His minimum criteria for subsequent entry into the active phase of labor are cervical dilatation rates of 1.2 cm/hr for nulliparas and 1.5 cm/hr for parous women. It is emphasized that these rates of cervical dilatation do not start at a specific dilatation. For example, Peisner and Rosen (1986), in an analysis of latent labor, found that 30 percent of women reached 5 cm dilatation before their dilatation rates conformed to the Friedman criteria for active phase labor. Conversely, other patients dilated more rapidly and had active labor phase cervical dilatation rates as early as at 3 cm. Thus, the latent phase commences with maternal perception of regular contractions, and in the presence of progressive, albeit slow, cervical dilatation ends at between 3 and 5 cm of dilatation, which is the threshold for the active phase transition. This threshold may be clinically useful, for it defines cervical dilatation limits beyond which active labor can be expected. For example, Rosen (1990) recommended that all women be classified as "in active labor" when at a maximum of 5 cm cervical dilatation, so that in the absence of progressive change, intervention should be considered.

Friedman and Sachtleben (1963) defined a **prolonged latent phase** to be greater than 20 hours in the nullipara and greater than 14 hours in the parous woman.

These were derived because they chose the 95 percentiles to define normalcy. In an earlier report, Friedman (1955) provided statistical data on the duration of latent phase labor in nulliparas. The mean duration of the latent phase was 8.6 hours and the range was 1 to 44 hours. The mean plus two standard deviations was 20.6 hours. Thus, the duration of latent phase of labor specified, 20 hours for nulliparous and 14 hours for parous women, represents a statistical maximum, with the majority of women exhibiting much shorter latent phases.

Factors that affect duration of the latent phase include excessive sedation or conduction analgesia, poor cervical condition (e.g., thick, uneffaced, or undilated), and false labor. Friedman claimed that either rest or oxytocin stimulation were equally efficacious and safe in correcting prolonged latent phases. Rest was preferable to active intervention because of the frequency of unrecognized false labor in these patients. Specifically, if rest was accomplished using strong sedatives, 85 percent of these women would commence active labor during or after awakening. Another 10 percent would cease contracting, and thus would have had false labor. Finally, 5 percent would experience recurrence of an abnormal latent phase and required oxytocin stimulation. Amniotomy was discouraged because of the 10 percent incidence of false labor.

Prolonged latent phases of labor are not common, and Sokol and colleagues (1977) reported a 3 to 4 percent incidence, regardless of parity. Importantly, Friedman (1972) reported that prolongation of the latent phase did not adversely influence fetal or maternal morbidity or mortality and cautioned against cesarean delivery as a primary therapy.

Friedman's introduction of the concept of a latent phase has great significance in attempting to understand normal human labor and thereby guide our clinical expectations. The normal progress of labor in primigravid women varies considerably depending on whether or not a latent phase is included. To better illustrate this, Figure 19–3 shows four labor curves from primigravidas where labor was diagnosed beginning with admission rather than with the parturient's recollection of when regular contractions commenced. When labor is defined to commence with admission, there is remarkable similarity of the individual labor curves. It is important to note that the principal difference between the labor curves, contingent upon when labor is defined to begin, is the presence or absence of a latent period in the slope of cervical dilatation plotted versus time. Hendricks and co-workers (1970) contended that Friedman's latent phase took place over the approximately 3 weeks antedating active labor requiring hospital admission. This process of slow outpatient cervical dilatation to about 3 cm when active labor commenced is shown in Figure 19–4 (also see Chap. 12). Clearly, clinical expectations for progress of labor are greatly influenced by the method used to define the commencement of labor.

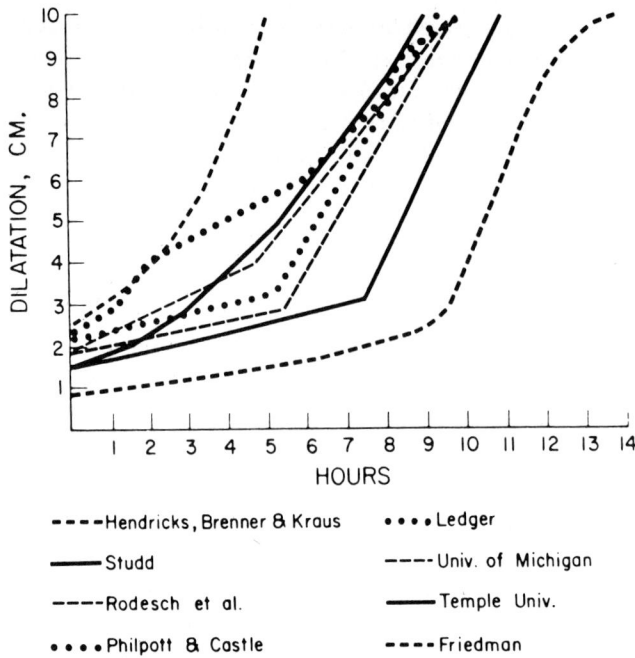

Fig. 19–3. Progress of labor in primigravid women from the time of admission. When the starting point on the abscissa begins with admission to the hospital, there is no latent phase observed. (From O'Connor and colleagues, 1976, with permission.)

Active Labor. As shown in Figure 19–3, the progress of labor in nulliparous women has particular significance because these curves all reveal a rapid change in the slope of cervical dilatation between 3 and 4 cm. That is, the "active" phase of labor, in terms of most rapid rates of cervical dilatation, consistently begins when the cervix is 3 to 4 cm dilated. These rather remarkable similarities in the onset timing of maximum rate of cervical dilatation serve to define the active phase of labor and provide useful guideposts in labor management. That is, cervical dilatation of 3 to 4 cm or more, in the presence

of uterine contractions, can be taken to reliably represent the threshold for the active phase of labor. Similarly, these curves permit the clinician to ask, given that labor can be reliably diagnosed to have commenced, how much time should elapse in normal active labor?

Turning again to Friedman's work (1955), the mean duration of active phase labor in primigravidas was 4.9 hours. The standard deviation of 3.4 hours is quite large, however. Hence, the active phase was reported to have a statistical maximum of 11.7 hours with considerable variation in the duration. This was due to the large range of normal rates of cervical dilatation shown as the slope of the labor curve. Indeed, rates of cervical dilatation ranged from 1.2 to 6.8 cm/hr. Thus, when the rate of cervical dilatation considered normal for active phase labor in the primigravida is reported to be 1.2 cm/hr, this is the minimum normal rate, not the maximum. Multiparas progress somewhat faster in active phase labor with a minimum normal rate of 1.5 cm/hr (Friedman, 1972). Friedman also reported that the active phase ended at about 8 to 9 cm when there was deceleration of cervical dilatation (Fig. 19–2). This deceleration phase is not typical of the other labor curves shown in Figure 19–3.

Another feature shared by the several labor curves depicted in Figure 19–3 is the remarkable tendency to similar duration for active phase labor. Specifically, primigravid women who enter the active phase at 3 to 4 cm reliably can be expected to reach 8 to 10 cm dilatation within 3 to 4 hours. This observation might have potential usefulness. For example, if cervical dilatation reaches 4 cm, the clinician could expect complete dilatation to be achieved in approximately 4 hours if spontaneous labor is "normal." Active labor phase abnormalities, however, are quite common, and Sokol and co-workers (1977) reported that 25 percent of nulliparous labors were complicated by active phase abnormalities while 15 percent of multigravidas developed this

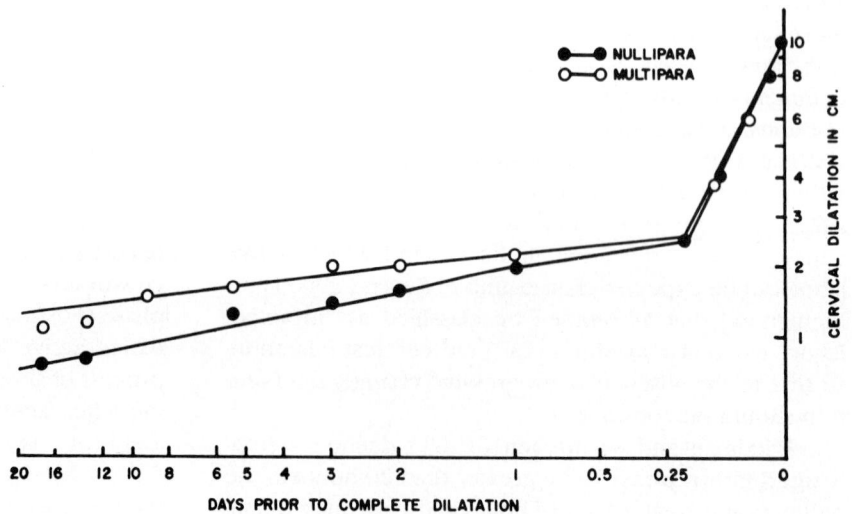

Fig. 19–4. Slow outpatient cervical change in the 3 weeks preceding active labor. (From Hendricks and co-workers, 1970).

problem. Indeed, active phase disorders are the most common abnormalities of labor.

Understanding Friedman's analysis of active phase labor is somewhat arduous because rates of fetal descent are considered in addition to cervical dilatation rates, and both of these indices of labor progress are occurring concomitantly (see Fig. 19–1). Descent begins in the later stage of active cervical dilatation and commences at about 7 to 8 cm in primigravidas and becomes most rapid after 8 cm. Moreover, Friedman (1972) further confounds active-phase abnormalities by subdividing problems during this phase into **protraction** and **arrest** disorders. He defined protraction as a slow *rate* of cervical dilatation or descent, which for nulliparas was less than 1.2 cm dilatation per hour or less than 1 cm descent per hour. For multiparas, protraction was defined as less than 1.5 cm dilatation per hour or less than 2 cm descent per hour. He defined arrest as a complete cessation of cervical dilatation or descent. **Arrest of dilatation** was defined as 2 hours with no cervical change and **arrest of descent** as 1 hour without fetal descent. The prognosis for protraction and arrest disorders differed considerably, and he found that about 30 percent of women with protraction disorders had cephalopelvic disproportion, whereas this was diagnosed in 45 percent of women in whom an arrest disorder developed. Abnormal labor patterns, diagnostic criteria, and methods of treatment according to Cohen and Friedman (1983) are summarized in Table 19–1.

Other associations or factors contributing to both protraction and arrest disorders were excessive sedation, conduction analgesia, and fetal malposition (e.g., persistent occiput posterior presentation). In both protraction and arrest disorders, Friedman recommended fetopelvic examination to diagnose cephalopelvic disproportion.

Recommended therapy for protraction disorders was expectant management, whereas oxytocin was advised for arrest disorders in the absence of cephalopelvic disproportion. Cephalopelvic disproportion is not defined precisely in Friedman's 1955 report, other than to note that 8 of 39 diagnosed cases of disproportion had x-ray pelvimetry evidence of pelvic incapacity, and the remaining 31 women were considered to have "relative disproportion for a variety of reasons such as persistent occiput posterior." Remarkably, of the 500 women studied, only 2 percent had cesarean deliveries. Put another way, cephalopelvic disproportion in Friedman's 1955 report did not equate with cesarean delivery. This fact must be kept in mind when considering the significance of Friedman's various labor abnormalities in the context of the current medicolegal implication that cephalopelvic disproportion mandates cesarean delivery. Alternatively, the great majority of active phase labor disorders described by Friedman in 1955 did not result in cesarean delivery. Given these observations, the significance of the many complexities in labor analysis introduced by Friedman must be questioned. Specifically, what do the various prolongation, protraction, and arrest disorders really mean?

Hendricks and co-workers (1970), contemporaries of Friedman, challenged his conclusions about the course of normal human labor. Their principal differences included (1) absence of a latent phase, (2) no deceleration phase, (3) brevity of labor, and (4) dilatation at similar rates for nulliparas and multiparas after 4 cm has been reached. Hendricks and associates disputed the concept of a latent phase because they observed that cervical dilatation and effacement occurred slowly during the 4 weeks preceding labor. Moreover, average cervical dilatation on diagnosis of active labor was 2.5 cm for nulli-

TABLE 19–1. ABNORMAL LABOR PATTERNS, DIAGNOSTIC CRITERIA, AND METHODS OF TREATMENT

| Labor Pattern | Diagnostic Criterion | | Preferred Treatment | Exceptional Treatment |
	Nulliparas	Multiparas		
Prolongation Disorder (Prolonged latent phase)	> 20 hr	> 14 hr	Therapeutic rest	Oxytocin or cesarean delivery for urgent problems
Protraction Disorders				
1. Protracted active phase dilatation	< 1.2 cm/hr	< 1.5 cm/hr		
2. Protracted descent	< 1.0 cm/hr	< 2 cm/hr	Expectant and support	Cesarean delivery for CPD[a]
Arrest Disorders				
1. Prolonged deceleration phase	> 3 hr	> 1 hr	Without CPD[a]: Oxytocin	Rest if exhausted
2. Secondary arrest of dilatation	> 2 hr	> 2 hr		
3. Arrest of descent	> 1 hr	> 1 hr	With CPD[a]: Cesarean delivery	Cesarean delivery
4. Failure of descent	No descent in deceleration phase or second stage of labor			

[a] CPD: Cephalopelvic disproportion.
Modified from Cohen and Friedman (1983).

paras and 3.5 for parous women. Thus, according to these investigators, Friedman's "latent phase" actually occurred over several weeks preceding active labor.

Hendricks and colleagues (1970) also observed that labor was relatively rapid, given the typical cervical dilatation of 2 to 4 cm at the time of admission. Specifically, the average time from admission to complete cervical dilatation was 4.8 hours for nulliparas and 3.2 hours for multiparas.

Second Stage of Labor. Second-stage labor begins when cervical dilatation is complete and ends with fetal expulsion. Its median duration is 50 minutes for nulliparas and 20 minutes for multiparas, but it is also highly variable (Kilpatrick and Laros, 1989). In a woman of higher parity with a previously dilated vagina and perineum, two or three expulsive efforts after full cervical dilatation may suffice to complete delivery. Conversely, in a woman with a contracted pelvis or a larger fetus, or with impaired expulsive efforts from conduction analgesia or intense sedation, the second stage may become abnormally long. Kilpatrick and Laros (1989) reported that average second-stage labor, prior to spontaneous fetal expulsion, was lengthened about 25 minutes by conduction analgesia. As previously noted, the pelvic or fetal descent division of labor largely occurs following complete cervical dilatation. Moreover, the second stage incorporates many of the cardinal movements of repositionings necessary for the fetus to negotiate the birth canal. Given the mechanical requirements of these fetal movements, it is logical for disproportion of the fetus and pelvis to become apparent during the second stage. Indeed, in earlier obstetrical times, cephalopelvic disproportion was diagnosed only after complete cervical dilatation had occurred and attempts to deliver the fetus with forceps had failed.

Today there are second-stage rules that limit its duration. Specifically, current recommendations for the length of the second stage in nulliparas is 2 hours, extended to 3 hours when conduction analgesia is used (American College of Obstetricians and Gynecologists, 1989a). For multiparas, 1 hour is the limit, extended to 2 hours with conduction analgesia. At Parkland Hospital, second-stage labors exceeding 2 hours are uncommon, and during 1991, only 5 percent of 5129 term deliveries in primiparous women were characterized as such. Importantly, labor epidural analgesia is seldom used at our hospital.

The origin of the second-stage rule, which in essence limits the duration of this phase of labor to 2 hours, cannot be assigned to any one individual (Hellman and Prystowsky, 1952). This rule seems to have been established fairly definitely in American obstetrics, however, by the turn of the century. The first edition of *Williams Obstetrics*, published in 1902, states that forceps are usually indicated if the second stage lasts more than 2 hours. This rule appears to have been derived

from concerns about fetal health, and indeed, the concept of prophylactic forceps delivery to shorten the second stage was popular during much of the 20th century (see Chap. 24, p. 559). This practice often led to the performance of difficult forceps operations, although the question was raised in the minds of many obstetricians whether prolongation of the second stage until such a time as an easy forceps delivery might be accomplished would be of some advantage. This more conservative attitude concerning the use of forceps is the contemporary practice.

Between 1937 and 1949, over 13,000 term deliveries at the Johns Hopkins Hospital were analyzed by Hellman and Prystowsky (1952) to evaluate the relationship between the duration of second-stage labor and pregnancy outcome. Prophylactic forceps delivery was practiced during this period at Johns Hopkins. A total of 1034 (8 percent) women were delivered after 2 hours in the second stage. A common cause of second-stage prolongation was persistent occiput posterior position. An interesting feature of pregnancies with a prolonged second stage was an excessive duration (beyond 20 hours) of the dilatation division of labor.

Maternal as well as fetal effects were attributed to prolongation of second-stage labor beyond 2 hours. Postpartum hemorrhage and infection were both linked to prolonged second-stage; however, the increases in their incidences were quite small, particularly when the length of the first stage of labor was taken into account. In the Hopkins study, infant mortality, corrected for the length of the first stage of labor, approximately doubled, from 5 per 1000 to 10 per 1000. Unfortunately, this report did not precisely define infant mortality, nor did it state the presumed cause(s) of perinatal deaths. These results were not reproduced in 1977 when Cohen investigated the fetal effects of second-stage labor length at Beth Israel Hospital. Cohen limited his investigation to 4403 term nulliparas in whom electronical fetal heart rate monitoring was performed. As shown in Table 19–2, infant mortality was not increased in women whose second-stage

TABLE 19–2. RELATIONSHIP BETWEEN INFANT MORTALITY AND DURATION OF SECOND-STAGE LABOR

Length of Second Stage (min)	Johns Hopkins Hospital[a] (1937–1949)		Beth Israel Hospital[b] (1977)	
	Women	Infant Deaths/1000	Women	Infant Deaths/1000
0–3	7138	2.5	623	0.0
31–60	3101	3.5	1257	2.4
61–90	1313	6.1	1007	3.0
91–120	746	5.4	599	0.0
121–180	645	10.9	662	0.0
181	389	15.4	255	0.0

[a] From Hellman and Prystowsky (1952).
[b] From Cohen (1977).

labor exceeded 2 hours. Epidural analgesia was used commonly, and this likely accounts for the large number of pregnancies with a prolonged second stage. These data likely also influenced recent recommendations by the American College of Obstetricians and Gynecologists (1989c) permitting an additional hour for the second stage when conduction analgesia is used.

Spontaneous Parturition. Our understanding of the normal duration of human parturition may be clouded by the many clinical variables that affect the conduct of labor in modern obstetrical units, and also by the complexities of the graphicostatistical labor curves discussed in the preceding sections. Specifically, how long is normal spontaneous labor and delivery?

Kilpatrick and Laros (1989) reported that the mean length of parturition was approximately 9 hours in nulliparous women without conduction analgesia, and that the 95th percentile upper limit was about 18.5 hours. Corresponding times for multiparous women were a mean of about 6 hours with a 95th percentile of about 13.5 hours. These investigators defined the onset of labor as the time when regular, painful contractions began occurring every 3 to 5 minutes, leading to cervical change. This time was determined by patient history. The extent of cervical dilatation present at admission is not stated. Leveno and co-workers (1992) studied spontaneous parturition in almost 25,000 women at term and found that parturition times did not follow a normal distribution and that use of parametric statistics (means) would falsely lengthen perceptions of the duration of human parturition. Parity (nulliparous versus multiparous) and cervical dilatation at admission were significant determinants of the length of spontaneous parturition. Almost 80 percent of women in this study were admitted with a cervical dilatation of 5 cm or less. The median time from admission to spontaneous delivery was 3.5 hours, and 95 percent of all women studied delivered within 10.1 hours. These results suggest that normal human parturition is relatively short in duration.

Summary. Normal human labor is characterized by brevity, considerable biological variation, and in our opinion, less complexity than anticipated based on contemporary graphic statistical interpretations. Table 19–3 summarizes average normal spontaneous parturition times according to parity and admission cervical dilatation. Active labor can be reliably diagnosed when cervical dilatation is 3 cm or more in the presence of uterine contractions. Once this cervical dilatation threshold is reached, normal progress to delivery can be expected, depending on parity in the ensuing 4 to 6 hours or so. Anticipated progress during a 1- to 2-hour second stage is governed by rules intended to ensure fetal safety. Finally, most women in spontaneous labor, regardless of parity and if left unaided, will deliver within approximately 10 hours after admission for spon-

TABLE 19–3. AVERAGE DURATION OF NORMAL SPONTANEOUS PARTURITION IN WOMEN AT TERM BASED UPON ACTIVE LABOR COMMENCING AT ≥ 3 CM CERVICAL DILATION

Labor Characteristic	Typical Normal Labor (Mean Time)
Kilpatrick and Laros (1989)	
First-stage length[a]	Nulliparous = 8.1 hr
	Parous = 5.7 hr
Second-stage length[a]	Nulliparous = 54 min
	Parous = 19 min
Leveno and associates (1992)	
Total duration of labor[b]	Nulliparous = 6.4 hr
	Parous = 4.6 hr

[a] Labor diagnosed based on patients' recollection of regular contractions.
[b] Labor diagnosed by admission time.

taneous labor. *When time breaches in normal labor boundaries are the only pregnancy complications, interventions other than cesarean delivery must be considered thoroughly before resorting to this method of delivery for failure to progress.* Insufficient uterine activity is a common and correctable cause of abnormal labor progress.

Uterine Dysfunction

As described above, the *first stage of labor* has commonly, but somewhat artificially, been divided into the *latent phase* and the *active phase*. Typically, the latent phase (*prodromal labor*) will be of several hours' duration, during which time the cervix undergoes softening and effacement but only slight dilatation. This phase of cervical change is characterized by uterine contractions of mild intensity, short duration, and variable frequency. The phase of more rapid cervical dilatation, or the active phase, follows. During the active phase, or what has long been called simply labor, the cervix dilates more rapidly and there is descent of the presenting part through the birth canal (Fig. 19–1).

Descent normally begins well before the cervix reaches full dilatation and proceeds until the presenting part reaches the perineum. **This pattern is highly variable.** The presenting part in nulliparous women may be at the + 1 or even + 2 station before the onset of labor, whereas in parous women, descent of the presenting part may not begin until the cervix nearly is dilated fully.

Failure of the cervix to dilate or of the presenting part to descend is cause for concern. Prolongation of either the *first or second stage of labor* may result in increased perinatal and maternal morbidity. Any delay in cervical dilatation during the first stage or prolongation of the second stage of labor should alert the obstetrician to possible danger.

Uterine dysfunction in any phase of cervical dilatation is characterized by lack of progress, for one of the prime characteristics of normal labor is its progression. The diagnosis of uterine dysfunction in the latent phase is difficult and sometimes can be made only in retrospect. One of the most common errors is to treat women for uterine dysfunction who are not yet in active labor.

There have been three significant advances in the treatment of uterine dysfunction: (1) realization that undue prolongation of labor may contribute to perinatal morbidity and mortality; (2) use of very dilute intravenous infusion of oxytocin in the treatment of certain types of uterine dysfunction; and (3) more frequent use of cesarean delivery rather than difficult midforceps delivery when oxytocin fails or its use is inappropriate (Table 19–4).

Types of Dysfunction. Reynolds and co-workers (1948) emphasized that uterine contractions of normal labor are characterized by a gradient of myometrial activity, being greatest and lasting longest at the fundus (fundal dominance) and diminishing toward the cervix. Caldeyro-Barcia and colleagues (1950) advanced the work of Reynolds by inserting small balloons into the myometrium at various levels (see Chap. 15, p. 419). With the balloons attached to strain-gauge transducers, they reported that in addition to a gradient of activity, there was a time differential in the onset of the contractions in the fundus, midzone, and lower uterine segments. Larks (1960) described the exciting stimulus as starting in one cornu and then several milliseconds later in the other, the excitation waves then joining and sweeping over the fundus and down the uterus.

The Montevideo group made another significant contribution to the understanding of uterine dysfunction. By inserting a polyethylene catheter through the abdominal wall into amnionic fluid, they ascertained that the lower limit of contraction pressure required to dilate the cervix is 15 mm Hg. This figure is in agreement with the findings of Hendricks and co-workers (1959), who reported that normal spontaneous contractions often exert pressures of about 60 mm Hg. From these observations, it is possible to define two types of uterine dysfunction. In one, **hypotonic uterine dysfunction,** there is no basal hypertonus and uterine contractions have a normal gradient pattern (synchronous), but the slight rise in pressure during a contraction is insufficient to dilate the cervix at a satisfactory rate. This type of uterine dysfunction usually occurs during the active phase of labor, after the cervix has dilated to more than 4 cm. In the other, **hypertonic uterine dysfunction** or **incoordinate uterine dysfunction,** either basal tone is elevated appreciably or the pressure gradient is distorted, perhaps by contraction of the midsegment of the uterus with more force than the fundus or by complete asynchronism of the impulses originating in each cornu, or a combination of these two. This type of dysfunction is typically encountered in the latent phase of labor.

In hypotonic uterine dysfunction, contractions become less frequent and the uterus is easily indentable even at the acme of a contraction. Contractions of the hypertonic or incoordinate variety are typically much more painful yet ineffective. As discussed below, hypotonic dysfunction often responds favorably to treatment with oxytocin. The opposite is most often true of the hypertonic variety, in which the abnormal pattern of uterine contractions is more likely to become accentuated and uterine tone increased. Exceptions have been documented, however, in which a uterus with basal hypertonus and frequent, incoordinate contractions did convert to orderly physiological contractions, apparently in response to intravenous oxytocin (Caldeyro-Barcia, 1957). In general, the likelihood of such a response is low and the risk of enhancing the hypertonus is considerable (Cohen and Friedman, 1983).

Uterine contractions less than 25 mm Hg in amplitude above baseline rarely cause cervical dilatation (Seitchik and Castillo, 1983). At first evidence of cervical dilatation, 95 percent of women will have three to five contractions every 10 minutes that are each greater than 25 mm Hg above baseline. However, "adequate labor" describes a wide range of uterine activities; the amplitude of each contraction varies from 25 to 75 mm Hg, and contractions occur over a total of 2 to 4.5 minutes in every 10 minute window, achieving from 95 to 395 Montevideo units (Fig. 19–5).

Etiology. Pelvic contraction and fetal malposition are common causes of uterine dysfunction. That moderate degrees of pelvic contraction and fetal malposition may cause hypotonic uterine dysfunction is of great clinical importance. Overdistention of the uterus, as with twins

TABLE 19–4. APGAR SCORES BY LABOR PATTERN IN NULLIPARAS AND PERINATAL MORTALITY BY DELIVERY METHOD

Labor Pattern	Percent of Apgar Scores Less than 5		Perinatal Mortality (per 1000)		
	At 1 Minute	At 5 Minutes	Spontaneous	Low Forceps	Midforceps
Normal	12.7	3.2	1.5	2.8	10.8[a]
Prolongation disorder	12.9	4.6	0.0	0.0	10.8[a]
Protraction disorders	23.7[a]	3.1	0.0	12.0[a]	28.5[a]
Arrest disorders	25.2[a]	8.0[a]	16.1[a]	24.4[a]	38.3[a]

[a] Statistically significant: $P < .01$.
Modified from Cohen and Friedman (1983).

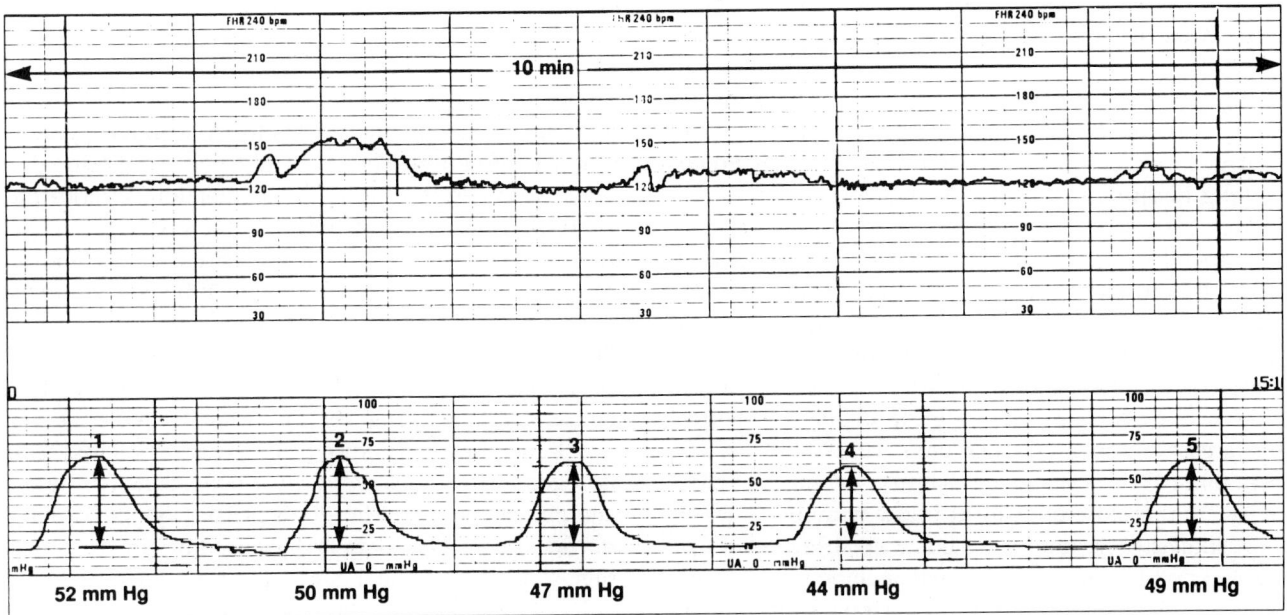

| 52 mm Hg | 50 mm Hg | 47 mm Hg | 44 mm Hg | 49 mm Hg |

Fig. 19–5. Montevideo units are calculated by subtracting the baseline uterine pressure from the peak contraction pressure for each contraction in a 10-minute window and adding the pressures generated by each contraction. In the example shown, five contractions occurred, producing pressure changes of 52, 50, 47, 44, and 49 mm Hg, respectively. The sum of these five contractions is 242 Montevideo units. (From the American College of Obstetricians and Gynecologists, 1989a).

and with hydramnios, may contribute to the condition. **In many—perhaps one half—of instances, however, the cause of uterine dysfunction is unknown** (Seitchik and co-workers, 1987). The main fault seldom lies within a cervix that is too rigid to dilate. In elderly nulliparas, and in women with cervical fibrosis from some cause, however, excessive rigidity of the cervix may be a factor in the production of dystocia.

Complications. Undue procrastination too often leads to an unfortunate outcome, whereas intervention too early results in needless cesarean deliveries. Fetal and neonatal deaths are accompaniments of intrauterine infection, which commonly develops in prolonged dysfunctional labor. Although it may be wise for the mother to be treated for these intrauterine infections with antibiotics, such therapy may be of less value for the fetus. Maternal exhaustion may occur if labor is greatly prolonged; however, supportive therapy with adequate intravenous fluids should be initiated and delivery effected before these complications appear. Difficult labors and deliveries are more likely to leave psychological scars on the mothers, as emphasized by Jeffcoate (1961) and Steer (1950). Both found that difficult labor exerted a definite deleterious effect upon future childbearing. These investigators showed that, although more than two thirds of their patients had additional children after spontaneous delivery, only one third did so after midforceps operations.

Dystocia

Under the broad category of dystocia is included a number of more specific terms, including cephalopelvic disproportion and failure to progress. The American College of Obstetricians and Gynecologists (1989a) defined *absolute* cephalopelvic disproportion as a disparity between the size of the maternal pelvis and the fetal head that precludes vaginal delivery, whether or not the fetal head presents optimal bony diameters. Similarly, *relative* cephalopelvic disproportion results when asynclitism or extension of the fetal head presents bony diameters too great to allow passage through the maternal pelvis. *Failure to progress* includes lack of progressive cervical dilatation and/or lack of descent of the fetal head. Ideally, the diagnosis of failure to progress should be explainable or at least attributable to excessive fetal size, malpresentation, or insufficient uterine expulsive forces.

Overdiagnosis. It is generally agreed that dystocia leading to cesarean delivery is overdiagnosed in the United States and elsewhere. However, factors leading to increased use of cesarean delivery for dystocia are controversial. Those implicated have included obstetrician convenience, incorrect diagnosis of dystocia, and fear of litigation (Fraser and co-workers, 1987). Perkins (1992) eloquently described contemporary obstetrical hazards in the management of labor: "It is not so much fun to await delivery any more because it used to represent a great relief to the patient and the beginning of life. It is now a great relief to the obstetrician and the ending of a slow 'death,' worrying about the possibility of an unexpectedly bad outcome that is unrelated to anything he/she did but at risk of being attributed to him/her."

Variability in the criteria for diagnosis of dystocia is likely a major determinant of the increase in cesarean deliveries for dystocia. Stewart and colleagues (1990) reported that 30 percent of 3740 women with labor in Ottawa were given a diagnosis of dystocia. Cesarean delivery for dystocia was done during all phases of labor. The largest number (40 percent) were done in the latent phase. They concluded that many cesarean deliveries were therefore done for dystocia without a trial of labor. Similarly, Cartmill and Thornton (1992) claimed that graphs of labor progress that included the latent phase, and thus appeared flat and portrayed long labor, erroneously influenced the early diagnosis of dystocia. DeMott and Sandmire (1992) reported that obstetricians with the lowest cesarean delivery rates for dystocia were those who used higher oxytocin dosages to stimulate labor, used oxytocin for longer durations, and started oxytocin at more advanced cervical dilatations. Moreover, cervical dilatation was more advanced when dystocia was diagnosed, and more women had reached complete dilatation with those obstetricians performing the fewest cesarean deliveries.

Diagnosis. Hauth and co-workers (1986, 1991) reported that to effectively induce or augment labor with oxytocin, most women (90 percent) achieve 200 to 224 Montevideo units, and 40 percent achieve at least 300 Montevideo units. These results suggest that there are certain minimums of uterine activity that should be achieved before diagnosing *failure to progress.* Accordingly, the American College of Obstetricians and Gynecologists (1989a) suggested that, before the diagnosis of arrest in the first stage of labor is made, both of these criteria should be met: (1) the latent phase of labor has been completed, with the cervix dilated 4 cm or more; and (2) a uterine contraction pattern of 200 Montevideo units or more in a 10-minute period has been present for 2 hours without cervical change. It is also important to emphasize that epidural analgesia can slow labor (American College of Obstetricians and Gynecologists, 1988).

ACTIVE MANAGEMENT OF LABOR. Other methods for management of labor and diagnosis of dystocia are in use, primarily in Europe, but also in other countries. O'Driscoll and Meagher (1980) promoted "active management of labor" as a solution for unnecessary cesarean deliveries for dystocia (see Chap. 14, p. 378). Active management of labor is a codified approach to labor diagnosis and management. Labor is diagnosed when painful contrac-

tions are accompanied by complete cervical effacement, bloody "show," or ruptured membranes. Women with such findings are committed to delivery within 8 hours. For example, a woman with painful uterine contractions and "show" is committed to delivery without regard to cervical condition. The onset of labor is considered to begin with admission. Pelvic examination is performed at regular intervals of 1 hour for the next 3 hours, and thereafter at 2-hour intervals. Progress is assessed for the first time 1 hour after admission. When dilatation has not increased by at least 1 cm, amniotomy is performed. Progress is assessed for the second time at 2 hours after admission. An oxytocin infusion is started at this time unless significant progress (i.e., 1 cm/hr) has occurred.

If membranes rupture prior to admission, oxytocin is begun for no progress at the 1-hour mark. No special equipment is used, either to dispense oxytocin or monitor its effects. Oxytocin is dispensed by simple gravity regulated by a personal nurse. The solution contains 10 units of oxytocin in 1 liter of dextrose and water; the total dose may not exceed 10 units and the rate of infusion may not exceed 60 drops (15 to 20 drops = 1 mL). Fetal blood sampling is used as the definitive test of fetal distress. Only in exceptional circumstances (unspecified) is a woman subjected to cesarean delivery, on the basis of a diagnosis of fetal distress without such scalp blood confirmation. Fetal heart monitors play little part in the care of the fetus, according to O'Driscoll and Meagher (1980).

More details are given in Chapter 14 (p. 378) for active management of labor. The World Health Organization adopted a labor "partogram" for use in developing countries (Dujardin and co-workers, 1992). Labor is divided into a latent phase, which should last no longer than 8 hours, and an active phase starting at 3 cm cervical dilatation, the rate of which should be no slower than 1 cm/hr. A 4-hour wait (lag time) is recommended before intervention when the active phase of labor is slow. The labor is graphed and analysis includes use of "alert" and "action" lines. Dujardin and co-workers (1992) described application of this partogram in Senegal in over 1000 parturients. Approximately 87 percent of the women had normal labors using this partogram. The incidence of intrapartum stillbirths in these normal labors was about 10 per 1000 births, and this increased to about 50 per 1000 births when labor was abnormal.

Maternal Position During Parturition. There is much disagreement in the obstetrical literature with respect to the potential influence of maternal position during labor on labor progress, pain perception, and fetal well-being (Carlson and associates, 1986). Miller (1983) reviewed the influence that maternal position has on the frequency and intensity of uterine contractions. He observed that uterine contractions occur more frequently but with less intensity with the mother in the supine position compared with lying on her side. Conversely, contraction frequency and intensity have been reported to increase while the parturient is sitting or standing. Lupe and Gross (1986) concluded, however, that there is no conclusive evidence that upright maternal posture or ambulation during the first stage improves labor. Both nulliparous and parous women preferred to lie on their side or sit in bed with individualized elevation of the head. Few chose to walk, fewer to squat, and none wanted the knee-chest position. They tended to assume fetal positions in the later stage of labor. Williams and co-workers (1980) found that 87 percent of women enthusiastic about ambulating requested to return to bed when active labor began. Carlson and associates (1986) studied the position elected by parturients and all returned to bed before the onset of the second stage.

Treatment of Insufficient Uterine Activity

Two questions must be answered before a treatment plan can be formulated: (1) Has the woman actually been in active labor? If there has been rhythmic uterine activity of sufficient intensity to produce some discomfort and the cervix has been observed to undergo distinct changes in effacement *and* in dilatation to 4 cm at least, it is correct to conclude that there has been real, albeit abnormal, labor. (2) Is there cephalopelvic disproportion? Uterine dysfunction is often a protection against some degree of pelvic contraction or abnormalities of fetal size or presentation. Fortunately, the uterus does not typically persist in spontaneous activity that would lead to rupture. Instead, the usual forces of labor are replaced by hypotonic uterine dysfunction.

Most often, once the diagnosis of active labor followed by hypotonic uterine dysfunction has been made and the head is well fixed in the pelvis, the membranes, if intact, should be ruptured and ideally an intrauterine pressure catheter and fetal scalp electrode placed. Close observation may be employed for 30 to 60 minutes to see if the amniotomy will improve the quality of contractions. Next, a decision must be made whether to stimulate labor with oxytocin or to effect cesarean delivery. The presence of meconium in the amnionic fluid may be an ominous sign, and this observation makes close monitoring of fetal heart rate and the uterine contraction pattern even more critical.

The choice of whether to augment labor with *hypotonic uterine dysfunction* has been for many years an empirical decision based largely upon clinical judgment as to fetal size, presentation, and position as well as clinical assessment of pelvic size. In practice, x-ray pelvimetry provides little help, and in some cases may result in an increased and unnecessary cesarean delivery rate (Bottoms and associates, 1987).

Oxytocin Stimulation. It should be ascertained that the birth canal is most likely adequate for the size of the

fetal head and that the fetal head is well flexed so as to utilize its smallest diameters to negotiate the birth canal (biparietal and suboccipitobregmatic diameters). A contracted pelvis is most *unlikely* when all of the following criteria are met:

1. The diagonal conjugate is normal.
2. The pelvic sidewalls are nearly parallel.
3. The ischial spines are not prominent.
4. The sacrum is not flat.
5. The subpubic angle is not narrow.
6. The occiput is known to be the presenting part.
7. The fetal head is engaged or descends through the pelvic inlet with fundal pressure (Hillis, 1938).

If these criteria are not met, the alternatives are cesarean delivery or possibly oxytocin stimulation. If oxytocin is used, it is mandatory that the fetal heart rate and the contraction frequency, intensity, duration, and timing in relation to the fetal heart rate be observed closely. The American College of Obstetricians and Gynecologists (1989b) recommends fetal heart rate and uterine contraction monitoring similar to that for any high-risk pregnancy.

Induction of labor implies stimulation of uterine contractions before the spontaneous onset of labor, with or without ruptured membranes. Elective induction of labor, defined as initiation of labor solely for convenience, is not recommended (American College of Obstetricians and Gynecologists, 1991). *Augmentation* refers to stimulation of uterine contractions when spontaneous contractions have been considered inadequate, with resultant failure of progressive cervical dilatation or descent of the fetus. Some also consider augmentation to include stimulation of contractions following spontaneous ruptured membranes without labor.

Technique for Intravenous Oxytocin. Oxytocin was the first polypeptide hormone synthesized (DuVigneaud and co-workers, 1953) and the Nobel Prize in chemistry (1955) was awarded for this achievement. A variety of methods for stimulation of uterine contractions with this synthetic posterior pituitary hormone have been employed. Seitchik and Castillo (1983) studied the pharmacokinetics of synthetic oxytocin in plasma and found that approximately 40 to 60 minutes are required to reach a steady-state concentration of oxytocin after initiating or altering the infusion rate. Response to oxytocin depends on pre-existing uterine activity, sensitivity, and cervical and fetal status, which are related to individual biological differences and to the duration of pregnancy. Caldeyro-Barcia and Poseiro (1960) reported that uterine response to oxytocin increases slowly from 20 to 30 weeks' gestation and is unchanged from 34 weeks until term, at which time sensitivity rapidly increases. Satin and co-workers (1992a) studied factors affecting the dose response to oxytocin for labor stimulation in 1773 pregnancies. Statistically important predictors of required oxytocin dosage included cervical dilatation, parity, and gestational age. However, the broad range of statistical confidence intervals precluded prediction of a given pregnancy's oxytocin requirement.

The mother should never be left alone while an oxytocin infusion is running. The goal of oxytocin administration is to effect uterine activity that is sufficient to produce cervical change and fetal descent while avoiding uterine hyperstimulation and fetal distress. Uterine contractions must be evaluated continually and oxytocin discontinued if contractions exceed 5 in a 10-minute period or last longer than 1 minute, or if the fetal heart rate decelerates significantly. When hyperstimulation occurs, immediate discontinuation of the oxytocin nearly always corrects the disturbances, preventing harm to mother and fetus. The oxytocin concentration in plasma rapidly falls, because the mean half-life of oxytocin is approximately 5 minutes. **Oxytocin has potent antidiuretic action.** Whenever 20 mU/minute or more of oxytocin is infused, free water clearance by the kidney decreases markedly. If aqueous fluids, especially dextrose in water, are infused in appreciable amounts along with oxytocin, water intoxication can occur, which may lead to convulsions, coma, and even death (see Chap. 14, p. 386).

Synthetic oxytocin is usually diluted into 1000 mL of a balanced salt solution that is administered via a controlled infusion pump. Oxytocin administration by any route other than in a dilute intravenous solution is not recommended for labor stimulation. To avoid bolus administration of oxytocin, the infusion should be inserted into the mainline intravenous line close to the venous puncture site. A typical oxytocin infusate consists of 10 units, USP (equivalent to 10,000 mU), mixed into 1000 mL of lactated Ringer solution, resulting in an oxytocin concentration of 10 mU/mL. In the United States, the prevailing obstetrical practice is to use low-dosage oxytocin regimens to induce labor or to correct ineffective labor. For example, Seitchik and Castillo (1983) began oxytocin at 0.5 to 1 mU/min and increased the dosage by 1 or 2 mU/min increments every 40 to 60 minutes depending upon uterine response. Similarly, Hauth and co-workers (1986) began oxytocin infusions at 1 or 2 mU/min and increased the dosage by 1 mU/min every 15 minutes as needed.

O'Driscoll and Meagher (1980) described success with a "high-dose" oxytocin regimen for labor stimulation in nulliparous women. Their method consists of diluting 10 units of synthetic oxytocin into 1000 mL of dextrose solution. The resulting solution (10 mU of oxytocin per mL) is infused by counting drops per minute. Approximately 15 to 20 drops are equivalent to 1 mL, and the infusion is begun at 10 drops per minute. The dosage is increased every 15 minutes by 10 drops per minute until a maximum of 60 drops per minute is reached. Converting to mU/min, the dosage of oxytocin

used at the outset is 5 to 6.6 mU/min, with incremental increases of the same magnitude every 15 minutes. Ferenchak and associates (1971) questioned the accuracy of infusions using the drop counting method and reported that drop size increased significantly as flow rates increased.

Parkland Hospital Protocol. At Parkland Hospital approximately 22 percent of labors are induced or augmented using oxytocin, and from 1983 to 1990, approximately 20,000 women were given oxytocin according to the following protocol:

1. Constant bedside attendance is provided by personnel experienced in oxytocin labor stimulation.
2. Continuous electronic monitoring of the fetal heart and uterine activity is conducted.
3. Use of oxytocin is avoided generally in cases of abnormal presentations of the fetus and of marked uterine overdistention such as pathological hydramnios, an excessively large singleton fetus, or multiple fetuses.
4. Women of high parity (6 or more) are generally not given oxytocin because uterine rupture occurs more readily than in women of lower parity (see Chap. 23, p. 548). Oxytocin is usually withheld from women with a previous uterine scar and a live fetus (see Chap. 26, p. 596).
5. Fetal condition must be good, as evidenced by heart rate and lack of thick meconium in amnionic fluid. A dead fetus is, of course, no contraindication to oxytocin unless there is overt fetopelvic disproportion or a transverse lie.
6. Oxytocin is infused initially at 1 mU/min. The dosage is titrated against uterine contractions using 1 mU/min, and 1 mU increments are increased every 20 minutes up to 8 mU/min. Thereafter, the infusion was increased in 2 mU/min increments up to a 20 mU/min dosage. Further increases to 40 mU/min were necessary in exceptional cases. Hyperstimulation or significant fetal heart rate change was managed by prompt discontinuation of oxytocin. The infusion could be restarted after reevaluation, usually at one half the dosage prior to hyperstimulation.

In late 1990 we changed the protocol for oxytocin stimulation of labor at Parkland Hospital to a higher dose regimen (Satin and co-workers, 1992b). The regimen described above was compared with a flexible high-dose protocol in nearly 2800 pregnancies. In the new protocol, oxytocin infusion was commenced at 6 mU/min, and this was increased as needed every 20 minutes by 6 mU/min, not to exceed a maximum dosage of 42 mU/min. Hyperstimulation occurred in approximately half of the pregnancies studied and resulted in discontinuation of oxytocin followed by resumption, when indicated, at onehalf the stopping dosage. Thereafter, dosage increases were at 3 mU/min every 20 minutes. When hyperstimulation persisted, 1 mU/min increments every 20 minutes were used. Labor augmentations were more than 3 hours shorter with the flexible high-dose regimen, and there were fewer cesarean deliveries for dystocia. Inductions failed less frequently but cesarean delivery for fetal distress was increased (6 versus 3 percent) when the flexible high-dose regimen was used. No adverse fetal effects were observed, however, in either the augmentation or induction group.

Risks Versus Benefits. Oxytocin is a powerful drug, and it has killed or maimed mothers through uterine rupture and even more babies through hypoxia from markedly hypertonic uterine contractions. The intravenous administration of oxytocin, however, has brought about a distinct advance in both its efficacy and safety. Failure to treat uterine dysfunction exposes the mother to increased hazards from maternal exhaustion, intrapartum infection, and traumatic operative delivery. At the same time, failure to treat uterine dysfunction may expose the fetus to an appreciably higher risk of death, whereas the risk from intravenous oxytocin should be negligible when used appropriately. Serious accidents, nevertheless, may accompany its use unless the precautions mentioned here are rigidly observed (Fig. 19–6).

One characteristic of intravenous oxytocin is that when successful, it acts promptly, leading to noticeable progress with little delay. Therefore, the drug need not

be used for an indefinite period of time to stimulate labor. It should be employed for no more than a few hours; if, by then, the cervix has not changed appreciably and if predictably easy vaginal delivery is not imminent, cesarean delivery should be performed. On the other hand, oxytocin should not be used to force cervical dilatation at a rate that exceeds normal (Cohen and Friedman, 1983). Ready resort to cesarean delivery in cases where oxytocin fails or in which there are contraindications to its use has served to appreciably diminish perinatal mortality and morbidity.

Stripping Membranes

Induction of labor by stripping the membranes is a relatively common practice, although there are few reports documenting the efficacy and safety of this practice. The potential for infection, bleeding from previously undiagnosed placenta previa, or low-lying placenta and accidental rupture of the membranes should be considered. McColgin and colleagues (1990) found in a randomized study involving 180 pregnancies that membrane stripping was safe and associated with a decreased incidence of postterm gestation. To date these results have not been confirmed by others.

Amniotomy

Artificial rupture of the membranes is an effective method of labor induction, particularly when the cervix is favorable. Amniotomy for the purpose of hastening spontaneous labor, however, has not proved effective (Fraser and co-workers, 1991). Several precautions to minimize the risk of cord prolapse should be observed when membranes are ruptured artificially. Care should be taken during amniotomy to avoid dislodging the fetal head. An assistant applying fundal and suprapubic pressure may reduce the risk of cord prolapse. The fetal heart rate should be assessed prior to and immediately after the procedure.

Ruptured Membranes Without Labor. Rupture of the membranes without spontaneous uterine contractions occurs in about 8 percent of term pregnancies (Duff and co-workers, 1984). Until recently, management generally included stimulation of contractions when labor did not commence after 6 to 12 hours of observation. This intervention evolved about 40 years ago because of maternal and fetal complications due to amnionitis (Calkins, 1952). Such routine intervention was the accepted practice until challenged by Kappy and co-workers (1979), when they reported excessive cesarean delivery in term pregnancies with ruptured membranes managed with labor stimulation compared with those managed by observation.

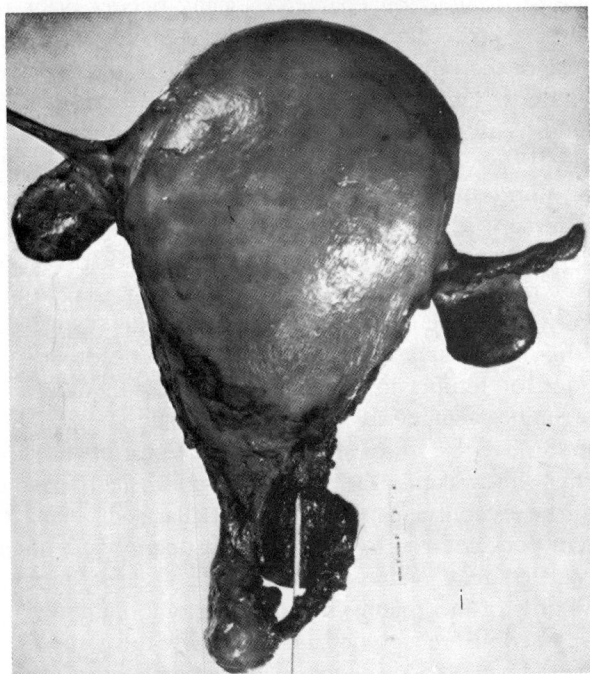

Fig. 19–6. Rupture of the lower uterine segment resulting from stimulation by dilute intravenous oxytocin in a 38-year-old multipara.

Duff and co-workers (1984) randomized 134 pregnancies of 36 weeks or more and an average of 5 hours' ruptured membranes to induction of labor or observation. Almost 75 percent of those randomized to observation entered labor spontaneously within 24 hours. The cesarean delivery rate almost was tripled in those receiving labor induction. In contrast, Wagner and associates (1989) randomized 182 pregnancies with 6 hours of ruptured membranes to immediate induction of labor or transfer to an antepartum unit to await spontaneous labor or evidence of infection. Those not in labor 24 hours after membrane rupture received labor inductions. Only 40 percent of those randomized to observation required inductions. These investigators concluded that there was no advantage to delaying intervention. Meikle and co-workers (1992) described that prostaglandin E_2 was successful in ripening the cervix in 146 women with ruptured membranes, no labor, and cervical dilatation of 2 cm or less.

Importantly, those recommending observation of ruptured membranes without labor at term are very careful. No other obstetrical or medical complications are permitted; the women are hospitalized until delivery; there is frequent surveillance of the fetal heart rate; a careful search is made for infection; and observation is generally limited to only those women with unfavorable cervices.

Prostaglandins. A variety of prostaglandins has been used, primarily outside the United States, for both cervical ripening and stimulation of labor. Most experiments in the United States have been with prostaglandin E_2 used for cervical ripening rather than labor induction. Typically, 20-mg prostaglandin E_2 (dinoprostone) vaginal suppositories have been modified by hospital pharmacies as doses in gel of 0.5 mg for intracervical use or up to 5 mg for vaginal use. None of the prostaglandins are currently approved by the Food and Drug Administration for cervical ripening or labor stimulation in the presence of a viable fetus. Lack of approval as reflected by a labeled indication for a drug does not contraindicate use of the same drug for unlabeled indications, provided there is an established policy and procedure for its use (U.S. Food and Drug Administration, 1982). Prostaglandin E_2 gel is currently under review for possible licensure for cervical ripening. Rayburn (1989) reviewed 16 reports published between 1978 and 1988 on prostaglandin E_2 gel for cervical ripening and concluded that because of its benefits, this drug should be made available commercially. Owen and co-workers (1991) were less enthusiastic about its efficacy.

A major difficulty in evaluating the safety and efficacy of cervical ripening with prostaglandin E_2 is the many regimens employed. For example, the incidence of uterine hyperstimulation varies considerably depending on the dosage of prostaglandin E_2 placed into the vagina or cervix. Egarter and co-workers (1990) studied nearly 3100 pregnancies treated with 3-mg intravaginal tablets or 2.5-mg and 0.5-mg intravaginal gels. The incidence of hyperstimulation was 7.3, 2.9, and 0.5 percent, respectively, as the dosage of prostaglandin E_2 was decreased. Overall, 6 percent of the women given prostaglandin E_2 developed hyperstimulation and three women had emergency cesarean deliveries. Perryman and associates (1992) compared quartered 20-mg E_2 suppositories to 5-mg doses of gel and discontinued the presumed 5-mg quartered suppositories because of unacceptable hyperstimulation. Maymon and co-authors (1991) reported a case of uterine rupture in association with application of 0.5 mg of intracervical prostaglandin E_2 gel.

Laminaria. Cervical ripening has been reported to be accomplished with use of laminaria as cervical dilators. Blumenthal and Ramanauskas (1990) compared a synthetic hydroscopic cervical dilator with *Laminaria japonicun* in 41 women with unripe cervices. As many dilators as could be comfortably tolerated were placed into the cervical canal the night before induction of labor. Approximately four synthetic cervical dilators were required and those given *laminaria* dilators required about 10 devices to fill the endocervical canal. The synthetic device was preferred because it appeared to work faster, but either dilator significantly ripened the cervix.

Treatment of Hypertonic Uterine Dysfunction. Hypertonic dysfunction is characterized by uterine pain that appears to be out of proportion to the intensity of contractions and certainly out of proportion to their effectiveness in effacing and dilating the cervix. This type of dysfunction characteristically occurs prior to the cervix reaching a dilatation of 4 cm or more. Because of the relative infrequency of this variety of dysfunctional labor, it has attracted little attention as a clinical entity, and thus its role in perinatal morbidity may be overlooked. **Placental abruption must always be considered as a possible cause of uterine hypertonus.**

Oxytocin is rarely indicated, if ever, in the presence of uterine hypertonus with a living fetus. Cesarean delivery should be employed if fetal distress is suspected. If the membranes are intact and there is no other evidence of fetopelvic disproportion, administration of morphine or meperidine will relieve pain and rest the mother as well as arrest the abnormal uterine activity. When she awakens, it is hoped that more effective labor will be established. It is important that such management does not lead to undue procrastination and unappreciated fetal distress, including passage of copious amounts of meconium into the amnionic fluid, and in turn, serious meconium aspiration by the fetus (see Chap. 44, p. 995). Tocolytic agents, such as ritodrine, have been used, presumably with some success, especially in other countries.

Inadequate Voluntary Expulsive Force

With achievement of full cervical dilatation, the great majority of women cannot resist the urge to "bear down" or "push" each time the uterus contracts. Typically, the laboring woman inhales deeply, closes her glottis, and contracts her abdominal musculature repetitively with vigor to generate increased intra-abdominal pressure throughout the time that the uterus is contracting. The combined force created by the contractions of the uterus and the abdominal musculature propels the fetus down the vagina and, in the case of spontaneous delivery, through the vaginal outlet.

Causes of Inadequate Expulsive Forces. At times, the magnitude of the force created by contractions of abdominal musculature is compromised sufficiently to prevent spontaneous vaginal delivery. Conduction analgesia—lumbar epidural, caudal, or intrathecal—is likely to reduce the reflex urge for the woman to "push," and at the same time may impair her ability to contract the abdominal muscles sufficiently. General anesthesia, with loss of consciousness, certainly imposes these adverse effects, as does *heavy* sedation.

In some instances, the inherent urge to "push" is overridden by the intensification of pain that is created by bearing down. Rarely, insufficient expulsive efforts may be the consequence of long-standing paralysis of the abdominal musculature, as may occur after poliomyelitis or transection of the spinal cord.

Management. Careful selection of the kind of analgesia and the timing of its administration are very important if compromise of voluntary expulsive efforts is to be avoided. With rare exception, intrathecal analgesia or general anesthesia should not be administered until all conditions for a safe, outlet forceps delivery have been met—that is, the fetal head is engaged, the sagittal suture is in the anteroposterior position, and the occiput distends the perineum and protrudes somewhat through the vaginal introitus with a contraction. With continuous epidural analgesia, it may be necessary to allow the paralytic effects to wear off so that the woman in response to coaching can generate intra-abdominal pressure sufficient to move the fetal head into position appropriate for outlet forceps delivery. The alternatives—a possibly difficult midforceps vaginal delivery or cesarean delivery—are unsatisfactory choices in the absence of any evidence of fetal distress.

For the woman who cannot bear down appropriately with each contraction because of great discomfort, analgesia is likely to be of considerable benefit. Perhaps the safest for both fetus and mother is nitrous oxide, mixed with an equal volume of oxygen and provided during the time of each uterine contraction. At the same time, appropriate encouragement and instruction are most likely to be of benefit.

Localized Abnormalities of Uterine Action

Pathological Retraction and Constriction Rings. Very rarely, localized rings or constrictions of the uterus develop in association with prolonged rupture of the membranes and protracted labors. The most common type is the so-called *pathological retraction ring of Bandl*, an exaggeration of the normal retraction ring described in Chapter 12 (p. 341). It is often, but not always, the result of obstructed labor, with marked stretching and thinning of the lower uterine segment. In such a situation, the ring may be seen clearly as an abdominal indentation and signifies impending rupture of the lower uterine segment (Fig. 20–11). Localized constrictions of the uterus are rarely seen today, because prolonged obstructed labor is no longer compatible with acceptable obstetrical practice. However, they may still occur occasionally as hourglass constrictions of the uterus following the birth of the first of twins. In such a situation, they can sometimes be relaxed and delivery effected with appropriate general anesthesia, but occasionally prompt cesarean delivery offers a better prognosis for the second twin (see Chap. 39, p. 911).

Precipitate Labor and Delivery

Precipitate—that is, extremely rapid—labor and delivery may result from an abnormally low resistance of the soft parts of the birth canal, from abnormally strong uterine and abdominal contractions, or *very rarely*, from the absence of painful sensations and thus a lack of awareness of vigorous labor.

Maternal Effects. Precipitate labor and delivery are seldom accompanied by serious maternal complications if the cervix is effaced appreciably and easily dilated, the vagina has been stretched previously, and the perineum is relaxed. However, vigorous uterine contractions combined with a long, firm cervix and a vagina, vulva, or perineum that resists stretch may lead to rupture of the uterus or extensive lacerations of the cervix, vagina, vulva, or perineum. It is in these latter circumstances that the rare condition *amnionic fluid embolism* is most likely to occur (see Chap. 37, p. 843). **The uterus that contracts with unusual vigor before delivery is likely to be hypotonic after delivery, with hemorrhage from the placental implantation site as the consequence** (see Chap. 27, p. 616).

Effects on Fetus and Neonate. Perinatal mortality and morbidity from precipitate labor may be increased considerably for several reasons. First, the tumultuous uterine contractions, often with negligible intervals of relaxation, prevent appropriate uterine blood flow and oxygenation of the fetal blood. Second, the resistance of the birth canal to expulsion of the head may cause intracranial trauma, although this must be rare. Moreover, Acker and colleagues (1988) reported that Erb–Duchenne palsy was associated with such labors in one third of cases. Third, during an unattended birth, the infant may fall to the floor and be injured or may need resuscitation that is not immediately available.

Treatment. Unusually forceful spontaneous uterine contractions are not likely to be modified to a significant degree by the administration of analgesia. The use of general anesthesia with agents that impair uterine contractibility, such as halothane and isofluvane, is often excessively heroic. Certainly, any oxytocic agents being administered should be stopped immediately. Tocolytic agents, such as ritodrine and parenteral magnesium sulfate, may prove effective. It is indefensible to lock the mother's legs or hold the baby's head back directly in attempts to delay delivery. Such maneuvers may damage the infant's brain.

References

Acker DB, Gregory KD, Sachs BP, Friedman EA: Risk factors for Erb-Duchenne palsy. Obstet Gynecol 71:389, 1988

American College of Obstetricians and Gynecologists: Induction and augmentation of labor. Technical bulletin no. 157, July 1991

American College of Obstetricians and Gynecologists: Dystocia. Technical bulletin no. 137, December 1989a

American College of Obstetricians and Gynecologists: Intrapartum fetal heart rate monitoring. Technical bulletin no. 132, September 1989b

American College of Obstetricians and Gynecologists: Obstetric forceps. ACOG Committee Opinion, no. 71, August 1989c

American College of Obstetricians and Gynecologists: Obstetric anesthesia and analgesia. Technical bulletin no. 112, January 1988

Blumenthal PD, Ramanauskas R: Randomized trial of Dilapan and laminaria as cervical ripening agents before induction of labor. Obstet Gynecol 75:305, 1990

Bottoms SF, Hirsch VJ, Sokol RJ: Medical management of arrest disorders of labor: A current overview. Am J Obstet Gynecol 156:939, 1987

Caldeyro-Barcia R: Oxytocin and pregnant human uterus. Paper presented at meeting of the 4th Pan-American Congress on Endocrinology, Buenos Aires, 1957

Caldeyro-Barcia R, Alvarez H, Reynolds SRM: A better understanding of uterine contractility through simultaneous recording with an internal and a seven channel external method. Surg Obstet Gynecol 91:641, 1950

Caldeyro-Barcia R, Poseiro JJ: Physiology of the uterine contraction. Clin Obstet Gynecol 3:386, 1960

Calkins LA: Premature spontaneous rupture of the membranes. Am J Obstet Gynecol 64:871, 1952

Carlson JM, Diehl JA, Murray MS, McRae M, Fenwick L, Friedman EA: Maternal position during parturition in normal labor. Obstet Gynecol 68:443, 1986

Cartmill RS, Thornton JG: Effect of presentation of partogram information on obstetric decision-making. Lancet 339:1520, 1992

Cohen W: Influence of the duration of second stage labor on perinatal outcome and puerperal morbidity. Obstet Gynecol 49:266, 1977

Cohen W, Friedman EA (eds): Management of Labor. Baltimore, University Park Press, 1983

DeMott RK, Sandmire HF: The Green Bay cesarean section study, II. The physician factor or a determinant of cesarean birth rates for failed labor. Am J Obstet Gynecol 166:1799, 1992

Duff P, Huff RW, Gibbs RS: Management of premature rupture of membranes and unfavorable cervix in term pregnancy. Obstet Gynecol 63:697, 1984

Dujardin B, DeSchampheleire I, Sene H, Ndiaye F: Value of the alert and action lines on the partogram. Lancet 339:1336, 1992

DuVigneaud V, Ressler C, Swan JM, Roberts CW, Katsoyannis PG, Gordon S: The synthesis of oxytocin. J Am Chem Soc 75:4879, 1953

Egarter CH, Hussein PW, Rayburn WF: Uterine hyperstimulation after low-dose prostaglandin E_2 therapy: Tocolytic treatment in 181 cases. Am J Obstet Gynecol 163:794, 1990

Ferenchak P, Collins JJ, Morgan A: Drop size and rate in parenteral infusion. Surgery 70:674, 1971

Fraser W, Sauve R, Parboosingh IJ, Fung T, Sokol R, Persaud D: A randomized trial of early amniotomy. Br J Obstet Gynaecol 98:84, 1991

Fraser W, Usher RH, McLean FH, Bossenberry C, Thomson ME, Kramer MS, Smith LP, Power H: Temporary variation in rates of cesarean section for dystocia: Does "convenience" play a role? Am J Obstet Gynecol 156:300, 1987

Friedman EA: Labor: Clinical Evaluation and Management, 2nd ed. New York, Appleton-Century-Crofts, 1978

Friedman EA: An objective approach to the diagnosis and management of abnormal labor. Bull NY Acad Med 48:842, 1972

Friedman EA: Primigravid labor. A graphicostatistical analysis. Obstet Gynecol 6:567, 1955

Friedman EA: The graphic analysis of labor. Am J Obstet Gynecol 68:1568, 1954

Friedman EA, Sachtleben MR: Amniotomy and the course of labor. Obstet Gynecol 22:755, 1963

Hauth JC, Hankins GD, Gilstrap III LC: Uterine contraction pressures achieved in parturients with active phase arrest. Obstet Gynecol 78:344, 1991

Hauth JC, Hankins GD, Gilstrap III LC, Strickland DM, Vance P: Uterine contraction pressures with oxytocin induction/augmentation. Obstet Gynecol 68:305, 1986

Hellman LM, Prystowsky H: The duration of the second stage of labor. Am J Obstet Gynecol 63:1223, 1952

Hendricks CH, Brenner WE, Kraus G: Normal cervical dilatation pattern in late pregnancy and labor. Am J Obstet Gynecol 106:1065, 1970

Hendricks CH, Quilligan EJ, Tyler AB, Tucker GJ: Pressure relationships between intervillous space and amniotic fluid in human term pregnancy. Am J Obstet Gynecol 77:1028, 1959

Hillis DS: Diagnosis of contracted pelvis. Ill Med J 74:131, 1938

Jeffcoate TNA: Prolonged labor. Lancet 2:61, 1961

Kappy KA, Cetrulo C, Knuppel RA: Premature rupture of membranes: Conservative approach. Am J Obstet Gynecol 134:655, 1979

Kilpatrick SJ, Laros RK: Characteristics of normal labor. Obstet Gynecol 74:85, 1989

Larks SD: Electrohysterography. Springfield, IL, Thomas, 1960

Leveno KJ, Satin AJ, Sherman ML, McIntire DD: Spontaneous parturition in 24,838 women. Presented at the Annual Meeting of the American Association of Gynecologists and Obstetricians, Hot Springs, VA, September, 1992

Lupe PJ, Gross TL: Maternal upright posture and mobility in labor: A review. Obstet Gynecol 67:727, 1986

Maymon R, Shulman A, Pomeranz M, Holtzinger M, Haimovich L, Bagary C: Uterine rupture at term pregnancy with the use of intracervical prostaglandin E$_2$ gel for induction of labor. Am J Obstet Gynecol 165:368, 1991

McColgin SW, Hampton HL, McCaul JF, Howard PR, Andrew ME, Morrison JC: Stripping membranes at term: Can it safely reduce the incidence of post-term pregnancy? Obstet Gynecol 76:678, 1990

Meikle SF, Bissell ME, Freedman WL, Gibbs RS: A retrospective review of the efficacy and safety of prostaglandin E$_2$ with premature rupture of the membranes at term. Obstet Gynecol 80:76, 1992

Miller FC: Uterine motility in spontaneous labor. Clin Obstet Gynecol 26:78, 1983

O'Connor TCF, Woods RE, Cavanaugh D: Indications for the simulation of labor. In Parke-Davis & Company: Oxytocin-induced Labor. Greenwich, CT, CPC Communications, 1976, p 10

O'Driscoll K, Meagher D: Diagnosis of labor. In Active Management of Labour. London, Saunders, 1980, p 23

Owen J, Winkler CL, Harris BA, Hauth JC, Smith MC: A randomized, double-blind trial of prostaglandin E$_2$ gel for cervical ripening and meta-analysis. Am J Obstet Gynecol 165:991, 1991

Peisner DB, Rosen MG: Transition from latent to active labor. Obstet Gynecol 68:448, 1986

Perkins RP: Discussions of The Green Bay cesarean section study, II. The physician factor as a determinant of cesarean birth rates for failed labor by RK DeMott, HF Landmire. Am J Obstet Gynecol 166:1799, 1992

Perryman D, Yeast JD, Holst V: Cervical ripening: A randomized study comparing prostaglandin E$_2$ gel to prostaglandin E$_2$ suppositories. Obstet Gynecol 79:670, 1992

Philpott RH, Castle WM: Cervicographs in the management of labour in primigravidae. J Obstet Gynaecol Br Commonw 79:592, 1972

Rayburn WF: Prostaglandin E$_2$ gel for cervical ripening and induction of labor: A critical analysis. Am J Obstet Gynecol 160:529, 1989

Reynolds SRM, Heard OO, Bruns P, Hellman LM: A multichannel strain-gauge tokodynamometer: An instrument for studying patterns of uterine contractions in pregnant women. Bull Johns Hopkins Hosp 82:446, 1948

Rodesch F, Ellinger LE, Wilkin P, Hubinont PO: Introduction, use and results of a new partogram. J Obstet Gynaecol Br Commonw 72:930, 1965

Rosen MG: Management of Labor. Physician Judgment and Patient Care. New York, Elsevier, 1990, p 52

Satin AJ, Leveno KJ, Sherman ML, Brewster DS, Cunningham FG: High- versus low-dose oxytocin for labor stimulation. Obstet Gynecol 80:111, 1992b

Satin AJ, Leveno KJ, Sherman ML, McIntire DD: Factors affecting the dose response to oxytocin for labor stimulation. Am J Obstet Gynecol 166:1260, 1992a

Seitchik J, Castillo M: Oxytocin augmentation of dysfunctional labor, II. Uterine activity data. Am J Obstet Gynecol 145:226, 1983

Seitchik J, Holden AE, Castillo M: Spontaneous rupture of the membrane, functional dystocia, oxytocin treatment, and the route of delivery. Am J Obstet Gynecol 156:125, 1987

Shiono PH, McNellis D, Rhoads GG: Reasons for the rising cesarean delivery rates: 1978–1984. Obstet Gynecol 1969:696, 1987

Sokol RJ, Stojkov J, Chik L, Rosen MG: Normal and abnormal labor progress, I. A quantitative assessment and survey of the literature. J Reprod Med 18:47, 1977

Steer CM: Effect of type of delivery on future childbearing. Am J Obstet Gynecol 60:395, 1950

Stewart PJ, Dulberg C, Arnill AC, Elmslie T, Hall PF: Diagnosis of dystocia and management with cesarean section among primiparous women in Ottawa-Carleton. Can Med Assoc J 142:459, 1990

Studd J: Partograms and nomograms of cervical dilatation in management of primigravid labour. Br Med J 4:451, 1973

U.S. Food and Drug Administration: Use of approved drugs for unlabeled indications. FDA Bull 12:4, 1982

Wagner MV, Chin VP, Peters CJ, Drexler B, Newman LA: A comparison of early and delayed induction of labor with spontaneous rupture of membranes at term. Obstet Gynecol 74:93, 1989

Williams RM, Thom MH, Studd JW: A study of the benefits and acceptability of ambulation in spontaneous labor. Br J Obstet Gynaecol 87:122, 1980

CHAPTER 20

Dystocia Due to Abnormalities in Presentation, Position, or Development of the Fetus

Breech Presentation

Incidence. Breech presentation is common remote from term, as demonstrated in Table 20–1. Most often, however, some time before the onset of labor the fetus turns spontaneously to a vertex presentation so that breech presentation persists in only about 3 to 4 percent of singleton deliveries. For example, 3 percent of 49,156 singleton infants delivered from 1983 through 1986 at Parkland Hospital presented as breech (Table 20–2).

Etiology. As term approaches, the uterine cavity, for reasons that are not entirely clear, most often accommodates the fetus in a longitudinal lie with the vertex presenting. Breeches are much more common at the end of the second trimester of pregnancy than at or near term (Table 20–1). Factors other than gestational age that appear to predispose to breech presentation include uterine relaxation associated with great parity, multiple fetuses, hydramnios, oligohydramnios, hydrocephalus, anencephalus, previous breech delivery, uterine anomalies, and tumors in the pelvis.

Implantation of the placenta in either cornual–fundal region of the uterus has been suspected of predisposing to breech presentation. Fianu and Vaclavinkova (1978) provided sonographic evidence of a much higher prevalence of placental implantation in the cornual–fundal region for breech presentations (73 percent) than for vertex presentations (5 percent). The frequency of breech presentation is also increased with placenta previa, but only a small minority of breech presentations are associated with placenta previa. No strong correlation has been shown between breech presentation and a contracted pelvis in most reports.

A live fetus is *not* required for a fetus to change presentations spontaneously. For example, a woman was admitted to Parkland Hospital at term with a fetus known to be dead, confirmed by real-time sonography examinations. The presentation was cephalic during the first oxytocin induction, which proved unsuccessful. Three days later, at the time of the second attempt at induction of labor, the fetus was in a breech presentation. Three days later, at the time of a third and successful induction of labor, the fetus was again in a cephalic presentation!

Significance. In the persistent breech presentation, an *increased* frequency of the following complications can be anticipated: (1) perinatal morbidity and mortality from difficult delivery; (2) low birthweight from preterm delivery, growth retardation, or both; (3) prolapsed cord; (4) placenta previa; (5) fetal, neonatal, and infant anomalies; (6) uterine anomalies and tumors; (7) multiple fetuses; and (8) operative intervention, especially cesarean delivery.

Diagnosis. The varying relations between the lower extremities and buttocks of breech presentations form the categories of frank, complete, and incomplete breech presentations (Figs. 10–2 to 10–4, pp. 274–275). With a **frank breech** presentation, the lower extremities are flexed at the hips and extended at the knees, and thus the feet lie in close proximity to the head. A **complete breech** presentation differs from a frank breech presentation in that one or both knees are flexed rather than both extended. With **incomplete breech** presentation, one or both hips are not flexed and one or both feet or knees lie below the breech, that is, a foot or knee is lowermost in the birth canal. The frank breech appears most commonly when the diagnosis is established radiologically near term.

Abdominal Examination. Typically, with the first maneuver of Leopold the hard, round, readily ballottable fetal head is found to occupy the fundus of the uterus (Fig. 20–1). The second maneuver indicates the back to be on one side of the abdomen and the small parts on the other. On the third maneuver, if engagement has not occurred—that is, if the intertrochanteric diameter of the fetal pelvis has not passed through the pelvic inlet—the breech is movable above the pelvic inlet. After engagement, the fourth maneuver shows the firm breech to be beneath the symphysis. The heart sounds of the fetus are usually heard loudest slightly above the umbilicus, whereas with engagement of the fetal head the heart sounds are loudest below the umbilicus.

Vaginal Examination. The diagnosis of a frank breech presentation is confirmed vaginally by palpating its characteristic components. Both ischial tuberosities, the sacrum, and the anus are usually palpable, and after further descent, the external genitalia may be distinguished. Especially when labor is prolonged, the but-

493

TABLE 20–1. FETAL PRESENTATION AT VARIOUS GESTATIONAL AGES DETERMINED SONOGRAPHICALLY

Gestation (wk)	Total Number	Percent		
		Cephalic	*Breech*	*Other*
21–24	264	54.6	33.3	12.1
25–28	367	61.9	27.8	10.4
29–32	443	78.1	14.0	7.9
33–36	638	88.7	8.8	2.5
37–40	463	91.5	6.7	1.7

From Scheer and Nubar (1976).

tocks may become markedly swollen, rendering differentiation of face and breech very difficult; the anus may be mistaken for the mouth, and the ischial tuberosities for the malar eminences. Careful examination, however, should prevent this error, because the finger encounters muscular resistance with the anus, whereas the firmer, less yielding jaws are felt through the mouth. Furthermore, the finger, upon removal from the anus, is sometimes stained with meconium. The mouth and malar eminences form a triangular shape, while the ischial tuberosities and anus are in a straight line. The most accurate information, however, is based on the location of the sacrum and its spinous processes, which establishes the diagnosis of position and variety.

In complete breech presentations, the feet may be felt alongside the buttocks, and in footling presentations, one or both feet are inferior to the buttocks (Fig. 20–2). In footling presentations, the foot can readily be identified as right or left on the basis of the relation to the great toe. When the breech has descended farther into the pelvic cavity, the genitalia may be felt; if not markedly edematous, they may permit identification of fetal sex.

X-ray, Computed Tomography, and Ultrasonic Examinations. Sonography should ideally be used to confirm a clinically suspected breech presentation and to identify, if possible, any fetal anomalies. Unfortunately, sonography usually cannot be used to identify the relationship of the lower extremities to the fetal pelvis, and this information is often essential in planning the route of delivery (see Chap. 25, p. 578).

TABLE 20–2. FETAL PRESENTATION IN 49,156 SINGLETON PREGNANCIES AT PARKLAND HOSPITAL, 1983–1986

Presentation	Number	Percent	Incidence
Cephalic	47,497	96.6	—
Breech	1468	3.0	1:33
Transverse	117	0.24	1:420
Face	41	0.08	1:1200
Compound	22	0.05	1:2235
Brow	11	0.02	1:4470

If cesarean delivery is planned without exception, there are few justifications for x-rays. If, however, the woman is in labor and vaginal delivery is considered, the type of breech presentation is of considerable importance (see Chap. 25, p. 578). In this instance, radiation exposure may be reduced considerably by using computed tomographic pelvimetry (Kopelman and associates, 1986). These imaging techniques can be used to provide information about the type of breech presentation, presence or absence of a flexed fetal head, and accurate measurements of the pelvis (see Chap. 11, p. 292).

Labor. There are fundamental differences between labor and delivery in cephalic and breech presentations, as described in Chapter 25. With a cephalic presentation, once the head is delivered, typically the rest of the body follows without difficulty. With a breech, however, successively larger and very much less compressible parts of the fetus are born.

Spontaneous complete expulsion of the fetus who presents as a breech, as described below, is seldom accomplished successfully. As a rule, either cesarean delivery (see Chap. 26) or vaginal delivery requires skilled participation by the obstetrician for a favorable outcome (see Chap. 25).

Prognosis. Both mother and fetus are at greater risk with breech presentation compared with cephalic presentation, but to nowhere near the same degree. In an analysis of 57,819 pregnancies in the Netherlands, Schutte and colleagues (1985) reported that even after correction for gestational age, congenital defects, and birthweight, perinatal mortality was higher in breech than in vertex infants. They concluded "it is possible that breech presentation is not coincidental but is a consequence of poor fetal quality, in which case medical intervention is unlikely to reduce the perinatal mortality associated with breech presentation to the level associated with vertex presentation."

The possibility that a breech presentation might be a factor identifying an already abnormal fetus had been suggested earlier by Hytten (1982) and by Susuki and Yamamuro (1985). This concept was strengthened even more by the report of Nelson and Ellenberg (1986), who observed that one third of the children with cerebral palsy who were in a breech presentation at birth had major noncerebral malformations.

Maternal. Because of the greater frequency of operative delivery, including cesarean delivery, there is a higher maternal morbidity and slightly higher mortality for pregnancies complicated by persistent breech presentation (Collea and co-authors, 1980). This risk is likely increased even more if an emergency operation is performed instead of an elective cesarean delivery (Bingham and Lilford, 1987). Labor is usually not prolonged;

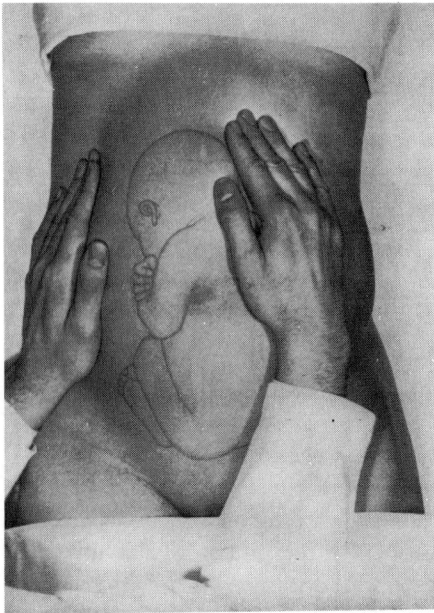

A

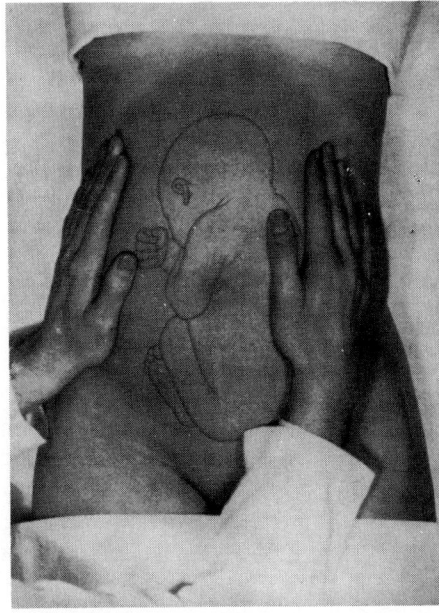

B

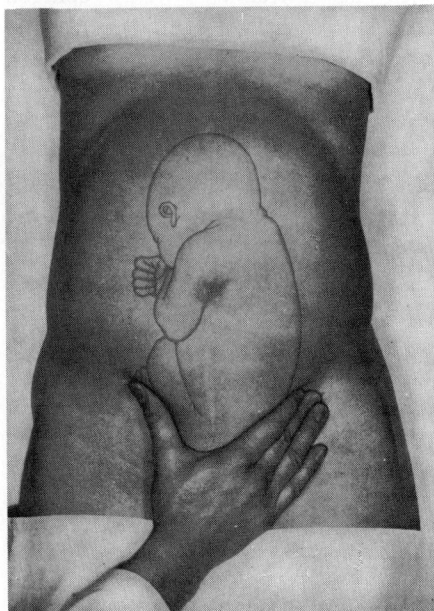

C

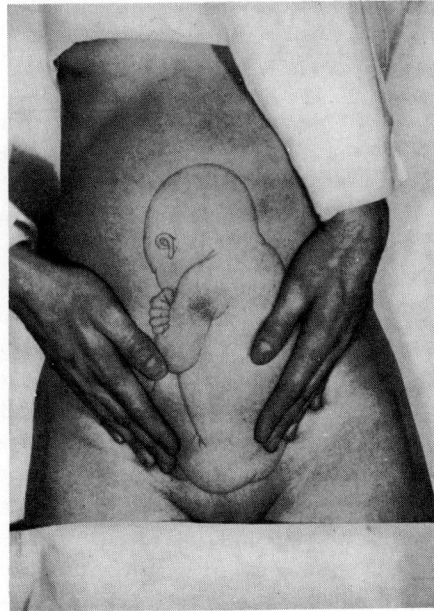

D

Fig. 20–1. Palpation in left sacroanterior position. **A.** First maneuver. **B.** Second maneuver. **C.** Third maneuver. **D.** Fourth maneuver.

Hall and Kohl (1956), in a large series of cases, reported the median duration of labor to be 9.2 hours for nulliparas and 6.1 hours for multiparas.

Fetus-Infant. **The prognosis for the fetus in a breech presentation is considerably worse than when in a vertex presentation.** The major contributors to perinatal loss are preterm delivery, congenital anomalies, and birth trauma. Brenner and associates (1974) provided a careful analysis of the characteristics and perils to the fetus from breech presentation. They determined the overall mortality rate for 1016 breech

deliveries to be 25 percent compared with 2.6 percent for nonbreech deliveries at the University Hospitals of Cleveland. At every stage of gestation, they identified antepartum, intrapartum, and neonatal deaths to be significantly greater among breeches and the average Apgar scores to be lower for those who survived. During the latter half of pregnancy, the birthweight at any gestational age was somewhat less for breech infants than for nonbreech infants. Congenital abnormalities were identified in 6.3 percent of breech deliveries compared with 2.4 percent in nonbreech deliveries.

Tank and associates (1971) examined the character

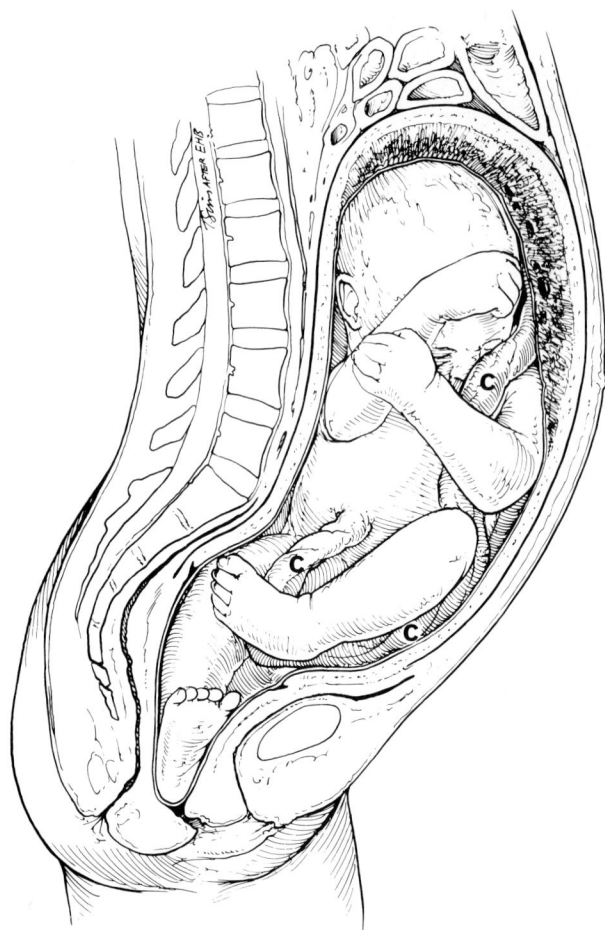

Fig. 20–2. Double-footling breech presentation in labor with membranes intact. Note possibility of umbilical cord accident at any instant, especially after rupture of membranes. (C = umbilical cord.)

of serious traumatic vaginal delivery. At autopsy, the organs most frequently found to be injured were, in order of frequency, the brain, spinal cord, liver, adrenal glands, and spleen. It is of interest that, in retrospective analysis of cases of "idiopathic" adrenal calcification, breech delivery was very common. Other sites of injuries from vaginal delivery included the brachial plexus; the pharynx, in the form of tears or pseudodiverticula from the obstetrician's finger in the mouth as part of the Mauriceau maneuver (see Fig. 25–7, p. 582); and the bladder, which might be ruptured if distended. Traction might injure the sternocleidomastoid muscle and, if not appropriately treated, lead to torticollis (see Chap. 44, p. 1044).

Similar results were reported from the Los Angeles Women's Hospital by Gimovsky and Paul (1982). They observed an overall mortality rate for all breech presentations of 8.5 percent compared with a 2.2 percent rate for cephalic presentations. These results were obtained despite a cesarean delivery rate of 75 percent for all breech presentations. Thus, even with liberal use of cesarean delivery and after exclusion of very preterm

fetuses or fetuses with severe congenital anomalies, there still remained a twofold risk for the infant delivered as a breech compared with the overall population.

Green and associates (1982) reported distressing results obtained for breeches managed during 1963 to 1972 at the Royal Victoria Hospital in Montreal compared with 1978 to 1979. In the decade 1963 to 1972, the cesarean delivery rate was 22 percent compared with 94 percent for 1978 to 1979. In spite of the significant increase in cesarean delivery rates, fetal asphyxia rates remained the same, despite a *trend* toward decreased fetal trauma and death. The authors concluded that cesarean delivery alone could not guarantee a good infant outcome because the "maneuvers of extracting a breech by cesarean delivery are similar to those associated with the delivery of a breech via the vaginal route." A similar warning that cesarean delivery alone cannot assure a better outcome was given by Calvert (1980), who urged a more liberal use of large uterine incisions for breeches.

Term Fetus. Collea and colleagues (1980) reported the results of a *prospective study* designed to identify the optimal method of delivery for the term frank breech fetus. Almost half of these women were excluded from further consideration because of possible fetopelvic disproportion based on x-ray pelvimetry. A total of 60 infants were eventually delivered vaginally, and all survived although 2 sustained brachial plexus injuries. There were no perinatal deaths, but half of the 148 women who had cesarean deliveries experienced significant morbidity compared with only 7 percent of 60 women who were delivered vaginally. Similar results were reported by Watson and Benson (1984) and by Flanagan and co-workers (1987).

Gimovsky and associates (1983) published the results of a prospective study designed to identify the optimal method of delivery for the term *nonfrank* breech fetus. There were 105 women in labor with nonfrank breech presentations entered into the study. Two thirds were placed in the group for a trial of labor and a third underwent elective cesarean delivery. Of those placed in the labor group, 31 (44 percent) delivered vaginally and 39 (56 percent) required cesarean delivery. The largest single reason for a cesarean delivery in the trial of labor group was inadequate pelvic dimensions observed by x-ray pelvimetry (60 percent). Neonatal morbidity assessed by Apgar scores, cord blood pH, birth injury, and hospital stay was essentially the same for infants delivered vaginally or by cesarean, except for one infant who died following a vaginal delivery. This infant death was attributed to inadequate resuscitation. Maternal morbidity in terms of fever, blood transfusions, wound infections, and length of hospital stay was greater among women with cesarean deliveries. This was an interesting evaluation of vaginal delivery of nonfrank breeches; however, the one perinatal death is of concern. This rate, if maintained, would be equivalent to a death rate of 32 per 1000.

In the retrospective study by Fortney and colleagues (1986), in which outcome variables were analyzed for nearly 11,000 breech deliveries from 86 hospitals throughout the world, the inescapable conclusion was that vaginal delivery of term footling breeches was associated with prohibitive perinatal mortality. They also reported that perinatal mortality increased significantly in vaginally delivered breeches weighing more than 3500 g, regardless of the type of breech.

Preterm Fetus. Vaginal delivery as a breech may be hazardous to the preterm infant. Ingemarsson and associates (1978) compared neonatal mortality and the frequency of subsequent developmental abnormalities in 42 preterm breech infants delivered by cesarean versus 48 preterm infants delivered vaginally. For those delivered vaginally, 6 succumbed, and developmental abnormalities were detected at 12 months of age in one fourth of the survivors. This compared with 2 deaths and 1 developmental abnormality among women undergoing cesarean delivery.

In a review of the method of delivery for very-low-birthweight infants, Westgren and Paul (1985b) summarized mortality rates in vaginally versus cesarean-delivered breech infants weighing less than 1500 g. Their summary included the results of their own study (Westgren and colleagues, 1985a) and those reported in 13 earlier studies. The mortality rate for over 5000 vaginally delivered infants was 45 percent; it was 18 percent for nearly 4300 infants delivered by cesarean. Furthermore, in each report, morbidity was greater in the vaginally delivered infants. Similarly, Morales and Koerten (1986) reported that intracranial hemorrhage and mortality were reduced significantly in abdominally delivered breech infants weighing less than 1500 g, when compared with those delivered vaginally. Bodmer and associates (1986) reported that head entrapment in vaginally delivered infants weighing less than 1000 g was a significant cause of neonatal mortality. Unfortunately, they also concluded that despite cesarean delivery, newborn depression and mortality were not always prevented.

The rather universal acceptance of primary cesarean delivery for infants less than 2000 g has been questioned by two groups of investigators. Cox and associates (1982) compared 1973 to 1974 and 1979 to 1980 morbidity and mortality figures for breech infants under 2500 g delivered at Coventry Maternity Hospital. They concluded that the perinatal mortality rate had decreased, but the increased survival rate was accounted for by the survival of handicapped infants. They speculated that the increased overall survival rate might have been the result of neonatal intensive care rather than the consequence of the increased cesarean delivery rate. Effer and associates (1983) reported that peri-

natal mortality decreased by 20 percent from 1976 to 1980 in very-low-birthweight infants. During the same time the cesarean delivery rate increased from 12 to 49 percent for these infants. They raised the possibility that the increased cesarean delivery rate might be incidental and in no way related to the observed improved outcome.

At Parkland Hospital, when delivery is indicated or when there is active labor, our practice is to perform a cesarean delivery for any live fetus presenting breech who weighs less than 2000 g and more than 700 g (26 weeks' gestation). We agree with Thiery (1987) and conclude that, despite the arguments advanced that no prospective study has been performed for breech fetuses in this weight range delivered vaginally versus by cesarean, the evidence presented above is sufficient to support this practice.

External Cephalic Version. Whenever a breech presentation is recognized during the third trimester, an attempt may be made to substitute a cephalic presentation by *external version* (see Chap. 25). This procedure, well known to our obstetrical predecessors, has received renewed interest in the past 2 decades coincident with the availability of ultrasound, electronic fetal heart rate monitoring, and β-mimetic uterine relaxants. It is likely that these developments have improved the maternal and fetal safety of external version compared with prior obstetrical eras.

Van Dorsten and co-workers (1981) rekindled interest in this procedure in the United States. They used ultrasound, fetal monitoring, and a uterine relaxant (terbutaline) in 25 pregnancies randomized to receive external version between 37 and 39 weeks' gestation and compared outcomes with 23 similar pregnancies managed without version. Approximately 70 percent of the versions were successful, resulting in a 30 percent cesarean delivery rate compared with 75 percent when version was not attempted. Several other reports concerning the efficacy of external version are summarized in Table 20–3. Hanss (1990) concluded that the overall impact was small because successful versions represented less than 10 percent of all breech deliveries at his hospital. Marchick (1988) also observed that not all women with breech presentations diagnosed before labor are being offered external version.

As experiences with external version have expanded in recent years, several investigators have attempted to refine the factors associated with success or failure. Hughey (1985) used ultrasound at 20, 30, and 36 weeks in nearly 1700 pregnancies and found that fetal presentations are unstable until about 36 weeks' gestation. Thus, attempts at external version much before 36 to 37 weeks are not warranted because of the likelihood that the fetus will spontaneously change its presentation. Other factors reported to improve success of external version include frank breech presentation,

TABLE 20–3. RESULTS OF EXTERNAL CEPHALIC VERSION FOR BREECH PRESENTATIONS PERFORMED LATE IN PREGNANCY

Study	Tocolysis	Attempts	Successes No. (%)	Successful Version Vertex at Delivery No. (%)	Control Patients Vertex at Delivery No. (%)	Complications
Brocks and colleagues (1984)	Yes	130	53 (41)	53 (100)	8/56 (14)	None
Dyson and associates (1986)	Yes	158	122 (77)	122 (100)	5/40 (12)	Fetal bradycardia during version (7)
Morrison and co-workers (1986)	Yes	304	207 (68)	201 (97)	Not done	None
Stine and co-authors (1985)	Yes	148	108 (73)	95/102 (93)[a]	4/23 (17)	Fetomaternal bleed (4%); unexplained fetal death (1); maternal mortality—amnionic fluid embolus (1)
Totals		740	490 (67)	471/483 (97)	17/119 (14)	

[a] Six patients lost to follow-up.

anteriorly located fetal spine, ample amnionic fluid volume, and parity (Donald and Barton, 1990; Hellstrom and co-workers, 1990). Fortunato and co-authors (1988) observed that descent of the breech into the pelvis was a factor associated with failed versions.

Frequent and sometimes serious fetal heart rate changes may result from external version. Phelan and associates (1984) reported that 40 percent of version attempts were associated with fetal heart rate changes. The most common changes were bradycardia, variable decelerations, and tachycardia, likely due to umbilical cord occlusion during fetal manipulation. All of these changes were transient, although two women were admitted because of prolonged bradycardia.

Complications. Chapman and associates (1978) described fetal spinal cord transection after an unsuccessful attempt at version. Marcus and associates (1975) identified significant fetomaternal hemorrhage in 6 of 100 pregnancies, and Gjode (1980) reported fetomaternal bleeds in 14 of 50 women during the first attempt at external version. He recommends that immunoprophylaxis with anti-D globulin be given *prior* to attempting external version in pregnant women who are D-negative (see Chap. 44, p. 1008).

Stine and co-workers (1985) reported a maternal death due to amnionic fluid embolus and one unexplained fetal death. Kasule and associates (1985) reported three perinatal deaths, two due to abruption and one to prematurely ruptured membranes and vaginal delivery. In this study, however, attempted versions were begun after 30 weeks' gestation. Petrikovsky and colleagues (1987) reported a case of fetal brachial plexus injury after a successful external version.

Problems with Vaginal Delivery. Major problems do arise from vaginal delivery of a fetus in a breech presentation. Delivery of the breech draws the umbilicus and attached cord into the pelvis, which compresses the cord. Therefore, once the breech has passed beyond the vaginal introitus, the abdomen, thorax, arms, and head must be delivered promptly. This involves the delivery of successively less readily compressible parts. With a term fetus, some degree of molding of the fetal head may be essential for the head to negotiate the birth canal successfully. In this unfortunate circumstance, the alternatives with vaginal delivery are both unsatisfactory; delivery may be delayed many minutes while the aftercoming head accommodates to the maternal pelvis, but hypoxia and acidosis become severe; or delivery may be forced, causing trauma from compression, traction, or both, to brain, spinal cord, skeleton, and abdominal viscera.

With a preterm fetus, the disparity between the size of the head and buttocks is even greater than with a larger fetus. At times, the buttocks and lower extremities of the preterm fetus will pass through the cervix and be delivered, and yet the cervix will not be dilated adequately for the head to escape without trauma to the infant (Bodmer and associates, 1986). In this circumstance, Dührssen incisions of the cervix may be attempted (see Chap. 24, p. 573). Even so, trauma to the fetus and mother may be appreciable, and fetal hypoxia may prove harmful.

The frequency of cord prolapse is increased when the fetus is small or when the breech is not frank. Collea and co-workers (1978) reviewed the incidence of cord prolapse in association with the various types of breech presentation. The incidence of cord prolapse with frank breech presentation was about 0.5 percent, which is similar to the incidence (0.4 percent) reported for cephalic presentations (Barrett, 1991). In contrast, the incidence of cord prolapse with footling presentation was 15 to 18 percent, and it was 4 to 6 percent with complete breech presentation. Interestingly, Soernes and Bakke (1986) confirmed earlier observations that the umbilical cord length is significantly shorter in breech compared with cephalic presentations. Moreover, multiple coils of cord entangling the fetus are more common in breech presentations (Spellacy and associates, 1966). These umbilical cord abnormalities likely play a role in the development of breech presentation as well as the relatively high incidence of fetal distress in labor. For example, Flanagan and co-workers (1987) selected 244 women with a variety of breech presentations (72 percent were frank breech) for a trial of labor, and there was a cord prolapse in 4 percent. Fetal distress not due to cord prolapse was diagnosed in another 5 percent of women selected for vaginal delivery. Overall, 10 percent of the women identified for vaginal birth underwent cesarean deliveries for fetal jeopardy in labor.

Neonatal Apgar scores of vaginally delivered breeches are generally lower than when elective cesarean delivery is done (Flanagan and co-workers, 1987). This is particularly true for the 1-minute Apgar score. Similarly, neonatal cord blood acid-base values are significantly different for vaginally delivered breech presentations. Christian and Brady (1991) reported that umbilical artery blood pH was lower, P_{CO_2} higher, and HCO_3 lower compared with cephalic deliveries. However, Socol and colleagues (1988) concluded that cesarean delivery could improve Apgar scores but not appreciably improve acid-base status of the vaginally delivered breech neonate. Flanagan and co-workers (1987) emphasized that ultimate infant outcome for breech birth was not worsened by these significant differences in Apgar scores or acid-base status at birth.

Recommendations for Delivery. A diligent search for any other complication, actual or anticipated, that might further justify cesarean delivery has become a feature of many obstetricians' philosophy for managing delivery of breech presentations. In attempts to minimize infant mortality and morbidity, cesarean delivery is now commonly used in the following circumstances to deliver all but the extremely immature fetus whose potential for survival is negligible: (1) a large fetus; (2) any degree of contraction or unfavorable shape of the pelvis; (3) a hyperextended head; (4) no labor, with maternal or fetal indications for delivery such as pregnancy-induced hypertension or ruptured membranes for 12 hours or more; (5) uterine dysfunction; (6) a footling presentation; (7) an apparently healthy but preterm fetus of 26 weeks or more, with the mother in either active labor or in need of delivery; (8) severe fetal growth retardation; (9) previous perinatal death or children suffering from birth trauma; and (10) a request for sterilization.

Large Fetus. Rovinsky and associates (1973) and Fortney and colleagues (1986) noted that fetal morbidity and mortality rates at term increased with birthweight. Therefore, the fetus estimated to weigh 3600 g or more often will benefit from cesarean delivery even though the pelvis appears adequate. This allows for underestimation of fetal weight, a relatively common phenome-

non when the fetus is large. With the head free in the uterine fundus, sonographic measurements of biparietal diameter to estimate fetal size are more likely to be erroneous than with a vertex presentation (Chap. 21, p. 521). Nonetheless, the obstetrician should feel more secure about estimates of fetal size if there is good agreement between the clinical and sonographic estimates.

Unfavorable Pelvis. In contrast to labor with a cephalic presentation, there is no time for molding of the aftercoming head. Therefore, a moderately contracted pelvis that had not previously caused problems in delivery of an average-size vertex fetus might prove dangerous with a breech. Rovinsky and colleagues (1973) urge not only accurate measurements of the pelvic dimensions but also precise evaluation of the pelvic architecture rather than reliance on pelvic indexes. Gynecoid (round) and anthropoid (elliptical) pelves are favorable configurations, but platypelloid (anteroposteriorly flat) and android (heart-shaped) pelves are not (see Chap. 11, p. 287). The platypelloid pelvis is typically narrowed anteroposteriorly, which is unfavorable for the aftercoming head. The android pelvis has a narrow forepelvis, which renders the inlet less favorable than indicated by the pelvic diameters.

Hyperextension of Fetal Head. In perhaps 5 percent of breech presentations at or near term, the fetal head may be in extreme hyperextension (Fig. 20–3). Most often, the cause of hyperextension is not apparent, but vaginal delivery may result in injury to the cervical spinal cord. In general, evidence for marked hyperextension of the fetal head after labor has begun is considered an indication of cesarean delivery (Svenningsen and associates, 1985).

No Labor or Uterine Dysfunction. Induction of labor in women with a breech presentation is defended by some and condemned by others. Brenner and associates (1974) noted no significant differences in mortality rates and Apgar scores between cases with induced labor and those with spontaneous labor. In instances in which oxytocin was used to augment labor, however, infant mortality rates were higher, and Apgar scores were lower. Gimovsky and Paul (1982) observed that augmentation of labor was followed by vaginal delivery in only 2 of 9 women, both multiparous. Moreover, one of the two deliveries resulted in entrapment of the aftercoming fetal head. The general policy at Parkland Hospital is to resort to cesarean delivery, rather than use oxytocin to induce or augment labor, unless the fetus is previable or has a severe anomaly.

Footling Breech Presentations. The possibility of compression of a prolapsed cord or a cord entangled around

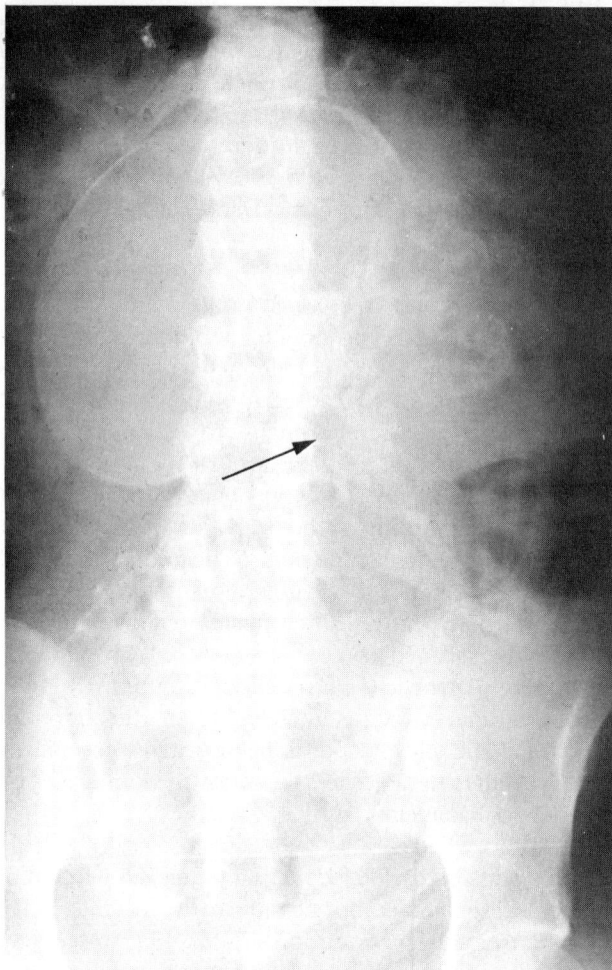

Fig. 20–3. Radiological demonstration of a complete breech presentation with a markedly hyperextended cervical spine (*arrow*) and head. Cesarean delivery resulted in a normal newborn infant.

the extremities as the breech fills the pelvis, if not before, is a threat to the fetus (Fig. 20–2).

Preterm Delivery. With a preterm fetus, the aftercoming head may be trapped by a cervix that is sufficiently effaced and dilated to allow passage of the thorax but not the less compressible head. The consequences of vaginal delivery in this circumstance all too often have been both hypoxia and physical trauma, both of which are especially deleterious to the preterm infant. Delivery of the apparently healthy, although preterm, fetus by cesarean reduces the risks of hypoxia, birth trauma, and their sequelae.

Previous Pregnancy Wastage. The compelling desire to minimize any likelihood of trauma to the fetus may lead to the decision for a cesarean delivery.

Desire for Sterilization. For the woman with a breech presentation who desires sterilization, the risk of cesar-

ean delivery and sterilization is no greater, and probably less, than the summation of risks from vaginal breech delivery followed by sterilization.

Vaginal Delivery. Vaginal delivery should be relatively safe for a frank breech presentation if the following conditions apply. (1) The pelvis is not contracted when examined by imaging pelvimetry. A previous cephalic delivery by itself is not proof that the pelvis may not be "contracted" for a breech delivery (Bistoletti and colleagues, 1981). (2) The fetus is judged not to be more than 3600 g when examined independently by two or more trained examiners or when estimated ultrasonically. (3) Spontaneous labor is demonstrated to effect orderly effacement and dilatation of the cervix and descent of the breech through the birth canal. (4) Individuals skilled in performing breech delivery, in providing appropriate anesthesia, and in infant resuscitation are in immediate attendance. Even when every attempt is made to fulfill these criteria, the outcome for the infant is not always as good as when a cesarean delivery is chosen (Collea and co-workers, 1980; Gimovsky and Paul, 1982; Schutte and colleagues, 1985).

The provider who might naively champion any childbirth outside of a hospital setting is either not aware of the hazards of breech delivery in such a setting or is totally insensitive to the welfare of the fetus and the mother. The techniques and precautions for vaginal delivery are detailed in Chapter 25.

Cesarean Delivery. There is little question that perinatal mortality and morbidity from trauma and hypoxia can be reduced by liberal use of cesarean delivery. Rovinsky and associates (1973) concluded that even for fetuses at term, defined as 2500 g or more, cesarean delivery improved fetal outcome. During the 17-year period studied, the use of cesarean delivery for breeches increased dramatically. This same trend in most training institutions toward cesarean delivery for the majority of breech fetuses means that one important criterion for safe vaginal delivery is becoming more and more difficult to fulfill; that is, most resident training programs within the near future will not provide sufficient opportunity for acquisition of skills essential for successful vaginal breech delivery.

Our policy at Parkland Hospital has been the liberal use of cesarean delivery for breech presentations. Even recently, the cesarean delivery rate for breech presentation has increased remarkably. For example, for singleton breech fetuses, the 75 percent rate in 1983 has increased progressively to 85 percent in 1991.

Summary. The fetus in a breech position is likely to benefit from cesarean delivery conducted early in labor but at the expense of an appreciable increase in maternal morbidity and a slight increase in maternal mortality. It is anticipated that the prevailing enthusiasm for offspring of the highest quality but of limited number will continue to result in the frequent use of cesarean delivery for breech presentations.

Face Presentation

In a face presentation, the head is hyperextended so that the occiput is in contact with the fetal back and the chin (mentum) is the presenting part. Duff (1981) extensively reviewed the diagnosis and management of face presentation.

Incidence. Cruikshank and White (1973) reported an incidence of 1 in 600, or 0.17 percent; the Obstetrical Statistical Cooperative identified a similar frequency of 0.2 percent. Of nearly 50,000 singleton infants delivered at Parkland Hospital from 1983 through 1986, 41—or 1 in 1200—were face presentations (Table 20–2).

Diagnosis. Although abdominal findings may be suggestive, the clinical diagnosis of face presentation is by vaginal examination. On palpation, the distinctive facial features are the mouth and nose, the malar bones, and particularly the orbital ridges. It is possible to mistake a breech for a face presentation, because the anus may be mistaken for the mouth and the ischial tuberosities for the malar prominences. The fetal anus is always on a line with the ischial tuberosities, whereas the fetal mouth and malar prominences form the corners of a triangle. The radiographic demonstration of the hyperextended head with the facial bones at or below the pelvic inlet is quite characteristic (Fig. 20–4).

Etiology. The causes of face presentations are numerous, generally stemming from any factor that favors extension or prevents flexion of the head. Extended positions, therefore, occur more frequently when the pelvis is contracted, or the fetus is very large. In a series of 141 face presentations studied by Hellman and coworkers (1950), the incidence of inlet contraction was 40 percent. This high incidence of pelvic contraction, as well as large infants, must be kept in mind when considering the successful management of a face presentation.

In multiparous women, a pendulous abdomen is another factor that predisposes to face presentation. It permits the back of the fetus to sag forward or laterally, often in the same direction in which the occiput points, thus promoting extension of the cervical and thoracic spine.

In exceptional instances, marked enlargement of the neck or coils of cord about the neck may cause extension. Anencephalic fetuses naturally present by the face because of faulty cranial development.

Mechanism. Face presentations are rarely observed above the pelvic inlet. The brow generally presents, and

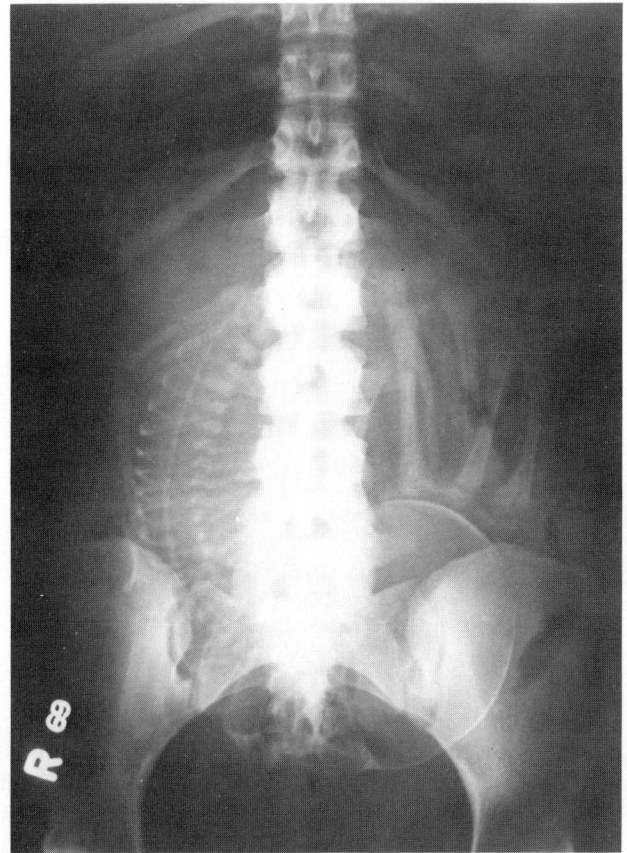

Fig. 20–4. Radiograph showing face presentation. Note marked hyperextension of head and spine of fetus.

it is usually converted into a face presentation after further extension of the head during descent through the pelvis. The mechanism of labor in these cases consists of the cardinal movements of descent, internal rotation, and flexion, and the accessory movements of extension and external rotation (Fig. 20–5). Descent is brought about by the same factors as in vertex presentations. Extension results from the relation of the fetal body to the deflected head, which is converted into a two-armed lever, the longer arm of which extends from the occipital condyles to the occiput. When resistance is encountered, the occiput must be pushed toward the back of the fetus while the chin descends (Fig. 20–6).

The object of internal rotation of the face is to bring the chin under the symphysis pubis. Unless the head is unusually small, natural delivery cannot otherwise be accomplished. Only in this way can the neck subtend the posterior surface of the symphysis pubis. If the chin rotates directly posteriorly, the relatively short neck cannot span the anterior surface of the sacrum, which measures about 12 cm in length (Fig. 20–6). Hence, the birth of the head is impossible unless the shoulders enter the pelvis at the same time, an event that is out of the question except when the fetus is extremely small or macerated. Internal rotation in a face presentation

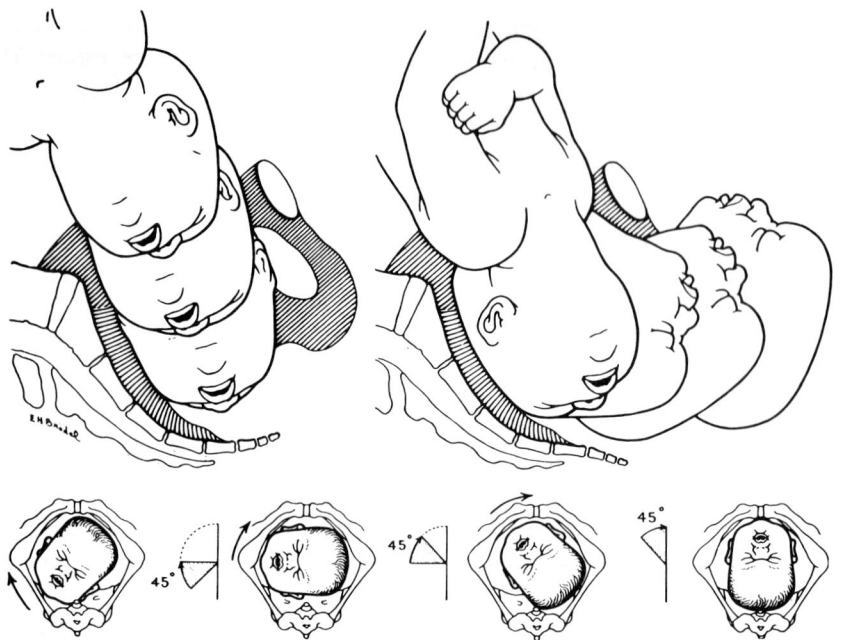

Fig. 20–5. Mechanism of labor for right mentoposterior position with subsequent rotation of mentum anterior and delivery.

results from the same factors as in vertex presentations.

After anterior rotation and descent, the chin and mouth appear at the vulva, the undersurface of the chin presses against the symphysis, and the head is delivered by flexion (Fig. 20–5). The nose, eyes, brow (bregma), and occiput then appear in succession over the anterior margin of the perineum. After birth of the head, the occiput sags backward toward the anus. In a few moments, the chin rotates externally to the side toward which it was originally directed, and the shoulders are born as in vertex presentations.

Edema may sometimes distort the face sufficiently to obliterate the features and lead to erroneous diagnosis of breech presentation (Fig. 20–7). At the same time, the skull undergoes considerable molding, manifested by an increase in length of the occipitomental diameter of the head (Fig. 20–6).

Treatment. In the absence of a contracted pelvis and with effective spontaneous labor and no evidence of

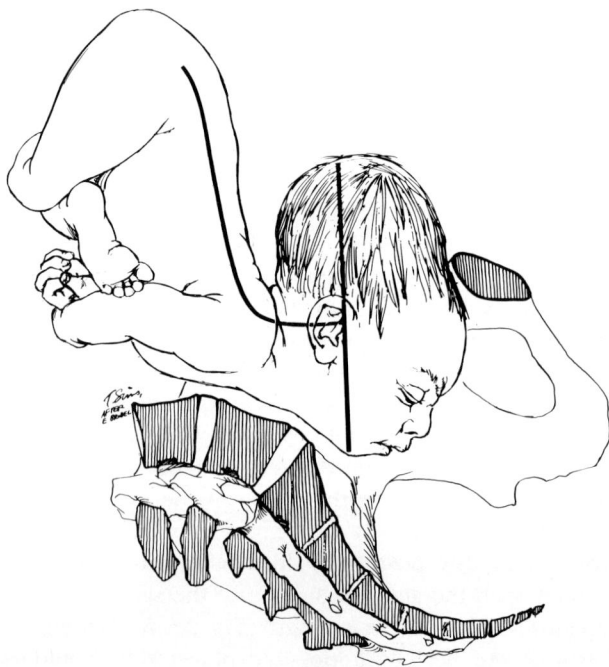

Fig. 20–6. Face presentation. The occiput is on the longer end of the head lever. The chin is directly posterior. Vaginal delivery is impossible unless the chin rotates anteriorly.

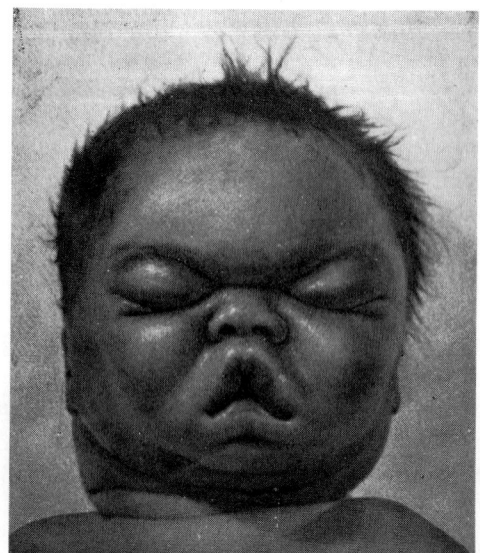

Fig. 20–7. Edema in face presentation.

fetal distress, successful vaginal delivery will usually follow. If labor is allowed, careful fetal heart rate monitoring is probably better done with external devices so as to avoid damage to the face and eyes. Because face presentations among term-size fetuses are more common when there is some degree of pelvic inlet contraction, cesarean delivery is frequently preferred.

Other methods of face presentation management rarely, if ever, are indicated in modern obstetrics. Attempts to convert a face manually into a vertex presentation, manual or forceps rotation of a persistently posterior chin to a mentum anterior position, and internal podalic version and extraction are obsolete and dangerous procedures.

Brow Presentation

Brow presentation is rare (Table 20–2). With it, that portion of the fetal head between the orbital ridge and the anterior fontanel presents at the pelvic inlet. As shown in Figure 20–8, the fetal head thus occupies a position midway between full flexion (occiput) and full extension (mentum or face). Except when the fetal head is small or the pelvis is unusually large, engagement of the fetal head and subsequent delivery cannot take place as long as the brow presentation persists.

Etiology. The causes of persistent brow presentation are the same as those for face presentation. A brow presentation is commonly unstable and often converts to a face or an occiput presentation. Cruikshank and White (1973), for example, observed either flexion to an occiput presentation or extension to a face presentation to take place in two thirds of cases that initially presented as a brow.

Diagnosis. The presentation may be recognized by abdominal palpation when both the occiput and chin can

Fig. 20–8. Brow posterior presentation.

be palpated easily, but vaginal examination is usually necessary. The frontal sutures, large anterior fontanel, orbital ridges, eyes, and root of the nose can be felt on vaginal examination. Neither mouth nor chin is within reach, however (Fig. 20–8).

Mechanism. The mechanism of labor varies greatly with the size of the fetus. With a very small fetus and a large pelvis, labor is generally easy. With larger fetuses, however, it is usually very difficult, because engagement is impossible until there is marked molding that shortens the occipitomental diameter or, more commonly, until there is either flexion to an occiput presentation or extension to a face presentation. The considerable molding essential for vaginal delivery of a persistent brow presentation characteristically deforms the head. The caput succedaneum is over the forehead, and it may be so extensive that identification of the brow by palpation is impossible. In these instances, the forehead is prominent and squared, and the occipitomental diameter is diminished.

Prognosis. In transient brow presentations, the prognosis depends upon the ultimate presentation. If the brow presentation persists, the prognosis is poor for vaginal delivery of an uncompromised infant unless the fetus is small or the birth canal is huge.

Treatment. The principles underlying the treatment of brow presentations are much the same as those for a face presentation. If, by chance, spontaneous labor is progressing without any evidence of distress in the closely monitored fetus and without unduly vigorous uterine contractions, no interference is necessary. If labor becomes either unduly vigorous or, more likely, ineffective, or if fetal distress is suspected, prompt cesarean delivery is indicated.

Transverse Lie

In this condition, the long axis of the fetus is approximately perpendicular to that of the mother. When the long axis forms an acute angle, an **oblique lie** results. An oblique lie is usually only transitory, because either a longitudinal or transverse lie commonly results when labor supervenes. For this reason, the oblique lie is called an *unstable lie* in Great Britain.

In transverse lies, the shoulder is usually over the pelvic inlet, with the head lying in one iliac fossa and the breech in the other. This condition is referred to as a **shoulder presentation.** The side of the mother toward which the acromion is directed determines the designation of the lie as right or left acromial. Moreover, because in either position the back may be directed anteriorly or posteriorly, superiorly or inferiorly, it is customary to distinguish varieties as dorsoanterior and dorsoposterior.

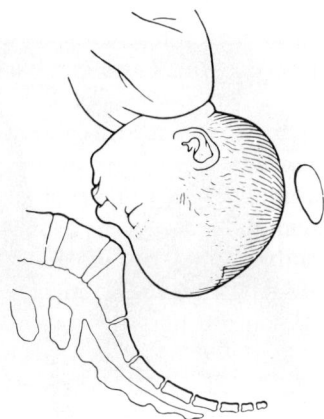

delivery. Once labor is well established, attempts at conversion to a longitudinal lie by abdominal manipulation will likely not be successful. Before labor or early in labor, with the membranes intact, attempts at external version are worthy of a trial in the absence of other obstetrical complications that point toward cesarean delivery. Phelan and co-workers (1986) recommend such an attempt only after 39 weeks because of the high (83 percent) spontaneous conversion to a longitudinal lie. If during early labor the fetal head can be maneuvered by abdominal manipulation into the pelvis, it should be held there during the next several contractions in an attempt to fix the head in the pelvis. The fetal heart rate must be closely checked during this time. If these measures fail in the woman in labor, cesarean delivery should be promptly performed.

Because neither the feet nor the vertex of the fetus occupy the lower uterine segment, a low transverse incision into the uterus may lead to difficulty in extraction of a fetus entrapped in the body of the uterus above the level of incision. Therefore, a vertical incision is usually performed. The treatment of neglected transverse lie entails support in the form of antimicrobials, fluid therapy, and transfusion, if needed. Delivery may be accomplished abdominally by cesarean delivery or cesarean hysterectomy, as indicated (see Chap. 26, pp. 591, 604).

Compound Presentation

In a compound presentation, an extremity prolapses alongside the presenting part, with both presenting in the pelvis simultaneously (Fig. 20–12).

Incidence and Etiology. Goplerud and Eastman (1953) identified a hand or arm prolapsed alongside the head once in every 700 deliveries. Much less common was prolapse of one or both lower extremities alongside a vertex presentation or a hand alongside a breech presentation. We have identified compound presentations in only 22 of nearly 50,000 singleton fetuses delivered from 1983 through 1986, an incidence of 1 in 2235 (Table 20–2).

As expected, the causes of compound presentations are conditions that prevent complete occlusion of the pelvic inlet by the fetal head. In the Goplerud and Eastman series, the incidence of preterm delivery was twice the expected rate. Often, however, no cause is demonstrable.

Prognosis and Management. Although the reported perinatal loss is increased, a major portion of the wastage is contributed by preterm delivery, prolapsed cord, and traumatic obstetrical procedures.

In most cases, the prolapsed part should be left alone, because most often it will not interfere with la-

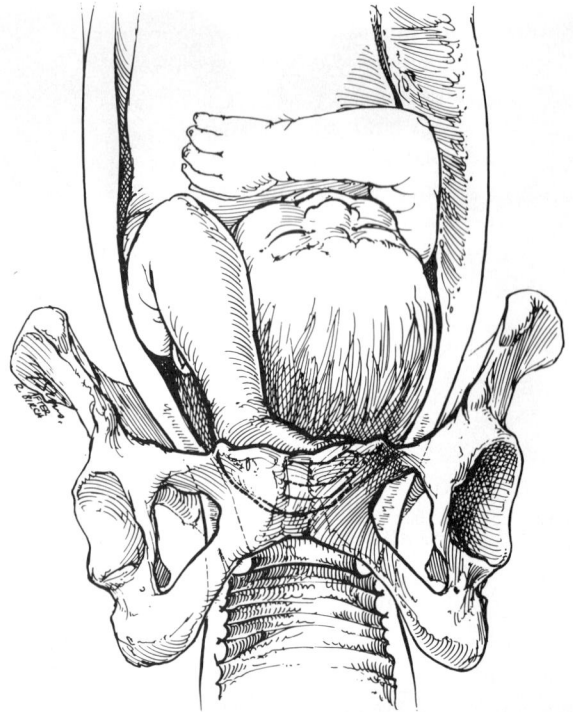

Fig. 20–12. Compound presentation. The left hand is lying in front of the vertex. With further labor, the hand and arm may retract from the birth canal and the head may then descend normally.

bor. Goplerud and Eastman (1953) described 50 cases not associated with a prolapsed cord; in almost half, normal delivery ensued with loss of only one infant. If the arm is prolapsed alongside the head, the condition should be closely observed to ascertain whether the arm rises out of the way with descent of the presenting part. If it fails to do so and if it appears to prevent descent of the head, the prolapsed arm should be gently pushed upward and the head simultaneously downward by fundal pressure. If there is fetal distress or uterine dysfunction, cesarean delivery is performed.

Persistent Occiput Posterior Positions

Most often, occiput posterior positions undergo spontaneous anterior rotation followed by uncomplicated delivery. In less than 10 percent of cases, spontaneous rotation does not occur. Although the precise reasons for failure of spontaneous rotation are not known, transverse narrowing of the midpelvis is undoubtedly a contributing factor.

The conduct of labor and delivery with the occiput posterior position need not differ remarkably from that with the occiput anterior position. The status of the fetus is probably best monitored, however, by continuous electronic techniques. Progress of labor may be ascertained by checking the rate and extent of cervical dilatation and the descent of the fetal head. In most instances, delivery can usually be accomplished without great difficulty once the head reaches the perineum.

The possibilities for vaginal delivery are (1) await spontaneous delivery, (2) forceps delivery with the occiput directly posterior, (3) forceps rotation of the occiput to the anterior position and delivery, or (4) manual rotation to the anterior position followed by spontaneous or forceps delivery.

Spontaneous Delivery. If the pelvic outlet is roomy and the vaginal outlet and perineum are somewhat relaxed from previous vaginal deliveries, rapid spontaneous delivery will often take place. If the vaginal outlet is resistant to stretch and the perineum is firm, the deceleration portion of the labor curve or the second stage of labor, or both, may be appreciably prolonged before spontaneous delivery occurs (Chap. 19, p. 482). During each expulsive effort, with the occiput posterior, the head is driven against the perineum to a much greater degree than when the occiput is anterior. Therefore, forceps delivery is often indicated. A generous episiotomy is usually needed for either a spontaneous or forceps delivery.

Forceps Delivery as an Occiput Posterior. The need for more traction compared with forceps deliveries from the occiput anterior position can be minimized by making a larger episiotomy. In most instances, a mediolateral incision should be made to avoid lacerations into the anus and rectum. The use of forceps and a large episiotomy warrant more complete analgesia than may be achieved with pudendal block and local perineal infiltration. The forceps are applied bilaterally along the occipitomental diameter, as described in Chapter 24 (p. 567).

It is important to identify the infrequent case in which protrusion of fetal scalp through the introitus is the consequence of marked elongation of the fetal head from molding combined with formation of a large caput. In this circumstance, the head may not even be engaged—that is, the biparietal diameter may not have passed through the pelvic inlet. Labor has characteristically been long in such a case and, in turn, descent of the head has been slow. Careful palpation above the symphysis may disclose the fetal head to be above the pelvic inlet. Prompt cesarean delivery is the appropriate action with such an occurrence. It may be necessary at the time of surgery to have an associate insert a sterile gloved hand into the vagina to dislodge the head upward.

Manual Rotation. The requirements for a forceps rotation must be met before doing a manual rotation. When the hand is introduced to locate the posterior ear and thus confirm the posterior position, the occiput often rotates toward the anterior position. The head

may be grasped with the fingers over the posterior ear and the thumb over the anterior ear and an attempt made to rotate the occiput to the anterior position (see Chap. 24, p. 565).

Forceps Rotation. If the head is engaged, the cervix fully dilated, and the pelvis adequate, forceps rotation may be attempted if the operator is sufficiently skilled. These circumstances are most likely to prevail when expulsive efforts of the mother during the second stage are ineffective, such as with continuous regional analgesia. Rotation by the Scanzoni maneuver or with Kielland forceps is described in Chapter 24 (p. 567).

Outcome. Phillips and Freeman (1974) reviewed the extensive experiences with occiput posterior positions at Grady Memorial Hospital in Atlanta. Basic management of the persistent occiput posterior position was similar to that for the occiput anterior position, namely, delivery without manual or forceps rotation. Compared with the occiput anterior position, labor was prolonged on the average 1 hour in parous women and 2 hours in nulliparous women. The perinatal mortality rate of 2.2 percent did not differ significantly from the 1.8 percent for the occiput anterior group. No significant increase in Apgar scores of less than 7 was found. Extension of the episiotomy, however, was increased appreciably. They stressed that midline episiotomies are not acceptable for occiput posterior deliveries and, instead, adequate mediolateral incisions should be made.

At Parkland Hospital, either manual rotation to the anterior position followed by forceps delivery, or forceps delivery from the occiput posterior position, is used to effect delivery. When neither can be done with relative ease, cesarean delivery is performed.

Persistent Occiput Transverse Position

In the absence of a pelvic architecture abnormality, the occiput transverse position is most likely a transitory one as the occiput rotates to the anterior position. If hypotonic uterine dysfunction, either spontaneous or the consequence of conduction analgesia, does not develop, spontaneous rotation is usually completed rapidly, thus allowing the choice of spontaneous delivery or delivery with outlet forceps.

Delivery. If rotation ceases because of lack of uterine action and in the absence of pelvic contraction, vaginal delivery can usually be accomplished readily in a number of ways: The occiput may be manually rotated anteriorly or posteriorly and forceps delivery carried out from either the anterior or posterior position. Another approach recommended by some is to apply forceps of the Kielland type to the head in the occiput transverse position (see Chap. 24, p. 567), rotate the occiput to the anterior position, and then deliver the head with either the same forceps or with standard outlet forceps. If the failure of spontaneous rotation is caused by hypotonic uterine dysfunction *without cephalopelvic disproportion*, dilute oxytocin may be infused while the fetal heart rate and uterine contractions are monitored closely.

The genesis of the occiput transverse position is not always so simple, or the treatment so benign. With the platypelloid (anteroposteriorly flat configuration) and the android (heart-shaped) pelves, there may not be adequate room for rotation of the occiput to either the anterior or the posterior position. With the android pelvis, the head may not even be engaged, yet the scalp may be visible through the vaginal introitus as the consequence of considerable molding and caput formation. This situation is fraught with danger to both the fetus and mother. If forceps are tried for delivery, it is imperative that undue force not be applied but, instead, a cesarean delivery be accomplished.

Fetal Macrosomia

Birthweights rarely exceed 11 pounds (5000 g). For example, at Parkland Hospital in 1991, only 23 infants, or 1.5 per 1000 births, weighed 5000 g or more. In 1979 the birth of an infant who weighed 16 pounds (7300 g) was widely publicized in the United States. Postpartum, delayed glucose metabolism was detected in the mother. She previously had delivered several infants who weighed 9 and 10 pounds. One of the largest infants on record weighed nearly 24 pounds (10,800 g), as reported by Beach in 1879 (Barnes, 1957). Between 1987 and 1991, almost 74,000 women were delivered at Parkland Hospital, and only 2 infants weighed 6000 g

or more, for a rate of 2.7 per 100,000 pregnancies (Fig. 20–13). The largest infant, who weighed 6050 g (13 lb 5½ oz), was delivered spontaneously.

Several factors, alone or in combination, may be operative in the genesis of macrosomia. These include (1) large size of the parents, especially the mother; (2) multiparity; (3) maternal diabetes; (4) maternal obesity; (5) prolonged gestation; and (6) previous delivery of an infant weighing more than 4000 g (Houchang and coworkers, 1980).

With large fetuses, dystocia may arise because the head not only becomes larger but harder and less moldable with increasing weight. Moreover, after the head has passed through the pelvic canal, dystocia may be caused by arrest of even larger shoulders at either the pelvic brim or outlet.

Incidence. According to the American College of Obstetricians and Gynecologists (1991a), it is reasonable to consider all newborn infants weighing 4500 g or more as macrosomic. Some, however, use 4000 g birthweight to define macrosomia. The incidence of infants who weighed 4000 g or more in over 104,000 deliveries in the Obstetrical Statistical Cooperative was 5.3 percent; the incidence of infants weighing 4500 g or more was 0.4 percent. Interestingly, in 1991 among the more than 15,000 deliveries at Parkland Hospital in often socioeconomically deprived, predominantly young women with a relatively low prevalence of diabetes, 7.7 percent of birthweights were 4000 g or more and approximately 1 percent of birthweights were 4500 g or more. Moreover, this number appears to be increasing.

Diagnosis. Because a clinical estimation of fetal size may be inaccurate, the diagnosis of macrosomia is often not made until after fruitless attempts at delivery. Nev-

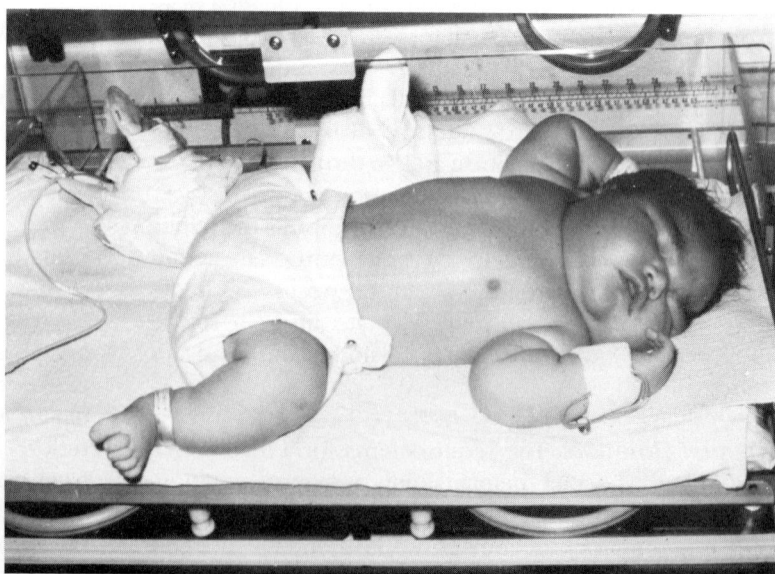

Fig. 20–13. Cesarean delivery was required for this 6065-g neonate. The mother had gestational diabetes.

ertheless, in the absence of maternal obesity, competent clinical examination should enable experienced examiners to arrive at fairly accurate estimates. Sonographic evaluation of the dimensions of the head, thorax, and abdomen often improves the estimate. Although ultrasound can identify a group of fetuses with significantly increased risk for macrosomia, no current formula has a sufficiently accurate predictive value to be used independently in making clinical decisions (American College of Obstetricians and Gynecologists, 1991a).

Serious dystocia may arise when an excessively large head attempts to pass through a normal pelvis, just as when the head of an average-size fetus is arrested by a definitely contracted pelvic inlet. At times, the head is delivered without great difficulty, but the large shoulder girdle becomes entrapped. Dystocia from a large shoulder girdle is discussed subsequently.

Prognosis. Because macrosomic infants are born more often to multiparous women and to those with diabetes, both maternal and fetal risks are increased. Langer and associates (1991) reviewed nearly 76,000 vaginal deliveries between 1970 and 1985, and the incidence of macrosomia, defined as birthweight 4000 g or greater, was 7.6 percent. Perinatal mortality was increased significantly when shoulder dystocia complicated delivery, and especially when maternal diabetes was also diagnosed. Spellacy and co-workers (1985) analyzed infant outcomes when birthweight was between 2500 and 3500 g compared with birthweights more than 4500 g. Perinatal mortality doubled from about 3.5 per 1000 births for smaller infants to approximately 8 per 1000 for those weighing 4500 g or more. Most of the increased mortality was related to birth trauma due to excessive fetal size.

Some investigators have suggested that fetuses estimated to weigh more than a specific number of grams should have routine cesarean deliveries in an attempt to avoid birth trauma due to macrosomia. For example, Acker and associates (1985) recommended cesarean delivery for diabetic gravidas with fetal weight estimates of 4000 g or greater. Similarly, they suggested that cesarean delivery should be considered with abnormal labor and a fetus estimated to weigh 4500 g or more. Spellacy and associates (1985) suggested that all fetuses estimated to weigh 4500 g or more should be delivered by elective cesarean. Langer and co-workers (1991) recommended elective cesarean deliveries for diabetic women with fetuses estimated to weigh 4250 g or more. In the absence of maternal diabetes, however, these investigators recommended attempted vaginal delivery for all fetuses expected to weigh 4000 g or more.

Unfortunately, accurate identification of large fetuses is an imperfect clinical skill. For example, Hirata and co-workers (1990) identified 141 fetuses estimated to weigh nearly 4000 g using Leopold examinations and then performed ultrasound examinations to test the ac-

curacy of several reported sonar methods. The actual birthweights ranged from 2920 to 5100 g, and 22 percent of the fetuses weighed less than 4000 g. These investigators concluded that the best sonographic estimates of fetal macrosomia were obtained using abdominal circumferences and femur length measurements. They also found that ultrasound-derived predictions of fetal macrosomia are prone to large inaccuracies, thus seriously compromising their usefulness. Delpapa and Mueller-Heubach (1991) analyzed pregnancy outcomes in 242 women with sonographic estimates of fetal macrosomia and concluded that cesarean delivery or early induction to avoid continued fetal growth were inappropriate when based solely upon ultrasound diagnosis.

Assuming that the weight of a macrosomic fetus could be uniformly and accurately estimated, electing cesarean delivery based upon certain fetal weight thresholds could result in many unnecessary cesareans. For example, in 1991 at Parkland Hospital, 1162 women were delivered of infants weighing 4000 g or more and 847 (73 percent) had uncomplicated vaginal births. Brachial plexus injuries of varying severity were diagnosed in 4 of 737 vaginal deliveries of infants weighing 4000 to 4500 g, and in 4 of 118 vaginally delivered neonates with weights exceeding 4500 g. Conversely, 99.5 percent of fetuses weighing between 4000 and 4500 g were delivered safely vaginally, as were 96.6 percent of those weighing more than 4500 g. Importantly, smaller birthweights do not preclude brachial plexus injury due to shoulder dystocia, because such injuries occurred in 8 infants weighing 2900 to 3900 g. Easily applied rules for governing use of cesarean delivery based on estimates of fetal weight remain elusive.

Shoulder Dystocia

The cited incidence of shoulder dystocia varies greatly depending on the criteria used for diagnosis. For example, Gross and co-authors (1987a) identified that 0.9 percent of almost 11,000 vaginal deliveries were coded for shoulder dystocia at the Toronto General Hospital. True shoulder dystocia, diagnosed because maneuvers were required to deliver the shoulders in addition to downward traction and episiotomy, occurred in only 24 (0.2 percent) births. Significant infant trauma was observed only in those shoulder dystocias requiring a maneuver to effect delivery. Acker and co-workers (1986) reported the incidence of shoulder dystocia to be as high as 2 percent in vaginal deliveries of infants weighing 2500 g or more when the diagnosis depended only on the judgement of the individual charting the diagnosis. There is some evidence that the incidence of shoulder dystocia has increased during the past two decades (Hopwood, 1982), and this is likely due to increasing birthweight (Modanlou and co-workers, 1982). These same investigators showed that neonates experiencing shoulder dystocia had significantly greater shoulder-to-head and chest-to-head disproportions compared to equally macrosomic infants delivered without dystocia.

Unfortunately, the etiology of shoulder dystocia is fetal macrosomia and not simply an increase in fetal weight to above an arbitrarily defined weight of 4000 g. Thus, fetal macrosomia is an *increase in body size in relation to head size*, the result often but not always being a larger shoulder girdle than fetal head. The ponderal index of such infants is most often increased, making a predictable diagnosis of fetal macrosomia extremely difficult and a *reliable prediction of shoulder dystocia* impossible. Any maternal or fetal factor that contributes to an increased incidence of fetal macrosomia also naturally increases the incidence of shoulder dystocia.

For convenience, factors that contribute to shoulder dystocia can be separated into antepartum and intrapartum considerations. It is important, however, to realize that in clinical practice each of these factors may influence the incidence of shoulder dystocia as an independent variable or in a multivariate manner. Unfortunately, clinical practice is rarely limited to a single variable, and thus single or isolated factors cannot be considered in making clinical decisions concerning the possibility of shoulder dystocia.

Antepartum Contributing Factors

Maternal Obesity. Maternal obesity alone is difficult to separate from gestational diabetes or overt diabetes; however, Johnson and colleagues (1987) reported that in pregnant women weighing more than 250 pounds the incidence of shoulder dystocia was 5.1 percent compared with 0.6 percent for control women who weighed less than 200 pounds. Spellacy and co-workers (1985) reported that for women weighing more than 90 kg, birthweight distribution was 8.2 percent for 2500- to 3500-g infants; 33 percent for 4500- to 5000-g infants; and 50 percent for infants who weighed more than 5000 g. Shoulder dystocia was identified in 0.3 percent of the 2500- to 3500-g infants; 7.3 percent of the 4500- to 5000-g infants; and 14.6 percent of the larger infants.

Diabetes Mellitus. The association of macrosomia with mild diabetes mellitus is well established and was a significantly important contributing factor to shoulder dystocia reported in the studies discussed above. Similar results have been reported by Berne and associates (1985) in Sweden, Klebe and co-workers (1986) in Denmark, and Cousins and colleagues (1985) in the United States. The incidences of shoulder dystocia in these studies were 2.5, 5, and 16.7 percent, respectively, versus 1.7 percent for controls. Keller and co-workers (1991) identified shoulder dystocia in 7 percent of pregnancies complicated by gestational diabetes, but

there was only one case of permanent brachial plexus injury. They concluded that a policy of cesarean delivery for all gestational diabetics would greatly increase the number of cesarean deliveries with minimal fetal benefit.

Postterm Pregnancy. The fact that many fetuses continue to grow after 42 weeks (see Chap. 38, p. 871) is now well recognized. The association of an increased incidence of shoulder dystocia in postterm pregnancy has been reported by Spellacy (1985), Acker (1985), Johnson (1987a), Eden (1987), and all their co-workers.

Intrapartum Contributing Factors. At least three intrapartum factors have been reported to be associated with an increased incidence of shoulder dystocia: (1) prolonged second stage of labor, (2) oxytocin induction or augmentation of labor, and (3) use of midforceps or a vacuum extraction during delivery. Acker and associates (1988) also reported that severe shoulder dystocia was increased in rapid second-stage labors. However, in another study, Gross and co-workers (1987) disputed that shoulder dystocia could be reliably predicted from labor abnormalities.

Prolonged Second Stage of Labor. Benedetti and Gabbe (1978) reported that with a prolonged second stage of labor and a midpelvic delivery (vacuum extraction or midforceps delivery), the incidence of shoulder dystocia was 4.6 percent compared with 0.16 percent in the absence of a prolonged second stage of labor. Acker and co-workers (1985) reported an increased incidence of shoulder dystocia in 4000 g and larger infants if there was a prolongation or arrest of labor. Acker and colleagues (1986) also reported an increased incidence of shoulder dystocia in normal weight infants (2500 to 3000 g) born to women in whom labor was complicated by an arrest disorder.

Oxytocin Induction. Because shoulder dystocia is the consequence of macrosomia, it is not surprising that oxytocin may be associated with an increased incidence. Large infants may be associated with dysfunctional labors, and oxytocin is frequently indicated in many forms of dysfunctional labor (see Chap. 19). Also, the treatment for postterm pregnancy is delivery, and this is accomplished by labor induction. Finally, a postterm gestation is often associated with increased macrosomia and shoulder dystocia.

Midforceps and Vacuum Extraction. For many of the same reasons discussed under oxytocin induction or augmentation, there is a significant increase in the incidence of shoulder dystocia with midforceps or vacuum extractions. As described earlier, Benedetti and Gabbe (1978) reported such an association, and subsequently other investigators have done so as well (Levine and co-workers, 1984; McFarland and associates, 1986).

Prediction and Prevention of Shoulder Dystocia.

There has been considerable evolution in obstetrical thinking about the preventability of shoulder dystocia in the last 10 to 15 years. During the 1970s, when the use of cesarean delivery was escalating rapidly, it was hoped that certain pregnancy risk factors could be used to identify women in need of abdominal delivery and thereby avoid shoulder dystocia. During the 1980s it became apparent, however, that the rate of cesarean delivery was excessive. It also became obvious that predicting, and therefore preventing, shoulder dystocia was not an easy task. While there are clearly several risk factors statistically associated with shoulder dystocia, actual identification of individual instances of shoulder dystocia before the fact has proven to be extremely difficult, if not impossible.

O'Leary and Leonetti (1990) believe that many cases of shoulder dystocia are preventable; others sharply disagree (Gimbel, 1990; Nagey, 1990). Indeed, O'Leary and Leonetti (1990) suggested that a high level of suspicion for shoulder dystocia is a reasonable indication for cesarean delivery if based on risk factors such as diabetes, obesity, postterm, and excessive fetal or maternal weight gain. They even suggested the mnemonic DOPE to remind clinicians of these risk factors. Presumably, this mnemonic was also selected to apply to those who dare overlook these risk factors. Despite this mnemonic, the preponderance of evidence is consistent with the view that most shoulder dystocia is not preventable without excessive use of cesarean delivery (Delpapa, 1991; Gross, 1987b; Keller, 1991; Langer, 1991; and their many co-workers). Jennett and associates (1992) provided evidence that brachial plexus impairment may occur even in the fetus prior to labor.

Fetal Consequences.

Shoulder dystocia, if not managed appropriately, may be associated with significant fetal morbidity and even mortality. Benedetti and Gabbe (1978) reported that of 19 neonates with shoulder dystocia, 5 had a fractured humerus or clavicle, 3 had Erb palsy, and 1 had an abnormal neurological examination. Similar results were reported by Spellacy (1985), McFarland (1986), and their co-workers. Hardy (1981) studied the prognosis of 36 infants diagnosed with brachial plexus injuries. Interestingly, shoulder dystocia had been reported in only 10 of these infants, and 2 of the infants without shoulder dystocia had been delivered abdominally. Nearly 80 percent of these children had made complete recoveries by 13 months of age, and none of those with residual defects had severe sensory or motor deficits in the hand. Prompt physiotherapy may improve brachial nerve damage in some but not all

cases of Erb palsy (see Chap. 44, p. 1021). Although fractures and brachial nerve damage are serious consequences, severe asphyxia and death also may result.

Maternal Consequences.

Postpartum hemorrhage, usually from uterine atony but also from vaginal and cervical lacerations, remains the major maternal risk (Benedetti and Gabbe, 1978; Parks and Ziel, 1978). Puerperal infection following cesarean section also remains a problem.

Management.

Because shoulder dystocia cannot be predicted, the practitioner of obstetrics *must* be well versed in the management principles of this occasionally devastating complication. Reduction in the interval of time from delivery of the head to delivery of the body is of great importance to survival. An initial gentle attempt at traction, assisted by maternal expulsive efforts, is recommended (American College of Obstetricians and Gynecologists, 1991b). Overly vigorous traction on the head or neck, or excessive rotation of the body, may cause serious damage to the infant.

Some have advocated performing a large episiotomy, and adequate analgesia is certainly ideal. The next step is to clear the infant's mouth and nose. Having completed the above steps, a variety of methods or techniques have been described to free the anterior shoulder from its impacted position beneath the maternal symphysis pubis. The most popular techniques include the following.

1. Resnik (1980), as well as others, recommended moderate **suprapubic pressure** by an assistant while downward traction is applied to the fetal head.
2. **The McRoberts maneuver** was described by Gonik and associates (1983). It is named for William A. McRoberts, Jr., who popularized its use at the University of Texas Health Science Center at Houston/Hermann Hospital. The maneuver consists of removing the legs from the stirrups and sharply flexing them upon the woman's abdomen (Fig. 20–14). This supposedly results in a straightening of the sacrum relative to the lumbar vertebrae with accompanying rotation of the symphysis pubis toward the patient's head and a decrease in the angle of pelvic inclination (see Chap. 11). This maneuver does not increase the dimensions of the pelvis, but the cephalic rotation of the pelvis frees the impacted anterior shoulder. Gonik and co-workers (1989) tested the McRoberts position objectively with laboratory pelvic and fetal models and found that the maneuver reduced fetal shoulder extraction forces. Pollack and associates (1985) reported the successful

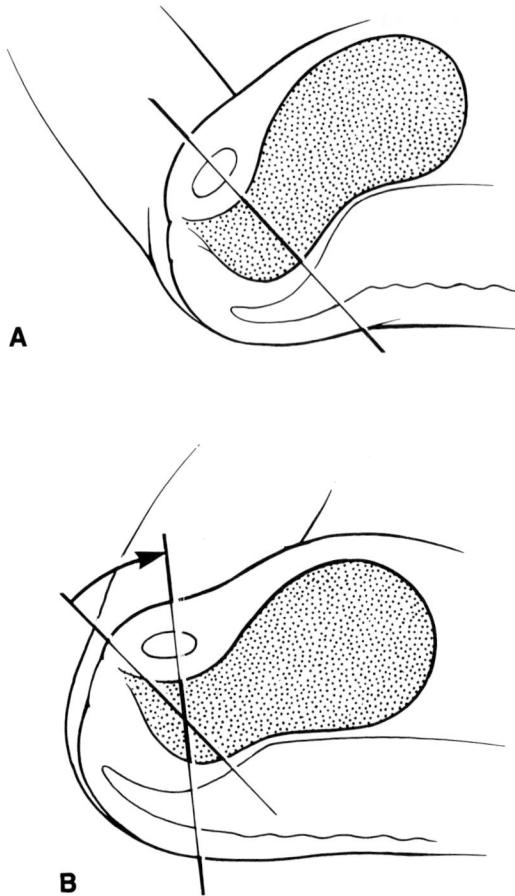

A

B

Fig. 20–14. The McRoberts maneuver. The maneuver consists of (**A**) removing the legs from the stirrups and (**B**) sharply flexing them upon the abdomen.

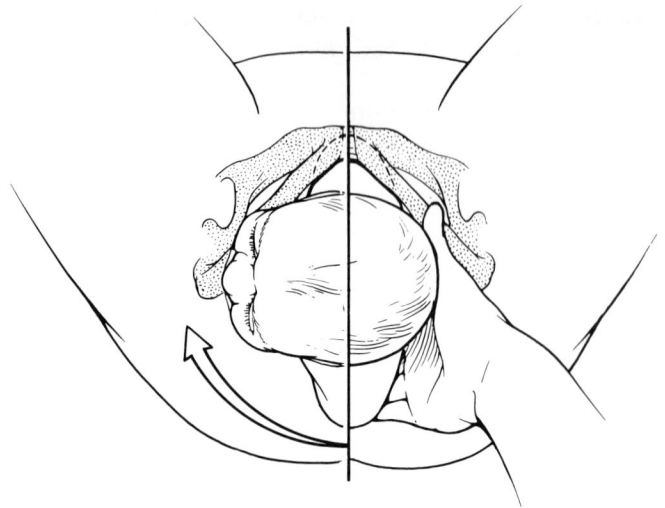

Fig. 20–15. Woods maneuver. The hand is placed behind the posterior shoulder of the fetus. The shoulder is then rotated progressively 180 degrees in a corkscrew manner so that the impacted anterior shoulder is released.

use of this maneuver in 24 of 25 cases of shoulder dystocia.

3. Woods (1943) reported that, by progressively rotating the posterior shoulder 180 degrees in a corkscrew fashion, the impacted anterior shoulder could be released. This is frequently referred to as the **Woods corkscrew maneuver** (Fig. 20–15).

4. **Delivery of the posterior shoulder** consists of carefully sweeping the posterior arm of the fetus across the chest, followed by delivery of the arm. The shoulder girdle is then rotated into one of the oblique diameters of the pelvis with subsequent delivery of the anterior shoulder (Fig. 20–16).

5. Rubin (1964) recommended two maneuvers. First, the fetal shoulders are rocked from side to side by applying force to the mother's abdomen. If this is not successful, the most easily accessible fetal shoulder is pushed toward the anterior surface of the chest. This most often results in abduction of both shoulders. This in

turn produces a smaller shoulder-to-shoulder diameter and displacement of the anterior shoulder from behind the symphysis pubis (Fig. 20–17).

6. Chavis (1979) described the use of a shoulder horn instrument consisting of a concave blade with a long handle, which is slipped between the symphysis and the impacted anterior shoulder. The instrument is then used like a shoehorn as a lever with the symphysis pubis as a fulcrum.

7. Hibbard (1982) recommended that pressure be applied to the infant's jaw and neck in the direction of the mother's rectum, with strong fundal pressure applied by an assistant as the anterior shoulder is freed. **This is a potentially dangerous procedure.** It must be remembered that strong fundal pressure applied at the wrong time may result in even further impaction of the anterior shoulder. Furthermore, Gross and associates (1987a) reported that fundal pressure in the absence of other maneuvers **"resulted in a 77 percent complication rate and was strongly associated with (fetal) orthopedic and neurologic damage."**

8. Sandberg (1988) reported the **Zavanelli maneuver** for cephalic replacement into the pelvis and then cesarean delivery. The first part of the maneuver consists of returning the head to the OA or OP position if the head has rotated from either position. The second step is to flex the head and slowly push it back into the va-

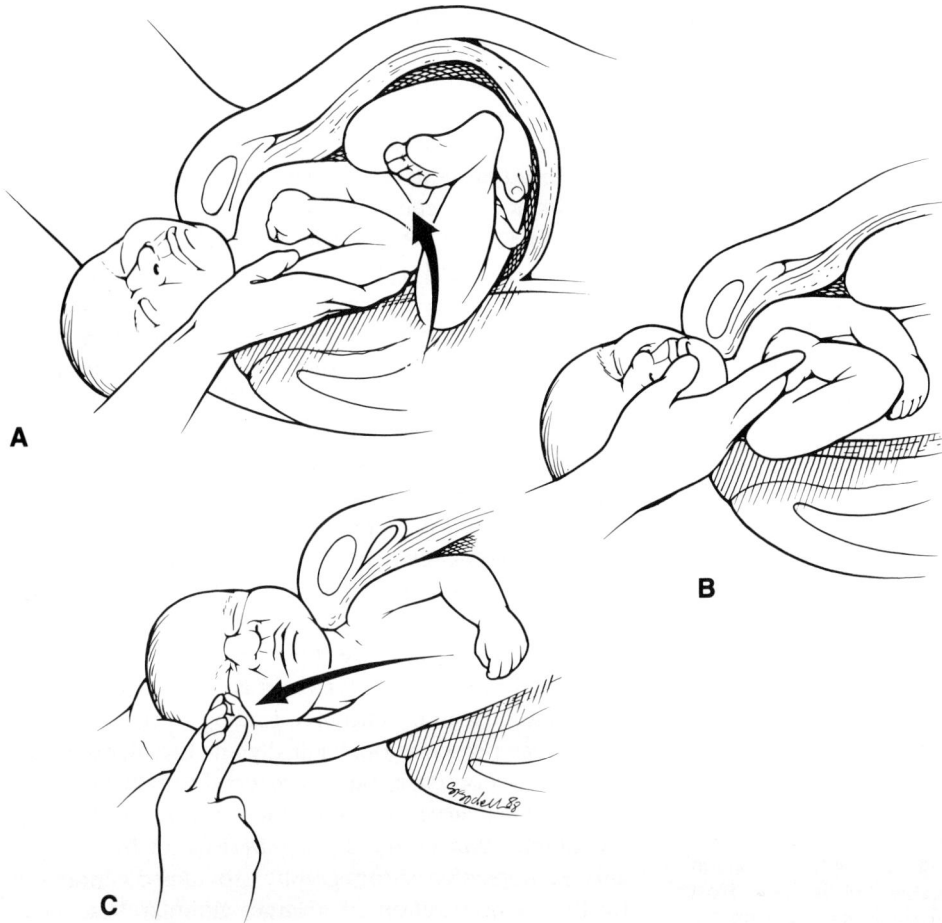

Fig. 20–16. Shoulder dystocia with impacted anterior shoulder of the fetus. **A.** The operator's hand is introduced into the vagina along the fetal posterior humerus, which is splinted as the arm is swept across the chest, keeping the arm flexed at the elbow. **B.** The fetal hand is grasped and the arm extended along the side of the face. **C.** The posterior arm is delivered from the vagina.

gina, following which a cesarean delivery is performed. O'Leary and Gunn (1985) reported success with the technique in 4 cases of shoulder dystocia. In 3 cases, they administered 0.25 mg of terbutaline subcutaneously to produce uterine relaxation. In contrast, Graham and colleagues (1992) resorted to use of the Zavanelli maneuver after all other methods failed. They found the Zavanelli procedure extremely difficult to accomplish because they were unable to totally replace the fetal head into the vagina despite both terbutaline and general anesthesia. The infant was finally delivered after a classical cesarean was performed in conjunction with reversed internal rotation accomplished vaginally. The infant weighed 3850 g and was delivered 15 minutes after shoulder dystocia was diagnosed. Umbilical artery blood pH was 7.17, and the infant was discharged without neurological sequelae.

9. Deliberate **fracture of the clavicle** by pressing the anterior clavicle against the ramus of the pubis can be done to free the shoulder impaction. The fracture will heal rapidly, and is not nearly as serious as a brachial nerve injury, asphyxia, or death.

10. **Cleidotomy** consists of cutting the clavicle with scissors or other sharp instruments, and is usually used on a dead fetus (Schramm, 1983). **Symphysiotomy** also has been applied successfully; the technique was described by Hartfield (1986).

Hernandez and Wendel (1990) suggested use of a "shoulder dystocia drill" to better organize emergency management of an impacted shoulder. The drill is a set of maneuvers performed sequentially as needed to complete vaginal delivery. The American College of Obstetricians and Gynecologists (1991b) recommends the following steps. The sequence of these maneuvers will depend on the experience and preference of the individual operator.

1. First, call for help. Mobilize assistants, an anesthesiologist, and a pediatrician. At this time, an initial gentle attempt at traction is made. Drain the bladder if it is distended.

2. A generous episiotomy (mediolateral or episioproctotomy) may afford room posteriorly.

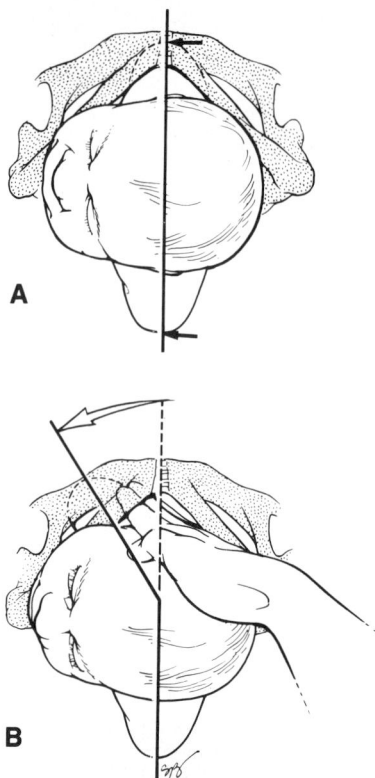

Fig. 20–17. Rubin (second) maneuver. **A.** The shoulder-to-shoulder diameter is shown as the distance between the two small arrows. **B.** The most easily accessible fetal shoulder (the anterior is shown here) is pushed toward the anterior chest wall of the fetus. Most often, this results in abduction of both shoulders, reducing the shoulder-to-shoulder diameter and freeing the impacted anterior shoulder.

3. Suprapubic pressure is utilized initially by most because it has the advantage of simplicity. Only one assistant is needed to provide suprapubic pressure while normal downward traction is applied to the fetal head.
4. The McRoberts maneuver requires two assistants. Each assistant grasps a leg and sharply flexes the maternal thigh against the abdomen.

These maneuvers will resolve most cases of shoulder dystocia. If they fail, however, the following steps may be attempted.

5. The Woods screw maneuver.
6. Delivery of the posterior arm is attempted, but if it is in a fully extended position, this is usually difficult to accomplish.
7. Other techniques generally should be reserved for cases in which all other maneuvers have failed. These include intentional fracture of the anterior clavicle or humerus and the Zavanelli maneuver.

Hydrocephalus as a Cause of Dystocia

Internal hydrocephalus, or excessive accumulation of cerebrospinal fluid in the ventricles of the brain with consequent enlargement of the cranium, occurs in about 1 in 2000 fetuses and accounts for about 12 percent of all severe malformations found at birth. Associated defects are common, with spina bifida occurring in about one third of cases. Not infrequently, the circumference of the head exceeds 50 cm, and sometimes it reaches 80 cm. The normal fetal head circumference at term ranges between 32 and 38 cm. The volume of fluid is usually between 500 and 1500 mL, but as much as 5 L may accumulate. Breech presentation is found in about one third of cases. Whatever the presentation, gross cephalopelvic disproportion is the rule, with serious dystocia the usual consequence (Figs. 20–18 and 20–19).

Diagnosis. In this condition particularly, an empty bladder facilitates both abdominal and vaginal examinations. In cephalic presentations, a broad, firm mass above the symphysis is evident from abdominal examination. The thickness of the abdominal wall usually prevents detection of the thin, elastic, hydrocephalic cranium. The high head forces the body of the infant upward, with the result that the fetal heart is often loudest above the umbilicus, a circumstance leading to the suspicion of a breech presentation. Vaginally, the broader dome of the head feels tense, but more careful palpation may disclose very large fontanels, wide suture lines, and an indentable, thin cranium characteristic of hydrocephalus. Radiography or sonography provides confirmation by the demonstration of a large, globular head (Fig. 20–20).

Hydrocephalus is somewhat more difficult to diag-

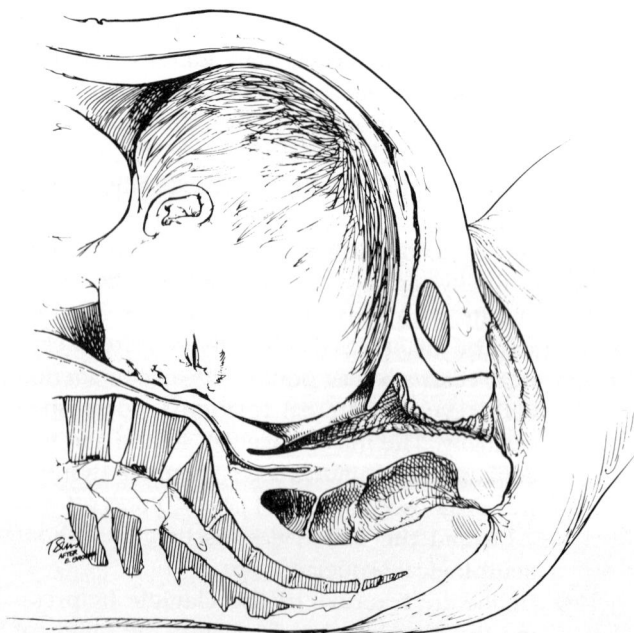

Fig. 20–18. Severe dystocia from hydrocephalus, cephalic presentation. Note the disparity between the small size of the face and the rest of the cranium.

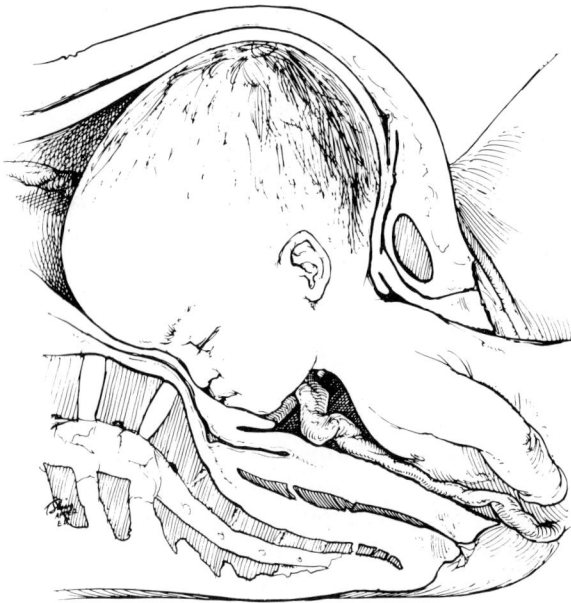

Fig. 20–19. Severe dystocia from hydrocephalus, breech presentation. Note the distention of the lower uterine segment.

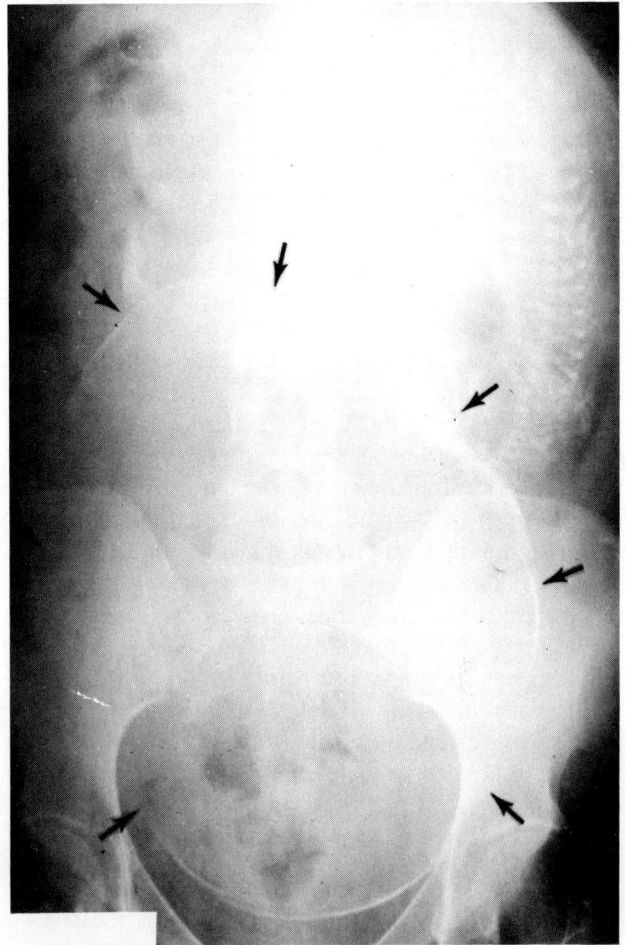

Fig. 20–20. Radiograph demonstrating severe hydrocephalus, further outlined by arrows; 2300 mL of cerebrospinal fluid were aspirated transvaginally.

nose radiographically with a breech presentation, because the radiographic outline of a normal fetal head often appears enlarged to a degree suggestive of hydrocephalus. This results from the fetal head lying more anterior than with a cephalic presentation and the divergence of x-rays inherent in diagnostic radiography. Therefore, in breech presentations hydrocephalus may not have been considered until it is found that the head cannot be extracted. The mistake may be avoided by paying particular attention to the following criteria: (1) the face of the hydrocephalic infant is small in relation to the large head; (2) the hydrocephalic cranium tends to be globular, whereas the normal head is ovoid; and (3) the shadow of the hydrocephalic cranium is often very thin or scarcely visible.

The difficulties inherent in radiological diagnosis are obviated by the use of sonography to compare the diameter of the lateral ventricles to the biparietal diameter of the head, and to evaluate the thickness of the cerebral cortex, as well as to compare the size of the head to that of the thorax and abdomen (Clark and associates, 1985).

Prognosis. Rupture of the uterus is a danger and may occur before complete dilatation of the cervix. Hydrocephalus predisposes to rupture not only because of the obvious disproportion but also because the great transverse diameter of the cranium overdistends the lower uterine segment.

Treatment. Most often, the size of the hydrocephalic head must be reduced if the head is to pass through the birth canal. Even with cesarean delivery, it may be de-

sirable to remove cerebrospinal fluid just before incising the uterus in order to circumvent dangerous extensions of a low transverse or vertical incision and to avoid deliberately creating a very long vertical incision in the uterus. The procedure for removal of cerebrospinal fluid is called cephalocentesis. Cephalocentesis was a mainstay in the historical management of fetal hydrocephalus with macrocephaly, but has come under considerable scrutiny in recent years. Chervenak and colleagues (1985) described results of cephalocentesis in 11 fetuses where the procedure was used to permit vaginal delivery or cesarean delivery. Ten of these fetuses died either in utero or within 3 hours of delivery, and 7 had intracranial bleeding at autopsy. The authors pointed out, however, that the procedure had been performed by several different operators at different hospitals. Chervenak and McCullough (1986) advocate that use of cephalocentesis be limited to fetuses with severe associated abnormalities. They recommended that all other cases be delivered abdominally. Such management requires precise knowledge of the extent of fetal malformations, which is not always possible. Antepartum identification and thorough evaluation of fetuses with hydrocephaly (see Chap. 40, p. 930) is paramount in guiding intrapartum management.

The procedure for cephalocentesis varies depending on the fetal presentation. With a cephalic presentation, as soon as the cervix is dilated 3 to 4 cm, the high ventricles may be tapped transvaginally with a needle. An 8-inch-long, 17-gauge needle has proved quite satisfactory for promptly removing appreciable volumes of cerebrospinal fluid. In the case illustrated in Figures 20–20 and 20–21, 2300 mL of cerebrospinal fluid were removed. With a breech presentation, labor can be allowed to progress and the breech and trunk may be delivered. With the head over the inlet and the face toward the mother's back, the needle is inserted transvaginally just below the anterior vaginal wall and into the aftercoming head through the widened suture line. To protect the birth canal from the needle as it is passed toward the head, the more distal part of the needle, including the point, may be covered with a segment of sterile plastic tubing about 6 inches long cut from an intravenous infusion set. Alternatively, fluid may be withdrawn through a needle inserted transabdominally into the fetal head. After the bladder is emptied and the skin is cleansed, the needle is inserted in the midline somewhat below the maternal umbilicus and inferior to the top of the fetal skull. The transabdominal approach to remove cerebrospinal fluid can also be used in the event of a cephalic presentation before trying to stimulate labor with oxytocin. The transabdominal approach has also been successfully applied in the breech fetus using ultrasound to guide the needle (Osathanondh, 1980).

Large Fetal Abdomen as a Cause of Dystocia

Enlargement of the fetal abdomen sufficient to cause grave dystocia is usually the result of a *greatly distended bladder* (Fig. 20–22), *ascites, or enlargement of the kidneys or liver.* Occasionally, the edematous fetal abdomen may attain such proportions that spontaneous delivery is impossible. Enlargement of the fetal abdomen may escape detection until fruitless attempts at delivery have demonstrated an obstruction. An enlarged abdomen and intra-abdominal accumulation of fluid can be diagnosed in utero by careful sonographic examination.

Treatment. If the abdominal enlargement is not discovered until the fetal head has been delivered, decompression of the fetal abdomen often becomes a necessity. The maternal bladder is emptied and the suprapubic area is cleansed. A long large-gauge needle, as described for hydrocephalus, is inserted through the midline of the maternal abdomen into the fetal abdomen. Fluid in the fetal bladder or peritoneal cavity promptly escapes. The decompression may be aided by use of continuous suction. As the fetal abdomen approaches normal dimensions, delivery is completed readily. At times, as with severe hydrops fetalis, ascites will be accompanied by such severe edema of the abdominal wall and so great an enlargement of the liver that removal of the peritoneal fluid provides insufficient decompression for easy delivery. Such cases, fortunately, are becoming extremely rare.

If the diagnosis of gross enlargement of the fetal abdomen is made before delivery, the decision must be made whether or not to perform an abdominal delivery (Clark and associates, 1985). In general, prognosis is very poor for the fetus with abdominal enlargement so marked as to cause dystocia, irrespective of route of delivery.

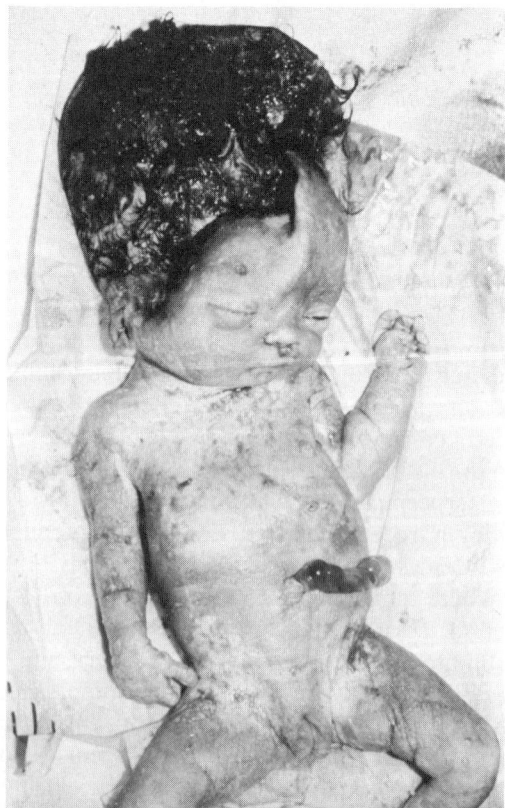

Fig. 20–21. Hydrocephalic infant delivered spontaneously after removal of 2300 mL of cerebrospinal fluid.

Conjoined Twins

The embryological basis of incomplete twinning is considered in Chapter 39. For practical purposes, three groups of conjoined twins may be distinguished: (1)

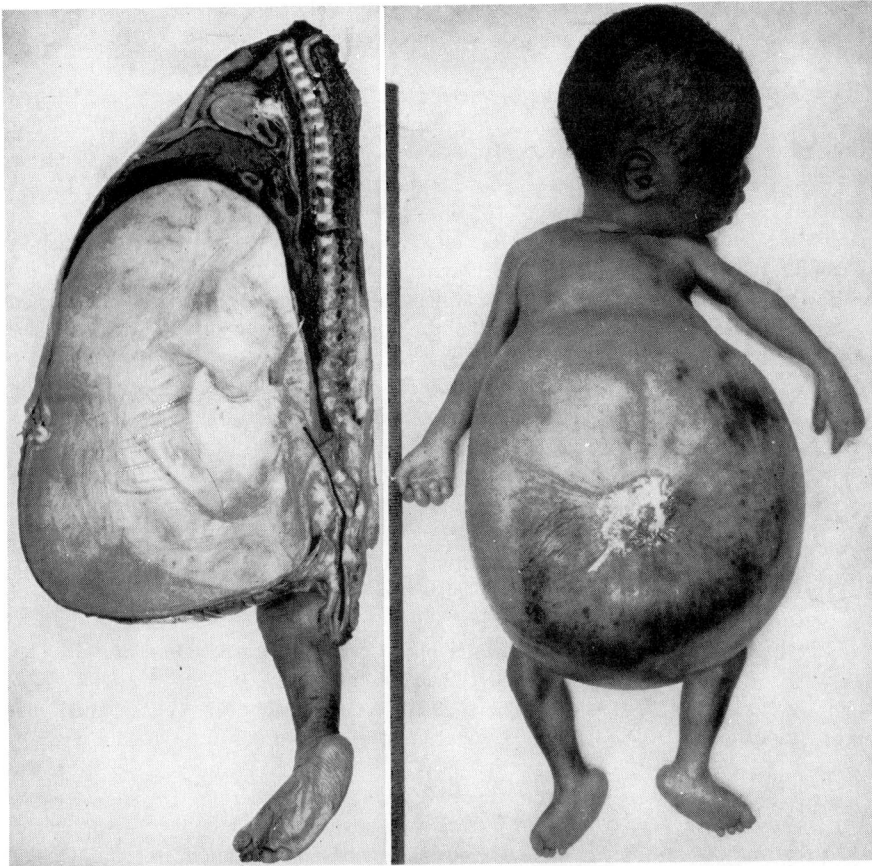

Fig. 20–22. Fetus at 28 weeks with immensely distended bladder. Delivery was made possible by expression of fluid from bladder through perforation at umbilicus. Median sagittal section shows interior of bladder and compression of organs of abdominal and thoracic cavities. A black thread has been laid in the urethra. (From Savage, 1935.)

incomplete double formations at the upper or lower half of the body (diprosopus dipygus); (2) twins that are united at the upper or lower end of the body (craniopagus, ischiopagus, or pygopagus); and (3) conjoined twins united at the trunk (thoracopagus and dicephalus).

Although twins may be diagnosed antenatally, conjoining is not always identified until difficulty is encountered at delivery. Because such pregnancies seldom go to term, conjoined twins may not greatly exceed the size of a normal fetus. Also, the connection between the halves is sometimes sufficiently flexible to allow vaginal delivery. Harper and co-workers (1980) reported a 300-year review of the obstetrical, morphopathological, neonatal, and surgical problems associated with xiphopagus conjoined twins.

References

Acker DB, Gregory KD, Sachs BP, Friedman EA: Risk factors for Erb-Duchenne palsy. Obstet Gynecol 71:389, 1988

Acker DB, Sachs BP, Friedman EA: Risk factors for shoulder dystocia in the average-weight infant. Obstet Gynecol 67:614, 1986

Acker DB, Sachs BP, Friedman EA: Risk factors for shoulder dystocia. Obstet Gynecol 66:762, 1985

American College of Obstetricians and Gynecologists: Fetal macrosomia. Technical bulletin no. 159, September 1991a

American College of Obstetricians and Gynecologists: Operative vaginal delivery. Technical bulletin no. 152, February 1991b

Barnes AC: An obstetric record from the Medical Record. Obstet Gynecol 9:237, 1957

Barrett JM: Funic reduction for the management of umbilical cord prolapse. Am J Obstet Gynecol 165:654, 1991

Benedetti TJ, Gabbe SG: Shoulder dystocia. A complication of fetal macrosomia and prolonged second stage of labor with mid-pelvic delivery. Obstet Gynecol 52:526, 1978

Berne C, Wibell L, Lindmark G: Ten-year experience of insulin treatment in gestational diabetes. Acta Paediatr Scand 320:85, 1985

Bingham P, Lilford RJ: Management of the selected term breech presentation: Assessment of the risks of selected vaginal delivery versus cesarean section for all cases. Obstet Gynecol 69:965, 1987

Bistoletti P, Nisell H, Palme C, Lagercrantz H: Term breech delivery: Early and late complications. Acta Obstet Gynecol Scand 60:165, 1981

Bodmer B, Benjamin A, McLean FH, Usher RH: Has use of cesarean section reduced the risks of delivery in the preterm breech presentation? Am J Obstet Gynecol 154:144, 1986

Brenner WE, Bruce RD, Hendricks CH: The characteristics and perils of breech presentation. Am J Obstet Gynecol 118:700, 1974

Brocks V, Philipsen T, Secher NJ: A randomized trial of external cephalic version with tocolysis in late pregnancy. Br J Obstet Gynaecol 91:653, 1984

Calvert JP: Intrinsic hazard of breech presentation. Br Med J 281:1319, 1980

Chapman GP, Weller RO, Normand ICS, Gibbens D: Spinal cord transection in utero. Br Med J 2:398, 1978

Chavis WM: A new instrument for the management of shoulder dystocia. Int J Gynaecol Obstet 16:331, 1979

Chervenak FA, Berkowitz RL, Tortona M, Hobbins JC: The management of fetal hydrocephalus. Am J Obstet Gynecol 151:933, 1985

Chervenak FA, McCullough LB: Ethical analysis of the intrapartum management of pregnancy complicated by fetal hydrocephalus with macrocephaly. Obstet Gynecol 68:720, 1986

Christian SS, Brady K: Cord blood acid–base values in breech-presenting infants born vaginally. Obstet Gynecol 78:778, 1991

Clark S, DeVore GR, Platt LD: The role of ultrasound in the aggressive management of obstructed labor secondary to fetal malformations. Am J Obstet Gynecol 152:1042, 1985

Collea JV, Chein C, Quilligan EJ: The randomized management of term frank breech presentation: A study of 208 cases. Am J Obstet Gynecol 137:235, 1980

Collea JV, Rabin SC, Weghorst GR, Quilligan EJ: The randomized management of term frank breech presentation: Vaginal delivery vs cesarean section. Am J Obstet Gynecol 131:186, 1978

Cousins L, Dattel B, Hollingsworth D, Hulbert D, Zettner A: Screening for carbohydrate intolerance in pregnancy: A comparison of two tests and reassessment of a common approach. Am J Obstet Gynecol 153:381, 1985

Cox C, Kendall AC, Hommers M: Changed prognosis of breech-presenting low birthweight infants. Br J Obstet Gynaecol 89:881, 1982

Cruikshank DP, White CA: Obstetric malpresentations: Twenty years' experience. Am J Obstet Gynecol 116:1097, 1973

Delpapa EH, Mueller-Heubach E: Pregnancy outcome following ultrasound diagnosis of macrosomia. Obstet Gynecol 78:340, 1991

Donald WL, Barton JJ: Ultrasonography and external cephalic version at term. Am J Obstet Gynecol 162:1542, 1990

Duff P: Diagnosis and management of face presentation. Obstet Gynecol 57:105, 1981

Dyson DC, Ferguson JE II, Hensleigh P: Antepartum external cephalic version under tocolysis. Obstet Gynecol 67:63, 1986

Eden RD, Seifert LS, Winegar A, Spellacy WN: Perinatal characteristics of uncomplicated postdate pregnancies. Obstet Gynecol 69:296, 1987

Effer SB, Saigal S, Rand C, Hunter DJS, Stoskopf B, Harper AC, Nimrod C, Milner R: Effect of delivery method on outcomes in the very low-birth weight breech infant: Is the improved survival related to cesarean section or other perinatal care maneuvers? Am J Obstet Gynecol 145:123, 1983

Fianu S, Vaclavinkova V: The site of placental attachment as a factor in the aetiology of breech presentation. Acta Obstet Gynecol Scand 57:371, 1978

Flanagan TA, Mulchahey KM, Korenbrot CC, Green JR, Laros RK Jr: Management of term breech presentation. Am J Obstet Gynecol 156:1492, 1987

Fortney JA, Higgins JE, Kennedy KI, Laufe LE, Wilkens L: Delivery type and neonatal mortality among 10,749 breeches. AJPH 76:790, 1986

Fortunato SJ, Mercer LJ, Guzick DS: External cephalic version with tocolysis: Factors associated with success. Obstet Gynecol 72:59, 1988

Gimbel GL: Can shoulder dystocia be predicted? Am J Obstet Gynecol 163:680, 1990

Gimovsky ML, Paul RH: Singleton breech presentation in labor. Am J Obstet Gynecol 143:733, 1982

Gimovsky ML, Wallace RL, Schifrin BS, Paul RH: Randomized management of the nonfrank breech presentation at term: A preliminary report. Am J Obstet Gynecol 146:34, 1983

Gjode P, Rasmussen K, Jorgensen J: Feto-maternal bleeding during attempts at external version. Br J Obstet Gynaecol 87:571, 1980

Gonik B, Allen R, Sorab J: Objective evaluation of the shoulder dystocia phenomenon: Effect of maternal pelvic orientation on force reduction. Obstet Gynecol 74:44, 1989

Gonik B, Stringer CA, Held B: An alternate maneuver for management of shoulder dystocia. Am J Obstet Gynecol 145:882, 1983

Goplerud J, Eastman NJ: Compound presentation: Survey of 65 cases. Obstet Gynecol 1:59, 1953

Graham JM, Blanco JD, Weu T, Magee KP: The Zavanelli maneuver: A different perspective. Obstet Gynecol 79:883, 1992

Green JE, McLean F, Smith LP, Usher R: Has an increased cesarean section rate for term breech delivery reduced the incidence of birth asphyxia, trauma, and death? Am J Obstet Gynecol 142:643, 1982

Gross SJ, Shime J, Farine D: Shoulder dystocia: Predictors and outcome: A five-year review. Am J Obstet Gynecol 156:334, 1987a

Gross TL, Sokol RJ, Williams T, Thompson K: Shoulder dystocia: A fetal–physician risk. Am J Obstet Gynecol 156:1408, 1987b

Hall JE, Kohl SG: Breech presentation: A study of 1456 cases. Am J Obstet Gynecol 72:977, 1956

Hanss Jr JW: The efficacy of external cephalic version and its impact on the breech experience. Am J Obstet Gynecol 162:1459, 1990

Hardy AE: Birth injuries of the brachial plexus: Incidence and prognosis. J Bone Joint Surg 63:98, 1981

Harper RG, Kenigsberg K, Sia CG, Horn D, Stern D, Bongiovi V: Xiphopagus conjoined twins: A 300-year review of the obstetric, morphopathologic, neonatal, and surgical parameters. Am J Obstet Gynecol 137:617, 1980

Hartfield VJ: Symphysiotomy for shoulder dystocia. Am J Obstet Gynecol 155:228, 1986

Hellman LM, Epperson JWW, Connally F: Face and brow presentation: The experience of the Johns Hopkins Hospital, 1896 to 1948. Am J Obstet Gynecol 59:831, 1950

Hellstrom AC, Nilsson B, Stange L, Nylund L: When does external cephalic version succeed? Acta Obstet Gynecol Scand 69:281, 1990

Hernandez C, Wendel GD: Shoulder dystocia. In Pitkin RM (ed): Clinical Obstetrics and Gynecology, Vol 33, Hagerstown, Lippincott, 1990, p 526

Hibbard LT: Coping with shoulder dystocia. Contemp Obstet Gynecol 20:229, 1982

Hirata GI, Medearis AL, Horenstein J, Bear MB, Platt LD: Ultrasonographic estimation of fetal weight in the clinically macrosomic fetus. Am J Obstet Gynecol 162:228, 1990

Hopwood HG: Shoulder dystocia: Fifteen years' experience in a community hospital. Am J Obstet Gynecol 144:162, 1982

Houchang D, Dorchester W, Thorosian A, Freeman RK: Macrosomia—maternal, fetal, and neonatal complications. Obstet Gynecol 55:420, 1980

Hughey MJ: Fetal position during pregnancy. Am J Obstet Gynecol 153:885, 1985

Hytten FE: Breech presentation: Is it a bad omen? Br J Obstet Gynaecol 89:879, 1982

Ingemarsson I, Westgren M, Svenningsen NW: Long-term follow-up of preterm infants in breech presentation delivered by caesarean section. A prospective study. Lancet 2:172, 1978

Jennett RJ, Tarby TJ, Kreinick CJ: Brachial plexus palsy: An old problem revisited. Am J Obstet Gynecol 166:1673, 1992

Johnson CE: Transverse presentation of the fetus. JAMA 187:642, 1964

Johnson SR, Kolberg BH, Varner MW: Maternal obesity and pregnancy. Surg Gynecol Obstet 164:431, 1987

Kasule J, Chimbira THK, Brown I McL: Controlled trial of external cephalic version. Br J Obstet Gynaecol 92:14, 1985

Keller JD, Lopez-Zeno JA, Dooley SL, Socol ML: Shoulder dystocia and birth trauma in gestational diabetes: A five-year experience. Am J Obstet Gynecol 165:928, 1991

Klebe JG, Espersen T, Allen J: Diabetes mellitus and pregnancy. A seven-year material of pregnant diabetics, where control during pregnancy was based on a centralized ambulant regime. Acta Obstet Gynecol Scand 65:235, 1986

Kopelman JN, Duff P, Karl RT, Schipul AH, Read JA: Computed tomographic pelvimetry in the evaluation of breech presentation. Obstet Gynecol 68:455, 1986

Langer O, Berkus MD, Huff RW, Samualhoff A: Shoulder dystocia: Should the fetus weighing ≥ 4000 grams be delivered by cesarean section? Am J Obstet Gynecol 165:831, 1991

Levine MG, Holroyde J, Woods JR, Siddiqi TA, Scott MacH, Miodovnik M: Birth trauma: Incidence and predisposing factors. Obstet Gynecol 63:792, 1984

Marchick R: Antepartum external cephalic version with tocolysis: A study of term singleton breech presentations. Am J Obstet Gynecol 158:1339, 1988

Marcus RG, Crewe-Brown H, Krawitz S, Katz J: Feto-maternal haemorrhage following successful and unsuccessful attempts at external cephalic version. Br J Obstet Gynaecol 82:578, 1975

McFarland LV, Raskin M, Daling JR, Benedetti TJ: Erb/Duchenne's palsy: A consequence of fetal macrosomia and method of delivery. Obstet Gynecol 68:784, 1986

Modanlou HD, Komatsu G, Dorchester W, Freeman RK, Bosu SK: Large-for-gestational-age neonates: Anthropometric reasons for shoulder dystocia. Obstet Gynecol 60:417, 1982

Morrison JC, Myatt RE, Martin JN Jr, Meeks GR, Martin RW, Bucovaz ET, Wiser WL: External cephalic version of the breech presentation under tocolysis. Am J Obstet Gynecol 154:900, 1986

Morales WJ, Koerten J: Obstetric management and intraventricular hemorrhage in very-low-birthweight infants. Obstet Gynecol 68:35, 1986

Nagey DA: Can shoulder dystocia be prevented? Am J Obstet Gynecol 163:1095, 1990

Nelson KB, Ellenberg JH: Antecedents of cerebral palsy: Multivariate analysis of risk. N Engl J Med 315:81, 1986

O'Leary JA, Gunn D: Cephalic replacement for shoulder dystocia. Am J Obstet Gynecol 153:592, 1985

O'Leary JA, Leonetti HB: Shoulder dystocia: Prevention and treatment. Am J Obstet Gynecol 162:5, 1990

Osathanondh R, Birnholz JC, Altman AM, Driscoll SG: Ultrasonically guided transabdominal encephalocentesis. J Reprod Med 25:125, 1980

Parks DG, Ziel HK: Macrosomia: A proposed indication for primary cesarean section. Obstet Gynecol 52:407, 1978

Petrikovsky BM, DeSilva HN, Fumia FD: Erb's palsy and fetal bruising after external cephalic version: Case report. Am J Obstet Gynecol 157:258, 1987

Phelan JP, Boucher M, Mueller E, McCart D, Horenstein J, Clark SL: The nonlaboring transverse lie: A management dilemma. J Reprod Med 31:184, 1986

Phelan JP, Stine LE, Mueller E, McCart D, Yeh S: Observations of fetal heart rate characteristics related to external cephalic version and tocolysis. Am J Obstet Gynecol 149:658, 1984

Phillips RD, Freeman M: The management of the persistent occiput posterior position: A review of 552 consecutive cases. Obstet Gynecol 43:171, 1974

Pollack NB, O'Leary JA: McRoberts maneuver for shoulder dystocia: A survey. Thesis, University Hospital of Jacksonville, FL, 1985, p 6

Resnik R: Management of shoulder girdle dystocia. Clin Obstet Gynecol 23:559, 1980

Rovinsky JJ, Miller JA, Kaplan S: Management of breech presentation at term. Am J Obstet Gynecol 115:497, 1973

Rubin A: Management of shoulder dystocia. JAMA 189:835, 1964

Sandberg EC: The Zavanelli maneuver extended: Progression of a revolutionary concept. Am J Obstet Gynecol 158:1347, 1988

Savage JE: Dystocia due to dilation of the fetal urinary bladder. Am J Obstet Gynecol 29:267, 1935

Scheer K, Nubar J: Variation of fetal presentation with gestational age. Am J Obstet Gynecol 125:269, 1976

Schramm M: Impacted shoulders—A personal experience. Aust NZ J Obstet Gynaecol 23:28, 1983

Schutte MF, van Hemel OJS, van de Berg C, van de Pol A: Perinatal mortality in breech presentations as compared to vertex presentations in singleton pregnancies: An analysis based upon 57,819 computer-registered pregnancies in the Netherlands. Eur J Obstet Gynecol Reprod Biol 19:391, 1985

Socol ML, Cohen L, Depp R, Dooley SL, Tamura RK: Apgar scores and umbilical cord arterial pH in the breech neonate. Int J Gynecol Obstet 27:37, 1988

Soernes T, Bakke T: The length of the umbilical cord in vertex and breech presentations. Am J Obstet Gynecol 154:1086, 1986

Spellacy WN, Gravem H, Fish RO: The umbilical cord complications of true knots, nuchal cords, and cord around the body. Am J Obstet Gynecol 94:1136, 1966

Spellacy WN, Miller MS, Winegar A, Peterson PQ: Macrosomia—Maternal characteristics and infant complications. Obstet Gynecol 66:158, 1985

Stine LE, Phelan JP, Wallace R, Eglinton GS, Van Dorsten JP, Schifrin BS: Update on external cephalic version performed at term. Obstet Gynecol 65:642, 1985

Susuki S, Yamamuro T: Fetal movement and fetal presentation. Early Hum Dev 11:255, 1985

Svenningsen NW, Westgren M, Ingemarsson I: Modern strategy for the term breech delivery—A study with a 4-year follow-up of the infants. J Perinat Med 13:117, 1985

Tank ES, Davis R, Holt JF, Morley GW: Mechanism of trauma during breech delivery. Obstet Gynecol 38:761, 1971

Thiery M: Management of breech delivery. Eur J Obstet Gynecol Reprod Biol 24:93, 1987

Van Dorsten JP, Schifrin BS, Wallace RL: Randomized control trial of external cephalic version with tocolysis in late pregnancy. Am J Obstet Gynecol 141:417, 1981

Watson WJ, Benson WL: Vaginal delivery for the selected frank breech infant at term. Obstet Gynecol 64:638, 1984

Westgren LMR, Songster G, Paul RH: Preterm breech delivery: Another retrospective study. Obstet Gynecol 66:481, 1985a

Westgren M, Paul RH: Delivery of the low birth weight infant by cesarean section. Clin Obstet Gynecol 28:752, 1985b

Woods CE: A principle of physics is applicable to shoulder delivery. Am J Obstet Gynecol 45:796, 1943

CHAPTER 21
Dystocia Due to Pelvic Contraction

Any contraction of the pelvic diameters that diminishes the capacity of the pelvis can create dystocia during labor. Pelvic contractions may be classified as follows:

1. Contraction of the pelvic inlet
2. Contraction of the midpelvis
3. Contraction of the pelvic outlet
4. Generally contracted pelvis (combinations of the above)

Contracted Pelvic Inlet

Definition. The pelvic inlet is usually considered to be contracted if its shortest *anteroposterior diameter is less than 10.0 cm or if the greatest transverse diameter is less than 12.0 cm*. The anteroposterior diameter of the pelvic inlet is commonly approximated by manually measuring the diagonal conjugate, which is about 1.5 cm greater. Therefore, inlet contraction is usually defined as a *diagonal conjugate of less than 11.5 cm*. The errors inherent in the use of this clinical measurement are discussed in Chapter 11 (p. 288).

Using clinical and, at times, imaging pelvimetry (Chap. 11, p. 290), it is important to identify the shortest anteroposterior diameter through which the fetal head must pass. Occasionally, the body of the first sacral vertebra is displaced forward so that the shortest distance may actually be between this false, or abnormal, sacral promontory and the symphysis pubis.

Prior to labor, the fetal biparietal diameter has been shown by sonography to *average* from 9.5 to as much as 9.8 cm in different clinical populations; therefore, it might prove difficult or even impossible for some fetuses to pass through an inlet with an anteroposterior diameter of less than 10 cm. Mengert (1948) and Kaltreider (1952), employing x-ray pelvimetry, demonstrated that the incidence of difficult deliveries is increased to a similar degree when either the anteroposterior diameter is less than 10 cm or the transverse diameter of the inlet is less than 12 cm. When both diameters are contracted, the incidence of obstetrical difficulty is much greater than when only one diameter is contracted. The configuration of the pelvic inlet is also an important determinant of the adequacy of any pelvis, independent of actual measurements of the anteroposterior and transverse diameters and of calculated "areas" (see Fig. 11–8, and "Caldwell–Moloy Classification," p. 286).

A small woman is likely to have a small pelvis, but at the same time she is more likely to have a small infant. Thoms (1937), in a study of 362 nulliparous women, found the average weight of offspring to be significantly lower (278 g) in women with small pelves than in those with medium or large pelves. In veterinary obstetrics, it has frequently been observed that in most species maternal size rather than paternal size is the important determinant of fetal size.

Size of Fetal Head. Clinical, radiological, and ultrasonic techniques have been used with varying degrees of success to identify the size of the fetal head relative to that of the pelvic inlet.

Clinical Estimation. Impression of the fetal head into the pelvis, as described by Müller (1880), may provide useful information. In an occiput presentation, the obstetrician grasps the brow and the suboccipital region through the abdominal wall with the fingers and makes firm pressure downward in the axis of the pelvic inlet. Fundal pressure by an assistant usually is helpful. The effect of the forces on the descent of the head can be evaluated by palpation with a sterile gloved hand in the vagina. If no disproportion exists, the head readily enters the pelvis, and vaginal delivery can be predicted. Inability to push the head into the pelvis, however, does not necessarily indicate that vaginal delivery is impossible. A clear demonstration of a flexed fetal head that overrides the symphysis pubis, however, is presumptive evidence of disproportion.

Radiological Estimation. Measurements of fetal head diameters using radiographic techniques have been disappointing.

Sonographic Measurements. The fetal biparietal diameter and head circumference can be measured precisely by ultrasonic means. The freely floating fetal head, as in breech presentations, unfortunately may move sufficiently during sonographic examination to invalidate the measurement. Additionally, the fetal head in a breech presentation may be dolichocephalic, that is, elongated in the occipitofrontal diameter (Kasby and Poll, 1982). This dolichocephalic, or so-called "breech head" (Fig. 21–1), may also be observed in multifetal gestations and in cases of oligohydramnios (Berkowitz and Hobbins, 1982). Such an observation may lead the sonographer to underestimate fetal weight and gestational age. When a dolichocephalic head is observed, a

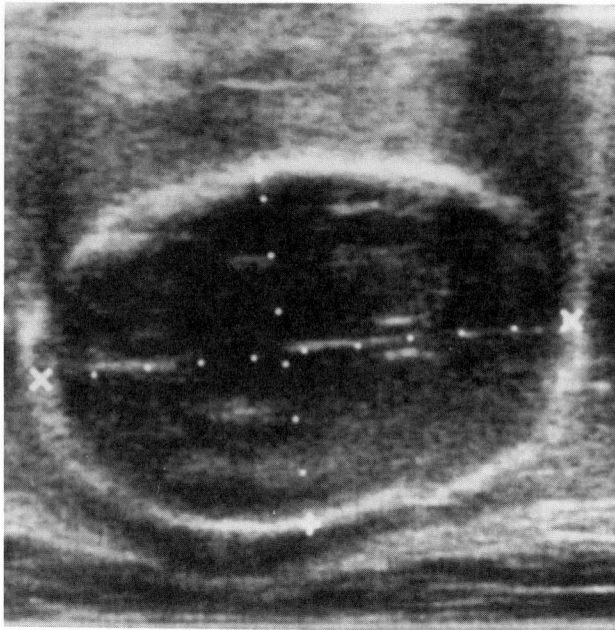

Fig. 21–1. Ultrasonic transverse scan of the head of a breech presenting fetus. The biparietal diameter is significantly smaller than the occipitofrontal diameter. This dolichocephalic configuration also may develop from crowding in multifetal gestation and from oligohydramnios. (Courtesy of Dr. R. Santos.)

head circumference measurement will result in a more accurate estimation of fetal size.

Fetal–Pelvic Index. Morgan and co-workers (1986) attempted to develop a standardized method for comparing fetal size with the respective maternal pelvis. They measured fetal head and abdominal circumferences using ultrasound. Maternal pelvic inlet and midpelvic circumferences were measured using x-ray pelvimetry. They computed a "fetal–pelvic index" number based upon differences in the pelvis and fetal circumferences. Maternal pelvic dimensions and fetal abdominal circumferences were related to cesarean deliveries for fetal–pelvic disproportion. Interestingly, fetal head circumference was not identified as a cause of dystocia. This finding challenges the concept of cephalopelvic disproportion as a common cause of dystocia. The fetal–pelvic index has been used successfully by this same group of investigators in several other types of labor complications (Morgan and Thurnau, 1988; Thurnau and associates, 1991).

Presentation and Position of the Fetus. A contracted pelvic inlet plays an important part in the production of abnormal presentations. In normal nulliparous women, the presenting part at term commonly descends into the pelvic cavity before the onset of labor. When the pelvic inlet is contracted considerably, however, descent usually does not occur until after the onset of labor, if at all. Cephalic presentations still pre-

dominate, but because the head floats freely over the pelvic inlet or rests more laterally in one of the iliac fossae, very slight influences may cause the fetus to assume other presentations. **For example, in women with contracted pelves, face and shoulder presentations occur three times more frequently, and prolapse of the cord and extremities occurs four to six times more frequently.**

Course of Labor. When a pelvic deformity is sufficiently severe to prevent the head from entering the inlet, the course of labor is prolonged and effective spontaneous labor is often never achieved. This obviously can result in serious maternal and fetal effects.

Maternal Effects. Although maternal and fetal effects resulting from inlet contraction are divided arbitrarily in the following discussion, bony dystocia may result in serious consequences to either or both patients.

Abnormalities in Cervical Dilatation. Normally, cervical dilatation is facilitated by hydrostatic action of the unruptured membranes or, after their rupture, by direct application of the presenting part against the cervix. In contracted pelves, however, when the head is arrested in the pelvic inlet, the entire force exerted by the uterus acts directly upon the portion of membranes that overlie the dilating cervix. Consequently, early spontaneous rupture of the membranes is more likely to result.

After rupture of the membranes, the absence of pressure by the fetal head against the cervix and lower uterine segment predisposes to less effective uterine contractions. Hence, further dilatation may proceed very slowly or not at all. Cibils and Hendricks (1965) reported that the mechanical adaptation of the fetal passenger to the bony passage plays an important part in determining the efficiency of uterine contractions. The better the adaptation, the more efficient are the contractions. Because adaptation is poor in the presence of a contracted pelvis, prolongation of labor often results. **With degrees of pelvic contractions incompatible with vaginal delivery, the cervix seldom dilates satisfactorily. Thus, cervical response to labor provides a prognostic view of the outcome of labor in women with inlet contraction.**

Danger of Uterine Rupture. Abnormal thinning of the lower uterine segment creates a serious danger during a prolonged labor. When the disproportion between fetal head and pelvis is so pronounced that engagement and descent do not occur, the lower uterine segment becomes increasingly stretched, and the danger of its rupture becomes imminent. In such cases, a **pathological retraction ring** may develop and may be felt as a transverse or oblique ridge extending across the uterus somewhere between the symphysis and the umbilicus. Whenever this condition is noted, immediate abdominal delivery is indicated. Unless cesarean delivery is employed, there is a great danger of uterine rupture and serious fetal compromise.

Fistula Formation. When the presenting part is firmly wedged into the pelvic inlet but does not advance for a considerable time, portions of the birth canal lying between it and the pelvic wall may be subjected to excessive pressure. Because the circulation was impaired, necrosis may result and become evident several days after delivery with the appearance of vesicovaginal, vesicocervical, or rectovaginal fistulas. Most often, pressure necrosis follows a very prolonged second stage of labor. Formerly, when operative delivery was deferred as long as possible, such complications were frequent, but today they are rarely seen except in undeveloped countries.

Intrapartum Infection. Infection is a serious danger to which mother and fetus are exposed in labors complicated by prolonged membrane rupture. These dangers are increased by repeated vaginal examinations and other intravaginal and intrauterine manipulations. If the amnionic fluid becomes infected, fever may or may not develop during labor.

Fetal Effects. Prolonged labor in itself may be deleterious to the fetus. In women with labors of more than 20 hours or in women with a second stage more than 3 hours, Hellman and Prystowsky (1952) reported significantly increased perinatal mortality rates. More recently, Rosen and co-workers (1989) studied brain damage after 2 years of age in 413 infants born after abnormal labors. Labor disorders, including arrests of descent and dilatation during active labor and protractions of the active phase of labor (see Chap. 19, p. 478),

were not associated with neurological morbidity. In contrast, Roemer and associates (1991) claimed that intelligence quotients (IQs) were about 10 points lower in infants subjected to more than 12 hours of labor compared with abdominally delivered siblings. However, these infants were delivered between 1952 and 1954 when intrapartum management was considerably different compared with current practices.

If the pelvis is contracted and there is associated prolonged rupture of membranes and intrauterine infection, fetal and maternal risks are compounded. Intrapartum infection is not only a serious maternal complication but also an important cause of fetal and neonatal death. This obtains because bacteria in amnionic fluid traverse the amnion and invade decidua and chorionic vessels, thus giving rise to maternal and fetal bacteremia. Fetal pneumonia, caused by aspiration of infected amnionic fluid, is another serious consequence.

Caput Succedaneum. If the pelvis is contracted, during labor a large *caput succedaneum* frequently develops on the most dependent part of the fetal head. As shown in Figure 21–2, this may assume considerable size and lead to serious diagnostic errors. **The caput may reach almost to the pelvic floor while the head is still not engaged. An inexperienced physician may make premature and unwise attempts at forceps delivery.** Typically, even a large caput disappears within a few days after birth.

Fetal Head Molding. Under the pressure of strong uterine contractions, cranial plates overlap one another at the major sutures, a process referred to as *molding* (Figs. 21–2, 44–15). As a rule, the median margin of the parietal bone that is in contact with the sacral promontory is overlapped by that of its fellow;

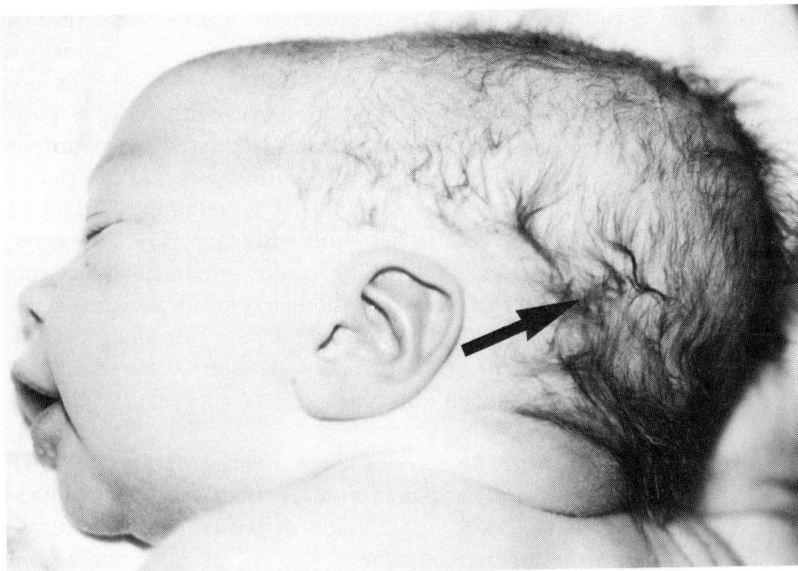

Fig. 21–2. Considerable molding of the head and caput formation in a very recently delivered infant. The arrow is directed toward the appreciable scalp edema that overlies the occiput, that is, caput succedaneum.

the same result occurs with the frontal bones. The occipital bone, however, is pushed under the parietal bones. These changes are frequently accomplished without obvious detriment to the child. Alternatively, when the distortion is marked, molding may lead to tentorial tears, laceration of fetal blood vessels, and fatal intracranial hemorrhage.

Sorbe and Dahlgren (1983) measured six fetal head diameters at birth and compared these with measurements obtained 3 days later. Molding was greatest in the subocciptobregmatic dimension and averaged 0.3 cm with a range up to 1.5 cm. The biparietal diameter was not affected by fetal head molding. Factors associated with molding included nulliparity, oxytocin labor stimulation, and delivery with a vacuum extractor. Carlan and colleagues (1991) described a locking mechanism by which the free edges of cranial bones are forced into one another, preventing further molding and presumably providing protection for the fetal brain. They also observed that severe fetal head molding could occur before labor. Holland (1922) observed that severe molding could lead to fatal subdural hemorrhage in the fetus due to tears involving the dura mater septa, especially the tentorium cerebelli. Such fetal tears were observed to occur in both normal and complicated deliveries.

Coincidental with molding, the parietal bone, which was in contact with the promontory, may show signs of being subjected to marked pressure, sometimes even becoming flattened. Accommodation more readily occurs when the bones of the head are imperfectly ossified. This important process may provide one explanation for the differences observed in the course of labor in two apparently similar cases in which the pelvis and the head present identical measurements. In one case, the head is softer and more readily molded, and spontaneous delivery results. In the other, the more ossified head retains its original shape and operative interference is required for delivery.

Characteristic pressure marks may form upon the scalp, covering the portion of the head that passes over the promontory of the sacrum. From their location, it is frequently possible to ascertain the movements that the head has undergone in passing through the pelvic inlet. Much more rarely, similar marks appear on the portion of the head that has been in contact with the symphysis pubis. Such marks usually disappear within a few days after birth, although in exceptional instances severe pressure may lead to scalp necrosis.

Skull fractures are occasionally encountered, usually following forcible attempts at delivery. As discussed in Chapter 44 (p. 1022), such fractures also may occur with spontaneous delivery or even with cesarean section (Skajaa and associates, 1987). The fractures are of two varieties, either a shallow groove or a spoon-shaped depression just posterior to the coronal suture (Fig. 21–3). The former is relatively common, but because it

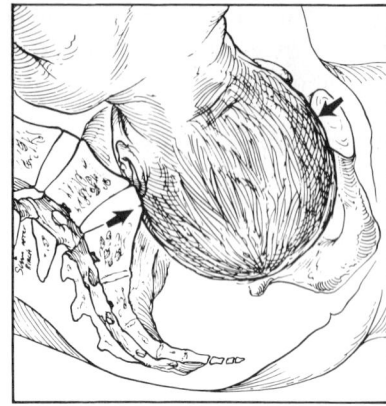

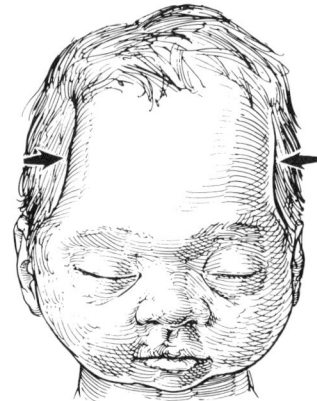

Fig. 21–3. Depression of the skull (*arrows*) caused by labor with a contracted pelvic inlet.

involves only the external plate of the bone, it is not very dangerous. The latter, however, if not surgically corrected, may lead to neonatal death, because it extends through the entire thickness of the skull and gives rise to inner surface projections that exert injurious pressure upon the brain and may cause hemorrhage. Accordingly, as soon as feasible after delivery, it is advisable to elevate or remove the depressed portion of the skull.

Umbilical Cord Prolapse. Prolapse of the cord is a serious fetal complication that is facilitated by imperfect adaptation between the presenting part and the pelvic inlet. Unless prompt delivery is accomplished, fetal death may result. Katz and associates (1988) noted, however, that rapid filling of the urinary bladder with 500 to 700 mL of normal saline to elevate the presenting fetal part and intravenous ritodrine to produce uterine relaxation prior to cesarean delivery resulted in improved neonatal outcomes.

Prognosis. In cases of severe inlet contraction with an anteroposterior diameter of less than 9 cm, the prognosis for successful vaginal delivery of a term-sized fetus is nearly hopeless. For the borderline group in which the anteroposterior diameter is slightly below 10 cm, the prognosis for vaginal delivery is influenced significantly by a number of variables, including the following:

1. Presentation is of extreme importance. All presentations but the occiput are unfavorable.
2. Fetal size is of obvious importance, but estimates of fetal size at term, especially the head, are often imprecise.
3. Pelvic inlet diameters and configuration play important roles. With an android configuration (Fig. 11–8), for any given anteroposterior diameter of the inlet, there is less available forepelvis space.
4. The frequency and intensity of spontaneous uterine contractions are informative. Uterine dysfunction, characterized by infrequent contractions of low intensity, is common with significant disproportion. The uterus does not often self-destruct.
5. Cervical response to labor has great prognostic significance. In general, orderly spontaneous progression to full dilatation indicates that vaginal delivery most likely will be successful.
6. Extreme asynclitism and appreciable molding of the fetal head without engagement are unfavorable prognostic signs.
7. Knowledge of previous labor and delivery outcomes at term is helpful as well as previous infant weights.
8. The prognosis for successful vaginal delivery is altered by coincidental conditions that impair uteroplacental perfusion, such as fetal growth retardation. In such circumstances, uterine contractions sufficient to dilate the cervix and propel the fetus through the birth canal are much more likely to further compromise already decreased placental perfusion to such a degree that the fetus is distressed.

Treatment. The management of inlet contraction is determined principally by the prognosis for safe vaginal delivery. If, on the basis of the criteria reviewed, a delivery that is safe for both mother and child cannot be anticipated, cesarean delivery is indicated. Today it is so rare to employ fetal craniotomy that even dead fetuses are often delivered abdominally in cases of pelvic contraction. Only in a minority of instances can a prognosis be reached before the onset of labor. A carefully managed trial of labor is desirable in most instances. Women with inlet contractions are particularly likely to have both weak uterine contractions during the first stage of labor and a need for vigorous voluntary expulsive efforts during the second stage. Therefore, the use of conduction analgesia should in general be approached with caution. The course of labor should be monitored closely and the prognosis established as soon as reasonably possible. Although signs of impending uterine rupture always should be looked for if contractions are strong, the danger of this accident occurring is remote in nulliparous women. With greater parity, however, the likelihood of uterine rupture increases. Finally, oxytocin administration in the presence of any form of pelvic contraction, unless the fetal head has unequivocally passed the point of obstruction, can be catastrophic for both fetus and mother.

Contracted Midpelvis

Definition. The obstetrical plane of the midpelvis extends from the inferior margin of the symphysis pubis, through the ischial spines, and touches the sacrum near the junction of the fourth and fifth vertebrae. A transverse line theoretically connecting the ischial spines divides the midpelvis into anterior and posterior portions. The former is bounded anteriorly by the lower border of the symphysis pubis and laterally by the ischiopubic rami. The posterior portion is bounded dorsally by the sacrum and laterally by the sacrospinous ligaments, forming the lower limits of the sacrosciatic notch.

Average midpelvis measurements are as follows: transverse (interspinous), 10.5 cm; anteroposterior (from the lower border of the symphysis pubis to the junction of the fourth and fifth sacral vertebrae), 11.5 cm; and posterior sagittal (from the midpoint of the interspinous line to the same point on the sacrum), 5 cm. Although the definition of midpelvic contractions has not been established with the same precision possible for inlet contractions, the midpelvis is likely contracted when the sum of the interischial spinous and posterior sagittal diameters of the midpelvis (normally, 10.5 plus 5 cm, or 15.5 cm) falls to 13.5 cm or below. This concept has been emphasized by Chen and Huang (1982) in evaluating possible midpelvic contraction. There is reason to suspect that midpelvic contraction exists whenever the interischial spinous diameter is less than 10 cm. When it is smaller than 8 cm, the midpelvis is contracted. The preceding definitions of midpelvic contraction do not, of course, imply that dystocia will necessarily occur in such a pelvis, but simply that it more likely will develop. Development of dystocia also depends upon the size and shape of the forepelvis and the size of the fetal head, as well as on the overall degree of midpelvic contraction.

Identification. Although there is no precise manual method of measuring midpelvic dimensions, a suggestion of midpelvic contraction can sometimes be obtained by ascertaining that the spines are prominent, the pelvic side walls converge, or the sacrosciatic notch is narrow. Eller and Mengert (1947), moreover, pointed out that the relationship between the intertuberous and interspinous diameters of the ischium is sufficiently constant that narrowing of the interspinous diameter can be anticipated when the intertuberous diameter is narrow. A normal intertuberous diameter, however, does not always exclude a narrow interspinous diameter (Chap. 11, p. 290).

Prognosis. Midpelvic contraction is probably more common than inlet contraction, and it is frequently a cause of transverse arrest of the fetal head. Such a contraction can potentially lead to a difficult midforceps operation or to a cesarean delivery.

Treatment. In the labor management of midpelvic contraction, the natural forces of labor should be allowed to push the biparietal diameter beyond the potential interspinous obstruction. Forceps operations may be very difficult when applied to a head whose greatest diameter has not yet passed a contracted midpelvis. This difficulty may be explained on two grounds: (1) pulling on the head with forceps destroys flexion, whereas pressure from above increases it; and (2) although the forceps blades occupy a space of only a few millimeters, the blades further diminish available space. Only when the head has descended to such an extent that the perineum is bulging and the vertex is actually visible is it reasonably certain that the head has passed the obstruction. It is then usually safe to apply forceps. Strong fundal pressure should not be used in attempts to force the head past the obstruction.

The use of forceps to affect delivery in midpelvic contraction, usually undiagnosed, has been responsible for much of the stigma attached to midforceps operations. Midforceps delivery, therefore, is contraindicated in any case of midpelvic contraction in which the fetal biparietal diameter has not passed beyond the level of contraction. Otherwise, perinatal mortality and morbidity rates associated with the operation are prohibitive.

The vacuum extractor (see Chap. 24, p. 571) has been reported to be of advantage in some cases of midpelvic contraction *after the cervix has become fully dilated.* Traction need not cause deflection of the fetal head, and the vacuum extractor does not occupy space, as do forceps. **As with forceps, however, the vacuum extractor should not be applied unless the biparietal diameter has passed the pelvic obstruction.** Oxytocin, of course, has no place in the treatment of dystocia caused by midpelvic contraction.

Contracted Pelvic Outlet

Definition and Incidence. Contraction of the pelvic outlet is usually defined as diminution of the interischial tuberous diameter to 8 cm or less. The pelvic outlet may be roughly likened to two triangles (Figs. 21–4 and 21–5). The interischial tuberous diameter constitutes

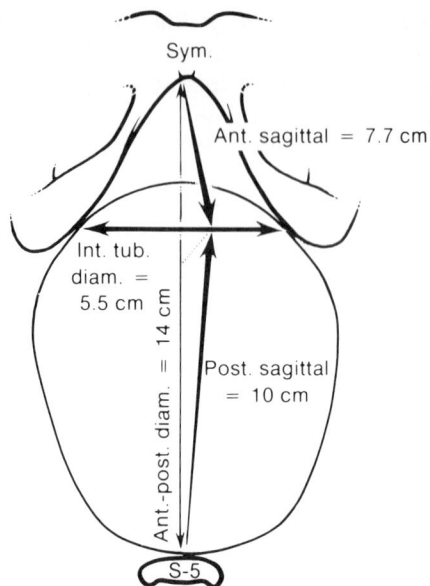

Fig. 21–4. Diagram of pelvic outlet of case shown in Figure 21–5. Even though the intertuberous diameter is quite narrow (5.5 cm), vaginal delivery is possible because of the long (10 cm) posterior sagittal diameter. (Int. tub. diam. = intertuberous diameter; Sym. = symphysis pubis; S-5 = fifth sacral vertebra.)

the base of both. The sides of the anterior triangle are the pubic rami, and its apex the inferior posterior surface of the symphysis pubis. The posterior triangle has no bony sides but is limited at its apex by the tip of the last sacral vertebra (not the tip of the coccyx). Floberg and associates (1987) reported that outlet contractions were found in 0.9 percent of over 1400 unselected term nulliparas cared for in their Stockholm hospital.

Maternal Position. Recently, considerable interest has been shown in alternative second-stage labor birth po-

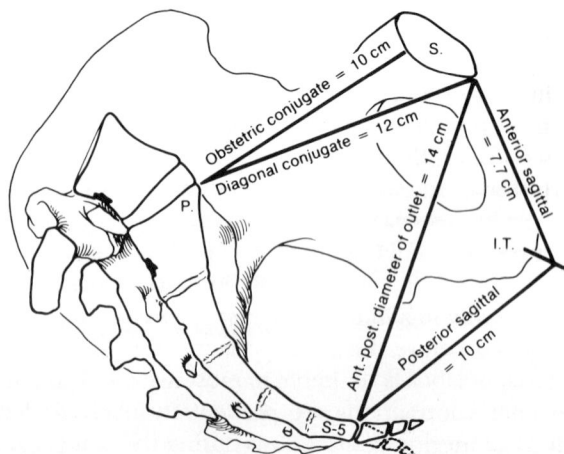

Fig. 21–5. Diagram of the lateral view of the same pelvis depicted in Figure 21–4. The long (10 cm) posterior sagittal diameter may allow the fetal head to negotiate the narrow (5.5 cm) intertuberous diameter (IT = ischial tuberosity; S = symphysis pubis; P = sacral promontory).

sitions. As reviewed by Gupta and co-workers (1991), several randomized controlled trials, with and without the use of specific birthing aids, have produced conflicting results and are confounded by observer bias. One reported advantage from avoiding the traditional lithotomy position is an increase in the dimensions of the pelvic outlet. Specifically, Russell (1969) described a 20 to 30 percent increase in the area of the pelvic outlet with squatting compared with the supine position. Gupta and co-workers (1991) compared the usual Western delivery position (recumbent with the head and shoulders up 30 degrees) with the squatting position and found no significant change in the dimensions of either the pelvic inlet or outlet. Crowley and associates (1991) randomized 634 women to deliver in an obstetrical birth chair and compared these with 596 women delivered in bed. There were no advantages with use of the birthing chair; however, hemorrhage was increased in the birth chair group. The parturients were questioned about their feelings of birthing in a chair versus a bed, and there were no differences in their overall assessment of their childbirth experience.

Prognosis. It is apparent from Figure 21–4 that diminution in the intertuberous diameter with consequent narrowing of the anterior triangle must inevitably force the fetal head posteriorly. Whether delivery can take place therefore partly depends on the size of the posterior triangle or, more specifically, the interischial tuberous diameter and the posterior sagittal diameter of the outlet. A contracted outlet may cause dystocia not so much by itself as through the often associated midpelvic contraction. *Outlet contraction without concomitant midplane contraction is rare.*

Even when the disproportion between the size of the fetal head and the pelvic outlet is not sufficiently great to give rise to severe dystocia, it may play an important part in the production of perineal tears. With increasing narrowing of the pubic arch, the occiput cannot emerge directly beneath the symphysis pubis but is forced increasingly farther down upon the ischiopubic rami. In extreme cases, the head must rotate around a line joining the ischial tuberosities. The perineum, consequently, must become increasingly distended and thus exposed to great danger of disruption. An extensive mediolateral episiotomy is usually indicated.

Pelvic Fractures and Pregnancy

Speer and Peltier (1972) reviewed their experiences and those of others with pelvic fractures and pregnancy. Trauma from automobile collisions was the most common cause of pelvic fractures. With bilateral fractures of the pubic rami, compromise of birth canal capacity by callus formation or malunion was very common. A history of pelvic fracture warrants careful review of previous x-rays and possibly computed tomographic pelvimetry later in pregnancy, unless cesarean delivery is performed for another reason (Chap. 11, p. 292).

Rare Pelvic Contractions

Due to the relative safety of cesarean delivery, rare pelvic contractions do not result in the same maternal and fetal consequences as in earlier times. Therefore, the descriptions and illustrations of these many and varied pelvic contractions have been omitted (see *Williams Obstetrics*, editions 10 through 17). It is important to note, however, that potentially lethal problems other than pelvic abnormalities may be encountered in dwarfs, and in women with poliomyelitis, kyphoscoliosis, and those who are small and dysmorphic. These dangers include, but *are not limited* to pulmonary and cardiovascular abnormalities.

References

Berkowitz RL, Hobbins JC: How head shape affects BPD. Contemp Obstet Gynecol 19:35, 1982

Carlan SJ, Wyble L, Lense J, Mastrogiannis DS, Parsons MT: Fetal head molding. Diagnosis by ultrasound and a review of the literature. J Perinatol 11:105, 1991

Chen H-Y, Huang SC: Evaluation of midpelvic contraction. Int Surg 67:516, 1982

Cibils LA, Hendricks CH: Normal labor in vertex presentation. Am J Obstet Gynecol 91:385, 1965

Crowley P, Elbourne D, Ashurst H, Garcia J, Murphy D, Duigan N: Delivery in an obstetric birth chair: A randomized controlled trial. Br J Obstet Gynaecol 98:667, 1991

Eller WC, Mengert WF: Recognition of mid-pelvic contraction. Am J Obstet Gynecol 53:252, 1947

Floberg J, Belfrage P, Ohlsén H: Influence of pelvic outlet capacity on labor: A prospective pelvimetry study of 1429 unselected primiparas. Acta Obstet Gynecol Scand 66:121, 1987

Gupta JK, Glanville JN, Johnson N, Lilford RJ, Dunahm RJ, Walters JK: The effect of squatting in pelvic dimensions. Eur J Obstet Gynecol Reprod Biol 42:19, 1991

Hellman LM, Prystowsky H: Duration of the second stage of labor. Am J Obstet Gynecol 63:1223, 1952

Holland E: Cranial stress in the foetus during labor. J Obstet Gynaecol Br Emp 29:549, 1922

Kaltreider DF: Criteria of midplane contraction. Am J Obstet Gynecol 63:392, 1952

Kasby CB, Poll V: The breech head and its ultrasound significance. Br J Obstet Gynaecol 89:106, 1982

Katz Z, Shoham Z, Lancet M, Blickstein I, Mogilner BM, Zalel Y: Management of labor with umbilical cord prolapse: A 5-year study. Obstet Gynecol 72:278, 1988

Mengert WF: Estimation of pelvic capacity. JAMA 138:169, 1948

Morgan MA, Thurnau GR: Efficacy of the fetal-pelvic index in patients requiring labor induction. Am J Obstet Gynecol 159:621, 1988

Morgan MA, Thurnau GR, Fishburne JI: The fetal–pelvic index as an indicator of fetal–pelvic disproportion: A preliminary report. Am J Obstet Gynecol 155:608, 1986

Müller: On the frequency and etiology of general pelvic contraction. Arch Gynaek 16:155, 1880

Roemer FJ, Rowland DY, Nuamali IF: Retrospective study of fetal effects of prolonged labor before cesarean delivery. Obstet Gynecol 77:653, 1991

Rosen MG, Debonne SM, Thompson K: Arrest disorders and infant brain damage. Obstet Gynecol 74:321, 1989

Russell JG: Moulding of the pelvic outlet. J Obstet Gynaecol Br Commonw 76:817, 1969

Skajaa K, Hansen ES, Bendix J: Depressed fracture of the skull in a child born by cesarean section. Acta Obstet Gynecol Scand 66:275, 1987

Sorbe B, Dahlgren S: Some important factors in the molding of the fetal head during vaginal delivery—a photographic study. Int J Gynaecol Obstet 21:205, 1983

Speer DP, Peltier LF: Pelvic fractures and pregnancy. J Trauma 12:474, 1972

Thoms H: The obstetrical significance of pelvic variations: A study of 450 primiparous women. Br Med J 2:210, 1937

Thurnau GR, Scates DH, Morgan MA: The fetal–pelvic index: A method of identifying fetal–pelvic disproportion in women attempting vaginal birth after previous cesarean delivery. Am J Obstet Gynecol 165:353, 1991

CHAPTER 22
Dystocia Due to Soft Tissue Abnormalities of the Reproductive Tract

Vulvar Abnormalities

Atresia. Complete *atresia of the vulva,* or the lower portion of the vagina, is usually congenital and, unless corrected, precludes conception. More frequently, vulvar atresia is incomplete, resulting from adhesions or scars following injury or infection. The defect may present a considerable obstacle to delivery, but the resistance usually is overcome eventually by continued pressure exerted by the fetal head. This may result in deep perineal tears unless prevented by an adequate episiotomy.

Edema. The vulva may become edematous, but dystocia rarely results from edema alone. Venous thromboses and hematomas may cause edema and significant pain and make an episiotomy difficult to perform; however, they seldom cause dystocia (see Chap. 29, p. 644).

Inflammatory Lesions. Inflammatory vulvar lesions have similar effects. Extensive perineal inflammation and scarring from *hidradenitis suppurativa, lymphogranuloma venereum,* or Crohn disease may create difficulty with vaginal delivery, episiotomy, and repair. A mediolateral episiotomy may prevent some of these difficulties and rectal lacerations.

BARTHOLIN ABSCESS. Aside from causing pain and discomfort, abscesses may be the starting point of a puerperal infection. For these reasons, drainage must be established whenever an abscess develops during pregnancy. After the contents are drained, the cut edges of the abscess cavity, if actively bleeding, are sutured with fine chromic catgut. A gauze drain should be inserted to keep the ostium open until granulation is complete. Both aerobic and anaerobic bacteria can be identified in pus from such abscesses, but *Neisseria gonorrhoeae* has been identified in less than 10 percent. A broad-spectrum antibiotic should be administered until the surrounding cellulitis responds to treatment.

BARTHOLIN CYSTS. Treatment of asymptomatic cysts, which are frequently the sequelae of abscesses, is best postponed until after delivery. Rarely is a labial cyst of sufficient size to cause difficulty at delivery. If so, needle aspiration will suffice as a temporary measure. Because of pregnancy-induced hyperemia, excision should not be attempted.

URETHRAL DIVERTICULAE, CYSTS AND ABSCESSES. Trauma to the urethra or infection of the periurethral glands may result in periurethral abscesses, cysts, and diverticulae. Abscesses usually resolve spontaneously, with cyst formation as a sequela. Most often, periurethral cysts are asymptomatic, do not result in dystocia, and are best not disturbed during pregnancy. A urethral diverticulum may fill with debris that empties intermittently through the urethra to give rise to proteinuria of obscure etiology. In general, surgical excision should not be done during pregnancy.

Condyloma Acuminata. Genital infection with the human papillomavirus results in condyloma acuminata, often called *venereal warts.* These sexually transmitted lesions are discussed in Chapter 59 (p. 1313). There is a strong association between several types of papillomaviruses and squamous carcinoma of the vulva, vagina, and cervix (see Chap. 57, p. 1273).

Genital condyloma may be so extensive that vaginal delivery is undesirable. Delivery usually can be accomplished, however, without extensive lacerations or hemorrhage, but predelivery eradication is preferable. This is done to prevent the lesions from expanding to cause dystocia. It also prevents secondary infection and hemorrhage, which may result in amnionitis, preterm labor, and episiotomy dehiscence (Ferenczy, 1989; Hankins and associates, 1989). There is no evidence that any therapy including surgical, chemical, laser, or immunological (alpha-interferon) will eradicate genital papillomavirus and prevent vertical transmission to a fetus-neonate (Hankins and co-workers, 1989; Patsner and associates, 1990). Although there is no proof that there is vertical transmission, there is compelling clinical and laboratory evidence to support this conclusion (Ferenczy, 1989; Rando and associates, 1989; Sedlacek and co-workers, 1989; Smith and colleagues, 1991). Current therapy does not cure genital papillomavirus infections, but reduction in mass may decrease the risk of neonatal infection (Patsner and colleagues, 1990).

Acceptable results during pregnancy can be accomplished using laser alone (Hankins and associates, 1989), locally applied 85 percent trichloracetic acid and laser vaporization (Schwartz and associates, 1988), or surgical excision and cryotherapy alone or in combination with electrocautery (Patsner and associates, 1990). Topically applied podophyllin and 5-fluorouracil are felt by many to be contraindicated during pregnancy, as are alpha-interferons (Patsner and associates, 1990). Some recommend that therapy during pregnancy should be withheld until after 32 weeks to prevent relapses and to ensure that if preterm labor ensues as a result of treatment, the fetus is sufficiently mature to survive (Ferenczy, 1984, 1989; Hankins and co-workers, 1989; Schwarz and associates, 1988).

Vaginal Abnormalities

Septa and Strictures. Occasionally, the vagina is divided by a *longitudinal septum,* which may be complete, extending from the vulva to the cervix. More often, it is incomplete and limited to either the upper or lower portion of the canal. Because such conditions frequently are associated with other abnormalities in development of the genital tract, their detection should prompt careful examination to ascertain whether there are coexistent uterine or renal deformities (see Chap. 33, p. 723). A complete longitudinal septum usually does not cause dystocia because the half of the vagina through which the fetus descends gradually dilates satisfactorily. An incomplete septum, however, occasionally interferes with descent, and the septum may become stretched around the presenting part as a band of varying thickness. Such structures usually tear spontaneously, but occasionally they are sufficiently resistant that either they must be divided or cesarean delivery must be performed.

Occasionally, the vagina may be obstructed by a congenital *annular stricture* or band. These are unlikely to interfere seriously with delivery because they usually soften during pregnancy and yield before the oncoming head. An incision rarely is required.

Sometimes the upper vagina is separated from the rest of the canal by a *transverse septum* with a small opening. Some of these are associated with in utero exposure to diethylstilbestrol (see Chap. 33, p. 725). Such a stricture is occasionally mistaken for the upper limit of the vaginal vault; and at the time of labor, the opening in the septum erroneously is considered to be an undilated external os. On careful examination, however, a finger usually can be passed through the opening and the cervix palpated; or on rectal examination, the cervix can be palpated above the level of the vaginal septum. After the external os has dilated completely, the head impinges upon the septum and causes it to bulge downward. If the septum does not yield, slight pressure upon its opening usually will lead to further dilatation, but occasionally cruciate incisions may be required to permit delivery.

Atresia. Complete congenital *vaginal atresia,* unless corrected operatively, forms an effective bar to pregnancy. Incomplete atresia either is a manifestation of faulty development or results from accidents such as scarring from injury or inflammation. Following an infection in which much of the lining of the vagina sloughs, the vaginal lumen may be obliterated almost entirely during the healing process. Atresia may result from the corrosive action of abortifacients inserted into the vagina. Injuries that lead to extensive scarring, such as the trauma that may ensue during rape of a child, also may cause vaginal atresia.

In most cases of atresia, because of pregnancy-induced tissue softening, obstructions gradually are overcome by the pressure exerted by the presenting part. Less often, manual or hydrostatic dilatation or incisions are necessary. If the structure is so resistant that spontaneous dilatation appears improbable, cesarean delivery is performed early in labor.

Cysts and Functional Abnormalities

GARTNER DUCT CYST. A Gartner duct cyst may protrude into the vagina and even through the introitus to such a degree that it may be confused with a cystocele. A *cystocele* may be managed successfully by emptying the bladder, using a catheter, and upward manual pressure on the prolapsed anterior vaginal wall. A Gartner duct cyst may or may not slip above the presenting part; if it does not, the cyst may be aspirated aseptically.

TETANIC CONTRACTION OF LEVATOR ANI. The functional abnormality of tetanic contraction of levator ani, analogous to vaginismus, occasionally interferes with descent of the presenting part by forming a thick, ringlike structure that completely encircles and constricts the vagina about midway between the cervix and the vulva. Ordinarily, the obstruction yields when epidural or spinal analgesia is administered.

Cervical Abnormalities

Atresia and Stenosis. Complete atresia of the cervix is incompatible with conception. Cicatrical *cervical stenosis* may follow extensive cauterization or difficult labor associated with infection and considerable tissue destruction (Cardwell, 1988; Melody, 1957). Of the 10 cases of severe cervical dystocia following cervical treatment reported by Gibbs and Moore (1968), previous conization was responsible in 6. Cryotherapy and laser therapy are less likely to produce stenosis. Rarely, cervical stenosis is caused by carcinoma or syphilitic ulceration and induration. Occasionally, it has resulted from corrosives, such as potassium permanganate tablets, used in attempts to induce abortion. Amputation of the cervix, with suturing to effect hemostasis and promote reepithelialization, may lead to stenosis, although cervical incompetence is much more likely.

Because softening of the tissues usually occurs during pregnancy, cervical stenosis gradually yields during labor. In rare instances, the stenosis may be so pronounced that dilatation appears improbable. In such cases, cesarean delivery is performed.

Due to cervical effacement at the time of labor, a *conglutinated cervix* may undergo complete obliteration, but the cervical os may not dilate. Thus, the presenting part often is separated from the vagina by only a thin layer of cervical tissue. Ordinarily, complete dilatation promptly follows pressure with a fingertip, although in rare instances manual dilatation or cruciate incisions may be required.

Carcinoma of the Cervix. Dystocia may be a consequence of extensive infiltration of the cervix by carcinoma because dilatation is likely to be inadequate even when uterine contractions remain forceful. With less involvement, the cervix usually will dilate. Carcinoma of the cervix complicating pregnancy is discussed in Chapter 57 (p. 1273).

Uterine Displacements

Anteflexion. Exaggerated degrees of anteflexion frequently are observed in the early months of pregnancy, but these are without significance. In later months, particularly when the abdominal walls are very lax, the uterus may fall forward. The sagging occasionally is so exaggerated that the fundus lies considerably below the lower margin of the symphysis pubis. Marked anteflexion of the enlarging pregnant uterus usually is associated with diastasis recti and a pendulous abdomen. When the abnormal position of the uterus prevents the proper transmission of the force of uterine contractions to the cervix, cervical dilatation, as well as engagement of the presenting part, is impeded. Marked improvement may follow maintenance of the uterus in an approximately normal position by means of a properly fitting abdominal binder.

Retroflexion. Uterine retroflexion is encountered during the first trimester in about 10 percent of women (Weekes and associates, 1976). These investigators also reported a higher frequency of early pregnancy bleeding in women with a retroflexed uterus, as well as an abortion rate of 16 percent compared with 9 percent in women with a normally positioned uterus. Most authorities do not regard the retroflexed uterus as a pathological finding in itself. Thus, no treatment is needed during pregnancy, except in the rare circumstance in which the growing retroflexed uterus remains incarcerated in the hollow of the sacrum (Fig. 22–1). Women with a retroflexed uterus should be evaluated frequently early in the second trimester to ensure that the uterus is not incarcerated.

Symptoms from an incarcerated uterus usually include abdominal discomfort and inability to void. As pressure from the full bladder increases, small amounts

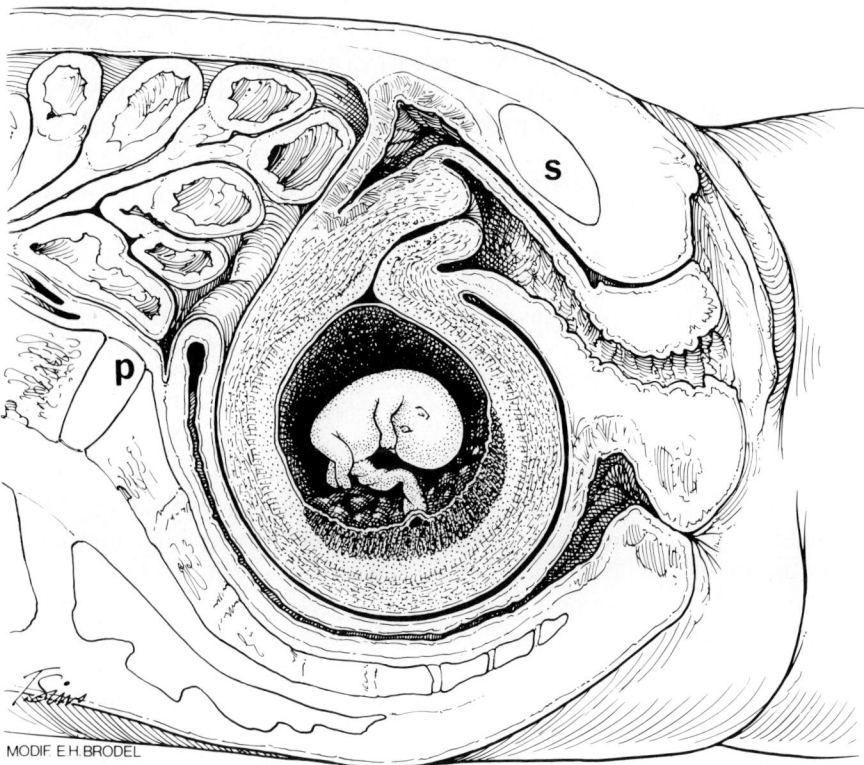

MODIF. E.H. BRODEL

Fig. 22–1. Incarcerated, retroflexed uterus.

of urine are passed involuntarily, but the bladder never empties entirely (*paradoxical incontinence*). Urinary obstruction can be so severe as to cause azotemia. With relief of obstruction, there may be a marked diuresis with loss of large amounts of sodium and potassium (Swartz and Komins, 1977). After bladder catheterization, the uterus usually can be pushed out of the pelvis when the woman is placed in the knee-chest position. Anesthesia seldom is necessary, but occasionally spinal analgesia or general anesthesia will be necessary to effect repositioning. A catheter is left in place until bladder tone returns. Insertion of a soft pessary usually will prevent reincarceration.

Sacculation of the Uterus. Persistent entrapment of the pregnant uterus in the pelvis by old inflammatory disease or endometriosis may result in an anterior uterine sacculation. Friedman and associates (1986) reported a posterior uterine sacculation following aggressive treatment for intrauterine adhesions (Asherman syndrome).

Rarely, the persistently entrapped uterus produces few symptoms, and yet extensive dilatation of the lower portion of the body of the uterus takes place to accommodate the fetus (Jackson and associates, 1988). In one case at Parkland Hospital, at the time of cesarean delivery, the Foley catheter bulb lay just above the urethra in the bladder at the level of the umbilicus. The cervix was at an equally high level. Most of the 2500 g—living fetus, amnionic fluid, and fetal membranes—were contained in a remarkably thin sacculation of the anterior wall of the lower segment. The fetal head was entrapped in the most superior part of the sacculation, along with three loops of cord, by a constricting ring of myometrium. The fundus of the uterus and the placenta were contained in the true pelvis beneath a sharp sacral promontory. After delivery, the uterus soon contracted and retracted to assume a more normal shape.

Spearing (1978) stressed the importance of describing the distorted anatomy. He suggested that the finding of an elongated vagina passing above the level of a fetal head deeply placed into the pelvis is suggestive of a sacculation or an abdominal pregnancy. He also recommended extension of the abdominal incision to above the umbilicus and delivery of the entire gravid uterus from the abdomen before an attempt was made to incise it. **This simple procedure will restore anatomy to the correct relationships and prevent inadvertent incisions into and through the vagina and bladder.** Weissberg and Gall (1972) reviewed the few published reports of sacculation of the pregnant uterus, and Engel and Rushovich (1984) reported the rare possibility of a true uterine diverticulum being confused with sacculation.

Prolapse of the Pregnant Uterus. The cervix, and occasionally a portion of the body of the uterus, may protrude to a variable extent from the vulva during the early months of pregnancy. As pregnancy progresses, however, the body of the uterus usually rises above the pelvis, and may draw the cervix up with it. If the uterus persists in its prolapsed position, symptoms of incarceration may appear during the third to fourth month of pregnancy.

Early in pregnancy, the uterus should be replaced and held in position with a suitable pessary. If, however, the pelvic floor is too relaxed to permit retention of the pessary, the woman should be kept recumbent as long as possible until after the fourth month of pregnancy. When the cervix reaches, or slightly protrudes from the vulva, scrupulous hygiene is mandatory. If much of the cervix persists outside the vulva and cannot be replaced, the pregnancy should be terminated.

Uterine prolapse of this degree is accompanied by prolapse of the bladder (cystocele) and rectum (rectocele) and the development of an enterocele with prolapse of intestinal loops (see below). During labor, all these structures may be forced down in front of the presenting part and interfere with its descent. In that event, they should be cleansed carefully and pushed back over the descending fetal part.

Cystocele and Rectocele. Attenuation of fascial support that normally is interposed between the vagina and the bladder leads to prolapse of the bladder into the vagina, or cystocele. Attenuation of fascia between the vagina and the rectum results in a rectocele. Urinary stasis associated with a large cystocele predisposes to urinary tract infection. A large rectocele may fill with feces that, at times, can only be evacuated manually. Both lesions can block the normal descent of the fetus through the birth canal unless they are emptied and pushed out of the way, as described above. A cystocele often is associated with *urinary stress incontinence* due to loss of the posterior urethrovesical angle. Such a defect is made worse during pregnancy by the increase in uterine weight and the resulting increase in intraabdominal pressure. These women have low urethral closing pressures that do not increase sufficiently to compensate for the progressive increase in bladder pressure induced by the enlarging uterus (Iosif and Ulmsten, 1981).

Enterocele. In rare instances, an enterocele of considerable size filled with loops of intestine may complicate pregnancy. If symptomatic, the protrusion should be replaced and the woman kept in a recumbent position. If the mass interferes with delivery, it should be pushed up or held out of the way.

Surgical repair of uterine prolapse, cystocele, rectocele, and enterocele should not be attempted during the antepartum or intrapartum periods. Definitive repair, often with vaginal hysterectomy for associated uterine prolapse and sterilization, should be carried out after pregnancy-induced pelvic hyperemia has subsided completely.

Torsion of the Pregnant Uterus.

Rotation of the pregnant uterus, most often to the right, is common during pregnancy. Torsion of sufficient degree to arrest uterine circulation and produce an acute abdominal catastrophe, however, is a rare accident of human gestation. Bakos and Axelsson (1987) reported a case of severe levotorsion associated with repeated fetal heart rate decelerations that prompted cesarean delivery. As a consequence of the extreme uterine torsion, the incision inadvertently was made in the posterior side of the uterus! As recommended by Spearing (1978), the uterus should be removed from the abdomen prior to making the uterine incision.

Previous Operative Correction.

Fortunately, routine operative "correction" of the retroflexed uterus has fallen into disrepute. Occasionally, therapy for extensive pelvic endometriosis requires uterine repositioning. Uterine suspension accomplished by shortening the round ligaments does not adversely affect subsequent labor. If, as part of the operation, the bladder is advanced on the anterior wall of the uterus, urinary frequency, as well as bladder discomfort, may be troublesome during pregnancy. When this situation exists, cesarean delivery must be carried out very carefully because of the distorted anatomy.

Pregnancy after fixation of the fundus of the uterus to the anterior abdominal wall may be complicated by considerable discomfort as the pregnant uterus enlarges. This procedure largely has been eliminated from contemporary gynecological surgery.

Uterine Leiomyomas

Uterine leiomyomas, or myomas, commonly are found during pregnancy. Rice and colleagues (1989) surveyed over 6700 pregnancies and found that 1.4 percent were complicated by myomas. Katz and associates (1989) found that 1 in 500 pregnant women were admitted for a complication related to a myoma.

Uterine myomas may be located immediately beneath the endometrial or decidual surface of the uterine cavity (*submucous myoma*), immediately beneath the uterine serosa (*subserous myoma*), or may be confined to the myometrium (*intramural myoma*). An intramural myoma, as it grows, may develop a significant subserous or submucous component, or both. Submucous and subserous myomas, at times, may be attached to the uterus by only a stalk (*pedunculated myoma*).

As in the nonpregnant state, pedunculated subserous myomas may undergo torsion with necrosis to the extent that the myoma is detached from the uterus. At times, a subserous myoma may become parasitic, and much or all of its blood is supplied through a highly vascularized omentum.

Myomas during pregnancy or the puerperium occasionally undergo "red," or "carneous," degeneration that is caused by *hemorrhagic infarction.* The symptoms and signs of degeneration are focal pain, with tenderness on palpation and sometimes low-grade fever. Moderate leukocytosis is common. On occasion, the parietal peritoneum overlying the infarcted myoma becomes inflamed and a peritoneal "rub" develops. Red degeneration is difficult to differentiate at times from appendicitis, placental abruption, ureteral stone, or pyelonephritis, but the imaging techniques discussed below likely will prove helpful. Treatment consists of analgesia such as codeine. Most often, the signs and symptoms abate within a few days.

Myomas may become infected during the course of puerperal metritis or septic abortion. They are especially likely to do so if the myoma is located immediately adjacent to the placental implantation site or if an instrument, such as a sound or curette, perforates the myoma. If the myoma is infarcted, the risk of infection is increased, and the likelihood of cure of the infection, except by hysterectomy, is reduced.

Effects of Pregnancy on Myomas.

Until recently, it was believed that myomas almost always increase in size during pregnancy, likely as a consequence of estrogen stimulation. Certainly, the stimulatory effects of estrogen on both uterine myoma growth and the pregnant uterus have been noted clinically for many years. These actions were assumed to be via estrogen and progesterone receptors that have been identified in normal uterine tissue and myomas (Soules and McCarty, 1982). Actually, the normal rapid uterine expansion that occurs during pregnancy is likely a more complex mechanism mediated, in part, by estrogen, progesterone, and some growth factors, especially *platelet-derived growth factor* (Mendoza and co-workers, 1990).

Estrogen receptors are reduced in number in normal myometrium during the secretory phase of the menstrual cycle and during pregnancy. In myomas, estrogen receptors are present throughout the menstrual cycle, but they are suppressed during pregnancy. Progesterone receptors are present in both myometrium and myomas throughout the menstrual cycle and pregnancy (Kawaguchi and associates, 1991). The Ki-67 cell proliferation-associated antigen is more abundant in myometrial cells during pregnancy, but it is even higher in myomas throughout the menstrual cycle and pregnancy (Kawaguchi and associates, 1991). Thus, factors that stimulate normal uterine growth during pregnancy appear to be estrogen, progesterone, various growth factors, and an increase in cells that have the Ki-67 antigen.

With respect to uterine myomas, stimulatory effects in the nonpregnant woman appear to be due to increased estrogen and estrogen receptors, progesterone and progesterone receptors, Ki-67 cells, and *epidermal growth factor* (Lumsden and associates, 1988). It is likely that epidermal growth factor is stimulated by estrogen, because in nonpregnant women, administration of a gonadotropin-releasing hormone agonist, which decreases estrogen, also decreases epidermal growth factor binding to myomas. Again in nonpregnant women, Rein and co-workers (1990) observed an increase in estrogen and progesterone receptors in myomas compared with normal myometrium. Paradoxically, they observed an even greater increase in estrogen receptors in myoma tissue following a decrease in estrogen induced by a gonadotropin-releasing hormone agonist. This increase in available estrogen receptors was likely due to the withdrawal of estrogen, thereby rendering all the receptors *available* for estrogen. Thus, with administration of a gonadotropin-releasing hormone agonist, estrogen was eliminated, resulting in a reduction in the size of the myomas but an apparent increase in myoma estrogen receptors because the receptors were now unoccupied. They hypothesized that after stopping therapy, the rapid increase in myoma regrowth is due to an increased estrogen transfer to myomas through more available estrogen receptors. This theory also is consistent with the concept that a return of estrogen also would favor myoma growth by increasing epidermal growth factor receptors.

Thus, clinical and laboratory observations support the concept that the same, or similar, hormonal and growth factors, that normally cause uterine growth during pregnancy, also stimulate growth of leiomyomas early in pregnancy. The paradoxical observations that large myomas remain unchanged or decreased in size late in pregnancy, may now be explained. It is likely that during pregnancy myoma estrogen receptors are **decreased** or down-regulated due to the massive amounts of estrogen. Without effective estrogen receptors and thus estrogen action in the myomas, epidermal growth factor binding is also decreased.

Lev-Toaff and co-workers (1987), using serial ultrasonic monitoring of myomas, observed that only half changed significantly in size during pregnancy (Table 22–1). Specifically, during the first trimester, myomas of all sizes either remained unchanged or increased in size (early response due to increased estrogen). During the second trimester, smaller myomas (2 to 6 cm) usually remained unchanged or *increased* in size, whereas larger myomas become smaller (start of down-regulation of estrogen receptors). Regardless of *initial* myoma size, during the third trimester, myomas usually remained unchanged or decreased in size (estrogen receptors down-regulated). The importance of these observations is that an accurate prediction of myoma growth in pregnancy cannot be made. After pregnancy, therapy with gonadotropin-releasing hormone agonists may prove useful in decreasing the size of myomas and in facilitating their surgical removal (see p. 536).

Effects of Myoma Size, Location, and Number on Pregnancy. Several investigators have attempted to assess the effects on pregnancy of myoma size, location, and number (Tables 22–2 and 22–3). With respect to size alone, Rice and associates (1987) concluded that women with myomas greater than 3 cm had significantly increased rates of preterm labor, placental abruption, pelvic pain, and cesarean delivery. Tumors less than 3 cm were not clinically significant. Lev-Toaff and colleagues (1987) noted that as both size and number of myomas increased, there was a significantly higher frequency of retained placentas, fetal malpresentations, and preterm contractions. Hasan and co-workers (1990) found no association with respect to myoma size except for an increased likelihood of obstructed labor when myoma size was more than 6 cm. Davis and associates (1990), however, observed no relationship of complications with myoma size, location, or number.

A review of Tables 22–2 and 22–3 shows that myomas are probably associated with an increased incidence of preterm labor, fetal malpresentation, and cesarean delivery. The likelihood of placental abruption appears to be increased if the placenta is in contact or covers a uterine myoma (Table 22–3). Abortion and postpartum hemorrhage were not increased unless the placenta was adjacent or implanted over a myoma. While the *incidence* of postpartum hemorrhage was not increased, if hemorrhage did occur, it was massive, unrelenting, and often only corrected by hysterectomy (Hasan and associates, 1990). Only Lev-Toaff and colleagues (1987) found an increased incidence of retained placenta in cases with lower uterine segment myomas. If

TABLE 22–1. ULTRASONICALLY MEASURED CHANGES IN MYOMAS DURING PREGNANCY

| Trimester | Small Myomas[a] (n = 111) | | | Large Myomas[b] (n = 51) | | |
	No Change No. (%)	Increase No. (%)	Decrease No. (%)	No Change No. (%)	Increase No. (%)	Decrease No. (%)
First	7 (58)	5 (42)	0	1 (20)	4 (80)	0
Second	42 (55)	23 (30)	11 (15)	11 (38)	4 (14)	14 (48)
Third	14 (61)	1 (4)	8 (35)	5 (29)	2 (12)	10 (59)

[a] Small myomas 2.0–5.9 cm.
[b] Large myomas 6.0–11.9 cm.
Modified from Lev-Toaff and co-workers (1987).

TABLE 22–2. PREGNANCY COMPLICATIONS ASSOCIATED WITH UTERINE MYOMAS

Study	Complication (%)								Cesarean Delivery	
	Antepartum Pain and/or Bleeding	Placental Abruption	Preterm Ruptured Membranes	Preterm Labor	Abortion	Fetal Malpresentation	Postpartum Hemorrhage	Obstructed Labor	Indicated	Elective
Winer-Muram and associates (1984)	Table 22–3[a]	NS	NS	5/79 (6)	10/89 (11)	NS	Table 22–3[a]	NS	11/79 (14)	—
Lev-Toaff and co-workers (1987)										
Uterine corpus	NS	NS	0/68	NS	6/68 (9)	NS	NS	1/68 (2)	11/68 (16)	10/68 (15)
Lower uterine segment	NS	NS	0/68	NS	0/68	NS	NS	8/45 (18)	15/45 (33)	9/45 (20)
Rice and associates (1989)[a]	Table 22–3	10/93 (11)	NS	20/93 (22)	NS	11/93 (NS)	NS	NS	26/93 (38)	—
Katz and co-workers (1989)	Increased	0/28	6/24 (25)	2/24 (8)	2/24 (8)	4/24 (17)	NS	NS	9/24 (38)	—
Hasan and associates (1990)	NS	NS	NS	16/60 (27)	NS	22/60 (37)	10/60 (17)	9/60 (21)	24/60 (40)	20/60 (33)
Davis and co-workers (1990)	NS	NS	6/85 (7)	15/85 (18)	NS	NS				

[a] Additional data presented in Table 22–3.
NS = not significant.

a placenta was retained, however, the consequences were significant (Gleeson and Onwude, 1990).

The issue of whether placental implantation over or adjacent to a myoma is clinically significant remains unresolved. Winer-Muram and associates (1984) and Rice and colleagues (1989) found that bleeding, abortion, preterm labor, postpartum hemorrhage, and placental abruption may be increased in such cases (Table 22–3). Lev-Toaff (1987), Davis (1990), and their co-workers could not identify such an association. If a placenta is implanted over or adjacent to a myoma, it seems prudent, at least, to consider this a *potential threat*.

The conclusions derived from these reports are clearly defined: (1) growth of myomas during pregnancy cannot be predicted; (2) placental implantation over or in contact with a myoma increases the likelihood of placental abruption, abortion, preterm labor, and postpartum hemorrhage; (3) multiple myomas are associated with an increased incidence of fetal malposition and preterm labor; (4) degeneration of myomas may be associated with a characteristic sonographic pattern; and (5) the incidence of cesarean delivery is increased. Serial ultrasonic examinations should be considered throughout pregnancy in women with uterine myomas, and prompt attention should be given to any complaints of bleeding, abdominal pain, or uterine contractions.

TABLE 22–3. PREGNANCY COMPLICATIONS AND RELATIONSHIP OF MYOMA TO PLACENTA

Study	Complication	Myoma (%)	
		No Contact with Placenta	Contact with Placenta
Winer-Muram and associates (1984)	Bleeding and pain	5/54 (9)	8/35 (23)
	Major complications		
	Abortion	1/54 (2)	9/35 (26)
	Preterm labor	0	5/35 (14)
	Postpartum hemorrhage	0	4/35 (11)
	Subtotal	6/54 (11)	26/35 (74)
Rice and associates (1989)	Pain	NS[a]	
	Major complications		
	Abortion		NS
	Preterm labor	19/79 (24)	NS 1/14 (7)
	Postpartum hemorrhage		NS
	Abruption	2/79 (3)	8/14 (57)
	Subtotal	21/79 (27)	9/14 (64)

[a] NS = not stated.

Cervical Myomas. Myomas in the cervix or in the lower uterine segment may obstruct labor and may be confused with the fetal head. Sonograms from such a case and a picture of the uterus are shown in Figures 22–2, and 22–3. Myomas that lie within or contiguous to the birth canal earlier in pregnancy may be carried upward as the uterus enlarges, with relief of obstruction to vaginal delivery. Even though relief was not provided in the case demonstrated in Figures 22–2 and 22–3, a decision regarding the method of delivery usually should not be made before the onset of labor.

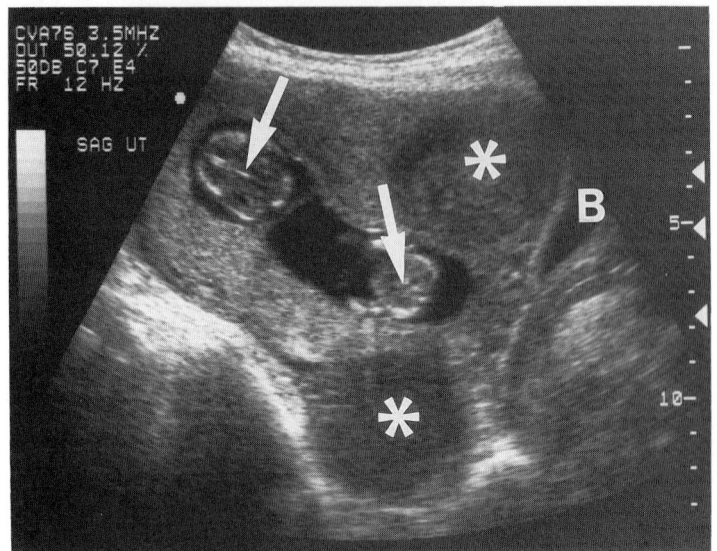

Fig. 22–2. Two uterine myomas (*), one posterior and one anterior, are seen in this 13-week pregnancy. Arrows point to fetal head and body. B = bladder. (Photo courtesy of Dr. R. Santos.)

Imaging Myomas. The critical issue to be resolved after the detection of an abdominopelvic mass is its etiology. Ultrasound has helped tremendously not only in correctly identifying such masses, but also in following the progression, regression, and response to therapy. Use of

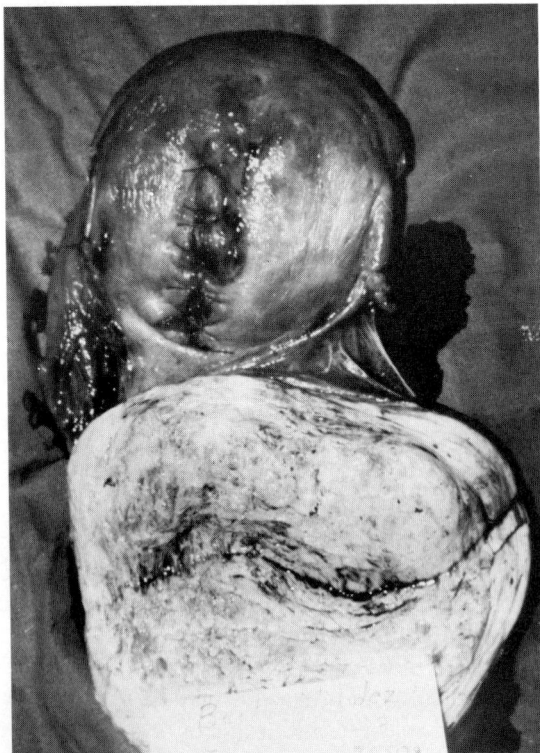

Fig. 22–3. Same case as shown in Figure 22–2. Cesarean hysterectomy specimen. The upper mass is the body of the uterus that was just emptied by cesarean delivery. The lower mass is a huge myoma arising low in the uterus and now incised. The infant weighed 3250 g, and the uterus with myoma weighed 2900 g. Red degeneration was not found. Delivery 2 years before also had been by cesarean.

sonography to identify and follow the natural progression of uterine myomas throughout pregnancy was discussed above (Aharonie and co-workers, 1988; Lev-Toaff and associates, 1987). More recently, however, the limitation of sonography in evaluating pelvic masses has been established (Baltarowich and co-workers, 1988; Borgstein and colleagues, 1989; Kier and co-workers, 1990). Ovarian masses (both benign and malignant), molar pregnancies, ectopic pregnancies, missed abortions, bowel abnormalities, and even fetal heads have all been confused with uterine myomas.

To improve accuracy, many recommend that magnetic resonance imaging supersede, or at least serve as an adjunct to ultrasound (al-Ahwani, 1991; Andreottii, 1988; Hamlin, 1985; Hricak, 1992; Karasick, 1992; Kier, 1990; Scoutt, 1990; and all their associates). Comparisons of ultrasound with magnetic resonance imaging have been made in the same patients, and magnetic resonance imaging is superior to ultrasound, especially in correctly identifying uterine myomas (Weinreb and associates, 1990; Zawin and colleagues, 1990). Even with magnetic resonance imaging, however, errors still are made in diagnosing uterine myomas (Brown and associates, 1990). This emphasizes again the importance and the difficulty in establishing a noninvasive diagnosis for an abdominopelvic mass, especially during pregnancy.

Myomectomy During Pregnancy. This procedure should be limited to myomas with a discrete pedicle that can be clamped and easily ligated (Burton and associates, 1989). Myomas should not be dissected from the uterus, during pregnancy or at the time of delivery, because bleeding may be profuse and, at times, hysterectomy may be required. While Glavind and associates (1990) maintain that a more aggressive approach will not increase pregnancy losses compared with nonsurgical controls, this remains to be confirmed. Bizarre nuclear changes often confused with sarcoma may be seen in myomas resected during pregnancy. Typically, myomas will undergo remarkable involution after delivery; therefore, myomectomy should be deferred until involution has occurred.

Treatment of Uterine Myomas in Nonpregnant Women. If the diagnosis of recurrent fetal wastage or morbidity due to uterine myomas has been established, the logical time to correct this abnormality is when the woman is not pregnant. Gonadotropin-releasing hormone agonists are powerful pharmacological drugs used to treat uterine myomas. Almost universally good results have been reported following their parenteral, inhaled, or intravaginal administration. Reduction in aggregate uterine size has been from 30 to 70 percent depending on the dose, agent, and duration of therapy (Adamson, 1992; Costantini, 1990; Friedman, 1987, 1989, 1991; Giorgino, 1991; Kessel, 1988; Letterie, 1989; Matta, 1989; Schlaff, 1989; Vollenhoven, 1990; and all of their co-investigators). **Unfortunately, with cessation of agonist therapy, uterine myomas rapidly regrow.** As discussed on page 534, rapid regrowth in uterine size likely is due to open availability of estrogen receptors in myoma tissue, the result of estrogen suppression during therapy. Nonmyoma uterine volume reduction and regrowth also might be responsible, at least in part, for these observed rapid increases in uterine volume (Schlaff and co-workers, 1989). Regardless, if permanent or sustained reduction in myoma size is the goal of therapy, early myomectomy should follow medical therapy. Matta and associates (1988), using Doppler ultrasound, reported that blood flow was decreased in uterine myomas after using a gonadotropin-releasing hormone agonist.

Myomectomy may be performed through an abdominal incision, but successful cases have been described using hysteroscopic resection alone or combined with laparoscopic techniques (Donnez and associates, 1989; Loffer, 1990). Short-term success for combined medical and surgical management generally has been favorable, but there are insufficient data to allow definite conclusions. There has been one report of short-term myoma recurrence following combined therapy (Fedele and associates, 1990). The 10-year cumulative risk of myoma recurrence following myomectomy alone is approximately 27 percent (Candiani and co-workers, 1991).

After myomectomy, there is a significant risk of uterine rupture during a subsequent pregnancy. Furthermore, rupture may occur early in gestation at a time remote from labor (Golan and associates, 1990). When a myomectomy results in a defect through or immediately adjacent to the endometrium, subsequent pregnancies should be delivered before active labor begins.

A new synthetic derivative of ethyl-nor-testosterone (Gestrinone) has been reported to be useful in suppressing myoma growth and decreasing uterine volume. A *possible* advantage over a gonadotropin-releasing hormone agonist is its reported longer suppression of myoma size (Continho and Gonçalves, 1989). Insufficient data are available to establish if this agent will be useful without surgery to treat myomas.

Ovarian Tumors

Benign Ovarian Tumors. Ovarian tumors may cause serious complications during pregnancy and postpartum. Some of these include adnexal torsion and obstruction to vaginal delivery. The most common ovarian tumors are cystic (Fig. 22–4). Beischer and associates (1971) described 164 ovarian tumors diagnosed during pregnancy; one fourth were cystic teratomas and one fourth were mucinous cystadenomas. Similar observations were reported by Sunoo and colleagues (1990). In the series reported by Beischer, 2.4 percent were malignant. Hopkins and Duchon (1986) reported an incidence of adnexal masses of 1 in 556 pregnancies. Benign cystic teratomas and corpus luteum cysts each accounted for about one third of these. Two women had corpus luteum cysts persisting into the third trimester, and one very large mass ruptured postpartum. Koonings and co-workers (1988) reported finding one adnexal neoplasm for every 197 cesarean deliveries.

The most frequent and most serious complication of benign ovarian cysts during pregnancy is torsion.

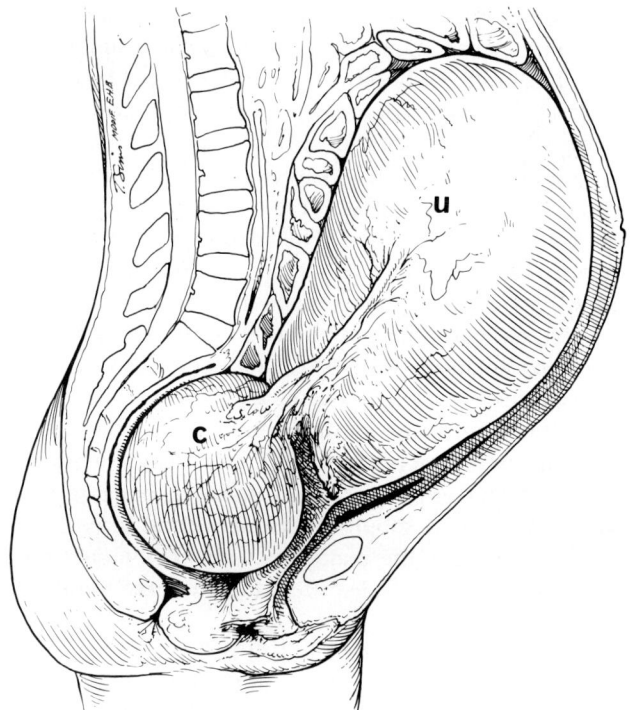

Fig. 22–4. Ovarian cyst filling most of true pelvis and causing dystocia. (c = ovarian cyst; u = pregnant uterus.)

Booth (1963) reported the incidence of this accident to be 12 percent. Torsion is most common in the first trimester, and may result in cyst rupture with extrusion of its contents into the peritoneal cavity. Cyst rupture also may occur during labor or during surgical removal. This event is not likely to be as devastating with serous cystadenomas as with dermoid cysts. When a tumor blocks the pelvis, it may lead to uterine rupture, or the tumor may be forced into the vagina, rectum, or rectovaginal septum.

Ovarian tumors complicating pregnancy often are entirely unsuspected (Stedman and Kline, 1988). Careful examination of all pregnant women would eliminate some, but not all, of these missed tumors. If an ovarian tumor does not occupy the pelvis, diagnosis through physical examination is especially difficult because abdominal enlargement may be attributed to a more advanced pregnancy, multiple fetuses, or hydramnios, and the true condition may not be recognized until after labor. Sonography often provides accurate differentiation between uterine enlargement and an extrauterine cystic mass.

Early in pregnancy, an ovary may be enlarged, creating a suspicion of neoplasm. Ovaries less than 6 cm in diameter usually are the consequence of corpus luteum formation. Thornton and Wells (1987) reported that with the advent of high-resolution sonography, a conservative approach to management of ovarian cysts might be adopted based upon their sonographic characteristics. They recommend resection of all cysts suspected of rupture, torsion, or obstruction of labor, and those over 10 cm in diameter because of the increased risk of cancer in large cysts. Cysts 5 cm or less could be left alone. Cysts between 5 and 10 cm in diameter also could be managed expectantly if they had a simple cystic appearance. If, however, the 5- to 10-cm cysts contained septae or nodules, or if there were solid components, the cysts should be resected. In contrast, Hess and colleagues (1988) recommend elective resection of any ovarian mass 6 cm or larger that persisted after 16 weeks' gestation. They reported a better fetal-neonatal outcome in such women compared with those in whom an emergency procedure was required for resection of a ruptured, twisted, or infarcted cyst. Fleischer and associates (1990) recommend observation in asymptomatic pregnant women with ovarian masses less than 5 cm. If a mass increases in size, becomes symptomatic, or has sonographic characteristics including irregular septae, papillary excrescences, or large solid areas, malignancy should be strongly considered.

In summary, the major questions to be answered once a pelvic mass is discovered include the following:

1. What is the mass and is it malignant?
2. Is there a good likelihood the mass will regress?
3. Will the mass result in dystocia and/or torsion and possible rupture?

Only time, careful serial surveillance with sonography, and labor will provide answers to the last two questions. As for the first question, Kier and associates (1990) reported that magnetic resonance imaging correctly identified the origin of unknown pelvic masses in 17 of 17 cases versus 12 of 17 cases (71 percent) using sonography. They concluded that magnetic resonance imaging was a valuable complement to sonography for preoperative evaluation of pelvic masses in pregnant women. Kurjak and Zalud (1990) claim that transvaginal color Doppler assessment of tumor vascularity can be used for better characterization of adnexal tumors and potentially may be useful as a screening test for ovarian malignancy. We recommend exploratory laparotomy if a reasonable doubt exists as to the possibility of malignancy.

Ovarian tumor markers rarely are helpful in doubtful cases. Frederiksen and associates (1991) and Montz and co-workers (1989) reported that elevated serum alpha-fetoprotein values obtained during routine screening for neural tube defects led to the diagnosis of an immature ovarian teratoma in two women. A similar discovery of an ovarian endodermal sinus tumor was reported (van der Zee and associates, 1991).

Laparotomy. In view of the high incidence of abortion during early pregnancy, the safest time to perform a laparotomy is alleged to be during the fourth month (Hess and associates, 1988; Struyk and Treffers, 1984). This is provided that the operation can be postponed until that time; surgery should not be delayed in cases of suspected malignancy. When the diagnosis is not made until late in pregnancy, it is advisable, except in the case of known or suspected malignancy, to delay laparotomy until fetal viability. If the ovarian cyst is not impacted, it usually is preferable to permit spontaneous labor and remove the tumor later. If the tumor is impacted in the pelvis, cesarean delivery is performed, along with tumor resection.

Carcinoma of the Ovary. Malignant ovarian neoplasms are unusual during pregnancy, but their incidence is probably increasing due to the recognition of borderline tumors of low malignant potential and the widespread use of ultrasound. The diagnosis and treatment of ovarian malignancies are discussed in Chapter 57 (p. 1275).

Pelvic Masses of Other Origins

Labor may be obstructed by pelvic masses of various origins sufficiently large to render delivery difficult or even impossible. A *distended bladder*, with or without a cystocele, may obstruct delivery. A less severely distended bladder, however, usually does not delay the normal progress of labor (Kerr-Wilson and co-workers,

1983; Read and colleagues, 1980). Bladder tumors may impede passage of the fetus, though rarely enough to require operative delivery. A *pelvic ectopic kidney* is a rare complication of pregnancy; however, a *transplanted kidney* usually is placed in the false pelvis. Although vaginal delivery is possible, such a kidney may block the birth canal and sustain injury during delivery. Most women with an ectopic kidney will deliver vaginally without hazard.

In rare instances, an enlarged spleen may prolapse into the pelvic cavity and obstruct labor. Echinococcal cysts have been found in the pelvis. An old extrauterine gestation may obstruct the birth canal, interfering with the delivery of a subsequent pregnancy. Tumors or inflammation arising from the lower part of the rectum or pelvic connective tissue also may give rise to dystocia.

References

Adamson GD: Treatment of uterine fibroids: Current findings with gonadotropin-releasing hormone agonists. Am J Obstet Gynecol 166:746, 1992

Aharoni A, Reiter A, Golan D, Paltiely Y, Sharf M: Patterns of growth of uterine leiomyomas during pregnancy. A prospective longitudinal study. Br J Obstet Gynaecol 95:510, 1988

al-Ahwani S, Assem M, Belal A, Abdel-Hamid H: Magnetic resonance imaging (MRI) of abnormal uterine masses. J Belge Radiol 74:19, 1991

Andreotti RF, Zusmer NR, Sheldon JJ, Ames M: Ultrasound and magnetic resonance imaging of pelvic masses. Surg Gynecol Obstet 166:327, 1988

Bakos O, Axelsson O: Pathologic torsion of the pregnant uterus. Acta Obstet Gynecol Scand 66:85, 1987

Baltarowich OH, Kurtz AB, Pennell RG, Needleman L, Vilaro MM, Goldberg BB: Pitfalls in the sonographic diagnosis of uterine fibroids. Am J Roentgenol 151:725, 1988

Beischer NA, Buttery BW, Fortune DW, Macafee CAJ: Growth and malignancy of ovarian tumors in pregnancy. Aust NZ J Obstet Gynecol 11:208, 1971

Booth RT: Ovarian tumors in pregnancy. Obstet Gynecol 21:189, 1963

Borgstein RL, Shaw JJ, Pearson RH: Uterine leiomyomata: Sonographic mimicry. Br J Radiol 62:1019, 1989

Brown JJ, Thurnher S, Hricak H: MR imaging of the uterus: Low-signal-intensity abnormalities of the endometrium and endometrial cavity. Magn Reson Imaging 8:309, 1990

Burton CA, Grimes DA, March CM: Surgical management of leiomyomata during pregnancy. Obstet Gynecol 74:707, 1989

Candiani GB, Fedele L, Parazzini F, Villa L: Risk of recurrence after myomectomy. Br J Obstet Gynaecol 98:385, 1991

Cardwell MS: Severe cervical stenosis with the twin-to-twin transfusion syndrome. South Med J 81:940, 1988

Costantini S, Anserini P, Valenzano M, Remorgida V, Venturini PL, De Cecco L: Luteinizing hormone-releasing hormone analog therapy of uterine fibroid: Analysis of results obtained with buserelin administered intranasally and goserelin administered subcutaneously as a monthly depot. Eur J Obstet Gynecol Reprod Biol 37:63, 1990

Coutinho EM, Gonçalves MT: Long-term treatment of leiomyomas with gestrinone. Fertil Steril 51:939, 1989

Davis JL, Ray-Mazumder S, Hobel CJ, Baley K, Sassoon D: Uterine leiomyomas in pregnancy: A prospective study. Obstet Gynecol 75:41, 1990

Donnez J, Schrurs B, Gillerot S, Sandow J, Clerckx F: Treatment of uterine fibroids with implants of gonadotropin-releasing hormone agonist: Assessment by hysterography. Fertil Steril 51:947, 1989

Engel G, Rushovich AM: True uterine diverticulum: A partial Müllerian duct duplication? Arch Pathol Lab Med 108:734, 1984

Fedele L, Vercellini P, Bianchi S, Brioschi D, Dorta M: Treatment with GnRH agonists before myomectomy and the risk of short-term myoma recurrence. Br J Obstet Gynaecol 97:393, 1990

Ferenczy A: HPV-Associated lesions in pregnancy and their complications. Clin Obstet Gynecol 32:191, 1989

Ferenczy A: Treating genital condyloma during pregnancy with the carbon dioxide laser. Am J Obstet Gynecol 148:9, 1984

Fleischer AC, Dinesh MS, Entman SS: Sonographic evaluation of maternal disorders during pregnancy. Radiol Clin North Am 28:51, 1990

Frederiksen MC, Casanova L, Schink JC: An elevated maternal serum alpha-fetoprotein leading to the diagnosis of an immature teratoma. Int J Gynaecol Obstet 35:343, 1991

Friedman A, DeFazio J, DeCherney A: Severe obstetric complications after aggressive treatment of Asherman syndrome. Obstet Gynecol 67:864, 1986

Friedman AJ, Barbieri RL, Benacerraf BR, Schiff I: Treatment of leiomyomata with intranasal or subcutaneous leuprolide, a gonadotropin-releasing hormone agonist. Fertil Steril 48:560, 1987

Friedman AJ, Harrison-Atlas D, Barbieri RL, Benacerraf B, Gleason R, Schiff I: A randomized, placebo-controlled, double-blind study evaluating the efficacy of leuprolide acetate depot in the treatment of uterine leiomyomata. Fertil Steril 51:251, 1989

Friedman AJ, Hoffman DI, Comit F, Browneller RW, Miller JD: Treatment of leiomyomata uteri with leuprolide acetate depot: A double-blind, placebo-controlled, multicenter study. Obstet Gynecol 77:720, 1991

Gibbs CE, Moore SF: The scarred cervix in pregnancy and labor. Gen Pract 37:85, 1968

Giorgino FL, Cetera C: The management of leiomyoma uteri by GnRH analogues. Clin Exp Obstet Gynecol 18:137, 1991

Glavind K, Palvio DHB, Lauritsen JG: Uterine myoma in pregnancy. Acta Obstet Gynecol Scand 69:617, 1990

Gleeson NC, Onwude JL: Uterine leiomyoma causing retained placenta. Br J Clin Pract 44:689, 1990

Golan D, Aharoni A, Gonen R, Boss Y, Sharf M: Early spontaneous rupture of the post myomectomy gravid uterus. Int J Gynecol Obstet 31:167, 1990

Hamlin DJ, Pettersson H, Fitzsimmons J, Morgan LS: MR imaging of uterine leiomyomas and their complications. J Comput Assist Tomogr 95:902, 1985

Hankins GDV, Hammond TL, Snyder RR, Gilstrap LC: Use of laser vaporization for management of extensive genital tract condyloma acuminata during pregnancy. J Infect Dis 159:1001, 1989

Hasan F, Arumugam K, Sivanesaratnam V: Uterine leiomyomata in pregnancy. Int J Gynaecol Obstet 34:45, 1990

Hess LW, Peaceman A, O'Brien WF, Winkel CA, Cruikshank DW, Morrison JC: Adnexal mass occurring with intrauterine pregnancy: Report of fifty-four patients requiring laparotomy for definitve management. Am J Obstet Gynecol 158:1029, 1988

Hopkins MP, Duchon MA: Adnexal surgery in pregnancy. J Reprod Med 31:1035, 1986

Hricak H, Finck S, Honda G, Göranson H: MR imaging in the evaluation of benign uterine masses: Value of gadopentetate dimeglumine-enhanced T_1-weighted images. AJR 158:1043, 1992

Iosif S, Ulmsten U: Comparative urodynamic studies of continent and stress incontinent women in pregnancy and in the puerperium. Am J Obstet Gynecol 140:645, 1981

Jackson D, Elliott JP, Pearson M: Asymptomatic uterine retroversion at 36 weeks' gestation. Obstet Gynecol 71:466, 1988

Karasick S, Lev-Toaff AS, Toaff ME: Imaging of uterine leiomyomas. AJR 158:799, 1992

Katz VL, Dotters DJ, Droegemueller W: Complications of uterine leiomyomas in pregnancy. Obstet Gynecol 73:593, 1989

Kawaguchi K, Fujii S, Konishi I, Iwai T, Nanbu Y, Nonogaki H, Ishikawa Y, Mori T: Immunohistochemical analysis of oestrogen receptors, progesterone receptors and Ki-67 in leiomyoma and myometrium during the menstrual cycle and pregnancy. Virchows Arch A Pathol Anat Histopathol 419:309, 1991

Kerr-Wilson RHJ, Parham GP, Orr JW Jr: The effect of a full bladder on labor. Obstet Gynecol 62:319, 1983

Kessel B, Liu J, Mortola J, Berga S, Yen SSC: Treatment of uterine fibroids with agonist analogs of gonadotropin-releasing hormone. Fertil Steril 49:538, 1988

Kier R, McCarthy SM, Scoutt LM, Viscarello RR, Schwartz PE: Pelvic masses in pregnancy: MR Imaging. Radiology 176:709, 1990

Koonings PP, Platt LD, Wallace R: Incidental adnexal neoplasms at cesarean section. Obstet Gynecol 72:767, 1988

Kurjak A, Zalud I: Transvaginal color Doppler for evaluating gynecologic pathology of the pelvis. Ultraschall Med 11:164, 1990

Letterie GS, Coddington CC, Winkel CR, Shawker TH, Loriaux DL, Collins RL: Efficacy of a gonadotropin-releasing hormone agonist in the treatment of uterine leiomyomata: Long-term follow-up. Fertil Steril 51:951, 1989

Lev-Toaff AS, Coleman BG, Arger PH, Mintz MC, Arenson RL, Toaff ME: Leiomyomas in pregnancy: Sonographic study. Radiology 164:375, 1987

Loffer FD: Removal of large symptomatic intrauterine growths by the hysteroscopic resectoscope. Obstet Gynecol 76:836, 1990

Lumsden MA, West CP, Bramley T, Rumgay L, Baird DT: The binding of epidermal growth factor to the human uterus and leiomyomata in women rendered hypo-oestrogenic by continuous administration of an LHRH agonist. Br J Obstet Gynaecol 95:1299, 1988

Matta WHM, Stabile I, Shaw RW, Campbell S: Doppler assessment of uterine blood flow changes in patients with fibroids receiving the gonadotropin-releasing hormone agonist Buserelin. Fertil Steril 49:1083, 1988

Matta WH, Shaw RW, Nye M: Long-term follow-up of patients

with uterine fibroids after treatment with the LHRH agonist buserelin. Br J Obstet Gynaecol 96:200, 1989

Melody GF: Obstructed cervix, a study of 100 patients. Obstet Gynecol 10:190, 1957

Mendoza AE, Young R, Orkin SH, Collins T: Increased platelet-derived growth factor A-chain expression in human uterine smooth muscle cells during the physiologic hypertrophy of pregnancy. Proc Natl Acad Sci USA 87:2177, 1990

Montz FJ, Horenstein J, Platt LD, d'Ablaing G, Schlaerth JB, Cunningham G: The diagnosis of immature teratoma by maternal serum alpha-fetoprotein screening. Obstet Gynecol 73:522, 1989

Patsner B, Baker DA, Orr JW: Human papillomavirus genital tract infections during pregnancy. Clin Obstet Gynecol 33:258, 1990

Rando RF, Lindheim S, Hasty L, Sedlacek TV, Woodland M, Eder C: Increased frequency of detection of human papillomavirus deoxyribonucleic acid in exfoliated cervical cells during pregnancy. Am J Obstet Gynecol 161:50, 1989

Read JA, Miller FC, Yeh SY, Platt LD: Urinary bladder distension: Effect on labor and uterine activity. Obstet Gynecol 56:565, 1980

Rein MS, Friedman AJ, Stuart JM, MacLaughlin DT: Fibroid and myometrial steroid receptors in women treated with gonadotropin-releasing hormone agonist leuprolide acetate. Fertil Steril 53:1018, 1990

Rice JP, Kay HH, Mahony BS: The clinical significance of uterine leiomyomas in pregnancy. Am J Obstet Gynecol 160:1212, 1989

Schlaff WD, Zerhouni EA, Huth JAM, Chen J, Damewood MD, Rock JA: A placebo-controlled trial of a depot gonadotropin-releasing hormone analogue (leuprolide) in the treatment of uterine leiomyomata. Obstet Gynecol 74:856, 1989

Schwartz DB, Greenberg MD, Daoud Y, Reid R: Genital condylomas in pregnancy: Use of trichloroacetic acid and laser therapy. Am J Obstet Gynecol 158:1407, 1988

Scoutt LM, McCarthy SM: Applications of magnetic resonance imaging to gynecology. Top Magn Reson Imaging 2:37, 1990

Sedlacek TV, Lindheim S, Eder C, Hasty L, Woodland M, Ludomirsky A, Rando R: Mechanism for human papillomavirus transmission at birth. Am J Obstet Gynecol 161:55, 1989

Smith EM, Johnson SR, Pignatari S, Cripe TP, Turek L: Perinatal vertical transmission of human papillomavirus and subsequent development of respiratory tract papillomatosis. Ann Otol Rhinol Laryngol 100:479, 1991

Soules MR, McCarty KS Jr: Leiomyomas: Steroid receptor content. Am J Obstet Gynecol 143:6, 1982

Spearing GJ: Uterine sacculation. Obstet Gynecol 51:11S, 1978

Stedman CM, Kline RC: Intraoperative complications and unexpected pathology at the time of cesarean section. Obstet Gynecol Clin North Am 15:745, 1988

Struyk AP, Treffers PE: Ovarian tumors in pregnancy. Acta Obstet Gynecol Scand 63:421:1984

Sunoo CS, Terada KY, Kamemoto LE, Hale RW: Adnexal masses in pregnancy: Occurrence by ethnic group. Obstet Gynecol 75:38, 1990

Swartz EM, Komins JI: Postobstructive diuresis after reduction of an incarcerated gravid uterus. J Reprod Med 19:262, 1977

Thornton JG, Wells M: Ovarian cysts in pregnancy: Does ultrasound make traditional management inappropriate? Obstet Gynecol 69:717, 1987 van der Zee AG, de Bruijn HW, Bouma J, Aalders JG, Oosterhuis JW, de Vries EG: Endodermal sinus tumor of the ovary during pregnancy: A case report. Am J Obstet Gynecol 164:504, 1991

Vollenhoven BJ, Shekleton P, McDonald J, Healy DL: Clinical predictors for buserelin acetate treatment of uterine fibroids: A prospective study of 40 women. Fertil Steril 54:1032, 1990

Weekes ARL, Atlay RD, Brown VA, Jordan EC, Murray SM: The retroverted gravid uterus and its effect on the outcome of pregnancy. Br Med J 1:622, 1976

Weinreb JC, Barkoff ND, Megibow A, Demopoulos R: The value of MR imaging in distinguishing leiomyomas from other solid pelvic masses when sonography is indeterminate. Am J Roentgenol 154:295, 1990

Weissberg SM, Gall SA: Sacculation of the pregnant uterus. Obstet Gynecol 39:691, 1972

Winer-Muram HT, Muram D, Gillieson MS: Uterine myomas in pregnancy. J Assoc Can Radiol 35:168, 1984

Zawin M, McCarthy S, Scoutt LM, Comite F: High-field MRI and US evaluation of the pelvis in women with leiomyomas. Magn Reson Imaging 8:371, 1990

CHAPTER 23
Injuries to the Birth Canal

Injuries to the Pelvic Floor and Vagina

Perineal Lacerations. All except the most superficial perineal lacerations are accompanied by varying degrees of injury to the lower portion of the vagina. Such tears may reach sufficient depth to involve the rectal sphincter and may extend to varying depths through the walls of the vagina. Bilateral lacerations into the vagina are usually unequal in length and separated by a tongue-shaped portion of vaginal mucosa (see Fig. 14–17). Their repair should form part of every operation for the restoration of a lacerated perineum. Suturing of just the external integument without approximation of underlying perineal and vaginal fascia and muscle may lead to relaxation of the vaginal outlet and may contribute to rectocele and cystocele formation, as well as uterine prolapse.

Vaginal Lacerations. Isolated lacerations involving the middle or upper third of the vagina but unassociated with lacerations of the perineum or cervix are observed less commonly. Vaginal lacerations in this location usually are longitudinal and frequently result from injuries sustained during a forceps or vacuum operation, but they may even develop with spontaneous delivery. Such lacerations frequently extend deep into the underlying tissues and may give rise to significant hemorrhage, which usually is controlled readily by appropriate suturing. They may be overlooked unless thorough inspection of the upper vagina is performed. **Bleeding while the uterus is firmly contracted is strong evidence of genital tract laceration, retained placental fragments, or both** (see Chap. 27, p. 615).

Lacerations of the anterior vaginal wall in close proximity to the urethra are relatively common. They often are superficial with little to no bleeding, and repair usually is not indicated. If such lacerations are large enough to require extensive repair, difficulty in voiding can be anticipated and an indwelling catheter placed.

Injuries to Levator Ani. Injuries to the levator ani muscle as a result of overdistention of the birth canal may result in separation of muscle fibers or in the diminution in their tonicity sufficient to interfere with the function of the pelvic diaphragm. In such cases, the woman may develop pelvic relaxation. If these injuries involve the pubococcygeus muscle, urinary incontinence also may develop.

Injuries to the Cervix

Etiology. Traumatic lesions of the upper third of the vagina are uncommon by themselves but are often associated with extensions of deep cervical tears. In rare instances, however, the cervix may be entirely or partially avulsed from the vagina, with colporrhexis in the anterior, posterior, or lateral fornices. Such lesions may follow difficult forceps rotations or deliveries performed through an incompletely dilated cervix with the forceps blades applied over the cervix. Rarely, cervical tears may extend to involve the lower uterine segment and uterine artery and its major branches, and even through the peritoneum. They may be totally unsuspected, but much more often they become manifest by excessive external hemorrhage or by the formation of a retroperitoneal hematoma that begins within the leaves of the broad ligaments. These extensive tears of the vaginal vault should be explored carefully. If there is question of perforation of the peritoneum, or of retroperitoneal or intraperitoneal hemorrhage, laparotomy should be performed. In the presence of damage of this severity, intrauterine exploration for possible rupture also is mandatory. Surgical repair usually is required and effective anesthesia, vigorous blood replacement, and capable assistance are mandatory for a satisfactory outcome.

Cervical lacerations up to 2 cm must be regarded as inevitable in childbirth. Such tears heal rapidly and rarely are the source of any difficulty. In healing, they cause a significant change in the round shape of the external os before cervical effacement and dilatation to that of appreciable lateral elongation after delivery.

Occasionally, during labor the edematous anterior lip of the cervix may be caught and compressed between the head and the symphysis pubis. If ischemia is severe, the cervical lip may undergo necrosis and separation. More rarely, the entire vaginal portion may be avulsed from the rest of the cervix. Such *annular* or *circular detachment of the cervix* is uncommon in modern obstetrics.

In all traumatic lesions involving the cervix, it is not uncommon for appreciable bleeding to manifest after delivery, when hemorrhage may then be profuse. Slight cervical tears heal spontaneously. Extensive lacerations have a similar tendency, but perfect union rarely results. As the consequence of such tears, eversion of the cervix with exposure of the delicate mucus-producing endocervical glands frequently is the cause of persistent leukorrhea. If the leukorrhea persists after the puerperium, treatment with cryotherapy usually is beneficial. If a Papanicolaou smear was not performed during pregnancy, then it should be done and the results reviewed before treatment is initiated.

Diagnosis. A deep cervical tear should always be suspected in cases of profuse hemorrhage during and after the third stage of labor, particularly if the uterus is firmly contracted. Thorough examination is necessary for definitive diagnosis. Because of the flabbiness of the cervix immediately after delivery, digital examination alone often is unsatisfactory. The extent of the injury can be fully appreciated only after adequate exposure and visual inspection of the cervix. The best exposure is gained by the use of right-angle vaginal retractors by an assistant while the operator grasps the patulous cervix with a ring forceps, as shown in Figure 23–1, and described below.

In view of the frequency with which deep tears follow major operative procedures, the cervix should be inspected routinely at the conclusion of the third stage after all difficult deliveries, even if there is no bleeding. Annular detachment of the vaginal portion of the cervix should be suspected whenever an irregular mass of tissue with a circular central opening is cast off before or after birth of the infant.

Treatment. Deep cervical tears require surgical repair, and treatment varies with their extent. When the laceration is limited to the cervix, or even when it extends somewhat into the vaginal fornix, satisfactory results are obtained by suturing the cervix after bringing it into view at the vulva. Visualization is best accomplished when an *assistant* makes firm downward pressure on the uterus while the operator exerts trac-

tion on the lips of the cervix with fenestrated ovum or sponge forceps. Right-angle vaginal wall retractors are often helpful (Fig. 23–1). Because the hemorrhage usually comes from the upper angle of the wound, it is advisable to apply the first suture just above the angle and suture outward toward the operator. Associated vaginal lacerations may be tamponaded with gauze packs to retard hemorrhage while cervical lacerations are repaired. Either interrupted or running absorbable sutures are suitable. Overzealous suturing in an attempt to restore the normal cervical appearance may lead to subsequent stenosis during uterine involution.

Rupture of the Uterus

Frequency. The incidence of uterine rupture may vary appreciably among institutions. Although the frequency of uterine rupture from all causes has probably not decreased remarkably during the past several decades, the etiology of rupture has changed appreciably and the outcome has improved significantly.

Eden and associates (1986) reviewed the experience with uterine rupture over a 53-year period at Duke University. Surprisingly, the incidence of uterine rupture did not decrease appreciably, and from 1931 to 1950 it was 1 in 1280 deliveries compared with 1 in 2250 from 1973 to 1983. Rachagan and colleagues (1991) reported a similar incidence of uterine rupture of about 1 in 3000 deliveries over a 21-year period. Rodriguez and colleagues (1989) reported an incidence of about 1 in 1650 in nearly 139,000 deliveries from Los Angeles County–University of Southern California Women's Hospital.

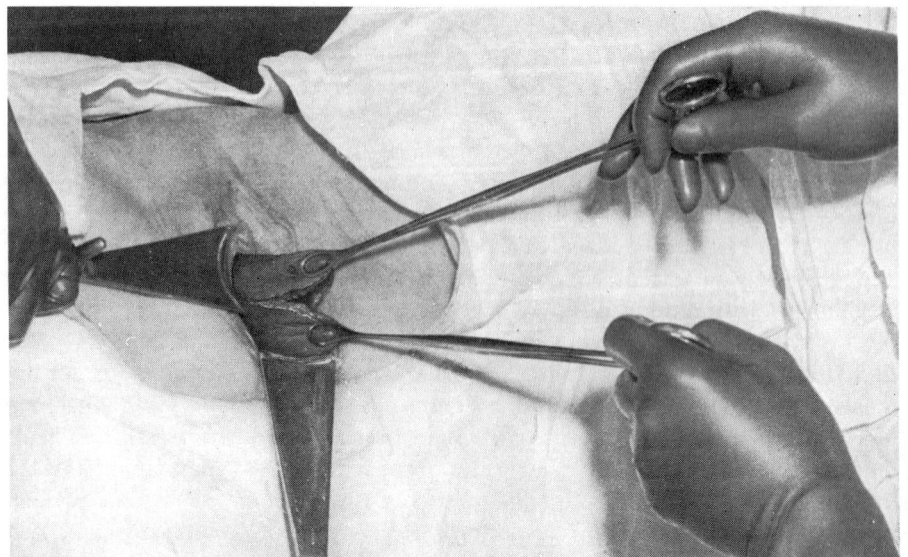

Fig. 23–1. Cervical laceration exposed for repair.

Etiology. Uterine rupture may develop as a result of preexisting injury or anomaly, it may be associated with trauma, or it may complicate labor in a previously unscarred uterus. A classification of the etiology of uterine rupture is presented in Table 23–1.

Currently, the most common cause of uterine rupture is separation of a previous cesarean section scar, and this probably is increasing with the developing trend of allowing a trial of labor following prior transverse cesarean section(s). Shiono and colleagues (1987) from the National Institutes of Health reported that in 1979 a trial of labor was allowed in 2.1 percent of women with prior cesarean delivery, and by 1984 this rate had increased to 8 percent. Flamm and colleagues (1988) reported that approximately one third of over 4900 women with a prior cesarean section underwent a trial of labor. Farmer and colleagues (1991) reported that two thirds of over 11,000 women with a prior cesarean section underwent such a trial. The incidence of overt uterine rupture in these two series was 0.2 and 0.8 percent, respectively.

Other common predisposing factors to uterine rupture are previous traumatizing operations or manipulations, such as uterine curettage or perforation (Fedorkow and colleagues, 1987). Deaton and associates (1989) described a fundal uterine rupture at 25 weeks in a woman who previously had sustained two fundal perforations at the time of hysteroscopically guided lysis of adhesions for Asherman syndrome. Excessive or inappropriate uterine stimulation with oxytocin, a previously common cause, has become very uncommon. Generally, the previously untraumatized, spontaneously laboring uterus will not persist in contracting so vigorously as to destroy itself.

From 1963 to 1983, there were 24 cases of uterine rupture at Duke University (Eden and colleagues, 1986). Only 21 percent had rupture of a previous cesarean section scar, and the remainder were about equally distributed among the following causes: midforceps delivery, breech version and extraction, precipitous delivery, inappropriate oxytocin administration, and prolonged labor. In the series of 34 cases of uterine rupture reported by Rachagan and associates (1991), approximately half were associated with rupture of a previous scar and only 10 percent with trauma. Of the 13 women with a spontaneous rupture, 9 were women of high parity; and in 6 of these labor was stimulated by oxytocin.

Definitions. Rupture of the uterus may communicate directly with the peritoneal cavity (*complete*) or may be separated from it by the visceral peritoneum over the uterus or that of the broad ligament (*incomplete*).

It is important to differentiate between *rupture versus dehiscence of a cesarean section scar*. Rupture refers to separation of the old uterine incision throughout most of its length, with rupture of the fetal membranes so that the uterine cavity and the peritoneal cavity communicate. In these circumstances, all or part of the fetus usually is extruded into the peritoneal cavity. In addition, there usually is bleeding, often massive, from the edges of the scar or from an extension of the rent into previously uninvolved uterus. By contrast, with dehiscence of a cesarean section scar, the fetal membranes are not ruptured and the fetus is not extruded into the peritoneal cavity. Typically, with dehiscence, the separation does not involve all of the previous uterine scar, the peritoneum overlying the defect is intact, and bleed-

TABLE 23–1. CLASSIFICATION OF CAUSES OF UTERINE RUPTURE

Uterine Injury or Anomaly Sustained Before Current Pregnancy	Uterine Injury or Abnormality During Current Pregnancy

1. Surgery involving the myometrium
    Cesarean section or hysterotomy
    Previously repaired uterine rupture
    Myomectomy incision through or to the endometrium
    Deep cornual resection of interstitial oviduct
    Metroplasty
2. Coincidental uterine trauma
    Abortion with instrumentation—curette, sounds
    Sharp or blunt trauma—accidents, bullets, knives
    Silent rupture in previous pregnancy
3. Congenital anomaly
    Pregnancy in undeveloped uterine horn
	1. Before delivery
	    Persistent, intense, spontaneous contractions
	    Labor stimulation—oxytocin or prostaglandins
	    Intra-amnionic instillation—saline, prostaglandins
	    Perforation by internal uterine pressure catheter
	    External trauma—sharp or blunt
	    External version
	    Uterine overdistention—hydramnios, multiple pregnancy
	2. During delivery
	    Internal version
	    Difficult forceps delivery
	    Breech extraction
	    Fetal anomaly distending lower segment
	    Vigorous uterine pressure during delivery
	    Difficult manual removal of placenta
	3. Acquired
	    Placenta increta or percreta
	    Gestational trophoblastic neoplasia
	    Adenomyosis
	    Sacculation of entrapped retroverted uterus

ing is absent or minimal. Dehiscence likely takes place gradually, whereas rupture very likely is symptomatic, and at times, fatal. With labor or intrauterine manipulations, a dehiscence may become a rupture.

Comparison of Classical and Lower-Segment Cesarean Section Scars.

The behavior of a vertical uterine incision through the body of the pregnant uterus—that is, a *classical scar*—in any subsequent pregnancy differs from that of a scar confined to the lower uterine segment. First, the probability of rupture of a classical scar is several times greater than that of a lower segment scar. Second, in about one third of cases, the classical scar ruptures before labor. Rupture not infrequently takes place several weeks before term. In an unusual case, Lazarus (1978) described disruption of a previous classical incision at 12 weeks' gestation with marked hemorrhage and hypovolemia. Thus, delivery by subsequent cesarean section will not prevent all such ruptures. Conversely, lower-segment scars *that are confined to the noncontractile portion of the uterus rarely,* if ever, rupture before labor.

The statistics available are insufficient to permit a precise calculation of the maternal mortality rate that attends rupture of a cesarean section scar. Rupture following a trial of labor in a woman with a prior transverse incision has not been associated with maternal deaths, and typically, perinatal loss is very low (Flamm and colleagues, 1988; Rachagan and associates, 1991). Conversely, in the 24 cases of uterine rupture principally unassociated with prior incisions, Eden and associates (1986) reported one maternal death and a 46 percent perinatal loss. Likewise, Rachagan and colleagues (1991) reported fetal mortality to be almost 70 percent with either spontaneous or traumatic uterine rupture compared with no losses in women with rupture of a previous incision.

Dehiscence of a lower-segment cesarean section scar is much more frequent than actual rupture, especially if the previous uterine incision was transverse. It is remarkable that these separated scars, often called *windows* and covered only by the peritoneum, in many instances appear to cause no difficulty in labor or subsequently.

Rupture of a Cesarean Section Scar

The current trend in obstetrical practice is to encourage a trial of labor in anticipation of vaginal delivery in women who previously have been delivered by one transverse cesarean section (American College of Obstetricians and Gynecologists, 1988). Even more recently, women with two and even three prior operations have been allowed to labor, either spontaneously or with oxytocin stimulation. The main drawback to this plan is that separation of the previous scar complicates

about 1 in 200 trials of labor. In most cases, the separation is only a dehiscence and of little consequence; however, ruptures may occur. Lee and Cass (1992) have described a case in which the bladder also ruptured along with the uterus in a woman undergoing a trial of labor.

The experience at Parkland Hospital has been that separation of the transverse uterine incision that develops antepartum or during early labor usually is limited to dehiscence without an appreciable increase in maternal or perinatal morbidity. From 1986 through 1990, there were a total of 7049 women at Parkland Hospital with prior cesarean sections, and 2044, or almost 30 percent, were allowed a trial of labor. Of the women undergoing such a trial, 1482 (73 percent) delivered vaginally. Uterine rupture with part of the fetus extruded outside of the uterus occurred in 3 women, for a rate of 1.5 per 1000. In the entire group, there were 2 stillbirths (1 per 1000) and 4 women required hysterectomy (2 per 1000). In another 307 women undergoing a trial of labor and who were given oxytocin, there were 3 uterine ruptures (10 per 1000).

Separation of a vertical scar is more likely to result in severe hemorrhage with increased perinatal morbidity and mortality. For example, in one case of uterine rupture at Parkland, a defect believed to be uterine was felt suprapubically during a uterine contraction. With her last two cesarean sections, a vertical uterine incision was made that apparently included some of the upper segment. At laparotomy, the separated vertical scar was covered by a hematoma of about 400 mL that was entrapped beneath the serosa and overlying adherent omentum. Blood also had infiltrated throughout the left broad ligament to the lateral pelvic wall. The 2950-g infant whose 5-minute Apgar score was 8 was delivered through the ruptured scar. Hysterectomy was performed with some difficulty because of dense adhesions (Fig. 23–2).

Another woman, in whom the cervix was fully dilated and the occiput at +2 station when she was admitted to the labor–delivery unit, was promptly delivered using forceps, although she had previously undergone cesarean section. **Immediate exploration of the uterus was conducted, as should be done in every case of previous cesarean section.** Extensive separation of the vertical cesarean section scar with appreciable hemorrhage was identified and the uterus was removed (Fig. 23–3). Both mother and infant survived.

Morbidity and Mortality.

There have been a considerable number of studies that espouse the benefits and safety of vaginal birth after cesarean section. Rosen and associates (1991) conducted a meta-analysis of 31 studies that included over 11,000 trials of labor after cesarean section, and concluded that it was safe and thus more women should undergo trials of labor after cesar-

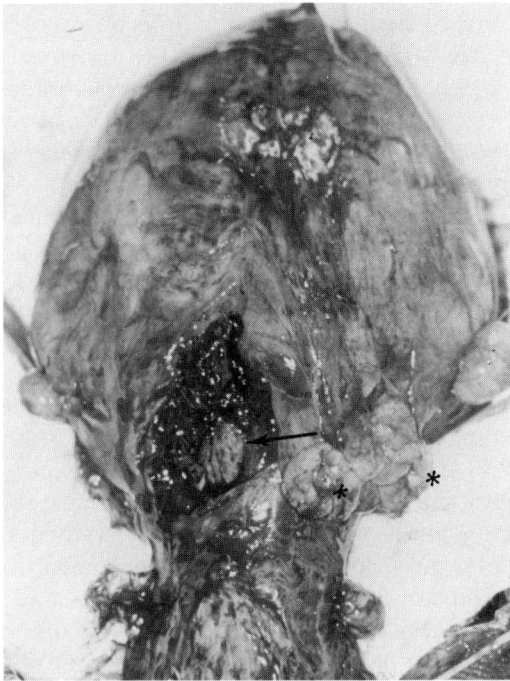

Fig. 23–2. Ruptured vertical cesarean section scar (*arrow*) identified at time of repeat cesarean section early in labor; asterisks indicate some of the sites of densely adherent omentum.

ean birth (Tables 23–2 and 23–3). They concluded further that the rate of uterine dehiscence was not related to the intended birth route, use of oxytocin, indication for cesarean, or unknown scar type (Table 23–2). The corrected perinatal mortality rate with a trial of

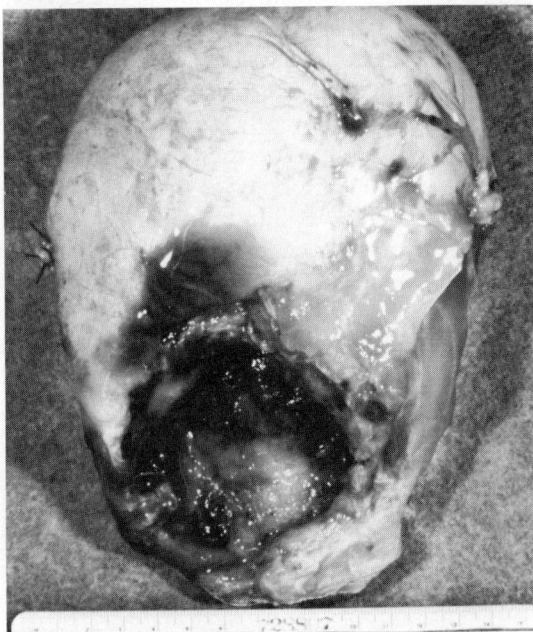

Fig. 23–3. Rupture of uterus identified immediately after vaginal delivery; the previous delivery was by cesarean section with a vertical uterine incision.

TABLE 23–2. META-ANALYSIS OF DEHISCENCE OR RUPTURES: VAGINAL BIRTH AFTER CESAREAN SECTION

Elements Studied	Ruptures or Dehiscences per 1000 Births	Summary Odds Ratio (95% CI)
All trials of labor (n = 2771)	18	0.8 (0.6–1.2)
Vaginal delivery successful (n = 1613)	12	0.7 (0.4–1.2)
Elective repeat cesarean (n = 361)	19	1.0 (—)
Failed trial of labor (n = 584)	33	2.8 (1.4–5.4)
Unknown vs low transverse (n = 1181 vs 2315)	22 vs 11	0.8 (0.4–1.8)
Oxytocin vs no oxytocin (n = 995 vs 2130)	23 vs 15	1.2 (0.7–2.1)
Recurrent vs nonrecurrent (n = 443 vs 607)	7 vs 26	0.4 (0.1–1.1)

Adapted from Rosen and colleagues (1991), with permission.

labor also was not significantly increased (Table 23–3). Finally, they reported that maternal febrile morbidity was decreased by half in women undergoing a trial of labor compared with those delivered by elective repeat cesarean section.

Thus, a trial of labor following a previous cesarean section, especially of the low transverse variety, indeed would appear to be a safe option for the woman. However, we agree with Pitkin (1991), who warns that "safety is relative" and that these women are neither normal nor low risk. Although maternal mortality is rare, significant morbidity still may accrue to both mother and fetus, even with a prior low transverse incision. Specifically, Jones and associates (1991) and Scott (1991) described a total of 20 cases of uterine rupture associated with a previous low segment cesarean scar. Among these 20 women, there were 4 perinatal deaths, at least 2 infants had long-term neurological sequelae, and 3 women required hysterectomy for hemostasis. Thus, while complete rupture of the uterus is uncom-

TABLE 23–3. META-ANALYSIS OF PERINATAL DEATHS: VAGINAL BIRTH AFTER CESAREAN SECTION

Elements Studied	Deaths per 1000 Births	Summary Odds Ratio (95% CI)
Trial of labor (n = 2585)	18	2.1 (1.3–3.4)
Elective repeat cesarean (n = 2945)	10	1.0 (—)
Excluding antenatal deaths, infants < 750 g, congenital anomalies		
Trial of labor (n = 2549)	3	0.8 (0.3–2.1)
Elective repeat cesarean (n = 2929)	4	1.0 (—)

Adapted from Rosen and colleagues (1991), with permission.

mon when a trial of labor is allowed after a prior low transverse cesarean section, when it occurs, the results may be disastrous for mother, fetus, or both. Unfortunately, assiduous observation during labor will not avoid these outcomes always.

Healing of the Cesarean Section Scar. There is little information that deals with healing of cesarean section scars. Williams (1921) believed that the uterus heals by regeneration of the muscular fibers and not by scar tissue formation. He based his conclusions on the histological examination of the incision site along with two principal observations: First, upon inspection of the un-opened uterus at the time of repeated cesarean sections there usually is no trace of the former incision, or at most, an almost invisible linear scar. Second, when the uterus is removed, often no scar is visible after fixation, or only a shallow vertical furrow in the external and internal surfaces of the anterior uterine wall is seen, with no trace of scar tissue between them. Conversely, Schwarz and co-workers (1938) concluded that healing occurs mainly by fibroblast proliferation. They studied the incision site in the human uterus some days after cesarean section, as well as in the uteri of guinea pigs, rabbits, and dogs, and they observed that as the scar shrinks, connective tissue proliferation becomes less obvious. Their conclusions appear to be justified by their histological studies, particularly in cases of adequate approximation of the myometrial edges. If the cut surfaces are closely apposed, the proliferation of connective tissue is minimal, and the normal relation of smooth muscle to connective tissue gradually is reestablished, accounting for the occasional absence of even a trace of a former incision. Even when the healing is so poor that marked thinning has resulted, the remaining tissue often is entirely muscular. The fundamental weakness appears to stem from failure to approximate the inner margins of the incision or from formation of a hematoma or abscess in the immediate vicinity. The impact of uterine infection following a previous cesarean section and rupture during subsequent pregnancy appears to be negligible.

Rupture of the Unscarred Uterus

Traumatic Rupture. Although the uterus is surprisingly resistant to blunt trauma, pregnant women sustaining blunt trauma to the abdomen should be watched carefully for signs of a ruptured uterus (see Chap. 47, p. 1076). The likelihood of a ruptured spleen or traumatic placental abruption is more common. Conversely, penetrating abdominal wounds are much more likely to involve the large pregnant uterus.

In the past, traumatic rupture during delivery most often was caused by internal podalic version and extraction. Other causes of traumatic rupture include difficult forceps delivery, breech extraction (Fig. 23–4), and un-usual fetal enlargement, such as hydrocephaly. Ruptured uterus caused by strong fundal pressure to try to accomplish vaginal delivery is particularly reprehensible.

Spontaneous Rupture. The previously intact uterus is more likely to rupture in women of high parity. Moreover, oxytocin stimulation of labor has been rather commonly associated with uterine rupture, especially in women of high parity (Rachagan and associates, 1991). Maymon and associates (1991) have reported a uterine rupture following vaginal delivery in a multiparous woman at term who had induction of labor with prostaglandin E_2 gel. Fuchs and colleagues (1985) reviewed pregnancy outcomes of nearly 5800 women who were para 7 or greater. They found that uterine rupture was 20 times more likely in these women compared with women of lower parity. For this reason, oxytocin rarely should be given to stimulate labor in women of high parity. Similarly, in women of high parity, a trial of labor in the presence of suspected cephalopelvic disproportion, or abnormal presentation such as a brow, may prove dangerous. Rarely, placenta accreta may result in uterine rupture (see Chap. 27, p. 620). Finally, Kyodo and colleagues (1988) reported complete separation with expulsion of a live fetus complicating a molar pregnancy.

Pathological Anatomy. The role in uterine rupture of excessive stretching of the lower uterine segment with the development of a pathological retraction ring is described in Chapter 19, p. 489. Rupture of the previously intact uterus at the time of labor most often involves the thinned-out lower uterine segment. The rent, when it is in the immediate vicinity of the cervix, frequently extends transversely or obliquely. Usually, the tear is longitudinal when it occurs in the portion of the uterus adjacent to the broad ligament (Fig. 23–4C). Although developing primarily in the lower uterine segment, it is not unusual for the laceration to extend further upward into the body of the uterus or downward through the cervix into the vagina. At times, the bladder may also be lacerated (Rachagan and colleagues, 1991). After complete rupture, the uterine contents escape into the peritoneal cavity, unless the presenting part is firmly engaged, when only a portion of the fetus may be extruded from the uterus.

Incomplete ruptures—that is, those in which the peritoneum remains intact—frequently extend into the broad ligament. In such circumstances, hemorrhage tends to be less severe than in complete rupture, and the blood accumulates between the leaves of the broad ligament. Such bleeding results in a large retroperitoneal hematoma that may involve sufficient blood loss to cause death. More frequently, fatal exsanguination supervenes after rupture of the hematoma relieves the tamponading effect of the intact broad ligament. With incomplete rupture, the products of conception may

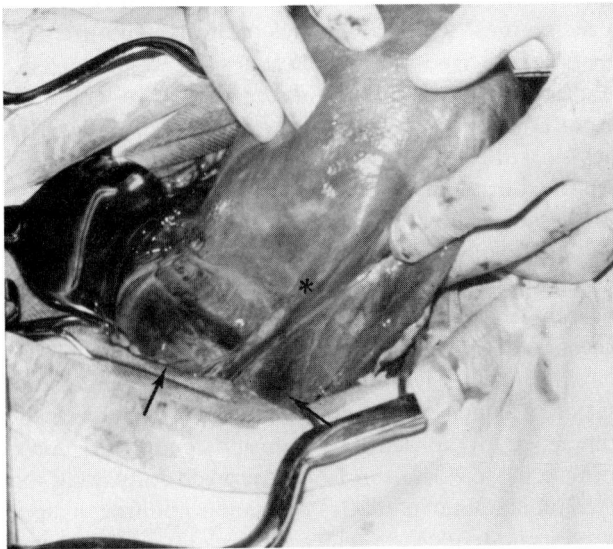

A

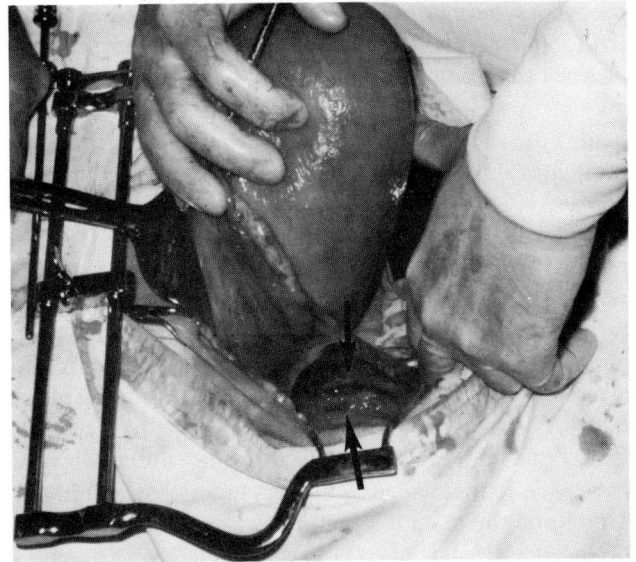

B

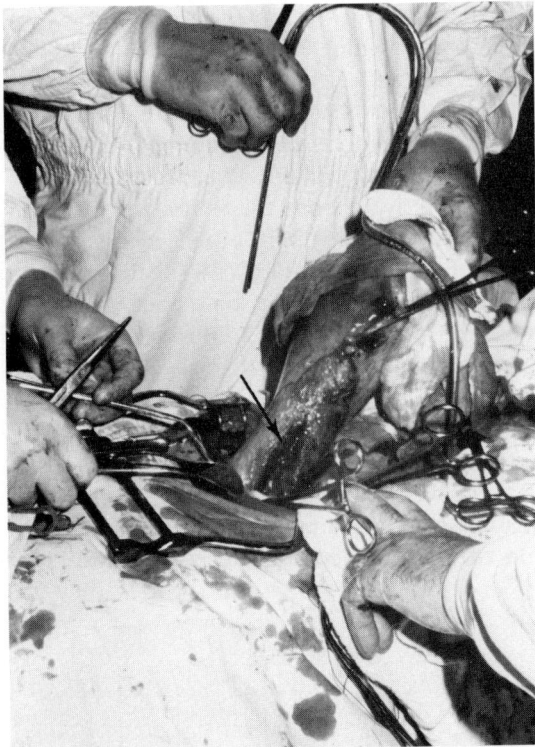

C

Fig. 23–4. A. Rupture of uterus with breech delivery; extensive bleeding beneath uterine serosa and bladder, and in left broad ligament (*arrow*). Asterisk identifies left round ligament. **B.** The broad ligament has been opened and the ureter (*upper arrow*) identified medial to the iliac vessels (*lower arrow*). **C.** Extent of rupture (*arrow*) of lateral wall of uterus is now apparent.

remain within the uterus or assume a position between the leaves of the broad ligament.

Apparent spontaneous rupture of the uterus at times may be associated with prior manipulations that may very well have caused unappreciated uterine injury. Three cases of rupture at our institution fall into this category. In one, the previous pregnancy had terminated in an induced septic abortion. During the next pregnancy, at laparotomy following rupture of the uterus, omentum was adherent to the fundus at the site

of uterine rupture, strongly suggesting that previous perforation of the uterus had occurred. In the second case, vigorous curettage had followed delivery of a hydatidiform mole and myometrial fragments were identified histologically in the curettings. In the next pregnancy, the uterus ruptured early in labor, the left uterine artery was severed, and rapid exsanguination followed. In the third case, an intrauterine device had been removed with considerable difficulty from the uterine fundus by use of a laparoscope. In the next pregnancy, a rent developed in the fundus early in labor, with expulsion of the fetus and placenta, causing fetal death. Taylor and Cummings (1979) described spontaneous rupture of the uterus of a primigravid woman before the onset of labor. The uterine fundus had been traumatized previously by a trocar inserted for laparoscopy.

Instances of uterine rupture have been observed in which hemorrhage was slight. The rupture did not involve large arteries and the emptied uterus contracted well after expulsion of the fetus and placenta into the peritoneal cavity. Less commonly, one or both uterine arteries have been totally avulsed, but spasm develops that prevents exsanguinating hemorrhage. In very rare cases, the fetus may be extruded into the peritoneal cavity while the placenta remains functional within the uterus and the gestation continues as a *uteroabdominal pregnancy* (Badwy, 1962).

Clinical Course. Prior to circulatory collapse from hemorrhage, the symptoms and physical findings may appear bizarre unless the possibility of uterine rupture is kept in mind. For example, hemoperitoneum from a ruptured uterus may result in irritation of the diaphragm and pain referred to the chest—leading one to a diagnosis of pulmonary or amnionic fluid embolus instead of uterine rupture.

If rupture occurs during labor, the woman, usually after a period of premonitory signs, at the acme of a uterine contraction suddenly complains of a sharp, shooting pain in the abdomen and may cry out that "something ripped" or "something tore" inside her. The so-called classical picture is that after these symptoms and signs have appeared, there is cessation of uterine contractions, and the woman, until that point in intense agony, suddenly experiences much relief. At the same time, there may be external hemorrhage, although often it is slight.

Recent observations indicate that few women experience these classical findings of uterine rupture. For example, Rodriguez and colleagues (1989) described data from 39 women with uterine rupture in whom an intrauterine pressure catheter was in place. In none of these was there a loss of intrauterine pressure or cessation of labor. Four women had increased baseline pressure associated with severe variable decelerations (Fig. 23–5). The most common finding in all of their 76 cases was fetal distress, and this was seen in almost 80 percent of cases. They concluded that intrauterine pressure monitoring added little to the diagnosis of uterine rupture.

In still other women, the appearance is identical to that of placental abruption. In others, rupture is unaccompanied by appreciable pain and tenderness. Also, because most women in labor are given something for discomfort, either narcotics or lumbar epidural analgesia, pain and tenderness may not be readily apparent and the condition becomes evident because of signs of fetal distress, maternal hypovolemia from concealed hemorrhage, or both.

In some cases in which the fetal presenting part had entered the pelvis with labor, there is *loss of station* detected by pelvic examination. If the fetus is partly or totally extrauterine, abdominal palpation or vaginal examination is helpful to identify the presenting part, which has moved away from the pelvic inlet. A firm contracted uterus may, at times, be felt alongside the fetus. Often fetal parts are more easily palpated than usual. On vaginal examination, it sometimes is possible to palpate a tear in the uterine wall through which the fingers can be passed into the peritoneal cavity. **Failure to detect the tear by no means proves its absence.** In suspected cases, it is imperative that thorough examination be performed by an experienced examiner before the suspicion is abandoned. Sonography, performed on site, may be useful. At times, either abdominal paracentesis in the flank or culdocentesis is indicated to

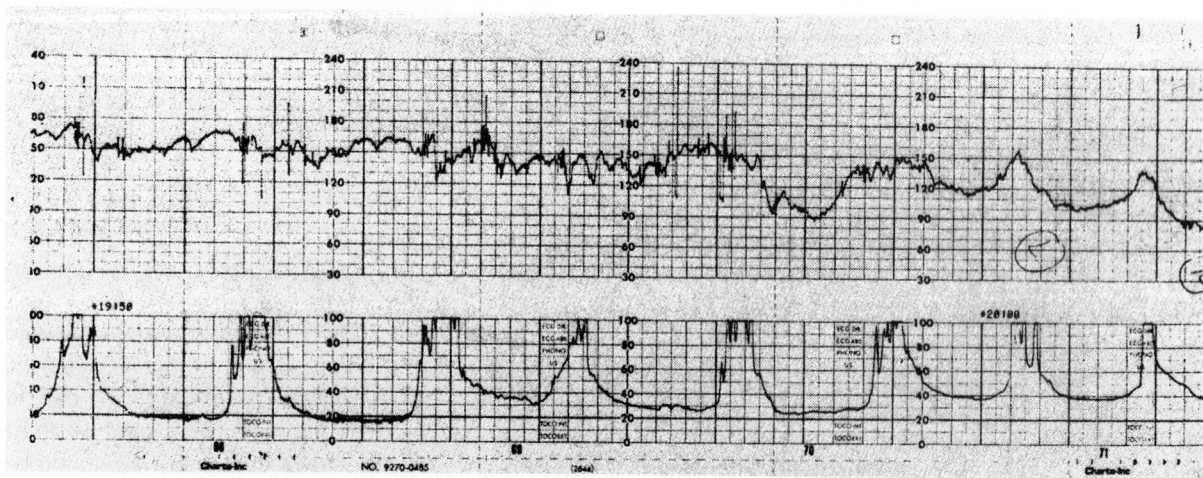

Fig. 23–5. Internal monitor tracing demonstrates fetal heart rate decelerations, increase in uterine tone, and continuation of uterine contractions in a woman with uterine rupture. (From Rodriguez and colleagues, 1989, with permission.)

identify hemoperitoneum. After delivery, culdocentesis can be performed through the posterior fornix.

Prognosis. The chances for fetal survival are dismal, and mortality rates reported in various studies range from 50 to 75 percent. If the fetus is alive at the time of the rupture, the only chance of continued survival is afforded by immediate delivery, most often by laparotomy. Otherwise, hypoxia from both placental separation and maternal hypovolemia is inevitable. If untreated, most of the women die from hemorrhage or, less often, later from infection, although spontaneous recovery has been noted in exceptional cases. Prompt diagnosis, immediate operation, the availability of large amounts of blood, and antimicrobial therapy have greatly improved the prognosis for women with a rupture of the pregnant uterus.

Immediate Treatment. The life of the woman will depend most often on the speed and efficiency with which hypovolemia can be corrected and hemorrhage controlled. Whenever uterine rupture is diagnosed, it is mandatory that the following functions be carried out, immediately and simultaneously:

1. Two effective, large-bore intravenous infusion catheters are established, and crystalloid solution, either lactated Ringer's or saline, is infused vigorously.
2. Type-specific whole blood is obtained in large quantities, beginning with at least 10 U if possible, and its rapid infusion is begun as soon as possible.
3. A surgical team, including anesthesia personnel, is assembled, with the operating room set up with instruments necessary to perform cesarean hysterectomy.
4. Pediatric personnel skilled in neonatal resuscitation are summoned.

It is emphasized that hypovolemic shock may not be quickly reversible until arterial bleeding has been surgically controlled; therefore, there should be no delay in starting surgery for these reasons. Instead, blood must be infused vigorously and the laparotomy begun. In desperate cases, compression applied to the aorta may help to reduce the bleeding. Oxytocin administered intravenously may incite contraction of the myometrium and, in turn, vessel constriction, thereby reducing the bleeding. Clamping the ovarian vessels immediately adjacent to the uterus will help to conserve blood. Techniques for monitoring the adequacy of the circulation, blood and blood-fraction replacement therapy, and the recognition and treatment of coagulation defects, are considered in detail in Chapter 37.

Hysterectomy Versus Repair. Hysterectomy usually is required, but in selected cases suture of the wound may be performed. Mokgokong and Marivate (1976), based on a review of 335 cases treated in Durban, South Africa, considered the merits of hysterectomy compared with uterine repair. Maternal mortality was 7 percent and fetal mortality was 80 percent. Three fourths of their cases involved women with previously unscarred uteri. Common specific causes of rupture of the previously unscarred uterus were cephalopelvic disproportion, fetal malpresentation, obstetrical instrumentation, oxytocin stimulation, and internal podalic version. The uterine tears were usually longitudinal and lateral, often involving the uterine artery or its major branches. They concluded that total hysterectomy, especially with longitudinal tears, is the surgical procedure of choice, although transverse lower segment lacerations may be dealt with adequately by repair of the rent. The frequency of subsequent successful pregnancies following repair of the rent was not provided. Martin and colleagues (1990) described a woman in whom recurrent uterine lateral fundal separation at 19 weeks' gestation was repaired using a Gore-Tex soft tissue patch. When delivered by cesarean section at 33 weeks, the patch was intact and epithelialized.

Sheth (1968) reported the findings in a series of 66 cases in which repair of a uterine rupture was elected rather than hysterectomy. In 25 instances, the repair was accompanied by tubal sterilization. Thirteen of the 41 mothers who did not have tubal sterilization had a total of 21 subsequent pregnancies, but uterine rupture recurred in 4 instances.

In the presence of a large hematoma in the broad ligament, identification and ligation of the uterine vessels can be extremely difficult. In general, efforts to control hemorrhage by clamping indiscriminately at the site of rupture involving the lower segment should be avoided. To do otherwise often leads to clamping and ligation of the ureter, bladder, or both. With uterine ruptures involving the lower uterine segment, bleeding vessels must be visualized free of surrounding tissue before clamping, or the ureter and bladder must be demonstrated to be remote from the tissue that is clamped. In some cases, the transected uterine artery has retracted laterally and is displaced to the pelvic sidewall by the hematoma that resulted. Placement of clamps to control bleeding carries little risk when rupture involves the body of the uterus remote from the ureters and bladder. The broad ligament may be entered and the ascending uterine artery and veins safely clamped. Usually, the ovarian vessels should be promptly clamped adjacent to the uterus.

Ligation of the internal iliac (hypogastric) arteries at times reduces the hemorrhage appreciably. This operation is more easily performed if the midline abdominal incision is extended upward above the umbilicus. With adequate exposure, ligation is accomplished by opening the peritoneum over the common iliac artery and dissecting down to the bifurcation of the external and in-

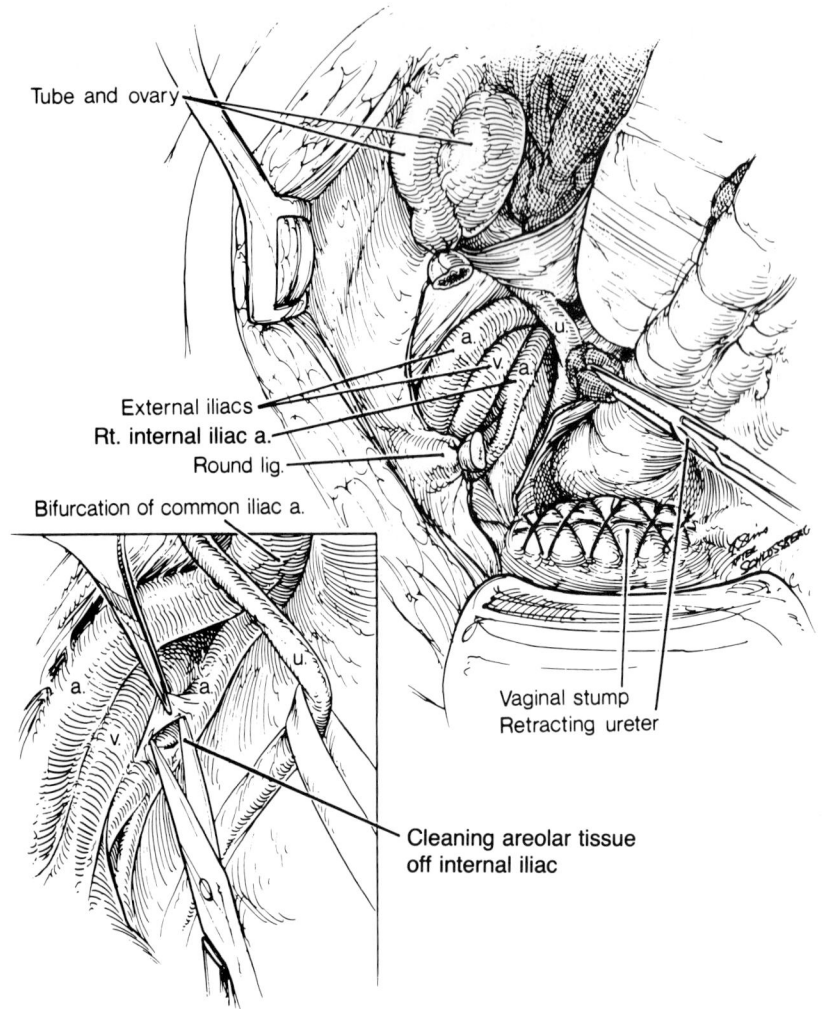

Fig. 23–6. Ligation of the right internal iliac artery. In the lower left insert, the areolar sheath covering the artery is being opened. (a. = artery; lig. = ligament; rt. = right; u. = ureter; v. = vein.)

ternal iliac arteries. The areolar sheath covering the internal iliac artery is incised longitudinally and a right-angle clamp is carefully passed just beneath the artery. Care must be taken not to perforate contiguous large veins, especially the internal iliac vein. Suture, usually nonabsorbable, is then inserted into the open clamp, the jaws are locked, the suture is carried around the vessel, and the vessel is securely ligated (Figs. 23–6 and 23–7). Pulsations in the external iliac artery, if present before tying the ligature, should be present afterward as well. If not, pulsations must be identified after arterial hypotension has been successfully treated, in order to assure that the blood flow through the external iliac vessel has not been compromised by the ligature. An important mechanism of action with internal iliac artery ligation is reduction of pulse pressure in those arteries distal to the ligation. It is of interest that bilateral ligation of these arteries does not appear in itself to interfere seriously with subsequent reproduction. Mengert and associates (1969) documented successful pregnancies in 5 women after bilateral internal iliac artery ligation. In 3, the ovarian arteries also were ligated.

In some women, pelvic vessel bleeding may con-

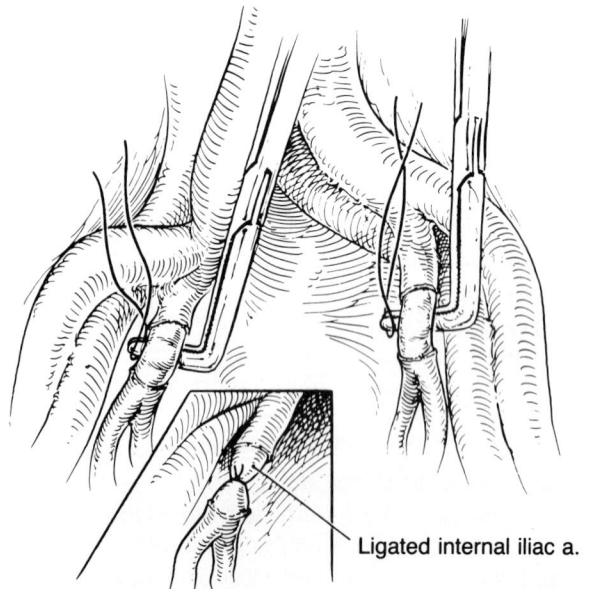

Fig. 23–7. Ligation of both internal iliac arteries. After the covering sheath has been opened and the artery has been carefully freed from the immediately adjacent veins, a ligature is carried beneath the artery with a right angle clamp and firmly tied. (a. = artery.)

tinue even after internal iliac artery ligation. In some cases, angiographically directed arterial embolization with Gelfoam or a similar substance has been described to successfully arrest hemorrhage (Greenwood and colleagues, 1987).

Genital Tract Fistulas from Parturition

In obstructed labor, the tissues of various parts of the genital tract may be compressed between the fetal head and the bony pelvis. If the pressure is brief, it is without significance; but if it is prolonged, necrosis results, followed in a few days by sloughing and perforation. In most such cases, the perforation develops between the vagina and the bladder, giving rise to a *vesicovaginal fistula*. Less frequently, the anterior cervical lip is compressed against the symphysis pubis, and an abnormal communication eventually is established between the cervical canal and the bladder, a *vesicocervical fistula*. If the woman has no infection, the fistula may heal spontaneously. More often it persists, requiring subsequent repair.

Rarely, the posterior wall of the uterus may be subjected to so much pressure against the promontory of the sacrum that necrosis results, and a fistula communicating with the cul-de-sac develops.

References

American College of Obstetricians and Gynecologists: Committee on Obstetrics: Maternal and Fetal Medicine: Guidelines for vaginal delivery after a previous cesarean birth. Number 64, October 1988

Badwy AH: Abdominal pregnancy in a previously ruptured uterus. Lancet 1:510, 1962

Deaton JL, Maier D, Andreoli Jr J: Spontaneous uterine rupture during pregnancy after treatment of Asherman's syndrome. Am J Obstet Gynecol 160:1053, 1989

Eden RD, Parker RT, Gall SA: Rupture of the pregnant uterus: A 53-year review. Obstet Gynecol 68:671, 1986

Farmer RM, Kirschbaum T, Potter D, Strong TH, Medearis AL: Uterine rupture during trial of labor after previous cesarean section. Am J Obstet Gynecol 165:996, 1991

Fedorkow DM, Nimrod CA, Taylor PJ: Ruptured uterus in pregnancy: A Canadian hospital's experience. Can Med Assoc J 137:27, 1987

Flamm BL, Lim OW, Jones C, Fallon D, Newman LA, Mantis JK: Vaginal birth after cesarean section: Results of a multicenter study. Am J Obstet Gynecol 158:1079, 1988

Fuchs K, Peretz B-A, Marcovici R, Paldi E, Timor-Tritsh I: The "grand multipara"—Is it a problem? A review of 5785 cases. Int J Gynaecol Obstet 23:321, 1985

Greenwood LH, Glickman MG, Schwartz PE, Morese SS, Denny DF: Obstetric and nonmalignant gynecologic bleeding: Treatment with angiographic embolization. Radiology 164:155, 1987

Jones RO, Nagashima AW, Hatnett-Goodman MM, Goodlin RC: Rupture of low transverse cesarean scars during trial of labor. Obstet Gynecol 77:815, 1991

Kyodo Y, Inatomi K, Abe T, Kudo K: A case report of destructive mole after uterine rupture. Am J Obstet Gynecol 158:1182, 1988

Lazarus EJ: Early rupture of the gravid uterus. Am J Obstet Gynecol 132:224, 1978

Lee JY, Cass AS: Spontaneous bladder and uterine rupture with attempted vaginal delivery after cesarean section. J Urol 147:3, 1992

Martin Jr JN, Brewer DW, Rush Jr LV, Martin RW, Hess LW, Morrison JC: Successful pregnancy outcome following midgestational uterine rupture and repair using Gore-Tex soft tissue patch. Obstet Gynecol 75:518, 1990

Maymon R, Shulman A, Pomeranz M, Holtzinger M, Haimovich L, Bahary C: Uterine rupture at term pregnancy with the use of intracervical prostaglandin E_2 gel for induction of labor. Am J Obstet Gynecol 165:368, 1991

Mengert WJ, Burchell RC, Blumstein RW, Daskal JL: Pregnancy after bilateral ligation of the internal iliac and ovarian arteries. Obstet Gynecol 34:664, 1969

Mokgokong ER, Marivate M: Treatment of the ruptured uterus. Afr Med J 50:1621, 1976

Pitkin RM: Once a cesarean? Obstet Gynecol 77:939, 1991

Rachagan SP, Raman S, Balasundram G, Balakrishnan S: Rupture of the pregnant uterus—A 21-year review. Aust NZ J Obstet Gynaecol 31:37, 1991

Rodriguez MH, Masaki DI, Phelan JP, Diaz FG: Uterine rupture: Are intrauterine pressure catheters useful in the diagnosis? Am J Obstet Gynecol 161:666, 1989

Rosen MG, Dickinson JC, Westhoff CL: Vaginal birth after cesarean: A meta-analysis of morbidity and mortality. Obstet Gynecol 77:465, 1991

Schwarz O, Paddock R, Bortnick AR: The cesarean scar: An experimental study. Am J Obstet Gynecol 36:962, 1938

Scott JR: Mandatory trial of labor after cesarean delivery: An alternative viewpoint. Obstet Gynecol 77:811, 1991

Sheth SS: Results of treatment of rupture of the uterus by suturing. J Obstet Gynaecol Br Commonw 75:55, 1968

Shiono PH, Fielden JG, McNellis D, Rhoads GG, Pearse WH: Recent trends in cesarean birth and trial of labor rates in the United States. JAMA 257:494, 1987

Taylor PJ, Cummings DC: Spontaneous rupture of a primigravid uterus. J Reprod Med 22:169, 1979

Williams JW: A critical analysis of 21 years' experience with cesarean section. Bull Johns Hopkins Hosp 32:173, 1921

■

CHAPTER 24
Forceps Delivery and Related Techniques

There is considerable controversy regarding the role of instrumental vaginal delivery in modern obstetrics. This controversy involves the definition and indications for such procedures, the influence of regional analgesia on the incidence of instrumental deliveries, and also the question of whether contemporaneously trained obstetrical residents are taught adequately to perform such procedures. In addition, there is no consensus regarding the association of operative vaginal delivery with adverse maternal or fetal and neonatal effects. Over the past several years, there have been attempts to elucidate some of these issues. An important consideration was addressed in 1988 when forceps applications were redefined by the Committee on Obstetrics of the American College of Obstetricians and Gynecologists. Additional information was forthcoming in the 1991 technical bulletin entitled *Operative Vaginal Delivery.*

FORCEPS DELIVERY

Obstetrical forceps are designed for extraction of the fetus. The intriguing history of the early development and use of these instruments is presented at the end of this chapter.

General Design. Forceps vary considerably in size and shape, but basically consist of two crossing *branches.* Each branch is maneuvered into appropriate relationship with the fetal head and then articulated. Each branch has four components: the *blade, shank, lock,* and *handle.* Each blade has two curves, the *cephalic* and *pelvic.* The cephalic curve conforms to the shape of the fetal head, and the pelvic curve with that of the birth canal. The blades are oval to elliptical in outline and

some varieties are fenestrated rather than solid to permit a more firm hold on the fetal head.

The cephalic curve (Fig. 24–1) should be large enough to grasp the fetal head firmly without compression. The pelvic curve (Fig. 24–1) corresponds more or less to the axis of the birth canal, but varies considerably among different instruments. The blades are connected to the handles by the shanks, which give the requisite length to the instrument. The shanks are either parallel as in Simpson forceps or crossing as in Tucker–McLane forceps.

The kind of articulation, or *forceps lock,* varies among different instruments. The common method of articulation consists of a socket located on the shank at the junction with the handle, into which fits a socket similarly located on the opposite shank (Figs. 24–1 and 24–2). This form of articulation is commonly referred to as the *English lock.* A *sliding lock* is used in some forceps, such as Kielland forceps (Fig. 24–3). The sliding lock allows the shanks to move forward and backward independently. The components of a quite different type of lock, the *French lock,* are a threaded eye bolt screwed partway into a threaded hole in the left shank and a notch in the right shank that articulates with the eye bolt. After each branch has been applied to the fetal head, the notch is moved over the stem of the eye bolt, and the eye bolt is tightened to lock the branches firmly together.

Definitions and Classification

Forceps used to aid in the delivery of a fetus presenting by the vertex are classified as follows, according to the level and position of the head in the birth canal at the time the blades are applied.

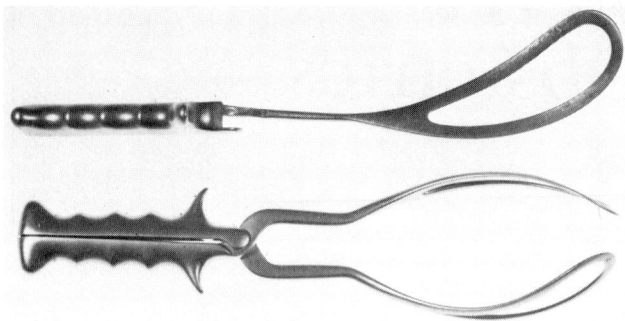

Fig. 24–1. Simpson forceps. Note the ample pelvic curve in the single blade above and cephalic curve evident in the articulated blades below. The fenestrated blade and the wide shank in front of the English-style lock characterize the Simpson forceps.

Classical Definitions. Classically, no distinction was made between **low forceps** and **outlet forceps,** which were defined as forceps applied to the fetal head in which the scalp was visible at the introitus without separating the labia, the skull had reached the pelvic floor, and the sagittal suture was in the anterior–posterior diameter of the pelvis.

Midforceps operations were defined as those in which forceps were applied before the criteria for low forceps were met but after engagement of the fetal head had taken place. Clinical evidence of engagement usually is afforded by the descent of the lowermost part of the skull to or below the level of the ischial spines, because the distance between the level of the ischial spines and the pelvic inlet is ordinarily greater than the distance from the biparietal diameter to the leading part of the fetal head (see Chap. 11, p. 289). Elongation of the fetal head from the combination of a marked degree of molding and caput formation may create the erroneous impression that the head is engaged, even though the biparietal diameter has not passed through the pelvic inlet (see Chap. 21, p. 523). Any rotation with the instrument, including those of less than 45 degrees, that is, left occiput anterior (LOA) and right occiput anterior

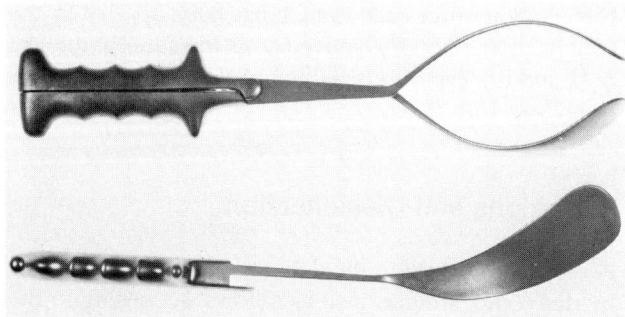

Fig. 24–2. Tucker–McLane forceps. The blade is solid and the shank is narrow.

(ROA), was considered a midforceps delivery. Moreover, under the classical definition, midforceps included many stations of the fetal head from engagement at zero station all the way to the perineum.

Because of the many different stations included in the classical definitions of midforceps operation, many clinicians chose to include a low midforceps operation in the classification. This was defined as forceps applied to the fetal head in which the biparietal diameter was at or below the level of the ischial spines, the head filled the sacral hollow, and the leading part of the head was within a fingerbreadth of the perineum between contractions (Dennen, 1952). Of interest is that this definition is very similar to the contemporaneous definition of low forceps. As emphasized by Richardson and colleagues (1983), the perinatal mortality reported for low forceps, low midforceps, and midforceps is significantly different.

Contemporaneous Classification. Because of the controversy regarding what constitutes a midforceps, the Maternal–Fetal Medicine Committee of the American College of Obstetricians and Gynecologists (1988) has reclassified outlet forceps, low forceps, and midforceps (Table 24–1). **It is emphasized that station here is measured in centimeters (0 to +5), rather than by dividing the lower pelvis into thirds** (see Chap. 14, p. 372). Thus, it is apparent that a +2 station under this new system is not exactly the same as a +2 station under the old system. This latter definition of +2 station probably better corresponds to 3 to 3.5 cm under the new system. At times, the fetal head, as the consequence of appropriate uterine contractions and voluntary expulsion efforts of the mother, will descend to lie firmly against the perineum with the sagittal suture anteroposterior; subsequent to anesthesia for delivery, however, the fetal head will recede somewhat from the perineum and the sagittal suture will revert to an oblique position. Forceps delivery with episiotomy in this circumstance is very likely to be a benign procedure.

High forceps operations are those in which forceps are applied before engagement. High pelvic delivery, either by forceps or vacuum, may be associated with significant morbidity in both mother and fetus and has no place in modern obstetrics.

Incidence. During much of the first half of this century, polarization of opinions over the use of forceps in obstetrics resulted in two very distinct schools of thought. One school vigorously maintained that forceps delivery should be accomplished as soon as the fetal head was engaged and the cervix fully dilated. The other contended with equal vigor that spontaneous delivery should be awaited. It was shown subsequently by objective analysis that there was increased perinatal mortality and morbidity and maternal morbidity from midforceps delivery. More recent studies do not con-

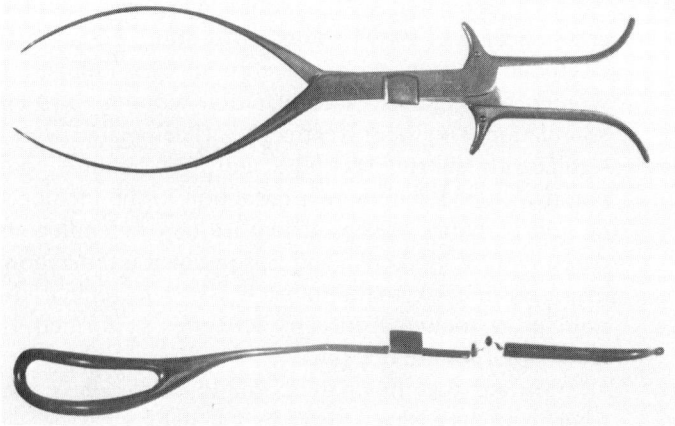

Fig. 24–3. Kielland forceps. The characteristic features are the sliding lock, minimal pelvic curvature, and light weight.

firm these associations, and there may be less perinatal and maternal morbidity with true outlet forceps delivery and an adequate episiotomy compared with delayed spontaneous delivery without episiotomy. In general, the incidence of forceps operations in any given institution will depend upon the attitude of the staff, kinds of analgesia and anesthesia used for labor and delivery, and parity of the obstetrical population. Of interest is that while the rate of forceps delivery generally has decreased in the United States in recent years, according to the National Institutes of Health (1981), the rate in Western European countries actually has increased.

Training for Obstetrical Forceps. There are few publications that address the status of forceps training in the United States. Healy and Laufe (1985), using the old definitions of forceps application, surveyed 144 obstetrical training programs in North America, and reported

that all of 105 responding hospitals reported utilization of outlet forceps. Moreover, 85 percent of the responding programs reported use of outlet forceps in 5 percent or more of all deliveries. The frequency of midforceps delivery in this survey ranged from 1 to 4 percent in more than 50 percent of respondents, and 16 percent of residency programs utilized midforceps in 5 percent or more of deliveries. Only one program reported not using midforceps in their residency training program. Healy and Laufe (1985) also found that hospitals with higher cesarean section rates generally performed more midforceps deliveries than hospitals with lower rates. Approximately two thirds of the program directors expressed the opinion that midforceps operations were important in modern day obstetrics.

More recently, Ramin and colleagues (1992) surveyed 295 residency training programs in the United States and Canada, of which 203 responded; these represented a minimal total of 458,000 deliveries for 1990. Although two programs were not familiar with the revised classification of the American College of Obstetrics and Gynecologists (1988), all but 20 percent of the remainder utilized these new definitions. All of the responding programs utilized outlet and low forceps. Approximately half of the programs utilized outlet forceps for 5 percent or more of their deliveries, while about one third utilized low forceps for 5 percent or more of their deliveries. Midforceps operations were much less prevalent, and 14 percent of programs reported no use, while another 60 percent performed these operations for fewer than 1 percent of deliveries. As with the earlier survey by Healy and Laufe (1985), hospitals with high cesarean section rates did not perform fewer midforceps operations. This decrease in midforceps rate from 99 percent in 1981 to 86 percent in 1990 may similarly reflect the newer, stricter definitions of this operation.

TABLE 24–1. CLASSIFICATION OF FORCEPS DELIVERY ACCORDING TO STATION AND ROTATION

Type of Procedure	Classification
Outlet forceps	1. Scalp is visible at the introitus without separating the labia 2. Fetal skull has reached pelvic floor 3. Sagittal suture is in anteroposterior diameter or right or left occiput anterior or posterior position 4. Fetal head is at or on perineum 5. Rotation does not exceed 45 degrees
Low forceps	Leading point of fetal skull is at station ≥ +2 cm, and not on the pelvic floor a. Rotation ≤ 45 degrees (left or right occiput anterior to occiput anterior, or left or right occiput posterior to occiput posterior) b. Rotation > 45 degrees
Midforceps	Station above +2 cm but head engaged
High	Not included in classification

From American College of Obstetricians and Gynecologists (1988, 1991), with permission.

Effects of Regional Analgesia on Instrumental Delivery. In their review, Kaminski and associates (1987) tabulated the results of 18 reports, most of which described increased frequently of instrumental deliveries with epidural analgesia. In the report by Hoult and colleagues (1977), 57 percent of 273 women who were given epidural analgesia had an instrumental delivery compared with only 11 percent of 275 women given other analgesia. Cox and colleagues (1987) reported that 28 percent of 296 women given epidural analgesia had forceps deliveries compared with only 4 percent of 822 women in the control group. Kaminski and associates (1987) reported a 50 percent instrumental delivery rate in 155 women given segmental epidural analgesia during labor and delivery, compared with a 20 percent incidence in 155 women in the control group who received either pudendal or local analgesia for delivery (Table 24–2). Importantly, significantly more women who were given epidural analgesia (26 percent) had a midforceps delivery compared with women in the control group (8 percent).

Epidural blockade may increase the frequency of malposition of the fetal head, especially the occiput posterior position, and this in turn may increase the frequency of instrumental delivery. For example, in the study by Kaminski and associates (1987), occiput posterior positions were documented in 27 percent of the women given epidural analgesia compared with only 8 percent of those not given epidural analgesia. However, considering delivery from the occiput anterior position only, 39 percent of women receiving epidural analgesia had an instrumental delivery compared with 13 percent of those in the control group (Table 24–2).

In an attempt to decrease the incidence of forceps

delivery associated with epidural analgesia, Saunders and colleagues (1989) compared routine second-stage oxytocin infusion with placebo in 225 nulliparous women who reached full dilatation without oxytocin stimulation. Oxytocin treatment was associated with a significantly shorter second stage (134 minutes compared with 151 minutes), a reduction in the incidence of nonrotational forceps deliveries (33 percent compared with 56 percent), and less perineal trauma; however, routine oxytocin infusion did not reduce the number of rotational forceps deliveries performed for malposition of the occiput.

The fact that the methods employed to relieve pain frequently necessitate instrumental delivery is not an indictment of the procedures, provided the obstetrician adheres strictly to the definition of outlet forceps for termination of labor in such cases.

Function and Choice of the Forceps

The forceps may be used as a tractor, rotator, or both. Its most important function is traction, although, particularly in transverse and posterior positions of the occiput, forceps may be employed successfully for rotation. Any properly shaped instrument will give satisfactory results, provided it is used intelligently. In general, Simpson forceps are used to deliver the fetus with a molded head, as is common in nulliparous women. The Tucker–McLane instrument is used for the fetus with a rounded head, which more characteristically is seen in multiparas. In some circumstances, more specialized forceps may be preferable, for example, in some cases of *deep transverse arrest* characterized by cessation of labor with the fetal head in the transverse position well down in the pelvis with the occiput below the spines. If there is no cephalopelvic disproportion, transverse arrest may be overcome with oxytocin stimulation, with resulting descent of the head to the perineum and spontaneous anterior rotation. **If, however, there are indications for prompt delivery, as in instances of a worrisome fetal heart rate pattern, but safe vaginal delivery without delay cannot be anticipated, then cesarean section should be performed.**

Forces Exerted by the Forceps. Obstetricians have long been interested in the forces exerted by the forceps blades on the fetal skull and maternal tissues. From experiments conducted on women in labor more than a century ago, Joulin (1867) estimated that a pull in excess of 60 kg might damage the fetal skull. These crude studies and subsequent ones have furnished only a gross approximation, for the force produced by the forceps on the fetal skull is a complex function of pull and compression by the forceps and friction produced by the maternal tissues.

TABLE 24–2. FREQUENCY OF INSTRUMENTAL AND MIDFORCEPS DELIVERIES IN WOMEN RECEIVING SEGMENTAL LUMBAR EPIDURAL ANALGESIA FOR LABOR AND DELIVERY[a]

Group	Nulliparous		Multiparous		All Women	
	No.	(%)	No.	(%)	No.	(%)
All Women						
Instrumental[b]						
Epidural	65	(52)	13	(43)	78	(50)
Control	29	(23)	2	(7)	31	(20)
Midforceps						
Epidural	33	(27)	4	(13)	37	(26)
Control	10	(8)	1	(4)	11	(8)
Occiput Anterior Position						
Instrumental						
Epidural	32	(40)	8	(32)	40	(39)
Control	12	(15)	1	(4)	13	(13)
Midforceps						
Epidural	10	(12)	1	(4)	11	(10)
Control	2	(2)	1	(4)	3	(3)

[a] $P < .05$ for comparison with patients in control group.
[b] Low forceps, midforceps, and vacuum extraction.
Data from Kaminski and colleagues (1987).

Indications for the Use of Forceps

The termination of labor by forceps, provided it can be accomplished safely, is indicated in any condition threatening the mother or fetus that is likely to be relieved by delivery. Such maternal indications include heart disease, acute pulmonary edema, intrapartum infection, certain neurological conditions, exhaustion, or a prolonged second stage of labor. Prolonged second-stage labor recently was redefined by the American College of Obstetricians and Gynecologists (1988, 1991) as more than 3 hours with and more than 2 hours without regional analgesia in the nulliparous woman. In the parous woman, this is more than 2 hours with regional analgesia and more than 1 hour without such analgesia. Utilizing the new classification of forceps delivery, midforceps rarely are indicated for labor termination specifically for maternal reasons. Thus, shortening of the second stage of labor for maternal reasons generally should be accomplished with outlet or low forceps procedures.

Fetal indications for operative vaginal delivery with either forceps or vacuum include prolapse of the umbilical cord, premature separation of the placenta, and a worrisome fetal heart rate pattern. Although "fetal distress" or "fetal jeopardy" are terms commonly used to define an indication for termination of labor, both terms are nonspecific and somewhat vague. In the case of a worrisome fetal heart rate pattern, which may or may not be associated with fetal distress or jeopardy, it is prudent to describe the fetal heart rate pattern and the station of the planned forceps application in a precisely written note.

Elective and Outlet Forceps. The vast majority of forceps operations performed in this country are elective and probably related to the frequent use of epidural analgesia. Forceps generally should not be used electively until the criteria for outlet forceps have been met. The fetal head must be on the perineal floor with the sagittal suture no more than 45 degrees from the anteroposterior diameter. In these circumstances, forceps delivery preceded by episiotomy is a simple and safe operation. By allowing the woman in labor ample time, the criteria for outlet forceps can usually be met despite the effects of analgesia. **However, if the head does not descend and rotate, the operation is not an outlet forceps procedure.** If anterior rotation is the only criterion not met for outlet forceps, then delivery usually can still be accomplished safely; however, in general, the head is higher before rotation occurs. In this latter circumstance, the operation is at least low forceps by the definition given in Table 24–1.

Prophylactic Forceps Delivery. In a minority of nulliparous women, marked resistance of the perineum and the vaginal introitus may sometimes present a serious obstacle to delivery of the fetus, even when the expulsive forces are normal. In such cases, an episiotomy and outlet forceps delivery may be beneficial to both mother and fetus. Because it was held widely at the time that prolonged pressure of the fetal head against a rigid perineum might result in fetal brain damage, DeLee (1920) recommended delivery by **prophylactic forceps.** There is no evidence that use of prophylactic forceps is beneficial in the otherwise normal labor and delivery. In a recent randomized, prospective study comparing prophylactic use of outlet forceps with spontaneous vaginal delivery in term pregnancies, Yancey and colleagues (1991) reported that outlet forceps had no immediate adverse effects on the newborn. Prophylactic outlet operations were associated with an increase in maternal perineal trauma in the nulliparous women, however, and did not significantly shorten the second stage of labor.

Prophylactic Low Forceps for Small Fetuses. Bishop and associates (1965), after analyzing data from the Collaborative Perinatal Project, suggested that prophylactic outlet forceps delivery improved neonatal outcome in low-birthweight infants. There appeared to be improved neurological function at 1 year of age in low-birthweight infants delivered by low forceps rather than spontaneously.

Subsequently, the practice of prophylactic forceps for the delivery of small fetuses has been questioned. Haesslein and Goodlin (1979) reported that the incidence of intraventricular hemorrhage in infants weighing 800 to 1350 g was two times greater in those delivered electively by low forceps compared with infants delivered spontaneously. O'Driscoll and associates (1981) reported that only preterm infants delivered by outlet forceps suffered traumatic intracranial hemorrhage. Both of these studies were retrospective and undoubtedly had inherent biases. For example, the effects of labor itself in the genesis of intraventricular hemorrhage must be considered (see Chap. 38, p. 868). Fairweather (1981) reported no significant differences in outcomes in neonates who weighed 500 to 1500 g delivered spontaneously or by low forceps. Schwartz and colleagues (1983) reported similar findings. Anderson and associates (1988) presented preliminary findings consistent with the view that forceps delivery was protective against progression of periventricular hemorrhage in vaginally delivered neonates who weighed less than 1750 g.

At present, there appears to be no obvious advantage to outlet forceps delivery of a small fetus. In such cases, the obstetrician should perform an appropriately large episiotomy in an attempt to increase the size of the vaginal outlet and perineum, thus hopefully ensuring the least trauma to the infant. If the perineum and vaginal introitus are already relaxed, an incision is not necessary.

Prerequisites for Forceps Application

There are at least six prerequisites for forceps successful application:

1. **The head must be engaged and preferably deeply engaged.** Whenever the blades are applied before the head has reached the perineal floor, it is common to find the head decidedly higher than was believed to be the case from the findings of vaginal examination. This is because of extensive caput succedaneum formation and molding. These difficulties of midforceps operation may be encountered even in the presence of a valid maternal indication for forceps delivery. For instance, it is generally agreed that women with heart disease should be spared, as much as safely possible, the effort of bearing down during the second stage of labor. Such efforts, however, may prove much less harmful than a difficult midforceps delivery. Therefore, forceps should not be used until the station of the head is low enough to ensure a safe operative procedure. The same generalization applies to forceps for a worrisome fetal heart rate pattern when the head is not close to the perineal floor. Granted that the fetal heart rate in such a case may suggest that the infant is in jeopardy, it may still be judicious to allow more time for the head to descend. If delivery is mandatory, cesarean section is preferable to a difficult and possibly damaging midforceps operation.

2. **The fetus must present either by the vertex or by the face with the chin anterior.**

3. **The position of the fetal head must be precisely known so that the forceps can be applied appropriately.** So-called pelvic application can be dangerous.

4. **The cervix must be completely dilated before application of forceps.** Even a small rim of cervix may offer great resistance when traction is applied, causing extensive cervical lacerations. If prompt delivery becomes imperative before complete dilatation of the cervix, cesarean section is preferable.

5. **Before forceps application, the membranes must be ruptured to permit a firm grasp of the head by the blades.**

6. **There should be no disproportion between the size of the head and that of the pelvic inlet or the midpelvis.**

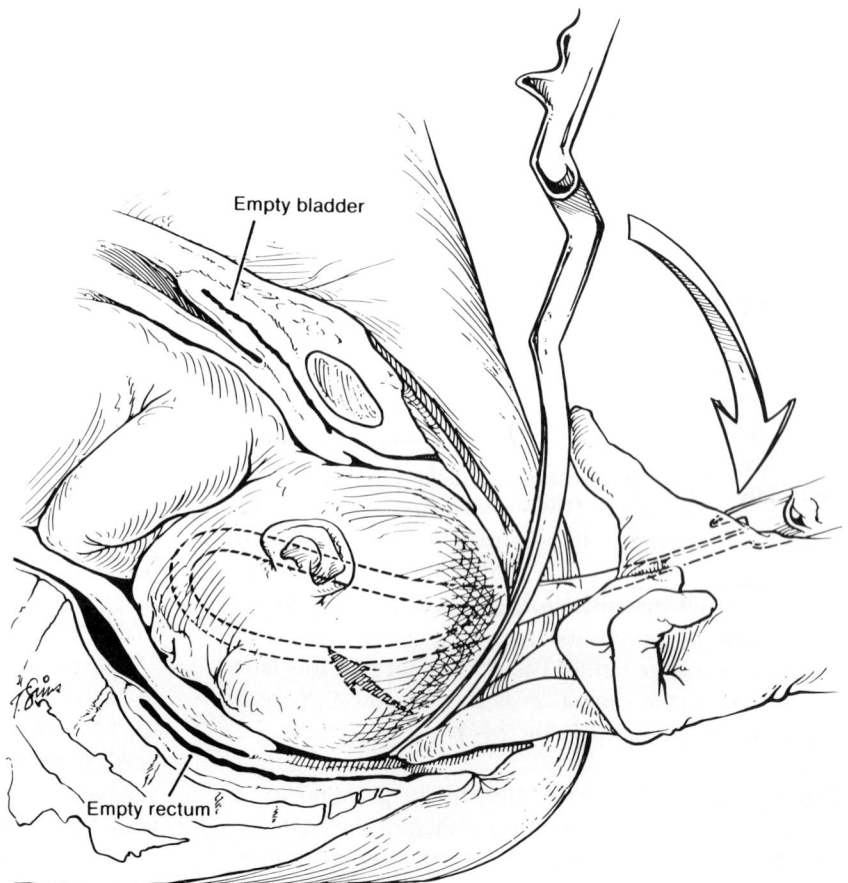

Fig. 24–4. The fetus is presenting as vertex with the occiput anterior and crowning. The application of the left blade of the Simpson forceps is shown. Next, the right blade is applied and the blades are articulated.

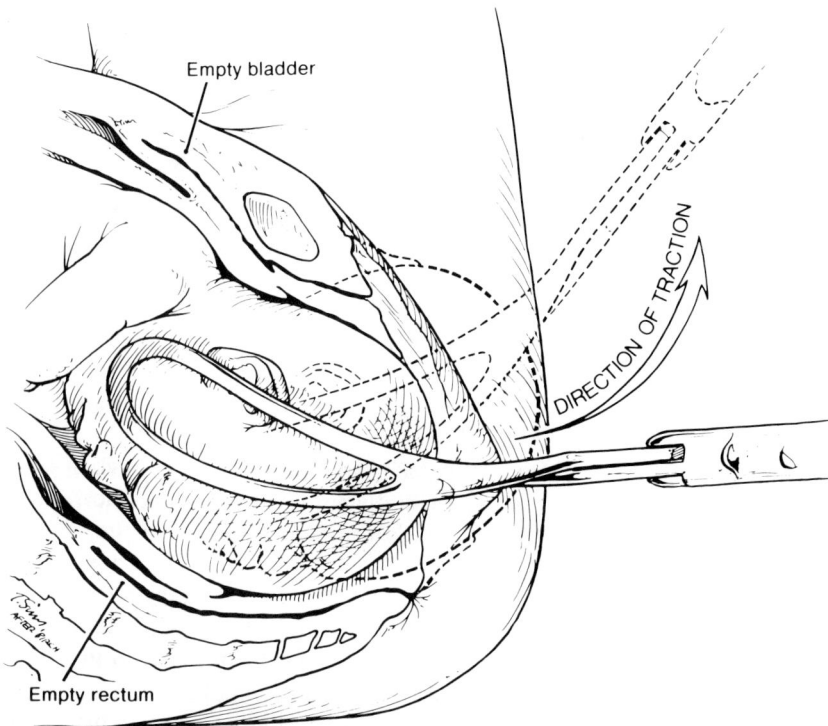

Fig. 24–5. Occiput anterior. Delivery by outlet forceps (Simpson). The direction of gentle traction for delivery of the head is indicated.

Techniques of Outlet Forceps Operations

Preparations for Operation. In the absence of previously instituted adequate conduction analgesia, a decision as to the type of analgesia or anesthesia is made based on factors addressed in Chapter 16. Although pudendal block may prove adequate for outlet forceps operations, either regional analgesia or general anesthesia is frequently required for low forceps or midpelvic procedures. The bladder should be emptied by catheterization if a low or midforceps delivery is planned. If spinal analgesia is to be used, the anesthetic agent is introduced before placing the woman in the lithotomy position for delivery. If general anesthesia is to be used, the woman is placed in the lithotomy position, the perineum is cleansed and draped, and the obstetrician is ready to perform the forceps delivery before anesthesia is induced.

Intravenously administered, ketamine may prove especially useful as an anesthetic for forceps delivery.

The usual dose is 1 to 2 mg per kg of body weight. This drug should be avoided in the woman with significant hypertension.

Application of Forceps. Forceps are constructed so that their cephalic curve is closely adapted to the sides of the fetal head (Fig. 24–4). The biparietal diameter of the fetal head corresponds to the greatest distance between the appropriately applied blades. Consequently, the head of the fetus is perfectly grasped only when the long axis of the blades corresponds to the occipitomental diameter, with the tips of the blade lying over the cheeks, while the concave margins of the blades are directed toward either the sagittal suture (occiput anterior position) or the face (occiput posterior position). Consideration must be given to the degree of molding. Thus applied, the forceps should not slip, and traction may be applied most advantageously as illustrated in Figure 24–5. When forceps are applied obliquely, however (Fig. 24–6), with one blade over the brow and the

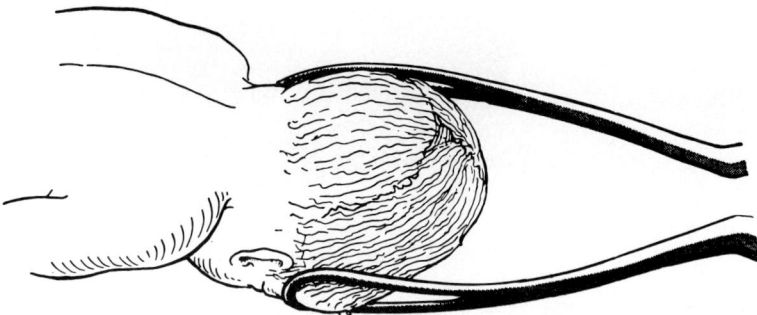

Fig. 24–6. Incorrect application of forceps over brow and mastoid region.

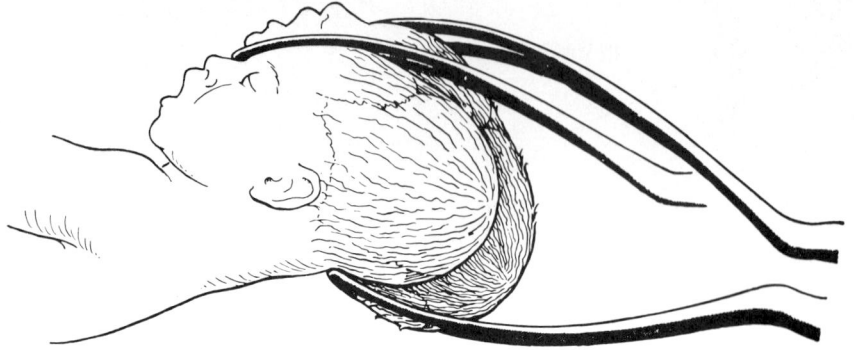

Fig. 24–7. Incorrect application of forceps, one blade over the occiput and the other over the brow. Forceps cannot be locked and the head is extended with tendency of blades to slip off with traction.

other over the opposite mastoid region, the grasp is less secure, and the fetal head is exposed to injurious pressure. With most forceps, if one blade is applied over the brow and the other over the occiput, the instrument cannot be locked or, if locked, the blades slip off when traction is applied. For these reasons, the forceps must be applied directly (Fig. 24–7) to the sides of the head along the *occipitomental diameter,* in what is termed the biparietal or bimalar application.

Identification of Position. **Precise knowledge of the exact position of the fetal head is essential to a proper cephalic application.** With the head low down in the pelvis, determination of position is made by examination of the sagittal suture and the fontanels; but when it is at a higher station, an absolute determination can be made by locating the posterior ear.

The term *pelvic application* is employed when the left blade is applied to the left and right blade to the right side of the pelvis, irrespective of the position of the fetal head. Pelvic application is likely to be injurious to the fetus and should not be practiced.

Outlet Forceps Delivery. Delivery by outlet forceps is illustrated in Figures 24–8 to 24–15. With the head at the low station required in the definition, the obstacle to delivery is usually insufficient expulsive forces, appreciable resistance of the perineum, or both. In such circumstances, the sagittal suture occupies the anteroposterior diameter of the pelvic outlet, with the small (posterior) fontanel directed toward either the symphysis pubis or the concavity of the sacrum. In either event, the forceps, if applied to the sides of the pelvis, grasps the head ideally. The left blade is introduced by the left hand into the left side of the pelvis, and then the right blade is introduced by the right hand into the right side of the pelvis, as follows: Two or more fingers of the right hand are introduced inside the left, posterior portion of

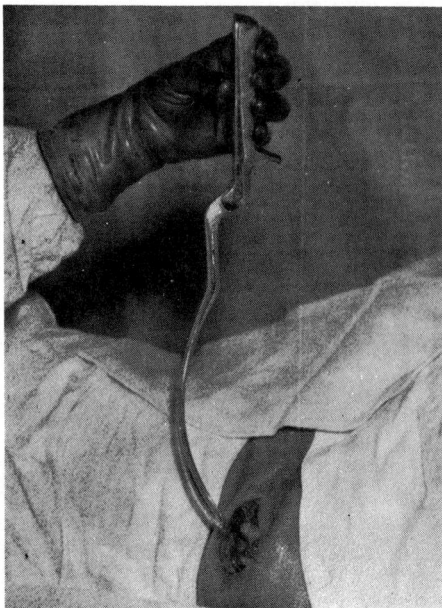

Fig. 24–8. The left handle held in the left hand. Simpson forceps.

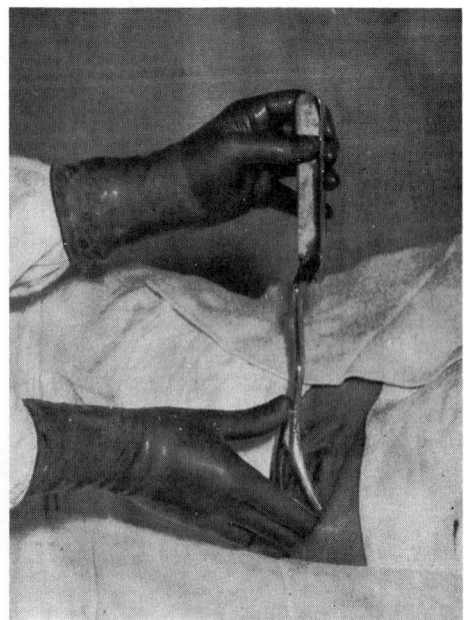

Fig. 24–9. Introduction of left blade into left side of pelvis.

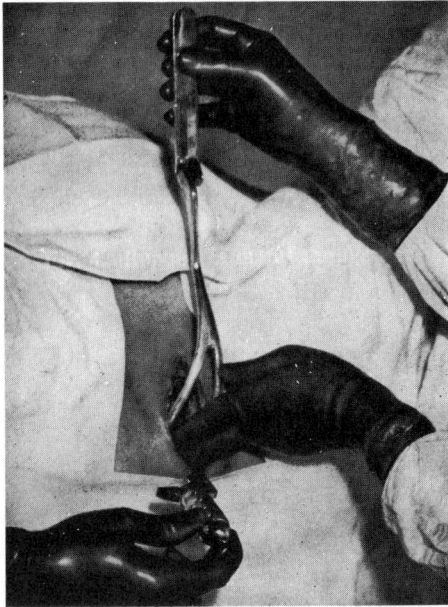

Fig. 24–10. Left blade in place; introduction of right blade by right hand.

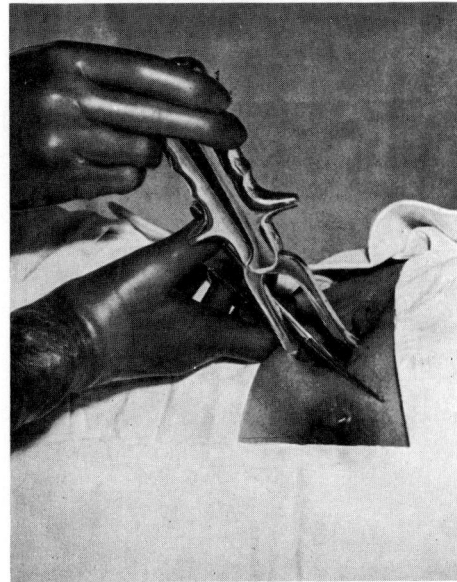

Fig. 24–12. Median or mediolateral episiotomy may be performed at this point. Left mediolateral episiotomy shown here.

the vulva and into the vagina beside the fetal head. The handle of the left branch is then grasped between the thumb and two fingers of the left hand, as in holding a pen, and the tip of the blade is gently passed into the vagina between the fetal head and the palmar surface of the fingers of the right hand, which serve as a guide. The handle and branch are held at first almost vertically; but

as the blade adapts itself to the fetal head, they are depressed, eventually to a horizontal position. The guiding fingers are then withdrawn, and the handle is left unsupported or held by an assistant. Similarly, two or more fingers of the left hand are then introduced into the right, posterior portion of the vagina to serve as a guide for the right blade, which is held in the right hand

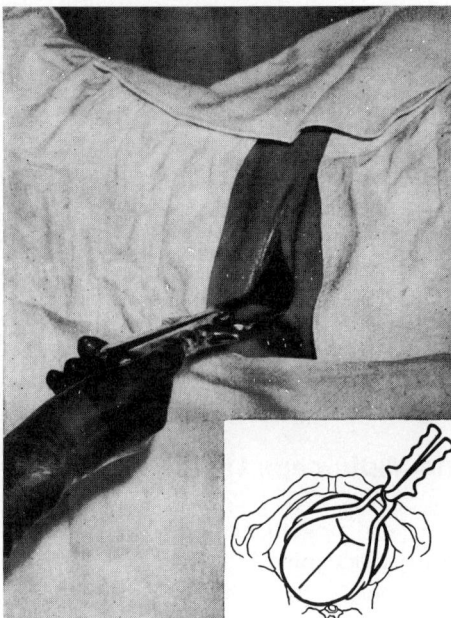

Fig. 24–11. Forceps have been locked. (Inset shows LOA.)

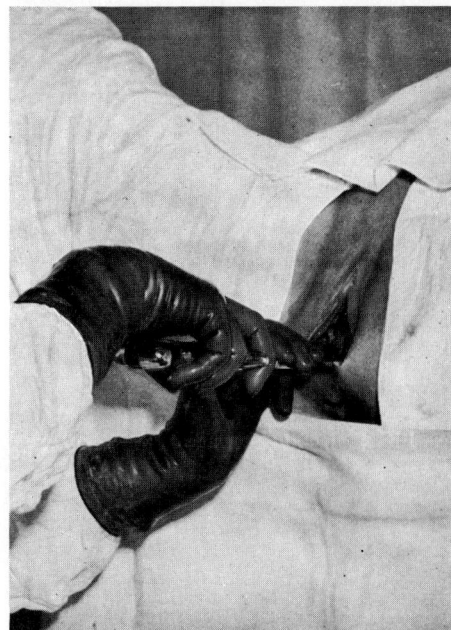

Fig. 24–13. Horizontal traction; operator seated.

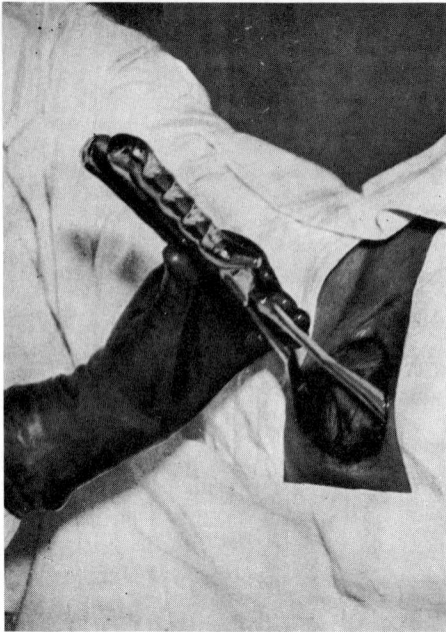

Fig. 24-14. Upward traction.

and introduced into the vagina. These guiding fingers are then withdrawn and the horizontally positioned branches are articulated. If necessary, one and then the other blade should be gently maneuvered until the handles are repositioned to effect easy articulation.

Appropriateness of Application. The application now is checked before any traction is applied. For the occiput

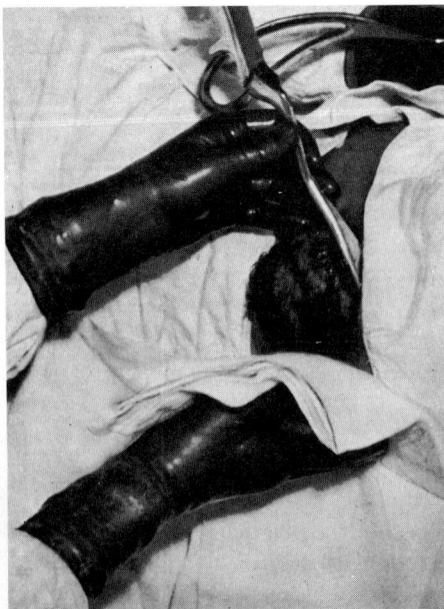

Fig. 24-15. Disarticulation of branches of forceps. Beginning modified Ritgen maneuver.

anterior position, appropriately applied blades are equidistant from the sagittal suture. In the occiput posterior position the blades are equidistant from the midline of the face and brow.

Traction with Forceps. When it is certain that the blades are placed satisfactorily and the cervix is not entrapped, gentle, intermittent, horizontal traction is exerted until the perineum begins to bulge. Traction with forceps is always applied gently and never with excessive force. As the vulva is distended by the occiput, the handles are gradually elevated, eventually pointing almost directly upward as the parietal bones emerge. With the fetal head in the occiput anterior position, this maneuver takes advantage of the smallest diameters of the fetal head and brings the suboccipital region beneath the symphysis. As the handles are raised, the head is extended. Episiotomy is performed most often when forceps traction on the head begins to distend the perineum. During upward traction, the four fingers should grasp the upper surface of the handles and shanks, while the thumb exerts the necessary force upon their lower surface (Fig. 24-14).

During the birth of the head, spontaneous delivery should be simulated as closely as possible. **Traction should therefore be intermittent, and the head should be allowed to recede in intervals, as in spontaneous labor.** Except when urgently indicated, as in severe fetal bradycardia, delivery should be sufficiently slow, deliberate, and gentle to prevent undue compression of the fetal head. It is preferable to apply traction with each uterine contraction.

After the vulva has been well distended by the head, and the brow can be felt through the perineum, the delivery may be completed in several ways. Some obstetricians keep the forceps in place, in the belief that the greatest control of the advance of the head is thus maintained. The thickness of the blades many times add to the distention of the vulva, however, thus increasing the likelihood of laceration or necessitating a large episiotomy. In such cases, the forceps are removed and delivery is completed by the modified Ritgen maneuver (Fig. 24-15), slowly extending the head by using upward pressure upon the chin through the posterior portion of the perineum, while covering the anus with a towel to minimize contamination from the bowel. If the forceps are removed prematurely, the modified Ritgen maneuver may prove to be a tedious and inelegant procedure.

Low and Midforceps Operations

When the head lies above the perineum, the sagittal suture usually occupies an oblique or transverse diameter of the pelvis. In such cases, the forceps should always be applied to the sides of the head. The application is best accomplished by introducing two or more fingers into the vagina to a sufficient depth to feel the posterior fetal ear, over which, whether right or left, the first blade should be applied.

Left Occiput Anterior Position. In the left occiput anterior positions, the right hand, introduced into the left posterior segment of the vagina, should identify the posteriorly located left ear and at the same time serve as a guide for introduction of the left branch of the forceps, which is held in the left hand and applied over the left ear. The handle is held by an assistant or left unsupported, the blade usually retaining its position without difficulty. Two fingers of the left hand are then introduced into the right posterior portion of the pelvis. The right branch of the forceps, held in the right hand, is then introduced along the left hand as a guide. It must then be applied over the anterior ear of the fetus by gently sweeping the blade anteriorly until it lies directly opposite the blade that was introduced first. Of the two branches, when articulated, one occupies the posterior and the other the anterior extremity of the left oblique diameter.

Right Occiput Anterior Position. In right positions, the blades are introduced similarly but in opposite directions, for in those cases the right ear of the fetus is the posterior ear, over which the first blade must be placed accordingly. After the blades have been applied to the sides of the head, the left handle and shank lie above the right. Consequently, the forceps do not immediately articulate. Locking of the branches is easily effected, however, by rotating the left around the right to bring the lock into proper position.

Occiput Transverse Positions. If the occiput is in a transverse position, the forceps are introduced similarly, with the first blade applied over the posterior ear and the second rotated anteriorly to a position opposite the first. In this case, one blade lies in front of the sacrum and the other behind the symphysis. The conventional Simpson or Tucker–McLane forceps (Figs. 24–1 and 24–2) or the specialized Kielland forceps (Fig. 24–3) may be used.

Rotation from Anterior and Transverse Positions. When the occiput is obliquely anterior, it gradually rotates spontaneously to the symphysis pubis as traction is exerted. When it is directly transverse, however, in order to bring it anteriorly a rotary motion of the forceps is required. The direction of rotation, of course, varies with the position of the occiput. Rotation counterclockwise from the left side toward the midline is required when the occiput is directed toward the left, and in the reverse direction when it is directed toward the right side of the pelvis. Infrequently, particularly when forceps are used in transverse positions in anteroposteriorly flattened (platypelloid) pelves, rotation should not

be attempted until the fetal head has reached or approached the pelvic floor. Premature attempts at anterior rotation under such conditions may result in injury to the fetus and maternal soft parts. Regardless of the original position of the head, delivery is eventually effected by exerting traction downward until the occiput appears at the vulva; the rest of the operation is completed as described.

In exerting traction before the head appears at the vulva, one or both hands may be employed. To avoid excessive force, the operator should sit with arms flexed and elbows held closely against the thorax, because the operator's body weight must not be applied.

Occiput Posterior Positions

As discussed previously, persistent occiput posterior position is more likely if epidural analgesia has been used for labor.

Obliquely Posterior Positions. Prompt delivery may at times become necessary when the small (occipital) fontanel is directed toward one of the sacroiliac synchondroses, namely, in right occiput posterior and left occiput posterior positions. When delivery is required in either instance, the head is often imperfectly flexed. In some cases, when the hand is introduced into the vagina to locate the posterior ear, the occiput rotates spontaneously toward the anterior, indicating that manual rotation of the fetal head might easily be accomplished.

Manual Rotation from Posterior Positions. The requirements for forceps must be met. A hand with the palm upward is inserted into the vagina and the fingers are brought in contact with the side of the fetal head that is to be pushed toward the anterior position, while the thumb is placed over the opposite side of the head (Fig. 24–16). With the occiput in a right anterior position, the left hand is used to rotate the occiput anteriorly in a clockwise direction; the right hand is used for the left occiput posterior position. At the beginning of the rotation, it may be helpful to dislodge the head *slightly* upward in the birth canal, but the head must not be disengaged. After the occiput has reached the anterior position, labor may be allowed to continue, or more commonly, forceps can be used to effect delivery. First one blade is applied to that side of the head that is held by the fingers to help maintain the occiput in the anterior position. The other blade is immediately applied and delivery accomplished as described for occiput anterior forceps delivery.

Forceps Delivery as Occiput Posterior. If manual rotation cannot be easily accomplished, application of the blades to the head in the posterior position and

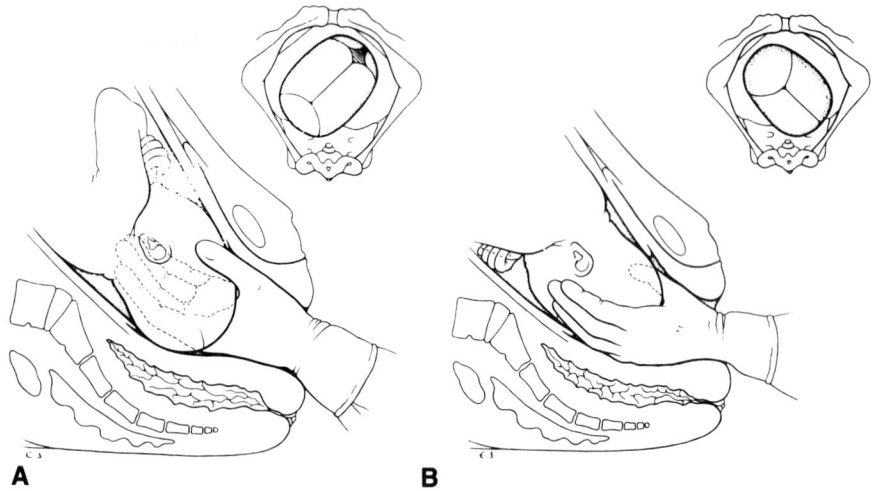

Fig. 24–16. A. Manual rotation, left hand in position grasping the head. **B.** Manual rotation accomplished to ROA. Note that with rotation to the ROA position the fetal head may become more flexed. (From Douglas and Stromme, 1976.)

delivery from the occiput posterior position may be the safest procedure (Fig. 24–17). In many cases, the cause of the persistent occiput posterior position and of the difficulty in accomplishing rotation is an anthropoid pelvis, the architecture of which predisposes to posterior delivery and opposes rotation. When the occiput is directly posterior, horizontal traction should be applied until the base of the nose is under the symphysis. The handles should then be slowly elevated until the occiput gradually emerges over the anterior margin of the perineum. Then, by imparting a downward motion to the instrument, the nose, face, and chin successively emerge

from the vulva. The extraction is more difficult than when the occiput is anterior, and because of greater distention of the vulva, a larger episiotomy may be needed. This may be accomplished with either a midline or mediolateral technique.

Forceps Rotations from Posterior Positions. Forceps rotations should be performed under the guidance of those who are experienced in these operations. Tucker–McLane, Simpson, or Kielland forceps may be used to try to rotate the fetal head. The oblique occiput may be rotated 45 degrees to the posterior position or

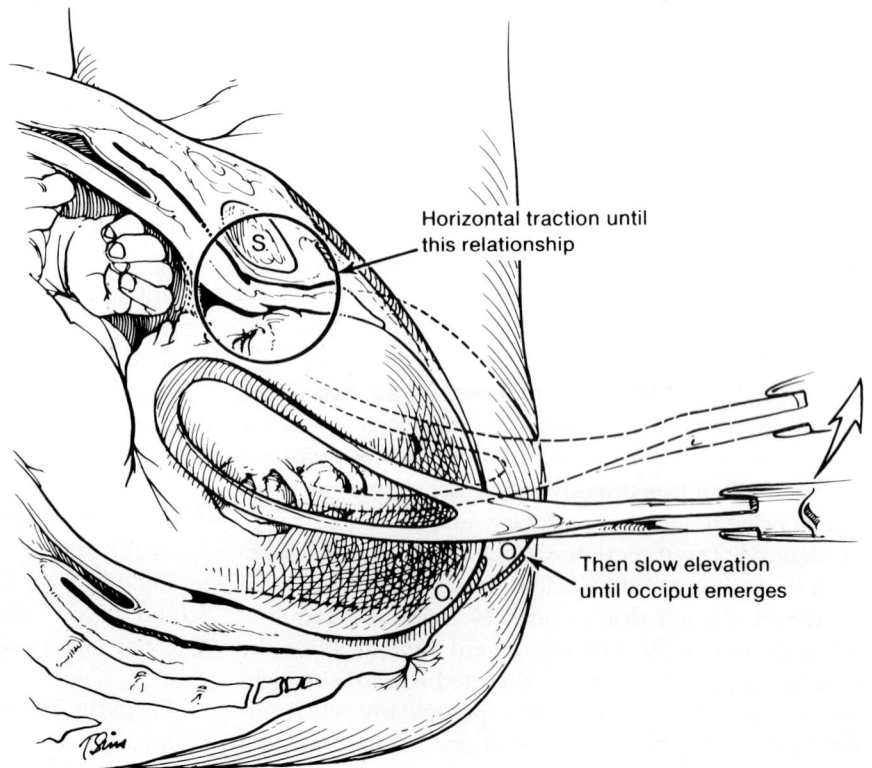

Fig. 24–17. Occiput directly posterior. Low forceps (Simpson) delivery as an occiput posterior. (O = occiput; S = symphysis). The *arrow* illustrates the point at which time the head should be flexed after the bregma passes under the symphysis. It is evident that to prevent serious perineal lacerations an extensive episiotomy is most often required.

Horizontal traction until this relationship

Then slow elevation until occiput emerges

135 degrees to the anterior (Fig. 24–18). If rotation is performed with Tucker–McLane or Simpson forceps, the head must be flexed, but this is not necessary with Kielland forceps because they have a more straightened pelvic curve. In rotating the occiput anteriorly with forceps, the pelvic curvature, originally directed upward, at the completion of rotation is inverted and directed posteriorly. Attempted delivery with the instrument in that position is likely to cause serious injury to maternal soft parts. To avoid such trauma, it is essential to remove and reapply the instrument as described below.

Special Forceps Maneuvers

Scanzoni–Smellie Maneuver. The double application of forceps, which was first described by Smellie (1752) and about a century later by Scanzoni (1853), has produced satisfactory results in some hands, although it is rarely necessary. Because the right posterior variety is much more frequent, the steps of the operation in that case are detailed.

In the first application, the blades of the forceps are applied to the sides of the head with the pelvic curve toward the face of the fetus, whereas in the second application the pelvic curve is directed toward the occiput. For the first application, the right hand is passed into the vagina posteriorly and the rear ear is located. The left blade is applied over the ear and held in position by an assistant, while the operator's left hand is passed into the right side of the vagina to control the introduction of the right blade, which is then rotated anteriorly until it lies over the left ear and opposite the first blade. The forceps are then locked and the handles elevated to flex the fetal head. Rotation may be facilitated by dislodging the fetal head very slightly upward. *The head must not be disengaged from the pelvis.* To compensate for the pelvic curvature in Tucker–McLane or Simpson forceps, the forceps handles are gently rotated clockwise through an arc that extends well lateral to the circumference of the birth canal (Fig. 24–18). This serves to rotate the fetal head about the occipitomental diameter. With an appropriate initial forceps application, it is often possible to rotate the head completely to the occiput anterior position without undue force.

Once the occiput is rotated anteriorly, it is necessary to remove and reapply the forceps as described for an occiput anterior delivery. The forceps are unlocked and the branch now on the left side of the pelvis (right branch) is removed by gently pulling the handle simultaneously downward and inward. During this maneuver, the other branch is held in position anteriorly by an assistant to help stabilize the occiput in an anterior position. The right branch is now inserted immediately after the remaining branch has been removed. During this time, the occiput typically will rotate back to a right occiput anterior position. After reapplication, some difficulty may arise in proper articulation, because the handle of the left branch lying above the right cannot be locked, but this can be readily overcome by rotating the handle of the left branch around the right to bring the lock into proper position. In left occiput posterior position, the blades are applied similarly but in the reverse order.

Rotation with Kielland Forceps. **Before attempts are made to perform any forceps operations, but especially with midforceps rotations, the station of the fetal head must be accurately ascertained to be at, or preferably below, the level of the ischial spines.** Too often in these cases there has been extreme molding of the fetal head, and the caput succedaneum has descended to below the ischial spines, giving the erroneous impression that the head is engaged when actually the occiput is above the spines. **Forceps application under these circumstances is classified as high and is never to be attempted under any circumstances.**

Kielland (1916) described forceps with narrow, somewhat bayonet-shaped blades that he claimed could be applied readily to the sides of the head in the occiput transverse position and surpassed all other models as a rotator (Fig. 24–3). He emphasized that his forceps were particularly useful when the station of the fetal head was high and when the sagittal suture was directed transversely. Kielland forceps have almost no pelvic curve, but they do have a sliding lock and are very light. On each handle is a small knob that indicates the direction of rotation.

There are two methods of applying the anterior blade of the Kielland forceps. In the first, the anterior blade is introduced first with its cephalic curve directed upward; after it has entered sufficiently far into the uterine cavity, it is turned through 180 degrees to adapt the cephalic curvature to the head. Kielland advised a safer **wandering** or **gliding** method of application for the anterior blade when the uterus is tightly contracted about the head and the lower uterine segment is stretched and thin. In the wandering or gliding method, the anterior blade is introduced at the side of the pelvis

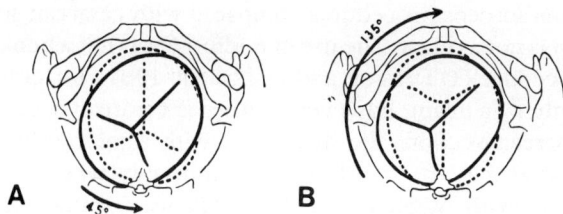

Fig. 24–18. Rotation of obliquely posterior occiput to sacrum (**A**) and symphysis pubis (**B**).

over the brow or face to an anterior position, with the handle of the blade held close to the opposite maternal buttock throughout the maneuver. The second blade is introduced posteriorly and the branches are locked. Because most cases amenable to Kielland forceps rotation are those in which there is deep transverse arrest (the fetal head is deep in the pelvis with the occiput well below the level of the ischial spines), rotation usually is accomplished by unwedging the fetal head from the pelvis by a small amount of upward pressure. From this slightly higher station, the rotation is accomplished. **The head should not be pushed high enough to allow disengagement because the cord may prolapse.**

Rubin and Coopland (1970) summarized the experiences with Kielland forceps rotation at Winnipeg General Hospital. Of the 1000 consecutive cases surveyed, almost exactly one half were occiput posterior and the remainder were occiput transverse. Rotation was accomplished successfully in 970. The same forceps were nearly always used for delivery, followed by reapplication when necessary. There were 8 perinatal deaths, including 4 with serious anomalies. Injuries to the infant were considered mostly minor for those contemporaneous times; however, there were 27 injuries that would not be considered minor today, including 7 infants with a fractured skull!

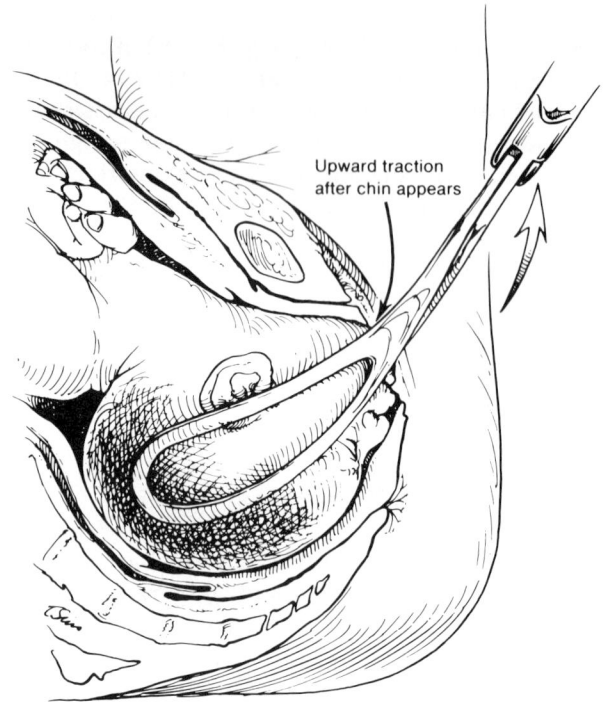

Fig. 24–19. Face presentation, mentum (chin) anterior. Delivery with low forceps (Simpson).

Forceps for Face Presentations

In the face presentation, with the chin directed toward the symphysis, the application of forceps is occasionally used to effect vaginal delivery. The blades are applied to the sides of the head along the occipitomental diameter, with the pelvic curve directed toward the neck. Downward traction is exerted until the chin appears under the symphysis. Then, by an upward movement, the face is slowly extracted, the nose, eyes, brow, and occiput appearing in succession over the anterior margin of the perineum (Fig. 24–19). Forceps should not be applied to the *mentum posterior presentation,* because vaginal delivery is impossible as such.

Morbidity from Forceps Operations

Maternal Morbidity. With any forceps application, and especially those that do not meet the criteria for outlet forceps and those in which rotations are done, serious trauma may result to both fetus and mother unless considerable care is exercised. In their review of midforceps delivery, Richardson and co-workers (1983) proposed three prerequisites for the use of midforceps: (1) midforceps must rationally be needed as an alternate method of delivery to cesarean section; (2) midforceps must be proven to be associated with a lower maternal morbidity rate than cesarean section; and (3)

midforceps should not result in fetal harm. With the revised classification of forceps by the American College of Obstetricians and Gynecologists (1988), the same three prerequisites might be proposed now for the use of *low forceps.*

There seems to be little question that the cesarean section rate has continued to rise in this country, with rates approaching 25 percent or higher in some hospitals (Chap. 26, p. 591). One of the major reasons for this increased rate of cesarean delivery is the generally held belief that it provides a safer route of delivery for the fetus than does operative vaginal delivery. Unfortunately, there is little scientific data to date to uniformly support this. With respect to the first requirement proposed by Richardson and associates (1983), there appears to be little doubt that there is a need for such a method in cases with a worrisome fetal heart rate pattern, maternal exhaustion, prolapsed umbilical cord, and cases of secondary labor arrest due to conduction analgesia.

The issue of maternal morbidity following the use of midforceps procedures compared with cesarean section is not as clear. The use of midforceps is not a benign procedure (O'Driscoll and associates, 1981) for either mother or infant; however, neither is cesarean section. Cesarean sections are associated with significantly increased maternal morbidity and mortality when compared with vaginal deliveries. Likewise, midforceps deliveries are associated with a higher incidence of maternal morbidity, usually assessed by lacerations and increased blood loss, when compared with women delivered by low or outlet forceps (Dierker and associates, 1985; Gilstrap and colleagues, 1984). Obviously the frequency and type of maternal morbidity will depend somewhat on classification of forceps utilized.

In a recent study by Bashore and associates (1990), they documented febrile morbidity in 25 percent of women following cesarean section compared with only 4 percent following midforceps deliveries. Moreover, the only cases of deep venous thrombosis and pulmonary embolus occurred in the cesarean section group. While 21 percent of women delivered by cesarean section had uterine incision extensions, 18 percent of those delivered by midforceps had cervical or vaginal lacerations, and 15 percent had third-degree and 12 percent fourth-degree extensions. Robertson and colleagues (1990), utilizing the 1988 forceps classification, reported maternal morbidity in 57 percent of women undergoing cesarean section compared with 25 percent of those delivered by midforceps. The maternal morbidity for low forceps was 33 percent compared with 70 percent for cesarean section of similar station and duration of second stage.

Thus, it must be concluded that low forceps and midforceps procedures carry less morbidity for the mother than does cesarean section. The same may not necessarily be true for the fetus.

Perinatal Morbidity. Forceps operations, especially those performed from the midpelvic level, have been reported associated with both short-term as well as long-term morbidity for the neonate. The immediate consequences of midforceps rotations have been reviewed by several investigators whose reports included control series. Chiswick and James (1979) reviewed neonatal morbidity and mortality following vaginal delivery with Kielland forceps compared with a matched group of babies born spontaneously. Birth trauma was evident in 15 percent of infants delivered with forceps. Neonatal mortality, most often from tentorial tears, occurred in 3 (3.5 percent) of 86 babies delivered with forceps and 2 of these were in babies delivered by emergency cesarean section after attempts at instrumental delivery. Factors significantly associated with the use of Kielland forceps were nulliparity, short maternal stature, induction of labor, late engagement of the fetal head, slow dilatation of the cervix, and epidural analgesia during labor.

Hughey and colleagues (1978) compared 458 midforceps operations with 17 cesarean section deliveries. The women delivered by cesarean section were selected when the cervix was completely dilated and the occiput failed to rotate to the anterior position from transverse or posterior position. Using a *perinatal morbidity index,* an unfavorable result of 30 percent was reported for the fetuses delivered by midforceps versus a zero percent morbidity with cesarean section. Bowes and

Bowes (1980) compared the fetal outcome in midforceps deliveries with fetal outcome in women delivered by cesarean section or vacuum extraction. Morbid events were identified in 14 of 71 midforceps deliveries (20 percent) compared with 2 morbid events in the 37 cesarean sections (5 percent) and 3 instances of fetal trauma in 15 vacuum extractions (20 percent).

There are several factors that must be taken into consideration when attempting to interpret the results of these studies. First and foremost, these studies were conducted prior to the redefined classification of forceps in 1988; thus, midforceps were not defined as clearly and included deliveries from relatively high stations (0 to +1) as well as difficult rotations. Secondly, spontaneous vaginal deliveries are not appropriate controls for midforceps as in the study by Chiswick and James (1979). Finally, as emphasized by Richardson and colleagues (1983), there is no uniformity in the criteria utilized to define immediate fetal morbidity.

Gilstrap and colleagues (1984) retrospectively compared immediate maternal and neonatal outcomes of 234 women delivered by midforceps with those of women delivered spontaneously, by outlet forceps, or by cesarean section. Importantly, forceps were not applied unless the fetal head was *below* zero station, or had descended to lower than +1 station (of 3 stations) in the case of transverse arrest. Almost 60 percent of women delivered by midforceps had epidural analgesia. These investigators assessed neonatal acid-base status by measuring cord blood pH, and found no difference in the incidence of neonatal acidosis between the groups when indications for delivery were matched. Likewise, they found no excessive trauma to fetuses delivered by midforceps.

Dierker and associates (1985) provided a retrospective review of 176 midforceps deliveries at Cleveland Metropolitan General Hospital from 1976 through 1982, and compared these with all other deliveries during the study period. Epidural analgesia was associated with slightly more than half of the midforceps deliveries. Although cephalohematomas were identified more commonly in neonates delivered by midforceps (7 percent), they found no increased incidence of low Apgar scores, seizures, shoulder dystocia, and brachial or facial nerve palsy when these infants were compared with the general obstetrical population. Conversely, Falco and Eriksson (1990) described 92 cases of seventh nerve palsy in over 44,000 newborns delivered from 1982 to 1987 at Brigham and Women's Hospital. Of these 92, 81 were acquired, and 74 (91 percent) of the 81 were associated with forceps delivery.

In the report by Bashore and associates (1990) cited above, these authors compared neonatal outcome in 358 midforceps deliveries with that of 486 infants delivered by cesarean section. They found no increase in significant neonatal morbidity in the forceps group, although 4 newborns had transient facial palsy. Conversely, Robertson and associates (1990) used the 1988 classification of forceps and reported significantly higher neonatal morbidity in the midforceps group compared with infants delivered by cesarean section. In this study, midforceps deliveries included those done at stations above +2 cm.

In a recent prospective study of 357 forceps deliveries classified by both the old and new systems, Hagadorn-Freathy and colleagues (1991) reported that neonatal morbidity was effectively stratified using the 1988 classification. For example, facial nerve palsy developed in 1.3 percent of infants delivered by outlet forceps and 3.2 percent of those delivered by midforceps using the 1965 classification. This compared favorably with 0.9 percent for outlet forceps, 1.7 percent for low forceps, and 9.2 percent for midforceps using the 1988 classification. Thus, the new classification of midforceps identifies a high-risk group for this complication.

Long-term Infant Morbidity. There has been significant controversy regarding possible associations of midforceps delivery with long-term morbidity for the newborn. Although some (Chefetz, 1965; Eastman and colleagues, 1962) have reported an increased frequency of cerebral palsy in association with the use of midforceps, others (Amiel-Tison, 1969; Steer and Boney, 1962) have not found such an association.

There is little question that of all the aspects of forceps use, none has engendered more controversy than the possible association with a decrease in the intelligence quotient (IQ) in the newborn. Unfortunately, the issue of intelligence following midforceps delivery is unsettled, but it is likely to remain so because of the multitude of variables affecting intelligence. Some of these, for example, include gender, mother's education, race, and socioeconomic status. Broman and co-workers (1975), controlling for socioeconomic status, race, and gender, but *not* for fetal weight, reported that infants delivered by midforceps had slightly higher intelligence scores at 4 years of age than children delivered spontaneously. There were no significant differences among the scores by type of delivery. Nilsen (1984) evaluated 18-year-old men drafted into the Norwegian Army and reported that those delivered by Kielland forceps had higher intelligence scores than those delivered spontaneously, by vacuum extraction, or by cesarean section.

The results published by Friedman and associates (1977, 1984) are in contrast to those reported by Broman and colleagues, and these have been the most controversial because data from the Collaborative Perinatal Project were used by both groups of investigators. In their second report, Friedman and co-workers (1984) described intelligence assessments at least up to 7 years of age, and concluded that those children who had been delivered by midforceps had lower mean IQs compared with children who were delivered by outlet forceps.

Dierker and colleagues (1986) assessed the long-term outcome of children delivered by midforceps in the study cited above and compared them with children who had been delivered by cesarean section performed for dystocia. These children were assessed at a minimum of 2 years of age, and the investigators found no increased morbidity associated with delivery by midforceps.

Seidman and colleagues (1991) studied over 52,000 persons who were examined by the Israeli Defense Forces draft board at age 17. They had been born between 1964 and 1972 in four West Jerusalem hospitals. Intelligence test scores were available through 1969, and data from these 32,425 deliveries are shown in Table 24–3. There was only one very small but statistically significant difference in intelligence test scores when persons delivered by cesarean section were compared with those born by spontaneous vaginal delivery. It is important to note that these data included all forceps deliveries, and the investigators concluded that midforceps use was probably limited because the incidence of vacuum extraction was double that for all forceps deliveries.

In a recent collaborative study of school-age children, Wesley and colleagues (1992) found no significant difference in standardized intelligent scores according to the method of delivery. There were 1746 children who were delivered spontaneously compared with 1351 children who had been delivered by either low or midforceps operations.

Conclusions Regarding Morbidity from Midforceps. There can be no doubt that midforceps delivery performed inappropriately, especially by an unsupervised inexperienced operator, can result in considerable adverse maternal as well as fetal effects. Studies in which these morbid events were reported to be increased substantively were done earlier and at times when cesarean section rates were still around 5 percent. Moreover,

TABLE 24–3. INTELLIGENCE TEST SCORES AT AGE 17 FOR SUBJECTS BORN IN JERUSALEM BETWEEN 1964 AND 1970

| Type of Delivery | Mean Intelligence Score (± SE) | |
	Unadjusted	Adjusted[a]
Spontaneous (n = 29,136)	105.4 (0.1)	105.7 (0.1)
Forceps (n = 567)	108.2[b] (0.7)	104.6 (0.4)
Vacuum extraction (n = 1207)	109.6[b] (0.5)	105.9 (0.4)
Cesarean section (n = 1335)	105.4 (0.4)	103.7[b] (0.1)

SE denotes standard error.
[a] Adjusted by multiple regression for confounding effects of sex, birthweight, ethnic origin, birth order, maternal age, and paternal and maternal education and social class.
[b] P < .0001 compared with spontaneous delivery.
From Seidman and associates (1991), with permission.

many of these earlier studies undoubtedly included forceps applications that would, in all likelihood, never be attempted today. By contrast, in two of the more recent studies, the authors appropriately emphasize that all (Gilstrap and colleagues, 1984) or the majority (Dierker and associates, 1986) of midforceps deliveries were done with the fetal vertex at +1 (of three stations) or lower station. It is unlikely that midforceps deliveries included in the Collaborative Perinatal Project during the 1960s were this conservative. Finally, the impact of the popular use of epidural analgesia on the incidence of low and midforceps deliveries cannot be discounted. The majority of such cases result from inadequate maternal expulsive forces against a relaxed pelvic sling, and thus they are not usually associated with true dystocia. Although it is prudent in these cases to allow a longer second stage of labor, in some women delivery is indicated. Low forceps rotations (formerly called midforceps) in such circumstances are likely to be safer than in women with prolonged labors and midpelvic arrest unassociated with conduction analgesia.

It seems reasonable to conclude that low forceps operations, classified according to the 1988 scheme, can be performed with safety for the mother and fetus if the basic guidelines set forth in this chapter are carefully observed. As previously described, the recent definition of low forceps corresponds very closely to the old definition of low midforceps. The operator must be experienced, and in general, forceps rotations or deliveries from zero station should be avoided. If the fetal head is at a lower station in the pelvis, then forceps may be used safely for those indications previously elucidated. In this scheme, *difficult* midforceps deliveries, especially those classified by the 1988 guidelines, are avoided, along with their adverse outcomes.

Trial Forceps and Failed Forceps. In *trial forceps,* the operator attempts low or midforceps delivery with the full knowledge that a certain degree of disproportion at the midpelvis may make the procedure incompatible with safety for the fetus. With an operating room both equipped and staffed for immediate cesarean section, and after a good forceps application has been achieved, firm downward pulls are made on the instrument. If there is no descent, the procedure is abandoned and cesarean section is performed. In a study of 122 women who had a trial of midcavity forceps or vacuum extraction in a setting with full preparations to proceed to cesarean section, Lowe (1987) found no significant difference in immediate neonatal or maternal morbidity compared with 42 women delivered for similar indications by cesarean section without such a trial of instrumentation. Conversely, neonatal morbidity was higher in 61 women who had "unexpected" forceps or vacuum failure in which there was no prior preparation for immediate cesarean section.

The term *failed forceps* usually is applied when a

forceps delivery was anticipated and a vigorous but unsuccessful attempt was made to deliver with forceps. The three fundamental factors responsible for such a failure are disproportion, incomplete cervical dilatation, and malposition of the fetal head. Some, but not all such cases stem from inexperience and ignorance of obstetrical fundamentals, and these cases are becoming less frequent. We certainly agree with Dennen (1989), especially when considering the present medicolegal climate in this country, that the term *failed forceps* should be discarded in favor of *trial forceps.*

While the term *failed forceps* frequently carries a pejorative connotation, it may also be used to describe abandonment of carefully planned *trial forceps.* Boyd and colleagues (1986) described 53 cases of failed forceps among 6524 nulliparas. By their definition, failed forceps included those cases in which there was difficulty with forceps application, and thus did not include any traction efforts. Over 75 percent of these nulliparous women had been given epidural analgesia for labor, and the incidence of midforceps was almost 20 percent, of which 4 percent were classified as failed forceps. They documented more adverse outcomes whenever any operative delivery was performed, but found no differences in outcomes of infants delivered successfully by midforceps when compared with those delivered by cesarean section following failed forceps or failure to progress in the second stage of labor.

Thus, as Lowe (1987) concluded, "a carefully conducted trial of instrumental delivery is an acceptable alternative to cesarean section for delay in the second stage due to a potentially difficult midcavity arrest." This includes performing such procedures in a setting in which preparations have been made for immediate cesarean section. Rather than using the term failed forceps, it seems preferable to instead place a detailed narrative report in the hospital record—which is better if typewritten—describing the indications for the attempted midforceps and the events that followed.

VACUUM EXTRACTOR

Simpson introduced the idea of vacuum extraction in the 1840s, and there have been numerous attempts since to attach a traction device by suction to the fetal scalp. In the United States, the device is referred to as the vacuum extractor, while commonly in Europe it is referred to as a **ventouse** (from French, literally, soft cup). The theoretical advantages of the vacuum extractor over forceps include the avoidance of insertion of space-occupying steel blades within the vagina and their positioning precisely over the fetal head, as is required for safe forceps delivery; the ability to rotate the fetal head without impinging upon maternal soft tissues; and less intracranial pressure during traction. All previously described instruments were unsuccessful until Malmström (1954) applied a new principle, namely, traction on a metal cap so designed that the suction creates an artificial caput, or *chignon*, within the cup that holds firmly and allows adequate traction.

Because of the reports of fetal damage—such as lacerations and abrasions of the scalp, cephalohematomas, intracranial hemorrhage, and infant death—the enthusiasm for vacuum utilizing a metal cup has waned. Certainly, in the United Sates, as well as other countries, the metal cup generally has been replaced by newer soft cup vacuum extractors. However, as emphasized by Duchon and associates (1988), high-pressure vacuum generates large amounts of force regardless of the cup used. The silastic cup vacuum device is a reusable instrument with a soft, 65 mm diameter cup. The Mityvac instrument utilizes a disposable 60 mm diameter cup (Fig. 24–20), and the CMI Tender Touch utilizes a 62 mm cup (Fig. 24–21). Little scientific evidence currently exists suggesting that any one of these new instruments is safer or more efficacious than the others.

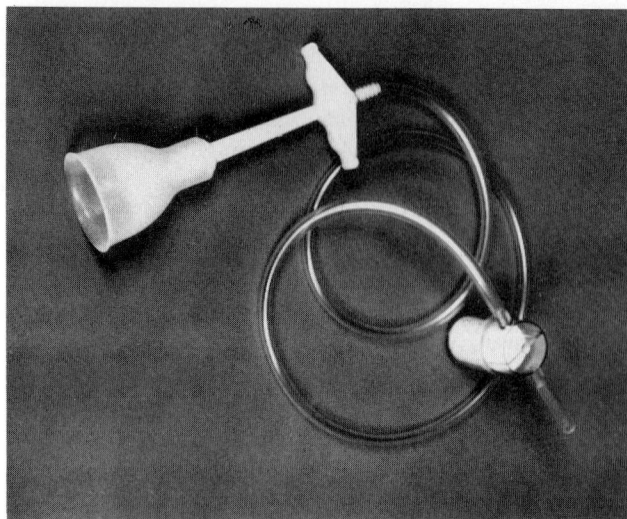

Fig. 24–21. CMI Tender Touch extractor cup. (Photograph reproduced with permission of Columbia Medical & Surgical, Inc, Bend, OR.)

INDICATIONS AND PREREQUISITES FOR VACUUM EXTRACTION

Generally, the indications and prerequisites for the use of the vacuum extractor for delivery are the same as for forceps delivery. The tendency to attempt vacuum deliveries at stations higher than usually attempted with forceps is worrisome. Broekhuizen and colleagues (1987) reported that 3.5 percent of vacuum deliveries were performed with the vertex above zero station, and another 20 percent were at zero station. If the vacuum instrument is to be used, the same indications for its use

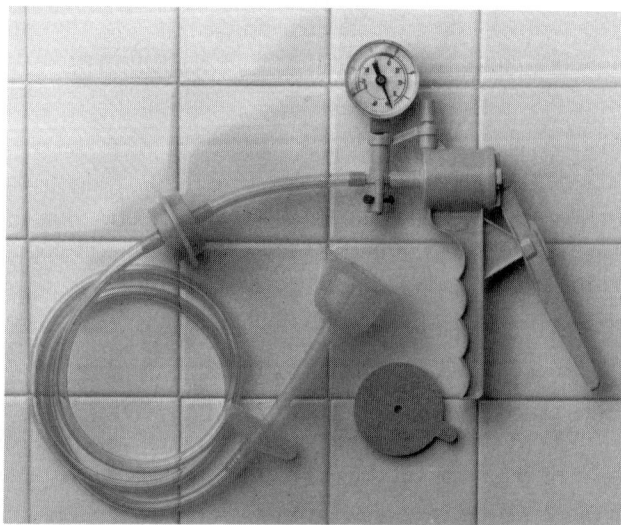

Fig. 24–20. Mityvac obstetrical vacuum delivery system includes extractor cup and pump. (Photograph reproduced with permission of Neward Enterprises, Inc, Rancho Cucamonga, CA.)

should be carefully applied as for any forceps delivery.

Relative contraindications for delivery using vacuum extraction include face or other nonvertex presentations, extreme prematurity, fetal coagulopathies, macrosomia, and following scalp blood sampling. Complications include scalp lacerations and bruising, cephalohematomas, intracranial hemorrhage, neonatal jaundice, subconjunctival hemorrhage, a higher incidence of shoulder dystocia, Erb palsy, retinal hemorrhage, and fetal death (Baerthelein, 1986; Berkus, 1985; Broekhuizen, 1987; Dell, 1985; McFarland, 1986; Meyer, 1987; Vacca, 1983, and their many colleagues). These complications appear to be higher with the metal cup instruments compared with the soft cup devices. For example, in a review by Plauche (1979) of the Malmström vacuum extractor, scalp injury ranged from 0.8 to 33 percent, cephalohematomas from 1 to 26 percent, and subgaleal hemorrhage from 0 to 10 percent. Berkus and associates (1985), on the other hand, found no increase in serious neonatal morbidity, including retinal hemorrhage, for the silastic vacuum extractor compared with spontaneous delivery.

COMPARISON OF VACUUM EXTRACTION WITH FORCEPS

There have been numerous studies comparing vacuum extraction with forceps deliveries. Vacca and associates (1983) conducted a randomized, prospective study comparing metal cup vacuum extraction to forceps delivery. They reported a higher frequency of maternal trauma and blood loss in the forceps group, but an increase in the incidence of neonatal jaundice in the vacuum group. There was no difference in serious neonatal morbidity between the groups. Berkus and colleagues (1985) in a prospective but nonrandomized study of the silastic vacuum cup compared with forceps, reported less maternal trauma with the vacuum and no significant difference in neonatal morbidity. Others have found decreased maternal trauma and similar neonatal morbidity in babies delivered by vacuum compared with forceps (Baerthlein and colleagues, 1986; Broekhuizen and co-workers, 1987; Dell and associates, 1985).

Unfortunately, published data are sparse regarding long-term neurological outcome in newborns delivered via vacuum extraction. In the report of an 18-year follow-up by Nilsen (1984), the mean intelligence score of 38 male infants delivered by vacuum was not different from the national average, although males delivered by rotational midforceps actually had significantly higher intelligence scores.

Conclusions Regarding Morbidity from Vacuum Extractors

It seems reasonable to conclude that delivery with the new soft cup vacuum extractors results in less maternal trauma and blood loss than forceps. It also appears that use of these new vacuum devices is not associated with an increase in serious neonatal morbidity when compared with forceps, although there is an increase in the frequency of cephalohematomas and retinal hemorrhage with the use of these instruments. Finally, considering that the indications and prerequisites for forceps and vacuum are the same, the choice of instruments must be based primarily on the experience of the operator. Neither instrument should be applied prior to the engagement of the fetal head.

Glossary

Dührssen (Cervical) Incisions

When immediate delivery is desirable before the cervix is fully dilated, multiple radial incisions may be made in the cervix and repaired immediately after delivery. These incisions are usually called Dührssen incisions, after the German obstetrician who described them in 1890. Although the complications may be formidable, the technique of the operation is simple: Three incisions, corresponding approximately to 2, 6, and 10 o'clock positions are made with scissors. Delivery is then effected by forceps or breech extraction, depending on the presentation. The operation should never be done unless the cervix is fully effaced and more than 7 cm dilated, lest profuse or even fatal hemorrhage result. The procedure is, of course, contraindicated in pla-

centa previa. Most obstetricians now consider the operation obsolete. It is included here only because of the rare possibility of its use in the presence of an ominous fetal heart rate pattern when the head of a fetus presenting as breech is trapped by the cervix deep in the pelvis and the cervix is almost fully dilated.

Symphysiotomy and Pubiotomy

Symphysiotomy is the division of the pubic symphysis with a wire saw or knife to effect an increase in the capacity of a contracted pelvis sufficient to permit passage of a living child. In pubiotomy, the pubis is severed a few centimeters lateral to the symphysis. Because of interference with subsequent locomotion, bladder injuries, and hemorrhage, and because of the greater safety of cesarean section, these two operations have been abandoned in the United States. Symphysiotomy is still performed in some third world countries, especially when it may be impossible to follow a patient in a subsequent pregnancy. Because, in these circumstances, a woman delivered by cesarean section for a mildly contracted pelvis might well die with a ruptured uterus in her next pregnancy, symphysiotomy may be indicated in such a case in an attempt to produce sufficient enlargement of the pelvis to allow vaginal delivery. Hartfield (1973) described a technique for subcutaneous symphysiotomy and summarized his experiences.

History of Forceps

Crude forceps are an ancient invention, several varieties having been described by Albucasis, who died in 1112. Because their inner surfaces were provided with teeth to penetrate the head, however, it appears that they were intended for use only on dead fetuses.

The true obstetrical forceps were devised in the latter part of the 16th century or the beginning of the 17th century by a member of the Chamberlain family. The invention was not made public at the time, but was preserved as a family secret through four generations, not becoming generally known until the early part of the 18th century. Previously, version had been the only method that permitted operative delivery of an unmutilated child. When that operation was impossible, imperative delivery was accomplished with hooks and crochets, which usually led to the destruction of the child. Thus, before the invention of forceps, the use of instruments was synonymous with the death of the child, and frequently of the mother as well.

William Chamberlain, a French physician who fled from France as a Huguenot refugee, landed at Southhampton in 1569. He died in 1596, leaving a large family. Two of his sons, both of whom were named Peter, and designated the elder and younger, studied medicine and settled in London. They soon became successful practitioners, devoting a large part of their attention to midwifery, in which they became very proficient. They attempted to control the instruction of midwives and, to justify their pretensions, claimed that they could successfully deliver women when all others failed.

The young Peter died in 1626 and the elder in 1631. The elder left no male children, but the younger was survived by several sons, one of whom, born in 1601, was likewise named Peter. To distinguish him from his father and uncle, he is usually spoken of as Dr. Peter, because the other two did not possess that title. He was well educated, having studied at Cambridge, Heidelberg, and Padua, and on his return to London was elected a Fellow of the Royal College of Physicians. He was most successful in his profession and his patients included many members of the royal family and nobility. Like his father and uncle, he attempted to monopolize control of the midwives, but his pretensions were set aside by the authorities. These attempts gave rise to much discussion, and many pamphlets were written about the mortality of women in labor attended by men. He answered them in a pamphlet entitled "A Voice in Ramah, or the Cry of Women and Children as Echoed Forth in the Compassions of Peter Chamberlain." He was a man of considerable ability, combining some of the virtues of a religious enthusiast with many of the devious qualities of a quack. He died at Woodham Mortimer Hall, Moldon, Essex, in 1683, the place remaining in the possession of his family until well into the succeeding century. He was formerly considered the inventor of the forceps, a fact now known to be incorrect.

Dr. Peter Chamberlain left a very large family, and three of his sons, Hugh, Paul, and John, became physicians who devoted special attention to the practice of midwifery. Of them, (Hugh 1630–?) was the most important and influential. Like his father, he was a man of considerable ability who took a practical interest in politics. Because some of his views were out of favor, he was forced to leave England for Paris, where in 1673 he attempted to sell the family secret to Mauriceau for 10,000 lires, claiming that with forceps he could deliver in a very few minutes the most difficult case. Mauriceau placed at his disposal a rachitic dwarf whom he had been unable to deliver, and Chamberlain, after several futile hours of strenuous effort, was obliged to acknowledge his inability to do so. Notwithstanding his failure, he maintained his friendly relations with Mauriceau, whose book he translated into English. In his preface he refers to the forceps in the following words: "My father, brothers, and myself (though none else in Europe as I know) have by God's blessing and our own industry attained to and long practiced a way to deliver women in this case without prejudice to them or their infants."

Some years later he went to Holland and sold his secret to Roger Roonhuysen. Shortly afterward the Medical–Pharmaceutical College of Amsterdam was given the sole privilege of licensing physicians to practice in Holland, to each of whom, under the pledge of secrecy, was sold Chamberlain's invention

for a large sum. The practice continued for a number of years until Fischer and Van de Poll purchased and made public the secret, whereupon it was discovered that the device consisted of only one blade of the forceps. Whether that was all Chamberlain sold to Roonhuysen, or whether the Medical–Pharmaceutical College had swindled the purchasers, is not known.

Hugh Chamberlain left a considerable family, and one of his sons, Hugh (1664–1728), practiced medicine. He was a highly educated, respected, and philanthropic physician, whose patients included members of the best families in England. He was a close friend of the Duke of Buckingham, who had a statue erected in Chamberlain's honor in Westminster Abbey. During the later years of his life he allowed the family secret to leak out, and the instrument soon came into general use.

For more than 100 years, Dr. Peter Chamberlain was considered the inventor of the forceps, but in 1813 Mrs. Kemball, the mother of Mrs. Codd, who was the occupant of Woodham Mortimer Hall at the time, found in the garret a trunk containing numerous letters and instruments, among them four pairs of forceps together with several levers and fillets. The forceps were in different stages of development (Fig. 24–22), one pair hardly applicable to the living woman, although the others were useful instruments. Aveling (1882), who carefully investigated the matter, believes that the three pairs of available forceps were used, respectively, by the three Peters, and that in all probability the first was devised by the elder Peter, son of the original William. The forceps came into general use in England during the lifetime of Hugh Chamberlain, the younger. The instrument was employed by Drinkwater, who died in 1728, and was well known to Chapman and Giffard.

In 1723, Palfyn, a physician of Ghent, exhibited before the Paris Academy of Medicine a forceps he designated *mains de fer*. It was crudely shaped and impossible to articulate. In the discussion following its presentation, De la Motte stated that it would be

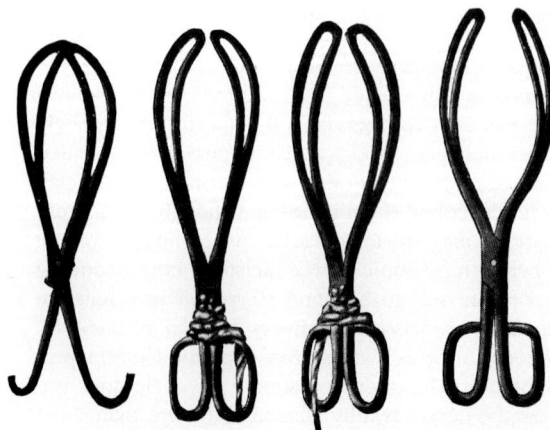

Fig. 24–22. Chamberlain forceps.

impossible to apply it to the living woman, and added that if by chance anyone should happen to invent an instrument that could be so used, and kept it secret for his own profit, he deserved to be exposed upon a barren rock and have his vitals plucked out by vultures. He had little knowledge that such an instrument had been in the possession of the Chamberlain family for nearly 100 years.

The Chamberlain forceps, a short, straight instrument with only a cephalic curve, is perpetuated in the short forceps of today. It was used, with but little modification, until the middle of the 18th century, when Levret, in 1747, and Smellie, in 1751, independently added the pelvic curve and increased the length of the instrument. Levret's forceps was longer, with a more decided pelvic curve than that of Smellie. From these two instruments, the long forceps of the present day are descended.

As soon as forceps became public property, they were subjected to various modifications. As early as 1798, Mulder's atlas included illustrations of nearly 100 varieties. The modifications attempted in improving the instrument are pictured in Witkowski's *Obstetrical Arsenal,* illustrating several hundred forceps but representing only a small fraction of those devised. The monograph of Das contains excellent historical sketches of the development of the instrument. It is remarkable, however, that little advance was made over the instruments of Levret and Smellie until Tarnier, in 1877, clearly enunciated the principle of axis traction. These forceps were designed to cope with very high stations of the fetal head and contracted pelves. Such problems today, however, are generally solved by other means. Episiotomy, furthermore, has eliminated many of the difficulties stemming from the pelvic curve, and severe traction at the fenestra, as in the axis-traction forceps, is therefore unnecessary and possibly undesirable.

Except for two specialized forceps, those of Barton and Kielland, very little that is both new and useful in modern obstetrics has been added to the development of the instrument in over 200 years.

References

American College of Obstetricians and Gynecologists, Committee on Obstetrics, Maternal and Fetal Medicine: Obstetric Forceps. No. 59, February 1988

American College of Obstetricians and Gynecologists: Operative vaginal delivery. Technical bulletin no. 152, February 1991

Amiel-Tison C: Cerebral damage in full-term newborns, etiological factors, neonatal status and long-term follow-up. Biol Neonatorum 14:234, 1969

Anderson GD, Bada HS, Sibai BM, Korone SB: Obstetrical factors related to progression of periventricular hemorrhage in the preterm newborn. Abstract 401, presented at the 35th annual meeting of the Society for Gynecologic Investigation, Baltimore, March 1988

Aveling JH: The Chamberlens and the Midwifery Forceps. London, Churchill, 1882

Baerthlein WC, Moodley S, Stinson SK: Comparison of maternal and neonatal morbidity in midforceps delivery and midpelvis vacuum extraction. Obstet Gynecol 67:594, 1986

Bashore RA, Phillips WH, Brankman CR III: A comparison of the morbidity of midforceps and cesarean delivery. Am J Obstet Gynecol 162:1428, 1990

Berkus MD, Ramamurthy RS, O'Connor PS, Brown K, Hayashi RH: Cohort study of silastic obstetric vacuum cup deliveries: I. Safety of the instrument. Obstet Gynecol 66:503, 1985

Bishop E, Israel L, Briscoe C: Obstetric influences on the premature infants' first year of development: A report from the Collaborative Study of Cerebral Palsy. Obstet Gynecol 26:628, 1965

Bowes WS, Bowes C: Current role of midforceps operations. Clin Obstet Gynecol 23:549, 1980

Boyd ME, Usher RH, McLean FH, Norman BE: Failed forceps. Obstet Gynecol 68:779, 1986

Broekhuizen FF, Washington JM, Johnson F, Hamilton PR: Vacuum extraction versus forceps delivery: Indications and complications, 1979 to 1984. Obstet Gynecol 69:338, 1987

Broman SH, Nichols PL, Kennedy WA: Preschool IQ: Prenatal and Early Developmental Correlates. Hillside, NJ, Erlbaum, 1975

Chefetz MD: Etiology of cerebral palsy: Role of reproductive insufficiency and the multiplicity of factors. Obstet Gynecol 25:635, 1965

Chiswick ML, James DK: Kielland's forceps: Association with neonatal morbidity and mortality. Br Med J 1:7, 1979

Cox SM, Bost JE, Faro S, Carpenter RJ: Epidural anesthesia during labor and the incidence of forceps delivery. Tex Med 83:45, 1987

DeLee JB: The prophylactic forceps operation. Am J Obstet Gynecol 1:34, 1920

Dell DL, Sightler SE, Plauche WC: Soft cup vacuum extraction: A comparison of outlet delivery. Obstet Gynecol 66:624, 1985

Dennen EH: A classification of forceps operations according to station of head in pelvis. Am J Obstet Gynecol 63:172, 1952

Dennen PC: Dennen's forceps deliveries, 3rd ed. Philadelphia, Davis, 1989

Dierker LJ, Rosen MG, Thompson K, Debanne S, Linn P: The midforceps: Maternal and neonatal outcomes. Am J Obstet Gynecol 152:176, 1985

Dierker LJ, Rosen MG, Thompson K, Lynn P: Midforceps deliveries: Long-term outcome of infants. Am J Obstet Gynecol 154:764, 1986

Douglas RB, Stromme WB: Operative Obstetrics, 3rd ed. New York, Appleton-Century-Crofts, 1976

Duchon MA, DeMund MA, Brown RH: Laboratory comparison of modern vacuum extractors. Obstet Gynecol 72:155, 1988

Dührssen A: On the value of deep cervical incisions and episiotomy in obstetrics. Arch Gynaekol 37:27, 1890

Eastman NJ, Kohl SG, Maisel JE, Kaveler F: The obstetrical background of 753 cases of cerebral palsy. Obstet Gynecol Surv 17:459, 1962

Fairweather D: Obstetric management and follow-up of the very low-birth-weight infant. J Reprod Med 26:387, 1981

Falco NA, Eriksson E: Facial nerve palsy in the newborn: Incidence and outcome. Plast Reconstr Surg 85:1, 1990

Friedman EA, Sachtleben MR, Bresky PA: Dysfunctional labor: XII. Long-term effects on the fetus. 127:779, 1977

Friedman EA, Sachtleben-Murray MR, Dahrouge D, Neff RK: Long-term effects of labor and delivery on offspring: A matched-pair analysis. Am J Obstet Gynecol 150:941, 1984

Gilstrap LC, Hauth JC, Schiano S, Connor KD: Neonatal acidosis and method of delivery. Obstet Gynecol 63:681, 1984

Haesslein H, Goodlin R: Survey of the tiny newborn. Am J Obstet Gynecol 134:192, 1979

Hagadorn-Freathy AS, Yeomans ER, Hankins GDV: Validation of the 1988 ACOG forceps classification system. Obstet Gynecol 77:356, 1991

Hartfield VJ: Subcutaneous symphysiotomy—Time for reappraisal? Aust NZ J Obstet Gynaecol 13:147, 1973

Healy DL, Laufe LE: Survey of forceps training in North American in 1981. Am J Obstet Gynecol 151:54, 1985

Hoult IJ, MacLennan AH, Carrier LES: Lumbar epidural analgesia in labour: Relation to fetal malposition and instrumental delivery. Br Med J 1:14, 1977

Hughey MJ, McElin JW, Lussky R: Forceps operation in perspective: I. Midforceps rotation operations. J Reprod Med 20:253, 1978

Joulin M: Study on the use of force in obstetrics. Arch Gen Med, 6th Series 9:149, 1867

Kaminski HM, Stafl A, Aiman J: The effect of epidural analgesia on the frequency of instrumental obstetric delivery. Obstet Gynecol 69:770, 1987

Kielland C: On the application of forceps to the unrotated head, with description of a new model of forceps. Monatsschrift fur Geburtshilfe und Gynkologie 43:48, 1916

Lowe B: Fear of failure: A place for the trial of instrumental delivery. Br J Obstet Gynaecol 94:60, 1987

Malmström T: The vacuum extractor, an obstetrical instrument. Acta Obstet Gynecol Scand 4(suppl):33, 1954

McFarland LV, Raskin M, Daling JR, Benedetti TJ: Erb/Duchenne's palsy: A consequence of fetal macrosomia and method of delivery. Obstet Gynecol 68:784, 1986

Meyer L, Mailloux J, Marcoux S, Blanchet P, Meyer F: Maternal and neonatal morbidity in instrumental deliveries with the Kobayashi vacuum extractor and low forceps. Acta Obstet Gynecol Scand 66:643, 1987

National Institutes of Health: Cesarean Childbirth. Bethesda, US Dept of Health and Human Services, pub. no. 82-2067, 1981

Nilsen ST: Boys born by forceps and vacuum extraction examined at 18 years of age. Acta Obstet Gynecol Scand 63:549, 1984

O'Driscoll K, Meagher D, MacDonald D, Geoghegan F: Traumatic intracranial hemorrhage in firstborn infants and delivery with obstetric forceps. Br J Obstet Gynaecol 88:577, 1981

Plauche WC: Fetal cranial injuries related to delivery with the Malmström vacuum extractor. Obstet Gynecol 53:750, 1979

Ramin S, Little B, Gilstrap L: Survey of operative vaginal delivery in North America in 1990. Abstract 578 presented at meeting of Society of Perinatal Obstetricians, Orlando, February 1992. Am J Obstet Gynecol 166:430, 1992

Richardson DA, Evans MI, Cibils LA: Midforceps delivery: A critical review. Am J Obstet Gynecol 145:621, 1983

Robertson PA, Laros RK, Zhao RL: Neonatal and maternal outcome in low-pelvic and mid-pelvic operative deliveries. Am J Obstet Gynecol 162:1436, 1990

Rubin L, Coopland AT: Kielland's forceps. Can Med Assoc J 103:505, 1970

Saunders NJSG, Spiby H, Gilbert L, Fraser RB, Hall JM, Mutton PM, Jackson A, Edmonds DK: Oxytocin infusion during second stage of labour in primiparous women using epidural analgesia: A randomized double blind placebo controlled trial. Br Med J 299:1423, 1989

Scanzoni FW: Lehrbuch der Geburtshülfe, 3rd ed. Vienna, Seidel, 1853, p 838

Schwartz DB, Miodovnik M, Lavin JP Jr: Neonatal outcome among low birth weight infants delivered spontaneously or by low forceps. Obstet Gynecol 62:283, 1983

Seidman DS, Laor A, Gale R, Stevenson DK, Mashiach S, Danon YL: Long-term effects of vacuum and forceps deliveries. Lancet 2:1583, 1991

Smellie W: A Treatise on the Theory and Practice of Midwifery. London, Wilson & Durham, 1752

Steer CM, Boney W: Obstetric factors in cerebral palsy. Am J Obstet Gynecol 83:526, 1962

Vacca A, Grant A, Wyatt G, Chalmers T: Portsmouth operative delivery trial: A comparison of vacuum extraction and forceps delivery. Br J Obstet Gynaecol 90:1107, 1983

Wesley B, Van den Berg B, Reece EA: The effect of operative vaginal delivery on cognitive development. Abstract 32 presented at meeting of Society of Perinatal Obstetricians, Orlando, February 1992. Am J Obstet Gynecol 166:288, 1992

Yancey MK, Herpelsheimer A, Jordan GD, Benson WL, Brady K: Maternal and neonatal effects of outlet forceps delivery compared with spontaneous vaginal delivery in term pregnancies. Obstet Gynecol 78:646, 1991

CHAPTER 25
Techniques for Breech Delivery

The indications for vaginal versus cesarean delivery for breech presentations were considered in Chapter 20 (p. 499). Labor and techniques for vaginal delivery of the breech presentation are considered in the present chapter.

Mechanism of Labor. Unless there is disproportion between the size of the fetus and the pelvis, engagement and descent of the breech in response to labor usually takes place with the bitrochanteric diameter of the breech in one of the oblique diameters of the pelvis. The anterior hip usually descends more rapidly than the posterior hip, and when the resistance of the pelvic floor is met, internal rotation usually follows, bringing the anterior hip toward the pubic arch and allowing the bitrochanteric diameter to occupy the anteroposterior diameter of the pelvic outlet. Rotation usually takes place through an arc of 45 degrees. If, however, the posterior extremity is prolapsed, it always rotates to the symphysis pubis, ordinarily through an arc of 135 degrees, but occasionally in the opposite direction past the sacrum and the opposite half of the pelvis through an arc of 225 degrees.

After rotation, descent continues until the perineum is distended by the advancing breech, while the anterior hip appears at the vulva and is stemmed against the pubic arch. By lateral flexion of the body, the posterior hip then is forced over the anterior margin of the perineum, which retracts over the buttocks, thus allowing the infant to straighten out when the anterior hip is born. The legs and feet follow the breech and may be born spontaneously, although the aid of the obstetrician usually is required.

After the birth of the breech, there is slight external rotation, with the back turning anteriorly as the shoulders are brought into relation with one of the oblique diameters of the pelvis. The shoulders then descend rapidly and undergo internal rotation, with the bisacromial diameter occupying the anteroposterior diameter of the inferior strait. Immediately following the shoulders, the head, which is normally sharply flexed upon the thorax, enters the pelvis in one of the oblique diameters and then rotates in such a manner as to bring the posterior portion of the neck under the symphysis pubis. The head then is born in flexion, with the chin, mouth, nose, forehead, bregma (brow), and occiput appearing in succession over the perineum.

The breech may engage in the transverse diameter of the pelvis, with the sacrum directed anteriorly or posteriorly. The mechanism of labor in the transverse position differs only in that internal rotation occurs through an arc of 90 degrees.

Infrequently, rotation occurs in such a manner that the back of the infant is directed toward the vertebral column instead of toward the abdomen of the mother. Such rotation should be prevented if possible. Although the head may be delivered by allowing the chin and face to pass beneath the symphysis, the slightest traction on the body may cause extension of the head. Extension, if uncorrected, increases the diameters of the head, which must pass through the pelvis (see Fig. 25–8 later in chapter).

Vaginal Delivery of Breech

There are three general methods of breech delivery through the vagina:

- **Spontaneous breech delivery.** The infant is expelled entirely spontaneously without any traction or manipulation other than support of the infant. This form of delivery in mature infants is rare.
- **Partial breech extraction.** The infant is delivered spontaneously as far as the umbilicus, but the remainder of the body is extracted.
- **Total breech extraction.** The entire body of the infant is extracted by the obstetrician.

Because the technique of breech extraction differs in complete and incomplete breeches on the one hand, and frank breeches on the other, it is necessary to consider these conditions in two separate sections later in the chapter. The varieties of breech presentation are illustrated in Figures 10–2 to 10–4.

Management of Labor. A woman admitted in labor with a breech presentation deserves the immediate attention of nursing and medical personnel, because both mother and fetus are at considerably increased risk compared with a woman with a cephalic presentation (Chap. 20, p. 494). A rapid assessment should be made to establish the stage of labor, status of the fetal membranes, and condition of the fetus. An intravenous infusion is established, the hematocrit determined, and a group and screen done to detect antibodies, because these women have a high likelihood of undergoing operative delivery. Close surveillance of fetal heart rate and uterine contractions is commenced, and we recommend using continuous electronic monitoring. An immediate recruitment of the necessary nursing and medical personnel to accomplish a vaginal or abdominal delivery should also be done.

Stage of Labor. Assessment of cervical dilatation and effacement and the station of the presenting part are essential in planning the route of delivery. If labor is too far advanced, there may not be sufficient time to obtain imaging pelvimetry, and this alone may force the decision for cesarean delivery.

Fetal Condition. The presence or absence of gross fetal abnormalities such as hydrocephaly or anencephaly can be rapidly ascertained with the use of sonography or x-ray. Such efforts will help to ensure that a cesarean delivery is not done under emergency conditions, thereby increasing maternal risks, for an anomalous infant with no chance of survival. If vaginal delivery is planned, the fetal head should be well flexed (Gimovsky and Petrie, 1992). Sometimes this is difficult to ascertain from sonography. Most often, digital radiographs using computed tomographic pelvimetry will be adequate to document flexion of the fetal head (Chap. 11, p. 292), but if not, a plain film of the abdomen will suffice.

Intravenous Infusion and Laboratory Values. An intravenous infusion through a venous catheter is begun as soon as the woman arrives in the labor suite. Possible emergency induction of anesthesia, or hemorrhage from lacerations or from uterine atony from halogenated anesthetics, are but two of many reasons that may require an immediate intravenous access route that can be used to administer medications or fluids, including blood.

Fetal Monitoring. Guidelines for monitoring the high-risk fetus are applied as discussed in Chapter 14 (p. 375). Thus, the fetal heart rate is recorded at least every 15 minutes. We prefer continuous electronic monitoring of fetal heart rate and uterine contractions. When membranes are ruptured, the risk of umbilical cord prolapse is appreciably increased (Chap. 20, p. 498). Therefore, a vaginal examination should be done following rupture of the membranes to check for umbilical cord prolapse. Special attention should be directed to the fetal heart rate for the first 5 to 10 minutes following membrane rupture, to ensure that there has not been an occult cord prolapse. After membrane rupture, internal electronic monitoring of fetal heart rate and uterine contractions is preferable, because of the more reliable information provided by these techniques.

Recruitment of Nursing and Medical Personnel. Additional help is required for managing labor and delivery of a breech. For labor, one-on-one nursing should be maintained due to the risk of umbilical cord prolapse or

occlusion, and the physician must also be readily available should there be an emergency.

Route of Delivery. Consideration for the route of delivery is given as soon as possible after admission. The choice of abdominal or vaginal delivery is based upon the type of breech, flexion of the head, fetal size, quality of uterine contractions, and size of the maternal pelvis. The indications and contraindications for vaginal delivery of a breech are discussed in detail in Chapter 20, p. 499.

Timing of Delivery. In general, preparations for breech extraction should be initiated when the buttocks or feet appear at the vulva. It is essential that the delivery team include (1) an obstetrician skilled in the art of breech extraction, (2) an associate to assist with the delivery, (3) an anesthesiologist who quickly can induce appropriate anesthesia when needed, (4) an individual trained to resuscitate the infant effectively, including tracheal intubation, and (5) someone to provide general assistance.

Delivery is easier and, in turn, perinatal morbidity and mortality are lower when the breech of the fetus is allowed to deliver spontaneously to the umbilicus. If fetal jeopardy or distress develop before this time, however, a decision must be made whether to perform total breech extraction or cesarean delivery. For a favorable outcome with any breech delivery, at the very minimum, the birth canal must be sufficiently large to allow passage of the fetus without trauma. Thus, the cervix must be fully dilated, and if not, then a cesarean delivery nearly always is the more appropriate method of delivery when fetal jeopardy develops.

Extraction of the Complete or Incomplete Breech. During total extraction of a complete or incomplete breech, the obstetrician's hand is introduced through the vagina and both feet of the fetus are grasped. The ankles are held with the second finger lying between them; the feet are brought with gentle traction through the vulva. If difficulty is experienced in grasping both feet, first one foot should be drawn into the vagina but not through the introitus; and then the other foot should be advanced in a similar fashion (Fig. 25–1). Now both feet are grasped and pulled through the vulva simultaneously. Unless there is considerable relaxation of the perineum, an *episiotomy* should be made. The episiotomy is an important adjunct to any type of breech delivery. A mediolateral episiotomy is usually preferred with a term-sized infant because it furnishes greater room and is less likely to extend into the rectum.

As the legs begin to emerge through the vulva, they should be wrapped in a sterile towel to obtain a firmer grasp, for the vernix caseosa renders them slippery and difficult to hold. Many obstetricians prefer the towel to be moistened. Downward gentle traction is then continued. As the legs emerge, successively higher portions are grasped, first the calves and then the thighs (Fig. 25–2). When the breech appears at the vulva, *gentle traction* is applied until the hips are delivered. As the buttocks emerge, the back of the infant usually rotates to the anterior. The thumbs of the operator are then placed over the sacrum and the fingers over the hips, and *gentle downward traction* is continued until the costal margins, and then the scapulas become visible (Fig. 25–3). As traction is exerted and the scapulas become visible, the back of the infant tends to turn spontaneously toward the side of the mother to which it was originally directed (Fig. 25–4). If turning is not spontaneous, slight rotation should be added to the traction, with the object of bringing the bisacromial diameter of the fetus into the anteroposterior diameter of the pelvic outlet.

A cardinal rule in successful breech extraction is to employ steady, gentle, downward traction until the lower halves of the scapulas are delivered outside the vulva, making no attempt at delivery of

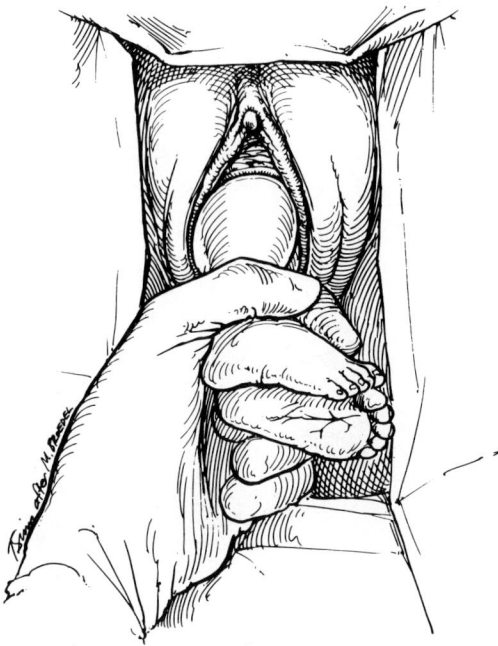

Fig. 25–1. Breech extraction. Traction on the feet and ankles.

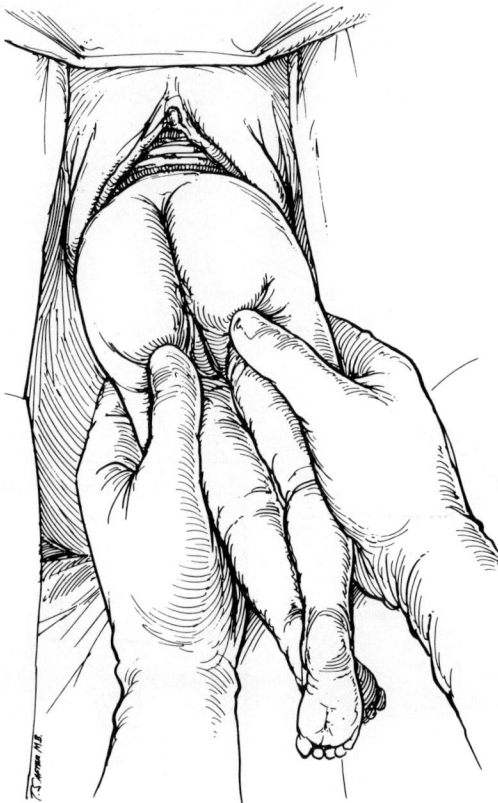

Fig. 25–2. Breech extraction. Traction on the thighs. A warm, moist towel is most often applied over the fetal parts to reduce slippage from vernix as traction is applied.

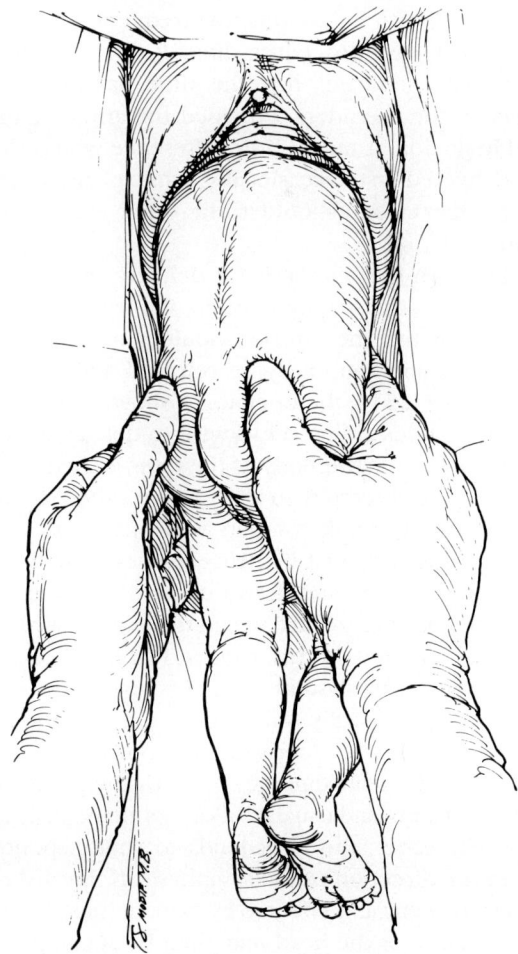

Fig. 25–3. Breech extraction. Extraction of the body. The hands are applied over, but not above, the infant's pelvis. Rotation is not attempted until the scapulas clearly are visible.

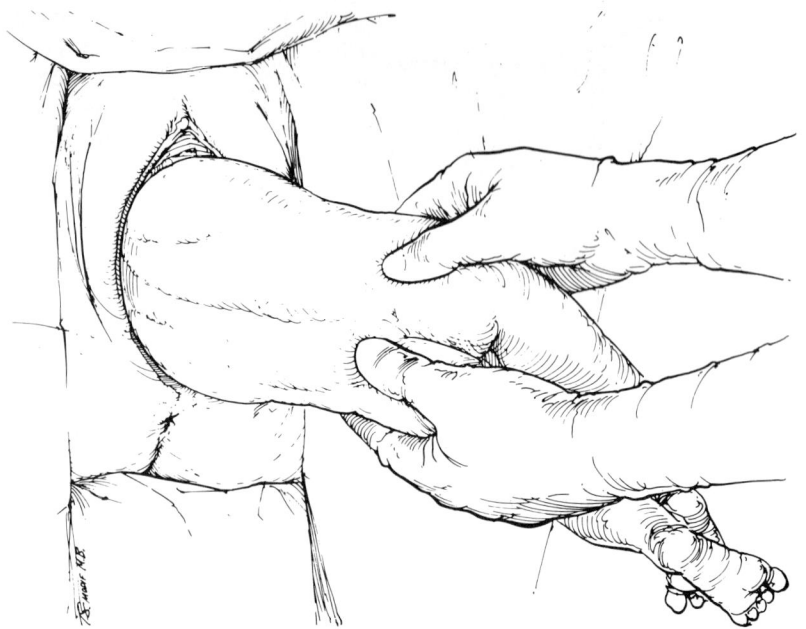

Fig. 25–4. Breech extraction. The scapulas are visible and the body is rotating.

the shoulders and arms until one axilla becomes visible. Failure to follow this rule frequently will make an otherwise easy procedure difficult. The appearance of one axilla indicates that the time has arrived for delivery of the shoulders. Provided the arms are maintained in flexion, it makes little difference which shoulder is delivered first. Occasionally, while plans are being made to deliver one shoulder, the other is born spontaneously.

There are two methods for delivery of the shoulders: (1) With the scapulas visible, the trunk is rotated in such a way that the anterior shoulder and arm appear at the vulva and can easily be released and delivered first. In Figure 25–4, the operator is shown rotating the trunk of the fetus counterclockwise to deliver the right shoulder and arm. The body of the fetus is then rotated in the reverse direction to deliver the other shoulder and arm. (2) If trunk rotation was unsuccessful, the posterior shoulder must be delivered first. The feet are grasped in one hand and drawn upward over the inner thigh of the mother toward which the ventral surface of the fetus is directed. In this manner, leverage is exerted upon the posterior shoulder, which slides out over the perineal margin, usually followed by the arm and hand (Fig. 25–5). Then, by depressing the body of the fetus, the anterior shoulder emerges beneath the pubic arch, and the arm and hand usually follow spontaneously (Fig. 25–6). Thereafter, the back tends to rotate spontaneously in the direction of the symphysis. If upward rotation fails to occur, it is effected by manual rotation of the body. Delivery of the head may then be accomplished.

Unfortunately, however, the process is not always so simple, and it is sometimes necessary first to free and deliver the arms. These maneuvers are much less frequently required today, presumably because of adher-

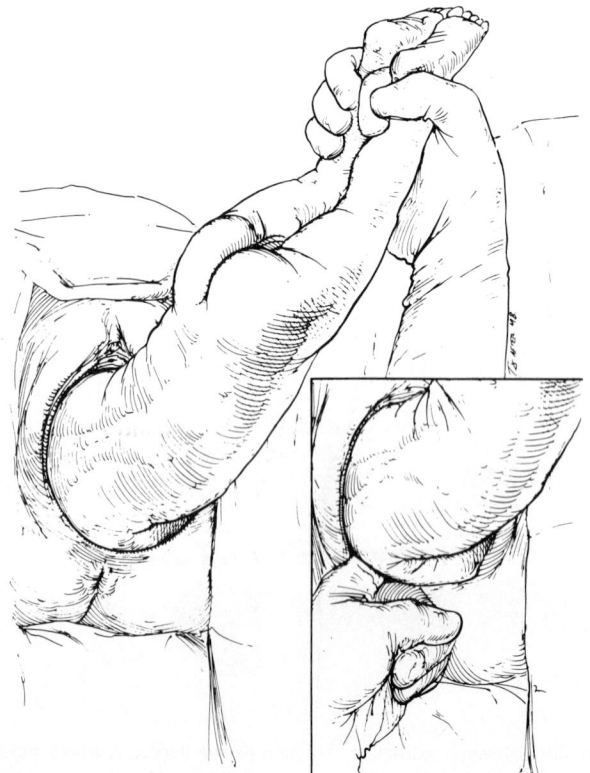

Fig. 25–5. Breech extraction. Upward traction to effect delivery of the posterior shoulder, followed by freeing the posterior arm (*inset*).

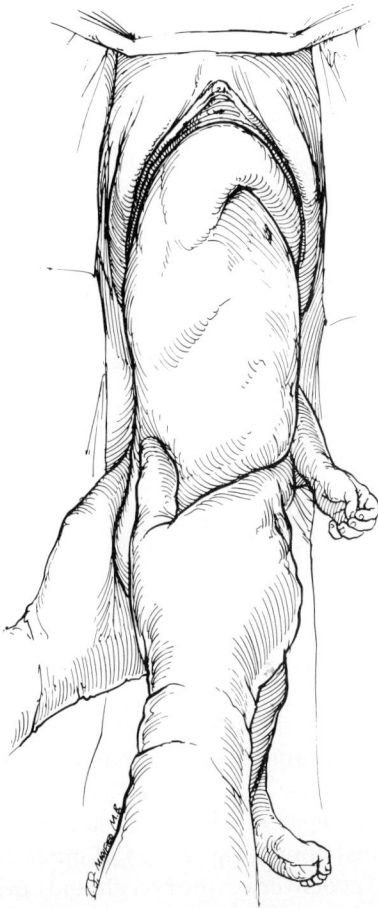

Fig. 25-6. Breech extraction. Delivery of the anterior shoulder by downward traction. The anterior arm then may be freed the same way as the posterior arm in Figure 25-5.

ence to the principle of continuing traction without attention to the shoulders until an axilla becomes visible. Attempts to free the arms immediately after the costal margins emerge should be avoided.

There is more space available in the posterior and lateral segments of the normal pelvis than elsewhere; therefore, in difficult cases, the posterior arm should be freed first. Because the corresponding axilla already is visible, upward traction upon the feet is continued, and two fingers of the obstetrician's other hand are passed along the humerus until the elbow is reached (Fig. 25-5, inset). The fingers are now used to splint the arm, which is swept downward and delivered through the vulva. To deliver the anterior arm, depression of the body of the infant is sometimes all that is required to allow the anterior arm to slip out spontaneously. In other instances, the anterior arm can be swept down over the thorax using two fingers as a splint. Occasionally, however, the body must be held with the operator's thumbs over the scapulas and rotated to bring the undelivered shoulder near the closest sacrosciatic notch. The legs then are carried upward to bring the ventral surface of the infant to the opposite inner thigh of the mother;

subsequently, the arm can be delivered as described previously.

If the arms have become extended over the head, their delivery, although more difficult, can usually be accomplished by the maneuvers just described. In so doing, particular care must be taken to carry the operator's fingers up to the elbow and to use the fingers as a splint, for if the operator's fingers are merely hooked over the fetal arm, the humerus or clavicle is exposed to great danger of fracture. Infrequently, one or both fetal arms is found around the back of the neck (*nuchal arm*), and delivery is still more difficult. If the nuchal arm cannot be freed in the manner described, extraction may be facilitated by rotating the fetus through half a circle in such a direction that the friction exerted by the birth canal will serve to draw the elbow toward the face. Should rotation of the fetus fail to free the nuchal arm, it may be necessary to push the fetus upward in an attempt to release it. If the rotation is still unsuccessful, the nuchal arm is often forcibly extracted by hooking a finger over it. In this event, fracture of the humerus or clavicle is very common. Fortunately, good union almost always follows appropriate treatment. Because of these frequently less than optimal outcomes associated with nuchal arms, Sherer and associates (1989) recommend radiological studies to identify, when possible, the presence of a nuchal arm during the first stage of labor. They recommend cesarean delivery if a nuchal arm is identified.

After the shoulders are born, the head usually occupies an oblique diameter of the pelvis with the chin directed posteriorly. The fetal head then may be extracted with forceps, as described later in the chapter, or by the *Mauriceau maneuver* (Fig. 25-7).

Mauriceau Maneuver

> The operator's index and middle finger of one hand are applied over the maxilla, to flex the head, while the fetal body rests upon the palm of the hand and forearm. The forearm is straddled by the fetal legs. Two fingers of the operator's other hand then are hooked over the fetal neck, and grasping the shoulders, downward traction is applied until the suboccipital region appears under the symphysis. Gentle *suprapubic pressure* simultaneously applied by an assistant helps keep the head flexed. The body of the fetus then is elevated toward the mother's abdomen, and the mouth, nose, brow, and eventually the occiput emerge successively over the perineum. *Gentle traction* should be exerted by the fingers over the shoulders. At the same time, appropriate suprapubic pressure applied by an assistant, as shown in Figure 25-7, is helpful in delivery of the head.

This maneuver was first practiced by Mauriceau (1721), but for some reason fell into disfavor. Much later Smellie (1876) described a similar procedure but rarely made use of it because he preferred forceps. Veit (1907) re-

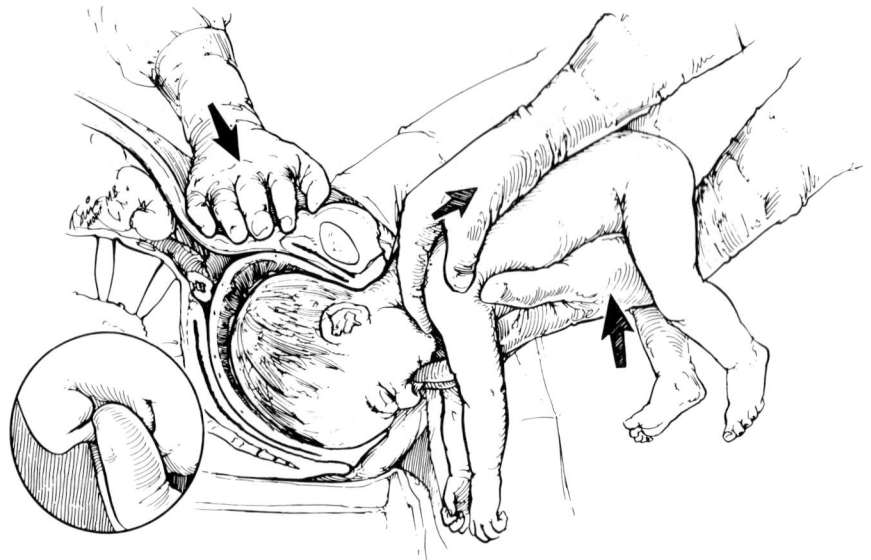

Fig. 25–7. Delivery of aftercoming head using the Mauriceau maneuver. Note that as the fetal head is being delivered, flexion of the head is maintained by suprapubic pressure provided by an assistant, and simultaneously by pressure on the maxilla (*inset*) by the operator as traction is applied.

directed attention to the Mauriceau maneuver, and in Germany the procedure frequently is named after Veit. The most accurate designation, however, is the Mauriceau–Smellie–Veit maneuver.

Prague Maneuver

Rarely, the back of the fetus fails to rotate to the anterior. When this occurs, rotation of the back to the anterior may be achieved by using stronger traction on the fetal legs. If the back still remains posteriorly, extraction may be accomplished using the Mauriceau maneuver and delivering the fetus back down. If this is impossible, the fetus still may be delivered using the *modified Prague maneuver*. This maneuver was recommended by Kiwisch (1846), who practiced in Prague. The maneuver had been described in London as early as 1754 by Pugh. The modified maneuver as practiced today consists of two fingers of one hand grasping the shoulders of the back-down fetus, from below, while the other hand draws the feet up over the abdomen of the mother (Fig. 25–8). Although the original Prague maneuver was employed in cases in which the fetal back was directed upward, this is not recommended.

Bracht Maneuver

In this maneuver, the breech is allowed to deliver spontaneously to the umbilicus. The fetal body then is held, but not pressed, against the maternal symphysis. This force is meant to be the equivalent of gravity (Bracht, 1936). The suspension of the fetus in this position, coupled with the effects of uterine contractions and moderate suprapubic pressure by an assistant, often results in a *spontaneous delivery*. Plental and Stone (1953) reviewed this maneuver in detail. Despite its popularity in Europe, there is no proof that its use is associated with better long-

term neurological outcomes (Krause and associates, 1991).

Extraction of Frank Breech. At times, extraction of a frank breech may be accomplished by *moderate* traction exerted by a finger in each groin and facilitated by a generous episiotomy (Fig. 25–9). If moderate traction does not effect delivery of the breech, and cesarean is not used, vaginal delivery can be accomplished only by *breech decomposition.* This procedure involves intrauterine manipulation to convert the frank breech into a footling breech. The procedure is accomplished more readily if the membranes have ruptured recently, but it becomes extremely difficult if considerable time has elapsed after the escape of amnionic fluid. In such cases, the uterus may have become tightly contracted over the fetus.

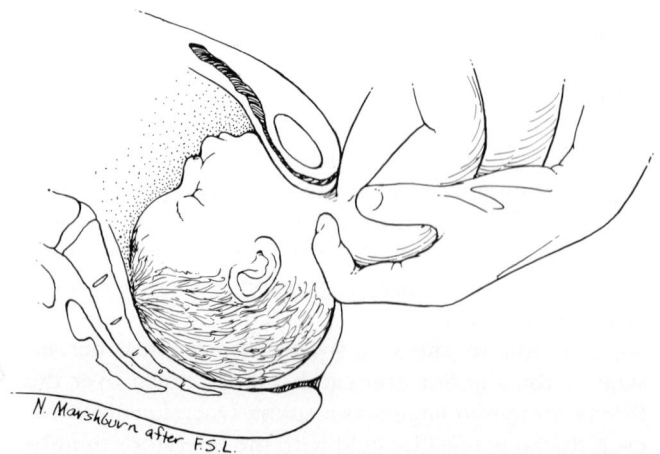

Fig. 25–8. Delivery of the aftercoming head using the modified Prague maneuver necessitated by failure of the fetal trunk to rotate anteriorly.

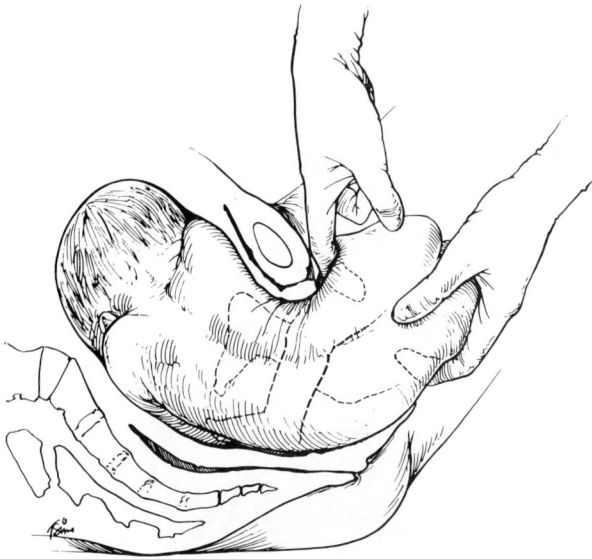

Fig. 25–9. Extraction of a frank breech using fingers in groins.

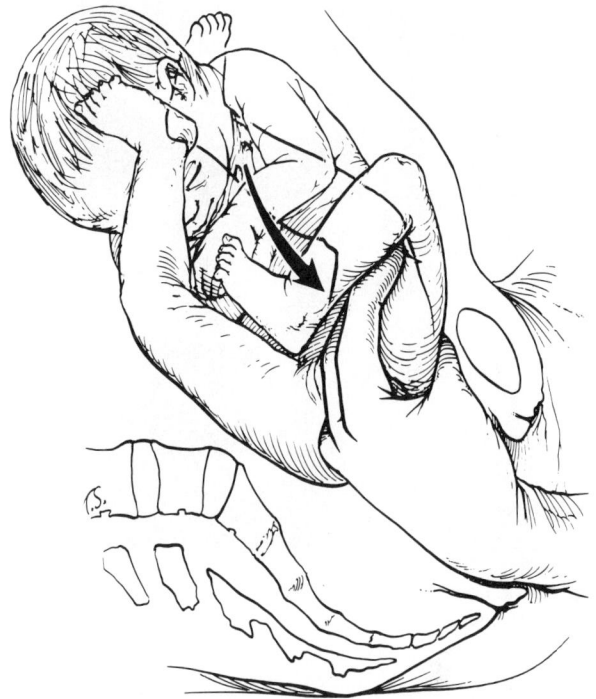

Fig. 25–10. Pinard maneuver, which is sometimes used in a case of a frank breech presentation to deliver a foot into the vagina.

Pinard Maneuver

In many cases, the *Pinard maneuver* (Pinard, 1889) aids in bringing the fetal feet within reach of the operator. In this maneuver, two fingers are carried up along one extremity to the knee to push it away from the midline. Spontaneous flexion usually follows, and the foot of the fetus is felt to impinge upon the back of the hand. The fetal foot then may be grasped and brought down (Fig. 25–10). As soon as the buttocks are born, first one leg and then the other is drawn out and extraction is accomplished as described under "Extraction of the Complete or Incomplete Breech" earlier in the chapter.

Forceps to Aftercoming Head. Piper forceps (Figs. 25–11 to 25–17) may be applied when the Mauriceau maneuver cannot be accomplished easily, or they may be applied electively and used instead of the Mauriceau maneuver. The blades of the forceps should not be applied to the aftercoming head until it has been brought into the pelvis by gentle traction, combined with supra-pubic pressure, and is engaged (Fig. 25–16). As shown in Figure 25–17, suspension of the body of the fetus in a towel keeps the arms out of the way and prevents excessive abduction of the trunk.

Entrapment of the Aftercoming Head. Occasionally, especially with small preterm fetuses, the incompletely dilated cervix will not allow delivery of the aftercoming head. Prompt action is necessary if a living infant is to be delivered. With gentle traction on the fetal body, the cervix, at times, may be manually slipped over the occiput, or the Bracht maneuver may be tried. If these actions are not rapidly successful, Dührssen incisions can be made in the cervix. This is one of the few indications for Dührssen incisions in modern obstetrics (see Chap. 24, p. 573).

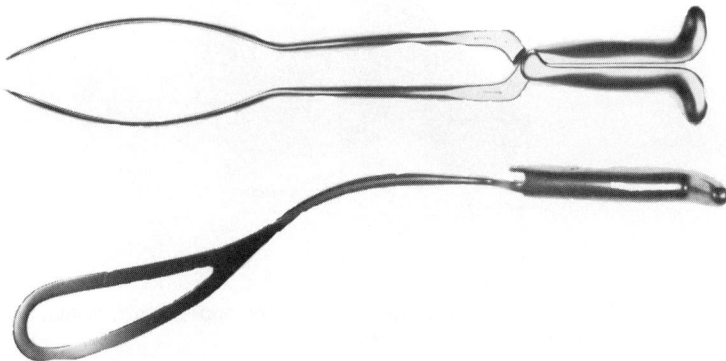

Fig. 25–11. Piper forceps.

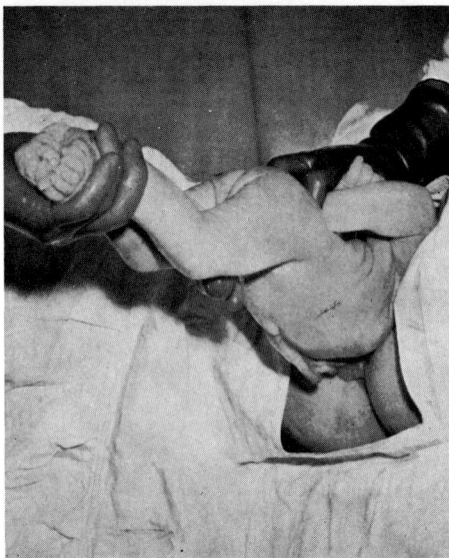

Fig. 25–12. Position of infant with head in pelvis prior to application of Piper forceps.

"Abdominal Rescue"

Iffy and colleagues (1986) described "abdominal rescue" for a 2050-g first twin whose fully deflexed head was entrapped after the arms had been delivered. An emergency classical cesarean delivery resulted in an Apgar 3/7 infant who remained neurologically normal despite a small subarachnoid hemorrhage detected by a computed tomographic scan. Sandberg (1988) has confirmed that replacement of the fetus higher into the vagina and uterus, followed by cesarean delivery, can be used successfully to rescue entrapped breeches that cannot be delivered vaginally.

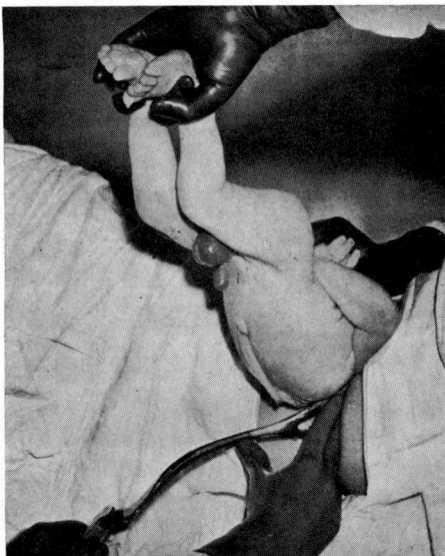

Fig. 25–14. Introduction of right blade, completing application.

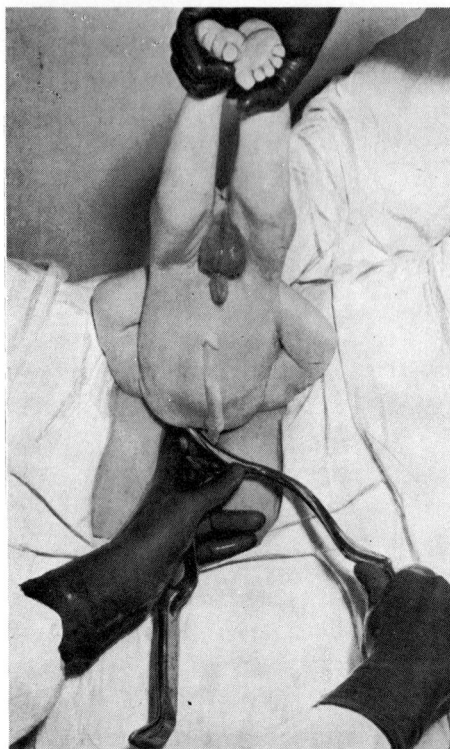

Fig. 25–13. Introduction of left blade to left side of pelvis.

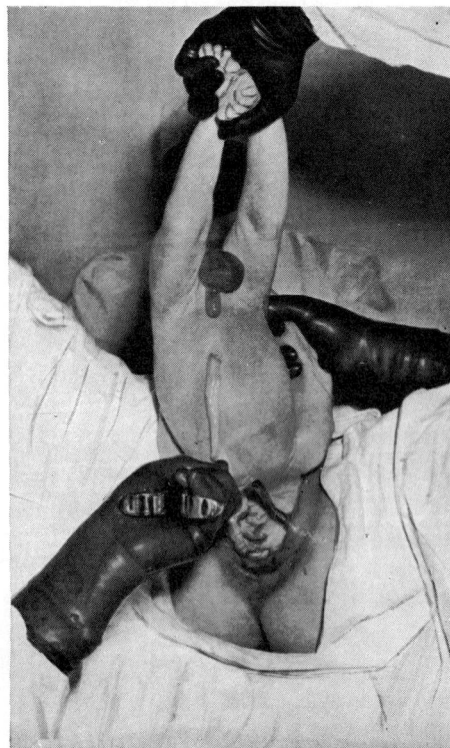

Fig. 25–15. Forceps locked and traction applied; chin, mouth, and nose emerging over perineum.

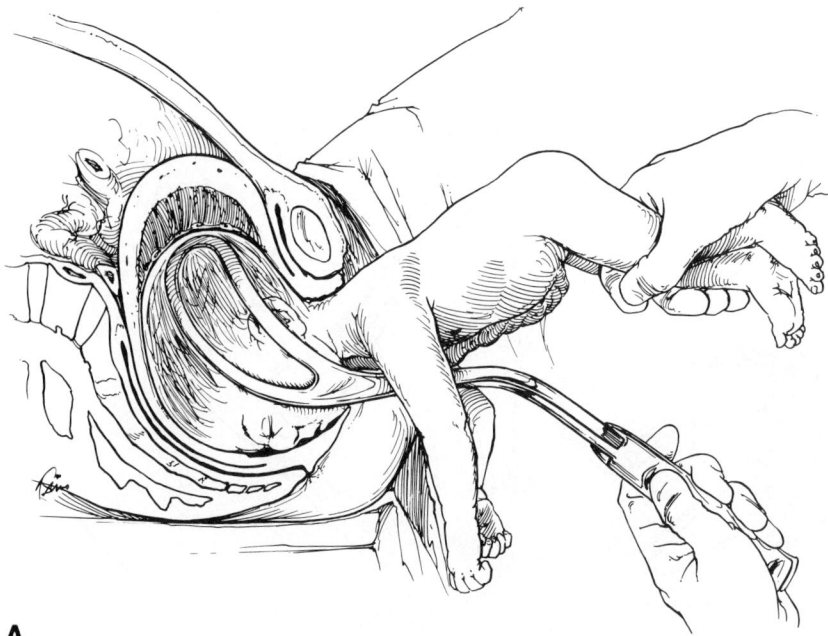

A

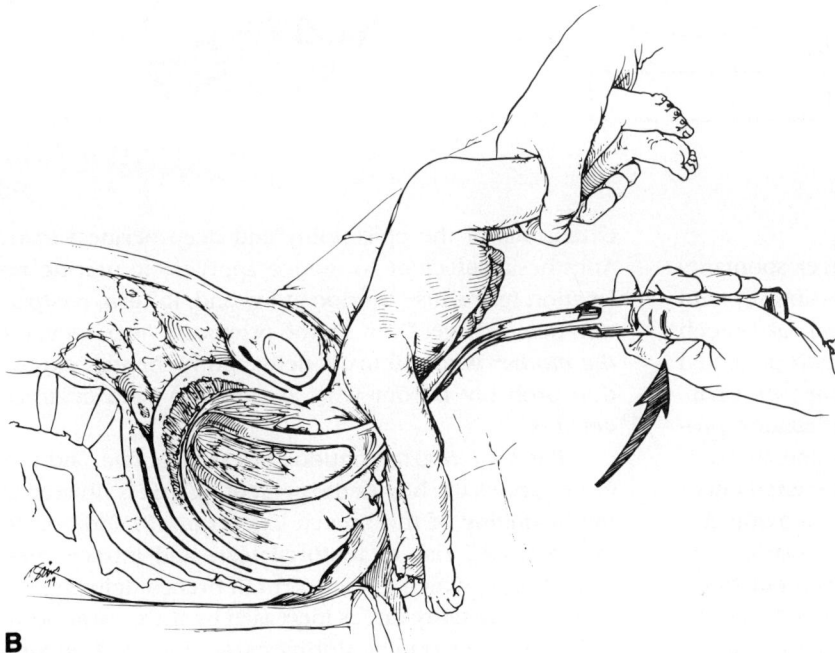

B

Fig. 25–16. A. Piper forceps applied to the aftercoming head. The head has entered the pelvis and forceps have been applied (see Figs. 25–11 to 25–15). **B.** Forceps delivery of aftercoming head. Note the direction of movement (*arrow*).

Analgesia and Anesthesia for Labor and Delivery.
Continuous epidural analgesia (see Chap. 16, p. 437) has been advocated by some as ideal for women in labor with a breech presentation. According to Crawford and Weaver (1982), such a block provides some protection for the fetal head during the second stage of labor as well as during delivery by abolishing the bearing-down reflex and by inducing pelvic muscle relaxation. Confino and colleagues (1985) reviewed the outcomes of 371 normally formed singleton breech fetuses delivered vaginally. About 25 percent of these women had been given continuous epidural analgesia, but it was quite worri-

some that oxytocin augmentation was necessary to effect delivery in half of them. Although first-stage labor was not longer than in a control group not given epidural analgesia, the second stage was prolonged significantly in women whose fetuses weighed more than 2500 g. In fact, it was doubled if the fetus weighed more than 3500 g. There was one neonatal death from trauma that followed full breech extraction for a prolapsed cord under epidural analgesia. Chada and associates (1992) observed similar outcomes but also noted an increased incidence of cesarean delivery. For the above reasons, we are reluctant to recommend continuous epidural

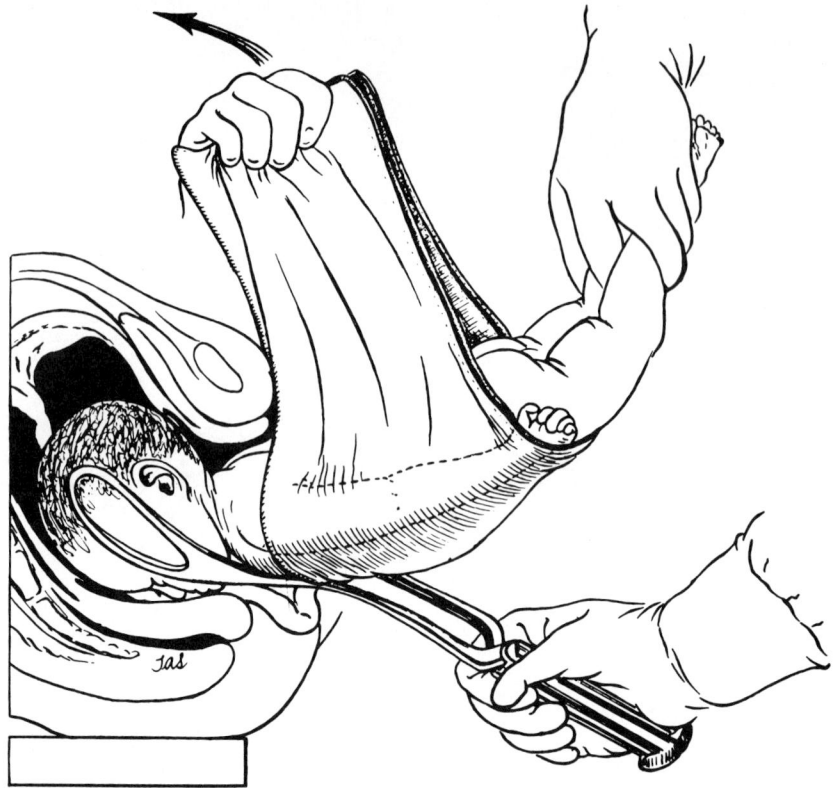

Fig. 25–17. Management of fetal arms in breech extraction.

analgesia for these women.

It is wise to allow the breech to deliver spontaneously to the umbilicus. Analgesia for episiotomy and intravaginal manipulations that are needed for breech extraction can usually be accomplished with pudendal block and local infiltration of the perineum (see Chap. 16, p. 431). Nitrous oxide plus oxygen inhalation provides further relief from pain. If general anesthesia is desired, it can be induced quickly with thiopental plus a muscle relaxant and maintained with nitrous oxide. Anesthesia for decomposition and extraction must provide sufficient relaxation to allow intrauterine manipulations. Although successful decomposition has been accomplished using epidural, caudal, or spinal analgesia, increased uterine tone may render the operation more difficult. Under such conditions, one of the halogenated anesthetic agents may be used to relax the uterus, as well as provide analgesia. The safeguards cited for the use of these agents in Chapter 16 (p. 427) must be followed.

Prognosis. With complicated breech deliveries, there are increased maternal risks. Manual manipulations within the birth canal increase the risk of maternal infection. Intrauterine maneuvers, especially with a thinned-out lower uterine segment, or delivery of the aftercoming head through an incompletely dilated cervix, may cause rupture of the uterus, lacerations of the cervix, or both. Such manipulations also may lead to

extensions of the episiotomy and deep perineal tears. Anesthesia sufficient to induce appreciable uterine relaxation may cause uterine atony and, in turn, postpartum hemorrhage. Even so, the prognosis, in general, for *the mother* whose fetus is delivered by breech extraction probably is somewhat better than with cesarean delivery.

For *the fetus,* the outlook is less favorable, and it is more serious the higher the presenting part is situated at the beginning of the breech extraction. In addition to the increased risk of tentorial tears and intracerebral hemorrhage, which are inherent in breech delivery, the perinatal mortality rate is increased by the greater probability of other trauma during extraction. With incomplete breech presentations, prolapse of the umbilical cord is much more common than in vertex presentations, and this complication further worsens the prognosis for the infant.

An adverse outcome for a breech vaginal delivery is not universally expected. In fact, Croughan-Minihane and associates (1990) reported that vaginally born infants were not at increased risk for adverse outcomes related to head trauma, neonatal seizures, cerebral palsy, mental retardation, or spasticity. Christian and colleagues (1990) reported no perinatal outcome differences for Apgar scores, hospital stay, neonatal complications, and cord blood gases between vaginally delivered frank breeches and those delivered by cesarean section. In this prospective study, all vaginal deliveries were in women with an adequate pelvis documented by computed tomographic pelvimetry. Vaginal deliveries were restricted to women with frank breech fetuses estimated to weigh between 2000 and 4000 g. Christian and Brady (1991), however, reported later that there were differences in cord acid-base studies between fetuses born vaginally as a breech versus a vertex presentation. Specifically, breech-presenting vaginally born infants, on the average, had a lower cord blood pH and higher PCO_2 than cephalic-presenting infants delivered vaginally. Hommel and associates (1989) reported no differences in the incidence of metabolic acidemia between vaginally and abdominally delivered breeches; however, the incidence of mixed respiratory–metabolic acidemia and pure respiratory acidemia were increased significantly in vaginally delivered breech infants. These observations emphasize the importance of measuring both umbilical cord gases as well as pH because it is likely that only metabolic acidemia of prolonged duration is associated with poor neurological outcomes (see Chap. 17, p. 446).

Fracture of the humerus and clavicle cannot always be avoided, and fracture of the femur may be sustained during difficult frank breech extractions. Such fractures are associated with both vaginal and cesarean deliveries (Vasa and Kim, 1990). Hematomas of the sternocleidomastoid muscles occasionally develop after delivery, though they usually disappear spontaneously. More serious problems, however, may follow separation of the epiphyses of the scapula, humerus, or femur. There is no evidence that the incidence of congenital hip dislocations is increased by vaginal delivery of a breech (Clausen and Nielsen, 1988), but minor hip abnormalities (best detected by sonography) may be more common in vaginally delivered breech neonates (Dorn, 1990; Walter and colleagues, 1992). Paralysis of the arm may follow pressure upon the brachial plexus by the fingers in exerting traction, but more frequently, it is caused by overstretching the neck while freeing the arms. When the fetus is extracted forcibly through a contracted pelvis, spoon-shaped depressions or actual

fractures of the skull may result. Occasionally, even the fetal neck may be broken when great force is employed. Perinatal morbidity and mortality are considered in greater detail in Chapter 20. Finally, testicular injury, in some cases severe enough to result in anorchia, may occur following vaginal delivery (Tiwary, 1989).

Version

Version, or turning, is an operation in which the presentation of the fetus is altered artificially, either substituting one pole of a longitudinal presentation for the other, or converting an oblique or transverse lie into a longitudinal presentation. According to whether the head or breech is made the presenting part, the operation is designated cephalic or podalic version, respectively. It is also named according to the method by which it is accomplished. Thus, in *external version,* the manipulations are performed exclusively through the abdominal wall; while in *internal version,* the entire hand is introduced into the uterine cavity.

External Cephalic Version. The object of this procedure is to convert a less favorable presentation into a vertex. The problems that have persisted until recently have not been whether an external cephalic version could be accomplished and by what technique, but rather, whether the procedure was necessary, safe, and cost effective. With respect to the first question, it appears from the results of randomized controlled studies shown in Table 25–1 that if version is not performed, approximately 80 percent of noncephalic presentations diagnosed in the late third trimester still will be present at delivery. This is compared only with 30 percent of those who underwent a successful version. Cesarean delivery rates in untreated women are more than twice the rate in those women in whom a version was performed (32 versus 15 percent).

The safety of external cephalic version with and without tocolytic agents remains a controversial area.

TABLE 25–1. RANDOMIZED STUDIES TO DETERMINE EFFECT OF CEPHALIC VERSION ON NONCEPHALIC BIRTHS AND CESAREAN DELIVERIES

| | Noncephalic at Delivery | | | | Cesarean Delivery | | | |
| | Treated | | Control | | Treated | | Control | |
Study	No.	(%)	No.	(%)	No.	(%)	No.	(%)
VanDorsten and colleagues (1981)	8/25	(32)	19/23	(83)	7/25	(28)	17/23	(74)
Hofmeyr (1983)	1/30	(3)	20/30	(67)	6/30	(20)	13/30	(43)
Brocks and associates (1984)	17/31	(55)	29/34	(85)	7/31	(23)	12/34	(35)
Van Veelen and co-workers (1989)	39/89	(44)	67/90	(74)	8/89	(9)	13/90	(14)
Mahomed and collaborators (1991)	18/103	(18)	87/105	(83)	13/103	(13)	35/105	(33)
Totals	83/278	(30)	222/282	(79)	41/278	(15)	90/282	(32)

Modified from Hofmeyr (1991).

According to their survey, Amon and Sibai (1988) reported that external version is thought by the majority of maternal–fetal medicine specialists to be a frequently successful technique that is associated with little morbidity (see Chap. 20, p. 497). Advocates believe that external version should be attempted in most noncephalic presentations to avoid maternal risks of cesarean delivery and perinatal morbidity and mortality associated with vaginal delivery (Hofmeyr, 1991). Results published to date support this conclusion, but the observed risks to this *elective procedure* include, and are not limited to, maternal mortality, placental abruption, uterine rupture, feto-maternal hemorrhage, isoimmunization, preterm labor, fetal distress necessitating emergency cesarean delivery, and fetal demise (see Chap. 20, p. 498).

Because of the fear of uterine rupture, women who had undergone cesarean delivery were excluded from most external cephalic version protocols. Flamm and co-workers (1991) reported no serious maternal or fetal complications associated with such attempts in women with previous low transverse uterine incisions. They were successful in 82 percent of 56 patients. At present, we are not performing external cephalic versions in women who have had previous uterine incisions.

The cost effectiveness of external cephalic version has not been established. Hanss (1990) reported that successful version represented less than 0.5 percent of all deliveries, and less than 10 percent of breech deliveries in his own institution in 1988. In a study from the Netherlands, van de Pavert and colleagues (1990) reached a similar conclusion. Specifically, they concluded that the "benefits of external version at term may not apply to populations with a low cesarean rate, unless versions are carried out with maximum efficiency."

Hofmeyr (1991), in a thoughtful commentary, makes a persuasive argument for universal external version. Using the data summarized in Table 25–1, he maintains that if external version were attempted in 2 percent of the 750,000 pregnancies delivered in the United Kingdom each year, the number of breech births would be decreased each year by 5100, and the number of cesarean deliveries would be decreased by 2100. Such a goal does not appear to be impossible in the United States. Morrison and co-workers (1986) attempted external cephalic version in 2.3 percent of pregnancies cared for at the University of Mississippi Medical Center between 1982 and 1984. Compared with the preceding 3 years at their institution, they decreased breech deliveries from 1.8 to 1.1 percent and cesarean deliveries performed for breeches from 2.8 to 1.6 percent.

Indications. If a breech or shoulder presentation (transverse lie) is diagnosed in the last weeks of pregnancy, its conversion to a vertex may be attempted by external maneuvers, provided there is no marked disproportion between the size of the fetus and the pelvis, and provided there is no placenta previa. If the fetus lies transversely, a change of presentation is the only alternative to cesarean delivery for a viable fetus (Hankins and colleagues, 1990).

According to Fortunato and colleagues (1988), external cephalic version using tocolysis is more likely to be successful if (1) the presenting part has not descended into the pelvis, (2) there is a normal amount of amnionic fluid, (3) the fetal back is not positioned posteriorly, and (4) the woman is not obese. After controlling for other variables, the first two factors listed had an independent effect on the success of the version. Hellstrom and colleagues (1990) reported their results from a similar study, and they identified only 3 of 16 significant variables to be associated with successful external cephalic version. The most important factor was parity, followed by fetal presentation and the amount of amnionic fluid. They found that a version appears to be more successful in a parous woman who has an unengaged fetus surrounded by a normal amount of amnionic fluid.

Technique. Cephalic version is performed solely by *external manipulations* (Fig. 25–18). Most investigators recommend that uterine relaxation be established with a tocolytic agent. Presentation and position of the fetus are ascertained carefully and documented by sonography, because Leopold maneuvers are less precise in breech presentations (Thorp and co-workers, 1991). Each hand then grasps one of the fetal poles. The pole that is to be converted into the presenting part then is gently stroked toward the pelvic inlet while the other is moved in the opposite direction. This procedure should always be performed with frequent fetal heart rate monitoring before, during, and after the procedure. Version probably is best attempted in a labor and delivery unit or close by, so that rapid cesarean delivery can be accomplished should fetal distress develop. After successful version, the fetus tends to return to the original position unless the presenting part is fixed in the pelvis. During labor, however, the head may be pressed into the pelvic inlet and held firmly until it becomes fixed under the influence of uterine contractions.

While most (Hofmeyr, 1983; Mahomed, 1991; Van Dorsten and co-workers, 1981, 1982) recommend tocolysis for external versions, not all agree that this is necessary (Scaling, 1988). Robertson and associates (1987) reported that ritodrine tocolysis did not improve their success. Similarly, Tan and colleagues (1989), in a prospective randomized trial, found that salbutamol did not improve their success rate.

Because such manipulations may cause fetomaternal bleeding, anti-D immune globulin prophylaxis should be given to all D-negative women in whom external cephalic version is attempted (see Chap. 20, p. 498 and Chap. 44, p. 1003).

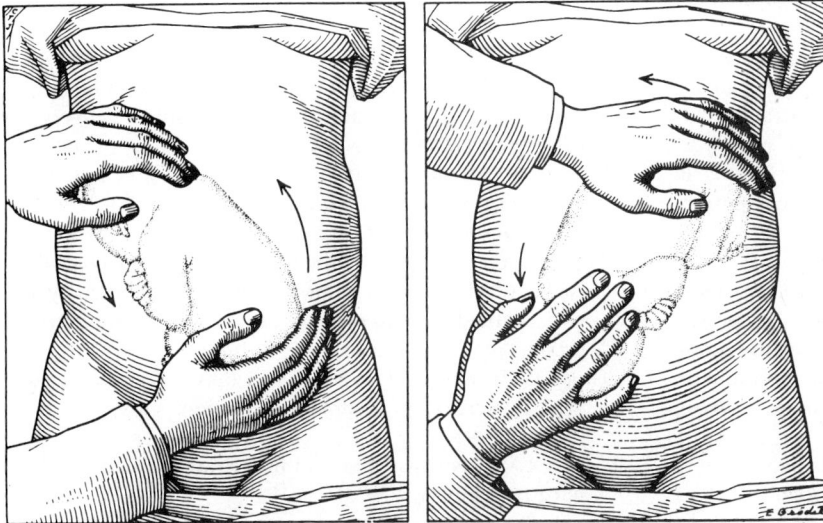

Fig. 25–18. External cephalic version.

Internal Podalic Version. This maneuver consists of the obstetrician turning the fetus by inserting a hand into the uterine cavity, seizing one or both feet, and drawing them through the cervix while pushing transabdominally the upper portion of the fetal body in the opposite direction. The operation is followed by breech extraction. Despite numerous attempts to defend or condemn this procedure, there is presently insufficient evidence to document its safety (Drew and associates, 1991). There is, however, a large amount of anecdotal information to support claims that the procedure may be associated with an increased fetal–neonatal risk of trauma and future neurological damage.

Indications. There are very few, if any, indications for internal podalic version other than for delivery of a second twin. The technique for delivering a second twin is described in Chapter 39 (p. 911). The possibility of serious trauma to the fetus and mother during internal podalic version of a cephalic presentation is apparent, as illustrated in Figures 39–20 and 39–21 (pp. 912, 913).

References

Amon E, Sibai BM, Anderson GD: How perinatologists manage the problem of the presenting breech. Am J Perinatol 5:247, 1988

Bracht E: Manual aid in breech presentation. Zeitschr Geburthshilfe Gynaekol 112:271, 1936

Brocks V, Philipsen T, Secher NJ: A randomized trial of external cephalic version with tocolysis in late pregnancy. Br J Obstet Gynaecol 91:653, 1984

Chadha YC, Mahmood TA, Dick MJ, Smith NC, Campbell DM, Templeton A: Breech delivery and epidural analgesia. Br J Obstet Gynaecol 99:96, 1992

Christian SS, Brady K: Cord blood acid-base values in breech-presenting infants born vaginally. Obstet Gynecol 78:778, 1991

Christian SS, Brady K, Read JA, Kopelman JN: Vaginal breech delivery: A five-year prospective evaluation of a protocol using computed tomographic pelvimetry. Am J Obstet Gynecol 163:848, 1990

Clausen I, Nielsen KT: Breech position, delivery route and congenital hip dislocation. Acta Obstet Gynecol Scand 67:595, 1988

Confino E, Ismajovich B, Rudick V, David MP: Extradural analgesia in the management of singleton breech delivery. Br J Anaesth 57:892, 1985

Crawford JS, Weaver JB: Anaesthetic management of twin and breech deliveries. Clin Obstet Gynecol 9:291, 1982

Croughan-Minihane MS, Petitti DB, Gordis L, Golditch I: Morbidity among breech infants according to method of delivery. Obstet Gynecol 75:821, 1990

Dorn U: Hip screening in newborn infants. Clinical and ultrasound results. Wiener Klinische Wochenschrift 181(suppl):3, 1990

Drew JH, McKenzie J, Kelly E, Beischer NA: Second twin: Quality of survival if born by breech extraction following internal podalic version. Aust NZ J Obstet Gynaecol 31:111, 1991

Flamm BL, Fried MW, Lonky NM, Giles WS: External cephalic version after previous cesarean section. Am J Obstet Gynecol 165:370, 1991

Fortunato SJ, Mercer LJ, Guzick DS: External cephalic version with tocolysis: Factors associated with success. Obstet Gynecol 72:59, 1988

Gimovsky ML, Petrie RA: Breech presentation: Alternatives to routine C/S. Contemporary Obstet Gynecol 37:35, 1992

Hankins GD, Hammond TL, Snyder RR, Gilstrap LC III: Transverse lie. Am J Perinatol 7:66, 1990

Hanss JW Jr: The efficacy of external cephalic version and its impact on the breech experience. Am J Obstet Gynecol 162:1459, 1990

Hellstrom AC, Nilsson B, Stange L, Nylund L: When does external cephalic version succeed? Acta Obstet Gynecol Scand 69:281, 1990

Hofmeyr GJ: Effect of external cephalic version in late pregnancy on breech presentation and cesarean section rate: A controlled trial. Br J Obstet Gynaecol 90:392, 1983

Hofmeyer GJ: External cephalic version at term: How high are the stakes? Br J Obstet Gynaecol 98:1, 1991

Hommel U, Bellee H, Link M: The validity of parameters in neonatal diagnosis and fetal monitoring of breech deliveries. 1. Neonatal status after breech delivery. Zentralblatt für Gynakologie 111:1293, 1989

Iffy L, Apuzzio JJ, Cohen-Addad N, Zwolska-Demczuk B, Francis-Lane M, Olenczak J: Abdominal rescue after entrapment of the aftercoming head. Am J Obstet Gynecol 154:623, 1986

Kiwisch FH: Beiträge zur Geburtskunde (Würzburg) 1:69, 1846

Krause W, Voigt C, Donczik J, Michels W, Gstottner H: Assisted spontaneous delivery vs Bracht manual aid within the scope of vaginal delivery in breech presentation. Late morbidity in children 5–7 years of age. Zeitschr Geburtshilfe Perinatol 195:76, 1991

Mahomed K, Seeras R, Coulson R: External cephalic version at term. A randomized controlled trial using tocolysis. Br J Obstet Gynaecol 98:8, 1991

Mauriceau F: The method of delivering the woman when the infant presents one or two feet first. In Traite des Maladies des Femmes Grosses, 6th ed. Paris, 1721, p 280

Morrison JC, Myatt RE, Martin JN, Meeks GR, Martin RW, Bucovarz ET, Wiser WL: External cephalic version of the breech presentation under tocolysis. Am J Obstet Gynecol 154:900, 1986

Pinard A: On version by external maneuvers. In Traite de Palper Abdominal. Paris, 1889

Plentl AA, Stone RE: Bracht maneuver. Obstet Gynecol Surv 8:313, 1953

Pugh A: Treatise on midwifery chiefly with regard to the operation. London, 1754

Robertson AW, Kopelman JN, Read JA, Duff P, Magelssen DJ, Dashow EE: External cephalic version at term: Is a tocolytic necessary? Obstet Gynecol 70:896, 1987

Sandberg EC: The Zavanelli maneuver extended: Progression of a revolutionary concept. Am J Obstet Gynecol 158:1347, 1988

Savage JE: Management of the fetal arms in breech extraction. Obstet Gynecol 3:55, 1954

Scaling ST: External cephalic version without tocolysis. Am J Obstet Gynecol 158:1424, 1988

Sherer DM, Menashe M, Palti Z, Aviad I, Ron M: Radiologic evidence of a nuchal arm in the breech-presenting fetus at the onset of labor: An indication for abdominal delivery. Am J Perinatol 6:353, 1989

Smellie W: Smellie's treatise on the theory and practice of midwifery. Vol 1, McClintock AH (ed), London, The New Sydenham Society, 1876, p 305

Tan GW, Jen SW, Tan SL, Salmon YM: A prospective randomised controlled trial of external cephalic version comparing two methods of uterine tocolysis with a non-tocolysis group. Singapore Med J 30, 155, 1989

Thorp JM Jr, Jenkins T, Watson W: Utility of Leopold maneuvers in screening for malpresentation. Obstet Gynecol 78:394, 1991

Tiwary CM: Testicular injury in breech delivery: Possible implications. Urology 34:210, 1989

van de Pavert R, Bennebroek Gravenhorst J, Keirse MJ: The benefit of external version in full-term breech presentation. Nederlands Tijdschrift Voor Geneeskunde 134:2245, 1990

VanDorsten JP: Safe and effective external cephalic version with tocolysis. Contemp Obstet Gynecol 19:44, 1982

VanDorsten JP, Schifrin BS, Wallace RL: Randomized control trial of external cephalic version with tocolysis in late pregnancy. Am J Obstet Gynecol 141:417, 1981

Van Veelen AJ, Van Cappellen AW, Flu PK, Straub MJ, Wallenburg HC: Effect of external cephalic version in late pregnancy on presentation at delivery: A randomized controlled trial. Br J Obstet Gynaecol 96:916, 1989

Vasa R, Kim MR: Fracture of the femur at cesarean section: Case report and review of literature. Am J Perinatol 7:46, 1990

Veit G: On version by external manipulation. Hamburgisches Magazin für die Geburtshilfe, 1907

Walter RS, Donaldson JS, Davis CL, Shkolnick A, Binns HJ, Carroll NC, Brouillette RT: Ultrasound screening of high-risk infants: A method to increase early detection of congenital dysplasia of the hip. Am J Dis Child 146:230, 1992

CHAPTER 26
Cesarean Section and Cesarean Hysterectomy

Cesarean Section

Cesarean section is defined as delivery of the fetus through incisions in the abdominal wall (laparotomy) and the uterine wall (hysterotomy). This definition does not include removal of the fetus from the abdominal cavity in case of rupture of the uterus or abdominal pregnancy.

Indications. The four most frequent indications for cesarean section are (1) repeat procedures, (2) dystocia or failure to progress in labor, (3) breech presentation, and (4) fetal distress. Repeat cesarean sections account for approximately one third of all operations, while failure to progress in labor is the most frequent indication for primary cesarean section in the United States (Neuhoff and associates, 1989; Rosen and colleagues, 1991).

Frequency. The rate for delivery by cesarean section has increased at an accelerated pace over the past 2 decades in the United States and other developed countries (Notzon and co-workers, 1987). In the United States, the rate increased from 4.5 percent in 1965, to 23 percent in 1985, to almost 25 percent in 1988 (Taffel and associates, 1991). According to the National Center for Health Statistics (1992), the rate is decreasing; it was 22.7 percent for the 4.18 million live births in 1990. Cesarean section is now one of the most commonly performed operations in this country. In 1990, the operation was performed 949,000 times. As shown in Figure 26–1, the cesarean section rate for the United States has reached a plateau and may be falling. Specifically, the rate of 23.8 percent in 1989 was not significantly different from the rates for the prior 3 years (Taffel and colleagues, 1991). Reasons for quadrupling of the section rate over about the past two decades are not completely understood, but some explanations include the following.

1. There is *reduced parity,* and almost half of pregnant women are nulliparas. Therefore, an increased number of cesarean sections might be expected for conditions that are more common in nulliparous women.
2. *Older women are having children.* In 1985, approximately 25 percent of births in the United States were in women 30 years or older (Taffel

and co-workers, 1987). The frequency of cesarean section increases with advancing age.
3. *Electronic fetal monitoring* is used extensively and there is little question that it is associated with an increased cesarean section rate compared with intermittent fetal heart rate auscultation.
4. *Breeches.* By 1989 almost 85 percent of all breeches were delivered abdominally (Taffel and associates, 1991).
5. The incidence of *midpelvic vaginal deliveries* has decreased. Between 1972 and 1980, forceps deliveries declined from 37 to 18 percent, while the cesarean section rate increased from 7 to 17 percent (Placek and colleagues, 1983).
6. It is a widely held belief that increased cesarean delivery rates will result in decreased **perinatal mortality.**
7. There is increasing concern for *malpractice litigation.* An apparently widely held belief is that cesarean section will in itself prevent or decrease the number of lawsuits. Unfortunately, obstetrical litigation cases have not decreased proportionately with the increased cesarean section rate.
8. *Socioeconomic factors* have a significant role in the cesarean section rate. Gould and associates (1989) reported that the primary section rate in Los Angeles County was 23 percent for women from areas with a median family income of more than $30,000 compared with 13 percent for women with a median income less than $11,000. Similarly, Stafford (1990) reported significantly lower vaginal births after a prior cesarean section comparing for-profit hospitals with university hospitals, patients with private insurance with indigent patients, and low-volume to high-volume hospitals.

Because failure to progress in labor or dystocia and repeat operations account for approximately two thirds of all cesarean deliveries, it seems logical to address these two areas if the cesarean section rate is to be reduced. Between 1980 and 1988, more than three fourths of the 16.5 to 24.7 percent increase in the cesarean section rate was the consequence of repeat sections and dystocia (Table 26–1). The contribution of

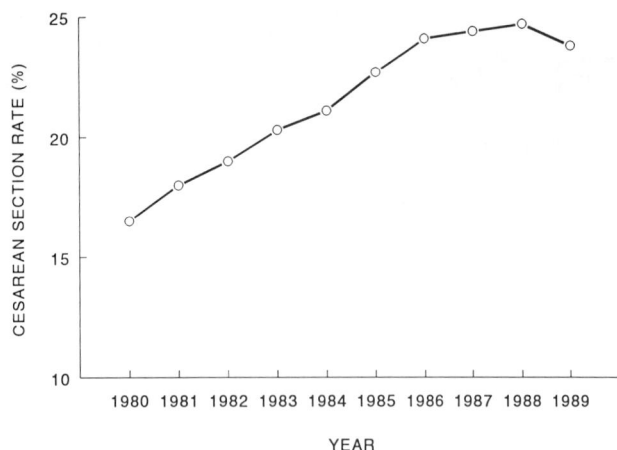

Fig. 26–1. The cesarean section rate for the United States, 1980 through 1989. (Adapted from Notzon and colleagues, 1987, and Taffel and associates, 1991).

TABLE 26–2. CESAREAN SECTION RATES FOR VARIOUS COMPLICATIONS

	Percentage of All Deliveries		Percent by Cesarean Section	
	1980	*1989*	*1980*	*1989*
Fetopelvic disproportion	4.1	4.2	96	99
Obstructed labor	1.1	4.3	26	66
Abnormal labor or inertia	3.0	7.4	54	43
Breech presentation	3.2	4.0	67	84
Fetal distress	1.7	8.8	67	46
Previous cesarean section	5.1	10.4	97	82

Adapted from Taffel and colleagues (1991).

each indication to the total section rate is a function of two variables: (1) the **change in incidence** of the indication and (2) the **change in the cesarean section rate** for the indication. In 1980, 51 percent of all deliveries had one or more complications, but by 1985 this had increased to 64 percent (Taffel and co-workers, 1987).

The cesarean section rates for various obstetrical complications are summarized in Table 26–2. Not surprisingly, almost all of the women with a diagnosis of fetopelvic disproportion were delivered by cesarean section in both 1980 and 1989. In 1989, 84 percent of the women with breech presentations were delivered by cesarean section compared with 67 percent in 1980. The section rate for three indications—fetal distress, and previous cesarean section, and abnormal labor or inertia—actually decreased from 1980 to 1989. This probably accounts for the leveling off of the current

cesarean section rate. Before this plateau was reached, it had been predicted that the cesarean rate would be as high as 40 percent by the year 2000 (Placek and colleagues, 1987).

Regardless of indications cited for cesarean section, its increased frequency has been accompanied by an absolute decrease in the perinatal mortality rate. Although the increased section rate may have contributed to this, many other factors were likely responsible, such as better prenatal care and advances in neonatal care. A report by O'Driscoll and Foley (1983) support the concept that the increased cesarean section rate was *not* responsible for decreased perinatal mortality. These authors studied the correlation of decreases in perinatal mortality and the increase in cesarean section rates from 1965 to 1980 in the United States and at the National Maternity Hospital in Dublin, Ireland (Fig. 26–2). They reported that while cesarean section rates were increasing in the United States, from less than 5 percent in 1965 to more than 15 percent in 1980, in Dublin the rate remained virtually unchanged, increasing from 4.1 to 4.8 percent from 1965 to 1980. Despite the nearly unchanged rate in Dublin, perinatal mortality fell from

TABLE 26–1. CESAREAN SECTION RATES[a] **FOR SELECTED INDICATIONS IN THE UNITED STATES**

	1980		1985		Increase 1980 to 1988	
Indication	*Rate*	*%*	*Rate*	*%*	*Rate*	*%*
Repeat section	4.9	30	9.0	36	4.1	50
Dystocia	4.8	30	7.6	31	2.8	34
Fetal distress	0.8	5	2.3	9	1.5	18
Breech	2.0	12	2.5	10	0.5	6
All other	4.0	24	3.3	13	−0.7	−8
Totals	16.5	100	24.7	100	8.2	100

[a] Cesarean sections per 100 deliveries for stated indication.
Modified from Taffel and associates (1987, 1991) and Myers and Gleicher (1990).

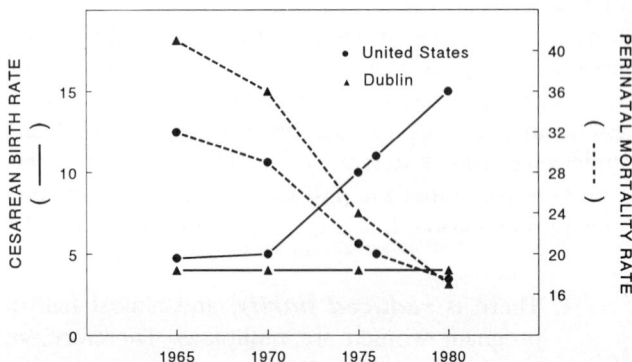

Fig. 26–2. Cesarean birth rates per 100 deliveries are represented by *solid lines* and perinatal mortality rates per 1000 deliveries by *broken lines* for the United States (*circles*), according to Bottoms and co-workers (1980), and for the National Maternity Hospital, Dublin (*triangles*). (Modified from O'Driscoll and Foley, 1983.)

42.1 to 16.8 per 1000 infants. The increased rate of cesarean sections reported in the United States supposedly did not significantly contribute to the simultaneously observed reduction in perinatal mortality rates.

The lower cesarean section rate in Dublin was attributed to lower frequencies of cesarean section for dystocia, repeat cesarean section, and breech delivery. O'Driscoll and associates (1969, 1973, 1984) attributed their apparent success to a more aggressive management of labor dystocias with oxytocin in the nulliparous woman whose uterus they considered to be *"almost immune to rupture except by manipulation."* Other major factors included allowing women with a previous transverse uterine incision a trial of labor, which proved successful in 60 percent of cases; and a liberal trial of labor policy for breech presentations. In 1983, O'Driscoll and Foley stated that "the high incidence of cesarean section now prevalent in the United States is not supported by results because by analogy with Dublin, the same perinatal mortality rates can be achieved with less than one third the number of sections now performed." In follow-up reports from the United States, Leveno and colleagues (1985, 1989) reported that there were marked differences between populations in certain parts of Ireland and the United States. For example, in a review of the perinatal mortality rates of the obstetrical services in Dublin and Parkland Hospital for 1983 through 1985, there were significantly more low birthweight infants born to the Dallas women (Table 26–3). As emphasized by these investigators, caution must be used when attempting to compare perinatal mortality between medical centers from different continents.

It seems unlikely that such low cesarean section rates as those reported from Dublin will be seen in the United States. One reason for this is the prevailing enthusiasm for small families, which will likely result in many women whose first infants were delivered by cesarean section electing to have a repeat section with tubal sterilization. Another reason is the reluctance to allow vaginal delivery for breech presentations. Even if the liberal standards applied to frank breech presentations recommended by Collea and associates (1980)

were applied, we would expect only a 15 to 30 percent decrease in the section rate for all breeches. However, vaginal delivery subsequent to cesarean section is safe and efficacious, in most cases, and it is becoming increasingly more popular (Taffel and associates, 1991).

The final answers with respect to the frequency, indications, and safety as well as the legal, ethical, and economical consequences of cesarean section are unlikely to become apparent for several years. To the credit of the obstetrical community, these questions continue to be addressed, and the literature is replete with articles that deal with them. There now are several reports by clinical investigators of successful attempts to reduce the incidence of cesarean section without increasing perinatal mortality and morbidity (Lopez-Zeno and colleagues, 1992; Neuhoff and associates, 1989).

Maternal Mortality. The most remarkable report of the safety of cesarean delivery is that from the Boston Hospital for Women by Frigoletto and associates (1980). These authors reported more than 10,000 consecutive cesarean deliveries with no maternal deaths. Certainly, maternal and perinatal mortality and morbidity typically are higher with cesarean section than with vaginal delivery, if for no other reason than because of the complication that led to the cesarean section, as well as because of increased risks inherent in abdominal delivery.

Sachs and co-workers (1988) attributed as a direct cause only 7 of 27 deaths following more than 121,000 cesarean sections performed in Massachusetts from 1976 through 1984. Although this mortality rate was 22 per 100,000 for all cesarean sections, it was only 5.8 per 100,000 for deaths directly due to cesarean delivery. More recently, Lilford and co-workers (1990) reported a relative risk of seven for maternal mortality with cesarean section compared with vaginal delivery. When significant complications associated with pregnancy were excluded, the relative risk was five. Of interest was that nonelective cesarean deliveries were associated with a relative risk of 2.3 for mortality compared with elective operations. This was decreased further to 1.4 after exclusions of complications. However, even a relatively low operative mortality rate must be considered excessive, because the majority of these deaths are in young, otherwise healthy women.

The major threats to women undergoing cesarean section have been anesthesia, infection with sepsis, and thromboembolic episodes. Aspiration pneumonia, which previously had been the leading cause of postoperative cesarean section deaths in many hospitals, has decreased significantly in frequency with the widespread use of preoperative antacids and regional analgesia. Despite such efforts to decrease mortality, it is unlikely that deaths from either cesarean or vaginal delivery can be further reduced in severely compromised women who elect, rightly or not, to pursue pregnancies despite their

TABLE 26–3. PERINATAL MORBIDITY RATES OF TWO OBSTETRICAL SERVICES IN DUBLIN, IRELAND AND DALLAS, TEXAS (1983–1985)

Factor	National Maternity Hospital	Parkland Memorial Hospital
Total births	23,590	36,001
Low-birthweight infants		
Incidence	39/1000	118/1000
Perinatal mortality	244/1000	115/1000
Birthweight 2500 g or more	22,661	31,770
Perinatal mortality	7/1000	3/1000

Adapted from Leveno and associates (1989).

already tenuous medical status. Therefore, it must be considered whether the death was related to a complication of the delivery itself, or was due at least in part to an underlying factor, such as heart disease.

Maternal Morbidity. Even when morbidity and mortality associated with the complication that led to cesarean section are excluded, maternal morbidity is more frequent and likely to be more severe following cesarean section than following vaginal delivery (Rubin and co-workers, 1981). The common causes of morbidity from cesarean delivery are infection, hemorrhage, and injury to the urinary tract.

Perinatal Mortality. The frequency of stillbirth and neonatal mortality will depend on the underlying reason for the cesarean section and the gestational age of the fetus. Although the decreasing perinatal mortality rate observed since the mid-1960s in many instances has been associated with, and has even been attributed to, the marked increase in cesarean section rates in the United States, O'Driscoll and Foley (1983) have questioned this assumption.

Perinatal Morbidity. It must be emphasized that cesarean section is not a guarantee against fetal injury. For example, the head of a preterm breech can be entrapped in a small transverse uterine incision that was judged incorrectly to be large enough for delivery. This may result in injury to the fetal spinal cord or brain, and may lead to extension of the uterine incision into the uterine vessels. The fetus may also be wounded during the incision into the uterus. Depressed skull fractures, femur fractures, and fractures of other limb bones may be found in newborns delivered by cesarean section (Alexander, 1987; Kaplan, 1987; Skajaa, 1987; Vasa, 1990, and their colleagues). The so-called *ping-pong fracture* of the fetal skull may occur when the head is being lifted out of the pelvis or pushed up from below at the time of cesarean section.

Although respiratory distress has been claimed to be higher for repeat cesarean section than for vaginal delivery, it is unlikely that there is a significant difference when gestational ages of the fetuses are identical and fetal hypoxia and acidosis are avoided.

Timing of Repeat Cesarean Section. There are advantages to a predetermined time for carrying out repeat cesarean sections. For example, the family can better arrange for assistance in caring for other children and for the care of the mother and infant after leaving the hospital. Importantly, an alert team can be assembled more easily to provide optimal care, including anesthesia, infant resuscitation if needed, and subsequent newborn care. Conversely, with emergency repeat cesarean section, an operating room may not be immediately available, or the mother may have very recently

eaten, which increases the anesthetic risk. Of considerable importance when dealing with a woman with a previous cesarean section is whether a vertical uterine incision was made that might rupture with the onset of labor, resulting in the death of the fetus and serious morbidity or even death of the mother. The likelihood of these disastrous consequences from rupture of a transverse scar in the lower uterine segment is very low.

Iatrogenic Preterm Delivery. Elective termination of pregnancy with the delivery of a preterm infant has been a major problem. This unfortunate circumstance has led some to routinely practice amniocentesis for pulmonary maturity studies before any elective delivery. It is now well established that amnionic fluid studies to assure fetal maturity are unnecessary in women with good gestational dating criteria. The Committee on Obstetrics of the American College of Obstetricians and Gynecologists (1990) has published guidelines for assessment of fetal pulmonary maturity prior to elective cesarean section or induction of labor. According to the committee, fetal maturity can be assumed if 39 weeks have elapsed since a "normal" last menstrual period and if the clinical criteria are supported by one of the laboratory parameters listed in Table 26–4.

For women with uncertain or unverified menstrual periods, and in whom early gestational dating by ultrasound was not performed, timing of delivery is best determined either by assuring pulmonary maturity with determination of the lecithin-sphingomyelin (L/S) ratio (Chap. 44, p. 993) or by awaiting spontaneous labor.

Vaginal Delivery Subsequent to Cesarean Section. There is no doubt that vaginal delivery will most often prove to be safe following a previous cesarean section. Moreover, the rate of vaginal births after cesarean section has increased in the United States from approximately 7 percent in 1985 to 18.5 percent in 1989 (Taffel and associates, 1991). Numerous reports have been published in the past decade that attest to the safety and efficacy of vaginal delivery in these women. Rosen and

TABLE 26–4. CLINICAL AND LABORATORY CRITERIA FOR FETAL MATURITY

Clinical Criteria
Documentation of fetal heart tones for 20 weeks with a fetoscope or up to 30 weeks with a Doppler
Establishment of uterine size by 16 weeks' gestation

Laboratory Criteria
36 weeks have elapsed since a positive urine pregnancy test
Ultrasound examination
   Crown–rump measurement at 6 to 12 weeks' gestation
   Estimation of gestational age prior to 24 weeks' gestation

---

Adapted from the American College of Obstetricians and Gynecologists (1990), with permission.

associates (1991), in an excellent review, summarized results from a meta-analysis of 31 studies totalling 11,417 women with prior cesarean sections. They concluded that uterine dehiscence or rupture is not significantly related to the intended birth route, the use of oxytocin, or the presence of an unknown uterine scar (Chap. 23, p. 546).

Even with the numerous reports of successful outcomes, several areas of management remain controversial:

1. How many cesarean sections can be done before it is unsafe to allow a trial of labor?
2. What is the incidence of uterine rupture or scar dehiscence?
3. Following vaginal delivery, should uterine exploration be performed routinely? If so, what should be done if a uterine defect is discovered?
4. If the woman had a cesarean section for a recurrent problem such as cephalopelvic disproportion, should a trial of labor be allowed?
5. Can epidural analgesia be used safely for a trial of labor?
6. Can oxytocin be used safely to induce or augment labor?
7. Should women with multifetal gestation be allowed a trial of labor?
8. Should women with a breech presentation be allowed a trial of labor?
9. What standards should be established for obstetrical services before a trial of labor is justified?

Attitudes and Practices. The American College of Obstetricians and Gynecologists completed a survey in 1990 regarding the attitude and practices of its Fellows with regard to vaginal birth after a previous cesarean section. According to this survey, 92 percent of the obstetricians surveyed encouraged their patients to attempt a vaginal birth after cesarean section. Of the patients offered a trial of vaginal delivery, approximately 58 percent accepted this option, and two thirds of these could be expected to successfully deliver vaginally. Perhaps not surprisingly, physicians less than 40 years of age and those in practice for less than 10 years tended to encourage vaginal delivery more often than older physicians and those in practice for longer than 10 years. Of interest, although almost half of all obstetrical malpractice claims in 1988 and 1989 involved cesarean sections, less than 1 percent were associated with a woman delivered vaginally after a prior cesarean section (American College of Obstetricians and Gynecologists, 1990).

Number and Type of Cesarean Sections. Vaginal delivery subsequent to a cesarean section can be carried out safely for women who have had one previous low transverse uterine incision without an extension. Studies have been published describing trials of labor in women with more than one cesarean section, and in most of these, the outcomes have been good and the complications minimal (Farmakides and associates, 1987; Phelan and colleagues, 1989; Pruett and coworkers, 1988). Phelan and associates (1989) reviewed the outcomes in 501 women who underwent a trial of labor following two previous cesarean deliveries. Of these, 69 percent delivered vaginally. The incidence of uterine dehiscence was 1.8 percent for women undergoing a trial of labor compared with 4.6 percent for those who did not. The one case of uterine rupture was in the "no trial of labor" group.

Uterine Scar Separation. The issue that has most often prevented physicians from allowing women to undergo a vaginal delivery following a cesarean section has been the fear of uterine rupture or dehiscence. O'Sullivan and co-workers (1981) reviewed over 8000 deliveries and added several hundred of their own patients. They reported that frank uterine rupture, or at least uterine dehiscence, occurred in 1.8 percent of women undergoing cesarean section compared with only 0.5 percent of women undergoing vaginal delivery. They concluded that vaginal delivery was not only as safe as an elective repeat cesarean section but was the preferred method of management in carefully selected women. Their conclusions were confirmed by the meta-analysis of Rosen and colleagues (1991), in which the rate of uterine rupture or dehiscence was 1.8 percent for all trials of labor, 1.2 percent for vaginal births after cesarean, and 1.9 percent for elective repeat cesarean.

However, as emphasized in three recent publications, when uterine rupture does occur in association with a trial of labor following a previous cesarean section, the results may be catastrophic, with an increase in the frequency of perinatal death, neurological sequelae in surviving neonates, and in the number of women requiring hysterectomy (Jones and co-workers, 1991; Pitkin, 1991; Scott, 1991). We also have experienced several catastrophic uterine ruptures in such women at Parkland Hospital undergoing a trial of labor. These often manifested by the sudden onset of fetal heart rate bradycardia requiring emergency cesarean section. Unfortunately, the outcome has not always been good in these cases (Chapter 23, p. 546).

Uterine Exploration. After vaginal delivery in a woman with a previous cesarean section, many recommend exploration of the uterine cavity. The issues to be assessed at the time of uterine exploration are whether there is a defect and, if so, whether it is connected with the peritoneal cavity. If it is contiguous with the peritoneal cavity and the woman manifests signs of hemodynamic instability, or if there is obvious excessive bleeding, laparotomy and either repair of the defect or hysterectomy is performed. If there is a defect discovered in the uterine wall that does not open into the peritoneal cavity, and it is small and not bleeding, repair probably is unnecessary. Under these circumstances, the woman is observed closely with frequent vital signs and serial hematocrit determinations. Most such patients do well without uterine repair. But what about a subsequent pregnancy in such a woman with a known uterine defect? Unfortunately, there is very little valid information available, and the decision to allow a trial of labor must be made on an individual basis (American College of Obstetricians and Gynecologists, 1988).

Recurrent Indications for Cesarean Section. The issue of whether or not an indication should be considered recurrent was controversial until Seitchik and Ramakrishna (1982) reported that women previously delivered by cesarean section for "dystocia" subsequently could be delivered vaginally. Flamm (1985) reviewed 13 studies and classified their indications for cesarean section as recurrent (cephalopelvic disproportion or failure to progress) or other nonrecurring causes. The success rate, defined as vaginal delivery, was 61 percent in 1064 women with recurring causes and 78 percent of 1808 with nonrecurring causes. Flamm and associates (1988) later confirmed these results. Table 26–5 summarizes five separate reports addressing this issue. The overall prognosis for vaginal delivery was 72 percent, and success could be anticipated in 63 percent of women who had cesarean sections for dystocia compared with 79 percent without recurring indications. Duff and colleagues (1988) confirmed these findings and reported that 68 percent of women with a prior cesarean section for dystocia delivered vaginally compared with 81 percent who had previously undergone abdominal delivery for other indications.

Epidural Analgesia. Most often, epidural analgesia is not withheld in women undergoing a trial of labor. Whereas Ruddick and co-workers (1984) reported a woman in whom uterine rupture was accompanied by pain despite epidural analgesia, Uppington (1983) reported another woman who felt no pain with rupture.

In both, oxytocin was given and fetal distress developed rapidly following uterine rupture, so that both were diagnosed promptly. The risk of epidural analgesia inhibiting maternal cardiovascular responses to hemorrhage from sympathetic blockade has not been adequately studied; however, the possibility is worrisome.

Flamm (1985) reported that 38 percent of 1692 women were given epidural analgesia for a trial of labor. There were no maternal or fetal deaths, but the two cases of uterine rupture cited above were recorded. These two fetuses survived because of early recognition of fetal distress in both. The incidence of forceps and vacuum deliveries is increased in women who are given epidural analgesia, and the need for oxytocin augmentation following an epidural block is increased appreciably. Farmer and colleagues (1991) reported 115 uterine ruptures or dehiscences in 7598 women undergoing a trial of labor after previous cesarean. Only 8 percent of these women had bleeding and abdominal pain. Prolonged fetal heart rate decelerations were present in 70 percent of the labors associated with scar separations.

If epidural analgesia is used, internal electronic monitoring of fetal heart rate and intrauterine pressure is recommended along with **continuous bedside attendance by an obstetrical nurse or the physician.**

Oxytocin. The issue of the safety of oxytocin induction or augmentation of labor is not clearly resolved. Flamm and co-workers (1987) reported 64 percent successful vaginal deliveries in 581 trials of labor in which oxytocin was given. There were no maternal or perinatal deaths, but there were two uterine ruptures. At Parkland Hospital, we reviewed 307 women with a previous cesarean section who underwent a trial of labor and were given oxytocin. There were 3 overt uterine ruptures, a rate of approximately 1 percent. In their meta-analysis, Rosen and associates (1991) found that oxytocin did not increase the risk of dehiscence or rupture. If oxytocin is used, strict criteria should be followed including internal electronic monitoring of fetal heart rate and

TABLE 26–5. TRIAL OF LABOR RELATED TO INDICATIONS FOR A PREVIOUS CESAREAN SECTION

Study	Overall Success for Trial of Labor No. (%)	Indication for Primary Cesarean Section			
		Dystocia[a] No. (%)	Breech No. (%)	Fetal Distress No. (%)	Other Nonrecurring No. (%)
Clark and colleagues, 1984	240/308 (78)	39/61 (64)	81/94 (86)	31/38 (61)	69/52 (75)
Jarrell and associates, 1985	142/216 (66)	42/78 (54)	54/72 (75)		
Mootabar and co-workers, 1984	161/296 (54)	77/163 (47)			75/123 (61)
Paul and collaborators, 1985	614/751 (82)	245/319 (77)	103/135 (91)	56/67 (84)	
Vengadasalam, 1986	176/271 (65)	38/82 (46)	33/42 (79)	68/91 (75)	37/56 (52)
Totals	1333/1842 (72)	441/703 (63)	291/343 (85)	155/196 (79)	181/271 (67)
Total nonrecurring = 627/810 (79)					

[a] Includes cephalopelvic disproportion and failure to progress.

intrauterine pressures and a limitation of the total dose of oxytocin (Clark and associates, 1984; Paul and colleagues, 1985; Vengadasalam, 1986).

Multifetal Gestation. Strong and associates (1989) reported 18 (72 percent) of 25 women with twin gestations and a previous cesarean section had a successful vaginal delivery of both infants. The dehiscence rate was 4 percent compared with 2 percent in these women with singleton pregnancies. There was no increase in either maternal or perinatal morbidity. Because any condition that results in uterine overdistension increases the risk of rupturing a uterine scar, it would seem reasonable to repeat the cesarean section in most women with twins. Those with multifetal gestations who choose to undergo an attempted vaginal birth should do so only with continuous bedside attendance by a physician or qualified attendant in a hospital capable of performing an emergency cesarean section.

Abnormal Presentation. With the possible exception of a frank breech presentation, repeat cesarean section generally is preferred by most clinicians for women with a previous cesarean section and with an abnormality in fetal lie or position. Ophir and colleagues (1989) have reviewed their experience with 71 breech deliveries after previous cesarean section. Of these, 47 (66 percent) were allowed a trial of labor and 37 delivered vaginally. Neonatal morbidity was not increased in the vaginal delivery group.

Flamm and associates (1991) have presented their experience with external cephalic version in 56 women with a prior cesarean delivery. The version was successful in 82 percent of women, and 65 percent of these had a successful vaginal delivery without serious complications.

Guidelines for a Trial of Labor. The question is not whether a woman can deliver vaginally following a previous cesarean section, but rather the criteria that should be applied and rigidly enforced in order to allow her to labor safely. Pitkin (1991) aptly stated: "Many women with previous cesarean can be delivered vaginally and thereby gain substantial advantage, but neither the decision for trial of labor nor management during labor should be arrived at in a cavalier or superficial manner." Specific guidelines have been revised by the Committee on Obstetrics (1988) of the American College of Obstetricians and Gynecologists. **Unlike prior recommendations, it is now felt that women with one prior transverse cesarean section should be counseled to undergo a trial of labor.** Those with two prior cesarean sections are not discouraged from a trial of labor provided there is no other contraindication. The committee further concluded that oxytocin induction or augmentation and epidural analgesia are not contraindicated. Unanswered issues include those of prior low vertical incisions (prior classical incisions contraindicate a trial of labor), twins, breeches, and the singleton fetus with an estimated weight of more than 4000 g.

If a woman is to undergo a trial of labor following a cesarean section, appropriate technical support must be available in the hospital. There should be an adequate blood bank continuously staffed. Electronic fetal heart rate and intrauterine pressure monitoring should be available. There should be adequate facilities and personnel to begin an emergency cesarean section.

The obstetrician in his or her zeal to abandon the old adage *"Once a cesarean section, always a cesarean section,"* should avoid substituting the even more inappropriate motto *"Once a cesarean delivery, never again a cesarean delivery!"*

Technique of Cesarean Section

Type of Uterine Incision. The so-called classical cesarean incision, a vertical incision into the body of the uterus above the lower uterine segment and reaching the uterine fundus, is seldom used today. Most always the incision is made in the lower uterine segment transversely (Kerr, 1926) or, less often, vertically (Krönig, 1912). The lower segment transverse incision has the advantage of requiring only modest dissection of the bladder from the underlying myometrium. If the incision extends laterally, the laceration may involve one or both of the uterine vessels. The low vertical incision may be extended upward so that in those circumstances where more room is needed, the incision can be carried into the body of the uterus; otherwise, it is a less desirable incision. More extensive dissection of the bladder is necessary to keep the vertical incision within the lower uterine segment. Moreover, if the vertical incision extends downward, it may tear through the cervix into the vagina and possibly involve the bladder. Importantly, during the next pregnancy the vertical incision is much more likely than is the transverse incision to rupture, especially during labor.

Lower Segment Transverse Incision. For a cephalic presentation, a transverse incision through the lower uterine segment is most often the operation of choice. Generally, the transverse incision (1) results in less blood loss, (2) is easier to repair, (3) is located at a site least likely to rupture with extrusion of the fetus into the abdominal cavity during a subsequent pregnancy, and (4) does not promote adherence of bowel or omentum to the incisional line.

Choice of Abdominal Incisions. An infraumbilical midline vertical incision is quickest to make. The incision should be of sufficient length to allow delivery of the infant without difficulty. Therefore, its length should correspond with the estimated fetal size. Sharp dissection is performed to the level of the anterior rectus sheath, which is freed of subcutaneous fat to expose a strip of fascia in the midline about 2 cm wide. Some surgeons prefer to incise the rectus sheath with the scalpel throughout the length of the fascial incision. Others prefer to make a small opening and then incise the fascial layer with scissors. The rectus and the pyramidalis muscles are separated in the midline by sharp and blunt dissection to expose transversalis fascia and peritoneum.

The transversalis fascia and preperitoneal fat are dissected carefully to reach the underlying peritoneum. The peritoneum near the upper end of the incision is opened carefully. Some elevate the peritoneum with two hemostats placed about 2 cm apart. The tented fold of peritoneum between the clamps is then visualized and palpated to be sure that omentum, bowel, or bladder are not adjacent. In women who have had previous intra-abdominal surgery, including cesarean section, omentum or even bowel may be adherent to the undersurface of the peritoneum. The peritoneum is incised superiorly to the upper pole of the incision and downward to just above the peritoneal reflection over the bladder.

With the modified **Pfannenstiel** incision, the skin and subcutaneous tissue are incised using a lower transverse, slightly curvilinear incision. The incision is made at the level of the pubic hairline and is extended somewhat beyond the lateral borders of the rectus muscles. After the subcutaneous tissue has been separated from the underlying fascia for 1 cm or so on each side, the fascia is incised transversely the full length of the incision. The superior and inferior edges of the fascia are grasped with suitable clamps and then elevated by the assistant as the operator separates the fascial sheath from the underlying rectus muscles by blunt dissection with the scalpel handle. Blood vessels coursing between the muscles and fascia are clamped, cut, and ligated. It is imperative that meticulous hemostasis be achieved. The separation is carried to near the umbilicus sufficient to permit an adequate midline longitudinal incision of the peritoneum. The rectus muscles are separated in the midline to expose the underlying peritoneum. The peritoneum is opened as discussed above. Closure in layers is carried out the same as with a vertical incision.

The cosmetic advantage of the transverse skin incision is apparent. Moreover, the incision is said to be stronger, with less likelihood of dehiscence or hernia formation. There are, nonetheless, disadvantages in its use. Exposure of the pregnant uterus and appendages in some women is not as good as with a vertical incision. Whenever more room is needed, the vertical incision can be rapidly extended around and above the umbilicus, whereas the Pfannenstiel incision cannot. If the woman is obese, the operative field is even more restricted. Therefore, Pfannenstiel incisions tend to be used for thin women by operators who have achieved technical expertise, while the vertical incision is often utilized whenever rapid delivery is indicated or the woman is obese. It is not appropriate to compare the vertical incision under these more adverse conditions to the transverse incision carried out under much more favorable circumstances. Importantly, at the time of repeat cesarean section, reentry through a Pfannenstiel incision is likely to be more time consuming because of scarring.

When a transverse incision is desired and more room is needed, the **Maylard incision** provides a safe option (Ayers and Morley, 1987). This latter incision also may be especially useful in women with significant scarring resulting from previous Pfannenstiel incisions. In the study by Ayers and Morley (1987), the mean incision length was 18.3 cm with the Maylard incision compared with 14.0 cm for the Pfannenstiel incision.

Uterine Incision. Commonly, the uterus is found to be dextrorotated so that the left round ligament is more anterior and closer to the midline than the right. Some operators prefer to lay a moistened laparotomy pack in each lateral peritoneal gutter to absorb amnionic fluid and blood that escape from the opened uterus. This technique may be beneficial, especially in the presence of thick meconium or infected amnionic fluid.

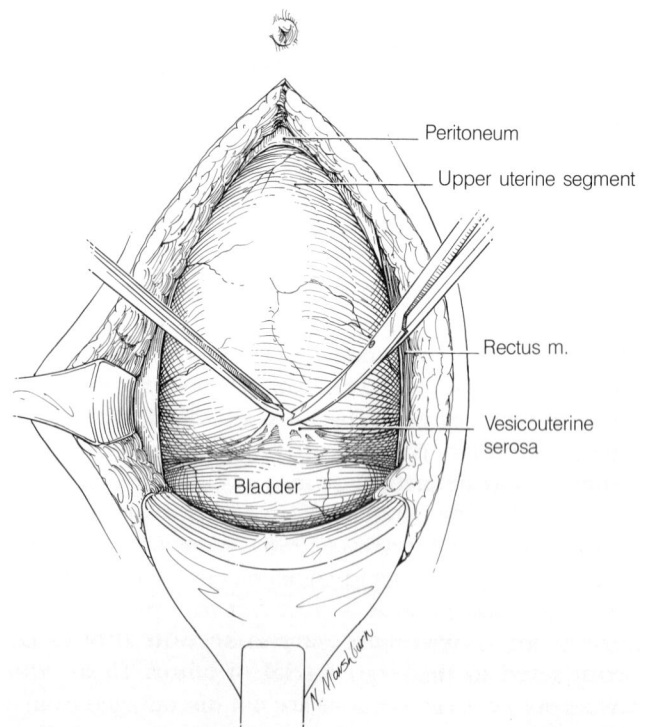

Fig. 26–3. The loose vesicouterine serosa is grasped with the forceps. The hemostat tip points to the upper margin of the bladder. The retractor is firm against the symphysis.

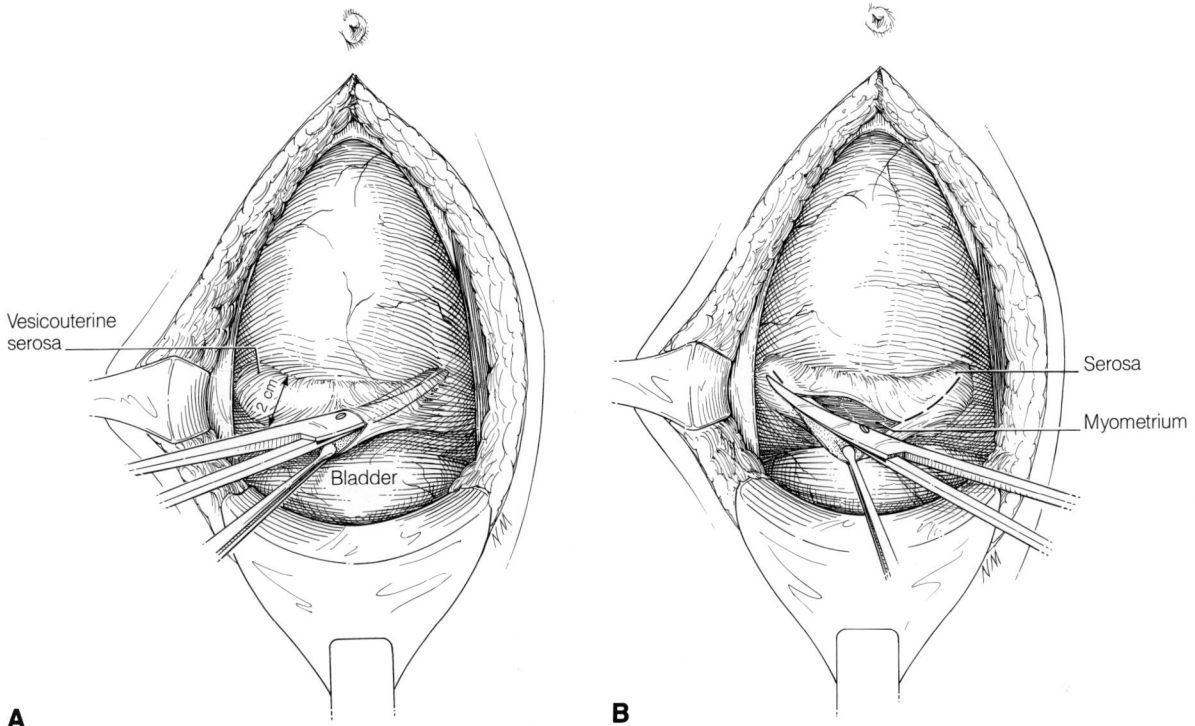

Fig. 26–4. The loose serosa above the upper margin of the bladder is elevated and incised laterally.

The typically rather loose reflection of peritoneum above the upper margin of the bladder and overlying the anterior lower uterine segment is grasped in the midline with forceps and incised with a scalpel or scissors (Fig. 26–3). Scissors are inserted between the serosa and myometrium of the lower uterine segment and are pushed laterally from the midline, while partially opening the blades intermittently, to separate a 2-cm-wide strip of serosa, which is then incised. As the lateral margin on each side is approached, the scissors are aimed somewhat more cephalad (Fig. 26–4). The lower flap of peritoneum is elevated and the bladder is gently separated by blunt or sharp dissection from the underlying myometrium (Fig. 26–5). In general, the separation of bladder should not exceed 5 cm in depth and usually less. It is possible, especially with an effaced, dilated cervix, to dissect downward so deeply as inadvertently to expose and then enter the underlying vagina rather than the lower uterine segment (Goodlin and co-workers, 1982).

The uterus is opened through the lower uterine segment about 2 cm above the detached bladder. The uterine incision can be made by a variety of techniques. Each is initiated by incising with a scalpel the exposed lower uterine segment transversely for 2 cm or so halfway between the lateral margins. This must be done carefully so as to cut completely through the uterine wall but not deeply enough to wound the underlying fetus (Fig. 26–6). Once the uterus is opened, the incision can be extended by cutting laterally and then slightly upward with bandage scissors; or when the

lower uterine segment is thin, the entry incision can be extended by simply spreading the incision, using lateral and upward pressure applied with each index finger (Fig. 26–7). *It is very important to make the uterine incision large enough to allow delivery of the head and trunk of the fetus without either tearing into or having to cut into the uterine arteries and veins that course through the lateral margins of the uterus.* If the placenta is encountered in the line of incision, it must either be detached or in-

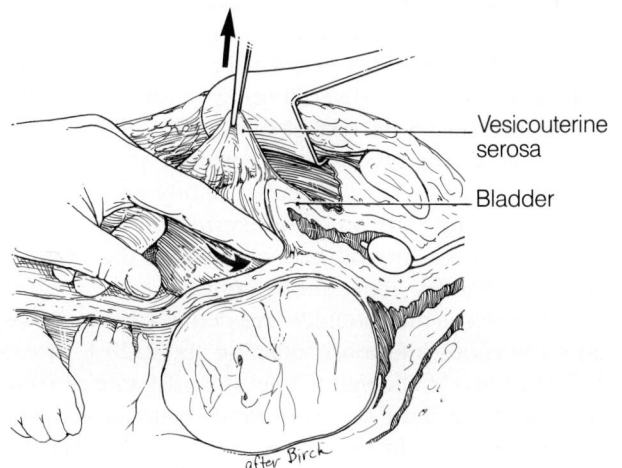

Fig. 26–5. Low-segment cesarean section. Cross section showing dissection of bladder off uterus to expose lower uterine segment.

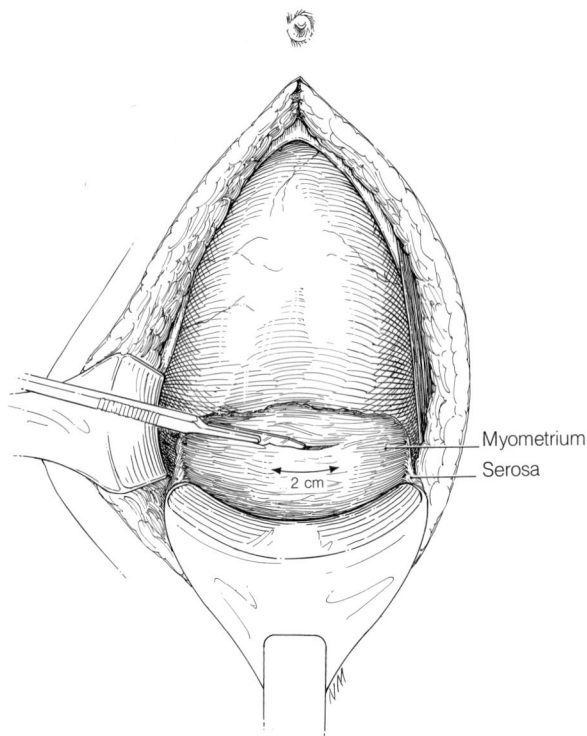

Fig. 26–6. The myometrium is being incised carefully to avoid cutting the fetal head.

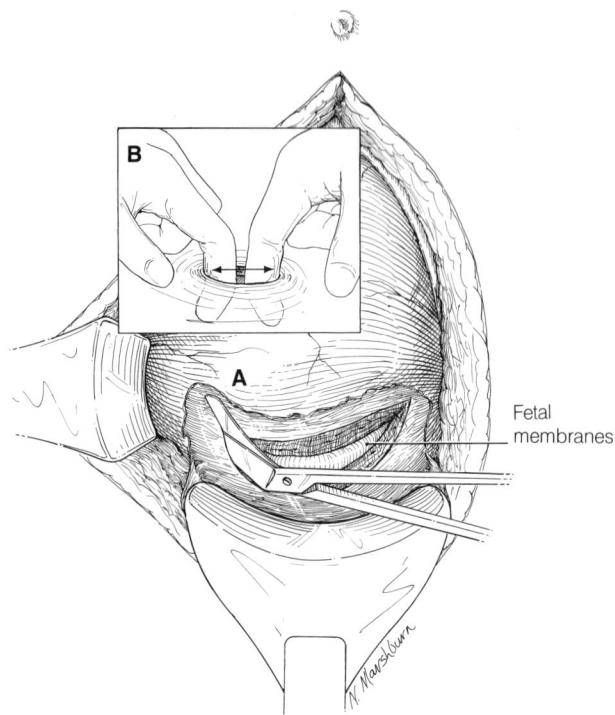

Fig. 26–7. After entering the uterine cavity, the incision is extended laterally with either fingers or bandage scissors.

cised. When the placenta is incised, fetal hemorrhage may be severe; thus, the cord should be clamped as soon as possible in such cases.

Delivery of the Infant. If the vertex is presenting, a hand is slipped into the uterine cavity between the symphysis and fetal head, and the head is elevated gently with the fingers and palm through the incision aided by modest transabdominal fundal pressure (Fig. 26–8). To minimize aspiration by the fetus of amnionic fluid and its contents, the exposed nares and mouth are aspirated with a bulb syringe before the thorax is delivered. The shoulders then are delivered using gentle traction plus fundal pressure. The rest of the body readily follows.

After a long labor with cephalopelvic disproportion, the fetal head may be rather tightly wedged in the birth canal. Upward pressure exerted through the vagina by an assistant will help to dislodge the head and allow its delivery above the symphysis.

As soon as the shoulders are delivered (Fig. 26–9), an intravenous infusion containing about 20 U of oxytocin per liter is allowed to flow at a brisk rate of 10 mL per minute until the uterus contracts satisfactorily, after which the rate can be reduced. The cord is clamped with the infant held at the level of the abdominal wall, and the infant is given to the member of the team who will conduct resuscitative efforts as they are needed.

If the fetus is not presenting as a vertex, or if there are multiple fetuses or a very immature fetus of a woman who has had no labor, a vertical incision through the lower segment may, at times, prove to be advantageous. The fetal legs must be carefully distinguished from the arms to avoid premature extraction of an arm and a difficult delivery of the rest of the fetus.

The uterine incision is observed for any vigorously bleeding sites. These should be promptly clamped with Pennington or ring forceps, or similar instruments. The placenta should be removed promptly manually, unless it is separating spontaneously (Fig. 26–10). Fundal massage, begun as soon as the fetus is delivered, reduces bleeding and hastens delivery of the placenta.

Repair of the Uterus. After delivery of the placenta, the uterus may be lifted through the incision onto the draped abdominal wall and the fundus covered with a moistened laparotomy pack. Although some clinicians prefer to avoid this latter step, uterine exteriorization often has advantages that outweigh any disadvantages. The relaxing uterus can be recognized quickly and massage applied. The incision and bleeding points are visualized more easily and repaired, especially if there have been extensions laterally. Adnexal exposure is superior and thus tubal sterilization is easier. The principal disadvantage is from discomfort and vomiting caused by

Low incision
in uterus

A

Hand pressure on fundus

B

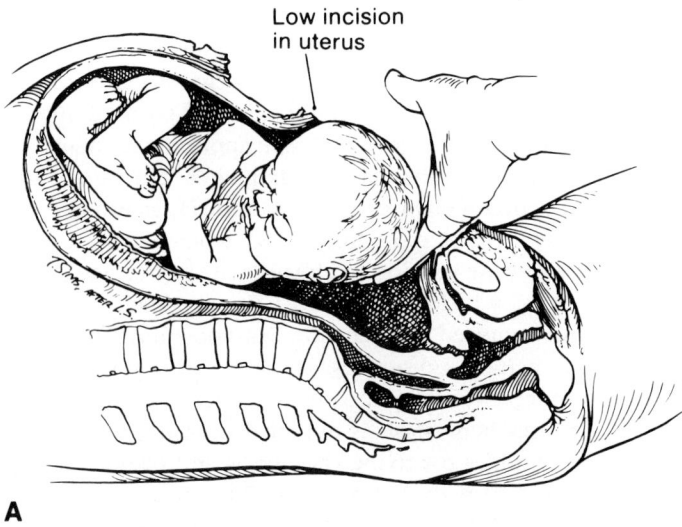

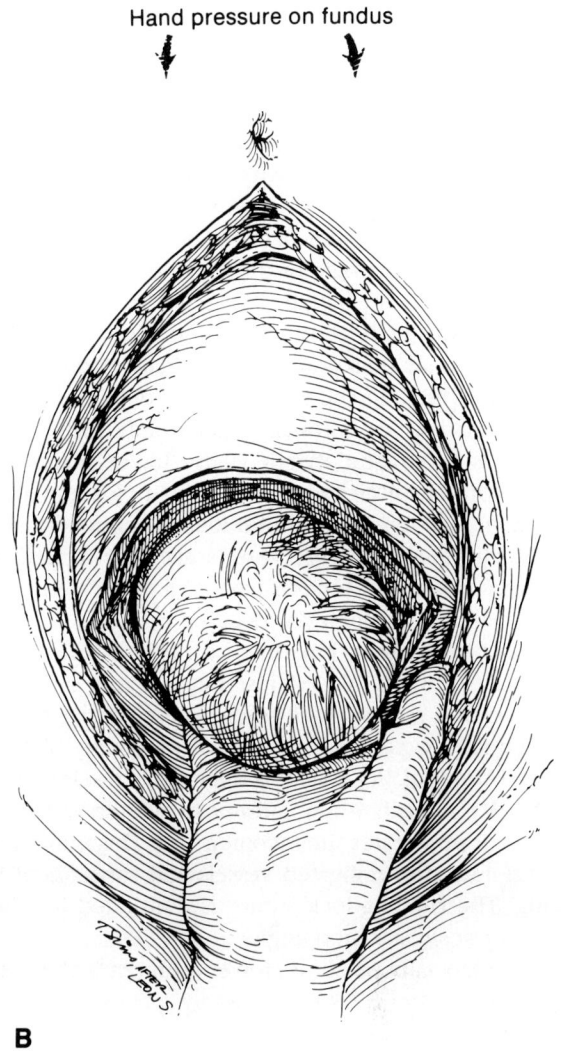

Fig. 26–8. A. Immediately after incising the uterus and fetal membranes, the operator's fingers are insinuated between the symphysis pubis and the fetal head until the posterior surface is reached. The head is lifted carefully anteriorly and, as necessary, superiorly to bring it from beneath the symphysis forward through the uterine and abdominal incisions. **B.** As the fetal head is lifted through the incision, pressure usually is applied to the uterine fundus through the abdominal wall to help expel the fetus.

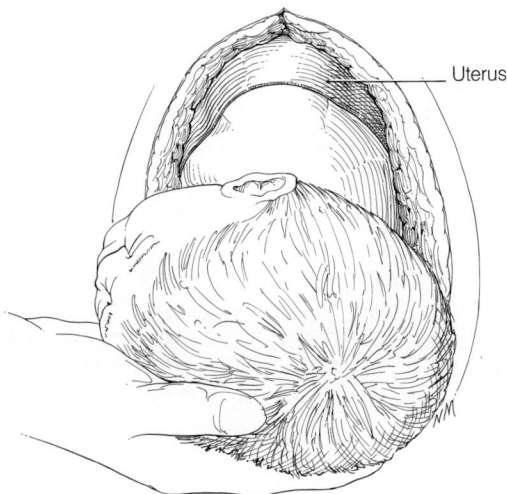

Uterus

Umbilical cord

Placenta

Lower margin of
uterine incision

Fig. 26–9. Just as shoulders are delivered, intravenous oxytocin is infused.

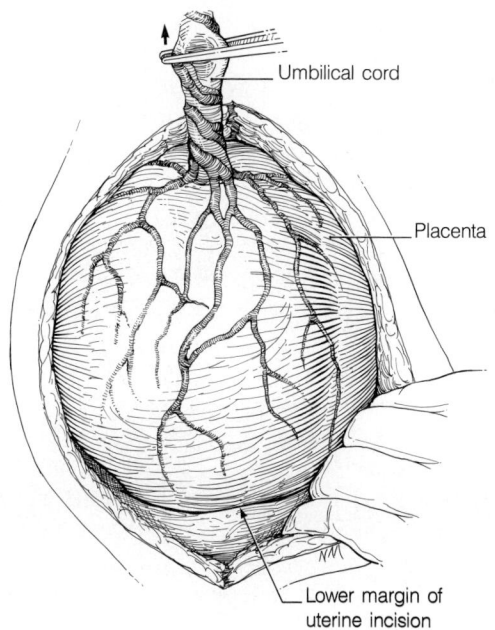

Fig. 26–10. Placenta bulging through the uterine incision as uterus contracts.

traction in the woman given spinal or epidural analgesia. Hershey and Quilligan (1978) reported that febrile morbidity was not increased if exteriorization for closure was performed routinely.

Immediately after delivery and inspection of the placenta, the uterine cavity is inspected and is wiped out with a gauze pack to remove avulsed membranes, vernix, clots, or other debris. The upper and lower cut edges and each angle of the uterine incision are examined carefully for bleeding vessels. The lower margin of an incision made through a thinned-out lower uterine segment may be so thin as to be inadvertently ignored. At the same time, the posterior wall of the lower uterine segment may occasionally buckle anteriorly in such a way as to suggest that it is the lower margin of the incision. The uterine incision may be closed with either one or two layers of continuous chromic suture. Individually clamped large vessels are best ligated with a suture ligature. Concern has been expressed by some that sutures through the decidua may lead to endometriosis in the scar, but this is a rare complication. The initial suture is placed just beyond one angle of the incision. A running-lock suture is then carried out, with each suture penetrating the full thickness of the myometrium (Fig. 26–11). It is important to select carefully the site of each stitch and not to withdraw the needle once it penetrates the myometrium. This minimizes the perforation of unligated vessels and subsequent bleeding. The running-lock suture is continued just beyond the opposite incision angle.

Especially when the lower segment is thin, satisfac-tory approximation of the cut edges usually can be obtained with one layer of suture. If approximation is not satisfactory after a single-layer continuous closure or if bleeding sites persist, either another layer of sutures may be placed so as to achieve approximation and hemostasis, or individual bleeding sites can be secured with figure-of-eight or mattress sutures. Hauth and colleagues (1992) randomized 761 women with a transverse uterine incision to closure with either one or two layers of #1 chromic suture. The single-closure technique required significantly less operating time and fewer hemostatic sutures. There were no differences in postoperative complications between the two groups.

After hemostasis is obtained from uterine closure, serosal edges overlying the uterus and bladder are approximated with a continuous 2-0 chromic catgut suture (Fig. 26–12). The lower edge of peritoneum should not be carried above the bladder, because this may lead to bladder discomfort and urinary frequency during later pregnancies. It also will make dissection of an unusually adherent overlapped peritoneum more difficult with subsequent cesarean section or hysterectomy.

If tubal sterilization is to be performed, it is now done. A partial mid-segment salpingectomy, described in Chapter 62 (p. 1353), is associated with a low failure rate.

Abdominal Closure. All packs are removed, and the gutters and cul-de-sac are emptied of blood and amnionic fluid by gentle suction. If general anesthesia is used, the upper abdominal organs may be palpated sys-

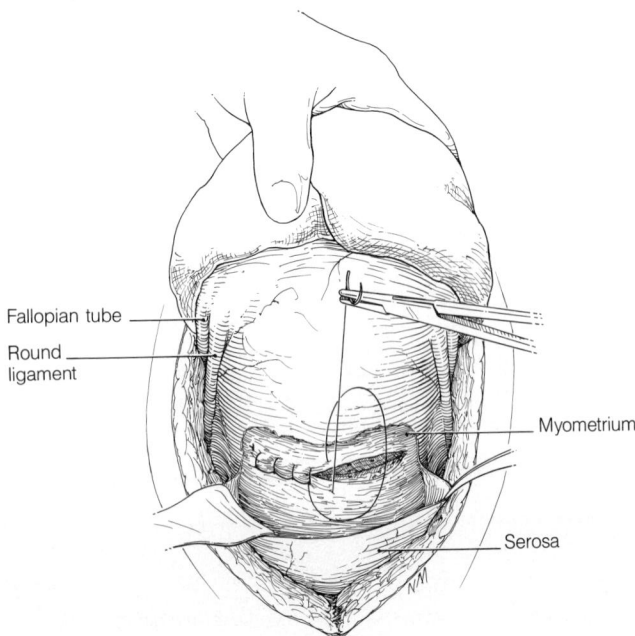

Fig. 26–11. The cut edges of the uterine incision are closed with a running-lock suture.

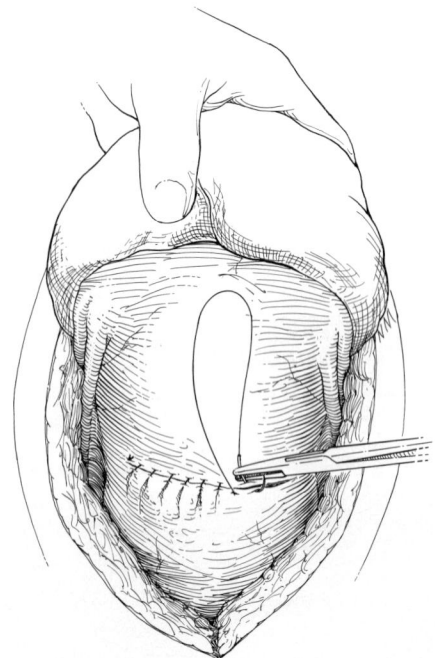

Fig. 26–12. The cut margins of the serosa are approximated to reperitonealize the uterus.

tematically. With conduction analgesia, however, this may produce considerable discomfort.

After the sponge and instrument counts are found to be correct, the abdominal incision is closed. As each layer is closed, bleeding sites are located, clamped, and ligated. Continuous 2-0 chromic catgut suture can be used to close the peritoneum, including the overlying transversalis fascia (Fig. 26–13). Not all surgeons approximate the peritoneum, and in two prospective studies, its nonclosure did not cause increased postoperative complications (Hull and Varner, 1991; Pietrantoni and associates, 1991). The rectus muscles are allowed to fall into place, and the overlying rectus fascia is closed either with interrupted 0 nonabsorbable sutures that are placed well lateral to the cut fascial edges and no more than 1 cm apart, or by continuous, nonlocking suture of a long-lasting absorbable or permanent type.

The subcutaneous tissue usually need not be closed separately if it is 2 cm or less in thickness, and the skin is closed with vertical mattress sutures of 3-0 or 4-0 silk or equivalent suture or skin clips. If there is more adipose tissue than this, or if clips or subcuticular closure are to be used, a few interrupted 3-0 plain catgut sutures will obliterate dead space and reduce tension on the skin edges. In a randomized prospective study of more than 1400 women undergoing cesarean section, Bohman and colleagues (1992) reported a significantly decreased frequency of superficial wound disruption when the subcutaneous layer was approximated.

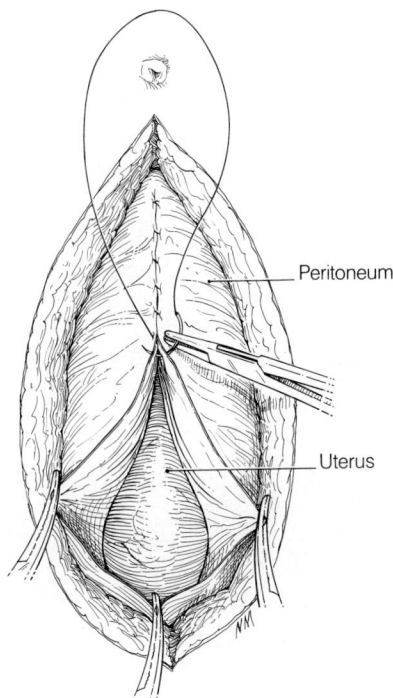

Fig. 26–13. The cut margins of the parietal peritoneum are elevated, and closure has been initiated.

Classical Cesarean Section. Occasionally it is necessary to use a classical cesarean section for delivery, for example: (1) if the lower uterine segment cannot be exposed or entered safely because the bladder is adherent densely from previous surgery, or if a myoma occupies the lower uterine segment, or if there is invasive carcinoma of the cervix; (2) when there is a transverse lie of a large fetus, especially if the membranes are ruptured and the shoulder is impacted in the birth canal; (3) in some cases of placenta previa with anterior implantation; (4) in some cases of very small fetuses, especially presenting as breech, in which the lower uterine segment is not thinned out; or (5) in some cases following renal transplantation in which the kidney is close to or obscuring the lower segment.

Incisions. The abdominal incision usually needs to extend somewhat higher than for a lower segment cesarean section. The vertical uterine incision is initiated with a scalpel beginning above the level of the attached bladder. Once sufficient room is made with the scalpel, the incision is extended cephalad with bandage scissors until it is sufficiently long to permit delivery of the fetus. Numerous large vessels that bleed profusely are commonly encountered within the myometrium. As soon as the fetus has been removed, these vessels may best be clamped and eventually ligated with chromic catgut sutures. As soon as the fetus has been delivered, oxytocin is administered and the placenta delivered, as described above under "Lower Segment Transverse Incision."

Uterine Repair. One method employs a layer of continuous 0- or 1-chromic catgut to approximate the inner halves of the incision. The outer half of the uterine incision then is closed with similar suture, using either a continuous stitch or figure-of-eight sutures. No unnecessary needle tracts should be made lest myometrial vessels be perforated with subsequent hemorrhage or hematomas. To achieve good approximation and to prevent the suture from tearing through the myometrium, it is essential that an assistant compress the myometrium on each side of the wound medially as each suture is placed and tied. The edges of the uterine serosa, if not already so, are approximated with continuous 2-0 chromic catgut. The operation is completed as described above under "Lower Segment Transverse Incision."

Extraperitoneal Cesarean Section. Early in this century, Frank (1907) and Latzko (1909) recommended extraperitoneal cesarean section rather than cesarean hysterectomy as a method of managing pregnancies with infected uterine contents. The goal of the operation was to open the uterus extraperitoneally by dissecting through the space of Retzius and then along one side and beneath the bladder to reach the lower uterine segment. Enthusiasm for the procedure has been transient, however, probably in large part because of the availability of a variety of effective antimicrobial agents.

Postmortem Cesarean Section. At times, cesarean section is performed on a woman who has just died, or who is expected to do so very soon. Both Weber (1970) and Arthur (1978) stressed that a satisfactory fetal outcome in such a situation is dependent upon (1) anticipation of death of the mother, (2) gestational age of fetus, (3) availability of personnel and appropriate equipment, (4) availability of continued postmortem ventilation and cardiac massage for the mother, and (5) prompt delivery and effective neonatal resuscitation. Although a few infants have survived with no apparent physical or intellectual compromise, others have not been so fortunate. In more recent years, the capability of life-support systems to maintain some level of vegetative function for long periods of time, and the reluctance of physicians to pronounce a mother dead, have further decreased the likelihood of delivering an infant that will survive and thrive following a postmortem cesarean section. However, Field and co-workers (1988) reported the successful delivery by cesarean section of an infant whose mother, though brain dead, was maintained for 10 weeks on life-support systems in order for fetal maturation to occur. The issue of cesarean delivery to aid in cardiopulmonary resuscitation of the mother is discussed in Chapter 47 (p. 1078).

Cesarean Hysterectomy

Indications. Indications for cesarean hysterectomy are discussed in connection with the various conditions for which the operation is indicated. A few of these include intrauterine infection; a grossly defective scar; a markedly hypotonic uterus that does not respond to oxytocin, prostaglandins, and massage; laceration of major uterine vessels; large myomas; and severe cervical dysplasia or carcinoma in situ. Placenta accreta or increta often may best be treated by immediate hysterectomy if cesarean section is performed. Major deterrents to cesarean hysterectomy are concern for increased blood loss and the frequency of urinary tract damage. A major factor in the complication rate appears to be whether the operation is performed as an elective procedure or as an emergency. For example, Gonsoulin and associates (1991) reported significantly increased blood loss, operative time, infection morbidity, and transfusion rate in women undergoing emergency cesarean hysterectomy compared with elective cases.

Technique. After delivery of the infant by cesarean section, supracervical or preferably total hysterectomy can be carried out according to standard operative techniques. Although all vessels are appreciably larger than those of the nonpregnant uterus, hysterectomy is usually facilitated by the ease of development of tissue

planes. Blood loss is commonly appreciable; however, with cesarean hysterectomy performed primarily for sterilization, blood loss averages about 1500 mL, or about 500 mL more than with cesarean section (Pritchard, 1965).

Following delivery, the major bleeding vessels are clamped and ligated quickly. The placenta is removed, and the uterine incision can be approximated with either a continuous suture or a few interrupted sutures. If the incision is not bleeding appreciably, closure is not necessary.

Next the round ligaments close to the uterus are divided between Heaney or Kocher clamps and doubly ligated. Either 0 or 1 sutures usually are used. The incision in the vesicouterine serosa, made to mobilize the bladder for cesarean section, is extended laterally and upward through the anterior leaf of the broad ligament to reach the incised round ligaments (Fig. 26–14). The posterior leaf of the broad ligament adjacent to the uterus is perforated just beneath the fallopian tubes, utero-ovarian ligaments, and ovarian vessels (Fig. 26–15A). These then are doubly clamped close to the uterus and severed (Fig. 26–15B); the lateral pedicle is doubly suture ligated. The posterior leaf of the broad ligament is divided inferiorly toward the uterosacral ligaments (Fig. 26–16). Next, the bladder and attached peritoneal flap are dissected from the lower uterine segment (Fig. 26–17) and retracted out of the operative field. If the bladder flap is unusually adherent, as it may be after previous cesarean sections, careful sharp dissection may be necessary.

Special care is necessary from this point on to avoid

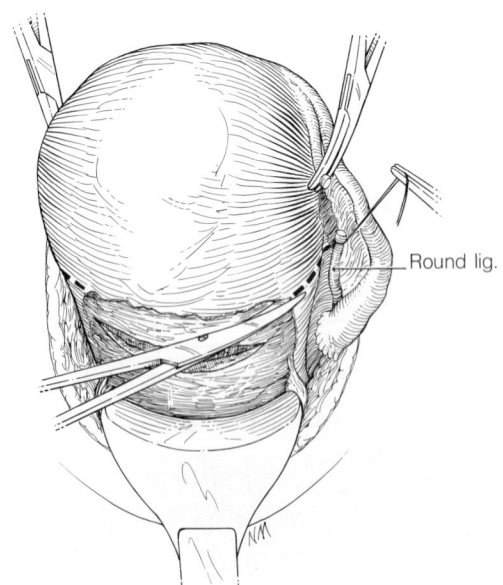

Fig. 26–14. The incision in the vesicouterine serosa is extended laterally and upward through the anterior leaf of the broad ligament to reach the incised round ligaments.

In rare cases of profuse hemorrhage, it may be more advantageous to clamp all of the vascular pedicles and remove the uterus before suture ligating the pedicles.

Supracervical Hysterectomy. To perform a subtotal hysterectomy, it is necessary only to amputate the body of the uterus at this level. The cervical stump may be closed with interrupted chromic sutures.

Total Hysterectomy. To perform a total hysterectomy, it is necessary to mobilize the bladder much more extensively in the midline and laterally. This will help carry the ureters caudad as the bladder is retracted beneath the symphysis and also will prevent laceration or suturing of the bladder during cervical excision and vaginal cuff closure. The bladder is dissected free for about 2 cm below the lowest margin of the cervix to expose the uppermost part of the vagina. If the cervix is effaced and dilated appreciably, the uterine cavity may be entered anteriorly in the midline either through the lower hysterotomy incision or through a stab wound made at the level of the ligated uterine vessels. A finger is directed inferiorly through the incision to identify the free margin of the dilated, effaced cervix and the anterior vaginal fornix. The contaminated glove is removed and the hand regloved. Another useful method to identify the cervical margins is to place transvaginally four metal skin clips at 12, 3, 6, and 9 o'clock positions on

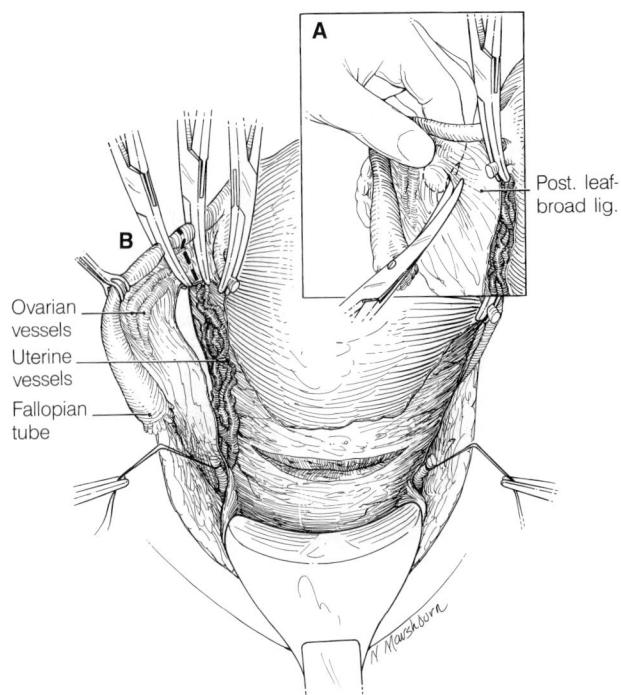

Fig. 26–15. A. The posterior leaf of the broad ligament adjacent to the uterus is perforated just beneath the fallopian tube, utero-ovarian ligaments, and ovarian vessels. **B.** These then are doubly clamped close to the uterus and severed.

injury to the ureters, which pass beneath the uterine arteries. The ascending uterine artery and veins on either side are identified and near their origin are doubly clamped immediately adjacent to the uterus and divided (Fig. 26–18). The vascular pedicle is doubly suture ligated.

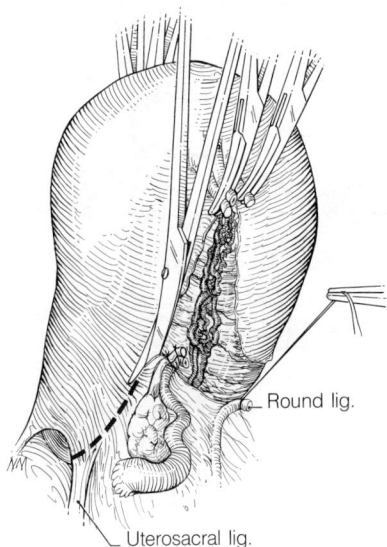

Fig. 26–16. The posterior leaf of the broad ligament is divided inferiorly toward the uterosacral ligament.

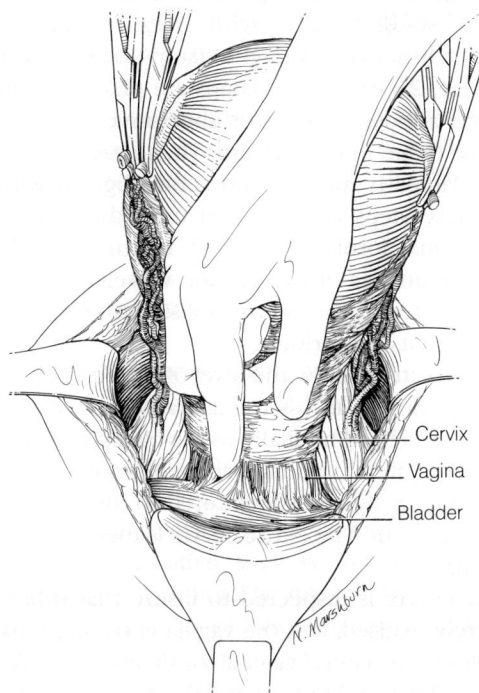

Fig. 26–17. The bladder is further dissected from the lower uterine segment by blunt dissection with pressure directed towards the lower segment and not bladder. Sharp dissection may be necessary.

(see Chap. 16, p. 429). This should be done routinely, even when conduction analgesia will be used; at times it is necessary to switch to, or at least supplement, the regional analgesia with inhalation anesthesia.

Intravenous Fluids. Requirements for intravenous fluids, including blood during and after cesarean section, can vary considerably. The woman of average size with a hematocrit of 30 or more and a normally expanded blood volume and extracellular fluid volume most often tolerates blood loss up to 1500 mL without difficulty. Unappreciated bleeding through the vagina during the procedure, bleeding concealed in the uterus after its closure, or both, commonly lead to underestimation. Blood loss averages about 1 L but is quite variable (Pritchard, 1965).

Intravenously administered fluids consist of either lactated Ringer solution or a similar solution with 5 percent dextrose. Typically, 1 to 2 L that contain electrolytes are infused during and immediately after the operation. Throughout the procedure, and subsequently while in the recovery area, the blood pressure and urine flow are monitored closely to ascertain that perfusion of vital organs is satisfactory.

Recovery Suite. In the recovery suite, the amount of bleeding from the vagina must be monitored closely, and the uterine fundus must be identified frequently by palpation to assure that the uterus is remaining firmly contracted. Unfortunately, as the woman awakens from general anesthesia or the conduction analgesia fades, palpation of the abdomen is likely to produce considerable discomfort. This can be made much more tolerable by giving an effective analgesic intramuscularly or intravenously, such as meperidine 75 mg or morphine 10 mg. A thick dressing with an abundance of adhesive tape over the abdomen interferes with fundal palpation and massage and later causes discomfort as the tape and perhaps skin are removed. Deep breathing and coughing are encouraged.

Once the mother is fully awake, bleeding is minimal, the blood pressure is satisfactory, and urine flow is at least 30 mL per hour, she may be returned to her room.

Subsequent Care

Analgesia. For the woman of average size, meperidine 75 mg is given intramuscularly as often as every 3 to 4 hours as needed for discomfort, or morphine 10 mg is similarly administered. If she is small, 50 mg, or if large, 100 mg of meperidine is more appropriate. An antiemetic, such as promethazine 25 mg, is usually given along with the narcotic.

Vital Signs. The patient is now evaluated at least hourly for 4 hours at the minimum, and blood pressure, pulse,

urine flow, amount of bleeding, and status of the uterine fundus are checked at these times. Thereafter, for the first 24 hours, these are checked at intervals of 4 hours, along with the temperature.

Fluid Therapy and Diet. Unless there has been pathological constriction of the extracellular fluid compartment from diuretics, sodium restriction, vomiting, fever, or prolonged labor without adequate fluid intake, the puerperium is characterized by excretion of fluid that was retained during pregnancy. Moreover, with the typical cesarean section or uncomplicated cesarean hysterectomy, significant extracellular fluid sequestration in bowel wall and bowel lumen does not occur, unless it was necessary to pack the bowel away from the operative field or peritonitis develops. Thus, the woman who undergoes cesarean section rarely develops fluid sequestration in the so-called third space. Quite the contrary, she normally begins surgery with a physiological third space that she acquired during pregnancy, namely, the physiological edema of pregnancy that she mobilizes and excretes after delivery. Therefore, large volumes of intravenous fluids during and subsequent to surgery are not needed to replace sequestered extracellular fluid. As a generalization, 3 L of fluid should prove adequate during the first 24 hours after surgery. If urine output falls below 30 mL per hour, however, the woman should be reevaluated promptly. The cause of the oliguria may range from unrecognized blood loss to an antidiuretic effect from infused oxytocin.

In the absence of extensive intra-abdominal manipulation or sepsis, the woman nearly always should be able to tolerate oral fluids or even a regular diet the day after surgery. By the second day after surgery, the great majority of women tolerate a general diet.

Bladder and Bowels. The bladder catheter most often can be removed by 12 hours after operation or, more conveniently, the morning after surgery. Subsequent ability to empty the bladder before overdistention develops must be monitored as with vaginal delivery. Bowel sounds may be hypoactive the day after surgery, but are usually normal by the third day. Gas pains from incoordinate bowel action may be troublesome the second and third postoperative days. Frequently, a rectal suppository provides appreciable relief.

Ambulation. In most instances, by the day after surgery the patient, with assistance, should get out of bed briefly at least twice. Ambulation can be timed so that a recently administered analgesic will minimize the discomfort. By the second day she may walk to the bathroom with assistance. With early ambulation, venous thrombosis and pulmonary embolism are uncommon.

Wound Care. The incision is inspected each day, and the skin sutures (or clips) are removed on the fourth day after surgery. By the third postpartum day, bathing by shower is not harmful to the incision.

Laboratory. The hematocrit is routinely measured the day after surgery. It is checked sooner when there was unusual blood loss or when there is oliguria or other evidence to suggest hypovolemia. If the hematocrit is decreased significantly from the preoperative level, it is repeated, and a search is instituted to identify the cause of the decrease. If the lower hematocrit is stable, the mother can ambulate without any difficulty, and if there is little likelihood of further blood loss, hematological repair in response to iron therapy is preferred to transfusion.

Breast Care. Breast feeding can be initiated by the day after surgery. If the mother elects not to breast feed, a breast binder that supports the breasts without marked compression will usually minimize discomfort (see Chap. 29, p. 646).

Discharge from the Hospital. Unless there are complications during the puerperium, the mother may be safely discharged from the hospital on the third or fourth postpartum day. Her activities during the following week should be restricted to self-care and care of her baby with assistance. It is advantageous to perform the initial postpartum evaluation during the third week after delivery rather than at the more traditional time of 6 weeks, for the reasons presented in Chapters 18 and 60.

Prophylactic Antimicrobial Therapy. Febrile morbidity is rather frequent after cesarean section and appears to be more common among indigent than affluent women. The literature is replete with reports of reduced febrile morbidity with antibiotics administered prophylactically.

At Parkland Hospital, without prophylactic antimicrobials, 85 percent of women in labor with membranes ruptured for longer than 6 hours who underwent cesarean delivery developed serious infection (Cunningham and associates, 1978). The incidence was much less (30 percent) in women who underwent cesarean section after laboring with membranes intact. Moreover, associated complications such as wound abscesses and pelvic phlegmons were encountered in less than 1 percent of women with intact membranes, compared with 30 percent of women whose membranes ruptured more than 6 hours before cesarean section. Finally, bacteremia was four times more common in those women whose membranes ruptured longer than 6 hours before surgery and who subsequently demonstrated infection.

Subsequently therapeutic intervention was evaluated for this high-risk group of nulliparous women who underwent cesarean delivery because of cephalopelvic disproportion (DePalma and colleagues, 1980, 1982). The administration of an antibiotic as soon as the cord

was clamped, followed by two more doses of the same medications given at intervals of 6 hours, resulted in a reduction in postoperative metritis from 85 to 20 percent. Associated complications, such as pelvic phlegmons, incisional abscesses, and pelvic thrombophlebitis, also decreased dramatically (Fig. 26–24).

Duff (1987) reviewed 25 randomized clinical trials in which it was demonstrated that one or three doses of an antimicrobial given at the time of cesarean section were found to decrease infection morbidity appreciably. For women in labor or with ruptured membranes, he recommends a single 2-g dose of ampicillin or a first-generation cephalosporin after delivery of the infant. A second dose in 3 to 4 hours is given if surgery is prolonged more than 90 minutes. For the majority of women, a single-dose of a cephalosporin or an extended-spectrum penicillin will prove efficacious.

In the very high-risk women addressed in Figure 26–24, almost 25 percent developed metritis despite the three-dose perioperative antimicrobial regimen. For women at lower risk, the clinical infection rate is correspondingly less. In most cases, women with failed prophylaxis have milder infections, which usually do not manifest until the third or fourth postoperative day. In a recent review of 1800 cesarean deliveries, Chang and Newton (1992) identified several predictors of prophylactic antibiotic failure to include the number of vaginal examinations, nulliparity, low gestational age, and use of cefazolin.

It is emphasized that the woman with clini-

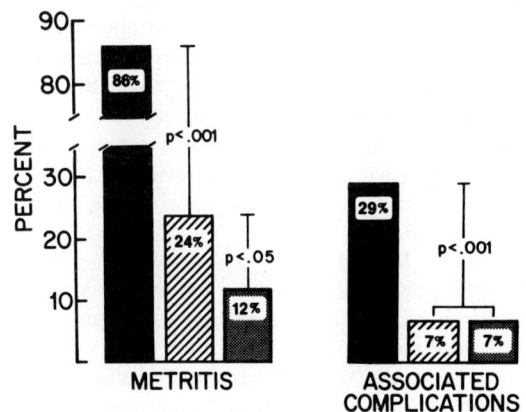

Fig. 26–24. Comparison of the incidence of metritis and its associated complications (pelvic phlegmons, incisional abscesses, and pelvic thrombophlebitis) according to treatment management in 642 high-risk women undergoing cesarean section. The *solid bars* represent infections in women not given prophylactic antimicrobials (n = 128). The *hatched bars* represent the outcomes following three-dose perioperative antimicrobials (n = 305). The *speckled bars* represent outcomes obtained by administering antimicrobials from the time of cesarean section until 4 days postpartum (n = 209). (From DePalma and associates, 1982.)

cally diagnosed chorioamnionitis should be given continuous antimicrobial therapy postoperatively until she is afebrile.

Historical Background

The origin of the term *cesarean section* is obscure. Three principal explanations have been suggested.

1. According to legend, Julius Caesar was born in this manner, with the result that the procedure became known as the "Caesarean operation." Several circumstances weaken this explanation. First, the mother of Julius Caesar lived for many years after his birth in 100 BC, and as late as the 17th century, the operation was almost invariably fatal. Second, the operation, whether performed on the living or dead, is not mentioned by any medical writer before the Middle Ages. Historical details of the origin of the family name Caesar are found in Pickrell's monograph (1935).

2. It has been widely believed that the name of the operation is derived from a Roman law, supposedly created by Numa Pompilius (eighth century BC), ordering that the procedure be performed upon women dying in the last few weeks of pregnancy in the hope of saving the child. This explanation then holds that this *lex regia*, as it was called at first, became the *lex caesarea* under the emperors, and the operation itself became known as the caesarean operation. The German term *Kaiserschnitt* ("Kaiser cut") reflects this derivation.

3. The word *caesarean* was derived sometime in the Middle Ages from the Latin verb *caedere*, "to cut." An obvious cognate is the word *caesura*, a cutting, or pause, in a line of verse. This explanation of the term *caesarean* seems most logical, but exactly when it was first applied to the operation is uncertain. Because "section" is derived from the Latin verb *seco*, which also means "cut," the term *caesarean section* seems tautological.

It is customary in the United States to replace the *ae* in the first syllable of *caesarean* with the letter *e*; in Great Britain and Australia, however, the "ae" is still retained.

From the time of Virgil's Aeneas to Shakespeare's Macduff, poets repeatedly have referred to persons "untimely ripped" from their mother's womb. Ancient historians, such as Pliny, moreover, say that Scipio Africanus (the conqueror of Hannibal), Martius, and Julius Caesar were all born by section. In regard to Julius Caesar, Pliny adds that it was from this circumstance that the surname rose by which the Roman emperors were known. Birth in this extraordinary manner, as described in ancient mythology and legend, was believed to confer supernatural powers and elevate the heroes so born above ordinary mortals.

In evaluating these references to abdominal delivery in antiquity, it is pertinent that no such operation is even mentioned by Hippocrates, Galen, Celsus, Paulus, Soranus, or any other medical writer of those periods. If cesarean section was actually employed, it is particularly surprising that Soranus, whose extensive work written in the second century AD covers all aspects of obstetrics, does not refer to cesarean section.

Several references to abdominal delivery appear in the Talmud, compiled between the second and sixth centuries AD, but whether they had any background in terms of clinical usage is conjectural. There can be no doubt, however, that cesarean section on the dead was first practiced soon after the Christian Church gained dominance, as a measure directed at baptism of the child. Faith in the validity of some of these early reports is rudely shaken, however, when they glibly state that a living, robust child was obtained 8 to 24 *hours* after the death of the mother.

Cesarean section on the living was first recommended, and the current name of the operation used, in the celebrated work of François Rousset (1581) entitled *Traité Nouveau de l'Hystérotomotokie ou l'Enfantement Césarien*. Rousset had never performed or witnessed the operation; his information was based chiefly on letters from friends. He reported 14 successful cesarean sections, a fact in itself difficult to accept. When it is further stated that 6 of the 14 operations were performed on the same woman, the credulity of the most gullible is exhausted.

The apocryphal nature of most early reports on cesarean section has been stressed because many of them have been accepted without question. Authoritative statements by dependable obstetricians about early use of the operation, however, did not appear in the literature until the mid-17th century, as for instance in the classical work of the French obstetrician, François Mauriceau, first published in 1668. These statements show without doubt that the operation was employed on the living in rare and desperate cases and that it was usually fatal. Details of the history of cesarean section are to be found in Fasbender's classical text (1906).

The appalling maternal mortality rate of cesarean section continued until the beginning of the 20th century. In Great Britain and Ireland, the maternal death rate from the operation had mounted in 1865 to 85 percent. In Paris, during the 90 years ending in 1876, not a single successful cesarean section had been performed. Harris (1879) noted that as late as 1889 cesarean section actually was more successful when performed by the patient herself or when the abdomen was ripped open by the horns of a bull! He collected from the literature 9 such cases with 5 recoveries, and contrasted them with 12 cesarean sections performed in New York City during the same period, with only 1 recovery.

The turning point in the evolution of cesarean section came in 1882, when Max Sänger, then a 28-year-old assistant of Credé in the University Clinic at Leipzig, introduced suturing of the uterine wall. The long neglect of so simple an expedient as uterine suture was not the result of oversight but stemmed from a deeply rooted belief that sutures in the uterus were superfluous as well as harmful by virtue of serving as the site for severe infection. In meeting these objections Sänger, who had himself used sutures in only one case, documented their value, not from the sophisticated medical centers of Europe but from frontier America. There, in outposts from Ohio to Louisiana, 17 cesarean sections had been reported in which silver wire sutures had been used, with the survival of 8 mothers, an extraordinary record in those days. In a table included in his monograph, Sänger gives full credit to these frontier surgeons for providing the supporting data for his hypothesis. The problem of hemorrhage was the first and most serious problem to be solved. Details are found in Eastman's review (1932).

Although the introduction of uterine sutures reduced the mortality rate of the operation from hemorrhage, generalized peritonitis remained the dominant cause of death; hence, various types of operations were devised to combat this scourge. The earliest was the Porro procedure (1876), in use before Sänger's time, that combined subtotal cesarean hysterectomy with marsupialization of the cervical stump. The first extraperitoneal operation was described by Frank in 1907 and, with various modifications, as introduced by Latzko (1909) and Waters (1940), was employed until recent years.

In 1912, Krönig contended that the main advantage of the extraperitoneal technique consisted not so much in avoiding the peritoneal cavity as in opening the uterus through its thin lower segment and then covering the incision with peritoneum. To accomplish this end, he cut through the vesical reflection of the peritoneum from one round ligament to the other and separated it and the bladder from the lower uterine segment and cervix. The lower portion of the uterus was then opened through a vertical median incision, and the child was extracted by forceps. The uterine incision was then closed and buried under the vesical peritoneum. With minor modifications, this low-segment technique was introduced into the United States by Beck (1919) and popularized by DeLee (1922) and others. A particularly important modification was recommended by Kerr in 1926, who preferred a transverse rather than a longitudinal uterine incision. The Kerr technique is the most commonly employed type of cesarean section today.

A monograph on the history of cesarean section by Trolle (1982) is recommended.

References

Alexander J, Gregg JE, Quinn MW: Femoral fractures at caesarean section. Case reports. Br J Obstet Gynaecol 94:273, 1987

American College of Obstetricians and Gynecologists, Vaginal birth after cesarean section: Report of a 1990 survey of ACOG's membership. August 1990

American College of Obstetricians and Gynecologists, Committee on Obstetrics, Maternal and Fetal Medicine: Assessment of fetal maturity prior to repeat cesarean delivery or elective induction of labor. No. 77, January 1990

American College of Obstetricians and Gynecologists, Committee on Obstetrics, Maternal and Fetal Medicine: Guidelines for vaginal delivery after a previous cesarean birth. No. 64, October 1988

Arthur RK: Postmortem cesarean section. Am J Obstet Gynecol 132:175, 1978

Ayers JWT, Morley GW: Surgical incision for cesarean section. Obstet Gynecol 70:706, 1987

Beck AC: Observations on a series of cases of cesarean section done at the Long Island College Hospital during the past six years. Am J Obstet Gynecol 79:197, 1919

Bohman VR, Gilstrap L, Leveno K, Ramin S, Santos-Ramos R, Goldaber K, Little B: Subcutaneous tissue: To close or not to close at cesarean section. Am J Obstet Gynecol 166:407, 1992. Abstract 481

Bottoms SF, Rosen MG, Sokol RJ: The increase in the cesarean birth rate. N Engl J Med 302:559, 1980

Burchell RC, Creed F, Rasoulpour M, Whitcomb M: Vascular anatomy of the human uterus and pregnancy wastage. Br J Obstet Gynaecol 85:698, 1978

Chang PL, Newton ER: Predictors of antibiotic prophylactic failure in post-cesarean endometritis. Obstet Gynecol 80:117, 1992

Clark SL, Eglinton GS, Beall M, Phelan JP: Effect of indication for previous cesarean section on subsequent delivery outcome in patients undergoing a trial of labor. J Reprod Med 29:22, 1984

Collea JV, Chein C, Quilligan EJ: The randomized management of term frank breech presentation: A study of 208 cases. Am J Obstet Gynecol 137:235, 1980

Cunningham FG, Hauth JC, Strong JD, Kappus SS: Infectious morbidity following cesarean section: Comparison of two treatment regimens. Obstet Gynecol 52:656, 1978

DeLee JB, Cornell EL: Low cervical cesarean section (laparotrachelotomy). JAMA 79:109, 1922

DePalma RT, Cunningham FG, Leveno KJ, Roark ML: Continuing investigation of women at high risk for infection following cesarean delivery: The three-dose perioperative antimicrobial therapy. Obstet Gynecol 60:53, 1982

DePalma RT, Leveno KJ, Cunningham FG, Pope T, Kappus SS, Roark ML, Nobles BJ: Identification and management of women at high risk for pelvic infection following cesarean section. Obstet Gynecol 55:185S, 1980

Duff P: Prophylactic antibiotics for cesarean delivery: A simple cost-effective strategy for prevention of postoperative morbidity. Am J Obstet Gynecol 157:794, 1987

Eastman NJ: The role of frontier America in the development of cesarean section. Am J Obstet Gynecol 24:919, 1932

Farmakides G, Duvivier R, Schulman H, Schneider E, Biordi J: Vaginal birth after two or more previous cesarean sections. Am J Obstet Gynecol 154:565, 1987

Farmer RM, Kirschbaun T, Potter D, Strong TH, Medearis AL: Uterine rupture during trial of labor after previous cesarean section. Am J Obstet Gynecol 165:996, 1991

Fasbender H: Geschichte der Geburtshilfe. Jena, 1906, p 979

Field DR, Gates EA, Creasy RK, Jonsen AR, Laros RK Jr: Maternal brain death during pregnancy. Medical and ethical issues. JAMA 260:816, 1988

Flamm BL: Vaginal birth after cesarean section: Controversies old and new. Clin Obstet Gynecol 28:735, 1985

Flamm BL, Fried MW, Lonky NM, Giles WS: External cephalic version after previous cesarean section. Am J Obstet Gynecol 165:370, 1991

Flamm BL, Goings JR, Fuelberth NJ, Fischermann E, Jones C, Hersh E: Oxytocin during labor after previous cesarean section: Results of a multicenter study. Obstet Gynecol 70:709, 1987

Flamm BL, Lim OW, Jones C, Fallon D, Newman LA, Mantis JK: Vaginal birth after cesarean section: Results of a multicenter study. Am J Obstet Gynecol 158:1079, 1988

Flamm BL, Newman LA, Thomas SJ, Fallon D, Yoshida MM: Vaginal birth after cesarean delivery: Results of a 5-year multicenter collaborative study. Obstet Gynecol 76:750, 1990

Frank F: Suprasymphysial delivery and its relation to other operations in the presence of contracted pelvis. Arch Gynaekol 81:46, 1907

Frigoletto FD Jr, Ryan KJ, Phillippe M: Maternal mortality rate associated with cesarean section: An appraisal. Am J Obstet Gynecol 136:969, 1980

Gilstrap LC III: Elective appendectomy during abdominal surgery. JAMA 265:1736 1991

Gonsoulin W, Kennedy RT, Guidry KH: Elective versus emergency cesarean hysterectomy cases in a residency program setting: A review of 129 cases from 1984 to 1988. Am J Obstet Gynecol 165:91, 1991

Goodlin RC, Scott JC Jr, Woods RE, Anderson JC: Laparoelytrotomy or abdominal delivery without uterine incision. Am J Obstet Gynecol 144:990, 1982

Gould JB, Davey B, Stafford RS: Socioeconomic differences in rates of cesarean section. N Engl J Med 321:233, 1989

Harris RP: Lessons from a study of the cesarean operation in the City and State of New York. Am J Obstet 12:82, 1879

Hauth JC, Owen J, Davis RO, Lincoln T, Piazza J: Transverse uterine incision closure: One versus two layers. Am J Obstet Gynecol 166:398, 1992. Abstract 444

Hershey DW, Quilligan EJ: Extraabdominal uterine exteriorization at cesarean section. Obstet Gynecol 52:189, 1978

Hull DB, Varner MW: A randomized study of closure of the peritoneum at cesarean delivery. Obstet Gynecol 77:818, 1991

Jones RO, Nagashima AW, Hatnett-Goodman MM, Goodlin RC: Rupture of low transverse cesarean scars during trial of labor. Obstet Gynecol 77:815, 1991

Kaplan M, Dollberg M, Wajntraub G, Itzchaki M: Fractured long bones in a term infant delivered by cesarean section. Pediatr Radiol 17:256, 1987

Kerr JMM: The technic of cesarean section with special reference to the lower uterine segment incision. Am J Obstet Gynecol 12:729, 1926

Krönig B: Transperitonealer Cervikaler Kaiserschnitt. In Doderlein A, Krönig B (eds): Operative Gynakologie, 1912, p 879

Latzko W: Ueber den extraperitonealen Kaiserschnitt. Zentralbl Gynaekol 33:275, 1909

Leveno KJ, Cunningham FG, Pritchard JA: Cesarean section:

The House of Horne revisited. Am J Obstet Gynecol 160:78, 1989

Leveno KJ, Cunningham FG, Pritchard JA: Cesarean section: An answer to the House of Horne. Am J Obstet Gynecol 153:838, 1985

Lilford RJ, Van Coeverden de Groot HA, Moore PJ, Bingham P: The relative risks of caesarean section (intrapartum and elective) and vaginal delivery: A detailed analysis to exclude the effects of medical disorders and other acute pre-existing physiological disturbances. Br J Obstet Gynaecol 97:883, 1990

Lopez-Zeno JA, Peaceman AM, Adashek JA, Socol ML: A controlled trial of a program for the active management of labor. N Engl J Med 326:450, 1992

Myers SA, Gleicher N: US Cesarean section rate: Good news or bad? N Engl J Med 323:200, 1990

Neuhoff D, Burke MS, Porreco RP: Cesarean birth for failed progress in labor. Obstet Gynecol 73:915, 1989

Notzon FC, Placek PJ, Taffel SM: Comparisons of national cesarean-section rates. N Engl J Med 316:386, 1987

O'Driscoll K, Foley M: Correlation of decrease in perinatal mortality and increase in cesarean section rates. Obstet Gynecol 61:1, 1983

O'Driscoll K, Foley M, MacDonald D: Active management of labor as an alternative to cesarean section for dystocia. Obstet Gynecol 63:485, 1984

O'Driscoll K, Jackson RJA, Gallagher JT: Prevention of prolonged labor. Br Med J 2:477, 1969

O'Driscoll K, Stronge JM, Minogue M: Active management of labour. Br Med J 3:135, 1973

Ophir E, Oettinger M, Yagoda A, Markovits Y, Rojansky N, Shapiro H: Breech presentation after cesarean section: Always a section? Am J Obstet Gynecol 161:25, 1989

O'Sullivan MJ, Fumia F, Holsinger K, McLeod AGW: Vaginal delivery after cesarean section. Clin Perinatol 8:131, 1981

Parsons AK, Sauer MY, Parsons MT, Tunca J, Spellacy WN: Appendectomy at cesarean section: A prospective study. Obstet Gynecol 68:479, 1986

Paul RH, Phelan JP, Yeh SY: Trial of labor in the patient with a prior cesarean birth. Am J Obstet Gynecol 151:297, 1985

Phelan JP, Ock Ahn M, Diaz F, Brar HS, Rodriguez MH: Twice a cesarean, always a cesarean? Obstet Gynecol 73:161, 1989

Pickrell K: An inquiry into the history of cesarean section. Bull Soc Med Hist (Chicago) 4:414, 1935

Pietrantoni M, Parsons MT, O'Brien WF, Collins E, Knuppel RA, Spellacy WN: Peritoneal closure or non-closure at cesarean. Obstet Gynecol 77:293, 1991

Pitkin RM: Once a cesarean? Obstet Gynecol 77:939, 1991

Placek PJ, Taffel SM, Keppel KG: Maternal and infant characteristics associated with cesarean section delivery. Department of Health and Human Services, pub. no. (PHS) 84-1232. Hyattsville, MD, National Center for Health Statistics, December 1983

Placek PJ, Taffel S, Liss T: The cesarean future. Ann Demogr 9:46, 1987

Pliny the Elder: Natural History. Cambridge, Harvard University Press, 1942, book VII, chap IX. Translated by H Rackham

Porro E: Della Amputazione Utero-ovarica. Milan, 1876

Pritchard JA: Changes in the blood volume during pregnancy and delivery. Anesthesiology 26:393, 1965

Pruett KM, Kirshon B, Cotton DB, Poindexter AN III: Is vaginal birth after two or more cesarean sections safe? Obstet Gynecol 72:163, 1988

Rosen MG, Dickinson JC, Westhoff CL: Vaginal birth after cesarean: A meta-analysis of morbidity and mortality. Obstet Gynecol 77:465, 1991

Rousset F: Traité Nouveau de l'Hystérotomotokie ou l'Enfantement Césaerien. Paris, Denys deVal, 1581

Rubin GL, Peterson HB, Rochat RW, McCarthy BJ, Terry JS: Maternal death after cesarean section in Georgia. Am J Obstet Gynecol 139:681, 1981

Ruddick V, Niv D, Hetman-Peri M, Geller E, Avni A, Golan A: Epidural analgesia for planned vaginal delivery following previous cesarean section. Obstet Gynecol 64:621, 1984

Sachs BP, Yeh J, Acker D, Driscoll S, Brown DAJ, Jewett JF: Cesarean section-related maternal mortality in Massachusetts, 1954–1985. Obstet Gynecol 71:385, 1988

Sänger M: Der Kaiserschnitt bei Uterusfibromen. Leipzig, 1882

Scott JR: Mandatory trial of labor after cesarean delivery: An alternative viewpoint. Obstet Gynecol 77:811, 1991

Seitchik J, Ramakrishna RV: Cesarean delivery in nulliparous women for failed oxytocin-augmented labor: Route of delivery in subsequent pregnancy. Am J Obstet Gynecol 143:393, 1982

Skajaa K, Hansen ES, Bendix J: Depressed fracture of the skull in a child born by cesarean section. Acta Obstet Gynecol Scand 66:275, 1987

Stafford RS: Alternative strategies for controlling rising cesarean section rates. JAMA 263:683, 1990

Strong TH, Phelan JP, Ahn MO, Sarno AP Jr: Vaginal birth after cesarean delivery in the twin gestation. Am J Obstet Gynecol 161:29, 1989

Taffel SM, Placek PJ, Liss T: Trends in the United States cesarean section rate for the 1980–1985 rise. Am J Public Health 77:955, 1987

Taffel SM, Placek PJ, Moien M, Kosary CL: 1989 US Cesarean section rate steadies—VBAC rises to nearly one in five. Birth 18:73, 1991

Trolle D: The History of Cesarean Section. Copenhagen, University Library, CA Reitzel Booksellers, 1982

Uppington J: Epidural analgesia and previous cesarean section. Anaesthesia 38:336, 1983

Vasa R, Kim MR: Fracture of the femur at cesarean section: Case report and review of literature. Am J Perinatol 7:46, 1990

Vengadasalam D: Vaginal delivery following cesarean section. Singapore Med J 37:396, 1986

Waters EG: Supravesical extraperitoneal cesarean section: Presentation of a new technique. Am J Obstet Gynecol 39:423, 1940

Weber CE: Postmortem cesarean section: Review of the literature and case reports. Am J Obstet Gynecol 110:158, 1970

Abnormalities of the Puerperium

■

CHAPTER 27

Abnormalities of the Third Stage of Labor

Postpartum Hemorrhage

Definition. Postpartum hemorrhage, the most common cause of serious hemorrhage in obstetrics, has most often been defined as blood loss in excess of 500 mL during the first 24 hours after delivery. Through quantitative measurements of puerperal blood loss, however, the incongruity of this definition has clearly been demonstrated, as blood loss resulting from vaginal delivery *frequently* is somewhat more than 500 mL (see Chap. 37, p. 819). Newton (1966), for example, measured the amount of hemoglobin shed by 105 women from the time of vaginal delivery through the next 24 hours, and ascertained that the average blood loss was about 550 mL. If appropriate allowance was made for the maternal blood discarded with the placenta, as well as that not measured because of incomplete recovery, blood loss during the first 24 hours averaged about 650 mL. Pritchard and associates (1962) and DeLeeuw and co-workers (1968) demonstrated that erythrocytes equivalent to approximately 600 mL of blood are lost from the maternal circulation during vaginal delivery and the next several hours.

Therefore, blood loss somewhat in excess of 500 mL by accurate measurement is not necessarily an abnormal event for vaginal delivery. Pritchard and associates (1962) noted that about 5 percent of women delivering vaginally lost more than 1000 mL of blood. They also observed that estimated blood loss is commonly only about half the actual loss. Based on an estimated blood loss greater than 500 mL, postpartum hemorrhage has been found in about 5 percent of deliveries. An estimated blood loss in excess of 500 mL in many institutions, therefore, may call attention to mothers who are bleeding excessively and warn the physician that dangerous hemorrhage is imminent. Hemorrhage after the first 24 hours is designated as *late postpartum hemorrhage* and is discussed in Chapter 29 (p. 644).

Duration of Third Stage. Occasionally, the placenta does not separate promptly. A question to which there is still no definite answer concerns the length of time that should elapse in the absence of bleeding before the placenta is removed manually. Obstetrical tradition has set somewhat arbitrary limits on third-stage duration in attempts to define *abnormally retained placenta*, and thus reduce blood loss due to excessively prolonged placental separation. Combs and Laros (1991) studied third-stage duration in 12,275 singleton vaginal deliveries without manual placental removal. The median third-stage duration was 6 minutes, and 3.3 percent lasted more than 30 minutes. They also investigated the relation between third-stage duration and hemorrhage. As shown in Figure 27–1, several measures of hemorrhage increased with third stages nearing 30 minutes or longer.

Methods of effecting placental delivery recently have included oxytocin administration into the umbilical vein to either prevent or treat retained placenta. Young and co-workers (1988) and Porter and colleagues (1991) performed randomized studies of prophylactic intraumbilical vein oxytocin and showed no benefits. Similarly, umbilical vein oxytocin administration to effect delivery of placentas retained 30 minutes or longer has been shown to be ineffective (Huber and co-workers, 1991).

Bullough and co-workers (1989) conducted a randomized trial in nearly 4400 deliveries to determine whether suckling immediately after birth reduced the frequency of postpartum hemorrhage. The overall incidence of postpartum hemorrhage was 8 percent, and such hemorrhage was not prevented by suckling.

Immediate Causes. The many factors of importance, singly or in combination, in the genesis of early postpartum hemorrhage are listed in Table 27–1. The two most common causes of immediate hemorrhage are hypotonic

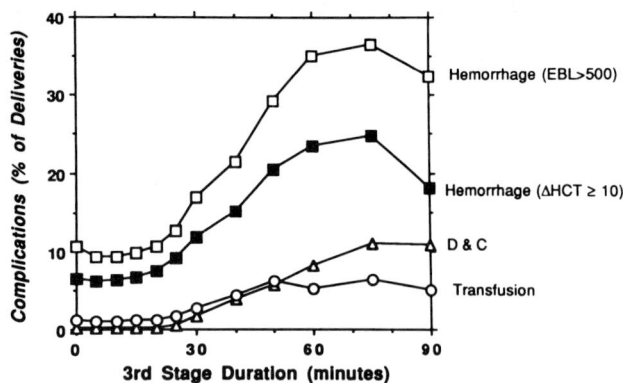

Fig. 27–1. Incidence of hemorrhage related to duration of the third stage of labor. (EBL = estimated blood loss; ΔHCT = change in hematocrit.) (From Combs and Laros, 1991, with permission.)

myometrium—**uterine atony**—and **lacerations of the vagina and cervix.** Retention of part or all of the placenta, a less common cause, may produce immediate or delayed hemorrhage, or both. It is uncommon for an episiotomy alone to cause severe postpartum hemorrhage, although blood so lost averages about 200 mL.

Predisposing Factors. As shown in Table 27–1, in many cases, postpartum hemorrhage can be predicted well in advance of delivery. Examples in which trauma is likely to lead to postpartum hemorrhage include delivery of a large infant, midforceps delivery, forceps rotation, any intrauterine manipulation, and perhaps vaginal delivery after cesarean section or other uterine incisions.

TABLE 27–1. PREDISPOSING FACTORS AND CAUSES OF IMMEDIATE POSTPARTUM HEMORRHAGE

Trauma to the Genital Tract
  Large episiotomy, including extensions
  Lacerations of perineum, vagina, or cervix
  Ruptured uterus

Bleeding from Placental Implantation Site
  Hypotonic myometrium—uterine atony
    Some general anesthetics—halogenated hydrocarbons
    Poorly perfused myometrium—hypotension
      Hemorrhage
      Conduction analgesia
    Overdistended uterus—large fetus, twins, hydramnios
    Following prolonged labor
    Following very rapid labor
    Following oxytocin-induced or augmented labor
    High parity
    Uterine atony in previous pregnancy
    Chorioamnionitis
  Retained placental tissue
    Avulsed cotyledon, succenturiate lobe
    Abnormally adherent—accreta, increta, percreta

Coagulation Defects
  Intensify all of the above

Uterine atony causing hemorrhage can be anticipated whenever excessive concentrations of halogenated anesthetic agents are used that will relax the uterus (Gilstrap and colleagues, 1987). The overdistended uterus very likely is to be hypotonic after delivery. Thus the woman with a large fetus, multiple fetuses, or hydramnios is prone to hemorrhage from uterine atony. Blood loss with delivery of twins, for example, averages nearly 1000 mL and may be much greater (Pritchard, 1965). The woman whose labor is characterized by uterine activity that is either remarkably vigorous or barely effective is also likely to bleed excessively from uterine atony after delivery.

Similarly, labor either initiated or augmented with oxytocin is more likely to be followed by postdelivery uterine atony and hemorrhage. The woman of high parity is at increased risk of hemorrhage from uterine atony. Fuchs and colleagues (1985) described the outcomes of nearly 5800 women para 7 or greater. They reported that the 2.7 percent incidence of postpartum hemorrhage in these women was increased fourfold compared with the general obstetrical population. However, Eidelman and colleagues (1988) found no such associations when they compared almost 900 women para 6 or more with their general population. Yet another risk is if the woman has previously suffered postpartum hemorrhage. Commonly, mismanagement of the third stage of labor involves an attempt to hasten delivery of the placenta short of manual removal. **Constant kneading and squeezing of the uterus that already is contracted likely will impede the physiological mechanism of placental detachment, causing incomplete placental separation and increased blood loss.**

Clinical Characteristics. Postpartum hemorrhage before placental delivery is called **third-stage hemorrhage.** Contrary to general opinion, whether bleeding occurs before or after placental delivery, or at both times, there may be no sudden massive hemorrhage but rather steady bleeding that at any given instant appears to be moderate, but persists until serious hypovolemia develops. Especially with hemorrhage after placental delivery, the constant seepage may, over a period of a few hours, lead to enormous blood loss. The effects of hemorrhage depend to a considerable degree upon the nonpregnant blood volume, magnitude of pregnancy-induced hypervolemia, and degree of anemia at the time of delivery. A treacherous feature of postpartum hemorrhage is the failure of the pulse and blood pressure to undergo more than moderate alterations until large amounts of blood have been lost, as emphasized in Chapter 37 (p. 821). The normotensive woman may actually become somewhat hypertensive in response to hemorrhage, at least initially. Moreover, the already hypertensive woman may be interpreted to be normotensive although remarkably hypovolemic. Tragically, the hypovolemia may not be recognized until very late.

As emphasized in Chapter 36 (p. 773), the woman with severe preeclampsia has usually lost her pregnancy-induced hypervolemia, and thus she frequently is very sensitive or even intolerant of what may be considered normal blood loss. **Therefore, when excessive hemorrhage is even suspected in the woman with severe pregnancy-induced hypertension, efforts should be made immediately to identify those clinical and laboratory findings that would prompt vigorous crystalloid and blood replacement.**

In instances in which the fundus has not been adequately monitored after delivery, the blood may not escape vaginally but instead may collect within the uterus. The uterine cavity may thus become distended by 1000 mL or more of blood while an inattentive attendant fails to identify the large uterus or, having done so, erroneously massages a roll of abdominal fat. The care of the postpartum uterus, therefore, must not be left to an inexperienced person.

Diagnosis. Except possibly when an intrauterine and intravaginal accumulation of blood is not recognized, or in some instances of uterine rupture with intraperitoneal bleeding, the diagnosis of postpartum hemorrhage should be obvious. The differentiation between bleeding from uterine atony and from lacerations is tentatively made on the condition of the uterus. If bleeding persists despite a firm, well-contracted uterus, the cause of the hemorrhage most probably is from lacerations. Bright red blood also suggests lacerations. **To ascertain the role of lacerations as a cause of bleeding, careful inspection of the vagina, cervix, and uterus is essential.**

Sometimes bleeding may be caused by both atony and trauma, especially after major operative delivery. In general, inspection of the cervix and vagina should be performed after every delivery to identify hemorrhage from lacerations. Anesthesia should be adequate to prevent discomfort during such an examination. Examination of the uterine cavity, the cervix, and all of the vagina is essential after breech extraction, after internal podalic version, and following vaginal delivery in a woman who previously underwent cesarean section. The same is true when unusual bleeding is identified during the second stage of labor.

Prognosis. Women with postpartum hemorrhage should not die, even though hysterectomy may be required in some instances. To obtain this objective requires assiduous attention to all women immediately postpartum, an effective blood bank, and alert action by an experienced obstetrical team. Although death from postpartum hemorrhage is currently rare in modern hospitals, it is common under less favorable conditions.

Other hazards associated with postpartum hemorrhage, discussed in Chapter 37 (p. 821), include renal failure from prolonged hypotension. Complications that follow treatment with blood include immediate reactions caused by donor–recipient incompatibilities. Late complications include bloodborne infections including hepatitis (Chap. 51, p. 1157) and human immunodeficiency virus infection (Chap. 59, p. 1310).

Sheehan Syndrome. Severe intrapartum or early postpartum hemorrhage is on rare occasions followed by Sheehan syndrome, which in the classical case is characterized by failure in lactation, amenorrhea, atrophy of the breasts, loss of pubic and axillary hair, superinvolution of the uterus, hypothyroidism, and adrenal cortical insufficiency. The exact pathogenesis is not well understood, because such endocrine abnormalities are not evident in most women who hemorrhage severely. In some but not all instances of Sheehan syndrome, varying degrees of anterior pituitary necrosis with impaired secretion of one or more of the pituitary's trophic hormones account for the endocrine abnormalities. The anterior pituitary of some women who develop hypopituitarism after puerperal hemorrhage does respond to various releasing hormones, which at the least implies impaired hypothalamic function. Moreover, confirmatory histological evidence of hypothalamic involvement was provided by Whitehead (1963), who identified specific atrophic changes in hypothalamic nuclei in some cases. Lactation after delivery usually, but not always, excludes extensive pituitary necrosis. In some women, failure to lactate may not be followed until many years later by other symptoms of pituitary insufficiency.

The incidence of Sheehan syndrome was originally estimated to be 1 per 10,000 deliveries (Sheehan and Murdoch, 1938). It appears to be equally rare today in the United States, although 100 cases were identified over two decades in a hospital in Puerto Rico (Haddock and colleagues, 1972). Application of the many tests of hypothalamic and pituitary function now available should identify milder forms of the syndrome are more prevalent (Grimes and Brooks, 1980). Bakiri and colleagues (1991) used computed tomography to study 54 women with documented Sheehan syndrome. In all of these, the appearance of the pituitary was abnormal, either the sella turcica was totally or partially empty.

Management of Third-Stage Bleeding. Some bleeding is inevitable during the third stage of every labor as the result of transient partial separation of the placenta. As the placenta separates, the blood from the implantation site may escape into the vagina immediately ("Duncan mechanism") or it may be concealed behind the placenta and membranes ("Schultze mechanism") until the placenta is delivered.

In the presence of any external hemorrhage during the third stage, the uterus should be massaged if it is not contracted firmly. If the signs of placental separation have appeared (see Chap. 14, p. 384), expression of the placenta should be attempted by manual fundal pressure. Descent of the placenta is indicated by the cord becoming slack. If bleeding continues, manual removal of the placenta is mandatory.

Technique of Manual Removal. When this operation is necessary, adequate analgesia or anesthesia is mandatory. Aseptic surgical technique should be employed and a sterile glove that covers the forearm to the elbow is recommended. After grasping the fundus through the abdominal wall with one hand, the other hand with the long glove is introduced into the vagina and passed into the uterus, along the umbilical cord. As soon as the placenta is reached, its margin is located and the ulnar border of the hand insinuated between it and the uterine wall (Fig. 27–2). Then with the back of the hand in contact with the uterus, the placenta is peeled off its uterine attachment by a motion similar to that employed in separating the leaves of a book. After its complete separation, the placenta should be grasped with the entire hand, which is then gradually withdrawn. Membranes are removed at the same time by carefully teasing them from the decidua, using ring forceps to grasp them as necessary. Some prefer to wipe out the uterine cavity with a sponge. If this is done, it is imperative that a sponge not be left in the uterus or vagina.

Management After Delivery of Placenta. The fundus should always be palpated following placental delivery to make certain that the uterus is well contracted. If it is not firm, vigorous fundal massage is indicated. In some institutions 0.2 mg of ergonovine (Ergotrate) or methylergonovine (Methergine) is administered routinely either intravenously or intramuscularly. More commonly,

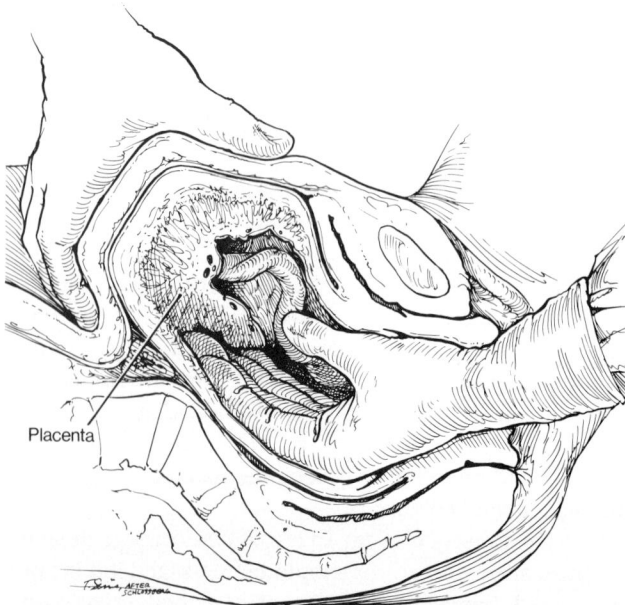

Placenta

Fig. 27–2. Manual removal of placenta. The fingers are alternately abducted, adducted, and advanced until the placenta is completely detached.

because hypertension occasionally develops following their administration, they are given only if there is excessive bleeding not controlled by an intravenous infusion of oxytocin and uterine massage. Most often 20 U of oxytocin in 1000 mL of lactated Ringers or normal saline solution proves effective when administered intravenously at approximately 10 mL per minute (200 μU of oxytocin per minute) simultaneously with effective uterine massage. Oxytocin should never be given as an undiluted bolus dose as serious hypotension may follow (see Chap. 14, p. 386).

ERGOT AND PROSTAGLANDIN DERIVATIVES. If oxytocin given by rapid infusion does not prove effective, some administer methylergonovine, 0.2 mg intramuscularly or intravenously. This may stimulate the uterus to contract sufficiently to control hemorrhage. Any superior therapeutic effects of ergot derivatives over oxytocin are speculative, and if intravenously administered they may cause dangerous hypertension, especially in the woman with preeclampsia.

In the mid 1980s, the 15-methyl derivative of prostaglandin $F_{2\alpha}$ (carboprost tromethamine) was approved by the Food and Drug Administration for treatment of postpartum hemorrhage from uterine atony. The initial recommended dose is 250 μg (0.25 mg) given intramuscularly, and this is repeated if necessary at 15- to 90-minute intervals up to a maximum of 8 doses. Oleen and Mariano (1990) studied use of carboprost for postpartum hemorrhage at 12 cooperating obstetrical units. Arrest of bleeding was considered successful in 208 of 237 (88 percent) women treated. An additional 17 women required other oxytocics for control of hemorrhage. The remaining 12 women in whom drug treatment failed required surgical intervention. Nelson and Suresh (1992) have suggested that such unrelenting immediate postpartum hemorrhage is due to lack of uterine artery reactivity.

In our experience, as well as that of others, continued bleeding after prostaglandin administration frequently results from unrecognized genital tract laceration, including, in some cases, uterine rupture. Carboprost is associated with side effects in about 20 percent of women (Oleen and Mariano, 1990). In descending order of frequency, these included diarrhea, hypertension, vomiting, fever, flushing, and tachycardia. At Parkland Hospital we have encountered serious hypertension in a few women so treated. Hankins and colleagues (1988) observed that intramuscular carboprost was associated with arterial oxygen desaturation that averaged 10 percent and developed within 15 minutes; they concluded that the decrease was because of pulmonary airway and vascular constriction.

If bleeding persists despite these procedures, no time should be lost in haphazard efforts to control hemorrhage, but the following management should be initiated immediately:

1. Employ bimanual uterine compression (Fig. 27–3). This procedure will control most hemorrhage.
2. Obtain help!
3. Begin blood transfusions. The blood group of every obstetrical patient should be known, if possible, before labor, and an indirect Coombs test done to detect erythrocyte antibodies. If the latter is negative, then cross-matching of blood is not necessary (Chap. 37, p. 822), but in an extreme emergency, type-specific whole blood is given.
4. Explore the uterine cavity manually for retained placental fragments or lacerations.
5. Thoroughly inspect the cervix and vagina after adequate exposure.
6. Add a second intravenous route using a large-bore intravenous catheter so that oxytocin is continued at the same time as blood is given.
7. Adequacy of cardiac output and arterial filling can be evaluated by monitoring urine output; a Foley catheter is inserted (see Chapter 37, p. 821).

The technique of bimanual compression consists simply of massage of the posterior aspect of the uterus with the abdominal hand and massage through the vagina of the anterior uterine aspect with the other fist, the knuckles of which contact the uterine wall (Fig. 27–3). Packing the uterus was an alternative procedure that formerly enjoyed greater popularity. **The recently pregnant uterus cannot be satisfactorily packed immediately after delivery because it dilates under the packing, with further concealed hemorrhage that may be fatal.**

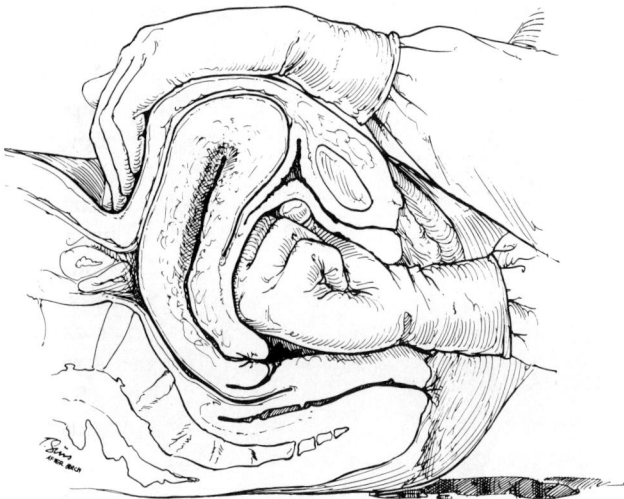

Fig. 27–3. Bimanual compression of the uterus and massage with the abdominal hand usually will effectively control hemorrhage from uterine atony.

Blood transfusion should be initiated immediately in any case of postpartum hemorrhage in which abdominal uterine massage and oxytocic agents fail to control the bleeding. With transfusion and simultaneous manual uterine compression and intravenous oxytocin, additional measures are rarely required. If the operator's hand tires, an associate can relieve.

Hemorrhage from Retained Placental Fragments. Immediate postpartum hemorrhage is seldom caused by retained small placental fragments, but a remaining piece of placenta is a common cause of bleeding late in the puerperium. Inspection of the placenta after delivery must be routine. If a portion of placenta is missing, the uterus should be explored and the fragment removed, particularly with continuing postpartum bleeding. Retention of a succenturiate lobe (see Figs. 5–15 and 5–16) is an occasional cause of postpartum hemorrhage. The late bleeding that may result from a placental polyp is discussed in Chapter 29 (p. 644).

Hemorrhage from Lacerations. If rupture of the uterus is identified, laparotomy, and usually hysterectomy, is mandatory for a favorable outcome (see Chap. 23, p. 551). Lacerations of the cervix and the vaginal vault sometimes cause profuse bleeding. **Anytime that bleeding persists in the presence of a firmly contracted intact uterus, hemorrhage from lacerations of the cervix, vagina, or uterus should be suspected.** In any case of protracted hemorrhage, moreover, even though uterine atony certainly is the cause, inspection of the birth canal is a necessary precaution to avoid overlooking a serious laceration. Uterine tears may cause persistent bleeding that distends the uterine cavity to cause in addition uterine atony. Proper exposure of the cervix and upper vagina to repair such lacerations usually requires an associate. Two retractors are inserted into the vagina, the walls of which are separated widely. Ring forceps are then placed on the anterior and posterior cervical lips, which are carefully inspected, especially laterally (see Chap. 23, Fig. 23–1). Lacerations that are bleeding should be repaired promptly. Either interrupted single sutures or figure-of-eight sutures are employed, with the highest one placed slightly above the apex of the tear, because bleeding from cervical lacerations usually arises from a vessel at this point.

If rupture of the uterus is identified, uterine repair, and oftentimes hysterectomy, is life-saving (see Chap. 23, p. 551). With an apparently intact uterus, and when other measures to combat postpartum hemorrhage fail, the question of hysterectomy arises. If performed without initiating blood replacement in a woman who is profoundly hypovolemic, hysterectomy may hasten death. On the other hand, hysterectomy should not be delayed unduly. Vigorous transfusion therapy should be initiated and surgery begun promptly. This approach will prevent deaths in cases in which all other measures to arrest hemorrhage fail. Cesarean hysterectomy technique is described in Chapter 26 (p. 604).

Vulvovaginal Hematomas. Puerperal hematomas may be associated with significant hemorrhage, both immediately after delivery and later in the postpartum course (see Chap. 29, p. 644). Hematomas may be classified according to their location in relation to the levator ani muscles. Those below the muscles are most commonly associated with vaginal delivery and present as a painful ischiorectal mass. These hematomas are limited superiorly by the levator ani and limited from spread onto the thigh by Colle's fascia and the fascia lata. The central tendon of the perineum prevents them from spreading across the midline. Supralevator or subperitoneal hematomas have the levator ani as their inferior border. These hematomas usually are associated with uterine rupture and dissect into the broad ligament and retroperitoneal space leading rapidly to hypovolemia. Management of vulvar hematomas is presented in Chapter 29 (p. 644).

Placenta Accreta, Increta, and Percreta

In most instances, the placenta separates spontaneously from its implantation site during the first few minutes after delivery of the infant. The precise reason for delay in detachment beyond this time is not obvious always, but quite often it seems to be due to inadequate uterine contraction. Very infrequently, the placenta is unusually adherent to the implantation site, with scanty or absent decidua, so that the physiological line of cleavage through the decidual spongy layer is lacking. As a consequence, one or more cotyledons are firmly bound to the defective decidua basalis or even to the myometrium. When the placenta is densely anchored in this fashion, the condition is called placenta accreta.

Definitions. The term **placenta accreta** is used to describe any placental implantation in which there is abnormally firm adherence to the uterine wall. As the consequence of partial or total absence of the decidua basalis and imperfect development of the fibrinoid layer *(Nitabuch layer)*, placental villi are attached to the myometrium in **placenta accreta** (Fig. 27–4), actually invade the myometrium in **placenta increta,** or penetrate through the myometrium in **placenta percreta** (Fig. 27–5). The abnormal adherence may involve all of the cotyledons (total placenta accreta), a few to several cotyledons (partial placenta accreta), or a single cotyledon (focal placenta accreta).

Significance. An abnormally adherent placenta, although an uncommon condition, assumes considerable significance clinically because of morbidity and, at times, mortality from severe hemorrhage, uterine perforation, and infection. The true frequencies of placenta accreta, increta, and percreta are unknown. For example, Breen and associates (1977) reviewed reports published since 1891. The incidence varied from 1 in 540 deliveries to 1 in 70,000 deliveries, with an average incidence of about 1 in 7000. Read and co-workers (1980) reported an incidence of about 1 per 2500 deliveries and con-

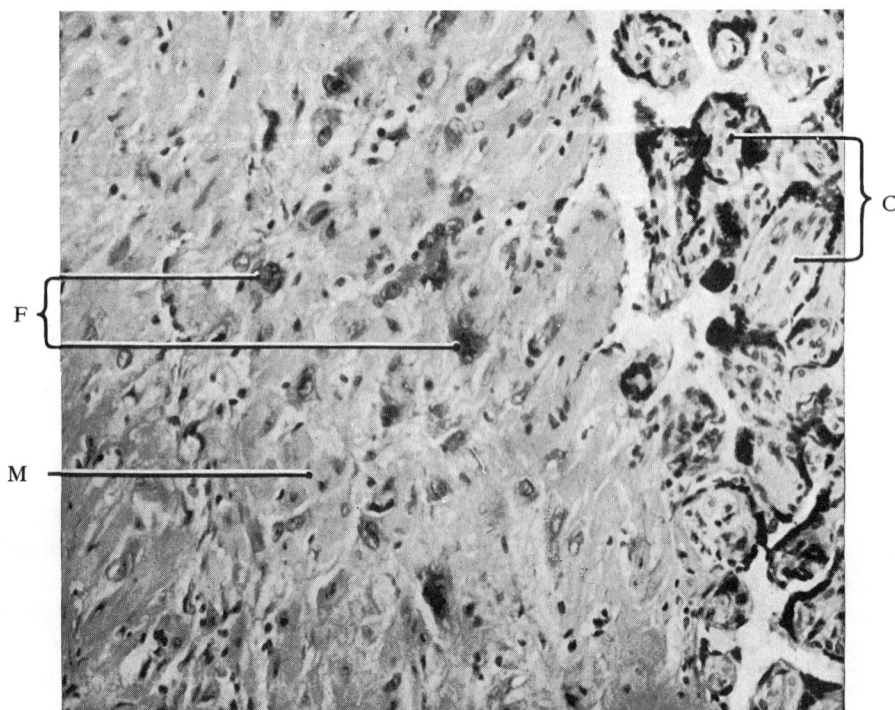

Fig. 27–4. Photomicrograph of uterine wall in a case of placenta accreta. Notice the absence of decidua with chorionic villi in contact with the myometrium. (C = chorionic villi; F = trophoblastic giant cells; M = myometrium.)

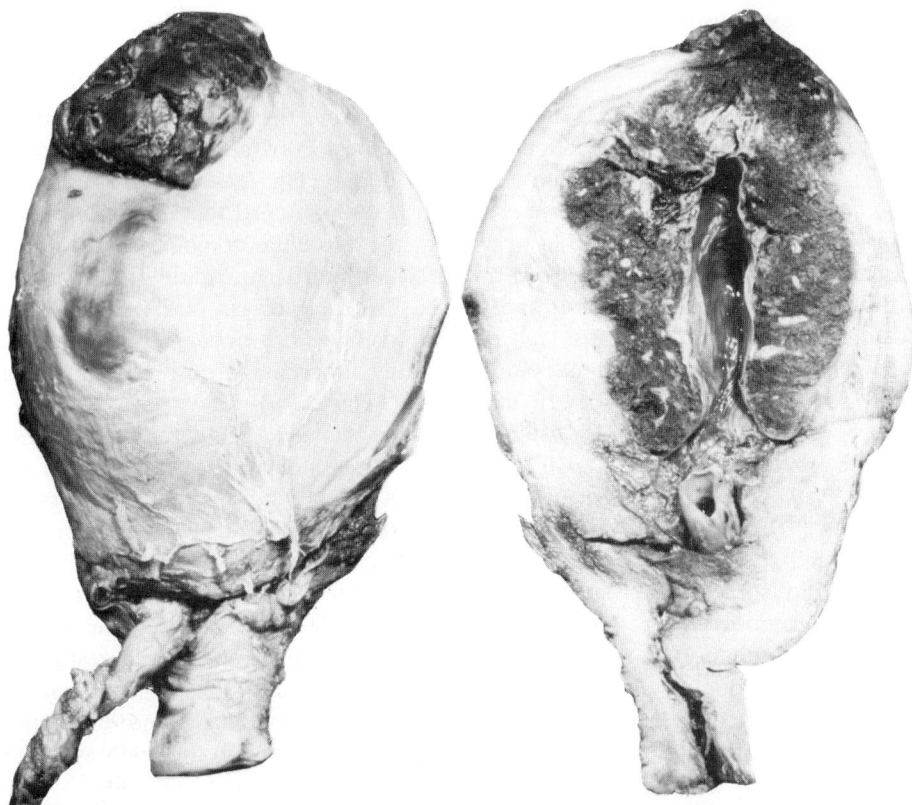

Fig. 27–5. Placenta percreta. On the left, the placenta is fungating through the fundus above the old classical cesarean section scar. In the opened specimen on the right, the variable penetration of the fundus by the placenta is evident. (From Morison, 1978.)

cluded that today there is a higher reported incidence, lower parity, and greater incidence of associated placenta previa, as well as decreasing maternal and perinatal mortality.

Etiological Factors. Abnormal placental adherence is found most often in circumstances where decidual formation was likely to have been defective. Associated conditions include implantation in the lower uterine segment, over a previous cesarean section scar, or other previous uterine incisions; or occurrence after uterine curettage. Fox (1972), in his review of 622 reported cases of placenta accreta collected between 1945 and 1969, noted the following characteristics: (1) placenta previa was identified in one third of affected pregnancies, (2) one fourth of the women had been delivered previously by cesarean section, (3) nearly one fourth previously had undergone curettage, and (4) one fourth were gravida 6 or more. Read and co-workers (1980) reported similar findings for women studied in the 1970s; however, the overall incidence and parity had decreased.

Clinical Course. Antepartum hemorrhage is common, but in the great majority of cases, antepartum bleeding is the consequence of coexisting placenta previa. Myometrial invasion by placental villi at the site of a previous cesarean section scar may lead to uterine rupture during labor or even before (Berchuck and Sokol, 1983).

Archer and Furlong (1987) described a woman who presented with an acute abdomen from massive hemoperitoneum caused by placenta percreta at 21 weeks' gestation. In women whose pregnancies go to term, however, labor most likely is to be normal in the absence of an associated placenta previa or an involved uterine scar.

The problems associated with delivery of the placenta and subsequent developments vary appreciably, depending upon the site of implantation, depth of myometrial penetration, and number of cotyledons involved. It is very likely that focal placenta accreta with implantation in the upper uterine segment develops much more often than is recognized. The involved cotyledon is either pulled off the myometrium with perhaps somewhat excessive bleeding, or the cotyledon is torn from the placenta and adheres to the implantation site with increased bleeding, immediately or later. This probably is the mechanism of formation of many so-called placental polyps which are further described in Chapter 29 (p. 644).

With more extensive involvement, however, hemorrhage becomes profuse as delivery of the placenta is attempted. Successful treatment depends upon immediate blood replacement therapy, as described in Chapter 37 (p. 822), and nearly always prompt hysterectomy.

With total placenta accreta, there may be very little or no bleeding, at least until manual placental removal is attempted. At times, traction on the umbilical cord will invert the uterus as described below. Moreover, usual attempts at manual removal will not succeed, because a cleavage plane between the maternal placental surface and the uterine wall cannot be developed. The safest treatment in this circumstance is prompt hysterectomy (Fig. 27–6).

In the 622 cases reviewed by Fox (1972), the most common form of "conservative" management was manual removal of as much placenta as possible and then packing of the uterus. **One fourth of the women died,** which was four times as many as when treatment consisted of immediate hysterectomy. So-called "conservative" treatment in at least 4 instances was followed by an apparently normal pregnancy.

The possibility exists that placenta increta might be diagnosed antepartum. Tabsh and co-workers (1982), as well as Cox and associates (1988), described a case of placenta previa in which they also were able to identify placenta increta ultrasonically from *the lack of the usual subplacental sonolucent space.* They hypothesize that the presence of this normal subplacental sonolucent area represents the decidual basalis and the underlying myometrial tissue. The absence of this sonolucent area is consistent with the presence of a placenta increta. Pasto and associates (1983) confirmed that the *absence* of a subplacental sonolucent or "hypoechoic retroplacental zone" is consistent with placenta increta.

Inversion of the Uterus

Etiology. Complete uterine inversion after delivery of the infant is almost always the consequence of strong traction on an umbilical cord attached to a placenta implanted in the fundus (Fig. 27–7). Contributing to uterine inversion is a tough cord that does not readily break away from the placenta, combined with fundal pressure and a relaxed uterus, including the lower segment and cervix. Placenta accreta may be implicated although uterine inversion can occur without the placenta being so firmly adherent. At times, the inversion may be incomplete (Fig. 27–8).

Shah-Hosseini and Evrard (1989) reported an incidence of about 1 in 6400 deliveries at the Women and Infant Hospital of Rhode Island. Of the 11 inversions identified, most were in primiparous women and immediate vaginal replacement of the inverted uterus was successful in 9 instances. Platt and Druzin (1981) reported 28 cases in over 60,000 deliveries, for an incidence of about 1 in 2100. These same investigators suggested that parenteral magnesium sulfate, which was administered to women with pregnancy-induced hypertension, might have played a role in the etiology of this complication.

Clinical Course. Uterine inversion is most often associated with immediate life-threatening hemorrhage, and

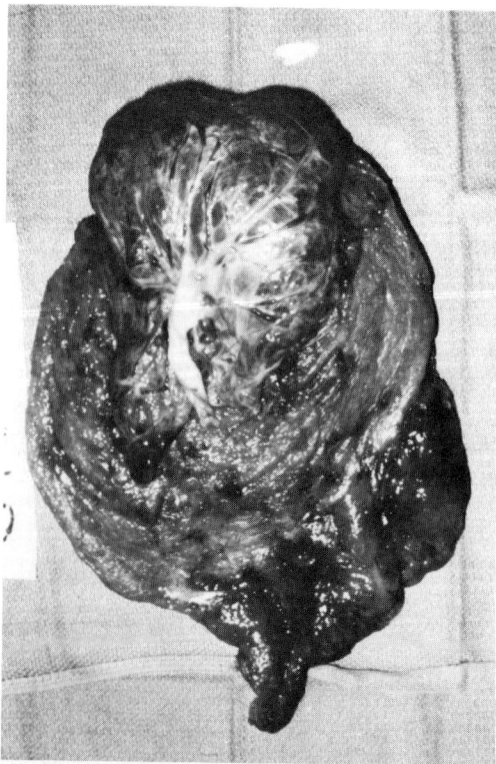

Fig. 27–6. Hysterectomy for placenta accreta. The uterus has been opened anteriorly to show the adherent placenta accreta in the fundal portion.

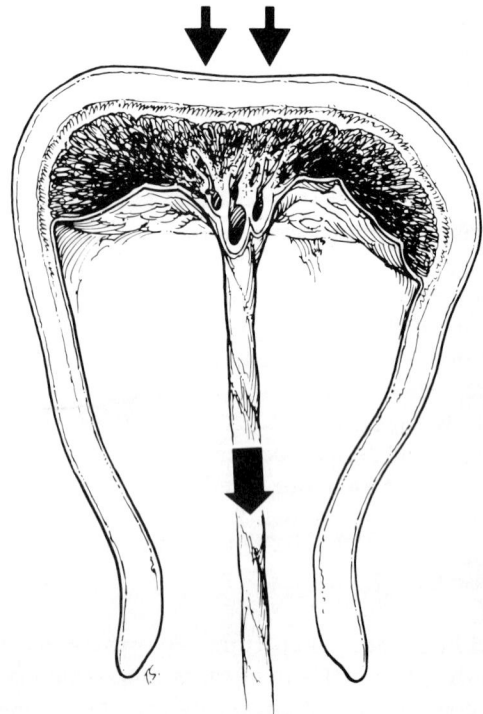

Fig. 27–7. Most likely site of placental implantation in cases of uterine inversion. With traction on the cord and the placenta still attached, the likelihood of inversion is obvious.

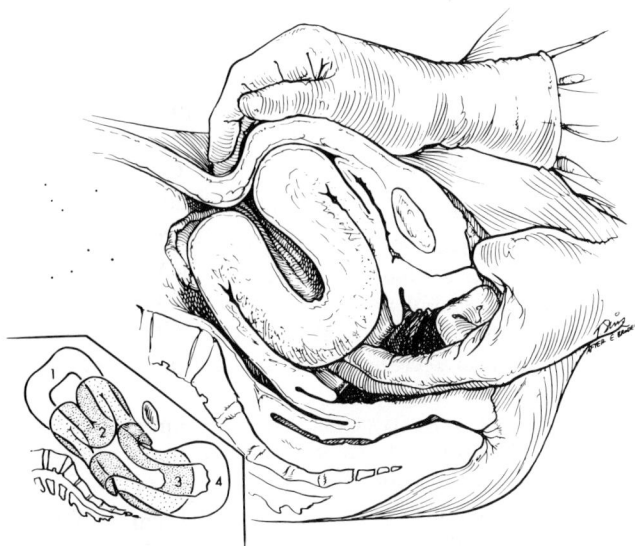

Fig. 27–8. Incomplete uterine inversion. The diagnosis is made by abdominal palpation of the craterlike depression and vaginal palpation of the fundal wall in the lower segment and cervix. Progressive degrees of inversion are shown in the *inset*.

without prompt treatment it may be fatal (Fig. 27–9). It has been stated that shock tends to be disproportionate to blood loss (Greenhill and Friedman, 1974). Careful evaluation of the effects from transfusion of large volumes of blood in such cases does not support this concept, but instead makes it very apparent that blood loss in such circumstances was often massive but greatly underestimated. It is not unusual even for the woman who has been given several units of blood because of hypotension to become anemic subsequently when isovolemic. Such outcomes are difficult to reconcile with

the concept of shock out of proportion to blood loss (Watson and associates, 1980).

Treatment. Delay in treatments increases the mortality rate appreciably. It is imperative that a number of steps be taken immediately and simultaneously:

1. Assistance, including an anesthesiologist, is summoned immediately.
2. The freshly inverted uterus with placenta already separated from it may often be replaced simply by immediately pushing up on the fundus with the palm of the hand and fingers in the direction of the long axis of the vagina.
3. Preferably two intravenous infusion systems are made operational, and lactated Ringer solution and whole blood are given to reverse hypovolemia.
4. If attached, the placenta is not removed until the infusion systems are operational, fluids are being given, and anesthesia, preferably halothane or forane, has been administered. More recently, tocolytic drugs have been used successfully for this purpose. Terbutaline, ritodrine, and magnesium sulfate have all been used for uterine relaxation and repositioning (Catanzarite and associates, 1986; Kovacs and DeVore, 1984; Thiery and Delbeke, 1985). To remove the placenta before this time increases the hemorrhage. In the meantime, the inverted uterus, if prolapsed beyond the vagina, is replaced within the vagina.
5. After removing the placenta, the palm of the hand is placed on the center of the fundus with the fingers extended to identify the margins of the cervix. Pressure is then applied with the hand so as to push the fundus upward through the cervix.
6. Oxytocin is *not* given until after the uterus is restored to its normal configuration.

As soon as the uterus is restored to its normal configuration, the agent used to provide relaxation is stopped and simultaneously oxytocin is started to contract the uterus while the operator maintains the fundus in normal relationship. Initially, bimanual compression, as illustrated in Figure 27–3, will aid in the control of further hemorrhage until uterine tone is recovered. After the uterus is well contracted, the operator continues to monitor the uterus transvaginally for any evidence of subsequent inversion, although this occurrence is quite unlikely.

Surgical Intervention. Most often, the inverted uterus can be restored to its normal position by the techniques described above. If the uterus cannot be reinverted by vaginal manipulation because of a dense constriction ring (Fig. 27–10), laparotomy is imperative. The fundus then may be simultaneously pushed upward from below

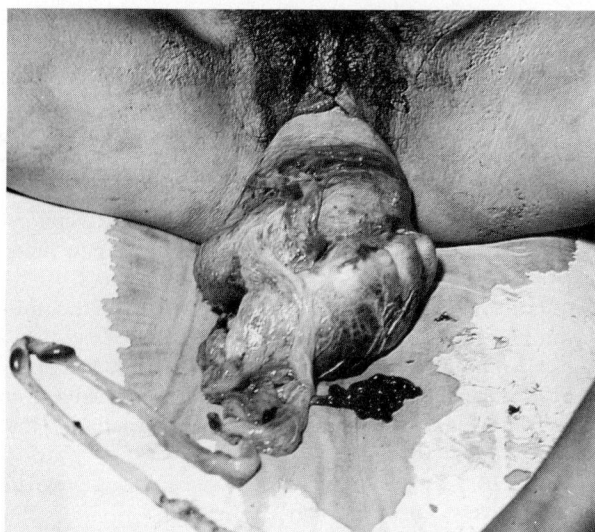

Fig. 27–9. A fatal case of inverted uterus associated with placenta accreta following delivery at home.

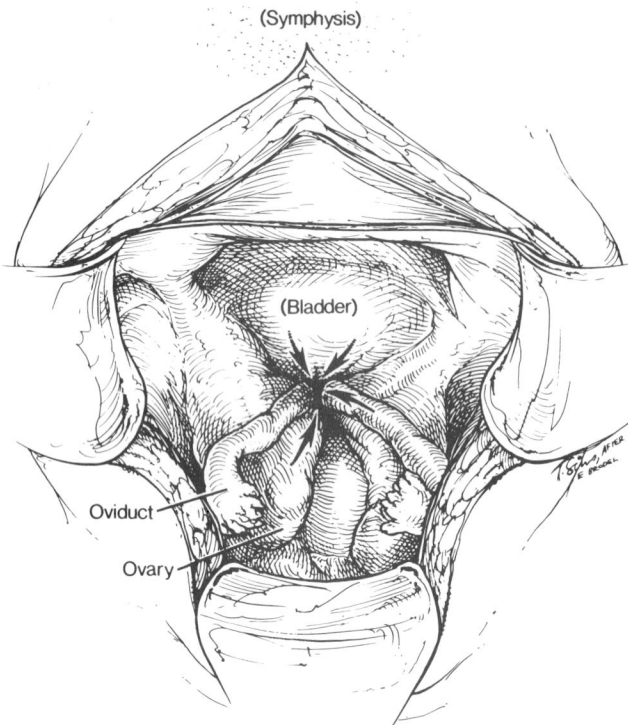

Fig. 27–10. Completely inverted uterus viewed from above.

and pulled from above. A traction suture well placed in the inverted fundus may be of aid. If the constriction ring still prohibits reposition, it is carefully incised posteriorly to expose the fundus. A graphic outline of this surgical technique was described by Van Vugt and associates (1981). After replacement of the fundus, the anesthetic agent used to relax the myometrium is stopped, oxytocin infusion is begun, and the uterine incision repaired. Following restoration of the uterus, the adjacent viscera are carefully examined for trauma.

References

Archer GE, Furlong LA: Acute abdomen caused by placenta percreta in the second trimester. Am J Obstet Gynecol 157:146, 1987

Bakiri F, Bendib SE, Maoui R, Bendib A, Benmiloud M: The sella turcica in Sheehan's syndrome: Computerized tomographic study in 54 patients. J Endocrinol Invest 14:193, 1991

Berchuck A, Sokol RJ: Previous cesarean section, placenta increta, and uterine rupture in second-trimester abortion. Am J Obstet Gynecol 145:766, 1983

Breen JL, Neubecker R, Gregori CA, Franklin JE Jr: Placenta accreta, increta, and percreta: A survey of 40 cases. Obstet Gynecol 49:43, 1977

Bullough CHW, Msuku RS, Karonde L: Early suckling and postpartum hemorrhagic controlled trial in deliveries by traditional birth attendants. Lancet 2:522, 1989

Catanzarite VA, Moffitt KD, Baker ML, Awadalla SG, Argubright KF, Perkins RP: New approaches to the management of acute puerperal uterine invasion. Obstet Gynecol 68:7S, 1986

Combs CA, Laros RK: Prolonged third stage of labor: Morbidity and risk factors. Obstet Gynecol 77:863, 1991

Cox SM, Carpenter RJ, Cotton DB: Placenta percreta: Ultrasound diagnosis and conservative surgical management. Obstet Gynecol 72:452, 1988

DeLeeuw NKM, Lowenstein L, Tucker EC, Dayal S: Correlation of red cell loss at delivery with changes in red cell mass. Am J Obstet Gynecol 84:1271, 1968

Eidelman AI, Kamar R, Schimmel MS, Bar-On E: The grandmultipara: Is she still a risk? Am J Obstet Gynecol 158:389, 1988

Fox H: Placenta accreta, 1945–1969. Obstet Gynecol Surv 27:475, 1972

Fuchs K, Peretz B-A, Marcovici R, Paldi E, Timor-Tritsh I: The "grand multipara"—Is it a problem? A review of 5785 cases. Int J Gynaecol Obstet 23:321, 1985

Gilstrap LC, Hauth JC, Hankins GDV, Patterson AR: Effect of type of anesthesia on blood loss at cesarean section. Obstet Gynecol 69:328, 1987

Greenhill JP, Friedman EA: Biological Principles and Modern Practice of Obstetrics. Philadelphia, Saunders, 1974, p 687

Grimes HG, Brooks MH: Pregnancy in Sheehan's syndrome. Report of a case and review. Obstet Gynecol Surv 35:481, 1980

Haddock L, Vega LA, Aguilo F, Rodriguez O: Adrenocortical, thyroidal and human growth hormone reserve in Sheehan's syndrome. Johns Hopkins Med J 131:80, 1972

Hankins GDV, Berry GK, Scott RT Jr, Hood D: Maternal arterial desaturation with 15-methyl prostaglandin F_2 alpha for uterine atony. Obstet Gynecol 65:605, 1988

Huber MG, Wildschut HI, Boer K, Kleiverda G, Hoek FJ: Umbilical vein administration of oxytocin for the management of retained placenta. Is it effective? Am J Obstet Gynecol 164:1216, 1991

Kovacs BW, DeVore GR: Management of acute and subacute puerperal uterine inversion with terbutaline sulfate. Am J Obstet Gynecol 150:784, 1984

Morison JE: Obstetrics and Gynecology Annual. New York, Appleton-Century-Crofts, 1978, p 113

Nelson SH, Suresh MS: Lack of reactivity of uterine arteries from patients with obstetric hemorrhage. Am J Obstet Gynecol 166:1436, 1992

Newton M: Postpartum hemorrhage. Am J Obstet Gynecol 94:711, 1966

Oleen MA, Mariano JP: Controlling refractory atonic postpartum hemorrhage with Hemabate sterile solution. Am J Obstet Gynecol 162:205, 1990

Pasto ME, Kurtz AB, Rifkin MD, Cole-Beuglet C, Wapner RJ, Goldberg BB: Ultrasonographic findings in placenta increta. J Ultrasound Med 2:155, 1983

Platt LD, Druzin ML: Acute puerperal inversion of the uterus. Am J Obstet Gynecol 141:187, 1981

Porter KB, O'Brien WF, Collins MK, Givens P, Knuppel R, Bruskivage L: A randomized comparison of umbilical vein and intravenous oxytocin during the puerperium. Obstet Gynecol 78:254, 1991

Pritchard JA: Changes in the blood volume during pregnancy and delivery. Anesthesiology 26:393, 1965

Pritchard JA, Baldwin RM, Dickey JC, Wiggins KM: Blood volume changes in pregnancy and the puerperium: II. Red blood cell loss and changes in apparent blood volume during and following vaginal delivery, cesarean section, and cesarean section plus total hysterectomy. Am J Obstet Gynecol 84:1271, 1962

Read JA, Cotton DB, Miller FC: Placenta accreta: Changing clinical aspects and outcome. Obstet Gynecol 56:31, 1980

Shah-Hosseini R, Evrard JR: Puerperal uterine inversion. Obstet Gynecol 73:567, 1989

Sheehan HL, Murdoch R: Postpartum necrosis of the anterior pituitary: Pathological and clinical aspects. Br J Obstet Gynaecol 45:456, 1938

Tabsh KMA, Brinkman CR III, King W: Ultrasound diagnosis of placenta increta. J Clin Ultrasound 10:288, 1982

Thiery M, Delbeke L: Acute puerperal uterine inversion: Two-step management with a β-mimetic and a prostaglandin. Am J Obstet Gynecol 153:891, 1985

Van Vugt PJH, Baudoin P, Blom VM, van Duersen TBM: Inversio uteri puerperalis. Acta Obstet Gynecol Scand 60:353, 1981

Watson P, Besch N, Bowes WA Jr: Management of acute and subacute puerperal inversion of the uterus. Obstet Gynecol 55:12, 1980

Whitehead R: The hypothalamus in post-partum hypopituitarism. J Pathol Bacteriol 86:55, 1963

Young SB, Martelly PD, Greb L, Considine G, Coustau DR: The effect of intraumbilical oxytocin on the third stage of labor. Obstet Gynecol 71:736, 1988

CHAPTER 28
Puerperal Infection

Puerperal infection is a general term used to describe any bacterial infection of the genital tract after delivery. Pelvic infections are the most common serious complications of the puerperium. Previously used but less satisfactory synonyms are puerperal fever, puerperal sepsis, and childbed fever. Infection, along with preeclampsia and obstetrical hemorrhage, for many decades of this century formed the lethal triad of causes of maternal deaths (Chap. 1, p. 4). Fortunately, more recently, maternal death from infection has become less common (Sachs and associates, 1988). The Maternal Mortality Collaborative (Rochat and colleagues, 1988) reported that about 4 percent of maternal deaths were caused by infection. In another review of 2644 maternal deaths from 1979 to 1986, infection was associated with about 8 percent of the total (Atrash and colleagues, 1990). During this time period there were approximately 0.6 maternal deaths from infection per 100,000 live births. Some of the more interesting historical aspects of puerperal infections are considered at the end of this chapter.

Puerperal Morbidity. Because most temperature elevations in the puerperium are caused by pelvic infection, the incidence of fever after childbirth is a reliable index of their incidence. For this reason, it has been customary to group all puerperal fevers under the general term *puerperal morbidity,* and to estimate the frequency of infection on this basis. Several definitions have been based on the degree of pyrexia. The Joint Committee on Maternal Welfare was convened in 1919 (Mussey and colleagues, 1935), and several years later it modified the European standards and defined puerperal morbidity as follows: *Temperature 38.0° C (100.4° F) or higher, the temperature to occur on any 2 of the first 10 days postpartum, exclusive of the first 24 hours, and to be taken by mouth by a standard technique at least four times daily.* This remains the most commonly employed definition in the United States, and while it suggests that all puerperal fevers are the consequence of pelvic infection, temperature elevations may be the result of other causes.

Differential Diagnosis of Fever. **Most persistent fevers after childbirth are caused by genital tract infection.** This is especially likely if the preceding labor was attended by extensive vaginal or uterine manipulation, prolonged membrane rupture, or intrauterine electronic monitoring. Regardless, every postpartum woman whose temperature rises to and persists at 38° C should be evaluated for extrapelvic causes of fever as well as for puerperal infection. Filker and Monif (1979) reported that only 21 percent of febrile women (first 24 hours) delivered vaginally were found to have infection, in contrast to 72 percent of those delivered by cesarean section. Some extragenital causes of puerperal fever include *respiratory complications, pyelonephritis, intense breast engorgement, bacterial mastitis, thrombophlebitis,* and in cases of laparotomy, *incisional wound abscess.*

Respiratory complications are most often seen within the first 24 hours following delivery, and almost invariably are in women delivered by cesarean section or given general anesthesia for vaginal delivery. Complications include atelectasis, aspiration pneumonia, or occasionally, bacterial pneumonia. Atelectasis is best prevented with the use of routine coughing and deep breathing on a fixed schedule, usually every 4 hours for at least 24 hours following the administration of general anesthesia. It is conjectural whether atelectasis alone causes fever. Because of severe sequelae, the possibility of aspiration must be suspected. These women most often will develop a high spiking fever, varying degrees of respiratory wheezing, and in most instances, obvious signs of hypoxemia (see Chap. 16, p. 430).

Pyelonephritis may be difficult to diagnose postpartum. In the typical case, bacteriuria, pyuria, costovertebral angle tenderness, and spiking temperature clearly indicate renal infection; however, the clinical picture varies. For example, in the puerperal woman the first sign of renal infection may be a temperature elevation, but costovertebral angle tenderness may not develop until later. The clinical diagnosis is confirmed by demonstrating bacteriuria microscopically and by urine culture. Empirical therapy is begun without waiting for culture results.

Breast engorgement commonly causes a brief temperature elevation. About 15 percent of all postpartum women develop fever from breast engorgement, which rarely exceeds 39° C in the first few postpartum days (Chap. 29, p. 646). The fever characteristically lasts no longer than 24 hours. In contrast, the elevated temperature of bacterial mastitis develops later and usually is sustained. It is associated with other signs and symptoms of breast infection that become overt within 24 hours.

Superficial or deep venous **thrombophlebitis** of the legs may cause temperature elevations in the puerperal woman. The diagnosis is made by the observation of a painful, swollen leg, usually accompanied by calf tenderness, or occasionally femoral triangle area tenderness. Treatment is given with intravenous heparin therapy (Chap. 49, p. 1115).

Postpartum Uterine Infection

Postpartum uterine infection has been called variously *endometritis, endomyometritis,* and *endoparametritis.* Because infection actually involves the decidua, myometrium, and parametrial tissues, we prefer the term **metritis with pelvic cellulitis.** Uterine infections are relatively uncommon following uncomplicated vaginal delivery, but they continue to be a major problem in women delivered by cesarean section. Thus, the route of delivery (e.g., cesarean section), is the single most significant risk factor for the development of postpartum uterine infection.

Wachsberg and Kurtz (1992) recently demonstrated that gas within the endometrial cavity following spontaneous vaginal delivery is not associated with uterine infection in most cases. Utilizing ultrasound, these authors studied 70 healthy women following uncomplicated vaginal delivery and demonstrated gas in the endometrial cavity in 20 percent within the first 3 days postpartum. Interestingly, 5 patients had gas in the endometrial cavity for more than 2 weeks after delivery. None of the women developed metritis.

Vaginal Delivery. Compared with cesarean section, metritis following vaginal delivery is relatively uncommon. Sweet and Ledger (1973) reported that the incidence of postpartum uterine infections after vaginal delivery was 2.6 percent. A 6-month survey during 1987 of nearly 5000 women delivered vaginally at Parkland Hospital showed that only 1.3 percent were given treatment for metritis. However, when women at high risk—defined by prolonged membrane rupture and labor, multiple cervical examinations, and internal fetal monitoring—were analyzed separately, the incidence of metritis after vaginal delivery was nearly 6 percent. The presence of intraamnionic infection (i.e., chorioamnionitis), also increases the risk of metritis following vaginal delivery to 13 percent (Maberry and colleagues, 1991). Finally, Monif (1991) has identified intrapartum bacteriuria to be a risk factor for metritis following vaginal delivery.

Cesarean Delivery. Delivery by cesarean section places the woman at extraordinary risk for developing uterine infection. The incidence of metritis following surgical delivery varies with socioeconomic factors, and over the years this has been altered substantively by the common use of perioperative antimicrobials (see Chap. 26, p. 609). Prior to common use of antimicrobial prophylaxis, Sweet and Ledger (1973) reported an overall

incidence of uterine infection of 13 percent among affluent women undergoing cesarean section at the University of Michigan Hospital; however, they reported the incidence to be 27 percent in indigent women delivered at Wayne County Hospital. Cunningham and associates (1978) found an overall incidence of about 50 percent in women delivered by cesarean section at Parkland Hospital. When risk factors for infection were analyzed, duration of labor and membrane rupture, multiple cervical examinations, and internal fetal monitoring were found to be important determinants of infection morbidity. Women with all of these factors delivered for cephalopelvic disproportion, who were not given perioperative prophylaxis, had an incidence of serious pelvic infection that was nearly 90 percent (DePalma and colleagues, 1982; Gilstrap and Cunningham, 1979).

Predisposing Causes. Besides the risk factors listed above, it is generally accepted that pelvic infection is much more common in women from populations of lower socioeconomic status compared with middle- or upper-class patients. The precise reasons for these differences are unclear. Anemia, poor nutrition, and sexual intercourse have also been considered to predispose to puerperal sepsis, although the evidence is mostly indirect.

The evidence that **anemia** increases the likelihood of infection is not conclusive (Cook and Lynch, 1986). The results obtained from both animal and in vitro experiments are consistent with the view that iron-deficiency anemia does not predispose to infection, and some believe it may actually prevent infection. For example, transferrin, which is increased in iron-deficiency anemia, appears to have significant antibacterial action. Moreover, growth of a variety of pathogenic bacteria in vitro is inhibited by lack of iron. Finally, there is no impairment of wound healing in animals previously made iron deficient. The role of **nutrition** in the genesis of infection is also unclear, although cell-mediated immunity is impaired in malnourished laboratory animals.

An increased incidence of puerperal infection resulting from **sexual intercourse** has not been clearly demonstrated. If, however, the membranes were ruptured at the time of coitus, or if they were to rupture very soon thereafter, the infection rate would most likely be increased. Moreover, preterm delivery has been reported to be more frequent in women who had intercourse late in gestation, and the etiology may possibly be the consequence of infection (Naeye, 1979).

Colonization of the lower genital tract with certain microorganisms such as group B Streptococcus, *Chlamydia trachomatis, Mycoplasma hominis,* and *Gardnerella vaginalis* has been reported to be associated with an increased risk of postpartum infection (Berenson and colleagues, 1990; Berman and associates, 1987; Minkoff and co-workers, 1982; Wager and colleagues, 1980). Recently, Watts and associates (1990) reported an increased risk of post-cesarean section metritis associated with bacterial vaginosis.

Bacteriology. Organisms that invade the placental implantation site, incisions, and lacerations that are the consequence of labor and delivery typically are those that normally colonize the cervix, vagina, and perineum. Most of these bacteria are of relatively low virulence, and seldom initiate infection in healthy tissues. Although more virulent bacteria may be introduced from exogenous sources, in modern obstetrics an epidemic of serious puerperal sepsis rarely develops, as virulent bacteria are usually not carried from person to person during labor, delivery, or early in the puerperium. However, at least one epidemic from group A β-hemolytic streptococcus has been well documented in the past 25 years (Jewett and associates, 1968). Moreover, there have been several recent reports of this organism in association with a toxic shock syndrome (Cone and associates, 1987; Dotters and Katz, 1991; Whitted and colleagues, 1990).

Common Pathogens. In the great majority of instances, bacteria responsible for pelvic infection are those that normally reside in the bowel and also commonly colonize the perineum, vagina, and cervix. Bacteria commonly responsible for female genital tract infections are shown in Table 28–1. Usually, multiple species of bacteria are isolated, and although typically considered to be of relatively low virulence, these bacteria may become pathogenic as a result of hematomas and devitalized tissue. Whatever the mechanism, their pathogenicity is now enhanced sufficiently to cause uterine infection with extensive pelvic cellulitis, abscesses, peritonitis, and suppurative thrombophlebitis.

Although the cervix and lower genital tract routinely harbor such bacteria, the uterine cavity is usually sterile before rupture of the amnionic sac. As the consequence of labor and delivery and associated manipulations, the amnionic fluid and perhaps the uterus commonly become contaminated with anaerobic and aerobic bacteria. For example, Gilstrap and Cunningham (1979), from cultures of amnionic fluid obtained at cesarean section performed in women in labor with membranes ruptured more than 6 hours, identified the following bacteria: anaerobic and aerobic organisms in 63 percent, anaerobes alone in 30 percent, and aerobes alone in 7 percent. Predominant anaerobic organisms were gram-positive cocci (*Peptostreptococcus* and *Peptococcus* species), 45 percent; *Bacteroides* species, 9 percent; and *Clostridium* species, 3 percent. Gram-positive aerobic cocci also were common (*Enterococcus*, 14 percent, and group B *Streptococcus*, 8 percent). *Escherichia coli* comprised 9 percent of isolates. An average of 2.5 organisms was identified from each specimen. These observations serve to emphasize the polymicrobial nature of genital tract infections associated with delivery, and especially cesarean section. Gibbs (1987) reemphasized the importance of these organisms, and reported an increasing prevalence of *Bacteroides bivius* as a cause of female pelvic infection. Walmer and colleagues (1988) provided evidence for the role of *Enterococcus* species in the pathogenesis of these infections.

Chlamydia trachomatis has been implicated as a cause of late-onset, indolent metritis that may develop in one third of women who had antepartum chlamydial cervical infection (Ismail and co-workers, 1985; Wager and colleagues, 1980). In a recent report by Berenson and colleagues (1990), *Chlamydia trachomatis* was isolated significantly more often from adolescents with post-cesarean section metritis compared with adults (21 versus 6 percent). Of interest, *Gardnerella vaginalis* was also isolated more often in the younger women. Whether these organisms are truly pathogenic or simply "markers" or risk factors for infection is unclear. For example, Gibbs and colleagues (1987) reported that *Gardnerella* lacked a pathogenic role in puerperal infections. The role of genital mycoplasmas is even less clear, but some have implicated these organisms in the etiology of puerperal metritis (Blanco and colleagues, 1983; Lamey and associates, 1982).

Bacterial Cultures. Precise identification of bacteria specifically responsible for any puerperal infection may be quite difficult. Even results of cultures of uterine specimens obtained by using double-lumen catheters are unclear. Using these techniques, Gibbs and associates (1975), like Hite and co-workers (1947) 3 decades before, cultured one or more pathogens from the uterine cavity in 70 percent or more of clinically healthy puerperal women. For these reasons, routine pretreatment genital tract cultures in women with puerperal infection are of little clinical utility, and we do not use them at Parkland Hospital.

TABLE 28–1. BACTERIA COMMONLY RESPONSIBLE FOR FEMALE GENITAL INFECTIONS

Aerobes
   Group A, B and D streptococci
   Enterococcus
   Gram-negative bacteria—*Escherichia coli*, *Klebsiella*, and *Proteus* species
   Staphylococcus aureus

Anaerobes
   Peptococcus species
   Peptostreptococcus species
   Bacteroides bivius, *B. fragilis*, *B. disiens*
   Clostridium species
   Fusobacterium species

Other
   Mycoplasma hominis
   Chlamydia trachomatis

From the American College of Obstetricians and Gynecologists (1988).

Appropriately performed anaerobic and aerobic blood cultures obtained before antimicrobials are given may be useful to identify some of these pathogens. Blood cultures were positive in 13 percent of women treated at Parkland Hospital for pelvic infections that followed cesarean section (Cunningham and colleagues, 1978), and 24 percent of those from Los Angeles County Hospital (diZerega and co-workers, 1979).

Pathogenesis. Puerperal uterine infection primarily involves the placental implantation site and the endometrium, or more exactly the decidua, and adjacent myometrium. Hence, the term *metritis* is more descriptive than endometritis. The appearance of the infected decidua varies widely. In some cases, the necrotic mucosa sloughs, the debris is abundant, and the discharge is foul, profuse, bloody, and sometimes frothy. In others, the discharge is scant. Uterine involution may be retarded. Microscopical sections may show a superficial layer of necrotic material containing bacteria and a thick zone of leukocytic infiltration.

As shown in Figure 28–1, the pathogenesis of uterine infection following cesarean section is that of an infected surgical incision. Bacteria that colonized the cervix and vagina gain access to amnionic fluid during labor, and postpartum they invade devitalized uterine tissue. Invariably, with uterine infections that follow cesarean sections, and probably in most of those after vaginal delivery, parametrial cellulitis develops. As shown in Figure 28–2, infection of the pelvic retroperitoneal fibroareolar connective tissue may then develop. It may be caused by the lymphatic transmission of organisms from an infected cervical laceration or uterine incision or laceration. Although perineal or vaginal lacerations may cause localized cellulitis, the process is usually limited to the paravaginal tissue and rarely extends deeply into the pelvis. Infection also may be caused by direct extension of cervical lacerations into the connective tissue at the base of the broad ligaments. This tissue may be exposed to direct invasion by pathogenic vaginal organisms. A similar outcome may be seen in cases of criminal abortion when a sharp instrument

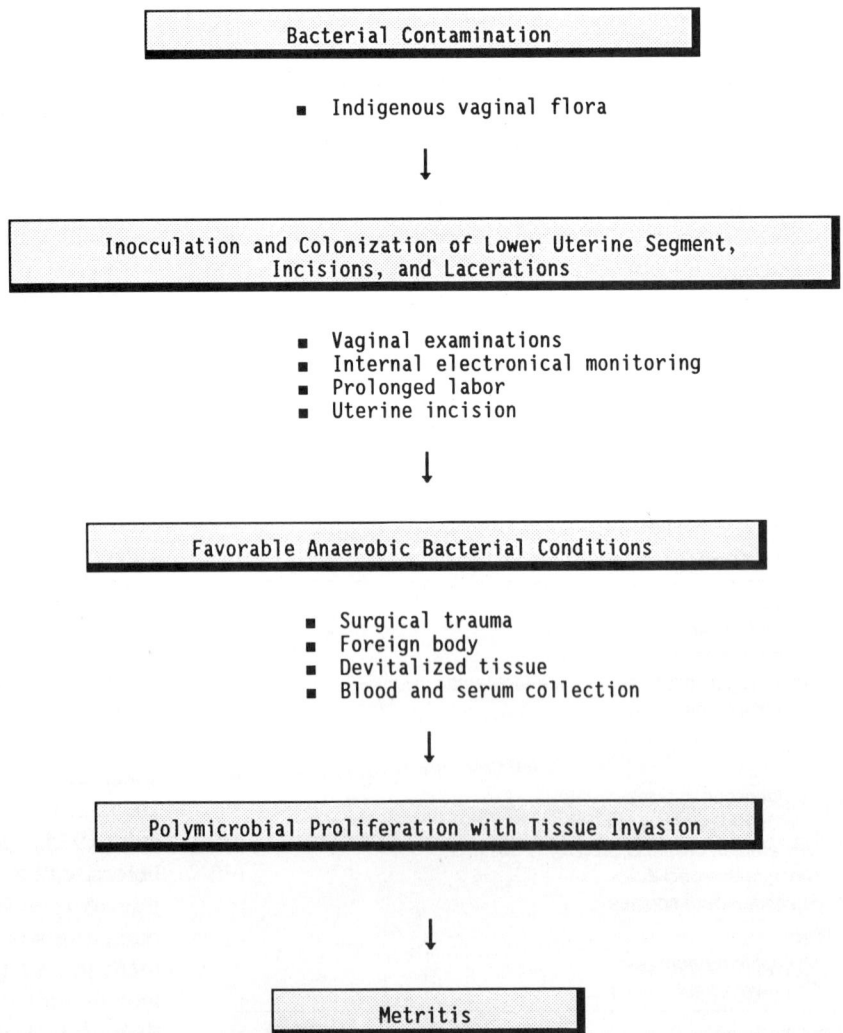

Fig. 28–1. Pathogenesis of metritis following cesarean section. (From Gilstrap and Cunningham, 1979.)

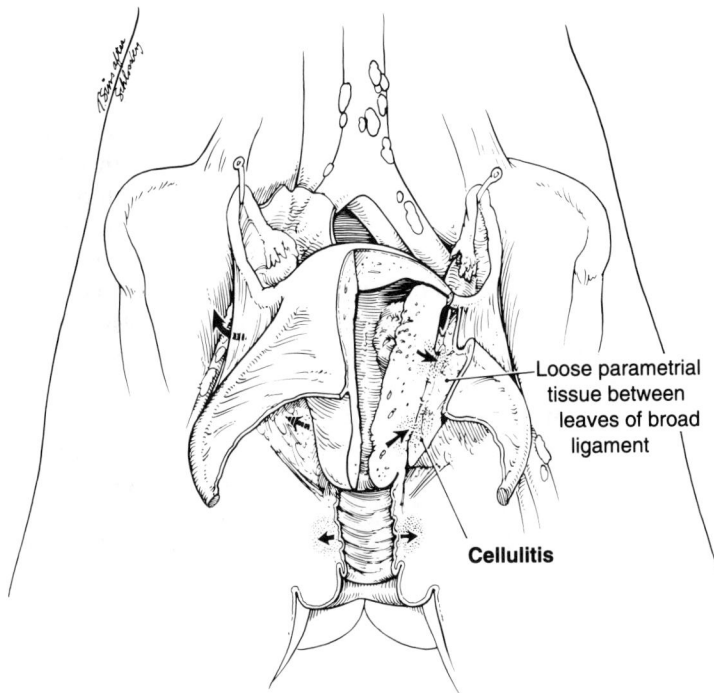

Fig. 28–2. Pelvic cellulitis (parametritis) from extension of puerperal infection. Bacteria may enter the parametrial tissue between the leaves of the broad ligament by direct extension or by lymphatic transmission from cervical lacerations or foci of trauma within the uterus, including placental implantation site or cesarean section incision. Bacterial spread may also develop across the wall of an infected vein. Lacerations of the perineum or vagina usually cause only localized cellulitis, but may extend to pelvic lymphatics.

has created a false passage into the paracervical connective tissue.

Clinical Course. The clinical picture of metritis varies with the extent of the disease; whenever fever persists postpartum, uterine infection should be suspected. The degree of temperature elevation is probably proportional to the extent of infection, and when confined to the endometrium (decidua) and superficial myometrium, the cases are mild and there is minimal fever. More commonly, the temperature exceeds 38.3° C. Chills may accompany fever and suggest bacteremia, which may be documented in nearly 20 percent of women with uterine infection following cesarean delivery. The pulse rate typically follows the temperature curve.

The woman usually complains of abdominal pain, and afterpains may be bothersome. There is tenderness on one or both sides of the abdomen, and parametrial tenderness is elicited upon bimanual examination. Even in the early stages, an offensive odor may develop, long regarded as an important sign of uterine infection. However, in many women, foul-smelling lochia without other evidence for infection is found. Conversely, some infections, and notably those due to group A β-hemolytic streptococci, are frequently associated with scanty, odorless lochia. Leukocytosis may range from 15,000 to 30,000 cells per μL, but in view of the physiological leukocytosis of the early puerperium, these findings are difficult to interpret.

If the process is localized to the uterus, the temperature may return to normal even without antimicro-

bial treatment. Indeed, localized metritis may be misdiagnosed as a urinary infection or incorrectly attributed to severe breast engorgement or pulmonary atelectasis. Without treatment, parametritis follows an indolent course and may ultimately undergo suppuration; however, with appropriate antimicrobial therapy, resolution usually is prompt.

Treatment of Metritis. Treatment for metritis is given with a broad-spectrum antimicrobial(s). For mild cases following vaginal delivery, an oral agent may suffice. However, for moderately to severely infected women, including most of those delivered by cesarean section, parenteral therapy is indicated. Improvement will follow in 48 to 72 hours in nearly 90 percent of women treated with one of the regimens discussed below. Persistence of fever after this interval mandates a careful search for causes of refractory pelvic infection, although nonpelvic sources are occasionally found. Complications of metritis that cause persistent fever despite appropriate therapy include parametrial phlegmons, surgical incisional and pelvic abscesses, and septic pelvic thrombophlebitis.

Following a successful response to the initial intravenous antimicrobial regimen, it became common practice in the past to send the woman home with oral antibiotics to complete a prearranged course of therapy. Data to support this are lacking, and the usual contemporaneous practice is to discharge the woman without further therapy after she has been afebrile for at least 24 hours. Indeed, Dinsmoor and colleagues (1991) found no differences in infection-related complications when oral antibiotic therapy was compared with placebo for women discharged following successful intravenous therapy.

Principles of Antimicrobial Treatment. Although few, if any, antimicrobial regimens are effective against all of these putative pathogens that cause pelvic infection, treatment is directed against at least most of the polymicrobial and mixed flora that are listed in Table 28–1 and that typically cause puerperal infections. Fortunately, selection of an agent(s) effective against those most common usually proves suitable. Because, as described above, material for culture frequently is impractical to obtain, antimicrobial therapy is empirical.

The spectra of **β-lactam antimicrobials** include activity against many anaerobic pathogens, and these antimicrobials have been used successfully for decades to treat such infections. Many of the popular and effective multi-agent regimens include a drug from this group, although some are effective when used alone. Examples include some cephalosporins (cefoxitin, cefoperazone, cefotetan, cefotaxime, and others) and extended-spectrum penicillins (piperacillin, ticarcillin, and mezlocillin). β-Lactam antimicrobials are inherently safe, and except for allergic reactions, they are free of major toxicity. Another advantage is the cost-effectiveness of administering only one drug. The **β-lactamase inhibitors** clavulinic acid and sulbactam have been combined with ampicillin, amoxicillin, and ticarcillin to extend their spectra, and these also have been proven effective.

In 1979, diZerega and colleagues compared the effectiveness of clindamycin plus gentamicin with penicillin G plus gentamicin given for treatment of pelvic infections following cesarean section. Women given the **clindamycin–gentamicin** regimen had a favorable response 95 percent of the time, and this regimen is now considered by most to be the standard by which others are measured. Unfortunately, clindamycin, like most other regimens effective against anaerobic flora, may induce **pseudomembranous colitis** by overgrowth of resistant enterotoxin-producing *Clostridium difficile*. If severe, such colitis may be life-threatening, and treatment with vancomycin or metronidazole is given along with supportive measures. Walmer and colleagues (1988) later provided evidence that enterococcal infections may be associated with clinical failure of the clindamycin–gentamicin regimen. While 93 percent of women from whom enterococci were not isolated responded to this regimen, only 82 percent with enterococcal infections responded. The incidence of wound infection was much higher in women with enterococcal infections compared with those without (16 versus 3 percent). Diligent monitoring of the impact of enterococcal isolates for these infections is needed.

Although many recommend that serum gentamicin levels be periodically monitored, we do not feel it necessary to measure peak and trough serum concentrations in most women. Because the potential for nephrotoxicity and ototoxicity are worrisome with gentamicin in the event of diminished glomerular filtration, we usually treat such women with a combination of clindamycin and a second-generation cephalosporin. Others have recommended a combination of clindamycin and aztreonam, a monobactam compound with activity against gram-negative aerobic pathogens similar to the aminoglycosides (American College of Obstetricians and Gynecologists, 1988).

Metronidazole has superior in vitro activity against most anaerobes, and it is recommended by some to be given intravenously in combination with either gentamicin or tobramycin, especially if an abscess is suspected. **Chloramphenicol** remains a potent antimicrobial in vitro against most anaerobes that cause pelvic infections. Given intravenously along with one of the β-lactam antimicrobials, it provides excellent coverage for severe pelvic sepsis. It can be given safely with impaired renal function, but unfortunately deaths due to irreversible bone marrow suppression follow in about 1 in 20,000 courses of therapy. As with any of these regimens, its benefits must be weighed against these adverse effects.

Imipenem is a carbapenem that has broad-spectrum coverage against the majority of organisms associated with metritis. It is used in combination with cilastatin, which inhibits the renal metabolism of imipenem. Although this antibiotic will most certainly be effective in the vast majority of cases of metritis following cesarean section, it seems reasonable to reserve it for more serious infections such as pelvic abscesses and for antibiotic failures.

Complications of Uterine Infections. In probably at least 90 percent of women, metritis responds within 48 to 72 hours to treatment with one of the regimens discussed above. In the others, any of a number of complications may arise.

Wound Infections. The incidence of abdominal incisional infections following cesarean section has been reported to range from 3 to 15 percent with an average of 7 percent (Faro, 1990). When prophylactic antibiotics are given, the incidence is probably 2 percent or less. Risk factors for abdominal wound infections include obesity, diabetes, corticosteroid therapy, immunosuppression, anemia, and poor hemostasis with hematoma formation.

Abdominal incisional abscesses that develop in women delivered by cesarean section usually cause fever beginning on about the fourth postoperative day. In most cases, these are preceded by uterine infection, and there is persistent fever despite adequate antimicrobial therapy. Erythema and drainage may also be present. Organisms causing these infections are usually the same as those isolated from amnionic fluid at the time of cesarean section, but hospital-acquired pathogens must be suspected (Emmons and colleagues, 1988; Gilstrap and Cunningham, 1979). Treatment is with antimicrobials and surgical drainage, with careful inspection to ensure that the fascia is intact; if not, secondary closure is performed. According to Soper and co-workers (1992), wound infection is the most common cause of antimicrobial failure in women given therapy for metritis.

Peritonitis. Uterine infection may extend by way of the lymphatics to reach the abdominal cavity and cause peritonitis. This complication is rarely seen today with prompt therapy, but may be encountered with infections following cesarean section when there is uterine incisional necrosis and dehiscence. Also rare, late in the course of pelvic cellulitis, a parametrial or adnexal abscess may rupture and produce catastrophic generalized peritonitis. This is a grave complication, and typically, fibrinopurulent exudate binds loops of bowel to one another, and locules of pus may form between the loops. The cul-de-sac and subdiaphragmatic space may then be sites for abscess formation.

Clinically, puerperal peritonitis resembles surgical peritonitis, except that abdominal rigidity usually is less prominent. Pain may be severe. Marked bowel distension is a consequence of paralytic ileus. It is important to identify the cause of the generalized peritonitis. If the infection began in the uterus and extended into the peritoneum, the treatment usually is medical. Conversely, peritonitis as the consequence of a bowel lesion or its appendages usually is best treated surgically. Antimicrobial therapy should include those agents most likely effective against *Peptostreptococcus, Peptococcus, Bacteroides, Clostridia,* and aerobic coliforms. Septicemic shock may supervene (see Chap. 47, p. 1072).

Intravenous fluid and electrolyte replacement are important because with generalized peritonitis large amounts of fluid are sequestered in the lumen, the wall of the gastrointestinal tract, and at times in the peritoneal cavity. Vomiting, diarrhea, and fever also contribute appreciably to fluid and electrolyte loss. The volumes of fluid and the amounts of electrolytes necessary to replace what is sequestered in the abdomen, aspirated from the gut, and lost through diaphoresis are usually quite large but must not be so massive as to produce circulatory overload. Because paralytic ileus is usually a prominent feature, the gastrointestinal tract should be decompressed by continuous nasogastric suction. Oral feeding is withheld throughout the course of treatment until bowel function returns and flatus is expelled.

Purulent exudate between loops of bowel, or between bowel and other organs, may cause intestinal kinking, following which symptoms of mechanical bowel obstruction will supervene. Surgical decompression may be necessary. Surgery is not indicated early in the course of the disease, although abscesses may form at various sites and need to be drained, and mechanical intestinal obstruction may need to be relieved.

Adnexal Infections. Most often with puerperal infections the fallopian tubes are involved only with perisalpingitis without subsequent tubal occlusion and sterility. An *ovarian abscess* rarely develops as a complication of puerperal infection, presumably from bacterial invasion through a rent in the ovarian capsule (Wetchler and Dunn, 1985). The abscess is usually unilateral and women typically present 1 to 2 weeks after delivery. In many cases, rupture causes peritonitis, which prompts surgical exploration. Unless peritonitis is apparent, initially intravenous antimicrobial agents are given, but surgical drainage usually becomes necessary.

Parametrial Phlegmon. In some women in whom metritis develops following cesarean delivery, parametrial cellulitis is intensive and forms an area of induration, termed a *phlegmon,* within the leaves of the broad ligament (Fig. 28–3). These infections are the most common cause of persistent fever despite prompt and adequate treatment of pelvic infections that complicate cesarean section (DePalma and colleagues, 1982). Such areas of cellulitis are more often unilateral, and while they frequently may remain limited to the base of the broad ligament, if the inflammatory reaction is more intense, cellulitis extends along natural lines of cleavage. The most common form of extension is directly laterally, along the base of the broad ligament, with a tendency to extend to the lateral pelvic wall. The uterus is pushed toward the opposite side and is fixed. Occasionally, high intraligamentous exudates spread from the region of the uterine cornua to the iliac fossa. Posterior extension may involve the rectovaginal septum with the development of a firm mass posterior to the cervix. Rarely, involvement of the connective tissue anterior to the cervix results in cellulitis of the space of Retzius, with extension upward and beneath the anterior abdominal wall.

Fortunately rare, intensive cellulitis of the uterine incision may cause necrosis and separation with extrusion of purulent material into the peritoneal cavity. Clinical findings then are as described in the previous section for peritonitis. Frequently, the first symptoms of peritonitis are those of *adynamic ileus,* which usually is absent or mild following uncomplicated cesarean section. Puerperal metritis with pelvic cellulitis is typically a retroperitoneal infection, and evidence for peritonitis should alert the physician to the possibility of uterine incisional necrosis with dehiscence, or less commonly a bowel injury or other lesion.

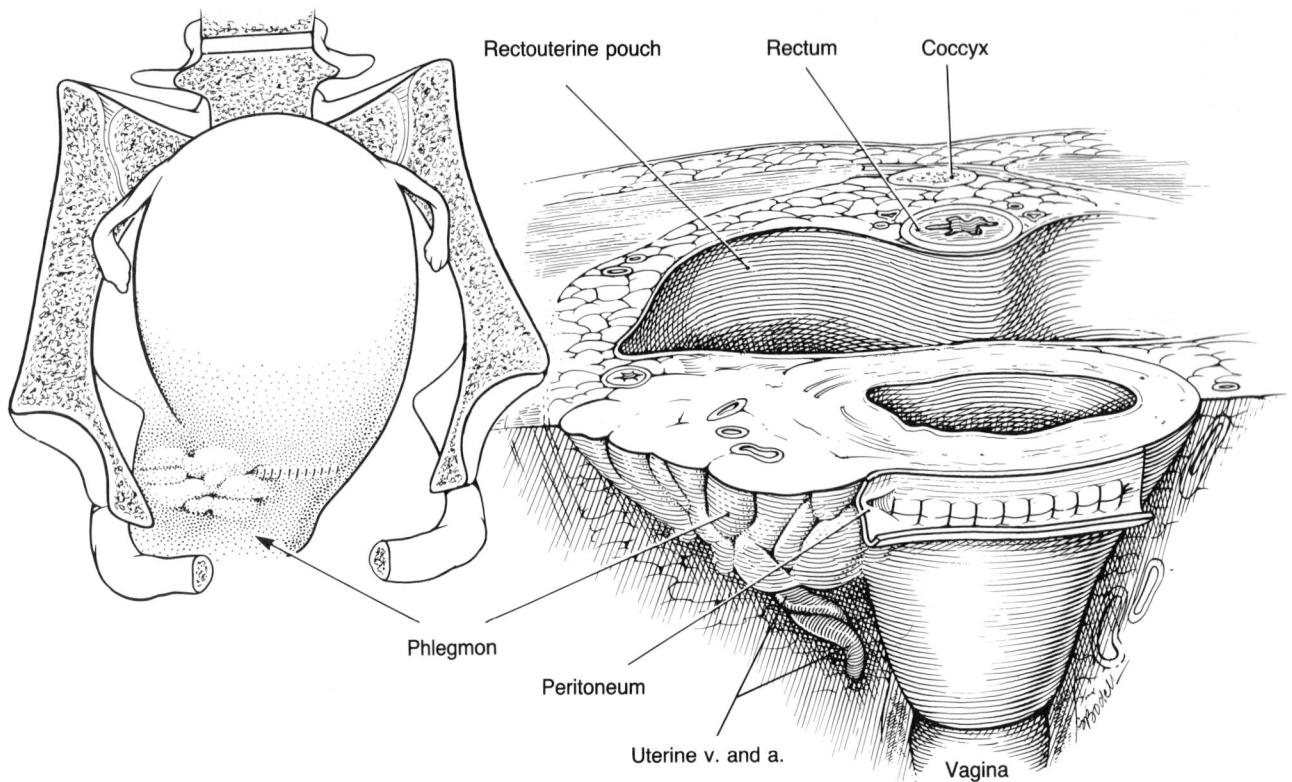

Fig. 28–3. Parametrial phlegmon. Cellulitis in the right parametrium begins adjacent to the cesarean section incision and extends to the pelvic sidewall. On pelvic examination, the phlegmon is palpable as a firm, three-dimensional mass.

TREATMENT. In the majority of women who develop a parametrial phlegmon, clinical response follows continued treatment with one of the intravenous antimicrobial regimens previously discussed. As long as the initial regimen has been appropriately chosen, and if there is no evidence for clinical deterioration, especially peritonitis, then the same regimen may be continued, or an alternate regimen chosen. Women with a phlegmon usually remain febrile for 5 to 7 days, and in some cases even longer. Absorption of the induration follows, but it may take several weeks to dissipate completely.

Surgery is reserved for women in whom uterine incisional necrosis is suspected. Hysterectomy and surgical debridement are usually difficult, and there is often appreciable blood loss. Frequently, the cervix and lower uterine segment are involved with an intensive inflammatory process that extends to the pelvic sidewall to encompass one or both ureters, and supracervical hysterectomy should be considered. The adnexae are seldom involved, and depending on their appearance, one or both ovaries may be conserved.

IMAGING STUDIES. Evaluation of persistent pelvic infections using sonography has been less than satisfactory for a variety of reasons. Frequently, these areas of cel-

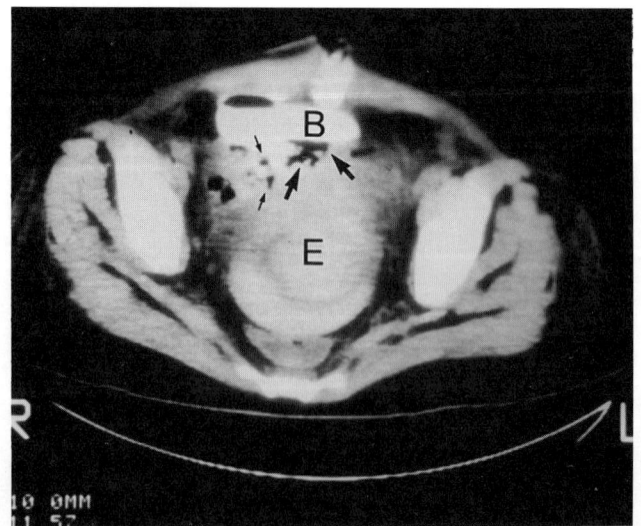

Fig. 28–4. Pelvic computed tomography showing uterine necrosis with gas (arrows) in the infected cesarean section incision. (B = bladder; E = endometrial cavity.)

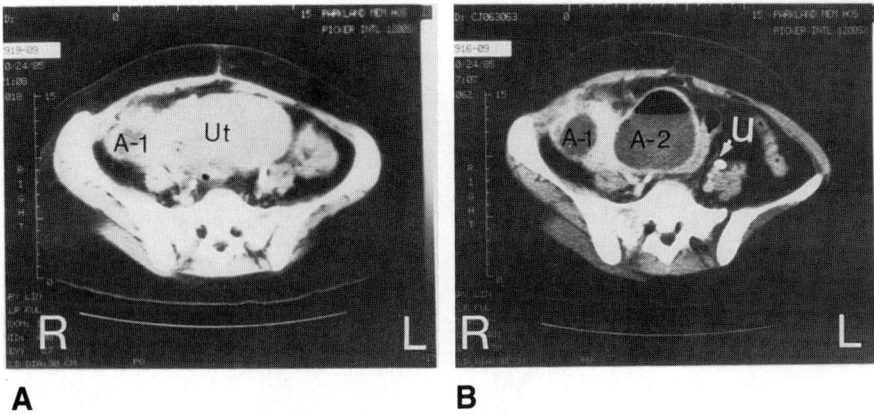

A   **B**

Fig. 28–5. Pelvic computed tomography showing two large pelvic abscesses. **A.** One abscess cavity (A-1) is within the right broad ligament adjacent to the puerperal uterus (Ut). **B.** The large abscess in the center (A-2) is bounded caudad by the uterine fundus and the smaller cavity (A-1) on the patient's right. The left ureter (U) is shown by the arrow.

lulitis have ultrasonic characteristics suggesting an abscess, but as discussed above, surgical drainage of a phlegmon is inadvisable. Brown and colleagues (1991) described the use of computed tomography in 74 women to assess refractory pelvic infections, and there was at least one abnormal radiological finding in three fourths of these women. Lev-Toaff and colleagues (1991) reported similar findings in 31 women utilizing ultrasound along with computed tomography or magnetic resonance imaging. Only 2 of these women had negative findings.

Sometimes evidence for uterine incisional dehiscence is detected (Fig. 28–4). It is important that these x-ray findings are interpreted along with the clinical course, because apparent uterine separations seen radiographically may resolve spontaneously. In that case, these are presumed to represent either infection without dehiscence or normal healing. Twickler and colleagues (1991) reported that myometrial incisional defects can be visualized radiographically in women after cesarean section who have no evidence for infection, dehiscence, or other complications.

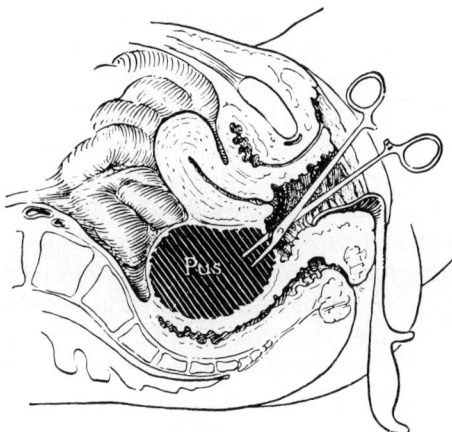

Fig. 28–6. Drainage of rectovaginal septal abscess by colpotomy.

Pelvic Abscess. Rarely, despite prompt and appropriate antimicrobial treatment given for metritis, a parametrial phlegmon will suppurate, forming a fluctuant broad ligament mass that may point above the Poupart ligament. In these circumstances the woman may not have worsening of symptoms, but fever persists. Should the abscess rupture into the peritoneal cavity, life-threatening peritonitis may develop, as previously described. More likely, these abscesses will dissect anteriorly and may be amenable to needle drainage directed by computed tomography (Fig. 28–5). Occasionally they dissect posteriorly through the retroperitoneal space to the rectovaginal septum, where surgical drainage is easily effected by colpotomy incision (Fig. 28–6).

Septic Pelvic Thrombophlebitis

Pathogenesis. Puerperal infection may extend along venous routes with resultant thrombophlebitis (Figs. 28–2 and 28–7). Halban and Köhler (1919) performed autopsies in 163 women who died from puerperal infection before the antimicrobial era, and reported that 82, or slightly more than half, had pelvic thrombophlebitis. In 36 women, it was the only mode of extension identified, whereas in 46 there was coexisting lymphangitis. Collins and colleagues (1951) cited the incidence to be 35 percent in women dying during the period from 1937 to 1946, which encompassed early use of chemotherapy.

Bacterial infection of the placental site causes thrombosed myometrial veins, which in turn support anaerobic bacteria proliferation. The ovarian veins may then become involved because they drain the upper uterus, which most often includes veins draining the placental site. The process is usually unilateral and probably more frequent on the right side, from where it may extend into the vena cava (Munsick and Gillanders, 1981). Septic phlebitis of the left ovarian vein may extend to the renal vein; Bahnson and colleagues (1985) have documented

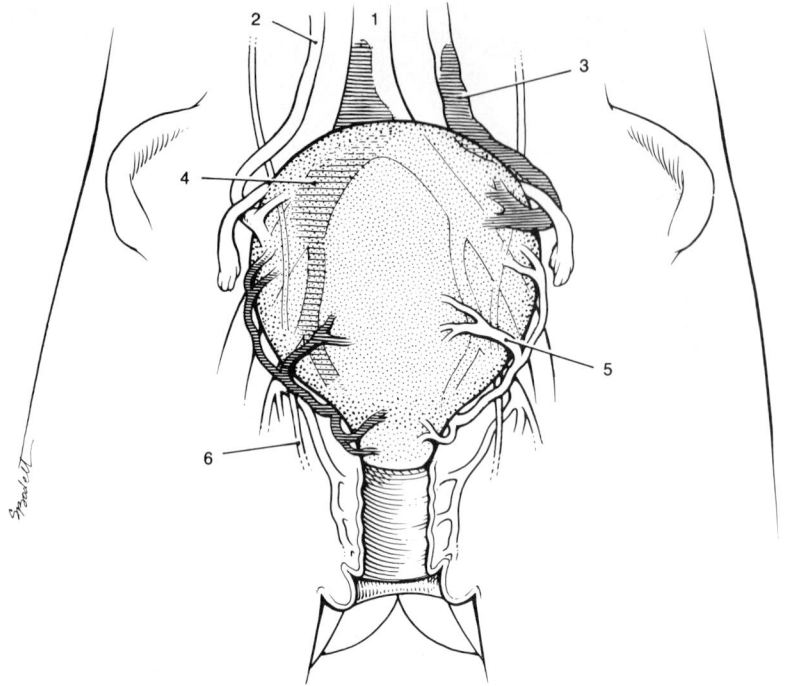

Fig. 28–7. Routes of extension of septic pelvic thrombophlebitis. Any pelvic vessels and the inferior vena cava may be involved: (1) inferior vena cava; (2) right ovarian vein; (3) clot in left ovarian vein; (4) clot in right common iliac vein, which extends from the uterine and internal iliac veins and into the inferior vena cava; (5) left uterine vein; and (6) right ureter.

such a case using computed tomography.

As described by Collins and co-workers (1951), other pelvic veins may be involved. Brown and colleagues (1986) reported 11 consecutive cases of septic thrombophlebitis diagnosed using computed tomography and magnetic resonance imaging over a 15-month period. In 5 of these women, the iliofemoral vessels were involved, usually along with the vena cava. In 6, an ovarian vein was thrombosed, such as that shown in Figure 28–8; but in only one woman was the ovarian vein involved along with iliofemoral vessels. Conversely, vena caval thrombosis was documented to accompany either ovarian or iliofemoral thrombophlebitis.

Clinical Findings. The usual clinical presentation of the woman with septic thrombophlebitis has been described by Gibbs (1976). These women usually experience most aspects of clinical improvement of their pelvic infection following antimicrobial treatment; however, they continue to have hectic fever spikes. They usually do not appear clinically ill, and are frequently asymptomatic unless chills accompany fever. This clinical picture was aptly termed *enigmatic fever* by Dunn and Van Voorhis (1967).

Munsick and Gillanders (1981) identified the following clinical features from review of cases of ovarian vein thrombophlebitis. The cardinal symptom was pain that developed typically on the second or third postpartum day with or without fever. Pain was present in the lower abdomen, the flank, or both. In some cases, but not all, a tender mass was palpable just beyond the uterine cornu.

Diagnosis and Treatment. Variable degrees of pelvic thrombophlebitis probably accompany most cases of metritis and parametrial cellulitis, and thus initial treatment is directed at both; usually it is successful. For women with persistent fever, with or without a palpable parametrial mass, computed tomography or magnetic resonance may disclose pelvic phlebitis (Figs. 28–9 and 28–10). Before these methods were available to confirm clinical suspicions of venous involvement, the *heparin challenge test* was advocated. Supposedly, after intravenous heparin was given, there was lysis of fever, and this was taken as diagnostic of pelvic phlebitis and heparin treatment continued (Duff and Gibbs, 1983; Josey and Staggers, 1974; Munsick and Gillanders, 1981). However, Brown and colleagues (1986) questioned this, because they showed that despite withholding heparin from 6 of 11 women with proven pelvic thrombophlebitis, continued antimicrobial therapy resulted in clinical resolution. Conversely, in 5 women given heparin along with antimicrobial drugs, the prolonged febrile course did not appear to be appreciably abbreviated, and in fact, 3 of these women had fever for more than 10 days after heparin was begun. Based on these experiences, we do not administer heparin routinely to these women.

In response to treatment, thrombosis of the in-

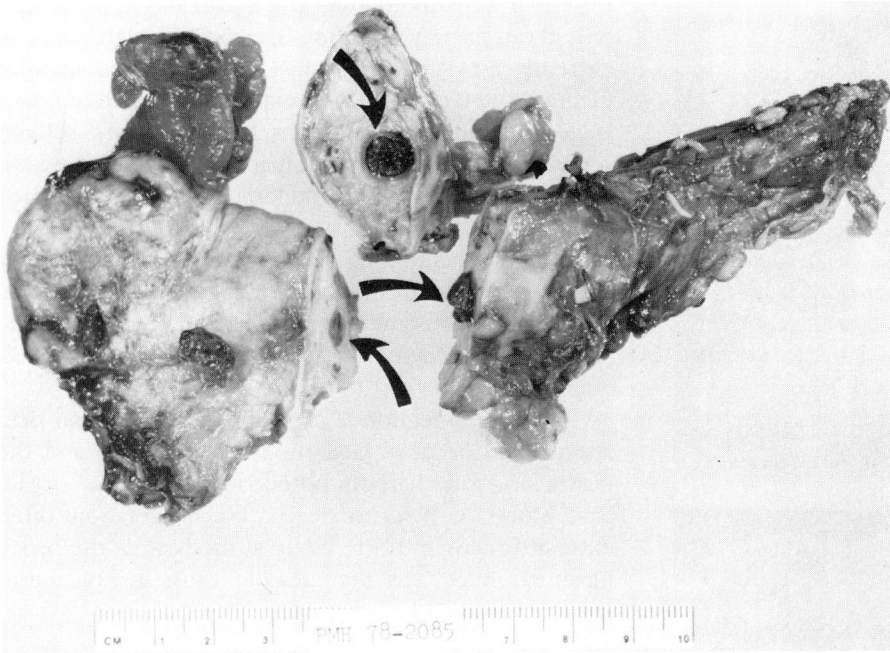

Fig. 28–8. Ovarian vein thrombophlebitis. Resected thrombosed right ovarian vein plus right oviduct.

volved veins usually limits the infection, and the clot undergoes organization. Rarely, the thrombus may suppurate, while the surrounding venous wall becomes edematous and necrotic. Pulmonary embolization, at least large enough to cause sudden death, is rare. In advanced cases, which are quite rare today, small septic emboli may reach the terminal branches of the pulmonary circulation, resulting in pleural effusions, pulmonary infarctions, and abscesses. In these cases, consideration should be given to a vena caval filter or surgical ligation as discussed in Chapter 49 (p. 1117).

Infections of the Perineum, Vagina, and Cervix

Surprisingly, infections of perineal wounds, including episiotomy incisions and repaired lacerations, are relatively uncommon considering the degree of bacterial contamination that accompanies delivery. Sweet and Ledger (1973) reported only 21 infected episiotomies (0.35 percent) among nearly 6000 women delivered vaginally at the University of Michigan and Wayne County Hospitals. From Parkland Hospital, Ramin and

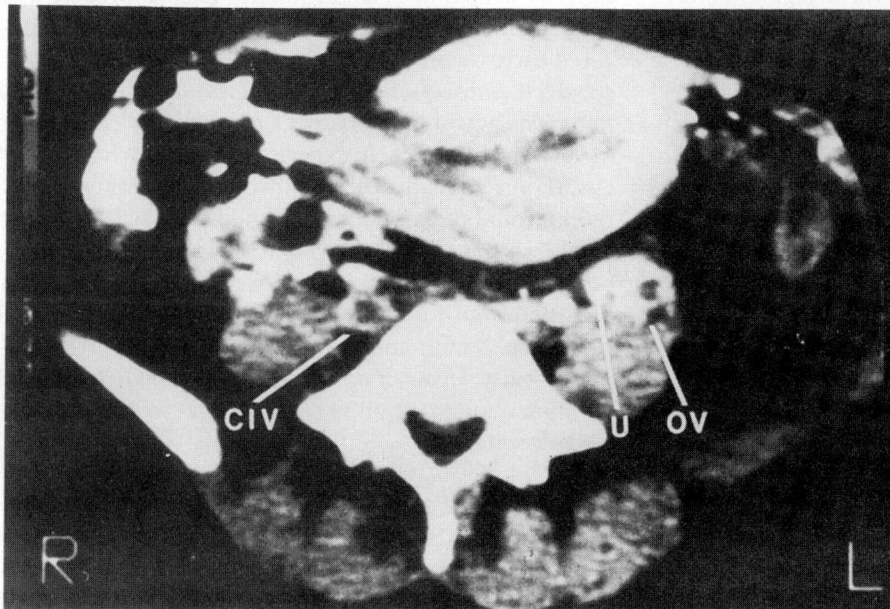

Fig. 28–9. Septic pelvic thrombophlebitis. Pelvic computed tomograph on day 13 from a woman with persistent fever since day 6 following vaginal delivery and manual removal of placenta. The left ureter (U) is filled with contrast, and there is the characteristic appearance of a thrombus in the right common iliac vein (CIV) and a thrombus with surrounding inflammation in the left ovarian vein (OV). (From Brown and colleagues, 1986.)

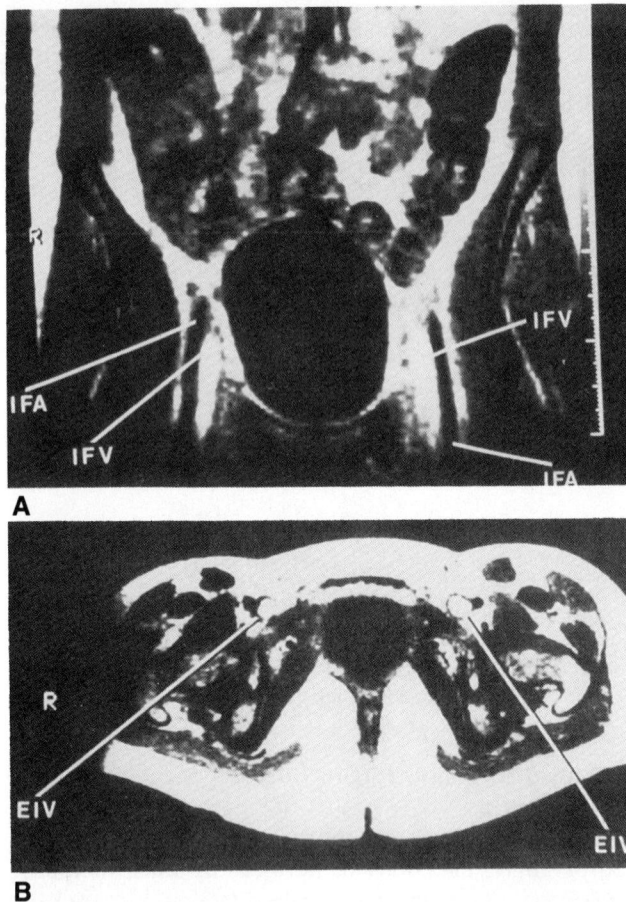

Fig. 28–10. A. Coronal magnetic resonance imaging section showing thrombi in both iliofemoral venous systems (IFV). By comparison, flowing blood in the iliofemoral arteries (IFA) appears dark (repetition time = 1.0 sec; echo time = 28 msec). **B.** Transverse magnetic resonance imaging section of **A** showing bilateral external iliac venous (EIV) thrombi (repetition time = 1.5 sec; echo time = 56 msec.) (From Brown and colleagues, 1986.)

colleagues (1992) reported a 0.5 percent incidence of episiotomy breakdown; almost 80 percent of these were due to infection. Perhaps not surprisingly, serious infection is more likely in women with fourth-degree lacerations. Goldaber and colleagues (in press) reported the clinical courses of 389 women delivered at Parkland Hospital and who sustained fourth-degree lacerations. These women represented 2 percent of all of those delivered vaginally. Almost 5 percent of these perineal wounds were complicated by infection, episiotomy breakdown, or both.

Pathogenesis and Clinical Course. Localized infection of the episiotomy wound is the most common puerperal infection of the external genitalia. The apposing wound edges become red, brawny, and swollen. The sutures then often tear through the edematous tissues, allowing the necrotic wound edges to gape, with the result that serous, serosanguineous, or frankly purulent material exudes. In this manner, complete breakdown of

the site frequently follows. Local pain and dysuria, with or without urinary retention, are common symptoms. In extreme cases, the entire vulva may become edematous, ulcerated, and covered with exudate. Provided drainage is good, superficial infections fortunately are seldom severe; however, if purulent material is confined within a closed space by suture, infection may be accompanied by chills and fever.

Vaginal lacerations may become infected directly or by extension from the perineum. The mucosa becomes edematous and hyperemic and may then become necrotic and slough. Parametrial extension may result in lymphangitis.

Cervical infection is probably more common than appreciated because lacerations are common and the cervix normally harbors potentially pathogenic organisms. Moreover, because deep cervical lacerations often extend directly into the tissue at the base of the broad ligament, infections may readily cause lymphangitis, parametritis, and bacteremia.

Treatment. Infected perineal wounds, like other infected surgical wounds, should be treated by establishing drainage. Sutures are removed and the infected wound opened. Failure to do this may lead not only to extension of the infection into the paracervical and paravaginal connective tissue, but to a worse ultimate anatomical result. A broad-spectrum antimicrobial regimen should be utilized. Relief of pain is afforded by effective analgesics and an indwelling bladder catheter if there is urinary retention.

Classically, it has been recommended that when an episiotomy dehiscence occurs, especially if associated with infection, a repair should not be attempted for at least 3 to 4 months (Mattingly and Thompson, 1985). It was postulated that such a delay would allow for adequate vascularization of the involved tissue and resolution of infection and cellulitis. This approach was challenged by Hauth and colleagues (1986), who advocated early repair after evidence of infection, if present, subsided. Subsequently, two large studies have attested to the efficacy of such practices. Hankins and co-workers (1990) described their experiences with early repair of episiotomy breakdown in 31 women. The average duration from breakdown to episiotomy repair was 6 days (range 1 to 11). All but 2 women had a successful repair; both developed a pinpoint rectovaginal fistula soon after repair and both were treated successfully with a small rectal flap. Ramin and colleagues (1992) reported successful early repair of episiotomy breakdown associated with infection in 32 of 34 (94 percent) women at Parkland Hospital.

Technique for Early Repair. **Prior to attempting early repair of episiotomy dehiscence, the surgical wound must be properly cleaned and free of infection.** Meticulous preparation is paramount for good results. The women must be afebrile before the operation is performed. A protocol for early repair is summarized in Table 28–2.

Necrotizing Fasciitis. A rare but frequently fatal complication of perineal and vaginal wound infections is deep soft tissue infection involving muscle and fascia. Such infections may extend from any infection adjacent to myofascial edges, and this includes surgical incisions or other wounds. They are also seen with vulvar infections in diabetic and immunocompromised women, but they rarely develop in otherwise healthy women. Shy and Eschenbach (1979) reported that necrotizing fasciitis infections were responsible for 20 percent of 15 maternal deaths in King County, Washington in the 1970s. Our experiences at Parkland Hospital indicate that these potentially fatal infections fortunately are quite rare.

Bacteria that cause these serious perineal infections appear to be similar to those that cause other pelvic infections, but anaerobes predominate. Gram-positive anaerobic cocci or *Clostridium perfringens* usually are isolated along with aerobic cocci or *Escherichia coli*, but group B streptococcus has been reported (Sutton and colleagues, 1985).

Necrotizing fasciitis of the episiotomy site may involve any of the several superficial or deep perineal fascial layers, and thus it may extend to the thighs, buttocks, and abdominal wall (Fig. 28–11). Although some infections may develop within a day of delivery, they more commonly do not cause symptoms until 3 to 5 days. Clinical symptoms vary, and it is frequently difficult to differentiate superficial perineal infections from deep fascial ones. A high index of suspicion, with surgical exploration if the diagnosis is uncertain, may be lifesaving. Stamenkovic and Lew (1984) recommend biopsy of the fascial edges with frozen section microscopical examination when the diagnosis is uncertain. Certainly, if myofasciitis progresses, the woman becomes very ill from septicemia, there is profound hemoconcentration from capillary leakage with circulatory failure, and death soon follows. Cases of marked vulvar

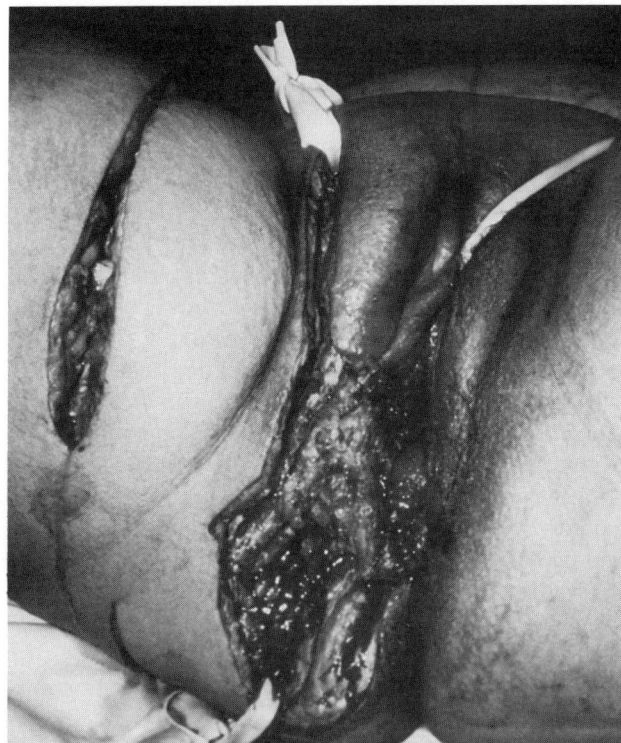

Fig. 28–11. Necrotizing fasciitis complicating episiotomy infection. Three days postpartum this woman had severe perineal pain and edema of the episiotomy site. Prompt extensive debridement was carried out. Bacteria cultured from the infected episiotomy included *Escherichia coli, Streptococcus viridans,* group D streptococcus, *Corynebacterium* species, *Bacteroides fragilis,* and *Clostridium* species. Blood cultures were positive for *Bacteroides fragilis.*

edema that have developed postpartum as described by Finkler and colleagues (1987) probably represent variants of this infection.

Aggressive surgical treatment is indicated and includes wide debridement of all infected tissue. As shown in Figure 28–11, this may include extensive vulvar debridement with unroofing and excision of abdominal, thigh, or buttock fascia. Split-thickness skin grafts later are used to repair the defects. **Mortality is virtually universal without surgical treatment, and it approaches 50 percent even if aggressive excision is performed.**

Similar infections may develop in abdominal surgical incisions following cesarean section. Prompt diagnosis and aggressive surgical debridement are likewise mandatory for survival.

Toxic Shock Syndrome

Although not typically a puerperal infection, toxic shock syndrome is considered here because it has been reported in the puerperium. This is an acute febrile illness with severe multisystem derangement and a case–fatality rate of 10 to 15 percent. The illness is usually

TABLE 28–2. PROTOCOL FOR EARLY REPAIR OF AN INFECTED EPISIOTOMY DEHISCENCE

Open wound completely
- Remove sutures
- Inspection for fasciitis
- Debridement
- Wound cleaning at least twice daily
- Sitz baths after bowel movements
- Antibiotics
- Oral electrolyte bowel prep day before surgery
- Secondary repair[a] when wound free of infection, cellulitis, and exudate and covered by granulation tissue

[a] Average of 6 days from breakdown.
Adapted from Hankins and colleagues (1990).

characterized by fever, headache, mental confusion, diffuse macular erythematous rash, subcutaneous edema, nausea, vomiting, watery diarrhea, and marked hemoconcentration. Renal failure followed by hepatic failure, disseminated intravascular coagulation, and circulatory collapse may follow in rapid sequence. During recovery, the rash-covered areas undergo desquamation. *Staphylococcus aureus* has been recovered from almost all of afflicted persons, and a staphylococcal exotoxin, termed *toxic shock syndrome toxin-1,* and formerly called both *enterotoxin F* and *pyrogenic exotoxin C,* causes the syndrome by provoking profound endothelial injury. Recently, McGregor and colleagues (1988) described almost identical findings in women with infection complicated by *Clostridium sordelli* colonization.

As mentioned previously, there have been several reports of a toxic shock syndrome associated with group A β-hemolytic streptococcus infection. For example, Whitted and colleagues (1990) reported such a case of toxic shock-like syndrome in a woman 2 weeks postpartum. Dotters and Katz (1991) reported a similar case in a 40-year-old woman following a spontaneous abortion. At Parkland Hospital, we have recently experienced similar cases of severe group A streptococcal infection in two postpartum women, one of whom died.

The syndrome develops most commonly in young women, and is usually associated with menstruating women who use tampons; however, it has been reported in a variety of other clinical situations (Reingold and co-workers, 1982). Nearly 10 percent of pregnant women have vaginal colonization with *S. aureus;* thus it is not surprising that the disease develops in postpartum women (Guerinot and co-workers, 1982; Lauter and Tom, 1982). It has also been described in a mother-and-newborn pair (Green and LaPeter, 1982).

Principal therapy for toxic shock is supportive, while allowing reversal of capillary endothelial injury. Treatment is similar to that for septic shock, discussed in Chapter 47 (p. 1073). In severe cases, it requires massive fluid replacement, mechanical ventilation with positive end-expiratory pressure, and renal dialysis. Antimicrobial therapy with specific antistaphylococcal drugs is given; however, their role in the resolution is uncertain.

History of Puerperal Infection

The earliest reference to puerperal infection is found in the 5th century BC works of Hippocrates. In his discussion of women, *De Muliebrum Morbis,* he described the condition and attributed it to retention of bowel contents. By 200 AD, Celsus and Galen had written in support of the theories of Hippocrates, and they recommended purgation. It was not until the late 1500s that lochial putrefaction or uterine inflammation were suspected as the cause of childbed fever, which had been linked to difficult labor.

William Harvey (1651) aptly described the placental implantation site as a "vast internal ulcer" that may lead to gangrene. In 1659, Willis wrote on the subject of *febris puerperarum,* although the English term *puerperal fever* was probably first employed by Strother in 1716.

The theory of *milk metastasis* of Puzos (1686) followed next and predominated for 100 years, but in the 1700s, uterine inflammation was again thought to cause febrile morbidity. John Leake (1772) first suggested the contagious nature of puerperal infection, and Alexander Hamilton embraced this in 1781. Alexander Gordon of Aberdeen, in a treatise on epidemic puerperal fever in 1795, discussed its infectious and contagious nature, antedating Holmes (1855) and Semmelweis (1861) by half a century. Charles White (1773) of Manchester postulated that puerperal fever was dependent on lochial stagnation, and advised complete isolation of infected women.

It was not until the mid-1800s that such views were becoming acceptable. In 1843, Oliver Wendell Holmes presented "Contagiousness of Puerperal Fever" before the Boston Society for Medical Improvement. He showed clearly that at least the epidemic forms of the infection could always be traced to the lack of proper precautions on the part of the physician or nurse. Four years later, Semmelweis, then an assistant at the Vienna Lying-In Hospital, began a careful inquiry into the causes of the frightful mortality rate following delivery in that institution, as compared with the relatively small number of women who died as a result of infection following home delivery. He concluded that the morbid process was essentially a wound infection caused by the introduction of septic material by the examining finger. He issued stringent orders that physicians, students, and midwives disinfect their hands with chlorine water, the forerunner of Dakin solution, before examining parturient women. Despite immediate and surprising results in which the mortality rate fell from over 10 percent to 1 percent, both his work and that of Holmes were ridiculed by many prominent physicians of the time. His discovery remained unappreciated until Lister's teachings in 1867 regarding antisepsis, and the development of bacteriology by Pasteur.

The history of puerperal infection is discussed in detail in the monographs of Eisenmann (1837), Burtenshaw (1904), and Peckham (1935). Willson (1988) provided a review of cesarean section infections.

References

American College of Obstetricians and Gynecologists: Antimicrobial therapy for obstetric patients. Technical Bulletin no. 117, June 1988

Atrash HK, Koonin LM, Lawson HW, Franks AL, Smith JC: Maternal mortality in the United States, 1979–1986. Obstet Gynecol 76:1055, 1990

Bahnson RR, Wendel EF, Vogelzang RL: Renal vein thrombosis following puerperal ovarian vein thrombophlebitis. Am J Obstet Gynecol 152:290, 1985

Berenson AB, Hammill HA, Martens MG, Faro S: Bacteriologic findings of post-cesarean endometritis in adolescents. Obstet Gynecol 75:627, 1990

Berman SM, Harrison HR, Boyce WT, Haffner WJJ, Lewis M, Arthur JB: Low birth weight, prematurity, and postpartum endometritis. JAMA 257:1189, 1987

Blanco JD, Gibbs RS, Malherbe H, Strickland-Cholmley M, St Clair PJ, Castaneda YS: A controlled study of genital mycoplasmas in amniotic fluid from patients with intra-amniotic infection. J Infect Dis 147:650, 1983

Brown CEL, Dunn DH, Harrell R, Setiawan H, Cunningham FG: Computed tomography for evaluation of puerperal infections. Surg Gynecol Obstet 172:285, 1991

Brown CEL, Lowe TW, Cunningham FG, Weinreb JC: Puerperal pelvic thrombophlebitis: Impact on diagnosis and treatment using x-ray computed tomography and magnetic resonance imaging. Obstet Gynecol 68:789, 1986

Burtenshaw JH: The fever of the puerperium. NY and Philadelphia Med J, June/July 1904

Collins CG, McCallum EA, Nelson EW, Weinstein BB, Collins JH: Suppurative pelvic thrombophlebitis: I. Incidence, pathology, etiology; II. Symptomatology and diagnosis; III. Surgical techniques: A study of 70 patients treated by ligation of the inferior vena cava and ovarian veins. Surgery 30:298, 1951

Cone LA, Woodard DR, Schlievert PM, Tomory GS: Clinical and bacteriologic observations of a toxic shock-like syndrome due to Streptococcus pyogenes. N Engl J Med 317:146, 1987

Cook JD, Lynch SR: The liabilities of iron deficiency. Blood 68:803, 1986

Cunningham FG, Hauth JC, Strong JD, Kappus SS: Infectious morbidity following cesarean: Comparison of two treatment regimens. Obstet Gynecol 52:656, 1978

DePalma RT, Cunningham FG, Leveno KJ, Roark ML: Continuing investigation of women at high risk for infection following cesarean delivery. Obstet Gynecol 60:53, 1982

Dinsmoor MJ, Newton ER, Gibbs RS: A randomized, double-blind placebo-controlled trial of oral antibiotic therapy following intravenous antibiotic therapy for postpartum endometritis. Obstet Gynecol 77:60, 1991

diZerega G, Yonekura L, Roy S, Nakamura RM, Ledger WJ: A comparison of clindamycin–gentamicin and penicillin–gentamicin in the treatment of post-cesarean section endomyometritis. Am J Obstet Gynecol 134:238, 1979

Dotters DJ, Katz VL: Streptococcal toxic shock associated with septic abortion. Obstet Gynecol 78:549, 1991

Duff P, Gibbs RS: Pelvic vein thrombophlebitis: Diagnostic dilemma and therapeutic challenge. Obstet Gynecol Surv 38:365, 1983

Dunn LJ, Van Voorhis LW: Enigmatic fever and pelvic thrombophlebitis. N Engl J Med 276:265, 1967

Eisenmann GE: Die Wundfieber und die Kindbettfieber. Erlangen, 1837

Emmons SL, Krohn M, Jackson M, Eschenbach DA: Development of wound infections among women undergoing cesarean section. Obstet Gynecol 72:559, 1988

Faro S: Soft tissue infections. In Gilstrap LC, Faro S (eds): Infections in Pregnancy. New York, Wiley-Liss, 1990, p 75

Filker R, Monif GRG: The significance of temperature during the first 24 hours postpartum. Obstet Gynecol 53:359, 1979

Finkler NJ, Safon LE, Ryan KJ: Bilateral postpartum vulvar edema associated with maternal death. Am J Obstet Gynecol 156:1188, 1987

Gibbs RS: Microbiology of the female genital tract. Am J Obstet Gynecol 156:491, 1987

Gibbs RS: Treatment of refractory postpartum fever. Clin Obstet Gynecol 19:83, 1976

Gibbs RS, O'Dell TN, MacGregor RR, Schwarz RH, Morton H: Puerperal endometritis: A prospective microbiologic study. Am J Obstet Gynecol 121:919, 1975

Gibbs RS, Weiner MH, Walmer K, St Clair PJ: Microbiologic and serologic studies of Gardnerella vaginalis in intra-amniotic infection. Obstet Gynecol 70:187, 1987

Gilstrap LC III, Cunningham FG: The bacterial pathogenesis of infection following cesarean section. Obstet Gynecol 53:545, 1979

Goldaber KG, Wendel PJ, McIntire DD, Wendel GD Jr: Postpartum morbidity after fourth degree perineal repair. Am J Obstet Gynecol (in press)

Gordon A: A Treatise on Epidemic Puerperal Fever of Aberdeen. London, CG & J Robinson, 1795

Green SL, LaPeter KS: Evidence for postpartum toxic-shock syndrome in a mother–infant pair. Am J Med 72:169, 1982

Guerinot GT, Gitomer SD, Sanko SR: Postpartum patient with toxic shock syndrome. Obstet Gynecol 59:43S, 1982

Halban J, Köhler R: Die pathologische Anatomie des Puerperalprozesses. Vienna and Leipzig, 1919

Hamilton A: A Treatise on Midwifery. London, 1781

Hankins GDV, Hauth JC, Gilstrap LC, Hammond TL, Yeomans ER, Snyder RR: Early repair of episiotomy dehiscence. Obstet Gynecol 75:48, 1990

Hauth JC, Gilstrap LC III, Ward SC, Hankins GDV: Early repair of an external sphincter ani muscle and rectal mucosal dehiscence. Obstet Gynecol 67:806, 1986

Hippocrates: Liber Prior de Muliebrum Morbis

Hite KE, Hesseltine HC, Goldstein L: A study of the bacterial flora of the normal and pathologic vagina and uterus. Am J Obstet Gynecol 53:233, 1947

Holmes OW: Puerperal Fever as a Private Pestilence. Boston, Ticknor & Fields, 1855

Ismail MA, Chandler AE, Beem ME: Chlamydial colonization of the cervix in pregnant adolescents. J Reprod Med 30:549, 1985

Jewett JF, Reid DE, Safon LE, Easterday CL: Childbed fever: A continuing entity. JAMA 206:344, 1968

Josey WE, Staggers SR Jr: Heparin therapy in septic pelvic thrombophlebitis: A study of 46 cases. Am J Obstet Gynecol 120:228, 1974

Lamey JR, Eschenbach DA, Mitchell SH, Blumhagen JM, Foy HM, Kenny GE: Isolation of mycoplasmas and bacteria from the blood of postpartum women. Am J Obstet Gynecol 143:104, 1982

Lauter CB, Tom WW: Spiking fever and rash in a postpartum patient. Hosp Pract, 17:163, 1982

Leake J: Practical Observations on the Child-bed Fever; Also on the Nature and Treatment of Uterine Haemorrhages, Convulsions, and Such Other Acute Disease as Are Most Fatal to Women During the State of Pregnancy. London, J Walter, 1772

Leigh J, Garite TJ: Amniocentesis and the management of premature labor. Obstet Gynecol 67:500, 1986

Lev-Toaff AS, Baka JJ, Toaff ME, Friedman AC, Radecki PD, Caroline DF: Diagnostic imaging in puerperal febrile morbidity. Obstet Gynecol 78:50, 1991

Lister J: On the antiseptic principle in the practice of surgery. Br Med J 2:246, 1867

Maberry MC, Gilstrap LC, Bawdon RE, Little BB, Dax JS: Anaerobic coverage for intra-amnionic infection: Maternal and perinatal impact. Am J Perinatol 8:338, 1991

Mattingly RF, Thompson JD: Anal incontinence and rectovaginal fistulas. In: TeLinde's Operative Gynecology, 6th ed. Philadelphia, Lippincott, 1985, p 669.

McGregor JA, Soper D, Lovell G: A toxic shock-like syndrome caused by *Clostridia sordelli* affecting postpartum women. Abstract 30 presented at meeting of Infectious Disease Society in Obstetrics and Gynecology, Aspen, CO, August 1988

Minkoff HL, Sierra MF, Pringle GF, Schwarz RH: Vaginal colonization with group B beta-hemolytic streptococcus as a risk factor for post-cesarean section febrile morbidity. Am J Obstet Gynecol 142:992, 1982

Monif GRG: Intrapartum bacteriuria and postpartum endometritis. Obstet Gynecol 78:245, 1991

Munsick RA, Gillanders LA: A review of the syndrome of puerperal ovarian vein thrombophlebitis. Obstet Gynecol Surv 36:57, 1981

Mussey RD, DeNormandie RL, Adair FL: The American Committee on Maternal Welfare, Inc: Its organization, purposes and activities. Am J Obstet Gynecol 28:754, 1935

Naeye RL: Coitus and associated amniotic fluid infections. N Engl J Med 301:1198, 1979

Peckham CH: A brief history of puerperal infection. Bull Hist Med 3:187, 1935

Puzos N: Première mémoire sur les depots laiteux. In: Traités des Accouchements. Paris, 1686, p 341

Ramin SM, Ramus R, Little B, Gilstrap LC: Early repair of episiotomy dehiscence associated with infection. Am J Obstet Gynecol 167:1104, 1992

Reingold AL, Shands KN, Dan BB, Broome CV: Toxic-shock syndrome not associated with menstruation: A review of 54 cases. Lancet 2:1, 1982

Rochat RW, Koonin LM, Atrash HK, Jewett JF, and the Maternal Mortality Collaborative: Maternal mortality in the United States: Report from the Maternal Mortality Collaborative. Obstet Gynecol 72:91, 1988

Sachs BP, Brown DA, Driscoll SG, Schulman E, Acker D, Ransil BJ, Jewett JF: Hemorrhage, infection, toxemia, and cardiac

disease, 1954–1985: Causes for their declining role in maternal mortality. Am J Public Health 78:671, 1988

Semmelweis IP: Die Aetiologie, der Begriff und die Prophylaxis des Kindbettfiebers. Pest, Vienna and Leipzig, 1861

Shy KK, Eschenbach DA: Fatal perineal cellulitis from an episiotomy site. Obstet Gynecol 52:293, 1979

Soper DE, Brockwell WJ, Dalton HP: The importance of wound infection in antibiotic failures in the therapy of postpartum endometritis. Surg Gynecol Obstet 174:265, 1992

Stamenkovic I, Lew PD: Early recognition of potentially fatal necrotizing fasciitis: The use of frozen-section biopsy. N Engl J Med 310:1689, 1984

Strother E: Critical Essay on Fevers. London, 1716

Sutton GP, Smirz LR, Clark DH, Bennett JE: Group B streptococcal necrotizing fasciitis arising from an episiotomy. Obstet Gynecol 66:733, 1985

Sweet RL, Ledger WJ: Puerperal infectious morbidity. A two-year review. Am J Obstet Gynecol 117:1093, 1973

Twickler DM, Setiawan AT, Harrell RS, Brown CEL: CT appearance of the pelvis after cesarean section. Am J Radiol 156:523, 1991

Wachsberg RH, Kurtz AB: Gas within the endometrial cavity after postpartum US: A normal finding after spontaneous vaginal delivery. Radiology 183:431, 1992

Wager GP, Martin DH, Koutsky L, Eschenbach DA, Daling JR, Chiang WT, Alexander ER, Holmes KK: Puerperal infectious morbidity: Relationship to route of delivery and to antepartum *Chlamydia trachomatis* infection. Am J Obstet Gynecol 138:1028, 1980

Walmer D, Walmer KR, Gibbs RS: Enterococci in post-cesarean endometritis. Obstet Gynecol 71:159, 1988

Watts DH, Krohn MA, Hillier SL, Eschenbach DA: Bacterial vaginosis as a risk factor for post-cesarean endometritis. Obstet Gynecol 75:52, 1990

Wetchler SJ, Dunn LJ: Ovarian abscess. Report of a case and a review of the literature. Obstet Gynecol Surv 40:476, 1985

White C: Treatise on the management of pregnancy and lying-in women and the means of curing but more especially of preventing the principal disorders to which they are liable. London, EC Dilly, 1773

Whitted RW, Yeomans ER, Hankins GDV: Group A β-hemolytic streptococcus as a cause of toxic shock. A case report. J Reprod Med 35:558, 1990

Willis T: Diatribae duae medico-philosophical ... de febribus ... London, T Raycroft, 1659

Willson JR: The conquest of cesarean section related infections: A progress report. Obstet Gynecol 72:519, 1988

CHAPTER 29
Other Disorders of the Puerperium

There are a number of abnormalities other than pelvic infection that may manifest during the puerperium. Some are quite common, and although distressing may be considered almost inconsequential; an example is breast engorgement. Others are very uncommon, but may be life-threatening; pulmonary embolism is an example.

Thromboembolic Disease

Thromboembolic disease traditionally was considered unique to the puerperium; however, this is no longer true. The frequency of thrombophlebitis complicating pregnancy and the puerperium has decreased in recent years, and now most cases are identified during the antepartum period. For these reasons, deep-vein thrombosis and pulmonary embolisms are discussed in Chapter 49 (p. 1111).

Pelvic Venous Thrombosis. During the puerperium, a thrombus may transiently form in any of the dilated pelvic veins, and possibly does so relatively often. Without associated thrombophlebitis, these thrombi likely do not incite clinical signs or symptoms unless the thrombosis is extensive or pulmonary embolism follows. Unfortunately, these vessels appear to be the source of many of the massive and fatal pulmonary emboli that develop without warning in the puerperium, although some undoubtedly arise from the deep venous system of the legs.

Symptomatic puerperal pelvic thrombosis is most commonly associated with uterine infection, and this is discussed in Chapter 28 (p. 628). The diagnosis of pelvic thrombophlebitis has improved remarkably with the use of computed tomography. As described by Brown and colleagues (1991), pelvic vein thrombosis may occur alone or in combinations of the ovarian, iliofemoral, and inferior caval venous systems. Most often this is associated with a septic course, and resolves with intensive antimicrobial therapy.

Diseases and Abnormalities of the Uterus

Subinvolution. *Subinvolution* describes an arrest or retardation of involution, the process by which the puerperal uterus is normally restored to its original proportions. It is accompanied by prolongation of lochial discharge and irregular or excessive uterine bleeding and sometimes by profuse hemorrhage. On bimanual examination, the uterus is larger and softer than normal for the particular period of the puerperium. Among the recognized causes of subinvolution are retention of placental fragments and pelvic infection. Because most cases of subinvolution result from local causes, they are usually amenable to early diagnosis and treatment. Ergonovine (Ergotrate) or methylergonovine (Methergine), 0.2 mg every 3 to 4 hours for 24 to 48 hours, is recommended by some, but its efficacy is questionable. On the other hand, metritis usually responds to oral antimicrobial therapy. Wager and colleagues (1980) reported that almost one third of cases of late postpartum uterine infection are caused by *Chlamydia trachomatis;* thus tetracycline therapy may be appropriate.

Andrew and colleagues (1989) described 25 cases of hemorrhage between 7 and 40 days postpartum associated with noninvoluted uteroplacental arteries. These abnormal arteries were characterized by no detectable endothelial lining and the vessels were filled with thrombi. Periauricular trophoblasts were also present in the walls of these vessels and the authors postulated that subinvolution, at least with regard to the placental vessels, may represent an aberrant interaction between uterine cells and trophoblast.

Postpartum Cervical Erosions. Cervical erosions, or eversions, are complications of the late postpartum period. Shallow cauterization or cryotherapy can be used to remove persistent exuberant granulations or the delicate exposed endocervical columnar epithelium, without causing stenosis of the endocervix.

Relaxation of the Vaginal Outlet and Prolapse of the Uterus. Extensive lacerations of the perineum during delivery, if not properly repaired, presumably are followed by relaxation of the vaginal outlet. Even when external lacerations are not visible, overstretching may lead to marked relaxation. Moreover, changes in the pelvic supports during parturition predispose to prolapse of the uterus and to urinary stress incontinence. These conditions may escape detection unless an examination is made at the end of the puerperium and unless there is long-term follow-up. In general, operative correction is postponed until childbearing is ended, unless, of course, serious disability, notably urinary stress incontinence, results in symptoms sufficient to require intervention.

Hemorrhages During the Puerperium

Puerperal Hematomas. In their review, Zahn and Yeomans (1990) found that the incidence of puerperal hematomas varied from 1 in 300 to 1 in 1500 deliveries. Episiotomy was the most commonly associated risk factor. In many other cases, however, hematomas develop following injury to a blood vessel without laceration of the superficial tissues. These may develop with spontaneous or operative delivery. Occasionally, the hemorrhage is delayed, perhaps as a result of sloughing of a vessel that had become necrotic from prolonged pressure.

Puerperal hematomas may be classified as vulvar, vaginal, vulvovaginal, or retroperitoneal. Vulvar hematomas most often involve branches of the pudendal artery, including the posterior rectal, transverse perineal, or posterior labial artery, while vaginal hematomas may involve the descending branch of the uterine artery (Zahn and Yeomans, 1990). Infrequently, the torn vessel lies above the pelvic fascia. In that event, the hematoma develops above it. In its early stages, the hematoma forms a rounded swelling that projects into the upper portion of the vaginal canal and may almost occlude its lumen. If the bleeding continues, it dissects retroperitoneally, and thus may form a tumor palpable above the Poupart ligament, or it may dissect upward, eventually reaching the lower margin of the diaphragm. Branches of the uterine artery may be involved with these types of hematomas.

Vulvar Hematomas. Vulvar hematomas, such as that shown in Figure 29–1, particularly those that develop rapidly, may cause excruciating pain, which often is the first symptom noticed. Hematomas of moderate size may be absorbed spontaneously. The tissues overlying the hematoma may give way as a result of necrosis caused

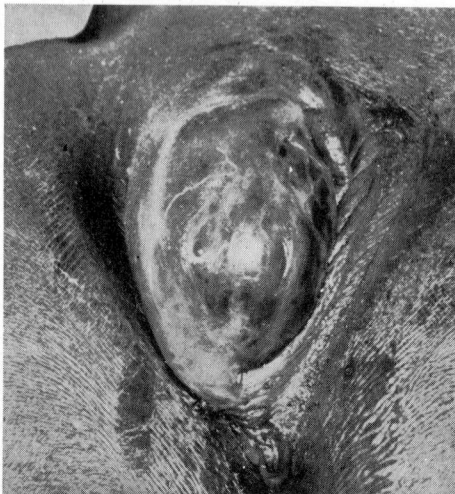

Fig. 29–1. Vulvar hematoma bulging into the right vaginal wall.

by pressure, and profuse hemorrhage may follow. In other cases, the contents of the hematoma may be discharged in the form of large clots.

In the subperitoneal variety, extravasation of blood beneath the peritoneum may be massive and occasionally fatal. Death may also follow secondary intraperitoneal rupture. Occasionally, rupture into the vagina leads to infection of the hematoma and potentially fatal sepsis.

A vulvar hematoma is readily diagnosed by severe perineal pain and the sudden appearance of a tense, fluctuant, and sensitive tumor of varying size covered by discolored skin. When the mass develops adjacent to the vagina, it may escape detection temporarily; but symptoms of pressure, if not pain, and inability to void should soon lead to a vaginal examination and the discovery of a round, fluctuant tumor encroaching on the lumen. When the hematoma extends upward between the folds of the broad ligament, it may escape detection unless a portion of the tumor can be felt on abdominal palpation or unless evidence of anemia or infection appears. The prognosis is usually favorable, although bleeding into very large hematomas has led to death.

Treatment. Smaller vulvar hematomas identified after leaving the delivery room may be treated expectantly. If, however, the pain is severe, or if it continues to enlarge, the best treatment is prompt incision and evacuation of blood and clots with ligation of bleeding points. The cavity can then be obliterated with mattress sutures. **With hematomas of the genital tract, blood loss is nearly always considerably more than the clinical estimate.** Hypovolemia and severe anemia should be prevented by adequate blood replacement. Broad-spectrum antibiotics are of value.

Subperitoneal and supravaginal hematomas are more difficult to treat. They can be evacuated by incision of the perineum; but unless there is complete hemostasis, which is difficult to achieve by this route, laparotomy is advisable.

Chin and colleagues (1989) described the technique of angiographic embolization for intractable puerperal hematomas. In one woman with a vulvovaginal hematoma, successful embolization was carried out with occlusion of the vaginal branch of the internal pudendal artery, uterine artery, and internal pudendal artery (Fig. 29–2). Similar bilateral embolization was successful in a second woman with a large vaginal wall hematoma previously that had been drained and packed.

Late Postpartum Hemorrhage. Serious uterine hemorrhage occasionally develops 1 to 2 weeks in the puerperium. Hemorrhage most often is the result of abnormal involution of the placental site, but it may also be caused by retention of a portion of the placenta. Usually, the retained piece of placenta undergoes necrosis with deposition of fibrin, and may eventually form a so-called *placental polyp*. As the eschar of the polyp

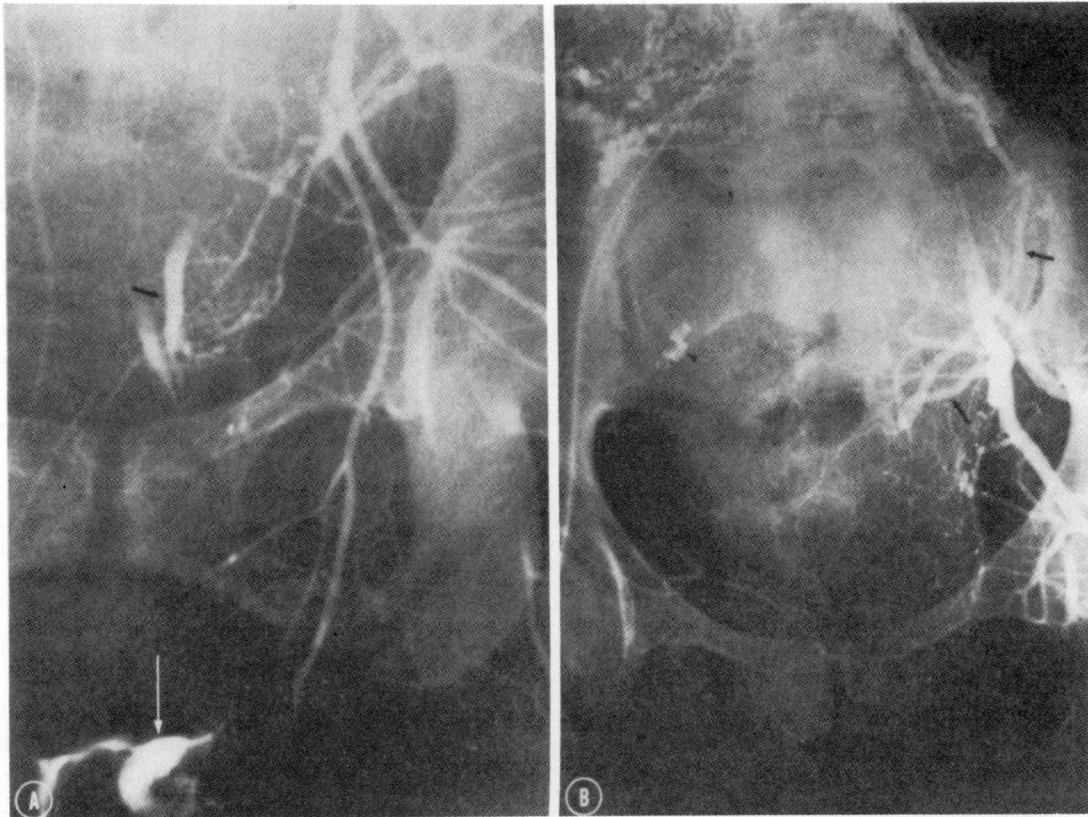

Fig. 29–2. A. Selective left internal iliac arteriogram before embolization. Note marked extravasation from vaginal (*black arrow*) and vulvar branches (*white arrow*) of left internal pudendal artery. **B.** After embolization. Now the branches of the left internal pudendal artery are occluded. There is patency of the left uterine artery (*arrows*) and coils in the right internal iliac artery (*arrowhead*).(From Chin and colleagues, 1989, with permission.)

detaches from the myometrium, hemorrhage may be brisk.

The observations of Lee and associates (1981) provide an estimate of the incidence of late postpartum hemorrhage. Of 3822 women delivered during a 1-year period at Henry Ford Hospital, 27 women, or 0.7 percent, had significant uterine bleeding after the first 24 postpartum hours. In 20 of these women the uterus was judged to be empty by sonographic evaluation, and importantly, only one woman had retained placental tissue.

It generally has been accepted that with late postpartum hemorrhage from the uterus, prompt curettage is necessary. However, curettage subsequent to late puerperal hemorrhage usually does not remove identifiable placental tissue, and hemorrhage frequently is intensified. The observations of Lee and co-workers (1981) support this and present evidence that sonography can exclude retained placental fragments as the cause of delayed postpartum hemorrhage in the majority of cases. Curettage, rather than reducing hemorrhage, is more likely to traumatize the implantation site and incite more bleeding, at times to such a degree that hysterectomy must be performed. Especially where there is good rea-

son to preserve the uterus for future childbearing, initial treatment may best be directed to control of the bleeding, using intravenous oxytocin, ergonovine, methylergonovine, or prostaglandins (Andrinopoulos and Mendenhall, 1983; Goldstein and co-workers, 1983). If the bleeding subsides, the woman is simply observed, and if the bleeding stops, she is discharged. In general, curettage is carried out only if appreciable bleeding persists or recurs after such management. It is imperative that the physician inform the woman that if a curettage is performed under these conditions, hysterectomy may be lifesaving. Furthermore, arrangements must be made for adequate blood replacement, appropriate anesthesia, and surgical assistance.

Disorders of the Urinary Tract

The puerperal bladder is not so sensitive to intravesical fluid tension as in the nonpregnant state. Moreover, it is commonplace in modern obstetrics to establish an intravenous infusion system during labor. After delivery, the infusion system is then used to administer oxytocin during the first hour or so after delivery, if not longer. Oxytocin induces potent antidiuresis until the time it is stopped, after which there is a prompt diuresis. The bladder then fills rapidly and may overdistend to a remarkable degree. General anesthesia, and especially conduction analgesia with temporarily disturbed neural bladder control, are important contributory factors. The woman in this circumstance may, in time, void small volumes of urine—*overflow incontinence*—misleading attendants into concluding that she is voiding normally. Inspection of the abdomen will disclose the uterine fundus to be much higher than it should be, with an overlying cystic mass, the distended bladder. **Genital tract trauma, especially with a large hematoma, may cause urinary retention, and pelvic examination should be performed whenever urinary retention is identified.**

The combination of residual urine and bacteriuria introduced by catheterization into a traumatized bladder presents the optimal conditions for the development of urinary infection. Initial symptoms include dysuria, frequency, and urgency. Signs and symptoms of infection will subsequently vary, depending upon whether the infection is localized to the bladder or ascends to involve the upper urinary tract. After urine has been obtained for culture, treatment should consist of appropriate antimicrobial or chemotherapeutic agents, as discussed in Chapter 50 (p. 1129).

In cases of bladder overdistention, it usually is best to leave an indwelling catheter in place for at least 24 hours, so as to empty the bladder completely and prevent prompt recurrence as well as to allow recovery of normal bladder tone and sensation. When the catheter is removed, it is necessary subsequently to demonstrate ability to void appropriately. If the woman cannot void after 4 hours, she should be catheterized and urine vol-ume measured. If there is more than 200 mL of urine, it is apparent that the bladder is not functioning appropriately. The catheter should be left in place and the bladder drained for another day. If less than 200 mL of urine are obtained, the catheter can be removed and the bladder rechecked subsequently as described.

In general, the first time the woman spontaneously voids after removal of an indwelling catheter inserted because of previous inability to void and gross overdistention, she should be immediately catheterized for residual urine. If the volume exceeds 200 mL, constant drainage should be reinstituted, and those steps in management just outlined should be resumed. Because bacteriuria may develop in women catheterized for postpartum urinary retention, it is our practice to give one-dose antimicrobial therapy at catheter removal.

Disorders of the Breasts

Breast Engorgement. For the first 24 to 48 hours after the development of the lacteal secretion, it is not unusual for the breasts to become distended, firm, and nodular. In some cases, such as that shown in Figure 29–3, this condition, commonly known as engorged breasts or *caked breasts,* often causes considerable pain and may be accompanied by a transient elevation of temperature. It represents an exaggeration of the normal venous and lymphatic engorgement of the breasts, which is a regular precursor of lactation. It is not the result of overdistention of the lacteal system with milk.

Puerperal fever from breast engorgement is common. Almeida and Kitay (1986) reported that 13 percent of all postpartum women had fever from this cause, and it ranged from 37.8 to 39° C. Fever seldom persists for longer than 4 to 16 hours. The incidence and sever-

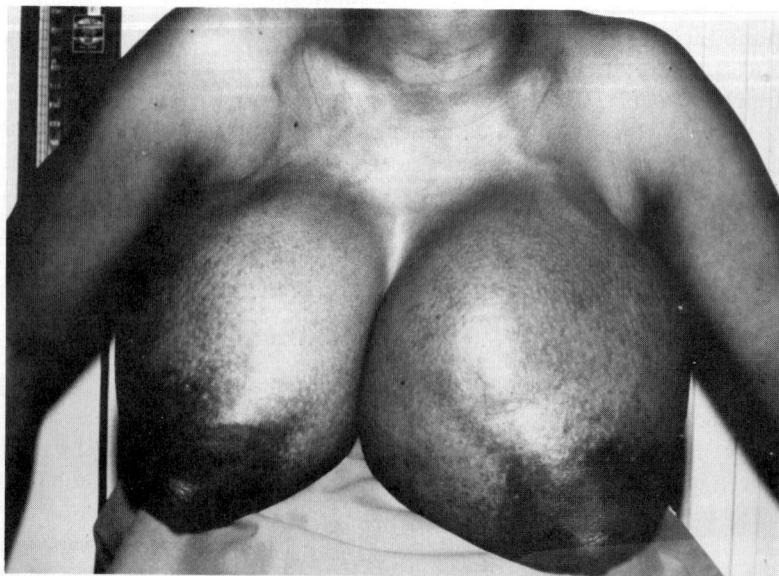

Fig. 29–3. Pathological breast engorgement 3 days after delivery. Pumping of the breasts, uplift support, and analgesia provided relief. (Courtesy of Dr. J. Duenhoelter.)

ity of breast engorgement, and fever associated with it, were lower if treatment was given for lactation suppression. Such fevers are particularly worrisome if infection cannot be excluded in women who have recently undergone cesarean delivery. **Other causes of fever, especially those due to infection, must be excluded.**

Treatment consists of supporting the breasts with a binder or brassiere, applying an ice bag, and if necessary, orally administering 60 mg of codeine sulfate or another analgesic. Pumping of the breast or manual expression of milk may be necessary at first, but in a few days the condition is usually alleviated and the infant is able to nurse normally.

Suppression of Lactation. When, for a variety of reasons, the infant is not to be breast fed, suppression of lactation becomes important. The simplest method consists of support with a comfortable binder, application of cold packs, and mild analgesics for pain. Usually, all signs and symptoms will disappear in 1 to 2 days if the breasts are not stimulated by pumping.

Hormones, particularly estrogens, either alone or combined with testosterone, formerly were widely used for this purpose; however, these have been shown to predispose to thromboembolism (Niebyl and colleagues, 1979; Turnbull, 1968). Moreover, their effect of lactation may be one of delay rather than effective suppression. Thus, these preparations seldom are used because of increased risk of thromboembolism and questionable benefit.

Bromocriptine, a dopamine agonist, stimulates the production of prolactin inhibitory factor, which in turn causes a fall in plasma prolactin and the suppression of lactation. When 2.5 mg of bromocriptine is given twice daily for 14 days, severe breast engorgement is prevented in 75 to 98 percent of women, but about one fourth have rebound engorgement when therapy is completed. An association has been reported with bromocriptine therapy and hypertension, seizures, stroke, and myocardial infarction (Katz and colleagues, 1985; Ruch and Duhring, 1989; Watson and associates, 1989). Considering the widespread use of the drug for lactation suppression, these complications fortunately are uncommon.

In 1988, the Maternal Health Advisory Committee of the Food and Drug Administration concluded that no drug should be routinely used to prevent postpartum lactation. An alternative regimen is to prescribe bromocriptine only after severe mammary engorgement develops. This method has not been evaluated objectively in clinical trials, but from our experiences at Parkland Hospital, it is very effective.

Although not available in the United States at this time, several long-acting parenteral forms of drugs are used elsewhere to prevent lactation. Kremer and colleagues (1990) recently reported the efficacy and safety of a depot form of bromocriptine (40 and 50 mg). This rapidly eliminated form of bromocriptine was successful in suppressing lactation in 98 percent of 61 postpartum women. Melis and co-workers (1988) described the efficacy of a single dose of the long-acting ergot derivative, cabergoline.

Mastitis. Parenchymatous infection of the mammary glands is a rare complication antepartum but is occasionally observed during the puerperium and lactation. Symptoms of suppurative mastitis seldom appear before the end of the first week postpartum and, as a rule, not until the third or fourth week. Infection almost invariably is unilateral and marked engorgement usually precedes the inflammation, the first sign of which is chills or actual rigor, soon followed by fever and tachycardia. The breast becomes hard and reddened, and the woman complains of pain. About 10 percent of women with mastitis develop an abscess, and constitutional symptoms attending a mammary abscess are severe. Local manifestations may be so slight as to escape observation; however, such cases are usually mistaken for pelvic infection. In still another group of women, the infection pursues a subacute or almost chronic course. The breast is somewhat harder than usual and more or less painful, but constitutional symptoms are either lacking or very slight. In such circumstances, the first indication of the true diagnosis often is afforded by the detection of fluctuation.

Thomsen and co-workers (1983, 1984) reported that if breast milk has a leukocyte count of more than 10^6 per mL in conjunction with more than 10^3 bacteria per mL identified by culture, infection was likely. Interestingly, in a third of asymptomatic women breast milk was colonized by more than 10^3 bacteria per mL.

Etiology. The most common offending organism is *Staphylococcus aureus;* Matheson and colleagues (1988) cultured this organism from 40 percent of women with mastitis. Other commonly isolated organisms are coagulase-negative staphylococci and viridans streptococci. Rench and Baker (1989) reported an unusual case in which mother and male infant both developed mastitis and the mother a breast abscess caused by group B streptococcus. The immediate source of the organisms that cause mastitis is almost always the nursing infant's nose and throat. At the time of nursing, the organism enters the breast through the nipple at the site of a fissure or abrasion, which may be quite small. Whether the bacteria commonly cause mastitis simply by entering the lactiferous ducts of the breast with completely intact integument is not clear. In cases of true mastitis, the offending organism can usually be cultured from breast milk. A case of toxic shock syndrome has been reported in a woman with a puerperal breast abscess from which *S. aureus* was cultured (Dixey and associates, 1982).

Suppurative mastitis among nursing mothers has at

times reached epidemic levels. Such outbreaks most often coincide with the appearance of a new strain of antibiotic-resistant *Staphylococcus*, an example being methicillin-resistant *S. aureus* (MRSA). Typically, the infant becomes infected after contact with nursery personnel who are colonized. Attendants' hands are the major source of contamination of the newborn. Especially in a crowded, understaffed nursery, it is a simple matter for the personnel to inadvertently transfer staphylococci from one colonized newborn infant to another. The colonization of staphylococci in the infant may be totally asymptomatic or may locally involve the umbilicus or the skin; but occasionally the organisms may cause a life-threatening systemic infection.

Prevention. Safeguards to prevent newborn colonization with virulent strains of staphylococci necessitate exclusion from the care of the infant and mother by all personnel with known or suspected staphylococcal infection or colonization. Also, as a matter of daily routine, close inspection should be made of every infant, with prompt isolation of any who appear to be developing an infection of the cord or of the skin. Frequent use of soap or detergent for handscrubbing by personnel is essential. At the first sign of an outbreak, all personnel should be checked with appropriate cultures and phage-typing of swabbings of the posterior nares to identify carriers of virulent staphylococci strains.

Treatment. Antimicrobials have improved markedly the prognosis of acute puerperal mastitis. Abscess formation is more common if *S. aureus* causes infection (Matheson and associates, 1988). Provided that appropriate therapy is started before suppuration begins, the infection usually resolves within 48 hours. Before initiating antimicrobial therapy, milk should be expressed from the affected breast onto a swab and cultured. By so doing, the organism can be identified and its antimicrobial sensitivities ascertained. Results of such cultures also provide information mandatory for a successful program for surveillance of nosocomial infections. The initial choice of antimicrobial will undoubtedly be influenced to a considerable degree by the current experiences with staphylococcal infections at the institution. Many staphylococcal infections are caused by organisms sensitive to penicillin or a cephalosporin. Erythromycin is given to women who are penicillin-sensitive. If the infection is caused by resistant, penicillinase-producing staphylococci, or if resistant organisms are suspected while awaiting the results of culture, an antimicrobial such as vancomycin, which is effective against methicillin-resistant staphylococci, should be given. It is important that treatment not be discontinued too soon. Even though clinical response may be prompt and striking, treatment should be continued for about 10 days.

Nursing should be discontinued when there is sup-purative mastitis, for it may be quite painful and the milk is infected; moreover, the infant usually harbors the organisms and therefore can cause reinfection. Because the infant is almost always colonized by the causative organism, close observation is necessary for signs of infection. Once established, resistant staphylococcal infections tend to spread and recur among the family for protracted periods of time.

Surgical drainage is essential for an abscess. General anesthesia usually is required. The incision should be made radially, extending from near the areolar margin toward the periphery of the gland, to avoid injury to the lactiferous ducts. In early cases, a single incision over the most dependent portion of the area of fluctuation is usually sufficient, but multiple abscesses require several incisions and a finger should be inserted to break up the walls of the locules. The resulting cavity is loosely packed with gauze, which should be replaced at the end of 24 hours by a smaller pack. If the pus has been thoroughly evacuated, the abscess cavity is obliterated and a complete cure is effected.

Galactocele. Very exceptionally, as the result of the clogging of a duct by inspissated secretion, milk may accumulate in one or more lobes of the breast. The amount is ordinarily limited, but an excess may form a fluctuant mass that may give rise to pressure symptoms. They may resolve spontaneously or require aspiration.

Supernumerary Breasts. One in every few hundred women has one or more accessory breasts *(polymastia)*. The supernumerary breasts may be so small as to be mistaken for pigmented moles, or, when without a nipple, for a lipoma. They rarely attain considerable size. They are likely to be situated in pairs on either side of the midline of the thoracic or abdominal walls, usually below the main breasts; they are also found in the axillae, and more rarely on other portions of the body such as the shoulder, flank, groin, or thigh. The number of supernumerary breasts varies greatly. When arranged symmetrically, 2 or 4 are most common, although 10 have been described.

Polymastia has no obstetrical significance, although occasionally the enlargement of supernumerary breasts in the axillae may result in considerable discomfort. Frequently, a tongue of mammary tissue extends out into the axilla from the outer margin of a normal breast, whereas an isolated fragment is sometimes found in the same location. Such structures may undergo hypertrophy during pregnancy. When lactation has been established, they may become swollen and painful. Ordinarily, they soon undergo regression and give no further trouble.

Abnormalities of the Nipples. The typical nipple is cylindrical, projecting well beyond the general surface of the breast; its exterior is slightly nodular but not fissured. Variations, however, are not uncommon, some sufficiently pronounced to seriously interfere with suckling.

In some women, the lactiferous ducts open directly into a depression at the center of the areola. In marked cases of depressed nipple, nursing is out of the question. When the depression is not very deep, the breast may occasionally be made available by use of a breast pump.

More frequently, the nipple, although not depressed, is so greatly inverted that it cannot be used for nursing. In such a case, daily attempts should be made during the last few months of pregnancy to draw the nipple out, using traction with the fingers. Because the maneuver is rarely successful, however, if the nipples cannot be made available by temporary use of an electric pump, suckling must be discontinued.

Nipples that are normal in shape and size may become fissured and therefore particularly susceptible to injury during suckling. In such cases, the fissures almost invariably render nursing painful, sometimes with a deleterious influence upon the secretory function. Moreover, such lesions provide a convenient portal of entry for pyogenic bacteria. For these reasons, every effort should be made to heal such fissures, particularly by protecting them from further injury with a nipple shield and topical medication. If such measures are of no avail, the child should not be permitted to nurse on the affected side. Instead, the breast should be emptied regularly with a suitable pump until the lesions are completely healed.

Abnormalities of Secretion. There are marked individual variations in the amount of milk secreted, many of which are dependent not upon the general health and appearance of the woman but upon the development of the glandular portions of the breasts. A woman with large breasts may produce only a small quantity of milk, whereas another with small, flat breasts may produce an abundant supply. Very rarely, there is complete lack of mammary secretion (*agalactia*). As a rule, it is possible to express a small amount from the nipple on the third or fourth day of the puerperium. Occasionally, the mammary secretion is excessive (*polygalactia*).

Formerly, persistent lactation or galactorrhea, together with amenorrhea and signs of estrogen deficiency, was referred to as the **Chiari–Frommel syndrome.** It was believed that this disorder was a pregnancy-induced derangement in the hypothalamic–pituitary control of prolactin and gonadotropin secretion. With the development of sensitive and accurate radioimmunoassays for prolactin and with the development of computed tomography for evaluating the contents of the sella turcica, it has been demonstrated that pituitary microadenomas are the most common cause of galactorrhea, amenorrhea, and estrogen deficiency.

Postpartum Psychosis. As discussed in Chapter 18 (p. 469), mild and transient depression, termed *postpartum blues*, is common within the first week or so after delivery. Frequently, this does not develop until the woman returns home, but in any case it is mild and self-limited. Depression thereafter, especially if severe, is not normal and it requires investigation. Episodes of previously diagnosed mental illness are likely to exacerbate postpartum (see Chap. 55, p. 1253). Importantly, women with previous postpartum psychosis are reported to have a 50 percent recurrence risk in subsequent pregnancies (Vandenbergh, 1980). Other risk factors include admission by the woman that her pregnancy was not wanted, or that she feels unloved by her mate. Signs and symptoms of postpartum depression are no different than those of other depressive disorders. Particularly worrisome are suicidal thoughts, paranoid delusions, and threats of violence to the woman's children (Vandenbergh, 1980).

As discussed in Chapter 55 (p. 1254), treatment of suspected serious mental illness is given in consultation with a psychiatrist familiar with these syndromes. Often, hospitalization is warranted, especially if severe depression is accompanied by suicidal ruminations.

Obstetrical Paralysis

Pressure on branches of the lumbosacral plexus during labor may be manifest by complaints of intense neuralgia or cramplike pains extending down one or both legs as soon as the head begins to descend the pelvis. As a rule, the compression is rarely severe enough to give rise to worrisome lesions. In some instances, however, the pain continues after delivery and is accompanied by paralysis of the muscles supplied by the external popliteal nerve. These include the flexors of the ankles and the extensors of the toes, and result in weakened ankle dorsiflexion and footdrop. Footdrop also may result from improper positioning of patients in stirrups or leg holders. Less commonly, the femoral, obturator, or sciatic nerves may be involved. In some instances, the gluteal muscles are affected.

Separation of the symphysis pubis or one of the sacroiliac synchondroses during labor may be followed by pain and marked interference with locomotion.

References

Adrinopoulos GC, Mendenhall HW: Prostaglandin F$_{2\alpha}$ in the management of delayed postpartum hemorrhage. Am J Obstet Gynecol 146:217, 1983

Almeida OD, Kitay DZ: Lactation suppression and puerperal fever. Am J Obstet Gynecol 154:940, 1986

Andrew AC, Bulmer JN, Wells M, Morrison L, Buckley CH: Subinvolution of the uteroplacental arteries in the human placental bed. Histopathology 15:375, 1989

Brown CEL, Dunn DH, Harrell R, Setiawan H, Cunningham FG: Computed tomography for evaluation of puerperal infection. Surg Gynecol Obstet 172:2, 1991

Chin HC, Scott DR, Resnik R, Davis GB, Lurie AL: Angiographic embolization of intractable puerperal hematomas. Am J Obstet Gynecol 160:434, 1989

Dixey JJ, Swanson DC, Williams TD, Rusin MH, Crook SJ, Midgley J, deSaxe MJ: Toxic-shock syndrome: Four cases in a London hospital. Br Med J 285:342, 1982

Goldstein AI, Kent DR, David A: Prostaglandin E_2 vaginal suppositories in the treatment of intractable late-onset postpartum hemorrhage: A case report. J Reprod Med 28:425, 1983

Katz M, Kroll D, Pak I, Osimoni A, Hirsch M: Puerperal hypertension, stroke, and seizures after suppression of lactation with bromocriptine. Obstet Gynecol 66:822, 1985

Kremer JAM, Rolland R, Van Der Heijden PFM, Schellekens LA, Vosmar MBJG, Lancranjan I: Lactation inhibition by a single injection of a new depot-bromocriptine. Br J Obstet Gynaecol 97:527, 1990

Lee CY, Madrazo B, Drukker BH: Ultrasonic evaluation of the postpartum uterus in the management of postpartum bleeding. Obstet Gynecol 58:227, 1981

Matheson I, Aursnes I, Horgen M, Aabø Ø, Melby K: Bacteriological findings and clinical symptoms in relation to clinical outcome in puerperal mastitis. Acta Obstet Gynecol Scand 67:723, 1988

Melis GB, Mais V, Paoletti AM, Beneventi F, Gambacciani M, Fioretti P: Prevention of puerperal lactation by a single oral administration of the new prolactin-inhibiting drug, cabergoline. Obstet Gynecol 71:311, 1988

Niebyl JR, Bell WR, Schaaf ME, Blake DA, Dubin NH, King TM: The effect of chlorotrianisene on postpartum lactation suppression on blood coagulation factors. Am J Obstet Gynecol 143:518, 1979

Rench MA, Baker CJ: Group B streptococcal breast abscess in a mother and mastitis in her infant. Obstet Gynecol 73:875, 1989

Ruch A, Duhring JL: Postpartum myocardial infarction in a patient receiving bromocriptine. Obstet Gynecol 74:448, 1989

Thomsen AC, Espersen T, Maigaard S: Course and treatment of milk stasis, noninfectious inflammation of the breast, and infectious mastitis in nursing women. Am J Obstet Gynecol 149:492, 1984

Thomsen AC, Hansen KB, Moller BR: Leukocyte counts and microbiologic cultivation in the diagnosis of puerperal mastitis. Am J Obstet Gynecol 146:938, 1983

Turnbull AC: Puerperal thromboembolism and the suppression of lactation. J Obstet Gynaecol Br Commonw 75:1321, 1968

Vandenbergh RL: Postpartum depression. Clin Obstet Gynecol 23:1105, 1980

Wager GP, Martin DH, Koutsky L, Eschenbach DA, Daling JR, Chiang WT, Alexander ER, Holmes KK: Puerperal infectious morbidity: Relationship to route of delivery and to antepartum *Chlamydia trachomatis* infection. Am J Obstet Gynecol 138:1028, 1980

Watson DL, Bhatia RK, Norman GS, Brindley BA, Sokol RJ: Bromocriptine mesylate for lactation suppression: A risk for postpartum hypertension? Obstet Gynecol 74:573, 1989

Zahn CM, Yeomans ER: Postpartum hemorrhage: Placental accreta, uterine inversion and puerperal hematomas. Clin Obstet Gynecol 33:422, 1990

SECTION VIII

Reproductive Success and Failure

CHAPTER 30

Pregnancy at the Extremes of Reproductive Life

The number of infants born in the United States in 1989 exceeded 4 million, the highest number reported since 1963; provisional statistics for 1990 indicate another 3 percent increase (National Center for Health Statistics, 1991). The largest increases in maternal age-specific birth rates, 6 to 8 percent, were observed in teenagers (15 to 19 years of age) and women 35 to 44 years of age (Fig. 30–1). This national trend began in the mid-1980s and has served as the impetus for this chapter.

Pregnancy in Teenagers

Since the 1980s, the continued rise in birth rates for women under age 20 has been associated with a rise in the proportion of teenagers who are sexually active (Centers for Disease Control, 1991). Among women aged 15 years, the proportion of those sexually active rose from 17 percent in 1980 to 20 percent in 1988. Similarly, among those aged 17 years, the proportion rose from 36 percent to 51 percent. Thus, an increasing proportion of teenagers are clearly at risk of becoming pregnant. Reports of abortion rates indicate little change among teenagers during the 1980s, and this coupled with increased birth rates, suggests that teenage pregnancy rates have risen (Henshaw and co-workers, 1991). According to McAnarney and Hendee (1989), compared with other developed countries, the United States exhibits significantly higher pregnancy, birth, and abortion rates within its adolescent population. It also is apparent that pregnancy in American teenagers is common in all social, economical, and racial groups.

In the 1960s, when the first prenatal programs for young mothers were established, societal attitudes were primitive, and little effort was made to search for solutions to early childbirth (Hollingsworth and Kreutner,

1980). During the 1970s, it became clear that teenage pregnancy was primarily a sociological problem with medical consequences. Obstetrical risks for older teenagers (16 to 18 years of age) were found to be poverty, inadequate nutrition, and poor health before pregnancy, rather than maternal age in itself (McAnarney and colleagues, 1978). These risk factors, when later analyzed by McAnarney (1987), were found to include poor nutrition, smoking, alcohol and drug abuse, and genital infections. In addition, there is particular concern that women 15 years of age or younger may experience pregnancy complications due to their physiological immaturity (Fielding, 1978).

Most reports of birth to teenagers indicate an increased risk of developing at least some complications of pregnancy and poor neonatal outcome, especially preeclampsia and low-birthweight infants. It is controversial whether biological or social inadequacies best explain these apparent reproductive disadvantages. They are frequently attributed to unspecified or variously defined factors under the rubric of "teenage pregnancy," both in the media and scientific literature. For example, *Time* magazine devoted 13 pages to "Teen Pregnancy in America" in a 1985 cover story and portrayed "teens" as those up to age 19. Hollingsworth and Kreutner (1980) summarized the medical literature and observed that obstetrical risks in older teenagers (16 to 18 years of age) were associated with social factors such as poverty rather than simply biological attributes of maternal age. In contrast, those 15 years or younger appeared to have pregnancy complications related to their young age. We have analyzed pregnancy outcomes in over 16,500 nulliparous women delivered at Parkland Hospital and found that preterm birth and pregnancy-induced hypertension were increased significantly among 1622 pregnancies in middle-school-age mothers

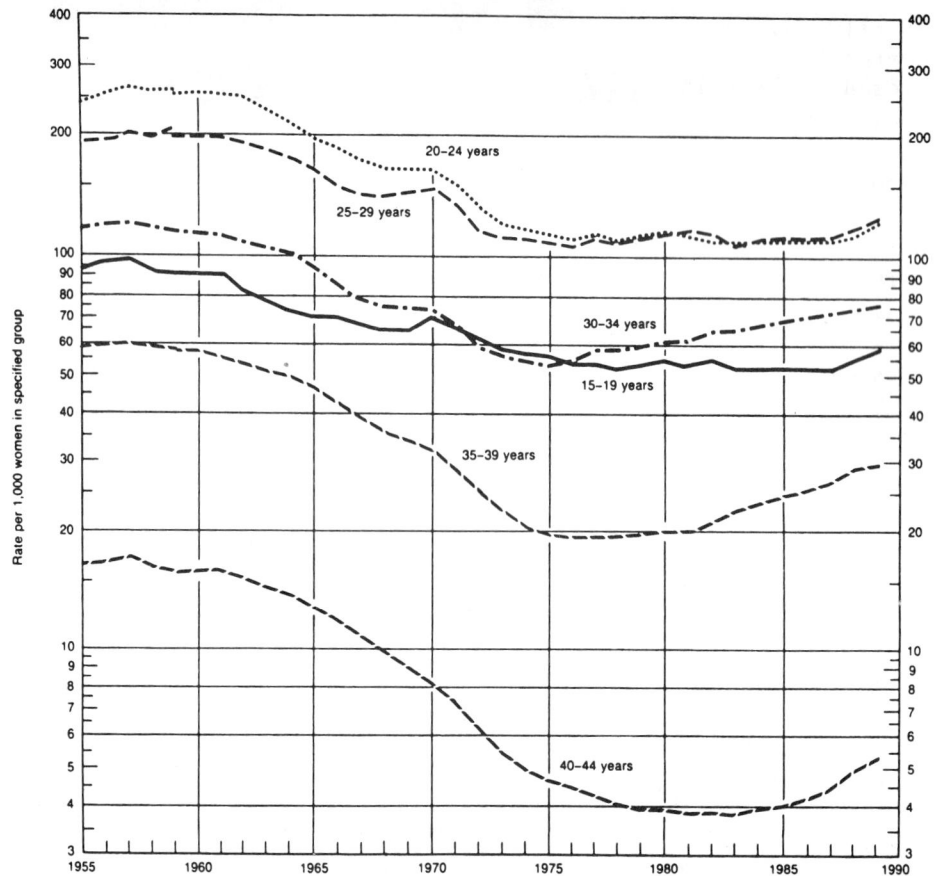

Fig. 30–1. Birthrates by age of mother, United States 1955–1989. (From National Center for Health Statistics, 1991.)

NOTE: Beginning with 1959, trend lines are based on registered live births; trend lines for 1955–59 are based on live births adjusted for underregistration

(11 to 15 years of age). High-school-age mothers (16 through 19 years of age) did not experience more complications compared with older first-time mothers (Satin and colleagues, in press).

Precocious Puberty. The youngest mother whose history is authenticated is Lina Medina, who was delivered by cesarean section in Lima, Peru, in 1939. Although her exact age is disputable, she was around 5 years old. Ms. Medina related to a writer from the *National Enquirer* in 1980 that she always knew that the child, who had been raised as her brother, had come from her own body, but she did not completely comprehend the significance of this until she was about 11. Gerardo, who was named for the doctor who performed the cesarean section, was 10 years old before he knew that Lina was his mother. He married at age 18, had two daughters, and died in 1979 of an apparent heart attack at age 40.

Although true precocious puberty is very uncommon, the average age of menarche and ovulation is appreciably lower than it was several decades ago (see Chap. 4, Fig. 4–6). The mean age of menarche in the United States is now estimated to be 12.3 years. As a consequence of this, and perhaps of greater sexual free-

dom, most obstetrical services have witnessed a marked increase in the number of extremely young pregnant women.

Teenage Fertility. From the postwar high of 3.8 births per woman at the peak of the baby boom, the total fertility rate in the United States had fallen to 1.8 in 1980, where it remained unchanged until 1985. This below-replacement level of fertility has, in recent decades, characterized most Western countries. Were it not for the continued infusion of immigrants, the United States population would stop growing and begin to decline before the middle of the next century.

One major exception to the very low fertility of the Western World is the high birthrate of teenagers in the United States. This birthrate temporarily declined in the first half of the 1980s, but only because of increasing abortions; the teenage pregnancy rate in fact was rising (Westoff, 1986). The rate of teenage births is especially high in the African-American population. An international comparison in 1980 found that the black teenage fertility rate was 2.3 times the white and 3.2 times the average rate in 30 advanced countries (Westoff and co-authors, 1983). Also, white US teenager birth rates were 40 percent higher than the average for other advanced countries. An intensive study of several countries with cultures similar to the United States, but with much lower teenage pregnancy rates, suggests that poverty, conflicting messages on sexuality, and the lack of contraceptive services play a major role (Jones and colleagues, 1985).

Maternal Mortality in Teens. In most industrialized nations, major causes of death in the second decade of life include motor vehicle accidents, other unintentional injuries, suicide, and homicide. However, for numerous developing nations, maternal mortality remains among the top three causes of teenage deaths (Blum, 1991). Most deaths are due to eclampsia, puerperal infection, and hemorrhage. Moreover, in nearly every country where it is illegal, abortion represents a major cause of teenage maternal mortality from both sepsis and hemorrhage.

Impact of Age on Pregnancy Outcome. Most studies of pregnancy complications in teenagers have yielded conflicting results. Either increased or decreased incidence in one or more of the following have been demonstrated: hypertension, anemia, uterine dysfunction, cephalopelvic disproportion, low-birthweight infants, certain congenital malformations, and perinatal mortality. The lack of agreement may be due in part to the various definitions used for "teenage pregnancy." For example, very young teenagers—those 15 years of age or less—are often indiscriminately compared with older teenagers. Some investigators have identified those teenagers 15 years or less as having increased risks of adverse pregnancy results (Duenhoelter and co-workers, 1975).

Young maternal age appears to be a health hazard for children born to teenage mothers. Specifically, high levels of postneonatal health problems such as accidents and infections have been linked to increased infant mortality (McCormick and co-workers, 1984). Similar problems in infancy have been observed in Britain and termed "transmitted deprivation."

Impact of Pregnancy on Teenagers. The psychosocial issues of adolescent pregnancy and childbearing are likely more overwhelming than the medical issues. Klein (1978) wrote of adolescent childbearing as "initiating a syndrome of failure: failure to complete one's education, failure in limiting family size, and failure to establish a vocation and become independent." Furstenberg and co-workers (1987) studied urban adolescent mothers and their children with follow-up interviews at 5 and 15 years subsequent to delivery. At the 5-year follow-up, many of the adolescent mothers were struggling to gain an education and to use contraceptives reliably, and approximately one third were receiving public assistance. At the 15-year follow-up, the situation was not so bleak. Those who fared better had remained in school, received family planning and financial assistance, and avoided another teenage birth.

Pregnancy After 35

During the last decade of this century, a rather impressive proportion of American women having babies are over 35, and many of these women will be pregnant for the first time. Now aged 30 to 40, these women were born during the post-World War II *baby boom.* In the years that followed, technological and social developments that reduced the death rate of the American population also reduced the birthrate (Garrett, 1988). Factors pivotal in the reduced birthrate underscore dramatic changes in the societal role of women. These changes have occurred as a result of rising education levels, effective means of birth control, and an increasing number of women in the work force. Indeed, families that include both male and female wage earners are quite typical in the United States today. Other factors affecting the birthrate include the higher costs of raising children and the availability of legal abortion.

As a net result of all these factors, in the 1990s there is a proportionately larger number of American women between the ages of 35 and 50. Combined with the trend documented by Ventura (1982), that many women are delaying childbearing, the age-specific birth rate for the 1990s is projected to show a dramatic increase for women over 35. According to Hansen (1986), the Census Bureau estimates that because of the higher fertility rate of women over 35, combined with the decrease in the number of women aged 20 to 29, the proportion of babies born to these older women will nearly double by the end of the century compared with the early 1980s. Specifically, the proportion of total births in women over 35 is projected to increase from 5 percent in 1982 to about 9 percent by 2000.

The trend among older, well-educated women to make up previously delayed childbearing has continued to intensify among women over 30. Conversely, the incidence of childlessness among women in their 30s has increased sharply over the past 2 decades (National Center for Health Statistics, 1991). For example, among women reaching 35 by the end of 1989, 20 percent had not had children, compared with just 9 percent of women aged 35 in 1970. Surveys show, however, that half of childless wives aged 30 to 34 expect to have at least one child (U.S. Bureau of the Census, 1989).

Women delaying childbearing continue to be disproportionately well educated. Among those aged 30 to 34 having their first child in 1988, 46 percent were college graduates, compared with 7 percent of women aged 20 to 24 and 33 percent of those aged 25 to 29 (National Center for Health Statistics, 1991). These patterns corroborate the widely held view that young, well-educated women have been delaying childbearing while their older counterparts have been making up for the childbearing they previously had postponed.

From the foregoing, it can be seen that older women are having more babies and more older women are having babies. There are numerous pregnancy complications, both maternal and perinatal, that may develop in these women over 35. Although there is no obvious age cutoff at which a woman becomes more susceptible to these complications, the age of 35 has previously been used, especially when referring to women pregnant for the first time. Thus, the indelicate term *elderly primigravida* is encountered frequently, and in fact this definition was adopted in 1959 by the International Federation of Obstetricians and Gynaecologists. More than 20 years ago, Kane (1967) argued that "the concept of the arbitrary age (35 years) at which maternal risk increases should be abandoned as myth, and the more logical concept of a sliding scale of difficulty should replace it."

Maternal Complications. Because the incidence of most chronic illnesses increase as a function of age, it is not surprising that medical complications are encountered more frequently in older pregnant women. It follows logically that the severity of many of these conditions increases along with their duration, and thus it is likely that older pregnant women will have more advanced chronic disorders. The best example of this concept is diabetes, because its incidence accrues with age, and most type II, or non-insulin-dependent, diabetics are aged 40 or older. Likewise, the horrific vasculopathic complications of diabetes are directly related to the length of time since the diabetes became clinically apparent.

Medical Complications

HYPERTENSION. As expected, chronic hypertension commonly complicates pregnancy in women over 35. It is difficult at times to clinically separate antecedent hypertensive disease from pregnancy-induced hypertension. Precision notwithstanding, the majority of reported studies cited a two- to fourfold increased incidence of hypertension when pregnancy outcomes in older women were compared with younger controls. In more recent studies, in which antecedent hypertension was identified more accurately, the incidence of chronic hypertension in pregnant women over 35 appears to be at least 10 percent. For example, Tuck and colleagues (1988) observed its incidence to be nearly 12 percent in 196 primigravid women, a threefold increase when compared with primigravidas between the ages of 20 and 25. In women aged 40 or older, Yasin and Beydoun

(1988) observed an incidence of 16 percent compared with about 2 percent in their general population, and Lehmann and Chism (1987) reported an incidence slightly over 20 percent. Importantly, perinatal mortality is amplified in older hypertensive women (Grimes and Gross, 1981).

PREECLAMPSIA. It is often difficult to separate antecedent chronic hypertension from pregnancy-induced hypertension. For example, the pattern of transient peripartum hypertension without proteinuria, especially in the multipara, probably signifies chronic hypertensive disease rather than preeclampsia (Chesley, 1985). Conversely, because chronic hypertension is so prevalent, proteinuric hypertension frequently signifies superimposed preeclampsia in many of these older women (see Chap. 36).

The findings in some of the more recent studies are at least suggestive that the incidence of preeclampsia is not increased substantively as a function of advanced maternal age unless chronic hypertension antedates pregnancy. For example, Yasin and Beydoun (1988), in a case-controlled study, found the incidence of "pure preeclampsia" to be about 5 percent in women in their 40s as well as in younger control women. Lehmann and Chism (1987), in a 3-year study from Charity Hospital, reported the incidence of preeclampsia to be about 13 percent in previously nonhypertensive women in their 40s, compared with 10 percent in their general obstetrical population. Tuck and colleagues (1988), reporting results from the Oxford Obstetric Data System, observed that the incidence of preeclampsia was lower in older primigravid women.

DIABETES. The incidence of as well as the complications due to type II, or *non-insulin-dependent,* diabetes accrues with age. Pregnancy in women over 35 is thus complicated by an increased incidence of *gestational diabetes* as well as overt disease (see Chap. 53, p. 1201). Most often, and especially in older studies, it is difficult to separate the incidence of the two because terminology has changed continuously in the past 20 years. With this caveat in mind, most studies are suggestive of at least a doubling of the incidence of some type of diabetes when women over 35 are compared with younger controls. Tysoe (1970) reviewed data from nearly 42,000 pregnancies at four Vancouver hospitals and observed that the incidence of diabetes increased from 0.3 percent in women aged 25 to 29 to 1 percent for women over 40. Kirz and colleagues (1985) observed a threefold increase in the incidence of diabetes when more than 1000 women older than 35 were compared with nearly 5350 control women aged 20 to 25.

GESTATIONAL DIABETES. The incidence of gestational diabetes increases with advancing maternal age. Mestman (1980) performed 3-hour glucose tolerance screening in 652 consecutive women attending prenatal clinic at Los Angeles County Women's Hospital and reported the following incidences of abnormal tests: 3.7 percent in women younger than 20, 7.5 percent for those 20 to 30, and 13.8 percent of women older than 30. Although O'Sullivan and colleagues (1973) reported earlier that older women with abnormal glucose tolerance tests had higher perinatal mortality rates, this finding was not substantiated by Gabbe and colleagues (1977) in a later investigation of 261 class A diabetic women.

OTHER DISEASES. A formidable number of other medical and surgical complications increase in incidence as well as in severity as a function of maternal age. This list includes, but is not limited to, cardiovascular, neurological, connective-tissue, renal, and pulmonary disorders, as well as diseases such as alcoholism and malignant neoplasms. As a result of these, as well as obstetrical complications discussed subsequently, the number of antepartum hospital admissions for older women is increased substantively (Yasin and Beydoun, 1988). Of 1984 admissions to the High Risk Pregnancy Unit at Parkland Hospital, only 5 percent of women younger than 30 were admitted for medical disorders, whereas 12 percent of those older than 30 had one of these complications.

As emphasized by Lehmann and Chism (1987), older women with medical complications are also at greater risk postpartum, especially for thrombotic complications and pulmonary edema. The high incidence of heart failure in these older women is related to chronic underlying hypertension (Cunningham and colleagues, 1986).

Late Pregnancy Bleeding. From his review, Hansen (1986) concluded that the incidence of maternal bleeding from both placental abruption and previa is increased in women older than 35. Fonteyn and Isada (1988) refuted this association. It seems logical that placental abruption is increased because older women have a higher incidence of chronic hypertension, a major risk factor. Although the risk for placenta previa increases with multiparity as well as advancing age, it is arguable which of these two is more important (see Chap. 37, p. 836).

Naeye (1980), citing data from the Collaborative Perinatal Project, reported that the incidence of abruption and previa increased with each of three 10-year maternal age increments. Tysoe (1970) reviewed nearly 42,000 births from four Vancouver hospitals and reported a similar trend. In a more recent study, Lehmann and Chism (1987) reported a 3.2 percent incidence of placental abruption in women aged 40 or older compared with 0.4 percent for their general obstetrical population. This incidence in older women was 3.7 percent if chronic hypertension was identified, but only 2 percent if the older women were normotensive when nonpregnant.

Cesarean Section. The cesarean birth rate is increased substantively in older women. This is the result of multiple factors, including increased hypertensive disorders, diabetes, preterm labor, and placental accidents. Most investigators have found that prolonged labor is more common in older women, especially nulliparas (Hansen, 1986).

Tuck and co-workers (1988) reported a cesarean section rate of 27 percent in women aged 40 or older compared with a rate of 7 percent in women aged 20 to 25. Martel and colleagues (1987) studied nearly 3500 consecutive births in Montreal and reported that the cesarean section rate in nulliparous women increased from 13 percent in those who were younger than 25 years old to nearly 28 percent for those 35 or older. A similar trend was reported for parous women; the rates were 3.4 and 10.1 percent for these two age groups.

Maternal Mortality. Given the multitude of medical and obstetrical complications that may complicate pregnancy in older women, it is not surprising that maternal mortality rates are increased. Rochat (1981) reviewed more than 5000 maternal deaths in the United States from 1968 through 1975, and reported that mortality rates for women aged 35 to 39 were increased fourfold compared with women aged 20 to 24. This disparity was even more marked in nonwhite women (Fig. 30–2). Buehler and colleagues (1986) reviewed maternal deaths reported to the Centers for Disease Control and concluded that by the mid-1980s, the mortality rate for women over 35 had decreased by 50 percent when compared with 1974 through 1978. They calculated a maternal mortality rate of 58 per 100,000 for women older than 35, which was again a fourfold increase over the rate for women aged 20 to 34.

Ectopic pregnancy continues to be a significant cause of maternal deaths in the United States, and its incidence is increased with advancing maternal age (see Chap. 32, p. 694). Rubin and associates (1983) cite a

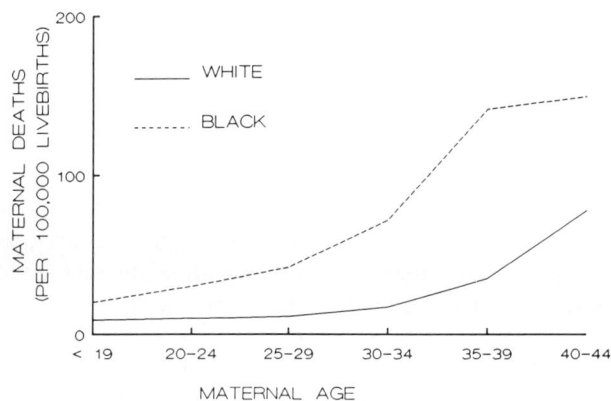

Fig. 30–2. Maternal mortality rates, United States 1974–1978. (Data from Buehler and colleagues, 1986.)

rate of 15.2 ectopic pregnancies per 1000 pregnancies for women aged 35 to 44 compared with a rate of 4.5 in women aged 15 to 24.

Fetal and Neonatal Complications. Perinatal morbidity and mortality are both increased in older women. Similarly, early pregnancy wastage is increased because of excessive spontaneous abortions and chromosomal anomalies. Preterm delivery, retarded fetal growth, and excessive fetal deaths contribute to substantively increased perinatal morbidity and mortality.

Abortion. The majority of epidemiological studies suggest that older women are at greater risk for having spontaneous abortions. Wilson and associates (1986) reviewed retrospectively 18,400 ultrasound examinations done between 7 and 12 weeks and in which an apparently normal embryo had been identified. Although only 1.4 percent of women younger than 30 had a spontaneous abortion subsequent to the ultrasound examination, this incidence was 4.3 percent for those over 35. Hansen (1986) reviewed five United States studies and one each from Canada and Hungary. He concluded that the spontaneous abortion rate increased in a fairly consistent fashion with age, with a two- to fourfold increase when women in their 40s were compared with those in their 20s.

Preterm Delivery and Retarded Fetal Growth. The incidence of low-birthweight infants is increased in women over 35 because of spontaneous and induced preterm delivery as well as increased fetal growth retardation. According to Hansen (1986), the aggregate of older studies suggests that the incidence of low-birthweight infants is increased by a factor of two in women over 35 compared with younger controls. Most of the more recent studies substantiate these findings. Tuck and colleagues (1988) reported that the relative risk for delivery before 37 weeks in primigravid women over 35 was increased fourfold compared with women aged 20 to 25 (incidence 6.1 versus 1.5 percent). Infants weighing less than 2500 g were born to 8.2 percent of older women compared with 3.6 percent of younger controls. The impact of hypertensive complications on low birthweight is illustrated by the data provided by Lehmann and Chism (1987). The incidence of infants who weighed less than 2500 g was 17 percent for women aged 40 or older, compared with 10 percent in the reference populations; however, when the older women with complications—usually hypertension, diabetes, or both—were analyzed separately, the incidence of low-birthweight infants was 32 percent.

Macrosomia. Large infants present substantive perinatal risks from difficult delivery, and *shoulder dystocia* is a principal cause of morbidity. Older women have a higher incidence of macrosomic babies when compared

with younger women. Presumably this results from the same factors that cause the substantial increase in diabetes as maternal age advances. Other common cofactors, some of which also are increased with advancing age, include large size of parents, especially maternal obesity; multiparity; prolonged gestation; and prior birth of a macrosomic infant (Modanlou and co-workers, 1980).

In their survey of nearly 27,000 births at Grady Memorial Hospital, Grimes and Gross (1981) reported that 9 percent of women aged 35 and older were delivered of infants who weighed more than 4000 g, compared with an incidence of 4 percent born to women younger than 35. Similarly, Lehmann and Chism (1987) reported a twofold increased incidence of babies who weighed more than 4000 g born to women older than 40 compared with their general obstetrical population.

Congenital Malformations. Chromosomal abnormalities constitute one of the principal identifiable risk factors for childbearing in later years. The association between maternal age and Down syndrome was observed many years ago. Collmann and Stoller (1962) described over 1100 cases of Down syndrome from Australia from 1942 to 1957. They reported an almost exponentially increased incidence with age beginning in the mid-30s. According to Hansen (1986), the incidence of abnormal chromosomal patterns has been reported to increase with age in studies of induced or spontaneous abortions, stillborns, midtrimester amniocentesis, and congenitally malformed liveborn infants. An inordinate increase in these aberrations was noted in women over age 40 (Fig. 30–3).

The association of age and congenital anomalies unrelated to morphological chromosomal aberrations is less clear. Hay and Barbano (1972) reviewed birth certificate data from 29 states. Excluding Down syndrome, there was only a slight maternal age effect on other

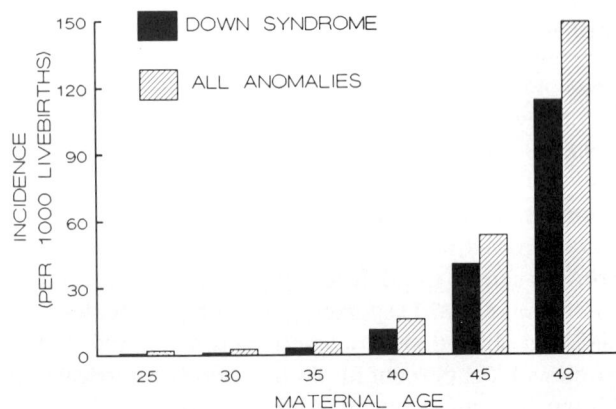

Fig. 30–3. Estimated incidence of Down syndrome and all chromosomal anomalies according to maternal age. (Data from Hansen, 1986, were derived from several published studies.)

malformations after age 40. Specifically, this rate was 8.8 per 1000 women over 40, compared with 6.6 for women younger than 35.

Perinatal Mortality. Perinatal mortality in older women is increased substantially, and stillbirths principally account for the increase. Shown in Table 30–1 are perinatal mortality statistics for Wisconsin from 1978 through 1984. Except for women over 45, the almost trebling of perinatal mortality in these nearly half million women was due to excess stillborns.

Grimes and Gross (1981) studied nearly 27,000 births at Grady Memorial Hospital from 1973 through 1978. They reported the perinatal mortality rate to be 28 per 1000 women younger than 35, while it was 47 per 1000 over 35. This risk was amplified in women with hypertension. In a more recent study from Women's Hospital of Long Beach, Kirz and colleagues (1985) reported no excessive perinatal mortality in 1023 women aged 35 or older, compared with 5343 women aged 20 to 25. They speculated that this may have been because of the efficacy of modern prenatal care given in a tertiary center.

INFANT MORTALITY. There is also increased infant mortality in older women. Infant mortality is calculated from infants born live who die in the first year. Friede and colleagues (1988) reported data from the National Infant Mortality Surveillance Project, which was a 1980 birth cohort that included 1.6 million births in women 25 to 49. While the risk of infant mortality was almost identical for women aged 25 to 29 compared with those aged 30 to 34, infants of mothers aged 35 to 39 had an 18 percent increased mortality risk while those born to mothers aged 40 to 49 had a 69 percent increased risk.

Parkland Hospital Experiences. In 1987 and 1988, 20,525 women who were 20 or older were delivered at Parkland Hospital. Approximately 39 percent were Hispanic, 33 percent African-American, and 26 percent white. The majority had previously given birth to one or more infants. Almost 900 (4.4 percent) were 35 or

older, and only 10 percent were primiparous. As shown in Figures 30–4 and 30–5, a number of adverse pregnancy outcomes were linked to a maternal age of 35 years or above.

Economic Considerations. Davidson and Fukushima (1985) emphasized that the complexity of care given to pregnant women aged 35 or older has resulted in increased costs. Specifically, they cite the increased need for high-technology prenatal care that includes genetic counseling and prenatal diagnosis, amniocentesis, ultrasonic examinations, and tests for fetal well-being. Increased costs seem inevitable given the higher incidence of preterm delivery and subsequent need for intensive neonatal care. While 7 percent of babies born to women younger than 30 were admitted to a special care nursery at Parkland Hospital, this number was 12 percent for women over 35. The twofold increased in-

TABLE 30–1. PERINATAL MORTALITY RATES BY MATERNAL AGE FOR WISCONSIN, 1978–1984

Maternal Age (yr)	Births (no.)[a]	Stillbirths (per 1000)	Neonatal Deaths (per 1000)	Perinatal Mortality (per 1000)
20–24	168,000	6.5	6.4	12.9
25–29	178,000	6.0	5.8	11.8
30–34	84,000	7.2	5.9	13.0
35–39	20,000	11.5	7.4	18.9
40–45	3,200	21.9	8.8	30.7
> 45	200	36.5	31.3	67.7

[a] Figures rounded off.
From Public Health Statistics, 1978–1984, Wisconsin DHHS.

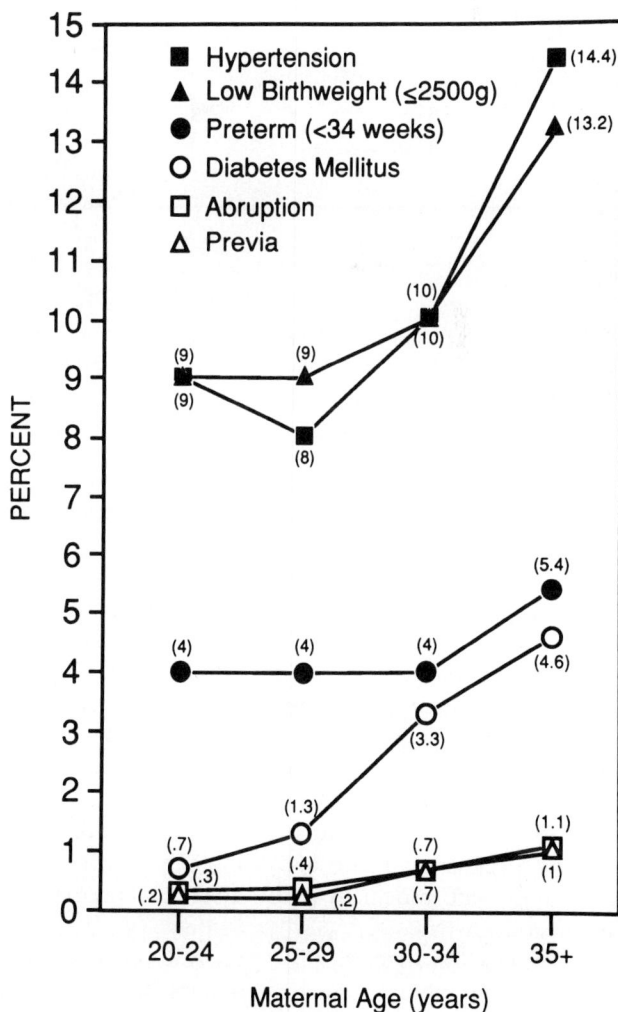

Fig. 30–4. Some pregnancy complications according to maternal age among 20,525 women 20 years or older who gave birth at Parkland Memorial Hospital in 1987 and 1988. (From Cunningham and Leveno, 1990.)

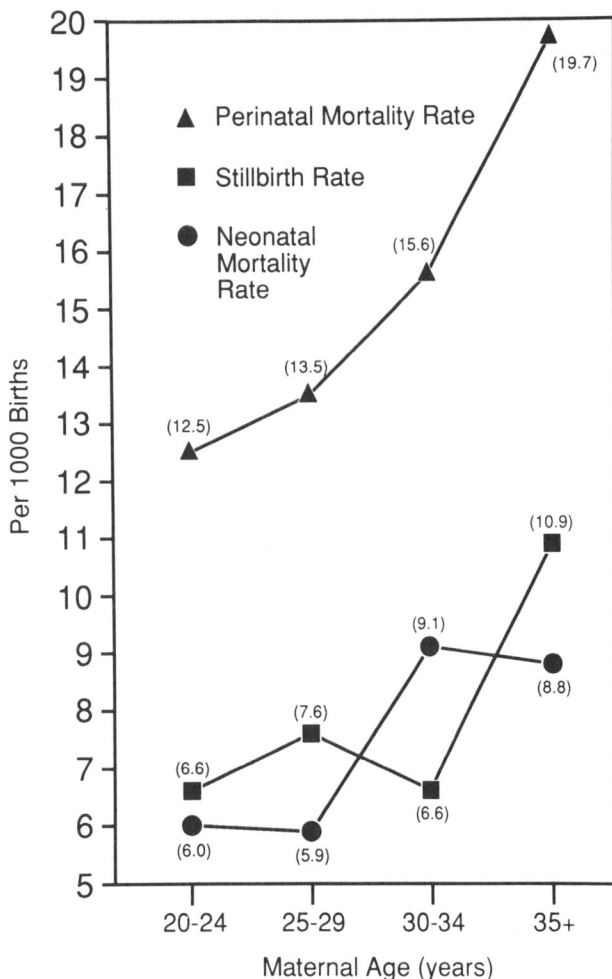

Fig. 30–5. Perinatal, stillbirth, and neonatal mortality rates according to maternal age. Actual rates are shown in parenthesis. (From Cunningham and Leveno, 1990.)

cidence of long-term antepartum hospitalization also contributes to higher medical costs.

Summary. One conclusion might be that pregnancy after the age of 35 is patently dangerous. Importantly, Berkowitz and co-authors (1990) reported that although pregnancy complications were more common in primiparous women 35 or older, the risk of poor neonatal outcome was not increased. Their study population was comprised of private patients who were predominantly white, married, and college-educated. Clearly, pregnancy in this age group can be concluded to be quite safe, especially in the absence of preexisting medical disorders.

Because of dramatically improved prospects for health, even when pregnancy occurs after age 35, women should realistically appraise the risks of pregnancy later in life, but should not necessarily fear delaying childbirth. Pregnancy after 35 is a fact of life in our society, and improved obstetrical care has made ad-

vanced maternal age compatible with successful pregnancy for the great majority of such women. Indeed, Resnik (1990) concluded that "The message is clear and optimistic."

References

Berkowitz GS, Shovnon ML, Lapinski RH, Berkowitz RL: Delayed childbearing and the outcome of pregnancy. N Engl J Med 322:659, 1990

Blum RW: Global trends in adolescent health. JAMA 265:2711, 1991

Buehler JW, Kaunitz AM, Hogue CJR, Hughes JM, Smith JC, Rochat RW: Maternal mortality in women aged 35 years or older: United States. JAMA 255:53, 1986

Centers for Disease Control: Premarital sexual experience among adolescent women: United States. 1970–SS. MMWR 39:929, 1991

Chesley LC: Diagnosis of preeclampsia. Obstet Gynecol 65:423, 1985

Collman RD, Stoller A: A survey of mongoloid births in Victoria, Australia, 1942–1957. Am J Publ Health 52:813, 1962

Cunningham FG, Leveno KJ: Maternal age and outcome of pregnancy. N Engl J Med 323:414, 1990

Cunningham FG, Pritchard JA, Hankins GDV, Anderson PL, Lucas MJ, Armstrong KF: Peripartum heart failure: Idiopathic cardiomyopathy or compounding cardiovascular events? Obstet Gynecol 678:157, 1986

Davidson EC Jr, Fukushima T: The age extremes for reproduction: Current implications for policy change. Am J Obstet Gynecol 152:467, 1985

Duenhoelter JH, Jimenez JM, Baumann G: Pregnancy performance of patients under fifteen years of age. Obstet Gynecol 46:49, 1975

Fielding JE: Adolescent pregnancy revisited. N Engl J Med 299:893, 1978

Fonteyn VJ, Isada NB: Nongenetic implications of childbearing after age thirty-five. Obstet Gynecol Surv 43:709, 1988

Friede A, Baldwin W, Rhodes PH, Buehler JW, Strauss LT: Older maternal age and infant mortality in the United States. Obstet Gynecol 72:152, 1988

Furstenberg F, Brooks-Gunn J, Morgan S: Adolescent mothers and their children in later life. Fam Plan Perspect 19:142, 1987

Gabbe SG, Mestman JH, Freeman RK, Anderson GV, Lowensohn RI: Management and outcome of class A diabetes mellitus. Am J Obstet Gynecol 127:465, 1977

Garrett WE: Historical Atlas of the United States. Washington, DC, National Geographic Society, 1988, p 62

Grimes DA, Gross GK: Pregnancy outcomes in black women aged 35 and older. Obstet Gynecol 58:614, 1981

Hansen JP: Older maternal age and pregnancy outcome: A review of the literature. Obstet Gynecol Surv 41:726, 1986

Hay S, Barbano H: Independent effects of maternal age and birth order on the incidence of selected congenital malformations. Teratology 5:271, 1972

Henshaw SM, Koonin LM, Smith JC: Characteristics of U.S. women having abortions, 1987. Fam Plan Perspect 23:2, 1991

Hollingsworth DR, Kreutner AK: Teenage Pregnancy. N Engl J Med 304:516, 1980

Jones EF, Forrest JD, Goldman N, Henshaw SK, Lincoln R, Rosoff JI, Westoff CF, Wulf D: Teenage pregnancy in developed countries: Determinants and policy implications. Fam Plan Perspect 17:53, 1985

Kane SH: Advancing age and the primigravida. Obstet Gynecol 29:409, 1967

Kirz DS, Dorchester W, Freeman RK: Advanced maternal age: The mature gravida. Am J Obstet Gynecol 152:7, 1985

Klein L: Antecedents of teenage pregnancy. Clin Obstet Gynaecol 21:1151, 1978

Lehmann DK, Chism J: Pregnancy outcome in medically complicated and uncomplicated patients aged 40 years or older. Am J Obstet Gynecol 157:738, 1987

Martel M, Wacholder S, Lippman A, Brohan J, Hamilton E: Maternal age and primary cesarean section rates: A multivariate analysis. Am J Obstet Gynecol 156:305, 1987

McAnarney ER: Young maternal age and adverse neonatal outcome. Am J Dis Child 141:1053, 1987

McAnarney ER, Hendee WR: Adolescent pregnancy and its consequences. 1989

McAnarney ER, Roghmann KJ, Adams BN, Tatelbaum RC, Kash C, Coulter M, Plume M, Charney E: Obstetric, neonatal, and psychosocial outcomes of pregnant adolescents. Pediatrics 61:199, 1978

McCormick MC, Shapiro S, Starfield B: High-risk mothers: Infant mortality and morbidity in four areas of the United States, 1973–1978. Am J Public Health 74:18, 1984

Mestman JH: Outcome of diabetes screening in pregnancy and perinatal morbidity in infants of mothers with mild impairment in glucose tolerance. Diabetes Care 3:447, 1980

Modanlou HD, Dorchester WL, Thorosian A, Freeman RK: Macrosomia—maternal, fetal, and neonatal implications. Obstet Gynecol 55:420, 1980

Naeye RL: Abruptio placentae and placenta previa: Frequency, perinatal mortality, and cigarette smoking. Obstet Gynecol 55:701, 1980

National Center for Health Statistics: Advance report of final natality statistics, 1989. Monthly Vital Statistics Report 40(suppl): 1, 1991, Washington, Government Printing Office, pub. no. (PHS) 92-1120

O'Sullivan JB, Charles D, Mahan CM, Dandrow RV: Gestational diabetes and perinatal mortality rate. Am J Obstet Gynecol 116:901, 1973

Public Health Statistics, 1978–1984. Wisconsin Department of Health and Human Services, Bureau of Health Statistics

Resnick R: The "elderly primigravida" in 1990. N Engl J Med 322:693, 1990

Rochat RW: Maternal mortality of the United States of America. World Health Stat Rep 34:2, 1981

Rubin GL, Peterson HB, Dorfman SF, Layde PM, Maze JM, Ory HW, Cates W: Ectopic pregnancy in the United States: 1970 through 1978. JAMA 249:1725, 1983

Satin AJ, Leveno KJ, Sherman ML, Reedy NJ, Lowe TW: Maternal youth and pregnancy outcomes: Middle school versus high school age groups compared to women beyond the teen years. JAMA, in press

Tuck SM, Yudkin PL, Turnbull AC: Pregnancy outcome in elderly primigravidae with and without a history of infertility. Br J Obstet Gynaecol 95:230, 1988

Tysoe FW: Effect of age on the outcome of pregnancy. Trans Pacif Coast Obstet Gynecol Soc 38:8, 1970

US Bureau of the Census. Fertility of American Women. Current Population Reports, series P-20, no. 436. Washington: US Department of Commerce, June 1989

Ventura SJ: Trends in birth to older mothers, 1970–79. National Center for Health Statistics Monthly Vital Statistics Report 31(suppl), 1982

Westoff CF: Fertility in the United States. Science 234:554, 1986

Westoff CF, Calot G, Foster AD: Teenage fertility in developed nations: 1971–1980. Fam Plan Perspect 15:105, 1983

Wilson RD, Kendrick V, Wittmann BK, McGillivray B: Spontaneous abortion and pregnancy outcome after normal first-trimester ultrasound examination. Obstet Gynecol 67:352, 1986

Yasin SY, Beydoun SN: Pregnancy outcome at greater than or equal to 20 weeks gestation in women in their 40s: A case-control study. J Reprod Med 33:209, 1988

CHAPTER 31
Abortion

Overview

For purposes of predicting reproductive success, and thereby the likelihood of reproductive failure in humans, an understanding of certain peculiarities of human reproduction is essential. In most mammalian species, the female is the limiting resource in reproduction; and this is the case in the human. But importantly, as Short (1976) observes, woman is the only mammal that has forsaken estrus, a condition when she instinctively is attractive and receptive to the male. In the human, this has been exchanged for a situation in which woman is attractive and potentially receptive at any time after puberty. Additionally, humans are the only primate in which puberty is delayed until the second decade of life; and humans are the only primate in which full breast development in females occurs at puberty (Milligan and associates, 1975). Therefore, because women at all times of the ovarian cycle are attractive to men, and because women are potentially receptive at all times of the ovarian cycle, humans seem to be adapted for low levels of continuous sexual activity (Short, 1984).

These are important considerations that constitute a perplexing and unique problem for human reproduction. Specifically, in other animals, estrus guarantees that spermatozoa are present in the fallopian tube at the time of ovulation. But in the human, spermatozoa may arrive late—and the life span of the fertilizable ovum may exceed the time during which fertilization will lead to a normal, healthy fetus (Adams, 1972). In the human, the advantages of family bonding that can result from continuous sexual activity may have been adapted in exchange for the risks that may accrue from late or absent fertilization of the ovum.

Predictions of Success and Failure in Human Reproduction. It is useful to predict the likelihood of success in human reproduction for many reasons. First, predictions are necessary to understand what factors contribute to the success. This is true if optimal strategies are to be devised for pregnancy prevention. Second, it is imperative to understand the natural limits of successful human reproduction in order to devise strategies for improving the likelihood of a liveborn infant. Third, it is essential to comprehend the likelihood of reproductive failure at each juncture of the reproductive process to understand the causes of pregnancy failure.

For these purposes, estimates have been developed of **the likelihood of pregnancy success and failure under optimal conditions.** An analysis is presented of the probable outcome of a given ovarian cycle in 1000 young (20 to 29 years), healthy, fertile women. It must be assumed there are normal viable spermatozoa in the fallopian tube at the time of ovulation (Fig. 31–1), that is, the male factor is not limiting. The likelihood of viable spermatozoa being present at the time the ovum enters the fallopian tube is decidedly less than 100 percent. During the course of several or even many ovarian cycles, this limitation is diminished, provided sexual intercourse with a fertile male occurs at reasonable intervals. Nonetheless, late fertilization of the ovum, that is, conception occurring in an ovum several hours after ovulation, may portend an unfavorable outcome of the resulting zygote (Adams, 1972). Thus, for the purpose of developing models to describe the natural course of human reproduction, this is a consideration of substantial weight. Namely, **what are the probabilities of conception (fertilization of the ovum), implantation of the blastocyst, and birth of a normal living infant during each ovarian cycle in fertile women in whom the presence of living spermatozoa in the fallopian tube at ovulation is not limiting?**

Life Span of Spermatozoa and Ova. The life span of liberated germ cells, both spermatozoa and ova, is short. Precise data are still not available for longevity of spermatozoa in the female reproductive tract or the fertilizable life span of ova. But, it is probable that few spermatozoa are capable of fertilization after more than 24 hours, and it is likely that the optimum time for fertilization of the ovum is substantially shorter, perhaps no more than 1 to 2 hours, or possibly less. Perhaps more importantly, as the liberated germ cells age, the likelihood of formation of an abnormal zygote increases. Provided these estimates are reasonable, it follows that viable spermatozoa must be present in the fallopian tube at the time of ovulation for optimal fertilization.

The time of intercourse, therefore, becomes more crucial in establishing the likelihood of successful conception with any given ovulation. This is especially important recognizing that semen volume and sperm density, even in normal men, declines when ejaculation occurs more often than every 48 hours.

Theoretical Basis for Predictions. For purposes of estimating **female fertility efficiency,** it is assumed that viable spermatozoa are in the fallopian tube at the time

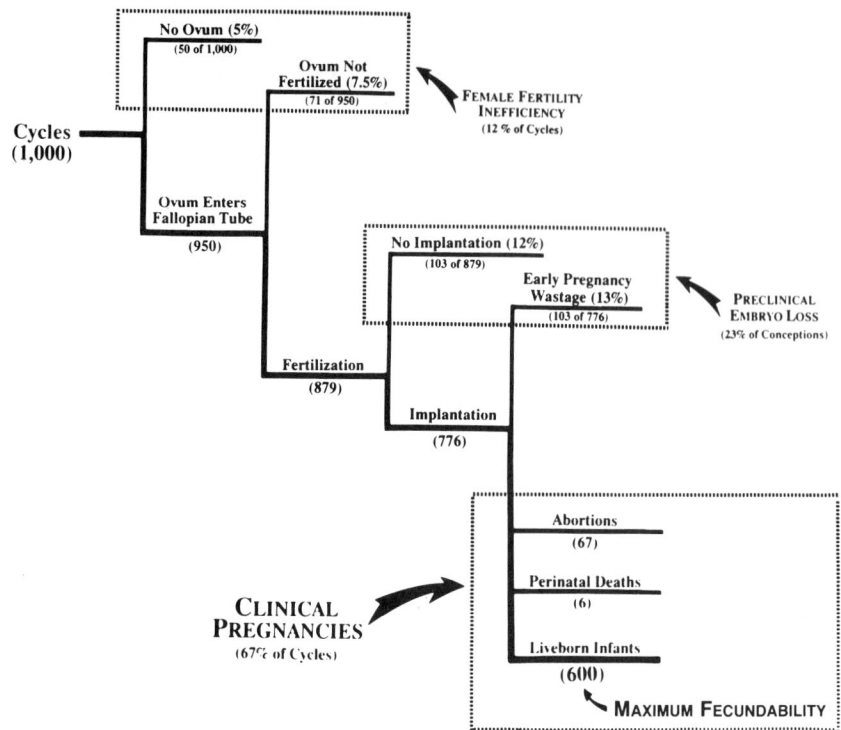

Fig. 31–1. Predictions of reproductive success and failure: Estimates were made on the basis of two assumptions. First, the population of women is young, healthy, and fertile. Second, spermatozoa capable of ovum fertilization are present in the fallopian tube at the time of ovulation.

of ovulation and fertilization takes place here. Based on these assumptions, reasonable estimates can be made of the likelihood of conception, pregnancy, early embryonic loss, and the number of live-born infants as a function of the number of menstrual cycles in young, healthy, fertile women. These estimates are useful in (1) predicting pregnancy success, (2) defining the contribution of both male and female infertility to pregnancy failures, (3) determining at what stage of reproduction the greatest risk of failure exists, (4) ascertaining the theoretical limits of success for therapy of fertility, and (5) devising strategies for contraception. By use of these approaches, estimates have been made of human reproductive success and failure at each step of the process from ovulation to live-born infant. The estimates were developed to describe the probability of the outcome of a given menstrual cycle in 1000 young, healthy, fertile women.

To develop estimates for each step in the reproductive process, it was necessary to make sure of the best sets of data available for some processes and thence to derive estimates of other processes by difference. For example, 1000 ovarian cycles were arbitrarily chosen by definition. The prediction ended with a theoretical maximum fecundability of 60 percent. In this theoretical circumstance, 60 percent of cycles would result in a living newborn infant. There is persuasive evidence to support the validity of this assumption. Nonetheless, this figure will come as a surprise to many.

Reproductive biologists are concerned extraordi-

narily with high pregnancy losses that seem to occur at every stage of human reproduction. Perinatal mortality rates of 40 per 1000 or more are not uncommon in some populations; yet among healthy young women with appropriate prenatal care and optimum newborn management, many medical centers now report perinatal mortality rates of less than 10 per 1000. Spontaneous abortion rates of nearly 25 percent are frequently reported; but in healthy, fertile women, abortion of clinically recognized pregnancies in the first trimester of pregnancy is probably no more than 10 percent.

Some investigators have reported extraordinarily high preclinical embryonic losses (i.e., early pregnancy wastage), that occurs after implantation but before or at the time of the next expected menses. But in some of these reports, definitive data were few or else estimates were made with essentially no data. In addition, many reports of high fetal wastage are based on studies of women who were acknowledged to be infertile; such data may not be directly relevant to estimates of reproductive success in normal, healthy, fertile women. Pregnancy failures are influenced by a number of factors—geographic, racial, ethnic, and environmental. For example, the incidence of hydatidiform mole in some areas of Southeast Asia is 1 per 100 pregnancies; in the United States, it is 1 per 2500. The incidence of anencephaly in Ireland is 5 to 10 times greater than in most other parts of the world.

To develop indices for deciphering the cause of fertility failure or loss of conceptuses, it is first helpful to attempt to estimate the ideal or the norm. The model presented is designed to address this goal.

Female Fertility Inefficiency.
Given that spermatozoa are not limiting for conception, *female fertility inefficiency* is attributable to (1) lack of ovum availability due to anovulation and failure of ova to enter the fallopian tube, that is, ovum recovery; or (2) nonfertilizability of the ovum.

Ovum Availability. The first delimiting step in human conception is ovum entry into the oviduct. Anovulation among young, fertile women is relatively uncommon, but not absent. Most investigators agree that, on occasion, all women experience an anovulatory cycle. This has been estimated to occur as often as once a year or about once in 13 cycles. This estimate seems a bit too high. In a study designed to evaluate early pregnancy wastage, Edmonds and colleagues (1982) found that only 9 of 207 cycles (4.3 percent) seemed to be anovulatory. In some cases, failure of ovulation may be associated with a luteinized follicle or "trapped ovum." Indeed, this may be one cause of the so-called short luteal phase.

There are inadequate data available to estimate the frequency of failure of the released ovum to enter the fallopian tube. Based on the findings of some studies involving the likelihood of transuterine migration of fertilized ova, however, this situation must exist. But in normal women, it probably is uncommon.

For these reasons, in about 95 percent of ovarian cycles of young, fertile women, an ovum actually will enter the fallopian tube; or conversely, in only 5 percent of cycles, there is no ovum to fertilize (Fig. 31–1). Therefore, in 1000 menstrual cycles in healthy, fertile, young women, 950 ova should be available for fertilization.

Fertilizable Ova. The second delimiting step in female fertility efficiency is the fertilizability of the ovum. There must be some number, albeit probably small, of ova that cannot be fertilized even by a normal spermatozoa. To make this estimate, it is assumed that fertilization in vivo is at least as likely as that which can be attained in vitro. Therefore, the number of nonfertilizable ova is small, perhaps about 7 to 8 percent of those that enter the fallopian tube.

Hence of 1000 ovarian cycles in young, fertile women, the maximum number of ova that could be fertilized would be 879, for a female fertility efficiency of 88 percent. Stated conversely, minimal female fertility inefficiency is about 12 percent (Fig. 31–1). These estimates are similar to those made by Hertig and associates (1959) based on a study of the presence of a conceptus in the uteruses removed from women during the luteal phase of the ovarian cycle.

Fecundability

Natural Fecundability. It is convenient to analyze the likelihood of pregnancy success (living newborn) per ovarian cycle (fecundability). One approach to such an estimate is to evaluate the number of living newborns that can be expected per ovarian cycle in young, healthy women desirous of pregnancy. This has been done in a number of studies, as reviewed by Short (1976). The results are expressed as the fecundability rate. This value is referred to here as the **natural fecundability rate,** because during some cycles, fertilization was precluded because of the absence of viable spermatozoa in the fallopian tube at the time of ovulation. In addition, absolute or relative infertility of the population under study may limit maximal natural fecundability. Nonetheless, the data available are very useful. In these studies, embryonic or fetal losses occurring at any time from conception are not considered; only living births are included in estimates of fecundability.

In rural French villages during the 18th century, the mean fecundability of women aged 20 to 29 was 23 percent. Several other studies have been conducted to ascertain how long it takes for a newlywed woman to conceive a pregnancy that results in a living newborn. In a study of 15,000 women who were contestants in a large-family competition in France after World War I, the peak in fecundability (27 percent) was observed in women at age 25. Similar values were obtained in studies of North American Hutterites believed to be reproducing at close to the maximum natural rate. The mean postnuptial fecundability in these women was 28 percent.

In other studies, Tietze and Potter (1962) calculated the probability of pregnancy in a given ovarian cycle as a function of different frequencies of intercourse. Their estimates ranged from a minimum probability of 28 percent at a coital frequency of 6 times per cycle to a maximum of 45 percent at a coital frequency of 12 times per cycle. Similar estimates were made by Lachenbruch (1967).

If it is assumed that absolute infertility affects 10 percent of married couples, and that relative infertility affects another 15 percent, it is obvious that even the estimates of 45 percent maximum natural fecundability are underestimates of the theoretical maximal fecundability in fertile women. Taking the 28 percent natural fecundability rate that is found most commonly in young, healthy women and correcting for absolute infertility (10 percent), the natural fecundability rate among fertile women is 31 percent. But this value is not corrected for (1) relative infertility or (2) absence of spermatozoa in the fallopian tube at the time of ovulation. Correcting for relative infertility (assuming 15 percent), natural fecundability in fertile women becomes 37 percent. Even in Hutterite women with a 28 percent fecundability and an average of 10.6 children, 33 percent have three or fewer offspring. Eliminating this group of relatively infertile Hutterite women may give rise to greater than 40 percent natural fecundability in this group.

Hertig and colleagues (1959) estimated fecundability as 43 percent in a group of presumably fertile women who were somewhat older, on average (33 years), than those women believed to be maximally fertile. And even in women of the studies of Hertig and co-workers, intercourse may have occurred only on the day after ovulation, a time unlikely to result in optimal rates of conception. Thus, the presence of spermatozoa in the fallopian tube at the time of ovulation is crucial in computing fecundability.

This same limitation exists for estimates of the corrected natural fecundability rate of 37 percent. These estimates were made from the findings of studies in which the number of ovulations were unknown that occurred when viable spermatozoa were not present in the fallopian tube. Even in couples for whom intercourse is frequent, spermatozoa will not always be present at the critical time. Moreover, frequent intercourse for several days prior to the 36 hours preceding ovulation will no doubt limit sperm supplies. A conservative estimate, we believe, is that spermatozoa are present in the fallopian tube at the time of 3 of 5 ovulations in the general population of young, fertile women desirous of pregnancy.

Therefore, theoretical maximal fecundability in young, fertile women is about 60 percent (37 percent divided by 0.6). Stated differently, of 1000 menstrual cycles in young, healthy, fertile women, 617 liveborn infants should result if viable spermatozoa were present in the fallopian tube at the time of ovum entry into the oviduct.

This estimate is also consistent with the probability that sperm regeneration time (42 to 48 hours) is about twice as long as is the fertilizable life span of the spermatozoa in the female reproductive tract (24 hours). Sperm motility likely persists longer than fertilizing capacity. Therefore, natural fecundability in a population of young, healthy, fertile women desirous of pregnancy (28 to 30 percent) is about one half the theoretical maximum fecundability in similar women if spermatozoa were not limiting.

Source of Pregnancy Losses. Defining pregnancy as commencing at the time of implantation, pregnancy wastage can take place at any time after implantation of the blastocyst. First, fetal loss may occur after the time of expected viability for reasons of preterm labor, fetal anomalies, and intrauterine or neonatal death. Second, spontaneous abortion may occur, usually within the first trimester of pregnancy. Third, the products of conception may be sloughed before or at about the time of the

next anticipated menstruation. In such cases, the pregnancy is not clinically recognized.

Late Pregnancy Wastage: Perinatal Mortality. A perinatal mortality rate of 10 per 1000 births, or 1 percent has been assumed in this model.

Early Clinical Pregnancy Wastage: Spontaneous First-trimester Abortion. An abortion rate of 10 percent has been assumed. The rate of spontaneous clinical abortion in young, healthy, fertile women is probably low compared with the rate of abortion in the general population of women.

Early Preclinical Loss of Conceptus

PREIMPLANTATION. Some number, albeit not precisely defined, of human conceptuses are lost early after fertilization. Some fertilized ova never undergo cleavage; and blastocysts may never implant. This naturally gives rise to fundamental inquiries as to the development and maturation of the ova as well as the genetics and environment of the zygote. It is becoming clear that **one of the limiting steps in the success of fertility is the quality of the fertilized ovum.**

EARLY POSTIMPLANTATION (PRECLINICAL) EMBRYONIC LOSS. After implantation, blastocysts may be lost before or at about the time of the next anticipated menstruation. Early embryonic wastage has also been referred to as *occult pregnancy,* because these losses are not interpreted as a pregnancy episode.

Recognizing that chorionic gonadotropin (hCG) begins to enter the maternal circulation on the day of implantation, several studies have been conducted to evaluate early pregnancy wastage by monitoring its levels in blood or urine of women during the luteal phase of the ovarian cycle. The detection of chorionic gonadotropin has been cited as evidence of "chemical" pregnancy. Other investigators have conducted similar investigations by use of other pregnancy-specific proteins, such as early pregnancy factor (EPF), which may also serve to identify the presence of a fertilized ovum before implantation.

In a prospective study of 226 ovulatory cycles in 91 healthy young women, Whittaker and associates (1983) detected chemical evidence (β-hCG in serum) of pregnancy in 92 cycles. Of these, 74 (80 percent) ended in the delivery of normal, living babies. In the model presented in Figure 31–1, 77 percent would have been predicted. About 12 percent terminated in spontaneous clinical abortion. In the model presented (Fig. 31–1), 8.6 percent would have been predicted. In 8 percent of cycles, chemical evidence of pregnancy was obtained, but these ended with apparently normal menstruation. In the model presented, 14 percent preclinical pregnancy losses would have been predicted. The criticism of the study of Whittaker and colleagues has been that β-hCG levels were determined only at weekly intervals and thus some early postimplantation embryo losses may have been missed.

In other studies, appreciably higher percentages of preclinical pregnancy wastage were observed. For example, Miller and associates (1980), in a study of β-hCG levels in urine during the luteal phase of the cycle, estimated a preclinical, postimplantation pregnancy loss of 33 percent. They concluded that a small portion of their population sample was relatively infertile.

In the classical morphological study of Hertig and colleagues (1959), they concluded that 10 of 34 embryos (29 percent) found in the fallopian tube or uterus would have aborted at some time, before or after the next menses. In the model presented in Figure 31–1, the postconception pregnancy loss predicted is 31 percent. Chartier and co-workers (1979) found a 21 percent postimplantation, preclinical pregnancy loss in infertile women, at least one third of whom were treated to induce ovulation and at least 10 percent of whom were pregnant with multiple fetuses.

In a prospective, pilot study of recruited volunteers, Sweeney and associates (1988) found that early pregnancy loss (1 to 91 days after implantation) was 18 percent. The model (Fig. 31–1) predicts 22 percent. Wilcox and associates (1988), in a study of 221 healthy women attempting to conceive, found a 22 percent postimplantation preclinical pregnancy wastage and a total (including spontaneous abortion) of 31 percent. In other studies, appreciably higher early embryonic losses were estimated. For example, Edmonds and co-workers (1982) presented evidence for total postimplantation loss of 62 percent based on the finding of β-hCG in urine samples of 82 women attempting to conceive.

Predictions of Pregnancy Outcome in Young, Healthy, Fertile Women.

The data presented and the computations made were evaluated and collated into the flowchart presented in Figure 31–1 to estimate the likelihood of pregnancy outcome in young women. It is important to emphasize that these predictions are based on the health, youth, and fertility of the women and upon the supposition that spermatozoa are present in the fallopian tube at the time of ovulation.

Conception. Based on these assumptions, fertilization of the human ovum occurs in 88 percent of the menstrual cycles of fertile, young women.

Postconceptional, Preclinical Embryo Loss. The fate of the 879 fertilized ova (of 1000 cycles) will be as follows: 206 (23 percent) will be lost, either as a consequence of failure of cleavage or failure of implantation or else by abortion before or at the time of the next expected menstruation. This estimate is appreciably lower than that produced in many different studies. One half of these losses were arbitrarily assigned to preimplantation failure and one half to postimplantation failure. It is likely that this arbitrary assignment is incorrect and that a greater proportion should be allocated to one category compared with the other. As yet, there are no data that permit a more rational assignment.

There is no doubt that the low estimate of postconception loss is caused by estimates of high fecundability among young, healthy, fertile women. On the other hand, it is probable that high estimates of early pregnancy wastage are derived from data assembled from studies of relatively infertile women. No doubt, high embryonic and fetal wastage contributes to absolute or relative infertility.

Clinical Pregnancy. Of 1000 cycles in young, healthy, fertile women, 673 clinically discernible pregnancies are predicted with an incidence of spontaneous clinical abortion of 10 percent and a perinatal mortality of 1 percent. Clinical evidence supports this conclusion. For example, once a pregnancy is recognized clinically, outcome is usually good. Indeed, Simpson and associates (1987) reported that in women with a sonographically confirmed live fetus at 8 weeks' gestation, subsequent fetal loss was only 3.2 percent. Similar clinical observations have been reported by Stabile and colleagues (1987) and Mackenzie and co-workers (1988).

Summary and Conclusions. The important features of the estimates presented by way of the diagram in Figure 31–1 are that the optimal fecundability in young, healthy, fertile women may be twice that observed in a general population of women of the same age who are desirous of pregnancy. Intercourse may occur frequently; but there is no doubt that viable spermatozoa are not in the fallopian tubes of all women at every ovulation time. Furthermore, there is no doubt that in a general population of young women, absolute and relative infertility affects a sizable number of couples.

SPONTANEOUS ABORTION

Definition. *Abortion* is the termination of pregnancy by any means before the fetus is sufficiently developed to survive. When abortion occurs spontaneously, the term *miscarriage* has been applied by laypersons. In the United States this definition is confined to the termination of pregnancy before 20 weeks' gestation based upon the date of the first day of the last normal menses. Another commonly used definition is the delivery of a fetus-neonate that weighs less than 500 g. In some European countries, this definition is less than 1000 g.

Pathology. Hemorrhage into the decidua basalis and necrotic changes in the tissues adjacent to the bleeding usually accompany abortion. The ovum becomes detached in part or whole and, presumably acting as a foreign body in the uterus, stimulates uterine contractions that result in expulsion. When the sac is opened, fluid is commonly found surrounding a small macerated fetus or, alternatively, there may be no visible fetus in the sac, the so-called *blighted ovum.* Visualized through the dissecting microscope, the placental villi often appear thick and distended with fluid, the ends of the villous branches resembling little sausage-shaped sacs. Such fluid-filled villi are undergoing molar degeneration with the imbibition of tissue fluid (see Chap. 35, p. 748).

Blood or carneous mole is an ovum that is surrounded by a capsule of clotted blood. The capsule is of varying thickness, with degenerated chorionic villi scattered through it. The small, fluid-containing cavity within appears compressed and distorted by thick walls of old blood clot. This type of specimen is associated with an abortion that occurs rather slowly, so that blood is allowed to collect between the decidua and chorion and to coagulate and form layers.

In abortions after the fetus has attained considerable size, several outcomes are possible. The retained fetus may undergo *maceration.* In such circumstances, the bones of the skull collapse, the abdomen becomes distended with blood-stained fluid, and the fetus takes on a dull reddish color. At the same time, skin softens and peels off in utero or at the slightest touch, leaving behind the corium. Internal organs degenerate and undergo necrosis, becoming friable and losing their capacity for histological stains. Amnionic fluid may be absorbed when the fetus becomes compressed upon itself and desiccated to form a *fetus compressus.* Occasionally, the fetus eventually becomes so dry and compressed that it resembles parchment, so-called *fetus papyraceous* (see Fig. 39–13, p. 902). This latter outcome is seen in twin pregnancy if one fetus has died at an early period and the other has gone on to full development.

Resumption of Ovulation. Ovulation may occur as early as 2 weeks after an abortion. Lähteenmäki and Luukkainen (1978) detected a surge of luteinizing hormone (LH) 16 to 22 days after abortion in 15 of 18 women studied. Moreover, plasma progesterone level, which had plummeted after the abortion, increased soon after the LH surge. These hormonal events are in temporal agreement with histological changes observed in endometrial biopsies and the rise in basal body temperature after abortion, as described by Boyd and Holmstrom (1972). Therefore, it is important that effective contraception be initiated soon after abortion. The use of various contraceptive techniques following abortion is discussed in Section XIV.

Etiologies of Spontaneous Abortion

More than 80 percent of abortions occur in the first 12 weeks of pregnancy, and the rate decreases rapidly thereafter (Harlap and associates, 1980a). Chromosomal anomalies cause at least half of these early abortions, and steadily and rapidly decrease thereafter (Fig. 31–2). The risk of spontaneous abortion appears to increase with parity as well as with maternal and paternal age (Warburton and Fraser, 1964; Wilson and associates, 1986). The frequency of clinically recognized abortion increases from 12 percent in women less than age 20 to 26 percent in those over age 40. The effect of advancing maternal age is illustrated in Figure 31–3. For the same paternal ages, the increase is from 12 to 20 percent. Finally, the incidence of abortion is increased if a woman conceives within 3 months of a live birth (Harlap and associates, 1980b).

The exact mechanisms responsible for abortion are not always apparent, but in the very early months of pregnancy, spontaneous expulsion of the ovum is nearly always preceded by death of the embryo or fetus. For this reason, etiological considerations of early abortion involve ascertaining whenever possible the cause of fetal death. In the subsequent months, the fetus frequently does not die in utero before expulsion and other explanations for its expulsion must be invoked. Fetal death may be caused by abnormalities in the ovum-zygote or by systemic disease of the mother, and, rarely perhaps, of the father.

Fetal Factors

Abnormal Zygote Development. The most common morphological finding in early spontaneous abortions is an abnormality of development of the zygote, embryo,

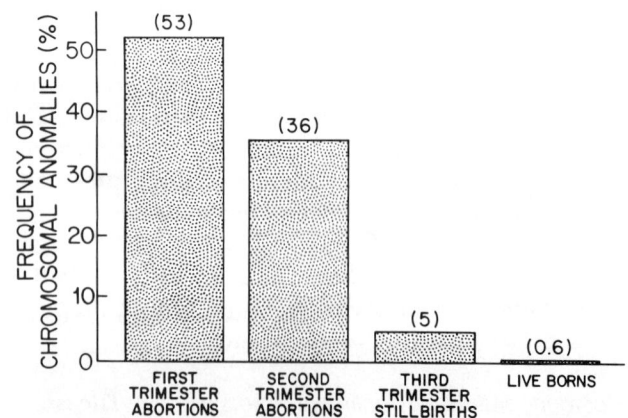

Fig. 31–2. Frequency of chromosomal anomalies in abortuses and stillbirths for each trimester compared with the frequency of chromosomal anomalies in live-born infants. The percentage for each group is shown in parentheses. (Data adapted from Warburton, 1980 and Fantel, 1980.)

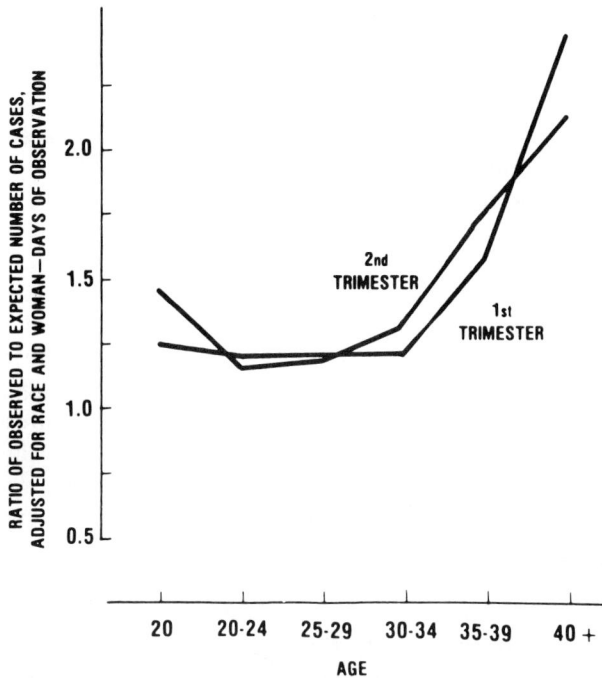

Fig. 31–3. First and second trimester spontaneous abortions by maternal age. (From Harlap and colleagues, 1980b, with permission.)

early fetus, or at times the placenta. In an analysis of 1000 spontaneous abortions, Hertig and Sheldon (1943) observed pathological ("blighted") ova in which the embryo was degenerated or absent in half (Fig. 31–4).

Poland and co-workers (1981) morphologically identified disorganization of growth in 40 percent of abortuses (both embryos and fetuses) that were ex-

pelled spontaneously before 20 weeks. Among embryos less than 30 mm crown to rump length, the frequency of abnormal morphological development was 70 percent. Of the embryos on which tissue culture and chromosomal analyses were performed, 60 percent had chromosomal abnormalities. For fetuses 30 to 180 mm crown to rump length, the frequency of chromosomal abnormalities was 25 percent.

Abnormal fetal development, especially in the first trimester, may be classified into that with an abnormal number of chromosomes (**aneuploidy**) or development with a normal chromosomal component (**euploidy**).

Aneuploid Abortion. Chromosomal abnormalities are common among embryos and early fetuses that are aborted spontaneously, and account for much or most of early pregnancy wastage. Approximately 50 to 60 percent of early spontaneous abortions are associated with a chromosomal anomaly of the conceptus (Table 31–1). Jacobs and Hassold (1980) reported that approximately one fourth of the chromosomal abnormalities were due to maternal gametogenesis errors and 5 percent paternal. Less than 10 percent were due to errors in fertilization and zygote divisions.

Autosomal trisomy is the most frequently identified chromosomal anomaly associated with first-trimester abortions (Table 31–1). It can be the result of an isolated nondisjunction, maternal or paternal **balanced translocation,** or balanced chromosomal inversion (Chap. 40, p. 923). Translocations may be identified in either parent and appropriate prenatal diagnostic procedures initiated

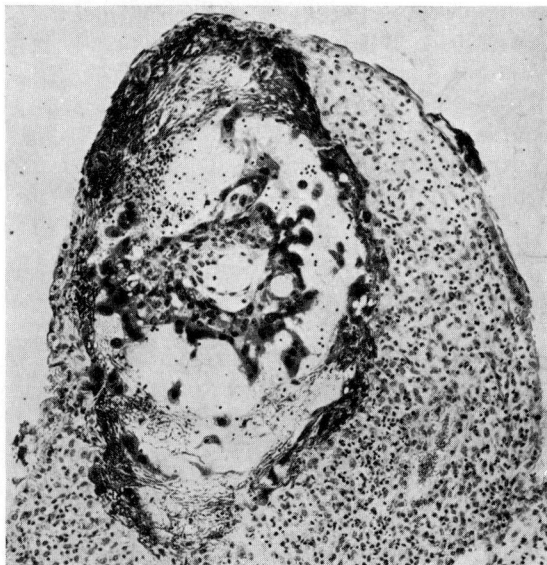

Fig. 31–4. Abnormal ovum. A cross section of a defective ovum showing an empty chorionic sac embedded within a polypoid mass of endometrium. (From Hertig and Rock, 1944.)

TABLE 31–1. CHROMOSOMAL FINDINGS IN HUMAN ABORTUSES

	Percent	
Chromosomal Studies	*Kajii and Associates (1980)*	*Simpson (1986)*
Normal (euploid), 46XY and 46XX	46	54
Abnormal (aneuploid)		
Autosomal trisomy	31	22
Monosomy X (45,X)	10	9
Triploidy	7	8
Tetraploidy	2	3
Structural anomaly	3	2
Double trisomy	2	0.7
Triple trisomy	0.4	NL
Others-XXY, monosomy 21	0.8	NL
Autosomal monosomy G	NL	0.1
Mosaic trisomy	NL	1.3
Sex chromosome polysomy	NL	0.2
Abnormality not specified	NL	0.9

NL = not listed.
From Kajii and associates (1980) and Simpson (1986).

in subsequent pregnancies to identify abnormal fetuses that may be aborted to prevent delivery of an abnormal infant. **Balanced chromosomal inversions** may also be identified in couples with recurrent abortions.

Trisomies for all autosomes except chromosome number 1 have been identified in tissue from abortuses, but autosomes 13, 16, 18, 21, and 22 are most common. These latter trisomies have been reported in live births, but many others have been reported in stillborns. Advancing maternal age is associated with an increased incidence of these defects, especially D and G group trisomies, and chorionic villus sampling or amniocentesis is indicated for prenatal diagnosis in women past 35 years of age (Chap. 41, p. 946).

Monosomy X (45,X) is the next most common chromosomal abnormality and is compatible with live-born (Turner syndrome) females who often thrive. It is not clear why some fetuses abort, but in those that do, there appear to be increased renal abnormalities. For reasons that also are not apparent, Turner syndrome is associated with a younger maternal age.

Triploidy is often associated with hydropic placental degeneration. Incomplete hydatidiform moles may have fetal development that is triploid or trisomic for chromosome number 16 (see Chap. 35, p. 749). The incomplete or partial hydatidiform mole is usually not malignant. Fetuses associated with these frequently abort early, and the few carried longer are all grossly malformed. Triploidy may be caused by (1) dispermy, which is likely the most common mechanism in the human; (2) failure in sperm meiosis resulting in a diploid sperm; or (3) failure in egg meiosis in which either the first or second polar body is retained. Interestingly, advanced maternal and paternal age do not appear to be associated with this abnormality.

Tetraploid abortuses are rarely live born and are most often aborted very early in gestation, so little morphological information is available.

Chromosomal structural abnormalities are unusual causes of abortion and have been identified only since the development of banding techniques. Some of these infants are live born with balanced translocations and can be normal. This is analogous in many respects to what is observed in 45,X fetuses.

Autosomal monosomy is extremely rare and is incompatible with life.

Sex chromosomal polysomy (47,XXX or 47,XXY) is unusual in abortus material but is commonly seen in live births. The 47,XXY variety is termed Kleinefelter syndrome and the 47,XXX variety is termed the *super female*. Both have well-described phenotypic and mental profiles.

Euploid Abortion. Chromosomally normal abortuses are usually lost later in gestation. Kajii and co-workers (1980) reported that three fourths of aneuploid abortions occurred at or before 8 weeks, while euploid abortions peaked at about 13 weeks. Stein and associates

(1980) presented evidence that the incidence of euploid abortions increases dramatically after a maternal age of 35 years. The reasons for this are unknown. In fact, the reason(s) for euploid abortions generally are unknown, but the following are possibilities: (1) a genetic abnormality such as an isolated mutation or polygenic factors, (2) various maternal factors, and (3) possibly some paternal factors.

An explanation of how an isolated euploid nonstructural genetic mutation or polygenic factors might result in an abortion was provided by Simpson (1980). He observed that approximately 0.5 percent of live-born infants have chromosomal abnormalities, while at least 2 percent of live births have diseases associated with a single-gene mutation or a polygenic mechanism of inheritance. He reasoned that these more common defects could produce abortions by altering various fetal functions or by altering differentiation.

Maternal Factors. Maternal diseases are usually associated with euploid abortion. In some cases an etiology that is amenable to correction may be established. Thus, an etiology should be sought for midtrimester abortions. A variety of medical disorders, mental conditions, and developmental abnormalities have been implicated in euploidic abortion, although the evidence is not convincing in all instances. Nevertheless, a brief discussion of many of these is presented, and emphasis is placed upon therapy in conditions where it has been shown to be efficacious.

Infections. Some chronic infections have either been implicated or are strongly suspected of causing abortion. *Brucella abortus* is a well known cause of chronic abortion in cattle, but it is not a significant cause of human abortion. The evidence that *Toxoplasma gondii* can cause abortion in humans is inconclusive. There is no evidence in humans that *Listeria monocytogenes* can produce abortions (Stray-Pedersen and Stray-Pedersen, 1984). Although *Chlamydia trachomatis* is sexually transmitted and can cause pelvic infection, there is no evidence that it causes subclinical disease that results in abortion (Quinn and associates, 1987). Herpes simplex has been associated with an increased incidence of abortion following genital infection in the first half of pregnancy or if pregnancy occurs within 18 months of a primary genital infection (Nahmias and associates, 1971; Naib and colleagues, 1970). Serological evidence supportive of a role for *Mycoplasma hominis* and *Ureaplasma urealyticum* in the genesis of abortion has been provided by Quinn and co-workers (1983b). They also reported improvement in pregnancy outcome following treatment with erythromycin (1983a). Their success rate of 85 percent is similar to what has been achieved repeatedly with widely varied treatment regimens. *Ureaplasma urealyticum* appears to be the major offender. Stray-Pedersen and associates (1978) demonstrated an increased incidence of positive uterine cultures for this organism in repeat aborters compared with control subjects (28 versus 7 percent). There were no differences in the organisms cultured from the cervix in the repeat aborters compared with control subjects. Treatment of these women and their sexual partners with doxycycline improved subsequent pregnancy outcomes, but a controlled study was not conducted. *Myoplasma hominis* was not demonstrated to be present in the reproductive tract of more women with abortions compared with controls.

Chronic Debilitating Diseases. In early pregnancy, chronic wasting diseases such as tuberculosis or carcinomatosis have seldom caused abortion; instead, the woman often dies undelivered. In later pregnancy, preterm labor may be induced by severe systemic maternal illness. Hypertension is seldom associated with abortion before 20 weeks' gestation, but rather may lead to fetal death and preterm delivery. Maternal diabetes has been found by some, but not others, to predispose to spontaneous abortion (see Chap. 53, p. 1207).

Endocrine Abnormalities

HYPOTHYROIDISM. There does not appear to be an increased incidence of abortion associated with clinical hypothyroidism (Montoro and associates, 1981). Thyroid autoantibodies, however, have been associated with an increased incidence of abortion despite the lack of overt hypothyroidism in these women (Stagnaro-Green and co-workers, 1990). Thus, autoantibodies may be markers and not causes of abortion.

DIABETES MELLITUS. Uncontrolled diabetes mellitus is associated with an increased incidence of abortion, but well-controlled diabetes is not (Sutherland and Pritchard, 1986). Crane and Wahl (1981) reported that with good insulin control both gestational and overt diabetics had the same incidence of abortion compared with matched control groups. In a prospective study, Mills and associates (1988) reported that early insulin control (within 21 days of conception) resulted in a similar spontaneous abortion rate compared with nondiabetic controls. Lack of glucose control, however, resulted in a marked increase in the abortion rate.

PROGESTERONE DEFICIENCY. Insufficient progesterone secretion by the corpus luteum or placenta has been associated with an increased incidence of abortion. Because progesterone maintains the decidua, its deficiency theoretically would interfere with nutrition of the conceptus and thus contribute to its death.

It has been suggested that abnormal levels of one or more hormones might help to forecast abortion or even serve as therapeutic guides. Unfortunately, reduced levels of these hormones are usually the consequence

rather than the cause of irreversible damage to the fetoplacental unit (Salem and co-workers, 1984). There are now well-documented cases of luteal phase defects (Horta and co-workers, 1977), but they appear to be uncommon. The issue of how to make the diagnosis either by serum progesterone measurements or endometrial biopsy, as well as the best therapy with either clomiphene citrate or progesterone, has been reviewed by Lee (1987). Briefly, the diagnosis is established by a midluteal progesterone peak of less than 9 ng/mL or an endometrial biopsy 3 days or more out of synchrony with menstrual dates during two separate menstrual cycles.

Check and co-workers (1987a,b) reported that progesterone administration alone is effective as long as there is ultrasonic evidence of normal follicular maturation and normal estrogen production. As yet, there is no convincing evidence in well-controlled, randomized studies that progesterone therapy is efficacious. Rock (1985), Ressequie (1985), Check (1986), and their co-workers presented evidence that *progesterone* therapy is not associated with increased fetal malformations.

Nutrition. Only very severe malnutrition predisposes to an increased likelihood of abortion. There is no conclusive evidence, however, that dietary deficiency of any one nutrient or moderate deficiency of all nutrients is an important cause of abortion. The nausea and vomiting that develop rather commonly during early pregnancy, and any inanition so induced, are rarely followed by spontaneous abortion. Most micronutrients have been reported at one time or another to have been of value in reducing the risk of spontaneous abortion. Evidence presented in support of such claims, however, has been weak to nonexistent.

Recreational Drugs and Environmental Factors. A variety of different agents has been reported to be associated with an increased incidence of abortion. As adequate information is gained, not all reports have been confirmed.

TOBACCO. Smoking has been associated with an increased risk of euploidic abortion (Armstrong and associates, 1992; Harlap and Shiono, 1980a). For women who smoked more than 14 cigarettes a day, the risk was approximately two times greater compared with controls and was independent of maternal age and alcohol ingestion (Kline and associates, 1980b). Armstrong and associates (1992) calculated that abortion risk increased in a linear fashion by a factor of 1.2 for each 10 cigarettes per day!

ALCOHOL. Spontaneous euploidic abortion was increased even when alcohol was consumed "in moderation" (Armstrong and associates, 1992; Harlap and Shiano, 1980a). Kline and co-workers (1980a,b) reported that the abortion rate was doubled in women drinking twice weekly and tripled in women who consumed alcohol daily compared with nondrinkers. Armstrong and colleagues (1992) computed that abortion increased by an average 1.3 for each drink per day. Although this increase was less than reported by Harlap and Shiano (1980a) and by Kline and co-workers (1980a), the results were significant. Increased euploidic abortion is strong evidence that both tobacco and alcohol are embryotoxins.

CAFFEINE. Coffee consumption greater than 4 cups of coffee per day appears to increase the risk of abortion slightly (Armstrong and associates, 1992). The risk also appears to increase with increasing amounts.

RADIATION. In sufficient doses, radiation is a recognized abortifacient. The human dose is not precisely known, but a minimum lethal dose on the day of implantation is believed to be about 5 rad (see Chap. 43, p. 982).

CONTRACEPTIVES. Oral steroidal contraceptives are alleged to be associated with an increased incidence of abortion; however, there is no evidence to support this (see Chap. 60, p. 1332). This is also true for oral contraceptives and spermicidal agents used in contraceptive creams and jellies (see Chap. 61, p. 1349). Intrauterine devices, however, are associated with an increased incidence of septic abortion after contraceptive failure (Chap. 61, p. 1344).

ENVIRONMENTAL TOXINS. *Anesthetic gases* have been implicated as causative agents of spontaneous abortion (see Chap. 16, p. 428). In some studies (Axelsson and associates, 1982), abortion rates in exposed women were *not* increased. In most instances, there is little valid information to indict any specific agent; however, there is good evidence that *arsenic, lead, formaldehyde, benzene,* and *ethylene oxide* may cause abortion (Barlow and Sullivan, 1982). *Video display terminals* and exposure to the accompanying electromagnetic fields do not increase the risk of abortion (Schnorr and co-workers, 1991). *Shortwaves* and *ultrasound* do not increase the risk of abortion in physiotherapists who are exposed to these physical forces (Taskinen and colleagues, 1990).

Immunological Factors

AUTOIMMUNE MECHANISMS. Autoimmune mechanisms are those by which a cellular or humoral response is directed against a specific site within the host. Connective-tissue disorders such as lupus erythematosus are associated with increased abortion and fetal death (Chap. 54, p. 1229).

Antiphospholipid antibodies, including the lupus anticoagulant and anticardiolipin antibodies, are examples of autoimmune disease that can cause recurrent abortion. These antibodies are directed against platelets and vascular endothelium and cause vascular damage, thrombosis, placental destruction, abortion, and fetal morbidity and death (Fig. 31–5). Antiphospholipid antibodies are IgG and IgM immunoglobulins. In most cases, only IgG antibodies are of clinical significance, but in high titers, IgM antibodies may cause disease. Because these antibodies are directed against glycerophospolipids, all of the phospholipid-dependent clotting tests are prolonged. For example, the *lupus anticoagulant* is most often identified by a prolonged activated partial thromboplastin time (APTT) that is not corrected by addition of normal plasma. The diagnosis is then confirmed if there is an abnormal tissue thromboplastin-inhibition test, platelet neutralization test, or dilute Russel viper venom time (dRVVT) (Ferro and co-workers, 1990; Gant, 1986).

The sensitivity of the activated partial thromboplastin time is impaired during pregnancy. Coagulation factors (fibrinogen, factors VIII, VII, X, and von Willebrand factors) are increased during normal pregnancy, and these may shorten the clotting time. Thus, the lupus anticoagulant may be masked by pregnancy. The dilute Russel viper venom time is confirmatory because the venom activates factor X and bypasses the extrinsic pathway (factor VII) and the intrinsic pathway (factor VIII). Pregnancy has no effect on this test.

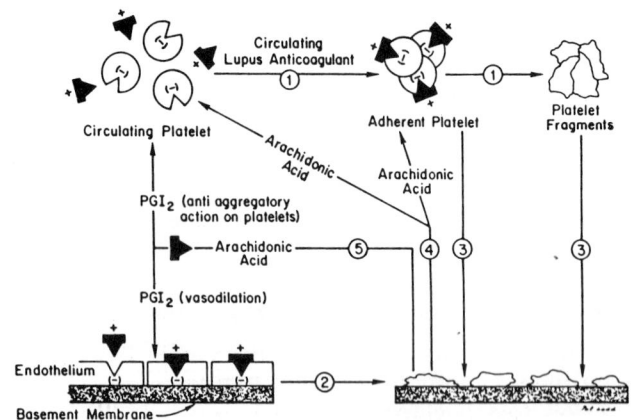

Fig. 31–5. Possible mechanism of thrombosis due to antiphospholipid antibodies: ① After exposure of the negatively charged platelet glycerophospholipid to the lupus anticoagulant, or anticardiolipin antibody, platelets may adhere into clumps and/or be destroyed and thus liberate thromboxanes. ② The antibodies directly damage endothelial cells, resulting in exposure of basement membrane. ③ Adherent and damaged platelets adhere to exposed basement membrane. ④ Damage to endothelial cells by the antibodies results in liberation of arachidonic acid, which increases platelet fragility. ⑤ Damage to the endothelial cells by antibodies results in liberation of arachidonic acid, which is converted to prostacyclin (PGI₂) unless blocked by antibodies, which then results in excess thromboxane, decreased prostacyclin, and vasospasm.

Anticardiolipin antibody is usually identified and titered as IgG or IgM by specific solid-phase or enzyme-linked immunoassays (Gant, 1986). The presence of a prolonged phospholipid-dependent clotting test is usually enough to make the diagnosis of the lupus anticoagulant if there is a history of recurrent abortion, fetal loss, or thromboembolic episodes. The diagnosis of the anticardiolipin antibody requires a similar history and a high titer of the specific IgG or IgM antibody.

Abortion and fetal wastage are more likely in women with antiphospholipid antibodies. Moreover, there is an overlap in the diagnosis of both antibodies and connective-tissue diseases (see Chap. 54, p. 1234) (Parke, 1989). Deleze and colleagues (1989) found that 80 percent of women with recurrent fetal loss and systemic lupus erythematosus had antiphospholipid antibodies compared with 15 percent of women who had systemic lupus erythematosus but no antiphospholipid antibodies. Infante-Rivard and colleagues (1991) emphasize that even when identified, antiphospholipid antibodies are not always the cause of spontaneous abortion or fetal loss. Conversely, Balasch and associates (1990) recommend routine screening in cases of recurrent abortion or fetal loss, and this is our practice.

Successful pregnancies have been achieved in a high percentage of these women using low-dose aspirin to inhibit thromboxane production by damaged platelets and endothelium. Low-dose aspirin allegedly does not inhibit prostacyclin production. Although low-dose aspirin has been used alone, most often heparin and/or high-dose corticosteroids are added. Heparin is given to inhibit thrombosis and corticosteroids to suppress antiphospholipid antibodies as well as inhibit their action on target antigens. More recently, immunoglobulin therapy has been used alone or as an adjunct to the previously mentioned drugs. A recent prospective, randomized, clinical trial was conducted to compare the efficiency of low-dose aspirin (80 mg per day) and low-dose heparin (10,000 units subcutaneously every 12 hours) with low-dose aspirin and prednisone 40 mg per day (Cowchock and associates, 1992). Women receiving the low-dose aspirin and heparin therapy had more live births and fewer preterm deliveries. The successes reported in women with recurrent abortions and fetal loss are indicative that other treatment regimens likely are successful (Balasch and co-workers, 1991; Branch and associates, 1985; Gant, 1986; Lockshin and co-workers, 1989; Lubbe and Liggins, 1985; Rosove and associates, 1990; Schiff and colleagues, 1989).

ALLOIMMUNE MECHANISMS. *Allogeneity* is used to describe genetic dissimilarities between animals of the same species. The human fetus is an allogenic transplant that is tolerated by the mother for reasons that are incompletely understood; however, several immunological mechanisms are reported to prevent fetal rejection.

These mechanisms include, but are not limited to, histocompatibility factors, circulating blocking factors, local suppressor factors, and maternal or antipaternal antileukocytotoxic antibodies (Scott and associates, 1987).

(1) *Histocompatibility locus antigens (HLA):* There is strong circumstantial evidence that maternal–fetal *histoincompatibility* is essential to successful human pregnancy, and that if mother and fetus are "too compatible," reproduction failure develops. In some cases of recurrent abortion, there is an increased sharing of maternal and paternal HLA sites. An association has been noted for A and B loci, but the strongest association is between the HLA-DR locus (Thomas and associates, 1985) and the HLA-DQ locus (Coulam and co-workers, 1987). Thomas and associates (1985) and Houwert-de Jong and colleagues (1989) believe, however, that the defect resulting in abortion might not be the consequence of a *too-similar immunological response,* but rather a genetic result from the sharing of alleles between husband and wife of recessive lethal genes near or linked to the HLA locus on chromosome 6.

Coulam and associates (1987) believe that the failure of Caudle and associates (1983) and Oksenberg and co-workers (1984) to document the HLA-DR and HLA-DQ similarities between couples is due to a small sample size and the fact that these investigators did not classify recurrent aborters into primary and secondary cases. The association between sharing the two HLA loci DQ and DR is greatest in couples with recurrent abortions who have no living children. This concept does not exclude the possibility of a lethal recessive gene near the HLA site being shared by both husband and wife.

(2) *Blocking antibodies:* Maternal blocking antibodies to paternal antigens appear to be essential to the maintenance of normal pregnancy. Failure to synthesize blocking antibodies that protect the fetus from her own antibodies directed against paternal antigens shared by the fetus might result in abortion. Blocking antibodies are apparently of immunoglobulin G origin and may act in several ways: (1) by being directed against maternal lymphocytes to prevent them from reacting with receptors in fetal tissue, (2) by reacting with antigen-specific receptors on the fetal allograft and thereby blocking recognition of the foreign antigens by maternal lymphocytes, or (3) anti-idiotypic blocking antibodies could bind to antigen receptors and block maternal lymphocytes from attacking the target fetal cells (Scott and colleagues, 1987).

(3) *Suppressor factors:* Local suppressor factors likely are essential to normal pregnancy and their absence may be involved in the mechanism of recurrent abortion. Suppressor T cells are lymphocytes that produce soluble factors that suppress immune responses. These are present in decidua of normal pregnancies but absent in some abortions (Daya and associates, 1985);

however, there currently is no clinical method of evaluating suppressor cells in the decidua of women with recurrent abortion.

(4) *Antipaternal antibodies:* Maternal antipaternal antileukocytotoxic antibodies increase in early pregnancy and then decrease near term (Taylor and Hancock, 1975). Scott and associates (1987) noted that it may be the failure of the mother to develop these antibodies that results in recurrent abortion. They emphasize, however, that it is unclear whether the absence of these maternal cytotoxic antibodies to paternal human lymphocyte antigens is a significant marker for women with recurrent abortion.

IMMUNOLOGICAL THERAPY. Therapeutic approaches for correction of the abnormal immune responses discussed above are directed at inducing normal maternal immune responses to paternal antigens or paternal HLA antigens inherited by the fetus. Two methods have been tried. In the first, immunizations are made against paternal leukocytes; in the second, third-party donor leukocytes or blood transfusions are used. This last procedure has all the current disadvantages of any blood transfusion, so other antigenic sources have been used, including trophoblastic membrane antigens (McIntyre and Faulk, 1986), frozen donor lymphocytes (Denegri and associates, 1986), and even sperm antigens (Johnson and coworkers, 1986).

Successes claimed for these methods have been questioned because of the lack of proper control subjects. Mowbray and co-workers (1985, 1987), however, used a paternal lymphocyte immunization regimen only in women without cytotoxic antibodies and those without other known causes for recurrent abortion. They reported significantly increased live births in treated versus untreated women. According to Scott and co-workers (1987), over 200 immunized women have been delivered of live infants without a marked increase in fetal abnormalities or pregnancy complications. In their excellent review they stressed that it still is unclear which women are most likely to benefit from immunotherapy, what source of antigen should be chosen for immunization, and how it should be administered. They emphasized that long-term consequences of such therapy are unknown and such studies should be conducted in research centers equipped to answer these questions.

Aging Gametes. The age of both sperm and egg may influence the spontaneous abortion rate. Guerrero and Rojas (1975) noted an increased incidence of abortion relative to successful pregnancies when insemination occurred 4 days before or 3 days after the time of shift in basal body temperature. They concluded, therefore, that aging of the gametes within the female genital tract before fertilization increased the chance of abortion. Dickey and colleagues (1992) reported that in infertility

patients over 35 there was a higher incidence of small amnionic sac syndrome and an increased incidence of euploidic abortion. Whether ovulation induction or in vitro fertilization result in aging of gametes prior to implantation is not known.

Laparotomy. The trauma of laparotomy may occasionally provoke abortion. In general, the nearer the site of surgery is to the pelvic organs, the more likely abortion is to occur. Ovarian cysts and pedunculated myomas may, however, generally be removed during pregnancy without interfering with the gestation. Peritonitis increases the likelihood of abortion.

Physical Trauma. Multiple examples of trauma that failed to interrupt the pregnancy are often forgotten. Only the particular event apparently related temporally to abortion is remembered. Most spontaneous abortions, however, occur some time after death of the embryo or fetus. If abortion were caused by trauma, it would not be a recent accident but an event that had occurred some weeks before the abortion.

Uterine Defects

ACQUIRED UTERINE DEFECTS

1. *Leiomyomas.* These benign uterine tumors may be associated with abortion. Even large and multiple uterine leiomyomas, however, usually do not cause abortion. When associated with abortion, their location is apparently more important than their size. Leiomyomas are discussed extensively in Chapter 22 (p. 533).

2. *Intrauterine adhesions.* Synechiae (Asherman syndrome) are most frequently the result of curettage for an infected or missed abortion or postpartum curettage (Schenker and Margalioth, 1982). It is caused by destruction of large areas of endometrium. This in turn results in amenorrhea and recurrent abortions believed to be due to insufficient endometrium to support implantation. The diagnosis can be made by a hysterosalpingogram that shows characteristic multiple filling defects, but the most accurate and direct diagnosis is made by hysteroscopy. The recommended treatment is lysis of the adhesions via hysteroscopy and placement of an intrauterine contraceptive device to prevent recurrence of synechiae. Continuous high-dose estrogen therapy is also recommended by some for 60 to 90 days. March and Israel (1981) reported a decrease in abortions from more than 80 percent to less than 15 percent with such therapy.

DEVELOPMENTAL UTERINE DEFECTS. These defects are the consequence of abnormal müllerian duct formation or fusion, and may occur spontaneously or be induced by in utero exposure to *diethylstilbestrol* (DES). Although these abnormalities are uncommon, some types are commonly associated with abortions (Barnes and colleagues, 1980; Cousins and co-workers, 1980; Herbst and associates, 1981; Mangan and colleagues, 1982). Müllerian abnormalities and their management are discussed in detail in Chapter 33.

Incompetent Cervix. The term *incompetent cervix* is applied to a discrete obstetrical entity. It is characterized by painless dilatation of the cervix in the second trimester or perhaps early in the third trimester, with prolapse and ballooning of membranes into the vagina, followed by rupture of membranes and expulsion of an immature fetus. Unless effectively treated, this sequence of events tends to repeat in each pregnancy. The presumptive diagnosis usually can be made if a woman has experienced appreciable cervical dilatation and spontaneous rupture of membranes without the usual discomforts of labor.

Attempts at a more precise diagnosis of cervical incompetence have not been successful. Numerous methods have been described in the nonpregnant woman to make the diagnosis, usually by documenting a more widely dilated internal cervical os than is normal. The methods have included hysterography, pull-through techniques of inflated Foley catheter balloons, and acceptance without resistance at the internal os of specifically sized cervical dilators (Ansari and Reynolds, 1987). During pregnancy, attempts have been made to predict premature dilation of the cervix using sonographic techniques with moderate success (Michaels and associates, 1989). The diagnosis, however, remains difficult and is a clinical one based upon specific sonographic criteria during pregnancy (see Chap. 33, p. 722) and a history of carefully observed and recorded events which include painless cervical dilatation and spontaneous rupture of the membranes.

ETIOLOGY. Although the cause of cervical incompetence is obscure, previous trauma to the cervix—especially in the course of dilatation and curettage, conization, cauterization, or amputation—appears to be a factor in many cases. In other instances, abnormal cervical development, including that following exposure to stilbestrol in utero (Chap. 33, p. 728), plays a role.

Cervical dilatation characteristic of this condition seldom becomes prominent before the 16th week, because before that time the products of conception are not sufficiently large to efface and dilate the cervix except when there are uterine contractions. Abortion from cervical incompetence is a distinct entity from spontaneous abortion in the first trimester, because it results from different factors, presents a different clinical picture, and requires different management. Whereas spontaneous abortion in the first trimester is an extremely

common complication of pregnancy, incompetence of the cervix is relatively rare.

TREATMENT. The treatment of cervical incompetence is surgical, consisting of reinforcement of the weak cervix by some type of pursestring suture. It is best performed after the first trimester but before cervical dilatation of 2 to 3 cm is reached. Bleeding, uterine contractions, or ruptured membranes are contraindications to surgery.

PREOPERATIVE EVALUATION. Cerclage should be delayed until after 14 weeks' gestation so that early abortions due to other factors will be completed. There is no general agreement as to how late in pregnancy the procedure should be performed. Certainly, the more advanced the pregnancy, the more likely surgical intervention will stimulate preterm labor or membrane rupture. For these reasons, some prefer bed rest rather than cerclage after midpregnancy. We seldom perform cerclage after 20 weeks, and certainly not after 26 weeks.

Sonography to exclude major fetal anomalies and to confirm a living fetus is mandatory. Cervical cytology should be negative. Obvious cervical infection should be treated, and cultures for gonorrhea, chlamydia, and group B streptococci are recommended. With a positive culture, treatment is given as described in Chapter 59 (p. 1303). For at least a week before and after surgery, there should be no sexual intercourse.

If there is a question as to whether cerclage should be performed, the woman is placed at decreased physical activity. Proscription of sexual intercourse is essential, and frequent cervical examinations should be conducted, preferably weekly, in order to assess cervical effacement and dilation. Some recommend weekly ultrasonic surveillance of the lower uterine cervicovaginal area between 14 and 27 weeks (Michaels and associates, 1989). Unfortunately, rapid effacement and dilation of the cervix can occur even with such precautions (Witter, 1984). Finally, cerclage does not prevent all preterm deliveries, and preterm labor may follow a cerclage as the result of infection or ruptured membranes induced by the procedure.

CERCLAGE PROCEDURES. Three types of operations are commonly used during pregnancy. One is a simple procedure recommended by McDonald (1963) and illustrated in Figure 31–6. The second is the more complicated Shirodkar operation (1955). The third is the modified Shirodkar shown in Figure 31–7 (Caspi and associates, 1990). There is less trauma and blood loss with the McDonald procedure during placement of the suture than with the Shirodkar procedure, but the modified Shirodkar procedure appears to be significantly less difficult to perform and is associated with less blood loss.

Success rates approaching 85 to 90 percent are achieved with both McDonald and the modified Shirod-

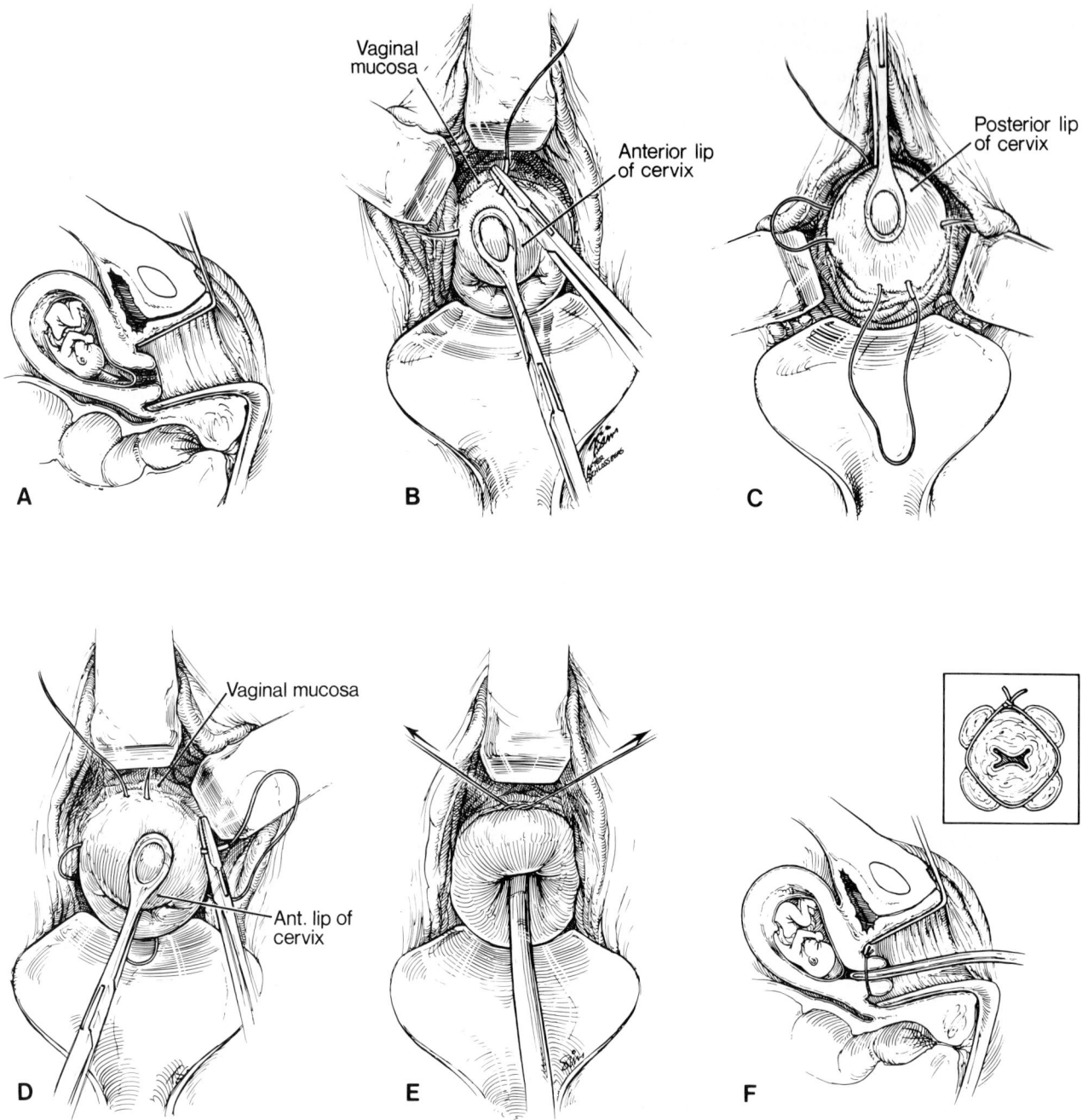

Fig. 31–6. Incompetent cervix treated with McDonald cerclage procedure. **A.** Somewhat dilated cervical canal and beginning prolapse of membranes (*arrow*). **B.** Start of the cerclage procedure with a suture of number 2 monofilament being placed superiorly in the body of the cervix very near the level of the internal os. **C.** Continuation of suture placement in the body of the cervix so as to encircle the os. **D.** Completion of encirclement. **E.** The suture is tightened around the cervical canal sufficiently to reduce the diameter of the canal to 5 to 10 millimeters. In the illustration the *small* dilator has been placed just through the level of ligation to maintain patency of the canal when the suture is tied. A second suture similarly placed but somewhat higher may be of value, especially if the first is not in close proximity to the internal os. **F.** The effect of the suture placement on the cervical canal is apparent.

kar techniques (Caspi and associates, 1990; Kuhn and Pepperell, 1977). Thus, there appears to be little reason for performing the more complicated original Shirodkar procedure. The modified Shirodkar procedure has been reserved for previous McDonald cerclage failures and structural abnormalities of the cervix. Success rates have been higher when cervical dilatation was slight and prolapse of the membranes was minimal to absent. Undoubtedly, some treated cases were not truly cases of cervical incompetence.

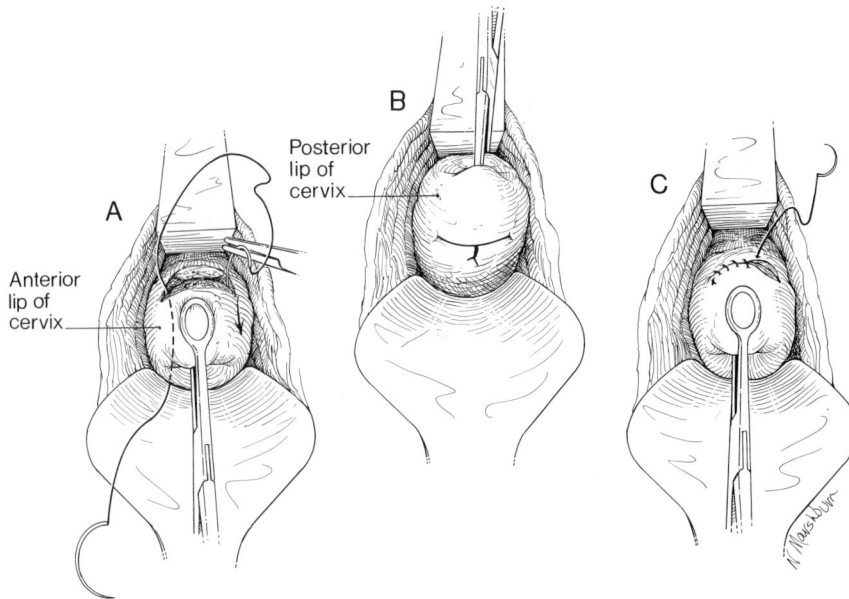

Fig. 31–7. Modified Shirodkar cerclage: **A.** After transverse cervical incision, bladder has been pushed cephalad. Double-needled ligature is passed anteriorly to posteriorly on each side of cervix. **B.** Ligature is tied posteriorly, usually around a 10-mm dilator. **C.** Cervical mucosa is run with chromic suture to bury the anterior pursestring suture.

COMPLICATIONS. Charles and Edward (1981) identified complications, especially infection, to be much less frequent when cerclage was performed by 18 weeks' gestation. When cerclage was performed much after 20 weeks, there was a high incidence of membrane rupture, chorioamnionitis, and intrauterine infection. Any suggestion of infection such as fever, uterine tenderness, or fetal or maternal tachycardia should be investigated. They recommend amniocentesis to substantiate a diagnosis of chorioamnionitis before antibiotic therapy. With clinical infection, the suture should be cut, and labor induced.

There is no good evidence that prophylactic antibiotics prevent infection, or progestational agents or beta-mimetic drugs, are of any adjunctive value (Thomason and co-workers, 1982). In the event that the operation fails and signs of imminent abortion or delivery develop, it is urgent that the suture be released at once, because failure to do so may result in grave sequelae. Rupture of the uterus or the cervix may be the consequence of vigorous uterine contractions with the ligature in place. If the membranes rupture in the absence of labor, the likelihood of serious infection in the fetus or the mother is increased appreciably if the suture is left in situ and delivery is delayed (Kuhn and Pepperell, 1977).

Following the Shirodkar operation, the suture can be left in place if it remains covered by mucosa, and cesarean delivery performed near term (a plan designed to prevent the necessity of repeating the cerclage procedure in subsequent pregnancies). Otherwise, the Shirodkar suture is released and vaginal delivery is permitted.

Treatment of an incompetent cervix by transabdominal cerclage placed at the level of the uterine isthmus has been recommended in some instances, especially in cases of cervical atresia or hypoplasia (Herron and Parer, 1988; Olsen and Tobiassen, 1982). The procedure requires laparotomy for placement of the suture and another laparotomy for its removal or for delivery of the fetus or both. We have had little experience with this operation. Obviously, the potential for trauma and other complications initially and subsequently is much greater with this procedure than with the McDonald or new Shirodkar procedure.

Paternal Factors. Little is known about paternal factors in the genesis of spontaneous abortion. Certainly, chromosome translocations in sperm can lead to a zygote with too little or too much chromosomal material, resulting in abortion.

Categories and Treatment of Spontaneous Abortion

It is convenient to consider the clinical aspects of spontaneous abortion under five subgroups: threatened, inevitable, incomplete, missed, and recurrent abortion. Treatment, when available will be discussed within each category.

Threatened Abortion. Threatened abortion is presumed when any bloody vaginal discharge or vaginal bleeding appears during the first half of pregnancy. Threatened abortion may or may not be accompanied by mild cramping pain resembling that of a menstrual period or by low backache. It is an extremely commonplace occurrence, because one out of four or five pregnant women has vaginal spotting or heavier bleeding during early gestation. Of those women who bleed in early pregnancy, approximately half will abort. The bleeding of threatened abortion frequently is slight, but it may persist for days or weeks. Unfortunately, an increased risk of suboptimal pregnancy outcome in the form of preterm delivery, low birthweight, and perinatal death persists (Batzofin and associates, 1984; Funderburk and colleagues, 1980). Importantly, the risk of a malformed infant does not appear to be increased.

Some bleeding about the time of expected menses may be physiological, analogous to the *placental sign* described by Hartman (1929) in the rhesus monkey, where there is always at least microscopic bleeding. Cervical lesions are likely to bleed in early pregnancy, especially after intercourse. Polyps presenting at the external cervical os as well as decidual reaction in the cervix tend to bleed in early gestation. Lower abdominal pain and persistent low backache do not accompany bleeding from these causes.

Because most physicians consider any bleeding in early pregnancy to be a sign of threatened abortion, any treatment of so-called threatened abortion has a considerable likelihood of success. Most women who actually are threatening to abort progress into the next stage no matter what is done. If, however, bleeding is attributable to one of the unrelated causes mentioned above, it is likely to disappear, regardless of treatment.

A woman should be instructed to notify her physician immediately whenever vaginal bleeding occurs during pregnancy. If bleeding is slight, and no cause is identified through careful inspection of the vagina and cervix, she should be so informed. If an intrauterine device is still present and the "string" is visible, the device should be removed for reasons cited in Chapter 61 (p. 1344).

Usually, bleeding begins first, and cramping abdominal pain follows a few hours to several days later. The pain of abortion may be anterior and clearly rhythmic, simulating mild labor; it may be a persistent low backache, associated with a feeling of pelvic pressure; or it may be a dull, midline, suprasymphyseal discomfort, accompanied by uterine tenderness. Whichever form the pain takes, prognosis for pregnancy continuation in the presence of bleeding and pain is poor. In some women with pain, however, bleeding ceases, pain resolves, and a normal pregnancy results. It is therefore reasonable not to intervene if the woman desires to continue the pregnancy. Little immediate harm should occur, but it is important to remember that higher perinatal mortality rates are observed in women whose pregnancies were complicated early by threatened abortion.

Each woman should be examined thoroughly, for there is always the possibility that the cervix already is dilated and abortion is inevitable, or there is a serious complication such as extrauterine pregnancy or torsion of an unsuspected ovarian cyst. The patient may be kept at home in bed with analgesia given to help relieve the pain, but in general if the symptoms are more severe, she should be hospitalized. If the bleeding persists, she must be reexamined and the hemoglobin concentration or hematocrit rechecked. If blood loss is sufficient to cause anemia, evacuation of the products of conception is generally indicated. If bleeding causes hypovolemia, termination of the pregnancy is mandatory.

Women with threatened abortion have been treated with progesterone intramuscularly or with a wide variety of synthetic progestational agents orally or intramuscularly. Some of the progestins, particularly those structurally related to testosterone, may result in virilization of a female fetus. Of even greater importance is the lack of evidence of effectiveness. "Success" from their use often results in no more than a missed abortion.

Occasionally, slight hemorrhage may persist for weeks. It then becomes essential to decide whether there is any possibility of continuation of the pregnancy. Vaginal sonography, serial serum quantitative chorionic gonadotropin titers (β-hCG), and serum progesterone values measured alone or in various combinations, have proven helpful in ascertaining if a live intrauterine pregnancy is present. Fossum and associates (1988) reported that a fetal sac can usually be seen using vaginal sonography between 33 and 35 days from the last menstrual period (Table 31–2). This was associated with chorionic gonadotropin titer of about 1000 mIU/mL. Thus, if a gestational sac can be seen and quantitative gonadotropin is less than 1000 mIU/mL, the gestation is likely not alive. If any doubt exists, however, gonadotropin levels should be measured. For example, if quantitative measurements do not increase by at least 65 percent every 48 hours, the outlook is almost always hopeless (Kadar and co-workers, 1981). Importantly, a single positive gonadotropin value in blood or urine does not indicate whether the fetus is alive or dead or its location, that is, uterine or extrauterine. Stovall and associates (1989, 1990, 1992) reported that only about 1 percent of abnormal pregnancies (spontaneous incomplete abortions and ectopic pregnancies) have a serum

TABLE 31–2. TEMPORAL VALUES FOR GESTATIONAL AGE, β-hCG LEVELS, AND VAGINAL ULTRASOUND FINDINGS IN NORMAL PREGNANCY

Days from Last Menses	β-hCG mIU/mL (2nd International Standard)	Vaginal Ultrasonography
34.8 ± 2.2[a]	914 ± 106	Fetal sac
40.3 ± 3.4[b]	3783 ± 683	Fetal pole
46.9 ± 6.0[b]	13,178 ± 2898[b]	Fetal heart activity

[a] ± Standard error of the mean.
[b] $P < 0.05$ when compared to fetal sac.
Modified from Fossum and colleagues (1988).

progesterone of 25 ng/mL or greater. They concluded that a serum progesterone value could be used as a screening test for an abnormal pregnancy. A serum progesterone value less than 5 ng/mL was associated with a dead conceptus, but this did not localize the pregnancy (uterine or extrauterine). Hahlin and colleagues (1990) noted that **no live intrauterine pregnancy** had a progesterone less than 10 ng/mL and that 88 percent of ectopic pregnancies and 83 percent of spontaneous abortions had lower values. Therefore, with a fetal sac clearly visible, a quantitative gonadotropin level less than 1000 mIU/mL, and a serum progesterone of less than 5 ng/mL, a live intrauterine pregnancy almost certainly does not exist. Finally, if the uterus, when accurately measured over a period of time, does not increase in size, or becomes smaller, it is safe to conclude that the fetus is dead. An increase in uterine size indicates that the fetus is still alive or that a hydatidiform mole is present (see Chap. 35, p. 748).

Sonographic demonstration of a distinct, well-formed gestational ring with central echoes from the embryo implies that the products of conception are reasonably healthy (Table 31–2). A gestational sac with no central echoes from an embryo or fetus implies strongly, but does not prove, death of the conceptus. When abortion is inevitable, mean gestational sac diameter is frequently smaller than appropriate for gestational age. Moreover, by approximately 45 days after the last menses and thereafter, fetal heart action should be discernible using real-time ultrasound. Most often, a single examination is insufficient to determine the likelihood of abortion. Serial sonographic observations to document lack of fetal growth are useful just as serial measurements of gonadotropin are useful. Recently, Emerson and associates (1992) and Pellerito and colleagues (1992) reported excellent results in identifying live intrauterine gestations using vaginal color and pulsed doppler flow imaging techniques (see Chap. 32, p. 701). After death of the conceptus, the uterus should be emptied. Some women choose abortion before fetal death is certain, rather than face further uncertainty and procrastination.

All tissue passed should be studied carefully to determine whether the abortion is complete as well as to ascertain gross normalcy of the products. Unless all of the fetus and placenta can be positively identified, curettage most often is indicated, and if neither are identified, ectopic pregnancy should be considered.

Women with threatened abortions probably should receive anti-D immunoglobulin. Von Stein and associates (1992) reported that more than 10 percent of their patients had significant fetomaternal hemorrhage (see Chap. 44, p. 1008).

Inevitable Abortion. Inevitability of abortion is signaled by gross rupture of the membranes in the presence of cervical dilatation. Under these conditions, abortion is almost certain. Rarely, a gush of fluid from the uterus occurs during the first half of pregnancy without serious consequence. The fluid may have collected previously between the amnion and chorion, to escape with rupture of the chorion while the initial defect in the amnion has healed completely. Most often, however, either uterine contractions begin promptly, resulting in expulsion of the products of conception, or infection develops.

With obvious gross rupture of the membranes during the first half of pregnancy, the possibility of salvaging the pregnancy is very unlikely. If in early pregnancy the sudden discharge of fluid, suggesting rupture of the membranes, occurs before any pain or bleeding, the woman may be put to bed and observed for further leakage of fluid, bleeding, cramping, or fever. If after 48 hours there has been no further escape of amnionic fluid, no bleeding or pain, and no fever, she may get up and, except for any form of vaginal penetration, continue her usual activities. If, however, the gush of fluid is accompanied or followed by bleeding and pain, or if fever ensues, abortion should be considered inevitable and the uterus emptied.

Incomplete Abortion. The fetus and placenta are likely to be expelled together in abortions occurring before the 10th week, but separately thereafter. When the placenta, in whole or in part, is retained in the uterus, bleeding ensues sooner or later, to produce the main sign of incomplete abortion. With abortions that are more advanced, bleeding is often profuse and occasionally may be massive to the point of producing profound hypovolemia. If the placenta is partly attached and partly separated, the splint-like action of the attached portion of the placenta interferes with myometrial contraction in the immediate vicinity. Vessels in the denuded segment of the placental site, deprived of the constriction provided by myometrial contractions, bleed profusely.

In instances of incomplete abortion, it is often unnecessary to dilate the cervix before curettage. In many cases, the retained placental tissue simply lies loose in the cervical canal and can be lifted from an exposed external os with ovum or ring forceps. Suction curettage, as described below, is effective for evacuating the uterus, especially if the procedure is to be performed only with local cervical and systemic analgesia. A woman with a more advanced pregnancy or a woman who is bleeding heavily should be hospitalized, and the retained tissue removed without delay. Hemorrhage from incomplete abortion is occasionally severe but rarely fatal. Treatment of obstetrical hemorrhage is described in Chapter 37 (p. 821). Fever is not a contraindication to curettage once appropriate antibiotic treatment has been started (see Septic Abortion, p. 686).

Missed Abortion. A missed abortion is defined as retention of dead products of conception in utero for several weeks. The rationale for an exact time period is not clear, and it serves no useful clinical purpose. In the typical instance, early pregnancy appears to be normal, with amenorrhea, nausea and vomiting, breast changes, and growth of the uterus. After fetal death, there may or may not be vaginal bleeding or other symptoms denoting a threatened abortion. For a time, the uterus seems to remain stationary in size, but mammary changes usually regress. The woman is likely to lose a few pounds. Thereafter, it becomes apparent that the uterus not only has ceased to enlarge but also has become smaller. Many women have no symptoms during this period except persistent amenorrhea. If the missed abortion terminates spontaneously, and most do, the process of expulsion is the same as in any abortion. The product, if retained several weeks after death, is a shriveled sac containing a macerated fetus (Fig. 31–8).

Occasionally, after prolonged retention of the dead products of conception, serious coagulation defects develop. This was more likely when the gestation had reached the second trimester before fetal death. The woman may note troublesome bleeding from the nose or gums and especially from sites of slight trauma. The pathogenesis and treatment of coagulation defects and any attendant hemorrhage in instances of prolonged retention of a dead fetus are considered in Chapter 37 (p. 841).

The reason some abortions do not terminate after fetal death, while others do, is not clear. The use of potent progestational compounds to treat threatened abortion, however, may contribute to a missed abortion. For example, Piver and colleagues (1967) treated 57 women for threatened abortion with injectable medroxyprogesterone acetate, following which more than one

third had a retained dead fetus for more than 8 weeks. Smith and co-workers (1978) observed that 73 percent of women who were given hormonal treatment because they threatened to abort did abort, but on the average 20 days later, whereas 67 percent of those who received no hormonal support aborted on the average 5 days later. They concluded that progestational agents did not improve outcome in threatened abortion, but instead delayed the inevitable.

Recurrent Spontaneous Abortion. Recurrent spontaneous abortion has been defined by various criteria of number and sequence, but probably the most generally accepted definition refers to *three or more consecutive spontaneous abortions.* Repeated spontaneous abortions are likely to be chance phenomena in the majority of cases. Support for this view is provided by the observation that the employment of any of a great variety of unrelated but presumed therapeutic modalities was followed by successful pregnancy outcome 70 to 90 percent of the time.

It is important to differentiate spontaneous abortions due to defective zygotes from those much less common abortions due to maternal factors. In early abortions, there is likely to be a nonrecurring aneuploidic abnormality of the conceptus that is responsible for the abortion. In late abortions, fetal development is more likely to have been euploidic with a maternal abnormality responsible for the abortion.

Most recommend parenteral karyotyping after three consecutive spontaneous abortions. Chromosomal banding techniques should be used in all karyotypes.

Prognosis. With the exception of antiphospholipid antibodies and an incompetent cervix, the apparent "cure rate" after as many as three consecutive spontaneous abortions will range between 70 and 85 percent regardless of treatment. That is, the loss rate will be higher, but not a great deal higher, than that anticipated for pregnancies in general. In fact, Warburton and Fraser (1964) reported that the likelihood of recurrent abortion was 25 to 30 percent regardless of the number of previous abortions. Poland and associates (1977) noted that if a woman had previously delivered a live-born infant, the risks for each recurrent abortion were approximately 30 percent. If, however, the woman had no live-born infants and had experienced at least one fetal loss (spontaneous abortion, fetal or neonatal death), the risk of abortion was 46 percent. Women with three or more spontaneous abortions are at increased risk in a subsequent pregnancy for preterm delivery, placenta previa, breech presentation, and fetal malformation (Thom and colleagues, 1992). Following a successful delivery, the likelihood of an abnormal child is not increased; but the risk for preterm and small for gestational age infants still is increased (Reginald and co-workers, 1987).

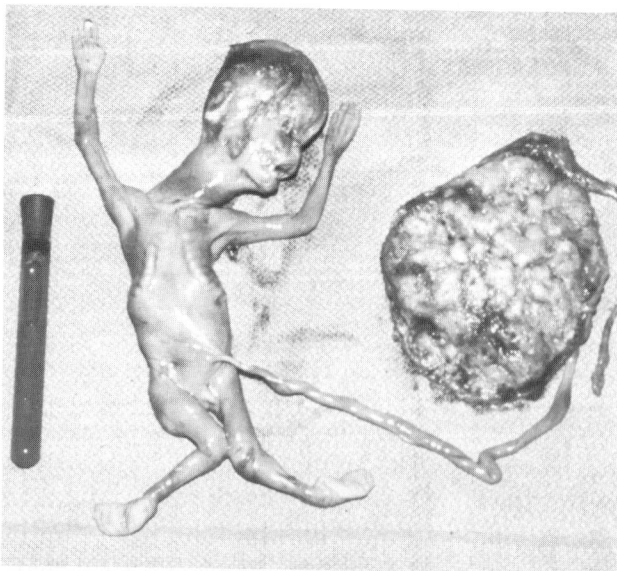

Fig. 31–8. Dead immature fetus retained in utero with placenta for many weeks. Characteristic thick, opaque amnionic fluid is contained in the stoppered tube.

INDUCED ABORTION

Therapeutic Abortion

Therapeutic abortion is the *termination of pregnancy before the time of fetal viability for the purpose of safeguarding the health of the mother.*

Legal Aspects. Until the United States Supreme Court decision of 1973, only therapeutic abortions could be performed legally in most states. The most common legal definition of therapeutic abortion until then was termination of pregnancy before the period of fetal viability for the purpose of saving the *life* of the mother. Not too long before the Supreme Court decision, a few states extended their laws to read "to prevent serious or permanent bodily injury to the mother" or "to preserve the life or health of the woman." A few states allowed abortion if pregnancy was likely to result in the birth of an infant with grave malformations.

Contrary to popular belief, the stringent abortion laws in effect until 1973 were of fairly recent origin. Abortion before *quickening*—the first definite perception of fetal movement, which most often occurs between 16 and 20 weeks' gestation—was either lawful or widely tolerated in both the United States and Great Britain until 1803. In that year, as part of a general restructuring of British criminal law, a statute was enacted that made abortion before quickening illegal. The Roman Catholic Church's traditional condemnation of abortion did not receive the ultimate sanction of universal law (excommunication) until 1869 (Pilpel and Norwich, 1969).

The British law of 1803 became a model for similar laws in the United States, but it was not until 1821 that Connecticut enacted the nation's first abortion law. Subsequently, throughout the United States, abortion became illegal except to save the life of the mother. Because therapeutic abortion *to save the life of the woman* is rarely necessary or definable, it follows that the great majority of such operations previously performed in this country went beyond the letter of the law.

Indications. Some indications for therapeutic abortion are discussed with the diseases that commonly lead to the operation. Well-documented indications are persistent heart disease after previous cardiac decompensation and advanced hypertensive vascular disease. Another is invasive carcinoma of the cervix. The American College of Obstetricians and Gynecologists (1987) established guidelines for therapeutic abortion, and according to this policy, therapeutic abortion may be performed for the following medical indications:

1. When continuation of pregnancy may threaten the life of the woman or seriously impair her health. In determining whether or not there is such a risk to health, account may be taken of her total environment, actual or reasonably foreseeable.
2. When pregnancy has resulted from rape or incest. In this case, the same medical criteria should be employed in evaluation of the woman.
3. When continuation of pregnancy is likely to result in the birth of a child with severe physical deformities or mental retardation.

Elective (Voluntary) Abortion

Definition. Elective or voluntary abortion is the interruption of pregnancy before viability at the request of the woman but not for reasons of impaired maternal health or fetal disease. Most abortions done today fall into this category; in fact, there is one elective abortion for every three live births in this country.

Legality

Roe versus Wade. The legality of elective abortion was established by the United States Supreme Court in its 1973 decision in the case of *Roe v Wade* (Supreme Court of the United States, 1973). The decision defined the extent to which states might regulate abortion:

(a) For the stage prior to approximately the end of the first trimester, the abortion decision and its effectuation must be left to the medical judgment of the pregnant woman's attending physician.

(b) For the stage subsequent to approximately the end of the first trimester, the State, in promoting its interest in the health of the mother, may, if it chooses, regulate the abortion procedures in ways that are reasonably related to maternal health.

(c) For the stage subsequent to viability the State, in promoting its interest in the potential of human life, may, if it chooses, regulate, and even proscribe, abortion, except where necessary, in appropriate medical judgment, for the preservation of the life or health of the mother.

Webster versus Reproductive Health Services. Since the *Roe v Wade* decision, many different pieces of legislation, both state and national, have been introduced and some enacted to regulate or even dismantle its three provisions. All such attempts were unsuccessful until the United States Supreme Court ruled in 1989 (*Webster v Reproductive Health Services*) that states could place restrictions interfering with provision of abortion services on such items as waiting periods, specific informed consent requirements, parenteral/spousal notification, and hospital requirements (Supreme Court of the United States, 1989). Based upon this decision, numerous challenges have arisen to limit a woman's choice and access to abortion services. Moreover, because this was a majority opinion, there is a possibility that *Roe v Wade* soon might be overturned. Justice Blackman, in his dissenting opinion to *Webster*, stated, "I fear for the future. I fear for the liberty and equality of the millions of women who have lived and come of age in the 16 years since *Roe v Wade* was decided. I fear for the integrity of, and the public esteem for, this Court. I dissent."

Planned Parenthood of Southeastern Pennsylvania versus Robert P. Casey. In 1992, the United States Supreme Court considered whether a state could require, prior to an abortion, a woman's informed consent, a 24-hour waiting period, spousal consent, parental consent in the case of a minor, and a physician's description of the fetus and the abortion technique to be employed. In a 5 to 4 decision, the court upheld a state's right to require all these except spousal consent. The court also reconsidered and reaffirmed the *Roe v Wade* decision by a 5 to 4 vote (Supreme Court of the United States, 1992).

Counseling Before Elective Abortion. There are only three choices available to the woman considering an abortion. These are continued pregnancy with its risks and responsibilities; continued pregnancy with its risks and arranged adoption; or the choice of abortion with its risks. In some instances, the pregnant woman may wish to avoid abortion and allow the pregnancy to continue if social and economic problems can be resolved. In any event, knowledgeable and compassionate counselors are invaluable.

Abortion Techniques

The techniques for performing abortion are outlined in Table 31–3. Prior to an elective abortion, bacterial vaginosis should likely be treated because treatment with metronidazole has been shown to reduce the postoperative infection rate (Larsson and colleagues, 1992).

Treatment of D-negative women after abortion with anti-D immunoglobulin is recommended, because about 5 percent of D-negative women become immunized after an abortion (Chap. 44, p. 1008).

Surgical Techniques for Abortion

The products of conception may be removed surgically through an appropriately dilated cervix or transabdominally by either hysterotomy or hysterectomy. These techniques have been reviewed by the American College of Obstetricians and Gynecologists (1987).

Dilatation and Curettage. Surgical abortion through the cervix is performed by first dilating the cervix and

TABLE 31–3. ABORTION TECHNIQUES

Surgical Techniques
Cervical dilatation followed by uterine evacuation
  1. Curettage
  2. Vacuum aspiration (suction curettage)
  3. Dilatation and evacuation
Menstrual aspiration
Laparotomy
  1. Hysterotomy
  2. Hysterectomy

Medical Techniques
Oxytocin intravenously
Intra-amnionic hyperosmotic fluid
  1. 20 percent saline
  2. 30 percent urea
Prostaglandins E_2, $F_{2\alpha}$, and prostaglandin analogues
  1. Intra-amnionic injection
  2. Extraovular injection
  3. Vaginal insertion
  4. Parenteral injection
  5. Oral ingestion
Antiprogesterones—RU 486 (mifepristone) and epostane
Various combinations of the above

then evacuating the products of conception by mechanically scraping out the contents (*sharp curettage*), by vacuum aspiration (*suction curettage*), or both. The likelihood of complications, including uterine perforation, cervical laceration, hemorrhage, incomplete removal of the fetus and placenta, and infection increases after the first trimester, and especially after about 14 to 16 weeks. For this reason, dilatation and curettage or vacuum aspiration should be performed before 14 weeks' gestation. After 16 weeks, **dilatation and evacuation (D&E)** is performed. This usually consists of wide cervical dilatation followed by mechanical destruction and evacuation of fetal parts. With complete removal of the fetus, a large-bore vacuum curette is used to remove the placenta and remaining products.

In the absence of maternal systemic disease, pregnancies are usually terminated by dilatation and curettage or evacuation without hospitalization. **When abortion is not performed in a hospital setting, it is imperative that capabilities for effective cardiopulmonary resuscitation be available, and that immediate access to hospitalization be possible.**

Hygroscopic Dilators. Mechanical dilatation of the undilated and uneffaced cervix is a potentially traumatic procedure. Trauma can be minimized by using an agent that will swell slowly and dilate the cervix. **Laminaria tents,** illustrated in Figure 31–9, are commonly used to help dilate the cervix. They are made from the stems of *Laminaria digitata* or *Laminaria japonica,* a brown seaweed obtained from northern ocean waters. The stems are cut, peeled, shaped, dried, sterilized, and packaged according to size (small, 3 to 5 mm in diameter; medium, 6 to 8 mm; and large, 8 to 10 mm). The

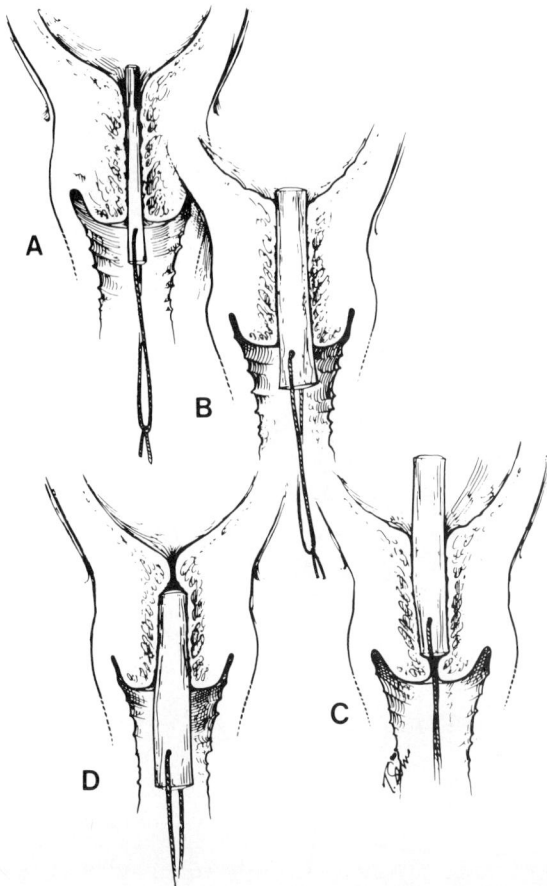

Fig. 31–9. Insertion of laminaria prior to dilatation and curettage. **A.** Laminaria immediately after being appropriately placed with its upper end just through the internal os. **B.** The swollen laminaria and dilated, softened cervix several hours later. **C.** Laminaria inserted too far through the internal os; the laminaria may rupture the membranes. **D.** Laminaria not inserted far enough to dilate the internal os.

strongly hygroscopic laminaria are thought to act by drawing water from proteoglycan complexes, causing them to dissociate and thereby allowing the cervix to soften and dilate.

A synthetic hygroscopic dilator made of hydrogel polymer has been used for some time. It has been claimed that it dilates the cervix more rapidly than dilators made of traditional seaweed (Blumenthal, 1988; Chvapil and co-workers, 1982). *Lamicel,* a polyvinyl alcohol polymer sponge impregnated with anhydrous magnesium sulfate ($MgSO_4$), has been used as a synthetic laminaria tent, and it is reported to be efficacious (Nicolaides and co-workers, 1983). The magnesium levels in plasma described by them before and during its use are probably too high to be compatible with life, but presumably they are erroneous because no complications were noted in the subjects.

The cleansed cervix is grasped anteriorly with a tenaculum. The cervical canal is carefully sounded, without rupturing the membranes, to identify the length of the canal. A laminaria of appropriate size is then inserted

so that the tip passes just beyond the internal os using a uterine packing forceps or a radium capsule forceps (Fig. 31–9). Later, usually after 4 to 6 hours, the laminaria will have swollen and thereby dilated the cervix sufficiently to allow easier mechanical dilatation and curettage. The laminaria may cause cramping but the pain can be easily managed with 60 mg of codeine orally every 3 to 4 hours.

Rather than using a laminaria to effect cervical softening and thereby minimize trauma from mechanical dilatation, prostaglandin pessaries (suppositories) have been inserted into the vagina against the cervix 3 hours or so before attempting dilatation. Chen and associates (1983) reported good results from applying 1 mg of prostaglandin E_1 methyl ester. Several newer prostaglandin products have been used to induce labor or to efface the cervix prior to labor induction. Many of these same products have also been used to prepare the cervix prior to mechanical dilatation for induction of abortion. These are discussed in Chapter 19 (p. 488).

Dilatation, Curettage, and Evacuation. At the time of abortion, the laminaria is removed by grasping the attached thread, and the vulva, vagina, and cervix are cleansed. The size and position of the uterus are reevaluated through bimanual examination. The anterior cervical lip is grasped with a multitoothed tenaculum and a local anesthetic is injected into the cervix. Commonly, 5 mL of 1 or 2 percent solution of lidocaine is injected bilaterally. Alternatively, a paracervical block may be used (see Chap. 16, p. 434). The usual precautions for use of local anesthetics must be observed because deaths have resulted from their use.

The uterus is sounded *carefully* to identify the status of the internal os and to confirm uterine size and position. The cervix is further dilated with Hegar or Pratt dilators until a vacuum aspirator suction curet of appropriate diameter can be inserted. As shown in Figure 31–10, the fourth and fifth fingers of the hand introducing the dilator should rest on the perineum and buttocks as the dilator is pushed through the internal os. This provides a further safeguard against uterine perforation.

Suction curettage then is used to aspirate pregnancy products. The vacuum aspirator is moved over the surface systematically in order eventually to cover all the uterine cavity. Once this is done and no more tissue is aspirated, the procedure is terminated. Gentle curettage with a sharp curet is then utilized if it is thought that any placenta or fetal fragments remain in the uterus. A sharp curet is more efficacious, and its dangers need not be greater than those of the dull instrument. Uterine perforations rarely occur on the downstroke of the curet, but they may occur when any instrument is introduced into the uterus. A curet, however, is a dangerous instrument if injudicious force is applied. As shown in Figure 31–11, manipulations

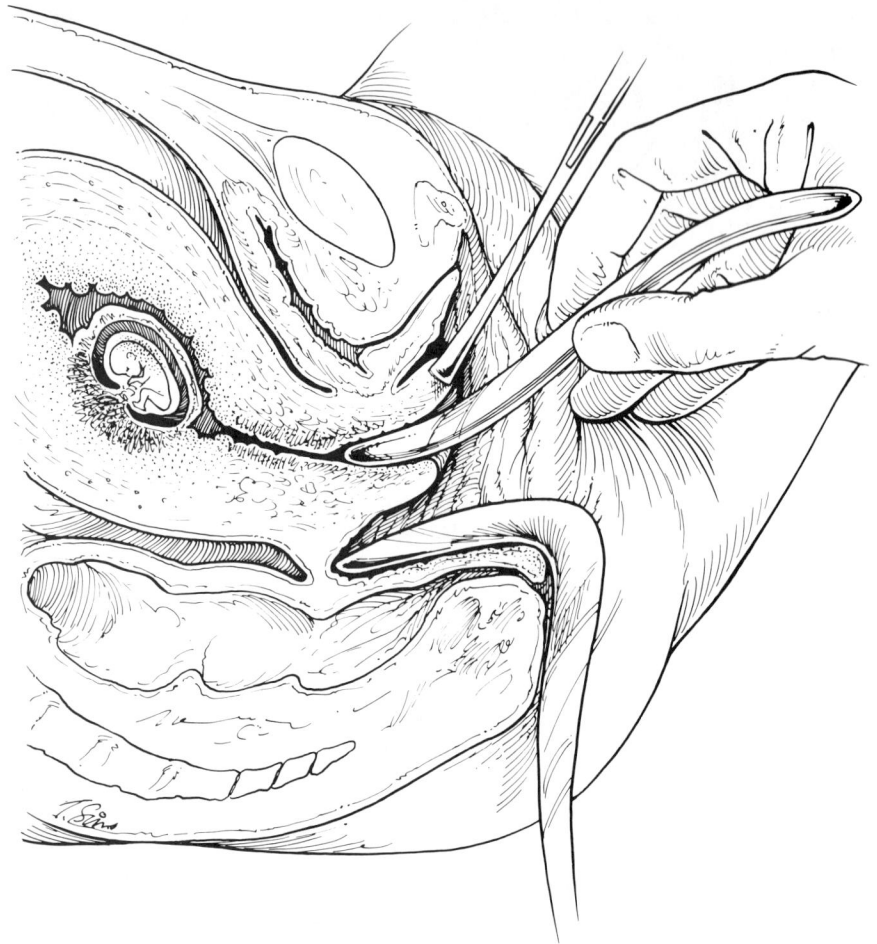

Fig. 31–10. Dilatation of cervix with Hegar dilator. Note that the fourth and fifth fingers rest against the perineum and buttocks, lateral to the vagina. This maneuver is a most important safety measure because if the cervix relaxes abruptly, these fingers prevent a sudden and uncontrolled thrust of the dilator, a common cause of uterine perforation.

should be carried out with the thumb and forefingers only.

In cases advanced past 16 weeks' gestation, the fetus is extracted, usually in parts, using Sopher forceps and other destructive instruments. The risks of uterine perforation and laceration are increased due to the larger fetus and the thinner uterine walls. These late abortions are unpleasant for medical and nursing personnel and more dangerous for the woman undergoing the procedure.

It is reemphasized that morbidity, immediate and remote, will be kept to a minimum if (1) the cervix is adequately dilated without trauma before attempting to remove products of conception, (2) removal of products of conception is accomplished without perforating the uterus, and (3) all of the products of conception, but not the decidua basalis, are removed.

Uterine Perforation. Accidental uterine perforation may occur during sounding of the uterus, dilatation, or curettage. The incidence of uterine perforation associated with elective abortion varies. Two important determinants of this complication are the skill of the physician and the position of the uterus, with a much greater

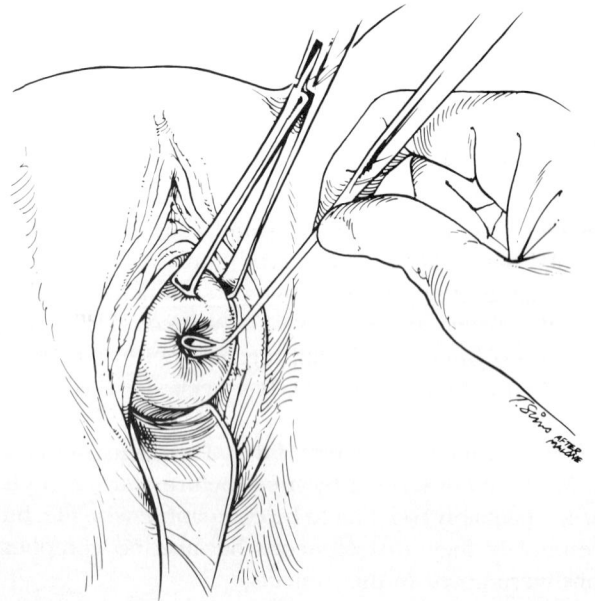

Fig. 31–11. Introduction of a sharp curet. Note that the instrument is held with the thumb and forefinger; in the upward movement of the curet, only the strength of these two fingers should be used.

likelihood of perforation if the physician is inexperienced and the uterus is retroverted.

Accidental uterine perforation is recognized easily, as the instrument passes without hindrance further than it should have. Observation may be sufficient therapy if the uterine perforation is small, as when produced by a uterine sound or narrow dilator. Small defects often heal without complication.

Considerable intra-abdominal damage can be caused by instruments passed through a uterine defect into the peritoneal cavity. This is especially true for suction and sharp curets. In this circumstance, laparotomy to examine the abdominal contents, especially the bowel, is the safest course of action. We have cared for a woman transferred to us after much of her right ureter had been removed at the time of attempted abortion using suction curettage! Similar cases have been observed by others (Keegan and Forkowitz, 1982). Nonetheless, vacuum aspiration is generally preferable to mechanical curettage for abortion because it is quicker, has a lower perforation rate, induces somewhat less blood loss at operation, and there are fewer infections afterward. In more advanced abortions, additional mechanical curettage as a second procedure may be necessary.

Some women may develop cervical incompetence or uterine synechiae. The possibility of these complications should be explained to those contemplating abortion. In general, the risk of these complications is very slight. Unfortunately, more advanced abortion performed by curettage may induce sudden, severe consumptive coagulopathy, which can prove fatal. This complication is further considered in Chapter 37 (p. 847).

Menstrual Aspiration. Aspiration of the endometrial cavity using a flexible 5- or 6-mm Karman cannula and syringe within 1 to 3 weeks after failure to menstruate has been referred to as menstrual extraction, menstrual induction, instant period, atraumatic abortion, and miniabortion. Problems include the woman not being pregnant, the implanted zygote being missed by the curet, failure to recognize an ectopic pregnancy, and rarely, uterine perforation.

A positive pregnancy test will serve to eliminate a needless procedure on a nonpregnant woman whose period has been delayed for other reasons. Munsick (1982) recommends the following technique for identifying placenta in the aspirate. First, the syringe contents are placed in a clear plastic container and examined with back lighting. Tap water is added and the bloodstained liquid is decanted until tissue becomes visible. The tissue is then removed and immersed in clear water. Placenta is macroscopically soft, fluffy, feathery, and villous. If there is doubt as to whether the tissue is placenta or decidua, microscopic examination of a small piece under a cover glass with high-light contrast will allow differentiation. Placental villi are obvious.

Laparotomy. In a few circumstances, *abdominal hysterotomy or hysterectomy* for abortion is preferable to either dilatation and curettage or medical induction. If significant uterine disease is present, hysterectomy may provide ideal treatment. If sterilization is to be performed, either hysterotomy with interruption of tubal continuity or hysterectomy on occasion may be more advisable than curettage or medical induction followed by tubal sterilization (see Chap. 62, p. 1358). At times, hysterotomy or hysterectomy becomes necessary because of failure of a medical induction during the second trimester.

The techniques employed for hysterotomy are similar to those for cesarean delivery (see Chap. 26, p. 597), except that the abdominal and uterine incisions are smaller. If further reproduction is anticipated, the smallest uterine incision that will allow removal of the fetus and placenta should be made in the lower uterine segment and the wound carefully repaired.

Following abortion by hysterotomy, the potential for rupture during subsequent pregnancies is appreciable, especially during labor. Therefore, in women with previous hysterotomies, cesarean delivery is indicated in subsequent pregnancies. After hysterotomy, Clow and Crompton (1973) identified 14 thin scars out of 31 evaluated in subsequent pregnancies. Higginbottom (1973) reviewed outcomes in 242 women in whom hysterotomy for abortion was performed; 12 required blood transfusion, 3 developed deep venous thrombosis, 1 had a pulmonary embolism, 1 had a repeat laparotomy for intestinal obstruction, and 2 subsequently required curettage for retained products. **Nottage and Liston (1975), based on a review of 700 hysterotomies, rightfully concluded that the operation is outdated as a routine method for terminating pregnancy.**

Medical Induction of Abortion

Throughout history, many naturally occurring substances have been tried as abortifacients by women desperate not to be pregnant. Most often, serious systemic illness or even death has been the result rather than abortion. Even today, there are only a few effective, safe abortifacient drugs.

Oxytocin. Successful induction of second-trimester abortion is possible with high doses of oxytocin administered in small volumes of intravenous fluids. One regimen we have found effective is to add 10 1-mL ampules of oxytocin (10 IU/mL) to 1000 mL of lactated Ringer solution. This solution contains 100 mU oxytocin/mL. An intravenous infusion is started at 0.5 mL/min (50 mU/min). The rate of infusion is increased at 30- to 40-minute intervals up to a maximum rate of 2 mL/min (200 mU/min). If effective contractions are not established at this infusion rate, the concentration of oxytocin is increased in the infused solution. It is safest to discard all but 500 mL of the remaining solution, which contains a concentration of 100 mU oxytocin/mL. To this 500 mL is added an additional 5 ampules of oxytocin. The resulting solution now contains 200 mU/mL, and the rate of infusion is reduced to 1 mL/min (200 mU/min). A resumption of a progressive rate increase is commenced up to a rate of 2 mL/min (400 mU/min) and left at this rate for an additional 4 to 5 hours, or until the fetus is expelled.

After each increase in infusion rate, careful attention must be directed to the frequency and intensity of uterine contractions, because each increase in infusion rate *markedly* increases the amount of oxytocin infused. If the induction is unsuccessful, serial inductions on a daily basis for 2 to 3 days are almost always successful. The chance of a successful induction with high-dose oxytocin is enhanced greatly by the use of laminaria tents (p. 680) inserted the night before induction. Once the cervix has undergone any degree of effacement and dilatation, either spontaneously or as the consequence of some other agent such as a prostaglandin, intravenously administered oxytocin is much more likely to prove effective.

There are complications from the use of oxytocin. If appreciable volumes of electrolyte-free solution are administered along with oxytocin, water intoxication may develop (see Chap. 14, p. 387). Rupture of the uterus from oxytocin infused during the first half of pregnancy has been documented in women of high parity (Peyser and Toaff, 1972) but is very unlikely. Rupture of the cervix or isthmus has been documented in instances in which oxytocin was given after intra-amnionic prostaglandin $F_{2\alpha}$. A large bolus of oxytocin intravenously may produce troublesome hypotension (see Chap. 14, p. 386).

Intra-Amnionic Hyperosmotic Solutions.

In order to effect abortion during the second trimester, 20 to 25 percent saline, or 30 to 40 percent urea, has been injected into the amnionic sac to stimulate uterine contractions and cervical dilatation. These techniques are used less often than before. In 1983, only 2 percent of abortions were induced by intra-amnionic instillation techniques (Centers for Disease Control, 1986).

According to the American College of Obstetricians and Gynecologists (1987), intra-amnionic instillation as a method of midtrimester abortion has been replaced by dilatation and evacuation. Benefits cited included speed, less cost, and less pain and emotional trauma.

Mechanism of Action.

The mechanism of action of hyperosmotic agents placed in the amnionic sac is not clear, but the likely mechanism appears to be prostaglandin mediated. Hypertonic solutions damage fetal membranes, likely resulting in liberation of phospholi-

pases. These lipases cleave arachidonic acid from storage sites in fetal membranes. The liberated arachidonic acid is then converted into prostaglandins (Chap. 12, p. 318).

Hypertonic Saline.

Intra-amnionically injected hypertonic saline may result in serious complications, including death. Other complications include (1) hyperosmolar crisis following entry of hypertonic saline into the maternal circulation, (2) cardiac failure, (3) septic shock, (4) peritonitis, (5) hemorrhage, (6) disseminated intravascular coagulation, and (7) water intoxication. Moreover, myometrial necrosis has followed injection of hypertonic saline into myometrium; cervical and isthmic fistulas and lacerations have been reported and gross rupture of the body of the uterus has been described (Horwitz, 1974). Use of laminaria tents to prevent such cervical trauma has been recommended, but fistula formations may still occur (Lischke and Gordon, 1974). Serious disruption of the coagulation mechanism characterized by changes of disseminated intravascular coagulation have been reported with use of hypertonic saline for abortion (see Chap. 37, p. 847).

Hyperosmotic Urea.

Urea, 30 to 40 percent, dissolved in 5 percent dextrose solution, has been injected into the amnionic sac, followed by intravenous oxytocin, about 400 mU per minute. Urea plus oxytocin is as efficacious as an abortifacient as hypertonic saline, but less likely to be toxic. Urea plus prostaglandin $F_{2\alpha}$ injected into the amnionic sac is similarly effective.

Prostaglandins.

Because of shortcomings of other medical methods of inducing abortion, prostaglandins are used extensively to terminate pregnancies, especially in the second trimester.

Mechanism of Action.

Compounds commonly used are prostaglandin E_2, prostaglandin $F_{2\alpha}$, and certain analogues, especially 15-methylprostaglandin $F_{2\alpha}$ methyl ester. The probable mode of action of the prostaglandins on the uterus and cervix is considered in detail in Chapter 12, p. 335).

Technique.

Prostaglandins can act effectively on the cervix and uterus when (1) placed in the vagina as a suppository or pessary immediately adjacent to the cervix, (2) administered as a gel through a catheter into the cervical canal and lowermost uterus extraovularly, or (3) injected into the amnionic sac by amniocentesis (Embrey, 1981). These three approaches reduce appreciably, but do not eliminate, the unpleasant systemic effects, especially gastrointestinal, that accompany oral or parenteral administration of prostaglandins. These routes of administration are effective, but repeated doses of prostaglandin may be required.

Prostaglandin vaginal suppositories applied to the

cervix are also used by some in a lower dose during the first and even early in the second trimesters to ripen or soften and dilate the cervix before terminating the pregnancy by curettage (MacKenzie and Fry, 1981; Niloff and Stubblefield, 1982). A troublesome feature with prostaglandin-induced abortions is the expulsion of a fetus with signs of life. The legal implications associated with expulsion of a living abortus may be profound. Although the purpose of abortion is to destroy the fetus before viability, statutes continue to be enacted to protect the abortus.

Antiprogesterone RU 486 (Mifepristone). The oral antiprogesterone RU 486 has been used to effect abortions in early human gestation, either alone (Grimes and associates, 1988) or in combination with oral prostaglandins (Baird and colleagues, 1992; Cameron and Baird, 1988). The effectiveness of the drug as an abortifacient is based upon its high receptor affinity for progesterone binding sites (Healey and colleagues, 1983). A single 600-mg dose of RU 486 administered prior to 6 weeks' gestation results in an 85 percent abortion rate. After this time, the agent is progressively less effective. The addition of various oral, vaginal, or injected prostaglandins to this regimen results in abortion rates over 95 percent.

Side effects of RU 486 include nausea, vomiting, and gastrointestinal cramping. The major risk *associated* with the agent is hemorrhage due to partial expulsion of the products of conception and due to intraabdominal hemorrhage from an early unsuspected ectopic pregnancy. The duration of vaginal bleeding is approximately 2 weeks after RU 486 alone and approximately 1½ weeks after RU 486 is given with a prostaglandin.

The risks and side effects from the often-used prostaglandins are not insignificant. These are discussed in more detail in Chapter 19 (p. 488). These risks should be taken seriously because respiratory deaths have occurred in asthmatic women who received prostaglandins and RU 486 in combination. **At present, RU 486 is not available in the United States for use as an abortifacient.** The Food and Drug Administration has placed RU 486 on the list of drugs an individual cannot bring into the United States even for personal use (Potts, 1992).

Epostane. Epostane is a 3β-hydroxysteroid dehydrogenase inhibitor that blocks the synthesis of endogenous progesterone. If administered within 4 weeks of the last menstrual period, the drug will induce an abortion in approximately 85 percent of women (Crooij and associates, 1988). Clinical responses are likely related to circulating endogenous progesterone levels. Nausea is a frequent side effect, and hemorrhage is a risk if the abortion is incomplete. **This drug is currently not available in the United States for use as an abortifacient.**

Consequences of Elective Abortion

Maternal Mortality. It is apparent that serious morbidity and even mortality have followed some elective abortions. Nonetheless, legally induced abortion is a relatively safe surgical procedure, especially when performed during the first 2 months of pregnancy. The risk of death from abortion performed during the first 2 months is about 0.6 per 100,000 procedures (Centers for Disease Control, 1986). The relative risk of dying as the consequence of abortion is approximately doubled for each 2 weeks of delay after 8 weeks' gestation. Atrash and colleagues (1988) reported that the proportion of abortion-related deaths caused by general anesthesia has increased from 8 percent in 1975 to 29 percent in 1985. This likely reflects an absolute decrease in deaths from nonanesthetic complications. LeBolt and co-workers (1982) estimated that, during the 1970s at least, overall risk of death from legal abortion was no more than one seventh the risk from childbirth.

Impact on Future Pregnancies. Hogue (1986), in a scholarly review of the impact of elective abortion upon subsequent pregnancy outcome, summarized data from more than 200 publications in 11 languages citing more than 150 studies from 21 countries. She emphasized that the method of inducing abortion must be considered, and that women chosen as control subjects should be primigravid because a parous woman has a reduced risk of complications in subsequent pregnancies. The following conclusions were derived from this and more recent data:

1. *Fertility* is not altered by an elective abortion. The only possible exception is the small risk from pelvic infection.
2. *Vacuum aspiration* for a first pregnancy results in no increased incidence of midtrimester spontaneous abortions, preterm deliveries, or low-birthweight infants in subsequent pregnancies when compared with primigravid controls.
3. *Dilatation and curettage* in primigravidas results in an increased risk for subsequent ectopic pregnancy, midtrimester spontaneous abortion, and low-birthweight infants.
4. *Subsequent ectopic* pregnancies are not increased if the first termination is done by vacuum aspiration. Possible exceptions are in women with preexisting *Chlamydia trachomatis* infection or those who develop postabortion infection.
5. *Multiple elective abortions* do not increase the incidence of preterm delivery and low-birthweight infants (Mandelson and associates, 1992).
6. *Placenta previa* has been reported to be increased following elective abortion (Barrett and

associates, 1981), but Hogue discounted the study because of a failure to control for maternal age.

7. *Induced midtrimester abortions* apparently carry little risk to subsequent pregnancies if injection techniques are used. The risk of a subsequent low-birthweight infant is increased following saline- versus prostaglandin-induced midtrimester terminations, but the difference is not significant (Meirik and Nygren, 1984). Similarly, the risk of subsequent low-birthweight infants is increased following *dilatation and evacuation;* however, this difference is also not significant. Unfortunately, there are not enough procedure-specific data available to form valid conclusions regarding the risks to future pregnancies following any midtrimester abortion.

Septic Abortion

Serious complications of abortion have most often been associated with criminal abortion. Severe hemorrhage, sepsis, bacterial shock, and acute renal failure have all developed in association with legal abortion but at a very much lower frequency. Sepsis from abortion is usually caused by pathogenic organisms of the bowel and vaginal flora. Metritis is the usual outcome, but parametritis, peritonitis (localized and general), and septicemia are not rare. In 300 septic abortions at Parkland Hospital, a positive blood culture was found in a fourth. The organisms identified are listed in Table 31–4.

Treatment of infection includes prompt evacuation of the products of conception. Although mild infections can be treated successfully with broad-spectrum antibiotics in the usual dosage, any serious infection should be treated vigorously from the start. For septic abortion complicated by persistent, apparently resistant infection, or with evidence of overwhelming sepsis, high-dose broad-spectrum antimicrobials are given intravenously (see Chap. 28, p. 632).

TABLE 31–4. BACTERIA RECOVERED FROM BLOOD CULTURES IN 76 CASES OF SEPTIC ABORTION

Organisms Cultured	Frequency (%)
Anaerobic	63
Peptostreptococcus species	41
Bacteroides species	9
Clostridium perfringens	4
Aerobic	37
Escherichia coli	14
Pseudomonas	9
β-hemolytic streptococcus	4
Enterococcus faecalis	3
Combination	7

From Smith and colleagues (1970).

Septic Shock. Endotoxemia and exotoxemia are likely to cause severe and even fatal shock. Septic shock, now rare, was previously seen most often in women of reproductive age in connection with induced and especially criminal abortions. This complication is discussed in detail in Chapter 47 (p. 1072).

Acute Renal Failure. Persistent renal failure complicating abortion usually stems from multiple effects of infection and hypovolemia. Less commonly, it has been induced by toxic compounds employed to produce abortion, such as soap, pHisohex, or Lysol. Whereas very severe forms of bacterial shock frequently are associated with intense renal damage, the milder forms rarely lead to overt renal failure. Early recognition of this very serious complication is most important (see Chap. 50, p. 1141).

Renal failure is likely to be most intense when the cause of the sepsis includes *Clostridium perfringens* with the production of a very potent hemolytic exotoxin. In our experience, whenever intense hemoglobinemia complicated clostridial infection, renal failure was the rule. At the outset, plans should be made to initiate effective dialysis early, before metabolic deterioration becomes severe.

References

Adams EC: Aging and reproduction. In Austin CR, Short RV (eds): Reproduction in Mammals: 4. Reproductive Patterns. Cambridge, Cambridge University Press, 1972, p 136

American College of Obstetricians and Gynecologists: Methods of midtrimester abortion. Technical Bulletin no. 109, October 1987

Ansari AH, Reynolds RA: Cervical incompetence: A review. J Reprod Med 32:161, 1987

Armstrong BG, McDonald AD, Sloan M: Cigarette, alcohol, and coffee consumption and spontaneous abortion. Am J Public Health 82:85, 1992

Atrash HK, Cheek TG, Hogue CJR: Legal abortion mortality and general anesthesia. Am J Obstet Gynecol 158:420, 1988

Axelsson G, Rylander R: Exposure to anesthetic gases and spontaneous abortion: Response bias in a postal questionnaire study. Int J Epidemiol 11:250, 1982

Baird DT, Norman JE, Thong KJ, Glasier AF: Misoprostol, mifepristone, and abortion. Lancet 339:313, 1992

Balasch J, Font J, López-Soto A, Cervera R, Jové I, Casals FJ, Vanrell JA: Antiphospholipid antibodies in unselected patients with repeated abortion. Hum Reprod 5:43, 1990

Balasch J, López-Soto A, Font J, Puerto B: Lupus anticoagulant as a marker of autoimmunity in recurrent pregnancy loss: A case report. Eur J Obstet Gynecol Reprod Biol 41:237, 1991

Barlow S, Sullivan FM: Reproductive hazards of industrial chemicals: An evaluation of animal and human data. New York, Academic Press, 1982

Barnes AB, Colton T, Gunderson J, Noller KL, Tilley BC, Strama T, Townsend DE, Hatab P, O'Brien PC: Fertility and outcome of pregnancy in women exposed in utero to diethylstilbestrol. N Engl J Med 302:609, 1980

Barrett JM, Boehm FH, Killam AP: Induced abortion: A risk factor for placenta previa. Am J Obstet Gynecol 141:769, 1981

Batzofin JH, Fielding WL, Friedman EA: Effect of vaginal bleeding in early pregnancy on outcome. Obstet Gynecol 63:515, 1984

Blumenthal PD: Prospective comparison of dilapan and laminaria for pretreatment of the cervix in second-trimester induction abortion. Obstet Gynecol 72:243, 1988

Boyd EF Jr, Holmstrom EG: Ovulation following therapeutic abortion. Am J Obstet Gynecol 113:469, 1972

Branch DW, Scott JR, Kochenour NK, Hershgold E: Obstetric complications associated with the lupus anticoagulant. N Engl J Med 313:1322, 1985

Cameron IT, Baird DT: Early pregnancy termination: A comparison between vacuum aspiration and medical abortion using prostaglandin (16,16 dimethyl-trans-Δ_2-PGE$_1$ methyl ester) or the antiprogestogen RU 486. Br J Obstet Gynaecol 95:271, 1988

Caspi E, Schneider DF, Mor Z, Langer R, Weinraub Z, Bukovsky I: Cervical internal os cerclage: Description of a new technique and comparison with Shirodkar operation. Am J Perinatol 7:347, 1990

Caudle MR, Rote NS, Scott JR, DeWitt C, Barney MF: Histocompatibility in couples with recurrent spontaneous abortion and normal fertility. Fertil Steril 39:793, 1983

Centers for Disease Control: Abortion surveillance: Preliminary analysis—United States, 1982–1983. MMWR 35:7SS, 1986

Charles D, Edward WR: Infectious complications of cervical cerclage. Am J Obstet Gynecol 141:1065, 1981

Chartier M, Roger M, Barrat J, Michelon B: Measurement of plasma human chorionic gonadotropin (hCG) and β-hCG activities in the late luteal phase: Evidence of the occurrence of spontaneous menstrual abortions in infertile women. Fertil Steril 31:134, 1979

Check JH, Adelson HG: The efficacy of progesterone in achieving successful pregnancy: II. In women with pure luteal phase defects. Int J Fertil 32:139, 1987a

Check JH, Chase JS, Wu CH, Adelson HG, Teichman M, Rankin A: The efficacy of progesterone in achieving successful pregnancy: I. Prophylactic use during luteal phase in anovulatory women. Int J Fertil 32:135, 1987b

Check JH, Rankin A, Teichman M: The risk of fetal anomalies as a result of progesterone therapy during pregnancy. Fertil Steril 45:575, 1986

Chen JK, Edler MG: Preoperative cervical dilatation by vaginal pessaries containing prostaglandin E$_1$ analogue. Obstet Gynecol 62:339, 1983

Chvapil M, Droegemueller W, Meyer T, Mascalka R, Stoy V, Suciu T: New synthetic laminaria. Obstet Gynecol 60:729, 1982

Clow WM, Crompton AC: The wounded uterus: Pregnancy after hysterotomy. Br Med J 1:321, 1973

Coulam CB, Moore SB, O'Fallon WM: Association between major histocompatibility antigen and reproductive performance. Am J Reprod Immunol Microbiol 14:54, 1987

Cousins L, Karp W, Lacey C, Lucas WE: Reproductive outcome of women exposed to diethylstilbestrol in utero. Obstet Gynecol 56:70, 1980

Cowchock FS, Reece EA, Balaban D, Branch DW, Plouffe L: Repeated fetal losses associated with antiphospholipid antibodies: A collaborative randomized trial comparing prednisone with low-dose heparin treatment. Am J Obstet Gynecol 166:1318, 1992

Crane JP, Wahl N: The role of maternal diabetes in repetitive spontaneous abortion. Fertil Steril 36:477, 1981

Crooij MJ, Coenraad CA, deNoyyer CCA, Rao BR, Berends GT, Gooren LJG, Janssens J: Termination of early pregnancy by the 3β-hydroxysteroid dehydrogenase inhibitor epostane. N Engl J Med 319:813, 1988

Daya S, Clark DA, Devlin C, Jarrell J: Preliminary characterization of two types of suppressor cells in the human uterus. Fertil Steril 55:778, 1985

Deleze M, Alarcon-Segovia D, Valdes-Macho E, Carmen VO, Ponce de Leon S: Relationship between antiphospholipid antibodies and recurrent fetal loss in patients with systemic lupus erythematosus and apparently healthy women. J Rheumatol 16:768, 1989

Denegri JF, Altin M, McConnachi P, Peterson J, Benny WB, Zouves CG, Wilson D: Immunotherapy of primary immunological aborters: Rationale for the use of pooled cyropreserved purified normal peripheral blood mononuclear cells. Am J Reprod Immunol Microbiol 12:65, 1986

Dickey RP, Olar TT, Taylor SN, Curole DN, Matulich EM: Relationship of small gestational sac-crown-rump length differences to abortion and abortus karyotypes. Obstet Gynecol 79:554, 1992

Edmonds DK, Lindsay KS, Miller JF, Williamson E, Wood PJ: Early embryonic mortality in women. Fertil Steril 38:447, 1982

Embrey MP: Prostaglandins in human reproduction. Br Med J 283:1563, 1981

Emerson DS, Cartier MS, Altieri LA, Felker RE, Smith WC, Stoval TG, Gray LA: Diagnostic efficacy of endovaginal color Doppler flow imaging in an ectopic pregnancy screening program. Radiology 183:413, 1992

Fantel AG, Shepard TH, Vadheim-Roth C, Stephens TD, Coleman C: Embryonic and fetal phenotypes: Prevalence and other associated factors in a large study of spontaneous abortion. In Porter IH, Hook EM (eds): Human Embryonic and Fetal Death. New York, Academic Press, 1980, p 71

Ferro D, Saliola M, Quintarelli C, Carlucci M, Valesini G, Violi F: Specificity and sensitivity of diluted aPTT and anticardiolipin antibodies towards thrombosis and miscarriages in patients with systemic lupus erythematosus. Thromb Res 59:609, 1990

Fossum GT, Davajan V, Kletzky OA: Early detection of pregnancy with transvaginal ultrasound. Fertil Steril 49:788, 1988

Funderburk SJ, Guthrie D, Meldrum D: Outcome of pregnancies complicated by early vaginal bleeding. Br J Obstet Gynaecol 87:100, 1980

Gant NF: Lupus erythematosus, the lupus anticoagulant, and the anticardiolipin antibody. Williams Obstetrics, 17th ed (suppl 6). Norwalk, CT, Appleton & Lange, May/June 1986

Grimes DA, Mishell DR Jr, Shoupe D, Lacarra M: Early abortion with a single dose of the antiprogestin RU-486. Am J Obstet Gynecol 158:1307, 1988

Guerrero R, Rojas OI: Spontaneous abortion and aging of human ova and spermatozoa. N Engl J Med 293:573, 1975

Hahlin M, Wallin A, Sjoblom P, Lindblom B: Single progesterone assay for early recognition of abnormal pregnancy. Hum Reprod 5:662, 1990

Harlap S, Shiono PH: Alcohol, smoking, and incidence of spontaneous abortions in the first and second trimester. Lancet 2:173, 1980a

Harlap S, Shiono PH, Ramcharan S: A life table of spontaneous abortions and the effects of age, parity and other variables. In Porter IH, Hook EB (eds): Human Embryonic and Fetal Death. New York, Academic Press, 1980b, p 145

Hartman CG: Uterine bleeding as an early sign of pregnancy in the monkey (*Macaca rhesus*), together with the observation on fertile period of menstrual cycle. Bull Johns Hopkins Hosp 44:155, 1929

Healy DL, Baulieu EE, Hodgen GD: Induction of menstruation by an antiprogesterone steroid (RU 486) in primates: Site of action, dose–response relationships, and hormonal effects. Fertil Steril 40:253, 1983

Herbst AL, Hubby MM, Azizi F, Makii MM: Reproductive and gynecologic surgical experience in diethylstilbestrol-exposed daughters. Am J Obstet Gynecol 141:1019, 1981

Herron MA, Parer JT: Transabdominal cerclage for fetal wastage due to cervical incompetence. Obstet Gynecol 71:865, 1988

Hertig AT, Rock J: On the development of the early human ovum, with special reference to the trophoblast of the previllous stage: A description of 7 normal and 5 pathologic human ova. Am J Obstet Gynecol 47:149, 1944

Hertig AT, Rock J, Adams EC, Menkin M: Thirty-four fertilized human ova, good, bad, and indifferent, recovered from 210 women of known fertility: A study of biologic wastage in early human pregnancy. Pediatrics 23:202, 1959

Hertig AT, Sheldon WH: Minimal criteria required to prove prima facie case of traumatic abortion or miscarriage: An analysis of 1,000 spontaneous abortions. Ann Surg 117:596, 1943

Higginbottom J: Termination of pregnancy by abdominal hysterotomy. Lancet 1:937, 1973

Hogue CJR: Impact of abortion on subsequent fecundity. Clin Obstet Gynaecol 13:95, 1986

Horta JLH, Fernandez JG, DeSota LB: Direct evidence of luteal insufficiency in women with habitual abortion. Obstet Gynecol 49:705, 1977

Horwitz DA: Uterine rupture following attempted saline abortion with oxytocin in a grand multiparous patient. Obstet Gynecol 43:921, 1974

Houwert-de Jong MH, Termijtelen A, Eskes TKAB, Mantingh A, Bruinse HW: The natural course of habitual abortion. Eur J Obstet Gynecol Reprod Biol 33:221, 1989

Infante-Rivard C, David M, Gauthier R, Rivard G-E: Lupus anticoagulants, anticardiolipin antibodies, and fetal loss. N Engl J Med 325:1063, 1991

Jacobs PA, Hassold TJ: The origin of chromosomal abnormalities in spontaneous abortion. In Porter IH, Hook EB (eds): Human Embryonic and Fetal Death. New York, Academic Press, 1980, p 289

Johnson PM, Chia KV, Risk JM: Immunological question marks in recurrent spontaneous abortion. In Clark DA, Croy BA (eds): Reproductive Immunology. New York, Elsevier, 1986, p 239

Kadar N, Caldwell BV, Romero R: A method of screening for ectopic pregnancy and its indications. Obstet Gynecol 58:162, 1981

Kajii T, Ferrier A, Niikawa N, Takahara H, Ohama K, Avirachan

S: Anatomic and chromosomal anomalies in 639 spontaneous abortions. Hum Genet 55:87, 1980

Keegan GT, Forkowitz MJ: A case report: Ureterouterine fistula as a complication of elective abortion. J Urol 128:137, 1982

Kline J, Stein ZA, Shrout P, Susser M: Drinking during pregnancy and spontaneous abortion. Lancet 2:176, 1980a

Kline J, Stein Z, Susser M, Warburton D: Environmental influences on early reproductive loss in a current New York City study. In Porter IH, Hook EB (eds): Human Embryonic and Fetal Death. New York, Academic Press, 1980b, p 225

Kuhn RPJ, Pepperell RJ: Cervical ligation: A review of 242 pregnancies. Aust NZ J Obstet Gynaecol 17:79, 1977

Lachenbruch P: Frequency and timing of intercourse: Its relation to the probability of conception. Popul Studies 21:23, 1967

Lähteenmäki P, Luukkainen T: Return of ovarian function after abortion. Clin Endocrinol 8:123, 1978

Larsson P-G, Platz-Christensen J-J, Thejls H, Forsum U, Påhlson C: Incidence of pelvic inflammatory disease after first-trimester legal abortion in women with bacterial vaginosis after treatment with metronidazole: A double-blind, randomized study. Am J Obstet Gynecol 166:100, 1992

LeBolt SA, Grimes DA, Cates W Jr. Mortality from abortion: Are the populations comparable? JAMA 248:188, 1982

Lee CS: Luteal phase defects. Obstet Gynecol Surv 42:267, 1987

Lischke JH, Gordon HR: Cervicovaginal fistula complicating induced midtrimester abortion despite laminaria tent insertion. Am J Obstet Gynecol 120:852, 1974

Lockshin MD, Druzin ML, Qamar T: Prednisone does not prevent recurrent fetal death in women with antiphospholipid antibody. Am J Obstet Gynecol 160:439, 1989

Lubbe WF, Liggins GC: Lupus anticoagulant and pregnancy. Am J Obstet Gynecol 153:322, 1985

MacKenzie IZ, Fry A: Prostaglandin E_2 pessaries to facilitate first trimester aspiration termination. Br J Obstet Gynaecol 88:1033, 1981

Mackenzie WE, Holmes DS, Newton JR: Spontaneous abortion rate in ultrasonographically viable pregnancies. Obstet Gynecol 71:81, 1988

Mandelson MT, Maden CB, Daling JR: Low birth weight in relation to multiple induced abortions. Am J Public Health 82:391, 1992

Mangan CE, Borow L, Burtnett-Rubin MM, Egan V, Giuntoli RL, Mikuta JJ: Pregnancy outcome in 98 women exposed to diethylstilbestrol in utero, their mothers, and unexposed siblings. Obstet Gynecol 59:315, 1982

March CM, Israel R: Gestational outcome following hysteroscopic lysis of adhesions. Fertil Steril 36:455, 1981

McDonald IA: Incompetent cervix as a cause of recurrent abortion. J Obstet Gynaecol Br Commonw 70:105, 1963

McIntyre JA, Faulk WP: Trophoblast antigens in normal and abnormal human pregnancy. Clin Obstet Gynecol 29:976, 1986

Meirik O, Nygren KG: Outcome of first delivery after 2nd trimester two-step induced abortion: Controlled historical cohort study. Acta Obstet Gynecol Scand 63:45, 1984

Michaels WH, Thompson HO, Schreiber FR, Berman JM, Ager J, Olson K: Ultrasound surveillance of the cervix during pregnancy in diethylstilbestrol-exposed offspring. Obstet Gynecol 73:230, 1989

Miller JF, Williamson E, Glue J, Gordon YB, Grudzinskas JG,

Sykes A: Fetal loss after implantation: A prospective study. Lancet 2:554, 1980

Milligan D, Brife JO, Short RV: Changes in breast volume during normal menstrual cycle and after oral contraceptives. Br Med J 4:494, 1975

Mills JL, Simpson JL, Driscoll SG, Jovanovic-Peterson L, Van Allen M, Aarons JH, Metzger B, Bieber FR, Knopp RH, Holmes LB: Incidence of spontaneous abortion among normal women and insulin-dependent diabetic women whose pregnancies were identified within 21 days of conception. N Engl J Med 319:1618, 1988

Montoro M, Collea JV, Frasier D, Mestman J: Successful outcome of pregnancy in women with hypothyroidism. Ann Intern Med 94:31, 1981

Mowbray JF, Gibbings C, Liddell H, Reginald PW, Underwood JL, Beard RW: Controlled trial of treatment of recurrent spontaneous abortion with paternal cells. Lancet 1:941, 1985

Mowbray JF, Underwood JL, Michel M, Forbes PB, Beard RW: Immunization with paternal lymphocytes in women with recurrent miscarriage. Lancet 1:680, 1987

Munsick RA: Clinical test for placenta in 300 consecutive menstrual aspirations. Obstet Gynecol 60:738, 1982

Nahmias AJ, Josey WE, Naib ZM, Freeman MG, Fernandez RJ, Wheeler JH: Perinatal risk associated with maternal genital herpes simplex virus infection. Am J Obstet Gynecol 11:825, 1971

Naib ZM, Nahmias AJ, Josey WE, Wheller JH: Association of maternal genital herpetic infection with spontaneous abortion. Obstet Gynecol 35:260, 1970

Nicolaides KH, Welch CC, Koullapis EN, Filshie GM: Cervical dilatation by Lamicel—Studies on the mechanism of action. Br J Obstet Gynaecol 90:1060, 1983

Niloff JM, Stubblefield PG: Low-dose vaginal 15 methyl prostaglandin $F_{2\alpha}$ for cervical dilatation prior to vacuum curettage abortion. Am J Obstet Gynecol 142:596, 1982

Nottage BJ, Liston WA: A review of 700 hysterectomies. Br J Obstet Gynaecol 82:310, 1975

Oksenberg JR, Persitz E, Amar A, Brautbar C: Maternal–paternal histocompatibility: Lack of association with habitual abortions. Fertil Steril 42:389, 1984

Olsen S, Tobiassen T: Transabdominal isthmic cerclage for the treatment of incompetent cervix. Acta Obstet Gynecol 61:473, 1982

Parke AL: Antiphospholipid antibody syndromes. Rheum Dis Clin North Am 15:275, 1989

Pellerito JS, Taylor KJW, Quedens-Case C, Hammers LW, Scoutt LM, Ramos IM, Meyer WR: Ectopic Pregnancy: Evaluation with endovaginal color flow imaging. Radiology 183:407, 1992

Peyser MR, Toaff R: Rupture of uterus in the first trimester caused by high-concentration oxytocin drip. Obstet Gynecol 40:371, 1972

Pilpel HF, Norwich KP: When should abortion be legal? New York, Public Affairs Committee, no. 429, 1969

Piver MS, Bolognese RJ, Feldman JD: Long-acting progesterone as a cause of missed abortion. Am J Obstet Gynecol 97:579, 1967

Poland BJ, Miller JR, Harris M, Livingston J: Spontaneous abortion: A study of 1961 women and their abortuses. Acta Obstet Gynecol Scand 102(suppl):1, 1981

Poland BJ, Miller JR, Jones DC, Trimble BK: Reproductive

counseling in patients who have had a spontaneous abortion. Am J Obstet Gynecol 127:685, 1977

Potts M: Access to mifepristone. Lancet 339:1161, 1992

Quinn PA, Petric M, Barking M, Butany J, Derzko C, Gysler M, Lie KI, Shewchuck AB, Shuber J, Ryan E, Chipman ML: Prevalence of antibody to *Chlamydia trachomatis* in spontaneous abortion and infertility. Am J Obstet Gynecol 156:291, 1987

Quinn PA, Shewchuk AB, Shuber J, Lie KI, Ryan E, Chipman ML, Nocilla DM: Efficacy of antibiotic therapy in preventing spontaneous pregnancy loss among couples colonized with genital mycoplasmas. Am J Obstet Gynecol 145:239, 1983a

Quinn PA, Shewchuk AB, Shuber J, Lie KI, Ryan E, Sheu M, Chipman ML: Serologic evidence of *Ureaplasma urealyticum* infection in women with spontaneous pregnancy loss. Am J Obstet Gynecol 145:245, 1983b

Reginald PW, Beard RW, Chapple J, Forbes PB, Liddell HS, Mowbray JF, Underwood JL: Outcome of pregnancies progressing beyond 28 weeks gestation in women with a history of recurrent miscarriage. Br J Obstet Gynaecol 94:643, 1987

Ressequie L, Hick JF, Bruen JA, Noller KL, O'Fallon WM, Kurland LT: Congenital malformations among offspring exposed in utero to progestins, Olmsted County, Minnesota, 1936–1974. Fertil Steril 43:514, 1985

Rock JA, Wentz AC, Cole KA, Kimball AW Jr, Zacur HA, Early SA, Jones GS: Fetal malformations following progesterone therapy during pregnancy: A preliminary report. Fertil Steril 44:17, 1985

Rosove MH, Tabsh K, Wasserstrum N, Howard P, Hahn BH, Kalunian KC: Heparin therapy for pregnant women with lupus anticoagulant or anticardiolipin antibodies. Obstet Gynecol 75:630, 1990

Salem HT, Ghaneimah SA, Shaaban MM, Chard T: Prognostic value of biochemical tests in the assessment of fetal outcome in threatened abortion. Br J Obstet Gynecol 91:382, 1984

Schenker JG, Margalioth EJ: Intrauterine adhesions: An updated appraisal. Fertil Steril 37:593, 1982

Schiff E, Peleg E, Goldenberg M, Rosenthal T, Ruppin E, Tamarkin M, Barkai G, Ben-Baruch G, Yahal I, Blankstein J, Goldman B, Mashiach S: The use of aspirin to prevent pregnancy-induced hypertension and lower the ratio of thromboxane A_2 to prostacyclin in relatively high risk pregnancies. N Engl J Med 321:351, 1989

Schnorr TM, Grajewski BA, Hornung RW, Thun MJ, Egeland GM, Murray WE, Conover DL, Halperin WE: Video display terminals and the risk of spontaneous abortion. N Engl J Med 324:727, 1991

Scott JR, Rote NS, Branch DW: Immunologic aspects of recurrent abortion and fetal death. Obstet Gynecol 70:645, 1987

Shirodkar VN: A new method of operative treatment for habitual abortions in the second trimester of pregnancy. Antiseptic 52:299, 1955

Short RV: Breast feeding. Sci Am 250:35, 1984

Short RV: The evolution of human reproduction. Proc R Soc Lond 195:3, 1976

Simpson JL: Genes, chromosomes, and reproductive failure. Fertil Steril 33:107, 1980

Simpson JL: Genetics. CREOG Basic Science Monograph in Obstetrics and Gynecology. Washington, DC, CREOG, 1986

Simpson JL, Mills JL, Holmes LB, Ober CL, Aarons J, Jovanovic L, Knopp RH: Low fetal loss rates after ultrasound-proved viability in early pregnancy. JAMA 258:2555, 1987

Smith C, Gregori CA, Breen JL: Ultrasonography in threatened abortion. Obstet Gynecol 51:173, 1978

Smith JW, Southern PM Jr., Lehmann JD: Bacteremia in septic abortion: Complications and treatment. Obstet Gynecol 35:704, 1970

Stabile I, Campbell S, Grudzinskas JG: Ultrasonic assessment of complications during first trimester of pregnancy. Lancet 2:1237, 1987

Stagnaro-Green A, Roman SH, Cobin RH, el-Harazy E, Alvarez-Marfany M, Davies TF: Detection of at-risk pregnancy by means of highly sensitive assays for thyroid antoantibodies. JAMA 264:1422, 1990

Stein Z, Kline J, Susser E, Shrout P, Warburton D, Susser M: Maternal age and spontaneous abortion. In Porter IH, Hook EB (eds): Human Embryonic and Fetal Death. New York, Academic Press, 1980, p 107

Stovall TG, Kellerman AL, Ling FW, Buster JE: Emergency department diagnosis of ectopic pregnancy. Ann Emerg Med 19:1098, 1990

Stovall TG, Ling FW, Carson SA, Burke JE: Serum progesterone and uterine curettage in differential diagnosis of ectopic pregnancy. Fertil Steril 57:456, 1992

Stovall TG, Ling FW, Cope BJ, Buster JE: Preventing ruptured ectopic pregnancy with a single serum progesterone. Am J Obstet Gynecol 160:1425, 1989

Stray-Pedersen B, Eng J, Reikvan TM: Uterine T-mycoplasma colonization in reproductive failure. Am J Obstet Gynecol 130:307, 1978

Stray-Pedersen B, Stray-Pedersen S: Etiologic factors and subsequent reproductive performance in 195 couples with a prior history of habitual abortion. Am J Obstet Gynecol 148:140, 1984

Supreme Court of the United States. *Planned Parenthood of Southeastern Pennsylvania v Robert P. Casey.* Opinion no. 91-744 and 91-902, June 29, 1992

Supreme Court of the United States. *William Webster v Reproductive Health Services.* Opinion no. 88-605, July 3, 1989

Supreme Court of the United States. *Jane Roe et al v Henry Wade,* District Attorney of Dallas County. Opinion no. 70-18, January 22, 1973

Sutherland HW, Pritchard CW: Increased incidence of spontaneous abortion in pregnancies complicated by maternal diabetes mellitus. Am J Obstet Gynecol 155:135, 1986

Sweeney AM, Meyer MR, Aarons JH, Mills JL, LaPorte RE: Evaluation of methods for the prospective identification of early fetal losses in environmental epidemiology studies. Am J Epidemiol 127:843, 1988

Taskinen H, Kyyrönen P, Hemminki K: Effects of ultrasound, shortwaves, and physical exertion on pregnancy outcome in physiotherapists. J Epidemiol Community Health 44:196, 1990

Taylor PV, Hancock KW: Antigenicity of trophoblast and possible antigen masking effects during pregnancy. Immunology 28:973, 1975

Thom DH, Nelson LM, Vaughan TL: Spontaneous abortion and subsequent adverse birth outcomes. Am J Obstet Gynecol 166:111, 1992

Thomas ML, Harger JH, Wagener DK, Rabin BS, Gill TJ III: HLA sharing and spontaneous abortion in humans. Am J Obstet Gynecol 151:1053, 1985

Thomason JL, Sampson MB, Beckman CR, Spellacy WN: The incompetent cervix: A 1982 update. J Reprod Med 27:187, 1982

Tietze C, Potter RG: Statistical evaluation of the rhythm method. Am J Obstet Gynecol 84:692, 1962

Von Stein GA, Munsick RA, Stiver K, Ryder K: Fetomaternal hemorrhage in threatened abortion. Obstet Gynecol 79:383, 1992

Warburton D, Fraser FC: Spontaneous abortion risks in man: Data from reproductive histories collected in a medical genetics unit. Am J Hum Genet 16:1, 1964

Warburton D, Stein Z, Kline J, Susser M: Chromosome abnormalities in spontaneous abortion: Data from the New York City study. In Porter IH, Hook EB (eds): Human Embryonic and Fetal Death. New York, Academic Press, 1980, p 261

Whittaker PG, Taylor A, Lind T: Unsuspected pregnancy loss in healthy women. Lancet 1:1126, 1983

Wilcox AJ, Weinberg CR, O'Connor JF, Baird DD, Schlatterer JP, Canfield RE, Armstrong EG, Nisula BC: Incidence of early pregnancy loss. N Engl J Med 319:189, 1988

Wilson RD, Kendrick V, Wittmann BK, McGillivray B: Spontaneous abortion and pregnancy outcome after normal first-trimester ultrasound examination. Obstet Gynecol 67:352, 1986

Witter FR: Negative sonographic findings followed by rapid cervical dilatation due to cervical incompetence. Obstet Gynecol 64:136, 1984

CHAPTER 32
Ectopic Pregnancy

The blastocyst normally implants in the endometrial lining of the uterine cavity. Implantation anywhere else is an ectopic pregnancy. More than 95 percent of ectopic pregnancies involve the oviduct, but tubal pregnancy is not synonymous with ectopic gestation. More than 1 in every 100 pregnancies in the United States is ectopic. The risk of death from an extrauterine pregnancy is 10 times greater than that for a vaginal delivery and 50 times greater than for an induced abortion (Dorfman, 1983). Moreover, prognosis for a successful subsequent pregnancy is reduced significantly in these women, especially if they are primigravid and over the age of 30. A clear understanding of the contributing factors responsible for ectopic pregnancies and of effective and modern methods for their earlier diagnosis is essential. With earlier diagnosis, both maternal survival and conservation of reproductive capacity are enhanced.

General Considerations

Etiology. Etiological factors associated with an increased incidence of ectopic pregnancy include those outlined in this section.

Mechanical Factors. Mechanical factors that prevent or retard passage of the fertilized ovum into the uterine cavity include the following.

1. *Salpingitis,* especially endosalpingitis, which causes agglutination of the arborescent folds of the tubal mucosa with narrowing of the lumen or formation of blind pockets (Brunham and colleagues, 1992; Coste and associates, 1991; Mäkinen and colleagues, 1989; Marchbanks and co-workers, 1988; Sherman and co-workers, 1990). Reduced ciliation of the tubal mucosa due to infection also may contribute to tubal implantation of the zygote.
2. *Peritubal adhesions* subsequent to postabortal or puerperal infection, appendicitis, or endometriosis (Coste and associates, 1991). These may cause kinking of the tube and narrowing of the lumen.
3. *Developmental abnormalities of the tube,* especially diverticula, accessory ostia, and hypoplasia. Such abnormalities are extremely rare but may occur following in utero exposure to diethylstilbestrol.

4. *Previous ectopic pregnancy.* After one, the chance of another is 7 to 15 percent (Brenner and colleagues, 1980; Coste and associates, 1991). The increased risk likely is due to previous salpingitis.
5. *Previous operations on the tube,* either to restore patency or, occasionally, the failure of tubal sterilization (Corson and Batzer, 1986; Coste and colleagues, 1991; Marchbanks and co-workers, 1988).
6. *Multiple previous induced abortions* may increase the risk of ectopic pregnancy. The risk is unchanged after one induced abortion; it is doubled after two induced abortions, likely due to small increases in the incidence of salpingitis (Levin and associates, 1982).
7. *Tumors that distort the tube,* such as uterine myomas and adnexal masses.
8. Tubal pregnancies are not increased by abnormal embryos (Sopelak and Bates, 1987).

Functional Factors. Functional factors that delay passage of the fertilized ovum into the uterine cavity include the following.

1. *External migration of the ovum* is probably not an important factor except in cases of abnormal müllerian development resulting in a hemiuterus with an attached noncommunicating rudimentary uterine horn (Chap. 33, p. 724). There also may be a slightly increased risk of ectopic pregnancy for the woman with one oviduct whenever she ovulates from the contralateral ovary (Sopelak and Bates, 1987).
2. *Menstrual reflux* has been suggested as a cause; however, there is little supporting evidence for this.
3. *Altered tubal motility* may follow changes in serum levels of estrogens and progesterone. A change in the number and affinity of adrenergic receptors in uterine and tubal smooth muscle is likely responsible (Jacobson and associates, 1987). The practical aspect is that an increased incidence of ectopic pregnancies has been reported with use of *progestin-only oral contraceptives* (Ory, 1981); with use of intrauterine devices (with and without progesterone) (Sivin, 1991; Tatum and Schmidt, 1977); after use of postovulatory high-dose estrogens to prevent

pregnancy ("morning after pill," see Chap. 60, p. 1335) (Morris and Van Wagenen, 1973); and after ovulation induction. There is an increased incidence of ectopic pregnancies in women who were exposed in utero to *diethylstilbestrol* (DES), possibly as a consequence of altered tubal motility rather than structural abnormalities (see Chap. 33, p. 728).

4. Cigarette smoking at the time of conception has been shown to increase the incidence of ectopic pregnancy (Coste and associates, 1991; Phillips, 1992). This probably occurs due to a change in adrenergic receptor number or affinity in tubal musculature.

Increased Receptivity of Tubal Mucosa to Fertilized Ovum. *Ectopic endometrial elements* may enhance tubal implantation. Although observers have reported foci of endometriosis in fallopian tubes, it is an uncommon finding.

Assisted Reproduction. Several forms of assisted reproduction have been reported to increase the incidence of ectopic pregnancy.

1. *Tubal pregnancy* has been reported to be increased following ovulation induction, gamete intrafallopian transfer (GIFT), and in vitro fertilization (IVF) and ovum transfer (Coste and associates, 1991; Guirgis and Craft, 1991; Marchbanks and colleagues, 1988). Herman and associates (1990) found this primarily in women with concurrent tubal disease, but McBain and associates (1980) reported ectopic gestation to be increased (12.5 percent) if urinary estrogen excretion exceeded 200 mg per day during ovulation induction with human pituitary and chorionic gonadotropin therapy.
2. *Heterotypic tubal pregnancy* is increased after in vitro fertilization and embryo transfer and ovulation induction (Bassil and associates, 1991; Dimitry and colleagues, 1990; Glassner and coworkers, 1990). *Heterotypic cervical pregnancy* is also increased following in vitro fertilization and embryo transfer (Bayati and associates, 1989).
3. *Abdominal pregnancy* has been reported following gamete intrafallopian transfer and in vitro fertilization and ovum transfer (Ferland and associates, 1991; Vignali and co-workers, 1990).
4. *Cervical pregnancy* may be increased after in vitro fertilization and embryo transfer (Bayati and associates, 1989; Weyerman and colleagues, 1989).

Failed Contraception. Failed contraception increases the incidence of ectopic pregnancies. With use of any

contraceptive, the actual number of ectopic pregnancies is decreased because pregnancy occurs less often. In contraceptive failures, however, there is an increased incidence of ectopic pregnancy following some forms of tubal sterilization and in women using intrauterine devices or taking progestin-only "minipills" (Sivin, 1991).

1. Relative risks for ectopic pregnancy overall are decreased in users of *intrauterine devices, oral contraceptives, and traditional barrier methods* compared with noncontraceptive users (Ory, 1981; Sivin, 1991).
2. Contraceptive failure following tubal *sterilization* has an ectopic pregnancy rate of 16 to 50 percent (McCausland, 1980; Tatum and Schmidt, 1977). The higher rates are seen following tubal sterilization using laparoscopic fulguration without accompanying tubal resection. McCann and Kessel (1978) also reported a 50 percent ectopic pregnancy rate after failure of tubal fulguration but only isolated cases following use of metal clips and silicon rings. With these techniques, a fistula does not form between the proximal tubal stump and the endometrial cavity. A fistula enables sperm to enter the peritoneal cavity and fertilize an ovum in the tubal ampulla. This results in a fertilized ovum trapped in the distal occluded part of the fallopian tube (Corson and Batzer, 1986; Shah and colleagues, 1977).
3. Tubal pregnancy may occasionally follow *hysterectomy.* Niebyl (1974) reviewed 21 such cases. In most instances, a recently fertilized ovum was trapped in the oviduct at the time of hysterectomy. More rarely, a fistula sufficient for passage of sperm developed between vagina and the severed end of the oviduct.

Epidemiology. There has been a marked increase in both the absolute number and rate of ectopic pregnancies in the United States in the past two decades. The actual number has increased out of proportion to population growth; in fact, it has more than quadrupled from 1970 to 1987 (Table 32–1). These rates may be calculated using three different methods:

1. Females 15 to 44 years: The number of ectopic pregnancies in women 15 to 44 years old per 10,000 females.
2. Live births: The number of ectopic pregnancies per 1000 live births.
3. Reported pregnancies: The number of ectopic pregnancies per 1000 reported pregnancies, which includes live births, legally induced abortions, and ectopic pregnancies.

Unfortunately, none of these rates is totally accurate because the numerator may be falsely low for all calcu-

TABLE 32–1. NUMBERS AND RATES OF REPORTED ECTOPIC PREGNANCIES IN THE UNITED STATES, 1970–1987

		Rates		
Year	Number[a]	Females 15–44 years[b]	Live Births[c]	Reported[d] Pregnancies
1970	17,800	—	—	4.5
1971	19,300	—	—	4.8
1972	24,500	5.5	7.5	6.3
1973	25,600	5.6	8.2	6.8
1974	26,400	5.7	8.4	6.7
1975	30,500	6.5	9.8	7.6
1976	34,600	7.2	11.0	8.3
1977	40,700	8.3	12.3	9.2
1978	42,400	8.5	12.8	9.4
1979	49,900	9.9	14.3	10.4
1980	52,200	9.9	14.5	10.5
1981	68,000	12.7	18.7	13.6
1982	61,800	11.5	17.0	12.3
1983	69,600	12.6	19.2	14.0
1984	75,400	13.6	20.6	14.9
1985	78,400	14.0	20.9	15.2
1986	73,700	—	—	14.3
1987	88,000	—	—	16.8
Total	877,400[e]	9.0	13.0	10.7

[a] Rounded to nearest hundred.
[b] Rate per 10,000 females.
[c] Rate per 1000 live births.
[d] Rate per 1000 reported pregnancies (live births, legally induced abortions, and ectopic pregnancies).
[e] Because of rounding, total differs from the sum of the numbers.
From Centers for Disease Control (1988); and Nederlof and associates (1990).

lations. For example, the number of ectopic pregnancies may be underestimated because the National Hospital Discharge Survey, from which these numbers are derived, does not include figures from federal hospitals. Also, an unknown number of ectopic pregnancies resolve spontaneously and thus are undiagnosed. Ectopic pregnancies certainly occur in women younger than 15 and older than 44. The denominator is falsely low in rates reported per live births, because stillbirth rates are not considered. Finally, the rate per reported pregnancies is an underestimate because it does not include stillbirths and spontaneous abortions, and likely does include an incorrect estimate of legal abortions. Regardless of the method used to calculate rates, all have increased three- to fourfold during the past 2 decades (Stock, 1988).

Care must be taken to insure that the rate method chosen to express a concept is not misinterpreted. For example, the rate using women 15 to 44 years of age as a denominator can be used as a public health device to estimate the magnitude of the problem in reproductive age women. This method should not be used, however, to ascertain risk factors for individual women because the denominator does not clearly define the population at risk. This is especially true when age as a risk factor is considered. For example, women 35 years and older are less likely to become pregnant than younger women. If

the denominator includes women who will not become pregnant, the ectopic pregnancy rate must fall and the true effect of increasing age on the incidence of ectopic pregnancy is lost! This is illustrated in Table 32–2, in which numbers and rates of ectopic pregnancies by age group using two different methods of calculation are listed. The increased incidence of ectopic pregnancy in older women also has been reported in Great Britain by Beral (1975) and in Sweden by Weström and associates (1981). Rates are expressed most often using the rate per 1000 reported pregnancies method.

The incidence of ectopic pregnancy is increased in nonwhite compared with white women (Table 32–3). Furthermore, rates for nonwhite women are higher in every age category than for whites, and this disparity increases with age. The combined factors of race and increasing age are at least additive. For example, nonwhite women 35 to 44 years were five times more likely to have an ectopic pregnancy than a white woman aged 15 to 24 years. Overall, in 1987 a nonwhite woman had a 1.4 times increased risk for ectopic pregnancy compared with a white woman (Nederlof and associates, 1990).

Thus, from 1970 through 1987, ectopic pregnancies rates in the United States increased by a factor of 4.9 (Table 32–1). This marked increase was greater for nonwhite than white women, and for both racial groups, the incidence increased with age (Ory, 1992). In 35- to 44-year-old white women, 1.75 of every 100 pregnancies was ectopic; this figure was 2.05 for nonwhite women. At Parkland Hospital, where the majority of obstetrical patients are less than 25 years old, the incidence of ectopic pregnancy has more than doubled in the past decade. At Magee-Womens Hospital, the incidence increased 3.7-fold from 1965 through 1985 (Stock, 1988).

Causes for Increased Rates of Ectopic Pregnancy. The reasons for increases in ectopic pregnancies in the United States are not entirely clear; however, similar increases have been reported from Eastern Europe, Scandinavia, and Great Britain (Tuomivaara and associ-

TABLE 32–2. NUMBERS AND RATES OF ECTOPIC PREGNANCY FOR THE UNITED STATES 1970–1978, EXPRESSED BY TWO CALCULATION METHODS

Age (yr)	No.	Rate per 1000 Reported Pregnancies[a]	Rate per 10,000 Women Aged 15–44 Years
15–24	92,400	4.5	5.3
25–34	138,700	9.7	10.3
35–44	30,600	15.2	2.9
Total	261,600	7.1	6.3

[a] Reported pregnancies include live births, legally induced abortions, and ectopic pregnancies.
Modified from Rubin and co-workers (1983).

TABLE 32–3. NUMBERS AND RATES OF ECTOPIC PREGNANCIES, BY RACE AND AGE GROUP, UNITED STATES 1970–1987

Race[a]	Age Group (yrs)	Number[b]	Rate[c]
White	15–44	620,600	9.7
	15–24	188,200	5.8
	25–34	367,700	13.1
	35–44	64,600	17.5
Black and other	15–44	256,800	14.2
	15–24	82,600	7.7
	25–34	142,400	22.2
	35–44	31,700	29.4
All races	15–44	877,400	10.7
	15–24	270,800	6.3
	25–34	510,200	15.0
	35–44	96,300	20.5

[a] Race "unknown" redistributed according to the percentage of race known. Redistribution and rounding sometimes cause the sum of individual cells not to equal the total.
[b] Rounded to the nearest hundred.
[c] Rate per 1000 pregnancies (live births, legally induced abortions, and ectopic pregnancies).
From Nederlof and associates (1990).

ates, 1986; Weström and co-workers, 1981). Although the reasons for this increase are multiple, some likely causes include (1) increased prevalence of sexually transmitted tubal infection (Brunham and associates, 1992; Maccato and colleagues, 1992); (2) popularity of contraception that prevents intrauterine but not extra-uterine pregnancies, that is, intrauterine devices and low-dose progestational agents; (3) unsuccessful tubal sterilizations; (4) induced abortion followed by infection; (5) assisted reproductive techniques; (6) previous pelvic surgery including salpingotomy for previous tubal pregnancy and tuboplasty; (7) exposure to DES in utero; and (8) better and earlier diagnostic techniques.

The reasons for the disproportionately increased incidence of ectopic pregnancies in nonwhite women is also not known. Possible explanations include the following: (1) health care is less available or acceptable to nonwhite women compared with white women (Atrash and colleagues, 1987b, 1990a), and (2) sexually transmitted diseases are reported more frequently in nonwhite compared with white women (Washington and associates, 1984).

Mortality. Deaths from ectopic pregnancy in the United States decreased from 63 in 1970, to 46 in 1980, and to 30 in 1987. Unfortunately, the percentage of all maternal deaths attributed to ectopic pregnancy increased from 8 percent in 1970 to 12 percent in 1987 (Atrash and colleagues, 1987b, 1991a, 1990b). From 1970 through 1987, 772 women died from ectopic pregnancies. The case–fatality rate, however, decreased 95 percent, from 35.5 per 10,000 ectopic pregnancies in 1970 to 3.4 per 10,000 in 1987 (Table 32–4). Moreover, the

fall in actual deaths and in mortality rates occurred in both white and nonwhite women (Atrash and co-workers, 1991a, 1990b; Nederlof and associates, 1990). This decline is remarkable in view of the increased incidence that occurred during the same time. Unfortunately, a nonwhite woman still has a 1.8 times greater chance of dying from an ectopic pregnancy compared with a white woman, and the highest mortality rate is in 15- to 19-year-old nonwhite women (Nederlof and colleagues, 1990). **Ectopic pregnancy remains the second leading case of maternal mortality in the United States** (Atrash and colleagues, 1991a, 1990b).

The dramatic decrease in deaths from ectopic pregnancies (Table 32–4) is probably due to improved diagnosis and management. Still, Dorfman and colleagues (1984) estimated that the death rate from ectopic pregnancies might be reduced another 50 percent by even more prompt diagnosis and treatment. They emphasized that another third of deaths might be prevented if the woman sought earlier care. In this carefully done analysis of ectopic mortalities in 1979 and 1980, they reported that 85 percent of women died from hemorrhage. Massive hemorrhage was often the result of abdominal and interstitial tubal pregnancies, which were likely to become symptomatic later in gestation and consequently have increased blood supply. The remaining major causes of death were infection in 5 percent and anesthesia complications in 2 percent. A more appalling consideration is the markedly high mortality rate in 15- to 19-year-old

TABLE 32–4. NUMBERS OF DEATHS DUE TO ECTOPIC PREGNANCY AND CASE–FATALITY RATES, BY RACE AND YEAR, UNITED STATES 1970–1987

Year	Number White	Number Black and Other	Number Total	Rate[a] White	Rate[a] Black and Other	Rate[a] Total
1970	28	35	63	21.7	72.1	35.5
1971	21	40	61	15.1	74.9	31.7
1972	28	20	48	16.2	27.7	19.6
1973	25	21	46	15.1	23.4	18.0
1974	20	31	51	10.1	47.0	19.4
1975	19	31	50	8.8	34.9	16.4
1976	11	28	39	4.4	28.7	11.3
1977	15	29	44	5.2	24.5	10.8
1978	13	24	37	4.4	18.7	8.7
1979	20	25	45	5.7	17.2	9.0
1980	22	24	46	6.0	15.4	8.8
1981	15	19	34	3.1	9.7	5.0
1982	19	24	43	3.8	19.3	7.0
1983	17	20	37	3.3	11.2	5.3
1984	14	15	29	2.7	10.8	5.2
1985	11	22	33	2.1	8.4	4.2
1986	17	19	36	3.3	7.6	4.9
1987	17	13	30	2.6	4.8	3.4
Total	332	440	772	5.3	17.5	8.9

[a] Deaths from ectopic pregnancy per 10,000 ectopic pregnancies.
From Nederlof and associates (1990).

nonwhite women (Nederlof and colleagues, 1990). This almost certainly is due in part to their lack of early prenatal care.

Anatomical Considerations. The fertilized ovum may develop in any portion of the oviduct, giving rise to *ampullary, isthmic, and interstitial tubal pregnancies* (see Fig. 3–18). In rare instances, the fertilized ovum may be implanted in the fimbriated extremity and occasionally even on the fimbria ovarica. The ampulla is the most frequent site of implantation and the isthmus the next most common. Interstitial pregnancy is very uncommon, occurring in only about 3 percent of all tubal gestations. From these primary types, certain secondary forms of tubo-abdominal, tubo-ovarian, and broad ligament pregnancies occasionally develop.

Zygote Implantation. The fertilized ovum does not remain on the surface but promptly burrows through the epithelium. As the zygote penetrates the epithelium, it comes to lie in the muscular wall, because the tube lacks a submucosa. At the periphery of the zygote is a capsule of rapidly proliferating trophoblast, which invades and erodes the subjacent muscularis. At the same time, maternal blood vessels are opened, and blood pours into the spaces, lying within the trophoblast or between it and the adjacent tissue.

The tube normally does not form an extensive decidua, although decidual cells usually can be recognized. Tubal wall in contact with the zygote offers only slight resistance to invasion by the trophoblast, which soon burrows through it, opening maternal vessels (Fig. 32–1). The embryo or fetus in an ectopic pregnancy is often absent or stunted.

Uterine Changes. In ectopic pregnancy, the uterus undergoes some of the changes associated with normal early pregnancy, including softening of the cervix and isthmus and an increase in size. Even so, of 1125 women with a proven ectopic pregnancy, 75 percent had a normal-sized uterus (Stabile and Grudzinskas, 1990). *These changes in the uterus do not exclude an ectopic pregnancy.*

The degree to which the endometrium is converted to decidua is variable. The finding of uterine decidua without trophoblast suggests ectopic pregnancy but is not an absolute indication. In 1954, Arias-Stella described, as had others before him, these changes in endometrium: Epithelial cells are enlarged and their nuclei are hypertrophic, hyperchromatic, lobular, and irregularly shaped. There is a loss of polarity, and abnormal nuclei tend to occupy the luminal portion of the cells. Cytoplasm may be vacuolated and foamy, and occasional mitoses are found. These endometrial changes have been collectively referred to as the *Arias-Stella reaction.* These cellular changes are not specific for ectopic pregnancy and also may occur with intrauterine gestations.

External bleeding, which is seen commonly in cases of tubal pregnancy, is uterine in origin and associated with degeneration and sloughing of the uterine decidua; hemorrhage is seldom severe. Soon after death of the fetus, the decidua degenerates and is usually shed in small pieces, but occasionally it is cast off intact, as a *decidual cast* of the uterine cavity. Absence of decidual tissue, however, does not exclude an ectopic pregnancy. Romney and co-workers (1950) identified secretory endometrium in 40 percent of cases of ectopic pregnancy, proliferative in 30 percent, and menstrual in 6 percent, while decidua was present in only 20 percent.

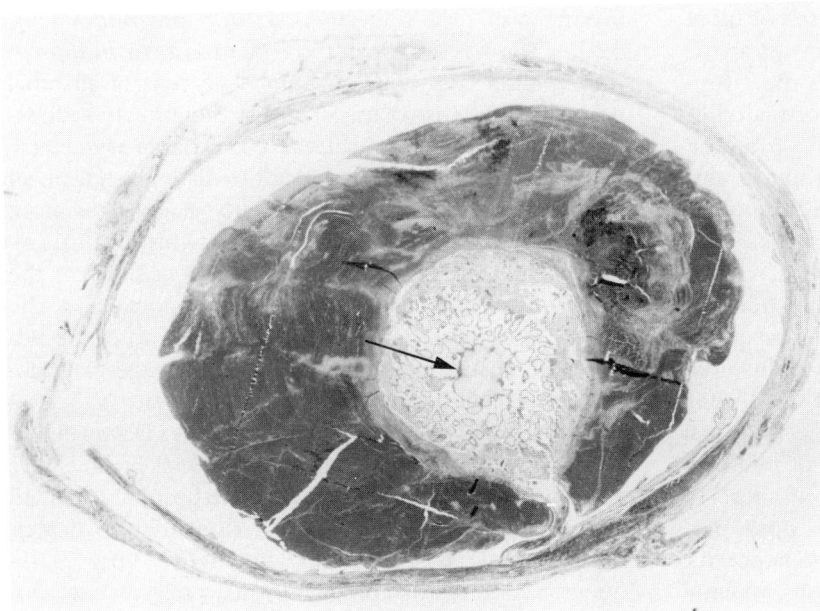

Fig. 32–1. Early tubal pregnancy. Amnionic sac (*arrow*) is surrounded by chorionic villi, which in turn are encased in blood clot. (Courtesy of Dr. Richard Voet.)

Natural History of Tubal Pregnancy

Tubal Abortion. A common termination of tubal pregnancy is separation of the conceptus from the implantation site and extrusion through the fimbriated end of the oviduct. The frequency of tubal abortion depends in part upon the site of implantation. Tubal abortion is common in ampullary tubal pregnancy, whereas rupture of the tube is the usual outcome with isthmic pregnancy. The immediate consequence of hemorrhage with tubal abortion is further disruption of the connection between the placenta and membranes and the tubal wall. If placental separation is complete, all of the products of conception may be extruded through the fimbriated end into the peritoneal cavity. At this point, hemorrhage may cease and symptoms disappear.

In cases of complete tubal abortion, when the zygote is retained within the oviduct and hemorrhage is moderate, the abortus may become infiltrated with blood and converted into a structure analogous to the blood mole observed in uterine abortion. Some bleeding usually persists as long as the products of conception remain in the oviduct, and blood slowly trickles from the tubal fimbria into the peritoneal cavity and typically pools in the rectouterine cul-de-sac. If the fimbriated extremity is occluded, the fallopian tube may gradually become distended by blood, forming a *hematosalpinx.*

After incomplete tubal abortion, pieces of the placenta or membranes may remain attached to the tubal wall and, after becoming surrounded by fibrin, give rise to a *placental polyp.* The process is similar to that which occurs in the uterus after an incomplete abortion.

Tubal Rupture. The invading, expanding products of conception may rupture the oviduct at any of several sites. Before sophisticated methods to measure chorionic gonadotropin were available, many cases of tubal pregnancy ended during the first trimester by intraperitoneal rupture. As a rule, whenever there is tubal rupture in the first few weeks, the pregnancy is situated in the isthmic portion of the tube a short distance from the cornu of the uterus. When the fertilized ovum is implanted well within the interstitial portion of the tube, rupture usually occurs later.

The immediate cause of rupture may be trauma associated with coitus or a bimanual examination, although in most cases rupture occurs spontaneously. With intraperitoneal rupture, the entire conceptus may be extruded from the tube, or if the rent is small, profuse hemorrhage may occur without extrusion. In either event, the woman commonly shows signs of collapse from hemorrhage and hypovolemia. Without surgery, the fate of the embryo or fetus will depend upon placental damage sustained during the rupture and upon its age. If an early conceptus is expelled essentially undamaged into the peritoneal cavity, it may reimplant almost anywhere, establish adequate circulation, survive, and grow. This outcome is most unlikely, however, because of damage during the transition. The conceptus, if small, may be resorbed or, if larger, may remain in the cul-de-sac for years as an encapsulated mass or even become calcified to form a *lithopedion.*

Abdominal Pregnancy. If only the fetus is extruded at the time of rupture, the effect upon the pregnancy will vary depending on the extent of injury sustained by the placenta. If the placenta is damaged appreciably, fetal death is inevitable; but if the greater portion of the placenta retains its attachment to the tube, further development is possible. The fetus may then survive for some time, giving rise to an *abdominal pregnancy.* Typically, in such cases, a portion of the placenta remains attached to the tubal wall and the periphery grows beyond the tube and implants on surrounding structures. Abdominal pregnancy is discussed later in the chapter.

Broad Ligament Pregnancy. When the original implantation of the zygote is toward the mesosalpinx, rupture may occur at the portion of the tube not immediately covered by peritoneum, and the contents of the gestational sac may be extruded into a space formed between the folds of the broad ligament. This condition is designated an intraligamentous or *broad ligament pregnancy.* It may terminate in fetal death and formation of a *broad ligament hematoma,* or the pregnancy may continue. Occasionally, the broad ligament sac ruptures at a later period, and the fetus is extruded into the peritoneal cavity while the placenta retains its position, forming an abdominal pregnancy.

Interstitial Pregnancy. Implantation of the fertilized ovum within the segment of tube that penetrates the uterine wall results in an *interstitial pregnancy* (Fig. 32–2). This has also been referred to as a *cornual pregnancy.* They account for about 3 percent of all tubal gestations. Because of the site of implantation, no adnexal mass is palpable; instead, there is variable asymmetry of the uterus that is often difficult to distinguish from an intrauterine pregnancy. Hence, early diagnosis is more frequently overlooked than in other types of tubal implantation. Because of the greater distensibility of the myometrium covering the interstitial portion of the tube, rupture occurs later, between the end of the 8th and 16th gestational weeks. The hemorrhage may rapidly prove fatal because the implantation site is located between the ovarian and uterine arteries (Dorfman and associates, 1984). In fact, tubal pregnancies in which the woman dies before she can reach the hospital often fall into this group. Because of the large uterine defect, hysterectomy is commonly necessary. Very infrequently, an interstitial pregnancy may convert to a tubo-uterine pregnancy, as described below.

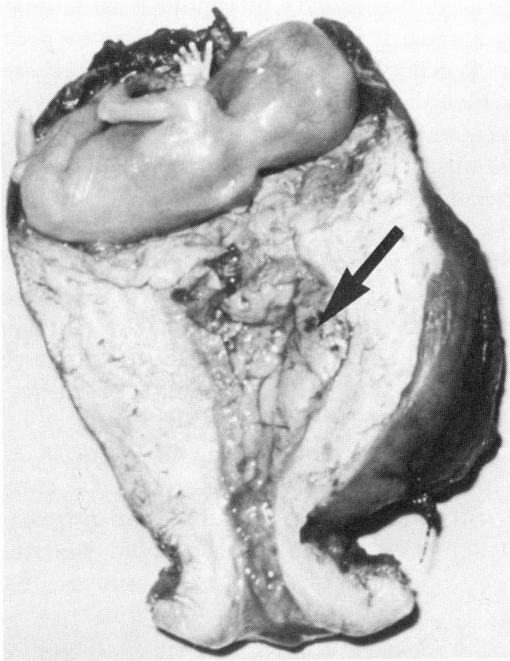

Fig. 32–2. Right interstitial tubal pregnancy. Fetus weighed 55 g and measured 90 mm crown to rump (14 to 15 weeks gestational age). Note abundant decidua (*arrow*) filling the uterine cavity. The patient sought medical help because of sudden severe abdominal pain with syncope following intercourse. Hysterectomy and 2000 mL blood transfusion were necessary.

Multifetal Ectopic Pregnancy

Heterotypic Ectopic Pregnancy. Tubal pregnancy may be complicated by a coexisting intrauterine gestation, a condition designated as *heterotypic pregnancy.* A heterotypic pregnancy is quite difficult to diagnose clinically. Typically, laparotomy is performed because of a tubal pregnancy. At the same time, the uterus is congested, softened, and somewhat enlarged. Although these features are suggestive of intrauterine pregnancy, they are commonly induced by a tubal pregnancy alone. Gestational products are ultrasonically demonstrable within the uterine cavity in practically all instances of heterotypic pregnancy.

Until recently, heterotypic pregnancies have been considered to be rare, that is, 1 per 30,000 intrauterine pregnancies (Glassner and associates, 1990). Today, in the general population, the incidence is likely 1 in 7000; and following ovulation induction, the incidence may be as high as 1 in 900 (Glassner and associates, 1990). In vitro fertilization and embryo transfer also increases the incidence (Bassil and associates, 1991; Dimitry and colleagues, 1990; Glassner and co-workers, 1990). Probably the ultimate example of a heterotypic pregnancy was an unfortunate woman described by Funderburk (1974) who had an ectopic pregnancy in the right and left fallopian tubes as well as an in utero fetus!

A heterotypic pregnancy is more likely, and should be considered (1) after assisted reproduction techniques; (2) with persistent or rising chorionic gonadotropin levels after dilation and curettage for an induced or spontaneous abortion; (3) when the uterine fundus is larger than menstrual dates; (4) with more than one corpus luteum; (5) with absence of vaginal bleeding in the presence of signs and symptoms of an ectopic pregnancy; and (6) when there is ultrasound evidence of uterine and extrauterine pregnancy (Kouyoumdjian and Kirkpatrick, 1990; Nugent, 1992). If such precautions are not observed, maternal mortality is increased appreciably. For example, Atrash and associates (1990b) reported that from 1972 through 1985, the death-to-case rate for ectopic pregnancies concurrent with induced abortion was 1.3 times higher than that for women not undergoing abortion.

Cervical heterotypic pregnancy was reported by Bayati and associates (1989) after in vitro fertilization and transcervical transfer of six embryos. Two apparent intrauterine sacs were identified sonographically, but one sac ultimately proved to be a cervical pregnancy.

Multifetal Ectopic Pregnancy. Twin tubal pregnancy has been reported with both embryos in the same tube, as well as with one in each tube. Arey (1923) concluded that single-ovum twins result in a far greater proportion of tubal than uterine pregnancies. He postulated that difficulties in migration and implantation retarded the growth of the zygote, which was somehow stimulated to form two identical embryos. Simultaneous pregnancy in both fallopian tubes is the rarest form of double-ovum twinning. *Quadruplet tubal pregnancy* in the same oviduct was described by Fujii and associates (1981). The ruptured oviduct contained four amnionic sacs covered by a single chorion, and the sacs contained embryos of widely different sizes.

Tubo-Uterine, Tubo-Abdominal, and Tubo-Ovarian Pregnancies. A tubo-uterine pregnancy results from the gradual extension into the uterine cavity of products of conception that originally implanted in the interstitial portion of the tube. Tubo-abdominal pregnancy is derived from a tubal pregnancy in which the zygote, originally implanted in the neighborhood of the fimbriated end of the tube, gradually extends into the peritoneal cavity. In such circumstances, the portion of the fetal sac projecting into the peritoneal cavity may form troublesome adhesions to surrounding organs. As a result, removal of the sac is much more difficult. Both of these conditions are very uncommon.

A *tubo-ovarian* pregnancy occurs when the fetal sac is adherent partly to tubal and partly to ovarian tissue. Such cases arise from the development of the zygote in a tubo-ovarian cyst or in a tube, the fimbriated extremity of which was adherent to the ovary at the time of fertilization or became so soon thereafter. Rarely, the fetus and placenta may achieve appreciable size before rupture occurs.

Clinical and Laboratory Features of Tubal Pregnancy

General Considerations. Clinical manifestations of a tubal pregnancy are diverse and depend on whether rupture has occurred. Commonly the woman believes she is normally pregnant or believes she is aborting an intrauterine pregnancy. Less often, she does not suspect she is pregnant. In "classical" cases, normal menstruation is replaced by variably delayed slight vaginal bleeding, which usually is referred to as "spotting." Suddenly, the woman is stricken with severe lower abdominal pain, frequently described as sharp, stabbing, or tearing in character. Vasomotor disturbances develop, ranging from vertigo to syncope. Abdominal palpation reveals tenderness, and vaginal examination, especially motion of the cervix, causes exquisite pain. The posterior fornix of the vagina may bulge because of blood in the cul-de-sac, or a tender, boggy mass may be felt to one side of the uterus. Symptoms of diaphragmatic irritation, characterized by pain in the neck or shoulder especially on inspiration, develop in perhaps 50 percent of women in whom there is sizable intraperitoneal hemorrhage. This is caused by intraperitoneal blood irritating cervical sensory nerves that supply the inferior surface of the diaphragm. The woman may or may not be hypotensive while lying supine. If she is not hypotensive when supine, she may become so when placed in a sitting position.

The diagnosis in such cases is not difficult to make. Even though symptoms and signs of ectopic pregnancy often range from indefinite to bizarre, more women are seeking medical care before the classical clinical picture develops. *The physician must make every reasonable effort to diagnose the condition before catastrophic events occur, but the task may not be simple.* The following symptoms, signs, and laboratory studies should be evaluated carefully.

Symptoms and Signs

Pain. The most frequently experienced symptoms of ectopic pregnancy are pelvic and abdominal pain (95 percent) and amenorrhea with some degree of vaginal spotting or bleeding (60 to 80 percent). Dorfman and associates (1984) also emphasized the importance of gastrointestinal symptoms (80 percent) and dizziness or light-headedness (58 percent). Symptoms are variable in their incidence of appearance due to the rate and extent of hemorrhage as well as the delay in diagnosis.

Pain may be anywhere in the abdomen. With a large hemoperitoneum, pleuritic chest pain may occur from diaphragmatic irritation. It has been assumed that abdominal pain associated with rupture of an ectopic pregnancy is caused by escape of blood into the peritoneal cavity. Pritchard and Adams (1957) observed that 500 mL of blood introduced into the peritoneal cavity most often caused abdominal tenderness, moderate intestinal distention, and especially pain in the top of the shoulder and the side of the neck from diaphragmatic irritation.

Amenorrhea. The absence of a missed menstrual period does not exclude tubal pregnancy. A history of amenorrhea is not obtained in a quarter or more of cases. Thus, the woman may mistake the uterine bleeding that frequently occurs with tubal pregnancy for a true menstrual period. This important source of diagnostic error can be eliminated in many cases by a carefully obtained menstrual history. It is extremely important that the character of the last menstrual period be elicited in detail with respect to time of onset, duration, and amount of bleeding, and it is advisable to ask whether it impressed her as abnormal in any way.

Vaginal Spotting or Bleeding. As long as placental endocrine function persists, uterine bleeding is usually absent; but when endocrine support for the endometrium declines, uterine mucosa bleeds. Bleeding is usually scanty, dark brown, and may be intermittent or continuous. Although profuse vaginal bleeding is suggestive of an incomplete abortion rather than an ectopic gestation, such bleeding can occur with tubal gestations.

Abdominal and Pelvic Pain. Exquisite tenderness on abdominal palpation and vaginal examination, especially on *motion of the cervix,* is demonstrable in over three fourths of women with ruptured or rupturing tubal pregnancies. However, such tenderness may be absent prior to rupture.

Uterine Changes. Because of placental hormones, in about one fourth of cases, the uterus grows during the first 3 months of a tubal gestation to nearly the same size as it would with an intrauterine pregnancy (Stabile and Grudzinskas, 1990). Its consistency, too, is similar as long as the fetus is alive. The uterus may be pushed to one side by an ectopic mass, or if the broad ligament is filled with blood, the uterus may be greatly displaced. Uterine casts (decidual casts) are passed by only 5 to 10 percent of women. Their passage may be accompanied by cramps similar to those with a spontaneous abortion.

Blood Pressure and Pulse. Early responses to moderate hemorrhage may range from no change in pulse and blood pressure to a slight rise in blood pressure, or a vasovagal response with bradycardia and hypotension. In a healthy young woman with an extrauterine pregnancy, blood pressure will fall and pulse rise only if bleeding continues and hypovolemia becomes intense.

Hypovolemia. There are two simple means for detecting significant hypovolemia before development of hypovolemic shock. The first is to compare blood pressure and pulse rates in the sitting and supine positions. A distinct decrease in blood pressure and rise in pulse rate in the sitting position are indicative of a sizable decrease in circulatory volume. Unfortunately, such changes may not develop until there is serious hypovolemia.

With the second method, urine flow is monitored carefully. Hypovolemia, in the absence of potent diuretic treatment, often causes oliguria before overt hypotension develops. The diagnosis and treatment of obstetrical hemorrhage are considered in detail in Chapter 37. Stabile and Grudzinskas (1990) reviewed several reports totalling almost 2400 women with surgically confirmed ectopic pregnancy. Almost one fourth presented in shock, but this ranged from 1 to 50 percent in various series.

Temperature. After acute hemorrhage, the temperature may be normal or even low. Temperatures up to 38° C may develop, but higher temperatures are rare in the absence of infection. Fever is important, therefore, in distinguishing a ruptured tubal pregnancy from acute salpingitis.

Pelvic Mass. A pelvic mass is palpable in about 20 percent of patients and varies in size, consistency, and position, ranging as a rule between 5 and 15 cm in diameter. Such masses are often soft and elastic. With extensive infiltration of blood into the tubal wall, however, the mass may be firm. It is almost always either posterior or lateral to the uterus. Pain and tenderness often preclude identification of the mass by palpation.

Pelvic Hematocele. Often there is gradual disintegration of the tubal wall followed by slow leakage of blood into the tubal lumen, the peritoneal cavity, or both. Signs of active hemorrhage are absent, and even mild symptoms may subside, but gradually the trickling blood collects in the pelvis, more or less walled off by adhesions, and a pelvic hematocele results. In some cases, the hematocele is eventually absorbed, and the patient recovers without operation. In others, it may rupture into the peritoneal cavity, or it may become infected and form an abscess. Most commonly, however, the hematocele causes continued discomfort, and the physician is finally consulted weeks or even months after the original rupture.

Laboratory Tests. Measurement of hemoglobin, hematocrit, and leukocyte count, as well as pregnancy tests and progesterone, are useful in certain cases if their *limitations* are understood.

Hemoglobin and Hematocrit. After hemorrhage, depleted blood volume is restored toward normal by hemodilution over the course of a few days. Even after a substantive hemorrhage, therefore, hemoglobin or hematocrit readings may at first show only a slight reduction. For the first few hours after an acute hemorrhage, a decrease in hemoglobin or hematocrit level while the patient is under observation is a more valuable index of blood loss than is the initial reading. This is true unless the initial reading is low and the anemia is normocytic. A normocytic anemia in this case is characteristic of recent blood loss. If the bleeding stops and the shed erythrocytes are free in the peritoneal cavity, reabsorption may help repair the anemia over several days. Hyperbilirubinemia usually does not develop (Pritchard and Adams, 1957).

Leukocyte Count. The leukocyte count varies considerably in ruptured ectopic pregnancy. In about half the patients, it is normal, but in the remainder, varying degrees of leukocytosis up to 30,000/μL may occur.

Pregnancy Tests. Ectopic pregnancy cannot be diagnosed by a positive pregnancy test alone. The key issue, however, is whether the woman is pregnant. In virtually all cases of ectopic gestation, chorionic gonadotropin will be detected in serum, but usually at markedly reduced concentrations compared with normal pregnancy. The problem then is how to detect this marker of pregnancy in the most clinically efficacious manner.

URINARY PREGNANCY TESTS. These most often are latex agglutination inhibition slide tests with sensitivities for chorionic gonadotropin in the range of 500 to 800 mIU/mL. Their ease of use and rapidity is offset by their small chance of being positive (50 to 60 percent) in a woman with an ectopic pregnancy (Barnes and associates, 1985). Even when tube-type tests are used (hemagglutination inhibition or latex agglutination inhibition), detection of the β-subunit of human chorionic gonadotropin (β-hCG) is within the 150 to 250 mIU/mL range, and the test is positive only in 80 to 85 percent of ectopic pregnancies. Tests using enzyme-linked immunosorbent assays (ELISA) are sensitive to 10 to 50 mIU/mL, and are positive in 90 to 96 percent of women with ectopic pregnancies (Barnes and associates, 1985; Cartwright and colleagues, 1986). These tests also have the advantages of rapidity and easy performance.

SERUM CHORIONIC GONADOTROPIN ASSAYS (β-hCG). Serum radioimmunoassay for β-hCG is the most precise method, and virtually any pregnancy event can be detected. In fact, because of the sensitivity of this assay, a pregnancy may be confirmed before there are pathological changes in the fallopian tube. Yaffe and associates (1979) first reported such an event in a woman 5 days overdue for a menstrual period who developed pelvic pain and in whom serum chorionic gonadotropin was detected. At laparoscopy no lesion was seen; however, when laparoscopy was repeated 7 days later, there was an ampullary pregnancy.

For practical purposes, absence of pregnancy can be established only when there is a negative test for serum chorionic gonadotropin with an assay sensitivity of 5 to 10 mIU/mL. Alternatively, a single positive pregnancy test does not exclude an ectopic pregnancy. Because of this, several different methods utilizing serial quantitative serum β-hCG values alone or in combination with sonography have been developed to establish the diagnosis of an extrauterine pregnancy.

Serum Progesterone. As previously noted, a single serum chorionic gonadotropin value cannot be used to establish or exclude a diagnosis of ectopic pregnancy because, most often, the precise duration of gestation is unknown. Because of this, several investigators have measured progesterone values in order to establish a diagnosis of normal pregnancy. Unfortunately, once again, a single hormone level cannot be used to confirm or exclude an ectopic pregnancy. Serum progesterone values, however, can often be used to establish that there is an abnormal pregnancy, that is, either an incomplete abortion or an ectopic pregnancy.

Yeko and associates (1987) and Mathews and colleagues (1986), in *retrospective* studies, reported that all ectopic pregnancies had serum progesterone values less than 15 ng/mL, and all live pregnancies had progesterone values of 20 ng/mL or higher. Stovall and co-workers (1989b, 1990a, 1992b) concluded that only about 1 percent of abnormal pregnancies (spontaneous incomplete abortions and ectopic pregnancies) are associated with a serum progesterone equal to or greater than 25 ng/mL. They also concluded that serum progesterone should be used only as a screening test for abnormal pregnancy. That is, a serum progesterone of less than 5 ng/mL only identifies a nonviable pregnancy, but it does not identify the location (uterine or ectopic). Hahlin and co-workers (1990) reported that no intrauterine pregnancy had progesterone levels less than 10 ng/mL, while 88 percent of ectopic pregnancies and 83 percent of spontaneous abortions had lower values. At Parkland Hospital, we have found serum progesterone values to be of little practical value; however, they might be useful if the uterus appears empty using vaginal sonography, and the quantitative β-hCG value is less than 2000 mIU/mL (see pp. 702, 703). Peterson and colleagues (1992) also have found serum progesterone values to be of little clinical use. A possible exception to these observations might be an abdominal pregnancy where, at least in late pregnancy, normal values have been observed for a variety of protein and steroid hormones, including progesterone (see p. 711).

Other Diagnostic Aids. A variety of diagnostic aids have been utilized. These include sonography, the combination of sonography and serial quantitative serum

β-hCG determinations, culdocentesis, curettage, colpotomy, laparoscopy, and laparotomy. **The essential diagnostic step in the identification of a suspected ectopic pregnancy is to establish or exclude the diagnosis of pregnancy.** If a sensitive pregnancy test such as an ELISA is positive, the diagnosis of pregnancy is established. A negative radioimmunoassay for serum β-hCG is required to exclude pregnancy.

Sonography

ABDOMINAL SONOGRAPHY. Identification of products of conception in the fallopian tube is difficult using abdominal sonography. If a gestational sac is clearly identified within the uterine cavity, it is unlikely an ectopic pregnancy coexists (see heterotypic pregnancy, p. 697). Moreover, with sonographic absence of an intrauterine pregnancy, a positive pregnancy test, fluid in the cul-de-sac, and an abnormal pelvic mass, ectopic pregnancy is almost certain (Robinson and associates, 1985; Romero and associates, 1988). Unfortunately, ultrasonic findings suggestive of early intrauterine pregnancy may be apparent in some cases of ectopic pregnancy. The sonographic appearance of a small sac (very early pregnancy) or a collapsed sac (dead fetus) may actually be a blood clot or decidual cast (Coleman and colleagues, 1985). The presence of an intrauterine pregnancy is usually not recognized using abdominal real-time ultrasound until 5 to 6 menstrual weeks (Coleman and colleagues, 1985) or 28 days after timed ovulation (Batzer and co-workers, 1983). Conversely, demonstration of an adnexal or cul-de-sac mass by sonography is not necessarily helpful. Corpus luteum cysts and matted bowel sometimes look like tubal pregnancies sonographically. Identification with real-time sonography of fetal heart action clearly outside the uterine cavity, however, provides firm evidence of an ectopic pregnancy (Fig. 32–3).

VAGINAL SONOGRAPHY. According to most investigators, vaginal compared with abdominal sonography is a more sensitive and specific technique to diagnose ectopic pregnancy (Bernaschek, 1988; Cacciatore, 1990a, b; de Crespigny, 1988; Nyberg, 1988; Timor-Tritsch, 1989; and their co-workers). With vaginal sonography, identification of both ovaries allows the operator to exclude conditions such as ovarian cysts or endometriomas and to detect directly tubal pathology. Nevertheless, even vaginal sonography can be misleading, and ectopic pregnancies can be missed when a tubal mass still is small or obscured by bowel. This happens in up to 10 percent of cases (Cacciatore and colleagues, 1990a).

Vaginal sonography results in earlier and more specific diagnoses of intrauterine pregnancy. The diagnostic criteria include identification of a 1 to 3 mm or larger gestational sac, eccentrically placed in the uterus, and surrounded by a decidual-chorionic reaction. A fetal pole within the gestational sac is diagnostic, especially

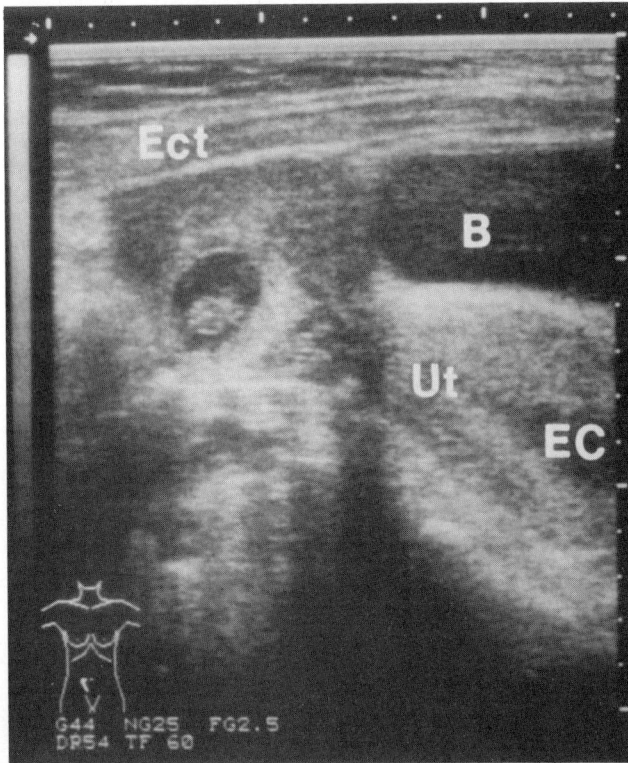

Fig. 32–3. Longitudinal midline abdominal sonogram showing a well-defined ectopic pregnancy (*Ect*) overlying the uterus (*Ut*). (B = bladder; EC = endometrial cavity.) (Courtesy of Dr. Rigoberto Santos.)

when accompanied by fetal heart action (Cacciatore and associates, 1990a; Mahoney and co-workers, 1985). An intrauterine collection of fluid can be confused for a gestational sac if these criteria are not followed rigidly.

Use of vaginal sonography alone can result in the correct diagnosis of ectopic pregnancy (Fig. 32–4) in

more than 90 percent of cases (Cacciatore and co-workers, 1990a). A more accurate clinical diagnosis, however, is based upon three possibilities. (1) An intrauterine pregnancy is identified as described above. (2) An empty uterus and an ectopic pregnancy are seen based upon the demonstration of an adnexal mass separate from two clearly identified ovaries. The adnexal mass must be complex, or contain a gestational sac-like adnexal ring with or without a fetal pole (fetal echoes or yolk sac). (3) The study may be nondiagnostic, that is, neither adnexal mass or intrauterine pregnancy sac is identified. *A heterotypic pregnancy is an exception to these diagnostic criteria* (Hirsch and associates, 1992).

In the event of a nondiagnostic study, two approaches are possible. Either repeat serial ultrasound studies or serial sonography along with serial quantitative β-hCG measurements (see below). Even with serial evaluations, careful clinical judgment is still required; and in doubtful cases, either laparoscopy or laparatomy may be necessary (Cacciatore and associates, 1990a).

VAGINAL COLOR AND PULSED DOPPLER ULTRASOUND. Recently, Emerson and associates (1992) and Pellerito and colleagues (1992) reported excellent results using vaginal color and pulsed Doppler flow imaging techniques to diagnose ectopic pregnancy. Briefly, the technique consists of identifying an intrauterine or extrauterine site of vascular color in a characteristic placental shape, the so-called "ring-of-fire" pattern, and a high-velocity low-impedance flow pattern in this site which is compatible with placental perfusion. If this pattern is seen outside the uterine cavity and the uterine cavity is "cold" with respect to blood flow, the diagnosis of ectopic pregnancy is apparent. The technique markedly improves the correct diagnosis of a viable intrauterine pregnancy and significantly improves the correct diagnosis of an ectopic pregnancy or an incomplete abortion (Emerson

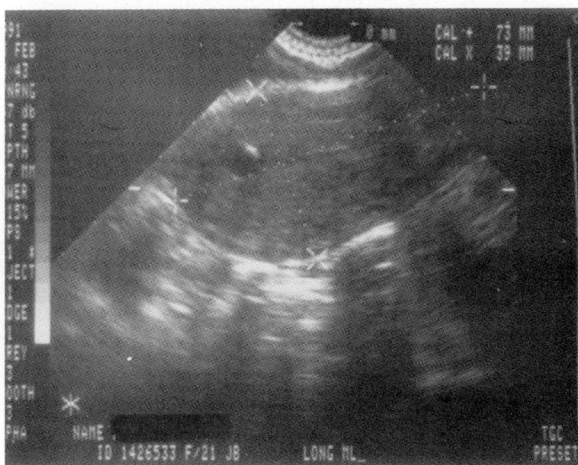

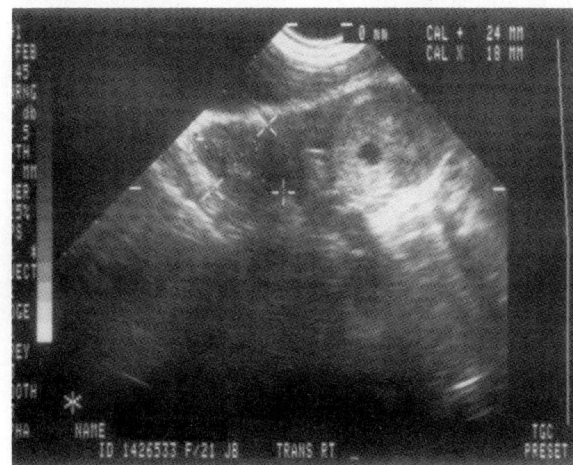

Fig. 32–4. Vaginal sonogram of ectopic pregnancy.

and colleagues, 1992). Unfortunately, the equipment is extremely expensive, and there is a steep learning curve associated with its use.

Quantitative β-hCG and Sonography. When pregnancy is diagnosed in a hemodynamically stable woman suspected of having an ectopic pregnancy, subsequent management is based upon serial quantitative serum β-hCG values and abdominal or vaginal sonograms. Kadar and associates (1981b) described four clinical possibilities based upon quantitative β-hCG values, and these have been modified by adding results achieved using vaginal or abdominal sonography:

1. When the β-hCG value is above 6000 mIU/mL and an intrauterine gestational sac is seen using abdominal sonography, normal pregnancy is virtually certain except for the unusual case of a heterotypic pregnancy. If vaginal sonography is used, the critical or **discriminatory β-hCG value** is between 1000 and 2000 mIU/mL (Cacciatore and associates, 1990a,b; Nyberg and co-workers, 1988).

2. When the β-hCG value is above 6000 mIU/mL (1000 to 2000 mIU/mL with vaginal sonogram) and there is an empty uterine cavity, an ectopic pregnancy is very likely.

3. When the β-hCG value is less than 6000 mIU/mL (1000 to 2000 mIU/mL with vaginal sonogram) and a definite intrauterine ring of pregnancy is visualized, then spontaneous abortion is likely now or very soon. Ectopic pregnancy is still a possibility because of the lack of ultrasonic resolution available with abdominal ultrasound machines, but it is much less likely using vaginal sonography. A serum progesterone value might be helpful in this instance (see p. 700).

4. When the β-hCG value is less than 6000 mIU/mL (1000 to 2000 mIU/mL with vaginal sonogram), and there is an empty uterus, no definitive diagnosis can be made. Failure to visualize a gestational sac within the uterus is not unusual using abdominal sonography prior to 5 weeks' gestation (Batzer and associates, 1983; Bryson, 1983; Coleman and colleagues, 1985). Vaginal sonography is more sensitive; but for practical purposes, precise gestational age is often unknown in a woman with suspected ectopic pregnancy. In these instances and during this *"20-day window,"* three events may occur. The woman may abort, may continue her pregnancy and develop a normal gestational sac, or may show evidence of an ectopic pregnancy (Figs. 32–3 and 32–4). Finally, the presence of serum β-hCG can confirm a pregnancy as early as 8 days past fertilization. Unfortunately, an intrauterine gestational sac cannot be reliably identified, even with vag-

inal ultrasound, until 28 days past conception; the time between 8 and 28 days results in the "20-day window" (Daus and colleagues, 1989). A serum progesterone value might also be helpful in this instance (see p. 700).

Cacciatore and associates (1990a) manage a suspected ectopic pregnancy based upon quantitative serum β-hCG and vaginal sonography. They reported their best results in diagnosing ectopic pregnancy when (1) the uterus was empty, (2) an adnexal mass clearly separate from the ovaries was present, and (3) the β-hCG level was greater than 1000 mIU/L (International Reference Preparation, or IRP). One International Standard unit per liter (1 IU/L) equals 1.8 International Reference Preparation units per liter (1.8 IRP/L). Using these criteria, the diagnosis in 200 women suspected of having an ectopic pregnancy had a sensitivity of 97 percent, specificity of 99 percent, positive predictive value of 98 percent, and negative predictive value of 98 percent. These are remarkable results, and similar results should be achievable in most hands.

Some, but certainly not all, feel that with an empty uterus and any proof of pregnancy, laparoscopy or laparotomy is indicated (Bryson, 1983). Another approach is to admit these women and perform serial hematocrits, frequent vital signs, and serial sonograms and quantitative β-hCG determinations. Such women will eventually continue with a normal pregnancy, abort, or develop clinical or ultrasonic evidence of ectopic pregnancy.

Kadar and co-workers (1981a) proposed another plan. They observed that in women with normal pregnancies, mean doubling time for β-hCG in serum was approximately 48 hours, and the lowest normal value for this increase was 66 percent (Table 32–5). They calculated this number by subtracting the initial value for β-hCG from the 48-hour value and dividing the result by the initial value, which is multiplied by 100 to obtain a percentage:

$$\frac{\beta\text{-hCG at 48 hours} - \text{initial }\beta\text{-hCG}}{\text{Initial }\beta\text{-hCG}} \times 100$$

Kadar and colleagues (1981a) cautioned that both β-hCG determinations must be performed simulta-

TABLE 32–5. LOWER NORMAL LIMITS FOR PERCENTAGE INCREASE OF SERUM β-hCG DURING EARLY UTERINE PREGNANCY

Sampling Interval (days)	Percent Increase in β-hCG from Initial Value
1	29
2	66
3	114
4	175
5	255

Modified from Kadar and co-workers (1981a).

neously, and that more reliable values could be obtained at 48-hour intervals. They concluded that a failure to maintain this rate of increased β-hCG production, along with an empty uterus, was suggestive evidence for ectopic pregnancy. They further acknowledged that this plan would delay surgery at least 48 hours, and the test still would falsely identify 15 percent of normal women as likely to have an ectopic pregnancy and 13 percent of women with an ectopic pregnancy as normal. Although Pittaway and co-workers (1985) did not confirm these observations, Kadar and Romero (1987) subsequently reported a larger series of patients with evidence to support the concept.

Yet another approach to this problem is to predict when a gestational sac and fetal signs can be seen by abdominal sonography when these anatomical features are compared with quantitative serum β-hCG levels. At least two groups have constructed such nomograms (Batzer and colleagues, 1983; Kadar and Romero, 1982). Despite their use, a more accurate prediction of uterine versus ectopic pregnancy is not always obtained.

Culdocentesis. The simplest technique for identifying hemoperitoneum is culdocentesis, because it can be performed without hospitalization. The cervix is pulled toward the symphysis with a tenaculum, and a long 16- or 18-gauge needle is inserted through the posterior vaginal fornix into the cul-de-sac. Fluid, if present can be aspirated. Failure to aspirate fluid can be interpreted only as unsatisfactory entry into the cul-de-sac. Fluid-containing fragments of old clots, or bloody fluid that does not clot, are compatible with the diagnosis of hemoperitoneum resulting from an ectopic pregnancy. If the blood subsequently clots, it may have been obtained from an adjacent perforated blood vessel rather than from a bleeding ectopic pregnancy. The very important exception to this generalization is brisk bleeding from the site of rupture, in which case the blood may be aspirated from the cul-de-sac before it has had time to clot. With bleeding of such intensity, culdocentesis is rarely necessary to establish the diagnosis of an intra-abdominal catastrophe. In most such instances, hypo-volemic shock is identified or will be apparent rapidly.

Culdocentesis may be unsatisfactory in women with previous salpingitis and pelvic peritonitis because the cul-de-sac may have been obliterated. **Thus, failure to obtain blood from the cul-de-sac does not exclude the diagnosis of hemoperitoneum and the presence of an ectopic pregnancy, either unruptured or ruptured.**

Curettage. Differentiation between threatened or incomplete abortion of an intrauterine pregnancy and a tubal pregnancy may be accomplished in many instances by curettage. Stovall and colleagues (1992a, b) recommend curettage in suspected cases of incomplete abortion versus ectopic pregnancy when serum progesterone is less than 5 ng/mL, β-hCG titers are rising abnormally (less than 2000 mU/mL), and an intrauterine pregnancy is not seen using transvaginal sonography. If embryo, fetus, or placenta are identified, a simultaneous tubal pregnancy is unlikely. When none of these structures is identified, tubal pregnancy is a probability and further follow-up with serial quantitative β-hCG titers and sonography is required. This may be useful during the "20-day window period" (p. 702) when an intrauterine pregnancy cannot be visualized using vaginal sonography. The identification of decidua alone in uterine curettings strongly implies extrauterine pregnancy, but decidua alone may also be found following complete abortion. The *Arias-Stella* endometrial reaction is also not diagnostic of an ectopic pregnancy. O'Connor and Kurman (1988) maintain, however, that intrauterine pregnancy can be diagnosed in the absence of villi by identifying the presence of intermediate trophoblast associated with enlarged vessels replaced by hyaline or with fragments of fibrinoid matrix.

Colpotomy. Direct visualization of the oviducts and ovaries can be accomplished by use of colpotomy unless pelvic inflammation has obliterated the cul-de-sac or the tubes are adherent to the broad ligaments or uterus to such a degree that they cannot be seen. This procedure has generally been abandoned because more satisfactory results can be obtained using laparoscopy.

Laparoscopy. Fiber-optic laparoscopy provides a means of visual diagnosis of pelvic disease, including ectopic pregnancy. Complete visualization of the pelvis, however, may be impossible if there is pelvic inflammation or active bleeding. At times, identification of an *early unruptured tubal pregnancy* may be difficult, even though the tube is fully visualized. Samuellson and Sjovall (1972) reported that 4 ectopic pregnancies out of 166 were not seen by laparoscopy, and that of 120 women with an intrauterine pregnancy, 6 were diagnosed as having an ectopic gestation. Such errors likely vary with operator experience and the degree of anatomical distortion encountered. The tube may show little change in shape and minimal change in color with early pregnancy. Moreover, demonstration of tubal patency by passage of dye through the tube does not exclude early tubal pregnancy (Yaffe and colleagues, 1976).

Advantages of diagnostic laparoscopy include (1) a definitive diagnosis, (2) a concurrent route to remove the ectopic mass using operative laparoscopy, or (3) a direct route to inject chemotherapeutic agents into the ectopic mass (see below).

Laparotomy. If any doubt remains, laparotomy should be performed. An unnecessary operation is far less tragic than death contributed to by indecision or delay. There is remarkably little morbidity associated with surgery that is limited to a carefully made and repaired suprapubic incision. It is imperative that laparotomy not be delayed while laparoscopy is performed in a woman with obvious pelvic or abdominal hemorrhage that requires immediate definitive treatment.

Differential Diagnosis. Prompt diagnosis of a ruptured tubal pregnancy may be lifesaving, and the earlier an unruptured tubal pregnancy is diagnosed, the greater will be the likelihood of a future successful pregnancy (p. 705). Unfortunately, there are few other disorders in obstetrics and gynecology that present so many diagnostic pitfalls (Jones, 1991). Brenner and associates (1980) reported that of 300 women with ectopic pregnancy, approximately one third had been seen once and 11 percent twice before the correct diagnosis was made. Dorfman and colleagues (1984), in an analysis of mortality from ectopic pregnancy in the United States in 1979 and 1980, concluded that more than half of the deaths might have been prevented had the woman or her physician(s) acted more expeditiously. The most commonly misdiagnosed conditions are listed in Table 32–6.

Conditions observed by us to be confused most frequently with tubal pregnancy are (1) acute or chronic salpingitis, (2) threatened or incomplete abortion of an intrauterine pregnancy, (3) rupture of a corpus luteum or follicular cyst with intraperitoneal bleeding, (4) torsion of an ovarian cyst, (5) appendicitis, (6) gastroenteritis, (7) discomfort from an intrauterine device, and (8) failure of tubal sterilization.

Gastrointestinal Disturbance. In some women with a ruptured ectopic pregnancy, the prominent symptoms are diarrhea, nausea, and vomiting, along with abdominal pain. The erroneous diagnosis of gastroenteritis has led to death (Dorfman and associates, 1984).

TABLE 32–6. MISDIAGNOSES FOR FATAL ECTOPIC PREGNANCIES IN THE UNITED STATES, 1979–1980

Misdiagnosis	Occurrences	
	(No.)	(%)
Gastrointestinal disorder	14	25
Normal pregnancy	10	18
Pelvic inflammatory disease	8	14
Psychiatric disorder	5	9
Spontaneous abortion	5	9
Complication of induced abortion	4	7
Urinary tract infection	4	7
Adnexal cyst	2	4
Dysfunctional uterine bleeding	2	4
Fetal death	1	2
Placenta previa or abruption	1	2
Total deaths	56	100[a]

[a] Total exceeds 100% due to rounding figures.
Modified from Dorfman and associates (1984).

Salpingitis. Salpingitis commonly is mistaken for ruptured tubal pregnancy. With salpingitis there is often a history of similar attacks. There is usually no missed period, and abnormal bleeding is not as common as the spotting characteristic of tubal gestation. Pain and tenderness are more likely to be bilateral. A pelvic mass in a tubal pregnancy, if palpable, is unilateral, whereas in salpingitis both fornices are likely to be equally resistant and tender. In fact, a unilateral mass with salpingitis should prompt consideration for an infected ectopic pregnancy. Dicker and associates (1984) reported a series of 8 such women who presented with a clinical picture of unilateral tubo-ovarian or pelvic abscess, and Kouyoumdjian and Kirkpatrick (1990) added an additional case. The correct preoperative diagnosis was made in each case by a positive β-hCG.

Temperature in acute salpingitis frequently exceeds 38° C. A positive urinary pregnancy test is important information, but a negative urinary pregnancy test does not exclude pregnancy. If there is any suspicion of an ectopic gestation, serum β-hCG should be measured.

Abortion of Intrauterine Pregnancy. In threatened or incomplete abortion, uterine bleeding is usually more profuse, and shock from hypovolemia, when present, is usually in proportion to the extent of vaginal hemorrhage. In tubal pregnancy, however, hypovolemic shock almost always is far in excess of observed vaginal blood loss. Abortion pain generally is less severe, likely to be rhythmic, and located low in the midline of the abdomen, whereas in tubal pregnancy it is unilateral or generalized. If embryo or placenta is found in the vagina or at the external cervical os, the diagnosis of abortion is confirmed. Shed decidua, however, may be abundant with an ectopic pregnancy, and unless carefully examined might be incorrectly considered to be products from an aborting intrauterine pregnancy. Combined extrauterine and intrauterine pregnancy should be considered. The marked histological variations in endometrium render an endometrial biopsy unreliable in ectopic pregnancy and may induce an unwanted abortion.

Rupture of a Corpus Luteum or Follicular Cyst. Intraperitoneal bleeding from an ovarian cyst may be difficult to distinguish from a ruptured tubal pregnancy. Even though identification of chorionic gonadotropin will sometimes help to make the diagnosis preoperatively, most often, the diagnosis is made only at the time of exploratory laparotomy (see Culdocentesis, p. 703).

Twisted Cyst or Appendicitis. In both ovarian cyst torsion and appendicitis, signs and symptoms of pregnancy, including amenorrhea, are usually lacking, and there is rarely a history of abnormal vaginal bleeding. The mass formed by a twisted ovarian cyst is more nearly discrete, whereas that of a tubal pregnancy is usually less well defined. With appendicitis, only rarely is there a mass found by vaginal examination, and pain on motion of the cervix is much less severe than with a ruptured tubal pregnancy. The pain from appendicitis, furthermore, often is localized higher, over McBurney's point. If either appendicitis or a twisted ovarian cyst is mistaken for a tubal pregnancy, the error is not costly because all three require prompt surgery.

Intrauterine Devices. Diagnosis of ectopic pregnancy is often more difficult in women with intrauterine devices. Cramping pelvic pain and uterine bleeding, both common features of ectopic pregnancy, may be caused by an intrauterine device. Moreover, in some women, the device predisposes to unilateral inflammation of the adnexa.

Previous Tubal Sterilization. Tatum and Schmidt (1977) reported that approximately 16 percent of pregnancies conceived after a failed tubal sterilization were ectopic. Following failed sterilization performed laparoscopically using electrocautery tubal fulguration, 50 percent of pregnancies may be ectopic (McCausland, 1980).

Tubal Pregnancy: Treatment and Prognosis

Treatment has most often been salpingectomy to remove a shattered, bleeding oviduct with or without ipsilateral oophorectomy. The goal of such treatment was and should remain the preservation of the woman's life. Recently, treatment has changed from salpingectomy to surgical and medical procedures that favor tubal conservation (Young and associates, 1991). Such conservative management is made possible by the earlier diagnosis of ectopic pregnancy using vaginal ultrasound and serum quantitative β-hCG determinations.

Surgical Management: Laparoscopy and Laparotomy

Salpingectomy. When removing the oviduct, it is advisable to excise a wedge no more than the outer third of the interstitial portion of the tube (so-called cornual resection) in an effort to minimize the rare recurrence of pregnancy in the tubal stump. Resection so extensive as to reach the cavity of the uterus must be avoided, lest the defect created lead to uterine rupture in a subsequent intrauterine pregnancy. Even with cornual resection, a subsequent interstitial pregnancy may not be prevented (Kalchman and Meltzer, 1966). Salpingectomy can be performed through an operative laparoscope and may be used for both ruptured and unruptured ectopic pregnancies.

Ipsilateral Oophorectomy. Removal of the adjacent ovary at the time of salpingectomy has been suggested as a means for both improving fertility and decreasing the likelihood of a subsequent ectopic pregnancy (Jeffcoate, 1967). Ovulation would always occur from the ovary immediately adjacent to the remaining oviduct. This should facilitate pickup of the ovum and avoid the possibility of external migration of the ovum resulting in an ectopic pregnancy. Removal of an otherwise normal-appearing ovary on these theoretical grounds, however, hardly seems justifiable.

Sterilization. If childbearing has been completed or if the ectopic pregnancy is the consequence of failed contraception, concomitant sterilization should be considered. Tubal sterilization can usually be performed via laparoscopy or laparotomy without increased risk. Conversely, all organs possible should be conserved in a woman of low parity with a strong desire for future pregnancies. She must know, however, that she has an increased risk of a subsequent ectopic pregnancy.

Fallopian Tube Conservation. Many factors must be considered in evaluating the success or failure of attempts at pregnancy following an ectopic pregnancy. These include, but are not limited to, age, parity, bilateral tubal disease, and whether the fallopian tube was ruptured. In general, women under age 30 and those of higher parity have significantly higher fertility rates and successful outcomes in subsequent pregnancies than older women of lower parity (Sherman and co-workers, 1982). A history of salpingitis and evidence of bilateral tubal disease are extremely bad prognostic signs. Finally, Sherman and co-workers (1982) reported that **subsequent pregnancy and lower recurrent ectopic pregnancy rates were observed in women in whom surgery was performed prior to rupture of the ectopic pregnancy.**

If the woman has no history of infertility and no gross evidence of previous salpingitis, then salpingotomy and salpingostomy result in equally favorable outcomes compared with salpingectomy. Sherman and associates (1982) reported intrauterine pregnancy rates for tubal-conservative surgery to be more than 80 percent (Table 32–7). If there is evidence for bilateral tubal disease, salpingostomy is clearly superior to salpingectomy, with subsequent intrauterine conception rates of 76 versus 44 percent, respectively. Similar results have been reported by DeCherney and Jones (1985), Reyniak (1985), and Vermesh (1989), who summarized results from several series.

Use of newer diagnostic techniques and surgical procedures to conserve damaged tubes will result in higher subsequent successful pregnancy outcomes. Several of the surgical approaches for tubal reconstruction are discussed below.

Salpingostomy. This technique is used to remove a small pregnancy that is usually less than 2 cm in length

TABLE 32–7. SURGICAL TREATMENTS AND SUBSEQUENT FERTILITY AMONG 151 WOMEN WITH A FIRST-EPISODE ECTOPIC PREGNANCY

Surgical Treatment[a]	No. Patients	Subsequent Outcomes (%)		
		Intrauterine	Repeat Ectopic	Sterility
(1) Conservative	21	16 (76)	1 (5)	4 (19)
Radical[b]	32	14 (44)	3 (9)	15 (47)
(2) Conservative	26	23 (88)	2 (8)	1 (4)
Radical[c]	72	61 (85)	3 (4)	8 (11)
(3) Totals[d]				
Conservative	47	39 (83)	3 (6)	5 (11)
Radical	104	75 (72)	6 (6)	23 (22)

[a] Radical surgery is salpingectomy and conservative surgery is fallopian tube conservation.
[b] These women had a history or operative findings consistent with coexisting sterility factors. The difference between conservative and radical were significant ($P = 0.04$).
[c] These women had a normal reproductive history and their other reproductive organs were normal at surgery. The difference between these groups was not significant ($P = 0.9$).
[d] All patients, conservative versus radical surgery, $P = 0.2$.
Modified from Sherman and co-workers (1982).

and located in the distal one third of the fallopian tube (Fig. 32–5). A linear incision, 2 cm in length or less, is made on the antimesenteric border immediately over the ectopic pregnancy. The ectopic usually will extrude from the incision and can be carefully removed. Small bleeding sites are controlled with needlepoint electrocautery or laser, and the incision is left unsutured to heal by secondary intention. Sherman and associates (1982) and Timonen and Neiminen (1967) reported

that salpingostomy is associated with a higher subsequent pregnancy rate than salpingectomy. This procedure is readily performed through a laparascope and is likely the preferred surgical method for an unruptured ectopic pregnancy.

Salpingotomy. This procedure was first described by Stromme in 1953. A longitudinal incision is made on the antimesenteric border of the fallopian tube directly over the ectopic pregnancy (Fig. 32–6). The products are removed with forceps or gentle suction, and the opened tube irrigated with lactated Ringer solution (not isotonic saline) so that bleeding sites are identified and controlled as described above. Most recommend one-layer closure with 7-0 interrupted vicryl sutures (De-Cherney and Jones, 1985). Reyniak (1985) additionally reported improved anatomical results with the use of optic magnification and microsurgical techniques. He also recommends that, when possible, the incision not be extended through the end of the tube into the ampulla. This procedure can also be performed through an operative laparoscope and may prove to be the preferred surgical method for unruptured tubal pregnancies.

Segmental Resection and Anastomosis. This is recommended for an unruptured pregnancy in the isthmic portion of the tube because salpingotomy or salpingostomy would likely cause scarring and subsequent narrowing of this small lumen (Stangel and associates, 1976). After the segment of the tube is exposed, the mesosalpinx beneath the tube is incised, and the tubal

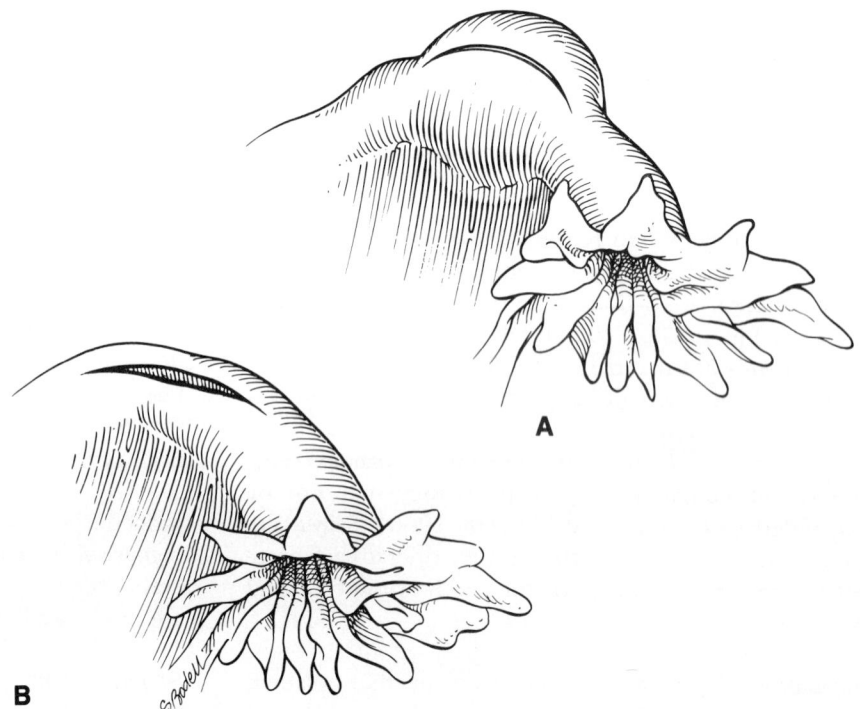

Fig. 32–5. A. Linear salpingostomy for removal of a small tubal pregnancy in distal third of fallopian tube. **B.** The incision is not sutured.

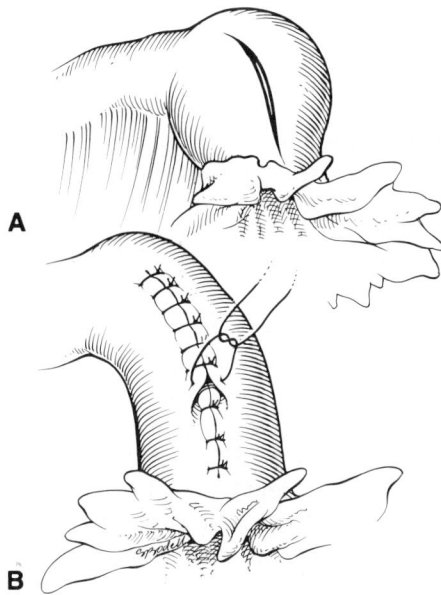

Fig. 32–6. A. Linear salpingotomy for removal of an ectopic pregnancy larger than 2 cm in length from distal third of fallopian tube. **B.** The incision is sutured, usually with a single layer of 7-0 interrupted sutures.

isthmus containing the ectopic mass is resected (Fig. 32–7). The mesosalpinx is sutured, thus reapproximating the tubal stumps. The segments of the tube are then anastomosed to one another in layers with interrupted 7-0 vicryl sutures, preferably using magnification. Three

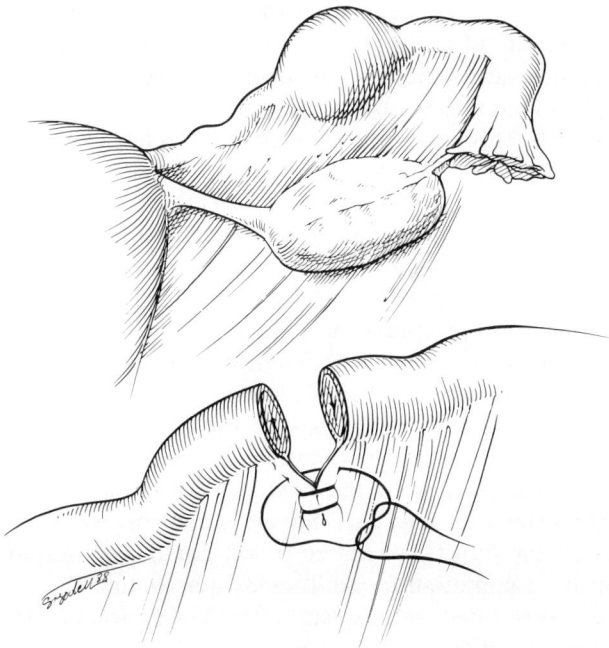

Fig. 32–7. Segmental resection and anastomosis of fallopian tube for an unruptured ectopic pregnancy. Closure of mesosalpinx results in reapproximation of tubal segments. Anastomosis is accomplished with interrupted 7-0 vicryl sutures (see text).

sutures are used in the muscularis and three in the serosa, with strict attention to avoid the tubal lumen. Suturing the serosal layer adds strength to the first layer. This procedure can be done at the initial surgery if the patient has stable vital signs, or it can be done at a subsequent laparotomy.

Fimbrial Evacuation. There is a temptation with distally implanted tubal pregnancies to evacuate the conceptual products by "milking" or "suctioning" the ectopic mass from the tubal lumen. **This is not recommended** because the practice is associated with an ectopic recurrence rate twice that of salpingotomy (Sherman and co-workers, 1982; Stromme, 1953). There is also a high rate of surgical reexploration for recurrent bleeding from persistent trophoblastic tissue (Bell and colleagues, 1987).

Other Techniques. *Fallopian tube reimplantation* into the uterine cornu, and the *Gepfert procedure* of everting the distal end of damaged fimbria or tubal mucosa, are associated with very poor pregnancy outcomes and are not recommended by DeCherney and Jones (1985). These and all of the previously mentioned techniques can be done at a later time if the woman is in shock. The first rule is rapid arrest of bleeding and cardiovascular resuscitation. If time and clinical circumstances warrant, the above procedures can be implemented.

If a second procedure is planned for a later time, it is logical to obtain hemostasis with the least amount of tubal damage. This obtains even when the opposite fallopian tube appears to be grossly normal. Unfortunately, many of the normal-appearing contralateral tubes have also been damaged by salpingitis, which is characteristically bilateral. If a tubal reconstructive procedure is done, all blood and debris should be irrigated from the abdomen and pelvis using lactated Ringer solution. Use of high-molecular-weight dextran has been recommended to decrease postoperative adhesion formation (Reyniak, 1985).

Persistent Trophoblast. There is a significant risk of persistent tubal or peritoneal trophoblastic tissue following a tubal evacuation procedure (Cartwright, 1991; DiMarchi and associates, 1987). Because of this, Bell and colleagues (1987) recommend that a quantitative serum β-hCG determination be performed 2 weeks postoperatively to compare with the original value. It is essential to establish that the value is falling. With persistent or increasing values, the choice of reexploration or chemotherapy with methotrexate must be made (Bengtsson and associates, 1992). Kamrava and co-workers (1983) reported that chorionic gonadotropin is usually undetectable by 12 days following resection of tubal pregnancies, but occasionally values are elevated even 3 weeks after surgery.

Obviously, none of these procedures guarantees subsequent tubal patency. Nonetheless, for women of low parity, they should be considered unless the tube is destroyed beyond repair. The results obtained using such techniques are presented in Table 32–7.

Medical Management

Methotrexate. Tanaka and associates (1982) recommended the use of methotrexate to treat interstitial pregnancy, and Miyazaki (1983) and Ory and colleagues (1986) reported the first clinical studies using it as first-line therapy for ectopic pregnancies. Since these initial reports, there have been numerous publications describing successful treatment of ectopic pregnancies (tubal, cornual, cervical, and abdominal) using different regimens of methotrexate both with and without leucovorin (folinic acid) rescue. In general, the following principles apply: Success is greatest if the gestation is less than 6 weeks, the tubal mass is not more than 3.5 cm in diameter, and the fetus is not alive (no fetal heart action). With more advanced gestations, success has been less frequent except after multicourse therapy, single high-dose therapy with folinic acid rescue, or fetal death induced by direct injection of potassium chloride and methotrexate into the amnionic sac using either transvaginal sonography or laparoscopy (Aboulghar and colleagues, 1990; Feichtinger and Kemeter, 1989; Kojima and associates, 1990; Kooi and co-workers, 1990; Ménard and colleagues, 1990).

PATIENT SELECTION. Candidates for methotrexate therapy must be hemodynamically stable with a normal hemogram and normal liver and renal function. Women given methotrexate are instructed that (1) medical therapy fails in 5 to 10 percent of patients, and this rate is higher in pregnancies past 6 weeks gestation or with a tubal mass greater than 3.5 cm in diameter; (2) failure of medical therapy means elective surgery, or if tubal rupture occurs (approximately a 5 percent chance), emergency surgery; (3) if treated as an outpatient, rapid transportation must be available for transfer to the hospital; (4) signs and symptoms of tubal rupture such as vaginal bleeding, abdominal and pleuritic pain, weakness, dizziness, or syncope must be reported promptly and should constitute a cause for immediate medical attention; (5) sexual intercourse is prohibited until after serum β-hCG is undetectable; (6) no alcohol can be consumed; and (7) multivitamins with folic acid should not be taken.

MONITORING METHOTREXATE TOXICITY. Although some investigators report minimal or no side effects, toxicity may develop suddenly and be severe. Fortunately, most reported treatment regimens, regardless of the dose, duration of therapy, and route administered, have been associated with minimal laboratory changes and mild symptoms. This is especially true with adjunctive use of folinic acid (citrovorum factor). Nevertheless, therapy should be stopped if significant increases are observed in serum hepatic enzyme levels or plasma creatinine. Treatment should also be stopped if there is evidence of bone marrow suppression reflected by thrombocytopenia or leukopenia. Evidence for dermatitis, stomatitis, gastritis, or pleuritis should also halt therapy (Stovall and Ling, 1992a).

MONITORING EFFICACY OF THERAPY. Various placental protein and steroid hormones have been used to monitor placental viability following medical and surgical therapy for ectopic pregnancies. The most widely used are serial quantitative β-hCG titers, but Carson and associates (1989) and Stovall and Ling (1992a) have also used serial titers of human placental lactogen (hPL).

The rationale for measuring serial β-hCG values is that after therapy the hormone usually disappears from plasma between 14 and 21 days. Occasionally, however, hormone levels remain elevated for 28 days (Feichtinger and Kemeter, 1989; Ménard and associates, 1990). Therefore, one of many effective follow-up schemes consists of measuring serial quantitative β-hCG levels on days 1, 2, 5, 10, and 15 and every 5 days thereafter if necessary. Vaginal sonography should be done on days 5, 10, 15 and every 5 days thereafter if necessary. Outpatient surveillance is preferred; but if there is any question of safety, hospitalization should be instituted. Failure is noted if there is no decline in β-hCG level, persistence of the ectopic mass, or any intraperitoneal bleeding.

Carson and associates (1989) reported two instances of tubal rupture in 21 women treated with methotrexate. In both, serum placental lactogen continued to increase, but both progesterone and β-hCG decreased. This interesting observation remains to be confirmed.

SYSTEMIC THERAPY. Stovall and associates (1989a) reported that, following systemic therapy with methotrexate, 34 of 36 patients (94 percent) had complete remission of tubal pregnancy. The other 2 ruptured, one 23 days after commencing methotrexate therapy and the other on day 14. The latter woman had fetal heart activity noted throughout most of therapy. Therapy consisted of alternating days of intramuscular methotrexate (1.0 mg/kg) followed the next day by intramuscular citrovorum (0.1 mg/kg). Daily measurements were obtained for β-hCG, complete blood count, and serum aspartate aminotransferase. Therapy was continued until there was a decline in quantitative β-hCG titers of 15 percent or more on two consecutive days. No patient was given more than 4 doses of methotrexate without a 1-week drug-free interval. After the last drug dose, serum β-hCG was measured 2 to 3 times weekly until it was less than 10 mIU/mL. There were no major side effects, and only 3 of 36 women had minor side effects. Two women developed transient hepatic enzyme elevation and one developed transient stomatitis after 4 doses of methotrexate.

Stovall and associates (1988, 1989a, 1991a, 1992a) expanded their multidose clinical trial to 100 patients and concluded that (1) methotrexate chemotherapy for asymptomatic ectopic pregnancy is effective and can be used in an outpatient setting, (2) tubal rupture can occur as late as 23 days after starting therapy, (3) fetal cardiac activity is a relative contraindication for chemotherapy, (4) chemotherapy is contraindicated in symptomatic women, and (5) chemotherapy offers no immediate advantages over laparoscopic surgery.

Stovall and co-workers (1991b, 1992a) now recommend single-dose therapy with intramuscular methotrexate, 50 mg/m^2, without citrovorum factor rescue. In their first 31 patients, 29 (97 percent) were treated successfully, and none had side effects. If a 15 percent decrease in serum β-hCG is not documented between days 4 and 7, then another identical dose is given. Of 75 women treated to date, only 2 required a second dose.

TUBAL PATENCY AND FERTILITY. Stovall and associates (1990b, 1992a) studied reproductive function in 57 successfully treated women given multidose methotrexate/citrovorum therapy. Both tubal anatomy and function were restored, and return of menses was not delayed. Nineteen of 23 women who had a hysterosalpingogram had patency in the ipsilateral tube. Subsequently, there have been 37 pregnancies (62 percent); 4 (11 percent) had another ectopic pregnancy, and 6 (16 percent) aborted spontaneously. The results compare favorably with those obtained using conservative surgical techniques (see Table 32–7).

SALPINGOCENTESIS THERAPY. Salpingocentesis is the aspiration of fluid from a fallopian tube. In this instance, amnionic fluid is aspirated from a tubal pregnancy followed by methotrexate injection into the amnionic sac or tubal mass. Treatment usually consists of a single 50 mg injection, but as little as 5 mg has been used successfully with prompt resolution of tubal pregnancy and documentation of patency (Feichtinger and Kemeter, 1989; Kojima and colleagues, 1990). If a 50 mg methotrexate dose is used, this usually is followed with a single oral dose of folinic acid to prevent systemic toxicity (Ménard and associates, 1990).

The technique most often used consists of introducing a 16-gauge needle through the cul-de-sac, and under sonographic guidance, directing the needle into the amnionic sac. Injection into the amnionic sac or tubal lumen also has been done through the laparoscope (Kooi and Kock, 1990). Material usually is aspirated for pathological examination, and methotrexate alone, or with potassium chloride, is injected into the sac. Both drugs are caustic to tubal epithelium; therefore, subse-

quent tubal patency and ultimately fertility may be compromised. Kojima and associates (1990) reported tubal patency in all 9 women treated with laparoscopically directed injection of methotrexate (5- to 25-mg doses) into the tubal mass. Direct injection methods are currently considered research techniques, but they are also being used successfully to treat cornual (interstitial) pregnancies (Timor-Tritsch and colleagues, 1992).

Prostaglandin and RU 486 Therapy. Egarter and Husslein (1989) treated unruptured ectopic pregnancies with prostaglandin-F$_{2\alpha}$ (5 to 10 mg) injected into the ectopic mass and 2 to 3 mg into the ipsilateral corpus luteum. Injections were laparoscopically directed. They followed with an oral prostaglandin E$_2$ analogue. Feichtinger and Kemeter (1989) also successfully injected 5 mg prostaglandin E$_2$ intraamnionically to treat an unruptured tubal pregnancy. Generally, while 85 to 90 percent effective, prostaglandin therapy has not been widely used because of side effects. These include cardiac arrthythmias, transient hypertension, pulmonary edema, and atrioventricular block, as well as usually expected nausea, vomiting, and diarrhea.

The antiprogesterone, RU 486, has been only marginally effective and is not generally available in the United States (Kenigsberg and associates, 1987).

Expectant Management. Mashiach and associates (1982) and Stovall and co-workers (1989a) have observed very early tubal pregnancies with stable or falling serum β-hCG levels. Stovall and Ling (1992a) restrict such action to women with these criteria: (1) decreasing serial quantitative β-hCG levels, (2) ectopic site restricted to fallopian tube, (3) no evidence of intraabdominal bleeding or rupture using vaginal sonography, and (4) diameter of the ectopic not greater than 3.5 cm. Although this is successful in selected cases, we do not manage patients in our own hospital using this technique, and Hochner-Celnikier and colleagues (1992) reported a ruptured tubal pregnancy in a woman managed expectantly who had chorionic gonadotropin levels below 10 mIU/mL.

Autotransfusion. Merrill and associates (1980) were enthusiastic for this procedure. With the newer red blood cell saving devices in use today, the procedure is usually warranted.

Anti-D Immune Globulin. If the woman is D-negative but not yet sensitized to D-antigen and the potential for reproduction persists, anti-D immune globulin should be administered to protect against isoimmunization. Moreover, if platelets are transfused, in all likelihood some contaminating D-positive red cells were also included. Therefore, D-negative patients also should receive anti-D immune globulin soon after platelet transfusion.

Resumption of Ovulation and Contraception. Following resection of an ectopic pregnancy, approximately 15 percent of women ovulate by 19 days and 65 percent by 24 days (Spirtos and associates 1987). By the 30th postoperative day, almost 75 percent have ovulated. **Contraception should ideally be commenced at the time of hospital discharge.**

Abdominal Pregnancy

Frequency. The incidence of abdominal pregnancy is influenced by the (1) frequency of ectopic gestation in the population, (2) availability of care early in pregnancy, (3) use of assisted reproductive techniques, and (4) degree of suspicion exercised by those providing care. Almost all cases of abdominal pregnancy follow early rupture or abortion of a tubal pregnancy into the peritoneal cavity. An incidence for abdominal pregnancy of 1 in 3337 births at Charity Hospital in New Orleans was reported by Beacham and colleagues (1962), compared with 1 in 7931 births at Indiana University Hospital (Strafford and Ragan, 1977). The Centers for Disease Control estimated that the incidence of abdominal pregnancy is 1 in 10,000 live births (Atrash and co-workers, 1987a). At Parkland Hospital, where ectopic pregnancy is common, advanced abdominal pregnancy is encountered in approximately 1 in 25,000 births.

Etiology. Typically, the growing placenta, after penetrating the oviduct wall, maintains its tubal attachment but gradually encroaches upon and implants in the neighboring serosa. Meanwhile, the fetus continues to grow within the peritoneal cavity. In such circumstances, the placenta is found in the general region of the oviduct and over the posterior aspect of the broad ligament and uterus (Fig. 32–8).

Even more rarely, the conceptus appears to have escaped after tubal rupture to reimplant elsewhere in the peritoneal cavity. Primary peritoneal implantation of the fertilized ovum is very rare, but conclusive proof of a case was provided by Studdiford (1942). The following criteria are required: (1) normal tubes and ovaries with no evidence of recent or remote injury, (2) absence of any evidence of uteroplacental fistula, and (3) presence of a pregnancy related exclusively to the peritoneal surface and young enough to eliminate the possibility of secondary implantation following primary nidation in the tube. Goldman and colleagues (1988) reported 5 cases of documented primary abdominal pregnancy, and Thomas and co-workers (1991a) reported a well-documented case of primary peritoneal pregnancy based upon Studdiford's revised criteria.

The incidence of abdominal pregnancy is increased after gamete intrafallopian transfer, in vitro fertilization and ovum transfer, and induced abortion (Ferland and

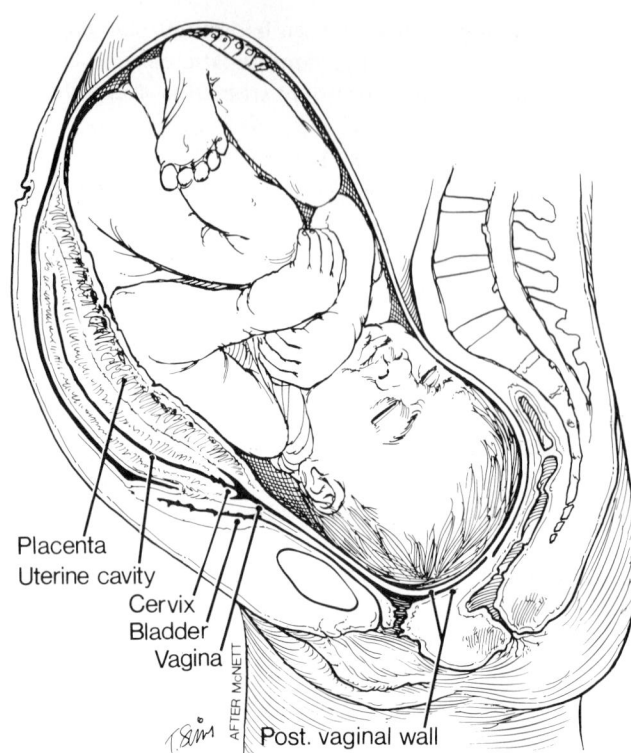

Fig. 32–8. Abdominal pregnancy at term. Placenta is implanted on posterior wall of uterus and broad ligament. The enlarged, flattened uterus is located just beneath the anterior abdominal wall. Cervix and vagina are dislodged anteriorly and superiorly by the large fetal head in the cul-de-sac.

associates, 1991; Vignali and co-workers, 1990). Endometriosis, tuberculosis, and intrauterine devices may also contribute to an increased incidence (Børlum and Blom, 1988; Durukan and co-workers, 1990; Goldman and associates, 1988; Vignali and colleagues, 1990).

Status of Fetus. Fetal viability in an abdominal pregnancy is exceedingly precarious, and the great majority succumb. In a world literature review, Ware (1948) cited a perinatal loss of 75 percent, but this figure may have been falsely low because of the tendency to report cases with good outcomes. Beachman and co-workers (1962) reported a perinatal loss in their own series of about 95 percent. Some authors report an incidence of congenital malformation in the infants as high as 50 percent.

If the pregnancy is diagnosed after 24 weeks' gestation, Cartwright and associates (1986) and Hage and colleagues (1988) await fetal viability with in-hospital expectant management. Such management carries a risk for sudden life-threatening intra-abdominal bleeding. In cases where amnionic fluid volume is minimal or absent, and in cases less than 24 weeks' gestation, treatment is probably indicated for maternal indications because fetal survival is extremely poor.

If the fetus dies after reaching a size too large to be

resorbed, it may undergo suppuration, mummification, calcification, or form an *adipocere*. Bacteria may gain access to the gestational products, particularly when they are adherent to intestine, resulting in suppuration. Eventually, the abscess ruptures, and if the woman does not die of peritonitis and septicemia, fetal parts may be extruded through the abdominal wall or more commonly into the intestine or bladder (Emembolu, 1989). Mummification and formation of a lithopedion occasionally ensue, and calcified products of conception may be carried for years without producing symptoms until they cause dystocia in a subsequent pregnancy or symptoms from pressure. There are instances in which a period of 20 to 50 years elapsed before removal of a lithopedion at operation or autopsy. Much more rarely, the fetus is converted into a yellowish, greasy mass to which the term *adipocere* is applied. The various bizarre terminations of abdominal pregnancy have been discussed, with illustrative cases graphically described by King (1954).

Diagnosis. Because early rupture or abortion of a tubal pregnancy is the usual antecedent of an abdominal pregnancy, in retrospect, a suggestive history can usually be obtained. Abnormalities likely to be recalled include spotting or irregular bleeding along with abdominal pain that usually was most prominent in one or both lower quadrants. Costa and associates (1991) presented an excellent and extensive review of this subject with numerous references.

Symptoms. Women with an abdominal pregnancy are likely to be uncomfortable but not sufficiently so to warrant thorough evaluation. Nausea, vomiting, flatulence, constipation, diarrhea, and abdominal pain may each be present in varying degrees. Multiparas may state that the pregnancy does not "feel right." Late in pregnancy, fetal movements may cause pain. Near term, the empty uterus has been alleged to go into spurious labor.

Physical Examination. Abnormal fetal positions can frequently be palpated, but the ease of palpating fetal parts is not a reliable sign. Fetal parts sometimes feel exceedingly close to the examining fingers even in normal pregnancies, especially in thin, multiparous women. *Abdominal massage over the pregnancy does not stimulate the mass to contract as it almost always does with advanced intrauterine pregnancy.* The cervix is usually displaced (see Fig. 32–8), depending in part on the fetal position, and it may dilate, but appreciable effacement is usually absent. The uterus may be outlined over the lower part of the pregnancy mass. Small parts or the fetal head may occasionally be palpated through the fornices and identified as clearly outside the uterus.

Laboratory Tests. An unexplained transient anemia early in pregnancy may accompany the initial tubal rup-

ture or abortion. Almost all other laboratory values, including those reflecting fetal well-being, are normal until fetal demise occurs. Urinary and plasma chorionic gonadotropin, estriol, estradiol, progesterone, human placental lactogen, Schwangerschafts-protein 1 (SP1), and alphafetoprotein (AFP) correspond to normal levels reported in pregnancy (Costa and associates, 1991; Kirkinen and colleagues, 1988). There have been 3 cases reported, however, of otherwise unexplained elevated maternal serum alphafetoprotein levels (Costa and associates, 1991). Doppler waveform analyses (S/D ratios) also have been reported to be normal in abdominal gestations (Hage and co-workers, 1988; Kirkinen and colleagues, 1988).

Oxytocin Stimulation. Cross and co-workers (1951) emphasized that oxytocin stimulation could be a valuable aid in the diagnosis of abdominal pregnancy. If no uterine activity is detected using a sensitive strain gauge applied over the products of conception while oxytocin is infused, the pregnancy almost certainly is extrauterine. Hertz and co-workers (1977) could detect no uterine activity while infusing oxytocin in excess of 50 mU/min because the empty uterus was inferior and posterior to the fetus. If the uterus were anterior, as in Figure 32–8, it might contract in response to oxytocin and possibly lead to the false diagnosis of intrauterine pregnancy.

Orr and associates (1979) reported that before the diagnosis of an abdominal pregnancy was made, the uterus contracted in response to oxytocin, and an oxytocin challenge test was interpreted as negative on two occasions. The growth-retarded fetus, who weighed 2000 g, expired undelivered one week later. The relationship between the abdominal wall, the uterus, and the extrauterine fetus was very similar to that depicted in Figure 32–8. Non-stress testing has been normal in most series, and as noted above, contraction stress testing may lead to varying results depending upon placental location (Costa and associates, 1991).

Radiological Examination. A strong suspicion of abdominal pregnancy may be confirmed by x-ray with a probe or radiopaque material in the uterus. The fetus then is shown clearly to lie outside the uterine cavity. Unfortunately, such techniques are not safe diagnostic procedures if the fetus is intrauterine. Other radiological signs that are not diagnostic include a cross-table view in which the fetal skull lies below the level of vertebral bodies.

Sonography. Ultrasonic findings with an abdominal pregnancy most often do not allow an unequivocal diagnosis to be made; however, in some suspected cases, these findings may be diagnostic. For example, if the fetal head is seen to lie immediately adjacent to the maternal bladder with no interposed uterine tissue, a specific diagnosis can be made (Kurtz and associates,

1982). Even with excellent equipment in well-trained hands, however, a sonographic diagnosis of abdominal pregnancy is missed in 50 percent of cases (Costa and associates, 1991).

Akhan and colleagues (1990) reported that the following sonographic criteria are suggestive of an abdominal pregnancy: (1) visualization of the fetus separate from the uterus, (2) failure to visualize uterine wall between the fetus and urinary bladder, (3) close approximation of fetal parts to the maternal abdominal wall, and (4) eccentric position (relation of fetus to uterus) or abnormal fetal attitude (relation of fetal parts to one another) and visualization of extrauterine placental tissue.

Magnetic Resonance Imaging. Magnetic resonance imaging has been used to confirm abdominal pregnancy following a suspicious sonographic examination, and the technique appears to be the most accurate and specific technique (Harris and associates, 1988; Murphy and associates, 1990). Even so, an abdominal pregnancy in our own institution was incorrectly diagnosed as a placenta previa.

Computed Tomography. Costa and associates (1991) maintain that computed tomography is superior to magnetic resonance imaging, but its use is limited because of fetal radiation effects. In cases of fetal demise, computed tomography may be diagnostic and should be considered (Glew and associates, 1989).

Treatment. Surgery for abdominal pregnancy may precipitate massive hemorrhage. Without massive blood transfusion, the outlook for many such women is hopeless. Hence, it is mandatory that at least 2000 mL of compatible blood be on hand in the operating room, with more readily available. Preoperatively, two intravenous infusion systems, each capable of delivering large volumes of fluid at a rapid rate, should be functioning. At the same time, techniques for monitoring the adequacy of the circulation should be employed, as described in Chapter 37. Whenever time allows, a mechanical bowel prep should be done.

The massive hemorrhage that often ensues in the course of operations for abdominal pregnancy is related to the lack of constriction of hypertrophied opened blood vessels after placental separation. It has been recommended by some that the operation be deferred until fetal viability is achieved (Hage and associates, 1988). Procrastination may be dangerous and undesirable, however, because partial separation of the placenta with hemorrhage occasionally occurs spontaneously while waiting. Moreover, even if the fetus has been dead several weeks, bleeding may still be torrential. For these reasons, surgery is indicated as soon as the diagnosis has been established and the appropriate preoperative steps have been completed.

Management of the Placenta. Because removal of the placenta always carries the risk of hemorrhage, blood vessels supplying the placenta should be ligated before removal of the organ. Partial separation can develop spontaneously or, more likely, in the course of the operation while attempting to locate the exact site of placental attachment. Therefore it is best to avoid unnecessary exploration of the surrounding organs. In general, the infant should be delivered, the cord severed close to the placenta, and the abdomen closed.

Unfortunately, the placenta, if left in the abdominal cavity, commonly causes complications in the form of infection, abscesses, adhesions, intestinal obstruction, and wound dehiscence (Martin and associates, 1988). *Although the complications of leaving the placenta are troublesome and usually lead to subsequent laparotomy, they may be less grave than the hemorrhage that sometimes results from placental removal during the initial surgery.*

If the placenta is left in situ, its involution may be monitored using ultrasound and a variety of placental hormones. Quantitative serum β-hCG levels are available in most areas, and the use of other markers has not proven to be superior (France and Jackson, 1980; Martin and associates, 1990b). For a short period of time, methotrexate was recommended to hasten involution and resorption. Unfortunately, this often led to accelerated placental destruction with accumulation of necrotic tissue and ultimately to infection and abscess formation (Rahman and associates, 1982). Presently, it is considered best not to use methotrexate. In most cases, placental function rapidly declines, and the placenta is resorbed (France and Jackson, 1980). In one case described by Belfar and associates (1986), placental resorption took over 5 years!

Selective Embolization of Bleeding Sites. Percutaneous femoral artery catheterization and pelvic angiography, followed by embolization of specific placental bleeding sites, has been lifesaving in instances of massive pelvic hemorrhage uncontrolled by conventional techniques. It also has been reported effective for massive bleeding from uterine atony, cervical and uterine lacerations, postabortion bleeding, uterine arteriovenous fistulas, and gynecological malignancies (Gilbert and co-workers, 1992; Haseltine and colleagues, 1984; Kivikoski and associates, 1988; Martin and colleagues, 1990b).

Briefly, the procedure consists of identification of the bleeding site(s) from a pelvic angiogram. A catheter tip is then advanced into the specific artery supplying the bleeding site, and the artery is embolized using small pieces of shredded Gelfoam dissolved in saline or angiography dye. Microspheres have been injected, and small pieces of wool have been pushed through the catheter to the bleeding site using a small steel wire. The last two methods result in permanent occlusion of the specific vessel(s), while Gelfoam is believed to occlude the vessel for only 7 to 21 days.

The worst complication of the technique is that bleeding may not be arrested. If bleeding is not controlled despite angiographic evidence of occlusion of the specific injured vessel(s), a collateral vessel is likely the source of continued bleeding. Other complications include necrosis of tissues distal to the embolized site such as colon and gluteal muscle. Finally, any angiographic procedure involves the risk of an allergic reaction to the dye as well as vascular spasm and arterial thrombosis; these procedures themselves are not without risk.

Prognosis. Strafford and Ragan (1977) cite a 6 percent maternal mortality and a 91 percent perinatal mortality. Two of the 10 cases described by Rahman and associates (1982) resulted in maternal deaths. Morbidity in surviving patients is excessive in many cases (Costa and colleagues, 1991; Martin and associates, 1988, 1990a, b).

Ovarian Pregnancy

In 1878, Spiegelberg formulated his criteria for diagnosis of ovarian pregnancy: (1) the tube on the affected side be intact, (2) the fetal sac must occupy the position of the ovary, (3) the ovary must be connected to the uterus by the ovarian ligament, and (4) definite ovarian tissue must be found in the sac wall. Bobrow and Winkelstein (1956) were able to collect 154 cases from the literature and added another that satisfied these criteria. Hallatt (1982) described 25 cases of primary ovarian pregnancy, and Grimes and co-workers (1983) reported 24 more. Shuster and associates (1990) reported an ovarian pregnancy that was diagnosed following an attempted midtrimester therapeutic abortion. It is not clear whether use of an intrauterine contraceptive device predisposes to ovarian pregnancy. Gray and Ruffolo (1978), for example, described 4 instances of ovarian pregnancy in which the women conceived with a Cu-7 device in situ.

Although the ovary can accommodate itself more readily than the tube to the expanding pregnancy, rupture at an early period is the usual consequence. Nonetheless, there are recorded cases in which the ovarian pregnancy went to term, and a few infants survived. Williams and associates (1982), while attempting a cesarean delivery because of a transverse lie at 41 weeks' gestation, found an ovarian pregnancy. The infant, who weighed about 3500 g, survived. The ovary, placenta, and membranes were resected, and the severed right ureter was reimplanted in the bladder.

Symptoms and Signs. Symptoms and physical findings are likely to mimic those of a tubal pregnancy or a

bleeding corpus luteum. At the time of operation, early ovarian pregnancies are likely to be considered corpus luteum cysts or a bleeding corpus luteum.

Management. Early ovarian pregnancies should be treated, when possible, by wedge resection or cystectomy; otherwise, oophorectomy is performed.

Cervical Pregnancy

Cervical pregnancy in the past has been a rare form of ectopic gestation. Dees (1966) estimated the incidence to be 1 in 18,000 pregnancies. In our experience, it is even less common, but the incidence appears to be increasing, in part due to newer forms of assisted reproduction, but especially after in-vitro fertilization and embryo transfer (Bayati and associates, 1989; Weyerman and colleagues, 1989).

In a typical case, the endocervix is eroded by trophoblast, and the pregnancy proceeds to develop in the fibrous cervical wall, as illustrated in Figure 32–9. The duration of the pregnancy and ultimately its capacity for growth is dependent upon the site of embryo implanta-

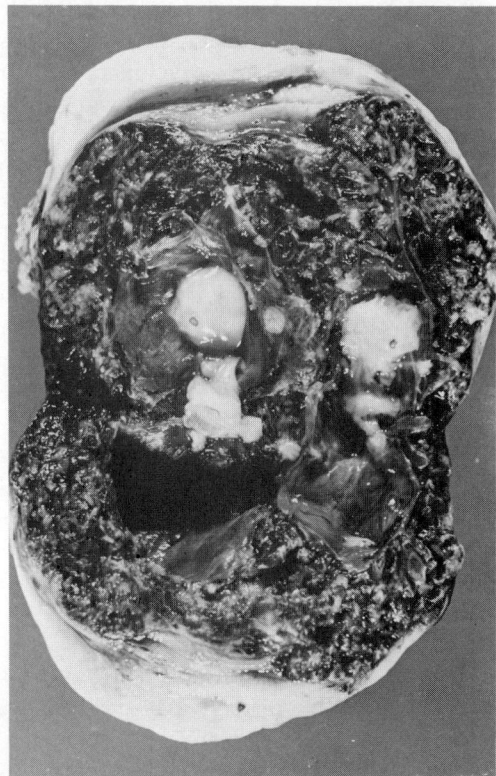

Fig. 32–9. Cervical pregnancy in situ removed by hysterectomy nearly 3 months after last normal menstrual period and 1 month after onset of vaginal bleeding. (Courtesy of Drs. D. Rubell and A. Brekken.)

tion. The higher it is implanted in the cervical canal, the greater is its capacity to grow *and bleed*.

Clinical Presentation and Diagnosis

Symptoms and Signs. Usually, painless bleeding appearing shortly after nidation is the first sign. As pregnancy progresses, a distended thin-walled cervix with the external os partially dilated may be evident. Bleeding without pain is the common clinical characteristic. Above the cervical mass, a slightly enlarged uterine fundus may be palpated. Gabbe and co-workers (1975) reported 2 women with a cervical pregnancy who had high fever that erroneously was initially attributed to an infected intrauterine pregnancy. Cervical pregnancy rarely goes beyond the 20th week of gestation and usually is surgically terminated because of bleeding.

Diagnosis. Diagnosis is based upon a high degree of suspicion and confirmed with either vaginal or abdominal sonography. A diagnosis is highly likely with an empty uterus and a gestation filling the cervical canal. If any doubt remains, magnetic resonance imaging most often confirms the diagnosis (Bader-Armstrong and associates, 1989; Rafal and co-workers, 1990).

Specific clinical diagnostic criteria for cervical pregnancy were established by Paalman and McElin (1959): (1) uterine bleeding without cramping after a period of amenorrhea, (2) softened cervix disproportionally enlarged to a size equal to or larger than the corpus, (3) complete confinement and firm attachment of the products of conception to the endocervix, and (4) a snug internal cervical os. In addition, there are pathological criteria that establish the diagnosis of cervical pregnancy (Rubin and co-workers, 1983): (1) cervical glands must be present opposite placental attachment, (2) attachment of placenta to cervix must be intimate, (3) the placenta must be below the entrance of uterine vessels or below the peritoneal reflection on the anteroposterior uterine surfaces, and (4) fetal elements must not be present in the uterine corpus.

Surgical Management.

In the past, hysterectomy was often the only choice available because of profuse hemorrhage that accompanied attempts at removal of the cervical pregnancy. Even with hysterectomy, hemorrhage was excessive and urinary tract injury frequent due to the enlarged barrel-shaped cervix.

Cerclage. Bernstein and associates (1981) successfully managed two cases by placing a heavy silk ligature around the cervix similar to a McDonald cerclage (see Chap. 31, p. 673). Since this report, the efficacy of this technique has been confirmed (Bachus and associates, 1990), and the prophalactic use of a Shirodkar cerclage and local injection of vasopressin has been recom-

mended by Wharton and Gore (1988) prior to evacuation of the productions of conception.

Foley Catheter. Nolan and associates (1989) and Thomas and co-workers (1991b) recommend placement of hemostatic cervical sutures at 3 and 9 o'clock. Suction curettage is then performed, followed immediately by insertion of a Foley catheter into the cervical canal. The 30-mL catheter bulb is inflated and the vagina is packed tightly with gauze to further tamponade bleeding. A suction catheter tip may be left above the vaginal packing to ensure adequate drainage and to monitor blood loss.

Uterine Artery Embolization. Lobel and colleagues (1990) and Simon and co-workers (1991) reported remarkable success with selective preoperative uterine artery embolization using Gelfoam. Despite this precaution, Simon and co-workers (1991) had one instance of heavy postcurettage bleeding that required an intracervical 30-mL Foley catheter and vaginal packing. Pliskow and colleagues (1991) had to perform a postcurettage laparotomy to repair a lower uterine laceration sustained during a curettage.

Nonsurgical Management.

Because of the risks of uncontrolled hemorrhage, nonsurgical methods utilizing methotrexate and other drug treatments have been developed. Today, nonsurgical techniques are the first line of therapy, and surgical techniques are generally used only when chemotherapy fails or in emergency conditions when a woman, usually undiagnosed, presents with life-threatening acute hemorrhage (Wolcott and associates, 1988).

Methotrexate. The anticancer drug methotrexate has been used successfully to treat cervical pregnancy. The general rules of its use have been described earlier (p. 708). In summary, the agent has been injected directly into the gestational sac with or without potassium chloride to induce fetal death; it has been given systemically in single high-dose therapy with folinic acid rescue; it has been given in lower-dose prolonged courses; and finally it has been given in various combinations, usually intraamnionically after failure of systemic therapy (Kaplan and associates, 1990; Oyer and colleagues, 1988; Palti and co-workers, 1989; Skannal and Burkman, 1989; Stovall and associates, 1988; Yankowitz and colleagues, 1990). More advanced pregnancies, that is, those greater than 6 weeks gestation generally require induction of fetal death (usually with KCl) or high-dose and prolonged therapy with methotrexate.

Combined Chemotherapy. Bakri and Badawi (1990) reported successful therapy using combined chemotherapy with methotrexate, actinomycin-D, and cyclophosphamide. This seems excessive during early gestation but might prove useful in more advanced cervical pregnancies.

Etoposide. This agent is a semisynthetic derivative of podophylotoxin that inhibits cell-cycle progression by inhibiting DNA synthesis (Sinkule, 1984). It has been used successfully to treat gestational trophoblastic disease (Wong and colleagues, 1986), and Segna and colleagues (1990) reported successful treatment of a 6-week cervical pregnancy with the agent. Treatment consisted of oral doses, 200 mg/m², administered 3 times a day for 5 days. It appears to be effective, convenient, and usable in an outpatient setting. Major side effects include myelosupression, usually mild reversible leukopenia; alopecia, reversible and present after two or three courses; and mild nausea (Wong and associates, 1986).

Other Sites of Ectopic Pregnancy

A primary *splenic pregnancy* has been reported by Mankodi and associates (1977). The symptoms and signs that led to laparotomy included pain in the epigastrium and left shoulder, hypotension, tachycardia, syncope, and tenderness in the vaginal fornices. At laparotomy considerable hemoperitoneum but normal pelvic organs were found. A rent in the hilar surface of the spleen prompted splenectomy. Microscopically, chorionic villi were identified in the splenic rent. A similar case was reported by Yackel and associates (1988). A few cases of primary *hepatic pregnancy* have been described, including one with lithopedion formation (Børlum and Blom, 1988; De Almeida Barbosa and associates, 1991; Luwuliza-Kirunda, 1978; Schlatter and colleagues, 1988).

References

Aboulghar MA, Mansour RT, Serour GI: Transvaginal injection of potassium chloride and methotrexate for the treatment of tubal pregnancy with a live fetus. Hum Reprod 5:887, 1990

Akhan O, Cekirge S, Senaati S, Besim A: Sonographic diagnosis of an abdominal ectopic pregnancy. Am J Radiol 155:197, 1990

Arey LB: The cause of tubal pregnancy and tubal twinning. Am J Obstet Gynecol 5:163, 1923

Arias-Stella J: Atypical endometrial changes associated with the presence of chorionic tissue. Arch Pathol 58:112, 1954

Atrash HK, Friede A, Hogue CJR: Abdominal pregnancy in the United States: Frequency and maternal mortality. Obstet Gynecol 69:333, 1987a

Atrash HK, Friede A, Hogue CJR: Ectopic pregnancy mortality in the United States, 1970–1983. Obstet Gynecol 70:817, 1987b

Atrash HK, Koonin LM, Lawson HW, Franks AL, Smith JC: Maternal Mortality in the United States, 1979–1986. Obstet Gynecol 76:1055, 1990a

Atrash HK, MacKay HT, Hogue CJR: Ectopic pregnancy concurrent with induced abortion: Incidence and mortality. Am J Obstet Gynecol 162:726, 1990b

Bachus KE, Stone D, Suh B, Thickman D: Conservative management of cervical pregnancy with subsequent fertility. Am J Obstet Gynecol 162:450, 1990

Bader-Armstrong B, Shah Y, Rubens D: Use of ultrasound and magnetic resonance imaging in the diagnosis of cervical pregnancy. J Clin Ultrasound 17:283, 1989

Bakri YN, Badawi A: Cervical pregnancy successfully treated with chemotherapy. Acta Obstet Gynecol Scand 69:655, 1990

Barnes RB, Roy S, Yee B, Duda MJ, Mishell DR Jr: Reliability of urinary pregnancy tests in the diagnosis of ectopic pregnancy. J Reprod Med 30:827, 1985

Bassil S, Pouly JL, Canis M, Janny L, Vye P, Chapron C, Bruhat MA: Advanced heterotopic pregnancy after in-vitro fertilization and embryo transfer, with survival of both the babies and the mother. Hum Reprod 6:1008, 1991

Batzer FR, Weiner S, Corson SL, Schlaff S, Otis C: Landmarks during the first forty-two days of gestation demonstrated by the β-subunit of human chorionic gonadotropin and ultrasound. Am J Obstet Gynecol 146:973, 1983

Bayati J, Garcia JE, Dorsey JH, Padilla SL: Combined intrauterine and cervical pregnancy from in vitro fertilization and embryo transfer. Fertil Steril 51:725, 1989

Beacham WD, Hernquist WC, Beacham DW, Webster HD: Abdominal pregnancy at Charity Hospital in New Orleans. Am J Obstet Gynecol 84:1257, 1962. (184 references cited)

Belfar HL, Kurtz AB, Wapner RJ: Long-term follow-up after removal of an abdominal pregnancy: Ultrasound evaluation of the involuting placenta. J Ultrasound Med 5:521, 1986

Bell OR, Awadalla SG, Mattox JH: Persistent ectopic syndrome: A case report and literature review. Obstet Gynecol 69:521, 1987

Bengtsson G, Bryman I, Thorburn J, Lindblom B: Low-dose oral methotrexate as second-line therapy for persistent trophoblast after conservative treatment of ectopic pregnancy. Obstet Gynecol 79:589, 1992

Beral V: An epidemiological study of recent trends in ectopic pregnancy. Br J Obstet Gynaecol 82:775, 1975

Bernaschek G, Rudelstorfer R, Csaicsich P: Vaginal sonography versus serum human chorionic gonadotropin in early detection of pregnancy. Am J Obstet Gynecol 158:608, 1988

Bernstein D, Holzinger M, Ovadia J, Frishman B: Conservative treatment of cervical pregnancy. Obstet Gynecol 58:741, 1981

Bobrow ML, Winkelstein LB: Intrafollicular ovarian pregnancy. Am J Surg 91:991, 1956

Børlum K-G, Blom R: Primary hepatic pregnancy. Int J Gynecol Obstet 27:427, 1988

Brenner PF, Ray S, Mishell DR: Ectopic pregnancy: A study of 300 consecutive surgically treated cases. JAMA 243:673, 1980

Brunham RC, Peeling R, Maclean I, Kosseim ML, Paraskevas M: *Chlamydia trachomatis*-associated ectopic pregnancy: Serologic and histologic correlates. J Infect Dis 165:1076, 1992

Bryson SCP: β-Subunit of human chorionic gonadotropin, ultrasound, and ectopic pregnancy: A prospective study. Am J Obstet Gynecol 146:163, 1983

Cacciatore B, Stenman UH, Ylöstalo P: Diagnosis of ectopic pregnancy by vaginal ultrasonography in combination with a discriminatory serum hCG level of 1000 IU/l (IRP). Br J Obstet Gynaecol 97:904, 1990a

Cacciatore B, Tiitinen A, Stenman UH, Ylöstalo P: Normal early pregnancy: Serum hCG levels and vaginal sonography findings. Br J Obstet Gynaecol 97:899, 1990b

Carson SA, Stoval TG, Unstot E, Andersen R, Ling F, Buster JE: Human chorionic somatomammotropin (HCS) predicts rising ectopic pregnancy rupture following methotrexate chemotherapy. Fertil Steril 51:593, 1989

Cartwright PS: Peritoneal trophoblastic implants after surgical management of tubal pregnancy. J Reprod Med 36:523, 1991

Cartwright PS, Brown JE, Davis RJ, Thieme GA, Boehm FH: Advanced abdominal pregnancy associated with fetal pulmonary hypoplasia: Report of a case. Am J Obstet Gynecol 155:396, 1986

Centers for Disease Control: Ectopic pregnancy—United States, 1984 and 1985. MMWR 37:637, 1988

Coleman BG, Baron RL, Arger PH, Arenson RL, Axel L, Mayer DP, Costello P: Ectopic embryo detection using real-time sonography. J Clin Ultrasound 13:545, 1985

Corson SL, Batzer FR: Ectopic pregnancy: A review of the etiologic factors. J Reprod Med 31:78, 1986

Costa SD, Presley J, Bastert G: Advanced abdominal pregnancy. Obstet Gynecol Surv 46:515, 1991

Coste J, Job-Spira N, Fernandez H, Papiernik E, Spira A: Risk factors for ectopic pregnancy: A case-control study in France, with special focus on infectious factors. Am J Epidemiol 133:839, 1991

Cross JB, Lester WM, McCain J: The diagnosis and management of abdominal pregnancy with a review of 19 cases. Am J Obstet Gynecol 62:303, 1951

Daus K, Mundy D, Graves W, Slade BA: Ectopic pregnancy. What to do during the 20-day window. J Reprod Med 34:162, 1989

De Almeida Barbosa A, Rodrigues de Freitas LA, Andrade Mota M: Primary pregnancy in the liver: A case report. Path Res Pract 187:329, 1991

DeCherney AH, Jones EE: Ectopic pregnancy. Clin Obstet Gynecol 28:365, 1985

de Crespigny L Ch: Demonstration of ectopic pregnancy by transvaginal ultrasound. Br J Obstet Gynaecol 95:1153, 1988

Dees HC: Cervical pregnancy associated with uterine leiomyomas. South Med J 59:900, 1966

Dicker D, Samuel N, Feldberg D, Goldman JA: Infected ectopic pregnancy presenting as unilateral tubo-ovarian abscess. Eur J Obstet Gynecol Reprod Biol 17:237, 1984

DiMarchi JM, Kosasa TS, Kobara TY, Hale RW: Persistent ectopic pregnancy. Obstet Gynecol 70:555, 1987

Dimitry ES, Subak-Sharpe R, Mills M, Margara R, Winston R: Nine cases of heterotopic pregnancies in 4 years of in vitro fertilization. Fertil Steril 53:107, 1990

Dorfman SF: Deaths from ectopic pregnancy, United States 1979 to 1980. Obstet Gynecol 62:344, 1983

Dorfman SF, Grimes DA, Cates W Jr, Binkin NJ, Kafrissen ME, O'Reilly KR: Ectopic pregnancy mortality, United States, 1979 to 1980: Clinical aspects. Obstet Gynecol 64:386, 1984

Durukan T, Urman B, Yarali H, Arikan Ü, Beykal Ö: An abdominal pregnancy 10 years after treatment for pelvic tuberculosis. Am J Obstet Gynecol 163:594, 1990

Egarter Ch, Husslein P: Treatment of ectopic pregnancy by means of prostaglandins. Prostaglandins Leukot Essent Fatty Acids 35:91, 1989

Emembolu JO: Celo-intestinal fistulae complicating advanced extra-uterine pregnancy. Int J Gynecol Obstet 28:177, 1989

Emerson DS, Cartier MS, Altieri LA, Felker RE, Smith WC, Stoval TG, Gray LA: Diagnostic efficacy of endovaginal color doppler flow imaging in an ectopic pregnancy screening program. Radiology 183:413, 1992

Feichtinger W, Kemeter P: Treatment of unruptured ectopic pregnancy by needling of sac and injection of methotrexate or PG E₂ under transvaginal sonography control. Report of 10 cases. Arch Gynecol Obstet 246:85, 1989

Ferland RJ, Chadwick DA, O'Brien JA, Granai CO III: An ectopic pregnancy in the upper retroperitoneum following in vitro fertilization and embryo transfer. Obstet Gynecol 78:544, 1991

France JT, Jackson P: Maternal plasma and urinary hormone levels during and after a successful abdominal pregnancy. Br J Obstet Gynaecol 87:356, 1980

Fujii S, Ban C, Okamura H, Nishimura T: Unilateral tubal quadruplet pregnancy. Am J Obstet Gynecol 141:840, 1981

Funderburk AG: Bilateral ectopic pregnancy with simultaneous intrauterine pregnancy. Am J Obstet Gynecol 119:274, 1974

Gabbe SG, Kitzmiller JL, Kosasa TS, Driscoll SG: Cervical pregnancy presenting as septic abortion. Am J Obstet Gynecol 123:212, 1975

Gilbert WM, Moore TR, Resnik R, Doemeny J, Chin H, Bookstein JJ: Angiographic embolization in the management of hemorrhagic complications of pregnancy. Am J Obstet Gynecol 166:493, 1992

Glassner MJ, Aron E, Eskin BA: Ovulation induction with clomiphene and the rise in heterotopic pregnancies. A report of two cases. J Reprod Med 35:175, 1990

Glew SS, Sivanesaratnam V: Advanced extrauterine pregnancy mimicking intrauterine fetal death: Case reports. Aust NZ J Obstet Gynecol 29:450, 1989

Goldman GA, Dicker D, Ovadia J: Primary abdominal pregnancy: Can artificial abortion, endometriosis and IUD be etiological factors? Eur J Obstet Gynecol Reprod Biol 27:139, 1988

Gray CL, Ruffolo EH: Ovarian pregnancy associated with intrauterine contraceptive devices. Am J Obstet Gynecol 132:134, 1978

Grimes HG, Nosal RA, Gallagher JC: Ovarian pregnancy: A series of 24 cases. Obstet Gynecol 61:174, 1983

Guirgis RR, Craft IL: Ectopic pregnancy resulting from gamete intrafallopian transfer and in vitro fertilization. Role of ultrasonography in diagnosis and treatment. J Reprod Med 36:793, 1991

Hage ML, Wall LL, Killam A: Expectant management of abdominal pregnancy. A report of two cases. J Reprod Med 33:407, 1988

Hahlin M, Wallin A, Sjoblom P, Lindblom B: Single progesterone assay for early recognition of abnormal pregnancy. Hum Reprod 5:662, 1990

Hallatt JG: Primary ovarian pregnancy: A report of twenty-five cases. Am J Obstet Gynecol 143:55, 1982

Harris MB, Angtuaco T, Frazier CN, Mattison DR: Diagnosis of a viable abdominal pregnancy by magnetic resonance imaging. Am J Obstet Gynecol 159:150, 1988

Haseltine FP, Glickman MG, Marchesi S, Spitz R, D'Lugi A, DeCherney AH: Uterine embolization in a patient with post-abortal hemorrhage. Obstet Gynecol 63:78S, 1984

Herman A, Ron-El R, Golan A, Weinraub Z, Bukovsky I, Caspi E: The role of tubal pathology and other parameters in ectopic pregnancies occurring in in vitro fertilization and embryo transfer. Fertil Steril 54:864, 1990

Hertz RH, Timor-Tritch I, Sokol RJ, Zador I: Diagnostic studies and fetal assessment in advanced extrauterine pregnancy. Obstet Gynecol 50(suppl):63, 1977

Hirsch E, Cohen L, Hecht BR: Heterotopic pregnancy with discordant ultrasonic appearance of fetal cardiac activity. Obstet Gynecol 79:824, 1992

Hochner-Celnikier D, Ron M, Goshen R, Zacut D, Amir G, Yagel S: Rupture of ectopic pregnancy following disappearance of serum beta subunit of hCG. Obstet Gynecol 79:826, 1992

Jacobson L, Riemer RK, Goldfien AC, Lykins D, Siiteri PK, Roberts JM: Rabbit myometrial oxytocin and alpha 2-adrenergic receptors are increased by estrogen but are differentially regulated by progesterone. Endocrinology 120:184, 1987

Jeffcoate TNA: Principles of Gynaecology, 3rd ed. New York, Appleton-Century-Crofts, 1967

Jones EE: Ectopic pregnancy: Common and some uncommon misdiagnoses. Obstet Gynecol Clin North Am 18:55, 1991

Kadar N, Caldwell BR, Romero R: A method of screening for ectopic pregnancy and its indications. Obstet Gynecol 58:162, 1981a

Kadar N, DeVore G, Romero R: The discriminatory hCG zone: Its use in the sonographic evaluation for ectopic pregnancy. Obstet Gynecol 58:156, 1981b

Kadar N, Romero R: Observations on the log human chorionic gonadotropin-time relationship in early pregnancy and its practical implications. Am J Obstet Gynecol 157:73, 1987

Kadar N, Romero R: The timing of a repeat ultrasound examination in the evaluation for ectopic pregnancy. J Clin Ultrasound 10:211, 1982

Kalchman GG, Meltzer RM: Interstitial pregnancy following homolateral salpingectomy: Report of 2 cases and a review of the literature. Am J Obstet Gynecol 96:1139, 1966

Kamrava MM, Taymor ML, Berger MJ, Thompson IE, Seibel MM: Disappearance of human chorionic gonadotropin following removal of ectopic pregnancy. Obstet Gynecol 62:486, 1983

Kaplan BR, Brandt T, Javaheri G, Scommegna A: Nonsurgical treatment of a viable cervical pregnancy with intra-amniotic methotrexate. Fertil Steril 53:941, 1990

Kenigsberg D, Porte J, Hull M, Spitz IM: Medical treatment of residual ectopic pregnancy. RU 486 and methotrexate. Fertil Steril 47:702, 1987

King G: Advanced extrauterine pregnancy. Am J Obstet Gynecol 67:712, 1954

Kirkinen P, Lauper U, Huch R, Huch A: Case Report. Normal placental function and fetoplacental blood circulation in advanced abdominal pregnancy. Acta Obstet Gynecol Scand 67:283, 1988

Kivikoski AI, Martin C, Weyman P, Picus D, Giudice L: Angiographic arterial embolization to control hemorrhage in abdominal pregnancy: A case report. Obstet Gynecol 71:456, 1988

Kojima E, Abe Y, Morita M, Motohiro I, Hirakawa S, Momose K: The treatment of unruptured tubal pregnancy with intratubal methotrexate injection and laparoscopic control. Obstet Gynecol 75:723, 1990

Kooi S, Kock HCLV: Treatment of tubal pregnancy by local injection of methotrexate after adrenaline injection into the mesosalpinx: A report of 25 patients. Fertil Steril 54:580, 1990

Kouyoumdjian A, Kirkpatrick J: Coexistence of an intrauterine pregnancy with both an ectopic pregnancy and salpingitis in the right fallopian tube. A case report. J Reprod Med 35:824, 1990

Kurtz AB, Dubbins PA, Wapner RJ, Goldberg BB: Problem of abnormal fetal position. JAMA 247:3251, 1982

Levin AA, Schoenbaum SC, Stubblefield PG, Zimicki S, Monson RR, Ryan KJ: Ectopic pregnancy and prior induced abortion. Am J Public Health 72:253, 1982

Lobel SM, Meyerovitz MF, Benson CC, Goff B, Bengtson JM: Preoperative angiographic uterine artery embolization in the management of cervical pregnancy. Obstet Gynecol 76:938, 1990

Luwuliza-Kirunda JMM: Primary hepatic pregnancy. Br J Obstet Gynaecol 85:311, 1978

Maccato M, Estrada R, Hammill H, Faro S: Prevalence of active *Chlamydia trachomatis* infection at the time of exploratory laparotomy for ectopic pregnancy. Obstet Gynecol 79:211, 1992

Mahoney BS, Filly RA, Nyberg DA, Callen PW: Sonographic evaluation of ectopic pregnancy. J Ultrasound Med 4:221, 1985

Mäkinen JI, Erkkola RU, Laippala PJ: Causes of the increase in the incidence of ectopic pregnancy. A study on 1017 patients from 1966 to 1985 in Turku, Finland. Am J Obstet Gynecol 160:642, 1989

Mankodi RC, Sankari K, Bhatt SM: Primary splenic pregnancy. Br J Obstet Gynaecol 84:634, 1977

Marchbanks PA, Annegers JF, Coulam CB, Strathy JH, Kurland LT: Risk factors for ectopic pregnancy. A population-based study. JAMA 259:1823, 1988

Martin JN Jr, McCaul JF IV: Emergent management of abdominal pregnancy. Clin Obstet Gynecol 33:438, 1990a

Martin JN Jr, Ridgway LE III, Connors JJ, Sessums JK, Martin RW, Morrison JC: Angiographic arterial embolization and computed tomography-directed drainage for the management of hemorrhage and infection with abdominal pregnancy. Obstet Gynecol 76:941, 1990b

Martin JN Jr, Sessums JK, Martin RW, Pryor JA, Morrison JC: Abdominal pregnancy: Current concepts of management. Obstet Gynecol 71:549, 1988

Mashiach S, Carp JHA, Serr DM: Nonoperative management of ectopic pregnancy: A preliminary report. J Reprod Med 27:127, 1982

Mathews CP, Coulson PB, Wild RA: Serum progesterone levels as an aid in the diagnosis of ectopic pregnancy. Obstet Gynecol 68:390, 1986

McBain JC, Evans JH, Pepperell RJ, Robinson HP, Smith MA, Brown JB: An unexpectedly high rate of ectopic pregnancy following the induction of ovulation with human pituitary and chorionic gonadotropin. Br J Obstet Gynaecol 87:5, 1980

McCann MF, Kessel E: International experience with laparoscopic sterilization: Follow-up of 8500 women. Adv Planned Parent 12:199, 1978

McCausland A: High rate of ectopic pregnancy following laparoscopic tubal coagulation failures. Am J Obstet Gynecol 136:97, 1980

Ménard A, Créquat J, Mandelbrot L, Hauuy JP, Madelenat P: Treatment of unruptured tubal pregnancy by local injection of methotrexate under transvaginal sonographic control. Fertil Steril 54:47, 1990

Merrill BS, Mitts DL, Rogers W, Weinberg PC: Autotransfusion. Intraoperative use in ruptured ectopic pregnancy. J Reprod Med 24:14, 1980

Miyazaki Y: Nonsurgical therapy of ectopic pregnancy. Hokkaido Iyaku Zasshi 58:132, 1983

Morris JM, Van Wagenen G: Interception: The use of postovulatory estrogens to prevent implantation. Am J Obstet Gynecol 115:101, 1973

Murphy WD, Feiglin DH, Cisar CC, Al-Malt AM, Bellon EM: Magnetic resonance imaging of a third trimester abdominal pregnancy. Magn Reson Imaging 8:657, 1990

Nederlof KP, Lawson HW, Saftlas AF, Atrash HK, Finch EL: Ectopic pregnancy surveillance, United States, 1970–1987. MMWR 39(suppl 4):9, 1990

Niebyl JR: Pregnancy following total hysterectomy. Am J Obstet Gynecol 119:512, 1974

Nolan TE, Chandler PE, Hess LW, Morrison JC: Cervical pregnancy managed without hysterectomy. A case report. J Reprod Med 34:241, 1989

Nugent PJ: Ruptured ectopic pregnancy in a patient with a recent intrauterine abortion. Ann Emerg Med 21:5, 1992

Nyberg DA, Mack LA, Laing FC, Brooke JR Jr: Early pregnancy complications: Endovaginal sonographic findings correlated with human chorionic gonadotropin levels. Radiology 167:619, 1988

O'Connor DM, Kurman RJ: Intermediate trophoblast in uterine currettings in the diagnosis of ectopic pregnancy. Obstet Gynecol 72:665, 1988

Orr JW Jr, Huddleston JF, Knox GE, Goldenberg RL, Davis RO: False negative oxytocin challenge test associated with abdominal pregnancy. Am J Obstet Gynecol 133:108, 1979

Ory HW: The woman's health study: Ectopic pregnancy and intrauterine contraceptive devices: New perspectives. Obstet Gynecol 57:137, 1981

Ory SJ: New options for diagnosis and treatment of ectopic pregnancy. JAMA 267:534, 1992

Ory SJ, Villanueva AL, Sand PK, Tamura RK: Conservative treatment of ectopic pregnancy with methotrexate. Am J Obstet Gynecol 154:1299, 1986

Oyer R, Tarakjian D, Lev-Toaff A, Friedman A, Chatwani A: Treatment of cervical pregnancy with methotrexate. Obstet Gynecol 71:469, 1988

Paalman RJ, McElin TW: Cervical pregnancy. Am J Obstet Gynecol 77:1261, 1959

Palti Z, Rosen NB, Goshen R, Ben-Chitrit A, Yagel S: Successful treatment of a viable cervical pregnancy with methotrexate. Am J Obstet Gynecol 161:1147, 1989

Pellerito JS, Taylor KJW, Quedens-Case C, Hammers LW, Scoutt LM, Ramos IM, Meyer WR: Ectopic pregnancy: Evaluation with endovaginal color flow imaging. Radiology 183:407, 1992

Peterson CM, Kreger D, Delgado P, Hung TT: Laboratory and clinical comparison of a rapid versus a classic progesterone radioimmunoassay for use in determining abnormal and ectopic pregnancies. Am J Obstet Gynecol 166:562, 1992

Phillips RS, Tuomala RE, Feldblum PJ, Schachter J, Rosenberg MJ, Aronson MD: The effect of cigarette smoking, *Chlamydia trachomatis* infection, and vaginal douching on ectopic pregnancy. Obstet Gynecol 79:85, 1992

Pittaway DE, Reish RL, Wentz AC: Doubling times of human chorionic gonadotropin increase in early viable intrauterine pregnancies. Am J Obstet Gynecol 152:299, 1985

Pliskow S, Herbst SJ, Cohn JM, Huber J, Ackerman RT: Preoperative angiographic uterine artery embolization for the management of cervical pregnancy. Am J Gynecol Health 5:19, 1991

Pritchard JA, Adams RH: The fate of blood in the peritoneal cavity. Surg Gynecol Obstet 105:621, 1957

Rafal RB, Kosovsky PA, Markisz JA: Case Report. MR appearance of cervical pregnancy. J Comput Assist Tomogr 14:482, 1990

Rahman MS, Al-Suleiman SA, Rahman J, Al-Sibai MH: Advanced abdominal pregnancy—observations in 10 cases. Obstet Gynecol 59:366, 1982

Reyniak JV: Conservative microsurgical management of gestation. Wiener Klinisch Wochenschrift 97:481, 1985

Robinson HP, deCrespigny LJC, Harvey J, Hay DL: Ectopic pregnancy—Potentials for diagnosis using ultrasound and urine and serum pregnancy tests. Aust NZ J Obstet Gynaecol 25:49, 1985

Romero R, Kadar N, Castro D, Jeanty P, Hobbins JC, DeCherney AH: The value of adnexal sonographic findings in the diagnosis of ectopic pregnancy. Am J Obstet Gynecol 158:52, 1988

Romney SL, Hertig AT, Reid DE: The endometria associated with ectopic pregnancy. Surg Gynecol Obstet 91:605, 1950

Rubin GL, Peterson HB, Dorfman SF, Layde PM, Maze JM, Ory HW, Cates W Jr: Ectopic pregnancy in the United States: 1970 through 1978. JAMA 249:1725, 1983

Samuellson S, Sjovall A: Laparoscopy in suspected ectopic pregnancy. Acta Obstet Gynecol Scand 51:31, 1972

Schlatter MC, DePree B, Vanderkolk KJ: Hepatic abdominal pregnancy: A case report. J Reprod Med 33:921, 1988

Segna RA, Mitchell DR, Misas JE: Successful treatment of cervical pregnancy with oral etoposide. Obstet Gynecol 76:945, 1990

Shah A, Courey NG, Cunanan RG: Pregnancy following laparoscopic tubal electrocoagulation and division. Am J Obstet Gynecol 129:459, 1977

Sherman D, Langer R, Sadovsky G, Bukovsky I, Caspi E: Improved fertility following ectopic pregnancy. Fertil Steril 37:497, 1982

Sherman KJ, Daling JR, Stergachis A, Weiss NS, Foy HM, Wang S-P, Grayston JT: Sexually transmitted diseases and tubal pregnancy. Sex Transm Dis 17:115, 1990

Shuster J, Alger L, Mighty H, Guzinski G, Crenshaw C Jr: Ovarian pregnancy diagnosed after a failed midtrimester therapeutic abortion. A case report. J Reprod Med 35:187, 1990

Simon P, Donner C, Delcour C, Kirkpatrick C, Rodesch F: Selective uterine artery embolization in the treatment of cervical pregnancy: Two case reports. Eur J Obstet Gynecol Reprod Biol 40:159, 1991

Sinkule JA: Etoposide: A Semisynthetic epipodophyllotoxin. Chemistry, pharmacology, pharmacokinetics, adverse effects and use as a neoplastic agent. Pharmacotherapy 4:61, 1984

Sivin I: Alternative estimates of ectopic pregnancy risks during contraception. Am J Obstet Gynecol 165:1900, 1991

Skannal D, Burkman RT: Cervical pregnancy treated with methotrexate. A case report. J Reprod Med 34:496, 1989

Sopelak VM, Bates GB: Role of transmigration and abnormal embryogenesis in ectopic pregnancy. Clin Obstet Gynecol 30:210, 1987

Spiegelberg O: Casuistry in ovarian pregnancy. Arch Gynaekol 13:73, 1878

Spirtos NM, Spirtos TW, Inouye C, Mishell DR Jr: Resumption of ovulation after ectopic pregnancy. Obstet Gynecol 69:933, 1987

Stabile I, Grudzinskas JG: Ectopic pregnancy: A review of incidence, etiology and diagnostic aspects. Obstet Gynecol Surv 45:335, 1990

Stangel JJ, Reyniak V, Stone ML: Conservative surgical management of tubal pregnancy. Obstet Gynecol 48:241, 1976

Stock RJ: The changing spectrum of ectopic pregnancy. Obstet Gynecol 71:885, 1988

Stovall TG, Kellerman AL, Ling FW, Buster JE: Emergency department diagnosis of ectopic pregnancy. Ann Emerg Med 19:1098, 1990a

Stovall TG, Ling FW: Some new approaches to ectopic pregnancy. Contemp Obstet Gynecol 37:35, 1992a

Stovall TG, Ling FW, Buster JE: Reproductive performance after methotrexate treatment of ectopic pregnancy. Am J Obstet Gynecol 162:1620, 1990b

Stovall TG, Ling FW, Buster JE: Outpatient chemotherapy of unruptured ectopic pregnancy. Fertil Steril 51:435, 1989a

Stovall TG, Ling FW, Carson SA, Buster JE: Serum progesterone and uterine curettage in differential diagnosis of ectopic pregnancy. Fertil Steril 57:456, 1992b

Stovall TG, Ling FW, Cope BJ, Buster JE: Preventing ruptured ectopic pregnancy with a single serum progesterone. Am J Obstet Gynecol 160:1425, 1989b

Stovall TG, Ling FW, Gray LA: Methotrexate treatment of unruptured ectopic pregnancy: A report of 100 cases. Obstet Gynecol 77:749, 1991a

Stovall TG, Ling FW, Gray LA: Single dose methotrexate for treatment of ectopic pregnancy. Obstet Gynecol 77:754, 1991b

Stovall TG, Ling FW, Smith WC, Felker R, Rasco BJ, Buster JE: Successful nonsurgical treatment of cervical pregnancy with methotrexate. Fertil Steril 50:672, 1988

Strafford JC, Ragan WD: Abdominal pregnancy: Review of current management. Obstet Gynecol 50:548, 1977

Stromme WB: Salpingotomy for tubal pregnancy. Obstet Gynecol 1:473, 1953

Studdiford WD: Primary peritoneal pregnancy. Am J Obstet Gynecol 44:487, 1942

Tanaka T, Hayashi H, Kutsuzawa T, Fujimoto S, Ichinoe K: Treatment of interstitial ectopic pregnancy with methotrexate: Report of a successful case. Fertil Steril 37:851, 1982

Tatum HJ, Schmidt FH: Contraceptive and sterilization practices and extrauterine pregnancy: A realistic perspective. Fertil Steril 28:407, 1977

Thomas JS Jr, Willie JO, Clark JFJ: Primary peritoneal pregnancy: A case report. J Natl Med Assoc 83:635, 1991a

Thomas RL, Gingold BR, Gallagher MW: Cervical pregnancy. A report of two cases. J Reprod Med 36:459, 1991b

Timonen S, Nieminen U: Tubal pregnancy, choice of operative method of treatment. Acta Obstet Gynecol Scand 46:327, 1967

Timor-Tritsch IE, Monteagudo A, Matera C, Veit CR: Sonographic evolution of cornual pregnancies treated without surgery. Obstet Gynecol 79:1044, 1992

Timor-Tritsch IE, Yeh MN, Peisner DB, Lesser KB, Slavik TA: The use of transvaginal ultrasonography in the diagnosis of ectopic pregnancy. Am J Obstet Gynecol 161:157, 1989

Tuomivaara L, Kauppila A, Puolakka J: Ectopic pregnancy—an analysis of the etiology, diagnosis and treatment in 552 cases. Arch Gynecol 237:135, 1986

Vermesh M: Conservative management of ectopic gestation. Fertil Steril 51:559, 1989

Vignali M, Busacca M, Brigante C, Doldi N, Spagnolo D, Belloni C: Abdominal pregnancy as a result of gamete intrafallopian transfer (GIFT) and subsequent treatment with methotrexate: Case report. Int J Fertil 35:280, 1990

Ware HH: Observations on thirteen cases of late extrauterine pregnancy. Am J Obstet Gynecol 55:561, 1948

Washington AE, Cates WJ, Zaidi AK: Hospitalizations for pelvic inflammatory disease: Epidemiology and trends in the United States, 1975 to 1981. JAMA 251:25, 1984

Weström L, Bengtsson LPH, Mardh P-A: Incidence, trends, and risks of ectopic pregnancy in a population of women. Br Med J: 282:15, 1981

Weyerman PC, Verhoevan A Th M, Alberda A Th: Cervical pregnancy after in vitro fertilization and embryo transfer. Am J Obstet Gynecol 161:1145, 1989

Wharton KR, Gore B: Cervical pregnancy managed by placement of a shirodkar cerclage before evacuation. A case report. J Reprod Med 33:227, 1988

Williams PC, Malvar TC, Kraft JR: Term ovarian pregnancy with delivery of a live female infant. Am J Obstet Gynecol 142:589, 1982

Wolcott HD, Kaunitz AM, Nuss RC, Benrubi GE: Successful pregnancy after previous conservative treatment of an advanced cervical pregnancy. Obstet Gynecol 71:1023, 1988

Wong LC, Choo YC, Ma HK: Primary oral etoposide therapy in gestational trophoblastic disease. Cancer 58:14, 1986

Yackel DB, Panton ONM, Martin DJ, Lee D: Splenic pregnancy—case report. Obstet Gynecol 71:471, 1988

Yaffe H, Navot D, Laufer N: Pitfalls in early detection of ectopic pregnancy. Lancet 1:277, 1979

Yaffe H, Sadovsky E, Beyth Y: Tubal pregnancy and tubal patency. Int J Gynaecol Obstet 14:265, 1976

Yankowitz J, Leake J, Huggins G, Gazaway P, Gates E: Cervical ectopic pregnancy: Review of the literature and report of a case treated by single-dose methotrexate therapy. Obstet Gynecol Surv 45:405, 1990

Yeko TR, Gorrill JM, Hughes LH, Rodi IA, Buster JE, Sauer MV: Timely diagnosis of ectopic pregnancy using a single blood progesterone measurement. Fertil Steril 48:1049, 1987

Young PL, Saftlas AF, Atrash HK, Lawson HW, Petrey FF: National trends in the management of tubal pregnancy, 1970–1987. Obstet Gynecol 78:749, 1991

CHAPTER 33
Developmental Abnormalities of the Reproductive Tract

A number of genitourinary defects may result from abnormalities in the embryological process. These may occur spontaneously or be induced by agents such as diethylstilbestrol. Although developmental anomalies of the female genital tract are not often encountered in obstetrics, even minor defects may result in an increased incidence of threatened abortion and abnormal fetal lie (Sorensen and Trauelsen, 1987). More serious defects often result in significant fetal and maternal hazards (Golan and Caspi, 1992; Kovacevic and associates, 1990; Stein and March, 1990). There is little familial tendency associated with these defects, which at most may represent polygenic or multifactorial traits (Elias and associates, 1984).

Spontaneous Developmental Abnormalities of the Reproductive Tract; Müllerian Anomalies

In order to understand the etiology of spontaneous developmental abnormalities, it is necessary to know how the structures are formed and where and when an interruption in these processes takes place. Briefly, development begins when the metanephric ducts emerge and connect with the cloaca between the third and fifth gestational weeks. Between the fourth and fifth weeks, two ureteric buds develop distally from the mesonephric ducts and begin to grow cephalad toward the mesonephros. Müllerian (paramesonephric) ducts form bilaterally between the developing gonad and the mesonephros. The müllerian ducts extend downward and laterally to the mesonephric ducts, and finally turn medially to meet and fuse together in the midline. The fused müllerian duct descends to the urogenital sinus to join the müllerian tubercle. **The close association between the müllerian and mesonephric ducts has clinical relevance, because damage to either duct system will most often be associated with damage to both (uterine horn, kidney, and ureter).**

The uterus is formed by the union of the two müllerian ducts at about the 10th week. The fusion begins in the middle of what will become the uterus, and then extends caudally and cephalad. The characteristic shape of the uterus is now formed, with cellular proliferation at the upper portion of the uterus and a simultaneous dissolution of cells at the lower pole, thus establishing the first uterine cavity. This cavity is at the lower pole with a thick wedge of tissue above. The upper thick wedge of tissue (septum) is dissolved slowly, creating the uterine cavity. This process is usually completed by the 20th week. It is reasonable to envision that any failure to fuse the two müllerian ducts or failure to resorb the cavity between them would result in separate uterine horns or some degree of persistent uterine septum.

The vagina forms between the urogenital sinus and the müllerian tubercle by a dissolution of the cell cord between the two structures. It is believed that this dissolution starts at the hymen and moves upward toward the cervix, which is also being canalized. A failure of this process will be associated with persistence of the cell cord, and agenesis of the vagina or lesser abnormalities of this process will result in varying degrees of vaginal septum formation.

Genesis and Classification of Müllerian Abnormalities. Because fusion of the two müllerian ducts forms the vagina, cervix, and uterine body, the principal groups of deformities arising from three types of embryological defects can be classified as follows:

1. Defective canalization of the vagina results in a transverse vaginal septum, or in the most extreme form, absence of the vagina.
2. Unilateral maturation of the müllerian duct with incomplete or absent development of the opposite duct results in defects associated with upper urinary tract abnormalities.
3. The most common abnormality is absent or faulty midline fusion of the müllerian ducts. Complete lack of fusion results in two entirely separate uteri, cervices, and vaginas. Incomplete resorption of the tissue between the two fused müllerian ducts results in a uterine septum.

Various classifications of these anomalies have been proposed, but none is completely satisfactory. The terminology is often so complicated and replete with Latin words that the relative obstetrical significance is obscured. One classification for müllerian duct abnormalities suggested by Buttram and Gibbons (1979) is based upon the failure of normal development. The classification separates a diversity of anomalies into groups with similar clinical characteristics, prognosis for pregnancy, and treatment (Table 33–1 and Figs. 33–1 to 33–6). The classification includes a category for abnormalities associated with fetal exposure to diethylstilbestrol (DES). The authors stressed that vaginal anomalies may exist alone or in association with other müllerian anomalies, but vaginal anomalies were not classified because they were not associated with fetal loss. Vaginal anomalies using their scheme were most often associated with classes III and IV.

There is in fact no simplified classification for uterine, cervical, and vaginal abnormalities. Toaff and coworkers (1984) proposed another classification, but it is complicated and further burdened with Latin titles and subtitles. They did, however, provide an excellent and complete set of anatomical drawings with their classification. We prefer the simplified classification for cervical and vaginal abnormalities outlined below.

Types of Cervices

1. *Single.* The normal cervix.
2. *Septate.* A cervix consisting of a single muscular ring partitioned by a septum. The septum may be confined to the cervix, or, more often, it may be the downward continuation of a uterine septum or the upward extension of a vaginal septum.
3. *Double.* Two distinct cervices, each resulting from separate müllerian duct maturation. Both septate and true double cervices frequently are associated with a longitudinal vaginal septum. Unfortunately, many septate cervices are classified erroneously as double. The diagnosis depends on careful visual and digital examination of the cervix, and it is of clinical importance.

TABLE 33–1. CLASSIFICATION OF MÜLLERIAN ANOMALIES

I. Segmental müllerian agenesis or hypoplasia
    A. Vaginal
    B. Cervical
    C. Fundal
    D. Combined anomalies
II. Unicornuate uterus
    A. With rudimentary horn
        1. With endometrial cavity
            a. Communicating
            b. Noncommunicating
        2. Without endometrial cavity
    B. Without rudimentary horn
III. Uterine didelphys
IV. Bicornuate uterus
    A. Complete (division down to internal os)
    B. Partial
    C. Arcuate
V. Septate uterus
    A. Complete (septum to internal os)
    B. Partial
VI. Diethylstilbestrol

Modified from Buttram and Gibbons (1979), with permission.

4. *Single hemicervix.* This arises from a unilateral müllerian maturation.

Types of Vaginas

1. *Single.* The normal vagina.
2. *Longitudinally septate.* More or less complete longitudinal septum.
3. *Double.* It is often difficult to distinguish the double from the completely septate vagina. The true double vagina includes a double introitus and resembles a double-barreled shotgun, with each passage terminating in a distinct, separate cervix. At times with double vaginas, one may end blindly.
4. *Transversely septate.* Transverse vaginal septa are of different developmental origin, resulting from faulty canalization of the united müllerian anlage rather than faulty longitudinal fusion.

Diagnosis. *Vaginal septa* are usually discovered during routine pelvic examinations or by the woman who notices that vaginal tampons are not always effective in absorbing menses.

Uterine malformations may be discovered by simple inspection or during bimanual examination. Frequently they are discovered at cesarean delivery or during manual exploration of the uterine cavity after vaginal delivery. Fundal notching, palpated abdominally, is most often indicative of a malformed uterus, and the clinical impression can be confirmed by laparoscopy. Ultrasonic screening for uterine anomalies, although 98 percent specific, has only a 43 percent sensitivity (Nicolini and associates, 1987). Without radiological examination, high-resolution sonography, direct visualization of the uterine cavity, and often laparoscopic examination, it is difficult to distinguish the septate from the bicornuate uterus. *Hysteroscopic examination* and *hysterography* are of value in ascertaining the configuration of the uterine cavity. When combined with a laparoscopic confirmation of the absence or presence of an external division of the uterus and the presence or absence of a rudimentary uterine horn, virtually all uterine abnormalities can be described and classified accurately.

A high index of suspicion is important for detection. Green and Harris (1976) identified 80 uterine developmental anomalies during the course of 31,836 deliveries. They emphasized that detection was greatest during a period when one especially interested staff member espoused uterine exploration at delivery, and when an anomaly was suspected, hysterosalpingography was performed 6 to 8 weeks postpartum.

Sonography may be used to identify abnormal uterine development, although it lacks the precision of diagnosis provided by hysteroscopy and hysterosalpingography. During actual or suspected pregnancy, however, sonographic examination can be quite informative, but

A. Vaginal

C. Fundal

B. Cervical

D. Tubal

E. Combined

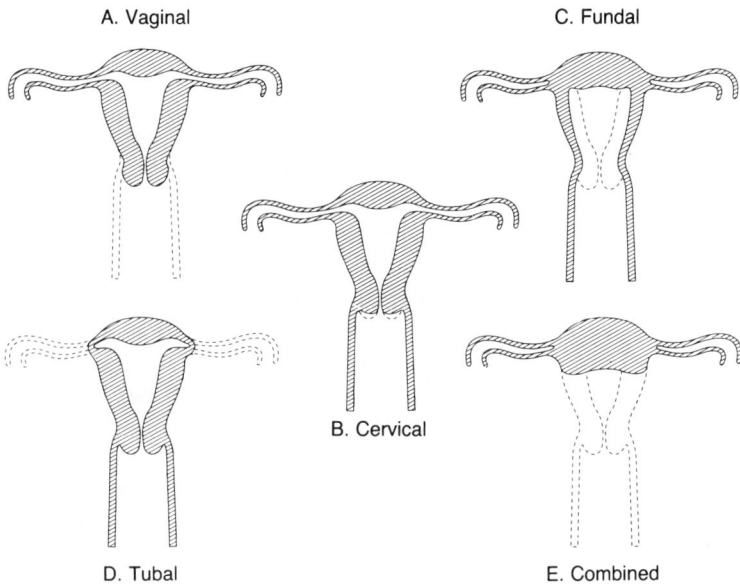

Fig. 33–1. Class I: Segmental müllerian agenesis or hypoplasia with subdivisions.

magnetic resonance imaging may be more specific (Kelley and associates, 1990).

Urological Evaluation. When asymmetrical development of the reproductive tract is found, urological evaluation is indicated because of the frequent association of urinary tract anomalies. When there is uterine atresia on one side or when one side of a double vagina terminates blindly, an ipsilateral urological anomaly is common (Fedele and associates, 1987; Heinonen, 1983, 1984; Toaff, 1974; Wiersma and colleagues, 1976; Woolf and Allen, 1953).

Auditory Evaluation. Up to a third of women with müllerian defects have been reported to have auditory defects (Letterie and Vauss, 1991). These are characterized as mild to severe sensorineural hearing defects in the high-frequency range. All 5 of the women described to date have bicornuate uteri and 3 of the 5 have renal anomalies, all right sided. Although these results are preliminary, some women with renogenital anomalies also appear to be at risk for accompanying auditory defects.

Obstetrical Significance of Müllerian Hypoplasia or Agenesis

Buttram and Gibbons Class I. The range of anomalies seen with müllerian agenesis is shown in Figure 33–1. Vaginal hypoplasia or agenesis renders pregnancy virtually impossible, and even in those rare cases in which a uterus is reattached surgically to a neovagina, successful pregnancy is extremely rare. The various types of vagi-

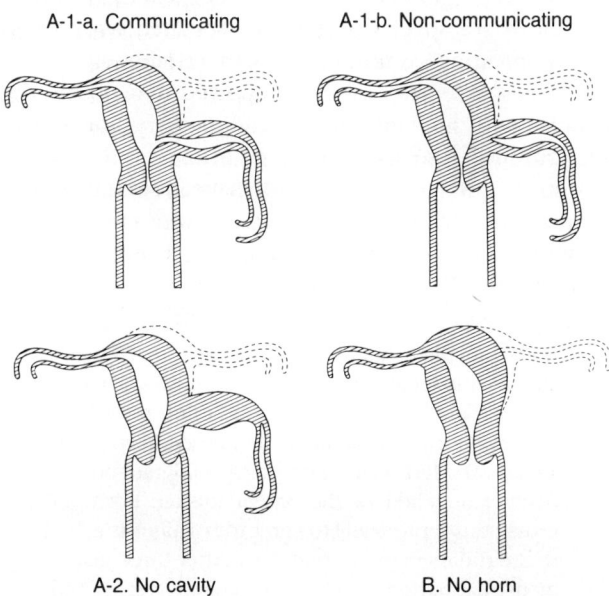

A-1-a. Communicating

A-1-b. Non-communicating

A-2. No cavity

B. No horn

Fig. 33–2. Class II: Unicornuate uterus with either rudimentary horn (A) or without rudimentary horn (B). Those with a rudimentary horn are divided into those with an endometrial cavity (A-1) or without an endometrial cavity (A-2). Those with an endometrial cavity either have a communication with the opposite uterine horn (A-1-a) or do not have a communication with the opposite horn (A-1-b).

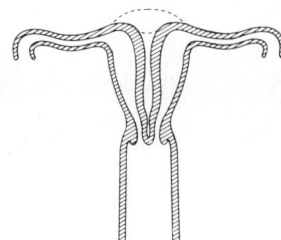

Fig. 33–3. Class III: Uterine didelphys.

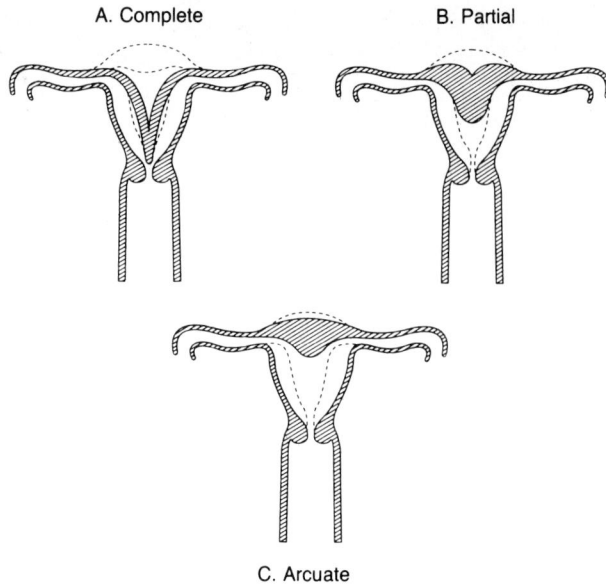

Fig. 33–4. Class IV: Bicornuate uterus in which the septum is complete down to the internal os (A), partial (B), or arcuate (C).

nal septa can be dilated, displaced, or surgically divided. The septate cervix functions remarkably well, but during labor, there is possible danger of rupture and hemorrhage.

Buttram and Gibbons Classes II Through V. Major obstetrical difficulties arise from uterine anomalies. The uterus must dilate and hypertrophy sufficiently to accommodate a term-sized fetus in a longitudinal lie; and at the proper time, it must contract efficiently to expel the fetus. Uterine defects that result from maturation of only one müllerian duct or from lack of fusion often give rise to a hemiuterus that fails to dilate and hypertrophy appropriately. This may result in a number of possible difficulties, including abortion, ectopic pregnancy, rudimentary horn pregnancy, preterm delivery, fetal growth retardation, abnormal fetal lie, uterine dysfunction, and even uterine rupture (Ben-Rafael and associates, 1991; Michalas, 1991). Surprisingly, even in conditions where only a uterine septum is present, abortion is increased

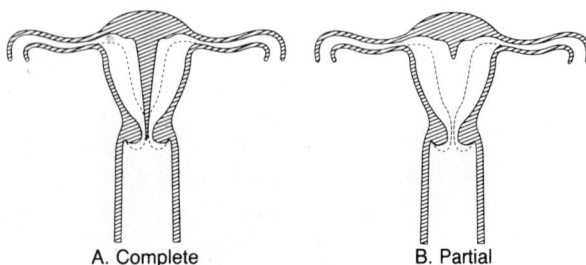

Fig. 33–5. Class V: Septate uterus with complete septum to the internal or external os (A) or partial septum (B).

(Buttram and Gibbons, 1979). Because of these obstetrical problems, each uterine defect is discussed within the classification suggested by Buttram and Gibbons (1979) and outlined in Table 33–1.

REPRODUCTIVE PERFORMANCE OF WOMEN WITH UNICORNUATE UTERUS (BUTTRAM AND GIBBONS CLASS II). The incidence of unicornuate uteri in a series of 1160 uterine anomalies was 14 percent (Zanetti and associates, 1978). This was likely an underestimate, because the major diagnostic technique used was hysterosalpingography, which cannot identify noncommunicating rudimentary horns. O'Leary and O'Leary (1963) estimated that in 90 percent of unicornuate uteri with rudimentary horns there was no communication between the horns. This information has both gynecological and obstetrical significance. Specifically, the increased incidence of infertility, endometriosis, and dysmenorrhea in such cases is certainly more easily understood (Buttram and Gibbons, 1979; Fedele and associates, 1987; Heinonen, 1983).

As shown in Table 33–2, pregnancy outcome is poor, likely due to anatomical defects (Fig. 33–2). For example, the increased incidence of abortion may be partially explained by smaller uterine size and the possible implantation of the zygote in a communicating rudimentary horn. The smaller hemiuterine size is almost certainly an explanation for the increased rates of preterm delivery, fetal growth retardation, breech presentation, abnormal uterine function in labor, and the increased incidence of cesarean delivery (Andrews and Jones, 1982; Fedele and associates, 1987; Heinonen, 1983).

Tubal pregnancies and pregnancies in the rudimentary horn are special problems associated with a noncommunicating rudimentary horn (Heinonen, 1983). Rolen and associates (1966) reported that in 70 pregnancies with implantations in rudimentary horns, uterine rupture usually occurred prior to 20 weeks' gestation. Intraperitoneal hemorrhage in such cases may be massive and life-threatening, but rare cases of fetal survival have been reported (Akhtar, 1988; Heinonen and Aro, 1988).

Pregnancy in a rudimentary uterine horn 15 weeks after the last menstrual period is shown in Figure 33–7. There was no connection between the rudimentary horn and the opposite uterine horn or the vagina. The fertilizing sperm had to migrate out the oviduct attached to the patent uterine horn and cross transperitoneally to enter the oviduct attached to the rudimentary uterine horn. After three missed menstrual periods, the woman complained of sudden, severe, cramping lower abdominal pain. A tender mass was felt to the left of a somewhat enlarged uterus. Fetal heart action was identified in this mass with Doppler ultrasound. At laparotomy, about 200 mL of blood was found free in the peritoneal cavity. A total hysterectomy and left salpingo-oophorec-

A. Constriction
bands

B. T-shaped

C. Widening of lower two-
thirds of uterine cavity

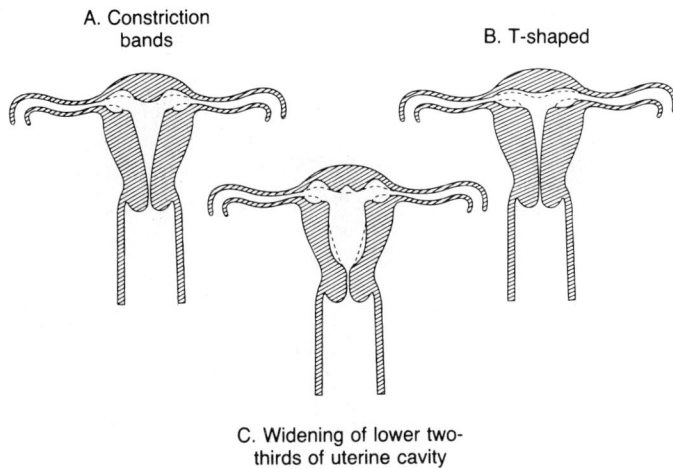

Fig. 33–6. Class VI: DES anomalies including uterus with luminal changes, such as constriction bands in the uterine cavity (A), T-shaped cavity (B), and widening of the lower two-thirds of the uterine cavity (C). (Modified from Buttram and Gibbons, 1979.)

tomy were performed. Her three previous pregnancies, all breech presentations, terminated with delivery of infants who weighed 750 g (expired), 1220 g (lived), and 2815 g (lived). The 2815-g infant was delivered by cesarean. Although a rudimentary horn was identified at that time, tubal patency to that horn was not interrupted.

REPRODUCTIVE PERFORMANCE IN WOMEN WITH UTERINE DIDELPHYS (BUTTRAM AND GIBBONS CLASS III). Uterine didelphys is distinguished from bicornuate and septate uteri by the presence of complete reduplication of cervices and hemiuterine cavities (Fig. 33–3). In a series of 26 such women, Heinonen (1984) reported that all had longitudinal vaginal septums as well. Although the problems associated with uterine didelphys are similar to those seen with a unicornuate uterus (except for ectopic and rudimentary horn pregnancies), Heinonen (1984) reported a better pregnancy outcome. The overall successful pregnancy outcome was 68 percent, with a 30 percent abortion rate and a perinatal mortality rate of only 4 percent.

Uterine didelphys, however, is not without significant problems. In addition to the 30 percent abortion rate, Heinonen (1984) observed preterm delivery in 21 percent, fetal growth retardation in 11 percent, breech presentation in 43 percent, and a cesarean delivery rate of 82 percent. The case shown in Figure 33–8 is illustrative of these complications.

Multifetal gestation is unusual but not rare in women with uterine didelphys (Heinonen, 1984; Hochner-Celnikier and colleagues, 1983). Mashiach and associates (1981) reported a case of triplets with a delivery interval of 72 days! Leiberman and co-workers (1980) also reported a delayed interval between delivery of fetuses from each hemiuterus.

REPRODUCTIVE PERFORMANCE IN WOMEN WITH BICORNUATE AND SEPTATE UTERI (BUTTRAM AND GIBBONS CLASSES IV AND V). In both classes IV and V (Figs. 33–4 and 33–5), there is a marked increase in abortions. The exception is for the arcuate uterus, which is merely a slight deviation from normal. Pregnancy losses in the first 20 weeks were

TABLE 33–2. PREGNANCY OUTCOME IN WOMEN WITH A UNICORNUATE UTERUS

Outcomes	Author						Totals
	Semmens (1962)	Beernink (1976)	Andrews (1982)	Heinonen (1982)	Buttram[a] (1979)	Fedele (1987)	
Patients	5	5	5	13	31	20	79
Conceptions	4	4	5	10	?	13	36
Pregnancies	11	8	13	15	60	29	136
Horn pregnancy	1	—	—	—	—	1	2
Abortion (%)	4 (36)	1 (12)	7 (54)	7 (47)	29 (48)	17 (59)	65 (48)
Preterm labor (%)[b]	?	3 (43)[c]	2 (33)	3 (37)	10 (33)	3 (25)	21 (30)
Term delivery[b]	?	4	4	5	21	8	42
Live births (%)[d]	63	75	45	40	40	38	45

[a] Partly personal data.
[b] Excludes abortions.
[c] One twin pregnancy.
[d] Of all pregnancies.
Modified from Fedele and co-workers (1987).

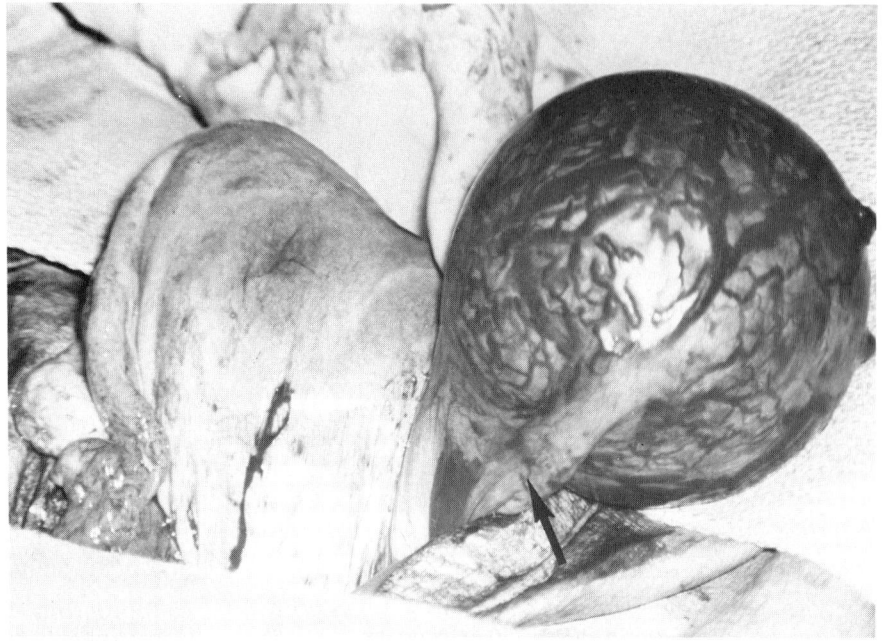

A

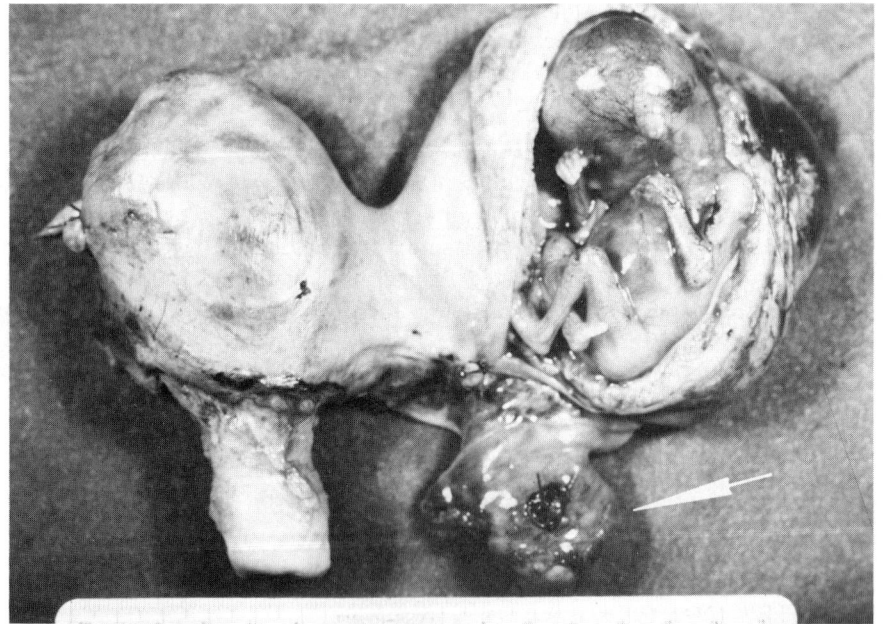

B

Fig. 33–7. A. Pregnancy of 15 weeks' gestational age in left rudimentary hemiuterus as seen at laparotomy. The tense, vascular rudimentary uterus was bleeding from veins over its extremely vascular surface. The attached oviduct (*arrow*) was patent and the adjacent left ovary contained the corpus luteum of pregnancy. **B.** Hysterectomy specimen from **A,** now with left hemiuterus opened to display the fetus and placenta. The inferior mass (*arrow*) consists of left tube and ovary. There is no cervix on the left and no communication with the right hemiuterus, which does have a cervix that communicated with the vagina.

observed by Buttram and Gibbons (1979) to be 70 percent for bicornuate and 88 percent for septate uteri. This extraordinarily high pregnancy wastage likely is due to partial or complete implantation on the largely avascular septum and failure of the conceptus to acquire an adequate blood supply (Fedele and co-workers, 1989; Gast and Martin, 1992). Once pregnancy is well established, overall outcome is associated with an increased incidence of preterm delivery, abnormal fetal lie, and cesarean delivery.

A hysterosalpingogram usually cannot be used alone to differentiate the septate and bicornuate uterus

because of the difficulty of establishing the presence or absence of an external division of the uterus. Buttram and Gibbons (1979) stressed the necessity of laparoscopy to establish the presence of an external uterine division.

Treatment. Abnormal fetal presentations, which are commonly seen with an abnormal uterus, are treated in the same way as when they are encountered in a normal uterus. Attempts at external podalic version, however, are less likely to be successful and may prove dangerous. If uterine dysfunction develops, it is unwise to stimulate

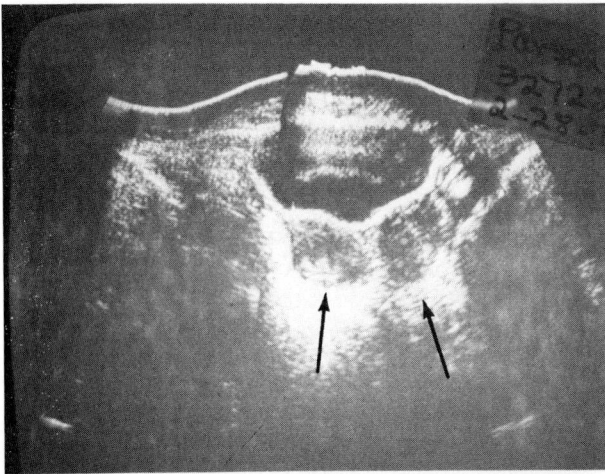

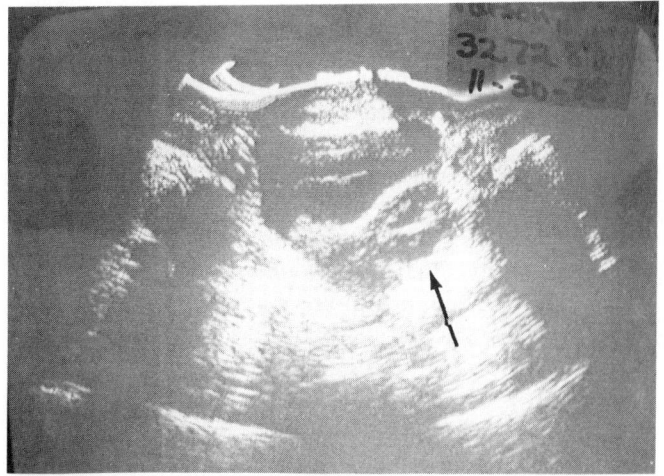

A   **B**

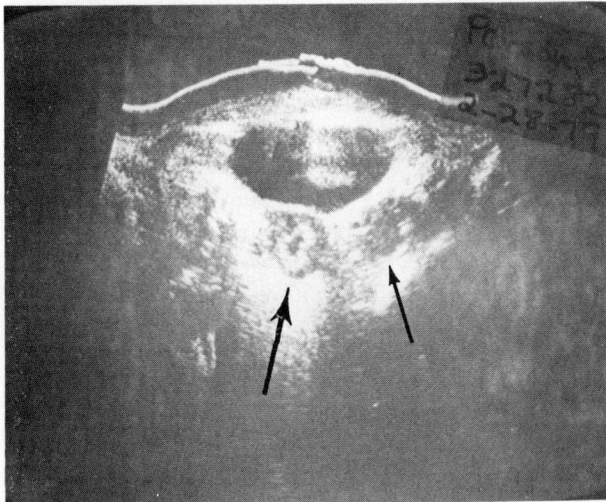

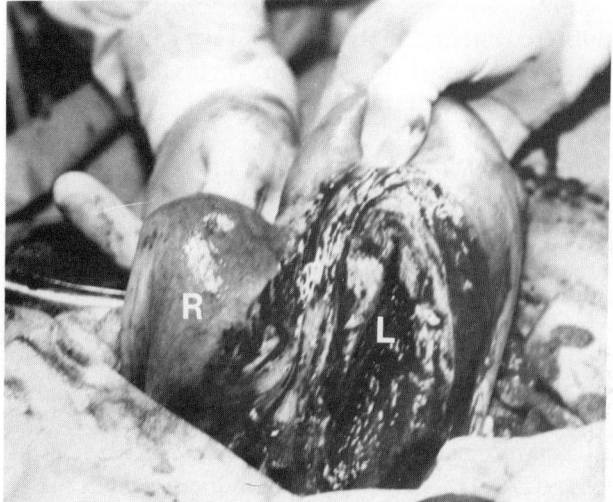

C   **D**

Fig. 33–8. Woman with uterine didelphys who had experienced seven consecutive abortions. In this 8th pregnancy, in transverse sonogram **A**, two uterine cavities are apparent above the arrows. In sonogram **B**, a pregnancy ring, probably abnormal, is seen in the left uterine cavity above the arrow. In sonogram **C**, made 90 days later, a normal pregnancy ring is seen in the right uterine cavity above the larger arrow but not in the left uterine cavity above the smaller arrow. A 2900 g healthy infant was delivered from the right uterus as a double footling breech by cesarean at 38 weeks' gestation. The left kidney was absent. Necrotic placental villi from the missed abortion were expelled from the left uterus 2 days postpartum. **D**. The same woman in **C** conceived again 3 years later in the left uterus (L). A growth-retarded fetus who thrived after cesarean birth was delivered at 37 weeks through a vertical uterine incision. The small right uterus (R) is larger than when nonpregnant.

these defective uteri with oxytocin. Cesarean delivery is safer, but unfortunately the diagnosis often is unexpected.

Cerclage. Therapeutic and prophylactic cervical cerclages are indicated in women with uterine didelphys and unicornuate or bicornuate uteri (Golan and associates, 1990; Maneschi and colleagues, 1988; Seidman and co-workers, 1991). Transabdominal cerclage offers the best hope of successful pregnancy outcome in women with partial cervical atresia or cervical hypoplasia (Hampton and colleagues, 1990; Welker and associates, 1988), but Caspi and associates (1990) have described

a modified Shirodkar cerclage that closes the internal os without resorting to an abdominal procedure. The new technique is performed by making a small transverse incision at the anterior vaginal–bladder junction and advancing the bladder up to the level of the internal os. A large round needle is used to insert a monofilament suture around either side of the cervix under the vaginal mucosa. The suture is brought out from under the vaginal mucosa in the cul-de-sac and ligated. The new procedure was performed in women with short or lacerated cervices and in women with previous McDonald cerclage failures. The results obtained were similar to those achieved with a Shirodkar cerclage, but operative time and blood loss were less. Importantly, the cerclage could be removed with less difficulty. Transvaginal cervical cerclage has been used successfully in DES-exposed women with cervical hypoplasia (Ludmir and co-workers, 1991). The question of whether to place a suture in both cervices of a uterine didelphys is unresolved (Heinonen, 1984). There appears to be no reason for cerclage with an arcuate uterus. Cerclage should not be needed after successful resection of a uterine septum (see below), but probably should still be used following abdominal metroplasties for uterine didelphys and bicornuate uteri. If active labor supervenes, procrastination in severing a cerclage ligature must be avoided because of the increased risk of uterine rupture (Chap. 31, p. 675).

Progestational agents and β-mimetic drugs administered either acutely or chronically have been used in attempts to prolong gestation. Their efficacy has not been established in these situations.

Metroplasty. Women with septate or bicornuate anomalies and poor reproductive outcomes are likely to benefit from uterine repair (Heinonen and associates, 1982; Musich and Behrman, 1978; Teti and colleagues, 1991). Ludmir and co-workers (1990) noted that bedrest and frequent obstetrical surveillance did not improve reproductive performance in women with bicornuate and septate uteri.

BICORNUATE UTERUS. Repair of a bicornuate uterus (classes IV A and IV B, Fig. 33–4) is by transabdominal metroplasty involving resection of the septum and recombination of the uterine fundi (Candiani and associates, 1990; Gitsch and colleagues, 1990; Kessler and co-workers, 1986). Following repair, uterine activity is normal if anatomically symmetrical uterine horns have been conjoined (Oliva and associates, 1992).

SEPTATE UTERUS. Repair of a septate uterus (class V, Fig. 33–5) is done best by hysteroscopic resection of the septum (Daly, 1989; Fayez, 1986; Guarino, 1989; Hassiakos, 1990; Israel, 1984; Maneschi, 1991; and all their co-workers). Excessive infusion of intrauterine dextran during these hysteroscopic procedures can result in life-threatening hypervolemic pulmonary edema and induce a severe coagulopathy (Vercellini and colleagues, 1992). Laser resection of the septum apparently only adds time and expense to the procedure when compared with microscissors (Candiani and associates, 1991). Postoperative intrauterine device insertion and hormonal therapy is not necessary to prevent septal fusion (Vercellini and associates, 1989).

UTERINE DIDELPHYS. Fedele and associates (1988) reported improved pregnancy outcomes following abdominal metroplasty to correct uterine didelphys (class

III, Fig. 33–3). Cerclage was used only once following uterine repair.

Induced Developmental Abnormalities of the Reproductive Tract; DES Exposure in Utero

For nearly a quarter of a century, until the early 1970s, diethylstilbestrol, a synthetic, nonsteroidal estrogen, was prescribed for an estimated 3 million women in the United States. Endorsements provided in early uncontrolled reports claimed the drug was useful in treating several forms of pregnancy complications, including abortion, preeclampsia and other hypertensive disorders, diabetes, and preterm labor.

The first serious problem to be linked to the use of DES (other than its lack of effectiveness) was the identification of vaginal clear cell adenocarcinoma in some daughters who were exposed in utero to diethylstilbestrol (Herbst and co-workers, 1971). It has been established that the risk of malignancy is slight but real (from 0.14 to 1.4 per 1000 exposed daughters observed through the age of 24 years). Subsequently, it was established that these women also had an increased risk of developing small cell carcinoma of the cervix. In at least one study, cervical intraepithelial neoplasia was more common among these women (Fowler and associates, 1981).

Several non-neoplastic abnormalities of the vagina and cervix have been reported; the most frequent are vaginal adenosis and cervical ectropion. Major structural abnormalities of the vagina, cervix, uterus, and fallopian tubes (all derived from the müllerian ducts) have also been reported. These structural abnormalities are associated with an increased incidence of poor reproductive performance (Managan and associates, 1982; Senekjian and co-workers, 1988).

Structural Abnormalities. One fourth to one half of women exposed to DES in utero have identifiable structural variations in the cervix and vagina. These include transverse septa, circumferential ridges involving the vagina and cervix, and collars over the cervix. The cervix may also be hypoplastic.

Anomalies of the uterine cavity are evident on hysterography in perhaps two thirds of exposed women (Kaufman and associates, 1980). Significantly smaller uterine cavities, shortened upper uterine segments, and T-shaped uterine cavities have also been described (Figs. 33–6 and 33–9). About half of women with uterine defects also have cervical defects, especially a hypoplastic cervix. Finally, a variety of abnormalities of the oviduct have been described, including shortening, narrowing, and absence of fimbriae.

In some women, vaginal adenosis, cervical ectropions, and cervical hoods have regressed, leaving an apparently normal-appearing cervix and vagina (Antonioli

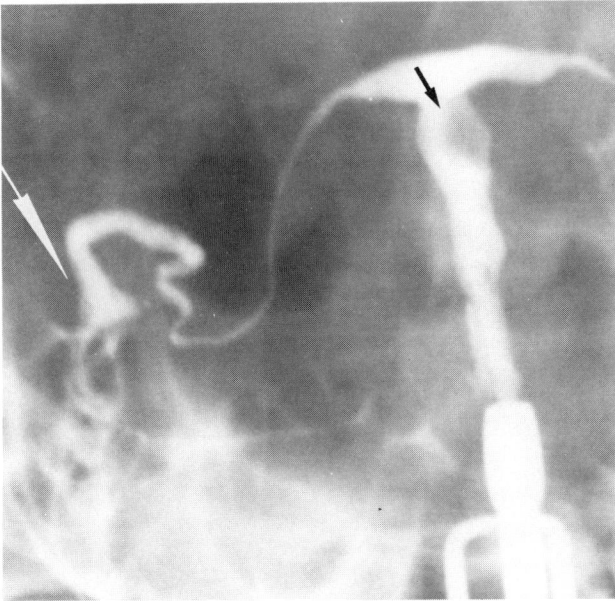

Fig. 33–9. Hysterosalpingogram from a woman who was exposed in utero to DES. Note the T-shaped uterine cavity filled with contrast material that also has spilled from the end of the right oviduct (*white arrow*), demonstrating tubal patency. The filling defect within the uterine cavity (*black arrow*) is probably hyperplastic myometrium, the consequence of the DES exposure. She has since been pregnant successfully. (Courtesy of Dr. Bruce R. Carr.)

and co-workers, 1980). Unfortunately, the major uterine and tubal anomalies are permanent.

Reproductive Performance. Lower conception rates are reported for women exposed to diethylstilbestrol in utero (Senekjian and co-workers, 1988). Of those who conceive, spontaneous abortions, ectopic pregnancies, and preterm births are increased (Herbst and co-workers, 1981, 1989; Kaufman and associates, 1984). The risk is greatest for women with demonstrated structural abnormalities.

Ectopic Pregnancy. The incidence of ectopic pregnancy is increased in women exposed to DES in utero, 7 percent compared with none for controls (Herbst and colleagues, 1989). The etiology is likely due to tubal anomalies, but decreased uterine size may also be a contributing factor (Kaufman and associates, 1980, 1984). Routine hysterosalpingographic studies are not recommended in these women, but all such women should be considered at risk for an ectopic pregnancy.

Abortion and Preterm Labor. The incidence of preterm labor is increased, likely due to uterine and cervical anomalies (de Hass and associates, 1991). The same is true for abortion, but the actual mechanism responsible for early abortion is not well understood. Cervical incompetence appears to be responsible for the increased incidence of midpregnancy abortions and preterm labor

(Ayers and associates, 1988; Ludmir and colleagues, 1987; Michaels and co-workers, 1989). This was shown graphically by Michaels and co-workers (1989) in their serial prospective sonographic study of DES-exposed women (Fig. 33–10). In 5 of 21 pregnancies, preterm cervical effacement and dilatation were identified using serial sonographic evaluations of the lower uterine segment, cervix, and vagina. A **cerclage** was applied in each of the 5 cases, and all pregnancies continued to at least 36 weeks' gestation.

Michaels and co-workers (1989) advise these women that they are at risk for preterm labor, and they are taught how to recognize the signs and symptoms of labor. They are followed weekly with serial ultrasound surveillance of the lower uterine–cervicovaginal area, beginning at 14 weeks and continuing through completion of the 27th week. If progressive cervical effacement and dilatation occur, cerclage is performed. Ayers and associates (1988) and Ludmir and co-workers (1987, 1991) recommend cervical cerclage in most of these women, but especially those with cervical hypoplasia. Hampton and colleagues (1990) recommend abdominal cerclage for women with partial atresia or hypoplasia of the cervix (see p. 727).

Infertility. Reduced fertility in these patients is poorly understood but is associated with cervical hypoplasia and atresia. Surgical correction with vaginal and cervical reanastomosis has been accomplished (Welker and co-workers, 1988). Successful pregnancies have been achieved using a variety of different zygote intrafallopian transfer techniques to avoid the damaged and poorly functioning cervix (Thijssen and associates, 1990).

Treatment. Treatment of DES-exposed women consists of continued surveillance for development of clear cell carcinoma of the vagina and cervix using vaginal and cervical cytology, colposcopy, iodine staining of the vagina and cervix, and biopsy, if indicated (Anonymous, 1992). Annual examinations are adequate for most women, but twice-yearly examinations should be made in women with extensive vaginal adenosis. Women with cervical or vaginal atypia should be examined as often as indicated. No specific therapy is recommended for adenosis in the absence of cellular atypia. Surgical management of structural anomalies is limited to cerclage.

The treatment of clear cell carcinoma of the vagina is gruesome, involving irradiation or radical extirpation. In a case of clear cell carcinoma discovered during pregnancy, the woman was delivered by cesarean section followed immediately by radical hysterectomy, vaginectomy, and pelvic node dissection (Jones and co-workers, 1981).

Fortunately, these problems from in utero exposure to DES should eventually disappear because the compound is no longer used during pregnancy.

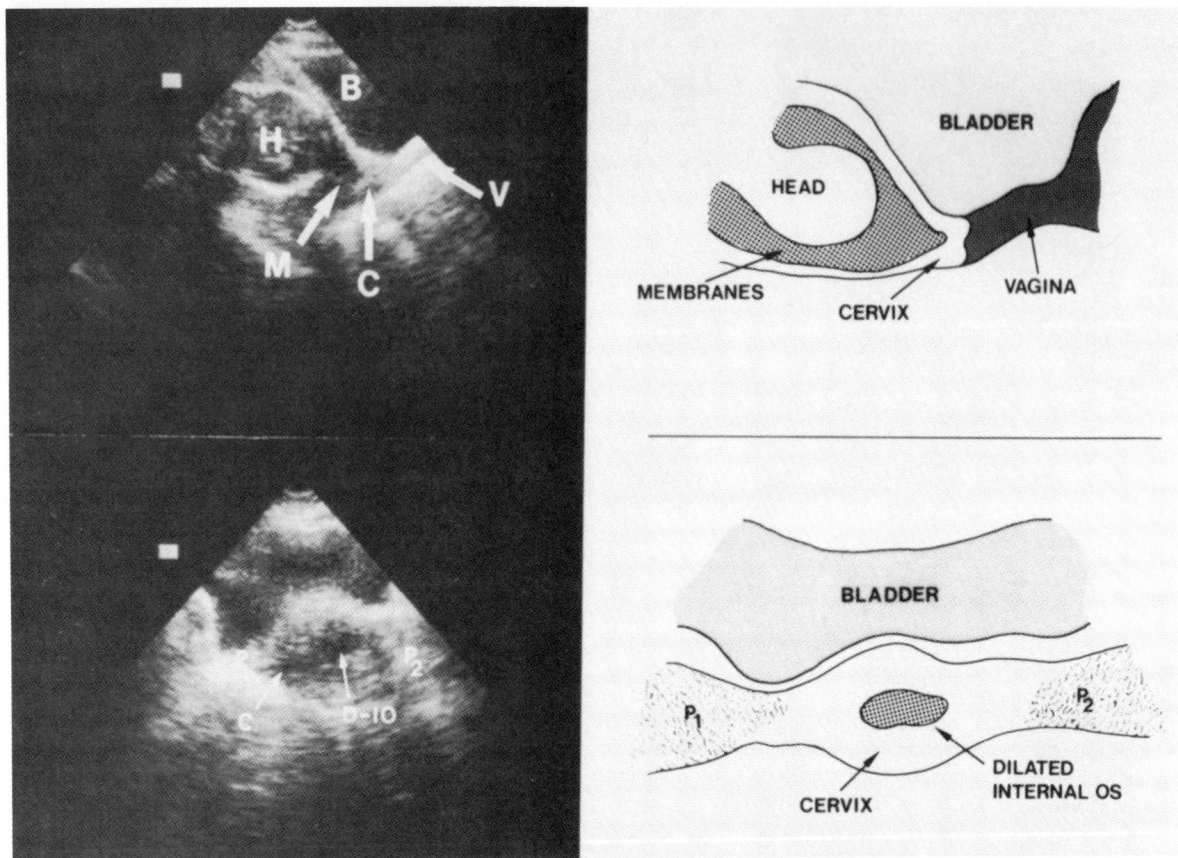

Fig. 33–10. Sonogram done in a woman exposed in utero to diethylstilbestrol. She is at 21 weeks' gestation. **Upper.** Longitudinal-view sonogram and illustration of the lower uterine–cervicovaginal area. Note the partially effaced cervix with membrane herniation. The cervix is 10 mm in length compared with 40 mm 1 week before. **Lower.** Transverse-view sonogram and illustration through the internal cervical os. Note the 20-mm dilated internal os. One week before, the cervix was "questionably dilated." (H = head; M = membrane herniation; V = vagina; C = cervix; B = bladder; P_1 = right parametrium; P_2 = left parametrium; D-IO = dilated internal os.) (From Michaels and associates, 1989, with permission.)

Miscellaneous Conditions

Endometriosis. Severe, active endometriosis is an uncommon complication of pregnancy. These women do become pregnant, however, and they sometimes exhibit bizarre and vexing clinical symptoms. For example, rupture of an endometrial cyst may result in clinical features suggestive of pyelonephritis, acute appendicitis, or tubal pregnancy (Rossman and associates, 1983). Rarely, an enlarging pelvic endometrioma may cause dystocia; but most women with endometriosis go through pregnancy and labor without complications.

Adenomyosis. Azziz (1986) reviewed the literature published for the prior 80 years and reported that adenomyosis and pregnancy coexisted in 17 percent of women over age 35. Although the condition was frequently encountered in pregnancy, it was rarely associated with obstetrical or surgical problems. For example, only 29 complications were reported over the 80-year period. When complications occurred, however, they were serious and included uterine rupture, ectopic pregnancy, uterine atony, and placenta previa.

References

Akhtar AZ: Term pregnancy in a rudimentary horn of a bicornuate uterus with foetal salvage: A case report. Asia Oceania J Obstet Gynaecol 14:143, 1988.

Andrews MC, Jones HW Jr: Impaired reproductive performance of unicornuate uterus: Intrauterine growth retardation, infertility and recurrent abortion in five cases. Am J Obstet Gynecol 144:173, 1982

Anonymous: DES-related cancers under renewed scrutiny. JNCI 84:560, 1992

Antonioli DA, Burke L, Friedman EA: Natural history of diethylstilbestrol-associated genital tract lesions: Cervical ectopy and cervicovaginal hood. Am J Obstet Gynecol 137:847, 1980

Ayers JWT, DeGrood RM, Compton AA, Barclay M, Ansbacher

R: Sonographic evaluation of cervical length in pregnancy: Diagnosis and management of preterm cervical effacement in patients at risk for premature delivery. Obstet Gynecol 71:939, 1988

Azziz R: Adenomyosis in pregnancy: A review. J Reprod Med 31:223, 1986

Beernink FJ, Beernink HE, Chinn A: Uterus unicornis with uterus solidaris. Obstet Gynecol 47:651, 1976

Ben-Rafael Z, Seidman DS, Recabi K, Bider D, Mashiach S: Uterine anomalies. A retrospective, matched-control study. J Reprod Med 36:723, 1991

Buttram VC, Gibbons WE: Müllerian anomalies: A proposed classification (an analysis of 144 cases). Fertil Steril 32:40, 1979

Candiani GB, Fedele L, Parazzini F, Zamberletti D: Reproductive prognosis after abdominal metroplasty in bicornuate or septate uterus: A life table analysis. Br J Obstet Gynaecol 97:613, 1990

Candiani GB, Vercellini P, Fedele L, Garsia S, Brioschi D, Villa L: Argon laser versus microscissors for hysteroscopic incision of uterine septa. Am J Obstet Gynecol 164:87, 1991

Caspi E, Schneider DF, Mor Z, Langer R, Weinraub Z, Bukovsky I: Cervical internal os cerclage: Description of a new technique and comparison with Shirodkar operation. Am J Perinatol 7:347, 1990

Daly DC, Maier D, Soto-Albors C: Hysteroscopic metroplasty: Six years' experience. Obstet Gynecol 73:201, 1989

de Haas I, Harlow BL, Cramer DW, Frigoleeto FD Jr: Spontaneous preterm birth: A case-control study. Am J Obstet Gynecol 165:1290, 1991

Elias S, Simpson JL, Carson SA, Malinak LR, Buttram VC Jr: Genetic studies in incomplete müllerian fusion. Obstet Gynecol 63:276, 1984

Fayez JA: Comparison between abdominal and hysteroscopic metroplasty. Obstet Gynecol 68:399, 1986

Fedele L, Dorta M, Brioschi D, Giudici MN, Candiani GB: Pregnancies in septate uteri: Outcome in relation to site of uterine implantation as determined by sonography. Am J Roentgenol 152:781, 1989

Fedele L, Zamberletti D, D'Alberton A, Vercellini P, Candiani GB: Gestational aspects of uterus didelphys. J Reprod Med 33:353, 1988

Fedele L, Zamberletti D, Vercellini P, Dorta M, Candiani GB: Reproductive performance of women with unicornuate uterus. Fertil Steril 47:416, 1987

Fowler WC Jr, Schmidt G, Edelman DA, Kaugman DG, Fenoglio CM: Risks of cervical intraepithelial neoplasia among DES exposed women. Obstet Gynecol 58:720, 1981

Gast MJ, Martin CM: Pregnancy in a woman with a uterine septum. J Reprod Med 37:85, 1992

Gitsch G, Riss P, Janisch H: Surgical correction of uterus abnormalities: Experiences with the Tompkins method. Geburtshilfe Frauenheilkd 50:467, 1990

Golan A, Caspi E: Congenital anomalies of the müllerian tract. Contemp Obstet Gynecol 37:39, 1992

Golan A, Langer R, Wexler S, Segev E, Niv D, David MP: Cervical cerclage—its role in the pregnant anomalous uterus. Int J Fertil 35:164, 1990

Green LK, Harris RE: Uterine anomalies: Frequency of diagnosis and associated obstetric complications. Obstet Gynecol 47:427, 1976

Guarino S, Incandela S, Maneschi M, Vegna G, D'Anna MR,

Leone S, Maneschi F: Hysteroscopic treatment of uterine septum. Acta Eur Fertil 20:321, 1989

Hampton HL, Meeks GR, Bates GW, Wiser WL: Pregnancy after successful vaginoplasty and cervical stenting for partial atresia of the cervix. Obstet Gynecol 76:900, 1990

Hassiakos DK, Zourlas PA: Transcervical division of uterine septa. Obstet Gynecol Surv 45:165, 1990

Heinonen PK: Uterus didelphys: A report of 26 cases. Eur J Obstet Gynecol Reprod Biol 17:345, 1984

Heinonen PK: Clinical implications of the unicornuate uterus with rudimentary horn. Int J Gynaecol Obstet 21:145, 1983

Heinonen PK, Aro P: Rupture of pregnant noncommunicating uterine horn with fetal salvage. Eur J Obstet Gynecol Reprod Biol 27:261, 1988

Heinonen PK, Saarikoski S, Pystynen P: Reproductive performance of women with uterine anomalies: An evaluation of 182 cases. Acta Obstet Gynecol Scand 61:157, 1982

Herbst AL, Hubby MM, Azizi F, Makii MM: Reproductive and gynecologic surgical experiences in diethylstilbestrol-exposed daughters. Am J Obstet Gynecol 141:1019, 1981

Herbst AL, Senekjian EK, Frey KW: Abortion and pregnancy loss among diethylstilbestrol-exposed women. Semin Reprod Endocrinol 7:124, 1989

Herbst AL, Ulfelder H, Poskanzer DC: Adenocarcinoma of the vagina. N Engl J Med 284:878, 1971

Hochner-Celnikier D, Yagel S, Beller U, Milwidsky A: Simultaneous pregnancy in each cavity of a double uterus: A case report. Int J Gynaecol Obstet 21:51, 1983

Israel R, March CM: Hysteroscopic incision of the septate uterus. Am J Obstet Gynecol 149:66, 1984

Jones WB, Woodruff JM, Erlandson RA, Lewis JL Jr: DES-related clear cell adenocarcinoma of the vagina in pregnancy. Obstet Gynecol 57:775, 1981

Kaufman RH, Adam E, Binder GL, Gerthoffer E: Upper genital tract changes and pregnancy outcome in offspring exposed in utero to diethylstilbestrol. Am J Obstet Gynecol 137:299, 1980

Kaufman RH, Noller K, Adam E, Irvine J, Gray M, Jeffries JJ, Hilton J: Upper genital tract abnormalities and pregnancy outcome in DES-exposed progeny. Am J Obstet Gynecol 148:973, 1984

Kelley JL III, Edwards RP, Wozney P, Vaccarello L, Laifer SA: Magnetic resonance imaging to diagnose a müllerian anomaly during pregnancy. Obstet Gynecol 75:521, 1990

Kessler I, Lancet M, Appelman Z, Borenstein R: Indications and results of metroplasty in uterine malformations. Int J Gynaecol Obstet 24:137, 1986

Kovacevic M, Lusic N, Vukic R: Congenital uterine anomalies in pregnancy. Jugosl Ginekol Perinatol 30:117, 1990

Leiberman JR, Schuster M, Piura B, Chaim W, Cohen A: Müllerian malformations and simultaneous pregnancies in didelphys uteri: Review and report of a case. Acta Obstet Gynecol Scand 59:89, 1980

Letterie GS, Vauss N: Müllerian tract abnormalities and associated auditory defects. J Reprod Med 36:765, 1991

Ludmir J, Jackson GM, Samuels P: Transvaginal cerclage under ultrasound guidance in cases of severe cervical hypoplasia. Obstet Gynecol 78:1067, 1991

Ludmir J, Landon MB, Gabbe SG, Samuels P, Mannuti MT: Management of the diethylstilbestrol-exposed pregnant patient: A prospective study. Am J Obstet Gynecol 157:665, 1987

Ludmir J, Samuels P, Brooks S, Mennuti MT: Pregnancy outcome of patients with uncorrected uterine anomalies managed in a high-risk obstetric setting. Obstet Gynecol 75:906, 1990

Managan CE, Borow L, Burtnett-Rubin MM, Egan V, Giuntoli RL, Mikuta JJ: Pregnancy outcome in 98 women exposed to diethylstilbestrol in utero, their mothers, and unexposed siblings. Obstet Gynecol 59:315, 1982

Maneschi F, Parlato M, Incandela S, Maneschi M: Reproductive performance in women with complete septate uteri. J Reprod Med 36:741, 1991

Maneschi M, Maneschi F, Fuc'a G: Reproductive impairment of women with unicornuate uterus. Acta Eur Fertil 19:273, 1988

Mashiach S, Ben-Rafael Z, Dor J, Serr DM: Triplet pregnancy in uterus didelphys with delivery interval of 72 days. Obstet Gynecol 58:519, 1981

Michaels WH, Thompson HO, Schreiber FR, Berman JM, Ager J, Olson K: Ultrasound surveillance of the cervix during pregnancy in diethylstilbestrol-exposed offspring. Obstet Gynecol 73:230, 1989

Michalas SP: Outcome of pregnancy in women with uterine malformation: Evaluation of 62 cases. Int J Gynaecol Obstet 35:215, 1991

Musich J Jr, Behrman SJ: Obstetric outcomes before and after metroplasty in women with uterine anomalies. Obstet Gynecol 52:63, 1978

Nicolini V, Bellotti M, Bannazzi B, Zamberletti D, Candiani GB: Can ultrasound be used to screen uterine malformations? Fertil Steril 47:89, 1987

O'Leary JL, O'Leary JA: Rudimentary horn pregnancy. Obstet Gynecol 22:371, 1963

Oliva GC, Fratoni A, Genova M, Romanini C: Uterine motility in patients with bicornuate uterus. Int J Gynaecol Obstet 37:7, 1992

Rolen AC, Choquette AJ, Semmens JP: Rudimentary uterine horn: Obstetric and gynecologic implications. Obstet Gynecol 27:806, 1966

Rossman F, D'Ablaing G III, Marrs RP: Pregnancy complicated by ruptured endometrioma. Obstet Gynecol 62:519, 1983

Seidman DS, Ben-Rafael Z, Bider D, Recabi K, Mashiach S: The role of cervical cerclage in the management of uterine anomalies. Surg Gynecol Obstet 173:384, 1991

Semmens JP: Congenital anomalies of female genital tract: Functional classification based on review of 56 personal cases and 500 reported cases. Obstet Gynecol 19:328, 1962

Senekjian EK, Potkul RK, Frey K, Herbst AL: Infertility among daughters either exposed or not exposed to diethylstilbestrol. Am J Obstet Gynecol 158:493, 1988

Sorensen SS, Trauelsen AGH: Obstetric implications of minor müllerian anomalies in oligomenorrheic women. Am J Obstet Gynecol 156:1112, 1987

Stein AL, March CM: Pregnancy outcome in women with müllerian duct anomalies. J Reprod Med 35:411, 1990

Teti G, Maffei S, Pippi E, Fioretti P: Reproductive capacity and outcome of pregnancy after metroplasty following the technique of Bret-Palmer partially modified in the pathological symmetric malformations of müllerian ducts. Clin Exp Obstet Gynecol 18:65, 1991

Thijssen RF, Hollanders JM, Willemsen WN, van der Heyden PM, van Dongen PW, Rolland R: Successful pregnancy after ZIFT in a patient with congenital cervical atresia. Obstet Gynecol 76:902, 1990

Toaff ME, Lev-Toaff AS, Toaff S: Communicating uteri: Review and classification with introduction of two previously unrecorded types. Fertil Steril 41:661, 1984

Toaff R: A major malformation—Communicating uteri. Obstet Gynecol 43:221, 1974

Vercellini P, Fedele L, Arcaini L, Rognoni MT, Candiani GB: Value of intrauterine device insertion and estrogen administration after hysteroscopic metroplasty. J Reprod Med 34:447, 1989

Vercellini P, Rossi R, Pagnoni B, Fedele L: Hypervolemic pulmonary edema and severe coagulopathy after intrauterine dextran instillation. Obstet Gynecol 79:838, 1992

Welker B, Krebs D, Lang N: Pregnancy following repair of a congenital atresia of the uterine cervix and upper vagina. Arch Gynecol Obstet 243:51, 1988

Wiersma AF, Peterson LF, Justema EJ: Uterine anomalies associated with renal agenesis. Obstet Gynecol 47:654, 1976

Woolf RB, Allen WM: Concomitant malformations: Frequent simultaneous occurrence of congenital malformations of the reproductive and urinary tracts. Obstet Gynecol 2:236, 1953

Zanetti E, Ferrari LR, Rossi G: Classification and radiographic features of uterine malformations: Hysterosalpingographic study. Br J Radiol 51:161, 1978

■ SECTION IX ■
Placental Disorders

■

CHAPTER 34

Diseases and Abnormalities of the Fetal Membranes

Diseases of the Amnion

Meconium Staining. The brownish-green discoloration of fetal membranes from meconium staining is characteristic. The presence of meconium is relatively common, and Wiswell and associates (1990) identified it in 12 percent of more than 175,000 live-born infants. At Parkland Hospital, this has been remarkably constant over the past 8 years. Of more than 100,000 women delivered during this period, about 20 percent had amnionic fluid that contained some meconium identified during labor or at delivery.

In a summary of 17 series, Katz and Bowes (1992) reported that the incidence of meconium passage ranged from 7 to 22 percent. Meconium passage is uncommon prior to 38 weeks, and it increases after 40 weeks (Table 34–1). Staining of the amnionic membranes occurs within 1 to 3 hours after meconium passage (Miller and colleagues, 1985). Fujikura and Klionsky (1975) identified meconium-stained membranes or fetus in about 10 percent of 43,000 live-born infants in the Collaborative Study of Cerebral Palsy. The neonatal mortality rate was 3.3 percent in the group with meconium-stained membranes compared with 1.7 percent in those without staining. Neonatal mortality associated with meconium primarily is the result of aspiration of thick, tenacious meconium (see Chap. 44, p. 995). Katz and Bowes (1992) have recently reviewed this subject.

Inflammation of the Amnion. In some cases, amnionitis is a manifestation of an intrauterine infection, and it is frequently associated with prolonged membrane rupture and long labors (Fox, 1978). When mononuclear and polymorphonuclear leukocytes infiltrate the chorion, the resulting microscopical finding is designated *chorioamnionitis*. These findings, however, may be nonspecific and are not associated always with other evidence for fetal or maternal infection. When organisms are isolated from amnionic fluid or membranes, they invariably are the same as those that normally colonize the vagina and cervix. The diagnosis and management of clinical chorioamnionitis is discussed in Chapter 38.

Clinically occult chorioamnionic infection caused by a wide variety of microorganisms has recently emerged as a possible explanation for many heretofore unexplained cases of ruptured membranes, preterm labor, or both.

Amnionic Cysts. Small cysts lined by typical amnionic epithelium are occasionally formed. The common variety results from fusion of amnionic folds, with subsequent retention of fluid.

Amnion Nodosum. These nodules in the amnion are sometimes called *squamous metaplasia* of the amnion or *amnionic caruncles*. They are most commonly seen in the amnion in contact with the chorionic plate, but they may also be found elsewhere. They usually appear near the insertion of the cord as elevations that are multiple, rounded or oval, and shiny grayish-yellow opaque; they vary from less than 1 mm to 5 mm in diameter. Bartman and Driscoll (1968) reported an association between amnion nodosum and multiple congenital abnormalities, especially hypoplastic kidneys with oligohydramnios. The nodules most likely are made up of fetal ectodermal debris, including vernix caseosa.

Amnionic Bands. Disruption of the amnion may lead to formation of bands or strings of amnion that adhere to the fetus and impair growth and development of the involved structure. Some conditions that appear to be

733

TABLE 34–1. MECONIUM PASSAGE AS FUNCTION OF GESTATIONAL AGE

Investigators	Infants with Meconium Passage (%)
Ostrea and Naqvi (1982)	
Less than 38 wk	4
39–42 wk	6
42 wk or greater	52
Eden and associates (1987)	
39 wk	14
40 wk	19
42 wk	26
Greater than 42 wk	29
Usher and colleagues (1988)	
39–40 wk	15
41 wk	27
42 wk or greater	32
Steer and co-workers (1989)	
Less than 36 wk	3
36–39 wk	13
40–41 wk	19
42 wk or greater	23

From Katz and Bowes (1992), with permission.

the consequence of this phenomenon, including intrauterine amputations, are considered in Chapter 44 (p. 1023).

Hydramnios

Hydramnios, sometimes called *polyhydramnios,* is excessive amnionic fluid. Normally, amnionic fluid volume increases to about 1 L, or somewhat more by 36 weeks, but decreases thereafter (Table 34–2). Postterm, there may be only a few hundred mL or even less. Somewhat arbitrarily, more than 2000 mL of amnionic fluid is considered excessive, or hydramnios. In rare instances, the uterus may contain an enormous quantity of fluid, with reports of as much as 15 L. In most instances, the increase in amnionic fluid is gradual, or *chronic hydramnios.* In *acute hydramnios,* the volume increases suddenly and the uterus may become markedly distended within a few days. Amnionic fluid in hydramnios is usually similar in appearance and composition to that in normal conditions.

TABLE 34–2. TYPICAL AMNIONIC FLUID VOLUME

Weeks Gestation	Fetus (g)	Placenta (g)	Amnionic Fluid (mL)	Percent Fluid
16	100	100	200	50
28	1000	200	1000	45
36	2500	400	900	24
40	3300	500	800	17

From Queenan (1991), with permission.

Incidence. Minor to moderate degrees of hydramnios—2 to 3 L—are rather common, but the more marked grades are not. Because of the difficulty of complete collection and measurement of amnionic fluid, the diagnosis is usually based on clinical impression (Fig. 34–1) or, more recently, sonographic estimation. Therefore, the frequency of the diagnosis varies appreciably with different observers, and it is not surprising that published data on its incidence have varied from 1 in about 60 deliveries to 1 in 750.

The carefully done studies of Hill and associates (1987) from the Mayo Clinic provide an accurate estimate of the incidence of hydramnios using ultrasonic measurements. More than 9000 regularly booked prenatal patients underwent routine ultrasonic evaluation near the end of the second or the beginning of the third trimester. They defined mild hydramnios as pockets of amnionic fluid measuring 8 to 11 cm in vertical dimension. Moderate hydramnios defined a pocket of fluid containing only small parts measured 12 to 15 cm deep. Finally, severe hydramnios was considered when a free-floating fetus was found in pockets of fluid of 16 cm or greater. Using these definitions, the overall incidence of hydramnios was 0.9 percent. The majority, almost 80 percent of these 85 cases, were mild; 17 percent were

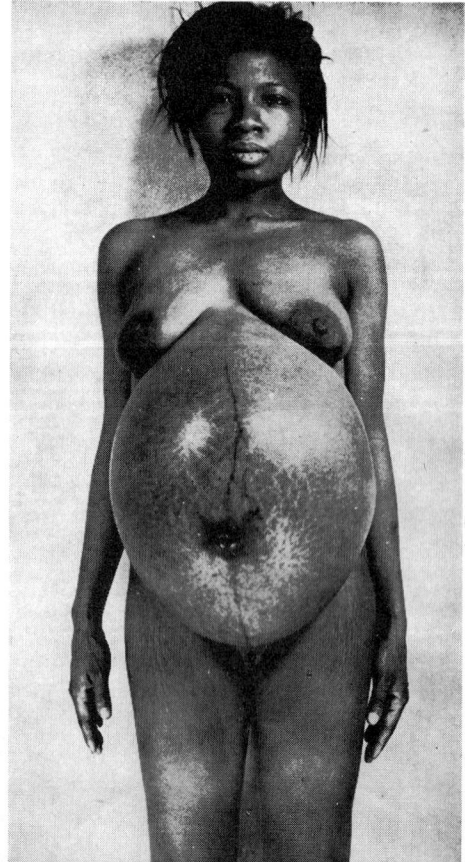

Fig. 34–1. Advanced degree of hydramnios—5500 mL of amnionic fluid was measured at delivery.

moderate; and in only 5 percent was hydramnios judged to be severe.

Significant hydramnios is frequently associated with fetal malformations, especially of the central nervous system and the gastrointestinal tract. For example, hydramnios accompanies about one half of the cases of anencephaly and esophageal atresia. According to Hill and colleagues (1987), the cause of mild hydramnios was identified in only about 15 percent of cases, whereas in cases with moderately or severely increased amnionic fluid, the cause was identified in more than 90 percent (Table 34–3). In almost one half of those cases with moderate and severe hydramnios, a fetal anomaly was identified.

More recently, the utilization of a single pocket of amnionic fluid 8 cm or more as an accurate quantitative definition of polyhydramnios has been questioned. Accordingly, Phelan and colleagues (1987) described the clinical utility of fluid quantification by the **amnionic fluid index.** This is calculated by adding the vertical depths of the largest pocket in each of four equal uterine quadrants. According to their calculations, significant polyhydramnios is defined by an index greater than 24 cm. Moore and Cayle (1990) reported normal values for the amnionic fluid index for 791 normal pregnancies from 16 to 42 weeks' gestation. Because of the skew of values at each gestational period, they used logarithmic transformations (Table 34–4). Interestingly, 25 cm or greater to define polyhydramnios corresponds to more than two standard deviations for all gestational ages.

Using 24 cm as the definition of hydramnios, some studies, but not all, indicate that perinatal mortality is increased substantively. In a report by Carlson and associates (1990) of 49 women with an amnionic fluid index of 24 cm or more, 22 (44 percent) had a recognized fetal malformation and 6 of these fetuses had aneuploidy. Moreover, there were 14 perinatal deaths among these 49 women. Brady and colleagues (1992) described findings with unexplained or idiopathic hydramnios, defined as an amnionic fluid index of 25 cm or greater, and reported 4 fetuses with chromosomal abnormalities, 2 with trisomy 18, and 2 with trisomy 21.

Smith and colleagues (1992) reported pregnancy

TABLE 34–3. ASSOCIATED FACTORS FOUND IN 102 CASES OF HYDRAMNIOS CLASSIFIED ACCORDING TO SEVERITY

Associated Factor	Number	Degree of Hydramnios		
		Mild	Moderate	Severe
Fetal anomalies	13	2	9	2
Overt diabetes	8	3	5	—
Gestational diabetes	7	7	—	—
Multifetal gestation	5	1	2	2
Idiopathic	68	66	2	—
Total	102	79	19	4

Modified from Hill and associates (1987), with permission.

TABLE 34–4. AMNIONIC FLUID INDEX VALUES (MM) FOR NORMAL PREGNANCIES

Week	Amnionic Fluid Index Percentile Values					Number
	2.5th	5th	50th	95th	97.5th	
16	73	79	121	185	201	32
17	77	83	127	194	211	26
18	80	87	133	202	220	17
19	83	90	137	207	225	14
20	86	93	141	212	230	25
21	88	95	143	214	233	14
22	89	97	144	216	235	14
23	90	98	146	218	237	14
24	90	98	147	219	238	23
25	89	97	147	221	240	12
26	89	97	147	223	242	11
27	85	95	146	226	245	17
28	86	94	146	228	249	25
29	84	92	145	231	254	12
30	82	90	145	234	258	17
31	79	88	145	238	263	26
32	77	86	144	242	269	25
33	74	83	143	245	274	30
34	72	81	142	248	278	31
35	70	79	140	249	279	27
36	68	77	138	249	279	39
37	66	75	135	244	275	36
38	65	73	132	239	269	27
39	64	72	127	226	255	12
40	63	71	123	214	240	64
41	63	70	116	194	216	162
42	63	69	110	175	192	30

From Moore and Cayle (1990), with permission.

outcomes in 97 women with mild, unexplained hydramnios defined by an amnionic fluid index of 24 to 40 cm (mean, 28.3 ± 4.7 cm). They found no increase in adverse perinatal outcomes in this group compared with pregnancies with normal amounts of fluid. Perhaps this should not be surprising; Moise (1991) emphasized that the normal range for the amnionic fluid index exceeds 24 cm between 26 and 39 weeks. He recommended that the best criterion for hydramnios is an index greater than three standard deviations, or the 97.5 percentile for gestational age (Table 34–4).

Etiology. Amnionic fluid volume is controlled in a number of ways. Early in pregnancy, the amnionic cavity is filled with fluid very similar in composition to extracellular fluid. During the first half of pregnancy, transfer of water and other small molecules takes place not only across the amnion but through the fetal skin. During the second trimester, the fetus begins to urinate, swallow, and inspire amnionic fluid (Abramovich and colleagues, 1979; Duenhoelter and Pritchard, 1976; Pritchard, 1966). These processes almost certainly have a significant modulating role in the control of fluid volume. Although the major source of amnionic fluid in hydramnios has most often been assumed to be the amnionic epithelium, no histological changes in amnion or chemical changes in amnionic fluid have been found.

Because the fetus normally swallows amnionic fluid, it has been assumed that this mechanism is one of the ways by which the volume is controlled. The theory gains validity by the nearly constant presence of hydramnios when swallowing is inhibited as, for example, in cases of esophageal atresia. Fetal swallowing is by no means the only mechanism for preventing hydramnios. Both Pritchard (1966) and Abramovich (1970) quantified this and found in some instances of gross hydramnios that appreciable volumes of fluid were swallowed.

In cases of anencephaly and spina bifida, increased transudation of fluid from the exposed meninges into the amnionic cavity may be an etiological factor. Another possible explanation in anencephaly, when swallowing is not impaired, is excessive urination caused either by stimulation of cerebrospinal centers deprived of their protective coverings, or lack of antidiuretic hormone. The converse is well established: fetal defects that cause anuria are nearly always associated with oligohydramnios.

In hydramnios associated with monozygotic twin pregnancy, the hypothesis has been advanced that one fetus usurps the greater part of the circulation common to both twins and develops cardiac hypertrophy, which in turn results in increased urine output (see Chap. 39, p. 898). Naeye and Blanc (1972) identified in this syndrome dilated renal tubules, enlarged bladder, and an increased urinary output in the early neonatal period, suggesting that increased fetal urine production is responsible for hydramnios. Conversely, donor members of parabiotic transplacental transfusion pairs had contracted renal tubules with oligohydramnios.

Hydramnios that rather commonly develops with maternal diabetes during the third trimester remains unexplained, and fetal urine formation is apparently normal (Wladimiroff and co-workers, 1975).

Naeye and Blanc (1972) described hypoplastic lungs commonly in neonates with hydramnios and questioned their role in the genesis of the hydramnios. The observations of Duenhoelter and Pritchard (1976) on both monkey and human fetuses establish that normal fetal lungs have the potential for the exchange of relatively large volumes of fluid as the consequence of inspiration. Hypoplastic lungs may compromise this pathway for removal of amnionic fluid.

The enlarged placenta may contribute to increased amnionic fluid. Prolactin may have a role in the control of its volume. Prolactin concentration in amnionic fluid is normally increased compared with that of maternal plasma, and prolactin receptors have been identified in chorion laeve. Healy and associates (1985) found that prolactin–receptor binding was less than normal in cases of idiopathic hydramnios, and they hypothesized that prolactin resistance owing to receptor deficiency may be the underlying cause of chronic hydramnios. Myhra and associates (1992) have linked maternal smoking to a 1.7-fold increase in hydramnios.

Symptoms. Major symptoms accompanying hydramnios arise from purely mechanical causes and result principally from pressure exerted within and around the overdistended uterus upon adjacent organs. The effects on maternal respiratory functions may be striking. When distension is excessive, the mother may suffer from severe dyspnea and, in extreme cases, she may be able to breathe only when upright. Edema, the consequence of compression of major venous systems by the very large uterus, is common, especially in the lower extremities, the vulva, and the abdominal wall. Rarely, severe oliguria may result from ureteral obstruction by the very large uterus (see Chap. 50, p. 1142). With *chronic hydramnios,* the accumulation of fluid takes place gradually and the woman may tolerate the excessive abdominal distension with relatively little discomfort. In *acute hydramnios,* however, distension may lead to disturbances sufficiently serious to be threatening. Acute hydramnios tends to develop earlier in pregnancy than does the chronic form, often as early as 16 to 20 weeks, and it may rapidly expand the hypertonic uterus to enormous size. Without treatment, pain is likely to become intense and the dyspnea so severe that the woman is unable to lie flat. As a rule, acute hydramnios leads to labor before 28 weeks, or the symptoms become so severe that intervention is mandatory. In the majority of cases of chronic hydramnios, and thus differing from acute hydramnios, the amnionic fluid pressure is not appreciably higher than in normal pregnancy.

Diagnosis. The primary clinical finding with hydramnios is uterine enlargement in association with difficulty in palpating fetal small parts and in hearing fetal heart tones. In severe cases, the uterine wall may be so tense that it is impossible to palpate any fetal parts (Fig. 34–1). Such findings call for ultrasonic examination to better quantify amnionic fluid and to identify multiple fetuses or fetal abnormalities.

Sonography. The differentiation among hydramnios, ascites, and a large ovarian cyst can usually be made without difficulty by ultrasonic evaluation. Large amounts of amnionic fluid can nearly always be readily demonstrated as an abnormally large echo-free space between the fetus and the uterine wall or placenta (Fig. 34–2). At times, a fetal abnormality such as anencephaly or other neural tube defects, or a gastrointestinal tract anomaly, may be seen.

Radiography. A large radiolucent area around the fetal skeleton suggests hydramnios, although a soft tissue mass such as a sacrococcygeal tumor may appear the same. Most often, anencephaly and other gross skeletal defects are easily diagnosed. *Amniography,* using contrast material such as Hypaque, may help identify excess amnionic fluid, soft tissue tumors projecting from the fetus, and the presence or absence of fetal swallowing.

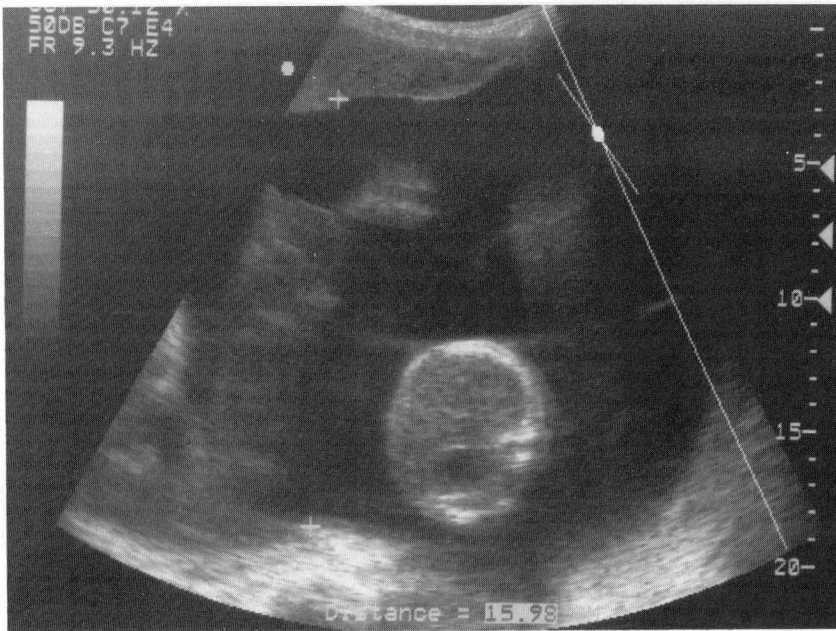

Fig. 34–2. Marked hydramnios in a 24-week twin gestation with twin–twin transfusion syndrome. (Courtesy of Dr. Diane Twickler.)

Radiography has largely been replaced by ultrasound scanning.

Prognosis. In general, the more severe the degree of hydramnios, the higher the perinatal mortality rate, so that the outlook for the infant in pregnancies with major degrees of hydramnios is poor. Even when sonography and x-ray show an apparently normal fetus, the prognosis is still guarded, because the incidence of fetal malformations is 15 to 20 percent and chromosomal abnormalities are more common. Perinatal mortality is increased further by preterm delivery, even with a normal fetus. Erythroblastosis, difficulties encountered by infants of diabetic mothers, prolapse of the umbilical cord when the membranes rupture, and placental abruption as the uterus rapidly decreases in size, add still further to bad outcomes.

The hazards imposed on the mother by hydramnios are significant but usually not life-threatening. The most frequent maternal complications are placental abruption, uterine dysfunction, and postpartum hemorrhage. Extensive premature separation of the placenta sometimes follows escape of massive quantities of amnionic fluid because of the decrease in the area of the emptying uterus beneath the placenta (see Chap. 37, p. 828). Uterine dysfunction and postpartum hemorrhage result from uterine atony consequent to overdistention. Abnormal presentations and operative intervention are also more common.

Treatment. Minor degrees of hydramnios rarely require treatment. Even moderate degrees with some discomfort usually can be managed without intervention until labor ensues or until the membranes rupture spontaneously. If there is dyspnea or abdominal pain, or if ambulation is difficult, hospitalization becomes necessary. There is no satisfactory treatment for symptomatic hydramnios other than removal of some of the amnionic fluid. Bed rest with sedation may make the situation endurable, but it rarely has any effect on fluid. Diuretics and water and salt restriction are likewise ineffective and potentially dangerous. Recently, indomethacin therapy has been utilized for symptomatic hydramnios.

Amniocentesis. The principal purpose of amniocentesis is to relieve maternal distress, and to that end it is transiently successful. At times, amniocentesis appears to initiate labor even though only a part of the fluid is removed; hence, relief of distress may not allow continuation of pregnancy. The volume of fluid removed at one time appears to be critical. Queenan (1970) and Pitkin (1976) described cases of recurrent severe hydramnios treated by amniocentesis. Whereas removal of a large volume of fluid at one time during the first pregnancy was soon followed by delivery of a very immature infant that succumbed, repeated amniocenteses with the frequent removal of smaller volumes during the next pregnancy resulted in delivery of an infant sufficiently mature to survive.

Technique

To remove amnionic fluid, a commercially available plastic catheter that tightly covers an 18-gauge needle (Angiocath) is inserted through the locally anesthetized abdominal wall into the amnionic sac, the needle is withdrawn, and an intravenous infusion set is connected to the catheter hub. The opposite end of the tubing is dropped into a graduated cylinder placed at floor level, and the rate of flow of amnionic fluid is controlled with the screw clamp so that about 500 mL/hr is withdrawn. After about 1500 to 2000 mL has been collected, the uterus has usually decreased in size sufficiently so that the plastic catheter may be withdrawn from the amnionic sac. At the same time, maternal relief is dramatic and the danger of placental separation from decompression is very slight. Using strict aseptic technique, this procedure can be repeated as necessary to make the woman comfortable.

Amniotomy. The disadvantages inherent in rupture of the membranes through the cervix is the possibility of cord prolapse and especially of placental abruption. Very slow removal of the fluid by amniocentesis helps to obviate these dangers.

Indomethacin Therapy. Several investigators have described the use of the prostaglandin synthase inhibitor, indomethacin, to treat hydramnios. In a review of several studies, Moise (1991) concluded that the most likely mechanism for the efficacy of indomethacin is decreased fetal urine production.

Cabrol and associates (1987) treated 8 women with idiopathic hydramnios from 24 to 35 weeks' gestation with indomethacin (2.2 to 3 mg/kg per day) for 2 to 11 weeks. Hydramnios, defined by at least one 8-cm fluid pocket, diminished in volume in all cases. There were no serious adverse effects and the outcome was good in all cases. Kirshon and associates (1990) treated 8 women (3 sets of twins) with hydramnios from 21 to 35 weeks' gestation. In all of these, two therapeutic amniocenteses had been done before indomethacin was given in a dose of 25 mg four times daily. Of 11 fetuses, 3 were stillborn, all associated with twin–twin transfusion syndrome, and 1 newborn died at 3 months of age. The remaining 7 infants did well. Mamopoulos and colleagues (1990) treated 15 women—11 were diabetic—who had hydramnios at 25 to 32 weeks' gestation. Hydramnios was defined by at least one vertical pocket with a depth over 8 cm. Indomethacin dose was 2 to 2.2 mg per kg, and amnionic fluid volume decreased in all women from a mean of 10.7 cm at 27 weeks to 5.9 cm after therapy. The outcome was good in all 15 newborns.

The major concern for the use of indomethacin is the potential for closure of the fetal ductus arteriosus. This was not demonstrated in the cases in the studies described above. Moreover, premature ductal closure with cardiopulmonary sequelae has not been described in two studies in which indomethacin was given for tocolysis (Dudley and Hardie, 1985; Niebyl and Witter, 1986). However, Moise and colleagues (1988) reported that 50 percent of 14 fetuses whose mothers received indomethacin had ductal constriction detected by Doppler ultrasound. They recommend monitoring for ductal constriction.

Oligohydramnios

In rare instances, the volume of amnionic fluid may fall far below the normal limits and occasionally be reduced to only a few mL of viscid fluid. The cause of this condition is not completely understood. Healy and colleagues (1985) reported that prolactin receptors in chorion laeve were normal in number in such cases. Diminished amnionic fluid may be found relatively often with pregnancies that have continued beyond term. Marks and Divon (1992) found oligohydramnios, defined as an amnionic fluid index of 5 cm or less, in 12 percent of 511 pregnancies 41 weeks or greater. In 121 women that they studied longitudinally, there was a mean decrease in the amnionic fluid index of 25 percent per week beyond 41 weeks. The risk of cord compression, and in turn fetal distress, is increased as the consequence of diminished fluid in all labors (Grubbs and Paul, 1992), but especially in postterm pregnancy (Leveno and colleagues, 1984).

Etiology and Prognosis. Oligohydramnios is almost always evident when there is either obstruction of the fetal urinary tract or renal agenesis. Therefore, anuria almost certainly has an etiological role in such cases of oligohydramnios. A chronic leak from a defect in the membranes may reduce the volume of fluid appreciably, but most often labor soon ensues. Exposure to angiotensin-converting enzyme inhibitors has been associated with oligohydramnios (see Chap. 42, p. 965). Shenker and colleagues (1991) reviewed the etiology of oligohydramnios, as well as its grave fetal prognosis, in a review of 80 women (Table 34–5).

Oligohydramnios early in pregnancy generally is associated with poor fetal outcome, because of both cause and effect. Mercer and Brown (1986) described 34 midtrimester pregnancies complicated by oligohydramnios diagnosed ultrasonically by the absence of amnionic-fluid pockets greater than 1 cm in any vertical plane. Nine of these fetuses (26 percent) had anomalies, and 10 of the 25 who were phenotypically normal ei-

TABLE 34–5. CAUSES OF OLIGOHYDRAMNIOS IN 80 WOMEN

Cause	Number	Survived No. (%)
Prematurely ruptured membranes	40	25 (62)
Fetal growth retardation	14	12 (84)
Fetal renal anomalies	9	0
Placental abruption	6	0
Twin–twin transfusion	3	0
Other congenital anomalies	2	0
Unknown	6	1 (18)
Total	**80**	**38 (48)**

Adapted from Shenker and associates (1991), with permission.

ther aborted spontaneously or were stillborn because of severe maternal hypertension, retarded fetal growth, or placental abruption. Of the 14 live-born infants, 8 were preterm and 7 died. The 6 infants who were delivered at term did well. Thus, there were only 7 surviving infants born to the 34 women with severe early-onset oligohydramnios.

Quetel and associates (1992) visualized ultrasonically 13 fetuses who had severe oligohydramnios after amnioinfusion with warm saline colored with indigo carmine. In 11, karyotyping was also obtained, and in all fetuses, anatomical assessment was possible after amnioinfusion. In most cases, they were able to make a definitive diagnosis.

Otherwise normal infants may suffer the consequences of severely diminished amnionic fluid, because adhesions between the amnion and fetal parts may cause serious deformities including amputation. Moreover, subjected to pressure from all sides, the fetus assumes a peculiar appearance, and musculoskeletal deformities such as clubfoot are observed frequently. Typically in cases of oligohydramnios, the skin of the fetus appears dry, leathery, and wrinkled. Oligohydramnios and decreased fetal urine production prior to labor may also be a marker for infants who may not tolerate labor well (Groome and associates, 1991). Significant oligohydramnios, defined by an amnionic fluid index of less than 2 cm, is also associated with an increased risk of prolonged fetal heart rate decelerations in labor (Grubb and Paul, 1992).

Pulmonary Hypoplasia. When amnionic fluid is scant, pulmonary hypoplasia is common. The possibilities to account for the hypoplasia are (1) compression of the thorax by the uterus in the absence of amnionic fluid, which prevents chest wall excursion and lung expansion; (2) lack of fluid to be inhaled into the terminal air sacs of the lung and, as a consequence, inhibition of lung growth; and (3) an intrinsic lung defect with failure of the lung to excrete fluid essential to maintenance of amnionic fluid volume. The appreciable volume of amnionic fluid demonstrated by Duenhoelter and Pritchard (1976) to be inhaled by the fetus is normally suggestive of a role for the inspired fluid in expansion, and in turn growth, of the lung. Fisk and colleagues (1992), however, concluded that fetal breathing impairment does not cause pulmonary hypoplasia with oligohydramnios.

References

Abramovich DR: Fetal factors influencing the volume and composition of liquor amnii. J Obstet Gynaecol Br Commonw 77:865, 1970

Abramovich DR, Garden A, Jandial L, Page KR: Fetal swallowing and voiding in relation to hydramnios. Obstet Gynecol 54:15, 1979

Bartman J, Driscoll SG: Amnion nodosum and hypoplastic cystic kidneys. Obstet Gynecol 32:700, 1968

Brady K, Pulzin WJ, Kopelman JN, Read JA: Risk of chromosomal abnormalities in patients with idiopathic polyhydramnios. Obstet Gynecol 79:234, 1992

Cabrol D, Landesman R, Muller J, Uzan M, Sureau C, Saxena BB: Treatment of polyhydramnios with prostaglandin synthetase inhibitor (indomethacin). Am J Obstet Gynecol 157:422, 1987

Carlson DE, Platt LD, Medearis AL, Hornestein J: Quantifiable polyhydramnios: Diagnosis and management. Obstet Gynecol 75:989, 1990

Dudley DK, Hardie MJ: Fetal and neonatal effects of indomethacin used as a tocolytic agent. Am J Obstet Gynecol 151:181, 1985

Duenhoelter JH, Pritchard JA: Fetal respiration: Quantitative measurements of amnionic fluid inspired near term by human rhesus fetuses. Am J Obstet Gynecol 125:306, 1976

Eden RD, Seifert LS, Winegar A, Spellacy W: Perinatal characteristics of uncomplicated postdate pregnancies. Obstet Gynecol 69:296, 1987

Fisk NM, Talbert DG, Nicolini U, Vaughan J, Rodeck CH: Fetal breathing movements in oligohydramnios are not increased by amnioinfusion. Br J Obstet Gynaecol 99:464, 1992

Fox H: Pathology of the placenta. Monograph, vol 7, Philadelphia, Saunders, 1978

Fujikura T, Klionsky B: The significance of meconium staining. Am J Obstet Gynecol 121:45, 1975

Groome LJ, Owen J, Neely CL, Hauth JC: Oligohydramnios: Antepartum fetal urine production and intrapartum fetal distress. Am J Obstet Gynecol 165:1077, 1991

Grubb DK, Paul RH: Amniotic fluid index and prolonged antepartum fetal heart rate decelerations. Obstet Gynecol 79:588, 1992

Healy DL, Herington AC, O'Herlihy C: Chronic polyhydramnios is a syndrome with a lactogen receptor defect in the chorion laeve. Br J Obstet Gynaecol 92:461, 1985

Hill LM, Breckle R, Thomas ML, Fries JK: Polyhydramnios: Ultrasonically detected prevalence and neonatal outcome. Obstet Gynecol 69:21, 1987

Katz VL, Bowes WA: Meconium aspiration: Reflections on a murky subject. Am J Obstet Gynecol 166:171, 1992

Kirshon B, Mari G, Moise KJ: Indomethacin therapy in the treatment of symptomatic polyhydramnios. Obstet Gynecol 75:202, 1990

Leveno KJ, Quirk JG Jr, Cunningham FG, Nelson SD, Santos-Ramos R, Toofanian A, DePalma RT: Prolonged pregnancy: I. Observations concerning the causes of fetal distress. Am J Obstet Gynecol 150:465, 1984

Mamopoulos M, Assimakopoulos E, Reece EA, Andreou A, Zheng XZ, Mantalenakis S: Maternal indomethacin therapy in the treatment of polyhydramnios. Am J Obstet Gynecol 162:1225, 1990

Marks AD, Divon MY: Longitudinal study of the amniotic fluid index in postdated pregnancy. Obstet Gynecol 79:229, 1992

Mercer LJ, Brown LB: Fetal outcome with oligohydramnios in the second trimester. Obstet Gynecol 67:840, 1986

Miller PW, Coen RW, Benirschke K: Dating the time interval from meconium passage to birth. Obstet Gynecol 66:459, 1985

Moise KJ: Indomethacin therapy in the treatment of symptomatic polyhydramnios. Clin Obstet Gynecol 34:310, 1991

Moise KJ, Huhta JC, Sharif DS, et al: Indomethacin in the treatment of premature labor: Effects on the fetal ductus arteriosus. N Engl J Med 319:327, 1988

Moore TR, Cayle JE: The amniotic fluid index in normal human pregnancy. Am J Obstet Gynecol 162:1168, 1990

Myhra W, Davis M, Mueller BA, Hickok D: Maternal smoking and the risk of polyhydramnios. Am J Public Health 82:176, 1992

Naeye RL, Blanc WA: Fetal renal structure and the genesis of amniotic fluid disorders. Am J Pathol 67:95, 1972

Niebyl JR, Witter FR: Neonatal outcome after indomethacin treatment for preterm labor. Am J Obstet Gynecol 155:747, 1986

Ostrea EM, Naqvi M: The influence of gestational age on the ability of the fetus to pass meconium in utero. Acta Obstet Gynecol Scand 61:275, 1982

Phelan JP, Smith CV, Broussard P, Small M: Amniotic fluid volume assessment with the four-quadrant technique at 36–42 weeks' gestation. J Reprod Med 32:540, 1987

Pitkin RM: Acute polyhydramnios recurrent in successive pregnancies. Obstet Gynecol 48:425, 1976

Pritchard JA: Fetal swallowing and amniotic fluid volume. Obstet Gynecol 28:606, 1966

Queenan JT: Polyhydramnios and oligohydramnios. Contemp Obstet Gynecol 36:60, 1991

Queenan JT: Recurrent acute polyhydramnios. Am J Obstet Gynecol 106:625, 1970

Quetel TA, Mejides AA, Salman FA, Torres-Rodriguez MM: Amnioinfusion: An aid in the ultrasonographic evaluation of severe oligohydramnios in pregnancy. Am J Obstet Gynecol 167:333, 1992

Shenker L, Reed KL, Anderson CF, Borjon JA: Significance of oligohydramnios complicating pregnancy. Am J Obstet Gynecol 164:1597, 1991

Smith CV, Plumbeck RD, Rayburn WF, Albaugh KJ: Relation of mild idiopathic polyhydramnios to perinatal outcome. Obstet Gynecol 79:387, 1992

Steer PJ, Eigbe F, Lissauer TJ, Beard RW: Interrelationships among abnormal cardiocograms in labor, meconium staining of the amniotic fluid, arterial cord blood pH and Apgar scores. Obstet Gynecol 74:715, 1989

Usher RH, Boyd ME, McLean FH, Kramer MS: Assessment of fetal risk in postdate pregnancies. Am J Obstet Gynecol 158:259, 1988

Wiswell TE, Tuggle JM, Turner BS: Meconium aspiration syndrome: Have we made a difference? Pediatrics 85:715, 1990

Wladimiroff JW, Barentsen R, Wallenburg HCS, Drogendijk AC: Fetal urine production in a case of diabetes associated with polyhydramnios. Obstet Gynecol 46:100, 1975

CHAPTER 35
Diseases and Abnormalities of the Placenta

Abnormalities of Placentation

Multiple Placentas with a Single Fetus. Occasionally, the placenta may be separated into lobes, most frequently two. When the division is incomplete and the vessels of fetal origin extend from one lobe to the other before uniting to form the umbilical cord, the condition is termed *placenta bipartita* or *bilobed placenta* (Fig. 35–1). Its reported incidence varies widely, and Fox (1978) cited it at about 1 of 350 deliveries. If the two lobes are separated entirely and the vessels remain distinct, the condition is designated *placenta duplex.* Occasionally, there is *placenta triplex,* with three distinct lobes.

Succenturiate Placenta. An important anomaly is *placenta succenturiata,* in which one or more small accessory lobes are developed in the membranes at a distance from the periphery of the main placenta, to which they usually have vascular connections of fetal origin (Fig. 35–1). Its incidence is about 3 percent. The accessory lobe may sometimes be retained in the uterus after expulsion of the main placenta and may subsequently give rise to serious hemorrhage. If, on placental examination, defects are seen in the membranes a short distance from the placental margin, retention of a succenturiate lobe should be suspected. The suspicion is confirmed if vessels extend from the placenta to the margins of the tear.

Ring-shaped Placenta. Ring-shaped placenta is a rare anomaly seen in fewer than 1 in 6000 deliveries. The placenta is annular in shape and sometimes a complete ring of placental tissue is present, but because of atrophy of a portion of the tissue of the ring, a horseshoe shape is more common. These abnormalities appear to be associated with a greater likelihood of antepartum and postpartum bleeding and fetal growth retardation. This anomaly may be a variant of membranaceous placenta (Fox, 1978).

Membranaceous Placenta. In rare circumstances, all of the fetal membranes are covered by functioning villi, and the placenta develops as a thin membranous structure occupying the entire periphery of the chorion. *Placenta membranacea* (Fig. 35–2) is also referred to as *placenta diffusa.* Although this abnormality seldom interferes with fetal nutrition, occasionally it gives rise to serious hemorrhage. Diagnosis can often be made using sonography. After delivery, the placenta may not separate readily from its attachment, and manual removal is sometimes very difficult in such cases. Bleeding resembles that seen in central placenta previa, and it may be necessary to perform a hysterectomy to control bleeding from the large area of implantation.

Fenestrated Placenta. *Fenestrated placenta* is a rare anomaly in which the central portion of a discoidal placenta is missing. In some instances, there is an actual hole in the placenta, but more often the defect involves villous tissue only, and the chorionic plate is intact. The clinical significance of this anomaly is that it may be mistakenly considered to represent a missing portion that has been retained in the uterus.

Extrachorial Placenta. In *extrachorial placenta,* the chorionic plate, which is on the fetal side of the placenta, is smaller than the basal plate, which is located on the maternal side. If the fetal surface of such a placenta presents a central depression surrounded by a thickened, grayish-white ring, it is called a *circumvallate placenta.* When the ring coincides with the placental margin, the condition is sometimes described as a marginate or *circummarginate placenta.* Within the ring, the fetal surface presents the usual appearance, gives attachment to the umbilical cord, and shows the usual large vessels, which terminate abruptly at the margin of the ring. In a circumvallate placenta, the ring is composed of a double fold of amnion and chorion, with degenerated decidua and fibrin in between. In a marginate placenta, the chorion and amnion are raised at the margin by interposed decidua and fibrin, without folding of the membranes. These relations are illustrated in Figure 35–3. The cause of circumvallate and circummarginate placentation is not understood. Antepartum hemorrhage, preterm delivery, perinatal deaths, and fetal malformations were reported to be increased for pregnancies with circumvallate placentas (Benirschke, 1974; Lademacher and co-workers, 1981).

Large Placentas. Although the normal-term placenta weighs on average about 500 g, in certain diseases, such as syphilis, the placenta may weigh up to one half as much as the fetus (see Fig. 59–2, p. 1301). The largest placentas are usually encountered in cases of *erythroblastosis fetalis* (see Fig. 44–9, p. 1008).

Placental Polyp. Occasionally, parts of a normal placenta or a succenturiate lobe may be retained after

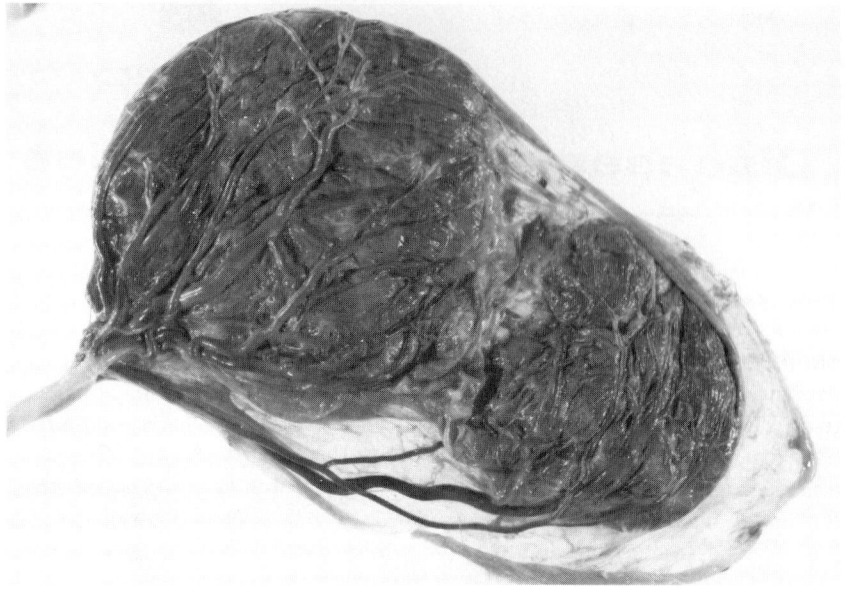

Fig. 35–1. Placenta demonstrating bilobed structure, marginal insertion of umbilical cord, and partial velamentous insertion of cord (fetal vessels traversing membranes to reach smaller placental lobe on right).

delivery. These may form polyps consisting of villi in varying stages of degeneration, and may be covered by regenerated endometrium. The clinical sequelae are often subinvolution of the uterus and late postpartum hemorrhage (see Chap. 29, p. 644).

Circulatory Disturbances

Placental Infarcts. The most common placental lesions, though of diverse origin, are referred to collectively as placental infarcts. The principal histopathological features include fibrinoid degeneration of the trophoblast, calcification, and ischemic infarction from occlusion of spiral arteries. Overclassification of these infarcts has led to unnecessary confusion. Small subchorionic and marginal foci of degeneration are present in every placenta. In simplest terms, degenerative lesions of the placenta have two etiological factors in common: (1) changes associated with aging of the trophoblast and (2) impairment of the uteroplacental circulation causing infarction.

Although the placenta is by no means a dying organ at term, there are morphological indications of aging. During the latter half of pregnancy, syncytial degeneration begins and *syncytial knots* are formed. At the same time, the villous stroma usually undergoes hyalinization. The syncytium may then break away, exposing the connective tissue directly to maternal blood. Clotting occurs as a result, and propagation of the clot may result in

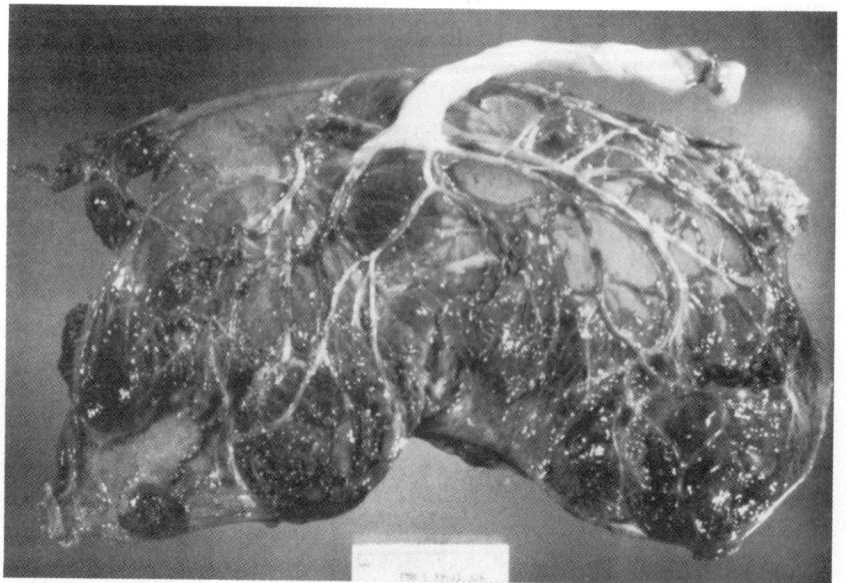

Fig. 35–2. Placenta membranacea. (Courtesy of Dr. Cristela Hernandez, from Ramin and Gilstrap, 1992, with permission.)

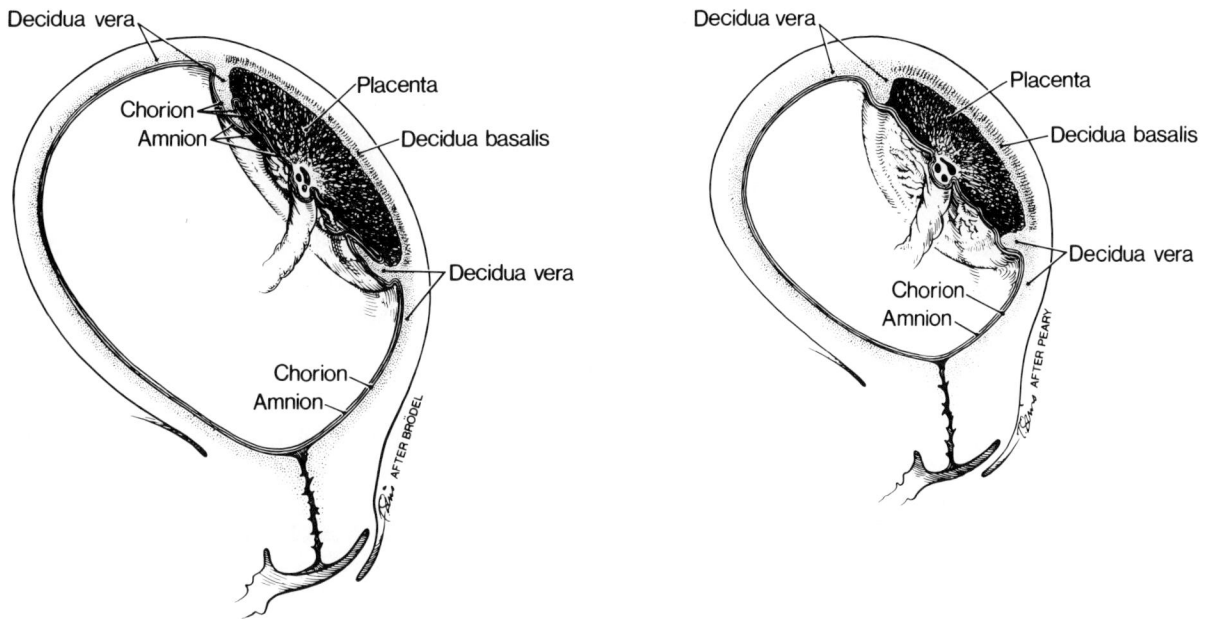

Fig. 35–3. Circumvallate (*left*) and marginate (*right*) varieties of extrachorial placentas.

the incorporation of other villi. Macroscopically, such a focus resembles closely an ordinary blood clot, but if not seen until it has become thoroughly organized, on section a firm, white island of tissue is seen.

Around the edge of nearly every term placenta there is a dense yellowish-white fibrous ring representing a zone of degeneration and necrosis, which usually is termed a *marginal infarct.* Underneath the chorionic plate, there are nearly always similar lesions, most often pyramidal shaped, ranging from 2 mm to 3 cm across the base, and extending downward with their apices in the intervillous space (*subchorionic infarcts*). Similar lesions may be noted about the intercotyledonary septa. Occasionally, these lesions meet and form a column of cartilage-like material extending from the maternal surface to the fetal surface. Less frequently, round or oval islands of similar tissue occupy the central portions of the placenta (Fig. 35–4).

Fox (1978) found that about one fourth of placentas from uncomplicated term pregnancies have infarcts, while those pregnancies complicated by severe hypertensive disease are infarcted in about two thirds of cases.

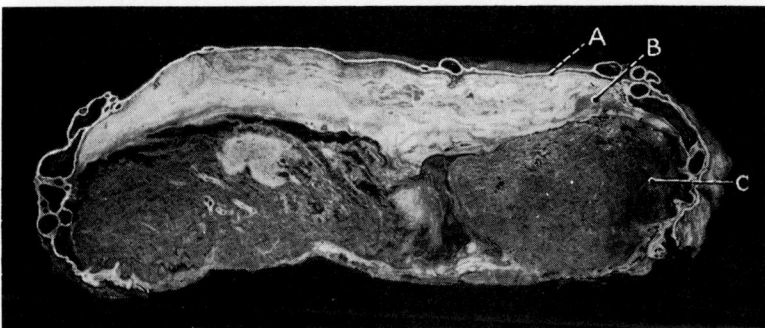

A

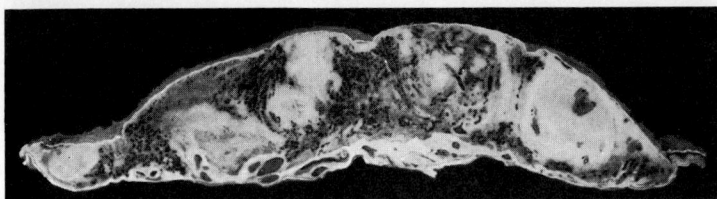

B

Fig. 35–4. A. Placental infarcts: A = chorioamnionic membrane; B = fibrin deposited locally beneath the chorion; C = normal placental tissue. In this instance, the infarct was unusually extensive, most likely contributing to the death of the fetus. **B.** Generalized fibrin deposition with little normal tissue remaining.

Calcification of the Placenta. Small calcareous nodules or plaques are frequently observed on the maternal surface of the placenta. In view of the widespread degenerative changes in the term placenta, calcification is not surprising. An extensive deposition of calcium is shown in Figure 35–5. Placental calcification may be visualized using sonography, and Spirit and colleagues (1982) reported that by 33 weeks more than half of placentas have some degree of calcification. As term approaches, the degree of calcification increases substantively. Placental calcification graded ultrasonically has been correlated with fetal lung maturity (Grannum and co-workers, 1979).

Villous (Fetal) Artery Thrombosis. Thrombosis of a fetal villous stem artery produces a sharply demarcated area of avascularity. Fox (1978) found single artery thrombosis in 4.5 percent of placentas from normal pregnancies and in 10 percent of those involving diabetic women. Benirschke and Driscoll (1974) observed an association between fetal artery thrombosis and an-

tiplatelet antibodies in maternal serum. Fox (1978) estimated that thrombosis of a single fetal stem artery will deprive only 5 percent of the villi of their blood supply. However, he also observed a few placentas from recent stillbirths in which 40 to 50 percent of the villi were so deprived.

Clinical Significance of Degenerative Changes in the Placenta. In general, placental infarcts caused either by local deposition of fibrin or by the more acute process of intervillous thrombosis, have little clinical significance. Nonetheless, in certain maternal diseases, notably severe hypertension, the reduction in functioning placenta through infarction, coupled with reduced blood flow to the uterus, may be sufficient to cause fetal death.

Villous (fetal) vessels may show endarteritic thickening and obliteration in association with fetal death. When the placental villi are excluded from their supply of maternal blood by fibrin deposits, hematomas, or direct blockage of the decidual circulation, they be-

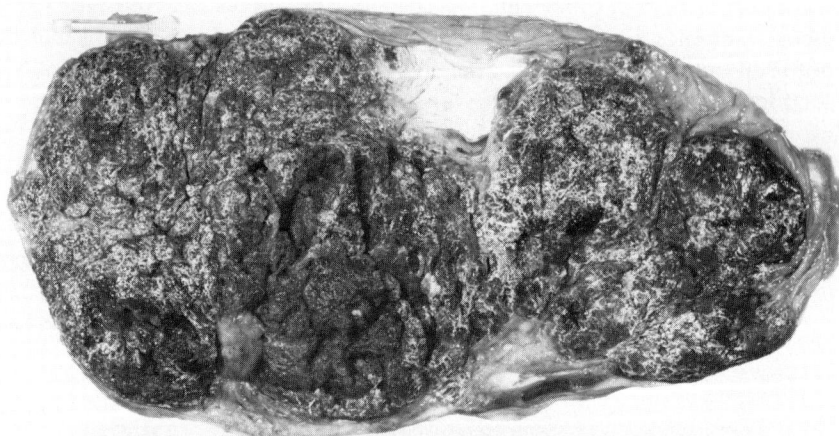

A

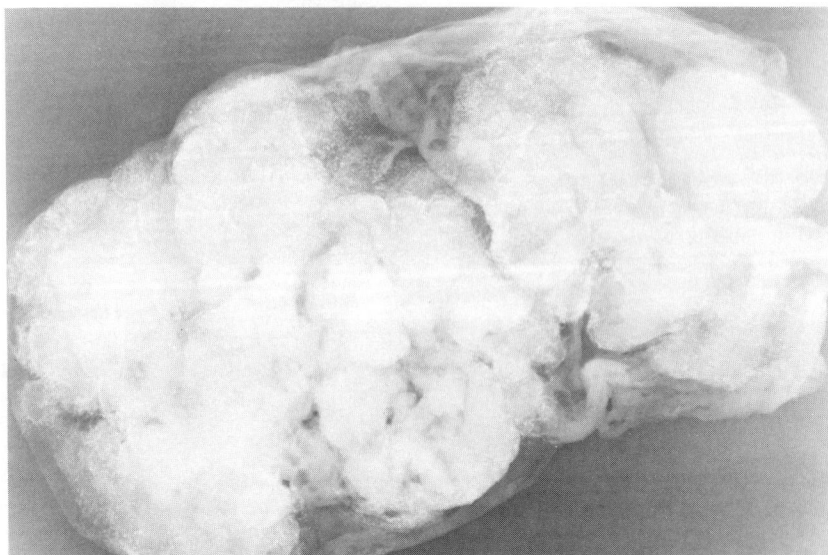

Fig. 35–5.A. Placental calcification is evident as gray plaques on the maternal surface of the placenta, a common finding at term. **B.** A radiograph of the same placenta emphasizes the extensive calcification.

B

come infarcted and die. Histologically, the compromised villi are characterized by fibrosis, obliteration of fetal vessels, and gradual disappearance of the syncytium. Shen-Schwarz and associates (1988) described hemorrhagic endovasculitis in less than 1 percent of placentas.

Hypertrophic Lesions of the Chorionic Villi.
Striking enlargement of the chorionic villi is commonly seen in association with severe erythroblastosis and fetal hydrops. It has also been described in diabetes and occasionally in severe fetal congestive heart failure.

Placental Abnormalities Detected by Microscopic Examination.
Beginning after the 32nd week of gestation, clumps of syncytial nuclei are found to project into the intervillous space, and these are called *syncytial knots*. By term, up to 30 percent of villi may be involved; however, formation of knots by more than one third of villi is considered abnormal (Fox, 1978). In prolonged pregnancies there are marked increases in syncytial knots and avascular villi as the consequence of fetal artery thrombosis. Generally, increased numbers of syncytial knots are found in placentas in which there may have been reduced uteroplacental blood flow, as, for example, with preeclampsia.

It is well recognized that the number of *cytotrophoblastic* cells becomes progressively reduced as pregnancy advances. In a normal mature placenta, cytotrophoblastic cells are found in about 20 percent of the villi (Fox, 1978). Most often, at this stage of pregnancy such cells are few and inconspicuous. However, numerous cytotrophoblastic cells are found in placentas of pregnant women with diabetes mellitus and erythroblastosis fetalis. Increased numbers of cytotrophoblasts have also been observed in placentas from women with pregnancy-induced hypertension.

Inflammation of the Placenta.
Changes that are now recognized as various forms of degeneration and necrosis were formerly described under the term *placentitis*. For example, small placental cysts with grumous contents were formerly thought to be abscesses. Nonetheless, especially in cases of prolonged rupture of the membranes, pyogenic bacteria do invade the fetal surface of the placenta, and after gaining access to the chorionic vessels, give rise to fetal infection.

Abnormalities of the Umbilical Cord (Funis)

Abnormalities in Cord Length.
Umbilical cord length varies appreciably, with the mean length being about 55 cm (Rayburn and associates, 1981). Extremes in cord length in abnormal instances range from apparently no cord (achordia) to lengths up to 300 cm. Vascular occlusion by thrombi and true knots are more common in excessively long cords, and they are more likely to pro-

lapse through the cervix. Rarely, excessively short umbilical cords may be instrumental in abruptio placenta and uterine inversion. They may rupture with hemorrhage, which can cause fetal death from exsanguination.

Determinants of cord length are intriguing. Studies performed on animals and experiments of nature in human pregnancy support the concept that cord length is positively influenced by the volume of amnionic fluid and by fetal mobility. Miller and associates (1981) identified the human umbilical cord to be shortened appreciably when there had been either chronic fetal constraint from oligohydramnios or decreased fetal movement because of limb dysfunction. Excessive cord length may be the consequence of entanglement of cord and fetus with stretching during fetal movement. Soernes and Bakke (1986) reported that the mean cord length in fetuses with breech presentations was about 5 cm shorter than those with vertex presentations.

Absence of One Umbilical Artery.
The absence of one umbilical artery, according to Benirschke and Dodds (1967), characterized 0.85 percent of all cords in singletons and 5 percent of the cords of at least one twin. **About 30 percent of all infants with one umbilical artery missing had associated congenital anomalies.** Bryan and Kohler (1975) identified the umbilical cords of 143 infants out of nearly 20,000 examined (0.72 percent), to have a single artery. Infants with a single-artery cord had an 18 percent incidence of major malformations, 34 percent were growth-retarded, and 17 percent delivered preterm. Bryan and Kohler (1975) followed 90 infants beyond infancy with a single umbilical artery and found previously unrecognized malformations in 10.

Peckham and Yerushalmy (1965) demonstrated a single umbilical artery twice as often in newborns of white women than in those of African-American women. The incidence is increased considerably in newborns of women with diabetes, a condition associated with a threefold increase in anomalous fetuses. Based on the finding of a high incidence of fetal malformations when a single umbilical artery exists, each umbilical cord should be examined carefully to ascertain the number of umbilical arteries present.

As expected, two-vessel cords are more frequently identified in fetuses aborted spontaneously, and Benirschke and Brown (1955) reported this to be 2.5 percent. Byrne and Blanc (1986) studied 879 consecutively aborted fetuses and identified a single umbilical artery in 1.5 percent. Eight of these 13 fetuses had serious malformations, most associated with chromosomal abnormalities.

Four-Vessel Cord.
Additional umbilical vessels are rarely apparent on casual examination; however, careful examination may disclose a venous remnant in 5 per-

cent of cases (Fox, 1978). It is unknown whether a true four-vessel cord is associated with an increased incidence of fetal anomalies.

Abnormalities of Cord Insertion. The umbilical cord usually, but not always, is inserted at or near the center of the fetal surface of the placenta.

Marginal Insertion. Insertion of the cord at the placental margin is sometimes referred to as a *battledore placenta.* Some have reported that such an insertion is more common in instances of preterm labor, but this opinion is not widely held (Robinson and co-workers, 1983).

Velamentous Insertion. Of considerable practical importance is velamentous insertion of the cord, because the umbilical vessels separate in the membranes at a distance from the placental margin, which they reach surrounded only by a fold of amnion (Figs. 35–1 and 35–6). This mode of insertion is noted in a little over 1 percent of singleton deliveries but much more frequently with twins, and it is almost the rule with triplets.

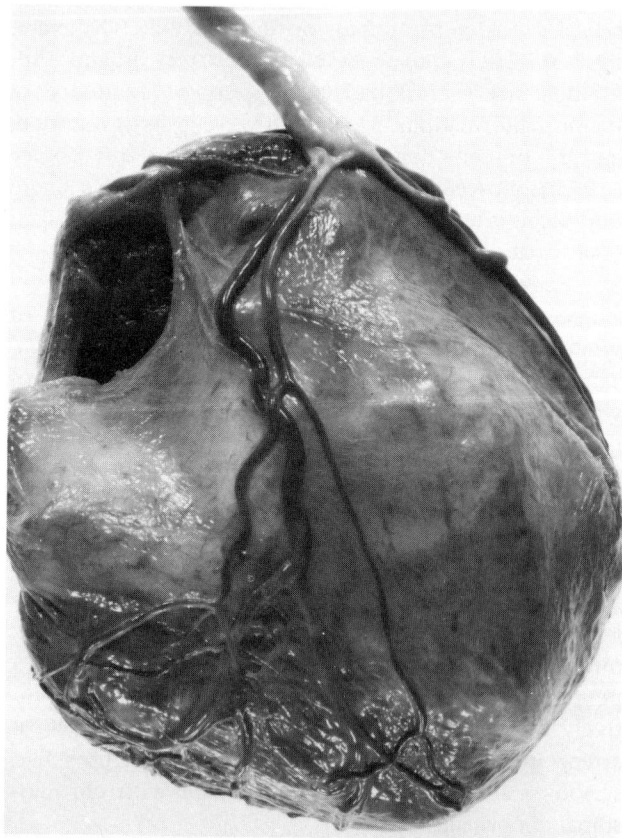

Fig. 35–6. Velamentous insertion of the cord. The placenta (*bottom*) and membranes have been inverted to expose the amnion. Note the large fetal vessels within membranes (*top*) and their proximity to the site of rupture of the membranes.

Vasa Previa. When with velamentous insertion, some of the fetal vessels in the membranes cross the region of the internal os and occupy a position ahead of the presenting part of the fetus, the condition is termed *vasa previa.* At times, the careful examiner will be able to palpate a tubular fetal vessel in the membranes overlying the presenting part. Compression of the vessels between the examining finger and the presenting part is likely to induce changes in the fetal heart rate. At times, the vessels may be visualized directly, or they may be seen on ultrasonic examination (Fig. 35–7). With vasa previa, there is considerable potential danger to the fetus, for rupture of the membranes may be accompanied by rupture of a fetal vessel, causing exsanguination.

Whenever there is hemorrhage antepartum or intrapartum, the possibility of vasa previa and a ruptured fetal vessel exists. Unfortunately, the amount of fetal blood that can be shed without killing the fetus is relatively small. Blood can be ascertained to be of fetal origin by demonstrating resistance of hemoglobin to denaturation with alkali. A quick, readily available approach is to smear the blood on glass slides, stain the smears with Wright stain, and examine for nucleated red cells, which normally are present in cord blood but not maternal blood. Messer and colleagues (1987) reported that of 107 obstetricians at medical schools and 52 at community hospitals who returned a survey questionnaire, only about 15 percent routinely tested for fetal blood in late pregnancy bleeding. The pessimism expressed by Kouyoumdjian (1980) for improving fetal salvage once a vessel is ruptured is probably justified.

Cord Abnormalities Capable of Impeding Blood Flow. Several mechanical and vascular abnormalities of the umbilical cord are capable of impairing fetal–placental blood flow.

Knots of the Cord. False knots, which result from kinking of the vessels to accommodate to the length of the cord, should be distinguished from *true knots,* which result from active fetal movements. In nearly 17,000 deliveries in the Collaborative Study on Cerebral Palsy, Spellacy and co-workers (1966) found an incidence of true knots of 1.1 percent. Perinatal loss was 6 percent in the presence of true knots. The incidence of true knots is especially high in monoamnionic twins.

Loops of the Cord. The cord frequently becomes coiled around portions of the fetus, usually the neck. In 1000 consecutive deliveries studied by Kan and Eastman (1957), the incidence of the umbilical cord around the neck ranged from one loop in 21 percent to three loops in 0.2 percent. Fortunately, coiling of the cord around the neck is an uncommon cause of fetal death. Typically, as labor progresses and the fetus descends the birth canal, contractions compress the cord vessels, which cause fetal heart-rate deceleration that persists until the

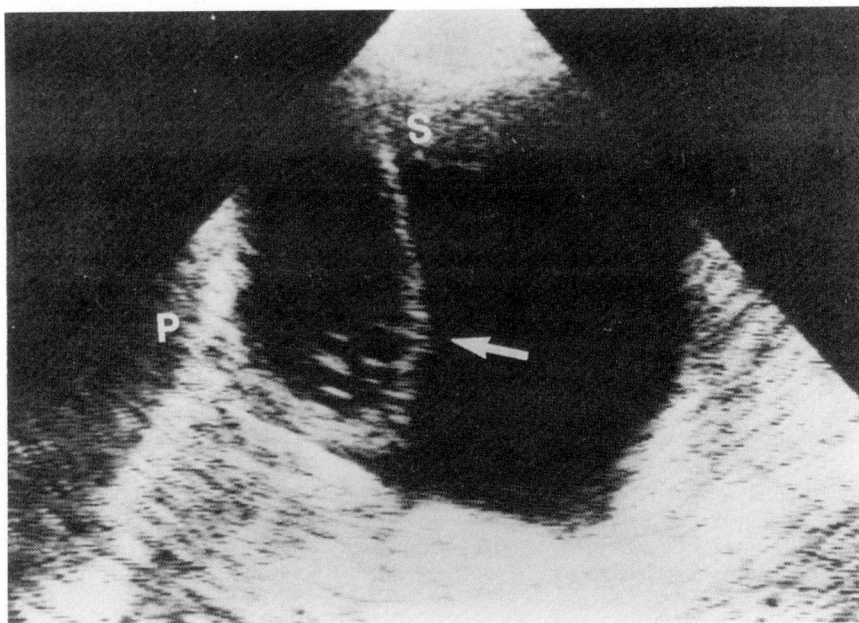

Fig. 35–7. Sonogram showing placenta (P), succenturiate lobe (S), and leading fetal vessels in *vasa previa* (*arrow*). (From Gianopoulos and colleagues, 1987, with permission.)

contraction ceases. Hankins and colleagues (1987a) reported 110 pregnancies in which labor at term was complicated by a nuchal cord. Compared with control infants, those with a nuchal cord had more moderate or severe variable fetal heart-rate decelerations in labor (20 versus 5 percent) and were more likely have a lower umbilical artery pH.

Torsion of the Cord. As a result of fetal movements, the cord normally becomes twisted. Occasionally, the torsion is so marked that fetal circulation is compromised. Extreme degrees of torsion may occur after the death of the fetus by a mechanism that is not understood. In monoamnionic twinning, a significant fraction of the high perinatal mortality rate is attributed to entwining of the umbilical cords before labor.

Because of the heightened interest in determining antepartum causes of cerebral palsy remote from delivery, it is tempting to speculate that cord entanglement may be related. In this scheme, intermittent cord occlusion causes sublethal cerebral hypoperfusion and hypoxia that leads to periventricular leukomalacia (see Chap. 44, p. 996).

Stricture of the Cord. Most, but not all, infants with cord stricture are stillborns; the stricture probably has a role in fetal death. Cord stricture, for unknown reasons, is associated with an extreme focal deficiency in Wharton jelly. Stricture is commonly associated, causally, with torsion.

Hematoma of the Cord. Hematomas occasionally result from the rupture of a varix, usually of the umbilical vein, with effusion of blood into the cord (Fig. 35–8). More recently, cord hematomas have been described as resulting from ultrasound-directed umbilical vessel venipuncture. Fox (1978), who reviewed the subject carefully, believes it unwise to attribute fetal death to a cord hematoma until other causes have been excluded.

Cysts of the Cord. Cysts are occasionally found along the course of the cord and are designated true and false, according to their origin. True cysts are quite small and may be derived from remnants of the umbilical vesicle or of the allantois. False cysts, which may attain considerable size, result from liquefaction of Wharton jelly. Such cysts may be detected by sonography but are difficult to identify precisely. For example, the cord cyst demonstrated in Figure 35–9 was thought possibly to be a meningocele when detected by sonography, because

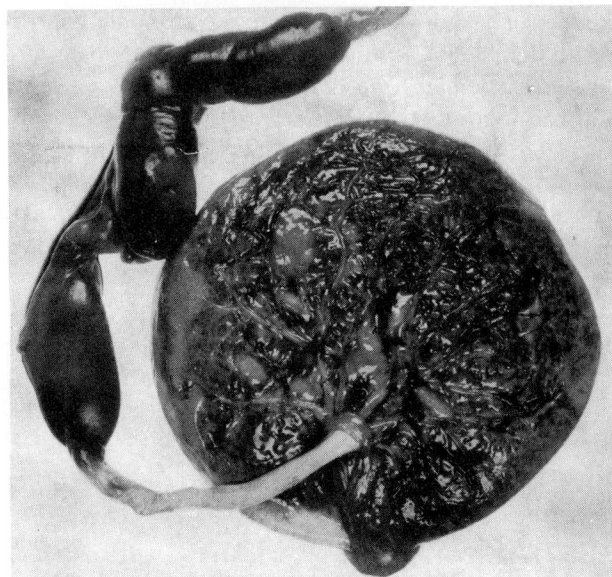

Fig. 35–8. Hematoma of the umbilical cord.

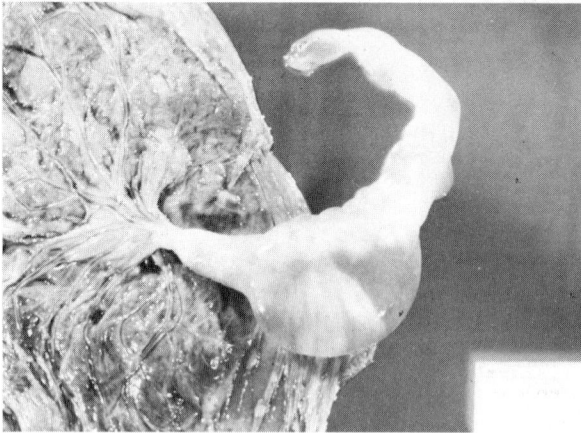
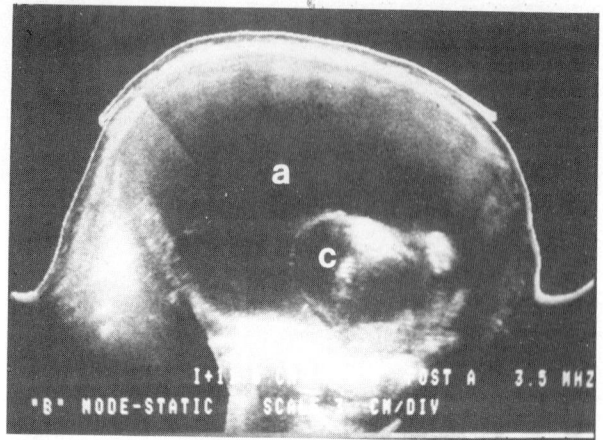

A   **B**

Fig. 35–9. A. Cyst of umbilical cord at 27 weeks' gestation in a monoamnionic twin pregnancy, further complicated by symptomatic acute hydramnios and marked discordance in the size of the fetuses. **B.** Sonogram from the same case demonstrating the cyst of the cord (c) and marked hydramnios (a). The possibility that the cyst was a meningocele was considered originally. (Courtesy of Dr. R. Santos.)

the cyst maintained a close and constant relationship over time with the lower spine of the fetus.

Edema of the Cord. Cord edema rarely occurs by itself but is frequently associated with edema of the fetus. It is very common with macerated fetuses.

Pathological Examination

The College of American Pathologists (1991) recommends routine pathological examination of the placenta with certain obstetrical and neonatal conditions. Conversely, the American College of Obstetricians and Gynecologists (1991) feels that there are insufficient data to support this recommendation.

Certainly, the placenta and cord—including the number of vessels—should be grossly examined following all deliveries. Although pathological examination of the placenta may be useful in the diagnosis of some unusual conditions, such as microabscesses seen with listeriosis, the possible correlation of specific placental pathological findings and both short- and long-term neonatal outcome is still unclear. Thus, routine placental examination on all births does not appear to be justified on either a scientific or cost-effective basis. With an increasing number of pathologists, obstetricians, and neonatologists with special interest and expertise in this field, such pathological examinations eventually may become enlightening. Pathological placental examination, as well as an autopsy of the fetus, often prove useful in the case of a stillbirth.

GESTATIONAL TROPHOBLASTIC DISEASE

Gestational trophoblastic disease refers to a spectrum of pregnancy-related trophoblastic proliferative abnormal-

ities, the classification of which for many years was based principally on histological criteria and included hydatidiform mole, invasive mole, and choriocarcinoma. In 1973, Hammond and colleagues proposed a clinical diagnostic spectrum for gestational trophoblastic diseases based principally upon clinical findings and serial determinations of chorionic gonadotropin, which is secreted by the abnormal tissue. Although these two classifications have caused some confusion, the clinical approach is now accepted.

The terminology utilized in the past for the definition and classification of gestational trophoblastic disease has been confusing. In 1983, the World Health Organization Scientific Group on Gestational Trophoblastic Diseases published specific recommendations regarding the terminology for the definition, classification, and staging of trophoblastic disease. Miller and Lurain (1988) have reviewed this subject. Basically, gestational trophoblastic disease can be divided into **hydatidiform mole** and **gestational trophoblastic tumors** (Table 35–1). The frequently utilized term, *gestational trophoblastic neoplasia,* should no longer be utilized because invasive moles are not true neoplasms (Miller and Lurain, 1988). As shown in Table 35–2, gestational trophoblastic tumors can be classified clinically as nonmet-

TABLE 35–1. CLINICAL CLASSIFICATION OF GESTATIONAL TROPHOBLASTIC DISEASE

Hydatidiform Mole
  Complete mole
  Partial mole

Gestational Trophoblastic Tumors
  Invasive mole
  Choriocarcinoma
  Placental-site tumor

Adapted from Miller and Lurain (1988).

TABLE 35–2. CLINICAL CLASSIFICATION OF GESTATIONAL TROPHOBLASTIC TUMORS

Nonmetastatic

Metastatic

Low-risk tumors
1. Chorionic gonadotropin
   a. Urine < 100,000 IU/24 hr, or
   b. Serum < 40,000 mIU/mL
2. Symptoms for less than 4 months
3. No brain or liver metastases
4. No prior chemotherapy
5. Pregnancy event not term delivery (rather a mole, ectopic pregnancy, or spontaneous abortion)

High-risk tumors
1. Chorionic gonadotropin
   a. Urine > 100,000 IU/24 hr, or
   b. Serum > 40,000 mIU/ml
2. Symptoms for more than 4 months
3. Brain or liver metastases
4. Prior chemotherapeutic failure
5. Antecedent term pregnancy

From the American College of Obstetricians and Gynecologists (1980).

TABLE 35–3. CHARACTERISTICS OF PARTIAL AND COMPLETE HYDATIDIFORM MOLES

Feature	Partial Mole	Complete Mole
Embryonic or fetal tissue	Present	Absent
Hydatidiform swelling of villi	Focal	Diffuse
Trophoblastic hyperplasia	Focal	Diffuse
Stromal inclusions	Present	Absent
Villous scalloping	Present	Absent
Karyotype	Paternal and maternal, 69,XXY or 69,XYY	Paternal, 46,XX (96%) or 46,XY (4%)
Trophoblastic tumors	~5% (choriocarcinoma rare)	~20%

From Berkowitz and co-workers (1986).

astatic and metastatic, and the latter are subdivided into low risk and high risk (Hammond and associates, 1973; Miller and Lurain, 1988).

Hydatidiform Mole (Molar Pregnancy)

Histologically, hydatidiform moles are characterized by abnormalities of the chorionic villi, consisting of varying degrees of trophoblastic proliferation and edema of villous stroma. Moles usually occupy the uterine cavity; however, they rarely may be located in the oviduct and even the ovary (Stanhope and associates, 1983). The presence or absence of a fetus or embryo has been used to classify them into *complete* and *partial* moles (Table 35–3).

Complete Hydatidiform Mole. The chorionic villi are converted into a mass of clear vesicles (Fig. 35–10). The vesicles vary in size from barely visible to a few centimeters in diameter and often hang in clusters from thin pedicles. The mass may grow large enough to fill the uterus to the size occupied by an advanced normal pregnancy.

The histological structure demonstrated in Figure 35–11 is characterized by (1) hydropic degeneration and swelling of the villous stroma, (2) absence of blood vessels in the swollen villi, (3) proliferation of the trophoblastic epithelium to a varying degree, and (4) absence of fetus and amnion.

Cytogenetic studies of complete molar pregnancies have identified the chromosomal composition most often, but not always, to be 46,XX, with the chromosomes completely of paternal origin. This phenomenon is referred to as *androgenesis*. Typically, the ovum has been fertilized by a haploid sperm, which then duplicates its own chromosomes after meiosis, and thus the chromosomes are homozygous. They may also be of heterozy-

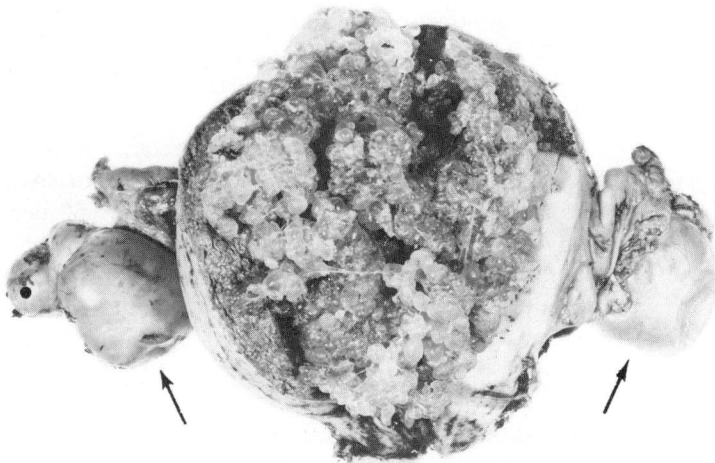

Fig. 35–10. A complete (classic) hydatidiform mole characterized grossly by abundance of edematous enlarged chorionic villi but no fetus or fetal membranes. Note theca-lutein cysts in each ovary (*arrows*).

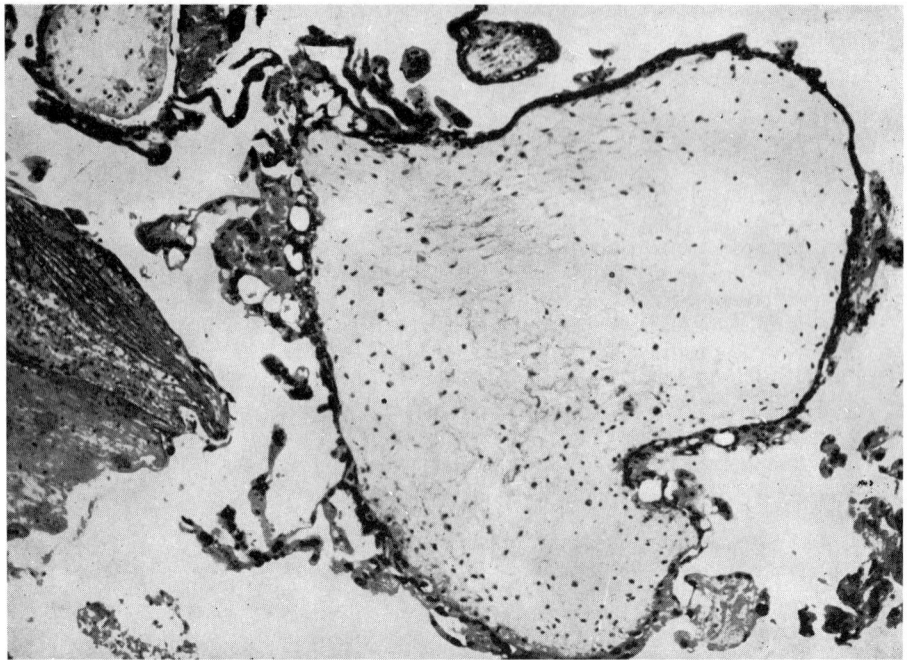

Fig. 35–11. Photomicrograph of a hydatidiform mole with slight to moderate trophoblastic hyperplasia, confined to the syncytium and considered as probably benign. (From Smalbraak, 1957.)

gous origin, with dispermy (Lawler and colleagues, 1991). The chromosomes of the ovum are either absent or inactivated. However, all complete hydatidiform moles are not so characterized, and infrequently, the chromosomal pattern in a complete mole may be 46,XY, that is, heterozygous (Bagshawe and Lawler, 1982).

Lawler and colleagues (1991) described 202 hydatidiform moles; 151 were complete and 49 partial moles (2 were unclassified). The genetic ploidy of these moles is summarized in Table 35–4. The majority (85 percent) of complete moles are diploid whereas most partial moles (86 percent) are triploid. Other variations have been described, such as 45,X. Thus, a morphologically complete mole can result from a variety of chromosomal patterns. The risk of trophoblastic tumors developing from a complete mole is approximately 20 percent (Table 35–3).

Partial Hydatidiform Mole. When the hydatidiform changes are focal and less advanced, and maybe a fetus or at least an amnionic sac is seen, the condition has been classified as a partial hydatidiform mole. There is slowly progressing hydatidiform swelling of some usu-

ally avascular villi, while other vascular villi with a functioning fetal–placental circulation are spared (Fig. 35–12). Trophoblastic hyperplasia is focal rather than generalized. As shown in Table 35–4, the karyotype typically is triploid—69,XXX, 69,XXY, or 69,XYY—with one maternal but usually two paternal haploid complements (Berkowitz and colleagues, 1986, 1991). The fetus of a partial mole typically has stigmata of triploidy, which includes multiple congenital malformations and growth retardation, and it is nonviable. In the report by Lawler and colleagues (1991), 86 percent of partial moles were triploid and 2 percent were diploid. A twin gestation with a complete mole and a normal twin and placenta is sometimes misdiagnosed as a diploid partial mole; this also may be confused with hydropic degeneration associated with an abortion (Berkowitz and colleagues, 1991). Hydropic or molar degeneration is not classified as trophoblastic disease.

The risk of choriocarcinoma arising from a partial hydatidiform mole is slight; however, nonmetastatic gestational trophoblastic tumors may follow in 4 to 8 percent of partial moles, according to Szulman and Surti (1982), Czernobilsky and colleagues (1982), and Berkowitz and colleagues (1986).

Vejerslev (1991) reviewed the outcomes of pregnancies reported with a hydatidiform mole coexistent with a normal fetus. Of 113 pregnancies, 52 (60 percent) of fetuses progressed to 28 weeks' gestation and the fetal survival was 70 percent. Thus, when providing counseling for women with a coexistent mole and a fetus, both cytogenetic and high-resolution ultrasound studies are of paramount importance.

Histological Diagnosis. Attempts to relate the histological structure of individual complete hydatidiform

TABLE 35–4. CHROMOSOMAL COMPOSITION OF 200 HYDATIDIFORM MOLES

Chromosomes	Complete (%) (n = 151)	Partial (%) (n = 49)
Haploid	1 (0.7)	—
Diploid	128 (85)	1 (2)
Triploid	3 (2)	42 (86)
Tetraploid	—	2 (4)
Unknown	19 (13)	4 (8)

Adapted from Lawler and colleagues (1991), with permission.

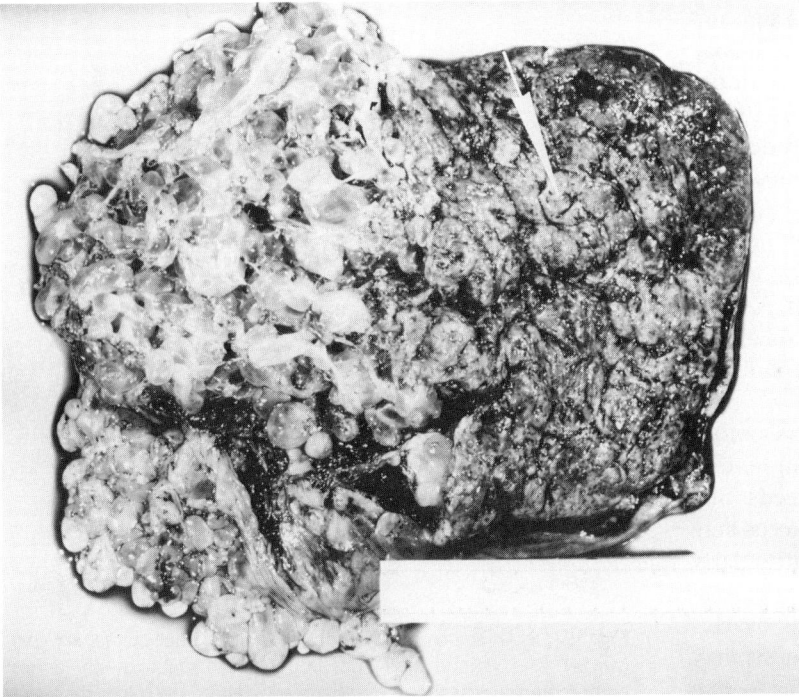

Fig. 35–12. Molar placenta on the left and normal placenta (*white arrow*) on the right. The molar placenta was identified by sonography late in pregnancy when the mother developed preeclampsia. A healthy fetus was delivered near term by cesarean section. Most likely, these were twins consisting of a placenta with a fetus from one ovum and a complete mole developing from the other ovum.

moles to their subsequent malignant tendencies generally have been disappointing. Novak and Seah (1954), for example, were unable to precisely establish such a relation in 120 cases of hydatidiform mole or in the molar tissue in 26 cases of choriocarcinoma following hydatidiform mole.

Ovarian Theca-Lutein Cysts. In many cases of hydatidiform mole, the ovaries contain multiple theca-lutein cysts (Fig. 35–10), which may vary from microscopic size to 10 cm or more in diameter. The surfaces of the cysts are smooth, often yellowish, and lined with lutein cells. The incidence of obvious cysts in association with a mole is reported to be from 25 percent to as high as 60 percent.

Theca-lutein cysts are thought to result from overstimulation of lutein elements by large amounts of chorionic gonadotropin secreted by proliferating trophoblast. In general, extensive cystic change is usually associated with larger hydatidiform moles and a long period of stimulation. Montz and colleagues (1988) reported that persistent trophoblastic disease was more likely in women with theca-lutein cysts, especially if bilateral. Theca-lutein cysts are not limited to cases of hydatidiform mole, and are associated with placental hypertrophy with fetal hydrops or multifetal pregnancy.

Very large cysts in particular may undergo torsion, infarction, and hemorrhage. However, oophorectomy should not be performed because of theca-lutein cysts; after delivery of the mole, the cysts regress.

Incidence. Hydatidiform mole develops in approximately 1 per 1000 pregnancies in the United States and

Europe. Although it has been reported to be more frequent in other countries, especially in parts of Asia, much of this information was based on hospital studies (Miller and associates, 1989). Based on population studies, the incidence in these countries is probably similar to that in the United States (Grimes, 1984; Miller and colleagues, 1989).

Age. There is a relatively high frequency of hydatidiform mole among pregnancies toward the beginning or end of the childbearing period. The most pronounced effect of age is seen in women older than 45, when the relative frequency of the lesion is more than 10 times greater than at ages 20 to 40. There are numerous authenticated cases of hydatidiform mole in women 50 years old and older, whereas normal pregnancy at such advanced ages is practically unknown (Jequier and Winterton, 1975).

Previous Mole. Recurrence of hydatidiform mole is uncommon, but it is seen in about 1 to 2 percent of cases (Miller and co-workers, 1989). Wu (1973) described a woman who had 9 consecutive molar pregnancies!

Clinical Course. In the very early stages of development of the mole, there are few characteristics to distinguish it from normal pregnancy; but later in the first trimester and during the second trimester the following changes are often evident. Symptoms are more likely to be dramatic with a complete mole. Schlaerth and colleagues (1988) reported complications in two thirds of 381 women with molar pregnancies.

Bleeding. Uterine bleeding is the most common sign and may vary from spotting to profuse hemorrhage. It may begin just before abortion or, more often, it may occur intermittently for weeks or even months. A dilutional effect from appreciable hypervolemia has been demonstrated in some women with larger moles. At times there may be considerable hemorrhage concealed within the uterus. Iron-deficiency anemia is a common finding and infrequently megaloblastic erythropoiesis is evident, presumably as a result of poor dietary intake because of nausea and vomiting coupled with increased folate requirement imposed by rapidly proliferating trophoblast.

Uterine Size. The growing uterus often enlarges more rapidly than usual. It is the most common finding, and in about half of cases, uterine size clearly exceeds that expected from the duration of gestation. The uterus may be difficult to identify precisely by palpation particularly in the nulliparous woman, because of its soft consistency beneath a firm abdominal wall. At times ovaries appreciably enlarged by multiple theca-lutein cysts may be difficult to distinguish from the enlarged uterus. The ovaries are likely to be tender.

Fetal Activity. Even though the uterus is enlarged sufficiently to reach well above the symphysis, typically no fetal heart action is detected. Rarely, there may be twin placentas with a complete molar pregnancy developing in one, while the other placenta and its fetus appear normal. Also, very infrequently there may be extensive but incomplete molar change in the placenta accompanied by a living fetus. Pregnancy outcomes reviewed by Vejerslev (1991) in 52 fetuses who had a coexistent mole and who progressed to 28 weeks were reviewed on page 750.

Pregnancy-induced Hypertension. Of special importance is the possible association of preeclampsia with molar pregnancies that persist into the second trimester. Because pregnancy-induced hypertension is rarely seen before 24 weeks, preeclampsia that develops before this time should at least suggest hydatidiform mole or extensive molar change.

Embolization. Variable amounts of trophoblast with or without villous stroma escape from the uterus in the venous outflow. The volume may be such as to produce signs and symptoms of acute pulmonary embolism and even a fatal outcome (Fig. 35–13). Such fatalities are rare. Hankins and colleagues (1987b) obtained hemodynamic measurements using a pulmonary artery catheter in 6 women with large molar pregnancies. They also searched for evidence of **trophoblastic deportation** before and during molar evacuation. Only small numbers of multinucleated giant cells and mononuclear cells, presumably trophoblasts, were identified. They found no evidence for acute cardiorespiratory changes,

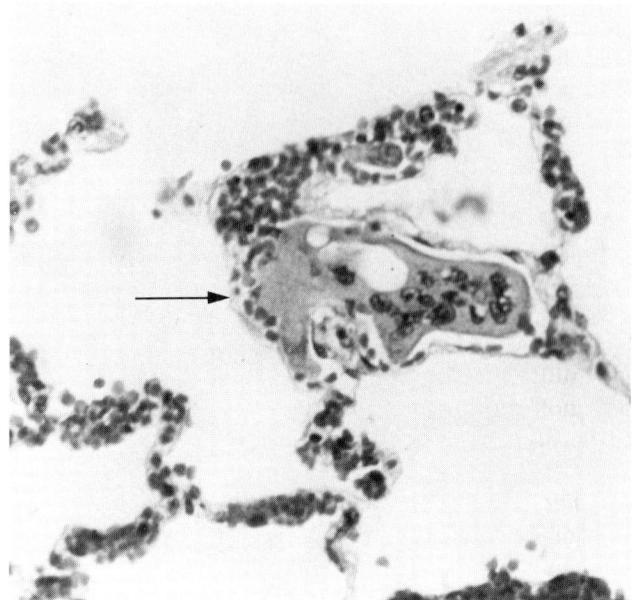

Fig. 35–13. An embolus of trophoblast within a small pulmonary vein (*arrow*). The woman died from trophoblastic embolization further complicated by massive hemorrhage soon after hysterotomy to evacuate a large hydatidiform mole.

and concluded that massive trophoblastic embolization with molar evacuation was probably infrequent.

Although it is generally believed that medical induction prior to evacuation of a hydatidiform mole may increase the risk of trophoblast embolization or persistent trophoblastic disease, Flam and associates (1991), in a retrospective study from Sweden of 266 women with trophoblastic disease, reported that stimulation of uterine contractions with prostaglandins did not increase the risk of persistent disease. Schlaerth and co-workers (1988) identified respiratory complications in 15 percent of women with a mole larger than 20-weeks' size. In many of their patients, pregnancy was terminated by hysterectomy or labor induction.

Even though trophoblast, with or without villous stroma, embolizes to the lungs in volumes too small to produce overt blockade of the pulmonary vasculature, these can subsequently invade the pulmonary parenchyma to establish metastases that are evident radiographically. The lesions may consist of trophoblast alone (metastatic choriocarcinoma) or trophoblast with villous stroma (metastatic hydatidiform mole). The subsequent course of such lesions is unpredictable, and some have been observed to disappear spontaneously either soon after uterine evacuation or even weeks to months later, while others proliferate and kill the woman unless she is treated effectively.

Thyroid Dysfunction. Plasma thyroxine levels in women with molar pregnancy are usually elevated appreciably, but clinically apparent hyperthyroidism is unusual. Amir and colleagues (1984) and Curry and associates (1975) identified hyperthyroidism in about 2 percent of cases. Plasma thyroxine elevation may be the effect primarily of estrogen, as in normal pregnancy, in which case free thyroxine levels are not elevated and the percentage of triiodothyronine bound by resin is increased. It remains controversial whether free thyroxine can be elevated as the consequence of the thyrotropin-like effect of chorionic gonadotropin, or whether variants of this hormone produce these effects (Amir and co-workers, 1984; Mann and colleagues, 1986).

Miller and Seifer (1990) recently reviewed the endocrinological aspects of gestational trophoblastic diseases.

Spontaneous Expulsion. Occasionally, hydatid vesicles, or grapes, are passed before the mole is aborted spontaneously or removed by operation. Spontaneous expulsion is most likely around 16 weeks and is rarely delayed beyond 28 weeks.

Diagnostic Features. Clinical findings of persistent bleeding and a uterus larger than the expected size arouse suspicion for a molar pregnancy. Consideration must be given to an error in menstrual data or a pregnant uterus further enlarged by myomas, hydramnios, or especially multiple fetuses.

Ultrasound. The greatest diagnostic accuracy is obtained from the characteristic ultrasonic appearance of hydatidiform mole (Fig. 35–14). The safety and precision of sonography make it the technique of choice. However, it must be kept in mind that some other structures may have an appearance similar to that of a mole, including uterine myoma with early pregnancy and pregnancies with multiple fetuses. A careful review of the history, coupled with careful sonar evaluation repeated in a week or two when necessary, should serve

to avoid the incorrect ultrasonic diagnosis of mole when the pregnancy is actually normal.

In summary, the clinical and diagnostic features of a complete hydatidiform mole are the following:

1. Continuous or intermittent bloody discharge evident by about 12 weeks, usually not profuse, and often more nearly brown rather than red.
2. Uterine enlargement out of proportion to the duration of pregnancy in about one half of the cases.
3. Absence of fetal parts on palpation and of fetal heart sounds even though the uterus may be enlarged to the level of the umbilicus or higher.
4. Characteristic ultrasonic appearance.
5. A very high serum chorionic gonadotropin level 100 days or more after the last menstrual period.
6. Preeclampsia–eclampsia developing before 24 weeks' gestation.

Prognosis. Current mortality from moles has been practically reduced to zero by more prompt diagnosis and appropriate therapy. With advanced molar pregnancies, these women are usually anemic and bleeding acutely. Intrauterine infection and sepsis in these cases may cause serious morbidity (Schlaerth and colleagues, 1988).

Nearly 20 percent of complete moles progress to gestational trophoblastic tumor. Lurain and colleagues (1983) reported follow-up results of 738 patients from 1962 to 1978 following evacuation of a hydatidiform mole. Spontaneous regression occurred in 596 women (81 percent), while gestational trophoblastic tumors developed in 142 (19 percent). Of this latter group, 125 (17 percent) had an invasive mole and 17 (2 percent) had choriocarcinoma. All 142 patients with trophoblastic tumors were cured and all 738 patients were free of disease at 4 to 18 years follow-up.

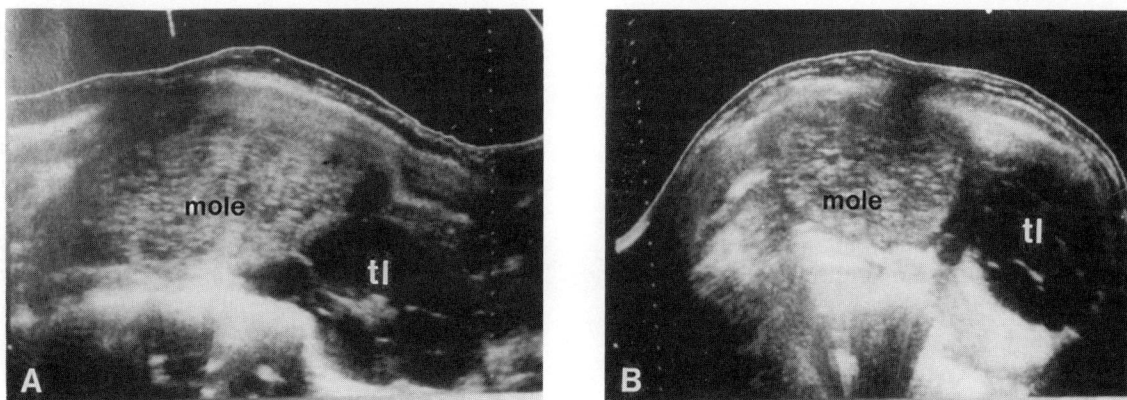

Fig. 35–14. A. Longitudinal sonogram demonstrating a complete hydatidiform mole that fills a uterus enlarged to well above the umbilicus. A large theca-lutein cyst (tl) is seen above the uterus. **B.** Transverse sonogram of the same woman. (Courtesy of Dr. R. Santos.)

Treatment. The treatment for hydatidiform mole consists of two phases, including the immediate evacuation of the mole and the subsequent follow-up for detection of persistent trophoblastic proliferation or malignant change. Initial evaluation prior to evacuation or hysterectomy includes at least a cursory search for metastatic disease. A chest radiograph should be done to look for pulmonary lesions. Although Mutch and colleagues (1986) showed that using computed tomography increased the likelihood of detecting metastatic disease, its routine use has not been evaluated and did not affect prognosis. Unless there is other evidence of extrauterine disease, computed tomography or magnetic resonance imaging to evaluate the liver or brain is not done routinely.

The rare circumstance of twinning with a complete hydatidiform mole plus a fetus and placenta presents an unusual therapeutic dilemma, especially in the absence of karyotypic aberrations or gross fetal anomalies. Neither the risks to the mother nor the likelihood of a healthy offspring have been established. Suzuki and associates (1980) and Vejerslev (1991) reviewed cases in which the outcome was good for both infant and mother (p. 750).

Termination of Molar Pregnancy. Because of greater awareness, and certainly because of better technique for diagnosis, especially sonography, moles now are terminated more often when they are still small, and under controlled circumstances rather than the chaos common when they abort spontaneously. Thus, there is time for adequate evaluation of the woman who may be anemic, hypertensive, or fluid depleted.

Prophylactic Chemotherapy. Although some advocate prophylactic chemotherapy for women with a hydatidiform mole, there is no evidence that such therapy improves the long-term prognosis. Not only will the majority of women experience a spontaneous regression of disease following evacuation, but the follow-up of all patients, including those receiving chemotherapy, is essentially the same. Moreover, the toxicity from prophylactic chemotherapy may be significant, including death (Curry and associates, 1975).

Vacuum Aspiration. Suction evacuation is the treatment of choice for hydatidiform mole, regardless of uterine size (Miller and colleagues, 1989). For large moles, compatible whole blood is made ready and an intravenous system is established for its rapid infusion, if needed. Unless the cervix is long, very firm, and closed—which is very unlikely—dilatation can be safely accomplished under general anesthesia to a diameter sufficient to allow insertion of a plastic suction curet. Anesthetic agents that relax the uterus, such as halothane, should be avoided in high concentrations.

After the great bulk of the mole has been removed by aspiration and oxytocin is given, and the myometrium has contracted, *thorough but gentle* curettage with a large sharp curet is usually performed. Care must be taken to neither perforate the uterus nor scrape so vigorously with the sharp curet as to deeply invade the myometrium and thereby weaken it. Facilities and personnel for immediate laparotomy are mandatory in case there is uncontrollable hemorrhage or serious trauma to the uterus.

Evacuation of all the contents of a large mole is not always easily accomplished, and intraoperative ultrasonic examination may be helpful to establish that the uterine cavity is empty.

Oxytocin, Prostaglandins, and Hysterotomy. Medical induction of labor rarely is utilized in this country for evacuation of hydatidiform moles, and there are many who feel that medical termination and hysterotomy have no role in the management (Curry and colleagues, 1975; Miller and co-workers, 1989; Stone and Bagshawe, 1979).

Hysterectomy. If the parity of the woman or her age are such that no further pregnancies are desired, then hysterectomy may be preferred to suction curettage. Hysterectomy is a logical procedure in women of 40 or over, because of the frequency with which malignant trophoblastic disease ensues in this age group. For example, Tow (1966) reported that 37 percent of women over age 40 with a complete mole went on to develop gestational trophoblastic tumor. Although hysterectomy does not eliminate trophoblastic tumor, it does appreciably reduce the likelihood of recurrent disease.

Follow-up Procedures. If the following important procedures are not adhered to carefully, some women will needlessly die of malignant trophoblastic tumor. The prime objective of follow-up is prompt detection of any change suggestive of malignancy. A general method of follow-up is the following:

1. Prevent pregnancy during the follow-up period—at a minimum, for 1 year.
2. Measure serum chorionic gonadotropin levels every 2 weeks using a specific radioimmunoassay. Although weekly assays are recommended by some, no distinct benefit has been demonstrated.
3. Withhold therapy as long as the serum chorionic gonadotropin levels continue to regress. A rise or persistent plateau in the serum level demands evacuation and usually treatment.
4. Once the level is normal—that is, once it has reached the lower limit of measurement—then test monthly for 6 months, and then every 2 months for a total of 1 year.
5. Follow-up may be discontinued and pregnancy allowed after 1 year.

Current follow-up and management centers on serial measurement of serum chorionic gonadotropin values to detect persistent trophoblastic tumor. Thus, any test must be sufficiently sensitive and specific to detect very low levels. As shown in Figure 35–15, chorionic gonadotropin levels should progressively fall to undetectable levels, otherwise trophoblast persists. An increase signifies trophoblastic proliferation that is most likely malignant unless the woman is again pregnant. Treatment of suspected persistent trophoblastic tumor is discussed subsequently.

Estrogen–progestin contraceptives have been used commonly to prevent a subsequent pregnancy and to suppress pituitary luteinizing hormone that cross-reacts with some tests for chorionic gonadotropin. Stone and co-workers (1976), however, observed that the need for chemotherapy for trophoblastic tumor was significantly increased among women who took oral contraceptives starting shortly after evacuation of a hydatidiform mole. Moreover, oral contraceptives appeared to delay the fall in chorionic gonadotropin levels in women who did not require treatment with chemotherapy. Subsequently, Yuen and Burch (1983) reported that neither the duration that chorionic gonadotropin persisted nor the frequency of invasive complications was increased in women after molar evacuation and who used an oral contraceptive that contained 50 μg of estrogen or less. Recently, Deicas and associates (1991)

studied the effect of contraception on subsequent development of postmolar gestational trophoblastic tumor in 162 women with hydatidiform mole and 137 with trophoblastic tumor. Of the women utilizing oral contraceptives, 33 percent developed gestational trophoblastic tumors compared with 57 percent who did not. The estrogen dose was not significant. They concluded that there was an apparent outcome advantage for women who took oral contraceptives after evacuation of a mole.

Although spontaneous disappearance of retained trophoblastic tissue is well known, the effectiveness of chemotherapeutic agents to treat trophoblastic neoplasia has led some to the routine use of these drugs in women with molar pregnancy. They are given to preclude development of malignancy and to hasten the disappearance of the retained trophoblast. Chemotherapeutic agents such as methotrexate are highly toxic and potentially lethal, and as previously mentioned, there are no data to suggest an improved long-term outcome.

Treatment of Persistent Trophoblastic Tumor. Following evacuation of a hydatidiform mole, about 20 percent of women will subsequently undergo further treatment for suspected persistent gestational trophoblastic tumor (Lurain and co-workers, 1983). If serum chorionic gonadotropin values have plateaued or are rising, if there is no evidence for disease beyond the uterus, and if the uterus is not important for future reproduction, hysterectomy will effect a cure in most cases. Often chorionic gonadotropin will disappear and the woman remains well. However, if the uterus is to be preserved, if there is radiographic evidence of lung lesions, or if there are vaginal metastases, chemotherapy is started at this time with or without curettage. Most often, such treatment has been successful in these circumstances.

Very small amounts of viable trophoblastic tumor can be detected by assay for the β-subunit of chorionic gonadotropin. Once gonadotropin activity has decreased to the limit of measurement, therapy can be stopped safely without likelihood of recurrence. Treatment is best carried out by experienced individuals in centers with appropriate facilities for precisely monitoring chorionic gonadotropin levels as well as bone marrow, hepatic, and renal function.

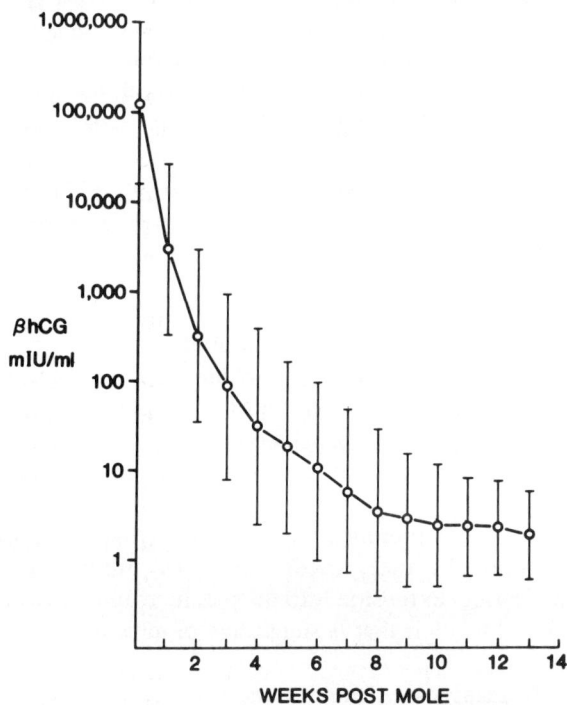

Fig. 35–15. The mean value and 95 percent confidence limits describing the normal postmolar β-subunit chorionic gonadotropin regression curve. (From Schlaerth and associates, 1981, with permission.)

Gestational Trophoblastic Tumors

Gestational trophoblastic tumor refers to persistent trophoblastic proliferation. It may follow molar pregnancy or normal pregnancy, or develop after abortive outcomes, including ectopic pregnancy. As shown in Table 35–2, gestational trophoblastic tumors are divided into two clinical categories, nonmetastatic and metastatic;

the latter is further divided into those women who are high risk and low risk with regard to prognosis.

Etiology. Gestational trophoblastic tumor most always develops with or follows some form of pregnancy. Very rarely, choriocarcinoma may arise from a teratoma. Approximately one half of cases follow a hydatidiform mole, 25 percent follow an abortion, and 25 percent develop after an apparently normal pregnancy. Of 48 fatal cases from the Brewer Trophoblastic Disease Center, only 14 (30 percent) developed in association with a hydatidiform mole (Lurain and co-workers, 1982). The remainder were associated with term or near-term pregnancies, abortions, or ectopic pregnancies.

Malignancy has been identified rarely in the placenta of a seemingly normal pregnancy. In a case described by Brewer and Mazur (1981), widespread malignant trophoblast was evident at 18 weeks' gestation, and a primary choriocarcinoma of the placenta was detected. A case in which malignant trophoblast metastasized to the fetus has also been described (Kruseman and colleagues, 1977).

Pathology. Clinical management is no longer dictated by histological findings. In most cases of gestational trophoblastic tumor, the diagnosis is made primarily by persistent chorionic gonadotropin. In most cases, no tissue is submitted for pathological study. In those cases with tissue submitted, either choriocarcinoma or invasive mole are most often found.

Choriocarcinoma. This extremely malignant form of trophoblastic tumor may be considered a carcinoma of the chorionic epithelium, although in its growth and metastasis it often behaves like a sarcoma. Factors involved in malignant transformation of the chorion are unknown. In choriocarcinoma, the predisposition of normal trophoblast to invasive growth and erosion of blood vessels is greatly exaggerated. The characteristic gross picture is that of a rapidly growing mass invading both uterine muscle and blood vessels, causing hemorrhage and necrosis (Fig. 35–16A). The tumor is dark red or purple and ragged or friable. If it involves the endometrium, then bleeding, sloughing, and infection of the surface usually occur early. Masses of tissue buried in the myometrium may extend outward, appearing on the uterus as dark, irregular nodules that eventually penetrate the peritoneum.

Microscopically, columns and sheets of trophoblast penetrate the muscle and blood vessels, sometimes in plexiform arrangement and at other times in complete disorganization, interspersed with clotted blood (Fig. 35–16B). An important diagnostic feature of choriocarcinoma, in contrast to hydatiform mole or invasive mole, is absence of a villous pattern. Both cytotrophoblast and syncytial elements are involved, although one or the other may predominate. Cellular anaplasia exists, often

in marked degrees, but is less valuable as a criterion of trophoblastic malignancy than in other tumors. The difficulty of cytological evaluation is one of the factors leading to error in the diagnosis of choriocarcinoma from examination of uterine curettings. Cells of normal trophoblast at the placental site have been erroneously diagnosed as choriocarcinoma.

Metastases often develop early and are generally blood-borne because of the affinity of trophoblast for blood vessels. The most common sites of metastasis are the lungs (over 75 percent) and the vagina (about 50 percent). The vulva, kidneys, liver, ovaries, brain, and bowel also contain metastases in many cases. Ovarian theca-lutein cysts are identified in over one third of the cases.

Invasive Mole. The distinguishing features of invasive mole are excessive trophoblastic overgrowth and extensive penetration by the trophoblastic elements, including whole villi, into the depths of the myometrium, sometimes to involve the peritoneum or the adjacent parametrium or vaginal vault. Such moles are locally invasive, but generally lack the pronounced tendency to widespread metastasis that is characteristic of choriocarcinoma.

Placental Site Trophoblastic Tumor. Very rarely, a trophoblastic tumor arises from the placental implantation site following either a normal term pregnancy or abortion. This tumor is characterized histologically by predominantly cytotrophoblastic cells, and immunohistochemical staining reveals many prolactin-producing cells and few gonadotropin-producing ones (Miller and associates, 1989). Thus, gonadotropin levels may be normal to elevated. Bleeding is the main presenting symptom.

Brewer and colleagues (1992) have recently described erythrocytosis associated with a placental-site trophoblastic tumor. The polycythemia resolved after hysterectomy.

Clinical History. Malignant trophoblastic disease may follow hydatidiform mole, abortion, ectopic pregnancy, or normal pregnancy. The most common, though not constant, sign is irregular bleeding after the immediate puerperium in association with uterine subinvolution. The bleeding may be continuous or intermittent, with sudden and sometimes massive hemorrhages. Uterine perforation by the growth may cause intraperitoneal hemorrhage. Extension into the parametrium may cause pain and fixation that is suggestive of inflammatory disease.

In many cases, the first indication may be a metastatic lesion. Vaginal or vulvar tumors may be found. The woman may complain of cough and have bloody sputum from pulmonary metastases. In a few cases it has been impossible to find choriocarcinoma in the uterus

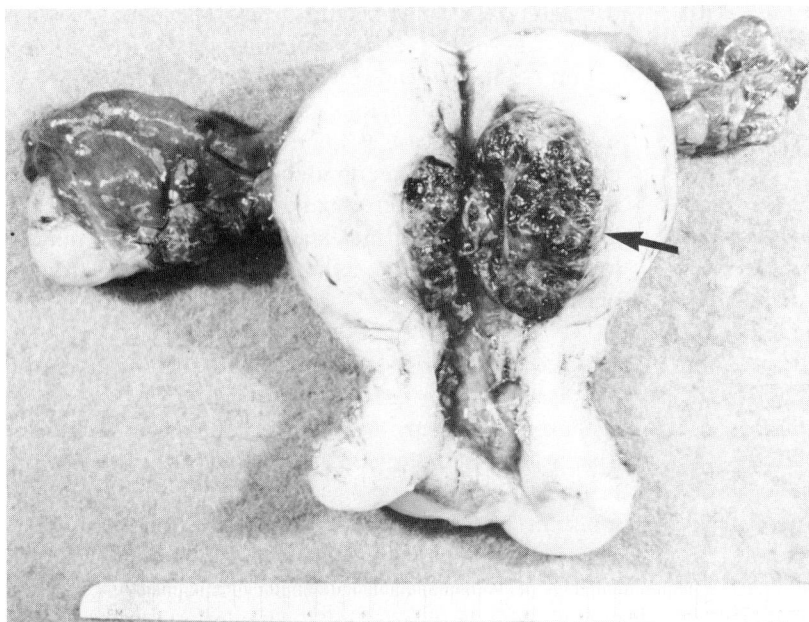

A

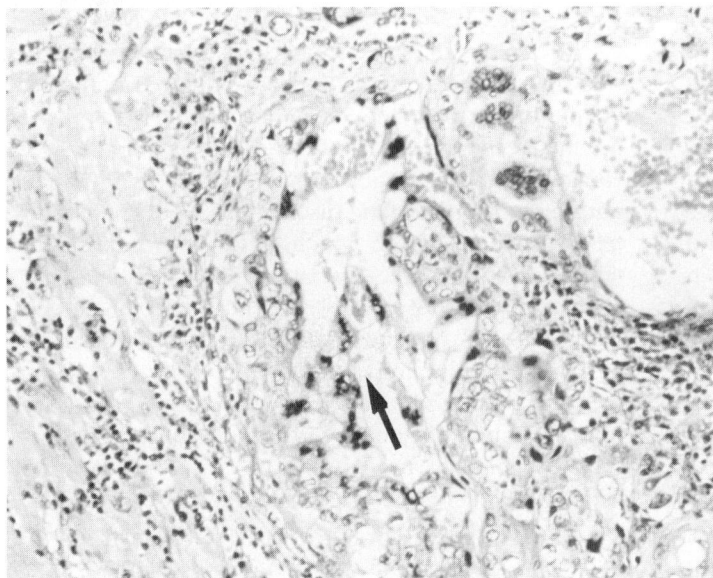

B

Fig. 35–16. A. Choriocarcinoma (*arrow*) invading the uterus. Persistent trophoblastic disease was demonstrated by curettage subsequent to the expulsion of a hydatidiform mole. Chemotherapy was given, consisting of repeated courses of actinomycin D, then methotrexate, and finally triple therapy with actinomycin D, 5-fluorouracil, and cyclophosphamide. When these failed to destroy the malignancy, hysterectomy and bilateral salpingo-oophorectomy were performed. The woman was known to be alive without detectable chorionic gonadotropin 10 years later. **B.** Histological characteristics of the choriocarcinoma demonstrated in **A.** Malignant syncytio- and cytotrophoblast without villous stroma invade the myometrium and vascular spaces (*arrow*) accompanied by necrosis and hemorrhage.

or pelvis, the original lesion having disappeared, leaving only distant metastases growing actively.

If unmodified by treatment, the course of choriocarcinoma is rapidly progressive, and death usually follows within a few months in the majority of cases. The most common cause of death is hemorrhage in various locations.

Diagnosis. Recognition of the possibility of the lesion is the most important factor in diagnosis. All women with a hydatidiform mole are at risk and need to be followed as described. Any case of unusual bleeding after term pregnancy or abortion should be investigated by curettage, but especially by measurements of chorionic gonadotropin, because absolute reliance cannot be placed on histological findings. Malignant tissue may be buried within the myometrium, inaccessible to the curette, or hidden in a distant metastasis.

Solitary or multiple nodules present in the chest radiograph that cannot be otherwise explained are suggestive of the possibility of choriocarcinoma. It should be kept in mind, however, that some nontrophoblastic tumors secrete small amounts of chorionic gonadotropin (Shane and Naftolin, 1975). Persistent or rising gonadotropin levels in the absence of pregnancy are indicative of trophoblastic tumor. Assay results should be confirmed before beginning medical or surgical therapy.

Other evaluation before treatment is given includes computed tomography to evaluate the brain, lungs, liver, and pelvis. Hricak and colleagues (1986) reported the use of magnetic resonance imaging in 9 women with malignant trophoblastic disease and concluded that this method was superior to sonography and computed tomography to evaluate the degree of uterine involvement.

Treatment. Current treatment for gestational trophoblastic tumor is much more successful than that used in the past. Formerly, the only hope for cure was hysterectomy or, even more remote, resection of a metastatic lesion. In 1956, Li and associates successfully treated a woman with metastatic gestational trophoblastic tumor by employing methotrexate. Since then, methotrexate and other agents effective against malignant tumors, especially actinomycin D, have been widely used with considerable success.

The pharmacology and clinical use of methotrexate have been reviewed extensively by Jolivet and colleagues (1983). The overall cure rate in past years for persistent gestational trophoblastic tumor of all severities has been about 90 percent (Lewis, 1980). Patients classified as having nonmetastatic tumors or good-prognosis gestational trophoblastic tumors have been cured virtually 100 percent of the time. As shown in Table 35–2, this category includes those women without metastases; and women with metastases whose duration of disease is less than 4 months, with serum chorionic gonadotropin levels less than 40,000 mIU/mL, no prior chemotherapy, and no brain or liver metastases. Cure usually has been achieved for these so-called low-risk patients following single-agent chemotherapy. Such treatment obviously reduces serious toxicity. Recently, Barter and associates (1987) reported success with methotrexate given orally; Homesley and associates (1988) reported similar results with weekly intramuscular methotrexate; and Petrilli and colleagues (1987) found that single-dose actinomycin D given every 2 weeks was highly effective in women with nonmetastatic disease. Fortunately, in those instances in which single-agent therapy proved ineffective, prompt treatment with combination chemotherapy, with or without radiotherapy, will most often provide a cure.

Patients are classified as high risk because they have metastatic tumor that is unlikely to be cured with single-agent chemotherapy based on the following risk factors: disease for more than 4 months, serum gonadotropin levels greater than 40,000 mIU/mL, liver or brain metastases, or previous chemotherapy without success. Some authorities, but not all, include choriocarcinoma developing in association with term pregnancy as having a poor prognosis. In these high-risk women, combination chemotherapy, in spite of increased toxicity, has produced the highest cure rate. Two recently used drugs, **etoposide** and **cisplatin,** are reported to be among the most active agents for treatment of trophoblastic disease (Jones, 1990). The combination of meth-

otrexate, dactinomycin, and cyclophosphamide (MAC) has for the most part been abandoned for new combination regimens centered around etoposide.

The most efficacious treatment for placental site trophoblastic disease is unknown, although Miller and colleagues (1989) recommend that most women are best treated by hysterectomy. Although chemotherapy is recommended for metastatic disease, it does not appear to be as effective as for other gestational trophoblastic tumors.

Prognosis. Women with nonmetastatic trophoblastic neoplasia have an extremely good prognosis if single-agent chemotherapy is started as soon as persistent disease is identified. Previously cited were the remarkable results of Lurain and colleagues (1983) of women with molar pregnancies from the Brewer Trophoblastic Disease Center of Northwestern University. From 1962 to 1978, 738 women with molar pregnancy were managed as generally outlined above. Chemotherapy was given for persistent disease in 19 percent, and all were living and disease-free 4 to 18 years later.

Women with low-risk metastatic gestational tumors who are treated aggressively with single- or multiagent chemotherapy in general do almost as well as those with nonmetastatic disease (DuBeshter and associates, 1987; Hammond and colleagues, 1980; Jones, 1987). Women with high-risk metastatic disease have appreciable mortality that depends on which factors were considered "high risk" (Soper and associates, 1988). Remission rates have been reported to vary from about 45 to 65 percent. Lurain (1987) analyzed 53 deaths from the Brewer Trophoblastic Center and concluded that the three factors primarily responsible were (1) extensive choriocarcinoma at initial diagnosis, (2) lack of appropriately aggressive initial treatment, and (3) failure of currently used chemotherapy.

There have been several prognostic scoring systems and an anatomical staging system reported (Bagshawe, 1976; Lurain and associates, 1991; Pettersson and colleagues, 1985; World Health Organization, 1983). Lurain and associates (1991) presented a simplified prognostic scoring system based on multivariate analysis of almost 400 women treated for gestational trophoblastic tumor. This system, known as the Brewer Score, is summarized in Table 35–5. This score is derived by adding the component scores for the three significant variables from the multivariate analysis. In the 168 women with metastatic trophoblastic tumors, survival was 100 percent with a score of 1, 88 percent for a score of 2, 63 percent for a score of 3, and only 30 percent for a score of 4.

Pregnancy After Trophoblastic Disease. After gestational trophoblastic disease, women are at increased risk for developing trophoblastic disease in a subsequent pregnancy. Berkowitz and colleagues (1987) re-

TABLE 35–5. THE BREWER SCORE FOR GESTATIONAL TROPHOBLASTIC TUMORS

Factor	Score
Lung and/or vaginal metastasis	0
One to four metastases	1
Metastasis other than lung and/or vaginal metastases, and prior chemotherapy	
Five to eight metastases	2
More than eight metastases	3

Adapted from Lurain and associates (1991), with permission.

ported that 1.3 percent of 1048 women treated at the New England Trophoblastic Disease Center for gestational trophoblastic disease had a recurrent molar pregnancy. Importantly, women who have been given chemotherapy do not have an increased risk for anomalous fetuses in subsequent pregnancies (Rustin and colleagues, 1984; Song and associates, 1988).

Other Tumors of the Placenta

Chorioangioma (Hemangioma). Various angiomatous tumors of the placenta ranging widely in size have been described, and because of the resemblance of their components to the blood vessels and stroma of the chorionic villus, the term *chorioangioma*, or *chorangioma*, has been considered the most appropriate designation. The tumors are most likely hamartomas of primitive chorionic mesenchyme. Their incidence has been reported to be about 1 percent. Larger chorioangiomas may be strongly suspected on the basis of sono-

graphic changes within the placenta. A dramatic example is provided in Figure 35–17.

Small growths are essentially asymptomatic, but large tumors may be associated with hydramnios or antepartum hemorrhage. Fetal death and malformations are uncommon complications, although there may be a positive correlation with low birthweight. Stiller and Skafish (1986) described a case with multiple placental chorioangiomas in which a blood group A fetus bled acutely into her O group mother. The mother showed evidence of acute hemolysis without anemia, and the fetus developed a sinusoidal heart rate pattern frequently seen in severe anemia. We have identified severe iron-deficiency anemia in the neonate as the consequence of chronic fetal to maternal hemorrhage associated with multiple small chorioangiomas. Large chorioangiomas provide an arteriovenous shunt in the fetal circulation that can lead to heart failure with all of its complications. With a large chorioangioma, consumptive coagulopathy and microangiopathic hemolytic anemia have also been observed in the fetus-infant. Figure 35–17 shows a placenta and a very large, discrete chorioangioma that led to heart failure, consumptive coagulopathy, and microangiopathic hemolysis in the fetus.

Tumors Metastatic to the Placenta. Metastases of malignant tumors are rare. The subject was reviewed by Read and Platzer (1981), who reported that malignant melanoma is the most common malignancy metastatic to the placenta; it makes up nearly one third of reported cases. Leukemias and lymphomas comprise another third. Interestingly, the fetus is involved with malignant tumor in about one fourth of reported cases. Any tumor with hematogenous spread is a potential source of pla-

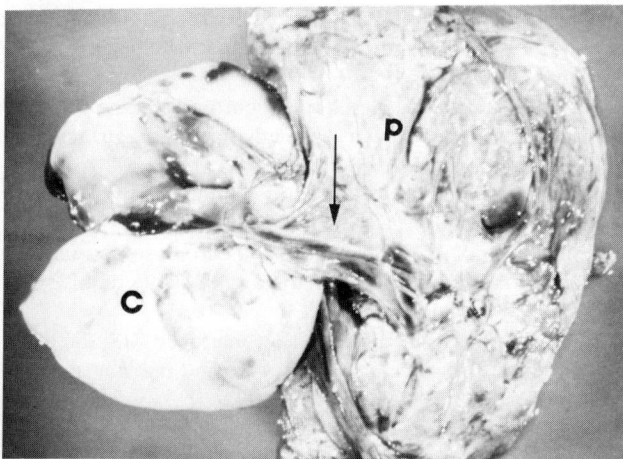

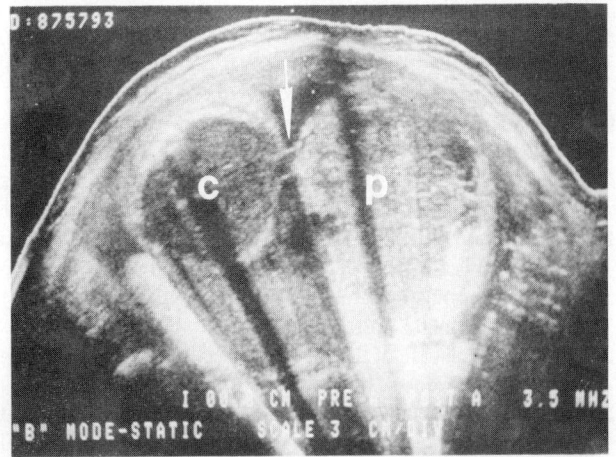

A   **B**

Fig. 35–17. A. Placenta (p) and discrete 450 g chorioangioma (c) connected to the placenta by vascular stalk (*arrow*). The 34-week fetus was identified by sonography to have marked hydrothorax. Demonstrated in cord blood were severe hypofibrinogenemia, thrombocytopenia, hypoprothrombinemia, and microangiopathic hemolysis. The infant had cardiomegaly, heart failure, pleural effusion, and hepatomegaly. After several cardiac arrests the infant succumbed 3 days after birth. **B.** Sonogram of the same placenta (p) and chorioangioma (c) connected by a short pedicle (*arrow*). (Courtesy of Dr. R. Santos.)

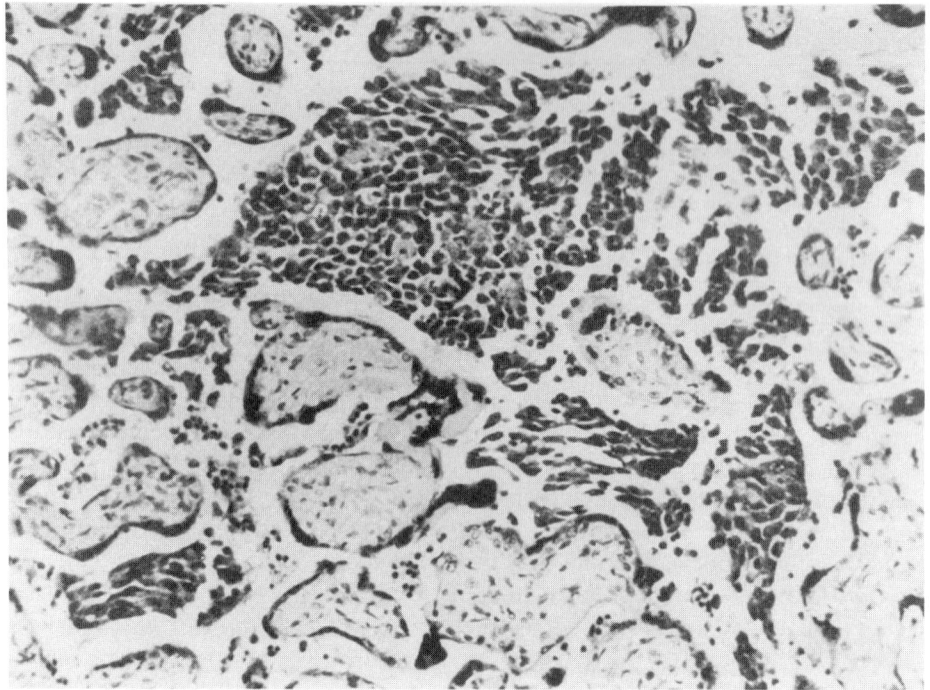

Fig. 35–18. Lung carcinoma metastatic to the placenta. (From Read and Platzer, 1981, with permission.)

cental metastases, as evidenced by the case of large-cell undifferentiated lung carcinoma metastatic to the placenta (Fig. 35–18). The mother succumbed but the child remained healthy by 16 months.

References

American College of Obstetricians and Gynecologists: Committee on Obstetrics: Maternal–Fetal Medicine. Placental pathology, no. 102, December 1991

American College of Obstetricians and Gynecologists: Management of gestational trophoblastic neoplasia. Technical bulletin no. 59, December 1980

Amir SM, Osathanondh R, Berkowitz RS, Goldstein DP: Human chorionic gonadotropin and thyroid function in patients with hydatidiform mole. Am J Obstet Gynecol 150:723, 1984

Bagshawe KD: Risk and prognostic factors in trophoblastic neoplasia. Cancer 38:1373, 1976

Bagshawe KD, Lawler SD: Commentary: Unmasking moles. Br J Obstet Gynaecol 89:255, 1982

Barter JF, Soong SJ, Hatch KD, Orr JW Jr, Partridge EC, Austin JM Jr, Shingleton HM: Treatment of nonmetastatic gestational trophoblastic disease with oral methotrexate. Am J Obstet Gynecol 157:1166, 1987

Benirschke K: Disease of the placenta. In Gluck L (ed): Modern Perinatal Medicine. Chicago, Year Book, 1974, p 99

Benirschke K, Brown WH: A vascular anomaly of the umbilical cord: The absence of one umbilical artery in the umbilical cords of normal and abnormal fetuses. Obstet Gynecol 6:399, 1955

Benirschke K, Dodds JP: Angiomyxoma of the umbilical cord with atrophy of an umbilical artery. Obstet Gynecol 30:99, 1967

Benirschke K, Driscoll SG (eds): The Pathology of the Human Placenta. New York, Springer-Verlag, 1974

Berkowitz RS, Goldstein DP, Bernstein MR: Advances in management of partial molar pregnancy. Contemp Obstet Gynecol 36:33, 1991

Berkowitz RS, Goldstein DP, Bernstein MR: Management of partial molar pregnancy. Contemp Obstet Gynecol 27:77, 1986

Berkowitz RS, Goldstein DP, Bernstein MR, Sablinska B: Subsequent pregnancy outcome in patients with molar pregnancy and gestational trophoblastic tumors. J Reprod Med 32:680, 1987

Block MF, Merrill JA: Hydatidiform mole with coexistent fetus. Obstet Gynecol 60:129, 1982

Brewer CA, Adelson MD, Elder RC: Erythrocytosis associated with a placental-site trophoblastic tumor. Obstet Gynecol 79:846, 1992

Brewer JI, Mazur MT: Gestational choriocarcinoma: Its origin in the placenta during a seemingly normal pregnancy. Am J Surg Pathol 5:267, 1981

Bryan EM, Kohler HG: The missing umbilical artery: II. Paediatric follow-up. Arch Dis Child 50:714, 1975

Byrne J, Blanc WA: Malformations and chromosome anomalies in spontaneously aborted fetuses with single umbilical artery. Am J Obstet Gynecol 151:340, 1985

College of American Pathologists: Conference XIX, the examination of the placenta: Patient care and risk management. Arch Pathol Lab Med 115:641, 1991

Curry SL, Hammond CB, Tyrey L, Creasman WT, Parker RT: Hydatidiform mole: Diagnosis, management, and long-time follow-up of 347 patients. Obstet Gynecol 45:1, 1975

Czernobilsky B, Barash A, Lancet M: Partial moles: A clinico-pathology study of 25 cases. Obstet Gynecol 59:75, 1982

Deicas RE, Miller DS, Rademaker AW, Lurain JR: The role of

contraception in the development of postmolar gestational trophoblastic tumor. Obstet Gynecol 78:221, 1991

DuBeshter B, Berkowitz RS, Goldstein DP, Cramer DW, Bernstein MR: Metastatic gestational trophoblastic disease: Experience at the New England Trophoblastic Disease Center, 1965 to 1985. Obstet Gynecol 69:390, 1987

Flam F, Lundstrom V, Petterson F: Medical induction prior to surgical evacuation of hydatidiform mole: Is there a greater risk of persistent trophoblastic disease? Eur J Obstet Gynecol Reprod Biol 42:57, 1991

Fox H: Pathology of the placenta. Monograph, vol 7. Philadelphia, Saunders, 1978

Gianopoulas J, Carver T, Tomich PG, Karlman R, Gadwood K: Diagnosis of vasa previa with ultrasonography. Obstet Gynecol 69:488, 1987

Grannum PAT, Berkowitz RL, Hobbins JC: The ultrasonic changes in the maturing placenta and their relation to fetal pulmonic maturity. Am J Obstet Gynecol 133:915, 1979

Grimes DA: Epidemiology of gestational trophoblastic disease. Am J Obstet Gynecol 150:309, 1984

Hammond CB, Borchert I, Tyrey I, Creasman WT, Parker RT: Treatment of metastatic trophoblastic disease: Good and poor prognosis. Am J Obstet Gynecol 115:451, 1973

Hammond CB, Weed JC, Currie JL: The role of operation in the current therapy of gestational trophoblastic disease. Am J Obstet Gynecol 136:844, 1980

Hankins GDV, Snyder RR, Hauth JC, Gilstrap LC III, Hammond T: Nuchal cords and neonatal outcome. Obstet Gynecol 70:687, 1987a

Hankins GDV, Wendel GW, Snyder RR, Cunningham FG: Trophoblastic embolization during molar evacuation: Central hemodynamic observations. Obstet Gynecol 69:368, 1987b

Homesley HD, Blessing JA, Rettenmaier M, Capizzi RL, Major FJ, Twiggs LB: Weekly intramuscular methotrexate for nonmetastatic gestational trophoblastic disease. Obstet Gynecol 72:413, 1988

Hricak H, Demas BE, Braga CA, Fisher MR, Winkler ML: Gestational trophoblastic neoplasm of the uterus: MR assessment. Radiology 161:11, 1986

Jequier AM, Winterton WR: Diagnostic problems of trophoblastic disease in women age 50 or more: Obstet Gynecol 42:378, 1975

Jolivet J, Cowan KH, Curt GA, Clendeninn NH, Chaber BA: The pharmacology and clinical use of methotrexate. N Engl J Med 309:1094, 1983

Jones WB: Gestational trophoblastic disease: What have we learned in the past decade? Am J Obstet Gynecol 162:1286, 1990

Jones WB: Current management of low-risk metastatic gestational trophoblastic disease. J Reprod Med 32:655, 1987

Kan PS, Eastman NJ: Coiling of the umbilical cord around the foetal neck. Br J Obstet Gynaecol 64:227, 1957

Kouyoumdjian A: Velamentous insertion of the umbilical cord. Obstet Gynecol 56:737, 1980

Kruseman AC, Lent MV, Blom AH, Lauw GP: Choriocarcinoma in mother and child, identified by immunoenzyme histochemistry. Am J Clin Pathol 67:279, 1977

Lademacher DS, Vermeulen RCW, Harten JJVD, Arts NFT: Circumvallate placenta and congenital malformation. Lancet 1:732, 1981

Lawler SD, Fisher RA, Dent J: A prospective genetic study of complete and partial hydatidiform moles. Am J Obstet Gynecol 164:1270, 1991

Lewis JL Jr: Treatment of metastatic gestational trophoblastic neoplasms. Am J Obstet Gynecol 136:163, 1980

Li MC, Hertz R, Spencer DB: Effect of methotrexate therapy upon choriocarcinoma and chorioadenoma. Proc Soc Exp Biol Med 93:361, 1956

Lurain JR: Causes of treatment failure in gestational trophoblastic disease. J Reprod Med 32:677, 1987

Lurain JR, Brewer JI, Mazur MT, Torok EE: Fatal gestational trophoblastic disease: An analysis of treatment failures. Am J Obstet Gynecol 144:391, 1982

Lurain JR, Brewer JI, Torek EE, Halpern B: Natural history of hydatidiform mole after primary evacuation. Am J Obstet Gynecol 145:591, 1983

Lurain JR, Casanova LA, Miller DS, Rademaker AW: Prognostic factors in gestational trophoblastic tumors: A proposed new scoring system based on multivariate analysis. Am J Obstet Gynecol 164:611, 1991

Mann K, Schneider N, Hoermann R: Thyrotropic activity of acidic isoelectric variants of human chorionic gonadotropin and trophoblastic tumors. Endocrinology 118:1558, 1986

Messer RH, Gomez AR, Yambao TJ: Antepartum testing for vasa previa: Current standard of care. Am J Obstet Gynecol 156:1459, 1987

Miller DS, Ballon SC, Teng NNH: Gestational trophoblastic diseases. In: Brody SA, Ueland K (eds): Endocrine Disorders in Pregnancy. Norwalk, CT, Appleton & Lange, 1989, p 451

Miller DS, Lurain JR: Classification and staging of gestational trophoblastic tumors. Obstet Gynecol Clin North Am 15:477, 1988

Miller DS, Seifer DB: Endocrinologic aspects of gestational trophoblastic diseases. Int J Fertil 35:137, 1990

Miller ME, Higginbottom M, Smith DW: Short umbilical cord: Its origin and relevance. Pediatrics 67:618, 1981

Montz FJ, Schlaerth JB, Morrow CP: The natural history of theca lutein cysts. Obstet Gynecol 72:247, 1988

Mutch DG, Soper JT, Baker ME, Bandy LC, Cox EB, Clarke-Pearson DL, Hammond CB: Role of computed axial tomography of the chest in staging patients with nonmetastatic gestational trophoblastic disease. Obstet Gynecol 68:348, 1986

Novak E, Seah CS: Choriocarcinoma of the uterus. Am J Obstet Gynecol 67:933, 1954

Peckham CH, Yerushalmy J: Aplasia of one umbilical artery: Incidence by race and certain obstetric factors. Obstet Gynecol 26:359, 1965

Petrilli ES, Twiggs LB, Blessing JA, Teng NNH, Curry S: Single-dose actinomycin-D treatment for nonmetastatic gestational trophoblastic disease: A prospective phase II trial of the Gynecologic Oncology Group. Cancer 60:2173, 1987

Pettersson F, Kolstad P, Ludwig H: Annual report on the results of treatment in gynecologic cancer. Stockholm: International Federation of Gynecology and Obstetrics, 1985

Ramin SM, Gilstrap LC III: Placental abnormalities: Previa, abruption and accreta. In: Plauche W, Morrison JC, O'Sullivan MJ (eds). Surgical Obstetrics. Philadelphia, Saunders, 1992, p 203

Rayburn WF, Beynen A, Brinkman DL: Umbilical cord length and intrapartum complications. Obstet Gynecol 57:450, 1981

Read EJ, Platzer PB: Placental metastasis from material carcinoma of the lung. Obstet Gynecol 58:387, 1981

Robinson LK, Jones KL, Benirschke K: The nature and structural defects associated with velamentous and marginal insertion of the umbilical cord. Am J Obstet Gynecol 146:191, 1983

Rustin GJ, Booth M, Dent J, Salt S, Rustin F, Bagshawe KD: Pregnancy after cytotoxic chemotherapy for gestational trophoblastic tumours. Br Med J 288:103, 1984

Schlaerth JB, Morrow CP, Kletzky OA, Nalick RH, D'Ablaing GA: Prognostic characteristics of serum human chorionic gonadotropin titer regression following molar pregnancy. Obstet Gynecol 58:478, 1981

Schlaerth JB, Morrow CP, Montz F, d'Ablaing G: Initial management of hydatidiform mole. Am J Obstet Gynecol 158:1299, 1988

Shane JM, Naftolin F: Aberrant hormone activity by tumors of gynecologic importance. Am J Obstet Gynecol 121:133, 1975

Shen-Schwarz S, Macpherson TA, Mueller-Heubach E: The clinical significance of hemorrhagic endovasculitis of the placenta. Am J Obstet Gynecol 159:48, 1988

Smalbraak J: Trophoblastic Growths. Haarlem, Netherlands, Elsevier, 1957

Soernes T, Bakke T: The length of the human umbilical cord in vertex and breech presentations. Am J Obstet Gynecol 154:1086, 1986

Song HZ, Wu PC, Wang YE, Yang XE, Dong SY: Pregnancy outcomes after successful chemotherapy for choriocarcinoma and invasive mole: Long-term follow-up. Am J Obstet Gynecol 158:538, 1988

Soper JT, Clarke-Pearson D, Hammond CB: Metastatic gestational trophoblastic disease: Prognostic factors in previously untreated patients. Obstet Gynecol 71:338, 1988

Spellacy WN, Gravem H, Fisch RO: The umbilical cord complications of true knots, nuchal coils and cords around the body. Am J Obstet Gynecol 94:1136, 1966

Spirit BA, Cohen WN, Weinstein HM: The incidence of placental calcification in normal pregnancies. Radiology 142:707, 1982

Stanhope CR, Stuart GCE, Curtis KL: Primary ovarian hydatidiform mole: Review of the literature and report of a case. Am J Obstet Gynecol 145:886, 1983

Stiller AG, Skafish PR: Placental chorioangioma: A rare cause of fetomaternal transfusion with maternal hemolysis and fetal distress. Obstet Gynecol 67:296, 1986

Stone M, Bagshawe KD: An analysis of the influence of maternal age, gestational age, contraceptive method, and the mode of primary treatment of patients with hydatidiform moles on the incidence of subsequent chemotherapy. Br J Obstet Gynaecol 86:782, 1979

Stone M, Dent J, Kardana A, Bogshawe KD: Relationship of oral contraception to development of trophoblastic tumour after evacuation of a hydatidiform mole. Br J Obstet Gynaecol 83:913, 1976

Suzuki M, Matsunobu A, Wakita K, Nishijima M, Osanai K: Hydatidiform mole with a surviving coexisting fetus. Obstet Gynecol 56:384, 1980

Szulman AE, Surti U: The clinicopathologic profile of the partial hydatidiform mole. Obstet Gynecol 59:597, 1982

Tow WSH: The classification of malignant growths of the chorion. Br J Obstet Gynaecol 73:1000, 1966

Vejerslev LO: Clinical management and diagnostic possibilities in hydatidiform mole with coexistent fetus. Obstet Gynecol Surv 46:577, 1991

World Health Organization Scientific Group on Gestational Trophoblastic Diseases: Gestational trophoblastic diseases. Technical report series no. 692. Geneva, World Health Organization, 1983

Wu FY: Recurrent hydatidiform mole: A case report of nine consecutive molar pregnancies. Obstet Gynecol 41:2000, 1973

Yuen BH, Burch P: Relationship of oral contraceptives and the intrauterine contraceptive devices to the regression of concentrations of the beta subunits of human chorionic gonadotropin and invasive complications after molar pregnancy. Am J Obstet Gynecol 145:214, 1983

Common Complications of Pregnancy

■

CHAPTER 36

Hypertensive Disorders in Pregnancy

Pregnancy can induce hypertension in normotensive women or aggravate already existing hypertension. Generalized edema, proteinuria, or both may also accompany pregnancy-induced or aggravated hypertension. If hypertension is untreated, convulsions may develop.

Hypertensive disorders complicating pregnancy are common and form one of the deadly triad, along with hemorrhage and infection, that results in a large number of maternal deaths. Rochat and colleagues (1988) reported that 12 percent of 601 maternal deaths from 1980 to 1985 in the United States were caused by hypertensive diseases. How pregnancy incites or aggravates hypertension remains unsolved despite decades of intensive research, and hypertensive disorders remain among the most important unsolved problems in obstetrics. The loss of maternal and infant lives to hypertension induced or aggravated by pregnancy can most often be prevented. With improved prenatal care and a rational approach to management, dramatic declines in maternal mortality rates have been reported (Lehmann and colleagues, 1987; Rochat and co-workers, 1988; Sachs and associates, 1987). Finally, early detection and appropriate treatment may prolong pregnancy long enough to ensure a satisfactory outcome for both mother and fetus.

GENERAL CONSIDERATIONS

Classification

Toxemia of pregnancy is an archaic term that was variously applied to any or all hypertensive disorders accompanied by proteinuria or edema and to a variety of other disorders including liver disease. In 1986, the American College of Obstetricians and Gynecologists published updated definitions and a newer classification. Previously, the criteria used were those of Hughes (1972), and these are similar to those of Davey and MacGillivray (1988). Unfortunately, no classification is adequate if etiology is unknown. Therefore, because of the confusion that has arisen from these classifications, we use the modified classification of the American College of Obstetricians and Gynecologists (1986) that is shown in Table 36–1. This was done to separate hypertension that is in some way induced by pregnancy from hypertension that merely coexists with it. Unfortunately, chronic hypertension may be aggravated by superimposition of preeclampsia or eclampsia.

The working group of the National High Blood Pressure Education Program (1990) recommends that the original classification of Hughes (1972) be used because *transient hypertension* is included. This category corresponds to pregnancy-induced hypertension without pathological edema or proteinuria (Table 36–1). The working group also cited current, quite complex classifications of the World Health Organization (1987) and the International Society for the Study of Hypertension in Pregnancy (Davey and MacGillivray, 1988).

Diagnosis of Pregnancy-induced Hypertension

Pregnancy-induced hypertension is divided into three categories: (1) hypertension alone, (2) preeclampsia, and (3) eclampsia (Table 36–1). **Preeclampsia** is diagnosed by development of hypertension plus proteinuria,

TABLE 36–1. CLASSIFICATION OF HYPERTENSIVE DISORDERS COMPLICATING PREGNANCY

Pregnancy-induced hypertension: Hypertension that develops as a consequence of pregnancy, and regresses postpartum
1. Hypertension without proteinuria or pathological edema[a]
2. Preeclampsia—with proteinuria and/or pathological edema
    a. Mild
    b. Severe
3. Eclampsia—proteinuria and/or pathological edema along with convulsions

Pregnancy-aggravated hypertension: Underlying hypertension worsened by pregnancy
1. Superimposed preeclampsia
2. Superimposed eclampsia

Coincidental hypertension: Chronic underlying hypertension that antecedes pregnancy or persists postpartum

[a] Corresponds to **transient hypertension,** defined as elevated blood pressure during pregnancy or in the first 24 hours postpartum without other signs of preeclampsia or coincidental hypertension.

or edema that is generalized and overt, or both. **Eclampsia** is diagnosed by convulsions precipitated by pregnancy-induced or aggravated hypertension. Only rarely does preeclampsia develop earlier than 20 weeks' gestation, and then usually in cases of hydatidiform mole or appreciable molar degeneration (see Chap. 35, p. 752). As emphasized by Chesley (1985), preeclampsia is almost exclusively a disease of nulliparous women. Although it more commonly affects teenagers or those older than 35, preeclampsia in the older woman is more likely pregnancy-aggravated hypertension. Pregnancy-induced hypertension is occasionally seen in the multipara with multifetal pregnancy or fetal hydrops. Pregnancy-aggravated hypertension is common in multiparas with vascular diseases, including chronic essential hypertension and diabetes mellitus, or those with coexisting renal disease.

Pregnancy-induced Hypertension. The diagnosis of pregnancy-induced hypertension is made when *blood pressure* is 140/90 mm Hg or greater. In the past, an increase of 30 mm Hg systolic or 15 mm Hg diastolic over baseline values on at least two occasions 6 or more hours apart was considered diagnostic for pregnancy-induced hypertension. In reality, these vague criteria have little practical clinical value. The real question is whether or not a change in systolic or diastolic blood pressure without an increase in blood pressure to at least 140/90 constitutes hypertension. According to Villar and colleagues (1989b), the answer is possibly. They reported that 30 percent of young nulliparas with a 15 mm Hg rise in diastolic pressure developed pregnancy-induced hypertension. For those without such a rise, the incidence was 15 percent. If the systolic pressure increased at least 30 mm Hg, more than 40 percent developed pregnancy-induced hypertension, compared with 17 percent in women without an increase. If both

systolic and diastolic pressures increased as defined, then more than 55 percent developed pregnancy-induced hypertension, compared with only 15 percent if there was no preceding increase.

Increases in systolic and diastolic blood pressure can either be normal physiological changes or signs of developing pathology. The separation of normal but profound pregnancy-induced physiological changes from those of disease is always difficult during prenatal care, but never more so than in this instance. The prudent physician can only increase surveillance and be aware of temporal changes in blood pressure and laboratory values, as well as the development of signs and symptoms discussed below.

Preeclampsia. The diagnosis of preeclampsia has traditionally required the identification of pregnancy-induced hypertension plus proteinuria *or* generalized edema. Today most authorities believe that edema, even of the hands and face, is such a common finding in pregnant women that its presence should not validate the diagnosis of preeclampsia any more than its absence should preclude the diagnosis (National High Blood Pressure Education Program, 1990; Redman and Jefferies, 1988). Indeed, Robertson (1971) reported that while one third of women developed generalized edema by 38 weeks, he was unable to show a significant correlation between edema and hypertension. Friedman and Neff (1976) identified perinatal mortality for women with edema alone to be 30 percent lower than for the general population. Edema of preeclampsia is pathological and not just dependent; it usually involves the face and hands and persists even after arising. A useful indicator of nondependent edema is a woman's complaint that her rings have become too tight.

Proteinuria is an important sign of preeclampsia and Chesley (1985) rightfully concluded that the diagnosis is questionable in its absence. Proteinuria is defined as 300 mg or more of urinary protein per 24 hours or 100 mg/dL or more in at least two random urine specimens collected 6 or more hours apart. The degree of proteinuria may fluctuate widely over any 24-hour period, even in severe cases. Therefore, a single random sample may fail to demonstrate significant proteinuria.

McCartney and co-workers (1971), in their extensive study of renal biopsy specimens obtained from hypertensive pregnant women, invariably found that proteinuria was present when the glomerular lesion considered to be characteristic of preeclampsia was evident. Importantly, both proteinuria and alterations of glomerular histology develop late in the course of pregnancy-induced hypertension. In fact, preeclampsia becomes evident clinically only near the end of an often protracted, covert pathophysiological process that may begin 3 to 4 months before hypertension develops.

The combination of proteinuria and hypertension during pregnancy markedly increases the risk of peri-

TABLE 36–2. FETAL DEATH RATE PER 100 BIRTHS ANALYZED ACCORDING TO DIASTOLIC PRESSURE AND PROTEINURIA

Diastolic Blood Pressure (mm Hg)	Proteinuria						
	None	Trace	1+	2+	3+	4+	Total
<65	15.5[a]	13.6	6.2	—	—	—	13.6
65–74	9.3	8.1	5.6	32.9[a]	41.5	—	8.8
75–84	6.2	7.4	6.2	19.2[a]	—	—	6.8
85–94	8.7	9.3	23.6[a]	—	22.3	—	10.2
95–104	19.2[a]	17.4[a]	26.7[a]	55.8[a]	115.3[a]	143[a]	25.2
105+	20.5[a]	27.9[a]	62.6[a]	68.8[a]	125.2[a]	111[a]	41.5[a]
Total	8.6	9.5	12.9	23.2[a]	42.0[a]	57[a]	

[a] $P < 0.01$.
Modified from Friedman and Neff (1976).

natal mortality and morbidity (Ferrazzani and associates, 1990; Friedman and Neff, 1976). In the 13-year prospective study reported by Friedman and Neff (1976), over 38,000 pregnancies with the following criteria were analyzed: (1) antepartum care before 28 weeks, (2) singleton fetus, (3) four or more antepartum visits, and (4) date of last menstrual period known. As shown in Table 36–2, hypertension alone, defined by diastolic blood pressure of 95 mm Hg or greater, was associated with a threefold increase in the fetal death rate. Worsening hypertension, especially if accompanied by proteinuria, was more ominous. Conversely, proteinuria without hypertension had little overall effect on the fetal death rate. Naeye and Friedman (1979) concluded that 70 percent of the excess fetal deaths in these same women were due to large placental infarcts, markedly small placental size, and abruptio placentae. They concluded that these microscopical placental lesions resulted from reduced uteroplacental perfusion.

When blood pressure rises appreciably during the latter half of pregnancy, it is dangerous, to the fetus especially, not to take action simply because proteinuria has not yet developed. As Chesley (1985) emphasized, 10 percent of eclamptic seizures develop before overt proteinuria. Thus, from pathophysiological and epidemiological perspectives, it is clear that hypertension is the *sine qua non* of preeclampsia; and when blood pressure begins to rise, both mother and fetus are at increased risk. Once blood pressure exceeds 140/90 mm Hg, pregnancy-induced hypertension is diagnosed and the woman treated accordingly. Proteinuria is a sign of worsening hypertensive disease, specifically preeclampsia; and when it is overt and persistent, maternal and fetal risks are increased even more.

Severity of Pregnancy-induced Hypertension. The severity of pregnancy-induced hypertension is assessed by the frequency and intensity of the abnormalities listed in Table 36–3. The more profound the frequency and intensity of these aberrations, the more likely is the need for pregnancy termination. **Importantly, the differentiation between mild and severe preeclampsia can-not be rigidly pursued, because apparently mild disease may progress rapidly to severe disease.**

Blood pressure alone is not always a dependable indicator of severity. For example, an adolescent woman may have 3+ proteinuria and convulsions while her blood pressure is 140/85 mm Hg, whereas most women with blood pressures as high as 180/120 mm Hg do not have seizures. Convulsions are usually preceded by an unrelenting severe headache or visual disturbances; thus, these symptoms are considered ominous.

Proteinuria is an important indicator of severity, because it usually develops late in the course of the disease. Certainly, persistent proteinuria of 2+ or more, or 24-hour urinary excretion of 4 g or more, is severe preeclampsia. With severe renal involvement, glomerular filtration may be impaired, and the plasma creatinine concentration may begin to rise.

Epigastric or right upper quadrant pain likely results from hepatocellular necrosis and edema that stretches Glisson's capsule. The characteristic pain is frequently accompanied by elevated serum liver enzymes, and usually it is a sign to terminate the pregnancy. Rarely, the pain presages liver rupture, or more correctly, catastrophic rupture of a hepatic subcapsular hematoma.

TABLE 36–3. PREGNANCY-INDUCED HYPERTENSION: INDICATIONS OF SEVERITY

Abnormality	Mild	Severe
Diastolic blood pressure	< 100 mg Hg	110 mm Hg or higher
Proteinuria	Trace to 1+	Persistent 2+ or more
Headache	Absent	Present
Visual disturbances	Absent	Present
Upper abdominal pain	Absent	Present
Oliguria	Absent	Present
Convulsions	Absent	Present (eclampsia)
Serum creatinine	Normal	Elevated
Thrombocytopenia	Absent	Present
Hyperbilirubinemia	Absent	Present
Liver enzyme elevation	Minimal	Marked
Fetal growth retardation	Absent	Obvious
Pulmonary edema	Absent	Present

Thrombocytopenia is characteristic of worsening preeclampsia, and probably is caused by microangiopathic hemolysis induced by severe vasospasm. Whatever the cause, evidence of gross hemolysis such as hemoglobinemia, hemoglobinuria, or hyperbilirubinemia is indicative of severe disease.

Other factors indicative of severe hypertension are most often associated with pregnancy-aggravated hypertension. These factors include cardiac dysfunction with pulmonary edema as well as fetal growth retardation.

Eclampsia. In neglected or, less often, fulminant cases of pregnancy-induced hypertension, eclampsia may develop. The seizures are grand mal and may appear before, during, or after labor. Any seizure that develops more than 48 hours postpartum is more likely the consequence of some other lesion in the central nervous system. Typical eclampsia, especially in primiparas, however, may be encountered up to 10 days postpartum (Brown and colleagues, 1987).

Diagnosis of Coincidental (Chronic) Hypertension

All *chronic hypertensive disorders,* regardless of their cause, predispose to development of superimposed preeclampsia or eclampsia. These disorders can create a difficult problem of diagnosis and management in women who are not seen until after midpregnancy. The diagnosis of coincidental or chronic underlying hypertension is suggested by the following: (1) hypertension (140/90 mm Hg or greater) antecedent to pregnancy, (2) hypertension (140/90 mm Hg or greater) detected before the 20th week of pregnancy (unless there is gestational trophoblastic disease), or (3) persistent hypertension long after delivery. Additional historical factors that help support the diagnosis are multiparity and hypertension complicating a previous pregnancy other than the first one.

The diagnosis of chronic hypertension may be difficult to make if the woman is not seen until the latter half of pregnancy, because blood pressure usually decreases during the second and early third trimesters in both normotensive and chronically hypertensive women. Thus, a woman with chronic vascular disease, who is seen for the first time at 20 weeks, will frequently have a normal blood pressure. During the third trimester, however, blood pressure returns to its former hypertensive level, presenting a diagnostic problem as to whether the hypertension is chronic or pregnancy induced.

There are many causes of hypertension that may be encountered during pregnancy (Table 36–4). Essential hypertension is the cause of underlying vascular disease in more than 90 percent of pregnant women. McCartney (1964) studied renal biopsies from women with "clinical preeclampsia," and found chronic glomerulo-

TABLE 36–4. UNDERLYING CHRONIC HYPERTENSIVE DISORDERS UPON WHICH PREECLAMPSIA MAY BE SUPERIMPOSED

Hypertensive Diseases
Essential familial hypertension
Renovascular hypertension
Coarctation of the aorta
Primary aldosteronism
Pheochromocytoma

Renal and Urinary Tract Disease
Glomerulonephritis (acute and chronic)
Nephrotic syndrome
Chronic renal insufficiency
Pyelonephritis
Lupus erythematosus
Scleroderma
Periarteritis nodosa
Acute renal failure
    Tubular necrosis
    Cortical necrosis
Polycystic kidney disease
Diabetic nephropathy

Modified from Sims (1970).

nephritis in 20 percent of nulliparas and in nearly 70 percent of multiparas. Fisher and co-workers (1969), however, did not confirm this high prevalence of chronic glomerulonephritis in their series.

Chronic hypertension causes morbidity whether or not a woman is pregnant. Specifically, chronic hypertension may lead to premature cardiovascular deterioration resulting in cardiac decompensation and/or cerebrovascular accidents. Intrinsic renal damage may also result from chronic hypertensive disease, but more commonly in young women, hypertension develops as a consequence of underlying renal parenchymal disease. Dangers specific to pregnancy complicated by chronic hypertension include the risk of pregnancy-aggravated hypertension, which may develop in as many as 20 percent of these women. Additionally, the risk of abruptio placentae is increased substantively. Moreover, the fetus of the woman with chronic hypertension is at increased risk for growth retardation and intrauterine death.

Pregnancy-aggravated Hypertension. Preexisting chronic hypertension worsens in some women, typically after 24 weeks' gestation. Such pregnancy-aggravated hypertension may be accompanied by proteinuria or pathological edema; the condition is then termed *superimposed preeclampsia.* Often, the onset of superimposed preeclampsia occurs earlier in pregnancy than pure preeclampsia, and it tends to be quite severe and accompanied in many cases by fetal growth retardation.

The diagnosis requires documentation of chronic underlying hypertension. Pregnancy-aggravated hypertension is characterized by at least a 15 mm Hg increase in diastolic or a 30 mm Hg rise in systolic blood pressure, and preeclampsia is accompanied by proteinuria, pathological edema, or both. Indicators of severity shown in Table 36–3 are also used to further characterize these disorders.

Incidence of Pregnancy-induced Hypertension

Pregnancy-induced hypertension more often affects nulliparous women. Older women, who accrue an increasing incidence of chronic hypertension with advancing age, are at greater risk of pregnancy-aggravated hypertension. Thus, women at either end of reproductive age have been considered in the past to be more susceptible (see Chap. 30, p. 653, 654). This traditional view was not supported by Guzick and associates (1987), who reported that younger-age women did not have a higher incidence of pregnancy-induced hypertension when parity was considered. Spellacy and associates (1986) reported that women over 40 had a threefold (10 versus 3 percent) increased incidence of hypertension compared with control women aged 20 to 30 years. Hansen (1986) reviewed several studies and reported a two- to threefold increase in the incidence of preeclampsia in nulliparas over 40 compared with those 25 to 29 years old (see Chap. 30, p. 654).

The incidence of preeclampsia is commonly cited to be about 5 percent, although remarkable variations are reported. The incidence is influenced by parity; it is related to racial—and thus to genetic—predisposition; and environmental factors may also have a role. About 13 percent of almost 50,000 women delivered at Parkland Hospital were diagnosed with pregnancy-induced or aggravated hypertension (Cunningham and Leveno, 1988). Almost 70 percent were nulliparous, but only half of these had proteinuria. The effects of parity were striking; nearly 20 percent of nulliparas had hypertension compared with an incidence of 7 percent in multiparas.

Racial and genetic factors are important because they contribute to the incidence of underlying chronic hypertension. Of over 5600 nulliparas delivered at Parkland Hospital, 18 percent of white women developed pregnancy-induced hypertension; this incidence was 20 percent in Hispanic and 22 percent in African-American women (Cunningham and Leveno, 1988). Only about half of these women had preeclampsia defined as proteinuric hypertension. The incidence of hypertension in multiparas was 6.2 percent in whites, 6.6 percent in Hispanics, and 8.5 percent in African-Americans, reflecting the increased incidence of underlying hypertension in African-Americans. Slightly more than half of these multiparous women with hypertension also had proteinuria and thus superimposed preeclampsia.

The tendency for preeclampsia–eclampsia is inherited. Chesley and Cooper (1986) studied the sisters, daughters, granddaughters, and daughters-in-law of eclamptic women delivered at the Margaret Hague Maternity Hospital from 1935 to 1984. They concluded that preeclampsia–eclampsia is highly heritable, and that the single-gene model, with a frequency of 0.25, best explained their observations. A multifactorial inheritance was also considered possible (see Chap. 40, p. 928). Kilpatrick and associates (1989) reported an association between human lymphocyte antigen (HLA) DR4 and proteinuric hypertension, but Hoff and colleagues (1990) and Hayward and co-workers (1992) observed no such association. Therefore, an appropriate genetic marker has not been identified.

Although Chesley (1974) disagrees, some have concluded that socioeconomically advantaged women have a lesser incidence of preeclampsia, even after racial factors are controlled. Regardless, when a socially affluent woman develops preeclampsia, it can be as severe and life-threatening as preeclampsia in a ghetto-dwelling teenager.

In general, eclampsia is preventable, and it has become less common in the United States, because most women now receive adequate prenatal care. For example, in the 17th edition of *Williams Obstetrics,* the incidence of eclampsia at Parkland Hospital was cited to be 1 in 700 deliveries for the past 25-year period. For the 4-year period 1983 to 1986, the incidence was 1 in 1150 deliveries, and for 1990 and 1991 the incidence was approximately 1 in 2300 deliveries. During this same time, there were proportionally more nulliparous women delivered in our hospital, and this should favor an increased rather than a decreased incidence of eclampsia.

Theories About the Cause of Pregnancy-induced Hypertension

Any satisfactory theory must account for the observation that pregnancy-induced or -aggravated hypertension is very much more likely to develop in the woman who (1) is exposed to chorionic villi for the first time; (2) is exposed to a superabundance of chorionic villi, as with twins or hydatidiform mole; (3) has preexisting vascular disease; or (4) is genetically predisposed to hypertension developing during pregnancy. Although chorionic villi are essential, they need not support a fetus or be located within the uterus.

The possibility that immunological as well as endocrine and genetic mechanisms are involved in the genesis of preeclampsia is intriguing. The risk of pregnancy-induced hypertension is appreciably enhanced in circumstances where formation of blocking antibodies to antigenic sites on the placenta *might* be impaired, such as during immunosuppressive therapy to protect a renal transplant; where effective immunization by a previous pregnancy is lacking, as in first pregnancies; or where the number of antigenic sites provided by the placenta is unusually great compared with the amount of antibody, as with multiple fetuses (Beer, 1978). Strickland and associates (1986), however, provided data that do not support "immunization" by a previous pregnancy. They analyzed the outcomes of over 29,000 pregnancies at Parkland Hospital and reported that pregnancy-induced hypertension was decreased only slightly (22 versus 25 percent) in women who previously had aborted and were now having their first baby. The immunization concept is supported, however, by the observation that preeclampsia develops more frequently in multiparous women impregnated by a new consort (Feeney and Scott, 1980) or by donor insemination (Need and colleagues, 1983). Cooper and associates (1988) and Jagadeesan (1988) found no association of complement fractions C3, C3^F, and CH50 with preeclampsia, and Hofmeyr and colleagues (1991) reported C4 concentrations to be reduced only in hypertensive pregnant women with proteinuria. Simon and co-workers (1988) reported no association of human lymphocyte antigens (HLA) A and B with preeclampsia. They did note, however, a higher incidence of recurrent hypertension in pregnancy in women with HLA DR4 phenotypes, an observation consistent with an increased incidence of chronic hypertension and not preeclampsia. Haeger and associates (1992) noted that complement, neutrophils, and macrophages are activated in women with severe preeclampsia. The role of these changes in the etiology or clinical course of preeclampsia has not been established. In summary, despite appealing theories that hypertension in pregnancy may be associated with an immunological disorder, convincing proof of clinical significance is lacking.

Chesley (1974) observed that everyone from allergist to zoologist has proposed a theory and suggested "rational therapy" based upon that theory. Such schemes have included mastectomy, oophorectomy, renal decapsulation, trephination, alignment of the woman with the earth's magnetic field, and a myriad of medical regimens. Everything from watermelon season to infestation with a worm (*Hydatoxi lualba*) has been claimed to be of importance. Chesley (1989)—tongue in cheek—even provided statistically sound evidence that the incidence of eclamptic deaths correlated with Baptist religion! The interested reader is urged to read the scholarly and entertaining review of various theories provided by Chesley (1978) in his elegant book, *Hypertensive Disorders in Pregnancy.*

Cooper and Liston (1979) examined the possibility that susceptibility to preeclampsia is dependent upon a single recessive gene. They calculated the expected first-pregnancy frequencies of daughters of women with eclampsia; daughters-in-law served as controls. The frequencies calculated by them and those actually observed by Chesley and co-workers (1968) in daughters and daughters-in-law of women with eclampsia are remarkably close in agreement. Subsequently, Chesley and Cooper (1986) concluded that the single-gene hypo-

thesis fits well, but multifactorial inheritance cannot be excluded.

Dietary deficiencies have been suspected as a cause of preeclampsia; however, this hypothesis lacks supportive data. For example, because pregnancy "depletes" a woman nutritionally, preeclampsia should be more common in multiparous women compared to nulliparas, but it is not. Moreover, various types of dietary supplementation do not decrease the frequency of hypertension (see Chap. 9, p. 258). Zlatnik and Burmeister (1983) provided convincing evidence that the incidence of preeclampsia is *not* related to the level of dietary protein. Calcium deficiency has been implicated by some (Belizán and colleagues, 1988; Marcoux and associates, 1991; Repke and Villar, 1991). Belizán and co-workers (1991) and López-Jaramillo and associates (1989) reported that after midpregnancy, dietary supplementation with 2 g of elemental calcium per day significantly reduced the incidence of hypertension. Certainly, a decreased urinary excretion of calcium has been documented in preeclamptic and future hypertensive women (August, 1992; Sanchez-Ramos, 1991; Taufield, 1987; and their co-workers). What remains to be established is whether there is a decreased dietary intake or altered calcium absorption (August and co-workers, 1992), or intrinsic renal tubular dysfunction (Frenkel and associates, 1991).

The apparent effectiveness of supplemental calcium may be explained by an overriding of impaired absorption or defective renal handling of calcium. Other possibilities exist, however, including changes in vasodilation and vascular reactivity mediated by increased prostacyclin or nitric oxide production (Gant and Gilstrap, 1990; López-Jaramillo and colleagues, 1990; St-Louis and Sicotte, 1992).

Endothelins are potent vasoconstrictors, and it is possible that they play a role in the etiology or response to pregnancy-induced hypertension. Three endothelins have been identified. *Endothelin-1* is the only endothelin produced by human endothelium. Endothelin-2 is of renal origin, and endothelin-3 is produced in neural tissue (Mastrogiannis and co-workers, 1991). Plasma endothelin-1 has been reported to be increased in normotensive laboring and nonlaboring women, and even higher levels have been reported in preeclamptic women (Clark, 1992; Mastrogiannis, 1991; Nova, 1991; Schiff, 1992; and their associates). Otani and colleagues (1991), however, did not observe increased plasma endothelin levels, and Barton and associates (in press) did not find increased urinary endothelin-1 levels in preeclamptic women.

Endothelium-derived relaxing factor (EDRF) appears to be identical in action to nitric oxide (Palmer and colleagues, 1987). It is synthesized by endothelial cells from L-arginine (Palmer and associates, 1988). The compound is a potent vasodilator whose absence or decreased concentration might also play a role in the etiology of pregnancy-induced hypertension. Inhibition of endothelium-derived relaxing factor has been shown to increase mean arterial pressure, decrease heart rate, and reverse the pregnancy-induced refractoriness to vasopressors in pregnant rats (Molnár and Hertelendy, 1992). Equally important, it appears to maintain the normal low-pressure vasodilated state characteristic of fetoplacental perfusion in the sheep, guinea pig, and human (Chang and colleagues, 1992; Myatt and co-workers, 1992; Weiner and associates, 1992).

Currently, endothelin-1 and endothelium-derived relaxing factor are being studied actively in both normal and hypertensive pregnancies. As yet, their exact roles in the etiology of pregnancy-induced hypertension, if any, remain to be established; however, the very nature of their production, their sites of action, and their apparent opposite effects are suggestive that if not etiological factors, they may still have important potential as therapeutic agents.

Wang and colleagues (1991a, 1991b) reported that normotensive pregnancies are characterized by progressive increases in the ratios of prostacyclin/thromboxane and vitamin E/lipid peroxides. They concluded that the vasodilating actions of prostacyclin and the antioxidant activity of vitamin E were favored progressively with advancing gestation. With increasing severity of preeclampsia, both ratios were progressively reversed. Thus, increased thromboxane resulted in increased vasospasm and platelet destruction, and increased lipid peroxides increased endothelial damage. Davidge and associates (1992), using a different assay, noted similar findings in antioxidant activity in preeclamptic women.

Wisdom and associates (1991) reported that free radical formation is increased in both normotensive women and women with pregnancy-induced hypertension. In normotensive women, red blood cell *lysate thiol levels* were elevated in a protective manner to clear free radicals. In contrast, these levels were not increased in hypertensive women. The authors did not know if these changes preceded the onset of hypertension.

Carefully controlled epidemiological studies of pregnancy have been conducted in Aberdeen, Scotland, where Baird (1969) found that the incidence of preeclampsia did not differ significantly among the five social classes. These classes range from the professional and well-to-do (class I) through unskilled laborers (class V). There was, however, a slightly increased incidence of hypertension in class III (skilled manual occupations).

PATHOPHYSIOLOGY OF PREECLAMPSIA–ECLAMPSIA

Vasospasm

Vasospasm is basic to the pathophysiology of preeclampsia–eclampsia. This concept, first advanced by

Volhard (1918), is based upon direct observations of small blood vessels in the nail beds, ocular fundi, and bulbar conjunctivae, and it has been surmised from histological changes seen in various affected organs (Hinselmann, 1924; Landesman and co-workers, 1954). Vascular constriction causes resistance to blood flow and accounts for the development of arterial hypertension. It is likely that vasospasm itself also exerts a damaging effect on vessels. Alternating segmental arteriolar dilatation and spasm probably contribute further to the development of vascular damage, because endothelial integrity may be compromised by the stretched dilated segments. Moreover, angiotensin II appears to have a direct action on endothelial cells, causing them to contract. These changes likely lead to interendothelial cell leaks through which blood constituents, including platelets and fibrinogen, are deposited subendothelially (Brunner and Gavras, 1975). The vascular changes, together with local hypoxia of the surrounding tissues, presumably lead to hemorrhage, necrosis, and other end-organ disturbances that have been observed at times with severe preeclampsia. With this scheme, fibrin deposition is then likely to be prominent, as seen in fatal cases (McKay, 1965).

Increased Pressor Responses. Normally pregnant women develop refractoriness to the pressor effects of infused angiotensin II (Abdul-Karim and Assali, 1961). Increased vascular reactivity to this and other pressor hormones in women with early preeclampsia has been identified by Raab and co-workers (1956) and Talledo and associates (1968) using either norepinephrine or angiotensin II, and by Dieckmann and Michel (1937) and Browne (1946) using vasopressin. Gant and co-workers (1973) demonstrated that increased vascular sensitivity to angiotensin II clearly preceded the onset of pregnancy-induced hypertension. As shown in Figure 36–1, normal nulliparas who remained normotensive were refractory to the pressor effect of infused angiotensin II, while women who subsequently became hypertensive lost this refractoriness weeks before the onset of hypertension. Of women who required more than 8 ng/kg per minute of angiotensin II to provoke a standardized pressor response, between 28 and 32 weeks, 90 percent remained normotensive throughout pregnancy. Conversely, among normotensive primigravidas who required less than 8 ng/kg per minute at 28 to 32 weeks, 90 percent subsequently developed overt hypertension. Similar results from 231 women were subsequently reported from Germany by Öney and Kaulhausen (1982).

A pressor response induced by having the woman assume the supine position after lying laterally recumbent was demonstrated in some pregnant women by Gant and co-workers (1974b). The majority of nulliparous women at 28 to 32 weeks who

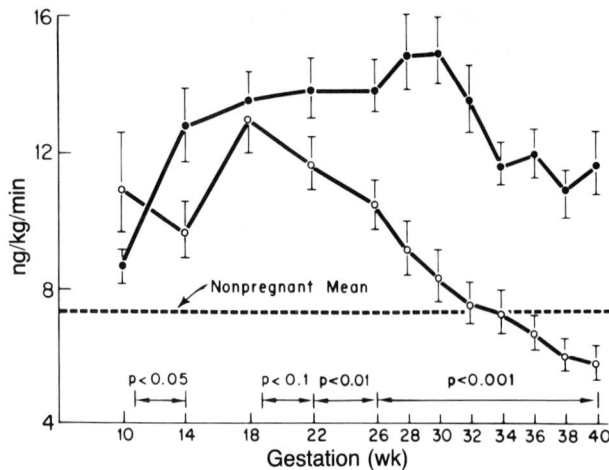

Fig. 36–1. Comparison of the mean angiotensin II infusion doses required to evoke a pressor response in 120 nulliparous women who remained normotensive (solid circles) and 72 who subsequently developed pregnancy-induced hypertension (open circles). (From Gant and co-workers, 1973.)

had increased diastolic pressure of at least 20 mm Hg when the maneuver was performed later developed pregnancy-induced hypertension. Conversely, most women whose blood pressure did not become elevated when this was done did not become hypertensive. Although not all investigators have reported equally good predictive results (Dekker and Sibai, 1991), this so-called "roll-over test" remains an effective screening test to identify asymptomatic women who will likely develop pregnancy-induced hypertension (O'Brien, 1990). As perhaps expected, those women who demonstrated a *supine pressor response* were also abnormally sensitive to infused angiotensin II, while those without a hypertensive response were normally refractory. The mechanism by which assuming the supine position incites a rise in blood pressure is not clear, but it is likely to be a manifestation of increased vascular responsivity of those who will later develop pregnancy-induced hypertension.

Women with underlying chronic hypertension have similar responses. An identically performed study of angiotensin II pressor responsiveness was conducted in women whose pregnancies were complicated by chronic hypertension (Gant and colleagues, 1977). Two groups were identified on the basis of clinical outcome and serial determinations of vascular reactivity to infused angiotensin II. All women were refractory to angiotensin II between 21 and 25 weeks; however, women who subsequently developed pregnancy-aggravated hypertension began to lose this refractoriness after 27 weeks.

It appears unlikely that the normally blunted pressor response to angiotensin II is due to down-regulation or decreased affinity of angiotensin II vascular smooth-muscle receptors (MacKanjee and associates, 1991).

Other factors may be operative, however, in mediating vascular refractoriness to angiotensin II. For example, aldosterone secretion is increased strikingly in pregnant women (Chap. 8, p. 238), and this is modulated by the effects of angiotensin II on the zona glomerulosa of the adrenal cortex. Based on the findings of a number of studies, it was concluded that the blunted pressor response was due principally to decreased vascular responsiveness mediated in part by vascular endothelial synthesis of prostaglandins or prostaglandin-like substances (Cunningham and associates, 1975; Gant and co-workers, 1974a). For example, refractoriness to angiotensin II in pregnant women is abolished by large doses of the prostaglandin inhibitors, indomethacin and aspirin (Everett and colleagues, 1978a). In some tissues, angiotensin II action is mediated by promoting accelerated synthesis, prostaglandin release, or both. It is interesting to speculate that pregnancy normally causes an increased capacity for endothelial prostaglandin synthesis with relatively greater synthesis of vasodilator than of vasoconstricting prostaglandins.

The exact mechanism by which prostaglandin(s) or related substances mediate vascular reactivity during pregnancy is unknown, but some findings have possibly elucidated mechanisms involved. Goodman and colleagues (1982) reported increased concentrations of vasodilating prostaglandins during normal pregnancy. Everett and colleagues (1978a) demonstrated that large doses of indomethacin and aspirin increased vascular sensitivity to infused angiotensin II, and they postulated that prostaglandin(s) synthesis was suppressed, returning the vascular system to a nonpregnant sensitive state. Sanchez-Ramos and colleagues (1987) documented a diminished vascular response within 2 hours of ingestion of 40 mg of aspirin likely due to a preferential suppression of the vasoconstrictor thromboxane.

Walsh (1985) showed that compared with normal pregnancy, placental production of prostacyclin is decreased significantly and thromboxane A_2 significantly increased in preeclampsia. Walsh (1988) reported subsequently that placental progesterone production is increased in vitro in placentas of preeclamptic pregnancies, and hypothesized that increased progesterone concentrations may inhibit prostacyclin production. Spitz and colleagues (1988) reported that 81 mg of aspirin given daily to future hypertensive women restored angiotensin II refractoriness by suppressing synthesis of thromboxane A_2 by about 75 percent; however, prostacyclin synthesis also was decreased by 20 percent and prostaglandin E_2 by 30 percent. Thus, arachidonic acid, an essential fatty acid, is converted by cyclooxygenase into prostacyclin, prostaglandin E_2, and thromboxane. In preeclamptic women, thromboxane is increased and prostacyclin and prostaglandin E_2 are decreased, resulting in vasoconstriction and sensitivity to infused angiotensin II.

Low-dose aspirin therapy markedly decreases

thromboxane production but only partially blocks prostacyclin and prostaglandin E_2 production, allowing these two vasodilating prostanoids to restore refractoriness to infused angiotensin II (Fig. 36–2). Brown and associates (1990) reported similar findings in angiotensin II-sensitive women rendered refractory to angiotensin II by low-dose aspirin; however, in women remaining sensitive despite aspirin, all three prostaglandins were reduced significantly by low-dose aspirin. These observations indicate that vessel reactivity may be mediated through a delicate balance of production and metabolism of at least these three vasoactive prostaglandins. In this scheme, preeclampsia may follow inappropriately increased production or destruction of one prostaglandin, diminished synthesis or release of the other, or perhaps both. Beaufils (1985), Wallenburg (1986), Hauth (in press), and their colleagues reported that chronic low-dose aspirin ingestion significantly decreased the incidence of proteinuric hypertension (preeclampsia). Sibai and colleagues (1993a, 1993b) could not confirm this observation. They did note, however, an increased incidence of placental abruption in women who received low-dose aspirin prophylaxis.

It appears that at least two vasoconstrictor mechanisms may be operative in women with pregnancy-induced hypertension. Specifically, in preeclampsia, arachidonic acid is converted via the cyclooxygenase pathway into thromboxane A_2 with an accompanying reduction of prostacyclin and prostaglandin E_2 (Catella and associates, 1990; Fitzgerald and colleagues, 1990; Mitchell and Koenig, 1991; Tannirandorn and co-workers, 1991). This pathway is responsive to low-dose aspirin therapy. The second route of arachidonic acid metabolism is via the lipoxygenase pathway, which results in an increased placental production of 15-hydroxyeicosatetraenioc acid (15-HETE); this inhibits prostacyclin production, resulting in further vasoconstriction (Mitchell and Koenig, 1991). Biagi and co-workers (1990) also reported an increased lipoxygenase pathway activation in placentas from hypertensive women.

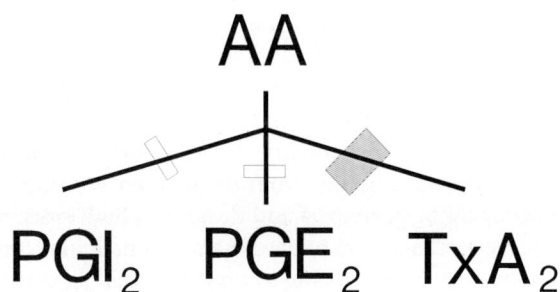

Fig. 36–2. Arachidonic acid (AA) may be converted into prostacyclin (PGI_2), prostaglandin E_2 (PGE_2), and thromboxane A_2 (TxA_2). Low-dose aspirin therapy usually blocks thromboxane A_2 production more than production of prostacyclin and prostaglandin E_2.

Maternal and Fetal Consequences of Preeclampsia–Eclampsia

Deterioration of function in a number of organs and systems, presumably as a consequence of vasospasm, has been identified in severe preeclampsia and eclampsia. For descriptive purposes, these effects are separated into maternal and fetal consequences; however, these aberrations often occur simultaneously.

Although there are many possible maternal consequences of pregnancy-induced hypertension, for simplicity these effects are considered by analysis of cardiovascular, hematological, endocrine and metabolic, and regional blood flow changes with subsequent end-organ derangements. The major cause of fetal compromise occurs as a consequence of reduced uteroplacental perfusion.

Cardiovascular Changes

Hemodynamic changes accompanying severe preeclampsia and eclampsia have been studied by a number of investigators. Key issues addressed include the cardiovascular status of these women before treatment, as well as volume expansion and pharmacological attempts to relieve vasospasm. Elucidation of the mechanisms that cause heart failure and pulmonary edema complicating the course of some women has also been pursued.

Clinical Assessment of Cardiac Function. In assessing cardiac function, four areas must be addressed: (1) preload—end-diastolic pressure and chamber volume, (2) afterload—intramyocardial systolic tension or resistance to ejection, (3) contractile or inotropic state of the myocardium, and (4) heart rate. These interactions are discussed in Chapter 47 (p. 1067).

Hemodynamic Changes. Hemodynamic values obtained in women with preeclampsia using invasive cardiovascular monitoring are listed in Table 36–5. The differences listed in this table in reported values for variables that define cardiovascular status range from high cardiac output with low vascular resistance to low cardiac output with high vascular resistance. Similarly, left ventricular filling pressures, estimated by pulmonary capillary wedge pressure determination, range from low to pathologically high. At least three factors may explain these differences: (1) women with preeclampsia might present with a spectrum of cardiovascular findings dependent upon both severity and duration, (2) chronic underlying disease may modify the clinical presentation, or (3) therapeutic interventions may significantly alter these findings. It is likely that in many of these women, more than one of these is operative.

The studies listed in Table 36–5 were separated into three groups, based upon clinical management

TABLE 36–5. SEVERE PREECLAMPSIA AND ECLAMPSIA: ASSOCIATED HEMODYNAMIC MEASUREMENTS

Therapy[a]	No.	Cardiac Output (L/min)	Pulmonary Capillary Wedge Pressure (mm Hg)	Left Ventricular Stroke Work Index (g/m/m^{-2})	Systemic Vascular Resistance (dyne/sec/cm^{-5})
No Therapy					
Cotton and associates (1984)	5	7.56	12.0	83	2256
Groenendijk and co-workers (1984)	10	4.66	3.3	44	1943
Magnesium, Hydralazine, and Fluid Restriction					
Benedetti and colleagues (1980a)	10	7.4	6.0	82	1322
Hankins and associates (1984)	8	6.7	3.9	66	1357
Magnesium, Hydralazine, and Volume Expansion					
Rafferty and Berkowitz (1980)	3	11.0	7.0	89	780
Phelan and Yurth (1982)	10	9.3	16.0	89	1042

[a] Values are those reported soon after pulmonary artery catheterization was performed, and are the means for each study.

prior to initial hemodynamic observations: (1) no therapy for preeclampsia, (2) magnesium sulfate and hydralazine without large volumes of intravenous fluid, and (3) magnesium sulfate and hydralazine plus intravenous volume loading. Ventricular function from the six studies listed in Table 36–5 is plotted in Figure 36–3. Cardiac function was hyperdynamic in all women, but filling pressures varied markedly.

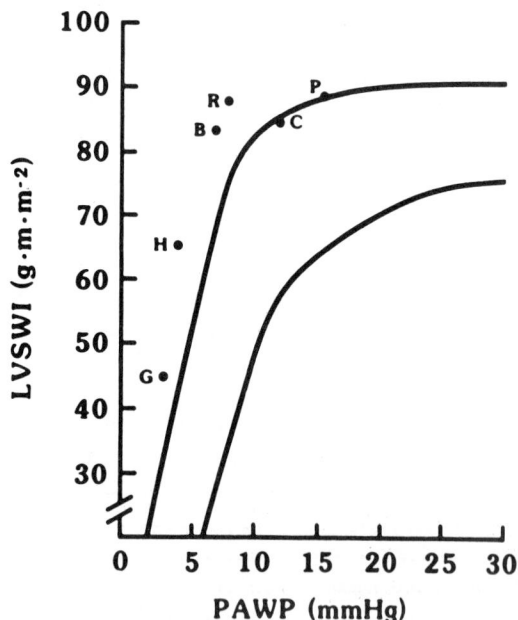

Fig. 36–3. Ventricular function in severe preeclampsia-eclampsia. Data plotted represent mean values obtained in each of 6 studies cited in Table 36–5. Left ventricular stroke work index (LVSWI) and pulmonary artery wedge pressure (PAWP) are plotted on a standard ventricular function curve. Points falling within the two solid lines represent normal function, while those below represent depressed function. Points above the solid lines represent hyperdynamic ventricular function. Each letter adjacent to the data points is the first initial of the last name of the investigator who reported this value.

Hemodynamic data obtained prior to active treatment of preeclampsia (Table 36–5) identified normal left ventricular filling pressures, high systemic vascular resistances, and hyperdynamic ventricular function. Benedetti (1980a), Hankins (1984), and their associates reported similar findings in women with severe preeclampsia or eclampsia who were being treated with magnesium sulfate, hydralazine, and intravenous crystalloid given at 75 to 100 mL/hour. Cardiac function in these women was appropriate, and the lower systemic vascular resistance was most likely secondary to hydralazine treatment.

Women similarly treated with magnesium sulfate and hydralazine plus aggressive intravenous therapy or volume expansion had the lowest systemic vascular resistances and highest cardiac outputs. A comparison of volume-restricted women with those hydrated aggressively shows hyperdynamic ventricular function in both groups, and two responses with respect to left ventricular stroke work index and pulmonary capillary wedge pressure (Fig. 36–4). Fluid restriction resulted in wedge pressures of less than 10 mm Hg, and most were less than 5 mm Hg. Thus, hyperdynamic ventricular function was largely a result of low wedge pressures and not a result of augmented left ventricular stroke work index, which more directly measures myocardial contractility. By comparison, women given appreciably larger volumes of fluid commonly had pulmonary capillary wedge pressures that exceeded normal; however, ventricular function remained hyperdynamic because of increased cardiac output. Subsequently, Cotton and co-workers (1988) reported findings from 45 women with severe preeclampsia or eclampsia and described high systemic vascular resistance and hyperdynamic ventricular function in most. It is reasonable to conclude that aggressive fluid administration given to women with severe preeclampsia causes normal left-sided filling pressures to become substantively elevated, while increasing an already normal cardiac output to supranormal levels.

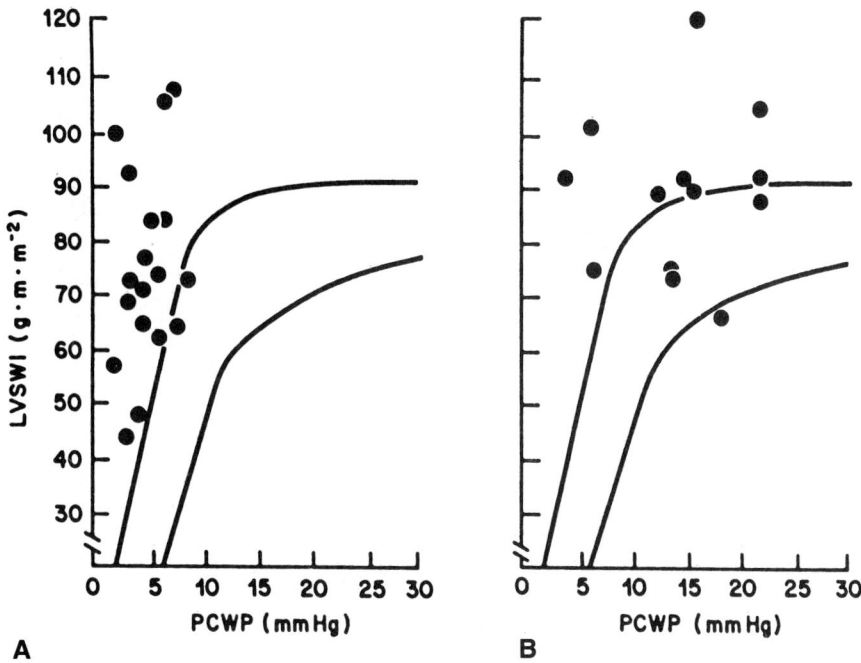

Fig. 36–4. Ventricular function in women with severe preeclampsia–eclampsia. Left ventricular stroke work index (LVSWI) and pulmonary capillary wedge pressure (PCWP) are plotted. **A.** Restricted intravenous fluids (Benedetti and colleagues, 1980a; Hankins and co-workers, 1984). **B.** Aggressive fluid therapy (Rafferty and Berkowitz, 1980; Phelan and Yurth, 1982). (From Hankins and colleagues, 1984.)

Easterling and colleagues (1990) provided evidence that preeclampsia is caused by high cardiac output. In their prospective longitudinal study of 179 nulliparas, they found that women who subsequently developed preeclampsia had elevated cardiac outputs throughout pregnancy. They challenged the concept of hypoperfusion as the hallmark of pathophysiology in preeclampsia. These intriguing results need to be corroborated.

Summary of Hemodynamic Changes. Five general observations can be made. (1) Myocardial contractility is rarely impaired prior to therapy, and ventricular function is usually within the normal to hyperdynamic range. (2) Afterload is elevated in the absence of therapeutic interventions. (3) Cardiac output predictably varies inversely with vascular resistance, and as blood pressure and afterload increase, cardiac output falls. (4) Medications that reduce peripheral vascular resistance, such as hydralazine, increase cardiac output. (5) Ventricular preload is usually normal or even low in severe preeclampsia in the absence of volume expansion.

Blood Volume. Hemoconcentration in women with eclampsia was emphasized by Dieckmann (1952) in *The Toxemias of Pregnancy*, and Pritchard and co-workers (1984) reported that in eclamptic women hypervolemia is usually absent (Table 36–6). Women of average size should have a blood volume of nearly 5000 mL during the last several weeks of a normal pregnancy, compared with about 3500 mL when nonpregnant. With eclampsia, however, much or all of the anticipated 1500 mL of blood normally present late in pregnancy is missing.

The virtual absence of an expanded blood volume is likely the consequence of generalized vasoconstriction, often made worse by increased vascular permeability. Either one or both mechanisms would account for the classical features, when compared with normal pregnancy, of too little fluid intravascularly and too much extravascularly.

Dieckmann (1952) believed that clinical improvement was characterized by hemodilution, as reflected by a fall in hematocrit. An acute fall in hematocrit is more likely the consequence of blood loss at delivery in the absence of normal pregnancy hypervolemia; or occasionally it is the result of intense erythrocyte destruction, as described below.

In the absence of hemorrhage, the intravascular compartment in eclamptic women usually is not underfilled. Vasospasm has contracted the space to be filled; the reduction persists until after delivery, when the vascular system typically dilates, blood volume increases, and hematocrit falls. **The woman with eclampsia, therefore, is unduly sensitive to vigorous fluid therapy**

TABLE 36–6. BLOOD VOLUMES IN 5 WOMEN MEASURED WITH ⁵¹CR-TAGGED ERYTHROCYTES DURING ANTEPARTUM ECLAMPSIA, AGAIN WHEN NONPREGNANT, AND AT A COMPARABLE TIME IN A SECOND NORMOTENSIVE PREGNANCY

	Eclampsia	Nonpregnant	Normal Pregnant
Blood volume (mL)	3530	3035	4425
Change (%)	+16		+47
Hematocrit	40.5	38.2	34.7

From Pritchard and colleagues (1984).

administered in an attempt to expand the contracted blood volume to normal pregnancy levels. She is sensitive as well to even normal blood loss at delivery. Management of blood loss in these circumstances is considered in Chapter 37 (p. 821).

Hematological Changes

The following hematological abnormalities may develop in some, but certainly not all, women who develop pregnancy-induced or pregnancy-aggravated hypertension: (1) thrombocytopenia may develop, and at times may become so severe as to be life threatening; (2) the level of some plasma clotting factors may be decreased; and (3) erythrocytes may be so traumatized that they display bizarre shapes and undergo rapid hemolysis.

Coagulation. Hematological changes consistent with intravascular coagulation, and less often erythrocyte destruction, may complicate preeclampsia and especially eclampsia (Pritchard and colleagues, 1954a, 1954b; Stahnke, 1922). Renewed interest in these changes has led to the concept by some investigators that disseminated intravascular coagulation is not only a characteristic feature of preeclampsia, but that it also plays a dominant role in its pathogenesis.

Since the early reports by Pritchard and coworkers (1954a, 1954b), we have found little evidence of an eclamptic coagulopathy. The results of some of these studies are presented in Table 36–7. Thrombocytopenia, infrequently severe, was the most common finding. Serum fibrin degradation products were elevated only occasionally, and unless some degree of placental abruption developed, plasma fibrinogen did not differ remarkably from levels found late in normal pregnancy. Similar results have been reported by Leduc and associates (1992). The *thrombin time* was somewhat prolonged in one third of the cases of eclampsia even when elevated levels of fibrin degradation products were not identified (Pritchard and colleagues, 1976). The reason for this elevation is not known, but it has been attributed to hepatic derangements discussed subsequently. The coagulation changes just described are also identified in women with severe preeclampsia, but certainly are no more common. These observations in eclampsia, as well as those reported by Kitzmiller and associates (1974) for preeclampsia, are most consistent with the concept that coagulation changes are the consequence of preeclampsia–eclampsia, rather than the cause.

Thrombocytopenia. Maternal thrombocytopenia can be induced acutely by preeclampsia–eclampsia; but after delivery, the platelet count will increase progressively to reach a normal level within a few days (Katz

TABLE 36–7. CHANGES IN COAGULATION FACTORS THAT IMPLY DISSEMINATED INTRAVASCULAR COAGULATION

	Intrapartum Primigravidas Normally Pregnant	Most Abnormal Value for Each Case of Eclampsia
Platelets[a] (per µL)		
Mean	278,000	206,000
−2 standard deviations	150,000	—
<150,000	0/20	24/91
<100,000	0/20	14/91
<50,000	0/20	3/91
Fibrin Degradation Products[b]		
8 µg/mL or less	17/20	51/59
16 µg/mL	3/20	6/59
>16 µg/mL	0/20	2/59
Plasma Fibrinogen[a]		
Mean (mg/dL)	415	413
−2 standard deviations	285	—
<285 mg/dL	0/20	7/89
Fibrin Monomer		
Positive	1/20	1/14

[a] Lowest value identified for each case of eclampsia.
[b] Highest value identified for each case of eclampsia.
From Pritchard and associates (1976).

and associates, 1990; Romero and colleagues, 1989). The frequency and intensity of maternal thrombocytopenia vary in different studies, apparently dependent upon the intensity of the disease process, the length of delay between the onset of preeclampsia–eclampsia and delivery, and the frequency with which platelet counts are performed (Leduc and associates, 1992).

Overt thrombocytopenia is a platelet count less than 100,000/µL. This is an ominous sign in women with preeclampsia, and delivery is usually indicated. Otherwise, the platelet count most often continues to decrease and may reach levels that can result in excessive blood loss during and after delivery, especially with cesarean delivery. The risk of maternal intracranial hemorrhage is also appreciably increased by severe thrombocytopenia.

The cause of the thrombocytopenia is not known. Immunological processes or simply platelet deposition at sites of endothelial damage may be the cause (Pritchard and colleagues, 1976). Samuels and colleagues (1987) performed direct and indirect antiglobulin tests and found that platelet-bound and circulating platelet-bindable immunoglobulin were increased in preeclamptic women and their neonates. They interpreted these findings to suggest platelet surface alterations. Burrows and colleagues (1987) reported that platelets from preeclamptic women were more likely to have platelet-associated IgG, even if thrombocytopenia did not develop (Fig. 36–5). Although they believed this

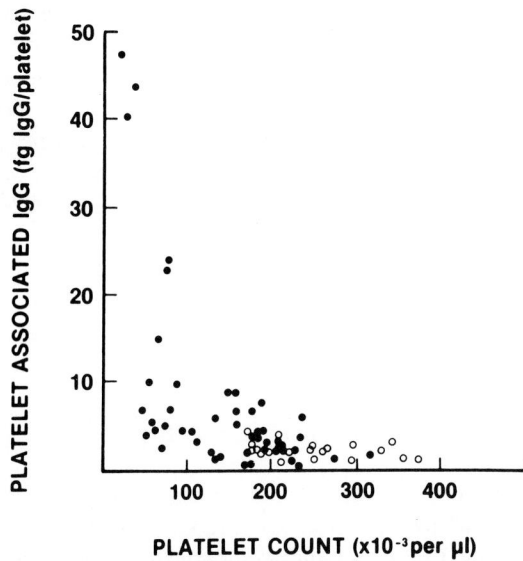

Fig. 36–5. The relationship of platelet-associated IgG to the platelet count in preeclamptic and in control women. The level of platelet-associated IgG is shown along the ordinate, and the platelet count along the abscissa. Women with preeclampsia are shown by solid dots and normally pregnant women by circles. (From Burrows and colleagues, 1987.)

ation in selecting the mode of delivery. They found no correlation between the maternal platelet count at delivery and the fetal platelet count. Weinstein (1985) later reported initial platelet counts to have been less than 150,000 per μL in 11 of the 46 infants whose mothers were thrombocytopenic as the consequence of preeclampsia–eclampsia. The exact times that the thrombocytopenia was identified after delivery were not stated, nor was the intensity of the thrombocytopenia described. Pritchard and colleagues (1987), however, did *not* observe severe thrombocytopenia in the fetus or infant at or very soon after delivery. In fact, no cases of fetal or neonatal thrombocytopenia were identified, despite severe maternal thrombocytopenia (Fig. 36–6). Thrombocytopenia did develop later in some of these infants after hypoxia, acidosis, and sepsis developed. Although overt thrombocytopenia has not been described, a general downward trend in platelet counts has been noted in cord blood from fetuses with abnormal Doppler umbilical flow waveforms (Wilcox and associates, 1989). These decreased platelet counts were observed in infants from both normotensive and hypertensive women with normal platelet counts.

mechanism implied an autoimmune process, they acknowledged that IgG could also be bound to platelets damaged by any mechanism.

These same investigators amplified their previous work (Kelton and colleagues, 1985) and again showed that thrombocytopenia with preeclampsia was frequently associated with a prolonged bleeding time. Moreover, they identified this even with normal platelet levels. They attributed this to impaired thromboxane synthesis.

Kilby and associates (1990) and Barr and colleagues (1989) found increased intracellular free calcium concentrations in platelets from preeclamptic women. Kilby and associates (1990) and Louden and colleagues (1991) interpret this and other evidence to mean that platelets from preeclamptic women are exhausted, that is, platelet aggregation and release are decreased.

The clinical significance of thrombocytopenia, in addition to the obvious impairment in coagulation, is that it reflects the severity of the pathological process. In general, the lower the platelet count, the greater are maternal and fetal morbidity and mortality (Leduc and co-workers, 1992; Verhaeghe and colleagues, 1991). The addition of elevated liver enzymes to this clinical picture is even more ominous (see p. 765, 780).

Neonatal Thrombocytopenia. Thiagarajah and co-workers (1984) reported severe thrombocytopenia in 2 of 10 neonates whose mothers had preeclampsia, and emphasized that these findings should be a consider-

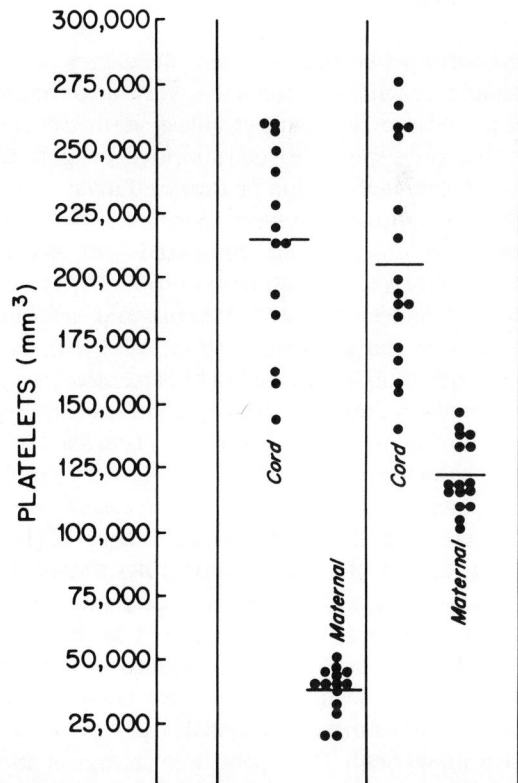

Fig. 36–6. Umbilical cord platelet counts in newborns of 14 eclamptic or severely preeclamptic mothers with platelet counts less than 50,000 per μL (mm³) are compared with those from 16 eclamptic or severely preeclamptic mothers with platelet counts of 100,000 to 150,000 per μL. The severity of the maternal thrombocytopenia had no demonstrable impact on the 31 cord platelet counts. (From Pritchard and associates, 1987.)

Hence, maternal thrombocytopenia in hypertensive women is not a fetal indication for cesarean delivery.

Fragmentation Hemolysis. Thrombocytopenia that accompanies severe preeclampsia and eclampsia may be accompanied by evidence of erythrocyte destruction characterized by hemolysis, schizocytosis, spherocytosis, reticulocytosis, hemoglobinuria, and occasionally hemoglobinemia (Pritchard and colleagues 1954a, 1954b, 1976). These derangements result in part from microangiopathic hemolysis, and human and animal studies are suggestive that intense vasospasm causes endothelial disruption, with platelet adherence and fibrin deposition. Cunningham and associates (1985) described these erythrocyte morphological characteristics using scanning electron microscopy. Women with eclampsia, and to a lesser degree those with severe preeclampsia, demonstrated schizocytosis and echinocytosis but not spherocytosis when compared with normally pregnant women. Miller and Keith (1988) reported similar observations in hypertensive pregnant sheep. It is likely that in preeclamptic women, plasma–erythrocyte membrane lipid changes are magnified by decreased serum albumin concentrations, and these changes intensify even more fragmentation hemolysis.

Other Clotting Factors. A severe deficiency of any of the soluble coagulation factors is very uncommon in severe preeclampsia–eclampsia unless another event coexists that predisposes to consumptive coagulopathy, such as placental abruption or ruptured liver.

Antithrombin III has been reported to be lower in women with preeclampsia compared with normally pregnant women and those with chronic hypertension (Saleh and associates, 1987; Weenik and colleagues, 1983; Weiner and associates, 1982, 1985). In fact, a normal antithrombin III value in a hypertensive pregnant woman might be used to identify a chronically hypertensive woman from one with preeclampsia (Leiberman and associates, 1988). *Fibronectin,* a glycoprotein associated with vascular endothelial cell basement membrane, is elevated in women with preeclampsia (Brubaker, 1992; Saleh, 1987, 1988; Stubbs, 1984; Taylor, 1991; and their associates). Moreover, Ballegeer and associates (1992), as well as others, have noted an increase in fibronectin and *laminin* 4 weeks prior to appearance of hypertension. These observations are consistent with other descriptions that preeclampsia causes vascular endothelial injury with subsequent hematological aberrations. The clinical utility of serial antithrombin III or fibronectin measurements for the prediction, diagnosis, and management of preeclampsia awaits further evaluation.

Thrombin levels are elevated in normal and preeclamptic women. This is likely due to an enhanced inactivation of *protein C* by α_1-antitrypsin, which is

increased in preeclampsia but not chronic hypertension (De Boer and co-workers, 1989; España and associates, 1991; Gilabert and colleagues, 1988). This results in an increased level of activated *protein C/α_1-antitrypsin complex.* Detection of an increased level of this complex might be used clinically to separate severe preeclampsia from chronic hypertension with superimposed preeclampsia. *Protein C inhibitor* also appears to be decreased by kallikrein, which is increased as a consequence of activation of the intrinsic coagulation pathway.

Endocrine and Metabolic Changes

Endocrine Changes. Plasma levels of *renin, angiotensin II,* and *aldosterone* are increased during normal pregnancy. Pregnancy-induced hypertension results in a decrease of these values toward the normal nonpregnant range (Weir and colleagues, 1973). With sodium retention, hypertension, or both, renin secretion by the juxtaglomerular apparatus decreases. Because renin is the enzyme that catalyzes the conversion of angiotensinogen to angiotensin I (which is then transformed into angiotensin II by converting enzyme), angiotensin II levels decline, resulting in a decrease in aldosterone secretion. Despite this, women with preeclampsia avidly retain infused sodium (Brown and colleagues, 1988b).

Another potent mineralocorticoid, *deoxycorticosterone* (DOC), is increased strikingly in third-trimester plasma (see Chap. 8, p. 238). Importantly, its increase is not the consequence of increased secretion by maternal adrenal glands. Treatment of pregnant women with dexamethasone to reduce corticotropin secretion does not decrease plasma deoxycorticosterone levels, and neither does corticotropin treatment of near-term pregnant women cause increased plasma levels. Because plasma progesterone is converted to deoxycorticosterone in nonadrenal tissues, it is reasonable to conclude that this pathway is not subject to control by angiotensin II. Thus, the amount formed from plasma progesterone is not reduced by sodium retention or hypertension, and it may play a role in the pathogenesis or perpetuation of preeclampsia.

> Winkel and co-workers (1980) found that the fractional conversion of plasma progesterone to deoxycorticosterone varied widely among individuals (0.002 to 0.22). Ordinarily, the fractional conversion of one steroid hormone to another seldom varies among normal individuals. Thus, in near-term pregnant women producing 250 mg of progesterone per day, DOC production from plasma progesterone could vary from 0.5 to 11 mg per 24 hours. Nonpregnant women produce, on average, 0.15 mg of DOC per day. Given the progesterone produced in women who are prone to develop preeclampsia—for example, women with diabetes, multiple fetuses, fe-

tal hydrops, and hydatidiform mole—the amount of DOC produced from plasma progesterone could be enormous.

Deoxycorticosterone production cannot be the only factor in the development of pregnancy-induced hypertension. Brown and co-workers (1972) reported that DOC levels in pregnant hypertensive women were not greater than were those in normotensive controls. Parker and colleagues (1980) measured the hormone throughout pregnancy and found that plasma DOC concentrations in primigravidas who ultimately developed preeclampsia were not greater than in primigravidas who remained normotensive. Winkel and co-workers (1983), however, subsequently reported that the conversion of progesterone into DOC was increased significantly in women who later developed pregnancy-induced hypertension. It may be that DOC has a local effect, and that it is produced and metabolized within the kidney so its plasma concentration need not be different in hypertensive women.

Increased *antidiuretic hormone* activity to account for oliguria has been suggested previously. In fact, normal (Elias and colleagues, 1988) or even low levels have been identified (J. Pritchard and J. Porter, unpublished). Plasma *chorionic gonadotropin* levels are elevated inconstantly; conversely, *placental lactogen* levels are reduced inconstantly.

Necrosis of the adrenal and the pituitary glands has been identified in some fatal cases of eclampsia (McKay, 1965). In our experience, compromised adrenal or pituitary function is rare in nonfatal cases.

Atrial natriuretic peptide is released upon atrial wall stretching from blood volume expansion. It is vasoactive and also promotes sodium and water excretion likely by inhibiting aldosterone, renin activity, angiotensin II, and vasopressin (Bond and colleagues, 1989). Thomsen and colleagues (1987), but not Hirai and associates (1988), reported that this peptide is increased in normal pregnancy. Both groups reported, however, that the atrial natriuretic peptide was increased substantively in women with preeclampsia (Fig. 36–7). With volume expansion, there is an augmented release of the compound in preeclamptic compared with normotensive pregnant women. Increases in atrial natriuretic peptide following volume expansion result in comparable increases in cardiac output and decreases in peripheral vascular resistance in both normotensive and preeclamptic women (Nisell and associates, 1992). This observation may in part explain observations of a fall in peripheral vascular resistance following volume expansion in preeclamptic women (see p. 772).

A more recently described compound, *ouabain-like natriuretic factor*, is being studied in pregnancy because the factor is elevated in essential hypertension. It cross-reacts with some anti-digoxin antibodies, and because of this, it also is called *digoxin-like immuno-*

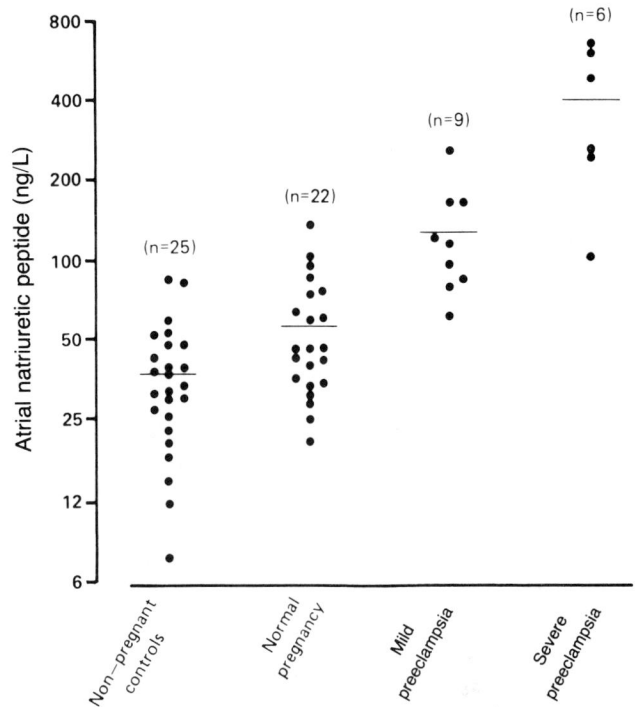

Fig. 36–7. Plasma immunoreactive atrial natriuretic peptide concentrations in normal nonpregnant and pregnant women, and preeclamptic women. Horizontal bars represent group means. (From Thomsen and colleagues, 1987.)

reactive substance. The factor inhibits the sodium-potassium-ATPase pump, which (1) increases intracellular sodium, resulting in increased intracellular calcium by inhibiting sodium-calcium exchanges; and (2) reduces the sodium electrochemical gradient, which results in increased neuronal release and decreased neuronal norepinephrine reuptake. These two mechanisms produce increased peripheral vascular resistance.

Ouabain-like natriuretic factor is increased in normal pregnancy. It is progressively more increased in women with pregnancy-induced hypertension alone, and even more increased in those with preeclampsia (Fievet, 1988; Gregoire, 1988; Kaminski, 1991; and their co-workers). The plasma concentration of digoxin-like immunoreactive substance increases progressively as pregnancy advances, but plasma values are not different in normal and future hypertensives prior to the onset of hypertension (Kerkez and associates, 1990). The compound is significantly increased in multifetal gestations compared with singleton pregnancies (Jakobi and co-workers, 1989).

Fluid and Electrolyte Changes. Commonly, the volume of *extracellular fluid* in women with severe preeclampsia–eclampsia has expanded beyond the normally increased volume that characterizes pregnancy. The mechanism responsible for the pathological expansion is not clear. Edema is evident at a time when, paradoxically, aldosterone levels are reduced compared with the remarkably elevated levels of normal pregnancy. As noted above, however, plasma deoxycorticosterone levels remain elevated, but they are not consistently greater than those in normotensive women. Electrolyte concentrations do not differ appreciably from those of normal pregnancy unless there has been vigorous diuretic therapy, dietary sodium restriction, or the administration of water with sufficient oxytocin to produce antidiuresis. Edema does not ensure a poor prognosis, and absence of edema does not ensure a favorable outcome for pregnancies complicated by preeclampsia–eclampsia.

Following an eclamptic convulsion, the *bicarbonate* concentration is lowered due to lactic acid acidosis and compensatory respiratory loss of carbon dioxide. The intensity of acidosis relates to the amount of lactic acid produced and its metabolic rate, as well as the rate at which carbon dioxide is exhaled.

The Kidney

During normal pregnancy, renal blood flow and glomerular filtration rate are increased appreciably (see Chap. 8, p. 230). With development of pregnancy-induced hypertension, renal perfusion and glomerular filtration are reduced. Levels that are much below normal nonpregnant values are the consequence of severe disease. Therefore, in milder cases plasma creatinine or urea concentration are seldom elevated above normal nonpregnant values. Plasma uric acid concentration is typically elevated, especially in women with more severe disease. The elevation in uric acid exceeds the reduction in glomerular filtration rate and creatinine clearance that accompanies preeclampsia (Chesley and Williams, 1945). Despite this, plasma uric acid measurements are generally of little practical value for diagnosis, management, or prognosis. Plasma uric acid values also can be elevated by thiazide diuretics.

In the majority of preeclamptic women, mild to moderately diminished glomerular filtration appears to result from a reduced plasma volume; thus, plasma creatinine seldom is below normal nonpregnant levels. In some cases of severe preeclampsia, however, renal involvement is profound, and plasma creatinine may be elevated two to three times over nonpregnant normal values. This is likely due to intrinsic renal changes caused by severe vasospasm (Pritchard and colleagues, 1984) because total renal perfusion does not appear to be reduced in preeclamptic women (Levine and associates, 1992). Lee and associates (1987) reported normal ventricular filling pressures in 7 severely preeclamptic women with oliguria, and concluded that this was consistent with intrarenal vasospasm. In most of these latter women, urine sodium concentration was elevated abnormally, suggesting an intrinsic renal etiology. Urine osmolality, urine–plasma creatinine ratio, and fractional excretion of sodium were also indicative that a prerenal mechanism was involved. *Importantly, intensive intravenous fluid therapy was not indicated for these women with oliguria.* Subsequently, this group infused dopamine into oliguric preeclamptic women, and this renal vasodilator caused increased urine output, fractional sodium excretion, and free water clearance (Kirshon and co-workers, 1988).

Taufield and associates (1987) reported that preeclampsia is associated with diminished urinary excretion of calcium because of increased tubular reabsorption. This mechanism would explain the decreased calcium excretion in hypertensive and future hypertensive pregnant women (see p. 768).

After delivery, in the absence of underlying chronic renovascular disease, complete recovery of renal function usually can be anticipated. This would not be the case, of course, if *renal cortical necrosis,* an irreversible but rare lesion, develops (Sibai and associates, 1990b).

Proteinuria. Some degree of proteinuria should be present to establish the diagnosis of preeclampsia–eclampsia (Chesley, 1985). Because proteinuria develops late in the course of the disease, however, some women may be delivered before it appears and thus still have actual preeclampsia without proteinuria.

Albuminuria is an incorrect term to describe proteinuria of preeclampsia. As with any other glomerulopathy, there is increased permeability to most large-molecular-weight proteins; thus, abnormal albumin excretion is accompanied by other proteins, such as hemoglobin, globulins, and transferrin. Normally, these large protein molecules are not filtered by the glomerulus, and their appearance in urine signifies a glomerulopathic process. Some of the smaller proteins that usually are filtered but reabsorbed also are detected in urine.

Because of the similarity with other renal diseases thought to be caused by immune-complex glomerulonephritis, it is tempting to regard these renal changes of preeclampsia as induced by immunological mechanisms. Certainly, if there is not underlying chronic renal disease, proteinuria gradually recedes following delivery and resolution of hypertension. This usually occurs within a week or so, even with heavy proteinuria and severe preeclampsia.

Microscopical Changes. Changes identifiable by light and electron microscopy are commonly found in the kidney. Sheehan (1950) observed that the glomeruli were enlarged by about 20 percent, often pouting into the neck of the tubule. The capillary loops variably are dilated and contracted. The endothelial cells are swollen, and deposited within and beneath them are fibrils that have been mistaken for thickening and reduplication of the basement membrane.

Sheehan's interpretations have been confirmed by electron microscopical studies of renal biopsies taken from women with preeclampsia. Most, but not all, of these studies are consistent with the view that the characteristic changes are glomerular capillary endothelial swelling. These changes, accompanied by subendothelial deposits of protein material, are called *glomerular capillary endotheliosis* by Spargo and associates (1959). The endothelial cells are often so swollen that they block or partially block the capillary lumens. Homogeneous deposits of an electron-dense substance are found between basal lamina and endothelial cells and within the cells themselves. Vassalli and co-workers (1963), on the basis of immunofluorescent staining, considered the material to be a fibrinogen derivative and regarded its presence as characteristic of preeclampsia. This observation, in part, led to a theory that the renal lesions of preeclampsia are the result of intravascular coagulation initiated by something, presumably thromboplastin, released from the placenta (Page, 1972). Lichtig and co-workers (1975), however, were able to identify deposited fibrinogen or its derivatives in only 13 of 30 renal biopsy specimens from women with preeclampsia, and the amount of fibrin was graded as more than a trace in only two. Kincaid-Smith (1991) has advanced a theory to explain this discrepancy. She noted that these deposits disappear progressively in the first week postpartum. Therefore, in order to identify such lesions, a renal biopsy must be done antepartum or soon after delivery. An alternative explanation for the renal lesion has been proposed by Petrucco and colleagues (1974), who detected IgM, IgG, and sometimes complement, in the glomeruli of preeclamptic women in proportion to the severity of disease. They suggested that an immunological mechanism was active in the production of the glomerular lesion.

The renal changes identified by electron microscopy have been advanced as being pathognomonic of preeclampsia. The uncertainties of clinical diagnosis are so great, however, as to preclude acceptance of such a one-to-one relation, except as an act of faith. The history of other alleged pathognomonic lesions in eclampsia engenders such skepticism.

Renal tubular lesions are common in women with eclampsia, but what has been interpreted as degenerative changes may represent only an accumulation within cells of protein reabsorbed from the glomerular filtrate. The collecting tubules may appear obstructed by casts from derivatives of protein, including, at times, hemoglobin.

Acute renal failure from *tubular necrosis* may develop. Although this is more common in neglected cases, it is invariably induced by hemorrhage, usually associated with delivery, for which adequate blood replacement is not given. Sibai and colleagues (1990b) noted that more than 50 percent of their patients with hypertension and acute renal failure also had a placental abruption, and more than 85 percent had postpartum hemorrhages. Rarely, *renal cortical necrosis* develops when the major portion of the cortex of both kidneys undergoes necrosis. Both cause acute renal failure characterized clinically by oliguria or anuria and rapidly developing azotemia. Renal cortical necrosis is irreversible, and although it develops in nonpregnant women and in men, the lesion has most often been associated with pregnancy (see Chap. 50, p. 1142).

An excellent review of renal disease and pregnancy was presented recently by Lindheimer and Abe (1991). The interested reader is referred to this review of the subject.

The Liver

With severe preeclampsia, there are at times alterations in tests of hepatic function and integrity, including delayed excretion of bromosulfophthalein and elevation of serum aspartate aminotransferase levels (Combes and Adams, 1972). Severe hyperbilirubinemia is uncommon with preeclampsia. Pritchard and colleagues (1976) reported that in 134 hypertensive women, including 45 with eclampsia, only 3 had a serum bilirubin greater than 1.2 mg/dL, with 2.3 mg/dL the highest value. Much of the increase in serum alkaline phosphatase is due to heat-stable alkaline phosphatase of placental origin.

Periportal hemorrhagic necrosis in the periphery of the liver lobule is the most likely reason for increased serum liver enzymes. In the past, this lesion was often identified at autopsy and was long considered to be the characteristic lesion of eclampsia. Such extensive lesions are seldom identified in nonfatal cases. Combes and Adams (1972) reported that liver histology was normal in biopsies from 6 preeclamptic and 12 eclamptic women. Because the specimen taken was small and thrombocytopenia was considered exclusionary, it is likely that women with some hepatocellular necrosis were missed. Most often abnormally elevated serum liver enzymes, and thus liver damage, are accompanied by thrombocytopenia (Sibai and colleagues, 1986c).

Bleeding from these lesions may cause *hepatic rupture* or they may extend beneath the hepatic capsule and form a *subcapsular hematoma*. Actually, such hemorrhages without rupture may be more common than previously suspected. Using computed tomography, Manas and colleagues (1985) showed that 5 of 7 women with preeclampsia and upper abdominal pain had hepatic hemorrhage (Fig. 36–8). Surgical repair was not necessary in any of these women, but 6 required blood and component transfusions. Subcapsular hemorrhage may be extensive enough to rupture the capsule, resulting in fatal intraabdominal hemorrhage. Prompt surgical intervention may be lifesaving. Smith and co-workers (1991) reviewed 28 published cases of spontaneous hepatic rupture associated with preeclampsia and added

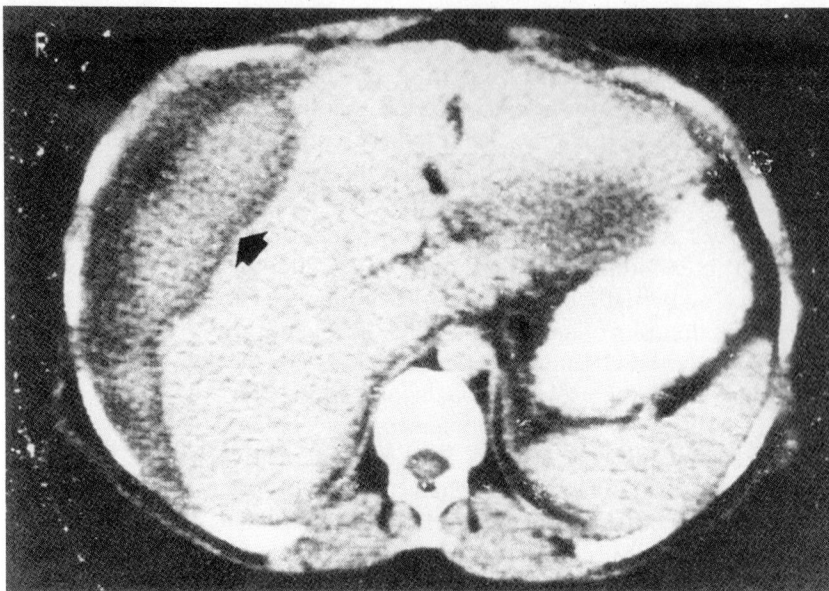

Fig. 36–8. Computed tomographic scan of liver showing a subcapsular hematoma (*arrow*) along the right margin of the liver. (From Manas and colleagues, 1985, with permission.)

7 cases from the affiliated hospitals of Baylor College of Medicine. The mortality rate was 30 percent, and they concluded that packing and drainage was superior to lobectomy. One such woman at Parkland Hospital survived after receiving blood and blood products from more than 200 donors.

Liver involvement in preeclampsia–eclampsia is serious and is frequently accompanied by evidence of other organ involvement, especially the kidney and brain, along with hemolysis and thrombocytopenia (De Boer, 1991; Neuman, 1990; Pritchard, 1954b; Sibai, 1986c; Weinstein, 1985; and their associates). Workers from Memphis identified this constellation in almost 10 percent of women with severe preeclampsia or eclampsia (Sibai and co-workers, 1986c). Other complications also were common, including placental abruption (20 percent), acute renal failure (8 percent), and pulmonary edema (5 percent). Two of the 112 women died.

The Brain

McCall (1953) reported that cerebral blood flow, oxygen consumption, and vascular resistance were not altered in women with preeclampsia, eclampsia, or essential hypertension; however, the possibility of focal cerebral hypoperfusion or hyperperfusion could not be excluded. Nonspecific electroencephalographic abnormalities can usually be demonstrated for some time after eclamptic convulsions. Sibai and colleagues (1985a) observed that 75 percent of 65 eclamptic women had abnormal electroencephalograms within 48 hours of seizures. Half of these abnormalities persisted past 1 week, but most were normal by 3 months. An increased incidence of electroencephalographic abnormalities has been described in family members of eclamptic women, a finding suggestive that some eclamptic women who convulse have an inherited predisposition to do so (Rosenbaum and Maltby, 1943).

The principal postmortem cerebral lesions are edema, hyperemia, focal anemia, thrombosis, and hemorrhage. Sheehan (1950) examined the brains of 48 eclamptic women very soon after their death, and hemorrhages, ranging from petechiae to gross bleeding, were found in 56 percent. According to Sheehan, if the brain is examined within an hour after death, most often it is as firm as normal, and there is no obvious edema. Govan (1961) investigated the cause of death in 110 fatal cases of eclampsia and concluded that cerebral hemorrhage was responsible in 39. Small cerebral hemorrhagic lesions were also found in 85 percent of the 47 women who died of cardiorespiratory failure. He further described as a regular finding fibrinoid changes in the walls of cerebral vessels. The lesions sometimes appeared to have been present for some time, as judged from the surrounding leukocytic response and hemosiderin-pigmented macrophages. These findings are consistent with the view that prodromal neurological symptoms and convulsions may be related to these lesions.

Using advanced equipment, Brown and colleagues (1988a) found that nearly half of eclamptic women studied had abnormal findings on cranial computed tomography scanning (Fig. 36–9). The most common findings were hypodense cortical areas, which corresponded to petechial hemorrhage and infarction sites reported at autopsy by Sheehan and Lynch (1973). These findings provide an explanation of why some women with preeclampsia convulse but others do not. It seems reasonable that the brain, like the liver and kidney, may be more

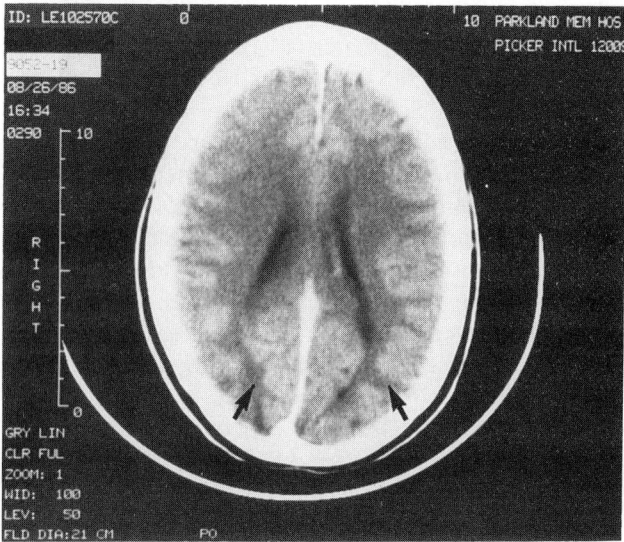

Fig. 36–9. Cranial computed tomograph of a woman with eclampsia. Radiographic hypodensities (*arrows*) are seen in the occipital and parietal areas. (From Brown and co-workers, 1988a.)

involved in some women than in others, and the extent of ischemic and petechial subcortical lesions, further altered by an inherent seizure threshold, influences the incidence of eclampsia.

Blindness. Although visual disturbances are common with severe preeclampsia, blindness, either alone or accompanying convulsions, is not. Some women with vary-

ing degrees of *amaurosis* are found to have radiographic evidence of extensive occipital lobe hypodensities; this is likely an exaggeration of the lesions described above and shown in Figure 36–9. Herzog and colleagues (1990) reported that magnetic resonance imaging was superior to computed tomography in identifying specific brain lesions responsible for this type of blindness. In most cases, the prognosis is good, and women usually recover within hours to 1 week (Nalliah and Thavarashah, 1989).

Retinal detachment may also cause altered vision, although it is usually one sided and seldom causes total visual loss as in some women with cortical blindness. Surgical treatment is seldom indicated; prognosis is good; and vision usually returns to normal within a week.

Coma. It is rare for a woman with eclampsia not to awaken after a seizure. It is also rare for a woman with severe preeclampsia to become comatose without an antecedent seizure. Prognosis for these women is good. In two such women, extensive cerebral edema was documented by computed tomography (Fig. 36–10). Thus, it does not appear that coma results from an extension of the ischemic and hemorrhagic lesions described above, because eclamptic women without coma have minimal cerebral edema (Brown and colleagues, 1988a). Because coma usually follows sudden and severe blood pressure elevations, it is more likely that this phenomena represents an inability to autoregulate cerebral blood flow with severe acute hypertension; the result is generalized cerebral edema.

Another cause of coma is *intracranial hemorrhage*

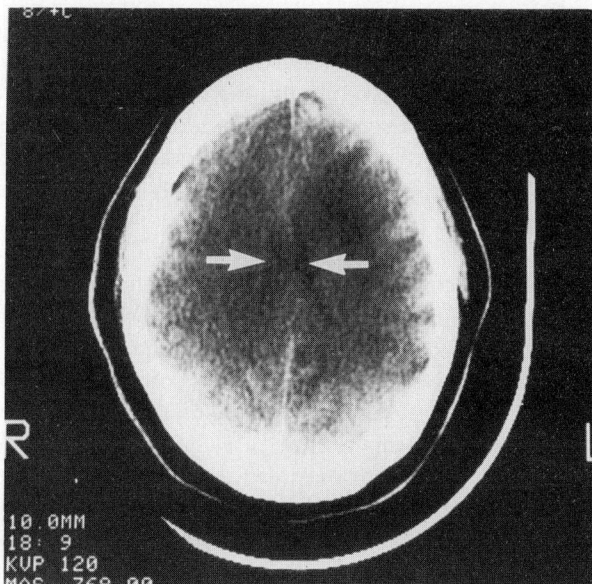

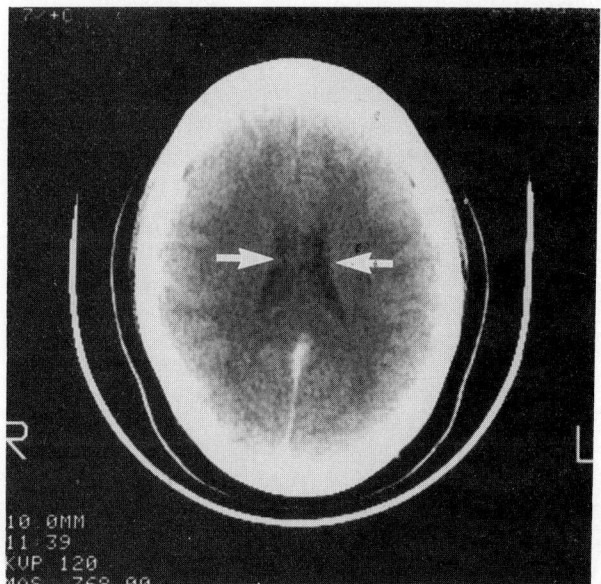

A   **B**

Fig. 36–10. Cranial computed tomographs of an eclamptic woman who was also comatose. **A.** Cerebral edema is characterized by loss of gyral configuration, as well as by much-narrowed lateral ventricles (*arrows*). **B.** After complete neurological recovery, about 4 weeks later, gyral architecture is better seen and ventricles are normal in size. (From Brown and colleagues, 1988a.)

from a ruptured intracerebral vessel, an arteriovenous malformation, or a berry aneurysm. Sheehan and Lynch (1973) reported that 6 of 76 women with fatal eclampsia had massive white matter hemorrhage that caused coma and death. They also reported a high mortality rate with bleeding into the basal ganglia or pons. These lesions have a much poorer prognosis than coma from cerebral edema, and the two should be differentiated by computed tomography or magnetic resonance imaging. Treatment is the same as for any nonpregnant woman.

Uteroplacental Perfusion

Compromised placental perfusion from vasospasm is almost certainly a major culprit in the genesis of increased perinatal morbidity and mortality associated with pregnancy-induced or pregnancy-aggravated hypertension.

Measurements of Placental Perfusion. Attempts to measure human maternal placental blood flow have been hampered by several obstacles, including inaccessibility of the placenta, the complexity of its venous effluent, and the unsuitability of certain investigative techniques for humans. Despite formidable problems, Assali and associates (1953) and Metcalfe and co-workers (1955) measured uterine blood flow in pregnant women and obtained reasonably consistent results. Both groups used a nitrous oxide Fick principle method that required cannulation of a uterine vein. Total uterine perfusion was measured, rather than maternal placental blood flow. Uterine blood flow in normal-term pregnant women was approximately 500 to 700 mL/min.

Browne and Veall (1953) estimated changes in maternal placental flow through the use of a ^{24}Na clearance technique. This method required needle insertion into the intervillous space. Browne and Veall (1953), Johnson and Clayton (1957), Morris and colleagues (1956), and Weis and associates (1958), all observed that ^{24}Na was cleared two to three times more rapidly in normotensive pregnant women than in preeclamptic women, implying a two- to threefold decrease in uteroplacental perfusion in hypertensive women compared with normotensive gravidas.

Indirect Methods. The consistent results and conclusions obtained from these early studies continue to be supported by other methods of investigation. For instance, Brosens and associates (1972) reported that the mean diameter of myometrial spiral arterioles of 50 normal pregnant women was 500 μm. The same measurement in 36 women with preeclampsia was 200 μm.

Dehydroisoandrosterone Sulfate Clearance. Everett and colleagues (1980) presented evidence that the clearance rate of dehydroisoandrosterone sulfate

through placental conversion to estradiol-17β was an accurate reflection of maternal placental perfusion. Fritz and colleagues (1985) reported that the technique paralleled uteroplacental perfusion in primates. Normally, as pregnancy advances, this measurement increases greatly. Moreover, in women destined to develop pregnancy-induced hypertension, the placental clearance rate of dehydroisoandrosterone sulfate is greater before the onset of hypertension than in control subjects, an intriguing observation in itself (Chap. 6, p. 149). The placental clearance rate decreases before the onset of overt hypertension (Worley and associates, 1975).

The placental clearance rate of dehydroisoandrosterone sulfate was measured in a study of the effect of *thiazide diuretics* on placental function and perfusion (Gant and associates, 1975; Shoemaker and co-workers, 1973). The clearance rate was computed for one woman with preeclampsia, another with chronic hypertension complicating pregnancy, and a third woman who had been hospitalized at 36 weeks simply because of excessive weight gain. The clearance rate was markedly lower during diuretic therapy in all three women. A similar reduction in uteroplacental perfusion was noted following furosemide (Gant and co-workers, 1976).

Gant and co-workers (1976) reported that intravenous administration of hydralazine to 8 chronically hypertensive women near term was followed by a 25 percent decrease in the metabolic clearance rate of dehydroisoandrosterone sulfate, apparently due to a 37 percent decrease in diastolic blood pressure and presumably reduced small vessel perfusion. Thus, even the intermittent administration of intravenous hydralazine, as described below, may decrease uteroplacental perfusion. Although the fetus in most normal pregnancies tolerates an appreciable decrease in placental perfusion without suffering profoundly, the fetus in a pregnancy complicated by severe preeclampsia or eclampsia, especially if growth-retarded, may not tolerate further reductions superimposed upon an already compromised uteroplacental perfusion.

Doppler Velocimetry. Doppler measurement of blood velocity through uterine arteries has been used to estimate uteroplacental blood flow (see Chap. 46, p. 1056). Vascular resistance is estimated by comparing arterial systolic and diastolic velocity waveforms. The uterine vascular bed is normally a low-resistance circuit, and flow continues throughout diastole. As resistance increases, diastolic velocity diminishes in relation to systolic velocity, and this relationship has been used to estimate decreased flow. Fleischer (1986), Trudinger (1985, 1990), and their colleagues reported an increased systolic–diastolic ratio in uterine arteries of women with preeclampsia. Conversely, Hanretty and colleagues (1988a) reported that technical factors severely limited data analysis obtained using these methods.

The absence of diastolic flow or actual reversal of flow is associated with increased fetal morbidity and mortality in hypertensive women (Fairlie, 1991; Kofinas, 1990; Lombardi, 1989; Pattinson, 1989; and their co-workers). In rare instances, diastolic flow has been restored with antihypertensive therapy (Hanretty and associates, 1988b). Nifedipine therapy and epidural analgesia have also been reported to decrease abnormally elevated systolic–diastolic ratios (Mires, 1990; Pirhonen, 1990; Puzey, 1991; Ramos-Santos, 1991; and their colleagues).

Ducey and associates (1987) described systolic–diastolic velocity ratios from both uterine and umbilical arteries in 136 pregnancies complicated by hypertension. Among 51 women considered to have preeclampsia, 20 percent had normal umbilical artery velocity ratios; 15 percent had normal umbilical but abnormal uterine artery ratios; and in 40 percent both ratios were abnormal. Kofinas and associates (1988, 1992) reported that in both normal and hypertensive women with unilateral placental locations, systolic–diastolic ratios were significantly lower in the ipsilateral uterine artery.

We have seldom encountered diminished uterine artery flow velocities in *uncomplicated* preeclampsia. This is true even with severely elevated blood pressures. With associated fetal growth retardation, however, aberrant flow velocities are often seen in both umbilical and aortic vessels (Cameron and colleagues, 1988). In some reports, such as that by Trudinger and colleagues (1985), women were studied *because of* growth retardation. Thus, it appears from these preliminary studies that preeclampsia alone may not be associated with significant changes in the uterine artery systolic–diastolic ratio. Aberrations in fetal blood flow velocities can be detected in hypertensive pregnancies, but these are much more likely if there is also retarded fetal growth (Lowery, 1990; Steel, 1988; Villar, 1989a; and their associates).

Although an increase in Doppler waveform ratio has been correlated with obliteration of placental stem arteries (Trudinger and associates, 1985), and waveform abnormalities have been shown to be related to uterine artery diameter (Adamson and colleagues, 1989), clinical usefulness of the technique has not been clearly established (Brown, 1990; Hanretty, 1988a, 1989; Kurmanavichius, 1990; Morrow, 1990; and their colleagues). We agree with Low (1991), who concluded that for now Doppler assessment of blood flow in pregnancy should be limited to an investigational setting.

Histological Changes in the Placental Bed. Hertig (1945) identified in preeclamptic pregnancies a lesion of uteroplacental arteries characterized by prominent lipid-rich foam cells. Zeek and Assali (1950) extended these observations and concluded that in preeclampsia there is a pathognomonic lesion of the uteroplacental vessels that they termed *acute atherosis*. Most investi-

gators are now in accord that there is a lesion, but they do not agree on its precise nature. Using electron microscopical studies of arteries taken from the uteroplacental implantation site, DeWolf and co-workers (1975) reported that early preeclamptic changes included endothelial damage, insudation of plasma constituents into vessel walls, proliferation of myointimal cells, and medial necrosis. They also found that lipid accumulates first in myointimal cells and then in macrophages. Robertson and colleagues (1986) provided a careful review of these microscopic vascular findings.

CLINICAL ASPECTS OF PREECLAMPSIA

Clinical Findings

The pregnant woman is usually unaware of the two most important signs of preeclampsia—hypertension and proteinuria. By the time symptoms such as headache, visual disturbances, or epigastric pain develop, the disorder is almost always severe. Hence, the importance of prenatal care in the early detection and management of preeclampsia is obvious.

Blood Pressure. The basic derangement in preeclampsia is arteriolar vasospasm, and the most dependable warning sign is an increase in blood pressure. Diastolic pressure is probably a more reliable prognostic sign than systolic, and any diastolic pressure of 90 mm Hg or more that persists is abnormal. The fifth Korotkoff sound is used by most clinical centers in the United States.

Weight Gain. A sudden increase in weight may precede the development of preeclampsia, and indeed, excessive weight gain in some women is the first sign. A weight increase of about 1 pound per week is normal, but when weight gain exceeds more than 2 pounds in any given week, or 6 pounds in a month, developing preeclampsia should be suspected. The suddenness of excessive weight gain is characteristic of preeclampsia rather than an increase distributed throughout gestation. Such a weight gain is due almost entirely to abnormal fluid retention and is usually demonstrable before visible signs of nondependent edema, such as swollen eyelids and puffy fingers. In cases of fulminating preeclampsia or eclampsia, fluid retention may be extreme; and in these women, a weight gain of 10 or more pounds per week is not unusual.

Obstetricians in the past often attempted to limit maternal weight gain to about 20 pounds, or even less, in the mistaken belief this would prevent preeclampsia. The total weight gained during pregnancy, however, probably has no relation to preeclampsia unless a large component of the gain is edema. Stringent restriction of weight gain is more likely to be detrimental rather than beneficial to both mother and fetus. The physician's scale, unfortunately, does not distinguish between edema fluid and the normal disposition of fluid in fetal and maternal tissues.

Proteinuria. The degree of proteinuria varies greatly in preeclampsia, not only from case to case but also in the same woman from hour to hour. The variability is suggestive of a functional (vasospasm) rather than an organic cause. In early preeclampsia, proteinuria may be minimal or entirely lacking; but in most severe forms, it is usually demonstrable. Proteinuria almost always develops later than hypertension and usually later than excessive weight gain.

Headache. Headache is unusual in milder cases but is increasingly frequent in more severe disease. It is often frontal but may be occipital, and it is resistant to relief from ordinary analgesics. **A severe headache almost invariably precedes the first eclamptic convulsion.**

Epigastric Pain. **Epigastric or right upper quadrant pain is often a symptom of severe preeclampsia and may be indicative of imminent convulsions.** It is probably due to stretching of the hepatic capsule, possibly by edema and hemorrhage (p. 779).

Visual Disturbances. These abnormalities are also ominous and were discussed previously (see p. 781).

Immediate Prognosis. The prognosis for mother and fetus is dependent to a considerable extent upon the gestational age of the fetus, whether improvement follows hospitalization, when and how delivery is accomplished, and whether eclampsia supervenes. Perinatal mortality rate is increased variably for pregnancies complicated by pregnancy-induced hypertension, as with other hypertensive disorders. It is primarily dependent upon the time of onset and the severity of the disease. Much of the neonatal loss is the consequence of preterm delivery, either from spontaneous labor or because of induced delivery necessitated by severe preeclampsia.

Prophylaxis and Early Treatment

Early Detection. Because women are usually asymptomatic and seldom notice the signs of incipient preeclampsia, its early detection demands careful observation at appropriate intervals, especially in women known to be predisposed to preeclampsia. Major predisposing factors are (1) nulliparity, (2) familial history of preeclampsia–eclampsia, (3) multiple fetuses, (4) diabetes, (5) chronic vascular disease, (6) renal disease, (7) hydatidiform mole, and (8) fetal hydrops.

Rapid weight gain any time during the latter half of pregnancy, or an upward trend in diastolic blood pressure, even while still in the normal range, is worrisome. Every woman should be examined at least weekly during the last month of pregnancy and every 2 weeks during the previous 2 months. At these visits, weight and blood pressure measurements are made. Furthermore, all women should be advised to report immediately any symptoms or signs of preeclampsia, such as headache, visual disturbances, and puffiness of hands or face. The reporting of any such symptoms calls for an immediate examination to confirm or exclude preeclampsia.

Diuretics and Sodium Restriction. Natriuretic drugs, such as chlorothiazide and its congeners, have been overused severely in the past. Although diuretics have been alleged to prevent preeclampsia, proof of their efficacy is tenuous. For example, the women studied by Kraus and associates (1966) took either a placebo or 50 mg of hydrochlorothiazide daily during at least the last 16 weeks of gestation. The incidence of preeclampsia was 6.7 percent in primigravid women given hydrochlorothiazide and the same in those who took the placebo. Moreover, the incidence of hypertension was not altered in multiparous women. Collins and colleagues (1985) reviewed the results of nine such studies that included more than 7000 women, and they concluded that perinatal mortality was not improved when diuretics were given to prevent preeclampsia. The failure of natriuretic drugs in the prevention of preeclampsia also raises serious doubt about the efficacy of rigid dietary sodium restriction.

Thiazide diuretics and similar compounds are not used in the treatment or prophylaxis of preeclampsia at Parkland Hospital. Although there is no clear evidence that they are of any value, there is evidence that diuretics reduce renal and uteroplacental perfusion (Gant and colleagues, 1975; Shoemaker and associates, 1973). Furthermore, thiazides can induce serious sodium and potassium depletion, hemorrhagic pancreatitis, and severe thrombocytopenia in some newborns.

Aspirin and Other Drugs. Wallenburg and co-workers (1986) reported their experiences with administration of either 60 mg of aspirin or placebo to primigravid women at 28 weeks' gestation. These women were sensitive to infused angiotensin II and judged to be at high risk for developing preeclampsia. The reduced incidence of preeclampsia in the treated group was attributed to selective suppression of thromboxane synthesis by platelets and sparing of endothelial prostacyclin production. In a group of women with prior bad pregnancy outcomes due to hypertension and placental insufficiency, Beaufils and colleagues (1985) reported that early prophylactic treatment with dipyridamole and aspirin reduced recurrence rates. They attributed their results to the antiplatelet actions of these drugs.

Spitz and colleagues (1988) reported that angiotensin II-sensitive women at high risk for developing pregnancy-induced hypertension could be rendered refractory to angiotensin II in most cases by a 1-week course of daily low-dose aspirin therapy (81 mg/day). They also confirmed that such low-dose aspirin therapy did significantly decrease thromboxane synthesis, likely by blocking the cyclooxygenase pathway of arachidonic acid conversion to thromboxane. The low-dose aspirin therapy did not spare prostacyclin and prostaglandin E_2 synthesis; they were also decreased 20 to 30 percent by therapy. Subsequently, the same group of investigators reported that approximately 20 percent of angiotensin II-sensitive pregnant women receiving low-dose aspirin therapy did not become refractory to angiotensin II, and all such women developed preeclampsia. The nonresponders to low-dose aspirin therapy, as expected, had a significant fall in thromboxane levels, but they also had significant declines in prostacyclin and prostaglandin E_2 levels (Brown and associates, 1990). Thus, daily 81-mg aspirin doses are not completely selective in blocking only thromboxane.

Low-dose aspirin therapy was apparently not effective in women already ill with mild pregnancy-induced hypertension (Schiff and associates, 1990); however, with moderate hypertension the opposite was true. Magness and colleagues (1991) observed that less than 20 percent of women with early-onset pregnancy-induced hypertension failed to become normotensive with hospitalization and restriction of physical activity; but in the 20 percent who remained hypertensive after hospitalization, low-dose aspirin therapy alone and with a linoleic acid food supplement significantly prolonged the duration of pregnancy compared with controls.

Low-dose aspirin may be effective in some, but not all, women in preventing the development of pregnancy-induced hypertension and fetal growth retardation. Such a qualified conclusion was reached by Imperiale and Petrulis (1991). In a meta-analysis of six different clinical trials of different doses and durations of low-dose aspirin therapy, they reported a significant decrease in the incidence of pregnancy-induced hypertension. Hauth and co-workers (in press) randomized 600 nulliparas to 60 mg aspirin or placebo beginning at 24 weeks. Only 1.7 percent of aspirin-treated women developed preeclampsia versus 5.6 percent of controls ($p = .009$). Conversely, studies from the National Institutes of Health sponsored Maternal–Fetal Medicine Network showed that aspirin prophylaxis did not significantly reduce preeclampsia (Sibai and colleagues, 1993a, 1993b). In the latter study, women who took aspirin had significantly more placental abruptions. Salutary effects or effects of low-dose aspirin therapy remain to be proven (Cunningham and Gant, 1989).

There are a variety of specific thromboxane inhibitors now available that spare prostacyclin while blocking thromboxane. These compounds are being tested in pregnant sheep with good results and without apparent adverse maternal or fetal effects (Cardin and associates, 1990; Keith and colleagues, 1989). Hopefully, within the next decade obstetricians will have the means to prevent pregnancy-induced hypertension.

Fetal Effects of Aspirin Therapy. Low-dose aspirin therapy appears to be safe for the fetus (Benigni, 1989; McParland, 1990; Schiff, 1989; Weinstein, 1990; and their co-workers). Although most clinical trials have resulted in no apparent maternal risks, Brown and colleagues (1990) noted a rapid clinical deterioration if therapy was stopped suddenly.

Objectives of Treatment

Basic management objectives for any pregnancy complicated by pregnancy-induced hypertension are (1) termination of pregnancy with the least possible trauma to mother and fetus, (2) birth of an infant who subsequently thrives, and (3) complete restoration of health to the mother. In certain cases of preeclampsia, especially in women at or near term, all three objectives are served equally well by careful induction of labor. **Therefore, the most important information that the obstetrician has for successful management of pregnancy, and especially a pregnancy that becomes complicated by hypertension, is precise knowledge of the age of the fetus** (see Chap. 9, p. 252).

Ambulatory Treatment. Excluding young nulliparas, some women without proteinuria and with blood pressure less than 140/90 mm Hg may be managed at home. Such management may continue as long as the disease does not worsen and if fetal growth retardation is not suspected. Bed rest throughout the greater part of the day is essential. Moreover, these women should be examined at least twice weekly, and they should be instructed in detail about reporting symptoms. With minor elevations of blood pressure, the response to this regimen is often immediate, but the woman must be cooperative and the obstetrician wary.

Hospital Management. Hospitalization is considered for women with pregnancy-induced hypertension if there is a sustained elevation in systolic blood pressure to or above 140 mm Hg or a sustained diastolic pressure to or above 90 mm Hg. With hospitalization, a systematic study should be instituted that includes the following:

1. A history and general physical examination followed by daily searches for development of signs and symptoms such as headache, visual disturbances, epigastric pain, and rapid weight gain.
2. Admittance weight and every day thereafter.
3. Admittance analysis for proteinuria and every 2 days thereafter.

4. Blood pressure readings with an appropriate-size cuff every 4 hours, except between midnight and morning, unless the midnight pressure has increased.

5. Measurements of plasma creatinine, hematocrit, platelets, and serum liver enzymes, the frequency to be determined by the severity of hypertension.

6. Frequent evaluation of fetal size and amnionic fluid volume by the same experienced examiner and by serial sonography if remote from term.

If these observations lead to a diagnosis of severe preeclampsia (Table 36–3), further management is the same as described for eclampsia (p. 793).

Bed rest, or at least reduced physical activity, throughout much of the day is beneficial. Ample, but not excessive, protein and calories should be included in the diet. Sodium and fluid intakes should not be limited or forced. Phenobarbital or other sedatives or tranquilizers have been used routinely by some; we do not recommend their use.

Further management of a pregnancy complicated by preeclampsia will depend upon (1) its severity, determined by the presence or absence of the conditions cited in Table 36–3, (2) duration of gestation, and (3) condition of the cervix. Fortunately, many cases prove to be sufficiently mild and near enough to term that they can be managed conservatively until labor commences spontaneously or until the cervix becomes favorable for labor induction. Complete abatement of all signs and symptoms, however, is uncommon until after delivery. *Almost certainly, the underlying disease persists until after delivery!*

Drug Therapy. The use of antihypertensive drugs in attempts to prolong pregnancy or modify perinatal outcomes in pregnancies complicated by various types and severities of hypertensive disorders has been of considerable interest, primarily in Western Europe, since Redman and colleagues (1976) first published their experiences with methyldopa. Theoretically, such antihypertensive therapy has potential usefulness when preeclampsia severe enough to warrant termination of pregnancy develops before neonatal survival is likely. Unfortunately, such management, based upon control of maternal hypertension with agents such as methyldopa and hydralazine, may be catastrophic. Sibai and colleagues (1985b) attempted to prolong pregnancy because of fetal immaturity in 60 women with severe preeclampsia diagnosed between 18 and 27 weeks' gestation. **The total perinatal mortality rate was 87 percent, and although no mothers died, 13 suffered placental abruption, 10 eclampsia, 5 consumptive coagulopathy, 3 renal failure, 2 hypertensive encephalopathy, 1 intracerebral hemorrhage, and 1 a ruptured hepatic hematoma.**

The development of β-blocker drugs has stimulated renewed interest in controlling maternal blood pressure in the interest of improving perinatal outcomes. Gallery and colleagues (1979) compared methyldopa and oxyprenolol and suggested that the latter offered a specific advantage because pregnancies treated with oxyprenolol resulted in infants of greater birthweight. In a randomized controlled study, Plouin and colleagues (1990) found no advantage of oxprenolol over nonpharmacological care in the treatment of a group of mixed-parity women with pregnancy-induced hypertension. Rubin and colleagues (1983) randomized 120 women of mixed parity who were mildly to moderately hypertensive during the last trimester, to be given atenolol or placebo. A total of 85 women completed the trial, and those given atenolol had significantly reduced blood pressures, less frequently developed proteinuria, and had fewer hospital admissions. There were no advantages found for infants born to mothers who completed the trial, and indeed, *the perinatal mortality was 35 per 1000.* The same investigators noted a marked increase in fetal growth retardation in chronically hypertensive women treated with atenolol (Butters and colleagues, 1990).

Collins and Wallenburg (1989) in a meta-analysis of several clinical trials concluded that treatment with β-blocking agents conferred no significant benefit. Redman (1991) went further; he concluded after a scholarly review that β-blocking agents are contraindicated for long-term treatment of hypertension. According to him, β-blocking agents are no more effective than methyldopa, and there is a significant risk of fetal growth retardation. Finally, the addition of other agents to β-blocker therapy apparently does not improve their safety or effectiveness. Constantine and co-workers (1987) reported that if nifedipine was added because of a poor response to atenolol, the perinatal mortality rate was 130 per 1000. Similar results were obtained by Högstedt and associates (1985), who used metoprolol plus hydralazine versus nonpharmacological management; they concluded that drug treatment was not mandatory for a good pregnancy outcome in cases of mild and moderate hypertension.

Plouin and colleagues (1988) reported that labetalol and methyldopa produced similar pregnancy outcomes in a group of women of mixed parity; they did not include a control group. Sibai and associates (1987a) reported their results from a well-designed randomized, comparative study done to evaluate the effectiveness of labetalol and hospitalization alone for 200 nulliparous women with proteinuric hypertension diagnosed between 26 and 35 weeks. Although women given labetalol had significantly lower mean blood pressures, there were no differences between the groups for mean pregnancy prolongation, gestational age at delivery, or birthweight (Table 36–8). The cesarean delivery rates were similar, as were the number of infants admitted to the special-care nurseries. **Importantly, growth-retarded infants were twice as frequent in the women given labetalol, compared with those treated by hospitalization alone (19 versus 9 percent).** In a randomized double-blind controlled trial of labetalol versus placebo, Pickles and associates (1989) observed that labetalol safely reduced blood pressures in a mixed-parity group of women with pregnancy-induced hypertension. They reported no significant fetal growth retardation, but **the incidence of fetal growth retardation was 9 percent in treated compared with 1 percent in controls.**

Phippard and colleagues (1991), in a prospective, randomized double-blind study, compared clonidine plus hydralazine with no drug treatment in 52 hospitalized nulliparous women with early third-trimester pregnancy-induced hypertension. There were no perinatal deaths, and good blood pressure control was obtained in the treated women. Proteinuria was present only in controls. Moreover, the incidence of preterm delivery and respiratory distress was increased in controls compared with treated women. They concluded that this therapy could prevent progression of disease and thereby decrease the incidence of preterm delivery. Although clonidine has been used for some time in pregnancy, there is new evidence that serious sleep disturbances and hyperactivity may develop in animals and children exposed in utero to the drug (Boutroy, 1989; Huisjes and co-workers, 1986; Mirmiran and colleagues, 1983).

Therapy of any pregnant woman with an angiotensin-converting-enzyme (ACE) inhibitor is contraindicated. These agents have been shown to cause fetal death, oligohydramnios, neonatal anuria, renal failure, fetal growth retardation, neonatal hypotension, and persistent ductus arteriosus (Kreft-Jais, 1988; Rosa, 1989; Scott, 1989; Tack, 1988; and their co-workers). In an editorial in the Lancet (Editorial, 1989), a recommendation was made that these agents not be given to pregnant women; we concur.

There have been no published studies that convince us to use antihypertensive drugs in women with pregnancy-induced hypertension in an effort to prolong gestation. With the exception of the studies by Sibai and colleagues (1987a) and Phippard and colleagues (1991), no effort has been made to distinguish pregnancy-induced hypertension from underlying chronic hypertension. Specifically, seldom was preeclampsia in the nullipara considered separately from probable chronic hypertension in the multipara. Importantly, antihypertensive therapy and nonintervention in pregnancies complicated by severe preeclampsia before fetal maturity benefits neither the fetus nor the mother—indeed, it places both in dire jeopardy. Thus, those pregnancies most in need of prolongation appear to be least served by the pharmacological attempt.

Severe Preeclampsia. Occasionally, fulminant or neglected preeclampsia is encountered, with blood pressure recordings in excess of 160/110 mm Hg, edema, and proteinuria. Headache, visual disturbances, or epi-

TABLE 36–8. MILD PREECLAMPSIA IN 200 NULLIPAROUS WOMEN: RESULTS OF TREATMENT WITH HOSPITALIZATION ALONE OR HOSPITALIZATION WITH LABETALOL TREATMENT

Factor	Hospitalization Alone (n = 100)	Hospitalization Plus Labetalol (n = 100)	Signficance
Entry (weeks)	32.4 ± 2.4	32.6 ± 2.4	NS
Delivery	35.5 ± 3.0	35.4 ± 3.0	NS
Prolongation (days)	21.3 ± 13	20.1 ± 14	NS
Blood pressure (means)			
Systolic (initial/treatment)	144/141	142/132[a]	$P < 0.0005$[a]
Diastolic (initial/treatment)	95/95	90/82[a]	$P < 0.005$[a]
Proteinuria (mg/day)			
Initial	565 ± 305	541 ± 303	NS
At delivery	1555 ± 1941	2032 ± 3135	NS
Increased excretion	58%	57%	NS
Decreased excretion	26%	20%	NS
Severe hypertension	15%	5%	$P < 0.05$
Placental abruption	0	2	NS
Cesarean delivery	32%	36%	NS
Perinatal outcomes			
Stillbirths	0	0	NS
Neonatal death	0	1	NS
Birthweight (mean)	2258 ± 762 g	2204 ± 765 g	NS
Fetal growth retardation	9%	19%	$P < .005$

NS = not significant.
[a] Initial blood pressure compared after treatment.
From Sibai and colleagues (1987a).

gastric pain are indicative that convulsions are imminent, and oliguria is another ominous sign. Severe preeclampsia demands anticonvulsant and usually antihypertensive therapy followed by delivery. Treatment is identical to that described below for eclampsia (p. 792). The prime objectives are to forestall convulsions, to prevent intracranial hemorrhage and serious damage to other vital organs, and to deliver a healthy infant.

In more severe cases of preeclampsia, as well as eclampsia, magnesium sulfate administered parenterally is the effective anticonvulsant agent. Magnesium sulfate may be given intramuscularly by intermittent injection or intravenously by continuous infusion. The dosage schedule for severe preeclampsia is the same as for eclampsia (p. 793). Because the period of labor and delivery is a more likely time for convulsions to develop, all women with pregnancy-induced hypertension at Parkland Hospital are treated with intramuscular magnesium sulfate during labor and for 24 hours postpartum. Intravenous hydralazine, administered in small intermittent doses, has proven to be an effective and safe antihypertensive agent. Its use is discussed in more detail below (p. 797).

Invasive cardiovascular monitoring is seldom used at Parkland Hospital even for severe preeclampsia and eclampsia. Such measures are usually reserved for women with accompanying severe cardiac disease and/or renal disease or in cases of refractory hypertension, oliguria, and pulmonary edema. Similar indications are apparently used by Clark and colleagues (1988) and Easterling and associates (1989b).

Conservative Management. Severe preeclampsia warrants consideration of prompt delivery, regardless of fetal age. To allow pregnancy to continue under these circumstances is dangerous for the mother at least, as well as for the fetus, assuming the fetus has reached viability. Cited above (p. 786) were the experiences of Sibai and colleagues (1985b), who delayed delivery in 60 women with severe preeclampsia because of extreme fetal immaturity. The women were managed conservatively with hospitalization, bed rest, and antihypertensive therapy; major life-threatening complications resulted. Fortunately, none of the women died, but more than half of the infants were stillborn. Only 8 neonates survived, resulting in a perinatal mortality of 87 percent.

Glucocorticoids. In attempts to enhance fetal lung maturation, glucocorticoids have been administered to severely hypertensive pregnant women remote from term. Treatment seems not to worsen maternal hypertension, and a decrease in the incidence of respiratory distress and improved fetal survival has been claimed. For example, Nochimson and Petrie (1979) administered betamethasone to 20 severely hypertensive women and

observed no untoward effect. Perinatal survival was 86 percent. Similar results have been reported by Semchyshyn and associates (1983) and Ruvinsky and colleagues (1984).

We do not use corticosteroids in these circumstances for three reasons: (1) their administration poses potential risks to the mother and the fetus-infant; (2) when the mother has severe preeclampsia requiring delivery, severe respiratory distress is uncommon even when the neonate is born preterm; and (3) there is a reduced incidence of germinal matrix hemorrhage even in preterm infants of hypertensive women (Kuban and colleagues, 1992).

Termination of Pregnancy. Delivery is the cure for preeclampsia. When the fetus is known or suspected to be preterm, however, the tendency is widespread to temporize in the hope that a few more weeks in utero will reduce the risk of neonatal death or serious morbidity. Such a policy is justified in milder cases. In severe preeclampsia, procrastination may be ill advised; preeclampsia itself may kill the fetus. Even for the fetus remote from term, the probability of fetal survival may be greater in a well-operated neonatal intensive care unit than in utero.

Assessments of fetal well-being and placental function have been attempted, especially when there is hesitation to deliver the fetus because of prematurity. The use of serial measurements of plasma or urinary estriol, or of placental lactogen, have been abandoned by most. Some recommend frequent performance of various tests currently used to assess fetal well-being, such as the *oxytocin challenge or contraction stress test,* the *biophysical profile,* or the *nonstress test* (see Chap. 45). Although they have not been demonstrated clearly to provide valuable information otherwise unavailable for management of pregnancies complicated by preeclampsia, some of the tests are helpful to verify appropriate fetal growth and amnionic fluid volume.

Failure of the fetus to grow or diminution of amnionic fluid volume, as estimated clinically and by sonography, are ominous signs of fetal jeopardy. Measurement of the lecithin–sphingomyelin ratio in amnionic fluid may provide evidence of lung maturity. Even when this ratio is less than 2.0, however, respiratory distress may not develop; and if it does, it is usually not fatal (see Chap. 44, p. 993).

With moderate or severe preeclampsia that does not improve after hospitalization, delivery is usually advisable for the welfare of both mother and fetus. Labor should be induced by intravenous oxytocin (see Chap. 19, p. 485). In severe cases this is often successful, even when the cervix is judged unfavorable for induction. Whenever it appears that labor induction almost certainly will not succeed, or attempts at induction of labor are not fruitful, cesarean delivery is indicated for the more severe cases. In women with severe preeclampsia and eclampsia, subarachnoid or epidural block for labor–delivery analgesia may induce hypotension detrimental to the fetus, as well as to the mother (see Chap. 16, p. 438). Spinal analgesia is felt to be contraindicated by most authorities, and if epidural analgesia is to be used, it should be administered by a physician with special expertise in obstetrical analgesia.

For a woman near term, with a soft, partially effaced cervix, even milder degrees of preeclampsia probably carry more risk to the mother and her fetus-infant than does induction of labor by carefully monitored oxytocin induction. This is not likely to be the case, however, if the preeclampsia is mild but the cervix is firm and closed, indicating that abdominal delivery might be necessary if pregnancy is to be terminated. The hazard of cesarean delivery may be greater than that of allowing the pregnancy to continue *under close observation* in the hospital until the cervix is more suitable for induction.

High-risk Pregnancy Unit

A high-risk pregnancy unit was established at Parkland Hospital in 1973 to provide care as just described; initial results were reported by Hauth (1976), Gilstrap (1978), and their colleagues. In the latter report 576 nulliparous women, usually teenage and often African-American, had been admitted because of hypertension remote from term. The perinatal mortality rate was 9 per 1000 in the 545 women who remained for care until delivery. In the 31 who left the unit before delivery, although advised not to, perinatal mortality was 130 per 1000. The mean birthweight of the infants whose mothers remained on the unit was 2975 g, with 83 percent weighing 2500 or more.

The majority of women hospitalized had a salutary response characterized by disappearance or improvement of hypertension (Table 36–9). **These women are not "cured," and thus they are not discharged. Indeed, nearly 90 percent of women who became normotensive after hospitalization had recurrent hypertension before or during labor.** Although these women became normotensive following hospitalization, they remained abnormally sensitive to infused angiotensin II (Whalley and colleagues, 1983). Moreover, using the placental clearance rate of dehydroisoandrosterone to estradiol-17β, Worley and colleagues (1975) showed that uteroplacental perfusion stayed persistently decreased despite amelioration of hypertension.

Through 1992, more than 3000 nulliparous women with mild to moderate early-onset pregnancy-induced hypertension have been managed on the High-Risk Pregnancy Unit as described above and with equally good results. The costs of providing the relatively simple physical facility, modest nursing care, no drugs other

TABLE 36–9. BLOOD PRESSURE RESPONSE IN 545 NULLIPAROUS WOMEN WITH PREGNANCY-INDUCED HYPERTENSION HOSPITALIZED ON THE HIGH-RISK PREGNANCY UNIT AT PARKLAND HOSPITAL

Initial Response		No.	(%)
Good			
Diastolic pressure decreased to < 90 mm Hg		441	(81)
Hypertension[a] recurred before labor	183	(41)	
Hypertension recurred during labor	199	(45)	
Remained normotensive through delivery	59	(13)	
Moderate			
Hypertensive[a] intermittently until delivery		70	(13)
Poor			
Hypertension[a] persisted until delivery		34	(6)

[a] Diastolic blood pressure 90 mm Hg or greater.
Modified from Gilstrap and colleagues (1978).

than iron supplement, and the very few laboratory tests that are essential are slight compared with the cost of neonatal intensive care for a preterm infant.

Home Health Care. Some argue that continued hospitalization for management of most women with mild pregnancy-induced hypertension is overly cautious and that further hospitalization is not warranted if hypertension abates within a few days. Unfortunately, many third-party payors even refuse hospital reimbursement under these circumstances. Indeed, many of the results cited above include single teenagers, and perhaps a married couple would be better motivated to have the woman follow instructions regarding limited activity at home. Another approach that has been evaluated on a limited basis is day-care. Tuffnell and colleagues (1992) randomized 54 women with non-proteinuric hypertension after 26 weeks to either day-care or routine management by their individual physicians. Hospitalizations, proteinuric hypertension, and labor inductions were significantly increased in the control group.

If this approach is elected, careful and frequent outpatient visits are mandatory to detect evidence of worsening of hypertension. Zuspan and Rayburn (1991) provided a description of a scheme for blood pressure self-monitoring. Outpatient management of the woman with proteinuric hypertension is not recommended. Because these approaches have never been studied in a systematic fashion, their impact on maternal and fetal morbidity and mortality are only speculative.

Postpartum

After delivery, there is usually rapid improvement, although at times hypertension may worsen transiently. If eclampsia develops, it will most likely occur during the first 24 hours postpartum, although otherwise typical eclampsia has been reported as late as 10 days (Brown and colleagues, 1987). At Parkland Hospital, magnesium sulfate therapy instituted before or during labor is continued for 24 hours postpartum, and intravenous hydralazine is given intermittently, if needed, to lower diastolic blood pressures of 110 mm Hg or higher.

The woman may be discharged, even though still hypertensive, if there is evidence that severe hypertension has abated, and she is otherwise well. Unless hypertension persists at dangerous levels during the puerperium, antihypertensive drugs are not prescribed; instead, the woman is reevaluated in 2 weeks. In those unusual instances where hypertension persists, a thiazide diuretic or a β-blocker drug have proven to be extremely effective and economical. Others recommend methyldopa, or in severe cases a calcium-channel blocker such as verapamil (Belfort and Moore, 1988; Griffis and associates, 1989). With such agents, care must be exercised not to produce profound and symptomatic hypotension in these women, as the pregnancy-induced hypertension spontaneously abates. Typically, but not always, hypertension induced by pregnancy dissipates spontaneously during the first 2 weeks postpartum. If so, the preeclampsia is not a contraindication for oral contraceptives (see Chap. 60, p. 1331). Conversely, hypertension persisting at this time usually signifies chronic vascular disease, often essential hypertension, and close follow-up is necessary to ascertain if antihypertension treatment is indicated or should be continued.

CLINICAL ASPECTS OF ECLAMPSIA

Eclampsia is characterized by generalized tonic–clonic convulsions that develop in some women with hypertension induced or aggravated by pregnancy. Coma without convulsions has also been called eclampsia; however, it is better to limit the diagnosis to women with convulsions and to regard fatal nonconvulsive cases as due to severe preeclampsia. As shown in Table 36–3, convulsions caused by cerebral involvement in pregnancy-induced hypertension are but one manifestation of severe preeclampsia; however, due to its associated high mortality, eclampsia is regarded with particular concern.

Clinical Course

Depending on whether convulsions appear before, during, or after labor, eclampsia is designated as antepartum, intrapartum, or postpartum. Eclampsia is most common in the last trimester and becomes increasingly more frequent as term approaches. Nearly all cases of postpartum eclampsia develop within 24 hours of delivery, but otherwise typical cases are seen up to 10 days

postpartum (Brown and colleagues, 1987). In 254 eclamptic women cared for at the University of Mississippi Medical Center, about 3 percent first developed seizures more than 48 hours postpartum (Miles and associates, 1990). **Another diagnosis should be considered in women with the onset of convulsions more than 48 hours postpartum.**

Almost without exception, preeclampsia precedes the onset of eclamptic convulsions. Isolated cases are occasionally cited of an eclamptic convulsion occurring without warning in women who were apparently in good health. Usually such a woman had not been examined by her physician for some days or—more likely—weeks previously, and she most likely had neglected to report symptoms of preeclampsia. Headache, visual disturbance, and epigastric or right upper quadrant pain are symptoms that should incite grave concern.

The convulsive movements usually begin about the mouth in the form of facial twitchings. After a few seconds, the entire body becomes rigid in a generalized muscular contraction. The face is distorted, the eyes protrude, the arms are flexed, the hands are clenched, and the legs are inverted. All muscles are now in a state of tonic contraction. This phase may persist for 15 to 20 seconds. Suddenly the jaws begin to open and close violently, and soon after, the eyelids as well. The other facial muscles and then all muscles alternately contract and relax in rapid succession. So forceful are the muscular movements that the woman may throw herself out of her bed, and almost invariably, unless protected, her tongue is bitten by the violent action of the jaws (Fig. 36–11). Foam, often blood tinged, exudes from the mouth. The face is congested and the conjunctivae are injected. This phase, in which the muscles alternately contract and relax, may last about a minute. Gradually, the muscular movements become smaller and less frequent, and finally the woman lies motionless. Throughout the seizure the diaphragm has been fixed, with respiration halted. For a few seconds the woman appears to be dying from respiratory arrest, but just when a fatal outcome seems almost inevitable, she takes a long, deep, stertorous inhalation, and breathing is resumed. Coma then ensues. She will not remember the convulsion or, in all probability, events immediately before and afterward.

The first convulsion is usually the forerunner of others, which may vary in number from 1 or 2 in mild cases to even 100 or more in untreated severe cases. In rare instances, convulsions follow one another so rapidly that the woman appears to be in a prolonged, almost continuous convulsion.

The duration of coma after a convulsion is variable. When the convulsions are infrequent, the woman usually recovers some degree of consciousness after each attack. As the woman arouses, a semiconscious combative state may ensue. In very severe cases, the coma persists from one convulsion to another, and death may result before she awakens. In rare instances, a single convulsion may be

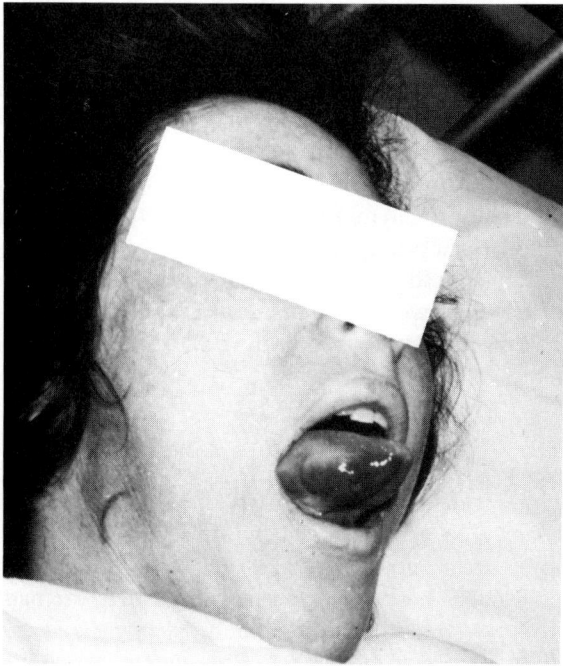

Fig. 36–11. Hematoma of tongue from laceration during eclamptic convulsion. Thrombocytopenia may have contributed to the bleeding.

followed by coma from which the woman may never emerge, although, as a rule, death does not occur until after frequent repetitive convulsions.

Respirations after an eclamptic convulsion are usually increased in rate and may be stertorous. The rate may reach 50 or more per minute, in response presum-

ably to hypercarbia from lactic acid acidemia, as well as to varying intensities of hypoxia. Cyanosis may be observed in severe cases. A temperature of 39° C or more is a very grave sign, because the fever is probably the consequence of a central nervous system hemorrhage.

Proteinuria is almost always present and frequently pronounced. Urine output is likely diminished appreciably, and occasionally anuria develops. Hemoglobinuria is common, but hemoglobinemia is observed only rarely. Some degree of edema is probably present in all women with eclampsia. Often (Fig. 36–12A) the edema is pronounced—at times, massive—but it may also be occult.

As with severe preeclampsia, after delivery an increase in urinary output is usually an early sign of improvement. Proteinuria and edema ordinarily disappear within a week (Fig. 36–12B). In most cases, blood pressure returns to normal within 2 weeks after delivery. The longer hypertension persists postpartum, the more likely that it is the consequence of chronic vascular or renal disease.

In antepartum eclampsia, labor may begin spontaneously shortly after convulsions ensue and progress rapidly to completion, sometimes before the attendants are aware that the unconscious or stuporous woman is having effective uterine contractions. If the attack occurs during labor, contractions may increase in frequency and intensity, and the duration of labor may be shortened. Because of maternal hypoxemia and lactic acidosis caused by convulsions, it is not unusual for fetal bradycardia to follow a seizure. This usually recovers within 3 to 5 minutes; if it persists more than 10 min-

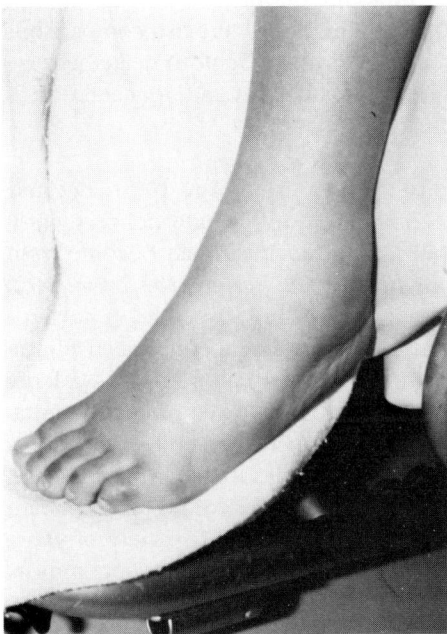

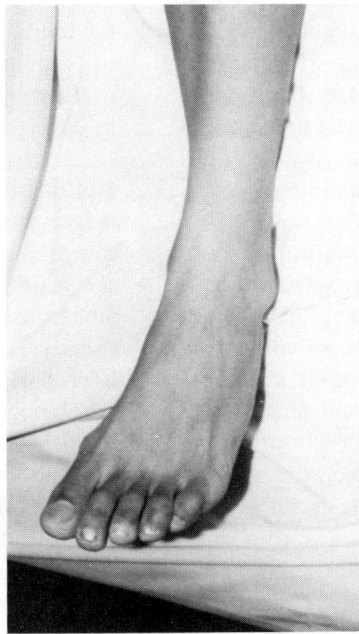

Fig. 36–12. A. Severe edema in a young primigravida with antepartum eclampsia and a markedly reduced blood volume compared with normal pregnancy. **B.** The same woman 3 days after delivery. The remarkable clearance of pedal edema, accompanied by diuresis and a 28-pound weight loss, was spontaneous and unprovoked by any diuretic therapy. (From Cunningham and Pritchard, 1984.)

A   **B**

utes, another cause must be considered, such as rapid labor or placental abruption.

> Very uncommonly, convulsions cease, the coma disappears, labor does not commence, and the woman becomes completely oriented. This improved state may continue for several days or longer, a condition known as *intercurrent eclampsia* (López-Llera, 1992). It has been claimed that such pregnancies may return entirely to normal with complete regression of hypertension and proteinuria, but such an event appears to be exceeding rare. Although convulsions and coma may subside entirely and blood pressure and proteinuria may decrease, most women continue to show substantial evidence of disease and are likely to convulse again unless they are given anticonvulsant treatment, and are delivered. A second attack may be much more severe than the first.

Pulmonary edema, which is a grave prognostic sign, may follow eclamptic convulsions. There are at least two sources. (1) Aspiration pneumonitis may follow inhalation of gastric contents if simultaneous vomiting accompanies convulsions. (2) Cardiac failure may be the result of a combination of severe hypertension and vigorous intravenous fluid administration.

In some women with eclampsia, sudden death occurs synchronously with a convulsion or follows shortly thereafter, as the result of a massive cerebral hemorrhage. Hemiplegia may result from sublethal hemorrhage. Cerebral hemorrhages are more likely in older women with underlying chronic hypertension; more rarely, they may be due to a ruptured berry aneurysm or arteriovenous malformation. Rarely, coma or substantively altered consciousness follows a seizure, or may even accompany preeclampsia without convulsions. At least in some cases (Fig. 36–10) this is due to extensive cerebral edema (Brown and colleagues, 1988a). The prognosis in our limited experience has been quite good, provided that a ruptured vessel is not the cause of the coma and appropriate supportive care is given until the woman regains consciousness. Uncal herniation also may cause death.

Blindness may follow a seizure, or it may arise spontaneously with preeclampsia (see p. 781). There are at least two causes: (1) varying degrees of retinal detachment; and (2) occipital lobe, ischemia, or infarction. Whether due to cerebral or retinal pathology, the prognosis for return of normal vision is good and usually complete within a week.

Rarely, eclampsia is followed by psychosis, and the woman becomes violent. This usually lasts for several days to 2 weeks, but the prognosis for return to normal is good, provided there was no preexisting mental illness. Chlorpromazine in carefully titrated doses has proved effective in the few cases of posteclampsia psychosis treated at Parkland Hospital.

Differential Diagnosis. Generally, eclampsia is much more likely to be diagnosed too frequently rather than overlooked, because epilepsy, encephalitis, meningitis, cerebral tumor, ruptured cerebral aneurysm, and even hysteria during late pregnancy and the puerperium may simulate eclampsia. Consequently, such conditions should be borne in mind whenever convulsions or coma develop during pregnancy, labor, or the puerperium, and they should be excluded. **Until other causes are excluded, however, all pregnant women with convulsions should be considered to be eclamptics.**

Treatment of Eclampsia

Treatment of eclampsia consists of (1) control of convulsions, (2) correction of hypoxia and acidosis, (3) blood pressure control, and (4) delivery after control of convulsions. Once delivery is accomplished, the pathological changes of eclampsia soon disappear and eventually are reversed completely. This generalization holds true for dysfunctions of the central nervous system, liver, and kidneys; for hematological abnormalities including thrombocytopenia and intense hemolysis; and usually for subsequent pregnancies.

Prognosis. The prognosis for eclampsia is always serious; this is one of the most dangerous conditions that can afflict a pregnant woman and her fetus. Fortunately, maternal mortality due to eclampsia has fallen in the past 3 decades. The maternal mortality rate reported since World War II for various methods of treatment applied in several countries is summarized in Table 36–10. In these reports, maternal mortality has ranged from less than 1 percent to as much as nearly 20 percent. At the same time, the perinatal mortality rate has ranged from 130 to 300 per 1000. Precise comparisons of perinatal mortality rates are difficult to make because of different definitions of stillbirths and neonatal deaths in different countries.

Historical Considerations. In the late 1920s, because of very poor outcomes from immediate delivery without medical stabilization, the slogan had become *treat the eclampsia medically and ignore the pregnancy.* Since this time, almost every drug suspected of having a sedative, hypotensive, or diuretic effect has been administered to the eclamptic woman (and her fetus). A large combination of drugs was usually employed simultaneously. Convulsions often were controlled, but coma persisted due to the medications rather than the disease. As the consequence of such empirical therapy, women with eclampsia have been treated in a variety of ways, especially in institutions where eclampsia is uncommon. Finally, without an organized plan in the hands of experienced health care teams, eclampsia is still a deadly disease (Redman, 1988). An example of this is the fail-

TABLE 36–10. MATERNAL MORTALITY FROM ECLAMPSIA

Authors	Treatment	Patients (no.)	Maternal Deaths (%)
Dewar and Morris (1947)	Tribromoethanol	44	4.5
Browne (1950)	Thiopental	26	7.6
Shears (1957)	Lytic cocktail	124	8.8
Menon (1961)	Lytic cocktail[a]	402	2.2
Llewellyn-Jones (1961)	Lytic cocktail	150	6.6
Bryant and Fleming (1962)	Magnesium sulfate and veratrum alkaloids	253	1.6
Zuspan and Ward (1964)	Magnesium sulfate	59	3.4
López-Llera (1982)			
A (1967)	Lytic cocktail	108	10.2
B (1970)	Lytic cocktail	120	11.7
C (1973)	Diazepam + reserpine	137	17.5
D (1976)	Furosemide, reserpine + volume expansion (albumin) + antithrombotic	160	12.5
E (1979)	Barbiturates + magnesium sulfate + reserpine and/or isoxsuprine	179	16.2
Total: A-E (1967–1979)	Those listed in A–E	704	13.9
Lean and co-workers (1968)	Chlordiazepoxide	90[b]	3.3
	Diazepam	60	5.0
Kawathekar and associates (1973)	Diazepam	16	6.3
Mojadidi and Thompson (1973)	Morphine + magnesium sulfate	30	6.7
Gedekoh and colleagues (1981)	Magnesium sulfate + hydralazine	52	5.8
Pritchard and associates (1984)	Magnesium sulfate + hydralazine + standardized regimen	245	0.4
Sibai and associates (1990a)	Magnesium sulfate + hydralazine	254	0.4

[a] Chlorpromazine, diethazine, and meperidine.
[b] Includes postpartum eclampsia (up to 14 days).

ure to decrease maternal mortality due to eclampsia in the United Kingdom between 1970 and 1981; three fourths of 36 maternal mortalities could have been prevented (Turnbull, 1987). Van Assche and colleagues (1989) also have presented a persuasive argument in favor of a consistent and effective management plan for the treatment of eclampsia.

Parkland Hospital Eclampsia Regimen

In 1955 Pritchard initiated a standardized treatment regimen at Parkland Hospital, and this has been used since then to manage women with eclampsia. The carefully analyzed results of treatment of 245 cases of eclampsia, typically the severest form of pregnancy-induced or -aggravated hypertension, were reported by Pritchard and associates in 1984. The specific plan of management is summarized below.

1. Control of convulsions with magnesium sulfate, using an intravenously administered loading dose and periodic intramuscular injections standardized in dose and frequency of administration.
2. Intermittent intravenous injections of hydralazine to lower blood pressure whenever the diastolic pressure is 110 mm Hg or higher.
3. Avoidance of diuretics and hyperosmotic agents.

4. Limitation of intravenous fluid administration unless fluid loss is excessive.
5. Delivery.

Magnesium Sulfate to Control Convulsions. Magnesium sulfate is used to arrest and prevent convulsions due to eclampsia without producing generalized central nervous system depression in either the mother or the fetus-infant. **Magnesium sulfate is not given to treat hypertension.** Based on the studies of Borges and Gücer (1978) cited below, as well as extensive clinical observations, the drug most likely exerts a rather specific anticonvulsant action on the cerebral cortex. Typically, the mother stops convulsing after the initial administration of magnesium sulfate, and within an hour or two regains consciousness sufficiently to be oriented as to place and time.

The magnesium sulfate dosage schedule is presented in Table 36–11, and the response in plasma magnesium levels is illustrated in Figure 36–13. Using this regimen, there has been no evidence of neonatal depression due to magnesium intoxication. In the unusual case in which the initial dose of 4 g intravenously plus 10 g intramuscularly has not arrested eclamptic convulsions, 2 g more, as a 20 percent solution, has been administered slowly intravenously. In a small woman, an additional 2 g dose may be used once, and twice if needed in a larger woman. In only 5 of the 245 women with eclampsia was it necessary to use supplementary medi-

TABLE 36–11. MAGNESIUM SULFATE DOSAGE SCHEDULE FOR SEVERE PREECLAMPSIA AND ECLAMPSIA

1. Give 4 g of magnesium sulfate (MgSO$_4$·7H$_2$O, USP) as a 20% solution intravenously at a rate not to exceed 1 g/min.
2. Follow promptly with 10 g of 50% magnesium sulfate solution, one half (5 g) injected deeply in the upper outer quadrant of both buttocks through a 3-inch-long 20-gauge needle. (Addition of 1.0 mL of 2% lidocaine minimizes discomfort.)

   If convulsions persist after 15 minutes, give up to 2 g more intravenously as a 20% solution at a rate not to exceed 1 g/min. If the woman is large, up to 4 g may be given slowly.
3. Every 4 hours thereafter give 5 g of a 50% solution of magnesium sulfate injected deeply in the upper outer quadrant of alternate buttocks, but only after assuring that
   a. The patellar reflex is present.
   b. Respirations are not depressed.
   c. Urine output the previous 4 hours exceeded 100 mL.
4. Magnesium sulfate is discontinued 24 hours after delivery.

cation to control convulsions. The agent used was sodium amobarbital given slowly intravenously in doses up to 250 mg. Maintenance magnesium sulfate therapy for eclampsia is continued intramuscularly every 4 hours for 24 hours after delivery. For eclampsia that develops postpartum, magnesium sulfate is administered for 24 hours after the onset of convulsions.

Parenterally administered magnesium is cleared almost totally by renal excretion, and magnesium intoxication is avoided by ensuring that before each dose (1) urine flow was at least 100 mL during the previous 4 hours, (2) the patellar reflex is present, and (3) there is no respiratory depression. Eclamptic convulsions are almost always prevented by plasma magnesium levels

maintained at 4 to 7 mEq/L. As discussed below, loss of the patellar reflex begins with plasma levels of 8 to 10 mEq/L and, importantly, respiratory arrest occurs at levels of 12 mEq/L or more. Calcium gluconate, 1 g **administered slowly** intravenously, and oxygen usually suffice for treatment of respiratory depression. If respiratory arrest occurs, prompt tracheal intubation and ventilation are lifesaving (McCubbin and associates, 1981).

Impaired Renal Function. Because magnesium is cleared almost exclusively by renal excretion, plasma magnesium concentration, using the doses described above, will be excessive if glomerular filtration is decreased substantively. Renal function is estimated by measuring plasma creatinine, and whenever it is 1.3 mg/dL or higher, we give only half of the maintenance magnesium sulfate dose outlined in Table 36–11. Thus, the woman with eclampsia who has impaired renal function is given a loading dose of 4 g intravenously in addition to the 10 g intramuscular dose, to be followed by 2.5 g intramuscularly every 4 hours. As shown in Figure 36–14, plasma magnesium levels are usually within the desired range of 4 to 7 mEq/L. Some prefer in these circumstances to give magnesium sulfate intravenously by continuous infusion. **With either method, when there is renal insufficiency, plasma magnesium levels must be checked periodically.**

PHARMACOLOGY AND TOXICOLOGY OF MAGNESIUM SULFATE. Magnesium sulfate USP is MgSO$_4$·7H$_2$O and not MgSO$_4$. When administered as described, the drug will practically always arrest eclamptic convulsions and prevent their recurrence. The initial intravenous infusion of 4 g

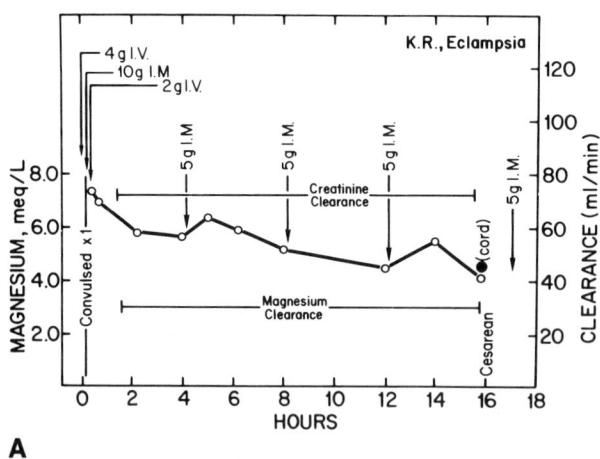

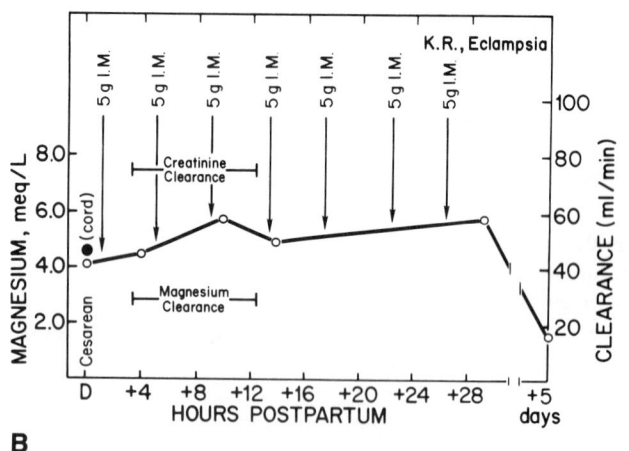

Fig. 36–13. A. Plasma magnesium levels are plotted for a woman with antepartum eclampsia in whom 4 g of magnesium sulfate intravenously and 10 g intramuscularly were administered at the outset. When she soon convulsed again, 2 g more were injected slowly followed by 5 g intramuscularly every 4 hours, as described in Table 36–11. She did not convulse again. **B.** The same woman as in **A.** Maternal magnesium levels during the first 28 hours postpartum and 4 days after magnesium sulfate was discontinued are plotted. Before and the day after delivery the renal clearance of magnesium remained relatively constant at about 35 percent of the somewhat depressed creatinine clearance. The mother recovered fully and the baby thrived. (From Pritchard and associates, 1984.)

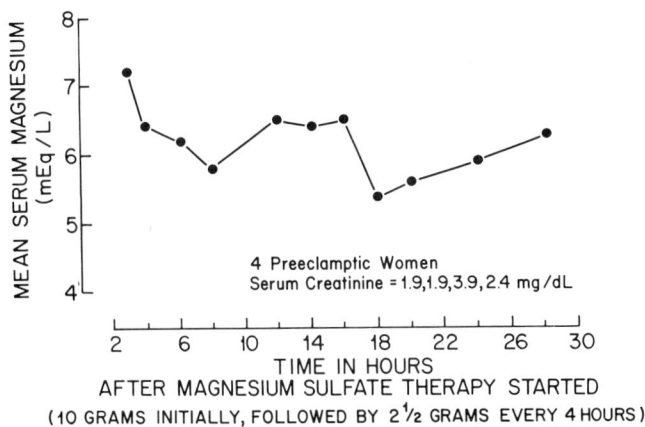

Fig. 36–14. Plasma magnesium levels in 4 women with chronic renal insufficiency. These women were given half of the usual maintenance dose.

is used to establish a prompt therapeutic level that is maintained by the nearly simultaneous intramuscular injection of 10 g of the compound, followed by 5 g intramuscularly every 4 hours, as long as there is no evidence of potentially dangerous hypermagnesemia. With this dosage schedule, therapeutically effective plasma levels of 4 to 7 mEq/L are achieved compared with pretreatment plasma levels of less than 2.0 mEq/L (Chesley and Tepper, 1957; Stone and Pritchard, 1970). Magnesium sulfate injected deeply into the upper outer quadrant of the buttocks, as described above, has not resulted in erratic absorption and consequent erratic plasma levels.

Sibai and co-workers (1984) performed a prospective study in which they compared continuous intravenous magnesium sulfate and intramuscular magnesium sulfate. There was no significant difference between mean magnesium levels observed after intramuscular magnesium sulfate and those observed following a maintenance intravenous infusion of 2 g/hour. However, the intramuscular regimen resulted in serum magnesium levels that were significantly higher than those obtained with a continuous intravenous maintenance dose of 1 g/hour (Fig. 36–15). It was concluded that there was no therapeutic advantage to the intravenous route of administration except for the avoidance of pain at the intramuscular injection site. When given intravenously, magnesium sulfate should be delivered by an infusion pump, and careful attention must be given to the solution concentration and the rate of delivery. Most recommend that 2 g/hour be given, to be followed by serial magnesium determinations to avoid toxicity. We favor the intramuscular route because of its safety.

Patellar reflexes disappear when the plasma magnesium level reaches 10 mEq/L, presumably because of a curariform action. This sign serves to warn of impending magnesium toxicity, because a further increase will lead to respiratory depression. Plasma cholinesterase activity

is decreased substantively in preeclamptic women, but this is not altered further by magnesium therapy (Kambam and associates, 1988).

When plasma levels rise above 10 mEq/L, respiratory depression develops, and at 12 mEq/L or more, respiratory paralysis and arrest follow. Treatment with calcium gluconate, 1 g intravenously, along with the withholding of magnesium sulfate usually reverses mild to moderate respiratory depression. Unfortunately, the effects of intravenously administered calcium may be short lived. For severe respiratory depression and arrest, prompt tracheal intubation and mechanical ventilation are lifesaving. Direct toxic effects on the myocardium from high levels of magnesium are very uncommon. In humans, it appears that a major cause of cardiac dysfunction is due to hypoxia, the consequence of respiratory arrest, rather than a direct effect of magnesium. With appropriate ventilation, cardiac action is satisfactory even when plasma levels are exceedingly high (McCubbin and associates, 1981).

Parenterally injected magnesium is filtered through the glomerulus and variably reabsorbed by the tubule. As plasma magnesium concentration increases, more magnesium is filtered and less is reabsorbed. Nonetheless, when glomerular filtration is impaired, so is magnesium clearance. Therefore, an appreciably elevated plasma creatinine level serves to warn of diminished capacity of the kidney to excrete magnesium (Fig. 36–14). Despite its antidiuretic action, concomitant oxytocin administration

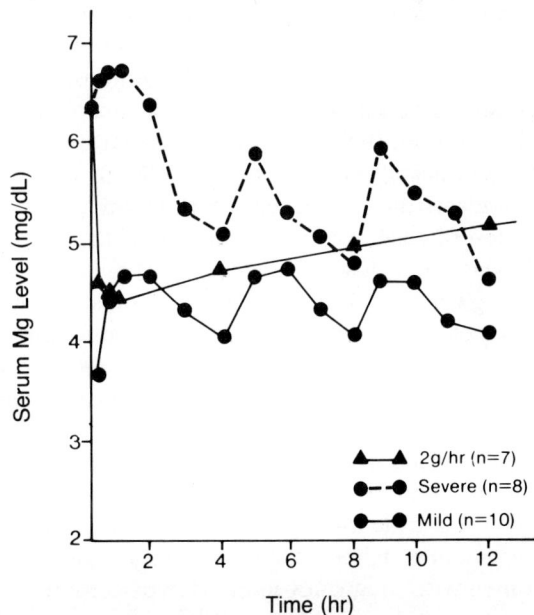

Fig. 36–15. Comparison of serum magnesium levels following (1) mild preeclampsia—10-g intramuscular loading dose of magnesium sulfate and a 5-g maintenance dose every 4 hours (● – ●), (2) severe preeclampsia—4-g intravenous loading dose followed by the same regimen as in (1) (● – – ●); compared with (3) 4-g intravenous loading dose followed by a continuous infusion of a 2 g per hour (▲–▲). (From Sibai and co-workers, 1984, with permission.)

does not alter plasma magnesium levels (Bloss and colleagues, 1987). A fraction of the injected magnesium is deposited reversibly into surface bone.

The acute cardiovascular effects of parenteral magnesium ion in women with severe preeclampsia have been studied by Cotton and associates (1984), who obtained data using pulmonary and radial artery catheterization. Following a 4-g intravenous dose given over 15 minutes, mean arterial blood pressure fell slightly, and this was accompanied by a 13 percent increase in cardiac index. Thus, magnesium decreased systemic vascular resistance and mean arterial pressure, and at the same time increased cardiac output, without evidence of myocardial depression. These findings were coincidental with transient nausea and flushing, and the cardiovascular effects persisted for only 15 minutes despite continued infusion of magnesium sulfate at 1.5 g/hour.

In monkeys with angiotensin-induced hypertension late in pregnancy, Harbert and co-workers (1969) demonstrated slightly increased uterine blood flow in response to the infusion of magnesium sulfate. At the same time, arterial blood pressure decreased minimally. Thiagarajah and colleagues (1985) infused magnesium into nonpregnant monkeys and found that while cardiac output was unchanged, uterine blood flow increased by 20 percent. They concluded that this was due to selectively decreased uterine vascular resistance.

Altura and colleagues (1983) observed that when isolated umbilical arteries and veins obtained from normal term infants were incubated with 0 to 9.6 mmol/L of magnesium, basal tension of the vessels increased in the absence of magnesium and decreased as the concentration of magnesium increased. They also observed that the absence of magnesium potentiated the contractile response of the vessels to bradykinin, angiotensin II, serotonin, and prostaglandin $F_{2\alpha}$. Watson and colleagues (1986) reported the effects of magnesium on cultured human umbilical vein endothelial cells. In concentrations similar to those achieved in plasma with therapeutic doses described above, magnesium stimulated prostacyclin release in a dose-dependent fashion. Plasma from women given magnesium sulfate therapy stimulated a two- to fivefold increase in prostacyclin production, compared with pretherapy plasma. Presumably also mediated by prostacyclin, magnesium enhanced the platelet aggregation inhibition characteristic of endothelial cells. In contrast, O'Brien and colleagues (1990) questioned the alleged magnesium stimulation of prostacyclin because they could not identify an increased renal excretion of prostaglandin metabolites following magnesium therapy in women with pregnancy-induced hypertension.

Somjen and co-workers (1966) induced in themselves, by intravenous infusion, marked hypermagnesemia, achieving plasma levels up to 15 mEq/L. **Predictably, at such high plasma levels, respiratory depression developed that necessitated mechanical ventilation, but depression of the sensorium**

was not dramatic as long as hypoxia was prevented. Thurnau and colleagues (1987) showed that there was a small but highly significant increase in cerebrospinal fluid magnesium concentration after magnesium therapy for preeclampsia. The magnitude of the increase was directly proportional to the corresponding serum concentration. Borges and Gücer (1978) provided convincing evidence that the magnesium ion exerts an effect on the central nervous system much more specific than generalized depression. They measured the actions of parenterally administered magnesium sulfate on epileptic neural activity induced in awake, unmedicated subhuman primates. The infused magnesium sulfate suppressed neuronal burst firing and interictal electroencephalographic spike generation in neuronal populations rendered epileptic by topically applied penicillin G. The degree of suppression increased as the plasma magnesium concentration increased and decreased as it fell. Therefore, even though elevated concentrations of plasma magnesium inhibit acetylcholine release in response to motor nerve impulses, reduce motor end-plate sensitivity to acetylcholine, and decrease motor end-plate potential, these actions do not account for, nor should they necessarily be implicated in, the explanation of the beneficial effects of magnesium sulfate in controlling the convulsions of eclampsia.

Goldman and Finkbeiner (1988) attribute therapeutic effects to neuronal calcium influx blocking through the glutamate channel. Cotton and associates (1992) induced seizure activity in the hippocampus region of rats because it is a region with a low seizure threshold and a high density of N-methyl-D-aspartate receptors. These receptors are linked to various models of epilepsy and can be blocked by magnesium. Because the hippocampal seizures could be blocked by magnesium, the investigators believed that this implicated the N-methyl-D-aspartate receptor in eclamptic seizures. Magnesium, therefore, has a central nervous system effect in blocking seizures.

Interestingly—and indeed, amazingly—Donaldson (1986, 1989) and other neurologists, for reasons that are hard to discern, have erroneously emphasized that magnesium sulfate is a peripherally acting anticonvulsant and therefore "bad medicine." They imply that the drug works only in concentrations that cause paralysis, and that consequently the woman with eclampsia so treated is "quiet on the outside but still convulsing on the inside." This conclusion obviously was not based on any direct experience with eclampsia and its control with parenterally administered magnesium! At the same time, Donaldson has urged other forms of anticonvulsant therapy, but cites no data. Most other drugs that effectively arrest and prevent eclamptic convulsions also cause appreciable general depression of the central nervous system in both mother and newborn. Donaldson (1986) later concluded that convulsions result from inability of cerebral blood flow autoregulation, and that nitroprusside, diazoxide, or hydralazine will prevent most seizures. Although dangerous hypertension most certainly must be treated, we have prevented further convulsions in more than 300 women with eclampsia by using magnesium sulfate as described, but perhaps only one third or so were given hydralazine to lower dangerously elevated blood pressure.

Magnesium ions in relatively high concentration will depress myometrial contractility both in vivo and in vitro. With the regimen described above and the plasma levels that have resulted, no evidence of myometrial depression has been observed beyond a transient decrease in activity during and immediately after the initial intravenous loading dose. Typically, as the cutaneous flushing from the intravenous dose disappeared, uterine activity returned to preinjection intensity.

Magnesium ions administered parenterally to the mother promptly cross the placenta to achieve equilibrium between mother and fetus. With a single large intravenous dose, but not with smaller doses, magnesium sulfate may transiently cause a loss of fetal heart rate beat-to-beat variability (Pritchard, 1979). Lenox and associates (1990) did not identify consistent fetal heart rate pattern changes with magnesium sulfate therapy in their series of hypertensive patients. The neonate may be depressed by magnesium only if *severe* hypermagnesemia exists at delivery. We have not observed neonatal compromise after intramuscular therapy with magnesium sulfate (Stone and Pritchard, 1970; Cunningham and Pritchard, 1984), nor have Green and associates (1983). The regimen used at Parkland Hospital, coupled with the safeguards observed before each injection, have prevented worrisome adverse effects from hypermagnesemia in newborns.

Hydralazine to Control Severe Hypertension.

Hydralazine is given intravenously whenever the diastolic blood pressure is 110 mm Hg or higher. It is administered in 5- to 10-mg doses at 15- to 20-minute intervals until a satisfactory response is achieved. A satisfactory response antepartum or intrapartum is defined as a decrease in diastolic blood pressure to 90 to 100 mm Hg, but not lower lest placental perfusion be compromised.

Hydralazine so administered has proven remarkably effective, and importantly, cerebral hemorrhage has been avoided. At Parkland Hospital, approximately 8 percent of all women with pregnancy-induced hypertension are given hydralazine as described; this drug has been administered to more than 3000 women to control acute peripartum hypertension. In none of these women was another antihypertensive agent needed because of poor response to hydralazine. In most European centers, hydralazine is also favored (Naden and Redman, 1985).

The tendency to give a larger initial dose of hydralazine when the blood pressure is higher must be avoided. The response to even 5- to 10-mg doses cannot be predicted by the level of hypertension; thus we always give 5 mg as the initial dose. An example of very severe hypertension in a woman with chronic hypertension complicated by superimposed eclampsia that responded to repeated intravenous injections of hydralazine is shown in Table 36–12. Hydralazine was injected more frequently than recommended in the protocol, and blood pressure decreased in less than 1 hour from 240–270/130–150 mm Hg to 110/80 mm Hg. Ominous fetal heart rate decelerations were evident when the pressure fell to 110/80 mm Hg, and the decelerations persisted until maternal blood pressure increased.

Other Antihypertensive Agents. Intravenously administered diazoxide has been championed by some for use in preeclampsia–eclampsia because of its very potent antihypertensive action. Unfortunately, intravenous diazoxide therapy is accompanied by many adverse side effects. For example, it likely is to arrest labor. It causes retention of sodium, water, and uric acid, and it causes serious hyperglycemia in mother and neonate. Importantly, it may produce irreversible, and therefore lethal, hypotension when administered with or after other antihypertensive agents. Diazoxide is seldom used in the United States, although some nonobstetricians continue to recommend it. The drug is used in the United Kingdom for blood pressure control, although it is reserved for the most extreme situations (Naden and Redman, 1985; Rubin, 1986). Undoubtedly many of the serious adverse reactions reported were associated with the standard 300-mg bolus dose recommended for nonpregnant patients; titration using intermittent small boluses of 30 to 60 mg is apparently safer. Diazoxide is not needed because hydralazine, given as described above, is effective.

A variety of other agents, such as nitroglycerin,

TABLE 36–12. INTRAVENOUS HYDRALAZINE FOR ACUTE CONTROL OF SEVERE HYPERTENSION

Time	Blood Pressure (mm Hg)	Fetal Condition
1140	240/150	Normal fetal heart rate
1145	Magnesium sulfate, 4 g IV and 10 g IM	
1155	270/130	
1156	Hydralazine, 5-mg IV bolus	
1200	200/120	
1201	Hydralazine, 5-mg IV bolus	
1205	230/130	
1206	Hydralazine, 10-mg IV bolus	
1210	185/120	
1220	180/120	
1221	Hydralazine, 5-mg IV bolus	
1230	150/105	
1235	150/105	
1250	110/80	Fetal bradycardia
1310	130/90	
1345	130/100	Return to normal
1430	150/105	of fetal heart
1500	150/90	rate

prazosin, and some β-blockers, have been used for acute hypertension control (Cotton and colleagues, 1986; Rubin, 1986). Mabie and associates (1987) compared intravenous hydralazine to labetalol for blood pressure control in 60 peripartum women with severe pregnancy-associated hypertension. Labetalol lowered blood pressure more rapidly, and associated tachycardia was minimal, but hydralazine lowered mean arterial pressure to safe levels more effectively. We have evaluated labetalol given intravenously for women with severe preeclampsia and our results are very similar.

Mabie and colleagues (1988b) later evaluated nifedipine administered sublingually to 34 women with peripartum hypertension. Because its antihypertensive effects were potent and rapid, 2 women developed worrisome hypotension. Toppozada and co-workers (1988) infused prostaglandin A_1 to lower blood pressure.

Persistent Postpartum Hypertension. The potential problem of antihypertensive agents causing serious compromise of placental perfusion and fetal well-being is obviated by delivery. If there is a problem after delivery in controlling severe hypertension and intravenous hydralazine is being used repeatedly early in the puerperium to control persistent severe hypertension, then intramuscular hydralazine is administered, usually in 10 mg doses at 4- to 6-hour intervals. Rarely are larger doses needed. Once repeated blood pressure readings remain near normal, hydralazine is stopped. If hypertension of appreciable intensity persists or recurs *in these postpartum women*, oral labetalol or a thiazide diuretic are given for as long as necessary. The persistence or refractoriness of hypertension is likely due to at least two mechanisms: (1) underlying chronic hypertension and/or (2) mobilization of edema fluid with redistribution into the intravenous compartment. Labetalol and a diuretic are effective treatment for both mechanisms.

Avoidance of Diuretics and Hyperosmotic Agents.
Potent diuretics further compromise placental perfusion, because their immediate effects include further intravascular volume depletion, which most often is already reduced compared with normal pregnancy (Shoemaker and colleagues, 1973; Gant and associates, 1975, 1976). Therefore, diuretics are not used to lower blood pressure lest they enhance the intensity of the maternal hemoconcentration and its adverse effects on the mother and the fetus (Zondervan and associates, 1988).

Once delivery is accomplished, in almost all cases of severe preeclampsia and eclampsia there is a spontaneous diuresis that usually begins within 24 hours and results in the disappearance of excessive extravascular extracellular fluid over the next 3 to 4 days, as demonstrated in Figure 36–12.

With infusion of hyperosmotic agents, the potential exists for an appreciable intravascular influx of fluid and, in turn, subsequent escape of intravascular fluid in the form of edema into vital organs, especially the lungs and brain. Moreover, an oncotically active agent that leaks through capillaries into lungs and brain promotes accumulation of edema at these sites. Most importantly, a sustained beneficial effect from their use has not been demonstrated. For all of these reasons, hyperosmotic agents have not been administered, and use of furosemide or similar drugs has been limited to the rare instances in which pulmonary edema was identified or strongly suspected.

Fluid Therapy. Lactated Ringer solution containing 5 percent dextrose, usually has been administered routinely at the rate of 60 mL to no more than 125 mL/hour unless there was unusual fluid loss from vomiting, diarrhea, or diaphoresis, or more likely, excessive blood loss at delivery. Oliguria, common in cases of severe preeclampsia and eclampsia, coupled with the knowledge that maternal blood volume is very likely constricted compared with normal pregnancy, makes it tempting to administer intravenous fluids more vigorously. The rationale for controlled, conservative fluid administration is that the typical eclamptic woman already has excessive extracellular fluid that is inappropriately distributed between the intravascular and extravascular spaces of the extracellular fluid compartment. Infusion of large fluid volumes could and does enhance the maldistribution of extracellular fluid and thereby appreciably increases the risk of pulmonary and cerebral edema (Benedetti and Quilligan, 1980b; Gedekoh and associates, 1981; Sibai and co-workers, 1981, 1987b).

Pulmonary Edema. Women with severe preeclampsia–eclampsia who develop pulmonary edema most often do so postpartum (Benedetti and colleagues, 1985; Cunningham and associates, 1986; Sibai and co-workers, 1987b). Aspiration of gastric contents, the result of convulsions or perhaps from anesthesia, should be excluded; however, the majority of these women have cardiac failure. Some normal pregnancy changes, magnified by preeclampsia, predispose to pulmonary edema. Importantly, and as discussed in Chapter 47 (p. 1071), plasma oncotic pressure decreases appreciably in normal term pregnancy because of decreases in serum albumin, and oncotic pressure falls even more with preeclampsia (Benedetti and Carlson, 1979; Zinaman and co-workers, 1985). Moreover, Oian and colleagues (1985, 1986) described increased extravascular fluid oncotic pressure in preeclamptic women, and this favors capillary fluid extravasation. Brown and associates (1989) verified increased capillary permeability in preeclamptic women. Bhatia and associates (1987) reported a correlation between plasma colloid osmotic pressure and fibronectin concentration; this suggested to them that vascular protein loss was the result of increased vascular permeability caused by vessel injury.

The frequent findings of hemoconcentration, and

more recently the identification of reduced central venous and pulmonary capillary wedge pressures in women with severe preeclampsia, have tempted some obstetricians to infuse various fluids, albumin concentrates, or both, in attempts to expand blood volume and thereby somehow to relieve vasospasm and reverse organ deterioration. Thus far, clear-cut evidence of benefits from this approach is lacking; however, serious complications, especially pulmonary edema, have been reported. López-Llera (1982) reported that vigorous volume expansion was associated with the highest incidence of pulmonary edema in his series of more than 700 eclamptic women. Benedetti and colleagues (1985) described pulmonary edema in 7 of 10 severely preeclamptic women who were given colloid therapy. Sibai and colleagues (1987b) cited excessive colloid and crystalloid infusions as causing most of 37 cases of pulmonary edema associated with severe preeclampsia–eclampsia. Finally, Lehmann and co-workers (1987) reported that pulmonary edema caused nearly one third of maternal deaths due to pregnancy-associated hypertension at Charity Hospital.

For these reasons, until it is understood how to contain more fluid within the intravascular compartment and, at the same time, less fluid outside the intravascular compartment, we remain convinced that, in the absence of marked fluid loss, fluids can be administered safely only in moderation. To date, no serious adverse effects have been observed from such a policy. Importantly, dialysis for renal failure was not required for any of the 245 cases of eclampsia so managed (Pritchard and colleagues, 1984). By comparison, in one large European renal dialysis center, eclampsia was identified as the leading associated cause of acute renal failure among women (Silke and co-workers, 1980). Finally, in the majority of eclamptic women managed at Parkland Hospital, sufficient follow-up has been achieved to establish that either normal renal function returned, or in those women with preexisting impaired renal function, subsequent plasma creatinine levels were no higher than before.

Invasive Hemodynamic Monitoring. As summarized in Table 36–5, much of what has been learned within the past decade about cardiovascular and hemodynamic pathophysiological alterations associated with severe preeclampsia–eclampsia has been made possible by invasive hemodynamic monitoring using a flow-directed pulmonary artery catheter. The need for clinical implementation of such technology for the woman with preeclampsia–eclampsia, however, has not been established. The subject has been reviewed by Hankins and Cunningham (1991), Wasserstrum and Cotton (1986), and Clark and Cotton (1988). Two conditions frequently cited as indications for such monitoring are preeclampsia associated with oliguria and preeclampsia associated with pulmonary edema. Perhaps somewhat paradoxically, it is usually vigorous treatment of the

former that results in most cases of the latter! The American College of Obstetricians and Gynecologists (1988a) does not list severe preeclampsia–eclampsia as an indication for pulmonary artery catheterization.

Because vigorous intravenous hydration and osmotically active agents are avoided at Parkland Hospital in women with severe preeclampsia and eclampsia, hemodynamic monitoring has not been used for the vast majority of these women. Oliguria associated with preeclampsia, unless also associated with blood loss, will improve after delivery, and thus vigorous hydration antepartum is unnecessary and potentially dangerous.

The routine use of such monitoring even if pulmonary edema develops is questionable. Most women who develop pulmonary edema from ventricular failure respond quickly to furosemide given intravenously. Afterload reduction with intermittent doses of intravenous hydralazine to lower blood pressure, as described above, may also be necessary, because women with chronic hypertension and severe superimposed preeclampsia are more likely to develop heart failure (Cunningham and associates, 1986). Obese women in these circumstances are even more likely to develop heart failure (Mabie and colleagues, 1988a).

Invasive monitoring should be considered for those women with multiple clinical factors such as intrinsic heart disease and/or advanced renal disease that might cause pulmonary edema by more than one mechanism. This is particularly relevant if pulmonary edema is inexplicable or refractory to treatment. Still, in most of these cases it is not necessary to perform pulmonary artery catheterization for clinical management. Finally, pulmonary artery catheterization may be associated with serious morbidity and even with mortality (see Chap. 47, p. 1068). Robin (1985) cited a major complication rate of 20 to 33 percent, with associated mortality of up to 4 percent.

Delivery. When the above treatment regimen was formulated in the 1950s, eclampsia immediately caused appropriate concern for maternal welfare. Therefore, to avoid maternal risks from cesarean delivery, steps to effect vaginal delivery were employed even in some circumstances in which it appeared the fetus might have been better served by cesarean delivery. It rapidly became apparent that labor often ensued spontaneously or could be induced successfully even in women remote from term without subjecting the fetus to greater risk. It also became apparent early on that a magic cure did not immediately follow delivery by any route, but serious morbidity was less common during the puerperium in women delivered vaginally. For these reasons, vaginal delivery is still attempted and is quite often successful. For example, labor culminating in vaginal delivery was accomplished in nearly 75 percent of 209 women with antepartum eclampsia (Cunningham and Pritchard, 1984). Moreover, labor often was induced successfully, and vaginal delivery accomplished even when the woman was remote from term. Therefore, labor is not impaired by magnesium sulfate (Pritchard, 1955; Stallworth and co-workers, 1981).

Blood Loss at Delivery. Hemoconcentration, or lack of normal pregnancy-induced hypervolemia, is an almost predictable feature of severe preeclampsia. **The woman with severe preeclampsia or eclampsia, who consequently lacks normal pregnancy hypervolemia, is much less tolerant of blood loss than is the normotensive pregnant woman.** It is of great importance to recognize that an appreciable fall in blood pressure very soon after delivery most often means excessive blood loss and not sudden dissolution of vasospasm. When oliguria follows delivery, the hematocrit should be evaluated frequently to help detect excessive blood loss that, if identified, should be treated appropriately by careful blood transfusion.

The average-sized normally pregnant woman can shed in the course of delivery almost all of the 1500 mL or so of blood that she had added to her nonpregnant volume without suffering an appreciable fall in hematocrit. The impact of comparable blood loss when pregnancy hypervolemia is seriously restricted is evident in the woman with eclampsia presented in Figure 36–16. Associated with her delivery was the loss of 405 mL of red blood cells, equivalent to 1100 mL of predelivery blood, primarily from uterine atony. Blood volume was restored by careful infusion of lactated Ringer solution. The hematocrit fell from 38 to 23, whereas if the blood volume had been normal for late pregnancy (about 45 percent greater than the nonpregnant volume, rather than 15 percent), it is anticipated that there

would have been no decrease in hematocrit. In fact, that was the sequence of events with her second pregnancy: an increase of blood volume of 43 percent followed by blood loss of a liter at delivery, but no fall in hematocrit.

Analgesia and Anesthesia. Intravenous or intramuscular meperidine, usually with promethazine, is given in moderation for discomforts of labor and after cesarean delivery. For women with severe preeclampsia and eclampsia, local or pudendal analgesia is used for nearly all vaginal deliveries. General anesthesia, using thiopental, succinylcholine, nitrous oxide, and oxygen, has been administered for cesarean delivery and indicated forceps deliveries. Hodgkinson and colleagues (1980) described a transient but severe hypertensive response to tracheal intubation and extubation in women with severe preeclampsia in whom general anesthesia was used. The hypertensive response may often be prevented by the intravenous administration of 5 mg of hydralazine just prior to anesthesia induction. Ramanathan and colleagues (1988) attenuated this response by administering labetalol intravenously. The hypotensive effect of labetalol appears to be by lowering cardiac output and not changing peripheral resistance. Although splanchnic circulation is decreased almost 20 percent, placental perfusion allegedly is not significantly reduced (Ahokas and associates, 1989).

Sublingual nifedipine has also been used for this purpose. It is reported not to reduce uterine blood flow acutely or change fetal heart rates in women or pregnant hypertensive rats (Ahokas, 1988; Lindow, 1988; Lurie, 1990; Seabe, 1989; and their co-workers). **Importantly, however, nifedipine and magnesium sulfate therapy together may cause profound hypo-**

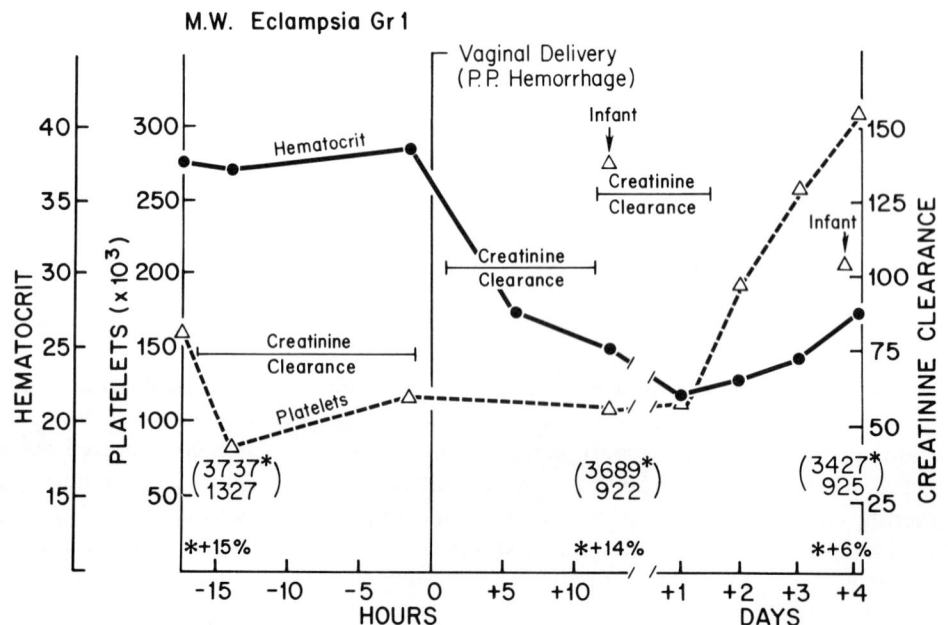

M.W. Eclampsia Gr 1

Fig. 36–16. Changes in maternal hematocrit and blood and red cell volumes determined using ^{51}Cr-labeled erythrocytes (numbers in parentheses), maternal and infant platelet counts, and maternal creatinine clearance in a woman with eclampsia who was delivered vaginally. Her blood volume was expanded only 15 percent over that when nonpregnant, and modest documented blood loss of only 1100 mL was followed by a fall in the hematocrit from 38 to 23. The creatinine clearance returned to normal soon after delivery, the maternal platelet count was normal by 2 days, and the newborn's platelet count always was normal.

tension (Waisman and colleagues, 1988). Nifedipine is not used for this purpose at Parkland Hospital because almost all hypertensive women are receiving parenteral magnesium sulfate therapy. Hydralazine remains our first choice for a prophylaxis against hypertension during tracheal intubation, and labetalol or nitroglycerin are also effective.

In the past, conduction analgesia has been avoided in women with severe preeclampsia and eclampsia because of concern for sudden, severe hypotension induced by splanchnic blockade and, in turn, the dangers from pressor agents or large volumes of intravenous fluid given to correct the iatrogenically induced hypotension. In many other centers, conduction analgesia is used to ameliorate vasospasm and to lower blood pressure. There is no doubt that lumbar epidural analgesia decreases peripheral vascular resistance and mean arterial blood pressure (Newsome and colleagues, 1986). However, because such vasodilatation results in hypovolemia that dangerously lowers uteroplacental perfusion, variable volumes of crystalloid must be infused either prior to or coincidentally with epidural injection to maintain cardiac output. This results in increased filling pressures that, as previously discussed, predispose to pulmonary and cerebral edema. Finally, even in the most experienced hands, and even with preload crystalloid, epidural analgesia still occasionally results in hypotension (see Chap. 16, p. 438). Attempts to restore blood pressure pharmacologically with vasopressors must be approached cautiously because these women are exquisitely sensitive to pressor agents. Montan and Ingemarsson (1989) reported that epidural analgesia in women with pregnancy-induced hypertension, preeclampsia, and chronic hypertension was associated with an almost threefold risk for ominous fetal heart rate patterns in labor when compared with normotensive women. **Moreover, the combination of epidural analgesia with antihypertensive drugs, especially β-blockers, was associated with a 50 percent incidence of ominous fetal heart rate patterns.** As cautioned by the American College of Obstetricians and Gynecologists (1988b) and Moore and associates (1985), if epidural analgesia is to be used, it should only be entrusted to the most experienced obstetrical anesthesiologists.

Other Treatment Agents. Although widely used to control convulsions from a variety of causes in nonpregnant individuals, **diazepam** therapy remains unproven for eclampsia. Crowther (1990), in a randomized trial, found magnesium sulfate superior to diazepam. It was worrisome that diazepam was associated with maternal aspiration pneumonitis. Apparently, larger doses of diazepam are often required to control eclamptic convulsions. Moreover, Cree and co-workers (1973) documented neonatal apnea persisting several hours after birth, hypotonia, drowsiness, and low Apgar scores, and impaired metabolic responses to cooling as a conse-

quence of maternal intrapartum administration of diazepam. We have observed one case of respiratory arrest in which diazepam was repeatedly given to a postpartum hypertensive woman in order to arrest convulsions so that computerized tomography could be performed.

Surprisingly, there are few published observations that describe **phenytoin** given to prevent or treat seizures of eclampsia. A number of investigators have provided preliminary data describing the pharmacokinetics of phenytoin in preeclamptic women (Appleton, 1991; Lucas, 1992; Ryan, 1989; and their colleagues). Slater and colleagues (1987) reported their experiences with a limited number of women with preeclampsia–eclampsia given intravenous phenytoin. Although the drug appeared to be effective for controlling convulsions, 6 of the 26 infants had 5-minute Apgar scores of 4 or less. Dommisse (1990) reported an opposite result. He treated 11 eclamptic women with magnesium sulfate and 11 eclamptic women with phenytoin. None of the women treated with magnesium sulfate had further convulsions, but 4 women treated with phenytoin continued to convulse. These 4 subsequently were treated effectively with magnesium sulfate.

Morphine and most sedatives will control convulsions only in doses that render the woman nearly unconscious. Such intense generalized central nervous system depression in the woman and her fetus should be avoided. Some other drugs that have been used in the treatment of eclampsia and severe preeclampsia are presented in Table 36–10. We have had little personal experience with most of them, and for further information the interested reader is referred to the various listed reports.

It should be pointed out that a tendency persists among some medical experts to group together for the purpose of treatment a variety of disease states that appear to have a common functional disturbance. So-called **hypertensive encephalopathy** is one that from time to time attracts interest and, in turn, incites recommendations for treatment broad in scope, without full appreciation of all the problems created by the disease or evoked by the proposed treatment. Too often, when eclampsia is included under the category of hypertensive encephalopathy, lack of concern for the impact of the recommended therapy on the fetus is apparent. Moreover, it is not unusual for the recommendations to have been based on little or no data.

The recurrent recognition occasionally of thrombocytopenia and rarely of other changes in the coagulation mechanism, with or without evidence of abnormal erythrocyte destruction (microangiopathic hemolysis), has led to the recommendation for treatment with heparin, fresh whole blood, fresh frozen plasma, platelets, fibrinogen, and other specific clotting factors. Merit, if any, from heparin treatment remains to be established, but heparin was reported not to be effective in ameliorating the clinical course of established preeclampsia

(Bonnar and associates, 1976; Howie and co-workers, 1975). The safety of deliberate anticoagulation with heparin in the presence of severe hypertension is illogical, dangerous, and cannot be recommended.

Long-term Consequences of Eclampsia

Reproduction After Eclampsia. Eclamptic women and their families are often quite concerned over the prognosis for future pregnancies. Chesley and co-workers (1962), through meticulous long-term follow-up of women with eclampsia at the Margaret Hague Maternity Hospital, reported that of 466 subsequent pregnancies in 189 of the eclamptic women, fetal survival was 75 percent. Much of the loss was from early abortion. Of the pregnancies that continued to 28 weeks or more, 93 percent resulted in infants who survived. Of subsequent pregnancies in the 189 previously eclamptic women, 25 percent were complicated by hypertension (Chesley, 1964). The hypertension, however, was severe in only 5 percent, while 2 percent were again eclamptic.

Chesley emphasized that many cases of recurrent pregnancy-associated hypertension represent nothing more than chronic hypertension. Some women have normal blood pressures between pregnancies and at follow-up, but in general, pregnancies following eclampsia are an excellent screening test for latent hypertensive disease. A large percentage of women who develop recurrent hypertension during subsequent pregnancies will develop chronic hypertension, whereas the prevalence of chronic hypertension is extremely low in those who are normotensive in later pregnancies.

Chesley and co-workers (1976) obtained follow-up data through 1974 in all but 3 of the 270 predominantly Caucasian women who survived eclampsia at the Margaret Hague Maternity Hospital from 1931 through 1952. Nulliparous eclamptic women who reached 28 or more weeks' gestation had no increase over the expected number of deaths. Multiparous eclamptic women, who undoubtedly had underlying chronic vascular disease, had three times the expected number of deaths.

The incidence of chronic hypertension is affected by racial factors and thus pregnancy-aggravated hypertension or superimposed preeclampsia. Sibai and colleagues (1992) reported subsequent pregnancy outcomes in 223 women whose index pregnancies were complicated by eclampsia. When the entire group of 223 women was considered, subsequent fertility was not impaired. There were 366 pregnancies in which 22 percent were preeclamptic, 1.9 percent were eclamptic, 2.5 percent were complicated by placental abruption, and 2.7 percent resulted in a perinatal death. Of 159 nulliparas, if eclampsia occurred before 37 weeks' gestation in the index pregnancy, there was a higher incidence of preeclampsia and poor perinatal outcome in subsequent pregnancies compared with those who had

eclampsia at or after 37 weeks. The highest incidence of subsequent obstetrical complications occurred in women who had had eclampsia at 30 or less weeks. At the time of followup, 20 of previously normotensive women had developed chronic hypertension. The highest subsequent incidence of chronic hypertension (18 percent) was observed in women who had eclampsia at less than 30 weeks, and the lowest (5 percent) incidence was in women with eclampsia after 37 weeks. Finally, women who were preeclamptic in subsequent pregnancies had a higher incidence of chronic hypertension compared with those who were normotensive in subsequent pregnancies (25 versus 2 percent).

Infant Outcome. Outcome for children of preeclamptic mothers is usually good if they are not born hypoxic or acidotic. There is, however, a slight delay in growth up to 1½ years in preterm infants born to preeclamptic women (Martikainen, 1989). Moreover, at age 6, infants of preeclamptic women have higher diastolic blood pressures (Palti and Rothschild, 1989). Unfortunately, longer follow-up studies are not available.

Relation of Preeclampsia–Eclampsia to Subsequent Hypertension. Whether preeclampsia and eclampsia actually cause ensuing chronic hypertension has been a subject of considerable debate. One point of view has been that preeclampsia and eclampsia represent an acute vascular disorder in the form of arteriolar muscle spasm that, if allowed to continue for several weeks, would result in a permanent structural injury to the vascular wall through hypoxia. This view led some to teach that permanent hypertension might be avoided by delivery of women within 3 weeks after the onset of preeclampsia. The problem has been confused by the erroneous diagnosis of pure preeclampsia in primigravid women who had underlying chronic renal disease or essential hypertension. Another problem was that in some studies a substantial proportion of multiparas were included, and only a few of these actually had true preeclampsia. To contribute to the confusion, at least 40 percent of women with essential hypertension have substantial decreases in blood pressure during much of pregnancy, and in most, these normal pressures are observed beginning early in gestation. Typically, blood pressure rises again early in the third trimester, and some edema and perhaps minimal proteinuria, may follow. In women in whom blood pressures before pregnancy are unknown, the erroneous diagnosis of preeclampsia is likely made.

The results of the long-term follow-up studies of Chesley and associates (1976), who have reexamined women repeatedly for up to 44 years after eclampsia in the first pregnancy, are consistent with the conclusion that the prevalence of hypertension is not increased over that in women matched for age and race. Tillman (1955) accumulated a series of 377 women whose blood pressures were recorded before, during, and at intervals after pregnancy. He could find no indication that normal, preeclamptic, or hypertensive pregnancies had any effect on the blood pressure at follow-up examination. He concluded that preeclampsia neither causes residual hypertension nor aggravates preexisting hypertension. Conversely, Sibai and associates (1986b), in the study discussed above, reported that young, predominately African-American primigravidas with severe preeclampsia–eclampsia have a threefold incidence of subsequent chronic hypertension. Like Chesley, they concluded that pregnancy was a screening test for chronic hypertension, rather than pregnancy being a cause of chronic hypertension.

CHRONIC HYPERTENSION

Hypertension that antedates pregnancy is one of the most common medical complications encountered during pregnancy. Its variable incidence and severity, along with the well-known proclivity for pregnancy to induce or aggravate hypertension, has caused much confusion concerning the management of pregnant hypertensive woman. For example, the majority of pregnant women with underlying chronic hypertension demonstrate improved blood pressure control and have largely uneventful pregnancies. Some, however, experience dangerous worsening of hypertension that is frequently accompanied by proteinuria, pathological edema, and convulsions, and except that chronic hypertension antedated pregnancy, they are indistinguishable from an otherwise healthy young nullipara with severe preeclampsia–eclampsia.

Diagnosis

A diagnosis of chronic hypertension complicating pregnancy is made whenever there is evidence that hypertension preceded pregnancy, or when a woman is hypertensive before 20 weeks' gestation (see p. 966). In addition to obvious chronic hypertension, there are instances of repeated pregnancies in which hypertension appears late in pregnancy, but blood pressure is normal between pregnancies. Many authors, notably Dieckmann (1952), regarded these recurrent episodes as evidence of latent hypertensive vascular disease. Others, however, concluded that they are repeated attacks of preeclampsia, and still others regarded recurrent hypertension as a separate entity. The results of the long-term follow-up studies of Chesley and co-workers (1976), as well as those of Sibai and colleagues (1986b, 1992), are supportive of Dieckmann's view.

In most women with chronic hypertensive vascular disease, increased blood pressure is the only demonstrable finding. A few women, however, have complications that are not only dangerous to pregnancy but also to life expectancy. These include hypertensive heart disease, ischemic heart disease, renal insufficiency, and retinal hemorrhages and exudates. Moreover, blood pressure may vary from levels scarcely above normal to extremes of 300 mm Hg systolic and 160 mm Hg or more diastolic.

Hypertensive vascular disease in pregnancy is encountered more frequently in older women. Obesity is another important predisposing factor; for example, 7 percent of pregnant women who weighed more than 200 pounds had chronic hypertension (Kliegman and Gross, 1985). As perhaps expected in older and commonly obese women, diabetes is also prevalent. Finally, heredity, which includes racial factors, plays an important role in the development of chronic hypertension. Hypertension is common in African-Americans, and frequently many members of the same family are hypertensive.

In most women with chronic hypertension, the blood pressure falls by the second trimester, but the decrement is usually temporary (Fig. 36–17). In most cases, the blood pressure rises during the third trimester to levels somewhat above those in early pregnancy. Adverse outcomes in these women are dependent largely upon whether superimposed preeclampsia develops. As discussed on page 770, most of these women destined to develop superimposed preeclampsia become abnormally sensitive to infused angiotensin II sometime after midpregnancy but before they are clinically hypertensive (Gant and colleagues, 1977). The incidence of pregnancy-aggravated hypertension or superimposed preeclampsia averages about 15 to 25 percent, and estimates are influenced largely by criteria used in making the diagnosis. Other factors that impact on its incidence are the severity of underlying disease, whether there is renal

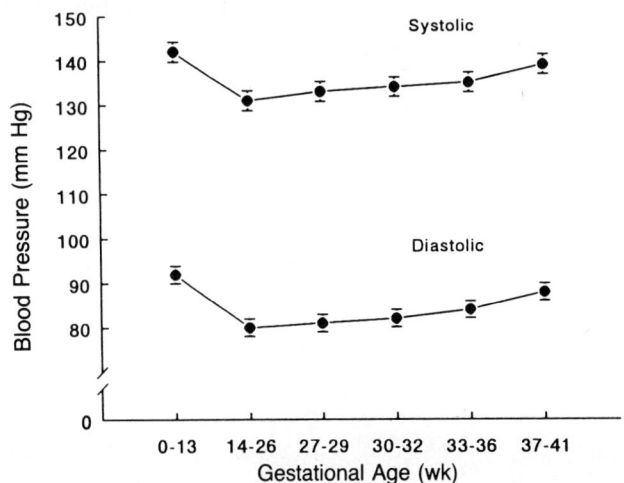

Fig. 36–17. Systolic and diastolic blood pressure changes during pregnancy in 90 chronically hypertensive women who were given no antihypertensive treatment. (Taken from Cunningham and Lowe, 1991, data from Sibai and colleagues, 1990c; shown as the mean ± standard error of the mean.)

disease (Cunningham and associates, 1990), and whether other conditions coexist, notably diabetes and obesity. Although adverse pregnancy outcomes are more likely in chronically hypertensive women who develop superimposed preeclampsia, they are also increased in those who remain normotensive throughout pregnancy. Some of the more common complications include hypertensive encephalopathy, heart failure, worsening of renal insufficiency, placental abruption, fetal growth retardation, and fetal death. Finally, the earlier the onset of hypertension in a pregnancy, the more likely the subsequent pregnancy will be hypertensive, and the more likely the woman is to have chronic hypertension, significant morbidity, and even maternal mortality (Sibai and colleagues, 1991).

Treatment During Pregnancy

The value of continued administration of antihypertensive drugs to pregnant women with chronic hypertension is debated. For example, although it may be beneficial to the hypertensive mother to reduce her blood pressure, a lower pressure may decrease uteroplacental perfusion and thereby jeopardize the fetus. Although it is not generally agreed whether antihypertensive therapy, as usually prescribed in the absence of pregnancy, is beneficial or detrimental to pregnancy outcome, there are now a few studies that can be used as clinical guides (Table 36–13).

Review of Studies. Redman and associates (1976) treated one group of hypertensive women with α-methyldopa and compared outcomes with those of a group of untreated women. They selected women of less than 28 weeks' gestation with blood pressures at or above 140/90 mm Hg but less than 170/100 mm Hg. Women with blood pressures of 170/100 mm Hg or higher were treated but not included in the study. A total of 101 women received α-methyldopa, and 107 did not. No diuretics were given, and both groups of women underwent early delivery at 37 to 38 weeks. In the control group, there was 1 stillbirth in a pregnancy complicated by superimposed preeclampsia and 1 neonatal death that

TABLE 36–13. CHRONIC HYPERTENSION AND SUPERIMPOSED PREECLAMPSIA—METHOD OF TREATMENT AND PERINATAL OUTCOME

Study and Treatment	Number	Superimposed Preeclampsia (%)	Perinatal Mortality (per 1000)
Chesley (1978)			
Chronic hypertension[a]			
No antihypertensives (1972–1974)	593	6	32
Superimposed preeclampsia[b]			
Hydralazine + α-methyldopa (1960–1974)	196	—	214
Redman (1980)[c]			
Chronic hypertension			
α-Methyldopa and/or hydralazine	184	25	16
Superimposed preeclampsia			
α-Methyldopa + others	69	—	145
Sibai and associates (1983)			
Chronic hypertension			
No antihypertensives	193	10	5
Superimposed preeclampsia			
α-Methyldopa and/or hydralazine	22	—	227
Mabie and associates (1986)			
Chronic hypertension, diastolic pressure			
< 90 mm Hg; no treatment	137	29	29
Chronic hypertension, diastolic pressure			
90–100 mm Hg; α-methyldopa	26	46	0
Sibai and associates (1986a)			
Severe chronic hypertension, 170/110 mm			
Hg or greater; α-methyldopa + hydralazine	44	52	250
Sibai and co-workers (1990c)			
Chronic hypertension			
No treatment	90	16	11
α-Methyldopa	87	18	11
Labetalol	86	16	12

[a] Three maternal deaths due to stroke, pulmonary embolus, and aspiration pneumonia.
[b] Two deaths due to stroke and postoperative infection.
[c] Data extracted from Table 1 from Ounsted and associates (1983), reporting on long term follow-up of children from the original and continuing study of treatment of chronic hypertension in pregnancy by Redman (1980).

was likely due to birth asphyxia and trauma. In the treatment group, there was 1 stillbirth in a pregnancy complicated by superimposed preeclampsia. The average birthweight and laboratory values were essentially the same for both groups. There were 4 abortions in the control group but none in the treatment group.

Sibai and colleagues (1983) reported their experiences with chronic hypertension in 211 consecutive women whose diastolic blood pressure was 90 to 110 mm Hg. Antihypertensive drugs were discontinued at the first prenatal visit, or they were not given, and all women were followed closely. Only 13 percent required antihypertensive therapy later in pregnancy for diastolic pressures exceeding 110 mm Hg, and the perinatal mortality was 28 per 1000. They concluded that factors other than chronic hypertension might be responsible for poor perinatal outcomes reported by others in such pregnancies.

Mabie and colleagues (1986) reported their experiences with pregnancies complicated by chronic hypertension at Charity Hospital of New Orleans. They stressed commonly associated conditions, which included obesity in one third and diabetes in 20 percent. Antihypertensive drugs, usually methyldopa, with or without a thiazide, were given to 82 women in whom diastolic pressure exceeded 90 mm Hg, while 82 women whose diastolic pressures remained less than 90 mm Hg were given no treatment. The perinatal mortality in each group was similar, but fetal growth retardation was increased fourfold in the treated group, presumably because of worse hypertension. Superimposed preeclampsia, defined as hypertension with either nondependent edema or proteinuria, developed in one third, but was more common in those women who were given treatment. The authors concluded that aggressive treatment did not improve perinatal outcome, and blood pressure control was but one aspect of management in these women.

The most carefully done study to date of chronic hypertension in pregnant women was reported by the Memphis group; the results are summarized in Table 36–14. In this randomized clinical trial, 263 women with mild to moderate hypertension that antedated pregnancy were allocated at 6 to 13 weeks to be given no antihypertensive treatment or to receive either labetalol or α-methyldopa. The aim of therapy was to keep blood pressure less than 140/90 mm Hg. Those not treated were initially given α-methyldopa if systolic blood pressure exceeded 160 mm Hg or if diastolic pressure exceeded 110 mm Hg. Although women treated throughout pregnancy had significantly lower blood pressure than control women not given treatment, the incidence of important complications was not altered by treatment. As perhaps expected, more women not given treatment eventually required antihypertensive therapy for serious hypertension, defined as blood pressure greater than 160/110 mm Hg.

To summarize some of these studies presented in Table 36–13, all investigators reported that superimposed preeclampsia or pregnancy-aggravated hypertension was a bad complication. It appears that treatment with antihypertensive medications decreases the incidence of this complication. Importantly, most pregnancy outcomes were good for women with chronic hypertension, whether or not antihypertensive treatment was given. The uncorrected perinatal mortality rates were low unless superimposed preeclampsia developed. Three maternal deaths reported in detail by Chesley warrant careful analysis. Death from stroke followed in a woman who was transferred from another hospital. She was in coma and died within 20 minutes of arrival. A second woman died of a pulmonary embolus after cesarean delivery of a 5000-g infant, followed by a complicated postoperative course and wound evisceration. The other death was the result of aspiration during anesthesia for a cesarean delivery.

Severe Chronic Hypertension. The prognosis for a pregnancy with chronic hypertension is related to the severity of disease before pregnancy. Many women with severe hypertension also have underlying renal disease (Cun-

TABLE 36–14. MATERNAL AND PERINATAL OUTCOMES IN 263 CHRONICALLY HYPERTENSIVE WOMEN RANDOMIZED TO NO TREATMENT OR TREATMENT WITH METHYLDOPA OR LABETALOL DURING PREGNANCY

Factor	No Treatment	Treatment Group	
		Methyldopa	*Labetalol*
Number of women	90	87	86
Additional drugs for hypertension (%)	11	6	6
Superimposed preeclampsia (%)	16	18	16
Abruptio placentae (%)	2	1	2
Preterm delivery (%)	10	12	12
Fetal growth retardation (%)	9	7	8
Perinatal mortality (per 1000)	11	11	12
Gestational age (wk)	39 ± 0.2	38.6 ± 0.2	38.7 ± 0.2
Birthweight (g)	3123 ± 69	3051 ± 73	3068 ± 71
Placental weight (g)	723 ± 23	716 ± 33	755 ± 69

From Sibai and co-workers (1990c).

ningham and colleagues, 1990). Sibai and co-workers (1986a) described 44 pregnancies in women whose blood pressure at 6 to 11 weeks was 170/110 mm Hg or higher (Table 36–13). They were given treatment with α-methyldopa and oral hydralazine to maintain blood pressures less than 160/110 mm Hg, and they were hospitalized for treatment with parenteral hydralazine if blood pressures exceeded 180/120 mm Hg. Half developed superimposed preeclampsia, and all adverse perinatal outcomes were in this group: all infants were preterm, nearly 80 percent were growth retarded, and the perinatal mortality rate was 48 percent. By contrast, in the women with severe hypertension who did not develop superimposed preeclampsia, only 5 percent of fetuses were growth retarded and all survived.

The use of α-methyldopa during early pregnancy has been questioned because of smaller head circumferences observed in male infants of women who received the drug between 16 and 20 weeks (Redman, 1980). However, long-term follow-up of the infants in Redman's 1976 and 1980 studies are reassuring. There have been no major adverse effects found in children followed for up to 7½ years (Cockburn and associates, 1982; Ounsted and co-workers, 1983).

Antihypertensive Drug Selection. Despite the relatively good results obtained with α-methyldopa, and the comparable results obtained without antihypertensive drugs, adrenergic blocking drugs are used extensively in England, Scotland, and Australia (Michael, 1982; Redman, 1982; Rubin, 1983; Walker, 1983; and their associates). The results of treatment with labetalol, a combined α- and β-adrenergic blocker, are consistent with the view that the drug offers no advantages over α-methyldopa (Sibai and colleagues, 1990c). Rubin and colleagues (1983) reported salutary results from a double-blind prospective study in which they compared placebo to the β-blocker atenolol given to 120 women with hypertension first apparent early in the third trimester. Because nearly 60 percent of their subjects were nulliparous, it was difficult to separate women with chronic hypertension from those with preeclampsia. The placebo group had worse perinatal outcomes, but there were more nulliparas assigned (67 versus 50 percent), and thus presumably more had preeclampsia at the outset. Moreover, the same group (Butters and colleagues, 1990) reported that atenolol treatment of chronically hypertensive women resulted in a higher incidence of growth-retarded neonates compared with untreated controls. Finally, β-blocker drugs are associated with an increased incidence of ominous fetal heart rate patterns during labor. Ominous patterns were reported in 20 percent of women receiving β-blocker therapy for hypertension (Montan and Ingemarsson, 1989). The incidence of ominous patterns was increased even more in growth-retarded fetuses and was seen in 50 percent of women given epidural analgesia.

Captopril or enalapril, angiotensin-I-converting-enzyme inhibitors, have been shown to reduce uteroplacental perfusion and often kill the fetuses of experimental animals (Broughton-Pipkin and associates, 1982; Ferris and Weir, 1983). Hanssens and colleagues (1991) reviewed the literature and found 85 pregnancies in which one of these drugs was given. Although low birthweight and respiratory distress were not increased, worrisome features, especially in preterm infants, have been the association with severe oligohydramnios, pulmonary hypoplasia, and neonatal anemia (see Chap. 42, p. 965). **This class of antihypertensive drugs is contraindicated during pregnancy.**

Recommendations for Therapy. The National High Blood Pressure Education Program Working Group (1990) stressed that there were limited data from which to draw conclusions whether to treat chronic hypertension in normotensive pregnant women. The group did, however, recommend therapy to prevent hypertensive vascular damage when maternal diastolic blood pressure reached 100 mm Hg. They also concluded that early treatment of hypertension would probably reduce the need for subsequent hospitalization during pregnancy. Certainly, Sibai and associates (1990c) found that subsequent treatment was needed for dangerous hypertension in 11 percent of women not given treatment, compared with only 6 percent in women given either α-methyldopa or labetalol earlier in pregnancy.

At Parkland Hospital, pregnancy complicated by chronic hypertension has not been treated with antihypertensive drugs or diuretics unless (1) blood pressure is above 150/110 mm Hg or (2) the woman was receiving antihypertensive medications prior to pregnancy and her hypertension is well controlled. If blood pressure increases rapidly and persists above 110 mm Hg diastolic, if significant proteinuria develops, if renal function deteriorates, or if fetal growth retardation is suspected, for the reasons that follow, the pregnancy is terminated as recommended above for severe preeclampsia and eclampsia.

Pregnancy-aggravated Hypertension

Diagnosis. The most common hazard faced by pregnant women with chronic hypertensive vascular disease is the superimposition of preeclampsia. The frequency of pregnancy-aggravated hypertension is difficult to specify precisely because the incidence varies with the diagnostic criteria employed. If the diagnosis is made only on the basis of (1) significant aggravation of the hypertension, (2) sustained proteinuria, and (3) generalized edema, the incidence will be relatively low because delivery is often accomplished before intense superimposed preeclampsia or eclampsia has developed. If, however, the diagnosis is made on the basis of a modest rise in blood pressure and minimal to modest proteinuria, the incidence will be much higher. For example, with mild chronic hypertension, the incidence of superimposed preeclampsia cited in the studies in Table 36–13 varied from 6 to 52 percent!

Pregnancy-aggravated hypertension typically becomes manifest by a sudden rise in blood pressure that almost always is complicated eventually by substantive proteinuria. Especially in neglected cases, extreme hypertension (systolic pressure greater than 200 mm Hg and diastolic pressure of 130 mm Hg or more), oliguria, and impaired renal clearance may rapidly ensue; the retina may contain extensive hemorrhages and cotton-wool exudates; and convulsions and coma are likely. Therefore, in its most severe form, the resultant syndrome is similar to hypertensive encephalopathy. With the development of superimposed preeclampsia or eclampsia, the outlook for both infant and mother is grave unless the pregnancy is rapidly terminated. The frequency of fetal growth retardation and preterm delivery is increased appreciably because of its relatively early onset in pregnancy, as well as the marked severity of the process itself (López-Llera and associates, 1972; Redman, 1980). If the infant is born alive and survives the perinatal period, however, long-term prognosis is good (Ounsted and colleagues, 1983).

References

Abdul-Karim R, Assali NS: Pressor response to angiotonin in pregnant and nonpregnant women. Am J Obstet Gynecol 82:246, 1961

Adamson SL, Morrow RJ, Bascom PAJ, Mo LYL, Ritchie JWK: Effect of placental resistance, arterial diameter, and blood pressure on the uterine arterial velocity waveform: A computer modeling approach. Ultrasound Med Biol 15:437, 1989

Ahokas RA, Mabie C, Sibai BM, Anderson GD: Labetalol does not decrease placental perfusion in the hypertensive term-pregnant rat. Am J Obstet Gynecol 160:480, 1989

Ahokas RA, Sibai BM, Mabie WC, Anderson GD: Nifedipine does not adversely affect uteroplacental blood flow in the hypertensive term-pregnant rat. Am J Obstet Gynecol 159:1440, 1988

Altura BM, Altura BT, Carella A: Magnesium deficiency-induced spasms of umbilical vessels: Relation to preeclampsia, hypertension, growth retardation. Science 221:376, 1983

American College of Obstetricians and Gynecologists: Invasive hemodynamic monitoring in obstetrics and gynecology. Technical bulletin no. 121, 1988a

American College of Obstetricians and Gynecologists: Obstetric Anesthesia and Analgesia. Technical bulletin no. 112, January 1988b

American College of Obstetricians and Gynecologists: Management of preeclampsia. Technical bulletin no. 91, February 1986

Appleton MP, Kuehl TJ, Raebel MA, Adams HR, Knight AB,

Gold WR: Magnesium sulfate versus phenytoin for seizure prophylaxis in pregnancy-induced hypertension. Am J Obstet Gynecol 165:907, 1991

Assali NS, Douglas RA, Baird WW: Measurement of uterine blood flow and uterine metabolism. Am J Obstet Gynecol 66:248, 1953

August P, Marcaccio B, Gertner JM, Druzin ML, Resnick LM, Laragh JH: Abnormal 1,25-dihydroxyvitamin D metabolism in preeclampsia. Am J Obstet Gynecol 166:1295, 1992

Baird D: Combined Textbook of Obstetrics and Gynaecology for Students and Practitioners. Edinburgh, Livingston, 1969, p 631

Ballegeer VC, Spitz B, DeBaene LA, Van Assche AF, Hidajat M, Criel AM: Platelet activation and vascular damage in gestational hypertension. Am J Obstet Gynecol 166:629, 1992

Barr SM, Lees KR, Butters L, O'Donnell A, Rubin PC: Platelet intracellular free calcium concentration in normotensive and hypertensive pregnancies in the human. Clin Sci 76:67, 1989

Barton JR, Sibai BM, Whybrew WD, Mercer BM: Urinary endothelin-1: Not a useful marker for preeclampsia. Am J Obstet Gynecol (in press)

Beaufils M, Uzan S, Donsimoni R, Colau JC: Prevention of preeclampsia by early antiplatelet therapy. Lancet 1:840, 1985

Beer AE: Possible immunologic bases of preeclampsia/eclampsia. Semin Perinatol 2:39, 1978

Belfort MA, Moore PJ: Verapamil in the treatment of severe postpartum hypertension. S Afr Med J 74:265, 1988

Belizán JM, Villar J, Gonzalez L, Campodonico L, Bergel E: Calcium supplementation to prevent hypertensive disorders of pregnancy. N Engl J Med 325:1399, 1991

Belizán JM, Villar J, Repke J: The relationship between calcium intake and pregnancy-induced hypertension: Up-to-date evidence. Am J Obstet Gynecol 158:898, 1988

Benedetti TJ, Carlson RW: Studies of colloid osmotic pressure in pregnancy-induced hypertension. Am J Obstet Gynecol 135:308, 1979

Benedetti TJ, Cotton DB, Read JC, Miller FC: Hemodynamic observations in severe preeclampsia with a flow-directed pulmonary artery catheter. Am J Obstet Gynecol 136:465, 1980a

Benedetti TJ, Kates R, Williams V: Hemodynamic observations in severe preeclampsia complicated by pulmonary edema. Am J Obstet Gynecol 152:330, 1985

Benedetti TJ, Quilligan EJ: Cerebral edema in severe pregnancy-induced hypertension. Am J Obstet Gynecol 137:860, 1980b

Benigni A, Gregorini G, Frusca T, Chiabrando C, Ballerini S, Valcamonico A, Orisio S, Piccinelli A, Pincirolli V, Fanelli R, Gastaldi A, Remuzzi G: Effect of low-dose aspirin on fetal and maternal generation of thromboxane by platelets in women at risk for pregnancy-induced hypertension. N Engl J Med 321:357, 1989

Bhatia RK, Bottoms SF, Saleh AA, Norman GS, Mammen EF, Sokol RJ: Mechanisms for reduced colloid osmotic pressure in preeclampsia. Am J Obstet Gynecol 157:106, 1987

Biagi G, De Rosa V, Pelusi G, Scagliarini G, Sani G, Coccheri S: Increased placental production of leukotriene B$_4$ in gestational hypertension. Thromb Res 60:377, 1990

Bloss JD, Hankins GDV, Hauth JC, Gilstrap LC: The effect of oxytocin infusion on the pharmacokinetics of intramuscular magnesium sulfate therapy. Am J Obstet Gynecol 157:156, 1987

Bond AL, August P, Druzin ML, Atlas SA, Sealey JE, Laragh JH: Atrial natriuretic factor in normal and hypertensive pregnancy. Am J Obstet Gynecol 160:1112, 1989

Bonnar J, Redman CWG, Denson KW: The role of coagulation and fibrinolysis in preeclampsia. In Lindheimer MD, Katz AI, Zuspan FP (eds): Hypertension in Pregnancy. New York, Wiley, 1976

Borges LF, Gücer G: Effect of magnesium on epileptic foci. Epilepsia 19:81, 1978

Boutroy MJ: Fetal effects of maternally administered clonidine and angiotensin-converting enzyme inhibitors. Dev Pharmacol Ther 13:199, 1989

Brosens IA, Robertson WB, Dixon HG: The role of the spiral arteries in the pathogenesis of preeclampsia. Obstet Gynecol Ann 1:177, 1972

Broughton-Pipkin F, Symonds EM, Turner SR: The effect of captopril upon mothers and fetuses in the chronically cannulated ewe and in the pregnant rabbit. J Physiol 323:415, 1982

Brown CEL, Cunningham FG, Pritchard JA: Convulsions in hypertensive, proteinuric primiparas more than 24 hours after delivery: Eclampsia or some other cause? J Reprod Med 32:499, 1987

Brown CEL, Gant NF, Cox K, Spitz B, Rosenfeld CR, Magness RR: Low-dose aspirin, II. Relationship of angiotensin II pressor responses, circulating eicosanoids, and pregnancy outcome. Am J Obstet Gynecol 163:1863, 1990

Brown CEL, Purdy PD, Cunningham FG: Head computed tomographic scans in women with eclampsia. Am J Obstet Gynecol 159:915, 1988a

Brown MA, Gallery EDM, Ross MR, Esber RP: Sodium excretion in normal and hypertensive pregnancy: A prospective study. Am J Obstet Gynecol 159:297, 1988b

Brown MA, North L, Hargood J: Uteroplacental Doppler ultrasound in routine antenatal care. Aust NZ J Obstet Gynaecol 30:303, 1990

Brown MA, Zammit VC, Lowe SA: Capillary permeability and extracellular fluid volumes in pregnancy-induced hypertension. Clin Sci 77:599, 1989

Brown RD, Strott CA, Liddle GW: Plasma deoxycorticosterone in normal and abnormal human pregnancy. J Clin Endocrinol Metab 35:736, 1972

Browne FJ: Sensitization of the vascular system in pre-eclamptic toxaemia and eclampsia. Br J Obstet Gynaecol 53:510, 1946

Browne JCM, Veall N: The maternal placental blood flow in normotensive and hypertensive women. J Obstet Gynaecol Br Emp 60:141, 1953

Browne O: The treatment of eclampsia. Br J Obstet Gynaecol 57:573, 1950

Brubaker DB, Ross MG, Marinoff D: The function of elevated plasma fibronectin in preeclampsia. Am J Obstet Gynecol 166:526, 1992

Brunner HR, Gavras H: Vascular damage in hypertension. Hosp Pract 10:97, 1975

Bryant RD, Fleming JG: Veratrum viride in the treatment of eclampsia. Obstet Gynecol 19:372, 1962

Burrows RF, Hunter DJS, Andrew M, Kelton JG: A prospective study investigating the mechanism of thrombocytopenia in preeclampsia. Obstet Gynecol 70:334, 1987

Butters L, Kennedy S, Rubin PC: Atenolol in essential hypertension during pregnancy. BMJ 301:587, 1990

Cameron AD, Nicholson SF, Nimrod CA, Harder JR, Davies DM: Doppler waveforms in the fetal aorta and umbilical artery in patients with hypertension in pregnancy. Am J Obstet Gynecol 158:339, 1988

Cardin JP Jr, Ross MG, Ervin MG, Schaffer AV, Douglas FL, Simke JP: Fetal and maternal response to intravenous infusion of a thromboxane synthetase inhibitor. Am J Obstet Gynecol 163:1345, 1990

Catella F, Lawson JA, Fitzgerald DJ, FitzGerald GA: Endogenous biosynthesis of arachidonic acid epoxides in humans: Increased formation in pregnancy-induced hypertension. Proc Natl Acad Sci 87:5893, 1990

Chang JK, Roman C, Heymann MA: Effect of endothelium-derived relaxing factor inhibition on the umbilical–placental circulation in fetal lambs in utero. Am J Obstet Gynecol 166:727, 1992

Chesley LC: Eclamptic deaths and Baptists. Am J Obstet Gynecol 160:1540, 1989

Chesley LC: Diagnosis of preeclampsia. Obstet Gynecol 65:423, 1985

Chesley LC: Superimposed preeclampsia or eclampsia. In Chesley LC (ed): Hypertensive Disorders in Pregnancy. New York, Appleton-Century-Crofts, 1978, pp 14, 302, 482

Chesley LC: A short history of eclampsia. Obstet Gynecol 43:599, 1974

Chesley LC, Annitto JE, Cosgrove RA: Long-term follow-up study of eclamptic women: Sixth periodic report. Am J Obstet Gynecol 124:446, 1976

Chesley LC, Annitto JE, Cosgrove RA: The familial factor in toxemia of pregnancy. Obstet Gynecol 32:303, 1968

Chesley LC, Annitto JE, Cosgrove RA: Prognostic significance of recurrent toxemia of pregnancy. Obstet Gynecol 23:874, 1964

Chesley LC, Cooper DW: Genetics of hypertension in pregnancy: Possible single gene control of pre-eclampsia and eclampsia in the descendants of eclamptic women. Br J Obstet Gynaecol 93:898, 1986

Chesley LC, Cosgrove RA, Annitto JE: A follow-up study of eclamptic women: Fourth periodic report. Am J Obstet Gynecol 83:1360, 1962

Chesley LC, Tepper I: Plasma levels of magnesium attained in magnesium sulfate therapy for preeclampsia and eclampsia. Surg Clin North Am April:353, 1957

Chesley LC, Williams LO: Renal glomerular and tubular function in relation to the hyperuricemia of pre-eclampsia and eclampsia. Am J Obstet Gynecol 50:367, 1945

Clark BA, Halvorson L, Sachs B, Epstein FH: Plasma endothelin levels in preeclampsia: Elevation and correlation with uric acid levels and renal impairment. Am J Obstet Gynecol 166:962, 1992

Clark SL, Cotton DB: Clinical indications for pulmonary artery catheterization in the patient with severe preeclampsia. Am J Obstet Gynecol 158:453, 1988

Cockburn J, Moar VA, Ounsted M, Redman CWG: Final report of study on hypertension during pregnancy: The effects of specific treatment on the growth and development of the children. Lancet 1:647, 1982

Collins R, Wallenburg HCS: Pharmacological prevention and treatment of hypertensive disorders in pregnancy. In Chalmers I, Enkin M, Keirse MJNC (eds): Effective Care in Pregnancy and Childbirth, Vol I. Oxford, Oxford University Press, 1989, p 512

Collins R, Yusuf S, Peto R: Overview of randomised trials of diuretics in pregnancy. BMJ 290:17, 1985

Combes B, Adams RH: Disorders of the liver in pregnancy. In Assali NS (ed): Pathophysiology of Gestation, Vol I. New York, Academic Press, 1972

Constantine G, Beevers DG, Reynolds AL, Luesley DM: Nifedipine as a second line antihypertensive drug in pregnancy. Br J Obstet Gynaecol 984:1136, 1987

Cooper DW, Deane EM, Marshall P, Gallery EDM: C3 allotypes in pregnancy hypertension and eclampsia. Hum Hered 38:52, 1988

Cooper DW, Liston WA: Genetic control of severe preeclampsia. J Med Genet 16:409, 1979

Cotton DB, Gonik B, Dorman KF: Cardiovascular alterations in severe pregnancy-induced hypertension: Acute effects of intravenous magnesium sulfate. Am J Obstet Gynecol 148:152, 1984

Cotton DB, Janusz CA, Berman RF: Anticonvulsant effects of magnesium sulfate on hippocampal seizures: Therapeutic implications in preeclampsia-eclampsia. Am J Obstet Gynecol 166:1127, 1992

Cotton DB, Jones MM, Longmire S, Korman KF, Tessem J, Joyce TH: Role of intravenous nitroglycerine in the treatment of severe pregnancy-induced hypertension complicated by pulmonary edema. Am J Obstet Gynecol 154:91, 1986

Cotton DB, Lee W, Huhta JC, Dorman KF: Hemodynamic profile of severe pregnancy-induced hypertension. Am J Obstet Gynecol 158:523, 1988

Cree JE, Meyer J, Hailey DM: Diazepam in labour: Its metabolism and effect on the clinical condition and thermogenesis of the newborn. Br Med J 4:251, 1973

Crowther C: Magnesium sulphate versus diazepam in the management of eclampsia: A randomized controlled trial. Br J Obstet Gynaecol 97:110, 1990

Cunningham FG, Cox K, Gant NF: Further observations on the nature of pressor responsivity to angiotensin II in human pregnancy. Obstet Gynecol 146:581, 1975

Cunningham FG, Cox SM, Harstad TW, Mason RA, Pritchard JA: Chronic renal disease and pregnancy outcome. Am J Obstet Gynecol 163:453, 1990

Cunningham FG, Gant NF: Prevention of preeclampsia—A reality. N Engl J Med 321:606, 1989

Cunningham FG, Leveno KJ: Management of pregnancy-induced hypertension. In Rubin PC (ed): Handbook of Hypertension. Vol X, Hypertension in Pregnancy. Amsterdam, Elsevier Science, 1988, p 290

Cunningham FG, Lowe TW: Cardiovascular diseases complicating pregnancy. Williams Obstetrics, 18th ed (suppl 14). Norwalk, CT, Appleton & Lange, 1991

Cunningham FG, Lowe T, Guss S, Mason R: Erythrocyte morphology in women with severe preeclampsia and eclampsia. Am J Obstet Gynecol 153:358, 1985

Cunningham FG, Pritchard JA: How should hypertension during pregnancy be managed? Experience at Parkland Memorial Hospital. Med Clin North Am 68:505, 1984

Cunningham FG, Pritchard JA, Hankins GDV, Anderson PL, Lucas MK, Armstrong KF: Idiopathic cardiomyopathy or compounding cardiovascular events? Obstet Gynecol 67:157, 1986

Davey DA, MacGillivray I: The classification and definition of the hypertensive disorders of pregnancy. Am J Obstet Gynecol 158:892, 1988

Davidge ST, Hubel CA, Brayden RD, Capeless EC, McLaughlin MK: Sera antioxidant activity in uncomplicated and preeclamptic pregnancies. Obstet Gynecol 79:897, 1992

De Boer K, Büller HR, Ten Cate JW, Treffers PE: Coagulation studies in the syndrome of haemolysis, elevated liver enzymes and low platelets. Br J Obstet Gynaecol 98:42, 1991

De Boer K, Ten Cate JW, Sturk A, Borm JJ, Treffers PE: Enhanced Thrombin generation in normal and hypertensive pregnancy. Am J Obstet Gynecol 160:95, 1989

Dekker GA, Sibai BM: Early detection of preeclampsia. Am J Obstet Gynecol 165:160, 1991

Dewar JB, Morris WIC: Sedation with rectal tribromoethanol (Avertin Bromethol) in the management of eclampsia. J Obstet Gynaecol Br Emp 54:417, 1947

DeWolf F, Robertson WB, Brosen I: The ultrastructure of acute atherosis in hypertensive pregnancy. Am J Obstet Gynecol 123:164, 1975

Dieckmann WJ: The Toxemias of Pregnancy, 2nd ed. St Louis, Mosby, 1952

Dieckmann WJ, Michel HL: Vascular–renal effects of posterior pituitary extracts in pregnant women. Am J Obstet Gynecol 33:131, 1937

Dommisse J: Phenytoin sodium and magnesium sulphate in the management of eclampsia. Br J Obstet Gynaecol 97:104, 1990

Donaldson JO: Eclampsia. In Neurology in Pregnancy, 2nd ed. Philadelphia, Saunders, 1989, p 269

Donaldson JO: Does magnesium sulfate treat eclamptic convulsions? Clin Neuropharmacol 9:37, 1986

Ducey J, Schulman H, Farmakides G, Rochelson B, Bracero L, Fleischer A, Guzman E, Winter D, Penny B: A classification of hypertension in pregnancy based on Doppler velocimetry. Am J Obstet Gynecol 157:680, 1987

Easterling TR, Benedetti TJ, Carlson KL, Watts DH: Measurement of cardiac output in pregnancy by thermodilution and impedance techniques. Br J Obstet Gynaecol 96:67, 1989a

Easterling TR, Benedetti TJ, Schmucker BC, Carlson KL: Antihypertensive therapy in pregnancy directed by noninvasive hemodynamic monitoring. Am J Perinatol 6:86, 1989b

Easterling TR, Benedetti TJ, Schmucker BC, Millard SP: Maternal hemodynamics in normal and preeclamptic pregnancies: A longitudinal study. Obstet Gynecol 76:1061, 1990

Editorial: Are ACE inhibitors safe in pregnancy? Lancet 1:482, 1989

Elias AN, Vaziri ND, Pandian MR, Powers DR, Domurat E: Atrial natriuretic peptide and arginine vasopressin in pregnancy and pregnancy-induced hypertension. Nephron 49:140, 1988

España F, Gilabert J, Aznar J, Estellés A, Kobayashi T, Griffin JH: Complexes of activated protein C with α_1-antitrypsin in normal pregnancy and in severe preeclampsia. Am J Obstet Gynecol 164:1310, 1991

Everett RB, Porter JC, MacDonald PC, Gant NF: Relationship of maternal placental blood flow to the placental clearance of maternal plasma dehydroisoandrosterone sulfate through placental estriol formation. Am J Obstet Gynecol 136:435, 1980

Everett RB, Worley RJ, MacDonald PC, Gant NF: Effect of prostaglandin synthetase inhibitors on pressor response to angiotensin II in human pregnancy. J Clin Endocrinol Metab 46:1007, 1978a

Everett RB, Worley RJ, MacDonald PC, Gant NF: Modification of vascular responsiveness to angiotensin II in pregnant women by intravenously infused 5α-dihydroprogesterone. Am J Obstet Gynecol 131:352, 1978b

Fairlie FM, Moretti M, Walker JJ, Sibai BM: Determinants of perinatal outcome in pregnancy-induced hypertension with absence of umbilical artery end-diastolic frequencies. Am J Obstet Gynecol 164:1084, 1991

Feeney JG, Scott JS: Pre-eclampsia and changed paternity. Eur J Obstet Gynaecol Reprod Biol 11:35, 1980

Ferrazzani S, Caruso A, De Carolis S, Martino IV, Mancuso S: Proteinuria and outcome of 444 pregnancies complicated by hypertension. Am J Obstet Gynecol 162:366, 1990

Ferris TF, Weir EK: Effect of captopril in uterine blood flow and prostaglandin E synthesis in the pregnant rabbit. J Clin Invest 71:809, 1983

Fievet P, Gregoire I, Fournier A, Roth D, Siegenthaler G, El Esper N, Favre H, DeBold A: Ouabain-like natriuretic factor and atrial natriuretic factor in pregnancy. Kidney Int 34 (suppl):89, 1988

Fisher ER, Pardo V, Paul R, Hayashi TT: Ultrastructural studies in hypertension, IV. Toxemia of pregnancy. Am J Pathol 55:901, 1969

Fitzgerald DJ, Rocki W, Murray R, Mayo G, FitzGerald GA: Thromboxane A$_2$ synthesis in pregnancy-induced hypertension. Lancet 335:751, 1990

Fleischer A, Schulman H, Farmakides G, Bracero L, Grunfeld L, Rochelson B, Koenigsberg M: Uterine artery Doppler velocimetry in pregnant women with hypertension. Am J Obstet Gynecol 154:806, 1986

Frenkel Y, Barkai G, Mashiach S, Dolev E, Zimlichman R, Weiss M: Hypocalciuria of preeclampsia is independent of parathyroid hormone level. Obstet Gynecol 77:689, 1991

Friedman EA, Neff RK: Pregnancy outcome as related to hypertension, edema, and proteinuria. In Lindheimer MD, Katz AI, Zuspan FP (eds): Hypertension in Pregnancy. New York, Wiley, 1976, p 13

Fritz MA, Stanczyk FZ, Novy MJ: Relationship of uteroplacental blood flow to the placental clearance of maternal dehydroepiandrosterone through estradiol formation in the pregnant baboon. J Clin Endocrinol Metab 61:1023, 1985

Gallery EDM, Saunders DM, Hunyor SN, Gyory AZ: Randomized comparison of methyldopa and oxyprenolol for treatment of hypertension in pregnancy. BMJ 1:1591, 1979

Gant NF, Chand S, Whalley PJ, MacDonald PC: The nature of pressor responsiveness to angiotensin II in human pregnancy. Obstet Gynecol 43:854, 1974a

Gant NF, Chand S, Worley RJ, Whalley PJ, Crosby UD, MacDonald PC: A clinical test useful for predicting the development of acute hypertension in pregnancy. Am J Obstet Gynecol 120:1, 1974b

Gant NF, Daley GL, Chand S, Whalley PJ, MacDonald PC: A study of angiotensin II pressor response throughout primigravid pregnancy. J Clin Invest 52:2682, 1973

Gant NF, Gilstrap LC III: Pharmacological approaches to prevent pregnancy-induced hypertension. Williams Obstetrics, 18th ed (suppl 5). Norwalk, CT, Appleton & Lange, 1990

Gant NF, Jimenez JM, Whalley PJ, Chand S, MacDonald PC: A prospective study of angiotensin II pressor responsiveness in pregnancies complicated by chronic essential hypertension. Am J Obstet Gynecol 127:369, 1977

Gant NF, Madden JD, Siiteri PK, MacDonald PC: The metabolic clearance rate of dehydroisoandrosterone sulfate, III. The effect of thiazide diuretics in normal and future preeclamptic pregnancies. Am J Obstet Gynecol 123:159, 1975

Gant NF, Madden JD, Siiteri PK, MacDonald PC: The metabolic clearance rate of dehydroisoandrosterone sulfate, IV. Acute effect of induced hypertension, hypotension, and natruresis in normal and hypertensive pregnancies. Am J Obstet Gynecol 124:143, 1976

Gedekoh RH, Hayashi TT, MacDonald HM: Eclampsia at Magee–Womens Hospital, 1970–1980. Am J Obstet Gynecol 140:860, 1981

Gilabert J, Fernandez JA, España F, Aznar J, Estelles A: Physiological coagulation inhibitors (protein S, protein C and antithrombin III) in severe preeclamptic states and in users of oral contraceptives. Thromb Res 49:319, 1988

Gilstrap LC, Cunningham FG, Whalley PJ: Management of pregnancy-induced hypertension in the nulliparous patient remote from term. Semin Perinatol 2:73, 1978

Goldman RS, Finkbeiner SM: Therapeutic use of magnesium sulfate in selected case of cerebral ischemia and seizure. N Engl J Med 319:1224, 1988

Goodman RP, Killam AP, Brush AR, Branch RA: Prostacyclin production during pregnancy: Comparison of production during normal pregnancy and pregnancy complicated by hypertension. Am J Obstet Gynecol 142:817, 1982

Govan ADT: The pathogenesis of eclamptic lesions. Pathol Microbiol 24:561, 1961

Green KW, Key TC, Coen R, Resnik R: The effects of maternally administered magnesium sulfate on the neonate. Am J Obstet Gynecol 146:29, 1983

Gregoire I, Roth D, Siegenthaler G, Fievet P, El Esper N, Favre H, Fournier A: A ouabain-displacing factor in normal pregnancy, pregnancy-induced hypertension and preeclampsia. Clin Sci 74:307, 1988

Griffis KR Jr, Martin JN Jr, Palmer SM, Martin RW, Morrison JC: Utilization of hydralazine or alpha-methyldopa for the management of early puerperal hypertension. Am J Perinatol 6:437, 1989

Groenendijk R, Trimbros JBM, Wallenburg HCS: Hemodynamic measurements in preeclampsia: Preliminary observations. Am J Obstet Gynecol 150:232, 1984

Guzick DS, Klein VR, Tyson JE, Lasky RE, Gant NF, Rosenfeld CR: Risk factors for the occurrence of pregnancy-induced hypertension. Clin Exp Hyper-Hyper Preg B6:281, 1987

Haeger M, Unander M, Norder-Hansson B, Tylman M, Bengtsson A: Complement, neutrophil, and macrophage activation in women with severe preeclampsia and the syndrome of hemolysis, elevated liver enzymes, and low platelet count. Obstet Gynecol 79:19, 1992

Hankins GDV, Cunningham FG: Severe preeclampsia and eclampsia: Controversies in management. Williams Obstetrics, 18th ed (suppl 12). Norwalk, CT, Appleton & Lange, 1991

Hankins GDV, Wendel GW Jr, Cunningham FG, Leveno KJ: Longitudinal evaluation of hemodynamic changes in eclampsia. Am J Obstet Gynecol 150:506, 1984

Hanretty KP, Primrose MH, Neilson JP, Whittle MJ: Pregnancy screening by doppler uteroplacental and umbilical artery waveforms. Br J Obstet Gynaecol 96:1163, 1989

Hanretty KP, Whittle MJ, Rubin PC: Doppler uteroplacental

waveforms in pregnancy-induced hypertension: A reappraisal. Lancet 1:850, 1988a

Hanretty KP, Whittle MJ, Rubin PC: Reappearance of end-diastolic velocity in a pregnancy complicated by severe pregnancy-induced hypertension. Am J Obstet Gynecol 158:1123, 1988b

Hansen JP: Older maternal age and pregnancy outcome: A review of the literature. Obstet Gynecol Surv 41:726,1986

Hanssens M, Keirse MJNC, Vankelecom F, VanAssche FA: Fetal and neonatal effects of treatment with angiotensin-converting enzyme inhibitors. Obstet Gynecol 78:128, 1991

Harbert GM Jr, Cornell GW, Thornton WN Jr: Effect of toxemia therapy on uterine dynamics. Am J Obstet Gynecol 105:94, 1969

Hauth JC, Goldenberg RL, Parker CR Jr, Philips JB III, Cooper RL, DuBard MB, Cutter GR: Low-dose aspirin therapy to prevent preeclampsia. Am J Obstet Gynecol (in press)

Hauth JC, Cunningham FG, Whalley PJ: Management of pregnancy-induced hypertension in the nullipara. Obstet Gynecol 48:253, 1976

Hayward C, Livingstone J, Holloway S, Liston WA, Brock DJH: An exclusion map for pre-eclampsia: Assuming autosomal recessive inheritance. Am J Hum Genet 50:749, 1992

Hertig AT: Vascular pathology in the hypertensive albuminuric toxemias of pregnancy. Clinics 4:602, 1945

Herzog TJ, Angel OH, Karram MM, Evertson LR: Use of magnetic resonance imaging in the diagnosis of cortical blindness in pregnancy. Obstet Gynecol 76:980, 1990

Hinselmann H: Die Eklampsie. Bonn, F Cohen, 1924

Hirai N, Yanaihara T, Nakayama T, Ishibashi M, Yamaji T: Plasma levels of atrial natriuretic peptide during normal pregnancy and in pregnancy complicated by hypertension. Am J Obstet Gynecol 159:27, 1988

Hodgkinson R, Husain FJ, Hayashi RH: Systemic and pulmonary blood pressure during cesarean section in parturients with gestational hypertension. Can Anaesth Soc J 27:389, 1980

Hoff C, Stevens RG, Mendenhall H, Peterson RDA, Spinnato JA: Association between risk for pre-eclampsia and HLA DR4. Lancet 335:660, 1990

Hofmeyr GJ, Wilkins T, Redman CWG: C4 and plasma protein in hypertension during pregnancy with and without proteinuria. BMJ 302:218, 1991

Högstedt S, Lindeberg S, Axelsson O, Lindmark G, Rane A, Sandström B, Lindberg BS: A prospective controlled trial of metoprolol-hydralazine treatment in hypertension during pregnancy. Acta Obstet Gynecol Scand 64:505, 1985

Howie PW, Prentice CRM, Forbes CD: Failure of heparin therapy to affect the clinical course of severe preeclampsia. Br J Obstet Gynaecol 82:711, 1975

Hughes EC (ed): Obstetric–Gynecologic Terminology. Philadelphia, Davis, 1972

Huisjes HJ, Haddres-Algra M, Touwen BCL: Is clonidine a behavioural teratogen in the human? Early Hum Dev 14:43, 1986

Imperiale TF, Petrulis AS: A meta-analysis of low-dose aspirin for the prevention of pregnancy-induced hypertensive disease. JAMA 266:260, 1991

Jagadeesan V: Serum complement levels in normal pregnancy and pregnancy-induced hypertension. Int J Gynecol Obstet 26:389, 1988

Jakobi P, Krivoy N, Weissman A, Paldi E: Digoxin-like immu-

noreactive factor in twin and pregnancy-associated hypertensive pregnancies. Obstet Gynecol 74:29, 1989

Johnson T, Clayton CG: Diffusion of radioactive sodium in normotensive and preeclamptic pregnancies. BMJ 1:312, 1957

Kambam JR, Perry SM, Entman S, Smith BE: Effect of magnesium on plasma cholinesterase activity. Am J Obstet Gynecol 159:309, 1988

Kaminski K, Rechberger T: Concentration of digoxin-like immunoreactive substance in patients with preeclampsia and its relation to severity of pregnancy-induced hypertension. Am J Obstet Gynecol 165:733, 1991

Katz VL, Thorp JM Jr, Rozas L, Bowes WA Jr: The natural history of thrombocytopenia associated with preeclampsia. Am J Obstet Gynecol 163:1142, 1990

Kawathekar P, Anusuya SR, Sriniwas P, Lagali S: Diazepam (Calmpose) in eclampsia: A preliminary report of 16 cases. Curr Ther Res 15:845, 1973

Keith JC Jr, Miller K, Eggleston MK, Kutruff J, Howerton T, Konczal C, McDaniels C: Effects of thromboxane synthetase inhibition on maternal–fetal homeostasis in gravid ewes with ovine pregnancy-induced hypertension. Am J Obstet Gynecol 161:1305, 1989

Kelton JG, Hunter DJS, Naeme PB: A platelet function defect in preeclampsia. Obstet Gynecol 65:107, 1985

Kerkez SA, Poston L, Wolfe CD, Quartero HW, Carabelli P, Petruckevitch A, Hilton PJ: A longitudinal study of maternal digoxin-like immunoreactive substances in normotensive pregnancy and pregnancy-induced hypertension. Am J Obstet Gynecol 162:783, 1990

Kilby MD, Broughton Pipkin F, Cockbill S, Heptinstall S, Symonds EM: A cross-sectional study of basal platelet intracellular free calcium concentration in normotensive and hypertensive primigravid pregnancies. Clin Sci 78:75, 1990

Kilpatrick DC, Liston WA, Gibson F, Livingstone J: Association between susceptibility to pre-eclampsia within families and HLA DR4. Lancet 2:1063, 1989

Kincaid-Smith P: The renal lesion of preeclampsia revisited. Am J Kidney Dis 17:144, 1991

Kirshon B, Lee W, Mauer MB, Cotton DB: Effects of low-dose dopamine therapy in the oliguric patient with preeclampsia. Am J Obstet Gynecol 159:604, 1988

Kitzmiller JL, Lang JE, Yelonosky PF, Lucas WE: Hematologic assays in preeclampsia. Am J Obstet Gynecol 118:362, 1974

Kliegman RM, Gross T: Perinatal problems of the obese mother and her infant. Obstet Gynecol 66:299, 1985

Kofinas AD, Penry M, Greiss FC Jr, Meis PJ, Nelson LH: The effect of placental location on uterine artery flow velocity waveforms. Am J Obstet Gynecol 159:1504, 1988

Kofinas AD, Penry M, Nelson LH, Meis PJ, Swain M: Uterine and umbilical artery flow velocity waveform analysis in pregnancies complicated by chronic hypertension or preeclampsia. South Med J 83:150, 1990

Kofinas AD, Penry M, Simon NV, Swain M: Interrelationship and clinical significance of increased resistance in the uterine arteries in patients with hypertension or preeclampsia or both. Am J Obstet Gynecol 166:601, 1992

Kraus GW, Marchese JR, Yen SSC: Prophylactic use of hydrochlorothiazide in pregnancy. JAMA 198:1150, 1966

Kreft-Jais C, Tchobroutsky C, Boutroy J: Angiotensin-converting enzyme inhibitors during pregnancy: A survey of 22 patients given captopril and nine given enalapril. Br J Obstet Gynaecol 95:420, 1988

Kuban KCK, Leviton A, Pagano M, Fenton T, Strassfeld R, Wolff M: Maternal toxemia is associated with reduced incidence of germinal matrix hemorrhage in premature babies. J Child Neurol 7:70, 1992

Kurmanavichius J, Baumann H, Huch R, Huch A: Uteroplacental blood flow velocity waveforms as a predictor of adverse fetal outcome and pregnancy-induced hypertension. J Perinat Med 18:255, 1990

Landesman R, Douglas RG, Holze E: The bulbar conjunctival vascular bed in the toxemias of pregnancy. Am J Obstet Gynecol 68:170, 1954

Lean, TH, Ratnam SS, Sivasamboo R: Use of benzodiazepines in the management of eclampsia. J Obstet Gynaecol Br Commonw 75:856, 1968

Leduc L, Wheeler JM, Kirshon B, Mitchell P, Cotton DB: Coagulation profile in severe preeclampsia. Obstet Gynecol 79:14, 1992

Lee W, Gonik B, Cotton DB: Urinary diagnostic indices in preeclampsia-associated oliguria: Correlation with invasive hemodynamic monitoring. Am J Obstet Gynecol 156:100, 1987

Lehmann DK, Mabie WC, Miller JM, Pernoll ML: The epidemiology and pathology of maternal mortality: Charity Hospital of Louisiana in New Orleans, 1965–1984. Obstet Gynecol 69:833, 1987

Leiberman JR, Hagay ZJ, Mazor M, Wiznitzer A, Aharon M, Nathan I, Dvilansky A: Plasma antithrombin III levels in pre-eclampsia and chronic hypertension. Int J Gynecol Obstet 27:21, 1988

Lenox JW, Ugura V, Cibils LA: Effects of hypertension on pregnancy monitoring and results. Am J Obstet Gynecol 163:1173, 1990

Levine AB, Lockwood CJ, Chitkara U, Berkowitz RL: Maternal renal artery doppler velocimetry in normotensive pregnancies and pregnancies complicated by hypertensive disorders. Obstet Gynecol 79:264, 1992

Lichtig C, Luger AM, Spargo BH, Lindheimer MD: Renal immunofluorescence and ultrastructural findings in preeclampsia. Clin Res 23:368A, 1975

Lindheimer MD, Abe S: Introduction and overview. Am J Kidney Dis 17:95, 1991

Lindow SW, Davies N, Davey DA, Smith JA: The effect of sublingual nifedipine on uteroplacental blood flow in hypertensive pregnancy. Br J Obstet Gynaecol 95:1276, 1988

Llewellyn-Jones D: The treatment of eclampsia. Br J Obstet Gynecol 68:33, 1961

Lombardi SJ, Rosemond R, Ball R, Entman SS, Boehm FH: Umbilical artery velocimetry as a predictor of adverse outcome in pregnancies complicated by oligohydramnios. Obstet Gynecol 74:338, 1989

López-Jaramillo P, Narvaez M, Felix C, Lopez A: Dietary calcium supplementation and prevention of pregnancy hypertension. Lancet 335:293, 1990

López-Jaramillo P, Narváez M, Weigel RM, Yépez R: Calcium supplementation reduces the risk of pregnancy-induced hypertension in an Andes population. Br J Obstet Gynaecol 96:648, 1989

López-Llera M: Main clinical types and subtypes of eclampsia. Am J Obstet Gynecol 166:4, 1992

López-Llera M: Complicated eclampsia: Fifteen years' experi-

ence in a referral medical center. Am J Obstet Gynecol 142:28, 1982

López-Llera M, Hernandez-Horta JL, Huttich FC: Retarded fetal growth in eclampsia. J Reprod Med 9:229, 1972

Louden KA, Broughton Pipkin F, Heptinstall S, Fox SC, Mitchell JRA, Symonds EM: Platelet reactivity and serum thromboxane B_2 production in whole blood in gestational hypertension and pre-eclampsia. Br J Obstet Gynaecol 98:1239, 1991

Low JA: The current status of maternal and fetal blood flow velocimetry. Am J Obstet Gynecol 164:1049, 1991

Lowery CL Jr, Henson BV, Wan J, Brumfield CG: A comparison between umbilical artery velocimetry and standard antepartum surveillance in hospitalized high-risk patients. Am J Obstet Gynecol 162:710, 1990

Lucas M, DePalma R, Peters M, Leveno K, Persons D, Cunningham FG: An easily administered phenytoin regimen for the management of preeclampsia. Abstract 66 presented at meeting of Society of Perinatal Obstetricians, Orlando, February, 1992

Lurie S, Fenakel K, Friedman A: Effect of nifedipine on fetal heart rate in the treatment of severe pregnancy-induced hypertension. Am J Perinatol 7:285, 1990

Mabie WC, Gonzalez AR, Sibai BM, Amon E: A comparative trial of labetalol and hydralazine in the acute management of severe hypertension complicating pregnancy. Obstet Gynecol 70:328, 1987

Mabie WC, Pernoll ML, Biswas MK: Chronic hypertension in pregnancy. Obstet Gynecol 67:197, 1986

Mabie WC, Ratts TE, Ramanathan KB, Sibai BM: Circulatory congestion in obese hypertensive women. A subset of pulmonary edema in pregnancy. Obstet Gynecol 72:553, 1988a

Mabie WC, Sibai BM, Anderson GD, Gonzalez-Ruiz AR, Moretti ML, Harvey CJ: Nifedipine in the treatment of severe peripartum hypertension. Abstract 87 presented at the eighth annual meeting of the Society of Perinatal Obstetricians, Las Vegas, February 1988b

MacKanjee HR, Shaul PW, Magness RR, Rosenfeld CR: Angiotensin II vascular smooth-muscle receptors are not down-regulated in near-term pregnant sheep. Am J Obstet Gynecol 165:1641, 1991

Magness RR, Cox K, Gant NF: Effects of low-dose aspirin (ASA) and linoleic acid (LA) on PGI_2 and TxA_2 and pregnancy outcome in preeclampsia (PE). Abstract 332 presented at the 38th annual meeting of the Society for Gynecologic Investigation, San Antonio, March 1991

Manas KJ, Welsh JD, Rankin RA, Miller DD: Hepatic hemorrhage without rupture in preeclampsia. N Engl J Med 312:426, 1985

Marcoux S, Brisson J, Fabia J: Calcium intake from diary products and supplements and the risks of preeclampsia and gestational hypertension. Am J Epidemiol 133:1266, 1991

Martikainen A: Growth and development at the age of 1.5 years in children with maternal hypertension. J Perinat Med 17:259, 1989

Mastrogiannis DS, O'Brien WF, Krammer J, Benoit R: Potential role of endothelin-1 in normal and hypertensive pregnancies. Am J Obstet Gynecol 165:1711, 1991

McCall ML: Cerebral circulation and metabolism in toxemia of pregnancy: Observations on the effects of veratrum viride and apresoline (1-hydrazinophthalazine). Am J Obstet Gynecol 66:1015, 1953

McCartney CP: Pathological anatomy of acute hypertension of pregnancy. Circulation 30(suppl 2):37, 1964

McCartney CP, Schumacher GFB, Spargo BH: Serum proteins in patients with toxemic glomerular lesion. Am J Obstet Gynecol 111:580, 1971

McCubbin JH, Sibai BM, Abdella TN, Anderson GD: Cardiopulmonary arrest due to acute maternal hypermagnesemia. Lancet 1:1058, 1981

McKay DG: Disseminated Intravascular Coagulation. New York, Harper & Row, 1965

McParland P, Pearce JM, Chamberlain GV: Doppler ultrasound and aspirin in recognition and prevention of pregnancy-induced hypertension. Lancet 335:1552, 1990

Menon MKK: The evolution of the treatment of eclampsia. J Obstet Gynaecol Br Commonw 68:417, 1961

Metcalfe J, Romney SL, Ramsey LH, Reid DE, Burwell CS: Estimation of uterine blood flow in normal human pregnancy at term. J Clin Invest 34:1632, 1955

Michael CA: The evaluation of labetalol in the treatment of hypertension complicating pregnancy. Br J Clin Pharmacol 127(suppl 1):127A, 1982

Miles JF, Martin JN Jr, Blake PG, Perry KG Jr, Martin RW, Meeks RG: Postpartum eclampsia: A recurring perinatal dilemma. Obstet Gynecol 76:328, 1990

Miller KW, Keith JC: Erythrocyte morphologic features and serum chemistry studies in ovine pregnancy-induced hypertension treated with thromboxane synthetase inhibitors. Am J Obstet Gynecol 159:1241, 1988

Mires GJ, Dempster J, Patel NB, Taylor DJ: Epidural analgesia and its effect on umbilical artery flow velocity waveform patterns in uncomplicated labour and labour complicated by pregnancy-induced hypertension. Eur J Obstet Gynecol Reprod Biol 36:35, 1990

Mirmiran M, Scholtens J, Van de Poll NE, Uylings HB, van der Gugten J, Boer GJ: Effects of experimental suppression of active (REM) sleep during early development upon adult brain and behaviour. Dev Brain Res 7:277, 1983

Mitchell MD, Koenig JM: Increased production of 15-hydroxyeicosatetraenoic acid by placentae from pregnancies complicated by pregnancy-induced hypertension. Prostaglandins Leukot Essent Fatty Acids 43:61, 1991

Mojadidi Q, Thompson RJ: Five years' experience with eclampsia. South Med J 66:414, 1973

Molnár M, Hertelendy F: Nω-Nitro-L-arginine, an inhibitor of nitric oxide synthesis, increases blood pressure in rats and reverses the pregnancy-induced refractoriness to vasopressor agents. Am J Obstet Gynecol 166:1560, 1992

Montan S, Ingemarsson I: Intrapartum fetal heart rate patterns in pregnancies complicated by hypertension. Am J Obstet Gynecol 160:283, 1989

Moore TR, Key TC, Reisner LS, Renick RR: Evaluation of the use of continuous lumbar epidural anesthesia for hypertensive pregnant women in labor. Am J Obstet Gynecol 152:104, 1985

Morris N, Osborn SB, Wright HP, Hart A: Effective uterine bloodflow during exercise in normal and pre-eclamptic pregnancies. Lancet 2:481, 1956

Morrow RJ, Adamson SL, Bull SB, Ritchie JWK: Hypoxic acidemia, hyperviscosity, and maternal hypertension do not affect the umbilical arterial velocity waveform in fetal sheep. Am J Obstet Gynecol 163:1313, 1990

Myatt L, Brewer AS, Langdon G, Brockman DE: Attenuation of the vasoconstrictor effects of thromboxane and endothelin by nitric oxide in the human fetal–placental circulation. Am J Obstet Gynecol 166:224, 1992

Naden RP, Redman CW: Antihypertensive drugs in pregnancy. Clin Perinatol 12:521, 1985

Naeye RL, Friedman EA: Causes of perinatal death associated with gestational hypertension and proteinuria. Am J Obstet Gynecol 133:8, 1979

Nalliah S, Thavarashah AS: Transient blindness in pregnancy induced hypertension. Int J Gynaecol Obstet 29:249, 1989

National High Blood Pressure Education Program Working Group Report on High Blood Pressure in Pregnancy. Am J Obstet Gynecol 163:1691, 1990

Need JA, Bell B, Meffin E, Jones WR: Pre-eclampsia in pregnancies from donor inseminations. J Reprod Immunol 5:329, 1983

Neuman M, Ron-El R, Langer R, Bukovsky I, Caspi E: Maternal death caused by HELLP syndrome (with hypoglycemia) complicating mild pregnancy-induced hypertension in a twin gestation. Am J Obstet Gynecol 162:372, 1990

Newsome LR, Bramwell RS, Curling PE: Severe preeclampsia: Hemodynamic effects of lumbar epidural anesthesia. Anesth Analg 65:31, 1986

Nisell H, Carlström K, Cizinsky S, Grunewald C, Nylund L, Randmaa I: Atrial natriuretic peptide concentrations and hemodynamic effects of acute plasma volume expansion in normal pregnancy and preeclampsia. Obstet Gynecol 79:902, 1992

Nochimson DJ, Petrie RH: Glucocorticoid therapy for the induction of pulmonary maturity in severely hypertensive gravid women. Am J Obstet Gynecol 133:449, 1979

Nova A, Sibai BM, Barton JR, Mercer BM, Mitchell MD: Maternal plasma level of endothelin is increased in preeclampsia. Am J Obstet Gynecol 165:724, 1991

O'Brien WF: Predicting preeclampsia. Obstet Gynecol 75:445, 1990

O'Brien WF, Williams MC, Benoit R, Sawai SK, Knuppel RA: The effect of magnesium sulfate infusion on systemic and renal prostacyclin production. Prostaglandins 40:529, 1990

Oian P, Maltau JM, Noddleland H, Fadnes HO: Transcapillary fluid balance in preeclampsia. Br J Obstet Gynaecol 93:235, 1986

Oian P, Maltau JM, Noddleland H, Fadnes HO: Oedema-preventing mechanisms in subcutaneous tissue of normal pregnant women. Br J Obstet Gynaecol 92:1113, 1985

Öney T, Kaulhausen H: The value of the angiotensin sensitivity test in the early diagnosis of hypertensive disorders of pregnancy. Am J Obstet Gynecol 142:17, 1982

Otani S, Usuki S. Saitoh T, Yanagisawa M, Iwasaki H, Tanaka J, Suzuki N, Fujino M, Goto K, Masaki T: Comparison of endothelin-1 concentrations in normal and complicated pregnancies. J Cardiovasc Pharmacol 17:S308, 1991

Ounsted M, Cockburn J, Moar VA, Redman CW: Maternal hypertension with superimposed pre-eclampsia: Effects on child development at 7 years. Br J Obstet Gynaecol 90:644, 1983

Page EW: On the pathogenesis of pre-eclampsia and eclampsia. J Obstet Gynaecol Br Commonw 79:883, 1972

Palmer RMJ, Ashton DS, Moncada S: Vascular endothelial cells synthesize nitric oxide from L-arginine. Nature 333:664, 1988

Palmer RMJ, Ferrige AG, Moncada S: Nitric oxide release accounts for the biological activity of endothelium-derived relaxing factor. Nature 327:524, 1987

Palti H, Rothschild E: Blood pressure and growth at 6 years of age among offsprings of mothers with hypertension of pregnancy. Early Hum Dev 19:263, 1989

Parker CR, Everett RB, Quirk JG, Whalley PJ, Gant NF, MacDonald PC: Hormone production during pregnancy in the primigravida, II. Plasma levels of deoxycorticosterone throughout pregnancy in normal women and women who developed pregnancy-induced hypertension. Am J Obstet Gynecol 138:626, 1980

Pattinson RC, Kriegler E, Odendaal HJ, Muller LMM, Kirsten G: Increased placental resistance and late decelerations associated with severe proteinuric hypertension predicts poor fetal outcome. S Afr Med J 75:211, 1989

Petrucco OM, Thomson NM, Lawrence JR, Weldon MW: Immunofluorescent studies in renal biopsies in pre-eclampsia. BMJ 1:473, 1974

Phelan JP, Yurth DA: Severe preeclampsia, I. Peripartum hemodynamic observations. Am J Obstet Gynecol 144:17, 1982

Phippard AF, Fischer WE, Horvath JS, Child AG, Korda AR, Henderson-Smart D, Duggin GG, Tiller DJ: Early blood pressure control improves pregnancy outcome in primigravid women with mild hypertension. Med J Aust 154:378, 1991

Pickles CJ, Symonds EM, Broughton Pipkin F: The fetal outcome in a randomized double-blind controlled trial of labetalol versus placebo in pregnancy-induced hypertension. Br J Obstet Gynaecol 96:38, 1989

Pirhonen JP, Erkkola RU, Ekblad UU: Uterine and fetal flow velocity waveforms in hypertensive pregnancy: The effect of a single dose of nifedipine. Obstet Gynecol 76:37, 1990

Plouin PF, Breart G, Llado J, Dalle M, Keller ME, Goujon H, Berchel C: A randomized comparison of early with conservative use of antihypertensive drugs in the management of pregnancy-induced hypertension. Br J Obstet Gynaecol 97:134, 1990

Plouin PF, Breart G, Maillard F, Papierrnik E, Relier JP, The Labetalol Methyldopa Study Group: Comparison of antihypertensive efficacy and perinatal safety of labetalol and methyldopa in the treatment of hypertension in pregnancy: A randomized controlled trial. Br J Obstet Gynaecol 95:868, 1988

Pritchard JA: The use of magnesium sulfate in preeclampsia–eclampsia. J Reprod Med 23:107, 1979

Pritchard JA: The use of the magnesium ion in the management of eclamptogenic toxemias. Surg Gynecol Obstet 100:131, 1955

Pritchard JA, Cunningham FG, Mason RA: Coagulation changes in eclampsia: Their frequency and pathogenesis. Am J Obstet Gynecol 124:855, 1976

Pritchard JA, Cunningham FG, Pritchard SA: The Parkland Memorial Hospital protocol for treatment of eclampsia: Evaluation of 245 cases. Am J Obstet Gynecol 148:951, 1984

Pritchard JA, Cunningham FG, Pritchard SA, Mason RA: How often does maternal preeclampsia–eclampsia incite thrombocytopenia in the fetus? Obstet Gynecol 69:292, 1987

Pritchard JA, Ratnoff OD, Weismann R Jr: Hemostatic defects and increased red cell destruction in preeclampsia and eclampsia. Obstet Gynecol 4:159, 1954a

Pritchard JA, Weisman R Jr, Ratnoff OD, Vosburgh G: Intravascular hemolysis, thrombocytopenia and other hematologic abnormalities associated with severe toxemia of pregnancy. N Engl J Med 250:87, 1954b

Puzey MS, Ackovic KL, Lindow SW, Gonin R: The effect of nifedipine on fetal umbilical artery Doppler waveforms in pregnancies complicated by hypertension. S Afr Med J 79:192, 1991

Raab W, Schroeder G, Wagner R, Gigee W: Vascular reactivity and electrolytes in normal and toxemic pregnancy. J Clin Endocrinol 16:1196,1956

Rafferty TD, Berkowitz RL: Hemodynamics in patients with severe toxemia during labor and delivery. Am J Obstet Gynecol 138:263, 1980

Ramanathan J, Sibai BM, Mabie WC, Chauhan D, Ruiz AG: The use of labetalol for attenuation of the hypertensive response to endotracheal intubation in preeclampsia. Am J Obstet Gynecol 159:650, 1988

Ramos-Santos E, Devoe LD, Wakefield ML, Sherline DM, Metheny WP: The effects of epidural anesthesia on the doppler velocimetry of umbilical and uterine arteries in normal and hypertensive patients during active term labor. Obstet Gynecol 77:20, 1991

Redman CWG: Controlled trials of antihypertensive drugs in pregnancy. Am J Kidney Dis 17:149, 1991

Redman CWG: Eclampsia still kills. BMJ 296:1209, 1988

Redman CWG: Controlled trials of treatment of hypertension during pregnancy. Obstet Gynecol Surv 37:523, 1982

Redman CWG: Treatment of hypertension in pregnancy. Kidney Int 18:267, 1980

Redman CWG, Beilin LJ, Bonnar J, Ounsted MK: Fetal outcome in a trial of antihypertensive treatment in pregnancy. Lancet 2:753, 1976

Redman CWG, Jefferies M: Revised definition of pre-eclampsia. Lancet 1:809, 1988

Repke JT, Villar J: Pregnancy-induced hypertension and low birth weight: The role of calcium. Am J Clin Nutr 54:237S, 1991

Robertson EG: The natural history of oedema during pregnancy. J Obstet Gynaecol Br Commonw 78:520, 1971

Robertson WB, Khong TY, Brosens I, DeWolf F, Sheppard BL, Bonnar J: The placental bed biopsy: Review from three European centers. Am J Obstet Gynecol 155:401, 1986

Robin ED: The cult of the Swan-Ganz catheter. Ann Intern Med 103:445, 1985

Rochat RW, Koonin LM, Atrash HK, Jewett JF, the Maternal Mortality Collaborative: Maternal mortality in the United States: Report from the Maternal Mortality Collaborative Obstet Gynecol 72:91, 1988

Romero R, Mazor M, Lockwood CJ, Emamian M, Belanger KP, Hobbins JC, Duffy T: Clinical significance, prevalence, and natural history of thrombocytopenia in pregnancy-induced hypertension. Am J Perinatol 6:32, 1989

Rosa FW, Bosco LA, Graham CF, Milstien JB, Dreis M, Creamer J: Neonatal anuria with maternal angiotensin-converting enzyme inhibition. Obstet Gynecol 74:371, 1989

Rosenbaum M, Maltby G: Cerebral dysrhythmia in relation to eclampsia. Arch Neurol Psychiatr 49:204, 1943

Rubin PC: Treatment of hypertension in pregnancy. Clin Obstet Gynaecol 13:307, 1986

Rubin PC, Butters L, Clark DM, Reynolds B, Summer DJ, Steedman D, Low RA, Reid JL: Placebo-controlled trial of atenolol in treatment of pregnancy-associated hypertension. Lancet 1:431, 1983

Ruvinsky ED, Douvas SG, Roberts WE, Martin JN Jr, Palmer SM, Rhodes PG, Morrison JC: Maternal administration of dexamethasone in severe pregnancy-induced hypertension. Am J Obstet Gynecol 149:722, 1984

Ryan G, Lange I, Naughler M: Clinical experience using phenytoin prophylaxis in severe preeclampsia. Am J Obstet Gynecol 161:1297, 1989

Sachs BP, Brown DAJ, Driscoll SG, Schulman E, Acker D, Ransil BJ, Jewett JF: Maternal mortality in Massachusetts—Trends and prevention. N Engl J Med 316:667, 1987

Saleh AA, Bottoms SF, Norman G, Farag A, Mammen EF: Hemostasis in hypertensive disorders of pregnancy. Obstet Gynecol 71:719, 1988

Saleh AA, Bottoms SF, Welch RA, Ali AM, Mariona FG, Mammen EF: Preeclampsia, delivery and the hemostatic system. Am J Obstet Gynecol 157:331, 1987

Samuels P, Main EK, Tomaski A, Mennuti MT, Gabbe SG, Cines DB: Abnormalities in platelet antiglobulin tests in preeclamptic mothers and their neonates. Am J Obstet Gynecol 157:109, 1987

Sanchez-Ramos L, Jones DC, Cullen MT: Urinary calcium as an early marker for preeclampsia. Obstet Gynecol 77:685, 1991

Sanchez-Ramos L, O'Sullivan MJ, Garrido-Calderone J: Effect of low-dose aspirin on angiotensin II pressor response in human pregnancy. Am J Obstet Gynecol 156:193, 1987

Schiff E, Barkai G, Ben-Baruch G, Mashiach S: Low-dose aspirin does not influence the clinical course of women with mild pregnancy-induced hypertension. Obstet Gynecol 76:742, 1990

Schiff E, Ben-Baruch G, Peleg E, Rosenthal T, Alcalay M, Devir M, Mashiach S: Immunoreactive circulating endothelin-1 in normal and hypertensive pregnancies. Am J Obstet Gynecol 166:624, 1992

Schiff E, Peleg E, Goldenberg M, Rosenthal T, Ruppin E, Tamarkin M, Barkai G, Ben-Baruch G, Yahal I, Blankstein J, Goldman B, Mashiach S: The use of aspirin to prevent pregnancy-induced hypertension and lower the ratio of thromboxane A_2 to prostacyclin in relatively high risk pregnancies. N Engl J Med 321:351, 1989

Scott AA, Purohit DM: Neonatal renal failure: A complication of maternal antihypertensive therapy. Am J Obstet Gynecol 160:1223, 1989

Seabe SJ, Moodley J, Becker P: Nifedipine in acute hypertensive emergencies in pregnancy. S Afr Med J 76:248, 1989

Semchyshyn S, Zuspan F, Cordero L: Cardiovascular response and complications of glucocorticoid therapy in hypertensive pregnancies. Am J Obstet Gynecol 145:530, 1983

Shears BH: Combination of chlorpromazine, promethazine, and pethidine in treatment of eclampsia. BMJ 2:75, 1957

Sheehan HL: Pathological lesions in the hypertensive toxaemias of pregnancy. In Hammond J, Browne FJ, Wolstenholme GEW (eds): Toxaemias of Pregnancy, Human and Veterinary. Philadelphia, Blakiston, 1950

Sheehan HL, Lynch JB (eds): Cerebral lesions. In: Pathology of Toxaemia of Pregnancy. Baltimore, Williams & Wilkins, 1973

Shoemaker ES, Gant NF, Madden JD, MacDonald PC: The effect of thiazide diuretics on placental function. Tex Med 69:109, 1973

Sibai BM: Eclampsia VI. Maternal-perinatal outcome in 254 consecutive cases. Am J Obstet Gynecol 163:1049, 1990a

Sibai BM, Abdella TN, Anderson GD: Pregnancy outcome in 211 patients with mild chronic hypertension. Obstet Gynecol 61:571, 1983

Sibai BM, Anderson GD: Pregnancy outcome of intensive therapy in severe hypertension in first trimester. Obstet Gynecol 67:517, 1986a

Sibai BM, Caritis S, Phillips E, Klebanoff M, McNellis D, Rocco L, and the NICHD-MFM Network: Prevention of preeclampsia: Low-dose aspirin in nulliparous women: A multicenter double-blind placebo controlled trial. Presented at the 13th annual meeting of the Society of Perinatal Obstetricians, San Francisco, 1993a

Sibai B, Caritis S, Phillips E, Klebanoff M, Paul R, Witter F, Depp R, Rosen M, Romero R, McNellis D, and the NICHD-MFM Network: Safety of low-dose aspirin in healthy nulliparous women: A double-blind placebo-controlled trial. Abstract 228 presented at the 40th annual meeting of the Society for Gynecologic Investigation, Toronto, Canada, 1993b

Sibai BM, El-Nazer A, Gonzalez-Ruiz A: Severe preeclampsia-eclampsia in young primigravid women: Subsequent pregnancy outcome and remote prognosis. Am J Obstet Gynecol 155:1011, 1986b

Sibai BM, Gonzalez AR, Mabie WC, Moretti M: A comparison of labetalol plus hospitalization versus hospitalization alone in the management of preeclampsia remote from term. Obstet Gynecol 70:323, 1987a

Sibai BM, Graham JM, McCubbin JH: A comparison of intravenous and intramuscular magnesium sulfate regimens in preeclampsia. Am J Obstet Gynecol 150:728, 1984

Sibai BM, Mabie BC, Harvey CJ, Gonzalez AR: Pulmonary edema in severe preeclampsia—eclampsia: Analysis of thirty-seven consecutive cases. Am J Obstet Gynecol 156:1174, 1987b

Sibai BM, Mabie WC, Shamsa F, Villar MA, Anderson GD: A comparison of no medication versus methyldopa or labetalol in chronic hypertension during pregnancy. Am J Obstet Gynecol 162:960, 1990c

Sibai BM, McCubbin JH, Anderson GD, Lipshitz J, Dilts PV Jr: Eclampsia: I. Observations from 67 recent cases. Obstet Gynecol 58:609, 1981

Sibai BM, Mercer B, Sarinoglu C: Severe preeclampsia in the second trimester: Recurrence risk and long-term prognosis. Am J Obstet Gynecol 165:1408, 1991

Sibai BM, Sarinoglu C, Mercer BM: Eclampsia VII. Pregnancy outcome after eclampsia and long-term prognosis. Am J Obstet Gynecol 166:1757, 1992

Sibai BM, Spinnato JA, Watson DL, Lewis JA, Anderson GA: Eclampsia, IV. Neurological findings and future outcome. Am J Obstet Gynecol 152:184, 1985a

Sibai BM, Taslimi M, Abdella TN, Brooks TF, Spinnato JA, Anderson GD: Maternal and perinatal outcome of conservative management of severe preeclampsia in midtrimester. Am J Obstet Gynecol 152:32,1985b

Sibai BM, Taslimi MM, El-Nazer A, Amon E, Mabie BC, Ryan GM: Maternal-perinatal outcome associated with the syndrome of hemolysis, elevated liver enzymes, and low platelets in severe preeclampsia-eclampsia. Am J Obstet Gynecol 155:501,1986c

Sibai BM, Villar MA, Mabie BC: Acute renal failure in hypertensive disorders of pregnancy. Am J Obstet Gynecol 162:777, 1990b

Silke B, Carmody M, O'Swyer WF: Acute renal failure in pregnancy. In Bonnar J, MacGillivray I, Symonds EM (eds): Pregnancy Hypertension. Baltimore, University Park Press, 1980, p 511

Simon P, Fauchet R, Pilorge M, Calvez C, Le Fiblec B, Cam G, Ang KS, Genetet B, Cloup B: Association of HLA DR4 with the risk of recurrence of pregnancy hypertension. Kidney Int 34:S125, 1988

Sims EAH: Pre-eclampsia and related complications of pregnancy. Am J Obstet Gynecol 107:154, 1970

Slater RM, Wilcos FL, Smith WD, Donnai P, Patrick J, Richardson T, Mawer GE, D'Souza SW, Anderton JM: Phenytoin infusion in severe preeclampsia. Lancet 2:1417, 1987

Smith LG Jr, Moise KJ Jr, Dildy GA III, Carpenter RJ Jr: Spontaneous rupture of liver during pregnancy: Current therapy. Obstet Gynecol 77:171, 1991

Somjen G, Hilmy M, Stephen CR: Failure to anesthetize human subjects by intravenous administration of magnesium sulfate. J Pharmacol Exp Ther 154:652, 1966

Spargo B, McCartney CP, Winemiller R: Glomerular capillary endotheliosis in toxemia of pregnancy. Arch Pathol 68:593, 1959

Spellacy WN, Miller SJ, Winegar A: Pregnancy after 40 years of age. Obstet Gynecol 68:452, 1986

Spitz B, Magness RR, Cox SM, Brown CEL, Rosenfeld CR, Gant NF: Low-dose aspirin, I. Effect on angiotensin II pressor responses and blood prostaglandin concentrations in pregnant women sensitive to angiotensin II. Am J Obstet Gynecol 159:1035, 1988

Stahnke E: Über das Verhalten der Blutplättchen bei Eklampsie. Zentralbl Gynaekol 46:391, 1922

Stallworth JC, Yeh SY, Petrie RH: The effect of magnesium sulfate on fetal heart rate variability and uterine activity. Am J Obstet Gynecol 140:702, 1981

Steel SA, Pearce JM, Chamberlain GV: Doppler ultrasound of the uteroplacental circulation as a screening test for severe pre-eclampsia with intra-uterine growth retardation. Eur J Obstet Gynecol Reprod Biol 28:279, 1988

St-Louis J, Sicotte B: Prostaglandin- or endothelium-mediated vasodilation is not involved in the blunted responses of blood vessels to vasoconstrictors in pregnant rats. Am J Obstet Gynecol 166:684, 1992

Stone SR, Pritchard JA: Effect of maternally administered magnesium sulfate on the neonate. Obstet Gynecol 35:574, 1970

Strickland DM, Guzick DS, Cox K, Gant NF, Rosenfeld CR: The relationship between abortion in the first pregnancy and the development of pregnancy-induced hypertension in the subsequent pregnancy. Am J Obstet Gynecol 154:146, 1986

Stubbs TM, Lazarchick J, Horger EO: Plasma fibronectin levels in preeclampsia: A possible biochemical marker for vascular endothelial damage. Am J Obstet Gynecol 150:885, 1984

Tack ED, Perlman JM: Renal failure in sick, hypertensive premature infants receiving captopril therapy. J Pediatr 112:805, 1988

Talledo OE, Chesley LC, Zuspan FP: Renin-angiotensin system in normal and toxemic pregnancies, III. Differential sensitivity to angiotensin II and norepinephrine in toxemia of pregnancy. Am J Obstet Gynecol 100:218, 1968

Tannirandorn Y, Sullivan MHF, Elder MG: Production of urinary 11-keto-thromboxane B_2 in normal and hypertensive pregnancies. Prostaglandins Leukot Essent Fatty Acids 42:91, 1991

Taufield PA, Ales KL, Resnick LM, Druzin ML, Gertner JM, Laragh JH: Hypocalcuria in preeclampsia. N Engl J Med 316:715, 1987

Taylor RN, Casal DC, Jones LA, Varma M, Martin JN Jr, Roberts JM: Selective effects of preeclamptic sera on human endothelial cell procoagulant protein expression. Am J Obstet Gynecol 165:1705, 1991

Thiagarajah S, Bourgeois FJ, Harbert GM, Caudle MR: Thrombocytopenia in preeclampsia: Associated abnormalities and management principles. Am J Obstet Gynecol 150:1, 1984

Thiagarajah S, Harbert GM, Bourgeois FJ: Magnesium sulfate and ritodrine hydrochloride: Systemic and uterine hemodynamic effects. Am J Obstet Gynecol 153:666, 1985

Thomsen JK, Storm T, Thamsborg G, de Nully M, Bodker B, Skouby S: Atrial natriuretic peptide concentrations in preeclampsia. BMJ 294:1508, 1987

Thurnau GR, Kemp DB, Jarvis A: Cerebrospinal fluid levels of magnesium in patients with preeclampsia after treatment with intravenous magnesium sulfate: A preliminary report. Am J Obstet Gynecol 157:1435, 1987

Tillman AJB: The effect of normal and toxemic pregnancy on blood pressure. Am J Obstet Gynecol 70:589, 1955

Toppozada MK, Ismail AA, Hegab HM, Kamel MA: Treatment of preeclampsia with prostaglandin A_1. Am J Obstet Gynecol 159:160, 1988

Trudinger BJ, Cook CM: Doppler umbilical and uterine flow waveforms in severe pregnancy hypertension. Br J Obstet Gynaecol 97:142, 1990

Trudinger BJ, Giles WB, Cook CM: Flow velocity waveforms in the maternal uteroplacental and fetal umbilical placental circulations. Am J Obstet Gynecol 152:155, 1985

Tuffnell DJ, Lilford RJ, Buchan PC, Prendiville VM, Tuffnell AJ, Holgate MP, Jones MDG: Randomised controlled trial of day care for hypertension in pregnancy. Lancet 339:224, 1992

Turnbull A: Maternal mortality and present trends. In Sharp F, Symmonds EM (eds): Hypertension in Pregnancy. London: Perinatology Press, 1987, p 135

Van Assche FA, Spitz B, Vansteelant L: Severe systemic hypertension during pregnancy. Am J Cardiol 63:22C, 1989

Vassalli P, Morris RH, McCluskey RT: The pathogenic role of fibrin deposition in the glomerular lesions of toxemia of pregnancy. J Exp Med 118:467, 1963

Verhaeghe J, Anthony J, Davey DA: Platelet count and liver function tests in proteinuric and chronic hypertension in pregnancy. S Afr Med J 79:590, 1991

Villar MA, Sibai BM, González AR, Emerson DP, Anderson GD: Plasma volume, umbilical artery Doppler flow, and antepartum fetal heart testing in high-risk pregnancies. Am J Perinatol 6:341, 1989a

Villar MA, Sibai BM, Moretti ML, Mundy DC, Tabb TN, Anderson GD: The clinical significance of elevated mean arterial blood pressure in the second trimester and a threshold increase in systolic and diastolic blood pressures during the third trimester. Am J Obstet Gynecol 160:419, 1989b

Volhard F: Die doppelseitigen haematogenen Nierenerkrankungen. Berlin, Springer, 1918

Waisman GD, Mayorga LM, Cámera MI, Vignolo CA, Martinotti A: Magnesium plus nifedipine: Potentiation of hypotensive effect in preeclampsia? Am J Obstet Gynecol 159:308, 1988

Walker JJ, Bonduelle M, Greer I, Calder AA: Antihypertensive therapy in pregnancy. Lancet 1:932, 1983

Wallenburg HCS, Dekker GA, Makovitz JW, Rotmans P: Low-dose aspirin prevents pregnancy-induced hypertension and preeclampsia in angiotensin-sensitive primigravidae. Lancet 1:1, 1986

Walsh SW: Preeclampsia: An imbalance in placental prostacyclin and thromboxane production. Am J Obstet Gynecol 152:335, 1985

Walsh SW: Progesterone and estradiol production by normal and preeclamptic placentas. Obstet Gynecol 71:222, 1988

Wang Y, Walsh SW, Guo J, Zhang J: The imbalance between thromboxane and prostacyclin in preeclampsia is associated with an imbalance between lipid peroxides and vitamin E in maternal blood. Am J Obstet Gynecol 165:1695, 1991a

Wang Y, Walsh SW, Guo J, Zhang J: Maternal levels of prostacyclin, thromboxane, vitamin E, and lipid peroxides throughout normal pregnancy. Am J Obstet Gynecol 165:1690, 1991b

Wasserstrum N, Cotton DB: Hemodynamic monitoring in severe pregnancy-induced hypertension. Clin Perinatol 13:781, 1986

Watson KV, Moldow CF, Ogburn PL, Jacob JS: Magnesium sulfate: Rationale for its use in preeclampsia. Proc Natl Acad Sci USA 83:1075, 1986

Weenik GH, Borm JJ, Ten Cate JW, Treffers PE: Antithrombin III levels in normotensive and hypertensive pregnancy. Gynecol Obstet Invest 16:230, 1983

Weiner CP, Brandt J: Plasma antithrombin III activity: An aid in the diagnosis of preeclampsia–eclampsia. Am J Obstet Gynecol 142:275, 1982

Weiner CP, Kwaan HC, Xu C, Paul M, Burmeister L, Hauck W: Antithrombin III activity in women with hypertension during pregnancy. Obstet Gynecol 65:301, 1985

Weiner CP, Thompson LP, Liu KZ, Herrig JE: Endothelium-derived relaxing factor and indomethacin-sensitive contracting factor alter arterial contractile responses to thromboxane during pregnancy. Am J Obstet Gynecol 166:1171, 1992

Weinstein EM, Cox K, Harris KC, Gant NF, Magness RR: Does low dose aspirin affect the fetal ductus arteriosus? Am J Cardiol 66:520, 1990. Abstract

Weinstein L: Preeclampsia–eclampsia with hemolysis, elevated liver enzymes, and thrombocytopenia. Obstet Gynecol 66:657, 1985

Weir, RJ, Fraser R, Lever AF, Morton JJ, Brown JJ, Kraszewski A, McIlevine GM, Robertson JIS, Tree M: Plasma renin, renin substrate, angiotensin II, and aldosterone in hypertensive disease of pregnancy. Lancet 1:291, 1973

Weis EB Jr, Bruns PD, Taylor ES: A comparative study of the disappearance of radioactive sodium from human uterine muscle in normal and abnormal pregnancy. Am J Obstet Gynecol 76:340, 1958

Whalley PJ, Everett RB, Gant NF, Cox K, MacDonald PC: Pressor responsiveness to angiotensin II in hospitalized primigravid women with pregnancy-induced hypertension. Am J Obstet Gynecol 145:481, 1983

Wilcox GR, Trudinger BJ, Cook CM, Wilcox WR, Connelly AJ: Reduced fetal platelet counts in pregnancies with abnormal Doppler umbilical flow waveforms. Obstet Gynecol 73:639, 1989

Winkel CA, Casey ML, Guerami A, Rawlins SC, Cox K, MacDonald SC, Parker CR: Ratio of plasma deoxycorticosterone (DOC) levels to plasma progesterone (P) levels in pregnant women who did not develop pregnancy-induced hypertension (PIH). Abstract 341 presented at the 30th annual meeting of the Society for Gynecologic Investigation, Washington, DC, March, 1983

Winkel CA, Milewich L, Parker CR Jr, Gant NF, Simpson ER, MacDonald PC: Conversion of plasma progesterone to deoxycorticosterone in men, nonpregnant and pregnant women, and adrenalectomized subjects: Evidence for steroid 21-hydroxylase activity in non-adrenal tissues. J Clin Invest 66:803, 1980

Wisdom SJ, Wilson R, McKillop JH, Walker JJ: Antioxidant systems in normal pregnancy and in pregnancy-induced hypertension. Am J Obstet Gynecol 165:1701, 1991

World Health Organization Study Group: The hypertensive disorders of pregnancy. WHO Technical Report Series No 758. Geneva: World Health Organization, 1987

Worley RJ, Everett RB, MacDonald PC, Gant NF: Placental clearance of dehydroisoandrosterone sulfate and pregnancy outcome in three categories of hospitalized patients with pregnancy-induced hypertension. Gynecol Obstet Invest 6:28, 1975

Zeek PM, Assali NS: Vascular changes in decidua associated with eclamptogenic toxemia of pregnancy. Am J Clin Pathol 20:1099, 1950

Zinaman M, Rubin J, Lindheimer MD: Serial plasma oncotic pressure levels and echoencephalography during and after delivery in severe pre-eclampsia. Lancet 1:1245, 1985

Zlatnik FJ, Burmeister LF: Dietary protein and preeclampsia. Am J Obstet Gynecol 147:345, 1983

Zondervan HA, Oosting J, Smorenberg-schoorl ME, Treffers PE: Maternal whole blood viscosity in pregnancy hypertension. Gynecol Obstet Invest 25:83, 1988

Zuspan FP, Rayburn WF: Blood pressure self-monitoring during pregnancy: Practical considerations. Am J Obstet Gynecol 164:2, 1991

Zuspan FP, Ward MC: Treatment of eclampsia. South Med J 57:954, 1964

General Considerations

Mortality from Hemorrhage. Obstetrics is "bloody business." Even though the maternal mortality rate has been reduced dramatically by hospitalization for delivery and the availability of blood for transfusion, death from hemorrhage remains prominent in the majority of mortality reports. The Centers for Disease Control analyzed 2067 nonabortion-related maternal deaths in the United States from 1974 through 1978 and reported that hemorrhage was a direct cause in at least 13 percent of these (Kaunitz and colleagues, 1985). Similarly, data from the Maternal Mortality Collaborative from 1980 through 1985 indicated that 11 percent of direct maternal deaths were caused by hemorrhage (Rochat and co-workers, 1988). There is evidence that great improvement in mortality from hemorrhage has followed modernization of American obstetrics. For example, Sachs and associates (1987) reported that maternal deaths from obstetrical hemorrhage in Massachusetts decreased tenfold from the mid-1950s to the mid-1980s. Obstetrical hemorrhage is most likely to be fatal to the mother in circumstances in which whole blood or blood components are not available immediately. The establishment and maintenance of facilities that allow prompt administration of blood are absolute requirements for acceptable obstetrical care. For pregnancies complicated by bleeding during the second and third trimesters, the rates of preterm delivery and perinatal mortality are at least quadrupled (Jouppilla, 1979).

Blood Loss at Parturition. Loss of 500 mL or more of blood after completion of the third stage of labor has persisted as the definition of postpartum hemorrhage. Nonetheless, nearly one half of all women who are delivered vaginally, and almost all who undergo cesarean delivery, shed that amount of blood or more, when measured quantitatively (Fig. 37–1).

The woman with normal pregnancy-induced hypervolemia usually increases her blood volume by 30 to 60 percent, which for an average-sized woman amounts to 1 to 2 L (Pritchard, 1965). Consequently, she will tolerate, without any remarkable decrease in postpartum hematocrit, blood loss at delivery that approaches the volume of blood she added during pregnancy. Data from a specific case that serve to illustrate the protective nature of pregnancy hypervolemia are presented in Table 37–1.

Conditions that Predispose to Obstetrical Hemorrhage. Because of inexact definitions used, the incidence of obstetrical hemorrhage is impossible to determine precisely. In one study of women delivered vaginally, Combs and colleagues (1991a) defined hemorrhage by a postpartum hematocrit drop of 10 vol percent or by need for transfusion. Using these criteria, which obviously encompass very severe hemorrhage, the incidence was 3.9 percent. In another study of women delivered by cesarean section, these same investigators reported an incidence of hemorrhage of 6.4 percent (Combs and associates, 1991b). Dickason and Dinsmoor (1992) reported an incidence of transfusion of 6.8 percent in women undergoing cesarean section. Certainly, the transfusion rate is an indicator of significant hemorrhage. Klapholz (1990) reviewed over 30,000 obstetrical cases at the Beth Israel Hospital from 1976 to 1986. Of these, 2.6 percent were given at least 1 unit of blood at delivery. About 10 percent were given 1 unit only, and 80 percent received 3 units or fewer. Only 4 percent of transfused patients required 8 units or more. As perhaps expected, the incidence of transfusion has decreased over the years; in 1976 it was 4.6 percent, but by 1986 it was 1.9 percent.

Listed in Table 37–2 are the many clinical circumstances in which risk of hemorrhage is appreciably increased. It is apparent that serious hemorrhage may occur at any time throughout pregnancy and the puerperium.

The time of bleeding in pregnancy is widely used to classify obstetrical hemorrhage; however, the term *third-trimester bleeding* is so imprecise for describing gestational age and, in turn, intelligent management of pregnancy, that it ought to be abandoned.

Uterine Bleeding Before Delivery. Slight bleeding through the vagina is common during active labor. This "bloody show" is the consequence of effacement and dilatation of the cervix, with tearing of small veins and, in turn, slight shedding of blood.

Uterine bleeding from a site above the cervix before delivery is cause for concern. The bleeding may be the consequence of some separation of a placenta implanted in the immediate vicinity of the cervical canal—that is, **placenta previa;** or from separation of a placenta located elsewhere in the uterine cavity—that is, **abruptio placentae.** Rarely, the bleeding may be the consequence of velamentous insertion of the umbilical cord

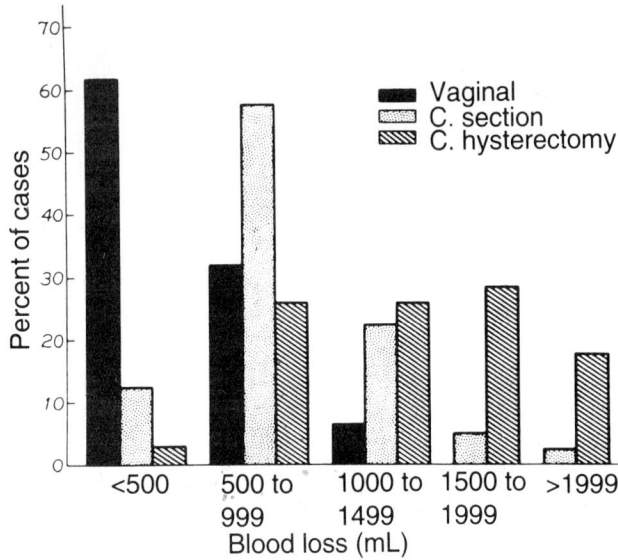

Fig. 37–1. Blood loss associated with vaginal delivery, repeat cesarean section, and repeat cesarean section plus total hysterectomy. (From Pritchard and associates, 1962, with permission.)

with rupture of a fetal blood vessel at the time of rupture of the membranes—**vasa previa**—with fetal hemorrhage (see Fig. 35–6, p. 746).

The source of uterine bleeding that originates above the level of the cervix is not always identified. In that circumstance, the bleeding typically begins with little or no other symptomatology, and then stops, and at delivery no anatomical cause is identified. Almost always the bleeding must have been the consequence of slight marginal separation of the placenta that did not

TABLE 37–1. PATIENT 37 WEEKS PREGNANT, CARCINOMA OF CERVIX, RADICAL HYSTERECTOMY, AND PELVIC LYMPHADENECTOMY

Day	Hematocrit	Blood Volume (mL)[a]		Blood Loss (mL)	
		Blood	Red Cells	Blood	Red Cells
− 1 Surgery	34.0	5440 Transfused 500 mL blood	1850		
+ 1	34.0	3835	1300	2200	750[b]
+ 2	30.5				
+ 4	30.5				
+ 6	29.0				
+ 8	31.0	4020	1250	2400	810[b]
+ 84	42.0	3760	1580		

[a] Blood volume calculated from apparent volume of distribution of ^{51}Cr-tagged red cells.
[b] Includes 200 mL of transfused red cells.

TABLE 37–2. CONDITIONS THAT PREDISPOSE TO OR WORSEN OBSTETRICAL HEMORRHAGE

Abnormal Placentation
Placental previa
Abruption placentae
Placenta accreta
Ectopic pregnancy
Hydatidiform mole

Trauma During Labor and Delivery
Episiotomy
Complicated vaginal delivery
Low- or mid-forceps delivery
Cesarean section or hysterectomy
Uterine rupture; risk increased by:
1. Previously scarred uterus
2. High parity
3. Hyperstimulation
4. Obstructed labor
5. Intrauterine manipulation
6. Midforceps rotation

Small Maternal Blood Volume
Small woman
Pregnancy hypervolemia not yet maximal
Pregnancy hypervolemia constricted
1. Severe preeclampsia
2. Eclampsia

Uterine Atony
Overdistended uterus
1. Large fetus
2. Multiple fetuses
3. Hydramnios
4. Distention with clots
Anesthesia or analgesia
1. Halogenated agents
2. Conduction analgesia with hypotension
Exhausted myometrium
1. Rapid labor
2. Prolonged labor
3. Oxytocin or prostaglandin stimulation
4. Chorioamnionitis
Previous uterine atony

Coagulation Defects– Intensify Other Causes
Placental abruption
Prolonged retention of dead fetus
Amnionic fluid embolism
Saline-induced abortion
Sepsis with endotoxemia
Severe intravascular hemolysis
Massive transfusions
Severe preeclampsia and eclampsia
Congenital coagulopathies
Anticoagulant treatment

expand. **It is emphasized that the pregnancy in which such bleeding occurs remains at increased risk for a poor outcome even though the bleeding soon stops and placenta previa appears to have been excluded by sonography.** Lipitz and colleagues (1991) reemphasized the importance of midtrimester uterine bleeding. They studied 65 consecutive women—almost 1 percent of their patients—who had uterine bleeding between 14 and 26 weeks' gestation. Almost one fourth had placental abruption or previa. Total fetal loss including abortions and perinatal deaths was 32 percent. Even in pregnancies with hemorrhage after 26 weeks that are not explained by placental abruption or previa, an adverse outcome was described by Ajayi and colleagues (1992) in one third of cases.

Etiology of Obstetrical Hemorrhage. Obstetrical hemorrhage is the consequence of excessive bleeding from the placental implantation site, trauma to the genital tract and adjacent structures, or both. Uterine atony and genital tract lacerations therefore account for most cases of postpartum obstetrical hemorrhage.

Bleeding from Placental Site. Near term, it is estimated that approximately 600 mL/min of blood flows through the intervillous space. With separation of the placenta, the many uterine arteries and veins that carry blood to and from the placenta are severed abruptly. Elsewhere in the body, hemostasis in the absence of surgical ligation depends upon intrinsic vasospasm and formation of blood clot locally. At the placental implantation site, most important for achieving hemostasis are contraction and retraction of the myometrium to compress the vessels and obliterate their lumens. Adherent pieces of placenta or large blood clots will prevent effective contraction and retraction of the myometrium and thereby impair hemostasis at the implantation site. Fatal postpartum hemorrhage can occur from a hypotonic uterus while the maternal blood coagulation mechanism is quite normal. Conversely, if the myometrium at and adjacent to the denuded implantation site contracts and retracts vigorously, fatal hemorrhage *from the placental implantation site* is unlikely even though the coagulation mechanism is severely impaired.

Bleeding from Lacerations. Lacerated or incised blood vessels in the reproductive tract, other than those in the body of the uterus, lack the unique mechanism for obliterating vessel patency provided by a vigorously contracting myometrium. Therefore, following delivery of an intact placenta, hemorrhage from the genital tract that persists with the uterus firmly contracted is almost certainly indicative of bleeding from lacerations.

Management of Hemorrhage

Whenever there is any suggestion of excessive blood loss from the genital tract, it is essential that steps be immediately taken to identify the presence of uterine atony, retained placental fragments, and lacerations of the genital tract. It is imperative that at least one—in the presence of frank hemorrhage, two—intravenous infusion systems of large caliber be established immediately to allow rapid administration of aqueous electrolyte solutions and blood. An operating room, surgical team, and an anesthesiologist should always be immediately available.

Estimation of Excessive Blood Loss

Visual Estimate. Visual inspection is most often resorted to but is notoriously inaccurate. In several reports, the amount of blood estimated by inspection to have been lost was on average about one half the actual measured loss. We have found that if estimated blood loss is "excessive" (i.e., more than average), final calculations usually show an actual loss of about three times the estimate! Finally, part or all of the hemorrhage may be concealed.

Blood Pressure and Pulse. Overt hypotension and tachycardia are signs of dangerous hypovolemia that cannot be ignored, but the converse is not necessarily true. Vital signs, if apparently normal, can be quite misleading. **A blood pressure reading in the normal range, or even hypertension, does not preclude imminently dangerous hypovolemia.** Hypertension, either pregnancy-induced or chronic, is not unusual in pregnant women, and therefore serious hemorrhage and the resultant hypovolemia may in this circumstance result in a fall in blood pressure only to normotensive levels. The normotensive reading may create a false sense of security, with delay in identification of compromised perfusion of vital organs.

The pulse rate may be equally misleading, because it may be elevated in circumstances in which the degree of hemorrhage is negligible, and normal or even slow in the presence of severe hypovolemia (Jansen, 1978).

"Tilt Test." The woman who has bled appreciably but whose blood pressure and pulse rate are normal when recumbent may, when placed in the sitting position, become hypotensive, develop tachycardia, or both. This so-called tilt test should be applied and interpreted with caution for the following reasons. (1) For the woman who is already hypotensive when recumbent, the tilt test is needless and potentially dangerous. (2) The parturient who has not yet fully recovered from the sympathetic blockade of conduction analgesia, may become hypotensive when placed in the sitting position, without necessarily having suffered serious hemorrhage. (3) The normally hypervolemic pregnant woman may lose a large amount of blood before demonstrating orthostatic hypotension, as illustrated by the following case.

The immediate effects from appreciable hemorrhage are demonstrated in Figure 37–2. The woman with sickle cell–hemoglobin C disease near term underwent phlebotomy for exchange transfusion. Using ^{51}Cr-tagged erythrocytes, her measured blood volume was 6000 mL and the hematocrit 38. After stabilization, 1000 mL of blood was removed over 8 minutes while she was very carefully observed lying on her side. During the 20 minutes following hemorrhage, until infusion of packed erythrocytes was begun, she was observed, first, laterally recumbent, then supine, and finally sitting. Her blood pressure was unchanged until she sat up, when it rose moderately, as did the maternal and fetal heart rates. Thus, the initial response to appreciable hemorrhage in this pregnant woman was a rise in blood pressure similar to that observed at times in normal nonpregnant individuals.

Urine Flow. **When carefully measured, the rate of urine formation, *in the absence of potent diuretics*, reflects the adequacy of renal perfusion and, in turn, the perfusion of other vital organs, be-**

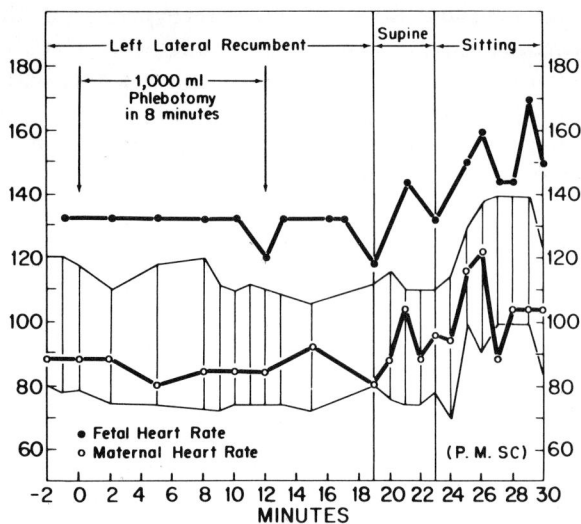

Fig. 37–2. Responses late in pregnancy to phlebotomy and changes in posture following phlebotomy. Partial exchange transfusion was being carried out in a woman with sickle-cell–hemoglobin C disease; her pregnancy-induced hypervolemia amounted to 1400 mL. Systolic and diastolic blood pressures are plotted as light lines and each reading is interconnected. The open circles connected by a heavy line demonstrate the maternal pulse rate, and the solid dots so connected are the fetal heart rates.

cause renal blood flow is especially sensitive to blood volume changes. With potentially serious hemorrhage, an indwelling catheter should be inserted promptly to measure all urine formed. Potent diuretics, such as furosemide, are very likely to invalidate the relationship between urine flow and renal perfusion. This need not be a problem in the management of the woman who is hemorrhaging, however, because there are no proven benefits from the use of furosemide in this setting. Actually, the reverse is more likely true, in that there is great potential for deleterious effects. An almost immediate effect of furosemide is venodilatation, which further reduces venous return to the heart, thereby further compromising cardiac output. The other dangerous effect is loss of fluid and electrolytes from the already seriously depleted intravascular compartment.

The antidiuretic agent to which the hemorrhaging woman is likely to be exposed is oxytocin. However, with the infusion of isotonic electrolyte solution, such as lactated Ringer solution, the amount of free water that is reabsorbed by the renal tubules is not greatly enhanced, and therefore *severe* oliguria does not develop as the consequence of oxytocin alone.

Fluid and Blood Replacement. Treatment of serious hemorrhage demands prompt and adequate refilling of the intravascular compartment. Two general guidelines have proven to be most valuable for determining the amounts and kinds of fluids that are needed to treat hypovolemia from obstetrical hemorrhage irrespective

of cause. **Lactated Ringer solution and whole blood are given in such amounts and in such proportions that (1) urine flow is at least 30 mL/hr and ideally approaches 60 mL/hr, and (2) the hematocrit is maintained at 30 percent.**

Considerable debate surrounds the hematocrit level or hemoglobin concentration that mandates blood transfusion. According to deliberations of a Consensus Development Conference (1988), cardiac output does not substantively increase until the hemoglobin concentration falls to about 7 g/dL. Although the committee noted that otherwise healthy anesthetized animals survived isovolemic anemia with hematocrit decreases down to 5 percent, it further found that significant functional deterioration occurred well before that point. Importantly, they recommended that good judgement be used for decisions regarding perioperative transfusions. Specifically, it cited factors for consideration including intravascular volume status, extent of operation, and probability for further massive blood loss.

Finally, because obstetrical hemorrhage at times can be torrential, a cushion is provided during acute resuscitation of hemorrhage if the hematocrit is kept at around 30 percent. Further support for these recommendations has been provided by Czer and Shoemaker (1978). In their series of 94 critically ill postoperative patients, mortality rates were lowest when hematocrit values were maintained between 27 and 33. Fortune and associates (1987) have shown that there are no cardiopulmonary advantages to maintaining the hematocrit over 30 percent.

For the woman who is isovolemic, physiologically stable, and in whom hemorrhage has abated and none further is expected, treatment of residual acute anemia differs from management of acute hemorrhage. Morrison and colleagues (1991), for example, reported no benefits of red cell transfusions given to women who had suffered postpartum hemorrhage and who were isovolemic but anemic with a hematocrit between 18 and 25 percent.

Blood and Component Replacement

Whole Blood. Compatible whole blood would appear to be ideal for treatment of hypovolemia from serious acute hemorrhage. The policy of the Obstetrics Service at Parkland Hospital, dictated by the practicalities of blood banking, is to treat hypovolemia from severe hemorrhage with any readily available whole blood that is compatible based on identification of the recipient's blood group and the absence of abnormal red cell antibodies in the recipient's plasma. The panel of red cells used to identify antibodies has been enzyme treated, and all incubations are performed at 37° C. Clinically significant antibodies have been detected only in 1 to 2 percent of cases. To date, this so-called *group and screen* technique has been used in more than 150,000 obstetrical and surgical cases at Parkland Hospital. In all cases in which transfusions were given, follow-up crossmatch disclosed no serious incompatibilities and there were no transfusion reactions.

Because of the practices of most blood banks for fractionation of donor units to provide component therapy, the availability of whole blood has diminished remarkably. Moreover, use of fresh-frozen plasma has increased tenfold within the past 15 years and is nearly 2 million units annually. Because there is little justification for the use of fresh-frozen plasma alone as a volume expander, and because each unit exposes the recipient to another additional source of transfusion-related infection, justifiable concerns have been raised over its use. A Consensus Development Conference to consider these issues was called by the National Institutes of Health and the Food and Drug Administration (1985). Unfortunately, while condemning the use of fresh-frozen plasma as a volume expander given for treatment of severe life-threatening hemorrhage and massive transfusion, the committee did not stress the need for whole blood for treatment of massive hemorrhage. Obstetrics notwithstanding, there appears to be a great need for availability of whole blood (Miller, 1985), and it is reasonable to hope that such conferences will stimulate more blood banks to provide whole blood. However, if whole blood is lacking, packed red cells plus recently thawed freshfrozen plasma are administered when serious hemorrhage is encountered.

In their classical study of massively transfused surgical patients, Counts and associates (1979) reported that it was unnecessary to supplement transfusions of whole blood with fresh-frozen plasma. However, the nonavailability of whole blood for life-threatening hemorrhage has caused obstetricians and trauma surgeons to "reconstitute" whole blood from components. Table 37–3 compares results for the obstetrical and surgical services at Parkland Hospital. In 1990 and 1991, the Surgical Service, which preferentially uses packed red cells for acute resuscitation, transfused 1 unit of freshfrozen plasma for every 3 units of red cells given. The Obstetrics Service, with the "whole blood policy" described above, was able to obtain whole blood in only about one half of cases, but gave fresh-frozen plasma for only 1 of 12 units of blood or red cells transfused. In 1987, when whole blood was more readily available, this ratio was 1 : 60.

AUTOLOGOUS TRANSFUSIONS. Under some circumstances, autologous blood storage for transfusion seems worthwhile (Herbert and associates, 1988). McVay and colleagues (1989) reported observations from 273 pregnant women in whom blood was drawn in the third trimester. Almost three fourths of these women donated only 1 unit. Minimal requirements were a hemoglobin concentration 11 g/dL or hematocrit of 34 percent. They reported no complications. Sherman and colleagues (1992) studied 27 women given two or more transfusions in over 16,000 deliveries. In only 40 percent was an antepartum condition identified. Andres and co-workers (1990) concluded that autologous transfusions likely were not cost effective.

Blood Fractions. Infusion of large volumes of packed red cells plus normal saline is not an appropriate substitute for whole blood being rapidly lost in large quantity. The deleterious effects of saline infused in large volume on coagulation factors, plasma proteins, and in turn, plasma oncotic pressure, are shown in Table 37–4. In normally pregnant women, the colloid oncotic pressure is already reduced because the plasma concentration of albumin is decreased about 25 percent.

At times, after the infusion of many units of stored blood, generalized bleeding may develop as a consequence of intense thrombocytopenia. If the platelet count confirms this, 6 to 10 units of platelets are administered. If the platelets from a D-positive donor are given to a D-negative recipient who might conceive again, anti-D immune globulin should be administered promptly.

Even with massive hemorrhage and blood replacement, it is highly unlikely that levels of factors V and VIII are sufficiently depressed to be clinically significant (Counts and associates, 1979). If these are identified, however, they can be readily corrected by infusion of fresh-frozen plasma.

Transfusion-related Infections. With each unit of blood or its component, the recipient is exposed to the risk of bloodborne infections. Fortunately, the most feared—infection with human immunodeficiency virus (HIV)—is the most rare. Ward and colleagues (1988) estimated that with donor screening for viral antibody the risk for infection is 1 per 40,000 transfusions. Cumming and colleagues (1989) estimate this risk to be about 1 in 310,000. Busch and co-workers (1991) addressed concerns that a seronegative donor may be incubating the

TABLE 37–3. TRANSFUSIONS BY THE OBSTETRICAL AND SURGICAL SERVICES AT PARKLAND HOSPITAL, 1990–1991

	Whole Blood	Packed Cells	Total Blood	Fresh-frozen Plasma (FFP)	Ratio Blood : FFP
Surgical Service "Packed cell policy"	85	8677	8792	2710	1:3
Obstetrical Service "Whole blood policy"	494	580	1074	90	1:12

TABLE 37–4. RUPTURED UTERUS WITH MASSIVE FATAL HEMORRHAGE TREATED VIGOROUSLY WITH ELECTROLYTE SOLUTION, CAUSING MARKED LOWERING OF COAGULATION FACTORS AND COLLOID ONCOTIC PRESSURE

	Plasma Proteins		Fibrinogen (mg/dL)	Platelets (μL)	Prothrombin Time (sec)	Partial Thromboplastin Time (sec)
	Total (g/dL)	Albumin (g/dL)				
Initial	6.4	3.4	324	187,000	11.3	28.3
Terminal	2.3	1.2	104	67,000	17.0	76.3

virus. They used polymerase chain reaction to detect incubating virus and reported that the probability of a seronegative donor being positive for HIV-I infection was about 1 in 60,000. Unfortunately, more than 60 percent of recipients of HIV-positive blood became seropositive, and half will have acquired immune deficiency syndrome by 7 years (Ward and associates, 1989).

Until recently, the transmission of non-A, non-B hepatitis virus was much more likely to complicate transfusion. The prevalence of hepatitis C is 1 to 2 percent of donors. In the past, most cases were undetected because they caused anicteric infection, although chronic hepatitis commonly resulted (see Chap. 51, p. 1160). Fortunately, a serological test for hepatitis C antibody is now available, and in 1990 the American Association of Blood Banks mandated hepatitis C testing for all donors.

Consumptive Coagulopathy

In 1901, DeLee reported that "temporary hemophilia" developed in a woman with a placental abruption and another with a long-dead macerated fetus. Observations that extensive placental abruption, as well as other accidents of pregnancy, were frequently associated with hypofibrinogenemia, stimulated interest in causes of intense intravascular coagulation. Although these observations were initially almost totally confined to obstetrical cases, subsequently they were made for almost all areas of medicine. These syndromes are commonly termed **consumptive coagulopathy** or **disseminated intravascular coagulation**.

Pregnancy Hypercoagulability. Pregnancy normally induces appreciable increases in the concentrations of coagulation factors I (fibrinogen), VII, VIII, IX, and X. Other plasma factors and platelets do not change so remarkably. Plasminogen levels are increased considerably, yet plasmin activity antepartum is normally decreased compared with the nonpregnant state. Various stimuli act to incite the conversion of plasminogen to plasmin, and one of the most potent is activation of coagulation.

Pathological Activation of Coagulation. In normal circumstances, there is not appreciable continuous

physiological intravascular coagulation. During pregnancy, there does appear to be increased activation of the platelet, clotting, and fibrinolytic mechanisms in vivo. Gerbasi and colleagues (1990) found significant increases in fibrinopeptide A, β-thromboglobulin, platelet factor 4, and fibrinogen–fibrin degradation products. They concluded that this compensated, accelerated intravascular coagulation may be for maintenance of uteroplacental interface.

In pathological states, coagulation may be activated via the extrinsic pathway by thromboplastin from tissue destruction and perhaps via the intrinsic pathway by collagen and other tissue components when there is loss of endothelial integrity. Another mechanism is by direct activation of factor X by proteases, for example, as present in mucin or produced by neoplasms. Still another mechanism is induction of procoagulant activity in lymphocytes, neutrophils, or platelets by stimulation with bacterial toxins.

Consumptive coagulopathy is almost always seen as a complication of an identifiable, underlying pathological process against which treatment must be directed to reverse defibrination. With pathological activation of procoagulants that triggers disseminated intravascular coagulation, there is consumption of platelets and coagulation factors in variable quantities. As a consequence, fibrin may be deposited in small vessels of virtually every organ system. Fortunately, this seldom causes organ failure. Small vessels are protected because coagulation typically incites the activation of plasminogen to plasmin, which then lyses fibrinogen, fibrin monomer, and fibrin polymers to form a series of fibrinogen–fibrin degradation products or split products as well as D-dimers.

Significance of Consumptive Coagulopathy. There are three possible clinical consequences of consumptive coagulopathy (Marder, 1990):

1. A bleeding tendency is created by consumption of platelets and clotting factors, potentiated by anticoagulant effects of fibrin degradation products.

2. Circulatory obstruction causes organ hypoperfusion and ischemic tissue damage may develop. Although there may be tubular necrosis or irreversible cortical necrosis, renal failure is usually

encountered in clinical situations with massive bleeding. Thus, undoubtedly there is a profound contribution from ischemia engendered by hypotension and hypovolemia. Other organs may be affected, and of critical interest is the development of the *adult respiratory distress syndrome,* which frequently is associated with clinical syndromes that also cause disseminated intravascular coagulation (see Chap. 47, p. 1069).

3. Consumptive coagulopathy may be associated with microangiopathic hemolysis, caused by mechanical disruption of the erythrocyte membrane within small vessels in which fibrin has been deposited. Varying degrees of hemolysis with anemia, hemoglobinemia, hemoglobinuria, and erythrocyte morphological changes are produced.

As the recognition of consumptive coagulopathy in nonobstetrical conditions advanced, so did undue emphasis of certain recommendations for management. Not infrequently, the precise nature of the underlying disease has not been thoroughly considered or has even been ignored. The use of heparin, for example, has been urged by some in circumstances in which the likelihood of benefit would appear to be slight but the risk of potentiating hemorrhage great, such as with placental abruption.

At the same time that these measures have been unduly stressed, the value of vigorous restoration and maintenance of the circulation to treat hypovolemia and persistent intravascular coagulation has not been given appropriate attention. With adequate perfusion of vital organs, activated coagulation factors and circulating fibrin and fibrin degradation products are promptly removed by the reticuloendothelial system. At the same time, hepatic and endothelial synthesis of procoagulants is promoted.

The likelihood of life-threatening hemorrhage in obstetrical situations complicated by defective coagulation will depend not only on the extent of the coagulation defects but—of great importance—on whether or not the vasculature is intact or disrupted. With gross derangement of blood coagulation, there may be fatal hemorrhage when vascular integrity is disrupted, yet no hemorrhage as long as all blood vessels remain intact.

Clinical and Laboratory Evidence of Defective Hemostasis. **Excessive bleeding at sites of modest trauma characterizes defective hemostasis.** Persistent bleeding from venipuncture sites, nicks shaving the perineum or abdomen, trauma from insertion of a catheter, and spontaneous bleeding from the gums or nose, are signs of possible coagulation defects. Purpuric areas at pressure sites may indicate incoagulable blood, or more commonly, clinically significant thrombocytope-

nia. A surgical incision provides the ultimate "bioassay" for intactness of coagulation. Continuous generalized oozing from the skin, subcutaneous and fascial tissues, and vascular retroperitoneal space, should at least suggest coagulopathy. Such evidence also may be gained by observing continuous oozing from episiotomy incisions or perineal lacerations.

Hypofibrinogenemia. In late pregnancy, plasma fibrinogen levels typically are 300 to 600 mg/dL. With activation of coagulation, these high levels may sometimes serve to protect against clinically significant hypofibrinogenemia. To promote clinical coagulation, fibrinogen levels must be at least about 100 mg/dL. Most clinical laboratories are able to measure plasma fibrinogen levels. If serious *hypofibrinogenemia* is present, the clot formed from whole blood in a glass tube may initially be soft but not necessarily remarkably reduced in volume. Then, over the next half hour or so, it becomes quite small, so that many of the erythrocytes are extruded and the volume of liquid clearly exceeds that of the clot. The addition of a drop of topical thrombin to hasten the conversion of circulating fibrinogen to fibrin has practical utility.

Fibrin and Fibrinogen Derivatives. Fibrin degradation products in serum may be detected by a number of sensitive test systems. More recently, monoclonal antibodies to the D-dimer have been used. With clinically significant consumption coagulopathy, these measurements are always abnormally high.

Thrombocytopenia. Serious thrombocytopenia is likely if petechiae are abundant, clotted blood fails to retract over a period of an hour or so, or if platelets are rare in a stained blood smear. Confirmation is provided by platelet count.

Prothrombin and Partial Thromboplastin Times. Prolongation of the partial thromboplastin time or prothrombin time may be the consequence of appreciable reductions in those coagulants essential for generating thrombin, a fibrinogen concentration below a critical level of about 100 mg/dL, or appreciable amounts of circulating fibrinogen–fibrin degradation products. Prolongation of the prothrombin time and partial thromboplastin time need not be the consequence of disseminated intravascular coagulation.

PLACENTAL ABRUPTION

Nomenclature. The separation of the placenta from its site of implantation before the delivery of the fetus has been variously called placental abruption, abruptio placentae, ablatio placentae, accidental hemorrhage, and premature separation of the normally implanted placenta.

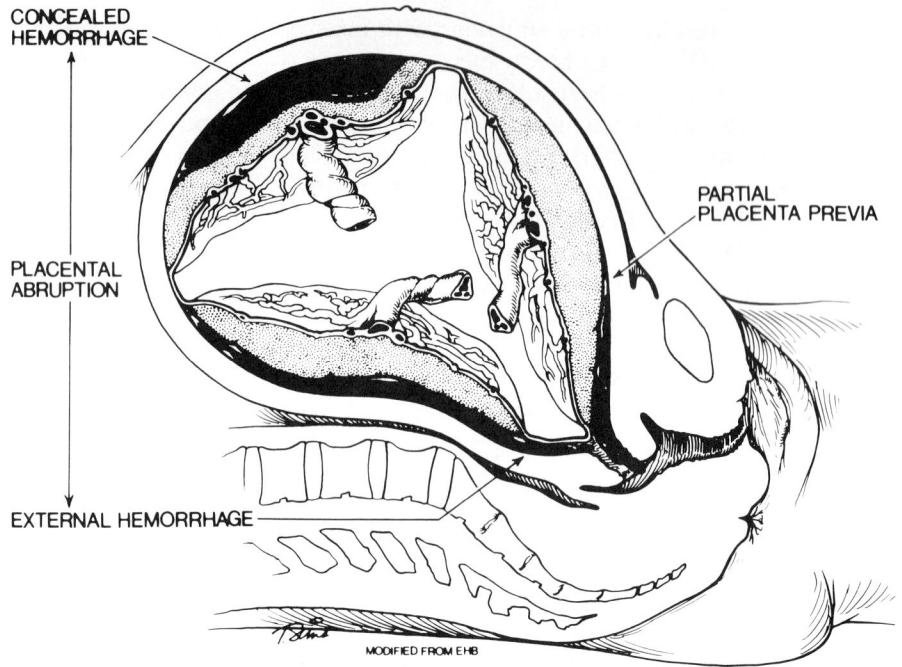

Fig. 37–3. Hemorrhage from premature placental separation. *Upper left:* Extensive placental abruption but with the periphery of the placenta and the membranes still adherent, resulting in completely concealed hemorrhage. *Lower:* Placental abruption with the placenta detached peripherally and with the membranes between the placenta and cervical canal stripped from underlying decidua, allowing external hemorrhage. *Right:* Partial placenta previa with placental separation and external hemorrhage.

The term *premature separation of the normally implanted placenta* is most descriptive, because it differentiates the placenta that separates prematurely but is implanted some distance beyond the cervical internal os, from one that is implanted over the cervical internal os—that is, placenta previa. It is cumbersome, however, and hence the shorter term **abruptio placentae,** or **placental abruption,** has been employed. The Latin *abruptio placentae,* which means "rending asunder of the placenta," denotes a sudden accident, a clinical characteristic of most cases of this complication. The term *ablatio placentae* means "a carrying away of the placenta" and is not used extensively. The term frequently employed in Great Britain is *accidental hemorrhage,* in the sense of an event that takes place without expectation, in contrast to the unavoidable hemorrhage of placenta previa.

Some of the bleeding of placental abruption usually insinuates itself between the membranes and uterus, and then escapes through the cervix, causing an *external hemorrhage* (Fig. 37–3). Less often, the blood does not escape externally but is retained between the detached placenta and the uterus, leading to *concealed hemorrhage* (Figs. 37–3 and 37–4). Placental abruption may be *total* (Figs. 37–3 and 37–4), or *partial* (Fig. 37–5). Placental abruption with concealed hemorrhage carries with it much greater maternal hazards, not only because the likelihood of intense consumptive coagulopathy is increased, but also because the extent of the hemorrhage is not appreciated.

Frequency, Intensity, and Significance. The frequency with which abruptio placentae is diagnosed will vary, because criteria employed for diagnosis differ. The intensity of the abruption will often vary depending on how quickly the woman seeks and receives care following the onset of symptoms. With delay, the likelihood of extensive separation causing death of the fetus is increased remarkably.

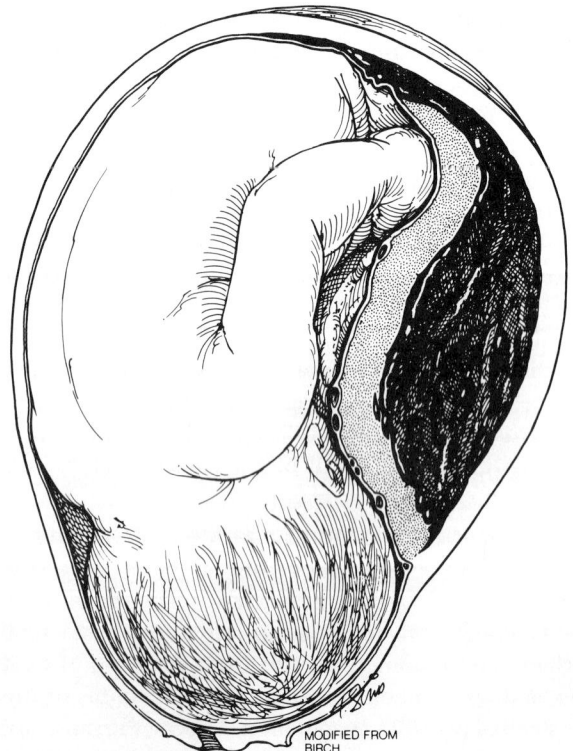

Fig. 37–4. Total placental abruption with concealed hemorrhage. The fetus is now dead.

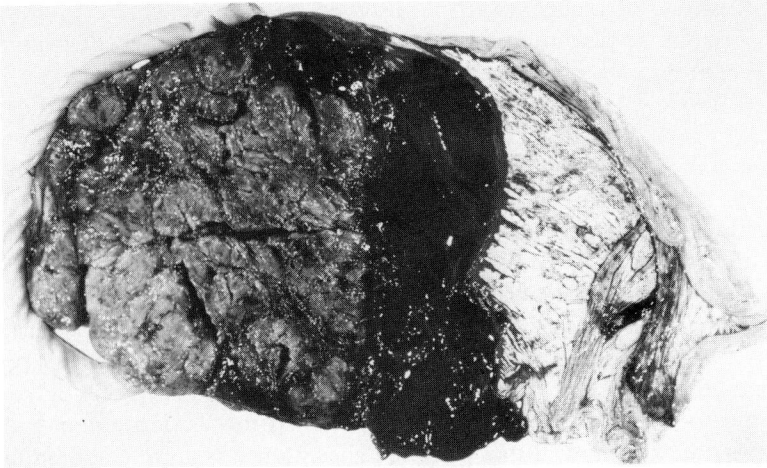

Fig. 37–5. Partial placental abruption with adherent clot.

The reported frequency for placental abruption varies but averages about 1 in 150 deliveries. In the largest study, Käregärd and Gennser (1986) surveyed 849,619 births in Sweden and reported that 3959 (0.44 percent, or 1 in 225) were complicated by abruptio placentae. The perinatal mortality rate in these cases was 20 percent. At the University of Tennessee the frequency of placental abruption was about 1 in 90 deliveries; the perinatal mortality rate was about 35 percent for all cases and 25 percent for infants who weighed 1000 g or more (Abdella and associates, 1984). Hurd and co-workers (1983) in Cincinnati have observed a frequency for abruptio placentae of about 1 per 75 deliveries, with a perinatal mortality rate of 30 percent, about equally divided between stillbirths and neonatal deaths. Krohn and associates (1987) reported that the perinatal mortality was 21 percent in 884 pregnancies complicated by placental abruption in Washington state.

According to Saftlas and colleagues (1991), who surveyed the National Hospital Discharge Survey, the rate of abruptio placentae increased significantly in the United States from 1979 to 1987. Conversely, at our hospital, the frequency of placental abruption is decreasing. In recent years at Parkland Hospital, the frequency of placental abruption of all degrees remains about 1 in 200 deliveries. Applying the criterion of placental separation so extensive as to kill the fetus, the incidence was 1 in 420 deliveries during 1956 through 1969 (Pritchard and Brekken, 1967). However, as the number of high-parity women cared for has decreased in more recent years, and community-wide availability of emergency transportation has increased, the frequency of placental abruption fatal to the fetus has dropped to about 1 in 830 deliveries (Pritchard and colleagues, 1991).

As stillbirths from other causes have decreased appreciably, those from abruptio placentae have become especially prominent. For example, of all third-trimester stillbirths at Parkland Hospital during 1990 and 1991,

10 percent were the consequence of placental abruption. This frequency is similar to that described recently by Fretts and associates (1992), who studied almost 89,000 births at the Royal Victoria Hospital in Montreal between 1961 and 1988. They observed that abruptio placentae had become the leading known cause of fetal death and accounted for 15 percent of all deaths.

Importantly, even if the infant survives, there may be adverse sequelae. Of the 182 infants who survived in the study by Abdella and associates (1984), 25 were identified to have significant neurological deficits within the first year of life. While maternal mortality is now uncommon, morbidity is common and may be severe.

Etiology. The primary cause of placental abruption is unknown, but there are several associated conditions. As shown in Figure 37–6, the incidence increases with age. In addition, Pritchard and colleagues (1991) have shown it to be higher in women of great parity, and it is more common in African-American women

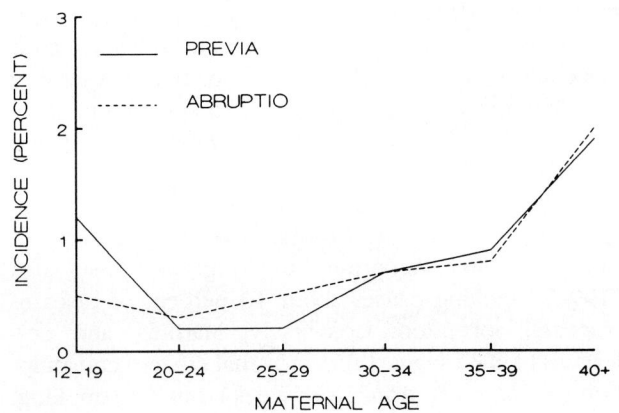

Fig. 37–6. Incidence of abruptio placentae and placenta previa plotted by age in 29,115 pregnancies delivered at Parkland Hospital, 1987 and 1988. (From Cunningham and Leveno, 1989.)

(1 : 595) than white (1 : 876) or Latin-American women (1 : 1473).

By far, the most commonly associated condition is either **pregnancy-induced or chronic hypertension.** In the Parkland Hospital study of 408 cases of placental abruption so severe as to kill the fetus, maternal hypertension was apparent in about half of the women once the depleted intravascular compartment was adequately refilled (Pritchard and co-workers, 1991). Half of the hypertensive women had chronic vascular disease; in the remainder, the hypertension appeared to be pregnancy induced. The high frequency of maternal hypertension has been observed by some others (Abdella and co-workers, 1984; Williams and associates, 1991a), but not by all. It appears that there is not an increased incidence of hypertension in pregnancies with lesser degrees of placental abruption (Sholl, 1987).

Preterm prematurely ruptured membranes have been associated with an increased incidence of premature placental separation. Vintzileos and colleagues (1987) reported that 6.3 percent of such patients developed placental abruption; about one fourth did so within 24 hours. Gonen and associates (1989) reported an incidence of 5.6 percent in 143 pregnancies less than 34 weeks that had prematurely ruptured membranes for more than 24 hours. We observed two cases of hydramnios with membrane rupture and sudden uterine decompression causing placental abruption (Pritchard and co-workers, 1991).

Lesser degrees of abruption may occur shortly before delivery of a singleton fetus when the amnionic fluid has drained from the uterus and the fetus has descended until the head is on the perineum. With twins, decompression following delivery of the first fetus may lead to premature separation of the placenta that endangers the second fetus (Chap. 39, p. 911).

External trauma could be implicated only in 3 of 207 cases of severe placental abruption cared for at Parkland Hospital. Our experiences are similar to those of Kettel (1988) and Stafford (1988) and their co-workers, who stress that abruption caused by relatively minor maternal trauma may cause fetal jeopardy that is not always associated with obvious clinical evidence for placental separation (see Chap. 47, p. 1075). A case of marginal abruption caused by percutaneous umbilical cord blood sampling was described by Feinkind and colleagues (1990).

Cigarette smoking was linked to an increased risk for abruption from the Collaborative Perinatal Project (Naeye, 1980). According to Voigt and associates (1990), smoking causes about 40 percent of cases of placental abruption. Conversely, Marbury and colleagues (1983) suggest that maternal ethanol consumption (14 or more drinks per week), but not smoking, predisposes to placental abruption.

Cocaine abuse has been associated with an alarming frequency of placental abruption. Chasnoff and col-

leagues (1985) observed the onset of labor with placental abruption in 4 of 23 women immediately after intravenous self-injection of cocaine. In another report of 50 women who abused cocaine during pregnancy, there were 8 stillbirths caused by placental abruption (Bingol and associates, 1987). Dombrowski and co-workers (1991) reported placental abruptions in almost 2 percent of 592 women known to have abused cocaine at some time during pregnancy. Hoskins and collaborators (1991) reported an astounding rate of placental abruption of 13 percent in 112 women with prior bad outcomes who were followed prospectively for cocaine abuse during pregnancy. Slutsker (1992) recently reviewed 10 studies that studied this association and all showed that placental abruption was more common in cocaine-using women than in controls.

Uterine leiomyoma, especially if located behind the placental implantation site, predispose to abruption (see Chap. 22, p. 534). Rice and associates (1989) reported that 8 of 14 women with retroplacental myomas developed placental abruption; in 4, fetal death ensued. By contrast, abruption developed in only 2 of 79 women whose myoma was not retroplacental.

Experimental obstruction of the inferior vena cava and ovarian veins was reported to produce placental abruption. There are, however, several recorded instances of ligation of ovarian veins and the inferior vena cava during the third trimester without subsequent placental abruption (Stone and colleagues, 1968).

Hibbard and Jeffcoate (1966) and others contended that folic acid deficiency played an etiological role in placental abruption (Chap. 9, p. 259). The hypothesis has been carefully examined by Whalley and associates (1969) and Alperin and colleagues (1969), who found no evidence to support such a relationship. More recently, we found that mean corpuscular volume in blood from 175 women with severe placental abruption was identical to that of controls.

Recurrence. The risk of recurrent abruption in a subsequent pregnancy is very high. Pritchard and co-workers (1970) identified a recurrence rate of 1 in 8 pregnancies, and Hibbard and Jeffcoate (1966) observed the remarkably high rate of 1 in 6 pregnancies. Käregärd and Gennser (1986) reported that the recurrent placental abruption risk was increased tenfold, from 0.4 to 4 percent, or 1 in 25. Importantly, of the 14 recurrent placental abruptions in the Parkland series, 8 were again fatal to the fetus.

Management of the subsequent pregnancy is made difficult by the fact that the placental separation may suddenly occur at any time, even remote from term. In the majority of cases, fetal well-being was normal beforehand, and thus currently available methods of fetal evaluation are usually not predictive. In an extreme example, Seski and Compton (1976) documented both a normal nonstress test and a normal contraction stress test done 4 hours before the onset of placental abruption that promptly killed the fetus.

Pathology. Placental abruption is initiated by hemorrhage into the decidua basalis. The decidua then splits, leaving a thin layer adherent to the myometrium. Consequently, the process in its earliest stages consists of the development of a decidual hematoma that leads to separation, compression, and the ultimate destruction of the placenta adjacent to it. In its early stage, there may be no clinical symptoms. The condition is discovered only upon examination of the freshly delivered organ, which will present on its maternal surface a circumscribed depression measuring a few centimeters in diameter, covered by dark, clotted blood. Undoubtedly, it takes several minutes for these anatomical changes to materialize. Thus, a very recently abrupted placenta may appear no different from a normal placenta at delivery.

In some instances, a decidual spiral artery ruptures to cause a retroplacental hematoma, which, as it expands, disrupts more vessels to separate more placenta. The area of separation rapidly becomes more extensive and reaches the margin of the placenta. Because the uterus is still distended by the products of conception, it is unable to contract sufficiently to compress the torn vessels that supply the placental site. The escaping blood may dissect the membranes from the uterine wall and eventually appear externally (Fig. 37–3), or may be completely retained within the uterus (Fig. 37–4).

Concealed Hemorrhage. Retained, or concealed, hemorrhage is likely when (1) there is an effusion of blood behind the placenta but its margins still remain adherent, (2) the placenta is completely separated yet the membranes retain their attachment to the uterine wall, (3) blood gains access to the amnionic cavity after breaking through the membranes, and (4) the fetal head is so closely applied to the lower uterine segment that the blood cannot make its way past it. In the majority of such cases, however, the membranes are gradually dissected off the uterine wall, and blood sooner or later escapes.

Chronic Placental Abruption. In a small minority of cases, hemorrhage with retroplacental hematoma formation is somehow arrested completely without delivery. We have been able to document this phenomenon by labeling maternal red cells with ^{51}chromium. This technique served to demonstrate that red blood cells concealed as clot within the uterus at delivery some days later contained no chromium and therefore were shed long before, even though separation at the time of introduction of labeled red cells had been so massive as to kill the fetus.

Fetal-to-Maternal Hemorrhage. Severe fetal-to-maternal hemorrhage associated with placental abruption has been very uncommon in our experience. In nontraumatic placental abruption, evidence for fetomaternal hemorrhage was found in 20 percent of 78 cases; however, in all instances it was less than 10 mL. Significant fetal bleeding is more likely seen with traumatic abruption (see Chap. 47, p. 1075, and Fig. 47–10A–C). Pearlman and associates (1990) found fetal bleeding that averaged 12 mL in one third of women with a traumatic abruption. Stettler and colleagues (1992) reported that there was fetomaternal hemorrhage of 80 to 100 mL in 3 of 8 cases of traumatic placental abruption.

Clinical Diagnosis

It is emphasized that the signs and symptoms with abruptio placentae can vary considerably. For example, external bleeding can be profuse, yet placental separation may not be so extensive as to compromise the fetus directly; or there may be no external bleeding but the placenta may be completely sheared off and the fetus dead as the direct consequence.

> In one very unusual case, a multiparous Mexican-American woman presented to the Parkland Hospital obstetrical emergency room because of nosebleed. She complained of no abdominal or uterine pain, and there was no tenderness or vaginal bleeding. Her fetus, which had moved the evening before, was dead, and her blood did not clot when placed in a tube containing thrombin. The plasma fibrinogen level was less than 25 mg/dL and fibrin–fibrinogen degradation products in serum were greater than 1000 µg/mL. Oxytocin induction was successful, and at delivery a total placental abruption with fresh clots was found.

Hurd and co-workers (1983), in a relatively small prospective study of abruptio placentae, identified the frequency of a variety of pertinent signs and symptoms (Table 37–5). **In 22 percent of cases idiopathic preterm labor was considered to be the diagnosis until subsequent fetal distress—including fetal death, se-**

TABLE 37–5. SIGNS AND SYMPTOMS DIAGNOSED PROSPECTIVELY IN 59 WOMEN WITH ABRUPTIO PLACENTAE

Sign or Symptom	Frequency (%)
Vaginal bleeding	78
Uterine tenderness or back pain	66
Fetal distress	60
High frequency contractions (17%) } Hypertonus (17%)	34
Idiopathic preterm labor[a]	22
Dead fetus	15

[a] All treated with tocolytic agents.
From Hurd and associates (1983), with permission.

rious bleeding, back pain, uterine tenderness, rapid uterine contractions, or persistent uterine hypertonus—were detected singly or more often in combination. These investigators were able to recognize a retroplacental hematoma sonographically in only 1 of 59 cases. Sholl (1987) described similar findings and could confirm the clinical diagnosis sonographically in only 25 percent of women with placental abruption. **Importantly, negative findings with ultrasound examination do not exclude life-threatening placental abruption.**

Shock. It was long held that the shock sometimes seen with placental abruption was out of proportion to the amount of hemorrhage. An explanation proposed for this disparity was that thromboplastin from decidua and placenta entered the maternal circulation at the site of placental separation and incited intravascular coagulation and, in turn, acute cor pulmonale. While certainly the sudden intravenous injection of large doses of thromboplastic material into experimental animals can cause profound shock (Schneider, 1954), the weight of evidence is that the intensity of shock is seldom out of proportion to maternal blood loss. Pritchard and Brekken (1967), for example, studied the blood loss in 141 women with placental abruption so severe as to kill the fetus and found that it often amounted to at least half of the pregnant blood volume.

Neither hypotension nor anemia is obligatory in cases of concealed hemorrhage even when the acute hemorrhage has achieved considerable magnitude. Fortunately, oliguria caused by inadequate renal perfusion but responsive to vigorous treatment of hypovolemia is frequently observed in these circumstances.

Differential Diagnosis. In severe cases of placental abruption, the diagnosis is generally obvious. Milder and more common forms of abruption are difficult to recognize with certainty, and the diagnosis is often made by exclusion. Therefore, with vaginal bleeding complicating a viable pregnancy, it often becomes necessary to rule out placenta previa and other causes of bleeding by clinical inspection and ultrasound evaluation. It has long been taught, perhaps with some justification, that painful uterine bleeding means abruptio placentae, while painless uterine bleeding is indicative of placenta previa. Unfortunately, the differential diagnosis is not that simple. Labor accompanying placenta previa may cause pain suggestive of abruptio placentae. On the other hand, abruptio placentae may mimic normal labor.

Unfortunately, there are neither laboratory tests nor diagnostic methods that accurately detect lesser degrees of placental separation. The cause of the vaginal bleeding at times remains obscure even after delivery. Witt and associates (1991) have reported observations on the utility of maternal serum CA-125 antigen levels as a marker for placental abruption. The origin of this antigen is thought from decidua. These investigators reported a sensitivity of 70 percent and a specificity of 94 percent in the diagnosis of abruption.

Early-onset Placental Abruption. Classical placental abruption with pain, shock, uterine rigidity, and absent fetal heart sounds may develop in the middle trimester. Oláh and colleagues (1988) described a woman with severe coagulopathy at 19 weeks. The fetus remained alive, the coagulopathy reversed, and delivery ensued at 26 weeks. From our experiences, these women may present the same complications as do those with more advanced pregnancies; thus, abruption may cause maternal death unless appropriate treatment is given.

Consumptive Coagulopathy. One of the most common causes of clinically significant consumptive coagulopathy in obstetrics is placental abruption. Overt *hypofibrinogenemia*—less than 150 mg/dL of plasma, along with elevated levels of fibrinogen–fibrin degradation products and variable decreases in other coagulation factors—is found in about 30 percent of women with placental abruption severe enough to kill the fetus. Such coagulation defects are much less common in those cases in which the fetus survives. Our experience has been that serious coagulopathy, when it develops, is usually evident by the time the symptomatic woman seeks care.

The major mechanism in the genesis of the coagulation defects is almost certainly the induction of coagulation intravascularly and, to a lesser degree, retroplacentally. Although an appreciable amount of fibrin is commonly deposited within the uterine cavity in cases of severe placental abruption and hypofibrinogenemia, the amounts are insufficient to account for all of the fibrinogen missing from the circulation (Pritchard and Brekken, 1967). Moreover, Bonnar and co-workers (1969) have observed, and we have confirmed, that the levels of fibrin degradation products are higher in serum from peripheral blood than in serum from blood contained in the uterine cavity. The reverse would be anticipated in the absence of significant intravascular coagulation.

An important consequence of intravascular coagulation is the activation of plasminogen to plasmin, which lyses fibrin microemboli, thereby maintaining patency of the microcirculation. In every instance of placental abruption severe enough to kill the fetus, we have identified clearly pathological levels (greater than 100 μg/mL) of fibrinogen–fibrin degradation products in maternal serum. At the outset, severe hypofibrinogenemia may or may not be accompanied by overt thrombocytopenia. After repeated blood transfusions, however, thrombocytopenia is common.

Renal Failure. Acute renal failure that persists for any length of time is rare with lesser degrees of placental abruption but is seen in severe forms when there is delayed or incomplete treatment of hypovolemia (see Chap. 50, p. 1141). Of 57 cases of acute renal failure in pregnant women described by Grünfeld and Pertuiset (1987), 23 percent were associated with placental abruption. Fortunately, reversible acute tubular necrosis accounts for three fourths of cases of renal failure (Grünfeld and Pertuiset, 1987; Turney and colleagues, 1989). Importantly, 7 of 19 women with acute cortical necrosis had a placental abruption (Grünfeld and Pertuiset, 1987).

The precise cause of renal damage that may be associated with placental abruption is not clear, but major factors very likely are seriously impaired renal perfusion from both reduced cardiac output and intra-renal vasospasm as the consequence of massive hemorrhage and, at times, coexisting acute or chronic hypertensive disorders. Severe preeclampsia frequently coexists with placental abruption. Even when placental abruption is complicated by severe intravascular coagulation, prompt and vigorous treatment of hemorrhage with blood and electrolyte solution will most often prevent clinically significant renal dysfunction.

During nearly 40 years at Parkland Hospital, more than 450 cases of placental abruption so severe as to kill the fetus have received fluid replacement therapy consisting of whole blood and lactated Ringer solution as discussed throughout this chapter. In only one instance has dialysis for renal failure been necessary, and in this woman, at least in retrospect, blood and crystalloid replacement were inadequate following delivery by cesarean section. Her course was further complicated postoperatively by occult intra-abdominal hemorrhage.

For unknown reasons, proteinuria is common, especially with more severe forms of placental abruption, but it usually clears soon after delivery.

Uteroplacental Apoplexy (Couvelaire Uterus). In the more severe forms of placental abruption, widespread extravasation of blood into the uterine musculature and beneath the uterine serosa is found (Fig. 37–7). This phenomenon of *uteroplacental apoplexy,* first described by Couvelaire early in this century, is now frequently called *Couvelaire uterus.* Such effusions of blood are also occasionally seen beneath the tubal serosa, in the connective tissue of the broad ligaments, and in the substance of the ovaries, as well as free in the peritoneal cavity, presumably from uterine bleeding through the oviducts or across the serosa. It is impossible to give a precise frequency of the incidence because it can only be demonstrated conclusively at laparotomy. These myometrial hematomas seldom interfere with uterine contractions sufficiently to produce severe postpartum hemorrhage; therefore, they are not an indication for hysterectomy.

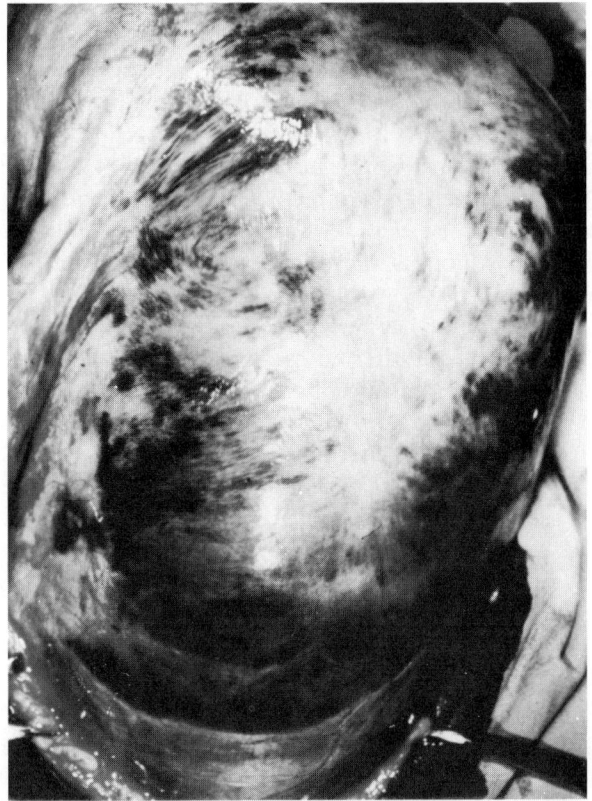

Fig. 37–7. Couvelaire uterus with total placental abruption before cesarean section. Blood had markedly infiltrated much of the myometrium to reach the serosa. After the infant was delivered and the uterus closed, the uterus remained well contracted despite extensive extravasation of blood into the uterine wall.

Management

Treatment for placental abruption will vary depending upon the status of the mother and fetus. With the development of massive external bleeding, intense therapy with blood plus electrolyte solution, and prompt delivery to try to control the hemorrhage, together are lifesaving for the mother and, hopefully, for the fetus. With blood loss occurring at a much slower rate, management will be considerably influenced by the status of the fetus. If the fetus is alive and there is no evidence of fetal compromise (persistent bradycardia, ominous decelerations, or a sinusoidal heart rate pattern), and if maternal hemorrhage is not causing serious hypovolemia or anemia, procrastination with very close observation, coupled with facilities for immediate intervention, can be practiced. This is likely to prove most beneficial when the fetus is immature.

Sholl (1987) provided observations from 130 women with clinically diagnosed placental abruption. Of the 72 women with pregnancies between 26 and 37 weeks, half were delivered within 3 days of admission because of progression to serious hemorrhage, fetal distress, or both. Interestingly, the cesarean section rate was about 50 percent for those delivered soon after admission, as well as those in whom delivery was postponed for at least 3 days. Likewise, Bond and associates (1989) expectantly managed 43 women with abruptio placentae before 35 weeks. Thirty-one were given tocolytic therapy. The mean time to delivery in all 43 was about 12 days and there were no stillborns. Three fourths were delivered by cesarean section.

Sonography has served in some cases to identify a blood clot in the uterine cavity formed as the consequence of placental abruption. **As emphasized earlier, failure to so identify such a clot does not exclude serious placental abruption.**

Lack of ominous decelerations does not guarantee the safety of the intrauterine environment for any period of time. The placenta may further separate at any instant and seriously compromise or kill the fetus unless delivery is performed immediately.

Some of the immediate causes of fetal distress from abruptio placentae are presented in Figure 37–8. It is important for the welfare of the distressed fetus that steps be initiated immediately to correct maternal hypovolemia, anemia, and hypoxia so as to restore and maintain the function of any placenta that is still implanted. Little can be done to favorably modify the other causes that contribute to fetal distress except to deliver the fetus. For example, serious fetal hemorrhage cannot be effectively treated until the fetus is delivered.

We have not been able to decrease uterine hypertonicity significantly with parenterally administered magnesium sulfate in doses given for preeclampsia. Ritodrine and other β-receptor agonists are not recommended, because they are likely to cause vasodilatation of the already underfilled vascular system. Astedt (1982) emphasized another potential risk from the use of β-receptor agonists to try to inhibit labor. In his experience these drugs can minimize the pain and uterine hypertonicity that typifies more extensive placental abruption. Thus, the abruption may go unrecognized for

a dangerously long period, especially in the absence of external hemorrhage. Hurd and associates (1983) have also encountered this problem. Sholl (1987) and Combs and co-workers (1992), on the other hand, provided data that tocolysis improved outcome in a highly selected group of preterm pregnancies complicated by partial abruption.

Cesarean Delivery. Rapid delivery of the fetus who is alive but in distress practically always means cesarean section. It is emphasized that an electrode applied directly to the fetus may provide misleading information, as in the case illustrated in Figure 37–9. At first impression at least, fetal bradycardia of 80 to 90 beats per minute, with a degree of beat-to-beat variability, seemed evident. The fetus, however, was dead. There were no audible fetal heart sounds, and the maternal pulse rate was identical to that recorded through the fetal scalp electrode. Cesarean section at this time would likely have proved dangerous for the mother because she was profoundly hypovolemic and she had severe hypofibrinogenemia.

If the fetus is alive but cesarean delivery is not carried out promptly, the fetus must be monitored for evidence of distress and be delivered immediately whenever distress is detected.

Vaginal Delivery. If placental separation is so severe that the fetus is dead, vaginal delivery is preferred unless hemorrhage is so brisk that it cannot be successfully managed even by vigorous blood replacement or there are other obstetrical complications that prevent vaginal delivery. Serious coagulation defects are likely to prove especially troublesome when delivery is accomplished transabdominally. The abdominal and uterine incisions are prone to bleed excessively when coagulation is impaired. Hemostasis at the placental implantation site depends primarily upon myometrial contraction. Therefore, with vaginal delivery, stimulation of the myometrium pharmacologically and by uterine massage will cause these vessels to be constricted so that serious hemorrhage is avoided even though coagulation defects persist. Moreover, bleeding that does occur is shed through the vagina. An example of an indication for abdominal delivery despite documented fetal demise is now illustrated:

Because rupture of a prior cesarean section incision could not be excluded, a 26-week stillborn fetus was delivered by repeat cesarean section (Fig. 37–10). She had profound hypofibrinogenemia and serious bleeding was encountered from all surgical incisions. Persistent bleeding necessitated hysterectomy followed by internal iliac artery ligation. Ringer's lactate solution was given along with 17 units of blood, 8 units of plasma, and 10 units of platelets to maintain perfusion and treat the coagulopathy, which finally resolved intraoperatively.

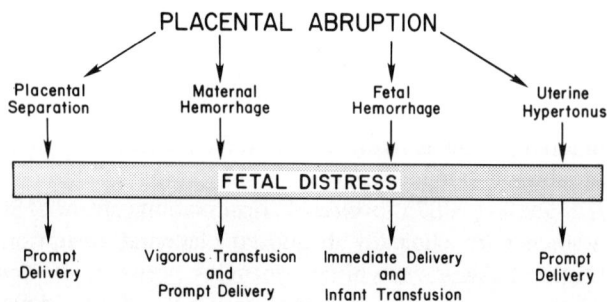

Fig. 37–8. Various causes of fetal distress from placental abruption and their treatment.

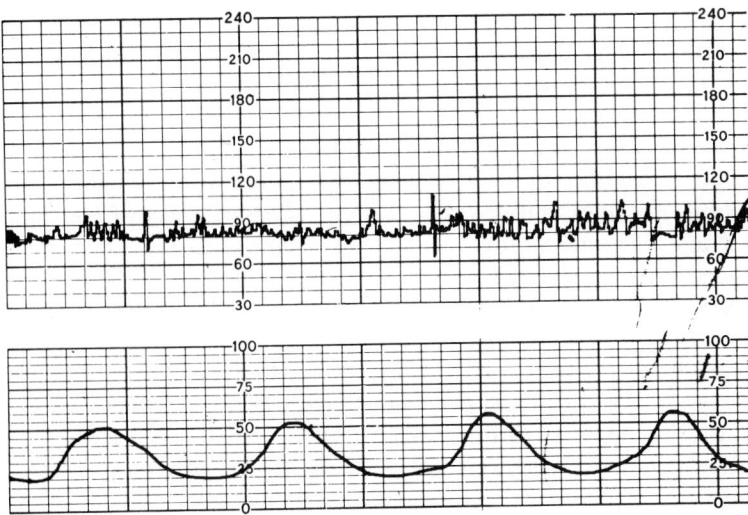

Fig. 37-9. A recording of uterine pressures and presumed fetal heart rate in a case of placental abruption so severe as to have killed the fetus. The scalp electrode conducted the maternal ECG signal. Note the increased uterine basal tone. Commonly, in cases of severe placental abruption both the basal tone and the maximum uterine pressure are greater than illustrated here.

Amniotomy. Rupture of the membranes as early as possible has long been championed in the management of placental abruption. The rationale for amniotomy is that the escape of amnionic fluid might both decrease bleeding from the implantation site and reduce the entry into the maternal circulation of thromboplastin and perhaps activated coagulation factors from the retroplacental clot. There is no evidence, however, that either is accomplished by amniotomy. If the fetus is reasonably mature, rupture of the membranes may hasten delivery. If the fetus is immature, the intact sac may be more efficient in promoting cervical dilatation than will a small fetal part poorly applied to the cervix.

Labor. With slight degrees of placental separation, uterine contractions are usually of normal frequency, duration, and intensity. With extensive placental abruption, the uterus will likely be persistently hypertonic. The baseline intra-amnionic pressure may be 25 to 50 mm

Hg or higher, with rhythmic increases up to 75 to 100 mm Hg. Because of persistent hypertonus, it is difficult at times to determine by palpation if the uterus is contracting and relaxing to any degree.

If severe placental abruption develops before cervical effacement and dilatation, the subsequent pattern of change in the cervix is typically one of progressive effacement with little dilatation until effacement is complete. Dilatation is then usually rapid.

Oxytocin. Although hypertonicity characterizes myometrial function in most cases of severe placental abruption, if no rhythmic uterine contractions are superimposed, then oxytocin is given in standard doses. Uterine stimulation to effect vaginal delivery provides benefits that override the risks. Care must be exercised not to provoke the uterus into self-destruction, especially in women of high parity or with fetopelvic disproportion. The use of oxytocin has been challenged on the basis that it might enhance the escape of thromboplastin into the maternal circulation and thereby initiate or enhance consumptive coagulopathy. There is no evidence to support this fear (Pritchard and Brekken, 1967).

Timing of Delivery After Severe Placental Abruption.
There is no evidence that setting an arbitrary time limit for delivery is necessary. Experiences at both the University of Virginia and Parkland Hospitals indicate that the outcome depends upon the diligence with which adequate fluid and blood replacement therapy is pursued, rather than upon the interval to delivery (Brame and associates, 1968; Pritchard and Brekken, 1967). At the University of Virginia Hospital, women with severe placental abruption who were transfused for 18 hours or more before delivery, experienced complications that were neither more numerous nor greater in severity than did the group in which delivery was accomplished sooner. Our observations are similar; Fig-

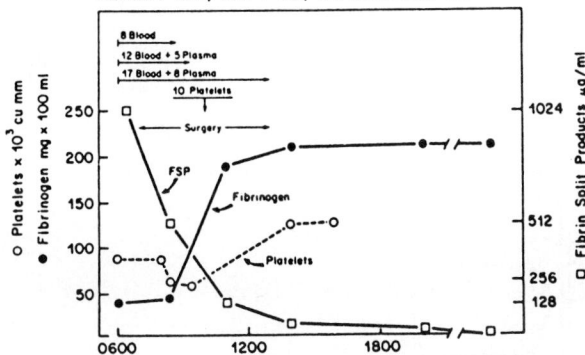

Fig. 37-10. Total placental abruption with severe consumptive coagulopathy at 26 weeks (C/S = cesarean section; TAH + SO = total abdominal hysterectomy, salpingo-oophorectomy; FSP = fibrin split products.)

ure 37–11 summarizes serial findings from one of the most severe cases in terms of the prolonged interval between the onset of symptoms and delivery and the necessity of transfusing a large volume of blood.

Hemorrhage and Hypovolemia. To combat hypovolemia successfully, blood must be available in large quantities, as demonstrated in Figure 37–11. More than 10 L of blood were administered to another woman with severe placental abruption who recovered at Parkland Hospital. **Basic rules for treating obstetrical hemorrhage are applied.** Blood and lactated Ringer solution are infused in such proportions that the hematocrit is maintained at 30 percent or slightly higher and urine flow is at least 30 mL/hr. For the oliguric patient, the dangers from furosemide outweigh any advantages. If *vigorous* fluid therapy does not relieve oliguria, some choose central venous pressure monitoring as more fluids are administered. Because central venous pressure measurement might not detect early pulmonary congestion, the woman must simultaneously be observed for other signs, especially dyspnea, cough, and rales. If pulmonary congestion were to develop, furosemide then would be beneficial.

Coagulation Defects. Much concern has been expressed over the rate of development of coagulation defects as well as their intensity. The extensive experiences at Parkland Hospital have been that coagulation defects most often develop within the first few hours,

and perhaps even minutes, after the onset of pain or bleeding. The coagulopathy usually does not worsen subsequently, except for dilutional effects from vigorous transfusion and crystalloid solution. We have observed a fibrinogen level of only 40 mg/dL less than 3 hours after the onset of intermittent pain thought to be labor and less than 2 hours after the onset of constant pain. Moreover, sufficient placenta remained attached so that the infant survived immediate delivery by cesarean section performed to try to save the distressed fetus (Table 37–6).

If the clot observation test yields a small or absent clot, the usual coagulation studies will be grossly abnormal and will provide very little immediately useful information. Although platelet counts are recommended to identify disseminated intravascular coagulation, hypofibrinogenemia may develop with placental abruption, and yet the platelet count may simultaneously be above 100,000/μL (Table 37–6). With extensive placental abruption, elevated fibrin degradation products are so common as to be anticipated; moreover, their measurement provides little help in clinical management.

Fibrinogen and Cryoprecipitate. In the past, concern—mostly theoretical in origin—was expressed that the use of fibrinogen simply "added fuel to the fire" of disseminated intravascular coagulation by imposing dire consequences of fibrin deposition and microcirculation obstruction in vital organs. There is no good evi-

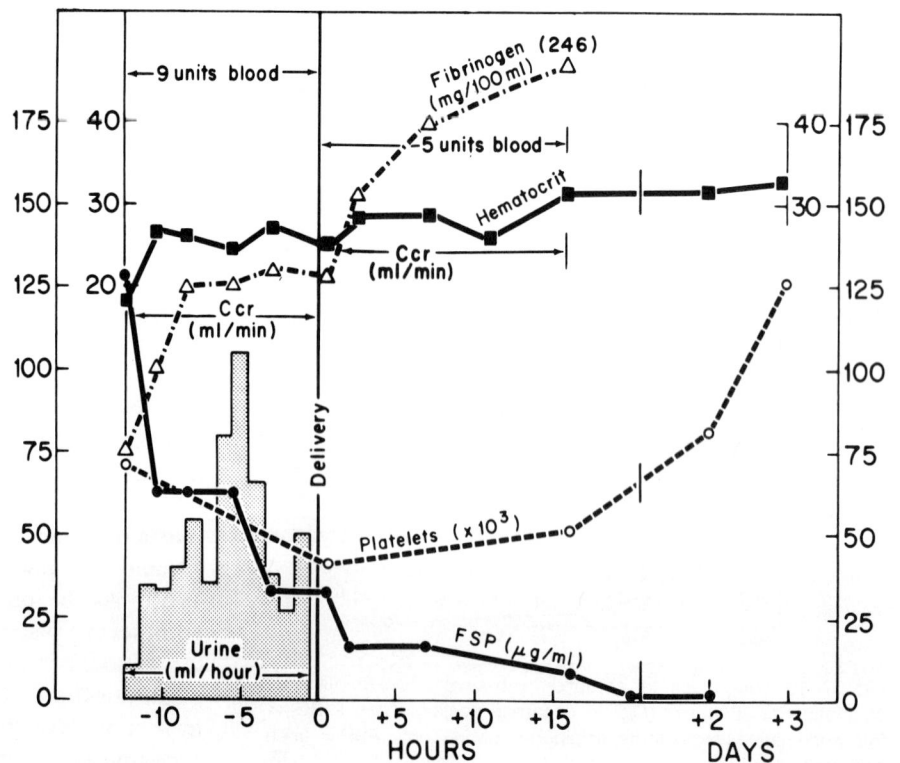

Fig. 37–11. Serial data from a case of placental abruption so extensive as to kill the fetus and induce serious consumptive coagulopathy. Symptoms of abruption began 2 hours before hospitalization and 14 hours before delivery. Note the normal creatinine clearances (Ccr). The patient left the hospital on the third postpartum day.

TABLE 37–6. PARTIAL ABRUPTIO PLACENTAE WITH RAPID SEVERE DEFIBRINATION YET DELIVERY OF AN INFANT WHO SURVIVED

Time	Hematocrit	Fibrinogen (mg/dL)	Fibrin Split Products (μg/mL)	Platelets (per μL)	Plasma Creatinine (mg/dL)
9 Oct					
0530		Onset of labor			
0630		Constant pain			
0805	34	43	1024	151,000	1.1
0808		Cesarean delivery			
0930	30	(2 units whole blood)			
1150	29	91	512		
		(2 units whole blood)			
1425	32	166	128	87,000	1.6
1700	32	178	64	85,000	
10 Oct					
0500	26	263	8	95,000	2.2
11 Oct	25	—	—	124,000	2.1
12 Oct	24	—	—	198,000	1.8
16 Oct	24	—	—	638,000	1.1

Oct = October.

dence, however, that effective doses of fibrinogen cause this. Typically, 4 g of fibrinogen is an effective dose and raises the plasma fibrinogen concentration by about 100 mg/dL.

Cryoprecipitate is currently the principal source of fibrinogen. Each unit or bag of cryoprecipitate carries a one-donor risk of hepatitis or other bloodborne infections. To supply 4 g of fibrinogen, 15 to 20 units must be given. According to the American Association of Blood Banks (1991), each bag contains *at least* 150 mg of fibrinogen.

For many years we have used cryoprecipitate very infrequently. With vaginal delivery, no episiotomy was made if the fetus was small or the perineum was relaxed; otherwise, a midline episiotomy was made and carefully repaired. The emptied and intact uterus was immediately stimulated with oxytocin, and the uterine fundus was monitored continuously and massaged when not firmly contracted. Even with cesarean delivery, cryoprecipitate has been given only if there was gross evidence of disruption of the coagulation mechanism, including uncontrolled bleeding from all sites of trauma. With lesser amounts of bleeding, ligation of all bleeding points with, at times, drainage of the abdominal incision subfascially has proved satisfactory.

Other Coagulation Factors. Massive transfusions using stored whole blood may occasionally result in lack of hemostasis from factor V and VIII deficiency. More often, thrombocytopenia is likely the cause, and if the platelet count is less than 50,000/μL, there may be troublesome oozing from surgical incisions. In these cases, 6 to 8 platelet packs are transfused.

Following delivery, the coagulation defects repair spontaneously within 24 hours or so, except for plate-

lets that, if very low, take 2 to 4 days to reach normal range (Fig. 37–11, Table 37–6).

Heparin. **The infusion of heparin to try to block disseminated intravascular coagulation associated with placental abruption is mentioned only to condemn its use.** The stimulus to activate intravascular coagulation ceases after delivery. Most importantly, excellent results have been achieved with the plan of management described above.

Epsilon-aminocaproic Acid. Epsilon-aminocaproic acid has been administered to try to control fibrinolysis by inhibiting the conversion of plasminogen to plasmin and the proteolytic action of plasmin on fibrinogen, fibrin monomer, and fibrin polymer (clot). Failure to clear fibrin polymer from the microcirculation could result in organ ischemia and infarction, such as renal cortical necrosis. Its use is **not** recommended.

Hysterectomy. In the presence of coagulation defects, the more extensive the surgery, the more likely the hemorrhage is to be intensified (Fig. 37–10). Therefore, hysterectomy to attempt prophylactically to minimize blood loss is unwise. At times, it must be performed because the uterus has been severely lacerated or simply will not contract to effect hemostasis at the implantation site. Supracervical hysterectomy, if the cervix is intact, will usually result in less blood loss than total hysterectomy. For reasons already considered, Couvelaire uterus is itself not an indication for hysterectomy.

Consumptive Coagulopathy in the Infant. Although we have never observed the phenomenon, changes in the coagulation mechanism of the newborn characteristic of those of intravascular coagulation have been described as accompanying placental abruption (Edson and colleagues, 1968; Nielsen, 1970). A variety of conditions predispose to neonatal disseminated intravascular coagulation in the absence of placental abruption, including trauma, prematurity, hypoxia, and sepsis.

PLACENTA PREVIA

Definition. In placenta previa, the placenta is located over or very near the internal os. Four degrees of the abnormality have been recognized:

1. **Total placenta previa.** The internal cervical os is covered completely by placenta (Fig. 37–12).
2. **Partial placenta previa.** The internal os is partially covered by placenta (Figs. 37–3 and 37–13).
3. **Marginal placenta previa.** The edge of the placenta is at the margin of the internal os.
4. **Low-lying placenta.** The placenta is implanted in the lower uterine segment such that the placental edge actually does not reach the internal os but is in close proximity to it.

The degree of placenta previa will depend in large measure on the cervical dilatation at the time of examination. For example, a low-lying placenta at 2 cm dilatation may become a partial placenta previa at 8 cm dilatation because the dilating cervix has uncovered placenta. Conversely, a placenta previa that appears to be total before cervical dilatation may become partial at 4 cm dilatation because the cervix dilates beyond the edge of the placenta (Fig. 37–13). **Digital palpation to try to ascertain these changing relations between the edge of the placenta and the internal os as the cervix dilates can incite severe hemorrhage!**

In both the total and partial placenta previa, a certain degree of spontaneous placental separation is an inevitable consequence of the formation of the lower uterine segment and cervical dilatation. Such separation is associated with hemorrhage from blood vessels so disrupted.

Frequency. The zygote that implants very low in the uterine cavity likely is to form a placenta that at the outset lies in very close proximity to the internal cervical os. The placenta so located usually migrates toward the fundus, or it may remain in situ, giving rise to placenta previa. Ultrasonic investigations of early pregnancies that subsequently aborted have disclosed an unexpectedly large number of low-lying embryos. Not all that do not abort eventuate in placenta previa, however. As the placenta and uterus both grow, the placental site is likely pulled further up into the uterus, and the placenta eventually becomes located some distance from the cervix.

Placenta previa that becomes apparent clinically is a serious but uncommon complication. In our experiences at Parkland Hospital, placenta previa is diagnosed about 1 in 200 deliveries, or 0.5 percent. Clark and co-workers (1985) reported an incidence of 0.3 percent in nearly 98,000 women admitted to labor and delivery at Los Angeles County/USC Medical Center. Nielsen and colleagues (1989) prospectively evaluated nearly 25,000 women admitted to their delivery unit in Sweden and documented an incidence of previa of 0.33 percent.

Contradictory statistics on the incidence of the various degrees of placenta previa mostly reflect the lack of precision in definition and identification for the reasons already discussed. A question difficult to answer is whether painless bleeding from focal separation of a placenta implanted in the lower uterine segment but away from a partially dilated cervical os should be classified as placenta previa or placental abruption. Obviously, it is both.

Etiology. Multiparity and advancing age increase the risk of placenta previa. As shown in Figure 37–6, in over 29,000 deliveries at Parkland Hospital in 1987 and 1988, the incidence of previa in women over 35 was 1 in 100 and for those over 40 it was 1 in 50. Conversely, this incidence was 1 in 300 for women aged 20 to 29 (Cunningham and Leveno, 1989). Prior cesarean delivery or

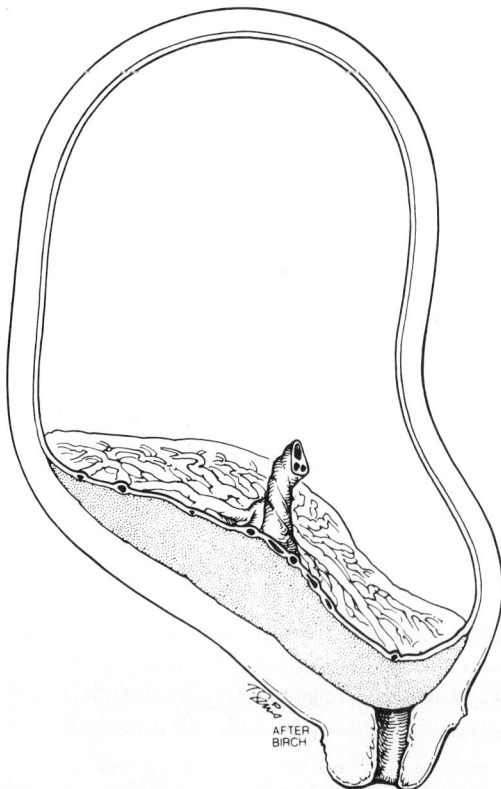

Fig. 37–12. Total placental previa. Even with the modest cervical dilatation illustrated, copious hemorrhage would be anticipated.

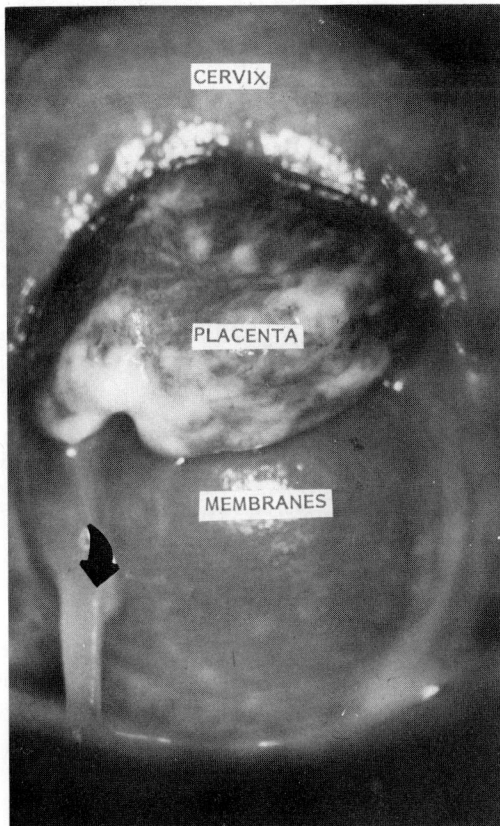

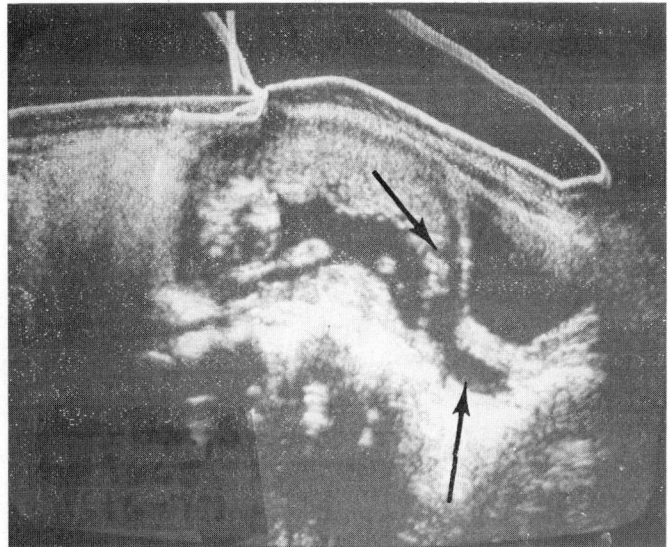

Fig. 37–13. A. Partial placenta previa seen through a cervix 3 to 4 cm dilated at 22 weeks' gestation. The arrow points to mucus dropping from the cervix. Uterine cramping was evident, but earlier intermittent bleeding had stopped 1 month before. The fetus weighed 410 g when delivered vaginally the next day. Blood loss was not massive. **B.** Gray scale longitudinal midline sonogram obtained the day after the photograph in **A.** The upper arrow points to a partial placenta previa from an anteriorly implanted placenta. The lower arrow points to the amnionic sac bulging through the cervix. (Courtesy of Dr. R. Santos.)

induced abortion increases the likelihood of placenta previa. Singh and associates (1981) identified placenta previa in 3.9 percent of women who had previously undergone cesarean delivery, compared with 1.9 percent for their general obstetrical population. Nielsen and colleagues (1989), in the Swedish study cited above, found a fivefold increased incidence of placenta previa with a prior cesarean section; 0.15 percent compared with 1.22 percent.

Defective decidual vascularization, the possible result of inflammatory or atrophic changes, has been implicated in the development of placenta previa. Williams and colleagues (1991b) found the relative risk of placenta previa to be increased twofold related to smoking. They theorized that carbon monoxide hypoxemia caused compensatory placental hypertrophy. Certainly, a large placenta, which spreads over a larger area of the uterus, as seen with erythroblastosis and with multiple fetuses, predisposes to previa.

Placenta previa may be associated with *placenta accreta* or one of its more advanced forms, *placenta increta* or *percreta* (Chap. 27, p. 620). Such abnormally firm attachment of the placenta might be anticipated because of poorly developed decidua in the lower uterine segment. Clark and colleagues (1985) found that 5 percent of women with a placenta previa also had a clinically significant placenta accreta. For women with a prior cesarean section, the incidence was almost 25 percent.

Clinical Findings

Signs and Symptoms. The most characteristic event in placenta previa is painless hemorrhage, which usually does not appear until near the end of the second trimester or after. Many abortions, however, probably result from such an abnormal location of the developing placenta.

Character of Bleeding. Frequently, bleeding from placenta previa has its onset without warning in a woman who had an uneventful prenatal course. Occasionally, it makes its first appearance while she is asleep, and on awakening, she is surprised to find herself lying in blood. Fortunately, the initial bleeding is rarely so profuse as to prove fatal. Usually, but certainly not always, it ceases spontaneously, only to recur. In some cases, particularly those with a placenta implanted near but not over the cervical os, bleeding does not appear until the onset of labor, when it may vary from slight to profuse hemorrhage.

The cause of hemorrhage is reemphasized. When the placenta is located over the internal os, the formation of the lower uterine segment and the dilatation of the internal os result inevitably in tearing of placental attachments. The bleeding is augmented by the inability of the myometrial fibers of the lower uterine segment to contract and thereby constrict the torn vessels.

As the result of abnormal adherence, such as is seen with placenta accreta, or an excessively large area of attachment, the process of placental separation is sometimes impeded, and then excessive hemorrhage is likely after delivery of the infant. Hemorrhage from the placental implantation site in the lower uterine segment may continue after delivery of the placenta, because the lower uterine segment is more prone to contract poorly than is the body. Bleeding may also result from lacerations in the friable cervix and lower uterine segment, especially with attempts at manual removal of a somewhat adherent placenta.

Coagulation Defects. Whereas coagulation defects characteristic of consumptive coagulopathy are rather common with placental abruption, they are rare with placenta previa even when extensive separation of the placenta from the implantation site has occurred. Presumably the inciters of intravascular coagulation that commonly characterize extensive abruptio placentae readily escape through the cervical canal rather than being forced into the maternal circulation.

Diagnosis. In women with uterine bleeding during the latter half of pregnancy, placenta previa or abruptio placentae should always be suspected. The possibility of placenta previa should not be dismissed until appropriate evaluation, including sonography, has clearly proved its absence. The diagnosis of placenta previa can seldom be established firmly by clinical examination unless a finger is passed through the cervix and the placenta is palpated. **Such examination of the cervix is never permissible unless the woman is in an operating room with all the preparations for immediate cesarean section, because even the gentlest examination of this sort can cause torrential hemorrhage.** Furthermore, such an examination should not be made unless delivery is planned, for it may cause bleeding of such a degree that immediate delivery becomes necessary even though the fetus is immature.

After the fetus has reached a gestational age of 37 weeks, the neonatal mortality rate is not greatly improved by further intrauterine development. In such cases, the cause of vaginal bleeding may be ascertained by pelvic examination but only under those conditions emphasized above. If placenta previa is identified, cesarean delivery should be accomplished forthwith.

Direct examination is withheld in women with preterm fetuses for whom delay of delivery is advisable. Placental location often can be obtained by careful

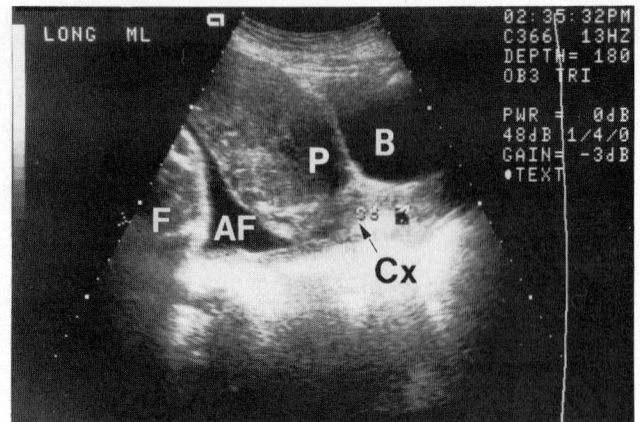

Fig. 37–14. Partial anterior placenta previa at 36 weeks' gestation. Placenta (P) extends anteriorly and downward towards cervix (C). Fetus (F), amnionic fluid (AF), and bladder (B) are seen. (Courtesy of Dr. R. Santos.)

sonography. Such information does not alter management remarkably, because those women who have bled must be carefully watched in any event. With proof that the placenta is normally located, the obstetrician may be more willing to discharge the mother.

Localization by Sonography. The simplest, most precise, and safest method of placental localization is provided by transabdominal sonography, which is used to locate the placenta with considerable accuracy (Figs. 37–13B, 37–14, 37–15). Accuracies of as high as 98 percent have been obtained (Table 37–7). **The false-positive results very likely were contributed to by bladder distention. Therefore, ultrasonic scans in apparently positive cases should be repeated after**

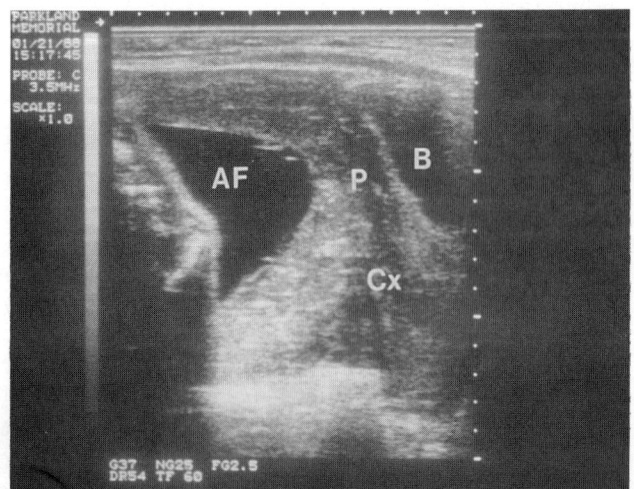

Fig. 37–15. Total placenta previa at 34 weeks' gestation. Placenta (P) completely overlies cervix (Cx). Bladder (B) and amnionic fluid (AF) are also visualized clearly. (Courtesy of Dr. R. Santos.)

TABLE 37–7. ACCURACY OF PLACENTAL LOCALIZATION BY ULTRASOUND

Authors	Year	Results
Gottesfeld and co-workers (Denver)	1966	112 cases: accuracy rate 97% 18 cesarean sections, 2 wrong predictions
Donald and Abdulla (Glasgow)	1968	613 cases: accuracy rate 94% 107 cesarean sections
Kobayashi and associates (Brooklyn)	1970	100 cases: accuracy rate 95% 92 cesarean sections, 4 errors 8 hysterotomies, 1 error
Sunden (Sweden)	1970	107 cases: accuracy rate 95% 45 cesarean sections, 2 wrong predictions
Santos and colleagues (Dallas)	1978	100 cases: accuracy rate 98% at cesarean section
Bowie and co-authors (Chicago)	1978	164 cases: accuracy rate 93% Missed 1 of 13 proven placenta previas
Leerentveld and associates (Rotterdam)	1990	100 cases—transvaginal sonography 93% positive predictive value
Total		1296 cases, average accuracy rate 94%

nearly emptying the bladder. An uncommon source of error has been identification of abundant placenta implanted in the uterine fundus but failure to appreciate that the placenta was large and extended downward all the way to the internal os of the cervix.

Farine and associates (1988) reported that the use of *transvaginal ultrasonography* has substantively improved diagnostic accuracy. They were able to visualize the internal cervical os in all cases with the transvaginal technique, in contrast to only 70 percent using transabdominal equipment. This is shown in Figure 37–16. Likewise, Leerentveld and colleagues (1990) studied

100 women suspected of having placenta previa. They reported a 93 percent positive predictive value and 98 percent negative predictive value for transvaginal ultrasonography. Hertzberg and associates (1992) demonstrated that *transperineal sonography* allowed visualization of the internal os in all 164 cases examined because transabdominal sonography disclosed a previa or was inconclusive. Placenta previa was correctly excluded in 154 women, and in 10 in whom it was diagnosed sonographically, 9 had a previa confirmed at delivery.

Magnetic Resonance Imaging. Preliminary investigation using magnetic resonance imaging to visualize placental abnormalities, including placenta previa, have been reported by several groups. Kay and Spritzer (1991) discussed the many positive attributes of such technology (Fig. 37–17). It is unlikely that this will replace ultrasonic scanning for routine evaluation in the near future.

Placental Migration. Since the report of King (1973), the peripatetic nature of the placenta has been appreciated. McClure and Dornal (1990) found a low-lying placenta in 25 percent of 1490 ultrasonic scans done at 18 weeks; however, at delivery, only 7 of these 385 previas persisted. Sanderson and Milton (1991) found that only 12 percent of placentas were low-lying in 4300 women surveyed ultrasonically at 18 to 20 weeks. Of those not covering the internal os, previa did not

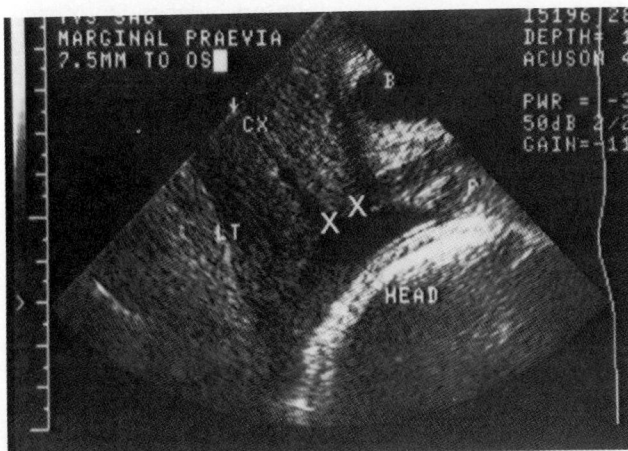

Fig. 37–16. Transvaginal ultrasonic scan at 34 weeks' gestation. Cervical canal is clearly visible (CX) and distance from internal os to placental edge, measured between calipers (X) is 0.75 cm. The patient was delivered by cesarean section 4 weeks later because of vaginal bleeding. (P = placenta; B = bladder.) (From Oppenheimer and colleagues, 1991, with permission.)

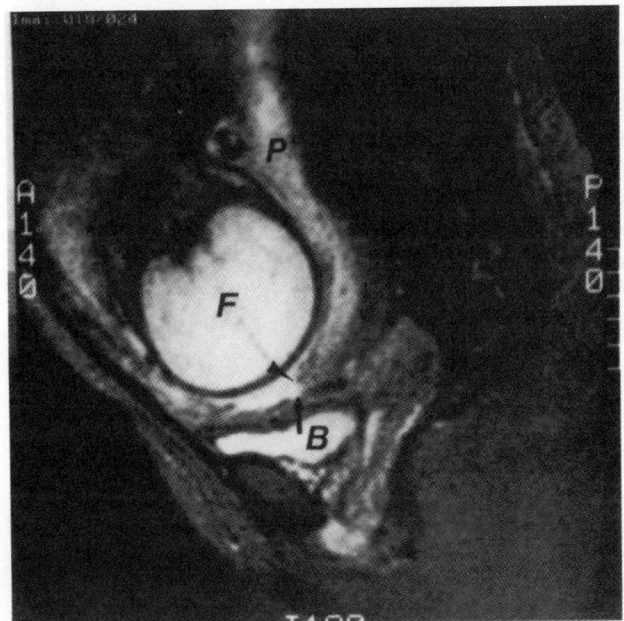

Fig. 37–17. A sagittal T2-weighted (2000/80 ms) image of a patient with a posterior marginal placenta previa. The arrowhead points to the placental edge and the arrow indicates the internal os. (F = fetal head; P = placenta; B = maternal bladder.) (From Kay and Spritzer, 1991, with permission.)

persist and hemorrhage was not encountered. Conversely, of those covering the os at midpregnancy, about 40 percent persisted as a previa. Therefore, placentas that lie close to the internal cervical os, but not over it, during the second trimester, or even early in the third trimester, are very likely to subsequently migrate toward the fundus.

The low frequency with which placenta previa persists when it has been identified sonographically before 30 weeks is shown in Table 37–8. It is apparent from these data that in the absence of any other abnormality, sonography need not be frequently repeated simply to follow placental migration. Because the great majority of cases of asymptomatic placenta previa found early are settled by placental migration, restriction of activity need not be practiced unless the previa persists beyond 30 weeks, or becomes clinically apparent before that time.

Management

Women with a placenta previa may be considered as follows: (1) those in whom the fetus is preterm but there is no pressing need for delivery, (2) those in whom the fetus is reasonably mature, (3) those in labor, and (4) those in whom hemorrhage is so severe as to mandate delivery despite fetal immaturity.

Management of the pregnancy complicated by placenta previa and a preterm fetus, but with no active bleeding, consists of procrastination in an environment that provides the greatest safety for both mother and fetus. Hospitalization would be ideal; however, in this practical world the woman is usually discharged after bleeding has ceased and the fetus is judged to be healthy. In this instance, the mother and her family must fully appreciate the problems of placenta previa and be prepared to transport her to the hospital immediately.

One of the benefits that may accrue from delayed delivery is sufficient placental migration from the cervix so that previa is no longer a major problem. To accomplish this, Arias (1988) described outstanding results from cervical cerclage done between 24 and 30 weeks in women with bleeding caused by placenta previa.

Delivery. Cesarean section is the accepted method of delivery in practically all cases of placenta previa, primarily for the welfare of the mother. When the placenta lies far enough posteriorly that the lower uterine segment can be incised transversely without encountering placenta, the transverse incision is preferred. If, however, such an incision were to be made through the placenta, bleeding, both maternal and fetal, could be severe, and extension of the incision to involve one or both uterine arteries could occur with surprising ease. Therefore, with anterior placenta previa, a vertical uterine incision may be safer.

When placenta previa is complicated by degrees of placenta accreta that render control of bleeding from the placental bed difficult by conservative means, other methods of hemostasis are necessary. Oversewing the implantation site with 0-chromic sutures may provide hemostasis. In some cases, bilateral uterine artery ligation is helpful and in others, bleeding ceases with internal iliac artery ligation. Cho and colleagues (1991) have described placing circular interrupted 0-chromic sutures around the lower segment, above and below the transverse incision, which controlled hemorrhage in all 8 women in whom this was employed. Druzin (1989) described 4 cases in which the lower uterine segment was tightly packed with gauze that successfully arrested hemorrhage. The pack was removed transvaginally 12 hours later.

If these methods fail, then hysterectomy is necessary. For women whose placenta is implanted anteriorly in the site of a prior cesarean section incision, there is an increased likelihood of associated placenta accreta and need for hysterectomy (Clark and colleagues, 1985).

Prognosis. A marked reduction in maternal mortality from placenta previa has been achieved, a trend that began in 1927 when Bill advocated adequate transfusion and cesarean section for its treatment. Since 1945, when Macafee and Johnson independently suggested expectant therapy for patients remote from term, a similar trend has been evident in perinatal loss. Although half of patients are near term when bleeding first develops, preterm delivery still poses a formidable problem for the remainder, because not all women with placenta previa and a preterm fetus can be treated expectantly.

Preterm delivery is a major cause of perinatal death even though expectant management of placenta previa is practiced. Serious fetal malformations are also somewhat more common. Moreover, for any fetal weight, perinatal mortality is likely to be somewhat greater with placenta previa than in the general population. The widely held belief is that fetal growth retardation is increased with placenta previa. For example, Brar and colleagues (1988) reported that the incidence was nearly 20 percent. Conversely, Wolf and associates (1991) performed a case-control study of 179 women with placenta previa matched with 171 control women for gestational age, race, parity, and fetal sex. The inci-

TABLE 37–8. SONOGRAPHIC IDENTIFICATION OF PLACENTA PREVIA AND SUBSEQUENT CLINICAL DISEASE

Gestational Age at Time of Sonography (wk)	Placenta Previa or Hemorrhage at Delivery (%)
< 20	2.3
20–25	3.2
25–30	5.2
30–35	23.9

Adapted from Comeau and associates (1983).

dence of small-for-gestational age infants in each group was about 5 percent.

FETAL DEATH AND DELAYED DELIVERY

Although in most women, spontaneous labor eventually ensues—most within 2 weeks—the psychological stress imposed by carrying a dead fetus, the dangers of coagulation defects that may develop, and the advent of more effective methods of labor induction have enhanced the desirability of early delivery. With the widespread availability of real-time ultrasound equipment, any doubts about fetal death can be resolved quickly and reliably.

Coagulation Changes. Weiner and associates reported in 1950 that some isoimmunized Rh-negative women who carried a dead fetus developed coagulation defects. A prospective study indicated that gross disruption of the maternal coagulation mechanism rarely developed before less than 1 month after fetal death (Pritchard, 1959, 1973). If the fetus was retained longer, however, about 25 percent of the women developed a coagulopathy. Thus the old wives' tale that the dead baby would poison the mother, proved to be true. Extrauterine pregnancy with fetal death and delayed delivery may also be complicated by acquired hypofibrinogenemia (Dehner, 1972).

Typically the fibrinogen concentration falls to levels that are normal for the nonpregnant state, and in some cases the decrease continues to reach potentially dangerous concentrations of 100 mg/dL or less (Pritchard, 1955, 1973). The rate of decrease commonly found is demonstrated in Figure 37–18. Simultaneously, fibrin

degradation products are elevated in serum. The platelet count tends to decrease in these instances, but in our experience, severe thrombocytopenia does not necessarily develop even if the fibrinogen level is quite low (Fig. 37–19). Although coagulation defects may be correct spontaneously before evacuation, this happens quite slowly (Pritchard, 1959).

Pathogenesis. It was clearly established that consumptive coagulopathy, presumably mediated by thromboplastin from the dead products of conception, is operational in these cases (Jimenez and Pritchard, 1968; Lerner and associates, 1967). Heparin infused alone over a few days corrected the coagulation defects, but ε-aminocaproic acid did not. Although these observations serve to establish the cause, they do not precisely identify the site where fibrinogen is converted to fibrin.

Use of Heparin. Correction of coagulation defects has been accomplished using heparin under carefully controlled conditions *in women with an intact circulation.* Heparin appropriately administered can block further pathological consumption of fibrinogen and other clotting factors and thereby allow spontaneous repair of the coagulation mechanism. Once correction has been accomplished and the heparin infusion is stopped, steps can be taken promptly to effect delivery (Jimenez and Pritchard, 1968). **For heparin to be used safely to block the consumptive coagulopathy, and thereby allow spontaneous repair of the coagula-**

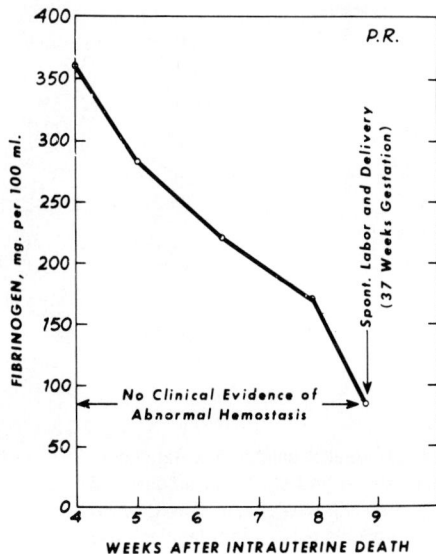

Fig. 37–18. Slow development of maternal hypofibrinogenemia following fetal death and delayed delivery. (From Pritchard, 1959, with permission.)

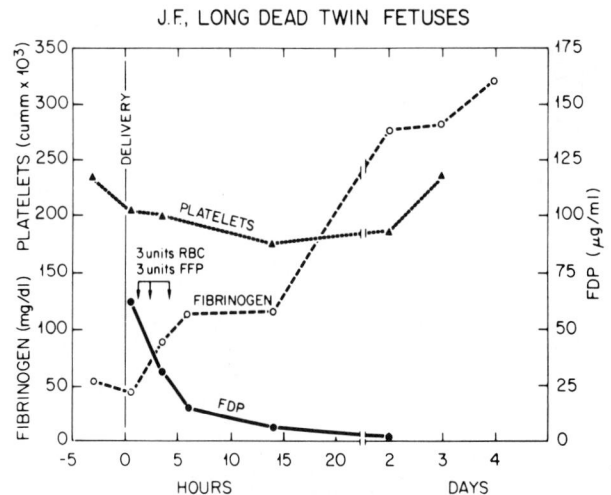

Fig. 37–19. Data from a case of fetal death and delayed delivery treated on an emergency basis at Parkland Hospital. The twin fetuses probably had been dead for 8 weeks or more. Spontaneous labor and delivery were followed by appreciable bleeding, which was treated with intravenous oxytocin, uterine massage, and blood transfusion. (Blood fractions were used because of nonavailability of type-specific blood.) Initially there was marked hypofibrinogenemia and elevation of fibrin split degradation products without thrombocytopenia. Recovery was uneventful; the hematocrit at discharge was 29. (FDP = fibrin degradation products.)

tion mechanism, it is essential that the maternal circulatory system be intact.

Fetal Death in Multifetal Pregnancy. There is a paucity of reports in which an obvious derangement in coagulation has been detected in a woman pregnant with multiple fetuses, some alive and some dead. Carlson and Towers (1989) described 642 multifetal gestations of which 3 percent were complicated by death of only one fetus. They reported no instances of maternal coagulopathy. Fusi and Gordon (1990) also found no evidence for coagulopathy in 11 of 485 twin pairs in which one fetus died. Chitkara and colleagues (1989) performed selective termination of the anomalous fetus of 17 twin pairs between 20 and 24 weeks. They monitored coagulation studies weekly and in no case was a coagulopathy detected. From their review, Landy and Weingold (1989) found only 3 such cases in which an antepartum maternal coagulopathy was managed prospectively. Chescheir and Seeds (1988) have observed, following death of one of twin fetuses and delayed delivery, a progressive but transient fall in maternal fibrinogen concentration and rise in fibrin split products. A similar case managed at Parkland Hospital is shown in Figure 37–20. Coagulation changes ceased spontaneously, and the surviving fetus, when delivered near term, was healthy. The placenta of the long-dead fetus was filled with fibrin.

A major concern is for the surviving twin who has been described at risk for multiple organ infarcts and emboli from material gaining access by placental anastomoses. To obviate this, Romero and colleagues (1984) recommended heparin administration because it resulted in prompt reversal of consumptive coagulopathy in a woman with one dead twin. It seems unlikely, however, that heparin would reverse any coagulopathy in the surviving fetus. Importantly, as discussed in Chapter 39 (p. 898), monochorionic multifetal gestation is associated with a high *a priori* risk of central nervous system infarctions, even if one fetus does not die. Fusi and Gordon (1990) reported that 3 of 8 surviving monochorionic twins developed severe neurological damage despite the absence of a maternal coagulopathy.

Treatment of Active Hemorrhage. If serious hemorrhage is encountered at delivery and overt hypofibrinogenemia and associated coagulation defects are identified, treatment with heparin almost certainly will enhance bleeding. In this circumstance, effective treatment initially is blood and lactated Ringer solution, according to the guidelines described under "Fluid and Blood Replacement" (p. 822). The consumptive coagulopathy stops once the products of conception are expelled, and repair soon follows. If there is excessive bleeding from lacerations or incisions, then cryoprecipitate, fresh-frozen plasma, and platelet packs, alone or in combination, coupled with careful ligation of all severed blood vessels, will prove effective in arresting hemorrhage.

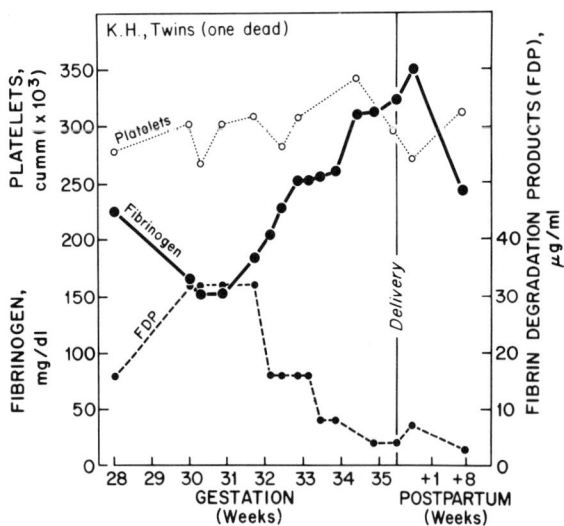

A

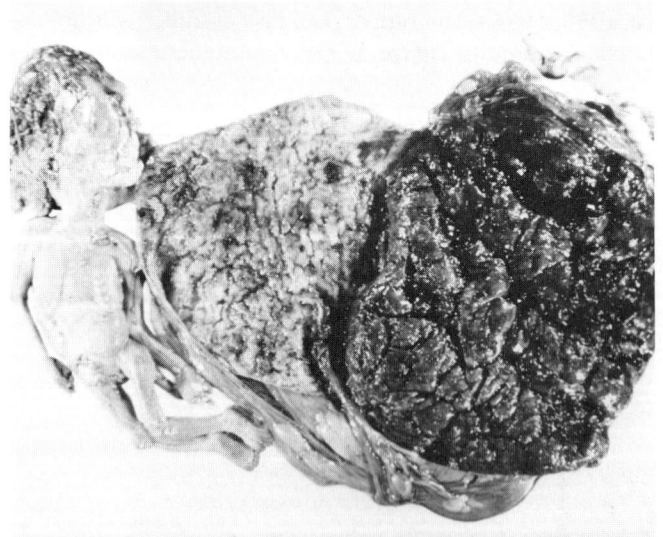

B

Fig. 37–20. A. Death of one twin was confirmed sonographically at 28 weeks' gestation. Coagulation studies then demonstrated a somewhat low plasma fibrinogen concentration and abnormal amounts of fibrin degradation products (FDP). These abnormalities became more intense 2 weeks later. Then, spontaneously, the fibrinogen concentration rose, and the fibrin degradation products fell in mirror fashion. The live-born infant was healthy, and coagulation studies on cord plasma and serum were normal. **B.** The fibrin-filled placenta of the long-dead fetus is apparent. Presumably, the fibrin curtailed the escape of thromboplastin from the dead products into the maternal circulation.

Pregnancy Termination with Dead Fetus. Near term, intravenously administered oxytocin is usually effective when given in a dose that stimulates uterine activity. Remote from term, however, it is less likely to prove effective unless given in high concentration and on more than one occasion. The oxytocin appears at times to influence the uterus subsequently to contract spontaneously, since during the next 24 hours or so after oxytocin infusion it is not rare, especially late in pregnancy, for spontaneous evacuation to take place. One or more laminaria tents placed in the cervical canal before the use of oxytocin may enhance expulsion of the dead products. The magnitude of risk of infection from use of laminaria in the presence of dead products of conception has not yet been quantified.

Prostaglandin E_2 given as a 20-mg suppository to induce labor in pregnancy complicated by fetal death is another option recommended by the American College of Obstetricians and Gynecologists (1986). After 28 weeks there is greater likelihood of uterine hyperstimulation and the possibility of uterine rupture increases; thus, special cautions must be used. These include careful clinical monitoring of the woman in labor. Almost all women develop nausea, vomiting, and diarrhea after prostaglandin suppositories are inserted intravaginally; fever is also common. Apparently rare complications that have been reported include uterine rupture and myocardial infarction.

Orr and co-workers (1979) emphasized that failure of prostaglandin E_2 suppositories to expel the dead products of conception must raise the question of extrauterine pregnancy, and they cite four such experiences. **Fetal death with delayed delivery should always provide the stimulus for asking if the pregnancy is extrauterine.**

The intra-amnionic injection of hypertonic saline is not recommended for evacuation of dead products of conception because the volume of amnionic fluid is often reduced, making the potentially highly toxic salt solution difficult to inject into the sac. Coagulation defects may be induced or enhanced by intra-amnionic hypertonic saline.

AMNIONIC FLUID EMBOLISM

Entry of amnionic fluid into the maternal circulation in some circumstances may prove fatal. Essential to the development of amnionic fluid embolism are (1) a rent through the amnion and chorion, (2) opened uterine or endocervical veins, and (3) a pressure gradient sufficient to force the fluid into the venous circulation. Marginal placental separation or laceration of the uterus or cervix serves to create an opening into the maternal circulation. Rapid or tumultuous labor is observed more commonly. These events may also distress the fetus, leading to defecation of meconium in utero, thereby markedly potentiating the toxic nature of amnionic fluid if it should enter the maternal circulation.

In the typical case of amnionic fluid embolism, the woman is being delivered when she develops varying degrees of respiratory distress and circulatory collapse. If she does not die immediately, serious hemorrhage with severe coagulation defects is soon evident from the genital tract and all other sites of trauma. In some presumably well-documented cases, acute cardiovascular collapse and other findings of amnionic fluid embolism may manifest for up to 48 hours after delivery (Clark, 1990).

Toxicity of Amnionic Fluid. The lethality of intravenously infused amnionic fluid appears to vary remarkably, depending especially upon the particulate matter it contains. The suddenness and intensity of cardiorespiratory problems that develop in many cases, and the histological findings in the pulmonary vessels at autopsy, strongly suggest that the likelihood of infused amnionic fluid proving lethal is greatest when it has been appreciably enriched with particulate debris, especially thick meconium.

Schneider (1955) showed that the lethal nature of human amnionic fluid infused intravenously into dogs was greatly enhanced by meconium. Under these circumstances, it is envisioned that particulate matter, including shed fetal squames (Fig. 37–21A), fetal lanugo hairs, vernix caseosa, and mucin, is pumped by vigorous contractions from the disrupted amnionic sac into a uterine vein. Severe pulmonary vascular obstruction from the particulate matter and possibly from fibrin formed intravascularly leads to *acute cor pulmonale.* Abruptly, hypoxia and reduced cardiac output develop, and if they are not immediately fatal, hemorrhage from coagulation defects is soon evident from disrupted blood vessels. Severe thrombocytopenia develops and the blood typically clots poorly, or a small, mushy clot forms that soon lyses. Plasma from such a patient, mixed with normal recalcified plasma or with thrombin added to form a clot, has been observed by us to lyse rapidly. Moreover, when fibrinogen was injected into the circulation, the thrombin–clottable protein promptly disappeared. These observations implicate intense fibrinolytic and even fibrinogenolytic activity, as well as consumptive coagulopathy.

Coagulation Initiated by Amnionic Fluid. The clot-accelerating activity of amnionic fluid is greatest at term. Even then, however, the activity normally is not great. The clot accelerator principle appears to behave more like Russell viper venom than tissue thromboplastin (Phillips and Davidson, 1972). Of significance, amnionic fluid at times contains appreciable amounts of mucus, which in the case of amnionic fluid embolism might incite or aggravate intravascular coagulation, apparently by activation of factor X. Lockwood and associates (1991) have also demonstrated substantive tissue factor

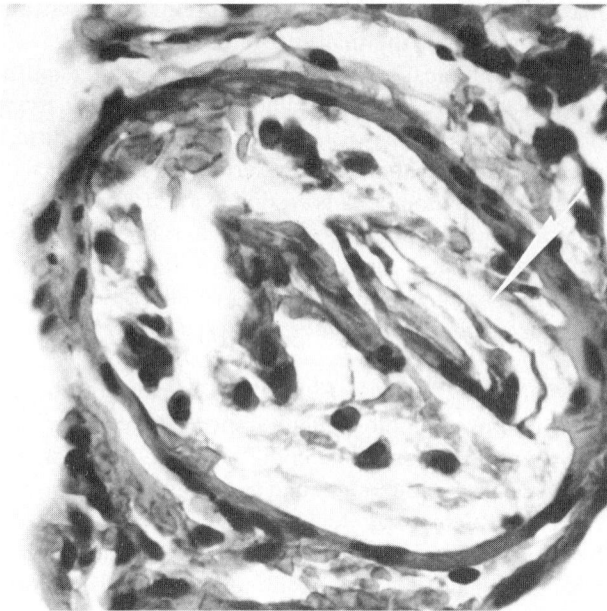

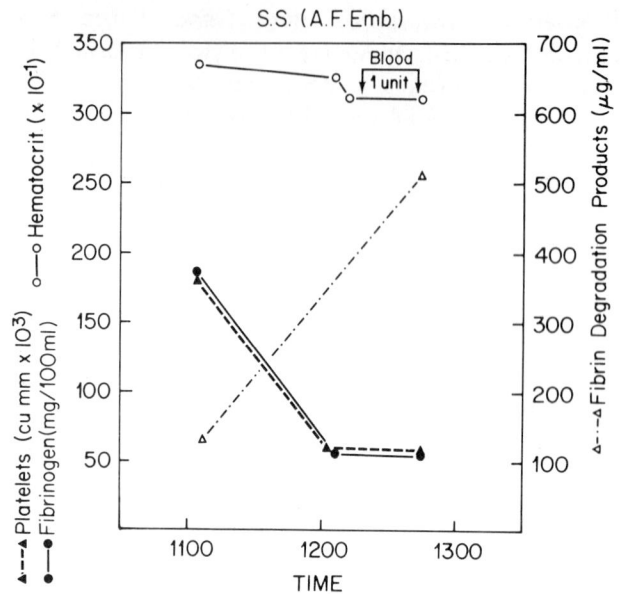

A

B

Fig. 37–21. A. Fetal squames (*arrow*) packed into a small pulmonary artery from a fatal case of amnionic fluid embolism. Most of the empty spaces within the vessel were demonstrated by appropriate staining for lipid to have been filled with vernix caseosa. **B.** Levels of fibrinogen, fibrinogen–fibrin degradation products, and platelets during fatal amnionic fluid embolism.

procoagulant activity in amnionic fluid, especially in late gestation.

Amnionic fluid contaminated with bacterial products, especially endotoxin, would almost certainly prove toxic if it were to enter the maternal circulation. The same is very likely true for amnionic fluid enriched with cytolytic products from a dead fetus.

EXPERIMENTAL AMNIONIC FLUID EMBOLISM. Problems associated with animal experiments to study amnionic fluid embolism have been analyzed in detail by Clark (1990) and Hankins and colleagues (in press). In the experiments of Halmagyi and co-workers (1962), after human amnionic fluid was injected into sheep, pulmonary hypertension, arterial hypoxia, and a marked fall in pulmonary compliance were noted. These changes, however, are similar to those found in pulmonary embolism of other causes. Importantly, they were not observed when the amnionic fluid was filtered and they were not completely prevented by heparin. Adamsons and associates (1971), as well as others, could not produce the syndrome in monkeys, nor could Spence and Mason (1974) do so in rabbits. While Attwood (1964) caused death in only 5 of 15 dogs by the intravenous injection of 50 mL of amnionic fluid, a suspension of human meconium injected into dogs was highly lethal (Schneider, 1955).

In carefully performed experiments, Hankins and colleagues (in press) obtained central hemodynamic measurements in goats injected intravenously with a variety of autologous amnionic fluid preparations. Although pressor responses were seen with raw as well as with filtered and boiled fluid, the greatest changes were recorded in animals given meconium-laden fluid. The latter produced acute but transient increases in systemic and pulmonary vascular resistance with concomitant hypertension, decreased cardiac output, and elevated pulmonary capillary wedge pressure, as well as hypoxia, arterial oxygen desaturation, and dysoxia.

Diagnosis. Fatal amnionic fluid embolism can be confirmed by the appearance of amnionic fluid debris, especially squames, vernix, mucin, and lanugo, widespread in small pulmonary blood vessels. Fatal amnionic fluid embolism has been encountered rarely at Parkland Hospital. A fairly typical case follows.

S.S., a young primigravida at term, felt no fetal movement for 12 hours before the onset of labor. When first evaluated 2 hours later, no fetal heart sounds were heard, but regular uterine contractions without uterine hypertonus or tenderness were identified clinically and electronically. The cervix was 2 cm dilated and 90 percent effaced. Neither amnionic fluid nor blood was visualized coming through the cervical canal until amniotomy, when brown meconium-laden fluid escaped. She was moderately hypertensive and received magnesium sulfate prophylactically. The hematocrit was 34, and a blood clot of appreciable size formed in a thrombin tube. The platelet count, prothrombin time, and partial thromboplastin time were normal. Two hours after admittance, her blood pressure began to fluctuate between 135/105 and 90/60 mm Hg. The hematocrit was now 29. She was given 2 units of whole blood for presumed abruptio placentae, although there was no uterine hypertonus or tenderness, no vaginal bleeding, and urine flow the previous hour was 60 mL. She suddenly became very quiet and then unresponsive; her blood pressure was undetectable, and the apical pulse dropped to 60 and then to zero. Tracheal intubation and cardiopulmonary resuscitation were initiated as a heavily meconium-stained, slightly macerated infant was delivered. The flattened placenta with the maternal surface covered with clot followed promptly.

The uterus contracted poorly and attempts at ventilation were thwarted by lack of pulmonary compliance. Cardiac function was maintained by closed chest compression, and hemorrhage from the flaccid uterus was combatted with blood transfusions. However, oxygenation was inadequate in spite of mechanical ventilation. She was pronounced dead.

Histologically, small blood vessels in the lungs were plugged by debris, including squames, mucin, and vernix caseosa, which accounted for the inability to oxygenate the patient (Fig. 37–21A). Serial values for plasma fibrinogen, serum fibrinogen–fibrin degradation products, and platelets are presented in Figure 37–21B. Abnormalities suggestive of modest consumptive coagulopathy were present when she was hospitalized. These changes had become severe when she demonstrated loss of consciousness, hypotension, and bradycardia, and they persisted until death. An unusual feature of this case is the presence of much meconium. In our considerable experience, meconium in amnionic fluid is rarely found with extensive placental abruption, even when severe enough to kill the fetus.

There almost certainly have been women who survived amnionic fluid embolism, although the diagnosis is always open to question without definite identification of obvious amnionic fluid debris within blood vessels in histological sections of lung or at least in the buffy coat of blood from the right side of the heart (Clark and associates, 1988). As emphasized by Clark (1990), squamous cells are frequently observed in maternal blood obtained through a pulmonary artery catheter placed for a variety of unrelated medical complications.

Intriguing, but in some ways troublesome, observations have been reported in recent years in which the buffy coat of blood drawn from the right side of the maternal heart or pulmonary artery has been identified morphologically to contain amnionic fluid debris—typically squames or vernix caseosa—many hours to even days after suspected amnionic fluid embolism.

Clinical Course and Management.

A successful outcome for the woman who suffers amnionic fluid embolism is probably related to its severity. From the observations reported above, it is reasonable to conclude that the clinical spectrum is varied and the incidence of amnionic fluid embolism is probably underestimated. If complicated by thick meconium, embolism seems to cause acute hypoxia, diminished pulmonary compliance, and rapid death. Vigorous and prompt treatment is mandatory and usually necessitates mechanical ventilation and blood replacement (Clark, 1990; Dashow and colleagues, 1989; Price and associates, 1985). The patient with cor pulmonale, however, tolerates any deficit or excess in blood volume very poorly. In one unusual case, Esposito and co-workers (1990) described a successful outcome in a woman treated by cardiopulmonary bypass and pulmonary arteriotomy with removal of a friable clot containing a high concentration of fetal squames.

With lesser degrees of meconium contamination, and probably to some extent with large amounts of mucus-containing but clear amnionic fluid, the pulmonary insult probably is less severe, and results in oxygen desaturation that is amenable to treatment. Simultaneously, intravascular coagulation is incited and may cause death from hemorrhage, but survival is possible if bleeding is arrested. Quance (1988) described a fatal case in a woman whose first finding was intraoperative oxygen desaturation detected by routine oximetry. Silent pulmonary edema soon followed, and 3 hours after delivery cardiac arrest ensued. From his review, Clark (1990) reported that a bleeding diathesis alone is the presenting manifestation in about 10 to 15 percent of cases.

Treatment is directed toward three goals: oxygenation, maintenance of cardiac output and blood pressure, and treatment of the coagulopathy (Clark, 1990). When amnionic fluid embolism is strongly suspected, use of a flow-directed pulmonary artery catheter, an arterial line to facilitate measurement of blood pressure and obtain blood samples, and instrumentation to record systemic, pulmonary artery and wedge pressures, cardiac output, and blood oxygenation, are likely to prove beneficial. Clark and associates (1988) used such instrumentation and concluded that there was little evidence for pulmonary circulatory obstruction. Indeed, these and other cases have emphasized the importance of left-ventricular failure and need for its correction to reverse hypotension. It is possible that findings of left-ventricular failure are late, because these studies were performed after resolution of acute events.

Whole blood or packed red cells and fresh-frozen plasma are given as described on page 822. Often hemorrhage is torrential because of uterine atony and incisional bleeding due to incoagulable blood. Use of fibrinogen or cryoprecipitate and other blood-component therapy, heparin, fibrinolytic agents, and antifibrinolytic agents has been described in case reports, but their efficacy is difficult to evaluate (Price and colleagues, 1985).

OTHER CAUSES OF OBSTETRICAL COAGULOPATHIES

Coagulation Defects Possibly Induced by Hemorrhage

Rarely, severe hemorrhage of itself can induce consumptive coagulopathy. In the case of massive fatal hemorrhage from rupture of the uterus considered in Table 37–3, the marked decrease in coagulation factors was the consequence primarily of hemodilution by electrolyte solution rather than of intense intravascular coagulopathy. Prompt treatment with blood and lactated Ringer solution, and at times, cryoprecipitate, fresh frozen plasma, and platelet packs, as described earlier in this chapter for placental abruption, has been effective in the few cases treated at Parkland Hospital.

Septicemia

Infections that lead to bacteremia and septic shock in obstetrics are most commonly due to septic abortion, antepartum pyelonephritis, or puerperal sepsis. Other aspects of septic shock are discussed in Chapter 47 (p. 1072).

Coagulopathy. The lethal properties of bacterial toxins, and especially endotoxins, are undoubtedly mediated largely by disruption of vascular endothelium. However, it is unclear whether this is the major mechanism that initiates consumptive coagulopathy. For ex-

ample, in experimental animals endothelial damage is greatest 24 hours after endotoxin is given, but intravascular coagulation can usually be identified during the first few hours. More likely, endotoxin initiates intrinsic clotting through activation of factor XII, or extrinsic clotting through release of thromboplastic activity from leukocytes or by platelet damage with release of platelet factor 3 (Marder, 1990).

As with any situation in which the blood is rendered incoagulable, surgical procedures become more hazardous. An example follows.

A 31-year-old primigravida was delivered by cesarean section for fetopelvic disproportion further complicated by chorioamnionitis (Fig. 37–22). Blood loss was massive from uterine atony plus incisional hemorrhages that resulted from severe hypofibrinogenemia, marked elevation of fibrin split products, and some degree of thrombocytopenia engendered by sepsis. During supracervical hysterectomy, blood, fresh-frozen plasma, and cryoprecipitate were given to maintain perfusion and to help correct the deficiencies in the coagulation mechanism. At the completion of the second surgical procedure, generalized bleeding from the various surfaces had abated.

Management. Therapy for women with septicemia from any cause is outlined in Chapter 47 (p. 1073). In general, treatment of the inciting cause will be followed by reversal of the coagulopathy. In some cases, especially if surgical procedures are performed before sepsis is controlled and the coagulopathy is reversed, treatment with fresh-frozen plasma, cryoprecipitate, and

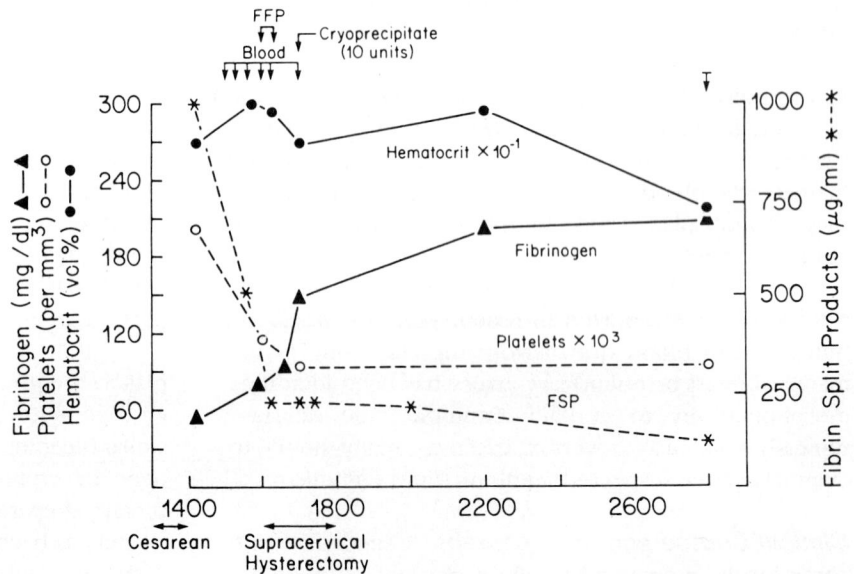

Fig. 37–22. Uterine atony with severe hemorrhage complicating cesarean section worsened by consumptive coagulopathy, the consequence of chorioamnionitis and sepsis. (CPD = cephalopelvic disproportion; FFP = fresh-frozen plasma; FSP = fibrin split products.)

platelet packs usually will arrest such bleeding. **Heparin therapy is dangerous and should not be given.**

Hemorrhage with Abortion

Etiology of Hemorrhage. Remarkable blood loss, especially acute hemorrhage but sometimes chronic, may occur as the consequence of abortion. Hemorrhage during the first trimester is less likely to be severe unless the abortion was induced and the procedure was traumatic. However, when the pregnancy is more advanced, the mechanisms responsible for the hemorrhage are most often the same as those described for placental abruption and placenta previa—that is, the disruption of a large number of maternal blood vessels at the site of placental implantation without myometrial contraction appropriate for mechanical constriction of these vessels.

Coagulation Defects. Serious disruption of the coagulation mechanism as the consequence of abortion may develop in the following circumstances: (1) prolonged retention of a dead fetus, as described above; (2) sepsis, a notorious cause; (3) the intrauterine instillation of hypertonic saline or urea solutions; (4) medical induction with a prostaglandin; and (5) during instrumental termination of the pregnancy.

The kinds of changes in coagulation that have been identified with abortion induced with *hypertonic solutions* imply at least that thromboplastin is released from placenta, fetus, decidua, or all three by the necrobiotic effect of the hypertonic solutions, which then initiates coagulation within the maternal circulation (Burkman and associates, 1977). Coagulation defects have been observed to develop rarely during induction of abortion with prostaglandin.

Consumptive coagulopathy has been an uncommon but serious complication among women with **septic abortion** cared for at Parkland Hospital. The incidence of coagulation defects in the past was highest in those with *Clostridium perfringens* sepsis and intense intravascular hemolysis (Pritchard and Whalley, 1971). In the presence of gross intravascular hemolysis, plasma fibrinogen concentrations ranged from normal to low, as did the platelet counts, while fibrin degradation products in serum were variably elevated. It has long been recognized that intense intravascular hemolysis is capable of inciting disseminated intravascular coagulation, which, if the circulatory system is not intact, contributes significantly to serious hemorrhage.

Prompt restoration and maintenance of the circulation and appropriate steps to control the infection, including evacuation of the infected products of conception, are most important for a successful outcome. There is no evidence that routine hysterectomy, rather than prompt curettage to remove infected products of conception in an intact uterus, improves the outcome.

Management is further described in Chapter 31 (p. 686).

Midtrimester abortion induced by *dilatation and evacuation* has also served to induce severe consumptive coagulopathy. There has been an array of cases reported, especially in the 1970s, in which midpregnancy abortions without prolonged fetal death were complicated by severe consumptive coagulopathy (Guidotti and co-workers, 1981; White and colleagues, 1983). Usually the etiology was ascribed to amnionic fluid embolism, although it has been our experience that amnionic fluid at or near midpregnancy contains very little particulate matter to obstruct the pulmonary microcirculation, and its capability for activating the coagulation mechanism is weak, at least in vitro.

We have observed at least 5 women in whom dilatation of the cervix and mechanical evacuation of the pregnancy at 15 to 21 weeks' gestation somehow induced severe consumptive coagulopathy with hypofibrinogenemia accompanied by high levels of fibrin degradation products. Four of the women were treated as described above for placental abruption and survived.

It seems plausible that in some of these cases, rather than amnionic fluid debris being the culprit, mechanical separation of the placenta during the course of the abortion allowed thromboplastic materials from injured placenta and decidua to enter the maternal circulation at the implantation site, thereby triggering intense consumptive coagulopathy. It seems unlikely that amnionic fluid of itself is the major culprit, for reasons considered under "Amnionic Fluid Embolism" (p. 843). In our experience, the coagulation defects are soon repaired and recovery is uneventful if perfusion of vital organs is maintained by appropriate refilling of the intravascular compartment, and if the products of conception are removed from the uterine cavity.

Miscellaneous Coagulation Defects

Coagulation defects caused by *eclampsia* or *severe preeclampsia* are discussed in Chapter 36. Inherited and other acquired coagulation defects that coincide with pregnancy are considered in Chapter 52 (p. 1192).

References

Abdella TN, Sibae BM, Hays JM Jr, Anderson GD: Perinatal outcome in abruptio placentae. Obstet Gynecol 63:365, 1984

Adamsons K, Mueller-Heubach E, Myers RE: The innocuousness of amniotic fluid infusion in the pregnant rhesus monkey. Am J Obstet Gynecol 109:988, 1971

Ajayi RA, Soothill PW, Campbell S, Nicolaides KH: Antenatal testing to predict outcome in pregnancies with unexplained antepartum haemorrhage. Br J Obstet Gynaecol 99:122, 1992

Alperin JB, Haggard ME, McGanity WJ: Folic acid, pregnancy, and abruptio placentae. Am J Clin Nutr 22:1354, 1969

American Association of Blood Banks: Circular of information for the use of human blood and blood components. ARC 1751, February 15, 1991

American College of Obstetricians and Gynecologists: Diagnosis and management of fetal death. Technical bulletin no. 98, November 1986

Andres RL, Piacquadio KM, Resnik R: A reappraisal of the need for autologous blood donation in the obstetric patient. Am J Obstet Gynecol 163:1551, 1990

Arias F: Cervical cerclage for temporary treatment of patients with placenta previa. Obstet Gynecol 71:545, 1988

Astedt B: Risk of β-receptor agonists delaying diagnosis of abruptio placentae. Acta Obstet Gynecol Scand 108(suppl):35, 1982

Attwood HD: A histological study of experimental amniotic-fluid and meconium embolism in dogs. J Pathol Bacteriol 88:285, 1964

Bill AH: The treatment of placenta previa by prophylactic blood transfusion and cesarean section. Am J Obstet Gynecol 14:523, 1927

Bingol N, Fuchs M, Diaz V, Stone RK, Gromish DS: Teratogenicity of cocaine in humans. J Pediatr 110:93, 1987

Bond AL, Edersheim TG, Curry L, Druzin ML, Hutson JM: Expectant management of abruptio placentae before 35 weeks gestation. Am J Perinatol 6:121, 1989

Bonnar J, McNicol GP, Douglas AS: The behavior of the coagulation and fibrinolytic mechanism in abruptio placentae. J Obstet Gynaecol Br Commonw 76:799, 1969

Bowie JD, Rochester D, Cadkin AV, Cooke WT, Kunzman A: Accuracy of placental localization by ultrasound. Radiology 128:177, 1978

Brame RG, Harbert GM Jr, McGaughey HS Jr, Thornton WN Jr: Maternal risk in abruption. Obstet Gynecol 31:224, 1968

Brar HS, Platt DL, DeVore GR, Horenstein J: Fetal umbilical velocimetry for the surveillance of pregnancies complicated by placenta previa. J Reprod Med 33:741, 1988

Burkman RT, Bell WR, Atienza MF, King TM: Coagulopathy with midtrimester induced abortion: Association with hyperosmolar urea administration. Am J Obstet Gynecol 127:533, 1977

Busch MP, Eble BE, Khayam-Bashi H, Heilbron D, Murphy EL, Kwok S, Sninsky J, Perkins HA, Vyas GN: Evaluation of screened blood donations for human immunodeficiency virus type 1 infection by culture and DNA amplification of pooled cells. N Engl J Med 325:1, 1991

Carlson NJ, Towers CV: Multiple gestation complicated by the death of one fetus. Obstet Gynecol 73:685, 1989

Chasnoff IJ, Burns WJ, Schnoll SH, Burns KA: Cocaine use in pregnancy. N Engl J Med 313:666, 1985

Chescheir NC, Seeds JW: Spontaneous resolution of hypofibrinogenemia associated with death of a twin in utero: A case report. Am J Obstet Gynecol 159:1183, 1988

Chitkara U, Berkowitz RL, Wilkins IA, Lynch L, Mehalek KE, Alvarez M: Selective second-trimester termination of the anomalous fetus in twin pregnancies. Obstet Gynecol 73:690, 1989

Cho JY, Kim SJ, Cha KY, Kay CW, Kim MI, Cha KS: Interrupted circular suture: Bleeding control during cesarean delivery in placenta previa accreta. Obstet Gynecol 78:876, 1991

Clark SL: New concepts of amniotic fluid embolism: A review. Obstet Gynecol Surv 45:360, 1990

Clark SL, Cotton DB, Gonik B, Greenspoon J, Phelan JP: Central hemodynamic alterations in amniotic fluid embolism. Am J Obstet Gynecol 158:1124, 1988

Clark SL, Koonings PP, Phelan JP: Placenta previa/accreta and prior cesarean section. Obstet Gynecol 66:89, 1985

Combs CA, Murphy EL, Laros RKL Jr: Factors associated with postpartum hemorrhage with vaginal birth. Obstet Gynecol 77:69, 1991a

Combs CA, Murphy EL, Laros RKL Jr: Factors associated with hemorrhage in cesarean deliveries. Obstet Gynecol 77:77, 1991b

Coombs CA, Nyberg DA, Mack LA, Smith JR, Benedetti TJ: Expectant management after sonographic diagnosis of placental abruption. Am J Perinatol 9:170, 1992

Comeau J, Shaw L, Marcell CC, Lavery JP: Early placenta previa and delivery outcome. Obstet Gynecol 61:577, 1983

Consensus Development Conference: Perioperative red cell transfusion. Bethesda, National Institutes of Health, June 27–29, 1988, vol. 7, no. 4

Consensus Development Conference: Fresh-frozen plasma: Indications and risks. JAMA 253:551, 1985

Counts RB, Haisch C, Simon TL, Maxwell NG, Heimbach DM, Carrico CJ: Hemostasis in massively transfused trauma patients. Ann Surg 190:91, 1979

Cumming PD, Wallace EL, Schorr JB, Dodd RY: Exposure of patients to human immunodeficiency virus through the transfusion of blood components that test antibody-negative. N Engl J Med 321:941, 1989

Cunningham FG, Leveno KJ: Pregnancy after 35. Williams Obstetrics, 18th ed(suppl 2). Norwalk, CT, Appleton & Lange, October/November 1989

Czer LSC, Shoemaker WC: Optimal hematocrit value in critically ill postoperative patients. Surg Gynecol Obstet 147:363, 1978

Dashow EE, Cotterill R, Benedetti TJ, Myhre S, Kovenda C, Sarrafan A: Amniotic fluid embolus: A report of two cases resulting in maternal survival. J Reprod Med 34:660, 1989

Dehner LP: Advanced extrauterine pregnancy and the fetal death syndrome. Obstet Gynecol 40:525, 1972

DeLee JB: A case of fatal hemorrhagic diathesis, with premature detachment of the placenta. Am J Obstet Gynecol 44:785, 1901

Dickason LA, Dinsmoor MJ: Red blood cell transfusion and cesarean section. Am J Obstet Gynecol 167:327, 1992

Dombrowski MP, Wolfe HM, Welch RA, Evans MI: Cocaine abuse is associated with abruptio placentae and decreased birth weight, but not shorter labor. Obstet Gynecol 77:139, 1991

Donald I, Abdulla U: Placentography by sonar. J Obstet Gynaecol Br Commonw 75:993, 1968

Druzin ML: Packing of lower uterine segment for control of postcesarean bleeding in instances of placenta previa. Surg Gynecol Obstet 169:543, 1989

Edson JR, Blaese RM, White JG, Krivit W: Defibrination syndrome in an infant born after abruptio placentae. Pediatrics 72:342, 1968

Esposito RA, Grossi EA, Coppa G, Giangola G, Ferri DP, Angelides EM, Andriakos P: Successful treatment of postpartum shock caused by amniotic fluid embolism with cardiopulmonary bypass and pulmonary artery thromboembolectomy. Am J Obstet Gynecol 163:572, 1990

Farine D, Fox HE, Jakobson S, Timor-Tritsch IE: Vaginal ultrasound for diagnosis of placenta previa. Am J Obstet Gynecol 159:566, 1988

Feinkind L, Nanda D, Delke I, Minkoff H: Abruptio placentae after percutaneous umbilical cord sampling: A case report. Am J Obstet Gynecol 162:1203, 1990

Fortune JB, Feustel PJ, Saifi J, Stratton HH, Newell JC, Shah DM: Influence of hematocrit on cardiopulmonary function after acute hemorrhage. J Trauma 27:243, 1987

Fretts RC, Boyd ME, Usher RH, Usher HA: The changing pattern of fetal death, 1961–1988. Obstet Gynecol 79:25, 1992

Fusi L, Gordon H: Twin pregnancy complicated by single intrauterine death: Problems and outcome with conservative management. Br J Obstet Gynaecol 97:511, 1990

Gerbasi FR, Bottoms S, Farag A, Mammen E: Increased intravascular coagulation associated with pregnancy. Obstet Gynecol 75:385, 1990

Gonen R, Hannah ME, Milligan JE: Does prolonged preterm premature rupture of the membranes predispose to abruptio placenta? Obstet Gynecol 74:347, 1989

Gottesfeld KR, Thompson HE, Holmes JH, Taylor ES: Ultrasound placentography: A new method for placental localization. Am J Obstet Gynecol 96:538, 1966

Grünfeld JP, Pertuiset N: Acute renal failure in pregnancy: 1987. Am J Kid Dis 9:359, 1987

Guidotti RJ, Grimes DA, Cates W Jr: Fatal amniotic fluid embolism during legally induced abortion, United States 1972 to 1978. Am J Obstet Gynecol 141:257, 1981

Halmagyi DR, Starzecki B, Shearman RP: Experimental amniotic fluid embolism: Mechanism and treatment. Am J Obstet Gynecol 84:251, 1962

Hankins GDV, Snyder RR, Clark SL, Schwartz L, Patterson WR, Butzin CA: Acute hemodynamic and respiratory effects of amniotic fluid embolism in the pregnant goat model. Am J Obstet Gynecol (in press)

Herbert WNP, Owen HG, Collins ML: Autologous blood storage in obstetrics. Obstet Gynecol 72:166, 1988

Hertzberg BS, Bowie JD, Carroll BA, Kliewer MA, Weber TM: Diagnosis of placenta previa during the third trimester: Role of transperineal sonography. AJR 159:83, 1992

Hibbard BM, Jeffcoate TNA: Abruptio placentae. Obstet Gynecol 27:155, 1966

Hoskins IA, Friedman DM, Frieden FJ, Ordorica SA, Young BK: Relationship between antepartum cocaine abuse, abnormal umbilical artery Doppler velocimetry, and placental abruption. Obstet Gynecol 78:279, 1991

Hurd WW, Miodovnik M, Hertzberg V, Lavin JP: Selective management of abruptio placentae: A prospective study. Obstet Gynecol 61:467, 1983

Jansen RPS: Relative bradycardia: A sign of acute intraperitoneal bleeding. Aust NZ J Obstet Gynaecol 18:206, 1978

Jimenez JM, Pritchard JA: Pathogenesis and treatment of coagulation defects resulting from fetal death. Obstet Gynecol 32:449, 1968

Johnson HW: The conservative management of some varieties of placenta previa. Am J Obstet Gynecol 50:248, 1945

Jouppilla P: Vaginal bleeding in the last two trimesters of pregnancy: A clinical and ultrasonic study. Acta Obstet Gynecol Scand 58:461, 1979

Käregärd M, Gennser G: Incidence and recurrence rate of abruptio placentae in Sweden. Obstet Gynecol 67:523, 1986

Kaunitz AM, Hughes JM, Grimes DA, Smith JC, Rochat RW, Kafrissen ME: Causes of maternal mortality in the United States. Obstet Gynecol 65:605, 1985

Kay HH, Spritzer CE: Preliminary experience with magnetic resonance imaging in patients with third-trimester bleeding. Obstet Gynecol 78:424, 1991

Kettel LM, Branch DW, Scott JR: Occult placental abruption after maternal trauma. Obstet Gynecol 71:449, 1988

King DL: Placental migration demonstrated by ultrasonography. Radiology 109:163, 1973

Klapholz H: Blood transfusion in contemporary obstetric practice. Obstet Gynecol 75:940, 1990

Kobayashi M, Hellman L, Fillisti L: Placenta localization by ultrasound. Am J Obstet Gynecol 106:279, 1970

Krohn M, Voigt L, McKnight B, Daling JR, Starzyk P, Benedetti TJ: Correlates of placental abruption. Br J Obstet Gynaecol 94:333, 1987

Landy HJ, Weingold AB: Management of a multiple gestation complicated by an antepartum fetal demise. Obstet Gynecol Surv 44:171, 1989

Leerentveld RA, Gilberts ECAM, Aronld MJCWJ, Wladimiroff JW: Accuracy and safety of transvaginal sonographic placental localization. Obstet Gynecol 76:759, 1990

Lerner R, Margolin M, Slate WG: Heparin in the treatment of hypofibrinogenemia complicating fetal death in utero. Am J Obstet Gynecol 97:373, 1967

Lipitz S, Admon D, Menczer J, Ben-Baruch G, Oelsner G: Midtrimester bleeding: Variables which affect the outcome of pregnancy. Gynecol Obstet Invest 32:24, 1991

Lockwood CJ, Bach R, Guha A, Zhou X, Miller WA, Nemerson Y: Amniotic fluid contains tissue factor, a potent initiator of coagulation. Am J Obstet Gynecol 165:1335, 1991

Macafee CHG: Placenta previa: A study of 174 cases. J Obstet Gynaecol Br Emp 52:313, 1945

Marbury MC, Linn S, Monson R, Schoenbaum S, Stubblefield PG, Ryan KJ: The association of alcohol consumption with outcome of pregnancy. Am J Public Health 73:1165, 1983

Marder VJ: Consumptive thrombohemorrhagic disorders. In Williams WJ, Beutler E, Erslev AJ, Lichtman MA (eds): Hematology, 4th ed. New York, McGraw-Hill, 1990, p 1523

McClure N, Dornal JC: Early identification of placenta praevia. Br J Obstet Gynaecol 97:959, 1990

McVay PA, Hoag RA, Hoag S, Toy PTCY: Safety and use of autologous blood donation during the third trimester of pregnancy. Am J Obstet Gynecol 160:1479, 1989

Miller RD: The National Institutes of Health Consensus Development Conference on fresh-frozen plasma: Indications and risks. Anesthesiology 62:379, 1985

Morrison JC, Martin RW, Dodson MK, Roberts WE, Morrison FS: Blood transfusions after postpartum hemorrhage due to uterine atony. J Matern Fetal Invest 1:209, 1991

Naeye RL: Abruptio placentae and placenta previa: Frequency, perinatal mortality, and cigarette smoking. Obstet Gynecol 55:701, 1980

Nielsen NC: Coagulation and fibrinolysis in mothers and their newborn infants following premature separation of the placenta. Acta Obstet Gynecol Scand 49:77, 1970

Nielsen TF, Hagberg H, Ljungblad U: Placenta previa and antepartum hemorrhage after previous cesarean section. Gynecol Obstet Invest 27:88, 1989

Oláh KS, Gee HY, Needham PG: The management of severe disseminated intravascular coagulopathy complicating placental abruption in the second trimester of pregnancy. Br J Obstet Gynaecol 95:419, 1988

Oppenheimer LW, Farine D, Ritchie JWK, Lewinsky RM, Telford J, Fairbanks LA: What is a low-lying placenta? Am J Obstet Gynecol 165:1035, 1991

Orr JW Jr, Huddleston JF, Goldenberg RL, Knox GE, Davis RO: Association of extrauterine fetal death with failure of prostaglandin E_2 suppositories. Obstet Gynecol 53(suppl):57, 1979

Pearlman MD, Tintinalli JE, Lorenz RP: A prospective controlled study of outcome after trauma during pregnancy. Am J Obstet Gynecol 162:1502, 1990

Phillips LL, Davidson EC Jr: Procoagulant properties of amniotic fluid. Am J Obstet Gynecol 113:911, 1972

Price TM, Baker VV, Cefalo RC: Amniotic fluid embolism: Three case reports with a review of the literature. Obstet Gynecol Surv 40:462, 1985

Pritchard JA: Haematological problems associated with delivery, placental abruption, retained dead fetus, and amniotic fluid embolism. Clin Haematol 2:563, 1973

Pritchard JA: Changes in the blood volume during pregnancy and delivery. Anesthesiology 26:393, 1965

Pritchard JA: Fetal death in utero. Obstet Gynecol 14:573, 1959

Pritchard JA, Baldwin RM, Dickey JC, Wiggins KM: Blood volume changes in pregnancy and the puerperium: II. Red blood cell loss and changes in apparent blood volume during and following vaginal delivery, cesarean section, and cesarean section plus total hysterectomy. Am J Obstet Gynecol 84:1271, 1962

Pritchard JA, Brekken AL: Clinical and laboratory studies on severe abruptio placentae. Am J Obstet Gynecol 97:681, 1967

Pritchard JA, Cunningham FG, Pritchard SA, Mason RA: On reducing the frequency of severe abruptio placentae. Am J Obstet Gynecol 165:1345, 1991

Pritchard JA, Mason R, Corley M, Pritchard S: Genesis of severe placental abruption. Am J Obstet Gynecol 108:22, 1970

Pritchard JA, Ratnoff OD: Studies of fibrinogen and other hemostatic factors in women with intrauterine death and delayed delivery. Surg Gynecol Obstet 101:467, 1955

Pritchard JA, Whalley PJ: Abortion complicated by *Clostridium perfringens* infection. Am J Obstet Gynecol 11:484, 1971

Quance D: Amniotic fluid embolism: Detection by pulse oximetry. Anesthesiology 68:951, 1988

Rice JP, Kay HH, Mahony BS: The clinical significance of uterine leiomyomas in pregnancy. Am J Obstet Gynecol 160:1212, 1989

Rochat RW, Koonin LM, Atrash HK, Jewett JF (the Maternal Mortality Collaborative): Maternal mortality in the United States: Report from the Maternal Mortality Collaborative. Obstet Gynecol 72:91, 1988

Romero R, Duffy TP, Berkowitz RL, Chang E, Hobbins JC: Prolongation of a preterm pregnancy complicated by death of a single twin in utero and disseminated intravascular coagulation: Effects of treatment with heparin. N Engl J Med 310:772, 1984

Sachs BP, Brown DAJ, Driscoll SG, Schulman E, Acker D, Ransil BJ, Jewett JF: Maternal mortality in Massachusetts: Trends and prevention. N Engl J Med 316:667, 1987

Saftlas AF, Olson DR, Atrash HK, Rochat R, Rowley D: National trends in the incidence of abruptio placentae, 1979–1987. Obstet Gynecol 78:1081, 1991

Sanderson DA, Milton PJD: The effectiveness of ultrasound screening at 18–20 weeks gestational age for predication of placenta previa. J Obstet Gynaecol 11:320, 1991

Santos R, Jimenez J, Duenhoelter J: Unpublished observations, 1978

Schneider CL: Coagulation defects in obstetric shock: Meconium embolism and heparin; fibrin embolism and defibrination. Am J Obstet Gynecol 69:758, 1955

Schneider CL: Obstetric shock: Some interdependent problems of coagulation. Obstet Gynecol 4:273, 1954

Seski JC, Compton AA: Abruptio placentae following a negative oxytocin challenge test. Am J Obstet Gynecol 125:276, 1976

Sherman SJ, Greenspoon JS, Nelson JM, Paul RH: Identifying the obstetric patient at high risk of multiple-unit blood transfusions. J Reprod Med 37:649, 1992

Sholl JS: Abruptio placentae: Clinical management in nonacute cases. Am J Obstet Gynecol 156:40, 1987

Singh PM, Rodrigues C, Gupta AN: Placenta previa and previous cesarean section. Acta Obstet Gynecol Scand 60:367, 1981

Slutsker L: Risks associated with cocaine use during pregnancy. Obstet Gynecol 79:778, 1992

Spence MR, Mason KG: Experimental amniotic fluid embolism in rabbits. Am J Obstet Gynecol 119:1073, 1974

Stafford PA, Biddinger PW, Zumwalt RE: Lethal intrauterine fetal trauma. Am J Obstet Gynecol 159:485, 1988

Stettler RW, Lutich A, Pritchard JA, Cunningham FG: Traumatic placental abruption: A separation from traditional thought. Paper presented at the American College of Obstetricians and Gynecologists Annual Clinical Meeting, Las Vegas, April 27, 1992

Stone SR, Whalley PJ, Pritchard JA: Inferior vena cava and ovarian vein ligation during late pregnancy. Obstet Gynecol 32:267, 1968

Sunden B: Placentography by ultrasound. Acta Obstet Gynecol Scand 49:179, 1970

Turney TH, Ellis CM, Parsons FM: Obstetric acute renal failure 1956-1987. Br J Obstet Gynaecol 96:679, 1989

Vintzileos AM, Campbell WA, Nochimson DJ, Weinbaum PJ: Preterm premature rupture of the membranes: A risk factor for the development of abruptio placentae. Am J Obstet Gynecol 156:1235, 1987

Voigt LF, Hollenbach KA, Krohn MA, Daling JR, Hickok DE: The relationship of abruptio placentae with maternal smoking and small for gestational age infants. Obstet Gynecol 75:771, 1990

Ward JW, Bush TJ, Perkins HA, Lieb LE, Allen JR, Goldfinger D, Samson SM, Pepkowitz SH, Fernando LP, Holland PV, Kleinman SH, Grindon AJ, Garner JL, Rutherford GW, Holmberg SD: The natural history of transfusion-associated infection with human immunodeficiency virus. Factors influencing the rate of progression to disease. N Engl J Med 321:947, 1989

Ward JW, Holmbert DS, Allen JR, Cohn DL, Critchley SE, Kleinman SH, Lenes BA, Ravenholt O, Davis JR, Quinn MG, Jaffee

HW: Transmission of human immunodeficiency virus (HIV) by blood transfusions screened as negative for HIV antibody. N Engl J Med 318:473, 1988

Weiner AE, Reid DE, Roby CC, Diamond LK: Coagulation defects with intrauterine death from Rh sensitization. Am J Obstet Gynecol 60:1015, 1950

Whalley PJ, Scott DE, Pritchard JA: Maternal folate deficiency and pregnancy wastage: I. Placental abruption. Am J Obstet Gynecol 105:670, 1969

White PF, Coe V, Dworsky WA, Margolis A: Disseminated intravascular coagulation following midtrimester abortions. Anesthesiology 58:99, 1983

Williams MA, Lieberman E, Mittendorf R, Monson RR, Schoenbaum SC: Risk factors for abruptio placentae. Am J Epidemiol 134:965, 1991a

Williams MA, Mittendorf R, Lieberman E, Monson RR, Schoenbaum SC, Genest DR: Cigarette smoking during pregnancy in relation to placenta previa. Am J Obstet Gynecol 165:28, 1991b

Witt BR, Miles R, Wolf GC, Koulianos GT, Thorneycroft IH: CA 125 levels in abruptio placentae. Am J Obstet Gynecol 164:1225, 1991

Wolf EJ, Mallozzi A, Rodis JF, Egan JFX, Vintzileos AM, Campbell WA: Placenta previa is not an independent risk factor for small for gestational age infant. Obstet Gynecol 77:707, 1991

CHAPTER 38

Preterm and Postterm Pregnancy and Fetal Growth Retardation

A fetus or newborn infant whose weight is appreciably above or below normal is at increased risk of dying or, if he or she survives, at increased risk of physical and intellectual impairment. Two distinct mechanisms are responsible for these increased risks: altered gestational age and inappropriate fetal growth. In the low-birthweight neonate, gestational age may have been shortened or the fetus may have failed to maintain a normal growth rate. In the excessively large neonate, gestational time may have been prolonged or the fetus may have exceeded the normal growth rate.

In any pregnancy it is essential to have a precise knowledge of the gestational age of the fetus; this knowledge is exceedingly important when the pregnancy is complicated. Gestational age must be known before any diagnosis of fetal growth retardation can be made. Unfortunately, for a variety of reasons, gestational age may be unknown or, worse, in error. It may be unknown as a consequence of the woman not obtaining prenatal care until long after events important for the identification of fetal age have passed or been forgotten. An error may result from an unrecognized ovulation delay, for example, following menses induced by withdrawal of an oral contraceptive. Regardless, without an accurate gestational age, the appropriateness of fetal growth *cannot* be established, and serious errors in patient management may result.

Establishment of Gestational Age

It is customary to estimate the time of delivery by adding 7 days to the date of the first day of the last normal spontaneous menses and subtracting 3 months (rule of Naegele, Chap. 9, p. 249). It is essential to establish that previous spontaneous menses were cyclically predictable and normal in length and that the last bleeding episode was *not* the consequence of oral contraceptive withdrawal.

Additional objective evidence can be established. A urinary pregnancy test (Chap. 32, p. 699) is useful to help document an early pregnancy if the test is positive during the first 6 weeks after the last normal menstrual bleeding began. The time of quickening as well as the detection of fetal heart sounds with a DeLee fetoscope between 17 and 19 weeks' gestation may be used as

reliable landmarks of gestational age when they coincide with menstrual history (Jimenez and co-workers, 1983). Measurement of fetal size by ultrasound before the 26th week provides reliable gestational age within days (Sholl and Sabbagha, 1984). Robinson and Fleming (1975) reported that fetal crown–rump measurements between 7 and 14 weeks had an error of only ± 1.2 mm and a range in gestational age of ± 4.7 days. O'Brien and associates (1981) reported that measurements of femur length between 12 and 22 weeks varied by only ± 1.6 mm and gestational age by ± 6.7 days. Biparietal diameter measurements between 17 and 26 weeks were reported to have an error in measurements of only ± 0.8 mm but a range of ± 10 days (Hughey and Sabbagha, 1978). After 26 weeks, gestational age assessment by ultrasound has a range of ± 14 to 21 days.

Goldenberg and co-workers (1989a) described the impact of ultrasonography on gestational age assessments in preterm, postterm, and fetal growth retardation. One result was an increase in births defined to be preterm and fewer postterm and growth-retarded infants. Other information is helpful, but does not narrow the gestational age estimate to less than 2 weeks. For example, the height of the uterine fundus corresponds in cm to weeks between the 18th and 30th weeks *when the bladder is empty* (Jimenez and co-workers, 1983). For practical purposes, if the uterine height in cm between 18 and 30 weeks is within 2 weeks of the estimated gestational age, based upon an accurate last normal spontaneous menstrual period, then there is sufficient evidence to establish a reasonable but not exact gestational age.

Chauham and colleagues (1992) suggested an interesting alternative for intrapartum assessment of fetal size—ask the mother! These investigators asked 106 parous women in labor with term pregnancies to estimate the birthweight of their fetus. The maternal estimates were equivalent in accuracy to clinical estimation by a physician or ultrasonic estimates based on fetal measurements.

Definitions

The fetus or newborn infant is referred to as a *fetus at term* or an *infant at term* during the interval from the

38th to the 42nd week after the onset of a menstrual period that was followed 2 weeks later by ovulation. The critical date for determining the age of the fetus is the date of ovulation or of fertilization. **The date of onset of the last normal menstrual period is of clinical importance for determining fetal age because it is usually known rather precisely, and when menstrual bleeding is spontaneous and previously regular, it is most often followed by ovulation and fertilization 2 weeks later.** Before the 38th week, **preterm** is the word best applied to categorize the fetus and the pregnancy; at 42 completed weeks and thereafter **postterm** is appropriate. Gestational (menstrual) age should be cited in weeks rather than months or trimesters.

In 1935, the American Academy of Pediatrics defined prematurity as a liveborn infant weighing 2500 g or less (Cone, 1985). These criteria were used widely until it became apparent that there were discrepancies between gestational age and birthweight because of retarded fetal growth. The World Health Organization in 1961 added gestational age as a criterion for premature infants defined as those born at 37 weeks or less. A distinction was made between *low birthweight* (2500 g or less) and *prematurity* (37 weeks or less).

With continued improved care of the preterm infant, other definitions have been developed. For example, the Collaborative Group on Antenatal Steroid Therapy (1981) reported that the great preponderance of mortality and serious morbidity from preterm birth is prior to 34 weeks. Moreover, low birthweight, defined as less than 2500 g, has been modified now to describe **very low birthweight,** infants weighing 1500 g or less; and **extremely low birthweight,** those who weigh 1000 g or less.

Although the term *premature* was used to designate the fetus or infant before the 38th week of gestational age, *premature* should be used to describe function. For example, an infant at birth may have a gestational age of 32 weeks and thus be chronologically preterm, yet from the standpoint of pulmonary function may demonstrate no respiratory difficulties because pulmonary function is mature. Such an infant probably should be described as preterm with mature pulmonary function. **Thus, it seems more appropriate to designate preterm and postterm to refer to age and maturity to refer to function.**

Postterm describes the fetus or newborn infant whose gestational age has exceeded 42 weeks. *Postdates* is another term that has achieved considerable usage, although the word seems to defy a precise definition as to the "dates" involved, other than perhaps the last menstrual period. Presumably, if the term *postdates* is acceptable, "predates" and "dates" are eligible for incorporation into the medical lexicon.

With respect to gestational age, a fetus or infant may be **preterm, term,** or **postterm.** With respect to size, the fetus or infant may be normally grown or *appropriate for gestational age,* small in size or *small for gestational age,* or overgrown and consequently *large for gestational age.* In recent years, the term *small for gestational age* has been used widely, especially by neonatologists, to categorize an infant whose birthweight is clearly below average and usually below the 10th percentile for its gestational age. Obstetricians have more often used the terms *fetal growth retardation* or the less precise term *intrauterine growth retardation.* The infant whose birthweight is above the 90th percentile has been categorized as *large-for-gestational-age,* and the infant whose weight is between the 10th and 90th percentiles is designated *appropriate for gestational age* (Fig. 38–1).

Typically, the fetus continues to grow after 36 weeks but at a slower rate (Fig. 38–2). When gestation is prolonged beyond term, some fetuses, perhaps the majority, continue to grow and some may achieve a remarkably large size. Those infants who do so have been referred to by some as *postmature* as well as *postterm.* Fetuses who become undernourished and demonstrate evidence of chronic distress in utero have been classified by some as **dysmature.** Unfortunately, some obstetricians and pediatricians use "postmature" to designate all fetuses and infants for whom the pregnancy is postterm, while others apply it only to the macrosomic "overgrown" postterm fetus or infant, and still others designate only the undernourished, postterm newborn infant as postmature. The term *postmature* literally means "after maturity," and probably should be reserved for those infants born with the features of prolonged gestation described later in the chapter.

It is more logical to consider time, size, and function as three distinctly different and frequently separate entities. With respect to size, a small-for-gestational-age infant may be *constitutionally* small for genetic reasons, such as small parents, or small as the consequence of an abnormality in function, that is, *growth retarded.* Therefore, *small for gestational age* is a descriptive term for *size* plotted as a function of *time. Constitutional* and *growth retardation* are functional terms used to describe the reasons for the small size. *Constitutional* implies a normal, nonpathological course, and *growth retardation* implies an abnormal process. Similarly, large-for-gestational-age infants may be *constitutionally large* because of large parents or they may be *macrosomic* as a consequence of a pathological process, such as diabetes mellitus. Finally, a neonate whose weight is appropriate for gestational age, that is, between the 10th and 90th percentiles, may still be growth retarded or macrosomic. Put another way, the neonate may be within a normal weight range but appear obese or too thin.

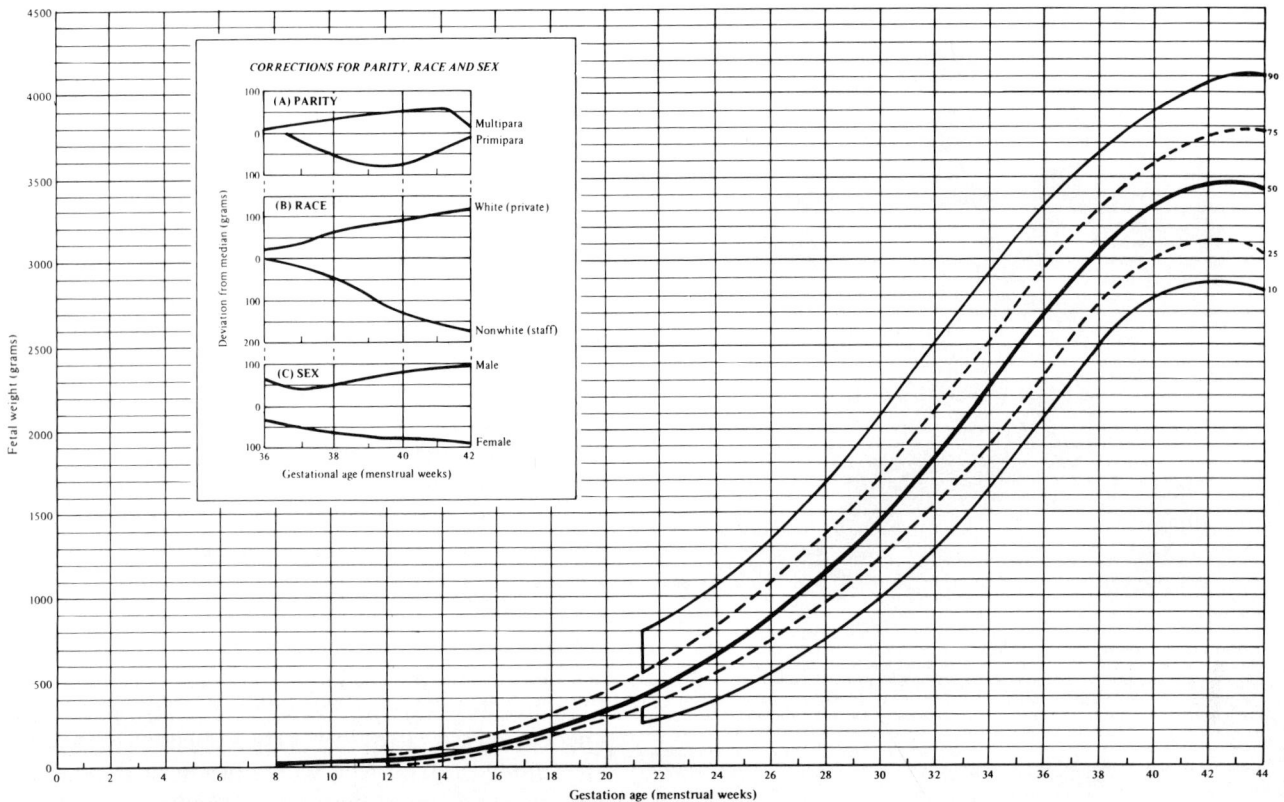

Fig. 38–1. Fetal weight. The 10th, 25th, 50th, 75th, and 90th percentiles of fetal weight in grams throughout pregnancy and correction factors for parity, race (socioeconomic status), and sex. Data obtained from 31,202 prostaglandin-induced abortions and spontaneous deliveries in Cleveland. (From Brenner and colleagues, 1976, with permission.)

Standards for Normal Fetal Growth and Development

By now, the practice of equating fetal size or maturation with fetal age, which unfortunately has been firmly ingrained into obstetrical and pediatric practices, should have been abandoned. For normal pregnancies, there is a strong correlation among these, but at times the fetus-infant who is very small at birth may be chronologically and functionally mature. This phenomenon is likely to be most dramatic when maternal chronic vascular disease complicates pregnancy (Fig. 38–3). Conversely, the infant of normal term size may be precariously preterm, as in some pregnancies complicated by gestational diabetes.

Fetal Weights at Various Gestational Ages. It is difficult to obtain precise standards for determining appropriate or inappropriate growth of the human fetus who is remote from term. In order to determine fetal weight directly, the fetus obviously must have been delivered and weighed, but the fetus of known gestational age who is born preterm is often not the product of a normal pregnancy. Persson and co-workers (1978a, 1978b) reported that fetal growth rate, as measured by serial ultrasonic determination of biparietal diameters, was somewhat retarded before preterm delivery when compared with measurements obtained in fetuses born at term. Nonetheless, several investigators have tabulated birthweights at various gestational ages, even though the data are not likely to be as precise as desired. For example, Goldenberg and colleagues (1989b) examined

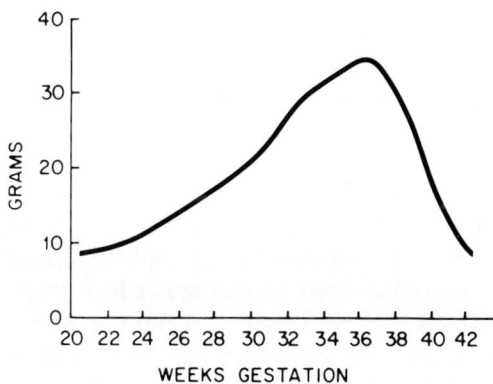

Fig. 38–2. Mean daily fetal growth during previous week of gestation (Adapted from Hendricks, 1964, with permission.)

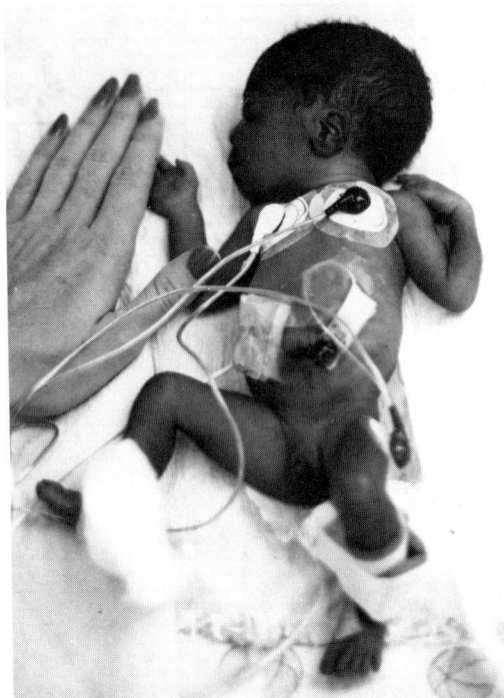

A

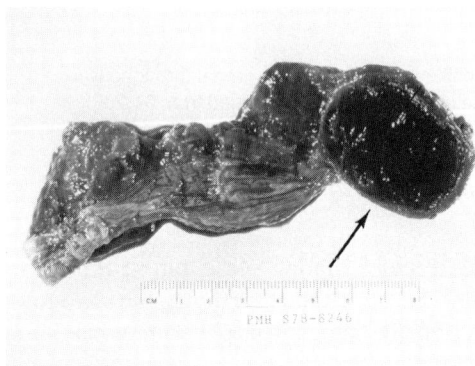

B

Fig. 38–3. A. The infant weighed 650 g when delivered at 29 to 30 weeks' gestation. The mother had become severely hypertensive. At delivery by cesarean section, there was a subchorial hematoma of many days' duration in the placenta. The infant thrived with no evidence of respiratory distress. **B.** Cross-sectional view of the subchorial hematoma (*arrow*) contained in the placenta of the severely growth-retarded, preterm infant.

several studies for American birthweight percentiles with particular attention to fetal growth retardation defined as births less than the 10th percentile. They found that this definition of fetal growth retardation could differ by several hundred grams at any gestational age. They called for a single national standard for fetal growth retardation.

There is general agreement that the following factors influence birthweight, at least in term pregnancies:

1. *Sex*: Boys weigh more than girls.

2. *Parity*: Birthweight increases with parity at least through para 2.
3. *Race*: White babies at term weigh more than black babies.

Ideally the standardization of birthweight for gestational age also should take into account maternal height and weight, because they may both influence birthweight. For example, Gardosi and associates (1992) showed that about 1 in 4 infants designated either small or large for gestational age were in fact within normal limits when corrective factors such as maternal weight were taken into account.

In four different studies in the United States, the mean birthweights identified at 40 weeks were similar for live-born infants (Brenner, 1976; Hoffman, 1974; Lubchenco, 1963; Naeye, 1978; and their associates). The mean birthweight at 40 weeks was 3335 g and ranged from 3280 to 3400 g. As gestational age decreased, however, the relative differences in mean birthweights increased more markedly, mostly because of the large weights recorded by Hoffman compared with the other three groups. The tabulation provided by Lubchenco and associates (1963) was obtained in Denver at an altitude of 5280 feet, which has been shown to reduce birthweight (Unger and co-authors, 1988). The information provided by Brenner and colleagues (1976) is likely to be more appropriate for sea level. Fetal weights throughout pregnancy, with correction factors for parity, race, and sex, are presented in Figure 38–1.

Physical Characteristics at Various Gestational Ages. A reasonably precise approximation of gestational age may be obtained in the delivery room or nursery by evaluating the infant's physical and neurological development. Examination is performed of the sole creases, breast nodule size, scalp hair, earlobe formation, posture, and in the male, size of the testes and scrotal rugae (Fig. 38–4A). A neurological examination done the day after delivery may be helpful as well (Fig. 38–4B).

Just as fetal or infant size cannot always be equated with age, neither can assessments of physical characteristics be used to assign in all neonates an accurate gestational age. At term there is indeed a strong correlation between gestational age and physical characteristics; however, a preterm, small-for-gestational-age infant may exhibit lung maturation as well as physical characteristics that appear earlier than usually expected. An excellent example of this was seen in the case of the Davis quintuplets (Chap. 39, p. 904). The delivery was by cesarean section at 31.5 weeks' gestation. The 3 largest infants were from separate ova, with the male infant being the heaviest at 1530 g and the 2 female infants weighing 1440 and 1420 g. The 2 female infants derived from a single ovum weighed 990 and 860 g. Only the largest infant, the male, developed

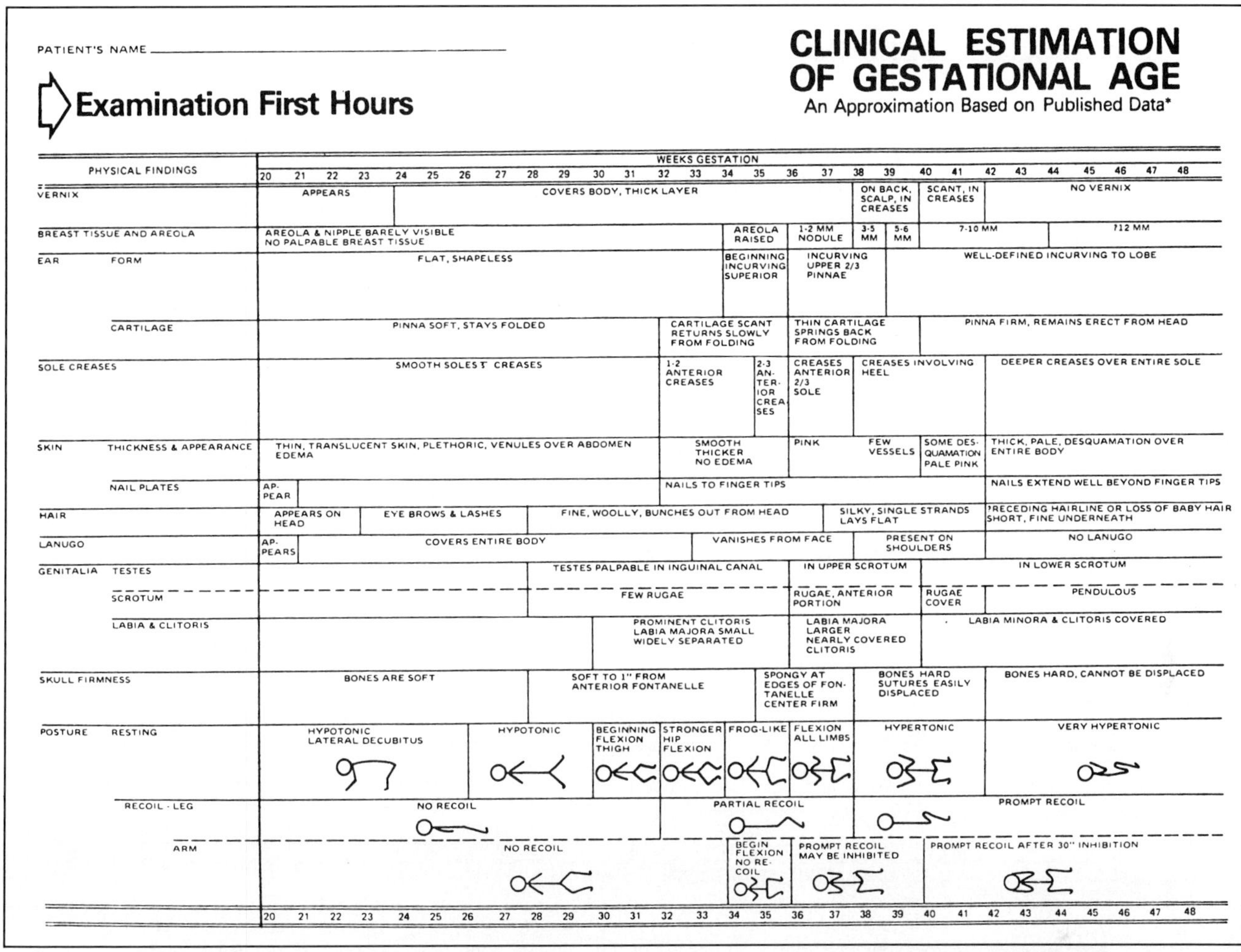

PATIENT'S NAME _____

▷ **Examination First Hours**

CLINICAL ESTIMATION OF GESTATIONAL AGE
An Approximation Based on Published Data*

WEEKS GESTATION: 20 21 22 23 24 25 26 27 28 29 30 31 32 33 34 35 36 37 38 39 40 41 42 43 44 45 46 47 48

PHYSICAL FINDINGS		Progression (20 → 48 weeks)
VERNIX		APPEARS → COVERS BODY, THICK LAYER → ON BACK, SCALP, IN CREASES → SCANT, IN CREASES → NO VERNIX
BREAST TISSUE AND AREOLA		AREOLA & NIPPLE BARELY VISIBLE NO PALPABLE BREAST TISSUE → AREOLA RAISED → 1-2 MM NODULE → 3-5 MM → 5-6 MM → 7-10 MM → ?12 MM
EAR	FORM	FLAT, SHAPELESS → BEGINNING INCURVING SUPERIOR → INCURVING UPPER 2/3 PINNAE → WELL-DEFINED INCURVING TO LOBE
	CARTILAGE	PINNA SOFT, STAYS FOLDED → CARTILAGE SCANT RETURNS SLOWLY FROM FOLDING → THIN CARTILAGE SPRINGS BACK FROM FOLDING → PINNA FIRM, REMAINS ERECT FROM HEAD
SOLE CREASES		SMOOTH SOLES ? CREASES → 1-2 ANTERIOR CREASES → 2-3 ANTERIOR CREASES → CREASES ANTERIOR 2/3 SOLE → CREASES INVOLVING HEEL → DEEPER CREASES OVER ENTIRE SOLE
SKIN	THICKNESS & APPEARANCE	THIN, TRANSLUCENT SKIN, PLETHORIC, VENULES OVER ABDOMEN EDEMA → SMOOTH THICKER NO EDEMA → PINK → FEW VESSELS → SOME DESQUAMATION PALE PINK → THICK, PALE, DESQUAMATION OVER ENTIRE BODY
	NAIL PLATES	APPEAR → NAILS TO FINGER TIPS → NAILS EXTEND WELL BEYOND FINGER TIPS
HAIR		APPEARS ON HEAD → EYE BROWS & LASHES → FINE, WOOLLY, BUNCHES OUT FROM HEAD → SILKY, SINGLE STRANDS LAYS FLAT → ?RECEDING HAIRLINE OR LOSS OF BABY HAIR SHORT, FINE UNDERNEATH
LANUGO		APPEARS → COVERS ENTIRE BODY → VANISHES FROM FACE → PRESENT ON SHOULDERS → NO LANUGO
GENITALIA	TESTES	TESTES PALPABLE IN INGUINAL CANAL → IN UPPER SCROTUM → IN LOWER SCROTUM
	SCROTUM	FEW RUGAE → RUGAE, ANTERIOR PORTION → RUGAE COVER → PENDULOUS
	LABIA & CLITORIS	PROMINENT CLITORIS LABIA MAJORA SMALL WIDELY SEPARATED → LABIA MAJORA LARGER NEARLY COVERED CLITORIS → LABIA MINORA & CLITORIS COVERED
SKULL FIRMNESS		BONES ARE SOFT → SOFT TO 1" FROM ANTERIOR FONTANELLE → SPONGY AT EDGES OF FONTANELLE CENTER FIRM → BONES HARD SUTURES EASILY DISPLACED → BONES HARD, CANNOT BE DISPLACED
POSTURE	RESTING	HYPOTONIC LATERAL DECUBITUS → HYPOTONIC → BEGINNING FLEXION THIGH → STRONGER HIP FLEXION → FROG-LIKE → FLEXION ALL LIMBS → HYPERTONIC → VERY HYPERTONIC
	RECOIL - LEG	NO RECOIL → PARTIAL RECOIL → PROMPT RECOIL
	ARM	NO RECOIL → BEGIN FLEXION NO RECOIL → PROMPT RECOIL MAY BE INHIBITED → PROMPT RECOIL AFTER 30" INHIBITION

Fig. 38–4. A. Clinical estimation of gestational age. (From Brazle and Lubchenco, 1974, with permission.)

respiratory distress. Interestingly, in all the neonates, including the male, physical characteristics were advanced by 2 to 4 weeks beyond what was expected. Moreover, these characteristics varied appreciably from infant to infant by as much as 3 weeks' gestational age. The time of conception was known precisely because the pregnancy was the result of induced ovulation. Thus, these 5 infants were certainly the same age, yet their physical characteristics were quite disparate.

PRETERM BIRTH

Obstetrical approaches to preterm labor and delivery are guided in large part by expectations the obstetrician has for survival of the premature or immature neonate, as well as the therapeutic alternatives available for management of preterm labor. That some very small infants do survive when provided with prolonged, very expensive intensive care has created serious problems in decision making for the obstetrician (Table 38–1). The obstetrician faces the challenge of effecting delivery in such a way

as to optimize the status of the fetus-infant at birth, in the event that intensive care will be applied. The neonatologist in turn must make a judgmental decision as how best to dispense the finite resources for medical care provided by the insurance carrier, the family, governmental agencies, the hospital, and the health care team.

Aside from the survival, another important issue is the quality of life achieved by quite immature, extremely-low-birthweight infants. It is apparent that appreciable compromise, both physical and intellectual, afflicts many such children. Given these concerns, at what time in gestation should obstetrical interventions be practiced? Although it is impossible to set precisely the earliest limit for neonatal survival, certain factors inevitably have an impact on the clinical decision-making process.

For example, the obstetrical perception of viability probably influences survival of extremely-low-birthweight infants. Goldenberg and colleagues (1982) surveyed physicians in Alabama in 1978 concerning their perceptions of survival for infants weighing 1500 g or less or who were at less than 32 weeks, and they found that the physicians tended to underestimate the potential for

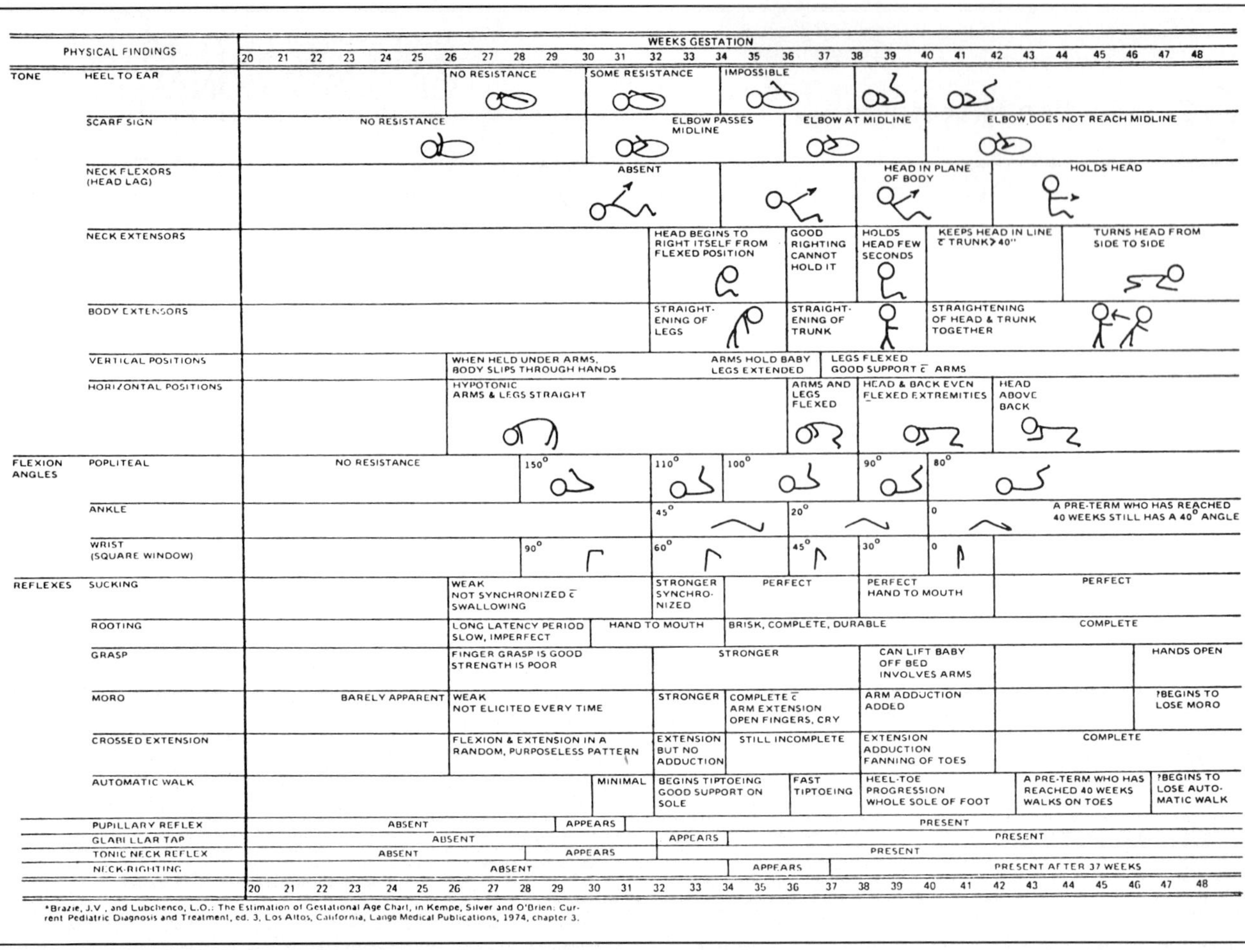

PHYSICAL FINDINGS		WEEKS GESTATION 20 21 22 23 24 25 26 27 28 29 30 31 32 33 34 35 36 37 38 39 40 41 42 43 44 45 46 47 48
TONE	HEEL TO EAR	NO RESISTANCE / SOME RESISTANCE / IMPOSSIBLE
	SCARF SIGN	NO RESISTANCE / ELBOW PASSES MIDLINE / ELBOW AT MIDLINE / ELBOW DOES NOT REACH MIDLINE
	NECK FLEXORS (HEAD LAG)	ABSENT / HEAD IN PLANE OF BODY / HOLDS HEAD
	NECK EXTENSORS	HEAD BEGINS TO RIGHT ITSELF FROM FLEXED POSITION / GOOD RIGHTING CANNOT HOLD IT / HOLDS HEAD FEW SECONDS / KEEPS HEAD IN LINE c̄ TRUNK > 40" / TURNS HEAD FROM SIDE TO SIDE
	BODY EXTENSORS	STRAIGHTENING OF LEGS / STRAIGHTENING OF TRUNK / STRAIGHTENING OF HEAD & TRUNK TOGETHER
	VERTICAL POSITIONS	WHEN HELD UNDER ARMS, BODY SLIPS THROUGH HANDS / ARMS HOLD BABY LEGS EXTENDED / LEGS FLEXED GOOD SUPPORT c̄ ARMS
	HORIZONTAL POSITIONS	HYPOTONIC ARMS & LEGS STRAIGHT / ARMS AND LEGS FLEXED / HEAD & BACK EVEN FLEXED EXTREMITIES / HEAD ABOVE BACK
FLEXION ANGLES	POPLITEAL	NO RESISTANCE / 150° / 110° / 100° / 90° / 80°
	ANKLE	45° / 20° / 0 / A PRE-TERM WHO HAS REACHED 40 WEEKS STILL HAS A 40° ANGLE
	WRIST (SQUARE WINDOW)	90° / 60° / 45° / 30° / 0
REFLEXES	SUCKING	WEAK NOT SYNCHRONIZED c̄ SWALLOWING / STRONGER SYNCHRONIZED / PERFECT / PERFECT HAND TO MOUTH / PERFECT
	ROOTING	LONG LATENCY PERIOD SLOW, IMPERFECT / HAND TO MOUTH / BRISK, COMPLETE, DURABLE / COMPLETE
	GRASP	FINGER GRASP IS GOOD STRENGTH IS POOR / STRONGER / CAN LIFT BABY OFF BED INVOLVES ARMS / HANDS OPEN
	MORO	BARELY APPARENT / WEAK NOT ELICITED EVERY TIME / STRONGER / COMPLETE c̄ ARM EXTENSION OPEN FINGERS, CRY / ARM ADDUCTION ADDED / ?BEGINS TO LOSE MORO
	CROSSED EXTENSION	FLEXION & EXTENSION IN A RANDOM, PURPOSELESS PATTERN / EXTENSION BUT NO ADDUCTION / STILL INCOMPLETE / EXTENSION ADDUCTION FANNING OF TOES / COMPLETE
	AUTOMATIC WALK	MINIMAL / BEGINS TIPTOEING GOOD SUPPORT ON SOLE / FAST TIPTOEING / HEEL-TOE PROGRESSION WHOLE SOLE OF FOOT / A PRE-TERM WHO HAS REACHED 40 WEEKS WALKS ON TOES / ?BEGINS TO LOSE AUTOMATIC WALK
	PUPILLARY REFLEX	ABSENT / APPEARS / PRESENT
	GLABELLAR TAP	ABSENT / APPEARS / PRESENT
	TONIC NECK REFLEX	ABSENT / APPEARS / PRESENT
	NECK-RIGHTING	ABSENT / APPEARS / PRESENT AFTER 37 WEEKS

*Brazie, J.V., and Lubchenco, L.O.: The Estimation of Gestational Age Chart, in Kempe, Silver and O'Brien: Current Pediatric Diagnosis and Treatment; ed. 3, Los Altos, California, Lange Medical Publications, 1974, chapter 3.

Fig. 38–4. B. Neurological examination to assess gestational age done after 24 hours. (From Brazle and Lubchenco, 1974, with permission.)

survival. Importantly, these estimations correlated with their management decisions. More recently, Amon and co-authors (1992) surveyed American obstetricians to determine their clinical opinions regarding intrapartum management of the severely preterm fetus requiring delivery. Intrapartum fetal heart rate monitoring was initiated at 23, 24, and 25 weeks by 10, 45, and 65 percent of respondents, respectively. Cesarean section was not performed at less than 24 weeks or less than 500 g fetal

weight. Ninety percent of respondents were willing to perform cesarean section for fetal distress or breech presentation at 26 weeks or 750 g fetal weight. Delivery management prior to 26 weeks or for fetuses smaller than 750 g was variable and individualized.

It is important to emphasize that the obstetrical decision not to perform cesarean section or use intrapartum electronic fetal monitoring does not necessarily imply that the fetus is "non-viable" or "written-off." For example, Kitchen and co-workers (1992) analyzed the outcomes of live births weighing 500 to 999 g and found that although 50 percent of the infants survived and only 7 percent were severely disabled, these outcomes were unrelated to the use of cesarean section or electronic monitoring.

Perceptions of the potential for survival are inevitably confused by difficulties incurred by imprecisely known gestational age, as discussed previously. Most survival data are based upon birthweight rather than fetal age, and individual birthweights vary appreciably between 24 and 26 weeks. For example, infants born between 24 and 26 weeks can vary in weight from 420 to 1320 g (Brenner and colleagues 1976).

TABLE 38–1. MORTALITY AND COST OF MEDICAL CARE FOR 247 INFANTS WEIGHING 500 TO 999 G AND DELIVERED BETWEEN 1977 AND 1981 IN PROVIDENCE, RHODE ISLAND

Birthweight (g)	Number of Infants	Mortality (%)	Cost of Care per Survivor
500–599	15	100	No survivors
600–699	38	97	$363,000
700–799	79	76	$116,000
800–899	50	62	$101,000
900–999	65	40	$ 41,000
Total	**247**	**68**	

From Walker and associates (1984), with permission.

The birthweight-linked survival rates for live births during 7 months of 1991 at Parkland Hospital are shown in Table 38–2. Chances for survival increase appreciably at or above 1000 g birthweight, whereas this likelihood decreases substantially for those weighing less. These data are consistent with the view that survival is possible for infants weighing 500 to 750 g. However, many of these extremely-low-birthweight infants were growth retarded and therefore of more advanced maturity. For example, the smallest survivor at Parkland Hospital, up to the present, weighed 520 g but was 28 weeks in chronological age (Fig. 38–5). Survival of a 380-g infant has been reported, but the gestational age was confirmed to be 25 3/7 weeks or considerably more advanced than predicted by birthweight (Ginsberg and associates, 1990). Clearly, expectations for neonatal survival are influenced by gestational age and maturity rather than simply by birthweight.

The frontier for infant survival has been progressively pushed earlier into gestation such that the current birthweight range that poses the greatest dilemma for both obstetrician and pediatrician is 500 to 800 g. For example, Kitchen and colleagues (1991) reported from Melbourne, Australia, on 149 live infants delivered between 24 and 29 weeks with follow-up to 8 years of age. Survival prospects increased progressively from 10 percent at 24 weeks to 90 percent at 29 weeks. Only 41 infants of 24 to 26 weeks' gestational age at birth were evaluated, but the prospects of a survivor at 8 years having a severe disability was reported to be zero!

Escobar and colleagues (1991) reviewed 1136 English language references in an attempt to determine the current prognosis for infants weighing less than 1500 g. They were interested not only in survival, but also in serious impairments. Escobar (1992) subsequently summarized this review:

What can we tell the parents of a very low-birthweight (< 1500 g) infant about their child's prognosis? One thing is certain: chances are the

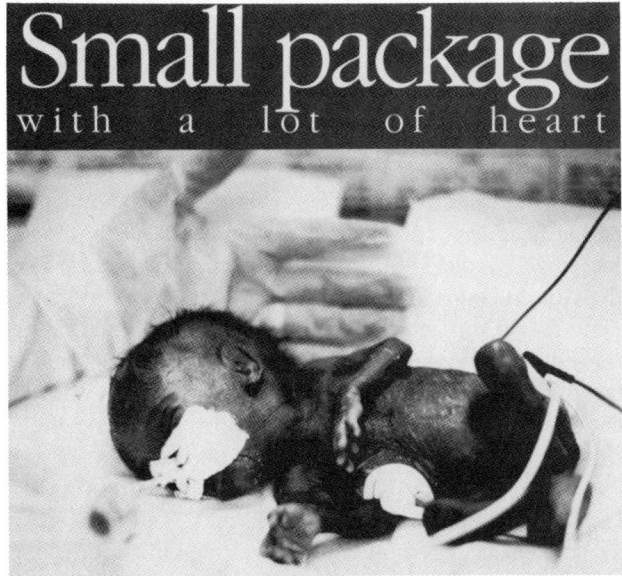

Fig. 38–5. Photograph from Parkland Hospital's bimonthly publication, *Highlights,* showing the smallest infant to survive at this institution. The severely growth-retarded infant weighed 520 g when delivered at 28 weeks' gestation because of severe maternal hypertension.

child will be discharged from the hospital alive. Of this the statistics leave no doubt: 74 percent of babies weighing less than 1500 g at birth survive to hospital discharge. But that does not dispel the darkness, for the question can be put differently: Will the child be handicapped? Will the child have cerebral palsy? Answers to these questions are less certain.

We turn to the literature, to multiple outcome studies describing the fate of these immature infants that have survived. When one first confronts such studies, one has the impression that definite answers are given: so and so says X percent of babies under 1500 g are entirely normal. If one looks a little harder, this impression is replaced by one of confusion: there seems to be so many of these studies, reporting all sorts of numbers, that no answer seems possible at all.... Nonetheless, ... certain inferences can be made. The most solid of these concerns is cerebral palsy. The median cerebral palsy rate among the ... studies ... was 7.7 percent which is 38 times the frequency in the general population (about 2 per 1000 livebirths). The median disability rate (eg. blindness, deafness, sudden infant death) ... was about 25 percent for infants followed to at least one year of age.... Hazy outlines with respect to certain outcomes begin to be described, but we remain largely in the dark and ... one cannot predict the fate of an individual baby.

During the past 20 years, a great variety of innovations in obstetrical care have been employed in attempts to prevent preterm birth. Throughout these two decades, expectations for neonatal outcome have improved progressively with increased availability and

TABLE 38–2. SURVIVAL RATES BY BIRTHWEIGHT FOR 23,774 INFANTS BORN FROM JANUARY 1, 1991 THROUGH JULY 31, 1992 AT PARKLAND HOSPITAL

Birthweight (g)	Number of Live Births	Number of Neonatal Deaths	Percent Survival
500–750	47	27	43
751–1000	93	26	72
1001–1250	93	3	96.8
1251–1500	135	8	94.1
1051–1750	189	9	95.2
1751–2000	326	11	96.6
2001–2500	1329	7	99.5
2501–3000	4854	11	99.8
3001–3500	9150	12	99.9
3501–4000	5738	3	99.9
>4000	1820	0	100
Total	**23,774**	**117**	**99.5**

continued innovation in neonatal care. Not only has the frontier for neonatal survival been pushed earlier into pregnancy, as already mentioned, but survival of larger preterm infants has become as good as that for term infants. Is there a birthweight or gestational age threshold after which attempts to delay delivery are unwarranted? In an effort to address this question, Robertson and colleagues (1992) analyzed neonatal outcomes between 1983 and 1986 from five tertiary care centers in the United States. A total of 20,680 carefully dated pregnancies without complications such as diabetes or hypertension were identified. Most thresholds—defined as the gestational week at which the incidence of complications attributable to preterm delivery became indistinguishable from term infants—were between 32 and 34 weeks. Respiratory distress syndrome, although decreasing precipitously between 33 and 34 weeks (31 to 13 percent, respectively) still developed in about 6 percent of births between 35 and 38 weeks. DePalma and co-workers (1992) found that the birthweight threshold for neonatal mortality was 1600 g and the threshold for neonatal morbidity due to complications of prematurity was approximately 1900 g. They concluded that aggressive obstetrical attempts to prevent preterm births for infants whose weights exceed 1900 g offer few apparent potential benefits.

Causes of Preterm Labor

In the majority of instances, the precise cause or causes of labor before term are not known. Listed below are some conditions that predispose to preterm labor and delivery:

1. **Spontaneous rupture of membranes.** Spontaneous labor remote from term is commonly preceded by spontaneous rupture of the membranes. Seldom is the cause of membrane rupture known, but local infection has been implicated in recent years.
2. **Amnionic fluid infection.** Although its exact incidence in the genesis of preterm labor is not known, there is mounting evidence that perhaps one third of the cases of preterm delivery are associated with chorioamnionic membrane infection. These cases are linked with preterm rupture of membranes as well as with idiopathic preterm labor.
3. **Anomalies of conception.** Malformations of the fetus or of the placenta not only predispose to fetal growth retardation but increase the likelihood of preterm labor as well.
4. **Previous preterm delivery or late abortion.** The woman who previously gave birth remote from term is more likely to do so again, even when no other predisposing factor is identified.
5. **Overdistended uterus.** Hydramnios, espe-

cially when acute and marked, or the presence of two or more fetuses, increases the risk of preterm labor, presumably as the consequence of uterine overdistension.
6. **Fetal death.** Death of a fetus remote from term is commonly, but not always, followed by spontaneous preterm labor.
7. **Cervical incompetency.** In a small percentage of women remote from term, an incompetent cervix effaces and dilates not as the result of increased uterine activity, but rather because of an intrinsic cervical weakness.
8. **Uterine anomalies.** Very uncommonly, anomalies of the uterus are identified in cases of preterm labor and delivery.
9. **Faulty placentation.** Abruptio placentae and placenta previa are more likely to be associated with preterm labor.
10. **Retained intrauterine device.** The likelihood of a preterm labor is increased appreciably when pregnancy and an intrauterine device coexist.
11. **Serious maternal disease.** Systemic disease in the mother, when it is severe, may cause preterm labor and delivery.
12. **Elective labor induction.** Incorrect estimation of gestational age can create undue concern over presumed prolonged gestation, or it can lead to considerable patient pressure for intervention. Induction of labor in some instances has been performed primarily for convenience, but the use of oxytocin specifically for **elective** induction has been disapproved by the Food and Drug Administration.
13. **Unknown causes.** Unfortunately, too many cases have to be so categorized.

Arias and Tomich (1982), in their study of 355 live-born infants weighing between 600 and 2500 g, reported the following causes of preterm birth: prematurely ruptured membranes (35 percent), preterm labor (30 percent), and other maternal fetal complications (35 percent). The latter included multifetal pregnancy, hypertensive disorders, congenital malformations, placental abruption, and placenta previa. Thus, approximately two thirds of preterm births are the result of either idiopathic preterm labor or preterm rupture of membranes. Leveno and associates (1985a) described a similar distribution of causes for preterm births before 34 weeks at Parkland Hospital. Savitz and co-authors (1991) reviewed the etiologies of preterm delivery.

Amnionic Fluid Infection

Chorioamnionic infection caused by a variety of microorganisms has emerged as a possible explanation for many heretofore unexplained cases of ruptured membranes and/or preterm labor. Although group B streptococcal cervical infection was associated with prematurity more than 25 years ago, there was renewed interest when Bobbitt and Ledger (1977) implicated subclinical amnionic fluid infection as a cause of preterm labor. The list of putative microorganisms has become extensive (Hillier and associates, 1988). The possibilities include many of the organisms that commonly comprise normal cervicovaginal flora, such as aerobic and anaerobic bacteria, mycoplasmas, chlamydia, and yeast. This extensive list is consistent with the view that a common mechanism may exist. Schwarz and co-workers (1976) suggested that term labor is initiated by activation of phospholipase A_2, which cleaves arachidonic acid from within fetal membranes, thereby making free arachidonic acid available for prostaglandin synthesis. Subsequently, Bejar and colleagues (1981) reported that many microorganisms produce phospholipase A_2, and thus, potentially at least, may initiate preterm labor. Bennett and Elder (1992) have shown that the common genital tract bacteria do not themselves produce the prostaglandins. Cox and associates (1989) provided data that are consistent with the view that bacterial endotoxin (lipopolysaccharide) in amnionic fluid stimulates decidual cells to produce cytokines and prostaglandins that may initiate labor. Romero and co-workers (1987, 1988) and Cox and associates (1988a) reported that endotoxin was present in the amnionic fluid when tested using the *Limulus* amebocyte assay.

It has now been established that endogenous host products secreted in response to infection are responsible for many of the effects of infection. In endotoxin shock, for example, bacterial endotoxins exert their deleterious effect through the release of endogenous indicators of the inflammatory response. Similarly, preterm parturition due to infection may be signaled by secretory products of macrophage activation. Cytokines, to include interleukin-1, tumor necrosis factor (cachectin), and interleukin-6, are such secretory products implicated in preterm labor (Gibbs and co-authors, 1992). However, the discovery of these secretory products of inflammation during preterm parturition has not eliminated the possibility that their presence is nothing more than a *result* of preterm labor rather than a *cause*. The role of interleukin-1 in disease has been reviewed by Dinarello and Wolff (1993).

Preterm Labor with Ruptured Membranes. An intense inflammatory reaction at the site of prematurely ruptured membranes was noted as early as 1950, and this suggested infection. More recently, McGregor and colleagues (1987) demonstrated that in vitro exposure to bacterial proteases reduced the bursting load of fetal membranes. Thus, microorganisms given access to fetal membranes may be capable of causing membrane rupture, preterm labor, or both.

The renewed interest in a possible microbial pathogenesis of preterm labor has prompted many investigators to evaluate amniocentesis for management of women with preterm labor or prematurely ruptured membranes. Garite and colleagues (1979) successfully performed sonar-directed amniocentesis in 30 of 59 women with ruptured membranes between 28 and 35 weeks. As none had clinical infection, their purpose was to establish fetal lung maturity while evaluating Gram stain and culture of amnionic fluid. Surprisingly, the fluids from 9 women (30 percent) contained bacteria; 6 of these women developed chorioamnionitis, and 2 neonates developed infection. The authors suggested that this approach might be reasonable when management choices included a substantial delay in delivery.

Several authors now have reported that bacteria, but not leukocytes, seen on stained amnionic fluid reliably correlate with infection. Moreover, mature lecithin–sphingomyelin ratios were found by Cotton and associates (1984a) in 62 percent of cases. Amniocentesis seems quite safe, although Broekhuizen and co-workers (1985) reported 1 case of heavy vaginal bleeding in 79 attempts. More recently, Gonik and colleagues (1985) reported that oligohydramnios identified by ultrasound was linked to antepartum clinical chorioamnionitis. Vintzileos and colleagues (1986) reported a similar association between oligohydramnios and bacterial colonization of amnionic fluid collected at amniocentesis. Vintzileos and colleagues (1985) also reported that fetal infection could be predicted reliably using daily biophysical profiles (see Chap. 45, p. 1039), but this observation was not confirmed by Miller and associates (1990) nor by Gauthier and co-workers (1992). Ohlsson and Wang (1990) reviewed antenatal tests to detect infection in preterm membrane rupture.

Despite these reports, it has not been shown that amniocentesis in the management of preterm rupture of the membranes is associated with improved pregnancy outcomes. For example, Feinstein and colleagues (1986) compared 73 cases of preterm ruptured membranes managed with the aid of amniocentesis with 73 matched historical controls. There were no differences in fetal condition at delivery, incidence of neonatal infection, or perinatal mortality.

Preterm Labor with Intact Membranes. In 8 of 31 pregnancies (25 percent) with preterm labor and intact membranes, amnionic fluid bacterial colonization was identified without clinical evidence of infection (Bobbitt and colleagues, 1981). Women from whom bacteria were identified almost always delivered within 48 hours despite tocolysis, in contrast to those with sterile amnionic fluids. Others since have confirmed "silent amnionitis" in some cases of preterm labor and have suggested that amniocentesis might be useful. Leigh and Garite (1986) observed that women with membrane rupture following amniocentesis were encountered only when amnionic fluid was colonized, and they suggested a bacterial pathogenesis for membrane rupture following the onset of preterm labor. As previously discussed, the efficacy of the routine use of amniocentesis in preterm labor has not been established.

Other approaches to defining a role for microorganisms include studies of the vaginal flora during pregnancy. Colonization versus *possible* infection with *Trichomonas vaginalis, Bacteroides* species (Minkoff and associates, 1984), *Chlamydia trachomatis* (Alger and associates, 1988; Gravett and co-workers, 1986), and mycoplasma (McCormack and colleagues, 1987) have been implicated by some as causes of preterm birth or low-birthweight infants.

Antimicrobial Therapy.

These observations on the bacterial pathogenesis of preterm delivery have led some to give antimicrobial treatment. McCormack and colleagues (1987) reported that erythromycin given after midpregnancy prevented most low-birthweight deliveries in mycoplasma-colonized women. The Infections and Prematurity Study Group (Eschenbach and associates, 1988) subsequently presented data that erythromycin given beginning at 23 to 26 weeks and continued until 36 weeks had no impact on pregnancy outcome in women colonized with *Ureaplasma urealyticum*. McGregor and associates (1988) reported that a 1-week course of erythromycin therapy given at 26 to 29 weeks to 200 women at high risk for preterm birth showed a trend to greater birthweight and gestational age, as well as reduced preterm ruptured membranes and preterm birth.

Gibbs and co-authors (1992) concluded that current antimicrobial trials allow no definite conclusion as to the efficacy of antimicrobials in prolonging pregnancy with either preterm labor or preterm ruptured membranes. Results of a recently completed randomized investigation of antimicrobial therapy versus placebo during expectant management of preterm ruptured membranes and performed at Parkland Hospital (Christmas and associates, 1992) indicated that such treatment did not significantly improve infant outcome.

Preterm Rupture of Membranes

Rupture of the membranes remote from term is better referred to as *preterm rupture of the membranes* rather than *premature rupture of the membranes*. Premature rupture of the membranes has been applied most commonly to rupture of the membranes at any time before the onset of labor irrespective of whether the duration of gestation at the time of rupture was 24 weeks or 44 weeks.

Preterm rupture of the membranes is defined as rupture of the membranes before 38 weeks' gestation and is an important cause of maternal and perinatal morbidity and mortality. Most often, rupture is sponta-

neous and for unknown reasons. Techniques for identification of rupture of the membranes are discussed in Chapter 14 (p. 373).

Natural History of Preterm Membrane Rupture.

Cox and associates (1988b) described the pregnancy outcomes of 298 consecutive women delivered following spontaneously ruptured membranes between 24 and 34 weeks. Although this complication was identified in only 1.7 percent of pregnancies, it contributed to 20 percent of all perinatal deaths during that time period.

Preterm membrane rupture was found to be associated with other obstetrical complications that affect perinatal outcome, including multifetal gestation, breech presentation, chorioamnionitis, and intrapartum fetal distress. As a consequence of these complications, cesarean sections were done in nearly 40 percent of the women. The most striking finding was the apparent inevitability of labor within a short time following membrane rupture. At admission, 75 percent of the women were already in labor, 5 percent were delivered for other complications, and another 10 percent were delivered following spontaneous labor within 48 hours. In only 7 percent was delivery delayed 48 hours or more after membrane rupture. This latter subgroup, however, appeared to benefit from delayed delivery, because no neonatal deaths occurred. This was in contrast to a neonatal death rate of 80 per 1000 in infants delivered within 48 hours of membrane rupture.

Unfortunately, perinatal outcome in surviving infants in whom labor is delayed is not always satisfactory (Moretti and Sibai, 1988). In a previous study from Parkland Hospital, Hankins and associates (1984) reported that 30 percent of 176 such infants required ventilator therapy. Overall, 13 percent died in the neonatal period and another 3 percent died before age 1. Care of these infants born preterm required over 5100 newborn hospital days (almost 14 years) and cost $2.3 million just for bed space. Importantly, follow-up to 4 years of age was carried out for 105 of these infants, and neurological abnormalities of varying degrees were found in 17. Based upon these experiences, it seems that of infants born to women with preterm ruptured membranes, and in whom labor was delayed, at least 30 percent either died or were neurologically damaged.

Management.

Attempts to avoid delivery when there is preterm ruptured membranes are of two primary forms: (1) nonintervention or *expectant management*, in which nothing is done and spontaneous labor is simply awaited; or (2) intervention that may include corticosteroids, given with or without tocolytic agents to arrest preterm labor in order that the corticosteroids have sufficient time to induce pulmonary maturation. Simple expectant management, apparently practiced widely in the 1950s, was again adopted during the 1970s, and most obstetricians today elect such management. Capeless and Mead (1987) conducted a national survey of management practices for preterm ruptured membranes and reported that 97 percent of respondents recommended expectant management. There was no consensus regarding use of corticosteroids for inducing lung maturation or tocolytics to forestall labor.

Despite an extensive literature concerning the management of preterm ruptured membranes, few prospective randomized studies have been performed. An exception is the study by Garite and colleagues (1981), who studied 160 pregnancies with preterm ruptured membranes between 28 and 34 weeks. The women were divided into two groups: (1) expectant management only or (2) corticosteroids plus tocolysis with either intravenous ethanol or magnesium sulfate. The authors concluded that active interventions did not improve perinatal outcomes and may have aggravated certain infection-related complications, such as maternal pelvic infections. Subsequent randomized studies by Garite and associates (1987) and Nelson and colleagues (1985) failed to show benefits for tocolysis, either with or without steroid therapy. Morales and co-workers (1989) studied 165 pregnancies with preterm ruptured membranes and lecithin:sphingomyelin ratios less than two. These were randomized to four treatment groups that included (1) expectant management only, (2) corticosteroids for fetal lung maturation, (3) ampicillin only, and (4) ampicillin plus corticosteroids. They concluded that ampicillin plus corticosteroids were beneficial because of less respiratory disease. However, neonatal survival was not ultimately affected by any intervention, nor was the length of gestation.

Thus, current data are consistent with a view that favors hospitalization with simple expectant management that includes close observation for evidence of maternal or fetal infection. At Parkland Hospital, pregnancy complicated by preterm rupture of the membranes is managed as follows:

1. One sterile speculum examination is performed to identify fluid coming from the cervix or pooled in the vagina. Demonstration of visible fluid or a positive Nitrazine test is indicative of ruptured membranes. Attempts are made to visualize the extent of cervical effacement and dilatation, but a digital examination is not performed. A cervicovaginal specimen is taken and culture sent for *Neisseria gonorrhoeae.*

2. Ultrasound examination is performed to help confirm gestational age, identify the presenting part, and assess amnionic fluid volume.

3. If the gestational age is 33 completed weeks or less and there are no other maternal or fetal indications for delivery, the woman is observed closely in Labor and Delivery, with continuous fetal heart rate monitoring to look for evidence

for cord compression, especially if labor supervenes.

4. If there is no evidence of fetal jeopardy, or if labor does not begin, the woman is transferred to the High-Risk Pregnancy Unit for close observation for signs of labor, infection, or fetal jeopardy. If gonococcal infection is identified by the culture taken at admission, then treatment is given.

5. If the gestational age is greater than 33 completed weeks and if labor has not begun spontaneously in 12 hours, a time period that provides for adequate evaluation, labor is carefully induced with an intravenous infusion of dilute oxytocin, avoiding hyperstimulation. A breech presentation or transverse lie are contraindications for induction. If induction fails, cesarean section is performed. At this and many other institutions, neonatal mortality is now very low for infants born after 33 weeks.

6. Labor and delivery are managed so as to minimize maternal hypotension and fetal hypoxia and acidosis, as well as infection, because these events are suspected to increase the likelihood of respiratory distress.

Overt Chorioamnionitis. Assuming that no untoward perinatal outcome results from an entangled or prolapsed cord or perhaps from placental abruption associated with oligohydramnios (Vintzileos and associates, 1987), the greatest concern of prolonged membrane rupture is for maternal and fetal infection. If chorioamnionitis is diagnosed, prompt efforts to effect delivery, preferably vaginally, are initiated. Unfortunately, fever is the only reliable indicator for making this diagnosis; a temperature of 38°C or higher accompanying ruptured membranes implies infection. Leukocytosis by itself has been found to be unreliable, at least by most investigators, and this has also been our experience.

With chorioamnionitis, fetal and neonatal morbidity are substantively increased. In a prospective study of nearly 700 women between 26 and 34 weeks with preterm ruptured membranes, Morales (1987) reported that 13 percent developed chorioamnionitis diagnosed by oral temperatures of 38°C and no other cause for fever. Infants born to women with chorioamnionitis had a fourfold increased neonatal mortality and a threefold increase in the incidence of respiratory distress, neonatal sepsis, and intraventricular hemorrhage.

Accelerated Maturation of Pulmonary Function

The infant who is born long before term is a candidate for the development of severe idiopathic *respiratory distress syndrome* (Chap. 44, p. 991). The intense hypoxia and acidosis that ensue as the consequence of inadequate alveolar–capillary exchange of oxygen and carbon dioxide may prove fatal. Moreover, some infants who survive severe respiratory distress may suffer lifelong physical or functional impairment. Because a major factor in the development of the respiratory distress syndrome is inadequate production of pulmonary surfactant, intense interest persists concerning those phenomena involved in surfactant production (Chap. 7, p. 186).

A variety of clinical events, some well defined and others not, have been proposed to accelerate maturation of surfactant production sufficient to protect against the development of respiratory distress. Gluck (1979) emphasized that surfactant production is likely to be accelerated remote from term in pregnancies complicated by the following conditions or stresses:

1. *Maternal*: Chronic renal or cardiovascular disease, long-standing pregnancy-induced hypertension, sickle cell disease, heroin addiction, or hyperthyroidism.
2. *Placenta and membranes*: Placental infarction, chronic focal retroplacental hemorrhage, chorioamnionitis, or ruptured membranes.
3. *Fetal*: The anemic member of parabiotic twins or the smaller member of nonparabiotic twins.

In contrast, Owen and associates (1990a) concluded that a "stressed" pregnancy (primarily pregnancy-associated hypertensive disease) conferred a negligible survival advantage to the fetus.

Glucocorticoid Therapy. The observations by Liggins and Howie of the effects of glucocorticoids on lung maturation have received considerable attention (Howie and Liggins, 1977; Liggins and Howie, 1974). On the basis of their previous observations that corticosteroids administered to the ewe accelerated lung maturation in the preterm fetus, they performed a well-designed study to evaluate the effects of maternally administered betamethasone to prevent respiratory distress in the subsequently delivered preterm infant. Infants born before 34 weeks had a significantly lowered incidence of respiratory distress and neonatal mortality from hyaline membrane disease if birth was delayed for at least 24 hours after completion of 24 hours of corticosteroids given to the mother and up to 7 days after completion of steroid therapy.

The mechanism by which betamethasone or other corticosteroids reduces the frequency of respiratory distress is not clear. Interestingly, the protective action likely is transient. Liggins and Howie (1974) noted that the frequency of respiratory distress increased when the infant was born more than 7 days after treatment with betamethasone, compared with that for infants delivered 1 to 7 days after completion of therapy. Moreover, Brown and associates (1979) observed in chronically catheterized fetal lambs that the increase in surfactant

that followed dexamethasone administration was transient, with surfactant levels falling to pretreatment values within 8 to 10 days. Therefore, if such compounds are used, retreatment may be considered whenever delivery has not occurred within 7 days of the initial treatment and the risk of early delivery persists.

Not all workers have reported salutary effects from corticosteroid administration. Quirk and co-workers (1979) identified no difference in fetal outcomes with and without the use of betamethasone. The incidence of respiratory distress (about 15 percent) and survival (about 87 percent) was similar in both groups of infants whose mothers were or were not given betamethasone. Subsequently, Simpson and Harbert (1985) reported that respiratory distress was significantly more frequent following the use of glucocorticoids in women with preterm ruptured membranes if the fetus was delivered after 48 hours.

Collaborative Study on Antenatal Steroid Therapy. A trial of corticosteroid therapy, funded by the National Institutes of Health, was initiated in 1976, and the results published in 1981. This double-blind collaborative trial was conducted at five centers, and of nearly 8000 women identified to be in preterm labor, 696 women at risk for preterm birth between 26 and 37 weeks were entered. Women randomized to steroid therapy were given intramuscular dexamethasone, 5 mg every 12 hours for a total of up to four doses. A total of 720 infants were available for analysis. A smaller number of infants, but significantly fewer, whose mothers were given dexamethasone, developed respiratory distress (13 versus 18 percent). Importantly, more than 80 percent in each study group did not develop respiratory distress. Neonatal mortality was not reduced by such corticosteroid treatment. Similar results were obtained from a multicenter randomized trial of betamethasone performed in the United Kingdom between 1975 and 1978 (Gamsu and colleagues, 1989).

In September 1985 a workshop on approaches for preventing neonatal respiratory distress was held in Washington, D.C., to review the results of the Collaborative Study (Avery and colleagues, 1986). The group agreed that no difference in terms of cognitive, motor, or neurological function were found when 406 of the study infants were followed to 36 months of age, suggesting that steroid treatment did not adversely effect the subsequent short-term neurological development (Collaborative Group, 1984). They further concluded that dexamethasone appeared beneficial only to a female fetus of more than 30 weeks' gestation and when the treatment to delivery interval exceeded 24 hours. Such therapy was not helpful in multiple gestations.

Other Studies of Corticosteroid Therapy. Garite and co-workers (1992) specifically studied the effects of betamethasone for the prevention of respiratory distress at 24 to 28 weeks with intact membranes. They were unable to demonstrate any beneficial effect. One benefit cited by others for corticosteroid treatment is a reduction in the incidence of bronchopulmonary dysplasia in preterm infants. Van Marter and colleagues (1990) retrospectively compared 72 preterm infants whose mother had received corticosteroids to 151 similar but untreated women and concluded that maternal therapy protected very low-birthweight infants from bronchopulmonary dysplasia. In contrast, Cummings and co-workers (1989) administered dexamethasone to the preterm infant rather than the mother in a randomized, double-blind, placebo-controlled trial. Dexamethasone therapy for 42 days improved pulmonary outcome. Similar results were obtained in a multicenter British study of dexamethasone therapy for chronic neonatal oxygen dependence (Collaborative Dexamethasone Trial Group, 1991). Thus it is apparent that there still are many unresolved issues regarding the efficacy of antenatal steroid treatment for the prevention of respiratory disease.

Other Treatment. Other strategies have been recently employed in efforts to reduce respiratory disease in premature infants. For example, **thyrotropin-releasing hormone** has been given to the mother in conjunction with corticosteroids (Ballard and co-workers, 1992). Such therapy was reported to reduce the incidence of bronchopulmonary dysplasia, although the mechanism for this result is uncertain. Finally, based on the observation that **inositol** is a component of membrane phospholipid involved with pulmonary surfactant, Hallman and associates (1992) provided inositol supplementation to preterm infants with respiratory distress. They observed less mortality, less severe respiratory disease, less bronchopulmonary dysplasia, and less retinopathy of prematurity when inositol supplementation was used.

Summary of Corticosteroid Use. Opinion as to the efficacy of glucocorticoid prophylaxis remains sharply divided in major perinatal centers. It is probably true that corticosteroids to enhance fetal lung function are avoided by most for preterm ruptured membranes and used in many but not all perinatal centers for preterm labor in the presence of intact fetal membranes. For all of these reasons, and especially because of their questionable benefits, at Parkland Hospital glucocorticoids have not been employed in women remote from term to try to reduce the risk of respiratory distress.

Identification of Women at Risk for Preterm Birth

Obstetrical approaches to preterm birth have traditionally been focused primarily on treatment interventions rather than earlier identification of women at risk. Papiernik and Kaminski (1974) and Creasy and associates (1980), however, have emphasized the potential importance of early risk identification, because many treatment interventions fail once labor firmly is established.

Risk-scoring Systems. A risk-scoring system devised by Papiernik and modified by Creasy and colleagues (1980) has been tested in several regions of the United States. In this system, scores of 1 through 10 are given to a variety of pregnancy factors, including socioeconomic status, reproductive history, daily habits, and current pregnancy complications. Women with scores of 10 or more are considered to be at high risk for preterm delivery. Although Creasy and associates (1980) and Covington and co-workers (1988) reported salutary results, the experiences of Main and colleagues (1989) in Philadelphia using this scoring system with indigent women was less satisfactory. Similar disappointing results in indigent women were obtained by Mueller-Heubach and Guzick (1989) and Owen and associates (1990b). Application of this scoring system to a wider population that included the north coast of California did not reduce the incidence of spontaneous preterm delivery (Konte and colleagues, 1988).

Although these scoring systems appear to have been unsuccessful in identifying pregnancies at risk for preterm labor, certain features included in the systems may be more useful than others in predicting the risk of preterm delivery and therefore warrant closer examination.

Prior Preterm Birth. A history of prior preterm delivery strongly correlates with subsequent preterm labor. Shown in Table 38–3 is the incidence of recurrent spontaneous preterm birth in over 6000 Scottish women. The risk of recurrent preterm delivery for those whose first delivery was preterm increased threefold compared with women whose first infant reached term. Strikingly, almost one third of women whose first two infants were preterm delivered preterm infants during their third pregnancies.

Cervical Dilatation. Asymptomatic cervical dilatation after midpregnancy has recently gained renewed atten-

TABLE 38–3. RECURRENT SPONTANEOUS PRETERM BIRTH ACCORDING TO PRIOR OUTCOME IN 6072 SCOTTISH WOMEN

First Birth	Second Birth	Next Birth Preterm (%)
Term	—	5
Preterm	—	15
Term	Preterm	24
Preterm	Preterm	32

From Carr-Hill and Hall (1985), with permission.

tion as a risk factor for preterm delivery. Some have considered such dilatation to be a normal anatomical variant, particularly in parous women; however, this no longer is universally accepted (Leveno, 1986a; Neilson, 1988; Papiernik, 1986; Stubbs, 1986; and their co-workers). Shown in Table 38–4 are the results of routine cervical examinations performed between 26 and 30 weeks in 185 women cared for at Parkland Hospital. Approximately one fourth of the women whose cervices were dilated 2 or 3 cm delivered prior to 34 weeks, either from unexplained labor or from labor that followed preterm rupture of membranes. Many of these women had experienced the same complication in earlier pregnancies. Similarly, Papiernik and colleagues (1986), in a study of cervical status before 37 weeks in 4430 women, found that precocious cervical dilatation increased the risk of preterm birth. Stubbs and colleagues (1986) performed cervical examinations in 191 women between 28 and 34 weeks and found that those with dilatation of 1 cm or more or effacement of more than 30 percent were at increased risk for preterm delivery.

Signs and Symptoms. In addition to painful or painless uterine contractions, symptoms such as pelvic pressure, menstrual-like cramps, watery or bloody vaginal discharge, and pain in the low back have been empirically associated with impending preterm birth. Such symptoms are thought by some to be common in normal pregnancy, and are therefore often dismissed by patients, physicians, and nurses. The importance of these signs and symptoms has been emphasized by several groups of investigators (Iams and associates, 1990; Katz and associates, 1990; Kragt and Keirse, 1990). Conversely, Cooper and colleagues (1990) did not find these signs and symptoms to be meaningful in the prediction of preterm delivery.

Fetal Fibronectin. Fibronectin is a polypeptide substance produced by a variety of cell types including hepatocytes, fibroblasts, endothelial cells, and fetal am-

niocytes. The role of fetal fibronectin is unclear but the other entities appear to play roles in the immunological responses to inflammation. Fetal fibronectin is abundant in amnionic fluid, and Eriksen and colleagues (1992) suggested that a qualitative enzyme-linked immunosorbent assay (ELISA) for fibronectin may be useful in the diagnosis of ruptured membranes. Moreover, Lockwood and co-workers (1991) reported that detection of fetal fibronectin in cervicovaginal secretions prior to membrane rupture may be a marker for impending preterm labor.

Ambulatory Uterine Contraction Testing. The diagnosis of preterm labor before it is irreversibly established is a goal of management. To this end, uterine activity monitoring, using tocodynamometry, has recently received considerable interest. Subsequent development and application of a new technology for sensing uterine contractions prompted Zahn (1973), Bell (1983), Katz (1986a, 1986b), and their co-workers to propose that ambulatory monitoring of uterine contractions might improve recognition of women destined to deliver preterm, and thus might lead to earlier and more effective interventions.

In 1957 Smyth described an external tocodynamometer with an innovative sensor that employed the so-called *guard-ring principle*. The abdominal wall is flattened by an outer ring, thus permitting the inner contraction-sensing transducer to be applied more directly to the underlying uterine wall. Several preterm birth-prevention programs incorporating a device using the guard-ring principle are now available for ambulatory uterine monitoring in women at risk for preterm labor. Patients wear the contraction sensor belted about their abdomens and connected to a small electronic recorder worn at the waist. This recorder is used to transmit uterine activity via phone on a daily basis to receiving centers. Patients are educated concerning signs and symptoms of preterm labor, and their attending physicians are kept apprised of their progress. The program is expensive; in Dallas in 1992 this service costs the patient between $100 and $140 per day (list price), depending on her risk of preterm birth.

The group from San Francisco reported that maternal perception of contractions is improved using the Term-Guard sensor, and they found that only 10 percent of women correctly perceived their contractions more than 50 percent of the time (Newman and associates, 1986). In addition, as shown in Figure 38–6, they found that women who subsequently had a preterm delivery experienced increased uterine activity beginning about 30 weeks (Katz and associates, 1986b). Subsequently, Katz and associates (1986a) reported outcomes in 60 women at risk for preterm birth who were managed using this system and compared them with 60 similar matched controls. Women with four or more contractions per hour were admitted for evaluation and given

TABLE 38–4. CERVICAL DILATATION BETWEEN 26 AND 30 WEEKS' GESTATION AND RISK OF DELIVERY BEFORE 34 WEEKS

	Total n = 185 (%)	Cervical Status at 26 to 30 Weeks		
		<1 cm n = 170 (%)	2–3 cm n = 15 (%)	Comparison
Prior low birthweight[a]	9 (5)	6 (4)	3 (20)	P < 0.001
Current pregnancy low birthweight	7 (4)	3 (2)	4 (27)	P < 0.002

[a] Less than 2200 g (50th percentile for 34 weeks).
From Leveno and associates (1986a), with permission.

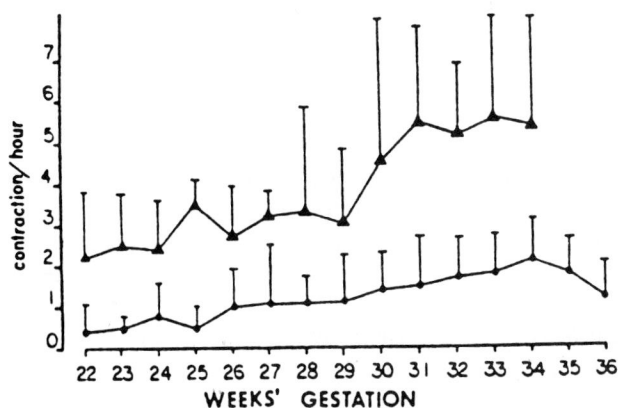

Fig. 38–6. Mean frequency (± SD) of contractions during pregnancy in women having preterm labor (▲) compared with those with term labor (●). (From Katz and colleagues, 1986b, with permission.)

either ritodrine or terbutaline if cervical changes accompanied regular contractions. Although no ultimate perinatal outcomes are described, the investigators noted that significantly fewer women enrolled in the Term-Guard system (7 percent) failed tocolysis, compared with controls (22 percent), and as a consequence there were fewer births prior to 36 weeks.

Widespread clinical application of home uterine contraction monitoring for the purpose of preventing preterm birth has provoked considerable controversy in the United States. Although many authorities consider home uterine contraction monitoring to be investigational, several companies are already successfully marketing this technology. For example, Tokos Medical Corporation in Santa Ana, California, had 1991 revenues totaling $115 million. Currently the American College of Obstetricians and Gynecologists (1992) continues to take the position that home uterine contraction monitoring should be considered investigational and cannot be recommended for routine use. Interestingly, the Food and Drug Administration has approved (April 4, 1990) only the *Genesis* system (Physiologic Diagnostic Service, Atlanta, GA) for detection of preterm labor. The Tokos *Term Guard* monitor system was deemed not approvable in May 1988, and the Healthdyne *Uterine Monitoring System* was rejected in March 1989 (Gray Sheet, 1990).

The dimensions of the controversy over the efficacy of home uterine contraction monitoring can be sensed by reading editorials or reviews that have appeared in major medical journals between 1989 and 1992. These include the *Journal of the American Medical Association* (Cole, 1989), *American Journal of Obstetrics and Gynecology* (Rhoads and co-authors, 1991), *New England Journal of Medicine* (Sachs and co-authors, 1991), and *Obstetrics and Gynecology* (Grimes and Schulz, 1992). The conclusion in all these reviews is that there is no consensus concerning the

effectiveness of home uterine contraction monitoring in the prevention of preterm birth. Grimes and Schulz (1992) have taken the position that "until the efficacy of this technology has been established, home uterine activity monitoring should not be used clinically."

There have been several randomized studies comparing the efficacy of home uterine contraction monitoring to intensive prenatal care. Morrison and associates (1987) randomized 67 pregnancies at risk for preterm delivery and concluded that contraction monitoring was beneficial. Iams and co-workers (1988) randomized 309 pregnancies and found contraction monitoring no better than nursing interventions. Mou and co-workers (1991) randomized 377 pregnancies and concluded that contraction monitoring was beneficial. Similar results were reported by Dyson and colleagues (1991) for twin gestations but not singletons. Most recently, Blondel and colleagues (1992) were unable to find benefits in a study performed in France and involving 168 pregnancies. Thus, among these five randomized studies, two reported benefits, two did not, and one was indeterminate.

Diagnosis of Preterm Labor

Early differentiation between true and false labor is often difficult before there is demonstrable cervical effacement and dilatation. Progressive dilatation, of course, is indicative of labor. A frequently used criterion for labor is that of uterine contractions with a frequency of at least once every 10 minutes and a duration of 30 seconds or more. Uterine function is often further evaluated by means of external tocography to record the frequency and duration of contractions. Uterine contractions alone can be misleading, however, because of *Braxton Hicks contractions*. These contractions, described as irregular, nonrhythmical, and either painful or painless, can cause considerable confusion in the diagnosis of preterm labor. Not infrequently, women who deliver before term have uterine activity that is attributed to Braxton Hicks contractions, prompting an incorrect diagnosis of false labor.

Because uterine contractions alone may be misleading, Herron and associates (1982) require the following criteria to document preterm labor: regular uterine contractions after 20 weeks or before 37 weeks, which are 5 to 8 minutes apart or less, and accompanied by one or more of the following: (1) progressive change in the cervix, (2) cervical dilatation of 2 cm or more, or (3) cervical effacement of 80 percent or more.

As a consequence of the confusion and imprecision as to the diagnosis of preterm labor, there has been corresponding uncertainty about the effectiveness of most preterm labor treatment regimens. For example, most attempts to prevent preterm delivery in patients with ruptured membranes are less than satisfactory. This is likely due to the considerable certainty of preterm delivery that follows. In other words, ruptured membranes definitively establish a diagnosis of impending preterm delivery, whereas uterine contractions alone may not be so predictive.

Management of Preterm Labor and Delivery

In general, the more immature the fetus, the greater the risks from labor and delivery. This is well established for breech delivery, which is a common presentation for the preterm fetus (Chap. 20, p. 497), and undoubtedly also is true to a degree for all immature fetuses regardless of presentation.

Labor. Whether labor is induced or spontaneous, abnormalities of fetal heart rate and uterine contractions should be sought, preferably by continuous electronical monitoring. If the fetal heart is not monitored continuously, it must be evaluated at very close intervals by adequately trained attendants (see Chap. 14, p. 376). Tachycardia, especially in the presence of ruptured membranes, is suggestive of sepsis.

Importantly, just as the markedly preterm infant is to be afforded special care in the neonatal intensive care unit, the mother and fetus should be observed very closely in the labor and delivery unit. Especially skilled physicians should monitor the labor and the delivery of the markedly preterm fetus.

Delivery. In the absence of a relaxed vaginal outlet, a liberal episiotomy for delivery is advantageous once the fetal head reaches the perineum. Argument persists as to the merits of spontaneous delivery versus forceps delivery to protect the more fragile preterm fetal head (Chap. 24, p. 559). It is doubtful whether use of forceps in most instances produces less trauma. Indeed, to compress and pull on the head of a grossly premature infant might be more traumatic than to push the fetus out by force applied from above to the buttocks. The use of outlet forceps of appropriate size may be of assistance when conduction analgesia is used and voluntary expulsion efforts are obtunded. Forceps should not be employed to pull the fetus through a vagina that is resistant to dilation or over a firm perineum.

Following the report of Bejar and colleagues (1980) that preterm infants frequently had germinal matrix bleeding that might extend to be more serious intraventricular hemorrhage, there was the idea that cesarean delivery to obviate trauma from labor and delivery might prevent these complications (see Chap. 44, p. 996). These initial observations have not been validated by all subsequent studies. From 1982 through 1987, 15 studies were published regarding the outcomes of preterm infants delivered from the cephalic presentation. In 12 of these reports the conclusion was

reached that there was no advantage of delivery by cesarean section for prematurity. Indeed, Malloy and co-authors (1989) concluded that the cesarean delivery rate for birthweights 500 to 1500 g increased from 24 percent to 44 percent in Missouri between 1980 and 1984 without apparent infant benefits.

A physician proficient in resuscitative techniques who has been fully oriented to the specific problems of the case should be present at delivery. **The principles of resuscitation described in Chapter 17 are applicable, including prompt tracheal intubation and ventilation.**

Methods Used To Arrest Preterm Labor

As previously mentioned, early differentiation between true and false labor often is difficult before there is cervical effacement and dilatation. Unfortunately, by this time, attempts to arrest labor are often ineffective. Successful arrest of preterm labor appears to require early implementation.

Before an attempt is made to arrest preterm labor, the question must be asked and correctly answered: *Is further intrauterine stay more likely to benefit or harm the fetus?* Many neonatal deaths continue to be the direct consequence of marked prematurity, and the number of such deaths undoubtedly could be reduced by delaying delivery. Not all fetuses, however, will benefit from a further intrauterine stay. This is borne out by an annual stillbirth rate in the United States that now exceeds the neonatal death rate. Obviously, some of these stillborn fetuses would have lived if only the fetus had been delivered earlier. For example, retarded fetal growth may be confused with a preterm fetus, and the malnourished fetus, to his or her detriment, may be left in a hostile uterine environment rather than a more favorable one provided by the nursery. Thus, the problem as to what is best for the fetus—as well as for the mother—is not so simple that the obstetrician can automatically attempt to delay delivery in all cases of presumed preterm labor. **The decision to attempt arrest of labor is made much easier if the gestational age is precisely known.**

Bed Rest. The treatment regimen that has been used most often is bed rest, with the mother lying more comfortably on her side. In the relatively few controlled studies of the effect of various treatment modalities, the control group most often was placed at bed rest and, at times, given a placebo. Satisfactory results in the prevention or arrest of preterm labor were often obtained in the control group. The success was attributable to bed rest and perhaps in part to the reassurance of the mother that she was being treated.

Magnesium Sulfate. It has been recognized for some time that ionic magnesium in a sufficiently high concentration can alter myometrial contractility in vivo as well as in vitro. The role of magnesium is presumably that of an antagonist of calcium.

Steer and Petrie (1977) concluded that intravenously administered magnesium sulfate, 4 g given as a loading dose followed by a continuous infusion of 2 g/hour, will usually arrest labor. Subsequent studies have been reported, some favorable and some not so favorable. Elliott (1983), in a retrospective study, found tocolysis with magnesium sulfate to be successful, inexpensive, and relatively nontoxic. He reported 87 percent success when the cervix was dilated 2 cm or less, but the period of arrest was as short as 48 hours. Spisso and co-workers (1982) were favorably impressed by the efficacy of magnesium sulfate when given intravenously in relatively large doses to women with intact membranes who had not begun the active phase of labor. They emphasized that for therapy to be effective it must be given in the early latent phase of labor. This seems to be true for all currently used tocolytic regimens.

Cotton and associates (1984b) compared magnesium sulfate with ritodrine as well as with a placebo, and they identified little difference in outcomes. Cox and associates (1990) randomized 156 women in preterm labor with intact fetal membranes to infusions of magnesium sulfate or normal saline. Magnesium sulfate was begun using a 4-g (20 percent solution) loading dose infusion followed by 2 g/hour intravenously. If contractions persisted after 1 hour, the infusion was increased to a maximum of 3 g/hour. The mean plasma magnesium concentration achieved was 5.5 mEq/L. No benefits for such magnesium sulfate therapy were found, and this method of tocolysis was abandoned at Parkland Hospital. Hollander and colleagues (1987) used an unprecedented infusion dose of magnesium sulfate that averaged 4.5 g/hour. They reported that such therapy was equal to ritodrine. Semchyshyn and associates (1983) failed to stop labor in a woman who inadvertently was given 17.3 g of magnesium sulfate in 45 minutes!

The woman must be monitored very closely for evidence of hypermagnesemia that might prove toxic to her and to her fetus-infant. Smith and associates (1992) reported that long-term (average 26 days) magnesium sulfate therapy for preterm labor markedly increased calcium losses, which may affect bone mineralization. The pharmacology and toxicology of parenterally administered magnesium are considered in more detail in Chapter 36 (p. 794).

β-Adrenergic Receptor Agonists.

Earlier in this century, epinephrine in low doses was demonstrated to exert a depressant effect on the myometrium of the pregnant uterus. Its tocolytic effects, however, proved to be rather weak, quite transient, and likely to be accompanied by troublesome cardiovascular effects. More recently, several compounds capable of reacting predominantly with β-adrenergic receptors have been investigated. Some of these now are extensively used in obstetrics, but only ritodrine hydrochloride has been approved (November 1980) by the Food and Drug Administration to treat preterm labor.

The adrenergic receptors are located on the outer surface of the smooth muscle cell membrane, where specific agonists can couple with them. Adenyl cyclase in the cell membrane is activated by the coupling of an agonist to the receptor. Adenyl cyclase enhances the conversion of adenosine triphosphate to cyclic AMP, which in turn initiates a number of reactions that reduce the intracellular concentration of ionized calcium and thereby prevent activation of the contractile proteins, as described in Chapter 12 (p. 311).

There are two classes of β-adrenergic receptors. The β_1 receptors are dominant in the heart and intestines, while β_2 receptors are dominant in the myometrium, blood vessels, and bronchioles. A number of compounds generally similar in structure to epinephrine have been evaluated in the search for one that ideally would provide optimal stimulation of β_2-adrenergic receptors on myometrial cells and thus inhibit uterine contractions, and simultaneously cause little or no adverse effects from stimulation of adrenergic receptors elsewhere. Thus far, no compound has exhibited these utopian properties. Compounds that have been or are being employed in attempts to arrest preterm labor include ritodrine, terbutaline, and fenoterol.

Ritodrine. In a multicenter study in the United States, infants whose mothers were treated with ritodrine for presumed preterm labor had a lower mortality rate, developed respiratory distress less often, and achieved a gestational age of 36 weeks or a birthweight of 2500 g more often than did infants whose mothers were not so treated (Merkatz and colleagues, 1980). Hesseldahl (1979), however, in a multicenter controlled study in Denmark, did not find any of several ritodrine regimens tested to be more efficacious than standard treatment, which consisted of bed rest and glucose infusion plus placebo tablets.

Because of concerns for the efficacy and safety of ritodrine, we evaluated the drug before we allowed its general use on the obstetrical service at Parkland Hospital (Leveno and associates, 1986b). Preterm labor was rigidly defined to include cervical dilation plus regular uterine contractions, and 106 women between 24 and 33 weeks were randomly allocated to receive either intravenous ritodrine or no tocolysis. Although ritodrine treatment significantly delayed delivery for 24 hours or less, it did not significantly modify the ultimate perinatal outcomes following preterm labor. Similar results in a randomized study involving 708 pregnancies were reported recently by the Canadian Preterm Labor Investigators Group (1992). A likely explanation for the transient uterine tocolytic effects of ritodrine and ultimate failure of such therapy may be the phenomenon of β-adrenergic receptor function densitization (Hausdorff and colleagues, 1990).

The infusion of ritodrine, as well as the other β-adrenergic agonists, has resulted in frequent and at times serious side effects. In the mother, tachycardia, hypotension, apprehension, chest tightness or actual pain, electrocardiographic S-T segment depression, pulmonary edema, and death have been observed. Maternal metabolic effects include hyperglycemia, hyperinsulinemia (unless diabetic), hypokalemia, and lactic and ketoacidosis. Less serious, but nonetheless troublesome, side effects include emesis, headaches, tremulousness, fever, and hallucinations.

A single mechanism has not been identified to explain the development of pulmonary edema, but maternal infection appears to increase the risk (Hatjis and Swain, 1988). The cause of the pulmonary edema appears to be multifactorial. Beta-adrenergic agonists have potent renal effects that cause the retention of sodium and water, and thus may lead to volume overload. In addition, the drugs have been implicated as a cause of increased capillary permeability, disturbances of cardiac rhythm, and myocardial ischemia. The simultaneous administration of potent glucocorticoids to try to hasten lung maturation may also contribute, although pulmonary edema has developed in their absence. The importance of these complications cannot be overstated, because they have been associated with at least 14 maternal deaths (Hankins, 1991). Caritis and associates (1983) summarized the pharmacodynamics of ritodrine in women during preterm labor.

Terbutaline. Terbutaline is commonly used to forestall preterm labor, and has been claimed by some, but certainly not by all, to inhibit myometrial contractions effectively even when cervical dilatation is far advanced. Toxicity, especially maternal pulmonary edema, and glucose intolerance have been evident with use of the drug (Angel and associates, 1988).

Lam and colleagues (1988) described long-term subcutaneous administration of low-dose terbutaline using a portable pump in 9 pregnancies. It was claimed that the lower dose of terbutaline used likely prevented β-adrenergic receptor desensitization, resulting in less "breakthrough tocolysis." To date there have been no other reports in the American literature except for a description of newborn myocardial necrosis after the mother had used the terbutaline pump for 12 weeks (Fletcher and colleagues, 1991). The Tokos Corporation began marketing this new approach to tocolysis in the fall of 1988. The current (1992) daily patient charge for use of the pump and uterine contraction monitoring is $447 (list price).

Fenoterol. Fenoterol is structurally very similar to ritodrine. It is not clear whether fenoterol is any more or less effective, or causes more or fewer adverse reactions, than do the other β-mimetic agents currently being used in several countries. Epstein and associates (1979) documented sustained hypoglycemia accompanied by elevated insulin levels in most infants who were delivered within 2 days after terminating the maternal fenoterol infusion. As mentioned above, a similar response has been documented for ritodrine and other β-adrenergic agonists.

The use of fenoterol has been extremely popular in West Germany. Kubli (1977), however, commented that despite the use of at least 1 million ampules and 6 million tablets of fenoterol annually for a birth rate of about 6 million, there had been no remarkable decrease in the number of low-birthweight infants.

Combined Therapy. To try to reduce the adverse effects of ritodrine while effectively arresting preterm labor, Ferguson and co-workers (1984) evaluated the response to magnesium sulfate and ritodrine administered together. They were forced to abandon the study because of the frequency and intensity of the maternal side effects that resulted from the use of this combination. Respiratory distress was troublesome, and both symptoms and electrocardiographic evidence of myocardial ischemia were common.

Hatjis and colleagues (1987) reported that ritodrine combined with magnesium sulfate was superior in arresting labor, compared with ritodrine alone, but Wilkins and associates (1988) could not confirm this observation.

Prostaglandin Inhibitors. Antiprostaglandins have been the subject of considerable interest since it was appreciated that prostaglandins are intimately involved in myometrial contractions that characterize normal labor (Chap. 12, p. 327). Antiprostaglandin agents may act by inhibiting the synthesis of prostaglandins or by blocking the action of prostaglandins on target organs.

A group of enzymes collectively called *prostaglandin synthase* are responsible for the conversion of free arachidonic acid to prostaglandins. Several drugs are known to block the prostaglandin synthase system, including aspirin and other salicylates, indomethacin, naproxen, and meclofenamic acid. Zuckerman and co-workers (1974) reported the successful treatment of preterm labor using indomethacin, but in their study no controls were used. Besinger and colleagues (1991) also reported good results using indomethacin. Unfortunately, indomethacin and other such prostaglandin synthase inhibitors may adversely affect the fetus by inducing major cardiovascular changes, especially premature closure of the ductus arteriosus (Eronen and colleagues, 1991).

Calcium-Channel Blocking Drugs. Smooth muscle activity, including myometrium, is directly related to free calcium within the cytoplasm, and a reduction in calcium concentration inhibits myometrial contraction. Calcium ions reach the cytoplasm through specific membrane portals or channels, and *calcium-channel blockers* act to inhibit, by a variety of different mechanisms, the entry of calcium through the cell membrane channels. Calcium-entry blockers, because of their smooth muscle arteriolar relaxation effects, are currently being used for the treatment of coronary artery disease and hypertension.

The possibility that calcium-channel blocking drugs might have applications in the treatment of preterm labor has been the subject of research in both animals and humans since the late 1970s. Forman and co-workers (1981) reported that nifedipine inhibited contractile activity in myometrial strips taken at cesarean section. Similarly, in women undergoing midtrimester abortion, nifedipine effectively inhibits uterine contractions induced by prostaglandin $F_{2\alpha}$. The first clinical trial in which nifedipine was given for preterm labor was reported from Denmark by Ulmsten and colleagues (1980). Nifedipine treatment postponed delivery at least 3 days in 10 women with preterm labor at 33 weeks or less. No serious maternal or fetal side effects were noted. Similarly, Read and Wellby (1986) compared orally administered nifedipine to either intravenous ritodrine or no treatment for preterm labor before 36 weeks. They concluded that nifedipine was more effective than ritodrine and was associated with fewer troublesome side effects. More recent reports have described nifedipine to be an effective tocolytic agent (Ferguson and associates, 1990; Murray and colleagues, 1992).

As promising as calcium-channel blockers may appear for treatment of preterm labor, some investigators caution that more research is needed to clarify the potential maternal or fetal dangers of such drugs. Parisi and colleagues (1986) reported that hypercapnia, acidosis, and possibly hypoxemia developed in fetuses of hypertensive ewes given nicardipine, another calcium-channel blocker. Similarly, Lirette and colleagues (1987) observed a fall in uteroplacental blood flow in pregnant rabbits (also see Chap. 5, p. 131). Finally, Duscay and co-workers (1987) reported fetal acidosis and hypoxemia in rhesus monkeys infused with nicardipine in doses sufficient for tocolysis. Drug-induced hepatotoxicity has been reported in pregnant women treated with nifedipine for preterm labor (Sawaya and Robertson, 1992).

Oxytocin Antagonists. A new class of drugs for inhibition of preterm uterine contractions is under development both in Europe and the United States. Melin and co-workers (1986) described a synthetic receptor antagonist that functions as a competitive inhibitor for oxytocin. Experience with oxytocin antagonists in humans has been limited to 13 pregnancies (Akerlund and associates, 1987). Hahn and colleagues (1987) and Wilson and associates (1990) described the effects of oxytocin antagonists in several animal species.

POSTTERM PREGNANCY

A postterm pregnancy is one that persists for 42 weeks or more from the onset of a menstrual period that was followed by ovulation 2 weeks later. Although this may include perhaps 10 percent of pregnancies, some may not be actually postterm but rather the result of an error in the estimation of gestational age. Once again the value of precise knowledge of the duration of gestation is evident, because in general the longer the truly postterm fetus stays in utero, the greater the risk of a severely compromised fetus and newborn infant (Shime and co-workers, 1984). Eden and associates (1987) compared nearly 3500 postterm pregnancies with over 8100 infants delivered at 40 weeks and reported that several adverse pregnancy outcomes were significantly increased (Table 38–5).

Causes. There are two categories of human pregnancies that reach 42 completed weeks: (1) those truly 40 weeks past conception and (2) those with less advanced gestations due to variations in the timing of ovulation. Munster and associates (1992) recently described that there is a high incidence of large menstrual cycle length variation in normal women. Indeed, although approximately 10 percent of human pregnancies reach 42 completed weeks, a relatively small proportion of such pregnancies evidence the fetal effects of *postmaturity* described below. Boyce and associates (1976) studied 317 French women with conceptional basal body temperature profiles and found that 70 percent of women who completed 42 postmenstrual weeks had less advanced gestations based on their ovulation dates. Thus, most pregnancies reliably 42 completed weeks beyond the last menses probably are not biologically prolonged. However, there is no method available currently to

TABLE 38–5. OUTCOMES IN POSTTERM PREGNANCIES COMPARED WITH THOSE DELIVERED AT 40 WEEKS

Factor[a]	40 wks (N = 8135) (%)	Postterm (N = 3457) (%)
First pregnancy	33	38
Meconium	19	27
Oxytocin induction	3	14
Shoulder dystocia	8	18
Cesarean section	0.7	1.3
Macrosomia (>4500 g)	0.8	2.8
Meconium aspiration	0.6	1.6
Congenital malformations	2	2.8

[a] For all comparisons between 40- and 42-week groups, $P < 0.05$.
From Eden and associates (1987), with permission.

identify these pregnancies. The obstetrician must, therefore, manage all pregnancies judged to be 42 completed weeks as if abnormally prolonged.

Some rare conditions associated with prolonged pregnancy include *anencephaly, fetal adrenal hypoplasia, absence of the fetal pituitary, placental sulfatase deficiency*, and *extrauterine pregnancy*. Although the etiology of prolonged pregnancy is not completely understood, these clinical conditions share a common feature: the lack of the usually high estrogen levels that characterize normal pregnancy (Chap. 6). In the case of fetal pituitary or adrenal insufficiency, the precursor hormone, dehydroisoandrosterone sulfate, is secreted in insufficient amounts for conversion to estradiol and indirectly to estriol in the placenta. A classical example of the deficiency of estrogen precursor is anencephaly (MacDonald and Siiteri, 1965).

Placental sulfatase deficiency is inherited as a sex-linked recessive trait (Ryan, 1980). In this condition, precursor hormone is produced by the fetal adrenal gland, but the placenta lacks the enzyme to cleave the sulfate from dehydroisoandrosterone sulfate, the initial enzymatic step in the conversion of this biologically weak androgen into estradiol and estriol (France and Liggins, 1969).

Effects on the Fetus-Infant.
The postterm fetus may continue to gain weight in utero and thus be an unusually large infant at birth. The fact that the fetus continues to grow serves as an indication of uncompromised placental function, with the implication he or she should tolerate the rigors of normal labor without problems. However, this *may not* be the result. For example, continued growth may have created fetopelvic disproportion, and consequently, labor may not progress normally. Moreover, as discussed below, oligohydramnios commonly develops as pregnancy advances past 42 weeks, and decreased amnionic fluid is associated with cord compression, which may lead to fetal distress, including defecation and aspiration of thick meconium (see Chap. 44, p. 995).

The infant affected by prolonged gestation presents a somewhat unique and characteristic appearance that was first described by Clifford (1954) and termed *postmature*. The infant is long but thin in girth and appears underweight from loss of subcutaneous tissues. Typically there are patchy areas of desquamation and the skin is stained with meconium, although rarely the latter feature may be absent. The ventral surfaces of the hands and feet are wrinkled and the nails are long and stained with meconium. Most such postmature infants are not growth retarded in the sense that their birthweight falls below the 10th percentile for gestational age. However, severe growth retardation, which logically must have preceded completion of 42 weeks' gestation, can occur.

Etiology of Fetal Jeopardy.
The reasons for the increased risks to postterm fetuses have been explained, at least partially, by Leveno and associates (1984). They reported that both antepartum fetal jeopardy and intrapartum fetal distress with postterm pregnancies was not due to placental insufficiency, but rather was the consequence of umbilical cord compression associated with oligohydramnios. This observation was subsequently confirmed by Phelan and co-workers (1984, 1985) and Bochner and associates (1987). Silver and colleagues (1987) reported that umbilical cord diameter, measured ultrasonically, was predictive of intrapartum fetal distress when decreased, and especially if further associated with oligohydramnios. **The exact role of placental insufficiency is unclear, but in our experience it has not been identified even in those fetuses who were obviously postterm and growth retarded.**

Antepartum Management of Postterm Pregnancy

Even in the absence of any recognizable maternal complication, there remains little doubt that some fetuses who stay in utero much beyond 42 weeks are in progressively greater danger of sustaining serious morbidity or even death. Therefore, it would be advantageous to such fetuses to deliver them by 42 weeks. Unfortunately, at least five difficult problems persist that serve to discourage a policy of delivering all fetuses whose gestational age is merely **suspected** to be at least 42 weeks:

1. Gestational age is not always known precisely, and thus the fetus may actually be less mature than believed.
2. It is very difficult to identify with precision those fetuses who are likely to die or to develop serious morbidity if left in utero.
3. The great majority of these fetuses fare rather well.
4. Induction of labor is not successful always.
5. Delivery by cesarean section appreciably increases the risk of serious maternal morbidity not only in this pregnancy, but also to a degree in subsequent ones.

In view of this list of problems, a definite plan of management should be established for all cases of prolonged gestation. It seems reasonable to decide as a first step whether gestational age is firmly established or is uncertain. Management is then directed at these two variations of postterm pregnancy. Finally, there must be equipment and personnel necessary to care for the woman in what may be a difficult labor and delivery. Pediatric personnel should also be present at delivery to render any necessary care required for the neonate.

It is now common practice in the antepartum management of postterm pregnancy to apply a variety of electronical and ultrasonic tests that have been championed to predict fetal well-being (see Chap. 45). Benedetti and Easterling (1988) reviewed the use of antepartum tests in postterm pregnancy. As long as these tests remain normal, the fetus is considered to be in minimal jeopardy and delivery is usually not attempted.

Oligohydramnios is increasingly being emphasized as a hallmark of perinatal pathological conditions in a large number of pregnancy complications, and is particularly relevant in prolonged pregnancies because the volume of amnionic fluid diminishes as gestation reaches term and beyond (Fig. 38–7). Several authors have suggested that the identification of diminished amnionic fluid determined by various ultrasonic methods may be helpful to identify a postterm fetus in jeopardy. There is no doubt that when amnionic fluid is decreased in a postterm pregnancy, or any pregnancy for that matter, the fetus is at increased risk. However, many different criteria for diagnosis of oligohydramnios with ultrasound have been proposed. For example, Crowley and co-workers (1984) defined this as "no single vertical pool of amnionic fluid measured greater than 30 mm." Phelan and co-workers (1985) divided women into three groups based upon an amnionic fluid volume: (1) adequate—amnionic fluid throughout the cavity, with the largest pocket greater than 1 cm in its vertical diameter; (2) adequate but decreased—a vertical amnionic fluid pocket greater than 1 cm but with the "overall im-

pression of the sonographer that fluid is decreased"; and (3) decreased—absence of amnionic fluid throughout the cavity and a single pocket equal to or less than 1 cm.

Regardless of the criteria used to diagnose oligohydramnios in postterm pregnancies, most investigators have found at least an increased incidence of fetal distress during subsequent labor. It therefore seems that oligohydramnios by most definitions is a clinically meaningful finding in postterm pregnancies. However, reassurance of continued fetal well-being in the presence of "normal" ultrasonic amnionic fluid volume seems tenuous because it is unknown how quickly pathological oligohydramnios may develop. For example, Clement and co-workers (1987) reported six postterm pregnancies in which amnionic fluid volume diminished abruptly over 24 hours and one fetus died.

Gestational Age Known. If gestational age is known, management by most includes delivery at the end of a fixed period of time, ranging from 42 to 44 weeks regardless of the cervical condition (Granados, 1984; Leveno and colleagues, 1985b; Shime and associates, 1984). If induction fails, many favor cesarean section.

In many institutions, management between 42 and 44 weeks consists of serial antepartum tests (see Chap. 45) directed especially at identifying fetal jeopardy while awaiting the onset of spontaneous labor. With documented or suspected fetal distress, the infant is delivered either by labor induction or by cesarean section, depending on obstetrical indications.

Leveno and associates (1985b) reported a more active approach in a prospective 3-year study of nearly 1400 women with suspected prolonged pregnancy as the *only* complication. Definitely prolonged pregnancy (42 completed weeks) was diagnosed in 376 women, and 994 others were designated as uncertain. Fetal jeopardy or well-being was evaluated by clinical assessment of amnionic fluid volume and maternal perception of fetal movement. During the first 2 years, labor was induced in all women who completed a definite 43 weeks, and at the end of 42 weeks during the last year of the study. Women with uncertain prolonged pregnancy were followed weekly, without intervention unless fetal jeopardy was identified by diminished amnionic fluid suspected clinically or by maternal perception of decreased fetal motion.

Induction of labor at 42 rather than 43 weeks in women with definitely prolonged pregnancy resulted in an increase in the number of inductions from 40 to 90 percent, but there was no increase in the cesarean section rate. By delivering all women at 42 weeks, the perinatal mortality rate was reduced from 10 per 1000 to zero. The perinatal mortality rate in the group of women with uncertain gestational age was 2 per 1000. These investigators concluded that:

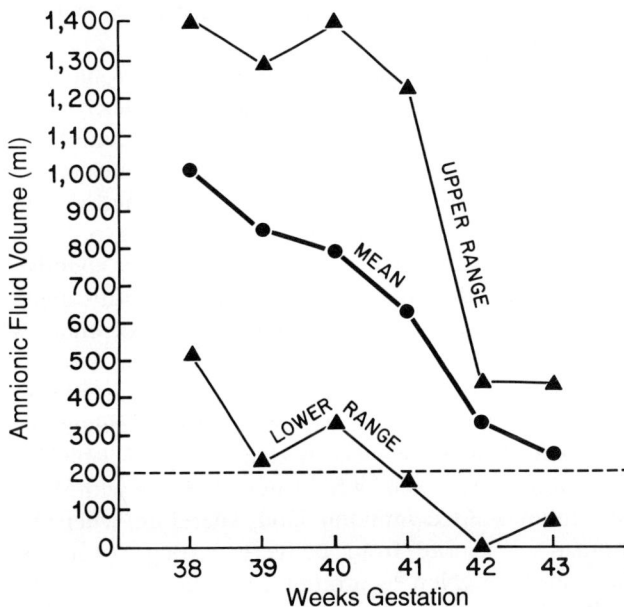

Fig. 38–7. Volume of amnionic fluid during the last weeks of pregnancy. (Adapted from Elliott and Inman, 1961, with permission).

1. Women with definite versus uncertain prolonged pregnancy represent two clinically separable groups with distinctly different perinatal risks.
2. Women with a definite prolonged pregnancy should be induced at 42 completed weeks.
3. More frequent induction attempts are not associated with an increased cesarean rate.

More recently, in some practices there has been a trend to begin labor induction or fetal surveillance at the end of 41, and even 40, completed weeks because of a small number of unexplained stillbirths (Bochner and coworkers, 1988).

From the preceding discussion, it becomes clear that there are two distinct approaches to the management of pregnancies determined to be 42 weeks or more. Should labor and delivery be induced or should antepartum tests of fetal health be employed and induction avoided? The importance of this question has prompted multicenter studies in both the United States and Canada. A randomized investigation comparing elective induction with antepartum tests— nonstress testing and ultrasonic estimation of amnionic fluid volume—was performed in 440 women with postterm pregnancies and cervices unfavorable for induction under the auspices of the National Institute of Child Health and Development (Medearis, 1990). No benefits were identified for either management strategy, and this was attributed to the very low incidence of adverse perinatal outcomes in postterm pregnancies. The Canadian study included over 3400 pregnancies at 41 or more completed weeks, and these were randomized to induction of labor or serial antenatal fetal testing (Hannah and colleagues, 1992). Women assigned to the fetal testing group were asked to count the number of times they felt the fetus kick over a 2-hour period each day, and they underwent nonstress testing three times weekly while ultrasonic assessment of amnionic fluid volume was performed two to three times per week. Induction of labor resulted in a significantly lower cesarean section rate (21 percent) compared with pregnancies managed with antepartum testing (25 percent). However, infant outcomes were equivalent in the two study subgroups.

Gestational Age Unknown. In many medical centers, if gestational age is unknown, clinical, electronic, or biochemical surveillance techniques, or various combinations of these (Chap. 45), are used after the best estimate of the 42nd week, and delivery is not induced unless there is evidence of fetal jeopardy. In these studies, because delivery dates most often are miscalculated, there generally is a favorable outcome. Leveno and associates (1985b) reported a perinatal mortality in these women of 2 per 1000 using only clinical methods of detecting fetal jeopardy (decreased amnionic fluid vol-

ume or decreased fetal movements perceived by the pregnant woman).

Medical or Obstetrical Complications. In the event of a medical or another obstetrical complication, it is generally unwise to allow a pregnancy to continue past 42 weeks. Indeed, in many such instances *early* delivery is indicated. Timing of delivery will depend on the individual complication. Examples include pregnancy-induced hypertension, prior cesarean delivery, diabetes, and many others.

Intrapartum Management of Postterm Pregnancy

Labor is a particularly dangerous time for the postterm fetus. Therefore, it is important that women whose pregnancies are known or suspected to be postterm come to the hospital as soon as they suspect they are in labor. Upon arrival, while being observed for possible labor, we recommend that electronic fetal heart rate and uterine contractions be monitored very closely for rate variations consistent with fetal distress (American College of Obstetricians and Gynecologists, 1987).

When to perform amniotomy is problematic. Further reduction in amnionic fluid volume following amniotomy can certainly enhance the possibility of cord compression, but on the other hand, amniotomy will likely identify thick meconium, which is dangerous to the fetus if aspirated. Moreover, once the membranes are ruptured, a scalp electrode and intrauterine pressure catheter can be placed, the use of which usually provides more precise data concerning fetal heart rate and uterine contractions than does external electronical monitoring.

Identification of *thick meconium* in amnionic fluid is particularly worrisome. The viscosity of such thick amnionic fluid probably signifies the lack of liquid and thus signifies oligohydramnios. Aspiration of thick meconium may cause severe pulmonary dysfunction and death during the newborn period (Chap. 44, p. 995). This may be minimized but not eliminated by effective suctioning of the pharynx as soon as the head is delivered but before the thorax is delivered. If meconium is identified, the trachea should be aspirated as soon as possible after delivery. Immediately thereafter, the infant should be ventilated as needed. The likelihood of successful vaginal delivery is reduced appreciably for the nulliparous woman who is in early labor with thick meconium-stained amnionic fluid. Therefore, when the woman is remote from delivery, strong consideration must be given to prompt cesarean section, especially when cephalopelvic disproportion is suspected or either hypotonic or hypertonic dysfunctional labor is evident. Many choose to avoid oxytocin use in these cases.

At times, the continued growth of the fetus post-term will result in a *postterm and large-for-gestational-age* infant, and shoulder dystocia may develop following delivery of the head. Freeman and associates (1981) reported a 25 percent incidence of fetal macrosomia (more than 4000 g) in their series of postterm pregnancies, and this was associated with a 2 percent incidence of shoulder dystocia. Likewise, Eden and colleagues (1987) reported that macrosomia of more than 4500 g was increased threefold and shoulder dystocia increased twofold in postterm pregnancies, compared with women delivered at 40 weeks (Table 38–5). Therefore, an obstetrician who is experienced in managing shoulder dystocia should be available to effect delivery (Chap. 20, p. 509).

Management of Postterm Pregnancy at Parkland Hospital. In women with definitely established gestational age, labor is induced at the completion of 42 weeks, or sooner if amnionic fluid volume is judged to be decreased or if she reports a decrease in fetal activity. Almost 90 percent of women are induced successfully, or enter labor within 2 days of attempted induction. For those who do not deliver with the first induction, a second induction is performed within 3 days. Almost all women will be delivered by this plan of management, but in the unusual few who are not delivered, a cesarean section may be justified.

This plan of active intervention, while increasing the number of inductions, has not resulted in an increased cesarean section rate, but has appreciably reduced fetal deaths (Leveno and co-workers, 1985b). Others also have reported that a comparable plan was beneficial for similar reasons (Barss and associates, 1985; Devoe and Sholl, 1983).

Women classified as having uncertain postterm pregnancies are followed on a weekly basis, without intervention unless fetal jeopardy is suspected. Fetal jeopardy is based upon the clinical or sonographic perception of decreased amnionic fluid volume. Equally worrisome is diminished fetal motion reported by the mother. If fetal jeopardy is suspected by either method, labor induction is carried out as described previously for the woman with a definite postterm gestation.

FETAL GROWTH RETARDATION

In both developed and developing countries, infant birthweight is probably the single most important factor affecting neonatal mortality, and it is a significant determinant of postneonatal infant mortality as well as later childhood morbidity (McCormick, 1985). Each year in the United States, approximately 250,000 babies are born weighing less than 2500 g (low birthweight). The National Institutes of Health estimated that approximately 40,000 are at term, but likely are growth re-

tarded (Frigoletto, 1986). The remaining infants include those who are preterm but may also be growth retarded. The actual number of growth-retarded neonates is unknown.

It was not until about 30 years ago that physicians first recognized that *runting*, or fetal growth retardation, was a human as well as an animal phenomenon. In 1961 Warkany and co-workers reported normal values for infant weights, lengths, and head circumferences and defined fetal growth retardation. Gruenwald (1963) reported that approximately one third of low-birthweight infants were *mature* and that their small size could be explained by *chronic fetal distress* probably due to *placental insufficiency*. These and observations by many others led to development of the concept that birthweight was governed not only by the length of gestation but also by the rate of fetal growth.

Definition

In 1963 Lubchenco and co-workers from Denver published detailed comparisons of gestational ages to birthweights in an effort to derive norms for expected fetal size and, therefore, growth, at a given gestational week. Battaglia and Lubchenco (1967) then classified *small-for-gestational-age* (SGA) infants as those whose weights were below the 10th percentile for their gestational age. *Large-for-gestational-age* (LGA) infants had weights above the 90th percentiles for their gestational ages. Infants between the 10th and 90th percentiles were classified as *appropriate for gestational age* (AGA). Thus, approximately 10 percent of human births were deemed "small" and another 10 percent "large." Those defined as *small-for-gestational-age* were shown to be at increased risk for neonatal death (Koops and associates, 1982). For example, the neonatal mortality rate of a small-for-gestational-age infant born at 38 weeks was 1 percent compared with 0.2 percent in those with appropriate birthweights. This served to equate *small for gestation age* with *abnormal*. In contrast, Usher and McLean (1969) proposed that fetal growth standards should be based on mean values with normal limits defined by ± 2 standard deviations because this definition would restrict small-for-gestational-age infants to 3 percent of births compared with 10 percent when percentiles were used.

Regardless of the birthweight percentile recommended, those infants deemed small for gestational age are also often considered to manifest *intrauterine fetal growth retardation* (IUGR). Although it seems awkward to reiterate that a *fetus* is, with extraordinarily rare exceptions such as abdominal pregnancy, inevitably an intrauterine creature, this description has become part of the contemporary lexicon. The phrase *fetal growth retardation* seems preferable. Moreover, not all infants with birthweights less than the 10th percentile are pathologically growth retarded. Some are small simply because of constitutional factors. Indeed, Gardosi and colleagues (1992) concluded that one fourth of babies conventionally diagnosed small for gestational age were in fact within normal limits when determinants of birthweight such as maternal ethnic group, parity, weight, and height were considered.

Birthweight standards for fetal growth have evolved considerably in the aftermath of the pioneering work done by Lubchenco and co-workers (1963) in Denver. The Denver fetal growth data were derived exclusively from white women who resided at high altitude. Infants born at high altitude are smaller than those born at sea level. For example, term infants average 3400 g at sea level, 3200 g at 5000 feet, and 2900 g at 10,000 feet altitude. Similarly, maternal race, parity, and infant sex also affect birthweight percentiles (Brenner and co-workers, 1976). The birthweight percentile information shown in Figure 38–1 is probably similar to that at our institution because the data are derived from white and black women living near sea level in Cleveland. It is likely that birthweight percentiles may differ for Hispanic women.

The impact of population differences on fetal growth standards cannot be overemphasized. Goldenberg and associates (1989b) reviewed studies on fetal growth published in the English literature since 1963, and in part due to population differences, concluded that there is currently no single national standard for fetal growth retardation. For example, if the 10th percentile is used to define "fetal growth retardation," the definition of abnormally grown infants could vary by several hundred grams at any given week of gestational age. Such observations attest to the considerable complexity inherent in attempting to define normal human fetal growth and departure from normal. Kramer (1987) reviewed 895 studies on fetal growth in English and French languages published between 1970 and 1984 and concluded that there was great confusion and controversy despite the profusion of studies.

Because of the foregoing, it seems prudent to consider that *small for gestational age* represents a mathematical description of small infants whereas *fetal growth retardation* should be reserved for those infants with clinical evidence of abnormal or dysfunctional growth. Unfortunately, diagnosis of which small-for-gestational-age infants are indeed growth retarded can be very imprecise. Moreover, the mathematical distributions of fetal size(s) at specific gestational ages just described, and which form the basis of our concepts of fetal growth, totally overlook the possibility that a fetus may have developed retarded growth during gestation but not severe enough to result in birthweight below the 10th percentile (Danielian and co-workers, 1992).

Mortality and Morbidity. Conventional obstetrical wisdom seems to pose a conflict when considering fetal growth retardation. It has long been considered that a growth-retarded *preterm* fetus seemingly has survival advantages, yet mortality is also reportedly increased. It is important to distinguish here between a preterm and term growth-retarded infant. Nonetheless, how can an advantaged fetus also be disadvantaged? Indeed, some investigators have challenged the concept that small-for-gestational-age birthweights accurately predict stillbirth (Myers and Ferguson, 1989), or other perinatal death between 36 and 41 weeks (Patterson and co-workers, 1986).

Advantages. A 1000-g infant born at 32 weeks and severely growth retarded physiologically functions differently in the nursery compared with a 1000 g but appropriately grown infant of 27 weeks. Obviously, the difference is due to chronological age, and in this sense fetal growth retardation *appears* to confer an advantage. However, there have also been numerous reports describing accelerated fetal pulmonary maturation in complicated pregnancies associated with growth retardation (Perelman and colleagues, 1985). One explanation for this phenomenon is that the fetus responds to a stressed environment by increasing adrenal glucocorticoid production, which leads to earlier or accelerated production of surface active phospholipids in the fetal lung (Laatikainen and associates, 1988). Although this concept pervades modern perinatal thinking, there is little clinical information to substantiate that pregnancy complications are a fetal advantage. Owen and associates (1990a) compared perinatal outcomes in a case-control study of 178 pregnancies delivered primarily because of hypertension with 159 pregnancies delivered because of spontaneous preterm labor or ruptured membranes. They concluded that a "stressed" pregnancy, which often resulted in small-for-gestational-age infants, did not confer an appreciable survival advantage.

Disadvantages. It is probably best to consider that it is not in the interests of a fetus for it to be small for gestational age. Although increasingly sophisticated neonatal care has probably eliminated most of the neonatal mortality associated with fetal growth retardation, morbidity remains a hazard. For example, because truly growth-retarded newborns have insufficient stores of glycogen and fat, they are unable to conserve heat and hypoglycemia is frequent. Indeed, the need for early feeding in growth-retarded infants because of hypoglycemia changed the pediatric policy of routinely withholding feedings to newborns.

Wennergren and co-workers (1988) analyzed the neonatal performance of 160 infants defined to be growth retarded because their birthweight was at or below two standard deviations from the mean. In most cases (83 percent), growth retardation had been suspected antenatally. Hypoglycemia and hypothermia occurred frequently, but these problems were managed satisfactorily in the nursery. The major hazards of growth retardation were stillbirth and fetal distress. Similar observations have been made by Villar and colleagues (1990) for fetal growth retardation at term and by Visser and associates (1986) between 25 and 34 weeks. Thus, most of the disadvantages of growth retardation accrue while the infant is still an intrauterine creature. Blair and Stanley (1990) reviewed the long-term neurological sequelae associated with growth retardation.

SYMMETRICAL VERSUS ASYMMETRICAL FETAL GROWTH. *Retardation* of growth could signify *suspension* of the potential for growth, as with placental insufficiency due to hypertension, or lack of the *potential* for growth, as from genetic causes. Indeed, autopsy findings in small-for-gestational-age infants have revealed two basic patterns of impaired fetal growth (Gruenwald, 1963; Naeye and Kelly, 1966). One of these is designated *symmetrical* growth retardation because all body organs tend to be proportionately reduced in size. Factors typically implicated in such proportional impaired fetal growth include malformations and congenital infection with rubella, cytomegalovirus, or toxoplasma. Other causes include severe chronic maternal malnutrition and smoking.

Asymmetrical fetal growth retardation implies that some body organs are more affected than others. For example, the fetal liver tends to be disproportionately small compared with the fetal brain, which is "spared." Such wasting of the liver is considered to represent loss of or diminished accumulation of glycogen stores. Consequently, fetal girth is often diminished out of proportion relative to head growth, and hence the description *asymmetrical*. Thus, head size is the last fetal dimension to be impacted, if at all, by impaired intrauterine growth. Muscle mass is also reduced, as are subcutaneous tissue fat stores. Asymmetrical fetal growth retardation is attributed to placental insufficiency due to a variety of hypertensive complications of pregnancy and advanced diabetes mellitus associated with impaired uteroplacental perfusion.

Recognition of symmetrical and asymmetrical patterns of impaired fetal growth has prompted considerable interest in the antepartum diagnosis of these two forms of compromised growth, because the pattern may reveal the cause. This has been particularly true in the ultrasonic evaluation of fetal growth retardation, where several dimensions of the fetus are now measurable and can be related to each other in an attempt to evaluate proportionality of fetal structures. However, accurate identification of the symmetrical versus asymmetrical fetus has in practice proved difficult. This is probably because the concept of brain sparing in asymmetrical growth retardation has proved difficult to document in all but the most extreme cases. Crane and Kopta (1980) analyzed several anthropometric measurements in growth-retarded newborns and concluded that the con-

cept of brain sparing was erroneous and could not be used to diagnose the cause of individual fetal growth retardation.

Causes of Small-for-Gestational-Age Fetuses

An etiological classification and brief description of some known causes of small-for-gestational-age fetuses are listed in the following sections. This selection is not and cannot be precise or complete, and hopefully soon will be rendered obsolete by a better understanding of the multiple etiologies of this clinical entity. Manning and Hohler (1991) estimated that about 75 percent of small-for-gestational-age infants will be constitutionally small, 15 to 20 percent will have suffered from uteroplacental insufficiency of various causes, and 5 to 10 percent have intrinsic impaired growth due to perinatal infections or malformations.

CONSTITUTIONALLY SMALL MOTHERS. Small women typically have smaller babies. If a woman begins pregnancy weighing less than 100 pounds, the risk of delivering a small-for-gestational-age infant is increased, at least by a factor of two (Simpson and colleagues, 1975). Data from the longitudinal study of all births in 1 week in 1958 in England, Wales, and Scotland indicate that there are intergenerational effects on birthweight that are transmitted through the maternal line (Emanuel and associates, 1992). Thus, there appear to be familial factors that significantly affect birthweight and likely explain why some infants are "constitutionally" small. In a small woman with a small pelvis, the birth of a small baby whose genetically determined weight is below the average for the entire population is not necessarily an undesirable event.

POOR MATERNAL WEIGHT GAIN. In the woman of average or low weight, lack of weight gain throughout pregnancy, or arrested weight gain after 28 weeks, are often associated with fetal growth retardation (Simpson and colleagues, 1975). If the mother is large and otherwise healthy, however, below-average maternal weight gain (Chaps. 8 and 9) without maternal disease is unlikely to be associated with appreciable fetal growth retardation. Marked restriction of weight gain during pregnancy should not be encouraged. During the last half of pregnancy, calories apparently have to be restricted to less than 1500 per day to cause fetal growth retardation (Lechtig and co-workers, 1975).

FETAL INFECTIONS. Viral, bacterial, protozoan, and spirochetal infections have all been associated with fetal growth retardation (Chap. 58, p. 1281). Certainly the best known of these are infections caused by rubella (Lin and Evans, 1984) and cytomegalovirus (Hanshaw,

1971; Stagno and associates, 1977). Hepatitis A and B are associated with preterm delivery but may also cause retarded fetal growth (Schweitzer, 1975; Waterson, 1979). Varicella and influenza rarely cause congenital infection and growth retardation (Varner and Galask, 1984). Listeriosis, tuberculosis, and syphilis have been reported to cause fetal growth retardation. Paradoxically, in cases of syphilis, the placenta is almost always increased in weight and size due to edema and perivascular inflammation (Varner and Galask, 1984). The protozoan infection most often associated with fetal growth retardation is toxoplasmosis, but congenital malaria may produce the same result (Varner and Galask, 1984).

CONGENITAL MALFORMATIONS. In general, the more severe the malformation, the more likely the fetus is to be small for gestational age. This is especially evident in fetuses with chromosomal abnormalities or those with serious cardiovascular malformations. For example, the anencephalic fetus is often growth retarded even when considering the missing brain and cranium (Honnebier and Swaab, 1973). Retarded growth of this degree is not seen in infants with spina bifida, but those infants are smaller than controls (Wald and associates, 1980).

CHROMOSOMAL ABNORMALITIES. The most severe forms of fetal growth retardation caused by chromosomal defects are trisomies, especially of chromosomes 13 and 18 (Larsen and Evans, 1984). Fetal growth retardation caused by trisomy 21 is less severe. Most often, trisomy 18 is associated with severe and early symmetrical fetal growth retardation and hydramnios. Trisomy 13 and Turner syndrome (45,X or gonadal dysgenesis) are also associated with some degree of retarded fetal growth (Larsen and Evans, 1984). Barlow (1973) reported that extra X chromosomes are associated with minimally decreased fetal weight.

DWARF SYNDROMES. Numerous inherited syndromes such as osteogenesis imperfecta and other such abnormalities are associated with fetal growth retardation.

TERATOGENS AND DRUGS. Any agent that causes a teratogenic injury is capable of producing fetal growth retardation. Some *anticonvulsants*, such as phenytoin and trimethadione, may produce specific and characteristic syndromes that include fetal growth retardation (Hanson and co-workers, 1976). *Tobacco* impairs fetal growth in a direct relationship with the number of cigarettes smoked (Dougherty and Jones, 1982; Meyer, 1978). *Narcotics* and related drugs act by decreasing maternal food intake and fetal cell number (Stone and associates, 1971). As discussed in Chapter 42 (p. 973), *alcohol* is a potent teratogen and acts in a linear dose-related fashion; 2 to 3 percent of infants born to moderate drinkers have the fetal alcohol syndrome even though their mothers are not alcoholics (Sokol and as-

sociates, 1980). There is a 10 percent incidence of the fetal alcohol syndrome in fetuses whose mothers are moderate drinkers (2 to 3 drinks per day), and up to a 30 percent incidence in fetuses whose mothers are heavy drinkers (5 or more drinks per day) (Hanson and co-workers, 1978).

SEVERE MALNUTRITION. Most often, the fetus grows normally despite significantly decreased maternal caloric intake. The best-documented effect of famine on fetal growth was in the winter of 1944 in Holland when the German Army enforced a restriction of approximately 600 kcal/day for pregnant women. The famine persisted for 28 weeks and there was an average birthweight decrease of 250 g per infant (Stein and colleagues, 1975). Although there was a small mean decrease, fetal mortality rates were increased significantly.

VASCULAR DISEASE. Chronic vascular disease, especially when further complicated by superimposed preeclampsia, commonly causes growth retardation. Conversely, pregnancy-induced hypertension without underlying vascular or renal disease is unlikely to be accompanied by fetal growth retardation (Robertson and associates, 1975).

CHRONIC RENAL DISEASE. Renal insufficiency may be accompanied by retarded fetal growth (Cunningham and colleagues, 1990; Katz and associates, 1980).

CHRONIC HYPOXIA. Fetuses of women who reside at high altitude usually weigh less than those born to women who live at a lower altitude. Fetuses of women with cyanotic heart disease are frequently growth retarded.

MATERNAL ANEMIA. Although maternal anemia has been implicated in the genesis of fetal growth retardation, in our experiences, this has been common only in fetuses of women with sickle cell disease or with other inherited anemias associated with serious maternal disease.

PLACENTAL AND CORD ABNORMALITIES. Chronic focal placental abruption, extensive infarction, or chorioangioma are likely to cause retarded fetal growth (Fig. 38–3). A circumvallate placenta or a placenta previa may impair growth, but usually the fetus is not markedly smaller than normal. Marginal insertion of the cord and especially velamentous insertions are more likely to be accompanied by a growth-retarded fetus (Chap. 35).

MULTIPLE FETUSES. Pregnancy with two or more fetuses is likely to be complicated by appreciable growth retardation of one or both fetuses, compared with normal singletons (Chap. 39).

EXTRAUTERINE PREGNANCY. Commonly, the fetus who has not been housed in the uterus is growth retarded. Similarly, some uterine malformations have been linked to impaired fetal growth.

Recent Insights into Human Fetal Growth Retardation. The technique of fetal blood sampling via the umbilical vein for karyotyping (see Chap. 41, p. 951) severely growth-retarded fetuses has permitted remarkable insights into the pathophysiology of fetal growth retardation. Much of this work has been done at King's College of Medicine in London and will be summarized here. Fetal growth retardation in these studies was diagnosed when the abdominal circumference, determined by ultrasound, was below the fifth percentile for gestational age.

Soothill and colleagues (1987) measured umbilical venous oxygen and carbon dioxide tensions, pH, lactate and glucose concentrations, nucleated red cell count, and hemoglobin concentrations in 38 growth-retarded fetuses. They found that the severity of fetal hypoxia correlated significantly with fetal hypercapnia, acidosis, lactic acidemia, hypoglycemia, and erythroblastosis. Subsequently, Economides and Nicolaides (1989a) found that the major cause of hypoglycemia in small-for-gestational-age fetuses is reduced supply rather than increased fetal consumption or decreased endogenous production of glucose. In a follow-up investigation, Economides and co-workers (1989b) found that these fetuses also had hypoinsulinemia, which they attributed to pancreatic dysfunction, as well as hypoglycemia. However, the degree of fetal smallness did not correlate with plasma insulin, suggesting that it is not the primary determinant of growth retardation.

In children with Kwashiorkor, the ratio of nonessential to essential amino acids is increased, presumably because of a decrease in intake of essential amino acids. Economides and colleagues (1989c) measured the glycine/valine ratio in umbilical vessel blood from growth-retarded fetuses and found that they had ratios similar to those observed in children with protein deprivation and Kwashiorkor. Moreover, protein deprivation correlated with fetal hypoxemia.

Economides and associates (1990) also measured plasma triglyceride concentrations in small- and appropriate-for-gestational-age fetuses. Growth-retarded fetuses demonstrated hypertriglyceridemia that was correlated with the degree of fetal hypoxemia. They hypothesized that hypoglycemic growth-retarded fetuses mobilize adipose tissue and that the hypertriglyceridemia is the result of lipolysis of fetal fat stores.

Other findings made possible because of cordocentesis included the observation that growth-retarded fetuses are thrombocytopenic, and the degree of platelet abnormality is correlated with the degree of fetal smallness, hypoxemia, and acidemia (Van den Hof and Nicolaides, 1990). Finally, fetal heart rate monitoring for 30 to 60 minutes was performed immediately before cordocentesis and results compared with fetal blood gases

(Visser and colleagues, 1990). Repetitive fetal heart rate decelerations best identified hypoxemic growth-retarded fetuses. However, several growth retarded infants with low normal Po_2 values still demonstrated acceleration of their heart rate.

Screening and Diagnosis of Fetal Growth Retardation

Identification through history of any of the above factors, as well as *a history of a previously growth-retarded fetus or fetal or neonatal death* should raise the possibility of growth retardation during the current pregnancy (Galbraith and associates, 1979). Early and meticulous establishment of gestational age and careful measurements of uterine height throughout pregnancy should serve to identify most instances of abnormal fetal growth; however, *definitive diagnosis* usually cannot be made until delivery.

The challenge remains primarily to identify the fetus who is inappropriately growing in utero. This difficulty is underscored by the fact that such identification is not always possible even in the nursery! Regardless, there are clinical techniques and high-technological equipment that may prove useful in helping to screen and hopefully to diagnose fetal growth retardation. Some of the widely used techniques, as well as those that are potentially useful, are described below.

Uterine Fundal Height. Carefully performed serial uterine fundal height measurements throughout gestation are a simple, safe, inexpensive, and reasonably accurate *screening* method that may be used to detect many small-for-gestational-age fetuses. The principal problem is the imprecision of such fundal height measurements. For example, Jensen and Larsen (1991) found that symphysis-to-fundus measurements helped to correctly identify only 40 percent of such infants. Thus, small-for-age infants were both overlooked and overdiagnosed. However, these results do not contravene carefully performed fundal height measurements as a simple screening method that is useful for suspecting many, but not all, instances of fetal growth retardation.

The method used in Parkland Hospital prenatal clinics was reported by Jimenez and colleagues (1983). Briefly this consists of a tape calibrated in centimeters being applied over the abdominal curvature from the top of the symphysis to the top of the uterine fundus, which is identified by palpation or percussion. The measurement is made after the bladder is emptied, and the tape is applied with the markings away from the examiner to avoid prejudice. Between 18 and 30 weeks, the uterine fundal height in centimeters roughly coincides with weeks of gestation. If the measurement is more than 2 cm from the expected height, inappropriate fetal growth is suspected.

Ultrasonic Measurements. Central to the debate over whether all pregnancies should routinely receive ultrasonic evaluations is the potential for diagnosis of fetal growth retardation (see Chap. 46, p. 1046). Typically, such routine screening incorporates an examination at 16 to 20 weeks to establish gestational age and then follow-up ultrasound imaging at 32 weeks or so to evaluate the rate of fetal growth. Benson and associates (1986) critically analyzed a large series of published ultrasonic criteria for identifying fetal growth retardation to ascertain the positive and negative predictive values. The study was drawn from 21 reports and included those from which sensitivity and specificity could be calculated. Predictive values were computed using Bayes theorem and based upon a 10 percent prevalence rate of fetal growth retardation. Seven of the nine techniques had positive predictive values of less than 50 percent. Thus, when one of these measurements was abnormal, a fetus was more likely to be normal than growth-retarded. The best predictive value, 62 percent, was obtained using the ratio of head to abdominal circumference. Benson and colleagues concluded that none of these methods allows for a confident antenatal diagnosis of fetal growth retardation.

More recently, Larsen and colleagues (1992) performed ultrasound after 28 weeks and every 3 weeks thereafter in 1000 pregnancies at risk for fetal growth retardation. They randomly withheld the results from the clinicians. Revealing the results of ultrasonic estimates of fetal growth during the third trimester significantly increased diagnosis of small-for-gestational-age fetuses. However, elective deliveries also increased, but without overall improvement in neonatal mortality or morbidity. Thus, this method of screening improved the diagnosis, but this was not followed by improved fetal outcome. Rather than an increase in diagnosis of fetal growth retardation, Goldenberg and colleagues (1989a) found that as the percentage of pregnancies receiving ultrasound increased, fetal growth retardation decreased. This was attributed to the gestational age information obtained using ultrasound.

An association between oligohydramnios and pathological fetal growth retardation has long been recognized and generally accepted. Several attempts, with varying success, have been made to use ultrasound estimates of amnionic fluid volume to improve identification of fetal growth retardation. For example, Philipson and associates (1983) found that 85 percent of small-for-gestational-age infants were preceded by oligohydramnios. Divon and associates (1986) found that an amnionic fluid pocket of 2 cm or less in diameter was highly suggestive of a small-for-gestational-age fetus when discovered in conjunction with poor growth of the fetal abdominal perimeter or femur length. However, even this contribution of fetal and amnionic fluid measurements did not permit detection of all affected fetuses. Patterson and colleagues (1987) reported similar experiences with the use of amnionic fluid volume in the prediction of fetal growth retardation.

Management of Fetal Growth Retardation

Once a small-for-gestational-age fetus is suspected, intensive efforts should be made to determine if growth retardation is present and, if so, its type and the etiology. Efforts are made to ensure delivery, when possible, of an infant who will subsequently thrive and grow to its normal potential. Finally, this must be done at the least cost to the patient in terms of finances and physical risk to herself and her fetus.

At Parkland Hospital, once a fetus is suspected of being growth retarded, an extensive ultrasonic survey is done to look for structural abnormalities. Anthropometric measurements are made, including head and abdominal circumferences, biparietal diameter, femur length, and the head circumference/abdominal circumference ratio. A clinical and ultrasonic assessment of amnionic fluid volume is also made. The gestational age is reconfirmed or, if not already known, established whenever possible. The condition of the cervix is assessed, and a decision is made as to whether or not to deliver the fetus.

Growth Retardation Near Term. Prompt delivery is likely to afford the best outcome for the fetus who is suspected of being growth retarded at or near term. Here, as in the management of such fetuses who are remote from term, growth retardation should be identified and antepartum and intrapartum care provided as outlined below.

Growth Retardation Remote from Term. A meticulous search should be made for fetal anomalies, and consideration should be given to obtaining umbilical blood for karyotyping, especially if a chromosomal anomaly is suspected (Chap. 41). Umbilical venous blood can be obtained by ultrasonically directed percutaneous umbilical blood sampling (see Chap. 41, p. 951). Although Pearce and Campbell (1985) recommend that screening be done for toxoplasmosis, rubella, cytomegalovirus, herpes, and other viral agents, we have not found this to be productive.

Often a diagnosis of structural or chromosomal abnormality is established too late for abortion; but even so, it is better that the parents, obstetrician, and pediatrician be forewarned. In some cases, such as with trisomy 13 or 18 fetuses who have multiple congenital anomalies and markedly attenuated life expectancies, cesarean section may be avoided.

Having excluded as nearly as possible structural, chromosomal, and possibly congenital infection, the woman is hospitalized, put at decreased physical activity, and given an adequate diet, and fetal surveillance is started. At a minimum, this includes fetal movement charts and clinical and sonographic assessment of fetal growth and amnionic fluid volume. Many recommend a battery of fetal surveillance tests, which includes, but certainly is not limited to, nonstress tests, contraction stress tests, biophysical profiles, serial Doppler velocity waveform measurements, and combinations thereof (see Chaps. 45 and 46). We follow fetal well-being with daily clinical evaluations of the woman, daily fetal movement counts, and frequent fetal heart rate monitoring. Most often, in the case of a seriously compromised fetus, the mother will notice decreased fetal activity or decreased amnionic fluid volume will be detected. In some cases, there may be a cessation of fetal growth detected by serial sonographic assessments.

In most instances of fetal growth retardation remote from term, there is no specific treatment that will ameliorate the condition. Possible exceptions are inadequate maternal nutrition, heavy smoking, use of street drugs, and possibly chronic alcoholism. Ideally, the use of tobacco, illicit drugs, and alcohol can be curtailed, and ingestion of an adequate diet should favorably influence fetal growth. Very sedentary living that approaches full-time bed rest may also favorably influence fetal growth and, at the same time, possibly reduce the risk of preterm labor.

It has been hypothesized that early antiplatelet therapy with low-dose aspirin may prevent uteroplacental thrombosis, placental infarction, and idiopathic fetal growth retardation in women with a history of recurrent severe fetal growth retardation (Wallenburg and Rotmans, 1987). Uzan and colleagues (1991) studied this hypothesis in a randomized double-blind trial in over 300 women at risk for recurrent fetal growth retardation. Although the incidence in the placebo group was twice that in the treated group, such aspirin therapy must be considered investigational and not for clinical use at this time.

Occasionally, the overtly growth-retarded fetus is in serious jeopardy irrespective of whether he or she remains in utero or is delivered. For the fetus who is severely growth retarded but remote from term, the decision to proceed with delivery becomes a matter of trying to ascertain the degree of risk from further uterine stay compared with the risks from preterm delivery. Confirmation of a lecithin–sphingomyelin (L–S) ratio of 2 or more, or identification of phosphatidylglycerol in amnionic fluid, is reassuring; however, a lower ratio or no detectable phosphatidylglycerol does not necessarily predict that respiratory distress will develop (Chap. 7).

Generally, delivery of an obviously growth-retarded fetus under the conditions outlined below, rather than procrastination with further fetal deterioration, offers the best chance for survival. By the time in gestation that fetal growth retardation has become severe, the fetus usually is mature enough to survive if (1) delivery is prompt rather than allowing the risk of further compromise, (2) there is close monitoring during labor to avoid further compromise or delivery is accomplished

by cesarean section, and (3) excellent neonatal care begins immediately after delivery.

The presence of maternal disease that is worsening as a consequence of the pregnancy, and thereby threatens the well-being of the mother as well as the fetus, should certainly influence the decision to deliver the severely growth-retarded fetus. Almost any maternal disease falls into this category when it is characterized by vascular disease, renal involvement, or both, and decidedly so if preeclampsia supervenes (see Chap. 36). With prompt delivery, fetal and neonatal salvage is likely to be improved compared to unduly delayed delivery, even though the L–S ratio is considered immature. At the same time, with prompt delivery, maternal deterioration is likely to be arrested.

Labor and Delivery

Throughout labor, spontaneous or induced, those fetuses who are suspected of being growth retarded should be monitored very closely for evidence of distress, including abnormalities of fetal heart rate and the presence of appreciable amounts of meconium in the amnionic fluid. The likelihood of severe fetal distress during labor is considerably increased. Fetal growth retardation is commonly the result of insufficient placental function as a consequence of faulty maternal perfusion, ablation of functional placenta, or both. These conditions are likely aggravated by vigorous labor. Importantly, lack of amnionic fluid predisposes to cord compression and its dangers. Consequently, the capabilities for immediate cesarean section should be available.

It can be anticipated that the infant at birth may need expert assistance in making a successful transition to air breathing. The fetus is at risk of being born hypoxic and of having aspirated meconium into the lungs, thus compromising chances of successful ventilation. As soon as the head is delivered from the vagina, or from the uterus during a cesarean section, the mouth, pharynx, and nares should be aspirated quickly. Moreover, it is essential that care for the newborn be provided immediately by someone who can skillfully clear the airway below the vocal cords, especially of meconium, and ventilate the infant as needed. The severely growth-retarded newborn is particularly susceptible to hypothermia and also may develop other metabolic derangements, especially serious hypoglycemia (Soothill and colleagues, 1987). Polycythemia and blood hyperviscosity may occasionally cause serious difficulty (Jones and Battaglia, 1977).

Subsequent Development of the Growth-retarded Fetus

Subsequent growth of the individual newborn who is growth retarded cannot be predicted reliably from an-

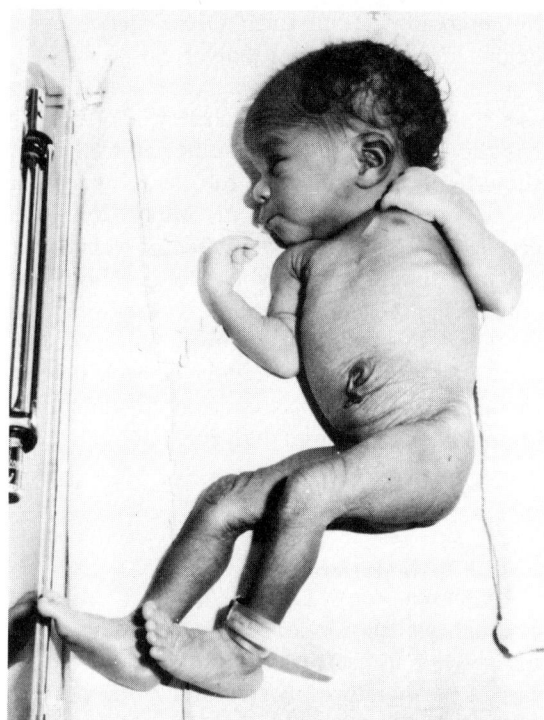

A

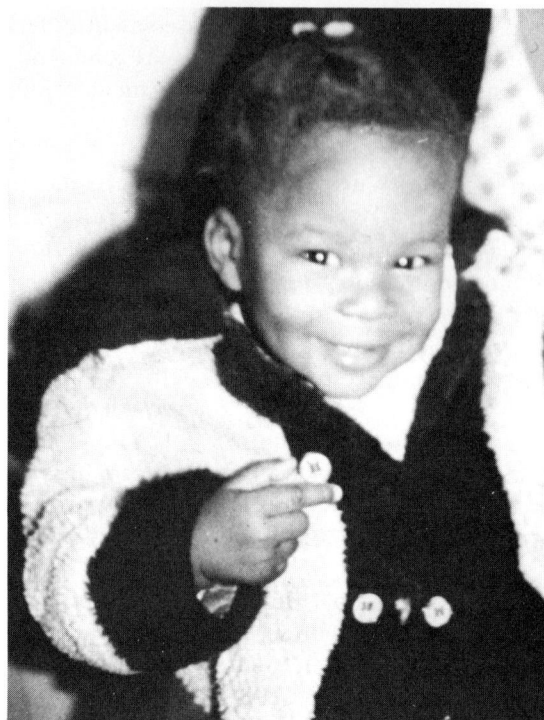

B

Fig. 38–8. A. A severely growth-retarded infant at 38 weeks but with a birthweight of only 1800 g. Delivery was by cesarean section. The chronically hypertensive mother had suffered two previous stillbirths. **B.** The same infant at 13 months of age. Physical and intellectual development was normal at that time.

thropometric measurements obtained at birth. In general, prolonged symmetrical, or generalized, growth retardation in utero is likely to be followed by slow growth after birth, whereas the asymmetrically growth-retarded fetus is more likely to catch up after birth (Fig. 38–8). Specifically, the infant whose weight is reduced can be expected to grow normally, but if length is also compromised, he or she is likely to remain small (Brook, 1983). Finally, infant sex and parental size play important roles in determining somatic size (Brook, 1983; Ounsted and associates, 1985).

The subsequent neurological and intellectual capabilities of the infant who was growth retarded in utero cannot be predicted precisely. The overall outcome is not bleak, however, and Vohr and associates (1979) reported that preterm, small-for-gestational-age infants had similar outcomes at 18 to 24 months, compared with appropriate-for-gestational-age preterm infants. A longer follow-up of preterm small-for-gestational-age infants also supports the view that a long-term favorable outcome may be expected (Vohr and Oh, 1983).

Fetal Growth Retardation in Subsequent Pregnancies

The risk of repeat instances of fetal growth retardation is increased in women in lower socioeconomic circum-

stances (Bakketeig and colleagues, 1986). This is especially true in women with a previous history of fetal growth retardation and a current medical complication (Patterson and colleagues, 1986).

References

Akerlund M, Stromberg PM, Hanksson A, Andersen LF, Lyndrup J, Trojnar J, Melin P: Inhibition of uterine contractions of premature labor with an oxytocin analogue. Results from a pilot study. Br J Obstet Gynaecol 94:1040, 1987

Alger LS, Lovchik JC, Hebel JR, Blackmon LR, Crenshaw MC: The association of *Chlamydia trachomatis, Neisseria gonorrhoea*, and group B streptococci with preterm rupture of the membranes and pregnancy outcome. Am J Obstet Gynecol 159:397, 1988

American College of Obstetricians and Gynecologists: Committee opinion: Home uterine activity monitoring. Committee on Obstetrics: Maternal and Fetal Medicine, no. 115, September 1992

American College of Obstetricians and Gynecologists: Committee opinion: Postterm pregnancy. Committee on Obstetrics: Maternal and Fetal Medicine, no. 57, October 1987

Amon E, Shyken JM, Sibai BM: How small is too small and how early is too early? A survey of American obstetricians specializing in high-risk pregnancies. Am J Perinatol 9:17, 1992

Angel JL, O'Brien WF, Knuppel RA, Morales WJ, Sims CJ: Carbohydrate intolerance in patients receiving oral tocolytics. Am J Obstet Gynecol 159:762, 1988

Arias F, Tomich P: Etiology and outcome of low birth weight and preterm infants. Obstet Gynecol 60:277, 1982

Avery ME, Aylward G, Creasy R, Little AB, Stripp B: Update on prenatal steroids for prevention of respiratory distress: Report of a conference—September 26–28, 1985. Am J Obstet Gynecol 155:2, 1986

Bakketeig LS, Bjerkedal T, Hoffman HJ: Small-for-gestational age births in successive pregnancy outcomes: Results from a longitudinal study of births in Norway. Early Hum Dev 14:187, 1986

Ballard RA, Ballard PL, Creasy RK, Padbury J, Polk DH, Bracken M, Moya FR, Gross I: Respiratory disease in very-low-birthweight infants after prenatal thyrotropin-releasing hormone and glucocorticoid. Lancet 339:510, 1992

Barlow P: The influence of inactive chromosomes on human development: Anomalous sex chromosome complements and the phenotype. Hum Genet 17:105, 1973

Barss VA, Frigoletto FD, Diamond F: Stillbirth after nonstress testing. Obstet Gynecol 65:541, 1985

Battaglia FC, Lubchenco LO: A practical classification of newborn infants by weight and gestational age. J Pediatr 71:159, 1967

Bejar R, Curbelo V, Coen RW, Leopold G, James H, Gluck L: Diagnosis and follow-up of intraventricular and intracerebral hemorrhages by ultrasound studies of infant's brain through the fontanelles and sutures. Pediatrics 66:661, 1980

Bejar R, Curbelo V, Davis C, Gluck L: Premature labor, II. Bacterial sources of phospholipase. Obstet Gynecol 57:479, 1981

Bell R: The prediction of preterm labour by recording spontaneous antenatal uterine activity. Br J Obstet Gynaecol 90:844, 1983

Benedetti TJ, Easterling T: Antepartum testing in postterm pregnancy. J Reprod Med 33:252, 1988

Bennett PR, Elder MG: The mechanisms of preterm labor: Common genital tract pathogens do not metabolize arachidonic acid to prostaglandins or to other eicosanoids. Am J Obstet Gynecol 166:1541, 1992

Benson CB, Doubilet PM, Saltzman DH: Intrauterine growth retardation: Predictive value of U.S. criteria for antenatal diagnosis. Radiology 160:415, 1986

Besinger RE, Niebyl JR, Keyes WG, Johnson TR: Randomized comparative trial of indomethacin and ritodrine for the long-term treatment of preterm labor. Am J Obstet Gynecol 164:981, 1991

Blair E, Stanley F: Intrauterine growth and spastic cerebral palsy. I. Association with birthweight for gestational age. Am J Obstet Gynecol 162:229, 1990

Blondel B, Bréart G, Berthoux Y, Berland M, Mellier G, Rudigoz RC, Thoulon JM: Home uterine activity monitoring in France: A randomized, controlled trial. Am J Obstet Gynecol 167:424, 1992

Bobbitt JR, Haslip CC, Damato JD: Amniotic fluid infection as determined by transabdominal amniocentesis in patients with intact membranes in premature labor. Am J Obstet Gynecol 140:947, 1981

Bobbitt JR, Ledger WJ: Unrecognized amnionitis and prematurity: A preliminary report. J Reprod Med 19:8, 1977

Bochner CJ, Medearis AL, Davis J, Oakes GK, Hobel CJ, Wade ME: Antepartum predictors of fetal distress in postterm pregnancy. Am J Obstet Gynecol 157:353, 1987

Bochner CJ, Williams J III, Castro L, Medearis A, Hobel CJ, Wade M: The efficacy of starting postterm antenatal testing at 41 weeks as compared with 42 weeks of gestational age. Am J Obstet Gynecol 159:550, 1988

Boyce A, Magaux MJ, Schwartz D: Classical and "true" gestational post maturity. Am J Obstet Gynecol 125:911, 1976

Brazle JV, Lubchenco LO: The estimation of gestational age chart. In Kenipe CH, Silver HK, O'Brien D (eds): Current Pediatric Diagnosis and Treatment, 3rd ed. Los Altos, CA, Lange Medical Publications, 1974

Brenner WE, Edelman DA, Hendricks CH: A standard of fetal growth for the United States of America. Am J Obstet Gynecol 126:555, 1976

Broekhuizen FF, Gilman M, Hamilton PR: Amniocentesis for Gram stain and culture in preterm premature rupture of the membranes. Obstet Gynecol 66:316, 1985

Brook CGD: Consequences of intrauterine growth retardation. BMJ 286:164, 1983

Brown ER, Nielsen H, Torday JS, Tauesch HW: Reversible induction of surfactant production in fetal lambs treated with glucocorticoids. Pediatr Res 13:491, 1979

Canadian Preterm Labor Investigators Group: Treatment of preterm labor with the beta-adrenergic agonist ritodrine. N Engl J Med 327, 308, 1992

Capeless EL, Mead PB: Management of preterm premature rupture of membranes: Lack of a national census. Am J Obstet Gynecol 157:11, 1987

Caritis SN, Lin LS, Toig G, Wong LK: Pharmacodynamics of ritodrine in pregnant women during preterm labor. Am J Obstet Gynecol 147:752, 1983

Carr-Hill RA, Hall MH: The repetition of spontaneous preterm labour. Br J Obstet Gynaecol 92:921, 1985

Chauham SP, Lutton PM, Bailey KJ, Guerrieri JP, Morrison JC: Intrapartum clinical, sonographic, and parous patients estimate of newborn birth weight. Obstet Gynecol 79:956, 1992

Christmas JT, Cox SM, Andrews W, Dax J, Leveno KJ, Gilstrap LC: Expectant management of preterm ruptured membranes: Effects of antimicrobial therapy. Obstet Gynecol 80:5, 1992

Clement D, Schifrin BS, Kates RB: Acute oligohydramnios in post date pregnancy. Am J Obstet Gynecol 157:884, 1987

Clifford SH: Postmaturity—with placental dysfunction. Clinical syndromes and pathologic findings. J Pediatr 44:1, 1954

Cole HM: Home monitoring of uterine activity. Questions and answers. JAMA 261:3027, 1989

Collaborative Dexamethasone Trial Group: Dexamethasone therapy in neonatal chronic lung disease: An international placebo-controlled trial. Pediatrics 88:421, 1991

Collaborative Group on Antenatal Steroid Therapy: Effects of antenatal dexamethasone administration in the infant: Long-term follow-up. J Pediatr 104:259, 1984

Collaborative Group on Antenatal Steroid Therapy: Effect of antenatal dexamethasone administration on the prevention of respiratory distress syndrome. Am J Obstet Gynecol 141:276, 1981

Cone JE: History of the Care and Feeding of the Premature Infant. Boston, Little, Brown, 1985, p 180

Cooper RL, Goldenberg RL, Davis RO, Cutter FR, DuBard MB, Corliss DK, Andrews JB: Warning symptoms, uterine contractions, and cervical examination findings in women at risk of preterm delivery. Am J Obstet Gynecol 162:748, 1990

Cotton DB, Hill LM, Strassner HT, Platt LD, Ledger WJ: Use of amniocentesis in preterm gestation with ruptured membranes. Obstet Gynecol 63:38, 1984a

Cotton DB, Strasner HT, Hill LM, Schifrin BS, Paul RH: Comparison between magnesium sulfate, terbutaline and a placebo for inhibition of preterm labor: A randomized study. J Reprod Med 29:92, 1984b

Covington DL, Carl J, Daley JG, Cushing D, Churchill MP: Effects of the North Carolina Prematurity Program among public patients delivering at New Hanover Memorial Hospital. Am J Public Health 78:1493, 1988

Cox SM, MacDonald PC, Casey ML: Cytokines and prostaglandins in amniotic fluid of preterm labor pregnancies: Decidual origin in response to bacterial toxins [lipopolysaccharide (LPS) and lipotechnoic acid (LTA)]. Abstract presented at the 36th annual meeting of the Society of Gynecologic Investigation, San Diego, March 1989

Cox SM, MacDonald PC, Casey ML: Assay of bacterial endotoxin (lipopolysaccharide) in human amniotic fluid: Potential usefulness in diagnosis and management of preterm labor. Am J Obstet Gynecol 159:99, 1988a

Cox SM, Sherman ML, Leveno KJ: Randomized investigation of magnesium sulfate for prevention of preterm birth. Am J Obstet Gynecol 163:767, 1990

Cox S, Williams ML, Leveno KJ: The natural history of preterm ruptured membranes: What to expect of expectant management. Obstet Gynecol 71:558, 1988b

Crane JP, Kopta MM: Comparative newborn anthropometric data in symmetric versus asymmetric intrauterine growth retardation. Am J Obstet Gynecol 138:518, 1980

Creasy RK, Gummer BA, Liggins GC: System for predicting spontaneous preterm birth. Obstet Gynecol 55:692, 1980

Crowley P, O'Herlihy C, Boylan P: The value of ultrasound measurement of amniotic fluid volume in the management of prolonged pregnancies. Br J Obstet Gynaecol 91:444, 1984

Cummings JJ, D'Eugenio DB, Gross SJ: A controlled trial of dexamethasone in preterm infants at high risk for bronchopulmonary dysplasia. N Engl J Med 320:1505, 1989

Cunningham FG, Cox SM, Harstad TW, Mason RA, Pritchard JA: Chronic renal disease and pregnancy outcome. Am J Obstet Gynecol 163:453, 1990

Danielian PJ, Allman AC, Steer PJ: Is obstetric and neonatal outcome worse in fetuses who fail to reach their own growth potential? Br J Obstet Gynaecol 99:452, 1992

DePalma RT, Leveno KJ, Kelly MA, Sherman ML, Carmody TJ: Birth weight threshold for postponing preterm birth. Am J Obstet Gynecol 167:4, 1992

Devoe LD, Sholl JS: Postdates pregnancy: Assessment of fetal risk and obstetric management. J Reprod Med 28:576, 1983

Dinarello CA, Wolff SM: The role of interleukin-1 in disease. N Engl J Med 328:106, 1993

Divon MY, Chamberlain PF, Lipos L, Manning FA, Platt LD: Identification of the small for gestational age fetus with the use of gestational age-independent indices of fetal growth. Am J Obstet Gynecol 155:1197, 1986

Dougherty CR, Jones AD: The determinants of birth weight. Am J Obstet Gynecol 144:190, 1982

Duscay CA, Thompson JS, Wu AT, Novy MJ: Effects of calcium entry blocker (nicardipine) tocolysis in rhesus macaques: Fetal plasma concentrations and cardiorespiratory changes. Am J Obstet Gynecol 157:1482, 1987

Dyson DC, Crites YM, Ray DA, Armstrong MA: Prevention of preterm birth in high-risk patients: The role of education and provider contact versus home uterine monitoring. Am J Obstet Gynecol 164:756, 1991

Economides DL, Crook D, Nicolaides KH: Hypertriglyceridemia and hypoxemia in small-for-gestational-age fetuses. Am J Obstet Gynecol 162:387, 1990

Economides DL, Nicolaides KH: Blood glucose and oxygen tension levels in small-for-gestational-age fetuses. Am J Obstet Gynecol 160:385, 1989a

Economides DL, Nicolaides KH, Gahl WA, Bernardini I, Bottoms S, Evans M: Cordocentesis in the diagnosis of intrauterine starvation. Am J Obstet Gynecol 161:1004, 1989c

Economides DL, Proudler A, Nicolaides KH: Plasma insulin in appropriate- and small-for gestational-age fetuses. Am J Obstet Gynecol 160:1091, 1989b

Eden RD, Seifert LS, Winegar A, Spellacy WN: Perinatal characteristics of uncomplicated postdate pregnancies. Obstet Gynecol 69:296, 1987

Elliott JP: Magnesium sulfate as a tocolytic agent. Am J Obstet Gynecol 147:277, 1983

Elliott PM, Inman WH: Volume of liquor amnii in normal and abnormal pregnancy. Lancet 2:835, 1961

Emanuel I, Alberman HFE, Evans SJ: Intergenerational studies of human birthweight from the 1958 birth cohort, I. Evidence for a multigenerational effect. Br J Obstet Gynaecol 99:67, 1992

Epstein MF, Nicholls E, Stubblefield PG: Neonatal hypoglycemia after beta-sympathomimetic tocolytic therapy. J Pediatr 94:449, 1979

Eriksen ML, Parisi VM, Daoust S, Flamm B, Garite TJ, Cox SM: Fetal fibronectin: A method for detecting the presence of amnionic fluid. Obstet Gynecol 80:451, 1992

Eronen M, Personen E, Kurki T, Ylikorkala O, Hallman M: The effects of indomethacin and a β-sympathomimetic agent on the fetal ductus arteriosus during treatment of premature labor: A randomized double-blind study. Am J Obstet Gynecol 164:141, 1991

Eschenbach DA, Gibbs RS, Martin DA, Rettig P, Regan J, Rao AY: Infectious and Prematurity Study Group: A randomized, placebo-controlled trial of erythromycin in pregnancy to prevent prematurity. Abstract presented at the 35th annual meeting of the Society for Gynecologic Investigation, Baltimore, March 1988

Escobar GJ: Prognosis of surviving very low-birthweight infants: still in the dark. Br J Obstet Gynaecol 99:1, 1992

Escobar GJ, Littenberg B, Petitti DB: Outcome among surviving very low-birthweight infants: A meta-analysis. Arch Dis Child 66:204, 1991

Feinstein SJ, Vintzileos AM, Lodiero JG, Campbell WA, Weinbaum PJ, Nochimson DJ: Amniocentesis with premature rupture of membranes. Obstet Gynecol 68:147, 1986

Ferguson JE, Dyson DC, Schutz T, Stevenson DK: A comparison of tocolysis with nifedipine or ritodrine: Analysis of efficacy and maternal, fetal, and neonatal outcome. Am J Obstet Gynecol 163:105, 1990

Ferguson JE II, Hensleigh PA, Kredenster D: Adjunctive use of magnesium sulfate with ritodrine for preterm labor tocolysis. Am J Obstet Gynecol 148:166, 1984

Fletcher SE, Fyfe DA, Case CL, Wiles HB, Newman RB, Upshur JK: Myocardial necrosis in a newborn after long-term maternal subcutaneous terbutaline infusion for suppression of preterm labor. Am J Obstet Gynecol 165:1401, 1991

Forman A, Andersson K-E, Ulmsten U: Inhibition of myometrial activity by calcium antagonists. Semin Perinatol 5:288, 1981

France JT, Liggins GC: Placental sulfatase deficiency. J Clin Endocrinol 29:138, 1969

Freeman RK, Garite TJ, Modanlou H, Dorchester W, Rommal C, Devaney M: Postdate pregnancy: Utilization of contraction stress testing for primary fetal surveillance. Am J Obstet Gynecol 140:128, 1981

Frigoletto F: Diagnostic Ultrasound Imaging in Pregnancy. US Department of Health and Human Services, Public Health Service, National Institutes of Health, publication no. 84667, 1986

Galbraith RS, Karchmar EJ, Piercy WN: The clinical prediction of intrauterine growth retardation. Am J Obstet Gynecol 133:281, 1979

Gamsu HR, Mullinger BM, Donnai P, Dash CH: Antenatal administration of betamethasone to prevent respiratory distress syndrome in preterm infants: Report of a UK multicentre trial. Br J Obstet Gynaecol 96:401, 1989

Gardosi J, Chang A, Kalyan B, Sahota D, Symonds EM: Customized antenatal growth charts. Lancet 339:283, 1992

Garite TJ, Freeman RK, Linzey EM, Braly PS: The use of amniocentesis in patients with premature rupture of membranes. Obstet Gynecol 54:226, 1979

Garite TJ, Freeman RK, Linzey EM, Braly PS, Dorchester WL: Prospective randomized study of corticosteroids in the management of premature rupture of the membranes and the premature gestation. Am J Obstet Gynecol 141:508, 1981

Garite TJ, Keegan KA, Freeman RK, Nageotte MP: A randomized trial of ritodrine tocolysis versus expectant management in patients with premature rupture of membranes at 24 to 30 weeks of gestation. Am J Obstet Gynecol 157:388, 1987

Garite TJ, Rumney PJ, Briggs GG, Harding JA, Nageotte MP, Towers CV, Freeman RK: A randomized placebo-controlled trial of betamethasone for the prevention of respiratory distress syndrome at 24 to 28 weeks gestation. Am J Obstet Gynecol 166:646, 1992

Gauthier DW, Meyer WJ, Bieniarz A: Biophysical profile as a predictor of amnionic fluid culture results. Obstet Gynecol 80:102, 1992

Gibbs RS, Romero R, Hillier SL, Eschenbach DA, Sweet RL: A review of premature birth and subclinical infection. Am J Obstet Gynecol 166:1515, 1992

Ginsberg HG, Goldsmith JP, Stedman CM: Survival of a 380-g infant. N Engl J Med 322:1753, 1990

Gluck L: Fetal lung maturity. Paper presented at the 78th Ross Conference on Pediatric Research, San Diego, May 30, 1979

Goldenberg RL, Cutter GR, Hoffman HJ, Foster JM, Nelson KG, Hanth JC: Intrauterine growth retardation: Standards for diagnosis. Am J Obstet Gynecol 161:271, 1989b

Goldenberg RL, Davis RO, Cutter GR, Hoffman HJ, Brumfield CG, Foster JM: Prematurity, postdates, and growth retardation: The influence of use of ultrasonography on reported gestational age. Am J Obstet Gynecol 160:462, 1989a

Goldenberg RL, Nelson KG, Dyer RL, Wayne J: The variability of viability: The effect of physicians' perceptions of viability on the survival of very-low-birth-weight infants. Am J Obstet Gynecol 143:678, 1982

Gonik B, Bottoms SF, Cotton DB: Amniotic fluid volume as a risk factor in preterm premature rupture of the membranes. Obstet Gynecol 65:456, 1985

Granados JL: Survey of the management of postterm pregnancy. Obstet Gynecol 63:651, 1984

Gravett MG, Nelson HP, DeRouen T, Critchlow C, Eschenbach DA, Holmes KK: Independent associations of bacterial vaginosis and Chlamydia trachomatis infection with adverse pregnancy outcome. JAMA 256:1899, 1986

Gray Sheet, vol 16, no 15, April 9, 1990. Published by F-D-C Reports, Chevy Chase, MD 20815

Grimes DA, Schulz KF: Randomized controlled trials of home uterine activity monitoring: A review and critique. Obstet Gynecol 79:137, 1992

Gruenwald P: Chronic fetal distress and placental insufficiency. Biol Neonate 5:215, 1963

Hahn DW, Demarest KT, Ericson E, Homm RE, Capetola RJ, McGuire JL: Evaluation of 1-deamino-[D-Tyr(Oethyl)^2, Thr^4, Orn^8] vasotocin, an oxytocin antagonist, in animal models of uterine contractility and preterm labor: A new tocolytic agent. Am J Obstet Gynecol 157:977, 1987

Hallman M, Bry K, Hopper K, Lappi M, Pohjavuori M: Inosital supplementation in premature infants with respiratory distress syndrome. N Engl J Med 326:1233, 1992

Hankins GDV: Complications of beta-sympathomimetic tocolytic agents. In Clark SL, Cotton DB, Hankins GDV, Phelan JP (eds): Critical Care Obstetrics, 2nd ed. Boston, Blackwell Scientific, 1991, p 231

Hankins GDV, Leveno KJ, Whalley PJ, DePalma RT, Williams ML, Nelson S: Maternal, fetal, neonatal, and infant outcomes with expectant management for preterm rupture of the membranes. Paper presented at the Society of Perinatal Obstetricians, San Antonio, February 2–4, 1984

Hannah ME, Hannah WJ, Hellman J, Hewson S, Milner R, Willan A, Canadian Multicenter Post-Term Pregnancy Trial Group: Induction of labor as compared with serial antenatal monitoring in post-term pregnancy. N Engl J Med 326:1587, 1992

Hanshaw JB: Congenital cytomegalovirus infection: A 15-year prospective study. J Infect Dis 123:555, 1971

Hanson JW, Myrianthopoulas NC, Harvey MAS, Smith DW: Risks to the offspring of women treated with hydantoin anticonvulsants, with emphasis on the fetal hydantoin syndrome. J Pediatr 89:662, 1976

Hanson JW, Streissguth AP, Smith DW: The effects of moderate alcohol consumption during pregnancy on fetal growth and morphogenesis. Pediatrics 92:457, 1978

Hatjis CG, Swain M: Systemic tocolysis for premature labor is associated with an increased incidence of pulmonary edema in the presence of maternal infection. Am J Obstet Gynecol 159:723, 1988

Hatjis CG, Swain M, Nelson LH, Meis PJ, Ernest JM: Efficacy of combined administration of magnesium sulfate and ritodrine in the treatment of premature labor. Obstet Gynecol 69:317, 1987

Hausdorff WP, Caron MG, Lefkowitz RJ: Turning off the signal: Densitization of β-adrenergic receptor function. FASEB J 4:2881, 1990

Hendricks CH: Patterns of fetal and placental growth: The second half of normal pregnancy. Obstet Gynecol 24:357, 1964

Herron MA, Katz M, Creasy RK: Evaluation of a preterm birth

prevention program: Preliminary report. Obstet Gynecol 59:452, 1982

Hesseldahl H: A Danish multicenter study of ritodrine in the treatment of pre-term labor. Danish Med Bull 25:126, 1979

Hillier SL, Martius J, Krohn M, Kiviat N, Holmes KK, Eschenbach DA: A case-control study of chorioamnionic infection and histologic chorioamnionitis in prematurity. N Engl J Med 319:972, 1988

Hoffman HJ, Stark CR, Lunden FE Jr, Ashbrook JD: Analyses of birth weight, gestational age, and fetal viability: U.S. births, 1968. Obstet Gynecol Surv 29:651, 1974

Hollander DI, Nagey DA, Pupkin MJ: Magnesium sulfate and ritodrine hydrochloride: A randomized comparison. Am J Obstet Gynecol 156:631, 1987

Honnebier WJ, Swaab DF: The influence of anencephaly upon intrauterine growth of fetus and placenta and upon gestational length. Br J Obstet Gynaecol 80:577, 1973

Howie RN, Liggins GC: Clinical trial of antepartum betamethasone therapy for prevention of respiratory distress in preterm infants: Proceedings of Fifth Study Group, Royal College of Obstetricians and Gynecologists, October 1977, p 281

Hughey M, Sabbagha RE: Cephalometry by real time imaging: A critical evaluation. Am J Obstet Gynecol 131:825, 1978

Iams JD, Johnson FF, O'Shaughnessy RW, West LC: A prospective random trial of home uterine activity monitoring in pregnancies at increased risk of preterm labor, II. Am J Obstet Gynecol 159:595, 1988

Iams JD, Stilson R, Johnson FF, Williams RA, Rice R: Symptoms that preceed preterm labor and preterm premature rupture of the membranes. Am J Obstet Gynecol 162:486, 1990

Jensen OH, Larsen S: Evaluation of symphysis fundus measurements and weighing during pregnancy. Acta Obstet Gynecol Scand 70:13, 1991

Jimenez JM, Tyson JE, Reisch J: Clinical measurements of gestational age in normal pregnancies. Obstet Gynecol 61:438, 1983

Jones MD Jr, Battaglia FC: Intrauterine growth retardation. Am J Obstet Gynecol 127:540, 1977

Katz AI, Davison JM, Hayslett JP, Singson E, Lindheimer MD: Pregnancy in women with kidney disease. Kidney Int 18:192, 1980

Katz M, Gill PJ, Newman RB: Detection of preterm labor by ambulatory monitoring of uterine activity for the management of oral tocolysis. Am J Obstet Gynecol 154:1253, 1986a

Katz M, Goodyear K, Creasy RK: Early signs and symptoms of preterm labor. Am J Obstet Gynecol 162:1150, 1990

Katz M, Newman RB, Gill PJ: Assessment of uterine activity in ambulatory patients at high risk of preterm labor and delivery. Am J Obstet Gynecol 154:44, 1986b

Kitchen WH, Doyle LW, Rickards AL, Ford G, Kelly E, Callahan C: Survivors of extreme prematurity—outcome at 8 years of age. Aust NZ J Obstet Gynaecol 31:337, 1991

Kitchen WH, Doyle LW, Rickards AL, Permezal MJ, Ford GW, Kelly EA: Changing obstetric practice and two-year outcome of the fetus of birthweight under 1000 g. Obstet Gynecol 79:268, 1992

Konte JM, Creasy RK, Laros RK: California north coast preterm birth prevention project. Obstet Gynecol 71:727, 1988

Koops BL, Morgan LJ, Battaglia FC: Neonatal mortality risk in relation to birthweight and gestational age: Update. J Pediatr 101:969, 1982

Kragt H, Keirse MC: How accurate is a woman's diagnosis of threatened preterm delivery? Br J Obstet Gynaecol 97:317, 1990

Kramer MS: Intrauterine growth and gestational duration determinants. Pediatrics 80:502, 1987

Kubli F: In Anderson A, Beard R, Brudenell JM, Dunn PM (eds): Preterm Labor. London, Royal College of Obstetricians and Gynaecologists, 1977, p 218

Laatikainen TJ, Raisanen IJ, Salminen KR: Corticotropin-releasing hormone in amnionic fluid during gestation and labor and in relation to fetal lung maturation. Am J Obstet Gynecol 59:891, 1988

Lam F, Gill P, Smith M, Kitzmiller JL, Katz M: Use of the subcutaneous terbutaline pump for long-term tocolysis. Obstet Gynecol 72:810, 1988

Larsen JW Jr, Evans MI: Genetic causes. In Lin C-C, Evans MI (eds): Intrauterine Growth Retardation. New York, McGraw-Hill, 1984, p 10

Larsen T, Larsen JF, Petersen S, Greisen G: Detection of small-for-gestation-age fetuses by ultrasound screening in a high risk population: A randomized controlled study. Br J Obstet Gynaecol 99:469, 1992

Lechtig A, Delgado H, Lasky RE, Yarbrough C, Klein RE, Habicht JP, Behar M: Maternal nutrition and fetal growth in developing societies. Am J Dis Child 129:434, 1975

Leigh J, Garite TJ: Amniocentesis and the management of premature labor. Obstet Gynecol 67:500, 1986

Leveno KJ, Cox K, Roark ML: Cervical dilatation and prematurity revisited. Obstet Gynecol 68:434, 1986a

Leveno KJ, Cunningham FG, Roark ML, Nelson SD, Williams ML: Prenatal care and the low birth weight infant. Obstet Gynecol 66:599, 1985a

Leveno KJ, Klein VR, Guzick DS, Young DR, Hankins DV, Williams ML: Single-centre randomised trial of ritodrine hydrochloride for preterm labour. Lancet 1:1293, 1986b

Leveno KJ, Lowe TW, Cunningham FG, Wendel GD, Nelson S: Management of prolonged pregnancy at Parkland Hospital. Proceedings of the Society for Gynecologic Investigation, abstract 290P, Phoenix, AZ, March 1985b

Leveno KJ, Quirk JG, Cunningham FG, Nelson SD, Santos-Ramos R, Toofanian A, DePalma RT: Prolonged pregnancy, I. Observations concerning the causes of fetal distress. Am J Obstet Gynecol 150:465, 1984

Liggins GC, Howie RN: The prevention of RDS by maternal steroid therapy. In Gluck L (ed): Modern Perinatal Medicine. Chicago, Year Book, 1974

Lin CC, Evans MI: Introduction. In Lin C-C, Evans MI (eds): Intrauterine Growth Retardation. New York, McGraw-Hill, 1984

Lirette M, Holbrook RH, Katz M: Cardiovascular and uterine blood flow changes during nicardipine HC1 tocolysis in the rabbit. Obstet Gynecol 69:79, 1987

Lockwood CJ, Senyei AE, Dische MR, Casal D, Shah KD, Thung SN, Jones L, Deligdisch L, Garite TJ: Fetal fibronectin in cervical and vaginal secretions as a predictor of preterm delivery. N Engl J Med 325:669, 1991

Lubchenco LO, Hansman C, Dressler M, Boyd E: Intrauterine growth as estimated from liveborn birth-weight data at 24 to 42 weeks of gestation. Pediatrics 32:793, 1963

MacDonald PC, Siiteri PK: Origin of estrogen in women pregnant with an anencephalic fetus. J Clin Invest 44:465, 1965

Main DM, Richardson DK, Hadley CB, Gabbe SG: Controlled trial of a preterm labor detection program: Efficacy and costs. Obstet Gynecol 74:873, 1989

Malloy MH, Rhoads GG, Schramm W, Land G: Increasing cesarean section rates in very-low-birthweight infants. JAMA 262:1475, 1989

Manning FA, Hohler C: Intrauterine growth retardation: diagnosis, prognostication, and management based on ultrasound methods. In Fleisher AC, Romero R, Manning FA, Jeanty P, James AE (eds): The Principles and Practices of Ultrasonography in Obstetrics and Gynecology, 4th ed. Norwalk, CT, Appleton & Lange, 1991, p 331

McCormack WM, Rosner B, Lee Y-H, Munoz A, Charles D, Kass EH: Effect on birth weight of erythromycin treatment of pregnant women. Obstet Gynecol 69:202, 1987

McCormick MC: The contribution of low birthweight to infant mortality and childhood morbidity. N Engl J Med 312:82, 1985

McGregor JA, French JI, Lawellin D, Franco-Buff A, Smith C, Todd JK: Bacterial protease-induced reduction of chorioamniotic membrane strength and elasticity. Obstet Gynecol 69:167, 1987

McGregor JA, French JI, Richter R, Vuchetich M, Bachus V, Franco-Buff A, Hillier S, Todd JK: Prospective, double-blinded, randomized, placebo-controlled trial of short-course erythromycin (E) base in women at high risk for preterm birth. Abstract 62 presented at the 35th annual meeting of the Society for Gynecologic Investigation, Baltimore, March 1988

Medearis AL: Postterm pregnancy: Active labor induction (PGE$_2$ gel) not associated with improved outcomes compared to expectant management. A preliminary report. Abstract 13 presented at 10th Annual Meeting of the NICHD Maternal Fetal Medicine Units, Network Society of Perinatal Obstetricians, Houston, January 23–27, 1990

Melin P, Trojnar J, Johansson B, Vilhardt H, Akerlund M: Synthetic antagonists of the myometrial response to oxytocin and vasopressin. J Endocrinol 111:125, 1986

Merkatz IR, Peter JB, Barden TP: Ritodrine hydrochloride: A betamimetic agent for use in preterm labor. II. Evidence of efficacy. Obstet Gynecol 56:7, 1980

Meyer MB: How does maternal smoking affect birth weight and maternal weight gain? Am J Obstet Gynecol 131:888, 1978

Miller J, Kho MS, Brown HL, Gabert HA: Clinical chorioamnionitis is not predicted by an ultrasonic biophysical profile in patients with premature rupture of membranes. Obstet Gynecol 76:1051, 1990

Minkoff H, Grunebaum AN, Schwarz RH, Feldman J, Cummings M, Crombleholme W, Clark L, Pringle G, McCormack WM: Risk factors for prematurity and premature rupture of membranes: A prospective study of the vaginal flora in pregnancy. Am J Obstet Gynecol 150:965, 1984

Morales WJ: The effect of chorioamnionitis on the developmental outcome of preterm infants at one year. Obstet Gynecol 70:183, 1987

Morales WJ, Angel JL, O'Brien WF, Knuppel RA: Use of ampicillin and corticosteroids in premature rupture of membranes: A randomized study. Obstet Gynecol 73:721, 1989

Moretti M, Sibai BM: Maternal and perinatal outcome of expectant management of premature rupture of membranes in the midtrimester. Am J Obstet Gynecol 159:390, 1988

Morrison JC, Martin JN Jr, Martin RW, Gookin KS, Wiser WL: Prevention of preterm birth by ambulatory assessment of uterine activity: A randomized study. Am J Obstet Gynecol 156:536, 1987

Mou SM, Sunderji SG, Gall S, How H, Patel V, Gray M, Kayne HL, Corwin M: Multicenter randomized clinical trial of home uterine activity monitoring for detection of preterm labor. Am J Obstet Gynecol 165:858, 1991

Mueller-Heubach E, Guzick DS: Evaluation of risk scoring in a preterm birth prevention study of indigent patients. Am J Obstet Gynecol 160:829, 1989

Munster K, Schmidt L, Helm P: Length and variation in the menstrual cycle—a cross-sectional study from a Danish county. Br J Obstet Gynaecol 99:422, 1992

Murray C, Haverkamp AD, Orleans M, Berga S, Pecht D: Nifedipine for treatment of preterm labor: A historic prospective study. Am J Obstet Gynecol 167:52, 1992

Myers SA, Ferguson R: A population study of the relationship between fetal death and altered fetal growth. Obstet Gynecol 74:325, 1989

Naeye RL, Dixon JB: Distortions in fetal growth standards. Pediatr Res 12:987, 1978

Naeye RL, Kelly JA: Judgement of fetal age. III. The pathologists' evaluation. Pediatr Clin North Am 13:849, 1966

Neilson JP, Verkuyl DAA, Crowther CA, Bannerman C: Preterm labor in twin pregnancies: Prediction by cervical assessment. Obstet Gynecol 72:719, 1988

Nelson LH, Meis PJ, Hatjis CG, Ernest JM, Dillard R, Schey HM: Premature rupture of membranes: A prospective, randomized evaluation of steroids, latent phase, and expectant management. Obstet Gynecol 66:55, 1985

Newman RB, Gill PJ, Wittreich P, Katz M: Maternal perception of prelabor uterine activity. Obstet Gynecol 68:765, 1986

O'Brien GD, Queenan JT, Campbell S: Assessment of gestational age in the second trimester by real-time ultrasound measurement of the femur length. Am J Obstet Gynecol 139:540, 1981

Ohlsson A, Wang E: An analysis of antenatal tests to detect infections in preterm premature rupture of the membranes. Am J Obstet Gynecol 162:809, 1990

Ounsted M, Moar VA, Scott A: Children of deviant birthweight: The influence of genetic and other factors on size at seven years. Acta Paediatr Scand 74:707, 1985

Owen J, Baker SL, Hauth JC, Goldenberg RL, Davis RO, Copper RL: Is indicated or spontaneous preterm delivery more advantageous for the fetus? Am J Obstet Gynecol 163:868, 1990a

Owen J, Goldenberg RL, Davis RO, Kirk KA, Copper RL: Evaluation of a risk scoring system as a predictor of preterm birth in an indigent population. Am J Obstet Gynecol 163:873, 1990b

Papiernik E, Bouyer J, Collin D, Winisdoerffer G, Dreyfus J: Precocious cervical ripening and preterm labor. Obstet Gynecol 67:238, 1986

Papiernik E, Kaminski M: Multifactorial study of the risk of prematurity at 32 weeks of gestation: A study for the frequency of 30 predictive characteristics. J Perinat Med 2:30, 1974

Parisi V, Salina J, Stockman E: Fetal cardiorespiratory responses to maternal administration of nicardipine in the hypertensive ewe. Abstract presented at meeting of the Society of

Perinatal Obstetricians, San Antonio, January 30–February 1, 1986

Patterson RM, Gibbs CE, Wood RC: Birthweight percentile and perinatal outcome: Recurrence of intrauterine growth retardation. Obstet Gynecol 68:464, 1986

Patterson RM, Prihoda JJ, Gibbs CE, Wood RC: Analysis of birthweight percentile as a prediction of perinatal outcome. Obstet Gynecol 68:459, 1986

Patterson RM, Prihoda TJ, Pouliot MR: Sonographic amniotic fluid measurements and fetal growth retardation: A reappraisal. Am J Obstet Gynecol 157:1406, 1987

Pearce JMF, Campbell S: Intrauterine growth retardation: Birth Defects 21:109, 1985

Perelman RH, Farrell PM, Engle MJ, Kemnitz JW: Development aspects of lung lipids. Ann Rev Physiol 47:803, 1985

Persson PH, Grennert L, Gennser G: Impact of fetal and maternal factors on the normal growth of biparietal diameter. Acta Obstet Gynecol Scand 78(suppl):21, 1978a

Persson PH, Grennert L, Gennser G: Diagnosis of intrauterine growth retardation by serial ultrasound cephalometry. Acta Obstet Gynaecol Scand 78(suppl):40, 1978b

Phelan JP, Platt LD, Yeh SY, Boussard P, Paul RH: The role of ultrasound assessment of amniotic fluid volume in the management of the postdate pregnancy. Am J Obstet Gynecol 151:304, 1985

Phelan JP, Platt LD, Yeh SY, Trujillo M, Paul RH: Continuing role of the nonstress test in the management of postdates pregnancy. Obstet Gynecol 64:624, 1984

Philipson EH, Sokol RJ, Williams MA: Oligohydramnios: Clinical associations and predictive value for intrauterine growth retardation. Am J Obstet Gynecol 146:271, 1983

Quirk JG, Raker RK, Petrie RH, Williams AM: The role of glucocorticoids, unstressful labor, and atraumatic delivery in the prevention of respiratory distress syndrome. Am J Obstet Gynecol 1134:768, 1979

Read MD, Wellby DE: The use of a calcium antagonist (nifedipine) to suppress preterm labor. Br J Obstet Gynaecol 93:933, 1986

Rhoads GG, McNellis DC, Kessel SS: Home monitoring of uterine contractility. Summary of a workshop sponsored by the National Institute of Child Health and Human Development. Am J Obstet Gynecol 165:2, 1991

Robertson PA, Laros RK, Heilbron D, Iams JD, Sniderman SH, Cowan R, Goldenberg RL, Creasy RK: Neonatal morbidity according to gestational age and birthweight from five tertiary care centers in the United States, 1983 through 1988. Am J Obstet Gynecol 166:1679, 1992

Robertson WB, Brosens I, Dixon G: Maternal uterine vascular lesions in the hypertensive complications of pregnancy. In Lindheimer M, Katz A, Zuspan F (eds): Hypertension in Pregnancy. New York, Wiley, 1975

Robinson HP, Fleming JEE: A critical evaluation of sonar crown–rump length measurements. Br J Obstet Gynaecol 82:702, 1975

Romero R, Kadar N, Hobbins JC, Duff GW: Infection and labor: The detection of endotoxin in amniotic fluid. Am J Obstet Gynecol 157:815, 1987

Romero R, Roslansky P, Oyarzun E, Wan M, Emamian M, Novitsky TJ, Gould MJ, Hobbins JC: Labor and infection. II. Bacterial endotoxin in amniotic fluid and its relationship to the onset of preterm labor. Am J Obstet Gynecol 158:1044, 1988

Ryan KJ: Placental synthesis of steroid hormones. In Tulchinsky D, Ryan KJ (eds): Maternal–Fetal Endocrinology. Philadelphia, Saunders, 1980

Sachs BP, Hellerstein S, Freeman R, Frigoletto F, Hauth JC: Home monitoring of uterine activity. Does it prevent prematurity? N Engl J Med 325:1374, 1991

Savitz DA, Blackmore CH, Thorp JM: Epidemiologic characteristics of preterm delivery: Etiologic heterogeneity. Am J Obstet Gynecol 164:467, 1991

Sawaya GF, Robertson PA: Hepatotoxicity with the administration of nifedipine for treatment of preterm labor. Am J Obstet Gynecol 167:512, 1992

Schwarz BE, Schultz FM, MacDonald PC: Initiation of human parturition, IV. Demonstration of phospholipase A_2 in the lysosomes of human fetal membranes. Am J Obstet Gynecol 125:1089, 1976

Schweitzer JL: Infection of neonates and infants with the hepatitis B virus. Prog Med Virol 20:27, 1975

Semchyshyn S, Zuspan FP, O'Shaughnessy R: Pulmonary edema associated with the use of hydrocortisone and a tocolytic agent for the management of premature labor. J Reprod Med 28:47, 1983

Shime J, Gare DJ, Andrews J, Bertrand M, Salgado J, Whillans G: Prolonged pregnancy: Surveillance of the fetus and the neonate and the course of labor and delivery. Am J Obstet Gynecol 148:547, 1984

Sholl JS, Sabbagha RE: Ultrasound detection. In Lin C-C, Evans MI (eds): Intrauterine Growth Retardation. New York, McGraw-Hill, 1984

Silver RK, Dooley SL, Tamura RK, Depp R: Umbilical cord size and amniotic fluid volume in prolonged pregnancy. Am J Obstet Gynecol 157:716, 1987

Simpson GF, Harbert GM Jr: Use of beta-methasone in management of preterm gestation with premature rupture of membranes. Am J Obstet Gynecol 66:168, 1985

Simpson JW, Lawless RW, Mitchell AC: Responsibility of the obstetrician to the fetus: II. Influence of prepregnancy weight and pregnancy weight gain on birth weight. Obstet Gynecol 45:481, 1975

Smith LG, Burns PA, Schanker RJ: Calcium homeostasis in pregnant women receiving long-term magnesium sulfate therapy for preterm labor. Am J Obstet Gynecol 167:45, 1992

Smyth CN: The guard-ring tocodynamometer: Absolute measurement of intra-amniotic pressure by a new instrument. J Obstet Gynaecol Br Commonw 64:59, 1957

Sokol RJ, Miller SI, Reed G: Alcohol abuse during pregnancy: An epidemiologic study. Alcoholism 4:135, 1980

Soothill PW, Nicolaides KH, Campbell S: Prenatal asphyxia, hyperlacticaemia, hypoglycaemia and erythroblastosis in growth retarded fetuses. BMJ 294:1046, 1987

Spisso KR, Harbert GM Jr, Thiagarajah S: The use of magnesium sulfate as the primary tocolytic agent to prevent premature delivery. Am J Obstet Gynecol 142:840, 1982

Stagno S, Reynolds DW, Hwang ES: Congenital cytomegalovirus infection. N Engl J Med 296:1254, 1977

Steer CM, Petrie RH: A comparison of magnesium sulfate and alcohol for the prevention of premature labor. Am J Obstet Gynecol 129:1, 1977

Stein Z, Susser M, Saenger G, Marolla F: Famine and Human Development: The Dutch Hunger Winter of 1944–1945. New York, Oxford University Press, 1975

Stone ML, Salerno LJ, Greene M, Zelson C: Narcotic addiction in pregnancy. Am J Obstet Gynecol 109:716, 1971

Stubbs TM, Van Dorsten P, Miller MC: The preterm cervix and preterm labor: Relative risks, predictive values, and change over time. Am J Obstet Gynecol 155:829, 1986

Ulmsten U, Andersson K-E, Wingerup L: Treatment of premature labor with the calcium antagonist nifedipine. Arch Gynecol 229:1, 1980

Unger C, Weiser JK, McCullough RE, Keefer S, Moore LG: Altitude, low birth weight, and infant mortality in Colorado. JAMA 259:3427, 1988

Usher R, McLean F: Intrauterine growth of live-born caucasian infants at sea level: Standards obtained from measurements in 7 dimensions of infants born between 25 and 44 weeks gestation. J Pediatr 74:901, 1969

Uzan S, Beaufils M, Breart G, Bazin B, Capitont C, Paris J: Prevention of fetal growth retardation with low-dose aspirin: Findings of the EPREDA trial. Lancet 337:1427, 1991

Van den Hof MC, Nicolaides KH: Platelet count in normal, small, and anemic fetuses. Am J Obstet Gynecol 162:730, 1990

Van Marter LJ, Leviton A, Kuban KC, Pagano M, Allred EN: Maternal glucocorticoid therapy and reduced risk of bronchopulmonary dysplasia. Pediatrics 86:331, 1990

Varner MW, Galask RP: Infectious causes. In Lin C-C and Evans MI (eds): Intrauterine Growth Retardation. New York, McGraw-Hill, 1984

Villar J, deOnis M, Kestler E, Bolanos F, Cerezo R, Bernedes H: The differential neonatal morbidity of the intrauterine growth retardation syndrome. Am J Obstet Gynecol 163:151, 1990

Vintzileos AM, Campbell WA, Nochimson DJ, Connolly ME, Fuenfer MM, Hoehn GJ: The fetal biophysical profile in patients with premature rupture of membranes—an early predictor of fetal infection. Am J Obstet Gynecol 152:510, 1985

Vintzileos AM, Campbell WA, Nochimson DJ, Weinbaum PJ: Preterm premature rupture of the membranes: A risk factor for the development of abruptio placentae. Am J Obstet Gynecol 156:1235, 1987

Vintzileos AM, Campbell WA, Nochimson DJ, Weinbaum PJ, Escoto DT, Mirochnick MH: Qualitative amniotic fluid volume versus amniocentesis in predicting infection in preterm premature rupture of the membranes. Obstet Gynecol 67:579, 1986

Visser GH, Huisman A, Saathof PW, Sinnige HA: Early fetal growth retardation: Obstetric background and recurrence rate. Obstet Gynecol 67:40, 1986

Visser GH, Sadovsky G, Nicolaides KH: Antepartum heart rate patterns in small-for-gestational-age third-trimester fetuses: Correlations with blood gas values obtained at cordocentesis. Am J Obstet Gynecol 162:698, 1990

Vohr BR, Oh W: Growth and development in preterm infants small for gestational age. J Pediatr 103:941, 1983

Vohr BR, Oh W, Rosenfield AG, Cowett RM, Berstein J: The preterm small-for-gestational-age infant: A two-year follow-up study. Am J Obstet Gynecol 133:425, 1979

Wald NJ, Cuckle HS, Boreham J, Althouse R: Birthweight of infants with spina bifida cystica. Br J Obstet Gynaecol 87:578, 1980

Walker D-JB, Feldman A, Vohr BR, Oh W: Cost–benefit analysis of neonatal intensive care for infants weighing less than 1,000 grams at birth. Pediatrics 74:20, 1984

Wallenburg HCS, Rotmans N: Prevention of recurrent idiopathic fetal growth retardation by low-dose aspirin and dipyridamole. Am J Obstet Gynecol 157:1230, 1987

Warkany JB, Monroe B, Sutherland BS: Intrauterine growth retardation. Am J Dis Child 102:24, 1961

Waterson AP: Virus infections (other than rubella) during pregnancy. BMJ 2:564, 1979

Wennergren M, Wennergren G, Vilbergsson G: Obstetric characteristics and neonatal performance in a four-year small for gestational age population. Obstet Gynecol 72:615, 1988

Wilkins IA, Lynch L, Mehalek KE, Berkowitz GS, Berkowitz RL: Efficacy and side effects of magnesium sulfate and ritodrine as tocolytic agents. Am J Obstet Gynecol 159:685, 1988

Wilson L Jr, Parsons MT, Ouano L, Flouret G: A new tocolytic agent: Development of an oxytocin antagonist for inhibiting uterine contractions. Am J Obstet Gynecol 163:195, 1990

Zahn V: Die Kontrole der Tokolyse durch ambulante Wehenmessung. In Dudenhausen JW, Saling E (eds): Perinatale Medizin. Stuttgart, George Ghieme, 1973, p 57

Zuckerman H, Reiss U, Robenstin I: Inhibition of human premature labor by indomethacin. Obstet Gynecol 44:787, 1974

CHAPTER 39
Multifetal Pregnancy

Morbidity and mortality are appreciably increased in pregnancies with multiple fetuses. It is not an overstatement, therefore, to consider a pregnancy with multiple fetuses to be a complicated pregnancy. Many of the complications more commonly encountered with multiple fetuses are:

1. Abortion
2. Perinatal mortality
3. Low birthweight
   Preterm delivery
   Fetal growth retardation
4. Malformations
5. Fetal–fetal hemorrhage
   Hypovolemia and anemia
   Hypervolemia and hyperviscosity
   Cerebral injury
6. Pregnancy-induced or aggravated hypertension
7. Maternal anemia
   Acute blood loss
   Iron deficiency
   Folate deficiency
8. Placental accidents
   Placental abruption
   Placenta previa
9. Other maternal hemorrhage
   Uterine atony
   Cesarean section
10. Cord accidents
    Prolapse
    Entwinement
    Vasa previa
11. Hydramnios
12. Complicated labor
    Preterm labor
    Ineffective labor
13. Abnormal fetal presentation

Etiology of Multiple Fetuses

Twin fetuses more commonly result from fertilization of two separate ova, that is, double-ovum, dizygotic, or "fraternal" twins. About one third as often twins arise from a single fertilized ovum that subsequently divides into two similar structures, each with the potential for developing into a separate individual, that is, single-ovum, monozygotic, or "identical" twins. Either or both processes may be involved in the formation of higher numbers of fetuses. Quadruplets, for example, may arise from one to four ova.

Fraternal Versus Identical Twins. Dizygotic twins are not in a strict sense true twins because they result from the maturation and fertilization of two ova during a single ovulatory cycle. Newman (1923) wrote: "Strictly speaking, twainning is twinning or twoing—the division of an individual into two equivalent and more or less completely separate individuals." Also, monozygotic or identical twins are not always identical. As discussed subsequently, the process of division of one fertilized zygote into two does not necessarily result in equal sharing of protoplasmic materials. In fact, dizygotic, or fraternal twins of the same sex, may *appear* more nearly identical at birth than do monozygotic twins; growth of monozygotic twin fetuses may be discordant and at times dramatically so.

Genesis of Monozygotic Twins. Valid hypotheses to explain single-ovum, or monozygotic, twinning are lacking. Monozygotic twins arise from division of the fertilized ovum at various early stages of development as follows:

1. If division occurs before the inner cell mass is formed and the outer layer of blastocyst is not yet committed to become chorion—that is, within the first 72 hours after fertilization—two embryos, two amnions, and two chorions will develop. There will evolve a *diamnionic, dichorionic,* monozygotic twin pregnancy. The frequency of two chorions with monozygotic twinning in various reports has ranged from 18 to 36 percent (MacGillivray, 1978). There may be two distinct placentas or a single fused placenta, as depicted in Figure 39–1A and B respectively.
2. If division occurs between the fourth and eighth day, after the inner cell mass is formed and cells destined to become chorion have already differentiated but those of the amnion have not, two embryos will develop, each in separate amnionic sacs. The two amnionic sacs will eventually be covered by a common chorion, thus giving rise to *diamnionic, monochorionic,* monozygotic twin pregnancy (Fig. 39–1C).
3. If, however, the amnion has already become established, which occurs about 8 days after fer-

Fig. 39–1. Placenta and membranes in twin pregnancies. **A.** Two placentas, two amnions, two chorions (from either dizygotic twins or monozygotic twins with cleavage of zygote during first 3 days after fertilization). **B.** Single placenta, two amnions, and two chorions (from either dizygotic twins or monozygotic twins with cleavage of zygote during first 3 days). **C.** One placenta, one chorion, two amnions (monozygotic twins with cleavage of zygote from the fourth to the eighth day after fertilization).

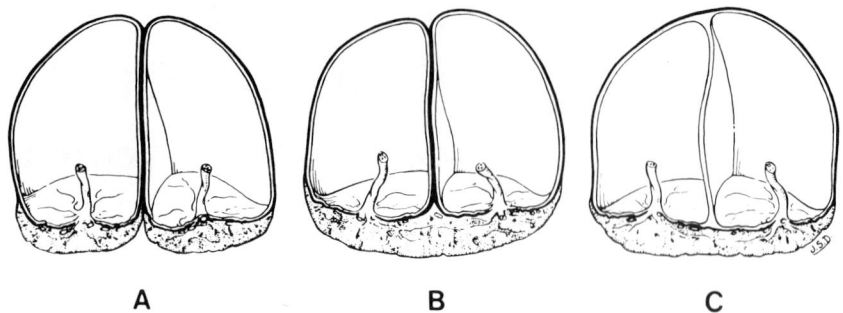

A   B   C

tilization, division will result in two embryos within a common amnionic sac, or *a monoamnionic, monochorionic,* monozygotic twin pregnancy.

4. If division is initiated even later—that is, after the embryonic disk is formed—cleavage is incomplete and conjoined twins are formed.

Frequency of Twins. The frequency of **monozygotic twinning** is relatively constant worldwide at approximately one set per 250 births and is largely independent of race, heredity, age, and parity. Until recently the frequency was thought to be independent of therapy for infertility; however, there is now evidence that the incidence of zygotic splitting is doubled following ovulation induction (Derom and colleagues, 1987). The incidence of **dizygotic twinning** is influenced remarkably by race, heredity, maternal age, parity, and especially, fertility drugs. The epidemiology of multifetal pregnancy was reviewed by MacGillivray (1986).

It is now apparent that the incidence of twin conceptions is much higher than indicated by figures based on the delivery of two fetuses. Robinson and Caines (1977), for example, by means of ultrasound performed during the first trimester, identified twin conceptions in 30 women, only 14 of whom eventually gave birth to two infants. Another 11 were delivered of a single fetus and a blighted ovum, four were diagnosed as having twin blighted ova, and one a blighted ovum and a missed abortion. Varma (1979) and others reported similar data. Undoubtedly, some "threatened" abortions have resulted in actual abortion of one embryo from an unrecognized twin gestation while the other embryo continued its growth and development (Jauniaux and coworkers, 1988).

Remarkably, fetal death as late as the end of the first trimester can be followed by complete fetal resorption, leaving no gross evidence at delivery that twins ever existed. Sonographic demonstration of such a case is presented in Figure 39–2.

Multiple embryos and fetuses may develop in varying degrees ectopically—that is, outside the uterus. Such multiple ectopic pregnancies, as well as *combined preg-*

nancies in which there are one or more embryos or fetuses extrauterine as well as one or more intrauterine, are considered in Chapter 32 (p. 697).

Race. The frequency of multiple fetal births varies significantly among different races (Table 39–1). For example, Myrianthopoulos (1970) identified in the Collaborative Cerebral Palsy Study the birth of twins in 1 of every 100 pregnancies among white women, compared with 1 out of 80 pregnancies for black women. In some areas of Africa the frequency of twinning is very high. Knox and Morley (1960), in a survey of one rural community in Nigeria, found that twinning occurred once in every 20 births! Twinning among Orientals is less common. In Japan, for example, among more than 10 million pregnancies analyzed, twinning was identified only once in every 155 births. These marked racial differences are the consequence of variations in the frequency of dizygotic twinning.

Heredity. As a determinant of twinning, the genotype of the mother is much more important than that of the father. White and Wyshak (1964), in a study of 4000 records of the General Society of the Church of Jesus Christ of Latter-day Saints, found that women who themselves were a dizygotic twin gave birth to twins at the rate of 1 set per 58 births. However, women not a twin but whose husbands were a dizygotic twin gave birth to twins at the rate of 1 set per 126 pregnancies. Bulmer (1960) reported that 1 out of 25 (4 percent) of twin's mothers was also a twin but only 1 out of 60 (1.7 percent) of their fathers was a twin.

Maternal Age and Parity. The positive effects of increasing maternal age and parity on the incidence of twinning have been well demonstrated by Waterhouse (1950). For any increase in age up to about 40, or parity up to 7, the frequency of twinning increased. Twin pregnancies were less than one third as common in women under 20 with no previous children than in women 35 to 40 years of age with four or more previous children. In Sweden, Pettersson and associates (1976) confirmed the remarkable increase in multiple birth rate associated with increased parity. In first pregnancies the frequency

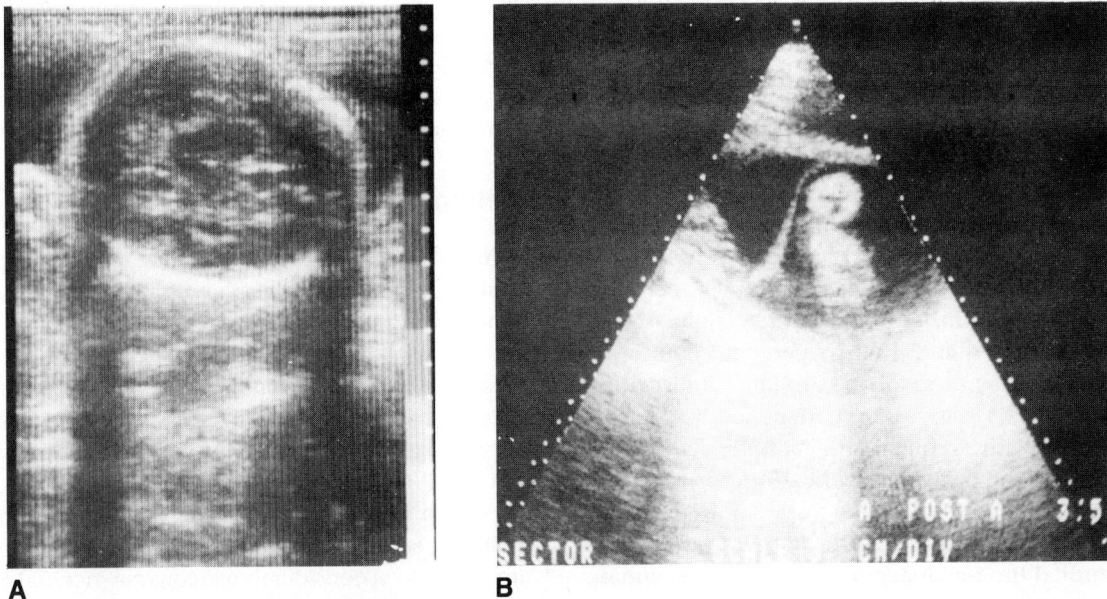

Fig. 39–2. Sonography at 27 weeks identified an appropriately grown fetus whose head is demonstrated in **A** accompanied by a gestational sac containing a dead 12-week fetus as estimated by crown-rump length in **B**. Four weeks later appropriate growth of one fetal head was ascertained and resorption of the dead fetus had occurred leaving an empty gestational sac. Three weeks later that sac was no longer visible sonographically and at delivery 1 week later no gross evidence of twins was found. (Courtesy of Dr. R. Santos.)

of multiple fetuses was 1.3 percent, compared with 2.7 percent in the fourth birth order.

In Nigeria, Azubuike (1982) identified the frequency of twinning to increase from 1 in 50 (2 percent) pregnancies among women pregnant for the first time to 1 in 15 (6.6 percent) for women pregnant six or more times!

Maternal Size. Dizygotic twinning is more common in large and tall women than in small women (MacGillivray, 1986). This may be related more to nutrition than to body size alone. During World War II, the incidence of dizygous twinning decreased in Europe when food deprivation was common. Even so, those women who had twins apparently did not consume more calories than those with singletons (Bulmer, 1959).

TABLE 39–1. TWINNING RATES PER 1000 BIRTHS BY ZYGOSITY

Country	Monozygotic	Dizygotic	Total
Nigeria	5.0	49	54
United States			
Black	4.7	11.1	15.8
White	4.2	7.1	11.3
England and Wales	3.5	8.8	12.3
India (Calcutta)	3.3	8.1	11.4
Japan	3.0	1.3	4.3

From MacGillivray (1986), with permission.

Endogenous Gonadotropin. Benirschke and Kim (1973) presented intriguing reasons for implicating elevated levels of endogenous follicle-stimulating hormone in the genesis of spontaneous dizygous twinning. A higher rate of dizygous twinning has been described for women who conceive within 1 month after stopping oral contraceptives, but not during subsequent months (Rothman, 1977). One possibility to account for the apparent increase is release of pituitary gonadotropin in amounts greater than usual during the first spontaneous cycle after stopping contraception. Another is increased fecundity among very recent users of oral contraceptives.

Infertility Agents. The number of triplets and higher-order multiple births increased dramatically (113 percent) in the United States between 1972 and 1989 (Kiely and co-authors, 1992). For example, an average of 930 per year higher-order multiple births was found in the early 1970s compared with 2150 per year in the late 1980s. Much of the increase in higher-order births has been observed in white women 30 through 39 years of age and is attributed to treatment of infertility.

The induction of ovulation by use of gonadotropins (follicle-stimulating hormone plus chorionic gonadotropin) or of clomiphene enhances remarkably the likelihood of multiple ovulations. The incidence of multiple fetuses following gonadotropin therapy is 20 to 40 percent, and in one instance as many as 11 fetuses were aborted (Jewelewicz and Vande Wiele, 1975). Nonuplet pregnancy with spontaneous labor 27 weeks after ovulation induction with human pituitary gonadotropin has been described by Garrett and associates (1976). None of the nine infants survived. Two of octuplets survived in Italy. Sextuplets after gonadotropin therapy survived in South Africa, as did five of the sextuplets born in Denver.

With clomiphene therapy, the likelihood of multiple fetuses is somewhat less than with human menopausal gonadotropin. Even so, among nearly 2400 conceptions following clomiphene, 165 (7 percent) were known to be twin, 11 (0.5 percent) triplet, 7 (0.3 percent) quadruplet, and 3 (0.13 percent) quintuplet (Merrell–National Laboratories Product Information Bulletin, 1972.) Harlap (1976) identified in smaller groups in Israel the frequency of multiple fetuses following clomiphene treatment to be 13 percent.

Ovulation induction likely increases both dizygotic and monozygotic twinning. Derom and colleagues (1987) studied the incidence of monozygotic twinning in almost 1000 twin-pairs delivered in East Flanders, Belgium, and reported that the incidence of zygotic splitting was doubled after induced ovulation. They also reported an alarming increase in monochorionic twinning in monozygotes conceived following induced ovulation.

IN VITRO FERTILIZATION. Twinning is more common in pregnancies that result from in vitro fertilization. The practice of some groups of attempting fertilization of all the ova collected after inducing superovulation and then depositing in utero more than one blastocyst when available accounts, in part at least, for the increased frequency of multifetal pregnancies (Bradshaw and colleagues, 1992). Liveborn quadruplets have been delivered in Australia and elsewhere following in vitro fertilization. Andrews and colleagues (1986) described their experiences with pregnancies resulting from in vitro fertilization performed at the Jones Institute for Reproductive Medicine. The average number of conceptuses transferred was three and there were 125 consecutive pregnancies that resulted. Excluding 30 preclinical pregnancies and 23 early abortions, 37 percent of pregnancies were multiple before 12 weeks, but by delivery only 22 percent were multiple. Thus, only about half of multiple pregnancies progressed to viability. In 10 of these 12 cases, reduction was accompanied by vaginal bleeding.

Sex Ratios with Multiple Fetuses. The percentage of male conceptuses in the human species decreases as the number of fetuses per pregnancy increases. Strandskov and co-workers (1946) found the sex ratio, or percentage of males, for 31 million singleton births in the United States to be 51.6 percent. For twins it was 50.9 percent; for triplets, 49.5 percent; and for quadruplets, 46.5 percent. Two explanations have been offered. First, the differential fetal mortality between the sexes is well known, as it is for the newborn infant, child, and adult. Survival is always in favor of the female and against the

male. The "population pressure" with multiple fetuses in utero may exaggerate the biological tendency noted in singleton pregnancies. A second possible explanation is that the female-producing zygote has a greater tendency to divide into twins, triplets, and quadruplets.

Determination of Zygosity

With the advent of organ transplantation, the zygosity of multiple fetuses from a single pregnancy has assumed more than theoretical importance.

Examination of Placenta. A knowledgeably performed examination of the placenta and membranes serves to establish zygosity promptly in about two thirds of cases (Benirschke and Kim, 1973). Moreover, it often serves to identify the zygosity of fetuses more firmly than do subsequent studies, which yield less precise information at considerable inconvenience and expense.

The following system for examination is recommended. As the first infant is delivered, one clamp is placed on the portion of the cord coming from the placenta. As the second infant is delivered, two clamps are placed on the cord toward the placental side. Three clamps are used to mark the cord of a third infant, and so on as necessary. Until the delivery of the last fetus is completed, it is important that each segment of cord attached to the placenta remain clamped lest fetal hemorrhage continues through anastomosed fetal vessels in the placenta.

Delivery of the placenta should be accomplished with care to preserve the attachment of the amnion and chorion to the placenta because identification of the relationship of the membranes to each other is critical. With one common amnionic sac, which is a rare finding, or with juxtaposed amnions not separated by chorion arising between the fetuses, the infants are monozygotic. If adjacent amnions are separated by chorion, the fetuses may be monozygotic, but more often are dizygotic (Figs. 39–1, 39–3, and 39–4). If the infants are of the same sex, blood group studies to identify zygosity may be initiated at this time on samples of blood obtained from the umbilical cords. A difference in major blood groups is indicative of dizygosity. If these simple procedures fail to identify zygosity, more complicated techniques, such as DNA "fingerprinting," can be used to look for differences. Azuma and associates (1989) and Kovacs and co-workers (1988) reported such DNA fingerprinting to be sufficiently reliable for molecular genetic determination of twin zygosity. Moreover, the method is rapid, permitting same-day results.

Sex and Zygosity. Although twins of opposite sex are almost always dizygotic, monozygotic twins rarely may be discordant for phenotypic sex. Schmidt and co-workers (1974), for example, described adolescent twins in whom concordance for 22 blood groups and

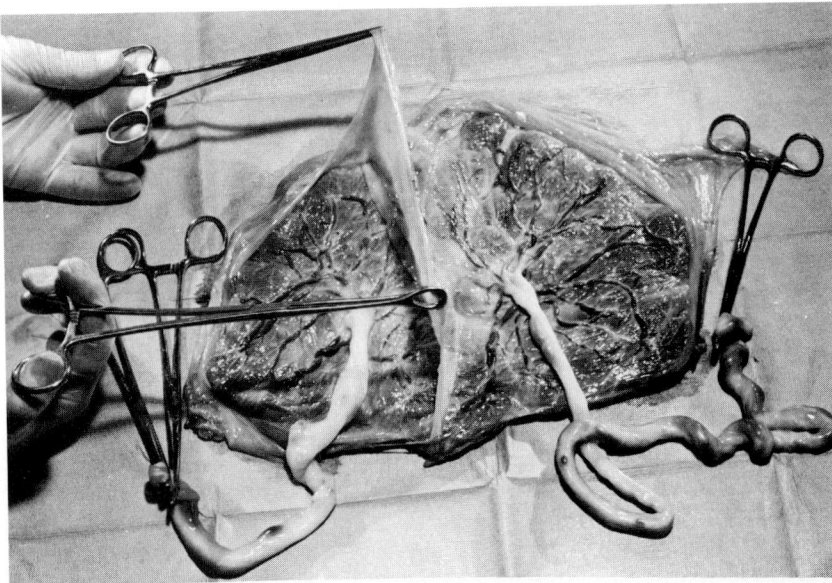

A

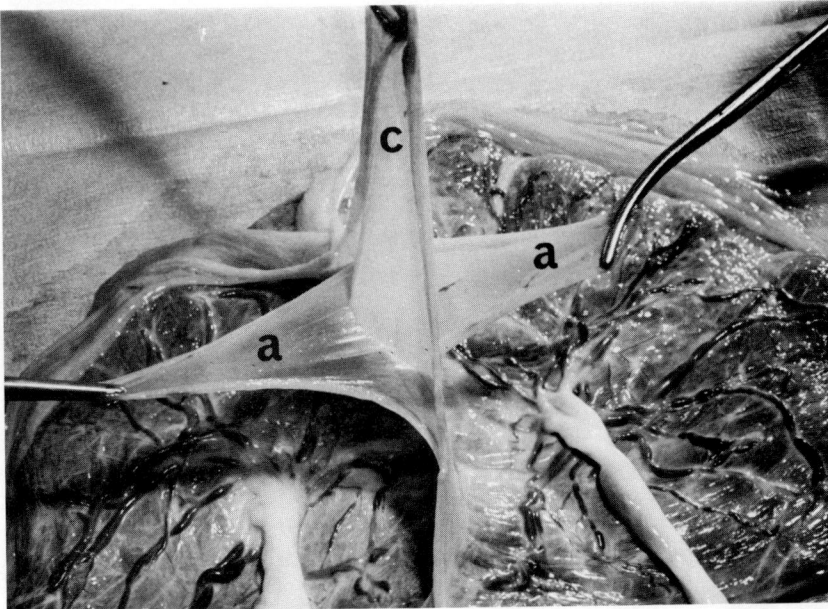

B

Fig. 39–3. A. The membrane partition that separated twin fetuses is elevated. **B.** The membrane partition consists of chorion (c) between two amnions (a).

other biochemical markers was demonstrated. The proband demonstrated classical features of Turner syndrome, including a single sex chromosome (karyotype 45,X), in tissue cultures from streak gonads. The karyotype of the other twin, a normal-appearing male, was 46,XY. Pedersen and associates (1980) summarized the salient features of 16 cases of monozygotic twins in whom one or both twins had gonadal dysgenesis and a 45,X karyotype, at least in some cells.

Conjoined Twins

In the United States, united or conjoined twins are commonly referred to as Siamese twins, after Chang and Eng Bunker of Siam (Thailand) who were displayed world-wide by P.T. Barnum. If twinning is initiated after the embryonic disc and the rudimentary amnionic sac have been formed, and if division of the embryonic disc is incomplete, conjoined twins result. When each of the joined twins is nearly complete, the commonly shared body site may be (1) anterior (*thoracopagus*), (2) posterior (*pyopagus*), (3) cephalic (*craniopagus*), or (4) caudal (*ischiopagus*). The majority are of the thoracopagus variety (Figs. 39–5 and 39–6).

When the bodies are duplicated only partly, the attachment more often is lateral. The incomplete division of the embryonic disc may begin at either or both poles and produce two heads; two, three, or four arms; two, three, or four legs; or some combination thereof. The frequency of conjoined twins is not well established. At Kandang Kerbau Hospital in Singapore, Tan

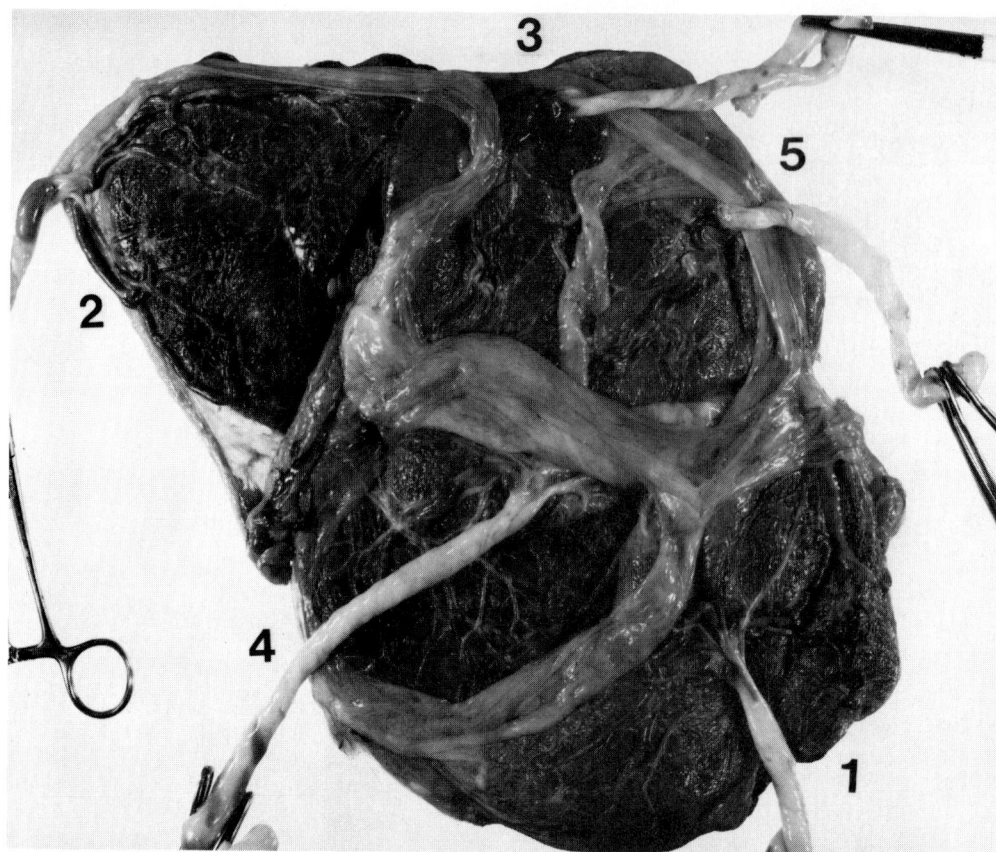

Fig. 39–4. Quintuplet placenta with five separate amnionic sacs delivered at 32 weeks. Amnionic sacs of numbers 3 and 5 were not separated by chorion and therefore those infants are monozygous. Infant birthweights ranged from a high of 1530 g (no. 1) to 860 g (no. 5). All of the infants survived.

and co-workers (1971) identified seven cases of conjoined twins among somewhat more than 400,000 deliveries (1 in 60,000).

The diagnosis of conjoined twins can frequently be made at midpregnancy by sonography (Fig. 39–6). The use of sonography to detect conjoined twins has been reviewed in some depth by Koontz and associates (1983).

Vaginal delivery of conjoined twins is possible because the union most often is somewhat pliable, although dystocia is common. If the fetuses are mature, vaginal delivery may be traumatic. Surgical separation of

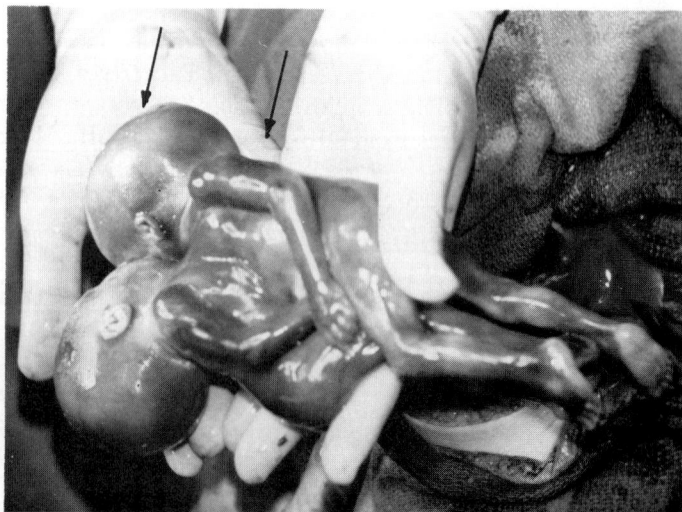

Fig. 39–5. Conjoined twins at delivery by hysterotomy.

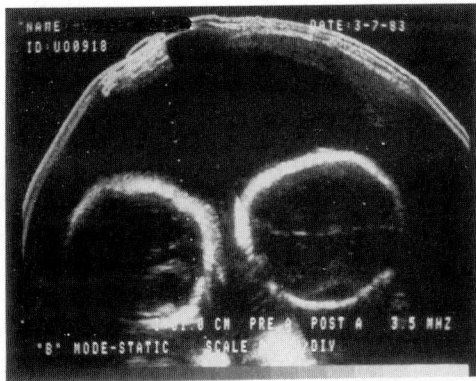
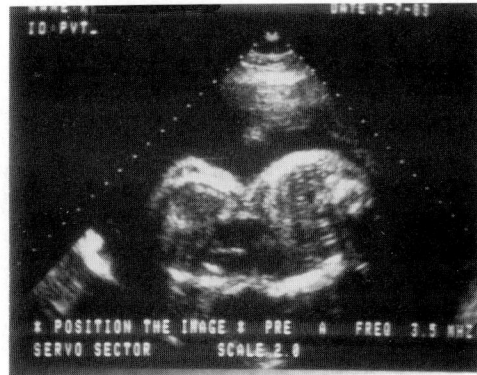
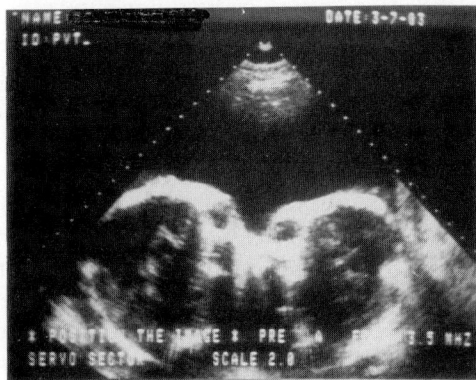
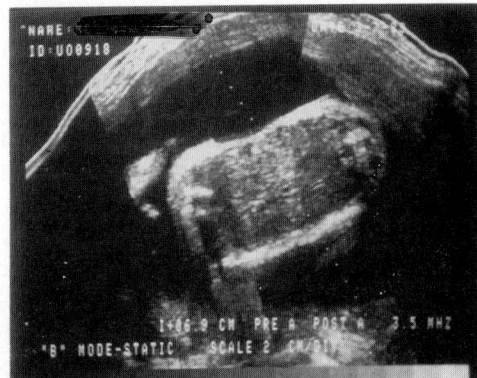

Fig. 39–6. Transverse sonograms of thoracopagus twins at about 28 weeks' gestation. **A.** Axial view of fetal heads. **B.** Fused thorax with conjoined hearts. **C.** Oblique view of the heads showing the proximity of the two faces. **D.** Fusion of the abdomen with a common liver. (Courtesy of Dr. R. Santos.)

conjoined twins may be successful when organs essential for life are not shared intimately.

Hydatidiform Mole

At times, twinning is expressed as a single fetus from one ovum plus a hydatidiform mole from another (see Chap. 35). Severe pregnancy-induced hypertension may develop at times before 24 weeks, but this is about as early as preeclampsia–eclampsia develops in the absence of a hydatidiform mole. The presence of a fetal heart action and hypertension earlier in pregnancy may cloud the etiology of the hypertension until the unsuspected mole is identified either by sonography or at delivery.

Vascular Communications Between Fetuses

Vascular anastomoses are frequently demonstrable in monochorionic placentas, either artery to artery, artery to vein (arteries are recognized as crossing over veins), or vein to vein (Fig. 39–7). Anastomoses rarely are de-

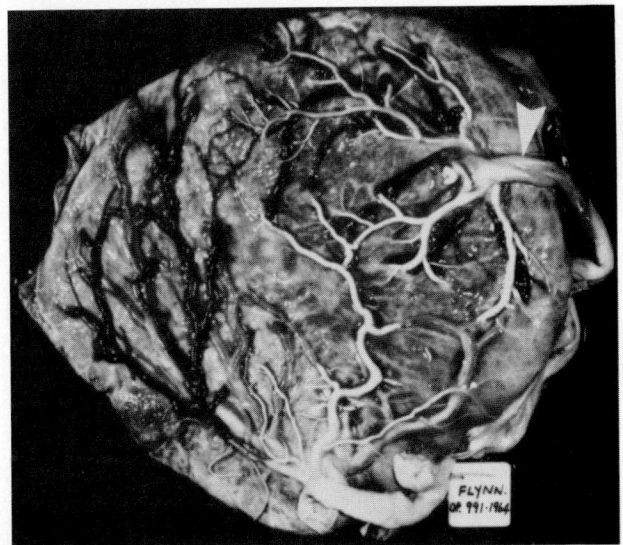

Fig. 39–7. Monochorionic twin placenta from which the amnion has been stripped. The arteries of cord 1 (*arrow*) have been injected with barium solution and a direct communication with an artery from cord 2 (*label*) is apparent. A major artery of cord 2 was injected with India ink and a communication with veins in placenta 1 is evident, indicating a deep vascular communication. (From Fox, 1978, with permission.)

monstrable in dichorionic placentas (Robertson and Neer, 1983). Arteriovenous anastomoses may develop quite early in pregnancy and may vary appreciably in number and in size. As emphasized by Benirschke and Kim (1973), the arteriovenous communication often proceeds through the capillary bed of a placental cotyledon. As the consequence of such anastomoses, blood is pumped from artery to vein, out of one fetus into the other.

Effects of Anastomotic Circulations. Effects from arteriovenous anastomoses can be profound. One monozygous twin may be very much smaller than the other as the consequence of chronic intrauterine malnutrition. Anatomical changes described by Naeye (1965) in the underperfused twin resemble those found in growth-retarded singletons whose placentas were extensively infarcted. In monozygotic twins with anastomosed circulations, the hemoglobin concentration may be 8 g/dL or less in the hypoperfused twin and as much as 27 g/dL in the other! Hypotension, microcardia, and generalized runting characterize the overtly affected hypovolemic "identical" donor twin, in contrast to hypertension and cardiac hypertrophy in the hypertransfused twin. Hydramnios, perhaps the consequence of increased renal perfusion, and, in turn, increased urine formation may accompany the hypervolemia and polycythemia in the typically larger recipient twin. At the same time, amnionic fluid may be scant to absent in the other sac, possibly as a result of marked oliguria in the underperfused donor twin. Death of one monozygotic fetus has been reported to precipitate serious consumption coagulopathy in the other fetus (p. 901).

The neonatal period may be complicated by dangerous circulatory overload with heart failure if severe hypervolemia and hyperviscosity are not identified promptly and treated by phlebotomy. Occlusive thrombosis is also much more likely to develop in this setting. Polycythemia may lead during the neonatal period to severe hyperbilirubinemia and, in turn, kernicterus (see Chap. 44, p. 1019).

Viewed from the maternal side, one portion of the placenta often appears quite pale compared with the rest of the placenta when there is anemia in one twin and polycythemia in the other. The vascular anastomoses can usually be visualized directly after the overlying amnion is removed, especially after injecting milk into an umbilical artery (Fig. 39–7).

Cerebral palsy, microcephaly, porencephaly, and multicystic encephalomalacia are found more frequently in preterm twins compared with preterm singletons (Bejar and co-workers, 1990). Explanations for such neurological damage include ischemic necrosis leading to cavitary brain lesions from emboli of thromboplastic material originating in a dead twin fetus. Fusi and co-workers (1991) observed that such ischemic antenatal brain damage may arise due to rapid hemodynamic

changes resulting from acute twin–twin anastomotic transfusion at the time of death of one twin fetus. Such twin sibling brain damage has been reported following death of one fetus as early as 16 weeks' gestation (Anderson and co-workers, 1990). Bejar and co-workers (1990) reviewed neonatal echoencephalographic studies in 89 twins and 12 triplets and diagnosed antenatal necrosis of cerebral white matter (when brain atrophy or cavities in the white matter were present by day 3 of life) in 15 percent of the infants (Fig. 39–8). Such neurological damage was linked to hydramnios, co-twin fetal death, hydrops, and multiple vascular connections. The most important factor appeared to be vein-to-vein anastomosis within the placenta because 90 percent of infants with such vascular connections had brain damage.

The prognosis for multiple gestations complicated by twin-to-twin transfusion syndrome is extremely guarded. Not only is brain damage a possibility, but antenatal death of one twin fetus as well as neonatal death due to preterm delivery are other hazards. Generally, the earlier in gestation that the diagnosis of twin–twin transfusion is established, the poorer the prognosis (Bebbington and Wittmann, 1989). Unfortunately, the most serious form of twin-twin transfusion syndrome with acute hydramnios in one sac and a **stuck twin** with almost total oligohydramnios in the other sac usually presents between 18 and 26 weeks' gestation. The survival rate for those diagnosed before 28 weeks has been reported to range between about 20 percent (Gonsoulin and co-workers, 1990) and 45 percent (Shah and Chaffin, 1989). Therapeutic serial amniocentesis to decompress the hydramnios and forestall preterm labor has been reported by some to be beneficial (Mahony and co-workers, 1990). In contrast, Gonsoulin and co-workers (1990) observed that amniocentesis for decompression failed to decrease perinatal mortality. De Lia and associates (1990) used fetoscopic laser occlusion of placental vessels in severe twin–twin transfusion syndrome.

The diagnostic criteria for twin–twin transfusion syndrome are problematic. Danskin and Neilson (1989) concluded that this syndrome cannot be established definitively if based solely upon birthweight or hemoglobin differences. Weinstrom and colleagues (1992) also concluded that twin birthweight and hemoglobin intrapair differences are so common as to preclude accurate diagnosis of twin–twin transfusion syndrome. Based on his review, Blickstein (1988) has proposed a rather extensive list of diagnostic criteria based upon both antenatal and postnatal findings.

Chimerism. A chimera is an individual with a mixture of genotypes from more than one ovum and sperm. Possible mechanisms include double fertilization of one ovum and, in cases of nonidentical fetuses, the transfer of genetic material from one to the other across chori-

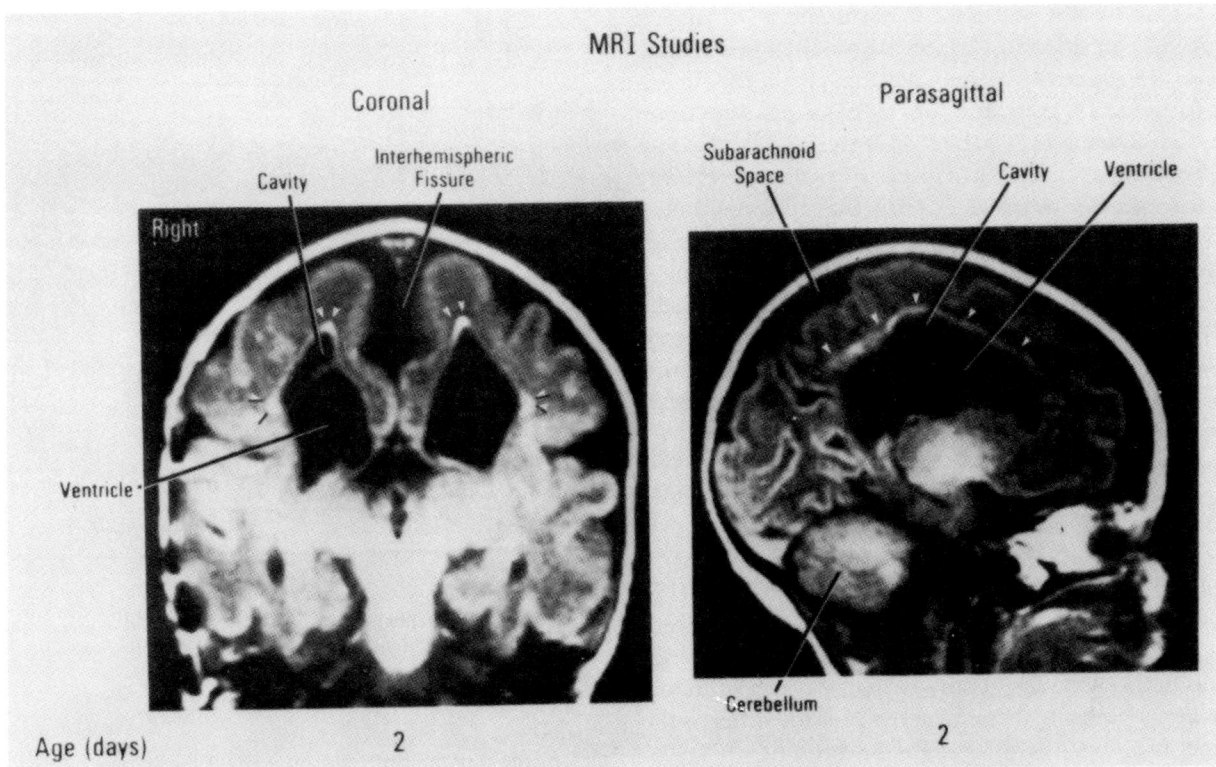

Fig. 39–8. Cranial magnetic resonance imaging study of diamnionic-monochorionic twin performed on day 2 of life. The subarachnoid space and lateral ventricles are markedly enlarged. There are large cavitary lesions in the white matter adjacent to the ventricles. The bright signals (*arrowheads*) in the periphery of the cavitary lesions most probably correspond to gliosis. (From Bejar and colleagues, 1990, with permission.)

onic vascular anastomoses. For example, the transfer of primitive blood cells from one dizygotic twin fetus through a vascular anastomosis to the other twin can lead to the production in the recipient of two populations of blood cells of quite dissimilar blood types, or *blood chimerism*. The transposed cells are not destroyed because exposure of the recipient twin to the dissimilar antigens of the donor twin early in fetal development renders the recipient twin tolerant to the donor twin's tissues. Blood chimerism has been most commonly discovered at the time of blood typing when discordant blood types are found (Benirschke, 1974).

Chimerism, in which cell lines are derived from different zygotes, is to be distinguished from *mosaicism*, in which two or more cell lines of different chromosomal composition arise from the same zygote as the consequence of nondisjunction during meiotic division.

Diagnosis of Multiple Fetuses

It is unfortunate that the diagnosis of twins has frequently not been made until late in pregnancy, often as late as the time of labor and delivery. Increasingly widespread use of prenatal ultrasound imaging has greatly changed the incidence of overlooked twin gestations.

Indeed, one argument in favor of routine ultrasound screening is earlier detection of multiple fetuses (see Chap. 46, p. 1046). Most contemporary reports on twin gestations where selective (based on indications) ultrasound examinations were performed indicate that about 80 percent of twins are diagnosed before labor using this approach (Andrews and colleagues, 1991; Kovacs and co-workers, 1989). Kemppaineu and co-workers (1990) diagnosed three fourths of twins by 21 weeks in over 4600 Helsinki women receiving clinically indicated ultrasound examinations, compared with the expected 100 percent in nearly 4700 women randomized to receive routine ultrasound. Although perinatal mortality was increased in twins diagnosed with indicated ultrasound, the trial did not have enough statistical power because of small numbers and because of the 75 percent detection rate in the group receiving clinically indicated ultrasound examinations. The identification of pregnancy complicated by multiple fetuses is missed not so much because it is unusually difficult but because the examiner fails to keep the possibility in mind.

History and Physical Examination. A familial history of twins by itself provides only a weak clue, but knowledge of recent administration of either clomiphene or pituitary gonadotropin provides a strong one. Physical examination with accurate measurement of fundal height, as described in Chapter 9 (p. 252), is essential. **During the second trimester, a discrepancy develops between gestational age determined from menstrual data and that from uterine size. The uterus that contains two or more fetuses clearly becomes larger than one with a single fetus.** In the case of a woman with a uterus that appears large for gestational age, the following possibilities are considered: (1) multiple fetuses, (2) elevation of the uterus by a distended bladder, (3) inaccurate menstrual history, (4) hydramnios, (5) hydatidiform mole, (6) uterine myomas or adenomyosis, (7) a closely attached adnexal mass, and (8) fetal macrosomia late in pregnancy.

Diagnostic Aids. A variety of techniques are utilized to identify multifetal gestation.

Fetal Parts. Before the third trimester, it is difficult to diagnose twins by palpation of fetal parts. It is apparent in Figure 39–9 that even late in pregnancy it may not always be possible to identify twins by transabdominal palpation, especially if one twin overlies the other, if the woman is obese, or if hydramnios is present.

Fetal Heart Sounds. Late in the first trimester, fetal heart action may be detected with generally available

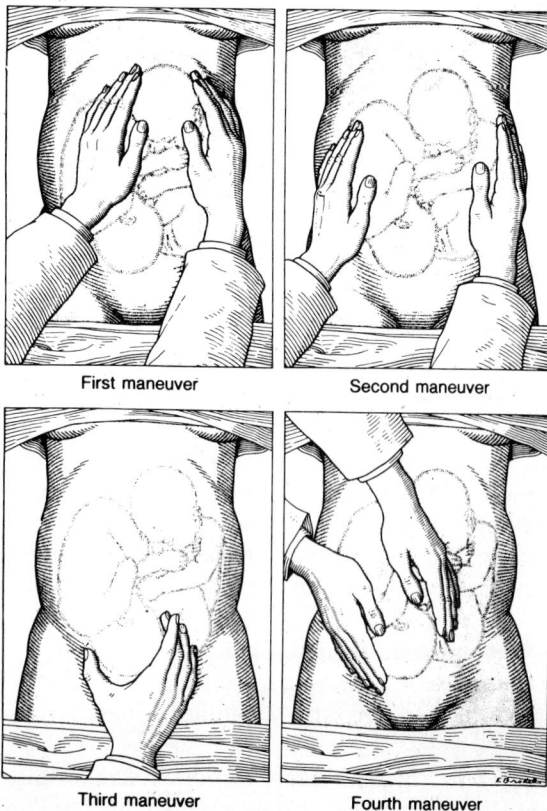

Fig. 39–10. Longitudinal sonogram demonstrating two gestational sacs, each containing a fetus, at 7 weeks menstrual age. (Courtesy of J. and J. Ackerman and Dr. R. Santos.)

Doppler ultrasonic equipment (see Chap. 2, p. 28). Sometime thereafter it becomes possible to identify the separate contractions of two fetal hearts if their rates are clearly distinct from each other as well as from that of the mother. It is possible by careful examination to identify fetal heart sounds with the usual aural fetal stethoscopes at 18 to 20 weeks.

Sonography. By careful ultrasonic examination, separate gestational sacs can be identified very early in twin pregnancy (Fig. 39–10). Subsequently, the identification of each fetal head should be made in two perpendicular

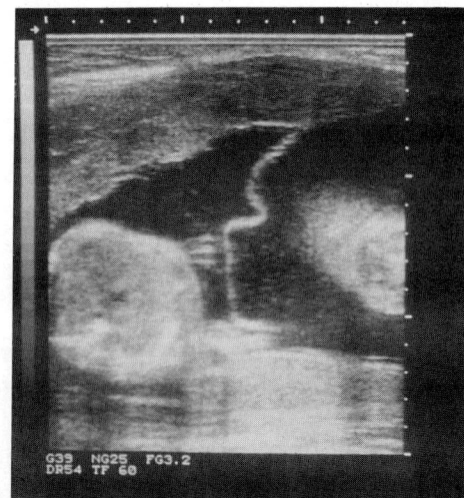

Fig. 39–9. Abdominal palpation in twin pregnancy. Cephalic presentation on the mother's right and frank breech on the left.

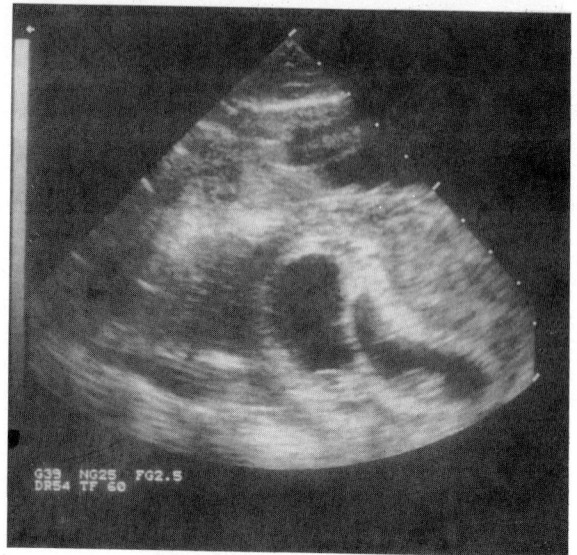

Fig. 39–11. Sonogram of twins at 18 weeks' gestational age. Two fetal poles are separated by intervening membranes that divide the amnionic sacs. (Courtesy of Dr. R. Santos.)

planes so as not to mistake a cross section of the fetal trunk for a second fetal head. A cross section of the fetal head remains nearly round in both planes, whereas the trunk does not. Carefully performed sonographic scanning should detect practically all sets of twins and even the presence of one amnionic sac or two (Fig. 39–11). Indeed, D'Alton and Dudley (1989) suggested that counting the number of layers seen in dividing fetal membranes during ultrasound examination is an accurate way of determining chorion relationships. Similarly, Winn and co-authors (1989) reported that dividing membranes measuring more than 2 mm are predictive of dichorionic twinning.

As the number of fetuses increases, the accuracy of diagnosis, both as to the number of fetuses and to the biparietal diameter of each head, decreases. In the case of quintuplets, demonstrated in the radiograph in Figure 39–12, only four fetuses were identified with certainty either by sonography or by radiography. It is not surprising that in the case of nonuplets studied by Kossoff and associates (1976) at 25 weeks, only six of the nine fetuses were identified by sonography. At times, sonographic examination will serve to identify conjoining of twins, as demonstrated in Figure 39–6.

In multifetal pregnancies, there is a general slowing of the rate of fetal growth compared with singleton pregnancies. Moreover, individual growth in the same multifetal gestation may be discordant. Significant discordance can usually be detected by careful ultrasonic measurement of the abdominal circumference as well as the biparietal diameter. Measurements of the biparietal diameters alone may provide misleading information because dolichocephaly in one fetal head may suggest erroneously growth discordance.

Radiological Examination. The indiscriminate use of x-ray should be avoided during pregnancy. Moreover, a radiograph of the maternal abdomen to try to demonstrate multiple fetuses in the following circumstances will provide no useful information and may be responsible for an incorrect diagnosis: (1) when taken before 18 weeks because the fetal skeletons are insufficiently radiopaque, (2) if the film is of poor quality from inappropriate exposure time or from malposition of the mother so that her upper abdomen and the fetus beneath are excluded from the x-ray, (3) when the mother is obese, (4) when there is hydramnios, and (5) if one fetus moves during the exposure. There are times, how-

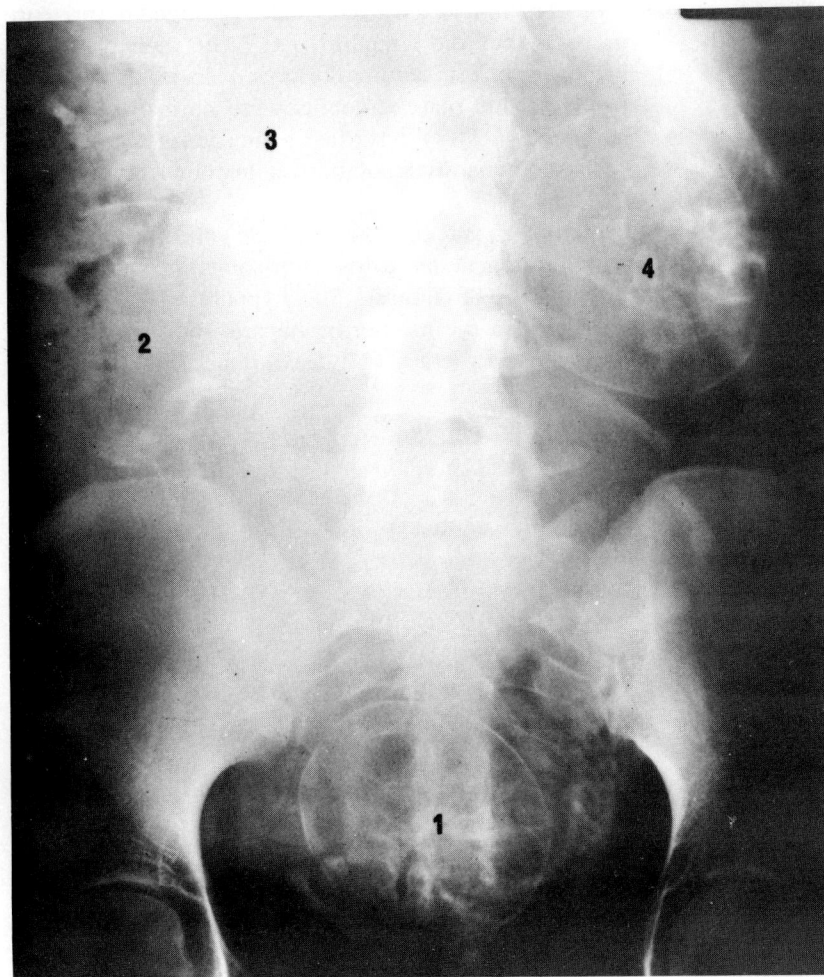

Fig. 39–12. Radiograph at 27 weeks' gestation that clearly demonstrates four fetal heads. A fifth fetus, not identifiable in this radiograph, weighed but 860 g when delivered 5 weeks later. (The placenta is shown in Figure 39–4.)

ever, when the importance of diagnosing the presence of multiple fetuses surely overrides the minimal risk associated with a carefully obtained and interpreted radiograph.

Biochemical Tests. The amounts of *chorionic gonadotropin* in plasma and in urine, on average, are higher than those found with a singleton pregnancy but not so high as to allow a definite diagnosis (Thiery and co-workers, 1976). Neither are the amounts of chorionic gonadotropin so low as to differentiate clearly between a twin pregnancy and a hydatidiform mole. *Placental lactogen* levels in maternal plasma average somewhat higher in a twin pregnancy than in a singleton pregnancy (Spellacy and colleagues, 1978). The *alpha-fetoprotein level* in maternal plasma commonly is higher in pregnancies with twins than in those with a single fetus. Even though Keilani and co-workers (1978) found that in 40 percent of twin pregnancies the level was above the 95th percentile of the normal range for singleton gestations, the measurement provides little help in diagnosing twins over that provided by careful clinical evaluation. There are also somewhat higher maternal plasma levels on the average for *estrogens, alkaline phosphatase,* and *leucine aminopeptidase* ("oxytocinase"), and in urine for *estriol* and *pregnanediol.* Thus far, however, there is no biochemical test that in any individual case will differentiate clearly between the presence of one and more than one fetus.

Pregnancy Outcome

Abortion. Abortion is more likely with multiple fetuses than with a single fetus. The demonstration sonographically of two gestational sacs with the subsequent disappearance of one or even both sacs is evidence that silent early abortion or resorption of one embryo is fairly common (p. 892). Both spontaneous abortion and surgically induced abortion have, on occasion, served to remove one embryo or fetus with the pregnancy nevertheless continuing until the birth of another fetus who survives.

Death of One Fetus. On occasion, one fetus succumbs remote from term, but the pregnancy continues with one living fetus. At delivery, the dead fetus with placenta and membranes may be identified readily but may be compressed appreciably (*fetus compressus*) or may be flattened remarkably through loss of fluid and most of the soft tissue (*fetus papyraceous*). A striking example is presented in Figure 39–13, in which the papyraceous fetus died at midpregnancy while the other fetus and placenta thrived. Sometimes the dead fetus will undergo complete resorption even though the conceptus had advanced well beyond the status of an embryo before succumbing, as demonstrated by serial sonography in Figure 39–2.

Theoretically, at least, acquired coagulation defects—disseminated intravascular coagulation, consumptive coagulopathy—could be triggered in the mother by the death of one of multiple fetuses. However, there is documented dangerous maternal hypofibrinogenemia and troublesome hemorrhage at delivery only when both of twin fetuses were dead in utero for a prolonged period (Chap. 37, p. 841 and Fig. 37–20A). We have observed transient, spontaneously corrected consumptive coagulopathy when one fetus died and was retained in utero along with the other who was alive. As concern mounted over the well-being of the mothers and their surviving fetuses, the fibrinogen concentration rose spontaneously and the level of serum fibrinogen–fibrin degradation products fell to normal. At delivery the portions of the placenta that supplied the living fetus appeared quite normal, whereas that which had once provided for the dead fetus was the site of massive fibrin deposition. This may have accounted directly for the fall in maternal fibrinogen and, in turn, an increase in fibrin degradation products, or it may have served to block the escape of thromboplastin from fetus and placenta into the maternal circulation and thereby prevented disseminated intravascular coagulation, or both mechanisms may have been operational until extensive fibrosis was achieved. The fetuses who were alive at the time of demise of the womb-mate continued to thrive in utero as they did after birth. At birth, their plasma fibrinogen levels, serum fibrinogen–fibrin degradation products, and platelet counts were normal. Chescheir and Leeds (1988) described a similar twin pregnancy with spontaneous resolution of maternal hypofibrinogenemia.

Romero and co-workers (1984) observed maternal hypofibrinogenemia to develop sometimes after death of one of twin fetuses. The hypofibrinogenemia was corrected in the mother by heparin infusion. The first time heparin therapy was discontinued the hypofibrin-

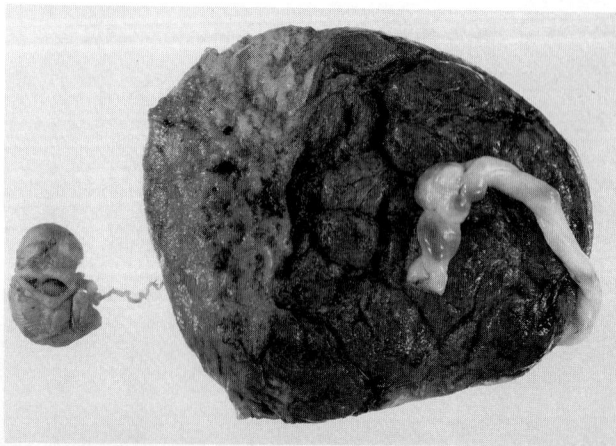

Fig. 39–13. To the left are a papyraceous fetus that died at midpregnancy, its cord, and its pale placenta. To the right are the normal placenta and cord of the healthy 3200 g twin.

ogenemia recurred, but the next time heparin was stopped hypofibrinogenemia did not recur. Presumably, by the second time, consumption coagulopathy in the mother was arrested by the sealing off of the maternal vascular bed with the fibrin. The liveborn infant appeared normal at 14 months of age.

The risk to a surviving fetus of developing serious consumptive coagulopathy may be enhanced if there are anastomoses between the fetal circulations, commonly found with monochorionic twins, as emphasized by Benirschke and Kim (1973). So far, however, we have not identified consumptive coagulopathy in cord blood of the living monozygotic twin when the other had been long dead. Cherouny and colleagues (1989) concluded that the risks of preterm delivery exceed the low risks related to continuation of multiple pregnancy after diagnosis of fetal death, and we agree with their recommendations of conservative management of the living fetus(es).

Perinatal Mortality. The perinatal mortality rate for pregnancies complicated by twin fetuses has been remarkably higher than for single fetuses. Spellacy and co-authors (1990) compared outcomes of 1253 twin pregnancies delivered in the Chicago area between 1982 and 1987 with that of singletons. The perinatal mortality rate was 54 per 1000 births for twins versus 10.4 per 1000 births in singletons. The perinatal mortality rate of twin B was 64 per 1000 births compared with 49 per 1000 births for first-born twins. Unlike singletons, where fetal and neonatal death rates were similar, neonatal mortality rates for twins clearly exceeded their stillbirth rates, thus implicating preterm birth as a relatively large cause of twin mortality. The twin pregnancies delivered earlier and the infants were smaller, had lower Apgar scores, and more often had congenital anomalies. Twin mortality increased in proportion to increasing differences in birthweights between twin A and B. For example, approximately 15 percent of twin pregnancies had intrapair birthweight differences of 25 percent or greater, and the perinatal mortality was 103 per 1000 births compared with 46 per 1000 births when twin siblings were closer to each other in size. Interestingly, low-birthweight twins (less than 2500 g) more often survived compared with low-birthweight singletons whereas larger twins did not fare as well compared with singletons with birthweights exceeding 2500 g.

The perinatal death rate for monozygotic twins is 2.5 times that for dizygotic twins (Kovacs and co-workers, 1989). There is an extremely high fetal death rate with the relatively rare variety of monozygous twinning in which both fetuses occupy the same amnionic sac—that is, *monoamnionic twins*. A common cause of death is intertwining of their umbilical cords, which has been estimated to complicate 50 percent or more of cases (Benirschke, 1983). An example is provided in Figure 39–14.

When only one amnionic sac can be identified sonographically because of the likelihood of death of one or both monoamnionic twins from cord entanglement, the destruction of one to try to protect the other has been considered by some. Following the death of the other twin, the possibility of an adverse effect on the "protected" twin, as a consequence of severe consumptive coagulopathy, has been raised (Benirschke, 1983).

We have observed a case of monozygous, monoamnionic twins in which at 31 weeks one twin was confirmed to be dead by real-time sonography while the other appeared to be thriving. Four weeks later, after spontaneous labor, an apparently healthy infant was delivered. In cord blood the levels of

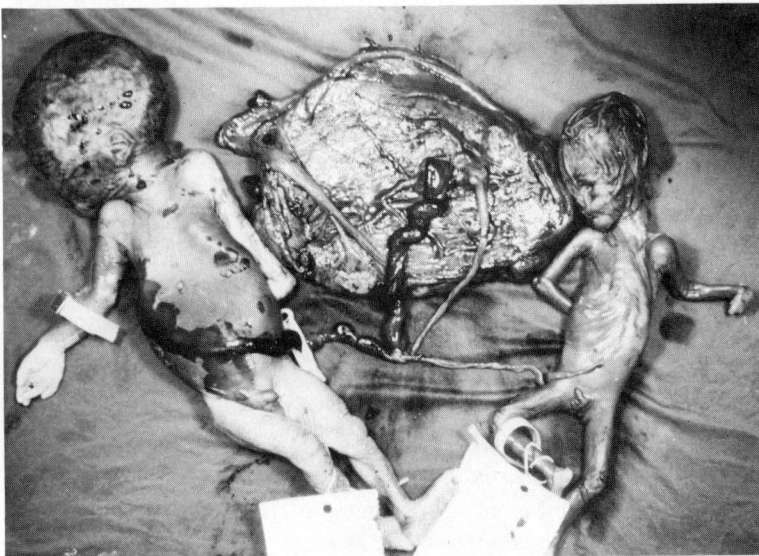

Fig. 39–14. Monozygotic twins in a single amnionic sac: the smaller fetus apparently died first and the second subsequently succumbed when the umbilical cords entwined.

fibrinogen, fibrin degradation products, and platelets were normal. The other fetus, badly decomposed and obviously dead in utero for more than 4 weeks, weighed 770 g. The two umbilical cords were in close proximity at their insertions into the single placenta. The cords were entwined for nine complete turns!

Approximately 1 percent of monozygotic twins are monoamnionic. Such twins have been reported in the older literature to have the highest perinatal mortality (30 to 70 percent) of any twin gestations, in part due to the intertwining of umbilical cords, but also due to preterm birth (Benirschke and Kim, 1973). Carr and co-authors (1990) reviewed 24 sets of monoamnionic twins where all the fetuses were known to be alive before 18 weeks' gestation. Seventy percent of the fetuses were alive at 30 weeks and no additional deaths occurred prior to delivery at an average of 36 weeks' gestation. These investigators concluded that the risks of early delivery to prevent cord accidents outweighed the risks of fetal death as a result of monoamnionic status alone. Similar experiences were reported by Tessen and Zlatnik (1991) in their description of 20 monoamnionic twin pregnancies at the University of Iowa Hospital between 1961 and 1989. No fetal death occurred after 32 weeks' gestation, suggesting that prophylactic preterm delivery may not be indicated in all cases. Moreover, unexplained rupture of the dividing membrane has been described and is associated with all the morbidity and mortality of true monoamnionic twins (Gilbert and colleagues, 1991).

Duration of Gestation. As the number of fetuses increases, the duration of gestation and birthweight decreases. McKeown and Record (1952) identified the mean duration of gestation for twins to be 260 days (37 weeks) and for triplets 247 days (35 weeks), compared with 281 days (40 weeks) for single fetuses. Caspi and associates (1976) precisely ascertained the time of ovulation for 111 pregnancies in women in whom ovulation was induced with pituitary plus chorionic gonadotropins. As shown in Table 39–2, the average duration of gestation decreased dramatically as the number of fetuses increased.

Birthweight. In an earlier review, Powers (1973) concluded that about half of all twins weigh less than 2500

TABLE 39–2. AVERAGE LENGTH OF GESTATION FOR PREGNANCIES WITH KNOWN TIME OF OVULATION AND 20 OR MORE WEEKS' GESTATION

No. of Fetuses	No. of Pregnancies	Weeks Completed[a]
Singleton	82	39
Twins	21	35
Triplets	5	33
Quadruplets	3	29

[a] Calculated from 2 weeks before ovulation.
From Caspi and co-workers (1976), with permission.

g. Retarded fetal growth and preterm delivery are both important etiologies of low birthweight in multifetal gestations. After the second trimester, growth of multiple fetuses as determined either by sonographic measurements or by birthweight is likely to be impaired compared with singleton fetuses. In general, the larger the number of fetuses, the greater the degree of growth retardation. Moreover, when two or more fetuses are derived from a single ovum, the degree of growth retardation is likely to be greater than when each fetus is derived from a different ovum. The differences in birthweight were dramatic in the quintuplets presented in Figure 39–15. When delivered at 31 weeks, the three infants from separate ova weighed 1420, 1530, and 1440 g, whereas the two derived from the same ovum weighed 990 and 860 g. Although the birthweights of these two monozygotic infants were nearly the same, remarkable differences have been observed. Marked discordance in size may also complicate pregnancies in which each fetus arose from a separate ovum. For example, dizygotic twins, one of whom weighed 2300 and the other 785 g, were delivered at Parkland Hospital (Fig. 39–16). Both survived but one remains appreciably smaller than the other.

Malformations. Kohl and Casey (1975) identified major malformations in approximately 2 percent of twin infants, compared with 1 percent of singletons delivered during the same times and in the same institutions. The frequency of minor malformation was approximately 4 percent in twins, compared with about 2.5 percent in singletons. The frequency of malformations is nearly twice as great in twins as in singletons. Malformations are more common among monozygotic than dizygotic twins. Rodis and associates (1990) reviewed chromosomal abnormalities in twin gestations and concluded that most evidence is suggestive of an increased incidence of aneuploidy.

Persistent or chronic hydramnios is more likely to be associated with fetal anomalies of one or both twins. Hashimoto and colleagues (1986) subjectively identified increased amnionic fluid in a fourth of twin pregnancies. In half, hydramnios at midpregnancy was transient and all of these fetuses were normal. In the 10 pregnancies in which hydramnios persisted, nine fetuses had anomalies.

Genetic Amniocentesis. Several debilities are best detected by examination of amnionic fluid. Most often there are two amnionic sacs and ideally fluid should be obtained separately from each. The technique for amniocentesis in twins is described in Chapter 41 (p. 947).

Subsequent Development. In Norway, Nilsen and associates (1984) evaluated the physical and intellectual development of male twins at 18 years of age. Compared with singletons, twice as many twins were found to be

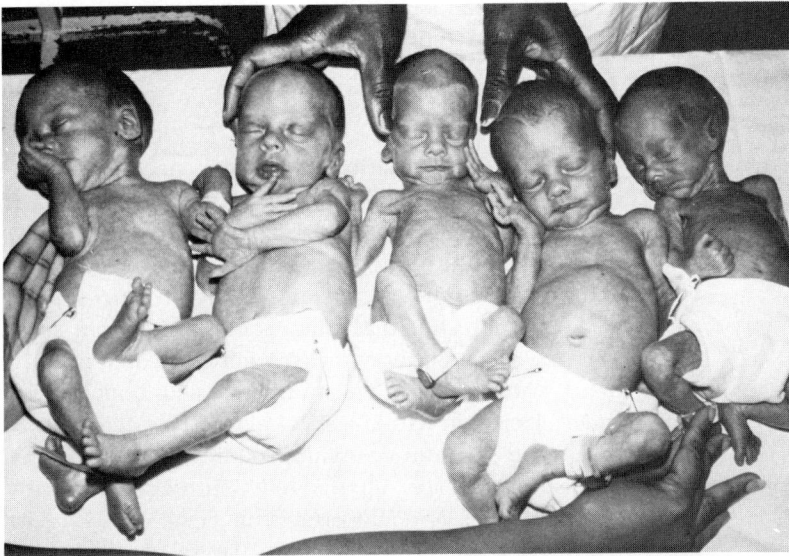

A

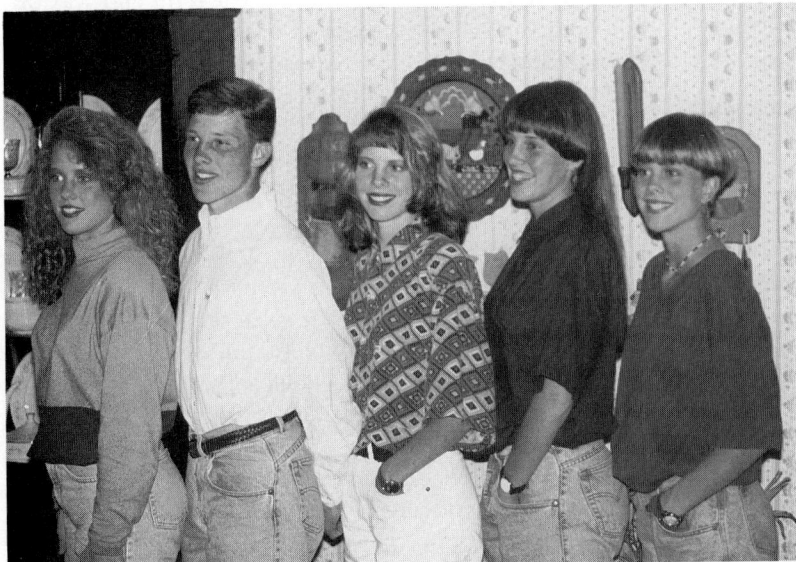

B

Fig. 39–15. A. Davis quintuplets at 3 weeks of age. The first, second, and fourth infants from the left each arose from separate ova, whereas the third and fifth infants are from the same ovum. **B.** Davis quintuplets at 17½ years of age.

physically unfit for military service. They attributed this to preterm delivery rather than twinning per se. General intelligence did not appear to differ between twins and singletons.

The pattern of subsequent development of the growth-retarded infant from a multifetal pregnancy varies. Babson and Phillips (1973), for example, reported that in monozygotic twins whose birthweights differed on the average by 35 percent, the twin who was smaller at birth remained so into adulthood. In their experience, height, weight, head circumference, and apparently intelligence often remained superior in the twin who weighed more at birth. Fujikura and Froelich (1974), however, failed to confirm a significant difference in mental and motor scores.

Baigts and co-workers (1982) studied 17-year-old monozygotic twins who had body frames that were quite similar but who were remarkably dissimilar in bodyweight, as they were at birth. The investigators documented hyperplasia of adipocytes in the heavier twin compared with her lighter sister. Their investigations excluded genetic differences through identity of the HLA system and eight other genetic markers and nutritional differences except for intrauterine nutrition. They suggested that perhaps, in the human, intrauterine nutritional status helps to determine adipocyte numbers and the way the body evolves. Others have concluded recently that genetic heritage in twins is more important than environment in determining body mass (Bouchard and co-workers, 1990; Stunkard and co-workers, 1990).

It seems reasonable to summarize that each fetus involved in a multifetal pregnancy is at some disadvantage from the outset compared with the singleton fetus. Those who do survive the newborn period may suffer

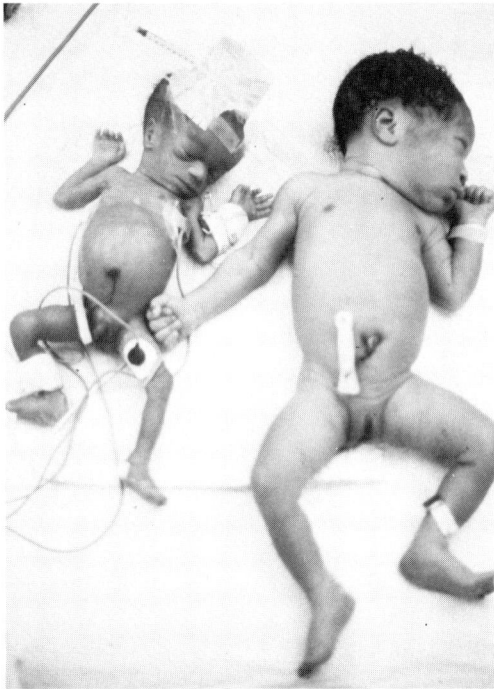

Fig. 39–16. Marked discordance in dizygotic twins. The larger infant weighed 2300 g, appropriate for gestational age. The markedly growth-retarded smaller infant weighed only 785 g. Both thrived.

some form of physical, intellectual, or psychological handicap, with the smaller usually at greater risk. Fortunately, in most instances their handicap will be minimal.

The outcome of twins reared apart often has been of considerable interest in debates over the relative significance of nature versus nurture in human development. The most notorious study of twins reared apart was undertaken by an English psychologist in the 1920s (NOVA, Public Broadcasting System, December 6, 1981). Twin research still is recovering from the scandal of Cyril Burt who used his twin studies to advance his theory that intelligence largely is inherited. On the basis of Burt's studies, an intelligence test was administered at age 11 to every English school child. The child's educational future rested on those test scores—it was either on to a university program or into a trade school. This tracked school system lasted from 1938 to 1967 when it was abandoned. After Burt's death, it was discovered he had fabricated some of his data!

Superfetation and Superfecundation. In superfetation, an interval as long as or longer than an ovulatory cycle intervenes between fertilizations. Superfetation has not been unequivocally demonstrated in women although it is theoretically possible until the uterine cavity is obliterated by the fusion of the decidua capsularis to the decidua vera. Thus, superfetation requires ovulation during the course of an established pregnancy, as yet unproven in humans though known to occur in

mares. Most authorities believe that the alleged cases of human superfetation result from marked inequality in growth and development of fetuses of the same gestational age, as described above.

Superfecundation refers to the fertilization of two ova within a short period of time but not at the same coitus, nor necessarily by sperm from the same man. It may be that, in many cases, twin ova are not fertilized by sperm from the same ejaculate, but the fact can be demonstrated only in exceptional circumstances.

It is interesting that John Archer, the first physician to receive a medical degree in America, related in 1810 that a white woman after intercourse with both a white and a black man within a short period was delivered of twins, one of whom was white and the other mulatto. A similar instance of superfecundation, documented by Harris (1982), is demonstrated in Figure 39–17. The mother was raped on the tenth day of her menstrual cycle and had intercourse one week later with her husband. She went into labor very near term and was delivered vaginally of a mulatto infant whose blood type was A and a white infant whose blood type was O. The blood type of both the mother and her husband was O. HLA typing was not done. Terasaki and co-workers (1978) described the use of HLA typing to establish that dizygotic twins were sired by different fathers.

Maternal Adaptation. In general, the degree of maternal physiological change is greater with multiple fetuses than with a single fetus. For example, the average increase in maternal blood volume induced during pregnancy with twin fetuses is significantly larger (Pritchard, 1965; Rovinsky and Jaffin, 1966). Whereas the average increase in late pregnancy is about 40 to 50 percent with a single fetus, the mean increase amounts to about 50 to 60 percent with twins. Measurements in the same

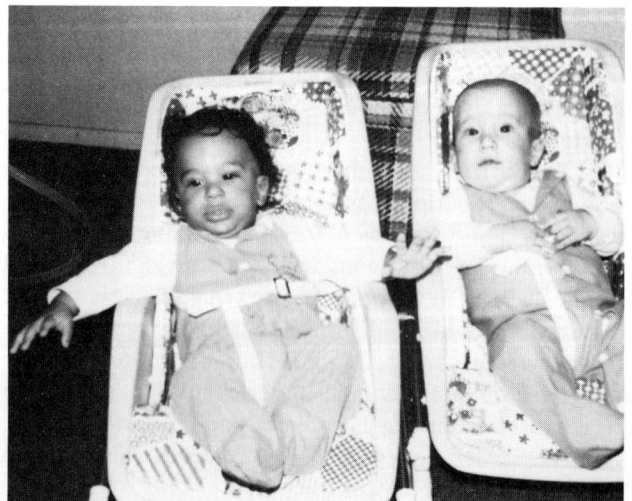

Fig. 39–17. An example of dizygotic twin boys as the consequence of superfecundation. (Courtesy of Dr. David Harris.)

woman late in one pregnancy with a single fetus and at the same time in another pregnancy with twins are indicative that, typically, maternal blood volume is about 500 mL greater with twins. Interestingly, the average blood loss with vaginal delivery of 25 sets of twins averaged 935 mL, or nearly 500 mL more than with delivery of a single fetus. Both the remarkable increase in maternal blood volume and the increased iron and folate requirements imposed by a second fetus predisposed to a greater prevalence of maternal anemia.

Veille and associates (1985) used M-mode echocardiography to assess cardiac function in women with twin pregnancies. As expected, cardiac output was increased compared with singleton pregnancy; however, end-diastolic ventricular dimensions were the same. During the third trimester, cardiac output was increased as a result of both increased pulse rate and increased stroke volume. Stroke volume was higher by virtue of an increased shortening fraction, which suggests increased contractility.

The larger size of the uterus with multiple fetuses intensifies the variety of mechanical effects that occur during pregnancy. The uterus and its contents may achieve a volume of 10 L or more and weigh in excess of 20 pounds! Especially with monozygotic twins, rapid accumulation of grossly excessive amounts of amnionic fluid—that is, *acute hydramnios*—may develop. In these circumstances it is easy to envision appreciable compression and displacement of many of the abdominal viscera as well as the lungs by the elevated diaphragm. The size and weight of the very large uterus may preclude more than a very sedentary existence for the woman pregnant with multiple fetuses.

In pregnancies with multiple fetuses further complicated by hydramnios, maternal renal function may become seriously impaired, most likely as the consequence of obstructive uropathy. Quigley and Cruikshank (1977), for example, described two pregnancies with twin fetuses plus acute and severe hydramnios in which oliguria and azotemia developed. Maternal urine output and plasma creatinine levels promptly returned to normal after delivery. In the case of gross hydramnios, transabdominal amniocentesis may be employed to provide relief for the mother and, it is hoped, to allow the pregnancy to continue (see Chap. 34, p. 734). Unfortunately, the hydramnios is often characterized by acute onset remote from term and by rapid reaccumulation following amniocentesis.

The various stresses of pregnancy on the mother and the likelihood of serious maternal complications will almost invariably be greater with multiple fetuses than with a singleton. This should be taken into account, especially when counseling the woman whose health is compromised and who is recognized early in pregnancy to have multiple fetuses. The same is true for a woman who is not pregnant but is considering treatment with agents used to induce ovulation.

Management of Pregnancies with Multiple Fetuses

To reduce significantly perinatal mortality and morbidity in pregnancies complicated by twins, it is imperative that (1) delivery of markedly preterm infants be prevented, (2) failure of one or both fetuses to thrive be identified and fetuses so afflicted be delivered before they become moribund, (3) fetal trauma during labor and delivery be eliminated, and (4) expert neonatal care be provided continuously from the time of birth. The first major step in fulfilling these goals is to identify early the pregnancy complicated by multiple fetuses. As soon as multiple fetuses (or embryos) are identified, meaningful efforts should be directed toward providing the fetuses with the best intrauterine environment possible.

Diet. The requirements for calories, protein, minerals, vitamins, and essential fatty acids are further increased in women with multiple fetuses. The Recommended Dietary Allowances made by the Food and Nutrition Board of the National Research Council for uncomplicated pregnancy should not only be met but also in most instances be exceeded (see Chap. 9, p. 253). Therefore, consumption of energy sources should be increased by another 300 kcal per day. Iron supplementation is essential; 60 to 100 mg per day is recommended. Folic acid, 1 mg per day, may prove beneficial, although a diet adequate in protein provided from a variety of sources should supply adequate amounts of folate. Sodium restriction is not beneficial.

Maternal Hypertension. Pregnancy-induced and pregnancy-aggravated hypertension are much more likely to develop in pregnancies with multiple fetuses (see Chap. 36, p. 764). Hypertension not only develops more often but also tends to develop earlier and to be more severe. In their analysis of 341 twin pregnancies at the University of Colorado, Thompson and associates (1987) reported that 18 percent were complicated by pregnancy-induced hypertension. Long and Oats (1987) reported that hypertension complicated 26 percent of 642 twin pregnancies: 35 percent in nulliparas and 20 percent in multiparas. Importantly, of those developing preeclampsia, it was identified before 37 weeks in nearly 70 percent of twin pregnancies, whereas it was found in only 25 percent of women with singleton pregnancies. In 284 twin pregnancies cared for at Parkland Hospital over a 22-month period, the incidence of pregnancy-induced hypertension was 17 percent compared with 11 percent in over 25,000 singleton pregnancies.

In singleton pregnancies, pregnancy-induced hypertension occurs less commonly in parous than in nulliparous women. This is not true, however, in multifetal pregnancies. At Parkland Hospital, pregnancy-induced hypertension developed in 10 percent of 204 multiparous women with twins, compared with 6 percent of over 15,000 multiparous women with singleton gestations.

Antepartum Surveillance of Fetal Growth. As discussed earlier (p. 901), fetal growth is slower in multifetal pregnancies than in singleton gestations, and moreover it may be unequal within a twin pair. Leveno and colleagues (1979) reported an average difference of 3.5 mm in biparietal diameters between 16 and 40 weeks. An important aspect of ultrasonic assessment of fetal growth is to identify *discordancy* between twin-pairs. This is most often defined by using the larger twin as the index. Brown and colleagues (1987) chose a 15 percent or greater birthweight difference and reported a 25 percent incidence of discordancy. Generally, as the weight difference within a twin pair increases, perinatal mortality increases proportionately. For example, Erkkola and co-authors (1985) described outcomes in 460 twin pregnancies and almost 10 percent were discordant, defined as a 25 percent difference in birthweight. **The perinatal mortality rate with discordancy of this magnitude was 97 per 1000 compared with 37 per 1000 for nondiscordant twin-pairs.** Blickstein and associates (1988) observed that the disadvantages for the growth-retarded discordant twin pertained only in preterm infants weighing less than 2500 g.

Although discordancy can be identified by disparity between biparietal diameters in twin-pairs, more recent evidence is consistent with the view that measurement of abdominal circumference improves identification of discordant twins. Using an intrapair difference in abdominal circumference of 20 mm or greater to predict 20 percent discordant growth, Storlazzi and colleagues (1987) reported a sensitivity of 80 percent, specificity of 85 percent, positive predictive value of 62 percent, and negative predictive value of 93 percent. When the abdominal circumference was correlated with the biparietal diameter to estimate fetal weight, the positive predictive value was now 80 percent, whereas the negative predictive remained 93 percent. Brown and colleagues (1987) found that the abdominal circumference was superior to the biparietal diameter to predict discordancy; however, they emphasized that more experience was needed before these techniques can be used alone to make clinical decisions. They also encouraged the liberal use of tests to establish fetal pulmonary maturation before effecting preterm delivery for suspected growth discordancy.

Doppler Velocimetry. Differences of vascular resistance estimated by blood flow velocity using continuous-wave Doppler ultrasound have been used to assess well-being in twin fetuses (Farmakides and colleagues, 1985; Giles and associates, 1985). Gerson and co-workers (1988) reported that the relationship between the systolic–diastolic ratio and gestational age is the same in single-

ton and twin pregnancies. As discussed in Chapter 46 (p. 1059), increased vascular resistance with diminished diastolic blood flow velocity may accompany retarded fetal growth. Gerson and co-workers (1987) used duplex Doppler ultrasound to measure umbilical venous blood flow and arterial systolic–diastolic velocity ratios. Normal studies correctly predicted 44 of 45 concordant twin-pairs and abnormal values, especially of the umbilical artery, correctly predicted 9 of 11 sets of discordant twins. Shah and colleagues (1992) reported similar results. Conversely, DiVou and co-workers (1989) reported that velocimetry alone was not uniformly successful in identifying twin discordance. These techniques need more extensive evaluation before they are applied routinely in clinical settings.

Prevention of Preterm Delivery. Several techniques have been applied in attempts to prolong multifetal gestations. These include considerable bed rest, especially through hospitalization, prophylactic administration of β-mimetic drugs, prophylactic cervical cerclage, and repeated injections of progestins.

Bed Rest. Several authors, but certainly not all, have claimed bed rest to be beneficial to twin fetuses, presumably by enhancing uterine perfusion and perhaps by reducing the physical forces that might act deleteriously on the cervix to hasten effacement and dilatation. Unfortunately, the benefits from bed rest are difficult to substantiate. Most recent evidence suggests that routine hospitalization is not beneficial. For example, Crowther and co-workers (1990) randomized hospitalization in 139 Zimbabwe women with twin pregnancies and found that hospitalization did not prolong pregnancy or improve infant survival, although bed rest incumbent with hospitalization did improve fetal growth. MacLennan and co-workers (1990) randomized 141 women with twins to hospitalization between 26 and 30 weeks and found no benefits. At Parkland Hospital, elective hospitalization at 26 weeks was compared longitudinally with outpatient management and no advantages were found for routine hospitalization (Andrews and colleagues, 1991). However, almost half of the twin pregnancies studied at Parkland Hospital required admission for specific indications such as hypertension or threatened preterm delivery. Currently at our hospital women with twins are managed as outpatients with frequent prenatal visits and prompt hospitalization for complications.

β-Mimetics. Most randomized trials of β-mimetics in twin pregnancies have not resulted in significant reductions in preterm delivery rates (Marivate and associates, 1977; O'Connor and co-workers, 1979). Skjaerris and Aberg (1982) claimed a reduction in the frequency of threatened preterm labor among pregnant women with twins who were given oral terbutaline prophylactically.

More recently, Ashworth and associates (1990) were unable to substantiate any benefits for prophylactic β-mimetic therapy with salbutamol in twin gestations.

Cerclage. No significant reduction in preterm delivery or perinatal deaths has been demonstrated from prophylactic cervical cerclage (Dor and associates, 1982; Weekes and co-authors, 1977).

Pulmonary Maturation. Pulmonary maturation measured by determination of the lecithin–sphingomyelin ratio usually is synchronous in twins (Leveno and associates, 1984). Moreover, although this ratio usually exceeds 2 by 36 weeks in singleton pregnancies, it often does so by about 32 weeks in multifetal pregnancy. In some cases, however, there may be marked disparity of pulmonary function. We observed the lecithin–sphingomyelin ratio with quintuplets to vary from less than 2 for the largest infant, who weighed 1530 g at 32 weeks and was of appropriate size for his gestational age, to greater than 5 for the severely growth-retarded smallest infant, who weighed 860 g. The largest infant developed appreciable respiratory distress, whereas the smallest infant did not.

Prolonged Gestation. Some investigators contend that the limit for twin postterm gestation should be set at 40 weeks, 2 weeks earlier than singletons (Dunn, 1969). The observation by Greenwald (1970) that peak mean birthweight of twins is reached at about 39 weeks compared with between 41 and 42 weeks in singletons suggests the possibility that twin gestation may be biologically shorter than in singletons. Unfortunately, there are not sufficient data to identify clearly the risks versus possible benefits from allowing a twin pregnancy to continue beyond 39 weeks.

Delivery of Multiple Fetuses

Labor. Many complications of labor and delivery, including preterm labor, uterine dysfunction, abnormal presentations, prolapse of the umbilical cord, premature separation of the placenta, and immediate postpartum hemorrhage, are encountered much more often with multiple fetuses. Therefore, the conduct of labor and delivery with multiple fetuses is an excellent test of the skills of the obstetrical team providing care for the woman and her fetuses.

To date, the capability is limited for safely arresting preterm labor in women pregnant with multiple fetuses. Pulmonary edema associated with the use of β-mimetic agents, for example, has been observed much more frequently in twin gestations. Bed rest, if not already being used, should be instituted. The problems of preterm labor and attempts to arrest it and of lack of fetal lung maturity and possible modification by corticosteroid therapy are considered elsewhere (see Chap. 38, p. 898).

As soon as it is apparent that labor has been established, immediate steps are taken to help assure a satisfactory outcome:

1. An appropriately trained obstetrical attendant remains with the mother throughout labor. Fetal heart rates are frequently monitored using any system of monitoring that, in the particular situation, will promptly identify significant changes in fetal heart rates. At times, continuous external electronical monitoring or, if the membranes are ruptured and the cervix dilated, evaluation of both fetuses by simultaneous internal and external electronical monitoring may prove quite satisfactory.
2. One liter of compatible whole blood or its equivalent in blood fractions is readily available.
3. A well-functioning intravenous infusion system capable of delivering fluid rapidly into the mother is established. In the absence of hemorrhage or metabolic disturbance during labor, lactated Ringer's with aqueous dextrose solution is infused at a rate of 60 to 120 mL/hour.
4. Two obstetricians are immediately available, and both are scrubbed and gowned at delivery. At least one should be skilled in intrauterine identification of fetal parts and intrauterine manipulation of the fetus.
5. An experienced anesthesiologist is immediately available in the event that intrauterine manipulation or cesarean delivery is necessary.
6. For *each* fetus, two people, one of whom is skilled in resuscitation and care of newborn infants, are appropriately informed of the case and remain immediately available.
7. The delivery area is immediately operational and provides adequate space for all members of the team to work effectively. Moreover, the site is appropriately equipped to take care of all possible maternal problems plus resuscitation and maintenance of each infant.

Presentation and Position. With twins, all possible combinations of fetal positions may be encountered. Either or both fetuses may present by the cephalic, breech, or shoulder. Compound, face, brow, and footling breech presentation are relatively common, especially when the fetuses are quite small, there is excess amnionic fluid, or maternal parity is high. Prolapse of the cord is fairly common in these circumstances.

The presentation can often be ascertained by real-time sonography. However, if any confusion about the relationship of the twins to each other or to the maternal pelvis persists, a single anteroposterior x-ray of the abdomen may be very helpful.

Induction or Stimulation of Labor. Even though labor, in general, is shorter with twins, both rupture of the membranes without effective labor and prolonged inefficient labor with or without previous rupture of the membranes do develop. These problems often are handled better by cesarean delivery unless there is little hope of salvaging the infants because of their gross immaturity. Termination of pregnancy is occasionally desirable before the spontaneous onset of labor, as, for example, with severe pregnancy-induced hypertension. In these circumstances, if the presenting part is well fixed in the pelvis and the cervix dilated somewhat, amniotomy often will initiate labor and effect delivery. There is no reluctance by some obstetricians to give oxytocin by dilute intravenous infusion to initiate or to stimulate labor in pregnancies complicated by multiple fetuses. The risks compared with the benefits to mother and fetuses of oxytocin to initiate and maintain labor and delivery, as contrasted with cesarean delivery, have not yet been adequately delineated in this circumstance.

Analgesia and Anesthesia. During labor and delivery of multiple fetuses, deciding what to use for analgesia and for anesthesia is unusually difficult because of the frequency of and, in turn, the problems imposed by (1) prematurity, (2) maternal hypertension, (3) desultory labor, (4) need for intrauterine manipulation, and (5) uterine atony and hemorrhage after delivery. There are undesirable effects from most forms of analgesia and anesthesia. Continuous epidural or caudal analgesia in hypertensive women, or those who have hemorrhaged, may cause hypotension with inadequate perfusion of vital organs, especially the placenta, which is dangerous to both the mother and her fetuses. The woman pregnant with multiple fetuses is even less tolerant of the supine position during labor and delivery. Moreover, conduction analgesia may cause or further aggravate desultory or prolonged labor and will not provide adequate uterine relaxation for intrauterine manipulation when such is necessary.

Epidural analgesia for vaginal delivery of twins has been described by Crawford (1987). In his series of 130 women with twins delivered vaginally, 105 who were given epidural analgesia had a significantly prolonged interval from complete dilatation until delivery. For women with epidural analgesia, the mean was about 90 minutes compared with 30 minutes for those without epidural analgesia. Interestingly, the mean delivery intervals between delivery of the first and second twins were not altered by epidural analgesia.

Use of narcotics, sedatives, and tranquilizers may lead to undue fetal depression if the fetuses are premature. Most forms of general anesthesia used for delivery also will depress the fetuses unless the anesthetic agents

are selected carefully and are skillfully administered with little delay between induction of anesthesia and delivery. Paracervical block may cause transient fetal bradycardia.

Either balanced general anesthesia or conduction analgesia, administered epidurally or in the subarachnoid space, has proved satisfactory at Parkland Hospital for cesarean delivery of twins. Pudendal block skillfully administered along with nitrous oxide plus oxygen provides appreciable relief of pain for spontaneous vaginal delivery. When intrauterine manipulation is necessary, as with internal podalic version, uterine relaxation is probably best accomplished with halothane or one of the other halogenated hydrocarbons. Although halothane provides effective relaxation for intrauterine manipulation, it commonly leads to an increase in blood loss during the third stage of labor until the uterus regains its ability to contract (see Chap. 16, p. 428).

Vaginal Delivery. In a study of 341 twin pregnancies, Thompson and associates (1987) reported a cephalic presentation in the first twin in 72 percent of cases (Fig. 39–18). In only about half of their cases was the presenting fetus the larger of the twin-pair. This twin typically bears the major brunt of dilating the cervix and the remaining soft tissues of the birth canal. Seldom with cephalic presentations are there unusual problems with delivery of the first infant. After appropriate episiotomy, spontaneous delivery or delivery assisted by the use of outlet forceps usually proves satisfactory.

When the first fetus presents as a breech, major problems are most likely to develop if (1) the fetus is unusually large and the aftercoming head taxes the capacity of the birth canal, (2) the fetus is quite small so that the extremities and trunk are delivered through a cervix inadequately effaced and dilated for the head to escape easily, or (3) the umbilical cord prolapses. When these problems are anticipated or identified, cesarean

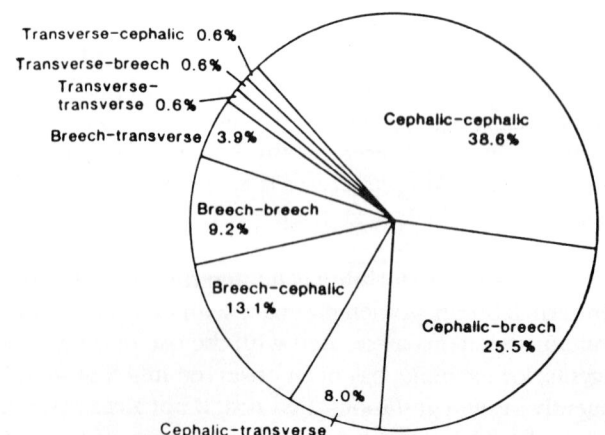

Fig. 39–18. Presentation of 341 twin-pairs at delivery. (From Thompson and colleagues, 1987, with permission.)

delivery will often be the better way to effect delivery except in those instances in which the fetuses are so immature that they will not survive. Otherwise, breech delivery may be accomplished as described in Chapter 25 (p. 577).

The safety of vaginal delivery for the second non-cephalic twin weighing more than 1500 g has been reported (Acker, 1982; Blickstein, 1987; Chervenak, 1985; Gocke, 1989; Laros and Dattel, 1988; and Rabinovici, 1987; and all their associates). For second twins weighing less than 1500 g, regardless of presentation, Davidson and co-workers (1992), Morales and associates (1989), and Rydhstrom (1990) reported that vaginal delivery was safe.

The phenomenon of *locked twins* is rare and according to Cohen and co-workers (1965) occurred only once in 817 twin gestations. For locking to occur, the first fetus must present by the breech and the second by the vertex. With descent of the breech through the birth canal, the chin of the first fetus locks in the neck and chin of the second cephalic fetus. If unlocking cannot be effected, either cesarean delivery before the body is delivered or decapitation must be performed.

Delivery of Second Twin. This demands experience that includes for some cases intrauterine manual dexterity. As soon as the first twin has been delivered, the presenting part of the second twin, size, and relationship to the birth canal are quickly ascertained by careful combined abdominal, vaginal, and, at times, intrauterine examination. Intrapartum real-time sonography has proved quite valuable in some cases. If the vertex or the breech is fixed in the birth canal, moderate fundal pressure is applied and membranes are ruptured. Immedi-

ately afterward, the examination is repeated to identify prolapse of the cord or other abnormality. Labor is allowed to resume while the fetal heart rate is monitored closely. With reestablishment of labor there is no need to hasten delivery unless there is ominous deceleration of the fetal heart rate, persistent bradycardia, or bleeding from the uterus. Bleeding from the uterus indicates placental separation, which can be deleterious to both the fetus and the mother. If contractions do not resume within approximately 10 minutes, dilute oxytocin may be used to stimulate appropriate myometrial activity leading to spontaneous delivery or delivery assisted by outlet forceps.

If the occiput or the breech presents immediately over the pelvic inlet but is not fixed in the birth canal, the presenting part can often be guided into the pelvis with a vaginal hand while a hand on the uterine fundus exerts moderate pressure. More recently, intrapartum external version of the noncephalic second twin has become popular. Using the method shown in Figure 39–19, the fetus who presents as breech or shoulder may be gently converted into a cephalic presentation. Once the presenting part is fixed in the pelvic inlet, membranes are ruptured and delivery is carried out as described above.

If the occiput or the breech is not over the pelvic inlet and cannot be so positioned by gentle pressure on the presenting part, or if appreciable uterine bleeding develops, the problem of delivery of the second twin assumes serious dimensions. So as to take maximum advantage of the very recently dilated cervix before the uterus contracts and the cervix retracts, procrastination must be avoided. An obstetrician skilled in intrauterine manipulation of the fetus and an anesthesiologist skilled

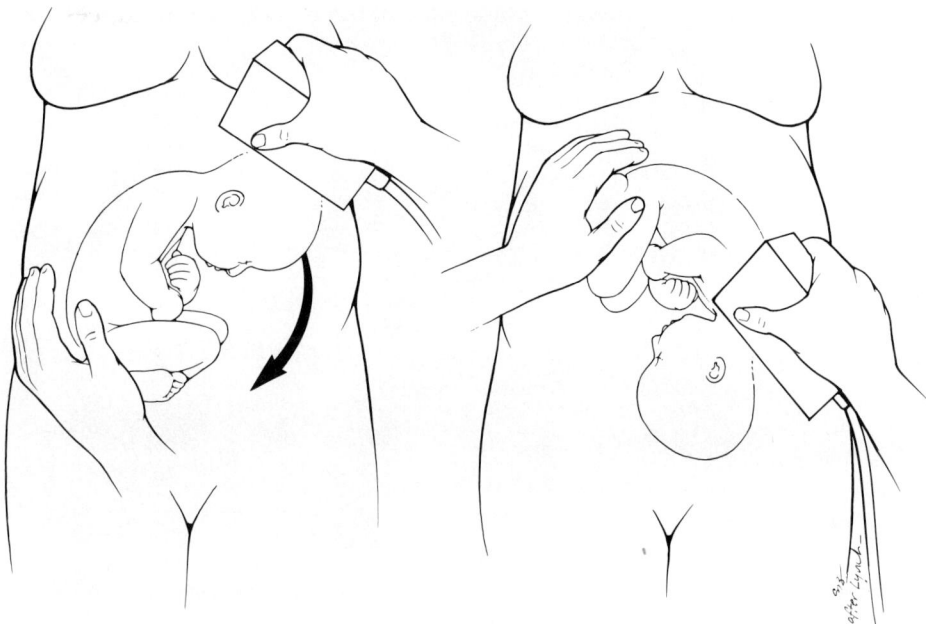

Fig. 39–19. External version of second breech twin fetus. Ultrasound transducer is being used to help guide vertex into pelvis. (Redrawn from Chervenak and colleagues, 1983, with permission.)

in providing anesthesia that will effectively relax the uterus are essential for vaginal delivery with a favorable outcome. Prompt delivery of the second fetus by cesarean delivery is the better choice if there is no one present who is skilled in the performance of internal podalic version (described below) or if anesthesia that will provide effective uterine relaxation is not immediately available.

In the past, the interval between delivery of the first and second twins was commonly cited to be safest if less than 30 minutes. Subsequently, as shown by Rayburn and colleagues (1984) as well as others, if continuous fetal monitoring is employed, there is a good outcome even if this interval is longer. Of 115 twin-pairs at 34 weeks or more, the mean interval between delivery of twins was 21 minutes, but it ranged from 1 to 134 minutes. In 60 percent, the interval was 15 minutes or less. Importantly, there was no excess trauma or evidence for fetal depression in those born after the 15-minute interval. As expected, the cesarean delivery rate was much higher if the interval was more than 15 minutes (18 percent) than if the interval was less than 15 minutes (3 percent).

In the circumstances where one of the fetuses has been expelled very preterm and uterine activity then ceased, the pregnancy has rarely been allowed to continue with delivery of another fetus days to even many weeks later. Cardwell and associates (1988) described delivery of triplets at 24, 24½, and 26 weeks. Wittmann and associates (1992) reviewed delayed delivery and reported an additional four cases with intervals ranging between 41 and 143 days.

Regardless of the route of delivery, respiratory distress is more common in the second twin. The reason is suspected but not proven to be depression of the second twin at birth. Arnold and colleagues (1987) studied 221 twin-pairs delivered between 27 and 36 weeks and they confirmed the higher incidence of respiratory distress in the second twin. They documented this to be independent of malpresentation or depression at birth. Because the incidence was identical in twin-pairs delivered by cesarean without labor, they hypothesized that the first twin benefitted disproportionately from the salutary effects of labor if delivered vaginally.

Internal Podalic Version. Through careful abdominal, vaginal, and intrauterine examinations, the various parts of the fetus can be identified. Typically, if the buttocks and legs are toward the left side of the mother or the right side of the obstetrician, a sterile intrauterine examining glove that covers the gown to above the elbow is drawn over the right hand and arm. The membranes are ruptured, both feet are accurately identified and grasped, and only then are they gently pulled toward the birth canal (Fig. 39–20). With the other hand applied to the abdomen, the vertex simultaneously is elevated gently (Fig. 39–21). An episiotomy is made or extended whenever more room is needed for uterine and vaginal manipulation. The legs of the fetus are drawn slowly through the birth canal until the buttocks are visible anteriorly just beyond the maternal symphysis. A moist, warm towel is applied to the buttocks and gentle traction is continued until the lower thirds of both scapulas are visible. Next, the trunk is slowly rotated with gentle traction until the shoulder and arm on one side of the fetus are delivered. The rotation of the fetal trunk now is gently reversed to deliver the other arm and shoulder into the vagina. The after-coming head may then be

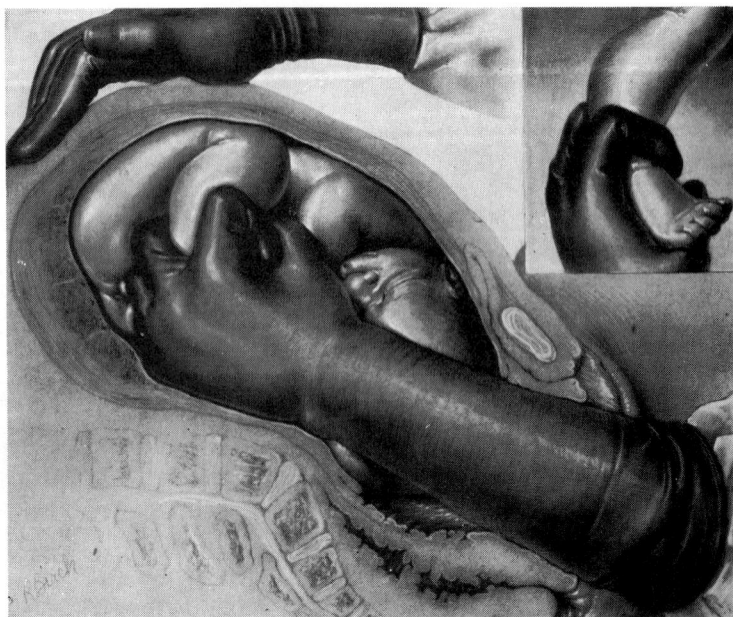

Fig. 39–20. Internal podalic version. Note the use of the long version gloves.

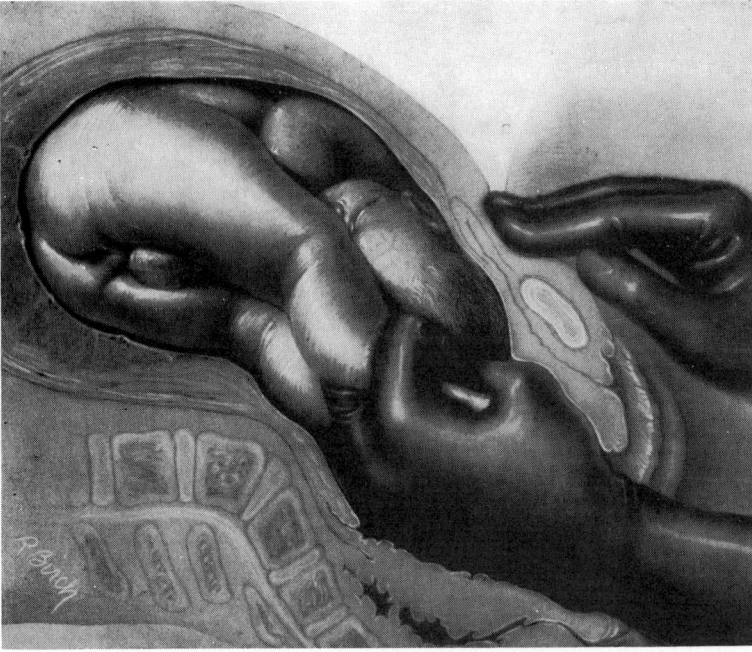

Fig. 39–21. Internal podalic version. Upward pressure on head is applied as downward traction is exerted on feet.

delivered either by simultaneous suprapubic external pressure to flex the head and gentle traction applied to the trunk, or by use of Piper forceps (see Chap. 25, p. 583).

The cord is clamped promptly with two clamps on the placental side to identify it as the cord of the second infant. The placenta or placentas are delivered immediately by manual removal, if necessary. The uterus is explored promptly for defects and for retained pregnancy products. As these steps are being carried out, the uterine-relaxing anesthetic agent is discontinued, and as soon as uterine exploration has been completed, oxytocin is administered through an intravenous infusion system. Fundal massage or, preferably, manual compression of the uterus with one hand in the vagina against the lower uterine segment and the other transabdominally over the uterine fundus is applied to hasten and enhance myometrial contraction.

The cervix, vagina, periurethral region, vulva, and perineum are inspected carefully. Lacerations likely to bleed are repaired along with the episiotomy.

Cesarean Delivery. There has been a recent trend for cesarean delivery of multiple fetuses. For example, Chervenak and colleagues (1985) reported a rate of 35 percent while Thompson and associates (1987) used cesarean delivery for 45 percent of both twins and another 10 percent of second twins by this route. At Parkland Hospital, approximately 50 percent of twin pregnancies are delivered by cesarean section. The most common indication was presentation other than cephalic by one or both fetuses. Other major indications were hypotonic uterine dysfunction, hypertension induced

or aggravated by the pregnancy, fetal distress, gross discordance in size of the fetuses with the smaller fetus the first candidate for vaginal delivery, and prolapsed cord.

Twin fetuses create other unusual problems. The mother is likely to be even less tolerant of the supine position and, therefore, it is important to rotate her position so as to move the uterus and its contents to one side (see Chap. 8, p. 229). A vertical incision in the lower uterine segment may be advantageous. If a fetus lies transversely and the arms are inadvertently delivered first, it is much easier and safer to extend a vertical uterine incision upward than to extend a transverse incision.

It is important that the uterus be well contracted during completion of the cesarean delivery and thereafter. Remarkable blood loss from the uterus may be concealed within the uterus and vagina and beneath the operating drapes during the time taken to close the incisions.

At times, attempts to deliver the second twin vaginally after vaginal delivery of first twin not only may be unwise but also impossible. This may occur, for example, when the second fetus is much larger than the first and is in a breech position or in a transverse lie. Or, even more perplexing, this may occur when the cervix promptly contracts and thickens after delivery of the first infant and does not dilate subsequently. Prompt cesarean delivery may be performed in these circumstances. The Colorado group (Thompson and colleagues, 1987) reported that 15 percent of second twins were delivered by cesarean section following vaginal delivery of the first twin. Of 29 such operations, 19 were for malpresentation, five for fetal distress, four for prolapsed cord, and one for arrested labor.

Three or More Fetuses. All of the problems of twin gestation are intensified remarkably by the presence of additional fetuses. With vaginal delivery the first infant commonly is born spontaneously or with little manipulation. Subsequent infants are delivered according to the presenting part. This may require complicated obstetrical maneuvers, such as total breech extraction or internal podalic version, followed by breech extraction, or this may even necessitate the addition of cesarean delivery. Associated with malposition of the fetuses is an increased incidence of cord prolapse and fetal collision. Moreover, reduced placental perfusion and hemorrhage from separating placentas are more likely during the intrapartum period. Therefore, speed of delivery is very important.

Several groups have described contemporary outcomes and management of pregnancies with three or more fetuses (Creinin, 1988; Lipitz, 1989; Newman, 1989; Sassoon, 1990; and all their colleagues). The general theme of these reports is that triplet outcomes have improved considerably so that a 95 percent infant survival rate can be expected. Collins and Bleyl (1990) and Lipitz and associates (1990) described a combined total of 79 quadruplet pregnancies. The majority of quadruplets were delivered after 28 weeks' gestation. Lipitz and associates (1990), however, observed that in quadruplets retarded growth occurred after 34 weeks. The great majority of triplets and quadruplets cited above were complicated by the same problems characteristic of twin gestation. Importantly, virtually all these triplets and quadruplet pregnancies were delivered by cesarean.

For all of the above reasons, we believe that delivery of pregnancies complicated by the presence of three or more fetuses is accomplished better by cesarean delivery. Vaginal delivery is reserved for those circumstances in which the fetuses are markedly immature or maternal complications make cesarean delivery hazardous to the mother.

Selective Termination

With high-resolution sonography, three and more fetuses can be identified at very early stages of pregnancy and fetal structural anomalies may be visualized precisely in many instances. With such diagnostic capabilities, it is not surprising that investigators have considered reducing the number of fetuses in some multifetal pregnancies to prevent many of the maternal and fetal complications described above. Certainly, the possibility of preventing the birth of one grossly abnormal fetus of a twin-pair has been considered since Bang and co-workers (1975) reported the first successful karyotyping of twin fetuses. In fact, they predicted the

inevitable medical and ethical dilemmas created by finding one abnormal and one normal fetus.

Twins Discordant for Abnormalities. With the identification of twin pregnancy discordant for structural or genetic abnormalities, three options are available: (1) abortion of both fetuses, (2) selective termination of the abnormal fetus, or (3) continuation of the pregnancy. Continuing the pregnancy most often results in delivery of a normal infant along with an abnormal one who may require tremendous familial and societal support. In other cases, the abnormal twin may jeopardize the normal one—for example, by pathological hydramnios developing around an anencephalic twin.

Identification of the Abnormal Fetus. Amnionic fluid can be obtained from each sac at the time of genetic amniocentesis (see Chap. 41, p. 947). This may be accomplished by injecting dye into the first sac sampled. Additionally, careful mapping of uterine structure, placental location, and fetal relationships are established so that if no dye is found later, the two fetuses still can be identified.

Grand Multifetal Pregnancies. The incidence of multifetal pregnancies with extremely large numbers of fetuses has increased during the past two decades because of newer techniques for ovulation induction and the placement of multiple embryos during in vitro fertilization (Evans and associates, 1988; Levene, 1986). Those with four or more embryos are commonly referred to as *grand multifetal pregnancies.* Unfortunately, pregnancy is often desired desperately and a successful outcome may be impossible. In contrast to one abnormal fetus of a twin-pair, the fetuses are most often normal but their number likely precludes successful pregnancy outcome unless selective termination is performed.

Selective reduction of quadruplet, quintuplet, and octuplet pregnancies to either twin or triplet pregnancies has been reported (Berkowitz, 1988; Brandes, 1987; Evans, 1988; Kanhai, 1986; and all their colleagues). There were no maternal complications and 24 out of a possible 45 infants survived to be delivered at or after 30 weeks. In one case reported by Evans and co-workers (1988), one fetus of the remaining pair was anephric (Potter syndrome) and the associated oliguria may have caused spontaneous abortion at 20 weeks. Intentional reduction of triplets to twins has been attempted but reportedly has not improved pregnancy outcomes (Melgar and co-workers, 1991; Porreco and colleagues, 1991).

In a recent review on the efficacy of transabdominal multifetal reduction in 463 completed pregnancies from several major medical centers, Evans and associates (in press) reported a technical success rate of 100 percent. There were 380 pregnancies reduced to twins, 57 reduced to singletons, and 26 reduced to triplets. Fetal loss was 3.9 percent at 2 weeks or less and 4.6 percent at 4 weeks or less.

Informed Consent for Selective Termination.

With twin pregnancies, there is always the risk of identifying one abnormal fetus. Prior to any attempt at prenatal diagnosis, genetic counseling should be conducted with this information provided to the couple (see Chap. 41, p. 939). Specific risks that are common to selective termination include but are not limited to (1) abortion of the remaining fetus(es), (2) abortion of the wrong (normal) fetus in twins, (3) retention of genetic or structurally abnormal fetuses after a reduction in number, (4) damage without death to a fetus, (5) preterm labor complicating pregnancies with the remaining fetus(es), (6) development of discordant twins or growth-retarded fetuses, or (7) maternal infection, hemorrhage, or possible disseminated intravascular coagulopathy owing to retained products of conception.

Techniques for Selective Termination.

These procedures are not easily performed and the technical skills and equipment required are formidable. They should be attempted only by those experienced in amniocentesis and high-resolution sonography. Dumez and Oury (1986) reported a transcervical suction technique to remove selectively any fetuses with a crown–rump length of up to 40 mm, or about 11 weeks. They reported that 9 of 11 pregnancies had gone to term. Berkowitz and colleagues (1988) described 11 women with 12 multifetal pregnancies and 32 embryos. Selective reduction was performed by transcervical aspiration or by fetal thoracic injection with potassium chloride. Three women spontaneously aborted but a total of 15 fetuses born after 30 weeks survived.

Ethics of Selective Termination.

The confusion surrounding ethical dilemmas associated with selective termination is best illustrated by listing its various names: (1) selective termination, (2) selective reduction, (3) selective fetocide, (4) selective embryocide, (5) selective abortion, and (6) selective birth. The ethical problems associated with these techniques are almost limitless and the interested reader is referred to the excellent review by Evans and co-workers (1988). In two earlier publications, the ethical problems associated with selective termination of one abnormal fetus of a twin pair was discussed (Motulsky and Murray, 1983; Silber, 1981).

References

Acker D, Lieberman M, Holbrook H, James O, Phillippe M, Edelin KC: Delivery of second twin. Obstet Gynecol 59:710, 1982

Anderson RL, Golbus MS, Curry CJ, Callen PW, Hastrup WH: Central nervous system damage and other anomalies in surviving fetus following second trimester antenatal death of co-twin. Prenat Diagn 10:513, 1990

Andrews MC, Muasher SJ, Levy DL, Jones HW Jr, Garcia JE, Rosenwaks Z, Jones GS, Acosta AA: An analysis of the obstetric outcome of 125 consecutive pregnancies conceived in vitro and resulting in 100 deliveries. Am J Obstet Gynecol 154:848, 1986

Andrews WW, Leveno KJ, Sherman ML, Mutz J, Gilstrap III LC, Whalley PJ: Elective hospitalization in the management of twin pregnancies. Obstet Gynecol 77:826, 1991

Archer J: Observations showing that a white woman, by intercourse with a white man and a Negro man, may conceive twins, one of which shall be white and the other mulatto. Medical Repository, 3d Hexade 1:319, 1810

Arnold C, McLean FH, Kramer MS, Usher RH: Respiratory distress syndrome in second-born versus first-born twins: A matched case-control analysis. N Engl J Med 317:1121, 1987

Ashworth MF, Spooner SF, Verkuyl DA, Waterman R, Ashurst HM: Failure to prevent preterm labour and delivery in twin pregnancy using prophylactic oral salbutamol. Br J Obstet Gynaecol 97:878, 1990

Azubuike JC: Multiple births in Igbo women. Br J Obstet Gynaecol 89:77, 1982

Azuma C, Kamiura S, Nobunaga T, Negoro T, Saji F, Tanizawa O: Zygosity determination of multiple pregnancy by deoxyribonucleic acid finger prints. Am J Obstet Gynecol 160:734, 1989

Babson SG, Phillips DS: Growth and development of twins dissimilar in size at birth. N Engl J Med 289:937, 1973

Baigts F, Dunica S, Fumeron F, Apfelbaum M: Birthweight difference in monozygous twins followed by differences in development of body weight. Lancet 2:274, 1982

Bang J, Nielsen H, Philip J: Prenatal karyotyping of twins by ultrasonically guided amniocentesis. Am J Obstet Gynecol 123:695, 1975

Bebbington MW, Wittmann BK: Fetal transfusion syndrome: Antenatal factors predicting outcome. Am J Obstet Gynecol 160:913, 1989

Bejar R, Vigliocco G, Gramajo H, Solana C, Benirschke K, Berry C, Coen R, Resnik R: Antenatal origin of neurological damage in newborn infants. II. Multiple gestations. Am J Obstet Gynecol 162:1230, 1990

Benirschke K: Chimerism and mosaicism—Two different entities. In Wynn RM (ed): Obstetrics and Gynecology Annual. New York, Appleton, 1974, p 33

Benirschke K: Personal communication, 1983

Benirschke K, Kim CK: Multiple pregnancy. N Engl J Med 288:1276, 1329, 1973

Berkowitz RL, Lynch L, Chitkara U, Wilkins IA, Mehalek KE, Alvarez E: Selective reduction of multifetal pregnancies in the first trimester. N Engl J Med 318:1043, 1988

Blickstein I, Schwartz-Shoham Z, Lancet M: Growth discordancy inappropriate for gestational age, term twins. Obstet Gynecol 72:582, 1988

Blickstein I, Schwartz-Shoham Z, Lancet M, Borenstein R: Vaginal delivery of the second twin in breech presentation. Obstet Gynecol 68:774, 1987

Bouchard C, Trembley A, Despres JP, Nadeau A, Lupien PJ, Teriault G, Dussault J, Moorjani S, Pinalt S, Fournier G: The response to long-term over feeding in identical twins. N Engl J Med 322:1477, 1990

Bradshaw KD, Marshburn PB, Cunningham FG: Assisted reproductive technology. Williams Obstetrics, 18th ed. (Suppl 17). Norwalk, CT, Appleton & Lange, April/May, 1992

Brandes JM, Itskovitz J, Timor-Tritsch IE, Drugan A, Frydman R: Reduction of the number of embryos in a multiple pregnancy: Quintuplet to triplet. Fertil Steril 48:326, 1987

Brown CEL, Guzick DS, Leveno KJ, Santos-Ramos R, Whalley PJ: Prediction of discordant twins using ultrasound measurement of biparietal diameter and abdominal perimeter. Obstet Gynecol 70:667, 1987

Bulmer MG: The effect of parental age, parity, and duration of marriage on the twinning rate. Ann Hum Genet 23:454, 1959

Bulmer MG: The familial incidence of twinning. Ann Hum Genet 24:1, 1960

Cardwell MS, Caple P, Baker CL: Triplet pregnancy with delivery on three separate days. Obstet Gynecol 71:448, 1988

Carr SR, Aronson MP, Coustan DR: Survival rates of monoamnionic twins do not decrease after 30 weeks' gestation. Am J Obstet Gynecol 163:719, 1990

Caspi E, Ronen J, Schreyer P, Goldberg MD: The outcome of pregnancy after gonadotropin therapy. Br J Obstet Gynaecol 83:967, 1976

Cherouny PH, Hoskins IA, Johnson TB, Niebyl JR: Multiple pregnancy with late death of one fetus. Obstet Gynecol 74:318, 1989

Chervanak FA, Johnson RE, Berkowitz RL, Hobbins JC: Intrapartum external version of the second twin. Obstet Gynecol 62:160, 1983

Chervanak FA, Johnson RE, Youcha S, Hobbins JC, Berkowitz RL: Intrapartum management of twin gestation. Obstet Gynecol 65:119, 1985

Chescheir NC, Leeds JW: Spontaneous resolution of hypofibrinogenemia associated with death of a twin in utero: A case report. Am J Obstet Gynecol 159:1183, 1988

Cohen M, Kohl SG, Rosenthal AH: Fetal interlocking complicating twin gestation. Am J Obstet Gynecol 91:407, 1965

Collins MS, Bleyl JA: Seventy-one quadruplet pregnancies: Management and outcome. Am J Obstet Gynecol 162:1384, 1990

Crawford JS: A prospective study of 200 consecutive twin deliveries. Anaesthesia 42:33, 1987

Creinin M, MacGregor S, Socol M, Hobart J, Ameli S, Keith LG: The Northwestern triplet study. Am J Obstet Gynecol 159:1140, 1988

Crowther CA, Neilson JP, Ashurst HM, Verkuyl DA, Bannerman C: The effects of hospitalization for rest on fetal growth, neonatal morbidity and length of gestation in twin pregnancy. Br J Obstet Gynaecol 97:872, 1990

D'Alton ME, Dudley DK: The ultrasonographic prediction of chorionicity in twin gestation. Am J Obstet Gynecol 160:557, 1989

Danskin FH, Neilson JP: Twin-to-twin transfusion syndrome: What are appropriate diagnostic criteria. Am J Obstet Gynecol 161:365, 1989

Davidson L, Easterling TR, Jackson JC, Benedetti TJ: Breech extraction of low-birth-weight second twins. Am J Obstet Gynecol 166:497, 1992

De Lia JE, Cruikshank DP, Keye WR: Fetoscopic neodymium: Yag laser occlusion of placental vessels in severe twin-twin transfusion syndrome. Obstet Gynecol 75:1046, 1990

Derom C, Derom R, Vlietinck R, Van den Berghe H, Thiery M: Increased monozygotic twinning rate after ovulation induction. Lancet 1:1237, 1987

DiVou MY, Girz BA, Sklar A, Guidetti DA, Langer O: Discordant twins—a prospective study of the diagnostic value of real time ultrasonography combined with umbilical artery velocimetry. Am J Obstet Gynecol 161:757, 1989

Dor J, Shalev J, Masiach J, Blankstein J, Serr DM: Elective cervical suture of twin pregnancies diagnosed ultrasonically in the first trimester following induced ovulation. Gynecol Obstet Invest 13:55, 1982

Dumez Y, Oury JF: Method for first trimester selective abortion in multiple pregnancy. Contrib Gynecol Obstet 15:50, 1986

Dunn PM: Some perinatal observations on twins. Dev Med Child Neurol 7:121, 1969

Erkkola R, Ala-Mello S, Piiroinen O, Kero P, Sillanpää M: Growth discordancy in twin pregnancies: A risk factor not detected by measurements of biparietal diameter. Obstet Gynecol 66:203, 1985

Evans MI, Dommergues M, Wapner RJ, Lynch L, Dumez Y, Goldberg JD, Zador IE, Nicolaides KH, Johnson MP, Golbus MS, Boulot P, Berkowitz RL: Efficacy of transabdominal multifetal pregnancy reduction: Collaborative experience among the world's largest centers. N Engl J Med (in press)

Evans MI, Fletcher JC, Zador IE, Newton BW, Quigg MH, Struyk CD: Selective first-trimester termination in octuplet and quadruplet pregnancies: Clinical and ethical issues. Obstet Gynecol 71:289, 1988

Farmakides G, Schulman H, Saldana LR, Bracero LA, Fleischer A, Rochelson B: Surveillance of twin pregnancy with umbilical arterial velocimetry. Am J Obstet Gynecol 153:789, 1985

Fox H: Pathology of the Placenta. London, Saunders, 1978, p 77

Fujikura T, Froelich LA: Mental and motor development in monozygotic co-twins with dissimilar birth weights. Pediatrics 53:884, 1974

Fusi L, McParland P, Fisk N, Nicolini U, Wigglesworth J: Acute twin-twin transfusion: A possible mechanism for brain-damaged survivors after intrauterine death of a monochorionic twin. Obstet Gynecol 78:517, 1991

Garrett WJ, Carey HM, Steven LM, Climie CR, Osborn RA: A case of nonuplet pregnancy. Aust N Z J Obstet Gynaecol 16:93, 1976

Gerson AG, Wallace DM, Bridgens NK, Ashmead GG, Weiner S, Bolognese RJ: Duplex Doppler ultrasound in the evaluation of growth in twin pregnancies. Obstet Gynecol 70:419, 1987

Gerson A, Johnson A, Wallace D, Bottalico J, Weiner S, Bolognese R: Umbilical arterial systolic/diastolic values in normal twin gestation. Obstet Gynecol 72:205, 1988

Gilbert WM, Davis SE, Kaplan C, Pretorius D, Merritt TA, Benirschke K: Morbidity associated with prenatal disruption of the dividing membrane in twin gestations. Obstet Gynecol 78:623, 1991

Giles WB, Trudinger BJ, Cook CM: Fetal umbilical artery flow velocity-time waveforms in twin pregnancies. Br J Obstet Gynaecol 92:490, 1985

Gocke SE, Nageotte MP, Garite T, Towers CV, Dorcester W: Management of the non-vertex second twin: Primary cesarean section, external version, or primary breech extraction. Am J Obstet Gynecol 161:111, 1989

Gonsoulin W, Moise KJ, Kirshon B, Cotton DB, Wheeler JM, Carpenter RJ: Outcome of twin-twin transfusion diagnosed before 28 weeks of gestation. Obstet Gynecol 75:214, 1990

Greenwald P: Environmental influences on twins apparent at birth. Biol Neonate 15:79, 1970

Harlap S: Ovulation induction and congenital malformations. Lancet 2:961, 1976

Harris DW: Letter to the editors. J Reprod Med 27:39, 1982

Hashimoto B, Callen PW, Filly RA, Laros RK: Ultrasound evaluation of polyhydramnios and twin pregnancy. Am J Obstet Gynecol 154:1069, 1986

Jauniaux E, Elkazen N, Leroy F, Wilkin P, Rodesch F, Hustin J: Clinical and morphologic aspects of the vanishing twin phenomenon. Obstet Gynecol 72:577, 1988

Jewelewicz R, Vande Wiele RL: Management of multifetal gestation. Contemp Obstet Gynecol 6:59, 1975

Kanhai HHH, Van Rijssel EJC, Meerman RJ, Bennebroek-Gravenhorst J: Selective termination in quintuplet pregnancy during first trimester. Lancet 2:1447, 1986

Keilani Z, Clarke PC, Kitau MJ: The significance of raised maternal plasma alpha-fetoprotein in twin pregnancy. Br J Obstet Gynaecol 85:510, 1978

Kemppaineu AS, Karjalainen O, Ylostalo P, Heinonen OP: Ultrasound screening and perinatal mortality: Controlled trial of systemic one-stage screening in pregnancy. Lancet 336:387, 1990

Kiely JL, Kleinman JC, Kiely M: Triplets and higher-order multiple births. Am J Dis Child 146:862, 1992

Knox G, Morley D: Twinning in Yoruba women. J Obstet Gynaecol Br Emp 67:981, 1960

Kohl SG, Casey G: Twin gestation. Mt Sinai J Med 42:523, 1975

Koontz WL, Herbert WNP, Seeds JW, Cefalo RC: Ultrasonography in the antepartum diagnosis of conjoined twins. J Reprod Med 28:627, 1983

Kossoff G, Garrett WJ, Radovanovich G: Ultrasonic examination of a nonuplet pregnancy. Aust N Z J Obstet Gynaecol 16:203, 1976

Kovacs BW, Kirschbaum TH, Paul RH: Twin gestations, I. Antenatal care and complications. Obstet Gynecol 74:313, 1989

Kovacs B, Shahbahrami B, Platt LD, Comings DE: Molecular genetic prenatal determination of twin zygosity. Obstet Gynecol 72:954, 1988

Laros RK, Dattel BJ: Management of twin pregnancy: The vaginal route is still safe. Am J Obstet Gynecol 158:1330, 1988

Levene MI: Grand multiple pregnancies and demand for neonatal intensive care. Lancet 2:347, 1986

Leveno KJ, Quirk JG, Whalley PJ, Herbert WNP, Trubey R: Fetal lung maturation in twin gestation. Am J Obstet Gynecol 148:405, 1984

Leveno KJ, Santos-Ramos R, Duenhoelter JH, Reisch JS, Whalley PJ: Sonar cephalometry in twins: A table of biparietal diameters for normal twin fetuses and a comparison with singletons. Am J Obstet Gynecol 135:727, 1979

Lipitz S, Frenkel Y, Watts C, Rafael ZB, Barkai G, Reichman B: High-order multifetal gestation—management and outcome. Obstet Gynecol 76:215, 1990

Lipitz S, Reichman B, Paret G, Modan M, Shaler J, Serr DM, Mashiach S, Frenkel Y: The improving outcome of triplet pregnancies. Am J Obstet Gynecol 161:1279, 1989

Long PA, Oats JN: Preeclampsia in twin pregnancy—Severity and pathogenesis. Aust NZ J Obstet Gynaecol 27:1, 1987

MacGillivray I: Epidemiology of twin pregnancy. Semin Perinatol 10:4, 1986

MacGillivray I: Twin pregnancies. In Wynn RM (ed): Obstetrics and Gynecology Annual. New York, Appleton, 1978 p 135

MacLennan AH, Green RC, O'Shea R, Brookes C, Morris D: Routine hospital admission in twin pregnancies between 26 and 30 weeks gestation. Lancet 335:267, 1990

Mahony BS, Petty CN, Nyberg DA, Luthy DA, Hickok DE, Hirsch JH: The "stuck twin" phenomenon: Ultrasonographic findings, pregnancy outcome, and management with serial amniocentesis. Am J Obstet Gynecol 163:1513, 1990

Marivate M, De Villiers KO, Fairbrother P: Effect of prophylactic outpatient administration of fenoterol on the time of onset of spontaneous labour and fetal growth rate in twin pregnancy. Am J Obstet Gynecol 128:707, 1977

McKeown T, Record RG: Observations on foetal growth in multiple pregnancy in man. J Endocrinol 5:387, 1952

Melgar CA, Rosenfeld DL, Rawlinson K, Greenberg M: Perinatal outcome after multifetal reduction to twins compared with non-reduced multiple gestations. Obstet Gynecol 78:763, 1991

Morales WJ, O'Brien WF, Knuppel RA, Gaylord S, Hayes P: The effect of mode of delivery on the risk of intraventricular hemorrhage in nondiscordant twin gestations under 1,500 g. Obstet Gynecol 73:107, 1989

Motulsky AG, Murray J: Will prenatal diagnosis with selective abortion affect society's attitude toward the handicapped? Prog Clin Biol Res 128:277, 1983

Myrianthopoulos NC: An epidemiologic survey of twins in a large prospectively studied population. Am J Hum Genet 22:611, 1970

Naeye RL: Organ abnormalities in a human parabiotic syndrome. Am J Pathol 46:829, 1965

Newman HH: The Physiology of Twinning. Chicago, Chicago University Press, 1923

Newman RB, Harner C, Miller MC: Outpatient triplet management: A contemporary review. Am J Obstet Gynecol 161:547, 1989

Nilsen ST, Bergsjo P, Nome S: Male twins at birth and 18 years later. Br J Obstet Gynaecol 91:122, 1984

NOVA, Public Broadcasting System, December 6, 1981. WGBH Educational Foundation, Boston.

O'Connor MC, Murphy H, Dalrymple IJ: Double blind trial of ritodrine and placebo in twin pregnancy. Br J Obstet Gynaecol 86:706, 1979

Pedersen IK, Philips J, Sele V, Starup J: Monozygotic twins with dissimilar phenotypes and chromosome complements. Acta Obstet Gynecol Scand 59:459, 1980

Pettersson F, Smedby B, Lindmark G: Outcome of twin birth: Review of 1636 children born in twin birth. Acta Paediatr Scand 64:473, 1976

Porreco RP, Burke MSB, Hendrix ML: Multifetal reduction of triplets and pregnancy outcome. Obstet Gynecol 78:335, 1991

Powers WF: Twin pregnancy: Complications and treatment. Obstet Gynecol 42:795, 1973

Pritchard JA: Changes in blood volume during pregnancy. Anesthesiology 26:393, 1965

Quigley MM, Cruikshank DP: Polyhydramnios and acute renal failure. J Reprod Med 19:92, 1977

Rabinovici J, Barkai G, Reichman B, Serr DM, Mashiach S: Randomized management of the second nonvertex twin:

Vaginal delivery or cesarean section. Am J Obstet Gynecol 156:52, 1987

Rayburn WF, Lavin JP Jr, Miodovnik M, Varner MW: Multiple gestation: Time interval between delivery of the first and second twins. Obstet Gynecol 63:502, 1984

Robertson EG, Neer KJ: Placental injection studies in twin gestation. Am J Obstet Gynecol 147:170, 1983

Robinson HP, Caines JS: Sonar evidence of early pregnancy failure in patients with twin conceptions. Br J Obstet Gynaecol 84:22, 1977

Rodis JF, Egan JF, Craffey A, Ciarleglio L, Greenstein RM, Scorza WE: Calculated risk of chromosomal abnormalities in twin gestations. Obstet Gynecol 76:1037, 1990

Romero R, Duffy TP, Berkowitz RL, Chang E, Hobbins JC: Prolongation of a preterm pregnancy complicated by death of a single twin in utero and disseminated intravascular coagulation: Effects of treatment with heparin. N Engl J Med 310:772, 1984

Rothman KJ: Fetal loss, twinning and birthweight after oral-contraceptive use. N Engl J Med 297:468, 1977

Rovinsky JJ, Jaffin H: Cardiovascular hemodynamics in pregnancy: III. Cardiac rate, stroke volume, total peripheral resistance, and central blood volume in multiple pregnancy: Synthesis of results. Am J Obstet Gynecol 95:787, 1966

Rydhstrom H: Prognosis for twins with birthweight < 1,500 g: The impact of cesarean section in relation to fetal presentation. Am J Obstet Gynecol 163:528, 1990

Sassoon DS, Castro LC, Davis JL, Hobel CJ: Perinatal outcome in triplet versus twin gestations. Obstet Gynecol 75:817, 1990

Schmidt R, Nitowsky HM, Sobel EH: Monozygotic twins discordant for sex. Pediatr Res 8:395, 1974

Shah DM, Chaffin D: Perinatal outcome in very preterm births with twin-twin transfusion syndrome. Am J Obstet Gynecol 161:1111, 1989

Shah YG, Gragg LA, Moodley S, Williams GW: Doppler velocimetry in concordant and discordant twin gestations. Obstet Gynecol 80:272, 1992

Silber TJ: Amniocentesis and selective abortion. Pediatr Ann 10:31, 1981

Skjaerris J, Aberg A: Prevention of prematurity in twin pregnancy by orally administered terbutaline. Acta Obstet Gynecol Scand Suppl 108:39, 1982

Spellacy WN, Buhi WC, Birk SA: Human placental lactogen levels in multiple pregnancies. Obstet Gynecol 52:210, 1978

Spellacy WN, Hondler A, Fene CD: A case-control study of 1,253 twin pregnancies from a 1982-1987 perinatal data base. Obstet Gynecol 75:168, 1990

Storlazzi E, Vintzileos AM, Campbell WA, Nochimson DJ, Weinbaum PJ: Ultrasonic diagnosis of discordant fetal growth in twin gestations. Obstet Gynecol 69:363, 1987

Strandskov HH, Edelen EW, Siemens GJ: Analysis of the sex ratios among single and plural births in the total "white" and "colored" U.S. populations. Am J Phys Anthropol 4:491, 1946

Stunkard AJ, Harris JR, Pedersen NL, McClearn GE: The body-mass index of twins who have been reared apart. N Engl J Med 322:1483, 1990

Tan KL, Goon SM, Salmon Y, Wee JH: Conjoined twins. Acta Obstet Gynecol Scand 50:373, 1971

Terasaki PI, Gjertson D, Bernoco D, Perdue S, Mickey MR, Bond J: Twins with two different fathers identified by HLA. N Engl J Med 299:590, 1978

Tessen JA, Zlatnik FJ: Monoamnionic twins: A retrospective controlled study. Obstet Gynecol 77:832, 1991

Thiery M, Dhont M, Vandekerckhove D: Serum HCG and HPL in twin pregnancies. Acta Obstet Gynecol Scand 56:495, 1976

Thompson SA, Lyons TL, Makowski EL: Outcomes of twin gestations at the University of Colorado Health Sciences Center, 1973–1983. J Reprod Med 32:328, 1987

Varma TR: Ultrasound evidence of early pregnancy failure in patients with multiple conceptions. Br J Obstet Gynaecol 86:290, 1979

Veille JC, Morton MJ, Burry KJ: Maternal cardiovascular adaptations to twin pregnancy. Am J Obstet Gynecol 153:261, 1985

Waterhouse JAH: Twinning in twin pedigrees. Br J Soc Med 4:197, 1950

Weekes AR, Menzies DN, deBoer CH: The relative efficacy of bed rest, cervical suture, and no treatment in the management of twin pregnancy. Br J Obstet Gynaecol 84:161, 1977

Weinstrom KD, Tessen JA, Zlatnik FJ, Sipes SL: Frequency, distribution, and theoretical mechanisms of hematologic and weight discordances in monochorionic twins. Obstet Gynecol 80:257, 1992

White C, Wyshak G: Inheritance in human dizygotic twinning. N Engl J Med 271:1003, 1964

Winn HN, Gabrielli S, Reece A, Roberts JA, Salafia C, Hobbins JC: Ultrasonographic criteria for the prenatal diagnosis of placental chorionicity in twin gestations. Am J Obstet Gynecol 161:1540, 1989

Wittmann BK, Farquharson D, Wong GP, Baldwin V, Wadsworth LD, Elit L: Delayed delivery of second twin: Report of four cases and review of the literature. Obstet Gynecol 79:260, 1992

Fetal Abnormalities: Inherited and Acquired Disorders

■

CHAPTER 40
Genetics

Three to 5 percent of all newborns have a recognizable birth defect (Shepard, 1986). Unfortunately, the causes of these anomalies are myriad and frequently not identifiable. Beckman and Brent (1986) suggested the following etiological categories and the estimated contribution of each to fetal damage:

Genetic—chromosomal and single-gene defects	20–25%
Fetal Infections—cytomegalovirus, syphilis, rubella, toxoplasmosis, and others	3–5%
Maternal diseases—diabetes, alcohol abuse, seizure disorders, and others	~ 4%
Drugs and medications	< 1%
Multifactorial or unknown	65–75%

Detection of functional congenital aberrations increases as the infant ages; thus the incidence ultimately increases to 6 or 7 percent in later childhood. Anomalies are increased in obstetrically abnormal pregnancies, and perhaps 50 percent of spontaneously aborted fetuses have a chromosomal abnormality. Preterm and stillborn infants more commonly have major malformations, and their detection is increased with performance of routine autopsies. Birth defects are the leading cause of infant deaths before age 1, accounting for 20 percent of such deaths (Oakley, 1986).

Teratogen-induced malformations—that is, those caused by drugs, medications, radiation, or infections—are discussed in detail in other chapters.

Probably no allied field has had more impact on the practice of obstetrics than medical genetics. Advances in molecular genetics and their application to prenatal diagnosis (Chap. 41), the introduction of maternal serum alpha-fetoprotein screening programs into clinical practice, and the rapid dissemination of genetic information to both lay public and health-care providers are examples of changes that have become important aspects of daily obstetrical care.

At least 20 to 25 percent of congenital malformations are the result of chromosomal abnormalities or single-gene defects. The majority—perhaps 65 to 75 percent—of birth defects are from unidentifiable causes; however, because of their patterns of inheritance, many are presumed to be the consequence of a complex interaction between genetic predisposition and fetal environmental factors, so-called *multifactorial inheritance*.

Chromosomal Abnormalities

The incidence of chromosomal abnormalities in live-born infants has been established in six studies to be 1 in 170 newborns (Jacobs and colleagues, 1974). The frequency among stillbirths and neonatal deaths is 6 to 7 percent (Boué and Boué, 1978). The incidence of various chromosomal abnormalities among live-born infants is presented in Table 40–1; and among stillbirths and neonatal deaths, in Table 40–2. Chromosomal abnormalities are identified in approximately 50 percent of early spontaneous abortions, and Turner syndrome (45,X) is the most common (Boué and associates, 1985).

Down syndrome, which was initially described in 1866, was the first chromosomal abnormality to be recognized when LeJuene and colleagues (1959) observed that an extra chromosome 21 was present. Since then, the specialty of cytogenetics has made both significant and rapid progress, with the addition of many sophisticated techniques to assist in the evaluation of chromo-

TABLE 40–1. INCIDENCE OF CHROMOSOMAL ABNORMALITIES IN 43,558 NEWBORNS

Chromosomal Anomaly	Approximate Incidence (per 1000 births)
Autosomal Trisomies	**1.2**
Trisomy 21	1.0
Trisomy 18	0.1
Trisomy 13	0.1
Sex Chromosome Abnormalities	**3.9**
Male (28,582)	2.6
XYY	0.9
XXY	1.0
Other	0.6
Female (14,976)	1.3
45, X	0.1
XXX	0.9
Other	0.3
Structural Rearrangements	**2.4**
Euploid (balanced)	1.9
Aneuploid (unbalanced)	0.5

Adapted from Jacobs and colleagues (1974).

somal disorders. Although details of techniques and terminology employed are beyond the scope of this textbook, the obstetrician must be familiar with certain basic principles and their application to patient care.

Techniques. Cytogenetic studies can be performed only on dividing cells in specialized laboratories. Thus, collection and handling of the specimen to insure viability are of the utmost importance. Peripheral blood and amnionic fluid are the most common sources of cells for cytogenetic evaluation. Also used are samples of chorionic villi, bone marrow, products of conception, and skin, as well as internal organs removed at surgery or autopsy. The cytogenetic laboratory should be consulted to ascertain the appropriate techniques for collection, transport, and shipping for each tissue.

The laboratory must establish cultures of cells from

TABLE 40–2. INCIDENCE OF VARIOUS CHROMOSOMAL ABNORMALITIES AMONG STILLBIRTHS AND NEONATAL DEATHS

Abnormality	Percent
Sex chromosome	1.2
Autosomal trisomies	
Trisomy 21	0.7
Trisomy 18	1.8
Trisomy 13	0.5
Structural anomalies	
Balanced	0.35
Unbalanced	0.5
Others	0.7
Triploidy	0.35
Total	6.1

Adapted from Boué and Boué (1978).

the sample, and maintain these until an adequate number of dividing cells are available for analysis. Through a variety of techniques, cells are induced to divide, captured in the process of chromosome division, fixed, stained, and analyzed under the light microscope. Individual nuclei are photographed, and the chromosomes are cut from the photograph and arranged on a karyotype chart (Fig. 40–1). Each chromosome is identified by its specific pattern of banding following staining. The number of chromosomes is determined, and each pair of chromosomes is analyzed for structural alterations. The chromosome study process can be aided by computerized equipment, but the ultimate responsibility for interpretation of the results rests on the highly trained laboratory personnel.

Each chromosome has its individual pattern of numbers corresponding to the dark and light bands produced by staining. Specific parts of a chromosome are identified by a combination of the chromosome number, arm, region (numbered from the centromere), band, and sub-band.

The normal or diploid number of chromosomes was shown by Tijo and Levan (1956) to be 46. There are a total of 44 autosomes, the pairs numbered from 1 to 22. The genes located on autosomes are involved, with few exceptions, in aspects of development and physiology that do not involve sex determination. The single pair of sex chromosomes, the X and the Y, determine sex, although the X chromosome also contains many genes crucial to other aspects of development. The Y chromosomes appear to carry only genes involved in the production of "maleness."

Chromosomal abnormalities can be divided into three basic categories:

1. Numerical—the number of chromosomes is either greater or less than 46; also referred to as *aneuploidy.*
2. Structural—chromosomal material is lost, gained, or rearranged. Structural alterations can involve a single or multiple chromosomes.
3. Mosaicism—two or more cytogenetically distinct cell lines are present in the same individual.

Numerical Autosomal Abnormalities. Numerical abnormalities are the result of **nondisjunction,** which is the uneven distribution of chromosomes at cell division. Nondisjunction can occur during meiosis or mitosis. The most common numerical abnormalities are trisomies, or the presence of an extra chromosome. Autosomal trisomies that involve chromosomes other than the X or Y invariably result in abnormal embryonic development and are associated with physical abnormalities and mental retardation. Most autosomal trisomies are never observed in live-born infants, but are identified in spontaneous abortions, suggesting that the imbalance of

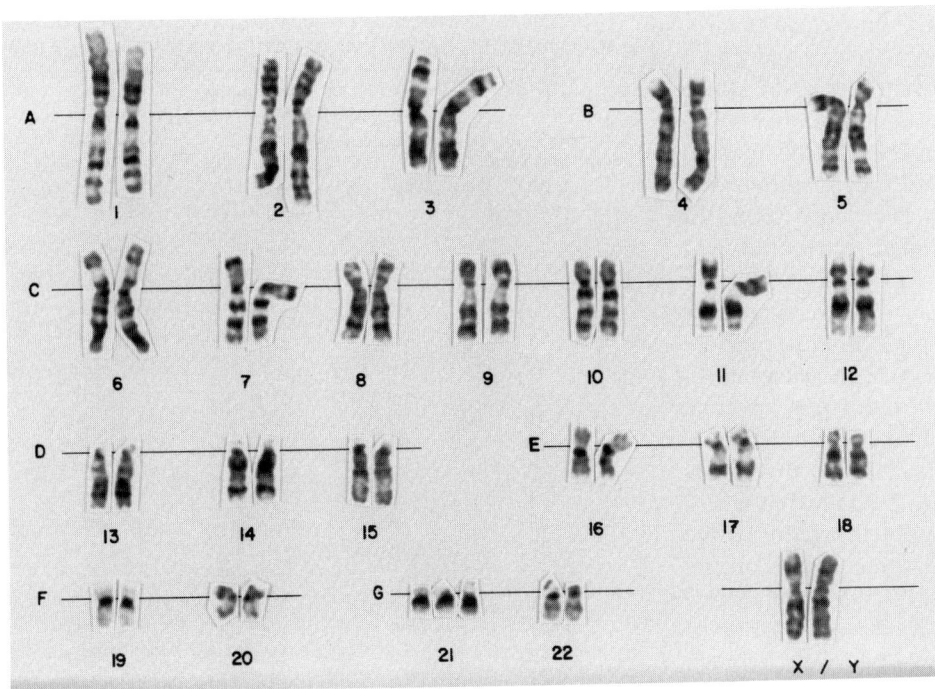

Fig. 40–1. Abnormal female karyotype with trisomy 21, consistent with Down syndrome: 47,XX,+21. (Courtesy of Dr. Nancy R. Schneider.)

genetic material is usually incompatible with normal development. Other autosomal trisomies are seen in live-born infants only in the mosaic state, with the presence of cytogenetically normal cells presumably modifying the effect of the abnormal cell line.

Trisomy 21. The most clinically significant autosomal trisomy is trisomy 21, and this is the cytogenetic finding in individuals with Down syndrome (Fig. 40–1). Down syndrome is associated with a characteristic facial appearance that may be striking in the newborn infant. The head is usually relatively small, with a flattened occiput. The nasal bridge is flat, the eyes appear wide-spaced due to epicanthal folds, the palpebral fissures are upslanting, and the tongue appears large for the mouth and often protrudes (Fig. 40–2). There is frequently loose skin at the nape of the neck, and the infants generally have poor tone. The fingers are short and stubby, and there is often a so-called *simian crease* on one or both palms. The fifth fingers are often incurved (*clinodactyly*) due to absence or hypoplasia of the middle phalanx. Associated major malformations include heart defects, particularly en-

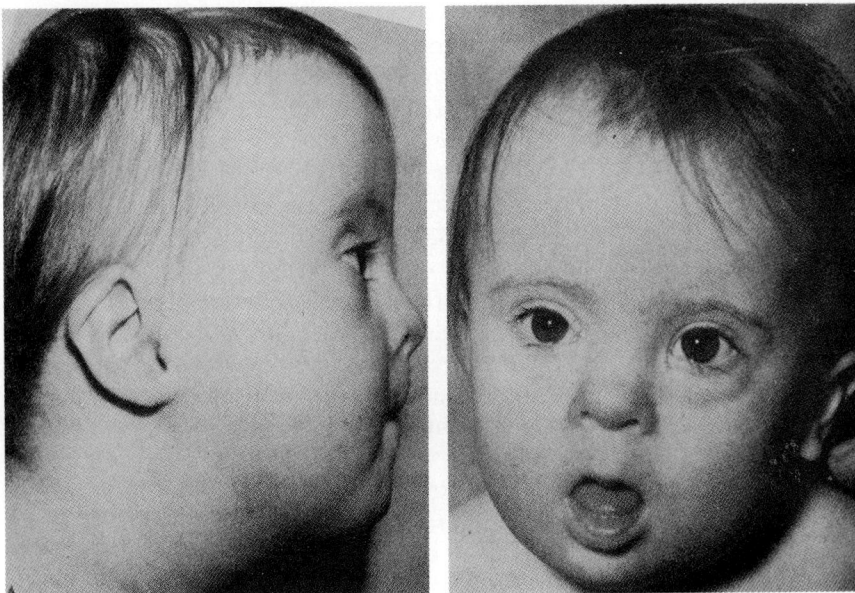

Fig. 40–2. Young infant with Down syndrome (trisomy 21). (From Jones, 1988, with permission.)

docardial cushion defects, and gastrointestinal atresias. There is an increased incidence of neonatal and childhood leukemia. The most significant feature of Down syndrome for most families is the associated mental retardation, which can vary greatly in severity. Infants with Down syndrome are often delayed only slightly compared with their peers, and they have been found to benefit from formal programs of infant stimulation and early childhood educational intervention.

Although the clinical diagnosis of Down syndrome is often suspected in the delivery room, chromosome studies must be performed to ascertain the exact chromosomal abnormality involved. Without this information, accurate genetic counseling is impossible. Trisomy 21 has a 1 to 2 percent recurrence risk in the subsequent children of a young mother. The recurrence risk for women 35 and older depends upon the maternal age at the time of conception. Chromosome studies on the parents of a child with trisomy 21 are not necessary.

The incidence of trisomy 21 increases with maternal age, with the likelihood of a 20-year-old woman having an affected child being approximately 1 in 1200, compared with a 1 in 70 risk for a 40-year-old woman. This increased risk is not limited to Down syndrome, but includes all aneuploidies with the exception of Turner syndrome (45,X). The incidence at conception of trisomy 21, and indeed of all cytogenetic abnormalities, is apparently much greater than live-birth statistics suggest, with one half to two thirds of affected conceptuses lost spontaneously (Table 40–3).

Effect of Paternal Age

Paternal age does not appear to be an important risk factor for Down syndrome or other chromosomal abnormalities, but the age of the father does play a role in the development of autosomal dominant genetic diseases. The relative frequency of new autosomal dominant mutations in offspring increases logarithmically with paternal age during the usual period of fatherhood (Friedman, 1981). For example, the majority of cases of the autosomal dominant condition known as achondroplasia, a type of short-limbed dwarfism, are new mutations, and paternal age is increased significantly among this group. The absolute frequency of autosomal dominant disease as the consequence of new mutations among newborns whose fathers are 40 years of age is at least 0.3 percent and presumably increases with age.

Pregnancy in a woman with Down syndrome is rare and is associated with a high incidence of Down syndrome. Bovicelli and associates (1982) reviewed the pregnancy experiences of 26 affected mothers. No male with Down syndrome is definitely known to have fathered a child.

Other Trisomies. Other clinically significant autosomal trisomies include trisomy 13 and trisomy 18. Both result

TABLE 40–3. INCIDENCE OF DOWN SYNDROME IN FETUSES AND LIVEBORN INFANTS IN RELATION TO MATERNAL AGE[a]

Maternal Age (yr)	Birth	Incidence Amniocentesis (16 wk)	Chorionic Villus Sampling (9–11 wk)
15–19	1/1250	—	—
20–24	1/1400	—	—
25–29	1/1100	—	—
30	1/900	—	—
31	1/900	—	—
32	1/750	—	—
33	1/625	1/420	—
34	1/500	1/325	—
35	1/350	1/250	1/240
36	1/275	1/200	1/175
37	1/225	1/150	1/130
38	1/175	1/120	1/100
39	1/140	1/100	1/75
40	1/100	1/75	1/60
41	1/85	1/60	1/40
42	1/65	1/45	1/30
43	1/50	1/35	1/25
44	1/40	1/30	1/20
45 and over	1/25	1/20	1/10

[a] Figures have been rounded and are approximate.
Data from Hook and colleagues (1983, 1988), modified from Thompson and associates (1991), with permission.)

in recognizable patterns of malformations and are frequently associated with life-threatening birth defects; stillbirths and neonatal deaths are common. Still, it is inaccurate to characterize these disorders as "lethal," because a minority of affected infants survive, sometimes into their teens. Profound mental retardation is associated with both trisomies. Their incidence also increases with advanced maternal age, and the conditions are occasionally encountered in prenatal diagnostic studies.

Other autosomal trisomies are very rarely seen in live-born infants. Mosaicism for several different autosomal trisomies has been reported, and characteristic malformation patterns have been described for specific trisomies. The obstetrician cannot be expected to recognize these rare conditions clinically, but any obstetrician should be aware that chromosomal studies are indicated on any newborn with multiple congenital anomalies. If an abnormal karyotype is identified, referral for genetic counseling should be arranged.

Monosomy. Monosomy, the absence of one member of a pair of chromosomes, is much less common than trisomy. With very rare exceptions, autosomal monosomy is lethal early in embryonic development. Sex chromosome monosomy is discussed below.

Structural Autosomal Abnormalities.
There are a variety of structural chromosomal alterations that include deletions and chromosomal rearrangements such as rings, inversions, and translocations.

Deletions. A deletion refers to a portion of a chromosome that is missing. For example, del (4p) refers to chromosome number 4 that is missing material from the short or "p" arm, while del (4q) refers to a material from the missing long or "q" arm of chromosome 4. Some chromosomal deletions are associated with a recognizable pattern of anomalies in the affected infant and have been given syndromic eponyms, such as *Wolf–Hirschhorn syndrome* for del (4p) and *cri du chat syndrome* for del (5p). The more recent literature uses the cytogenetic nomenclature to describe the precise deleted chromosome portion. Any member of the 23 pairs of chromosomes may incur a deletion, and the amount of material missing can vary greatly from patient to patient, yielding different phenotypes. Deletions may occur spontaneously, or may be the result of meiotic distribution of an inherited rearrangement; thus chromosome studies should always be performed on the parents of an infant found to have a chromosomal deletion.

Translocations. Rearrangement of material between chromosomes results in a translocation (or insertion). Translocations are the clinically most significant type of chromosomal rearrangement, and they result when portions of two or more chromosomes have broken and rejoined to form "new" chromosomes. This type of rearrangement may interfere with normal segregation of chromosomes during meiosis, which in turn may have significant clinical implications. The two common types are Robertsonian and reciprocal translocations.

Robertsonian translocations always involve the acrocentric chromosomes, and are thought to be caused by centric fusion after loss of the satellite region of the short arms of the original acrocentric chromosomes. This type of rearrangement involves the entire long arms of the chromosomes involved (Fig. 40–3). There is no significant loss of genetic material because the satellites contain ribosomal DNA present in multiple copies on other chromosomes.

The clinical phenotype of Down syndrome can result from translocation of chromosome number 21 material onto another chromosome. The affected individual has a total of 46 chromosomes, but in effect has three copies of chromosome 21. This arrangement results in Down syndrome features that are indistinguishable from those from trisomy 21. Such translocations commonly involve chromosome 14, but any of the acrocentric chromosomes (13, 14, 15, 21, or 22) can be involved. These Robertsonian translocations may be spontaneous events, but they can also be inherited from a carrier parent. The karyotype of a parent who carries a balanced translocation of this type will appear to have only 45 chromosomes. The full complement of genetic material is present, however, and there are no clinical effects.

Chromosome studies should be obtained on both parents of an infant found to have Down syndrome due to a translocation. The recurrence risk in future pregnancies depends upon whether the translocation is spontaneous, in which case the recurrence risk is similar to that for trisomy 21, or approximately 1 percent. The recurrence risk for an inherited translocation depends upon the specific chromosomes involved, which can be determined by cytogenetic techniques and the sex of the transmitting parent. In general, the risk is greater

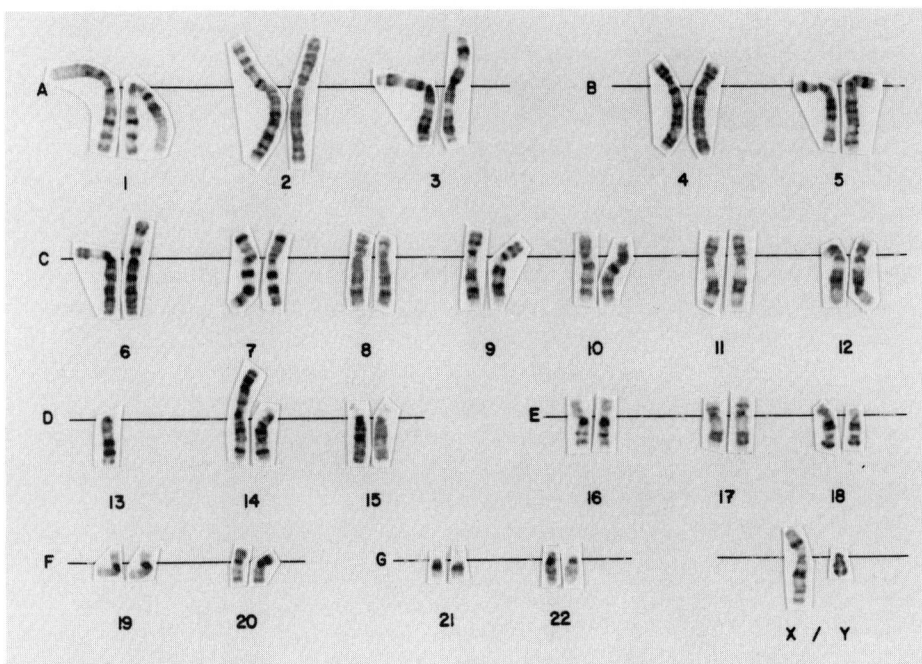

Fig. 40–3. Karyotype of a male carrier of a Robertsonian translocation: 45,XY,t(13q14q). (Courtesy of Dr. Nancy R. Schneider.)

when the mother carries the translocation. There is also an increased risk of reduced fertility or early pregnancy loss due to the presence of a translocation in either parent, as some of the possible meiotic products are incompatible with survival.

In the event of an inherited 21/21 translocation, the couple faces a dilemma that is rare in human genetics. It is impossible for the carrier parent to produce a normal gamete, and all conceptions will result in abnormal embryos. Pregnancy will either result in a child with 21/21 translocation Down syndrome or monosomy 21, a lethal condition that usually causes early spontaneous abortion. Oocyte donation is the only alternative when this condition is present in the woman.

Reciprocal translocations can involve any two or more chromosomes, and occur when there is breakage and reunion of portions of the involved chromosomes to yield new products (Fig. 40–4). In contrast to the situation with Robertsonian translocations, carriers of balanced reciprocal translocations have 46 chromosomes, with both rearranged derivative chromosomes present. Their offspring who receive an unbalanced meiotic product usually also have 46 chromosomes, but have only one of the derivative chromosomes present. This results in partial monosomy for one chromosome, and partial trisomy for another. The clinical effect of such unbalanced rearrangements ranges from embryonic death to viability with relatively mild physical and developmental abnormalities.

Cytogenetic studies of couples with recurrent pregnancy loss show approximately 2 to 3 percent incidence of balanced Robertsonian or reciprocal translocations in one of the partners (DeWald and Michels, 1986). Iden-

tification of such translocations has implications for other family members, and translocation carriers should be encouraged to inform their parents and siblings of the desirability of chromosome evaluation.

Rings and Inversions. Rearrangements of chromosomal material within the chromosome itself can result in rings and inversions. When there is a deletion from both ends of a chromosome, the ends may unite, forming a **ring chromosome.** The clinical significance of this rearrangement primarily depends on the amount and significance of material lost. This configuration may interfere with normal segregation of chromosomes and may be inherited from a parent who is mosaic for the presence of this ring.

Chromosome inversions result from the breakage and rejoining of a chromosome loop during interphase of the cell. Inversions may involve the centromere, so-called *pericentric inversions;* or may occur distal to the centromere, so-called *paracentric inversions.* Both types of inversions interfere with normal meiotic pairing of chromosomes, and this can result in abnormal gametes that may be either nonviable or abnormal.

Mosaicism. Mosaicism is the presence of two or more cytogenetically distinct cell lines in the same individual. It is believed to arise through nondisjunction during early mitotic divisions of the zygote, resulting in two distinct cell lines. Depending upon the ultimate embryonic "fate" of the cytogenetically abnormal cells, mosaicism may involve the placenta, fetus, or both. Detection of mosaicism often requires the study of more than the usual number of cells as well as different tissue speci-

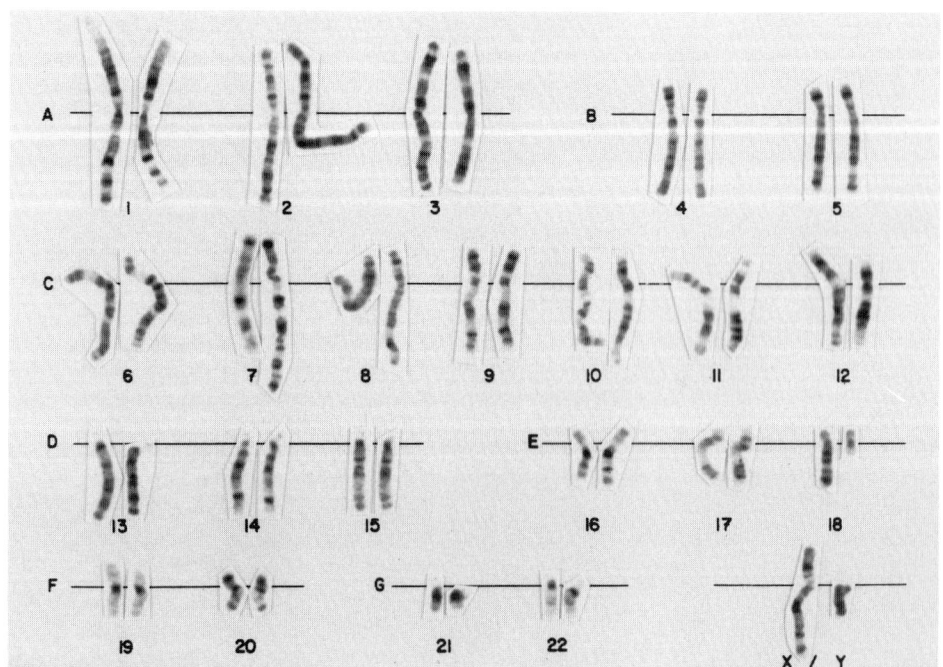

Fig. 40–4. Karyotype of a male carrier of a balanced (or reciprocal) translocation: 46,XY,t(7;18)(q36;q11.2). (Courtesy of Dr. Nancy R. Schneider.)

mens. Mosaicism is never excluded completely by a cytogenetic study, because the abnormal cell line may be confined to tissues that cannot be studied cytogenetically. **Placental mosaicism** may play a role in the survival of some cytogenetically abnormal fetuses. In these cases, normal placental cells may be able to compensate to some degree for the impaired function of the abnormal cells. Conversely, some cytogenetically normal but severely growth-retarded infants have been found to have placental chromosomal abnormalities that presumably impair normal function (Kalousek and Dill, 1983). **Gonadal mosaicism** is an important risk factor for recurrence of both cytogenetic abnormalities and disorders of Mendelian inheritance. A parent who carries an abnormal cell line in the gonad may have multiple affected offspring. This phenomenon may account for the observed recurrence risk for Down syndrome and other autosomal trisomies.

Sex Chromosome Abnormalities. The majority of sex chromosome disorders involve abnormalities in number, or *aneuploidy.* Klinefelter syndrome, Turner syndrome, XYY genotype, and trisomy X are among the most commonly encountered sex chromosomal abnormalities. monosomy X or Turner syndrome is the most common cytogenetic aberration identified in spontaneous abortions.

Turner Syndrome (45,X). Sex chromosome monosomy occurs as monosomy X or Turner syndrome (45,X). Monosomy X is also prenatally lethal in most cases, with approximately half of cytogenetically abnormal spontaneous abortions having this chromosomal finding. The incidence of monosomy X does not appear to be associated with increased maternal age. It is usually the paternal sex chromosome that is absent, suggesting that nondisjunction in the spermatogonium may be the underlying mechanism in the majority of cases. Monosomy Y is never observed; presumably, the presence of at least one X chromosome is required for early embryonic development. Loss of the long arm of one X chromosome results in streaked ovaries and amenorrhea, while loss of the short arm results in short stature.

Infants with Turner syndrome of 45,X monosomy have a characteristic pattern of growth and physical characteristics that often results in a clinical diagnosis in the newborn period. They are short, may have marked lymphedema of the hands and feet, and frequently have webbing of the neck as the sequelae of cystic hygromas that develop in the nuchal region during fetal life. Cardiac defects, especially aortic coarctation, are relatively common, as are renal and urinary tract abnormalities. Intelligence is usually normal, although specific areas of learning difficulties have been documented. The ovaries are usually represented by gonadal streaks, and puberty does not ensue without hormone replacement. Mosaicism is common, and some mosaic individuals may

reproduce. There is speculation that all live-born 45,X individuals have mosaicism, which may not be apparent in lymphocytes or skin cells, the tissues that are usually studied.

Deletions and mosaic patterns are also encountered. For example, deletions or absence of the short arm of the X chromosome result in some of the stigmata of Turner syndrome. The same is true for an isochromosome of the long arm of the X chromosome with duplication of the long ("q") arm and absence of the short ("p") arm.

Extra X Chromosomes. Females with one extra X chromosome (47,XXX) may be indistinguishable from those with a normal 46,XX karyotype, although decreased fertility and an increased risk for nondisjunction may lead to reproduction problems. Females with more than three X chromosomes (48,XXXX; 49,XXXXX) have an increased incidence of physical abnormalities that may be apparent at birth, and they exhibit varying degrees of mental retardation.

Klinefelter Syndrome (47,XXY). Additional X chromosomes to the normal male XY karyotype are relatively common polysomies, seen in about 1 in 1000 male infants. Males with 47,XXY constitute the most frequent abnormality of sexual differentiation and, except for some mosaics, are invariably infertile. They have testicular atrophy, azoospermia, and elevated serum gonadotropin levels. There may be associated somatic abnormalities, especially gynecomastia and truncal obesity. This syndrome is generally not recognized until puberty. Mild mental deficiency is common. In syndromes caused by more than two X chromosomes, both physical and developmental abnormalities are common.

Extra Y Chromosomes. Males with the 47,XYY complement may have increased height and an increased frequency of severe acne. Intelligence does not appear to be affected in most individuals, but learning disabilities are common. Although this condition was initially reported increased in prison populations, the precise association of this karyotype with criminal or antisocial behavior has never been confirmed. The incidence at birth is about 1 per 1000 (Table 40–1). Males with more than two extra Y chromosomes (48,XYYY) or with both additional X and Y chromosomes (48,XXYY; 49,XXXYY) have obvious physical abnormalities and significant mental retardation.

Single-gene Defects

Single-gene mutations cause disorders that are characterized by Mendelian inheritance patterns. Mendelian disorders cause phenotypic abnormalities in 1 percent of all newborns. The prevalence in the population is much higher, as many such disorders do not become manifest until after the newborn period. Individual disorders are rare, but the number so far catalogued—nearly 4000—underscores their importance (McKusick, 1990). As with any Mendelian inheritance, their clinical presentation can be classified into autosomal dominant, autosomal recessive, and X-linked. Some of the more common Mendelian disorders are shown in Table 40–4.

Modes of Autosomal Inheritance

Dominant Inheritance. A mutant gene producing its effects when present in a single copy is referred to as a

TABLE 40–4. SOME RELATIVELY FREQUENT MENDELIAN DISORDERS AFFECTING ADULTS

Autosomal dominant
Achondroplasia
Acute intermittent porphyria
Adult polycystic kidney disease
Familial hypercholesterolemia
Hereditary spherocytosis
Huntington chorea
Idiopathic hypertrophic subaortic stenosis
Marfan syndrome
Myotonic dystrophy
Neurofibromatosis
Noonan syndrome
Osteogenesis imperfecta tarda
Polydactyly
Tuberous sclerosis
von Willebrand disease

Autosomal recessive
Albinism
Congenital adrenal hyperplasia
Cystic fibrosis
Deafness
Familial mediterranean fever
Friedrich ataxia
Hemochromatosis
Hereditary emphysema
Homocystinuria
Phenylketonuria
Sickle cell anemia
Tay–Sach disease
α-Thalassemia
β-Thalassemia
Wilson disease

X linked
Chronic granulomatous disease
Color blindness
Fabry disease
Glucose-6-phosphate deficiency
Hemophilia A and B
Hunter syndrome
Hypophosphatemic rickets
Ichthyosis
Lesch–Nyhan syndrome
Muscular dystrophy
Nephrogenic diabetes insipidus
Ocular albinism
Testicular feminization

Modified from Goldstein and Brown (1991).

dominant gene, and nearly 1200 have been identified (McKusick, 1990). A dominantly inherited disease caused by a single gene is transmitted from one generation to the next in a direct line—so-called *vertical transmission*—so that each affected individual has an affected parent and there are no skipped generations, although reduced penetrance of the clinical effects of the gene may make it seem to "skip" a generation. There is a 50 percent chance that an affected parent will transmit the gene to each of his or her offspring. The affected child will in turn transmit the defect to half of his or her offspring.

Some autosomal dominant diseases have a delayed age of onset and may show variability in clinical expression. Other characteristics include penetrance, imprinting, and expressivity.

PENETRANCE. A dominant gene with recognizable phenotypic expression in all individuals who carry the gene is said to have 100 percent penetrance. If not phenotypically expressed in some individuals, who have the gene, the gene is not penetrant. The degree of penetrance may be quantitatively expressed as the ratio of carriers who show the trait to the total number of individuals who have the gene. A gene that is 80 percent penetrant is expressed in only 80 percent of the individuals who have that gene.

IMPRINTING. The expression of a particular disease also may depend on whether the mutant gene was of paternal or maternal origin, a condition known as imprinting (Hall, 1992).

EXPRESSIVITY. The degree to which the same gene may express itself is known as the expressivity of the condition. The expressivity of a gene ranges from complete or severe manifestation of the condition to mild expression.

Autosomal Recessive Inheritance. An autosomal recessive disorder is expressed when two copies of a mutant gene are inherited, one from each parent. The affected individual is homozygous. The carrier parents who have one mutant and one normal gene are heterozygous and are clinically unaffected. More than 600 disorders have been described (McKusick, 1990). Common examples are shown in Table 40–4. Most inherited enzyme defects are recessive.

Either sex may be similarly affected. Parents and more remote carrier ancestors are usually clinically unaffected. Because the disease is present in only one generation, this type of inheritance is often referred to as *horizontal transmission*. The probability of a subsequent child being affected after the birth of one affected child is one in four. The likelihood that a normal sibling of an affected child is a carrier of the gene is two out of three. The carrier child will not produce affected children, however, except by mating with another carrier or an affected individual. If the recessive gene is rare, there is only a small chance that unrelated carriers will mate.

UNIPARENTAL DISOMY. It is a well-established genetic dogma that fertilization unites two genetically equal gametes, each of which carries 23 chromosomes, one from each pair of parental chromosomes. The existence of *uniparental disomy* has recently been recognized in humans, as well as in experimental animals, in which both members of one pair of chromosomes are inherited from the same parent. This appears to occur as the result of "correction" of a trisomic zygote by loss of a chromosome, leaving the correct number of chromosomes, but a same-parent origin for both members of one pair.

Uniparental disomy was first recognized in humans when molecular studies of DNA of a patient with cystic fibrosis and unusually short stature indicated that both number 7 chromosomes had been inherited from the mother; no paternal number 7 was present (Spence and colleagues, 1988). This resulted in homozygosity for any mutant autosomal recessive genes that might be present on the mother's chromosome 7, even though the father was not a carrier for the mutation. Nonpaternity was ruled out by the DNA testing.

Other examples of uniparental disomy in the human involve syndromes that sometimes, but not always, are associated with a detectable chromosomal deletion, which almost always involves the parental chromosome. Prader–Willi syndrome, characterized by obesity, mental retardation, and a distinctive physical appearance, occurs when there is a deletion of a specific region of paternal chromosome 15. A similar deletion in maternal chromosome 15 results in Angelman syndrome, a phenotypically different mental retardation disorder (Knoll and colleagues, 1989, 1991). Cases of Prader–Willi syndrome with no detectable deletion of chromosome 15 at the cytogenetic or molecular level have been shown to have uniparental disomy for chromosome 15, with both copies being maternal; there is thus the equivalent of a paternal deletion of chromosome 15 (Mascari and colleagues, 1992; Nicholls and co-workers, 1989).

Animal studies have shown that uniparental disomy is frequently associated with early pregnancy wastage, abortion, stillbirth, and neonatal death; pregnancy outcome may differ with the parental origin of the disomic chromosome. This may prove to be an explanation for much of the human pregnancy loss that is currently of unknown etiology.

CONSANGUINITY. Consanguinity or kinship increases the likelihood that a couple will share autosomal recessive genes. First cousins share 1/8 of their genes; second cousins share 1/16. If there is a family history of an autosomal recessive disorder, it is possible to calculate the mathematical risk that the couple will have an affected child, and in some cases, prenatal diagnosis may be appropriate. With a negative family history, there is still an increased risk that both members of the couple are carriers for a deleterious gene. Genetic counseling for such a couple must emphasize that there is an increased risk for genetic disorders, miscarriage, and stillbirth in the offspring of first cousin matings, but that the risk is relatively low, approximately double the risk for non-consanguineous couples.

Incest, the mating of individuals more closely related than first cousins, involves significant risks of congenital anomalies in the offspring (Reed, 1963), and this practice is proscribed by law. Several investigators have estimated the risk for anomalous children of brother–sister or parent–child matings to be as high as 50 percent.

INBORN ERRORS OF METABOLISM. Among the autosomal recessive disorders are several rare but heritable inborn errors of metabolism, most of which result in the absence of crucial enzymes, and in incomplete metabolism of proteins, sugars, or fats. High blood levels of these toxic metabolites cause mental retardation and other defects. *Phenylketonuria*, a classic example of such a defect, is due to a diminished *phenylalanine hydroxylase* activity. This results in the inability to metabolize phenylalanine appropriately to tyrosine. It has been reported in 1 in 10,000 to 15,000 white infants, but much less often in African-American infants. Early diagnosis is important, because optimal early treatment with limitation of phenylalanine consumption may result in normal intelligence (Williamson and associates, 1981). All states now require a newborn screening test for phenylketonuria. As an example, about 10 cases are identified annually by the Texas Newborn Screening program.

Women with phenylketonuria adequately managed by diet during childhood may still have poor pregnancy outcomes, including high frequencies of spontaneous abortion, microcephaly, and mental retardation. These abnormalities are induced by excessive maternal phenylalanine concentrations, and women who wish to conceive should be advised to adhere to a diet low in phenylalanine before conception and throughout pregnancy (Ghavami and associates, 1986; Rohr and colleagues, 1987). Unfortunately, even then a normal outcome cannot be guaranteed (Lenke and Levy, 1982).

Modes of Sex-linked Inheritance.
Sex-linked disorders are in reality all X linked. These are classified as dominant, recessive, or fragile.

X-linked Dominant Disorders.
The X-linked dominant disorders tend to be lethal in male offspring. Examples of some dominant X-linked disorders include focal dermal hypoplasia, vitamin D-resistant rickets, and incontinentia pigmenti.

X-linked Recessive Disorders. The majority of sex-linked disorders are recessive. Several recessive X-linked disorders are shown in Table 40–4. Perhaps the best known are color blindness, hemophilia A (classical hemophilia or factor VIII deficiency), and Duchenne muscular dystrophy. X-linked recessive inheritance is known as *oblique transmission* because only male offspring are affected primarily. Half of male offspring of a carrier mother will be affected and half of the daughters will be carriers; however, females heterozygous for the affected X-linked gene may still manifest some aspects of the abnormal phenotype. This may result from *lyonization* (inactivation of one of the X chromosomes early in embryogenesis), in which case there is inactivation of a relatively greater percentage of the X chromosomes carrying the normal allele. In general, X-chromosome inactivation occurs in a random fashion but is present in all future cell lines.

Fragile X Syndrome. This X-chromosome abnormality is the most commonly inherited cause of mental retardation (Rousseau and colleagues, 1991). The prevalence in the general population is estimated at 1 in 2000 males, with a heterozygous prevalence in females of 1 in 1000 (Chudley and Hagerman, 1987). The prevalence in severely mentally retarded, usually institutionalized, populations varies from 2 to 6 percent.

The male with fragile X syndrome typically has before puberty a long or triangular face and prominent ears. Macroorchidism may develop after puberty; but newborn genitalia appear normal. Other organ system abnormalities are common and are apparently due to connective tissue dysplasia—for example, aortic dilation and mitral valve prolapse. There are a number of behavioral and speech patterns, and the degree of mental retardation is variable. Autism is common, and about 8 percent of autistic males are found to have fragile X syndrome (Brown and colleagues, 1986).

This condition is the only known genetic disorder associated with *fragile sites*, that is, specific chromosome regions that fail to condense normally during mitosis. On karyotyping, these chromosomes are characterized by a nonstaining gap or constriction. Interestingly, only 5 to 50 percent (average 20 percent) of cells from affected males have a demonstrable fragile site (Chudley and Hagerman, 1987). Carrier females may fail to demonstrate the fragile site in cultures cells.

In the past, the diagnosis of the fragile X syndrome or obligate heterozygous female has been primarily via cytogenetic techniques involving cell cultures grown in the absence of folate. Not only is the cytogenetic analysis difficult, but it may also result in both false positive and negative diagnoses (Jenkins and associates, 1991; Sutherland and associates, 1991). Recent molecular techniques have allowed for the direct diagnosis of the fragile X syndrome and for the carrier status of a cytogenetically normal woman, as well as for prenatal diag-

nosis in the fetus (Rousseau and colleagues, 1991; Sutherland and co-workers, 1991). The underlying mutation now appears to be a large increase in the number of CGG repeats in a gene on chromosome X (Pergolizzi and associates, 1992). Pergolizzi and colleagues (1992) have recently described a polymerase chain reaction method for screening at-risk populations and for prenatal diagnosis of affected individuals.

Multifactorial Inheritance

In multifactorial inheritance, characteristic Mendelian patterns are not found, but there is increased frequency of the disorder or phenotypes in families. Multifactorial inheritance is thought to involve multiple genes in concert with environmental factors. Common multifactorial conditions include congenital heart lesions, neural-tube defects, cleft lip and palate, pyloric stenosis, clubfoot, and congenital hip dislocation. Some multifactorial traits are more common in one sex—that is, it takes "fewer genes to produce the phenotype"; for example, pyloric stenosis is much more common in males. In general, the recurrence risk of multifactorial disorders after one affected offspring is 1 to 5 percent.

Neural-tube Defects. Neural-tube defects result from failure of tubal closure by day 26 to 28 of embryonic life. This produces a spectrum of cranial and spinal canal defects that range from anencephaly to very slight vertebral defects. Some of the more common neural-tube anomalies are listed in Table 40–5. The prenatal diagnosis of neural-tube defects is discussed in Chapter 41.

Anencephaly. Anencephaly is characterized by absence of the cranium along with cerebral hemispheres that are either rudimentary or absent (Fig. 40–5). There is also extreme diminution in adrenal gland size. Anencephaly is probably the most common cause of gross hydramnios, which occasionally may be sufficiently massive to require therapeutic amniocentesis (Chap. 34, p. 734). Breech and face presentations are common. The condi-

TABLE 40–5. INCIDENCE OF VARIOUS NEURAL-TUBE DEFECTS IN THE UNITED STATES

Type	Incidence (per 1000 births)	Neonatal Deaths (%)	Long-term Disability[a] (%)
Anencephaly	0.6–0.8	100	0
Open spina bifida	0.5–0.8	33	65
Closed spina bifida	0.1–0.14	7	10
Total	**1.2–1.7**	**60**	**60**

[a] Includes lower limb paralysis, sensory loss, bladder and bowel problems, clubfoot, scoliosis, meningitis, hydrocephaly, and mental retardation.
From American College of Obstetricians and Gynecologists (1986), with permission.

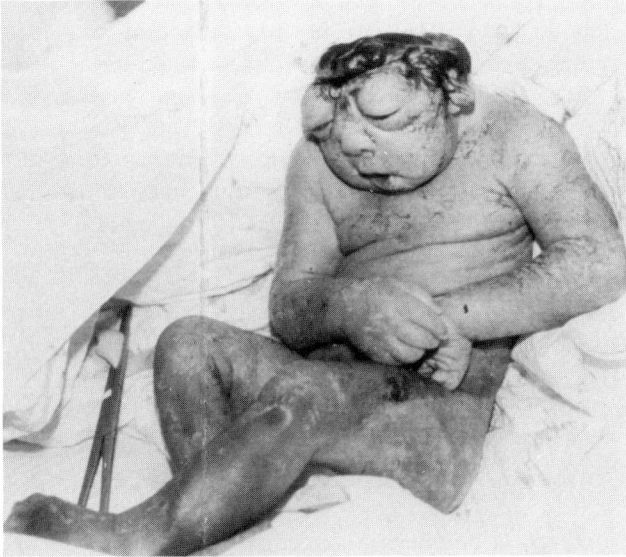

Fig. 40–5. Anencephalic infant.

tion is lethal, although survival for a period of months has been reported.

The most frequent practical question posed by a pregnancy complicated by anencephaly is whether to initiate labor as soon as the diagnosis is confirmed. The uterus containing an anencephalic fetus may be refractory to oxytocin. Late in pregnancy, when severe hydramnios is almost always the rule, the slow aspiration of 2 to 3 L of excess amnionic fluid may reduce the risk of placental abruption following spontaneous rupture of the membranes with sudden loss of amnionic fluid and marked uterine decomposition. Moreover, the myo-

metrium appears to contract more effectively after slow removal of some fluid.

The duration of anencephalic pregnancies, especially in the absence of hydramnios, may be remarkably long. In the well-authenticated case of Higgins (1954), for example, the duration of pregnancy was 1 year and 24 days after the last menstrual period, and fetal movements were perceived until the moment of delivery.

Spina Bifida and Meningomyelocele. Spina bifida consists of a hiatus, usually in the lumbosacral vertebrae, through which a meningeal sac may protrude, forming a *meningocele.* If the sac contains spinal cord as well, the anomaly is called *meningomyelocele* (Fig. 40–6). If the defect is in the skull and part of the brain protrudes into the sac, a *meningoencephalocele* results. In the presence of complete rachischisis, the spinal cord is represented by a ribbon of spongy, red tissue lying in a deep groove. Associated malformations, particularly hydrocephaly, anencephaly, and clubfoot, are common. In case of open neural-tube defects, alphafetoprotein near midpregnancy is unusually high in both amnionic fluid and maternal plasma.

Folic Acid Supplementation and Neural-tube Defects. As discussed in Chapter 9, preconception folic acid supplementation may decrease recurrences of neural-tube defects in women with a prior affected infant. Not all investigators have documented such benefits from folic acid supplementation. As discussed in Chapter 9 (p. 259), until the issue is resolved, it seems reasonable to supplement women at risk with folic acid, 4 mg daily, according to the Centers for Disease Control guidelines (1991).

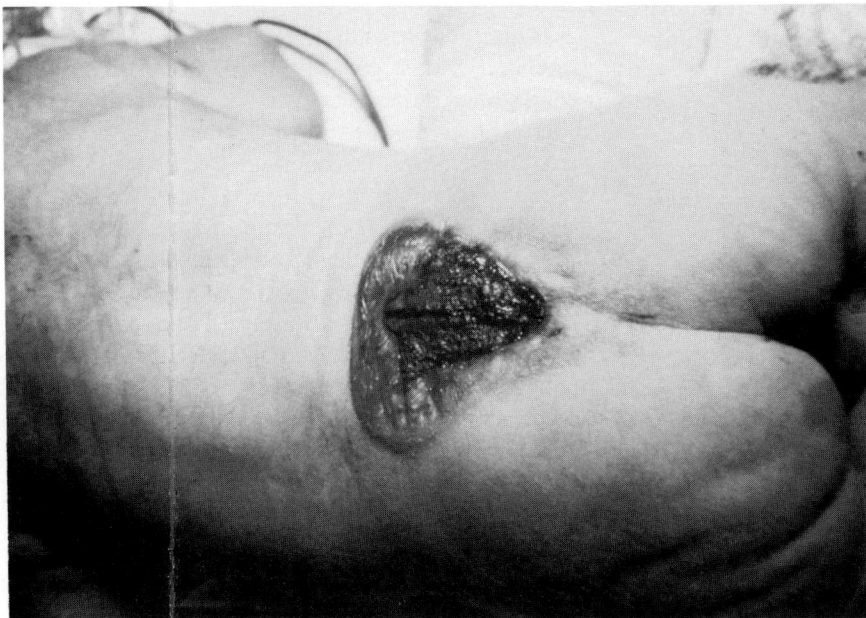

Fig. 40–6. Large lumbar meningomyelocele. (Courtesy of Dr. Victor Klein.)

Congenital Heart Disease. The incidence of congenital heart disease is unknown, but it has been estimated at about 0.5 to 1.0 percent (Nora and Nora, 1988). The majority of isolated congenital heart defects are multifactorial. The recurrence risk for such lesions depends on the specific defect and the family history (Table 40–6.) **It is of paramount importance to distinguish isolated defects from those that are only part of a syndrome that may carry a significantly higher risk of recurrence.**

Orthopedic Anomalies

Clubfoot (Talipes Equinovarus). Clubfoot is observed in about 1 in 1000 births. Because the borderline between normal and pathological is not sharp in this malformation, early orthopedic consultation is essential. Many such defects may actually be related to position in utero (i.e., deformation) rather than to a genetic cause.

Congenital Hip Dislocation. Hip dislocation is a fairly common malformation, more frequent in females than in males. It has geographic variations; for example, it is found with unusual frequency in northern Italy. It is rarely seen in African-American infants. Carter (1963) found concordance in 40 percent of monozygous twins but in only 3 percent of dizygous twins with congenital hip dislocations. Only 1 percent of subsequent male siblings, but 5 percent of later female siblings, were affected.

Cleft Lip and Cleft Palate. Cleft lip, either unilateral or bilateral, may be isolated or may be associated with a cleft palate. It is one of the most frequent congenital deformities and has an incidence of 1.3 per 1000 births. Because of difficulties in feeding, it is advisable to surgically correct a cleft lip as soon as the infant's condition permits. A cleft palate may represent even greater difficulties in feeding, requiring the use of a prosthesis until around age 2 years.

The risk of cleft lip in a second child of unaffected parents is about 4 percent. If both children are affected, the risk of the third child having a cleft lip is 10 percent. If one parent has a cleft lip, the risk of the first child

being affected is also about 4 percent. Identification of cleft lip and cleft palate has been made at or before midpregnancy using real-time ultrasonography (Seeds and Cefalo, 1983).

Pyloric Stenosis. Pyloric stenosis, a multifactorial disorder, is more common in males than females. However, the risk of pyloric stenosis in the offspring of an affected parent is much greater if that parent is female (Carter, 1976). This is because it takes more "abnormal genes" to cause the defect in the female; thus it seems logical that with an affected mother, more of these genes are available to pass on to the next generation.

Congenital Anomalies of Unknown Etiology

There are a number of congenital anomalies of uncertain etiology, especially when they occur as isolated lesions. Examples include hydrocephaly, certain urinary tract anomalies, and abdominal wall defects. **These anomalies may be part of a genetic syndrome or due to a chromosomal anomaly, in which case their risk of recurrence would be increased significantly.**

Hydrocephaly. Hydrocephaly is common, with a frequency of 0.3 to 0.8 per 1000 births (Habib, 1981). Its etiology is varied and includes genetic alterations, infections, and neoplasms. In many cases, the etiology of the obstruction is unknown; however, most cases of hydrocephaly are associated with other abnormalities. For example, in a review of 53 consecutive cases, Chervenak and colleagues (1985) found that 44 (83 percent) were associated with neurological, cardiovascular, renal, gastrointestinal, or skeletal anomalies. Almost 10 percent were associated with chromosomal abnormalities.

Certain forms of hydrocephaly are more likely to be associated with a genetic etiology than others. It has been estimated that as many as 25 percent of males with aqueductal stenosis may have inherited this condition by X-linked recessive inheritance (Burton, 1979). Hydrocephaly associated with the Dandy–Walker malformation may occur as the result of autosomal dominant and recessive syndromes as well as major chromosomal alterations (Murray and associates, 1985).

The characteristic ultrasonic finding is dilatation of the lateral ventricles (Fig. 40–7). Hydrocephaly is seldom identified at or before midpregnancy; but if so, pregnancy termination is an option.

Because of the bleak outlook for normal intellectual development in fetuses with substantive degrees of ventricular distention, considerable enthusiasm developed among several groups of investigators to perform in utero shunts for cerebrospinal fluid. Emphasizing a team approach, and taking careful steps to first exclude fetuses with other anomalies by careful ultrasonic imaging

TABLE 40–6. RECURRENCE RISK (%) FOR CONGENITAL HEART DEFECTS IF SIBLINGS OR PARENTS ARE AFFECTED

	Father	Mother	1 Sibling	2 Siblings
Ventricular septal defects	2	6–10	3	10
Atrial septal defects	1.5	4–4.5	2.5	8
Fallot tetralogy	1.5	2.5	2.5	8
Pulmonary stenosis	2	4–6.5	2	6
Aortic stenosis	3	13–18	2	6
Coarctation	2	4	2	6

Adapted from Nora and Nora (1988), with permission.

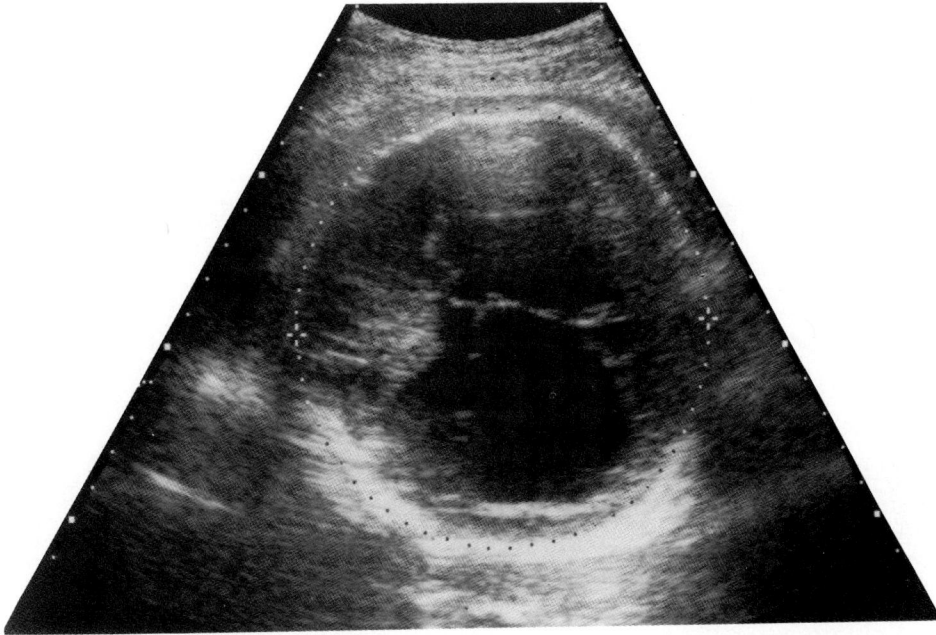

Fig. 40–7. Hydrocephaly in a 38-week fetus with an arachnoid cyst near the third ventricle. The biparietal diameter measured 107 mm. (Courtesy of Dr. Rigoberto Santos.)

and fetal karyotyping, plans were made to place shunts surgically in those fetuses with isolated progressive ventriculomegaly. The results of such procedures, unfortunately, have been discouraging. Manning and co-workers (1986) described results from the first 44 cases reported to the International Fetal Surgery Registry. Although 83 percent of the fetuses survived, the procedure-related death rate was 10 percent. Of the survivors, more than half had severe neurological handicaps, and only 35 percent are developing normally. A protocol for management of congenital hydrocephaly, including incidence, epidemiology, embryology, pathophysiology, and genetic counseling, has been provided by Vintzileos and associates (1983).

Urinary Tract Anomalies

Renal Agenesis. The incidence of complete absence of the kidneys is about 1 in 4000 births (Potter, 1965). This malformation is more frequent in males and is characteristically accompanied by oligohydramnios. Renal agenesis and the associated changes due to oligohydramnios are commonly referred to as the *Potter sequence.* The infant has prominent epicanthal folds, a flattened nose, and large, low-set ears. The skin is loose and the hands often seem large. One third of infants are stillborn. The longest reported survival is 48 hours, because pulmonary hypoplasia is almost invariably found. Renal agenesis should be suspected when sonographic evidence exists of scant to absent amnionic fluid and neither kidneys nor a filled bladder are observed.

Urinary Tract Obstruction. Persistent obstruction of the fetal urinary-collecting system will destroy the kidneys unless relieved. Therefore, when obstruction of the

lower urinary tract has been detected, relief may be accomplished in some circumstances by providing drainage from the bladder. Persistent obstruction is almost certainly accompanied by oligohydramnios. With normal amounts of amnionic fluid, obstruction is most likely intermittent and probably does not warrant attempts at drainage in utero. Results with urinary diversion for obstructive uropathy have been more encouraging than shunts done for hydrocephaly. Evaluation is similar for both procedures, and careful ultrasonic examination is done to look for other congenital anomalies as well as pulmonary hypoplasia from oligohydramnios. Determination of amnionic fluid alphafetoprotein and fetal karyotyping should be performed. In those fetuses with lower tract obstruction from a posterior urethral valve, a catheter is guided transabdominally (Fig. 40–8). Manning and colleagues (1986) described the results obtained in the first 73 shunt procedures done for obstructive uropathy and reported to the International Fetal Surgery Registry. The procedure-related death rate was 5 percent, and 41 percent of fetuses survived. Most of deaths were due to pulmonary hypoplasia. **Importantly, 8 percent of fetuses had a karyotype abnormality and 7 percent had renal dysplasia.**

Elder and associates (1987) reviewed 57 reported cases of fetal urinary tract drainage and found a 44 percent complication rate. Only 6 of 28 fetuses survived when there was associated oligohydramnios. They concluded that a prospective, randomized trial should be undertaken.

Abdominal-wall Defects. *Omphalocele* and *gastroschisis* are relatively common ventral-wall defects. An omphalocele is a defect in the umbilical ring from which

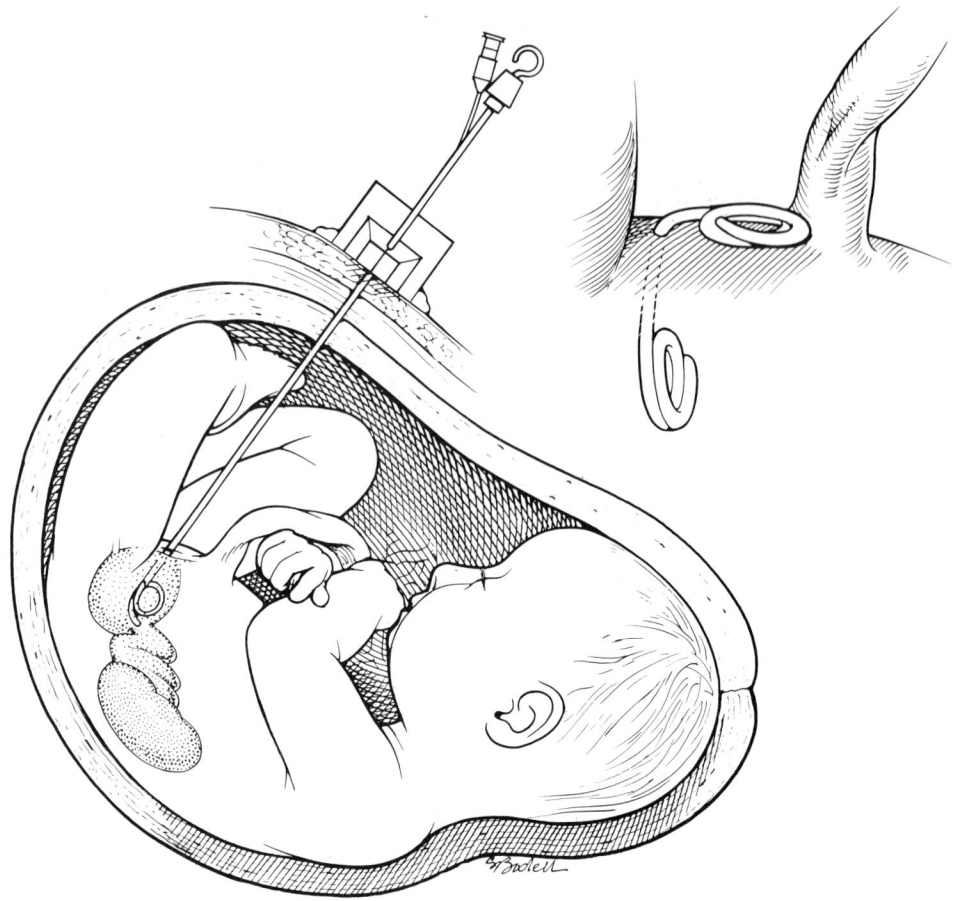

Fig. 40–8. Intrauterine catheter placement to relieve fetal urinary obstruction. (Redrawn from Williamson, 1987.)

protrudes a sac, covered with amnion and peritoneum, and into which abdominal contents have typically herniated (Fig. 40–9). It is the more common of the two, and is seen in about 1 in 4000 live births. Gastroschisis is intestinal herniation through a defect in the anterior abdominal wall, usually to the right of the umbilicus. There is no sac and the intestines are covered with a thickened inflammatory exudate. This anomaly is identified in perhaps 1 in 10,000 births.

Associated congenital anomalies contribute to a high mortality rate for either condition (Hasan and Hermansen, 1986; Sermer and colleagues, 1987), but an omphalocele is associated with other anomalies in up to 70 percent of cases. Gilbert and Nicolaides (1987) performed karyotyping in 35 fetuses with an omphalocele at 16 to 36 weeks. They reported that 54 percent had chromosomal abnormalities. Omphaloceles containing only bowel appear to have the highest association with an abnormal karyotype. Getachew and associates (1991) reported that 87 percent of fetuses with an omphalocele containing only bowel also had abnormal karyotypes, contrasted to only 9 percent in which the sac contained liver. Most cases of gastroschisis occur sporadically and chromosomal anomalies are less common; however, about one third of affected fetuses have associated anom-

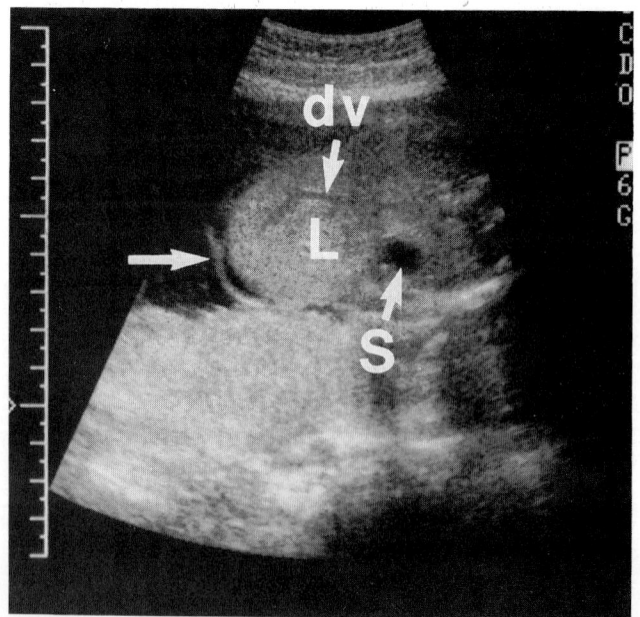

Fig. 40–9. Transverse sonogram of a fetus with a large hepato-omphalocele with the covering abdominoperitoneal membrane (*long arrow*). The ductus venosus (dv), liver (L), and stomach bubble (S) are seen. (Courtesy of Dr. R. Santos.)

alies. These include genitourinary, cardiac, musculoskeletal, and gastrointestinal abnormalities.

Preterm labor and delivery complicate over half of pregnancies associated with a fetal abdominal wall defect. The corresponding mortality rate is 60 percent for omphalocele and 40 percent for gastroschisis. The prognosis is good for the fetus who weighs more than 1500 g and has no associated anomalies, provided surgical correction is achieved rapidly. Although there is no evidence that cesarean delivery improves survival (Hasan and Hermansen, 1986), Fitzsimmons and colleagues (1988) emphasize that elective timing of delivery optimizes neonatal surgical care.

Diaphragmatic Hernia. The incidence of congenital diaphragmatic hernia was cited to be about 1 in 3700 in a review by Wenstrom and colleagues (1991). Its etiology is generally unknown. Most cases are probably multifactorial, but they are also associated with chromosomal aberrations. An autosomal recessive genetic form of the condition has been described. In cases detected prenatally, the perinatal mortality is high and about three fourths of affected fetuses or neonates die (Sharland and associates, 1992). The high incidence of associated severe malformations or chromosomal anomalies undoubtedly contributes to this high perinatal mortality. Wenstrom and colleagues (1991) reported a 55 percent survival rate for newborns with an uncomplicated diaphragmatic hernia. Survival may be improved with extracorporeal membrane oxygenation (Finer and associates, 1992), and the isolated defect has been repaired successfully in utero (Harrison and colleagues, 1990).

Molecular Genetics

During the past decade there have been significant advances in DNA technology that now allow for the isolation and sophisticated analysis of human genes. It seems reasonable to believe that in the foreseeable future the make-up of most, if not all, of the human genome will be known. As summarized recently, the physical mapping and nucleotide sequencing of the human genome is now underway in an effort referred to as the **Human Genome Project** (Friedman, 1990; Green and Waterston, 1991). Watson (1991) cautions, however, that "Our descendants will be working for hundreds if not thousands of years to fully understand all the information contained in the three billion DNA base pairs that constitute the human genome." The following is a cursory review of the molecular genetics related to obstetrics and prenatal diagnosis discussed in Chapter 41.

Genes. A gene represents the total sequence combination of four purine and pyrimidine bases in DNA that specifies the amino acid sequence for a single polypep-

tide chain of a protein molecule (Goldstein and Brown, 1991). The human chromosome contains approximately 3 billion base pairs of DNA (Green and Waterston, 1991). Their complexity is emphasized by Weatherall (1985), who estimated that DNA from each cell nucleus, if uncoiled, would stretch 2 meters! The relative sizes of genomes, chromosomes, and cloned DNA segments are summarized in Table 40–7 (Green and Waterston, 1991).

There are between 50,000 and 100,000 genes in each human nucleus. Of these, almost 2000 have been assigned to a particular chromosome and over 500 have been cloned (Green and Waterston, 1991).

Transmission of Genetic Material. Enzymes and other biologically important proteins are composed of one or more polypeptide chains that are genetically determined through inheritance of specific DNA segments or genes. In the nucleus, genetic information is transcribed onto *messenger RNA,* which in the cytoplasm translates this information by forming a template for ribosomal protein synthesis. *Transcription* generates a single-stranded RNA identical in sequence with one of the strands of the DNA helix (Fig. 40–10). *Translation* converts the RNA-nucleotide sequence into the amino-acid sequence that constitutes a protein.

A *mutation* is an alteration of DNA sequencing that is passed on to future progeny. These can be visible alterations of chromosomes, such as deletions, or they may involve a single change in just one of the purine or pyrimidine bases of a single gene, resulting in a *point* or *single-gene mutation,* such as that causing sickle cell anemia.

Analytical Techniques

Complementary DNA. *Reverse transcriptases* are enzymes isolated from tumor viruses, which are used to synthesize a DNA copy from messenger RNA isolated from human cell nuclei. These copies, called *complementary DNA* or *cDNA,* are labeled by inserting radio-

TABLE 40–7. RELATIVE SIZE OF GENOMES, CHROMOSOMES, AND CLONED DNA

	Size (base pairs)
Size	
Human genome	3,000,000,000
Human chromosome (average)	130,000,000
Yeast genome	15,000,000
Escherichia coli genome	5,000,000
Cloning Capacity	
YAC (yeast artificial chromosome)	1,000,000
Cosmid	45,000
Bacteriophage	25,000

Adapted from Green and Waterston (1991), with permission.

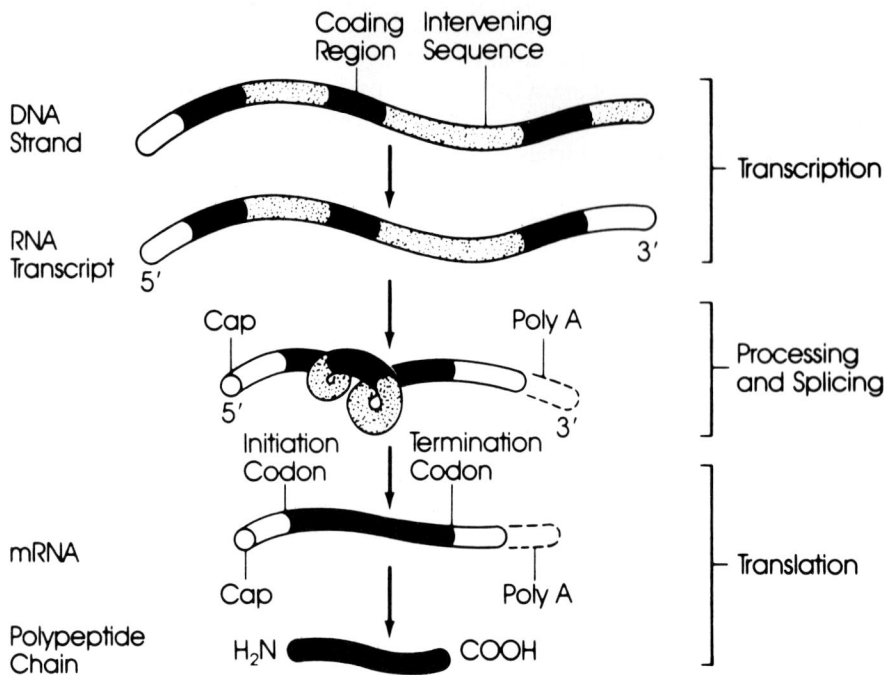

Fig. 40–10. Expression of an idealized gene. Schematic diagram of the genetic control of protein synthesis, illustrating the flow of genetic information from the base sequence of DNA to the RNA transcript (*transcription*) to the mRNA (*processing*) to the polypeptide chain of a protein molecule (*translation*). Only one of the two strands of DNA is used as a template for transcribing the RNA transcript. Solid sections represent coding regions in DNA, RNA transcript, mRNA, and amino acid sequence in polypeptide chain; dotted sections represent intervening sequences in DNA and RNA transcript. (From Goldstein and Brown, 1991, with permission.)

active bases into the sequences, and the resulting labeled cDNA probe is used to look for complementary sequences of DNA isolated on nitrocellulose filters by Southern blotting. These probes are very specific in combining with their complementary single-stranded DNA from the cell nucleus to be analyzed, and the radioactive label allows for detection of this binding. Relatively large fragments of DNA can be produced via either cloning or polymerase chain reaction.

CLONING. DNA initially was cloned primarily by utilizing bacterial plasmids. More recently, DNA fragments have been cloned in bacteriophages, cosmids (modified plasmids), and yeast systems (Green and Waterston, 1991). *Yeast artificial chromosomes* (YAC) are artificial chromosome vectors utilized for cloned DNA (Burke and colleagues, 1987; Schlessinger, 1990).

POLYMERASE CHAIN REACTION. The polymerase chain reaction (PCR) is an in vitro technique in which large amounts of specific DNA sequences can be synthesized over a relatively short period of time. Unlike other techniques, the chain reaction utilizes very minute quantities of DNA; however, either the gene sequence or a sequence in its region must be known. The first step involves separating double-stranded DNA into single-stranded fragments via heat treatment. The oligonucleotide primers are then allowed to anneal to the 3′ ends of the separated DNA and, with the addition of a heat-stable DNA polymerase, new strands of DNA are synthesized. The process is repeated and DNA is increased in a geometric fashion (Layman, 1992). In short, this technique allows for a millionfold increased

amplification of the desired DNA segment (Green and Waterston, 1991).

Restriction Endonucleases and Southern Blotting. DNA fractionation became possible with isolation of bacterial enzymes termed *restriction endonucleases*, which cleave a specific sequence of base pairs. More than 200 restriction enzymes have been identified. As shown in Figure 40–11, some enzymes recognize sequences of four nucleotides, some six, and others seven. Depending on the types and numbers of enzymes used, hundreds of thousands of fragments are produced with varying numbers of nucleotides. These DNA fragments are then separated by electrophoresis into single strands and hybridized with their radiolabeled complementary DNA probe, using the technique known as *Southern blotting*, which can be identified by autoradiography (Fig. 40–12). Known sequences, or probes, are used to determine if these same sequences are present in the patient's genome, and in this way abnormal sequences (mutations) can be identified.

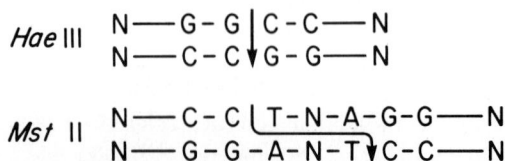

Fig. 40–11. Restriction endonucleases. *Hae* III (*H influenzae III*) cleave a four-base sequence. *Mst* II (*Microcoleus*) cleaves a seven-base sequence, the center of which is a nonspecific nucleotide, shown here as N.

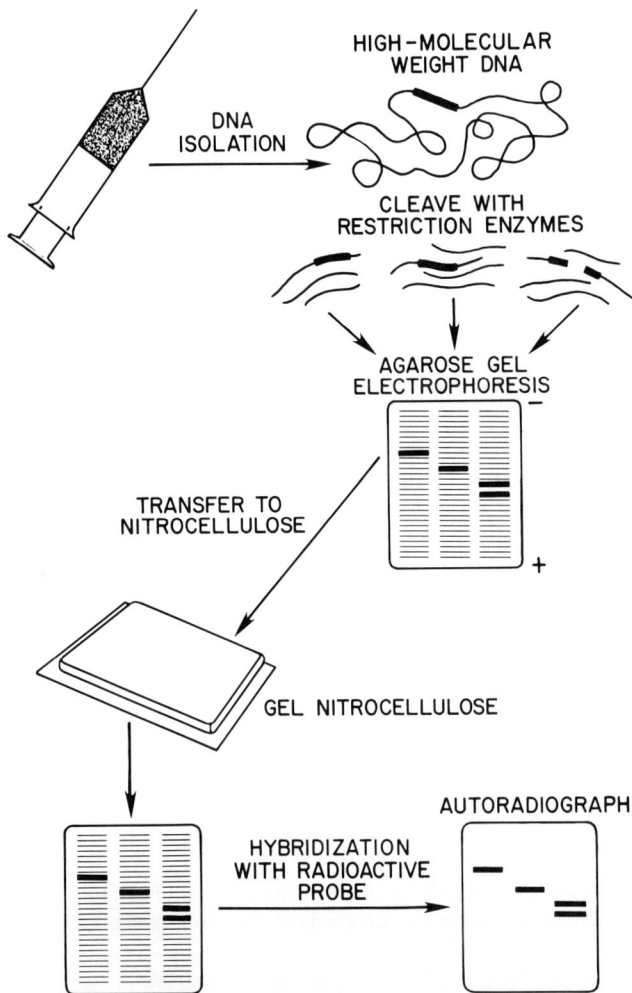

Fig. 40–12. Southern blotting analysis. Genomic DNA is isolated from leukocytes or amniocytes and digested with a restriction enzyme. This yields a series of reproducible fragments that are separated by agarose gel electrophoresis. DNA is then transferred to a nitrocellulose membrane that binds DNA. The membrane is treated with a solution containing a radioactive single-stranded nucleic acid probe, which forms a double-stranded nucleic acid complex at membrane sites when homologous DNA is present. These regions are then detected using x-ray film.

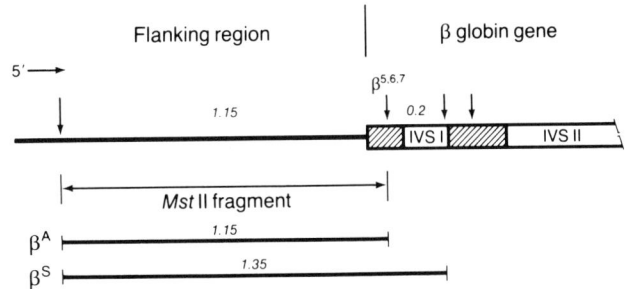

Fig. 40–13. *Mst* II restriction enzyme used to identify hemoglobin A and S. Arrows indicate the *Mst* II restriction sites, including the one corresponding to amino acids 5, 6, and 7. Using the ^{32}P-labeled 1.15-kilobase *Mst* II fragment probe indicated in the diagram, the 1.15-kilobase fragment was seen as DNA from hemoglobin A, and the 1.35 kilobase fragment was seen in sickle hemoglobin DNA. Southern blotting analysis using the appropriate beta-globin fragment as a DNA probe then allows for identification of AS, AA, and SS genotypes. (From Chang and colleagues, 1982, with permission.)

An example of an exciting aspect of genetics using molecular technology involves sickle cell anemia. In 1982 Chang and Kan described an assay with the restriction enzyme *Mst* II for direct prenatal diagnosis of sickle cell mutations. This technique, which provides accurate diagnosis of sickle cell anemia, can be performed on chorionic villus specimens or amnionic fluid. The normal beta-globin gene is separated into two fragments by *Mst* II, 1.15 and 0.2 kilobase long (Fig. 40–13). The sickle mutation at the sixth amino acid changes the amino acid from glutamic acid to valine with a corresponding change in DNA sequence. This causes a loss of the *Mst* II recognition site and results in a single 1.35-kilobase fragment. By using Southern blotting analysis and the 1.15-kilobase *Mst* II fragment as a probe, they found 1.15-kilobase fragments in the AA genotype, the 1.35-kilobase fragment with SS, and both fragments in patients with AS.

Linkage Analysis. Another advantage of restriction endonucleases is use of the technique called *linkage analysis,* an extremely valuable method of analyzing genetic diversity. Not all abnormal genes are associated with an identifiable alteration in a restriction endonuclease cleavage site. Diagnosis may still be possible, however, because mutations are frequently linked to other DNA sequences that vary from person to person. Consequently, digested pieces of DNA generated by restriction endonucleases differ so often in a population that it is frequently possible to associate a mutant gene with a nearby restriction enzyme site. Although the abnormal gene is not identified, a *marker gene* is found closely linked to the mutant gene. Such *restriction fragment length polymorphisms (RFLPs)* are inherited in a Mendelian fashion. A change in DNA sequence that affects or changes a restriction site is detected by a difference in restriction fragments. It is through such linkage analysis that many hereditary conditions, heretofore not amenable to detection, have become identifiable. Examples include α_1-antitrypsin deficiency (Hejtmancik and co-workers, 1986), carriers of hemophilia A (Antonarakis and colleagues, 1985), and Huntington disease (Quarrell and colleagues, 1987). It is important to bear in mind that with chromosomal crossover events, linkage analysis may not correctly identify the chromosome associated with the phenotype of concern.

Allele-specific Oligonucleotides. Allele-specific oligonucleotides (ASO) are utilized to detect point mutation or changes of only a few base pairs (Layman, 1992; Phillips, 1990). These "areas" can be detected utilizing allele-specific oligonucleotides or ASO probes (15 to 25

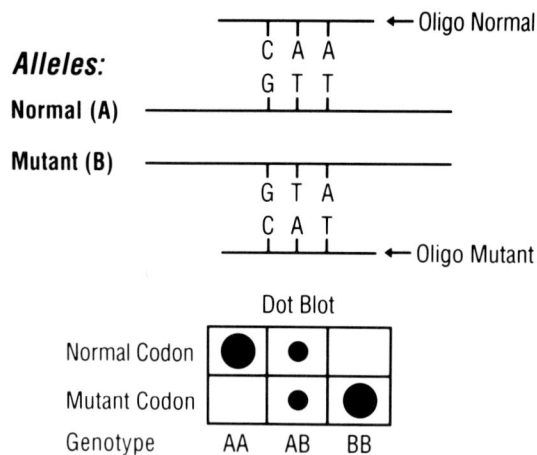

Fig. 40–14. A dot blot is shown using allele-specific oligonucleotide probes. Note that the normal allele A differs from B by one base pair (GTT versus GTA). This difference can be used to construct probes that should only hybridize to the complementary strand. (From Layman, 1992, with permission.)

bases in length), which will anneal differentially to the normal and mutant alleles. This annealization can be detected via a dot blot (Fig. 40–14).

Positional Cloning. Positional cloning, formerly called "reverse genetics," refers to the arduous task of attempting to clone the actual gene of a specific disease without knowing the nature of the gene product. This is possible once the gene has been localized to a specific part of a given chromosome (Gelehrter and Collins, 1990). Because localization or mapping of the abnormal gene to a specific chromosome region still involves over a million base pairs, it is helpful if the affected patient also has a cytogenetic abnormality such as a chromosomal deletion (Gelehrter and Collins, 1990). Examples of genes that have been cloned using this technique include cystic fibrosis and Duchenne muscular dystrophy. Gelehrter and Collins (1990) recently reviewed this genetic strategy for cloning of genes.

References

American College of Obstetricians and Gynecologists: Prenatal detection of neural tube defects. Technical bulletin no. 99, December 1986

Antonarakis SE, Waber PG, Kittur SD, Patei AS, Kazazian HH Jr, Mellis MA, Counts RB, Stamatoyannopoulos G, Bowie EJ, Fass DN, Pittman DD, Wozney JM, Toole JJ: Hemophilia A: Detection of molecular defects and of carriers by DNA analysis. N Engl J Med 313:842, 1985

Beckman DA, Brent RL: Mechanism of known environmental teratogens: Drugs and chemicals. Clin Perinatol 13:649, 1986

Boué A, Boué J: Chromosomal abnormalities associated with fetal malformations. In Schrimgeout J (ed): Towards the Prevention of Fetal Malformation. Edinburgh, Edinburgh University Press, 1978

Boué A, Boué J, Gropp A: Cytogenetics of pregnancy wastage. Annu Rev Genet 14:1, 1985

Bovicelli L, Orsini LF, Rizzo N, Montacuti V, Bacchetta M: Reproduction in Down's syndrome. Obstet Gynecol 59:135, 1982

Brown WT, Jenkins EC, Cohen IL, Fisch GS, Wolf-Schein EG, Gross A, Waterhouse L, Fein D, Mason-Brothers A, Ritvo E: Fragile X and autism: A multicenter survey. Am J Med Genet 23:341, 1986

Burke DT, Carle G, Olson MV: Cloning of large segments of exogenous DNA into yeast by means of artificial chromosome vectors. Science 236:806, 1987

Burton BK: Recurrence risks for congenital hydrocephalus. Clin Genet 16:47, 1979

Carter CO: Genetics of common single malformations. Br Med Bull 32:21, 1976

Carter CO: Genetic factors in congenital dislocation of the hip. Proc R Soc Med 56:803, 1963

Centers for Disease Control: Use of folic acid for prevention of spina bifida and other neural tube defects—1983–1991. MMWR 40:513, 1991

Chang JC, Kan YW: A sensitive new prenatal test for sickle cell anemia. N Engl J Med 307:30, 1982

Chervenak FA, Berkowitz RL, Tortora M, Hobbins JC: The management of fetal hydrocephalus. Am J Obstet Gynecol 151:933, 1985

Chudley AE, Hagerman RJ: Fragile X syndrome. J Pediatr 110:821, 1987

DeWald GW, Michels VV: Recurrent miscarriages: Cytogenetic causes and genetic counseling of affected families. Clin Obstet Gynecol 29:865, 1986

Elder JS, Duckett JW Jr, Snyder HM: Intervention for fetal obstructive uropathy: Has it been effective? Lancet 2:1007, 1987

Finer NN, Tierney AJ, Hallgren R, Hayashi A, Peliowski A, Etches PC: Neonatal congenital diaphragmatic hernia and extracorporeal membrane oxygenation. Can Med Assoc J 146:501, 1992

Fitzsimmons J, Nyberg DA, Cyr DR, Hatch E: Perinatal management of gastroschisis. Obstet Gynecol 71:910, 1988

Friedman JM: Genetic disease in the offspring of older fathers. Obstet Gynecol 57:745, 1981

Friedman T: Opinion: The human genome project—Some implications of extensive "reverse genetic" medicine. Am J Hum Genet 46:407, 1990

Gelehrter TD, Collins FS: Anatomy of the human genome: Gene mapping and linkage. In Gelehrter TD, Collins FS (eds): Principles of Medical Genetics. Baltimore, Williams & Wilkins, 1990, p 193

Getachew MM, Goldstein RB, Edge V, Goldberg JD, Filly RA: Correlation between omphalocele contents and karyotypic abnormalities: Sonographic study in 37 cases. AJR 158:133, 1991

Ghavami M, Levy HL, Erbe RW: Prevention of fetal damage through dietary control of maternal hyperphenylalaninemia. Clin Obstet Gynecol 29:580, 1986

Gilbert WM, Nicolaides KH: Fetal omphalocele: Associated malformations and chromosomal defects. Obstet Gynecol 70:633, 1987

Goldstein JC, Brown MS: Genetic aspects of disease. In Wilson JD, Braunwald E, Isselbacher KJ, Petersdorf RG, Martin JB, Fauci AS, Root RK (eds): Harrison's Principles of Internal Medicine, 12th ed. New York, McGraw-Hill, 1991, p 21

Green ED, Waterston RH: The human genome project: Prospects and implications for clinical medicine. JAMA 266:1966, 1991

Habib Z: Genetics and genetic counseling in neonatal hydrocephalus. Obstet Gynecol Surv 36:529, 1981

Hall JG: Genomic imprinting and its clinical implications. N Engl J Med 326:827, 1992

Harrison MR, Adzick NS, Longaker MT, Goldberg JD, Rosen MA, Filly RA, Evans MI, Golbus MS: Successful repair in utero of a fetal diaphragmatic hernia after removal of herniated viscera from left thorax. N Engl J Med 322:1582, 1990

Hasan S, Hermansen MC: The prenatal diagnosis of ventral abdominal wall defects. Am J Obstet Gynecol 155:842, 1986

Hejtmancik JF, Ward PA, Mansfield T, Sifers RN, Harris S, Cox DW: Prenatal diagnosis of α_1-antitrypsin deficiency by restriction fragment length polymorphisms, and comparison with oligonucleotide probe analysis. Lancet 2:767, 1986

Higgins LG: Prolonged pregnancy. Lancet 2:1154, 1954

Hook EB, Cross PK, Jackson LG, Pergament E, Brambati B: Maternal age specific rates of 47, +21 and other cytogenetic abnormalities diagnosed in the first trimester of pregnancy in chorionic villus biopsy specimens: Comparison with rates expected from observations at amniocentesis. Am J Human Genet 42:797, 1988

Hook EB, Cross PK, Schreinemachers DM: Chromosomal abnormality rates of amniocentesis and in liveborn infants. JAMA 249:2034, 1983

Jacobs PA, Melville M, Ratcliff S, Keay AJ, Syme J: A cytogenetic survey of 11,680 newborn infants. Ann Human Genet 37:359, 1974

Jenkins EC, Krawczun MS, Stark-Houck SL, Duncan CJ, Kunaporn S, Gu H, Schwartz-Richestein C, Howard-Peebles PN, Gross A, Sherman SL, Brown WT: Improved prenatal detection of Fra(X)(q27.3): Methods for prevention of false negatives in chorionic villus and amniotic fluid cell cultures. Am J Med Genet 38:447, 1991

Jones KL: Recognizable patterns of malformations. In Jones KL (ed): Smith's Recognizable Patterns of Human Malformation, 4th ed. Philadelphia, Saunders, 1988, p 14

Kalousek DK, Dill FJ: Chromosomal mosaicism confined to the placenta in human conceptions. Science 221:665, 1983

Knoll JHM, Glatt KA, Nicholls RD, Malcolm S, Lalande M: Chromosome 15 uniparental disomy is not frequent in Angelman Syndrome. Am J Hum Genet 41:16, 1991

Knoll JHM, Nicholls RD, Magenis RE, Graham JM Jr, Lalande M, Satt SA: Angelman and Prader-Willi syndromes share a common chromosome 15 deletion but differ in parental origin of the deletion. Am J Med Genet 32:285, 1989

Layman LC: Basic concepts of molecular biology as applied to pediatric and adolescent gynecology. Obstet Gynecol Clin North Am 19:1, 1992

Lejeune J, Gautier M, Turpin R: Étude des chromosomes somatique de neuf enfants mongoliens. CR Acad Sci (Paris) 248:1720, 1959

Lenke RR, Levy HL: Maternal phenylketonuria—results of dietary therapy. Am J Obstet Gynecol 142:548, 1982

Manning FA, Harrison MR, Rodeck C, and Members of the International Fetal Medicine and Surgery Society: Catheter shunts for fetal hydronephrosis and hydrocephalus—Report of the International Fetal Surgery Registry. N Engl J Med 315:336, 1986

Mascari MJ, Gottlieb W, Rogan PK, Butler MG, Waller DA, Armour JA, Jeffreys AJ, Ladda RL, Nicholls RD: The frequency of uniparental disomy in Prader-Willi syndrome. N Engl J Med 326:1599, 1992

McKusick VA: Mendelian Inheritance in Man: Catalogs of Autosomal Dominant, Autosomal Recessive, and X-linked Phenotypes, 9th ed. Baltimore, Johns Hopkins University Press, 1990

Murray JC, Johnson JA, Bird TD: Dandy-Walker malformation: Etiologic heterogeneity and empiric recurrence risks. Clin Genet 28:272, 1985

Nicholls RD, Knoll JH, Butler MJ, Karam S, Lalande M: Genetic imprinting suggested by maternal heterodisomy in nondeletion Prader-Willi syndrome. Nature 342:281, 1989

Nora JJ, Nora AH: Updates on counseling the family with a first-degree relative with a congenital heart defect. Am J Med Genet 29:137, 1988

Oakley GP: Frequency of human congenital malformation. Clin Perinatol 13:545, 1986

Pergolizzi RG, Goonewardena P, Erster SH, Brown WT: Detection of full fragile X mutation. Lancet 339:271, 1992

Phillips JA: Diagnosis at the bedside by gene analysis. South Med J 83:868, 1990

Potter EL: Bilateral absence of ureters and kidneys: A report of 50 cases. Obstet Gynecol 25:3, 1965

Quarrell OWJ, Meredith AL, Tyler A, Youngman S, Upadhyaya M, Harper PS: Exclusion testing for Huntington's disease in pregnancy with a closely linked DNA marker. Lancet 2:1281, 1987

Reed SC: Counseling in Medical Genetics, 2nd ed. Philadelphia, Saunders, 1963

Rhor RJ, Doherty LB, Waisbren SE, Bailey IV, Ampola MG, Benacerraf B, Levy HL: New England Maternal PKU Project: Prospective study of untreated and treated pregnancies and their outcomes. J Pediatr 110:391, 1987

Rousseau F, Heitz D, Biancalana V, Blumenfeld S, Kretz C, Boué J, Tommerup N, Van Der Hagen C, CeLozier-Blanchet C, Croquette MF, Gilgenkrantz S, Jalbert P, Voelckel MA, Oberlé I, Mandel JL: Direct diagnosis by DNA analysis of the fragile X syndrome of mental retardation. N Engl J Med 325:1673, 1991

Schlessinger D: Yeast artificial chromosomes: tools for mapping and analysis of complex genomes. Trends Genet 6:248, 1990

Seeds JW, Cefalo RC: Technique of early sonographic diagnosis of bilateral cleft lip and palate. Obstet Gynecol 62S:2, 1983

Sermer M, Benzie RJ, Pitson L, Carr M, Skidmore M: Prenatal diagnosis and management of congenital defects of the anterior abdominal wall. Am J Obstet Gynecol 156:308, 1987

Sharland GK, Lockhart SM, Heward AJ, Allan LD: Prognosis in fetal diaphragmatic hernia. Am J Obstet Gynecol 166:9, 1992

Shepard TH: Human teratogenicity. Adv Pediatr 33:225, 1986

Spence JE, Percioccante RG, Greig GM, Willard HF, Ledbetter DH, Hejtmancik JF, Pollak MS, O'Brien WE, Beaudet AL: Uniparental disomy as a mechanism for human genetic disease. Am J Hum Genet 42:217, 1988

Sutherland GR, Gedeon A, Kornman L, Donnelly A, Mulley JC, Kremer E, Lynch M, Pritchard M, Yu S, Richards RI: Prenatal diagnosis of fragile X syndrome by direct detection of the unstable DNA sequence. N Engl J Med 325:1720, 1991

Thompson MW, McInnes RR, Willard HF: Genetics in Medicine, 5th ed. Philadelphia, Saunders, 1991

Tijo JH, Levan A: The chromosome number in man. Hereditas 42:1, 1956

Vintzileos AM, Ingardia CJ, Nochimson DJ: Congenital hydrocephalus: A review and protocol for perinatal management. Obstet Gynecol 62:529, 1983

Watson JD: The human genome initiative: A statement of need. Hosp Pract October 15, 1991

Weatherall DJ: The New Genetics and Clinical Practice, 2nd ed. Oxford, Oxford University Press, 1985

Wenstrom KD, Weiner CP, Hanson JW: A five-year statewide experience with congenital diaphragmatic hernia. Am J Obstet Gynecol 165:838, 1991

Williamson JL, Kock R, Azen C, Chang C: Correlates of intelligence test results in treated phenylketonuric children. Pediatrics 68:161, 1981

Williamson RA, Pringle KC: Correcting hydrocephalus and fetal uropathy: How good are the prospects? Contemp Obstet Gynecol 30:77, 1987

CHAPTER 41

Prenatal Diagnosis and Invasive Techniques to Monitor the Fetus

In the past 20 years there has been incredible development of techniques that allow for early and accurate prenatal diagnosis for a myriad of fetal disorders. Beginning with simple cytogenetic techniques to determine gross chromosomal abnormalities in amnionic fluid cells, there now are methods that permit rapid detection of mutant genes by using minute quantities of fetally derived DNA, obtained by direct sampling of chorionic tissue or fetal blood. These techniques, coupled with those of molecular genetics (Chap. 40, p. 933), allow detection of an ever-expanding list of inherited conditions.

Of paramount importance is the ability to provide parents with counseling regarding various screening and diagnostic techniques available. In addition, risks and consequences of such procedures, as well as options available, are explained. Genetic counseling regarding pregnancy may be preconceptional, prenatal, or post-delivery.

GENETIC COUNSELING

Along with the current trend for smaller families is the concern that children be born healthy and free of birth defects and inherited disorders. A malformed child often precipitates the request for guidance, although other problems that frequently lead to consultation include inheritable diseases, birth defects in the family, advanced maternal age, teratogen exposure, and consanguinity. Genetic counseling is becoming increasingly complex with the rapid accumulation of new information, and amateurish advice, particularly if unjustifiably optimistic, may produce tragic results. Genetic counseling is now a well-recognized specialty.

Preconceptional Counseling

The ideal time for genetic counseling is before attempting pregnancy. Genetic screening tests can be discussed if an individual has a positive screening test, and he or she can be advised of risks for an affected child if conception is with another carrier. The costs and feasibility of prenatally detecting an affected fetus, and the possibility of pregnancy interruption, can be introduced.

Age-related risks and malformation risks associated with various maternal conditions such as diabetes, seizures disorders, and associated medications (for example, anticonvulsants) can also be discussed at this time. The family history should also be reviewed.

Prenatal Counseling

In addition to the routine history obtained from all pregnant women, specific questions such as those listed in Figure 41–1 should be asked to help identify the woman whose fetus is at unusual risk of having a genetic disorder or birth defect. The completed record also serves to document that the mother was informed of any unusual risks, or that referral for further genetic counseling was advised.

Although a thorough genetic history provides useful information, it is often necessary to obtain medical records of other family members to confirm a diagnosis and decide whether a disease follows a recognized inheritance pattern or represents an isolated congenital defect. Often, further steps to identify the fetus at risk for a serious disorder and to counsel the expectant parents are best handled through a specialized genetics center with established expertise in counseling and quality control of laboratory procedures.

In addition to supplying positive information, appropriate genetic studies and subsequent counseling help dispel many misapprehensions and ill-founded rumors concerning congenital malformations. They also help relieve guilt feelings that frequently follow the birth of a malformed child. If a woman chooses not to terminate a pregnancy with an abnormal conceptus, then prenatal counseling may help prepare her mentally and emotionally for its birth.

Evaluation of Malformed Infants Who Die in the Perinatal Period. A *detailed history* of events from before conception through delivery should be obtained. Times of exposure to potential teratogens are especially important. *Photographs* should be made of the face, body, and all anomalies. A *radiographic skeletal survey* may prove valuable. *Chromosomal analysis* is carried out on 2 to 3 mL of blood collected aseptically from a large vessel or the heart; or on sterile skin, umbilical cord, amnion, or lung. If the diagnosis of fetal death is made prior to fetal membrane rupture, amniocentesis

THE UNIVERSITY OF TEXAS
Southwestern Medical Center
AT DALLAS

MEDICAL GENETICS QUESTIONNAIRE

PAST PREGNANCY HISTORY:

1. How many times have you been pregnant? (Counting this pregnancy.)   _____

2. How many live-born babies have you had?   _____

3. Are all of your liveborn children still living?   No___Yes___

4. Have you had any of the following:

   a. Miscarriage?   No___Yes___
   b. Stillborn baby?   No___Yes___
   c. Children born with birth defects?   No___Yes___
      (example: spinal defect, heart defect, limb defect, Down syndrome)

FAMILY HISTORY:

   Your Family

5. Anyone in your family:

   a. mentally retarded?   No___Yes___
   b. had a child with birth defects?   No___Yes___

6. Are there any diseases that "run" in your family?   No___Yes___

   Baby's Father's Family

7. How old is this baby's father?   _____

8. Anyone in his family:

   a. mentally retarded?   No___Yes___
   b. had a child with birth defects?   No___Yes___

9. Are there any diseases that "run" in his family?   No___Yes___

ETHNICITY:

10. Are you or the baby's father of:

    a. Eastern European Jewish origin (Ashkenazi)?   No___Yes___
    b. Italian, Greek or Southeast Asian origin?   No___Yes___
    c. African origin? (example: Black American,   No___Yes___
       Ethiopian, Haitian, Nigerian, West Indian, Other)

TESTING

11. Have you or the baby's father been tested for:

    a. Tay-Sachs disease: No___Yes___
    b. Thalassemia?   No___Yes___
    c. Sickle Cell disease?   No___Yes___

CURRENT PREGNANCY:

12. Will you be age 35 or older when this baby is born?   No___Yes___

13. Do you:

    a. smoke?   No___Yes___
    b. drink?   No___Yes___
    c. use "recreational" or street drugs?   No___Yes___

14. Do you have any chronic health problem?   No___Yes___
    (diabetes, heart disease, epilepsy)

15. During this pregnancy have you had:

    a. any type of illness?   No___Yes___
    b. a high fever (102°F or greater)?   No___Yes___

16. Do you take medicines on a regular basis?   No___Yes___

    a. prescription?   No___Yes___
    b. non-prescription?   No___Yes___
       (medicines you can buy without a doctor's prescription)

17. During this pregnancy have you taken any:

    a. prescription medication?   No___Yes___
    b. non-prescription?   No___Yes___

18. Do you:

    a. take vitamins?   No___Yes___
    b. follow any special diet?   No___Yes___
       (example: vegetarian, macrobiotic, etc.)?

19. Have you had any X-rays or any type of surgery during   No___Yes___
    this pregnancy?

20. Have you been exposed to any possibly toxic chemicals   No___Yes___
    at home or at work?

Fig. 41–1. Sample prenatal diagnosis questionnaire. (Courtesy of Drs. Mary Jo Harrod and Barbara Cambridge.)

should be considered to obtain cells for chromosome analysis. A complete autopsy is done looking for all malformations, both external and internal.

Postpartum Counseling

After birth of a fetus with a genetic disorder or congenital abnormality, the mother is provided with information regarding the specific condition(s) and with an opportunity to ask questions during the early postpartum period. Follow-up genetic counseling is provided at a later date—after she has had ample time to adjust to the initial event. Not surprisingly, many women will not remember much of the initial counseling session. Follow-up not only affords the couple the opportunity to ask questions concerning the etiology of the abnormal fetus, but offers the opportunity to obtain information regarding risks for such an outcome in future pregnancies and the availability and option of prenatal diagnosis.

SCREENING PROGRAMS

There are screening programs to identify some of the more common autosomal recessive disorders; examples include sickle cell anemia, Tay–Sachs disease, cystic fibrosis, and the thalassemias. These programs raise many social, ethical, economical, and legal questions, including the possible psychological stigmata of carrying "bad genes." Important to the success of such screening programs is an intensive education program for persons undergoing testing, and this, unfortunately, is where many programs have typically failed. Without careful planning and education, such a program may cause more harm than good.

All states have laws for newborn screening for phenylketonuria and congenital hypothyroidism. A variable number of states mandate newborn screening for sickle cell disease, galactosemia, maple syrup urine disease, homocystinuria, or other conditions that may be ameliorated by early treatment.

Screening Programs for Prenatal Diagnosis. Some screening programs play a significant role in assessing candidates for prenatal counseling and, equally important, prenatal diagnosis. Besides the screening programs for various disorders listed above, maternal age is a screening device (Chap. 40, p. 922), as is the questionnaire shown in Figure 41–1. The most common prenatal screening test for inherited disorders for pregnant women is maternal serum alphafetoprotein determination.

Alphafetoprotein Screening Programs

Alphafetoprotein (AFP) is a glycoprotein synthesized by the fetus early in gestation by the yolk sac and later by the gastrointestinal tract and liver. It has a molecular weight of approximately 70,000 and, although its function is unknown, it is the major serum protein of the embryo and early fetus. The concentration of AFP is highest in both fetal serum and amnionic fluid around the 13th week (Fig. 41–2). Concentration in fetal serum (mg) is about 150 times that in amnionic fluid (μg). The major source of AFP in amnionic fluid is fetal urine. Some protein crosses fetal membranes to enter the maternal circulation, but AFP concentrations in maternal serum (ng) are only approximately 1/1000th those of fetal serum. After 13 weeks' gestation, both fetal serum and amnionic fluid levels normally decrease rapidly in parallel fashion while those in maternal serum continue to rise until late in pregnancy. Detection of AFP in maternal serum forms the basis of maternal serum AFP screening for both neural-tube defects (elevated levels) and Down syndrome (low levels).

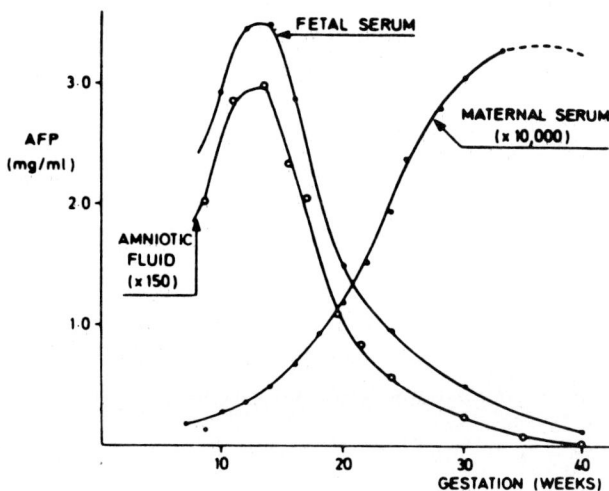

Fig. 41–2. Maternal and fetal serum and amnionic fluid alphafetoprotein levels corresponding with gestational age. (From Roberts and Dunn, 1983, with permission.)

Elevated AFP Levels. The AFP level in amnionic fluid, maternal serum, or both, may be elevated in a great variety of circumstances in which fetal integument is not intact, and the protein leaks from the capillaries into the amnionic fluid (Table 41–1). Levels also are increased in circumstances in which the amount leaked by the fetal kidney is increased, and whenever the placenta contains increased numbers of thin-walled fetal vessels.

Open Neural-tube Defects. In 1972, Brock and colleagues reported an association of anencephaly and elevated maternal serum AFP at 16 weeks' gestation. Soon after, there were two reports supporting the efficacy of maternal serum AFP screening programs in detecting neural-tube defects (Macri and associates, 1976; U.K. Collaborative Study on Alpha-fetoprotein, 1977). Experiences with screening for open neural-tube defects are now extensive, especially in the United Kingdom, where such defects are much more common (approximately 1 in 100 births). Considerable enthusiasm has been generated for measuring near midpregnancy the level of serum AFP. When levels are elevated sufficiently to suspect the possibility of a neural-tube defect, amniocentesis is then performed to look for distinctly elevated levels in amnionic fluid. Moreover, the fetus is usually carefully surveyed by ultrasound for evidence of abnormality, especially anencephaly and spina bifida.

The AFP level at which amniocentesis is performed is based on statistical possibilities whether a fetus will

TABLE 41–1. SOME CONDITIONS ASSOCIATED WITH ABNORMAL MATERNAL SERUM ALPHAFETOPROTEIN CONCENTRATIONS

Elevated Levels
Neural-tube defects
Pilonidal cysts
Esophageal or intestinal obstruction
Liver necrosis
Cystic hygroma
Sacrococcygeal teratoma
Abdominal wall defects—omphalocele, gastroschisis
Urinary obstruction
Renal anomalies—polycystic or absent kidneys
Congenital nephrosis
Osteogenesis imperfecta
Congenital skin defects
Cloacal exstrophy
Low birthweight
Oligohydramnios
Multifetal gestation
Decreased maternal weight
Underestimated gestational age

Low Levels
Chromosomal trisomies
Gestational trophoblastic disease
Fetal death
Increased maternal weight
Overestimated gestational age

be affected at that level. It is customary to report values as *multiples of the median,* because serum AFP levels do not follow a Gaussian distribution. Shown in Figure 41–3 is a schematic of this concept. **Regardless of the cutoff point chosen as "abnormal," there will always be false-positive and false-negative results.** Most laboratories routinely test for AFP levels in all midtrimester amnionic fluid samples, regardless of the indication for which the fluid was obtained.

Amnionic Fluid Acetylcholinesterase Activity. Elevated levels of acetylcholinesterase activity in amnionic fluid accompany most open neural-tube defects. By demonstrating the absence of an acetylcholinesterase band in amnionic fluid using the technique of slab gel electrophoresis, Milunsky and Sapirstein (1982) were able to reclassify correctly 89 percent of the normal pregnancies in which they had found spuriously high AFP levels in the amnionic fluid. It is especially useful for detecting falsely elevated amnionic fluid AFP levels from fetal blood contamination (American College of Obstetricians and Gynecologists, 1991a).

Maternal Serum AFP Screening. Routine screening for neural-tube defects by measuring AFP levels in maternal serum currently is employed widely in the United States. Indeed, some states mandate that it be made available to all prenatal patients. After initial controversy surrounding its implementation, the American College of Obstetricians and Gynecologists (1991a) now recommends that such screening programs be established, but only within a coordinated system that includes quality control, counseling, follow-up, and high-resolution sonographic facilities.

If the procedure is accepted after informed consent

is obtained, initial serum screening is usually done at 16 to 18 weeks' gestation. About 2.5 to 5 percent of all women will have abnormally high levels, defined by most as greater than 2.5 multiples of the median determined for the population under study. Repeat serum testing eliminates 2 percent of the total, and ultrasound evaluation is performed for the remaining 3 percent. In approximately 1 percent of the total, multiple gestation, inaccurate gestational age estimation, or missed abortion are identified. Thus, 1.5 to 2 percent of all women screened will be candidates for amniocentesis so that amnionic fluid AFP concentration can be measured, and only a small fraction of these will be found to have abnormally elevated levels (Fig. 41–4).

Richards and colleagues (1988) reported that the likelihood of a neural-tube defect associated with an abnormal serum screening value is decreased by 90 percent if the ultrasound examination is normal. This is because about half of neural-tube defects are anencephaly, virtually 100 percent detectable using ultrasound; and the other half are spina bifida, 80 percent of which can be diagnosed by ultrasound. In a recent review of 234 fetuses with spina bifida from nine different reports, Watson and associates (1991) reported that 99 percent had some type of cranial anomaly detected by ultrasound. These included frontal notching ("lemon sign"), ventriculomegaly, obliteration of the cisterna magna, small biparietal diameter, or cerebellar changes. They concluded that a woman with an elevated serum AFP should be counseled that the risk is reduced by 95 percent if high-resolution ultrasound is normal. Likewise, Nadel and colleagues (1990) reported close to a 100 percent accuracy of detection of neural-tube defects with ultrasound. Conversely, others have emphasized that as many as 10 to 25 percent of neural-tube defects may be missed if amniocentesis is not performed routinely for elevated maternal serum levels accompanied by a normal ultrasonic examination (Drugan and colleagues, 1988; Evans and associates, 1992).

It seems reasonable to counsel women with confirmed elevated maternal serum AFP that the risk of a fetus with an open neural-tube defect can be reduced significantly when high-resolution ultrasound is normal, but the risk is not zero. It also is important to emphasize that a growing number of conditions other than neural-tube defects have been recognized to be associated with both abnormally elevated as well as low serum AFP concentrations (Table 41–1). In a review of more than 225,000 pregnancies from several screening studies, Katz and colleagues (1990) reported that up to 38 percent of pregnancies associated with unexplained maternal serum AFP elevations had adverse pregnancy outcomes, including perinatal mortality and placental abruption. Waller and colleagues (1991) likewise reported an increase in fetal deaths in association with unexplained elevation of maternal serum AFP. Unfortunately, neither the etiology of these elevated values nor

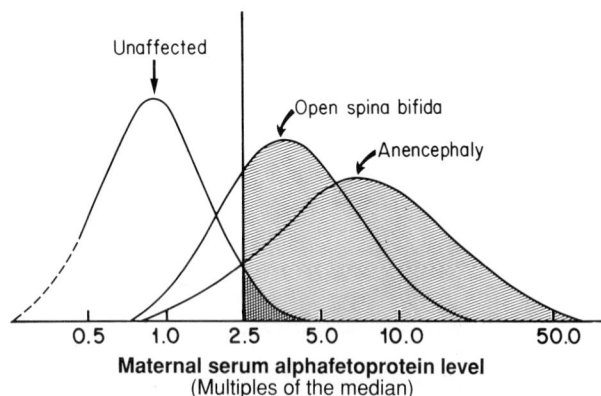

Fig. 41–3. Maternal serum alphafetoprotein levels in singleton gestations 16 to 18 weeks. The cutoff value of 2.5 multiples of the median results in both false-positive and false-negative diagnosis. Any cutoff point chosen, however, would result in false-positive (cross-hatched area) and false-negative rates. (Redrawn from American College of Obstetricians and Gynecologists, 1986, with permission.)

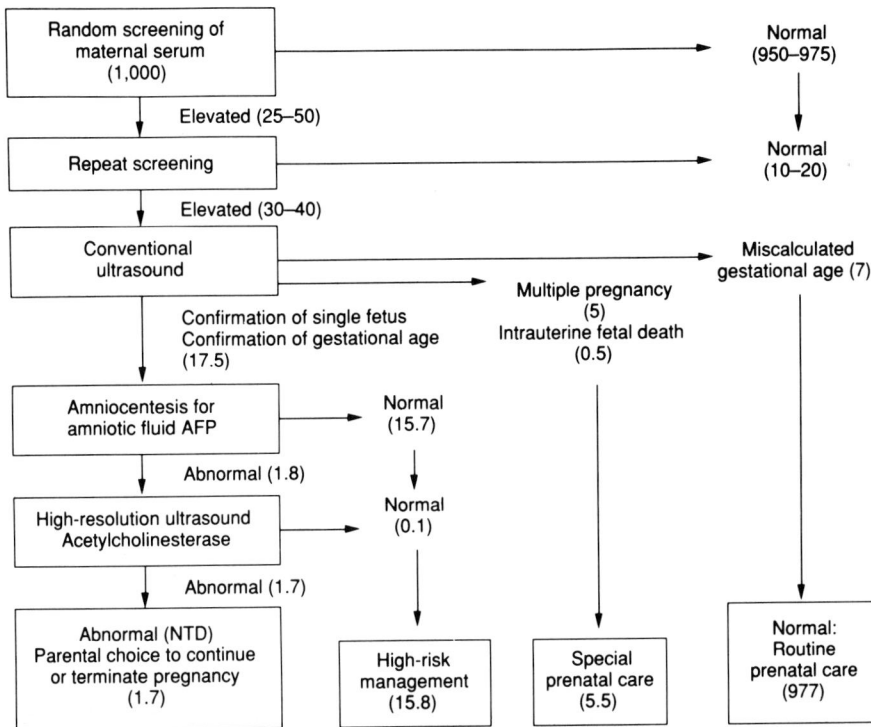

Fig. 41–4. Anticipated results of elevated maternal serum alphafetoprotein (AFP) screening of 1000 prenatal patients at 16 to 18 weeks' gestation to detect neural-tube defects (NTD). (From American College of Obstetricians and Gynecologists, 1991a, with permission.)

the most appropriate management protocols for these women is clear (Cunningham and Gilstrap, 1991).

Family History of Neural-tube Defects. Patients with a family history of neural-tube defects have an increased risk for having an affected child (Chap. 40, p. 928). There is a 2 to 3 percent risk of having another child with a neural-tube defect following the birth of one affected child if one parent is affected. These women should be offered high-resolution ultrasonography as well as amniocentesis at 16 to 18 weeks (American College of Obstetricians and Gynecologists, 1991a).

Abnormally Low AFP Concentrations. Following the observations of Merkatz (1984), Cuckle (1984), and their colleagues that serum AFP concentrations were abnormally low in women bearing chromosomally abnormal fetuses, it is now appreciated that the value of screening is greatly enhanced. Simpson and colleagues (1986) reported results from screening of over 1400 women, of which 9 percent had abnormally low serum levels, defined as less than 0.4 multiples of the median. Half of these women still had low values when repeated, and 3 of 49 who underwent amniocentesis had a chromosomally triploid fetus. These workers appropriately emphasized that the yield of 6 percent was much greater than for routine amniocentesis in women who were 35 years old. Moreover, 80 percent of Down syndrome fetuses are born to women under age 35.

Low serum AFP values can be used in conjunction with maternal age to predict risks for Down syndrome,

and amniocentesis is generally recommended when the risk approaches that for a 35-year-old woman, that is, 1 in 270 (American College of Obstetricians and Gynecologists, 1991a). In a report of over 77,000 screened pregnant women under age 35 from the New England Regional Genetics Group (1989), 25 percent of all fetuses with Down syndrome were identified using AFP screening with age to determine when to perform amniocentesis. One case of Down syndrome was detected for every 89 amniocenteses. Thus, by providing amniocentesis to women age 35 and older and for those less than 35 who have a low serum AFP level, about 45 to 50 percent of all Down syndrome fetuses can be identified prenatally. The outcome in 1000 hypothetical cases screened for low maternal serum AFP is summarized in Figure 41–5.

Other Markers. To increase the sensitivity of maternal serum AFP as a screening tool for Down syndrome, some investigators have recommended the addition of two other serum markers—unconjugated estriol and chorionic gonadotropin (Wald and co-workers, 1988). Women with a Down syndrome fetus are more likely to have "low" maternal serum AFP along with low unconjugated estriol and elevated chorionic gonadotropin. Utilizing the so-called *triple screen*, some report that up to 60 percent of Down syndrome fetuses can be detected prenatally (MacDonald and colleagues, 1991; Wald and associates, 1988). Others are less optimistic concerning the efficacy of these three serum markers to predict Down syndrome (Evans and colleagues, 1992;

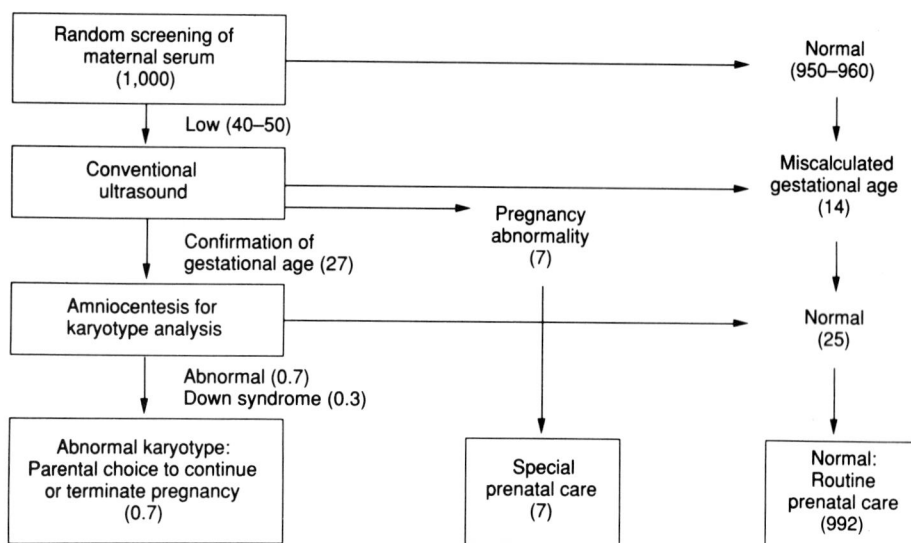

Fig. 41–5. Anticipated results of low maternal serum alphafetoprotein screening of 1000 prenatal patients at 16 to 18 weeks' gestation. (From the American College of Obstetricians and Gynecologists, 1991a, with permission.)

Macri and associates, 1990). There have also been reports of an association with markedly low serum chorionic gonadotropin levels and trisomy 18 and 13 pregnancies (Barkai, 1991; Crossley, 1991; Johnson, 1991; Kratzer, 1991; and their colleagues).

The clinical utility of a low serum chorionic gonadotropin as a marker for trisomy 18 and 13 is unclear at this time. Currently, the American College of Obstetricians and Gynecologists (1991a) recommends that the use of the combination markers be considered investigational.

Hemoglobinopathies

Sickle cell disease is a common hemoglobinopathy, and approximately 1 of every 12 African-Americans is heterozygous for the sickle cell gene (see Chap. 52, p. 1179). The thalassemias are common in individuals of Mediterranean or Oriental descent. However, in a screening program involving more than 18,000 prenatal patients in Rochester, 7 percent of the subjects with a positive sickle screen were not black, and 22 percent of those with β-thalassemia were not Mediterranean, Asian, or black (Bowman, 1991; Rowley and associates, 1991). Although total population screening for hemoglobinopathies certainly can be questioned on an efficacy and economical basis, it is reasonable to offer screening to high-risk groups. For example, if a pregnant woman is positive for sickle trait, sickle screening is offered for her partner. If he is positive, or if screening is unavailable, then she can be offered prenatal diagnosis by either chorionic villus sampling or amniocentesis (see Chap. 40, Fig. 40–13). Prenatal diagnosis is also available for other hemoglobinopathies (Maberry and associates, 1990).

Tay–Sachs Disease

An autosomal recessive lysosomal storage disorder, Tay–Sachs disease results from an enzyme deficiency of hexosaminidase A. The heterozygous state occurs in approximately 1 in 30 Ashkenazi Jews (Eastern and Central Europe) and approximately 1 in 150 non-Jewish individuals. The adult carrier state can be determined by measuring hexosaminidase A activity in blood. However, in pregnancy it is usually necessary to utilize a special leukocyte assay for ascertaining maternal levels (American College of Obstetricians and Gynecologists, 1991b). If both parents test positive, or if the paternal status is unknown, prenatal diagnosis usually can be accomplished by measuring the enzyme level in fetal cells obtained by chorionic villus sampling or amniocentesis. If one of the two parents is negative, then prenatal diagnosis is not necessary. Nonpaternity may be an important consideration in some cases when the male partner is negative.

Cystic Fibrosis

Cystic fibrosis is one of the most common autosomal recessive disorders in the Caucasian population, occurring in approximately 1 in 2500 live births. It has been estimated that approximately 1 in 25 Caucasians is a carrier for cystic fibrosis. Recently, the gene locus for this disease has been shown to be on chromosome 7, and the major cystic fibrosis gene has been sequenced (Kerem, 1989; Riordan, 1989; Rommens, 1989; and their colleagues). There are several mutations that cause cystic fibrosis, and one of the most common mutations, occurring in 75 percent of Caucasians, is referred to as ΔF508, which is a three-base pair deletion resulting in the loss of phenylalanine at amino acid position 508. This specific mutation is found in only 25 to 30 percent of the Jewish and non-Caucasian carrier population. Four other relatively common mutations include G542X, F5510, R553X, and N1202K. Along with ΔF508 mutation, these five account for about 85 percent of the alleles in affected and carrier individuals (Asch and colleagues, 1992). Screening is currently recommended for anyone with a family history of cystic fibrosis. Asch and co-workers (1992) recently reviewed the various alternative ways to report the results of heterozygous screening (Table 41–2).

Various molecular techniques may be utilized to diagnose both the carrier state and the affected fetus. These include allele-specific oligonucleotide probes (ASO) with the polymerase chain reaction (PCR) and with linkage analysis of affected families and restriction fragment polymorphisms (RFLPs) and Southern blotting (see Chap. 40, p. 935).

PRENATAL DIAGNOSIS

Indications for Prenatal Counseling and Diagnosis

Probably the most common indications for prenatal counseling and diagnosis are advanced maternal age and an abnormal maternal serum AFP screening test. Indications for counseling include the following circumstances:

1. Pregnancies in women 35 years of age or older.
2. A previous pregnancy that resulted in the birth of a chromosomally abnormal offspring.
3. Chromosomal abnormality in either parent, including
   a. Balanced translocation carrier and other structural rearrangements.
   b. Aneuploidy.
   c. Mosaicism.
4. Down syndrome or other chromosomal abnormality in a close family member.
5. Pregnancies at risk of a serious Mendelian disorder.
6. A previous child or a parent with a neural-tube defect or an abnormally low or high maternal serum AFP level obtained during routine screening.
7. Abnormal fetus identified by sonographic examination.
8. A previous infant with multiple major malformations in whom no cytogenetic study was performed.
9. Fetal sex determination in pregnancies at risk of a serious X-linked hereditary disorder for which specific prenatal diagnosis is not available (this is better accomplished using the new DNA techniques to identify Y-chromosomal material).
10. Positive answer to questions listed in Figure 41–1.

With the virtual "explosion" in molecular biology technology, it is anticipated that prenatal screening and diagnosis will be available for the majority of common genetic disorders in the very near future.

Techniques for Prenatal Diagnosis

Techniques utilized for prenatal diagnosis include x-ray, sonography, magnetic resonance imaging, amniocentesis, chorionic villus sampling, and percutaneous umbilical cord sampling.

TABLE 41–2. RISKS FACED BY COUPLES UNDERGOING CYSTIC FIBROSIS CARRIER SCREENING USING THREE ALTERNATIVE REPORTING SYSTEMS

Reporting System	Screening Result	Risk of Offspring with Cystic Fibrosis
Both partners tested and results reported	1. Both partners positive	1/4
	2. One partner positive	1/640
	3. Neither partner positive	1/104,000
Second partner tested only if first is positive	1. Both partners positive	1/4
	2. First partner positive, second partner negative	1/640
	3. First partner negative, second partner not screened	1/16,000
Report as negative screen unless both partners positive	1. Both partners positive	1/4
	2. First partner positive, second partner negative; or first partner negative, second partner not screened	1/9000

Adapted from Asch and colleagues (1992), with permission.

Radiography and Ultrasonography. X-ray has been used to identify gross skeletal anomalies, but it is seldom utilized today. High-resolution ultrasound, especially after 18 weeks' gestation, is useful to identify many fetal anomalies (Table 41–3), and for the most part, it has replaced x-ray for the diagnosis of such anomalies. Recently, Quashie and colleagues (1992) reported that it is possible to demonstrate the majority of major fetal structures by 13 weeks utilizing a transvaginal approach (Table 41–4). Ultrasound is discussed in further detail in Chapter 46.

Magnetic Resonance Imaging. Equipment essential for organ and body imaging using magnetic resonance is available in many medical centers. This technology has been used for imaging of structural and anatomical fetal defects (Lowe, 1985; Powell, 1988; Smith, 1983; Symonds, 1984; and their co-workers). **It especially is useful for definition of maternal anatomy with suspected intraabdominal or retroperitoneal disease.**

As discussed in Chapter 43 (p. 987), magnetic resonance imaging during pregnancy appears to be safe. The National Institutes of Health Consensus Development Conference (Marx, 1987), however, concluded that "pregnant women, especially early in pregnancy, should not undergo the procedure unless they have a clear medical need that cannot be resolved by other means."

Amniocentesis. Amniocentesis is the most commonly performed invasive test for prenatal diagnosis of genetic disease. Amniocentesis is also utilized for measuring other markers of fetal health, such as lung maturity (Chap. 44).

Midtrimester Amniocentesis. Amniocentesis for prenatal diagnosis has most often been performed at 16 to 18 weeks' gestation, when it is likely there are sufficient fetal cells to allow successful culture. Cultured amnionic fluid cells can be utilized for cytogenetic studies as well as enzyme and DNA analysis. The success rate for amnionic fluid cell growth and cytogenetic studies approaches 98 to 99 percent. The fluid itself can be utilized for measuring a variety of substances such as AFP or acetylcholinesterase, which may provide useful clues as to the presence or absence of fetal disorders.

The three major risks of amniocentesis include maternal or fetal trauma, infection, and abortion or preterm labor. Surgical asepsis is mandatory to avoid infection not only in the mother and fetus but also in the aspirated amnionic fluid. As well as causing hemorrhage into the placenta and into the amnionic sac, perforation of the placenta may lead to significant transfer of fetal blood to the mother, which may incite or enhance maternal isoimmunization. Sonographic localization of the placenta before amniocentesis will reduce, but not eliminate, the likelihood of placental perforation. There-

TABLE 41–3. HIGH-RESOLUTION ULTRASONOGRAPHY FOR DETECTION OF FETAL ANOMALIES

Head Anomalies
Anencephaly
Ventriculomegaly/hydrocephaly
Encephalocele
Intracranial lesions

Neck Anomalies
Cystic hygroma
Branchial cleft-cysts
Teratomas

Spinal Anomalies
Myelomeningocele
Sacrococcygeal teratomas

Chest Anomalies
Diaphragmatic hernia
Pleural effusion

Gastrointestinal Anomalies
Duodenal atresia
Omphalocele
Gastroschisis

Urinary Tract Anomalies
Bilateral renal agenesis
Polycystic kidneys
Multicystic kidneys

Skeletal Anomalies
Achondroplasia
Agenesis or hypoplasia of bones
Osteogenesis imperfecta
Camptomelic dysplasia

Cardiac Anomalies[a]

[a] Frequently require echocardiography.
Adapted from Vintzileos and colleagues (1987), with permission.

TABLE 41–4. SUMMARY OF ANATOMICAL SURVEY

Structures	Menstrual Weeks When Structure Usually Visualized					
	8	9	10	11	12	13
Biparietal diameter			----	----	----	----
Head circumference			----	----	----	----
Anterior abdominal wall				----	----	----
Extremities		----	----	----	----	----
Digits					----	----
Cord insertion				----	----	----
Diaphragm			----	----	----	----
Fetal spine			----	----	----	----
Choroid plexus			----	----	----	----
Cerebellum					----	----
Ventricles		----	----	----	----	----
Orbits				----	----	----
Facial profile				----	----	----
Jaw					----	----
Stomach bubble				----	----	----
Bladder					----	----
Kidneys				----	----	----
Doppler			----	----	----	----

From Quashie and colleagues (1992), with permission.

fore, anti-D globulin is administered to nonsensitized D-negative women at the time of amniocentesis (see Chap. 44).

Several reports quantify the overall risk of amniocentesis performed near midpregnancy. In the study by the National Institute of Child Health and Human Development (1976), no significant differences were found in fetal loss rate, birthweight, birth defects, neonatal complications, or growth and development at 1 year of age. The overall fetal loss was 3.5 percent for the amniocentesis group and 3.2 percent for the control group. The overall accuracy of prenatal diagnosis was 99.4 percent. Similar results were obtained in a Canadian study (Simpson and colleagues, 1976). The Working Party on Amniocentesis (1978), in Great Britain, however, reported a significantly higher fetal loss rate—2.6 percent —in the amniocentesis group, compared with an unusually low value of 1.1 percent for the control group. In all studies, complications were greater when an 18-gauge or larger needle was used, and when more than two attempts were needed to obtain fluid.

In our recent experience of over 1000 midtrimester procedures, the complication rate was less than 0.5 percent above the background pregnancy loss of 2 to 3 percent. In an earlier review of over 1200 second-trimester genetic amniocenteses, Hankins and colleagues (1984) reported that 83 (7 percent) had either green or brown discolored fluid. Interestingly, there were no significant differences in the incidence of pregnancy loss, abnormal fetal karyotype, newborn abnormalities, or other pregnancy complications when these 83 women were compared with matched controls. Free hemoglobin measurement showed that the fluid discoloration was from blood breakdown products. Blood contaminating amnionic fluid may inhibit the replication in culture of fetal cells. Moreover, blood may change the apparent level of various constituents of amnionic fluid under study. Minute amounts of fetal blood can lead to falsely high levels of amnionic fluid AFP. Acetylcholinesterase levels are helpful when amnionic fluid AFP values are falsely elevated by blood.

TECHNIQUE. The technique of midtrimester amniocentesis is relatively simple and easy to master. After locally anesthetizing the abdominal wall, a 20- or 22-gauge needle, 3 to 6 inches long, depending upon the thickness of the abdominal wall, the size of the uterus, and the site of puncture, is inserted carefully into the amnionic cavity under sonographic guidance. When cells from amnionic fluid are desired for culture, 20 to 30 mL of fluid will usually prove satisfactory.

Amniocentesis is relatively easy to perform in twin gestations. Elias and colleagues (1980) reported successful results in 19 of 20 twin cases. These authors utilized indigo carmine dye (1 to 3 mL of 0.8 percent dye diluted with sterile water for a final concentration of 0.08 percent) to distinguish the separate sacs (Fig. 41–6).

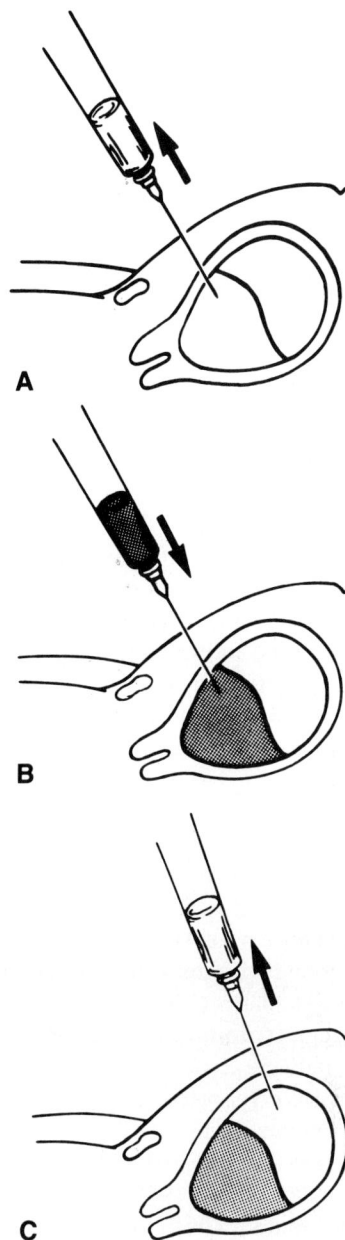

Fig. 41–6. Technique for amniocentesis in twin gestation, performed immediately after ultrasonic examination. **A.** Fluid aspirated from the first amnionic sac. **B.** Indigo carmine injected into the first sac. **C.** Second tap in the ultrasonically determined location of the second fetus. Clear fluid confirms that the second sac was aspirated successfully. (From Elias and colleagues, 1980, with permission.)

More recently Bahado-Singh and colleagues (1992) described a technique of amniocentesis in twins that entails identifying the separating membrane with a curvilinear or linear transducer. The first needle and transducer are left in place during the insertion of the second needle. This technique is illustrated in Figure 41–7. Beekhuis and associates (1992) described another technique utilizing maternal hemoglobin as a dye marker to differentiate between the two sacs.

Methylene blue is not recommended as a dye as it

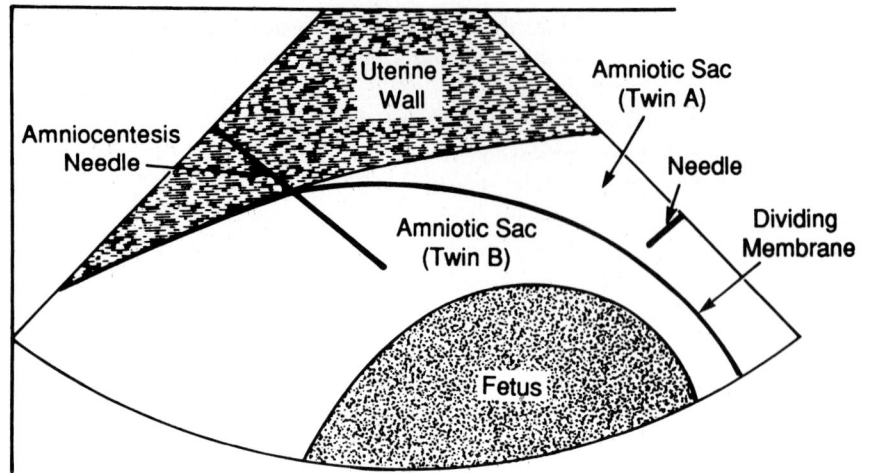

Fig. 41–7. Technique for amniocentesis in twins. The separating fetal membrane is identified. (From Bahado-Singh and associates, 1992, with permission.)

has been reported to cause hemolytic anemia or methemoglobinemia (Twickler and co-workers, 1992). An association with fetal intestinal obstruction and jejunal atresia and the use of methylene blue dye for amniocentesis in twins has been reported (Nicolini and Monni, 1990; Van der Pol and collaborators, 1992).

Early Amniocentesis. The trend is to perform amniocentesis earlier than 16 to 18 weeks. Hanson and colleagues (1990) described their experiences with 527 procedures performed before 15 weeks, and they reported a pregnancy loss of 0.8 percent within 2 weeks. In a review of 505 cases of amniocentesis prior to 16 weeks, Stripparo and associates (1990) reported a pregnancy loss of 3.2 percent within the first 28 weeks, excluding elective terminations; 2 percent were in the first two weeks. Others have reported similar results with early amniocentesis, some of which have included procedures as early as 9 weeks (Elejalde, 1990; Evans, 1989; Hackett, 1991; Nevin, 1990; Penso, 1990; and their colleagues). Assel and colleagues (1992) recently compared outcomes of early versus midsecond trimester amniocentesis (Table 41–5). Although this was a non-randomized study, all procedures were accomplished by a single operator. In each group, outcomes were similar.

The technique for early amniocentesis is similar to that for amniocentesis at 16 to 20 weeks. The success of obtaining fluid is surprisingly high and exceeds 95 percent in most reports. Drugan and co-workers (1988) reported normal amnionic fluid values for AFP and acetylcholinesterase in 476 samples obtained between 10 and 15 weeks. The cytogenetic success is also high, approaching 99 to 100 percent (Penso and Frigoletto, 1990).

In a recent report by Iwanicki and colleagues (1992), the failed cell culture rate for fluid obtained from 11 to 14 weeks was only 0.6 percent. Because most reports include few, if any, patients at 9 to 10 weeks'

gestation, it seems reasonable to conclude that early amniocentesis is best accomplished at 11 to 14 weeks.

Chorionic Villus Biopsy. Since its development beginning in the early 1970s, chorion sampling has become a widely accepted first-trimester alternative to amniocentesis for prenatal diagnosis. The chorion is of fetal origin, and cells obtained by villus biopsy can be examined using the same techniques as for amniocytes obtained by amniocentesis. The primary difference is that amniocentesis must be used for assays for which amnionic fluid is integral, an example being AFP concentration. The major advantage of villus biopsy is that fetal cells are obtained earlier and lengthy culture procedures are unnecessary because chorion cells divide very rapidly. Thus, a diagnosis is made earlier and, if chosen, pregnancy can be terminated sooner and with greater safety. However, because chorionic villus sampling is done earlier, the likelihood of finding a cytogenetic abnormality is greater (see Chap. 40, Table 40–3). A major concern with chorionic villus sampling

TABLE 41–5. COMPARISON OF EARLY VERSUS MID-SECOND TRIMESTER AMNIOCENTESIS

Factor	Early[a] (%)	Midsecond Trimester[a] (%)
Failed sampling	5/300 (1.7)	2/567 (0.4)
Confirmation requested	2/295 (0.7)	3/565 (0.4)
Termination	11/300 (3.7)	11/567 (1.9)
Pregnancy loss		
Less than 4 wk	5/276 (1.8)	2/542 (0.4)
More than 4 wk	1/271 (0.4)	4/540 (0.7)
Preterm births	10/270 (3.7)	35/537 (6.5)
Perinatal death rate	7.4 per 1000	11.1/1000

[a] All comparisons not significant.
From Assel and colleagues (1992), with permission.

is whether it is as safe as amniocentesis. There also is some controversy regarding the best approach to this procedure, i.e., transcervical versus transabdominal.

Safety and Efficacy of Chorionic Villus Sampling.

There are three large collaborative studies in which the safety and efficacy of chorionic villus sampling were compared with amniocentesis—the United States study sponsored by the National Institute of Child Health and Development (USNICHD Collaborative CVS Study Group, 1990), the European study sponsored by the Medical Research Council (MRC Working Party on the Evaluation of Chorionic Villus Sampling, 1991), and the Canadian Collaborative CVS-Amniocentesis Clinical Trial Group (1989; Lippman and colleagues, 1992). Some of their reported results are summarized in Table 41–6. Although it appears that chorionic villus sampling is *relatively* safe, it is associated with a slightly higher pregnancy loss than amniocentesis.

The initial report from the United States study (Rhoads and associates, 1989) included 2235 attempted chorionic villus sampling procedures and 651 amniocenteses. Ledbetter and colleagues (1990) described follow-up of 6033 women who had a successful villus biopsy and 862 who underwent amniocentesis. In the most recent report from this group (Ledbetter and coworkers, 1992), cytogenetic results are presented for 11,473 chorionic villus sampling procedures. In this report, a successful cytogenetic result was obtained in 99.7 percent of women; 1.1 percent required a second procedure.

In the Canadian Collaborative Trial (1989), laboratory failure was identified in 2.3 percent of the chorionic villus group versus 0.1 percent of the amniocentesis group. A cytogenetic abnormality was detected in 5.6 percent of the villus sampling group and 3.4 percent of the amniocentesis group. Prenatal cytogenetic diagnosis was 97.5 percent accurate for villus sampling and 99.8 percent accurate for amniocentesis. In the European Col-

laborative Study (MRC Working Party, 1991), a successful procedure was accomplished in 89 percent of 1609 women allocated to chorionic villus sampling and 89 percent of 1592 in the amniocentesis group. Cytogenetic abnormalities were detected in 5.6 percent of the former and 3.9 percent of the latter groups.

Transcervical Versus Transabdominal.

Initially, most chorionic villus sampling was performed transcervically (Fig. 41–8). This procedure is generally performed between 9 and 11 weeks under ultrasonographic guidance. Following cleansing of the cervix and ascertainment of the uterine position, a small-diameter catheter (usually polyethylene) is introduced through the ectocervix to the center of the chorion and a sample is obtained via aspiration with a syringe containing nutrient medium (Jackson, 1991). The transabdominal approach is similar to the technique for amniocentesis except that the 18- to 20-gauge "thin-walled" needle is inserted into the chorionic bed instead of amnionic fluid. The specimen obtained by either procedure should be inspected for villi under high magnification.

There is no consensus as to which procedure is best. The transcervical technique appears to be somewhat easier when the placenta is located posteriorly, while the transabdominal technique might be best when the placenta is anterior. In a randomized trial of transabdominal versus transcervical techniques at 7 to 12 weeks' gestation, Brambati and associates (1991) reported that the overall fetal loss rate was 16.5 percent for the transabdominal approach and 15.5 percent for the transcervical approach. These numbers are high because they include spontaneous abortions prior to and after villus biopsy, as well as elective terminations. More women in the transcervical group required a second device insertion compared with the transabdominal group (10.3 versus 3.3 percent). Complications were identified in 6.4 percent of the transcervical group and 3.8 percent of the transabdominal group.

In the United States Collaborative Study (Jackson and colleagues, 1992), the pregnancy loss rate was similar in both groups (Table 41–7). Post-procedure bleeding, however, was significantly greater in the transcervical group. As Golbus (1992) emphasizes, the "learning curve" is greater for the transcervical approach than with other procedures. For example, the fetal loss rate was 5.1 percent during the first 3000 cases at the University of California at San Francisco and decreased to 2.9 percent after 5000 procedures. The corresponding rate for the latter time period for the transabdominal procedure was 3.1 percent.

In a series of 515 transabdominal chorionic villus sampling procedures performed at the University of Texas Southwestern Medical Center at Dallas and Parkland Hospital, there were 18 (3.5 percent) fetal losses (Peters and Courtney, unpublished observations).

TABLE 41–6. COMPARISON OF PREGNANCY LOSSES WITH CHORIONIC VILLUS SAMPLING AND AMNIOCENTESIS

Study[a]	Chorionic Villus Sampling	Amniocentesis[a]
United States[b]	164/2278 (7.2%)	38/671 (5.7%)
Canadian[c]	89/1164 (7.6%)	82/1169 (7.1%)
European[d]	220/1609 (14%)	144/1592 (9.0%)

[a] Includes elective terminations, stillborns, and neonatal deaths.
[b] Adapted from Rhoads and associates (1989).
[c] From Lippman and colleagues (1992).
[d] From Medical Research Council European Trial of Chorion Villus Sampling (1991).

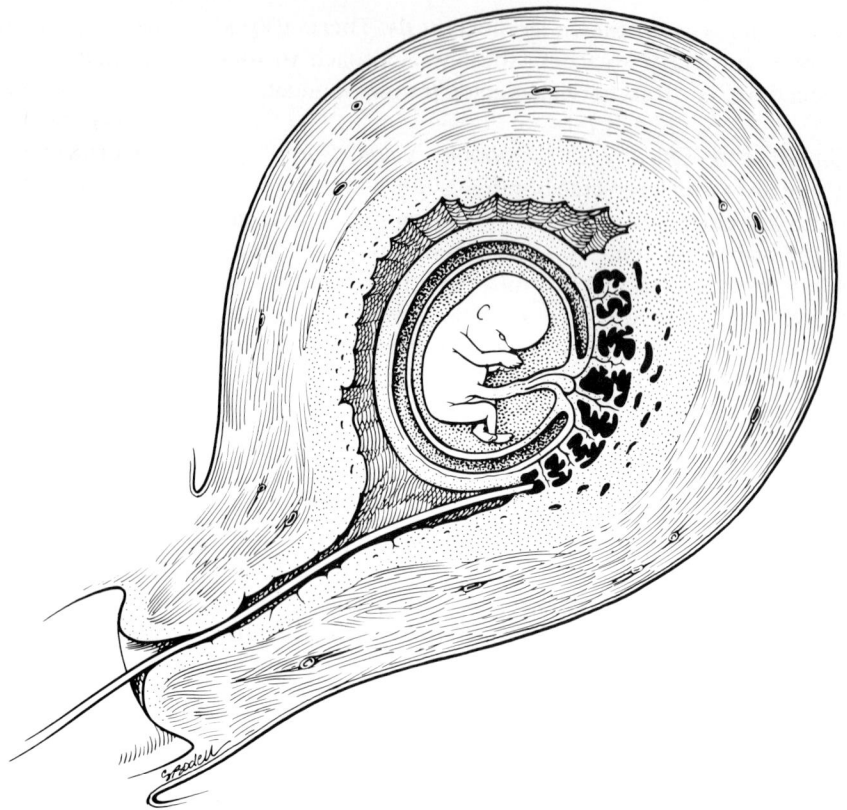

Fig. 41–8. Transcervical chorionic villus sampling.

TABLE 41–7. OUTCOME AFTER CHORIONIC VILLUS SAMPLING FOR WOMEN WITH GENETICALLY NORMAL PREGNANCIES

Pregnancy Outcome	Assigned Procedure	
	Transcervical Sampling (n = 1846) (%)	Transabdominal Sampling (n = 1816) (%)
Losses at ≤ 28 Weeks' Gestation[a]		
Fetal loss between sampling and 16 weeks' gestation	25 (1.4)	27 (1.5)
Fetal loss, stillbirth, or neonatal death at 17–28 weeks	24 (1.3)	20 (1.1)
Elective abortion of chromosomally normal fetus	21 (1.1)	21 (1.2)
Losses After 28 Weeks' Gestation		
Stillbirth	3 (0.2)	3 (0.2)
Neonatal death	1 (0.1)	1 (0.1)
Live Births	1772 (96.0)	1744 (96.0)

[a] Exclusions: 91 transcervical and 103 transabdominal group women with abnormal or unusual karyotypes, or biochemical or molecular diagnosis indicating affected or high probability of affected fetus. Also excluded: 7 transcervical and 10 transabdominal women lost to follow-up.
From Jackson and co-workers (1992), with permission.

Late Chorionic Villus Procedures. Holzgreve and colleagues (1990) reported the outcomes of over 2000 cases of chorionic villus sampling after 12 weeks' gestation. This is sometimes referred to as *placental biopsy.* The rate of cytogenetic abnormalities was 21 percent if the procedure followed a suspicious ultrasound compared with 6 percent without such findings. Likewise, pregnancy losses were higher (10 percent) in the former group compared with the latter (2 percent). This procedure may prove especially useful for cytogenetic diagnosis in the woman with fetal demise or oligohydramnios.

Chorionic Villus Sampling in Twins. Pergament and colleagues (1992) reported the results of a multicenter study of chorionic villus sampling in 126 twin and two triplet pregnancies. An adequate sample was obtained in 99 percent. Cytogenetic analysis was obtained in all cases and total pregnancy loss was 5 percent for multifetal gestations compared with 4 percent for singleton pregnancies. Cell contamination was identified in 2.3 percent of the samples, and fetal sex was assessed incorrectly in two (0.8 percent) cases.

Placental Mosaicism. One of the major technical problems with chorionic villus sampling is the increased frequency of chromosomal mosaicism that ultimately will not be found in the fetus upon further testing. The frequency of mosaicism is approximately 1 to 2 percent.

In the review by Johnson and colleagues (1990), chromosomal mosaicism was present in 55 of 4319 (1.3 percent) chorionic villus samples.

Although the majority of fetuses will be normal and not manifest mosaicism, there is a reported association of placental mosaicism and poor pregnancy outcome, which includes growth retardation and perinatal losses (Goldberg and colleagues, 1990; Johnson and associates, 1990; Leschot and Wolf, 1991). For example, Johnson and colleagues (1990) reported perinatal loss to be 16.7 percent for the mosaic group compared with 2.7 percent for those without such findings. Another problem is maternal cell contamination, which is found in a significant number of specimens (Cheung and colleagues, 1987; Hogge and associates, 1985).

In the recent report from the United States collaborative (Wapner and associates, 1992), placental mosaicism was found in 108 (1 percent) of 11,403 villus samples. Pregnancy loss was significantly higher in those with placental mosaicism compared with those with normal cytogenetic results (8.6 versus 3.4 percent, respectively). However, there were no significant differences between these two groups with regard to preterm delivery, growth retardation, pregnancy-induced hypertension, abruptio placentae, or depressed newborns.

Limb Abnormalities and Chorionic Villus Sampling. Firth and colleagues (1991) were among the first to report an increased risk for severe limb abnormalities associated with chorionic villus sampling. These were found with transabdominal procedures performed between 56 and 66 days' gestation. Although increased limb abnormalities were not found in the United States Collaborative Study (Mahoney, 1991), 88 percent of the sampling procedures were accomplished after 66 menstrual days. More recently, Burton and associates (1992) reported 3.3 percent major anomalies out of 394 fetuses whose mothers had undergone chorionic villus sampling. Of particular concern was that 1 percent of the infants had limb deformities. Importantly, the gestational age at the time of the procedure ranged from 67 to 79 days.

Golbus (1992) concluded that transcervical and transabdominal chorionic villus sampling performed at 8 to 9 weeks are both associated with an increased risk for fetal limb defects. He added that villus sampling at the standard time of 9 to 12 menstrual weeks is not associated with severe limb abnormalities, but it may be associated with increased minor nail or phalangeal hypoplasia. Although the exact risk of this complication is unknown, it seems reasonable to counsel women that either transcervical or transabdominal chorionic villus sampling may be associated with an increase in limb anomalies.

Chorionic Villus Sampling for Biochemical and Molecular Diagnosis. Tissue obtained by chorionic villus sampling can be utilized for the diagnosis of many inherited

diseases that are determined on a gene level. In a report from the United States Collaborative Study (Desnick and associates, 1992), villus sampling was used for diagnosis in 283 pregnancies with possible biochemical disorders that included lysosomal storage diseases (Tay–Sachs, Gaucher, and Niemann–Pick), amino acid disorders, urea cycle defects, and other conditions (congenital adrenal hypoplasia). Of these 283, 20 percent of fetuses were subsequently shown to be affected.

In this same report, tissue obtained by villus sampling was subjected to a variety of molecular techniques in 318 women in an attempt to diagnose fetal conditions that included hemoglobinopathies, cystic fibrosis, hemophilia A and B, and Duchenne or Becker muscular dystrophy. Of these, one fourth were subsequently shown to be affected. Although other techniques such as amniocentesis or fetal blood sampling were necessary in some women because of inconclusive results, chorionic villus samples usually provided rapid and accurate diagnosis for both biochemical and molecular-based diagnoses (Desnick and associates, 1992).

Chorionic Villus Sampling for Diagnosis of Fetal Infection. Villus sampling may also be utilized as an adjunct for the early diagnosis of some fetal infections. Foulon and colleagues (1990) reported successful diagnosis of congenital toxoplasmosis utilizing in vitro cell culture of material obtained by chorionic villus sampling and early amniocentesis. Isada and co-workers (1991) found evidence for varicella-zoster virus infection using polymerase chain reaction for DNA obtained by first-trimester villus sampling. However, infection was not confirmed in either of the fetuses (one aborted and one was normal). They concluded that the presence of varicella-zoster DNA sequences in the placenta does not correlate with fetal infection.

Percutaneous Umbilical Blood Sampling (Cordocentesis). In 1982, Bang and associates reported umbilical vein blood sampling and direct transfusion of a severely anemic D-isoimmunized fetus. They also obtained umbilical blood at 23 weeks from another fetus with a known chromosomal anomaly. Subsequently, the Paris group further developed fetal blood sampling techniques and expanded indications for its use (Daffos and associates, 1983; Forestier and colleagues, 1988).

Technique for Umbilical Cord Blood Sampling. Daffos and colleagues (1983) use a 20-gauge spinal needle, 10 to 13 cm in length, filled with a 3.8-percent sodium citrate solution with an attached 2-mL disposable syringe containing 0.1 mL of the same anticoagulant. The anterior abdominal wall is prepared and a local anesthetic is injected into the skin and anterior abdominal wall. With a real-time transducer held stationary, the needle is inserted through the abdominal and uterine walls, and the progress of the needle tip is followed into the umbilical vein.

Hobbins and associates (1985) use a 25-gauge spinal needle with a stylet. They stress the importance of identifying the site of insertion of the umbilical cord into the placenta. Rotating the ultrasound transducer 90 degrees to the long axis of the umbilical cord allows a cross-sectional view approximately 1 to 2 cm from its placental insertion. The operator then may follow the needle tip directly into the umbilical vein.

There are three basic approaches to the umbilical cord (Fig. 41–9): (1) with the placenta anterior, the needle is introduced transplacentally, without entering the amnionic cavity, to puncture the umbilical cord at its base; (2) with a posterior placenta, the needle passes through the amnionic fluid to penetrate the umbilical cord 1 to 2 cm from its insertion; and (3) when the placenta is fundal and lateral, the needle passes transplacentally and through the amnionic fluid before puncturing the umbilical cord 1 to 2 cm from its insertion. An initial 0.5 mL sample of blood is obtained with a heparinized syringe and discarded. Either the umbilical vein or artery may be utilized, although complications such as bleeding and fetal bradycardia appear to be greater with umbilical artery sampling (Meizner and Glezerman, 1992; Nicolaides and Snijders, 1992).

After blood is obtained, a second syringe without anticoagulant is attached to the needle, and blood is aspirated and transferred to appropriate tubes. Surprisingly, after needle withdrawal, the duration of bleeding from the umbilical cord is usually very short and can be monitored ultrasonically. Daffos and co-workers (1985) recommend continuous fetal heart rate monitoring for a few minutes after the procedure and a repeat ultrasound examination one hour later to ensure that there is no further bleeding or hematoma formation. In cases of oligohydramnios, the cord can be punctured at any site because it is less likely to move away as the needle is introduced. Confirmation that fetal blood has been obtained is made using a Coulter Channelyzer to detect larger fetal red blood cells.

Using a 20-gauge needle, Daffos and associates (1985) reported a 1.1 percent fetal death rate and a 0.8 percent abortion rate with the first 606 umbilical cord samplings. They were successful on the first attempt in 588 cases (97 percent), and a second attempt was suc-

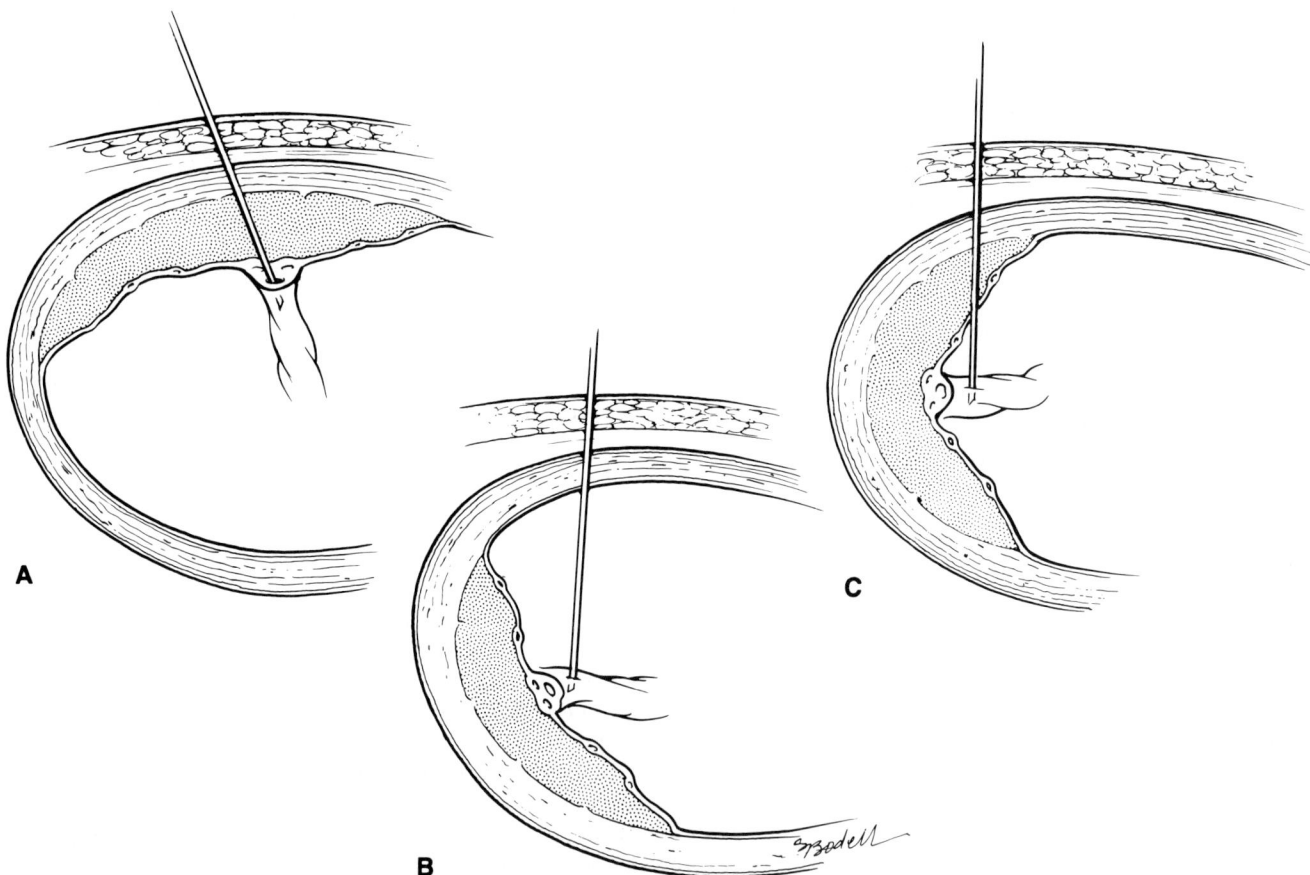

Fig. 41–9. Umbilical cord blood sampling. Access to the umbilical artery or vein varies, depending upon both the placental location and the position of cord insertion into the placenta. **A.** With an anterior placenta, the needle may traverse the placenta. **B.** With a posterior implantation, the needle usually passes through the amnionic fluid before penetrating an umbilical vessel. **C.** With a lateral or fundal placenta, the needle may pass through the placenta and amnionic cavity to enter the umbilical vessel. (Redrawn after Queenan and King, 1987.)

cessful in the remaining 18 cases. In a recent review of 928 cases for prenatal diagnosis, Nicolaides and Snijders (1992) reported 1 percent early fetal losses including death or spontaneous abortion within 2 weeks, and 1 percent fetal deaths within 4 to 20 weeks after cordocentesis.

Normal Fetal Blood Values. One of the many advantages of this technique is the ability to establish normal fetal blood values throughout gestation. Fetal hemoglobin values from 16 through 26 weeks' gestation are shown in Figure 44–12 (Chap. 44). Soothill and colleagues (1986) reported that fetal blood gas and acid-base values also change with gestational age. Furthermore, fetal values may be altered if the mother has been sedated (Soothill and colleagues, 1986). It is likely that other fetal blood values will vary with gestational age. Fetal blood carbon dioxide tension and plasma lactate concentrations increase with gestational age, but normal preterm values have not been established (Soothill and associates, 1987a, 1987b).

Indications for Fetal Blood Sampling. Percutaneous umbilical blood sampling has revolutionized the fields of fetal physiology, diagnosis, and therapy. The indications for its application are increasing rapidly, and any list will be outdated by the time of its publication. Although genetic indications are expanding most rapidly, diagnostic and treatment techniques for fetal hypoxia, isoimmunization, and infection are also being developed. These and other current indications are presented in Table 41–8.

ISOIMMUNIZATION AND PLATELET DISORDERS. The earliest attempts at umbilical blood sampling arose from a need to evaluate the hemoglobin concentration of the D-isoimmunized fetus and to have intravenous access for fetal transfusion (Bang and associates, 1982). Today, one accepted management of fetal hemolytic disease includes fetal blood sampling and direct intraumbilical vein transfusion (Berkowitz, 1986; deCrespigny, 1985; Grannum, 1986; Nicolaides, 1986b, 1992; Seeds, 1986; and their colleagues) (see Chap. 44, p. 1012).

Cordocentesis also has been utilized in the diagnosis of both autoimmune and alloimmune thrombocytopenia (Daffos, 1984c, 1988b; Moise, 1988; Scioscia, 1988; and their associates). This procedure has also been used for fetal therapy of alloimmune thrombocytopenia (Kaplan and co-workers, 1988; Nicolini and colleagues, 1988). The diagnosis and management of thrombocytopenia in pregnancy is discussed in more detail in Chapter 52 (p. 1187).

CONGENITAL INFECTIONS. As summarized in Table 41–8, fetal blood sampling may be utilized as an aid to diagnose a variety of viral infections including rubella (Boulot, 1990; Daffos, 1984a; Orlandi, 1990; and their col-

TABLE 41–8. SOME INDICATIONS FOR FETAL BLOOD SAMPLING

Prenatal Diagnosis of Blood Disorders
Hemoglobinopathies
Hemophilia A and B
Autoimmune thrombocytopenia
Von Willebrand disease
Isoimmunization
CDE disease
Kell and other red cell antibodies
Alloimmune thrombocytopenia
Metabolic Disorders
Fetal Infection
Toxoplasmosis
Rubella
Cytomegalovirus
Varicella
Parvovirus B19
Fetal Karyotyping
Placental mosaicism
Need for rapid karyotype
Fetal malformation by ultrasound
Fetal growth retardation
Evaluation of Fetal Hypoxia
Fetal Therapy
Red cell and platelet transfusion
Monitor fetal drug therapy

Adapted from Copel and associates (1990), Meizner and Glezerman (1992), Nicolaides and Snijders (1992), and Weiner (1988).

leagues); cytomegalovirus infection (Lamy and associates, 1992; Meisel and colleagues, 1990); varicella (Cuthbertson and colleagues, 1987; Grose and coworkers, 1989); and toxoplasmosis (Boulot and colleagues, 1990; Daffos and co-workers, 1984b, 1988a, 1988b). Diagnosis and management of these infections are discussed in detail in Chapter 58.

GENETIC DISEASES. There are several Mendelian or single-gene disorders that can be diagnosed by fetal blood sampling. These include hemophilia A and B, von Willebrand disease, sickle cell disease, and α- and β-thalassemia, as well as several metabolic disorders (Daffos, 1985; Hobbins, 1985; Nicolaides, 1992; and their colleagues). With rapid advances in molecular biology techniques, many of these conditions can be diagnosed even earlier with chorionic villus sampling.

Fetal blood obtained by cordocentesis also may be utilized for karyotyping. We currently offer this technique to women who present for care near the limits for legal abortion when a rapid diagnosis is of paramount importance. This technique also is useful for karyotyping in later pregnancy when a malformation or significant growth retardation is detected by ultrasound. In their review of over 1700 fetuses with malformations or growth retardation, Nicolaides and Snijders (1992) reported that 15 percent of the fetuses had chromosomal abnormalities.

FETAL CONDITION. Cordocentesis has been utilized to evaluate fetal condition (Nicolaides and associates, 1986c), especially in the growth-retarded fetus (Pearce and Chamberlain, 1987). A variety of laboratory studies on fetal blood such as hemolytic indices and acid-base status may prove helpful in the evaluation of the fetus suspected to be compromised or hypoxic. Meizner and Glezerman (1992) recently reviewed this subject in detail.

Other Techniques. Both fetal skin and liver biopsy techniques have been utilized for prenatal diagnosis. Skin samples may be useful for the diagnosis of ichthyosis and epidermolysis bullosa, while liver tissue may be utilized for prenatal diagnosis of ornithine transcarbamylase deficiency, carbamyl phosphate synthetase deficiency, and von Gierke disease (Chueh and Golbus, 1992; Golbus and associates, 1989). Golbus and colleagues (1989) reported successful results in 7 out of 8 liver biopsies and 14 of 15 skin biopsies.

References

American College of Obstetricians and Gynecologists: Alphafetoprotein. Technical Bulletin no. 154, April 1991a

American College of Obstetricians and Gynecologists: Screening for Tay–Sachs disease. Committee on Obstetrics: Maternal–Fetal Medicine no. 93, March 1991b

American College of Obstetricians and Gynecologists: Prenatal detection of neural tube defects. Technical Bulletin no. 99, December 1986

Asch DA, Patton JP, Hershey JC, Mennuti MT: Reporting the results of cystic fibrosis carrier screening. Am J Obstet Gynecol (in press)

Assel BG, Lewis SM, Dickerman LH, Park VM, Jassani MN: Single-operator comparison of early and mid-second trimester amniocentesis. Obstet Gynecol 79:940, 1992

Bahado-Singh R, Schmitt R, Hobbins JC: New technique for genetic amniocentesis in twins. Obstet Gynecol 79:304, 1992

Bang J, Bock JE, Trolle D: Ultrasound-guided fetal intravenous transfusion for severe rhesus haemolytic disease. Br Med J 284:373, 1982

Barkai G, Chaki R, Sochat M, Goldman B: Human chorionic gonadotropin and trisomy 18. Am J Med Genet 41:52, 1991

Beekhuis JR, De Bruijn HWA, Van Lith JMM, Mantingh A: Second trimester amniocentesis in twin pregnancies: Maternal haemoglobin as a dye marker to differentiate diamniotic twins. Br J Obstet Gynaecol 99:126, 1992

Berkowitz RL, Chitkara U, Goldberg JD, Wilkins I, Chervenak FA, Lynch L : Intrauterine intravascular transfusions for severe red blood cell isoimmunization: Ultrasound-guided percutaneous approach. Am J Obstet Gynecol 155:574, 1986b

Boulot P, Deschamps F, Lefort G, Sarda P, Mares P, Hedon B, Laffargue F, Viala JL: Pure fetal blood samples obtained by cordocentesis: Technical aspects of 322 cases. Prenat Diag 10:93, 1990

Bowman JE: Invited editorial: Prenatal screening for hemoglobinopathies. Am J Hum Genet 48:433, 1991

Brambati B, Terzian E, Tognoni G: Randomized clinical trial of transabdominal versus transcervical chorionic villus sampling methods. Prenat Diag 11:285, 1991

Brock DJH, Sutcliffe RG: Alpha-fetoprotein in the antenatal diagnosis of anencephaly and spina bifida. Lancet 2:197, 1972

Burton BK, Schulz CJ, Burd LI: Limb anomalies associated with chorionic villus sampling. Obstet Gynecol 79:726, 1992

Canadian Collaborative CVS–Amniocentesis Clinical Trial Group: Multicentre randomized clinical trial of chorionic villus sampling and amniocentesis. Lancet 1:1, 1989

Cheung SW, Crane JP, Beaver HA, Burgess AC: Chromosome mosaicism and maternal cell contamination in chorionic villi. Prenat Diag 7:535, 1987

Chueh J, Golbus MS: Fetal invasive procedures. In Plauche WC, Morrison JC, O'Sullivan MJ (eds): Surgical Obstetrics. Philadelphia, Saunders, 1992, p 477

Copel JA, Cullen MT, Grannum PA, Hobbins JC: Invasive fetal assessment in the antepartum period. Obstet Gynecol Clin North Am 17:201, 1990

Crossley JA, Aitken DA, Connor JM: Prenatal screening for chromosome abnormalities using maternal serum chorionic gonadotropin, alpha-fetoprotein, and age. Prenat Diag 11:83, 1991

Cuckle HS, Wald NJ, Lindenbaum RH: Maternal serum alphafetoprotein measurement: A screening test for Down syndrome. Lancet 1:926, 1984

Cunningham FG, Gilstrap LC: Maternal serum alphafetoprotein screening. N Engl J Med 325:55, 1991. Editorial

Cuthbertson G, Weiner CO, Giller RH, Grose C: Prenatal diagnosis of second trimester congenital varicella syndrome by virus-specific IgM. J Pediatr 111:592, 1987

Daffos F, Capella-Pavlovsky M, Forestier F: Fetal blood sampling during pregnancy with the use of a needle guided by ultrasound: A study of 606 consecutive cases. Am J Obstet Gynecol 153:655, 1985

Daffos F, Capella-Pavlovsky M, Forestier F: A new procedure for fetal blood sampling in utero: Preliminary results of 53 cases. Am J Obstet Gynecol 146:985, 1983

Daffos F, Forestier F, Capella-Pavlovsky M: Fetal blood sampling during the third trimester of pregnancy. Br J Obstet Gynaecol 91:118, 1984a

Daffos F, Forestier F, Capella-Pavlovsky M, Thulliez P, Aufrant C, Valenti D, Cox WL: Prenatal management of 746 pregnancies at risk for congenital toxoplasmosis. N Engl J Med 318:271, 1988a

Daffos F, Forestier F, Grangeot-Keros L, Capella-Pavlovsky M, Lebon P, Chartier M: Prenatal diagnosis of congenital toxoplasmosis. Lancet 2:1, 1984b

Daffos F, Forestier F, Kaplan C, Cox W: Prenatal diagnosis and management of bleeding disorders with fetal blood sampling. Am J Obstet Gynecol 158:939, 1988b

Daffos F, Forestier F, Muller JY, Reznikoff-Etievant M, Habibi B, Capella-Pavlovsky M, Maigret P, Kaplan C: Prenatal treatment of alloimmune thrombocytopenia. Lancet 2:632, 1984c

deCrespigny L, Robinson HP, Quinn M, Doyle L, Ross A, Cauchi M: Ultrasound-guided fetal blood transfusion for severe rhesus isoimmunization. Obstet Gynecol 66:529, 1985

Desnick RJ, Schuette JL, Golbus MS, Jackson L, Lubs HA, Ledbetter DH, Pergament E, Simpson JL, Zachary JM, Fowler SE, Rhoads GG, de la Cruz F: First-trimester biochemical and molecular diagnoses using chorionic villi: High accuracy in the U.S. Collaborative Study. Prenat Diag 12:357, 1992

Drugan A, Zador IE, Syner FN, Sokol RJ, Sacks AJ, Evans MI: A normal ultrasound does not obviate the need for amniocentesis with elevated levels of maternal serum alphafetoprotein. Obstet Gynecol 72:627, 1988

Elejalde BR, deElejalde MM, Acuna JM, Thelen D, Trujillo C, Karrmann M: Prospective study of amniocentesis performed between 9 and 16 weeks of gestation; its feasibility, risks, complications, and use in early genetic prenatal diagnosis. Am J Med Genet 35:188, 1990

Elias S, Gerbie AB, Simpson JE, Nadler HL, Sabbagha RE, Shkolnik A: Genetic amniocentesis in twin gestations. Am J Obstet Gynecol 138:169, 1980

Evans MI, Drugan A, Koppitch FC III, Zador IE, Sacks AJ, Sokol RJ: Genetic diagnosis in the first trimester; the norm for the 1990s. Am J Obstet Gynecol 160:1332, 1989

Evans MI, Dvorin E, O'Brien JE, Moody JL, Drugan A: Alphafetoprotein and biochemical screening. In Evans MI (ed): Reproductive Risks and Prenatal Diagnosis. Norwalk, CT, Appleton & Lange, 1992, p 223

Firth HV, Boyd PA, Chamberlain P, MacKenzie IZ, Lindenbaum RH, Huson SM: Severe limb abnormalities after chorion villus sampling at 56–66 days' gestation. Lancet 337:762, 1991

Forestier F, Cox WL, Daffos F, Rainaut M: The assessment of fetal blood samples. Am J Obstet Gynecol 158:1184, 1988

Foulon W, Naessens A, de Catte L, Amy JJ: Detection of congenital toxoplasmosis by chorionic villus sampling and early amniocentesis. Am J Obstet Gynecol 163:1511, 1990

Golbus MS: Invited editorial. Prenat Diag 12:313, 1992

Golbus MS, McGonigle KJ, Goldberg JD, Filly RA, Callen PW, Anderson RL: Fetal tissue sampling: The San Francisco experience with 190 pregnancies. West J Med 150:423, 1989

Goldberg JD, Porter AE, Golbus MS: Current assessment of fetal losses as a direct consequence of chorionic villus sampling. Am J Med Genet 35:174, 1990

Grannum PA, Copel JA, Plaxe SC, Scioscia AL, Hobbins JL: In utero exchange transfusion by direct intravascular injection in severe erythroblastosis fetalis. N Engl J Med 314:1431, 1986

Grose C, Itani O: Pathogenesis of congenital infection with three diverse viruses: Varicella–zoster virus, human parvovirus, and human immunodeficiency virus. Semin Perinatol 13:278, 1990

Hackett GA, Smith JH, Rebello MT, Gray CTH, Rooney DE, Beard RW, Loeffler FE, Corman DV: Early amniocentesis at 11–14 weeks gestation for the diagnosis of fetal chromosomal abnormality—a clinical evaluation. Prenat Diag 11:311, 1991

Hankins GDV, Rowe J, Quirk JC, Trubey R, Strickland DM: Significance of brown and/or green amniotic fluid at the time of second trimester genetic amniocentesis. Obstet Gynecol 64:353, 1984

Hanson FW, Happ RL, Tennant FR, Hune S, Peterson AG: Ultrasonography guided early amniocentesis in singleton pregnancies. Am J Obstet Gynecol 162:1376, 1990

Hobbins JC, Grannum PA, Romero R, Reece EA, Mahoney MJ: Percutaneous umbilical blood sampling. Am J Obstet Gynecol 152:1, 1985

Hogge WA, Schonberg SA, Golbus MS: Prenatal diagnosis by chorionic villus sampling: Lessons of the first 600 cases. Prenat Diag 5:393, 1985

Holzgreve W, Miny P, Schloo R, Participants of the "Late CVS" Registry: "Late CVS" international compilation of data from 24 centres. Prenat Diag 10:159, 1990

Isada NB, Paar DP, Johnson MP, Evans MI, Holzgreve W, Qureshi F, Straus SE: In utero diagnosis of congenital varicella zoster virus infection by chorionic villus sampling and polymerase chain reaction. Am J Obstet Gynecol 165:1727, 1991

Iwanicki S, Pattinson M, Cox D, Pattinson H, King D: Early amniocentesis—reliability and safety. A longitudinal follow-up to delivery in 400 consecutive cases. Am J Obstet Gynecol 166:356, 1992. SPO abstract 285

Jackson LG: Fetal genetic diagnosis by chorionic villus sampling. Sem Perinatol 15:43, 1991

Jackson LG: Transcervical and transabdominal chorionic villus sampling are comparably safe procedures for first trimester prenatal diagnosis. USNICHD Collaborative CVS Study Group. Am J Hum Genet 47:A278, 1990

Jackson LG, Zachary JM, Fowler SE, Desnick RJ, Golbus MS, Ledbetter DH, Mahoney MU, Pergament E, Simpson JL, Black S, Wapner RJ: A randomized comparison of transcervical and transabdominal chorionic villus sampling. N Engl J Med 327:594, 1992

Johnson A, Cowchock FS, Darby M, Wapner R, Jackson LG: First trimester maternal serum alphafetoprotein and chorionic gonadotropin in aneuploid pregnancies. Prenat Diag 11:443, 1991

Johnson A, Wapner RJ, Davis GH, Jackson LG: Mosaicism in chorionic villus sampling: An association with poor perinatal outcome. Obstet Gynecol 75:573, 1990

Kaplan C, Daffos F, Forestier F, Cox WL, Lyon-Caen D, Dupuy-Montbrun MC, Salmon C: Management of allo-immune thrombocytopenia: Antenatal diagnosis and in utero transfusion of maternal platelets. Blood 72:340, 1988

Katz VL, Chescher NC, Cefalo RC: Unexplained elevations of maternal serum alpha-fetoprotein. Obstet Gynecol Surv 45:719, 1990

Kerem B, Rommens JM, Buchanan JA, Markiewicz D, Cox TK, Chakravarti A, Buchwald M, Tsui LC: Identification of the cystic fibrosis gene: Genetic analysis. Science 245:1073, 1989

Kratzer PG, Golbus MS, Monroe SE, Finkelstein DE, Taylor RN: First-trimester aneuploidy screening using serum human chorionic gonadotropin (hCG), free ahCG, and protesterone. Prenat Diag 11:751, 1991

Lamy ME, Mulongo KN, Gadisseux JF, Lyon G, Gaudy V, Van-Lierde M: Prenatal diagnosis of fetal cytomegalovirus infection. Am J Obstet Gynecol 166:91, 1992

Ledbetter DH, Martin AO, Verlinsky Y, Pergament E, Jackson L, Yang-Feng T, Schonberg SA, Gilbert F, Zachary JM, Barr M, Copeland KL, DiMaio MS, Fine B, Rosinsky B, Schuette J, de la Cruz FF, Desnik RJ, Elias S, Golbus MS, Goldberg JD, Lubs HA, Mahoney MJ, Rhoads GG, Simpson JL, Schlesselman SE: Cytogenetic results of chorionic villus sampling: High success rate and diagnostic accuracy in the United States Collaborative Study. Am J Obstet Gynecol 162:495, 1990

Ledbetter DH, Zachary JM, Simpson JL, Golbus MS, Pergament E, Jackson L, Mahoney MJ, Desnick RJ, Sculman J, Copeland KL, Verlinsky Y, Yang-Feng T, Schonberg SA, Babu A, Tharapel A, Dorfmann A, Lubs HS, Rhoads GG, Fowler E, de la Cruz F: Cytogenetic results from the U.S. Collaborative Study on CVS. Prenat Diag 12:317, 1992

Leschot NJ, Wolf H: Is placental mosaicism associated with poor perinatal outcome? Prenat Diag 11:403, 1991

Lippman A, Tomkins DJ, Shime J, Hamerton JL on behalf of the Canadian Collaborative CVS-Amniocentesis Clinical Trial Group: Canadian multicentre randomized clinical trial of chorion villus sampling and amniocentesis: Final report. Prenat Diag 12:385, 1992

Lowe TW, Weinreb J, Santos-Ramos R, Cunningham FG: Magnetic resonance imaging in human pregnancy. Obstet Gynecol 66:629, 1985

Maberry MC, Klein VR, Boehm C, Warren TC, Gilstrap LC: Alpha-thalassemia: Prenatal diagnosis and neonatal implications. Am J Perinatol 7:356, 1990

MacDonald ML, Wagner RM, Slotnick RN: Sensitivity and specificity of screening for Down syndrome with alpha-fetoprotein, hCG, unconjugated estriol, and maternal age. Obstet Gynecol 77:63, 1991

Macri JN, Kasturi RV, Krantz DA, Cook EJ, Sunderji SG, Larsen JW: Maternal serum Down syndrome screening: Unconjugated estriol is not useful. Am J Obstet Gynecol 162:672, 1990

Macri JN, Weiss RR, Tillitt R, Balsam D, Elligers KW: Prenatal diagnosis of neural tube defects. JAMA 236:1251, 1976

Mahoney MJ for the USNICHD Collaborative CVS Study Group: Limb abnormalities and chorionic villus sampling. Lancet 337:1422, 1991

Marx JL: Imaging technique passes muster. Science 238:888, 1987

Meisel RL, Alvarez M, Lunch L, Chitkara U, Emanuel DJ, Berkowitz RL: Fetal cytomegalovirus infection: A case report. Am J Obstet Gynecol 162:663, 1990

Meizner I, Glezerman M: Cordocentesis in the evaluation of the growth-retarded fetus. Clin Obstet Gynecol 35:126, 1992

Merkatz IR, Nitowsky HM, Macri JN, Johnson WE: An association between low maternal serum alpha-fetoprotein and fetal chromosome abnormalities. Am J Obstet Gynecol 148:886, 1984

Milunsky A, Sapirstein VS: Prenatal diagnosis of open neural tube defects using the amniotic fluid acetylcholinesterase assay. Obstet Gynecol 59:1, 1982

Moise KJ, Carpenter RJ Jr, Cotton DB, Wasserstrum N, Kirshon B, Cano L: Percutaneous umbilical cord blood sampling in the evaluation of fetal platelet counts in pregnant patients with auto-immune thrombocytopenia purpura. Obstet Gynecol 72:346, 1988

MRC Working Party on the Evaluation of Chorion Villus Sampling: Medical Research Council European Trial of chorion villus sampling. Lancet 337:1491, 1991

Nadel AS, Green NK, Holmes LB, Frigoletto FD, Benacerraf BR: Absence of need for amniocentesis in patients with elevated levels of maternal serum alpha-fetoprotein and normal ultrasonographic examinations. N Engl J Med 323:557, 1990

National Institute of Child Health and Human Development, National Registry for Amniocentesis Study Group: Midtrimester amniocentesis for prenatal diagnosis: Safety and accuracy. JAMA 236:1471, 1976

Nevin J, Nevin NC, Dornan JC, Sim D, Armstrong MJ: Early amniocentesis: Experience of 222 consecutive patients, 1987–1988. Prenat Diag 10:79, 1990

New England Regional Genetics Group Prenatal Collaborative Study of Down Syndrome Screening: Combining maternal serum AFP and age to screen in pregnant women under age 35. Am J Obstet Gynecol 160:575, 1989

Nicolaides KH, Rodeck CH, Gosden CM: Rapid karyotyping in non-lethal malformations. Lancet 1:283, 1986a

Nicolaides KH, Rodeck CH, Mibashan RS, Kemp JR: Have Liley charts outlived their usefulness? Am J Obstet Gynecol 155:90, 1986b

Nicolaides KH, Rodeck CH, Soothill PW, Campbell S: Ultrasound-guided sampling of umbilical cord and placental blood to assess fetal wellbeing. Lancet 1:1065, 1986c

Nicolaides KH, Snijders RJM: Cordocentesis. In Evans MI (ed): Reproductive Risks and Prenatal Diagnosis. Norwalk, CT, Appleton & Lange, 1992, p 201

Nicolini U, Monni G: Intestinal obstruction in babies exposed in utero to methylene blue. Lancet 336:1258, 1990

Nicolini U, Rodeck CH, Kochenour NK, Greco P, Fisk NM, Letsky E, Lubenko A: In utero platelet transfusion for allo-immune thrombocytopenia. Lancet 2:506, 1988

Orlandi F, Damiani G, Jakil C, Lauricella S, Bertolino O, Maggio A: The risks of early cordocentesis (12–21 weeks): Analysis of 500 procedures. Prenat Diag 10:425, 1990

Pearce JM, Chamberlain GVP: Ultrasonically guided percutaneous umbilical blood sampling in the management of intrauterine growth retardation. Br J Obstet Gynaecol 94:318, 1987

Penso CA, Frigoletto FD: Early amniocentesis. Semin Perinatol 14:465, 1990a

Penso CA, Sandstrom MM, Garber M-F, Ladoulis M, Stryker JM, Benacerraf BB: Early amniocentesis: Report of 407 cases with neonatal follow-up. Obstet Gynecol 76:1037, 1990

Pergament E, Schulman JD, Copeland K, Fine B, Black SH, Ginsberg NA, Frederiksen MC, Carpenter RJ: The risk and efficacy of chorionic villus sampling in multiple gestations. Prenat Diag 12:377, 1992

Powell MC, Worthington BS, Buckley JM, Symonds EM: Magnetic resonance imaging (MRI) in obstetrics, II. Fetal anatomy. Br J Obstet Gynaecol 95:38, 1988

Quashie C, Weiner S, Bolognese R: Efficacy of first trimester transvaginal sonography in detecting normal fetal development. Am J Perinatol 9:209, 1992

Queenan JT, King JC: Intrauterine transfusion for severe Rh-EBF. Contemp Obstet Gynecol 30:51, 1987

Rhoads GG, Jackson LG, Schlesselman SE, de la Cruz FF, Desnick RJ, Golbus MS, Ledbetter DH, Lubs HA, Mahoney MJ, Pergament E, Simpson JL, Carpenter RJ, Elias S, Ginsberg NA, Goldberg JD, Hobbins JC, Lynch L, Shiono PH, Wapner WJ, Zachary JM: The safety and efficacy of chorionic villus sampling for early prenatal diagnosis of cytogenetic abnormalities. N Engl J Med 320:609, 1989

Richards DS, Seeds JW, Katz VL, Lingley LH, Albright SG, Cefalo RC: Elevated maternal serum alpha-fetoprotein with normal ultrasound: Is amniocentesis always appropriate? A review of 26,069 screened patients. Obstet Gynecol 71:203, 1988

Riordan JR, Rommens JM, Kerem BS, Alon N, Rozmahel R, Grzelczak Z, Zielinski J, Lpk S, Plavsic N, Chou JL, et al: Identification of the cystic fibrosis gene: Cloning and characterization of complementary DNA. Science 245:1066, 1989

Roberts NS, Dunn LK, Weiner S, Godmilow L, Miller R: Midtrimester amniocentesis: Indications, technique, risks and potential for prenatal diagnosis. J Reprod Med 28:167, 1983

Rommens JM, Iannuzzi MC, Kerem BS, Drumm ML, Melmer G, Dean M, Rozmahel R, Cole JL, Kennedy D, Hidaka N, et al: Identification of the cystic fibrosis gene: Chromosome walking and jumping. Science 245:1059, 1989

Rowley PT, Loader S, Sutera CJ, Walden M, Kozyra A: Prenatal screening for hemoglobinopathies, I. A prospective regional trial. Am J Hum Genet 48:439, 1991

Scioscia AL, Grannum PA, Copel JA, Hobbins JC: The use of percutaneous blood sampling in immune thrombocytopenia purpura. Am J Obstet Gynecol 159:1066, 1988

Seeds JW, Bowes WA Jr: Ultrasound-guided fetal intravascular transfusion in severe rhesus isoimmunization. Am J Obstet Gynecol 154:1105, 1986

Simpson H, Dallaire L, Miller J, Simonovitch L, Hamerton J: Prenatal diagnosis of genetic disease in Canada: Report of a collaborative study. Can Med Assoc J 115:739, 1976

Simpson JL, Baum LD, Marder R, Elias S, Ober C, Martin AO: Maternal serum alpha-fetoprotein screening: Low and high values for detection of genetic abnormalities. Am J Obstet Gynecol 155:593, 1986

Smith FW, Adam AH, Phillips WDP: NMR imaging in pregnancy. Lancet 1:61, 1983

Soothill PW, Nicolaides KH, Campbell S: Prenatal asphyxia, hyperlacticaemia, hypoglycaemia, and erythroblastosis in growth retarded fetuses. Br Med J 294:1051, 1987a

Soothill PW, Nicolaides KH, Rodeck CH, Campbell S: The effect of gestational age on blood gas and acid-base values in human pregnancy. Fetal Ther 1:166, 1986

Soothill PW, Nicolaides KH, Rodeck CH, Clewell WH, Lindridge J: Relationship of fetal hemoglobin and oxygen content to lactate concentration in Rh isoimmunized pregnancies. Obstet Gynecol 69:268, 1987b

Stripparo L, Buscaglia M, Longatti L, Ghisoni L, Dambrosio F, Guerneri S, Rosella F, Lituania M, Cordone M, DeBasio P, et al: Genetic amniocentesis: 505 cases performed before the sixteenth week of gestation. Prenat Diag 10:359, 1990

Symonds EM, Johnson IR, Kean DM, Worthington BS, Pipkin FB, Hawkes RC, Gyngell M: Imaging the pregnant human uterus with nuclear magnetic resonance. Am J Obstet Gynecol 148:1136, 1984

Twickler DM, Gilstrap LC, Little BB: Use of diagnostic agents during pregnancy. In Gilstrap LC III, Little BB (eds): Drugs and Pregnancy. New York, Elsevier, 1992, p 327

U.K. Collaborative Study on Alpha-fetoprotein in Relation to Neural Tube Defects: Maternal serum-alpha-fetoprotein measurement in antenatal screening for anencephaly and spina bifida in early pregnancy. Lancet 1:1323, 1977

USNICHD Collaborative CVS Study Group: Transcervical and transabdominal chorionic villus sampling are comparably safe procedures for first trimester prenatal diagnosis: Preliminary analysis. Am J Hum Genet 47:A278, 1990

Van der Pol JG, Wolf H, Boer K, Treffers PE, Leschot NJ, Hey HA, Vos A: Jejunal atresia related to the use of methylene blue in genetic amniocentesis in twins. Br J Obstet Gynaecol 99:141, 1992

Vintzileos AM, Campbell WA, Nochimson DJ, Weinbaum PJ: Antenatal evaluation and management of ultrasonically detected fetal anomalies. Obstet Gynecol 69:640, 1987

Wald NJ, Cuckle HS, Densem JW, Nanchahal K, Canick JA, Haddow JE, Knight GJ, Palomaki GE: Maternal serum unconjugated oestriol as an antenatal screening test for Down's syndrome. Br J Obstet Gynaecol 95:334, 1988

Waller DK, Lustig LS, Cunningham GC, Golbus MS, Hook EB: Second-trimester maternal serum alpha-fetoprotein levels and the risk of subsequent fetal death. N Engl J Med 325:6, 1991

Wapner RJ, Simpson JL, Golbus MS, Zachary JM, Ledbetter DH, Desnick RJ, Fowler SE, Jackson LG, Lubs H, Mahoney RJ, Pergament E, Rhoads GG, Shulman JD, de la Cruz F: Chorionic mosaicism: Association with fetal loss but not with adverse outcome. Prenat Diag 12:347, 1992

Watson WJ, Chescher NC, Katz VL, Seeds JW: The role of ultrasound in evaluation of patients with elevated maternal serum alpha-fetoprotein: A review. Obstet Gynecol 78:123, 1991

Weiner CP: The role of cordocentesis in fetal diagnosis. Clin Obstet Gynecol 31:285, 1988

Working Party on Amniocentesis: An assessment of the hazards of amniocentesis: Report to the MRC. Br J Obstet Gynaecol 85(suppl):2, 1978

CHAPTER 42
Drugs and Medications During Pregnancy

Women commonly ingest medications or drugs while pregnant. The Centers for Disease Control (1987) surveyed 492 pregnant women in New York State and found that 90 percent averaged taking 3.8 prescription or over-the-counter drugs from 48 different classes. In a study of almost 9000 Medicaid prenatal patients in Michigan, Piper and colleagues (1987) reported that they were given an average of 3.1 prescriptions for drugs other than vitamins.

Besides prenatal vitamin and mineral supplements, commonly used drugs include antiemetics, antacids, antihistamines, analgesics, antimicrobials, tranquilizers, hypnotics, and diuretics. Although some of these are prescribed, many are taken either without physician advice or prior to realization of pregnancy. Both patient and physician are primarily concerned with whether a drug or medication causes congenital anomalies or is a *teratogen.* Although almost any drug with systemic effects in the mother will cross the placenta to reach the embryo or fetus, most drugs do not appear to adversely affect the fetus.

Principles of Human Teratology

Teratogens. A teratogen is any agent or factor to which embryofetal exposure produces a permanent alteration in form or function of the offspring (Shepard, 1986). Of premier importance is the time period in pregnancy during which there was fetal exposure. For these purposes, gestation is divided into three periods: (1) the *ovum,* from fertilization to implantation; (2) the *embryonic period,* from the second through the eighth week; and (3) the *fetal period,* from after 8 completed weeks until term.

The embryonic period is the most critical with regard to malformations because it encompasses organogenesis. By way of example, a drug ingested during late pregnancy cannot cause malformations such as limb reduction defects. Although uncommon, certain drugs do have adverse effects when taken during the second half of pregnancy. For example, tetracyclines may cause yellow or brown discoloration of deciduous teeth. There is virtually no information regarding possible long-term effects, such as learning or behavioral problems, that might result from chronic prenatal medication ingestion. In some instances, teratogenicity may not be apparent for years. For example, diethylstilbestrol may cause müllerian anomalies, as well as vaginal adenosis and carcinoma—problems that do not become apparent until reproductive age.

Whether a chemical or a drug and its metabolites have fetal access in quantities sufficient to cause developmental anomalies is important. Maternal absorption and metabolism, protein binding and storage, molecular size, electrical charge, and lipid solubility are factors that may determine the degree of placental transfer. Also important is the concept that some agents are harmful only if given in sufficient amounts over prolonged periods. Given the plethora of drugs and medications available, as well as these complex factors, it is understandable that there is a paucity of information regarding the majority of drugs and their potential detrimental effects.

Known Teratogens. The number of drugs or medications that are strongly suspected or proven human teratogens is surprisingly small (Table 42–1). Included are alcohol, thalidomide, some folic acid antagonists, the vitamin A isomers isotretinoin and etretinate, and some of the sex steroids such as diethylstilbestrol. Other drugs or medications considered by either some teratologists or the manufacturer to have substantive fetal risk include androgens, various anticonvulsants, some live-virus vaccines such as rubella, radioactive iodine, and some synthetic estrogens. Although there is no consensus regarding the teratogenicity of some of these latter medications, they should be avoided during pregnancy when possible. Fortunately, if inadvertently taken during pregnancy, fetal outcome is usually favorable with no significant adverse effects or malformations. **This list is not all inclusive, and the number of agents will likely increase as more information becomes available.** Radiation can be a potent teratogen; radioactive medications and their effects are discussed in Chapter 43.

An important aspect of human teratology is that teratogenic medications administered after the vulnerable period usually will not cause structural malformations. For example, agents administered after the critical period for closure of the posterior and anterior neuropores are not capable of inducing neural-tube defects regardless of their known potential for inducing such congenital anomalies.

Animal Studies. Although studies of teratogenic effects of drugs in animals must be conducted before prescribing during human pregnancy, unfortunately

TABLE 42–1. DRUGS OR SUBSTANCES SUSPECTED OR PROVEN TO BE HUMAN TERATOGENS

ACE inhibitors[a]	Etretinate
Alcohol	Isotretinoin
Aminopterin	Lithium
Androgens	Methimazole
Busulfan	Methotrexate
Carbamazepine	Penicillamine
Chlorbiphenyls	Phenytoin
Coumarins	Radioactive iodine
Cyclophosphamide	Tetracycline
Danazol	Trimethadione
Diethylstilbestrol (DES)	Valproic acid

[a] Angiotension converting enzyme inhibitors
Adapted from Shepard (1986, 1989).

there is not always an obvious one-to-one relationship. The best example is the hypnotic drug thalidomide, which causes very few malformations in animals but is now one of the best-documented and potent human teratogens. The converse is more likely, and most small laboratory animals commonly employed for these experiments are generally very susceptible to teratogenic effects. Shepard (1986) emphasized that of nearly 1600 drugs tested in animals, probably half cause teratogenic effects, although there are only approximately 30 documented human teratogens.

Criteria for Human Teratogens. Identification of human teratogens requires careful interpretation of data obtained from several kinds of studies, as shown in Table 42–2. The first evidence that an agent is teratogenic in humans often comes from clinical case reports. Although case reports are important in raising causal hypotheses, most are subsequently proven incorrect.

Epidemiological studies provide the only means of obtaining quantitative estimates regarding the strength

TABLE 42–2. CRITERIA FOR AN AGENT TO BE RECOGNIZED AS A HUMAN TERATOGEN

1. Proven exposure to agent at critical time(s) in prenatal development (prescriptions, medical records, dates).
2. Consistent findings by two or more epidemiological studies of high quality, (i.e., control of confounding factors, sufficient numbers of exposed pregnancies, exclusion of positive and negative bias factors); prospective studies; or relative risk of 6 or more.
3. Careful delineation of the clinical cases attempting to isolate a specific defect or syndrome.
4. Rare environmental exposure associated with rare defect. Probably three or more cases; examples, oral anticoagulants and warfarin syndrome, methimazole and scalp defects (?), and heart block and maternal connective-tissue diseases.
5. The association should make biological sense.

From Shepard (1989), with permission.

and statistical significance of associations between agent exposures in pregnant women and abnormalities in their offspring. In **cohort studies,** the frequencies of certain anomalies are compared in the offspring of women exposed and unexposed to the substance. In **case-control studies,** the frequency of prenatal exposure to the agent is compared among children with and without a given anomaly.

Potential Litigation. Although not validated by scientific evidence, legal declarations of teratogenicity have prompted cessation of manufacture of some very useful drugs. An example is Bendectin, which was safe and effective for treatment of nausea and vomiting in early pregnancy. It is estimated that more than 30 million women used this drug worldwide (Brent, 1983). Despite contrary scientific evidence, Bendectin was declared a "legal teratogen" by the court, and manufacture ceased (Holmes, 1983).

Another worrisome example of judicial disregard for scientific proof lies in the *Wells v Ortho* decision in which a judge-directed $5.1 million verdict was upheld by an appellate court. As summarized by Mills and Alexander (1986), the court ruled that a spermicidal jelly was a teratogen, despite "the overwhelming body of evidence to the contrary," as well as the Food and Drug Administration's decision that no warning label concerning possible teratogenicity was necessary. The case prompted Brent (1985) to classify the spermicide as a *litogen*—a drug that does not cause malformations but does cause lawsuits!

Food and Drug Administration Classification of Medications

In 1979, the Food and Drug Administration established five categories for drugs and medications with regards to possible adverse fetal effects.

Category A. Category A drugs are those for which controlled studies in humans have demonstrated no fetal risks. There are few category A drugs, and examples include multivitamins or prenatal vitamins but not "megavitamins."

Category B. With category B drugs, animal studies indicate no fetal risks, but there are no human studies; or adverse effects have been demonstrated in animals, but not in well-controlled human studies. Several classes of commonly used drugs, an example of which is the penicillins, are in this category.

Category C. Drugs for which there are no adequate studies, either animal or human, or drugs in which there are adverse fetal effects in animal studies but no available human data, are classified in category C. Many drugs or medications commonly taken during pregnancy are in this category.

Category D. Category D drugs are those for which there is evidence of fetal risk, but benefits are thought to outweigh these risks. Carbamazepine and phenytoin are examples.

Category X. Category X is used for drugs with proven fetal risks that clearly outweigh any benefits. The acne medication isotretinoin, which may cause multiple central nervous system, facial, and cardiovascular anomalies, is an example of a category X drug.

The classifications of some of the more commonly encountered drugs and medications are summarized in Table 42–3. These categories are intended to provide therapeutic guidance considering potential benefits and maternal and fetal risks of using a drug during pregnancy. Not all agree that this classification is best. For example, Friedman and colleagues (1990) showed that the pregnancy categories have no correlation with teratogenic risk using a system designed to assess the risk of anomalies from medication exposure during pregnancy. One reason that the categories have no relation to teratogenic risk is that they combine into a single assessment several risk statements that include congenital anomalies, fetal effects, perinatal risks, and therapeutic risk : benefit ratio.

Drugs Given for Specific Conditions

Pregnant women commonly have associated conditions or complications for which specific drug therapy is indicated. They should be counseled about the possible teratogenic risks from the condition itself—for example, diabetes, epilepsy, or alcoholism—as well as any known fetal risks from drug therapy. Ideally, they should be counseled before attempting pregnancy. In actual practice, however, they have frequently already taken medications chronically during the critical period of organogenesis when they are first seen for prenatal care. Fortunately, but with a few notable exceptions, most drugs and medications prescribed for common medical and surgical diseases can be used with relative safety. Moreover, the untreated disease or condition itself may pose more serious risks to both mother and fetus than any theoretical risks from these medications. It is emphasized that the absence of reports concerning potential adverse drug effects is not "proof" of safety. Certainly, alcohol, thalidomide, valproic acid, phenytoin, and warfarin were used for years without apparent adverse effects.

Infections. A number of bacterial, viral, fungal, and parasitic infections are commonly encountered during

TABLE 42–3. CLASSIFICATION BY INDICATION OF SOME DRUGS AND MEDICATIONS USED DURING PREGNANCY[a]

Asthma	**Hormones**	**Nausea and Vomiting**
Albuterol C	Clomiphene X	
Corticosteroids B,C,D	Contraceptives X	Chlorpromazine C
Cromolyn B	Estrogens X	Cyclizine C
Ephedrine C	Progestins D	Meclizine B
Epinephrine C	**Infections**	Prochlorperazine C
Metaproterenol C	Acyclovir C	Promethazine C
Terbutaline B	Amphotericin B	Trimethobenzamide C
Theophylline C	Aztreonam C	**Pain and Inflammation**
Cancer	Cephalosporins B	Acetaminophen B
Azathioprine	Chloroquine C	Aspirin C
Chlorambucil D	Erythromycin B	Codeine C
Cisplatin D	Lindane B	Ibuprofen B/D
Cyclophosphamide D	Mebendazole C	Indomethacin B/D
Fluorouracil D	Metronidazole B	Meperidine B
Melphalan D	Miconazole B	Morphine B
Methotrexate D	Nitrofurantoin B	**Psychiatric Disorders**
Procarbazine D	Nystatin B	Amitriptyline D
Vincristine D	Penicillins B	Chlordiazepoxide D
Cardiovascular	Pyrantel C	Diazepam D
β-blockers C	Quinine D	Imipramine D
Captopril D	Sulfonamides B	Lithium D
Coumarins D	Tetracyclines D	Nortriptyline D
Digoxin C	Trimethoprim C	Phenothiazines C
Enalapril D	Vancomycin C	
Furosemide C	Zidovudine C	
Heparin C	**Miscellaneous**	
Methyldopa C	Antihistamines B,C	
Procainamide C	Barbiturates C	
Quinidine C	Caffeine B	
Thiazides D	Cocaine C	
Verapamil C	Cyclosporine C	
Convulsive Disorders	Dextroamphetamine C	
Carbamazepine C	Etretinate X	
Phenobarbital D	Guaifenesin C	
Phenytoin D	Heroin B/D	
Trimethadione D	Insulin B	
Valproic acid D	Isotretinoin X	
	Thioureas D	
	Thyroid A	

[a] Categories according to Food and Drug Administration guidelines, either by manufacturer or according to Briggs and colleagues (1990).

pregnancy. Virtually all antimicrobial and chemotherapeutic agents utilized for these infections readily cross the placenta.

Antibacterial Agents. A large number of antimicrobial agents are available, but there have been few studies regarding their efficacy and safety during pregnancy. Many compounds from the various classes have been used empirically in a large number of pregnant women without apparent adverse embryofetal effects.

Penicillins have been used for many years, and as a group they are probably the "safest" antimicrobial to use during pregnancy. Penicillins with newer broad-spectrum activity such as piperacillin and mezlocillin, as well as those combined with the β-lactamase inhibitors, clavulanic acid and sulbactam, are included in this group. As with most antibiotics, serum penicillin levels from a given dose are usually lower in pregnant women (Landers and colleagues, 1983).

Erythromycin is often given to penicillin-allergic patients, especially for treatment of syphilis and community-acquired pneumonia. The fetus is not always treated effectively when erythromycin is given for maternal syphilis because only small amounts of the drug gain fetal access (see Chap. 59, p. 1300).

These are numerous oral and parenteral **cephalosporins** available. When given during pregnancy, all cross the placenta, although their half-life may be shorter compared with nonpregnant women because of increased renal clearance (Gilstrap and colleagues, 1988; Landers and associates, 1983). Few studies have been published regarding the safety of cephalosporins during pregnancy, although they are some of the most commonly used antibiotics during pregnancy. Certainly, limited data suggest no adverse embryofetal effects.

The **tetracyclines,** including doxycycline and minocycline, should generally be avoided during pregnancy. They have been reported to cause yellow-brown discoloration of the deciduous teeth (Kutscher and associates, 1966). Tetracyclines are also deposited in fetal long bones, although this does not appear to inhibit growth. Tetracycline has been reported to cause acute fatty liver changes in pregnant women with renal insufficiency (Whalley and colleagues, 1964). Perhaps one use of tetracycline during pregnancy is for the treatment of maternal syphilis in the penicillin-allergic woman for whom desensitization is impractical or impossible.

Aztreonam is a member of a relatively new class of antibiotics, the **monobactams.** It is used primarily as an aminoglycoside alternative, but it is not associated with either renal or ototoxicity. Although there are no well-controlled studies in humans, aztreonam is not teratogenic for rodents according to its manufacturer.

Aminoglycosides readily cross the placenta to result in significant fetal cord blood levels (Gilstrap and co-workers, 1988). One of the earliest compounds, streptomycin, was reported to be associated with fetal eighth nerve damage when given to the mother for protracted periods (Conway, 1965). The risk of ototoxicity with any of the aminoglycosides appears to be about 1 to 2 percent, and while this appears minimal, these antibiotics are usually reserved for serious maternal infections resistant to other antibiotics.

Clindamycin readily crosses the placenta and may result in significant fetal blood levels (Gilstrap and associates, 1988). There have been no studies of potential adverse embryofetal effects from its use during pregnancy, although clinical experience suggests that this drug seems relatively safe.

Chloramphenicol readily crosses the placenta and results in significant fetal blood levels. In one review of almost 100 infants exposed to this antibiotic in early pregnancy, the frequency of congenital anomalies was not increased compared with controls (Heinonen, 1977). The *gray baby syndrome,* manifested by cyanosis, vascular collapse, and death, has been reported with large doses of chloramphenicol given to the preterm neonate, but it seems unlikely that fetal levels obtained from maternal administration would cause this syndrome.

Sulfonamides readily cross the placenta but fetal blood levels appear to be lower than maternal (Reid and colleagues, 1975). There have been no studies exploring a possible association of sulfa drugs with congenital anomalies. These drugs compete for bilirubin-binding sites, and may be associated with hyperbilirubinemia if used near delivery, especially in the preterm infant (Landers and colleagues, 1983). **Trimethoprim** is often used in association with a sulfonamide, and because it is a folate antagonist in bacteria, some caution against its use during pregnancy. In studies of infants exposed to trimethoprim–sulfamethoxazole during early pregnancy, the frequency of congenital anomalies was not increased (Brumfitt and Pursell, 1973).

Nitrofurantoin is used commonly for uncomplicated urinary infections during pregnancy, and in a prospective study of 100 women treated with this drug, congenital anomalies were not increased (Lenke and colleagues, 1983). Nitrofurantoin has been associated with hemolytic anemia in women with glucose-6-phosphate dehydrogenase deficiency, and this theoretically could affect fetuses deficient in this enzyme. In our experiences from Parkland Hospital with more than 10,000 pregnant women who have been given this drug for asymptomatic bacteriuria, hemolytic anemia has not been observed in either the mother or the fetus.

Vancomycin is used primarily for bacterial endocarditis prophylaxis in penicillin-allergic patients. It also is the drug of choice for *Clostridium difficile* pseudomembranous colitis (see Chap. 51, p. 1152). Although there are no available human reproductive studies, vancomycin is associated with maternal nephrotoxicity and ototoxicity, and theoretically it may cause these in the embryo or fetus (Hermans, 1987).

Fluoroquinolones are relatively new antimicrobials that are especially useful for the treatment of urinary infections. Ciprofloxacin and norfloxacin are two that are used commonly. Although there are no well-controlled studies in pregnant women, fluoroquinolones are reported by their manufacturer to be associated with irreversible arthropathy in immature dogs and should not be used during pregnancy unless needed for resistant infections.

Commonly used **tuberculostatic** drugs include rifampicin, isoniazid, and ethambutol (see Chap. 49, p. 1119). Snyder and associates (1980) reviewed studies of several hundred pregnant women given these drugs, and reported no increase in the frequency of congenital anomalies.

Imipenem, a **carbapenem**, is a relatively new antimicrobial effective against both aerobic and anaerobic organisms commonly isolated from intra-abdominal and female pelvic infections. Although there are no available human data regarding the safety of this drug during pregnancy, there are few indications for its use. Exceptions would be life-threatening conditions such as perforative appendicitis during pregnancy.

Antifungal Agents. Vaginal candidiasis is common during pregnancy, and three commonly used agents for its treatment are **clotrimazole, miconazole,** and **nystatin.** In one report there was no increase in congenital malformations reported with their use (Rosa and associates, 1987a). **Butoconazole** is a relatively new antifungal agent, and although there are no human studies regarding its use during early pregnancy, it is not teratogenic in rodents, according to the package insert.

Amphotericin B is used primarily to treat systemic mycotic infections such as histoplasmosis, coccidioidomycosis, cryptococcosis, and candidiasis. In a review by Ismail and Lerner (1982), there was no evidence for congenital anomalies based on case reports. **Griseofulvin** is given orally principally for the treatment of mycotic infections of the skin, nails, and scalp. There is one report of its possible association with conjoined twins (Rosa and associates, 1987b). Animal studies indicate increased anomalies of the central nervous system and skeleton in offspring, and thus, griseofulvin should be used with extreme caution during pregnancy.

Antiviral Agents. Development of antiviral medications is in its infancy, and this is reflected by the small number of available drugs listed in Table 42–4. Knowledge of their use during pregnancy is limited. There is ample reason for concern regarding use of antiviral drugs during pregnancy because their mechanism of action is by inhibition of host-intracellular viral replication through action at the molecular level on RNA or DNA substrates. Although these purportedly are designed to be highly organism-specific, in high concentration they can inhibit mitosis of normal mammalian cells.

Zidovudine, previously called azidothymidine or AZT, is a thymidine analog that inhibits DNA synthesis. It is used specifically to treat human immunodeficiency virus infections, including acquired immune deficiency syndrome (AIDS). More recently it has been given to delay the onset of clinical disease in asymptomatic seropositive persons, or it is given prophylactically following accidental viral exposure. Transplacental passage has been documented (Pons and colleagues, 1991). MacGregor (1991) has suggested that zidovudine might also decrease the risk of transplacental immunodeficiency viral infection. There are recent animal data regarding

TABLE 42–4. MECHANISMS OF ACTION OF SOME ANTIVIRAL MEDICATIONS

Medication	Mechanism of Action
Acyclovir, ganciclovir	Viral DNA polymerase is inhibited by competitive inhibition with deoxyguanosine triphosphate.
Amantadine, ramantadine	Appears to block late stages of viral assembly, and perhaps through inhibition of DNA polymerase.
Idoxuridine	Interrupts normal transcriptions of DNA viruses through a triphosphate derivative.
Interferon	Mechanism unknown, but may be related to mRNA inhibition or interrupted translation.
Ribavirin	Viral RNA polymerase inhibited by competitive inhibition of GTP.
Trifluridine	Inhibits viral DNA synthesis by unknown means.
Vidarabine	Competitive inhibition of thymidine triphosphate, affecting DNA polymerase activity.
Zidovudine	Viral RNA-dependent DNA polymerase inhibited (reverse transcriptase).

the prevention of maternal transmission of retroviruses by zidovudine therapy (Sharpe and co-workers, 1989). Taylor and associates (1992) reported observations from 10 women who were given zidovudine while pregnant, and no fetal anomalies were noted. According to its manufacturer, zidovudine is not teratogenic for several animal species. Despite the paucity of information regarding its efficacy or safety during pregnancy, it seems logical to treat infected pregnant women because of the universally fatal outcome of symptomatic infection.

Dideoxyinosine (ddI) and **dideoxycitidine (ddC)** are two new drugs used for immunodeficiency viral infections. They are still in initial evaluation phases and there is no information regarding their use in pregnancy.

Acyclovir and **ganciclovir** are effective in treating primary herpes and possibly varicella infections. In a summary of the Acyclovir in Pregnancy Registry, Andrews and colleagues (1992) reported the outcome of 239 pregnancies in which this agent was given during the first trimester. There were 47 induced and 24 spontaneous abortions. Of 168 live-born infants, 159 (95 percent) had no congenital anomalies. Of the 9 infants with anomalies, there was no distinctive pattern of abnormalities. Topical administration of acyclovir results in minimal systemic absorption, which probably reduces unknown risks considerably. Ganciclovir has greater toxicity than acyclovir in laboratory animals, but it has not been studied during pregnancy.

Amantadine is used to prevent or modify influenza infections. This drug has been studied in human pregnancy, but anecdotal experience with 20 pregnancies in which amantadine was given during the first trimester resulted in two abortions and 18 normal live births.

Ribavirin is given by inhalation of an aerosol to treat respiratory syncytial viral infections in infants and young children. No studies of ribavirin in human pregnancy have been published; however, based upon well-conducted animal studies, the drug appears to have significant teratogenic potential. It consistently produces hydrocephalus and limb abnormalities in rodent models. A concern is that pregnant women are exposed to the drug while working in intensive care nurseries.

Interferon-α is approved for treating hairy cell leukemia, and it is effective for some viral infections. Experience with interferon in pregnant women has not been reported. Animal teratology studies indicate that interferon has a very low potential for toxicity.

Idoxuridine is effective against adenovirus, cytomegalovirus, varicella, and vaccinia viral infections. **Trifluridine** is effective in treating herpes virus infections, and **vidarabine** is effective against herpes virus and pox virus infections. **Idoxuridine** has not been investigated in human pregnancy, and may have the same potential for damage as other cytotoxic drugs, such as, trifluridine and vidarabine, which were developed originally as antineoplastics.

Antiparasitic Agents. Parasitic infections during pregnancy are quite common. Because they are usually asymptomatic, in general most do not need to be treated until after delivery. **Metronidazole** is a nitroimidazole and is the only effective agent currently available for treatment of vaginal trichomoniasis. Because the drug is carcinogenic in rodents and mutagenic in certain bacteria, many do not recommend its use in early pregnancy (Hammill, 1989). However, in a study of over 1000 infants born to women who used metronidazole during the first trimester, there was no increase in the frequency of congenital anomalies (Rosa and colleagues, 1987a). Moreover, the drug has not been shown to be teratogenic for animals given five times the usual human dose (Hammill, 1989). Because of medicolegal implications of first-trimester metronidazole use, it is prudent not to use this agent if possible. In the case of inadvertent exposure in early pregnancy, the woman can generally be assured that there is a very low risk, if any, from this exposure.

Lindane is used topically for the treatment of *pediculosis pubis* and scabies. Although there are no adequate human reproduction studies of this drug, according to the manufacturer lindane was not teratogenic for a variety of animals given several times the usual human dose. In adults, although a significant amount of lindane is absorbed systemically, this rarely causes central nervous system toxicity (Orkin and Maibach, 1983). Because of this, some recommend that a combination of pyrethrins and piperonal butoxide be used as initial treatment of *pediculosis pubis* during pregnancy, with lindane reserved for resistant infections. Likewise, crotamiton (10 percent lotion or cream) or 6 percent sulfur in petrolatum can be used as first-line treatment for scabies during pregnancy.

Malaria is endemic in many parts of the world, and is encountered in the United States in Southeast Asian and Central American refugees. **Chloroquine** is a valuable first-line antimalarial. There was no increase in congenital anomalies in over 150 offspring of mothers who received this drug during pregnancy (Wolfe and Cordero, 1985). In much lower doses, it is also used for chemoprophylaxis against malaria in pregnant women who must travel to or live in countries in which malaria is endemic. Although **quinine** is widely used for chloroquine-resistant falciparum malaria, there are no large studies regarding its safety during pregnancy. An increased frequency of congenital anomalies was reported during the 1930s when large doses were used to attempt to induce abortion. Quinine should not be withheld in severely ill women with chloroquine-resistant malaria.

Pyrimethamine is an antiparasitic folic acid antagonist used to treat malaria and toxoplasmosis. There is little information regarding its safety during pregnancy; however, Hengst (1972) reported no increased frequency of malformations in 64 newborns whose mothers took this drug in early pregnancy. **Spiramycin** has been used to treat toxoplasmosis, and has been used extensively in Europe during the first trimester with no adverse embryofetal effects. Sulfadiazine also has been used for toxoplasmosis, usually in conjunction with pyrimethamine. Unfortunately, the efficacy of all of these agents for either the prevention or amelioration of embryofetal effects of toxoplasmosis is uncertain, and despite therapy, newborns may have chorioretinitis, hydrocephalus, and intracranial calcifications (Foulon and colleagues, 1990).

Mebendazole is effective for treatment of a variety of helminths including enterobiasis (pinworm), trichuriasis (whipworm), ascariasis (roundworm), and uncinariasis (hookworm). According to its manufacturer, mebendazole is teratogenic for laboratory animals given several times the usual human adult dose; however, no reports of use in human pregnancy has been published. **Thiabendazole** is a broad-spectrum antihelmintic similar to mebendazole. It is used primarily to treat strongyloidiasis, trichinosis, and cutaneous larval migrans. It is also used as second-line therapy to treat pinworm, whipworm, roundworm, and hookworm infections. It has not been reported to be teratogenic for animals and there are no adequate human reproduction studies. **Pyrantel pomoate** is primarily used for the treatment of ascariasis and enterobiasis. It has not been reported as teratogenic for animals and there are no adequate human studies.

Cardiovascular Diseases. As discussed in Chapter 48, almost 1 percent of pregnant women have some form of heart disease. They are often given a myriad of drugs and medications, the majority of which are safe during pregnancy.

Heart Failure and Arrhythmias. The use of cardiac glycosides is declining. They are prescribed for heart failure, atrial fibrillation or flutter, and other supraventricular tachycardias. **Digoxin** is the most commonly used preparation, and although it rapidly crosses the placenta, there is no convincing evidence that it causes adverse fetal effects. Antiarrhythmic drugs have been maternally administered in attempts to control fetal tachycardias (Harrigan and colleagues, 1981; Kerenyi and associates, 1980).

Quinidine is commonly used to treat supraventricular tachycardias and some ventricular arrhythmias. The drug readily crosses the placenta and has been given to the mother to treat fetal supraventricular tachycardias (Killeen and Bowers, 1987). There are no epidemiological studies of congenital anomalies following its use during the first trimester, but it is relatively safe during later pregnancy (Rotmensch and colleagues, 1987).

Other antiarrhythmic drugs include **lidocaine, procainamide, verapamil, propranolol, disopyramide, amiodarone, bretylium, encainide, flecainide, adenosine,** and **nifedipine.** All cross the placenta and many have been used to treat fetal arrhythmias (Dumesic and colleagues, 1982; Rey and associates, 1985). There are no well-documented human reproduction studies for these commonly used drugs.

Propranolol is a β-adrenergic blocker used to treat supraventricular and ventricular tachycardias, as well as chronic hypertension and hyperthyroidism during pregnancy. It was reported earlier to be associated with fetal growth retardation; however, in a review of five prospective studies of propranolol and oxprenolol given during pregnancy, fetal growth retardation was identified in only 4 percent (Rotmensch and colleagues, 1983).

Antihypertensive Drugs. **Methyldopa** is widely used during pregnancy for the treatment of chronic hypertension. Although there are no large epidemiological studies in early pregnancy, its many years of use attest to its safety. **Hydralazine** is commonly utilized to treat hypertension in women in the latter half of pregnancy without apparent adverse fetal effects. There are no human reproduction studies of **sodium nitroprusside;** however, this drug readily crosses the placenta (Lewis and colleagues, 1977). Theoretically, use of nitroprusside may result in the accumulation of cyanide in the fetal liver resulting from metabolism of the drug, and this could adversely effect embryofetal development. **Clonidine,** an α-adrenergic blocker, has been used to treat hypertension in pregnant women without apparent adverse fetal effects (Horvath and co-workers, 1985).

A number of **β-adrenergic blocking agents** are used primarily for the treatment of chronic hypertension. These include propranolol, labetalol, atenolol, metoprolol, nadolol, and timolol. Some also are useful for the chronic treatment of angina pectoris, some cardiac arrhythmias, and occasionally for treatment of hyperthyroidism. There is little information regarding their use in early gestation; however, several have been used without apparent adverse effects in pregnant women in the United Kingdom. In two American studies, Sibai and associates (1987, 1990) reported that labetalol therapy for preeclampsia or chronic hypertension did not improve perinatal outcome compared with untreated hypertensive control women. Importantly, more infants of women with preeclampsia given labetalol were growth retarded, but this was not found in the chronically hypertensive women who took the drug.

Calcium-channel-blocking agents are also commonly used to treat chronic hypertension. Verapamil is used to treat hypertension, angina, and supraventricular tachycardias. Although verapamil is commonly utilized for the treatment of hypertension in pregnant women without apparent adverse effects, it should be used with caution as it may cause a decrease in uterine blood flow (Murad and colleagues, 1985). Moreover, it has also been reported to be associated with fetal cardiac depression and arrest when utilized transplacentally for treatment of fetal supraventricular tachycardias (Kleinman and Copel, 1991). Whether nifedipine is associated with similar adverse effects is unclear at this time. Recently, Sibai and associates (1992) reported their experiences with nifedipine for the treatment of women with preeclampsia remote from term. Although no adverse fetal effects were noted, there was also no improvement in perinatal outcome associated with its use.

The **angiotensin-converting enzyme inhibitors,** captopril and enalapril, have been reported to be associated with congenital hypocalvaria, renal anomalies, nephrotoxicity, and neonatal anuria (Barr and Cohen, 1991; Boutroy, 1989; Pryde and associates, 1992). Because of these reasons they are listed in Table 42–1 with other strongly suspected teratogens.

Diuretics. Diuretics are prescribed during pregnancy for some women with chronic hypertension, and are also given acutely or chronically to treat pulmonary edema caused by heart failure. In the past, **thiazide diuretics** were commonly used, and the frequency of congenital anomalies was not increased among over 60 women who took chlorothiazide in the first trimester, or among over 5000 who took it after this (Heinonen, 1977). Similarly, hydrochlorothiazide use during early pregnancy was not associated with an increased frequency of congenital anomalies (Heinonen, 1977; Jick and colleagues, 1981). Thiazides have been reported to be associated with neonatal thrombocytopenia when given near the time of delivery.

Acetazolamide is a carbonic anhydrase inhibitor, and there is little information regarding its use during pregnancy. In two reports of only 31 pregnancies exposed during the first trimester, malformations were not increased in one and only questionably increased in the other (Heinonen, 1977). On the other hand, the drug has been consistently reported to be associated with an unusual type of limb abnormality in animals (Hirsch and colleagues, 1983). It seems prudent to avoid carbonic anhydrase inhibitors during pregnancy.

Spironolactone is a commonly used potassium-sparing diuretic that has not been studied in human pregnancy. Theoretically at least, spironolactone could cause feminization of male fetuses because of its antiandrogenic effects (Messina and colleagues, 1979).

Ethacrynic acid and **furosemide,** loop diuretics, have not been extensively studied in human pregnancy despite common use of the latter. There have been no reports of association with congenital anomalies and these drugs given in early pregnancy.

Anticoagulants. Deep vein thrombosis or pulmonary embolus is estimated to complicate about 1 in 2500 pregnancies (Cunningham and Lowe, 1991). **Heparin** is the mainstay of treatment for both, and it may be given intravenously, either continuously or intermittently, or by subcutaneous injection (see Chap. 49, p. 1115). Heparin is a large, highly-polar molecule that does not cross the placenta. Its protracted use may cause maternal osteoporosis and thrombocytopenia. Large studies indicate that heparin is not associated with congenital anomalies, and it is the anticoagulant of choice for pregnant women.

In contrast, **coumarin** derivatives are of much smaller molecular weight and readily cross the placenta to cause significant adverse embryo and fetal effects. Their genesis is probably from hemorrhage into any of several organs, such as the brain. The *fetal warfarin syndrome* is identified in 15 to 25 percent of fetuses exposed during the first trimester (Hall and associates, 1980; Stevenson and colleagues, 1980). The two most consistent findings are nasal hypoplasia (Fig. 42–1) and stippled vertebral and femoral epiphyses seen on radiographs. Other adverse effects that may follow second- or third-trimester fetal exposure are listed in Table 42–5. Spontaneous abortion, stillbirth, and neonatal death are also increased when warfarin is given. The period of greatest susceptibility of the embryo to the effects of warfarin appears to be between the sixth and ninth postmenstrual weeks.

Asthma. Asthma complicates 1 to 2 percent of pregnancies and severe disease may be associated with poor maternal and perinatal outcome (see Chap. 49, p. 1108).

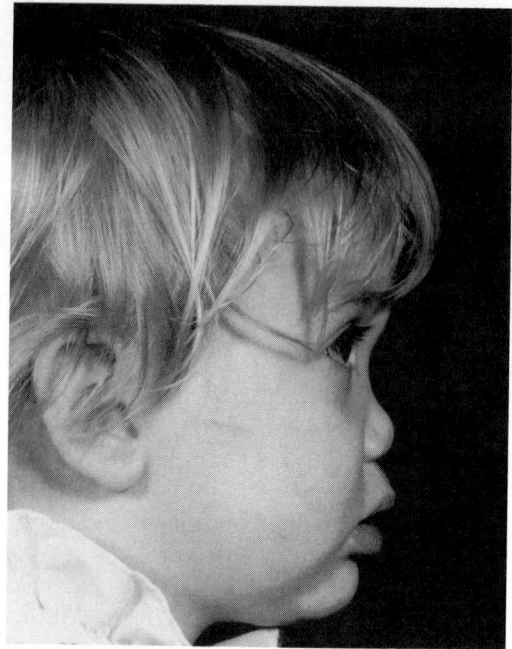

Fig. 42–1. Warfarin embryopathy or fetal warfarin syndrome: nasal hypoplasia and depressed nasal bridge. (Photograph courtesy of Dr. Mary Jo Harrod.)

Most medications for treatment of asthma can be used with apparent safety during pregnancy. The most commonly used bronchodilators are **β-adrenergic blockers.** During an acute asthma attack, epinephrine may be given subcutaneously, and there is little evidence that this causes adverse fetal effects. Terbutaline has potent bronchodilator activity, and although commonly used for threatened preterm labor, it is not approved by the Food and Drug Administration for this purpose. There is no evidence that terbutaline given during early pregnancy causes congenital anomalies, and in one long-term study of infants exposed in utero, Wallace and colleagues (1978) reported no increased adverse effects. Metaproterenol and albuterol are self-administered by inhalation and there is little information regarding their possible teratogenicity following first-trimester use.

Theophylline salts are commonly used broncho-

TABLE 42–5. ADVERSE FETAL EFFECTS OF MATERNAL WARFARIN INGESTION

Nasal hypoplasia
Stippled bone epiphyses
Hydrocephaly
Microcephaly
Ophthalmological abnormalities
Fetal growth retardation
Developmental delay

From Hall and colleagues (1980).

dilators; however, there are no large studies of their use during pregnancy. Aminophylline is the only salt available for parenteral use, but there are numerous oral forms, many of which contain other bronchodilators, such as ephedrine. **Cromolyn** inhibits mast cell histamine release and is given chronically for asthma prophylaxis. There are no large studies in pregnant women, nor are there reports of congenital anomalies after its first-trimester use.

Corticosteroid use has become common for asthma treatment. Preparations include beclomethasone, betamethasone, and prednisone. Because severe asthma may be dangerous to the mother, glucocorticoids should be given if indicated. Although there are no adequate studies of their use in early pregnancy, no association with congenital anomalies or with adverse fetal effects has been reported.

Seizure Disorders. Epilepsy is encountered in about one of every 200 pregnancies, and its management during pregnancy may be difficult (see Chap. 55, p. 1244). Although the precise pathophysiology has not been elucidated, it is well established that women with epilepsy who take anticonvulsant medications have a two- to threefold increased risk of malformed fetuses compared with non-epileptics. Kelly (1984), in a review of over 750,000 pregnancies from 13 cohort studies, calculated a malformation rate of 70 per 1000 for infants of epileptic mothers compared with 30 per 1000 for infants born to non-epileptic control women. Because offspring of epileptic mothers not taking anticonvulsants are also at risk for increased anomalies, it remains unclear whether epilepsy in itself causes the increased malformations, or whether anticonvulsant exposure does. More likely, it is the combination of a potentially teratogenic drug working in concert with a genetic predisposition. Some characteristics of the anticonvulsant embryopathies are given in Table 42–6. It has been postulated that the teratogenicity of various anticonvulsant medications are mediated via toxic intermediary metabolites and that inability to metabolize these is related to a genetic defect in arene oxide detoxification (Stickler and colleagues, 1985). Jones and associates (1989) reported a carbamazepine embryopathy similar to the fetal hydantoin syndrome and suggested the possibility that the epoxide intermediate for both drugs was toxic because the arene oxide pathway is common to each.

An intriguing link to a genetic etiology was described by Buehler and associates (1990), who reported that the characteristic features of the hydantoin syndrome developed only in fetuses who demonstrated decreased *epoxide hydrolase* activity. This enzyme is necessary for elimination of various phenytoin epoxide metabolites. Enzyme activity measured in cultured amniocytes obtained by amniocentesis from 100 normal pregnancies showed a distribution suggestive of two re-

TABLE 42–6. SOME ASPECTS OF ANTICONVULSANT EMBRYOPATHIES

Hydantoin Syndrome	Carbamazepine Syndrome	Trimethadione Syndrome
Craniofacial abnormalities	Craniofacial abnormalities	Craniofacial abnormalities
Cleft lip/palate	Upslanting palpebral fissures	Cleft palate
Broad nasal bridge	Short nose	V-shaped eyebrows
Hypertelorism	Epicanthal folds	Irregular teeth
Epicanthal folds		Epicanthal folds
		Backward-sloped ears
Limb defects	Limb defects	Speech difficulty
Hypoplasia of distal phalanges, nails	Hypoplasia of distal phalanges, nails	Simian creases
		Hearing loss
		Cardiac anomalies
Growth deficiency	Growth deficiency	Growth deficiency
		Mental deficiency
Mental deficiency	Mental deficiency	Microcephaly

From Hansen and Smith (1975), Jones and colleagues (1989); Zackai and co-workers (1975).

cessive alleles. These investigators hypothesized that fetuses homozygous for the recessive allele had low enzyme activity and were thus at risk for phenytoin toxicity. Importantly, it may become possible to determine which fetus is at risk for anticonvulsant embryopathy because enzyme activity can be measured prenatally.

Anticonvulsant Medications. **Phenytoin,** a hydantoin, is the most commonly prescribed anticonvulsant. Other hydantoin anticonvulsants are mephenytoin and ethotoin. In 1975 Hansen and Smith described the *fetal hydantoin syndrome,* which is characterized by craniofacial and limb malformations accompanied by mental deficiency (Table 42–6 and Fig. 42–2). In a review of studies that included 460 women taking anticonvulsants, Kelly (1984) reported that as many as 30 percent of fetuses exposed to phenytoin had minor craniofacial and digital anomalies.

Carbamazepine, another commonly prescribed anticonvulsant, at least initially appeared to be less teratogenic than phenytoin. Indeed, for many years it was felt by many that carbamazepine was the drug of choice to treat pregnant epileptics. Niebyl and colleagues (1979) reviewed 94 exposed infants and found that only 4 had malformations, a rate similar to that of the general population. A decade later, however, Jones and co-workers (1989) reported findings that strongly suggest that carbamazepine is teratogenic and causes significant malformations (Table 42–6).

Trimethadione, and closely related paramethadione, are oral anticonvulsants used to treat petit mal seizures. A characteristic pattern of malformations called the *fetal trimethadione syndrome* (Table 42–6) is found among children of women treated with trimetha-

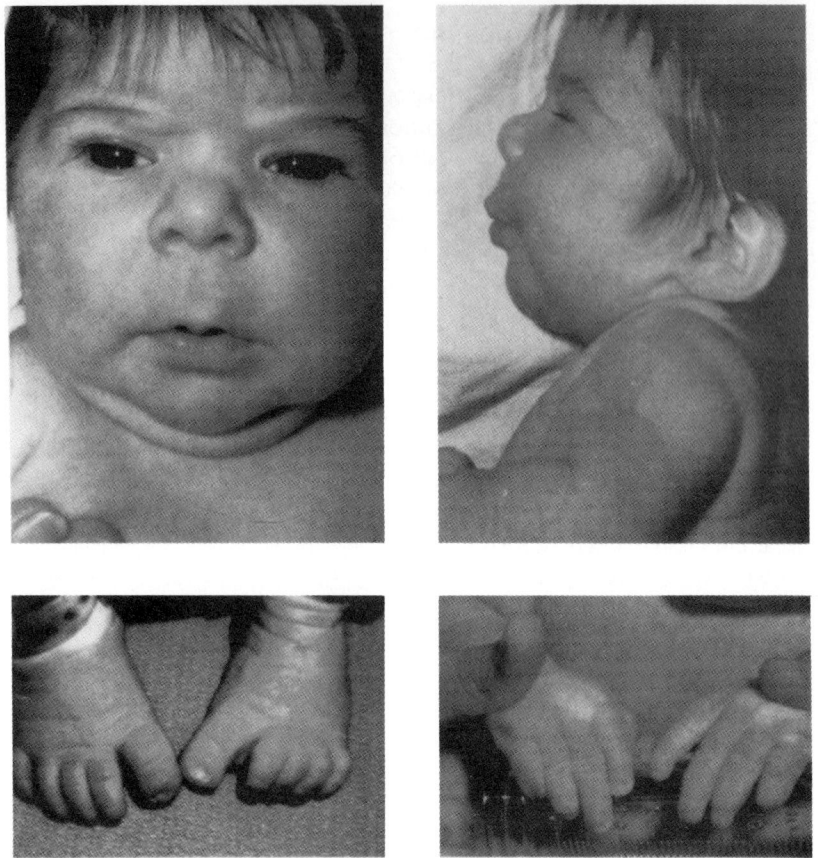

Fig. 42–2. Fetal hydantoin syndrome. (*Upper*) Facial features including upturned nose, mild midfacial hypoplasia, and long upper lip with thin vermilion border. (*Lower*) Distal digital hypoplasia. (From Buehler and colleagues, 1990, with permission.)

dione or paramethadione during pregnancy (German and associates, 1970; Zackai and co-workers, 1975).

Valproic acid is a commonly used anticonvulsant. In a case-control study that included 150 affected children, the drug was associated with an increased frequency of spina bifida among infants whose mothers used the drug in the first trimester (Robert and colleagues, 1983). The best available estimate of the risk for spina bifida in the offspring of women treated with valproic acid during early pregnancy is 1 to 2 percent. The *fetal valproate syndrome* has been described as a distinctive pattern of minor anomalies of the face and digits (Dalens and colleagues, 1980; DiLiberti and associates, 1984; Jager-Roman and co-workers, 1986). This pattern has not been delineated completely, but appears to involve brachycephaly with a high forehead, shallow orbits, ocular hypertelorism, small nose, small mouth, low-set posteriorly rotated ears, long, overlapping fingers and toes, and hyperconvex fingernails. Cleft palate and congenital heart disease have occasionally been described in babies exposed to valproic acid during embryogenesis (Thomas and Buchanan, 1981).

Phenobarbital is frequently used in combination with other anticonvulsant agents. It has also been used for many decades in pregnant women for other indications. Over 1000 mother–infant pairs of first-trimester exposure to phenobarbital were included in the Collab-

orative Perinatal Project database; the frequency of either minor or major birth defects was not increased compared with unexposed controls (Heinonen, 1977).

Ethosuximide and **methsuximide** are succinimide anticonvulsants utilized primarily for petit mal seizures. There are no human reproduction studies available or reports of malformations attributed solely to either of these agents.

Psychiatric Conditions. Medications used to treat psychiatric illness include sedatives, hypnotics, tranquilizers, antidepressants, and antipsychotics. Some of these conditions are outlined in Chapter 55.

Sedatives, Tranquilizers, and Hypnotics. **Barbiturates** are not commonly used as sedatives today, although they were in the past. There is no evidence that phenobarbital, secobarbital and butalbital are teratogenic. **Diazepam** use in some studies (Aarskog, 1975; Saxen and Saxen, 1975), but not others (Rosenberg and associates, 1983; Shiono and Mills, 1984), has been associated with cleft lip in children whose mothers took this medication during the first trimester. The drug has been associated with hypotonia, respiratory depression, and hypothermia in newborns whose mothers were given large doses during labor. Neither **chlordiazepoxide** nor **meprobamate** were found to be associated with an increased frequency of malformations in the Collaborative Perinatal Project database (Heinonen and colleagues, 1977).

Antidepressant Drugs. **Tricyclic antidepressants** such as amitriptyline and imipramine have been associated with limb-reduction defects in some reports (Morrow, 1972), however, others have not confirmed these findings (Crombie and co-workers, 1972; Heinonen and colleagues, 1977). **Fluoxetine** is classified as B by its manufacturer, but there is very limited experience with human pregnancy.

Lithium and its salts, especially lithium carbonate, are used for treatment of affective mental illness. An association has been observed between maternal lithium carbonate treatment and fetal cardiovascular malformations, especially Ebstein anomaly. Weinstein (1980) reported that 8 percent of 225 lithium-exposed infants reported to an international registry had serious congenital cardiovascular anomalies. Six of the affected infants, or 2.7 percent of the total, had Ebstein anomaly, a cardiac malformation with an expected incidence of only about 1 per 20,000. Noncardiovascular malformations were observed in 3 percent of the 225 infants, a frequency not different from background risk. More recently, Jacobson and colleagues (1992b) reported their prospective follow-up study of 148 women given lithium in the first trimester. They reported a 2.8 percent major congenital malformation rate, which was similar to the 2.4 percent observed in controls. There was one fetus with Ebstein anomaly. They concluded that lithium is not a major teratogen, and recommend continuation of pregnancy if the fetus appears normal on ultrasonic and echocardiographic examination.

Antipsychotic Medications. The **phenothiazine** group of major tranquilizers is commonly used to treat psychotic illnesses. Chlorpromazine has been used extensively and was not found to be associated with an increased malformations in two studies involving several thousand women (Heinonen and associates, 1977; Farkas and Farkas, 1971). Currently, haloperidol is used even more commonly, and although it has been associated in isolated reports with limb-reduction defects, most studies attest to its safety (Briggs and colleagues, 1990). Heinonen and associates (1977) found no association between congenital anomalies and first-trimester use of prochlorperazine and perphenazine.

There are no large epidemiological studies regarding some of the other antipsychotic drugs such as thiothixene, loxapine, clozapine, molindone, or chlorprothixene.

Analgesics

Salicylates and Acetaminophen. In one review of over 1000 women, Streissguth and colleagues (1987) reported that almost half of pregnant women utilized salicylates and acetaminophen during pregnancy. Most investigators have found no association between maternal salicylate ingestion and fetal anomalies (Heinonen, 1977; Slone, 1976; Turner, 1975; and their associates). Aspirin is a potent prostaglandin synthase inhibitor and it has been reported to be associated with oligohydramnios, premature closure of the ductus arteriosus, and pulmonary hypertension (Levin and associates, 1978; Sibai and Amon, 1988).

Acetaminophen was not found to be associated with an increased risk of fetal anomalies in over 500 offspring from two reports (Aselton and colleagues, 1985; Heinonen and associates, 1977). It has not been associated with ductal closure, pulmonary hypertension, or oligohydramnios; however, liver toxicity and fetal demise may result from maternal overdose (Haibach and colleagues, 1984).

Nonsteroidal Anti-inflammatory Drugs. There are a variety of nonsteroidal anti-inflammatory drugs with analgesic action, and **ibuprofen** and **naproxen** have been the most commonly used to date. **Indomethacin** has been used as a tocolytic agent to treat preterm labor (Niebyl and colleagues, 1980). These drugs are considered to be nonteratogenic. Of concern are reports of possible closure of the fetal ductus arteriosus with subsequent pulmonary hypertension (Csaba and associates, 1978; Levin and co-workers, 1978). At least theoretically, any nonsteroidal anti-inflammatory drug could cause premature ductal closure because of prostaglandin synthase inhibition. Of interest, some of these agents have been associated with decreased amnionic fluid volume when they were used for tocolysis (Hickok and colleagues, 1989). Because of these observations, these agents generally are not recommended for use in pregnant women after 34 weeks.

Narcotic Analgesics. Meperidine and morphine are **opioids.** Heinonen and colleagues (1977) found no association with either of these drugs and congenital anomalies. As with all narcotics, chronic maternal ingestion may be associated with a neonatal withdrawal syndrome. Neither **codeine** nor **propoxyphene** were found to be associated with congenital anomalies in one study of several hundred patients (Heinonen and colleagues, 1977). There is little information regarding the use of **butorphanol, hydrocodone,** or **hydromorphone** during early pregnancy.

Anesthesia

General Anesthesia. It has been estimated that as many as 50,000 pregnant women undergo emergency surgery each year, and many operations are performed prior to the recognition of pregnancy (Friedman, 1988). Virtually all anesthetic agents cross the placenta at least to some degree, and many result in significant fetal blood concentrations. Two commonly used parenteral anesthetic agents are thiopental and ketamine. Of 152 women who were given **thiopental** in early pregnancy and studied by the Collaborative Perinatal Project, the frequency of congenital malformations was not increased (Heinonen and colleagues, 1977). There are no large studies regarding the use of **ketamine** in pregnant women.

A wide variety of inhalation agents are utilized for general anesthesia. The most commonly used is **nitrous oxide,** and although there have been reports of increased fetal losses and malformations in rodent studies, the frequency of malformations was not increased in offspring of mothers exposed during the first 4 months of pregnancy (Friedman, 1988; Heinonen and co-workers, 1977). Halogenated agents commonly are used to supplement nitrous oxide during general anesthetic procedures. **Halothane** has been reported to be teratogenic in some animal studies, but not in others (Friedman, 1988). It was not associated with increased malformations in the offspring of 25 women who were given this agent in the first 4 months of pregnancy (Heinonen and colleagues, 1977). There are no epidemiological studies regarding the use of either **isoflurane** or **methoxyflurane** during pregnancy.

The two most commonly used muscle relaxants during general anesthesia are **curare** and **succinylcholine.** There are no large human studies regarding their use during pregnancy.

Local Anesthesia. A variety of local anesthetic agents may be used for spinal or epidural analgesia in pregnant women. **Lidocaine** is probably the most frequently used local anesthetic. In one review of almost 300 children whose mothers were given lidocaine in the first trimester, the frequency of congenital malformations was not greater than expected (Heinonen and colleagues, 1977). The frequency of malformations in offspring who were exposed to either **tetracaine** or **procaine** during early pregnancy was not greater than expected in the general population; however, malformations were increased twofold in the offspring of 82 women who were given **bupivacaine** during the first 16 weeks of pregnancy (Heinonen and collaborators, 1977). Whether there is a "cause and effect" from bupivacaine is unclear, but it is unlikely that it is a potent teratogen (Friedman, 1988).

Hyperemesis. Nausea and vomiting are common complaints, especially in early pregnancy, and until recently antiemetics were probably the most commonly prescribed group of drugs. Bendectin has probably received more attention, especially from a litigation standpoint, than any other drug given during pregnancy (see p. 960). The drug is a combination of doxylamine and pyridoxine, but is no longer available in the United States, not because it was a proven teratogen but rather

a "most popular litogen" (Brent, 1985; Holmes, 1983). Brent has aptly chronicled this in his editorial, *The Bendectin Saga: Another American Tragedy.*

There is a variety of other antiemetics that may be used during pregnancy, such as the **piperazines** (meclizine, cyclizine, and others) and **phenothiazines** (chlorpromazine, prochlorperazine, and promethazine). There is no evidence that any of the antiemetics are associated with an increased risk of congenital anomalies after exposure during organogenesis. Specifically, cyclizine, meclizine, promethazine, and Bendectin taken during the first trimester were not associated with increased risk for congenital anomalies (Farkas and Farkas, 1971; Heinonen and colleagues, 1977).

Antineoplastic Agents. Malignancy is relatively uncommon during pregnancy, but as discussed in Chapter 57, common cancers encountered are breast carcinoma, cutaneous melanomas, lymphomas, and leukemias. A large number of antineoplastic agents are used to treat cancer in pregnant women, and of the small list of known or highly suspected teratogens (Table 42–1), four belong to this class of medications. Busulfan and cyclophosphamide are alkylating agents and methotrexate and aminopterin are folate antagonist antimetabolites.

Cyclophosphamide is an alkylating agent, and although no adequate epidemiological studies have been published, at least 8 infants with anomalies have been born to women who were given the drug during early pregnancy. The most common defects reported were missing digits from hands and feet with hypoplastic development of other digits. Other concomitant defects included cleft palate, single coronary artery, imperforate anus, and fetal growth retardation with microcephaly (Kirshon and colleagues, 1988; Murray and associates, 1984). Although antineoplastic agents in general are associated with growth retardation, the deletion of digits, arterial systems, and imperforate anus appear to cluster among infants whose mothers were given cyclophosphamide during pregnancy.

A very uncommon but strikingly similar pattern of congenital anomalies has been observed in at least 8 children after exposure during embryogenesis to **aminopterin** (Char, 1979; Warkany, 1978). Features of this syndrome include short stature, delayed calvarial ossification, craniosynostosis, hydrocephalus, abnormal auricles, ocular hypertelorism, micrognathia, and cleft palate. Similar features have been observed in babies born after first-trimester maternal exposure to **methotrexate** (Milunsky and co-workers, 1968).

Doll and associates (1989) have summarized the outcome in 139 pregnancies with first-trimester exposure to antineoplastic agents. A total of 17 percent of these newborns had malformations. The highest rate of malformations—24 percent—was from aminopterin, methotrexate, or polydrug exposures in the first trimester. The frequency of malformations from second-trimester exposure was only 1 to 5 percent. Because most antineoplastic drugs interfere with cell growth in the embryo, they may also be associated with fetal growth retardation with exposure after early pregnancy (Yazigi and Cunningham, 1990).

Immunosuppressant Drugs. Immunosuppressive agents are given to pregnant women primarily for the treatment of autoimmune disease and for organ transplantation maintenance. **Corticosteroids** are the most commonly used. Although steroids have been associated with cleft lip in animals, first-trimester exposure was not associated with an increased risk for malformations in the Collaborative Perinatal Project database (Heinonen and colleagues, 1977).

Azathioprine is primarily used to prevent organ transplant rejection or to treat inflammatory bowel disease. Although teratogenic for animals, most investigators have found the drug safe for use during human pregnancy (Briggs and colleagues, 1990). Neonatal hematological abnormalities, including fatal pancytopenia, have been described in association with maternal therapy (Davidson and co-workers, 1985; DeWitte and associates, 1984).

Cyclosporine is an antibiotic used as an immunosuppressive agent for the prevention of organ transplant rejection. It is widely used for liver and heart allografts, and has recently also been used for renal transplantation. Cyclosporine may result in significant maternal toxicity, especially nephrotoxicity. There are no large epidemiological reports regarding its use in pregnancy, but it appears to be safe for the fetus.

Retinoids. Retinoids are vitamin A isomers used primarily for dermatological disorders (see Chap. 56, p. 1264). **Isotretinoin** (13-*cis*-retinoic acid) is used to treat cystic acne and other dermatological diseases. An uncommon but strikingly similar pattern of anomalies has been observed in children exposed during embryonic development (Centers for Disease Control, 1984; Lammer and colleagues, 1985; Thompson and Cordero, 1989). Characteristic features include microtia or anotia, micrognathia, cleft palate, conotruncal heart and great vessel defects, thymic abnormalities, eye anomalies, and brain malformations (Fig. 42–3). In 57 pregnancies with first-trimester isotretinoin exposure, 16 percent spontaneously aborted and 19 percent resulted in infants with major malformations (Lammer and co-workers, 1985, 1987). The drug has an average serum half-life of 10 to 12 hours and the frequency of congenital anomalies does not appear to be increased among the children of women who discontinue isotretinoin therapy prior to conception (Dai and colleagues, 1989).

Etretinate is an orally administered retinoid used to treat psoriasis. The drug has an extremely long elimination time and it has been detected in the serum more than 2 years after cessation of therapy (DiGiovanna and colleagues, 1984). The length of time that any teratogenic effects of etretinate persist after therapy discontinuation is unknown. There are no epidemiological studies of infants of women treated with etretinate during pregnancy. However, at least 4 cases of neural-tube and other central nervous system defects and 3 cases of craniofacial and skeletal abnormalities have been observed (Happle and colleagues, 1984; Rosa and co-workers, 1986). These anomalies appear generally similar to those in offspring of animals treated with etretinate. A woman who conceived 4 months after cessation of etretinate therapy delivered an infant with hypoplasia of one leg (Grote and colleagues, 1985). Another whose therapy ended 51 weeks before conception gave birth to a baby with a central nervous system

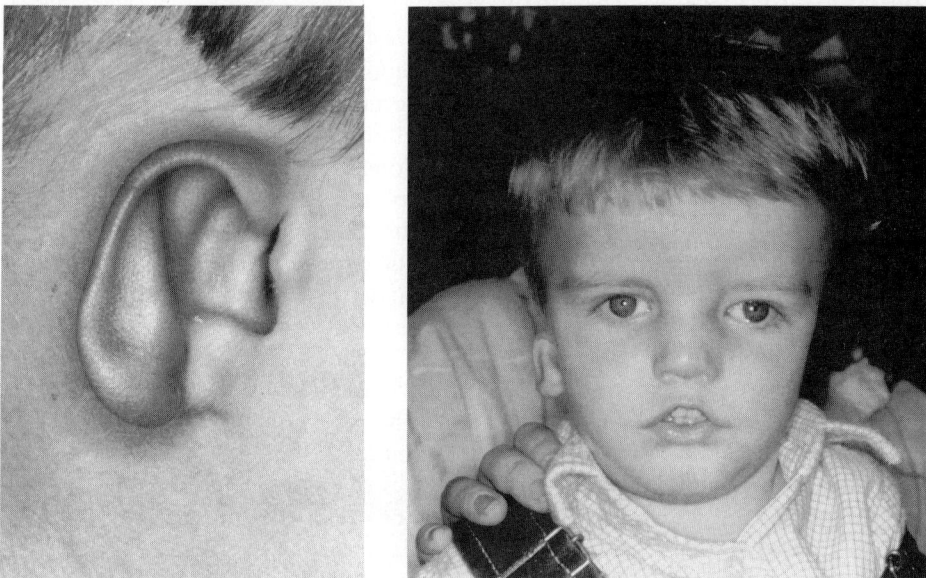

Fig. 42–3. Isotretinoin embryopathy: Bilateral microtia or anotia with stenosis of external ear canal (*left*). Flat depressed nasal bridge, ocular hypertelorism (*right*). (Photograph courtesy of Dr. Edward Lammer.)

anomaly and craniofacial features consistent with retin-oic acid embryopathy (Lammer, 1988). These observations raise concern that the teratogenic potential of etretinate may be manifested long after maternal therapy has ended.

Interestingly, **tretinoin** (*all-trans*-retinoic acid), another retinoid prescribed for treatment of acne vulgaris, has not been found teratogenic in experimental animals. This is probably because tretinoin is available only in topically applied gel, and the skin metabolizes most of the drug with no apparent absorption because systemic concentrations are undetectable. Although listed in Category B by its manufacturer, because of little human experience, its use is not recommended during pregnancy.

Hormones. Both androgens and the nonsteroidal synthetic estrogen, diethylstilbestrol, may be associated with congenital anomalies (Table 42–1).

Androgens. Prenatal maternal **testosterone** treatment may cause virilization of the external genitalia in female fetuses (Grumbach and Ducharme, 1960; Schardein, 1985). Affected fetuses have varying degrees of phallic enlargement and labioscrotal fusion. Phallic enlargement may be produced by exposure to testosterone and its analogs anytime after the genitalia have developed; labioscrotal fusion is seen only with first-trimester exposure. In general, the degree of virilization is greater with exposure to larger doses. Other structural abnormalities have not been observed. Surgical correction of the genital defect may occasionally be necessary. Normal female maturation can be anticipated at puberty in affected girls.

Danazol is a derivative of ethinyltestosterone with weak androgenic activity that acts as a pituitary–ovarian axis inhibitor. It is primarily used to treat endometriosis, and its use during early pregnancy has been reported in 47 cases (Quagliarello and Greco, 1985; Rosa, 1984). Of the 18 female fetuses exposed to danazol during the period of sensitivity to androgenic substances (eighth week of embryogenesis and thereafter), 13 had virilization that included clitoromegaly and partial labial fusion. In only 2 fetuses were the internal genitalia affected. Virilization was not observed among any embryos exposed before the eighth week (Rosa, 1984).

Diethylstilbestrol. Diethylstilbestrol (DES) is a nonsteroidal synthetic estrogen that was approved by the Food and Drug Administration in 1942 to prevent miscarriages. It was not until 1971 that the first report was published of clear-cell adenocarcinoma of the vagina and cervix in the daughters of women who were treated with DES early in pregnancy. It is estimated that between 500,000 and 2 million pregnant women took this drug. In a registry that includes more than 400 cases of this rare tumor diagnosed in the United States since

1971, DES treatment was verified in at least 65 percent of patients in whom the maternal history was available (Herbst and colleagues, 1981). In 80 percent of these cases, mothers who took DES did so prior to 12 weeks. The age at which malignancy was diagnosed ranged from 7 to 30 years, with a median of 19 years. It has been calculated that about 1 per 1000 DES-exposed daughters will develop clear-cell adenocarcinoma of the vagina or cervix by age 24.

Nonmalignant genital tract abnormalities, especially adenosis, are common among the daughters of women treated with DES. Gross structural abnormalities of the cervix or vagina are identified in about one fourth and abnormalities of the vaginal epithelium in up to half (Herbst and colleagues, 1975; Robboy and associates, 1981, 1984). Malformations such as T-shaped uterus, constricting bands of the uterine cavity, uterine hypoplasia, or paraovarian cysts also are found with increased frequency (Kaufman and co-workers, 1984). As discussed in Chapter 33 (p. 728), preterm delivery, spontaneous abortions, and ectopic pregnancy also appear to be more common than expected in these women (Barnes and colleagues, 1980; Herbst and co-workers, 1980; Sandberg and colleagues, 1981). Finally, epididymal cysts, hypoplastic testes, and cryptorchidism have been observed with increased frequency in the sons of women who were treated with DES during pregnancy (Stillman, 1982).

Oral Contraceptives. Initial data from the Collaborative Perinatal Project indicated that oral contraceptives were associated with an increased fetal risk for cardiovascular and limb-reduction defects. Subsequent analysis, however, has shown no difference when compared with control women (Wiseman and Dodds-Smith, 1984). In 1988, the Food and Drug Administration approved the removal of this rejoinder in the package insert that warned against birth defects and oral contraceptives (Brent, 1989).

Thalidomide. Thalidomide is an anxiolytic and sedative drug that is the most notorious human teratogen. Several teratological principles were forcefully demonstrated by the thalidomide "epidemic." One is that there is extreme variability in species susceptibility to thalidomide. Another is that there is a very close relationship between the time of exposure during embryogenesis and the presence and type of congenital defect. The types of defects observed in children correlated well with the timing of embryonic exposure (Knapp and co-workers, 1962). Mothers whose children had phocomelic defects took the drug only between the 27th and 40th days. Furthermore, thalidomide ingestion during the 27th to 30th days of embryogenesis was associated with a preponderance of upper limb phocomelia, while treatment during the 30th to 33rd days was associated with a predominance of lower limb phocomelia. The appearance of the upper limbs buds at 27 days and lower limb buds at about the 30th day in the human embryo correlated well with these observations. Thalidomide-associated external ear defects occur earlier in embryogenesis, at approximately days 21 to 27.

Social and Illicit Substance Use

Social, or so-called recreational, drug use is virtually epidemic in the United States. Richards (1985) estimated that 70 to 90 percent of Americans 15 to 40 years old had used mood-altering chemicals. Many of these users are women of childbearing age, and substance abuse is relatively common in pregnant women. In one survey of 715 pregnant women screened for alcohol, opiates, cocaine, and cannabinoids, 15 percent had positive urine toxicological tests (Chasnoff and associates, 1990). Moreover, it has been estimated that from 350,000 to over 700,000 infants may be exposed to illicit substances in utero each year (Chasnoff, 1991; Gomby and Shiono, 1991).

Factors Affecting Substance Abuse

Polydrug Use. **Illicit drug users seldom abuse one drug.** For example, alcohol abuse is commonplace in women who use illicit drugs. In a review of patterns of substance abuse during pregnancy, Little and colleagues (1990b) analyzed the use of methamphetamine, cocaine, heroin, and "t's and blues" in a primarily indigent population. Overall, 75 percent of these women reported that they abused more than one drug during pregnancy.

The concomitant use of several substances may increase the risk of potential adverse effects. For example, fetal growth retardation appears to be more severe and the frequency of congenital anomalies is probably increased in offspring whose mothers abuse multiple substances (Oro and Dixon, 1987). As already mentioned, alcohol is frequently a common co-factor and it increases the risk of congenital anomalies and growth retardation. For example, infants born to women who abuse "t's and blues" are at a 3- to 14-fold risk of alcohol-induced embryofetal damage than infants born to abusers of other drugs (Little and co-workers, 1990b).

Impurities and Dilutants. Because there is little interest in quality control, many illegal substances contain impurities and contaminants. Examples include lead, cyanide, cellulose, herbicides, and pesticides. Many substances are utilized as dilutants, including fine glass beads, powdered sugar, finely ground sawdust, strychnine, arsenic, and antihistamines. Coumadin has also been utilized to "cut" heroin. Some of these dilutants and impurities may have serious adverse effects on both the mother and her fetus.

Specific Substances. Unfortunately, there are not enough data concerning substance use during pregnancy to allow full assessment of risks, especially to the embryo-fetus. Available information is usually confounded by factors that include poor maternal health, malnutrition, infectious diseases, and especially by the use of a myriad of substances.

Alcohol. Ethyl alcohol is a potent teratogen (Table 42–1). It is the most commonly used central nervous system depressant, and as many as 70 percent of Americans imbibe alcohol socially. During pregnancy, alcohol use varies considerably depending on the population studied. In one review, the prevalence was reported to be 1.4 percent (Little and colleagues, 1989). One beer, glass of wine, or mixed drink contains about half an ounce of absolute alcohol, and moderate alcohol abuse is characterized by daily consumption of 4 to 6 drinks, or 2 to 3 ounces of alcohol. Jones (1988) has defined overt alcoholism as ingestion of 8 or more drinks, or 4 ounces or more of absolute alcohol per day.

The *fetal alcohol syndrome* was first described in the human by Jones and colleagues (1973). Subsequently, this association was confirmed by others (Clarren and Smith, 1978; Streissguth and co-workers, 1985). The syndrome is characterized by prenatal and postnatal growth deficiency, mental retardation, behavioral disturbances, and an atypical facial appearance (Fig. 42–4 and Table 42–7). Congenital heart defects and brain anomalies are common, and other major congenital anomalies, such as spina bifida, limb defects, and genitourinary defects, are seen less frequently. This syndrome occurs in 30 to 40 percent of newborns born to women who are frank alcoholics (Jones, 1988).

Although the threshold dose can only be approximated, the fetal alcohol syndrome is usually seen among children of women who drink more than 3 ounces of absolute alcohol daily throughout pregnancy. Lesser amounts may be associated with a variety of less severe manifestations in children called *fetal alcohol effects* (American Medical Association, 1983; Mills and colleagues, 1984). Minor anomalies, moderate growth deficiency, mild mental deficits, and subtle behavioral abnormalities are seen more frequently among children of women who averaged more than 2 to 4 alcoholic drinks daily during pregnancy. Jacobson and colleagues (1992a) recently presented evidence of a "threshold" of prenatal alcohol exposure and impaired neurobehavioral function in offspring. They reported that 30 percent of offspring exposed to 14 ounces of absolute alcohol or greater periconceptionally, or 3.5 ounces or greater during pregnancy, had impaired neurobehavioral functions.

Pragmatically, no safe level for maternal drinking during pregnancy has been established, and the effects of episodic or "binge" drinking have not been clearly defined. Nonhuman primates given a single dose of 4

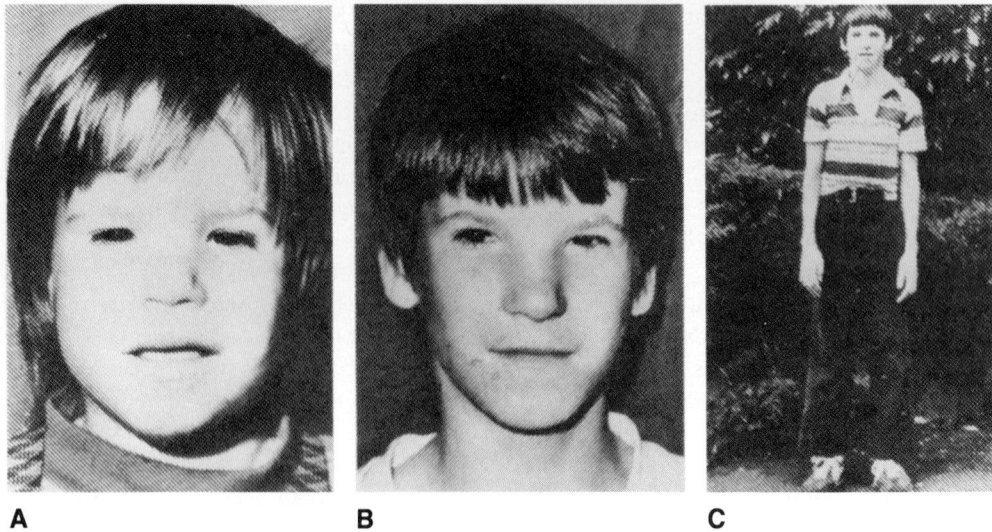

Fig. 42–4. Fetal alcohol syndrome. Male child. **A.** At 2 years 6 months. **B, C.** At 12 years. Note persistence of short palpebral fissures, epicanthial folds, flat midface, hypoplastic philtrum, and thin upper vermilion border. He also has the short, lean prepubertal stature characteristic of young adolescent males with fetal alcohol syndrome. (From Streissguth and colleagues, 1985, with permission.)

ounces of absolute alcohol frequently have pregnancy failures as well as offspring with facial anomalies and central nervous system dysfunction similar to that seen with human fetal alcohol syndrome (Clarren and colleagues, 1987, 1988). These studies at least imply that binge drinking during pregnancy may carry significant risks for congenital and developmental abnormalities.

Autti-Rämö and colleagues (1992) have stressed the importance of identifying and treating women who consume large amounts of alcohol in early pregnancy. In a prospective follow-up of 60 children exposed to alcohol in utero, they identified no adverse effects on either mental or language development in those children who had been exposed to heavy drinking only in the first trimester. Children exposed to heavy drinking through-

out pregnancy, however, had significantly lower scores when tested in these two areas.

The American Medical Association Council on Scientific Affairs (1983) estimated that as many as 1 in 300 live-born infants have stigmata of the fetal alcohol syndrome. Excluding genetic causes, **alcohol ingestion is the most commonly identifiable cause of mental retardation** (Clarren and Smith, 1978).

Tobacco. In a dose-related fashion, maternal smoking appears to be related to an increased frequency of spontaneous abortion, low birthweight, perinatal mortality, and placental abruption (Stillman and colleagues, 1986; Voight and colleagues, 1990). Possible effects of maternal smoking on the incidence of congenital anomalies have been investigated in several studies that included thousands of infants. In the bulk of investigations, the frequency of major congenital anomalies was not increased among infants born to mothers who smoked during pregnancy.

Marijuana. Marijuana or hashish is used by nearly 15 percent of pregnant women (Abel and Sokol, 1988; Chasnoff and colleagues, 1990). The active ingredient is delta-9-tetrahydrocannabinol (THC), which in high doses is teratogenic for animals; however, there is no evidence that marijuana is associated with any adverse human effects (Greenland and colleagues, 1983). In one cohort study, the frequency of major congenital anomalies in 1246 infants born to mothers who smoked marijuana during pregnancy was no greater than background risk (Linn and colleagues, 1983). Although in one study birthweight was lower in infants of mothers who smoked

TABLE 42–7. FEATURES OF FETAL ALCOHOL SYNDROME

Congenital Anomalies
Brain defects
Cardiac defects
Spinal defects

Craniofacial Anomalies
Absent to hypoplastic philtrum
Broad upper lip
Flattened nasal bridge
Hypoplastic upper lip vermilion
Micrognathia
Microphthalmia
Short nose
Short palpebral tissues
Prenatal or postnatal growth retardation

From Jones (1988), with permission.

marijuana than controls, studies with larger sample sizes failed to corroborate this (Greenland and colleagues, 1983; Linn and co-workers, 1983).

Amphetamines. **Dextro-amphetamine** is a sympathomimetic agent used as a central nervous system stimulant, an anorectic, and to treat narcolepsy. It is used illicitly as a stimulant. In three cohort studies of 766 women who took amphetamine during early pregnancy, the frequencies of major and minor congenital anomalies were no greater than in control infants (Heinonen and colleagues, 1983; Milkovich and van den Berg, 1977; Nora and co-workers, 1967).

Methamphetamines are used medically to treat obesity, narcolepsy, and hyperkinetic children. This is also a popular class of "recreational drug," and they are often used to dilute other illicit drugs. In one cohort study of medically supervised methamphetamine use, the frequency of congenital anomalies was not increased compared with controls (Heinonen and co-workers, 1977). In another investigation, symmetric fetal growth retardation was increased compared with control women, but the frequency of congenital anomalies was not different (Little and colleagues, 1988).

Cocaine. Cocaine is derived from the leaves of the South American tree, *Erythroxylon coca.* The drug is a highly effective topical anesthetic and local vasoconstrictor. Through sympathomimetic action by dopamine potentiation it also is a central nervous system stimulant, and currently is one of the most widely abused drugs. The true incidence of cocaine abuse during pregnancy is unknown, and utilization of either a single urine toxicology screen or interview is probably inadequate to assess prevalence (Lowery and associates, 1992). Callahan and colleagues (1992) recently reported that radioimmunoassay of infants' hair and gas chromatography–mass spectrometry of meconium are sensitive methods for detecting fetal cocaine exposure during the last half of pregnancy. As summarized by the American College of Obstetricians and Gynecologists (1990), cocaine may result in numerous maternal medical complications that include acute myocardial infarction, arrhythmias, aortic rupture, strokes, seizures, bowel ischemia, hyperthermia, and sudden death. Additionally, there is an impressive number of adverse pregnancy sequelae evidently caused by cocaine abuse. One of the first reported was abruptio placentae, which frequently resulted in fetal death (Acker, 1983; Bingol, 1987; Chasnoff, 1985; and their colleagues). It is thought that premature placental separation is due to the vasoconstrictive and hypertensive effects of cocaine (see Chap. 37, p. 828). Vascular disruption within the embryo, fetus, or placenta may occur any time after implantation, and it has been suggested that this is particularly hazardous after the first trimester (Hoyme and associates, 1990).

There have been a number of congenital anomalies

TABLE 42–8. CONGENITAL ANOMALIES POSSIBLY RELATED TO COCAINE ABUSE

Segmental intestinal atresia
Limb-reduction defects
Disruptive brain anomalies
Congenital heart defects
Prune-belly syndrome
Urinary tract anomalies

directly attributed to vascular disruption from cocaine (Table 42–8). Five infants with segmental intestinal atresia, 7 with limb-reduction defects, and 21 with disruptive brain anomalies have been described (Chasnoff and colleagues, 1988; MacGregor and co-workers, 1987; Hoyme and associates, 1990). One mechanism by which brain defects may develop is shown in Figure 42–5. All of these embryofetal defects are consistent with well-documented cocaine-induced infarctions in children and adults; other anomalies raise the possibility of vascular-induced lesions. Little and colleagues (1989) reported that 12 percent of 53 exposed infants had a congenital heart defect. Prune-belly anomaly has been reported by several investigators (Bingol and co-workers, 1986; Chasnoff and colleagues, 1985, 1988). A significantly increased risk of urinary tract anomalies among 276 infants whose mothers used cocaine was found in one case-control study (Chavez and colleagues, 1988). Lutiger and colleagues (1991) conducted a meta-analysis of 20 studies and reported a higher rate of genitourinary tract malformations in offspring of cocaine abusers versus those with no drug use.

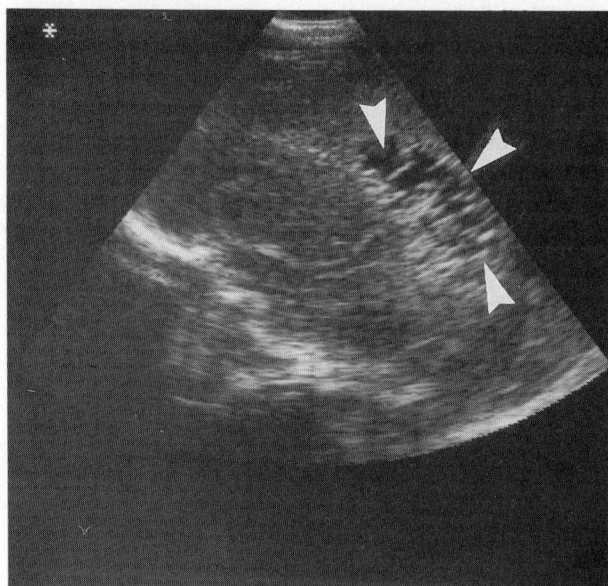

Fig. 42–5. Cocaine-induced fetal brain infarction causing periventricular leukomalacia. Arrows indicate large area of multiocular cavitation that was posterior and lateral to lateral ventricles. (Sonogram courtesy of Dr. Jeff Perlman.)

Heroin. Heroin is an opiate narcotic that is abused worldwide. In most studies, the frequency of congenital anomalies is not higher among infants born to heroin-addicted mothers (Little and associates, 1990c; Naeye and colleagues, 1973). Although the frequency of anomalies was increased in one cohort study of 830 infants born to heroin-addicted mothers, the frequency of 2.4 percent was similar to background risk (Ostrea and Chavez, 1979).

Although congenital anomalies are not increased in these infants, other morbidity is common. Specifically, fetal growth retardation, perinatal death, and a variety of other perinatal complications are observed with high frequency in the offspring of narcotic-addicted mothers (Lifschitz and colleagues, 1983; Little and co-workers, 1990c). It is not clear whether these effects are due to fetal heroin exposure or to generally poor maternal health. Postnatal growth of these children appears to be normal in most cases, although the average head circumference was smaller than that of unexposed children (Lifschitz and co-workers, 1983). In addition, Chasnoff and colleagues (1986), as well as others, have reported mild developmental delay or behavioral disturbances in the children of narcotic-addicted women.

Withdrawal symptoms in exposed neonates are common. Tremors, irritability, sneezing, vomiting, fever, diarrhea, and occasionally seizures are observed in 40 to 80 percent of infants born to heroin-addicted women (Alroomi and colleagues, 1988). Although these symptoms can be of prolonged duration, they usually persist for less than 3 weeks.

Methadone. Methadone is a synthetic opiate narcotic that structurally resembles propoxyphene. Its principal use medically is maintenance therapy for heroin addiction. The frequency of congenital anomalies was not increased above the background rate in cohort studies and clinical series of infants born to heroin-addicted women who were treated with methadone (Stimmel and Adamsons, 1976). Briggs and colleagues (1990) found that infants born to methadone users did not have an increased frequency of congenital anomalies, but withdrawal symptoms frequently developed and birthweight was significantly lower than in unexposed infants. Chasnoff and co-workers (1987) compared 52 cocaine-using pregnant women to 73 women who were former heroin addicts maintained on methadone, and found a significantly higher rate of preterm labor, precipitous labor, abruptio placentae, and meconium staining among cocaine users.

Lysergic Acid Diethylamide (LSD). Lysergic acid amides or lysergides, classically known as lysergic acid diethylamide, are amine alkaloids obtained only through chemical synthesis. There is little evidence that this drug is a human teratogen. Some investigators, but not all, have found increased frequencies of chromosomal breakage in somatic cells of individuals who used lysergic acid, among infants born to women who used the drug, or in human cells incubated in vitro with the drug (Long, 1972). Regardless, changes in somatic cells cannot be extrapolated to the risk for congenital anomalies in children of parents who used lysergic acid.

Phencyclidine (PCP). Phencyclidine (PCP) is no longer manufactured legally, although it is still used "recreationally." Wachsman and cohorts (1989) described 57 infants whose mothers used phencyclidine throughout pregnancy, including embryogenesis, and reported the frequency of congenital anomalies to be no greater than background. Neonatal withdrawal characterized by tremors, jitteriness, and irritability was observed in more than half of exposed infants.

T's and Blues. "T's and blues" is the name given to a street mixture of the narcotic analgesic pentazocine (Talwin) and the over-the-counter antihistamine tripelennamine (Pyribenzamine). Since 1972 this mixture has gained popularity in urban centers among lower socioeconomic groups as a less costly substitute for heroin. Effects of t's and blues abuse by pregnant women have been reported for only 86 women (Chasnoff and colleagues, 1983; Little and co-workers, 1990a; von Almen and Miller, 1984). Infants are more likely to have fetal growth retardation and often suffer from withdrawal symptoms; however, an increased frequency of congenital anomalies was not reported.

References

Aarskog D: Association between maternal intake of diazepam and oral clefts. Lancet 2:921, 1975

Abel EL, Sokol RJ: Marijuana and cocaine use during pregnancy. In Niebyl J (ed): Drug Use in Pregnancy, 2nd ed. Philadelphia, Lea & Febiger, 1988, p 223

Acker D, Sachs BP, Tracey KJ, Wise WE: Abruptio placentae associated with cocaine use. Am J Obstet Gynecol 146:220, 1983

Alroomi LG, Davidson J, Evans TJ, Galea P, Howat R: Maternal narcotic abuse and the newborn. Arch Dis Child 63:81, 1988

American College of Obstetricians and Gynecologists. Cocaine Abuse: Implications for pregnancy. ACOG committee opinion no. 81, March 1990

American Medical Association, Council on Scientific Affairs: Fetal effects of maternal alcohol use. JAMA 249:2517, 1983

Andrews EB, Yankaskas BC, Cordero JF, Schoeffler K, Hampps: Acyclovir in pregnancy registry: Six years experience. Obstet Gynecol 79:7, 1992

Aselton P, Jick H, Milunsky A, Hunter JR, Stergachis A: First trimester drug use and congenital disorders. Obstet Gynecol 65:451, 1985

Autti-Rämö I, Korkman M, Hilakivi-Clark L, Lehtonen M, Halmesmäki E, Granström ML: Mental development of 2-year-old children exposed to alcohol in utero. J Pediatr 120:740, 1992

Barnes AB, Colton T, Gundersen J, Noller KL, Tilley BC, Strama T, Townsend DE, Hatab P, O'Brien PC: Fertility and outcome of pregnancy in women exposed in utero to diethylstilbestrol. N Engl J Med 302:609, 1980

Barr M, Cohen MM: ACE inhibitor fetopathy and hypocalvaria: The kidney–skull connection. Teratology 44:485, 1991

Bingol N, Fuchs M, Diaz V, Stone RK, Gromisch DS: Teratogenicity of cocaine in humans. J Pediatr 110:93, 1987

Bingol N, Fuchs M, Holipas N, Henriquez R, Pagan M, Diaz V: Prune belly syndrome associated with maternal cocaine abuse. Am J Hum Gen 39:A51, 1986

Boutroy MJ: Fetal effects of maternally administered clonidine and angiotensin-converting enzyme inhibitors. Dev Pharmacol Ther 13:199, 1989

Brent RL: Editorial comment: Kudos to the Food and Drug Administration: Reversal of the package insert warning for birth defects for oral contraceptives. Teratology 39:93, 1989

Brent RL: Teratogen update: Bendectin. Teratology 31:429, 1985. Editorial

Brent RL: The Bendectin saga: Another American tragedy. Teratology 27:283, 1983. Editorial

Briggs GG, Freeman RK, Yaffe SJ: Drugs in Pregnancy and Lactation, 3rd ed. Baltimore, Williams & Wilkins, 1990

Brumfitt W, Pursell R: Trimethoprim/sulfamethoxazole in the treatment of bacteriuria in women. J Infect Dis 128:657, 1973

Buehler BA, Delimont D, van Waes M, Finnell RH: Prenatal prediction of risk of the fetal hydantoin syndrome. N Engl J Med 322:1567, 1990

Callahan CM, Grant TM, Phipps P, Clark G, Novack AH, Streissguth AP, Raisys VA: Measurement of gestational cocaine exposure: Sensitivity of infants' hair, meconium, and urine. J Pediatr 120:763, 1992

Centers for Disease Control: Use of supplements containing high-dose vitamin A—New York. MMWR 36:80, 1987

Centers for Disease Control: Isotretinoin—A newly recognized human teratogen. MMWR 33:171, 1984

Char F: Denouement and discussion: Aminopterin embryopathy syndrome. Am J Dis Child 133:1189, 1979

Chasnoff IJ: Drugs, alcohol, pregnancy, and the neonate: Pay now or pay later. JAMA 266:1567, 1991. Editorial

Chasnoff IJ, Burns KA, Burns WJ: Cocaine use in pregnancy: Perinatal Morbidity and Mortality. Neurotoxicol Teratol 9:291, 1987

Chasnoff IJ, Burns KA, Burns WJ, Schnoll SH: Prenatal drug exposure: Effects on neonatal and infant growth development. Neurobehav Toxicol Teratol 8:357, 1986

Chasnoff IJ, Burns WJ, Schnoll SH, Burns KA: Cocaine use in pregnancy. N Engl J Med 313:666, 1985

Chasnoff IJ, Chisum GM, Kaplan WE: Maternal cocaine use and genitourinary tract malformations. Teratology 37:201, 1988

Chasnoff IJ, Hatcher R, Burns WJ, Schnoll SH: Pentazocine and Tripelennamine (t's and blue's): Effects on the fetus and neonate. Dev Pharmacol Ther 6:162, 1983

Chasnoff IJ, Landress HJ, Barrett ME: The prevalence of illicit drug or alcohol use during pregnancy and the discrepancies in mandatory reporting in Pinellas County, Florida. N Engl J Med 322:1202, 1990

Chavez GF, Mulinare J, Cordero JF: Maternal cocaine use and the risk for genitourinary tract defects: An epidemiologic approach. Am J Hum Genet 43:A43, 1988

Clarren SK, Astley SJ, Bowden DM: Physical anomalies and developmental delays in nonhuman primate infants exposed to weekly doses of ethanol during gestation. Teratology 37:561, 1988

Clarren SK, Bowden DM, Astley SJ: Pregnancy outcomes after weekly oral administration of ethanol during gestation in the pig-tailed macaque (Macaca nemestrina). Teratology 35:345, 1987

Clarren SK, Smith DW: The fetal alcohol syndrome. N Engl J Med 298:1063, 1978

Conway N, Birt DN: Streptomycin in pregnancy: Effect on the foetal ear. BMJ 2:260, 1965

Cordero JF, Oakley GP: Drug exposure during pregnancy: Some epidemiologic considerations. Clin Obstet Gynecol 26:418, 1983

Crombie DL, Pinsent R, Fleming D: Imipramine in pregnancy. BMJ 1:745, 1972

Csaba I, Sulyok FE, Ertl T: Relationship of maternal treatment with indomethacin to persistence of fetal circulation syndrome. J Pediatr 92:484, 1978

Cunningham FG, Lowe TW: Cardiovascular diseases complicating pregnancy. Williams Obstetrics, 18th ed(suppl 14). Norwalk, CT, Appleton & Lange, October/November 1991

Dai WS, Hsu MA, Itri LM: Safety of pregnancy after discontinuation of isotretinoin. Arch Dermatol 125:362, 1989

Dalens B, Raynaud EJ, Gaulme J: Teratogenicity of valproic acid. J Pediatr 97:332, 1980

Davidson JM, Dallagrammatikas H, Parkin JM: Maternal azathioprine therapy and depressed hemopoiesis in the babies of renal allograft patients. Br J Obstet Gynaecol 92:233, 1985

DeWitte DB, Buick MK, Cyran SE, Maisels MJ: Neonatal pancytopenia and severe combined immunodeficiency associated with antenatal administration of azathioprine and prednisone. J Pediatr 105:625, 1984

DiGiovanna JJ, Zezh LA, Ruddel ME, Gantt G, McClean SW, Gross EG, Peck GL: Etretinate: Persistent serum levels of a potent teratogen. Clin Res 32:579A, 1984

DiLiberti JH, Farndon PA, Dennis NR, Curry CJR: The fetal valproate syndrome. Am J Med Genet 19:473, 1984

Doll DC, Ringenberg S, Yarbro JW: Antineoplastic agents and pregnancy. Semin Oncol 16:337, 1989

Dumesic DA, Silverman NH, Tobias S, Golbus MS: Transplacental cardioversion of fetal supraventricular tachycardia with procainamide. N Engl J Med 307:1128, 1982

Farkas VG, Farkas G: Teratogenic action of hyperemesis in pregnancy and of medication used to treat it. Zentralbl Gynaekol 93:325, 1971

Food and Drug Administration Drug Bulletin: Pregnancy categories for prescription drugs. September 1979

Foulon W, Naessens A, Mahler T, deWaele M, deCatte L, deMeuter F: Prenatal diagnosis of congenital toxoplasmosis. Obstet Gynecol 76:769, 1990

Friedman JM: Teratogen update: Anesthetic agents. Teratology 37:69, 1988

Freidman JM, Little BB, Brent RL, Cordero JF, Hanson JW, Shepard TH: Potential human teratogenicity of frequently prescribed drugs. Obstet Gynecol 75:594, 1990

German J, Kowal A, Ellers KH: Trimethadione and human teratogenesis. Teratology 3:349, 1970

Gilstrap LC, Bawdon RE, Burris JS: Antibiotic concentration in maternal blood, cord blood, and placental membranes in chorioamnionitis. Obstet Gynecol 72:124, 1988

Gomby DS, Shiono PH: Estimating the number of substance-exposed infants. Future Child 1:17, 1991

Greenland S, Richwald GA, Honda GD: The effects of marijuana use during pregnancy: II. A study in a low-risk home-delivery population. Drug Alcohol Depend 11:359, 1983

Grote W, Harms D, Janig U, Kietzmann H, Ravens U, Schwarze I: Malformation of fetus conceived 4 months after termination of maternal etretinate treatment. Lancet 1:1276, 1985

Grumbach MM, Ducharme JR: The effects of androgens on fetal sexual development. Androgen-induced female pseudohermaphrodism. Fertil Steril 11:157, 1960

Haibach H, Akhter JE, Muscato MS, Cary PL, Hoffmann MF: Acetaminophen overdose with fetal demise. Am J Clin Pathol 82:240, 1984

Hall JG, Pauli RM, Wilson K: Maternal and fetal sequelae of anticoagulation during pregnancy. Am J Med 68:122, 1980

Hammill H: Metronidazole, clindamycin, and quinolones. Obstet Gynecol North Am 16:317, 1989

Hansen JW, Smith DW: The fetal hydantoin syndrome. J Pediatr 87:285, 1975

Happle R, Traupe H, Bounameaux Y, Fisch T: Teratogenicity of etretinate in humans. Dtsch Med Wochenschr 109:1476, 1984

Harrigan JT, Kangos JJ, Sikka KR, Spisso KR, Natarajan N, Rosenfeld D, Leiman S, Korn D: Successful treatment of fetal congestive failure secondary to tachycardia. N Engl J Med 304:1527, 1981

Heinonen OP, Slone D, Shapiro S: Birth Defects and Drugs in Pregnancy. Littleton, MA, Publishing Sciences Group, 1977

Heinonen OP, Slone D, Shapiro S: Birth Defects and Drugs in Pregnancy. Littleton, MA, John Wright–Publishing Sciences Group, 1983

Hengst VP: Investigations of the teratogenicity of Daraprim (pyrimethamine) in humans. Zentralbl Gynakol 94:551, 1972

Herbst AL: Clear cell adenocarcinoma and the current status of DES-exposed females. Cancer 48:484, 1981

Herbst AL, Hubby MM, Azizi F, Makii MM: Reproductive and gynecologic surgical experience in diethylstilbestrol-exposed daughters. Am J Obstet Gynecol 141:1019, 1981

Herbst AL, Hubby MM, Blough RR, Azizi F: A comparison of pregnancy experience in DES-exposed and DES-unexposed daughters. J Reprod Med 24:62, 1980

Herbst AL, Poskanzer DC, Robboy SJ, Friedlander L, Scully RE: Prenatal exposure to stilbestrol: A prospective comparison of exposed female offspring with unexposed controls. N Engl J Med 292:334, 1975

Hermans PE, Wilhelm MP: Vancomycin. Mayo Clin Proc 62:901, 1987

Hickok DE, Hollenbach KA, Reilley SF, Nyberg DA: The association between decreased amniotic fluid volume and treatment with nonsteroidal anti-inflammatory agents for preterm labor. Am J Obstet Gynecol 160:1525, 1989

Hirsch KS, Wilson JG, Scott WJ, O'Flaherty EJ: Acetazolamide teratology and its association with carbonic anhydrase inhibition in the mouse. Teratogenesis Carcinog Mutagen 3:133, 1983

Holmes LB: Teratogen update: Bendectin. Teratology 27:277, 1983

Horvath JS, Phippard A, Korda A, Henderson-Smart DS, Child A,

Tiller DJ: Clonidine hydrochloride: A safe and effective antihypertensive agent in pregnancy. Obstet Gynecol 66:634, 1985

Hoyme HE, Jones KL, Dixon SD, Jewett T, Hanson JW, Robinson LK, Msaii ME, Allanson JE: Prenatal cocaine exposure and fetal vascular disruption. Pediatrics 85:743, 1990

Ismail MA, Lerner SA: Disseminated blastomycosis in a pregnant woman. Am Rev Respir Dis 126:350, 1982

Jacobson JL, Jacobson SW, Sokol RS, Martier SS, Ager JW: Prenatal alcohol exposure and neurobehavioral function in infancy: Evidence for threshold and differential vulnerability. Am J Obstet Gynecol 166:346, 1992a

Jacobson SJ, Jones K, Johnson K, Ceolin L, Kaur P, Sahn D, Donnenfeld AE, Rieder M, Santelli R, Smythe J, Pastuszak A, Einarson T, Koren G: Prospective multicentre study of pregnancy outcome after lithium exposure during the first trimester. Lancet 339:530, 1992b

Jager-Roman E, Deichl A, Jakob S, Hartmann A-M, Koch S, Rating D, Steldinger R, Nau H, Helge H: Fetal growth, major malformations, and minor anomalies in infants born to women receiving valproic acid. J Pediatr 108:997, 1986

Jick H, Holmes LB, Hunter JR, Madsen S, Stergachis A: First-trimester drug use and congenital disorders. JAMA 246:343-6, 1981

Jones KL: Smith's Recognizable Patterns of Human Malformation, 4th ed. Philadelphia, Saunders, 1988

Jones KL, Lacro RV, Johnson KA, Adams J: Patterns of malformations in the children of women treated with carbamazepine during pregnancy. N Engl J Med 320:1661, 1989

Jones KL, Smith DW, Ulleland CN, Streissguth AP: Patterns of malformation in offspring of chronic alcoholic mothers. Lancet 1:1267, 1973

Kaufman RH, Noller K, Adam E, Irwin J, Gray M, Jeffries JA, Hilton J: Upper genital tract abnormalities and pregnancy outcome in diethylstilbestrol-exposed progeny. Am J Obstet Gynecol 148:973, 1984

Kelly TE: Teratogenicity of anticonvulsant drugs: I. Review of the literature. Am J Med Gen 19:413, 1984

Kerenyi TD, Gleicher N, Meller J, Brown E, Steinfeld L, Chitkara U, Raucher H: Transplacental cardioversion of intrauterine supraventricular tachycardia with digitalis. Lancet 2:393, 1980

Killeen AA, Bowers LD: Fetal supraventricular tachycardia treated with high-dose quinidine: Toxicity associated with marked elevation of the metabolite, 3(S)-3-hydroxy-quinidine. Obstet Gynecol 70:445, 1987

Kirshon B, Wasserstrum N, Willis R, Herman GE, McCabe ERB: Teratogenic effects of first trimester cyclophosphamide therapy. Obstet Gynecol 72:462, 1988

Kleinman CS, Copel JA: Electrophysiological principles and fetal antiarrhythmic therapy. Ultrasound Obstet Gynecol 1:286, 1991

Knapp K, Lenz W, Nowack E: Multiple congenital abnormalities. Lancet 2:725, 1962

Kutscher AH, Zegarelli EV, Tovell HM, Hochberg B, Hauptman J: Discoloration of deciduous teeth induced by administration of tetracycline antepartum. Am J Obstet Gynecol 96:291, 1966

Lammer EJ: Embryopathy in infant conceived one year after termination of maternal etretinate. Lancet 2:1080, 1988

Lammer EJ, Chen DT, Hoar RM, Agnish ND, Benke PJ, Braun JT, Curry CJ, Fernhoff PM, Griz AW Jr, Lott IT, Richard JM,

Sun SC: Retinoic acid embryopathy. N Engl J Med 313:837, 1985

Lammer EJ, Hayes AM, Schunior A, Holmes LB: Risk for major malformation among human fetuses exposed to isotretinoin (13-cis-retinoic acid). Teratology 35:68A, 1987

Landers DV, Green JR, Sweet RL: Antibiotic use during pregnancy and the postpartum period. Clin Obstet Gynecol 26:391, 1983

Lenke RR, VanDorsten JP, Schifrin BS: Pyelonephritis in pregnancy: A prospective randomized trial to prevent recurrent disease evaluating suppressive therapy with nitrofurantoin and close surveillance. Am J Obstet Gynecol 146:953, 1983

Levin D, Fixler D, Morriss F, Tyson J: Morphologic analysis of the pulmonary vascular bed in infants exposed in utero to prostaglandin synthetase inhibitors. J Pediatr 92:478, 1978

Lewis PE, Cefalo RC, Naulty JS, Rodkey FL: Placental transfer and fetal toxicity of sodium nitroprusside. Gynecol Invest 8:46, 1977

Lifschitz MH, Wilson GS, Smith EO, Desmond MM: Fetal and postnatal growth of children born to narcotic-dependent women. J Pediatr 102:686, 1983

Linn S, Schoenbaum SC, Monson RR, Rosner R, Stubblefield PC, Ryan KJ: The association of marijuana use with outcome of pregnancy. Am J Public Health 73:1161, 1983

Little BB, Gilstrap LC III: Drug overdoses during pregnancy. In Little BB, Gilstrap LC III (eds): Drugs and Pregnancy. New York, Elsevier, 1992

Little BB, Snell LM, Gilstrap LC: Methamphetamine abuse during pregnancy: Outcome and infant effects. Obstet Gynecol 72:541, 1988

Little BB, Snell LM, Gilstrap LC, Breckenridge JD, Knoll KA: Effects of t's and blues abuse during pregnancy on maternal and infant health status. Am J Perinatol 7:359, 1990a

Little BB, Snell LM, Gilstrap LC, Gant NF, Rosenfeld CR: Alcohol abuse during pregnancy: Changes in frequency in a large urban hospital. Obstet Gynecol 74:547, 1989

Little BB, Snell LM, Gilstrap LC, Johnston WL: A review of patterns of substance abuse during pregnancy: Implications for the mother and fetus. South Med J 83:507, 1990b

Little BB, Snell LM, Klein VR, Gilstrap LC: Cocaine abuse during pregnancy: Maternal and fetal implications. Obstet Gynecol 73:157, 1989

Little BB, Snell LM, Klein VR, Gilstrap LC, Knoll KA, Breckenridge JD: Maternal and fetal effects of heroin addiction during pregnancy. J Reprod Med 35:159, 1990c

Long SY: Does LSD induce chromosomal damage and malformations? A review of the literature. Teratology 6:75, 1972

Lowery CL, Crone C, Kirby R, Valentine J: Anonymous drug screening of prenatal patients by paired urine collection and drug history. Am J Obstet Gynecol 166:314, 1992

Lutiger B, Graham K, Einarson TR, Koren G: Relationship between gestational cocaine use and pregnancy outcome: A meta-analysis. Teratology 44:405, 1991

MacGregor SN: Human immunodeficiency virus infection in pregnancy. Clin Perinatol 18:33, 1991

MacGregor SN, Keith LG, Chasnoff IJ, Rosner MA, Chisum GM, Shaw P, Minogue JP: Cocaine use during pregnancy: Adverse perinatal outcome. Am J Obstet Gynecol 157:686, 1987

Messina M, Biffignandi P, Ghigo E, Jeantet MG, Molinatti GM: Possible contraindication of spironolactone during pregnancy. J Endocrinol Invest 2:222, 1979

Milkovich L, van den Berg BJ: Effects of antenatal exposure to anorectic drugs. Am J Obstet Gynecol 129:637, 1977

Mills JL, Alexander D: Teratogens and "litogens." N Engl J Med 315:1234, 1986

Mills JL, Graubard BI, Harley EE, Rhoads GG, Berendes HW: Maternal alcohol consumption and birth weight. How much drinking during pregnancy is safe? JAMA 252:1875, 1984

Milunsky A, Graef JW, Gaynor MF: Methotrexate-induced congenital malformations. J Pediatr 72:790-95, 1968

Morrow AW: Imipramine and congenital abnormalities. NZ Med J 75:228, 1972

Murad SH, Tabsh KM, Shilyanski G, Kapur PA, Ma C, Lee C, Conklin KA: Effects of verapamil on uterine blood flow and maternal cardiovascular function in the awake pregnant ewe. Anesth Analg 64:7, 1985

Murray CL, Reichert JA, Anderson J, Twiggs LB: Multimodal cancer therapy for breast cancer in first trimester of pregnancy. JAMA 252:2607, 1984

Naeye RL, Blanc W, Leblanc W, Khatamee MA: Fetal complications of maternal heroin addiction: Abnormal growth, infections, and episodes of stress. J Pediatr 83:1055, 1973

Niebyl JR, Blake DA, Freeman JM, Luft RD: Carbamazepine levels in pregnancy and lactation. Obstet Gynecol 53:139, 1979

Niebyl JR, Blake D, White R, Kumor KM, Dubin NH, Robinson JC, Egnor PG: The inhibition of premature labor with indomethacin. Am J Obstet Gynecol 136:1014, 1980

Nora JJ, McNamara DG, Fraser FC: Dexamphetamine sulfate and human malformations. Lancet 1:570, 1967

Orkin M, Maibach HI: Scabies and pediculosis pubis. Dermatol Clin 1:111, 1983

Oro AS, Dixon SP: Perinatal cocaine and methamphetamine exposure: Maternal and neonatal correlates. J Pediatr 111:571, 1987

Ostrea EM, Chavez CJ: Perinatal problems (excluding neonatal withdrawal) in maternal drug addiction: A study of 830 cases. J Pediatr 94:292, 1979

Piper JM, Baum C, Kennedy DL: Prescription drug use before and during pregnancy in a Medicaid population. Am J Obstet Gynecol 157:148, 1987

Pons JC, Taburet AM, Singlas E, Delfraissy JF, Papiernik E: Placental passage of azathiothymidine (AZT) during the second trimester of pregnancy: Study by direct fetal blood sampling under ultrasound. Eur J Obstet Gynecol Reprod Biol 40:229, 1991

Pryde PG, Nugent CE, Sedman AB: ACE inhibitor fetopathy. Am J Obstet Gynecol 166:348, 1992

Quagliarello J, Greco MA: Danazol and urogenital sinus formation in pregnancy. Fertil Steril 43:939, 1985

Reid DWJ, Caille G, Kaufmann NR: Maternal and transplacental kinetics of trimethoprim and sulfamethoxazole, separately and in combination. Can Med Assoc J 112:675, 1975

Rey E, Duperron L, Gauthier R, Lemay M, Grignon A, LeLorier J: Transplacental treatment of tachycardia-induced fetal heart failure with verapamil and amiodarone: A case report. Am J Obstet Gynecol 153:311, 1985

Richards LG: Demographic Trenda and Drug Abuse, 1980–1985. NIDA research monograph 35. Department of Health and Human Services, Washington, DC, May 1985

Robboy SJ, Noller KL, O'Brien P, Kaufman RH, Townsend D, Barnes AB, Gundersen J, Lawrence D, Bergstrahl E, McGorray S, Tilley BC, Anton J, Chazen G: Increased incidence of cervical and vaginal dysplasia in 3,980 diethylstilbestrol-exposed young women. Experience of the National Collaborative Diethylstilbestrol Adenosis Project. JAMA 252:2979, 1984

Robboy SJ, Szyfelbein WM, Goellner JR, Kaufman RH, Taft PD, Richard RM, Gaffey TA, Prat J, Virata R, Hatab PA, McGorray SP, Noller KL, Townsend D, Labarthe D, Barnes AB: Dysplasia and cytologic findings in 4,589 young women enrolled in Diethylstilbestrol-Adenosis (DESAD) project. Am J Obstet Gynecol 140:579, 1981

Robert E, Robert JM, Lapras C: Is valproic acid teratogenic? Rev Neurol 139:445, 1983

Rosa FW: Virilization of the female fetus with maternal danazol exposure. Am J Obstet Gynecol 149:99, 1984

Rosa FW, Baum C, Shaw M: Pregnancy outcomes after first trimester vaginitis drug therapy. Obstet Gynecol 69:751, 1987a

Rosa FW, Hernandez C, Carlo WA: Griseofulvin teratology, including two thoracopagus conjoined twins. Lancet 1:171, 1987b

Rosa FW, Wilk AL, Kelsey FO: Teratogen update: Vitamin A congeners. Teratology 33:355, 1986

Rosenberg L, Mitchell AA, Parsells JL, Pashayan H, Louik C, Shapiro S: Lack of relation of oral clefts to diazepam use during pregnancy. N Engl J Med 309:1282, 1983

Rotmensch HH, Elkayam U, Frishman W: Antiarrhythmic drug therapy during pregnancy. Ann Intern Med 98:487, 1983

Rotmensch HH, Rotmensch S, Elkayam U: Management of cardiac arrhythmias during pregnancy: Current concepts. Drugs 33:623, 1987

Sandberg EC, Riffle NL, Higdon JV, Getman CE: Pregnancy outcome in women exposed to diethylstilbestrol in utero. Am J Obstet Gynecol 140:194, 1981

Saxen I, Saxen L: Association between maternal intake of diazepam and oral clefts. Lancet 2:498, 1975

Schardein JL: Chemically Induced Birth Defects. New York, Marcel Dekker, 1985

Sharpe AH, Hunter JJ, Ruprecht RM, Jaenisch R: Maternal transmission of retroviral disease and strategies for preventing infection of the neonate. J Virol 63:1049, 1989

Shepard TH: Catalog of Teratogenic Agents, 6th ed. Baltimore, Johns Hopkins University Press, 1989

Shepard TH: Human teratogenicity. Adv Pediatr 33:225, 1986

Shiono PH, Mills JL: Oral clefts and diazepam use during pregnancy. N Engl J Med 311:919, 1984

Sibai BM, Amon EA: How safe is aspirin use during pregnancy? Contemp Obstet Gynecol 32:73, 1988

Sibai BM, Barton JR, Sarinoglu C, Mercer BM: A randomized prospective comparison of nifedipine and bed rest alone in the management of preeclampsia remote from term. Am J Obstet Gynecol 166:280, 1992

Sibai BM, Gonzalez AR, Mabie WC, Moretti M: A comparison of labetalol plus hospitalization versus hospitalization alone in the management of preeclampsia remote from term. Obstet Gynecol 70:323, 1987

Sibai BM, Mabie WC, Shamsa F, Villar GD: A comparison of no medication versus methyldopa or labetalol in chronic hypertension during pregnancy. Am J Obstet Gynecol 162:960, 1990

Slone D, Siskind V, Heinonen OP, Monson RR, Kaufman DW, Shapiro S: Aspirin and congenital malformations. Lancet 1:1372, 1976

Snyder DE, Layde PM, Johnson MW, Lyle MA: Treatment of tuberculosis during pregnancy. Am Rev Respir Dis 122:65, 1980

Stevenson RE, Burton M, Ferlauto GJ, Taylor HA: Hazards of oral anticoagulants during pregnancy. JAMA 243:1549, 1980

Stickler SM, Dansky LV, Miler MA, Seni MH, Andermann E, Spielberg SP: Genetic predisposition to phenytoin-induced birth defects. Lancet 2:746, 1985

Stillman RJ: In utero exposure to diethylstilbestrol: Adverse effects on the reproductive tract and reproductive performance in male and female offspring. Am J Obstet Gynecol 142:905, 1982

Stillman RJ, Rosenberg MJ, Sachs BP: Smoking and reproduction. Fertil Steril 46:545, 1986

Stimmel B, Adamsons K: Narcotic dependency in pregnancy. Methadone maintenance compared to use of street drugs. JAMA 235:1121, 1976

Streissguth AP, Clarren SK, Jones KL: Natural history of the fetal alcohol syndrome: A 10-year follow-up of eleven patients. Lancet 2:85, 1985

Streissguth AP, Treder RP, Barr HM, Shepard TH, Bleyer WA, Sampson PD, Martin DC: Aspirin and acetaminophen use by pregnant women and subsequent child IQ and attention decrements. Teratology 35:211, 1987

Taylor U, Bardeguez A: Antiretroviral therapy during pregnancy and postpartum. Am J Obstet Gynecol 166:390, 1992

Thomas D, Buchanan N: Teratogenic effects of anticonvulsants. J Pediatr 99:163, 1981

Thomson EJ, Cordero JF: The new teratogens: Accutane and other vitamin-A analogs. MCN 14:244, 1989

Turner G, Collins E: Fetal effects of regular salicylate ingestion in pregnancy. Lancet 2:338, 1975

Voight LF, Hollenbach KA, Krohn MA, Daling JR, Hickok DE: The relationship of abruptio placentae with maternal smoking and small-for-gestational-age infants. Obstet Gynecol 75:771, 1990

von Almen WF, Miller JM: "T's and blues" in pregnancy. J Reprod Med 31:236, 1984

Wachsman L, Schuetz S, Chan LS, Wingert WA: What happens to babies exposed to phencyclidine (PCP) in utero? Am J Drug Alcohol Abuse 15:31, 1989

Wallace R, Caldwell D, Ansbacher R, Otterson W: Inhibition of premature labor by terbutaline. Obstet Gynecol 51:387, 1978

Warkany J: Aminopterin and methotrexate: Folic acid deficiency. Teratology 17:353, 1978

Weinstein MR: Lithium treatment of women during pregnancy and in the post-delivery period. In Johnson FN (ed): Handbook of Lithium Therapy. Baltimore, University Park Press, 1980, p 421

Whalley PJ, Adams RH, Combes B: Tetracycline toxicity in pregnancy: Liver and pancreatic dysfunction. JAMA 189:357, 1964

Wiseman RA, Dodds-Smith IC: Cardiovascular birth defects and antenatal exposure to female sex hormones: A reevaluation of some basic data. Teratology 30:359, 1984

Wolfe MS, Cordero JF: Safety of chloroquine in chemosuppression of malaria during pregnancy. BMJ 290:1466, 1985

Yazigi R, Cunningham FG: Cancer and pregnancy. Williams Obstetrics, 18th ed (suppl 4), February/March, 1990

Zackai EH, Mellman WJ, Neiderer B, Hanson JW: The fetal trimethadione syndrome. J Pediatr 87:280, 1975

CHAPTER 43
Imaging Modalities During Pregnancy

Imaging modalities used as an adjunct for both diagnosis and therapy during pregnancy include ultrasound, magnetic resonance imaging, and x-ray. Of these, x-ray is the most worrisome to both the obstetrician and the patient with regard to its safety for the fetus. Many radiological procedures are performed during early pregnancy prior to the time pregnancy is diagnosed. These procedures are frequently undertaken because of emergencies such as trauma or life-threatening illness. Fortunately, most diagnostic x-ray procedures are associated with little or no known significant fetal risks. However, as with drugs and medications, radiological procedures done during pregnancy may lead to litigation if there is an adverse pregnancy outcome, including therapeutic abortion because of patient or physician anxiety.

Ionizing Radiation

Radiation is a poorly understood term that often is applied not only to x-rays, but also to microwaves, ultrasound, diathermy, and radiowaves. The latter four energy forms have rather long wavelengths and are of low energy (Brent, 1989). Conversely, x-rays and gamma rays have short wavelengths with very high energy, and are forms of *ionizing radiation*. The types of radiation and their biological effects are summarized in Table 43–1.

Thus, ionizing radiation from x-rays and gamma rays, with their high energy, is of primary concern from a biological standpoint. Ionizing radiation refers to waves or particles (photons) of significant energy that can break chemical bonds, such as those in DNA, or create free radicals or ions capable of causing tissue damage (Hall, 1991). Methods of measuring x-ray effects are summarized in Table 43–2. The standard terms used are the exposure (in air), the dose (to tissue), and the relative effective dose (to tissue). In the range of energies for diagnostic x-rays, the dose, expressed in *rad*, and the relative effective dose expressed in *rem*, are the same, so that these units can be used interchangeably. For the sake of consistency, all doses to follow will be expressed in rad, the traditional unit, or Gray (Gy), the modern unit.

X-Ray Dose Estimation. When calculating the dose of ionizing radiation such as that from x-ray, several factors are considered: (1) the type of study, (2) the type and age of equipment, (3) the distance of the organ in question from the source of radiation, (4) the thickness of the body part penetrated, and (5) the method or technique employed for the study (Wagner and colleagues, 1985). When evaluating dose estimates, consideration is given not only to the mathematical model used, but also to when the data were compiled. The use of faster screen–film combinations, higher frequency x-ray generators, and other technical improvements have contributed significantly to reduced radiation exposures in recent years.

Estimates of dose to the uterus and embryo for a variety of commonly used radiological examinations (plain film) are summarized in Table 43–3. These data are based on measurements made with an anthropometric phantom and do not account for differences in size and build of individual patients. These estimates are also made without consideration for usual gonadal shielding during the study. Radiological studies of maternal body parts at the greatest distances from the uterus—for example, the head—result in a very small dose of scattered radiation to the developing embryo or fetus. The specific anthropometric features of the woman, x-ray techniques used, and performance parameters of the equipment should all be considered. Thus, data presented in the tables should serve only as a guideline. When the dose of radiation for a specific individual is required, a medical physicist may be consulted.

Potential Adverse Fetal Effects. The harmful effects of ionizing radiation can be direct or indirect with three principal biological effects; (1) cell death, which affects embryogenesis; (2) carcinogenesis; and (3) genetic effects of future generations from germ cell mutations (Brent, 1989; Hall, 1991). The harmful fetal effects of ionizing radiation have been extensively studied in the case of cell damage with resultant dysfunction of embryogenesis, both in the animal model as well as from human studies of Japanese atomic bomb survivors. Interestingly, adverse radiation effects in animals appear to be somewhat different than in humans.

Animal Studies. A number of animal studies have addressed potential embryopathological effects of ionizing radiation (Brent, 1971, 1989; Russell and Russell, 1950, 1954; Wilson and colleagues, 1953). Several conclusions can be drawn: (1) large-dose ionizing radiation is most likely to be lethal to the embryo during the pre-implantation stage (i.e., the pre-blastocyst); the embryo is very insensitive to teratogenic or other effects of radiation at this time; (2) during the period of embryo-

TABLE 43–1. COMPARATIVE ASPECTS OF VARIOUS FORMS OF RADIATION

Type	Physical Characteristics	Biological Effects
X-rays, γ-rays	Short-wavelength electromagnetic waves, highly penetrating, with the capacity of producing ionization within tissues and subsequent electrochemical reactions.	Electrochemical reaction. Can result in tissue damage with high exposures that result in cell death, mutation, cancer, and developmental defects. Effects are dose related.
Microwaves, radar, diathermy	Longer electromagnetic waves with variable ability to penetrate, but no ability to produce ionization within tissues.	The primary biological effect is hyperthermia, although possible nonthermal effects are being investigated. Cataract development is the most widely known complication of extensive microwave or radar exposure.
Ultrasound	Sound waves with a frequency above the audible range, which produce mechanical compression and rarefactions in matter, and with *no* capability of producing ionization.	If the energy is high enough, sound waves can cause tissue disruption by the production of cavitation and streaming as well as hyperthermia. None of these effects occur with energies used in diagnostic ultrasonography.

From Brent (1989), with permission.

TABLE 43–2. SOME MEASURES OF IONIZING RADIATION

Exposure	The number of ions produced by x-rays per kg of air. Unit: Roentgen (R)

Dose	The amount of energy deposited per kg of tissue
	    Traditional unit: rad[a]
	    Modern unit: Gray (Gy) [1 Gy = 100 rad]

Relative effective dose	The amount of energy deposited per kg of tissue normalized for biological effectiveness
	    Traditional unit: rem[a]
	    Modern unit: Sievert (Sv) [1 Sv = 100 rem]

[a] For diagnostic x-rays, 1 rad = 1 rem.

genesis (i.e., organogenesis), such radiation is more likely to cause teratogenicity, growth retardation, or lethal effects; (3) during the fetal period, the fetus will more likely manifest central nervous system effects and growth retardation.

Various organs may manifest teratogenic effects in the animal model, whereas in the human, growth retardation and central nervous system anomalies are the most common following high-dose ionizing radiation. Most of these studies involved large doses—100 to 200 rad (1 to 2 Gy)—and a threshold phenomenon was demonstrated (Brent, 1989). The effects of 200 rad of ionizing radiation in the mouse are summarized in Figure 43–1. Unfortunately, as with drugs and medications, it is not always possible to extrapolate animal data directly to the human.

Human Data. Possible adverse human fetal effects of high-dose ionizing radiation are principally derived from

two sources. One source is the earlier reports of large-dose radiation given to treat women for a variety of reasons that included malignancy, menorrhagia, or uterine myomas. (Brent, 1989). Goldstein and Murphy (1929) reported the adverse effects of an estimated radiation exposure of more than 100 rad. They described either microcephaly or hydrocephaly in 19 of 75 exposed embryos. Other adverse effects included mental retardation, abnormal genitalia, growth retardation, microphthalmia, and cataracts. Dekaban (1968) reported 22 infants with microcephaly, mental retardation, or both following exposure to an estimated 250 rad in the first half of pregnancy. In both of these studies, other organ malformations were not found unless there was microcephaly, eye abnormalities, or growth retardation (Brent, 1989).

The second and most often quoted human data are derived from multiple studies of atomic bomb survivors from Hiroshima and Nagasaki (Miller and Blot, 1972; Miller and Mulvihill, 1982; Otake, 1986; Otake and co-workers, 1987). Yamazaki and Schull (1990) recently summarized the adverse effects from in utero exposure to fallout from the atomic bomb in these two cities. As shown in Figure 43–2, there is an increased risk of microcephaly and severe mental retardation with high exposure at certain gestational ages. The risk is greatest at 8 to 15 weeks, and larger doses were necessary at 16 to 25 weeks to cause equivalent percentages of mental retardation. Another important observation is the suggestion of a nonthreshold linear relationship of radiation dose at 8 to 15 weeks' gestation, so that even very low doses will cause a slight increase in mental retardation compared with the general population (Hall, 1991). There is no documented increased risk of mental retardation in humans at gestational ages less than 8 weeks or greater than 25 weeks, even with doses exceeding 50 rad (Committee on Biological Effects, 1990).

The effect of ionizing radiation on intelligence quotient (IQ) scores in children exposed in utero is also dependent on gestational age as well as radiation dose (Fig. 43–3). The highest risk again is at 8 to 15 weeks, followed by 16 to 25 weeks for doses greater than 50 rad.

The implications of these findings seem straightfor-

TABLE 43–3. DOSE TO THE UTERUS FOR COMMON RADIOLOGICAL PROCEDURES OF CONCERN IN OBSTETRICS

Study	View	Dose[a]/ View (mrad)	Films/Study[b]	Dose/Study (mrad)
Skull[c]	AP, PA	< 0.01		
	Lat	< 0.01	4.1	< 0.05
Chest	AP, PA[c]	0.01–0.05		
	Lat[d]	0.01–0.03	1.5	0.02–0.07
Mammogram[d]	CC	0.1–0.5		
	Lat	3–5	4.0	7–20
Lumbar spine	AP[e] (7 × 17″)	30–58		
	(14 × 17″)	33–65		
	Lat[d]	11–32	2.9	51–126
Lumbosacral spine	AP[c]	92–187		
	PA[d]	40–97		
	Lat[d]	12–33	3.4	168–359
Abdomen	AP[c]	80–163		
	PA[d]	23–55		
	Lat[d]	29–82	1.7	122–245
Intravenous pyelogram[b]	AP	130–264		
	PA	43–104		
	Lat	13–37	5.5	686–1398
Retrograde pyelogram	AP[e]	109–220	1.0	
Hip[b] (single)	AP	72–140		
	Lat	18–51	2.0	103–213

AP denotes anterior–posterior; PA, posterior–anterior; Lat, lateral; CC, cranial–caudal.
[a] Calculated for x-ray beams with half-value layers ranging from 2 to 4 mm Al equivalent. Calculated using the methodology of Rosenstein (1988).
[b] Based on data and methods reported by Laws and Rosenstein (1978).
[c] Entrance exposure data from Conway (1989).
[d] Authors' estimates based on compilation of above data.
[e] Based on NEXT data reported in National Council on Radiation Protection and Measurements (1989).

ward. At 8 to 15 weeks' gestation, the embryo is most susceptible to radiation-induced mental retardation. This risk is probably a nonthreshold linear function of dose, with the risk of severe mental retardation being as low as 4 percent for 10 rad and as high as 60 percent for 150 rad (Committee on Biological Effects, 1990; Hall, 1991). These doses are obviously much higher than those used for diagnostic purposes. **According to the American College of Radiology, no single diagnostic procedure results in a radiation dose significant**

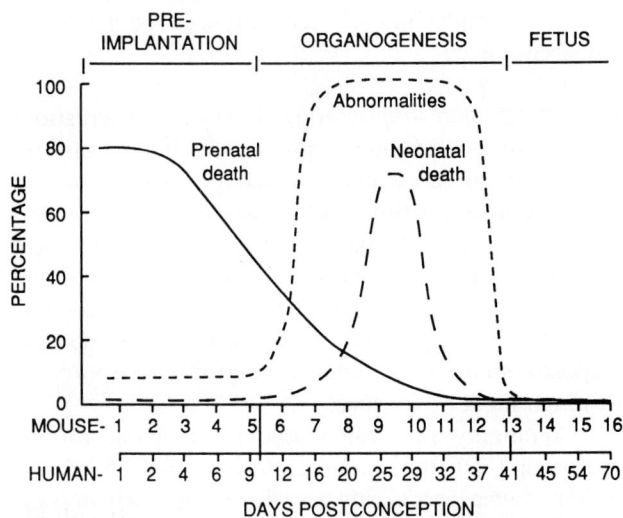

Fig. 43–1. Effects of ionizing radiation in mice exposed to 200 rad. There was a high death rate during preimplantation days 0 to 5, fetal abnormalities between days 5 and 13, and neonatal deaths at exposures between days 8 and 11. Human equivalent days are noted below mouse days. (Data from Russell and Russell, 1954, with permission.)

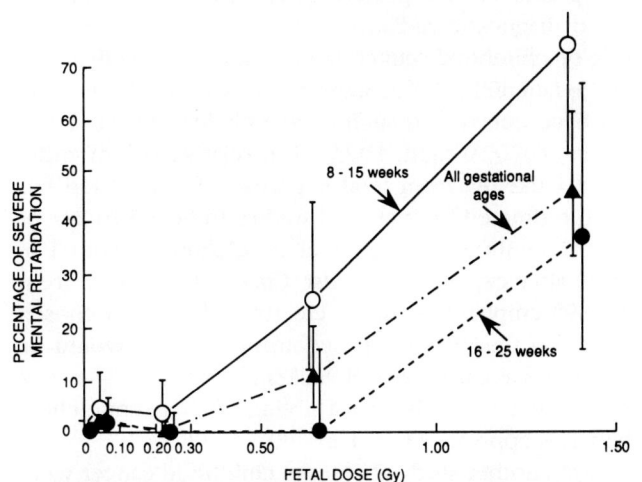

Fig. 43–2. Effects of ionizing radiation on severe mental retardation in fetuses exposed at various gestational ages to the atomic bomb in Hiroshima and Nagasaki (1 Gy = 100 rad). The bar lines represent 90-percent confidence levels. (Data from Otake and associates, 1987, with permission.)

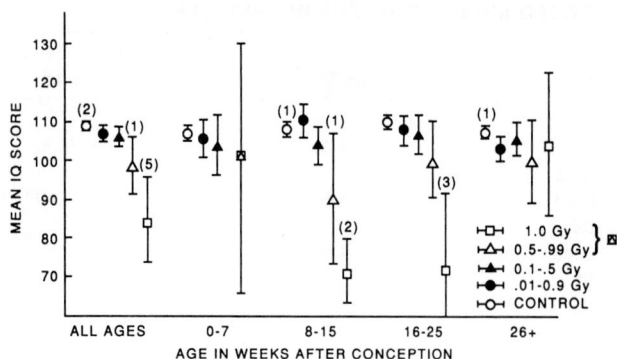

Fig. 43–3. Effects of various doses of ionizing radiation on mean intelligence quotient (IQ) scores as a function of gestational age. These children were exposed in utero to the atomic bomb explosion (1 Gy = 100 rad). Numbers in parentheses are those children with scores less than 64. (Data from Schull and Otake, 1986, with permission.)

enough to threaten the well-being of the developing embryo and fetus (Hall, 1991). Cumulative doses from multiple procedures may enter that harmful range, however, especially at 8 to 15 weeks' gestation. At 16 to 25 weeks, the risk is less, and there is no proven risk in humans at 0 to 8 weeks or greater than 25 weeks (Committee on Biological Effects, 1990).

As summarized by Brent (1989), current evidence suggests that there is no increased risk to the fetus with regard to congenital malformation, growth retardation, or abortion from ionizing radiation at a dose of less than 5 rad. The risk of spontaneous abortion, malformations, and fetal growth retardation in the general population not exposed to diagnostic radiation is much greater than that which can be theorized from exposure to 1 to 5 rad.

Oncogenic Effects of Ionizing Radiation. Several investigators have reported an association between in utero diagnostic radiation exposure and an increased risk of childhood leukemia (Diamond and colleagues, 1973; Lilienfeld, 1966; Stewart and Kneale, 1970). Others have questioned such an association (Brent, 1989; Miller, 1970; Wright, 1973). The relative risk of childhood leukemia from fetal exposure of 1 to 2 rad has been estimated from several studies to be 1.5 to 2.0, or from 1 in 3000 in the general population to about 1 in 2000 after exposure (see also Chap. 11, p. 292). Brent (1989) emphasizes that if elective abortion is chosen based on this, 1999 exposed-normal fetuses would be aborted for each case of leukemia prevented—a risk much lower than that for a sibling of a leukemic child, which is approximately 1 in 700.

In another study, 2 cases of childhood cancer were detected among 1630 atomic bomb survivors, each of whom had high exposure (Committee on Biological Effects, 1990; Yoshimoto and colleagues, 1988). The data are not yet available on whether atomic bomb survivors are at risk for adult cancers, but late-occurring carcinogenic effects have been observed in laboratory mice exposed to high radiation doses (Covelli and associates, 1984).

Diagnostic Radiation. As previously discussed, therapeutic abortion is not indicated solely because of fetal exposure to a single diagnostic x-ray procedure. To put the fetal risk into perspective, it is important to be aware of the dosimetry of x-ray procedures, realizing that averages are very crude estimates.

Plain Films. Doses for standard plain film x-rays are presented in Table 43–3. Maternal indications for film x-rays are extensive, and one most commonly used is the chest x-ray. Fetal exposure is exceptionally small (0.07 mrad), even for two views of the chest, and it is far below any significant risk for any gestational age. The single abdominal film is a higher-dose examination because the embryo or fetus is directly in the x-ray beam. Thus, its average exposure is approximately 100 mrad. Three films taken for a lumbosacral spine series increase the exposure to 300 mrad. The intravenous pyelogram may exceed 1 rad because of the number of films taken. For this reason, as discussed in Chapter 50 (p. 1127), the one-shot pyelogram may be useful. Most "trauma series," such as x-rays of an extremity, skull, or rib series, deliver low doses because of the fetal distance from the target area. The single hip film is the highest of these, films at 200 mrad.

Fetal indications for plain film studies are very limited; the most common is evaluation of breech presentation. As discussed in Chapter 11, at many institutions pelvimetry is now done using computed-tomographic scanning. A suspected fetal skeletal anomaly is an uncommon indication when the ultrasonic diagnosis is unclear. Examples include caudal regression syndrome and sirenomelia.

Fluoroscopy and Angiography. Dosimetry calculations for fluoroscopy and angiography are much more difficult because of variations in the number of x-ray films obtained, fluoroscopy time, and the amount of fluoroscopy time the fetus is in the radiation field. As shown in Table 43–4, the range is quite variable. Although the Food and Drug Administration limits exposure rate for conventional fluoroscopy, such as barium studies, special-purpose systems such as angiography units have potential for much higher exposure.

Commonly performed studies involving routine fluoroscopy are the upper gastrointestinal series and barium enema. Frequently, these are done early in pregnancy during the period of preimplantation or early organogenesis and most often before the woman is aware that she is pregnant. As expected, the upper gastrointestinal series has significantly less exposure to the fetus than a barium enema. Because of this exposure,

TABLE 43–4. REPRESENTATIVE DOSES TO UTERUS/EMBRYO FROM COMMON FLUOROSCOPIC PROCEDURES

Procedure	Total Dose to Uterus (mrad)	Fluoroscopic Exposure Time (sec)	Cinegraphic Exposure Time (sec)
Cerebral angiography[a]	< 10	—	—
Cardiac angiography[b,c]	65	223 (SD = 118)	49 (SD = 9)
Single vessel PTCA[b,c]	60	1023 (SD = 952)	32 (SD = 7)
Double vessel PTCA[b,c]	90	1186 (SD = 593)	49 (SD = 13)
Upper gastrointestinal series[d]	56	136	—
Barium swallow[b,e]	6	192	—
Barium meal[b,e]	8	228	—
Barium enema[b,f,g]	1945–3986	289–311	—
Small bowel series with upper gastrointestinal series[b,h]	2132 (SD = 2700)	684 (SD = 282)	—

PTCA = percutaneous transluminal coronary angioplasty.
[a] Wagner and associates (1985), p 90.
[b] Calculations based on data of Gorson and colleagues. Table 18 (1984). Doses calculated for 168 cm^2 radiation field at tabletop with beam quality 3.5 mm aluminum equivalent half-value layer. Thickness of mother = 22 cm, depth of embryo 6 cm from anterior surface.
[c] Finci and co-workers (1987).
[d] From Suleiman and colleagues (1991).
[e] Based on female data from Rowley and associates (1987).
[f] Assumes embryo in radiation field for entire examination.
[g] Based on data from Bednarek and co-workers (1983).
[h] Based on data from Thoeni and Gould (1991).

gastrointestinal endoscopy is commonly used when a pregnant woman needs evaluation (see Chap. 51, p. 1145).

Angiography occasionally may be necessary in pregnancy for serious maternal complications. As in the case of plain film x-rays, the farther the distance from the embryo or fetus, the less the exposure risk. Angiographic procedures should be performed when the information obtained alters pregnancy management.

Computed Tomography. Computed tomography, or **CT scanning,** has become an important imaging modality for evaluation of all organ systems. In simple terms, it involves multiple exposures of very thin x-ray beams in a 360-degree circle with computerized interpretations of these exposures. The result is an axial (and occasionally sagittal) image of a portion of the body, referred to as a slice. Multiple slices of the target body part are obtained along the length of the entire organ or area in question.

Newer-generation tomography equipment is more sensitive than older systems. As a result, higher resolution scanning may be associated with higher radiation exposure in the area scanned. On the other hand, because there is less scatter with newer equipment, areas not directly scanned have less exposure. For example, skin exposure from a head tomographic scan will typically be as high as 5 to 6 rad along the area scanned. In the body, doses typically range from approximately 5 rad at the skin surface to 2 rad in the center of the slice.

Many variables in each study affect calculation of radiation doses, especially slice thickness and number of cuts obtained. If a study is performed with and without contrast, twice as many images will be obtained, and the

dose to the target area is therefore doubled. Fetal radiation exposure is also dependent on factors such as the size of the mother and the size and position of the fetus (Ragossino and colleagues, 1986). Finally, the closer the target area is to the fetus, the greater the fetal radiation exposure. Estimated maximal fetal doses from CT scans are summarized in Table 43–5.

Cranial CT scanning is the most commonly requested study in pregnant women. Nonenhanced CT scanning is the best imaging technique to detect acute hemorrhage within the epidural, subdural, or subarachnoid spaces, and is usually the initial procedure performed in emergency situations. An enhanced scan should not be performed first, because it may mask identification of acute hemorrhage. Cranial CT in women with eclampsia are discussed in Chapter 36 (p. 780).

Computed tomography pelvimetry is performed to evaluate maternal pelvic bony dimension for breech vaginal delivery (see Chap. 11, p. 292 and Chap. 11, p. 290). Depending on exposure parameters, fetal dose may approach 1.5 rad, but utilizing a low-exposure technique, this dose can be reduced to 250 mrad (Moore and Shearer, 1989).

Nuclear Medicine Studies. Ventilation–perfusion scans, thyroid scans, and thallium heart scans require the intravenous injection of a radioisotope, which in turn emits radiation that is detected by sensitive cameras. Nuclear medicine studies are performed by "tagging" a radioactive element to a chemical agent. For instance, technetium[99m] is a radioisotope that can be tagged to red blood cells, sulphur colloid, or pertechnetate, as well as many other agents. The method used to tag the

TABLE 43–5. ESTIMATED MAXIMUM FETAL DOSES FROM CT SCANS

| | Fetal Dose[a] (rad) at Gestational Age (weeks)[b] | | | | | | | | | |
| | 0–14 | | 15–24 | | 25–29 | | 30–34 | | 35–42 | |
Study	Head	Abdomen	Head	Abdomen	Head	Abdomen	Head	Abdomen	Head	Abdomen
Head (10 slices × 10 mm thick)	< 0.05	< 0.05	< 0.05	< 0.05	< 0.05	< 0.05	< 0.05	< 0.05	< 0.05	< 0.05
Chest (10 slices × 10 mm thick)	< 0.10	< 0.10	< 0.10	< 0.10	< 0.10	< 0.10	< 0.10	< 0.10	< 0.10	< 0.10
Abdomen (10 slices × 10 mm [5 mm gaps])	2.6	2.6	2.2	2.4	2.3	2.3	2.1	2.0	1.7	1.7
Lumbar spine (5 slices × 10 mm thick)	3.5	3.5	2.8	3.2	3.0	3.0	2.7	2.6	2.3	2.3
Pelvimetry[c] (1 slice × 10 mm thick, including lateral scout)	—	—	—	—	—	—	—	—	0.25	0.25

[a] Doses based on calculations derived from computed tomography dose index measurements (CTDI) as described in Shope and colleagues (1981). Doses are derived from the average of the CTDI values reported by the manufacturers of the GE 8800, Picker 1200SX, Toshiba TCT-900S, and Philips Tomoscan LX-models of CT scanners.
[b] Thickness of mother and position of fetus at gestational intervals based on measurements of Ragossino and co-workers (1986).
[c] Radiographic technique and dose for GE 9800 CT scanner, adapted from Moore and Shearer (1989).

agent will determine fetal radiation exposure, particularly if it crosses the placenta, or if it is excreted to urine, whereby fetal proximity to the maternal bladder increases exposure. The measurement of this radioactive substance is based on its decay, and the units used are the curie (Ci) or the becquerel (Bq). Doses usually are expressed in milliCurie (mCi).

Depending on the physical and biochemical properties of a radioisotope, an average fetal exposure can be calculated (Mettler and Guiberteau, 1991; Wagner and associates, 1985). Commonly used radiopharmaceuticals and the estimated absorbed fetal doses are given in Table 43–6.

RADIOIODINE. Radioiodine readily crosses the placenta, and fetal thyroidal uptake begins late in the 11th week of gestation, with uptake between 12 and 20 weeks' gestation higher than that of adults (Mettler and Moseley, 1985). Sodium iodine[123] results in an absorbed dose of 0.32 to 0.35 mrad/mCi. In this low-exposure range, the fetal risk is minimal. Iodine[131] is most often used for its therapeutic thyrotoxic effects to treat maternal thyroid disease. Stabin and colleagues (1991) suggest uptake of ^{131}I by the embryo is highest from 0 to 8 weeks of embryonic development, earlier than other reports, and noted that embryonic uptake of ^{131}I is inversely proportional to maternal uptake. The estimated uptake by the fetal thyroid is significantly greater after 13 weeks' gestation. Fetal hypothyroidism from maternal ingestion of therapeutic doses of radioiodine has been reported (Fisher and associates, 1963; Green and colleagues, 1971; Mettler and Moseley, 1985). It is a Category X drug and therefore contraindicated in pregnancy (see Chap. 42, p. 960).

TECHNETIUM. Technetium[99m] is tagged to various radiopharmaceuticals for nuclear procedures such as bone

scans, renal filtration, blood flow, lung perfusion, erythrocyte tagging for assessment of cardiac blood pool, gastrointestinal bleeding, and venous thrombosis. The distribution of the radiopharmaceutical will predict the fetal exposure, in addition to any drug excreted into the bladder.

TABLE 43–6. RADIOPHARMACEUTICALS USED IN NUCLEAR MEDICINE STUDIES

Examination	Estimated Activity Administered per Examination (mCi)	Dose to Uterus/Embryo per Pharmaceutical (mrad)
Brain	20 mCi ^{99m}Tc pentetic acid	440
	20 mCi [99m]Tc O$_4$	440
Hepatobiliary	50 mCi ^{99m}Tc iminodiacetic acid	170
	50 mCi ^{99m}Tc sulfur colloid	40
Bone	20 mCi ^{99m}Tc phosphate	440
Respiratory		
Perfusion	5 mCi ^{99m}Tc macroaggregated albumin	40
Ventilation	10 mCi ^{133}Xe gas	10
Thyroid[a]	5 mCi [99m]Tc O$_4$	110
	0.1 mCi [131]I	13
	0.3 mCi [123]I	10
Renal	20 mCi ^{99m}Tc pentetic acid	440
	0.25 mCi ^{131}I hippurate	< 10
Abscess or tumor	3 mCi ^{67}Ga citrate	840
Cardiovascular	20 mCi ^{99m}Tc labeled blood cells	80
	3 mCi [210]Tl chloride	111
	20 mCi ^{99m}Tc phosphate	44

[a] Prior to 10–12 weeks' gestational age, iodine is not taken up by the fetal thyroid.
Adapted from National Council on Radiation Protection and Measurements (1989).

Fetal radiation exposure for most technetium studies is 30 to 60 mrad/mCi and has little clinical significance. Free technetium[99m] pertechnetate crosses the placenta, and fetal exposure may be up to 450 mrad, with even greater uptake to the fetal thyroid, stomach, and colon (Mettler and Moseley, 1985). Because of its limited body distribution, fetal radiation exposure is low (40 mrad) from maternal lung perfusion scanning utilizing technetium tagged to macroaggregated albumin (Ginsburg and colleagues, 1989). During this imaging procedure, macroalbumin injected intravenously is sequestered in the lung, with little entering the maternal systemic circulation (see Chap. 49, p. 1114).

XENON. Xenon[127] and xenon[133] gases are used for pulmonary ventilation scans to augment perfusion scans described above. Fetal radiation exposure is extremely low with ventilation scans because the physiological half-life of xenon is exceedingly short (Ginsburg and co-workers, 1989).

Ultrasound

Ultrasound employs sound wave transmission at certain frequencies. At very high intensities, there is a potential for human tissue damage from heat and cavitation (Dakins, 1991; Merritt, 1989; Wells, 1986). In the low-intensity range of real-time imaging, however, no fetal risks have been demonstrated in more than 25 years of use (AIUM, 1983, 1984, 1988).

Recent advances in technology have introduced Doppler-shift imaging coupled with gray-scale imaging to localize spectral waveforms and superimpose color mapping. Higher energy intensities are utilized with this duplex Doppler imaging. For this reason, the Food and Drug Administration has arbitrarily limited ultrasound energy exposure to 94 milliwatts/cm^2 during fetal imaging. Doppler imaging is most commonly utilized to evaluate blood flow in suspected fetal growth retardation.

There is no contraindication to ultrasound imaging of maternal organs during pregnancy. To date, no documented harmful fetal effects have been reported from ultrasound imaging, nor would such effects be predicted from this nonionizing imaging modality. Clinical uses of ultrasound are discussed further in Chapter 46 as well as in most other sections of this book.

Magnetic Resonance Imaging

Magnetic resonance imaging (MRI) has emerged as a major imaging modality in recent years because of its resolution, ability to characterize tissue, and its reproduction of information in three planes (axial, sagittal, and coronal). Rather than ionizing radiation, this technique employs powerful magnets to temporarily alter the energy state of hydrogen protons in molecules, especially water. Through a series of acquisitions, information about the location and characteristics of these hydrogen protons can be obtained as they return to their normal state (Curry and associates, 1990).

There have been several studies attesting to the safety of MRI. To date, no harmful effects in pregnancy have been reported (McRobbie and Foster, 1985), nor have there been mutagenic effects (Geard and colleagues, 1984; Schwartz and Crooks, 1982; Thomas and Morris, 1981). No deleterious effects have been observed in diagnostic systems using less than 2 tesla (a measure of magnetic field strength) in three areas of magnetic resonance imaging studied (Wagner and associates, 1985). Nonetheless, the National Radiological Protection Board advises against imaging in the first trimester unless termination of the pregnancy is probable (Garden and co-workers, 1991).

There have been several studies that explore the applications of MRI for management of complications of pregnancy (Angtuaco and associates, 1992; McCarthy, 1985; Weinreb and colleagues, 1985, 1986). Because this technique does not use ionizing radiation, it is preferred over computed tomography in the case of pelvic masses during pregnancy. Also, such techniques may allow for better visualization because of multiplanar potential as well as better tissue characterization using both T_1- and T_2-weighted images in many organ systems. For example, pelvimetry provides images in the sagittal plane that are superior to the lateral computed tomographic film (Stark and associates, 1985).

Fetal indications for MRI have been reported, particularly in reference to central nervous system anomalies (Angtuaco and associates, 1992; Williamson and colleagues, 1989) and fetal growth retardation, with or without oligohydramnios (Brown and Weinreb, 1988). Garden and colleagues (1991) recently reported that new fast-scan imaging provides improved fetal visualization with less degradation from fetal movement. To be clinically effective, however, MRI must provide better information than that obtained with ultrasound, and at a reasonable cost. Currently, ultrasound with its superior fetal imaging ability, real-time capabilities, and lower cost is the preferred modality in the vast majority of circumstances.

References

AIUM (American Institute of Ultrasound in Medicine): AIUM bioeffects committee. J Ultrasound Med 2:R14, 1983

AIUM (American Institute of Ultrasound in Medicine): AIUM statement on clinical safety. J Ultrasound Med 3:R10, 1984

AIUM (American Institute of Ultrasound in Medicine): AIUM bioeffects considerations for the safety of diagnostic ultrasound. J Ultrasound Med 7:S1, 1988

Angtuaco TL, Shah HR, Mattison DR, Quirk JG: MR imaging in high-risk obstetric patients: A valuable complement to US. Radiographics 12:91, 1992

Bednarek DR, Rudin S, Wong R, Andres ML: Reduction of fluoroscopic exposure for the air-contrast barium enema. Br J Radiol 56:823, 1983

Brent RL: The effect of embryonic and fetal exposure to x-ray, microwaves, and ultrasound: Counseling the pregnant and nonpregnant patient about these risks. Semin Oncol 16:347, 1989

Brent RL: The response of the 9½ day-old rat embryo to variations in exposure rate of 150 R X-irradiation. Radiat Res 45:127, 1971

Brown CEL, Weinreb JC: Magnetic resonance imaging appearance of growth retardation in a twin pregnancy. Obstet Gynecol 71:987, 1988

Committee on Biological Effects of Ionizing Radiation, National Research Council: Other somatic and fetal effects. In Beir V: Effects of Exposure to Low Levels of Ionizing Radiation. Washington, National Academy Press, 1990

Conway BJ: Nationwide evaluation of x-ray trends: Tabulation and graphical summary of surveys 1984 through 1987. Frankfort, KY, Conference of Radiation Control Program Directors, 1989

Covelli V, Di Majo V, Bassani B, Rebessi S, Coppola M, Silini G: Influence of age on life shortening and tumor induction after x-ray and neutron irradiation. Radiat Res 100:348, 1984

Curry TS III, Dowdey JE, Murry RC Jr: Christensen's Physics of Diagnostic Radiology, 4th ed. Philadelphia, Lea & Febiger, 1990, pp 1, 470

Dakins DR: US output deliberations hinge on thermal effects. Diag Imaging May:91, 1991

Dekaban AS: Abnormalities in children exposed to x-irradiation during various stages of gestation: Tentative timetable of radiation injury to the human fetus. J Nucl Med 9:471, 1968

Diamond EL, Schmerler H, Lilienfeld AM: The relationship of intrauterine radiation to subsequent mortality and development of leukemia in children. A prospective study. Am J Epidemiol 97:283, 1973

Finci L, Meier B, Steffenino G, Roy P, Rutishauser W: Radiation exposure during diagnostic catheterization and single- and double-vessel percutaneous transluminal coronary angioplasty. Am J Cardiol 60:1401, 1987

Fisher WD, LoVorhees M, Gardener LT: Congenital hypothyroidism in infants following maternal I[131] therapy. J Pediatr 62:132, 1963

Garden AS, Griffiths RD, Weindling AM, Martin PA: Fast-scan magnetic resonance imaging in fetal visualization. Obstet Gynecol 164:1190, 1991

Geard CR, Osmak RS, Hall EJ, Simon HE, Maudsley AA, Hilal SK: Magnetic resonance imaging and ionizing radiation: A comparative evaluation in-vitro of oncogenic and genotoxic potential. Radiology 152:199, 1984

Ginsberg JS, Hirsh J, Rainbow AJ, Coates G: Risks to the fetus of radiologic procedures used in the diagnoses of maternal venous thromboembolic disease. Thromb Haemost 61:189, 1989

Goldstein L, Murphy DP: Etiology of the ill-health in children born after maternal pelvic irradiation. II. Defective children born after postconception pelvic irradiation. Am J Roentgenol 22:322, 1929

Gorson RO, Lassen M, Rosenstein M: Patient dosimetry in diagnostic radiology. In Waggener RG, Kereiakes JG, Shalek R (eds): Handbook of Medical Physics, vol II. Boca Raton, CRC Press, 1984

Green HG, Gareis FJ, Shepard TH, Kelley VC: Cretinism associated with maternal sodium iodine[131] therapy during pregnancy. Am J Dis Child 122:247, 1971

Hall EJ: Scientific view of low-level radiation risks. Radiographics 11:509, 1991

Laws PW, Rosenstein M: A somatic index for diagnostic radiology. Health Phys 35:629, 1978

Lilienfeld AM: Epidemiological studies of the leukemogenic effects of radiation. Yale J Biol Med 39:143, 1966

McCarthy SM, Stark DD, Filly RA, Callen PW, Hricak H, Higgins CB: Obstetrical magnetic resonance imaging: Maternal anatomy. Radiology 154:421, 1985

McRobbie D, Foster MA: Pulsed magnetic field exposure during pregnancy and implications for NMR foetal imaging: A study with mice. Magn Reson Imaging 3:231, 1985

Merritt CRB: Ultrasound safety: What are the issues? Radiology 173:304, 1989

Mettler FA, Guiberteau MJ: Essentials of Nuclear Medicine Imaging. Philadelphia, Saunders, 1991, p 320

Mettler FA, Moseley RD: Medical Effects of Ionizing Radiation. New York, Grune & Stratton, 1985, p 202

Miller RW: Epidemiological conclusions from radiation toxicity studies. In Fry RJM, Grahn D, Griem ML, et al (eds): Late Effects of Radiation. London, Taylor & Francis, 1970

Miller RW, Blot WJ: Small head size after exposure to the atomic bomb. Lancet 2:784, 1972

Miller RW, Mulvihill JJ: Small head size after atomic radiation. Teratology 14:355, 1982

Moore MM, Shearer DR: Fetal dose estimates for CT pelvimetry. Radiology 171:265, 1989

National Council on Radiation Protection and Measurements: Exposure of the US population from diagnostic medical radiation. Bethesda, National Council on Radiation Protection, report no. 100, 1989, p 26

Otake M, Schull WJ: Analysis and interpretation on deficits of the central nervous system observed in the in utero exposed survivors of Hiroshima and Nagasaki. Jpn J Appl Stat 15:163, 1986

Otake M, Yoshimaru H, Schull WJ: Severe mental retardation among the prenatally exposed survivors of the atomic bombing of Hiroshima and Nagasaki: A comparison of the old and new dosimetry systems. Radiation Effects Research Foundation, technical report no. 16-87, 1987

Ragossino MW, Breckle R, Hill LM, Gray JE: Average fetal depth in utero: Data for estimation of fetal absorbed radiation dose. Radiology 158:513, 1986

Rosenstein M: Handbook of selected tissue doses for projections common in diagnostic radiology. Rockville, Department of Health and Human Services, Food and Drug Administration. DHHS pub no. (FDA) 89-8031, 1988

Rowley KA, Hill SJ, Watkins RA, Moores BM: An investigation into the levels of radiation exposure in diagnostic examinations involving fluoroscopy. Br J Radiol 60:167, 1987

Russell LB, Russell WL: An analysis of the changing radiation response of the developing mouse embryo. J Cell Comp Physiol 43:103, 1954

Russell LB, Russell WL: The effects of radiation on the preimplantation stages of the mouse embryo. Anat Res 108:521, 1950

Schull WJ, Otake M: Effects on intelligence of prenatal exposure to ionizing radiation. Radiation Effects Research Foundation, technical report no. 7-86, 1986

Schwartz JL, Crooks LE: NMR imaging produces no observable mutations or cytotoxicity in mammalian cells. Am J Radiol 139:5, 1982

Shope TG, Gagne RM, Johnson GC: A method for describing the doses delivered by transmission x-ray computed tomography. Med Phys 8:488, 1981

Stabin MG, Watson EE, Marcus CS, Salk RD: Radiation dosimetry for the adult female and fetus from iodine-131 administration in hyperthyroidism. J Nucl Med 32:808, 1991

Stark DD, McCarthy SM, Filly RA, Callen PW, Hricak H, Parer JT: Intrauterine growth retardation: Evaluation by magnetic resonance. Radiology 155:425, 1985

Stewart A, Kneale GW: Radiation dose effects in relation to obstetric x-rays and childhood cancers. Lancet 1:1185, 1970

Suleiman OH, Anderson J, Jones B, Rao GUV, Rosenstein M: Tissue doses in the upper gastrointestinal examination. Radiology 178:653, 1991

Thoeni RF, Gould RG: Enteroclysis and small bowel series: Comparison of radiation dose and examination time. Radiology 178:659, 1991

Thomas A, Morris PG: The effects of NMR exposure on living organisms, a microbial assay. Br J Radiol 55:615, 1982

Wagner LK, Lester RG, Saldana LR: Exposure of the Pregnant Patient to Diagnostic Radiation. Philadelphia, Lippincott, 1985, pp 40, 61

Weinreb JC, Brown CE, Lowe TW, Cohen JM, Erdman WA: Pelvic masses in pregnant patients: MR and US imaging. Radiology 159:717, 1986

Weinreb JC, Lowe TW, Santos-Ramos R, Cunningham FG, Parkey R: Magnetic resonance imaging in obstetric diagnosis. Radiology 154:157, 1985

Wells PNT: The prudent use of diagnostic ultrasound. Brit J Radiol 59:1143, 1986

Williamson RA, Weiner CP, Yuh WTC, Abu-Yousef MM: Magnetic resonance imaging of anomalous fetuses. Obstet Gynecol 73:952, 1989

Wilson JG, Brent RL, Jordan HC: Differentiation as a determinant of the reaction of rat embryos on x-irradiation. Proc Soc Exp Biol Med 82:67, 1953

Wright FW: Diagnostic radiology and the fetus. BMJ 3:693, 1973

Yamazaki JN, Schull WJ: Perinatal loss and neurological abnormalities among children of the atomic bomb. Nagasaki and Hiroshima revisited, 1949 to 1989. JAMA 264:605, 1990

Yoshimoto YH, Kato H, Schull WJ: Risk of cancer among in utero children exposed to A-bomb radiation 1950–1984. Radiation Effects Research Foundation, technical report no. 4-88, 1988

CHAPTER 44

Diseases and Injuries of the Fetus and Newborn Infant

The fetus and newborn are subject to a great variety of diseases, some of which are the direct consequence of maternal disease, which has been considered along with the maternal illness. This chapter provides an introduction to other fetal and neonatal diseases and injuries of major clinical importance. Congenital malformations are considered in Chapters 41 and 42 and neonatal infections in Chapters 58 and 59.

DISEASES OF THE FETUS AND NEWBORN

Hyaline Membrane Disease

To provide prompt blood-gas exchange after birth, the infant's lungs must rapidly fill with air while clearing them of fluid, and the volume of blood that perfuses the lungs must increase remarkably. Some of the fluid is usually expressed as the chest is compressed during vaginal delivery, and the remainder is absorbed through the pulmonary lymphatics. Of great importance is the presence of appropriate surfactant synthesized by the type II pneumonocytes to stabilize the air-expanded alveoli by lowering surface tension and thereby preventing lung collapse during expiration.

If the alveoli cannot be maintained in an expanded state because of inappropriate surfactant action, obvious respiratory distress develops. This is characterized by the formation of hyaline membranes in the distal bronchioles and alveoli and considerable cardiopulmonary shunting of blood.

Hyaline membrane disease has decreased as a cause of neonatal deaths in the United States. According to Malloy and colleagues (1987), from 1969 to 1973, 19 in 1000 liveborns died from respiratory distress, but from 1979 to 1983, this number was 12 in 1000. It would appear that the rate of death from hyaline membrane diseases has continued to decline with significant drops from 1989 to 1990. Surfactant therapy probably is responsible for much of this decrease (Wegman, 1991). Boys are more prone than girls to develop these problems, and white infants appear to be more often and more severely affected than are black infants.

Diagnosis. Clinically these infants exhibit an increased respiratory rate and severe chest wall retraction during inspiration. Expiration is often accompanied by a whimper and grunt. Grunting is common in the newborn whenever there is uneven expansion of the lungs or lower airway obstruction. Progressive shunting of blood through nonventilated lung areas contributes to the hypoxemia and metabolic and respiratory acidosis. Finally, poor peripheral circulation and systemic hypotension may be evident.

Other forms of respiratory insufficiency that may be confused with idiopathic respiratory distress syndrome include respiratory failure caused by sepsis, pneumonia, meconium aspiration, pneumothorax, diaphragmatic hernia, and heart failure. Common causes of cardiac decompensation in the early newborn period are patent ductus arteriosus and primary myocardial disease. In case of idiopathic respiratory distress, the chest x-ray shows a diffuse reticulogranular infiltrate throughout the lung fields with an air-filled tracheobronchial tree (air bronchogram).

Pathology. In the fatal case, the atelectatic lungs on gross examination resemble liver. Histologically, many alveoli are collapsed while some are dilated widely, hyaline membranes of fibrin-rich protein and cellular debris line the dilated alveoli and terminal bronchioles, and the epithelium underlying the membrane is necrotic.

Treatment. The establishment of appropriately staffed and equipped neonatal intensive-care units has served to reduce dramatically the number of deaths from idiopathic respiratory distress. Similarly, advances in respiratory therapy and ventilatory support have been crucial. An arterial PO_2 below 40 mm Hg is indicative of the need for effective oxygen therapy. Oxygen concentration administered to these infants should be sufficient to relieve hypoxia and acidosis, but not higher. Arterial oxygen tensions of 50 to 70 mm Hg are adequate. Humidification of inspired air is also important. The infant from the time of birth must be kept warm, because chilling increases oxygen consumption.

The use of oxygen-enriched air under pressure to prevent the collapse of unstable alveoli, or *continuous positive airway pressure*, has brought about an appreciable reduction in the mortality rate. Successful ventilation usually allows reduction of high inspired oxygen concentrations and thereby reduces pulmonary and retinal oxygen toxicity. Disadvantages are that venous return to the heart may be impaired, causing a fall in cardiac output. Moreover, there is always the possibility of barotrauma, characterized by rupture of the lung with interstitial emphysema and pneumothorax or pneumomediastinum. These complications are not always the consequence of overzealous resuscitation and ventilation, and are encountered even with low ventilatory pressures. Although vigorous mechanical ventilation has undoubtedly improved survival, it is probably an important factor in the genesis of bronchopulmonary dysplasia.

Surfactant Treatment. Since the early 1980s, when Fujiwara and colleagues (1980) demonstrated that aerosolized surfactant treatment appeared to ameliorate the severity of the respiratory distress syndrome, there have been a number of clinical trials to study its efficacy. Berry (1991) described preparations that have been used to include biological or animal surfactants such as bovine (Survanta), calf (calf lung surfactant extract or CLSE), porcine (Curosurf), human, or synthetic surfactant (Exosurf).

Surfactant has been utilized both for prophylaxis as well as a "rescue" agent for respiratory distress syndrome. It is now well established that surfactant therapy results in a reduction in neonatal oxygen requirements and the frequency of pneumothoraces. It also appears that neonatal mortality, especially from respiratory distress syndrome, is significantly reduced with surfactant therapy (Berry, 1991; Morley, 1991). Conversely, surfactant, given either prophylactically or as rescue therapy, is less efficacious to prevent other complications such as persistent ductus arteriosus, bronchopulmonary dysplasia, and intraventricular hemorrhage.

Morley (1991) recently reviewed the results from 15 controlled clinical trials—eight were with prophylactic therapy and seven involved rescue therapy. He emphasized that it is not appropriate to compare results from prophylaxis with rescue therapy because the former includes all babies at risk whereas the latter includes only seriously ill neonates. Similarly, Berry (1991) summarized the results of several controlled studies of surfactant utilized either as prophylaxis or rescue therapy (Table 44–1). The reduction in mortality in infants given prophylaxis was 6.6 percent and for the rescue group it was 10.4 percent.

Preliminary data indicate that surfactant treatment is beneficial for the very-low-birthweight infant. In a recent report of the comparison of surfactant as immediate prophylaxis and as rescue therapy in newborns less than 30 weeks' gestation, Kendig and colleagues (1991) reported increased survival for infants (especially at 26 weeks or less) in the prophylactic group. The frequency of pneumothorax in the very premature infant also was significantly lower in this group. Stevenson and associates (1992) also reported significantly decreased neonatal deaths from respiratory distress in

TABLE 44–1. NEONATAL MORTALITY AND OTHER COMPLICATIONS (IN PERCENT) FOR RESCUE THERAPY OR PROPHYLAXIS WITH SURFACTANT

Factor	Prophylaxis		Rescue Therapy	
	Surfactant (n = 548)	*Controls (n = 542)*	*Surfactant (n = 606)*	*Controls (n = 578)*
Mortality	8.2	14.8	18.8	29.2
Pneumothorax	8.8	13.3	16.2	32.9
Bronchopulmonary dysplasia	20.6	23.8	16.9	23.7
Grades 3 or 4 intracranial hemorrhage	12.6	14.9	14.5	16.1

Adapted from Berry (1991), with permission.

neonates weighing 500 to 699 g who were given a single prophylactic dose of synthetic surfactant compared with controls. Unfortunately, overall mortality was not decreased.

COMPLICATIONS. Potential adverse effects associated with surfactant therapy include tracheal tube blockage and pulmonary hemorrhage (Fetus and Newborn Committee, 1992). Long and colleagues (1992) reported an incidence of pulmonary hemorrhage of 1.9 percent in newborns receiving synthetic surfactant compared with 1 percent of controls in the American Exosurf Neonatal Study Group. There was no evidence for a generalized bleeding diathesis in the surfactant group. Van Houten and colleagues (1992) from the same study group reported that the diagnosis of pulmonary hemorrhage at autopsy was not increased in newborns who received synthetic surfactant.

LONG-TERM FOLLOW-UP. Long-term benefits of surfactant therapy remain undefined. Dunn and colleagues (1988) performed a 2-year follow-up of 55 survivors from their randomized trial. They reported that neurodevelopmental handicaps were not lessened by surfactant therapy. Vaucher and associates (1988) reported similar findings in 46 survivors evaluated at 12 to 24 months.

Complications. Oxygen therapy is not innocuous. Persistent hyperoxia likely injures the lung, especially the alveoli and capillaries. If hyperoxemia is sustained, the infant is at risk of developing **retrolental fibroplasia**, now called commonly **retinopathy of prematurity.** Therefore, the concentration of oxygen administered must be reduced appropriately as the arterial Po_2 rises. Tracheal tubes after prolonged use cause erosion and serious infection of the upper airway, and they must be removed as soon as possible. **Bronchopulmonary dysplasia,** or oxygen toxicity lung disease, may develop in infants treated for severe respiratory distress with high oxygen concentrations given at high pressures.

This is a chronic lung condition characterized by hypoxia, hypercarbia, and oxygen dependence as the consequence of alveolar and bronchiolar epithelial damage followed by peribronchial and interstitial fibrosis. Pulmonary hypertension is also a frequent complication. Hallman and colleagues (1992) reported that inositol administered via parenteral nutrition to preterm infants with respiratory distress increased survival without bronchopulmonary dysplasia and with a decreased incidence of retinopathy.

Prevention. There are several approaches to the prevention of respiratory distress syndrome. Obviously, the best approach would be to assure pulmonary maturation prior to delivery of a woman with an uncertain gestational age. Approaches in the preterm infant include antenatal glucocorticoid therapy (see Chap. 38, p. 864) and surfactant prophylaxis immediately after birth.

Amniocentesis for Fetal Lung Maturity. Amniocentesis is often utilized to determine the relative concentration of surfactant-active phospholipids to confirm fetal lung maturity. The technique is similar to that described for second trimester amniocentesis (see Chap. 41, p. 946) and is often performed suprapubically (Fig. 44–1).

The specific lecithin, dipalmitoyl phosphatidylcholine, plus phosphatidylinositol and especially phosphatidylglycerol are important in the formation and stabilization of the surface-active layer that prevents alveolar collapse and the development of respiratory distress.

Several tests used to estimate pulmonary surfactant, and thus to predict respiratory distress, have been reviewed in detail by Weiner and Weinstein (1987).

Lecithin-to-Sphingomyelin (L–S) Ratio. Before 34 weeks, lecithin and sphingomyelin are present in amnionic fluid in similar concentrations. At about 34 weeks, the concentration of lecithin relative to sphingomyelin begins to rise (Fig. 44–2).

Gluck and co-workers (1971) reported that the risk of neonatal respiratory distress is very slight whenever the concentration of lecithin is at least twice that of sphingomyelin (L–S ratio). Conversely, there is increased risk of respiratory distress when this ratio is below 2. Harvey and colleagues (1975) combined the data from 25 reports in which lecithin–sphingomyelin ratios were measured by similar techniques on amnionic fluid collected within 72 hours of delivery. When the ratio was greater than 2, the risk of respiratory distress was found to be slight unless the mother had diabetes (see Chap. 53, p. 1203). If the ratio was 1.5 to 2.0, respiratory distress was identified in 40 percent, and if below 1.5, it was 73 percent. Importantly, although 73 percent of infants developed respiratory distress when the ratio was below 1.5, it was fatal in only 14 percent. There are times when the risk to the fetus from a hostile intrauterine environment are greater than the risk of

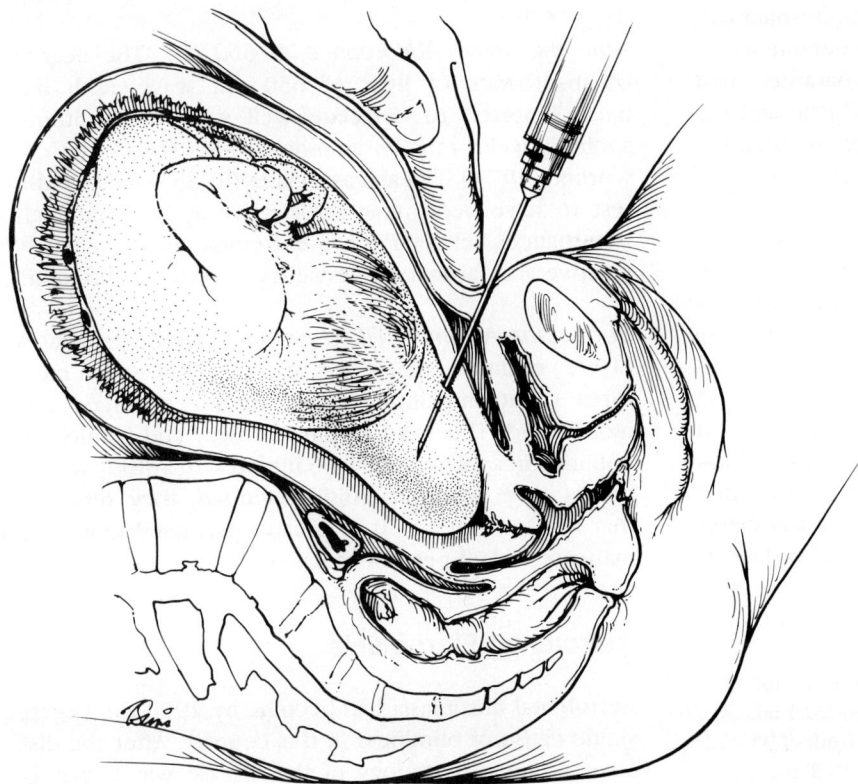

Fig. 44–1. Amniocentesis late in pregnancy, performed suprapubically.

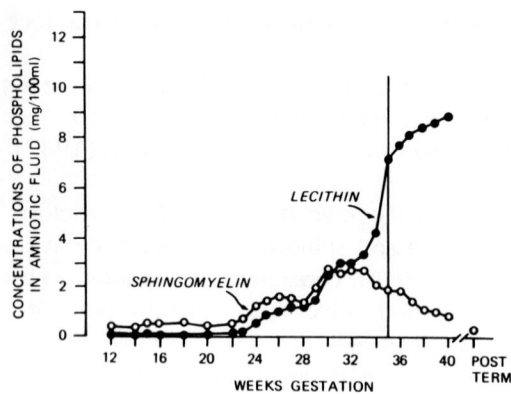

Fig. 44–2. Changes in mean concentrations of lecithin and sphingomyelin in amnionic fluid during gestation in normal pregnancy. (From Gluck and Kulovich, 1973, with permission.)

death from respiratory distress, even though the ratio is less than 2.

Unfortunately, with some pregnancy complications, for example, class A and B maternal diabetes (Quirk and Bleasdale, 1986), erythroblastosis fetalis, fetal-neonatal sepsis, or most any event that causes the infant to be metabolically seriously compromised at birth, a lecithin–sphingomyelin ratio of 2 does not preclude necessarily the development of respiratory distress.

Phosphatidylglycerol. Surfactant action insufficient to prevent respiratory distress, even though the lecithin–sphingomyelin ratio is 2, is thought to be due in part to lack of phosphatidylglycerol and its enhancement of surface-active properties. Identification of phosphatidylglycerol in amnionic fluid provides considerable assurance, but not necessarily an absolute guarantee, that respiratory distress will not develop (Whittle and co-workers, 1982). Phosphatidylglycerol has not been detected in blood, meconium, or vaginal secretions; consequently, these contaminants do not confuse the interpretation. Importantly, the absence of phosphatidylglycerol is not necessarily a strong indicator that respiratory distress is likely to develop after delivery; its absence serves only to indicate that the infant *may* develop respiratory distress.

Foam Stability (Shake) Test. To reduce the time and effort inherent in precise measurement of the lecithin–sphingomyelin ratio, the foam stability test, or so-called **shake test**, was introduced by Clements and associates (1972). The test depends upon the ability of surfactant in amnionic fluid, when mixed appropriately with ethanol, to generate stable foam at the air-liquid interface.

> Into one chemically clean 13 × 100-mm glass tube with a Teflon-lined plastic screw cap are added 1 mL of recently collected amnionic fluid and 1 mL of 95 percent ethanol (prepared by diluting 19.0 parts absolute alcohol with 1 part of distilled water); 0.5

mL of amnionic fluid, 0.5 mL of 0.9 percent saline, and 1 mL of the 95 percent ethanol are added to another tube. Each tube is vigorously shaken for 15 seconds and placed upright in a rack for 15 minutes. The persistence of an intact ring of bubbles at the air-liquid interface after 15 minutes is considered a positive test.

If the ring of foam persists for 15 minutes, the risk of respiratory distress is very low. For example, Schlueter and co-workers (1979) identified only one instance of respiratory distress developing out of 205 pregnancies in which the test was positive for amnionic fluid diluted with an equal volume of saline. There are two problems with the test: (1) slight contamination of amnionic fluid, reagents, or glassware, or errors in measurement, may alter the tests results, and (2) a false-negative test is rather common. In our experience, a lecithin-sphingomyelin ratio of 4 to 6 or higher is necessary for a positive shake test.

Lumadex-FSI Test. This test is based on the principle of foam stability to identify surfactant activity in amnionic fluid. It has also been found to be reliable (Herbert and associates, 1984; Sher and Statland, 1983).

Fluorescent Polarization (Microviscometry). The microviscosity of lipid aggregates in amnionic fluid may be assayed by mixing the fluid with a specific fluorescent dye that incorporates into the hydrocarbon region of the surfactant lipids. The intensity of the fluorescence induced by polarized light then is measured. The technique is rapid and appears simple to perform, but the instrument is expensive (Barkai and associates, 1982).

Amnionic Fluid Absorbance at 650 nm. The degree of absorbance of light of 650 nm wavelength has been reported to correlate well with the lecithin–sphingomyelin ratio in amnionic fluid (Sbarra and co-workers, 1977). Tsai and associates (1983) reported the test to have been most informative at low and high absorbance; between these extremes, however, false-positive and false-negative values proved troublesome.

Surfactant–Albumin Ratio. Steinfeld and associates (1992) evaluated a new test, the TDx-FLM which measures surfactant–albumin ratio in uncentrifuged amnionic fluid. This is an automated assay and results are obtained in approximately 30 minutes. In a study of 374 consecutive amnionic fluid specimens, they reported that a TDx value of 50 or greater predicted fetal lung maturity in 100 percent of cases.

Retrolental Fibroplasia

Retrolental fibroplasia had become by 1950 the largest single cause of blindness in this country. After the discovery that the etiology of the disease was hyperoxemia, its frequency decreased remarkably.

Pathology. The retina vascularizes centrifugally from the optic nerve starting about the fourth month of gestation and continuing until shortly after birth. During the time of vascularization, retinal vessels are easily damaged by excessive oxygen. The temporal portion of the retina, which is the last to be vascularized, is most vulnerable. Oxygen induces severe vasoconstriction, endothelial damage, and vessel obliteration. When the oxygen level is reduced, there is new vessel formation at the site of previous vascular damage. The new vessels penetrate the retina and extend intravitreally, where they are prone to leak proteinaceous material or burst with subsequent hemorrhage. Adhesions then form which detach the retina.

Prevention. Precise levels of hyperoxemia that can be sustained without causing retrolental fibroplasia are not known. Unfortunately, a cooperative study did not provide answers to many difficult but important questions concerning arterial PO_2 levels and retrolental fibroplasia (Kinsey and colleagues, 1977). Most pediatricians feel that inhalation of air enriched with oxygen to no more than 40 percent will not cause retrolental fibroplasia.

Very small immature infants who develop respiratory distress will most likely require ventilation with high oxygen concentrations to maintain life until respiratory distress clears. During this period, it is important that overzealous treatment not lead to dangerous hyperoxemia and, in turn, retrolental fibroplasia. Frequent measurements of PO_2, therefore, may be necessary first to assure adequate oxygen and then to prevent hyperoxemia.

Vitamin E has been administered to very-low-birthweight infants to try to prevent or minimize the development of retrolental fibroplasia. It is generally believed that the preterm infant is deficient in vitamin E. However, the results of administration of relatively large doses of vitamin E to prevent anemia, retrolental fibroplasia, bronchopulmonary dysplasia, and intraventricular hemorrhage have been conflicting (Mino, 1992).

Meconium Aspiration

The aspiration of some amnionic fluid before birth is most likely a physiological event. Unfortunately, this normal process can be the cause of inhalation of amnionic fluid containing thick meconium, which, in some cases, leads to subsequent respiratory distress and hypoxia with many complications described above. Some neonates inhale meconium at birth. Thus, **meconium aspiration syndrome** may follow delivery in otherwise normal labor, but it is more often encountered in postterm pregnancy or in those complicated by fetal growth retardation. The common feature of these pregnancy complications appears to be reduced amnionic fluid volume into which the fetus defecates copious amounts of meconium. From the observations of Leveno and colleagues (1984) on prolonged pregnancy, these events likely follow transient episodes of umbilical-cord compression in the otherwise healthy fetus, an event more likely if there is oligohydramnios.

Dooley and co-workers (1985) conducted a study to determine if intrapartum meconium aspiration was more common in labors complicated by evidence of fetal hypercarbia or hypoxia. They used meconium visualized beneath the vocal cords as being indicative of aspiration, and they found that 20 percent of fetuses from 272 pregnancies with meconium-stained amnionic fluid had aspirated some meconium. This incidence was not predicted by variable, saltatory, or late fetal heart decelerations during labor. Importantly, they reported that liberal cesarean section (60 percent) for labors complicated by meconium and fetal heart rate abnormalities did not alter the frequency of meconium found beneath the cords. Moreover, the single death was not prevented by aggressive pulmonary toilet.

Mitchell and colleagues (1985), in a study of 53 women with moderate to thick meconium, found meconium below the vocal cords only in those infants who had metabolic acidemia at birth. However, they utilized an umbilical arterial pH cut-off of 7.25 to define acidemia.

In a study of 323 pregnancies with meconium-stained amnionic fluid, Yeomans and associates (1989) reported that 31 percent of those with meconium below the cords versus 18 percent without had acidemia at birth, defined as an umbilical cord pH less than 7.20 (Table 44–2). Only 3 percent of these infants developed meconium aspiration syndrome, one with an umbilical artery pH less than 7.2 and five with a pH greater than 7.2. None of the 323 newborns had an umbilical artery pH less than 7.0, a frequently used cut-off to define severe acidemia (see Chap. 17, p. 446).

TABLE 44–2. FREQUENCY OF MECONIUM BELOW VOCAL CORDS AND MECONIUM ASPIRATION IN RELATION TO UMBILICAL ARTERY pH IN 323 NEONATES

Factor	No. (%)	Umbilical Artery pH (%)				
		≥ *7.25*	> *7.20*	< *7.20*	< *7.15*	< *7.00*
Meconium below the cords	74 (23)	39 (53)	51 (69)	12 (31)	8 (11)	0
Meconium aspiration syndrome	6 (3)		5 (83)	1 (17)		0
No meconium below cords	249 (77)	138 (55)	204 (82)	45 (18)	13 (5)	0

From Yeomans and associates (1989), with permission.

In a recent review of 40 term pregnancies not in labor with meconium found at amniocentesis or at elective cesarean section, Ramin and colleagues (in press) found no significant differences in the frequency of acidemia when compared with 40 normal controls.

Pathology. Meconium aspiration likely causes both mechanical obstruction of the airways and chemical pneumonitis. There is also evidence that the free fatty acids in meconium strip away alveolar surfactant (Clark and colleagues, 1987). Atelectasis, consolidation, and barotrauma may prove fatal unless treated vigorously. Even with prompt and appropriate therapy, seriously affected infants frequently die.

Marshall and associates (1978) found no evidence of persistent chronic lung disease among survivors of meconium aspiration; however, two of three infants who developed seizures while acutely ill subsequently demonstrated psychomotor retardation.

Recently, Katz and Bowes (1992) have questioned the etiology of meconium aspiration syndrome. They reviewed recent data that support the hypothesis that the etiology of the syndrome is fetal asphyxia rather than direct damage from meconium. They postulate that asphyxia causes pathophysiological changes of pulmonary vascular damage, pulmonary hypertension, persistent fetal circulation, and severe hypoxemia.

Diagnosis and Management. At Parkland Hospital, whenever meconium has been identified in amnionic fluid before or during delivery, someone skilled in resuscitative techniques is present at delivery. To prevent further aspiration, the mouth and nares are carefully suctioned before the shoulders are delivered, or as the mouth is visualized through the uterine incision at cesarean delivery. As soon as possible after delivery, all meconium-stained fluid that remains above the vocal cords is aspirated and the cords are visualized. Tracheal intubation and suction are then performed and as much meconium as possible is aspirated from the trachea. The stomach is emptied to avoid the possibility of further meconium aspiration. **It is emphasized that ventilation must not be delayed unduly while these procedures are carried out.**

These practices have been questioned recently (Katz and Bowes, 1992). Falciglia (1988) and Linder and colleagues (1988) reported that tracheal suctioning of meconium did not reduce the incidence or severity of respiratory distress from aspiration.

Suction Bulb Versus DeLee Trap. Locus and colleagues (1987) studied 80 women whose labors were complicated by moderate to thick meconium-stained amnionic fluid. Fetus-infants were randomly assigned to undergo suction at delivery of the head by either bulb or DeLee trap. They quantified meconium recovered from below the cords at tracheal suctioning and found that both methods were equally efficacious. Importantly, even with careful suctioning, 5 percent of these infants developed meconium aspiration syndrome, although none died.

Intraventricular Hemorrhage

Intraventricular hemorrhage, or hemorrhage into the germinal-matrix tissues, which then may extend into the ventricular system and brain parenchyma, is a common problem in preterm neonates. Although these lesions usually are seen in infants born at less than 34 weeks, they may develop later and are occasionally seen in term neonates. Most hemorrhages will develop within 72 hours of birth; however, they have been observed as late as 24 days (Perlman and Volpe, 1986). Although external perinatal and postnatal influences undoubtedly alter the incidence and severity of these lesions, the greatest impact is that of preterm birth. Unfortunately, because their onset is usually within 3 days of delivery, their genesis is often attributed erroneously to birth events.

Pathology. Central to the pathological process is damage to the germinal-matrix capillary network that predisposes to subsequent extravasation of blood into the surrounding tissue. Hemorrhage usually develops within 72 hours after delivery, and this may be influenced by several factors.

Less severe forms of intraventricular hemorrhage are generally associated with low mortality and are unlikely to cause significant long-term disability. However, if death does not follow from extensive hemorrhage, or from other complications of preterm birth, these lesions sometimes, but not always, are associated with major neurodevelopmental handicaps (Morales, 1987; Papile and co-workers, 1983). Interestingly, DeVries and colleagues (1985) attribute long-term sequelae to cystic areas, or **periventricular leukomalacia,** that develop more commonly as a result of ischemic lesions, and less commonly to hemorrhages per se.

Incidence and Severity. The incidence undoubtedly depends upon the level of immaturity, and about half of all neonates born before 34 weeks will have evidence of some hemorrhage. Interestingly, Hayden and colleagues (1985) reported that 4 percent of asymptomatic term neonates have sonographic evidence of subependymal hemorrhage. Perlman and Volpe (1986) have shown that very-low-birthweight infants have the earliest onset of hemorrhage, the greatest likelihood for progression into parenchymal tissue, and the highest mortality rate. Morales and Koerten (1986) reported similar experiences with 488 infants born weighing between 500 and 1500 g, and the incidence of associated mortality and intraventricular hemorrhage is shown in Figure 44–3.

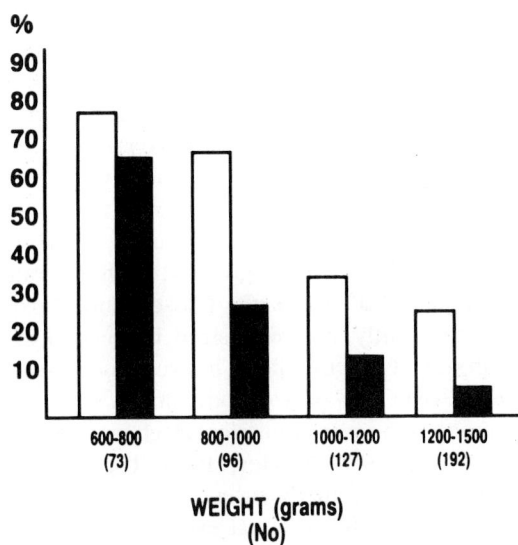

Fig. 44–3. Incidence of intraventricular hemorrhage (*white bars*) and mortality (*black bars*) according to birthweight groupings. (From Morales and Koerten, 1986, with permission.)

The severity of intraventricular hemorrhage can be assessed by ultrasound and computed tomography, and various grading schemes are used to quantify the extent of the lesion. The following scheme was proposed by Papile and colleagues (1978) and is commonly used:

Grade I—Hemorrhage limited to the germinal-matrix

Grade II—Intraventricular hemorrhage

Grade III—Hemorrhage with ventricular dilatation

Grade IV—Parenchymal extension of hemorrhage

In a report of neonatal outcomes of 1765 very-low-birthweight infants delivered at seven centers in the National Institute of Child Health and Human Development Neonatal Intensive Care Network, the incidence of intraventricular hemorrhage was 45 percent. About 20 percent had grades III or IV hemorrhage (Hack and colleagues, 1991).

It is emphasized that events that predispose to germinal-matrix hemorrhage are multifactorial and complex. Factors other than immaturity itself that predispose low-birthweight infants to such hemorrhages appear to be those events that lead to hypoxia. Morales and Koerten (1986) showed that an umbilical cord pH of less than 7.2 and severe respiratory distress were associated with significantly increased severe hemorrhages. Luthy and co-workers (1987) reported a three-fold increased risk for grade III or IV hemorrhage when the cord arterial pH was less than 7.2. Respiratory distress syndrome and mechanical ventilation commonly are associated factors. Lesko and colleagues (1986) reported that heparin used to maintain vascular catheter patency in intensive-care units was associated with a fourfold increased risk of germinal-matrix hemorrhage. Obviously, other factors that cause hypoxia and acido-sis, a prime example being sepsis, must be important.

In a review of 232 very low-birthweight-infants (less than 1500 g), Wallin and co-workers (1990) reported postnatal factors related to periventricular or intraventricular hemorrhage included respiratory distress syndrome, ventilator therapy, a $PaCO_2$ of 60 mm Hg or greater, a PO_2 less than 40 mm Hg at 2 hours of life or greater, and pneumothorax.

Prevention and Treatment. There is no evidence that routine cesarean delivery for the preterm fetus presenting vertex will decrease the incidence of periventricular hemorrhage (Morales and Koerten, 1986; Newton and colleagues, 1986; Tejani and co-workers, 1987; Welch and Bottoms, 1986). Moreover, Strauss and colleagues (1985) found no association with the presence of labor or its duration. In a recent study of 106 preterm infants weighing less than 1750 g, Anderson and associates (1992) found no significant difference in the overall frequency of intraventricular hemorrhage in infants whose mothers were not in labor compared with those in either latent or active labor. There was, however, an increased frequency of grade III or IV hemorrhage in infants of women in active labor.

Avoiding hypoxic episodes after delivery is of paramount importance. Administration of muscle relaxants appears to diminish some of the cerebral blood-flow fluctuations, and thus hemorrhage (Perlman and colleagues, 1985). Phenobarbital, administered either to the neonate or to the mother during labor, has been shown to diminish the frequency and severity of these hemorrhages (Donn and colleagues, 1981; Morales and Koerten, 1986). Similarly, vitamin K_1 given intramuscularly to women with preterm labor improved neonatal prothrombin activity and significantly decreased the frequency of intraventricular hemorrhage (Pomerance and colleagues, 1987). Vitamin E injections given to these neonates may decrease the incidence and severity of hemorrhage, but not mortality (Chiswick and colleagues, 1991; Sinha and associates, 1987). Indomethacin given to neonates weighing less than 1000 g was associated with a similar incidence of hemorrhage, but a higher mortality rate than untreated controls (Hanigan and colleagues, 1988).

Morales (1991) has recently reviewed antenatal pharmacological therapy for prevention of intraventricular hemorrhage.

Brain Disorders

In 1862, a London orthopedist, William Little, described 47 children with spastic rigidity, and he concluded that virtually nothing other than abnormalities of birth could cause this clinical picture. Although others have suggested that prenatal events may be causal factors, Paneth (1986) stated that the *presumed* birth-injury etiology for cerebral palsy has endured and has influenced the opinions and practices of countless obstetricians and pediatricians. Unfortunately, this presumption likely accounts in part for the high malpractice premiums among those who deliver and care for newborns.

In 1985, a report was published by a panel of experts assembled by the National Institutes of Child Health and Human Development and the National Institute of Neurologic and Communicative Disorders and Stroke (Freeman, 1985). This information has done much to enhance our knowledge of brain disorders that were previously assumed to be due to intrapartum factors. Importantly, the report set some guidelines that are crucial to resolving some medicolegal issues that invariably surround children with brain disorders that includes cerebral palsy, mental retardation, learning disabilities, and seizure disorders. Unfortunately, many clinicians have a poor understanding as to what antepartum, intrapartum, and neonatal factors are, and—possibly more important—*are not* associated with neurological abnormalities and cerebral palsy. Thus, many obstetricians, pediatricians, and neurologists erroneously attribute most cases of cerebral palsy to intrapartum or perinatal asphyxia. Unfortunately, "asphyxia" itself is an imprecise term, and its diagnosis is frequently based on low Apgar scores alone, which may be caused by other factors such as preterm birth, maternal sedation, anesthesia, the person assigning the score, vigorous suctioning or intubation, congenital malformations, and newborn muscle, neurological, or cardiorespiratory disease (Gilstrap and Cunningham, 1989).

Cerebral Palsy. The National Institutes of Health panel defined cerebral palsy as a nonprogressive motor disorder of early infant onset, involving one or more limbs, with resulting muscular spasticity or paralysis. Although epilepsy and mental retardation may be associated with cerebral palsy, these two conditions rarely, if ever, are associated with perinatal asphyxia in the absence of cerebral palsy (American College of Obstetricians and Gynecologists, 1992; Freeman and Nelson, 1988). The major types of cerebral palsy are spastic quadriplegia (increased association with mental retardation and seizure disorders), diplegia (common in preterm or low-birthweight infants), hemiplegia, choreoathetoid types, and mixed varieties (Freeman and Nelson, 1988). In a recent review of the literature Rosen and Dickinson (1992) reported that approximately 34 percent of the cases of cerebral palsy were of the diplegia type, 30 percent were hemiplegia, 20 percent quadriplegia, and 16 percent were of the extrapyramidal type. Moreover, significant mental retardation (I.Q. < 50) was associated with 25 percent of cerebral palsy cases, 18 percent in infants less than 2500 grams, and 30 percent for infants 2500 grams or greater (Rosen and Dickinson, 1992).

Incidence and Causes. The incidence of cerebral palsy is approximately 1 to 2 per 1000 live births (American College of Obstetricians and Gynecologists, 1992). In a recent review of eleven studies published from 1985 through 1990, the average cumulative rate for cerebral palsy at ages 5 to 7 years was 2.7 per 1000 livebirths (Rosen and Dickinson, 1992). The rate for low birthweight (less than 2500 g) infants was 15 per 1000 and for survivors, if 500 to 1500 grams at birth, the rate was 13 to 90 per 1000 livebirths (Rosen and Dickinson, 1992). Importantly, as emphasized by several groups, the incidence of cerebral palsy has remained essentially unchanged over the past decade, and it may actually have increased in some countries (Hagberg, 1984; Jarvis, 1985; Pharoah, 1987; Stanley, 1988; Torfs, 1990; and their colleagues). In many cases, cerebral palsy is erroneously attributed to perinatal events. Contrary to earlier dogma, it is now well established that only about 10 percent of cerebral palsy in term infants is associated with perinatal asphyxia (Blair and Stanley, 1988; Freeman and Nelson, 1988). **As emphasized by the American College of Obstetricians and Gynecologists, (1992), it is of paramount importance to understand that "it is erroneous to believe that the observed asphyxia caused the cerebral palsy in all cases."**

The antecedents and possible associated factors of cerebral palsy have been examined extensively by Nelson and Ellenberg (1984, 1985, 1986a, 1986b), who described findings from the Collaborative Perinatal Project. They reported that maternal mental retardation, birthweight less than 2000 g, and fetal malformations were leading predictors of cerebral palsy, whereas obstetrical complications were not strongly predictive. Only 21 percent of affected children had markers for perinatal asphyxia, and over half of these had associated congenital malformations, low birthweight, microcephaly, or another explanation for the brain disorder. **They concluded that the causes are unknown for most cases of cerebral palsy.** Thus, "no foreseeable single intervention is likely to prevent a large proportion of cerebral palsy" (Nelson and Ellenberg, 1986a).

Torfs and associates (1990) have presented data which confirm these observations. They reported an incidence of cerebral palsy of 0.3 percent among 19,044 liveborn children from the California Child Health and Development Studies database. Of the 55 children with cerebral palsy, 14 (25 percent) had neural-tube defects or obvious postnatal causes, that is, infection or injury. There were only nine (22 percent) infants with cerebral palsy who had perinatal asphyxia defined as a time to cry longer than 5 minutes. Importantly, all nine of these infants had birth defects, gestational risk factors, or both. The strongest predictors for cerebral palsy were the presence of a major or minor congenital anomaly, low birthweight, low placental weight, or abnormal fetal position, that is, face, breech, or transverse lie. The factors were similar to those factors identified in the Collaborative Perinatal Project (Table 44–3). Interestingly, instrumental delivery, including low, mid, or even high forceps, or cesarean delivery did not correlate with the presence of cerebral palsy.

Intraventricular hemorrhage is a potent risk factor for cerebral palsy. Recall that cerebral palsy is more common in preterm infants. Luthy and colleagues (1987) reported that more than 40 percent of low-birthweight infants with cerebral palsy had grade III or IV hemorrhages. They computed a 16-fold increased risk for cerebral palsy when these infants were compared with those either with no hemorrhage or those with grade I or II hemorrhage. Graham and associates (1987) reported that multiple cystic areas following periventricular hemorrhage were strongly associated with subsequent cerebral impairment.

Apgar Scores. Nelson and Ellenberg (1984) studied the interaction between obstetrical complications and a low Apgar score as a predictor of poor neurological outcome. A variety of late pregnancy complications were identified in 62 percent of pregnancies, and when considered alone, they were not associated strongly with cerebral palsy. However, in infants with complicated births who also had 5-minute Apgar scores of 3 or less, the incidences of mortality and cerebral palsy were increased appreciably. In the absence of complications, low Apgar scores alone were not associated with a high level of risk. Dijxhoorn and colleagues (1986) reported similar findings and concluded that most neonatal neurological abnormalities were due to factors other than perinatal hypoxia. Luthy and associates (1987) reported that in low-birthweight infants with 1-minute Apgar scores of 3 or less, the incidence of death was increased five-fold and the incidence of cerebral palsy was increased three-fold.

TABLE 44–3. PRENATAL AND PERINATAL RISK FACTORS IN CHILDREN WITH CEREBRAL PALSY

Risk Factors	Risk Ratio	95% CI
Long menstrual cycle (> 36 days)[a]	9.0	2.2–37.1
Hydramnios[a]	6.9	1.0–49.3
Premature placental separation[a]	7.6	2.7–21.1
Intervals between pregnancies < 3 months or > 3 years	3.7	1.0–4.4
Birthweight < 2000 g[a]	4.2	1.8–10.2
Breech, face, or transverse lie[a]	3.8	1.6–9.1
Severe birth defect[a]	15.6	8.1–30.0
Non-severe birth defect	6.1	3.1–11.8
Time to cry more than 5 minutes[a]	9.0	4.3–18.8
Low placental weight[a]	3.6	1.5–8.4

[a] Also associated with cerebral palsy in the Collaborative Perinatal Project (Nelson and Ellenberg, 1985, 1986a, 1986b).
Adapted from Torfs and associates (1990), with permission.

The American College of Obstetricians and Gynecologists (1986a) has summarized the use and misuse of the Apgar score to assess asphyxia and to predict future neurological deficit (see Chap. 17, p. 445). It was concluded that low scores at 1 and 5 minutes are excellent indicators for identification of those infants who need resuscitation. It further was concluded that low Apgar scores alone are not evidence for sufficient hypoxia to result in neurological damage. In a child found to have cerebral palsy, low 1- or 5-minute Apgar scores provide insufficient evidence that the damage was due to hypoxia.

Electronic Fetal Heart Rate Monitoring. It is now well established that continuous electronic fetal heart rate monitoring neither predicts nor reduces the risk of cerebral palsy when compared with intermittent auscultation (American College of Obstetricians and Gynecologists, 1992; Freeman, 1990; Freeman and Nelson, 1988; Grant and associates, 1989; Shy and coworkers, 1990). In a randomized, prospective study of over 13,000 pregnancies, MacDonald and associates (1985) compared continuous electronic monitoring (n = 6527) with intermittent auscultation (n = 6552); Grant and colleagues (1989) later found three infants in each group with cerebral palsy at age 4.

Neonatal Acidosis. As summarized in Chapter 17 (p. 446), an important criterion in the definition of asphyxia is metabolic acidosis, and it is unlikely that there is significant intrapartum asphyxia in its absence. Although there has been significant enthusiasm for the clinical use of umbilical cord acid-base determinations, when utilized alone, they have proven no more useful than the 1- and 5-minute Apgar scores in predicting long-term neurological sequelae. For example, Dijxhoorn and associates (1986), in a study of 805 term newborns delivered vaginally, reported that the largest number of neurologically abnormal infants had a normal umbilical arterial pH but low Apgar score. **These authors concluded that intrapartum hypoxia was not a major cause of neurological morbidity.** Others have reported that neither pH measurements nor acidemia correlated with long-term neurological outcome in term infants (American College of Obstetricians and Gynecologists, 1992; Fee and associates, 1990; Freeman and Nelson, 1988; Ruth and Raivio, 1988). Subsequently, it was reported that the pH cut-off for clinically significant acidemia most likely is less than 7.0 instead of less than 7.2, especially the degree of acidosis which might be associated with neurological sequelae (Gilstrap, 1989; Goldaber, 1991; Winkler, 1991; and their colleagues).

Neonatal Encephalopathy. Seizures and recurrent apnea are important predictors of cerebral palsy and future cognitive defects. Low and colleagues (1985) studied 303 high-risk preterm and term neonates, 30 percent of whom had newborn encephalopathy. *Mild* encephalopathy was defined as hyperalertness, irritability, jitteriness, and hypertonia and hypotonia. *Moderate* encephalopathy included lethargy, severe hypertonia, and occasional seizures. *Severe* encephalopathy was defined by coma, multiple seizures, and recurrent apnea. Cognitive and motor deficits were more likely in infants with mild or moderate (25 percent) or severe (55 percent) encephalopathy, compared with those without neonatal seizures (17 percent). Neonatal respiratory complications were the most commonly identifiable risk factor, but in 72 percent of those with mild to moderate encephalopathy, there were no risk factors identified (Fig. 44–4). Perinatal hypoxia was associated with, or contributed to, 26 percent of cases of mild to moderate encephalopathy and 66 percent of those with severe encephalopathy.

In the report by Robertson and Finer (1985), 100 percent of newborns with mild hypoxic encephalopathy, 80 percent with moderate encephalopathy, and none with severe encephalopathy had normal neurological outcome.

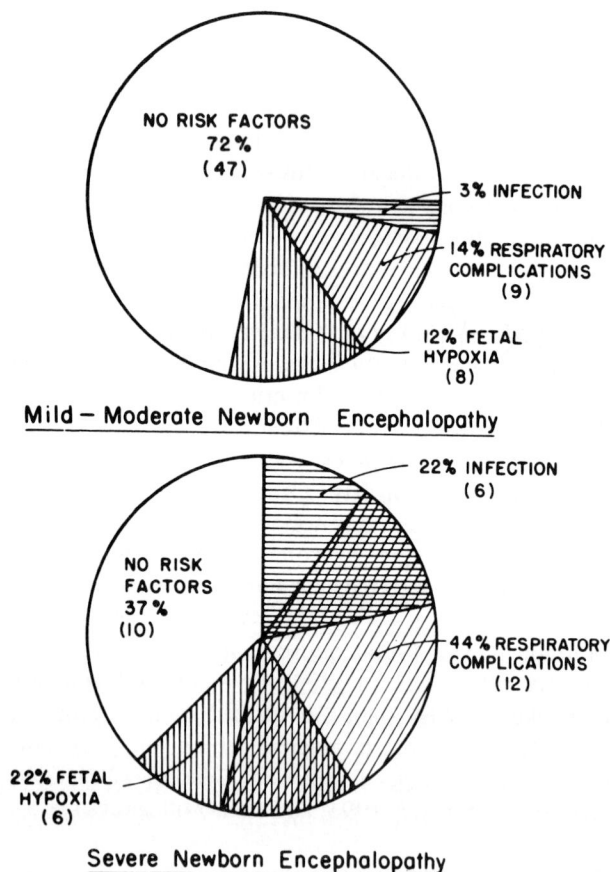

Mild – Moderate Newborn Encephalopathy

Severe Newborn Encephalopathy

Fig. 44–4. Incidence of significant biological risk factors observed in high-risk preterm and term neonates with mild-to-moderate and severe neonatal encephalopathy. (From Low and colleagues, 1985, with permission.)

Neuroradiological Imaging and Timing of Injury. Imaging techniques (computed tomography and magnetic resonance imaging) performed later in childhood have been utilized to define the neuropathology and timing of cerebral palsy (Perlman and Cunningham, 1993). In the first sets of studies, Wiklund and colleagues (1991a, 1991b) used computed tomography to study 28 preterm infants and 83 term infants with hemiplegic cerebral palsy between 5 and 16 years of age. In the preterm infants, 50 percent had evidence for periventricular leukomalacia, 20 percent had brain maldevelopment indicative of brain injury early in fetal life, and in 25 percent of cases computed tomography was normal. In term infants, computed tomography findings suggested a prenatal origin of injury in over half of the cases, that is, periventricular atrophy in 37 percent and maldevelopment in 17 percent. Cortical and subcortical injury suggestive of a perinatal injury was found in 19 percent, whereas in 27 percent computed tomography was normal (Table 44–4).

In another study, 11 preterm and 29 term infants were evaluated with magnetic resonance imaging (Truwit and colleagues, 1992). The predominant finding in preterm infants was evidence of periventricular white matter damage in more than 80 percent, indicative of hypoxic ischemic brain injury. It was difficult to distinguish the exact chronology of onset with this lesion. In contrast, in term infants, 50 percent of imaging findings were consistent with antenatal brain damage (gyral abnormalities suggestive of polymicrogyri consistent with mid-second trimester injury, and isolated periventricular leukomalacia) (Table 44–5). In approximately 25 percent of these cases, magnetic resonance imaging findings coupled with clinical events were suggestive of hypoxic ischemic injury at the time of birth. This figure is similar to that obtained in the several large epidemiological studies of cerebral palsy noted previously (Blair, 1988; Grant, 1989; Nelson, 1986a, 1986b; Torfs, 1990; and their colleagues).

An example of the use of neuroimaging in timing of neurological injury is given below:

> A 1150 g infant was born at 27 weeks to a mother whose pregnancy was uncomplicated until the onset of vaginal bleeding. The diagnosis of placental abruption was made and emergency cesarean section performed. Arterial blood from the umbilical cord had a pH of 7.05, PCO_2 of 80 mm Hg, PO_2 of 7

TABLE 44–4. COMPUTED TOMOGRAPHY FINDINGS IN 83 TERM INFANTS WITH HEMISPHERIC CEREBRAL PALSY

Type of Lesion	Percent of Total
Maldevelopment	17
Periventricular atrophy	37
Cortical/subcortical atrophy	19
Normal	27

Adapted from Wiklund and colleagues (1991), with permission.

TABLE 44–5. MAGNETIC RESONANCE IMAGING FINDINGS IN TERM INFANTS WITH CEREBRAL PALSY

Type of Lesion	Percent of Total
Migration abnormalities	31
Periventricular leukomalacia	21
Hydrencephaly	3
Cortical/subcortical injury	17
Others	28

Adapted from Truwit and colleagues (1992), with permission.

mm Hg, and a base deficit of -14 mEq/L. The infant was intubated in the delivery room because of poor respiratory effort. The Apgar scores were 5 at one minute and 6 at five minutes. The infant's postnatal course was complicated by severe respiratory distress syndrome necessitating surfactant replacement, pneumothorax, and hypotension requiring volume expanders. A head ultrasound scan performed on the first day showed small bilateral cysts in periventricular white matter and bilateral germinal matrix hemorrhages (Fig. 44–5A). A repeat scan performed on day 3 showed bilateral intraventricular hemorrhage and a large intraparenchymal echodensity on the right (Fig. 44–5B). The bilateral cysts noted on the first scan were not identified on the repeat scan.

The clinical findings are typical of a preterm infant who develops periventricular-intraventricular hemorrhage with an associated intraparenchymal echodensity (Perlman and Cunningham, 1993; Volpe, 1987). The head ultrasound performed on the first postnatal day showed bilateral cystic periventricular leukomalacia. This lesion

was not seen on the scan performed two days later. The ultrasonic evolution of cysts takes from days to weeks to occur. The head ultrasound obtained on the first day of life was critical in diagnosing antenatal brain injury. Intraventricular hemorrhage, although common to the preterm infant, was a secondary insult. The infant's urine tested positive for cocaine. Chronic cocaine exposure probably caused cystic periventricular leukomalacia and may have contributed to the placental abruption.

Another case which illustrates the importance of neuroimaging is given below:

A 2965 g infant was born to a woman at term. Pregnancy was complicated by a viral infection during the early third trimester. On the day of admission, she complained of decreased fetal movement. When the membranes ruptured, meconium was noted in the amnionic fluid, and fetal heart rate tracing was nonreactive with a rate of 160 beats per minute. Emergency cesarean section was performed and the infant was delivered with Apgar scores of 2 at one minute and 3 at five minutes. The umbilical arterial cord pH was 7.10 with a base deficit of − 15mEq/L. Intubation was performed and positive pressure ventilation initiated. The infant was oliguric in the first 36 hours of life. Newborn examination disclosed a full anterior fontanel in an unresponsive infant with absent cortical and brain stem function. The only response obtained was episodic reflex withdrawal to painful stimuli in the left lower extremity. A computed tomography scan was performed that demonstrated a grade III intraventricular hemorrhage (Fig. 44–6A). An ultrasound scan confirmed the intraventricular hemorrhage (Fig. 44–6B). In addition, bilateral cystic periven-

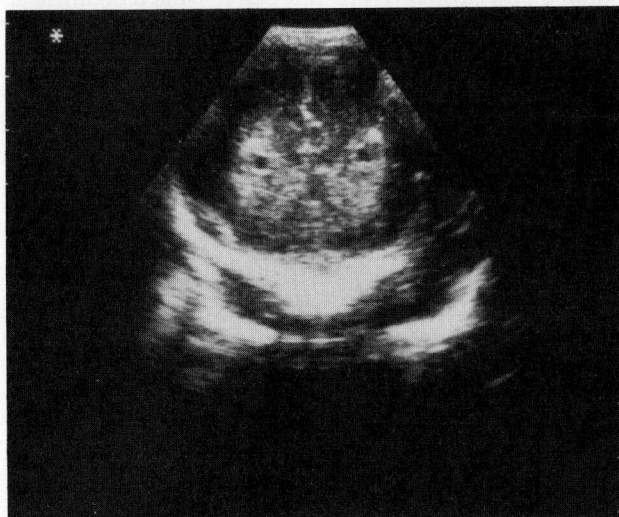

A

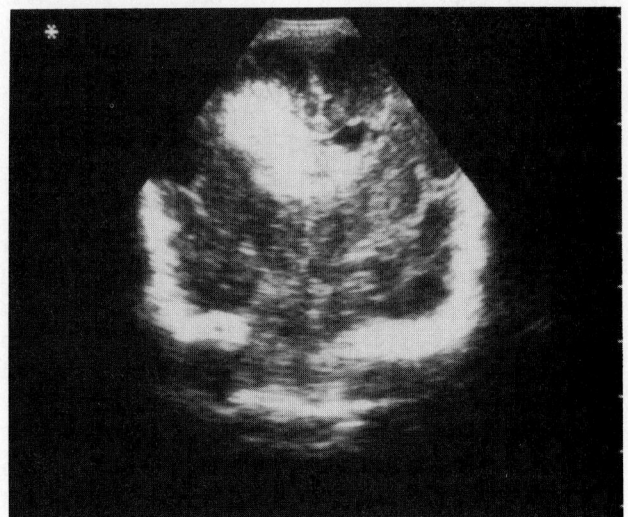

B

Fig. 44–5. Preterm infant delivered at 27 weeks because of placental abruption. **A.** Head ultrasound performed on the first postnatal day shows small bilateral cysts in periventricular white matter and bilateral germinal matrix hemorrhages. These findings indicate a much older lesion than one due to perinatal asphyxia. **B.** Repeat ultrasound of same infant on day 3 of life showed bilateral intraventricular hemorrhage and a large intraparenchymal echodensity on the right. (Courtesy of Dr. Jeffrey Perlman.)

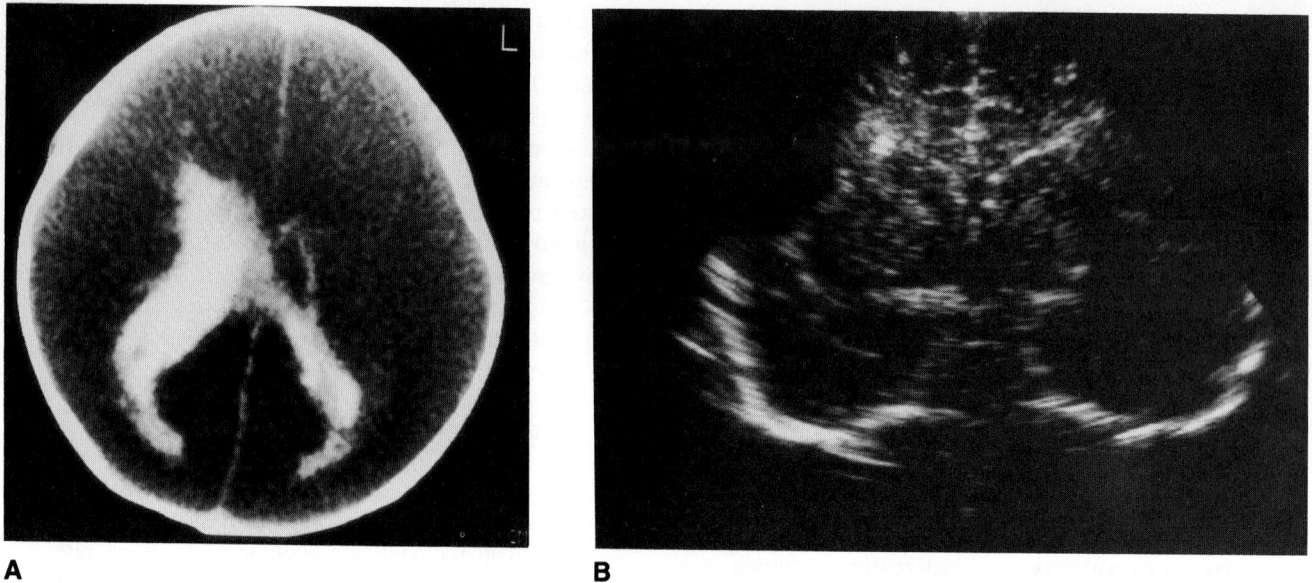

A   **B**

Fig. 44–6. Term infant born depressed. **A.** Computed tomography scan demonstrates a grade III intraventricular hemorrhage. **B.** Ultrasound scan confirmed intraventricular hemorrhage and, in addition, bilateral cystic periventricular leukomalacia was seen which was not observed on the computed tomography scan. These findings documented a severe antenatal brain insult of 4 to 5 weeks duration. (From Perlman and Cunningham, 1993.)

tricular leukomalacia was noted. This was not observed on the computed tomography scan.

These clinical findings are consistent with severe brain injury secondary to a perinatal insult, that is, low Apgar score, acidemia in cord blood, and a markedly abnormal neurological examination. However, neuroimaging proved the presence of antenatal brain injury. Based on the vascular development and the usual occurrence of periventricular leukomalacia, which is between 28 and 34 weeks, the ultrasonic findings suggest that the injury was sustained approximately 4 to 5 weeks prior to delivery. The perinatal lesion, intraventricular hemorrhage, was a secondary event. This case also illustrates a potential limitation of computed tomography—the inability to detect cystic periventricular leukomalacia.

Mental Retardation. Etiological factors for severe mental retardation, which has a prevalence of 3 per 1000 children, are shown in Table 44–6. In the National Institutes of Health report, the panel ascertained that isolated mental retardation—that is, mental retardation without epilepsy or cerebral palsy—was associated with perinatal hypoxia in only 5 percent of cases.

Seizure Disorders. Unless manifest in association with cerebral palsy, seizure disorders or epilepsy are not related to perinatal hypoxia. Nelson and Ellenberg (1986b) determined that the major predictors of seizure disorders were fetal malformations (cerebral and noncerebral), family history of seizure disorders, and neonatal seizures.

Cerebral Palsy Attributable to Perinatal Asphyxia. As emphasized by Freeman and Nelson (1988), the condition of the neonate in the nursery and early neonatal period is of paramount importance in attempting to ascertain whether intrapartum events, such as perinatal asphyxia, were related to cerebral palsy. They state that "The term infant who was in the normal nursery, who went out to feed with mother, or who was discharged at the usual time cannot have shown evidence of serious hypoxic-ischemic encephalopathy early in the nursery course and probably did not suffer sufficient intrapartum hypoxia to result in permanent neurologic deficit." These authors also emphasize that even when the newborn does have signs of moderate to severe encephalopathy, this does not necessarily mean that the infant has suffered intrapartum asphyxia—other conditions

TABLE 44–6. SOME ETIOLOGICAL FACTORS FOR SEVERE MENTAL RETARDATION

Factor	Percent
Prenatal	73
Chromosomal	36
Mutant genes	7
Multiple congenital anomalies	20
Acquired—infections, diabetes, dysmaturity	10
Perinatal	10
Asphyxia/hypoxia	5
Unidentified causes	5
Postnatal	11
Unknown	6

Modified from Rosen and Hobel (1986), with permission.

such as metabolic, genetic, structural, and trauma may cause encephalopathy (Freeman and Nelson, 1988).

The criteria for diagnosing perinatal asphyxia to a degree which might be associated with neurological sequelae, including cerebral palsy, has recently been reviewed by the American College of Obstetricians and Gynecologists (1992) and is summarized in Chapter 17 (p. 445).

CONCLUSIONS REGARDING CEREBRAL PALSY AND PERINATAL AS-PHYXIA. There is now almost universal agreement concerning the poor correlation between intrapartum events, perinatal asphyxia, and cerebral palsy. This was best summarized by an editorial in the *Lancet* (Anonymous, 1989) and a recent technical bulletin from the American College of Obstetricians and Gynecologists (1992). In the former, it was stated that "... the continued willingness of doctors to reinforce the fable that intrapartum care is an important determinant of cerebral palsy can only be regarded as shooting the specialty of obstetrics in the foot."

Anemia

Diagnosis. The diagnosis of anemia in the newborn infant is not always simple. After 35 weeks' gestation, the mean cord hemoglobin concentration is about 17 g/dL and values much below 14 g/dL may be regarded as pathologically low. During the first several hours of life, the hemoglobin value may rise by as much as 20 percent, especially when cord clamping was delayed, and as the consequence, an appreciable volume of blood was expressed from the placenta through the cord into the infant. Alternatively, if the placenta was cut or torn, a fetal vessel was perforated or lacerated, or the infant was held well above the level of the placenta for some time before cord clamping, the hemoglobin concentration more likely falls after delivery.

Fetal-to-Maternal Hemorrhage. The presence of fetal red cells in the maternal circulation may be identified by use of the acid elution principle first described by Kleihauer, Brown, and Betke, or any of several modifications. Very small volumes of red cells commonly escape from the fetal intravascular compartment across the placental barrier into the maternal intervillous space. Large bleeds are uncommon, and Bowman (1985) reported that only 21 of 9000 women had fetal hemorrhage at delivery exceeding 30 mL. Although the bleed is usually small, it may incite maternal iso-immunization, as discussed later. Stedman and colleagues (1986), using the erythrocyte rosette test, reported hemorrhage of this magnitude in only 6 of 1000 women.

Rarely, fetal-to-maternal hemorrhage may be so severe as to kill the fetus (Fig. 44–7). The hypovolemic or

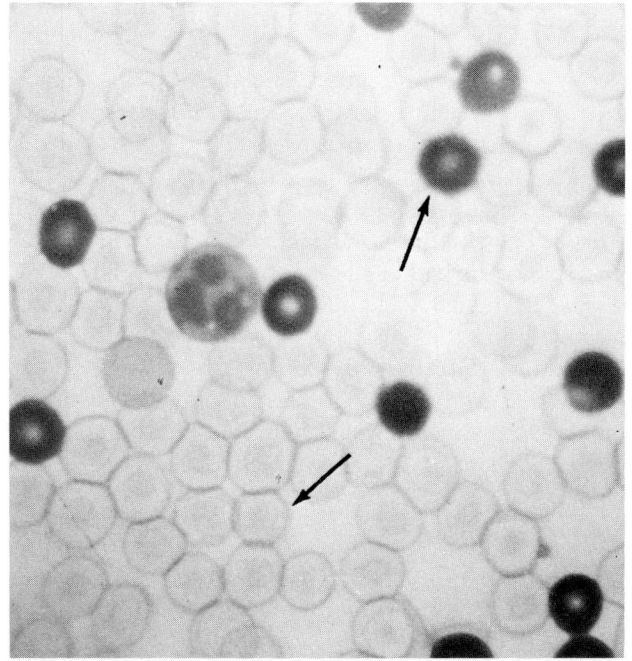

Fig. 44–7. Massive fetal-to-maternal hemorrhage. After acid-elution treatment, fetal red cells rich in hemoglobin F stain darkly (*upper arrow*), whereas maternal red cells with only very small amounts of hemoglobin F stain lightly (*lower arrow*).

severely anemic fetus-infant may be salvaged if the condition is recognized and treatment with blood, red cells, or both, is promptly initiated. The fetus who is severely anemic is more likely to demonstrate an ominous heart rate pattern. On occasion, the hemorrhage may have been chronic and so severe as to produce evidence of iron deficiency in the fetus. Maternal anemia, however, even when severe, is not accompanied by anemia in the fetus.

With larger fetal-to-maternal hemorrhages, a placental lesion—for example, a chorioangioma—is likely the cause. We know of two instances of severe fetal-to-maternal hemorrhage in which the mothers were later found to have choriocarcinoma. Placental abruption, in our experience, does not commonly cause appreciable fetal-to-maternal hemorrhage, although if due to trauma, the likelihood is increased (see Chap. 37, p. 829).

At Parkland Hospital, for some time maternal blood has been studied for fetal red cells in each instance of stillbirth whenever a cause was not readily apparent, and massive bleeds have been found in only a small minority of stillborn infants.

Large fetal-to-maternal hemorrhages may also prove dangerous to the mother. It is possible for up to 400 mL of fetal blood to be transferred from the fetoplacental circulation into the maternal circulation. A transfusion reaction may then develop in the mother whenever A or B antigens are present in fetal, but not maternal, erythrocytes.

Hemolysis from Isoimmunization

In 1892, Ballantyne established clinicopathological criteria for the diagnosis of **hydrops fetalis**. In 1932, Diamond, Blackfan, and Baty reported that fetal anemia characterized by numerous circulating erythroblasts was associated with this syndrome. Certainly ranking as a major contribution to medicine is the subsequent delineation of the pathogenesis of most cases of hemolytic disease in the fetus and newborn, including the related discovery of the rhesus factor by Landsteiner and Weiner in 1940. In 1941, Levine and associates confirmed that erythroblastosis was due to maternal isoimmunization with paternally inherited fetal factors, and the subsequent development of effective maternal prophylaxis was attributed to Finn and associates (1961) in England, and Freda and co-workers (1963) in the United States.

Isoimmunization. Originally, the Rh concept was defined by one antiserum and two blood group factors, namely Rh-positive and Rh-negative. The Rh factors, however, have become increasingly complex, and more than 400 other red cell antigens have been identified. Although some of them are immunologically and genetically important, fortunately many are so rare as to be of little clinical significance.

Individuals who lack a specific red cell antigen can potentially produce an antibody when exposed to that antigen. The antibody may prove harmful to the individual in the case of a blood transfusion or to a fetus when a woman conceives. The vast majority of humans have at least one such factor inherited from their father and lacking in their mother. In these cases, the mother could be sensitized if enough erythrocytes from the fetus were to reach her circulation to elicit an immune response. That the disease is identified in very few pregnancies is a result of several circumstances. These include (1) the varying rates of occurrence of the offending red cell antigens, (2) their variable antigenicity, (3) insufficient transplacental passage of antigen from fetus to mother, (4) the variability of maternal response to the antigen, (5) protection from isoimmunization by ABO incompatibility of fetus and mother, and (6) lack of transfer of antibody across the placenta from mother to fetus in amounts sufficient to affect the fetus.

To best illustrate the likelihood of Rh or D-isoimmunization, the report of Bowman (1985) is cited. A D-negative woman delivered of a D-positive, ABO-compatible infant, has a likelihood of isoimmunization of 16 percent. About 2 percent of such women will be immunized by the time of delivery, another 7 percent will have anti-D antibody by 6 months postpartum, and the remaining 7 percent will demonstrate D-isoimmunization when challenged in a subsequent pregnancy by another D-positive fetus. ABO incompatibility confers some protection against D-isoimmunization because fetal red cells entering the mother usually are rapidly destroyed before they elicit an antigenic response. The D-negative woman delivered of a D-positive, but ABO-incompatible, infant has only a 2 percent chance of D-isoimmunization by 6 months postpartum.

CDE (Rhesus) Blood Group System. The CDE, or rhesus, blood group system is of considerable clinical importance because the majority of individuals who lack its major antigenic determinant, D or Rho, become immunized after a single exposure to erythrocyte antigen. Several nomenclature systems currently are used; however, the CDE grouping system seems best, especially to describe the non-D antigens and their respective antibodies, anti-C, anti-c, anti-E, and anti-e.

The CDE antigens are inherited independent of other blood group antigens and are located on the short arm of chromosome 1. There is apparently no difference in the distribution of the CDE antigens with regard to sex; however, there are important racial differences. American Indians and Chinese and other Asiatic peoples are almost all D-positive (99 percent). Among African-Americans there is a lesser incidence of D-negative individuals (7 to 8 percent) than among white Americans (13 percent). Of all racial and ethnic groups studied thus far, the Basques show the highest incidence of D-negativity (34 percent).

CDE antigens other than D have low immunogenicity and typically are ignored unless the pregnant woman has already formed an antibody to them. **All pregnant women should be tested routinely for the presence or absence of D (Rho) antigen on their erythrocytes and for other irregular antibodies in their serum.** Barss and colleagues (1988) have argued convincingly that this be done only once in D-positive women.

ABO Blood Group System. The major blood group antigens A and B are the most common, but are not the most serious cause of hemolytic disease in the newborn. For example, group O women may from early life have anti-A and anti-B isoagglutinins, which may be augmented by pregnancy, particularly if the fetus is a secretor. Although about 20 percent of all infants have an ABO maternal blood group incompatibility, only 5 percent of them show overt signs of hemolytic disease. Moreover, when they do, the disease almost always is much milder than that with D-isoimmunization. **Unlike Rh hemolytic disease, the incidence of stillbirths among ABO-incompatible pregnancies is not increased.**

Thus, ABO isoimmunization will cause hemolytic disease of the newborn, but it does not cause hydrops fetalis. The reasons for this probably are at least two-fold. First, most species of isoantibodies to A and B antigens are immunoglobulin M, and thus not likely to gain access to fetal erythrocytes. Second, fetal red cells have a diminished number of A and B antigenic sites, at least when compared with later in life.

Black infants are more likely to develop ABO disease than are white infants (Kirkman, 1977). Desjardins and co-workers (1979) studied a large number of infants of blood group O mothers to try to identify a relationship between the degree of red cell sensitization by antibody and the cord blood hemoglobin and bilirubin concentrations. They found that when the infant blood type was A or B, the bilirubin was higher and hemoglobin was lower than in cord blood from blood group O infants, even when no antibody was identified on the type A or B red cells. They concluded that ABO incompatibility represents a spectrum of hemolytic disease that ranges from those with little laboratory evidence of red cell sensitization to those with severe hemolytic disease.

The usual criteria for diagnosis of hemolysis due to ABO incompatibility include: (1) the mother is major blood group O, with anti-A and anti-B in her serum, while the fetus is group A, B, or AB; (2) there is onset of jaundice within the first 24 hours; (3) there are varying degrees of anemia, reticulocytosis, and erythroblastosis; and (4) there has been careful exclusion of other causes of hemolysis. Unlike the result in rhesus hemolytic disease, the Coombs antiglobulin test in ABO incompatibility may be negative, although it is usually positive.

Because there is no adequate method of antenatal diagnosis, careful observation is essential in the neonatal period if cases are to be detected. Unlike Rh hemolytic disease, ABO disease is frequently seen in infants of primigravidas, and it is likely to recur in subsequent pregnancies. Katz and co-workers (1982) identified a recurrence rate of 87 percent, and 62 percent of the affected infants required treatment, but this was most often limited to phototherapy for hyperbilirubinemia.

The principles of management of the newborn with ABO hemolytic disease are similar to those for the infant born with Rhesus isoimmunization, particularly with reference to the behavior of hemoglobin and bilirubin. For simple transfusion or exchange transfusion, group O blood is used. Because the incidence of stillbirths among ABO-incompatible pregnancies is not increased, there is no justification for early labor induction or for performing amniocentesis.

Other Blood Group Incompatibilities. D-antigen incompatibility and ABO heterospecificity account for approximately 98 percent of all cases of hemolytic disease. For each red cell antigen there is the potential for hemolytic disease in the fetus and infant if the fetus has the antigen but the mother does not, the antibody is of IgG type and can cross the placenta, and the antibody does so in amounts sufficient to cause hemolysis.

The possibility of hemolytic disease from rarer blood groups may be suspected from the results of the indirect Coombs test done to screen for abnormal antibodies in maternal serum. Listed in Table 44–7 are a number of red cell antigens and their capacity for causing hemolytic disease.

An idea of the frequency of some of these antibodies comes from the report of Bowell and colleagues (1986a), who screened 70,000 pregnant women over a 2-year period. They identified 677 pregnancies with atypical red cell antibodies, for an incidence of nearly 1 percent. One fourth of these were from the Lewis system, which do not cause fetal hemolysis because the antigens do not develop on erythrocytes until a few weeks after birth. Of the remaining 544 antibodies, 72 percent were of the CDE group, and anti-D was most common (158), followed by anti-E (130), anti-c (49), and anti-C (19). Antibodies to the Kell system antigens also were common (76).

Bowman and colleagues (1992a) recently reviewed their experiences from Manitoba with 459 pregnancies from 311 Kell-immunized women. Of these, 63 ended in abortion or stillbirth unrelated to anti-Kell sensitization. Of the remaining infants, 376 were unaffected. Of 20 who were affected, 12 newborns required no therapy. There were four perinatal deaths; one from kernicterus and three from hydrops. As emphasized by these authors, although Kell hemolytic disease is rare, it may be severe and cause death; thus when the maternal anti-Kell titer is 8 or greater, it must be investigated by amniocentesis or fetal blood sampling.

The clinical importance of anti-c isoimmunization recently has been emphasized by Wenk (1986) and Bowell (1986b) and their colleagues. This antibody was the next most common cause of clinically significant isoimmunization following anti-D. Although anti-c isoimmunization most commonly resulted from previous pregnancies, those fetuses whose mothers had been transfused were more likely to have moderate to severe hemolysis.

Bowman and colleagues (1992b) recently reviewed their experiences with 80 women in Manitoba with either anti-C or anti-Ce alloimmunization. Of 120 pregnancies, 22 ended in abortion or stillbirth unrelated to isoimmunization. Of 33 affected fetuses, only eight required treatment after birth and none had severe disease.

Mother as Provider of Rare Type Red Cells. Following maternal isoimmunization with a rare blood type, the possibility exists of hemolytic disease in the fetus and neonate. This could create a need for red cells devoid of the antigen or antigens to which the mother is isoimmunized. Moreover, the mother herself may require red cells, for example, because of a complication of hemorrhage at delivery. For such circumstances, even while pregnant, she can successfully donate her own red cells, which are then appropriately frozen for subsequent use, as demonstrated by the following case:

G.D., a 17-year-old gravida 2, P1, lacked immunological evidence of all Rhesus antigens except D, and had acquired antibodies during the previous pregnancy to C, c, E, and e. Compatible red cells

TABLE 44–7. SOME RED CELL ANTIGENS AND THEIR PROPENSITY TO CAUSE HEMOLYTIC DISEASE IN THE FETUS-INFANT WHOSE MOTHER IS ISOIMMUNIZED

Blood Group System	Antigen	Severity of Hemolytic Disease	Proposed Management
CDE (Rh)	D	Mild to severe with hydrops fetalis	Amnionic fluid studies
	C	Mild to moderate	Amnionic fluid studies
	c	Mild to severe	Amnionic fluid studies
	E	Mild to severe	Amnionic fluid studies
	e	Mild to moderate	Amnionic fluid studies
I		Not a proven cause of hemolytic disease	
Lewis		Not a proven cause of hemolytic disease	
Kell	K	Mild to severe with hydrops fetalis	Amnionic fluid studies
	k	Mild to severe	Amnionic fluid studies
Duffy	Fy^a	Mild to severe with hydrops fetalis	Amnionic fluid studies
	Fy^b	Not a cause of hemolytic disease	
Kidd	Jk^a	Mild to severe	Amnionic fluid studies
	Jk^b	Mild to severe	Amnionic fluid studies
MNSs	M	Mild to severe	Amnionic fluid studies
	N	Mild	Expectant
	S	Mild to severe	Amnionic fluid studies
	s	Mild to severe	Amnionic fluid studies
	U	Mild to severe	Amnionic fluid studies
Lutheran	Lu^a	Mild	Expectant
	Lu^b	Mild	Expectant
Diego	Di^a	Mild to severe	Amnionic fluid studies
	Di^b	Mild to severe	Amnionic fluid studies
Xg	Xg^a	Mild	Expectant
P	$PP_{1Pk(Tja)}$	Mild to severe	Amnionic fluid studies
Public Antigens	Yt^a	Moderate to severe	Amnionic fluid studies
	Yt^b	Mild	Expectant
	Lan	Mild	Expectant
	En^a	Moderate	Amnionic fluid studies
	Ge	Mild	Expectant
	Jr^a	Mild	Expectant
	Co^a	Severe	Amnionic fluid studies
Private Antigens	Co^{a-b}	Mild	Expectant
	Batty	Mild	Expectant
	Becker	Mild	Expectant
	Berrens	Mild	Expectant
	Biles	Moderate	Amnionic fluid studies
	Evans	Mild	Expectant
	Gonzales	Mild	Expectant
	Good	Severe	Amnionic fluid studies
	Heibel	Moderate	Amnionic fluid studies
	Hunt	Mild	Expectant
	Jobbins	Mild	Expectant
	Radin	Moderate	Amnionic fluid studies
	Rm	Mild	Expectant
	Ven	Mild	Expectant
	$Wright^a$	Severe	Amnionic fluid studies
	$Wright^b$	Mild	Expectant
	Zd	Moderate	Amnionic fluid studies

Modified with permission from the American College of Obstetricians and Gynecologists (1986b).

available in the United States were limited to two units frozen in Portland, Oregon. Therefore, repeated phlebotomies were performed during pregnancy and the red cells promptly frozen for possible subsequent use. In spite of her small size (67 inches tall and 109 pounds, nonpregnant), she tolerated quite well the removal of six units (3000 mL total) of blood at the rate of 500 mL every 3 to 5 weeks. Iron was provided orally and parenterally along with supplementary folic acid. Oral iron alone, if taken regularly, would have provided sufficient iron. Her measured blood volume of 3800 mL was 47 percent above the nonpregnant state.

Repeat cesarean delivery was accomplished without incident. Hemolytic disease in the newborn was treated with exchange transfusions using all of the red cells harvested and stored from the six phlebotomies plus the two frozen units from Portland.

Pathological Changes in Hemolytic Disease. In D-positive fetuses, maternal antibodies are both adsorbed to the D-positive erythrocytes and exist unbound in fetal serum. The adsorbed antibodies act as hemolysins, leading to an accelerated rate of red cell destruction.

Maternal antibodies detectable at birth gradually disappear from the infant's circulation over a period of 1 to 4 months. Their rate of disappearance is influenced to some extent by exchange transfusion. Detection of adsorbed antibodies is best accomplished by the direct Coombs test. If D red cells coated with anti-D antibody are typed with an anti-D saline agglutinin, they may be reported incorrectly as D-negative because of the blocking effect produced by the adsorbed antibody. Therefore, erythrocytes reported to be D-negative from an infant whose mother may be isoimmunized must always be checked by the direct Coombs test.

Immune Hydrops. The pathological changes in the organs of the fetus and newborn infant vary with the severity of the process. The severely affected fetus or infant may show considerable subcutaneous edema as well as effusion into the serous cavities—**hydrops fetalis.** At times, the edema is so severe that the diagnosis can be easily identified using sonography (Fig. 44–8). In these cases, the placenta is also markedly edematous, appreciably enlarged and boggy, with large, prominent cotyledons and edematous villi. Excessive and prolonged hemolysis serves to stimulate marked erythroid hyperplasia of the bone marrow as well as large areas of *extramedullary hematopoiesis*, particularly in the spleen and liver, which may in turn cause hepatic dysfunction (Nicolini and associates, 1991). Histological examination of the liver may also disclose fatty degenerative parenchymal changes as well as deposition of

hemosiderin and engorgement of hepatic canaliculi with bile. There may be cardiac enlargement and pulmonary hemorrhages. The ascites, and to a lesser degree hepatomegaly and splenomegaly, may be so massive as to lead to severe dystocia as the consequence of the greatly enlarged abdomen. Hydrothorax may be so severe as to compromise respirations after birth.

The pathophysiology of hydrops remains obscure. Theories of its causation include heart failure from profound anemia, capillary leakage caused by hypoxia from severe anemia, portal and umbilical venous hypertension from hepatic parenchymal disruption by extramedullary hematopoiesis, and decreased colloid oncotic pressure from hypoproteinemia caused by liver dysfunction. To study this, Nicolaides and colleagues (1985) performed percutaneous umbilical artery blood sampling in 17 severely D-isoimmunized fetuses at 18 to 25 weeks' gestation. All fetuses with hydrops had hemoglobin values of less than 3.8 g/dL as well as plasma protein concentrations less than 2 standard deviations from the mean for normal fetuses of the same age. The hydropic fetuses also had substantive protein concentrations in ascitic fluid collected at fetoscopy. Conversely, all nonhydropic fetuses had hemoglobin values that exceeded 4 g/dL; however, 6 of 10 had hypoproteinemia of the same magnitude as the hydropic fetuses. These investigators concluded that the degree and duration of anemia influence the severity of ascites, and this is made worse by hypoproteinemia. They also hypothesized that severe chronic anemia causes tissue hypoxia with resultant capillary endothelial leakage with protein loss.

Fetuses with hydrops may die in utero from profound anemia and circulatory failure (Fig. 44–9). A sign of severe anemia and impending death is a *sinusoidal fetal heart rate* pattern (Chap. 15, p. 403). The liveborn hydropic infant appears pale, edematous, and limp at birth, often requiring resuscitation. The spleen and liver are enlarged, and there may be widespread ecchymoses or scattered petechiae. Dyspnea and circulatory collapse are common.

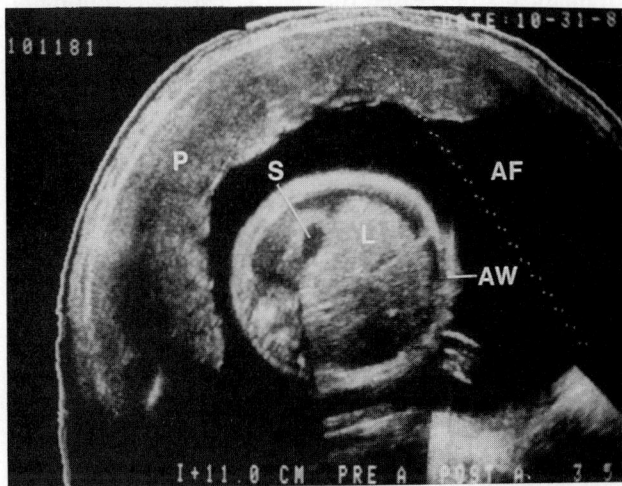

Fig. 44–8. Transverse sonogram of a hydropic fetus. Illustrated are the edematous fetal abdominal wall (AW) and the fetal liver (L) and stomach (S). Increased amnionic fluid (AF) is apparent, and there is also a large placenta (P). (Courtesy of Dr. R. Santos.)

Hyperbilirubinemia. Less severely affected infants may appear well at birth, only to become jaundiced within a few hours. Marked hyperbilirubinemia, if untreated, may lead to central nervous system damage, especially to the basal ganglia or *kernicterus*, which will be discussed subsequently.

Anemia, in part resulting from impaired erythropoiesis, may persist for many weeks to months in the infant who had demonstrated hemolytic disease at birth. In the absence of hypoxia, erythrocyte production normally falls after birth, especially in the preterm infant.

Mortality. The number of perinatal deaths from hemolytic disease caused by D-isoimmunization has dramatically dropped for the following reasons:

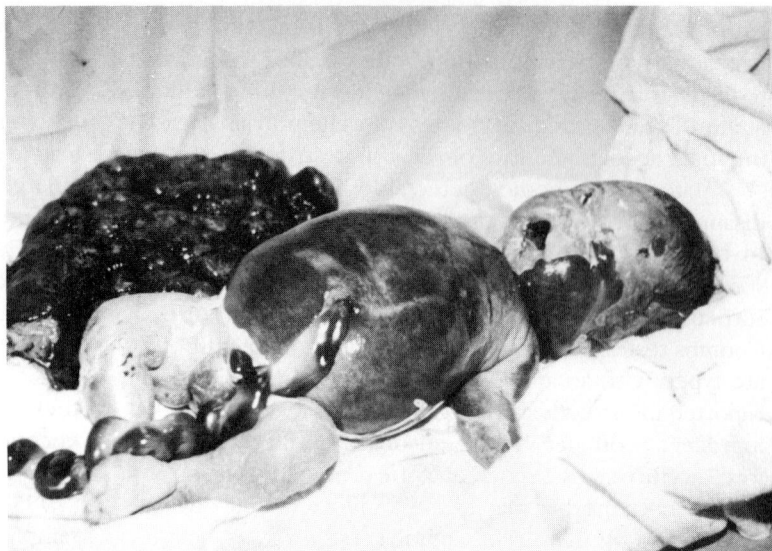

Fig. 44–9. Severe erythroblastosis fetalis. Hydropic macerated stillborn infant and characteristically large placenta.

1. Pregnant women who are D-negative and who are isoimmunized can be identified readily.
2. Hemolysis in the fetus of the sensitized D-negative woman can be predicted with considerable accuracy.
3. The fetus who most likely is to be seriously affected can be treated by intraperitoneal or direct intravascular transfusions or be delivered preterm.
4. The appropriate administration to the D-negative mother of D-immune globulin during or immediately after pregnancy has eradicated most D-isoimmunization.

The favorable impact on reducing perinatal mortality as the consequence of these procedures is exemplified by experiences in Manitoba. In that Canadian province, the number of perinatal deaths from hemolytic disease decreased from 29 in 1964 to only 1 in 1975 (Bowman and colleagues, 1977).

Immune Globulin Prophylaxis for the D-Negative, Nonsensitized Mother. Anti-D immune globulin is a 7S immune globulin G extracted by cold alcohol fractionation from plasma containing high-titer D-antibody. Each dose provides not less than 300 μg of D-antibody as determined by radioimmunoassay.

Freda and co-workers (1975) summarized their 10 years of clinical experience with D-immune globulin, confirming their original observations that such globulin given to the previously unsensitized D-negative woman within 72 hours of delivery is highly protective. D-negative women undergoing abortion should also be treated, because up to 2 percent having spontaneous abortions and 5 percent having elective terminations become isoimmunized without D-immune globulin. Likewise, women with ectopic pregnancies or hydatidiform moles should be treated. The observation of

Blajchman and co-workers (1974) of detectable fetal-maternal hemorrhage after 6 percent of amniocenteses has provided support for a policy that all unsensitized D-negative women suspected of having a D-positive fetus should receive D-immune globulin following such a procedure.

D-negative women who receive blood or blood fractions are at risk of becoming sensitized. Red cells can supply massive amounts of foreign antigen if the cells are D-positive and their recipient is D-negative. Moreover, platelet transfusions and plasmapheresis can provide sufficient D-antigen to cause sensitization, which can be prevented by an injection of D-antiglobulin. **Freda (1973), as well as Bowman (1985), emphasize that when in doubt whether to give anti-D immune globulin, then it should be given.**

Although adherence to the above guidelines has dramatically decreased the risk of maternal isoimmunization, the problem has not been eliminated. For example, Bowman and Pollock (1978) identified 1.8 percent of women who became isoimmunized in spite of adherence to the above recommendations. They deduced that most often the failures were the consequence of spontaneous silent fetal-maternal bleeds before delivery and before the administration postpartum of D-immune globulin. Therefore, to try to avoid isoimmunization from fetal-maternal bleeds remote from term, 300 μg of antibody routinely was administered intramuscularly to all nonsensitized D-negative women at 28 weeks, again at 34 weeks, as well as at the time of amniocentesis or uterine bleeding. If the infant was D-positive, a third dose of the immunoglobulin was administered to the mother after delivery. This program was followed by a reduction in the incidence of D-isoimmunization during pregnancy from 1.8 percent to 0.07 percent. A single dose at about 28 weeks proved to be almost as effective as were the two doses antepartum, and only 2 of 1799

D-negative women developed D-isoimmunization despite antenatal prophylaxis.

The small amount of antibody that crosses the placenta results at times in a weakly positive direct Coombs test in cord and infant blood; however, none of the infants showed evidence of anemia or exaggerated hyperbilirubinemia.

Chavez and associates (1991) in a recent review of the epidemiology of Rh hemolytic disease in the United States estimated an incidence of 10.6 per 10,000 livebirths. They concluded that Rh hemolytic disease still contributed significantly to both neonatal morbidity and mortality. Thus, it is apparent that the availability of immunoglobulin prophylaxis has not resulted in eradication of this condition.

Appropriate concern has been raised for the possibility that the human immunodeficiency virus may be transmitted by plasma-derived products such as D-immunoglobulin. Up to 5 years ago, more than 350,000 women each year were given 500,000 doses of D-immune globulin, and there has been no verified case of immunodeficiency transmission (Centers for Disease Control, 1987).

Recommendations. A single intramuscular dose of 300 μg of D-immunoglobulin is administered routinely to all D-negative, *nonimmunized* women at 28 to 32 weeks' gestation, and again within 72 hours of the birth of a D-positive infant. A similar dose is also given at the time of amniocentesis and whenever there is uterine bleeding, unless the routine dose at 28 to 32 weeks had been given very recently. If a massive fetal-maternal hemorrhage is recognized, more immune globulin should be given, as described below. One dose of 300 μg will protect the mother against a bleed of up to 15 mL of D-positive red cells, or 30 mL of fetal blood.

The report by Ness and colleagues (1987) provided data for the incidence of excessive fetal-maternal hemorrhage that may cause isoimmunization despite postpartum immune globulin administration. Using the enzyme-linked antiglobulin test, they studied almost 800 D-negative mothers giving birth to D-positive infants, and found evidence in 1 percent of the mothers for fetal bleeding in excess of 30 mL. Another 5.6 percent of these pregnancies had fetal-maternal bleeds of between 11 and 30 mL. Thus, at least 1 percent, and perhaps more, of susceptible mothers would have been given insufficient immune globulin if not tested. Importantly, they identified no risk factors that predicted excess bleeding, and recommended that all women be tested at delivery. Stedman and co-workers (1986), utilizing the erythrocyte rosette test, reported similar results.

At Parkland Hospital, our policy for many years was to verify free circulating D-antibody, using the indirect Coombs test, 24 hours after immune globulin was given postpartum. More recently, we have replaced this with the rosette test. This will detect excessive fetomaternal hemorrhage at delivery. If the test is positive, then the Kleinhauer-Betke test is done for qualification.

Whether to provide routinely D-antiglobulin prophylaxis for D^u-positive women is controversial. Bowman (1985) cites five instances in 750,000 pregnancies in which a D^u-positive mother produced anti-D antibody. Fortunately, in none of these was the fetus severely affected. If there is any doubt about D-antigen status, then globulin should be given.

Large Fetal-to-Maternal Bleed. In the case of a larger fetal-maternal hemorrhage, the D-positive erythrocytes may, by careful examination, be identified at times as clumps in the crossmatch of the erythrocytes from maternal blood and the D-immune globulin. However, the acid-elution technique for identifying erythrocytes that contain appreciable hemoglobin is best used to identify a major bleed and to approximate its magnitude.

When the acid-elution test is performed, red cells rich in fetal hemoglobin are easy to identify (Fig. 44–7). A careful differential count will serve to approximate closely the percentage of fetal cells in the maternal blood. From this value, multiplied by maternal hematocrit and by maternal blood volume, an estimate of the volume of fetal red cells in the maternal circulation can be made. Maternal blood volume will average about 5 L before delivery and 4 L shortly afterwards. The volume of fetal red cells calculated is then divided by 15 (volume of red cells effectively neutralized by 300 μg of antibody), and this provides a reasonable estimate of the number of 300 μg ampules of D-immune globulin required for protection. If the estimate is doubled, almost certainly more than adequate protection would be afforded. In practice, in cases of fetal-maternal hemorrhage, sensitization of the mother can be prevented by injecting sufficient D-immune globulin intramuscularly to provide demonstrable free antibody in the maternal serum.

> In a case of massive fetal-maternal hemorrhage successfully treated at Parkland Hospital, 14 vials of D-immune globulin (at least 4200 μg) were injected intramuscularly over 48 hours to maintain a clearly demonstrable excess of antibody after delivery of a recently exsanguinated, very large infant. From the differential count of erythrocytes of maternal and fetal origin identified by Kleinhauer-Betke staining of maternal blood, at least 150 mL of type O, D-positive fetal erythrocytes were demonstrated to have entered the maternal circulation (Fig. 44–7). The mother subsequently gave birth to three unaffected type O, D-positive infants, including a set of twins.

Maternal-Fetal Bleed. Rarely, the D-negative woman will have been exposed in utero to D-antigen from her mother and become sensitized as the consequence. As with fetal-maternal bleeds, a major blood group (ABO) incompatibility offers appreciable protection against D-sensitization. Jennings and Clauss (1978), in a study of 105 D-negative infants born to D-positive mothers, identified a maternal-fetal bleed in only two instances. Jennings and Clauss (1978) and Bowman (1985), on the basis of their extensive studies, do not believe that D-immune globulin prophylaxis is warranted for D-negative babies born to D-positive mothers.

Management. The management of isoimmunization, except for ABO incompatibility, is similar regardless of the inciting antigen. Since D-isoimmunization is most common, general management for this clinical situation is discussed.

The mother who is sufficiently immunized to produce enough antibody to cause overt hemolytic disease in the fetus and newborn will have detectable D-antibody in her serum by 36 weeks' gestation. Most often, if appropriate techniques are used, the antibody will be demonstrable much earlier. According to Freda (1973), if no treatment is given for the pregnancy of a sensitized D-negative woman with a D-positive fetus, the perinatal mortality rate will be about 30 percent. With aggressive management, including diagnostic amniocenteses or studies performed on fetal blood obtained by percutaneous sampling, repeated ultrasound examinations, intrauterine transfusions in selected cases, and early delivery in most cases, the perinatal mortality rate can be lowered remarkably (Harman and co-workers, 1983; Queenan and King, 1987).

For optimal outcome, management is individualized and aided by the following information:

1. Past obstetrical history, with emphasis on fetal outcome and how that outcome was achieved.
2. Accurate knowledge of fetal age.
3. The paternal D-antigen status, because if he is negative, then the fetus cannot be affected.
4. Maternal antibody determinations repeated throughout pregnancy.
5. Spectrophotometric analyses of amnionic fluid, or sonographically-directed fetal blood sampling.
6. Identification of other pregnancy complications.

An antibody titer, performed using the indirect Coombs test, that is no higher than 1 : 16 almost always means that the fetus will not die in utero from hemolytic disease. A titer higher than this indicates the *possibility* of severe hemolytic disease. It is emphasized that the titer in the previously sensitized woman may, during a subsequent pregnancy, rise infrequently to high levels even though her fetus is D-negative, the so-called *amnestic response*. Whenever the antibody titer is sufficiently elevated to be clinically significant, fetal evaluation is warranted. In most institutions this **critical titer** is considered to be 1 : 16 or greater; however, in

some centers, if the titer remains below 1 : 32, then a good fetal outcome is anticipated.

Until recently, indirect evaluation of fetal hemolytic disease was accomplished by determining the amount of bilirubin pigment in amnionic fluid by spectrophotometric analysis. There is now reasonable experience with sonographically-directed fetal blood sampling to assess the degree of hemolysis and anemia, as well as identifying the presence or absence of the suspected antigen.

Amniocentesis. The absorbance of breakdown pigments, mostly bilirubin, in the supernatant of amnionic fluid, when measured in a continuously recording spectrophotometer, is demonstrable as a hump with maximum absorbance at 450 nm wavelength, as shown in Figure 44–10. Because the *change* in optical density is measured, this is referred to as ΔOD_{450}. The magnitude of the increase in optical density above baseline at 450 nm most often, but not always, correlates well for any gestational age with the intensity of the hemolytic disease.

Liley (1964) constructed a graph that provides for reasonably precise prediction of the severity of hemolysis, a modification of which is demonstrated in Figure 44–11. Depending on the severity of disease, amniocenteses are repeated at 1- to 3-week intervals (American College of Obstetricians and Gynecologists 1986b). For pregnancies at 26 weeks or less, there are no accurate data to assess the severity of fetal involvement by amnionic fluid analysis. For this reason, most recommend that fetal blood be obtained directly by cordocentesis and tested for hemoglobin concentration (see below).

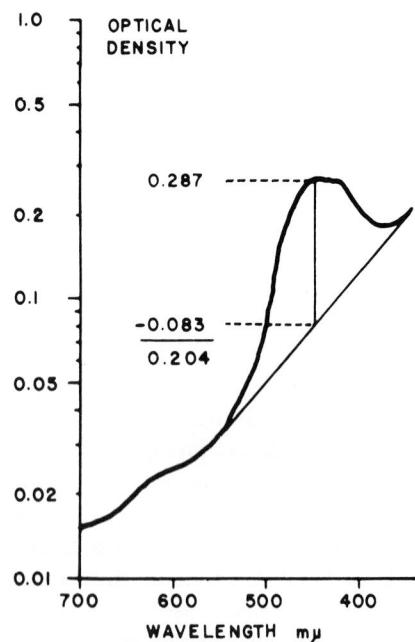

Fig. 44–10. Spectral absorption curve of amnionic fluid in hemolytic disease. (From Liley, 1964, with permission.)

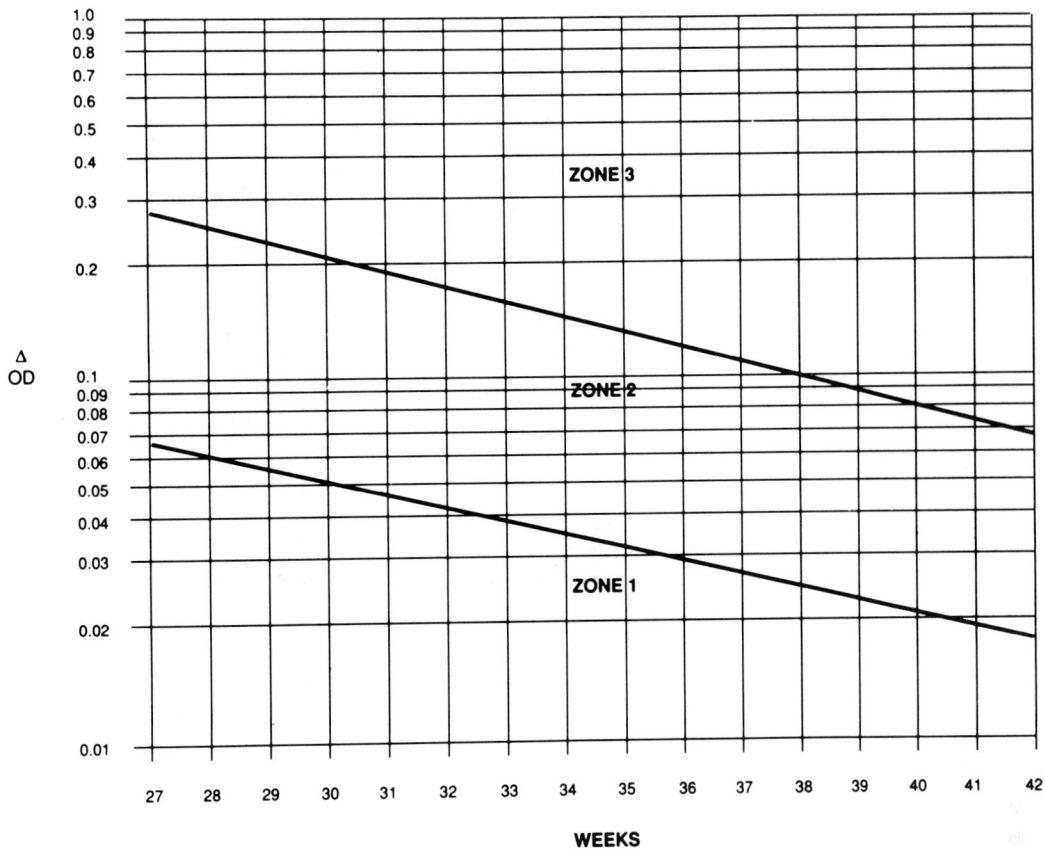

Fig. 44–11. Liley graph used to depict severity of fetal hemolysis with red cell isoimmunization. (From Liley, 1961, with permission.)

Although the information obtained by amnionic fluid analysis in isoimmunized women may not be as precise and accurate as fetal blood sampling (especially for earlier pregnancies), optical density values in zone 1 generally indicate an unaffected fetus or one who will only have mild disease. A D-negative fetus is also a possibility. Values in zone 3 indicate a severely affected fetus, and death within 1 week to 10 days may be expected. Transfusion or delivery is indicated. In zone 2, the prognosis is less accurate, but the fetus is at moderate to severe risk and repeated amniocentesis or fetal blood sampling may be required to establish the actual condition of the fetus. In lower zone 2, the expected fetal hemoglobin concentration is between 11.0 and 13.9 g/dL, whereas in upper zone 2, the anticipated hemoglobin level ranges from 8.0 to 10.9 g/dL.

Ananth and Queenan (1989), in a study of 32 women with D-isoimmunized pregnancies at 16 to 20 weeks, reported that amnionic fluid ΔOD_{450} values greater than 0.15 were predictive of severe fetal hemolysis, while those less than 0.09 had mild or no disease. Values between these two were not predictive and require further evaluation.

Fetal Blood Sampling. Nicolaides and colleagues (1986) studied 59 D-isoimmunized pregnancies at 18 to 25 weeks, and reported poor correlation in nonhydropic fetuses between the degree of fetal anemia and the trend in amnionic fluid analysis using the Liley graph. Nicolaides and Snijders (1992) have concluded that the only reliable method to determine severity in the second trimester is direct measurement of fetal hemoglobin. Nicolaides and co-workers (1988) recommend that transfusions be commenced when the hemoglobin deficit exceeds 2 g/dL from the mean for normal fetuses of corresponding gestational age (Fig. 44–12).

Intraperitoneal Fetal Transfusions. The refinement in prognostic precision furnished by amnionic fluid analysis led Liley (1963) to try, in apparently hopeless cases, intrauterine blood transfusion into the fetal peritoneal cavity. With such transfusions, the overall survival rate in more recent years was probably about 50 percent. The team in Winnipeg, however, has been much more successful. They reported 100 percent survival of nonhydropic fetuses and 75 percent survival of hydropic fetuses when treated with intrauterine transfusion, or an overall survival rate of 92 percent (Harman and co-

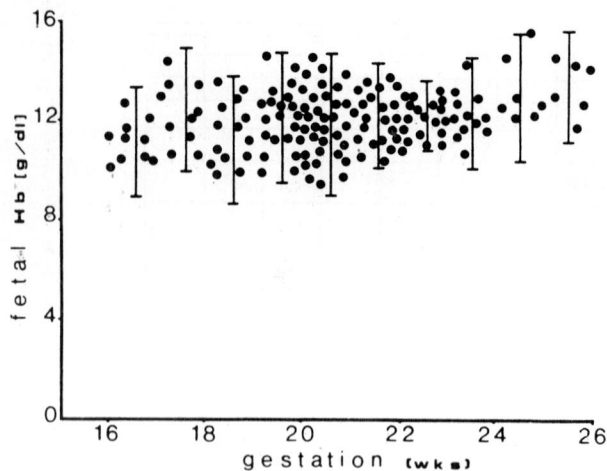

Fig. 44–12. Reference range (mean + 2SD) and distribution of individual values for fetal hemoglobin concentration from 153 pregnancies not complicated by fetal hemolysis. (From Nicolaides and colleagues, 1986, with permission.)

workers, 1983). Watts and colleagues (1988) reported similar results. Both groups emphasized improved fetal evaluation through the use of real-time sonography before, during, and after fetal transfusion.

At Winnipeg Center, 731 fetal transfusions have been carried out on 302 fetuses since the first transfusion was attempted in 1964. Mortality has decreased progressively as follows: 1964 to 1968, 55 percent; 1968 to 1972, 34 percent; 1972 to 1976, 34 percent; 1976 to 1980, 29 percent; and the recent study cited above, 8 percent. Importantly, the publicly funded anti-D prophylaxis program in Manitoba has lowered the risk of sensitization of mothers in that province from 13 percent to 0.18 percent, and, in turn, the frequency of intrauterine transfusions.

In a comparison of 44 intraperitoneal versus 44 intravascular transfusions, Harman and colleagues (1990) reported that the intravascular approach resulted in significantly more surviving infants (91 versus 66 percent), less infants with Apgar scores of less than 7 at 5 minutes (14 versus 38 percent), and increased frequency of vaginal delivery (83 versus 50 percent). They concluded that although intraperitoneal transfusion should not be abandoned, it was relegated a second-choice procedure for very limited circumstances (Harman and colleagues, 1990).

Intravascular Fetal Transfusions. In 1981, the group from Lewisham Hospital in London described a technique for direct intravascular blood transfusion using fetoscopy (Rodeck and colleagues, 1981). Subsequent to this (1984), they reported results from 25 severely D-isoimmunized fetuses, including 15 with hydrops, who were given intravascular transfusions between 19

and 32 weeks. They again used fetoscopy, but some of these transfusions were now accomplished using sonographically-directed needle placements. Those fetuses in whom treatment was begun before 25 weeks had a remarkable 84 percent survival. Since this time, investigators from Yale (Grannum and colleagues, 1986, 1988) and Mount Sinai in New York (Berkowitz and co-workers, 1988) have also reported their successes with the method, which is depicted in Figure 44–13. In many centers, this procedure has largely replaced the intraperitoneal technique for transfusion.

Ney and co-workers (1991) reported an overall survival of 85 percent with intravascular transfusion in severely isoimmunized fetuses. Survival was not significantly different comparing hydropic fetuses to non-hydropic fetuses in their study. Weiner and colleagues (1991a) reported an overall survival rate of 96 percent when intravascular transfusion was given for severe fetal anemia defined as a hematocrit of 30 percent or less.

Nicolini and associates (1990) reported their results from fetal blood sampling and intravascular transfusion utilizing the fetal intrahepatic vein. A fetal blood sample was successfully obtained in 91 percent of attempts, and the fetal hematocrit was raised to satisfactory levels in approximately 90 percent of the transfusions. The survival rate in 42 fetuses who were transfused was 86 percent.

Although intravascular transfusion is a relatively safe procedure, it is not without risk. In a review of 594 diagnostic cordocenteses and 156 intravascular transfusions, Weiner and associates (1991b) reported that duration of bleeding was greater with arterial than venous puncture and with intravascular transfusions compared

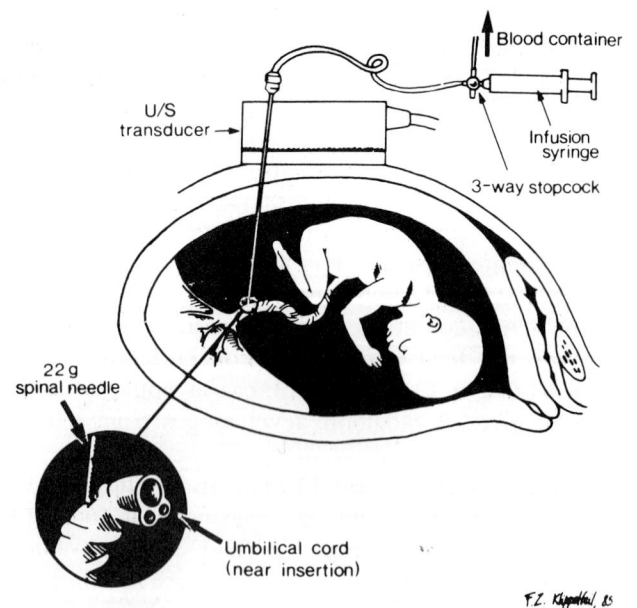

Fig. 44–13. Diagrammatic view of direct fetal intravascular transfusion. U/S = ultrasound. (From Grannum and colleagues, 1986, with permission.)

with diagnostic venipuncture. Preterm prematurely ruptured membranes and amnionitis developed overall in 0.4 percent and 0.5 percent of procedures, respectively. Fetal bradycardia was identified in 7 percent of all cases, and the perinatal loss rate as 0.8 percent. Other complications include hyperkalemia (Thorp and associates, 1990), development of a porencephalic cyst (Dildy and colleagues, 1991), and depressed neonatal erythropoiesis (Millard and co-workers, 1990; Thorp and collaborators, 1991). Radunovic and co-workers (1992) have reported increased mortality in hydropic fetuses who had acute hematocrit increases associated with intravascular transfusions.

Subsequent Child Development.
In Bowman's experience (1978), the great majority of fetal transfusion survivors developed normally; 74 of 89 tested when 18 months of age or older were completely normal, four were abnormal, whereas development in 11 appeared to be somewhat delayed, perhaps because of preterm birth.

Other Methods to Try to Minimize Fetal Hemolysis.
In an attempt to prevent D-antibody formation, to remove antibody already formed, or to block antibody action on the red cell, a number of techniques have been tried without consistent success. *Plasmapheresis* does not appear to provide benefits that outweigh the risks and the costs. *Promethazine* in large doses has been cited by some as being beneficial (Charles and Blumenthal, 1982); however, this is unproven. D-positive *erythrocyte membrane* in enteric coated capsules has been administered orally to sensitized women throughout pregnancy on the basis that such treatment might induce T-suppressor cell formation that would, in turn, reduce antibody response to challenges by the antigen. This also does not appear to provide any benefit (Gold and co-workers, 1983). Attempts at immunosuppression with corticosteroids were once considered by some to be beneficial, but were subsequently proven to be of no benefit.

Delivery Before Term.
In many circumstances, as previously alluded to, delivery somewhat before term is advantageous. When it is considered necessary to administer transfusions, delivery rather than further attempts at fetal transfusion is desirable provided that sufficient maturity has been achieved to forecast an excellent chance of survival.

Sinusoidal fetal heart rate and repetitive decelerations have been identified in a number of circumstances, including erythroblastosis fetalis. These changes in the presence of D-isoimmunization serve to imply, at least, that there is severe fetal anemia. Thus, their message is ominous and should stimulate strong consideration for either transfusion or prompt delivery (Lowe and colleagues, 1984).

Whenever a decision is reached to terminate pregnancy before term, skilled personnel, blood, and equipment should be immediately available in or adjacent to the delivery room.

Method of Delivery.
The fetus who is to be delivered remote from term because of evidence of hemolytic disease will sometimes benefit from cesarean section. By doing so, the time of birth is set and the most experienced neonatologists and laboratory personnel can be assembled to provide for precise neonatal evaluation and optimal treatment. Moreover, the likelihood of a difficult, prolonged, or unsatisfactory induction of labor is avoided.

Exchange Transfusion in the Newborn.
Examination of cord blood should be carried out immediately for any pregnancy in which the D-negative mother is known to be sensitized. The cord blood hemoglobin concentration and the direct Coombs test are of considerable importance when the infant is D-positive. If the infant is overtly anemic, it is often best to carry out the initial exchange promptly to correct anemia. Type O, D-negative red cells, recently collected, are used.

For infants who are not overtly anemic, the need for exchange transfusion is determined by the rate of increase in bilirubin concentration, the maturity of the infant, and the presence or absence of other complications.

Hyperbilirubinemia

Disposal of Bilirubin.
Before birth, unconjugated or free bilirubin is readily transferred across the placenta from the fetal to the maternal circulation (and vice versa, if the maternal plasma level of unconjugated bilirubin is high). Whereas bilirubin glucuronide is water soluble and normally is excreted into the bile by the liver and into the urine by the kidney when the plasma level is elevated, unconjugated bilirubin is not excreted in the urine or to any extent in the bile. Glucuronic acid is made available for this reaction by transfer from uridine diphosphoglucuronic acid catalyzed by the microsomal enzyme uridine diphosphoglucuronyl transferase. Conjugated bilirubin is secreted from the hepatocytes through the canalicular apparatus into the biliary tree and then into the small intestine.

Kernicterus.
The great concern over unconjugated hyperbilirubinemia in the newborn is its association with *kernicterus*. This complication occurs with greater frequency in preterm infants. The yellow staining of the basal ganglia and hippocampus is indicative of profound degeneration in these regions. Surviving infants show spasticity, muscular incoordination, and varying degrees of mental retardation. There is a positive correlation

between kernicterus and unconjugated bilirubin levels above 18 to 20 mg/dL, although kernicterus may develop at lower concentrations, especially in very premature infants.

Factors other than the serum bilirubin concentration contribute to the development of kernicterus. Hypoxia and acidosis enhance bilirubin toxicity. Both hypothermia and hypoglycemia predispose the infant to kernicterus by raising the level of nonesterified fatty acids, which compete with bilirubin for the binding sites on albumin and inhibit bilirubin conjugation. Sepsis contributes to kernicterus, although the mechanism of action is not clear. Although it is extremely unlikely that they lead to kernicterus, sulfonamides and salicylates may increase the level of bilirubin because they compete with unconjugated bilirubin for protein-binding sites. Sodium benzoate, in injectable diazepam, furosemide, and gentamicin, displaces bilirubin from albumin. Excessive doses of vitamin K analogues may be associated with hyperbilirubinemia. The importance of the serum albumin concentration and the binding sites so provided is obvious.

Breast Milk Jaundice. Breast feeding can cause nonphysiological jaundice in the otherwise normal newborn. The jaundice has been attributed to the excretion of pregnane-3α,20β-diol into breast milk by some mothers. This steroid was reported by Arias and colleagues (1964) to block bilirubin conjugation by inhibiting glucuronyl transferase activity. Breast milk samples from mothers of infants with hyperbilirubinemia have been described to have an unusually high lipolytic activity and liberate large quantities of fatty acids that inhibit bilirubin conjugation (Foliot and co-workers, 1976). Another explanation is that bilirubin is broken down in the intestine to form free bilirubin, which can be reabsorbed. Usually, bovine milk and human milk appear to block the reabsorption of free bilirubin, whereas the milk of mothers with jaundiced offspring does not, and may even enhance its reabsorption.

With breast milk jaundice, the serum bilirubin level rises from about the fourth day after birth to a maximum by 15 days. If breast feeding is continued, the high levels persist for another 10 to 14 days and slowly decline over the next several weeks. No cases of overt bilirubin encephalopathy have been reported caused by this phenomenon (Maisels, 1979).

Physiological Jaundice. By far the most common form of unconjugated nonhemolytic jaundice is so-called *physiological jaundice*. In the mature infant, the serum bilirubin increases for 3 to 4 days to achieve serum levels up to 10 mg/dL or so and then falls rapidly. In preterm infants, the rise is more prolonged and may be more intense.

Jaundice in the newborn should not be ignored as being physiological in the following circumstances:

1. The infant is visibly jaundiced in the first 24 hours after birth.
2. The total bilirubin concentration in serum is increasing daily by more than 5 mg/dL.
3. The total bilirubin concentration is above 15 mg/dL.
4. Jaundice is visible for more than 1 week in a term infant or 2 weeks in a preterm infant.

Treatment. *Exchange transfusion* for severe hyperbilirubinemia is not an innocuous procedure, but the mortality rate is less than 1 percent when moribund, hydropic, and kernicteric infants are excluded from analysis.

Phototherapy is now widely used to treat hyperbilirubinemia. In most instances, its use leads to a lower bilirubin level from its oxidation. Light that penetrates the skin also increases peripheral blood flow, which enhances photo-oxidation. By some unknown mechanism, light seems to promote hepatic excretion of unconjugated bilirubin. A common situation in which phototherapy is justified, besides that of the infant with hemolytic disease, is the jaundiced low-birthweight infant who appears otherwise well.

As much of the infant's surface as possible should be exposed, and the infant should be turned every 2 hours with close temperature monitoring to prevent dehydration. The fluorescent bulbs must be appropriate wavelength and the eyelids should be closed and completely shielded from the light. The serum bilirubin should be monitored for at least 24 hours after discontinuance of phototherapy.

Phenobarbital has been shown to induce microsomal enzymes and thereby increase hepatic bilirubin conjugation and excretion.

Nonimmune Hydrops Fetalis

Hutchison and associates (1982) reported an incidence of nonimmune hydrops of 1 in 3700 pregnancies. Undoubtedly, hydrops is identified in utero much more frequently since high-resolution sonography has become universally available. For example, in a review of 12,572 pregnant women referred for ultrasound examination, Santolaya and colleagues (1992) identified 76 fetuses (0.6 percent) with hydrops fetalis (Fig. 44–14). Commonly identifiable fetal malformations were cystic hygroma, heart abnormalities, and multiple malformations.

The formation and accumulation of serous fluid in body cavities and subcutaneous edema have been attributed to a great variety of causes, many of which were tabulated by Holzgreve and associates (1984) and are presented in Table 44–8. There also appears to be a category of transient idiopathic hydrops, and we, as well as Mueller-Heubach and Mazer (1983), have observed

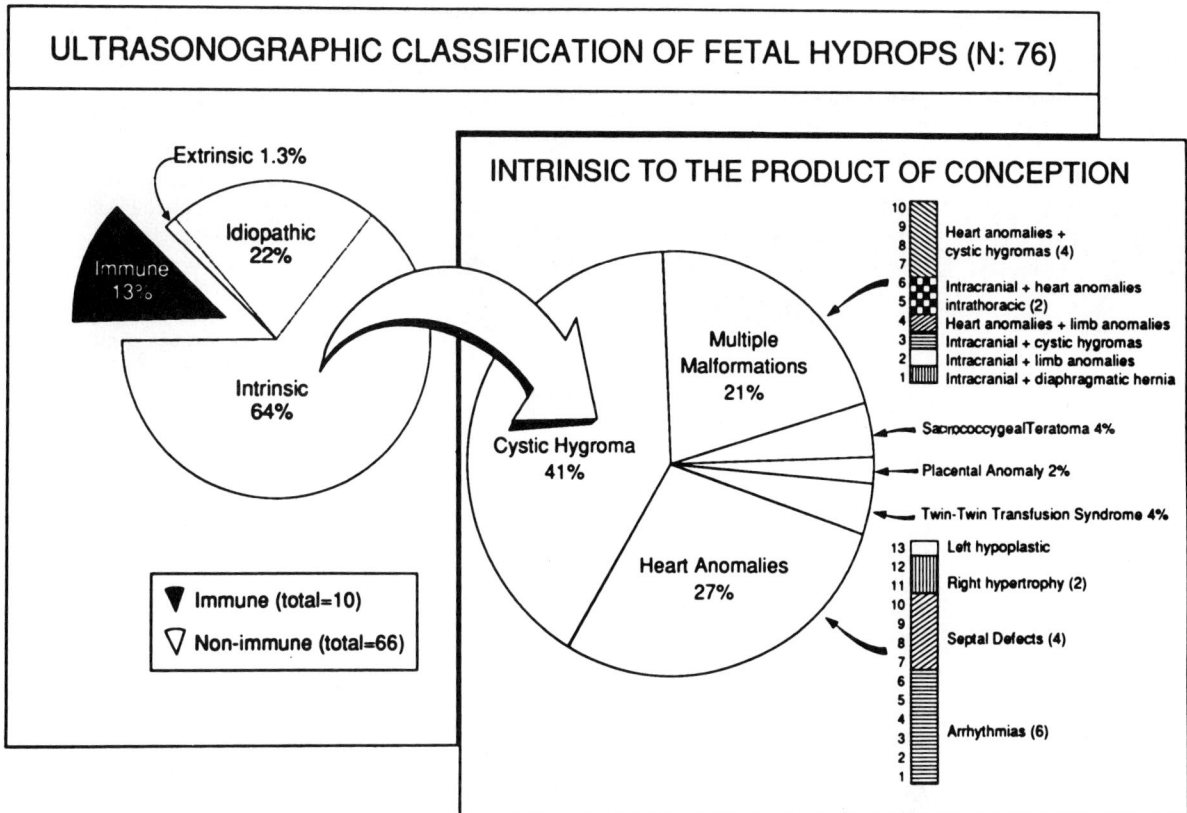

Fig. 44–14. Classification and cause in 76 cases of fetal hydrops in which the etiology could be diagnosed by ultrasound. (From Santolaya and associates, 1992, with permission.)

sonographic evidence of fetal hydrops, especially ascites, remote from term, only to have the ascites resolve and the fetus be normal at birth.

The precise incidence of these various causes of hydrops is unclear and there are definite population biases. For example, the San Francisco group reported a 10 percent incidence of hydrops caused by α-thalassemia (Holzgreve and colleagues, 1984). From their data, as well as those of Allan (1986), Gough (1986), Castillo (1986), and Santolaya (1992) and their many co-workers, cardiac abnormalities, either structural or rhythm related, or both, are associated with 20 to 45 percent of cases of nonimmune hydrops. Approximately 35 percent are due to chromosomal anomalies or other malformations, and 10 percent are associated with twin-twin transfusions. Those cases previously labeled idiopathic are less common, occurring in 22 percent of cases reported by Santolaya and colleagues (1992).

Previously unknown causes continue to be reported. Anand and colleagues (1987) documented hydrops from maternal-fetal *parvovirus* infection. Pryde and co-workers (1992) recently reported two pregnancies with parvovirus-related hydrops in which the hydrops resolved spontaneously without intervention. Both infants were healthy at birth.

Diagnosis. Ultrasonic evaluation is the most useful method for evaluating pregnancy complicated by fetal hydrops; however, other noninvasive steps should be taken (Gough and co-workers, 1986; Holzgreve and colleagues, 1984). After immunological hydrops has been excluded, hematological, chemical, and serological studies are done to look for maternal causes such as severe anemia, diabetes, or syphilis. A Kleihauer-Betke stain of maternal blood may disclose evidence for significant fetomaternal hemorrhage. If these and detailed sonar evaluation fail to disclose the apparent cause, then fetal echocardiography is done to search again for cardiac abnormalities. If still no cause is found, then some recommend amniocentesis or sonographically directed fetal blood sampling for karyotyping or other tests appropriate for the specific cause. Appelman and colleagues (1988) have detected bilirubin in Liley zone 3 in three pregnancies with nonimmune hydrops.

Treatment. Treatment will vary considerably and is dependent upon the cause of the hydrops. Because most lesions associated with these syndromes ultimately prove fatal for the fetus or newborn, knowledge of the cause is important in planning the route of delivery. In general, when hydrops persists and the fetus is mature enough that survival is likely, then delivery should be

TABLE 44–8. CAUSES OF NONIMMUNE HYDROPS FETALIS AND ASSOCIATED CLINICAL CONDITIONS.

Category	Condition	Category	Condition
Cardiovascular	Tachyarrhythmia	Urinary	Urethral stenosis or atresia
	Congenital heart block		Posterior neck obstruction
	Anatomical defects (atrial		Spontaneous bladder
	septal defect, ventricular		perforation
	defect, hypoplastic left heart,		Neurogenic bladder with reflux
	pulmonary valve		Ureterocele
	insufficiency, Ebstein's	Gastrointestinal	Jejunal atresia
	subaortic stenosis, dilated		Midgut volvulus
	heart, atrioventricular canal		Malrotation of intestines
	defect, single ventricle,		Duplication of intestinal tract
	tetralogy of Fallot, premature		Meconium peritonitis
	closure of foramen ovale,	Liver	Hepatic calcifications
	subendocardial fibroelastosis,		Hepatic fibrosis
	dextrocardia in combination		Cholestasis
	with pulmonic stenosis)		Polycystic disease of liver
	Calcified aortic valve		Biliary atresia
	Coronary artery embolus		Hepatic vascular malformations
	Myocarditis (coxsackie virus)		Familial cirrhosis
	Atrial hemangioma	Maternal	Severe diabetes mellitus
	Intracardial rhabdomyoma		Severe anemia
	Endocardial teratoma		Hypoproteinemia
Chromosomal	Down syndrome (trisomy 21)	Medications	Antepartum indomethacin
	Other trisomies		(taken to stop preterm labor,
	Turner syndrome		causing fetal ductus closure
	Triploidy		and secondary non-immune
Malformation syndromes	Thanatophoric dwarfism		hydrops fetalis)
	Arthrogryposis multiplex	Placenta–umbilical cord	Chorioangioma
	congenita		Chorionic vein thrombosis
	Asphyxiating thoracic dystrophy		Fetal–maternal transfusion
	Hypophosphatasia		Placental and umbilical vein
	Osteogenesis imperfecta		thrombosis
	Achondrogenesis		Umbilical cord torsion
	Neu–Laxova syndrome		True cord knots
	Recessive cystic hygroma		Angiomyxoma of umbilical cord
	Saldino–Noonan syndrome		Aneurysm of umbilical artery
	Pena–Shokeir type I syndrome	Infections	Cytomegalovirus
			Toxoplasmosis
Hematological	α-Thalassemia		Syphilis
	Arteriovenous shunts (vascular		Congenital hepatitis
	tumors)		Rubella
	Kasabach-Merritt syndrome		Parvovirus
	In utero closed-space		Leptospirosis
	hemorrhage		Chaga disease
	Caval, portal, or femoral	Miscellaneous	Congenital lymphedema
	thrombosis		Congenital hydrothorax or
Twin pregnancy	Twin–twin transfusion		chylothorax
	syndrome		Polysplenia syndrome
	Parabiotic (acardiac) twin		Congenital neuroblastoma
	syndrome		Tuberous sclerosis
Respiratory	Diaphragmatic hernia		Torsion of ovarian cyst
	Cystic adenoma of lung		Fetal trauma
	Hamartoma of lung		Sacrococcygeal teratoma
	Mediastinal teratoma		

Modified from Holzgreve and co-workers (1984).

accomplished. When hydrops appears to be the consequence of heart failure from supraventricular tachyarrhythmia, conversion is attempted by maternal administration of digoxin, a beta-blocker, or verapamil. If heart failure is due to structural lesions, reversal of failure is less likely, and the prognosis is much worse.

There have been several reports of intrauterine transfusion for the treatment of nonimmune hydrops. For example, Sahakian and associates (1991) reported a successful outcome following an intravascular transfusion of a 20-week fetus with parvovirus B-19 infection. Hydrops associated with this viral infection also may spontaneously resolve (Pryde and colleagues, 1992). Others have reported the successful use of intravascular transfusion for nonimmune hydrops caused by fetomaternal hemorrhage (Rouse and Weiner, 1990; Thorp and colleagues, 1992).

Maternal complications include an increased incidence of preeclampsia, which may develop early and necessitate delivery. Preterm labor is common because about half the cases are complicated by hydramnios. Finally, postpartum hemorrhage is common and is related to uterine overdistension as well as retained placenta.

Fetal Cardiac Arrhythmias

Recognition of fetal cardiac rhythm disturbances has become more common because of extensive use of Doppler ultrasound technology. Whereas most of these arrhythmias are transient and benign, and usually are isolated extrasystoles, some tachyarrhythmias, if sustained, result in congestive heart failure, nonimmune hydrops, and fetal death. Sustained bradycardia, although less often associated with hydrops, may signify underlying cardiac pathology that includes structural lesions or autoimmune myocarditis.

Kleinman and associates (1985) summarized their experiences with fetal arrhythmias, which are shown in Table 44–9. They emphasize that sustained supraventricular tachycardia, usually more than 200 beats per minute, is most likely to cause cardiac failure, and they have documented fetal ascites developing after only 36 hours. Treatment, usually with digoxin, almost always is successful if there are no underlying heart lesions. Battiste and colleagues (1992) recently described in utero conversation of supraventricular tachycardia with digoxin and procainamide in a fetus with hydrops at 17 weeks. The infant was normal at birth.

Rajadurai and Menahem (1992) described eight cases of fetal arrhythmias over a 3-year period. Five had tachyarrhythmias, two had atrial or ventricular extrasys-

TABLE 44–9. TYPES OF ARRHYTHMIAS IN 198 FETUSES FROM PREGNANCIES REFERRED TO YALE UNIVERSITY

Arrhythmias (Number)
Isolated extrasystoles (164)
Atrial (145)
Ventricular (19)
Sustained arrhythmias (34)
Supraventricular tachycardia (15)
Complete heart block (8)
Atrial flutter or fibrillation (5)
Ventricular tachycardia (2)
Second-degree heart block (2)
Sinus bradycardia (2)

From Kleinman and colleagues (1985).

toles, and one had complete heart block. Three of the five cases of tachyarrhythmias presented with nonimmune hydrops.

The prognosis for the fetus with bradycardia from heart block is less promising. Taylor and colleagues (1986) demonstrated that half of the mothers of children with congenital heart block have antibodies to fetal myocardial tissue. Many of these women have, or subsequently develop, lupus erythematosus or another connective-tissue disease (see Chap. 54, p. 1232). A serological marker for congenital myocarditis is the anti-SS-A (anti-Ro) antibody, and as many as 1 in 20 fetuses born to women positive for this have cardiac disease (Ramsey-Goldman and colleagues, 1986). Fetal cardiac antigens to which anti-SS-A affixes are not confined to the conduction system as once thought, and if there is extensive carditis, the prognosis is poor. Of seven infants described by Ramsey-Goldman and colleagues (1986), three died within 9 months, two required permanent pacemaking, and two underwent cardiac surgery. Only one infant had no problems.

Cameron and associates (1988) and Shenker and colleagues (1987) recently reported that fetal cardiac anomalies are common with heart block in the absence of connective-tissue disease. Their recommended work-up includes fetal echocardiography and consideration for karyotyping.

Hemorrhagic Disease of the Newborn

Hemorrhagic disease of the newborn is a syndrome characterized by spontaneous internal or external bleeding accompanied by hypoprothrombinemia and very low levels of other vitamin K–dependent coagulation factors (V, VII, IX, and X). Bleeding may begin any time after birth but is typically delayed for a day or two. The infant may be mature and healthy in appearance, although there is a greater incidence of the disease in preterm infants.

The prothrombin and partial thromboplastin times are greatly prolonged. The coagulation changes of vitamin K deficiency, especially if accompanied by a lowered platelet count, might lead to an erroneous diagnosis of disseminated intravascular coagulation, which has a much poorer prognosis (Lane and Hathaway, 1985). In the differential diagnosis, hemophilia, congenital syphilis, bacterial sepsis, thrombocytopenic purpura, erythroblastosis, and intracranial hemorrhage must be considered.

Hypoprothrombinemia in the neonate appears to be the consequence of poor placental transport of vitamin K_1 to the fetus. Plasma vitamin K_1 levels are somewhat lower in pregnant women than in nonpregnant adults, and the vitamin is undetectable in cord plasma (Shearer and associates, 1982). When 1 mg of vitamin K_1 was administered intravenously to mothers shortly before delivery, maternal plasma levels were remarkably raised, but cord plasma levels still were very low. However, Pomerance and colleagues (1987) reported that prothrombin activity was improved in preterm neonates whose mothers were given intramuscular vitamin K_1 during labor.

The main cause of hemorrhagic disease of the newborn from vitamin K deficiency appears to be a dietary deficiency of vitamin K as the consequence of small amounts of the vitamin in breast milk in an infant already depleted at birth. The prothrombin time 24 hours after the start of feedings with cow's milk is comparable to that found 24 hours after vitamin K administration, whereas in infants fed with breast milk it remains prolonged (Keenan and colleagues, 1971).

Serious reduction of vitamin K–dependent clotting factors during the first week after birth in infants of women with epilepsy treated with anticonvulsant drugs has been described by Mountain and associates (1970). These drugs apparently have a mechanism similar to warfarin and act by depressing hepatic synthesis of several coagulation factors (VII, IX, and X).

Prophylaxis. As prophylaxis against hemorrhagic disease of the newborn, the intramuscular injection of 1 mg of vitamin K_1 has proved very efficacious. For treatment of active bleeding, the vitamin is injected intravenously. Abnormalities in clotting usually are corrected over several hours.

The toxic effects of menadione, a synthetic vitamin K, and its derivatives in causing hyperbilirubinemia were the consequence of unnecessarily large doses, particularly to preterm infants. There is no evidence that the small but effective dose of 1 mg of vitamin K_1 (phytonadione) to the infant, or 2.5 to 5 mg given to the mother before delivery, are associated with significant hyperbilirubinemia.

Thrombocytopenia

A number of diseases or conditions are associated with neonatal thrombocytopenia of varying degrees. It tends to be more severe in preterm fetuses, especially those with respiratory distress and hypoxia or sepsis.

Antiplatelet IgG antibody transferred from mother to fetus and causing thrombocytopenia in the fetus-neonate can be suspected when the mother has thrombocytopenia from an autoimmune disease, especially **immunological thrombocytopenic purpura** (see Chap. 52, p. 1187). Avoidance of traumatic delivery and appropriate corticosteroid therapy to try to improve hemostasis are important to a successful outcome. Maternally produced antibody most often is directed against almost all platelets; thus donor platelet transfusions are of little benefit. Corticosteroids or intravenous immune globulin given to the infant may be helpful; in desperation, exchange transfusion and platelet replacement may be tried.

Neonatal thrombocytopenia has been suggested by some to result from **preeclampsia–eclampsia.** However, in a large number of infants born to women with pregnancy-induced hypertension at Parkland Hospital, we identified no case where neonatal thrombocytopenia correlated with maternal thrombocytopenia (Pritchard and colleagues, 1987). Instead, thrombocytopenia commonly developed after delivery in low-birthweight infants who were hypoxic or who had evidence for sepsis.

Isoimmune Thrombocytopenia. Isoimmunization to fetal platelet antigens may develop in a manner similar to D-antigen isoimmunization. The incidence is reported to be approximately 2 to 5 per 10,000 livebirths (Nicolaides and Snijders, 1992). In this condition, thrombocytopenia follows maternal isoimmunization against fetal platelet antigens, usually Pl^{A1}, which is found in 98 percent of the population. Thus, the mother lacks the common platelet antigen and becomes immunized when exposed to the antigen by fetal platelets that enter the maternal circulation. Even though diagnostic tests to type platelet antigens are not commonly available, the diagnosis most often can be made correctly on clinical grounds: (1) the mother has a normal platelet count and there is no evidence of a disorder which causes autoimmune thrombocytopenia, and (2) the infant has thrombocytopenia without evidence of other disease.

In the case of active bleeding, treatment ideally includes transfusion with platelets compatible with those of the mother. Unfortunately, most of the donor population will have the platelet antigen to which the maternal antibody is directed. However, maternal platelets are appropriate because they lack the inciting antigen, and platelets collected from the mother by plasmapheresis and differential centrifugation are likely to be of greatest benefit. When one infant has been affected, there is appreciable likelihood that subsequent infants will also be affected. The incidence of intraventricular hemorrhage has been estimated to be as high as 10 to 30 percent in affected neonates (Bussel and colleagues, 1988). Cesarean section to minimize birth trauma will likely be advantageous for the affected fetus-infant, yet of little added risk to the mother, because she is not thrombocytopenic.

It has become appreciated over the past decade that fetal central nervous system hemorrhage may be common. Morales and Stroup (1985) described a case in which the fetus apparently suffered massive spontaneous intraventricular hemorrhage at 34 weeks. Because of this eventuality, fetal treatment has been considered. Kaplan and colleagues (1988) described fetal platelet transfusions using sonographically-directed umbilical vein catheterization. Bussel and co-workers (1988) reported that maternal intravenous gamma globulin increased fetal platelet counts in seven cases. Nicolaides and Snijders (1992) have recommended that cordocentesis be considered as early as 20 weeks' gestation. If the fetus is thrombocytopenic, consideration can be given for intrauterine platelet transfusions (Kaplan, and associates, 1988; Nicolaides and Snijders, 1992; Nicolini and colleagues, 1988).

Polycythemia and Hyperviscosity

Several conditions predispose to neonatal polycythemia and blood hyperviscosity. These include *chronic hypoxia* in utero and *placental transfusion* from a twin or, much more rarely, from the mother. As the hematocrit rises above 65, blood viscosity markedly increases. Signs and symptoms include plethora, cyanosis, and neurological aberrations. Laboratory findings include hyperbilirubinemia, thrombocytopenia, fragmented erythrocytes, and hypoglycemia. Treatment consists of prompt recognition and lowering of the hematocrit by partial exchange transfusion with plasma.

Necrotizing Enterocolitis

This condition commonly presents with clinical findings of abdominal distention, ileus, and bloody stools, along with radiological evidence of *pneumatosis intestinalis*, caused by intestinal wall gas as the consequence of invasion by gas-forming bacteria and bowel perforation.

The disease is primarily seen in low-birthweight infants, but occasionally it is encountered in mature neonates. Various causes have been suggested for necrotizing enterocolitis, including perinatal hypotension, hypoxia, or sepsis, as well as umbilical catheters, exchange transfusions, and the feeding of cow's milk and hypertonic solutions (Kliegman and Fanaroff, 1984). The disease tends to occur in clusters, and coronaviruses have been suspected of having an etiological role. Kanto and colleagues (1987) reported that 5.7 percent of 2123 preterm infants developed necrotizing enterocolitis. The incidence of the disease was related to birthweight, but not to other perinatal factors. They concluded that gastrointestinal immaturity, and not ischemia, is the major causative factor for necrotizing enterocolitis. Orally administered immunoglobulin was shown to prevent enterocolitis when given to preterm infants (Eibl and associates, 1988).

Abdominal distention or blood in the stools may signal developing enterocolitis. Usually, further oral feeding is withheld until the condition clears, although at times it is so severe that bowel resection is necessary. The prognosis appears to be improving with such management (Walsh and Kliegman, 1986).

INJURIES OF THE FETUS AND NEWBORN

Considered here are several varieties of birth injuries. Others are described elsewhere in connection with specific obstetrical complications that led to or contributed to the injury.

Intracranial Hemorrhage

Hemorrhage within the head of the fetus-infant may be located at any of several sites: subdural, subarachnoid, cortical, white matter, cerebellar, intraventricular, and periventricular. Intraventricular hemorrhage into the germinal matrix is the most common type of intracranial hemorrhage encountered, and as previously discussed, it usually is a result of prematurity and not a traumatic injury. Hayden and colleagues (1985) reported that nearly 4 percent of otherwise normal newborns at term have sonographic evidence for subependymal germinal matrix hemorrhages unrelated to obstetrical factors.

Birth trauma may cause intracranial hemorrhage, but it is no longer a common cause. The head of the fetus may undergo appreciable molding during passage through the birth canal. The skull bones, the dura mater, and the brain itself permit considerable alteration in the shape of the fetal head without untoward results. The dimensions of the head are changed, with lengthening especially of the occipitofrontal diameter of the skull (Fig. 44–15). Bridging veins from the cerebral cortex to the sagittal sinus may tear as the consequence of severe molding and marked overlap of the parietal bones or of difficult forceps delivery. Less common are rupture of the internal cerebral veins, the vein of Galen at its junction with the straight sinus, or the tentorium itself. Compression of the skull can stretch the tentorium cerebelli and may tear the vein of Galen or its tributaries. Wigglesworth and Pape (1980) have provided lucid descriptions of the pathophysiology of intracranial hemorrhages in the newborn.

Illingworth (1979), an English pediatrician, rightfully contended that because of superficial thinking, obstetricians have been blamed unjustifiably for causing brain damage and other injuries, the genesis of which

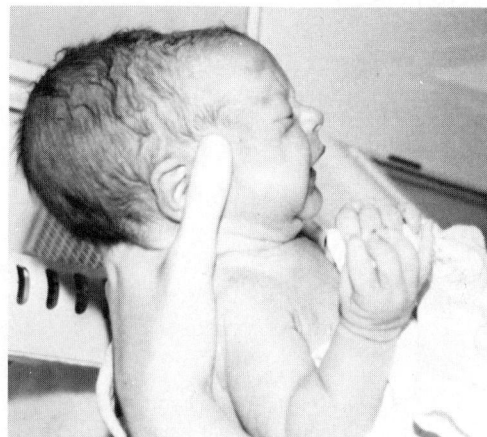

Fig. 44–15. Molding of the head in normal newborn.

was not limited just to difficulties during labor and delivery, but involved prenatal factors, including those that were genetic and environmental in nature. Nonetheless, the elimination of difficult forceps operations, the use of cesarean section when there was cephalopelvic disproportion, and the correct management of breech delivery all contributed significantly to a reduction in the incidence of all birth injuries, including intracranial hemorrhage.

Clinical Findings. Commonly, infants suffering intracranial hemorrhage from mechanical injury are born depressed but their conditions appear to improve until about 12 hours of age. Then drowsiness, apathy, feeble cry, pallor, failure to nurse, dyspnea, cyanosis, vomiting, and convulsions may become evident. Atelectasis, hypoxia, acidosis, and meconium aspiration may be associated findings. To help rule out diaphragmatic hernia, congenital heart disease, atelectasis, idiopathic respiratory distress, and pneumonia, prompt radiographic examination of the chest is useful. In recent years, head scanning using sonography and computed tomography not only has proved of diagnostic value but has also contributed appreciably to an understanding of the etiology of some forms of intracranial hemorrhage and the frequency with which they occur (Perlman and Cunningham, 1993). For example, periventricular and intraventricular hemorrhages occur often in infants born quite preterm and these hemorrhages usually develop without birth trauma.

Treatment. Therapy includes oxygen when there is dyspnea and cyanosis as well as sedation to control convulsions. The blood can be removed from some sub-

dural hematomas by careful needle aspiration. In other instances, surgical intervention may be required. The value of administering plasma clotting factors to infants with intracranial hemorrhage is not clear; however, prompt intramuscular administration of vitamin K to all newborn infants is indicated.

Cephalohematoma

A cephalohematoma (Figs. 44–16 and 44–17) usually is caused by injury to the periosteum of the skull during labor and delivery, although it may develop in the absence of birth trauma when hemostasis is defective. The incidence is 2.5 percent according to the 10-year review by Thacker and colleagues (1987). The subperiosteal hemorrhages may develop over one or both parietal bones. The periosteal limitations with definite palpable edges differentiate the cephalohematoma from *caput succedaneum*. The latter lesion consists of a focal swelling of the scalp from edema fluid that overlies the periosteum (Fig. 44–16). Furthermore, a cephalohematoma may not appear for hours after delivery, often growing larger and disappearing only after weeks or even months (Fig. 44–17). In contrast, caput succedaneum is maximal at birth, grows smaller, usually and disappears within a few hours if small and within a few days even when very large.

Increasing size of the hematoma and other evidence of extensive hemorrhage are indications for additional investigation, including radiographic studies of the skull and assessment of coagulation factors, since the infant may have defective blood clotting, such as may be seen with severe thrombocytopenia.

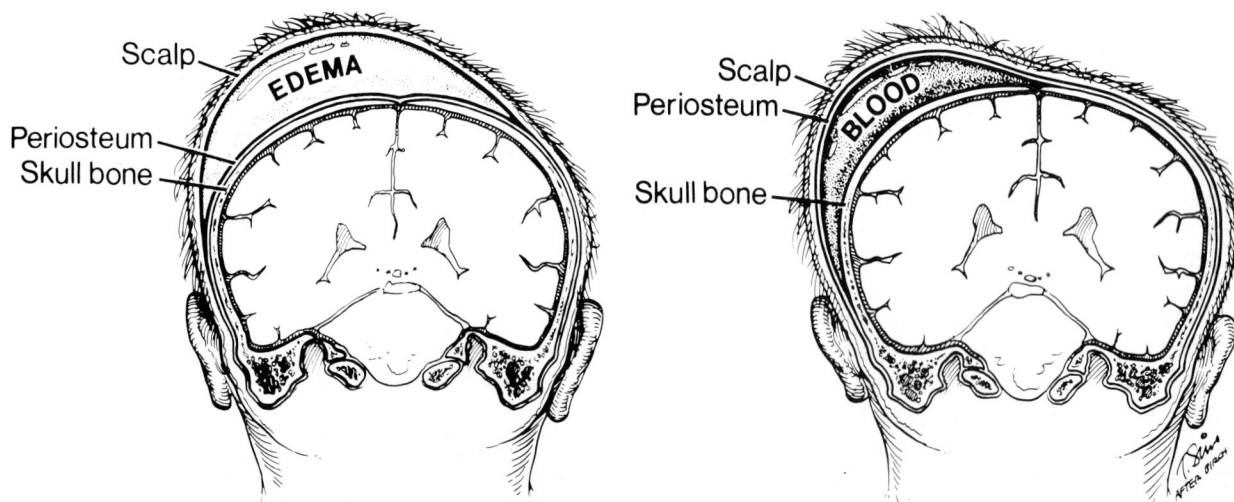

Fig. 44–16. Difference between a large caput succedaneum (*left*) and cephalohematoma (*right*). In a caput succedaneum, the effusion overlies the periosteum and consists of edema fluid; in a cephalohematoma, it lies under the periosteum and consists of blood.

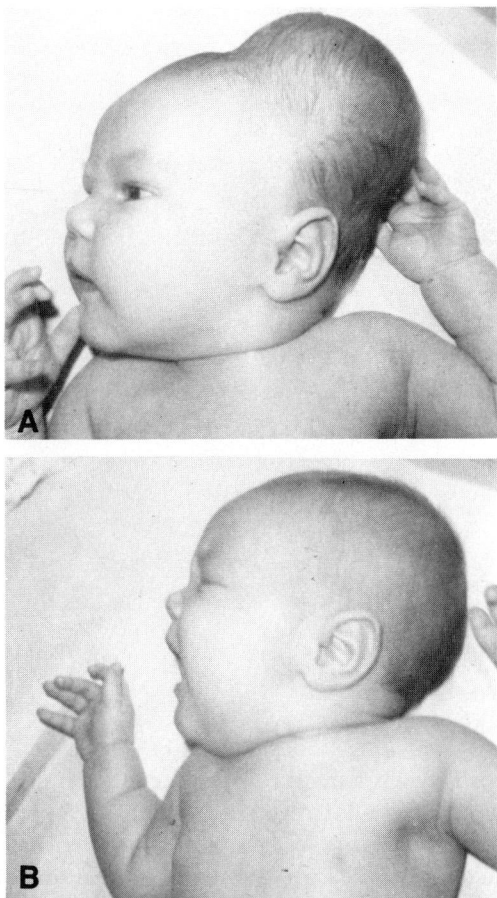

Fig. 44–17. A. A very large cephalohematoma photographed 2 weeks after delivery. **B.** The same infant 4 weeks later. (Courtesy of Dr. William Austin.)

Nerve Injuries

Spinal Injury. Overstretching the spinal cord and associated hemorrhage may follow excessive traction during a breech delivery, and there may be actual fracture or dislocation of the vertebrae. Complete data on such lesions are lacking, because even the most careful autopsy seldom includes thorough examination of the spine.

Brachial Plexus Injury. Brachial plexus injuries are common and encountered in nearly 1 in 500 term births (Levine and colleagues, 1984). In a review of over 14,000 liveborn infants in Finland, Salonen and Uüsitalo (1990) described brachial plexus injury in approximately 1 in 1000 births. In a review of over 21,500 livebirths, Oppenheim and colleagues (1990) reported 58 clavicular fractures (2.7 per 1000), three of which were associated with Erb palsy. In a prospective study of over 26,000 Malaysian neonates, Boo and associates (1991) found 42 brachial plexus injuries (1.6 per 1000). Increasing birthweight and breech de-

liveries were the most significant risk factors. The injury usually follows a difficult delivery, but it occurs not infrequently after an apparently easy one, and the infant is born with a paralyzed arm.

Duchenne, or **Erb paralysis,** involves paralysis of the deltoid and infraspinatus muscles, as well as the flexor muscles of the forearm, causing the entire arm to fall limply close to the side of the body with the forearm extended and internally rotated. The function of the fingers usually is retained. The lesion results from stretching or tearing of the upper roots of the brachial plexus, which is readily subjected to extreme tension as a result of pulling laterally upon the head, thus sharply flexing it toward one of the shoulders. Because traction in this direction is frequently employed to effect delivery of the shoulders in normal vertex presentations, Erb paralysis may result without the delivery appearing to be difficult. In extracting the shoulders, therefore, care should be taken not to impose excessive lateral flexion of the neck. Most often, in the case of cephalic presentations, the afflicted fetus is unusually large, typically weighing 4000 g or more. Other risk factors reported by Levine and coworkers (1984) and McFarland and associates (1986) are prolonged labor, forceps delivery, and shoulder dystocia.

In breech extractions, particular attention should be devoted to preventing the extension of the arms over the head. Extended arms not only materially delay breech delivery but also increase the risk of paralysis. The prognosis is usually good with prompt, appropriate physiotherapy. Occasionally, however, the arm may remain permanently paralyzed.

Less frequently, trauma is limited to the lower nerves of the brachial plexus, which leads to paralysis of the hand, or **Klumpke paralysis.**

Facial Paralysis. According to Levine and colleagues (1984), the incidence of facial nerve injury was 7.5 per 1000 term births; however, this has decreased recently. In the report by Salonen and Uüsitalo (1990), there was only one case of facial nerve palsy in over 14,000 livebirths. Facial paralysis may be apparent at delivery or it also may develop shortly after birth (Fig. 44–18). It is usually seen with delivery of an infant in which the head has been seized obliquely with forceps. The injury is caused by pressure exerted by the posterior blade of the forceps on the stylomastoid foramen, through which the facial nerve emerges. Facial marks from the forceps may be obvious (Fig. 44–19). Not every case of facial paralysis following forceps delivery should be attributed to the operation, however, because the condition is also encountered after spontaneous delivery. In fact, Levine and co-workers (1984) reported that one third of cases of facial palsy followed spontaneous delivery. Spontaneous recovery within a few days is the rule (Fig. 44–18).

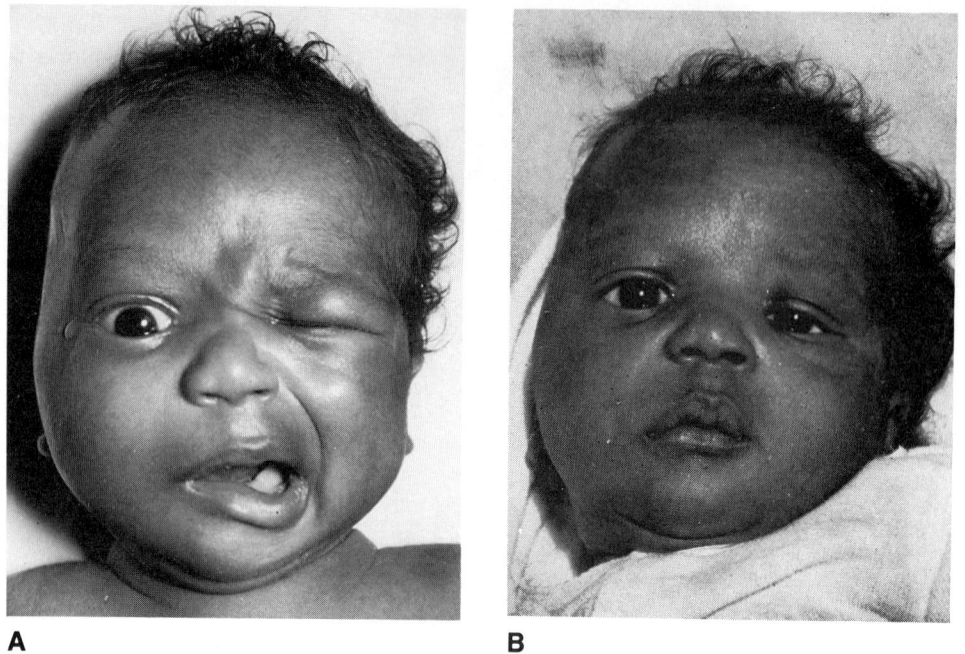

Fig. 44–18. A. Paralysis of right side of face 15 minutes after forceps delivery. **B.** Same infant 24 hours later. Recovery was complete in another 24 hours.

A   **B**

Skeletal and Muscle Injuries

Fractures. Fractures of the clavicle are identified in from 2 to 3 per 1000 livebirths (Levine and associates, 1984; Oppenheim and colleagues, 1990; Salonen and Uüsitalo, 1990). Humeral fractures are less common. Difficulty encountered in the delivery of the shoulders in cephalic deliveries and extended arms in breech deliveries are the main factors in the production of such fractures. A fractured femur is relatively uncommon and is usually associated with breech delivery. Upper extremity fractures associated with delivery are often of the greenstick type, although complete fracture with overriding of the bones may occur. Palpation of the

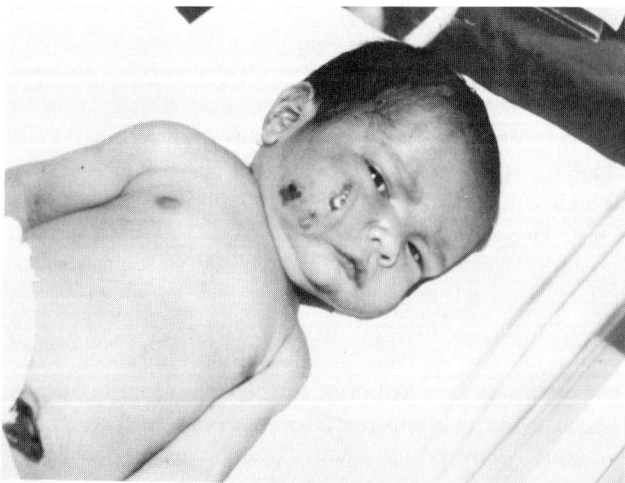

Fig. 44–19. Healing abrasions and lacerations from a difficult forceps delivery. Palsy of the right facial nerve has nearly cleared.

clavicles and long bones should be performed on all newborns when a fracture is suspected, and any crepitation or unusual irregularity should prompt radiographic examination. It is also important to seek evidence of brachial palsy so that treatment can be instituted.

Fracture of the skull may follow forcible attempts at delivery, especially with forceps, spontaneous delivery, or even cesarean section (Saunders and colleagues, 1979; Skajaa and associates, 1987). In the radiograph presented in Figure 44–20, a focal, but marked, depressed skull fracture is apparent. Labor was characterized by vigorous contractions, full dilatation of the cervix, and arrest of descent of the head, which was tightly wedged in the pelvis. The fracture was the consequence of compression of the skull against the sacral promontory of the mother, or perhaps from pressure from an assistant's hand in the vagina or as the head was pushed upwards out of the birth canal at cesarean delivery. Surgical decompression was successful. Saunders and colleagues (1979) reported successful use of the obstetrical vacuum extractor to apply negative pressure to reduce these fractures.

Muscular Injuries. Injury to the sternocleidomastoid muscle may occur, particularly during a breech delivery. There may be a tear of the muscle or possibly of the fascial sheath, leading to a hematoma and gradual cicatricial contraction. As the neck lengthens in the process of normal growth, the child's head is gradually turned toward the side of the injury, because the damaged muscle is less elastic and does not elongate at the same rate as its normal contralateral counterpart, thus producing *torticollis*. Roemer (1954) reported that 27 of

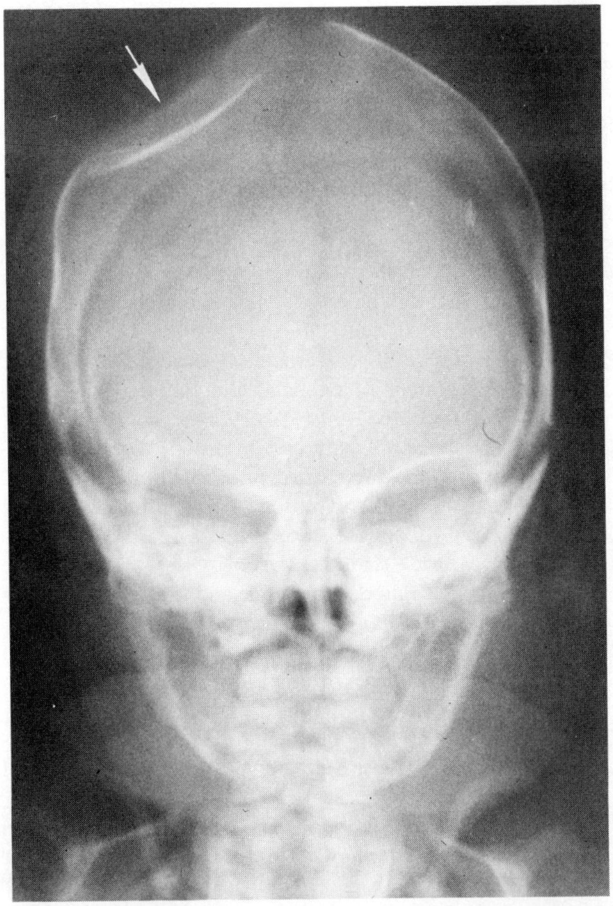

Fig. 44–20. Depressed skull fracture evident immediately after birth. Delivery followed vigorous but obstructed labor and dislodgement upward of the fetal head from the birth canal by an assistant's hand in the vagina at the time of cesarean section.

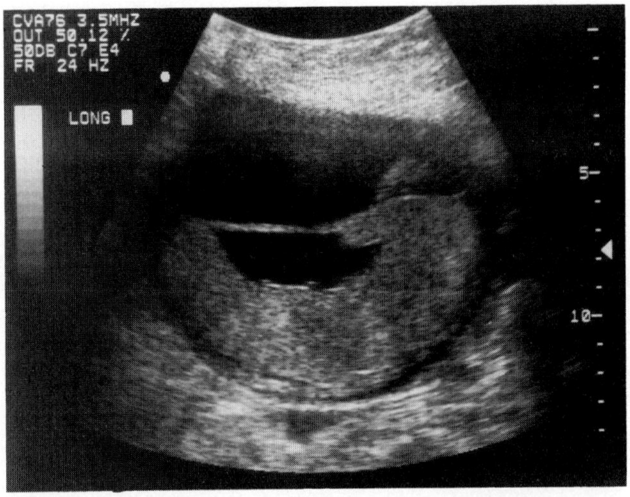

Fig. 44–21. Sonogram showing amnionic band extending from one side of placenta to the other. (Courtesy of Dr. R. Santos.)

explicable by band disruptions. An example of an amnionic band is shown in Figure 44–21.

Congenital Postural Deformities. Mechanical factors arising from chronically low volumes of amnionic fluid and restrictions imposed by the small size and inappropriate shape of the uterine cavity may mold the growing fetus into distinct patterns of deformity, including talipes (clubfoot), scoliosis, hip dislocation, limb reduction, and body wall defects (Miller and co-workers, 1981). Hypoplastic lungs also can result from oligohydramnios.

44 infants showing this deformity had been delivered by breech or internal podalic version. He postulated that lateral hyperextension sufficient to rupture the sternocleidomastoid may occur as the aftercoming head passes over the sacral promontory.

Congenital Injuries

Amnionic Band Syndrome. Focal ring constrictions of the extremities and actual loss of a digit or a limb are rare complications. Their genesis is debated. Streeter (1930), and others since, maintain that localized failure of germ plasm usually is responsible for the abnormalities. Torpin (1968) and others contend that the lesions are the consequence of early rupture of the amnion, which then forms adherent tough bands that constrict and, at times, actually amputate an extremity of the fetus. Occasionally, the amputated part may be found within the uterus. Although this mechanism is favored currently, Hunter and Carpenter (1986) recently reported four cases with associated anomalies not entirely

Coincidental Injuries

Experience at Parkland Hospital, with a very large trauma service, has been that trauma to the fetus inflicted at the time of severe trauma to the mother is less common than might be expected. Because the fetus is floating in amnionic fluid, it is likely to be shielded from forces that cause serious injury to adjacent maternal structures. Fetal traumatic injuries are considered in Chapter 49.

References

Allan LD, Crawford DC, Sheridan R, Chapman MG: Aetiology of non-immune hydrops: The value of echocardiography. Br J Obstet Gynaecol 93:223, 1986

American College of Obstetricians and Gynecologists: Committees on Obstetrics, Maternal and Fetal Medicine and on the Fetus and Newborn: Use and misuse of the Apgar score. November, 1986a

American College of Obstetricians and Gynecologists: Fetal

and neonatal neurologic injury. Technical bulletin no. 163, January 1992

American College of Obstetricians and Gynecologists: Management of isoimmunization in pregnancy. Technical bulletin no. 90, January 1986b

American College of Obstetricians and Gynecologists: Perinatal Viral and Parasitic Infections. Technical bulletin no. 114, March 1988

Anand A, Gray ES, Brown T, Clewley JP, Cohen BJ: Human parvovirus infection in pregnancy and hydrops fetalis. N Engl J Med 316:183, 1987

Ananth U, Queenan JT: Does midtrimester ΔOD_{450} of amniotic fluid reflect severity of Rh disease? Am J Obstet Gynecol 161:47, 1989

Anderson GD, Bada HS, Shaver DC, Harvey CJ, Korones SB, Wong SP, Arheart KL, Magill HL: The effect of cesarean section on intraventricular hemorrhage in the preterm infant. Am J Obstet Gynecol 166:1091, 1992

Anonymous: Cerebral palsy, intrapartum care and a shot in the foot. Editorial. Lancet 2:1251, 1989

Appelman Z, Blumberg BD, Golabi M, Golbus MS: Nonimmune hydrops fetalis may be associated with an elevated ΔOD_{450} in the amniotic fluid. Obstet Gynecol 71:1005, 1988

Arias IM, Gartner LM, Seifter S, Furman M: Prolonged neonatal unconjugated hyperbilirubinemia associated with breast feeding and steroid, pregnane-3α,20β-diol in maternal milk that inhibits glucuronide formation in vitro. J Clin Invest 43:2037, 1964

Ballantyne JW: The Diseases and Deformities of the Foetus. Oliver and Boyd, 1892–1895

Barkai G, Mashiach S, Lanzer D, Kayam Z, Brish M, Goldman B: Determination of fetal lung maturity from amniotic fluid microviscosity in high-risk pregnancy. Obstet Gynecol 59:615, 1982

Barss VA, Frigoletto FD, Konugres A: The cost of irregular antibody screening. Am J Obstet Gynecol 159:428, 1988

Battiste CE, Neff TW, Evans JE, Cline BW: In utero conversion of supraventricular tachycardia with digoxin and procainamide at 17 weeks' gestation. Am J Perinatol 9:302, 1992

Berkowitz RL, Chitkara U, Wilkins IA, Lynch L, Plosker H, Bernstein HH: Intravascular monitoring and management of erythroblastosis fetalis. Am J Obstet Gynecol 158:783, 1988

Berry DD: Neonatology in the 1990's: Surfactant replacement therapy becomes a reality. Clin Pediatr 30:167, 1991

Blair E, Stanley FJ: Intrapartum asphyxia: A rare cause of cerebral palsy. J Pediatr 112:515, 1988

Blajchman MA, Maudsley RF, Uchida I, Zipursky A: Diagnostic amniocentesis and fetal-maternal bleeding. Lancet 1:993, 1974

Boo NY, Lye MS, Kanchanamala M, Ching CL: Brachial plexus injuries in Malaysian neonates: Incidence and associated risk factors. J Trop Pediatr 37:327, 1991

Bowell PJ, Allen DL, Entwistle CC: Blood group antibody screening tests during pregnancy. Br J Obstet Gynaecol 93:1038, 1986a

Bowell PJ, Brown SE, Dike AE, Inskip MJ: The significance of anti-c alloimmunization. Br J Obstet Gynaecol 93:1044, 1986b

Bowman JM: Controversies in Rh prophylaxis: Who needs Rh immune globulin and when should it be given? Am J Obstet Gynecol 151:289, 1985

Bowman JM: The management of Rh-isoimmunization. Obstet Gynecol 52:1, 1978

Bowman JM, Chown B, Lewis M, Pollock J: Rh isoimmunization, Manitoba, 1963–1975. Can Med Assoc J 116:282, 1977

Bowman JM, Pollock JM: Antenatal Rh prophylaxis: 28 week gestation service program. Can Med Assoc J 118:622, 1978

Bowman JM, Pollock JM, Manning FA, Harman CR: Severe anti-C hemolytic disease of the newborn. Am J Obstet Gynecol 166:1239, 1992b

Bowman JM, Pollock JM, Manning FA, Harman CR, Menticoglou S: Maternal Kell blood group alloimmunization. Obstet Gynecol 79:239, 1992a

Bussel JB, Berkowitz RL, McFarland JG, Lynch L, Chitkara U: Antenatal treatment of neonatal alloimmune thrombocytopenia. N Engl J Med 319:1374, 1988

Cameron A, Nicholson S, Nimrod C, Harder J, Davies D, Fritzler M: Evaluation of fetal cardiac dysrhythmias with two-dimensional, M-mode, and pulsed Doppler ultrasonography. Am J Obstet Gynecol 158:286, 1988

Castillo RA, Devoe LD, Hadi HA, Martin S, Giest D: Nonimmune hydrops fetalis: Clinical experience and factors related to a poor outcome. Am J Obstet Gynecol 155:812, 1986

Centers for Disease Control: Lack of transmission of human immunodeficiency virus through $Rh_o(D)$ immune globulin (human). MMWR 36:728, 1987

Charles AG, Blumenthal LS: Promethazine hydrochloride therapy in severe Rh-sensitized pregnancies. Obstet Gynecol 60:627, 1982

Chavez GF, Mulinare J, Edmonds LD: Epidemiology of Rh hemolytic disease of the newborn in the United States. JAMA 265:3270, 1991

Chiswick M, Gladman G, Sinha S, Toner N, Davies J: Vitamin E supplementation and periventricular hemorrhage in the newborn. Am J Clin Nutr 53:370S, 1991

Clark DA, Nieman GF, Thompson JE, Paskanik AM, Rokhar JE, Bredenberg CE: Surfactant displacement by meconium free fatty acids: An alternative explanation for atelectasis in meconium aspiration syndrome. J Pediatr 110:765, 1987

Clements JA, Platzker ACG, Tierney DF, Hobel CL, Creasy RK, Margolis AJ, Thibeault DW, Tooley WH, Oh W: Assessment of the risk of respiratory distress syndrome by a rapid test for surfactant in amniotic fluid. N Engl J Med 286:1077, 1972

Desjardins L, Blajchman MA, Chintu G, Gent M, Zipursky A: The spectrum of ABO hemolytic disease of the newborn infant. J Pediatr 95:447, 1979

DeVries LS, Dubowitz V, Lary S, Whitelaw A, Dubowitz LMS, Kaiser A, Silverman M, Wigglesworth JS: Predictive value of cranial ultrasound in the newborn baby: A reappraisal. Lancet 2:137, 1985

Diamond LK, Blackfan KP, Baty JM: Erythroblastosis fetalis and its association with universal edema of the fetus, icterus gravis neonatorum and anemia of the newborn. J Pediatr 1:269, 1932

Dildy GA, Smith LG Jr, Moise KJ Jr, Cano LE, Hesketh DE: Porencephalic cyst: A complication of fetal intravascular transfusion. Am J Obstet Gynecol 165:76, 1991

Dijxhoorn MJ, Visser GHA, Fidler VJ, Touwen BCL, Huisjes HJ: Apgar score, meconium and acidaemia at birth in relation to neonatal neurological morbidity in term infants. Br J Obstet Gynaecol 86:217, 1986

Donn SM, Roloff DW, Goldstein GW: Prevention of intraventricular hemorrhage in preterm infants by phenobarbitone. Lancet 2:215, 1981

Dooley SL, Pesavento DJ, Depp R, Socol ML, Tamura RK, Wiringa KS: Meconium below the vocal cords at delivery: Correlation with intrapartum events. Am J Obstet Gynecol 153:767, 1985

Dunn MS, Shennan AT, Hoskins EM, Lennox K, Enhorning G: Two-year follow-up of infants enrolled in a randomized trial of surfactant replacement therapy for prevention of neonatal respiratory distress syndrome. Pediatrics 82:543, 1988

Eibl MM, Wolf HM, Fürnkranz H, Rosenkranz A: Prevention of necrotizing enterocolitis in low-birth-weight infants by IgA-IgG feeding. N Engl J Med 319:1, 1988

Falciglia HS: Failure to prevent meconium aspiration syndrome. Obstet Gynecol 71:349, 1988

Fee SC, Malee K, Deddish R, Minogue JP, Min D, Socol ML: Severe acidosis and subsequent neurologic status. Am J Obstet Gynecol 162:802, 1990

Fetus and Newborn Committee, Canadian Paediatric Society: Neonatal surfactant replacement therapy. Can Med Assoc J 8:146, 1992

Finn R, Clarke CA, Donohoe W, McConnell RB, Sheppard PM, Lehane D, Kulke W: Experimental studies on the prevention of Rh haemolytic disease. BMJ 1:1486, 1961

Foliot A, Ploussard JP, Housset E, Christoforov B: Breast milk jaundice: In vitro inhibition of rat liver bilirubin-uridine diphosphate glucuronyltransferase activity and Z protein-bromosulfonphthalein binding by human breast milk. Pediatr Res 10:594, 1976

Freda V: Hemolytic disease. Clin Obstet Gynecol 16:72, 1973

Freda VJ, Gorman JG, Pollack W: Successful prevention of sensitization to Rh with an experimental anti-Rh gamma$_2$ globulin antibody preparation. Fed Proc 22:374, 1963

Freda VJ, Gorman JG, Pollack W, Bowe E: Prevention of Rh hemolytic disease: Ten years' clinical experience with Rh immune globulin. N Engl J Med 292:1014, 1975

Freeman J (ed): Prenatal and Perinatal Factors Associated with Brain Disorders. US Department of Health and Human Services, Public Health Service, National Institutes of Health, NIH publication no. 85-1149, 1985

Freeman JM, Nelson KB: Intrapartum asphyxia and cerebral palsy. Pediatrics 82:240, 1988

Freeman R: Intrapartum fetal monitoring—a disappointing story. N Engl J Med 322:624, 1990

Fujiwara T, Maeta H, Shida S, Morita T, Watabe Y, Abe T: Artificial surfactant therapy in hyaline-membrane disease. Lancet 1:55, 1980

Gilstrap LC, Cunningham FG: Umbilical cord blood acid-base analysis. Williams Obstetrics, 18th ed (suppl 1). Appleton & Lange, Norwalk, CT, Aug/Sept 1989

Gilstrap LC III, Leveno KJ, Burris J, Williams ML, Little BB: Diagnosis of asphyxia on the basis of fetal pH, Apgar score, and newborn cerebral dysfunction. Am J Obstet Gynecol 161:825, 1989

Gluck L, Kulovich MV: Lecithin/sphingomyelin ratios in amniotic fluid in normal and abnormal pregnancy. Am J Obstet Gynecol 115:539, 1973

Gluck L, Kulovich MV, Borer RC Jr, Brenner PH, Anderson GG, Spellacy WN: Diagnosis of the respiratory distress syndrome by amniocentesis. Am J Obstet Gynecol 109:440, 1971

Gold WR Jr, Queenan JT, Woody J, Sacher RA: Oral desensitization in Rh disease. Am J Obstet Gynecol 146:980, 1983

Goldaber KJ, Gilstrap LC, Leveno KJ, Dax JS, McIntire DD: Pathologic fetal acidemia. Obstet Gynecol 78:1103, 1991

Gough JD, Keeling JW, Castle B, Iliff PJ: The obstetric management of non-immunological hydrops. Br J Obstet Gynaecol 93:226, 1986

Graham M, Trounce JQ, Levene MI, Rutter N: Prediction of cerebral palsy in very low birthweight infants: Prospective ultrasound study. Lancet 2:593, 1987

Grannum PA, Copel JA, Moya FR, Scioscia AL, Robert JA, Winn HN, Coster BC, Burdine CB, Hobbins JC: The reversal of fetal hydrops by intravascular intrauterine transfusion in severe isoimmune fetal anemia. Am J Obstet Gynecol 158:914, 1988

Grannum PA, Copel JA, Plaxe SC, Scioscia AL, Hobbins JC: In utero exchange transfusion by direct intravascular injection in severe erythroblastosis fetalis. N Engl J Med 314:1431, 1986

Grant A, O'Brien N, Joy MT, Hennessy E, MacDonald D: Cerebral palsy among children born during the Dublin randomised trial of intrapartum monitoring. Lancet 2:1233, 1989

Hack M, Horbar JD, Malloy MH, Tyson JE, Wright E, Wright L: Very low birth weight outcomes of the National Institute of Child Health and Human Development Neonatal Network. Pediatrics 87:587, 1991

Hagberg B, Hagberg G, Olow I: The changing panorama of cerebral palsy in Sweden, IV. Epidemiological trends 1959-78. Acta Paediatr Scand 73:433, 1984

Hallman M, Bry K, Hoppu K, Lappi M, Pohjavuori M: Inositol supplementation in premature infants with respiratory distress syndrome. N Engl J Med 326:1233, 1992

Hanigan WC, Kennedy G, Roemisch F, Anderson R, Cusack T, Powers W: Administration of indomethacin for the prevention of periventricular-intraventricular hemorrhage in high-risk neonates. J Pediatr 112:941, 1988

Harman CR, Bowman JM, Manning FA, Menticoglou SM: Intrauterine transfusion—intraperitoneal versus intravascular approach: A case control comparison. Am J Obstet Gynecol 162:1053, 1990

Harman CR, Manning FA, Bowman JM, Lange IR: Severe Rh disease—Poor outcome is not inevitable. Am J Obstet Gynecol 145:823, 1983

Harvey D, Parkinson CE, Campbell S: Risk of respiratory-distress syndrome. Lancet 1:42, 1975

Hayden CK, Shattuck KE, Richardson CJ, Ahrendt DK, House R, Swischuk LE: Subependymal germinal matrix hemorrhage in full-term neonates. Pediatrics 75:714, 1985

Herbert WNP, Chapman JE, Cefalo RC: Reliability of the foam stability index test in assessing fetal lung maturation. Presented at the meeting of the Society of Perinatal Obstetricians, San Antonio, February, 1984

Holzgreve W, Curry CJR, Golbus MS, Callen PW, Filly RA, Smith JC: Investigation of nonimmune hydrops fetalis. Am J Obstet Gynecol 150:805, 1984

Hunter AGW, Carpenter BF: Implications of malformations not due to amniotic bands in the amniotic band sequence. Am J Med Genet 24:691, 1986

Hutchison AA, Drew JH, Yu VYH, Williams ML, Fortune DW, Beischer NA: Nonimmunologic hydrops fetalis: A review of 61 cases. Obstet Gynecol 59:347, 1982

Illingworth RS: Why blame the obstetrician?: A review. BMJ 1:797, 1979

Jarvis SN, Holloway JS, Hey EN: Increase in cerebral palsy in normal birthweight babies. Arch Dis Child 60:1113, 1985

Jennings ER, Clauss B: Maternal-fetal hemorrhage: Its incidence and sensitizing effects. Am J Obstet Gynecol 131:725, 1978

Kanto WP Jr, Wilson R, Breart GL, Zierler S, Purohit DM, Peckham GJ, Ellison RC: Perinatal events and necrotizing enterocolitis in premature infants. Am J Dis Child 141:167, 1987

Kaplan C, Daffos F, Forestier F, Cox WL, Lyon-Caen D, Dupuy-Montbrun MC, Salmon CH: Management of alloimmune thrombocytopenia: Antenatal diagnosis and in utero transfusion of maternal platelets. Blood 72:340, 1988

Katz LV, Bowes WA: Meconium aspiration syndrome: Reflections on a murky subject. Am J Obstet Gynecol 166:171, 1992

Katz MA, Kanto WP Jr, Korotkein JH: Recurrence rate of ABO hemolytic disease of the newborn. Obstet Gynecol 59:611, 1982

Keenan WJ, Jewitt T, Glueck HI: Role of feeding and vitamin K in hypoprothrombinemia of the newborn. Am J Dis Child 121:271, 1971

Kendig JW, Notter RH, Cox C, Reubens LJ, Davis JM, Maniscalco WM, Sinkin RA, Bartoletti A, Dweck HS, Horgan MJ, Risemberg H, Phelps DL, Shapiro DL: A comparison of surfactant as immediate prophylaxis and as rescue therapy in newborns of less than 30 weeks' gestation. N Engl J Med 324:865, 1991

Kinsey VE, Arnold HJ, Kalina RE, Stern L, Stahlman M, Odell G, Driscoll J, Elliott J, Payne J, Patz A: Pao$_2$ levels and retrolental fibroplasia: A report of the cooperative study. Pediatrics 60:655, 1977

Kirkman HN Jr: Further evidence for a racial difference in the frequency of ABO hemolytic disease. J Pediatr 90:717, 1977

Kleinman CS, Copel JA, Weinstein EM, Santulli TV, Hobbins JC: In utero diagnosis and treatment of fetal supraventricular tachycardia. Semin Perinatol 9:113, 1985

Kliegman RM, Fanaroff AA: Necrotizing enterocolitis. N Engl J Med 310:1093, 1984

Landsteiner K, Weiner AS: An agglutinable factor in human blood recognized by immune sera for rhesus blood. Proc Soc Exper Biol Med 43:223, 1940

Lane PA, Hathaway WE: Vitamin K in infancy. J Pediatr 106:351, 1985

Lesko SM, Mitchell AA, Epstein MF, Louik C, Giacoia GP, Shapiro S: Heparin use as a risk factor for intraventricular hemorrhage in low-birth-weight infants. N Engl J Med 314:1156, 1986

Levine MG, Holroyde J, Woods JR, Siddiqi TA, Scott M, Miodovnik M: Birth trauma: Incidence and predisposing factors. Obstet Gynecol 63:792, 1984

Levine P: Isoimmunization in pregnancy and the pathogenesis of erythroblastosis fetalis. In Karsner HT, Hooker SB (eds): 1941 Yearbook of Pathology and Immunology. Chicago, Yearbook Publishers, 1941, p 505

Leveno KJ, Quirk JG, Cunningham FG, Nelson SD, Santo-Ramos R, Toofanian A, DePalma RT: Prolonged pregnancy, I. Observations concerning the causes of fetal distress. Am J Obstet Gynecol 150:465, 1984

Liley AW: Intrauterine transfusion of foetus in hemolytic disease. BMJ 2:1107, 1963

Liley AW: Amniocentesis and amniography in hemolytic disease. In Greenhill JP (ed): Yearbook of Obstetrics & Gynecology, 1964–1965 Series. Chicago, Year Book, 1964, p 256

Liley AW: Liquor amnii analysis in management of pregnancy complicated by rhesus sensitization. Am J Obstet Gynecol 82:1359, 1961

Linder N, Aranda JV, Tsur M, Matoth I, Yatsiv I, Mandelberg H, Rottem M, Feigenbaum D, Ezra Y, Tamir I: Need for endotracheal intubation and suction in meconium-stained neonates. J Pediatr 112:613, 1988

Locus P, Yeomans E, Crosby U: The efficacy of bulb versus DeLee suction at deliveries complicated by meconium-stained amniotic fluid. Presented at the District VII meeting of the American College of Obstetricians and Gynecologists, October 1987

Long W, Corbet A, Allen A, McMillan D, Boros S, Vaughan R, Gerdes J, Houle L, Edwards K, Schiff D, and the American Exosurf Neonatal Study Group I, and the Canadian Exosurf Neonatal Study Group: Retrospective search for bleeding diathesis among premature newborn infants with pulmonary hemorrhage after synthetic surfactant treatment. J Pediatr 120:S45, 1992

Low JA, Galbraith RS, Muir DW, Killen HL, Karchmar EJ: The relationship between perinatal hypoxia and newborn encephalopathy. Am J Obstet Gynecol 152:256, 1985

Lowe TW, Leveno KJ, Quirk JG Jr, Santos-Ramos R, Williams ML: Sinusoidal fetal heart rate pattern after intrauterine transfusion. Obstet Gynecol 64:21S, 1984

Luthy DA, Shy KK, Strickland D, Wilson J, Bennett FC, Brown ZA, Benedetti TJ: Status of infants at birth and risk for adverse neonatal events and long-term sequelae: A study in low birthweight infants. Am J Obstet Gynecol 157:676, 1987

MacDonald D, Grant A, Sheridan-Pereira M, Boylan P, Chalmers I: The Dublin randomized control trial of intrapartum fetal heart rate monitoring. Am J Obstet Gynecol 152:524, 1985

Maisels MJ: Neonatal jaundice, III. Breast feeding and jaundice. Perinat Press 3:19, 1979

Malloy MH, Hartford RB, Kleinman JC: Trends in mortality caused by respiratory distress syndrome in the United States, 1969–83. Am J Public Health 77:1511, 1987

Marshall R, Tyrala E, McAlister W, Sheehan M: Meconium aspiration syndrome: Neonatal and follow-up study. Am J Obstet Gynecol 131:672, 1978

McFarland LV, Raskin M, Daling JR, Benedetti TJ: Erb/Duchenne's palsy: A consequence of fetal macrosomia and method of delivery. Obstet Gynecol 68:784, 1986

Millard DD, Gidding SS, Socol ML, MacGregor SN, Dooley SL, Ney JA, Stockman JA: III: Effects of intravascular, intrauterine transfusion on prenatal and postnatal hemolysis and erythropoiesis in severe fetal isoimmunization. J Pediatr 117:447, 1990

Miller ME, Graham JM Jr, Higginbotton MC, Smith DW: Compression-related defects from early amnion rupture: Evidence for mechanical teratogenesis. J Pediatr 98:292, 1981

Mino M: Clinical uses and abuses of vitamin E in children. Proc Soc Exp Biol Med 200:266, 1992

Mitchell J, Schulman H, Fleischer A, Farmakides G, Nadeau D: Obstet Gynecol 65:352, 1985

Morales WJ: Antenatal therapy to minimize neonatal intraventricular hemorrhage. Clin Obstet Gynecol 34:328, 1991

Morales WJ: Effect of intraventricular hemorrhage on the one-year mental and neurologic handicaps of the very low birth weight infant. Obstet Gynecol 70:111, 1987

Morales WJ, Koerten J: Prevention of intraventricular hemorrhage in very low birth weight infants by maternally administered phenobarbital. Obstet Gynecol 68:295, 1986

Morales WJ, Stroup M: Intracranial hemorrhage in utero due to isoimmune neonatal thrombocytopenia. Obstet Gynecol 65:20S, 1985

Morley CJ: Surfactant treatment for premature babies—a review of clinical trials. Arch Dis Child 66:445, 1991

Mountain K, Hirsh J, Gallus AS: Neonatal coagulation defect and maternal anti-convulsant treatment. Lancet 1:265, 1970

Mueller-Heubach E, Mazer J: Sonographically documented disappearance of fetal ascites. Obstet Gynecol 61:253, 1983

Nelson KB, Ellenberg JH: Antecedents of cerebral palsy: Multivariate analysis of risk. N Engl J Med 315:81, 1986a

Nelson KB, Ellenberg JH: Antecedents of seizure disorders in early childhood. Am J Dis Child 140:1053, 1986b

Nelson KB, Ellenberg JH: Antecedents of cerebral palsy: Univariate analysis of risks. Am J Dis Child 139:1031, 1985

Nelson KB, Ellenberg JH: Obstetric complications as risk factors for cerebral palsy or seizure disorders. JAMA 251:1843, 1984

Ness PM, Baldwin ML, Niebyl JR: Clinical high-risk designation does not predict excess fetal-maternal hemorrhage. Am J Obstet Gynecol 156:154, 1987

Newton ER, Haering WA, Kennedy JL, Herschel M, Cetrulo C, Feingold M: Effect of mode of delivery on morbidity and mortality of infants at early gestational age. Obstet Gynecol 67:507, 1986

Ney JA, Socol ML, Dooley SN, MacGregor SW, Silver RK, Millard DO: Perinatal outcome following intravascular transfusion in severely isoimmunized fetuses. Int J Gynecol Obstet 35:41, 1991

Nicolaides KH, Clewell WH, Mibashan RS, Soothill PW, Rodeck CH, Campbell S: Fetal haemoglobin measurement in the assessment of red cell isoimmunization. Lancet 1:1073, 1988

Nicolaides KH, Rodeck CH, Mibashan RS, Kemp JR: Have Liley charts outlived their usefulness? Am J Obstet Gynecol 155:90, 1986

Nicolaides KH, Snijders RJM: Cordocentesis. In Evans MI (ed): Reproductive Risks and Prenatal Diagnosis. Norwalk, CT, Appleton & Lange, p 201, 1992

Nicolaides KH, Warenski JC, Rodeck CH: The relationship of fetal plasma protein concentration and hemoglobin level to the development of hydrops in rhesus isoimmunization. Am J Obstet Gynecol 152:341, 1985

Nicolini U, Nicolaides P, Fisk NM, Tannirandorn Y, Rodeck CH: Fetal blood sampling from the intrahepatic vein: Analysis of safety and clinical experience with 214 procedures. Obstet Gynecol 76:47, 1990

Nicolini U, Nicolaides P, Tannirandorn Y, Fisk N, Nasrat H, Rodeck CH: Fetal liver dysfunction in Rh alloimmunization. Br J Obstet Gynaecol 98:287, 1991

Nicolini U, Rodeck CH, Kochenour NK, Greco P, Fisk NM, Letsky E, Lubenko A: In utero platelet transfusion for alloimmune thrombocytopenia. Lancet 2:506, 1988

Oppenheim WL, Davis A, Growdon WA, Dorey FJ, Davlin LB: Clavicle fractures in the newborn. Clin Orthop 250:176, 1990

Paneth N: Birth and the origins of cerebral palsy. N Engl J Med 315:124, 1986

Papile L-A, Burstein J, Burstein R, Koffler H: Incidence and evolution of subependymal and intraventricular hemor-

rhage: A study of infants with birth weights less than 1500 gm. J Pediatr 92:529, 1978

Papile L-A, Munsick-Bruno G, Schaefer A: Relationship of cerebral intraventricular hemorrhage and early childhood neurologic handicaps. J Pediatr 103:273, 1983

Perlman JM, Cunningham FG: Fetal and neonatal hypoxic ischemic cerebral injury. Williams Obstetrics, 18th ed (suppl 21). Norwalk, CT, Appleton & Lange, Dec/Jan 1993

Perlman JM, Goodman S, Kreusser KL, Volpe JJ: Reduction in intraventricular hemorrhage by elimination of fluctuating cerebral blood-flow velocity in preterm infants with respiratory distress syndrome. N Engl J Med 312:1353, 1985

Perlman JM, Volpe JJ: Intraventricular hemorrhage in extremely small premature infants. Am J Dis Child 140:1122, 1986

Pharoah POD, Cooke T, Rosenbloom I, Cooke RWI: Trends in birth prevalence of cerebral palsy. Arch Dis Child 62:379, 1987

Pomerance JJ, Jeal JG, Gogolok JF, Brown S, Stewart ME: Maternally administered antenatal vitamin K_1: Effect on neonatal prothrombin activity, partial thromboplastin time and intraventricular hemorrhage. Obstet Gynecol 70:235, 1987

Pritchard JA, Cunningham FG, Pritchard SA, Mason RA: How often does maternal preeclampsia-eclampsia incite thrombocytopenia in the fetus? Obstet Gynecol 69:292, 1987

Pryde PG, Nugent CE, Pridjian G, Barr M Jr, Faix RG: Spontaneous resolution of nonimmune hydrops fetalis secondary to human parvovirus B19 infection. Obstet Gynecol 79:859, 1992

Queenan JT, King JC: Intrauterine transfusion for severe Rh-EBF—Past and future. Contemp Ob/Gyn 30:51, 1987

Quirk JG, Bleasdale JE: Fetal lung maturation in the pregnancy complicated by diabetes mellitus. In DiRenzo GC, Hawkins PR (eds): Perinatal Medicine: Updates and Controversies. New York, Cortina International, 1986, p 117

Rajadurai VS, Menahem S: Fetal arrhythmias: A 3-year experience. Aust NZ J Obstet Gynaecol 32:28, 1992

Radunovic N, Lockwood CJ, Alvarez M, Plecas D, Chitkara U, Berkowitz RL: The severely anemic and hydropic isoimmune fetus: Changes in fetal hematocrit associated with intrauterine death. Obstet Gynecol 79:390, 1992

Ramin SM, Gilstrap LC, Leveno KJ, Dax JS, Little BB: The acid-base significance of meconium discovered prior to labor. Am J Perinatol (in press)

Ramsey-Goldman R, Hom D, Deng J, Ziegler GC, Kahl LE, Steen VD, LaPorte RE, Medsger TA Jr: Anti-SS-A antibodies and fetal outcome in maternal systemic lupus erythematosus. Arthritis Rheum 29:1269, 1986

Robertson C, Finer N: Term infants with hypoxic-ischemic encephalopathy: Outcome at 3.5 years. Dev Med Child Neurol 27:473, 1985

Rodeck CH, Holman CA, Karicki J, Kemp JR, Whitmore DN, Austin MA: Direct intravascular fetal blood transfusion by fetoscopy in severe rhesus isoimmunization. Lancet 1:625, 1981

Rodeck CH, Nicolaides KH, Warsof SL, Fysh WJ, Gamsu HR, Kemp JR: The management of severe rhesus isoimmunization by fetoscopic intravascular transfusions. Am J Obstet Gynecol 150:769, 1984

Roemer RJ: Relation of torticollis to breech delivery. Am J Obstet Gyncol 67:1146, 1954

Rosen MG, Dickinson JC: The incidence of cerebral palsy. Am J Obstet Gynecol 167:417, 1992

Rosen MG, Hobel CJ: Prenatal and perinatal factors associated with brain disorders. Obstet Gynecol 68:416, 1986

Rouse D, Weiner C: Ongoing fetomaternal hemorrhage treated by serial fetal intravascular transfusions. Obstet Gynecol 76:974, 1990

Ruth VJ, Raivio KO: Perinatal brain damage: Predictive value of metabolic acidosis and the Apgar score. BMJ 297:24, 1988

Sahakian V, Weiner CP, Naides SJ, Williamson RA, Scharosch LL: Intrauterine transfusion treatment of nonimmune hydrops fetalis secondary to human parvovirus B19 infection. Am J Obstet Gynecol 164:1090, 1991

Salonen IS, Uüsitalo R: Birth injuries: Incidence and predisposing factors. Zeitschr fur Kinderch 45:133, 1990

Santolaya J, Alley D, Jaffe R, Warsof SL: Antenatal classification of hydrops fetalis. Obstet Gynecol 79:256, 1992

Saunders BS, Lazoritz S, McArtor RD, Marshall P, Bason WM: Depressed skull fracture in the neonate. J Neurosurg 50:512, 1979

Sbarra AJ, Michlewitz H, Selvaraj RJ, Mitchell GW, Cetrulo CL, Kelley EC, Kennedy JL, Herschell MJ, Paul BB, Louis F: Relation between optical density at 650 nm and L/S ratio. Obstet Gynecol 50:273, 1977

Schlueter MA, Phibbs RH, Creasy RK, Clements JA, Tooley WH: Antenatal prediction of graduated risk of hyaline membrane disease by amniotic fluid foam test for surfactant. Am J Obstet Gynecol 134:761, 1979

Shearer MJ, Barkhan P, Rahim S, Stimmler L: Plasma vitamin K_1 in mothers and their newborn babies. Lancet 2:460, 1982

Shenker L, Reed KL, Anderson CF, Marx GR, Sobonya RE, Graham AR: Congenital heart block and cardiac anomalies in the absence of maternal connective tissue disease. Am J Obstet Gynecol 157:248, 1987

Sher G, Statland BE: Assessment of fetal pulmonary maturity by the Lumadex foam stability index test. Obstet Gynecol 61:444, 1983

Shy KK, Luthy DA, Bennett FC, Whitfield M, Larson EB, van Belle G, Hughes JP, Wilson JA, Stenchever MA: Effects of electronic fetal heart rate monitoring, as compared with periodic auscultation, on the neurologic development of premature infants. N Engl J Med 322:588, 1990

Sinha S, Davies J, Toner N, Bogle S: Vitamin E supplementation reduces frequency of periventricular hemorrhage in very preterm babies. Lancet 1:466, 1987

Skajaa K, Hansen ES, Bendix J: Depressed fracture of the skull in a child born by cesarean section. Acta Obstet Gynecol Scand 66:275, 1987

Stanley FJ, Watson L: The cerebral palsies in Western Australia: trends, 1968 to 1981. Am J Obstet Gynecol 158:89, 1988

Stedman CM, Baudin JC, White CA, Cooper ES: Use of the erythrocyte rosette test to screen for excessive fetomaternal hemorrhage in Rh-negative women. Am J Obstet Gynecol 154:1363, 1986

Steinfeld JD, Samuels P, Bulley MA, Cohen AW, Goodman DBP, Senior MB: The utility of the TDx test in the assessment of fetal lung maturity. Obstet Gynecol 79:460, 1992

Stevenson D, Walther F, Long W, Sell M, Pauly T, Gong A, Easa D, Pramanik A, LeBlanc M, Anday E, Dhanireddy R, Burchfield D, Corbet A, and the American Exosurf Neonatal Study Group: Controlled trial of a single dose of synthetic surfac-

tant at birth in premature infants weighing 500 to 699 grams. J Pediatr 120:S3, 1992

Strauss A, Kirz D, Modanlou HD, Freeman RK: Perinatal events and intraventricular/subependymal hemorrhage in the very low-birth weight infant. Am J Obstet Gynecol 151:1022, 1985

Streeter GL: Contrib Embryol 22:1, 1930

Taylor PV, Scott JS, Gerlis LM, Esscher E, Scott O: Maternal antibodies against fetal cardiac antigens in congenital complete heart block. N Engl J Med 315:667, 1986

Tejani N, Verma U, Hameed C, Chayen B: Method and route of delivery in the low birth weight vertex presentation correlated with early periventricular/intraventricular hemorrhage. Obstet Gynecol 69:1, 1987

Thacker KE, Lim T, Drew JH: Cephalhaematoma: A 10-year review. Aust NZ J Obstet Gynaecol 27:210, 1987

Thorp JA, Cohen GR, Yeast JD, Perryman D, Welsh C, Honssinger N, Stephenson S, Hedrick J: Nonimmune hydrops caused by massive fetomaternal hemorrhage and treated by intravascular transfusion. Am J Perinatol 9:22, 1992

Thorp JA, O'Connor T, Callenbach J, Cohen GR, Yeast JD, Albin J, Plapp F: Hyporegenerative anemia associated with intrauterine transfusion in rhesus hemolytic disease. Am J Obstet Gynecol 165:79, 1991

Thorp JA, Plapp FV, Cohen GR, Yeas JD, O'Kell RT, Stephenson S: Hyperkalemia after irradiation of packed red blood cells: Possible effects with intravascular fetal transfusion. Am J Obstet Gynecol 163:607, 1990

Torfs CP, van den Berg B, Oechsli FW, Cummins S: Prenatal and perinatal factors in the etiology of cerebral palsy. J Pediatr 116:615, 1990

Torpin R: Fetal Malformations Caused By Amnion Rupture During Gestation. Springfield, IL, Thomas, 1968

Truwit CL, Barkovich AJ, Koch TK, Ferriero DM. Cerebral palsy: MR findings in 40 patients. AJNR 13:67, 1992

Tsai MY, Josephson MW, Knox GE: Absorbance of amniotic fluid at 650 nm as a fetal lung maturity test: A comparison with the lecithin/sphingomyelin ratio and tests for desaturated phosphatidylcholine and phosphatidylglycerol. Am J Obstet Gynecol 146:963, 1983

Van Houten J, Long W, Mullett M, Finer N, Derleth D, McMurray B, Peliowski A, Walker D, Wold D, Sankaran K, Corbet A, and the American Exosurf Neonatal Study Group I, and the Canadian Exosurf Neonatal Study Group: Pulmonary hemorrhage in premature infants after treatment with synthetic surfactant: An autopsy evaluation. J Pediatr 120:S40, 1992

Vaucher YE, Merritt TA, Hallman M, Jarvenpaa A, Telsey AM, Jones BL: Neurodevelopmental and respiratory outcome in early childhood after human surfactant treatment. Am J Dis Child 142:927, 1988

Volpe JJ: Neurology of the Newborn, 2nd ed. Philadelphia, Saunders, 1987

Wallin LA, Rosenfeld CR, Laptook AR, Maravilla AM, Strand C, Campbell N, Dowling S, Lasky RE: Neonatal intracranial hemorrhage, II. Risk factor analysis in an inborn population. Early Hum Dev 23:129, 1990

Walsh MC, Kliegman RM: Necrotizing enterocolitis: Treatment based on staging criteria. Pediatr Clin North Am 33:179, 1986

Watts DH, Luthy DA, Benedetti TJ, Cyr DR, Easterling TR, Hickok D: Intraperitoneal fetal transfusion under direct ultrasound guidance. Obstet Gynecol 71:84, 1988

Wegman ME: Annual summary of vital statistics–1990. Pediatrics 88:1081, 1991

Weiner CP, Wenstrom KD, Sipes SL, Williamson RA: Risk factors for cordocentesis and fetal intravascular transfusion. Am J Obstet Gynecol 165:1020, 1991a

Weiner CP, Williamson RA, Wenstrom KD, Sipes SL, Widness JA, Grant SS, Estle L: Management of fetal hemolytic disease by cordocentesis, II. Outcome of treatment. Am J Obstet Gynecol 165:1302, 1991b

Weiner SA, Weinstein L: Fetal pulmonary maturity and antenatal diagnosis of respiratory distress syndrome. Obstet Gynecol Surv 42:75, 1987

Welch RA, Bottoms SF: Reconsideration of head compression and intraventricular hemorrhage in the vertex very-low-birth-weight fetus. Obstet Gynecol 68:29, 1986

Wenk RE, Goldstein P, Felix JK: Alloimmunization by hr' (c), hemolytic disease of newborns, and perinatal management. Obstet Gynecol 67:623, 1986

Whittle MJ, Wilson AI, Whitfield CR, Paton RD, Logan RW: Amniotic fluid phosphatidylglycercol and the lecithin/sphingomyelin ratio in the assessment of fetal lung maturity. Br J Obstet Gynaecol 89:727, 1982

Wigglesworth JS, Pape KE: Pathophysiology of intracranial hemorrhage in the newborn. J Perinat Med 8:119, 1980

Wiklund LM, Uvebrant P, Flodmark O. Computed tomography as an adjunct in etiological analysis of hemiplegic cerebral palsy, I. Children born preterm. Neuropediatrics 22:50, 1991a

Wiklund LM, Uvebrant P, Flodmark O. Computed tomography as an adjunct in etiological analysis of hemiplegic cerebral palsy, II. Children born at term. Neuropediatrics 22:121, 1991b

Winkler CL, Hauth JC, Tucker JM, Owen J, Brumfield CG: Neonatal complications at term as related to the degree of umbilical artery acidemia. Am J Obstet Gynecol 164:637, 1991

Yeomans E, Gilstrap LC, Leveno KJ, Burris JS: Meconium-stained amniotic fluid and neonatal acid-base status. Obstet Gynecol 73:175, 1989

Techniques Used to Assess Fetal Health

■

CHAPTER 45
Antepartum Fetal Testing

TECHNIQUES TO EVALUATE FETAL HEALTH

The rate of foetal heart is subject to considerable variations which afford us a fairly reliable means of judging as to the well-being of the child.
                                    J. Whitridge Williams

The brief statement above is the total extent of text devoted to judging fetal well-being in the 1908 Second Edition of *Williams Obstetrics.* At that time, the mother was the patient for whom care was given and the fetus was simply a transient maternal organ. During the past two decades, remarkably intimate knowledge of the human fetus along with technological developments have prompted a new phenomenon in medicine: forecasts of fetal health. The fetus is no longer dealt with as a maternal appendage ultimately to be shed, but has achieved the status of a second patient who faces greater risks of serious morbidity and mortality than does the mother. Indeed, the technological boundary for fetal assessment has even been extended to the embryonic period of human development. As an example, Achiron and colleagues (1991) found that embryonic heart rates may be predictive of early abortion!

In this chapter we consider the evolution of several techniques employed to forecast fetal well-being. We will focus principally on contemporary testing procedures that depend upon physical fetal activities, including movement, breathing, and heart rate. Hormonal methods occupy a position of historical importance in the evolution of fetal tests of well-being but, because they have been largely abandoned, they are not discussed. Examples include measurement of human pla-

cental lactogen in maternal plasma and estriol in maternal plasma or urine.

Fetal Movements

The detection of fetal movements by the mother has long been recognized as a sign of pregnancy. Women typically first feel fetal movements—*quickening*—between 16 and 20 weeks, although fetal activity has been shown to occur as early as 6 weeks when rolling movements were observed using sophisticated ultrasonic devices (Stephens and Birnholz, 1977). As might be expected, mothers do not detect all fetal movements. For example, beyond 36 weeks, mothers perceived only 15 percent of fetal body movements recorded by a Doppler device. Fetal motions lasting more than 20 seconds were identified more accurately by the mother compared with shorter episodes of fetal activity (Johnson and colleagues, 1990).

It has also been taught for many years that diminished movement may be a harbinger of impending fetal death and lack of movement a sign of death. Current interest in maternally discerned fetal motion as an indicator of health followed clinical observations that decreasing movements sometimes indicated impending fetal death. Rovinsky and Guttmacher (1965), Mathews (1973), and Sadovsky and Yaffe (1973) observed that fetal movements subsided prior to fetal death in pregnancies complicated by placental insufficiency due to preeclampsia. The latter investigators proposed using a *daily fetal movement record* in high-risk pregnancies in which placental insufficiency was suspected. Importantly, they stressed the need for daily movement records for each woman because each fetus has its own rhythm and rate of movement compounded by variable perceptiveness on the part of the mother. These vagaries of fetal motion prompted Sadovsky and Yaffe (1973) to measure movements from 8 AM to 8 PM and to calculate the sum of movements during the 12-hour period to determine the *daily fetal movement record.*

The first half of human pregnancy is characterized by rapid emergence of a wide variety of fetal movements of relatively high frequency but little neurological organization (DeVries and co-workers, 1982). During the second half of pregnancy, these movements become organized (Pillai and associates, 1992). Figure 45–1 shows fetal movements during the last half of gestation in 127 pregnancies with normal outcomes. The mean number of weekly movements calculated from 12-hour daily recording periods increased from about 200 in the 20th week to a maximum of 575 movements in the 32nd week. Weekly fetal movements then declined to an average of 282 at 40 weeks. Normal weekly counts of fetal movements ranged between 50 and 950, with large daily variations that included counts as low as 4 to 10 per 12-hour day in normal pregnancies.

An important determinant of fetal activity appears to be sleep-awake cycles, which are independent of the maternal sleep-awake state. This cyclicity also has some importance in the interpretation of the nonstress test as discussed below. "Sleep" cyclicity of the fetus has been described to vary from about 20-minutes to as much as 2-hour intervals. For example, Timor-Tritsch and associates (1978) reported that the mean length of the quiet or inactive state for term fetuses was about 23 minutes; Sterman (1967) reported it to be 40 to 60 minutes; van Geijn and colleagues (1980) 30 to 70 minutes; and Granat and co-workers (1979) 40 to 80 minutes per cycle interval. Patrick and associates (1982) measured gross fetal body movements with real-time ultrasound for 24-hour periods in 31 normal pregnancies and found that

the longest observed period of inactivity was 75 minutes.

Not only are sleep-awake cycles and daily or weekly fluctuations in fetal movement hallmarks of such activity, but several investigators also have reported diurnal and circadian rhythms. For example, Goodlin and Lowe (1974) reported two peaks of fetal activity, with one such peak identified between 9 PM and 1 AM. However, others have been unable to confirm such diurnal variations (Birkenfeld and co-workers, 1980).

Some investigators have associated rapid eye movements (REMs), signifying relative wakefulness in the fetus, with body movement cycles (Goodlin and Lowe, 1974). Indeed, the wakefulness cycle has considerable influence not only upon body movement, but also upon other behavioral states used to monitor fetal health. Relative fetal wakefulness associated with low-voltage brain waves is accompanied by rapid eye movements, respiratory activity, body movement, and corresponding acceleration of heart rate. Thus, the wakefulness of the fetus is an important determinant of movement patterns and behavioral state in general.

Sadovsky and colleagues (1979b) studied the type of fetal movements in 120 normal pregnancies and classified the movements into three categories according to both maternal perceptions and independent recordings using piezoelectric sensors. Weak, strong, and rolling movements were described, and their relative contributions to total weekly movements throughout the last half of pregnancy were quantified. As pregnancy advances, weak movements decrease and are superseded by more vigorous movements, which increase for several weeks then subside at term. Presumably, declining amnionic fluid and uterine volume account for this diminishing fetal activity at term.

A somewhat astounding array of other determinants of fetal activity has been described, including maternal meals and blood glucose concentration, smoking, audible stimuli, ultrasound, light, maternal position, and amnio-

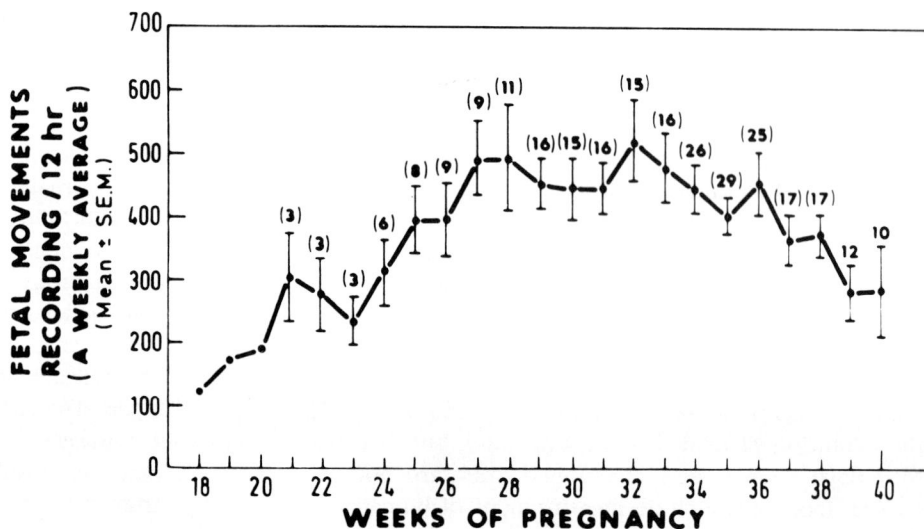

Fig. 45–1. Weekly average fetal movements calculated from "daily fetal movement records" during normal pregnancy. The mean ± standard error are shown. (From Sadovsky, 1979a, with permission.)

centesis, as well as the mother's character, occupation, and readiness to cooperate! As a result of the extreme multiplicity of determinants affecting fetal activity, Sadovsky (1981) concluded that it was incorrect to evaluate fetal motion with only brief observation periods. He recommended observing movements for at least 30 minutes three times a day and extending these periods of observation when fetal movement is reported to decline.

Clinical Application of Fetal Movement Assessment. Since Sadovsky and Yaffe (1973) described seven case reports of pregnancies with decreased fetal activity that preceded fetal death, there have been various methods described to discern and quantify fetal movement for the purpose of prognosticating fetal well-being. Methods used to document fetal activity include use of a tocodynamometer, visualization with real-time ultrasound, and maternal subjective perceptions. Most investigators have reported excellent correlation between maternally perceived fetal motion and movements documented by instrumentation. For example, Rayburn (1980) found that 80 percent of all movements seen during ultrasonic monitoring were perceived by the mother. Even with the wide range of normal activity observed in human fetuses, some investigators have attempted to quantify fetal movements in order to prognosticate fetal well-being. Pearson and Weaver (1976) used 12-hour daily maternal counts of fetal movement in 122 complicated pregnancies and defined abnormal activity as less than 10 movements per 12-hour study interval. Of 14 fetuses who had abnormal movement counts, one third were stillborn, whereas all 108 with normal counts were liveborn. These investigators concluded that low fetal movement counts were associated with chronic fetal asphyxia and that movements rapidly diminished and stopped 12 to 48 hours before death.

Rayburn (1982) defined reassuring maternally perceived fetal activity as an average of four or more movements per hour when counting was performed at least one hour per day. Three or fewer movements per hour for two consecutive days was defined to be abnormal. Fetal death occurred in 16 of 46 inactive fetuses, whereas death occurred in only 7 of 1115 active fetuses. Most of the inactive fetuses were chronically ill, as evidenced by growth retardation. However, fetal death also occurred, albeit much less frequently, in fetuses exhibiting normal activity as a result of umbilical cord entanglements, placental abruption, oligohydramnios, and uterine rupture. Rayburn concluded that normal activity was generally reassuring but that fetal inactivity required further assessment. Because decreased activity was not necessarily ominous, he suggested further fetal evaluation in such cases, with methods described in the following sections.

Moore and Piacquadio (1989) described a novel method of evaluating maternal perception of fetal movements. The woman was instructed to record the elapsed time required to appreciate 10 fetal movements during the evening hours (7 to 11 PM). The mean elapsed time interval was 21 minutes. Those women who required 2 hours or more to appreciate 10 fetal motions (less than 1 percent of women) were evaluated promptly with other antepartum fetal tests. The fetal mortality rate decreased from 44 per 1000 to 10 per 1000 with application of this fetal movement screening program.

Fetal Breathing

After decades of uncertainty as to whether the fetus normally breathes, Dawes and co-workers (1972) showed small inward and outward flows of tracheal fluid indicating fetal thoracic movement in sheep. These chest wall movements differed from those following birth in that they were discontinuous. Another interesting feature of fetal respiration was *paradoxical chest wall movement*. As shown in Figure 45–2, during inspiration, the chest wall paradoxically collapses and the abdomen protrudes (Johnson and co-authors, 1988). In the newborn or adult, the opposite occurs. One interpretation of the paradoxical respiratory motion might be coughing to clear amnionic fluid debris.

Two types of respiratory movements were identified: (1) *gasps* (or *sighs*), which occurred at a frequency of 1 to 4 per minute, and (2) *irregular bursts of breathing* occurring at rates up to 240 cycles per minute (Dawes, 1974). The latter rapid respiratory movements were associated with REMs. The possibility that assessment of fetal respiratory movement might be useful in evaluating fetal well-being was raised by the observation that a mild degree of hypoxia greatly reduced or even arrested respiratory efforts. Similarly, apnea and gasping were terminally reported in animal fetuses before death (Chapman and co-workers, 1978).

A method utilizing ultrasound for detecting human fetal chest wall movements was devised by Boddy and Robinson (1971). Similar methods were used to determine the rate and physiological control of human breathing in utero (Dawes, 1974). The results are consistent with the view that fetal hypoxia was also associated with diminished breathing movements in humans. The fre-

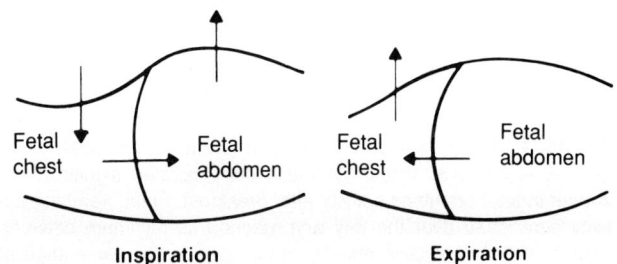

Fig. 45–2. Paradoxical chest movement with fetal respiration. (From Johnson and co-workers, 1988, with permission.)

quency of breathing and the appearance of gasping were viewed as a potentially useful guide to fetal condition.

Subsequently, many investigators examined human fetal breathing movements utilizing real-time ultrasound to determine whether monitoring chest wall movements might be of benefit in the evaluation of fetal health. Many variables other than hypoxia were found to affect human fetal respiratory movements. Examples included labor (during which it is normal for respiration to cease), hypoglycemia, sound stimuli, cigarette smoking, amniocentesis, impending preterm labor, gestational age, and the fetal heart rate itself. Paradoxically, insofar as interpretation of biophysical features is concerned, cardiac acceleration coincident with fetal body motion may be associated with cessation of fetal respiration (Dawes and colleagues, 1981).

Because fetal breathing movements are episodic, interpretation of fetal condition when respirations are absent may be tenuous. Patrick and associates (1980a) performed continuous 24-hour periods of observations using real-time ultrasonography in an effort to characterize fetal breathing patterns during the last 10 weeks of pregnancy. A total of 1224 hours of fetal observation was completed in 51 pregnancies. Figure 45–3 shows the percentage of time human fetuses spent breathing near term. Clearly, there is diurnal variation, because breathing substantively diminishes during the night. In addition, breathing activity increases somewhat following maternal meals. Total absence of breathing was observed in some of these normal fetuses for up to 122 minutes, thus indicating that fetal evaluation to diagnose absent respiratory motion may require very long periods of observation. In an effort to deal with these exigencies of normal fetal breathing cycles, Patrick and co-workers (1980b) more closely studied maternal postprandial periods and observed no normal periods of apnea in excess of 45 minutes during the second and third hours after meals. They concluded these hours could be useful time periods for observation of fetal condition.

Clinical Application of Fetal Breathing. The potential for fetal breathing activity to be an important marker of fetal health appears to be somewhat unfulfilled owing to the multiplicity of factors that affect breathing in normal fetuses. Few reports have described the use of fetal breathing alone as an index of fetal condition (Lewis and Boylan, 1979). Most clinical applications have included assessment of other fetal biophysical indices, such as heart rate. More recently, as discussed below, fetal breathing has become a component of the *biophysical profile*. It thus appears that evaluation of fetal breathing activity alone has not been very useful in predicting fetal condition.

Contraction Stress Testing

It was not long after the discovery that fetal heart rate deceleration following uterine contractions (late deceleration) is associated with uteroplacental insufficiency that oxytocin was given to antepartum women at risk for placental insufficiency in an effort to unmask fetal jeopardy from compromised placental function (Kubli and co-workers, 1969). As amnionic fluid pressure increases with uterine contractions, myometrial pressure exceeds collapsing pressure for vessels coursing through uterine muscle, ultimately isolating the intervillous space. Brief periods of impaired oxygen exchange result and, if uteroplacental pathology is present, these elicit late fetal heart rate decelerations (see Chap. 15, p. 405).

Ray and colleagues (1972) used this concept and developed what they termed the **oxytocin challenge test.** Results of these tests in 66 complicated pregnancies were not known to the attending obstetrician. The criteria for a positive (abnormal) test were uniform fetal heart rate deceleration, which reflected the uterine contraction waveform and had an onset at or beyond the acme of a contraction, and similar heart rate changes following subsequent contractions. The tests were generally repeated on a weekly basis, and 24-hour urinary estriol excretions also were monitored. They concluded that negative (normal) oxytocin challenge tests forecast fetal health and that abnormal tests may indicate that the fetus is in an unfavorable environment. One disadvantage cited was that the average oxytocin challenge test required 90 minutes to complete. Such "stressed" (by induced contractions) antepartum fetal testing rapidly captured national attention, as attested by a 1975 survey of residency programs, which found that 94 percent of

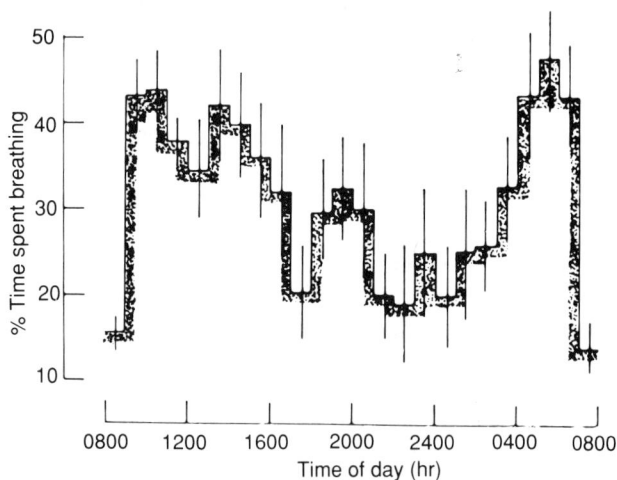

Fig. 45–3. The percentage of time spent breathing (± SEM) by 11 fetuses at 38 to 39 weeks gestation demonstrated significant increase in fetal breathing activity after breakfast. Fetal breathing activity diminished over the day and reached its minimum between 1900 and 2400 hours. A significant increase in the percentage of time spent breathing occurred between 0400 and 0700 hours when mothers were asleep. (From Patrick and co-workers, 1980a, with permission.)

programs were teaching this method of testing (Dilts, 1976).

Freeman (1975) subsequently reported a much larger experience with 1500 oxytocin challenge tests in 600 pregnancies at risk for placental insufficiency. Contractions lasting 40 to 60 seconds and occurring at least three per 10 minutes were defined arbitrarily as adequate uterine activity for a "challenge." Spontaneous uterine contractions meeting these criteria were also considered acceptable. Testing was performed on a weekly basis because only one fetal death was observed within a week of a normal test result. Interpretation criteria were expanded to include five separate categories (Table 45–1). Peck (1980) used these definitions to evaluate the subjectivity of interpretation of the oxytocin challenge test. He evaluated 50 tests, 33 of which were originally read as positive; all were reinterpreted by five obstetricians with expertise in maternal-fetal medicine. There was considerable disagreement among these readers and, indeed, two physicians agreed on interpretation in only one half of the cases!

Freeman (1975) also introduced the terms **non-stressed antepartum monitoring** to describe fetal heart rate deceleration in response to spontaneous fetal movement as a sign of fetal health. He proposed combining oxytocin challenge tests with 24-hour urinary estriol measurements, the former presumably a test of placental *respiratory function* and the latter an index of *nutritive function*. Importantly, both tests used in combination were considered superior to either alone, because false positives for either test were cross-checked. One fourth of the pregnancies with positive oxytocin challenge tests tolerated subsequent labor, and these were thus considered false-positive (Freeman and co-workers, 1976). Others reported much higher false-positive rates. For example, Gauthier and colleagues (1979) experienced a 75 percent false-positive rate and similar results were reported by Bissonnette and colleagues (1979). Difficulties with the meaningfulness of positive oxytocin challenge tests have prompted most investigators to perform these tests hoping for a normal (negative test) result because this permits the clinician to avoid intervention.

Several groups have reported successful substitution of the **nipple stimulation test** in the performance of contraction stress tests (Huddleston and associates, 1984; Lenke and colleagues, 1984; MacMillan and co-workers, 1984). Advantages include reduced cost and shortened testing times. Success at achieving a satisfactory contraction stress test with nipple stimulation alone has been reported in 60 to 100 percent of tests attempted. Several techniques of nipple stimulation have been described and include manual stimulation with moist, warm towels, and a variety of breast pumps (Curtis and co-authors, 1986). Although Schellpfeffer and associates (1985) reported unpredictable uterine hyperstimulation with fetal distress, others did not find excessive nipple–stimulated induced uterine activity to be harmful (Frager and Miyazaki, 1987). In our limited experiences, this method is awkward for both the patient and for those performing the test.

Some investigators have taken issue with the value of stress tests. For example, Staisch and colleagues (1980) performed 435 tests on 217 high-risk pregnancies and blinded the results. This study is unusual in the history of the oxytocin challenge test as it was performed specifically to investigate the prognostic value of the test in the absence of physician bias. They found that a given fetus at risk could not be identified with a high degree of accuracy. Indeed, two thirds of the tests were false positive and 15 percent were false negative. They stressed the limitations of the oxytocin challenge test and emphasized the importance of clinical judgment in the management of high-risk pregnancies.

Nonstress Testing

By the end of the 1970s, the oxytocin challenge test appeared to have been supplanted by the nonstress test as the primary method of testing fetal health. The nonstress test is much easier to perform and normal results were increasingly used to further discriminate false-positive oxytocin challenge tests (Evertson and Paul, 1978). Currently, the nonstress test has become the most widely used primary testing method for assessment of fetal well-being.

This contemporary mainstay for assessing fetal health is done by using Doppler-detected fetal heart rate recording, using acceleration in response to movement as an index of well-being. Simplistically, the nonstress test is primarily a test of *fetal condition* and it differs

TABLE 45–1. OXYTOCIN CHALLENGE TEST: DEFINITION OF TEST RESULTS

Outcome	Definition
Negative	No periodic decelerations with satisfactory recordings and at least three contractions lasting 40 to 60 sec within 10 min
Positive	Persistent and consistent late decelerations noted with most (> half) of the adequate contractions
Suspicious	Late decelerations with < half of any adequate contractions noted during monitoring
Hyperstimulation	Late decelerations occurring with or following a period of excessive uterine contractions (contraction[s] > 90 sec or occurring more frequently than every 2 min); no late decelerations with excessive contractions is considered negative
Unsatisfactory	Adequate contractions are not achieved or the fetal heart rate tracing is inadequate for interpretation

From Freeman, (1975), with permission.

from the contraction stress test, which is a test of *utero-placental function.*

As stress testing became more widely used in the United States, fetal heart rate accelerations observed during such tests were reported to portend fetal health (Freeman, 1975; Lee and co-workers, 1975). Actually, according to Lavery (1982), *unstressed antepartum cardiography* was a European concept that can be traced to the observations of Hammacher and colleagues (1968). These latter investigators observed that fetal movements frequently stimulated very brief heart rate accelerations. Although they did not specifically describe accelerations in response to movements as a fetal test, they did observe that the absence of baseline oscillation was ominous. They concluded that normal baseline fluctuation or oscillation with the absence of contractions precluded demise of the fetus and that oxytocin challenge testing was rarely necessary.

Lee and colleagues (1975) observed that accelerations were responses of the healthy fetus and that such accelerations were the most frequent fetal heart rate response found in electronic fetal heart rate monitoring. One year later, Lee and co-workers (1976) described good correlation between fetal movement and acceleration of the heart rate in 410 pregnancies in whom the oxytocin challenge test was conducted. These investigators concluded that acceleration in response to movement signified good fetal health.

In his review, Lavery (1982) observed that a plethora of studies subsequently appeared, all in support of the conclusion that fetal heart rate acceleration associated with movement was a simple predictor of fetal well-being. Although a normal response—acceleration—suggested a good outcome, absence of satisfactory acceleration was difficult to interpret. Generally speaking, normal fetal heart rate responses to movements were far more prognostic than absence of acceleration.

Physiology of Fetal Heart Rate Acceleration. Fetal cardiac response normally is affected by neural and humoral factors. Sympathetic cardiac accelerator nerve fibers arise in the upper thoracic segments of the spinal cord and function as a *cardioaccelerator center* which is subordinate to higher centers in the hypothalamus (Lavery, 1982). During early fetal development, sympathetic dominance prevails, and with maturation parasympathetic influence slows the heart rate. Thus, normal human fetal cardiac development is characterized by progressive dominance of the parasympathetic system as maturation proceeds. Pillai and James (1990) studied the development of fetal heart rate acceleration patterns during normal pregnancy. The percentage of body movements accompanied by acceleration and the amplitude of these accelerations increased with gestational age (Fig. 45–4). Johnson and co-workers (1992) claimed that black fetuses have baseline heart rates about 10 beats per minute higher than white fe-

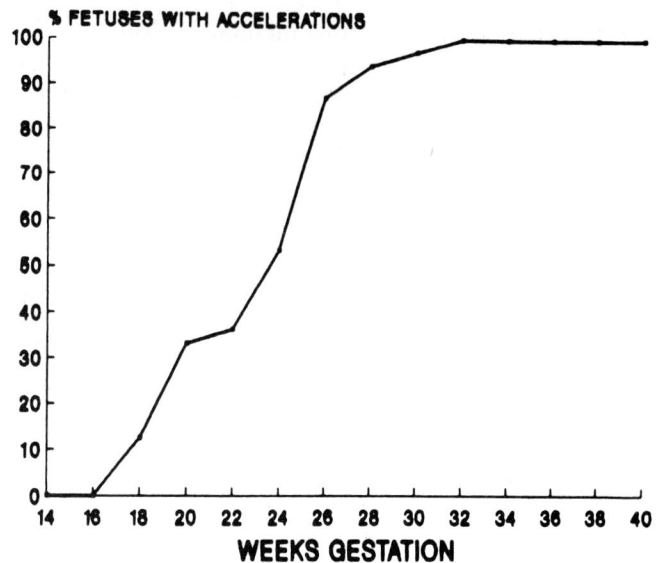

Fig. 45–4. Percentage of fetuses with at least one acceleration (15 beats per minute sustained for 15 seconds) with movement. (From Pillai and James, 1990, with permission.)

tuses and speculated this might affect nonstress test results.

Moment-to-moment heart rate is influenced primarily by the aortic and carotid baroreceptor reflexes, which reflect systemic blood pressure. Similarly located chemoreceptors may be stimulated by arterial oxygen tension. Acute hypoxia produces increased variability whereas chronic hypoxia results in decreased variability of the heart rate. Smith and colleagues (1988) observed a decrease in the number of accelerations in preterm human fetuses subsequently found to have lower umbilical artery blood Po_2 values compared with those fetuses who had normal fetal heart rate characteristics. Thus, nonstress testing is considered to reflect the chronic condition of the fetus.

Definition of Normal Nonstress Tests. There have been many different interpretations of the normal fetal heart rate response to movement. Shown in Table 45–2 are 10 such definitions, and this is but a partial compilation. The definitions may vary as to the number, amplitude, and duration of acceleration, as well as the test duration itself. Figure 45–5 gives an example of a nonstress test showing acceleration of the fetal heart rate in response to spontaneous fetal movements.

Although a normal number and amplitude of accelerations by any of these interpretations seems to reflect adequately fetal well-being, "insufficient acceleration" does not invariably predict fetal compromise. Indeed, some investigators have reported false-positive nonstress test rates in excess of 50 percent when fetal heart rate acceleration was considered insufficient. Because healthy fetuses may not move for periods up to 75 minutes, Brown and Patrick (1981) considered that a

TABLE 45–2. SOME REPORTED DEFINITIONS OF NORMAL (REACTIVE) NONSTRESS TEST RESULTS

Investigator	Accelerations			Maximum Test Duration (min)	Other
	No.	*Amplitude (beats/min)*	*Duration (sec)*		
Evertson and Paul, 1978	1	10	Not stated	30	Fetal manipulation, > 10 beats per minute
Lee and Drukker, 1979	3	10	Not stated	"Extended"	Fetal manipulation
Pratt and associates, 1979	2	15	30	30	None
Schifrin and co-workers, 1979	2	15	15	40	In 10 minute period, including contractions
Amankwah and colleagues, 1980	"Any"	10	10	60	None
Mendenhall and associates, 1980	1	10	Not stated	30	Fetal manipulation
O'Leary and co-workers, 1980	1	15	15	5	Auscultation
DeVoe and colleagues, 1980	3	15	15	30	None
Koller and Curet, 1978	3–4	10	Not stated	15	Fetal manipulation
Trudinger and Boylan, 1980	Not stated	15	Not stated	20	Variability > 5 beats per minute

From Leveno and Cunningham (1988).

longer duration of nonstress testing might increase the positive predictive value of an abnormal, or nonreactive test. They concluded that either the test became reactive during a period of time up to 80 minutes or that the test remained nonreactive for 120 minutes and the fetus was very sick.

Not only are there many different definitions of normal nonstress test results, but reproducibility of in-terobserver interpretation is problematic. For example, Hage (1985) mailed five nonstress tests, blinded to specific patient clinical data, to a national sample of obstetricians for their interpretations. He concluded that although nonstress testing is very popular, the reliability of the test interpretation needs improvement. Bobitt (1979) reviewed five fetal deaths that followed after nonstress testing and cited failure to obtain satisfactory

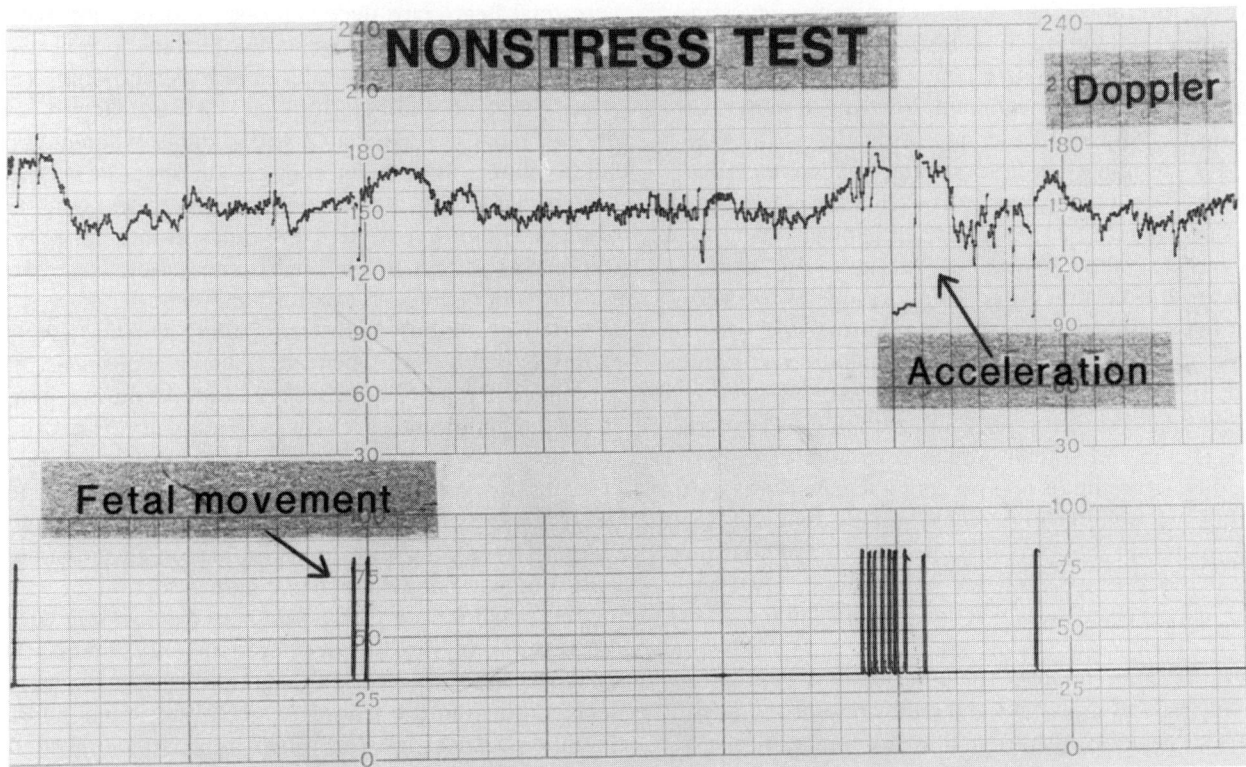

Fig. 45–5. Reactive nonstress test. Notice increase of fetal heart rate to more than 15 beats per minute for longer than 15 seconds following fetal movements, indicated by the vertical marks on the lower part of the recording.

fetal heart rate tracings and to recognize actual abnormal fetal heart rate as pitfalls of antepartum monitoring programs. He also concluded that test interpretation should be based on strict criteria. Some of this intraobserver and interobserver variation in interpretation may be due to fetal monitors with autocorrelation technology (see Chap. 15, p. 398). Dawes and associates (1990) found that erroneous or doubtful accelerations were present in 10 percent of antepartum fetal heart rate tests.

These admittedly arbitrary normal standards for fetal reactivity aside, there are abnormal nonstress test patterns that reliably forecast severe fetal jeopardy. Hammacher and co-workers (1968) described not only acceleration in response to movement, but also antepartum cardiotocograms with what he termed a *silent oscillatory pattern.* This pattern consisted of a fetal heart rate baseline that oscillated less than 5 beats per minute and presumably indicated absent acceleration as well as beat-to-beat variability. Hammacher considered this pattern ominous. Rochard and co-workers (1976), using phonocardiography, found that absence of accelerations coupled with less than 6 beats per minute variability of the baseline were associated with a 40 percent perinatal mortality. Likewise, Farahani and Fenton (1977) found a high correlation between tests showing less than 10 beats per minute fetal heart rate acceleration and perinatal pathology. In their report, less than 10 beats per minute acceleration in response to movements was linked to uteroplacental-insufficiency–type decelerations during contraction stress testing of 38 fetuses with these antepartum heart rate characteristics. Moreover, 90 percent had thick meconium, low Apgar scores, or dysmaturity. Similarly, Visser and associates (1980) described a "terminal cardiotocogram," which included (1) absent baseline irregularity or oscillation of less than 5 beats per minute, (2) absent accelerations in response to movements, and (3) late decelerations with spontaneous uterine contractions. These results were very similar to experiences from our own institution in which absence of accelerations during an 80-minute recording period in 27 pregnancies was associated consistently with evidence of uteroplacental pathology (Leveno, 1983). This included fetal growth retardation (75 percent), oligohydramnios (80 percent), fetal acidosis (40 percent), meconium (30 percent), and evidence of placental infarction (93 percent). We concluded that inability of the fetus to accelerate its heart rate, when not due to maternal sedation, was an ominous finding.

INTERVAL BETWEEN TESTING. The interval between tests, originally rather empirically and arbitrarily set at 7 days, appears to have been shortened as experience evolved with nonstress testing. For example, Barrett and associates (1981) concluded that twice-weekly testing was necessary in certain high-risk pregnancies to avoid fetal death following a reactive test within 7 days. Indeed,

some clinicians apparently perform nonstress tests as often as daily or even more frequently. The most recent nuance in nonstress testing is for the patient to record fetal heart rate data while at home and then use telephone links to transmit the results elsewhere (Lindsay and associates, 1990; Reece and co-workers, 1992).

Decelerations During Nonstress Testing. Fetal movements may produce heart rate decelerations as well as accelerations during antepartum testing. The significance of such decelerations has received increased attention. Timor-Tritsch and co-authors (1978) reported that fetal heart rate decelerations may be observed during nonstress testing in one half to two thirds of tracings, depending on the vigor of the fetal motion. Such a high incidence of decelerations inevitably makes interpretation of their significance problematic. Indeed, Meis and co-workers (1986) reported that variable fetal heart rate decelerations during nonstress tests were not a sign of fetal compromise. In contrast, O'Leary and co-workers (1980) observed persistent mild variable fetal heart rate decelerations in 8 percent of nonstress test tracings and linked these to intrapartum umbilical cord problems. Similar observations were made by Phelan and Lewis (1981) who also observed that 75 percent of pregnancies with decelerations during a nonstress test passed the test in the sense that adequate accelerations also were present.

Druzin and co-workers (1981) described more severe fetal heart rate decelerations in association with fetal movements during nonstress testing. Specifically, they found that prolonged decelerations (see Chap. 15, p. 407) predicted intrapartum fetal distress (50 percent of cases) that was associated with diminished amnionic fluid volume. Bourgeois and co-workers (1984) reported that fetal heart rate deceleration to less than 90 beats per minute for 1 to 10 minutes during nonstress testing was potentially ominous because there were two stillbirths in eight such cases. Similar experiences were reported by Dashow and Read (1984). Druzin (1989) reported that prompt delivery following diagnosis of prolonged fetal heart rate decelerations during nonstress testing did not prevent cerebral palsy in two instances.

Hoskins and associates (1991) attempted to refine interpretation of nonstress tests showing variable decelerations by adding ultrasonic estimation of amnionic fluid volume. The incidence of cesarean section for fetal distress in labor progressively increased coincident with the severity of variable decelerations and diminished amnionic fluid volume. For example, severe variable decelerations during a nonstress test plus an amnionic fluid index of 5 or less (see Chap. 46, p. 1047) resulted in a 75 percent rate of cesarean section for intrapartum fetal distress. However, fetal distress in labor also frequently developed in those pregnancies with variable decelerations but with normal amounts of amnionic fluid. Similar results were reported by Grubb and Paul in 1992.

False-normal Nonstress Tests. Smith and associates (1987) performed a detailed analysis of the causes of fetal death within 7 days of normal nonstress tests. The most common indication for testing was prolonged pregnancy. The mean interval between test and death was 4 days with a range of 1 to 7 days. The single most common autopsy finding was meconium aspiration, of which seven had some type of umbilical cord abnormality. These investigators interpreted these findings to suggest an acute asphyxial insult that produced fetal gasping. They concluded that the nonstress test was not adequate to preclude an acute asphyxial event and that other biophysical characteristics might be beneficial adjuncts. For example, assessment of amnionic fluid volume was considered likely to be of some value. Other ascribed frequent causes of fetal death included intrauterine infection, abnormal cord position, malformations, and placental abruption. Smith and co-workers (1987) concluded: "The concept of a single best test of fetal well-being may be erroneous." They also emphasized that the search continues for the best test.

Acoustic Stimulation Tests

It has long been known that the fetus responds to sound (Sontag and Wallace, 1935). More recently, Benzaquen and co-workers (1990) and Richards and colleagues (1992) used miniaturized hydrophones to study the intrauterine sound environment during parturition. External low frequency sounds (less than 125 Hz) are enhanced, but sounds of greater frequency are attenuated with maximum attenuation at 4000 Hz. Intrauterine sound levels of the maternal voice were enhanced at an average of 5 dB whereas external male or female voices were attenuated by 2 to 3 dB. Maternal cardiovascular sounds as well as bowel sounds are audible inside the uterus. Uterine contractions did not affect the fetal sound environment. The background noise level was about 60 dB and consisted primarily of low frequency sounds (that is, less than 100 Hz). This investigation indicates that the intrauterine environment is relatively quiet. The devices used to stimulate the fetus acoustically generate sound pressures considerably above those just described. For example, Gagnon and co-workers (1988), who have extensively studied the fetal biophysical consequences of sound stimulation, used a device that produced 110 dB sound levels at 10,000 Hz. Kisilevsky and colleagues (1989) determined that only those sounds of 100 to 105 dB or more discernibly provoke fetal movements.

Read and Miller (1977) were the first to suggest that acoustic stimulation could be used to examine fetal health. They performed paired contraction stress tests

and acoustic stimulation in 39 pregnancies. By 1988, Romero and co-authors, in their review of acoustic stimulation as an antenatal test for fetal well-being, recommended vigorous clinical evaluation before such testing becomes a part of standard obstetrical care. The sound intensities used for acoustic stimulation ranged from 82 to 126 dB in their review of the literature.

Biophysical Profile

Manning and colleagues (1980) proposed the combined use of five fetal biophysical variables as a more accurate means of assessing fetal health than any single variable used alone. They concluded that consideration of five variables could significantly reduce both false-positive and false-negative single test rates. Required equipment included a real-time ultrasound device and Doppler ultrasound to record fetal heart rate. Typically, these tests require 30 to 60 minutes examiner time. Five biophysical variables (see Table 45–3) were assessed in 216 complicated pregnancies. These were (1) fetal heart rate acceleration, (2) fetal breathing, (3) fetal movements, (4) fetal tone, and (5) amnionic fluid volume. Normal variables were assigned a score of two each and abnormal variables a score of zero. Thus, the highest score possible for a normal fetus was 10.

Manning and colleagues (1987) tested over 19,000 pregnancies using the biophysical profile interpretation and management shown in Table 45–4. They reported a false-normal test rate, defined as an antepartum death of a structurally normal fetus, of approximately 1 per 1000. Importantly, more than 97 percent of the pregnancies tested had normal test results.

Manning and co-workers (1990a) have subsequently described the outcomes of 29 fetuses with complete absence (score of zero) of all the components of the biophysical profile. These 29 fetuses were identified after more than 70,000 biophysical profiles were performed in nearly 30,000 pregnancies. Fourteen of the fetuses died (11 stillbirths and three neonatal deaths), thus attesting to the ominous sequelae of such low biophysical profile scores. Similarly, Manning and colleagues (1990b) analyzed abnormal infant outcomes associated with higher biophysical profile scores. The incidence of adverse outcomes increased as the scores decreased from six to zero. However, scores of four to six were considered equivocal. Scores of seven or greater were not linked to abnormalities. However, Manning and colleagues (1990c) subsequently emphasized that not all abnormal biophysical profile scores are equal. The nonstress test, fetal breathing movements, and amnionic fluid volume components were more predictive of pregnancy outcomes compared with fetal tone and fetal movements. DeVoe and colleagues (1992) also evaluated the implications of combinations of biophysical test components. The many potential pitfalls of bio-

TABLE 45–3. COMPONENTS AND THEIR SCORES OF THE BIOPHYSICAL PROFILE

Variable	Score 2	Score 0
Fetal breathing movements	The presence of at least 30 sec of sustained fetal breathing movements in 30 min of observation	Less than 30 sec of fetal breathing movements in 30 min
Fetal movements	Three or more gross body movements in 30 min of observation; simultaneous limb and trunk movements	Two or less gross body movements in 30 min of observation
Fetal tone	At least one episode of motion of a limb from position of flexion to extension and rapid return to flexion[a]	Fetus in position of semi- or full-limb extension with no return or slow return to flexion with movement; absence of fetal movement counted as absent tone
Fetal reactivity	Two or more fetal heart rate accelerations of at least 15 beats/min and lasting at least 15 sec and associated with fetal movement in 20 min	No acceleration or less than two accelerations of fetal heart rate in 20 min of observation
Qualitative amnionic fluid volume	Pocket of amnionic fluid that measures at least 1 cm in two perpendicular planes	Largest pocket of amnionic fluid measures < 1 cm in two perpendicular planes

[a] Opening and closing of hand considered normal tone.
From Manning and colleagues (1985), with permission.

physical profile scoring are highlighted by the discussants of these reports. For example, interpretation of the biophysical score is dependent on gestational age because the capacity of the fetus to perform the various components is linked to its maturity.

Platt and associates (1985) performed a randomized prospective trial of the biophysical profile versus the nonstress test. They managed 279 pregnancies using a biophysical profile protocol and 373 with nonstress tests. They recommended further study because, although there was a trend suggesting the biophysical profile to be more predictive in diagnosing fetal condition, statistical significance was not recorded for all measured perinatal outcome variables.

Vintzileos and co-workers (1987a) examined relationships among components of the biophysical profile and umbilical cord pH in 124 pregnancies delivered by cesarean section. They reported that the first manifestations of fetal acidosis, defined by an umbilical artery blood pH of less than 7.20, were abnormal nonstress tests and loss of fetal breathing. In advanced acidemia,

fetal movements and tone also were compromised. They proposed a new protocol of antepartum fetal evaluation based on individual biophysical components rather than numerical scores (Vintzileos and co-workers, 1987b). Complexity of such protocols has caused some to propose computerization of biophysical testing (DeVoe and colleagues, 1980). Goodlin (1988) described reliance upon such protocols as "... another example of cookbook medicine that has so often plagued obstetrics."

Current Antenatal Testing Recommendations

According to the American College of Obstetricians and Gynecologists (1992), there is no unanimity of opinion regarding the best antenatal test to evaluate fetal well-being. All three testing systems—contraction stress test, nonstress test, and biophysical profile—have different end points that may be considered, depending on the clinical situation requiring fetal testing. The most important consideration in deciding when to begin an-

TABLE 45–4. MODIFIED BIOPHYSICAL PROFILE SCORE, INTERPRETATION, AND PREGNANCY MANAGEMENT

Biophysical Profile Score	Interpretation	Recommended Management
10	Normal nonasphyxiated	No fetal indication for intervention; repeat test weekly except in diabetic patient and postterm pregnancy (twice weekly)
8/10 normal fluid 8/8	Normal nonasphyxiated fetus	No fetal indication for intervention; repeat testing per protocol
8/10 decreased fluid	Chronic fetal asphyxia suspected	Deliver
6	Possible fetal asphyxia	If amnionic fluid volume abnormal, deliver. If normal fluid at > 36 weeks with favorable cervix, deliver. If < 36 weeks or lecithin–sphingomyelin < 2/1 or cervix unfavorable, repeat test in 24 hr. If repeat test ≤, deliver. If repeat test > 6, observe and repeat per protocol
4	Probable fetal asphyxia	Repeat testing same day; if biophysical profile score ≤ 6, deliver
0 to 2	Almost certain fetal asphyxia	Deliver

From Manning and colleagues (1987), with permission.

tepartum testing is the prognosis for neonatal survival. The severity of maternal disease is another important consideration. In general, with most high-risk pregnancies, most recommend that testing should begin by 32 to 34 weeks when indicated. Pregnancies with severe complications might require testing as early as 26 to 28 weeks. The frequency for repeating tests has been arbitrarily set at 7 days; however, more frequent testing often is used.

At Parkland Hospital, antepartum fetal heart rate recordings have been limited to about 700 women admitted to the High-Risk Pregnancy Unit each year. Fetal heart rate recordings are often obtained several times throughout the week (for example, Monday, Wednesday, Friday) in these pregnancies. The primary focus of fetal heart rate assessments is detection of decelerations; delivery is not withheld simply because accelerations are witnessed. Clinical and ultrasonic estimations of amnionic fluid volume also are used to assess fetal jeopardy. Despite this extremely limited use of antepartum testing, the fetal death rate in structurally normal infants is quite low and is 3.5 per 1000 among more than 13,500 low- and high-risk women with prenatal care who are delivered each year at our hospital. Most of the antepartum fetal deaths at Parkland Hospital are now occurring in low-risk pregnancies and are attributable to unpreventable placental abruptions and umbilical cord accidents.

Significance of Fetal Testing

Does antenatal fetal forecasting really make a difference? Platt and co-workers (1987) reviewed the impact of fetal testing between 1971 and 1985 at one of the largest obstetrical services in the United States. During the 15-year period reviewed, more than 200,000 pregnancies were managed at Los Angeles County Hospital and nearly 17,000 of these underwent antepartum testing of various types. Fetal surveillance increased from less than 1 percent of pregnancies in the early 1970s to 15 percent more recently. They concluded that such testing was clearly beneficial because the fetal death rate was significantly less in the tested high-risk pregnancies compared with the rate in those not tested.

A contrasting opinion on the benefits of antenatal fetal testing was offered by Thacker and Berkelman (1986). It was their view that efficacy is best evaluated in randomized controlled trials. After reviewing 600 reports, they found only four such trials, all performed with the nonstress test and none with the contraction stress test. The numbers in these four trials were considered too small to detect important benefits. They projected that the costs of such testing exceeded $200 million per year and that published studies did not support the use of either test method.

Another important and unanswered question is,

"Does antenatal electronic fetal heart rate monitoring identify fetal asphyxia early enough to prevent brain damage?" Until recently, the medical literature contained no reports on the question of long-term neurological damage after antenatal fetal heart rate testing (Niswander, 1989). However, Todd and co-workers (1992) attempted to correlate cognitive development in infants up to 2 years following either abnormal Doppler velocimetry or nonstress tests. The latter were associated with marginally poorer cognitive outcomes but not those with abnormal Doppler velocimetry. Importantly, these investigators concluded that by the time fetal compromise is diagnosed with antenatal testing, fetal damage has already occurred.

Antenatal forecasts of fetal health clearly have been the focus of intense interest for almost two decades. When such testing is reviewed, several themes emerge. First, the methods of fetal forecasting have evolved continually, a phenomenon that itself suggests dissatisfaction with the efficacy of any given method. Second, the biophysical performance of the human fetus is characterized by wide ranges of normal variation resulting in difficulty determining when such performance should be considered abnormal. *How many movements, respirations, or accelerations? In what time period?* Unable to easily quantify normal fetal biophysical performance, most investigators have resorted to somewhat arbitrary answers for such questions. Third, despite the invention of increasingly complex testing methods, abnormal results are seldom reliable, prompting most clinicians to use antenatal testing to forecast fetal *wellness* rather than *illness*. Considering that the overall stillbirth rate is less than 10 per 1000 births, it seems a rather safe bet to forecast to a pregnant woman, *Your baby will be alive for X days!* Despite the statistical safety of such predictions, we remain uneasy with this forecast.

References

Achiron R, Tadmor O, Mashiach S: Heart rate as a predictor of first-trimester spontaneous abortion after ultrasound-proven viability. Obstet Gynecol 78:330, 1991

Amankwah KS, Kaufmann RC, Roller RW, Prentice RL: A new definition of the nonstress test. Obstet Gynecol 56:48, 1980

American College of Obstetricians and Gynecologists: Guidelines for perinatal care, 3rd ed. Washington, DC, 1992, p 65

Barrett JM, Salyer SL, Boehm FH: The nonstress test: An evaluation of 1,000 patients. Am J Obstet Gynecol 141:153, 1981

Benzaquen S, Gagnon R, Hunse C, Foreman J: The intrauterine sound environment of the human fetus during labor. Am J Obstet Gynecol 163:484, 1990

Birkenfeld A, Laufer N, Sadovsky E: Diurnal variation of fetal activity. Obstet Gynecol 55:417, 1980

Bissonnette JM, Johnson K, Toomey C: The role of a trial of labor with a positive contraction stress test. Am J Obstet Gynecol 135:292, 1979

Bobitt JR: Abnormal antepartum fetal heart rate tracings, failure to intervene, and fetal death: Review of five cases reveals potential pitfalls of antepartum monitoring programs. Am J Obstet Gynecol 133:415, 1979

Boddy K, Robinson JS: External method for detection of fetal breathing in utero. Lancet 2:1231, 1971

Bourgeois FJ, Thiagarajah S, Harbert GN: The significance of fetal heart rate decelerations during nonstress testing. Am J Obstet Gynecol 150:213, 1984

Brown R, Patrick J: The nonstress test: How long is enough? Am J Obstet Gynecol 141:646, 1981

Chapman RLK, Dawes GS, Rurak DW, Wilds PL: Intermittent breathing before death in fetal lambs. Am J Obstet Gynecol 131:894, 1978

Curtis P, Evans S, Resnick J, Rimer R, Lynch K, Carlson JR: Uterine responses to three techniques of breast stimulation. Obstet Gynecol 67:25, 1986

Dashow EE, Read JA: Significant fetal bradycardia during antepartum heart rate testing. Am J Obstet Gynecol 148:187, 1984

Dawes GS: Breathing before birth in animals and man. An essay in medicine. Physiology Med 290:557, 1974

Dawes GS, Fox HE, Leduc BM, Liggins GC, Richards RT: Respiratory movements and rapid eye movement sleep in the foetal lamb. J Physiol 220:119, 1972

Dawes GS, Moulden M, Redman WG: Limitations of antenatal fetal heart rate monitors. Am J Obstet Gynecol 162:170, 1990

Dawes GS, Visser GHA, Goodman JDS, Levine DH: Numerical analysis of the human fetal heart rate: Modulation by breathing and movement. Am J Obstet Gynecol 140L535, 1981

DeVoe LD: Clinical implications of prospective antepartum fetal heart rate testing. Am J Obstet Gynecol 137:983, 1980

DeVoe LD, Yousef AA, Gardner P, Dear C, Murray C: Defining the biophysical profile with risk-related evaluation of test performance. Am J Obstet Gynecol 167:346, 1992

DeVries JP, Visser GH, Prechtl HF: The emergence of fetal behaviour, I. Qualitative aspects. Early Hum Dev 7:301, 1982

Dilts PV: Current practices in antepartum and intrapartum fetal monitoring. Am J Obstet Gynecol 126:491, 1976

Druzin ML: Fetal bradycardia during antepartum testing, further observations. J Reprod Med 34:47, 1989

Druzin ML, Gratacos J, Keegan KA, Paul RH: Antepartum fetal heart rate testing: VII. The significance of fetal bradycardia. Am J Obstet Gynecol 139:194, 1981

Evertson LR, Paul RH: Antepartum fetal heart rate testing: The nonstress test. Am J Obstet Gynecol 132:895, 1978

Farahani G, Fenton AN: Fetal heart rate acceleration in relation to the oxytocin challenge test. Obstet Gynecol 49:163, 1977

Frager NB, Miyazaki FS: Intrauterine monitoring of contractions during breast stimulation. Obstet Gynecol 69:767, 1987

Freeman RK: The use of the oxytocin challenge test for antepartum clinical evaluation of uteroplacental respiratory function. Am J Obstet Gynecol 121:481, 1975

Freeman RK, Goebelsman U, Nochimson D, Cetrulo C: An evaluation of the significance of a positive oxytocin challenge test. Obstet Gynecol 47:8, 1976

Gagnon R, Huuse C, Carmichael L, Fellows F, Patrick J: Fetal heart rate and fetal activity patterns after vibratory acoustic stimulation at thirty to thirty-two weeks' gestational age. Am J Obstet Gynecol 75:9, 1988

Gauthier RJ, Evertson LR, Paul RH: Antepartum fetal heart rate testing, II. Intrapartum fetal heart rate observation and newborn outcome following a positive contraction stress test. Am J Obstet Gynecol 133:34, 1979

Goodlin RC: Cookbook obstetrics. Am J Obstet Gynecol 159:266, 1988

Goodlin RC, Lowe EW: Multiphasic fetal monitoring, Am J Obstet Gynecol 119:341, 1974

Granat M, Lavie P, Adar D, Sharf M: Short-term cycles in human fetal activity, I. Normal pregnancies. Am J Obstet Gynecol 134:696, 1979

Grubb DK, Paul RH: Amnionic fluid index and prolonged antepartum fetal heart rate decelerations. Obstet Gynecol 79:558, 1992

Hage ML: Interpretation of nonstress tests. Am J Obstet Gynecol 153:490, 1985

Hammacher K, Hüter KA, Bokelmann J, Werners PH: Foetal heart frequency and perinatal condition of the foetus and newborn. Gynaecologia 166:349, 1968

Hoskins IA, Frieden FJ, Young BK: Variable decelerations in reactive nonstress tests with decreased amnionic fluid index predict fetal compromise. Am J Obstet Gynecol 165:1094, 1991

Huddleston JF, Sutliff JG, Robinson D: Contraction stress test by intermittent nipple stimulation. Obstet Gynecol 63:669, 1984

Johnson MJ, Paine LL, Mulder HH, Cezar C, Gegor C, Johnson TRB: Population differences of fetal biophysical and behavioral characteristics. Am J Obstet Gynecol 166:138, 1992

Johnson T, Besigner R, Thomas R: New clues to fetal behavior and well-being. Contemp Ob/Gyn, May, 1988

Johnson TB, Jordan ET, Paine LL: Doppler recordings of fetal movement, II. Comparison with maternal perception. Obstet Gynecol 76:42, 1990

Kisilevsky BS, Muir DW, Low JA: Human fetal responses to sound as a function of stimulus intensity. Obstet Gynecol 73:971, 1989

Koller WS, Curet LB: Fetal activity determinations and oxytocin challenge tests for assessment of fetal well-being. Obstet Gynecol 52:176, 1978

Kubli FW, Kaeser O, Hinselmann M: Diagnostic management of chronic placental insufficiency. In Pecile A, Finzi C (eds): The Foeto-Placental Unit. Amsterdam, Excerpta Medica, 1969, p 323

Lavery JP: Nonstress fetal heart rate testing. Clin Obstet Gynecol 25:689, 1982

Lee CY, DiLoreto PC, Logrand B: Fetal activity acceleration determination for the evaluation of fetal reserve. Obstet Gynecol 48:19, 1976

Lee CY, DiLoreto PC, O'Lane JM: A study of fetal heart rate acceleration patterns. Obstet Gynecol 45:142, 1975

Lee CY, Drukker B: The nonstress test for the antepartum assessment of fetal reserve. Am J Obstet Gynecol 134:460, 1979

Lenke RR, Nemes JM: Use of nipple stimulation to obtain contraction stress test. Obstet Gynecol 63:345, 1984

Leveno KJ, Cunningham FG: Forecasting fetal health. Williams Obstetrics, 17th ed (suppl 14). Norwalk, CT, Appleton & Lange, 1988

Leveno KJ, Williams ML, DePalma RT, Whalley PJ: Perinatal outcome in the absence of antepartum fetal heart rate acceleration. Obstet Gynecol 61:347, 1983

Lewis P, Boylan P: Fetal breathing: A review. Am J Obstet Gynecol 134:587, 1979

Lindsay PC, Beveridge R, Tayob Y, Irvine LM, Vellacott ID, Giles JA, Hussain SY, O'Brien PM: Patient-recorded domiciliary fetal monitoring. Am J Obstet Gynecol 162:466, 1990

MacMillan JB III, Hale RW: Contraction stress testing with mammary self-stimulation. J Reprod Med 29:219, 1984

Manning FA, Morrison I, Harman CR, Lange IR, Menticoglou S: Fetal assessment based on fetal biophysical profile scoring: Experience in 19,221 referred high-risk pregnancies, II. An analysis of false-negative fetal deaths. Am J Obstet Gynecol 157:880, 1987

Manning FA, Harman CR, Morrison I, Menticoglou S: Fetal assessment based on biophysical profile scoring, III. Positive predictive accuracy of the very abnormal test. Am J Obstet Gynecol 162:398, 1990a

Manning FA, Harman CR, Morrison I, Menticoglou S: Fetal assessment based on fetal biophysical profile scoring, IV. An analysis of perinatal morbidity and mortality. Am J Obstet Gynecol 162:703, 1990b

Manning FA, Harman CR, Morrison I, Menticoglou S: The abnormal fetal biophysical profile scoring, V. Predictive accuracy according to score composition. Am J Obstet Gynecol 162:918, 1990c

Manning FA, Morrison I, Lange IR, Harman CR, Chamberlain PFC: Fetal assessment based on fetal biophysical profile scoring: Experience in 12,620 referred high-risk pregnancies, I. Perinatal mortality by frequency and etiology. Am J Obstet Gynecol 151:343, 1985

Manning FA, Platt LD, Sipos L: Antepartum fetal evaluation: Development of a fetal biophysical profile. Am J Obstet Gynecol 136:787, 1980

Mathews DD: Fetal movements and fetal well-being. Lancet 1:1315, 1973

Meis PJ, Ureda JR, Swain M, Kelly RT, Penry M, Sharp P: Variable decelerations during nonstress tests are not a sign of fetal compromise. Am J Obstet Gynecol 154:586, 1986

Mendenhall HW, O'Leary JA, Phillips KO: The nonstress test: The value of a single acceleration in evaluating the fetus at risk. Am J Obstet Gynecol 136:87, 1980

Moore TR, Piacquadio K: A prospective evaluation of fetal movement screening to reduce the incidence of antepartum fetal death. Am J Obstet Gynecol 160:1075, 1989

Niswander KR: Can electronic fetal heart rate monitoring predict neurologic damage? In Zuspan FP (ed): Obstetrics/Gynecology Report, Vol. 1, No. 2. St. Louis, Mosby, 1989, p 128

O'Leary JA, Andrinopoulos GC, Giordano PC: Variable decelerations and the nonstress test: An indication of cord compromise. Am J Obstet Gynecol 137:704, 1980

Patrick J, Campbell K, Carmichael L, Natale R, Richardson B: A definition of human fetal apnea and the distribution of fetal apneic intervals during the last ten weeks of pregnancy. Am J Obstet Gynecol 136:471, 1980b

Patrick J, Campbell K, Carmichael L, Natale R, Richardson B: Patterns of gross fetal body movements over 24-hour observation intervals during the last 10 weeks of pregnancy. Am J Obstet Gynecol 142:363, 1982

Patrick J, Campbell K, Carmichael L, Natale R, Richardson B: Patterns of human fetal breathing during the last 10 weeks of pregnancy. Obstet Gynecol 56:24, 1980a

Pearson JF, Weaver JB: Fetal activity and fetal well-being: An evaluation. BMJ 1:1305, 1976

Peck TM: Physicians' subjectivity in evaluating oxytocin challenge tests. Obstet Gynecol 56:13, 1980

Phelan JP, Lewis PE: Fetal heart rate decelerations during a nonstress test. Obstet Gynecol 57:228, 1981

Pillai M, James D: The development of fetal heart rate patterns during normal pregnancy. Obstet Gynecol 76:812, 1990

Pillai M, James DK, Parker M: The development of ultradian rhythms in the human fetus. Am J Obstet Gynecol 167:1727, 1992

Platt LD, Paul RH, Phelan J, Walla CA, Broussard P: Fifteen years of experience with antepartum fetal testing. Am J Obstet Gynecol 156:1509, 1987

Platt LD, Walla CA, Paul RH, Trujillo ME, Loesser CV, Jacobs ND, Broussard PM: A prospective trial of the fetal biophysical profile versus the nonstress test in the management of high–risk pregnancies. Am J Obstet Gynecol 153:624, 1985

Pratt D, Diamond F, Yen H, Bieniarz J, Burd L: Fetal stress and nonstress tests: An analysis and comparison of their ability to identify fetal outcome. Obstet Gynecol 54:419, 1979

Ray M, Freeman R, Pine S, Hesselgesser R: Clinical experience with the oxytocin challenge test. Am J Obstet Gynecol 114:1, 1972

Rayburn WF: Clinical implications from monitoring fetal activity. Am J Obstet Gynecol 144:967, 1982

Rayburn WF: Clinical significance of perceptible fetal motion. Am J Obstet Gynecol 138:210, 1980

Read JA, Miller FC: Fetal heart rate acceleration in response to acoustic stimulation as a measure of fetal well-being. Am J Obstet Gynecol 129:512, 1977

Reece EA, Hagay Z, Garofalo J, Hobbins JC: A controlled trial of self-nonstress test versus assisted nonstress test in the evaluation of fetal well-being. Am J Obstet Gynecol 166:489, 1992

Richards DS, Frentzen B, Gerhardt KJ, McCann ME, Abrams RM: Sound levels in the human uterus. Obstet Gynecol 80:186, 1992

Rochard F, Schifrin BS, Goupil F, Legrand H, Blottiere J, Sureau C: Nonstress fetal heart rate monitoring in the antepartum period. Am J Obstet Gynecol 126:699, 1976

Romero R, Mazor M, Hobbins JC: A critical appraisal of fetal acoustic stimulation as an antenatal test for fetal well-being. Obstet Gynecol 71:781, 1988

Rovsinsky JJ, Guttmacher AP: Medical, Surgical and Gynecological Complications of Pregnancy. Baltimore, Williams & Wilkins, 1965, p 805

Sadovsky E: Fetal movements and fetal health. Semin Perinatol 5:131, 1981

Sadovsky E, Evron S, Weinstein D: Daily fetal movement recording in normal pregnancy. Riv Obstet Ginecol Practica Med Perinatal 59:395, 1979a

Sadovsky E, Laufer N, Allen JW: The incidence of different types of fetal movement during pregnancy. Br J Obstet Gynaecol 86:10, 1979b

Sadovsky E, Yaffe H: Daily fetal movement recording and fetal prognosis. Obstet Gynecol 41:845, 1973

Schellpfeffer MA, Hoyle D, Johnson JWC: Antepartal uterine hypercontractility secondary to nipple stimulation. Obstet Gynecol 65:588, 1985

Schifrin BS, Foye G, Amato J, Kates R, MacKenna J: Routine

fetal heart rate monitoring in the antepartum period. Obstet Gynecol 54:21, 1979

Smith CV, Nguyen HN, Kovacs B, Mccart D, Phelan JP, Paul RH: Fetal death following antepartum fetal heart rate testing: A review of 65 cases. Obstet Gynecol 70:18, 1987

Smith JH, Anand KJ, Cotes PM, Dawes GS, Harkness RA, Howlett TA, Rees LH, Redman CW: Antenatal fetal heart rate variation in relation to the respiratory and metabolic status of the compromised human fetus. Br J Obstet Gynaecol 95:980, 1988

Sontag LW, Wallace RF: The movement response of the human fetus to sound stimuli. Child Dev 6:253, 1935

Staisch KJ, Westlake JR, Bashore RA: Blind oxytocin challenge test and perinatal outcome. Am J Obstet Gynecol 138:399, 1980

Stephens JD, Birnholz KC: Presented at the meeting of the American College of Obstetricians and Gynecologists, Chicago, May 11, 1977

Sterman MB: Relationship of intrauterine fetal activity to maternal sleep state. Exp Neurol 19:98, 1967

Thacker SB, Berkelman RL: Assessing the diagnostic accuracy and efficacy of selected antepartum fetal surveillance techniques. Obstet Gynecol Surv 41:121, 1986

Timor–Tritsch IE, Dierker LJ, Hertz RH, Deogan NC, Rosen MG: Studies of antepartum behavioral state in the human fetus at term. Am J Obstet Gynecol 132:524, 1978

Todd AL, Tridinger BJ, Cole MJ, Cooney GH: Antenatal tests of fetal welfare and development at age 2 years. Am J Obstet Gynecol 167:66, 1992

Trudinger BJ, Boylan P: Antepartum fetal heart rate monitoring: Value of sound stimulation. Obstet Gynecol 55:265, 1980

van Geijn H, Jongsma HW, de Haan J, Eskes TKAB, Prechtl HFR: Heart rate as an indicator of the behavioral state. Studies in the newborn infant and prospects for fetal heart rate monitoring. Am J Obstet Gynecol 136:1061, 1980

Vintzileos AM, Gaffney SE, Salinger LM, Campbell WA, Nochimson DJ: The relationship between fetal biophysical profile and cord pH in patients undergoing cesarean section before the onset of labor. Obstet Gynecol 70:196, 1987a

Vintzileos AM, Cambell WA, Nochimson DJ, Weinbaum PJ: The use and misuse of the biophysical profile. Am J Obstet Gynecol 156:527, 1987b

Visser GHA, Redman CWG, Huisjes HJ, Turnbull AC: Nonstressed antepartum heart rate monitoring: Implications of decelerations after spontaneous contractions. Am J Obstet Gynecol 138:429, 1980

Williams JW: Obstetrics, 2nd ed. New York, D. Appleton, 1908, p 182

CHAPTER 46
Ultrasound in Obstetrics

Ultrasonography

The impact of the use of ultrasonography on the practice of obstetrics has been profound. Given but one choice from the many biochemical and biophysical techniques that have been developed in more recent years to try to improve pregnancy outcome, sonography would seem the best. Methods for evaluating the health of the fetus that apply pulse-echo ultrasound are now employed widely for many reasons summarized below and illustrated frequently throughout this book. Sonographic techniques that are now available, when performed carefully and interpreted accurately, can supply vital information about the status of the fetus, with no known risks from ultrasound. Reece and co-authors (1990) reviewed available information concerning the safety of obstetrical ultrasound and concluded that there are no confirmed biological hazards.

Technology. Intermittent high-frequency sound waves are generated by applying an alternating current to a transducer made of a piezoelectric material. The transducer is "connected" to the abdominal wall by placing a coupling agent, usually water-soluble gel, on the skin to diminish the loss of ultrasound waves at the interface between the transducer and the skin. In static systems, the transducer so applied emits a pulse of sound waves that passes through soft tissue until an interface between the structures of different tissue densities is reached. When this occurs, some of the energy, proportional to the difference in densities at the interface, is reflected, or echoed, back to the transducer. This, in turn, stimulates the transducer while in the listening state to generate a small electrical voltage that is then amplified and displayed on a screen.

With real-time ultrasonography, the transducers employed generate multiple pulse-echo systems that are activated in sequence and thereby detect movement, including breathing, cardiac actions, and vessel pulsations.

Clinical Applications. Sonography has proved valuable for monitoring pregnancy in a variety of ways. To name a few:

1. Very early identification of intrauterine pregnancy.
2. Demonstration of the size and the rate of growth of the amnionic sac and the embryo, and, at times, resorption or expulsion of the embryo.
3. Identification of multiple fetuses, including conjoined twins.
4. Measurements of the fetal head, abdominal circumference, femur, and other anatomical landmarks to help identify the duration of gestation for the normal fetus or, when measured sequentially, to help identify the growth-retarded fetus.
5. Comparison of fetal head and chest or abdominal circumference to identify hydrocephaly, microcephaly, or anencephaly.
6. Detection of fetal anomalies such as abnormal distention of the fetal bladder, ascites, polycystic kidneys, renal agenesis, ovarian cysts, intestinal obstruction, diaphragmatic hernia, meningomyelocele, and intracranial, cardiac, or limb defects.
7. Demonstration of hydramnios or oligohydramnios.
8. Identification of the location and size of the placenta.
9. Demonstration of placental abnormalities such as hydatidiform mole, molar degeneration, and anomalies such as chorioangioma.
10. Identification of uterine tumors or anomalous development.
11. Detection of a foreign body such as an intrauterine device, blood clot, or retained placental fragments.

Guidelines for Real-time Sonography. Since the first obstetrical application of ultrasound imaging by Donald and co-workers (1958), ultrasound use during pregnancy has steadily increased in the United States and other countries. In this country, Read and co-workers (1983) reported that antenatal ultrasound imaging use increased from 20 percent of all pregnancies in 1975 to 35 percent in 1978. By 1989, at least 45 percent of pregnancies resulting in liveborn infants—almost 1.7 million women in the United States—received diagnostic ultrasound (National Center for Health Statistics, 1992). There has been similar expansion of ultrasound imaging throughout all disciplines of American medicine (Wagner, 1992). Indeed, health-care providers spent $1 billion on diagnostic ultrasound equipment in 1991 and marketing analysts expect this amount to steadily increase through 1997.

The already widespread use of sonography in obstetrics and its potential for identification of fetal abnormalities and for providing reassurance of fetal well-being have stimulated several questions that are difficult to answer: Should sonography be used in all pregnancies and, if so, when should it be initiated, how often should it be repeated, and how vigorous an examination for possible fetal abnormalities should be carried out? Who should perform the examination? Who should directly supervise the examination? Who should interpret the results of the examination? What should be the responsibilities of the practicing obstetrician? In what circumstances should sonography be performed under the supervision of and interpreted by a certified obstetrical or radiological specialist highly trained in sonography?

Some of these questions have been addressed and partially answered. The American College of Obstetricians and Gynecologists (1991) recommended that ultrasound examinations be performed by a "a trained professional," and that **targeted examinations,** which are done for suspected defective fetuses, should be performed by an operator with "expertise in more sophisticated scanning." Shown in Table 46–1 are the guidelines recommended for a *basic* obstetrical ultrasound examination. Vaginal sonography may be necessary during the first trimester if abdominal scanning is insufficient to identify these specified components. Similarly, complete second or third trimester fetal anatomical surveys may not be possible in the presence of oligohydramnios, hyperflexed fetus, engaged fetal head, or compression of fetal body parts and maternal obesity. There are exceptions when it is unnecessary to perform a full fetal survey. Some examples include placental localization during antepartum hemorrhage, determination of fetal presentation in labor, determination of multiple gestation, amniocentesis, antenatal fetal testing (see Biophysical Profile, Chap. 45, p. 1039), and estimation of amnionic fluid volume.

The American Institute of Ultrasound in Medicine (1991) has also provided similar guidelines for the performance of antepartum ultrasound examinations. They differ somewhat in that the American Institute makes specific recommendations for the content of fetal anatomical surveys. Specifically, the anatomical survey is

TABLE 46–1. COMPONENTS OF BASIC ULTRASOUND EXAMINATION ACCORDING TO TRIMESTER OF PREGNANCY

First Trimester	Second and Third Trimesters
1. Gestational sac location	1. Fetal number
2. Embryo identification	2. Presentation
3. Crown–rump length	3. Fetal heart motion
4. Fetal heart motion	4. Placental location
5. Fetal number	5. Amnionic fluid volume
6. Uterus and adnexal evaluation	6. Gestational age; at least two fetal parameters
	7. Survey of fetal anatomy

Modified from American College of Obstetricians and Gynecologists (1991).

recommended to include the cerebral ventricles, four-chamber view of the heart, spine, stomach, urinary bladder, umbilical cord insertion on the abdominal wall, and renal region.

Selected Versus Routine Ultrasound. The question of whether all pregnant women should receive ultrasound screening remains unanswered. Advantages of routine screening have included less frequent labor induction for postterm pregnancy, detection of fetal growth retardation, and identification of malformed fetuses. The British Royal College of Physicians (1989) concluded that most structural fetal malformations could be detected if mid-trimester sonography was done during all pregnancies. Luck (1992) performed routine ultrasound scanning at 19 weeks in over 8800 British women and concluded that this approach reduced perinatal morbidity and mortality because of pregnancy termination in 25 fetuses with crippling or lethal malformations.

Thacker (1985) reviewed the four randomized studies published between 1982 and 1984 concerning the effectiveness of universal ultrasound screening. He concluded that the results failed to support the usefulness of universal screening for all pregnant women. Since then, there have been at least four subsequent randomized studies that addressed the efficacy of routine sonography. Waldenstrom and colleagues (1988), using a single scan at approximately 15 weeks in nearly 2500 Swedish women, found that the incidence of labor inductions was 5.9 percent in the screened versus 9.1 percent in the control women. Secher and associates (1987) performed fetal ultrasound measurements before 22 weeks and again at 32 weeks in nearly 2800 Danish women and then randomized management of those fetuses identified to be small-for-gestational-age. They found no significant benefits for this management scheme. Ewigman and co-workers (1990) randomized over 900 American women with low-risk pregnancies to routine ultrasound or normal prenatal care and also found no benefits for routine sonography. In contrast, Kemppaineu and colleagues (1990) randomized over 9300 Finnish women to routine ultrasound between 16 and 20 weeks or routine antenatal care. The perinatal mortality rate was significantly lower in the sonography group because of pregnancy terminations for malformed fetuses.

In the United States, sonography is not used routinely in all clinics. The National Institutes of Health Consensus Conference (1984) concluded that ultrasonic studies during pregnancy appeared to be safe, but that they should be performed only when specifically indicated.

Fetal and Amnionic Fluid Measurements. The literature contains many tables and nomograms that describe the normal growth of various fetal dimensions. Among the most commonly measured dimensions are

TABLE 46–2. PREFERRED[a] FETAL DIMENSION FOR ESTIMATION OF GESTATIONAL AGE AT VARIOUS STAGES OF PREGNANCY

	Weeks' Gestation		
7–10	*10–14*	*15–28*	*29*
Crown–rump length	Crown–rump length	Biparietal diameter	Femur length
	Biparietal diameter	Femur length	Humerus length
	Femur length	Humerus length	Binocular distance
	Humerus length	Head circumference	Biparietal diameter[b]
		Binocular distance	Other long bones
			Head circumference

[a] In decreasing order of preference.
[b] Only if cephalic index (biparietal diameter divided by occipital frontal diameter) is normal (76 to 84 percent); otherwise, the fetal head may be dolichocephalic or brachycephalic.
Modified from Jeanty (1991).

crown–rump length, biparietal diameter, abdominal circumference, and femur length. There also are nomograms for other fetal dimensions such as head circumference, length of the humerus, ulna, tibia, and clavicle, and binocular distance. As emphasized by Jeanty (1991), deciding which table(s) to use can be difficult. It also is important to emphasize that most predictions of gestational age are based upon the 50th percentile measurement observed in normal fetuses. However, there is a wide range of normal percentiles (5th through 95th) for a given fetal dimension. For example, a biparietal diameter of 40 mm could represent a fetus of 14 weeks (5th percentile) or 20 weeks (95th percentile) as compared with 17 weeks when the 50th percentile is used. Jeanty (1991) has reviewed thoroughly the many considerations necessary in the selection of appropriate nomograms for estimating gestational age and fetal size. Importantly, most ultrasound machines now are available with microcomputers and software that permit instantaneous calculation of fetal indices such as fetal weight estimates.

Different fetal dimensions have different reliability and ease of measurement at different gestational ages. Shown in Table 46–2 are the preferred fetal measurements at various stages of pregnancy (Jeanty, 1991).

Shown in Tables 46–3 and 46–4 are commonly used gestational age nomograms for crown–rump length, biparietal diameter, head circumference, abdominal circumference, and femur length. Shepard and co-workers (1982) have reported formulae frequently used for estimation of fetal weight using the biparietal diameter and abdominal circumference.

TABLE 46–3. ASSESSMENT OF GESTATIONAL AGE IN WEEKS PLUS DAYS FROM THE CROWN–RUMP LENGTH

mm	Percentile[a]			mm	Percentile		
	5th	*50th*	*95th*		*5th*	*50th*	*95th*
10	6+5	7+3	8	30	9+5	10+2	11
11	6+6	7+4	8+2	31	9+5	10+3	11+1
12	7+1	7+5	8+3	32	9+6	10+4	11+2
13	7+2	8	8+4	33	10	10+5	11+2
14	7+3	8+4	8+6	34	10+1	10+6	11+3
15	7+4	8+2	9	35	10+2	10+6	11+4
16	7+5	8+3	9+1	36	10+2	11	11+5
17	8	8+4	9+2	37	10+3	11+1	11+6
18	8+1	8+5	9+3	38	10+4	11+2	11+6
19	8+2	8+6	9+4	39	10+5	11+2	12
20	8+3	9	9+5	40	10+5	11+3	12+1
21	8+4	9+1	9+6	41	10+6	11+4	12+1
22	8+5	9+2	10	42	11	11+4	12+2
23	8+6	9+3	10+1	43	11	11+5	12+3
24	8+6	9+4	10+2	44	11+1	11+6	12+3
25	9	9+5	10+3	45	11+2	11+6	12+4
26	9+1	9+6	10+4	46	11+2	12	12+5
27	9+2	10	10+5	47	11+3	12+1	12+5
28	9+3	10+1	10+5	48	11+4	12+1	12+6
29	9+4	10+2	10+6	49	11+4	12+2	13

[a] Week of gestational age (weeks plus days) from the crown–rump length.
From Robinson and Fleming (1975) with permission.

TABLE 46–4. AVERAGE PREDICTED FETAL MEASUREMENTS AT SPECIFIC MENSTRUAL AGES

Menstrual Age (wks)	Biparietal Diameter (cm)	Head Circum- ference	Abdominal Circum- ference (cm)	Femur Length (cm)
12.0	1.7	6.8	4.6	0.7
12.5	1.9	7.5	5.3	0.9
13.0	2.1	8.2	6.0	1.1
13.5	2.3	8.9	6.7	1.2
14.0	2.5	9.7	7.3	1.4
14.5	2.7	10.4	8.0	1.6
15.0	2.9	11.0	8.6	1.7
15.5	3.1	11.7	9.3	1.9
16.0	3.2	12.4	9.9	2.0
16.5	3.4	13.1	10.6	2.2
17.0	3.5	13.8	11.2	2.4
17.5	3.8	14.4	11.9	2.5
18.0	3.9	15.1	12.5	2.7
18.5	4.1	15.8	13.1	2.8
19.0	4.3	16.4	13.7	3.0
19.5	4.5	17.0	14.4	3.1
20.0	4.6	17.7	15.0	3.3
20.5	4.8	18.3	15.6	3.4
21.0	5.0	18.9	16.2	3.5
21.5	5.1	19.5	16.8	3.7
22.0	5.3	20.1	17.4	3.8
22.5	5.5	20.7	17.9	4.0
23.0	5.6	21.3	18.5	4.1
23.5	5.8	21.9	19.1	4.2
24.0	5.9	22.4	19.7	4.4
24.5	6.1	23.0	20.2	4.5
25.0	6.2	23.5	20.8	4.6
25.5	6.4	24.1	21.3	4.7
26.0	6.5	24.6	21.9	4.9
26.5	6.7	25.1	22.4	5.0
27.0	6.8	25.6	23.0	5.1
27.5	6.9	26.1	23.5	5.2
28.0	7.1	26.6	24.0	5.4
28.5	7.2	27.1	24.6	5.5
29.0	7.3	27.5	25.1	5.6
29.5	7.5	28.0	25.6	5.7
30.0	7.6	28.4	26.1	5.8
30.5	7.7	28.8	26.6	5.9
31.0	7.8	29.3	27.1	6.0
31.5	7.9	29.7	27.6	6.1
32.0	8.1	30.1	28.1	6.2
32.5	8.2	30.4	28.6	6.3
33.0	8.3	30.8	29.1	6.4
33.5	8.4	31.2	29.5	6.5
34.0	8.5	31.5	30.0	6.6
34.5	8.6	31.8	30.5	6.7
35.0	8.7	32.2	30.9	6.8
35.5	8.8	32.5	31.4	6.9
36.0	8.9	32.8	31.8	7.0
36.5	8.9	33.0	32.3	7.1
37.0	9.0	33.3	32.7	7.2
37.5	9.1	33.5	33.2	7.3
38.0	9.2	33.8	33.6	7.4
38.5	9.2	34.0	34.0	7.4
39.0	9.3	34.2	34.4	7.5
39.5	9.4	34.4	34.8	7.6
40.0	9.4	34.6	35.3	7.7

From Hadlock and co-workers (1984), with permission.

Estimation of amnionic fluid volume using ultrasound has emerged as an important method of fetal assessment (see Chap. 34, p. 734). Many different definitions of diminished amnionic fluid volume (oligohydramnios) and excessive fluid (hydramnios) have been proposed, depending on the method used to quantify the volume of fluid. Originally, Manning and co-workers (1980) proposed that a "pocket" of fluid measuring 1 cm less in the vertical dimension signified pathological oligohydramnios. Other investigators have proposed broadened criteria for pocket size. For example, Crowley and co-workers (1984) used a 4-cm pocket dimension to predict fetal distress in postterm pregnancies. Subjective estimations of "decreased" amnionic fluid volume during ultrasound scanning have also been reported to be useful (Phelan and co-workers, 1985).

More recently, Phelan and co-workers (1987) introduced the increasingly popular technique termed the **amnionic fluid index.** This technique begins by dividing the maternal abdomen into four quadrants. Using the umbilicus as one reference during the third trimester, the uterus is divided into upper and lower halves. The linea nigra is then used as the midline, with the uterus now divided into right and left halves. The ultrasound transducer head is then placed on the maternal abdomen along the longitudinal axis and the transducer is kept perpendicular to the floor. The vertical diameter of the largest amnionic fluid pocket in each quadrant is measured and the sum calculated in total centimeters. Moore and Cayle (1990) have described the amnionic fluid index values in percentiles for pregnancies between 16 and 42 weeks; these are shown in Table 46–5.

Fetal Anatomy. Most attempts to survey fetal anatomy using ultrasound take place during the early second trimester or later. Although some investigators have reported success with imaging various fetal structures during the first trimester, Green and Hobbins (1988) generally were unable to identify fetal structures transabdominally before 9 weeks; their success rate improved remarkably, however, as gestation progressed. By 12 weeks, they were able to visualize the stomach in 95 percent, the anterior abdominal wall in 80 percent, the adrenal glands in 100 percent, the kidneys in 100 percent, and the bladder in 60 percent. Similarly, Timor-Tritsch and associates (1990) reported consistent success at imaging the skull, brain, spine, limbs, and anterior abdominal wall in 35 fetuses examined transvaginally between 9 and 14 weeks. By 11 weeks, they were able to visualize the fingers and feet.

Although there are increasing numbers of case reports that describe detection of a variety of fetal anomalies during the first trimester, and in spite of the obvious potential for identifying congenital fetal malformations at this point, caution is recommended for several reasons: (1) Normal first-trimester embryological development may mimic pathological changes in the second

TABLE 46–5. AMNIONIC FLUID INDEX VALUES IN NORMAL PREGNANCY

Week	Amnionic Fluid Index Percentile Values				
	2.5th	*5th*	*50th*	*95th*	*97.5th*
16	73	79	121	185	201
17	77	83	127	194	211
18	80	87	133	202	220
19	83	90	137	207	225
20	86	93	141	212	230
21	88	95	143	214	233
22	89	97	145	216	235
23	90	98	146	218	237
24	90	98	147	219	238
25	89	97	147	221	240
26	89	97	147	223	242
27	85	95	146	226	245
28	86	94	146	228	249
29	84	92	145	231	254
30	82	90	145	234	258
31	79	88	144	238	263
32	77	86	144	242	269
33	74	83	143	245	274
34	72	81	142	248	278
35	70	79	140	249	279
36	68	77	138	249	279
37	66	75	135	244	275
38	65	73	132	239	269
39	64	72	127	226	255
40	63	71	123	214	240
41	63	70	116	194	216
42	63	69	110	175	192

Modified from Moore and Cayle (1990), with permission.

and third trimesters; for example, physiological anterior wall herniation may mimic an omphalocele. (2) Grossly abnormal embryos may appear normal; for example, with anencephaly. (3) Some abnormal embryos may manifest only with a crown–rump length that is less than expected for their gestational age (Levi and associates, 1990).

Cardiac Anomalies. Congenital heart disease has been the most commonly recognized birth defect with a reported frequency of 8 per 1000 livebirths and 27 to 77 per 1000 stillborns (Hoffman and Christianson, 1978; Mitchell and associates, 1971). Interestingly, the reported frequency of specific heart defects varies significantly between studies done on liveborns, stillborns, and fetuses in whom heart lesions were identified in utero (see Chap. 48, p. 1092). Perone (1988) recommends that women with any of the following risk factors undergo a detailed ultrasound examination of the fetal heart: nonimmune hydrops, suspected abnormality seen by screening sonogram, teratogen exposure, parental or sibling heart defects, aneuploidy, extracardiac anomalies, maternal diabetes, and fetal arrhythmias. The recurrence risk for congenital heart defects if siblings or parents are affected is shown in Table 40–6 (p. 930).

Congenital heart defects are frequently associated with aneuploidy, and Copel and co-workers (1988a) reported that 11 of 34 fetuses (32 percent) with cardiac anomalies detected prenatally had an abnormal karyotype. Additionally, associated extracardiac structural abnormalities are present in 25 to 45 percent of such fetuses (Copel and associates, 1986).

Although heart motion can be visualized sonographically in a 6- to 7-week embryo, detailed cardiac evaluation is usually not possible until at least 18 weeks. Even at this time, adequate anatomical cardiac assessment is dependent on factors that include fetal position and activity, maternal size, and amnionic fluid volume. The detail of such examinations depends on the availability of proper equipment and expertise, and the study may be time-consuming and require pediatric cardiological collaboration.

Visualization of a four-chamber view is central to fetal cardiac assessment (Fig. 46–1). This view is obtained by imaging a transverse plane through the fetal thorax at a level just above the diaphragm and allows evaluation of the size, location, and orientation of the fetal heart. Additionally, the atrial and ventricular chambers can be assessed, the interatrial and interventricular septa viewed, and the atrioventricular valves observed. Normally, the two atria are similar in size as are the two ventricles. The apex of the heart typically forms a 45-degree angle with the left anterior chest wall (Comstock, 1987).

The importance of the four-chamber view was demonstrated by Copel and colleagues (1987), who reported that 71 of 74 fetuses (96 percent) with sonographically detectable heart defects had abnormal four-chamber views. As reviewed by Perone (1988), at times other cross-sectional views may be required, either to demonstrate fetal heart integrity or to characterize abnormalities. In addition to these, **M-mode echocardiography**

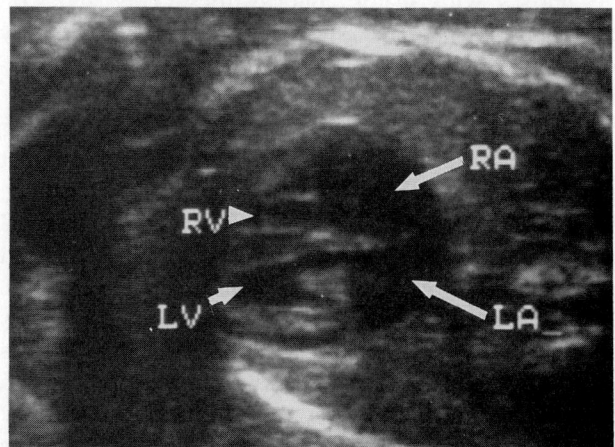

Fig. 46–1. Transverse sonogram through the thorax of a 23-week fetus demonstrating a four-chamber cardiac view. Seen are the right atrium (RA), left atrium (LA), right ventricle (RV), and left ventricle (LV). (From Lowe and colleagues, 1990.)

may be required to measure chamber size, wall thickness, and wall and valve motion, and to facilitate assessment of cardiac arrhythmias (DeVore and co-workers, 1982, 1987). **Pulse Doppler** and, more recently, **real-time Doppler color-flow mapping** have been used to define normal or abnormal blood flow in the fetal cardiovascular system (DeVore and associates, 1987; Shenker and colleagues, 1988).

Given these technological considerations, what accuracy should be expected of an ultrasound examination to detect fetal cardiac disease? Crawford and colleagues (1988) reported their experiences with almost 1000 women at high risk for having children with cardiac abnormalities. They performed over 1750 fetal echocardiograms and successfully identified 74 of 91 anomalies (80 percent). In almost half of those with cardiac anomalies, chromosomal or extracardiac structural defects were also found. Crawford and colleagues (1988) emphasized that heart disease diagnosed prenatally is usually severe and is associated with a poor long-term prognosis. By contrast, Benacerraf and associates (1987) studied a group of women who underwent sonographic studies for multiple reasons. Although 49 fetuses subsequently were found to have 66 cardiac defects, only 33 (50 percent) of these were detected antenatally. According to both of these reports, ventricular septal defects, anomalous pulmonary venous return, and aortic or pulmonic stenosis especially were likely to be missed by fetal ultrasound evaluation.

Central Nervous System Abnormalities. Prenatal sonography has proven an excellent method to detect and characterize fetal central nervous system abnormalities. This is especially important because of the frequency of these abnormalities as well as their potential for causing severe disability or death. By adopting a systematic approach to the ultrasound evaluation of the central nervous system, it is possible to identify virtually all fetuses with major abnormalities (Filly and colleagues, 1989). Such early identification allows timely consideration of prognosis and therapeutic options, including pregnancy termination.

Three routine transverse (or axial) sonographic views are recommended by Nyberg (1989) to depict the fetal brain and cranium. The transthalamic view (Fig. 46–2), which is used to measure biparietal diameter and head circumference, includes the thalamus, cavum septi pellucidae, and the frontal horns of the lateral ventricle. Moving superiorly yields the transventricular view (Fig. 46–3), which contains the lateral cerebral ventricles and the echogenic choroid plexus and also allows visualization of cranial contour. The transcerebellar view (Fig. 46–4) is obtained by angling through the posterior fossa in the suboccipital bregmatic plane and demonstrates the cerebellum and cisterna magna. Normal transverse cerebellar diameters for fetuses between 13 and 40 weeks have been reported by Goldstein and associates (1987).

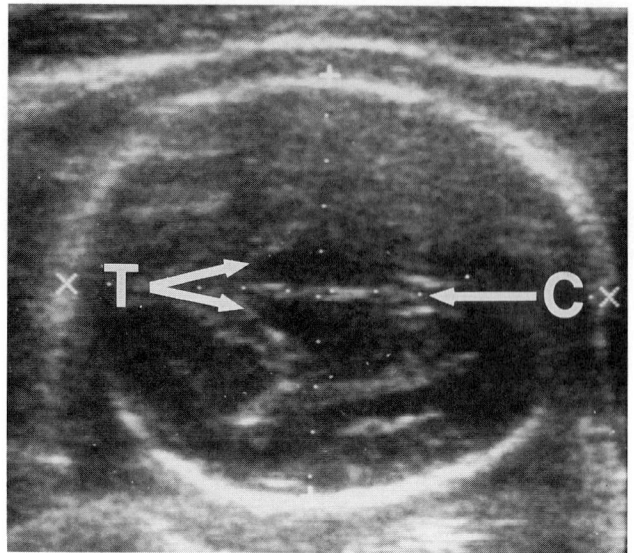

Fig. 46–2. Transthalamic view in a 23-week fetus. Depicted are thalami (T) and cavum septum pellucidum (C). (From Lowe and colleagues, 1990.)

Filly and colleagues (1989) reported their experiences with 137 fetuses between 15 and 39 weeks who had sonographically diagnosed central nervous system abnormalities. Of these, 25 had obvious anencephaly and 99 had a ventricular atrial diameter larger than 10 mm. Seven of the remaining 13 fetuses had a cisterna magna either smaller than 2 mm or larger than 11 mm in size. Using this sequence of evaluation, only 6 of 137 fetuses with abnormal nervous systems were not identified; however, in three of these fetuses, other grossly apparent abnormalities were seen. Thus, using a relatively simple sequence of evaluation, 134 of 137 fetuses with central nervous system abnormalities would have

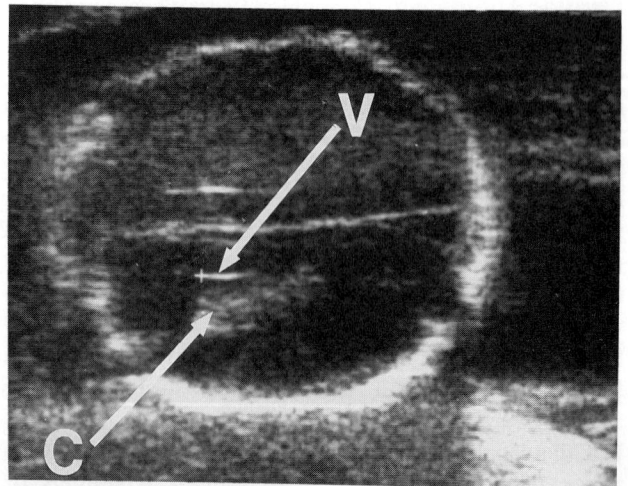

Fig. 46–3. Transventricular view in a 20-week fetus. Note choroid plexus (C) in ventricular atrium (V). (From Lowe and associates, 1990.)

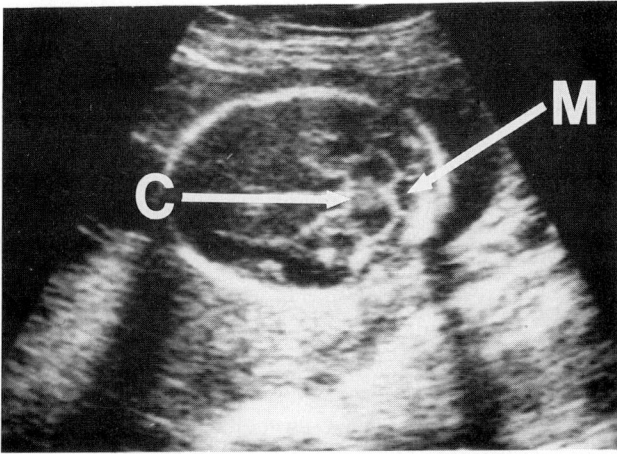

Fig. 46–4. Transcerebellar view in a 20-week fetus. The cisterna magna (M) and cerebellum (C) are depicted. (From Lowe and co-workers, 1990.)

been identified. This same group also studied 150 normal fetuses between 15 and 40 weeks and found that the ventricular atrium could be identified and measured in 99 percent and the cisterna magna in 90 percent.

Hydrocephalus. The incidence of hydrocephalus ranges from 0.3 to 0.8 per 1000 births (Chap. 40, p. 930). Fetuses who are diagnosed prenatally have other intracranial or extracranial malformations or chromosomal abnormalities in 85 percent of cases and appear to have a very poor prognosis for normal long-term development (Chervenak and colleagues, 1983; Nyberg and associates, 1987a; Pretorius and associates, 1985).

Initially, hydrocephalus was diagnosed sonographically by identifying an abnormally large fetal head. This method was found to be inadequate and was later replaced by determining the lateral ventricular ratio. To calculate this ratio, a transverse plane through the fetal vertex is visualized at a point where the lateral ventricular walls parallel the midline. The lateral ventricular width, measured from the middle of the midline echo to the lateral wall of the lateral ventricle, is then divided by the hemispheric width, measured on the same image from the middle of the midline echo to the inner table of the calvarium. Benacerraf (1988) has reported that the echogenic line originally thought to represent the lateral ventricular wall in reality represents reflections from vascular structures adjacent to the ventricle and thus yields only an approximation of ventricular size. The lateral ventricular ratio may be normally as high as 71 percent at 15 weeks but decreases to 33 percent by 24 weeks. After 24 weeks, a ratio greater than 50 percent is considered abnormal. In the normal fetus, the diameter of the lateral ventricular atrium is relatively constant from 6 to 9 mm between 18 and 35 weeks (Cardoza and colleagues, 1988a). An atrial diameter greater than 10 mm suggests ventriculomegaly. This observation may be especially useful, as dilatation of the

ventricular atrium and occipital horns is thought to be an early event in the development of fetal hydrocephalus.

Cardoza and associates (1988b) examined the relationship between the choroid plexus and the lateral wall of the dependent lateral ventricle. They compared 50 normal fetuses at 15 to 38 weeks with 25 hydrocephalic fetuses at 18 to 39 weeks. Mahony and colleagues (1988) reported preliminary findings in which they quantified the anatomical relationship between the choroid plexus and the medial wall of the dependent lateral ventricle. The findings of these two studies are promising and may facilitate the early diagnosis of fetal hydrocephalus for the following reasons: (1) Typically, the choroid plexus is easy to visualize sonographically throughout the second and third trimesters. (2) The choroid plexus normally fills the lateral ventricular body posterior to the foramen of Monro. (3) In the presence of hydrocephalus, the heavy choroid plexus in the dependent lateral ventricle will separate from the medial ventricular wall and remain in contact with the lateral ventricular wall through the action of gravity. Cardoza and associates (1988b) have used the term *dangling choroid plexus* to describe this separation.

Other disorders that may mimic hydrocephalus include holoprosencephaly, agenesis of the corpus callosum, hydranencephaly, porencephalic cysts, and cerebral atrophy from destruction of cerebral tissue by intrauterine infection.

Neural-tube Defects. Neural-tube defects result from failure of tube closure by the 6th gestational week (embryonic age 26 to 28 days). A more detailed account of common neural-tube anomalies is found in Chapter 40 and their incidence is cited in Table 40–5.

Anencephaly was the first fetal malformation to be diagnosed prenatally by using sonography. Although its diagnosis is theoretically possible as early as 8 weeks, it can be missed by experienced sonographers in the first trimester (Levi and associates, 1990). In the second trimester, however, if an adequate ultrasound examination can be performed, anencephaly is diagnosed with virtually 100 percent accuracy. Sonographically, anencephaly is characterized by absence of the cranial vault and brain above the base of the skull and orbits.

Hydramnios, secondary to impaired fetal swallowing (Pritchard, 1965), commonly accompanies anencephaly but typically is a late finding. Goldstein and Filly (1988) reported increased amnionic fluid in 85 percent of anencephalic fetuses after 25 weeks, but in only about 10 percent before. Associated fetal anomalies are common but have not been described extensively because anencephaly itself is uniformly fatal.

Encephalocele defines the condition in which the meninges and cerebrospinal fluid, usually in association with brain tissue, herniate through a cranial defect. This lesion most commonly results from an occipital midline defect. Sonographically, encephaloceles vary in size and are characterized by either a cystic or solid appearance depending on which fetal structures are involved. Encephaloceles commonly are associated with either hydrocephaly or microcephaly. The presence of an encephalocele is an important feature of **Meckel–Gruber syndrome** and frequently accompanies **amnionic band syndrome.** An occipital encephalocele usually can be detected utilizing transthalamic and transcerebellar views.

Spina bifida consists of a hiatus, usually in the lumbosacral vertebrae, through which a meningeal sac may protrude, forming a **meningocele.** If the sac contains neural elements, as it does in 90 percent of cases, the anomaly is called a **meningomyelocele.** Roberts and colleagues (1983) reported their 6-year experience with the ultrasound diagnosis of spina bifida in a group of women at high risk for an affected fetus. All studies were performed before 20 weeks, and in the first 3 years they correctly diagnosed only 6 of 18 defects while they falsely diagnosed a defect in 49 of 1243 normal fetuses. In the second three years of their study, they correctly diagnosed 16 of 20 defects and misdiagnosed only 4 of 1171 normal fetuses. The importance of experience is apparent.

The fetal spine should be examined by sonography with sagittal, transverse, and coronal views (Fig. 46–5) whenever possible. These provide the best opportunity to detect the presence and extent of defects in the fetal spine and overlying soft tissues. It is emphasized that fetal movement of the lower extremities and urination may be seen despite the presence of neurologically significant spina bifida.

Because of the difficulty in detecting small spinal defects, especially during the second trimester, the as-

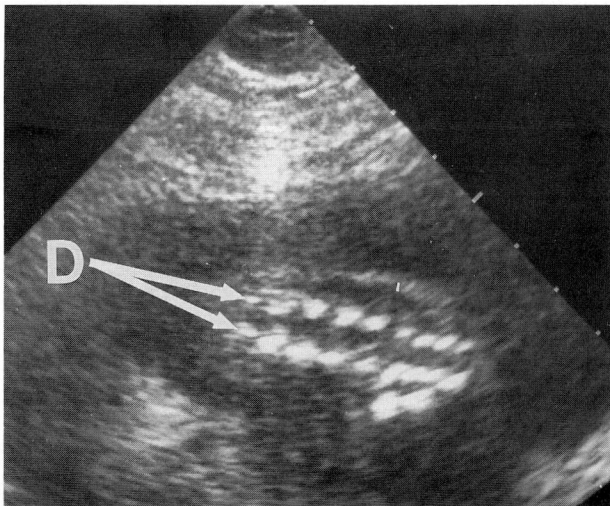

Fig. 46–5. Coronal view of the lumbosacral spine in a 20-week fetus. Paired dorsal ossification centers (D) are depicted. (From Lowe and colleagues, 1990.)

sociation of cranial abnormalities with spina bifida recently has been the subject of intense investigation. For example, spina bifida is commonly, if not invariably, accompanied by the **Arnold–Chiari malformation.** While the exact cause of this malformation is unclear, its pathology is well characterized: the medulla and fourth ventricle are elongated and, in combination with a portion of the cerebellum, extend through the foramen magnum into the upper cervical spinal canal. The Arnold–Chiari malformation is felt to be responsible for sonographically detectable fetal abnormalities that include cerebral ventriculomegaly, frontal bone scalloping (*lemon sign*), abnormal curvature of the cerebellum (*banana sign*), decreased cerebellar size, and failure to visualize the cerebellum and obliteration of the cisterna magna.

Cerebral ventriculomegaly has been reported in approximately 80 percent of fetuses with spina bifida. Although it generally is mild to moderate, it tends to worsen with advancing gestational age (Goldstein and colleagues, 1989; Nyberg and co-workers, 1988a). Benacerraf and co-workers (1989) reported that a cerebellar **banana sign** was present in 22 of 23 fetuses diagnosed with spina bifida between 16 and 27 weeks. In a larger study, Van den Hof and associates (1990) presented findings from 130 fetuses with sonographically diagnosed spina bifida. A banana sign was found in 74 of 107 affected fetuses (70 percent) before 24 weeks, and another 29 had an "absent cerebellum." After 24 weeks, only 4 of the 23 fetuses with spina bifida demonstrated a banana sign, but another 17 had an absent cerebellum. It is important to note that when the data from these two studies are combined, a total of 1405 fetuses subsequently proven not to have spina bifida were examined with ultrasound because of maternal risk factors for neural-tube defects, and none had an abnormal cerebellum. In a related observation, Goldstein and colleagues (1989) evaluated a group of fetuses between 17 and 38 weeks who were at risk for neural-tube defects. They obtained an adequate view of the posterior fossa in 19 of 20 fetuses with spina bifida. In 18 of these fetuses the cisterna magna was completely effaced, and in one it measured 2 mm. In all 33 of the nonaffected fetuses, the cisterna magna measured 4 to 9 mm.

Normally, when visualized in the transthalamic or transventricular planes, the frontal contour of the fetal cranium is convex. The presence of a concave or flattened frontal contour has been termed the **lemon sign.** In the study by Van den Hof and associates (1990), 105 of the 107 fetuses less than 24 weeks with spina bifida had this sign compared with only 3 of 23 after 24 weeks. Similarly, Nyberg and associates (1988a) found a lemon sign in 24 of 27 affected fetuses before 24 weeks, compared with 8 of 25 fetuses later in gestation. Combining the two studies, however, only 12 of 1497 fetuses evaluated because they were at increased risk for neural-tube defects had a lemon sign in the absence of spina bifida.

Choroid Plexus Cysts. Choroid plexus cysts have been identified in 1 to 3 percent of second-trimester fetuses (Benacerraf and co-workers, 1990; Chinn and associates, 1990). Usually, these cysts are transient and of no clinical significance. In some situations, however, they have been associated with trisomy 18, and this association recently has been subject to intense scrutiny. Nicolaides and colleagues (1986) found choroid plexus cysts in four fetuses between 18 and 24 weeks, and three of these had trisomy 18. All three trisomic fetuses had other sonographic abnormalities.

Chitkara and associates (1988) detected choroid plexus cysts measuring 2 to 20 mm in 40 fetuses between 16 and 21 weeks. Approximately half were bilateral. Of the 40 cysts, 33 resolved by 23 to 24 weeks, and another four by 26 to 28 weeks. One fetus with large bilateral cysts and additional ultrasound abnormalities had trisomy 18. Chan and co-workers (1989) prospectively studied 513 women who underwent genetic amniocentesis between 16 and 24 weeks. Thirteen fetuses had choroid plexus cysts between 3 and 10 mm. Approximately one third were bilateral. All 13 fetuses had normal karyotypes. Conversely, of the 500 fetuses without choroid plexus cysts, five had trisomy 21 and two had trisomy 18.

Benacerraf and co-workers (1990) calculated that if all second-trimester fetuses with no ultrasound abnormalities except choroid plexus cysts underwent genetic amniocentesis, 478 procedures would have to be done to identify each case of trisomy 18.

Gastrointestinal Abnormalities. Using high-resolution diagnostic sonography, the integrity of the abdominal wall, umbilical cord insertion, and intraabdominal anomalies can be assessed with confidence (Fig. 46–6). The liver, spleen, gallbladder, and bowel can be identified in most pregnancies. Normally, the appearance of the fetal bowel changes with gestational age and considerable overlap exists between normal and pathological conditions (Nyberg and co-workers, 1987b). Pretorius and colleagues (1988) reported successfully visualizing the fetal stomach in 98 percent of fetuses after 14 weeks. Moreover, nonvisualization was associated with an abnormal outcome in 55 percent of fetuses studied after 14 weeks and 100 percent after 19 weeks. They suggested that repeat sonograms should be obtained in all cases of stomach nonvisualization.

Diaphragmatic Hernia. Congenital diaphragmatic hernia results from incomplete fusion of the pleuroperitoneal membrane, occurs more frequently on the left, and has a frequency of 1 in 2000 to 3000 births (Romero and associates, 1988a). On ultrasound examination, a cystic structure, usually behind the left atrium, is seen

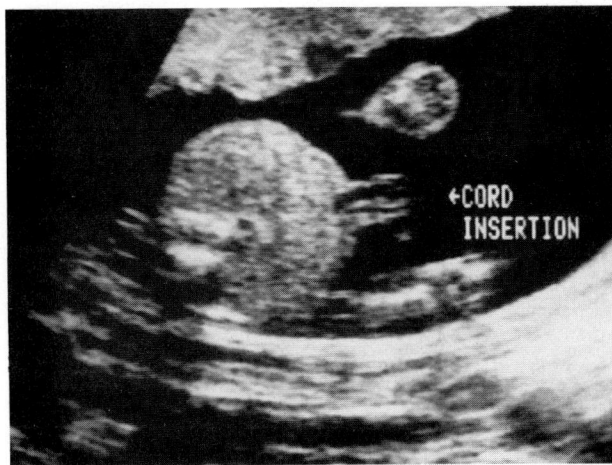

Fig. 46–6. Transverse sonogram of a second-trimester fetus with an intact anterior abdominal wall and normal cord insertion. (From Lowe and associates, 1990.)

on an axial image at the level of the four-chamber cardiac view. Associated findings include absence of an intra-abdominal stomach bubble, a mediastinal shift usually with a normal cardiac axis, and a small abdominal circumference. The most specific finding is peristalsis in the fetal chest. Associated hydramnios also is common and was identified in 75 percent of affected fetuses studied by Adzick and co-workers (1985).

Diaphragmatic hernia is associated with other major anomalies in almost half of all cases, and chromosomal abnormalities are found in up to 20 percent of affected infants (Benacerraf and Adzick, 1987; Romero and associates, 1988a). Importantly, Benacerraf and Adzick (1987) reported an overall survival rate of only 10 percent despite accurate prenatal diagnosis and optimal neonatal management in a tertiary-care hospital. Adzick and co-workers (1985) found that survival is related to defect size and noted that nonsurvivors may have more abdominal viscera displaced into the chest earlier in gestation. They also reported that survival was 55 percent when there was normal amnionic fluid volume, compared with 10 percent when hydramnios was present. Neonatal death generally results from respiratory failure secondary to pulmonary hypoplasia or from associated lethal anomalies. Although diaphragmatic hernias usually are repaired after delivery, Harrison and associates (1990) have attempted repair in utero.

Abdominal Wall Defects. Anterior abdominal wall defects as a group are relatively common malformations. The two most common are **omphalocele** and **gastroschisis,** and each has a frequency of approximately 1 in 5000 livebirths. Because of maternal serum alphafetoprotein screening programs, these two defects can be ascertained early in pregnancy. Although these defects have many similarities, it is important to recognize that they differ markedly in developmental pathology, association with other major abnormalities, and prognosis.

OMPHALOCELE. An omphalocele is a congenital midline defect in the anterior abdominal wall that results when the lateral abdominal folds fail to fuse. This condition has been diagnosed accurately as early as 12 weeks (Curtis and Watson, 1988). The defect results in herniation of intra-abdominal structures into the base of the umbilical cord. The hernia sac is continuous with the umbilical cord and must be differentiated from the physiological herniation that may be apparent normally until 14 weeks. The diagnosis is made when a sac containing intraabdominal structures is imaged outside the abdomen (see Fig. 40–9). The umbilical cord should be seen inserting into the hernia sac. The defect size varies and the sac may contain any of the intra-abdominal organs. Nyberg and associates (1989) classified 26 fetuses with omphaloceles based on whether or not the sac contained liver. When the liver was intracorporeal, all eight fetuses studied were chromosomally abnormal. By contrast, only 2 of 18 (11 percent) with an extracorporeal liver had karyotypic abnormalities. It is important to note that associated major malformations are found in about half of fetuses with an omphalocele (Hughes and colleagues, 1989; Nyberg and associates, 1989). The prognosis depends largely on other major malformations or chromosomal abnormalities as emphasized by Hughes and colleagues (1989).

GASTROSCHISIS. With gastroschisis, intra-abdominal organs herniate through a defect in the anterior abdominal wall. The defect is caused by interruption of the right omphalomesenteric artery and is located usually to the right of the umbilicus and spares the rectus muscle (Hoyme and associates, 1981). Gastroschisis has been diagnosed as early as 13 weeks using transvaginal sonography (Kushnir and associates, 1990). Mabogunje and Mahour (1984) found herniation of the small bowel in 90 percent of cases, the large bowel in 70 percent, the stomach in 55 percent, and a portion of the liver in only 5 percent. Sonographically, extracorporeal bowel has a typical *cauliflower* appearance. Herniated organs float freely in the amnionic fluid with no covering membrane, and the umbilical cord insertion is normal. Gastroschisis is associated with other anomalies in 20 to 40 percent of cases (Hoyme and associates, 1981; Mabogunje and Mahour, 1984). These commonly involve stenosis or atresia of some portion of the gastrointestinal tract, presumably with a vascular etiology.

Bond and colleagues (1988) reported their experiences with 11 cases of gastroschisis diagnosed prenatally. They found that sonographically detected small-bowel dilatation and mural thickening correlated with severe intestinal damage in four neonates and suggested that these findings indicate the need for early delivery. Others have been unable to confirm the utility of this

approach (Chambers and associates, 1990; Lenke and co-workers, 1990), and it seems likely that their findings are significant prognostically, but are related to the original vascular injury and not to subsequent events.

Gastrointestinal Atresia. Ultrasound can be used to diagnose abnormalities in the hollow gastrointestinal tract. Most of these anomalies are caused by obstruction with subsequent proximal bowel dilatation. In general, the more proximal the obstruction, the more likely it will be associated with hydramnios. **Esophageal atresia** and **tracheoesophageal fistula** cannot be diagnosed reliably in utero, although they may be suspected when hydramnios is found in the absence of a fluid-filled stomach. However, Pretorius and colleagues (1987), in a retrospective review, reported that only 7 of 22 infants born with a tracheoesophageal fistula had both hydramnios and a nonvisualizing stomach. In an additional seven pregnancies, hydramnios and a fetal stomach were both present sonographically. None of these women developed hydramnios before 24 weeks, and other abnormalities were present in 12 of the 22 infants.

Duodenal atresia is diagnosed prenatally by the demonstration of the *double-bubble sign*, which represents the distention of the stomach and the first part of the duodenum. Demonstrating continuity between these two structures will differentiate duodenal atresia from other cystic structures in the upper abdomen. The diagnosis of duodenal atresia generally is not possible before 24 weeks, although it has been made as early as 19 weeks (Romero and associates, 1988b). This anomaly has been associated with trisomy 21 in approximately 30 percent of infants and may be even more common in cases diagnosed prenatally (Romero and associates, 1988a). Obstructions in the lower small bowel usually result in multiple dilated loops, and these may show increased peristaltic activity. Large bowel obstructions and anal atresia are less readily diagnosed in utero because hydramnios is not a typical feature and the bowel may not be significantly dilated.

Genitourinary Tract. Using transabdominal sonography, the fetal kidneys are visualized as paraspinous masses frequently as early as 14 weeks, and routinely by 18 weeks (Patten and co-workers, 1990). Normal kidneys appear elliptical in parasagittal planes (Fig. 46–7) and circular in transverse planes (Fig. 46–8). Initially, fetal kidneys uniformly are hypoechoic; however, as pregnancy advances, more detail is visualized. The renal cortex, which is echogenic, surrounds the hypoechoic medullary pyramids and is outlined by perinephric fat and the renal capsule. The renal pelvis is centrally located and anechoic.

Nomograms have been developed that describe normal fetal kidney dimensions throughout pregnancy (Grannum and colleagues, 1980; Sagi and associates, 1987). Although kidney length increases linearly

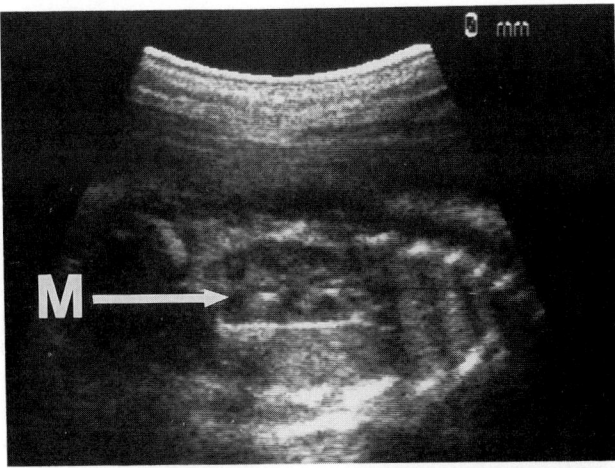

Fig. 46–7. Longitudinal sonogram of a fetal kidney. The hypoechoic medullary pyramids (M) are depicted. (From Lowe and associates, 1990.)

throughout pregnancy, the ratio of kidney circumference, measured in a transverse plane, to the corresponding abdominal circumference remains constant between 0.28 and 0.30.

Urine production normally begins late in the first trimester, and consequently the fetal bladder can be observed as an anechoic area in the pelvis early in the second trimester. Fetal urine production increases from 5 mL/hour at 20 weeks to about 50 mL/hour at 40 weeks (Rabinowitz and co-workers, 1989). In the normal fetus, the bladder fills and empties every 20 to 45 minutes.

Assessment of amnionic fluid volume provides important information regarding fetal renal function. Often, significant fetal urinary tract abnormalities result in oligohydramnios. Conversely, normal amnionic fluid volume suggests urinary tract patency with at least one functioning kidney, especially in the second half of pregnancy when fetal urine is an increasingly important

component of the amnionic fluid. Sivit and colleagues (1986) reported 16 women identified to have severe oligohydramnios between 16 and 30 weeks. When studied after pregnancy termination or delivery, 10 of these infants had urinary tract anomalies. Before 16 to 20 weeks, there may be normal amnionic fluid volume despite absent renal function, although otherwise unexplained oligohydramnios still suggests a urinary abnormality.

There have been at least two large prospective antenatal sonographic screening programs from which the frequency and type of fetal urinary tract abnormalities can be ascertained. Helin and Persson (1986) performed 24,000 ultrasound examinations in nearly 12,000 women at 17 and again at 33 weeks. They identified urinary tract anomalies in 33 fetuses (0.27 percent), and were able to confirm an abnormality in 23 neonates. Only 3 of 33 anomalies were detected at 17 weeks, and the remainder were identified at 33 weeks. By contrast, Livera and co-workers (1989) performed sonograms on nearly 6300 women at 28 weeks and diagnosed fetal renal abnormalities in 92 (1.5 percent). Postnatal studies confirmed abnormalities in 42 neonates, and 13 had bilateral disease. There were four perinatal deaths, and all of these had bilateral disease. Seven infants (0.11 percent) thought to be normal as assessed by fetal sonography were diagnosed to have renal abnormalities after they developed urinary infections during the first year of life. Some of the neonatal abnormalities reported in these two studies are listed in Table 46–6.

Callan and colleagues (1990) reported findings from 55 fetuses identified to have genitourinary abnormalities in women referred to Johns Hopkins Hospital for ultrasound evaluation. More than half (57 percent) of these fetuses had bilateral involvement. They undertook no interventional therapy in utero, and there were 35 survivors (66 percent), of whom 22 underwent surgical therapy postnatally. Factors that portended a poorer prognosis were bilateral disease, oligohydramnios, and associated anomalies.

Obstructive Uropathy. Fetal urinary tract obstruction may develop at the ureteropelvic junction, the ure-

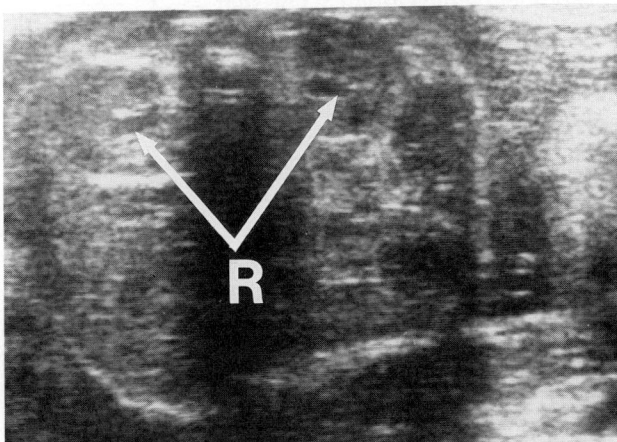

Fig. 46–8. Transverse sonogram of a fetus demonstrating kidneys. Note anechoic renal pelves (R). (From Lowe and associates, 1990.)

TABLE 46–6. FREQUENCY OF SELECTED URINARY TRACT ABNORMALITIES DIAGNOSED IN 72 NEONATES

Abnormality	No.	% of Total
Hydronephrosis and hydroureter	27	38
Renal cystic disease	13	18
Vesicoureteric reflux	9	12
Unilateral renal agenesis or hypoplasia	5	7
Duplication of collecting system	4	6
Urethral valves	3	4
Bilateral renal agenesis	2	3
Others	9	12

Adapted from Helin and Persson (1986) and Livera and co-workers (1989).

terovesical junction, or at the urethra. The severity and location of the obstruction can be determined by assessing amnionic fluid volume as well as the distribution of any resulting urinary tract dilatation. As a general rule, fetal ureters are not visualized, thus their identification indicates hydroureter. By contrast, after 20 weeks the fetal renal pelves normally may have an anteroposterior diameter of up to 1 cm. The ratio of the anteroposterior renal pelvis diameter and kidney diameter measured in a transverse plane also has been evaluated, and a normal ratio is less than 50 percent (Arger and co-workers, 1985).

Brown and colleagues (1987) described 142 neonates evaluated for hydronephrosis over 6 years and reported that 110 were first identified by antenatal sonography. Of the fetuses diagnosed with hydronephrosis, almost 50 percent had ureteropelvic junction obstruction, 25 percent distal ureteral obstruction, 15 percent duplication of the collecting system, and 5 percent had a posterior urethral valve. Ghidini and cohorts (1990) reported results from 70 fetuses with ureteropelvic junction obstruction. Those with renal pelvis dilatation less than 1 cm uniformly did well, whereas those with dilatation more than 2 cm required postnatal pyeloplasty in three fourths of the cases. Those with dilatation of 1 to 2 cm—about half of the total—did well if the findings were bilateral; about 10 percent with unilateral dilatation of this magnitude eventually required pyeloplasty postnatally.

RENAL AGENESIS. Bilateral renal agenesis has an incidence of about 1 in 4000 births. No kidneys will be visualized sonographically at any point during gestation. Because there is no urine production, severe oligohydramnios ultimately develops. In this situation, the fetal adrenal glands appear to enlarge, and care must be taken to avoid mistaking them for kidneys (McGahan and Myracle, 1986). Death invariably follows, either in utero or shortly after birth, and the infant exhibits pulmonary hypoplasia, limb deformities, loose skin, and typical facies of the **Potter syndrome.** Associated anomalies, especially cardiac, are common.

CYSTIC RENAL DISEASE. Depending on the timing and severity of urinary obstruction, secondary cystic changes may develop in the fetal kidneys. In the extreme, this results in the formation of a classic multicystic dysplastic kidney sometimes referred to as **Potter type II.** Sonographically, the kidney is replaced by randomly oriented cysts of varying size and normal renal contour is lost. Obstruction of lesser severity or shorter duration or both may result in peripheral cysts with increased echogenicity of the renal cortex. Because the renal pelvis and ureter are preserved in the latter circumstance, prenatal differentiation from simple hydronephrosis is difficult or even impossible.

Doppler Velocimetry

Ultrasound technology has evolved from only producing images of the pregnancy to now include methods for measurement of both maternal and fetal circulatory functions. The phenomenon of *Doppler shift* of ultrasonic echoes forms the technical basis for acquisition of information on the maternal–fetal hemodynamic circulations.

Johann Christian Doppler was an Austrian physicist who taught in Prague during the mid-1800s (White, 1982). He suggested that when a sound source (for example, red blood cells in fetal umbilical circulation) is moving relative to an observer (for example, an ultrasound transducer), the perceived pitch will vary from the true pitch. In accordance with the Doppler shift principle, echoes returning from moving structures are altered in frequency and the amount of shift is directly proportional to the velocity of the moving structure. The frequencies of echoes returning from structures moving toward the transducer are higher than the frequency originally transmitted by the transducer. In contrast, the frequencies of echoes returning from structures moving away from the transducer are lower. The primary uses of these Doppler echo shifts in obstetrics have been to detect and measure blood flow. The sound of moving blood cells within the vasculature generates an effective Doppler shift which serves as the basis of Doppler velocimetry studies of maternal and fetal circulations. There are two methods of estimating circulatory hemodynamics: (1) direct measurement of the volume of blood flow, and (2) indirect estimation of flow velocity using wave form analysis.

Determination of Blood Volume Flow. Doppler-shifted sound frequencies depend on a number of factors as shown in Figure 46–9 and summarized in the following equation:

$$\text{Frequency deviation } (f_d) \text{ or shift} = 2f_o \frac{v \cos \theta}{c}.$$

In this equation, f_o is the original frequency of the ultrasound beam (in obstetrical imaging this is usually 3 to 5 MHz), v is the velocity of blood cells in the vessel studied, θ is the incident angle (angle of insonance) between the ultrasound beam and the vessel, and c is the speed of sound (in tissue, equal to 1540 m/sec). The cosine remains close to 1 as long as the angle is kept low, but at higher angles of insonance, especially those more than 60 degrees, considerable error in measurement is introduced.

The equation in Figure 46–9 includes a factor (v) for the velocity of blood in the vessel studied. To solve for v, and to thus estimate the velocity of red blood cells, the following equation is used:

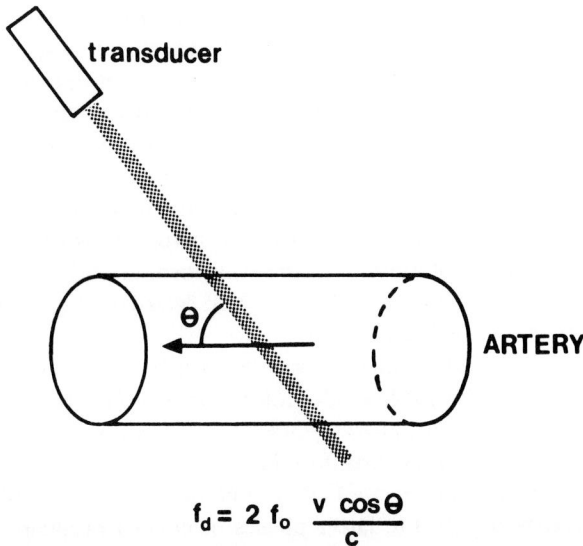

Fig. 46-9. Doppler equation: ultrasound emanating from transducer with initial frequency f_o strikes blood moving at velocity. Reflected frequency f_d is dependent on angle θ between beam of sound and vessel. (From Copel and associates, 1988.)

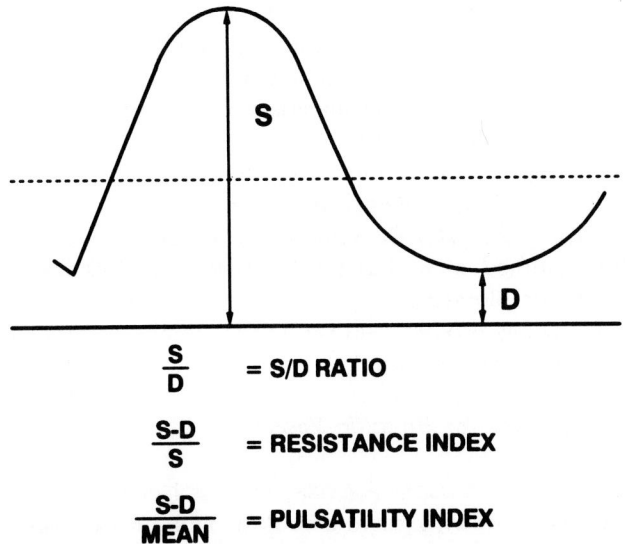

Fig. 46-10. Doppler systolic–diastolic waveform indices of blood flow velocity. S = systole. D = diastole. Mean is calculated from computer digitized waveforms. (From Low, 1991, with permission.)

$$\text{Velocity} = \frac{(f_d \times c)}{2 f_o \times \cos \theta}.$$

Because volume flow (mL/minute) is simply velocity times cross-sectional area of the blood vessel (area equals pi times the square of the radius), it is possible to calculate volume flow by measuring the blood vessel diameter using ultrasound. However, there are several technical difficulties with measurement of vessel diameters. For example, the vessels are dynamic with changing diameters during the cardiac cycle. The many technical difficulties inherent in Doppler blood volume flow measurements result in high error rates for this methodology. Estimates of error up to 15 percent have been reported with the most careful attention to methodology (Gill, 1985) and errors up to 50 percent are not uncommon (Burns, 1987). Because of these methodological problems, blood volume flow measurements have been largely abandoned in clinical applications (Low, 1991).

Waveform Analysis of Blood Velocity. From the foregoing, the errors encountered in volume flow estimation may be profound. Thus indirect indices of flow have been developed that might provide useful information about flow without engendering excessive errors. These indices are independent of the angle of insonation and do not require measurement of the diameter of the vessel.

Perhaps the most simple of these indices to compute is the systolic–diastolic ratio, or **S–D ratio** (Fig. 46–10). The maximal systolic shift is divided by the end-diastolic shift. This may be measured from the ma-

ternal uterine or fetal umbilical artery. In both vessels, the index gradually decreases as gestation progresses. Because of the low diastolic velocities seen in more central fetal vessels, such as the descending aorta, the S–D ratio is not useful elsewhere in the fetal circulation.

Similar in ease of calculation is the **Pourcelot index,** or the **resistance index** (see Fig. 46–10). To calculate this index, the difference in systolic and diastolic shifts is divided by the systolic value ([S − D]/S, also expressed as 1 − [D/S]). This ratio is also applicable only to the umbilical and the uterine arteries, and low diastolic values limit its usefulness in the fetal aorta or other central vessels.

Of the widely used indices, the most complicated to measure is the **pulsatility index** (see Fig. 46–10). It requires a digitized waveform for calculating the mean of the maximal frequencies represented. Because of the mean value in the denominator, this index can be computed using flow data from the fetal descending aorta without encountering excessive variation caused with division by small numbers as with the other two indices. Doppler arterial waveforms in nonpregnant humans are characterized by high systolic velocity and little or no diastolic velocity. Exceptions are the carotid and cerebral vessels, which have continuous diastolic blood flow seen on waveform analysis. During pregnancy, maternal and fetal vessels perfusing the placenta assume waveforms indicative of continuous diastolic flow.

Doppler waveforms of vessels have been described in a variety of ways, but all are based upon the relationship between systole and diastole. The most common measurements are some variation of the S–D ratio. These measurements are intended to relate peak flow at systole to that at end-diastole, and the ratio is calculated from the height of the systolic and diastolic peaks.

Waveforms with a high flow in diastole accompany low downstream vessel impedance. In contrast, waveforms with little diastolic flow, or reversed flow, are seen when vascular impedance downstream is abnormally high (e.g., placental insufficiency). Figure 46–11 illustrates several of the vessels in which S–D ratios have been studied, as well as the corresponding S–D waveforms for blood velocity in these vessels. Blood flow velocity has also been studied in the umbilical vein and fetal cerebral circulation.

Techniques for Specific Vessels

Uterine and Arcuate Arteries. Placental circulation is characterized by high volume flow, with an extensive diastolic component. Uterine blood flow increases from

50 mL/minute shortly after conception, to 500 to 750 mL/minute by term. Its Doppler waveform shape is unique, characterized by high diastolic velocities similar to those in systole and highly turbulent flow, with many different velocities apparent (see Fig. 46–11). With this degree of diastolic flow, indices *decrease* as term approaches—that is, diastolic velocity increases with advancing gestation. A failure of this pattern to appear or the presence of a notch in the waveform at end-systole has been reported with fetal growth retardation (Schulman and associates, 1986).

The external iliac arteries are easily identified because they do not have diastolic flow (see Fig. 46–11). For other vessels, any absence of late-diastolic flow, or reversal of flow, is considered abnormal. As mentioned, the various indices applied to umbilical artery analysis *decrease* during the latter phases of normal pregnancy (Hendricks and co-workers, 1989).

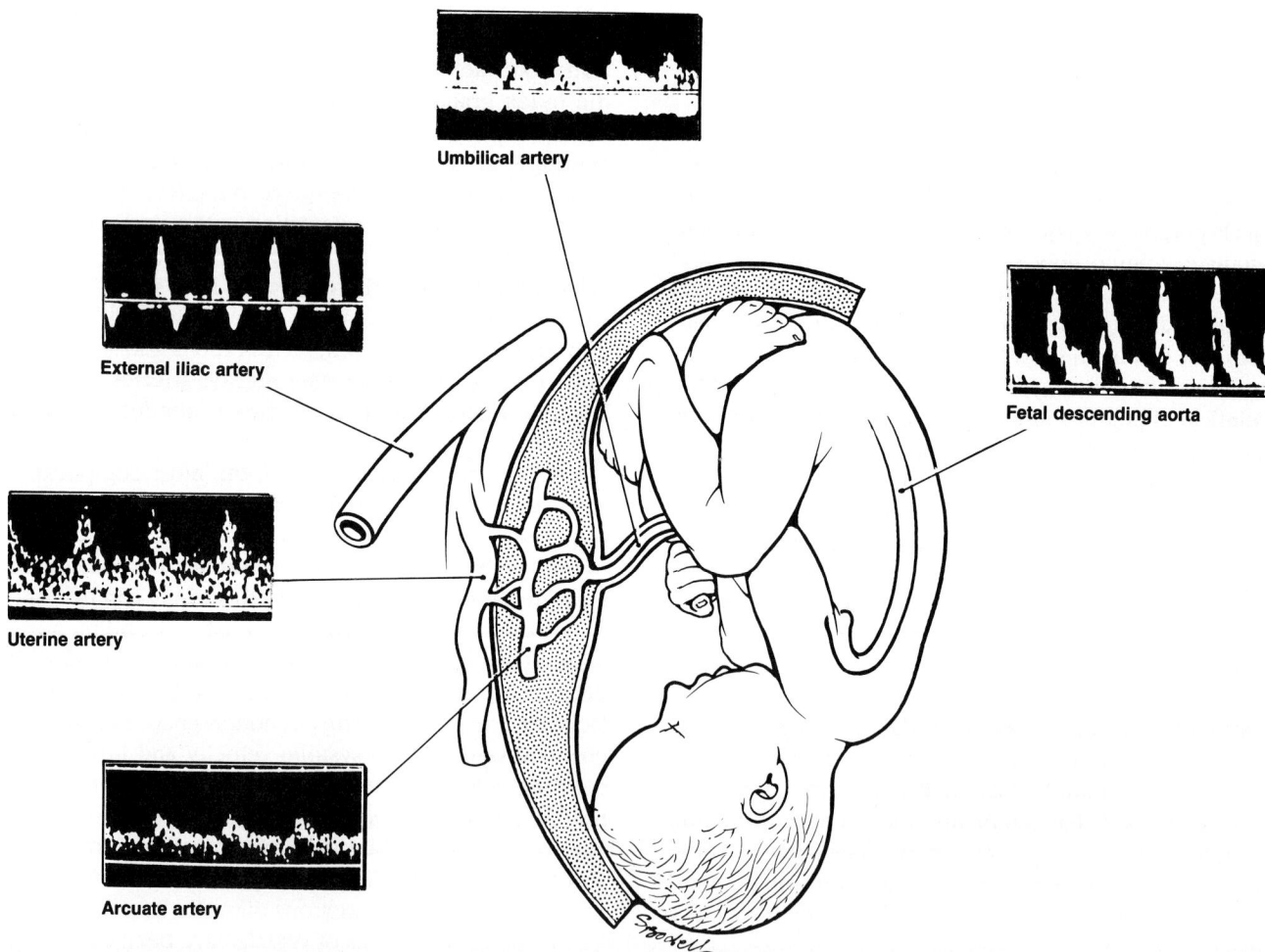

Fig. 46–11. Doppler waveforms from normal pregnancy. Shown clockwise are normal waveforms from the maternal arcuate, uterine, and external iliac arteries, and from the fetal umbilical artery and descending aorta. Reversed end-diastolic flow velocity is apparent in the external iliac artery, whereas continuous diastolic flow characterizes the uterine and arcuate vessels. Finally, note the greatly diminished end-diastolic flow in the fetal descending aorta. (From Copel and colleagues, 1988b.)

Umbilical Vein. The intra-abdominal portion of the umbilical vein is relatively straight and the flow tends to be constant rather than pulsating. Therefore, the umbilical vein is a reasonable vessel for measuring volume flow rather than indexed flow. Umbilical vein blood-flow measurements range from 108 to 153 mL/kg per minute with decreasing flows as gestation advances (Gerson and co-workers, 1987).

Fetal Descending Aorta. The fetal descending aorta receives the majority of right-ventricular output via the ductus arteriosus, while the majority of left-ventricular output supplies the fetal head and upper arms. Flow in the descending aorta is highly pulsatile, with little diastolic flow. The straight course of the aorta also makes it amenable to volume flow studies. Waveform flow measurement is limited to the pulsatility index because of the lack of diastolic flow. Measurements of fetal descending aorta blood flow range from 185 to 246 mL/kg per minute (Eik-Nes and co-workers, 1982; Griffin and associates, 1985).

Carotid Artery and Cerebral Blood Flow. Attempts have been made to measure fetal cerebral blood flow to explain why fetal head growth is spared in some forms of fetal growth retardation. If there is preferential blood flow to the brain, there should be maintenance, or even augmentation, of cerebral blood flow. Currently, the carotid arteries are the only cerebral vessels that can be identified reliably, but they are too narrow to measure accurately. Thus, preliminary findings are interpreted with caution since it is not always possible to be sure that comparable vessels are studied.

Potential Clinical Applications of Doppler Velocimetry

Applications of this technology are discussed in relation to its use in the diagnosis and management of a variety of pregnancy complications and their management is presented throughout this book.

Fetal Cardiac Function. The measurement of fetal cardiac function may have immediate clinical importance as well as research implications.

Cardiac Output. Doppler techniques that measure fetal cardiac output are extremely difficult to apply because of fetal movement and technical factors discussed above. However, with combined use of two-dimensional ultrasound and Doppler echocardiography, initial results appear promising. Reed and colleagues (1986a, 1986b) reported that mean right-ventricular output was 307 mL/kg per minute and left-ventricular output was 232 mL/kg per minute (right to left ventricular output ratio 55:45). DeSmedt and associates (1987) reported a slightly higher value for combined ventricular output.

Ductus Arteriosus. Functional applications of fetal Doppler echocardiography have been reported by Huhta and colleagues (1987). They assessed ductus arteriosus constriction in both lamb and human fetuses. Reversible ductal constriction was observed in three fetuses whose mothers received indomethacin for treatment of preterm labor. Such changes were not observed in 25 normal pregnancies.

Fetal Arrhythmias. Using a variety of techniques, fetal cardiac arrhythmias can be diagnosed and appropriately treated. In most instances these diagnostic techniques consist of two-dimensional real-time ultrasound examinations to identify cardiac anatomy and accurate placement of M-mode echocardiographic beams. M-mode echocardiography appears to be useful especially in diagnosing fetal cardiac arrhythmias and in assessing ventricular wall function. Functional outputs by atria and ventricles as well as timing of these events can be measured using pulsed-Doppler methods. Reed and associates (1987) presented evidence of improved (ventricular) cardiac output after conversion of supraventricular tachycardias to normal sinus rhythms. They also were able to confirm that the Frank–Starling mechanism (increased diastolic volume results in increased stroke volume) is operative even in the fetus!

Other Fetal Cardiac Applications. Silverman and associates (1985) used combined cardiac ultrasound examinations, cross-sectional M-mode echocardiography, and pulsed Doppler to diagnose arterioventricular valvar incompetence in fetuses with nonimmune hydrops. These workers were also able to diagnose some congenital structural cardiac anomalies that caused hydrops.

Fetal Well-being. A recurring theme in the potential practical applications of Doppler ultrasound is the search to distinguish normal from abnormal pregnancies. Of particular interest have been predictions of growth retardation, fetal hypoxia, and fetal distress. It has also been proposed that abnormal uteroplacental waveforms may identify women at risk for pregnancy-induced hypertension.

Fetal Growth Retardation. Low (1991) has reviewed prediction of fetal growth retardation using Doppler waveform analysis. Fetal aortic or umbilical artery circulations as well as uteroplacental waveforms have been studied in attempts to predict fetal growth retardation. False-positive results have been common and the test sensitivity of velocimetry has been unsatisfactory. He concluded that there is little evidence that Doppler velocimetry is useful as a screening test for fetal growth retardation. Miller and Gabert (1992) concluded that ultrasonic estimates of fetal weight were superior to Doppler velocimetry in the prediction of small-for-age fetuses.

Some investigators have used Doppler velocimetry in efforts to predict fetal hemodynamic condition in pregnancies complicated by severe erythroblastosis fetalis (Copel and associates, 1988; Rightmire and colleagues, 1986).

Fetal Distress. A test to predict fetal asphyxia before or during labor would be of great value and attempts have been made to apply Doppler velocimetry in this capacity. Unfortunately, velocimetry has not yet been proved to be a good predictor of antepartum or intrapartum fetal condition because of wide random variations in Doppler results.

Several randomized investigations on the potential clinical usefulness of Doppler velocimetry in the prediction of fetal jeopardy have been reported. Trudinger and colleagues (1987) randomized 300 complicated pregnancies and concluded that the availability of Doppler velocimetry led to better obstetrical management decisions. Tyrrell and associates (1990) randomized 250 pregnancies and concluded that neonatal outcome was improved when Doppler velocimetry was used. In contrast, Newnham and colleagues (1991) and Hofmeyr and co-workers (1991) were unable to demonstrate benefits for Doppler velocimetry in the management of a combined total of over 1400 complicated pregnancies. Davies and co-workers (1992) also reported no benefits in 2475 randomized pregnancies.

Prediction of Hypertension. It has been proposed that abnormal uteroplacental waveforms may reflect the raised vascular resistance due to maternal hypertension in the spiral arterioles that support the placental circulation (McParland and co-workers, 1990). Harretty and colleagues (1988), however, have shown that pregnancies with or without hypertension may have abnormal uteroplacental waveforms.

Summary. The first report of Doppler velocimetry in the analysis of human fetal blood flow was published in 1977 by Fitzgerald and Drumm and since then multiple studies have been reported. At present, the clinical utility of Doppler velocimetry has not been proven conclusively. It is likely that Doppler velocimetry may considerably aid investigation of perinatal pathophysiology yet not be applicable in the clinical management of individual pregnancies. Low (1991) has thoroughly reviewed the many potential applications of Doppler assessment of blood flow in pregnancy and concluded that such velocimetry should be considered investigational.

References

Adzick NS, Harrison MR, Glick PL, Nakayama DK, Manning FA, deLorimier AA: Diaphragmatic hernia in the fetus: Prenatal diagnosis and outcome in 94 cases. J Pediatr Surg 20:357, 1985

American College of Obstetricians and Gynecologists: Ultrasound imaging in pregnancy. Committee opinion, no. 96, August 1991

American Institute of Ultrasound in Medicine: Guidelines for performance of the antepartum obstetrical ultrasound examination. Rockville, MD, 1991

Arger PH, Coleman BG, Mintz MC, Snyder HP, Camardese T, Arenson RL, Gabbe SG, Aquino L: Routine fetal genitourinary tract screening. Radiology 156:485, 1985

Benacerraf BR: Fetal hydrocephalus: Diagnosis and significance. Radiology 169:858, 1988

Benacerraf BR, Adzick NS: Fetal diaphragmatic hernia: Ultrasound diagnosis and clinical outcome in 19 cases. Am J Obstet Gynecol 156:573, 1987

Benacerraf BR, Harlow B, Frigoletto F: Should amniocentesis be done for second trimester choroid plexus cysts? Abstract No. 1602, official proceedings of the 34th annual convention, American Instutite of Ultrasound in Medicine, New Orleans, March, 1990

Benacerraf BR, Pober BR, Sanders SP: Accuracy of fetal echocardiography. Radiology 165:847, 1987

Benacerraf BR, Stryker J, Frigoletto FD: Abnormal US appearance of the cerebellum (banana sign): Indirect sign of spina bifida. Radiology 171:151, 1989

Bond SJ, Harrison MR, Filly RA, Callen PW, Anderson RA, Golbus MS: Severity of intestinal damage in gastroschisis: Correlation with prenatal sonographic findings. J Pediatr Surg 23:520, 1988

British Royal College of Physicians Report: Prenatal diagnosis in genetic screening. London, Royal College of Physicians, 1989, p 14

Brown T, Mandell J, Lebowitz RL: Neonatal hydronephrosis in the era of sonography. AJR 148:959, 1987

Burns PN: Doppler flow estimations in the fetal and maternal circulations: Principles, techniques and some limitation. In Maulik D, McNellis D (eds): Reproductive and Perinatal Medicine. Doppler Ultrasound Measurement of Maternal–Fetal Hemodynamics. Ithica, NY, Perinatology Press, 1987, vol 8, p 43

Callan NA, Blakemore K, Park J, Sanders RC, Jeffs RD, Gearhart JP: Fetal genitourinary tract anomalies: Evaluation, operative correction, and follow-up. Obstet Gynecol 75:67, 1990

Cardoza JD, Filly RA, Podrasky AE: The dangling choroid plexus: A sonographic observation of value in excluding ventriculomegaly. AJR 151:767, 1988b

Cardoza JD, Goldstein RB, Filly RA: Exclusion of fetal ventriculomegaly with a single measurement: The width of the lateral ventricular atrium. Radiology 169:711, 1988a

Chambers M, Zwiebel W, Palumbos J, Ward K: Prenatal ultrasound findings in gastroschisis do not predict neonatal course. Abstract No. 508, 10th annual meeting of the Society of Perinatal Obstetricians, Houston, January, 1990

Chan L, Hixson JL, Laifer SA, Marchese SG, Martin JG, Hill LM: A sonographic and karyotypic study of second-trimester fetal choroid plexus cysts. Obstet Gynecol 73:703, 1989

Chervenak FA, Berkowitz RL, Romero R, Tortora M, Mayden K, Duncan C, Mahoney MJ, Hobbins JC: The diagnosis of fetal hydrocephalus. Am J Obstet Gynecol 147:703, 1983

Chinn D, Worthy L, Towers C, Miller E: Fetal choroid plexus cysts: Incidence and prediction of trisomy 18. Abstract No. 1621, official proceedings of the 34th annual convention of the American Institute of Ultrasound in Medicine, New Orleans, March, 1990

Chitkara U, Cogswell C, Norton K, Wilkins IA, Mehalek K, Berkowitz RL: Choroid plexus cysts in the fetus: A benign anatomic variant or pathologic entity? Report of 41 cases and review of the literature. Obstet Gynecol 72:185, 1988

Comstock CH: Normal fetal heart axis and position. Obstet Gynecol 70:255, 1987

Copel JA, Cullen M, Green JJ, Mahoney MJ, Hobbins JC, Kleinman CS: The frequency of aneuploidy in prenatally diagnosed congenital heart disease: An indication for fetal karyotyping. Am J Obstet Gynecol 158:409, 1988a

Copel JA, Grannum PA, Hobbins JC, Cunningham FG: Doppler ultrasound in obstetrics. Williams Obstetrics, 17th ed (suppl 16). Norwalk, CT, Appleton & Lange, 1988b

Copel JA, Pilu G, Green J, Hobbins JC, Kleinman CS: Fetal echocardiographic screening for congenital heart disease: The importance of the four-chamber view. Am J Obstet Gynecol 157:648, 1987

Copel JA, Pilu G, Kleinman CS: Congenital heart disease and extracardiac anomalies: Associations and indications for fetal echocardiography. Am J Obstet Gynecol 154:1121, 1986

Crawford DC, Chita SK, Allan LD: Prenatal detection of congenital heart disease: Factors affecting obstetric management and survival. Am J Obstet Gynecol 159:352, 1988

Crowley P, O'Herlihy C, Boylan P: The value of ultrasound measurement of amniotic fluid volume on the management of prolonged pregnancies. Br J Obstet Gynaecol 91:444, 1984

Curtis JA, Watson l: Sonographic diagnosis of omphalocele in the first trimester of fetal gestation. J Ultrasound Med 7:97, 1988

Davies JA, Gallivan S, Spencer JA: Randomized controlled trial of Doppler ultrasound screening of placental perfusion during pregnancy. Lancet 340:1299, 1992

deSmedt MCH, Visser GHA, Meijboom EJ: Fetal cardiac output estimated by Doppler echocardiography during mid- and late gestation. Am J Cardiol 60:338, 1987

DeVore GR, Donnerstein RL, Kleinman CS, Platt LD, Hobbins JC: Fetal echocardiography, I. Normal anatomy as determined by real-time-directed M-mode ultrasound. Am J Obstet Gynecol 144:249, 1982

DeVore GR, Horenstein J, Siassi B, Platt LD: Fetal echocardiography, VII. Doppler color flow mapping: A new technique for the diagnosis of congenital heart disease. Am J Obstet Gynecol 156:1054, 1987

Donald I, MacVicar J, Brown TG: Investigation of abdominal masses by pulsed ultrasound. Lancet 7032:1188, 1958

Eik-Nes SH, Marsal K, Brubakk AO, Kristofferson K, Ulstein M: Ultrasonic measurement of human fetal blood flow. J Biomed Eng 4:28, 1982

Ewigman B, LeFevre M, Hessler J: A randomized trial of routine prenatal ultrasound. Obstet Gynecol 76:189, 1990

Filly RA, Cardoza JD, Goldstein RB, Barkovich AJ: Detection of fetal central nervous system anomalies: A practical level of effort for a routine sonogram. Radiology 172:403, 1989

Fitzgerald DE, Drumm JE: Noninvasive measurement of human fetal circulation using ultrasound. A new method. BMJ 2:1450, 1977

Gerson AG, Wallace DM, Stiller RJ, Paul D, Weiner S, Bolognese RJ: Doppler evaluation of umbilical venous and arterial flow in the second and third trimester of normal pregnancy. Obstet Gynecol 70:672, 1987

Ghidini A, Sirtori M, Bergani P, Orsenigo E, Tagliabue P, Parravicini E: Ureteropelvic junction obstruction in utero and ex utero. Obstet Gynecol 75:805, 1990

Gill RW: Measurement of blood flow by ultrasound accuracy and source of error. Ultrasound Med Biol 11:625, 1985

Goldstein I, Reece EA, Pilu G, Bovicelli L, Hobbins JC: Cerebellar measurements with ultrasonography in the evaluation of fetal growth and development. Am J Obstet Gynecol 156:1065, 1987

Goldstein RB, Filly RA: Prenatal diagnosis of anencephaly: Spectrum of sonographic appearances and distinction from the amniotic band syndrome. AJR 151:547, 1988

Goldstein RB, Podrasky AE, Filly RA, Callen PW: Effacement of the fetal cisterna magna in association with myelomeningocele. Radiology 172:409, 1989

Grannum P, Bracken M, Silverman R, Hobbins JC: Assessment of fetal kidney size in normal gestation by comparison of ratio of kidney circumference to abdominal circumference. Am J Obstet Gynecol 136:249, 1980

Green JJ, Hobbins JC: Abdominal ultrasound examination of the first-trimester fetus. Am J Obstet Gynecol 159:165, 1988

Griffin DR, Teague MJ, Tallet P, Wilson K, Bilardo C, Massin L, Campbell S: A combination ultrasonic linear array scanner and pulsed Doppler velocimeter for the estimation of blood flow in the foetus and adult abdomen, II. Clinical evaluation. Ultrasound Med Biol 11:37, 1985

Hadlock FP, Deter RL, Harrist RB, Park SK: Estimating fetal age: Computer-assisted analysis of multiple fetal growth parameters. Radiology 152:497, 1984

Harretty KP, Whittle MJ, Rubin PC: Doppler uteroplacental waveforms in pregnancy-induced hypertension: A reappraisal. Lancet 1:850, 1988

Harrison MR, Langer JC, Adzick NS, Golbus MS, Filly RA, Anderson RL, Rosen MA, Callen PW, Goldstein RB, deLorimier AA: Correction of congenital diaphragmatic hernia in utero, V. Initial clinical experience. J Pediatr Surg 25:47, 1990

Helin I, Persson PH: Prenatal diagnosis of urinary tract abnormalities by ultrasound. Pediatrics 78:879, 1986

Hendricks SK, Sorensen TK, Wang KY, Breshnell JM, Seguin EM, Zingheim RW: Doppler umbilical artery waveform indices—Normal values from fourteen to forty-two vessels. Am J Obstet Gynecol 161:761, 1989

Hoffman JIE, Christianson R: Congenital heart disease in a cohort of 19,502 births with long-term follow-up. Am J Cardiol 42:641, 1978

Hofmeyr GJ, Pattinson R, Buckley D, Jennings J, Redmon CWG: Umbilical artery resistance index as a screening test for fetal well-being, II. Randomized feasibility study. Obstet Gynecol 78:359, 1991

Hoyme HE, Higginbottom MC, Jones KL: The vascular pathogenesis of gastroschisis: Intrauterine interruption of the omphalomesenteric artery. J Pediatr 98:228, 1981

Hughes MD, Nyberg DA, Mack LA, Pretorius DH: Fetal omphalocele: Prenatal US detection of concurrent anomalies and other predictors of outcome. Radiology 173:371, 1989

Huhta JC, Moise KJ, Fisher DJ, Sharif Ds, Wasserstrum N, Martin C: Detection and quantitation of constriction of the fetal ductus arteriosus by Doppler echocardiography. Circulation 75:406, 1987

Jeanty P: Fetal biometry. In Fleischer AC, Romero R, Manning FA, Jeanty PJ, James AE (eds): The Principles and Practice of

Ultrasonography in Obstetrics and Gynecology, 4th ed. Norwalk, CT, Appleton & Lange, 1991, p 93

Kemppaineu AS, Karjalaineu O, Ylostalo P, Heinoneu OP: Ultrasound screening and perinatal mortality: Controlled trial of systematic one-stage screening in pregnancy. Lancet 336:387, 1990

Kushnir O, Izquierdo L, Vigil D, Curet LB: Early transvaginal sonographic diagnosis of gastroschisis. J Clin Ultrasound 18:194, 1990

Lenke RR, Persutte WH, Weaver M: Ultrasonographic assessment of intestinal damage in fetuses with gastroschisis; is it of clinical value? Abstract No. 376, 10th annual meeting of the Society of Perinatal Obstetricians, Houston, January, 1990

Levi CS, Lyons EA, Lindsay DJ: Ultrasound in the first trimester of pregnancy. Radiol Clin North Am 28:19, 1990

Livera LN, Brookfield DSK, Egginton JA, Hawnaur JM: Antenatal ultrasonography to detect fetal renal abnormalities: A prospective screening programme. BMJ 298:1421, 1989

Low JA: The current status of maternal and fetal blood flow velocimetry. Am J Obstet Gynecol 164:1049, 1991

Lowe TW, Peters MT, Twickler D, Cunningham FG: Obstetrical sonography update, 1990. Williams Obstetrics, 18th ed (suppl 6). Norwalk, CT, Appleton & Lange, 1990

Luck CA: Value of routine ultrasound scanning at 19 weeks: A four-year study of 8,849 deliveries. BMJ 304:1474, 1992

Mabogunje OA, Mahour GH: Omphalocele and gastroschisis: Trends and survival across two decades. Am J Surg 148:679, 1984

Mahony BS, Nyberg DA, Hirsch JH, Petty CN, Hendricks SK, Mack LA: Mild idiopathic lateral cerebral ventricular dilatation in utero: Sonographic evaluation. Radiology 169:715, 1988

Manning FA, Platt LD, Sipos L: Antepartum fetal evaluation: Development of a fetal biophysical profile. Am J Obstet Gynecol 136:787, 1980

McGahan JP, Myracle MR: Adrenal hypertrophy: Possible pitfall in the sonographic diagnosis of renal agenesis. J Ultrasound Med 5:265, 1986

McParland P, Pearce JM, Chamberlain GVP: Doppler ultrasound and aspirin in recognition and prevention of pregnancy-induced hypertension. Lancet 335:1552, 1990

Miller JM, Gabert HA: Comparison of dynamic image and pulsed Doppler ultrasonography for the diagnosis of the small-for-gestational-age fetus. Am J Obstet Gynecol 166:1870, 1992

Mitchell SC, Korones SB, Berendes HW: Congenital heart disease in 56,109 births: Incidence and natural history. Circulation 43:323, 1971

Moore TR, Cayle JE: Amnionic fluid index in normal human pregnancy. Am J Obstet Gynecol 162:1168, 1990

National Center for Health Statistics: Advance report of new data from the 1989 birth certificate. In U.S. Public Health Service: Monthly Vital Statistics Report, Publication no. (PHS) 92-1120, Vol. 40, no. 12(S), April 1992, p 1

National Institutes of Health: Diagnostic ultrasound imaging in pregnancy, 1984. U.S. Department of Health and Human Services: No. 84-667, 1984

Newnham JP, O'Dea MR, Reid KP, Diepeveen DA: Doppler low velocimetry waveform analysis in high risk pregnancies: A randomized controlled trial. Br J Obstet Gynaecol 98:956, 1991

Nicolaides KH, Rodeck CH, Gosden CM: Rapid karyotyping in non-lethal fetal malformations. Lancet 1:283, 1986

Nyberg DA: Recommendations for obstetric sonography in the evaluation of the fetal cranium. Radiology 172:309, 1989

Nyberg DA, Fitzsimmons J, Mack LA, Hughes M, Pretorius DH, Hickok D, Shepard TH: Chromosomal abnormalities in fetuses with omphalocele: Significance of omphalocele contents. J Ultrasound Med 8:299, 1989

Nyberg DA, Mack LA, Hirsch J, Mahony BS: Abnormalities of fetal cranial contour in sonographic detection of spina bifida: Evaluation of the "lemon" sign. Radiology 167:387, 1988a

Nyberg DA, Mack LA, Hirsch J, Pagon RO, Shepard TH: Fetal hydrocephalus: Sonographic and clinical significance of associated anomalies. Radiology 163:187, 1987a

Nyberg DA, Mack LA, Laing FC, Jeffrey RB: Early pregnancy complications: Endovaginal sonographic findings correlated with human chorionic gonadotropin levels. Radiology 167:619, 1988b

Nyberg DA, Mack LA, Patten RM, Cyr DR: Fetal bowel—Normal sonographic findings. J Ultrasound Med 6:3, 1987b

Patten RM, Mack LA, Wang KY, Cyr DR: The fetal genitourinary tract. Radiol Clin North Am 28:115, 1990

Perone N: A practical guide to fetal echocardiography. Contemp Obstet Gynecol 1:55, 1988

Phelan JP, Ahn MO, Smith CV, Rutherford SE, Anderson E: Amnionic fluid index measurements during pregnancy. J Reprod Med 32:601, 1987

Phelan JP, Platt LD, Yeh SY, Broussard P, Paul RH: The role of ultrasound assessment of amniotic fluid volume in the management of the post date pregnancy. Am J Obstet Gynecol 151:304, 1985

Pretorius DH, Davis K, Manco-Johnson ML, Manchester D, Meier PR, Clewell WH: Clinical course of fetal hydrocephalus: 40 cases. AJNR 6:23, 1985

Pretorius DH, Drose JA, Dennis MA, Manchester DK, Manco-Johnson ML: Tracheoesophageal fistula in utero: Twenty-two cases. J Ultrasound Med 6:509, 1987

Pretorius DH, Gosink BB, Clautice-Engle T, Leopold GR, Minnick CM: Sonographic evaluation of the fetal stomach: Significance of nonvisualization. AJR 151:987, 1988

Pritchard JA: Deglutition by normal and anencephalic fetuses. Obstet Gynecol 25:289, 1965

Rabinowitz R, Peters MT, Vyas S, Campbell S, Nicolaides KH: Measurement of fetal urine production in normal pregnancy by real-time ultrasonography. Am J Obstet Gynecol 161:1264, 1989

Read JL, Stern RS, Thibudeau LA, Geer DE, Klapholz H: Variation in antenatal testing over time and between clinic settings. JAMA 249:1605, 1983

Reece EA, Assimakopoulos E, Zheng XZ, Hagay Z, Hobbins JC: The safety of obstetric ultrasonography: Concern for the fetus. Obstet Gynecol 76:139, 1990

Reed KL, Meijboom EJ, Sahn DJ, Scagnelli SA, Valdez-Cruz LM, Shenker L: Cardiac Doppler flow velocities in human fetuses. Circulation 73:41, 1986a

Reed KL, Sahn DJ, Marx GR, Anderson CF, Shenker L: Cardiac Doppler flow during fetal arrhythmias: Physiological consequences. Obstet Gynecol 70:1, 1987

Reed KL, Sahn DJ, Scagnelli S, Anderson CF, Shenker L: Doppler echocardiographic studies of diastolic function in the human fetal heart: Changes during gestation. J Am Coll Cardiol 8:391, 1986b

Rightmire DA, Nicolaides KH, Rodeck CH, Campbell S: Fetal blood velocities in Rh isoimmunization: Relationship to gestational age and to fetal hematocrit. Obstet Gynecol 68:233, 1986

Roberts CJ, Hibbard BM, Roberts EE, Evans KT, Laurence KM, Robertson IB: Diagnostic effectiveness of ultrasound in detection of neural tube defect. Lancet 2:1068, 1983

Robinson HP, Fleming JEE: A critical evaluation of sonar crown–rump length measurements. Br J Obstet Gynaecol 82:702, 1975

Romero R, Ghidini A, Costigan K, Touloukian R, Hobbins JC: Prenatal diagnosis of duodenal atresia: Does it make any difference? Obstet Gynecol 71:739, 1988b

Romero R, Pilu G, Jeanty P, Ghidini A, Hobbins JC: Prenatal Diagnosis of Congenital Anomalies. Norwalk, CT, Appleton & Lange, 1988a, p 211

Sagi J, Vagman I, David MP, Van Dongen LGR, Goudie E, Butterworth A, Jacobson MJ: Fetal kidney size related to gestational age. Gynecol Obstet Invest 23:1, 1987

Schulman H, Fleischer A, Farmakides G, Bracero L, Rochelson B, Grunfeld L: Development of uterine artery compliance in pregnancy as detected by Doppler ultrasound. Am J Obstet Gynecol 155:1031, 1986

Secher NJ, Kern Hansen P, Lenstrup C, Eriksen PS, Morsing G: A randomized study of fetal abdominal diameter and fetal weight estimation for detection of light-for-gestation infants in low-risk pregnancies. Br J Obstet Gynaecol 94:105, 1987

Shenker L, Reed KL, Marx GR, Donnerstein RL, Allen HD, Anderson CF: Fetal cardiac Doppler flow studies in prenatal diagnosis of heart disease. Am J Obstet Gynecol 158:1267, 1988

Shepard NJ, Richards VA, Berkowitz FL, Warsof SL, Hobbins JC: An evaluation of two equations for predicting fetal weight by ultrasound. Am J Obstet Gynecol 142:47, 1982

Silverman NH, Kleinman CS, Rudolph AM, Copel JA, Weinstein EM, Enderlein MA, Golbus M: Fetal atrioventricular valve insufficiency associated with non-immune hydrops: A two-dimensional echocardiographic and pulsed Doppler ultrasound study. Circulation 72:825, 1985

Sivit CJ, Hill MC, Larsen JW, Kent SG, Lande IM: The sonographic evaluation of fetal anomalies in oligohydramnios between 16 and 30 weeks gestation. AJR 146:1277, 1986

Thacker SB: Quality of controlled clinical trials. The case of imaging ultrasound in obstetrics: A review. Br J Obstet Gynaecol 92:437, 1985

Timor-Tritsch IE, Monteagudo A, Peisner DB: High frequency transvaginal sonographic examination and malformation workup of the 9–14 week fetus. Abstract No. 374, 10th annual meeting of the Society of Perinatal Obstetricians, Houston, January, 1990

Trudinger BJ, Cook CM, Giles WB, Connelly A, Thompson RS: Umbilical artery flow velocity waveforms in high-risk pregnancy. Randomized controlled trial. Lancet 1:188, 1987

Tyrrell SW, Lilford RJ, MacDonald HN, Nelson EJ, Porter J, Gupta JK: Randomized comparison of routine vs highly selective use of Doppler ultrasound and biophysical scoring to investigate high risk pregnancies. Br J Obstet Gynaecol 97:909, 1990

Van den Hof MC, Nicolaides KH, Campbell J, Campbell S: Evaluation of the lemon and banana signs in one hundred thirty fetuses with open spina bifida. Am J Obstet Gynecol 162:322, 1990

Wagner M: Ultrasound evaluation. Mod Health April 6, 1992, p 26

Waldenstrom U, Nilsson S, Fall O, Axelsson O, Eklund G, Lindeberg S, Sjodin Y: Effects of routine one-stage ultrasound screening in pregnancy: A randomized controlled trial. Lancet 2:585, 1988

White DN: Johann Christian Doppler and his effect. Ultrasound Med Biol 8:853, 1982

Medical and Surgical Complications in Pregnancy

■

CHAPTER 47
Critical Care and Trauma

A wealth of information and technology that has been developed over the past 25 years has resulted in the evolution of the concept of *critical care obstetrics*. Women with a broad spectrum of pathophysiological conditions, some of which may have previously precluded pregnancy, may be benefitted by technology and expertise in critical care obstetrics. Examples include women with structural cardiac lesions or prosthetic heart valves causing them to be classified with functional class III or IV heart disease, women with acute or chronic pulmonary injuries, or those with complications of severe preeclampsia or septic shock syndrome. Moreover, the pregnant woman is not spared multiple causes of trauma, including automobile accidents and aggravated and sexual assaults, which may include gunshot and knife wounds. Because the pregnant woman and her fetus have unique considerations for critical care, it is imperative that obstetricians have a working knowledge of some of these concepts.

Basic Considerations. The most practical, efficient, and economical means of caring for the critically ill obstetrical patient who requires invasive monitoring or ventilatory support will depend upon the number of pregnant women cared for at a particular facility, including those referred. While a few clinical services have a sufficient volume and acuity of such patients, most encounter fewer than 20 such women per year. Accordingly, arrangements are needed to either care for these women in surgical or medical intensive care units or to have specialized rooms designated in the obstetrical suite where necessary equipment is readily available to provide appropriate care.

The type of unit necessarily will be reflected by the medical, surgical, or obstetrical conditions of women admitted. For example, Mabie and Sibai (1990) reported that 0.9 percent of women delivered at their hospital in Memphis were admitted to the obstetrical intensive care unit. Kilpatrick and Matthay (1992) reported that only 0.4 percent of obstetrical patients were transferred to the medical–surgical intensive care unit at the University of California, San Francisco. With appropriate development, either type of unit should be satisfactory for care of the critically ill pregnant women (Kirshon and colleagues, 1990).

For the woman who is undelivered, ideal care is best provided by specially trained obstetricians and obstetrical nurses with extensive knowledge and experience in critical care medicine. In their absence, a team of physicians and nurses is assembled to include those with special expertise sufficient to deal with all problem areas. Physician members of the team include obstetricians, anesthesiologists, pulmonologists, cardiologists, and intensivists. Whereas the obstetrical team may be intimidated somewhat by ventilators, pulmonary artery catheters, pressure transducers, and alarms, the intensive care team is equally intimidated by the large uterus, the fetus, and fetal monitors! Even in circumstances in which a primary obstetrical intensive care unit is in operation, consultation with other medical and surgical specialists may be necessary.

Use of data flow sheets common to intensive care units is encouraged. These facilitate quick assessment of the woman's condition. Key components of such flow sheets include assessment of hemodynamic parameters, ventilator settings, blood gas analyses, temperature, medications, intake and output (to include specific fluids infused), and daily weight.

Patient care standards that have been established for both obstetrical as well as intensive care areas must be met. Proper equipment is a basic prerequisite. Any equipment that may be needed in the obstetrical suite also may be needed in the intensive care unit. Standard critical care equipment also is necessary. Provisions must be made for initial neonatal resuscitation and stabilization.

Application of Invasive Technologies

Pulmonary Artery Catheter. Development of the flow-directed pulmonary artery catheter (Fig. 47–1) transformed an instrument that previously had been limited to cardiac catheterization and research laboratories into a clinical bedside instrument to monitor continuously cardiovascular status and function (Swan and associates, 1970). Information obtained from its use may facilitate diagnosis, management, and evaluation of therapeutic decisions. Indications for the use of invasive hemodynamic monitoring are principally the same in obstetrics as in other areas of medicine, and it is reasonable to expect that similar results can be gained from its use in pregnant women.

Pulmonary artery catheterization has been used to diagnose or manage a number of cardiac complications complicating pregnancy, including myocardial infarction, cardiomyopathy, and mitral stenosis (Clark and associates, 1985b, Cunningham and colleagues, 1986; Hankins and colleagues, 1985), adult respiratory distress syndrome, (Cunningham and co-workers, 1987), amnionic fluid embolism (Clark and colleagues, 1985a), and severe preeclampsia–eclampsia (Clark and colleagues, 1988; Hankins and co-workers, 1984). Perhaps even more importantly, understanding of the pathophysiology of these as well as other conditions unique to obstetrics has been advanced significantly by invasive monitoring. Examples include pulmonary edema associated with the use of β-agonists and the hemodynamic alterations of preeclampsia–eclampsia. Ironically, with improved understanding of this pathophysiology, the need for invasive monitoring is reduced.

The decision to use invasive monitoring includes an assessment of the personnel to insert the catheter and availability of support staff for equipment maintenance. Some indications are shown in Table 47–1.

VENOUS ACCESS. Invasive monitoring is usually initiated through the internal or external jugular vein or the

TABLE 47–1. SOME INDICATIONS FOR INVASIVE HEMODYNAMIC MONITORING

Sepsis with refractory hypotension or oliguria
Unexplained or refractory pulmonary edema, heart failure, or oliguria
Severe pregnancy-induced hypertension with persistent pulmonary edema or oliguria
Unexplained intraoperative or intrapartum cardiovascular decompensation
Selected cases with massive blood and volume loss or replacement
Adult respiratory distress syndrome
Persistent shock of undefined etiology
Some chronic conditions, particularly when associated with labor or major surgery:
   NYHA[a] class III or IV cardiac disease
   Peripartum or perioperative coronary artery disease

[a] NYHA = New York Heart Association.
Modified after American College of Obstetricians and Gynecologists (1992).

subclavian vein. The femoral and antecubital veins are used less frequently because of greater difficulty in positioning the catheter. However, in the woman with a coagulopathy, the antecubital approach may be prudent. Use of the inguinal area in pregnant women may limit access and catheter manipulation at critical times, such as during delivery.

Arterial Lines. Intra-arterial lines are frequently used for critically ill patients because they allow continuous monitoring of systemic blood pressure as well as easy access to arterial blood samples. The latter is important if sequential blood gas and pH determinations are anticipated.

Data Collection. Continuous central venous and pulmonary artery pressures and intermittent pulmonary capillary wedge pressure measurements are obtained by the pulmonary artery catheter. Cardiac output can be measured by the thermodilution technique. Both heart rate and rhythm are observed and may be recorded through continuous electrocardiographic monitoring. Systemic arterial pressure can be measured noninvasively by manual or automatic sphygmomanometers or by arterial catheterization.

Several mean pressures are measured: filling pressures include central venous and pulmonary capillary

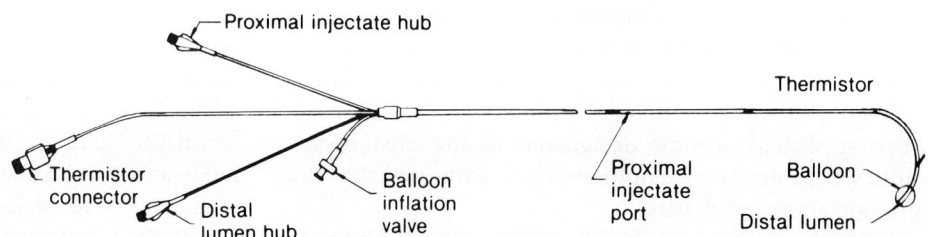

Fig. 47–1. The pulmonary artery catheter. (From Clark and colleagues, 1991, with permission.)

Proximal injectate hub

Thermistor

Thermistor connector

Distal lumen hub

Balloon inflation valve

Proximal injectate port

Balloon

Distal lumen

wedge pressures; arterial pressures are those of the pulmonary and systemic circulations. These can be determined by electronic dampening or they can be calculated (Table 47–2). Various other hemodynamic values that reflect cardiac function and vascular resistance can be calculated or derived. **Stroke volume** is a measure of the amount of blood pumped per cardiac contraction. Both cardiac output and stroke volume may be corrected for body size by division of the values by body surface area to obtain **cardiac index** and **stroke index.** Body surface area nomograms have not been developed for pregnant women, thus adult nomograms are used. Resistance to flow can be calculated from right and left ventricles through determinations of the pulmonary and systemic vascular resistance. Clark and colleagues (1989) have reported normal hemodynamic parameters for healthy nonpregnant and pregnant women, as shown in Table 47–3.

Data Interpretation. Cardiac function is assessed in four areas: (1) preload, (2) afterload, (3) inotropic state, and (4) heart rate.

Preload is determined by intraventricular pressure and volume, thus setting the initial myocardial muscle fiber length. Clinically, the right and left ventricular end-diastolic filling pressures are assessed by central venous pressure and pulmonary capillary wedge pressure, respectively. Cardiac output plotted against central venous or pulmonary capillary wedge pressure constructs a cardiac function curve for the respective ventricle. The ventricular function curve demonstrates that a failing heart requires a higher preload or filling

TABLE 47–3. CENTRAL HEMODYNAMIC CHANGES INDUCED BY PREGNANCY

Measurement	Non-pregnant	Term Pregnant	Change (%)
Cardiac output (L/min)	4.3 ± 0.9	6.2 ± 1.0	+ 44
Heart rate (beats/min)	71 ± 10.0	83 ± 10.0	+ 17
Mean arterial pressure (mm Hg)	86.4 ± 7.5	90.3 ± 5.8	+ 4
Systemic vascular resistance (dyne × cm × sec^{-5})	1530 ± 520	1210 ± 266	− 21
Pulmonary vascular resistance (dyne × cm × sec^{-5})	119 ± 47.0	78 ± 22	− 35
Pulmonary capillary wedge pressure (mm Hg)	6.3 ± 2.1	7.5 ± 1.8	+ 18
Central venous pressure (mm Hg)	3.7 ± 2.6	3.6 ± 2.5	− 2
Left ventricular stroke work index (g × m × m^{-2})	41 ± 8	48 ± 6	+ 17
Colloid oncotic pressure (mm Hg)	20.8 ± 1.0	18.0 ± 1.5	− 14
Colloid oncotic/wedge pressure gradient (mm Hg)	14.5 ± 2.5	10.5 ± 2.7	− 28

From Clark and colleagues (1989), with permission.

pressure to achieve the same cardiac output as a normally functioning heart (Fig. 47–2). Therapeutic manipulation of ventricular filling pressures and simultaneous measurement of cardiac output allows calculation of optimal preload at the bedside. Preload can be increased

TABLE 47–2. FORMULAS FOR DERIVING VARIOUS CARDIOPULMONARY PARAMETERS

Mean pressure (mm Hg) = [Systolic pressure + 2 (diastolic pressure)] ÷ 3

Stroke index (SI) (mL/beat/m^2) = stroke volume/BSA

Pulmonary vascular resistance (PVR) (dynes × sec × cm^{-5}) = [(MPAP − PCWP)/CO] × 80

Stroke volume (SV) (mL/beat) = CO/HR

Cardiac index (CI) (L/min/m^2) = CO/BSA

Systemic vascular resistance (SVR) (dynes × sec × cm^{-5}) = [(MAP − CVP)/CO] × 80

Oxygen content: arterial or mixed venous = [(Hb–g%) (1.39) (%Sat) + PaO$_2$ × .0031)]

Oxygen delivery = CO[(Hb–g%) (1.39) (%Sat) + (PaO$_2$ × .0031)]

Lung compliance:

$$\text{Static} = \frac{\text{tidal volume}}{\text{plateau inspiratory pressure}}$$

$$\text{Dynamic} = \frac{\text{tidal volume}}{\text{peak inspiratory pressure}}$$

BSA = body surface area (m^2); CO = cardiac output (L/min); CVP = central venous pressure (mm Hg); HR = heart rate (beats/min); MAP = mean systemic arterial pressure (mm Hg); MPAP = mean pulmonary artery pressure (mm Hg); PCWP = mean pulmonary capillary wedge pressure (mm Hg); Hb–g% = hemoglobin, gram percentage; %Sat = percentage of saturation; PaO$_2$ = arterial pressure of oxygen (mm Hg).

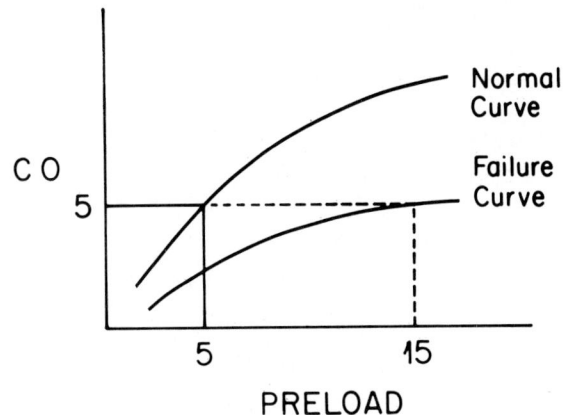

Fig. 47–2. Ventricular function (Starling) curve for the normal heart and the heart in failure. Pulmonary capillary wedge pressure or central venous pressure represents fiber length, and cardiac output (CO) represents fiber shortening. To maintain cardiac output, the failing heart is required to function at higher preloads measured by pulmonary capillary wedge and central venous pressures. In this example, a preload of 15 mm Hg is required by the failing heart to achieve the same cardiac output that the normal heart could at a preload of 5 mm Hg. (Adapted from Hankins and associates, 1983, with permission.)

by the administration of crystalloid, colloid, or blood, and it can be decreased by the use of a diuretic, a vasodilator, or by phlebotomy.

Afterload is defined as ventricular wall tension during systole and is dependent on end-diastolic ventricular radius, aortic diastolic pressure, and ventricular wall thickness. The extent to which right or left intraventricular pressures rise during systole depends primarily on the pulmonary or systemic vascular resistance (Fig. 47–3). With heart failure, afterload increases worsen failure by decreasing both stroke volume and cardiac output. Afterload, like preload, can be increased or decreased therapeutically. Increases are mediated through α-adrenergic stimulation, for example, with phenylephrine. Decreases in afterload or systemic vascular resistance can be achieved with numerous agents. Sodium nitroprusside by continuous intravenous infusion is commonly used in medical intensive care units, whereas hydralazine is used most commonly in obstetrics. The intermittent intravenous administration of small incremental doses of hydralazine, without continuous arterial pressure monitoring, has been proven safe for both mother and fetus.

The **inotropic** state of the heart is defined as the force and velocity of ventricular contractions when preload and afterload are held constant. In low-output cardiac failure, both preload and afterload should be optimized through therapeutic manipulation. If this fails to restore cardiac output to an acceptable level, attention should be directed to improving myocardial contractility. Beta-agonists such as dopamine, dobutamine, and isoproterenol are effective in improving cardiac output acutely. Digitalis may be used either short-term or long-term.

Heart rate is important, and may cause problems if too fast or too slow. Cardiac output can be compromised if the rate is too slow. In this circumstance, either treatment with atropine or cardiac pacing is indicated. Conversely, sustained tachycardia can lead to congestive heart failure because of shortened systolic ejection and diastolic filling times or myocardial ischemia, especially with valvar heart disease (Clark and colleagues, 1985b). The pathophysiological basis of tachycardia should be determined and corrected; common causes include fever, hypovolemia, and pain.

Efficacy of Invasive Hemodynamic Monitoring. Although the pulmonary artery catheter gained widespread acceptance and use in medicine and surgery in the mid-1970s and in obstetrics in the mid-1980s, studies demonstrating its effect to improve patient outcome significantly or to reduce mortality are lacking. Tuchschmidt and Sharma (1987) reported observations from a medical intensive care unit and found in only one third of patients that data collected from the catheter actually was used to alter treatment. Bush and colleagues (1989) found that the pulmonary artery catheter was associated with a higher mortality rate than that of controls matched to the same level of illness by acuity score (APACHE II score). Similar results were reported by Gore and associates (1987) among a large series of patients with verified acute myocardial infarctions. To date no similar studies comparing results in pregnant women with and without the use of these technologies exist.

Admission to the intensive care unit is itself a bad prognostic sign. It has been demonstrated that with single-organ system failure necessitating a one-day stay in the intensive care unit that mortality is about 50 percent. Mortality becomes progressively higher with each additional organ system failure. For example, in the patient with pulmonary and renal failure, the mortality is 90 percent. Among patients with three organ systems in failure for three days, mortality exceeds 99 percent. Given these odds, it is not surprising that any technology or medication will be associated with a high failure rate.

Complications of Invasive Hemodynamic Monitoring. Important risks of invasive monitoring concern overinterpreting or misinterpreting data. Other complications are summarized in Table 47–4. Although most complications arise from gaining venous access and can be reduced by attention to detail and experience, there remains a minimal risk inherent to any invasive monitoring.

Peripheral arterial cannulation may be complicated by hematoma, infection, and vessel thrombosis. Serious complications from use of arterial lines, such as gangrene and loss of a digit or extremity, develop in less than 1 percent of cases.

Whereas complications as the result of attempts to

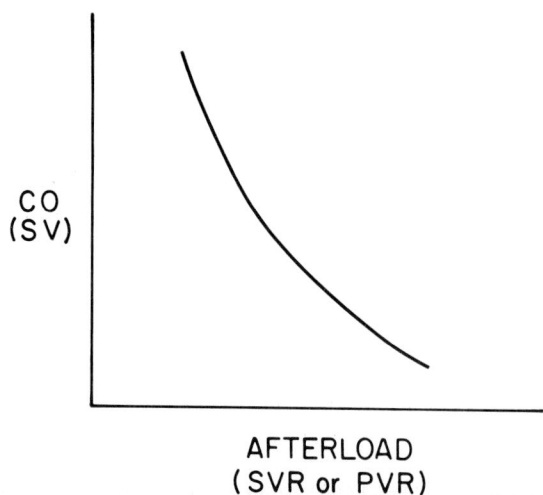

Fig. 47–3. Relationship of afterload—systemic vascular resistance (SVR) or pulmonary vascular resistance (PVR)—to cardiac output (CO) or stroke volume (SV) at a constant preload. (From Hankins and colleagues, 1983, with permission.)

TABLE 47–4. SOME COMPLICATIONS OF PULMONARY ARTERY CATHETERIZATION

Complication	Incidence (%)
Premature ventricular contractions	15–27
Arterial puncture	8
Superficial cellulitis	3
Pulmonary infarction/ischemia	1–7
Pneumothorax	1–2
Catheter-related sepsis	1
Balloon rupture	<1
Pulmonary artery rupture	<1
Catheter knotting	<1
Thromboembolism	?

Data from Buchbinder and Ganz (1976); Clark and associates (1985b); Moser and Spragg (1983); Robin (1985).

TABLE 47–5. SOME CAUSES OF ACUTE LUNG INJURY AND RESPIRATORY FAILURE IN PREGNANT WOMEN

Pneumonia	Embolism
Aspiration	Amnionic fluid
Bacterial	Trophoblastic
Viral	Septic
Sepsis	Air
Chorioamnionitis	Connective Tissue Disease
Pyelonephritis	Substance Abuse
Puerperal infection	Heroin
Hypovolemia	Placidyl
Shock	Methadone
Massive transfusion therapy	Irritant Inhalation and Burns
	Pancreatitis
	Pheochromocytoma

gain vascular access are similar with pulmonary artery and central venous catheters, complications resulting from the monitoring itself are far greater with the pulmonary artery catheter. The catheter itself may incite a variety of ventricular and supraventricular **arrhythmias. Hemorrhage** may result from disconnection of the catheter or introducer from their associated intravenous lines or from pulmonary artery rupture. This latter complication results in acute and massive hemoptysis and, in most instances, death. Lethal **intrathoracic bleeding** has been reported during attempts at subclavian vein cannulation with injuries to either arteries or veins. Rare complications include knotting of the catheter, thromboembolism, and balloon rupture.

Given a broad range of medical and surgical patients with conditions necessitating invasive monitoring, 3 percent will sustain a major complication, including death. Experience reported to date in obstetrics indicates fewer complications in the pregnant woman, probably as a direct reflection of her overall better health compared with that of other populations reported.

Acute Respiratory Failure

A number of disorders that have been reported to cause or be associated with acute pulmonary injury in pregnancy are listed in Table 47–5. Although most of these are coincidental, some are unique to pregnancy. The importance of recognizing these conditions lies in early diagnosis and treatment. Final outcome is determined by the extent of the original lung injury, the success of initial resuscitation and support, and avoidance of further injury and complications. The usual mortality rate is 50 to 60 percent in nonpregnant patients and increases to 90 percent if acute respiratory failure was triggered or complicated by sepsis.

Adult Respiratory Distress Syndrome (ARDS). Adult respiratory distress syndrome is a pathophysiological diagnosis. It includes both primary lung alveolar epithelial injuries sustained via the airways and endothelial injuries sustained via the pulmonary vasculature. A number of mediators, probably related to neutrophil accumulation, initiate tissue injury (Repine, 1992). This results in increased pulmonary capillary permeability, loss of lung volume, and shunting with resultant arterial hypoxemia (Ashbaugh and colleagues, 1967; Petty, 1982). Physiological criteria required for diagnosis of the syndrome are listed in Table 47–6. In nonpregnant patients, sepsis and diffuse infectious pneumonia are the most common single-agent causes of pulmonary failure (Petty, 1982). This also has been our experience with pregnant women at Parkland Hospital. More than 70 percent of patients, however, have some combination of sepsis, shock, trauma, fluid overload, or aspiration that causes injury. Indeed, multiplicity of causes is the rule with acute and severe lung injury.

Clinical Course. The clinical condition depends largely on the magnitude of the insult, the ability to compensate for it, and the stage of the disease. For example, if the woman presents soon after the initial injury, there are commonly no physical findings except hyperventilation. Arterial oxygenation usually is adequate initially. Normal pregnancy-induced metabolic al-

TABLE 47–6. PHYSIOLOGICAL CRITERIA FOR DIAGNOSIS OF ADULT RESPIRATORY DISTRESS SYNDROME

PO_2 <50 mm Hg with FIO_2 >0.6
Pulmonary capillary wedge pressure ≤ 12 mm Hg
Total respiratory compliance <50 mL/cm (usually 20 to 30 mL/cm)
Functional residual capacity reduced
Shunt (Q_s/Q_t) >30%
Dead space (V_D/V_T) >60%
Alveolar–arterial gradient with FIO_2 1.0 ≥ 350 mm Hg

PO_2 = partial pressure of oxygen; FIO_2 = fraction of inspired oxygen; Q_s = blood flow to nonventilated areas; Q_t = total blood flow to both ventilated and nonventilated areas; V_D = dead space; V_T = tidal volume.
From Pontoppidan and colleagues (1972b), with permission.

kalosis may be accentuated because of hyperventilation. With continued insult, or with time, auscultatory and radiological evidence for pulmonary disease becomes more obvious. There usually will be decreased lung compliance and increased intrapulmonary blood shunting. There is progressive alveolar and interstitial edema with extravasation of erythrocytes and inflammatory cells into the interstitium.

Ideally, pulmonary injury will be identified at this early stage, the insult terminated, and specific therapy directed at the injury. If not, then further progression results in acute respiratory failure characterized by marked dyspnea, tachypnea, and hypoxemia. Further loss of lung volume results in worsening of both pulmonary compliance and increasing intrapulmonary shunts. The chest radiograph characteristically demonstrates bilateral lung involvement (Fig. 47–4), while auscultation also shows diffuse abnormalities. At this phase, injury has progressed to a point that ordinarily will be lethal in the absence of treatment with high inspired oxygen concentrations. The institution of positive airway pressure, whether by mask or by intubation, frequently is necessary at this stage.

During the final phase of the respiratory distress syndrome, **intrapulmonary shunts** in excess of 30 percent result in severe and refractory hypoxemia. The marked increase in dead space, often exceeding 60 percent of tidal volume, leads to hypercapnia and an inability to provide ventilation and oxygenation. Metabolic and respiratory acidosis result in myocardial irritability and dysfunction, which often leads to cardiac arrest. Microscopically, intra-alveolar fibrosis and fibroblastic infiltration of the alveolar septum combine to form massive tissue plates that completely mask the original architecture of the lung parenchyma during end-stage disease.

Management. In acute and severe lung injury, attempts are made to ensure adequate oxygenation of peripheral tissues while ensuring that therapeutic maneuvers do not aggravate lung injury further. Oxygen delivery is best evaluated by using several simultaneously measured parameters, including arterial and mixed venous oxygen saturations, oxygen content, and oxygen differences. Optimal tissue extraction of oxygen may require therapeutic maneuvers designed to shift the oxyhemoglobin dissociation curve to maximize arterial oxygen content and delivery. Pulmonary compliance and intrapulmonary shunt fractions are valuable indices, obtainable at the bedside, to assess day-to-day status of the lung injury.

Three critical points are worth emphasis: (1) Oxygen delivery is directly proportional to cardiac output; if cardiac output falls by 50 percent, then so does oxygen delivery. Conversely, doubling cardiac output doubles oxygen delivery. (2) The overwhelming majority of transported oxygen is bound to hemoglobin and is *not* in solution. Accordingly, oxygen delivery can be improved by correction of anemia because each gram of hemoglobin carries 1.35 mL of oxygen when 97 percent saturated and 1.25 mL when 90 percent saturated. (3) Increasing the arterial pressure of oxygen (Pao_2) above 100 mm Hg has very little effect on oxygen delivery. Because oxygen may aggravate lung injury further if given at high inspired concentrations, tissue oxygen delivery should be increased primarily by optimization of cardiac output and hemoglobin concentration and only secondarily by increasing the inspired oxygen concentration. Reasonable goals in caring for the woman with severe lung injury are to obtain a Pao_2 of 60 mm Hg or 90 percent oxyhemoglobin saturation as determined by pulse oximetry.

Oxyhemoglobin Dissociation Curve. The propensity of the hemoglobin molecule to release oxygen is described by the oxyhemoglobin dissociation curve. Simplistically, as shown in Figure 47–5, the curve can be divided into an upper oxygen association curve (representing the alveolar–capillary environment) and a lower oxygen dissociation portion (representing the tissue capillary environment). Shifts of the curve have their greatest impact at the steep portion because they affect oxygen delivery. A rightward shift is associated with decreased hemoglobin affinity for oxygen and hence increased tissue–capillary oxygen interchange. Rightward shifts are produced by hypercapnia, metabolic acidosis, increased body temperature, and increased 2,3-diphosphoglycerate levels. During pregnancy, the intraerythrocyte concentration of 2,3-diphosphoglycerate is increased by approximately 30 percent compared with nonpregnant

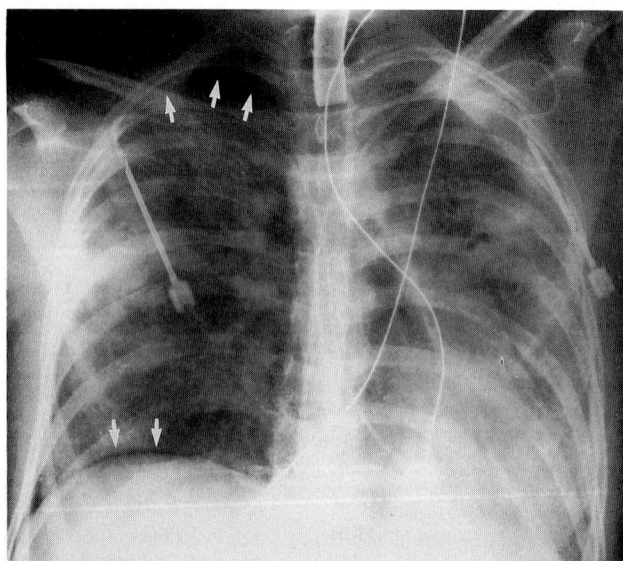

Fig. 47–4. Severe adult respiratory distress syndrome with diffuse infiltrates and right pneumothorax (*arrows*) caused by positive pressure ventilation. (Courtesy of Dr. Michael Landay.)

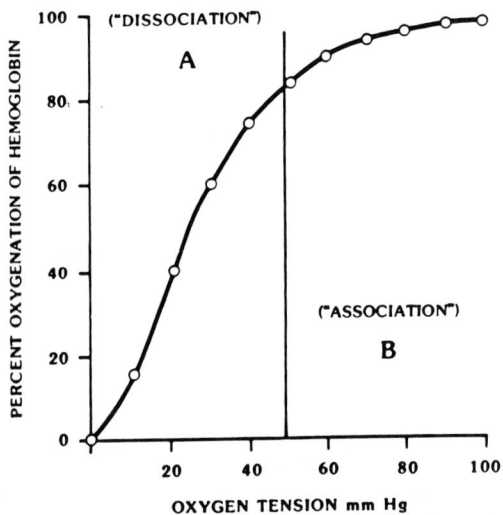

Fig. 47–5. Oxyhemoglobin dissociation curve. Mixed venous oxygen saturations operate on the "dissociation" or linear phase of the curve and are very sensitive to physiological instability. (From Clark and colleagues, 1991, with permission.)

values. This favors oxygen delivery to both the fetus and peripheral maternal tissues (Rorth and Bille-Brahe, 1971).

Fetal hemoglobin has a higher oxygen affinity than adult hemoglobin and its curve is positioned to the left of the adult curve (Bauer and associates, 1961). At a level of 50 percent hemoglobin saturation, the maternal Pa_{O_2} is 27 mm Hg compared with 19 mm Hg in the fetus. Under normal physiological conditions, fetal conditions constantly are on the dissociation, or tissue, portion of the curve. Even with severe maternal lung disease and very depressed maternal Pa_{O_2} levels, oxygen displacement to fetal hemoglobin is favored. This has been confirmed by studies of pregnant women and their fetus at high altitude, where despite a maternal Pa_{O_2} of only 60 mm Hg, the fetal Pa_{O_2} is equivalent to that at sea level (Subrevilla and colleagues, 1971).

Mechanical Ventilation. In an attempt to protect the fetus, early intubation and assisted ventilation is advised in the pregnant woman if respiratory failure appears to be imminent. Invasive hemodynamic monitoring also may be indicated to avoid any iatrogenic worsening of the pulmonary injury and to better assess therapeutic manipulations. Mechanical ventilation for acute respiratory failure usually requires a volume-cycled ventilator. After initial settings, including 100 percent inspired oxygen, an arterial blood sample is analyzed and the ventilator adjusted to obtain a Pa_{O_2} greater than 60 mm Hg, or a hemoglobin saturation of 90 percent and a Pa_{CO_2} of 35 to 45 mm Hg. Assessment of changes in shunt, mixed venous oxygen saturation, compliance, and cardiac output allow adjustments for tidal volume or respiratory rate to maintain adequate minute ventilation. The nor-

mal Pa_{CO_2} in pregnancy is 30 to 35 mm Hg, and levels lower than this should be avoided because they can affect placental perfusion adversely (Levinson and co-workers, 1974).

Positive End-Expiratory Pressure (PEEP). With severe lung injury and high intrapulmonary shunt fractions, it may not be possible to provide adequate oxygenation with usual pressures, even on 100 percent oxygen. Positive pressure is usually successful in decreasing the shunt by recruiting collapsed alveoli. Moreover, at low levels (for example, 5 to 15 cm H_2O), positive pressure can usually be employed safely without invasive cardiovascular monitoring. At the higher levels, however, right-sided venous return can be impaired, resulting in decreased cardiac output. Recall that oxygen delivery is directly proportional to cardiac output; thus, oxygen availability to peripheral tissues, including the uteroplacental circulation, can be decreased. High levels of positive pressure can also result in overdistention of alveoli, falling compliance, and barotrauma.

Perhaps the greatest benefit of positive pressure is that prompt institution arrests the early stages of injury and limits oxygen exposure and toxicity. Pressures should be adjusted, in increments of about 5 cm H_2O, whether increasing or decreasing the level, with its effects documented prior to further adjustments. Additionally, the positive pressure *should not be* discontinued when collecting hemodynamic information, such as pulmonary capillary wedge pressure measurements. Such sudden changes in pressures can result in significant clinical deterioration.

Fluid Therapy. Treatment of critically ill patients who have acute respiratory failure requires assiduously detailed attention to fluid balance because fluid overload further compromises pulmonary status. In the intensive care setting, intake and output records should be supplemented with daily weights. A mechanically ventilated patient retains an extra liter of fluid per day. Because the syndrome is characterized by a pulmonary permeability defect, fluid leaks into the interstitium, even at normal pressures. Thus, it is best to maintain the lowest pulmonary capillary wedge pressure possible while avoiding decreased cardiac output.

Some pregnancy-induced physiological changes may predispose the woman to a greater risk of lung injury from fluid therapy. Robertson (1969) demonstrated a continuous decline in the colloid oncotic pressure (COP) across pregnancy; it fell from 28 mm Hg nonpregnant to 23 mm Hg at term. Benedetti and Carlson (1979) later demonstrated a further decline to 17 mm Hg in the puerperium. Women with preeclampsia had an even lower oncotic pressure; it was 16.1 mm Hg antepartum and 13.8 mm Hg postpartum (Zinaman and co-workers, 1985). The importance of these changes is their impact on the **colloid oncotic pressure/wedge**

pressure gradient. Under normal conditions, this gradient exceeds 8 mm Hg; however, reductions to 4 mm Hg or less are associated with increased risks for pulmonary edema.

Weaning and Extubation. Weaning and extubation are not attempted until all other organ system failures or compromises are resolved. Because both high inspired oxygen concentrations and high positive pressures have associated complications, these variables should be tapered first. As a rule, extubations are accomplished in the early morning. This allows the woman to be well rested and monitored thoroughly by a fully staffed unit during the first several hours after extubation. Continued serial blood gas monitoring is required postextubation and supplemental oxygen is provided by face shield.

Bacteremia and Septicemic Shock

Infections that most commonly cause bacteremia and septicemic shock in obstetrical patients are septic abortion (see Chap. 31, p. 686), antepartum pyelonephritis (see Chap. 50, p. 1130), and puerperal sepsis (see Chap. 28, p. 633).

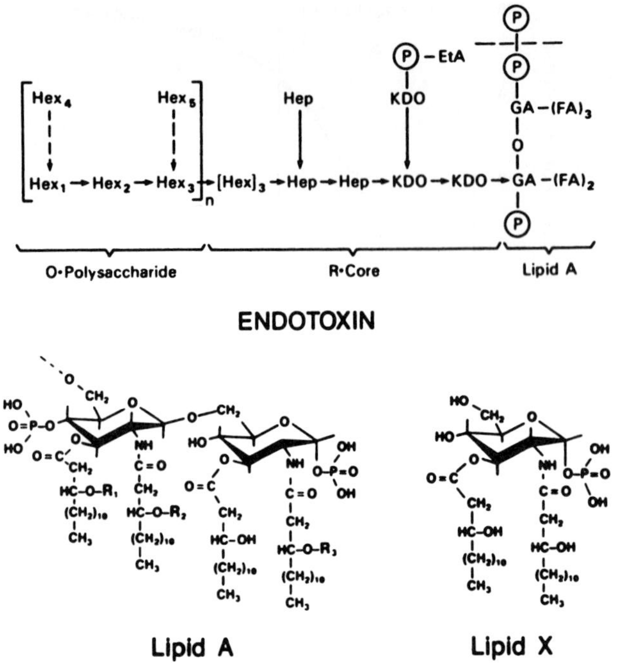

Etiology. Most pelvic infections are polymicrobial; thus, septic shock may be caused by a number of pathogens. Most commonly, bacteria that cause shock are from members of the endotoxin-producing *Enterobacteriaceae* family, especially *Escherichia coli*. Pathogens that less often cause shock are aerobic and anaerobic streptococci and *Bacteroides* and *Clostridium* species.

Pathogenesis. **Endotoxin** is a lipopolysaccharide that is released upon lysis of the cell wall of gram-negative bacteria (Fig. 47–6). There are probably other bacterial substances that result in mediator release with activation of complement, kinins, or the coagulation system (see Chap. 37, p. 824). Bacterial **exotoxins** also can cause shock and death (Parrillo and colleagues, 1990). Examples include exotoxin A from *Pseudomonas aeruginosa* or toxic shock syndrome toxin from *Staphylococcus aureus* (Glauser and colleagues, 1991). More recently we, as well as others, have encountered a virulent toxic-shock-like syndrome caused by group A streptococcal infection. Extensive tissue necrosis and gangrene, especially of the postpartum uterus, may cause maternal death.

Release of vasoactive mediators produces selective vasodilation with maldistribution of blood flow. Leukocyte and platelet aggregation cause capillary plugging. Vascular endothelial injury causes profound capillary leakage and interstitial fluid accumulation. The end results of this cascade of pathophysiological events, shown in Figure 47–7, cause the **septic shock syndrome.** Clinical shock, as described by Parker and Parrillo

Fig. 47–6. Chemical structures of endotoxin, lipid A, and lipid X. (From Parrillo and colleagues, 1990, with permission.)

(1983), results primarily from decreased systemic vascular resistance which is not compensated fully by increased cardiac output. Hypoperfusion results in lactic acidosis, decreased oxygen extraction, and end-organ dysfunction (Table 47–7). This is also referred to as **multiple organ failure syndrome.**

Hemodynamic Changes in Septic Shock. A greater understanding of the septic shock syndrome has been made possible by technology discussed earlier that allows direct hemodynamic measurements. The pathophysiology of sepsis has been elucidated by the elegant clinical studies of Parker and Parrillo and their colleagues (1983, 1987, 1990) from the National Institutes of Health. According to their observations, if initially circulating volume is restored, then septic shock can be characterized as a high-cardiac-output, low-vascular-resistance condition. Concomitantly, pulmonary hypertension develops. Paradoxically, patients with severe sepsis are likely to have myocardial depression despite high cardiac output (Ognibene and co-workers, 1988). An elevated cardiac index with decreased systemic vascular resistance are the most common cardiovascular manifestations of septic shock and may have prognostic significance (Parker and colleagues, 1987; Parrillo and co-workers, 1990).

Most generally healthy women with sepsis complicating obstetrical infections respond well to fluid resuscitation, given along with intensive antimicrobial therapy and, if indicated, removal of infected tissue. If hypotension is not corrected following vigorous fluid

NIDUS OF INFECTION ⟶ ORGANISMS ⟶ EXOGENOUS TOXINS ⟶ ENDOGENOUS MEDIATORS

Pneumonitis
Peritonitis
Cellulitis
Abscess
Other infection sites

Organism
Structural Component
Exotoxin (TSST-1, Toxin A)
Endotoxin

CYTOKINES
 • Interleukin 1,2...6
 • Tumor Necrosis Factor (TNF)
PLATELET ACTIVATING FACTOR (PAF)
ARACHIDONIC ACID METABOLITES
HUMORAL DEFENSE SYSTEMS
 • Complement
 • Kinins
 • Coagulation
OTHERS
 • Myocardial Depressant Substance (MDS)
 • Endorphins
 • Histamine

SEVERE DECREASE SVR
HYPOTENSION
DEPRESSED CO
DEATH
MOSF
MULTIPLE ORGAN SYSTEM FAILURE
CARDIOVASCULAR INSUFFICIENCY
RECOVERY

MYOCARDIUM
 • Depression
 • Dilatation

VASCULATURE
 • Vasodilatation
 • Vasoconstriction
 • Maldistribution of Blood Flow
 • Endothelial Destruction

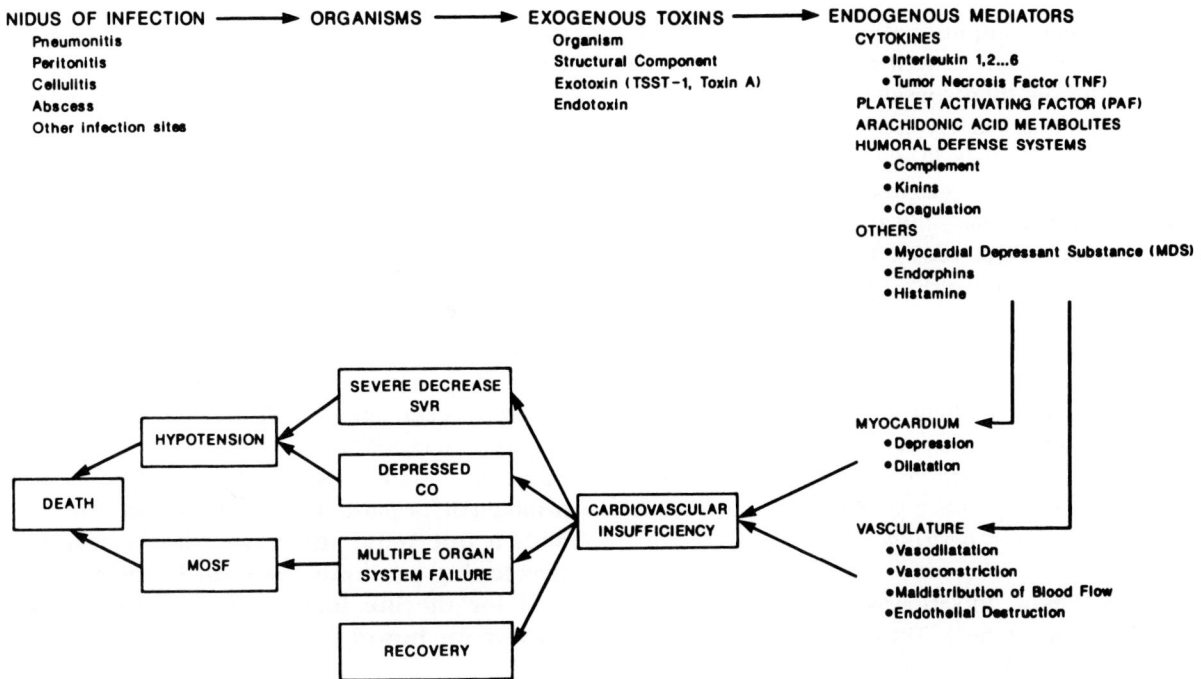

Fig. 47–7. Sequence of pathogenetic steps leading from a nidus of infection to cardiovascular dysfunction and shock during human sepsis. SVR = systemic vascular resistance; CO = cardiac output; MOSF = multiple organ system failure. (From Parrillo and associates, 1990, with permission.)

infusion, then the prognosis is poor. Lack of response may be due to severe and unresponsive vascular insufficiency, or it may be due to myocardial depression. Lee and colleagues (1988) described two maternal deaths in 10 women with low cardiac output unresponsive to fluid resuscitation. Another poor prognostic sign is continued end-organ dysfunction, that is, renal, pulmonary, and cerebral failure, although hypotension has been corrected.

TABLE 47–7. MULTIPLE ORGAN EFFECTS WITH SEPSIS AND SHOCK

Organ/System	Clinical and Laboratory Findings
Central nervous	Confusion
Hypothalamus	Hypothermia, hyperthermia
Cardiovascular	Vasodilation and hypotension, increased cardiac output (early), myocardial depression (decreased ejection fraction), hypotension, tachyarrhythmias
Pulmonary	Arteriovenous shunting with hypoxemia and tachypnea, alveolar–capillary leakage with pulmonary edema
Gastrointestinal	Vomiting, diarrhea
Liver	Toxic hepatitis, jaundice
Kidney	Oliguria, renal failure
Hematological	Thrombocytopenia, leukopenia, leukocytosis, consumptive coagulopathy

Modified from American College of Obstetricians and Gynecologists (1984), with permission.

Diagnosis. Whenever serious bacterial infection is suspected, blood pressure and urine flow should be monitored closely. Septic shock, as well as hemorrhagic shock, should be considered whenever there is evidence of hypotension or oliguria. In the absence of evidence for active hemorrhage, if hypotension and oliguria are not improved by the rapid administration of at least a liter of lactated Ringer solution, it is likely that shock is caused by infection-related agents.

Treatment. When shock from sepsis is suspected, prompt and aggressive treatment includes the following: (1) careful monitoring of vital signs and urinary output, (2) vigorous intravenous fluid infusion to restore circulating volume, (3) administration of empirical antimicrobial drugs selected to provide a spectrum that includes all suspected pathogens, and, if indicated, (4) surgical intervention after the woman's condition has been stabilized.

Rapid infusion with as many as 4 to 6 L of crystalloid fluids may be required to restore renal perfusion in severely affected women. Because of the vascular leak, these women usually are hemoconcentrated, and if the hematocrit is 30 or less, then blood is given along with crystalloid to maintain the hematocrit at about 30 or perhaps slightly higher. A hemodynamic algorithm for managing obstetrical septic shock has been presented by Lee and associates (1988).

If aggressive volume replacement is not promptly

followed by urinary output of at least 30 mL and preferably 50 mL per hour, as well as other indicators of improved perfusion, then consideration is given for insertion of a pulmonary artery catheter (see p. 1066). In women who are seriously ill, the pulmonary capillary endothelium is also likely damaged, with alveolar leakage and pulmonary edema—the **adult respiratory distress syndrome** (see p. 1069). This must be differentiated from circulatory overload from overly vigorous fluid therapy.

Broad-spectrum antimicrobials are administered in large doses after appropriate cultures are taken. These include blood cultures, along with specimens of exudates that are not contaminated by normal flora. For women with infected abortions or those with deep fascial infections, a Gram-stained smear may be helpful in identifying *Clostridium perfringens.*

Surgical Treatment. In seriously ill women, continuing sepsis may prove fatal. Thus, debridement of necrotic tissue or drainage of purulent material is crucial to their survival. Therefore, a meticulous search is made for such foci.

For women with infected abortions, the products of conception must be removed promptly by curettage. According to Pritchard and Whalley (1971), as well as others, hysterectomy seldom is indicated unless the uterus has been lacerated or is obviously intensely infected (Fig. 47–8). Bacterial shock may become clinically apparent several hours after evacuation of infected products from the uterus.

For women with pyelonephritis, continuing sepsis usually is from urinary obstruction caused by calculi or a perinephric abscess or phlegmon, and flank exploration may be indicated (see Chap. 50, p. 1131). In some cases, end-stage pyonephrosis is found as a source of continuing sepsis and nephrectomy must be performed.

Puerperal infections that cause sepsis which may be amenable to surgical treatment are those in which there is appreciable infection of devitalized tissue. In addition to clostridial infections, we have recently encountered several women with massive uterine myonecrosis from group A β-hemolytic streptococci; the mortality rate has been high. Other examples include deep myofascial infections of the episiotomy site or abdominal surgical incision (see Necrotizing Fasciitis, Chap. 28, p. 639). In women with persistent infections following cesarean section, the uterine incision may undergo necrosis and dehiscence with subsequent peritonitis. Another source may be from a ruptured parametrial or intra-abdominal abscess. **Any woman with a puerperal infection who is suspected of developing peritonitis should be carefully evaluated for uterine incisional necrosis and separation or for bowel perforation.**

Adjunctive Therapy

Pressor Agents. Vasoactive drugs are not given unless aggressive fluid treatment fails to correct hypotension and perfusion abnormalities. If central filling pressure measurements indicate that fluid replacement is adequate, then vasoactive drugs are given. One commonly used is dopamine hydrochloride, which when given in doses of 2 to 10 μg/kg per minute stimulates cardiac β-receptors to increase cardiac output. Doses of 10 to 20 μg/kg per minute cause α-receptor stimulation and increase blood pressure. At doses of more than 20 μg/kg per minute, α-receptor stimulation predominates, but dopamine is seldom needed at these higher doses. If there

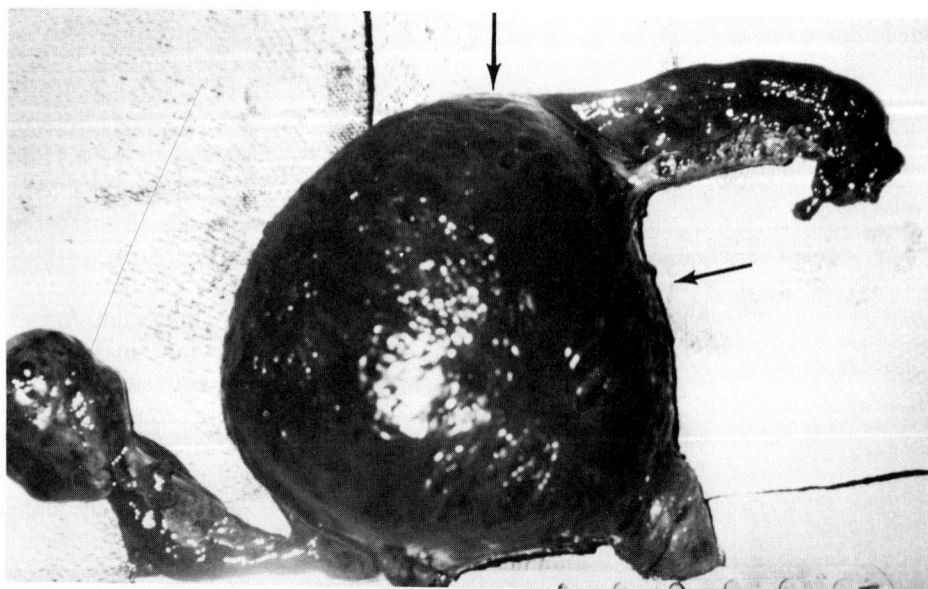

Fig. 47–8. The numerous rents in the uterine serosa (*arrows*) were the consequence of gas formation plus intensive necrosis from *Clostridium perfringens.*

is no response to dopamine, then dobutamine or isoproterenol may be of benefit (Lee and colleagues, 1988).

Oxygenation and Ventilation. Oxygen is administered by mask in an attempt to improve ongoing tissue hypoxia. As the septic shock syndrome progresses, and intravascular volume is restored, there may be substantive pulmonary capillary endothelial damage with leakage into alveoli. Resultant pulmonary edema causes hypoxemia, which worsens tissue hypoxia and acidosis. When this is severe, and adequate oxygenation cannot be maintained by increased oxygen delivered by a nonrebreathing mask, then tracheal intubation and mechanical ventilation that delivers positive pressure may prove to be lifesaving.

Adrenal Corticosteroids. If control of the infection by antimicrobials and the infusion of blood and aqueous fluids do not result in prompt improvement, corticosteroids are recommended by some. Results of two large clinical studies have shown that methylprednisolone given in large doses within a few hours of sepsis did not improve early or late morbidity or mortality (Bone and colleagues, 1987; Veterans Administration Study Group, 1987).

Anti-endotoxin Antibodies. There have been several recent studies with adjunctive immunotherapy (anti-endotoxin antibody serum) for gram-negative sepsis or septic shock. Greenman and colleagues (1991) used E5 murine monoclonal IgM endotoxin antibody to treat 316 patients with gram-negative sepsis. Antibody treatment did not result in increased survival for all patients, but there was a two-fold greater survival for treated patients with gram-negative sepsis who were not in shock. This subset of patients also had more frequent resolution of organ failure.

Ziegler and associates (1991) described treatment of gram-negative bacteremia with a human monoclonal IgM antibody (HA–1A) that binds to lipid A. Among the 200 patients with gram-negative bacteremia, there were 50 percent deaths in the placebo group compared with 30 percent in the HA–1A treatment group. Antibody treatment was of no proven benefit in the 343 septic patients without demonstrable gram-negative bacteremia.

These preliminary studies suggest that anti-endotoxin antibody therapy may be of some benefit in some patients with sepsis, especially those not in shock when treatment is begun (Cohen and Glauser, 1991; Wenzel, 1992). Because of marginal benefits, high cost ($4000 per dose), and the known difficulties in clinically diagnosing sepsis, some urge that such treatment be considered experimental (Warren and colleagues, 1992). Obviously, more data is needed before the widespread use of immunotherapy can be recommended for all patients with presumed sepsis.

Trauma in Pregnancy

Trauma and similar violent events are the leading cause of death in young women. According to the American College of Obstetricians and Gynecologists (1991b), one in every 12 pregnancies will be complicated by physical trauma. In Cook County, Illinois, traumatic events caused nearly half of 95 maternal deaths from 1986 through 1989 (Fildes and colleagues, 1992).

Blunt Trauma. Automobile accidents cause most cases of blunt trauma to the pregnant woman. The use of three-point restraints has been shown effective to prevent many severe maternal injuries (American College of Obstetricians and Gynecologists, 1991a). Other common causes of trauma are falls and aggravated assaults. As emphasized by the Council on Scientific Affairs of the American Medical Association (1992), as well as Newberger and colleagues (1992), the latter deserves especial attention because of its increasing frequency. Serious intra-abdominal injuries are of particular concern and, probably related to the markedly increased pelvic and abdominal vascularity, retroperitoneal hemorrhage is encountered more commonly compared with nonpregnant women. Conversely, bowel injuries are less frequent because of the protective effect of the large uterus. Splenic, liver, and kidney injuries also may be sustained.

Traumatic Placental Abruption. There are obvious concerns for uterine injuries in the pregnant woman. Particularly worrisome is the specter of placental abruption, which complicates 1 to 6 percent of "minor" injuries and up to 50 percent of major injuries (Crosby and associates, 1971; Goodwin and colleagues, 1990; Pearlman and co-workers, 1990a, 1990b). Crosby and associates (1968) have hypothesized that abruption is likely caused by deformation of the elastic myometrium around the relatively inelastic placenta.

In many cases, findings are similar to those discussed in Chapter 37 (p. 829). Stettler and associates (1992) reviewed our experiences with 13 women with a traumatic abruption at Parkland Hospital and reported that although 11 had uterine tenderness, only five had vaginal bleeding. Other common findings are uterine contractions; evidence for fetal compromise such as fetal tachycardia, late decelerations, and acidosis; and fetal death. Because placental abruption associated with trauma may be concealed, the incidence of associated severe coagulopathy is higher than with nontraumatic abruption. We found that almost two thirds of these women had clinically significant hypofibrinogenemia compared with only one third of women with a nontraumatic abruption (Stettler and associates, 1992).

Kettel and co-workers (1988) stress that abruption may be occult and not associated with uterine pain, tenderness, and bleeding. According to Pearlman and associates (1990b), detection of uterine contractile activity using electronic monitoring is suggestive of abruption. For these reasons, β-agonists to treat preterm labor is considered inadvisable for most of these women.

Uterine Rupture. Rupture of the uterus is uncommon with blunt trauma and is found in less than 1 percent of cases. It is usually associated with a direct impact of substantive force. Findings may be identical to those for placental abruption, and maternal and fetal deterioration are soon inevitable. Dash and Lupetin (1991) described a 24-week pregnancy in which traumatic uterine rupture was confirmed using computed tomography.

Fetal Injury. According to Kissinger and co-workers (1991), fetal death is more likely with direct fetoplacental injury, maternal shock, pelvic fracture, maternal head injury, and hypoxia. Although fetal injury and death are uncommon, there are many interesting case reports that describe it. Fetal skull and brain injury are most common and are more likely if the head is engaged and the maternal pelvis is fractured on impact. Conversely, fetal head injuries, presumably from a *contrecoup* effect, may be sustained in unengaged vertex or nonvertex presentations (Fries and Hankins, 1989). Weyerts and colleagues (1992) described a newborn with paraplegia and contractures associated with a motor vehicle accident several months before birth.

Penetrating Trauma. Knife and gunshot wounds are the most common penetrating injuries and may be associated with aggravated assaults, suicide attempts, or attempts to cause abortion. When the uterus is injured by penetrating wounds, the fetus is more likely to be injured (Fig. 47–9). Indeed, although the fetus sustains

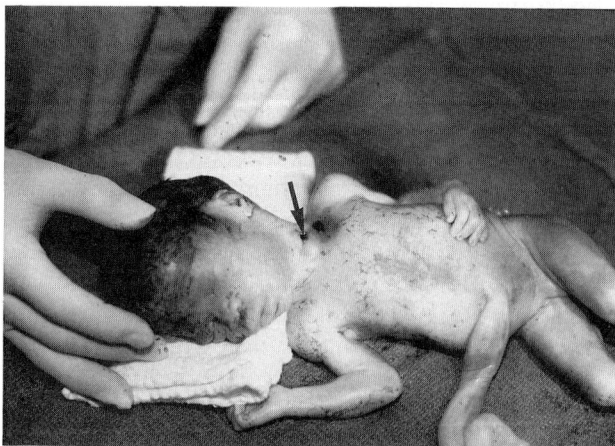

Fig. 47–9. Twenty-five-week fetus with fatal gunshot wound to neck. The .22 caliber bullet entered the uterine fundus anteriorly and exited posteriorly in the lower uterine segment just underneath serosa. (Photograph courtesy of Dr. R. Santos.)

injury in two thirds of such cases, visceral injuries to the mother are seen in only 20 percent (Buchsbaum, 1979).

Management. With minimal restrictions, treatment priorities are directed toward the injured pregnant woman as they are for nonpregnant patients. Primary goals are evaluation and stabilization of maternal injuries. Attention to fetal assessment during the acute evaluation may divert attention from life-threatening maternal injuries (American College of Obstetricians and Gynecologists, 1991b). Basic rules are applied to resuscitation, including establishing ventilation and arrest of hemorrhage along with treatment for hypovolemia with crystalloid and blood products. **An important aspect is deflection of the large uterus away from the great vessels to diminish their effect on decreased cardiac output.** Hoff and associates (1991), as well as Scorpio and colleagues (1992), documented that fetal death is related to the severity of maternal injury. They found close correlation of low maternal serum bicarbonate level with fetal demise.

Following emergency resuscitation, evaluation is continued for fractures, internal injuries, bleeding sites, as well as uterine and fetal injuries. Esposito and colleagues (1989) and Scorpio and associates (1992) have found that open peritoneal lavage is worthwhile in the pregnant woman, if indicated. Penetrating injuries in most cases must be evaluated using radiography (see Chap. 43, p. 984). Because clinical response to peritoneal irritation is blunted during pregnancy, an aggressive approach to exploratory celiotomy is pursued for abdominal trauma (American College of Obstetricians and Gynecologists, 1991b). Whereas exploration is mandatory for abdominal gunshot wounds, some advocate close observation for stab wounds (Grubb, 1992).

The necessity for cesarean delivery of a live fetus depends on several factors. Certainly, laparotomy itself is not an indication for cesarean section. Some considerations include gestational age, fetal condition assessed by antepartum evaluation, extent of uterine injury, and whether the large uterus hinders adequate treatment or evaluation of other intraabdominal injuries.

Electronic Monitoring. As for many other acute or chronic maternal conditions, fetal well-being may reflect the status of the mother, and thus, fetal monitoring is another "vital sign" to help evaluate extent of maternal injuries. Even if the mother is stable, the use of electronic monitoring may be predictive of placental abruption. Pearlman and associates (1990b) observed that no woman was found to have an abruption if no uterine contractions were detected, or if their frequency was less than every 10 minutes, 4 hours after trauma was sustained. Importantly, 20 percent of those who had more frequent contractions had an associated placental abruption. In these cases, abnormal monitor tracings also were common and included fetal tachycardia and late decelerations. Up to one third of these women have uterine contractions (Williams and colleagues, 1990).

Because placental abruption usually develops early following trauma, fetal monitoring is begun as soon as the maternal condition is stabilized. It is continued as long as there are uterine contractions, a nonreassuring fetal heart pattern, vaginal bleeding, uterine tenderness or irritability, serious maternal injury, or ruptured membranes (American College of Obstetricians and Gynecologists, 1991b). According to Goodwin and Breen (1990), an observation period of 2 to 6 hours is sufficient if there are no other ominous signs such as contractions, uterine tenderness, or bleeding. Rarely, abruptio placentae occurs days after trauma (Higgins and Garite, 1984; Lavin and Miodovnik, 1981).

Fetomaternal Hemorrhage. If there is considerable abdominal force associated with trauma, and especially if the placenta is lacerated, life-threatening fetomaternal hemorrhage may be encountered (Pritchard and associates, 1991). Some degree of bleeding from the fetal to maternal circulation is found in 10 to 30 percent of trauma cases (Goodwin and Breen, 1990; Pearlman and associates, 1990b; Rose and colleagues, 1985). In 90 percent of these cases, however, hemorrhage is inconsequential and less than 15 mL. We encountered three cases of massive fetomaternal hemorrhage in eight women with a traumatic abruption (Stettler and associates, 1992). Two cases were associated with a placental laceration and their infants were stillborn. An example of massive and fatal hemorrhage follows:

> At 33 weeks' gestation, the mother was forcefully thrown against the steering wheel during an auto accident, even though she was wearing an over-the-shoulder seat belt. The fetal heart was not heard on arrival 20 minutes later. Spontaneous labor developed 22 hours after the accident. At that time, the maternal blood contained at least 75 mL of fetal erythrocytes, or 175 mL of fetal blood, calculated from the percentage of fetal red cells found in maternal blood (4.5 percent, as demonstrated in Fig. 47-10), the maternal blood volume, and hematocrit. The macerated fetus weighed 2140 g. The placenta contained a long rent that extended to the chorionic plate. The clot adherent to the placenta at the site of partial placental abruption contained nearly all maternal red cells. Moreover, these red cells had been shed before the onset of labor, because they contained none of the radiolabeled [51] chromium used to measure the maternal blood volume at the onset of labor.

These findings raise pragmatic concerns with the D-negative woman who has sustained trauma. It seems reasonable to administer 300 μg of anti-D immunoglobulin as described in Chapter 44 (p. 1008). It also seems reasonable to determine the number of fetal cells in maternal blood by use of the Kleihauer–Betke stain or an equivalent test. It is unclear, however, if their routine use will modify adverse outcomes associated with fetal anemia, cardiac arrhythmias, and death (American College of Obstetricians and Gynecologists, 1991b). Del Valle and colleagues (1992) described a 28-week pregnancy complicated by a motor vehicle accident. The fetal heart pattern was sinusoidal and cordocentesis confirmed fetal anemia. Direct intravascular transfusion was performed with resolution of the abnormal heart rate pattern. Unfortunately, when the infant was delivered at 37 weeks, microcephaly was evident, presumably due to cerebral damage incurred at 28 weeks.

Thermal Injury

Although Parkland Hospital is a major burn center for the United States, we have not seen a large number of pregnant women with severe burns. It has become apparent, however, that pregnant women who suffer chemical pneumonitis from smoke inhalation tolerate this poorly, as they do most all forms of pneumonitis.

On the basis of experience with 50 burned pregnant women, Matthews (1982) recommended that women in the second or third trimester with burns over 50 percent of their body should be delivered immediately because maternal death otherwise almost is certain and fetal survival rate is not improved by waiting. He emphasized that, if undelivered, the maternal prognosis is markedly worse than for a nonpregnant woman suffering otherwise comparable burns. Conversely, Amy and colleagues (1985) reported that pregnancy did not alter maternal outcome compared with nonpregnant women of similar age. They, as well as Rayburn and co-workers (1984), noted that fetal survival usually parallels the percentage of burned surface area and survival of the mother.

Thus, for severely burned women, fetal prognosis is poor. Usually the woman enters labor spontaneously within several days to a week, and often delivers a stillborn infant. Contributory factors are hypovolemia, pulmonary injury, septicemia, and the intensely catabolic state. Rode and associates (1990) conducted a multicenter retrospective review of five South African burn centers and reported similar results from 33 women with an average burn area of 30 percent. Maternal mortality was 70 percent for burns exceeding 50 percent total body surface area. They reserved cesarean delivery for the unusual case when the gravely ill woman's condition jeopardized the viable fetus.

Skin Contractures. Skin contracture following serious abdominal burns may be painful during a subsequent pregnancy and even may necessitate surgical decompression and split skin autografts (Matthews, 1982). Widgerow and colleagues (1991) described two women

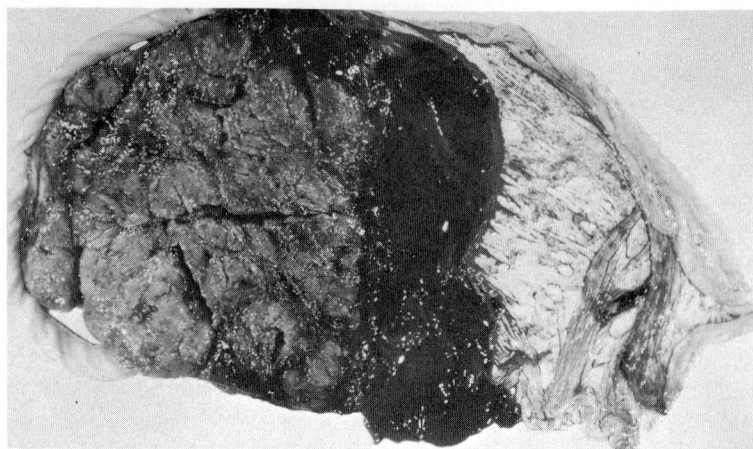

Fig. 47–10. A. Partial placental abruption with adherent blood clot. The fetus died from massive hemorrhage, chiefly into the maternal circulation. **B.** The adherent blood clot has been removed. Note the laceration of the placenta. **C.** Kleihauer–Betke stain of a smear of maternal blood after fetal death. The dark cells (4.5 percent) are fetal red cells, whereas the empty cells are maternal in origin.

A

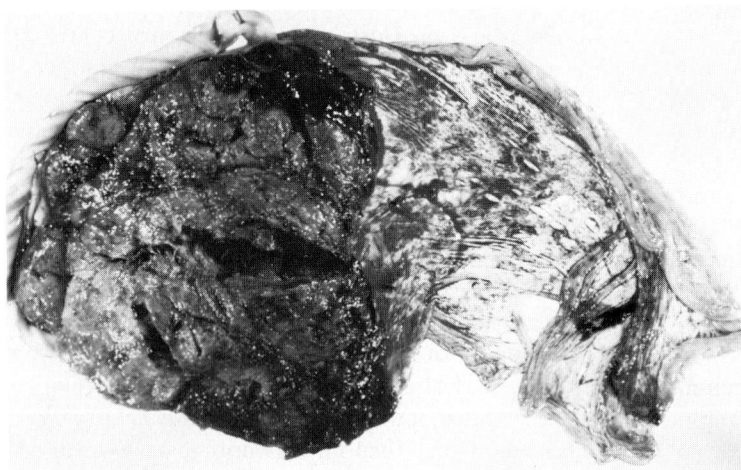

B

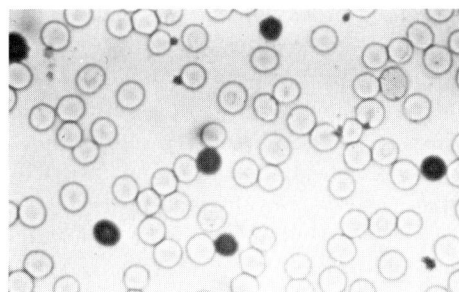

C

in whom surgical release without covering the resulting defect was sufficient. McCauley and colleagues (1991) followed seven woman with severe circumferential truncal burns sustained at a mean age of 7.7 years. All of 14 subsequent pregnancies were delivered at term without major complications. In one instance, there was breakdown of scar tissue in late pregnancy. It has been our limited experience that the burn scar during pregnancy undergoes considerable softening and therefore can stretch appreciably.

Loss or distortion of nipples may cause problems in breast feeding. Daw and Mohandas (1983) described cases in which breast feeding was satisfactory from one breast without problems in the contralateral breast without a nipple.

Sexual Assault

According to the Federal Bureau of Investigation of the United States Department of Justice (1988), the inci-

dence of sexual assault has increased four-fold compared with other crimes in the United States. It generally is held that only 10 to 20 percent of sexual assaults are reported. Until recently, there has been limited published experiences of rape in pregnancy.

Satin and co-workers (1991) reviewed over 5700 sexual assaults that were committed in Dallas County over 6 years, and found that 2 percent of the victims were pregnant. Perhaps surprisingly, associated physical trauma was less common than in nonpregnant rape victims, and only a third of assaults took place after 20 weeks' gestation. From a forensic standpoint, evidence collection was not altered because of pregnancy. The importance of psychological counselling for the rape victim and her family cannot be overemphasized.

Cardiopulmonary Resuscitation

Cardiac arrest fortunately is rare during pregnancy. There are special considerations for cardiopulmonary resuscitation (CPR) conducted in the second half of pregnancy. In nonpregnant women, external chest compression results in a cardiac output of only 30 percent of normal (Satin and Hankins, 1991). Cardiac output is even less in advanced pregnancy when aortocaval compression from the enlarged uterus may impede resuscitative efforts by diminishing forward flow as well as venous return. **Thus, uterine displacement is paramount to accompany other resuscitative efforts.** Left lateral displacement can be accomplished manually by a member of the team, by tilting the operating table laterally, by placing a wedge under the right hip, or by using the Cardiff resuscitation wedge (Satin and Hankins, 1991). Rees and Willis (1988) showed with a manikin that resuscitation with the Cardiff wedge was as efficient as resuscitation in the supine position. Between 25 and 32 weeks, when there is likelihood of fetal viability, Lee and colleagues (1986) recommend thoracotomy and open-chest massage if there is no response to cardiopulmonary resuscitation within 15 minutes. If this is not successful by 5 minutes, or if the woman is 32 weeks or greater, then they recommend emergency cesarean section. They emphasize that the hemodynamics of resuscitation in pregnant humans or animals have not been evaluated systematically. Oates and colleagues (1988) reported a case and cited the Royal College of Physicians' support of emergency cesarean section to facilitate resuscitation. We have found that during resuscitation, deflection of the pregnant uterus away from the great vessels allows sufficient venous return despite the low arterial pressures generated by chest compression.

Another special consideration is sodium bicarbonate administration. Because bicarbonate diffuses slowly across the placenta, rapid correction of maternal acidosis results in increased P_{CO_2} which also raises fetal P_{CO_2}. Thus, fetal pH decreases even more.

References

American College of Obstetricians and Gynecologists: Automobile passenger restraints for children and pregnant women. Technical bulletin no. 151, January 1991a

American College of Obstetricians and Gynecologists: Guidelines for Perinatal Care, 3rd ed. Washington DC, 1992

American College of Obstetricians and Gynecologists: Septic shock. Technical bulletin no. 75, March 1984

American College of Obstetricians and Gynecologists: Invasive hemodynamic monitoring in obstetrics and gynecology. Technical bulletin no. 175, December 1992

American College of Obstetricians and Gynecologists: Trauma during pregnancy. Technical bulletin no. 161, November 1991b

Amy BW, McManus WF, Goodwin CW, Mason A, Pruitt BA: Thermal injury in the pregnant patient. Surg Gynecol Obstet 161:209, 1985

Ashbaugh DG, Bigelow DB, Petty TL, Levine BE: Acute respiratory distress in adults. Lancet 2:319, 1967

Bauer C, Ludwig M, Ludwig I, Bartels H: Factors governing the oxygen affinity of human adult and foetal blood. Respir Physiol 7:271, 1961

Benedetti TJ, Carlson RW: Studies of colloid osmotic pressure in pregnancy-induced hypertension. Am J Obstet Gynecol 135:308, 1979

Bone RC, Fisher CJ Jr, Clemmer TP, Slotman GJ, Metz CA, Balk RA: A controlled clinical trial of high-dose methylprednisolone in the treatment of severe sepsis and septic shock. N Engl J Med 317:653, 1987

Buchbinder N, Ganz W: Hemodynamic monitoring: Invasive techniques. Anesthesiology 45:146, 1976

Buchsbaum HJ: Trauma in Pregnancy. Philadelphia, Saunders, 1979

Bush HS, Taylor RW, Thoi L: Does invasive hemodynamic monitoring improve survival in a medical intensive care unit? Crit Care Med 17:S137, 1989

Clark SL, Cotton DB: Clinical indications for pulmonary artery catheterization in the patient with severe pregnancy-induced hypertension. Am J Obstet Gynecol 158:453, 1988

Clark SL, Cotton DB, Hankins GDV, Phelan JP: Critical Care Obstetrics, 2nd ed. Boston, Blackwell Scientific Publications, 1991

Clark SL, Cotton DB, Lee W, Bishop C, Hill T, Southwick J, Pivarnik J, Spillman T, DeVore GR, Phelan J, Hankins GDV, Benedetti TJ, Tolley D: Central hemodynamic assessment of normal term pregnancy. Am J Obstet Gynecol 161:1439, 1989

Clark SL, Montz FJ, Phelan JP: Hemodynamic alterations in the patient with amniotic fluid embolism: A reappraisal. Am J Obstet Gynecol 151:617, 1985a

Clark SL, Phelan JP, Greenspoon J, Aldahl D: Labor and delivery in the presence of mitral stenosis: Central hemodynamic observations. Am J Obstet Gynecol 152:948, 1985b

Cohen J, Glauser MP: Septic shock: Treatment. Lancet 338:736, 1991

Crosby WM, Costiloe JP: Safety of lap-belt restraint for pregnant victims of automobile collisions. N Engl J Med 284:632, 1971

Crosby WM, Snyder RG, Snow CC, Hanson PG: Impact injuries in pregnancy, I. Experimental studies. Am J Obstet Gynecol 101:100, 1968

Council on Scientific Affairs, American Medical Association: Violence against women. Relevance for medical practitioners. JAMA 267:3184, 1992

Cunningham FG, Lucas MJ, Hankins GDV: Pulmonary injury complicating antepartum pyelonephritis. Am J Obstet Gynecol 156:797, 1987

Cunningham FG, Pritchard JA, Hankins GDV, Anderson P, Lucas J, Armstrong K: Peripartum heart failure: A specific pregnancy-induced cardiomyopathy or the consequence of coincidental compounding cardiovascular events? Obstet Gynecol 67:157, 1986

Dash N, Lupetin AR: Uterine rupture secondary to trauma: CT findings. J Comput Assist Tomogr 15:329, 1991

Daw E, Mohandas I: Pregnancy in patients after severe abdominal burns. Br J Obstet Gynaecol 90:69, 1983

Del Valle GO, Joffe GM, Izquierdo LA, Smith JF, Kasnic T, Gilson GJ, Chatterjee MS, Curet LB: Acute posttraumatic fetal anemia treated with fetal intravascular transfusion. Am J Obstet Gynecol 166:127, 1992

Esposito JT, Gens DR, Smith LG, Scorpio R: Evaluation of blunt abdominal trauma occurring during pregnancy. J Trauma 29:1628, 1989

Fildes J, Reed L, Jones N, Martin M, Barrett J: Trauma: The leading cause of maternal death. J Trauma 32:643, 1992

Fries MH, Hankins GDV: Motor vehicle accidents associated with minimal maternal trauma but subsequent fetal demise. Ann Emerg Med 18:301, 1989

Glauser MP, Zanetti G, Baumgartner JD, Cohen J: Septic shock: Pathogenesis. Lancet 338:732, 1991

Goodwin TM, Breen MT: Pregnancy outcome and fetomaternal hemorrhage after noncatastrophic trauma. Am J Obstet Gynecol 162:665, 1990

Gore JM, Goldberg RJ, Spodick DH, Alpert JS, Dalen JE: A community-wide assessment of the use of pulmonary artery catheters in patients with acute myocardial infarction. Chest 92:721, 1987

Greenman RL, Schein RMH, Martin MA, Wenzel RP, MacIntyre NR, Emmanuel G, Schmel H, Kohler RB, McCarthy M, Plouffe J, Russell JA, and the XOMA Sepsis Study Group: A controlled clinical trial of E5 murine monoclonal IgM antibody to endotoxin in the treatment of gram-negative sepsis. JAMA 266:1097, 1991

Grubb DK: Nonsurgical management of penetrating uterine trauma in pregnancy: A case report. Am J Obstet Gynecol 166:583, 1992

Hankins GDV, Wendel GD, Cunningham FG, Leveno KJ: Longitudinal evaluation of hemodynamic changes in eclampsia. Am J Obstet Gynecol 150:506, 1984

Hankins GDV, Wendel GD, Leveno KJ, Stoneham J: Myocardial infarction during pregnancy. A review. Obstet Gynecol 65:139, 1985

Hankins GDV, Wendel GW Jr, Whalley PJ, Quirk JG Jr: Cardiovascular monitoring in the high risk pregnancy. Perinatol Neonatol 7:29, 1983

Higgins SD, Garite TJ: Late abruptio placentae in trauma patients: Implications for monitoring. Obstet Gynecol 63(suppl 3):10S, 1984

Hoff WS, D'Amelio LF, Tinkoff GH, Lucke JF, Rhodes M, Diamond DL, Indeck M, Smith SJ Jr: Maternal predictors of fetal demise in trauma during pregnancy. Surg Gynecol Obstet 172:175, 1991

Kettel LM, Branch DW, Scott JR: Occult placental abruption after maternal trauma. Obstet Gynecol 71:449, 1988

Kilpatrick SJ, Matthay MA: Obstetric patients requiring critical care: A five-year review. Chest 101:1407, 1992

Kirshon B, Hinkley CM, Cotton DB, Miller J: Maternal mortality in a maternal–fetal medicine intensive care unit. J Reprod Med 35:25, 1990

Kissinger DP, Rozycki GS, Morris JA Jr, Knudson MM, Copes WS, Bass SM, Yates HK, Champion HR: Trauma in pregnancy: Predicting pregnancy outcome. Arch Surg 126:1079, 1991

Lavin JP, Miodovnik M: Delayed abruption after maternal trauma as a result of an automobile accident. J Reprod Med 26:621, 1981

Lee RV, Rodgers BD, White LM, Harvey RC: Cardiopulmonary resuscitation of pregnant women. Am J Med 81:311, 1986

Lee W, Clark SL, Cotton DB, Gonik B, Phelan J, Faro S, Giebel R: Septic shock during pregnancy. Am J Obstet Gynecol 159:410, 1988

Levinson G, Shnider SM, DeLorimier AA, Steffenson JL: Effects of maternal hyperventilation on uterine blood flow and fetal oxygenation and acid–base status. Anesthesiology 40:340, 1974

Mabie WC, Sibai BM: Treatment in an obstetric intensive care unit. Am J Obstet Gynecol 162:1, 1990

Matthews RN: Old burns and pregnancy. Br J Obstet Gynaecol 89:610, 1982

McCauley RL, Stenberg BA, Phillips LG, Blackwell SJ, Robson MC: Long-term assessment of the effects of circumferential truncal burns in pediatric patients on subsequent pregnancies. J Burn Care Rehabil 12:51, 1991

Moser KM, Spragg RG: Use of the balloon-tipped pulmonary artery catheter in pulmonary disease. Ann Intern Med 98:53, 1983

Newberger EH, Barkan SE, Lieberman ES, McCormick MC, Yllo K, Gary LT, Schechter S: Abuse of pregnant women and adverse birth outcome: Current knowledge and implications for practice. JAMA 267:2370, 1992

Oates S, Williams GL, Rees GAD: Cardiopulmonary resuscitation in late pregnancy. Br Med J 297:404, 1988

Ognibene FP, Parker MM, Natanson C, Shelhamer JH, Parrillo JE: Depressed left ventricular performance. Response to volume infusion in patients with sepsis and septic shock. Chest 93:903, 1988

Parker MM, Parrillo JE: Septic shock: Hemodynamics and pathogenesis. JAMA 250:3324, 1983

Parker MM, Shelmamer JH, Natanson C, Alling DW, Parrillo JE: Serial cardiovascular variables in survivors and nonsurvivors of human septic shock: Heart rate as an early predictor of prognosis. Crit Care Med 15:923, 1987

Parrillo JE, Parker MM, Natanson C, Suffredini AF, Danner RL, Cunnion RE, Ognibene FP: Septic shock in humans: Advances in the understanding of pathogenesis, cardiovascular dysfunction, and therapy. Ann Intern Med 113:227, 1990

Pearlman MD, Tintinalli JE, Lorenz RP: Blunt trauma during pregnancy. N Engl J Med 323:1609, 1990a

Pearlman MD, Tintinalli JE, Lorenz RP: A prospective controlled study of outcome after trauma during pregnancy. Am J Obstet Gynecol 162:1502, 1990b

Petty TL: Adult respiratory distress syndrome. Semin Respir Med 3:219, 1982

Pontoppidan H, Geffin B, Lowenstein E: Acute respiratory failure in the adult. N Engl J Med 287:690, 1972a

Pontoppidan H, Geffin B, Lowenstein E: Acute respiratory failure in the adult. N Engl J Med 287:743, 1972b

Pontoppidan H, Geffin B, Lowenstein E: Acute respiratory failure in the adult. N Engl J Med 287:799, 1972c

Pritchard JA, Cunningham G, Pritchard SA, Mason RA: On reducing the frequency of severe abruptio placentae. Am J Obstet Gynecol 165:1345, 1991

Pritchard JA, Whalley PJ: Abortion complicated by *Clostridium perfringens* infection. Am J Obstet Gynecol 111:484, 1971

Rayburn W, Smith B, Feller I, Varner M, Cruiskshank D: Major burns during pregnancy: Effects on fetal well being. Surg Gynecol Obstet 63:392, 1984

Rees GAD, Willis BA: Resuscitation in late pregnancy. Anaesthesia 43:347, 1988

Repine JE: Scientific perspectives on adult respiratory distress syndrome. Lancet 339:466, 1992

Robertson EG: Oedema in normal pregnancy. J Reprod Fertil 9(suppl):27, 1969

Robin ED: The cult of the Swan–Ganz catheter. Ann Int Med 103:445, 1985

Rode H, Millar AJW, Cywes S, Bloch CE, Boes EGM, Theron EJ, Lodder JV, van der Merwe AE, deKock M: Thermal injury in pregnancy—The neglected tragedy. S Afr Med J 77:346, 1990

Rorth M, Bille-Brahe NE: 2,3-Diphosphoglycerate and creatine in the red cells during pregnancy. Scand J Clin Lab Invest 28:271, 1971

Rose PG, Strohm PL, Zuspan FP: Fetomaternal hemorrhage following trauma. Am J Obstet Gynecol 153:844, 1985

Satin AJ, Hankins GDV: Cardiopulmonary resuscitation in pregnancy. In Clark SL, Cotton DB, Hankins GDV, Phelan JP (eds): Critical Care Obstetrics, 2nd ed. Boston, Blackwell Scientific Publications, 1991, p 579

Satin AJ, Hemsell DL, Stone IC Jr, Theriot S, Wendel GD Jr: Sexual assault in pregnancy. Obstet Gynecol 77:710, 1991

Scorpio RJ, Esposito TJ, Smith LG, Gens DR: Blunt trauma during pregnancy. Factors affecting fetal outcome. J Trauma 32:213, 1992

Shoemaker WC: Use and abuse of the balloon tip pulmonary artery (Swan–Ganz) catheter: Are patients getting their money's worth? Crit Care Med 18:1294, 1990

Stettler RW, Lutich A, Pritchard JA, Cunningham FG: Traumatic placental abruption: A separation from traditional thought. Presented at the annual clinical meeting of American College of Obstetricians and Gynecologists, Las Vegas, NV, May 1992

Subrevilla LA, Cassinelli MT, Carcelen A, Malaga JM: Human fetal and maternal oxygen tension and acid–base status during delivery at high altitude. Am J Obstet Gynecol 111:1111, 1971

Swan HJ, Ganz W, Forrester J, Marcus H, Diamond G, Chonette D: Catheterization of the heart in man with use of a flow-directed balloon-tipped catheter. N Engl J Med 283:447, 1970

Tuchschmidt J, Sharma OP: Impact of hemodynamic monitoring in a medical intensive care unit. Crit Care Med 15:840, 1987

United States Department of Justice, Federal Bureau of Investigation: Uniform crime reports for the United States. Washington, DC, United States Government Printing Office, 46, 1988

Veterans Administration Systemic Sepsis Cooperative Study Group: Effect of high-dose glucocorticoid therapy on mortality in patients with clinical signs of systemic sepsis. N Engl J Med 317:659, 1987

Warren HS, Danner RL, Munford RS: Anti-endotoxin monoclonal antibodies. N Engl J Med 326:1153, 1992

Wenzel RP: Anti-endotoxin monoclonal antibodies—A second look. N Engl J Med 326:1151, 1992

Widgerow AD, Ford TD, Botha M: Burn contracture preventing uterine expansion. Ann Plast Surg 27:269, 1991

Williams JK, McClain L, Rosemurgy AS, Colorado NM: Evaluation of blunt abdominal trauma in the third trimester of pregnancy: Maternal and fetal considerations. Obstet Gynecol 75:33, 1990

Weyerts LK, Jones MC, James HE: Paraplegia and congenital contractures as a consequence of intrauterine trauma. Am J Med Genet 43:751, 1992

Ziegler EJ, Fisher CJ Jr, Sprung CL, Straube RC, Sadoff JC, Foulke GE, Wortel CH, Fink MP, Dellinger RP, Teng NNH, Allen IE, Berger HJ, Knatterud GL, LoBuglio AF, Smith CR, and the HA–1A Sepsis Study Group: Treatment of gram-negative bacteremia and septic shock with HA–1A human monoclonal antibody against endotoxin: A randomized, double-blind, placebo-controlled trial. N Engl J Med 324:429, 1991

Zinaman M, Rubin J, Lindheimer MD: Serial plasma oncotic pressure levels and echoencephalography during and after delivery in severe pre-eclampsia. Lancet 1:1245, 1985

CHAPTER 48
Cardiovascular Diseases

HEART DISEASE IN PREGNANCY

Heart disease complicates about 1 percent of pregnancies. Rheumatic heart disease formerly accounted for the majority of cases, and more than 90 percent of women with heart disease cared for at the Boston Lying-in Hospital from 1921 to 1938 had rheumatic lesions (Hamilton and Thomson, 1941). This incidence has changed remarkably as rheumatic fever has almost disappeared in this country. An additional factor is that better medical management, together with a number of newer surgical techniques, has enabled more girls with congenital heart disease to reach childbearing age. As a result of these factors, congenital heart lesions now constitute at least half of all cases of heart disease encountered during pregnancy (Bitsch and colleagues, 1989; McFaul and associates, 1988). Hypertensive heart disease contributes a few cases of organic heart disease in pregnancy, whereas other varieties are even less common; these include coronary, thyroid, syphilitic, and kyphoscoliotic cardiac disease, as well as idiopathic cardiomyopathy, cor pulmonale, constrictive pericarditis, various forms of heart block, and isolated myocarditis.

Sachs and associates (1988) reported that maternal mortality from cardiac disease fell from 5.6 to 0.3 per 100,000 live births in Massachusetts from 1954 through 1985. Unfortunately, heart disease still significantly contributes to maternal mortality, and Dorfman (1990) reported that 8 percent of maternal deaths in New York City from 1981 through 1983 were caused by cardiac disease.

Physiological Considerations. The marked hemodynamic changes stimulated by pregnancy have a profound effect on underlying heart disease in the pregnant woman. These physiological changes are detailed in Chapter 8 (p. 225). The most important consideration is that during pregnancy cardiac output is increased by as much as 30 to 50 percent. Cardiac output is maximized by midpregnancy. Using noninvasive methods, Capeless and Clapp (1989) have shown that almost half of the total increase has occurred by 8 weeks' gestation, and that it can be attributed to augmented stroke volume. This apparently results from decreased vascular resistance, which is accompanied by diminished blood pressure. Later in pregnancy, there is also an increased resting pulse, and stroke volume is even more increased, presumably related to increased diastolic filling from the augmented blood volume.

As discussed in Chapter 47 (p. 1067), using right-sided heart catheterization, Clark and colleagues (1989) measured hemodynamic function in 10 healthy primigravid women. Pregnancy values were compared with values measured again 11 to 13 weeks postpartum (Table 48–1). At or near term, cardiac output in the lateral recumbent position was increased 43 percent by virtue of elevated pulse rate (17 percent) and stroke volume (27 percent). Because vascular resistance concomitantly decreased by 21 percent, there was no change in intrinsic left-ventricular contractility. As shown in Figure 48–1, normal pregnancy is characterized by normal left-ventricular function, not hyperdynamic function as once thought. These investigators concluded that maintenance of normal left-ventricular filling pressures comes about as the result of ventricular dilatation.

Because significant hemodynamic alterations are apparent early in pregnancy, the woman with clinically significant cardiac dysfunction may experience worsening of heart failure before midpregnancy.

Prognosis. The likelihood of a favorable outcome for the mother with heart disease depends upon the (1) functional capacity of her heart, (2) likelihood of other complications that further increase the cardiac load, and (3) quality of medical care provided. Psychological and socioeconomical factors also may assume great importance, because for some women, hospitalization with complete bed rest may be required throughout pregnancy.

In the past, it was incorrectly concluded that maternal hemodynamic burden peaked some weeks before term, following which the risk of cardiac failure dropped dramatically. Considerable emphasis was placed, for example, on the apparent reduction in cardiac output after 32 weeks (see Chap. 8, p. 229). Importantly, the misconception that cardiac decompensation would seldom develop after this time is not supported by clinical observations. Most investigators have not shown a decrease in blood volume of any appreciable magnitude during the last several weeks. **Cardiac failure is just as likely to develop during the last few weeks of pregnancy, or during labor and the puerperium.** Of 542 women whose pregnancies were complicated by heart disease, 8 of 10 maternal deaths were during the puerperium (Etheridge and Pepperell, 1977).

TABLE 48–1. HEMODYNAMIC CHANGES IN 10 NORMAL PREGNANT WOMEN AT TERM COMPARED WITH POSTPARTUM VALUES

Parameter	Change
Cardiac output	+ 43 percent
Heart rate	+ 17 percent
Left ventricular stroke work index	+ 17 percent
Vascular resistance	
Systemic	− 21 percent
Pulmonary	− 34 percent
Mean arterial pressure	+ 4 percent
Colloid osmotic pressure	− 14 percent

Adapted from Clark and colleagues (1989).

Congenital Heart Disease in Offspring. Many congenital heart lesions appear to be inherited as polygenic characteristics (see Chap. 40, p. 930). Thus it might be expected that some women with congenital lesions would give birth to similarly affected infants. Shime and colleagues (1987) found congenital cardiovascular lesions, including Marfan syndrome, in 3 percent of 87 infants born to women with congenital heart lesions.

Diagnosis of Heart Disease

Many of the physiological changes of normal pregnancy tend to make the diagnosis of heart disease more difficult (Chap. 8, p. 225). For example, in normal pregnancy, functional systolic heart murmurs are quite common. Moreover, as the uterus enlarges and the diaphragm is elevated, the heart is elevated and rotated so that the apex is rotated laterally while the heart is moved closer to the anterior chest wall. Respiratory effort in normal pregnancy is accentuated, at times suggesting dyspnea. Presumably this change is brought about in large part by a stimulatory effect of progesterone on the respiratory center. Edema, a further source of confusion, is often prevalent, especially in the lower extremities during the latter half of pregnancy. Importantly, the physician must be quite careful not to diagnose heart disease during pregnancy when none exists, and at the same time not fail to detect and appropriately treat heart disease when it does exist. Shown in Table 48–2 are a number of symptoms and clinical findings that may indicate heart disease. Pregnant women who have none of these findings rarely have serious heart disease.

Diagnostic Studies. Most cardiovascular diagnostic studies are noninvasive and can be conducted quickly and efficiently in pregnant women. Certainly, clinical suspicion of heart disease warrants further investigation, because confirmation of the diagnosis may alter pregnancy management. In most cases, conventional testing to include electrocardiography, echocardiography, and chest radiography will provide the necessary data. If indicated, right-heart catheterization can be performed without x-ray guidance. On rare occasions, it may be necessary to perform left-heart catheterization.

Electrocardiography. As the diaphragm is elevated in advancing pregnancy, there is an average 15-degree left-axis deviation seen in the electrocardiogram, and mild ST changes may be seen in the inferior leads. Atrial and ventricular premature contractions are relatively fre-

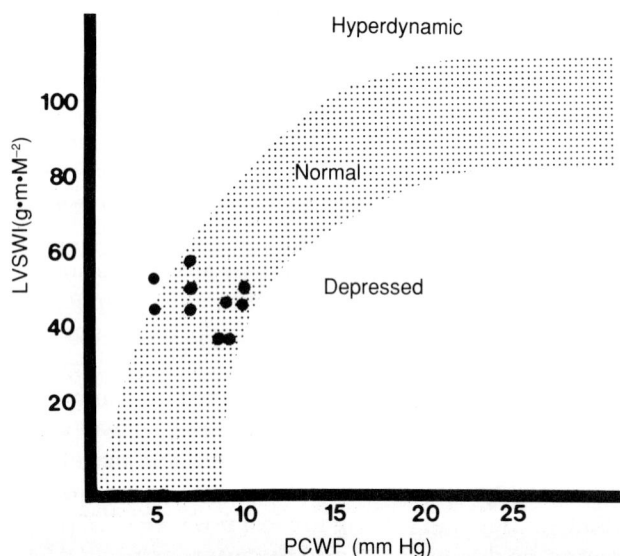

Fig. 48–1. Left ventricular function in the late third trimester in normotensive women. (PCWP = pulmonary capillary wedge pressure; LVSWI = left ventricular stroke work index.) (From Clark and colleagues, 1989, with permission.)

TABLE 48–2. SOME CLINICAL INDICATORS OF HEART DISEASE DURING PREGNANCY

Symptoms
Severe or progressive dyspnea
Progressive orthopnea
Paroxysmal nocturnal dyspnea
Hemoptysis
Syncope with exertion
Chest pain related to effort or emotion
Clinical Findings
Cyanosis
Clubbing of fingers
Persistent neck vein distension
Systolic murmur greater than grade 3/6
Diastolic murmur
Cardiomegaly
Sustained arrhythmia
Persistent split second sound
Criteria for pulmonary hypertension
   Left parasternal lift
   Loud P_2

Adapted from Metcalfe and colleagues (1986).

quent (Carruth and colleagues, 1981). Pregnancy does not alter voltage findings.

Chest X-ray. Anterior–posterior and lateral chest radiographs may be very useful when heart disease is suspected clinically. When used with an abdominal lead apron shield, fetal radiation exposure is reduced (see Chap. 43, p. 984). Minimal heart enlargement cannot be detected accurately by x-ray because the heart silhouette is larger in normal pregnancy; however, gross cardiomegaly can be excluded.

Echocardiography. The widespread use of echocardiography has been beneficial to better diagnose heart disease during pregnancy, as well as to provide data on normal pregnancy-induced hemodynamic and cardiovascular changes. However, there is justifiable concern regarding its overuse. These tests are expensive, they may be anxiety-provoking, and their results may be misinterpreted in light of pregnancy-induced hemodynamic changes. For example, during normal pregnancy, there is a high prevalence of tricuspid regurgitation (Limacher and co-workers, 1985), and left-atrial size and left-ventricular outflow cross-sectional area are increased significantly. None of these considerations, however, should prevent echocardiographic evaluation in a pregnant woman with suspected heart disease.

Clinical Classification. There is no clinically applicable test for accurately measuring functional capacity of the heart. A helpful clinical classification, however, was first published in 1928 by the New York Heart Association, and was revised for the eighth time in 1979. One important change was the addition of an assessment of the woman's cardiac status after all data have been reviewed. Thus, the classification is no longer based only on clinical symptoms. Still, for use in pregnancy, a functional classification is important. The following is based on past and present disability and is uninfluenced by the presence or absence of physical signs.

- **Class I.** Uncompromised: Patients with cardiac disease and *no limitation of physical activity.* These patients do not have symptoms of cardiac insufficiency, nor do they experience anginal pain.
- **Class II.** Slightly compromised: Patients with cardiac disease and *slight limitation of physical activity.* These women are comfortable at rest, but if ordinary physical activity is undertaken, discomfort results in the form of excessive fatigue, palpitation, dyspnea, or anginal pain.
- **Class III.** Markedly compromised: Patients with cardiac disease and *marked limitation of physical activity.* These women are comfortable at rest, but less than ordinary activity causes discomfort in the form of excessive fatigue, palpitation, dyspnea, or anginal pain.

- **Class IV.** Severely compromised: Patients with cardiac disease and *inability to perform any physical activity without discomfort.* Symptoms of cardiac insufficiency or of the anginal syndrome may develop even at rest, and if any physical activity is undertaken, discomfort is increased.

Preconceptional Counseling. Women with serious heart disease probably should not become pregnant. Maternal mortality varies directly with functional classification; moreover, some lesions carry a much graver prognosis, pregnancy notwithstanding. Conversely, in some women, life-threatening cardiac abnormalities can be reversed by corrective surgery and subsequent pregnancy is less dangerous. In some cases, fetal considerations predominate. For example, women with a mechanical prosthetic valve generally must take warfarin compounds, which are known to be teratogenic. Therefore, during pregnancy, heparin is usually substituted for warfarin.

The American College of Obstetricians and Gynecologists (1992a) has recently classified women in three groups according to risks for death during pregnancy (Table 48–3). These were comprised to aid in counseling the patient regarding advisability of conception or continuation of pregnancy.

TABLE 48–3. RISKS FOR MATERNAL MORTALITY CAUSED BY VARIOUS HEART DISEASES

Cardiac Disorder	Mortality (%)
Group 1	0–1
Atrial septal defect	
Ventricular septal defect	
Patent ductus arteriosus	
Pulmonic or tricuspid disease	
Fallot tetralogy, corrected	
Bioprosthetic valve	
Mitral stenosis, NYHA[a] class I and II	
Group 2	5–15
2A: Mitral stenosis, NYHA[a] class III and IV	
Aortic stenosis	
Aortic coarctation without valvar involvement	
Fallot tetralogy, uncorrected	
Previous myocardial infarction	
Marfan syndrome, normal aorta	
2B: Mitral stenosis with atrial fibrillation	
Artificial valve	
Group 3	25–50
Pulmonary hypertension	
Aortic coarctation with valvar involvement	
Marfan syndrome with aortic involvement	

[a] New York Heart Association.
From the American College of Obstetricians and Gynecologists (1992a), with permission.

GENERAL MANAGEMENT

Treatment of heart disease during pregnancy is dictated by the functional capacity of the heart. Excessive weight gain, **abnormal** fluid retention, and **anemia** should be prevented when possible. Increased bodily bulk increases cardiac work, and anemia with its compensatory rise in cardiac output also predisposes to cardiac failure. The development of **pregnancy-induced hypertension** is hazardous, for in this circumstance cardiac output can be maintained only by an increase in cardiac work commensurate with increased afterload. At the same time, hypotension is undesirable, especially in women with stenotic valvar lesions, septal defects, or patent ductus arteriosus. Each of these allow shunting of blood from right to left heart chambers and from the pulmonary artery to aorta. **Infection** increases cardiac workload appreciably, and should be prevented if possible, and treated vigorously when it develops.

McAnulty and colleagues (1988) pose a list of six questions that should be asked whenever a woman with heart disease is encountered:

1. Is the hemodynamic status optimal?
2. Is antimicrobial prophylaxis against endocarditis indicated?
3. Is antimicrobial prophylaxis for prevention of rheumatic fever required?
4. Is anticoagulation necessary?
5. Is the presenting symptom due to the underlying heart disease?
6. Should diagnostic or therapeutic plans be changed because a woman is pregnant or contemplating pregnancy?

Management of Classes I and II

With rare exceptions, women in class I and most in class II go through pregnancy without morbidity. Throughout pregnancy and the puerperium, however, special attention should be directed toward both prevention and early recognition of heart failure. As emphasized by Sugrue and associates (1981), a more favorable functional classification at the outset should not engender any relaxation in vigilance of management. Almost 40 percent of their Class I patients developed frank cardiac failure. According to Sullivan and Ramanathan (1985), maternal mortality is 0.4 percent in classes I and II, but McFaul and co-workers (1988) encountered no maternal deaths in 445 such women.

A specific routine that assures adequate rest should be outlined for each woman. The recommendations of Hamilton and Thomson (1941) are still pertinent: The pregnant woman should rest in bed 10 hours each night, and she should lie down for half an hour after each meal. Light housework and walking without climbing stairs are permitted. She should do no heavy work. Items rich in sodium should be avoided. Weight gain should not exceed the 24 pounds or so that are accounted for by physiological changes induced by normal pregnancy. In essence, the pregnant woman must learn to spare herself all unnecessary effort and must rest as much as possible.

Not infrequently, infection has proved to be an important factor in precipitating cardiac failure. Each woman should receive instructions to avoid contact with persons who have respiratory infections, including the common cold, and to report at once any evidence of an infection. Pneumococcal and influenza vaccines are recommended.

Cigarette smoking is to be vigorously prohibited, both because of its cardiac effects as well as the propensity to cause upper respiratory infections. Alcohol use is contraindicated for fetal reasons (Chap. 42, p. 973). Illicit drug use may be particularly harmful, as with the cardiovascular effects of cocaine or amphetamines, as well as the propensity for intravenous use of any illegal substance to cause infective endocarditis.

The onset of congestive heart failure is often gradual. The first warning sign of cardiac failure is likely to be persistent rales at the base of the lungs, frequently accompanied by a cough. To be significant, rales must persist after two or three deep breaths, because rales that are sometimes heard in normal pregnant women usually disappear after one or two deep inspirations. A sudden diminution in the woman's ability to carry out her household duties, increasing dyspnea on exertion, attacks of smothering with cough, and hemoptysis, are other signals warning of serious heart failure, as are progressive edema and tachycardia.

Home Health Care and Hospitalization. Admission remote from delivery of women with class II cardiac disease was once common practice. Unfortunately, rising health costs have made this cost prohibitive, and managed home health care with encouraged bed rest is a contemporaneous substitute.

Labor and Delivery. Delivery should be accomplished vaginally unless there are obstetrical indications for cesarean delivery. In spite of the physical effort inherent in labor and vaginal delivery, less morbidity and mortality are associated with it. In some women with severe heart disease, **pulmonary artery catheterization** may be indicated for continuous hemodynamic monitoring (American College of Obstetricians and Gynecologists, 1992b). This may be performed electively when labor begins or planned cesarean delivery is performed.

Relief from pain and apprehension without undue depression is especially important during labor and delivery. For many multiparous women, analgesics in moderate doses provide satisfactory pain relief. For others, especially nulliparas, continuous epidural analgesia often proves valuable for reducing pain and apprehension. The major danger of conduction analgesia is maternal hypotension (see Chap. 16, p. 435). This is especially dangerous in women with intracardiac shunts, in whom flow may be reversed with blood passing from the right to the left side of the heart or the aorta, thereby bypassing the lungs. For example, in women with pulmonary hypertension, aortic stenosis, or hypertrophic cardiomyopathy, general anesthesia is usually given if needed for delivery.

During labor, the mother should be kept in a semirecumbent position. Measurements of the pulse and respiratory rates should be made between contractions at least four times every hour during the first stage of labor, and every 10 minutes during the second stage. Increases in the pulse rate much above 100 per minute or in the respiratory rate above 24, particularly when associated with dyspnea, suggest impending ventricular failure. With any evidence of cardiac decompensation, intensive medical management must be instituted immediately. Only in the presence of the completely dilated cervix and an engaged presenting part may these changes be taken as an indication for immediate delivery. With the cervix only partially dilated and the mother showing obvious evidence of cardiac embarrassment, there is no method of delivery that will not first intensify rather than relieve heart failure.

For vaginal delivery, pudendal analgesia given along with intravenous sedation often suffices; however, epidural analgesia is preferable if forceps are used to shorten the second stage. Subarachnoid blockade (spinal analgesia, saddle block) is not recommended in women with significant heart disease. For cesarean delivery, epidural blockade provides excellent surgical anesthesia; however, if unavailable or inadvisable, the combination of thiopental, succinylcholine, nitrous oxide, and at least 30 percent oxygen, with an endotracheal tube placed after previously neutralizing gastric juice, has also proved satisfactory (see Chap. 16, p. 429).

Intrapartum Heart Failure. Immediate medical treatment usually consists of morphine, oxygen, intravenously administered furosemide, and the Fowler position. Morphine will serve not only to reduce the elevated respiratory rate, but in the second stage of labor it will reduce reflex abdominal muscular activity associated with uterine contractions. In the presence of pulmonary edema, oxygen is given by intermittent positive-pressure breathing to promote adequate oxygenation and to help clear alveolar edema. Digitalis in the form of a rapidly acting glycoside may be given intravenously.

Furosemide, given intravenously in a dose of 20 to 50 mg, promptly stimulates diuresis. It also relaxes capacitance vessels, which in turn decreases preload by reducing venous return. Intrapulmonary and left atrial blood pressures are reduced, and this reduces pulmonary congestion. A common precipitating event of heart failure is pregnancy-induced hypertension, and if severe, hydralazine is given to reduce cardiac afterload.

Hypotension further reduces cardiac output, and its cause must be identified. If coincidental hemorrhage is the cause—for example, from severe placental abruption with concealed hemorrhage—then careful blood replacement and arrest of the hemorrhage are important. Successful therapy is reflected by a satisfactory hematocrit and adequate urinary output. If hypotension is the consequence of a severely impaired myocardium, treatment is more difficult. Specifically, if there is no improvement after instituting the treatment just outlined, invasive cardiac monitoring with a pulmonary artery catheter is begun in order to obtain serial hemodynamic measurements that may be essential in decision-making involving further therapy.

Puerperium. Women who have shown little or no evidence of cardiac distress during pregnancy, labor, or delivery may still decompensate after delivery. Therefore, it is important that the same meticulous care provided during the antepartum and intrapartum periods be continued into the puerperium. Postpartum hemorrhage, anemia, infection, and thromboembolism are much more serious complications in the woman with heart disease. Indeed, we have observed that these factors frequently act in concert to precipitate postpartum heart failure in women with underlying heart disease (Cunningham and associates, 1986).

If there was no evidence of cardiac compromise during labor, delivery, and the early puerperium, breast feeding is usually not contraindicated. If tubal sterilization is to be performed, it should be delayed for several days until it is obvious that the mother is afebrile, not anemic, and has demonstrated that she can ambulate without evidence of distress. Women who do not undergo tubal sterilization should be given detailed contraceptive advice.

Management of Class III

Women with class III cardiac disease present difficult problems that demand expert medical care. Maternal mortality for classes III and IV has been reported to be 4 to 7 percent (McFaul and colleagues, 1988; Sullivan and Ramanathan, 1985). The important question is whether pregnancy should be undertaken. If women choose to become pregnant, they must understand the risks and cooperate fully with planned care. If seen early enough, women with class III cardiac disease should consider pregnancy interruption unless they can be hospitalized for the duration of pregnancy.

Gorenberg and Chesley (1958) concluded that any woman with heart disease seen early in gestation can be carried through pregnancy successfully if she and her family are willing to abide by certain strict rules. Their recommended regimen included hospitalization and bed rest throughout pregnancy for any woman with class III disease. Application of this basic principle, together with good medical and obstetrical care in more than 1000 women, reduced the maternal death rate to not much more than that of the general obstetrical population. The absolute importance of rigid adherence to their rules is demonstrated by the fact that cardiac disease was the leading cause of maternal death at their hospital, but those who died were not women attending their cardiac clinic.

As with women in classes I and II, the preferred method of delivery is vaginal, and cesarean section is limited to obstetrical indications. These very sick women tolerate major surgical procedures poorly.

Management of Class IV

Treatment of women with class IV heart disease is essentially that of cardiac failure in pregnancy, labor, and the puerperium. In the presence of cardiac failure, delivery by any method carries a high maternal mortality rate. Accordingly, treatment of heart failure in pregnancy is primarily medical rather than obstetrical. In some cases, surgical intervention during pregnancy may be done to repair an underlying cardiac defect, such as tight mitral stenosis. The prime objective is to correct the decompensation, for only then will delivery be less dangerous.

Remote Prognosis

Although it is well established that the woman with cardiac disease who receives appropriate care rarely dies during pregnancy or the puerperium, the possibility has been raised that pregnancy in some way might accelerate the rate of deterioration of cardiac function and shorten life span. The conclusions derived from the comprehensive long-term studies by Chesley (1980) of a large number of pregnant women observed over a long period are consistent with the view that pregnancy has no deleterious remote effect on the course of rheumatic heart disease.

SURGICALLY CORRECTED HEART DISEASE

To improve cardiac function, several kinds of procedures have been performed on the heart and large vessels, with many cases requiring open heart surgery and bypass. Morris and Menashe (1991) reviewed mortality statistics for over 2700 children having corrective cardiac surgery in Oregon from 1958 through 1989. At 25 years, more than 75 percent were still alive. With successful repair, many of these women now are likely to

attempt pregnancy. In some instances, surgical corrections of cardiac lesions have been performed even during pregnancy.

Valve Replacement

A number of reproductive-age women have had a cardiac valvar prosthesis implanted to replace a severely damaged mitral or aortic valve. Reports of subsequent pregnancy outcomes are now quite numerous, and indeed, successful pregnancies have followed replacement of even three heart valves by prostheses (Nagorney and Field, 1981).

Effect on Pregnancy. Severe complications can arise during pregnancy when the mother has a prosthetic valve. Other than thromboembolism and hemorrhage from anticoagulation, there may be deterioration in cardiac function. Spontaneous abortions, stillborns, low-birthweight infants, and malformed fetuses are more common. Pregnancy is to be undertaken in these women only after serious consideration.

With use of a mechanical valve prosthesis, these women must be maintained on anticoagulant therapy, and at least when not pregnant, warfarin is recommended. There are reports that describe a higher incidence of thromboembolic complications with prostheses during pregnancy. Sareli and co-workers (1989) summarized 442 reported cases and identified 12 with thrombotic obstruction of the prosthesis and 14 with systemic embolization despite anticoagulation. In another series, Ismail and colleagues (1986) reported 4 maternal deaths in 50 women during 76 pregnancies.

Two reports outline many of the specific problems encountered in these pregnancies. In the first, Iturbe-Alessio and colleagues (1986) provide an estimate of risk for both mother and fetus. They studied prospectively 72 women with cardiac valve prostheses. In some women, warfarin derivatives were given throughout pregnancy, while in others 5000 U of heparin was administered subcutaneously twice daily and substituted for coumarin from the 6th through 12th weeks, after which coumarin therapy again was given. Three of 35 women taking low-dose heparin suffered a massive thrombosis of a Björk–Shiley mitral prosthesis, and 2 of them died. On the other hand, while the women taking warfarin had no thromboses, there was evidence for embryopathy in 28 percent of their fetuses. Although they did not study the effects of full anticoagulation with heparin, these investigators concluded that pregnancy was inadvisable in women with such prostheses.

In the other report, Sareli and associates (1989) described their experiences with 50 pregnancies in women with valvar prostheses. They elected to continue warfarin therapy during early pregnancy with plans to substitute heparin anticoagulation at 36 weeks. There were no maternal valve thromboses during pregnancy. Nine (18 percent) of these women "aborted" prior to 28 weeks, but importantly, of the 38 other fetuses exposed to warfarin, 6 were stillborn, 2 infants died of intracranial hemorrhage, and another 2 had warfarin embryopathy. These investigators attributed the low incidence of maternal thromboembolic episodes to the newer-model prostheses that were used, and indeed 46 were Medtronic Hall or St. Jude Medical prostheses, which are generally associated with fewer thrombotic complications.

Deviri and colleagues (1985) observed no thrombi in 22 pregnancies in 11 unanticoagulated women with porcine xenografts. Unfortunately, although less thrombogenic, such bioprostheses are not as durable as mechanical prostheses.

Management. If women who have undergone valve replacement choose to risk pregnancy, then full anticoagulation is recommended with either warfarin or heparin after the woman is apprised of the respective risks. We recommend full heparinization during pregnancy. Heparin does not cross the placenta, and pregnant women usually can be instructed to inject heparin satisfactorily. Heparin is given as described in Chapter 49 (p. 1115) to prolong the partial thromboplastin time by 1½ to 2½ times baseline values. Just before delivery, heparin is stopped. If delivery supervenes while the anticoagulant is still effective, and extensive bleeding is encountered, protamine sulfate is given. Anticoagulant therapy with warfarin or heparin may be restarted the day following vaginal delivery, usually with no problems. Following cesarean delivery, however, we begin partial heparinization on the day following surgery, but withhold full anticoagulation for 4 or 5 days.

Contraception. Because of their possible thrombogenic action, oral contraceptives containing estrogen and a progestin are contraindicated in women with prosthetic valves. Satisfactory contraception can be achieved, however, using traditional barrier techniques. Sterilization should be considered because of problems encountered during pregnancy.

Valve Replacement During Pregnancy

Open-heart surgery usually is postponed until after pregnancy, but occasionally valve replacement during pregnancy may be lifesaving. Bernal and Miralles (1986) reviewed the outcomes of 21 pregnant women in whom open-heart surgery had been performed while using cardiopulmonary bypass. Almost half of these women had mitral or aortic valve replacements. Surprisingly, these women tolerated the procedures well, and there was only one stillborn infant and one instance of preterm

labor and delivery. Westaby and associates (1992) reviewed 115 cardiac surgeries using cardiopulmonary bypass from 1959 through 1990. They reported 2 maternal deaths and a 17 percent fetal death rate.

Strickland and colleagues (1991) reported the Mayo Clinic experience with cardiac or valvar surgical procedures performed during 10 pregnancies. There was 1 maternal death and 1 stillborn associated with cardiopulmonary bypass times ranging from 18 to 154 minutes. The fetal response to cardiopulmonary bypass was usually bradycardia, and it was recommended that high-flow, normothermic perfusion be used if possible so that any theoretical risk of fetal hypoxia could be obviated. Burke and colleagues (1990) described a 24-week fetus, who despite its mother's normothermic, high-flow cardiopulmonary bypass procedure, exhibited a persistent sinusoidal pattern with a heart rate of 120 to 150 beats per minute.

Mitral Valvotomy. Schenker and Polishuk (1968) reported a total of 325 pregnancies in 182 women who previously had undergone mitral valvotomy. They emphasized that good clinical results following valvotomy do not guarantee an uncomplicated labor and delivery, and heart failure developed in 42 percent of these women at some point during their first postoperative pregnancy. This percentage increased with successive pregnancies, and women suffering heart failure in one pregnancy inevitably had the same experience in subsequent pregnancies. Coexisting atrial fibrillation was especially ominous and commonly was associated with heart failure, thromboembolic disease, and death. Surprisingly, spontaneous abortion, preterm delivery, and perinatal mortality were similar when compared with noncardiac controls.

Mitral Valvotomy During Pregnancy. The efficacy and relative safety of closed mitral valvotomy during pregnancy has been addressed by several authors, and some of the studies are listed in Table 48–4. Following surgery, functional classification was usually downgraded from class III or IV to class I. There were no maternal deaths, and the fetal death rate was 7 percent. Mitral valvotomy is the most common open-heart surgery performed during pregnancy at Parkland Hospital. These women usually have done well, and heart failure is often relieved immediately.

Heart Transplantation

By 1989, the Registry of the International Society for Heart Transplantation had compiled data from more than 10,000 heart and heart–lung transplant operations (Heck and co-workers, 1989). It was inevitable that some of these women would become pregnant, and Löwenstein and associates (1988) reported the first suc-

TABLE 48–4. RESULTS OF CLOSED MITRAL VALVOTOMY PERFORMED DURING PREGNANCY

Investigators	Patients	Preoperative Status NYHA[a] Classes III and IV No. (%)	Postoperative Status NYHA[a] Class I No. (%)	Maternal Deaths	Fetal Deaths No. (%)
El-Maraghy and co-workers (1983)	42	42 (100)	32 (76)	0	1 (2)
Vosloo and Reichart (1987)	41	35 (85)	32 (78)	0	5 (12)
Pavankumar and associates (1988)	126	115 (91)	106 (84)	0	8 (7)
Total	209	192 (92)	170 (81)	0	14 (7)

[a] New York Heart Association.

cessful pregnancy in a woman who previously had undergone heart transplantation. Hedon and colleagues (1990) described a twin pregnancy with successful outcome. Key and associates (1989) provided detailed data to show that the transplanted heart responded normally to pregnancy-induced changes.

Kirk (1991) reviewed the physiological adaptations to transplantation, along with concerns for potential teratogenic effects of immunosuppressive drugs given to prevent rejection. Complex medical and psychosocial problems are frequently encountered in these patients.

VALVE DISEASES

Rheumatic fever is uncommon in the United States because of less crowded living conditions, availability of penicillin, and evolution of nonrheumatogenic streptococcal strains. Still, it remains the chief cause of serious valvar disease. During epidemics of streptococcal pharyngitis, as many as 3 percent of untreated young adults may develop rheumatic fever. In 1986, the estimated prevalence of rheumatic fever and heart disease was 1.7 million persons, or 7 per 1000. Thus, as many as 0.5 to 1 percent of childbearing-age women may have rheumatic valvar disease.

Mitral Stenosis

Rheumatic endocarditis is the most common cause of mitral stenosis, which is the most important lesion hemodynamically. Mitral valve stenosis impedes blood flow from the left atrium to its ventricle. With tight mitral stenosis, the left atrium is dilated, as shown in Figure 48–2. Thus, left atrial pressure is chronically elevated and may result in significant passive pulmonary hypertension if not surgically corrected. The increased preload of normal pregnancy, as well as other factors that stimulate increased cardiac output, may cause ventricular failure with pulmonary edema. Indeed, 25 percent of women with mitral stenosis have cardiac failure for the first time during pregnancy (Sullivan and Ramanathan, 1985). This may be confused with idiopathic

peripartum cardiomyopathy (Cunningham and colleagues, 1986).

The normal mitral valve surface area is 4.0 cm^2. When stenosis narrows this to less than 2.5 cm^2, symptoms usually develop. The most prominent complaint is dyspnea due to pulmonary venous hypertension. Other common symptoms are fatigue, palpitations, and hemoptysis. Frequently, symptoms of heart failure appear suddenly. Atrial fibrillation is common with mitral valve stenosis. Because rapid ventricular response may precipitate heart failure, digoxin prophylaxis is usually given to slow ventricular response. Tachycardia shortens ventricular filling time and increases the mitral gradient, which raises left atrial and pulmonary venous and capillary pressures even more. Thus, atrial tachyarrhythmias are treated aggressively with cardioversion if necessary. Atrial fibrillation also predisposes to mural thrombosis formation and aortic embolization causing stroke (see Chap. 55, p. 1246).

For women who develop intractable heart failure,

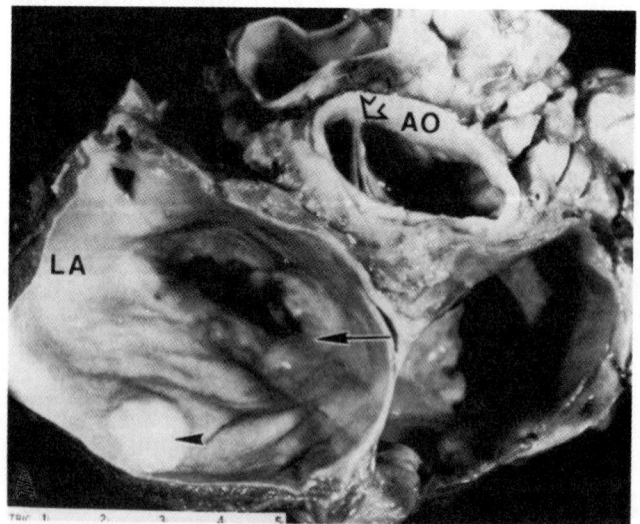

Fig. 48–2. Superior view of heart of a patient with rheumatic mitral stenosis showing fibrous adhesions and narrowing of mitral valve (*arrow*). The left atrium (LA) is dilated. The arrowhead points to focal endocardial fibrosis and the open arrow shows mild fibrosis of the valve of the aorta (AO). (From Brady and Duff, 1989, with permission.)

mitral valvotomy may provide dramatic relief of heart failure (p. 1089). Percutaneous transluminal balloon dilatation of the mitral valve has also been described during pregnancy (Smith and colleagues, 1989).

Management. Limited physical activity is recommended, as discussed earlier under "General Management." If symptoms of pulmonary congestion develop, activity is restricted even more, dietary sodium is restricted, and a diuretic is administered. Some recommend a β-blocker drug to slow heart rate response to activity and anxiety. Using either propranolol or atenolol, Al Kasab and associates (1990) treated 25 pregnant women with mitral stenosis. Their mean heart rate was decreased from 86 to 78 beats per minute, and 92 percent had significant symptomatic improvement as measured by reassignment to a lower New York Heart Association classification. If new-onset atrial fibrillation develops, intravenous verapamil, 5 to 10 mg, is given, or electrocardioversion is done.

Labor and delivery are particularly stressful for women with tight mitral stenosis. Pain, work, and anxiety cause tachycardia, with increasing chances of rate-related heart failure. Epidural analgesia for labor, with strict attention to avoid intravenous fluid overload, is ideal. As shown in Figure 48–3, pulmonary capillary wedge pressures usually increase even more immediately postpartum. Clark and colleagues (1985) hypothesize that this is likely due to loss of the low-resistance placental circulation as well as "autotransfusion" from the now-empty uterus. Abrupt increases in preload may lead to increased pulmonary capillary wedge pressure and edema. Thus, care must be taken to avoid fluid overload.

Vaginal delivery is preferable, and some recommend elective induction so that labor and delivery can be monitored and attended by the most knowledgeable team. In cases of severe stenosis with chronic heart failure, insertion of a pulmonary-artery catheter will help guide management decisions. Intrapartum endocarditis prophylaxis is required (see p. 1098).

Mitral Insufficiency

Mitral regurgitation develops when there is improper coadaption of mitral valve leaflets during systole, and this is eventually followed by left-ventricular dilatation and hypertrophy. Chronic mitral regurgitation may be due to a number of causes, including rheumatic fever, mitral valve prolapse, or left-ventricular dilatation of any etiology (for example, dilated cardiomyopathy). Less common causes include a calcified mitral annulus, connective-tissue diseases, and in older women, ischemic heart disease. Acute mitral insufficiency is caused by rupture of a chordae tendineae, infarction of papillary muscle, or by leaflet perforation from infective endocarditis.

In nonpregnant patients, symptoms from mitral valve incompetence are rare, and valve replacement is seldom indicated, except for infective endocarditis. Likewise, mitral regurgitation is well tolerated during pregnancy, probably due to decreased systemic vascular resistance, which actually results in less regurgitation. Heart failure only rarely develops during pregnancy, and occasionally tachyarrhythmias need to be treated. Prophylaxis against bacterial endocarditis is given intrapartum.

Aortic Stenosis

In a woman less than 30 years old, aortic stenosis is most likely due to a congenital lesion. This is the result of the decline in incidence of rheumatic diseases. The most common stenotic lesion is a bicuspid valve. Stenosis reduces the normal 2 to 3 cm^2 aortic orifice and creates resistance to ejection. A systolic pressure gradient de-

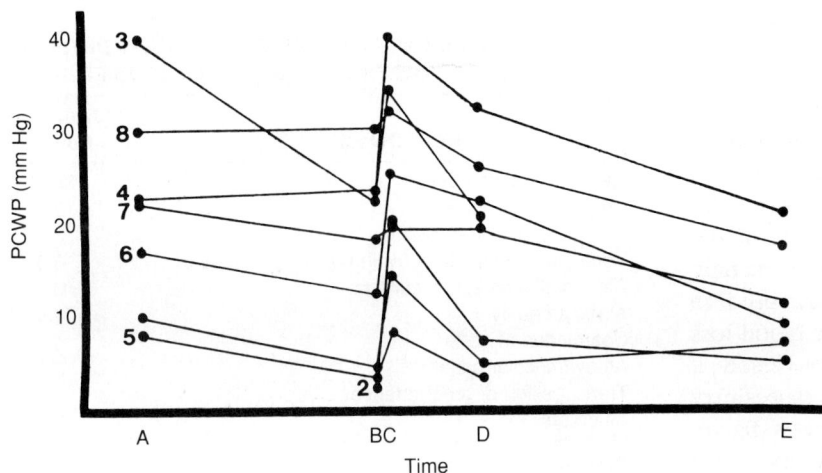

Fig. 48–3. Intrapartum alterations in pulmonary capillary wedge pressure (PCWP) in eight women with mitral stenosis. **A.** First-stage labor. **B.** Second-stage labor, 15 to 30 minutes before delivery. **C.** Postpartum 5 to 15 minutes. **D.** Postpartum 4 to 6 hours. **E.** Postpartum 18 to 24 hours. (From Clark and colleagues, 1986, with permission.)

velops between the left ventricle and the systemic arterial outflow tract. Concentric left-ventricular hypertrophy follows, and if severe, end-diastolic pressures become elevated, ejection fraction declines, cardiac output is reduced, and pulmonary hypertension eventually develops. Characteristic clinical manifestations develop late and include chest pain, syncope, heart failure, and sudden death from arrhythmias. Life expectancy after exertional chest pain develops averages only 5 years, and valve replacement is indicated for symptomatic patients.

Clinically significant aortic stenosis is uncommonly encountered during pregnancy. Mild to moderate degrees of stenosis are well tolerated, but severe disease is life threatening. The principal underlying hemodynamic problem is the fixed cardiac output associated with severe stenosis. During pregnancy, a number of factors may be encountered that commonly decrease preload further and thus aggravate the fixed cardiac output. Some examples include blood loss, regional analgesia, and vena caval occlusion. Importantly, all of these decrease cardiac, cerebral, and uterine perfusion. Because of these considerations, severe aortic stenosis may be extremely dangerous during pregnancy; indeed, Arias and Pineda (1978) reported a 17 percent mortality rate with severe disease.

Management in Pregnancy. For the asymptomatic pregnant woman, no treatment except close observation is required. Management of the symptomatic woman includes strict limitation of activity and prompt treatment of infections. If symptoms persist despite bed rest, valve replacement or valvotomy using cardiopulmonary bypass must be considered. Angel and colleagues (1988), as well as McIvor (1991), described percutaneous balloon valvoplasty at midpregnancy for women with severe symptomatic aortic stenosis. Anesthesia and cardiopulmonary bypass were obviated, and they calculated that fetal radiation exposure associated with the procedure was acceptable.

For women with critical stenosis, intensive monitoring during labor is important. Pulmonary-artery catheterization may be helpful because of the narrow margin separating fluid overload from hypovolemia. During labor, pain is relieved with liberal doses of narcotics, and epidural analgesia is usually avoided. Easterling and colleagues (1988) described their experiences with 5 women with severe aortic stenosis. Although they used epidural analgesia without maternal mortality, they demonstrated the immediate and profound effects of decreased filling pressures associated with its use. Pushing is discouraged, and if necessary, forceps are used to shorten the second stage of labor. Excessive blood loss must be treated to avoid hypotension, but conversely, if blood loss is minimal, postpartum filling pressures may cause pulmonary congestion, requiring diuresis. Bacterial endocarditis prophylaxis is given at delivery.

Aortic Insufficiency

Aortic regurgitation is the diastolic flow of blood from the aorta into the left ventricle. Because the prevalence of rheumatic fever has declined, major causes of aortic valvar incompetence are connective-tissue abnormalities and congenitally acquired lesions. For example, with Marfan syndrome, the aortic root may dilate, resulting in aortic insufficiency. Acute insufficiency may develop with bacterial endocarditis or aortic dissection. With chronic disease, left-ventricular hypertrophy and dilatation develop. This is followed by delayed symptoms of fatigue, dyspnea, and edema, although rapid deterioration usually follows.

Generally, aortic insufficiency is well tolerated during pregnancy, and like mitral valve incompetence, diminished peripheral vascular resistance is thought to improve the lesion (Lang and Borow, 1991; McAnulty and associates, 1988). Development of symptoms necessitates therapy for heart failure including bed rest, sodium restriction, and diuretics. Epidural analgesia is used for labor pain and vaginal or cesarean delivery. Intrapartum bacterial endocarditis prophylaxis is given.

CONGENITAL HEART DISEASE

The incidence of congenital heart disease in the United States is approximately 8 per 1000 live-born infants. About one third of these infants have critical disease that requires cardiac catheterization or surgery, or they die within the first year (Nugent and associates, 1990). Estimates of incidence of specific lesions will depend on the age group surveyed, viz, newborns versus autopsy studies, and some of these data are cited in Table 48–5.

Lang and Borow (1991) divide congenital heart lesions that complicate pregnancy into three groups: (1) volume overload or left-to-right shunts, examples of which include atrial or ventricular septal defects; (2) pressure overload, such as aortic and pulmonary steno-

TABLE 48–5. INCIDENCE OF CONGENITAL HEART DEFECTS IN 103,590 NEWBORNS FROM 5 COLLECTED STUDIES

Heart Defect	Averaged Percent
Ventricular septal defect	28.3
Pulmonary stenosis	9.5
Patent ductus arteriosus	8.7
Ventricular septal defect with pulmonary stenosis	6.8
Atrial septal defect, secundum	6.7
Aortic stenosis	4.4
Coarctation of aorta	4.2
Atrioventricular canal	3.5
Transposition of great arteries	3.4
All others	7.4

Modified with permission from Nugent and colleagues (1990).

sis, aortic coarctation, and hypertrophic subaortic stenosis; and (3) cyanotic lesions or right-to-left shunts that include Fallot tetralogy and Eisenmenger syndrome.

Septal Defects

Atrial septal defect is the second most common cardiac abnormality in adults after bicuspid aortic valve. Many of these lesions are asymptomatic. The secundum type defect accounts for 70 percent of all cases, and associated mitral valve myxomatous abnormalities with prolapse are common. Unless the lesion is large, findings of right atrial and ventricular dilatation are clinically inconsequential. Pregnancy is well tolerated unless pulmonary hypertension has developed, and this is rare before the third decade. If congestive heart failure or an arrhythmia develops, treatment is commenced. Bacterial endocarditis prophylaxis is felt by most to be unnecessary, unless the defect was repaired with a patch.

Ventricular septal defect is the most common cardiac anomaly found at birth (Table 48–5). In adults it follows bicuspid aortic valve, atrial septal defect, and pulmonic stenosis in frequency. Almost 75 percent of defects are paramembraneous, and physiological derangements are related to their size. Most defects are small and close spontaneously by 10 years of age; however, in children when the effective size of the defect is greater than the aortic valve orifice, symptoms rapidly develop. Many of these children undergo surgical repair before pulmonary hypertension develops, and they do well. Those with unrepaired defects of longer duration develop pulmonary hypertension, and they also have a high incidence of bacterial endocarditis. In general, if the defect is less than 1.25 cm^2, pulmonary hypertension and heart failure do not develop.

Pregnancy is well tolerated with small to moderate left-to-right shunts and even with moderate pulmonary hypertension. When pulmonary arterial pressures reach systemic levels, however, there is reversal or bidirectional flow. This is called the **Eisenmenger syndrome.** When this develops, maternal mortality is 30 to 50 percent. Thus, pregnancy is contraindicated, and therapeutic abortion is advised if contraception fails. Bacterial endocarditis is common with unrepaired defects, and prophylaxis is recommended.

Persistent Ductus Arteriosus

Like other shunts, the physiological consequences of a persistent ductus arteriosus are related to its size. Most significant-sized lesions are repaired in childhood; however, some women with an unrepaired persistent ductus develop pulmonary hypertension. Occasionally, heart failure develops in these women. Moreover, if systemic blood pressure falls, reversal of blood flow from the pulmonary artery into the aorta may occur, and this results in cyanosis. Sudden drops in blood pressure at delivery, as with conduction analgesia or hemorrhage, may lead to fatal collapse. Therefore, hypotension should be avoided whenever possible and treated vigorously if it develops. Prophylaxis for bacterial endocarditis should be given at delivery.

Cyanotic Heart Disease

When congenital heart lesions are associated with right-to-left shunting of blood past the pulmonary capillary bed, then cyanosis develops. The classical and most commonly encountered lesion in pregnancy is the **Fallot tetralogy.** This is characterized by a large ventricular septal defect, right ventricular hypertrophy, and an overriding aorta. The magnitude of the shunt varies inversely with systemic vascular resistance. Hence, during pregnancy, when peripheral resistance decreases, the shunt increases and cyanosis worsens. Women who have undergone repair, and in whom cyanosis did not reappear, do well in pregnancy.

Some women with **Ebstein anomaly** of the tricuspid valve may reach reproductive age. Right-ventricular failure from volume overload and appearance or worsening of cyanosis are common during pregnancy. If there is no cyanosis, these women usually tolerate pregnancy well.

Effect on Pregnancy. Women with cyanotic heart disease do poorly during pregnancy. With uncorrected Fallot tetralogy, for example, maternal mortality approaches 10 percent. Any disease complicated by severe maternal hypoxemia is likely to lead to abortion, preterm labor and delivery, or fetal death. There is a relationship between chronic hypoxemia and the polycythemia it causes with the outcome of pregnancy. Whittemore and colleagues (1980) reported fetal wastage of 36 percent in women with cyanotic congenital heart disease. When hypoxemia is intense enough to stimulate a rise in hematocrit above 65 percent, pregnancy wastage is virtually 100 percent. Shime and associates (1987) reported that 13 of 23 women with cyanotic heart disease developed functional deterioration during pregnancy, and 7 had cardiac failure. Three of these 23 infants (13 percent) died, and low-birthweight infants were common. Patton and colleagues (1990) described 6 such pregnancies; all were complicated by preterm delivery and fetal growth retardation.

With satisfactory surgical correction prior to pregnancy, maternal risks are decreased dramatically, and fetal environment is improved (Whittemore, 1982). Singh and associates (1982), on the basis of 40 pregnancies in 27 patients with surgically corrected tetralogy of

Fallot, concluded that a woman with no major residual defects after surgery may be reassured that pregnancy will be well tolerated, and delivery can be accomplished in a normal manner.

Vaginal delivery of a woman with cyanotic heart disease is preferred unless there is an obstetrical indication for cesarean delivery. Pulmonary artery catheter monitoring has limitations because of the sometimes bizarre anatomical abnormalities. Care must be taken to avoid sudden blood pressure decreases, and most approach the use of epidural analgesia with caution (Patton and colleagues, 1990).

Eisenmenger Syndrome. The Eisenmenger syndrome develops with any cardiac lesion in which pulmonary vascular resistance becomes equal to or greater than systemic resistance and in whom at least some right-to-left shunting occurs at rest or with exercise. These women may survive for decades with relatively few symptoms (Nugent and colleagues, 1990).

The prognosis for pregnancy complicated by these lesions is poor, as it is whenever there is pulmonary hypertension from any cause. Gleicher and associates (1979) reported that both maternal and perinatal mortality rates for Eisenmenger syndrome were about 50 percent. Shime and colleagues (1987) later described 19 pregnancies in 9 such women; half were terminated by spontaneous or therapeutic abortion, and there were only 4 term births. Three women developed heart failure and one died. These women tolerate hypotension poorly, and the cause of death usually is right-ventricular failure with cardiogenic shock.

OTHER CARDIOVASCULAR LESIONS OR CONDITIONS

Pulmonary Hypertension

Pulmonary hypertension is generally secondary to cardiac or pulmonary disease, and common causes are persistent and prolonged left-to-right shunting (as discussed above under "Eisenmenger syndrome"). Other causes are recurrent pulmonary emboli and drug abuse. **Primary pulmonary hypertension,** characterized by medial hypertrophy and plexiform lesions, is usually idiopathic, but some previously unexplained cases may be due to antiphospholipid antibodies (Chap. 54, p. 1234).

Effects on Pregnancy. Whether pulmonary hypertension is primary or secondary, maternal mortality is appreciable. Thus, with severe disease, pregnancy is contraindicated, but milder degrees of secondary pulmonary hypertension probably go unnoticed. For example, with the more common use of pulmonary artery catheterization in women with heart disease, we have identified women with mild to moderate pulmonary hypertension who tolerated pregnancy, labor, and delivery quite well.

Management of labor and delivery is particularly problematic. **These women are at greatest risk when there is diminished venous return and right ventricular filling; this is associated with most maternal deaths.** Treatment of symptomatic pregnant women includes limitation of activity, avoidance of the supine position in late pregnancy, careful attention to blood loss at delivery, avoidance of epidural analgesia, and consideration for pulmonary-artery catheterization during labor and delivery. Pollack and colleagues (1990), as well as others, have reported successful labor analgesia without significant cardiovascular effects from morphine administered intrathecally.

Mitral Valve Prolapse

As many as 5 percent of otherwise normal young women have mitral valve prolapse. Although the condition appears to be inherited, prolapse is commonly associated with a wide variety of other cardiac disorders, including atrial septal defect, Marfan syndrome, Epstein anomaly, and hypertrophic cardiomyopathy. The etiology of *myxomatous degeneration* is unknown.

Most women with mitral valve prolapse are asymptomatic, and they are diagnosed by routine physical examination or as an incidental finding at echocardiography. The small percentage of women with symptoms have anxiety, palpitations, dyspnea, atypical chest pain, and syncope. Nishimura and colleagues (1985) identified only those patients with redundant mitral valve leaflets to be at increased risk of sudden death, infective endocarditis, or cerebral embolism. Artal and colleagues (1988) described such a woman who developed transient cerebral ischemia during pregnancy.

Effects on Pregnancy. Pregnant women with mitral valve prolapse rarely have cardiac complications. In fact, pregnancy-induced hypervolemia may improve alignment of the mitral valve (Rayburn and colleagues, 1987). For women who are symptomatic, β-blocking drugs are given to decrease sympathetic tone, relieve chest pain and palpitations, and reduce the risk of life-threatening arrhythmias. In our experience, mitral valve prolapse has not been deleterious to pregnancy; however, we manage these women as if not pregnant and prescribe β-blocker drugs for symptoms. Mitral valve prolapse is considered by some, but certainly not all, to be a significant risk factor for development of bacterial endocarditis. Women should be given antibiotic prophylaxis if there is mitral valve regurgitation, valvular damage, or any of the risk factors discussed above (Degani and associates, 1989).

Peripartum Cardiomyopathy

A common time for women to develop heart failure is during labor or shortly after delivery. The term peripartum cardiomyopathy is now used widely to describe women with peripartum heart failure with no readily apparent etiology; however, it is doubtful that there is a cardiomyopathy unique to pregnancy. Although 28 women with peripartum heart failure of obscure etiology were initially thought to have idiopathic cardiomyopathy, heart failure in 21 was ultimately attributed to chronic hypertension, unrecognized mitral stenosis, obesity, or viral myocarditis (Cunningham and associates, 1986).

Underlying hypertension, especially with superimposed preeclampsia, is a common finding in otherwise inexplicable peripartum heart failure (Fig. 48–4). Obesity is a common co-factor. Although it commonly coexists with chronic hypertension, obesity alone was correlated with increased left-ventricular mass in the Framingham Heart Study (Lauer and colleagues, 1991).

Regardless of the underlying condition that causes cardiac dysfunction, women who develop peripartum heart failure often have superimposed preeclampsia, and

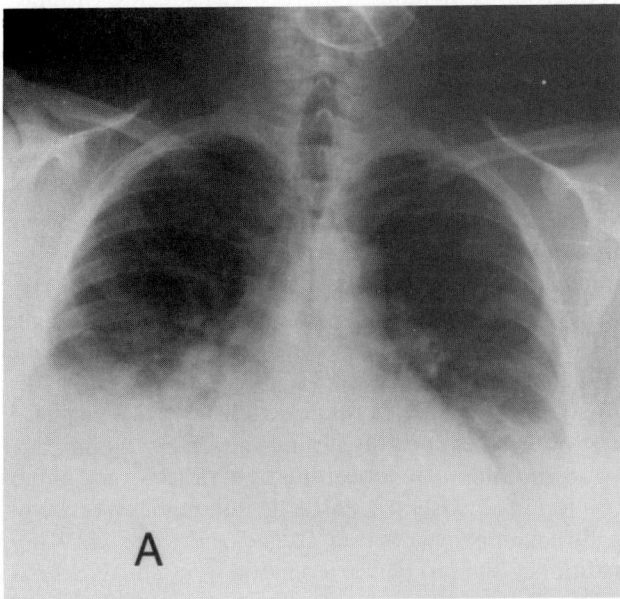

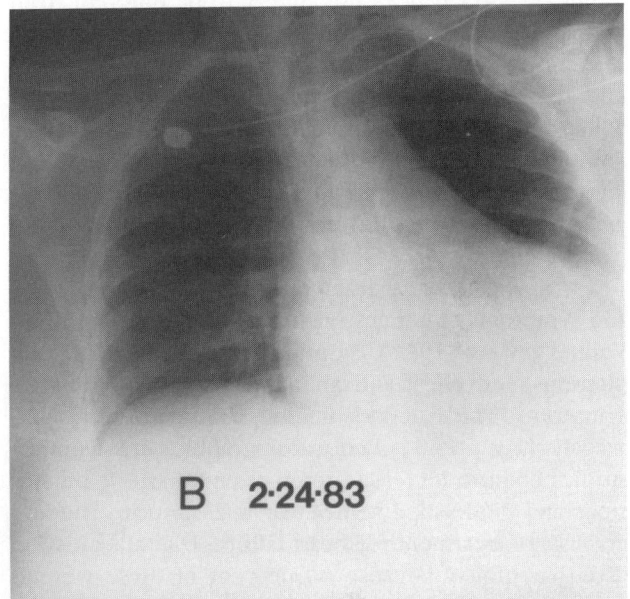

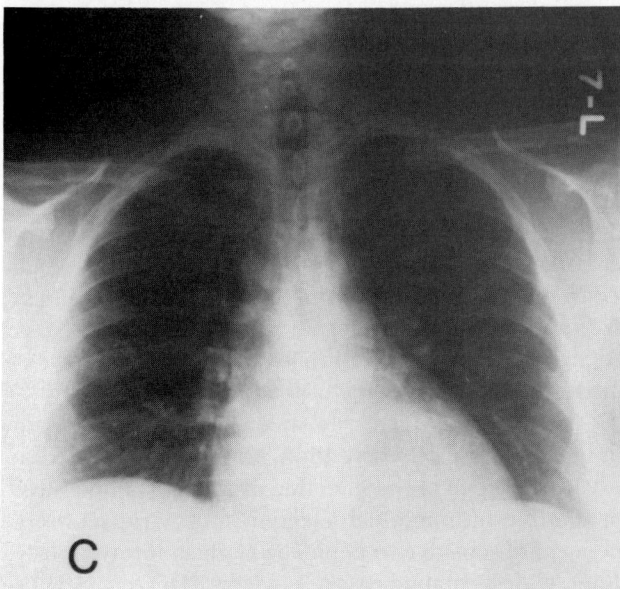

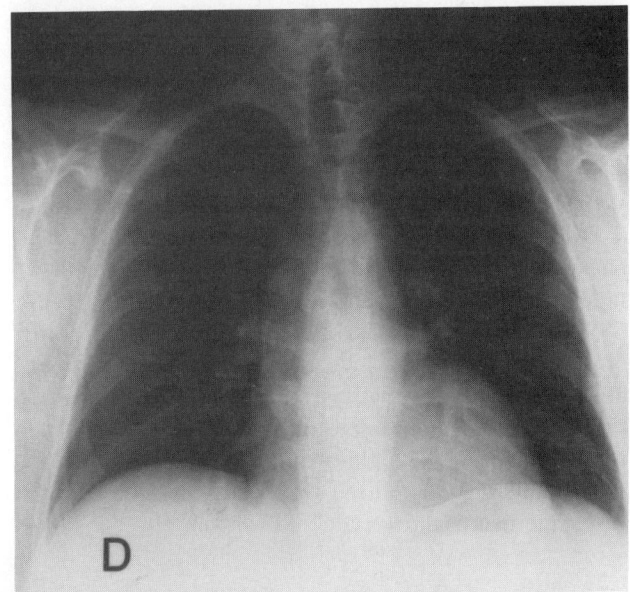

Fig. 48–4. An obese 36-year-old Hispanic multipara with heart failure. **A.** She presented at term with severe preeclampsia, cardiomegaly, and pulmonary edema. **B.** One day later, pulmonary edema resolved but cardiomegaly persisted. Cardiomegaly improved in 2 days **(C)**, and almost completely resolved in 3 days **(D)**. (From Cunningham and associates, 1986, with permission.)

they usually have other obstetrical complications that either contribute to or precipitate heart failure. Factors commonly associated with heart failure include anemia and infection. Anemia likely magnifies compromised ventricular function. Similarly, infection and the accompanying fever increase cardiac output and oxygen utilization.

Idiopathic Cardiomyopathy. In some women after a thorough but unsuccessful search for an underlying cause for heart failure, idiopathic cardiomyopathy may be considered. This was identified in about 1 in 15,000 deliveries at Parkland Hospital (Cunningham and colleagues, 1986). It does not appear to be different from idiopathic cardiomyopathy in nonpregnant young women. In some cases, it may be caused by clinically undetected **myocarditis** (James 1983; Sanderson and colleagues, 1988). O'Connell and colleagues (1986) found that almost 30 percent of pregnant women with idiopathic cardiomyopathy had biopsy evidence of myocarditis compared with only 10 percent of nonpregnant patients.

Women with cardiomyopathy present with signs and symptoms of congestive heart failure. According to Veille's review (1984), dyspnea, orthopnea, cough, palpitations, and chest and abdominal pain are common symptoms. The hallmark finding is impressive cardiomegaly (Fig. 48–5). Echocardiographic and Doppler studies confirm increased internal end-diastolic dimensions and diminished ventricular wall motion. Therapy consists of treatment for heart failure. Digitalis must be given cautiously because 60 percent of these women have complex ventricular arrhythmias (O'Connell and colleagues, 1986). Diuretics are also given, and sodium intake is limited while avoiding hypokalemia. Afterload reduction has been recommended; however, angiotensin-converting enzyme inhibitors should be avoided if the woman is undelivered (see Chap. 42, p. 965). Because there is a high incidence of associated pulmonary embolism, anticoagulation with heparin is recommended.

The distinction between peripartum heart failure from explicable causes versus idiopathic is important, because prognosis for the latter is poor (Fig. 48–5). Indeed, in the study by O'Connell and associates (1986), 6 of 14 women with peripartum idiopathic cardiomyopathy were dead by 1 year. In nonpregnant patients, idiopathic cardiomyopathy eventually results in death in over 75 percent from unrelenting cardiomegaly and failure (Homans, 1985). Unfortunately, heart transplantation is the only definitive treatment for women with end-stage heart failure (Lee and Cotton, 1989).

Infective Endocarditis

Infective endocarditis involves cardiac endothelium and produces vegetations that usually deposit on a valve. While the incidence of rheumatic fever has diminished, that of bacterial endocarditis has become more common. This is most often because children and adults who survive corrective surgery for congenital heart disease are at greatest risk. Indeed, except for acute bacterial endocarditis associated with illicit drug use, about 75 percent of adult patients have a known preexisting heart lesion. The relative risks of endocarditis with some lesions are shown in Table 48–6.

Subacute bacterial endocarditis usually is due to a low-virulence bacterial infection superimposed on an underlying lesion. Organisms that cause subacute, indolent bacterial endocarditis are most commonly streptococci, including α-hemolytic or viridans group or those from group D including *Enterococcus* species. Group B streptococcal endocarditis can be subacute or acute. Gallagher and Watanakunakorn (1986) noted that almost 10 percent of such cases reported since 1962 were in pregnant women. Acute endocarditis is usually caused by coagulase-positive staphylococci, and the predominant organism in intravenous drug abusers is *Staphylococcus aureus.* This organism, along with *Streptococcus pneumoniae* and *Neisseria gonorrheae,* causes acute, fulminating disease. Bataskov and colleagues (1991) recently described the third case of fatal gonococcal endocarditis complicating pregnancy. Deger and Ludmir (1992) described the first case of infective endocarditis caused by *Neisseria sicca* and we have had a maternal death due to endocarditis from *Neisseria mucosa.*

Symptoms of endocarditis are variable and often develop insidiously. Fever, chills, and night sweats typically accompany anorexia, fatigue, and weakness. Constitutional symptoms are common, and the illness is frequently described as "flu-like." Other findings are manifestations of embolic lesions, including focal neurological manifestations (see Chap. 55, p. 1246), chest or abdominal pain, and ischemia in an extremity. In some cases, heart failure may develop. In the usual case, symptoms usually persist for 4 to 8 weeks before the diagnosis is made (Durack, 1990). Thus, a high index of suspicion is necessary to consider endocarditis. Diagnosis is confirmed by excluding other causes of febrile illnesses and recovering positive blood cultures for typical organisms. Echocardiography and two-dimensional sector scanning are useful, but lesions only 3 to 4 mm in size or those on the tricuspid valve may be missed. **A negative echocardiographic study does not exclude endocarditis.**

Treatment is primarily medical with appropriate timing of surgical intervention if this becomes necessary. Knowledge of the infecting organism is imperative for sensible antimicrobial selection. Most viridans streptococci are sensitive to penicillin G given intravenously along with gentamicin for 2 weeks (Durack, 1990). Women with complicated infections are treated longer, and those allergic to penicillin are either desensitized or given intravenous ceftriaxone or vancomycin for 4 weeks. Staphylococci, enterococci, and other organisms are treated according to microbial sensitivity for 4 to 6

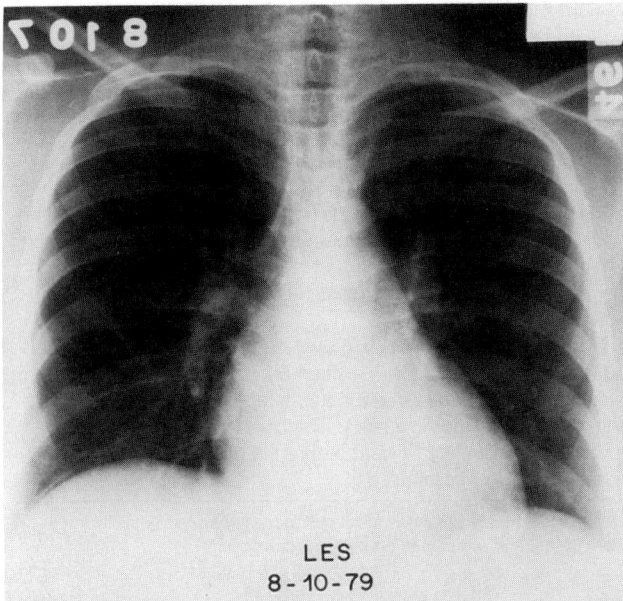

A

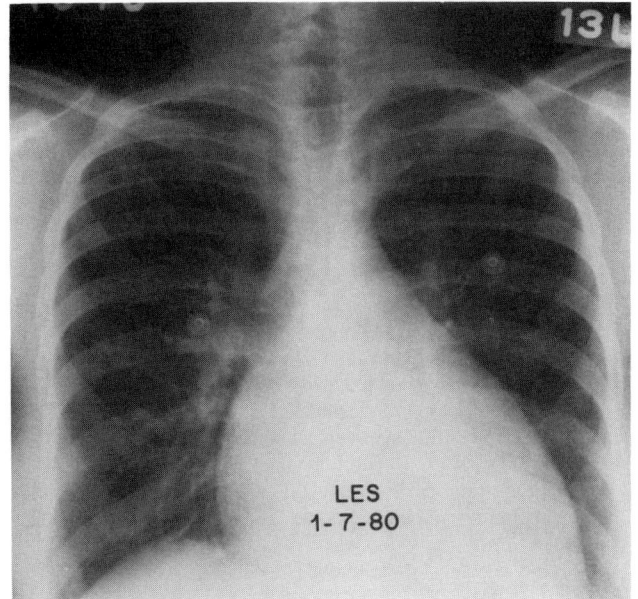

B

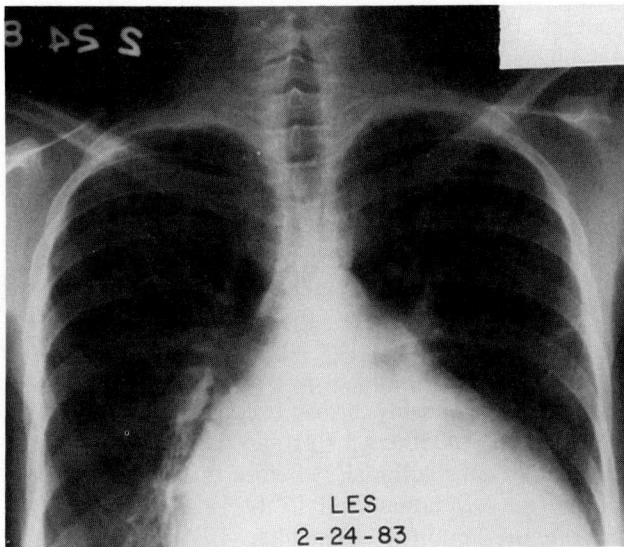

C

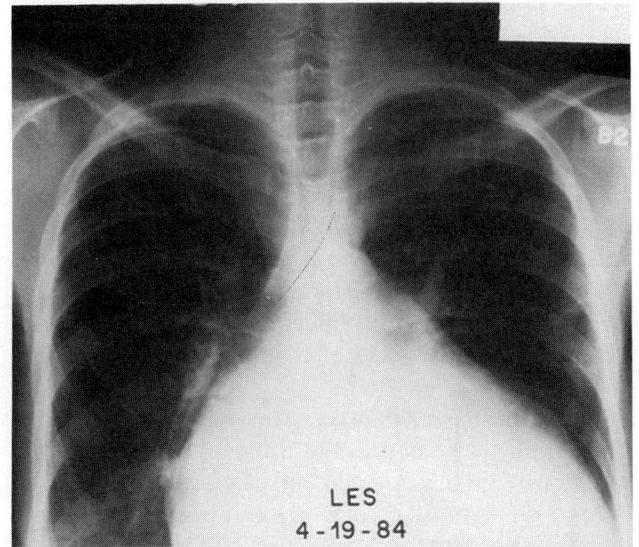

D

Fig. 48–5. Idiopathic peripartum cardiomyopathy. This woman developed peripartum heart failure without any identifiable underlying cardiac disease and no associated preeclampsia. Despite an initially good symptomatic response and clearing of pulmonary edema, mild cardiomegaly persisted 3 months postpartum (**A**). Over the ensuing 5 years (**B–D**) cardiomegaly worsened, and she died of end-stage heart failure at age 23. (From Cunningham and colleagues, 1986, with permission.)

weeks or longer. Carefully timed surgical intervention may be necessary to eradicate infection or to reverse heart failure. Persistent native valve infection may require replacement, and this is even more commonly indicated with an infected prosthetic valve.

Endocarditis in Pregnancy. Bacterial endocarditis, acute or subacute, is uncommon during pregnancy and the puerperium. Pastorek and colleagues (1983) cited an incidence of 1 in 4000 to 8000 during pregnancy. Seaworth and Durack (1986) reviewed the literature and reported a 33 percent maternal mortality rate. Cox

and Leveno (1989) cited a maternal mortality of 20 to 25 percent in their review, but found this to be no different than for nonpregnant women. Endocarditis has contributed appreciably to maternal deaths at Parkland Hospital in recent years. Most often the pregnant women were taking illicit drugs intravenously, then developed bacterial endocarditis, and died from valvar incompetence or cerebral emboli. Over 7 years, the incidence of endocarditis at Parkland Hospital was about 1 in 16,000 deliveries (Cox and associates, 1988). Two of 7 women died.

Surgical intervention with prosthetic valve replace-

TABLE 48–6. ESTIMATES OF RELATIVE RISKS FOR INFECTIVE ENDOCARDITIS WITH VARIOUS TYPES OF CARDIAC LESIONS

High Risk	Intermediate Risk	Low or Negligible Risk
Prosthetic heart valves	Mitral valve prolapse	Atrial septal defect
Aortic valve disease	Mitral stenosis	Arteriosclerotic plaques
Mitral insufficiency	Tricuspid valve disease	Coronary artery disease
Patent ductus arteriosus	Pulmonary valve disease	Syphilitic aortitis
Ventricular septal defect	Previous infective endocarditis	Pacemakers
Aortic coarctation	Asymmetrical septal hypertrophy	Surgically corrected lesions without prosthesis
Marfan syndrome	Calcific aortic stenosis	
	Intravenous lines into right atrium	
	Nonvalvar intracardiac prosthesis	

Modified from Durack (1990).

TABLE 48–7. 1990 AMERICAN HEART ASSOCIATION GUIDELINES FOR BACTERIAL ENDOCARDITIS PROPHYLAXIS FOR GENITOURINARY AND GASTROINTESTINAL PROCEDURES

Standard regimen—ampicillin, gentamicin, and amoxicillin:
 Intravenous or intramuscular ampicillin, 2 g, plus gentamicin, 1.5 mg/kg (not to exceed 80 mg), 30 minutes before the procedure; then amoxicillin, 1.5 g orally, 6 hours after the initial dose. Alternatively, the parenteral regimen may be repeated 8 hours after the initial dose.
Regimen for penicillin-allergic patients–vancomycin and gentamicin:
 Intravenous vancomycin, 1 g over 1 hour, plus intravenous gentamicin, 1.5 mg/kg (not to exceed 80 mg), 1 hour before the procedure; may be repeated 8 hours after the initial dose.
Alternate regimen for low-risk patients[a]—amoxicillin:
 Oral amoxicillin, 3 g, 1 hour before the procedure, then 1.5 g 6 hours after the initial dose.

[a] Also recommended regimen for dental procedures.
From Dajani and colleagues (1990), with permission.

ment of the destroyed valve along with antimicrobial therapy and meticulous supportive care may prevent a fatal outcome. Cavalieri and associates (1982) described a woman in whom a ruptured, abscessed aortic valve was replaced early in the puerperium and the mother discharged after 6 weeks of antibiotic therapy.

Antimicrobial Prophylaxis. The efficacy of antimicrobial prophylaxis to prevent bacterial endocarditis is questionable. Only 13 percent of cases arising in patients with high-risk cardiac lesions do so after a procedure (van der Meer and associates, 1992). Despite a low incidence of disease, the American Heart Association recommends that one of the antimicrobial regimens shown in Table 48–7 be given prophylactically during high-risk procedures in order to minimize the risk of bacterial endocarditis and infective arteritis in certain patients (Dajani and colleagues, 1990). These are those with valvar prostheses, previous bacterial endocarditis, most congenital heart abnormalities, rheumatic or acquired valvar disease, hypertrophic cardiomyopathy, or mitral valve prolapse with regurgitation. Those high- and intermediate-risk lesions listed in Table 48–6 constitute indication for endocarditis prophylaxis.

Obstetrical Procedures. The 1990 guidelines include a long list of invasive procedures for which prophylaxis is recommended, but the only obstetrical indication is vaginal delivery in the presence of infection. Specifically, cesarean section is excluded. The incidence of transient bacteremia at delivery is about 5 to 10 percent

(Durack, 1990). Although there is meager evidence that a significant number of cases of bacterial endocarditis have been prevented with antimicrobial prophylaxis given for uncomplicated delivery, its risk and costs are not great (McFaul and associates, 1988; Seaworth and Durack, 1986). Individualization seems appropriate. For example, with premature or prolonged membrane rupture, manual placental removal, or fourth-degree perineal lacerations in women with high-risk lesions, prophylaxis is recommended. According to the American College of Obstetricians and Gynecologists (1992), it would be appropriate to provide prophylaxis for all pregnant women with cardiac lesions.

Current guidelines for prophylaxis include an initial dose of antimicrobial(s) before the procedure and another several hours later (Table 48–7). Obviously, accurate prediction of vaginal delivery time is problematic to timely administration of the first dose.

Arrhythmias

Cardiac arrhythmias are commonly encountered during pregnancy, labor and delivery, and the puerperium. It is debated whether arrhythmias are more common during pregnancy, but in our experiences, their detection is probably increased because of closer observation. Perhaps the normal but mild hypokalemia of pregnancy induces arrhythmias. Most arrhythmias in young women are not associated with organic heart disease, and most often their treatment in pregnancy is not different from that for nonpregnant patients.

Bradyarrhythmias, including complete heart block, are compatible with a successful pregnancy outcome. Some women with complete heart block will have syncope during labor and delivery and occasionally temporary cardiac pacing is necessary. Women with permanent artificial pacemakers usually tolerate pregnancy well (Jaffe and associates, 1987). With fixed-rate devices, cardiac output apparently is increased by augmented stroke volume.

Tachyarrhythmias are relatively common. Whenever these arrhythmias are encountered, underlying cardiac disease should be considered; for example, Wolff–Parkinson–White syndrome may first appear during pregnancy (Gleicher and associates, 1981). In some cases, these women have been documented to have an increased incidence of tachycardia during pregnancy (Widerhorn and co-workers, 1992). **Paroxysmal supraventricular tachycardia** is encountered most frequently. If vagal maneuvers do not stimulate conversion, treatment consists of digoxin, β-blocker drugs, or calcium-channel blocking drugs. Although these drugs cross the placenta, they do not appear to harm the fetus (Rotmensch and colleagues, 1983). We have had success with intravenous adenosine when these arrhythmias were refractory to calcium-channel blocking drugs. Cardioversion is not contraindicated by pregnancy in itself. **Ventricular tachycardia** is uncommon in healthy young women without underlying heart disease. Brodsky and associates (1992) described 7 pregnant women with new-onset ventricular tachycardia and reviewed 23 previously published reports. Most of these women were not found to have structural heart disease, and in 60 percent, arrhythmias were stimulated by physical exercise or psychological stress. Of those remaining, 2 had myocardial infarction, 2 had a prolonged QT interval, and anesthesia provoked tachycardia in another. In 6 of 26, no precipitating event was found. The investigators concluded that pregnancy events probably precipitated tachycardia and recommended β-blocker therapy for control.

Atrial flutter or fibrillation are more likely associated with underlying disease, such as thyrotoxicosis. Major complications include thromboembolism. Thus, heparin is recommended by some if fibrillation is chronic, was identified before pregnancy, and persists during pregnancy. If atrial fibrillation is associated with mitral stenosis, pulmonary edema may develop in late pregnancy if the ventricular rate is increased. Digitalis is given to diminish ventricular response, and quinidine may prevent its recurrence.

Diseases of the Aorta

Marfan syndrome and coarctation of the aorta are two aortic diseases that place the pregnant woman at increased risk for **aortic dissection.** Other risk factors are bicuspid aortic valve and Turner or Noonan syndrome. The initiating event is an aortic intimal tear, and following medial hemorrhage, rupture may occur. Although the mechanism(s) involved are unclear, half of all aortic dissections in women under age 40 develop during late pregnancy (Lang and Borow, 1991). Pertinent to this may be the observations by Easterling and colleagues (1991) that aortic diameter increased significantly over the course of pregnancy. This was even greater for women who developed preeclampsia.

In most cases, women with aortic dissection present with severe chest pain described as ripping, tearing, or stabbing in nature. Diminution or loss of peripheral pulses in conjunction with a recently acquired murmur of aortic insufficiency are important physical findings. According to DeSanctis and colleagues (1987), the differential diagnosis of aortic dissection includes myocardial infarction, pulmonary embolism, pneumothorax, and aortic valve rupture. Lang and Borow (1991) rightfully add obstetrical catastrophes to the list, especially placental abruption and uterine rupture.

Over 90 percent of patients have an abnormal chest x-ray. Although aortic angiography is the most definitive method for confirming the diagnosis, noninvasive imaging with sonography, computed tomography, and magnetic-resonance imaging are being used more frequently. The urgency of the clinical situation frequently will dictate which procedure is best. Initial treatment is medical to lower blood pressure. Proximal dissections most often need to be resected, along with aortic valve replacement if indicated. Distal dissections are more complex, and many may be treated medically (DeSanctis and colleagues, 1987).

Marfan Syndrome. This syndrome is usually inherited as an autosomal dominant trait with a high degree of penetrance. It is caused by an abnormal fibrillin gene located on chromosome 15q. It is characterized by a generalized weakness of connective tissue, which can result in dangerous cardiovascular complications. Progressive aortic dilatation causes aortic valve insufficiency, and there may be infective endocarditis, mitral valve prolapse, and mitral insufficiency. Aortic dilatation and dissecting aneurysm are the most serious abnormalities. Early death is due either to valvar insufficiency and heart failure or to a dissecting aneurysm.

Effect of Pregnancy. As discussed above, deaths due to dissecting aortic aneurysm are more common during pregnancy in women with Marfan syndrome. Previous grave concerns, however, of the effects of pregnancy were overestimated. Pyeritz (1981) reviewed the literature and found that 20 of 32 women with Marfan syndrome who became pregnant either died or had aortic dissection during or shortly after pregnancy. Most of these were case reports, which he inferred constituted significant bias. Indeed, only 1 of his own 26 patients from the Johns Hopkins Hospital died postpartum from infective endocarditis, and this woman had severe pre-existing heart disease. He concluded that women with aortic dilatation more than 40 mm in diameter or mitral valve dysfunction are at high risk for life-threatening cardiovascular complications during pregnancy. Conversely, women with minimal or no dilatation, and those with normal cardiac function by echocardiography, are counseled regarding the small but potential risk of aortic dissection.

From their review, Mor-Yosef and colleagues (1988) likewise concluded that there were no contraindications to conception in women with Marfan syndrome who had no cardiovascular manifestations. During pregnancy, they recommended monthly echocardiographic aortic diameter measurement. Although Marfan syndrome alone is not an indication for abdominal delivery, they recommended cesarean delivery using epidural analgesia and pulmonary-artery catheter monitoring for women with aortic involvement. Finally, unless complications ensued, repair was delayed until 4 to 6 weeks postpartum.

Coarctation of the Aorta. Aortic coarctation is a relatively rare lesion often accompanied by lesions of other large arteries. For example, a bicuspid aortic valve is demonstrated by echocardiography in approximately 25 percent of affected patients, and about 10 percent also have cerebral artery aneurysms. Other associated lesions are persistent ductus arteriosus, septal defects, and Turner syndrome. The collateral circulation arising above the level of the coarctation expands, often to a striking extent, to cause localized erosion of rib margins by hypertrophied intercostal arteries. Typical findings on physical examination are hypertension in upper extremities but normal or reduced blood pressures in lower extremities.

Aortic Coarctation in Pregnancy. The major complications of coarctation are congestive heart failure after long-standing severe hypertension, bacterial endocarditis of the **bicuspid aortic valve,** and rupture of the aorta. Reported maternal mortality rates average about 3 percent (McAnulty, 1990). Because hypertension may worsen in pregnancy, antihypertensive therapy using β-blocking drugs is usually required. Aortic rupture is more likely to occur late in pregnancy or early in the puerperium. Rupture may be associated with changes in the media that are histologically similar to those of Erdheim idiopathic medial cystic necrosis. Cerebral hemorrhage from **circle of Willis aneurysms** may also develop.

Congestive heart failure demands vigorous efforts to improve cardiac function and may warrant pregnancy interruption. It has been recommended by some that resection of the coarctation be undertaken during pregnancy to protect against the possibility of a dissecting aneurysm and aortic rupture. The operation, however, has significant risks. This is especially true for the fetus, because all the collaterals must be clamped for variable periods of time during the procedure, possibly leading to serious fetal hypoxia.

Some authorities recommend cesarean delivery to prevent transient arterial blood pressure elevations that commonly accompany labor. It is speculated that such blood pressure increases might lead to rupture of either the aorta or coexisting cerebral aneurysms. Available evidence, however, is consistent with the conclusion that cesarean delivery should be limited to obstetrical indications. Bacterial endocarditis prophylaxis should be given at delivery.

Coarctation of the aorta has a familial tendency, and about 2 percent of infants born to an affected patient will have the lesion.

Ischemic Heart Disease

Ischemic heart disease, which may lead to **myocardial infarction,** is a rare complication of pregnancy. The collective incidence of myocardial infarction complicating pregnancy is cited to be 1 in 10,000 (Lang and Borow, 1991). Our experiences at Parkland Hospital indicate that it is much less common. Frequently, women with coronary artery disease have classical risk factors such as cigarette smoking, familial hyperlipidemia, obesity, hypertension, or diabetes. Reece and associates (1986) documented unusually high mortality in pregnant diabetics who suffered myocardial infarction.

Treatment of infarction is similar to that for the nonpregnant patient, and concerns are directed to whether the infarct was sustained before or during pregnancy. Surprisingly, infarction is reported to be more common during pregnancy. Some women who have no preexisting coronary artery disease have sustained infarctions associated with prostaglandin E_2 suppositories to induce labor (Meyer and associates, 1991), ergonovine given for postpartum hemorrhage (Liao and associates, 1991), or bromocriptine given to suppress lactation (Ruch and During, 1989).

Effect of Pregnancy. The advisability of pregnancy after a myocardial infarction is unclear. Ischemic heart disease is characteristically progressive; and because it is usually associated with hypertension, pregnancy seems inadvisable. Certainly, pregnancy increases cardiac workload; therefore, symptoms as well as adequacy of ventricular function prior to contraception will determine outcome.

Frenkel and colleagues (1991) reviewed the 20 reported cases of pregnancy in women who had sustained an infarction remote from pregnancy. They added their experiences with 4 women. Although none of the 24 women died, 4 had congestive heart failure and 4 had worsening angina during pregnancy. They concluded that ventricular performance should be assessed prior to conception using ventriculography, radionuclide studies, echocardiography, and coronary angiography. If there is no significant ventricular dysfunction, pregnancy will likely be tolerated. For the woman who becomes pregnant before these studies are performed, echocardiography should be done. Exercise tolerance testing may be indicated, and radionuclide ventriculography results in very little radiation exposure for the fetus (see Chap. 43, p. 986).

The prognosis for myocardial infarction during pregnancy is serious, but fortunately it also is quite rare. Hankins and co-workers (1985) reviewed pregnancy outcomes in 68 cases and reported an overall maternal mortality rate of 30 to 35 percent. In a more recent review, Hands and colleagues (1990) found an overall mortality of 30 percent. Of 50 women who sustained infarction in the third trimester, 40 percent died, compared with only 20 percent of the other 35 women who had an infarction earlier in pregnancy. Women who sustain an infarction less than 2 weeks prior to labor appear to be at especially high risk of death.

Management. For women with myocardial infarction diagnosed during pregnancy, there should be strict limitation of activity throughout pregnancy, with usual medical treatment given for signs and symptoms of coronary insufficiency or ventricular dysfunction (Hands and associates, 1990; Hankins and colleagues, 1985). Nitrates and calcium-channel or β-blockers are given if indicated. Cesarean delivery is reserved for obstetrical indications, and epidural analgesia is administered to reduce pain during labor.

In some women, invasive or surgical procedures may be indicated because of unrelenting disease. Hands and associates (1990) reported successful use of percutaneous transluminal coronary angioplasty in a 36-week pregnant woman. Majdan and colleagues (1983) performed aortocoronary bypass grafting in a woman at 14 weeks' gestation. Cardiopulmonary bypass time was 90 minutes; no complications were encountered; and she delivered at term. Saxena and co-workers (1992) described balloon angioplasty done in a diabetic woman 3 days following cesarean delivery.

Hypertrophic Cardiomyopathy

Although concentric left ventricular hypertrophy commonly develops after long-standing hypertension, there is a familial as well as a sporadic form not related to hypertension called **idiopathic hypertrophic subaortic stenosis.** The condition is commonly associated with pheochromocytoma, Friedreich ataxia, Turner syndrome, and neurofibromatosis. In the half of cases that are inherited, about 50 percent are autosomally dominant disorders (Baughman, 1992). The abnormality is in the myocardial muscle, and it is characterized by idiopathic left ventricular myocardial hypertrophy that may provide a pressure gradient to left ventricular outflow (Lang and Borow, 1990). Diagnosis is confirmed by Doppler echocardiography.

The majority of affected women are asymptomatic, but dyspnea, anginal or atypical chest pain, syncope, and arrhythmias may develop. Complex arrhythmias may progress to sudden death, which is the most common form of death. Asymptomatic patients with runs of ventricular tachycardia are especially prone to sudden death. Symptoms are usually worsened by exercise.

Management in Pregnancy. There is little published experience with hypertrophic aortic stenosis complicating pregnancy. Although limited reports suggest that pregnancy is well tolerated, congestive heart failure may develop. Oakley and colleagues (1979) reviewed the outcomes of 53 pregnancies. Although pronounced shortness of breath developed in about one fourth, this usually responded to bed rest and diuretic therapy. Only 2 women had symptoms of angina during pregnancy. In a report of 3 patients, van Kasteren and associates (1990) described a woman with worsening dyspnea controlled with limited activity during two successive pregnancies.

Strenuous exercise is prohibited during pregnancy. Abrupt positional changes are avoided to prevent reflex vasodilation and decreased preload. Likewise, drugs that evoke diuresis or diminish vascular resistance are not used. If symptoms develop, especially angina, β-adrenergic or calcium-channel blocking drugs are given. The route of delivery is determined by obstetrical indications and epidural analgesia is usually avoided. Endocarditis prophylaxis is given at delivery. Infants rarely demonstrate inherited lesions at the time of birth.

Kyphoscoliotic Heart Disease

During pregnancy, severe degrees of kyphoscoliosis commonly cause serious cardiopulmonary problems, sometimes referred to as **kyphoscoliotic heart disease.** In these circumstances, some regions of the lungs in the markedly deformed thoracic cage may be quite emphysematous, while others are atelectatic, with both lesions contributing to an inadequate ventilatory capacity. In addition, chronic hypercapnia and hypoxemia may induce pulmonary vasoconstriction, leading to right ventricular hypertrophy and pulmonary hypertension with **cor pulmonale.**

The increased oxygen demands and cardiac work imposed by pregnancy and delivery must be taken into account when counseling these women. For example, if pulmonary function studies indicate that the vital capacity is not appreciably reduced, then pregnancy outcome is most often favorable. Sawicka and associates (1986) described 6 cases of pregnancy and severe kyphoscoliosis characterized by vital capacities from 20 to 40 percent of predicted values. In all women, breathlessness worsened during pregnancy, and cyanosis and the need for mechanical ventilation were common. In women with marked degrees of kyphoscoliosis and markedly impaired pulmonary function, therapeutic abortion probably is indicated.

Frequently, the bony pelvis is so distorted that cesarean delivery is necessary. Kopenhager (1977) reported that 40 percent of 49 women with kyphoscoliosis had to have cesarean deliveries because of cephalopelvic disproportion. The supine position during delivery may result in serious hypotension. Commonly used analgesics such as meperidine should be given carefully, because respiratory depression is tolerated very poorly. During and after delivery, meticulous care should be directed toward prevention of further atelectasis, which could rapidly lead to severe hypoxia and death. Intermittent positive-pressure breathing is helpful when used with appropriate concentrations of oxygen and mucolytic agents. Sterilization is often indicated.

Cardiopulmonary Resuscitation

Cardiac arrest fortunately is rare during pregnancy. Special considerations for resuscitation are described in detail in Chapter 47 (p. 1078).

References

Al Kasab SM, Sabag T, Al Zaibag M, Awaad M, Al Bitar I, Halim MA, Abdullah MA, Shahed M, Rajendran V, Sawyer W: β-Adrenergic receptor blockade in the management of pregnant women with mitral stenosis. Am J Obstet Gynecol 163:37, 1990

American College of Obstetricians and Gynecologists: Cardiac disease in pregnancy. Technical bulletin no. 168, June 1992a

American College of Obstetricians and Gynecologists: Invasive hemodynamic monitoring in obstetrics and gynecology. Technical bulletin no. 175, December 1992

Angel JL, Chapman C, Knuppel RA, Morales WJ, Sims CJ: Percutaneous balloon aortic valvuloplasty in pregnancy. Obstet Gynecol 72:438, 1988

Arias F, Pineda J: Aortic stenosis and pregnancy. J Reprod Med 20:229, 1978

Artal R, Greenspoon JS, Rutherford S: Transient ischemic attack: A complication of mitral valve prolapse in pregnancy. Obstet Gynecol 71:1028, 1988

Bataskov KL, Hariharan S, Horowitz MD, Neibart RM, Cox MM: Gonococcal endocarditis complicating pregnancy: A case report and literature review. Obstet Gynecol 78:494, 1991

Baughman KL: Hypertrophic cardiomyopathy. JAMA 267:846, 1992

Bernal JM, Miralles PJ: Cardiac surgery with cardiopulmonary bypass during pregnancy. Obstet Gynecol Surv 41:1, 1986

Bitsch M, Johansen C, Wennevold A, Osler M: Maternal heart disease: A survey of a decade in a danish university hospital. Acta Obstet Gynecol Scand 68:119, 1989

Brady K, Duff P: Rheumatic heart disease in pregnancy. Clin Obstet Gynecol 32:21, 1989

Brodsky M, Doria R, Allen B, Sato D, Thomas G, Sada M: New-onset ventricular tachycardia during pregnancy. Am Heart J 123:933, 1992

Burke AB, Hur D, Bolan JC, Corso P, Resano FG: Sinusoidal fetal heart rate pattern during cardiopulmonary bypass. Am J Obstet Gynecol 163:17, 1990

Capeless EL, Clapp JF: Cardiovascular changes in early phase of pregnancy. Am J Obstet Gynecol 161:1449, 1989

Carruth JE, Mivis SB, Brogan DR, Wenger NK: The electrocardiogram in normal pregnancy. Chest 102:1075, 1981

Cavalieri RL, Watkins L, Abraham RA, Berkay HS, Niebyl JR: Acute bacterial endocarditis with postpartum aortic valve replacement. Obstet Gynecol 59:124, 1982

Chesley LC: Severe rheumatic cardiac disease and pregnancy: The ultimate prognosis. Am J Obstet Gynecol 136:552, 1980

Clark SL, Cotton DB, Lee W, Bishop C, Hill T, Southwick J, Pivarnik J, Spillman T, DeVore GR, Phelan J, Hankins GDV, Benedetti TJ, Tolley D: Central hemodynamic assessment of normal term pregnancy. Am J Obstet Gynecol 161:1439, 1989

Clark SL, Phelan JP, Greenspoon J, Aldahl D, Horenstein J: Labor and delivery in the presence of mitral stenosis: Central hemodynamic observations. Am J Obstet Gynecol 152:984, 1985

Cox SM, Hankins GDV, Leveno KJ, Cunningham FG: Bacterial endocarditis: A serious pregnancy complication. J Reprod Med 33:671, 1988

Cox SM, Leveno KJ: Pregnancy complicated by bacterial endocarditis. Clin Obstet Gynecol 32:48, 1989

Cunningham FG, Pritchard JA, Hankins GDV, Anderson PL, Lucas MK, Armstrong KF: Idiopathic cardiomyopathy or compounding cardiovascular events. Obstet Gynecol 67:157, 1986

Dajani AS, Bisno AL, Kyung JC, Durack DT, Freed M, Gerber MA, Karchmer AW, Millard HD, Rahimtoola S, Shulman ST, Watanakunakorn C, Taubert KA: Prevention of bacterial endocarditis. Recommendations of the American Heart Association. JAMA 264:2919, 1990

Degani S, Abinader EG, Scharf M: Mitral valve prolapse and pregnancy: A review. Obstet Gynecol Surv 44:642, 1989

Deger R, Ludmir J: Neisseria sicca. Endocarditis complicating pregnancy. J Reprod Med 37:473, 1992

DeSanctis RW, Doroghazi RM, Austen WG, Buckley MJ: Aortic dissection. N Engl J Med 317:1060, 1987

Deviri E, Levinsky L, Yechezkel M, Levy MJ: Pregnancy after valve replacement with porcine xenograft prothesis. Surg Gynecol Obstet 160:437, 1985

Dorfman SF: Maternal mortality in New York City, 1981–1983. Obstet Gynecol 76:317, 1990

Durack DT: Infective and noninfective endocarditis. In Hurst JW, Schlant RC, Rackley CE, Sonnenblick EH, Wenger NK (eds): The Heart, 7th ed. New York, McGraw-Hill, 1990, p 1230

Easterling TR, Benedetti TJ, Schmucker BC, Carlson K, Millard SP: Maternal hemodynamics and aortic diameter in normal and hypertensive pregnancies. Obstet Gynecol 78:1073, 1991

Easterling TR, Chadwick HS, Otto CM, Benedetti TJ: Aortic stenosis in pregnancy. Obstet Gynecol 72:113, 1988

El-Maraghy M, Abou Senna I, El-Tehewy F, Bassiouni M, Ayoub

A, El-Sayad H: Mitral valvotomy in pregnancy. Am J Obstet Gynecol 145:708, 1983

Etheridge MJ, Pepperell RJ: Heart disease and pregnancy at the Royal Women's Hospital. Med J Aust 2:277, 1977

Frenkel Y, Barkai G, Reisin L, Rath S, Mashiach S, Battler A: Pregnancy after myocardial infarction: Are we playing safe? Obstet Gynecol 77:822, 1991

Gallagher PG, Watanakunakorn C: Group B streptococcal endocarditis: Report of seven cases and review of the literature, 1962–1985. Rev Infect Dis 8:175, 1986

Gleicher N, Meller J, Sandler RZ, Sullum S: Wolff–Parkinson–White syndrome in pregnancy. Obstet Gynecol 58:748, 1981

Gleicher N, Midwall J, Hochberger D, Jaffin H: Eisenmenger's syndrome and pregnancy. Obstet Gynecol Surv 34:721, 1979

Gorenberg H, Chesley LC: Rheumatic heart disease in pregnancy: The remote prognosis in patients with "functionally severe" disease. Ann Intern Med 49:278, 1958

Hamilton BE, Thomson KJ: The Heart in Pregnancy and the Childbearing Age. Boston, Little, Brown, 1941

Hands ME, Johnson MD, Saltzman DH, Rutherford JD: The cardiac, obstetric, and anesthetic management of pregnancy complicated by acute myocardial infarction. J Clin Anesth 2:258, 1990

Hankins GD, Wendel GD Jr, Leveno KJ, Stoneham J: Myocardial infarction during pregnancy: A review. Obstet Gynecol 65:138, 1985

Heck CF, Shumway SJ, Kaye MP: The registry of the International Society of Heart Transplantation: Sixth official report, 1989. J Heart Transplant 8:271, 1989

Hedon B, Montoya F, Cabrol A: Twin pregnancy and vaginal birth after heart transplantation. Lancet 335:476, 1990

Homans DC: Peripartum cardiomyopathy. N Engl J Med 312:1432, 1985

Ismail MB, Abid F, Trabelsi S, Taktak M, Fekih M: Cardiac valve prostheses, anticoagulation, and pregnancy. Br Heart J 55:101, 1986

Iturbe-Alessio I, Fonseca MDC, Mutchinik O, Santos MA, Zajarias A, Salazar E: Risks of anticoagulant therapy in pregnant women with artificial heart valves. N Engl J Med 315:1390, 1986

Jaffe R, Gruber A, Fejgin M, Altaras M, Ben-Aderet N: Pregnancy with an artificial pacemaker. Obstet Gynecol Surv 42:137, 1987

James TN: Myocarditis and cardiomyopathy. N Engl J Med 308:39, 1983

Johnson RA, Palacios I: Dilated cardiomyopathies of the adult. N Engl J Med 307:1119, 1983

Key TC, Resnik R, Kittrich HC, Reisner LS: Successful pregnancy after cardiac transplantation. Am J Obstet Gynecol 160:367, 1989

Kirk EP: Organ transplantation and pregnancy: A case report and review. Am J Obstet Gynecol 164:1629, 1991

Kopenhager T: A review of 50 pregnant patients with kyphoscoliosis. Br J Obstet Gynaecol 84:585, 1977

Lang RM, Borow KM: Heart Disease. In Barron WM, Lindheimer MD (eds): Medical Disorders During Pregnancy. St. Louis, Mosby Yearbook, 1991, p 148

Lauer MS, Anderson KM, Kannel WB, Levy D: The impact of obesity of left ventricular mass and geometry: The Framingham Heart Study. JAMA 266:231, 1991

Lee W, Cotton DB: Peripartum cardiomyopathy: Current con-cepts and clinical management. Clin Obstet Gynecol 32:54, 1989

Liao KJ, Cockrill BA, Yurchak PM: Acute myocardial infarction after ergonovine administration for uterine bleeding. Am J Cardiol 68:823, 1991

Limacher MC, Ware JA, O'Meara ME, Fernandez GC, Young JB: Tricuspid regurgitation during pregnancy: Two-dimensional and pulsed Doppler echocardiographic observations. Am J Cardiol 55:1059, 1985

Löwenstein BR, Vain NW, Perrone SV, Wright DR, Boullón FJ, Favaloro RG: Successful pregnancy and vaginal delivery after heart transplantation. Am J Obstet Gynecol 158:589, 1988

Majdan JF, Walinsky P, Cowchock SF, Wapner RJ, Plzak L Jr: Coronary artery bypass surgery during pregnancy. Am J Cardiol 52:1, 1983

McAnulty JH, Metcalfe J, Ueland K: Heart Disease and Pregnancy. In Hurst JW, Schlant RC, Rackley CE, Sonnenblick EH, Wenger NK (eds): The Heart, 7th ed. New York, McGraw-Hill, 1990, p 1465

McAnulty JH, Morton MJ, Ueland K: The heart and pregnancy. Curr Probl Cardiol 13:589, 1988

McFaul PB, Dornan JC, Lamki H, Boyle D: Pregnancy complicated by maternal heart disease. A review of 519 women. Br J Obstet Gynaecol 95:861, 1988

McIvor RA: Percutaneous balloon aortic valvuloplasty during pregnancy. Int J Cardiol 32:1, 1991

Metcalfe J, McAnulty JH, Ueland K (eds): Burwell and Metcalfe's Heart Disease and Pregnancy, 2nd ed. Boston, Little, Brown, 1986

Meyer WJ, Benton SL, Hoon TJ, Gauthier DW, Whiteman VE: Acute myocardial infarction associated with prostaglandin E_2. Am J Obstet Gynecol 165:359, 1991

Mor-Yosef S, Younis J, Granat M, Kedari A, Milgalter A, Schenker JG: Marfan's syndrome in pregnancy. Obstet Gynecol Surv 43:382, 1988

Morris CD, Menashe VD: 25-year mortality after surgical repair of congenital heart defect in childhood. JAMA 266:3447, 1991

Nagorney DM, Field CS: Successful pregnancy 10 years after triple cardiac valve replacement. Obstet Gynecol 57:386, 1981

Nishimura RA, McGoon MD, Shub C, Miller FA, Ilstrup DM, Tajik AJ: Echocardiographically documented mitral-valve prolapse: Long-term follow-up of 237 patients. N Engl J Med 313:1305, 1985

Nugent EW, Planter WH, Edwards JE, Williams WH: The pathology, abnormal physiology, clinical recognition, and medical and surgical treatment of congenital heart disease. In Hurst JW, Schlant RC, Rackley CE, Sonnenblick EH, Wenger NK (eds): The Heart, 7th ed. New York, McGraw-Hill, 1990, p 655

Oakley GDG, McGarry K, Limb DG, Oakley CM: Management of pregnancy in patients with hypertrophic cardiomyopathy. BMJ 1:1749, 1979

O'Connell JB, Costanzo-Nordin MR, Subramanian R, Robinson JA, Wallis DE, Scanlon PJ, Gunnar RM: Peripartum cardiomyopathy: Clinical, hemodynamic, histologic and prognostic characteristics. J Am Coll Cardiol 8:52, 1986

Pastorek JG III, Plauche WC, Faro S: Acute bacterial endocarditis. J Reprod Med 28:611, 1983

Patton DE, Lee W, Cotton DB, Miller J, Carpenter RJ Huhta J,

Hankins G: Cyanotic maternal heart disease in pregnancy. Obstet Gynecol Surv 45:594, 1990

Pavankumar P, Venugopal P, Kaul U, Iyer KS, Das B, Sampathkumar A, Airon B, Rao IM, Sharma ML, Bhatia ML, Gopinath N: Closed mitral valvotomy during pregnancy: A 20 year experience. Scand J Thorac Cardiovasc Surg 22:11, 1988

Pollack KL, Chestnut DH, Wenstrom KD: Anesthetic management of a parturient with Eisenmenger's syndrome. Anesth Analg 70:212, 1990

Pyeritz RE: Maternal and fetal complications of pregnancy in the Marfan syndrome. Am J Med 71:784, 1981

Rayburn WF, LeMire MS, Bird JL, Buda AJ: Mitral valve prolapse: Echocardiographic changes during pregnancy. J Reprod Med 32:185, 1987

Reece EA, Egan JFX, Coustan DR, Tamborlane W, Bates SE, O'Neill TM, Fitzpatrick JG: Coronary artery disease in diabetic pregnancies. Am J Obstet Gynecol 154:150, 1986

Rotmensch HH, Elkayam U, Frishman W: Antiarrhythmic drug therapy during pregnancy. Ann Intern Med 98:487, 1983 Ruch A, Duhring JL: Postpartum myocardial infarction in a patient receiving bromocriptine. Obstet Gynecol 74:448, 1989

Sachs BP, Brown DAJ, Driscoll SG, Schulman E, Acker D, Ransil BJ, Jewett JF: Hemorrhage, infection, toxemia, and cardiac disease, 1954–85: Causes for their declining role in maternal mortality. Am J Public Health 78:671, 1988

Sanderson JE, Olsen EGJ, Gatei D: Peripartum heart disease: An endomyocardial biopsy study. Br Heart J 56:285, 1986

Sareli P, England MJ, Berk MR, Marcus RH, Epstein M, Driscoll J, Meyer T, McIntyre J, van Gelderen C: Maternal and fetal sequelae of anticoagulation during pregnancy in patients with mechanical heart valve protheses. Am J Cardiol 63:1462, 1989

Sawicka EH, Spencer GT, Branthwaite MA: Management of respiratory failure complicating pregnancy in severe kyphoscoliosis: A new use for an old technique? Br J Dis Chest 80:191, 1986

Saxena R, Nolan TE, Dohlen TV, Houghton JL: Postpartum myocardial infarction treated by balloon coronary angioplasty. Obstet Gynecol 79:810, 1992

Schenker JG, Polishuk WZ: Pregnancy following mitral valvotomy—A survey of 182 patients. Obstet Gynecol 32:214, 1968

Seaworth BJ, Durack DT: Infective endocarditis in obstetric and gynecologic practice. Am J Obstet Gynecol 154:180, 1986

Shime J, Mocarski EJM, Hastings D, Webb GD, McLaughlin PR: Congenital heart disease in pregnancy: Short- and long-term implications. Am J Obstet Gynecol 156:313, 1987

Singh H, Bolton PJ, Oakley CM: Pregnancy after surgical correction of tetralogy of Fallot. BMJ 285:168, 1982

Smith R, Brender D, McCredie M: Percutaneous transluminal balloon dilation of the mitral valve in pregnancy. Br Heart J 61:551, 1989

Strickland RA, Oliver WC, Chantigian RC, Ney JA, Danielson GK: Anesthesia, cardiopulmonary bypass, and the pregnant patient. Mayo Clin Proc 66:411, 1991

Sugrue D, Blake S, MacDonald D: Pregnancy complicated by maternal heart disease at the National Maternity Hospital, Dublin, Ireland, 1969 to 1978. Am J Obstet Gynecol 139:1, 1981

Sullivan JM, Ramanathan KB: Management of medical problems in pregnancy: Severe cardiac disease. N Engl J Med 313:304, 1985

van der Meer JTM, Van Wijk W, Thompson J, Vandenbroucke JP, Valkenburg HA, Michel MF: Efficacy of antibiotic prophylaxis for prevention of native-valve endocarditis. Lancet 339:135, 1992

van Kasteren YM, Kleinhout J, Smit MA, van Vugt JMG, van Geijn JP: Hypertrophic cardiomyopathy and pregnancy: A report of three cases. Eur J Obstet Gynecol Reprod Biol 38:63, 1990

Veille JC: Peripartum cardiomyopathies: A review. Am J Obstet Gynecol 148:806, 1984

Vosloo S, Reichart B: The feasibility of closed mitral valvotomy in pregnancy. J Thorac Cardiovasc Surg 93:675, 1987

Westaby S, Parry AJ, Forfar JC: Reoperation for prosthetic valve endocarditis in the third trimester of pregnancy. Ann Thorac Surg 53:263, 1992

Whittemore R, Hobbins JC, Engle MA: Pregnancy and its outcome in women with and without surgical treatment of congenital heart disease. Am J Cardiol 50:641, 1982

Whittemore R, Wright MR, Leonard MF, Johnson M: Results of pregnancy in women with congenital heart defects. Pediatr Res 14:452, 1980

Widerhorn J, Widerhorn ALM, Rahimtoola SH, Elkayam U: WPW syndrome during pregnancy: Increased incidence after supraventricular arrhythmias. Am Heart J 123:796, 1992

CHAPTER 49
Pulmonary Disorders

There are a number of important pregnancy-induced changes in the respiratory system. In addition, pregnancy may alter the course of underlying lung disease, and there is evidence that pregnant women do not tolerate some acute pulmonary disorders as well as when not pregnant.

Pulmonary Physiology. The important and sometimes marked changes in the respiratory system induced by pregnancy are discussed in detail in Chapter 8 (p. 230). Because of their importance to the clinical approach of lung disease complicating pregnancy, some of these are now reiterated. There are four lung volumes and four lung capacities that are used commonly to describe pulmonary physiology. Except for residual volume and lung capacities derived therefrom, these can be measured using direct spirometric techniques. The physiological changes induced by pregnancy have been summarized by de Swiet (1991):

1. **Vital capacity** may be increased by 100 to 200 mL.
2. **Inspiratory capacity** increases by about 300 mL by late pregnancy.
3. **Expiratory reserve volume** decreases from a total of 1300 mL to about 1100 mL.
4. **Residual volume** decreases from a total of 1500 mL to about 1200 mL.
5. **Functional residual capacity,** the sum of expiratory reserve and residual volumes, is reduced considerably by about 500 mL.
6. **Tidal volume** increases considerably from about 500 to 700 mL.
7. **Minute ventilation** increases 40 percent, from 7.5 L to a total of 10.5 L/min; this is primarily due to increased tidal volume because the respiratory rate is unchanged.

The sum of these changes is substantively increased ventilation due to deeper but not more frequent breathing. Presumably these changes are induced to help supply increased basal oxygen consumption, which increases incrementally by 20 to 40 mL per minute in the second half of pregnancy. As a result, arterial Po_2 falls very slightly, Pco_2 averages 28 mm Hg, plasma pH is slightly alkalotic at 7.45, and bicarbonate decreases to about 20 mEq/L.

Dyspnea During Pregnancy. Pregnant women are frequently aware of the need to breathe. The common complaint of "shortness of breath" is not associated with exercise, and frequently is worse when the woman is sitting down. Milne and associates (1978) reported that about half of women notice dyspnea at rest by midpregnancy, and three fourths complained of this by 31 weeks. Although its exact mechanisms are unclear, dyspnea has been attributed to alveolar hyperventilation and a response to substantively decreased Pco_2 as well as a consequence of anatomical changes in the thorax that accompany normal pregnancy.

Pneumonia

Pneumonia is inflammation affecting the lung parenchyma distal to the larger airways and involving the respiratory bronchioles and alveolar units. Bronchopneumonia refers to patchy and diffuse areas of involvement, and at least implies a less severe form of pneumonitis because there is no consolidation seen radiographically. Pneumonitis causing an appreciable loss of ventilatory capacity is tolerated less well by women during pregnancy. This generalization seems to hold true regardless of the etiology of the pneumonia. Moreover, hypoxemia and acidosis are poorly tolerated by the fetus, and they frequently lead to preterm labor after midpregnancy. Therefore, it is important to the pregnant woman and her fetus that pneumonia be diagnosed as soon as possible. Because many cases of pneumonia follow common viral upper respiratory illnesses, worsening or persistence of symptoms should prompt consideration for the diagnosis of pulmonary parenchymal infection. **Any pregnant woman suspected of having pneumonia should undergo anteroposterior and lateral chest radiography.**

Bacterial Pneumonia. Bacteria usually reach the lung by inhalation or by aspiration of nasopharyngeal secretions. Some bacterial organisms that cause community-acquired pneumonia, such as *Streptococcus pneumoniae,* are part of the normal resident flora. Viruses usually are not present. There are a number of factors that can upset the symbiotic relationship between colonizing bacteria and the mucosal and phagocytic defenses of the nasopharynx and bronchial tree. For example, there may be acquisition of a new virulent and invasive strain, or infection may follow a viral infection. Importantly, cigarette smoking and chronic bronchitis favor colonization with *S. pneumoniae, Haemophilus influenzae,* and *Legionella.*

Causes of Pneumonia. Foy and colleagues (1973) reported an overall incidence of 7 to 17 cases per 1000 for all adults. There are no extensive epidemiological studies concerning the incidence of various etiologies of pneumonias in young adults. At least two thirds of adult pneumonias are bacterial, and *S. pneumoniae* causes two thirds of these. Other common causes are *Mycoplasma pneumoniae* and influenza A. The British Thoracic Society (Research Committee, 1987) prospectively studied the clinical courses of 453 adults of all age groups admitted to 25 hospitals for pneumonia. In two thirds of cases, a microbial etiology was determined; *S. pneumoniae* was found in 34 percent, *Mycoplasma pneumoniae* in 18 percent, and influenza A virus in 7 percent. In most of the unclassified one third of cases, there was indirect evidence that pneumococcal infection was the cause of pneumonia.

Although these studies included adults of all age groups, it seems reasonable to conclude that most cases of community-acquired pneumonias in young adults are caused by pneumococci. Also, because mycoplasmal pneumonias are much more common in young adults than in older patients, it seems likely that these infections are commonly encountered in pregnant women. The **TWAR organism,** now termed *Chlamydia pneumoniae,* has been shown to cause perhaps 20 percent of pneumonias in college students (Grayston and associates, 1990). Although not studied specifically, it seems reasonable that this organism causes pneumonia during pregnancy. Finally, *Legionella pneumophilia* occasionally causes outbreaks or sporadic cases of **Legionnaire's disease** in young adults.

Diagnosis and Management. Typical symptoms of pneumonia include productive cough, fever, chest pain, and dyspnea. Mild upper respiratory symptoms and malaise usually precede these symptoms. There is usually mild leukocytosis. The chest x-ray is essential to the diagnosis, although its appearance does not predict the etiology accurately. Most recommend examination of Gram-stained sputum to search for pneumococci or staphylococci. Additionally, sputum or urine testing for pneumococcal antigen and serum testing for mycoplasma-specific immunoglobulin M may be helpful.

Hospitalization is recommended for the pregnant woman with pneumonia. Because the majority of adult pneumonias are caused by pneumococci or mycoplasmas, erythromycin therapy is the logical choice. The usual dose is 500 to 1000 mg every 6 hours, and this is usually given intravenously, at least initially. If staphylococcal or *Haemophilus* pneumonia is suspected, then cefotaxime, ceftizoxime, or cefuroxime is given instead. Clinical improvement usually is rapid. If fever persists, follow-up radiography should be considered. A pleural effusion can be demonstrated in about 20 percent of cases of pneumococcal pneumonia, and if fever persists, thoracentesis for drainage may be necessary. We have encountered a number of cases in which thoracostomy tube drainage was necessary.

Pneumococcal vaccine has been shown to be about 60 to 70 percent protective against vaccine-related serotypes. It is recommended by the Advisory Committee on Immunization Practices (1988) for immunocompromised adults including those with human immunodeficiency virus infection. It also is given to those who have underlying diabetes, cardiac, pulmonary, or renal disease.

Effect of Pneumonia on Pregnancy. Benedetti and associates (1982) summarized their experiences with 39 cases of pneumonia in pregnant women caused by a variety of organisms, but most often *Streptococcus pneumoniae* was isolated. Management included prompt hospitalization, antimicrobial therapy, and oxygen therapy when indicated. All of the mothers survived. One fetus expired whose mother also had sickle cell anemia.

In contrast, Madinger and colleagues (1989) reported frequent maternal and fetal complications in their review of 25 cases of pneumonia among more than 32,000 deliveries at Cedars–Sinai Medical Center. For example, 20 percent required tracheal intubation and mechanical ventilation, and 16 percent had empyema, pneumothorax, or pericardial tamponade. Underlying disease was associated with increased maternal complications, and the one maternal death was a woman with cystic fibrosis and *Pseudomonas* pneumonia. Preterm labor was diagnosed in 44 percent of these women, and there were 3 perinatal deaths.

Berkowitz and LaSala (1990) described their experiences with 26 cases of radiographically proven antepartum pneumonia complicating nearly 10,000 deliveries at Sloane Hospital for Women. Again, *S. pneumoniae* was most commonly isolated. Perinatal outcome was good despite severe infection, including 2 women with asthma who required tracheal intubation. These authors reported a much higher incidence of cocaine abuse and human immunodeficiency virus infection in these women.

Richey and colleagues (1993) described 55 women admitted because of pneumonia to Parkland Hospital from 1989 to 1991. There were two maternal deaths; preterm labor ensued in four of these women and there were two fetal deaths. These and the above outcomes underscore the severity of the problem and also serve to emphasize the value of prompt diagnosis and effective treatment.

Viral Pneumonia

Influenza Pneumonia. Influenza is an acute respiratory infection caused by ribonucleic acid viruses. Some of their serological characteristics are reviewed in detail in Chapter 58 (p. 1284). Influenza outbreaks occur virtually every year, with global pandemics every 10 to 15 years. The virus is spread by aerosolized droplets and quickly infects ciliated columnar epithelium, alveolar cells, mucus gland cells, and macrophages. If uncomplicated, the usual clinical course is 2 to 5 days.

Pneumonia is the most common complication of influenza. Primary pneumonitis is the most severe form, and it is characterized by sparse sputum production and radiographic interstitial infiltrates. Secondary bacterial pneumonia is more common, and usually caused by streptococci or staphylococci. Secondary infection usually manifests after 2 to 3 days of clinical improvement.

During the 1918 to 1919 and 1957 to 1958 influenza pandemics, it was accepted widely that pregnant women had excess mortality compared with nonpregnant individuals. Evidence from subsequent epidemics was less convincing, and currently, the Advisory Committee on Immunization Practices (1989) does not recommend that pregnant women be routinely given influenza immunization. **Certainly, women who are at high risk because of underlying disease such as diabetes or heart disease should be vaccinated against influenza.** There is no evidence that influenza vaccine is teratogenic (Chap 9, p. 264).

Clinically, it is difficult to distinguish viral from bacterial pneumonia, especially infection caused by *Mycoplasma pneumoniae.* The virus can be isolated by throat swab cultures or serological confirmation can be performed. Peripheral blood leukocyte counts are variable, but seldom exceed 15,000/μL. Treatment generally is symptomatic, but **amantadine** (pregnancy category C) may be effective in reducing the severity of infection if begun within 48 hours of symptoms. It may also be given prophylactically to nonimmunized exposed women in whom it will prevent 50 to 90 percent of clinical infection (Douglas, 1990).

Varicella Pneumonia. Varicella–zoster virus is a member of the herpesvirus family, and at least three fourths of adults are immune. Primary infection causes **chickenpox,** which has an attack rate of 90 percent in seronegative individuals. In the healthy patient, the typical maculopapular and vesicular rash is accompanied by constitutional symptoms and fever for 3 to 5 days.

Although secondary skin infection with streptococci or staphylococci is the most common complication of chickenpox, varicella pneumonia is the most serious. It develops in up to 20 percent of adults. It usually appears 3 to 5 days into the course of the illness and is characterized by tachypnea, cough, dyspnea, fever, and pleuritic chest pain. Chest x-ray discloses the characteristic nodular infiltrates and interstitial pneumonitis shown in Figure 49–1. Although resolution of pneumonitis parallels that of the skin lesions, fever and compromised pulmonary function may persist for weeks.

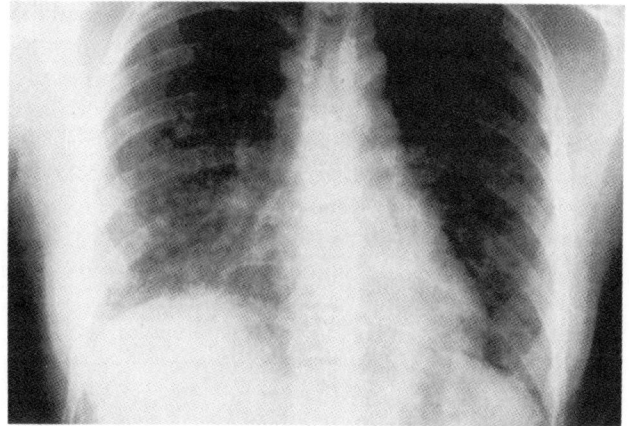

Fig. 49–1. Varicella pneumonia. (From Haake and colleagues, 1990, with permission.)

According to the review by Haake and colleagues (1990), varicella pneumonia in pregnancy has a 35 percent mortality rate compared with only 10 percent in otherwise healthy nonpregnant adults. Paryani and Arvin (1986) reported observations from 43 pregnant women with chickenpox. Four (10 percent) of these women developed pneumonia, and of the 2 women who required ventilatory support, 1 died. Clark and associates (1991) reported a 12-week pregnant woman who was treated successfully with extracorporeal membrane oxygenation (ECMO).

MANAGEMENT. In an attempt to lower the high mortality rate with varicella pneumonitis, many recommend the use of intravenous acyclovir. In one retrospective study, nonpregnant patients given acyclovir for pneumonia within 36 hours of admission had improved oxygenation by the sixth day compared with untreated controls (Haake and co-workers, 1990). These same authors, as well as others (Broussard and colleagues, 1991; Smego and associates, 1991), reviewed published cases of pregnant women with varicella pneumonia who were given acyclovir treatment, and they found an average 15 percent mortality rate. Given these high figures of mortality without treatment, and the possibly lowered mortality with treatment, it seems reasonable to use acyclovir. The dose is 5 to 15 mg/kg, given intravenously every 8 hours. Its efficacy, however, has yet to be proved.

As discussed in Chapter 58 (p. 1282), because of the apparent severe morbidity, some recommend passive immunization for susceptible pregnant women if they are significantly exposed to persons with chickenpox. Current Centers for Disease Control (1984) guidelines do not include varicella–zoster immune globulin for the exposed pregnant woman unless she is immunocompromised.

Aspiration Pneumonitis. Aspiration of acidic gastric contents during anesthesia for delivery can cause severe chemical pneumonitis, primarily as the consequence of the necrotizing effects of hydrochloric acid. The aspiration of gastric contents is not limited to anesthesia for delivery. For example, treatment of eclampsia with large doses of morphine, barbiturates, or diazepam has been followed by the aspiration of gastric contents and a bad outcome. In one study done to evaluate diazepam given for eclampsia, Crowther (1990) reported that 3 of 27 women developed pneumonic infiltrates, presumably from aspiration while heavily sedated!

Some aspects of the pathophysiology, prophylaxis, and treatment of aspiration pneumonitis are discussed in detail in Chapter 16 (p. 429).

Fungal and Parasitic Pneumonia. Fungal and parasitic pulmonary infections are usually of greatest consequence in the immunocompromised host, especially the woman with acquired immunodeficiency syndrome.

Pneumocystis Pneumonia. The most common pneumonia in women with acquired immunodeficiency syndrome is caused by the parasite, *Pneumocystis carinii.* This is a life-threatening infection and its symptoms include dry cough, tachypnea, and dyspnea. The characteristic radiographic finding is a diffuse infiltrate. Although the organism can be identified by sputum culture, bronchoscopy with lavage or biopsy may be necessary. Although Stratton and colleagues (1992) reported that 35 pregnant women with pneumocystis pneumonia had been treated through the AIDS Clinical Trials Centers, details were not given. Treatment is with trimethoprim–sulfamethoxazole or pentamidine. Both drugs are category C.

For some immunodeficiency virus-positive patients, the Centers for Disease Control (1989) has recommended prophylaxis against pneumocystis infection with aerosolized pentamidine or oral trimethoprim–sulfamethoxazole. These include persons who previously had pneumocystis infections, those with CD4+ lymphocyte counts less than 200/μL, or those in whom CD4+ cells constitute less than 20 percent of lymphocytes. Although they did not consider such prophylaxis advisable for pregnant women because of limited experience with these drugs, we agree with Sperling and colleagues (1992) that the same guidelines should be applied to pregnant women.

Fungal Pneumonia. Any of a number of fungi can cause pneumonia during pregnancy, especially histoplasmosis, coccidioidomycosis, and blastomycosis (see Chap. 58, p. 1294). Their spores are found in soil, and although infection is common, it usually is mild and self-limited. Infection is characterized by cough and fever; only rarely is there dissemination.

Histoplasmosis and blastomycosis are not believed to be more common or more severe during pregnancy. Conversely, many have considered that coccidioidomy-cosis more commonly undergoes dissemination during pregnancy when compared with nonpregnant women (Schmidt and Hall, 1991). This may be related to findings from *in vitro* studies, which have shown a stimulatory effect of the organism by estradiol-17β (Powell and associates, 1983). Wack and colleagues (1988) analyzed 10 cases among more than 47,000 pregnant women who lived in Tucson, Arizona, an endemic area. They concluded that the disease was rare, and that unless contracted in late pregnancy, there was not an increased risk for dissemination.

Treatment of disseminated fungal infections is with intravenous amphotericin B (category B) or ketoconazole (category C). Although amphotericin B is a toxic drug, its use for these infections in pregnant women has usually been successful (Cantanzaro, 1984; McGregor and associates, 1986; Wack and colleagues, 1988).

Asthma

Asthma affects about 3 to 4 percent of the general population (Smith, 1988). According to the Centers for Disease Control (1990a), the prevalence of asthma increased during the years 1980 to 1987. Asthma causes nearly 4000 deaths annually in the United States, and the mortality rate ranges from 1 to 3 percent (Corre and Rothstein, 1985). Because the disease is less common in women from 20 to 65, it complicates only 0.5 to 1.5 percent of pregnancies, and status asthmaticus complicates about 0.2 percent (Hernandez and colleagues, 1980; Mabie and associates, 1992).

Effects of Pregnancy on Asthma. There is no evidence that pregnancy has a predictable effect on underlying asthma. Turner and colleagues (1980) reviewed nine studies of 1054 pregnancies complicated by asthma. They reported that in 50 percent asthma was unchanged, in 30 percent it improved, and in 20 percent it worsened. Schatz and colleagues (1988) prospectively studied both symptoms and spirometry measurements throughout pregnancy and the puerperium in 366 asthmatic women. They reported that 28 percent were improved, 33 percent remained unchanged, 35 percent clearly worsened, and 4 percent had equivocal changes. In another prospective study of 198 pregnancies by Stenius-Aarniala and associates (1988), almost 40 percent of women required more intensive therapy for their asthma at some time during the pregnancy. **Thus, it appears that about one third of asthmatic women can expect worsening of disease at some time during pregnancy.**

Women beginning pregnancy with severe asthma are more likely to experience worsening disease than are those with mild disease. In about 60 percent of women, asthma behaves similarly with successive pregnancies. About 10 percent will have an exacerbation during labor and delivery (Schatz and colleagues, 1988). Importantly, Mabie and associates (1992) reported an 18-fold increased risk of exacerbation following cesarean delivery compared with vaginal delivery.

Effects of Asthma on Pregnancy. Asthma, especially when severe, can substantively affect pregnancy outcome. Several investigators have noted increased incidences of abortions, preterm labor, low-birthweight infants, and neonatal hypoxia (Bahna and Bjerkedal, 1972; Sims and colleagues, 1976). Severity of asthma is important, and Schatz and associates (1990) showed a small but significant correlation between measurements of maternal pulmonary function and birthweight. Among 277 women with asthma from the Collaborative Study of Cerebral Palsy, perinatal mortality was twice that of control women (Gordon and co-workers, 1970). Fetal complications, including death, are increased with severe disease (Fitzsimons and colleagues, 1986; Greenberger and Patterson, 1988).

Severe uncontrolled asthma also has maternal risks. Among the 16 women with severe asthma from the Collaborative Perinatal Project, 4 women died (Gordon and associates, 1970). Maternal deaths may be associated with **status asthmaticus.** Life-threatening complications include pneumothorax, pneumomediastinum, acute cor pulmonale, cardiac arrhythmias, and muscle fatigue with respiratory arrest (Woolcock, 1988). Mortality rates exceed 40 percent when asthma requires mechanical ventilation (Scoggin and co-workers, 1977).

Pathophysiology. The hallmarks of asthma are bronchial smooth muscle contraction, mucus hypersecretion, and mucosal edema. Biochemical effectors of these changes include *primary mediators,* such as histamines, which are released from lung tissue immediately upon challenge with an allergen. *Secondary mediators* include prostaglandins, thromboxane, and leukotrienes.

A number of allergens, respiratory infections, strenuous exercise, or aspirin may precipitate asthma (Schatz and Zeiger, 1991). Because F-series prostaglandins and ergonovine exacerbate asthma, these commonly used obstetrical drugs should be avoided if possible.

Clinical Course. Clinically, asthma represents a broad spectrum of illness ranging from mild wheezing to severe bronchoconstriction capable of causing respiratory failure, severe hypoxia, and death. The functional result of acute bronchospasm is airway obstruction and decreased air flow. The work of breathing progressively increases and patients present with chest tightness, wheezing, or breathlessness. Subsequent alterations in oxygenation primarily reflect ventilation–perfusion mismatching as the distribution of airway narrowing is uneven (Rodriguez-Roisin and colleagues, 1989; Woolcock, 1988).

The clinical stages of asthma are summarized in Table 49–1. With mild disease, hypoxia is initially well compensated by hyperventilation, as reflected by a normal arterial oxygen tension and decreased carbon dioxide tension with resultant respiratory alkalosis. As airway narrowing worsens, ventilation–perfusion defects increase and arterial hypoxemia ensues. With severe obstruction, ventilation becomes impaired sufficiently to result in early CO_2 retention. Because of hyperventilation, this may only be seen initially as an arterial CO_2 tension returning to the normal range. Finally, with critical obstruction, respiratory failure follows, characterized by hypercapnia and acidemia.

Although these changes in pulmonary function generally are reversible and well tolerated in the healthy, nonpregnant individual, even the early stages of asthma may pose grave risk to the pregnant woman and her fetus. The smaller functional residual capacity and the increased effective shunt render her more susceptible to develop hypoxia and hypoxemia.

Fetal Effects. Both animal and human studies suggest that maternal alkalosis may cause fetal hypoxemia well before maternal oxygenation is compromised (Moya and colleagues, 1965; Rolston and associates, 1974). Fetal compromise is hypothesized to result from a combination of factors to include decreased uterine blood flow, decreased maternal venous return, and an alkaline-induced leftward shift of the oxyhemoglobin dissociation curve (Bartels, 1962; Rolston, 1974; Wulf, 1972; and their associates). Once the mother can no longer maintain normal oxygen tension and hypoxemia develops, the fetus responds with decreased umbilical blood flow, increased systemic and pulmonary vascular resistance, and finally decreased cardiac output. Realization that the fetus may be seriously compromised before maternal disease is severe underscores the need for aggressive management of all pregnant women with acute asthma. Monitoring the fetal response, in effect, becomes an indicator of maternal compromise.

Clinical Evaluation. The subjective impression by the patient of the severity of asthma frequently does not correlate with objective measures of airway function or ventilation. Clinical examination is also inaccurate in

TABLE 49–1. CLINICAL STAGES OF ASTHMA

Stage	P_{O_2}	P_{CO_2}	pH	FEV$_1$ (% predicted)
Mild respiratory alkalosis	Normal	↓	↑	65–80
Respiratory alkalosis	↓	↓	↑	50–64
Danger zone	↓	Normal	Normal	35–49
Respiratory acidosis	↓	↑	↓	< 35

Modified after Barth and Hankins (1991), with permission.

predicting severity, but helpful signs include labored breathing, tachycardia, pulsus paradoxus, prolonged expiration, and use of accessory respiratory muscles. Signs of a potentially fatal attack include central cyanosis and altered level of consciousness (Summer, 1985).

Arterial blood gas analysis provides direct objective assessment of maternal oxygenation, ventilation, and acid-base status. With this information, the severity of an acute attack can be classified (Table 49–1). Care must be taken, however, to compare the results to normal values for pregnancy (see Chap. 8, p. 230). For example, a Pco_2 greater than 35 mm Hg with a pH less than 7.35 is consistent with hyperventilation and CO_2 retention in a pregnant woman.

Pulmonary function testing has become routine, and sequential measurements of the forced expiratory volume in one second (FEV_1) or peak expiratory flow rate (PEFR) are the most useful tests to monitor airway obstruction. An FEV_1 less than 1 L, or less than 20 percent of that predicted, correlates with severe disease as manifest by hypoxia, poor response to therapy, and a high relapse rate (Corre and Rothstein, 1985; Noble and colleagues, 1988).

Management of Acute Asthma. Treatment of acute asthma during pregnancy is similar to that of the nonpregnant asthmatic. An exception is a significantly lowered threshold for hospitalization of the pregnant woman. Most will benefit from intravenous hydration to help clear pulmonary secretions. Supplemental oxygen is given by mask after a blood gas sample is obtained.

First-line pharmacological therapy of acute asthma includes use of a **β-adrenergic agonist,** either epinephrine, isoproterenol, terbutaline, albuterol, isoetharine, or metaproterenol (National Heart, Lung and Blood Institute, 1991). The more commonly used agents, their dosages, and routes of administration are listed in Table 49–2. These drugs bind to specific cell-surface receptors and activate adenyl cyclase, which increases intracellular cyclic AMP to modulate bronchial smooth muscle relax-

ation (Woolcock, 1988). They are given by inhalation or orally and are also used for maintenance therapy of outpatients.

Recently, it has been recognized that **corticosteroids** should be given early to all patients in the course of severe acute asthma (National Heart, Lung and Blood Institute, 1991; Noble and colleagues, 1988). According to Reed (1991), the recognition of asthma as an inflammatory disease has led to more frequent use of corticosteroids, especially those topically administered by inhalation. **Because their onset of action is several hours, it is emphasized that steroids, whether given intravenously or by aerosol, are given along with β-agonists for treatment of acute asthma.** Commonly used corticosteroids and their respective dosages and routes of administration are listed in Table 49–3.

Management of Chronic Asthma. For outpatients, treatment depends on the severity of disease. In general, β-agonists are administered by inhalation every 3 to 4 hours as needed. Corticosteroid therapy is usually given for recalcitrant cases. A quickly tapered dose of prednisone has been shown effective, and corticosteroids administered by inhalation are preferred because of minimal side effects.

Theophylline is a methylxanthine, and its various salts are bronchodilators. **Aminophylline** is the diethyleneamine salt of theophylline and the only form available for parenteral use. In the past, aminophylline was used for severe acute asthma as initial therapy or as an adjunct to β-adrenergic therapy, but currently it is being replaced by corticosteroids. Although aminophylline is no longer the mainstay of therapy for severe acute asthma, theophylline derivatives continue to be useful for oral maintenance therapy of outpatients who do not respond optimally to inhaled β-agonists and corticosteroids.

Cromolyn sodium (category B), which stabilizes mast cell membranes, has a preventive effect on asthma mediators and is used chronically. Two puffs adminis-

TABLE 49–2. ADRENERGIC DRUGS USED FOR TREATMENT OF ASTHMA

Drug	Receptor	Administration	Recommended Dosages
Epinephrine	α, β₁, β₂	Subcutaneous	0.3–0.5 mL of a 1:1000 solution q 20 min × 3
		Inhaled	200–300 μg/puff; 1–2 puffs q 4 hr
Isoetharine	β₂	Inhaled	340 μg/puff, 3–7puffs q 3–4 hr
		Metered dose	3–7 puffs q 3–4 hr
		Aerosolized	0.5 mL of 1% solution, diluted 1:3 with saline
Isoproterenol	β₁, β₂	Inhaled	1:100 solution, 3–7 inhalations q 4–6 hr
			1:200 solution, 5–15 inhalations q 4–6 hr
		Intravenous	0.5–5 μg/min by infusion
Metaproterenol	β₂	Inhaled	
		Metered dose	650 μg/puff, 2–3 puffs q 3–4 hr
		Nebulizer	0.3 mL of 5% solution q 4 hr
Terbutaline	β₂	Subcutaneous	250 μg q 15 min × 3
		Oral	2.5 mg q 4–6 hr

TABLE 49–3. ADRENAL CORTICOSTEROID REGIMENS USED FOR TREATMENT OF ACUTE ASTHMA

Drug	Relative Potency	Adminis-tration	Recom-mended Dosages
Hydrocor-tisone	1	Intravenous	2 mg/kg loading dose, then q 4 hr or followed by 0.5 mg/kg/hr by infusion
Methylpred-nisolone	5	Intravenous	60–80 mg q 6–8 hr
Prednisone	3.5	Oral	60 mg initially, then 60–120 mg daily, tapered over several days

Modified from National Heart, Lung and Blood Institute (1991).

tered by an inhaler are given four times daily for added therapy in women with moderate to severe chronic asthma. **Immunotherapy** or desensitization therapy is safe in pregnancy, but its effects have not been evaluated. Medications with potential adverse fetal effects include **iodide-containing preparations** given primarily as expectorants. They are associated with neonatal hypothyroidism, goiter, and occasionally critical upper-airway obstruction; thus, they should not be used (Hassan and colleagues, 1968).

Status Asthmaticus and Respiratory Failure. Severe asthma of any type not responding after 30 to 60 minutes of intensive therapy is termed status asthmaticus. In nonpregnant patients with status asthmaticus, Braman and Kaemmerlen (1990) have shown that modern management in an intensive care unit will result in a good outcome in almost all cases. During pregnancy, consideration should be given to early intubation when the maternal respiratory status continues to decline despite aggressive treatment (see Table 49–1). Fatigue, carbon dioxide retention, or hypoxemia are indications for intubation and mechanical ventilation.

Management of Labor and Delivery. Stress-dose corticosteroids should be considered for any woman given steroid therapy within the preceding 9 months. In choosing an analgesic for labor, a nonhistamine-releasing narcotic, such as fentanyl, may be preferable to meperidine or morphine. For surgical delivery, some prefer to avoid general anesthesia because tracheal intubation can trigger severe bronchospasm. Thus, consideration should be given for regional analgesia techniques.

In the event of refractory postpartum hemorrhage, prostaglandin E_2 and other uterotonics should be used in lieu of prostaglandin $F_{2\alpha}$, which has been associated with significant bronchospasm in asthmatic patients given these compounds for midtrimester abortion (Kreisman and associates, 1975). Moreover, oxygen desatura-

tion following 15-methyl $PGF_{2\alpha}$ given for postpartum hemorrhage has been reported in women without reactive airway disease (Hankins and colleagues, 1988).

Thromboembolic Disease

According to the Consensus Conference sponsored by the National Institutes of Health (1986), the likelihood of venous thromboembolism in normal pregnancy and the puerperium is increased by a factor of five when compared to nonpregnant women of similar age. Certainly, venous thrombosis and pulmonary embolism remain a major cause of maternal death in the United States. Kaunitz and colleagues (1985) found that thrombotic pulmonary embolism caused 13 percent of 2067 nonabortion-related direct maternal deaths in the United States from 1974 through 1978. Sachs and associates (1987) reported that pulmonary embolism is now the second most common cause of maternal mortality in Massachusetts.

In the past, thromboembolic diseases were considered unique to the puerperium; however, this is no longer true. In recent years, there has been a decrease in the frequency of deep venous thrombosis and thromboembolism during the puerperium, but perhaps an increase antepartum. For example, Henderson and co-workers (1972) described 20 cases that developed antepartum among 29,770 pregnancies, but during the same period, only 16 were identified postpartum. Our observations from Parkland Hospital indicate even more of a propensity for antepartum disease. During the 3-year period ending in 1992, 20 of 24 cases of deep venous thrombosis or pulmonary embolism were identified antepartum.

Undoubtedly, the frequency of venous thromboembolic disease during the puerperium decreased remarkably when early ambulation became widely practiced. **Stasis is probably the strongest single predisposing event to deep vein thrombosis, and therefore should be kept to a minimum.** Venous thrombosis with a significant potential for generating pulmonary emboli may originate in the deep veins of the leg, thigh, or pelvis. A thrombosis that involves only the superficial veins of the leg or thigh is very unlikely to generate a pulmonary embolus. Antecedent events that might possibly predispose to deep vein thrombosis during the antepartum period include the use of oral contraceptives before conception and the great prevalence of women working during pregnancy at jobs in which they sit for long periods of time.

More recently, attention has been directed to a number of isolated deficiencies of proteins involved either in coagulation inhibition or in the fibrinolytic system (see Chap. 52, p. 1194). In some women these deficiencies can lead to hypercoagulability and recurrent venous thromboembolism. For example, according to Hellgren and associates (1989), up to 70 percent of pregnancies in women with hereditary deficiency of antithrombin-III may experience thromboembolic complications. To address this, Heijboer and colleagues (1990) studied the prevalence of isolated coagulation protein deficiencies in 277 consecutive nonpregnant outpatients with venographically proven acute deep vein thrombosis. Overall, 8.3 percent of these patients had deficiencies of **antithrombin-III, protein C, protein S,** or **plasminogen,** compared with 2.2 percent of age- and sex-matched controls without thrombosis. They concluded that such screening was not cost effective.

Superficial Venous Thrombosis. Antepartum or postpartum thrombosis limited strictly to the superficial veins of the saphenous system is treated with analgesia, elastic support, and rest. If it does not soon subside, or if deep venous involvement is suspected, appropriate diagnostic measures are taken, and heparin is given if deep vein involvement is confirmed. Superficial thrombophlebitis is typically seen in association with superficial varicosities or as a sequela to intravenous catheterization.

Deep Venous Thrombosis. In a carefully conducted prospective investigation in which thrombosis was confirmed by venography, Bergqvist and colleagues (1983) from Sweden reported that the incidence of antepartum deep venous thrombosis was 7 per 1000. The experience, however, of most American and other European workers is that the incidence is much lower. Barss and colleagues (1985) confirmed by venography 11 cases at Brigham and Women's Hospital from 1981 to 1984, during which time 27,000 women were delivered; thus, the incidence was about 1 in 2500. Our experiences are similar, and we have observed that the incidence of deep venous thrombosis, both antepartum and postpartum, has decreased. For example, in the 3-year period ending 1991, nearly 42,000 women were delivered at Parkland Hospital; in these, we identified 17 cases of deep venous thrombosis, an incidence of about 1 in 2000. This low incidence of proven thrombosis, both in Boston as well as in Dallas, is likely due in part to improved techniques to confirm as well as exclude thrombosis suspected clinically.

The signs and symptoms of deep venous thrombosis involving the lower extremity vary greatly, depending in large measure upon the degree of occlusion and the intensity of the inflammatory response. Ginsberg and colleagues (1992) reported an amazing tendency for left-leg involvement in pregnant women. Indeed, of 60 consecutive antepartum women, 58 had isolated left-leg thrombosis, and it was bilateral in the other two. Classical puerperal thrombophlebitis involving the lower extremity, sometimes called *phlegmasia alba dolens* or *milk leg,* is abrupt in onset, with severe pain and

edema of the leg and thigh. The thrombus typically involves much of the deep venous system from the foot to the iliofemoral region. Occasionally, reflex arterial spasm causes a pale, cool extremity with diminished pulsations. More likely, there may be appreciable volume of clot yet little reaction in the form of pain, heat, or swelling. Importantly, calf pain, either spontaneous or in response to squeezing, or to stretching the Achilles tendon (Homans sign), may be caused by a strained muscle or a contusion. The latter may be common during the early puerperium as the consequence of inappropriate contact between the calf and the delivery table leg holders.

Diagnosis. **Venography** or **phlebography** remains the standard for confirmation of the clinical diagnosis of deep venous thrombosis. In most studies, it has been shown that by using this technique at least half of clinically suspected cases do not have a thrombosis, thereby obviating the need for anticoagulation and its hazards. Venography is not without complications, and indeed the method itself may induce thrombosis (Fig. 49–2). Because of this, there has been renewed interest in noninvasive methods to confirm the clinical diagnosis.

In nonpregnant patients, **impedance plethysmography** apparently has promise, both as a screening method and for diagnosis. In a study from Amsterdam (Huisman and colleagues, 1986), 471 consecutive patients in whom deep venous thrombosis was clinically suspected were screened with serial impedance plethysmography, and if positive, they underwent venography. The positive predictive was 92 percent, and all patients in whom plethysmography was normal did well without treatment. Hull and colleagues (1985) presented similarly optimistic data, but emphasized that *serial* plethysmography was imperative when deep venous thrombosis was suspected clinically, the initial exami-

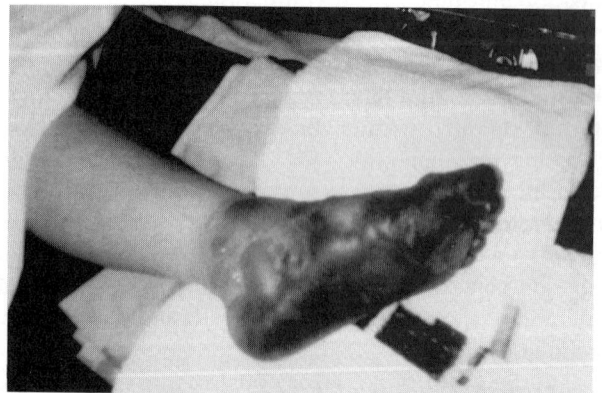

Fig. 49–2. Aseptic gangrene of the foot that followed extravasation of contrast material injected intravenously under pressure preparatory to performing ascending venography. Partial foot amputation later was necessary. The patient did not have a venous thrombosis. (Photograph courtesy of Dr. Tom Lowe.)

nation was negative, and venography was not to be performed. They also reported that calf-vein thrombosis likely would be missed using plethysmography alone.

Hull and associates (1990b) later reported their experiences with serial plethysmography in 152 pregnant women referred for clinically suspected deep vein thrombosis. Plethysmography was abnormal in only 13 women (9 percent); 12 of these 13 subsequently underwent venography, and proximal-vein thrombosis was confirmed in 11. Importantly, none of the 139 with negative findings had venous thromboembolism on long-term follow-up. From these findings, it seems reasonable to use impedance plethysmography for screening in pregnant women in whom thrombosis is suspected, but if the examination is abnormal, then a confirmatory study is recommended.

Real-time B-mode ultrasonography, during which venous compressibility is assessed, is yet another noninvasive method to detect proximal deep vein thrombosis. Lensing and colleagues (1989) evaluated 220 consecutive nonpregnant patients with clinically suspected deep venous thrombosis. They compared contrast venography with real-time ultrasonography and evaluated the *common femoral and popliteal veins* for full compressibility (no thrombosis) and noncompressibility (thrombosis). Both of these vessels were fully compressible in 142 of 143 patients with normal venograms (specificity, 99 percent). All 66 patients with proximal-vein thrombosis had noncompressible femoral or popliteal veins, or both (sensitivity, 100 percent). Lensing and co-workers further reported that intraluminal echogenicity and venous distension during the Valsalva maneuver were relatively inaccurate. Although they found ultrasonography to be highly accurate and simple, they cautioned against its widespread clinical use as the sole diagnostic test for clinically suspected thrombosis until the safety of withholding anticoagulation in patients with negative tests was evaluated.

With the addition of duplex and color Doppler ultrasound technology, similar sensitivities can be found with shorter examination times (Scott and colleagues, 1990). Real-time sonography, coupled with duplex and color Doppler ultrasound, has tremendous potential to diagnose deep venous thrombosis of the lower extremities, but its role in the evaluation of pelvic vein thrombosis is less clear. **In pregnant women, thrombosis frequently originates in the iliac veins.** Using real-time and Doppler ultrasound along with impedance plethysmography, complete but not partial iliac vein occlusion can be detected (Hull and colleagues, 1990b). In a recent prospective evaluation of color-flow imaging in conjunction with compression ultrasonography, Polak and Wilkinson (1991) reported an incidence of symptomatic deep venous thrombosis of 7 per 10,000 deliveries, which was similar to the incidence in a retrospective cohort group (11 of 26,196 deliveries) in which the diagnosis was confirmed by venography.

Magnetic resonance imaging has also been utilized more recently for diagnosis of symptomatic deep venous thrombosis. This technique allows for excellent delineation of anatomical detail above the inguinal ligament, and phase images can be used to diagnose the presence or absence of pelvic vein flow. An additional advantage is the ability to image in coronal and sagittal planes. Erdman and co-workers (1990) reported that magnetic resonance imaging was 100 percent sensitive and 90 percent specific for detection of venographically proven deep venous thrombosis in nonpregnant patients. Furthermore, in 44 percent of patients without deep venous thrombosis, they were able to demonstrate nonthrombotic conditions to explain the clinical findings that originally had suggested venous thrombosis. Examples include cellulitis, edema, hematomas, or superficial phlebitis.

Computed-tomographic scanning may also be used to assess these findings. It is more widely available but it requires contrast agents and ionizing radiation (see Chap. 43, p. 985).

Pulmonary Embolism. In many cases, but certainly not all, clinical evidence for deep venous thrombosis of the legs precedes pulmonary embolization. In others, especially those that arise from deep pelvic veins, the woman is usually asymptomatic until symptoms of embolization develop (Fig. 49–3). The mortality rate of treated acute pulmonary embolism is about 3 percent, and most of these are fatal within the first week (Carson and associates, 1992). The incidence of pulmonary embolism associated with pregnancy has varied widely, and has been reported to be from 1 in 2700 deliveries (Stamm, 1960) to less than 1 in 7000 deliveries (Mengert, 1945). Our recent experiences from Parkland Hospital are more consonant with Mengert's earlier observations and indicate that pulmonary embolism is quite uncommon. Indeed, in the past 3 years, during which time nearly 40,000 women gave birth, we encountered only 4 cases of pulmonary embolism; 2 were antepartum and 2 were postpartum, one immediately after delivery and another 4 weeks later. Unfortunately, the latter woman succumbed to a massive saddle embolism.

Diagnosis. Chest discomfort, shortness of breath, air hunger, tachypnea, or obvious apprehension are signs and symptoms that should alert the physician to a strong likelihood of pulmonary embolism. The most common abnormality in one study was a respiratory rate of greater than 16 per minute (Bell and associates, 1977). Its frequency was so striking that a lower respiratory rate was felt to exclude the diagnosis. Examination of the chest may yield findings such as an accentuated pulmonic closure sound, rales, or friction rub. Right axis deviation may or may not be evident in the electrocardiogram. Even with massive pulmonary embolism, signs,

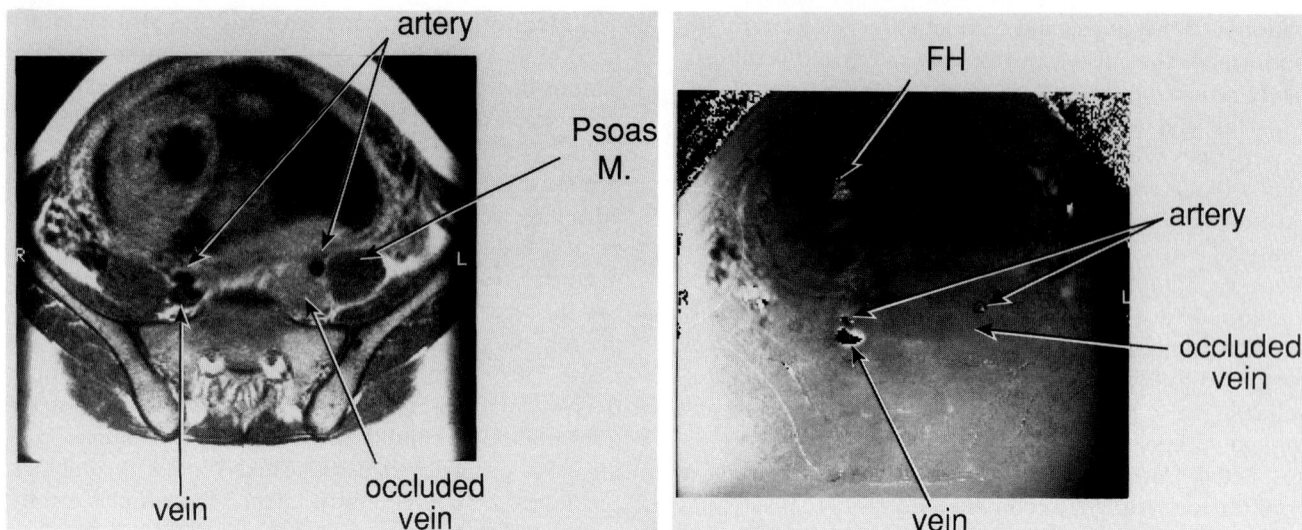

Fig. 49–3. Magnetic resonance images through the pelvis of a 26-week pregnant woman who presented with symptoms of pulmonary embolism but without clinically apparent deep venous thrombosis of the lower extremities. Left, T$_1$-weighted image showing occlusion of left common iliac vein. Right, phase image which demonstrates flow and therefore shows right common iliac artery and vein patency, arterial patency on the left, but lack of signal from the occluded left common iliac vein. Because flow is detected by this method, fetal heart motion (FH) is also visualized. (Photographs courtesy of Dr. Diane Twickler.)

symptoms, and laboratory data to support the diagnosis of pulmonary embolism may be deceivingly unspecific. In one study, pulmonary angiography was used to identify 90 patients with a massive embolism (Wenger and colleagues, 1972). Although at least two lobar arteries were obstructed, the classic triad of hemoptysis, pleuritic chest pain, and dyspnea was noted in only 20 percent of patients.

Controversy still exists regarding the safest, least invasive technique that can accurately diagnose pulmonary embolism. Some investigators believe that **ventilation–perfusion scintigraphy** is adequate. These scans use a small dose of a radioactive agent, usually technetium (^{99m}Tc) macroaggregated albumin administered intravenously. A lung scan may not provide a definite diagnosis because many other conditions—for example, pneumonia or local bronchospasm—can cause perfusion defects. Ventilation scans with inhaled xenon 133 or ^{99m}Tc were added to perfusion scans in the hope that ventilation would be abnormal, but perfusion normal, in areas of pneumonia or hypoventilation. Reporting data from the Hamilton District Thromboembolism Programme, Hull and associates (1990b) concluded that ventilation scanning increased the probability of an accurate diagnosis of pulmonary embolus in patients with *large perfusion defects and ventilation mismatches,* but that a ventilation–perfusion match was *not* helpful in ruling out pulmonary embolism. They reported that pulmonary angiography was necessary in most patients with perfusion abnormalities because the diagnosis of pulmonary embolism could not be made or excluded with sufficient accuracy in such patients.

Because of these uncertainties, the National Heart, Lung and Blood Institute commissioned the Prospective Investigation of Pulmonary Embolism Diagnosis (PIOPED, 1990). This study was designed to determine the sensitivities and specificities of ventilation–perfusion scans to diagnose pulmonary embolism. This prospective investigation included 933 patients of whom 931 underwent scintigraphy and 755 pulmonary angiography; 33 percent of the 755 patients studied angiographically had pulmonary embolism. Although almost all patients with an embolism had abnormal scans of high, intermediate, or low probability, so did most without embolism (sensitivity, 98 percent; specificity, 10 percent). Of 116 patients with high-probability scans, 88 percent had an embolism seen on angiography, but only a minority of patients with a pulmonary embolism had a high-probability scan (sensitivity, 41 percent; specificity, 97 percent). Of 322 with intermediate-probability scans, 33 percent had an embolism on angiography; for those with a low-probability scan, the figure was 12 percent. **Importantly, 4 percent of patients with a near normal to normal scan had pulmonary embolism detected by angiography.**

The PIOPED investigators concluded that a high-probability scan usually indicates pulmonary embolism, but that only a small number of patients with emboli have a high-probability scan. A low-probability scan combined with a strong clinical impression that embolism is unlikely makes the possibility of pulmonary embolism remote. Similarly, near-normal or normal scans make the diagnosis very unlikely. Finally, an intermediate-probability scan is of no help in establishing the diagnosis.

Thus, the scan combined with clinical assessment permits a noninvasive diagnosis or exclusion of pulmonary embolism for a minority of patients. Bone (1990) suggested that diagnostic accuracy could be improved by combining the results of ventilation–perfusion scans with noninvasive studies of the deep leg veins. He emphasized that when there is significant doubt, pulmonary angiography should be done. **Because half of pulmonary emboli during pregnancy arise from the pelvic veins, this approach using leg vein studies clearly has limitations.** As discussed previously, magnetic resonance imaging shows great promise for visualizing thromboses arising in pelvic veins (Erdman and colleagues, 1990).

It is our practice to pursue vigorously verification of the clinical diagnosis of pulmonary embolism. Initial evaluation includes a chest radiograph, and if this is not suggestive of another diagnosis, then a ventilation–perfusion lung scan is performed. If the scan is completely normal, this is taken as evidence against embolism, and the workup is considered complete. Conversely, a high-probability scan such as that shown in Figure 49–4, in concert with a chest radiograph showing no corresponding abnormalities—for example, a pneumonic infiltrate—is considered diagnostic of embolization, and therapy is begun. For cases in which the diagnosis is still in doubt after these measures, pulmonary angiography is performed.

Although there is often great reluctance on the part of some to perform the various diagnostic procedures to confirm thromboembolic disease, the actual amount of

fetal radiation exposure is quite small (see Chap. 43, p. 985). Ginsberg and associates (1989) have estimated such exposure from a perfusion scan utilizing technetium to be from 6 to 18 mrad; for a ventilation scan with xenon this is 4 to 19 mrad. The radiation exposure to the fetus from pulmonary angiography is estimated at 220 to 370 mrad via the femoral route and less than 50 mrad using the brachial route. The estimated exposure for limited venography is also less than 50 mrad.

Management of Postpartum Thromboembolism

Deep Venous Thrombosis. Treatment of deep venous thrombosis consists of heparin, bed rest, and analgesia. Most often, the pain is soon relieved by these measures. After the signs and symptoms have completely abated, graded ambulation should be started with the legs fitted with elastic stockings, and the heparin continued. Recovery to this stage usually takes about 7 to 10 days.

Anticoagulation is achieved initially with intravenous heparin such that the activated partial thromboplastin time is prolonged to 1.5 to 2.5 times the laboratory control value (Hirsh, 1991a). Hull and co-workers (1986) reported the results of a randomized clinical trial in which they compared continuous intravenous heparin with intermittent subcutaneous heparin for proximal vein thrombosis in 115 nonpregnant patients. Although each group received a total of approximately 30,000 units of heparin per day, most of those given the drug subcutaneously had an initial anticoagulant response below the target range, and importantly, nearly 20 percent had recurrent thromboembolism compared with only 5 percent of those given heparin intravenously. All patients in this study were given warfarin beginning on the sixth or seventh day of heparin therapy, and heparin was continued for a total of 10 days. More recently, the Ontario group (Hull and associates, 1990a) demonstrated that if intravenous heparin and oral warfarin are initiated simultaneously, then heparin can be safely discontinued after only 5 days.

LOW-MOLECULAR-WEIGHT HEPARIN. Soon to be released for clinical use, low-molecular-weight heparin (about 4000 d compared with about 15,000 d for conventional heparin) has been shown safe and effective for treatment of proximal-vein thrombosis in nonpregnant patients (Hull and co-workers, 1992). It has not been used in pregnant women.

Pulmonary Embolism. Treatment for pulmonary embolism is similar to that for deep venous thrombosis, but with less well documented results. In general, heparin is given in a similar fashion for deep venous thrombosis or pulmonary embolism, whether antepartum or postpartum. Considerable controversy exists as to which regimen is best, and several are widely used, effective, and

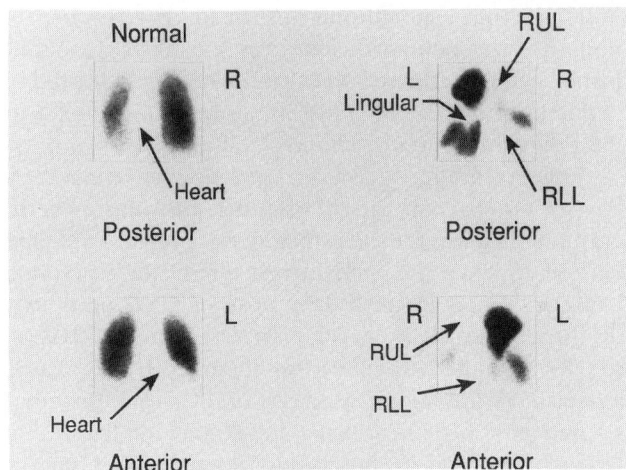

Fig. 49–4. Abnormal ventilation–perfusion scintigraphy showing pulmonary emboli in a 26-week pregnant woman compared with a normal scan. Left, anterior-posterior view of normal ventilation scan showing homogenous distribution of ^{133}Xe. Right, anterior-posterior view of perfusion scan showing large nonperfused areas (*arrows*). There is virtually no perfusion of the right upper and lower lobes, and very little perfusion of the right middle lobe. The absence of lingular lobe perfusion is evident on the left side. (Photographs courtesy of Dr. Diane Twickler.)

considered acceptable (Mohr and colleagues, 1988; Weiner, 1985). Heparin is commonly administered by continuous intravenous infusion, and most recommend starting with a dose of 1000 U/hr after an initial bolus dose of 5000 U. Intermittent intravenous injections of 5000 U every 4 hours or 7500 U every 6 hours are preferred by others. Finally, heparin may be given subcutaneously in doses of 10,000 U every 8 hours or 20,000 U every 12 hours. The common theme of these regimens is that the total daily heparin dose is between 25,000 and 40,000 U.

The most serious complication with any of these regimens is hemorrhage, which is more likely if there has been recent surgery or lacerations, such as with delivery. Troublesome bleeding is also more likely if the heparin dosage is excessive. Conversely, thrombus extension or embolization are more likely if the heparin dosage is inadequate. Unfortunately, many management schemes using laboratory testing to identify whether heparin dosage is sufficient to inhibit further thrombosis, yet not cause serious hemorrhage, have been discouraging (Moser, 1991).

Whole blood clotting times have long been used; more recently measurement of the plasma partial thromboplastin time has been popularized. The two tests often correlate poorly. An important test that will aid in detecting hemorrhage is the frequent measurement of the hematocrit. Clinical improvement without hemorrhage is the desired goal. It is important to remember that heparin is being administered whenever blood is to be drawn or medications are ordered to be given parenterally. Serious hemorrhage may occur, especially when arterial blood is drawn for blood gas analyses.

Therapy with heparin as described may be discontinued in the postpartum woman after 10 days to 2 weeks if the disease process has clearly abated and there is no evidence of underlying chronic venous abnormalities that would predispose to venous thrombosis and no evidence of underlying cardiopulmonary dysfunction. If a switch to warfarin therapy is the plan, heparin is discontinued after the prothrombin time is considered therapeutically prolonged (Gallus and colleagues, 1986).

Long-term Therapy. During the past several years, considerable controversy has arisen concerning the most effective agent and its duration of use for long-term therapy to prevent recurrent thromboembolism (Hirsh, 1991a,b). In nonpregnant patients, Hull and co-workers (1982a) reported that heparin was as effective as oral warfarin when heparin was administered subcutaneously every 12 hours with the dose adjusted to prolong the activated partial thromboplastin time to 1½ times the control value when measured 6 hours after injection. Furthermore, heparin therapy was associated with a lower risk of bleeding. Subsequently, Hull and colleagues (1982b) reported that by decreasing the dosage

of warfarin, bleeding complications could be reduced to the level achieved with heparin and yet the effectiveness of the two agents remained comparable.

In the absence of pregnancy, it seems reasonable to consider warfarin the drug of choice for long-term treatment or prophylaxis when appropriate consideration is given to the cost of heparin, the problem of administration, and the possibility of heparin-induced thrombocytopenia or osteoporosis (Hirsh, 1991a). The exact incidence of these latter two with heparin use is unclear. Thrombocytopenia probably occurs in less than 6 percent of patients given porcine heparin, while osteoporosis appears to be associated with heparin doses of greater than 20,000 units per day for periods longer than 6 months (Hirsch, 1991a).

Management of Antepartum Thromboembolism. Antepartum thrombosis involving the deep venous system is especially difficult to manage satisfactorily. As discussed above, confirmation of the diagnosis is imperative; otherwise, the woman will either have to undergo prolonged anticoagulation with its attendant risks, or run the risk of pulmonary embolism.

As with postpartum venous thrombosis, therapy with intravenous heparin usually controls active disease; but thrombosis, perhaps with embolization, may recur antepartum, intrapartum, or postpartum unless anticoagulation is continued throughout these periods. Initially, full heparinization by continuous intravenous infusion is preferred by most. One recommended dose for nonpregnant patients is 5000 units by bolus injection, followed by 30,000 units per 24 hours given by continuous infusion (Hirsh, 1991a). If subcutaneous heparin is given, Hirsh (1991a) recommends that the 5000-unit intravenous bolus dose be followed by 17,500 units given subcutaneously every 12 hours. In either instance, it is recommended that the dose be adjusted to maintain activated partial thromboplastin time at 1.5 to 2.5 times the laboratory control value.

After symptoms have abated following acute therapy for antepartum thrombosis, it is probably wise to continue heparin for the remainder of pregnancy. Some choose to have the woman self-administer **low-dose heparin** subcutaneously in a dose of 5000 units two or three times daily. A regimen that provides 10,000 to 15,000 units of heparin subcutaneously per day is associated with an increased risk of recurrent thrombosis and possibly embolism compared with that using larger heparin doses, but a much lower risk of hemorrhage.

Barss and colleagues (1985) reported the use of a subcutaneous pump to deliver heparin continuously to 6 women for a mean of 20 weeks before delivery. The heparin dose was adjusted to maintain the partial thromboplastin time 1 to 1.5 times baseline, and the mean daily dose was nearly 40,000 U. Significant bleeding complications developed in 4 women and 3 were given blood transfusions. They concluded that further studies of optimum dose and duration were needed.

Aspirin and other drugs that impair platelet function increase the risk of hemorrhage, even with low-dose heparin, and therefore should be avoided. Warfarin and related compounds that inhibit the synthesis of vitamin K-dependent coagulation factors cross the placenta and thereby also impair the coagulation mechanism of the fetus. Moreover, as discussed in Chapter 42 (p. 966), warfarin is teratogenic, and if given during the first 8 weeks of gestation it may result in congenital malformations, which include nasal hypoplasia, ophthalmological abnormalities, and retarded development (Hall and colleagues, 1980). Whether the malformations are the consequence of microhemorrhages in embryonic cartilage or a more complex teratogenic action is not known. Central nervous system abnormalities have also been reported with second- and third-trimester coumarin exposure. Finally, a variety of drugs act to enhance or inhibit the action of warfarin.

Because of the mechanical forces that develop during labor, the fetus is at increased risk of bleeding, especially from intracranial hemorrhage. Therefore, if warfarin has been used as an anticoagulant during the antepartum period, the drug should be stopped several weeks before the anticipated time of delivery and anticoagulation with heparin initiated.

Anticoagulation and Abortion. The treatment of deep venous thrombosis with heparin does not preclude termination of pregnancy by careful curettage (see Chap. 31, p. 681). After the products of conception are removed without trauma to the reproductive tract, heparin can be restarted in several hours in therapeutic doses without undue risk. If abdominal hysterotomy is to be performed, those precautions presented below for cesarean section are applicable. Experiences are lacking in which hypertonic saline or a prostaglandin has been used as an abortifacient in the presence of effective anticoagulation. The safety of laparoscopic tubal sterilization is also unknown for a heparinized patient.

Anticoagulation and Delivery. Labor and delivery may induce severe hemorrhage in the fetus if the mother has recently been treated with warfarin. The effects of warfarin may be reversed by the slow intravenous administration of vitamin K_1 in a dose of 10 mg. The activities of the vitamin K-dependent clotting factors usually increase to safe levels within 8 hours in the mother, but less rapidly in the fetus. Maternal transfusion of fresh-frozen plasma will correct the deficiency immediately in the mother but, unfortunately, not in the fetus. Hepatitis and other blood-borne diseases may be transmitted with this plasma fraction.

Heparin does not cross the placenta. Its effects on blood loss at delivery will depend upon a number of variables, including: (1) the dose, route, and time of administration; (2) the magnitude of incisions and lacerations; (3) the intensity of myometrial contraction and retraction once the products of conception have been delivered; and (4) the presence of other coagulation defects. Measured blood loss is not greatly increased with vaginal delivery if the midline episiotomy is modest in depth, there are no lacerations of the genital tract, and the uterus promptly becomes firmly contracted and remains so after delivery of the placenta. Such ideal circumstances do not always prevail during and after vaginal delivery. For example, Mueller and Lebherz (1969) described 10 women with antepartum thrombophlebitis treated with heparin. Three who continued to receive heparin during labor and delivery bled remarkably and developed severe postpartum hemorrhage with large hematomas. Blood replacement of 1500, 2500, and 4500 mL was essential, as was repeated drainage of the hematomas.

Therefore, in general, heparin therapy should be stopped during the time of labor and delivery. If the uterus is well contracted and there has been negligible trauma to the lower genital tract, it can be restarted within several hours. Otherwise, a delay of 1 or 2 days may be prudent. Protamine sulfate administered intravenously will generally reverse the effect of heparin promptly and effectively, but of course will be of no benefit for hematomas already formed. Protamine sulfate should not be given in excess of the amount needed to neutralize the heparin, because excess protamine has an anticoagulant effect.

The woman who has very recently suffered a pulmonary embolism and who must be delivered by cesarean section presents a serious problem, because reversal of anticoagulation may be followed by another embolus, and surgery while she is fully anticoagulated frequently results in life-threatening hemorrhage or troublesome hematomas. In this situation, consideration should be given before surgery for placement of a vena caval filter device. These may be placed using either the jugular or femoral approach as discussed subsequently. With either treatment, strong consideration should be given to tubal sterilization because of the risk of recurrence with subsequent pregnancy.

Serious bleeding is likely when heparin in usual therapeutic doses is administered to a woman who has undergone cesarean section within the previous 72 hours. Again, preexisting defects in the hemostatic mechanism, such as thrombocytopenia, or impaired platelet function as induced by aspirin, enhance the likelihood of hemorrhage with heparin.

Vena Caval Filters. In the very infrequent circumstances where heparin therapy fails to prevent recurrent pulmonary embolism from the pelvis or legs, or when embolism develops from these sites despite heparin given for their treatment, then vena caval interruption is indicated. In the past, vena caval ligation or plication was preferred; however, this procedure, which requires extensive surgical dissection in an area that is highly vascular during pregnancy, has been largely replaced by use of a *vena caval filter.* Greenfield and Michna (1988) recommend suprarenal placement during pregnancy and Hux and colleagues (1986) described the use of the Greenfield filter in 5 pregnant women and another who was 3 days postpartum. Their indications for filter placement, which is inserted through either the jugular or femoral vein, were bleeding, thrombocytopenia, or recurrent embolization in women who were anticoagulated with heparin.

Our experiences have been good with the **bird's-nest filter,** such as that shown in Figure 49–5. In a multi-institutional trial, Roehm and colleagues (1988) described its use in 568 nonpregnant patients at risk for pulmonary embolism. The prevalence of clinically suspected recurrent embolism was 2.7 percent and that of inferior vena caval occlusion was 2.9 percent.

Thromboembolism in Previous Pregnancy. There are insufficient data to conclude which regimen is best to provide the safest maximal effect against recurrent antepartum pulmonary embolism. This was considered in detail at the National Institutes of Health Consensus Conference (1986), and it was concluded that the woman with either deep venous thrombosis or pulmonary embolism in a *prior* pregnancy should be given prophylactic subcutaneous heparin in doses of 5000 U, either two or three times daily throughout pregnancy.

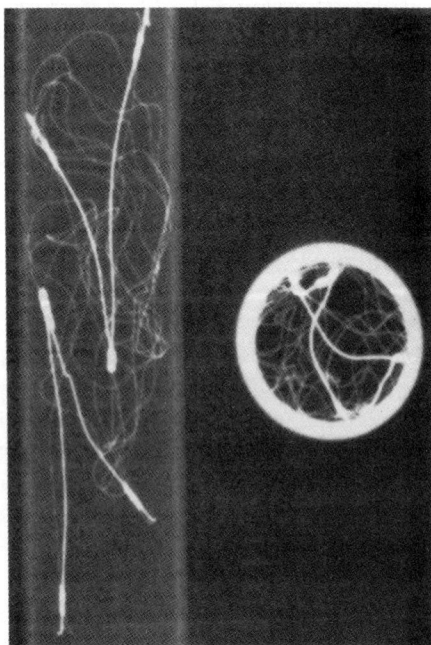

Fig. 49–5. Lateral and axial radiographs of modified bird's-nest filter that has been placed into a 2.5-cm-diameter plastic tube. (From Roehm and colleagues, 1988, with permission.)

One Swedish study would indicate that such prophylaxis is not effective. Tengborn and colleagues (1989) reported outcomes in 87 pregnancies in women who had prior thromboembolic disease. Despite heparin prophylaxis, usually 5000 U twice daily, 3 of 20 (15 percent) women developed antepartum recurrence, compared with 8 of 67 (12 percent) not given heparin. Postpartum, 3 of 57 (5 percent) who were given low-dose prophylaxis, and 3 of 30 (10 percent) receiving no prophylaxis, had recurrent thrombosis.

Our practice at Parkland Hospital for many years for women recovering from antepartum pulmonary embolism has been to administer subcutaneous heparin, 5000 units twice daily. With this regimen, the recurrence of documented embolization has been rare.

Tuberculosis

While still a major worldwide concern, tuberculosis has become less common in the United States in recent decades, and in 1988, the rate was about 10 per 100,000 persons aged 25 to 44 (Centers for Disease Control, 1992). Almost 20 percent of cases reported from 1986 to 1989 were in foreign-born persons. Indeed, the disease in this country is one of the elderly, the urban poor, minority groups, and patients with acquired immunodeficiency syndrome. Acquisition of infection is via inhalation of *Mycobacterium tuberculosis,* which incites a granulomatous pulmonary reaction. In over 95 percent of patients the infection is contained and lies dormant for long periods. In some patients, especially those who are immunocompromised or who have other diseases, tuberculosis becomes reactivated to cause clinical disease.

While patients with tuberculosis may be asymptomatic, clinical manifestations usually include cough with minimal sputum production, low-grade fever, hemoptysis, and weight loss. Chest x-ray discloses a variety of infiltrative patterns, and there may be associated cavitation or mediastinal lymphadenopathy. Acid-fast bacilli are seen on repeated stained smears of sputum in about two thirds of culture-positive patients. Extrapulmonary tuberculosis may occur in any organ.

Tuberculosis in Pregnancy. The considerable influx of women into the United States from Southeast Asia, Mexico, and Central America has been accompanied by an increased frequency of tuberculosis in pregnant women. Although in the past some recommended tuberculin-skin testing for all pregnant women, this currently is not necessary. A reasonable alternative is to skin test women in high-risk groups, as recommended by the Centers for Disease Control (1990b) and shown in Table 49–4. The preferred antigen is purified protein derivative (PPD) in the intermediate-strength of 5 tuberculin units. If the intracutaneously applied PPD is

TABLE 49–4. HIGH-RISK GROUPS RECOMMENDED FOR TUBERCULOSIS SCREENING BY THE ADVISORY COMMITTEE FOR ELIMINATION OF TUBERCULOSIS

1. Persons infected with the human immunodeficiency virus.
2. Close contacts of persons known or suspected to have tuberculosis, sharing the same household or other closed environment.
3. Persons with medical risk factors known to increase the risk of disease if infection has occurred.
4. Foreign-born persons from countries with a high tuberculosis prevalence.
5. Medically underserved low-income populations, including high-risk racial or ethnic minority populations—for example, blacks, hispanics, and Native Americans.
6. Alcoholics and intravenous drug users.
7. Residents of long-term-care facilities, correctional institutions, mental institutions, nursing homes/facilities, and other long-term residential facilities.

From Centers for Disease Control (1990b).

negative, no further evaluation is needed. A positive skin test is interpreted according to risk factors (American Thoracic Society/Centers for Disease Control, 1990). For *very high-risk* patients (i.e., those who are HIV-positive, those with abnormal chest radiography, or those who have a recent contact with an active case), 5 mm is considered positive. For those at *high risk* (i.e., foreign-born, intravenous drug users who are HIV-negative, low-income populations, or those with medical conditions that increase the risk for tuberculosis), 10 mm is considered positive. For persons with none of these risk factors, 15 mm is defined as positive. If the chest radiograph is negative, then no treatment is necessary until after delivery, when isoniazid chemoprophylaxis usually is given for 1 year. Patients who have been vaccinated with bacillus Calmette–Guérin (BCG) pose special problems with interpretation of skin testing (Medchill and Gillum, 1989).

Pregnancy does not alter the course of active tuberculosis; however, evaluation of the degree of activity of pulmonary disease radiographically may at times be difficult. As pregnancy advances and the diaphragm rises, the lungs undergo some degree of compression, which may mask the extent of lesions. In the absence of seriously impaired pulmonary infection, analgesia and anesthesia for labor and delivery can usually be accomplished as for normal pregnancy.

Tuberculosis is seldom an indication for therapeutic abortion unless there is disseminated tuberculosis or severely compromised cardiopulmonary function.

Rifampin, which has usually been used in combination with isoniazid, may impair the efficacy of oral contraceptives.

Treatment. In nonpregnant tuberculin-positive patients who are less than 35, and who have no evidence of active disease, isoniazid, 300 mg daily, is given for 1 year. In pregnant women, most recommend that this not be started until after delivery. Exceptions include known recent convertors in whom the incidence of active infection is 3 percent in the first year, and women exposed to active infection in whom the incidence of infection is 0.5 percent per year, and women seropositive for immunodeficiency virus. Selwyn and associates (1989) reported that active tuberculosis developed in 4 percent of HIV-positive tuberculin-positive nonpregnant drug users over a 21-month period of observation. It seems reasonable to treat those that are pregnant. Isoniazid is a category C drug, and it is considered safe during pregnancy (Briggs and colleagues, 1990). An alternative is to withhold therapy until after 12 weeks gestation in these asymptomatic women (Medchill and Gillum, 1989).

Active disease is always treated with at least two tuberculostatic drugs. Fortunately, several first-line tuberculostatic drugs do not appear to adversely affect the fetus (Snider and colleagues, 1980). There seems to be general agreement that the orally prescribed regimen for pregnant women should include **isoniazid,** 5 mg/kg, not to exceed 300 mg daily, along with **pyridoxine,** 50 mg daily, both for 9 months. The American Thoracic Society and Centers for Disease Control (1986) recommend that the isoniazid regimen be given along with **rifampin,** 10 mg/kg daily for 9 months. Others recommend instead that isoniazid be combined with **ethambutol,** 15 to 25 mg/kg per day. Both regimens apparently are safe and efficacious.

The safety of other regimens is less well known. An attenuated 6-month course of isoniazid and rifampin, given along with **pyrazinamide** for the first 2 months, has been shown effective for nonpregnant patients (Combs and colleagues, 1990). Unfortunately, experience in pregnancy with pyrazinamide, although a category C drug, is limited at this time. **Streptomycin** is not recommended during pregnancy, because auditory and vestibular abnormalities, including severe deafness, have been identified in about 15 percent of exposed infants.

Neonatal Tuberculosis. Although **congenital tuberculosis** is rare, it can prove fatal (Myers and co-workers, 1981). Infection is often acquired hematogenously and it usually is in the liver. Some infants are infected by aspiration of infected secretions at delivery. Neonatal infection is unlikely if the mother with active disease has been treated for at least 2 weeks before delivery, or if her sputum culture is negative. Because the newborn is quite susceptible to tuberculosis, most recommend isolation from the mother suspected of having active disease. If untreated, the risk of disease in the infant born to a woman with active infection is 50 percent in the first year (Jacobs and Abernathy, 1988). Therefore, 3-months of isoniazid chemoprophylaxis is recommended for the infant, with or without BCG vaccination.

Sarcoidosis

Sarcoidosis is a chronic, multisystem disease of unknown etiology characterized by an accumulation of T lymphocytes and phagocytes within noncaseating granulomas. Pulmonary involvement is most common, followed by the skin, eyes, and lymph nodes. Its prevalence in the United States is 10 to 40 per 100,000, with equal sex distribution but a 10- to 20-fold predilection for African-Americans (Crystal, 1991). Clinical presentation varies, but most commonly dyspnea and a dry cough without constitutional symptoms develop insidiously over months. In about one fourth of patients, disease onset is abrupt, and 10 percent are asymptomatic at discovery.

Interstitial pneumonitis as demonstrated on chest x-ray is the hallmark of pulmonary involvement. About half of affected patients develop permanent radiological changes. **Lymphadenopathy,** especially of the mediastinum, is present in at least 75 percent of cases; 25 percent have **uveitis;** and 25 percent have skin involvement, usually manifest as **erythema nodosum.** Confirmation of diagnosis is not possible without biopsy, and because the lung may be the only involved organ, tissue acquisition is often difficult.

The overall prognosis for sarcoidosis is good, and in half of the affected patients the disease resolves without treatment. About 10 percent of patients die because of their disease. Glucocorticoids are the most widely used treatment; however, permanent organ derangement is seldom reversed by their use. Thus, the decision to treat is based on symptoms, physical findings, chest x-ray, and pulmonary function tests. Unless respiratory symptoms are prominent, therapy is usually withheld for a several-month observation period, and if inflammation does not subside, then prednisone, 1 mg/kg is given daily for 4 to 6 weeks (Crystal, 1991).

Sarcoidosis and Pregnancy. There is no evidence that sarcoidosis impairs fertility. Because of very low prevalence, however, sarcoidosis uncommonly complicates pregnancy. De Regt (1987) described 14 cases over a 12-year period at Downstate Medical Center, during which time nearly 20,000 women were delivered. Beneficial effects of pregnancy on sarcoidosis have been reported, but because of its tendency to improve spontaneously, these benefits are questionable. Likewise, the available evidence is suggestive that sarcoidosis seldom affects pregnancy adversely unless there is severe preexisting disease, (de Regt, 1987; O'Leary, 1968; Schmidt and Hall, 1991). De Regt reported two fatal cases due to extensive disease, one with multiple lung abscesses and the other with severe interstitial fibrosis. We have cared for one pregnant woman who died because her severe pulmonary sarcoidosis and extensive hilar adenopathy were further complicated by placenta previa, extreme obesity, and aspiration of gastric contents.

Selroos (1990) reviewed 655 patients with sarcoidosis referred to the Mjölbolsta Hospital District in southern Finland. Of 252 women between 18 and 50, 15 percent had sarcoidosis during pregnancy, or within 1 year postpartum. Active disease complicated 26 pregnancies; 3 aborted spontaneously, and the other 23 women were delivered at term. There was no evidence for disease progression. Similarly, in the 18 pregnancies in 12 women with inactive disease, pregnancy outcome was good and there was no evidence of disease activation. These experiences are similar to those reported by Agha and colleagues (1982) for 35 pregnancies cared for at the University of Michigan Hospital.

Active sarcoidosis is treated using the same guidelines as for the woman who is not pregnant. Severe disease warrants serial determination of pulmonary function. Symptomatic uveitis, constitutional symptoms, and pulmonary symptoms are treated with prednisone, 1 mg/kg per day.

Cystic Fibrosis

Cystic fibrosis is one of the most common serious genetic disorders in whites (see Chap. 41, p. 944). Its frequency is estimated to be 1 per 1500 white births and 1 per 17,000 African-American births. The median survival is about 20 to 25 years, and because of improvements in diagnosis and treatment, nearly 80 percent of girls with cystic fibrosis now survive to adulthood. Although many are infertile because of delayed sexual development and perhaps abnormal cervical mucus production, pregnancy is still not uncommon. Males who survive to adulthood often have aspermia.

Cystic fibrosis is characterized by exocrine gland dysfunction with production of thick, viscid secretions. Almost all affected patients have lung involvement, which is also the most common cause of death. Bronchial gland hypertrophy with mucous plugging and small-airway obstruction leads to subsequent infection that ultimately causes chronic bronchitis and bronchiectasis. Three bacteria are found to colonize the respiratory tract in these patients: *Pseudomonas aeruginosa* is identified in over 90 percent, and *Staphylococcus aureus* and *Haemophilus influenzae* are recovered in a minority. Acute and chronic parenchymal inflammation ultimately causes extensive fibrosis, and along with airway obstruction there is a ventilation–perfusion mismatch. Pulmonary insufficiency is the end result. Eccrine sweat gland abnormalities provide the basis for the diagnostic **sweat test,** characterized by elevated sodium, potassium, and chloride levels in sweat.

Cystic Fibrosis and Pregnancy. Pulmonary involvement in cystic fibrosis can prove very deleterious to pregnancy because of chronic lung disease with hypoxia and frequent pulmonary infections. **Cor pulmonale** is common, and Cohen and associates (1980) reported that 13 percent of pregnant women with cystic fibrosis developed heart failure. **Pancreatic dysfunction** also can contribute significantly to poor maternal nutrition. Cohen and associates (1980), in a survey of cystic fibrosis centers, obtained information on 129 pregnancies and reported that increased maternal and perinatal mortality were related to severe pulmonary infection. These authors suggested that pregnancy be discouraged except for the healthiest women. They used the **Shwachman–Kulezycki** or **Taussig scores of severity,** which are based on radiological and clinical criteria. These scores range from 0 to 100, and a score of 50 or less in nonpregnant patients portends an overall bad prognosis, while a score of 90 or more predicts a good outcome. These investigators concluded that pregnancy should be discouraged unless the score was at least 80.

More recently, Canny and co-workers (1991) presented their experiences from Toronto with 38 pregnancies in 25 women with cystic fibrosis. Prepregnancy treatment was continued, including pancreatic enzyme replacement in the 12 women with pancreatic insufficiency, oral antibiotics, aerosolized bronchodilators, chest physiotherapy, and nutritional support. Although none of these women developed heart failure, admission was required for pulmonary complications during 30 percent of pregnancies. Three women developed gestational diabetes and another had postpartum pancreatitis. Of 34 completed pregnancies, outcomes were generally good. There were 2 preterm deliveries and one 31-week neonate died of sepsis. One growth-retarded infant was delivered at term to a mother who had severe obstructive lung disease. Only one mother died within two years of delivery, in contrast to 18 percent reported in the survey by Cohen and colleagues (1980). Canny and associates (1991) stressed that the women they described were not as ill as many patients with cystic fibrosis. For example, they had a relatively late age at diagnosis and a high incidence of pancreatic sufficiency, both good prognostic factors.

Management. Prepregnancy counseling is important. Women who become pregnant should be followed closely with serial pulmonary function testing, surveillance for superimposed infection, and for heart failure. Careful attention is given to postural drainage and bronchodilator therapy. Preliminary findings indicate that recombinant human DNase, administered by inhalation, improves lung function by reducing the viscosity of sputum produced by these patients (Aitken and colleagues, 1992; Hubbard and associates, 1992). Pancreatic insufficiency is treated by oral pancreatic enzyme replacement. Hospitalization is recommended if complications develop. Treatment of cor pulmonale consists of bronchodilators, oxygen, and diuretics (Palevsky and Fishman, 1990). Genetic counseling regarding this disease is discussed in Chapter 41 (p. 944).

Pulmonary Resection

The effect of pulmonary resection, usually for bronchiectasis or tuberculosis, will depend upon the functional capacity of the remaining pulmonary tissue. Gaensler and associates (1953) studied pulmonary function during 9 pregnancies in 7 women in whom operative collapse of one lung or pneumonectomy had been performed for tuberculosis. They compared these findings with those of 19 normal pregnant women. The stimulus for increased ventilation was not as great in women with impaired pulmonary function, and indeed, those with severely impaired function increased ventilation by increasing the respiratory rate rather than the depth of breathing. All of these women tolerated pregnancy well. In general, it can be concluded that if pulmonary function is equivalent to one normal lung, and active pulmonary disease does not persist, then pregnancy is tolerated without undue risk to the mother and with a good likelihood of delivery of a healthy infant (Laros, 1980).

Carbon Monoxide Poisoning

Carbon monoxide is ubiquitous, and most nonsmoking adults have a carbon monoxyhemoglobin saturation of 1 to 3 percent. In cigarette smokers, levels may be as high as 5 to 10 percent (Farrow and associates, 1990). Toxic levels are frequently encountered from inadequately ventilated areas warmed by space heaters that utilize natural fuels. Carbon monoxide is an odorless, tasteless gas that has a high affinity and binding for hemoglobin, thus displacing oxygen and impeding its transfer.

The pregnant woman, and especially her fetus, do not tolerate excessive carbon monoxide inhalation. Symptoms usually appear when carboxyhemoglobin concentration is 20 to 30 percent, and concentrations over 50 to 60 percent produce severe symptoms and may be fatal to the mother. Presumably, lesser concentrations are fatal for the fetus. Because hemoglobin F has a higher affinity for carbon monoxide, fetal carboxyhemoglobin levels are 10 to 15 percent higher than those in the mother (Longo, 1977).

At room air, the half-life of carbon monoxide is 4 to 6 hours, but in 100 percent oxygen it is about 1 hour. Thus, treatment of poisoning is supportive along with administration of inspired 100 percent oxygen. Hollander and colleagues (1987) have reported the successful use of hyperbaric oxygen to treat an affected pregnant woman. The half-life of carbon monoxide in hyperbaric oxygen is only 15 to 30 minutes.

References

Advisory Committee on Immunization Practices: Prevention and control of influenza: 1. Vaccines. MMWR 38:297, 1989

Advisory Committee on Immunization Practices: Pneumococcal polysaccharide vaccine. MMWR 5:64, 1988

Agha FP, Vade A, Amendola MA, Cooper RF: Effects of pregnancy on sarcoidosis. Surg Gynecol Obstet 155:817, 1982

Aitken ML, Burke W, McDonald G, Shak S, Montgomery AB, Smith A: Recombinant human DNase inhalation in normal subjects and patients with cystic fibrosis. A phase 1 study. JAMA 267:1947, 1992

American Thoracic Society/Centers for Disease Control: Diagnostic standards and classification of tuberculosis. Am Rev Respir Dis 142:725, 1990

American Thoracic Society: Treatment of tuberculosis and tuberculosis infection in adults and children. Am Rev Respir Dis 134:355, 1986

Bahna SL, Bjerkedal T: The course and outcome of pregnancy in women with bronchial asthma. Acta Allerg 27:397, 1972

Bartels H, Moll W, Metcalfe J: Physiology of gas exchanges in the human placenta. Am J Obstet Gynecol 84:1714, 1962

Barss VA, Schwartz PA, Green MF, Phillippe M, Saltzman D, Frigoletto FD: Use of the subcutaneous heparin pump during pregnancy. J Reprod Med 30:899, 1985

Bell WR, Simon TL, DeMets DL: The clinical features of submassive and massive pulmonary emboli. Am J Med 62:355, 1977

Benedetti TJ, Valle R, Ledger WJ: Antepartum pneumonia in pregnancy. Am J Obstet Gynecol 144:413, 1982

Bergqvist A, Bergqvist D, Hallbook T: Deep vein thrombosis during pregnancy. A prospective study. Acta Obstet Gynecol Scand 62:443, 1983

Berkowitz K, LaSala A: Risk factors associated with the increasing prevalence of pneumonia during pregnancy. Am J Obstet Gynecol 163:981, 1990

Bone RC: Ventilation/perfusion scan in pulmonary embolism. "The emperor is incompletely attired." JAMA 263:2794, 1990

Braman SS, Kaemmerlen JT: Intensive care of status asthmaticus. A 10-year experience. JAMA 264:366, 1990

Briggs GG, Freeman RK, Yaffee SJ: Drugs in Pregnancy and Lactation, 3rd ed. Baltimore, Williams & Wilkins, 1990

Broussard RC, Payne K, George RB: Treatment with acyclovir of varicella pneumonia in pregnancy. Chest 99:1045, 1991

Canny GJ, Corey M, Livingstone RA, Carpenter S, Green L, Levison H: Pregnancy and cystic fibrosis. Obstet Gynecol 77:850, 1991

Carson JL, Kelley MA, Duff A, Weg JG, Fulkerson WJ, Palevsky HI, Schwartz JS, Thompson BT, Popovich J, Hobbins TE, Spera MA, Alavi A, Terrin ML: The clinical course on pulmonary embolism. N Engl J Med 326:1240, 1992

Catanzaro A: Pulmonary mycosis in pregnant women. Chest 86:14S, 1984

Centers for Disease Control: Tuberculosis morbidity in the United States: Final data, 1990. MMWR 40:23, 1992

Centers for Disease Control: Asthma—United States, 1980–1987. MMWR 39:493, 1990a

Centers for Disease Control: Screening for tuberculosis and tuberculous infection in high-risk populations. Recommendations of the Advisory Committee for Elimination of Tuberculosis. MMWR 39:1, 1990b

Centers for Disease Control: Guidelines for prophylaxis against

Pneumocystis carinii pneumonia for persons infected with immunodeficiency virus. MMWR 38:1, 1989

Centers for Disease Control: Varicella–zoster immune globulin distribution—United States and other countries, 1981–1983. MMWR 33:81, 1984

Clark GPM, Dobson PM, Thickett A, Turner NM: Chickenpox pneumonia, its complications and management: A report of three cases, including the use of extracorporeal membrane oxygenation. Anaesthesia 46:376, 1991

Cohen LF, di Sant Agnese PA, Friedlander J: Cystic fibrosis and pregnancy: A national survey. Lancet 2:842, 1980

Combs DL, O'Brien RJ, Geiter LJ: USPHS tuberculosis short-course chemotherapy trial 21: Effectiveness, toxicity, and acceptability. The report of final results. Ann Intern Med 112: 397, 1990

Corre KA, Rothstein RJ: Assessing severity of adult asthma and need for hospitalization. Ann Emerg Med 14:45, 1985

Crowther C: Magnesium sulphate versus diazepam in the management of eclampsia: A randomized controlled trial. Br J Obstet Gynaecol 97:110, 1990

Crystal RG: Sarcoidosis. Chapter 227. In Wilson JD, Braunwald E, Isselbacher KJ, Petersdorf RG, Martin JB, Fauci AS, Root RK (eds): Harrison's Principles of Internal Medicine, 12th ed. New York, McGraw-Hill, 1991, p 1463

de Regt RH: Sarcoidosis and pregnancy. Obstet Gynecol 70:369, 1987

de Swiet M: The Respiratory System. In Hytten F, Chamberlain G (eds): Clinical Physiology in Obstetrics, 2nd ed. London, Blackwell Scientific Publications, 1991, p 83

Douglas RG Jr: Drug Therapy: Prophylaxis and treatment of influenza. N Engl J Med 322:443, 1990

Erdman WA, Jayson HT, Redman HC, Miller GL, Parkey RW, Peshock RW: Deep venous thrombosis of extremities: Role of MR imaging in the diagnosis. Radiology 174:425, 1990

Farrow JR, Davis GJ, Roy TM, McCloud LC, Nichols GR II: Fetal death due to nonlethal maternal carbon monoxide poisoning. J Forensic Sci 35:1448, 1990

Fitzsimons R, Greenberger PA, Patterson R: Outcome of pregnancy in women requiring corticosteroids for severe asthma. J Allergy Clin Immunol 78:349, 1986

Foy HM, Cooney MK, McMahan R, Grayston JT: Viral mycoplasmal pneumonia in a prepaid medical care group during an eight-year period. Am J Epidemiol 97:93, 1973

Gaensler EA, Patton WE, Verstraeten JM, Badger TL: Pulmonary function in pregnancy, III. Serial observations in patients with pulmonary insufficiency. Am Rev Tuberc 67:779, 1953

Gallus A, Jackaman J, Tillett J, Mills W, Wycherley A: Safety and efficacy of warfarin started early after submassive venous thrombosis or pulmonary embolism. Lancet 2:1293, 1986

Ginsberg JS, Brill-Edwards P, Burrows RF, Bona R, Prandoni P, Büller HR, Lensing A: Venous thrombosis during pregnancy: Leg and trimester of presentation. Thromb Haemost 67:519, 1992

Ginsberg JS, Hirsh J, Rainbow AJ, Coates G: Risks to the fetus of radiologic procedures used in the diagnoses of maternal venous thromboembolic disease. Thromb Haemost 61:189, 1989

Gordon M, Niswander KR, Berendes H, Kantor AG: Fetal morbidity following potentially anoxigenic obstetric conditions: Bronchial asthma. Am J Obstet Gynecol 106:421, 1970

Grayston JT, Campbell LA, Kuo CC, Mordhorst CH, Saikku P, Thom DH, Wang SP: A new respiratory tract pathogen: *Chlamydia pneumoniae* strain TWAR. J Infect Dis 161:618, 1990

Greenberger PA, Patterson R: The outcome of pregnancy complicated by severe asthma. Allergy Proc 9:539, 1988

Greenfield LJ, Michna BA: Twelve-year clinical experience with the Greenfield vena caval filter. Surg 104:706, 1988

Haake DA, Zakowski PC, Haake DL, Bryson YJ: Early treatment with acyclovir for varicella pneumonia in otherwise healthy adults: Retrospective controlled study and review. Rev Infect Dis 12:788, 1990

Hall JG, Pauli RM, Wilson KM: Maternal and fetal sequelae of anticoagulation during pregnancy. Am J Med 68:122, 1980

Hankins GDV, Berryman GK, Scott RT, Hood D: Maternal arterial desaturation with 15-methyl prostaglandin F$_2$ alpha for uterine atony. Obstet Gynecol 72:367, 1988

Hassan AI, Aref GH, Kassem AS: Congenital iodide-induced goiter with hypothyroidism. Arch Dis Child 43:702, 1968

Heijboer H, Brandjes DPM, Buller HR, Sturk A, ten Cate WJ: Deficiencies of coagulation-inhibiting and fibrinolytic proteins in outpatients with deep-vein thrombosis. N Engl J Med 323:1512, 1990

Hellgren M, Trenhgborn L, Abildgaard U: Pregnancy in women with congenital antithrombin III deficiency: Experience of treatment with heparin and antithrombin. Gynecol Obstet Invest 14:127, 1989

Henderson SR, Lund CJ, Creasman WT: Antepartum pulmonary embolism. Am J Obstet Gynecol 112:476, 1972

Hernandez E, Angell CS, Johnson JWG: Asthma in pregnancy: Current concepts. Obstet Gynecol 55:739, 1980

Hirsh J: Heparin. N Engl J Med 324:1565, 1991a

Hirsh J: Oral anticoagulant drugs. N Engl J Med 324:1865, 1991b

Hollander DI, Nagey DA, Welch R, Pupkin M: Hyperbaric oxygen therapy for the treatment of acute carbon monoxide poisoning in pregnancy. A case report. J Reprod Med 32:615, 1987

Hubbard RC, McElvaney NG, Birrer P, Shak S, Robinson WW, Wu CJM, Chernick MS, Crystal RG: A preliminary study of aerosolized recombinant human deoxyribonuclease I in the treatment of cystic fibrosis. N Engl J Med 326:812, 1992

Huisman MV, Büller HR, Ten Cate JW, Vreeken J: Serial impedance plethysmography for suspected deep venous thrombosis in outpatients: The Amsterdam general practitioner study. N Engl J Med 314:823, 1986

Hull R, Delmore T, Carter C, Hirsh J, Genton E, Gent M, Turpie G, Laughlin D: Adjusted subcutaneous heparin versus warfarin sodium in the long-term treatment of venous thrombosis. N Engl J Med 306:189, 1982a

Hull R, Hirsh J, Jay R, Carter C, England C, Gent M, Turpie AGG, Loughlin D, Dodd P, Thomas M, Raskob G, Ockelford P: Different intensities of oral anticoagulant therapy in the treatment of proximal-vein thrombosis. N Engl J Med 307:1676, 1982b

Hull RD, Hirsh J, Carter CJ, Jay RM, Ockelford PA, Buller HR, Turpie AG, Powers P, Kinch D, Dodd PE: Diagnostic efficacy of impedance plethysmography for clinically suspected deep-vein thrombosis. A randomized trial. Ann Intern Med 102:21, 1985

Hull RD, Raskob GE, Carter CJ: Serial impedance plethysmography in pregnant patients with clinically suspected deep-vein thrombosis. Clinical validity of negative findings. Ann Intern Med 112:664, 1990a

Hull RD, Raskob GE, Hirsh J, Jay RM, Leclerc JR, Geerts WH, Rosenbloom D, Sackett DL, Anderson C, Harrison L: Continuous intravenous heparin compared with intermittent subcutaneous heparin in the initial treatment of proximal-vein thrombosis. N Engl J Med 315:1109, 1986

Hull RD, Raskob GE, Pineo GF, Green D, Trowbridge AA, Elliott CG, Lerner RG, Hall J, Sparling T, Brettell HR, Norton J, Carter CJ, George R, Merli G, Ward J, Mayo W, Rosenbloom D, Brant R: Subcutaneous low-molecular-weight heparin compared with continuous intravenous heparin in the treatment of proximal-vein thrombosis. N Engl J Med 326:975, 1992

Hull RD, Raskob GE, Rosenbloom D, Panju AA, Bull-Edwards P, Ginsberg JS, Hirsh J, Martin GJ, Green D: Heparin for 5 days as compared with 10 days in the initial treatment of proximal venous thrombosis. N Engl J Med 322:1260, 1990b

Hux CH, Wapner RJ, Chayen B, Rattan P, Jarrell B, Greenfield L: Use of the Greenfield filter for thromboembolic disease in pregnancy. Am J Obstet Gynecol 155:734, 1986

Jacobs RF, Abernathy RS: Management of tuberculosis in pregnancy and the newborn. Clin Perinatol 15:305, 1988

Kaunitz AM, Hughes JM, Grimes DA, Smith JC, Rochat RW, Kafrissen ME: Causes of maternal mortality in the United States. Obstet Gynecol 65:605, 1985

Kreisman H, de Wrel WV, Mitchell CA: Respiratory function during prostaglandin-induced labor. Am Rev Respir Dis 111:564, 1975

Larcos KD: The postpneumonectomy mother. Respiration 39:185, 1980

Lensing AWA, Prandoni P, Brandjes D, Huisman PM, Vigo M, Tomasella G, Krekt J, Wouter TCJ, Huisman MV, Buller HR: Detection of deep-vein thrombosis by real-time B-mode ultrasonography. N Engl J Med 320:342, 1989

Longo L: The biologic effects of carbon monoxide on the pregnant woman, fetus and newborn infant. Am J Obstet Gynecol 129:69, 1977

Mabie WC, Barton JR, Wasserstrum N, Sibai BM: Clinical observations on asthma in pregnancy. J Mat Fet Med 1:45, 1992

Madinger NE, Greenspoon JS, Ellrodt AG: Pneumonia during pregnancy: Has modern technology improved maternal and fetal outcome? Am J Obstet Gynecol 161:657, 1989

Mathison DA: Asthma in adults: Diagnosis and treatment. In Middleton E, Reed CE, Ellis EF (eds): Allergy: Principles and Practice, 3rd ed. St. Louis, Mosby, 1988, p 1063

McGregor JA, Kleinschmidt-DeMasters BK, Ogle J: Meningoencephalitis caused by *Histoplasma capsulatum* complicating pregnancy. Am J Obstet Gynecol 154:925, 1986

Medchill MT, Gillum M: Diagnosis and management of tuberculosis during pregnancy. Obstet Gynecol Surv 44:81, 1989

Mengert WF: Venous ligation in obstetrics. Am J Obstet Gynecol 50:467, 1945

Milne JA, Howie AD, Pack AI: Dyspnoea during normal pregnancy. Br J Obstet Gynaecol 85:260, 1978

Mohr DN, Rhu JH, Litin SC, Rosenow EC III: Recent advances in the management of venous thromboembolism. Mayo Clin Proc 63:281, 1988

Moser KM: Pulmonary thromboembolism. In Wilson JD, Braunwald E, Isselbacher JK, Petersdorf RG, Martin JB, Fauci

AS, Root RK (eds): Harrison's Principles of Internal Medicine, 12 ed. New York, McGraw-Hill, 1991, p 1090

Moya F, Morishima HO, Shnider SM, James LS: Influence of maternal hyperventilation on the newborn infant. Am J Obstet Gynecol 91:76, 1965

Mueller MJ, Lebherz TB: Antepartum thrombophlebitis. Obstet Gynecol 34:867, 1969

Myers JP, Peristein PH, Light IJ, Towbin RB, Dincsoy HP, Dincsoy MY: Tuberculosis in pregnancy with fatal congenital infection. Pediatrics 67:89, 1981

National Heart, Lung and Blood Institute: National Asthma Education Program, expert panel report. Guidelines for the diagnosis and management of asthma. Pediatr Asthma Allergy Immunol 5:57, 1991

National Institutes of Health Consensus Development Conference: Prevention of venous thrombosis and pulmonary embolism. JAMA 256:744, 1986

Noble PW, Lavee AE, Jacobs NM: Respiratory diseases in pregnancy. Obstet Gynecol Clin North Am 15:391, 1988

O'Leary JA: A continuing study of sarcoidosis and pregnancy. Am J Obstet Gynecol 101:610, 1968

Palevsky HI, Fishman AP: Chronic cor pulmonale. Etiology and management. JAMA 263:2347, 1990

Paryani SG, Arvin AM: Intrauterine infection with varicella–zoster virus after maternal varicella. N Engl J Med 314:1542, 1986

PIOPED Investigators: Value of the ventilation/perfusion scan in acute pulmonary embolism: Results of the Prospective Investigation of Pulmonary Embolism Diagnosis (PIOPED). JAMA 263:2753, 1990

Polak JF, Wilkinson DL: Ultrasonographic diagnosis of symptomatic deep venous thrombosis in pregnancy. Am J Obstet Gynecol 165:625, 1991

Powell BL, Drutz DJ, Huppert M, Sun SH: Relationship of progesterone- and estradiol-binding proteins in *Coccidioides immitis* to coccidioidal dissemination in pregnancy. Infect Immun 40:478, 1983

Reed CE: Aerosol steroids as primary treatment of mild asthma. N Engl J Med 325:425, 1991

Research Committee of the British Thoracic Society: Community-acquired pneumonia in adults in British hospitals in 1982–1983: A survey of aetiology, mortality, prognostic factors and outcome. BMJ 62:195, 1987

Richey SD, Ramin KD, Ramin SM, Cunningham FG: Pneumonitis in pregnancy—not a benign condition. Presented at the meeting of American College of Obstetricians and Gynecologists, Washington, DC, May 1993

Rodriguez-Roisin R, Ballester E, Roca J, Torres A, Wagner PD: Mechanisms of hypoxemia in patients with status asthmaticus requiring mechanical ventilation. Am Rev Respir Dis 139:731, 1989

Roehm JOF, Johnsrude IS, Barth MH, Gianturco C: The bird's nest inferior vena cava filter. Progress report. Radiology 168:745, 1988

Rolston DH, Shnider SM, de Lorimer AA: Uterine blood flow and fetal acid-base changes after bicarbonate administration to the pregnant ewe. Anesthesiology 40:348, 174

Sachs BP, Brown DA, Driscoll SG, Schulman E, Acker D, Ransil BJ, Jewett JF: Maternal mortality in Massachusetts: Trends and prevention. N Engl J Med 316:667, 1987

Schatz M, Harden K, Forsythe A, Chilingar L, Hoffman C, Sperling W, Zeiger RS: The course of asthma during pregnancy, postpartum, and with successive pregnancies: A prospective analysis. J Allergy Clin Immunol 81:509, 1988

Schatz M, Zeiger RS: The management of asthma, rhinitis, and anaphylaxis during pregnancy. In Lee RV (ed): Current Obstetric Medicine. St. Louis, Mosby, 1991, p 65

Schatz M, Zeiger RS, Hoffman CP, Kaiser Permanente Asthma and Pregnancy Study Group: Intrauterine growth is related to gestational pulmonary function in pregnant asthmatic women. Chest 98:389, 1990

Schmidt GA, Hall JB: Pulmonary Disease. In Barron WM, Lindheimer MD (eds): Medical Disorders During Pregnancy. St. Louis, Mosby Yearbook, 1991, p 197

Scoggin CH, Sahn SA, Petty TL: Status asthmaticus. A nine-year experience. JAMA 238:1158, 1977

Scott LM, Zawin ML, Taylor KJW: Doppler US: II. Clinical applications. Radiology 174:310, 1990

Selroos O: Sarcoidosis and pregnancy: A review with results of a retrospective survey. J Int Med 227:221, 1990

Selwyn PA, Hartel D, Lewis VA, Schoenbaum EE, Vermund SH, Klein RS, Walker AT, Friedland GH: A prospective study of the risk of tuberculosis among intravenous drug users with human immunodeficiency virus infection. N Engl J Med 320:544, 1989

Sims CD, Chamberlain GVP, de Swiet M: Lung function tests in bronchial asthma during and after pregnancy. Br J Obstet Gynaecol 83:434, 1976

Smego RA, Asperilla MO: Use of acyclovir for varicella pneumonia during pregnancy. Obstet Gynecol 78:1112, 1991

Smith JM: Epidemiology and natural history of asthma, allergic rhinitis and atopic dermatitis. In Middleton E Jr, Reed CE, Ellis E (eds): Allergy: Principles and Practice, 3rd ed. St. Louis, Mosby, 1988, p 899

Snider DE Jr, Layde PM, Johnson MW, Lyle MA: Treatment of tuberculosis during pregnancy. Am Rev Respir Dis 122:65, 1980

Sperling RS, Stratton P: Treatment options for human immunodeficiency virus-infected pregnant women. Obstet Gynecol 79:443, 1992

Stamm H: Obstetrical and gynecological mortality due to embolism in Central Europe and Scandinavia. Geburtshilfe Frauenheilkd 20:675, 1960

Stenius-Aarniala B, Pririla P, Teramo K: Asthma and Pregnancy: A prospective study of 198 pregnancies. Thorax 43:12, 1988

Stratton P, Mofenson LM, Willoughby AD: Human immunodeficiency virus infection in pregnant women under care at AIDS Clinical Trials Centers in the United States. Obstet Gynecol 79:364, 1992

Summer WR: Status asthmaticus. Chest 87:87s, 1985

Tengborn L, Bergqvist D, Matzsch T, Bergqvist A, Hedner U: Recurrent thromboembolism in pregnancy and puerperium Is there a need for thromboprophylaxis? Am J Obstet Gynecol 160:90, 1989

Turner ES, Greenberger PA, Patterson R: Management of the pregnant asthmatic. Ann Intern Med 6:905, 1980

Wack EE, Ampel NM, Galgiani JN, Bronnimann DA: Coccidioidomycosis during pregnancy: An analysis of ten cases among 47,120 pregnancies. Chest 94:376, 1988

Weiner CP: Diagnosis and management of thromboembolic disease during pregnancy. Clin Obstet Gynecol 28:107, 1985

Wenger NK, Stein PD, Willis PW III: Massive acute pulmonary

embolism: The deceivingly nonspecific manifestations. JAMA 220:843, 1972

Wilkins I, Mexrow G, Lynch L, Bottone EJ, Berkowitz RL: Amnionitis and life-threatening respiratory distress after percutaneous umbilical blood sampling. Am J Obstet Gynecol 160:427, 1989

Wulf KH, Kunze IW, Lehman V: Clinical aspects of placental gas exchange. In Respiratory Gas Exchange and Blood Flow in the Placenta. Bethesda, MD, National Institutes of Health, Public Health Service, 1972, pp 505–521

Woolcock AJ: Asthma. In Murray JF, Nadel JA (eds): Textbook of Respiratory Medicine. Philadelphia, Saunders, 1988, p 1030

CHAPTER 50
Renal and Urinary Tract Diseases

Some diseases of the kidney and urinary tract may be associated with pregnancy by chance and be little affected by it. Conversely, pregnancy often predisposes to the development of urinary tract disorders, an example being acute pyelonephritis. In other cases, pregnancy may predispose to worsening of renal disease and its sequelae, as with lupus nephritis with hypertension. In the not too distant past, obstetrical dogma was that pregnancy was contraindicated in the woman with significant underlying renal disease. However, as reported experience was gained, it appears that the prognosis for these women and their pregnancies is not invariably bleak. Indeed, most women with these disorders negotiate pregnancy without serious sequelae.

Urinary Tract Changes During Pregnancy. Pregnancy exerts profound effects on renal function as well as causing significant anatomical changes in the urinary system (see Chap. 8, p. 230). Urinary tract dilation is one of the most significant anatomical alterations induced by pregnancy. It involves dilatation of the renal calyces and pelves, as well as the ureters. These changes, which are more prominent on the right side, are mediated by hormonal but especially mechanical obstructive factors, create urinary stasis, and may lead to serious upper urinary infections. Another factor predisposing to infection is increased vesicoureteral reflux. These changes also may lead to erroneous interpretation of studies done to evaluate suspected pathological obstruction.

Evidence for hypertrophy of renal function is apparent very soon after conception. It appears to be mediated by pregnancy-induced intrarenal vasodilatation. Effective renal plasma flow and glomerular filtration are increased on the average by 40 and 65 percent, respectively. These changes have clinical relevance when interpreting renal function studies; for example, serum concentrations of creatinine and urea are decreased substantively. Other normal pregnancy-induced renal physiological alterations include those related to maintaining normal acid-base homeostasis, osmoregulation, and fluid and electrolyte retention.

Assessment of Renal Disease During Pregnancy. Interpretation of the **urinalysis** is essentially unchanged during pregnancy, except for occasional glucosuria that is discovered. Although protein excretion normally is increased, it seldom reaches levels to be detected by usual screening methods. Davison (1985) measured serial 24-hour protein excretion in 10 normal women throughout pregnancy. Their prepregnancy mean was about 100 mg/day, and this increased to about 150 mg/day during the first trimester and about 200 mg/day in the second and third trimesters. Although probably a high estimate, most agree that proteinuria must exceed 500 mg/day to be considered abnormal for pregnancy (Baylis and Davison, 1991). Unless precautions are taken to prevent contamination, there usually is admixture of vaginal secretions when the specimen is collected; thus, a clean-catch specimen should be taken to verify any pathological proteinuria detected.

Unless prerenal factors are present, if the serum creatinine persistently exceeds 0.9 mg/dL (75 μmol/L), then intrinsic renal disease should be suspected. A carefully collected timed urine specimen can be used to estimate the glomerular filtration rate by creatinine clearance. Ultrasonography provides imaging of renal size and relative consistency, as well as elements of obstruction. Full-sequence **intravenous pyelography** is not done routinely, but injection of contrast media with one or two abdominal x-rays may be indicated by the clinical situation (see Chap. 43, p. 984). The usual clinical indications for **cystoscopy** are followed. Although Packham and Fairley (1987) reported **renal biopsy** to be safe and helpful in guiding treatment in 111 pregnant women with renal disease, we agree with most others that this procedure can usually be postponed until pregnancy is completed (Baylis and Davison, 1991; Lindheimer and Davison, 1991).

Orthostatic Proteinuria. Abnormal amounts of protein sometimes are detectable in urine formed while the pregnant woman is ambulatory but not when recumbent. No other evidence for renal disease is apparent. Such orthostatic or *postural proteinuria* has been observed in up to 5 percent of normal young adults. The pregnant woman with orthostatic proteinuria should be evaluated for bacteriuria, abnormal urinary sediment, reduced glomerular filtration rate, and hypertension. In the absence of these abnormalities, and if protein excretion is not constant, then it probably is inconsequential.

Pregnancy After Unilateral Nephrectomy. Because the excretory capacity of two kidneys is much in excess of ordinary needs, and because the surviving kidney usually undergoes hypertrophy with increased excretory capacity, women with one normal kidney most often have no difficulty in pregnancy. Indeed, pregnancy in these women is associated with significant augmentation of renal hemodynamics (Baylis and Davison, 1991). However, before advising a woman with one kidney about the risk of future pregnancy, a thorough functional evaluation of the remaining organ is essential, even in asymptomatic women.

Urinary Tract Infections

Infections of the urinary tract are the most common bacterial infections encountered during pregnancy. Although **asymptomatic bacteriuria** is more common, symptomatic infection may involve the lower tract to cause **cystitis,** or it may involve the renal calyces, pelvis, and parenchyma to cause **pyelonephritis.**

Organisms that cause urinary infections are those from the normal perineal flora. There is now evidence that some strains of *Escherichia coli* have pili that enhance their virulence (Svanborg-Eden, 1982). Also called *adhesins* or *P-fimbriae,* these appendages allow bacterial attachment to glycoprotein receptors on uroepithelial cell membranes. Although pregnancy does not seem to enhance these virulence factors, urinary stasis apparently does, and along with vesicoureteral reflux in some women, it predisposes to symptomatic upper urinary infections.

In the early puerperium, bladder sensitivity to intravesical fluid tension is often decreased as the consequence of the trauma of labor as well as analgesia, especially epidural or spinal blockade. After these effects dissipate, sensations of bladder distension are likely diminished by discomfort caused by a large episiotomy, periurethral lacerations, or vaginal wall hematomas. Moreover, starting immediately after delivery, oxytocin is commonly infused with an appreciable volume of fluid at rates that cause antidiuresis. When the oxytocin is stopped, a diuresis often follows with copious urine production and bladder distension. Overdistension, coupled with catheterization to provide relief, commonly leads to urinary infection.

Asymptomatic Bacteriuria. Asymptomatic or covert bacteriuria refers to persistent actively multiplying bacteria within the urinary tract without symptoms. The reported prevalence of bacteriuria during pregnancy varies from 2 to 7 percent, and depends on parity, race, and socioeconomic status. The highest incidence has been reported in African-American multiparas with sickle cell trait, and the lowest incidence has been found in affluent white women of low parity.

Bacteriuria typically is present at the time of the first prenatal visit, and after an initial negative urine culture, only about 1 percent of women develop urinary infection (Whalley, 1967). A clean-voided specimen containing more than 100,000 organisms of the same species per mL is considered evidence for infection.

Although smaller numbers of bacteria may represent contamination during collection, Stamm and colleagues (1980) showed that lower colony count may represent active infection.

Significance. If asymptomatic bacteriuria is not treated, about 25 percent of infected women subsequently develop acute symptomatic infection during that pregnancy. Eradication of bacteriuria with antimicrobial agents has been shown to prevent most of these clinically evident infections. Although it is reasonable to perform routine screening for bacteriuria in women at high-risk, screening may not be cost effective when the prevalence is low (Campbell-Brown and associates, 1987). One-time screening does not allow prevention of all symptomatic infections. For example, at Parkland Hospital, women who had sterile screening cultures constitute about one third of those admitted for antepartum pyelonephritis.

In addition to causing symptomatic infection, covert bacteriuria has been associated in some studies with a number of other adverse pregnancy outcomes. In early studies by Kass (1962, 1965), the incidence of preterm births, defined as a birthweight of 2500 g or less, was 27 percent among 95 bacteriuric women given a placebo during pregnancy, whereas it was only 7 percent among 84 women treated with antimicrobial agents. The corresponding perinatal death rates were 14 and 0 percent, respectively. Kincaid-Smith and Bullen (1965) also reported an increased incidence of low-birthweight infants among untreated bacteriuric women, but they were unable to reduce this with antimicrobial therapy.

Other investigators did not corroborate a relationship between bacteriuria and low-birthweight infants (Table 50–1). Romero and colleagues (1989) performed meta-analysis of several studies and concluded that covert bacteriuria was associated with preterm delivery and low-birthweight infants. They were unable to address the effects of prevention of acute pyelonephritis on preterm labor and delivery. From evidence currently available, however, it seems unlikely that bacteriuria is a

TABLE 50–1. INCIDENCE OF LOW-BIRTHWEIGHT INFANTS BORN TO WOMEN WITH AND WITHOUT BACTERIURIA

Study	Bacteriuric Patients		Nonbacteriuric Patients	
	No.	(%)[a]	No.	(%)[a]
Gilstrap and colleagues (1981b)	248	(12)	248	(13)
Little (1966)	141	(9)	4735	(8)
Norden & Kilpatrick (1965)	114	(15)	109	(13)
Whalley (1967)	176	(15)	176	(12)
Wilson and associates (1966)	230	(11)	6216	(10)

[a] Numbers in parentheses indicate percent of low-birthweight infants.

prominent factor in the genesis of low-birthweight or preterm infants.

In other studies, bacteriuria has been linked to an increased incidence of pregnancy-induced hypertension and anemia. However, Gilstrap and colleagues (1981b) compared pregnancy outcomes in 248 pregnant woman in whom they localized asymptomatic infection to the bladder or kidney. As shown in Table 50–2, there was no association of bacteriuria with anemia or pregnancy-induced hypertension, as well as low-birthweight infants from growth retardation or preterm delivery.

Bacteriuria persists after delivery in many of these women, and there is also a significant number of women with pyelographic evidence of chronic infection, obstructive lesions, or congenital urinary abnormalities (Kincaid-Smith and Bullen, 1965; Whalley and associates, 1965, 1967).

Treatment. Women with asymptomatic bacteriuria may be given treatment with any of several antimicrobial regimens. Selection can be chosen on the basis of in vitro susceptibilities, if performed. At Parkland Hospital, we do not perform these studies routinely, as they add substantive costs. Empirical treatment for 10 days with nitrofurantoin macrocrystals, 100 mg once daily, has proved effective in most women. Other regimens include ampicillin or a cephalosporin given four times daily for 7 to 10 days. The recurrence rate for all of these regimens is about 30 percent.

More recently, single-dose antimicrobial therapy for bacteriuria has been used with success. Andriole and Patterson (1991) reviewed some of these regimens: amoxicillin in a 3-g dose alone or a 2-g dose given with probenecid, 1 g; nitrofurantoin, 200-mg single dose; sulfisoxazole, 2-g single dose; cephalexin as a 3-g single dose or 2 g given with probenecid, 1 g; or trimethoprim-sulfamethoxazole, 320 mg/1600 mg, given as a single dose. They emphasized that studies showing efficacy of these regimens were limited by small numbers of patients.

TABLE 50–2. ADVERSE PREGNANCY OUTCOMES: COMPARISON OF 248 WOMEN WITH RENAL OR BLADDER BACTERIURIA WITH CONTROL WOMEN

	Bacteriuric Women (%)[a]		Control Women (%)[a]
	Renal	*Bladder*	
Pregnancy Complication	*(n = 114)*	*(n = 134)*	*(n = 248)*
Hematocrit less than 30	2.6	3.7	2.1
Hypertension	12	15	14
Low-birthweight infants	10	13	13
Fetal growth retardation	8	8	8
Preterm delivery	4	8	5

[a] All values not significant when compared for each group.
Modified after Gilstrap and colleagues (1981b).

Cystitis and Urethritis. There is evidence that bladder infection during pregnancy develops without antecedent covert bacteriuria (Harris and Gilstrap, 1981). Typically, cystitis is characterized by dysuria, urgency, and frequency. There are few associated systemic findings. Usually there is pyuria as well as bacteriuria. Erythrocytes are commonly found in the sediment, and occasionally there is gross hematuria. Although cystitis usually is uncomplicated, it is presumed that the upper urinary tract may become involved by ascending infection. Certainly, 40 percent of pregnant women with acute pyelonephritis have preceding symptoms of lower-tract infection (Gilstrap and associates, 1981a).

Treatment. Women with bacterial cystitis respond readily to any of several regimens. Harris and Gilstrap (1981) reported a 97 percent cure rate with a 10-day ampicillin regimen. Sulfonamides, nitrofurantoin, or a cephalosporin also are effective when given for 10 days. Recently, there has been a trend to use shorter courses of therapy (3 to 5 days), especially in nonpregnant patients. Single-dose therapy as described for asymptomatic bacteriuria has been shown effective for both nonpregnant and pregnant women. Because 40 percent of women with early pyelonephritis initially have lower-tract symptoms, renal infection must be confidently excluded before one-dose therapy is given.

Frequency, urgency, dysuria, and pyuria accompanied by a "sterile" urine culture may be the consequence of urethritis caused by *Chlamydia trachomatis,* a common pathogen of the genitourinary tract. Frequently, mucopurulent cervicitis coexists (see Chap. 59, p. 1304). Erythromycin therapy usually is effective. *Eosinophilic cystitis* may cause persistent symptoms despite seemingly adequate therapy for bacterial cystitis. Chamberlin (1992) recently described a case complicating pregnancy.

Acute Pyelonephritis. Acute pyelonephritis is the most common serious medical complication of pregnancy, occurring in 1 to 2 percent of pregnant women. According to the Professional Activities Study Database (1987), more than 85,000 pregnant women were hospitalized in the United States in 1985 for this complication. The population incidence varies and depends on the prevalence of covert bacteriuria and whether it is treated. For example, at Parkland Hospital, nearly 90 percent of women attend prenatal clinics where bacteriuria screening is performed and treatment given for the 8 percent who are infected. Before we began routine screening, nearly 3 percent of pregnancies were complicated by pyelonephritis; but with screening and attempts to eradicate bacteriuria, acute renal infection now complicates only about 1 percent of pregnancies.

Pyelonephritis is more common after midpregnancy, it is unilateral and right-sided in more than half of cases, and bilateral in one fourth. In most women, renal parenchymal infection is caused by bacteria that ascend from the lower tract. Between 75 and 90 percent of renal infections are caused by bacteria that have P-fimbriae adhesins (Stenqvist and associates, 1987; Väisänen and colleagues, 1981).

Clinical Findings. The onset of pyelonephritis is usually rather abrupt. Symptoms include fever, shaking chills, and aching pain in one or both lumbar regions. There may be anorexia, nausea, and vomiting. The course of the disease may vary remarkably with fever to as high as 40° C or more and hypothermia to as low as 34° C. Tenderness usually can be elicited by percussion in one or both costovertebral angles. The urinary sediment frequently contains many leukocytes, frequently in clumps, and numerous bacteria. In a survey of 190 women admitted during 1986 and 1987 to Parkland Hospital, *E. coli* was isolated from the urine in 77 percent, *Klebsiella pneumoniae* in 11 percent, and *Enterobacter* or *Proteus* each in 4 percent (Cunningham, 1988). Culture results from 121 women with antepartum pyelonephritis treated at Madigan Army Medical Center were similar (Dunlow and Duff, 1990). **Importantly, about 15 percent of women with acute pyelonephritis also have bacteremia.**

Although the diagnosis usually is apparent, pyelonephritis may be mistaken for labor, chorioamnionitis, appendicitis, placental abruption, or infarction of a myoma, and, in the puerperium, for metritis with pelvic cellulitis.

Management. Almost all clinical findings in these women are ultimately caused by endotoxemia, and so are the serious complications of acute pyelonephritis. A frequent and sometimes dramatic finding is thermoregulatory instability characterized by high spiking fever followed by hypothermia. Commonly, temperatures fluctuate from as low as 34° C to as high as 42° C (Fig. 50–1). This reaction is mediated, probably in the anterior hypothalamus, by *cytokines* that are elaborated by macrophages in response to endotoxin. These include *interleukin-1,* previously termed *endogenous pyrogen,* or *tumor necrosis factor* (Michie and colleagues, 1988).

Pregnant women with acute pyelonephritis need prompt treatment. The management scheme that we have found satisfactory at Parkland Hospital is shown in Table 50–3. **Intravenous hydration to insure adequate urinary output is essential.** Because 15 percent of these women have bacteremia, during the first day or so of therapy they should be watched carefully to detect symptoms of bacterial shock or its sequelae (see Chap. 47, p. 1072). Urinary output, blood pressure, and temperature should be monitored closely. High fever should be treated, usually with a cooling blanket.

Plasma creatinine should be measured early in the course of therapy. As shown in Figure 50–2, acute pyelonephritis in some pregnant women causes a consider-

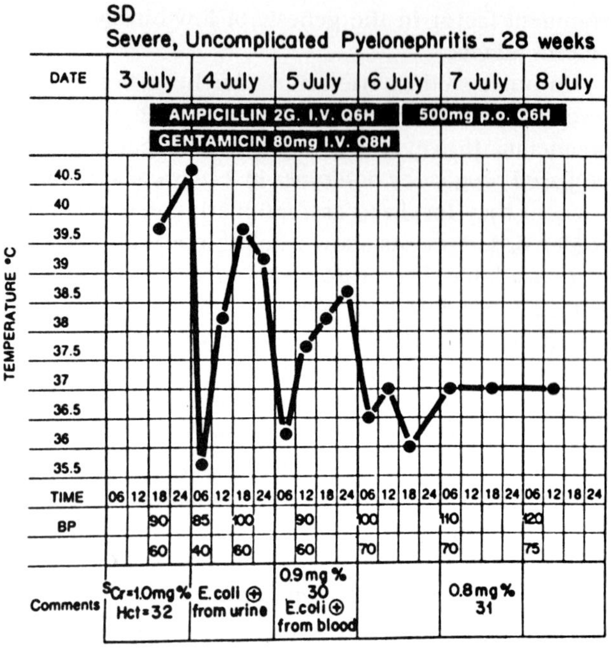

Fig. 50–1. Vital signs graphic chart from a 25-year-old primigravida with acute pyelonephritis at 28 weeks' gestation. (From Cunningham and colleagues, 1987, with permission.)

able reduction in glomerular filtration rate that is reversed by effective treatment and recovery (Whalley and co-workers, 1975). Up to 2 percent of women with antepartum pyelonephritis develop varying degrees of respiratory insufficiency caused by endotoxin-induced alveolar injury and pulmonary edema (Cunningham and associates, 1987). Ridgway and colleagues (1991) observed that plasma colloid osmotic pressure reaches a nadir in these women 24 hours after treatment is begun. In some women, pulmonary injury is severe with resultant **adult respiratory distress syndrome** (see Chap. 47, p. 1069). Occasionally, tracheal intubation and mechanical ventilation is lifesaving (Fig. 50–3). Endotoxin-

TABLE 50–3. MANAGEMENT OF THE PREGNANT WOMAN WITH ACUTE PYELONEPHRITIS AT PARKLAND HOSPITAL

1. Hospitalization
2. Urine and blood cultures
3. Complete blood count, serum creatinine, and electrolytes
4. Monitor vital signs frequently, including urinary output (place indwelling bladder catheter if necessary)
5. IV hydration to establish urinary output to at least 30 mL/hr
6. IV antimicrobial therapy
7. Chest x-ray if there is dyspnea or tachypnea
8. Repeat hematology and chemistry studies in 48 hours
9. Change to oral antimicrobials when afebrile
10. Discharge after afebrile 24 hours, continue antimicrobials for 7 to 10 days
11. Urine culture 1 to 2 weeks after antimicrobial therapy completed

Modified from Cunningham and colleagues (1987).

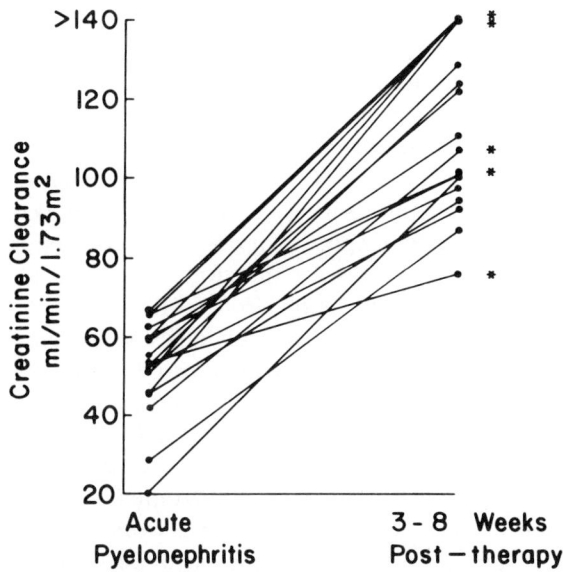

Fig. 50–2. Endogenous creatinine clearance values in 18 pregnant women during and 3 to 8 weeks after an attack of acute pyelonephritis. Asterisk indicates patients reevaluated while still pregnant. (From Whalley and colleagues, 1975.)

induced **hemolysis** is also common in these women, and about one third develop acute anemia (Cox and colleagues, 1991).

These serious urinary infections usually respond quickly to intravenous hydration and antimicrobial therapy. The choice of drug is empirical, and ampicillin, a cephalosporin, or an extended-spectrum penicillin is

satisfactory (Cox and Cunningham, 1988b). Antimicrobial resistance of *E. coli* to ampicillin has often been encountered, and Duff (1984) reported a 27 percent clinical failure rate in 131 women given ampicillin. For these reasons, many prefer to give gentamicin or tobramycin along with ampicillin. Serial determinations of serum creatinine are important if nephrotoxic drugs are given. For these reasons, some prefer a cephalosporin or extended-spectrum penicillin, which have been shown effective in 96 percent of such women (Cox and Cunningham, 1988b; Dunlow and Duff, 1990; Faro and colleagues, 1984).

Clinical symptoms for the most part resolve during the first 2 days of therapy; but even though the symptoms promptly abate, many recommend therapy for a total of 7 to 10 days. Cultures of urine usually become sterile within the first 24 hours. Because changes in the urinary tract induced by pregnancy persist, reinfection is possible. If subsequent cultures of the urine are positive remote from the time of therapy, suppressive treatment is indicated. We give nitrofurantoin, 100 mg at bedtime.

Angel and associates (1990) described a randomized clinical trial in which they compared oral versus intravenous antimicrobial therapy for 90 women with antepartum pyelonephritis. Their purpose was to simulate outpatient therapy. They excluded women with underlying medical complications, those who could not tolerate oral medications, those with possible sepsis, and at least retrospectively, those 15 percent with bacteremia. These women generally did well, and one in each group developed a serious complication; one had

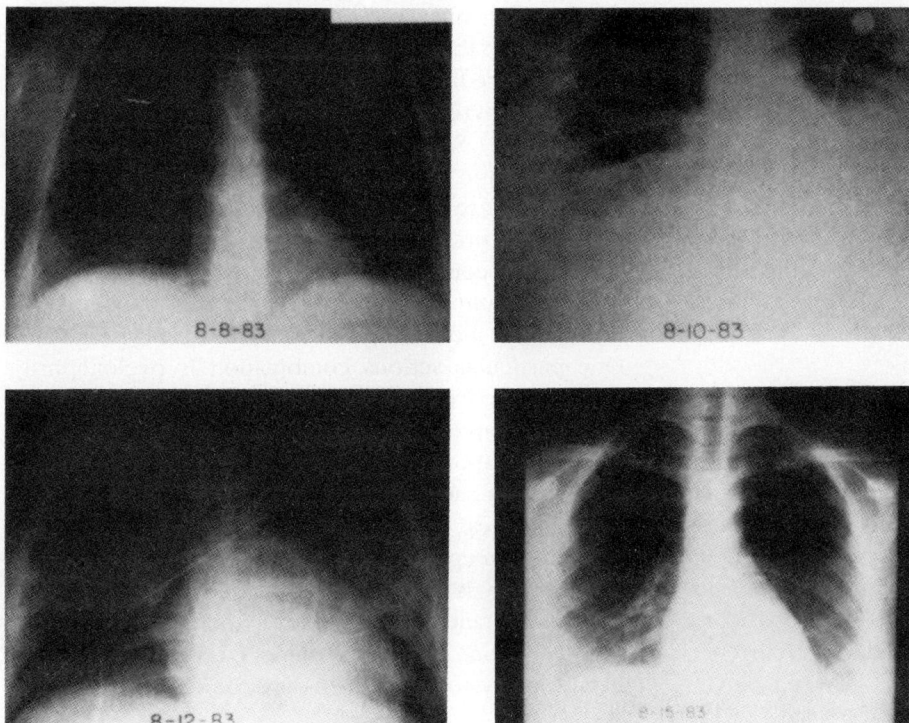

Fig. 50–3. An 18-year-old multipara with acute pyelonephritis at 20 weeks' gestation had a normal radiograph when admitted 8-8-83. Respiratory distress 20 hours later was accompanied by a left-sided pulmonary infiltrate, which progressed to bilateral infiltrates by 8-10-83. The infiltrates improved, and she had a normal x-ray by 8-15-83. (From Cunningham and colleagues, 1987.)

permeability pulmonary edema and the other developed hemolytic anemia. Although their results can be interpreted to support home care for these women, they also projected significant cost savings from limiting hospital stay to 24 hours. In either case, careful home managed health care and close observation would be mandatory if these women are discharged before they are afebrile.

Management of Nonresponders. If clinical improvement is not obvious by 48 to 72 hours, then the woman should be evaluated for urinary tract obstruction. A search is made for abnormal ureteral or pyelocaliceal distension. In many cases, this is caused by calculi, but some women with continuing infection have serious sequelae without any evidence for obstruction. Most prefer renal sonography to detect underlying lesions, but its sensitivity is decreased in pregnancy and stones may not be visualized (Maikranz and colleagues, 1987). Pyelocaliceal dilatation, urinary calculi, and possibly an intrarenal or perinephric abscess or phlegmon may be visualized (Cox and Cunningham, 1988a). Sonar is not always successful in localizing these lesions; thus a negative examination should not prompt cessation of the workup in a woman with continuing urosepsis.

In some cases, a plain abdominal radiograph is indicated because nearly 90 percent of renal stones are radiopaque. Possible benefits far outweigh any minimal fetal risk from radiation. If negative, then intravenous pyelography, modified by the number of radiographs taken after contrast injection, is recommended (see Chap. 43, p. 984). The "one-shot pyelogram," in which a single radiograph is obtained 30 minutes after contrast injection, usually provides adequate imaging of the collecting system so that stones or structural anomalies can be detected.

Passage of a double-J ureteral stent will relieve the obstruction in most cases (Krieger, 1986; Rodriguez and Klein, 1988). If unsuccessful, then percutaneous nephrostomy is done. If this fails, surgical removal of renal stones is required for resolution of infection. Retrograde pyelography may disclose an end-stage obstructed kidney with pyonephrosis as a cause of continuing sepsis. In these cases, calculi frequently coexist, and nephrectomy may be lifesaving.

Follow-up. Recurrent infection, both covert and symptomatic, is common and can be demonstrated in 30 to 40 percent of these women following completion of treatment for pyelonephritis (Cunningham and associates, 1973; Van Dorsten and colleagues, 1987). Unless measures are taken to insure urine sterility, then nitrofurantoin, 100 mg at bedtime, is given for the remainder of the pregnancy. Van Dorsten and co-workers (1987) reported that this regimen reduces recurrence of bacteriuria to 8 percent.

Chronic Pyelonephritis. Chronic interstitial nephritis, which is thought to be caused by bacterial infection, is termed chronic pyelonephritis. In contrast to acute pyelonephritis, chronic infection frequently is not symptomatic, and in advanced cases, symptoms are those of renal insufficiency. Fewer than half of women with chronic pyelonephritis have a clear history of preceding cystitis, acute pyelonephritis, or obstructive disease. The pathogenesis of this disease therefore is obscure, but it is doubtful that it is simply from persistent bacterial infection. Certainly, very few individuals with recurrent clinical episodes of urinary infections develop chronic infections or progressive renal involvement.

As in all chronic progressive renal diseases, the maternal and fetal prognosis in a particular case depends on the extent of renal destruction. Women with hypertension or renal insufficiency have a worse prognosis (see p. 1136). Conversely, women with adequate renal function and no hypertension usually tolerate pregnancy without serious complications. Regardless of the extent of renal destruction, when chronic pyelonephritis or any other chronic renal lesion is complicated by bacteriuria during pregnancy, there is an associated risk of superimposed acute pyelonephritis. This, in turn, may lead to further deterioration of renal function. Martinell and colleagues (1990) found that almost half of women with renal scarring following childhood urinary infection had bacteriuria when pregnant.

Nephrolithiasis

Urinary stones are more common in men than women, and their average age of onset is in the third decade. Calcium salts make up about 75 percent of renal stones, and in half of these, idiopathic hypercalciuria is the most common predisposing cause (Coe and Favus, 1991). Hyperparathyroidism should be excluded (see Chap. 53, p. 1217). Struvite stones are associated with infection, and often *Proteus* is cultured from the urine. Uric acid stones are even less common.

During pregnancy, symptoms of pain and hematuria are far less common than in the nonpregnant patient. Although stones do not cause infection, infection may coexist, and indeed is quite common during pregnancy. One particular serious combination is pyelonephritis superimposed on urinary obstruction from stone disease (see above). After a stone is formed, others usually will follow about every 2 to 3 years. Patients with calcium stones caused by hypercalciuria respond to thiazide diuretics. Patients with stone disease should be advised to keep well hydrated.

Therapy is medical or surgical depending on clinical circumstances. In general, if there are symptoms, then the stone should be removed. Placing a flexible basket via cystoscopy to ensnare the calculus has been used with the greatest frequency, and this method is reasonable for use in pregnant women. In the recent past, **lithotripsy** has replaced surgical removal of stones. This relatively noninvasive method employs shock waves delivered in an extracorporeal bath, or by placing an ultrasonic transducer near the stone either via cystoscopy or percutaneously. Understandably, there is little information concerning the use of lithotripsy during pregnancy and it is not recommended.

Stone Disease During Pregnancy. Because of their predilection for men and older patients, renal and ureteral lithiasis are relatively uncommon complications of pregnancy. From their review of 14 series, Hendricks and co-workers (1991) cite an incidence of abut 1 per 2000 pregnancies. Because pregnancy creates some of the cardinal prerequisites for stone formation (urinary stasis and infection), the incidence might be expected to be higher were it not for the relatively short duration of pregnancy.

Pregnant women have fewer symptoms and pass stones more efficiently, presumably because of urinary tract dilatation. For example, Hendricks and colleagues (1991) reported observations from 15 pregnant women in whom the most common presenting symptom was infection (60 percent), while flank and abdominal pain (27 percent) and hematuria (13 percent) were less common. To take advantage of this phenomenon, Mikkelsen and associates (1988) treated 24 males and nonpregnant females who had stone disease with hydroxyprogester-

one. By 4 to 6 weeks, 60 percent of stones had passed spontaneously, a rate much greater than in historic controls.

As discussed above, women who have formed renal stones previously are at risk of doing so again; however, Maikranz and associates (1987) have found no evidence that pregnancy increased that risk. Moreover, stone disease does not appear to have any adverse effects on pregnancy outcome except for an increased frequency of urinary infections. **Although urinary calculi seldom cause severe symptomatic obstruction during pregnancy, persistent pyelonephritis despite adequate antimicrobial therapy should prompt a search for renal obstruction, which most frequently is due to nephrolithiasis.**

Diagnosis and Management. Sonography is usually helpful to confirm a suspected renal stone, but pregnancy hydronephrosis sometimes obscures these findings. Hendricks and associates (1991) were able to visualize stones in two thirds of affected pregnant women (Fig. 50–4). However, if there is abnormal dilatation without stone visualization, then x-rays may be performed. Stones are identified in most women by carefully performed and limited radiography, with or without contrast media (see Chap. 43, p. 984).

Treatment depends on the symptoms and the duration of pregnancy. Intravenous hydration and analgesics are given. Associated infection is treated vigorously. In over half of the cases, the stone passes spontaneously,

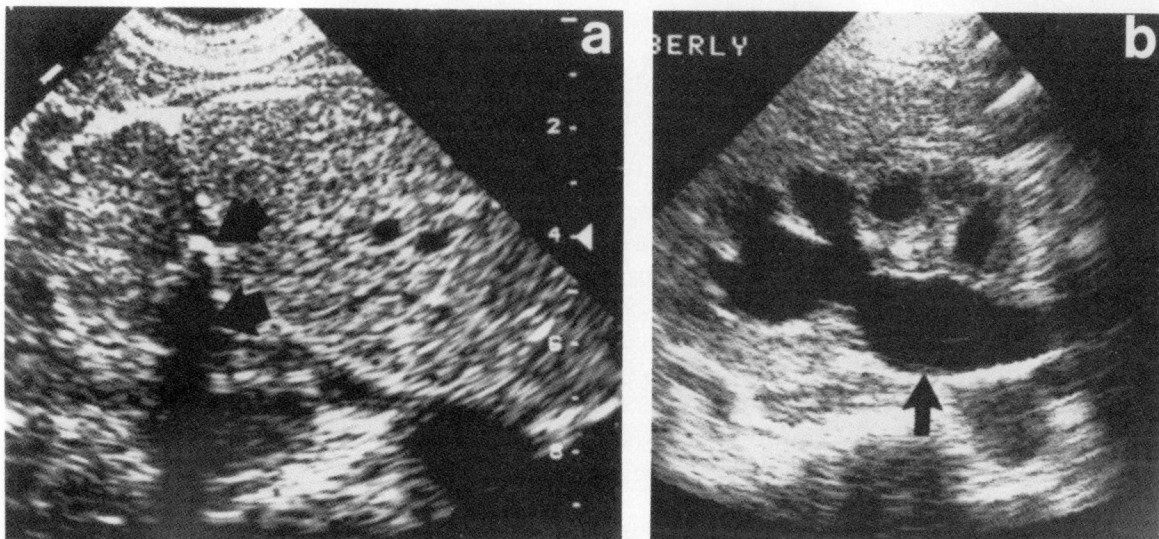

Fig. 50–4. This 23-year-old multipara with a history of recurrent urinary infections and hypertension was referred to the high-risk obstetrical clinic at 6 weeks' gestation. **A.** Ultrasound examination shows a right renal calculus (*upper arrow*) with typical acoustic shadowing (*lower arrow*). **B.** At 24 weeks, she presented with right flank pain, nausea and vomiting. Repeat ultrasonography demonstrated right hydronephrosis (*arrow*), but the previously identified calculus was no longer visible, suggesting that it had descended into the ureter. (From Hendricks and associates, 1991, with permission.)

but about one third of pregnant women with symptomatic stones will need cystoscopy, ureteral catheterization, percutaneous nephrostomy, basket extraction, or surgical exploration (Hendricks and co-workers, 1991; Maikranz and colleagues, 1987). Loughlin and Bailey (1986) reported that ureteral double-J stents, placed via cystoscopy under local anesthesia, relieved persistent symptoms from ureteral calculi in 8 pregnant women. As shown in Figure 50–5, this method has been used to avoid more invasive procedures, including percutaneous nephrostomy, basket extraction, nephrolithotomy, and even nephrectomy. However, if symptoms persist, especially infection, then surgical exploration may be lifesaving.

Glomerulopathies

The kidney, especially the glomerulus and its capillaries, is subject to a large number and variety of acute and chronic diseases. These may result from a single stimulus such as poststreptococcal glomerulonephritis, or from a multisystem disease such as systemic lupus erythematosus. According to Glasscock and Brenner (1991), there are five major glomerulopathic syndromes: acute and chronic glomerulonephritis, rapidly progressive glomer-

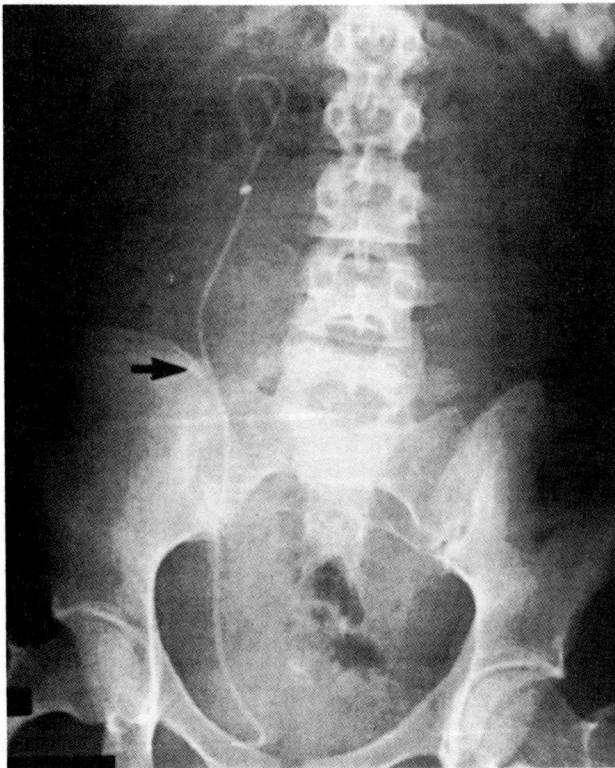

Fig. 50–5. Abdominal x-ray in a 24-week-pregnant woman after passage of double-J stent to relieve obstruction caused by a right ureteral calculus (*arrow*). The fetus is also visualized. (From Hendricks and associates, 1991, with permission.)

ulonephritis, the nephrotic syndrome, and those caused by asymptomatic urinary abnormalities. The majority of these diseases are encountered in young women of childbearing age, and thus they may complicate pregnancy. Many of these disorders first become apparent because of chronic renal insufficiency.

Acute Glomerulonephritis. Like most glomerulopathies, acute glomerulonephritis may result from any of several causes, including those following infectious diseases, multisystem diseases, or primary disorders unique to the glomerulus (Table 50–4). All are characterized by an abrupt onset of hematuria and proteinuria accompanied by varying degrees of renal insufficiency and salt and water retention causing edema, hypertension, and circulatory congestion.

Acute poststreptococcal glomerulonephritis is prototypical of these syndromes. Although it rarely develops acutely during pregnancy, its management is similar to acute glomerulonephritis from any cause. Acute glomerulonephritis, especially that which arises during the second half of pregnancy, is in most cases clinically indistinguishable from preeclampsia. Renal biopsy might be of value in unusual circumstances to try to exclude preeclampsia and identify the type of glomerular disease (Madaio and Harrington, 1983).

In general, the treatment of acute poststreptococcal glomerulonephritis is the same as in the nonpregnant woman. There are insufficient data to predict fetal or maternal prognosis. The prognosis and treatment of the other causes of acute glomerulonephritis listed in Table 50–4 depend on their etiology. Renal biopsy may be helpful in determining etiology as well as to direct management. For example, Yankowitz and colleagues (1992) reported successful management of a pregnancy complicated by *Goodpasture syndrome,* characterized by pulmonary hemorrhage, glomerulonephritis, and autoantibodies to basement membrane antigens.

Women with a history of poststreptococcal glomer-

TABLE 50–4. SOME CAUSES OF ACUTE GLOMERULONEPHRITIS

Infectious Diseases
Poststreptococcal[a]
Nonstreptococcal
   Bacterial: infective endocarditis,[a] sepsis,[a] and others
   Viral: hepatitis B and others
   Parasitic: malaria, toxoplasmosis

Multisystem Diseases
Systemic lupus erythematosus[a]
Vasculitis[a]
Henoch–Schönlein purpura[a]

Primary Glomerular Diseases
Berger disease (IgA nephropathy)[a]
Mesangial glomerulonephritis

[a] Common cause.
Modified from Glasscock and Brenner (1991), with permission.

ulonephritis that subsequently has healed may undergo additional pregnancies without any appreciable increase in the incidence of complications. Some patients with acute glomerulonephritis never completely recover, and **rapidly progressive glomerulonephritis** leads to end-stage renal failure. Up to half of adults with sporadic poststreptococcal disease develop **chronic glomerulonephritis** with slowly progressive renal disease.

Effect of Glomerulonephritis on Pregnancy. Most cases of glomerulonephritis are not caused by poststreptococcal infection. In some cases, the underlying etiology is not found. Whatever the cause, glomerulonephritis has a profound effect on pregnancy outcome. Packham and colleagues (1989) reported the results of 395 pregnancies in 238 women who had been previously diagnosed with *primary* glomerulonephritis. The most common lesions on biopsy were membranous glomerulonephritis, IgA glomerulonephritis, and diffuse mesangial glomerulonephritis. Most of these women had normal renal function before becoming pregnant. The overall fetal loss was 26 percent, including perinatal mortality rate after 28 weeks' gestation of 80 per 1000. Preterm delivery was effected in 25 percent, and 15 percent of fetuses were growth retarded. Overall, about half of these women developed hypertension; one quarter did so before 32 weeks, and it was severe in three fourths of these. Proteinuria worsened in 60 percent of these women. Factors that portended the worst perinatal prognosis included impaired renal function, early or severe hypertension, and nephrotic-range proteinuria.

Rapidly Progressive Glomerulonephritis. In some cases, acute glomerulonephritis does not resolve, and rapidly progressive glomerulonephritis progresses to end-stage renal failure within weeks to months. Because extensive extracapillary or **crescenteric glomerulonephritis** is commonly identified, the two terms are often used interchangeably (Glasscock and Brenner, 1991).

Common causes of rapidly progressive disease include poststreptococcal glomerulonephritis, infective endocarditis, lupus erythematosus, Henoch–Schönlein purpura, systemic vasculitis, and Goodpasture syndrome. Their management depends on the underlying cause.

Chronic Glomerulonephritis. Chronic glomerulonephritis is characterized by progressive renal destruction over a period of years or decades, eventually producing the **end-stage kidney.** Usually, persistent proteinuria and hematuria accompany a gradual decline in renal function. In many cases the cause is unknown, but it may follow almost any type of acute glomerulonephritis or the nephrotic syndrome. Microscopically, the renal lesions are categorized as proliferative, sclerosing, or membranous.

According to Glasscock and Brenner (1991), chronic glomerulopathies may be detected in any of several ways: (1) Some patients may remain asymptomatic for years, and proteinuria or abnormal urinary sediment are detected by screening. (2) It may be discovered in some women during the course of evaluation for chronic hypertension. (3) The disease may first manifest as the nephrotic syndrome. (4) It may exacerbate, and the clinical presentation may be quite similar to acute glomerulonephritis. (5) Renal failure may be the first manifestation. (6) A woman with symptoms and signs of preeclampsia–eclampsia, but without their resolution, may be found to have chronic glomerulonephritis.

The evolution, management, and prognosis of chronic glomerulonephritis depends on its etiology. In some patients, 10 to 20 years may elapse before end-stage renal failure supervenes. Renal biopsy may be helpful to establish prognosis.

Nephrotic Syndrome. The nephrotic syndrome, or **nephrosis,** is also a spectrum of renal disorders of many causes. In its overt form, it is characterized by proteinuria in excess of 3 to 4 g per day, hypoalbuminemia, hyperlipidemia, and edema. Most patients have microscopical renal abnormalities and many have accompanying evidence for renal dysfunction. The defects in the barriers of the glomerular capillary wall that allow excessive filtration of plasma proteins are caused by primary glomerular disease, or they may follow immunological or toxic injury or metabolic or vascular diseases. Some of these are shown in Table 50–5, and the overlap with causes of acute glomerulonephritis in Table 50–4 is obvious.

Management of the nephrotic syndrome depends on its etiology. Edema is managed cautiously, especially during pregnancy. Dietary protein of high biological value is encouraged. Thromboembolism occurs with some frequency, and includes arterial as well as venous thromboses. Renal vein thrombosis is particularly worrisome. Some cases of nephrosis from primary glomer-

TABLE 50–5. SOME CAUSES OF THE NEPHROTIC SYNDROME

Primary Glomerular Disease
Minimal change disease (lipoid nephrosis, nil lesion)
Berger disease (IgA nephropathy)
Focal and segmental glomerulonephritis
Mesangiocapillary glomerulonephritis

Secondary to Other Diseases
Infections: poststreptococcal glomerulonephritis, hepatitis B, and many others
Drugs: heroin and many others
Neoplasia
Multisystem: lupus, Henoch–Schönlein purpura, amyloidosis, and others
Heredofamilial: diabetes and others

Modified from Glasscock and Brenner (1991), with permission.

ular disease will respond to corticosteroid or cytotoxic drug therapy. In most of those cases caused by infection or drugs, proteinuria recedes when these are treated or withdrawn. Response of the nephrotic syndrome due to multisystem disease will depend on response of the underlying condition.

Nephrotic Syndrome Complicating Pregnancy. When the nephrotic syndrome complicates pregnancy, the maternal and fetal prognosis, as well as the appropriate treatment, depend on the underlying cause of the disease and the extent of renal insufficiency. For example, we identified two women with antepartum syphilis that likely caused the nephrotic syndrome, because after penicillin therapy, nephrosis cleared and pregnancy outcomes were satisfactory. Whenever possible, the specific cause should be ascertained and renal function assessed. In this regard, when the cause is not apparent, percutaneous renal biopsy, usually after pregnancy, may be of value.

Chronic proteinuria usually increases during pregnancy. Katz and associates (1980) observed that nearly half of women with chronic renal disease either developed proteinuria, or it worsened. Moreover, in two thirds of those with proteinuria, excretion exceeded 3 g per day. Similarly, Packham and colleagues (1989) reported that 60 percent of women with one of the primary glomerulopathies had increased proteinuria during pregnancy. However, in women without appreciably diminished renal function, there usually is some augmentation of renal function (Cunningham and colleagues, 1990).

A review of reported cases of nephrosis indicates that the majority of women who are not hypertensive and do not have severe renal insufficiency will usually have a successful pregnancy outcome, particularly since glucocorticoids have been available. In other cases, however, in which there is evidence for renal insufficiency, moderate to severe hypertension, or both, the prognosis for mother and fetus is poor. Our experiences from Parkland Hospital with women who had proteinuria antecedent to pregnancy indicate that it is not a benign association (Stettler and colleagues, 1992). Protein excretion in 65 pregnancies averaged 4 g/day, and one third had classical nephrotic syndrome. Some degree of renal insufficiency was found in three fourths of the women, 40 percent had chronic hypertension, and 25 percent had persistent anemia. Importantly, preeclampsia developed in 62 percent, and 43 percent of infants were delivered preterm. When abortions were excluded, however, 53 of 57 infants were born alive. In all 21 women who subsequently underwent renal biopsy, histological evidence of renal disease was found. Long-term follow-up indicated that at least 20 percent of women had progressed to end-stage renal disease, requiring dialysis or transplantation.

Polycystic Kidney Disease

Polycystic kidney disease is an inherited disease in which the cortex and medulla are filled with thin-walled cysts that are millimeters to centimeters in diameter, and these cause renal enlargement and dysfunction. It is an autosomally dominant disease linked to the α-hemoglobin gene complex and the phosphoglycerate kinase genes on the short arm of chromosome 16. The condition is genetically heterogeneous, and prenatal diagnosis now is available, with a 1 to 5 percent error rate (Breuning and associates, 1990). The disease is found in 1 in 500 autopsies, accounts for 1 in 3000 hospital admissions, and causes 10 percent of all end-stage renal disease (Coe and Kathpalia, 1991).

Symptoms usually appear in the third or fourth decade. Flank pain, hematuria, nocturia, and associated calculi are frequent findings. Proteinuria and associated infection are also common. Hypertension develops in three fourths of patients, and progression to end-stage renal disease is a major problem. Superimposed acute renal failure results from infection or obstruction from ureteral angulation by cyst displacement.

Asymptomatic hepatic cysts coexist in 30 percent of patients with polycystic kidneys. Hossack and colleagues (1988) studied 163 nonpregnant patients and reported substantively increased cardiac valvar lesions detected by echocardiography. The incidence of mitral valve prolapse was increased 13-fold over that of the control group, and there was excessive mitral, aortic, and tricuspid incompetence. Importantly, about 10 percent of patients die from an associated intracranial berry aneurysm.

Polycystic Kidney Disease and Pregnancy. As with most chronic renal diseases, pregnancy outcome in women with polycystic kidney disease will depend on the degree of associated hypertension and renal insufficiency. An in-depth study of the apparent effects of this disease on pregnancy and vice versa was provided by Milutinovic and co-workers (1983). Of 137 women at risk of having inherited the autosomal dominant gene, 55 percent demonstrated multiple renal cysts. Fertility, spontaneous abortion, stillbirth, and symptomatic urinary tract infection were comparable in both groups. Although hypertension was more common in women with polycystic disease, both when pregnant and nonpregnant, there was no evidence that pregnancy had an adverse effect on the disease.

Chronic Renal Disease

A number of kidney diseases listed in Tables 50–4 and 50–5 may become chronic. Surprisingly, even with chronic disease, renal function may be entirely normal, and disease is manifest by varying degrees of hypertension, proteinuria, or an abnormal urinary sediment. Thus, **chronic renal disease** does not address function, and when there is impairment, then **chronic renal insufficiency** or **chronic renal failure** is said to exist.

Because the treatment of many causes of glomerulonephritis has improved in the past few decades, these are no longer the most common reasons for renal failure. According to the Health Care Financing Administration, in 1985 the most common causes of end-stage renal disease were diabetes (30 percent), hypertension (25 percent), glomerulonephritis (20 percent), and polycystic kidney disease (4 percent).

In many cases of chronic renal disease, biopsy will be necessary to determine the underlying cause. Packham and Fairley (1987) performed 111 percutaneous biopsies in 104 pregnant women before the third trimester and reported a 5 percent complication rate. Lindheimer and Davison (1987) emphasize that such good outcomes are unusual and attributable to the experience of the Australian group. We agree with them that biopsy is usually best reserved until after pregnancy, unless it is perceived that biopsy results will significantly alter the management of renal disease.

Pregnancy Complicated by Chronic Renal Disease.

Most women with chronic renal disease complicating pregnancy have reasonably normal renal function. There is good evidence that the degree of renal insufficiency is more important than the type of lesion in determining pregnancy outcome. Importantly, preexisting hypertension is also predictive of pregnancy outcome. **However, in women with chronic renal disease, even if renal function is normal and the woman normotensive, pregnancy outcome is still not always good.** In a large number of pregnancies complicated by primary glomerulonephritis reported from Melbourne by Packham and colleagues (1989), the fetal loss rate was 15 percent even without impaired renal function, early or severe hypertension, or nephrotic-range proteinuria.

Physiological Changes.

In women with mild renal insufficiency, pregnancy is usually accompanied by a rise in renal plasma flow and glomerular filtration rate (Katz and colleagues, 1980). These changes are thought to be induced by renal vasodilation, and because this already is maximal with advanced renal disease, they are less evident in women with more severe renal dysfunction. In pregnant women studied at Parkland Hospital, only half of those with moderate renal insufficiency (serum creatinine 1.4 to 2.5 mg/dL) demonstrated augmented glomerular filtration rate (Cunningham and colleagues, 1990). None of those with severe disease (serum creatinine greater than 2.5 mg/dL) showed augmentation of renal function.

Nonpregnant women with chronic renal insufficiency have normal blood volumes. During pregnancy, blood volume expansion is dependent on the severity of

their disease, and it is proportional to the serum creatinine (Fig. 50–6). In women with mild to moderate dysfunction, there is normal pregnancy-induced hypervolemia that averages 50 percent (Cunningham and associates, 1990). However, in women with severe renal insufficiency, volume expansion is attenuated, and averages only 23 percent. Finally, although there is some degree of pregnancy-induced erythropoiesis in these women, it is not proportional to the plasma volume increase; thus, preexisting anemia is intensified.

Pregnancy Outcome with Chronic Renal Disease.

There are a number of studies that allow an estimation of risk of pregnancy for the woman with chronic renal disease. In most of these, all women with evidence for chronic renal disease were evaluated. In a few studies, however, women were included only if there was evidence for chronic renal insufficiency.

Katz and associates (1980) reviewed pregnancy outcomes in 89 women who had chronic renal disease but generally good renal function. Excluding abortions, of 121 pregnancies, perinatal mortality was 11 percent, 20 percent of infants were delivered preterm, and 24 percent were growth retarded. Superimposed preeclampsia was common and abruptio placentae developed in 3 instances. Surian and colleagues (1984) described the clinical course of 123 pregnancies in 86 women with biopsy-proven glomerular disease. Only a few of these women had renal dysfunction. In 40 percent there were obstetrical or renal complications, or both. Hypertension developed in 20 percent, and it persisted in one half of these postpartum. In 8 percent of the women, renal function deteriorated, and this persisted in one half.

Packham and co-workers (1989), in a study cited

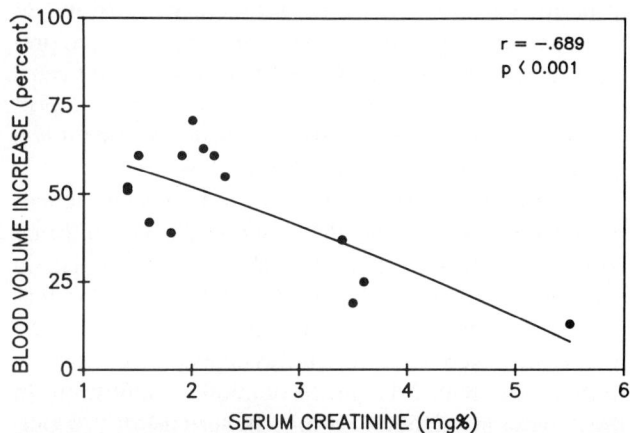

Fig. 50–6. Blood volume expansion during pregnancy plotted as function of serum creatinine concentration. As renal insufficiency worsens (i.e., serum creatinine increases), the percent of blood volume expansion during pregnancy is less. (From Cunningham and colleagues, 1990, with permission.)

previously, described their vast experiences from Melbourne with 238 women and 395 pregnancies complicated by preexisting primary glomerulonephritis. Only a few had preexisting renal insufficiency. All had undergone biopsy and diffuse mesangial proliferative disease, and IgA nephritis comprised 70 percent of the lesions. During pregnancy, 15 percent of these women had impaired renal function and 60 percent had worsening proteinuria. Although only 12 percent had hypertension antedating pregnancy, over half became hypertensive during pregnancy. Hypertension before 20 weeks complicated 25 percent of these pregnancies, and 20 percent of all pregnancies had severe hypertension. Five percent developed irreversible worsening of renal function during pregnancy. The overall fetal loss was 26 percent; the overall perinatal mortality rate was 140 per 1000, and after 28 weeks it was 80 per 1000. Factors associated with increased perinatal mortality and preterm delivery were impaired renal function, early or severe hypertension, and nephrotic-range proteinuria. In the absence of these factors, perinatal mortality was still 50 per 1000.

Other retrospective studies from Japan (Abe, 1991a, 1991b, 1992) and France (Jungers and colleagues, 1991) of large numbers of pregnancies in women with chronic primary glomerulonephritis substantiate these conclusions.

Pregnancy Outcome and Chronic Renal Insufficiency. There have been two studies in which pregnancies in women with chronic renal insufficiency were reported. In the first, Hou and colleagues (1985) described the outcomes of 25 pregnancies in 23 women studied because of moderate renal insufficiency defined by baseline serum creatinine ranging from 1.2 to 1.7 mg/dL. Pregnancy-induced or aggravated hypertension developed in slightly more than half of these women, and because of this, early delivery frequently was indicated. Although 92 percent of the fetuses were live born and 84 percent survived, nearly 60 percent were delivered preterm. Pregnancy was associated with accelerated renal dysfunction in about one third of these women. Importantly, pregnancy-aggravated hypertension was identified in most women whose renal function worsened.

In the second study, we reported our experiences from Parkland Hospital with 37 pregnancies complicated by moderate to severe renal insufficiency (Cunningham and associates, 1990). Moderate renal dysfunction was defined by serum creatinine concentration of 1.4 to 2.5 mg/dL and severe impairment was defined by concentrations greater than 2.5 mg/dL. Common complications in these women included chronic hypertension (70 percent), anemia (75 percent), preeclampsia (60 percent), fetal growth retardation (30 percent), and preterm delivery (35 percent). Perinatal outcome was surprisingly good, and of 31 pregnancies reaching 26 weeks' gestation, 30 resulted in live-born infants and all survived.

Birthweight correlated inversely and significantly with serum creatinine concentration.

Management. Careful observation is accorded women with chronic renal disease who become pregnant. Frequent prenatal visits are necessary to determine blood pressure trends. Serial measurements, the intervals determined by severity of findings, are done to estimate renal function, and protein excretion is monitored if indicated. Bacteriuria must be detected and eradicated to prevent pyelonephritis. Although protein-restricted diets are prescribed for nonpregnant patients with chronic renal disease, we do not recommend this during pregnancy. Anemia associated with chronic renal insufficiency responds to recombinant erythropoietin given subcutaneously; however, hypertension is a well-documented side effect. The appearance of hypertension is managed as described in Chapter 36 (p. 785), and suspected fetal growth retardation as in Chapter 38 (p. 880).

Except for an increased risk of hypertension and superimposed preeclampsia, women with relatively normal renal function and no hypertension before pregnancy usually have a relatively normal pregnancy. As renal impairment worsens, so does the likelihood of pregnancy complications. At least half of women with renal insufficiency will develop hypertension. Worsening of hypertension or superimposed preeclampsia develops in 80 percent of those with moderate insufficiency and 86 percent who have severe disease (Cunningham and co-workers, 1990; Packham and associates, 1989).

Follow-up. A long-standing unresolved issue is whether pregnancy accelerates chronic renal insufficiency. Jungers and associates (1991) found no adverse effect of pregnancy on actuarial survival in women with chronic renal disease. Conversely, Abe (1991a) concluded that pregnancy may accelerate antecedent disease in women with moderate dysfunction. We are of the view that, at least in most women, **in the absence of superimposed preeclampsia or severe placental abruption,** pregnancy does not appreciably accelerate deterioration in renal function. Importantly, because of the inevitable likelihood of long-term progression of the chronic disease, the ultimate maternal prognosis is guarded. In the study from Parkland Hospital, at least 20 percent of women with moderate to severe disease had developed end-stage renal failure by a mean of 4 years (Cunningham and colleagues, 1990).

Pregnancy After Renal Transplantation

Renal transplantation for end-stage kidney failure has become commonplace, and over 100,000 patients have undergone these procedures in the United Stated in the past 25 years. The first-year survival for cadaveric grafts exceeds 80 percent, and ovulation promptly returns in most women. Murray and associates in 1963 reported two successful pregnancies in a woman who had a kidney transplanted from her identical twin sister. Since that time there have probably been more than 2500 pregnancies in women who previously had received a kidney from immunologically nonidentical donors.

Davison (1991) reviewed the outcomes in 2309 pregnancies in 1594 women, 80 percent of whom had had cadaveric transplants. The incidence of spontaneous and therapeutic abortion was 40 percent. Of the pregnancies that continued beyond the first trimester, over 90 percent had a successful outcome. As shown in Figure 50–7, beginning early in pregnancy, the glomerular filtration rate in these women usually increases in proportion to that seen in normal women. Although proteinuria developed in 40 percent of these women, it was not significant in the absence of hypertension.

In pregnancies reviewed by Davison (1985), preeclampsia developed in 30 percent and signs of kidney rejection were observed in about 10 percent. Without renal biopsy, however, rejection may be difficult to distinguish from acute pyelonephritis, recurrent glomerulopathy, or severe preeclampsia. Serious infections, most likely related to immunosuppressive therapy, complicated some pregnancies. Urinary infections were diagnosed in 40 percent and viral infections were increased. Prematurely ruptured membranes and preterm labor were common, and about half of live-born infants were delivered preterm. Fetal growth retardation averaged 20 to 30 percent. Fortunately, although respiratory distress syndrome was common among the preterm infants, it was seldom fatal. Fetal malformations were identified in

only 2 percent, and no specific type predominated. The newborns, as well as the mother, were at increased risk of infection because of maternal immunosuppressive therapy.

Hou (1989) reached similar conclusions after reviewing the studies summarized in Table 50–6. From these experiences, recommendations have been formulated for factors requisite before pregnancy should be attempted. These include good general health without severe hypertension for at least 2 years after transplantation, because graft rejection is more common during this period. There should be no evidence of graft rejection or persistent proteinuria. Even so, the effects of pregnancy are unpredictable and not necessarily related to previous rejection episodes, lack of problems in previous pregnancies, or human leukocyte-antigen typing. If stable, prednisone dosage should be maintained at 15 mg/day or less, and azathioprine at 2 mg/kg per day or less. We and others have observed azathioprine hepatotoxicity with severe jaundice developing during pregnancy. A reduction in dosage is likely to improve hepatic function. Although not considered teratogenic, azathioprine is listed in category D. Cyclosporine is not given routinely in renal transplant recipients, but its use has special concerns. Specifically, it decreases the glomerular filtration rate and also may cause hypertension. The drug has been associated with what appears to be excessive fetal growth retardation, but it is not considered to be teratogenic, and it is listed as category C (Briggs and colleagues, 1990).

Concern persists over the possibility of late effects in the offspring subjected to immunosuppressive therapy in utero. These include malignancy, germ cell dysfunction, and malformations in the offspring's children.

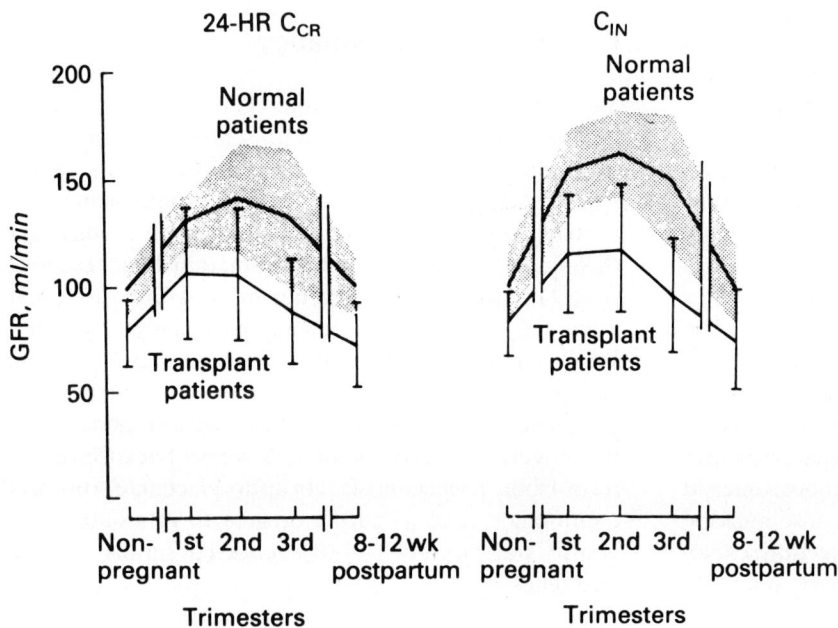

Fig. 50–7. Serial 24-hour creatinine (C_{Cr}) and inulin (C_{In}) clearances (mean ± SD) during 10 pregnancies in 8 women with renal transplants. Values from 10 normal women (mean ± SD) are shown in the shaded areas. (From Davison, 1985, with permission.)

TABLE 50–6. MATERNAL AND FETAL OUTCOMES IN 678 PREGNANCIES IN WOMEN WHO HAD UNDERGONE RENAL TRANSPLANTATION

Study	Pregnancies	Maternal Complications				Pregnancy Outcomes				
		Decreased Glomerular Filtration (%)	Graft Rejected	Worsening Hypertension (%)	Death	Abortion (182)		Perinatal Mortality (453)		
						Spontaneous	Therapeutic	Stillborn	Neonatal Death	Live Born
Rifle and Traeger (1975)	120	6	0	28	2	9	22	0	—	86
Rudolph and associates (1979)	440	6	4	30	1	23	105	6	10	279
Penn and Makowski (1980)	56	7	3	32	0	1	7	1	2	44
O'Donnell and colleagues (1985)	38	13	2	27	0	9	6	1	—	—
Marushak and co-workers (1986)	24	8	0	25	0	0	0	0	—	24
Total	678	~ 6	9	~ 30	3	42 (6%)	140 (20%)	8	12	433 (95%)

Data modified from Hou (1989), with permission.

Penn and colleagues (1980) reported that 58 of 60 babies sired by fathers who had undergone renal transplant were normal. One infant was born with a meningomyelocele, hip dislocation, and talipes equinovarus. The other infant with congenital anomalies, including microcephaly and polycystic kidneys, died at birth.

Finally, although theoretically pregnancy-induced renal hyperfiltration may impair long-term graft survival, Sturgiss and Davison (1992) found no evidence for this in a case-controlled study of 36 allograft recipients followed for a mean of 12 years.

Management. Close surveillance is necessary. Covert bacteriuria must be treated, and if recurrent, suppressive treatment for the remainder of pregnancy is given with nitrofurantoin, 100 mg at bedtime. Serial serum hepatic enzyme concentrations and blood counts are monitored for toxic effects of azathioprine. Gestational diabetes is more common if corticosteroids are taken; thus, glucose tolerance testing is done at about 26 weeks. Overt diabetes must be excluded.

Renal function is monitored, at first with serum creatinine determinations, but if abnormal, determination of glomerular filtration rate is preferable. Hou (1989) suggests that a decline of less than 30 percent in the glomerular filtration rate during the third trimester is normal and need not be evaluated aggressively. The observations of Davison (1985), shown in Figure 50–7, are in accordance with these recommendations. Moreover, Sturgiss and Davison (1991) observed that renal function in women with adverse perinatal outcomes was no different than in women with good outcomes. If a significant decline is detected, then its cause must be determined. Possibilities include acute rejection, cyclosporine toxicity, preeclampsia, and urinary tract obstruction. Imaging studies and possibly even kidney biopsy may be indicated.

Throughout pregnancy, the woman is carefully monitored for development or worsening of underlying hypertension, and especially superimposed preeclampsia. Management of hypertension during pregnancy is the same as for nontransplanted patients (see Chap. 36, p. 785). Evidence for graft infection or rejection should prompt admission for aggressive management.

Because of the significantly increased incidences of fetal growth retardation and preterm delivery, vigilant fetal surveillance is conducted using techniques described in Chapters 45 and 46. Although cesarean section is reserved for obstetrical indications, occasionally the transplanted kidney will obstruct labor. In the review by Hou (1989), the reported cesarean rate for all indications averaged almost 50 percent.

Dialysis During Pregnancy

Most often, significantly impaired renal function is accompanied by infertility. With chronic hemodialysis or peritoneal dialysis, however, fertility may be restored. A few women undergoing chronic hemodialysis have become pregnant and have been so managed throughout pregnancy, but with marginal success. Hou (1987) reported the outcomes in 37 women in whom hemodialysis was used during pregnancy. Hypertension complicated half of the pregnancies and placental abruption developed in four. Only one fourth of the pregnancies resulted in live-born infants and half of these were delivered before 36 weeks because of preterm labor, preeclampsia, abruptio placentae, ruptured membranes, fetal jeopardy, or growth retardation. Nageotte and Grundy (1988) reported similar adverse outcomes.

Elliott and colleagues (1991) reported observations from 7 pregnancies in women with varying degrees of renal insufficiency in whom chronic ambulatory peritoneal dialysis was utilized. Two infants died presumably from placental abruption, but the other 5 lived. Severe hypertension and fetal growth retardation were common. Fetal jeopardy prompted cesarean delivery in all live-born infants. Jakobi and co-workers (1992) successfully managed a similar case in which preterm labor was stimulated by peritonitis that complicated dialysis at 34 weeks.

All of these investigators reported that an increased frequency of dialysis was required during pregnancy, but even with such management it was unclear if there was improved fetal survival. In our experiences, the likelihood of salutary pregnancy outcome with a chronically dialysed woman is very low.

Acute Renal Failure

Acute renal failure associated with pregnancy has become less common, but it certainly has not been eliminated. Of all cases of acute renal failure referred for dialysis, 10 to 20 percent are related to pregnancy (Grünfeld and Pertuiset, 1987; Krane, 1988; Turney and colleagues, 1988). As shown in Table 50–7, the most common obstetrical causes of acute renal failure are abruptio placentae and eclampsia. Importantly, one third of these 57 women developed cortical necrosis and 14 percent died.

Data from the Renal Unit in Leeds, England underscore the changing indications for dialysis in obstetrical patients for acute renal failure (Turney and colleagues, 1988). Whereas, in early years obstetrical cases comprised 35 percent of patients requiring dialysis, more recently only 10 percent did. Almost all of the 142 obstetrical cases they described were contributed to or caused by abortion (25 percent), hemorrhage (35 percent), or preeclampsia (50 percent). The immediate mortality rate with acute renal failure was 20 percent. Importantly, after legalization of abortion in England in 1968, cases of obstetrical acute renal failure decreased by 30 percent.

Sibai and associates (1990) reported observations from 31 women with acute renal failure complicating

hypertensive disorders of pregnancy. Although 18 had "pure" preeclampsia, the remainder had antecedent chronic hypertension, parenchymal renal disease, or both. Half required dialysis and 3 of these women died as a direct cause of renal failure. About half of these women had suffered placental abruption and almost 90 percent had postpartum hemorrhage. They emphasized that early identification and proper management of renal failure in women with pure preeclampsia does not result in residual renal damage.

Management. Identification of acute renal failure and, in turn, its cause(s) is important. In all but a few women, renal failure develops postpartum, so management is usually not complicated by fetal considerations. Appropriate therapy initiated promptly will minimize the intensity and duration of functional impairment. Oliguria is an important sign of acutely impaired renal function. Unfortunately, potent diuretics such as furosemide can increase urine flow without correcting but rather intensifying some causes of oliguria. Moreover, their use may negate the value of various urinary indices that might be used to try to differentiate prerenal from intrarenal or postrenal causes of acute renal failure. For example, a urine to plasma creatinine ratio of greater than 20 is strongly suggestive of prerenal azotemia, as is an elevated urine to plasma osmolality ratio of more than 1.5. Also, with prerenal azotemia, most filtered sodium is reabsorbed so that the urinary concentration typically is less than 20 mEq/L. In obstetrical cases, however, both prerenal and intrarenal factors are commonly operative. For example, with total placental abruption, severe hypovolemia is common from massive concealed hemorrhage. Moreover, chronic hypertension with superimposed preeclampsia is frequent, and these women may have diminished sodium resorption (see Chap. 36, p. 778). Finally, intense consumptive coagulopathy commonly triggered by abruption might impede the intrarenal microcirculation, but causes even more blood loss from lacerations and surgical incisions.

Acute Tubular Necrosis. This clinical entity may often be prevented by the following means: (1) prompt and vigorous replacement of blood in instances of massive hemorrhage, as in placental abruption, placental previa, uterine rupture, and postpartum uterine atony, following the guidelines described in Chapter 37 (p. 821); (2) termination of pregnancies complicated by severe preeclampsia and eclampsia with careful blood replacement if loss is excessive; (3) close observation for early signs of septic shock, especially in women with pyelonephritis, septic abortion, amnionitis, or sepsis from other pelvic infections; (4) avoidance of potent diuretics to treat oliguria before initiating appropriate efforts to assure cardiac output adequate for renal perfusion; and (5) avoidance of vasoconstrictors to treat hypotension, unless pathological vasodilation unequivocally is the cause of the hypotension.

TABLE 50–7. PRINCIPAL CAUSES AND OUTCOMES OF ACUTE RENAL FAILURE IN 57 PREGNANT WOMEN

Primary Cause of Renal Failure	Number	Cortical Necrosis	Death
Abruptio placentae	13	7	2
Preeclampsia–eclampsia	12	1	0
Prolonged fetal death	6	5	2
Idiopathic postpartum	5	3	2
Hemorrhage	4	2	0
Other causes	17	1	2
Total	**57**	**19 (33%)**	**8 (14%)**

Modified from Grünfeld and Pertuiset (1987), with permission.

When azotemia is evident and severe oliguria persists, hemodialysis should be initiated before marked deterioration of general well-being occurs. Early dialysis appears to appreciably reduce mortality and may enhance the extent of recovery of renal function. After healing has taken place, renal function usually returns to normal or near normal. Future pregnancies are therefore not necessarily contraindicated.

Renal Cortical Necrosis. Compared with acute tubular necrosis, bilateral necrosis of the renal cortex is uncommon. When cortical necrosis has developed, however, it is widely held to be associated with pregnancy. For example, among 38 cases studied by Kleinknecht and co-workers (1973), 26 were obstetrical. Cortical necrosis complicates between 15 and 30 percent of all cases of acute renal failure associated with obstetrical causes (Grünfeld and Pertuiset, 1987; Turney and colleagues, 1989). Most of the reported cases in pregnant women have followed such complications as placental abruption, preeclampsia–eclampsia, or endotoxin-induced shock. Histologically, the lesion appears to result from thrombosis of segments of the renal vascular system. The lesions may be focal, patchy, confluent, or gross. Clinically, renal cortical necrosis follows the course of acute renal failure with oliguria or anuria, uremia, and generally death within 2 to 3 weeks unless dialysis is initiated. Differentiation from acute tubular necrosis during the early phase is not possible. The prognosis depends on the extent of the necrosis, because recovery is a function of the amount of renal tissue spared.

Obstructive Renal Failure. Rarely, bilateral ureteral compression by a very large pregnant uterus is greatly exaggerated, causing ureteral obstruction and, in turn, severe oliguria and azotemia. Brandes and Fritsche (1991) reviewed 13 cases that described this phenomenon as the consequence of a markedly overdistended gravid uterus. They described a woman with twins who developed anuria and serum creatinine of 12.2 mg/dL at 34 weeks. After amniotomy, urine flow at 500 mL/hr was followed by rapid return to normal of serum creatinine. Eckford and Gingell (1991) described 10 women in whom ureteral obstruction was relieved by stenting. These were left in place for a mean of 15.5 weeks and removed 4 to 6 weeks postpartum.

We have observed this phenomenon on several occasions (Satin and colleagues, 1992). Partial ureteral obstruction may be accompanied by fluid retention and significant hypertension. When the obstructive uropathy is relieved, diuresis ensues and hypertension dissipates. For example, in one woman with massive hydramnios (9.4 L) and an anencephalic fetus, amniocentesis and removal of some of the amnionic fluid was followed promptly by diuresis, lowering of the plasma creatinine concentration, and improvement of hypertension. In another instance, progressive oliguria and azotemia were identified during two successive pregnancies early in the third trimester in a woman who as a child had had reimplantation of both ureters into the bladder to try to prevent reflux. During the second pregnancy at 23 weeks, ureteral catheters were teased through the markedly narrowed ureteral lumens and provided significant relief from the obstructions and reversal of hypertension (Laverson and colleagues, 1984). In our experiences, women with previous urinary tract surgery are more likely to have such obstructions. Austenfeld and Snow (1988) also emphasized the high incidence of urinary infections in women who have undergone ureteral reimplantation. Conversely, Vordermark and associates (1990) reviewed published experiences with pregnancy following major urinary reconstruction, and found minimal complications.

Thrombotic Microangiopathies

In 1968, Robson and associates described what they believed to be a new syndrome of **acute irreversible renal failure** that developed within the first 6 weeks postpartum. Pregnancy and delivery appeared to have been normal in the 7 cases reported and none of the known causes of renal failure was found. The pathological changes identified by renal biopsy were necrosis and endothelial proliferation in glomeruli, plus necrosis, thrombosis, and intimal thickening of the arterioles. No vascular abnormalities were demonstrated in the other visceral organs in the 4 cases in which autopsy was performed. Morphological changes in the erythrocytes consistent with microangiopathic hemolysis and thrombocytopenia were usually present. These findings are similar to those reported for the **postpartum hemolytic uremic syndrome.** Moreover, they are also similar to those in which renal failure is identified as part of the syndrome of **thrombotic thrombocytopenic purpura.** It is obvious that these disorders are not limited to the kidneys, and in most cases there is widespread arteriolar hyalinization and evidence for endothelial damage. Although these three syndromes may be due to different etiologies, it is currently difficult to separate them, at least clinically (Hayslett, 1985). Treatment consists of plasmapheresis, red cell transfusions, and dialysis for renal failure. These syndromes are considered in detail in Chapter 52 (p. 1190).

References

Abe S: An overview of pregnancy in women with underlying renal disease. Am J Kidney Dis 17:112, 1991b

Abe S: Pregnancy in IgA nephropathy. Kidney Int 40:1098, 1991b

Andriole VT, Patterson TF: Epidemiology, natural history, and management of urinary tract infections in pregnancy. Med Clin North Am 75:359, 1991

Angel JL, O'Brien WF, Finan MA, Morales WJ, Lake M, Knuppel

RA: Acute pyelonephritis in pregnancy: A prospective study of oral versus intravenous antibiotic therapy. Obstet Gynecol 76:28, 1990

Austenfeld MS, Snow BW: Complications of pregnancy in women after reimplantation for vesicoureteral reflux. J Urol 140:1103, 1988

Baylis C, Davison J: The urinary system. In Hytten F, Chamberlain G (eds): Clinical Physiology in Obstetrics, 2nd ed. London, Blackwell, 1991, p 245

Brandes JC, Fritsche C: Obstructive acute renal failure by a gravid uterus: A case report and review. Am J Kidney Dis 18:398, 1991

Breuning MH, Snijdewint FGM, Dauwerse JG, Saris JJ, Bakker E, Pearson PL, van Ommen GJB: Two-step procedure for early diagnosis of polycystic kidney disease with polymorphic DNA markers on both sides of the gene. J Med Genet 27:614, 1990

Briggs GG, Freeman RK, Yaffee SJ: Drugs in Pregnancy and Lactation, 3rd ed. Baltimore, Williams & Wilkins, 1990

Campbell-Brown M, McFadyen IR, Seal DV, Stephenson ML: Is screening for bacteriuria in pregnancy worthwhile? BMJ 294:1579, 1987

Chamberlin RO: Eosinophilic cystitis during pregnancy. Am J Obstet Gynecol 166:28, 1992

Coe FL, Favus MJ: Nephrolithiasis. Chapter 232. In Wilson JD, Braunwald E, Isselbacher KJ, Petersdorf RG, Martin JB, Fauci AS, Root RK (eds): Harrison's Principles of Internal Medicine, 12th ed. New York, McGraw-Hill, 1991

Coe FL, Kathpalia S: Polycystic renal disease in adults. Chapter 231. In Wilson JD, Braunwald E, Isselbacher KJ, Petersdorf RG, Martin JB, Fauci AS, Root RK (eds): Harrison's Principles of Internal Medicine, 12th ed. New York, McGraw-Hill, 1991

Cox SM, Cunningham FG: Acute focal pyelonephritis (lobar nephronia) complicating pregnancy. Obstet Gynecol 71:510, 1988a

Cox SM, Cunningham FG: Ureidopenicillin therapy for acute antepartum pyelonephritis. Curr Ther Res 44:1029, 1988b

Cox SM, Shelburne P, Mason R, Guss S, Cunningham FG: Mechanisms of hemolysis and anemia associated with acute antepartum pyelonephritis. Am J Obstet Gynecol 164:587, 1991

Cunningham FG: Urinary tract infections complicating pregnancy. Clin Obstet Gynecol 1:891, 1988

Cunningham FG, Cox SM, Harstad TW, Mason MT, Pritchard JA: Chronic renal disease and pregnancy outcome. Am J Obstet Gynecol 163:453, 1990

Cunningham FG, Lucas MJ, Hankins GDV: Pulmonary injury complicating antepartum pyelonephritis. Am J Obstet Gynecol 156:797, 1987

Cunningham FG, Morris GB, Mickal A: Acute pyelonephritis of pregnancy: A clinical review. Obstet Gynecol 42:112, 1973

Davison JM: Dialysis, transplantation, and pregnancy. Am J Kid Dis 17:127, 1991

Davison JM: The effect of pregnancy on kidney function in renal allograft recipients. Kidney Int 27:74, 1985

Davison JM, Lindheimer MD: Pregnancy in renal transplant recipients. J Reprod Med 27:613, 1982

Duff P: Pyelonephritis in pregnancy. Clin Obstet Gynecol 27:17, 1984

Dunlow S, Duff P: Prevalence of antibiotic-resistant uropathogens in obstetric patients with acute pyelonephritis. Obstet Gynecol 76:241, 1990

Eckford SD, Gingell JC: Ureteric obstruction in pregnancy—diagnosis and management. Br J Obstet Gynaecol 98:1137, 1991

Elliott JP, O'Keeffe DF, Schon DA, Cherem LB: Dialysis in pregnancy: A critical review. Obstet Gynecol Surv 46:319, 1991

Faro S, Pastorek JG, Plauche WC, Korndorffer FA, Aldridge KE: Short-course parenteral antibiotic therapy for pyelonephritis in pregnancy. South Med J 77:455, 1984

Gilstrap LC III, Cunningham FG, Whalley PJ: Acute pyelonephritis in pregnancy: An anterospective study. Obstet Gynecol 57:409, 1981a

Gilstrap LC III, Leveno KJ, Cunningham FG, Whalley PJ, Roark ML: Renal infection and pregnancy outcome. Am J Obstet Gynecol 141:708, 1981b

Glasscock RJ, Brenner BM: The major glomerulopathies. Chapter 227. In Wilson JD, Braunwald E, Isselbacher KJ, Petersdorf RG, Martin JB, Fauci AS, Root RK (eds): Harrison's Principles of Internal Medicine, 12th ed. New York, McGraw-Hill, 1991, p 1170

Grünfeld JP, Pertuiset N: Acute renal failure in pregnancy: 1987. Am J Kidney Dis 9:359, 1987

Harris RE, Gilstrap LC III: Cystitis during pregnancy: A distinct clinical entity. Obstet Gynecol 57:578, 1981

Hayslett JP: Current concepts: Postpartum renal failure. N Engl J Med 312:1556, 1985

Hayslett JP, Lynn RI: Effect of pregnancy in patients with lupus nephropathy. Kidney Int 18:207, 1980

Hendricks SK, Ross SO, Krieger JN: An algorithm for diagnosis and therapy of management and complications of urolithiasis during pregnancy. Surg Gynecol Obstet 172:49, 1991

Hossack KF, Leddy CL, Johnson AM, Schrier RW, Gabow PA: Echocardiographic findings in autosomal dominant polycystic kidney disease. N Engl J Med 319:907, 1988

Hou S: Pregnancy in organ transplant recipients. Med Clin North Am 73:667, 1989

Hou S: Pregnancy in women requiring dialysis for renal failure. Am J Kidney Dis 9:368, 1987

Hou SH, Grossman SD, Madias NE: Pregnancy in women with renal disease and moderate renal insufficiency. Am J Med 78:185, 1985

Jakobi P, Ohel G, Szylman P, Levit A, Lewin M, Paldi E: Continuous ambulatory peritoneal dialysis as the primary approach in the management of severe renal insufficiency in pregnancy. Obstet Gynecol 79:808, 1992

Jungers P, Houillier P, Forget D, Henry-Amar M: Specific controversies concerning the natural history of renal disease in pregnancy. Am J Kidney Dis 17:116, 1991

Kass EH: Progress in pyelonephritis. Philadelphia, FA Davis, 1965

Kass EH: Pyelonephritis and bacteriuria. Ann Intern Med 56:46, 1962

Katz AI, Davison JM, Hayslett JP, Singson E, Lindheimer MD: Pregnancy in women with kidney disease. Kidney Int 18:192, 1980

Katz M, Quagiorello J, Young BK: Severe polycystic kidney disease in pregnancy. Obstet Gynecol 53:119, 1979

Kincaid-Smith P, Bullen M: Bacteriuria in pregnancy. Lancet 1:395, 1965

Kleinknecht D, Grünfeld JP, Gomez PC, Moreau JF, Garcia-Torres R: Diagnostic procedures and long-term prognosis in bilateral renal cortical necrosis. Kidney Int 4:390, 1973

Krane NK: Acute renal failure in pregnancy. Arch Intern Med 148:2347, 1988

Krieger JN: Complications and treatment of urinary tract infections in pregnancy. Urol Clin North Am 13:685, 1986

Laverson PL, Hankins GD, Quirk JG Jr: Ureteral obstruction during pregnancy. J Urol 131:327, 1984

Lindheimer MD, Davison JM: Renal biopsy during pregnancy: "To b... or not to b...?" Br J Obstet Gynaecol 94:932, 1987

Little PJ: The incidence of urinary infection in 5000 pregnant women. Lancet 2:925 1966

Loughlin KKR, Bailey RB: Internal ureteral stents for conservative management of ureteral calculi during pregnancy. N Engl J Med 315:1647, 1986

Madaio MP, Harrington JT: The diagnosis of acute glomerulonephritis. N Engl J Med 309:1299, 1983

Maikranz P, Coe FL, Parks J, Lindheimer MD: Nephrolithiasis in pregnancy. Am J Kidney Dis 9:354, 1987

Martinell JF, Jodel U, Lidin-Janson G: Pregnancies in women with and without renal scarring after urinary infections in childhood. BMJ 300:840, 1990

Marushak A, Weber T, Bock J: Pregnancy following kidney transplantation. Acta Obstet Gynaecol Scand 65:557, 1986

Michie HR, Manogue KR, Spriggs DR, Revhaug A, O'Dwyer S, Dinarello CA, Cerami A, Wolff SM, Wilmore DW: Detection of circulating tumor necrosis factor after endotoxin administration. N Engl J Med 318:1482, 1988

Mikkelsen AL, Meyhoff HH, Lindahl F, Christensen J: The effect of hydroxyprogesterone on ureteral stones. Int Urol Nephrol 20:257, 1988

Milutinovic J, Fialkow P, Agodoa LY, Phillips LA, Bryant JI: Fertility and pregnancy complications in women with autosomal dominant polycystic kidney disease. Obstet Gynecol 61:566, 1983

Murray JE, Reid DE, Harrison JH, Merrill JP: Successful pregnancies after human renal transplantation. N Engl J Med 269:341, 1963

Nageotte MP, Grundy HO: Pregnancy outcome in women requiring chronic hemodialysis. Obstet Gynecol 72:456, 1988

Norden CW, Kilpatrick WH: Bacteriuria of pregnancy. In Kass EH (ed): Progress in Pyelonephritis. Philadelphia, Davis, 1965, p 64

O'Donnell D, Sevitz H, Seggie J: Pregnancy after renal transplantation. Aust NZ Med 15:320, 1985

Packham D, Fairley KF: Renal biopsy: Indications and complications in pregnancy. Br J Obstet Gynaecol 94:935, 1987

Packham DK, North RA, Fairley KF, Kloss M, Whitworth JA, Kincaid-Smith A: Primary glomerulonephritis and pregnancy. Q J Med 71:537, 1989

Penn I, Makowski EL, Harris P: Parenthood following renal transplant. Kidney Int 2:221, 1980

Professional Activities Study Database. Ann Arbor, Commission on Professional and Hospital Activities, 1987

Ridgway LE, Martin RW, Hess LW, Buchanan J, Whitworth NS, Martin JN Jr: Acute gestational pyelonephritis: The impact on colloid osmotic pressure, plasma fibronectin, and arterial oxygen saturation. Am J Perinatol 8:222, 1991

Rifle G, Traeger J: Pregnancy after renal transplantation: An international survey. Transplant Proc 7:723, 1975

Robson JS, Martin AM, Ruckley VA, MacDonald MK: Irreversible postpartum renal failure. Q J Med 37:423, 1968

Rodriguez PN, Klein AS: Management of urolithiasis during pregnancy. Surg Gynecol Obstet 155:103, 1988

Romero R, Oyarzun E, Mazor M, Sirtori M, Hobbins JC, Bracken M: Meta-analysis of the relationship between asymptomatic bacteriuria and preterm delivery/low birth weight. Obstet Gynecol 73:576, 1989

Rudolph JE, Schweizer RT, Bar SA: Pregnancy in renal transplant patients. Transplantation 27:26, 1979

Sibai BM, Villar MA, Mabie BC: Acute renal failure in hypertensive disorders of pregnancy. Pregnancy outcome and remote prognosis in thirty-one consecutive cases. Am J Obstet Gynecol 162:777, 1990

Stamm WE, Wagner KF, Amsel R, Alexander R, Turck M, Counts GW, Holmes KK: Causes of the acute urethral syndrome in women. N Engl J Med 303:409, 1980

Stenqvist K, Sandberg T, Lidin-Janson G, Orskov F, Orskov I, Svanborg-Eden C: Virulence factors of *Escherichia coli* in urinary isolates from pregnant women. J Infect Dis 156:870, 1987

Stettler RW, Cunningham FG: Natural history of chronic proteinuria complicating pregnancy. Am J Obstet Gynecol 167:1219, 1992

Sturgiss SN, Davison JM: Effect of pregnancy on long-term function of renal allografts. Am J Kidney Dis 19:167, 1992

Sturgiss SN, Davison JM: Perinatal outcome in renal allograft recipients: Prognostic significance of hypertension and renal function before and during pregnancy. Obstet Gynecol 78:573, 1991

Surian M, Imbasciati E, Cosci P, Banfi G, di Belgiojoso B, Brancaccio D, Minetti L, Ponticelli C: Glomerular disease and pregnancy: A study of 123 pregnancies in patients with primary and secondary glomerular diseases. Nephron 36:101, 1984

Svanborg-Eden C, Hagberg L, Leffler H, Lonberg H: Recent progress in the understanding of the role of bacterial adhesion in the pathogenesis of urinary tract infection. Infection 10:327, 1982

Turney JH, Ellis CM, Parsons FM: Obstetric acute renal failure 1956-1987. Br J Obstet Gynaecol 96:679, 1989

Väisänen V, Elo J, Tallgren LG, Siitonen A, Makela PH, Svanborg-Eden C, Kallenius G, Svenson SB, Hultbert H, Korhonen T: Mannose-resistant haemagglutination and P antigen recognition are characteristic of *Escherichia coli* causing primary pyelonephritis. Lancet 2:1366, 1981

Van Dorsten JP, Lenke RR, Schifrin BS: Pyelonephritis in pregnancy: The role of in-hospital management and nitrofurantoin suppression. J Reprod Med 32:897, 1987

Vordermark JS, Deshon GE, Agee RE: Management of pregnancy after major urinary reconstruction. Obstet Gynecol 75:564, 1990

Whalley PJ: Bacteriuria of pregnancy. Am J Obstet Gynecol 97:723, 1967

Whalley PJ, Cunningham FG, Martin FG: Transient renal dysfunction associated with acute pyelonephritis of pregnancy. Obstet Gynecol 46:174, 1975

Whalley PJ, Martin FG, Peters PC: Significance of asymptomatic bacteriuria detected during pregnancy. JAMA 198:879, 1965

Wilson MG, Jewitt WI, Monzon OT: Effect of bacteriuria on the fetus. N Engl J Med 275:1115, 1966

Yankowitz J, Kuller JA, Thomas RL: Pregnancy complicated by Goodpasture syndrome. Obstet Gynecol 79:806, 1992

CHAPTER 51

Gastrointestinal Disorders

During normal pregnancy the gastrointestinal (GI) tract and its appendages undergo changes, both anatomical and functional, that can appreciably alter the criteria for diagnosis and treatment of several diseases to which they are susceptible. For example, nausea and vomiting are frequent symptoms early in normal pregnancy, but if these symptoms are erroneously attributed to a normal physiological change, then GI disease can be overlooked. Conversely, persistent nausea and vomiting in late pregnancy always should prompt a search for underlying pathology. In another example, heartburn is reported in half of women at some time during pregnancy, especially in late gestation. **During advanced pregnancy, GI symptoms become difficult to assess, and physical findings are greatly obtunded by the large uterus and its contents.**

Most obstetricians, but not most internists or gastroenterologists, are aware that upper abdominal pain—epigastric or right upper quadrant—can be an ominous sign of severe preeclampsia. An ultrasonic examination negative for gallstones, or a normal serum amylase value, does not serve to exclude serious disease, but rather supports the diagnosis of severe preeclampsia or eclampsia.

Although many of these disorders are best managed by medical treatment, laparotomy and surgical treatment may be lifesaving for certain conditions, acute appendicitis being the most common. Allen and colleagues (1989) reported that they performed abdominal surgery in 90 women during nearly 41,500 pregnancies cared for at their institution over a 17-year period. The figures for Parkland Hospital are similar; from 1989 through 1991, 62 abdominal operations unrelated to pregnancy were carried out in nearly 45,000 pregnant women. Although about half of these were for adnexal masses, most of the remainder were for GI lesions.

Diagnostic Techniques. Confirmative diagnosis of most GI lesions cannot be made by physical examination alone. Radiography is usually avoided during pregnancy. The advent of fiber-optic endoscopic instruments for examination of the upper GI tract as well as the colon has revolutionized the diagnosis and management of many of these conditions. It is particularly well-suited for use in the pregnant woman. **Endoscopy** permits evaluation of the esophagus, stomach, and duodenum. With specialized instruments, the proximal jejunum can be studied, and the ampulla of Vater can be cannulated to perform retrograde cholangiopancreatography.

Colonoscopy is used to view the entire colon and the distal ileum, and is invaluable in diagnosis and management of inflammatory bowel disease. Diagnostic and therapeutic uses of endoscopy were reviewed by Morrissey and Reichelderfer (1991).

There are a number of sophisticated noninvasive imaging techniques to evaluate GI diseases. Of these, abdominal ultrasonography has a crucial role in evaluation of some of these diseases, especially those involving the gallbladder. Although frequently useful, **computed tomography** must be limited in its application because of radiation exposure (see Chap. 43, p. 981). **Magnetic resonance imaging** has proved invaluable for evaluating the abdomen and retroperitoneal space during pregnancy. The principal drawback of this technique is its great expense and limited availability.

The limitations of these techniques must be realized, along with the knowledge that their use during pregnancy for evaluation of many GI disorders has not been validated. However, although none should be considered routine during pregnancy, they likewise should not be withheld if indicated.

Parenteral Nutrition. For some of the disorders that will be discussed, parenteral feeding, or **hyperalimentation,** may be considered. Its purpose is to provide nutrition when the intestinal tract must be kept quiescent. Peripheral venous access may be adequate for short-term supplemental nutrition, which derives calories from isotonic fat solutions. Jugular or subclavian venous catheterization is necessary for **total parenteral nutrition,** because its hyperosmolarity requires rapid dilution in a high-flow system. These solutions provide up to 24 to 40 kcal/kg, principally as hypertonic glucose solution. They cause thrombophlebitis if infused by peripheral vein. Madan and colleagues (1992) reported that these hyperosmolar solutions may be infused through a peripheral vein with a low risk of thrombophlebitis if an ultra-fine-bore silicone catheter is used.

A number of complications are associated with parenteral nutrition (Howard, 1991). Major mechanical complications include pneumothorax, hemothorax from injury to subclavian vessels, brachial plexus injury, and catheter malpositions. Greenspoon and colleagues (1989b) described a maternal death from cardiac tamponade 7 days after successful placement of a subclavian venous catheter for hyperalimentation in a woman with hyperemesis gravidarum. Metabolic complications may be avoided by slowly increasing the dietary prescription to avoid fluid overload, osmotic diuresis, and massive electrolyte shifts due to insulin secretion. Late metabolic complications include gallstones and hepatic cholestasis. Catheter-induced sepsis is an important source of morbidity.

Total Parenteral Nutrition During Pregnancy. Kirby and colleagues (1988) reviewed the use of total parenteral nutrition (TPN) for a variety of indications in 55 pregnant women (Table 51–1). Gastrointestinal disorders were the most common indication, and the duration of parenteral feeding ranged from conception to delivery, with a mean of 4.8 weeks. Their observations were similar to those reported earlier in reviews by Catanzarite and associates (1986) and Lee and colleagues (1986). Complications were identified in about one third of these women, and one that is particularly worrisome is the reversible **Wernicke–Korsakoff psychosis,** which may complicate up to 10 percent of cases. Lee and colleagues (1986) emphasize that parenteral nutrition for the woman with diabetic gastroenteropathy is particularly hazardous, and they reported 1 antepartum maternal death and 4 women with deteriorating renal function. Sepsis is also common. Currently at Parkland Hospital, nutritional support costs about $400 per day, and Catanzarite and colleagues (1986) rightly caution that careful informed consent with patient participation in decision making is important.

DISORDERS OF THE UPPER GASTROINTESTINAL TRACT

Hyperemesis Gravidarum

Nausea and vomiting of moderate intensity are especially common complaints from early pregnancy until about 16 weeks (see Chap. 9, p. 265). Klebanoff and colleagues (1985) reported observations from more

TABLE 51–1. SOME REPORTED CONDITIONS IN WHICH PARENTERAL NUTRITION HAS BEEN USED DURING PREGNANCY

Anorexia nervosa	Hyperemesis gravidarum
Appendiceal rupture	Jejunoileal bypass
Bowel obstruction	Leukemia
Burns	Pancreatic cancer
Cholecystitis	Pancreatitis
Crohn disease	Paroxysomal nocturnal
Cystic fibrosis	hemoglobinuria
Diabetic complications	Partial hepatectomy
Esophageal injury	Persistent abdominal pain
Esophagocolonogastrostomy	Short bowel syndrome
	Ulcerative colitis

Modified from Kirby and colleagues (1988), with permission.

than 9000 women enrolled during the first trimester into the Collaborative Perinatal Project. They found that slightly over half of these women had vomiting in early pregnancy. They also found that vomiting was more likely during the first pregnancy in younger women, and that it usually recurred in subsequent gestations. Intriguingly, women with early-pregnancy vomiting had better outcomes than women without vomiting.

Fortunately, hyperemesis gravidarum has become uncommon. This syndrome is defined as vomiting sufficiently pernicious to produce weight loss, dehydration, acidosis from starvation, alkalosis from loss of hydrochloric acid in vomitus, and hypokalemia. Its pathogenesis is unknown, but it has been related to high or rapidly rising serum levels of chorionic gonadotropin or estrogens. In a study of 35 women with hyperemesis from the Collaborative Perinatal Project, Depue and associates (1987) found that total serum estradiol, but not chorionic gonadotropin, was elevated compared with control women. Hyperemesis may lead to evidence of hepatic dysfunction manifest by elevation of serum transaminases and slight jaundice, both of which return to normal with hydration and feeding (p. 1153).

Management. Management of pernicious vomiting of pregnancy comprises treatment of dehydration with correction of fluid and electrolyte deficits and acidosis or alkalosis. This requires appropriate amounts of sodium, potassium, chloride, lactate or bicarbonate, glucose, and water, which should be administered parenterally until the vomiting has been controlled. A number of antiemetics may be given to alleviate nausea and vomiting. These include the category C phenothiazine derivatives such as promethazine, prochlorperazine, and chlorpromazine. For severe disease, we have given metoclopramide parenterally. This is a category B drug that stimulates motility of the upper intestinal tract without stimulating gastric, biliary, or pancreatic secretions. Its antiemetic properties apparently result from central antagonism of dopamine receptors. **With persistent vomiting, appropriate steps are taken to diagnose other diseases, such as gastroenteritis, cholecystitis, pancreatitis, hepatitis, peptic ulcer, pyelonephritis, and fatty liver of pregnancy.**

In many instances, social and psychological factors contribute to the illness. With these circumstances, the woman usually improves remarkably while hospitalized, only to relapse after discharge. Positive assistance with psychological and social problems is beneficial.

Godsey and Newman (1991) studied 140 women admitted for hyperemesis on 220 occasions to the Medical University of South Carolina Hospital. In 27 percent of these women, multiple admissions were necessary. In some women with persistent and severe disease, parenteral nutrition had been used. Levine and Esser (1988) have studied the use of parenteral alimentation during early pregnancy and concluded that it is safe and effective. More recently, enteral nutrition has been successfully used after acute nausea and vomiting subside (Boyce, 1992).

Reflux Esophagitis

Heartburn, also called pyrosis, from regurgitation of gastric contents, is a common symptom in late pregnancy. The retrosternal burning sensation is caused by esophagitis from gastroesophageal reflux related to relaxation of the lower esophageal sphincter (Hytten, 1991). Castro (1967) demonstrated that instillation of hydrochloric acid into the lower esophagus in pregnant women with heartburn mimicked the characteristic pain whereas women who were asymptomatic remained so with acid application.

Management. Common heartburn during pregnancy is seldom severe enough to warrant diagnostic investigation. Raising the head of the bed and ingestion of oral antacids will usually suffice to relieve symptoms. If severe symptoms persist despite these simple measures, then endoscopy should be considered. If severe esophagitis is demonstrated, then an H_2-receptor antagonist is prescribed. Both cimetidine and ranitidine are category B drugs (Briggs and associates, 1990).

Hiatal Hernia

Rigler and Eneboe (1935) performed upper GI radiological examinations in 195 unselected women in the last trimester of pregnancy. Among 116 multiparas, 18 percent had hiatal hernias; and among 79 primigravidas, 5 percent had such findings. When 10 of these women with a pregnancy-associated hernia were reexamined 1 to 18 months postpartum, only 3 had a persistent hernia. These types of hernias encountered during pregnancy may be produced by an intermittent but prolonged increase in intra-abdominal pressure.

The relationship of hiatal hernia with reflux esophagitis, and thus symptoms, is not clear. Cohen and Harris (1971) demonstrated no relationship between reflux and hernia, and showed that the lower esophageal sphincter functioned effectively even when displaced intrathoracically. Nevertheless, during pregnancy these hernias may cause vomiting, epigastric pain, and even bleeding from ulceration.

Diaphragmatic Hernia

Symptomatic diaphragmatic hernias rarely complicate pregnancy. These are herniations of abdominal contents through either the foramen of Bochdalek or the foramen of Morgagni. Kurzel and associates (1988) surveyed the literature and found 18 cases of symptomatic diaphragmatic hernia complicating pregnancy. These women had acute obstruction, and maternal mortality was 45 percent. They recommend repair during pregnancy even if the woman is asymptomatic.

Achalasia

Achalasia is a motor disorder of esophageal smooth muscle in which the lower sphincter does not relax properly with swallowing and there are abnormal esophageal contractions. The cause is defective innervation of the smooth muscle of the esophagus and lower esophageal sphincter. Symptoms are dysphagia, chest pain, and regurgitation. Diagnosis is usually confirmed by demonstrating a "bird's beak" narrowing at the distal esophagus via barium esophagogram (Satin and colleagues, 1992). Endoscopy may also be helpful. Evaluation demonstrates esophageal dilatation and manometry is confirmatory. Endoscopy is used to rule out secondary causes, particularly gastric carcinoma.

Achalasia has received little attention as a pregnancy complication. Mayberry and Atkinson (1987) described clinical findings in 20 such women and reported no excessive reflux esophagitis compared with nonpregnant women with achalasia. Of 16 women who became pregnant after symptoms developed, 11 had no change in symptomatology, 2 improved, and 3 worsened.

Management. Soft foods and anticholinergic drugs are prescribed. If symptoms persist, then balloon dilatation is used to reduce lower esophageal sphincter pressure by rupturing muscle fibers. Almost 85 percent of nonpregnant patients respond to such treatment. Satin and colleagues (1992) reported a successful outcome with the use of pneumatic dilation and hyperalimentation in a woman with achalasia in late pregnancy. Thus, although there is little experience reported in pregnant women, it seems reasonable to attempt such therapy if the woman is symptomatic. Complications of dilatation include perforation and hemorrhage.

Peptic Ulcer

There are conflicting data regarding gastric physiology during pregnancy. According to Hytten (1991), there is consensus that gastric secretion is reduced, motility is reduced, and there is considerably increased mucus secretion. From these observations, it is not surprising that active peptic ulcer disease is uncommon during pregnancy. In the past 20 years at Parkland Hospital, during which time we have cared for nearly 200,000 pregnant women, we have encountered very few women with presumed symptomatic peptic ulcer. Obviously, complications such as perforation or hemorrhage are even more rare. Published experiences indicate that women with a symptomatic peptic ulcer most often note considerable improvement during pregnancy. Clark (1953) studied 313 pregnancies in 118 women with proven ulcer disease and reported a clear remission in almost 90 percent. These benefits were short lived, and within 3 months of delivery symptoms had recurred in over half. By the end of 2 years, almost every woman had suffered a recurrence.

Upper Gastrointestinal Bleeding

Occasionally, especially during early pregnancy, nausea and vomiting may be accompanied by worrisome upper GI bleeding. The obvious concern is that there is a bleeding peptic ulceration; however, in our experiences, most of these women have minute linear mucosal tears near the gastroesophageal junction, or so-called **Mallory–Weiss** tears. These women usually respond promptly to conservative measures that include iced-saline irrigations, topical antacids, and intravenously administered cimetidine. In some instances, blood transfusions are needed. **Endoscopy, if indicated, should not be withheld because of pregnancy.** It may be important to distinguish this from the more dangerous **Boerhaave syndrome,** which is esophageal rupture caused by greatly increased esophageal pressure from retching.

DISORDERS OF THE SMALL BOWEL AND COLON

Physiology. The small bowel has diminished motility during pregnancy. Parry and associates (1970) showed that small intestinal transit time was about 60 hours in women 12 to 20 weeks' pregnant compared with 52 hours in nonpregnant controls. They showed that the colon undergoes muscular relaxation as well, and this was accompanied by increased absorption of water and sodium. Both of these predispose towards constipation.

Constipation. According to Anderson and Whichelow (1985), almost 40 percent of women complain of constipation at some time during pregnancy, and 20 percent do so in the third trimester. Such symptoms are usually only mildly bothersome, but we have on several occasions encountered pregnant women at Parkland Hospital who developed megacolon from impacted stool. Although these women almost invariably had abused stimulatory laxatives, Sheld (1987) described a woman with recurrent megacolon during pregnancy related to **Hirschsprung disease.** As discussed in Chapter 9 (p. 263), preventative measures include a high-fiber diet along with prescription of bulk-forming laxatives when there is mild constipation.

Inflammatory Bowel Disease

Inflammatory bowel disease refers to at least two forms of intestinal inflammation, **ulcerative colitis** and **Crohn disease.** The latter also is known as regional enteritis, Crohn ileitis, and granulomatous colitis. As shown in Table 51–2, these two diseases share common factors, and sometimes it is impossible to distinguish the two if Crohn disease involves the colon. The etiology of both is enigmatic, but their pathogenesis has been partially elucidated. There appears to be a genetic predisposition towards both diseases with increased incidence

TABLE 51–2. SOME DIFFERENTIATING CHARACTERISTICS OF ULCERATIVE COLITIS AND CROHN DISEASE

Characteristic	Ulcerative Colitis	Crohn Disease
Epidemiology	Equal prevalence	Equal prevalence but increasing
Genetic factors		
Concordance with twins	Increased	High
First-degree relatives	10-fold risk	10-fold risk
HLA association	HLA-Bw35, HLA-B27	HLA-A2, HLA-B27
Natural history		
Bowel involvement	Large bowel mucosa and submucosa	Small and large bowel mucosa and deeper layers; transmural involvement common
	Continuous involvement beginning at rectum	Small or large bowel only, or both; segmental involvement
Colonoscopy	Mucosal granularity and friability with superficial ulceration	Patchy involvement
Symptoms	Bloody diarrhea	Abdominal pain and diarrhea, obstructive symptoms
Clinical course	Exacerbations and remissions	Exacerbations and remissions; surgery commonly required
Complications	Toxic megacolon	Fistula formation
	Reactive arthritis	Reactive arthritis
	Sclerosing cholangitis	Toxic megacolon
	Cancer 1% per year	Cancer 6-fold increased
Management	Medical	Medical
	Proctocolectomy curative	Segmental resection if indicated

Data from Podolsky (1991a,b).

in twins and first-degree relatives. In some studies, an association with inflammatory bowel disease has been found with certain HLA alleles. Although suspected, neither an infectious nor an immune-mediated etiology has been proved.

Clinical Features. In general, the salient clinical and laboratory features of ulcerative colitis and Crohn disease shown in Table 51–2 permit a confident diagnostic differentiation between these two inflammatory bowel diseases.

Ulcerative Colitis. Ulcerative colitis is confined to the superficial layers of the colon, typically beginning at the rectum and extending proximally for a variable distance. As shown in Figure 51–1, sigmoidoscopic findings include mucosal granularity and friability, which are interspersed with mucosal ulcerations and a mucopurulent exudate. The extent of inflammation is proportional to symptoms and **bloody diarrhea** is the cardinal presenting finding. The disease is characterized by exacerbations and remissions. **Toxic megacolon** is a particularly dangerous complication necessitating emergency colectomy. **Extraintestinal manifestations** include arthritis, uveitis, and erythema nodosum. The risk of **cancer** is high and approximates about 1 percent per year.

Management of ulcerative colitis is medical, and sulfasalazine is given to reduce both the frequency and severity of attacks. Other agents containing 5-aminosalicylic acid have shown promise and have fewer side effects because they are "sulfa-free" (Courtney and colleagues, 1992). Prednisone is used for active disease. Immunosuppressive drugs including azathioprine and 6-mercaptopurine have been used in nonpregnant patients with success, and more recently cyclosporine has been used to treat severe, active disease (Lichtiger and Present, 1990). Proctocolectomy is performed for recalcitrant disease, with permanent ileostomy or an ileoanal anastomosis with one of the newly devised continent ileal pouches.

Crohn Disease. Crohn disease has more protean manifestations than ulcerative colitis. It involves not only the bowel mucosa but also the deeper layers, as well as having transmural involvement (Table 51–2). The disease is typically segmental. About 40 percent of patients have small bowel involvement, 30 percent have isolated colon involvement, and the remainder have both, usually with the terminal ileum and colon involved (Podolsky, 1991a).

Complaints include abdominal pain and diarrhea, and obstructive symptoms are common. Clinical symptoms are diverse and frequently have been present several years before presentation for care. The disease is chronic and marked by exacerbations and remissions. Almost 30 percent of patients require surgery during the first year after the diagnosis is made; thereafter, 5 percent per year require surgery (Podolsky, 1991b). Complications include fistula formation, and particularly distressing are perineal communications that interfere with vaginal delivery. Reactive arthritis is common and the risk of cancer is increased substantively.

Prednisone therapy controls active disease and sulfasalazine is used for colonic disease. Immunosuppressive drugs, including azathioprine and 6-mercaptopurine, have been used successfully. Brynskov and colleagues (1989) reported that oral cyclosporine was effective to control corticosteroid-resistant active disease. Because cure is unlikely with resection of affected bowel, conservative surgery is indicated for complications.

Inflammatory Bowel Disease and Pregnancy. Chronic inflammatory bowel disease, either ulcerative colitis or Crohn disease, is relatively common in women of childbearing age, and thus either may complicate pregnancy. Donaldson (1985) addressed four questions concerning these disorders and concluded the following: (1) Pregnancy does not increase the likelihood of an attack of inflammatory bowel disease. If the disease is quiescent in early pregnancy, then flares are uncommon, but if they develop, they may be severe. (2) Active disease at conception increases the likelihood of poor pregnancy outcome. (3) Diagnostic evaluations, including limited radiological studies, should not be postponed if their results are likely to affect management in a substantive way. (4) Many of the usual treatment regimens, including corticosteroids, may be continued during pregnancy, and if indicated, surgery should be performed.

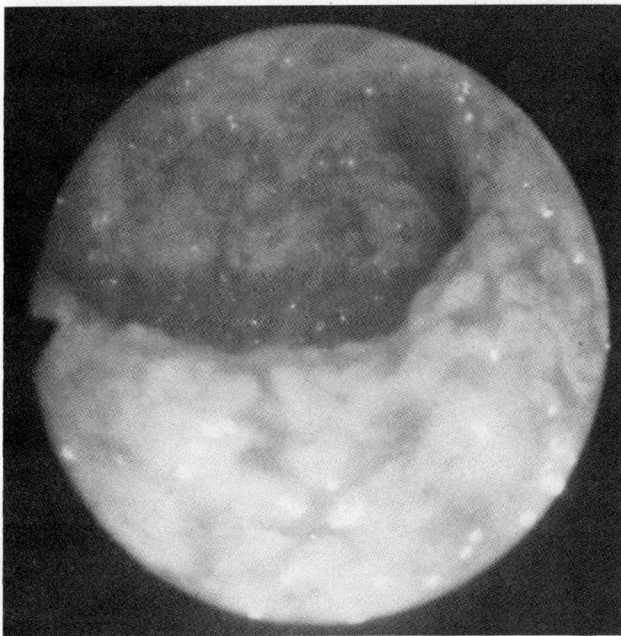

Fig. 51–1. Sigmoid colonoscopy in a patient with severe ulcerative colitis. Note mucosal ulceration, mucopurulent exudate, and mucosal bleeding. (From Podolsky, 1991a, with permission.)

The effects of inflammatory bowel disease on pregnancy outcome are unclear. Porter and Stirrat (1986) reported similar pregnancy outcomes when 82 women with disease were matched with normal women for age and parity. Conversely, Fedorkow and colleagues (1989) reported in a retrospective controlled study that women with inflammatory bowel disease had a threefold increased incidence of preterm delivery as well as a twofold increased risk for fetal growth retardation. These risks were increased if the disease exacerbated during pregnancy. Likewise, Baird and associates (1990) reported a threefold increased risk of preterm birth.

Ulcerative Colitis. In an analysis of one of the largest series reported, Crohn and associates (1956) found that ulcerative colitis that was quiescent at the beginning of gestation was reactivated during pregnancy, usually in the first trimester, in about half the cases. If the colitis was already active at the time of conception, it was materially aggravated in three fourths of the cases. They also emphasized the excessive and prolonged severity of postpartum recurrences.

In an extensive review of more than 1000 cases, Miller (1986) reported that ulcerative colitis quiescent at conception worsened during pregnancy in about one third of cases (Table 51–3). He also found that women with active disease at the time of conception had a worse prognosis.

When ulcerative colitis becomes worse in gestation, the etiological factor may be psychogenic rather than related to any intrinsic effect of pregnancy. Reassurance is therefore an important part of management. Parenteral nutrition can be employed in women with severe and prolonged exacerbations. In the very few cases at Parkland Hospital in which emergency surgery for **toxic megacolon** was performed during pregnancy, the results have been poor, and one woman died from sepsis. Watson and Gaines (1987) described such a case in a 28-week pregnant woman in whom cecal perforation complicated corticosteroid-resistant disease. She survived, but preterm labor ensued shortly after surgery.

TABLE 51–3. EFFECT OF PREGNANCY ON INFLAMMATORY BOWEL DISEASE

Condition	Improved (%)	No Change (%)	Worse (%)
Inactive disease at conception			
Ulcerative colitis (n = 528)	—	66	34
Crohn disease (n = 186)	—	73	27
Active disease at conception			
Ulcerative colitis (n = 227)	27	24	45
Crohn disease (n = 93)	34	32	33

From Miller (1986).

Crohn Disease. There is no evidence that pregnancy exerts adverse effects on the course of Crohn disease. Miller (1986) reported findings very similar to those described above with ulcerative colitis; thus, disease quiescent at conception carries a good prognosis (Table 51–3). Woolfson and colleagues (1990) reported similar results, and they found that abdominal surgery was required during 5 percent of pregnancies. Although Homan and Thorbjarnarson (1976) observed relapses in one fourth of women postpartum, abortion, preterm delivery, and stillbirths were not increased.

Parenteral hyperalimentation has been used successfully for women with severe recurrences of inflammatory bowel disease during pregnancy (Kirby and associates, 1988; Lee and colleagues, 1986).

Ostomy and Pregnancy. Women with a colostomy or an ileostomy may develop complications during pregnancy. Gopal and colleagues (1985) described 82 pregnancies in 66 women following ostomy, usually done for inflammatory bowel disease. Although stomal dysfunction was common, it responded to conservative management in all cases. Bowel obstruction developed in 6 women, and in 3 surgery was necessary. Ileostomy prolapse was surgically corrected in 3 women during pregnancy or at cesarean section, and in a fourth postpartum. The cesarean section rate was 37 percent, and one third of these were done because of prior abdominoperineal resection.

Intestinal Obstruction

The incidence of bowel obstruction during pregnancy is probably not different from that for the general population. According to Davis and Bohon (1983), since 1940 the incidence of intestinal obstruction during pregnancy was between 1 in 2500 to 1 in 3500 deliveries. Our experiences from Parkland Hospital indicate that it is much less common than this. Most cases—probably 60 to 70 percent—are due to adhesions from previous pelvic surgery, and after cesarean section omental adhesions to the uterine incision may cause obstruction. Volvulus is another common cause, and as discussed above, complications of Crohn disease include small bowel obstruction.

Intestinal obstruction is a grave complication of pregnancy and usually results from pressure of the growing uterus on intestinal adhesions. According to Davis and Bohon (1983), there are three times when obstruction is most likely: (1) around midpregnancy, when the uterus becomes an abdominal organ; (2) at term, when the fetal head descends; and (3) immediately postpartum, when there is an acute change in the uterine size. Nausea and vomiting are common. Abdominal pain, either continuous or colicky, is present in 85 percent of cases of intestinal obstruction during pregnancy. Although characteristic high-pitched intestinal rushes may be heard, this finding is unreliable.

The mortality rate with intestinal obstruction can be very high, principally because of errors in diagnosis, delayed diagnosis, reluctance to operate during pregnancy, and inadequate preparation for surgery. Limited x-ray examinations, including plain abdominal films, and those following administration of soluble contrast medium, either orally or by enema, should be performed if indicated.

Ludmir and associates (1989) reported a case of spontaneous small bowel obstruction in a woman with triplets. Kohn and colleagues (1944) reported a remarkable case in which the same woman was operated upon for **volvulus** four times, three of the operations having been performed in the course of two pregnancies. In one third of the cases reported by Harer and Harer (1958), delivery by cesarean section was necessary to obtain proper exposure. Volvulus, especially of the cecum, has been observed early in the puerperium after cesarean section (Pratt and colleagues, 1981).

Pseudo-obstruction of the colon, or **Ogilvie syndrome,** is caused by adynamic colonic ileus, and about 10 percent of all reported cases follow delivery. The syndrome is characterized by massive abdominal distention with cecal dilation found on x-ray studies. Although unusual, the large bowel may rupture, and decompression is recommended when the bowel becomes distended to 10 to 12 cm. Laparotomy or cecostomy may be indicated, but colonoscopy for decompression has been described in a woman 2 days following cesarean section (Moore and associates, 1986).

Appendicitis

Pregnancy does not predispose to appendicitis, but reflects the general prevalence of the disease. Mazze and Källén (1991) described findings from 720,000 Swedish registry deliveries and reported that 778—about 1 in 1000 pregnancies—of these women underwent appendectomy during pregnancy. Appendicitis was confirmed in 64 percent, or 1 in 1440 pregnancies.

Reasons that pregnancy often makes diagnosis of appendicitis more difficult include the following. (1) Anorexia, nausea, and vomiting that accompany normal pregnancy are fairly common symptoms of appendicitis. (2) As the uterus enlarges, the appendix commonly moves upward and outward toward the flank, so that pain and tenderness may not be prominent in the right lower quadrant (Fig. 51–2). (3) Some degree of leukocytosis is the rule during normal pregnancy. (4) During pregnancy especially, other diseases may be readily confused with appendicitis, such as pyelonephritis, renal colic, placental abruption, and degeneration of a uterine myoma. (5) Pregnant women, especially those late in gestation, frequently do not have symptoms considered "typical" for nonpregnant patients with appendicitis.

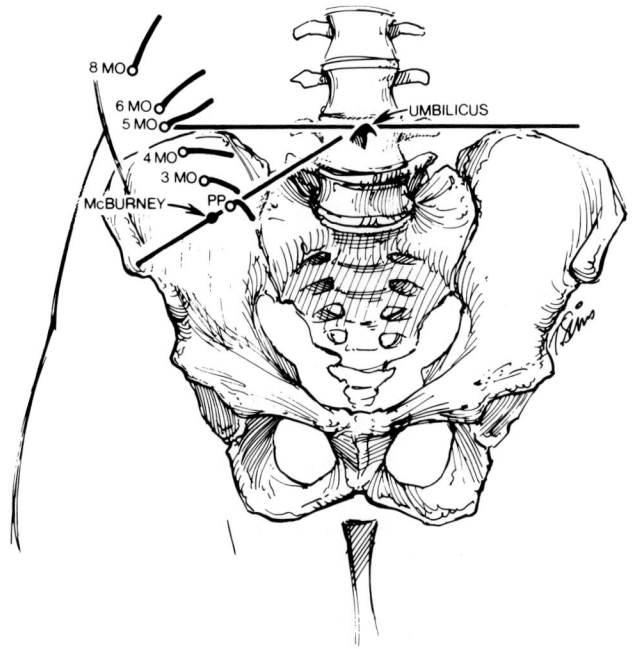

Fig. 51–2. Changes in position of the appendix as pregnancy advances. (MO = month, PP = postpartum). (Modified from Baer and associates, 1932, with permission.)

As the appendix is pushed progressively higher by the growing uterus, containment of infection by the omentum becomes increasingly unlikely and appendiceal rupture causes generalized peritonitis. These complications are more common if treatment is delayed and gangrene supervenes. Acute appendicitis in the last trimester, therefore, may carry a poor prognosis, and it is worth emphasizing that in some series **maternal mortality approaches 5 percent** (DeVore and colleagues, 1980). Increased mortality is due to surgical delay (Cunningham and McCubbin, 1975).

Effects on Pregnancy Outcome. Appendicitis increases the likelihood of abortion or preterm labor, especially if there is peritonitis. Pregnancies further advanced are at greater risk. For example, Mazze and Källén (1991) found that spontaneous labor ensued with greater frequency if surgery for appendicitis was performed after 23 weeks' gestation. Fetal loss is increased in most series, and overall it is about 15 percent. In the Swedish study, fetal loss was 22 percent if surgery was performed after 23 weeks' gestation (Mazze and Källén, 1991).

Management. Persistent abdominal pain and tenderness are the most reproducible findings. If appendicitis is suspected, then treatment, regardless of the stage of gestation, is immediate surgical exploration. **Even though diagnostic errors sometimes lead to the removal of a normal appendix, it is better to operate unnecessarily than to postpone intervention**

until generalized peritonitis has developed. In most reports, the diagnosis is verified in about half of women who undergo surgical exploration. In the Swedish study of 778 women operated for suspected appendicitis, the diagnosis was confirmed in 64 percent (Mazze and Källén, 1991). In the first trimester, 77 percent of diagnoses were correct; however, in the latter two trimesters, only 57 percent of diagnoses were confirmed at surgery.

It is important during surgery and recovery that both hypoxia and hypotension are avoided. Intravenous antimicrobials are given if there is gangrene, perforation, or a periappendiceal phlegmon. If generalized peritonitis does not develop, then the prognosis is quite good. Seldom is cesarean section indicated at the time of appendectomy, and aside from local tenderness, a recent abdominal incision presents no problem during labor and vaginal delivery. Uterine contractions are common if there is peritonitis. Although many recommend tocolytic agents for these women, we caution against their use, because there is evidence that pulmonary permeability edema is increased when they are given to women with sepsis (see Chap. 47, p. 1072).

In our experiences from Parkland Hospital, undiagnosed appendicitis stimulated labor in some women, and in many of these, it was before term. The large uterus helped to contain infection locally, but after delivery when the uterus rapidly empties, the walled-off infection is disrupted with spillage of free pus into the peritoneal cavity. In these cases, an acute surgical abdomen is encountered within a few hours postpartum.

Simply because it is coincidental, appendicitis during the early puerperium is rare. In some cases, especially with early appendicitis, diagnosis is particularly difficult because of the normally robust leukocytosis as well as the frequency of other puerperal disorders with similar signs and symptoms. Anorexia with any evidence of peritoneal irritation, such as distension and adynamic ileus, should suggest appendicitis. **Puerperal pelvic infections typically do not cause peritonitis** (see Chap. 28, p. 633).

Acute Colitis

A number of infectious agents can cause acute inflammation of the colon. In many cases, the principal diagnostic dilemma is to exclude new-onset inflammatory bowel disease, or to rule out superimposed disease in women with chronic ulcerative colitis or Crohn disease. **Infectious colitis** often presents with bloody diarrhea, but its hallmark is the demonstration of numerous leukocytes in the stool.

Traveler's diarrhea, usually due to enterotoxigenic *Escherichia coli,* afflicts as many as one third of foreign travelers. Symptoms appear abruptly, with urgent diarrhea, abdominal cramping, nausea, and low-grade fever. Fluid loss may be impressive and treatment is to insure adequate hydration given along with bismuth subsalicylate. Women with severe diarrhea are also given trimethoprim-sulfamethoxasole. **Amebiasis** may present as colitis and bloody diarrhea, and the diagnosis should be suspected in foreign-born nationals or in women who have recently traveled outside of the United States (see Chap. 58, p. 1294).

Acute bacillary dysentery is caused by *Shigella,* nontyphoidal *Salmonellae,* or *Campylobacter* species. These invasive organisms characteristically affect the colon and terminal ileum and destroy segments of mucosa. Along with numerous small-volume stools of blood, pus, and mucus, they also usually have associated systemic symptoms. Diagnosis is by stool culture. Intravenous hydration is provided, and unless symptoms are severe, most do not recommend antibacterial and antiperistaltic agents.

Antibiotic-associated colitis, which in its worst form is termed **pseudomembranous colitis,** is caused by the toxin of *Clostridium difficile,* which overgrows after treatment is given with any of a large number of antimicrobials. Treatment for the clostridial colonization is with vancomycin or metronidazole.

DISEASES OF THE LIVER

It has become customary to divide liver diseases into those coincidental to pregnancy, those specifically related to pregnancy, and chronic liver disease upon which pregnancy supervenes. Liver diseases complicating pregnancy more often than not are coincidental, as with acute viral hepatitis or drug-induced hepatic failure. There are some diseases that are induced by pregnancy that disappear following termination of gestation. These include intrahepatic cholestasis of pregnancy with or without icterus gravidarum, acute fatty liver of pregnancy, hepatocellular damage of varying intensity that is the direct consequence of severe preeclampsia and eclampsia, and hepatic dysfunction associated with hyperemesis gravidarum. Finally, pregnancy may be superimposed on chronic hepatitis or cirrhosis, or more recently, may follow liver transplantation.

Hepatic Physiology in Pregnancy. Pregnancy normally induces appreciable changes in many of the tests as well as some physical findings that are usually employed to assess liver function (Table 51–4). In some women, palmar erythema and spider angiomas develop. Histological findings of liver biopsy specimens taken from normal pregnant women have disclosed no changes when compared with nonpregnant subjects (Ingerslev and Teilum, 1945).

TABLE 51–4. RESULTS OF SOME TESTS OF LIVER FUNCTION DURING PREGNANCY

Test	Effects of Pregnancy
Enzymes	
Alkaline phosphatase	Markedly increased
Aminotransferases	Unchanged
Lactic acid dehydrogenase	Unchanged
Bilirubin	Unchanged
Proteins	
Albumin	Decreased by 1 g/dL
Globulin	Slightly increased
Ceruloplasmin	Elevated
Hormone binding proteins	Elevated
Transferrin	Elevated
Lipids	
Triglycerides	Elevated
Cholesterol	Doubled
Clotting factors	
Fibrinogen	Elevated
Factors VII, VIII, X	Elevated
Clotting times	Unchanged

Hyperemesis Gravidarum

Pernicious nausea and vomiting are discussed on p. 1146. Abnormal liver function tests may be encountered in these women. For example, hyperbilirubinemia and sulfobromophthalein retention have been described, and serum hepatic transaminase levels are elevated in 15 to 25 percent of women who are hospitalized (Combes and colleagues, 1968; Morali and Braverman, 1990). Enzyme levels seldom exceed three to four times upper limit normal values and are more likely elevated if there is ketonuria.

Intrahepatic Cholestasis of Pregnancy

Intrahepatic cholestasis of pregnancy has also been referred to as **recurrent jaundice of pregnancy, cholestatic hepatosis,** and **icterus gravidarum.** It is characterized clinically by pruritus, icterus, or both. The major histological lesion is intrahepatic cholestasis with centrilobular bile staining without inflammatory cells or proliferation of mesenchymal cells. The cause of cholestasis is unknown, but it appears to be stimulated in susceptible persons by high estrogen concentrations. There is evidence that it may be an autosomal dominantly inherited condition (Holzbach and colleagues, 1983). It has been identified as especially common among Scandinavian women and members of a tribe of Chilean Indians (Burroughs and colleagues, 1982; Steven, 1981). Because of genetic influences, the incidence of cholestasis varies, but it is probably about 1 in 500 to 1000 pregnancies (Fisk and colleagues, 1988; Schorr-Lesnick and associates, 1991).

Pathogenesis. Estrogen-induced changes account for cholestasis in susceptible women. Some drugs that similarly decrease the canicular transport maximum for bile acids will aggravate the disease. For example, we have seen cholestatic jaundice in pregnant women who were taking azathioprine following renal transplantation.

Bile acids are cleared incompletely by the liver and accumulate in plasma of women with cholestasis. Levels typically are much greater than in normal pregnancy, and total bile acids may be elevated 10- to 100-fold. Lunzer and associates (1986) studied serial plasma levels of the glycine conjugate of cholic acid, cholylglycine, during normal pregnancy in 297 women. They observed a threefold elevation as pregnancy progressed. About 10 percent of these women had an abrupt rise of cholylglycine beginning early in the third trimester, and half of these had sustained pruritus until delivery. Other factors are involved, because 20 percent of those with normally elevated cholylglycine levels had significant pruritus.

Modest hyperbilirubinemia mainly results from retention of conjugated pigment, but total bilirubin plasma concentrations rarely exceed 4 to 5 mg/dL. The serum alkaline phosphatase is usually more elevated than for normal pregnancy. Serum aminotransferase activities are normal to moderately elevated, and seldom exceed 250 U/L. Liver biopsy shows mild cholestasis with intracellular bile pigments and canalicular bile plugging without necrosis. These changes disappear after delivery, but often recur in subsequent pregnancies or when an oral contraceptive containing estrogen is taken.

Clinical Presentation. Most women with cholestasis develop pruritus in late pregnancy although the syndrome occasionally occurs in the second trimester, and even as early as 8 weeks' gestation. Generalized pruritus is usually the presenting symptom, but there are no accompanying skin changes unless there are excoriations from scratching (see Chap. 56, p. 1259). A minority of women develop jaundice within several days following pruritus. There are no constitutional symptoms.

Several other disorders should be considered. The absence of hypertension and proteinuria militate against liver disease associated with preeclampsia. Ultrasound examination will often serve to exclude biliary obstruction by gallstones. If the serum aminotransferase levels are not appreciably elevated and the woman is asymptomatic, then viral hepatitis is not likely.

Management. Pruritus associated with cholestasis is caused by elevated serum bile salts, and may be quite troublesome. Orally administered **antihistamines** may provide some relief. **Cholestyramine** has been reported to be effective; however, Fisk and colleagues (1988) and Shaw and associates (1982) did not find this to be so. This too has been our experience at Parkland Hospital, and frequently there is only marginal clinical improvement despite 20 g of cholestyramine administered daily. Prolonged therapy may be beneficial. Absorption of fat-soluble vitamins, already impaired, is worsened with cholestyramine. Thus, impaired coagulation as the consequence of vitamin K deficiency may develop unless supplemental vitamin K is provided.

Hirvioja and colleagues (1992) reported prompt relief of pruritis in 10 women given **dexamethasone,** 12 mg daily for 7 days. They postulated that associated diminished estrogen synthesis caused relief of pruritis as well as lowered serum hepatic enzyme levels.

Preliminary trials with **S-adenosyl-L-methionine** for cholestatic disorders, including obstetrical cholestasis, have been reported (Schorr-Lesnick and colleagues, 1991). The compound alters hepatocyte membrane fluidity or bile acid metabolism, and it may increase methylation of toxic catechol estrogens. The drug lowers serum bilirubin and bile acid levels. Palma and associates (1992) likewise reported preliminary observations using **ursodeoxycholic acid,** which quickly relieved pruritus and lowered serum hepatic enzyme levels in 8 women. Use of these drugs in pregnancy is not currently recommended.

Effect of Cholestasis on Pregnancy. The majority of reported evidence indicates that adverse pregnancy outcomes are increased in women with cholestatic jaundice. Reid and associates (1976) reported 5 stillbirths and 1 neonatal death among 56 pregnancies, intrapartum asphyxia was observed in 5 infants, 18 infants were delivered preterm, and 5 mothers had postpartum hemorrhage. Likewise, Fisk and Storey (1988) reported 2 stillbirths and 1 neonatal death in 86 affected pregnancies, which also were complicated by meconium staining (45 percent), preterm labor (44 percent), and intrapartum fetal distress (22 percent).

Johnston and Baskett (1979) observed much lower pregnancy wastage but found an abnormally high incidence of preterm births and postpartum hemorrhage. It has been postulated that malabsorption of vitamin K may be associated with increased hemorrhage. Fisk and Storey (1988) reported that perinatal mortality fell from 107 per 1000 to 35 per 1000 when close monitoring of fetal well-being was employed along with delivery once lung maturity was achieved.

Acute Fatty Liver of Pregnancy

Acute liver failure may be caused by fulminant viral hepatitis, drug-induced hepatic toxicity, or acute fatty liver of pregnancy. The latter is also called **acute fatty metamorphosis** or **acute yellow atrophy,** and fortunately it is a rare complication of pregnancy that often has proved fatal for both mother and fetus. According to the reviews by Schorr-Lesnick and colleagues (1991) and Watson and Seeds (1990), its incidence is about 1 in 10,000 to 15,000 pregnancies. Gross examination of the liver in fatal cases shows a small, soft, yellow, and greasy organ. The prominent histological abnormalities consist of swollen hepatocytes in which the cytoplasm is filled with microvesicular fat with central nuclei and periportal sparing and minimal hepatocellular necrosis (Fig. 51–3). The disorder may not be limited to the liver, and there is also lipid accumulation within renal tubular cells (Slater and Hague, 1984).

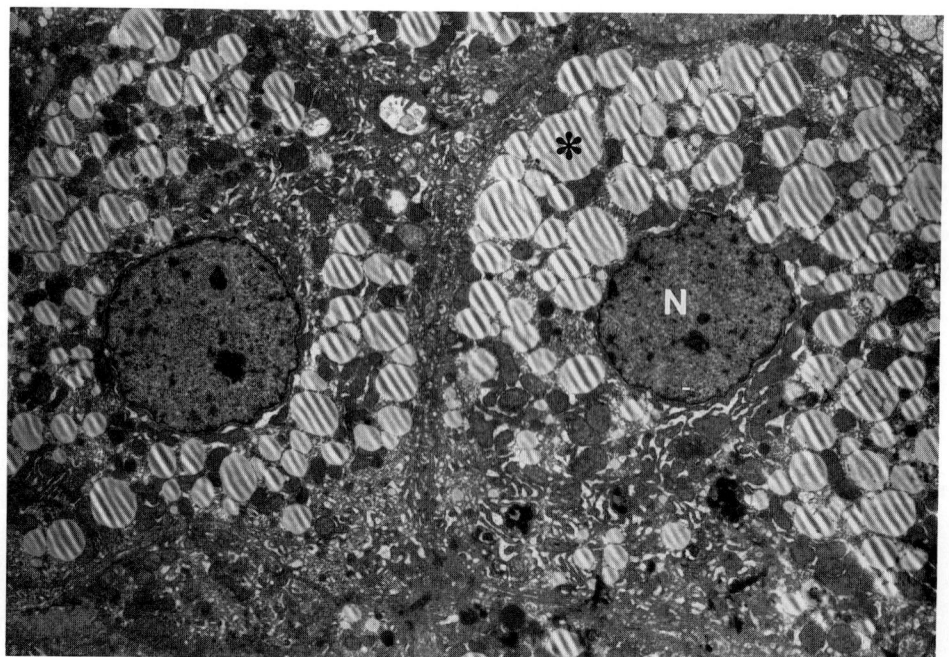

Fig. 51–3. Fatty liver of pregnancy. Electron photomicrograph of two hepatocytes containing numerous microvesicular fat droplets (*). The nuclei (N) remain centered within the cells, unlike with the case of macrovesicular fat deposition. (Courtesy of Dr. Don Wheeler.)

Pathogenesis. The mechanism by which pregnancy incites fatty liver changes is not known. Excessive doses of tetracycline, especially in women with impaired renal function, can cause these histological changes and clinical picture in nonpregnant individuals, as well as pregnant women. Although fatty metamorphosis has been linked with preeclamptic liver disease, the current consensus is that they are different syndromes. Despite this, Minakami and co-workers (1988) described some hepatic microvesicular fat deposition in all 41 Japanese women with preeclampsia who underwent liver biopsy. Other disorders in nonpregnant subjects are characterized by hepatic microvesicular fat changes similar to those of fatty liver of pregnancy include Reye syndrome, hepatotoxicity with sodium valproate, salicylate intoxication in children, and those seen with carnitine deficiency.

Riely (1987) suggests that acquired abnormalities in mitochondria, intermediary metabolism of fatty acids, or both, may be the cause of fatty liver. According to Snyder and Hankins (1986), similar hepatic changes have not been found in fetuses born to affected mothers. The disease seldom recurs, and only one woman has been described with a recurrence in a subsequent pregnancy (Barton and colleagues, 1990).

Clinical Findings. Acute fatty liver of pregnancy almost always develops late in pregnancy. Although unusual, it has been reported as early as 26 weeks' gestation. It is more common in nulliparas, and it probably is more common with a male fetus or with multifetal gestation. Typically, there is onset over several days to weeks of malaise, anorexia, nausea and vomiting, epigastric pain, and progressive jaundice. In many women, vomiting is the major symptom. In perhaps half of these women, there is hypertension, proteinuria, and edema—signs suggestive of preeclampsia. Laboratory abnormalities include prolonged clotting studies, hyperbilirubinemia of usually less than 10 mg/dL, and serum transaminase levels

of 300 to 500 U/L. Peripheral blood shows hemoconcentration and leukocytosis, frequently mild thrombocytopenia, and evidence for hemolysis.

Various imaging techniques have been used to confirm the clinical diagnosis of acute fatty metamorphosis (Farine and colleagues, 1990; Van Le and Podrasky, 1990; Watson and Seeds, 1990). Although sonography, computed-tomographic scanning, and magnetic resonance imaging have been used, experience with them is currently limited.

In many woman, the syndrome worsens after diagnosis. Marked hypoglycemia is common, and obvious hepatic coma develops in 60 percent, severe coagulopathy in 55 percent, and there is evidence for renal failure in about half (Schorr-Lesnick and associates, 1991). Fetal death is common at this severe stage. Fortunately, either the disease is self-limited, or as generally accepted, delivery arrests rapid deterioration of liver function. During recovery, evidence for acute pancreatitis is common and ascites is almost universal. Recovery usually is complete and recurrence is very rare.

We have concluded that there is a spectrum of liver aberrations, and that liver failure is not universal, but rather it represents the most extensive involvement. Probably many milder cases of this syndrome go unnoticed, and are attributed to preeclampsia or mild hepatitis.

Coagulopathy. The pathogenesis of the coagulopathy that complicates fatty liver of pregnancy almost certainly results from increased consumption of procoagulants as well as their impaired production by the liver. Shown in Table 51–5 are laboratory data suggestive of consumptive coagulopathy in 9 women with idiopathic acute fatty liver of pregnancy cared for at Parkland Hospital. All had low plasma fibrinogen levels, and in some this was marked. The hypofibrinogenemia was accompanied by variable elevations of fibrin split products in serum. These observations are compatible with a com-

TABLE 51–5. CONSUMPTIVE COAGULOPATHY AND ERYTHROCYTE CHANGES IN 9 WOMEN WITH ACUTE FATTY LIVER OF PREGNANCY

Patient	Plasma Fibrinogen[a] (mg/dL)	Serum FSP[b] (μg/mL)	Platelets[a] (per μL)	Reticulocytes (%)	Peripheral Erythrocytes (% Totals)		
					Abnormal	Echinocytes	Schizocytes
1	178	32	ND[c]	4.8	37	35	2
2	< 20	128	73,000	2.6	ND	ND	ND
3	182	128	103,000	1.2	60	59	1
4	89	16	150,000	ND	10	9	1
5	95	16	189,000	ND	9	8	1
6	45	128	198,000	1.0	36	35	1
7	200	16	108,000	4.1	ND	ND	ND
8	116	128	170,000	3.8	24	22	—
9	215	16	50,000	3.0	26	25	1

[a] Lowest value recorded.
[b] FSP = Fibrin split products—highest value recorded.
[c] ND = Not done.

bination of decreased production and increased destruction of fibrinogen. Severe thrombocytopenia was not identified, but in some of these women, there was evidence for microangiopathic hemolysis. Echinocytes were the predominant red cell abnormality, presumably caused by impaired hepatic synthesis of various lipid components of the erythrocyte membrane (Cunningham and colleagues, 1985).

Effects on Pregnancy. Maternal mortality was quite high in earlier reports and approached 75 percent. When there is severe hepatic dysfunction, there is frequently severe maternal hypovolemia and acidosis. In these circumstances, fetal death is common, or if labor supervenes, fetal distress is likely. Correspondingly, fetal mortality was reported to be nearly 90 percent. This undoubtedly was related to selection of the worst cases for reporting. More recently, maternal mortality rates of 25 percent or less have been described, along with fetal mortality less than 50 percent. Again, this probably includes the most severe cases, and there appears to be a spectrum of disease that includes mild liver dysfunction to overt hepatic failure.

Management. Because spontaneous resolution usually follows delivery, many assume that delivery is essential for cure. It would follow that early diagnoses would improve both maternal and fetal outcomes. Some recommend cesarean delivery to minimize the time until restoration of hepatic function begins. Although immediate delivery is also likely to benefit the often-distressed fetus, cesarean section in the presence of a severe coagulopathy may prove dangerous for the mother. Other problems might be encountered with an abdominal incision in circumstances in which severe hypoproteinemia and ascites are likely complications. Transfusions with variable amounts of fresh-frozen plasma, cryoprecipitate, whole blood, packed red cells, and platelets are usually necessary if surgery is performed.

Because of maternal acidosis that develops from liver failure in severe cases, some fetuses are dead by the time the diagnosis is made, and many others poorly tolerate the stresses of even normal labor. Procrastination in effecting delivery can increase the risk of coma and death from hyperammonemia usually further complicated by hypoglycemia, renal failure, acidosis, and severe hemorrhage.

Either coincidental with delivery, or with time, hepatic dysfunction resolves. In the interim, intensive medical support is required. Maternal deaths are reported to be caused by sepsis, aspiration, renal failure, circulatory collapse, pancreatitis, or GI bleeding (Snyder and Hankins, 1986). Therapy is directed towards these complications. If hepatic failure does not resolve, liver transplantation is an alternative (Ockner and associations, 1990). Diabetes insipidus, presumably due to elevated vasopressinase concentrations, has been reported (Krege and colleagues, 1989), and in our experiences, it is identified in over half of these women. Interestingly, subsequent pregnancies in an appreciable number of women who previously had severe acute fatty liver of pregnancy have proved to be totally benign. One exception described by Barton and associates (1990) was cited previously.

The Liver in Preeclampsia–Eclampsia

The liver may be involved in women with severe preeclampsia and eclampsia (see Chap. 36, p. 779). Both the degree of dysfunction and the histological changes that develop can vary considerably. Typically, upper abdominal pain—epigastric or right upper quadrant—signals potentially dangerous liver involvement. Thrombocytopenia commonly accompanies elevations in serum transaminase levels. Although aspartate aminotransferase levels vary from 50 to 3000 U/L, typically they are less than 500 U/L. Serum bilirubin levels sometimes are mildly elevated. Intrahepatic and subcapsular hemorrhage may develop and become so intense as to rupture the liver and produce extensive and fatal hemorrhage.

Pathogenesis. The liver changes associated with preeclampsia and eclampsia are enigmatic. It is generally agreed that the liver is not involved primarily, but rather is a target organ for severe disease. Most of the underlying pathological lesions of preeclampsia are explicable on the basis of arterial spasm and subsequent ischemia. However, the liver receives only about one third of its blood supply from the hepatic artery, and in fact this vessel can be ligated with impunity (Riely, 1986). Indeed, the portal venous system is the major source of blood to the liver.

The incidence of liver involvement with preeclampsia is unknown, but it seems to be related to the severity of disease as it affects other organs. For example, elevated serum transaminase levels are more common if thrombocytopenia is identified. In some cases however, the liver may be the only organ with obvious major involvement. Certainly, as illustrated by data shown in Table 51–6, liver involvement is common in fatal cases. Rolfes and Ishak (1986) reviewed autopsy findings at the Armed Forces Institute of Pathology from 97 women who died from preeclampsia–eclampsia. Hepatic infarction was common (13 percent), and there were hepatic histological abnormalities in 72 percent. Characteristic findings were periportal fibrin deposition, hemorrhage, and hepatocellular necrosis.

Clinical Presentation. The signs and symptoms of preeclampsia are discussed in detail in Chapter 36 (p. 783). In most women with preeclamptic liver disease, there will be obvious pregnancy-induced hypertension. Although the liver is more likely to be affected if there

TABLE 51–6. LABORATORY AND ANATOMICAL HEPATIC FINDINGS IN 97 WOMEN WHO DIED FROM PREECLAMPSIA–ECLAMPSIA

Finding	Prevalence (%)
Hepatic symptoms	42/97 (43)
Serum transaminases (n = 26)	350–3720 U/L
Gross appearance	
Normal	28/97 (29)
Preeclampsia	10/20 (50)
Eclampsia	18/71 (25)
Infarction	13/97 (13)
Hematoma	2/97 (2)
Histological appearance	
Pure fibrin deposition	33/97 (34)
Primary hemorrhage	9/97 (9)
Fibrin deposition and hemorrhage	31/97 (32)
Bile inspissation	10/97 (10)

Data from Rolfes and Ishack (1986).

is epigastric pain, most women have no symptoms relating to the liver, and laboratory assessment discloses elevated serum transaminase levels. In most cases, these are only modestly elevated, and seldom exceed 200 to 500 U/L (Watson and Seeds, 1990). Similarly, serum bilirubin levels seldom exceed 2 to 4 mg/dL. Hepatic failure with encephalopathy and consumptive coagulopathy are not usual features of preeclamptic liver disease. Indeed, in the 97 fatal cases described by Rolfes and Ishak (1986), hepatic failure was diagnosed in only 4.

When the diagnosis of pregnancy-induced hypertension is equivocal, preeclamptic liver involvement must be differentiated from fatty liver and hepatitis. As discussed, women with fatty liver of pregnancy often have hypertension and proteinuria, and the degree of liver dysfunction is the differentiating factor. Women with hepatitis usually do not have hypertension.

Management of women with preeclampsia and liver involvement almost always includes prompt delivery. Laboratory abnormalities usually peak by 24 to 48 hours postpartum, and hepatic enzyme abnormalities, lactic dehydrogenase, and platelet counts begin to normalize typically within about 2 to 3 days (Martin and colleagues, 1991).

Hepatic Hematoma and Rupture. Hemorrhage with hepatic and subcapsular hematomas with rupture are two feared complications of liver involvement with preeclampsia. Smith and colleagues (1991) reported an incidence of 1 in 45,000 pregnancies cared for at Baylor College of Medicine. Although liver rupture may develop spontaneously in the otherwise normal pregnant woman, the decided majority of cases are associated with preeclampsia and eclampsia (Neerhof and colleagues, 1989; Rolfes and Ishak, 1986). The hematoma usually develops on the diaphragmatic surface of the right lobe. There is usually right upper quadrant pain

and tenderness and the diagnosis can be confirmed by computed tomography (Manas and colleagues, 1985).

If the hematoma is intrahepatic and intact, close observation seems reasonable as proposed by Manas and colleagues (1985). In some cases, however, liver rupture will cause hemorrhagic shock and a distended abdomen will prompt surgical intervention before diagnostic studies can be performed. In these cases, management includes correction of any associated coagulopathy along with oversewing of the liver laceration, and packing. For resistant cases, hepatic artery ligation and partial hepatic resection are performed. Smith and associates (1991) reported that packing was associated with an overall 80 percent survival compared with 25 percent if lobectomy was done. Bleeding can be severe, and we have encountered an eclamptic woman who suffered rupture of an hepatic hematoma intrapartum. She required many surgical procedures for hemostasis and was given over 200 units of blood and blood products. Fortunately, she survived.

Viral Hepatitis

Hepatitis is the most common serious liver disease encountered in pregnant women. There are at least five distinct types of viral hepatitis: hepatitis A; hepatitis B; the hepatitis B-associated delta agent; and two types of non-A, non-B hepatitis, one bloodborne (termed hepatitis C), and the other enterically transmitted. During their acute phases, these forms of hepatitis are often clinically similar; however, long-term complications in the mother and the risks to the fetus and infant are quite different.

With all of these forms of hepatitis, symptoms may precede jaundice by 1 to 2 weeks. These include nausea and vomiting, headache, and malaise. Low-grade fever is more common with hepatitis A. When jaundice develops, symptoms usually improve, and there may be pain and tenderness over the liver. Serum aminotransferase levels vary, and their peaks do not correspond with disease severity. Peak levels of 400 to 4000 U/L are usually reached by the time jaundice develops (Dienstag and associates, 1991). Serum bilirubin levels usually peak at 5 to 20 mg/dL, and typically continue to rise despite falling aminotransferase levels. Complete clinical and biochemical recovery usually occurs within 1 to 2 months in all cases of hepatitis A and most cases of hepatitis B and C.

The Centers for Disease Control have issued guidelines to minimize infectivity of patients hospitalized for viral hepatitis. They recommend that feces, secretions, and bedpans and other articles in contact with the intestinal tract be handled with glove-protected hands. These precautions need not be continued once hepatitis A is excluded. Extra precautions, such as double gloving during delivery, are wise in cases of hepatitis B and C.

Complications. The case fatality rate for nonpregnant patients with acute hepatitis is 0.1 percent, and for those ill enough to be hospitalized it is as high as 1 percent. Most fatalities are due to **fulminant hepatic necrosis,** which in later pregnancy must be distinguished from acute fatty liver. About half of patients with fulminant hepatitis have infection with B virus, and many of these are associated with the delta agent. **Hepatic encephalopathy** is the usual presentation of patients with fulminant hepatitis, and mortality is 80 percent.

A small number of patients with hepatitis A infection have **relapsing hepatitis,** in which there is recurrence of symptoms and biochemical abnormalities weeks to months after recovery from acute infection. Some form of chronic hepatitis B infection follows acute disease in 5 to 10 percent of cases. Most of these patients will be **asymptomatic carriers,** but others have low-grade **chronic persistent hepatitis** or **chronic active hepatitis with or without cirrhosis.** Transfusion-related hepatitis C infection is associated with a high incidence of persistently abnormal biochemical tests, chronic active hepatitis, and cirrhosis.

Hepatitis A. Viral hepatitis A was previously referred to as **infectious hepatitis.** It is caused by a 27-nm RNA picornavirus classified as enterovirus type 72. It is transmitted by the fecal–oral route. Individuals developing this disease shed virus in their feces, and during the relatively brief period of viremia their blood is also infectious. The infection is usually spread by ingestion of contaminated blood or water, and the incubation period is about 2 to 7 weeks. The signs and symptoms are not very specific, and it may go undiagnosed or be considered an influenza-like illness unless jaundice is detected; however, the majority of cases are anicteric.

Serological confirmation can be done even when serum transaminase levels are still elevated. Early detection is by identification of IgM antibody (Table 51–7). Although this indicates acute infection, it may persist for several months. During convalescence, IgG antibody predominates; it persists and is responsible for immu-

nity from subsequent hepatitis A infection. A formalin-inactivated vaccine has been licensed in the United Kingdom, Switzerland, Belgium, Austria, and Iceland, and is reported to be 97 percent effective (Editorial, 1992).

Hepatitis A and Pregnancy. In developed countries, the effects of hepatitis A on pregnancy are not dramatic. However, at least in some underprivileged populations, both perinatal and maternal deaths are substantively increased. Treatment consists of a well-balanced diet and diminished activity. We have long followed the policy of hospitalizing all pregnant women with hepatitis until it is clear that they are able to eat and drink, and that liver function is improving, or at least, not continuing to deteriorate. Women with less severe illness may be managed as outpatients (American College of Obstetricians and Gynecologists, 1992b).

There is no evidence that hepatitis A virus is teratogenic. Risk of transmission to the fetus is negligible, and to the newborn infant it is quite small. The risk of preterm birth appears to be increased somewhat for pregnancies complicated by hepatitis A (Steven, 1981).

The pregnant woman who has been recently exposed to hepatitis A should be given gamma globulin prophylactically (see Chap. 9, p. 264).

Hepatitis B. Viral hepatitis B, once referred to as **serum hepatitis,** is found worldwide but is endemic in some regions, especially in Asia and Africa. Hepatitis B is a DNA hepadnavirus type 1.

Hepatitis B infection is a major cause of acute hepatitis as well as its serious sequelae, namely chronic hepatitis, cirrhosis, and hepatocellular carcinoma. The latter is so common that the World Health Organization considers hepatitis B to be second only to tobacco among human carcinogens. The most serious consequences are the result of chronic infection, which occurs in 5 to 10 percent of infected adults and 70 to 90 percent of infected infants. According to the Centers for Disease Control (1991), there are approximately 300,000 cases of acute hepatitis B in the United States annually, but only half are icteric and symptomatic. There are an estimated 1 million chronic carriers.

A variety of immunological markers to hepatitis B have been identified in patients with acute or chronic disease, in those who have had the disease and now are immune, and in chronic carriers. The hepatitis B virus (Dane particle), core antigen (HB_cAg), surface antigen (HB_sAg), e antigen (HB_eAg), and their corresponding antibodies are all detectable by various techniques. The virus is unique in that concentrations of viral antigen and particles in serum and other body fluids may reach 10 trillion per mL.

Hepatitis B infections are found most often among intravenous drug abusers, homosexuals, health care personnel, and patients who have been treated often with

TABLE 51–7. SIMPLIFIED DIAGNOSTIC APPROACH IN PATIENTS WITH HEPATITIS

Diagnosis	Serological Test		
	HB_sAG	IgM Anti-HAV	IgM Anti-HB_c
Acute hepatitis B	+	−	+
Chronic hepatitis B	+	−	−
Acute hepatitis A with chronic hepatitis B	+	+	−
Acute hepatitis A and B	+	+	+
Acute hepatitis A	−	+	−
Compatible with non-A, non-B hepatitis	−	−	−

Modified from Dienstag and associates (1991).

blood products, such as hemophiliacs. It is transmitted by infected blood or blood products, and in saliva, vaginal secretions, and semen; thus, it is a sexually transmitted disease. The e antigen correlates with infectivity and the presence of intact viral particles.

After infection with hepatitis B, the first virological marker is HB_sAg (Fig. 51–4). Hepatitis B infection is diagnosed by detection of HB_sAg in serum, and only rarely is this test falsely negative. Although HB_cAg invariably is present during early acute hepatitis, its persistence indicates chronic infection. Approximately 90 percent of persons with hepatitis B infections recover completely.

Hepatitis B and Pregnancy. The course of hepatitis B infection in the mother does not seem to be altered by pregnancy, at least in developed countries. As discussed, **fulminant hepatitis** may occasionally complicate hepatitis B infections, but does not seem to be more prevalent during pregnancy. Treatment is supportive. As with hepatitis A, the likelihood for preterm delivery is increased.

Transplacental viral transfer from the mother to the fetus is thought to be rare (Goudeau and co-workers, 1983). Instead, infection of the fetus or infant is by ingestion of infected material during delivery or exposure subsequent to birth. The infant may possibly obtain the virus through breast feeding. Some infected infants are asymptomatic, but others develop fulminant disease and succumb. The majority, nearly 85 percent, become chronic carriers who can infect others. They are also at appreciable risk for later development of hepatocellular carcinoma, cirrhosis, or both.

The discovery of the e antigen of hepatitis B virus and its correlation with the number of circulating viral particles led to recognition that vertical transmission of hepatitis B correlates closely with the maternal e anti-

gen status. Mothers with hepatitis B surface antigen and e antigen are very likely to transmit the disease to their infants, whereas those who are negative for e antigen but positive for anti-HB_c antibody do not appear to transmit the infection.

Prevention of Neonatal Infection. The Centers for Disease Control (1990) estimates that about 18,000 infants were born in the United States in 1987 to HB_sAg-positive women. Without immunoprophylaxis given at delivery, nearly 4000 will become chronically infected with hepatitis B. Infection of the newborn whose mother chronically carries the virus can usually be prevented by the administration of hepatitis B immune globulin very soon after birth, followed promptly by hepatitis B vaccine (Beasley and associates, 1983; Hsu and co-workers, 1988). **For these reasons, the Centers for Disease Control (1988), as well as the American College of Obstetricians and Gynecologists (1992a, 1992b), recommend hepatitis B serological screening for all prenatal patients.** If positive, and especially if e antigen is identified in the mother, the offspring should be given hepatitis B immune globulin and recombinant vaccine. A second and third dose of vaccine are given at 1 and 6 months of age. We test only for Hb_sAg and vaccinate infants of all positive mothers. Importantly, for high-risk mothers who test antigen-negative, vaccine can be provided during pregnancy.

PRENATAL HEPATITIS SCREENING. Cruz and colleagues (1987), Kumar and associates (1987), and Wetzel and Kirz (1987) have provided data that justify the cost effectiveness of hepatitis carrier screening for inner-city lower socioeconomic women in Gainesville, Cleveland, and Chicago. Butterfield and colleagues (1990) reached similar conclusions for a military population. Surface antigen positivity prevalence in all of these studies was about 1 percent, but risk factors were not predictive. Greenspoon and colleagues (1989a) and Dinsmoor and Gibbs (1990) reported a lower rate (3 to 4 per 1000) for Mexican-American women in Los Angeles and San Antonio; however, because risk factors in these women were not predictive, they perform routine screening.

Wetzel and Kirz (1987) emphasized that one case of hepatitis B antigenemia costs only half as much to detect as one case of syphilis. Arevalo and Washington (1988) reviewed the literature and calculated that routine screening of all American women would result in net savings of $105 million annually. Conversely, Koretz (1989) estimated the cost to be $180,000 to prevent a clinically important case of hepatitis B in infants born to mothers with no risk factors. This cost was 15 times that for neonates born to women with risk factors, and he concluded that routine screening was not cost effective. Christian and Duff (1989) performed a serosurvey in another military population and found 0.66 percent of women to be seropositive. All of these women had high

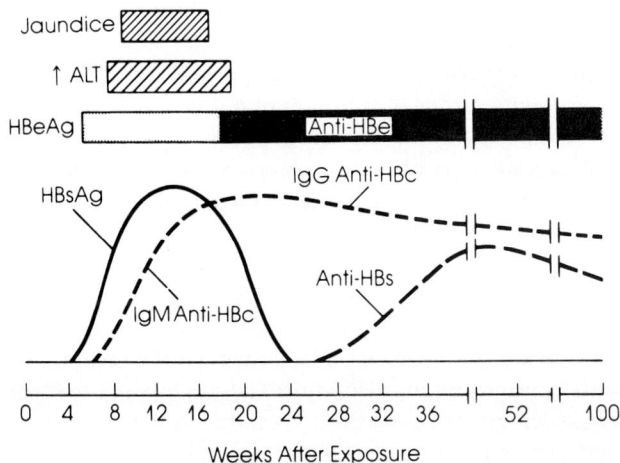

Jaundice

↑ ALT

HBeAg   Anti-HBe

HBsAg

IgG Anti-HBc

IgM Anti-HBc

Anti-HBs

0 4 8 12 16 20 24 28 32 36   52   100
Weeks After Exposure

Fig. 51–4. Acute hepatitis B—Appearance of various antigen and antibodies. (From Dienstag and associates, 1991, with permission.)

risk factors; thus, they concluded that it would be advisable and cost effective to selectively screen only high-risk mothers.

Delta Hepatitis. Delta hepatitis is a "defective" RNA virus that is a hybrid particle with a hepatitis B surface antigen coat and a delta core. The virus must co-infect with hepatitis B and cannot persist in serum longer than hepatitis B virus. Anti-delta antibody is produced only transiently unless chronic infection develops.

Transmission is similar to hepatitis B viral infection. Simultaneous infection with B and delta hepatitis is usually not more virulent than B alone; however, particularly virulent epidemics in homosexuals and parenteral drug abusers have been associated with a case fatality rate of 5 to 10 percent (Dienstag and colleagues, 1991; Lettau and colleagues, 1987). Neonatal transmission has been reported, but it seems reasonable to assume that hepatitis B vaccination will prevent delta hepatitis.

Hepatitis C. Hepatitis C virus is an RNA virus of the family flaviviridae. Its recent identification was made possible by development of an assay to detect anti-hepatitis C antibody. There may be two major types of non-A, non-B hepatitis, but hepatitis C virus is thought to be responsible for 80 percent of infections caused by bloodborne non-A, non-B infections. Conversely, hepatitis C virus does not seem to be the agent responsible for enterically transmitted non-A, non-B infections. The Centers for Disease Control (1991) estimate that there are about 150,000 new infections annually and that about one fourth develop icterus or other symptoms of hepatitis. If hepatitis C is acquired through transfusion, about 40 percent of patients have evidence of chronic hepatitis at 5 years; however, if infection is community acquired, then this is less than 20 percent.

Transmission of hepatitis C infection appears to be identical to hepatitis B, and thus it is more prevalent in intravenous drug abusers and hemophiliacs, and is sexually transmitted. After acute infection, anti-C antibody is not detected for an average of 15 weeks, and in some cases it is not detectable for a year. Unfortunately, current antibody assays do not differentiate between infectious and noninfectious persons, and it must be presumed that all antibody-positive patients are capable of transmitting infection.

The incidence of persistent disease is common after hepatitis C infection. As many as 50 percent of patients with transfusion-related non-A, non-B (and presumably C) infections have abnormal biochemical liver tests for more than a year. In most of these, liver biopsy shows chronic active hepatitis, which in 20 percent will progress to cirrhosis within 10 years (Dienstag and associates, 1991). Interferon-α has been used with some success for treatment.

Screening of blood donors should markedly decrease the incidence of posttransfusion hepatitis. In the past, nearly 90 percent of individuals who developed hepatitis after blood or its products had non-A, non-B hepatitis. In one study, 18 of 842 cardiac surgery patients developed posttransfusion hepatitis, and 14 were attributed to non-A, non-B hepatitis (Cossart and colleagues, 1982). Most cases are anicteric and are not diagnosed.

Hepatitis C also may be contracted from an infected sexual partner, and the injection of some preparations of human immunoglobulin has been implicated in the causation of non-A, non-B hepatitis (Lane, 1983).

Effect on Pregnancy. There is little published experience with the clinical course of hepatitis C complicating pregnancy, but there is no reason to believe that it is different compared with that in nonpregnant women. Thaler and colleagues (1991) have demonstrated that hepatitis C is transmitted vertically at birth. Bohman and colleagues (1992) reported our experiences from Parkland Hospital with asymptomatic pregnant women who were seropositive for anti-C antibody. The prevalence of antibody was 2.3 percent, and risk factors included intravenous drug use, sexually transmitted diseases, increased age and parity, history of transfusions, multiple sex partners, and sex partners who used intravenous drugs. Perinatal outcome was not adversely affected in seropositive women compared with seronegative controls.

According to the Centers for Disease Control (1990), studies to evaluate immune serum globulin for prophylaxis against non-A, non-B hepatitis have been equivocal. Until such data are conclusive, it seems reasonable to administer immune globulin to the newborn of the mother who has anti-C antibody, because it may prevent disease acquisition by the offspring.

Chronic Active Hepatitis

Chronic active hepatitis is a disorder of varying etiology that is characterized by continuing hepatic necrosis, active inflammation, and fibrosis that may lead to cirrhosis and liver failure. Most cases are due to chronic infection with either B or non-A, non-B hepatitis. Another cause is autoimmune chronic hepatitis, characterized by high serum titers of homogeneous antinuclear antibodies. In both forms, there is evidence that a cellular immune reaction is interactive with a genetic predisposition.

The diagnosis is suspected clinically, but must be confirmed by liver biopsy. Clinical characteristics of the disease are an insidious onset over weeks to months with intermittent malaise, anorexia, and low-grade fever with recurrent or persistent jaundice. In some patients, cirrhosis is the presenting finding. The course is variable, sometimes with long periods of clinical remission; however, progression to cirrhosis is the rule.

Chronic Hepatitis and Pregnancy. The effect of pregnancy on chronic active hepatitis, as well as the effects of the disease on pregnancy outcome, will depend in large part on the intensity of the disease and whether there is portal hypertension or hepatic failure. Pregnancy is uncommon when disease is severe because anovulation is common. However, corticosteroids, alone or combined with azathioprine, have increased both fertility and survival in women with autoimmune chronic hepatitis. The beneficial effects of therapy in asymptomatic women is unclear, and neither drug is effective in patients with hepatitis B-associated chronic infection. Although interferon-α produces serological remission in up to 50 percent of carriers of chronic hepatitis B and C infections, whether this agent is effective to prevent or treat chronic active hepatitis remains to be determined.

Steven and associates (1979) concluded that with chronic active hepatitis (1) fertility is reduced, but pregnancies can proceed without serious detriment to the mother if corticosteroid treatment is maintained; (2) fetal loss will be increased; and (3) preterm delivery will be common but malformations are not increased. The few women who we have managed have done well, but because their long-term prognosis is poor, they should be counseled regarding abortion and sterilization.

Cirrhosis

Hepatic cirrhosis is characterized by irreversible chronic injury to the liver parenchyma with extensive fibrosis and regenerative nodules. In all patients, chronic exposure to alcohol is the most common cause. In young women, however—and thus most pregnant women—postnecrotic cirrhosis from hepatitis is the most common cause. Other causes include biliary cirrhosis from long-standing obstruction and cardiac cirrhosis from chronic right-sided heart failure. Although cirrhosis is the final common pathway for a variety of hepatic injuries, the clinical manifestations are inseparable. These include jaundice, edema, coagulopathy, metabolic abnormalities, and portal hypertension along with its sequelae of gastroesophageal varices and splenomegaly.

Cirrhosis and Pregnancy. Women with cirrhosis are very likely to be infertile. Cheng (1977) reviewed pregnancy outcomes and concluded that perinatal loss is high and maternal prognosis grave. Esophageal varices were prone to bleed, with fatal hemorrhage as the consequence. Schreyer and associates (1982) confirmed the high morbidity and appreciable mortality associated with cirrhosis. They reviewed 69 pregnancies in 60 women without shunts and 28 pregnancies in 23 women who had undergone portal decompression shunting. Severe variceal hemorrhage was increased sevenfold in non-

shunted women compared with those who had undergone such procedures (24 versus 3.3 percent). The authors suggested that the high incidence of esophageal hemorrhage, and in turn the high mortality rate, might be decreased by prophylactic portal-systemic shunting. They also hastened to emphasize that the procedure and its sequelae are not benign.

Esophageal Varices

Esophageal varices may complicate portal venous hypertension that results from cirrhosis or from extrahepatic portal vein obstruction. Postnecrotic hepatitis and chronic alcoholism account for almost all cases of portal hypertension due to liver disease in young women. A seeming equal number of cases of esophageal varices, at least in pregnant women, are caused by **extrahepatic portal hypertension.** About half of these are idiopathic, but a number arise as a complication of umbilical vein catheterization in the neonate. With increasing salvage of very small preterm infants who survive to childbearing age, this entity is expected to be encountered more commonly during pregnancy.

Whatever its underlying cause, portal vein pressure rises from its normal value of 10 to 15 mm Hg to exceed 30 mm Hg. This leads to formation of collateral circulation, which carries blood to the systemic circulation. Drainage is via the gastric, intercostal, and other veins ultimately to the esophageal system, where varices develop. Bleeding from varices is usually near the gastroesophageal junction. Bleeding can be torrential, and whole blood and clotting factors are given as needed (see Chap. 37, p. 821). In some cases, bleeding can be stopped with a triple-lumen tube, but this is not always successful. Emergency shunting procedures may be necessary, but these are associated with high mortality. Recently, endoscopically guided **sclerotherapy** for control of acute hemorrhage has been used for acute hemorrhage, and some have found it preferential in preventing subsequent bleeding episodes.

Varices in Pregnancy. Bleeding from esophageal varices causes much of the maternal mortality associated with cirrhosis. Britton (1982) reviewed outcomes in 160 pregnancies complicated by cirrhosis, varices, or both (Table 51–8). Bleeding was common when pregnancy was complicated by varices, regardless of whether there was cirrhosis. Conversely, mortality depended heavily on varices associated with cirrhosis. They showed that maternal mortality from bleeding in women with cirrhosis was 18 percent, but in those without cirrhosis it was only 2 percent. As expected, perinatal mortality was common.

Sclerotherapy. In recent years, endoscopically directed injection of a sclerosing solution has been used to con-

TABLE 51-8. OUTCOMES IN 160 PREGNANCIES COMPLICATED BY CIRRHOSIS, ESOPHAGEAL VARICES, OR BOTH

Outcome	Cirrhosis	Varices without Cirrhosis
Patients	53	38
Varices	35/53	38/38
Pregnancies	83	77
Bleeding during pregnancy at risk	13/21 (62%)	25/54 (46%)
Operation during pregnancy	5	2
Pregnancy outcome		
Losses		
Abortions	14	10
Stillborn	4	5
Neonatal death	3	2
Vaginal delivery	59	43
Cesarean section	11	11
Maternal mortality	7	2

Modified from Britton (1982), with permission.

trol variceal bleeding. Such sclerotherapy is at least 90 percent effective in controlling hemorrhage in nonpregnant patients. When used repeatedly, it decreases the number of subsequent bleeding episodes. This has now been successfully used during pregnancy (Kochhar and colleagues, 1990; Pauzner and associates, 1991). Our preliminary results with sclerotherapy have also been successful for esophageal variceal bleeding but less so for gastric varices.

Acute Acetaminophen Overdosage

Acetaminophen is commonly used during pregnancy. Acute overdosage with suicidal attempts is relatively common, and may lead to acute liver failure. Early symptoms of overdosage are nausea, vomiting, diaphoresis, malaise, and pallor. After a latent period of 24 to 48 hours, liver failure begins to manifest, and usually begins to resolve in 5 days.

The antidote is *N*-acetylcysteine and it must be given promptly. The drug is thought to act by increasing glutathione levels, which facilitates metabolism of the toxic metabolite. The need for treatment is based on projections of possible plasma hepatotoxic levels as a function of the time of acute ingestion. Many use the nomogram established by Rumack and Matthew (1975). Plasma levels are obtained 4 hours after ingestion, and if greater than 120 μg/mL, treatment is given. If plasma determinations are not available, empirical treatment is given if the dose exceeded 7.5 g. An oral loading dose of 140 mg/kg of *N*-acetylcysteine is followed by 17 maintenance doses of 70 mg/kg every 4 hours for 72 hours total treatment time.

After 14 weeks, the fetus has some cytochrome P-450 activity, which is necessary for metabolism of acetaminophen to the toxic metabolite. Riggs and colleagues (1989) reported data from the Rocky Mountain Poison and Drug Center and described follow-up experiences in 60 such women. The likelihood of maternal and fetal survival was better if the antidote was given soon after overdosage. The one mother who died was not treated until 16 to 24 hours after ingestion. At least one 33-week fetus appears to have died as a direct result of hepatotoxicity 2 days after ingestion.

Liver Transplantation

Liver transplantation was first performed in the United States in 1963, and the first successful pregnancy in a recipient in 1972 was reported by Walcott and associates (1978). According to Starzl and colleagues (1989a,b) the number of liver transplants done in the United States in 1988 was 1600, but as many as 50,000 may be indicated.

Because of its growing use, it is not surprising that a number of women have had pregnancies following liver transplantation. The Pittsburgh group reported their experiences with 19 pregnancies in 17 such women (Scantlebury and colleagues, 1990). Most of these women had stable serum hepatic transaminase levels during pregnancy. Four women with mild enzyme elevations did well, and 3 with moderate elevation had acute or chronic rejection or hepatitis. Including the one set of twins, all 20 infants were born alive, but pregnancy complications included hypertension in 50 percent, anemia in 25 percent, and preterm delivery in 60 percent. Neuropsychiatric complications were also common. At 2 to 18 years after transplantation, 16 of 17 mothers were still living. These investigators cited concern for side effects of immunosuppressive treatment with corticosteroids and cyclosporine. In another report, they showed efficient transfer of cyclosporine from mother to fetus, and cord serum levels of the drug were about half of those obtained in maternal serum (Venkataramanan and associates, 1988).

Contraception. Hill and colleagues (1991) reported that 5 of 10 spontaneous conceptions after liver transplantation occurred within 12 months of the operation. They emphasized the need for contraception in these women, and recommended that pregnancy be delayed for at least a year because this is the period at greatest risk for complications. Whether oral contraceptive are contraindicated is conjectural. Laifer and colleagues (1990) advise against their use because of the high incidence of hypertension in these women. They also emphasized the known hepatic effects of contraceptive steroids, as well as their effect on cyclosporine elimination, which potentiates its hepatotoxicity.

DISEASES OF THE GALLBLADDER AND PANCREAS

Cholelithiasis and Cholecystitis

In the United States, 20 percent of women over 40 have gallstones. Over 80 percent of stones contain cholesterol, and its oversecretion into bile is thought to be a major factor in their pathogenesis. *Biliary sludge,* which may increase during pregnancy, is an important precursor to gallstone formation. The cumulative risk of a patient with silent gallstones to require surgery for symptoms or complications is about 1 to 2 percent per year; it is 10 percent at 5 years, 15 percent at 10 years, and 18 percent at 15 years (Greenberger and Isselbacher, 1991). For these reasons, many feel that prophylactic cholecystectomy is not warranted for asymptomatic stones.

A number of nonsurgical approaches have been used for gallstone disease. These include oral bile acid therapy with chenodeoxycholic acid, extracorporeal shock wave lithotripsy, and contact dissolution with methyl tert-butyl ether placed directly into the gallbladder. There is no experience with any of these methods during pregnancy, and they are currently not recommended.

Acute cholecystitis usually develops when there is obstruction of the cystic duct. Bacterial infection plays a role in 50 to 85 percent of these acute inflammatory conditions. In over half of patients with acute cholecystitis, a history of previous right-upper-quadrant pain from cholelithiasis is elicited. With acute disease, pain is accompanied by anorexia, nausea and vomiting, low-grade fever, and mild leukocytosis. Ultrasonography can be used to visualize stones as small as 2 mm, and false-positive and false-negative rates for diagnosing gallstones is about 2 to 4 percent (Greenberger and Isselbacher, 1991). Ultrasonic examination confirms gallstones in about 90 percent of patients (Fig. 51–5).

About 75 percent of nonpregnant patients with acute cholecystitis respond to medical therapy consisting of nasogastric suction, intravenous fluids and antimicrobials, and analgesics (Greenberger and Isselbacher, 1991). The remaining 25 percent require cholecystectomy for persistent pain or gangrene, empyema, or perforation of the gallbladder.

Gallbladder Disease During Pregnancy. Gallbladder kinetics during pregnancy using real-time sonography have been investigated by Braverman and associates (1980). After the first trimester, both gallbladder volume during fasting and residual volume after contracting in response to a test meal were twice as great as in nonpregnant subjects. Incomplete emptying may result in retention of cholesterol crystals, a prerequisite for cholesterol gallstones. These findings are supportive of the view that pregnancy increases the risk of gallstones. Presumably, the very high progesterone levels that characterize the second and third trimester, are responsible for diminished gallbladder motility. Singletary and colleagues (1986) established that gallbladder tissue has both nuclear and cytosolic receptors for estrogens and progesterone. Progesterone has been shown to impair the gallbladder response to exogenously administered cholecystokinin in experimental animals. *Biliary sludge,* probably a forerunner to gallstones, was immediately seen ultrasonically in one fourth of nearly 300 postpartum women. A year later, only 4 percent had persistent sludge.

Management. In general, acute cholecystitis during pregnancy or the puerperium is managed in a manner similar as for nonpregnant women. Landers and colleagues (1987) reported their experiences with 30 women with acute cholecystitis complicating pregnancy. The incidence was about 1 in 1000 deliveries. Gallstones were successfully visualized in 96 percent of women undergoing ultrasonic scanning. Although 21 of these women presented for care before the third trimes-

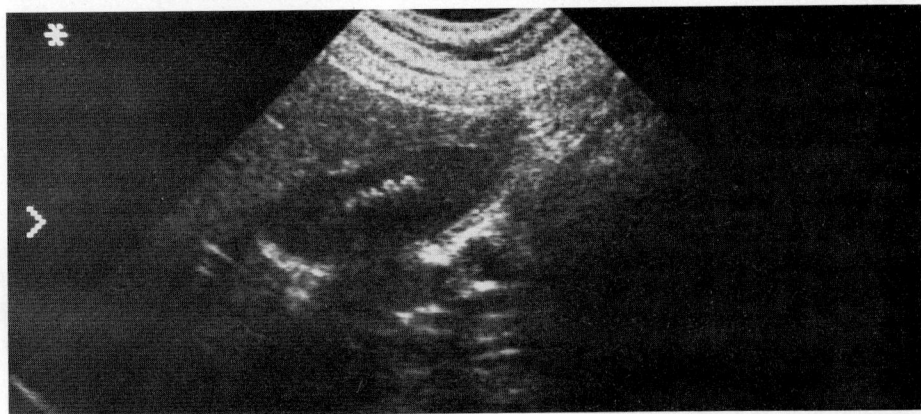

Fig. 51–5. Mulitple floating gallstones visualized in a 26-week pregnant woman. (Photograph courtesy of Dr. Diane Twickler.)

ter, these investigators elected medical therapy in 25. Such therapy was successful in 21, and the other 4 women required cholecystectomy for persistent or worsening pain. In 5 of 30 women, cholecystectomy was performed primarily.

Dixon and colleagues (1987) preferred more aggressive surgical management, and performed cholecystectomy in 18 of 44 women with acute cholecystitis or cholelithiasis with biliary colic. The women treated surgically did well; in contrast, 15 of the 26 managed medically had recurrent disease during pregnancy. Multiple hospitalizations were common in the latter group, and 2 women required prolonged parenteral nutrition during late pregnancy. Similarly, Hiatt and associates (1986) performed cholecystectomy and cholangiography during pregnancy in 9 of 26 women with acute cholecystis. These women all did well.

It seems reasonable to consider cholecystectomy for acute cholecystitis diagnosed during pregnancy. If cholecystectomy is to be performed during pregnancy, many consider the second trimester to be the optimal time, because the risk of abortion is lower and that of preterm labor and delivery is reduced; moreover, the uterus is not yet large enough to impinge on the operative field. **Regardless, when surgery is thought to be indicated in the pregnant woman, procrastination should be avoided.** Delay can only place the woman and her fetus in greater jeopardy. At times, gallbladder drainage may be the procedure of choice. Recent surgery does not complicate labor except for incisional discomfort.

Asymptomatic Gallstones During Pregnancy. Because of their prevalence in the general population, it is perhaps expected that gallstones would be relatively common findings in asymptomatic pregnant women. Indeed, an incidence of ultrasonically visualized asymptomatic stones of 2.5 to 5 percent during pregnancy or the puerperium has been reported in over 800 women (Chesson, 1985; Maringhini, 1987; Stauffer, 1982; and their colleagues). Although ideal treatment for silent stones is debated, pregnancy is not the appropriate time for surgical removal if they remain asymptomatic.

Other Treatment for Gallstone Disease. Stones obstructing the common bile duct can be removed using **endoscopic retrograde cholangiopancreatography (ERCP)** along with sphincterotomy. This procedure has been used in pregnant women, but experiences are limited (Baillie and colleagues, 1990). **Laparoscopic cholecystectomy** is evolving in this country as the primary operation for gallbladder disease, but there is currently little experience with the technique during pregnancy. Although Gadacz and Talamini (1991) list pregnancy as an absolute contraindication, laparoscopic cholecystectomy has been used without complication in a 31-week pregnant woman (Pucci and Seed, 1991).

Acute Pancreatitis

In nonpregnant patients, acute pancreatitis is most likely associated with chronic alcohol ingestion; but during pregnancy, cholelithiasis is a more common predisposing condition. Why inflammation is triggered is unclear, but there is activation of pancreatic enzymes followed by autodigestion characterized by cellular membrane disruption and proteolysis, edema, hemorrhage, and necrosis. There are a number of associated causes. In addition to alcohol abuse and cholelithiasis, pancreatitis is encountered more commonly in the postoperative patient, and it is associated with trauma, certain metabolic conditions including acute fatty liver of pregnancy, familial hypertriglyceridemia, and some viral infections; or it may be drug-associated.

Clinically, acute pancreatitis is characterized by mild to incapacitating epigastric pain, nausea and vomiting, and abdominal distension. Patients are usually in distress and have low-grade fever and tachycardia; hypotension is common. Findings include abdominal tenderness, and up to 10 percent of patients have associated pulmonary findings. Serum amylase levels three times upper normal values are confirmatory, but there is no correlation with their degree of elevation and severity of disease. In fact, usually by 48 to 72 hours, serum amylase levels return to normal despite evidence for continuing pancreatitis. Other conditions may cause hyperamylasemia, and measurement of serum lipase activity increases the diagnostic yield. There is usually leukocytosis, and 25 percent of patients have hypocalcemia. Serum bilirubin and aspartate aminotransferase levels are usually elevated somewhat.

A number of prognostic factors may be used to predict severity of the disease. These include respiratory failure, shock, need for massive colloid replacement, hypocalcemia of less than 8 mg/dL, or dark hemorrhagic fluid on paracentesis. If three of the first four features are documented, survival is only 30 percent.

Management is medical and includes analgesics for pain, intravenous hydration, and measures to decrease pancreatic secretion by proscribing oral intake. Nasogastric suction has not been shown to improve the outcome in mild to moderate disease. Antimicrobials are not indicated unless there is evidence of established infection. In most patients, acute pancreatitis is self-limited and in 90 percent inflammation subsides within 3 to 7 days after treatment. For patients with unrelenting disease, intensive supportive therapy is given, and laparotomy with debridement and drainage may be life-saving.

Complications. In some cases, a pancreatic **phlegmon** develops. Imaging studies may be necessary to distinguish this from a pseudocyst or abscess. Sonography will usually confirm a **pseudocyst,** but differentiation between an abscess and phlegmon is more difficult, even if computed tomography is used. A **pancreatic abscess** must be drained or mortality is high. Pseudocysts develop in perhaps 15 percent of all patients following acute inflammation, and although at least half subside spontaneously, persistent pseudocysts should be drained because they may rupture subsequently with disastrous results.

Pancreatitis During Pregnancy. Pregnancy does not predispose to pancreatitis, and its incidence reflects that of otherwise healthy young women. At Parkland Hospital, pancreatitis complicates about 1 in 3000 pregnancies (Ramin and colleagues, 1993). Unlike nonpregnant patients, these women seldom have associated alcoholism; however, cholelithiasis commonly coexists (Block and Kelly, 1989). Certainly, the predisposition of pregnancy toward gallstone formation may indirectly link pregnancy with pancreatitis. In a small number of pregnant women with pancreatitis, there is an associated familial hyperlipidemic syndrome, usually hypertriglyceridemia (Nies and Dreiss, 1990). Sanderson and colleagues (1991) described a woman in whom aggressive dietary therapy and intermittent intravenous glucose feedings ostensibly prevented recurrent pancreatitis in her fourth term pregnancy. Watts and associates (1992) described two pregnant women with hypertriglyceridemia due to familial lipoprotein lipase deficiency.

The diagnosis of pancreatitis during pregnancy is made using the same criteria as in nonpregnant patients. Abdominal pain is almost always present. Despite earlier reports, Strickland and colleagues (1984) found no significant change in serum amylase levels in 413 normal women studied at various stages of gestation and again 6 weeks postpartum. Ordorica and associates (1991) confirmed these findings, and showed also that serum lipase levels were not changed during pregnancy. Serial determinations of serum amylase and lipase activity remain the best methods to confirm the clinical diagnosis of pancreatitis. Block and Kelly (1989) reported that in all 21 pregnant or recently pregnant women with pancreatitis, serum amylase values exceeded 1500 IU/L. Of 35 pregnant women with pancreatitis admitted to Parkland Hospital, the mean amylase level was 1370 IU/L and the mean lipase level was 7975 IU/L (Ramin and associates, 1993). Importantly, amylase values do not correlate with the severity of disease.

Management. The principles of therapy are the same as for nonpregnant patients; thus, primary treatment is medical. Mild inflammation usually subsides in response to conservative therapy. Because most cases are associated with gallstone disease, consideration is given to cholecystectomy after inflammation subsides. Block and Kelly (1989) described their experiences with 11 women with antepartum gallstone pancreatitis. One woman required cholecystectomy shortly after admission for persistent pancreatitis. Women in whom pancreatitis was encountered before the third trimester underwent cholecystectomy after acute inflammation subsided. In 4 of 5 women in the third trimester, surgery was postponed until after delivery. In women with severe disease, fetal loss is high because of associated hypovolemia, hypoxia, and acidosis.

Chronic Pancreatitis

Symptoms of chronic pancreatitis are similar to those of acute disease, and in fact, chronic disease may be represented by exacerbations of acute inflammation. Although alcoholism is common, chronic relapsing pancreatitis is often idiopathic. In many cases, the serum amylase concentration and lipase activity may be normal. Diffuse pancreatic calcifications frequently are seen using sonography or computed tomography. In about one third of cases, such calcifications are found, along with steatorrhea from exocrine insufficiency and diabetes.

There is little experience with chronic pancreatic disease during pregnancy. Exocrine insufficiency complicating **cystic fibrosis** is common and is discussed in Chapter 49 (p. 1120).

Pancreatic Transplantation

According to the International Pancreas Transplant Registry, there were about 3000 pancreatic transplantations done in the 4-year period ending in 1990 (Östman, 1991). Although the 1-year graft survival has recently been almost 70 percent, there is far improved survival when a combined pancreas and kidney are grafted; thus, most operations include both organs. Diabetes accounts for about one fourth of cases of renal failure leading to kidney transplantation (see Chap. 50, p. 1138). Currently, many such patients receiving transplanted kidneys are also undergoing pancreatic transplantation; thus, it should be encountered with some frequency in pregnant women.

Tydén and colleagues (1989) described 4 women in whom pancreatic–kidney transplantation was followed in 1 to 2 years by pregnancy. Because of pelvic placement of the pancreatic graft, there was concern that the enlarging uterus or labor might cause pancreatitis, but this did not occur. Glucose homeostasis was well-maintained throughout pregnancy. Of concern is the one woman who suffered pancreatic graft acute rejection postpartum. Prior to this time, the graft had functioned well for 3 years.

Obesity

Obesity is not easy to define. The etiology of obesity is usually multifactorial, and although it is not a GI disorder, it is considered here. One acceptable method for ascertaining the definition of obesity is by using the **body mass index** derived from weight in kilograms divided by height in meters squared. The 1985 National Institutes of Health consensus panel on obesity defined obesity as a 20 percent increase in body weight or a body mass index greater than the 85th percentile, which is 27.3 for women aged 20 to 29. Using this latter definition, in the United States, 30 percent of young adult men and almost 40 percent of young adult women are obese. Morbidity of obesity is from risks involved for diabetes, hypertension, and heart disease. For example, although only a minority of obese individuals have type II diabetes, almost 90 percent of those with maturity-onset diabetes are obese.

Effects of Obesity on Pregnancy.

Marked obesity is a hazard to the pregnant woman and her fetus. Because there are no standardized definitions of obesity, investigators have used a variety of classifications. Calandra and colleagues (1981) assessed pregnancy performance in women whose weight was above the 95th percentile. They reported a 10-fold increased incidence of chronic hypertension and a 17 percent incidence of gestational diabetes. Garbaciak and associates (1985) defined morbid obesity as greater than 150 percent of ideal weight. They too found that chronic hypertension was increased about 10-fold and gestational diabetes was found in about 10 percent of these women. As expected, in both studies infants were larger in the obese women.

Johnson and colleagues (1987) described the pregnancy outcomes of 588 women who weighed more than 250 pounds and who were cared for at the University of Iowa from 1961 to 1980. Complications were common, and those found to be significantly different when compared with a group of control women who weighed less than 200 pounds are shown in Table 51–9. The incidences of hypertension, diabetes, and postterm pregnancy were increased substantively. These factors led to a higher oxytocin induction and augmentation rate, as well as a doubled primary cesarean rate. Moreover, anesthetic and postoperative complications are increased. Our experiences at Parkland Hospital are similar, and we also have identified obesity, further complicated by hypertension, to be a cause of peripartum heart failure (Cunningham and associates, 1986). Finally, Wolfe and colleagues (1990) reported difficulty in sonographic fetal visualization in women whose body mass index was greater than the 90th percentile.

Management.

Management of obesity during pregnancy is a challenge. The usual net caloric increase during normal pregnancy ranges from 20,000 to 40,000 kcal and about 3.6 kg of gained weight is fat (Kliegman and Gross, 1985). A program of weight reduction is probably unrealistic, but if such a regimen is chosen, it is mandatory that the quality of the diet be monitored closely and that ketosis be avoided. The effects of caloric control in the obese woman with gestational diabetes are considered in Chapter 53 (p. 1205).

Surgical Procedures for Obesity

Gastric Surgery.

Various means to surgically decrease gastric volume have been devised to treat morbid obesity. **Gastroplasty** creates a narrow channel through the stomach by using stapling devices. **Gastric bypass** excludes the lower 90 percent of stomach by creating an upper gastrojejunostomy. Printen and Scott (1982) have described their experiences with 51 pregnancies in 45 women who underwent gastric bypass surgery because of morbid obesity. Of the 46 infants delivered, fetal growth retardation was not a problem, but one had a serious malformation. They concluded that neither the mother nor the developing fetus is endangered unduly by a pregnancy conceived subsequent to the period of rapid postoperative weight loss.

Richards and colleagues (1987) reported similar experiences from 57 pregnancies cared for at the University of Utah. These women weighed an average of 194 pounds before and 147 after surgery. Using pregnancies before gastric bypass as controls, they showed that the mean birthweight decreased from 3600 to 3200 g. They also found that only 16 percent of the women after bypass surgery had large-for-gestational age infants compared with an incidence of 37 percent before surgery. Importantly, the incidence of hypertension complicating pregnancy fell from 46 to 9 percent in women who had lost weight.

Jejunoileal Bypass.

Jejunoileal bypass has been followed by significant long-term morbidity and mortality, and the operation has been abandoned by most. Knudsen and Källén (1986) reported results of the Danish–

TABLE 51–9. PERCENTAGE OF COMPLICATIONS THAT WERE SIGNIFICANTLY INCREASED IN 588 OBESE (> 250 LB) WOMEN COMPARED TO 588 NONOBESE (< 200 LB) CONTROLS

Complications	Obese	Nonobese
Diabetes		
All types	10	2
Gestational	8	0.7
Hypertension	28	3
Postterm pregnancy	15	4
Oxytocin induction	23	8
Oxytocin augmentation	17	8
Macrosomic infant	24	7
Shoulder dystocia	5	0.6
Primary cesarean section	13	6
Wound infection	38	10
Excessive blood loss	38	14

Modified from Johnson and colleagues (1987).

Swedish registry of 77 pregnancies after intestinal bypass. They described a lower mean birthweight, shorter gestations, and more small-for-gestational-age infants when compared to normal control women.

At least 10 pregnant women with a jejunoileal bypass have been cared for at Parkland Hospital. Most of the pregnancies were quite benign. All of the women were given supplemental iron, folic acid, vitamin B_{12}, and a commercially available prenatal vitamin–mineral preparation. All but one infant were appropriately grown and in good health.

References

Allen JR, Helling TS, Langenfeld M: Intraabdominal surgery during pregnancy. Am J Surg 158:567, 1989

American College of Obstetricians and Gynecologists, Committee on Obstetrics: Maternal and Fetal Medicine: Guidelines for hepatitis B virus screening and vaccination during pregnancy. No. 111, May 1992a

American College of Obstetricians and Gynecologists: Hepatitis in Pregnancy. Technical bulletin no. 174, November, 1992b

Anderson AS, Whichelow MJ: Constipation during pregnancy: Dietary fibre intake and the effect of fibre supplementation. Hum Nutr Appl Nutr 39A:202, 1985

Arevalo JA, Washington E: Cost-effectiveness of prenatal screening and immunization for hepatitis B virus. JAMA 259:365, 1988

Baer JL, Reis RA, Arens RA: Appendicitis in pregnancy with changes in position and axis of normal appendix in pregnancy. JAMA 98:1359, 1932

Baillie J, Cairns SR, Putnam WS, Cotton PB: Endoscopic management of choledocholithiasis during pregnancy. Surg Gynecol Obstet 171:1, 1990

Baird DD, Narendranathan M, Sandler RS: Increased risk of preterm birth for women with inflammatory bowel disease. Gastroenterology 99:987, 1990

Barton JR, Sibai BM, Mabie WC, Shanklin DR: Recurrent acute fatty liver of pregnancy. Am J Obstet Gynecol 163:534, 1990

Beasley RP, Lee GCY, Roan CH, Hwang LY, Lan CC, Huang FY: Prevention of perinatally transmitted hepatitis B virus infections with hepatitis B immune globulin and hepatitis B vaccine. Lancet 2:1099, 1983

Block P, Kelley TR: Management of gallstone pancreatitis during pregnancy and the postpartum period. Surg Gynecol Obstet 168:426, 1989

Bohman V, Stettler RW, Little BB, Wendel G, Sutor LJ, Cunningham FG: Seroprevalence and risk factors for hepatitis C virus antibody in pregnant women. Obstet Gynecol 80:609, 1992

Boyce RA: Enteral nutrition in hyperemesis gravidarum: A new development. J Am Diet Assoc 92:733, 1992

Braverman DZ, Johnson ML, Kern F Jr: Effects of pregnancy and contraceptive steroids on gallbladder function. N Engl J Med 302:362, 1980

Briggs GG, Freeman RK, Yaffee SJ: Drugs in Pregnancy and Lactation, 3rd ed. Baltimore, Williams & Wilkins, 1990

Britton RC: Pregnancy and esophageal varices. Am J Surg 143:421, 1982

Brynskov J, Freund L, Rasmussen SN, Lauritsen K, de Muckadell OS, Williams N, MacDonald AS, Tanton R, Molia F, Campanini MC, Bianchi P, Ranzi T, Di Palo FQ, Malchow-Moller A, Thomsen OO, Tage-Jensen U, Binder V, Riis P: A placebo-controlled, double-blind, randomized trial of cyclosporin therapy in active chronic Crohn's disease. N Engl J Med 321:845, 1989

Burroughs AK, Seong NH, Dojcinov DM, Scheur PJ, Sherlock SVP: Idiopathic acute fatty liver of pregnancy in 12 patients. Q J Med 51:481, 1982

Butterfield CR, Shockley M, San Miguel G, Rosa C: Routine screening for hepatitis B in an obstetric population. Obstet Gynecol 76:25, 1990

Calandra C, Abell DA, Beischer NA: Maternal obesity in pregnancy. Obstet Gynecol 57:8, 1981

Castro LDP: Reflux esophagitis as the cause of heartburn in pregnancy. Am J Obstet Gynecol 98:1, 1967

Catanzarite VA, Arguright K, Mann BA, Brittain VL: Malnutrition during pregnancy: Consider parenteral feeding. Contemp Obstet Gynecol 27:110, 1986

Centers for Disease Control: Public health service interagency guidelines for screening donors of blood, plasma, organs, tissues, and semen for evidence of hepatitis B and hepatitis C. MMWR 40:1, 1991

Centers for Disease Control: Protection against viral hepatitis. Recommendations of the Immunization Practices Advisory Committee. MMWR 39:1, 1990

Centers for Disease Control: Prevention of perinatal transmission of hepatitis B virus. Recommendations of the Immunization Practices Advisory Committee: Prenatal screening of all pregnant women for hepatitis B surface antigen. MMWR 37:341, 1988

Cheng YS: Pregnancy in liver cirrhosis and/or portal hypertension. Am J Obstet Gynecol 128:812, 1977

Chesson RR, Gallup DG, Gibbs RL, Jones BE, Thomas B: Ultrasonographic diagnosis of asymptomatic cholelithiasis in pregnancy. J Reprod Med 30:921, 1985

Christian SS, Duff P: Is universal screening for hepatitis B infection warranted in all prenatal populations? Obstet Gynecol 74:259, 1989

Clark DH: Peptic ulcer in women. BMJ 2:1254, 1953

Cohen S: The sluggish gallbladder of pregnancy. N Engl J Med 302:397, 1980

Cohen S, Harris LD: Does hiatus hernia affect competence of the gastroesophageal sphincter? N Engl J Med 284A:1053, 1971

Combes B, Adams R, Gordon J, Trammell V, Shibata H: Hyperemesis gravidarum, II. Alterations in sulfobromophthalein sodium-removal mechanisms from blood. Obstet Gynecol 31:665, 1968

Cossart YE, Kirsch S, Ismay SL: Post-transfusion hepatitis in Australia. Lancet 1:208, 1982

Courtney MG, Nunes DP, Bergin CF, O'Driscoll M, Trimble V, Keeling PWN, Weir DG: Randomised comparison of olsalazine and mesalazine in prevention of relapses in ulcerative colitis. Lancet 339:1279, 1992

Crohn BB, Yarnis H, Walter RI, Gabrilov JL, Crohn EB: Ulcerative colitis as affected by pregnancy. NY J Med 56:2651, 1956

Cruz C, Frentzen BH, Behnke M: Hepatitis B: A case for prenatal screening of all patients. Am J Obstet Gynecol 156:1180, 1987

Cunningham FG, Lowe TW, Guss S, Mason R: Erythrocyte morphology in women with severe preeclampsia and eclampsia. Am J Obstet Gynecol 153:358, 1985

Cunningham FG, McCubbin JH: Appendicitis complicating pregnancy. Obstet Gynecol 45:415, 1975

Cunningham FG, Pritchard JA, Hankins GDV, Anderson PL, Lucas MK, Armstrong KF: Idiopathic cardiomyopathy or compounding cardiovascular events? Obstet Gynecol 67:157, 1986

Davis MR, Bohon CJ: Intestinal obstruction in pregnancy. Clin Obstet Gynecol 26:832, 1983

Depue RH, Bernstein L, Ross RK, Judd HL, Henderson BE: Hyperemesis gravidarum in relation to estradiol levels, pregnancy outcome, and other maternal factors: A seroepidemiologic study. Am J Obstet Gynecol 156:1137, 1987

DeVore GR: Acute abdominal pain in the pregnant patient due to pancreatitis, acute appendicitis, cholecystitis, or peptic ulcer disease. Clin Perinatol 7:349, 1980

Dienstag JL, Wands JR, Isselbacher KJ: Acute hepatitis. Chapter 252 in Wilson JD, Braunwald E, Isselbacher KJ, Petersdorf RG, Martin JB, Fauci AS, Root RK (eds): Harrison's Principles of Internal Medicine, 12th ed. New York, McGraw-Hill, 1991, p 1322

Dinsmoor MJ, Gibbs RS: Prevalence of asymptomatic hepatitis B infection in pregnant Mexican-American women. Obstet Gynecol 76:239, 1990

Dixon NF, Faddis DM, Silberman H: Aggressive management of cholecystitis during pregnancy. Am J Surg 154:294, 1987

Donaldson RM: Management of medical problems in pregnancy—inflammatory bowel disease. N Engl J Med 312:1618, 1985

Editorial: Hepatitis A: A vaccine at last. Lancet 339:1198, 1992

Farine D, Newhouse J, Owen J, Fox HE: Magnetic resonance imaging and computed tomography scan for the diagnosis of acute fatty liver of pregnancy. Am J Perinatol 4:316, 1990

Fedorkov DM, Persaud D, Nimrod MB: Inflammatory bowel disease: A controlled study of late pregnancy outcome. Am J Obstet Gynecol 160:998, 1989

Fisk NM, Bye WB, Storey GNB: Maternal features of obstetric cholestasis: 20 years experience at King George V Hospital. Aust NZ J Obstet Gynecol 28:172, 1988

Fisk NM, Storey GNB: Fetal outcome in obstetric cholestasis. Br J Obstet Gynaecol 95:1137, 1988

Gadacz TR, Talamini MA: Traditional versus laparoscopic cholecystectomy. Am J Surg 161:336, 1991

Garbaciak JA Jr, Richter M, Miller S, Barton JJ: Maternal weight and pregnancy complications. Am J Obstet Gynecol 152:238, 1985

Godsey RK, Newman RB: Hyperemesis gravidarum: A comparison of single and multiple admissions. J Reprod Med 36:287, 1991

Gopal KA, Amshel AL, Shonberg IL, Levinson BA, Vanwert M, Vanwert J: Ostomy and pregnancy. Dis Colon Rectum 28:912, 1985

Goudeau A, Yvonnet B, Lesage G, Barin F, Denis F, Coursaget P, Chiron JP: Lack of anti-HBc IgM in neonates with HBs Ag carrier mothers argues against transplacental transmission of hepatitis B virus infection. Lancet 2:1103, 1983

Greenberger NJ, Isselbacher KJ: Diseases of the gallbladder and bile ducts. In Wilson JD, Braunwald E, Isselbacher KJ, Petersdorf RG, Martin JB, Fauci AS, Root RK (eds): Harrison's Principles of Internal Medicine, 12th ed. New York, McGraw-Hill, 1991, p 1358

Greenspoon JS, Martin J, Greenspoon RL, McNamara BT: Necessity for routine obstetric screening for hepatitis B surface antigen. J Reprod Med 34:655, 1989a

Greenspoon JS, Masaki DI, Kurz CR: Cardiac tamponade in pregnancy during central hyperalimentation. Obstet Gynecol 73:465, 1989b

Harer WB Jr, Harer WB Sr: Volvulus complicating pregnancy and the puerperium: A report of three cases and review of the literature (37 references cited). Obstet Gynecol 12:399, 1958

Hiatt JR, Hiatt JCG, Williams RA, Klein SR: Biliary disease in pregnancy: Strategy for surgical management. Am J Surg 151:263, 1986

Hill NCW, Morris NH, Shaw RW, Mathur S, Rolles K, Burroughs AK: Pregnancy after orthotopic liver transplantation. Case report. Br J Obstet Gynaecol 98:719, 1991

Hirvioja ML, Tuimala R, Vuori J: The treatment of intrahepatic cholestasis of pregnancy by dexamethasone. Br J Obstet Gynaecol 99:109, 1992

Holzbach RT, Sivak DA, Braun WE: Familial recurrent intrahepatic cholestasis of pregnancy: A genetic study providing evidence for transmission of a sex-limited, dominant trait. Gastroenterology 85:175, 1983

Homan WP, Thorbjarnarson B: Crohn disease and pregnancy. Arch Surg 111:545, 1976

Howard LJ: Parenteral and enteral nutrition therapy. Chapter 75, in Wilson JD, Braunwald E, Isselbacher KJ, Petersdorf RG, Martin JB, Fauci AS, Root RK (eds): Harrison's Principles of Internal Medicine, 12th ed. New York, McGraw-Hill, 1991, p 427

Hsu HM, Chen DS, Chuang CH, Lu JCF, Jwo DM, Lee CC, Lu HC, Cheng SH, Wang YF, Wang CC, Lo KJ, Shih CJ, Sung JL: Efficacy of a mass hepatitis B vaccination program in Taiwan: Studies on 3463 infants of hepatitis B surface antigen-carrier mothers. JAMA 260:2231, 1988

Hytten FE: The alimentary system. In Hytten F, Chamberlain G (eds): Clinical Physiology in Obstetrics. London, Blackwell Scientific, 1991, p 137

Ingerslev M, Teilum G: Biopsy studies on the liver in pregnancy, II. Liver biopsy on normal pregnant women. Acta Obstet Gynaecol Scand 25:352, 1945

Johnson SR, Kolberg BH, Varner MW, Railsback LD: Maternal obesity and pregnancy. Surg Gynecol Obstet 164:431, 1987

Johnston WG, Baskett TF: Obstetric cholestasis. Am J Obstet Gynecol 133:299, 1979

Kirby DF, Fiorenza V, Craig RM: Intravenous nutritional support during pregnancy. JPEN 12:72, 1988

Klebanoff MA, Koslowe PA, Kaslow R, Rhoads GG: Epidemiology of vomiting in early pregnancy. Obstet Gynecol 66:612, 1985

Kliegman RM, Gross T: Perinatal problems of the obese mother and her infant. Obstet Gynecol 66:299, 1985

Knudson LB, Källén B: Intestinal bypass operation and pregnancy outcome. Acta Obstet Gynecol Scand 65:831, 1986

Kochhar R, Goenka MK, Mehta SK: Endoscopic sclerotherapy during pregnancy. Am J Gastroenterol 85:1132, 1990

Kohn SG, Briele HA, Douglass LH: Volvulus complicating pregnancy. Am J Obstet Gynecol 48:398, 1944

Koretz RL: Universal prenatal hepatitis B testing: Is it cost-effective? Obstet Gynecol 74:808, 1989

Krege J, Katz VL, Bowes WA: Transient diabetes insipidus of pregnancy. Obstet Gynecol Surv 44:789, 1989

Kumar ML, Dawson NV, McCullough AJ, Radivoyevitch M, King KC, Hertz R, Kiefer H, Hampson M, Cassidy R, Tavill AS: Should all pregnant women be screened for hepatitis B? Ann Intern Med 107:273, 1987

Kurzel RB, Naunheim KS, Schwartz RA: Repair of symptomatic diaphragmatic hernia during pregnancy. Obstet Gynecol 71:869, 1988

Laifer SA, Darby MJ, Scantlebury, VP, Harger JH, Caritis SN: Pregnancy and liver transplantation. Obstet Gynecol 76:1083, 1990

Landers D, Carmona R, Crombleholme W, Lim R: Acute cholecystitis in pregnancy. Obstet Gynecol 69:131, 1987

Lane RS: Non A–non B hepatitis from intravenous immunoglobulins. Lancet 2:974, 1983

Lee RV, Rodgers BD, Young C, Eddy E, Cardinal J: Total parenteral nutrition during pregnancy. Obstet Gynecol 68:563, 1986

Lettau LA, McCarthy JG, Smith MH, Hadler SC, Morse LJ, Ukena T, Bessette R, Gurwitz A, Irvine WG, Fields HA, Grady GF, Maynard JE: Outbreak of severe hepatitis due to delta and hepatitis B viruses in parenteral drug abusers and their contacts. N Engl J Med 317:1256, 1987

Levine MG, Esser D: Total parenteral nutrition for the treatment of severe hyperemesis gravidarum: Maternal nutritional effects and fetal outcome. Obstet Gynecol 72:102, 1988

Lichtiger S, Present DH: Preliminary report: Cyclosporin in treatment of severe active ulcerative colitis. Lancet 336:16, 1990

Ludmir J, Samuels P, Armson BA, Torosian MH: Spontaneous small bowel obstruction associated with a spontaneous triplet gestation. A case report. J Reprod Med 34:985, 1989

Lunzer M, Barnes P, Byth K, O'Halloran M: Serum bile acid concentrations during pregnancy and their relationship to obstetric cholestasis. Gastroenterology 91:825, 1986

Madan M, Alexander DJ, McMahon MJ: Influence of catheter type on occurrence of thrombophlebitis during peripheral intravenous nutrition. Lancet 339:101, 1992

Manas KJ, Welsh JD, Rankin RA, Miller DD: Hepatic hemorrhage without rupture in preeclampsia. N Engl J Med 312:435, 1985

Maringhini A, Marcenò MP, Lanzarone F, Caltagirone M, Fusco G, DiCuonzo G, Cittadini E, Pagliaro L: Sludge and stones in gallbladder after pregnancy: Prevalence and risk factors. J Hepatol 5:218, 1987

Martin JN Jr, Blake PG, Perry KG Jr, McCaul JF, Hess LW, Martin RW: The natural history of HELLP syndrome: Patterns of disease progression and regression. Am J Obstet Gynecol 164:1500, 1991

Mayberry JF, Atkinson M: Achalasia and pregnancy. Br J Obstet Gynaecol 94:855, 1987

Mazze RI, Källén B: Appendectomy during pregnancy: A Swedish registry study of 778 cases. Obstet Gynecol 77:835, 1991

Miller JP: Inflammatory bowel disease in pregnancy: A review. J Roy Soc Med 79:221, 1986

Minakami H, Oka N, Sato T, Tamada T, Yasuda Y, Hirota N: Preeclampsia: A microvesicular fat disease of the liver? Am J Obstet Gynecol 159:1043, 1988

Moore JG, Gladstone NS, Lucas GW, Ravry MJR, Ansari AH: Successful management of post-cesarean-section acute pseudoobstruction of the colon (Ogilvie's syndrome) with colonoscopic decompression. A case report. J Reprod Med 31:1001, 1986

Morali GA, Braverman DZ: Abnormal liver enzymes and ketonuria in hyperemesis gravidarum. A retrospective review of 80 patients. J Clin Gastroenterol 12:303, 1990

Morrissey JF, Reichelderfer M: Gastrointestinal endoscopy. N Engl J Med 325:1142, 1991

Neerhof MG, Zelman W, Sullivan T: Hepatic rupture in pregnancy. Obstet Gynecol Surv 44:407, 1989 Nies BM, Dreiss RJ: Hyperlipidemic pancreatitis in pregnancy: A case report and review of the literature. Am J Perinatol 7:166, 1990

Ockner SA, Brunt EM, Cohn SM, Krul ES, Hanto DW, Peters MG: Fulminant hepatic failure caused by acute fatty liver of pregnancy treated by orthotopic liver transplantation. Hepatology 11:59, 1990

Ordorica SA, Frieden FJ, Marks F, Hoskins IA, Young BK: Pancreatic enzyme activity in pregnancy. J Reprod Med 36:359, 1991

Östman JIC: Update of pancreatic transplantation. Ann Med 23:101, 1991

Palma J, Reyes H, Ribalta J, Iglesias J, Gonzalez MC, Hernandez I, Alvarez C, Molina C, Danitz AM: Effects of ursodeoxycholic acid in patients with intrahepatic cholestasis of pregnancy. Hepatology 15:1043, 1992

Parry E, Shields R, Turnbull AC: Transit time in the small intestine in pregnancy. J Obstet Gynaecol Br Commonwealth 77:900, 1970

Pauzner D, Wolman I, Niv D, Ber A, David MP: Endoscopic sclerotherapy in extrahepatic portal hypertension in pregnancy. Am J Obstet Gynecol 164:152, 1991

Podolsky DK: Inflammatory bowel disease (part 1). N Engl J Med 325:928, 1991a

Podolsky DK: Inflammatory bowel disease (part 2). N Engl J Med 325:1009, 1991b

Porter RJ, Stirrat GM: The effects of inflammatory bowel disease on pregnancy: A case-controlled retrospective analysis. Br J Obstet Gynaecol 93:1124, 1986

Pratt AT, Donaldson RC, Evertson LR, Yon JL Jr: Cecal volvulus in pregnancy. Obstet Gynecol 57(suppl):37, 1981

Printen KJ, Scott D: Pregnancy following gastric bypass for the treatment of morbid obesity. Am Surg 48:363, 1982

Pucci RO, Seed RW: Case report of laparoscopic cholecystectomy in the third trimester of pregnancy. Am J Obstet Gynecol 165:401, 1991

Ramin K, Richey R, Ramin S, Cunningham FG: Acute pneumonitis in pregnancy. (abstract) Presented at the annual clinical meeting of American College of Obstetricians and Gynecologists, Washington, DC, May 1993

Reid R, Ivey KJ, Rencoret RH, Storey B: Fetal complications of obstetric cholestasis. BMJ 1:870, 1976

Richards DS, Miller DK, Goodman GN: Pregnancy after gastric bypass for morbid obesity. J Reprod Med 32:172, 1987

Riely CA: Acute fatty liver of pregnancy. Semin Liver Dis 7:47, 1987

Riely CA: The liver in preeclampsia/eclampsia: The tip of the iceberg. Am J Gastroenterol 81:1218, 1986

Riggs BS, Bronstein AC, Kulig K, Archer PG, Rumack BH: Acute acetaminophen overdose during pregnancy. Obstet Gynecol 74:247, 1989

Rigler LG, Eneboe JB: Incidence of hiatus hernia in pregnant women and its significance. J Thorac Surg 4:262, 1935

Rolfes DB, Ishak KG: Liver disease in toxemia of pregnancy. Am J Gastroenterol 81:1138, 1986

Rumack BH, Matthew H: Acetaminophen poisoning and toxicity. Pediatrics 55:871, 1975

Sanderson SL, Iverius PH, Wilson DE: Successful hyperlipemic pregnancy. JAMA 265:1858, 1991

Satin AJ, Twickler D, Gilstrap LC: Esophageal achalasia in late pregnancy. Obstet Gynecol 79:812, 1992

Scantlebury V, Gordon R, Tzakis A, Koneru B, Bowman J, Mazzaferro V, Stevenson WC, Todo S, Iwatsuki S, Starzl TE: Childbearing after liver transplantation. Transplantation 49:317, 1990

Schorr-Lesnick B, Lebovics E, Dworkin B, Rosenthal WS: Liver diseases unique to pregnancy. Am J Gastroenterol 86:659, 1991

Schreyer P, Caspi E, El-Hindi JM, Eschar J: Cirrhosis—Pregnancy and delivery: A review. Obstet Gynecol Surv 37:304, 1982

Shaw D, Frohlich J, Wittmann BA, Williams M: A prospective study of 18 patients with cholestasis of pregnancy. Am J Obstet Gynecol 142:621, 1982

Sheld HH: Megacolon complicating pregnancy. J Reprod Med 32:239, 1987

Singletary BK, Van Thiel DH, Eagon PK: Estrogen and progesterone receptors in human gallbladder. Hepatology 6:574, 1986

Slater DN, Hague WM: Renal morphological changes in idiopathic acute fatty liver of pregnancy. Histopathology 8:567, 1984

Smith LG, Moise KJ Jr, Dildy GA III, Carpenter RJ Jr: Spontaneous rupture of liver during pregnancy: Current therapy. Obstet Gynecol 77:171, 1991

Snyder RR, Hankins GDV: Etiology and treatment of acute fatty liver of pregnancy. Clin Perinatol 13:813, 1986

Starzl TE, Demetris AJ, Van Theil D: Liver transplantation (part 1). N Engl J Med 321:1014, 1989a

Starzl TE, Demetris AJ, Van Thiel D: Liver transplantation (part 2). N Engl J Med 321:1092, 1989b

Stauffer RA, Adams A, Wygal J, Lavery JP: Gallbladder disease in pregnancy. Am J Obstet Gynecol 144:661, 1982

Steven MM: Progress report: Pregnancy and liver disease. Gut 22:592, 1981

Steven MM, Buckley JD, Mackay IR: Pregnancy in chronic active hepatitis. Q J Med 48:519, 1979

Strickland DM, Hauth JC, Widish J, Strickland K, Perez R: Amylase and isoamylase activities in serum of pregnant women. Obstet Gynecol 63:389, 1984

Thaler MM, Park CK, Landers DV, Wara DW, Houghton M, Veereman-Wauters G, Sweet RL, Han JH: Vertical transmission of hepatitis C virus. Lancet 338:17, 1991

Tydén G, Brattström C, Björkman U, Landgraf R, Baltzer J, Hillebrand G, Land W, Calne R, Brons GM, Squifflet JP, Ghysen J, Alexandre GPJ: Pregnancy after combined pancreas–kidney transplantation. Diabetes 38:43, 1989

Van Le L, Podrasky A: Computed tomographic and ultrasonographic findings in women with acute fatty liver of pregnancy. J Reprod Med 35:815, 1990

Venkataramanan R, Koneru B, Wang CCP, Burckart GJ, Caritis SN, Starzl TE: Cyclosporine and its metabolites in mother and baby. Transplantation 40:468, 1988

Walcott WO, Derick DE, Jolley JJ, Synder DL, Schmid R: Successful pregnancy in a liver transplant patient. Am J Obstet Gynecol 132:340, 1978

Watson WJ, Gaines TE: Third-trimester colectomy for severe ulcerative colitis. J Reprod Med 32:869,1987

Watson WJ, Seeds JW: Acute fatty liver of pregnancy. Obstet Gynecol Surv 45:585, 1990

Watts GF, Morton K, Jackson P, Lewis B: Management of patients with severe hypertriglyceridaemia during pregnancy: Report of two cases with familial lipoprotein lipase deficiency. Br J Obstet Gynaecol 99:163, 1992

Wetzel AM, Kirz DS: Routine hepatitis screening in adolescent pregnancies: Is it cost effective? Am J Obstet Gynecol 156:166, 1987

Wolfe HM, Sokol RJ, Martier SM, Zador IE: Maternal obesity: A potential source of error in sonographic prenatal diagnosis. Obstet Gynecol 76:339, 1990

Woolfson K, Cohen Z, McLeod RS: Crohn's Disease and pregnancy. Dis Colon Rectum 33:869, 1990

CHAPTER 52
Hematological Disorders

Pregnancy induces physiological changes that often confuse the diagnosis of several hematological disorders and the assessment of their treatment. This is especially true for anemia.

Physiological Changes. A number of marked hematological changes are induced by pregnancy, and these are discussed in detail in Chapter 8 (p. 221). One of the most significant changes is that of blood volume expansion by a mean of 50 percent. Plasma volume increases disproportionately compared with red cell mass, resulting in physiological decrease in hematocrit. During this time, iron requirements for mother and fetus average nearly 1000 mg.

Definition of Anemia. A precise definition of anemia in women is complicated by normal differences in the concentrations of hemoglobin between women and men, between white and black women, between women who are pregnant and those who are not, and between pregnant women who receive iron supplements and those who do not.

Extensive hematological measurements have been made in healthy nonpregnant women, none of whom were iron deficient because each had histochemically proven iron stores, and none were folate deficient because marrow erythropoiesis remained normoblastic. On the basis of data presented in Table 52–1, anemia in nonpregnant women is defined as hemoglobin concentration less than 12 g/dL and less than 10 g/dL during pregnancy or the puerperium. The hemoglobin concentration is lower in midpregnancy, and as shown in Figure 52–1, early in pregnancy and again near term, the hemoglobin level of most healthy women with iron stores is 11 g/dL or higher. For these reasons, the Centers for Disease Control (1990) defined anemia as less than 11 g/dL in the first and third trimesters, and less than 10.5 g/dL in the second trimester.

The modest fall in hemoglobin levels observed during pregnancy in healthy women not deficient in iron or folate is caused by a relatively greater expansion of plasma volume compared with the increase in hemoglobin mass and red cell volume. The disproportion between the rates at which plasma and erythrocytes are added to the maternal circulation is normally greatest during the second trimester. Late in pregnancy, plasma expansion essentially ceases while hemoglobin mass continues to increase (see Chap. 8, p. 221).

During the puerperium, in the absence of excessive blood loss, hemoglobin concentration is not appreciably less than predelivery. After delivery the hemoglobin level typically fluctuates to a modest degree around the predelivery value for a few days and then rises to the somewhat higher nonpregnant level. The rate and magnitude of increase early in the puerperium are the result of the amount of hemoglobin added during pregnancy and the amount lost by hemorrhage at delivery and modified by a puerperal decrease in plasma volume.

Frequency of Anemia. Although anemia is somewhat more common among indigent pregnant women, it is by no means restricted to them. The frequency of anemia during pregnancy varies considerably, depending primarily upon whether supplemental iron is taken during pregnancy. For example, at Parkland Hospital the hemoglobin level at the time of delivery among women who took iron supplements averaged 12.4 g/dL, whereas it was only 11.3 g/dL among those who were not taking iron. Moreover, in none of the group receiving iron supplements was the hemoglobin less than 10 g/dL, but it was below this level in 16 percent of those who took no supplements (see Chap. 9, p. 257). Taylor and associates (1982) reported similar observations, that is, hemoglobin levels at term averaged 12.7 g/dL among women who received supplemental iron compared with 11.2 g/dL for women who did not.

Etiology of Anemia. The causes of anemia during pregnancy are the same as those encountered in nonpregnant women. Any anemia common to childbearing age women may complicate pregnancy. A classification based primarily on etiology and including most of the common causes of anemia in pregnant women is shown in Table 52–2. Although laboratory error as a cause of apparent anemia has not been included, the results from clinical laboratories may sometimes be inaccurate. A common source of error during pregnancy stems from the rapid erythrocyte sedimentation rate, which is induced by hyperfibrinogenemia of normal pregnancy. If the specimen of blood is not mixed immediately before sampling, the results will likely be inaccurate. Most automated devices used currently have constant mixing features that obviate this problem.

The observed differences between hemoglobin concentrations in pregnant and nonpregnant women, coupled with the well-recognized phenomenon of hypervolemia induced by normal pregnancy, have led to the use of the term **physiological anemia.** This is a

TABLE 52–1. HEMOGLOBIN CONCENTRATIONS IN 85 HEALTHY WOMEN WITH PROVEN IRON STORES

Hemoglobin	Non-pregnant	Mid-pregnancy	Late Pregnancy
Mean	13.7 g/dL	11.5 g/dL	12.3 g/dL
Less than 12.0	1%	72%	36%
Less than 11.0	None	29%	6%
Less than 10.0	None	4%	1%
Lowest	11.7 g/dL	9.7 g/dL	9.8 g/dL

From Scott and Pritchard (1967), with permission.

TABLE 52–2. CAUSES OF ANEMIA DURING PREGNANCY

Acquired
Iron-deficiency anemia
Anemia caused by acute blood loss
Anemia of inflammation or malignancy
Megaloblastic anemia
Acquired hemolytic anemia
Aplastic or hypoplastic anemia

Hereditary
Thalassemias
Sickle cell hemoglobinopathies
Other hemoglobinopathies
Hereditary hemolytic anemias

poor term for describing a normal process and should be discarded because there is virtually no anemia during normal pregnancy if anemia is defined as decreased hemoglobin mass.

Effects of Anemia on Pregnancy. The etiology of anemia is important when evaluating its effects on pregnancy outcome. For example, maternal and perinatal outcomes are altered markedly in women with sickle cell anemia. Conversely, there is no evidence that adverse outcomes are related to the anemia per se, but rather to the vascular complications of sickling.

Most studies of the effects of anemia on pregnancy, such as those discussed in Chapter 9 (p. 257), describe large populations, and at least ostensibly deal with nutritional anemias, specifically those due to iron deficiency. Murphy and colleagues (1986) reported findings from the Cardiffs Birth Survey of over 54,000 singleton pregnancies and reported excessive perinatal mortality with *high* hemoglobin concentrations. Specifically, women whose hemoglobin concentration exceeded 13.2 g/dL at 13 to 18 weeks had excessive perinatal mortality, low-birthweight infants, and preterm delivery,

as well as preeclampsia in nulliparas. Lu and associates (1991) studied the relationship between hematocrit and pregnancy outcome in over 17,000 iron- and folate-supplemented women and found a relationship between fetal growth retardation and a high hematocrit. Klebanoff and co-workers (1991) studied nearly 27,000 women and found a slightly increased risk of preterm birth with mid-trimester anemia. Lieberman and collaborators (1987) found a positive association with low hematocrit and preterm birth in black women and suggested that anemia was a marker for nutritional deficiencies.

Iron-deficiency Anemia

The two most common causes of anemia during pregnancy and the puerperium are iron deficiency and acute blood loss. Not infrequently, the two are intimately related, because excessive blood loss with its concomitant loss of hemoglobin iron and exhaustion of iron stores in one pregnancy can be an important cause of iron-deficiency anemia in the next pregnancy.

As discussed elsewhere (see Chap. 8, p. 222 and Chap. 9, p. 257), the iron requirements of pregnancy are considerable, and unfortunately the majority of American women have reduced stores. In a typical gestation with a single fetus, the maternal need for iron induced by pregnancy averages close to 800 mg; about 300 mg for the fetus and placenta and about 500 mg, if available, for maternal hemoglobin mass expansion. Approximately 200 mg more are shed through the gut, urine, and skin. This total amount—1000 mg—exceeds considerably the iron stores of most women. Unless the difference between the amount of stored iron available to the mother and the iron requirements of normal pregnancy cited above is compensated for by absorption of iron from the gastrointestinal tract, iron-deficiency anemia develops.

With the rather rapid expansion of blood volume during the second trimester, iron lack is often manifested by an appreciable drop in hemoglobin concentration. Although the rate of expansion of blood volume

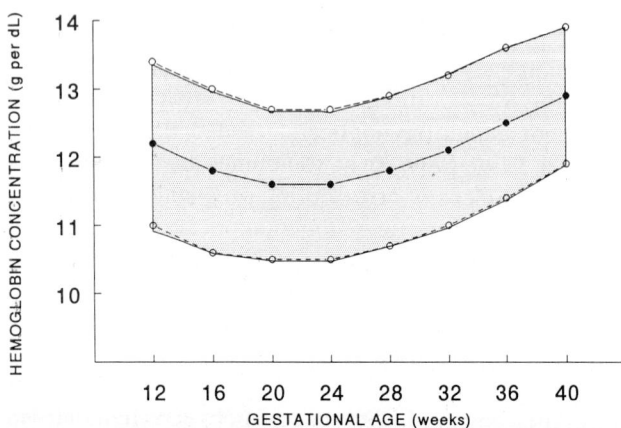

Fig. 52–1. Mean hemoglobin concentrations (●—●) and 5th and 95 (○---○) percentiles for healthy pregnant women taking iron supplements. (Data from Centers for Disease Control, 1989.)

is not so great in the third trimester, the need for iron is still increased because augmentation of maternal hemoglobin mass continues, and considerable iron is now transported to the fetus. Because the amount of iron diverted to the fetus from an iron-deficient mother is not much different from the amount normally transferred, the newborn infant of a severely anemic mother does not suffer from iron-deficiency anemia. Iron stores in the infant are influenced much more by when and how the cord is clamped rather than by maternal iron stores (see Chap. 14, p. 383).

Diagnosis. Classical morphological evidence of iron-deficiency anemia—erythrocyte hypochromia and microcytosis—is less prominent in the pregnant woman compared with the nonpregnant woman with the same hemoglobin concentration. Moderate iron-deficiency anemia during pregnancy, for example, a hemoglobin concentration of 9 g/dL, usually is not accompanied by obvious morphological changes in erythrocytes. With this degree of anemia from iron deficiency, however, serum ferritin levels are lower than normal, and there is no stainable bone marrow iron. The serum iron-binding capacity is elevated, but by itself is of little diagnostic value, because it also is elevated during normal pregnancy in the absence of iron deficiency. Moderate normoblastic hyperplasia of the bone marrow also is found to be similar to that in normal pregnancy. **Thus, iron-deficiency anemia during pregnancy is the consequence primarily of expansion of plasma volume without normal expansion of maternal hemoglobin mass.**

The initial evaluation of a pregnant woman with moderate anemia should include measurements of hemoglobin, hematocrit, and red cell indices, careful examination of a well-prepared smear of the peripheral blood, a sickle cell preparation if the woman is of African origin, and the measurement of the serum iron concentration or serum ferritin level, or both. Carriaga and colleagues (1991) reported that normal serum ferritin concentration excludes iron deficiency but that decreased values do not confirm it. In their study, the mean serum ferritin concentration during pregnancy was 14.3 μg/L, compared with 25 to 30 μg/L in nonpregnant women. They also found that transferrin receptor concentration on erythrocytes was not altered by pregnancy in iron-sufficient women, but that levels were raised in iron-deficient women. Examination of the bone marrow at this point is seldom done, although the demonstration of hemosiderin rules out iron deficiency. The diagnosis of iron deficiency in moderately anemic pregnant women usually is presumptive and based largely on the exclusion of other causes of anemia.

When the pregnant woman with moderate iron-deficiency anemia is given adequate iron therapy, a hematological response is detected by an elevated reticulocyte count. The rate of increase of hemoglobin

concentration or hematocrit varies considerably, but usually it is slower than in nonpregnant women. The reason is related largely to the differences in blood volumes, and during the latter half of pregnancy, newly formed hemoglobin is added to the characteristically much larger volume (Fig. 52–2). There is no evidence that pregnancy per se depresses erythropoiesis to any degree.

Treatment. The objectives of treatment are correction of the deficit in hemoglobin mass and eventually restitution of iron stores. Both of these objectives can be accomplished with orally administered, simple iron compounds—ferrous sulfate, fumarate, or gluconate—that provide a daily dose of about 200 mg of **elemental iron.** There is no need to prescribe ascorbic acid or fruit juices or to withhold food to enhance iron absorption, nor is there any advantage from delayed-release or sustained-release medication. If the woman cannot, or will not, take oral iron preparations, then parenteral therapy is given. To replenish iron stores, oral therapy should be continued for 3 months or so after the anemia has been corrected.

Folic acid may be given along with the iron as a safeguard against folate deficiency, although the response of pregnant women with iron-deficiency anemia treated with iron and folic acid is not appreciably better than when iron is given alone. Similarly, there is no good

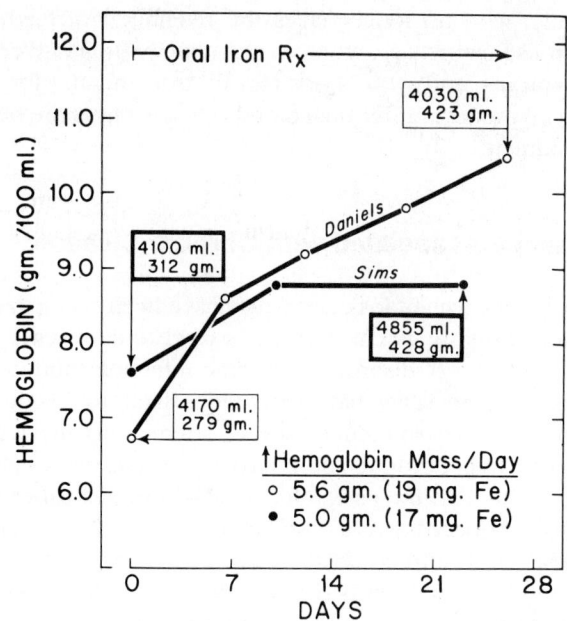

Fig. 52–2. Two pregnant women with iron-deficiency anemia, when treated with the same simple iron compound, responded by increasing their hemoglobin mass at similar rates but not their hemoglobin concentrations. The excellent response in Sims treated late in the second trimester was masked by a simultaneous increase in blood volume of nearly 20 percent. The blood volume did not increase in Daniels who was treated late in pregnancy, and thus blood volume expansion already was maximal.

evidence that the addition of cobalt, copper, molybdenum, or ascorbic acid to the iron tablet is advantageous.

Transfusions of red cells or whole blood seldom are indicated for the treatment of iron-deficiency anemia unless hypovolemia from blood loss coexists or an emergency operative procedure must be performed on a *severely* anemic woman.

Anemia from Acute Blood Loss

Anemia resulting from recent hemorrhage is more likely to be evident during the puerperium. Both abruptio placentae and placenta previa may be sources of serious blood loss and of anemia before as well as after delivery. Earlier in pregnancy, anemia caused by acute blood loss is common in instances of abortion, ectopic pregnancy, and hydatidiform mole.

Treatment. Massive hemorrhage demands immediate blood replacement with whole blood or packed red cells and volume expanders in amounts that restore and maintain adequate perfusion of vital organs (see Chap. 37, p. 821). Even though the amount of blood replaced commonly does not completely repair the hemoglobin deficit created by the hemorrhage, in general, once dangerous hypovolemia has been overcome and hemostasis has been achieved, the residual anemia should be treated with iron. For the moderately anemic woman whose hemoglobin is more than 7 g/dL, whose condition is stable, who no longer faces the likelihood of further serious hemorrhage, who can ambulate without adverse symptoms, and who is not febrile, iron therapy for at least 3 months rather than blood transfusions is the best treatment.

Anemia Associated with Chronic Disease

Weakness, weight loss, and pallor have been recognized since antiquity as characteristics of chronic disease. A wide variety of disorders—chronic infections and neoplasms, especially—have been identified to produce moderate and sometimes severe anemia, usually with slightly hypochromic and microcytic erythrocytes (Erslev, 1990). In the past, infections—especially tuberculosis, endocarditis, or osteomyelitis—were common causes, but antimicrobial therapy has decreased their incidences significantly. Today, infections, inflammation, and neoplasia are the three categories of disease that cause these disorders (Sears, 1992). Examples of chronic inflammatory diseases include connective tissue disorders and inflammatory bowel disease.

In nonpregnant patients with chronic inflammatory diseases, the hemoglobin concentration rarely is less than 7 g/dL. Typically, bone marrow cellular morphology is not altered markedly. Serum iron concentration is de-

creased, and serum iron-binding capacity, while lower than in normal pregnancy, is not much below the normal nonpregnant range. Serum ferritin levels usually are normal. These anemias, although slightly different from each other mechanistically, appear to share similar features which include varying degrees and combinations of alterations in reticuloendothelial function, iron metabolism, and decreased erythropoiesis. Iron released from senescent erythrocytes often is retained rather than returned to plasma and reuse by erythroblasts. The fate of iron administered in therapeutic doses is similar. The life span of the erythrocyte usually is shortened by 20 to 30 percent by extracorpuscular factors. In some instances, anemia results from a combination of decreased erythropoiesis and a slightly increased destruction. A diminished response to erythropoietin also is thought to explain some types of relative bone marrow failure.

During pregnancy, a number of chronic diseases may cause anemia. Some of these are chronic renal disease, suppuration, inflammatory bowel disease, systemic lupus erythematosus, granulomatous infections, malignant neoplasms, and rheumatoid arthritis. As expected, anemia is intensified as plasma volume expands out of proportion to red cell mass expansion. At least some cases of so-called **refractory anemia of pregnancy** are the consequence of one of these diseases which has gone unrecognized. The anemia of infection, renal disease, and malignancy is refractory in the sense that it is not corrected by treatment with iron, folic acid, vitamin B_{12}, or any other hematinic agent. Nonetheless, prophylaxis with iron and folic acid usually is desirable to offset any deficiency induced by pregnancy.

Kidney Disease and Anemia of Pregnancy. Chronic renal insufficiency is characterized by anemia of variable severity, and usually is due to erythropoietin deficiency. There is, however, an element of anemia of chronic disease (Sears, 1992). During pregnancy, red cell mass is augmented in some of these women, but less so than in normal pregnancy (Cunningham and associates, 1990). The degree of red cell mass expansion corresponds to the degree of renal impairment, and because total blood volume expansion usually is normal in these women, preexisting anemia is intensified.

Recombinant erythropoietin has been used to treat anemia of chronic renal disease with low endogenous erythropoietin production (Humpheries, 1992). It also is used successfully to treat anemia of chronic disorders characterized by normal erythropoietin production. Experience with its use during pregnancy is limited. McGregor and colleagues (1991) treated a woman with severe renal insufficiency requiring hemodialysis during pregnancy. The dose of erythropoietin given was 4000 units subcutaneously three times weekly. Her hemoglobin concentration increased from about 7 g/dL to almost 10 g/dL. We have treated only a few pregnant women whose anemia was due to chronic renal insufficiency, but red cell mass usually increased over several weeks. A worrisome side effect of the drug is hypertension, which is already prevalent in these women (Chap. 50, p. 1138).

Women with severe **acute pyelonephritis,** but not those with asymptomatic bacteriuria or cystitis, often develop overt anemia. The genesis of this anemia appears to be increased red cell destruction, coupled with impaired production that may persist for some weeks (Cox and associates, 1991; Cunningham, 1988).

Megaloblastic Anemia

Megaloblastic anemias are a family of hematological disorders whose characteristic blood and bone marrow abnormalities are caused by impaired DNA synthesis. The prevalence of megaloblastic anemia during pregnancy varies considerably throughout the world, and it is now rare in the United States.

Folic Acid Deficiency. In this country, megaloblastic anemia beginning during pregnancy almost always results from folic acid deficiency, and in the past was referred to as **pernicious anemia of pregnancy.** It usually is found in women who do not consume fresh green leafy vegetables or foods with a high content of animal protein. Women with megaloblastic anemia may have developed troublesome nausea, vomiting, and anorexia during pregnancy. As the folate deficiency and anemia worsen, anorexia often becomes more intense, further aggravating the dietary deficiency. In some instances, excessive ethanol ingestion either is the cause or contributes to its development.

Herbert and co-workers (1962) estimated that in normal nonpregnant women the daily folate requirements expressed as folic acid are in the range of 50 to 100 μg per day. During pregnancy, requirements for folic acid are increased. Deficiency of metabolically active forms of folic acid induces many biochemical and hematological changes. The sequence of changes from folate deficiency probably is unaltered by pregnancy. The earliest biochemical evidence is low folic acid activity in plasma. The earliest morphological evidence usually is hypersegmentation of neutrophils. As anemia develops, the newly formed erythrocytes, now being produced in reduced numbers, are macrocytic, even when there has been previous iron deficiency with microcytosis. With preexisting iron deficiency, the more recently formed macrocytic erythrocytes cannot be detected by measurement of the mean corpuscular volume of the erythrocytes. Careful examination of a smear of peripheral blood, however, usually will demonstrate some macrocytes. As the anemia becomes more intense, an occasional nucleated erythrocyte appears in the peripheral blood. If smears of the buffy coat from peripheral blood are made, several such cells with the distinct features of megaloblasts usually are demonstrable. At the same time, examination of the bone marrow discloses megaloblastic erythropoiesis. As maternal folate deficiency and, in turn, the anemia become severe, thrombocytopenia, leukopenia, or both also may develop.

The fetus and placenta extract folate from maternal circulation so effectively that the fetus is not anemic even when the mother is severely anemic from folate deficiency. Cases have been recorded in which newborn hemoglobin levels were 18 g/dL or more, while maternal values were as low as 3.6 g/dL (Pritchard and co-workers, 1970).

Treatment. The treatment of pregnancy-induced megaloblastic anemia should include folic acid, a nutritious diet, and iron. As little as 1 mg of folic acid administered orally once daily produces a striking hematological response. By 4 to 7 days after beginning treatment, the reticulocyte count is increased appreciably, and leukopenia and thrombocytopenia are corrected promptly. Sometimes the rate of increase in hemoglobin concentration or hematocrit is disappointing, especially when compared with the usual exuberant reticulocytosis that starts soon after therapy has been initiated. Severe megaloblastic anemia during pregnancy typically is accompanied by an appreciably smaller blood volume than that of a normal pregnancy, but soon after folic acid therapy has been started, the blood volume usually increases considerably. Therefore, even though hemoglobin is being rapidly added to the circulation, the hemoglobin concentration does not reflect precisely the total amount of additional hemoglobin because of the simultaneous expansion of blood volume.

Women who develop megaloblastic anemia during pregnancy commonly are also deficient in total body iron. Paradoxically, ineffective erythropoiesis resulting from the folate deficiency and, in turn, a decreased amount of iron being incorporated into hemoglobin, induce a considerable elevation of the plasma iron and even some accumulation of storage iron. With the onset of effective erythropoiesis, however, the concentration of iron in plasma falls precipitously and any stored iron is exhausted rapidly. Iron then may become the limiting factor in production of hemoglobin.

Megaloblastic anemia may recur in subsequent pregnancies, very likely because of persistence of dietary inadequacies and perhaps in part because of a peculiarity in absorption or utilization of folic acid. Congenital folate malabsorption has been identified (Poncz and associates, 1981).

Prevention. A great deal of attention has been devoted to the frequency of maternal folate deficiency and megaloblastic anemia in pregnancy and the puerperium, the possible role of folate deficiency in various forms of reproductive failure, and the value of prophylactic administration of folic acid throughout pregnancy (see

Chap. 9, p. 259 and Chap. 40, p. 929). A good case can be made for supplemental folic acid in circumstances where folate requirements are unusually excessive, for example, multifetal pregnancy or hemolytic anemia. Other indications include Crohn disease, alcoholism, and some inflammatory skin disorders. There is evidence that women who previously have had infants with neural-tube defects have a lower recurrence rate if folic acid, 4 mg daily, is given prior to and through early pregnancy. Most recently, Czeizel and Dudás (1992) provided periconceptional folic acid (0.8 mg) supplementation to over 2000 Hungarian women who became pregnant. There were 23 congenital malformations per 1000 compared with 13 per 1000 in women given a trace-element supplement. These findings led the Centers for Disease Control (1992) to recommend that childbearing-age women consume at least 0.4 mg of folic acid daily.

Vitamin B$_{12}$ Deficiency. Megaloblastic anemia caused by lack of vitamin B$_{12}$ during pregnancy is exceedingly rare. **Addisonian pernicious anemia** is characterized by the failure to absorb vitamin B$_{12}$ because of lack of intrinsic factor. It is an extremely uncommon autoimmune disease in women of reproductive age, and typically has its onset in women over 40. Moreover, unless women with this disease are treated with vitamin B$_{12}$, infertility may be a complication. In our limited experience, vitamin B$_{12}$ deficiency in pregnant women is more likely encountered following partial or total gastric resection. Other causes are Crohn disease, ileal resection, and bacterial overgrowth in the small bowel.

Serum vitamin B$_{12}$ levels are measured by radioimmunoassay. During pregnancy, these normally are lower than nonpregnant values because of decreased serum concentrations of B$_{12}$-carrier proteins, the **transcobalamins** (Zamorano and colleagues, 1985). Women who have had a total gastrectomy should be given 1000 μg of cyanocobalamin (vitamin B$_{12}$) intramuscularly at monthly intervals. Those with a partial gastrectomy usually do not need such therapy, but vitamin B$_{12}$ levels during pregnancy should be measured. There is little reason for withholding folic acid during pregnancy simply out of fear of jeopardizing the neurological integrity of women who might be pregnant and simultaneously have unrecognized, and therefore untreated, Addisonian pernicious anemia.

Breast-fed infants of mothers who suffer vitamin B$_{12}$ deficiency, either as the consequence of lack of intrinsic factor or because of chronic ingestion of a strict vegetarian diet, may develop megaloblastic anemia during infancy (see Chap. 9, p. 260).

Acquired Hemolytic Anemias

Autoimmune Hemolytic Anemia. Autoimmune hemolysis is an uncommon condition mediated by the patient's own immunological mechanisms. The cause for aberrant antibody production is unknown. Anemias caused by these factors may be due to warm-active autoantibodies (80 to 90 percent), cold-active antibodies, or a combination. These syndromes also may be classified as primary or idiopathic versus secondary autoimmune hemolysis caused by underlying diseases or other factors. Examples of the latter include lymphomas and leukemias, connective-tissue diseases, some infections, chronic inflammatory diseases, or drug-induced factors. In some cases classified initially as idiopathic, careful follow-up may allow detection of an underlying disease.

With autoimmune hemolytic anemia, typically both the direct and indirect antiglobulin (Coombs) tests are positive. Hemolysis and the positive antiglobulin tests may be the consequence of either IgM or IgG anti-erythrocyte antibodies. Spherocytosis and reticulocytosis are characteristic of the peripheral blood smear. Cold-agglutinin disease may be induced by *Mycoplasma pneumoniae* or infectious mononucleosis.

Women with autoimmune hemolytic anemia sometimes demonstrate marked acceleration of hemolysis during pregnancy. Glucocorticoids usually are effective as in the nonpregnant state, and treatment is with prednisone, 1 mg/kg per day, or its equivalent. Coincidental thrombocytopenia usually is corrected by therapy.

IgM antibodies do not cross the placenta and thus fetal red cells are not affected; however, IgG antibodies, especially subclasses IgG$_1$ and IgG$_3$, do cross. The most common example of adverse fetal effects from maternally produced IgG antibodies is maternal D isoimmunization with hemolytic disease in the fetus and neonate. Whenever IgG antibodies are detected in the mother, the fetus should be considered at risk for serious hemolytic disease and appropriate steps should be taken to gauge its intensity (see Chap. 44, p. 1010).

Transfusion of red cells for the mother with severe autoimmune hemolytic disease is complicated by the presence of circulating anti-erythrocyte antibodies. Warming the donor cells to body temperature decreases their destruction by cold agglutinins.

Pregnancy-induced Hemolytic Anemia. Unexplained hemolytic anemia during pregnancy is a rare but apparently distinct entity in which severe hemolysis develops early in pregnancy and resolves within months after delivery. It is characterized by no evidence for an immune mechanism or for any intraerythrocytic or extraerythrocytic defects (Starksen and associates, 1983). Because the fetus-infant also may demonstrate transient hemolysis, an immunological cause is suspected. Maternal corticosteroid treatment usually is effective. We have observed one woman with recurrent hemolysis during several pregnancies, and in each instance, intense severe hemolytic anemia was controlled by prednisone given until delivery. Her children appear to be normal.

Paroxysmal Nocturnal Hemoglobinuria. Although commonly regarded as a hemolytic anemia, paroxysmal nocturnal hemoglobinuria is a hemopoietic stem cell disorder characterized by formation of defective platelets, granulocytes, and erythrocytes. Paroxysmal nocturnal hemoglobinuria is not familial. It appears to arise from one abnormal clone of cells, much like a neoplasm. Clinical disease is the consequence of a defect in the erythrocyte and granulocyte membrane which makes them unusually susceptible to lysis by complement and in vitro by acid treatment. The defect is seen in discrete red cell populations and already exists in newly formed cells rather than being acquired after entering the circulation.

Its clinical manifestation is that of acquired hemolytic anemia that has an insidious onset and a chronic course. Hemoglobinuria develops at irregular intervals and is not necessarily nocturnal. Hemolysis may be initiated by transfusions, infections, or surgery. The severity of disease ranges from mild to lethal. Complications include those from chronic anemia, which is exacerbated by iron deficiency from urinary loss of iron. Bleeding is encountered if severe thrombocytopenia develops. Venous thromboses are unusually common, and the Budd–Chiari syndrome caused by hepatic vein thrombosis has been observed (see Chap. 51, p. 1161). Renal abnormalities and hypertension also are common.

Except possibly for marrow transplantation, no definitive treatment exists. Heparin therapy, in general, has been disappointing, but is used for thrombotic complications. Corticosteroids may sometimes be of value to diminish hemolysis. Transfusions should be limited to compatible, washed red cells. Iron loss from hemoglobinuria can be high and iron-deficiency anemia frequently co-exists.

Effects on Pregnancy. Paroxysmal nocturnal hemoglobinuria is a serious and unpredictable disease and pregnancy may be dangerous. Greene and colleagues (1983) reviewed 31 cases in pregnancy and found that complications developed in over three fourths of these. They cited a maternal death rate of 10 percent. Postpartum, almost half of the women had deep-vein thrombosis, including Budd–Chiari syndrome or cerebral vein thrombosis. Solal-Céligny and co-workers (1988) later reported their experiences with eight pregnancies in six women. Only half of the pregnancies resulted in surviving infants. Despite this outcome, they concluded that successful outcomes are possible with close medical supervision. In a multicenter study, De Gramont and colleagues (1987) reported that the condition was complicated in two thirds of 38 pregnancies. Although they observed no maternal deaths, life-threatening complications were common, especially from hemolysis and hemorrhage.

Venous thromboembolism is particularly worrisome. Hurd and associates (1982) reported a pregnant woman with severe anemia who developed skin lesions characteristic of purpura fulminans. Heparin proved to be of no benefit. Cesarean delivery was performed primarily because of maternal thrombocytopenia and demonstration of maternal platelet antibody which caused concern for the fetus; however, his platelet count at birth was normal. After a stormy postpartum course, which included a splenectomy, the mother survived.

Drug-induced Hemolytic Anemia. Drug-induced hemolysis is occasionally encountered during pregnancy. It must be differentiated from other forms of autoimmune hemolytic anemia. Hemolysis typically is mild; it resolves upon withdrawing the drug, and it can be prevented by the drug's avoidance. Mechanisms of actions differ, but generally they are mechanisms of drug-mediated immunological injury to red cells (Packham and Leddy, 1990). The drug acts as a high-affinity hapten with a red cell protein to which antidrug antibodies attach, for example IgM anti-penicillin antibodies. It may act as a low-affinity hapten and adhere to cell membrane proteins. Finally, drugs actually may induce anti-erythrocyte antibodies. Some drugs incriminated in these reactions that might be used during pregnancy are shown in Table 52–3.

The severity of symptoms depends on the degree of hemolysis. Usually there is mild to moderate chronic hemolysis, but some drugs that act as low-affinity haptens may precipitate severe acute hemolysis. The direct antiglobulin test is positive, there is spherocytosis and reticulocytosis, and there may be thrombocytopenia and leukopenia. In most cases, withdrawing the offending drug results in reversal of symptoms. Corticosteroids are of questionable efficacy and transfusions are given only if there is severe anemia. Especially in African-American women, drug-induced hemolysis much more often is related to a congenital erythrocyte enzymatic defect, for example severe **glucose-6-phosphate dehydrogenase (G6PD) deficiency** (p. 1186).

TABLE 52–3. SOME DRUGS ASSOCIATED WITH POSITIVE RED CELL ANTIGLOBULIN TESTS

Drug	Immune Injury
Acetaminophen	Uncertain
Cephalosporins	High-affinity hapten
Chlorpromazine	Uncertain
Erythromycin	Uncertain
Ibuprofen	Uncertain
Isoniazid	Uncertain
Methyldopa	Autoantibody induction
Penicillins	Hapten
Probenecid	Low-affinity hapten
Quinidine	Low-affinity hapten
Rifampin	Low-affinity hapten
Thiopental	Low-affinity hapten

Modified from Packham and Leddy (1990).

Other Acquired Anemias. As described by Pritchard and associates (1976), overt fragmentation (microangiopathic) hemolysis with visible hemoglobinemia infrequently complicates **preeclampsia–eclampsia** (see Chap. 36, p. 776). The most fulminant acquired hemolytic anemia encountered during pregnancy is caused by the exotoxin of *Clostridium perfringens* and may prove fatal (see Chap. 31, p. 686). More recently, we encountered two cases of severe hemolytic anemia caused by exotoxin of Group A β-hemolytic streptococcus. Finally, as discussed on page 1175, Gram-negative bacterial endotoxin, or lipopolysaccharide, especially with severe acute pyelonephritis, may be accompanied by evidence of hemolysis and mild to moderate anemia (Cox and colleagues, 1991).

Aplastic or Hypoplastic Anemia

Although rarely encountered during pregnancy, aplastic anemia is a grave complication. The diagnosis is made when anemia, usually with thrombocytopenia, leukopenia, and markedly hypocellular bone marrow is demonstrated. Although *Fanconi anemia* is an autosomally recessive inherited variety, aplastic anemia is more commonly induced by drugs and other chemicals, infection, irradiation, leukemia, and immunological disorders. In over half of cases, a cause cannot be determined. The basic functional defect appears to be a marked decrease in committed marrow stem cells. There is considerable evidence that it is immunologically mediated. With severe disease, defined as bone marrow hypocellularity of less than 25 percent, the 1-year survival rate is only 20 percent.

Aplastic Anemia During Pregnancy. In most cases, aplastic anemia and pregnancy appear to have been a chance association. Because about a third of women improved following termination of pregnancy, it is postulated that pregnancy induces erythroid hypoplasia in some way (Aitchison and colleagues, 1989). Certainly, in a very few women, hypoplastic anemia has been identified first during a pregnancy and then improved or even resolved when the pregnancy terminated, only to recur with a subsequent pregnancy (Snyder and colleagues, 1991).

The two great risks to the pregnant woman with aplastic anemia are hemorrhage and infection. In cases reported since 1960, mortality during or after pregnancy has been 50 percent, and almost invariably, mortality is due to bleeding or sepsis (Snyder and colleagues, 1991). Fanconi anemia appears to be associated with a better prognosis. Alter and colleagues (1991) reviewed the literature and described 18 surviving children born to 19 women. They concluded that women who become pregnant had less severe disease.

Management. None of the erythropoietic agents that predictably produce remission in other anemias are effective. The treatment for severe aplastic anemia that is most likely to be effective is **bone marrow transplantation.** Corticosteroids are possibly of value, as are large doses of testosterone or other androgenic steroids. The effects from the administration of large doses of potent androgens during pregnancy are unknown. The women almost certainly would become virilized. The female fetus may develop the stigmata of androgen excess (pseudohermaphroditism), depending upon the compound, dose, and capacity of the placenta to aromatize the androgen. Liver toxicity has been a common complication of therapy with large doses of androgens. **Antithymocyte globulin** may be the best available therapy for patients who do not have a suitable marrow donor (Aitchison and co-workers, 1989; Camitta and co-workers, 1982).

A continuous search for infection should be made, and when found, specific antimicrobial therapy should be started promptly. Granulocyte transfusions are given only during actual infection. Red cell transfusions are given for symptomatic anemia, and we transfuse routinely to maintain the hematocrit at about 20. If the platelet count is very low, platelet transfusions may be needed to control hemorrhage. Vaginal delivery performed so as to minimize incisions and lacerations will lessen blood loss if the uterus is stimulated to contract vigorously after delivery. Even when thrombocytopenia is intense, the risk of severe hemorrhage can be minimized by vaginal delivery performed to avoid lacerations and an extensive episiotomy.

Bone Marrow Transplantation. Bone marrow transplantation typically requires immunosuppressive therapy for some months after marrow infusion. Unfortunately, previous blood transfusions, and even pregnancy, enhance the risk of graft rejection. In patients who have not been transfused, survival rates of 80 percent are to be expected with transplantation. Acute and chronic graft-versus-host disease is a serious complication following marrow transfusion. Fertility is common if transplantation is done for nonmalignant conditions, but it is rare if the indication is a hematological malignancy (Storb and Champlin, 1991).

Deeg and co-workers (1983), Hinterberger-Fischer and associates (1991), as well as others, have described pregnancies in women who previously had undergone bone marrow transplantation. In most cases, these pregnancies have been uneventful. We have followed only one woman in whom marrow transplantation was done at age 12 for hypoplastic anemia. At age 20, when first seen at 30 weeks, she had normal hemoglobin, platelet, and leukocyte values, and her reticulocyte count was 2.3 percent. She delivered a normal infant without complications at term.

Sickle Cell Hemoglobinopathies

Sickle hemoglobin (hemoglobin S) results from a single β-chain substitution of glutamic acid by valine because of an A for T substitution at codon 6 of the β-globin gene. Sickle cell anemia (SS disease), sickle cell–hemoglobin C disease (SC disease), and sickle cell–β-thalassemia disease (S–β-thalassemia disease) are the most common of the sickle hemoglobinopathies. Maternal morbidity and mortality, abortion, and perinatal mortality are all increased with these hemoglobinopathies.

Pathophysiology. Red cells with hemoglobin S undergo sickling when they are deoxygenated and the hemoglobin aggregates. Constant sickling and desickling causes membrane damage, and the cell may become irreversibly sickled. Clinically, the hallmark of sickling episodes are periods during which there is ischemia and infarction within various organs. These changes produce clinical symptoms, predominately pain, and are called "sickle crisis." To emphasize the importance of severe pain in sickle cell disease, Platt and colleagues (1991) observed that African cultures have named the disease for its painful episodes. For example, in the Ga language of Ghana, the disease is known as *chwech-weechwe*, for relentless repetitive chewing often seen in patients with excruciating pain. In addition to painful episodes, there may be aplastic, megaloblastic, sequestration, and hemolytic crises.

Chronic and acute changes from sickling include bony abnormalities, renal medullary damage, autosplenectomy by adulthood in homozygous SS patients and splenomegaly in other variants, hepatomegaly, ventricular hypertrophy, pulmonary infarctions, cerebrovascular accidents, leg ulcers, and a propensity to infection and sepsis with Gram-positive organisms.

Inheritance of Sickling Syndromes. The inheritance of the gene for S hemoglobin from each parent results in sickle cell anemia (SS disease). In the United States, 1 of 12 African-Americans has the sickle cell trait, which results from inheritance of one gene for the production of S hemoglobin and one for normal hemoglobin A. The theoretical incidence of sickle cell anemia among African Americans is 1 in 576 ($1/12 \times 1/12 \times 1/4 = 1/576$), but the disease is not so common during pregnancy because of an earlier high mortality rate, especially during early childhood.

About 1 in 40 African-Americans has the gene for hemoglobin C. Therefore, the probability of hemoglobin S and C traits in a black couple is about 1 in 500 ($1/40 \times 1/12$), and the probability of their child coinheriting the gene for hemoglobin S and an allelic gene for hemoglobin C is 1 in 4. As the consequence of these genetic frequencies, about 1 of 2000 ($1/12 \times 1/40 \times$ $1/4$) pregnant African-American women are expected to have SC disease.

The inheritance of the gene for hemoglobin S from one parent and the allelic gene for β-thalassemia from the other results in sickle cell–β-thalassemia disease. Because the incidence of β-thalassemia minor is about 1 in 40 to 50, S–β-thalassemia has a prevalence of about 1 in 2000.

Effect on Pregnancy. Pregnancy is a serious burden to women with sickle hemoglobinopathies. This is especially true for those with hemoglobin SS disease in whom anemia often becomes more intense, vasoocclusive episodes with severe pain—so-called **sickle cell crisis**—usually become more frequent, and infections and pulmonary complications are more common. Powars and colleagues (1986), in an extensive review, compared maternal and perinatal outcomes from before and after 1972. They reported that maternal mortality fell from 6 to 1 percent in these two periods. As shown in Table 52–4, in addition to excessive maternal mortality, more than one third of pregnancies terminated in abortion, stillbirth, or neonatal death. Although perinatal mortality with contemporaneous management probably is less than the 180 per 1000 shown in Table 52–4, it continues to be excessive. Morbidity from fetal growth retardation likewise is common.

In nonpregnant women, morbidity and mortality from sickle cell–hemoglobin C disease are appreciably lower than from sickle cell anemia. Indeed, less than half of women with SC disease have ever been symptomatic prior to pregnancy. During pregnancy and the puerperium, however, attacks of severe bone pain and episodes of pulmonary infarction and embolization become fairly common (Cunningham and associates, 1983). A particularly worrisome pulmonary complication is related to embolization of necrotic bone marrow, both fat and cellular, and acute respiratory insufficiency may develop. In an 18-year anterospective study at Parkland

TABLE 52–4. PREGNANCY OUTCOMES REPORTED SINCE 1956 FOR WOMEN WITH SICKLE CELL ANEMIA AND HEMOGLOBIN SC DISEASE

	Sickle Cell (SS) Disease	Hemoglobin SC Disease
Women	747	211
Pregnancies	1478	605
Maternal deaths (per 100,000)	2570	2310
Spontaneous abortions (%)	18	16
Perinatal mortality (per 1000)	180	75

Data from Carache (1980); El-Shafei (1992); Milner (1980); Poddar (1986); Powars (1986); and their many colleagues.

Hospital, the maternal mortality rate for women with hemoglobin SC disease was close to 2 percent (Pritchard and co-workers, 1973). As shown in Table 52–4, maternal deaths with hemoglobin SC disease were as common as with SS disease. Powars and associates (1986) reported that maternal mortality at their institution decreased from 6 percent before 1972 to zero since that time. Also as shown in Table 52–4, the perinatal mortality rate is somewhat greater than that of the general population but nowhere as great as with sickle cell anemia.

Management. Adequate management of pregnant women with sickle cell anemia or other sickle cell hemoglobinopathies necessitates close observation with careful evaluation of all symptoms, physical findings, and laboratory studies. One rather common danger is that the symptomatic woman may categorically be considered to be suffering from a sickle cell crisis. As a result, ectopic pregnancy, placental abruption, pyelonephritis, appendicitis, cholecystitis, or other serious obstetrical or medical problems that cause pain or anemia, or both, may be overlooked. **The term sickle cell crisis should be applied only after all other possible causes of pain or fever or reduction in hemoglobin concentration have been excluded.**

In the absence of infection or nutritional deficiency, the hemoglobin concentration usually does not fall below 7 g/dL. Because these women maintain their hemoglobin concentration by intense hemopoiesis to compensate for the markedly shortened erythrocyte life span, any factor that impairs erythropoiesis or increases red cell destruction, or both, aggravates the anemia. The folic acid requirements during pregnancy complicated by sickle cell anemia are considerable and supplementary folic acid of 1 mg per day is given.

There are special circumstances during pregnancy that increase appreciably the morbidity of these women. Covert bacteriuria and acute pyelonephritis are increased substantively, and careful surveillance for bacteriuria and its eradication is important to prevent most urinary symptomatic infections. If pyelonephritis develops, these erythrocytes are extremely susceptible to endotoxin, which can cause dramatic and rapid red cell destruction while simultaneously suppressing erythropoiesis. Pneumonia, especially due to *Streptococcus pneumoniae*, is common, and the woman with advanced pregnancy may not tolerate severe pulmonary infections. Most authorities recommend polyvalent pneumococcal vaccine for these women.

Women with sickle cell disease seldom die of heart failure; however, the basal hemodynamic state is characterized by high cardiac output, which is further augmented by pregnancy. There is now abundant evidence that they have myocardial dysfunction at rest which is augmented by exercise. Thus, although most of these women tolerate the changes of normal pregnancy well, when complications such as severe preeclampsia or serious infection develop, ventricular failure becomes likely (Cunningham and associates, 1986). More recently, the extent of chronic lung disease, both restrictive and associated with arteriolar vasculopathy, has been appreciated (Powars and colleagues, 1988).

Intense sequestration of sickled erythrocytes with infarction in various organs may develop acutely, especially late in pregnancy, during labor and delivery, and early in the puerperium. Acute infarction is usually accompanied by severe pain, and because the bone marrow is frequently involved, intense bone pain is common. Anyaegbunam and colleagues (1991) reported observations obtained during 39 sickling crises in 24 women. In almost 60 percent they demonstrated reversible nonreactive stress tests and all had increases in the uterine artery systolic–diastolic ratio. Conversely, they found no changes in the umbilical artery systolic–diastolic ratios, suggesting that transient effects of crises did not compromise umbilical blood flow.

Relief of pain from intravascular sickling is not afforded by heparinization or dextran. Intravenous hydration is provided, and for severe pain, meperidine or morphine are administered parenterally. Red cell transfusions administered after the onset of severe pain, in our experience, have no dramatic effect on the intensity or the duration of the pain. Conversely, prophylactic red cell transfusions almost eliminate pain by preventing these vaso-occlusive episodes.

Because of the high incidence of fetal growth retardation, as well as increased perinatal mortality, careful fetal assessment is necessary. Perry and Morrison (1990) recommend weekly nonstress testing beginning at 32 weeks, along with serial ultrasonography to monitor fetal growth and amnionic fluid. Fetal surveillance techniques are described in Chapter 45.

Labor and delivery in women with hemoglobin SS disease should be managed the same way as for women with cardiac disease (see Chap. 48, p. 1086). The woman should be kept comfortable but not oversedated. Epidural analgesia is ideally suited. Compatible blood should be available. If a difficult vaginal or cesarean delivery is contemplated, and the hematocrit is less than 20 percent, the hemoglobin concentration should be increased by packed erythrocyte transfusions. At the same time, care must be taken to prevent circulatory overload from ventricular failure and pulmonary edema.

Prophylactic Red Cell Transfusions. There currently is controversy over the use of prophylactic erythrocyte transfusions during pregnancy for women with sickle cell anemia, sickle cell–hemoglobin C disease, or sickle cell–β-thalassemia disease. Among the more than 100 pregnancies complicated by sickle hemoglobinopathy so managed at Parkland Hospital, morbidity has been minimal, but there has been one maternal death. The degree of relief from chronically debilitating sickle cell anemia provided one woman by transfusion during pregnancy is illustrated in Figure 52–3.

The most dramatic impact of prophylactic transfusions is on maternal morbidity (Cunningham and associates, 1983). Although perinatal outcome has improved substantively, it has been emphasized that other management advances have contributed significantly. Despite occasional worrisome evidence of a compromised intrauterine environment in the form of fetal growth retardation, meconium staining, and ominous fetal heart rate decelerations during labor, perinatal mortality now is remarkably low when compared with previous experiences (Cunningham and associates, 1979, 1983).

The hazards of transfusions are obvious and intuitively should be avoided. To address this, Koshy and colleagues (1988) randomized 72 pregnant women with sickle cell disease to be given either prophylactic red cell transfusions or to be transfused only if indicated. They too cited significantly decreased maternal morbidity in women transfused; however, they reported that perinatal outcomes were not improved, and they concluded that transfusion therapy was not necessary.

Morbidity from transfusions has proved troublesome, especially isoimmunization and hepatitis. We calculated that the incidence of isoimmunization per unit of blood transfused at Parkland Hospital was 3 percent (Cox and associates, 1988). Vichinsky and co-workers (1990) reported that almost 30 percent of all chronically transfused sickle patients were isoimmunized.

They noted that more extensive typing of donor erythrocytes would decrease this incidence. Finally, although the spectre of iron overload and transfusion hemochromatosis is worrisome, we found no evidence of this in liver biopsies performed in 40 such women transfused during pregnancy (Yeomans and co-workers, 1990).

Experimental Therapy. Increasing the production of hemoglobin S may be harmful to patients with sickle cell anemia because blood viscosity increases with hematocrit. Conversely, induction of hemoglobin F by stimulating gamma-chain synthesis appears to be a promising form of chronic treatment for sickling and some thalassemia syndromes. For example, 5-azacytidine and hydroxyurea selectively increase hemoglobin F production (Rodgers and associates, 1990). Preliminary studies indicate that patients who respond to hydroxyurea with increased F-cell production have less sickling. Unfortunately, the dose of drug given also was myelosuppressive (Goldberg and colleagues, 1990). Hydroxyurea is a category D drug, and there is limited experience with its use in pregnancy. Finally, Perrine and co-workers (1993) have shown that butyrate infusions stimulate fetal-globin production in nonpregnant persons.

Contraception and Sterilization. Because of the chronic debility from sickle cell anemia, the further complications caused by pregnancy, and the predictably shortened life span of women with sickle cell anemia, sterilization, or at least a very effective means of contraception, is indicated, even for women of low parity.

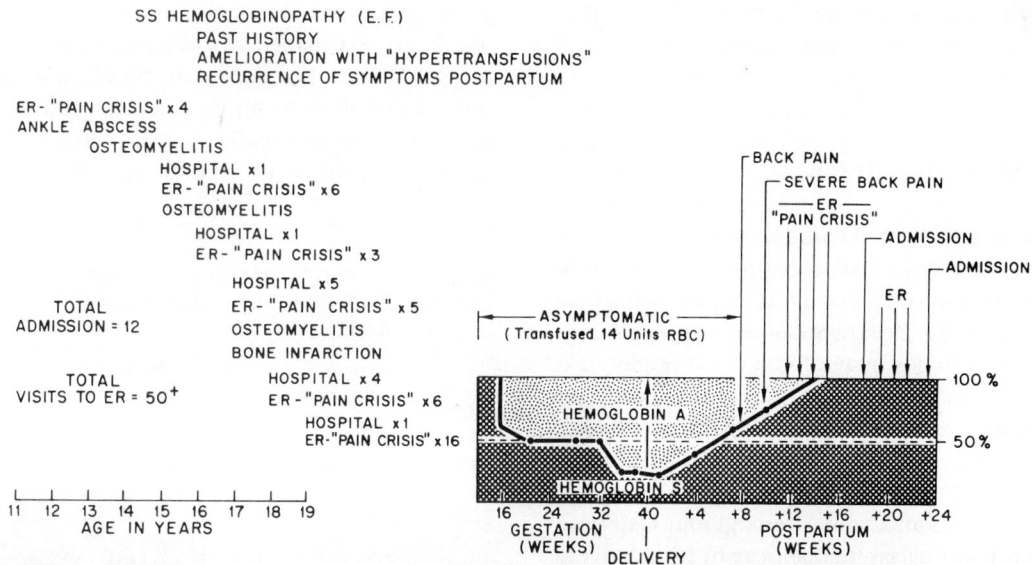

Fig. 52–3. Patient E.F., who has sickle cell anemia. Debility before her first pregnancy is summarized on the left. To the right, the reduction in hemoglobin S level as the consequence of transfusion of 14 units of packed red cells, and the recurrence of severe pain 9 weeks after delivery are emphasized (ER = Emergency Room). (From Cunningham and Pritchard, 1979.)

Estrogen–progestin oral contraceptives are relatively contraindicated in women with sickle hemoglobinopathies (see Chap. 60, p. 1333).

Sickle Cell Trait. The inheritance of the gene for hemoglobin S from one parent and for hemoglobin A from the other results in sickle cell trait. The amount of S hemoglobin is distinctly less than the amount of A hemoglobin. In a survey of nearly 250,000 people in the United States, the frequency of red cell sickling among African-Americans was reported to be about 8 percent (Schneider and co-workers, 1976). We tested almost 50,000 black women attending Parkland Hospital prenatal and family planning clinics and also determined that 8 percent had sickle trait.

Extensive studies of the effect, or lack of effect, of sickle cell trait on pregnancy have been reported (Pritchard and associates, 1973; Tuck and co-workers, 1983). Sickle cell trait did not influence unfavorably the frequency of abortion, perinatal mortality, low birthweight, or pregnancy-induced hypertension. Urinary infection, however, was about twice as common in the group with sickle cell trait. Subsequent investigations disclosed that twice as many pregnant women with sickle cell trait had asymptomatic bacteriuria as did black women whose erythrocytes did not sickle (Whalley, 1967).

Sickle cell trait should not be considered a deterrent to pregnancy on the basis of increased risks to the mother. The probability, however, for a serious sickle cell hemoglobinopathy in her offspring is 1 in 4 whenever the father carries a gene for an abnormal hemoglobin or for β-thalassemia. Prenatal diagnosis of sickle cell disease through amniocentesis or chorionic villus sampling now is available (see Chap. 41, p. 948). In a 1987 survey, Rowley (1989) reported that prenatal diagnosis was performed in only 4 percent of pregnancies at risk.

Other Hemoglobinopathies

Hemoglobin C and C–β-Thalassemia. Hemoglobin C results from a single β-chain substitution of glutamic acid by lysine at position 6. It is quite common in West Africa, but only about 2 percent of African-Americans have the mutant gene for hemoglobin C. Hemoglobin C trait does not cause anemia, nor does it predispose to adverse pregnancy outcomes. When co-inherited with sickle cell trait, the resultant hemoglobin SC causes problems discussed on page 1179.

Pregnancy and homozygous hemoglobin C disease or hemoglobin C–β-thalassemia appear to be relatively benign associations. Maberry and colleagues (1990b) reported our experiences at Parkland Hospital with 72 pregnancies complicated by C-hemoglobinopathies. The degree of anemia was usually mild to moderate, and the mean late pregnancy hematocrit was 27 percent (range

21 to 33) for 49 pregnancies complicated by hemoglobin CC disease and 30 percent (range 28 to 33) for 23 pregnancies complicated by C–β-thalassemia. Blood volume expansion in these women averaged about 35 percent compared with their nonpregnant volumes.

Pregnancy outcomes, shown in Table 52–5, were not different in women with C hemoglobin syndromes compared with the general obstetrical population at Parkland Hospital. When severe anemia is identified, iron or folic acid deficiency or some other superimposed cause should be suspected. Supplementation with folic acid and iron, unless blood is transfused, is likely to prove of value in pregnant women with any hemoglobinopathy.

Hemoglobin E. Hemoglobin E results from a single β-chain substitution of lysine for glutamic acid at codon 26. The hemoglobin is susceptible particularly to oxidative stress. The prevalence of hemoglobin E trait is common in Southeast Asia, and is very close to that for hemoglobin S in the United States. Homozygous inheritance gives rise to hemoglobin E disease. This hemoglobinopathy has become more prevalent in the United States since the influx of a large number of Southeast Asians after 1970. Hurst and co-workers (1983) identified homozygous hemoglobin E, hemoglobin E plus α-thalassemia, or hemoglobin E trait in 36 percent of Cambodian children and 25 percent of Laotians, but in only 1 percent of Vietnamese. Alpha- and β-thalassemia traits were prevalent in all groups.

Despite its frequency, there has been little reported about the homozygous state for hemoglobin E. In our limited experience, it appears to be characterized by hypochromia, marked microcytosis, and erythrocyte targeting. These women may not even be anemic, or only mildly so. Pregnancies in women homozygous for hemoglobin E do not appear to be at increased risk. Hemoglobin E–β-thalassemia, however, has been reported to cause severe anemia that may require transfusion during pregnancy (Ferguson and Reilly, 1985; Hsia,

TABLE 52–5. OUTCOMES IN 72 PREGNANCIES COMPLICATED BY HEMOGLOBIN CC AND C–β-THALASSEMIA

	Hemoglobin CC	C–β-thalassemia
Women	15	5
Pregnancies	49	23
Maternal complications[a]	0	0
Spontaneous abortions	7	1
Birthweight (g)		
Mean	2990	2960
Range	1145–4770	2320–3980
Stillbirths	0	2
Neonatal deaths	1	0
Surviving infants	42	20

[a] Excluding mild to moderate anemia.
From Maberry and colleagues (1990b), with permission.

1991). It is not clear whether sickle cell–hemoglobin E disease is as ominous during pregnancy as sickle cell–hemoglobin C disease or sickle–β-thalassemia disease. Ramahi and colleagues (1988) described a woman with SE hemoglobinopathy. Even though she had only mild anemia and no history of clinical sickling, they elected to treat her with exchange transfusions during pregnancy.

Iron-deficiency anemia as the consequence of intestinal parasites, repeated pregnancies, or both, may coexist with E hemoglobinopathy. We are providing supplements of folic acid as well as iron for pregnant women identified to have homozygous hemoglobin E or hemoglobin E–thalassemia.

Hemoglobinopathy in the Newborn. Hemolytic anemias characteristic of many hemoglobinopathies are not operational in utero or at birth because most of the erythrocyte hemoglobin is fetal (F). After birth, as newly synthesized red cells contain more abnormal hemoglobin, the disease becomes clinically apparent. Newborn infants with sickle cell anemia, sickle cell–hemoglobin C disease, and homozygous hemoglobin C disease can be identified accurately at birth by electrophoresis performed on hemoglobin obtained from uncontaminated cord blood (Nussbaum and colleagues, 1984). In many states, such screening is performed routinely on blood submitted for phenylketonuria and hypothyroidism screening (Chap. 40, p. 927). Vichinsky and colleagues (1988) described the benefits of early diagnosis of sickle cell disease provided by screening of nearly 85,000 newborns in California.

Genetic Counseling. Identification of the common hemoglobinopathies and their traits involves relatively simple laboratory procedures, and the genetic aspects of these diseases are straightforward. Therefore, genetic counseling can be provided readily. On the average, 1 of 4 children will be afflicted with the disease whenever both parents have a trait form. If one parent has the hemoglobinopathy and the other only the trait, then half of their children can be expected to inherit the hemoglobinopathy and the other half the trait. If both parents have a hemoglobinopathy, so will all their children.

Remarkable technical advances have been made in identifying the fetus who is genetically destined to develop sickle syndromes, especially sickle cell anemia. Early procedures required the collection of fetal red cells whose capabilities for synthesizing abnormal β-globin chains were then measured in vitro. It was next demonstrated that desquamated fetal amniocytes cultured from amnionic fluid could be treated with a **restriction endonuclease** enzyme that would cleave DNA into fragments (Chang and Kan, 1982). Thus the gene on chromosome 11 for β-globin chain synthesis could be identified. Initially, linkage analysis was used, and this was followed by direct analysis of the fragments, which served to identify prenatally fetuses who were destined to develop sickle cell anemia. Assays using DNA amplification techniques by polymerase chain reaction have been developed that are so sensitive that restriction endonuclease MstII can be applied immediately to cells obtained from 10 to 20 mL of amnionic fluid without prior culture, thereby avoiding the delay that had been imposed by cell culture (Kazazian and colleagues, 1989).

Hemoglobin C cannot be identified using the MstII enzyme, but hemoglobin C and most instances of β-thalassemia can be identified by analysis of DNA polymorphism or by identifying in vitro the kinds of globin chains synthesized by fetal red cells obtained from the fetus or placenta. The usefulness of DNA polymorphisms in circumstances where the inheritance of these diseases cannot be determined directly is borne out by the experiences of Boehm and associates (1983).

Chorionic villus biopsy during the first trimester has been used to identify fetal sickle cell anemia or β-thalassemia (Chap. 41, p. 944). DNA extracted from the trophoblast without prior culture is treated with an appropriate restriction enzyme and oligonucleotide analysis is performed (Monni and colleagues, 1987; Old and co-workers, 1986).

Thalassemias

The genetically determined hemoglobinopathies that are classified as thalassemias are characterized by an impaired production rate of one or more of the peptide chains that are normal components of globin. The abnormal synthesis rates may result in ineffective erythropoiesis, hemolysis, and varying degrees of anemia. The different forms of thalassemia are classified according to the globin chain which is deficient in amount compared to its partner chain. Literally hundreds of thalassemia syndromes have been described (Weatherall, 1990). The two major forms of thalassemias involve either impaired production of alpha peptide chains causing α-thalassemia, or of beta chains to cause β-thalassemia. The incidence of these traits during pregnancy for all races is probably 1 in 300 to 500 (Gehlbach and Morgenstern, 1988).

Alpha-Thalassemias. Because there are two α-globin genes, the genetics of α-thalassemia is more complicated than for β-thalassemia. Four clinical syndromes, the consequence of impaired α-globin chain synthesis, have been identified. For each syndrome, a close correlation has been established between clinical severity and the degree of impairment of synthesis of α-globin chains. In most populations the α-globin chain "cluster" or gene loci are duplicated on chromosome 16 and thus the normal genotype for diploid cells can be expressed as αα/αα. There are two main groups of α-thalassemia determinants: α°-thalassemia is characterized by the deletion of both loci from one chromosome (—/$\alpha\alpha$), whereas α^+-thalassemia is characterized by the loss of a single locus from one chromosome (-α/$\alpha\alpha$, heterozygote) or both (-α/-α, homozygote). The α^+ thalassemias may be deletion or nondeletion types. All α° and α^+ thalassemias are extremely heterogenous at the molecular level (Weatherall, 1990).

There are two major phenotypes. The deletion of all four α-globin chain genes (—/—) characterizes homozygous α-thalassemia. Because α-chains make up fetal hemoglobin, the fetus is affected. Without α-globin chains, hemoglobin Bart (γ_4) and hemoglobin H (β_4) are formed as abnormal tetramers. Hemoglobin Bart has an appreciably increased affinity for oxygen. The fetus dies either in utero or very soon after birth and demonstrates the typical clinical features of nonimmune hydrops fetalis shown in Figure 52–4 (see Chap. 44, p. 1014). Hemoglobin Bart disease is a common cause of stillbirths in Southeast Asia. Hsieh and associates (1989) studied 20 hydropic fetuses at 17 to 35 weeks' gestation by funipuncture and reported that blood contained 65 to 98 percent Bart hemoglobin.

The compound heterozygous state for α° and α^+ thalassemia results in the deletion of three of four genes(—/-α), leaving only one functional α-globin gene per diploid genome. This is referred to as hemoglobin H disease (β_4), and it is compatible with extrauterine life. The abnormal red cells at birth contain a mixture of hemoglobin Bart (γ_4), hemoglobin H (β_4), and hemoglobin A. The neonate appears well at birth, but after early infancy, hemolytic anemia develops. Most, if not all, of the 20 to 40 percent of hemoglobin Bart present at birth is replaced postnatally by hemoglobin H. In the adult, 5 to 30 percent of hemoglobin is H. The disease is characterized by hemolytic anemia of varying severity and, in some patients, disease severity is similar to β-thalassemia major. Anemia in these women usually is worsened during pregnancy.

A deletion of two genes results clinically in **α-thalassemia minor,** which is characterized by minimal to moderate hypochromic microcytic anemia. These may be due to α°- or α^+-thalassemia traits. Thus, genotypes may be -α/-α or —/$\alpha\alpha$. Because there is no associated clinical abnormality with α-thalassemia minor, it often goes unrecognized. Hemoglobin Bart is present at birth, but as it dissipates, it is not replaced by hemoglobin H. Red cells are hypochromic and microcytic, and the hemoglobin concentration is normal to slightly depressed. Women with α-thalassemia minor appear to tolerate pregnancy quite well.

The single gene deletion (-α/$\alpha\alpha$) is the **silent carrier state.** No clinical abnormality is evident in the individual with a single gene deletion.

Frequency. The relative frequency of α-thalassemia minor, hemoglobin H disease, and hemoglobin Bart disease varies remarkably among racial groups. All of these variants are encountered in Orientals. In individuals of African descent, however, even though α-thalassemia minor is demonstrated in about 2 percent, hemoglobin H disease is extremely rare and hemoglobin Bart disease is unreported. The reason for the discrepancy is that Orientals usually have α°-thalassemia minor with both

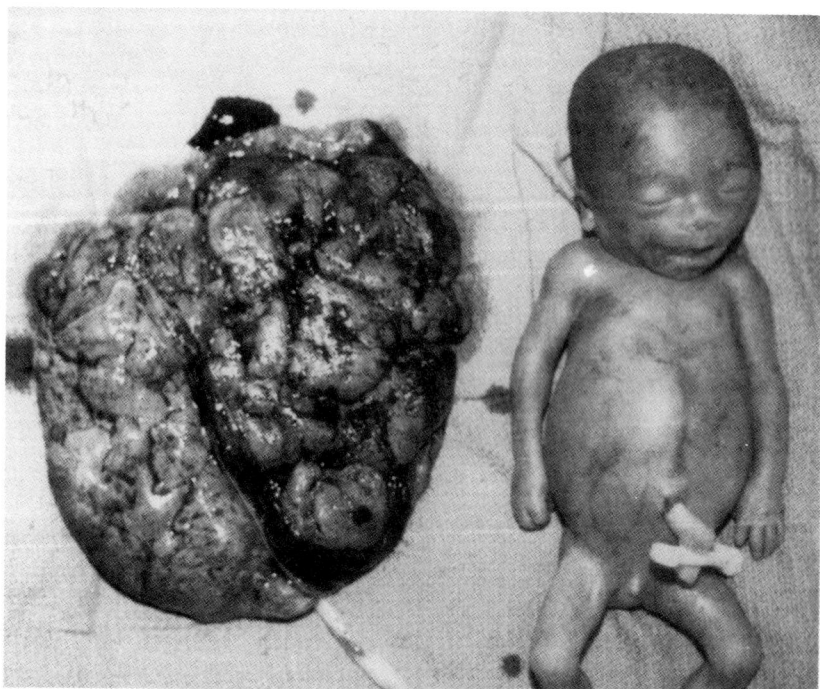

Fig. 52–4. Stillborn hydropic fetus with extremely large placenta caused by homozygous α-thalassemia. (From Hsia, 1991, with permission.)

gene deletions typically from the same chromosome (—/αα), whereas in blacks with α$^+$-thalassemia minor, one gene is deleted from each chromosome (-α/-α). The α-thalassemia syndromes appear sporadically in other racial and ethnic groups. Diagnosis of α-thalassemia minor, as well as α-thalassemia major in the fetus, can be accomplished by DNA analysis using molecular techniques (Hsia, 1991; Maberry and colleagues, 1990a).

Beta-Thalassemias. The β-thalassemias are the consequence of impaired production of β-globin chains, and the molecular pathology for the defective production is quite complex. Kazazian and Boehm (1988) described 51 point mutations in the β-globin gene. Most are single nucleotide substitutions that produce transcription defects, RNA splicing or modification, translation, or highly unstable hemoglobins. Thus, deletional and nondeletional mutations affect the transcription, processing, or translation of β-globin RNA. The δγβ— gene "cluster" is on chromosome 11.

With β-thalassemia there is decreased β-chain production and excess α-chains precipitate to cause cell membrane damage. These basic defects lead to the panorama of pathology that characterizes homozygous β-thalassemia, so-called β-thalassemia major or Cooley anemia. With heterozygous β-thalassemia minor, hypochromia, microcytosis, and slight to moderate anemia develop without the intense hemolysis that characterizes the homozygous state. The hallmark of the common β-thalassemias is an elevated hemoglobin A$_2$ level.

In the typical case of **thalassemia major,** the neonate is healthy at birth, but as the hemoglobin F level falls, the infant becomes severely anemic and fails to thrive. If children are entered into an adequate transfusion program, they develop normally until the end of the first decade when effects of iron loading become apparent. Those females who do survive beyond childhood usually are sterile, and life expectancy with transfusion therapy is to the third decade. They seldom become pregnant, but successful outcomes have been reported (Mordel and colleagues, 1989). Transfusion therapy must be continued. Lucarelli and associates (1990) evaluated bone marrow transplantation for patients with thalassemia major. They reported a 3-year survival of 94 percent with no recurrences in patients who had no hepatomegaly or portal fibrosis.

With **β-thalassemia minor,** A$_2$ hemoglobin (comprised of two α- and two δ-globin chains) is increased to more than 3.5 percent and hemoglobin F (two α- and two γ-globin chains) is usually increased to more than 2 percent. The red cells are hypochromic and microcytic but anemia is mild. The hemoglobin concentration typically is 8 to 10 g/dL late in the second trimester, with an increase to between 9 and 11 g/dL near term, compared with a hemoglobin level of 10 to 12 g/dL in the nonpregnant state (Alger and colleagues, 1979; Pritchard, 1962). There is usually pregnancy-induced augmentation of erythropoiesis and, using ^{51}chromium-tagged erythrocytes, we have documented normal blood volume expansion with slightly subnormal red cell mass expansion.

There is no specific therapy for β-thalassemia minor during pregnancy. Most often, the outcomes for the mother and fetus are satisfactory (Pritchard, 1962; Smith and associates, 1975). Blood transfusions are seldom indicated except for hemorrhage. Prophylactic iron and folic acid in daily doses of about 30 mg and 1 mg, respectively, are given. Any disease that depresses hemopoiesis or increases erythrocyte destruction naturally intensifies the anemia. Therefore, infections should be identified promptly and treated. The modest anemia, when not correctly diagnosed, has led to overzealous treatment, especially with parenteral iron and at times with blood transfusions.

The potential exists for the fetus to inherit the serious problem of β-thalassemia major or sickle–β-thalassemia. Prenatal diagnosis of β-thalassemia may be difficult and is successful in only 80 percent of cases. Techniques include a combination of site-specific restriction endonuclease analysis, restriction fragment polymorphism linkage analysis, and oligonucleotide probes (Antonarakis, 1989; Old and colleagues, 1986).

The term **β-thalassemia intermedia** has been applied commonly to the clinical condition of individuals whose disease was nowhere near as intense as in β-thalassemia major but obviously more severe than that of β-thalassemia minor. Weatherall (1990) described several possibilities that explain this intermediate condition, including that it may be a mild form of β-thalassemia major. Co-inheritance of α-thalassemia, δβ-thalassemia, or inheritance of *extra* α-globin genes are known to modify the clinical syndrome.

Hemolytic Anemias Caused by Inherited Erythrocyte Membrane Defects

The normal erythrocyte is shaped like a biconcave disc, and there is a redundancy of membrane surface area relative to volume. This allows numerous cycles of reversible deformations as the erythrocyte withstands shearing forces created in arteries and negotiations through splenic slits a fraction of its cross-sectional diameter. A number of inherited red cell membrane defects result in destabilization of the membrane lipid bilayer. This leads to loss of lipids from the erythrocyte membrane, surface area deficiency, and poorly deformable cells that undergo hemolysis resulting in varying degrees of anemia. Some of these inherited membrane defects that will cause accelerated destruction are hereditary spherocytosis, pyropoikilocytosis, and ovalocytosis.

Hereditary Spherocytosis. There are several inherited erythrocyte membrane protein deficiencies that give rise to the syndrome of hereditary spherocytosis. Although most are due to autosomally dominant variably penetrant **spectrin** deficiency, others are autosomally recessive and may be caused by **ankyrin** or **protein 4.2** deficiency or combinations thereof (Agre, 1989; Chasis and co-workers, 1988). These disorders are characterized clinically by varying degrees of anemia and jaundice as the consequence of hemolysis of microspherocytic red cells (Fig. 52–5). Confirmation of diagnosis is by documentation of spherocytes on peripheral smear, reticulocytosis, and increased osmotic fragility.

Hemolysis with corresponding anemia is dependent upon an intact spleen, which is usually enlarged. Splenectomy, although not correcting the membrane defect, spherocytosis, or increased osmotic fragility, does greatly reduce hemolysis, anemia, and jaundice. So-called **crisis,** characterized by severe anemia from accelerated red cell destruction or more likely failure of production, or both, may develop in the woman with a functioning spleen. Infection must be detected and vigorously treated.

Pregnancy. In general, women with hereditary spherocytosis do well during pregnancy. Maberry and associates (1992) reported our experiences from Parkland Hospital with 50 pregnancies in 23 women with spherocytosis. In late pregnancy, their hematocrits varied from 23 to 41 percent (mean 31) and reticulocyte counts ranged from 1 to 23 percent. There was minimal maternal morbidity. There were eight abortions, and 4 of 42 infants were born preterm but none were growth retarded. Infection in four women intensified hemolysis and three required transfusions. A previously normal pregnancy does not preclude sudden development of severe anemia in a subsequent pregnancy (Ventura, 1982). Folic acid supplementation avoids the risk of megaloblastic erythropoiesis.

The newborn infant who has inherited hereditary spherocytosis may or may not demonstrate hyperbilirubinemia and anemia during the neonatal period. We observed the hemoglobin level to fall to as low as 5.0 g/dL by 5 weeks of age in the daughter of a woman with hereditary spherocytosis.

Red Cell Enzyme Deficiencies. A number of erythrocyte enzymes are necessary for anaerobic utilization of glucose by the red cell. A deficiency of many but certainly not all of these enzymes may cause **hereditary nonspherocytic anemia.** Most of these are inherited as autosomal recessive traits. **Glucose-6-phosphate dehydrogenase deficiency,** by far the most commonly identified enzyme deficiency, is a well-known exception that is X-linked. There are over 400 variants of this enzyme (Beutler, 1991). In the A-variant, inherited by about 2 percent of African-American women, erythrocytes are markedly deficient in normal enzyme activity. In this the deficient or homozygous state, both X chromosomes are affected. The heterozygous state, with one deficient and one normal X chromosome, is identified in 10 to 15 percent of African-American women. The defect probably confers some degree of protection against malarial infection. Random X-chromosome inactivation results in a variable deficiency of enzyme activity. Infections or several oxidant drugs may induce hemolysis in some heterozygous as well as homozygous women. Thus, anemia is episodic, although some variants induce chronic nonspherocytic hemolysis. Since young erythrocytes contain more enzyme activity than do older erythrocytes, in the absence of bone marrow depression, anemia ultimately stabilizes and is corrected soon after the drug is discontinued.

Pyruvate kinase deficiency, although unusual, is probably the next most common enzyme deficiency. It is inherited as an autosomal recessive trait. In addition to these enzyme deficiencies, there are a number of very rare enzyme abnormalities that may cause hemolysis, and some that do not. Although the degree of chronic hemolysis varies, most episodes of severe anemia with all of these enzyme deficiencies are induced by drugs or infections as previously discussed.

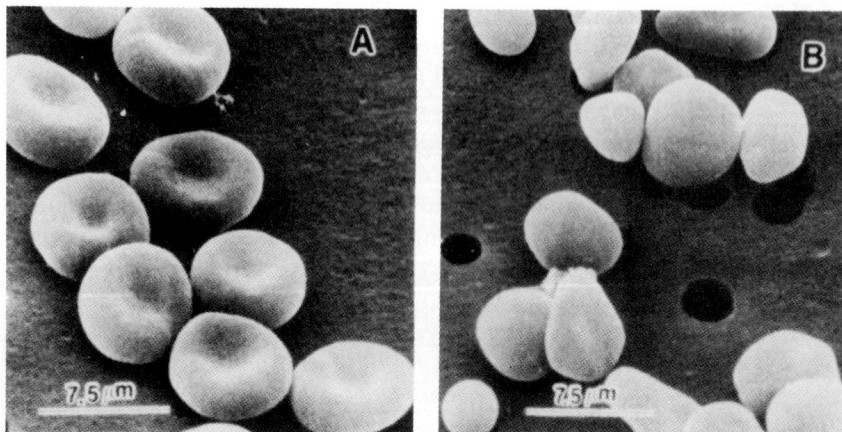

Fig. 52–5. Scanning electron micrograph showing normal-appearing erythrocytes from a heterozygous carrier of recessive spherocytosis (**A**) and her daughter, a homozygote with severe anemia (**B**). (From Agre, 1989, with permission.)

During pregnancy, we prescribe iron and folic acid routinely for these women. Oxidant drugs are avoided, and bacterial infections are treated promptly. Transfusions with red cells are given only if the hematocrit falls below 20, unless there is evidence for heart failure or hypoxia.

Polycythemia

Erythrocytosis during pregnancy is usually of the secondary type related to chronic hypoxia, most often from congenital cardiac disease or a pulmonary disorder. Occasionally it follows heavy cigarette smoking. We have encountered otherwise healthy young women who were heavy smokers who had chronic bronchitis and whose hematocrits were 55 to 60 percent! If polycythemia is severe, the probability of a successful pregnancy outcome is remote.

Brewer and colleagues (1992) described a woman with persistent erythrocytosis associated with a placental site tumor. The hematocrit remained around 55 to 60 percent until hysterectomy was done. Serum erythropoietin concentration was normal.

Polycythemia vera is a hemopoietic stem cell disorder characterized by excessive proliferation of erythroid, myeloid, and megakaryocytic precursors. Symptoms are related to increased blood viscosity, and thrombotic complications are common. It is a condition of older patients and rarely coexists with pregnancy. Ruch and Klein (1964) described a woman whose nonpregnant hematocrit was as high as 63. During each of two pregnancies, however, her hematocrit ranged from a low of 35 during the second trimester to 44 at term. Fetal loss seems to be high in women with polycythemia vera.

Koeffler and Goldwasser (1981) reported that measurement of serum erythropoietin by radioimmunoassay will differentiate polycythemia vera (low values) from secondary polycythemia (high values). No experiences during pregnancy were noted.

Thrombocytopenias

Thrombocytopenia may appear clinically to be idiopathic or, more often, to be associated with one of the following disorders: acquired hemolytic anemia, severe preeclampsia or eclampsia, severe obstetrical hemorrhage with blood transfusions, consumptive coagulopathy from placental abruption or similar hypofibrinogenemic states, septicemia, lupus erythematosus, antiphospholipid antibodies, megaloblastic anemia caused by severe folate deficiency, drugs, viral infections, allergies, aplastic anemia, or excessive irradiation.

An enormous number of drugs and naturally occurring foods can cause platelet dysfunction (George and Shattil, 1991). Aspirin is a prototype. Rarely, platelet dysfunction causes bleeding much like thrombocytopenic syndromes. The **Bernand–Soulier syndrome** is characterized by lack of platelet membrane glycoprotein (gpIb/IX) and severe dysfunction. Peng and colleagues (1991) described an affected woman who during four pregnancies had episodes of postpartum hemorrhage, gastrointestinal hemorrhage, and fetal thrombocytopenia because of maternal IgG antiplatelet antibodies to the missing glycoprotein. Saade and associates (1991) described another woman who had two uneventful pregnancies, yet another with early postpartum hemorrhage, and a fourth with intrapartum and late postpartum bleeding.

Occasionally, thrombocytopenia may be inherited. Chatwani and associates (1992) described a woman with autosomally dominant **May–Hegglin** anomaly. Because fetal inheritance could not be excluded, they performed cesarean section at term. The infant was not affected.

The definition used for thrombocytopenia is important. Burrows and Kelton (1990b) reported that 7.6 percent of pregnant women had a platelet count of less than 150,000 per μL, but in only 0.9 percent was it less than 100,000 per μL. They divided 513 women whose platelet counts were less than 150,000 per μL into three groups: healthy women with incidental thrombocytopenia (65 percent), healthy women with an obstetrical condition such as preterm labor or a medical condition such as diabetes (13 percent), and women with hypertension or immune thrombocytopenia (21 percent). The incidence of neonatal thrombocytopenia in all of these 513 women was 4 percent, a rate identical to infants born to healthy nonthrombocytopenic women.

Immunological Thrombocytopenic Purpura. The entity long referred to as **idiopathic thrombocytopenic purpura** is the consequence most often of an immune process in which antibodies are directed against platelets. Acute idiopathic thrombocytopenic purpura most often is a childhood disease that follows a viral infection. Most cases resolve spontaneously, although perhaps 10 percent become chronic. Conversely, chronic immunological thrombocytopenic purpura is primarily a disease of adults and rarely resolves spontaneously. Familial occurrence is rare. Secondary forms of chronic thrombocytopenia must be ruled out. These are seen with other immune-mediated diseases, for example, systemic lupus erythematosus, as well as lymphomas, leukemias, or a number of systemic diseases.

Antibody-coated platelets are destroyed prematurely in the reticuloendothelial system, especially the spleen. The mechanism of production of these platelet-associated immunoglobulins (PAIgG, PAIgM, PAIgA) is not known, and although unproven, they usually are considered to be autoantibodies.

About 10 percent of adults with idiopathic thrombocytopenia recover spontaneously. For those who do not, platelet counts usually range from 5000 to 75,000 per μL. About 2 percent have positive serological tests for lupus, and some cases are associated with high titers of anticardiolipin antibodies. In those whose platelet counts remain less than 50,000 per μL, treatment with prednisone, 1 mg/kg, will raise the platelet count in about 90 percent. Glucocorticoids exert their action by suppressing phagocytic activity of the splenic monocyte–macrophage system.

For patients in whom remission is not induced by 2 to 3 weeks, or those in whom massive doses of steroids are needed to sustain remission, splenectomy is indicated. This often results in substantive improvement as the consequence of decreased removal of platelets by the spleen and reduced antibody production. Massive doses—400 mg/kg—of gamma globulin given intravenously over 5 days results in satisfactory platelet count elevation in two thirds of patients (Bierling and colleagues, 1982). According to the NIH Consensus Conference (1990), this compound likely works by short-term reticuloendothelial blockade with diminished platelet sequestration. It was concluded that such therapy may be useful in patients with life-threatening thrombocytopenia refractive to other therapy, or preoperatively before splenectomy. Its mechanisms of action were reviewed recently by Dwyer (1992). Immunosuppressive drugs, including azathioprine, cyclophosphamide, vinca alkaloids, and cyclosporine, also have been used with some success in cases refractory to corticosteroids and splenectomy.

Immunological Thrombocytopenia and Pregnancy. Pregnancy is especially challenging to women with immune thrombocytopenia and to their fetuses and newborn infants. Some feel that pregnancy may increase the risk of relapse in women previously in remission and make the condition worse in women with active disease. It is certainly not unusual for women who have been in clinical remission for several years to have recurrent thrombocytopenia during pregnancy; however, this may be because of closer surveillance. The reason(s) for possible deleterious effects from pregnancy are unknown but hyperestrogenemia has been suggested.

There is no contraindication to the use of corticosteroids during pregnancy. Large doses may be required for improvement and most likely treatment will have to be continued for the remainder of pregnancy. Corticosteroid therapy usually produces amelioration; but in refractory women, splenectomy may be effective. Late in pregnancy, the procedure technically is more difficult and cesarean delivery may be necessary to improve exposure. At the same time, the fetus who may be severely thrombocytopenic avoids trauma from vaginal delivery.

The efficacy, if any, of high-dose immunoglobulin for correcting severe thrombocytopenia in pregnancy is not known. It is possible that the risk from thrombocytopenia to the fetus-infant, as well as the mother, could be reduced appreciably by maternal administration of this maternal and placental transfer of IgG to the fetus. Such therapy is expensive, and at our hospital in 1992, patient charges for a 5-day course of treatment totalled about $6000.

Effects on Fetus. Major concerns have been expressed for the fetus of the woman with immunological thrombocytopenia. Platelet-associated IgG antibodies can cross the placenta and cause thrombocytopenia in the fetus-neonate. The frequency and severity of this has been the subject of much attention recently. The severely thrombocytopenic fetus is at increased risk of serious hemorrhage, especially intracranial hemorrhage, as the consequence of labor and delivery.

Considerable attention has been directed at identifying the fetus with potentially dangerous thrombocytopenia. All investigators have concurred that there is not a strong correlation between fetal and maternal platelet counts. Unfortunately, the conclusion of Karpatkin and associates (1981) was incorrect that the administration of corticosteroids to the mother assures an adequate platelet count in the fetus-infant. It cannot be substantiated by either the findings demonstrated in the infant shown in Figure 52–6, or by observations of others (Cines, 1982; Cook, 1991; Kaplan, 1990; Kelton, 1982; Samuels, 1990; Scott, 1983; and their numerous colleagues). To test this hypothesis further, Christiaens

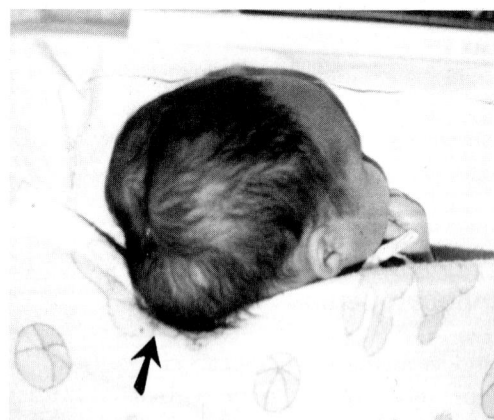

Fig. 52–6. Newborn with extensive cephalohematomas, especially over the occipital bone (*arrow*). The mother had chronic immunological thrombocytopenic purpura for which splenectomy had been performed years earlier. Severe thrombocytopenia developed in this pregnancy and she was treated with prednisone. Her platelet count at the time of cesarean section was 115,000 per μL, and the cord blood platelet count was 17,000 per μL. When it decreased to 3000 per μL, the infant was treated with corticosteroids and platelet transfusions and did well.

and colleagues (1990) randomized 41 pregnant women with immunological thrombocytopenia to betamethasone therapy versus no treatment beginning at 36 weeks and until delivery. Neonatal thrombocytopenia in both groups was similar; but importantly, maternal corticosteroid therapy did not prevent severe neonatal thrombocytopenia.

Because fetal platelet counts do not correlate accurately with maternal values, several investigators have attempted to quantify the relationship between maternal IgG circulating platelet antibody, platelet-associated antibody, and fetal platelet count. Cines and associates (1982) reported that monitoring circulating platelet antibody, but not platelet-associated antibody, may help identify a fetus with severe thrombocytopenia. Conversely, Kelton and colleagues (1982) reported that measurement of platelet-associated antibody could be used to predict fetal thrombocytopenia.

Samuels and colleagues (1990) showed that detection of indirect platelet antiglobulin was helpful to estimate the risk of neonatal thrombocytopenia. In their study, 28 percent of 162 mothers had a negative indirect antiglobulin test; none of these gave birth to an infant whose platelet count was less than 50,000 per μL. In women with a positive test, historical information was important in establishing neonatal risk (Fig. 52–7). Specifically, only those women who had a positive indirect antiglobulin test and who historically had immune thrombocytopenia had infants whose platelet counts were less than 50,000 per μL. Women in whom thrombocytopenia was first diagnosed during pregnancy, that

is, those without a history of immunological thrombocytopenia antedating pregnancy, had a low risk of infants with thrombocytopenia. In none of these 74 was the platelet count less than 50,000 per μL.

Kaplan and associates (1990) used this technique to assess 64 pregnancies complicated by thrombocytopenia. They found no correlation between maternal antiplatelet antibodies and neonatal disease, but found that a third of fetuses whose mothers had chronic immune thrombocytopenia had thrombocytopenia; importantly, 10 percent of all of these had severe disease. About 13 percent of women with asymptomatic gestational thrombocytopenia had thrombocytopenic fetuses, and one of these four had severe disease. They reported no complications with fetal testing. These investigators concluded that all women with moderate or severe thrombocytopenia—platelet counts less than 100,000 per μL—should undergo fetal platelet estimation.

Earlier, Scott and co-workers (1983) concluded that no antepartum maternal clinical characteristic or laboratory test would accurately predict the fetal platelet count. They recommended the use of intrapartum platelet counts made on blood obtained from the fetal scalp once the cervix was 2 to 3 cm dilated and the membranes were ruptured. Whenever the platelet count in scalp blood was identified to be less than 50,000 per μL, they performed immediate cesarean delivery. Daffos and colleagues (1985) did direct umbilical cord blood sampling and platelet counts in fetuses whose mothers had immune thrombocytopenia and were in labor.

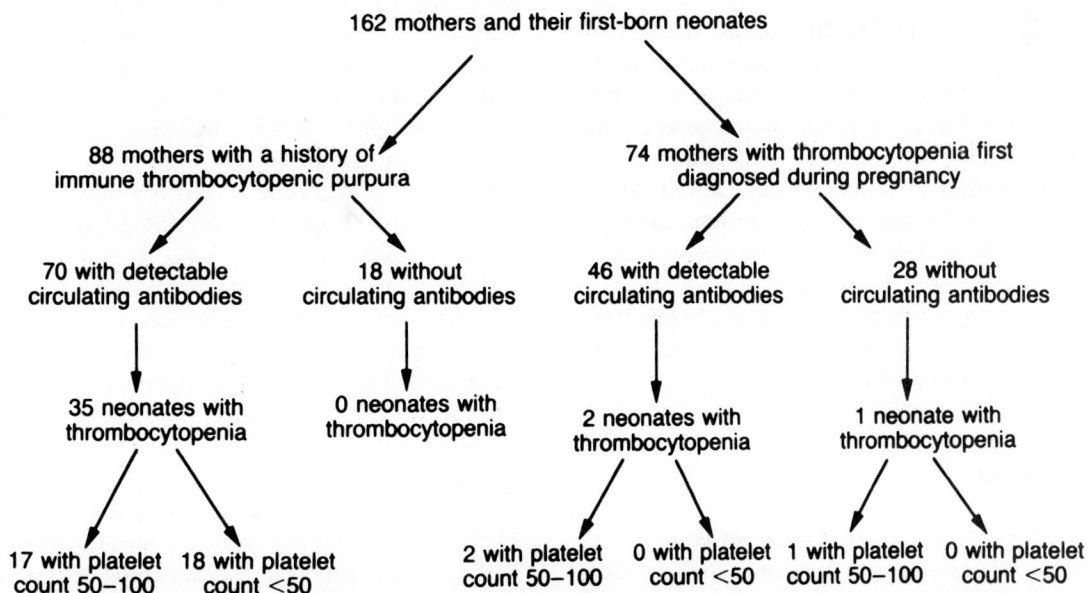

Fig. 52–7. Identification of high-risk and low-risk neonates born to women with thrombocytopenia. The relation between the neonatal platelet counts after the index pregnancy, the maternal history, and the results of indirect antiglobulin tests for all 162 women are shown. Platelet counts indicated are × 10⁹ per liter. (From Samuels and associates, 1990, with permission.)

Management. For the women with an adequate stable platelet count and who is not taking corticosteroids, cesarean delivery is unlikely to be any more a risk than for the normal woman. The administration of large doses of steroids increases somewhat the risks of poor wound healing and infection. The obstetrician faces the dilemma that the route of delivery that may be best for the fetus-infant is likely to be bad for the mother. Indeed, the mother with severe thrombocytopenia who undergoes cesarean delivery is at increased risk for serious morbidity and even mortality. Blood loss at and after vaginal delivery, however, will not be massive when delivery is managed to avoid lacerations and to minimize episiotomy size and maximize myometrial contraction. Platelet transfusions most often are ineffective because donor platelets are coated by antibody and rapidly cleared from the circulation.

As summarized above, most evidence suggests that neonates at risk are born to women with chronic immunological thrombocytopenia recognized before pregnancy. Indeed, these fetuses have about a 20 percent risk of severe disease (Samuels and colleagues, 1990) and about 3 percent of moderately to severely affected neonates have intracranial hemorrhage (Cook and associates, 1991). Because indirect antiglobulin testing is not standardized or widely available (Aster, 1990), it seems reasonable to consider some type of fetal testing for women with documented chronic disease, or those with severe "incidental" gestational thrombocytopenia. Burrows and Kelton (1990a) on the other hand, because of the low incidence of severe neonatal thrombocytopenia and lack of morbidity in their study, have quit performing fetal platelet determinations.

Isoimmune Thrombocytopenia. Platelet isoimmunization can develop in a manner identical to erythrocyte antigen isoimmunization. Its incidence may be as high as 1 in 2000 to 3000 births. If fetal platelet antigens for which maternal platelets are negative gain access to her circulation, the mother then may produce antibodies in subsequent pregnancies that will destroy fetal platelets that have this antigen. The most common antibody is against Pl^{A1} platelet-specific antigen. The first pregnancy is affected in about half of cases. This disorder was reviewed by Deaver and colleagues (1986) and is discussed in Chapter 44 (p. 1018).

Thrombocytosis

Thrombocytosis, or thrombocythemia, generally is defined as platelets persisting in numbers greater than 400,000 per μL. Common causes of secondary or reactive thrombocytosis are malignant tumors, iron deficiency, hemorrhage, inflammatory diseases, and connective-tissue disorders. Platelet counts seldom exceed 800,000 per μL in these secondary disorders, and myeloprolifer-

ative disorders account for most cases in which the counts exceed 1 million per μL. Thrombocytosis usually is asymptomatic, but venous thrombosis may develop. The prognosis depends on the underlying disease.

Sparse evidence from case reports indicates that pregnancies associated with thrombocytosis have excessive spontaneous abortions, placental infarctions, and preterm delivery (Falconer and colleagues, 1987; Mercer and co-workers, 1988). Beard and co-workers (1991), however, challenged this and described nine pregnancies in six women with primary thrombocytopenia whose mean platelet count was 1.25 million per μL. One woman aborted and eight pregnancies were delivered at term. One woman had superficial thrombophlebitis antepartum and also developed postpartum hemorrhage. Jones and associates (1988) reported a woman whose platelet count declined during pregnancy to near-normal levels. Treatment that has been suggested during pregnancy includes aspirin, dipyridamole, heparin, or plateletpheresis, or combinations thereof (Johnson and colleagues, 1989).

Thrombotic Microangiopathies

The original description in 1925 by Moschcowitz of **thrombotic thrombocytopenic purpura** was characterized by the pentad of thrombocytopenia, fever, neurological abnormalities, renal impairment, and hemolytic anemia. In 1955, Gasser and colleagues described the **hemolytic uremic syndrome,** which was similar to thrombotic thrombocytopenic purpura but with more profound renal involvement and fewer neurological aberrations. In 1968, Robson and Wagoner and their colleagues described **postpartum renal failure** characterized by uremia associated with microangiopathic hemolytic anemia and thrombocytopenia.

Although it is likely that there are different etiologies to account for the variable findings within these syndromes, at this time it usually is impossible to separate them, at least clinically (Hayslett, 1985; Moake, 1991; Ruggenenti and Remuzzi, 1990). It seems indisputable that there is a pure form of the hemolytic uremic syndrome in children, incited by viral or bacterial infection; however, its sporadic adult form differs little from thrombotic thrombocytopenic purpura except for the severity of renal involvement. Moreover, there is no evidence that postpartum renal failure differs remarkably from the hemolytic uremic syndrome except that the woman recently had been pregnant. Finally, it seems likely that these syndromes account for the occasional case of severe preeclampsia accompanied by hemolysis and thrombocytopenia that does not respond to delivery (Martin and colleagues, 1990).

Pathogenesis. Microthrombi develop within arterioles and capillaries, consisting of hyaline material made up of platelets and small amounts of fibrin. These aggregates produce fluctuating ischemia or infarctions in various organs. The general consensus is that intravascular platelet aggregation stimulates the cascade of events leading to end-organ failure, and although there is evidence for endothelial damage, it is unknown whether this is a consequence or a cause. Neither the precise pathogenesis of the disease, nor the mechanisms by which cure now often is achieved, are understood. In one scheme, endothelial stimulation or injury causes release of unusually large von Willebrand factor multimers that stimulate platelet aggregation. Another hypothesis is that a plasma factor, which somehow inhibits platelet aggregation, is deficient. One such suspected deficient factor is prostacyclin (prostaglandin I_2), although an excess of its natural antagonist, thromboxane A_2, also has been implicated as an inciting factor. Defective endothelial prostacylin synthesis has been found consistently in both thrombotic thrombocytopenic purpura as well as the hemolytic uremic syndrome (Ruggenenti and Remuzzi, 1990).

Clinical Presentation.
Thrombotic microangiopathies are characterized by thrombocytopenia, fragmentation hemolysis, and variable organ dysfunction (Table 52–6). A viral prodrome may precede up to 40 percent of cases. Neurological abnormalities include headache, altered consciousness, focal findings, convulsions, or stroke. Neurological symptoms are present at discovery in 60 percent of patients and up to 90 percent of those with thrombotic thrombocytopenic purpura will de-

TABLE 52–6. FREQUENCY OF CLINICAL AND LABORATORY FINDINGS WITH THROMBOTIC THROMBOCYTOPENIC SYNDROMES

Findings	%
Symptoms at presentation	
Neurological	60
Hemorrhagic	44
Malaise, fatigue	25
Nausea, vomiting	24
Fever	20
Clinical findings	
Fever	98
Hemorrhage	96
Pallor	96
Neurological	92
Jaundice	42
Weakness	34
Laboratory findings	
Thrombocytopenia	100
Red cell fragmentation	100
Anemia	96
Renal involvement	88
Leukocytosis	60
Hyperbilirubinemia	60
Fibrin split products	60

Modified from Bell (1991), with permission.

velop these. These features also are common with the hemolytic uremic syndrome. Moreover, up to 75 percent of patients with thrombotic thrombocytopenia have renal abnormalities, and these observations make the two syndromes difficult to separate (Moake, 1991). Renal abnormalities include proteinuria, microscopical hematuria, and renal failure. The latter is more severe with the hemolytic uremic syndrome, and in half of the cases, dialysis is required.

Hematological Abnormalities. Thrombocytopenia usually is severe. Fortunately, even with very low platelet counts, spontaneous severe hemorrhage is uncommon. Microangiopathic hemolysis is associated with moderate to marked anemia, and transfusions frequently are necessary. The blood smear is characterized by erythrocyte fragmentation with schizocytosis. The reticulocyte count is high, and nucleated red blood cells are numerous. Consumptive coagulopathy, although common, usually is subtle and clinically insignificant.

Treatment. Treatment of these syndromes until recently has been controversial. Glucocorticoids are considered by many to be ineffective. Heparin administration is of no benefit, and platelet transfusions may even worsen the disease. Antiplatelet agents have been tried with variable success.

More recently, plasma infusion or exchange transfusion with normal plasma and plasmapheresis, usually in combination, has remarkably improved the outcome for these formerly commonly fatal diseases. Preceding therapy with corticosteroids and antiplatelet agents, especially aspirin and dipyridamole, has obfuscated their exact utility. Rock and colleagues (1991) described results from the Canadian national prospective trial in which plasma exchange was found to be superior to plasma infusion in nonpregnant patients. Overall mortality was 30 percent. Bell and co-workers (1991) reported their experiences with 108 patients treated at Johns Hopkins Hospital; 9 percent of these patients were pregnant. Those with minimal neurological symptoms were given prednisone, 200 mg daily, but if there were neurological abnormalities or rapid clinical deterioration, plasmapheresis and plasma exchange were performed daily. About one fourth of patients with mild disease responded to prednisone alone. Of those requiring plasmapheresis, relapses were common but overall survival was 91 percent.

Vincristine or splenectomy, alone or in combination, has been said to cause amelioration of disease that does not respond to plasma exchange. Bell and associates (1991), however, reported that splenectomy was not beneficial in six patients who did not respond to plasmapheresis.

Transfusions with red blood cells are imperative to counteract life-threatening anemia. Unless surgery is contemplated, or there is active bleeding, the hematocrit is maintained at about 20 or somewhat higher. Hemodialysis may be necessary, and placement of an arteriovenous shunt for this procedure also greatly facilitates repeated plasmaphereses.

Pregnancy and Thrombotic Microangiopathy.

There is no firm evidence that pregnancy predisposes women to develop thrombotic microangiopathies, although almost 10 percent of the 108 patients described by Bell and associates (1991) were pregnant. In the past 20 years, we have encountered perhaps 10 pregnant women with these syndromes, or their presumed variants, among the nearly 200,000 women delivered at Parkland Hospital. Because their frequency has not been greater than that in our general hospital population, the question persists concerning the role, if any, of pregnancy and puerperium in the genesis of these syndromes. Our experiences support the thesis that they are coincidental and thus represent an example of sporadic thrombotic microangiopathy that developed during pregnancy. It is possible that some pregnancy-related event may contribute to their development, such as bacterial sepsis, viral infections, and possibly some drugs, for example ergot alkaloids.

As discussed above, the concept of faulty endothelial prostacyclin production currently is popular, and in this respect there is a similarity to severe preeclampsia–eclampsia (Chap. 36, p. 769). It is not surprising that severe preeclampsia and eclampsia complicated further by thrombocytopenia and overt hemolysis have been confused with thrombotic thrombocytopenic purpura and vice versa (Martin and co-workers, 1990; Schwartz and colleagues, 1985; Vandekerckhove and associates, 1984; Weiner, 1987). As described below and in Chapter 36, delivery with supportive care appropriate for severe preeclampsia and eclampsia soon results in the disappearance of both severe thrombocytopenia and the evidence of hemolysis, and is followed by complete recovery. Otherwise, the disease process is not preeclampsia–eclampsia.

It is not established whether pregnancy worsens the prognosis for these syndromes characterized by thrombocytopenic microangiopathy, or whether termination of the pregnancy improves the prognosis. Unless the diagnosis is unequivocally one of these thrombotic microangiopathies, rather than severe preeclampsia or eclampsia, the response to pregnancy termination should be evaluated before resorting to massive-dose glucocorticoid therapy, exchange transfusion, plasmapheresis, or antiplatelet drug therapy. **Plasmapheresis is not indicated for preeclampsia–eclampsia complicated by hemolysis and thrombocytopenia.**

Maternal and fetal outcomes in reported cases have been dismal. Weiner (1987) reviewed 65 cases in which he tried carefully to exclude women with preeclampsia. Perinatal mortality was 80 percent. With plasma therapy, maternal salvage was excellent, but without such

therapy, mortality was 68 percent. Watson and colleagues (1990) provided a scholarly review of the use of plasmapheresis during pregnancy.

In a few instances, thrombotic thrombocytopenic purpura has developed so early in pregnancy that preeclampsia could be excluded. In five cases summarized by Ambrose and colleagues (1985), a variety of therapeutic regimens allowed prolongation of pregnancy until fetal viability. Alternatively, in at least one other woman, termination of early pregnancy was followed by amelioration of the disease on two occasions (Natelson and White, 1985).

In one woman managed at Parkland Hospital, recurrent hemolysis and thrombocytopenia developed peripartum in two successive pregnancies, but delivery had no ameliorative effect. Repeated plasmapheresis, and ultimately splenectomy after the second pregnancy were necessary to induce remission. In at least two other women in whom the syndrome was identified in early pregnancy, termination did not reverse the disease process. In one woman whose recurrent disease manifest at 18 weeks, plasmapheresis with more than 500 donor plasma and red cell units was necessary to control severe thrombocytopenia and hemolysis that persisted despite termination of pregnancy at 23 weeks. The course of the second woman is shown in Table 52–7.

Inherited Coagulation Defects

Obstetrical hemorrhage, a common event, is rarely the consequence of an inherited defect in the coagulation mechanism. There are a number of syndromes, however, that are particularly important in obstetrics.

Hemophilia A.

Hemophilia A is characterized by a marked deficiency of small component antihemophilic factor (factor VIII:C). It is rare among women compared with men. With few exceptions, the homozygous state that results from the inheritance of two abnormal X chromosomes is the requisite for classic hemophilia A in women. In men, one affected X chromosome, the heterozygous state, is responsible for the disease. In a few instances hemophilia A appears to have developed in women spontaneously, presumably as the consequence of a newly mutant gene.

The degree of risk is influenced markedly by the level of circulating factor VIII:C. If the level is at or very close to zero, the risk is major, but if the level is higher, the risk is reduced. Factor VIII:C activity increases appreciably during normal pregnancy. Such an increase is likely in hemophiliacs who can synthesize some factor VIII:C. The risk of grave hemorrhage at and after delivery is reduced by avoiding lacerations, minimizing episiotomy, and maximizing postpartum myometrial contractions and retraction.

Vaginal delivery of a fetus who inherited hemo-

TABLE 52–7. THROMBOTIC MICROANGIOPATHY COMPLICATING EARLY PREGNANCY

	Hematocrit	Platelets	Reticulocytes (%)	Creatinine (mg/dL)	Comments
7 weeks	18	75,000	4	0.9	Normotensive; 2 RBC transfusions
8 weeks	12	60,000	—	1.5	RBC transfusions; prednisone; BP 160/90, 3 + proteinuria; 10 RBC transfused
Transferred to Parkland Hospital					
15 weeks	20	13,000	11	1.3	Plasmapheresis with 10–15 U FFP 9 times over 14 days. RBC transfusions continued
17 weeks	20	10,000	10	1.4	Therapeutic abortion; RBC transfusions continued
Postabortion					
1 week	20	11,000	13	1.4	
2 weeks	18	18,000	16		Splenectomy
3 weeks	30	55,000	5	1.5	Discharged; given total of 17 U RBC and 150 U FFP
Discharged					
1 month	27	110,000		1.5	No transfusions since discharge; severe hypertension; no proteinuria
1 year	37	250,000	1.0	1.6	Severe hypertension
7 years	39	260,000	1.0	1.6	Severe hypertension

RBC = packed red blood cells; FFP = fresh-frozen plasma.

philia A usually has not resulted in perinatal bleeding. After delivery the risk of hemorrhage in the neonate increases, especially if circumcision is attempted. Why labor and vaginal delivery do not commonly incite serious bleeding in the fetus and neonate is not clear because maternal factor VIII:C does not cross the placenta.

Whenever the mother has hemophilia A, all of her sons will have the disease, and all of her daughters will be carriers. If she is a carrier, half of her sons will inherit the disease and half of her daughters will be carriers.

Prenatal diagnosis of hemophilia A is now possible in some families using chorionic villus biopsy (Chap. 41, p. 948). The identification of fetal sex identifies those at risk of inheriting hemophilia A, namely, male fetuses.

Factor VIII Inhibitor. Rarely, antibodies directed against factor VIII are acquired and may lead to life-threatening hemorrhage. This phenomenon has been identified in women during the puerperium. The prominent clinical feature is severe, protracted, repetitive hemorrhage from the reproductive tract starting a week or so after an apparently uncomplicated delivery (Reece and associates, 1982). The activated partial thromboplastin time is markedly prolonged. Treatment has included multiple transfusions of whole blood and plasma, huge doses of cryoprecipitate, large volumes of an admixture of activated coagulation factors, immunosuppressive therapy, and attempts at various surgical procedures, especially curettage and hysterectomy.

Hemophilia B. The genetic and clinical features of severe deficiency of factor IX (Christmas disease or hemophilia B) are quite similar to those for hemophilia A. The homozygous state, essential for severe disease in women, is rare. Rust and associates (1975) described a

pregnancy with a favorable outcome. A successful vaginal delivery was accomplished, and no replacement therapy was given despite a persistently low factor IX activity. The male newborn appeared to tolerate labor and vaginal delivery without hemorrhage.

Von Willebrand Disease. Clinically, von Willebrand disease is a heterogenous group of functional disorders involving aberrations of factor VIII complex and platelet dysfunctions. These abnormalities are the most commonly inherited bleeding disorders and may be identified in as many as 1 in 1000 patients. Most of the more than 10 variants of von Willebrand disease are inherited as autosomal dominant traits, but type III, which is the most severe, is phenotypically recessive.

The von Willebrand factor (vWF) is a large multimeric glycoprotein. It is essential for normal platelet adhesion to subendothelial collagen and formation of a primary hemostatic plug at the site of blood vessel injury. It also plays a major role in the stabilization of the coagulant properties of factor VIII. The procoagulant component is the antihemophilic factor or factor VIII:C, which is a glycoprotein synthesized by the liver. Conversely, von Willebrand factor, which is present in platelets as well as plasma, is synthesized by endothelium and megakaryocytes under the control of autosomal genes on chromosome 12. The von Willebrand factor antigen (vWF:Ag) is the antigenic determinant measured by immunoassays.

Clinical Presentation. The possibility of von Willebrand disease is usually considered in women with bleeding suggestive of a chronic disorder of coagulation. The classical autosomal dominant form usually is symptomatic in the heterozygous state. The less common but clinically more severe autosomal recessive form is manifest when inherited from both parents, both of whom demonstrate little or no disease. Type I, the most common form of von Willebrand disease, is characterized clinically by easy bruising, epistaxis, mucosal hemorrhage, and excessive bleeding with trauma, including surgery. Its laboratory features are usually a prolonged bleeding time, prolonged partial thromboplastin time, decreased von Willebrand factor antigen, decreased factor VIII immunological as well as coagulation-promoting activity, and inability of platelets in plasma from an affected person to react to a variety of stimuli.

Effect of Pregnancy. During pregnancy, women with von Willebrand disease often develop normal levels of factor VIII coagulant activity as well as von Willebrand factor antigen, although the bleeding time still may be prolonged. Conti and associates (1986) summarized 38 cases, and in a fourth of these, bleeding was reported at the time of abortion, delivery, or the puerperium. Similarly, Greer and colleagues (1991) reported that 8 of 14 pregnancies in such women were complicated by postpartum hemorrhage. In five, this was despite cryoprecipitate treatment. Moreover, in the three in whom factor VIII:C had been measured, it was normal.

Although the hemostatic defects characteristically improve during pregnancy, if factor VIII activity is very low, administration of factor VIII-rich cryoprecipitate is recommended for delivery. Factor VIII concentrate does not contain some multimers of VIII:vWF and thus is ineffective. With significant bleeding, 15 or 20 units of cryoprecipitate must be given every 12 hours. Worrisome hemorrhage, however, still may be encountered in women with severe disease (Chediak and colleagues, 1986; Greer and associates, 1991). In some patients, usually those with type I disease, but none with type III disease, infusion of desmopressin will stimulate release of von Willebrand factor.

Most persons with von Willebrand disease are heterozygous and have only a mild bleeding disorder. When both parents have the disorder, their offspring may, if homozygous, develop a serious bleeding disorder. Mullaart and colleagues (1991) documented evidence for periventricular hemorrhage in a 32-week fetus who inherited type IIa von Willebrand disease from her father. Chorionic villus biopsy with DNA analysis to detect the missing genes has been accomplished (see Chap. 40, p. 935). Some authorities recommend cesarean delivery to avoid trauma to a possibly affected fetus if the mother has had severe disease.

Other Inherited Coagulation Factor Deficiencies.
Factor VII deficiency is a rare autosomal recessive disorder, the gene for which is on chromosome 13. Normally, factor VII increases during pregnancy, but it may do so only mildly in factor VII-deficient patients (Fadel and Krauss, 1989).

Factor XI deficiency probably is the consequence of an autosomal trait that is manifested as severe disease

in the homozygous individuals but a minor defect in the heterozygote. This deficiency state is most prevalent in Ashkenazi Jews, and it seldom is encountered in pregnancy. Musclow and colleagues (1987) described 41 deliveries in 17 women with factor XI deficiency, and in none were transfusions required. They also described a 37-week pregnant woman who developed a spontaneous hemarthrosis. Steinberg and associates (1986), however, described hematoma formation requiring treatment with blood and fresh-frozen plasma in both obstetrical and gynecological patients.

Factor XII deficiency is another autosomal recessive disorder that rarely complicates pregnancy. An increased incidence of thromboembolism is encountered in nonpregnant patients with this deficiency. Lao and colleagues (1991) reported an affected pregnant woman in whom placental abruption developed at 26 weeks.

Inherited abnormalities of fibrinogen usually involve the formation of a functionally defective fibrinogen, commonly referred to as **dysfibrinogenemia.** Familial hypofibrinogenemia as a recessive disorder has been described very infrequently. Our experiences suggest that the condition represents a heterozygous autosomal dominant state with 50 percent of the offspring affected. Typically, thrombin-clottable protein has ranged from 80 to 110 mg/dL when nonpregnant and this increases by 40 or 50 percent in normal pregnancy. Those pregnancy complications that give rise to acquired hypofibrinogenemia, that is, placental abruption, were more common in our cases, but the existence of such conditions provided the impetus for study. Reports of pregnancy experiences for women with congenital afibrinogenemia are rare. Goodwin (1989) reviewed the literature and reported a high incidence of third-trimester placental abruption and postpartum hemorrhage. Trehan and Fergusson (1991) described a successful outcome in a woman in whom fibrinogen infusions were given weekly throughout pregnancy.

Regulatory Protein Deficiencies.
A number of important regulatory proteins inhibit clotting. Examples include antithrombin III and protein C and its cofactor, protein S. Deficiencies of these inhibitory proteins may be associated with recurrent thromboembolism, and a few cases in which pregnancy was complicated by them have been reported. Heijboer and colleagues (1990) studied the prevalence of isolated coagulation-inhibiting proteins in 277 nonpregnant patients with venographically proven deep-vein thrombosis. Their incidence combined was 8.3 percent compared with 2.2 percent for normal controls.

Conard and co-workers (1990) reported that half of 63 pregnancies with **antithrombin III deficiency** were complicated by thrombosis either antepartum or postpartum. Nelson and colleagues (1985) described the pregnancy courses of two women with such a deficiency, and although these were uneventful, one woman had suffered numerous thrombotic episodes before pregnancy. Baudo and associates (1990) described a woman who at 35 weeks had a massive pulmonary embolism associated with antithrombin III deficiency for which they gave treatment with recombinant tissue plasminogen activator. Heat-treated, plasma-derived antithrombin III also is available.

Protein C deficiency is an autosomal dominant disease. The heterozygous trait, which results in plasma protein C levels of 55 to 65 percent of normal, has an incidence of about 1 in 200 to 300 (Miletich and associates, 1987). Homozygotes, or double heterozygotes, have severe deficiency usually manifest as purpura fulminans in the neonate. It is estimated that about half of heterozygotes will suffer venous thrombotic episodes by adulthood. Conard and colleagues (1990) reported that 25 percent of 93 pregnancies complicated by protein C deficiency had deep-vein thrombosis. Brenner and co-workers (1987) reported a pregnant woman with deep vein thrombosis who had placental infarctions and preeclampsia, as well as multiple episodes of venous thromboses. In their case, continuous heparinization did not prevent preeclampsia and fetal growth retardation. Roos and co-workers (1990) described a woman with functional protein C deficiency who suffered a sagittal sinus thrombosis 10 days postpartum. Conversely, Vogel and colleagues (1989), as well as Bertault and associates (1991) described a total of three women in whom heparin therapy may have contributed to successful pregnancies.

Protein S is a cofactor for protein C activity. According to Comp and colleagues (1986), total protein S plasma concentrations, as well as functional protein S activity, are diminished substantively during normal pregnancy. Because these levels are similar to those seen in nonpregnant patients with protein S deficiency, diagnosis during pregnancy may be difficult. Conard and associates (1990) described thrombosis in 5 of 29 pregnancies with protein S deficiency. One woman had a cerebral vein thrombosis. Rose and associates (1986) described a woman with protein S deficiency who elected termination because of warfarin ingestion. Because of the thrombotic tendency, these investigators recommend that anticoagulation with heparin be given during pregnancy; however, many of these patients already are receiving warfarin when they conceive. Chronic warfarin ingestion is associated with several fetal anomalies (Chap. 42, p. 966).

References

Agre P: Hereditary spherocytosis. JAMA 262:2887, 1989

Aitchison RGM, Marsh JCW, Hows JM, Russel NH, Gordon-Smith EC: Pregnancy associated aplastic anaemia: A report of five cases and review of current management. Br J Haematol 73:541, 1989

Alger LS, Golbus MS, Laros RK Jr: Thalassemia and pregnancy: Results of an antenatal screening program. Am J Obstet Gynecol 134:662, 1979

Alter BP, Frissora CL, Halpérin DS, Freedman MH, Chitkara U, Alvarez E, Lynch L, Adler-Brecher B, Auerbach AD: Fanconi's anaemia and pregnancy. Br J Haematol 77:410, 1991

Ambrose A, Welham RT, Cefalo RC: Thrombotic thrombocytopenic purpura in early pregnancy. Obstet Gynecol 66:267, 1985

Antonarakis SE: Diagnosis of genetic disorders at the DNA level. N Engl J Med 320:153, 1989

Anyaegbunam A, Morel M-I G, Merkatz IR: Antepartum fetal surveillance tests during sickle cell crisis. Am J Obstet Gynecol 165:1081, 1991

Aster RH: "Gestational" thrombocytopenia: A plea for conservative management. N Engl J Med 323:264, 1990

Baudo F, Caimi TM, Redaelli R, Nosari AM, Mauri M, Leonardi G, de Cataldo F: Emergency treatment with recombinant tissue plasminogen activator of pulmonary embolism in a pregnant woman with antithrombin III deficiency. Am J Obstet Gynecol 163:1274, 1990

Beard J, Hillmen P, Anderson CC, Lewis SM, Pearson TC: Primary thrombocythaemia in pregnancy. Br J Haematol 77:371, 1991

Bell W: Thrombotic thrombocytopenic purpura. JAMA 265:91, 1991

Bell WR, Braine HG, Ness PM, Kickler TS: Improved survival in thrombotic thrombocytopenic purpura–hemolytic uremic syndrome. Clinical experience in 108 patients. N Engl J Med 325:398, 1991

Bertault D, Mandelbrot L, Tchobroutsky C, Sultan Y: Unfavourable pregnancy outcome associated with congenital protein C deficiency. Case reports. Br J Obstet Gynaecol 98:934, 1991

Beutler E: Glucose-6-phosphate dehydrogenase deficiency. N Engl J Med 324:169, 1991

Bierling P, Farcet JP, Dveradi N, Rochant H, Mondor HH: Gamma globulin for idiopathic thrombocytopenic purpura. N Engl J Med 307:1150, 1982

Boehm CD, Antonarakis SE, Phillips JA III, Stetten G, Kazazian HH Jr: Prenatal diagnosis using DNA polymorphisms. N Engl J Med 308:1054, 1983

Brenner B, Shapira A, Bahari C, Haimovich L, Seligsohn U: Hereditary protein C deficiency during pregnancy. Am J Obstet Gynecol 157:1160, 1987

Brewer CA, Adelson MD, Elder RC: Erythrocytosis associated with a placental-site trophoblastic tumor. Obstet Gynecol 79:846, 1992

Burrows RF, Kelton JG: Incidentally detected thrombocytopenia in healthy mothers and their infants. N Engl J Med 319:142, 1988

Burrows RF, Kelton JG: Low fetal risks in pregnancies associated with idiopathic thrombocytopenic purpura. Am J Obstet Gynecol 163:1147, 1990a

Burrows RF, Kelton JG: Thrombocytopenia at delivery: A prospective survey of 6715 deliveries. Am J Obstet Gynecol 162:731, 1990b

Camitta BM, Storb R, Thomas ED: Aplastic anemia: Pathogenesis, diagnosis, treatment, and prognosis. N Engl J Med 306:645, 712, 1982

Carache S, Scott J, Niebyl J, Bonds D: Management of sickle cell disease in pregnant patients. Obstet Gynecol 55:407, 1980

Carriaga MT, Skikne BS, Finley B, Cutler B, Cook JD: Serum transferrin receptor for the detection of iron deficiency in pregnancy. Am J Clin Nutr 54:1077, 1991

Centers for Disease Control: Anemia during pregnancy in low-income women—United States, 1987. MMWR 39:73, 1990

Centers for Disease Control: CDC criteria for anemia in children and childbearing-aged women. MMWR 38:400, 1989

Centers for Disease Control: Recommendations for the use of folic acid to reduce the number of cases of spina bifida and other neural tube defects. MMWR 41(RR-14), 1992

Chang JC, Kan YW: A sensitive new prenatal test for sickle cell anemia. N Engl J Med 307:30, 1982

Chasis JA, Agre P, Mohandas N: Decreased membrane mechanical stability and in vivo loss of surface area reflect spectrin deficiencies in hereditary spherocytosis. J Clin Invest 82:617, 1988

Chatwani A, Bruder N, Shapiro T, Reece A: Am J Obstet Gynecol 166:143, 1992

Chediak JR, Alban GM, Maxey B: Von Willebrand's disease and pregnancy: Management during delivery and outcome of offspring. Am J Obstet Gynecol 155:618, 1986

Christiaens GCML, Nieuwenhuis HK, Von Dem Borne AEGK, Ouwehand WH, Helmerhorst FM, Van Dalen CM, Van Der Tweel I: Idiopathic thrombocytopenic purpura in pregnancy: A randomized trial on the effect of antenatal low dose corticosteroids on neonatal platelet count. Br J Obstet Gynaecol 97:893, 1990

Cines DB, Dusak B, Tomaski A, Mennuti M, Schreier AD: Immune thrombocytopenic purpura and pregnancy. N Engl J Med 306:826, 1982

Comp PC, Thurnau GR, Welsh J, Esmon CT: Functional and immunologic protein S levels are decreased during pregnancy. Blood 68:881, 1986

Conard J, Horellou MH, Van Dreden P, Lecompte T, Samama M: Thrombosis and pregnancy in congenital deficiencies in AT III, protein C or protein S: Study of 78 women. Thromb Haemost 63:319, 1990

Conti M, Mari D, Conti E, Muggiasca L, Mannucci PM: Pregnancy in women with different types of von Willebrand disease. Obstet Gynecol 68:282, 1986

Cook RL, Miller RC, Katz VL, Cefalo RC: Immune thrombocytopenic purpura in pregnancy: A reappraisal of management. Obstet Gynecol 78:578, 1991

Cox JV, Steane E, Cunningham G, Frenkel EP: Risk of alloimmunization and delayed hemolytic transfusion reactions in patients with sickle cell disease. Arch Intern Med 148:2485, 1988

Cox SM, Shelburne P, Mason R, Guss S, Cunningham FG: Mechanisms of hemolysis and anemia associated with acute antepartum pyelonephritis. Am J Obstet Gynecol 164:587, 1991

Cunningham FG: Urinary tract infections complicating pregnancy. Clin Obstet Gynecol 1:891, 1988

Cunningham FG, Cox SM, Harstad TW, Mason RA, Pritchard JA: Chronic renal disease and pregnancy outcome. Am J Obstet Gynecol 163:453, 1990

Cunningham FG, Pritchard JA: Prophylactic transfusions of normal red blood cells during pregnancies complicated by sickle cell hemoglobinopathies. Am J Obstet Gynecol 135:994, 1979

Cunningham FG, Pritchard JA, Hankins GDV, Anderson PL, Lucas MK, Armstrong KF: Idiopathic cardiomyopathy or compounding cardiovascular events. Obstet Gynecol 67:157, 1986

Cunningham FG, Pritchard JA, Mason R: Pregnancy and sickle hemoglobinopathy: Results with and without prophylactic transfusions. Obstet Gynecol 62:419, 1983

Czeizel AE, Dudás I: Prevention of the first occurrence of neural-tube defects by periconceptional vitamin supplementation. N Engl J Med 327:1832, 1992

Daffos F, Capella-Pavlovsky M, Forestier F: Fetal blood sampling during pregnancy with the use of a needle guided by ultrasound: A study of 606 consecutive cases. Am J Obstet Gynecol 153:655, 1985

De Gramont A, Krulik M, Debray J: Paroxysmal nocturnal haemoglobinuria and pregnancy. Lancet 1:868, 1987

Deaver JE, Leppert PC, Zaroulis CG: Neonatal alloimmune thrombocytopenic purpura. Am J Perinatol 3:127, 1986

Deeg HJ, Kennedy MS, Sanders JE, Thomas ED, Storb R: Successful pregnancy after marrow transplantation for severe aplastic anemia and immunosuppression with cyclosporine. JAMA 250:647, 1983

Dwyer JM: Manipulating the immune system with immune globulin. N Engl J Med 326:107, 1992

El-Shafei AM, Dhaliwal JK, Sandhu AK: Pregnancy in sickle cell disease in Bahrain. Br J Obstet Gynaecol 99:101, 1992

Erslev AJ: Anemia of chronic disorders. In Williams WJ, Beutler E, Erslev AJ, Lichtman MA (eds): Hematology. New York, McGraw-Hill, 1990, p 540

Fadel HE, Krauss JS: Factor VII deficiency and pregnancy. Obstet Gynecol 73:453, 1989

Falconer J, Pineo G, Blahey W, Bowen T, Docksteader B, Jadusingh I: Essential thrombocythemia associated with recurrent abortions and fetal growth retardation. Am J Hematol 25:345, 1987

Ferguson JE II, O'Reilly RA: Hemoglobin E and pregnancy. Obstet Gynecol 66:136, 1985

Gasser C, Gautier E, Steck A, Siebenmann RE, Dechslin R: Hamolytasch-uramisch syndrome: Bilaterale Nierenrindennekrosen bie akuten erworbenin haemolytischen Amamien. Schweiz med Wochenschr 85:905, 1955

Gehlbach DL, Morgenstern LL: Antenatal screening for thalassemia minor. Obstet Gynecol 71:801, 1988

George JN, Shattil SJ: The clinical importance of acquired abnormalities of platelet function. N Engl J Med 324:27, 1991

Goldberg MA, Brugnara C, Dover GJ, Schapira L, Charache S, Bunn HF: Treatment of sickle cell anemia with hydroxyurea and erythropoietin. N Engl J Med 323:366, 1990

Goodwin TM: Congenital hypofibrinogenemia in pregnancy. Obstet Gynecol Surv 44:157, 1989

Greene MF, Frigoletto FD Jr, Claster SZ, Rosenthal D: Pregnancy and paroxysmal nocturnal hemoglobinuria: Report of a case and review of the literature. Obstet Gynecol Surv 38:591, 1983

Greer IA, Lowe GDO, Walker JJ, Forbes CD: Haemorrhagic problems in obstetrics and gynaecology in patients with congenital coagulopathies. Br J Obstet Gynaecol 98:909, 1991

Hayslett JP: Current concepts: Postpartum renal failure. N Engl J Med 312:1556, 1985

Heijboer H, Brandjes DPM, Büller HR, Sturk A, ten Cate JW:

Deficiencies of coagulation-inhibiting and fibrinolytic proteins in outpatients with deep-vein thrombosis. N Engl J Med 323:11512, 1990

Herbert V, Cunneen N, Jaskiel L, Kopff C: Minimal daily adult folate requirement. Arch Intern Med 110:649, 1962

Hinterberger-Fischer M, Kier P, Kalhs P, Marosi C, Geissler K, Schwarzinger I, Pabinger I, Huber J, Spona J, Kolbabek H, Koren H, Müller G, Hawliczek R, Lechner K, Hayek-Rosenmayr A, Hinterberger W: Fertility, pregnancies and offspring complications after bone marrow transplantation. Bone Marrow Transplant 7:5, 1991

Hsia YE: Detection and prevention of important α-thalassemia variants. Semin Perinatol 15:35, 1991

Hsieh FJ, Chang FM, Ko TM, Kuo PL, Chang DY, Chen HY: The antenatal blood gas and acid–base status of normal fetuses and hydropic fetuses with Bart hemoglobinopathy. Obstet Gynecol 74:722, 1989

Humpheries JE: Anemia of renal failure. Use of erythropoietin. Med Clin North Am 76:711, 1992

Hurd WW, Miodovnik M, Stys SJ: Pregnancy associated with paroxysmal nocturnal hemoglobinuria. Obstet Gynecol 60:742, 1982

Hurst D, Little B, Kleman KM, Emburg SH, Lubin GH: Anemia and hemoglobinopathies in Southeast Asian refugee children. J Pediatr 102:692, 1983

Johnson PM, Davies JM, Rand J: Thromobcythaemia and recurrent miscarriage. Br J Obstet Gynaecol 96:1231, 1989

Jones EC, Mosesson MW, Thomason JL, Jackson TC: Essential thrombocythemia in pregnancy. Obstet Gynecol 71:501, 1988

Kaplan C, Daffos F, Forestier F, Tertain G, Catherine N, Pons JC, Tchernia G: Fetal platelet counts in thrombocytopenic pregnancy. Lancet 336:979, 1990

Karpatkin M, Porges RF, Karpatkin S: Platelet counts in infants of women with autoimmune thrombocytopenia. N Engl J Med 305:936, 1981

Kazazian H Jr, Boehm C: Molecular basis and prenatal diagnosis of β-thalassemia. Blood 72:1107, 1988

Kazazian HH, Phillips DG, Dowling CE, Boehm CD: Prenatal diagnosis of sickle cell anemia—1988. Ann NY Acad Sci 565:44, 1989

Kelton JG, Inwood MJ, Barr RM, Effer SB, Hunter D, Wilson WE, Ginsburg DA, Powers PJ: The prenatal prediction of thrombocytopenia in infants of mothers with clinically diagnosed immune thrombocytopenia. Am J Obstet Gynecol 144:449, 1982

Klebanoff MA, Shiono PH, Selby JV, Trachtenberg AI, Graubard BI: Anemia and spontaneous preterm birth. Am J Obstet Gynecol 164:59, 1991

Koeffler HP, Goldwasser E: Erythropoietin radioimmunoassay in evaluating patients with polycythemia. Ann Intern Med 94:44, 1981

Koshy M, Burd L, Wallace D, Moawad A, Baron J: Prophylactic red-cell transfusions in pregnant patients with sickle cell disease: A randomized cooperative study. N Engl J Med 319:1447, 1988

Lao TT, Lewinsky RM, Ohlsson A, Cohen H: Factor XII deficiency and pregnancy. Obstet Gynecol 78:491, 1991

Lieberman E, Ryan KJ, Monson RR, Schoenbaum SC: Risk factors accounting for racial differences in the rate of premature birth. N Engl J Med 317:743, 1987

Lu ZM, Goldenberg RL, Cliver SP, Cutter G, Blankson M: The relationship between maternal hematocrit and pregnancy outcome. Obstet Gynecol 77:190, 1991

Lucarelli G, Galimberti M, Polchi P, Angelucci E, Baronciani D, Giardini C, Politi P, Durazzi SMT, Muretto P, Albertini F: Bone marrow transplantation in patients with thalassemia. N Engl J Med 322:417, 1990

Maberry MC, Klein VR, Boehm C, Warren TC, Gilstrap LC III: Alpha-thalassemia: Prenatal diagnosis and neonatal implications. Am J Perinatol 7:356, 1990a

Maberry MC, Mason RA, Cunningham FG, Pritchard JA: Pregnancy complicated by hemoglobin CC and C–β-thalassemia disease. Obstet Gynecol 76:324, 1990b

Maberry MC, Mason RA, Cunningham FG, Pritchard JA: Pregnancy complicated by hereditary spherocytosis. Obstet Gynecol 79:735, 1992

Martin JN Jr, Files JC, Blake PG, Norman PH, Martin RW, Hess LW, Morrison JC, Wiser WL: Plasma exchange for preeclampsia, I. Postpartum use for persistently severe preeclampsia–eclampsia with HELLP syndrome. Am J Obstet Gynecol 162:126, 1990

McGregor E, Stewart G, Junor BJR, Rodger RSC: Successful use of recombinant human erythropoietin in pregnancy. Nephrol Dial Transplant 6:292, 1991

Mercer B, Drouin J, Jolly E, d'Anjou G: Primary thrombocythemia in pregnancy: A report of two cases. Am J Obstet Gynecol 159:127, 1988

Miletich J, Sherman L, Broze G Jr: Absence of thrombosis in subjects with heterozygous protein C deficiency. N Engl J Med 317:991, 1987

Milner PF, Jones BR, Döbler J: Outcome of pregnancy in sickle cell anemia and sickle cell–hemoglobin C disease. Am J Obstet Gynecol 138:239, 1980

Moake JL: TTP—Desperation, empiricism, progress. N Engl J Med 325:426, 1991

Monni G, Ibba RM, Olla G, Rosatelli C, Cao A: Chorionic villus sampling by rigid forceps: Experience with 300 cases at risk for thalassemia major. Am J Obstet Gynecol 156:921, 1987

Mordel N, Birkenfeld A, Goldfarb AN, Rachmilewitz EA: Successful full-term pregnancy in homozygous β-thalassemia major: Case report and review of the literature. Obstet Gynecol 73:837, 1989

Moschcowitz E: An acute febrile pleochromic anemia with hyaline thrombosis of the terminal arterioles and capillaries. Arch Intern Med 31:89, 1925

Mullaart RA, Van Dongen P, Gabreëls FJM, van Oostrom C: Fetal periventricular hemorrhage in von Willebrand's disease: Short review and first case presentation. Am J Perinatol 8:190, 1991

Murphy JF, O'Riordan J, Newcombe RG, Coles EC, Pearson JF: Relation of haemoglobin levels in first and second trimester to outcome of pregnancy. Lancet i:992, 1986

Musclow CE, Goldenberg H, Bernstein EP, Abbot D: Factor XI deficiency presenting as hemarthrosis during pregnancy. Am J Obstet Gynecol 157:178, 1987

NIH Consensus Conference: Intravenous immunoglobin: Prevention and treatment of disease. JAMA 264:3189, 1990

Natelson EA, White D: Recurrent thrombotic thrombocytopenia purpura in early pregnancy: Effect of uterine evacuation. Obstet Gynecol 55:545, 1985

Nelson DM, Stempel LE, Brandt JT: Hereditary antithrombin III deficiency and pregnancy: Report of two cases and review of the literature. Obstet Gynecol 65:848, 1985

Nussbaum RL, Powell C, Graham HL, Caskey CT, Fernbach DJ: Newborn screening for sickle hemoglobinopathies: Houston, 1976 to 1980. Am J Dis Child 138:44, 1984

Old JM, Fitches A, Heath C, Thein SL, Weatherall DJ, Warren R, McKenzie C, Rodeck CH, Modell B, Petrou M, Ward RHT: First-trimester fetal diagnosis for haemoglobinopathies: Report on 200 cases. Lancet 2:763, 1986

Packham CH, Leddy JP: Drug-related immunologic injury of erythrocytes. In Williams WJ, Beutler E, Erslev AJ, Lichtman MA (eds): Hematology. New York, McGraw-Hill, 1990, p 681

Peng TC, Kickler TS, Bell WR, Haller E: Obstetric complications in a patient with Bernard–Soulier syndrome. Am J Obstet Gynecol 165:425, 1991

Perrine SP, Ginder GD, Faller DV, Dover GH, Ikuta T, Wikowska HE, Cai S-P, Vichinsky EP, Olivieri NF: A short-term trial of butyrate to stimulate fetal-globin-gene expression in the β-globin disorders. N Engl J Med 328:81, 1993

Perry KG, Morrison JC: The diagnosis and management of hemoglobinopathies during pregnancy. Semin Perinatol 14:90, 1990

Platt OS, Thorington BD, Brambilla DJ, Milner PF, Rosse WF, Vichinsky E, Kinney TR: Pain in sickle cell disease: Rates and risk factors. N Engl J Med 325:11, 1991

Poddar D, Maude GH, Plant MJ, Scorer H, Serjeant GR: Pregnancy in Jamaican women with homozygous sickle cell disease: Fetal and maternal outcome. Br J Obstet Gynaecol 93:927, 1986

Poncz M, Colman N, Herbert V, Schwartz E, Cohen AR: Therapy of congenital folate malabsorption. J Pediatr 98:76, 1981

Powars D, Weidman JA, Odom-Maryon T, Niland JC, Johnson C: Sickle cell chronic lung disease: Prior morbidity and the risk of pulmonary failure. Medicine 67:66, 1988

Powars DR, Sandhu M, Niland-Weiss J, Johnson C, Bruce S, Manning PR: Pregnancy in sickle cell disease. Obstet Gynecol 67:217, 1986

Pritchard JA: Hereditary hypochromic microcytic anemia in obstetrics and gynecology. Am J Obstet Gynecol 83:1193, 1962

Pritchard JA, Cunningham FG, Mason RA: Coagulation changes in eclampsia: Their frequency and pathogenesis. Am J Obstet Gynecol 124:855, 1976

Pritchard JA, Scott DE: Iron demands in pregnancy. In Hallberg L, Harwerth H-G, Vanotti A (eds): Iron Deficiency Pathogenesis, Clinical Aspects, Therapy. New York, Academic Press, 1970

Pritchard JA, Scott DE, Whalley PJ, Cunningham FG, Mason RA: The effects of maternal sickle cell hemoglobinopathies and sickle cell trait on reproductive performance. Am J Obstet Gynecol 117:662, 1973

Ramahi AJ, Lewkow LM, Dombrowski MP, Bottoms SF: Sickle cell E hemoglobinopathy and pregnancy. Obstet Gynecol 71:493, 1988

Reece EA, Coustan DR, Hayslett JP, Holford T, Coulehan J, O'Connor TZ, Hobbins JC: Diabetic nephropathy: Pregnancy performance and fetomaternal outcome. Am J Obstet Gynecol 159:56, 1988

Robson JS, Martin AM, Ruckley VA, MacDonald MK: Irreversible postpartum renal failure. Q J Med 37:423, 1968

Rock GA, Shumak KH, Buskard NA, Blanchette VS, Kelton JG, Nair RC, Spasoff RA, and The Canadian Apheresis Study Group: Comparison of plasma exchange with plasma infusion in the treatment of thrombotic thrombocytopenic purpura. N Engl J Med 325:393, 1991

Rodgers GP, Dover GJ, Noguchi CT, Schechter AN, Nienhius AW: Hematologic responses of patients with sickle cell disease to treatment with hydroxyurea. N Engl J Med 322:1037, 1990

Roos KL, Pascuzzi RM, Kuharik MA, Shapiro AD, Manco-Johnson MJ: Postpartum intracranial venous thrombosis associated with dysfunctional protein C and deficiency of protein S. Obstet Gynecol 76:492, 1990

Rose PG, Essig GF, Vaccaro PS, Brandt JT: Protein S deficiency in pregnancy. Am J Obstet Gynecol 155:140, 1986

Rowley PT: Prenatal diagnosis for sickle cell disease: A survey of the United States and Canada. Ann NY Acad Sci 565:48, 1989

Ruch WA, Klein RL: Polycythemia vera and pregnancy. Obstet Gynecol 23:107, 1964

Ruggenenti P, Remuzzi G: Thrombotic thrombocytopenic purpura and related disorders. Hematol Oncol Clin North Am 4:219, 1990

Rust LA, Goodnight SH, Freeman RK, Johnson CS: Pregnancy and delivery in a woman with hemophilia B. Obstet Gynecol 46:483, 1975

Saade G, Homsi R, Seoud M: Bernard–Soulier syndrome in pregnancy; a report of four pregnancies in one patient, and review of the literature. Eur J Obstet Gynecol Reprod Biol 40:149, 1991

Samuels P, Bussel JB, Braitman LE, Tomaski A, Druzin ML, Mennuti MT, Cines DB: Estimation of the risk of thrombocytopenia in the offspring of pregnant women with presumed immune thrombocytopenic purpura. N Engl J Med 323:229, 1990

Schneider RG, Hightower B, Hasty TS, Ryder H, Tomlin G, Atkins R, Brimhall B, Jones RT: Abnormal hemoglobins in a quarter million people. Blood 48:629, 1976

Schwartz ML, Brenner W: Severe preeclampsia with persistent postpartum hemolysis and thrombocytopenia treated by plasmapheresis. Obstet Gynecol 65:53S, 1985

Scott DE, Pritchard JA: Iron deficiency in healthy young college women. JAMA 199:147, 1967

Scott JR, Rote NS, Cruikshank DP: Antiplatelet antibodies and platelet counts in pregnancies complicated by autoimmune thrombocytopenic purpura. Am J Obstet Gynecol 145:932, 1983

Sears DA: Anemia of chronic disease. Med Clin North Am 76:567, 1992

Smith MB, Whiteside MG, DeGaris CN: An investigation of the complications and outcome of pregnancy in heterozygous beta-thalassaemia. Aust NZ J Obstet Gynecol 15:26, 1975

Snyder TE, Lee LP, Lynch S: Pregnancy-associated hypoplastic anemia: A review. Obstet Gynecol Surv 46:264, 1991

Solal-Céligny P, Tertian G, Fernandez H, Pons J-C, Lambert T, Najean Y, Clauvel J-P, Papiernik E, Tchernia G: Pregnancy and paroxysmal nocturnal hemoglobinuria. Arch Intern Med 148:593, 1988

Starksen NF, Bell WR, Kickler TS: Unexplained hemolytic anemia associated with pregnancy. Am J Obstet Gynecol 146:617, 1983

Steinberg MH, Saletan S, Funt M, Baker D, Coller BS: Management of factor XI deficiency in gynecologic and obstetric patients. Obstet Gynecol 68:130, 1986

Storb R, Champlin RE: Bone marrow transplantation for severe aplastic anemia. Bone Marrow Transplant 8:69, 1991

Taylor DJ, Mallen C, McDougal N, Lind T: Effect of iron supplementation on serum ferritin levels during and after pregnancy. Br J Obstet Gynaecol 89:1011, 1982

Trehan AK, Fergusson ILC: Congenital afibrinogenaemia and successful pregnancy outcome. Case report. Br J Obstet Gynaecol 98:722, 1991

Tuck SM, Studd JWW, White JM: Pregnancy in women with sickle cell trait. Br J Obstet Gynaecol 90:108, 1983

Vandekerckhove F, Noems L, Coldardyn F, Thiery M, Delbarge W: Thrombotic thrombocytopenic purpura mimicking toxemia of pregnancy. Am J Obstet Gynecol 150:320, 1984

Ventura CS: Hereditary spherocytosis with haemolytic crisis during pregnancy. Aust NZ J Obstet Gynaecol 22:50, 1982

Vichinsky EP, Earles A, Johnson RA, Hoag S, Williams A, Lubin B: Alloimmunization in sickle cell anemia and transfusion of racially unmatched blood. N Engl J Med 322:1617, 1990

Vichinsky E, Hurst D, Earles A, Kleman K, Lubin B: Newborn screening for sickle cell disease: Effect on mortality. Pediatrics 81:749, 1988

Vogel JJ, de Moerloose PA, Bounameaux H: Protein C deficiency and pregnancy: A case report. Obstet Gynecol 73:455, 1989

Wagoner RD, Holley KE, Johnson WJ: Accelerate nephrosclerosis and postpartum acute renal failure in normotensive patients. Ann Intern Med 69:237, 1968

Watson WJ, Katz VL, Bowes WA: Plasmapheresis during pregnancy. Obstet Gynecol 76:451, 1990

Weatherall DJ: The thalassemias. In Williams WJ, Beutler E, Erslev AJ, Lichtman MA, (eds): Hematology. New York, McGraw-Hill, 1990, p. 510

Weiner CP: Thrombotic microangiopathy in pregnancy and the postpartum period. Semin Hematol 24:119, 1987

Whalley PJ: Bacteriuria of pregnancy. Am J Obstet Gynecol 97:723, 1967

Yeomans E, Lowe TW, Eigenbrodt EH, Cunningham FG: Liver histopathologic findings in women with sickle cell disease given prophylactic transfusion during pregnancy. Am J Obstet Gynecol 163:958, 1990

Zamorano AF, Arnalich F, Sánchez Casas E, Sicilia A, Solis C, Vázquez JJ, Gasalla R: Levels of iron, vitamin B_{12}, folic acid and their binding proteins during pregnancy. Acta Haemat 74:92, 1985

CHAPTER 53
Endocrine Disorders

A variety of endocrine disorders can complicate pregnancy and vice versa. The most common of these, diabetes mellitus, is made more difficult to manage by pregnancy and increases appreciably the risk of a number of pregnancy complications. With some other conditions, for example, thyrotoxicosis, pregnancy often only appears to worsen the endocrinopathy by increasing the concentration of circulating thyroxine, but not necessarily the amount of free, or active, hormone.

Diabetes Mellitus

Before the isolation of insulin in 1921, most diabetic women were too ill to conceive. For example, Williams (1915), after 13 years as Chief of Obstetrics at the Johns Hopkins Hospital, and with a large consulting practice, had encountered only one case of pregnancy complicated by diabetes. The exact cause of infertility during the preinsulin era is not clear, but the incidence of amenorrhea has been estimated to be as high as 50 percent. Of the infrequent pregnancies, about one fourth of the mothers and half of the fetuses and infants died. With the discovery of insulin in 1921, childbearing in severely diabetic women became a reality. Indeed, Kjaer and co-workers (1992) studied fertility in 245 women with insulin-dependent diabetes and found that their ability to conceive was normal but that they intentionally had fewer pregnancies. The fascinating history of diabetes treatment with insulin was recounted recently by Gabbe (1992). Currently, with optimal care, and excluding major congenital malformations, maternal and perinatal mortality in these women is equivalent almost to that of normally pregnant women.

Pathogenesis. The National Diabetes Data Group (1979) classifies diabetes into primary and secondary forms. Primary diabetes implies that there is no associated disease whereas secondary disease is due to a number of conditions, for example, chronic pancreatitis and pheochromocytoma. Although **type 1** diabetes is often used synonymously with insulin-dependent diabetes, it may be misleading because patients with apparent noninsulin-dependent disease later become fully insulin dependent and ketoacidosis prone. **Type 2** implies noninsulin dependent disease. These terms do not imply that all diabetics taking insulin are type 1; only those who would develop ketoacidosis with its withdrawal are

so classified. Some differentiating characteristics between types 1 and 2 are shown in Table 53–1.

The lack of agreement about the minimal requirements for the diagnosis of diabetes makes it difficult to assess its prevalence. By diagnostic criteria acceptable to most, it is estimated that 1 percent of the general population of childbearing-age women now has overt diabetes, and about one fourth of these have type 1 insulin-dependent disease (Foster, 1991). Type 2 noninsulin-dependent diabetes accrues with age; thus its prevalence will be modified by the population studied. For example, pregnant women as a group are young, thus there will be an inordinately high ratio of type 1 disease compared with all diabetics in the general population.

Type 1 diabetes is immune-mediated and develops in genetically susceptible persons. This predisposition is permissive rather than causal and disease presumably is triggered by a viral infection. There is inflammatory *insulitis* with lymphocytic infiltration of islets. Subsequently, there is β-cell surface modification and immune stimulation of antibodies against the "abnormal" β-cell. The β-cell membrane becomes susceptible to autoimmune cytotoxic antibodies, which leads to eventual destruction of the cell and resultant diabetes. The genetics of type 1 diabetes is complex, but there is general agreement that there is an association with the HLA-D histocompatibility complex located on chromosome 6. There is a low vertical transmission rate in type 1 disease. Moreover, the concordance rate for diabetes in monozygous twins, rather than being nearly 100 percent if diabetes were solely genetic in origin, is less than 50 percent (Foster, 1991).

There has been no HLA association discovered with type 2 noninsulin-dependent diabetes. The disease has a familial occurrence and concordance in monozygotic twins is 100 percent. Nearly 40 percent of siblings and a third of offspring develop abnormal glucose tolerance or obvious diabetes (Foster, 1991). Its pathophysiology is abnormal insulin secretion and insulin resistance in target tissues. Most patients are overtly obese, and there is speculation that peripheral resistance induced by obesity leads to β-cell exhaustion. Conversely, the majority of massively obese persons are not diabetic.

Classification During Pregnancy. Women whose pregnancies are complicated by diabetes can be separated into those who were known to have diabetes before pregnancy and those with gestational diabetes. The

TABLE 53–1. SOME GENERAL CHARACTERISTICS OF INSULIN-DEPENDENT (TYPE 1) AND NONINSULIN-DEPENDENT (TYPE 2) DIABETES MELLITUS

Characteristic	Type 1 (Insulin-Dependent)	Type 2 (Noninsulin-Dependent)
Genetic locus	Chromosome 6	Chromosome 11 (?)
Age at onset	Young (< 40)	Older (> 40)
Habitus	Normal to wasted	Obese
Plasma insulin	Low to absent	Normal to high
Plasma glucagon	High, suppressible	High, resistant
Acute complication	Ketoacidosis	Hyperosmolar coma
Insulin therapy	Responsive	Responsive to resistant
Sulfonylurea therapy	Unresponsive	Responsive

From Foster (1991), with permission.

White classification (1978) was designed originally to prognosticate pregnancy outcome, because infant survival decreased with increasing severity of diabetes. Shown in Table 53–2 is the classification suggested by the American College of Obstetricians and Gynecologists (1986). The salient features of this classification, which encompasses that of White (1978), are that the duration of diabetes relates to the severity of end-organ derangement, especially the eyes, kidneys, and cardiovascular system.

Diagnosis During Pregnancy. The woman with high plasma glucose levels, glucosuria, and ketoacidosis presents no problem in diagnosis. The woman at the opposite end of the spectrum, with only minimal metabolic derangement, may be difficult to identify. The likelihood of impaired carbohydrate metabolism is increased appreciably in women who have a strong familial history of diabetes, have given birth to large infants, demonstrate persistent glucosuria, or have unexplained fetal losses.

Reducing substances are commonly found in the urine of pregnant women. Unless a method that is specific for glucose is used, often the material identified is lactose, which is not a source of concern. Commercially available dipsticks may be used to identify glucosuria while avoiding a positive reaction from lactose. Even then, glucosuria most often does not reflect impaired glucose tolerance, but rather augmented glomerular filtration (see Chap. 8, p. 230). Nonetheless, the detection of glucosuria during pregnancy warrants further investigation.

Effect of Pregnancy on Diabetes. The diabetogenic effects of pregnancy are borne out by the fact that some women who have no evidence for diabetes when not pregnant develop distinct abnormalities of glucose tolerance during pregnancy and, at times, overt diabetes.

Most often these changes are reversible. After delivery, evidence for either the induction of or a worsening of diabetes usually disappears rapidly, and the ability of the mother to metabolize carbohydrate returns to the prepregnancy status.

In normal women, insulin secretion during pregnancy is maintained, and there is enhanced glucagon suppression. As discussed in Chapter 8 (p. 217), physiological changes of pregnancy impair peripheral insulin action. The insulin antagonism that develops during pregnancy is probably the consequence of the actions of *placental lactogen*, which is secreted in enormous quantities, and to lesser degrees those actions of *estrogens* and *progesterone*. There is no sound evidence that *placental insulinase* contributes to pregnancy-induced diabetogenicity.

During pregnancy, control of diabetes usually is made more difficult by a variety of complications. Nausea and vomiting may lead on the one hand to hypoglycemic shock and, on the other, to insulin resistance if starvation is severe enough to cause ketosis. The pregnant woman is more prone to develop metabolic acidosis than when nonpregnant. Presumably, placental lactogen is responsible for this tendency by virtue of its carbohydrate-sparing and lipolytic actions. With diabetes, the likelihood of severe metabolic acidosis is increased appreciably. Infection during pregnancy commonly results in insulin resistance and ketoacidosis unless it is recognized promptly and both the infection and diabetes treated. The exertion of labor accompanied by the ingestion of little or no carbohydrate also may result in troublesome hypoglycemia unless the amount of insulin given is reduced accordingly or glucose is provided by intravenous infusion.

After delivery, the need for exogenous insulin most often decreases at a rapid rate and to a considerable degree. Puerperal infection, however, may blunt this response. Presumably, the rapid decrease in insulin requirements that is usually seen in the absence of other complications stems from the rapid disappearance of those pregnancy factors cited above.

Effects of Diabetes on Pregnancy. Diabetes may be deleterious to pregnancy in a number of ways. Because of a number of complications that may arise, both maternal and perinatal morbidity and mortality are increased compared with normally pregnant women.

Maternal Effects of Diabetes. Adverse maternal effects associated with diabetic pregnancy include the following:

1. The likelihood of **preeclampsia–eclampsia** is increased about fourfold. This incidence is increased even in the absence of demonstrated preexisting vascular or renal disease.

TABLE 53–2. CLASSIFICATION OF DIABETES COMPLICATING PREGNANCY

Pregestational Diabetes				Gestational Diabetes			
Class	Age of Onset	Duration (Years)	Vascular Disease	Therapy	Class	Fasting Plasma Glucose		Postprandial Plasma Glucose
A	Any	Any	None	A-1, diet only	A-1	< 105 mg/dL	and	< 120 mg/dL
B	Over 20	< 10	None	Insulin	A-2	> 105 mg/dL	and/or	> 120 mg/dL
C	10 to 19	or 10 to 19	None	Insulin				
D	Before 10	or > 20	Benign retinopathy	Insulin				
F	Any	Any	Nephropathy	Insulin				
R	Any	Any	Proliferative retinopathy	Insulin				
H	Any	Any	Heart disease	Insulin				

From American College of Obstetricians and Gynecologists (1986), with permission.

2. Some **bacterial infections** are more common in diabetic pregnancy.
3. The fetus can be **macrosomic,** and this may lead to difficult delivery with injury to the birth canal.
4. Because of substantively increased perinatal jeopardy, as well as the possibility of dystocia, the rate of **cesarean delivery** is increased and maternal risks imposed by surgery are increased correspondingly.
5. **Hydramnios** is common, and at times the large volume of amnionic fluid, coupled with fetal macrosomia, may cause cardiorespiratory symptoms in the mother.
6. **Maternal mortality** is increased because of complications of diabetes as well as an increased risk for hypertension, infection, and cesarean delivery.

Fetal and Neonatal Effects. Maternal diabetes adversely affects the fetus and newborn infant in several ways:

1. In the absence of excellent diabetes and pregnancy management, the **perinatal death rate** is increased considerably compared with that of the general population.
2. **Major anomalies** are increased at least threefold in fetuses of women with overt diabetes.
3. The incidence of **preterm delivery,** in many cases induced because of hypertension, is increased two- to three-fold.
4. **Neonatal morbidity** is common. In some instances, morbidity is direct and results from birth injury as the consequence of fetal macrosomia. In other instances, it is indirect and takes the form of severe respiratory distress and metabolic derangements that include hypoglycemia and hypocalcemia.
5. The infant may inherit at least a **predisposition to diabetes.**

Except for the brain, most fetal organs are affected by macrosomia that commonly, but not always, characterizes the fetus of the diabetic woman. At the same time, body fat is increased (Fig. 53–1). The mechanisms responsible for the extra fetal growth are not well defined. In several studies, however, the degree of fetal macrosomia appeared to correlate well with the degree of maternal hyperglycemia and lack of maternal vascular disease. Both favor the transfer of excessive glucose to the fetus. This stimulates fetal insulin secretion, which is a potent growth factor. Insulin concentration in amnionic fluid and cord blood is increased in diabetic pregnancy, and this has been presumed to be entirely of fetal origin because the placenta is impermeable to free insulin. However, Menon and co-workers (1990) have observed that anti-

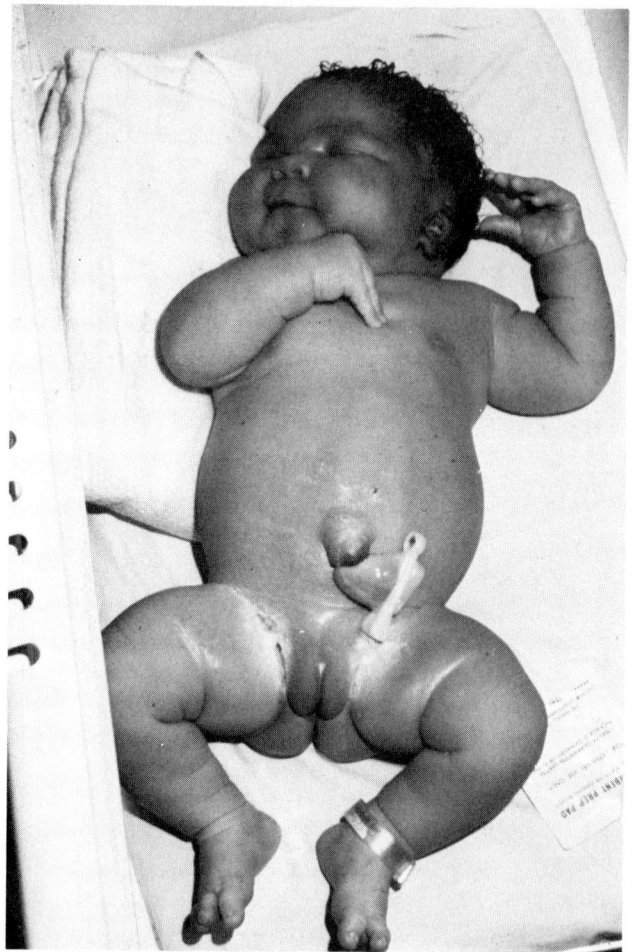

Fig. 53–1. This macrosomic infant who weighed 6050 g was born to a woman with gestational diabetes.

body bound to animal insulin is transferred from mother to fetus in some women with overt diabetes. They also observed that excessive fetal growth was correlated with increased animal insulin concentrations in cord blood.

Thus, it is envisioned that hyperglycemia and hyperinsulinemia in concert enhance glycogen synthesis, lipogenesis, and protein synthesis. There is abundant experimental evidence that insulin is a potent fetal growth factor. Mintz and co-workers (1972) injected streptozotocin into the pregnant monkey to destroy maternal islet β-cells and the subsequent maternal diabetes resulted in fetal macrosomia. Cheek (1968) injected streptozotocin into the monkey fetus to destroy its capacity to make insulin and, conversely, fetal size was reduced appreciably. Moreover, marked fetal growth retardation with very poor development of striated muscle and near absence of adipose tissue has been observed in a newborn infant whose plasma and vestigial pancreas contained no insulin (Hill, 1978).

Neonatal **cardiomyopathy,** characterized by cardiomegaly, respiratory distress, and heart failure has been associated with maternal diabetes. Its cause is unknown, but it appears to be reversible. Veille and coworkers (1992) reported ventricular septal hypertrophy in 75 percent of fetuses of diabetic mothers studied with M-mode echocardiography. They attribute this to a specific diabetic cardiomyopathy.

A common finding at autopsy in the infant of a diabetic mother is hypertrophy and hyperplasia of the islets of Langerhans. Although the changes are not specific—for example, they also are seen in erythroblastotic infants—they are sufficiently characteristic to suggest that the mother had impaired glucose metabolism. It has been suggested that maternal hyperglycemia and, in turn, fetal hyperglycemia are responsible for the striking increase in the size, and sometimes the number, of islets.

Gestational Diabetes

"Gestational" diabetes implies that this disorder is induced by pregnancy, perhaps due to exaggerated physiological changes in glucose metabolism (see Chap. 8, p. 217). An alternative pathophysiological explanation is that gestational diabetes is not induced by pregnancy, but instead may be maturity-onset diabetes unmasked during pregnancy. For example, Harris (1988) found that the prevalence of undiagnosed glucose intolerance in nonpregnant American women between the ages of 20 and 44 years was virtually identical to the prevalence of gestational diabetes.

The American Diabetes Association convened three workshop–conferences on gestational diabetes between 1979 and 1990. These conferences and the published proceedings have been major influences on current management of gestational diabetes in the United States. In 1990, the Third International Workshop–Conference on Gestational Diabetes (1991) was held in Chicago. Gestational diabetes was defined as carbohydrate intolerance of variable severity with onset or first recognition during the current pregnancy. This definition did not exclude the possibility that glucose intolerance may have antedated pregnancy. Use of the diagnostic term **gestational diabetes** was encouraged in order to communicate the need for increased surveillance and to convince women of the need for further testing postpartum. It also was concluded that gestational diabetes is a heterogeneous disorder with varied worldwide prevalence. In the United States, the prevalence of gestational diabetes is between 1 and 3 percent. During this time, there was no international agreement on the most appropriate diagnostic criteria. An important confounding factor is obesity, and Johnson and colleagues (1987) reported that 8 percent of 588 women who weighed more than 250 pounds had gestational diabetes compared with less than 1 percent of women who weighed

less than 200 pounds. Age also is an important factor; Mestman (1980) reported that the incidence of gestational diabetes was 3.7 percent in women younger than 20, 7.5 percent for those 20 to 30, and 13.8 percent for women older than 30.

It was concluded at the 1990 Workshop that widespread testing and identification of gestational diabetes as well as intensive management appear to have been associated with a decrease in overall *morbidity* in the infant of the mother with gestational diabetes. The likelihood of fetal death in the woman with appropriately treated gestational diabetes was found to be no different than in the general population. The most important perinatal concern in offspring of mothers with gestational diabetes was excessive fetal growth, which is observed two to three times more often than expected and may result in birth trauma. Importantly, more than half of women with gestational diabetes ultimately develop overt diabetes, and there is mounting evidence for long-range complications that include obesity and diabetes in offspring born to these women.

As shown in Table 53–2, the current classification of gestational diabetes includes two subgroups—class A_1 and class A_2—which are differentiated based upon fasting blood glucose values.

Screening. There is no international agreement as to the appropriate and globally acceptable diagnostic criteria for gestational diabetes. Moreover, screening for gestational diabetes within the United States is controversial. For example, the 1990 Workshop–Conference continued to recommend that all pregnant women should be screened using a 50-g oral glucose tolerance test between 24 and 28 weeks' gestation without regard to time of day or last meal, and that a plasma value at 1 hour exceeding 140 mg/dL be used as the cutoff for performing a 100-g 3-hour oral glucose tolerance test. Values used are the same as those recommended originally by O'Sullivan and Mahan (1964), and abnormal values for the 100-g test, administered after an 8- to 14-hour overnight fast, are shown in Table 53–3. Test strips and reflectance meters are not sufficiently precise for screening and diagnosis. About 15 percent of all pregnant women have an abnormal 1-hour screening test and 15 percent of these will be found to have

TABLE 53–3. CRITERIA FOR DIAGNOSIS OF GESTATIONAL DIABETES USING 100 G OF GLUCOSE TAKEN ORALLY

Timing of Glucose Measurement	Whole Venous Blood (mg/dL)	Plasma (mg/dL)
Fasting	90	105
1-hour	165	190
2-hour	145	165
3-hour	125	145

From Second International Workshop–Conference on Gestational Diabetes (1985).

gestational diabetes defined by at least two abnormal values using the 3-hour glucose tolerance test. If the screening test is repeated at 34 weeks, Watson (1989) reported that 8 percent of previously negative tests will now be positive.

In contrast, the American College of Obstetricians and Gynecologists (1986) recommends screening only for women considered to be at risk: age over 30; family history of diabetes; a prior macrosomic, malformed, or stillborn infant; obesity; hypertension; or glucosuria. Additionally, some drugs impair glucose utilization. For example, Angel and colleagues (1988) reported a 12 percent incidence of impaired carbohydrate tolerance in 86 women taking oral terbutaline for preterm labor. Proponents of universal screening cite data that one third to one half of women with gestational diabetes will be missed if these traditional risk factors are used for screening (Coustan and co-workers, 1989).

Two factors are central to the controversy regarding universal screening for glucose intolerance. Firstly, there is no evidence that detection will lower perinatal mortality because it is not excessive in these women (Ales and Santini, 1989). Secondly, although fetal macrosomia is linked to abnormal glucose tolerance, maternal obesity is a prominent co-factor, and it is not possible to separate the two. Put another way, fetal size depends on maternal size, and it is not always directly related to the level of glucose control (Jacobson and Cousins, 1989; Larsen and colleagues, 1990).

Adverse Effects. There has been an important shift in focus concerning adverse fetal consequences of gestational diabetes. Importantly, unlike in women with overt diabetes, fetal anomalies are not increased (Reece and Hobbins, 1986). Similarly, whereas pregnancies in women with overt diabetes are at greater risk for fetal death, this danger is not apparent for those with postprandial hyperglycemia only, that is, class A_1. In contrast, gestational diabetes with elevated fasting glucose (class A_2), has been associated with unexplained stillbirth similar to pregnancies complicated by overt diabetes (Johnstone and colleagues, 1990).

The perinatal focal point now is avoidance of difficult delivery due to macrosomia, with concomitant neonatal morbidity from birth trauma. Although women with gestational diabetes have a higher incidence of macrosomic fetuses, a separate effect of co-existing obesity cannot be distinguished (Maresh and colleagues, 1989). Still, one alleged advantage of identifying gestational diabetes is increased awareness of potential shoulder dystocia. Unfortunately, as discussed in detail in Chapter 20 (p. 509), precise identification of macrosomic infants currently is not possible. In fact, Bochner and colleagues (1987) reported that the predictive value for macrosomia was only 56 percent when the fetal abdominal circumference was greater than the 90th percentile.

Management. Pregnant women without persistent fasting hyperglycemia (Class A_1), but with an abnormal oral glucose tolerance test, are treated typically by diet alone. Mild dietary restriction has been shown to reduce plasma glucose levels in women with gestational diabetes but without inducing ketosis (Buchanan and co-workers, 1990). A liberal exercise program is encouraged. Jovanovic-Peterson and associates (1989) have shown that a program of cardiovascular-conditioning exercise improves glycemic control when compared with diet alone. Exercise prescriptions, according to the 1990 Workshop, should be individualized and conducted under careful supervision until it is established that they are effective and accepted by most women with gestational diabetes.

An acceptable diet is that recommended by the American Diabetes Association in amounts that provide 30 to 35 kcal/kg of ideal body weight each day. The utility of self-monitoring of capillary blood glucose in women with mild gestational diabetes and not requiring insulin, although reasonable and logical, has not been proven. In general, for women with gestational diabetes who do not require insulin, early delivery seldom is required. Labor induction at 40 weeks, although ideal, is not done unless the cervix is favorable.

Beneficial effects of prophylactic insulin to decrease complications related to macrosomia have not been proven. Participants at the Workshop–Conference (1991) observed that although insulin now is recommended widely when standard dietary management does not consistently maintain normal fasting plasma glucose (105 mg/dL or less) or the 2-hour postprandial glucose less than 120 mg/dL, or both, such therapy requires additional cost–benefit studies. Coustan and Imarah (1984) concluded from a nonrandomized study that routine insulin treatment given to women with gestational diabetes decreased the incidence of macrosomia, midforceps and cesarean deliveries, and birth trauma from shoulder dystocia. Langer and colleagues (1989) compared birthweight with glucose levels obtained throughout pregnancy. In women whose mean capillary blood glucose exceeded 105 mg/dL, the incidence of large-for-gestational age infants was increased 20-fold compared with women whose mean glucose levels were 85 mg/dL or lower (24 versus 1.4 percent). Thompson and colleagues (1990) randomized 108 gestational diabetics to diet alone or diet plus insulin and showed a significant birthweight reduction in the insulin-treated group. In contrast, Nordlander and co-workers (1989) randomized 261 gestational diabetics to diet or diet plus insulin and found no neonatal benefits for insulin therapy.

Beta-agonists given to forestall preterm labor will aggravate gestational diabetes (see Chap. 38, p. 870). Lindenbaum and associates (1992) reported that although terbutaline did not increase its incidence, gestational diabetes treatment invariably required insulin if subcutaneous terbutaline was given by pump. Half of women taking the drug orally needed insulin for diabetes control.

As discussed previously, there is no evidence that perinatal mortality in infants of women with gestational diabetes is greater than that for the general obstetrical population (Ales and Santini, 1989). If the diabetes worsens as pregnancy advances, however, the prognosis for the fetus-infant also worsens. Adverse outcome also is more likely if there was a prior stillbirth, or if pregnancy-induced hypertension develops (Gabbe, 1985). Therefore, throughout the remainder of pregnancy, periodic checks of fasting plasma glucose concentration are essential to detect the 10 to 15 percent of women who possibly may develop overt diabetes.

Postpartum Consequences. Participants at the 1990 Workshop–Conference recommended that women diagnosed to have gestational diabetes receive postpartum evaluation with a 75-g oral glucose tolerance test at an unspecified time during the puerperium. According to the National Diabetes Data Group (1979), diabetes is diagnosed in nonpregnant adults when the following criteria are met after a 75-g oral glucose load: fasting plasma glucose 140 mg/dL or higher, or 1-hour value 200 mg/dL plus 2-hour value greater than 200 mg/dL.

Glucose intolerance persists for a variable period of time after delivery. Oats and colleagues (1990) demonstrated that an abnormal glucose tolerance test persisted in about 30 percent of gestational diabetics for up to 7 days after delivery. In 246 women with gestational diabetes, Kjos and associates (1990a) showed that about 20 percent had a persistent abnormal glucose tolerance test between 5 and 8 weeks postpartum. In a longer-term follow-up study by Metzger and co-workers (1985), about one fourth of women with gestational diabetes without fasting hyperglycemia had persistent diabetes at 1 year, and another 15 percent had abnormal glucose tolerance. Moreover, according to the 1984 Workshop–Conference, if followed longer, about half of gestational diabetics will ultimately develop overt diabetes. If fasting hyperglycemia is identified during pregnancy, diabetes is more likely to persist postpartum; for women with fasting glucose levels of 105 to 130 mg/mL, this figure is 43 percent (Metzger and colleagues, 1985). When fasting glucose exceeded 130 mg/dL during pregnancy, 86 percent of women remained overtly diabetic.

Recurrence of gestational diabetes in subsequent pregnancies was documented in 20 of 30 women reported by Philipson and Super (1989). Obese women were more likely to have impaired glucose intolerance in subsequent pregnancies.

Overt Diabetes

The likelihood of successful outcomes for the fetus-infant and the overtly diabetic mother is related somewhat to the degree of diabetes control, but more importantly, to the intensity of any underlying maternal cardiovascular or renal disease. Therefore, as the letter classification shown in Table 53–2 advances, the likelihood of a good pregnancy outcome lessens.

The criteria for diagnosis of diabetes during pregnancy is the identification of fasting hyperglycemia on two or more occasions. During pregnancy, this has been defined as a **plasma** level of 105 mg/dL or higher, compared with 140 mg/dL or higher in nonpregnant individuals. The decision to establish a lower value during pregnancy was influenced, in part, by the fact that plasma glucose levels in women are lower during much of normal pregnancy than when nonpregnant (Gabbe, 1985).

Management Before Conception. Overtly diabetic women have a significantly increased risk of a fetus with a birth defect. Reece and Hobbins (1986) described a threefold increased incidence of offspring with congenital malformations in these women. Becerra and colleagues (1990) reported results from the Atlanta Birth Defects Case-Control Study and described an eight-fold relative risk for insulin-treated women compared with nondiabetic mothers. At Parkland Hospital, Lucas and associates (1989) found that 9 percent of 87 insulin-treated diabetic women had infants with major malformations. Heart defects are the most common congenital lesions, and their incidence is increased 5 to 18-fold over the general population. Neural-tube defects are encountered in 20 to 50 per 1000 pregnancies (Becerra and colleagues, 1990; Reece and Hobbins, 1986). Minor anomalies also are increased substantively. Although Lucas and co-workers (1989) found that 7 percent of fetuses had such defects, Rosenn and colleagues (1990) reported their incidence to be nearly 20 percent. Maternal insulin-dependent diabetes is not associated with increased risk for fetal chromosomal abnormalities (Henriques and colleagues, 1991).

It is generally believed that the increased frequency of severe malformations is the consequence of poorly controlled diabetes both preconceptionally as well as early in pregnancy. The retrospective study from Miller and co-workers (1981) suggested that women with lower glycosylated hemoglobin values at the time of conception have a reduced incidence of anomalous fetuses compared with women with abnormally high values. Lucas and colleagues (1989) found that high levels of glycosylated hemoglobin correlated with a higher incidence of anomalies when considered along with severity and duration of disease as determined by the White classification. Data reported by Mills and colleagues (1988a) from the Diabetes in Early Pregnancy Study did not corroborate these findings. This investigation included over 600 diabetic women, and it was concluded that a normal glycosylated hemoglobin did not guarantee that diabetes-associated anomalies were absent. Conversely an elevated level did not necessarily indicate an increased risk for such anomalies. Despite this, they observed that women in whom periconceptional glucose control was optimized had 4.9 percent fetal malformations compared with 9 percent in the group who did not present for care until after organogenesis was complete.

Kitzmiller and associates (1991) tested the effectiveness of intensive periconceptional glycemic management by recruiting 84 women into their study prior to conception. They compared pregnancy outcomes in these tightly controlled women with those of 110 diabetics who presented for care between 6 and 30 weeks' gestation. Only 1.2 percent of the well-controlled mothers had a fetus with a major anomaly compared with 11 percent of those who enrolled late. These investigators reconciled their data vis-a-vis those of Mills and colleagues (1988a) because their patients had evidence for much tighter glucose control. Thus, it would appear that tighter periconceptional glucose control lowers the congenital malformation rate, but that this rate still is higher than in nondiabetic women.

Early pregnancy loss also is increased in poorly controlled diabetics. Again, reporting data from the Diabetes in Early Pregnancy Study, Mills and colleagues (1988b) found that spontaneous abortion was increased in women with elevated blood glucose and glycosylated hemoglobin levels. Likewise, Rosenn and co-workers (1991) reported that early pregnancy loss was reduced three-fold in a group of women who presented for preconceptional control.

Perinatal and Maternal Mortality. In several reports of overtly diabetic pregnancies published in the past 15 years, if substantively increased congenital malformations are disregarded, perinatal mortality rates have not been much higher than those for the general population. For example, the perinatal mortality rate was reported to be 4.6 percent by Gabbe and associates (1977), 3.6 percent by Kitzmiller and co-workers (1978), 4.5 percent by Leveno and co-workers (1979), 3.7 percent by Schneider and associates (1980), 4 percent by Coustan and associates (1980), and 3.9 percent by Martin and colleagues (1987). Severe congenital malformations accounted for much of the excess perinatal mortality.

The Vanderbilt University group (Diamond and colleagues, 1987) reported that Pederson's prognostically bad signs still are applicable for pregnant diabetics. Specifically, ketoacidosis, pregnancy-induced hypertension, pyelonephritis, or maternal neglect were associated with a perinatal mortality rate of 17 percent compared with only 7 percent in insulin-dependent diabetic women without any of these complications. Reece and associates (1988) reported that women with diabetic nephropathy who had good care had pregnancy outcomes comparable to such women without renal disease.

Hypertension is more common in diabetic women, and its incidence increases with severity of classification. Diabetic women have higher systolic and diastolic blood pressures throughout pregnancy when compared with nondiabetic control women (Peterson and colleagues, 1992). In most recent studies that address this issue specifically, pregnancy-induced hypertension is increased two- to three-fold in diabetic women compared with nondiabetic controls. These figures vary widely, probably because of difficulties in differentiating pregnancy-induced changes from those of underlying chronic hypertension. Garner and colleagues (1990) reported an incidence of 10 percent in diabetic patients compared with 4 percent in their control population. Siddiqi and co-workers (1991) found this comparison to be 15 versus 6 percent. Greene and associates (1989) reported a 26 percent incidence of pregnancy-induced hypertension in 420 diabetics compared with 10 percent in nondiabetic controls. At Parkland Hospital, the incidence of any hypertension in all diabetics, including those with class A, is 18 percent, compared with about 10 percent in all pregnant women.

Although generally it was felt that women with overt diabetes suffer disproportionate mortality, there were no maternal deaths reported in the above-cited studies of nearly 600 pregnancies. **Still, as emphasized by Cousins (1987), maternal mortality is increased 10-fold in diabetic women, most often as a result of ketoacidosis, underlying hypertension, preeclampsia, and pyelonephritis.**

Management During Pregnancy. In all of the reports cited above regarding management, early diagnosis of pregnancy and meticulous management of diabetes were stressed. It was emphasized that, ideally, the maternal glucose level should be kept as close to normal as possible. The pregnancy should continue until the fetus is functionally mature, unless the intrauterine environment is deteriorating. With evidence of deterioration, the fetus most often is better delivered even though preterm. The specific techniques emphasized by the several investigators to provide control of the diabetes and to monitor fetal well-being differed, yet the perinatal outcomes were nearly identical.

A precise knowledge of fetal age is important to a successful pregnancy outcome. A carefully obtained menstrual history and accurate measurements of uterine height during the second trimester provide useful information (see Chap. 38, p. 879). Ultrasonic confirmation of fetal age is of value. Midpregnancy ultrasonic examination performed to identify fetal malformations should be performed in conjunction with maternal serum alphafetoprotein screening at 16 to 18 weeks. Sonographic evaluation later in pregnancy may serve to document either fetal macrosomia, a common phenomenon with less severe diabetes, or growth retardation, a complication seen especially when the mother has underlying vascular disease. Data from the Diabetes in Early Pregnancy Study (Brown and colleagues, 1992) examined the predictability of early fetal growth delay— between 10 and 15 weeks' gestation—and found no correlation with congenital malformations or fetal growth retardation at term.

Effective maternal counseling is an extremely important function of prenatal care. The woman should be seen often and instructed carefully to recognize and deal with problems that may arise in the interim. She must be encouraged to report immediately any of a variety of events. For example, respiratory or urinary infections—rather common occurrences during pregnancy—can precipitate diabetic ketoacidosis that is tolerated poorly by the fetus. Otherwise normal nausea and vomiting of pregnancy may lead to the characteristic hypoglycemic reactions, and when more severe and prolonged, starvation may lead to both serious acidosis and insulin resistance much sooner than in the nonpregnant woman.

Similar to normal pregnancy, glucosuria is likely to increase as the consequence of pregnancy-induced glomerular hyperfiltration (see Chap. 8, p. 231). In a few centers, diabetes control is still evaluated by glucosuria. If the pregnant diabetic increased her insulin dosage to a level that avoids glucosuria, symptomatic hypoglycemia would likely develop. In general, glucosuria is a signal to evaluate carefully the plasma glucose levels. Overt acetonuria should never be ignored and most often means that the insulin dosage should be increased.

The intelligent, well-coached, highly motivated pregnant woman with relatively stable diabetes, who conscientiously follows her appropriate diet, which may have to be ingested in as many as five meals a day, and who takes multiple forms of insulin two or more times a day, has the best chance for achieving normoglycemia. In actuality, many women who attempt such rigid control commonly run the risk of hypoglycemic episodes that are dangerous not only to themselves but also to their fetuses. Frequent measurements of plasma glucose, especially before meals, and adjustment of insulin dosage and of diet on the basis of these measurements will help achieve the goal of avoiding both serious hyperglycemia and hypoglycemia.

Within the past decade, there has been an impetus to monitor the effects of insulin therapy by blood glucose levels determined several times daily at home. At her first evaluation, the woman is taught to use glucose oxidase reagent strips, preferably with a reflectance meter (Bourgeois and Duffer, 1990; Landon and Gabbe, 1985). Blood is obtained by finger prick, and glucose concentration is estimated upon arising in the morning, then again before each meal, and at bedtime. Combinations of intermediate-acting and regular insulin then are adjusted to achieve desired levels.

Schneider and co-workers (1980) and later Bourgeois and Duffer (1990) described a method of management that emphasizes ambulatory care throughout pregnancy until delivery. The woman is taught self-measurement of blood glucose using a reflectance meter and, depending upon the results, either the alterations to make in insulin dosage and diet, or how to obtain expert advice immediately. The management team included physicians especially knowledgeable in obstetrics and diabetes. The low perinatal mortality rate in both of these studies is meritorious.

Hemoglobin A₁c. Glycosylated hemoglobin A, commonly referred to as hemoglobin A_{1c}, is often elevated in diabetes, and the magnitude of the elevation generally correlates inversely with the degree of long-term control of plasma glucose concentration. Some investigators measure the total hemoglobin A_1 fraction, which includes A_{1a}, A_{1b}, and A_{1c}. Morris and colleagues (1985) also have shown a good correlation between glycosylated serum protein and blood glucose control over a 1-week period. Brans and colleagues (1982) found no correlation between maternal hemoglobin A_{1c} levels measured at the time of delivery and either infant birthweight or neonatal hypoglycemia. It has been emphasized that there are several pitfalls in the analysis of glycosylated hemoglobin (Garlick and co-workers, 1983).

Insulin Pump. Subcutaneous insulin infusion by a calibrated pump may be used during pregnancy. The pump has both advantages and disadvantages, and as emphasized by Kitzmiller and associates (1985) and Leveno and colleagues (1988), any salutary pregnancy effects have yet to be determined.

Oral Hypoglycemic Agents. Tolbutamide and other oral hypoglycemic agents are not used during pregnancy. Insulin is given instead. Oral agents are avoided because of the possibility of fetal teratogenesis and prolonged serious neonatal hypoglycemia. Piacquadio and co-investigators (1991), in an analysis of 20 pregnancies in Mexican-American women who were taking oral hypoglycemic agents during early pregnancy, concluded that malformations, especially involving the ear, and neonatal hypoglycemia were linked to such therapy. However, a large prospective study is needed to exclude the confounding effect of maternal metabolic derangement secondary to diabetes.

Hospitalization. Because of increased hospitalization costs, as well as reluctance of third-party payers for reimbursement, routine antepartum hospitalization for the overt diabetic woman is no longer commonly practiced. With a predominantly indigent population at Parkland Hospital, conversion to predominately outpatient management was associated with a doubling of the perinatal mortality rate (Table 53–4). Specifically, for 266 insulin-dependent pregnant women routinely admitted

TABLE 53–4. CHANGES IN PERINATAL MORTALITY IN 398 OVERTLY DIABETIC WOMEN RELATED TO THE TIME OF ROUTINE ADMISSION TO THE PARKLAND HOSPITAL HIGH-RISK PREGNANCY UNIT

Time	Policy	Stillbirths (%)	Neonatal Deaths (%)	Perinatal Mortality (%)
1972–1982 (n = 266)	Routine admission at 32 weeks	2.6	1.9	4.5
1982–1985 (n = 132)	Routine admission at 36–37 weeks	7.6	1.6	9.0[a]

[a] Increase due to unexplained stillbirths.

to the High-Risk Pregnancy Unit at 32 weeks from 1972 through 1982, the perinatal mortality was 4.5 percent. Because of budgeting cutbacks, bed space in this unit then was decreased, and from 1982 through 1985, diabetic women were not routinely admitted until 36 to 37 weeks. For these 132 women, the perinatal mortality rate was 9 percent. This doubling of perinatal mortality was due solely to unexplained fetal deaths that typically occurred at about 36 weeks.

Diabetic Retinopathy. Eye complications are the leading cause of blindness for adults in the United States (Merimee, 1990). Virtually all patients with type 1 disease for 25 years have some form of retinopathy. These lesions comprise a spectrum ranging from background retinopathy to proliferative retinopathy characterized by *neovascularization* (Fig. 53–2A). These latter lesions cause visual impairment from vitreous hemorrhage or tractional retinal detachment. Siddiqi and colleagues (1991) reported that almost one third of 175 insulin-dependent pregnant diabetics examined by 10 weeks' gestation had diabetic background retinal changes or proliferative retinopathy. The effects of pregnancy on

worsening of diabetic retinopathy are controversial (Elman and colleagues, 1990; Jovanovic-Peterson and Peterson, 1991a, 1991b). Laser photocoagulation reduces by half the rate of progression of visual loss and blindness and it is indicated during pregnancy for affected women (Fig. 53–2B). Thus, careful ophthalmological evaluation is integral to good prenatal care.

Diabetic Nephropathy. Renal disease from diabetes causes 30 percent of all end-stage renal disease in the United States (Selby and associates, 1990). Moreover, almost half of both type 1 and type 2 diabetics develop this complication. *Microproteinuria* is the first manifestation of nephropathy, but it is not detectable by the usual diagnostic testing. Once *macroproteinuria* develops, gradual decline in renal function follows. The incidence of renal involvement in pregnant women varies and undoubtedly is dependent upon the age of the population. Kitzmiller and colleagues (1981) diagnosed nephropathy in 10 percent of 366 pregnant diabetics cared for at the Joslin Clinic from 1975 through 1978. Siddiqi and associates (1991) reported that 6 percent of 175 insulin-dependent pregnant diabetics had protei-

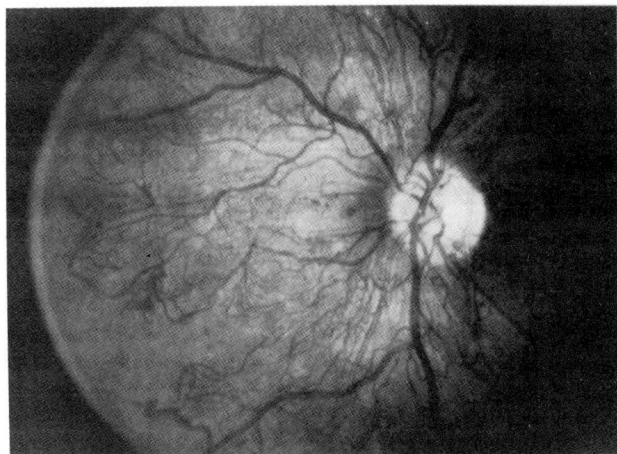

A

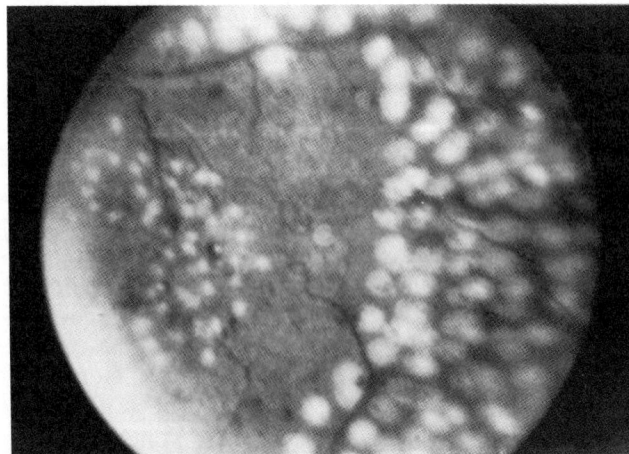

B

Fig. 53–2. Retinal photographs from 30-year-old diabetic woman. **A.** Optic nerve head showing severe proliferative retinopathy characterized by extensive networks of new vessels surrounding the optic disc. **B.** A portion of the acute photocoagulation full "scatter" pattern following argon laser treatment. (From Elman and colleagues, 1990, with permission.)

nuria by 10 weeks' gestation. When nephropathy is identified, pregnancy complications appear to be worsened. In the Boston study (Kitzmiller and co-workers, 1981), almost three fourths of patients had third-trimester hypertension, and proteinuria worsened in 70 percent of all women. Combs and Kitzmiller (1991) reviewed pregnancy outcomes in four studies describing 108 women with diabetic nephropathy characterized by overt proteinuria. During pregnancy, proteinuria usually worsened, and in one study, it exceeded 6 g per 24 hours in 60 percent of women. Preeclampsia was identified in 40 percent of women. Adverse perinatal outcomes, including preterm delivery in half, and fetal growth retardation in 20 percent, were not substantively different from a group of nondiabetic women with intrinsic renal disease. Management of women with chronic renal disease is discussed in Chapter 50 (p. 1138).

Timing of Delivery. Ideally, delivery of the overtly diabetic woman should be accomplished near term. At Parkland Hospital, because of experiences related above, currently these women are requested to enter the hospital at 34 weeks' gestation and to stay until delivered. Typically the lecithin–sphingomyelin ratio in amnionic fluid is measured at about 37 weeks and, if 2.0 or greater, delivery is effected during the 38th week. For women whose gestational age is known for certain, tests to determine fetal pulmonary maturation are not done, and delivery is planned after 38 completed weeks. If severe hypertension develops, delivery is carried out even though the lecithin–sphingomyelin ratio is less than 2.0. Of 118 liveborn infants who were delivered according to this policy, all survived except one who had trisomy 18. Of the four stillbirths during the same period, one who died in utero at 34 weeks might have been salvaged if delivery had been performed even earlier (Leveno and co-workers, 1979). A lecithin–sphingomyelin ratio of 2.0 or more, measured in our laboratory, has served to exclude severe respiratory distress and its serious sequelae in infants of insulin-treated diabetic mothers. It has become evident, however, from the experiences of others that in some circumstances identification of such a ratio does not always assure fetal lung maturity, especially in pregnancies complicated by gestational diabetes (Gabbe, 1985; Leveno and Whalley, 1982).

Others who report very favorable success rates have emphasized other plans of management in an effort to optimize the time selected for delivery. Most employ various tests of fetal well-being, as described in Chapters 45 and 46. Landon and Gabbe (1991) recently reviewed application of such tests in diabetic pregnancies. Gabbe (1985), as well as the American College of Obstetricians and Gynecologists (1986), recommend that serial non-stress tests be performed weekly beginning at 28 to 30 weeks. Landon and Gabbe (1991) recommend twice weekly testing after 32 weeks. If nonreactive, then a contraction stress test or biophysical profile is performed.

At Parkland Hospital, for women hospitalized on the High-Risk Unit, but not those followed as outpatients, assessment of fetal heart rate activity is done weekly. It is emphasized that acceleration with movement, although signifying a contemporaneously healthy fetus, does not predict good fetal health for 7 days. Similarly, a reassuring test should not dissuade the physician to effect delivery in a woman whose clinical condition is deteriorating, as in the case of severe preeclampsia or rapidly developing hydramnios.

Method of Delivery. In the diabetic woman with an A or B White classification, cesarean section has commonly been used to avoid traumatic delivery of a large infant at or near term. In women with advanced classes of diabetes, especially those associated with vascular disease, the reduced likelihood of inducing labor safely remote from term also has contributed appreciably to an increased cesarean delivery rate. Labor induction may be attempted when the fetus is not excessively large, and the cervix is considered favorable for induction. In the reports cited above with low perinatal mortality, the cesarean section rate was more than 50 percent in Melbourne (Martin and colleagues, 1987), 55 percent in Los Angeles (Gabbe and colleagues, 1977), 69 percent in Boston (Kitzmiller and associates, 1978), 70 percent in a midwestern multicenter study (Schneider and co-workers, 1980), and 81 percent in Dallas (Leveno and associates, 1979). At Parkland Hospital, the cesarean delivery rate for all diabetic women, including class A, was 45 percent from 1988 through 1991, but for overtly diabetic women, it has remained at about 80 percent for the past 20 years.

Peripartum Insulin Administration. It is important to reduce considerably or delete the dose of long-acting insulin given on the day of delivery. Regular insulin should be used to meet most or all of the insulin needs of the mother at this time, because insulin requirements typically drop markedly after delivery. We have found that constant insulin infusion by calibrated pump is most satisfactory. During and after either cesarean section or labor and delivery, the mother should be hydrated adequately intravenously as well as given glucose in sufficient amounts to maintain normoglycemia. Plasma glucose levels should be checked frequently, and regular insulin administered accordingly. It is not unusual for the woman to require virtually no insulin for the first 24 hours or so and then for insulin requirements to fluctuate markedly during the next few days after delivery. Infection must be detected quickly and treated promptly.

Perinatal Morbidity. Even though perinatal mortality among infants of diabetic mothers has been reduced remarkably in recent years, troublesome morbidity persists. The most frequent morbidity is from severe *congenital malformations*. As discussed above, it is hoped that more assiduous preconceptional metabolic control and maintenance during embryogenesis will reduce the frequency and severity of these malformations. More recently, Rizzo and colleagues (1991) presented data to indicate that behavioral and intellectual development of offspring of diabetic mothers may be impaired with poor metabolic control.

Preterm delivery is common in overtly diabetic women. In many, induction or cesarean section is mandated by the development of preeclampsia. Greene and co-workers (1989) reported that one fourth of 420 insulin-requiring diabetic women were delivered before 37 completed weeks. *Hypoglycemia* is commonplace in the newborn infant, presumably due in part to hyperplasia of the fetal β-islet cells by chronic hyperglycemia. *Hypocalcemia* and *hyperbilirubinemia* also are common complications of the newborn period. Fortunately, these three problems are readily treatable. *Polycythemia* was reported in 40 percent of fetuses of diabetics in whom cordocentesis was performed 24 hours before elective delivery (Salvesen and associates, 1992). *Idiopathic respiratory distress* is likely to be somewhat more common among infants of diabetic mothers compared with other infants of the same gestational age. This is controversial; for example, Gabbe (1977) and Leveno (1979) and their co-workers did not find this to be a major problem.

Contraception. The two most common forms of reversible contraception, estrogen-progestin oral contraceptives and the intrauterine device, are best avoided if possible in women who have overt diabetes when nonpregnant. Combination oral contraceptives likely worsen diabetes. Moreover, steroidal oral contraceptives may worsen complications from vascular disease that often accompanies diabetes (see Chap. 60, p. 1328). On the other hand, in women with prior gestational diabetes (class A_1 or A_2), short-term use of low-dose oral contraceptives did not have any adverse effects on carbohydrate or lipid metabolism (Kjos and co-workers, 1990b). These investigators recommended, however, that serum lipids and glucose tolerance be monitored. The newly released *progestin implant* system (Norplant) has minimal effects on carbohydrate metabolism and may be ideal for contraception in diabetic women. These are discussed in Chapter 60 (p. 1334). Progestin-only oral contraceptives also may be utilized. The risk of pelvic infection from an *intrauterine device* very likely is increased in the diabetic woman. In many of these women, barrier methods also are an excellent choice for reversible contraception, followed by sterilization once it is certain that the woman wants no more children.

THYROID DISEASES

The interactions between pregnancy and the thyroid gland are fascinating from at least three aspects. First, there are the now well-known and seemingly aberrant changes in tests of thyroid function induced by pregnancy, and, indeed, there may be actual functional changes. Second, there is an intimate relationship between maternal and fetal thyroid function, and although the latter is largely autonomous even early in pregnancy, drugs that affect the maternal gland also affect the fetal gland. Third, there are a number of related abnormal pregnancy and thyroid conditions that at least appear to interact. For example, clinical thyrotoxicosis may be caused by gestational trophoblastic disease. Thyroid autoantibodies have been associated with increased early pregnancy wastage, and uncontrolled thyrotoxicosis and untreated hypothyroidism are both associated with adverse pregnancy outcomes. Finally, there is evidence that while the severity of some autoimmune thyroid disorders is ameliorated during pregnancy, these same disorders may be exacerbated postpartum.

Thyroid disease is common in the general population, and especially in young women. The incidence of sporadic nontoxic goiter is estimated to be up to 5 percent of the North American population. Importantly, the incidence of thyrotoxicosis, hypothyroidism, and thyroiditis probably approaches 1 percent for each condition.

Thyroid Physiology. The impact of pregnancy on maternal thyroid physiology is substantial. There are changes in the structure and function of the gland that can cause confusion in the diagnosis of thyroid abnormalities. Consequently, evaluation of thyroid disorders and proper interpretation of thyroid function tests during pregnancy requires an understanding of these changes. These are discussed in detail in Chapter 8 (p. 236) and are now summarized.

Anatomically, there is moderate thyroid enlargement as a result of glandular hyperplasia and increased vascularity. Histologically, the appearance of the gland is consistent with active formation and secretion of thyroid hormone. Thyroid gland volume determined ultrasonographically increases during pregnancy, although its echostructure and echogenicity remain unchanged (Brander and Kivisaari, 1989; Rasmussen and colleagues, 1989). Conversely, pregnancy usually does not cause impressive thyromegaly, and thus any goiter or nodule should be approached as if pathological.

During pregnancy, there is increased uptake of radioiodine by the maternal thyroid gland. Beginning as early as the second month of pregnancy, total serum thyroxine and triiodothyronine concentrations rise sharply. Contrary to conventional teaching, substantial amounts of thyroxine are transferred from mother to fetus, at least in those cases of fetal thyroid agenesis. During pregnancy, the serum concentration of the major thyroid hormone carrier protein, thyroid-binding globulin, is increased considerably. Thyroid-releasing hormone secretion does not appear to be altered during normal pregnancy, but it does cross the placenta.

Thyrotropin is not bound by carrier proteins, its concentration is unchanged during pregnancy, and it does not cross the placenta. Although a thyrotropic substance has been isolated from human placenta, the role of chorionic gonadotropin as the **chorionic thyrotropin,** if any, in thyroid stimulation is unclear (Kennedy and associates, 1992; Kennedy and Darne, 1991; Hershman, 1992). Kimura and co-workers (1990) presented evidence that in early pregnancy, coincidental with maximum chorionic gonadotropin levels, serum free thyroxine levels increase, and those of thyrotropin decrease. During most of pregnancy, however, serum levels of free thyroxine and triiodothyronine, as well as thyrotropin, are maintained within a narrow normal range, and thus there is not overt functional hyperthyroidism.

Hyperthyroidism

Thyrotoxicosis complicates about 1 in 1000 to 1500 pregnancies. As perhaps expected, mild thyrotoxicosis is difficult to diagnose during pregnancy. Some helpful signs include: (1) tachycardia that exceeds the increase associated with normal pregnancy, (2) an abnormally elevated sleeping pulse rate, (3) thyromegaly, (4) exophthalmos, and (5) failure in a nonobese woman to gain weight despite normal or increased food intake. In most cases, the serum thyroxine levels are markedly elevated, even when compared with the elevated but normal values induced by pregnancy. At the same time, in vitro binding tests fail to demonstrate the appreciably decreased uptake of triiodothyronine characteristic of normal pregnancy. Rarely, hyperthyroidism may be associated with normal serum thyroxine values but abnormally high serum triiodothyronine levels, so-called **T$_3$-toxicosis.**

Graves Disease and Pregnancy. The overwhelming majority of cases of thyrotoxicosis in pregnancy are caused by **Graves disease,** an organ-specific autoimmune process usually associated with thyroid-stimulating antibodies. These autoantibodies mimic thyrotropin in its ability to stimulate thyroid function; consequently, they appear to be responsible for both thyroid hyperfunction and growth in Graves disease. Interestingly, it has been reported that thyroid-stimulating antibody activity in Graves disease usually declines during pregnancy (Hardisty and Munro, 1983; Zakarija and McKenzie, 1983). As shown in Figure 53–3, Amino and colleagues (1982b) reported chemical remission during almost all of 41 pregnancies complicated by

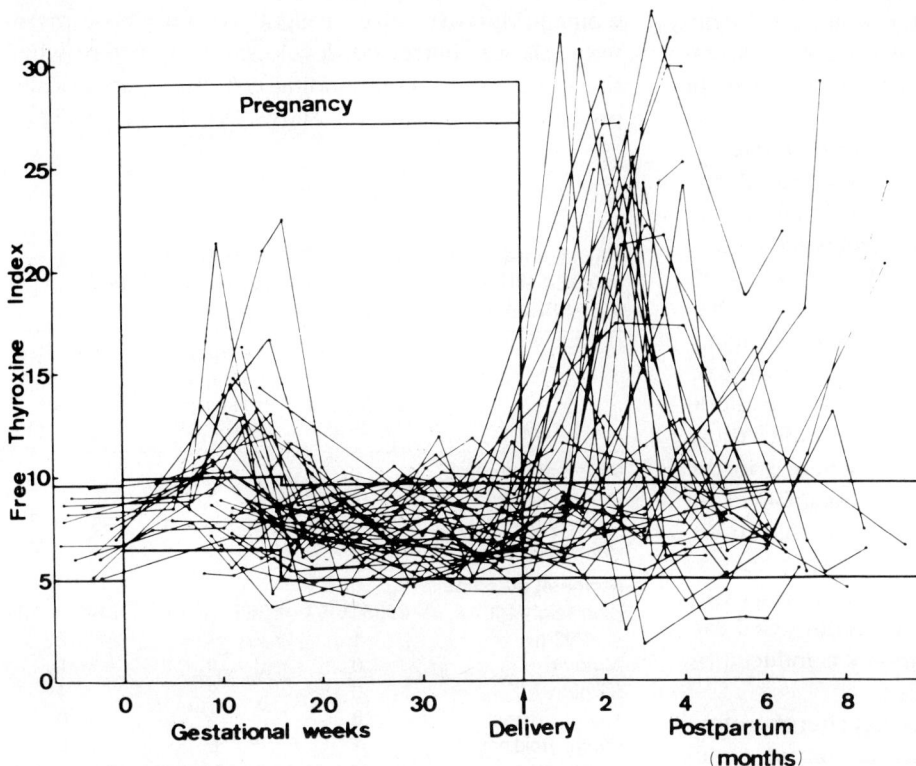

Fig. 53–3. Early pregnancy and postpartum exacerbation of Graves disease during 41 pregnancies in 35 untreated women considered to be in remission. Spontaneous sequential changes in free thyroxine index are plotted as a function of pregnancy duration. (From Amino and colleagues, 1982a, with permission.)

Graves disease. The early pregnancy hyperthyroxinemia in these women was not associated with increased thyroid-stimulating antibody and was presumed to be due to exaggerated response to chorionic gonadotropin stimulation (Kimura and colleagues, 1990). Although this is consistent with the widely held belief that women with Graves disease tend to experience remission during pregnancy, clinical observations do not support this.

Jansson and associates (1987) explored the relationship between Graves disease and pregnancy in a different fashion. They evaluated 93 consecutive women between 20 and 40 years of age who had new-onset Graves disease. The preponderance of these women had given birth within a year of the time Graves disease was discovered, suggesting that pregnancy in some way may have initiated or precipitated thyrotoxicosis.

Treatment. Thyrotoxicosis during pregnancy is treated medically, or medically until such time as the mother is nearly euthyroid, and then surgically. Hyperthyroidism nearly always can be controlled by thioamide drugs. Medical treatment has the potential for causing fetal complications because both **propylthiouracil** and **methimazole** readily cross the placenta and are at least capable of inducing fetal hypothyroidism and goiter. It is difficult to ascribe all cases of neonatal thyroid abnormalities to thiourea drugs because thyrotropin-blocking antibodies also cross the placenta and may bind to the fetal thyroid gland.

A regimen employing propylthiouracil without replacement thyroid hormone has been followed at Parkland Hospital for nearly three decades with very satisfactory pregnancy outcomes for women who become euthyroid (Davis and associates, 1989). As emphasized by Becks and Burrow (1991), the dose of propylthiouracil is empirical, and depending upon symptoms, the starting dose is 300 to 450 mg daily. If necessary, this dose should be increased until the woman appears clinically to be only minimally thyrotoxic, and the total serum thyroxine level is reduced to the upper normal range for pregnancy. In our experiences, metabolic control requires higher doses than those recommended previously (Davis and colleagues, 1989). Of more than 50 women with Graves thyrotoxicosis given an initial mean propylthiouracil dose of 600 mg, only a third underwent remission. In another third, it was necessary to increase the dose, whereas in the remaining third, this 600-mg dose was maintained. In only 10 percent of these women were we able to decrease the dose to 150 mg by the end of pregnancy as recommended by some authorities. These clinical experiences are at variance with observations discussed earlier suggesting that remission commonly is induced by pregnancy.

Thyroidectomy may be carried out after thyrotoxicosis has been brought under medical control. Opinions differ as to the wisdom of surgical treatment during the first trimester—a time when abortion is relatively common—or during the third trimester—when preterm labor may ensue. From the beginning of the second trimester until early in the third trimester, however, for elective treatment, or for women who cannot adhere to medical treatment, or for women in whom drug therapy proves toxic, subtotal thyroidectomy may be the treatment of choice after appropriate pharmacological control is achieved.

Pregnancy Outcome. Pregnancy outcomes in thyrotoxic women depend upon whether metabolic control is achieved. In women who remain hyperthyroid despite therapy, and in those whose disease is untreated, there is a higher incidence of preeclampsia and heart failure, as well as adverse perinatal outcomes (Table 53–5). Sherif and colleagues (1991) reported a perinatal mortality of 6 percent in 92 women with thyrotoxicosis, even though most were controlled with thiourea drugs before conception.

Thyroid Storm or Heart Failure. Thyroid storm is encountered only rarely in untreated women (Davis and associates, 1989). Much more likely, and perhaps simulating storm, is heart failure apparently caused by the long-term myocardial effects of thyroxine. Easterling and colleagues (1991) documented the hyperdynamic cardiovascular state of thyrotoxic pregnant women. This may be intensified by other pregnancy complications that include severe preeclampsia, infection, or anemia (Hankins and co-workers, 1984). In our experiences, heart failure developed in 12 percent of 60 thyrotoxic women. Moreover, five of eight women whose thyrotoxicosis was untreated developed heart failure when there were other confounding conditions, specifically, preeclampsia, anemia, or sepsis. As shown in Figure

TABLE 53–5. PREGNANCY OUTCOMES IN 60 WOMEN WITH OVERT THYROTOXICOSIS CARED FOR AT PARKLAND HOSPITAL

Factor	Treated and Euthyroid (n = 36)	Thyrotoxic Despite Therapy (n = 16)	Untreated Thyrotoxicosis (n = 8)
Maternal outcome			
Preeclampsia	2	3	2
Delivery (wk)	38.6 ± 0.5	38.8 ± 1.1	33.1 ± 1.5
Heart failure	1	1	5
Neonatal outcome			
Birthweight (g)	2905 ± 97	2665 ± 155	2140 ± 164
< 2000 g	1	1	2
Abortion	0	0	1
Stillbirth	0	2	4
Thyrotoxicosis	0	1	0
Hypothyroidism	1	0	0

Adapted from Davis and associates (1989).

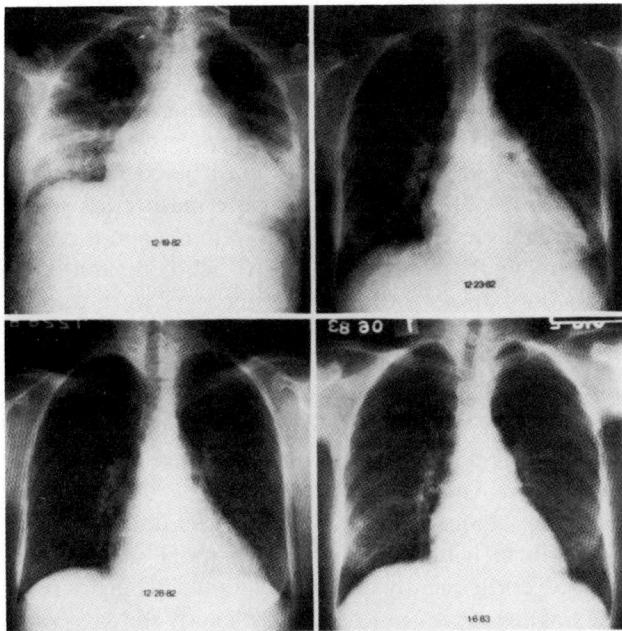

Fig. 53–4. Serial chest radiographs demonstrating the 18-day resolution of pulmonary edema and cardiomegaly in a 27-year-old thyrotoxic woman with septic abortion and heart failure at 20 weeks' gestation. (From Hankins and colleagues, 1984, with permission.)

53–4, thyroxine-induced cardiomyopathy is reversed with treatment.

If thyroid storm or heart failure is suspected, treatment consists of 1 g each of propylthiouracil and potassium iodide given orally or through a nasogastric tube. Some authorities give propranolol intravenously, but this must be done with caution if there is heart failure. A principal directive of therapy is aggressive treatment of serious hypertension, infection, and anemia.

Effects of Thyrotoxicosis on the Neonate. Earlier estimates of adverse fetal effects induced by thiourea drugs may have been erroneously large. In the 52 women treated at Parkland Hospital, there was evidence for hypothyroidism in only one infant (Davis and colleagues, 1989). Momotani and associates (1986) reported that cord serum thyroxine levels were lower in neonates born to thyrotoxic mothers who were taking propylthiouracil up until delivery when compared with mothers in whom the drug had been discontinued earlier. They found no dose-response relationship, however, and none of these infants were hypothyroid. Davidson and colleagues (1991) described a case of Graves disease in which the mother was overtreated with propylthiouracil and the fetus developed a goiter by 28 weeks. Blood obtained by percutaneous umbilical vein sampling confirmed fetal hypothyroidism and thyroxine injected intraamnionically at 35, 36, and 37 weeks caused rapid resolution of the goiter.

Burrow and associates (1978) carried out a long-term study of the intellectual and physical development, including thyroid function, of children born to thyrotoxic mothers treated with propylthiouracil during pregnancy. They found no adverse effects on subsequent growth and development.

Even after being rendered euthyroid by surgery or radiation, women with Graves disease may give birth to infants with manifestations of thyrotoxicosis, including goiter and exophthalmos. Matsuura and colleagues (1988) presented evidence that neonatal thyrotoxicosis results from the transplacental passage of maternal thyroid-stimulating antibodies. Based on detailed autopsy findings, there is good evidence that fetal thyrotoxicosis from transplacental passage of maternal thyroid-stimulating antibodies can cause fetal demise (Houck and associates, 1988; Page and co-workers, 1988). Because of this, Porreco and Bloch (1990) and Wenstrom and colleagues (1990) advocate cord blood sampling by funipuncture to assess fetal thyroid status. If thyrotoxic, thiourea treatment is given.

Thyroid Dysfunction with Gestational Trophoblastic Disease. Serum thyroxine levels in women with molar pregnancy usually are elevated appreciably, but clinically apparent hyperthyroidism is less common (see Chap. 35, p. 752). Amir and colleagues (1984) identified thyrotoxicosis in about 2 percent of such cases.

Hypothyroidism

Hypothyroidism is diagnosed if the expected rise in serum thyroxine during pregnancy fails to take place, and the thyrotropin level is elevated. Overt hypothyroidism complicating pregnancy is uncommon, probably because it is often associated with infertility. Montoro and colleagues (1981) reported one fetal death and one infant with anomalies in 11 pregnancies in hypothyroid women. From our experiences, hypothyroid women who do become pregnant have a high incidence of preeclampsia and placental abruption with a correspondingly inordinate number of low-birthweight and stillborn infants (Table 53–6). Heart failure also is encountered with increased frequency in hypothyroid women.

Although replacement therapy is imperative in these women, the optimal dose of thyroid hormone is more controversial. Traditional teaching is that hypothyroid women receiving a maintenance dose of thyroid hormone before pregnancy rarely require an increased dose during pregnancy. However, Mandel and colleagues (1990), as well as Tamaki and associates (1990), have recently presented evidence that pregnancy is associated with a significant, albeit small, increase in thyroxine requirements. Certainly, the thyroxine replacement dose should be adjusted so that the serum thyrotropin level is within the normal range.

TABLE 53–6. PREGNANCY OUTCOMES IN 28 WOMEN WITH OVERT AND SUBCLINICAL HYPOTHYROIDISM

Factor	Hypothyroidism	
	Overt (n = 16)	Subclinical (n = 12)
Mean age (yr)	28 ± 2.3	24 ± 1.8
Mean gestational age at delivery (wk)	35.7 ± 1.6	36 ± 2.9
Thyroxine therapy (wk)		
When initiated	21.8 ± 4.2	19.5 ± 4.6
Duration to delivery	14.5 ± 3.4	16.4 ± 4.8
Pregnancy complications		
Preeclampsia	7	2
Abruptio placentae	3	0
Hematocrit < 26 percent	5	0
Postpartum hemorrhage	3	2
Cardiac dysfunction	1	1
Birthweight < 2000 g	5	1[a]
Stillbirths	2	1[b]

[a] Class F diabetes.
[b] Due to syphilis.
Modified from Davis and colleagues (1988).

Subclinical hypothyroidism is much more common. It is characterized by a lack of clinical symptoms in conjunction with elevated serum thyrotropin levels and normal serum thyroxine and triiodothyronine levels. Its effects on pregnancy outcome are unknown, but thyroxine replacement is recommended. Jovanovic-Peterson and associates (1988) reported a high incidence of subclinical hypothyroidism in 51 pregnant women with type 1 diabetes, all of whom had normal thyroxine levels before conception. During the first trimester, 26 of the 51 women were found to have elevated thyrotropin levels, microsomal autoantibodies, or both. Of these 26 women, eight subsequently developed abnormally low serum thyroxine levels, decreased insulin requirements, and nephrotic-range proteinuria. After thyroid replacement, insulin requirements increased to the expected level in these eight women.

Effect of Hypothyroidism on the Fetus and Infant.

In general, infants of hypothyroid mothers appear healthy without evidence of thyroid dysfunction (Montoro and co-workers, 1981). In some situations, however, the infant of a hypothyroid mother may be similarly afflicted. For example, if maternal hypothyroidism was caused by radioiodine therapy (not tracer doses) during pregnancy, destruction of the fetal thyroid gland also may have resulted. Any infant whose mother was so treated during pregnancy must be carefully evaluated and probably treated prophylactically for hypothyroidism. Abortion should be considered.

Environmental factors also may be important in fetal hypothyroidism. Thilly and associates (1978) reported their experiences with a group of women from a region in Africa where severe endemic goiter is common because of dietary iodine deficiency, dietary goi-

trogens, or both. Women whose iodine deficiency was corrected prenatally had significantly higher thyroxine levels and lower thyrotropin levels at delivery compared with women not receiving iodine supplementation. Similar results were obtained when thyroxine and thyrotropin were measured in cord blood from these two groups. Most impressively, the mean cord serum thyrotropin level in infants born to mothers not receiving supplementation was 19.6 μU/mL compared with 9.4 μU/mL in newborns whose mothers were treated. This same group now has shown that iodine supplementation in young children with cretinism will restore a biochemically euthyroid state (Vanderpas and colleagues, 1986). Thus, iodine supplementation seems reasonable for all pregnant women in areas of endemic iodine deficiency.

The clinical diagnosis of **congenital hypothyroidism** in neonates is difficult to make and is often missed; consequently mass population newborn screening was introduced in 1974. Because early and aggressive thyroxine replacement therapy is critical to these infants, biochemical screening of all newborns is mandatory in all states. According to various reports based on mass screening of newborns, congenital hypothyroidism is detected with a frequency of about 1 in 4000 to 7000 infants. Based on 5- to 7-year follow-up results of infants identified by the earliest screening programs and treated promptly and adequately with thyroid hormone, it appears that most, if not all, sequelae of congenital hypothyroidism, including intellectual impairment, are preventable (Fisher and Foley, 1989). Unfortunately, Grant and colleagues (1992) reported that 8 percent of 449 infants with congenital hypothyroidism also had major congenital anomalies.

Nodular Thyroid Disease

In nonpregnant patients, evaluation of a thyroid nodule commonly includes radioisotope scanning to demonstrate hyperfunctioning or hypofunctioning. Because radioiodine usually is used, most authorities believe thyroid scanning to be contraindicated in pregnancy, although the likelihood of fetal injury seems remote (see Chap. 43, p. 986). Ultrasound examination reliably detects nodules greater than 0.5 cm and their solid or cystic nature also can be determined. Although cystic lesions are associated with a lower incidence of malignancy compared with solid masses, the diagnosis can easily be made using fine-needle aspiration. Whereas the utility of diagnostic ultrasound in distinguishing benign and malignant nodules currently is unclear, fine-needle aspiration has false-positive rates of up to 2 percent and false-negative rates of 1 to 3 percent for distinguishing malignant from benign disease.

Current evidence seems to indicate that with the assistance of an experienced cytopathologist, fine-needle aspiration of thyroid nodules is a reasonable method of assessment during pregnancy. Rosen and Walfish (1986) provided data from 30 pregnant women assessed for neoplasia because of palpable thyroid nodular disease, and many of these underwent fine-needle aspiration. Thirteen of these 30 were found to have a malignancy, 11 had an adenoma, and 6 were described simply as having a goiter. They recommended that surgery be performed for women with neoplasms either during midpregnancy or after delivery. Although most thyroid carcinomas are well differentiated and pursue an indolent course, the purposeful delay in surgical therapy seems difficult to justify except in unusual circumstances.

Postpartum Thyroiditis

Transient postpartum hypothyroidism or thyrotoxicosis associated with autoimmune thyroiditis is common. When women are carefully scrutinized postpartum, clinical and biochemical evidence of thyroid dysfunction has been found consistently in 5 to 10 percent regardless of their geographic locale (Roti and Emerson, 1992). Nevertheless, postpartum thyroiditis is diagnosed infrequently, largely because it typically develops after the traditional postpartum examination and because it results in vague and nonspecific symptoms (Ramsay, 1986). These factors should not lead to an underestimation of its clinical importance. Hayslip and colleagues (1988) reported that such women were significantly more likely than euthyroid women to manifest troublesome symptoms that included depression, carelessness, and memory concentration impairment 3 to 5 months after delivery.

Pathogenesis. Although the precise cause of postpartum thyroiditis is unknown, it has been well characterized histologically as a destructive, lymphocytic thyroiditis (Roti and Emerson, 1992). The majority of women who develop postpartum thyroid dysfunction have a positive assay for microsomal autoantibodies (Jansson and co-workers, 1988). Thus, postpartum thyroid dysfunction is an autoimmune disorder in which thyroid microsomal autoantibodies apparently play a central role (Vargas and colleagues, 1988). Presumably, preexisting subclinical autoimmune thyroid disease is susceptible to exacerbation because of changes in the immunoregulatory system that develop postpartum (Stagnaro-Green and colleagues, 1992). It can be anticipated that women at increased risk for postpartum thyroid dysfunction include those who have experienced it before and those who have a personal or family history of autoimmune disease. Iodide deficiency also may play a role (Glinoer and associates, 1992).

Thyroid Autoantibodies. Thyroid microsomal autoantibodies have been identified in 7 to 10 percent of women

either early in pregnancy or shortly following delivery (Jansson and associates, 1988; Hayslip and colleagues, 1988). Stagnaro-Green and collaborators (1990) found that the incidence was 20 percent in 552 consecutive women studied before 13 weeks' gestation. While 17 percent of these autoantibody-positive women aborted, only 8 percent of control women did so. When microsomal autoantibody titers are followed sequentially in seropositive women during pregnancy and the puerperium, a characteristic pattern emerges. As shown in Figure 53-5, titers decrease somewhat during pregnancy, rise to a peak 4 to 6 months after delivery, and then decline to early pregnancy levels by 10 to 12 months postpartum. Detection of microsomal autoantibodies either early in pregnancy or shortly after delivery may identify women at high risk for developing postpartum thyroid dysfunction.

An association between maternal serum thyroid autoantibodies and fetal **Down syndrome** has long been suspected. Cuckle and colleagues (1988) measured thyroglobulin and microsomal autoantibodies using both enzyme-linked immunosorbent assay and hemagglutination assay. They studied 77 pregnancies complicated by fetal Down syndrome and 385 unaffected control pregnancies during the mid-trimester. They identified both types of thyroid autoantibodies more frequently in affected pregnancies, although the differences were not significant.

Clinical Manifestations. Between 1 and 4 months postpartum, approximately 4 percent of all women develop transient **thyrotoxicosis** (Walfish and Chan, 1985). The onset is abrupt and a small, painless goiter is commonly found. Although there may be many symptoms, only fatigue and palpitations are more frequent in these thyrotoxic women compared with normal postpartum women. Thyrotoxicosis results from excessive

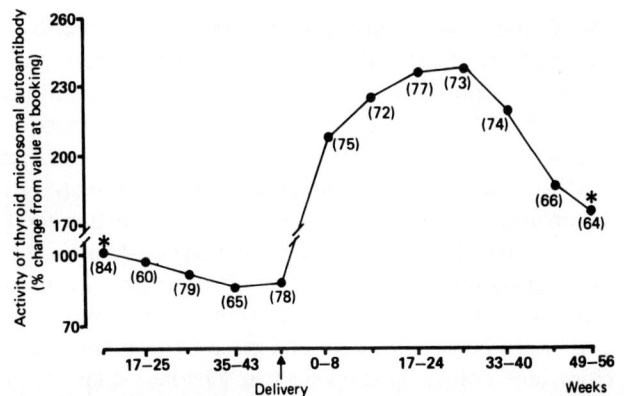

Fig. 53-5. Changes in serum activity of thyroid microsomal autoantibody during pregnancy and up to 12 months postpartum in 84 women. Numbers in parentheses indicate women assessed at each time point. ($p < 0.001$ when compared with values at delivery). (From Fung and colleagues, 1988, with permission.)

release of preformed hormone secondary to glandular disruption (*destruction-induced thyrotoxicosis*), rather than excessive hormone production. Antithyroid medications such as propylthiouracil and methimazole are ineffective in this condition, and they may even hasten the development of a subsequent hypothyroid phase. Treatment usually is not given, but if symptoms due to excessive thyroid hormone are severe, a β-adrenergic blocker may be useful. Approximately two thirds of these women return directly to a euthyroid state, but the other third subsequently experience hypothyroidism.

Between 4 and 8 months postpartum, 2 to 5 percent of all women develop **hypothyroidism** (Jansson and co-workers, 1988). At least one third of these women will previously have experienced the thyrotoxic phase of postpartum thyroid dysfunction. Goiters, as well as clinically significant symptoms, are common and are more prominent than during the thyrotoxic phase. Hypothyroidism can develop rapidly in these women, sometimes in over one month. Thus, women at risk for postpartum hypothyroidism should be evaluated regularly; and at least in selected situations, thyroid function tests performed. If hypothyroidism develops and the severity of symptoms warrants, thyroxine replacement is initiated. It has been suggested that thyroxine be continued until 12 to 18 months after delivery, then gradually withdrawn (Jansson and colleagues, 1988).

Women who experience postpartum thyroiditis are at risk of developing permanent hypothyroidism. Although the exact frequency is unknown, it has been estimated to be between 10 and 30 percent. The incidence may be even greater if subclinical disease is considered (Jansson and associates, 1988; Tachi and colleagues, 1988). The importance of long-term follow up in these women is apparent.

PARATHYROID DISEASE

The function of parathyroid hormone is to maintain extracellular fluid calcium concentration. The 115-amino acid hormone acts directly on bone and kidney and indirectly on small intestine through its effects on synthesis of vitamin D ($1,25(OH)_2D$) to increase serum calcium. Parathyroid hormone secretion is regulated by serum ionized calcium concentration, a negative feedback system. **Calcitonin** is a potent hypocalcemic hormone produced by the thyroid gland. It acts in many ways as a physiological parathyroid hormone antagonist. The interrelationships between these hormones and calcium metabolism is discussed in Chapter 8 (p. 237). Because of substantive fetal needs—300 mg per day late in pregnancy—and increased renal losses of calcium due to augmented glomerular filtration, parathyroid hormone levels are increased in pregnant women.

Hyperparathyroidism

Hypercalcemia is caused by hyperparathyroidism or cancer in 90 percent of cases. In most tumor-related cases, the malignancy is not occult, and the cause of increased serum calcium is obvious. Primary hyperparathyroidism is common, and its incidence peaks between the third and fifth decades. Because many automated laboratory test systems include measurement of serum calcium, cases of hyperparathyroidism that previously would have been undiagnosed are being detected. Almost 80 percent of cases are caused by a solitary adenoma and another 15 percent by generalized chief cell hyperplasia. Symptoms of hypercalcemia include fatigue, depression, and confusion; anorexia, nausea, and vomiting; constipation; reversible renal tubular defects; and electrocardiographic abnormalities with occasional arrhythmias. Generally, symptoms are not apparent until the serum calcium exceeds 12 mg/dL in the nonpregnant person.

Hyperparathyroidism in Pregnancy. Although hyperparathyroidism is more common than once thought, only about 100 women with this disease complicating pregnancy have been reported (Kelly, 1991; Patterson, 1987; Pitkin, 1985). It is presumed that many hypercalcemic pregnant women with hyperparathyroidism either were not detected or reported. As in nonpregnant patients, hyperparathyroidism usually is caused by a parathyroid adenoma, but it can be due to ectopic parathyroid hormone production, or rarely to parathyroid carcinoma (Parham and Orr, 1987). Symptoms include hyperemesis, generalized weakness, renal calculi, pancreatitis, and psychiatric disorders. Whalley (1963) described a woman who had parathyroid storm characterized by hypercalcemia and convulsions which were co-existent with chronic pyelonephritis and hypertension. The combination of these might erroneously have been considered to be eclampsia.

Pregnancy theoretically will improve hyperparathyroidism because of significant calcium shunting to the fetus as well as augmented renal excretion. When the protective effects of pregnancy are withdrawn, there is significant danger of postpartum hypercalcemia and possible crisis (Shangold and colleagues, 1982).

Pitkin (1985) reported that adverse pregnancy outcomes are likely. Earlier reports described excessive stillbirths and preterm deliveries in hyperparathyroid women. With earlier detection and better management, the incidence of adverse effects is lower (Shangold and associates, 1982). Certainly, if asymptomatic hypercalcemic women are included, adverse perinatal outcomes certainly will be less likely.

Management. Definitive management is surgical removal of the parathyroid adenoma. Elective neck exploration is tolerated well by pregnant women. Higgins and Hisley (1988) described two women in whom parathyroid adenomas were localized using sonography and removed at 28 weeks in one and 12 weeks in the other. An alternative is to treat the asymptomatic women with oral phosphate, 1 to 1.5 g daily in divided doses. This may lower serum calcium, thus allowing parathyroidectomy to be postponed until delivery.

For women with dangerously elevated serum calcium levels, or in those who are mentally obtunded, emergency treatment is instituted. Intravenous hydration with normal saline to evoke diuresis is the first step. Urine flow should exceed 150 mL per hour. Furosemide given in conventional doses will block tubular reabsorption of calcium. Careful attention to prevent hypokalemia and hypomagnesemia is important. Adjunctive therapy includes mithramycin, which inhibits bone resorption; calcitonin, which decreases skeletal calcium release; and oral phosphorus. Intravenous phosphate phosphorus may be used in life-threatening emergencies, but its use is exceedingly dangerous. Corticosteroids may be effective if hypercalcemia is caused by a malignancy or sarcoidosis; however, they are ineffective for primary hyperparathyroidism.

Neonatal Effects. Cord blood calcium levels are greater than those in the mother. These elevated levels suppress fetal parathyroid function resulting in a fall in serum calcium levels that reaches a nadir at 24 to 48 hours after birth. Accordingly, 15 to 25 percent of these newborns develop severe hypocalcemia with or without tetany (Moltich, 1992). Thus, it is not surprising that tetany has been occasionally noted in newborns of mothers with hyperparathyroidism. At times, neonatal tetany alone has led to a search that identified a maternal parathyroid adenoma.

Hypoparathyroidism

The most common cause of hypocalcemia is hypoparathyroidism; it usually follows parathyroid or thyroid surgery. Chronically hypocalcemic pregnant women may have a fetus with skeletal demineralization. Treatment with 1-25-dihydroxyvitamin D_3 (calcitriol), dihydrotachysterol, or large doses of vitamin D (50,000 to 150,000 U/day), together with calcium gluconate or calcium lactate (3 to 5 g daily), and a diet low in phosphates, usually prevents symptomatic hypocalcemia. The risk to the fetus from large doses of vitamin D has not been established. Caplan and Beguin (1990) reported their experiences with five pregnancies complicated by hypoparathyroidism. They observed that whereas the calcitriol dose was increased during the second half of pregnancy, it was reduced during lactation.

DISEASES OF THE ADRENAL GLANDS

Pregnancy has profound effects on adrenal gland cortical secretion and its control or stimulation. These interrelationships are discussed in detail in Chapter 8 (p. 238). Briefly, serum corticotropin levels increase after a marked reduction in early pregnancy. The considerable increase in plasma cortisol is explained by increased transcortin production and binding. In addition, plasma renin increases, which stimulates angiotensin and, in turn, aldosterone secretion. Baseline adrenal medullary hormone secretion probably is unaffected. Although there is no evidence that pregnancy causes any adrenal-specific disorders, a number of adrenal disorders may co-exist with pregnancy.

Pheochromocytoma

Pheochromocytomas are chromaffin tumors that secrete catecholamines. Most are located in the adrenal medulla, but 10 percent are found as tumors in sympathetic ganglia. There is an association with medullary thyroid carcinoma and hyperparathyroidism in some of the **multiple endocrine neoplasia syndromes (MENS),** as well as neurofibromatosis and von Hippel–Lindau disease. Pheochromocytomas are common but frequently are not diagnosed. St. John Sutton and colleagues (1981) found their incidence at autopsy to be 1 in 750 at the Mayo Clinic. In three fourths of these patients, the tumor was not diagnosed until after death. Moreover, only 0.1 percent of hypertensive patients have a pheochromocytoma. In adults, they are sometimes called the "10-percent tumor" because 10 percent are bilateral, 10 percent are extraadrenal, and about 10 percent are malignant.

Symptoms usually are paroxysmal and manifest as hypertensive crisis, seizure disorders, or anxiety attacks. Hypertension is sustained in 60 percent of patients, but half of these patients also have paroxysmal crises. Other symptoms during paroxysmal attacks are headaches, profuse sweating, palpitations, and apprehension. Chest pain, nausea and vomiting, and pallor or flushing also are common. There usually is severe hypertension and tachycardia.

Diagnosis is confirmed by measurement of 24-hour urine vanillylmandelic acid (VMA), metanephrines, or unconjugated catecholamines. Adrenal localization usually is successful with computed tomography or magnetic resonance imaging. Extra-adrenal tumors may be localized using these, but often abdominal arteriography (after α-blockade is accomplished) or ^{131}I-metaiodobenzylguanidine (MIBG) scanning are necessary for localization.

Pheochromocytoma Complicating Pregnancy.
Pheochromocytoma is a rare but dangerous complication of pregnancy. Geelhoed (1983) cited an earlier

review of 89 cases in which 43 mothers died. Maternal death was much more common (58 versus 18 percent) if the tumor was not diagnosed antepartum. Because of improved diagnostic methods and management, maternal survival has improved. Harper and colleagues (1989) analyzed 42 cases reported from 1980 through 1987 and added five cases of their own. Overall maternal mortality was 17 percent, and it was zero if the diagnosis was made antepartum. Still, in only half of these cases was this accomplished.

Diagnosis is the same as for nonpregnant patients and a 24-hour urine specimen is assayed for VMA, metanephrines, or unconjugated catecholamines. Measuring two, or even three, of these increases the accuracy of diagnosis (Daly and Landsberg, 1992). Plasma catecholamine levels technically are difficult and are not recommended currently for screening. Tumor localization during pregnancy is possible using computed tomography or magnetic resonance imaging as shown in Figure 53–6. In general, for nonpregnant patients, computed tomography will localize 95 percent of adrenal tumors, whereas magnetic resonance imaging is helpful particularly for extra-adrenal tumors (Daly and Landsberg, 1992).

In some cases, the principal challenge is to differentiate preeclampsia from the hypertensive crises caused by a pheochromocytoma. Combs and colleagues (1989) have shown that during paroxysmal hypertension, cardiac output falls substantively. They expressed appropriate concerns for adverse fetal effects of even mild hypertensive paroxysms.

Management. In all cases, medical management of hypertension and symptoms with an α-adrenergic blocking drug such as phenoxybenzamine is imperative. Only after α-blockade is achieved, can β-blockers be given for tachycardia. In some cases, surgical exploration and tumor removal may be performed during pregnancy. Favorable outcomes have been described for women in whom the diagnosis was made late in pregnancy and the blood pressure controlled pharmacologically during cesarean section and tumor resection (Burgess, 1979; Harper and colleagues, 1989; Schenker and Granat, 1982).

Recurrent tumors are troublesome. We have cared for three women in whom recurrent pheochromocytoma was identified during pregnancy. Pharmacological control of hypertension with phenoxybenzamine was induced successfully in all three. Two infants were healthy, but a third was stillborn in a mother with a massive tumor load who was receiving phenoxybenzamine, 100 mg daily. In all three women, resection of the tumor was carried out postpartum, one at the time of cesarean section and in the others at 2 and 6 months postpartum. Lyons and Colmorgen (1988) reported a similar case in which they controlled symptoms of a recurrent extra-adrenal tumor by using phenoxybenzamine and atenolol beginning at 10 weeks' gestation. A healthy infant was delivered by cesarean section at 35 weeks. Despite α- and β-blockade, dangerous peripartum hypertension developed.

Addison Disease

Primary adrenocortical insufficiency, or Addison disease, is rare. More than 90 percent of the glands must be destroyed for symptoms to develop. Whereas in the past, chronic granulomatous disease such as tuberculosis and histoplasmosis caused most cases, currently, **id-**

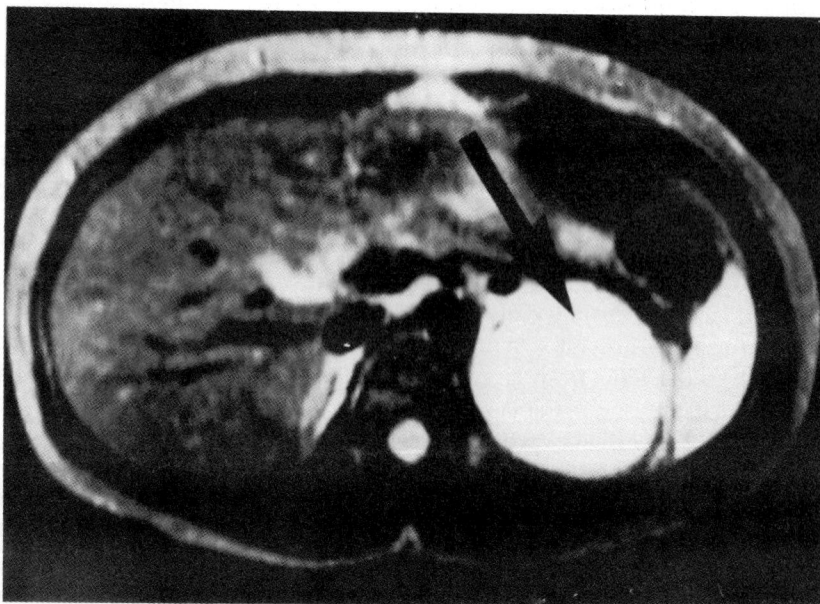

Fig. 53–6. Magnetic resonance imaging of left adrenal gland pheochromocytoma (*arrow*) in a 17-week pregnant woman. (From Combs and colleagues, 1989, with permission.)

iopathic autoimmune adrenalitis is responsible for the majority. There is an increased incidence of concurrent Hashimoto thyroiditis, premature ovarian failure, type 1 diabetes, and Graves disease. These **polyglandular autoimmune syndromes** also include pernicious anemia, vitiligo, alopecia, nontropical sprue, and myasthenia gravis.

Pregnancy. Before 1953, only 50 published cases of Addison disease in pregnancy had been identified, suggesting that untreated adrenal hypofunction caused sterility. With the synthesis of cortisone and related compounds, pregnancy has become much more common in these women. Fetal prognosis in general parallels maternal health. Because serum cortisol levels are increased, the diagnosis made during pregnancy should include documentation of a lack of response to infused corticotropin (O'Shaughnessy and Hackett, 1984). Seaward and colleagues (1989) found only five cases published since 1972. They reported a woman with unrecognized Addison disease who suffered a placental abruption and fetal death associated with Addisonian crisis. Albert and associates (1989) reported six successful pregnancy outcomes in six women in whom adrenal insufficiency had been diagnosed before conception.

Management. During pregnancy and the puerperium, it is essential to observe the woman with adrenal insufficiency closely for evidence of either inadequate or excessive steroid replacement. Except at times of stress, replacement therapy need not be greater than in the nonpregnant state. There may be little need during pregnancy for potent mineralocorticoid compounds. During labor and after delivery or after a surgical procedure, steroid replacement must be increased appreciably to approximate the normal adrenal response. Hydrocortisone, 100 mg usually is given intravenously every 8 hours. It is important that shock from causes other than adrenocortical insufficiency be recognized and treated promptly, especially that caused by hemorrhage or bacterial septicemia.

Cushing Syndrome

The most common cause of Cushing syndrome is iatrogenic from treatment with corticosteroids. Endogenous Cushing syndrome is caused by increased adrenal cortisol production. Most cases are due to bilateral adrenal hyperplasia stimulated by corticotropin-producing pituitary adenomas or by abnormal amounts of hypothalamic corticotropin releasing factor. Hyperplasia also is caused by nonendocrine tumors that produce polypeptides similar to either corticotropin-releasing factor or corticotropin. A fourth of cases of Cushing syndrome are caused by an adrenal adenoma; these usually are bilateral and half are malignant.

Almost all patients have the typical body habitus caused by adipose tissue deposition, which characteristically results in *moon facies, a buffalo hump,* and truncal obesity. Fatiguability and weakness, hypertension, hirsutism, amenorrhea, cutaneous striae, and easy bruisability are each encountered in 70 to 80 percent of cases. Diagnosis is by confirmation of elevated plasma cortisol that cannot be suppressed by dexamethasone.

Pregnancy and Cushing Syndrome. Because most women have amenorrhea, pregnancy associated with Cushing syndrome is rare and only 70 or so cases have been reported (Aron and associates, 1990a; Buescher and co-workers, 1992; Koerten and colleagues, 1986). From these reviews, it was found that over half of the cases were caused by adrenal tumors of which 80 percent were benign. They stressed the difficulties in diagnosis of Cushing syndrome because of pregnancy-induced increases in plasma cortisol, corticotropin, and corticotropin-releasing factor.

Most cases described in pregnant women are the classical picture of Cushing syndrome. In some cases, symptoms may be exacerbated. Maternal complications include hypertension in 60 to 90 percent of cases and gestational diabetes in 30 to 60 percent. Heart failure is common during pregnancy, and there have been three maternal deaths in 65 pregnancies (Buescher and associates, 1992). Perinatal morbidity and mortality are correspondingly high. Preterm delivery was reported in 60 percent of cases. In most series, perinatal mortality is cited at about 25 percent.

Management. Long-term medical therapy for Cushing syndrome usually is ineffective. During pregnancy, medical therapy of hypertension in mild cases may suffice until delivery (Martin and associates, 1989). This also is recommended for cases diagnosed late in pregnancy. Aron and colleagues (1990b) reported a well-documented case of Cushing syndrome diagnosed during pregnancy and treated with *cyproheptadine.* Postpartum, all clinical and biochemical evidence of disease resolved spontaneously by 2 months.

Pricolo and co-workers (1990) reviewed outcomes in seven women in whom unilateral adrenalectomy was performed during pregnancy for an adenoma. Direct attempts to treat Cushing syndrome were reported in 16 cases summarized by Aron and associates (1990a). In six, unilateral adrenalectomy was done for an adenoma, in five bilateral resection was done for hyperplasia, four were treated with *metyrapone, aminoglutethimide,* or *cyproheptadine,* and one underwent pituitary irradiation. Amado and co-workers (1990) reported rapid control of adrenal hyperfunction in a women treated with oral *ketoconazole* given beginning at 32 weeks. The drug also blocks testicular steroidogenesis, and its use in a woman with a male fetus is worrisome.

Primary Aldosteronism

A few cases of primary aldosteronism associated with pregnancy have been reported. In view of the very high levels of aldosterone in normal pregnancies, it is not surprising that there may be amelioration of symptoms as well as of electrolyte abnormalities during pregnancy (Biglieri and Slaton, 1967). Lotgering and colleagues (1986) reported a woman who at midpregnancy presented with severe hypertension and hypokalemia. She was treated with aldosterone antagonists and antihypertensives, and at 36 weeks cesarean delivery resulted in a severely growth-retarded but otherwise normal female infant without clitoromegaly. An adrenal adenoma was resected 2 months later.

In many cases, hypertension responds to *spironolactone*, but labetalol or nifedipine also may be given. Neerhof and colleagues (1991) reported a woman with idiopathic hyperaldosteronism whose hypertension was refractory to several conventional agents. She developed a placental abruption at 26 weeks and her 720-g infant succumbed.

PITUITARY DISEASES

Prolactinomas

With the advent of serum prolactin assay in the 1970s, the relative common frequency of pituitary prolactinomas became appreciated. Almost simultaneously, the ergot derivative, *bromocriptine*—a dopamine-receptor stimulator—was developed as a powerful prolactin inhibitor. Amenorrhea, galactorrhea, and hyperprolactinemia caused by pituitary microadenomas were found to be amenable to therapy with bromocriptine. Subsequently, many pregnancies were observed in women treated with bromocriptine. Fortunately, it does not appear to affect the fetus adversely (Nader, 1990; Turkalj and associates, 1982).

Prolactinomas and Pregnancy. Pituitary prolactinomas are classified arbitrarily by their size, as determined by computed tomography or magnetic resonance imaging. By convention, a microadenoma is 10 mm or less and a macroadenoma is greater than 10 mm. Because symptoms induced by pregnancy-induced pituitary enlargement are much more frequent with macroadenomas, most authorities recommend definitive therapy with surgery or irradiation before pregnancy is attempted (Nader, 1990).

The experiences of pregnancy with prolactin-secreting pituitary adenomas has been reviewed. Moltich (1985) described outcomes in almost 250 women with previously untreated **microadenomas** who became pregnant. Only four of these women developed enlargement during pregnancy, and another 11, who were asymptomatic, had radiographic evidence for enlargement. In a review of 352 pregnancies, Albrecht and Betz (1986) reported 2.3 percent with visual disturbances, 4.8 percent with headaches, and 0.6 percent with diabetes insipidus.

Symptomatic tumor enlargement is more common with **macroadenomas.** According to Moltich (1985), 15 percent of 45 such women developed headaches or visual field defects during pregnancy. Albrecht and Betz (1986) reported that of 144 patients, 15 percent had visual disturbances, 15 percent headaches, and 1.4 percent developed diabetes insipidus.

Serial serum prolactin concentrations and visual field testing have not been found to be effective, and Moltich (1992) recommends computed tomography during pregnancy only if symptoms develop. Symptomatic tumor enlargement during pregnancy is treated immediately with bromocriptine. Surgery is undertaken for women with no response to this drug. According to Nader (1990), as of 1987 more than 2500 pregnant women have taken bromocriptine at some time during pregnancy and there have been no adverse effects. Briggs and colleagues (1990) reached similar conclusions after their review of more than 1500 pregnancies.

Acromegaly

Acromegaly is caused by excessive growth hormone, usually from an acidophilic or chromophobic pituitary adenoma. Diagnosis is confirmed by the failure of a glucose-tolerance test to suppress growth hormone. Pregnancy is rare in acromegalic women. Development of acromegaly in a pregnant woman and in turn her fetus-infant has been described by Fisch and associates (1974). The mother was treated with x-rays to the pituitary fossa during the third trimester. The newborn infant presented a constellation of skeletal anomalies. In two women previously treated by transsphenoidal adenomectomy, Beckers and colleagues (1990) demonstrated that persistently elevated growth hormone was not suppressed during pregnancy. Yap and co-workers (1990) described a woman with an acidophilic tumor who was diagnosed with acromegaly at midpregnancy. Bromocriptine corrected visual-field defects and suppressed prolactin but not growth hormone levels.

Diabetes Insipidus

Diabetes insipidus is a rare complication of pregnancy. Only a few cases have been cared for in the last 35 years at Parkland Hospital, during which time there were nearly 250,000 deliveries. This incidence is remarkably close to that cited by Hime and Richardson (1978). As long as the woman takes vasopressin appropriately for replacement therapy, there should be no serious pregnancy complications. The specific agent of choice is the synthetic analogue of vasopressin, 1-deamino-8-D-arginine vasopressin (DDAVP). Most women with diabetes insipidus require increased doses during pregnancy, likely because of an increased metabolic clearance rate stimulated by placental vasopressinase (Dürr, 1987). Because of this same mechanism, subclinical diabetes insipidus may become symptomatic during pregnancy (Barron and co-workers, 1984). Krege and associates (1989) reviewed 17 such cases. Iwasaki and colleagues (1991) showed that pregnancy unmasked subclinical forms of both nephrogenic as well as central diabetes insipidus. Raziel and colleagues (1991) described two cases of transient diabetes insipidus that developed postpartum.

In a few instances of diabetes insipidus, there appeared to have been an impairment of labor, possibly caused by diminished or absent endogenous oxytocin (Hime and Richardson, 1978). Sende and associates (1975) were unable to detect oxytocin by radioimmunoassay in plasma of a pregnant woman with diabetes insipidus before labor, but during labor and puerperium there was a surge of oxytocin. A woman described by Chau and associates (1969) lactated normally, with measured milk ejection pressures comparable to those of normal lactating women.

In our experiences, transient diabetes insipidus more likely is encountered with **acute fatty liver of pregnancy** (see Chap. 51, p. 1156). This association was described by Cammu and colleagues (1987) as being nephrogenic; however, the syndrome may be due to altered vasopressinase clearance rate by the diseased liver. If this is indeed the case, diabetes insipidus should respond to desmopressin, which is more resistant to inactivation than naturally occurring vasopressin. Harper and associates (1987) described similar findings in a 38-week pregnant woman with biopsy-proven viral hepatitis.

Diabetes insipidus with or without anterior pituitary deficiency characteristic of **Sheehan syndrome** has been described following massive obstetrical hemorrhage and prolonged shock (Dürr, 1987).

References

Albert E, Dalaker K, Jorde R, Berge LN: Addison's disease and pregnancy. Acta Obstet Gynecol Scand 68:185, 1989

Albrecht BH, Betz G: Prolactin-secreting pituitary tumors and pregnancy. In Olefshy JM, Robinson RJ (eds): Contemporary Issues in Endocrinology and Metabolism: Prolactinomas, Vol 2. New York, Churchill Livingston, 1986, p 195

Ales KL, Santini DL: Should all pregnant women be screened for gestational glucose intolerance? Lancet 1:1188, 1989

Amado JA, Pesquera C, Gonzalez EM, Otero M, Freijanes J, Alvarez A: Successful treatment with ketoconazole of Cushing's syndrome in pregnancy. Postgrad Med J 66:221, 1990

American College of Obstetricians and Gynecologists: Management of diabetes mellitus in pregnancy. Technical bulletin no. 92, May 1986

Amino N, Mori H, Iwatani Y, Tanizawa O, Kawashima M, Tsuge I, Ibaragi K, Kumahara Y, Miyai K: High prevalence of transient post-partum thyrotoxicosis and hypothyroidism. N Engl J Med 306:849, 1982a

Amino N, Tanizawa O, Mori H, Iwatani Y, Yamada T, Kurachi K, Kumahara Y, Miyai K: Aggravation of thyrotoxicosis in early pregnancy and after delivery in Graves' disease. J Clin Endocrinol Metab 55:108, 1982b

Amir SM, Osathanondh R, Berkowitz RS, Goldstein DP: Human chorionic gonadotropin and thyroid function in patients with hydatidiform mole. Am J Obstet Gynecol 150:723, 1984

Angel JL, O'Brien WF, Knuppel RA, Morales WJ, Sims CJ: Carbohydrate intolerance in patients receiving oral tocolytics. Am J Obstet Gynecol 159:762, 1988

Aron DC, Schnall AM, Sheeler LR: Cushing's syndrome and pregnancy. Am J Obstet Gynecol 162:244, 1990a

Aron DC, Schnall AM, Sheeler LR: Spontaneous resolution of Cushing's syndrome after pregnancy. Am J Obstet Gynecol 162:472, 1990b

Barron WM, Cohen LH, Ulland LA, Lassiter WE, Fulghum EM, Emmanouel D, Robertson G, Lindheimer MD: Transient vasopressin-resistant diabetes insipidus of pregnancy. N Engl J Med 310:442, 1984

Becerra JE, Khoury MJ, Cordero JF, Erickson JD: Diabetes mellitus during pregnancy and the risks for specific birth defects: A population-based case-control study. Pediatrics 85:1, 1990

Beckers A, Stevenaert A, Foidart J-M, Hennen G, Frankenne F: Placental and pituitary growth hormone secretion during pregnancy in acromegalic women. J Clin Endocrinol Metab 71:725, 1990

Becks GP, Burrows GN: Thyroid disease and pregnancy. Med Clin North Am 75:121, 1991

Biglieri EG, Slaton PE Jr: Pregnancy and primary aldosteronism. J Clin Endocrinol Metab 27:1628, 1967

Bochner CJ, Medearis AL, Williams J III, Castro L, Hobel CJ, Wade ME: Early third-trimester ultrasound screening in gestational diabetes to determine the risk of macrosomia and labor dystocia at term. Am J Obstet Gynecol 157:703, 1987

Bourgeois FJ, Duffer J: Outpatient obstetric management of women with type I diabetes. Am J Obstet Gynecol 163:1065, 1990

Brander A, Kivisaari L: Ultrasonography of the thyroid during pregnancy. J Clin Ultrasound 17:403, 1989

Brans YW, Huff RW, Shannon DL, Hunter MA: Maternal diabetes and neonatal macrosomia. Pediatrics 70:576, 1982

Bravo FI, Gifford RW Jr: Pheochromocytoma: Diagnosis, localization and management. N Engl J Med 311:1298, 1984

Briggs GG, Freeman RK, Yaffee SJ: Drugs in Pregnancy and Lactation, 3rd ed. Baltimore, Williams & Wilkins, 1990

Brown ZA, Mills JL, Metzger BE, Knopp RH, Simpson JL, Jovanovic-Peterson L, Scheer K, Van Allen MI, Aarons JH, Reed GF, National Institute of Child Health and Human Development Diabetes in Early Pregnancy Study: Early sonographic evaluation for fetal growth delay and congenital malformations in pregnancies complicated by insulin-requiring diabetes. Diabetes Care 15:613, 1992

Buchanan TA, Metzger BE, Freinkel N: Accelerated starvation in late pregnancy: A comparison between obese women with and without gestational diabetes mellitus. Am J Obstet Gynecol 162:1015, 1990

Buescher MA, McClamrock HD, Adashi EY: Cushing syndrome in pregnancy. Obstet Gynecol 79:130, 1992

Burgess GE: Alpha blockade and surgical intervention of pheochromocytoma in pregnancy. Obstet Gynecol 53:266, 1979

Burrow GN, Klatskin EH, Genel M: Intellectual development in children whose mothers received propylthiouracil during pregnancy. Yale J Biol Med 51:151, 1978

Cammu H, Velkeniers B, Charels K, Vincken W, Amy JJ: Idiopathic acute fatty liver of pregnancy associated with transient diabetes insipidus. Br J Obstet Gynaecol 94:173, 1987

Caplan RH, Beguin EA: Hypercalcemia in a calcitriol-treated hypoparathyroid woman during lactation. Obstet Gynecol 76:485, 1990

Chau SS, Fitzpatrick RJ, Jamieson B: Diabetes insipidus and parturition. Br J Obstet Gynaecol 76:444, 1969

Cheek DB (ed): Human Growth. Philadelphia, Lea & Febiger, 1968

Combs CA, Easterling TR, Schmucker BC, Benedetti TJ: Hemodynamic observations during paroxysmal hypertension in a pregnancy with pheochromocytoma. Obstet Gynecol 74:439, 1989

Combs CA, Kitzmiller JL: Diabetic nephropathy and pregnancy. Clin Obstet Gynecol 34:505, 1991

Cousins L: Pregnancy complications among diabetic women: Review 1965–1985. Obstet Gynecol Surv 42:140, 1987

Coustan DR, Berkowitz RL, Hobbins JC: Tight metabolic control of overt diabetes in pregnancy. Am J Med 68:845, 1980

Coustan DR, Imarah J: Prophylactic insulin treatment of gestational diabetes reduces the incidence of macrosomia, operative delivery, and birth trauma. Am J Obstet Gynecol 150:836, 1984

Coustan DR, Nelson C, Carpenter MW, Carr SR, Rotondo L, Widness JA: Maternal age and screening for gestational diabetes: A population-based study. Obstet Gynecol 73:557, 1989

Cuckle H, Wald N, Stone R, Densem J, Haddow J, Knight G: Maternal serum thyroid antibodies in early pregnancy and fetal Down's syndrome. Prenat Diagn 8:439, 1988

Daly PA, Landsberg L: Pheochromocytoma: Diagnosis and management. Bailliére's Clin Endocrinol Metab 6:143, 1992

Davidson KM, Richards DS, Schatz DA, Fisher DA: Successful in utero treatment of fetal goiter and hypothyroidism. N Engl J Med 324:543, 1991

Davis LE, Leveno KL, Cunningham FG: Hypothyroidism complicating pregnancy. Obstet Gynecol 72:108, 1988

Davis LE, Lucas MJ, Hankins GDV, Roark ML, Cunningham FG: Thyrotoxicosis complicating pregnancy. Am J Obstet Gynecol 160:63, 1989

Diamond MP, Salyer SL, Vaughn WK, Cotton R, Boehm FH: Reassessment of White's classification and Pedersen's prognostically bad signs of diabetic pregnancies in insulin-dependent diabetic pregnancies. Am J Obstet Gynecol 156:599, 1987

Dürr JA: Diabetes insipidus in pregnancy. Am J Kidney Dis 9:276, 1987

Easterling TR, Schmucker BC, Carlson KL, Millard SP, Benedetti TJ: Maternal hemodynamics in pregnancies complicated by hyperthyroidism. Obstet Gynecol 78:348, 1991

Elman KD, Welch RA, Frank RN, Gyoert GL, Sokol RJ: Diabetic retinopathy in pregnancy: A review. Obstet Gynecol 75:119, 1990

Fisch RO, Prem KA, Feinberg SB, Gehrz RC: Acromegaly in a gravida and her infant. Obstet Gynecol 43:861, 1974

Fisher DA, Foley BL: Early treatment of congenital hypothyroidism. Pediatrics 83:785, 1989

Foster DW: Diabetes mellitus. In Wilson JD, Braunwald E, Isselbacher KJ, Petersdorf RG, Martin JB, Fauci AS, Root RK (eds): Harrison's Principles of Internal Medicine, 12th ed. New York, McGraw-Hill, 1991, p 1739

Fung HY, Kologlu M, Collison K, John R, Richards CJ, Hall R, McGregor AM: Postpartum thyroid dysfunction in Mid Glamorgan. BMJ 296:241, 1988

Gabbe SG: A story of two miracles: The impact of the discovery of insulin on pregnancy in women with diabetes mellitus. Obstet Gynecol 79:295, 1992

Gabbe SG: Management of diabetes mellitus in pregnancy. Am J Obstet Gynecol 153:824, 1985

Gabbe SG, Mestman JH, Freeman RK, Goebelsmann UT, Lowensohn RI, Nochimson D, Cetrulo C, Quilligan EJ: Management and outcome of diabetes mellitus, classes B–R. Am J Obstet Gynecol 129:723, 1977

Garlick RL, Mazer JS, Higgins PJ, Bunn HF: Characterization of glycosylated hemoglobins. J Clin Invest 71:1062, 1983

Garner PR, D'Alton ME, Dudley DK, Huard P, Hardie M: Preeclampsia in diabetic pregnancies. Am J Obstet Gynecol 163:505, 1990

Geelhoed GW: Surgery of the endocrine glands in pregnancy. Clin Obstet Gynecol 26:865, 1983

Glinoer D, Lemone M, Bourdoux P, DeNayer P, Delange F, Kinthaert J, Lejeune B: Partial reversibility during late postpartum of thyroid abnormalities associated with pregnancy. J Clin Endocrinol Metab 74:453, 1992

Grant DB, Smith I, Fuggle PW, Tokar S, Chapple J: Congenital hypothyroidism detected by neonatal screening: Relationship between biochemical severity and early clinical features. Arch Dis Child 67:87, 1992

Greene MF, Hare JW, Krache M, Phillippe M, Barss VA, Saltzman DH, Nadel A, Younger MD, Heffner L, Scherl JE: Prematurity among insulin-requiring diabetic gravid women. Am J Obstet Gynecol 161:106, 1989

Hankins GDV, Lowe TW, Cunningham FG: Dilated cardiomyopathy and thyrotoxicosis complicated by septic abortion. Am J Obstet Gynecol 149:85, 1984

Hardisty CA, Munro DS: Serum long acting thyroid stimulator protector in pregnancy complicated by Graves' disease. Br Med J 286:934, 1983

Harper M, Hatjis CG, Appel RG, Austin WE: Vasopressin-resistant diabetes insipidus, liver dysfunction, and hyperuricemia and decreased renal function. J Reprod Med 32:862, 1987

Harper MA, Murnaghan GA, Kennedy L, Hadden DR, Atkinson AB: Pheochromocytoma in pregnancy. Five cases and a review of the literature. Br J Obstet Gynaecol 96:594, 1989

Harris MI: Gestational diabetes may represent discovery of preexisting glucose intolerance. Diabetes Care 11:402, 1988

Hayslip CC, Fein HG, O'Donnell VM, Friedman DS, Klein TA, Smallridge RC: The value of serum antimicrosomal antibody testing in screening for symptomatic postpartum thyroid dysfunction. Am J Obstet Gynecol 159:203, 1988

Henriques CU, Damm P, Tabor A, Goldstein H, Mostsed-Pedersen L: Incidence of fetal chromosome abnormalities in insulin dependent diabetic women. Acta Obstet Gynecol Scand 70:295, 1991

Hershman JM: Editorial: Role of human chorionic gonadotropin as a thyroid stimulator. J Clin Endocrinol Metab 74:258, 1992

Higgins RV, Hisley JC: Primary hyperparathyroidism in pregnancy: A report of two cases. J Reprod Med 33:726, 1988

Hill DE: Effect of insulin on fetal growth. Semin Perinatol 2:319, 1978

Hime MC, Richardson JA: Diabetes insipidus and pregnancy: Case report, incidence, and review of literature. Obstet Gynecol Surv 3:375, 1978

Houck JA, Davis RE, Sharma HM: Thyroid-stimulating immunoglobulin as a cause of recurrent intrauterine fetal death. Obstet Gynecol 71:1018, 1988

Iwasaki Y, Oiso Y, Kondo K, Takagi S, Takatsuki K, Hasegawa H, Ishikawa K, Fujimura Y, Kazeto S, Tomita A: Aggravation of subclinical diabetes insipidus during pregnancy. N Engl J Med 324:522, 1991

Jacobson JD, Cousins L: A population-based study of maternal and perinatal outcome in patients with gestational diabetes. Am J Obstet Gynecol 161:981, 1989

Jansson R, Dahlberg PA, Karlsson FA: Postpartum thyroiditis. Bailliéres Clin Endocrinol Metab 2:619, 1988

Jansson R, Dahlberg PA, Winsa B, Meirik O, Säfwenberg J, Karlsson A: The postpartum period constitutes an important risk for the development of clinical Graves' disease in young women. Acta Endocrinol Suppl (Copenh) 116:321, 1987

Johnson SR, Kolberg BH, Vance MW, Railsback LD: Maternal obesity and pregnancy. Surg Gynecol Obstet 164:431, 1987

Johnstone FD, Nasrat AA, Prescott RJ: The effect of established and gestational diabetes on pregnancy outcome. Br J Obstet Gynaecol 97:1009, 1990

Jovanovic-Peterson L, Durak EP, Peters CM: Randomized trial of diet versus diet plus cardiovascular conditioning on glucose levels in gestational diabetes. Am J Obstet Gynecol 161:415, 1989

Jovanovic-Peterson L, Peterson CM: De novo clinical hypothyroidism in pregnancies complicated by type I diabetes, subclinical hypothyroidism, and proteinuria: A new syndrome. Am J Obstet Gynecol 159:442, 1988

Jovanovic-Peterson L, Peterson CM: Diabetic retinopathy. Clin Obstet Gynecol 34:516, 1991a

Jovanovic-Peterson L, Peterson CM: Sweet success, but an acid aftertaste? N Engl J Med 325:959, 1991b

Jovanovic-Peterson L, Peterson CM, Reed GF, Metzger BE, Mills JL, Knopp RH, Aarons JH, National Institute of Child Health and Human Development Diabetes in Early Pregnancy Study: Maternal postprandial glucose levels and infant birth weight. Am J Obstet Gynecol 164:103, 1991

Kelly TR: Primary hyperparathyroidism during pregnancy. Surgery 110:1028, 1991

Kennedy RL, Darne J: The role of hCG in regulation of the thyroid gland in normal and abnormal pregnancy. Obstet Gynecol 78:298, 1991

Kennedy RL, Darne J, Cohn M, Price A, Davies R, Blumsohn A, Griffiths H: Human chorionic gonadotropin may not be responsible for thyroid-stimulating activity in normal pregnancy serum. J Clin Endocrinol Metab 74:260, 1992

Kimura M, Amino N, Tamaki H, Mitsuda N, Miyai K, Tanizawa O: Physiologic thyroid activation in normal early pregnancy is induced by circulating hCG. Obstet Gynecol 75:775, 1990

Kitzmiller JL, Brown ER, Phillippe M, Stark AR, Acker D, Kaldany A, Singh S, Hare JW: Diabetic nephropathy and perinatal outcome. Am J Obstet Gynecol 141:741, 1981

Kitzmiller JL, Cloherty JP, Younger MD, Tabatabaii A, Rothchild SB, Sosenkol I, Epstein MF, Singh S, Neff RK: Diabetic pregnancy and perinatal outcome. Am J Obstet Gynecol 131:560, 1978

Kitzmiller JL, Gavin LA, Gin GD, Jovanovic-Peterson L, Main EK, Zigrang WD: Preconception care of diabetes: Glycemic control prevents congenital anomalies. JAMA 265:731, 1991

Kitzmiller JL, Younger MD, Hare JW, Phillippe M, Vignati L, Fargnoli B, Grause A: Continuous subcutaneous insulin therapy during early pregnancy. Obstet Gynecol 65:606, 1985

Kjaer K, Hagen C, Sando SH, Eshoj O: Infertility and pregnancy outcome in an unselected group of women with insulin-dependent diabetes mellitus. Am J Obstet Gynecol 166:1412, 1992

Kjos SL, Buchanan TA, Greenspoon JS, Montoro M, Bernstein GS, Mestman JH: Gestational diabetes mellitus: The prevalence of glucose intolerance and diabetes mellitus in the first two months post partum. Am J Obstet Gynecol 163:93, 1990a

Kjos SL, Shoupe D, Donyou S, Friedman RL, Bernstein GS, Mestman JH, Mishell DR Jr: Effect of low-dose oral contraceptives on carbohydrate and lipid metabolism in women with recent gestational diabetes: Results of a controlled, randomized, prospective study. Am J Obstet Gynecol 163:1822, 1990b

Koerten JM, Morales WJ, Washington SR III, Castaldo TW: Cushing's syndrome in pregnancy: A case report and literature review. Am J Obstet Gynecol 154:626, 1986

Krege J, Katz VL, Bowes WA Jr: Transient diabetes insipidus of pregnancy. Obstet Gynecol Surv 44:789, 1989

Landon MB, Gabbe SG: Fetal surveillance in the pregnancy complicated by diabetes mellitus. Clin Obstet Gynecol 34:535, 1991

Landon MB, Gabbe SG: Glucose monitoring and insulin administration in the pregnant diabetic patient. Clin Obstet Gynecol 3:496, 1985

Langer O, Levy J, Brustman L, Anyaegbunam A, Merkatz R, Divon M: Glycemic control in gestational diabetes mellitus—How tight is tight enough: Small for gestational age versus large for gestational age? Am J Obstet Gynecol 161:646, 1989

Larsen CE, Serdula MK, Sullivan KM: Macrosomia: Influence of maternal overweight among a low-income population. Am J Obstet Gynecol 162:490, 1990

Leveno KJ, Fortunato SJ, Raskin P, Williams ML, Whalley PJ: Continuous subcutaneous insulin infusion during pregnancy. Diabetes Res Clin Pract 4:257, 1988

Leveno KJ, Hauth JC, Gilstrap LC III, Whalley PJ: Appraisal of "rigid" blood glucose control during pregnancy in the overtly diabetic woman. Am J Obstet Gynecol 135:793, 1979

Leveno KJ, Whalley PJ: Dilemmas in the management of pregnancy complicated by diabetes. Med Clin North Am 66:1325, 1982

Lindenbaum C, Ludmir J, Teplick FB, Cohen AW, Samuels P: Maternal glucose intolerance and the subcutaneous terbutaline pump. Am J Obstet Gynecol 166:925, 1992

Lotgering FK, Derkx FMH, Wallenburg HCS: Primary hyperaldosteronism in pregnancy. Am J Obstet Gynecol 155:986, 1986

Lucas MJ, Leveno KJ, Williams ML, Raskin P, Whalley PJ: Early pregnancy glycosylated hemoglobin, severity of diabetes, and fetal malformations. Am J Obstet Gynecol 161:426, 1989

Lyons CW, Colmorgen GHC: Medical management of pheochromocytoma in pregnancy. Obstet Gynecol 72:450, 1988

Mandel SJ, Larsen PR, Seely EW, Brent GA: Increased need for thyroxine during pregnancy in women with primary hypothyroidism. N Engl J Med 323:91, 1990

Maresh M, Beard RW, Bray CS, Elkeles RS, Wadsworth J: Factors predisposing to and outcome of gestational diabetes. Obstet Gynecol 74:342, 1989

Martin FR, Health P, Mountain KR: Pregnancy in women with diabetes. Fifteen year's experience: 1973–1985. Med J Aust 146:187, 1987

Martin RW, Lucas JA, Martin JN, Morrison JC, Cowan BD: Conservative management of Cushing's syndrome in pregnancy. A case report. J Reprod Med 34:493, 1989

Matsuura N, Fujieda K, Iida Y, Fujimoto S, Konishi J, Kasagi K, Hagisawa M, Fukushi M, Takasugi N: TSH-receptor antibodies in mothers with Graves' disease and outcome in their offspring. Lancet 1:14, 1988

Menon RK, Cohen RM, Sperling MA, Cutfield WS, Mimouni F, Khoury JC: Transplacental passage of insulin in pregnant women with insulin-dependent diabetes mellitus. N Engl J Med 323:309, 1990

Merimee TJ: Diabetic retinopathy: A synthesis of perspectives. N Engl J Med 322:978, 1990

Mestman JH: Outcome of diabetes screening in pregnancy and perinatal morbidity in infants of mothers with mild impairment in glucose tolerance. Diabetes Care 3:447, 1980

Metzger BE, Bybee DE, Freinkel N, Phelps RL, Radvany RM, Vaisrub N: Gestational diabetes mellitus: Correlations between the phenotypic and genotypic characteristics of the mother and abnormal glucose tolerance during the first year postpartum. Diabetes 34:111, 1985

Miller E, Hare JW, Cloherty JP, Dunn PJ, Gleason RE, Soeldner JS, Kitzmiller JL: Elevated maternal hemoglobin A_{1c} in early pregnancy and major congenital anomalies in infants of diabetic mothers. N Engl J Med 304:1331, 1981

Mills JL, Knopp RH, Simpson JL, Jovanovic-Peterson L, Metzger BE, Holmes LB, Aarons JH, Brown Z, Reed GF, Bieber FR, Van Allen M, Holzman I, Ober C, Peterson CM, Witham JM, Duckles A, Mueller-Heubach E, Polk BF, National Institute of Child Health and Human Development Diabetes in Early Pregnancy Study: Lack of relation of increased malformation rates in infants of diabetic mothers to glycemic control during organogenesis. N Engl J Med 318:671, 1988a

Mills JL, Simpson JL, Driscoll SG, Jovanovic-Peterson L, Van Allen M, Aarons JH, Metzger B, Bieber FR, Knopp RH, Holmes LB, Peterson CM, Witham-Wilson M, Brown Z, Ober C, Harley E, MacPherson TA, Duckles A, Mueller-Heubach E, National Institute of Child Health and Human Development Diabetes in Early Pregnancy Study: Incidence of spontaneous abortion among normal women and insulin-dependent diabetic women whose pregnancies were identified within 21 days of conception. N Engl J Med 319:1617, 1988b

Mintz DH, Chez RA, Hutchinson DL: Subhuman primate pregnancy complicated by streptozotocin-induced diabetes mellitus. J Clin Invest 51:837, 1972

Molitch ME: Endocrine emergencies in pregnancy. Bailliére's Clin Endocrinol Metab 6:167, 1992

Molitch ME: Pregnancy and the hyperprolactinemic woman. N Engl J Med 312:1364, 1985

Momotani N, Noh J, Oyanagi H, Ishikawa N, Ito K: Antithyroid drug therapy for Graves' disease during pregnancy: Optimal regimen for fetal thyroid status. N Engl J Med 315:24, 1986

Montoro M, Collea JV, Frasier SD, Mestman JH: Successful outcome of pregnancy in women with hypothyroidism. Ann Intern Med 94:31, 1981

Morris MA, Grandis AS, Litton J: The correlations of glycosylated serum protein and glycosylated hemoglobin concentrations with blood glucose in diabetic pregnancy. Am J Obstet Gynecol 153:257, 1985

Nader S: Pituitary disorders and pregnancy. Semin Perinatol 14:24, 1990

National Diabetes Data Group: Classification and diagnosis of diabetes mellitus and other categories of glucose intolerance. Diabetes 28:1039, 1979

Neerhof MG, Shlossman PA, Poll DS, Ludomirsky A, Weiner S: Idiopathic aldosteronism in pregnancy. Obstet Gynecol 78:489, 1991

Nordlander E, Hanson U, Persson B: Factors influencing neonatal morbidity in gestational diabetic pregnancy. Br J Obstet Gynaecol 96:671, 1989

Oats JN, Beischer NA: The persistence of abnormal glucose tolerance after delivery. Obstet Gynecol 75:397, 1990

O'Shaughnessy RW, Hackett KJ: Maternal Addison's disease and fetal growth retardation. J Reprod Med 29:752, 1984

O'Sullivan JB, Mahan CM: Criteria for the oral glucose tolerance test in pregnancy. Diabetes 13:278, 1964

Page DV, Brady K, Mitchell J, Pehrson J, Wade G: The pathology of intrauterine thyrotoxicosis: Two case reports. Obstet Gynecol 72:479, 1988

Parham GP, Orr JW Jr: Hyperparathyroidism secondary to parathyroid carcinoma in pregnancy. J Reprod Med 32:123, 1987

Peterson CM, Jovanovic-Peterson L, Mills JL, Conley MR, Knopp RH, Reed GF, Aarons JH, Holmes LB, Brown Z, Van Allen M, Schmeltz R, Metzger BE, National Institute of Child Health and Human Development Diabetes in Early Pregnancy Study: Changes in cholesterol, triglycerides, body weight, and blood pressure. Am J Obstet Gynecol 166:513, 1992

Patterson R: Hyperparathyroidism in pregnancy. Obstet Gynecol 70:457, 1987

Philipson EH, Super DM: Gestational diabetes mellitus: Does it recur in subsequent pregnancy? Am J Obstet Gynecol 160:1324, 1989

Piacquadio K, Hollingsworth DR, Murphy H: Effects of in-utero exposure to oral hypoglycemic drugs. Lancet 338:866, 1991

Pitkin RM: Calcium metabolism in pregnancy and the perinatal period: A review. Am J Obstet Gynecol 151:99, 1985

Porreco RP, Bloch CA: Fetal blood sampling in the management of intrauterine thyrotoxicosis. Obstet Gynecol 76:509, 1990

Pricolo VE, Monchik JM, Prinz RA, DeJong S, Chadwick DA, Lamberton RP: Management of Cushing's syndrome secondary to adrenal adenoma during pregnancy. Surgery 108:1072, 1990

Ramsay I: Postpartum thyroiditis—An underdiagnosed disease. Br J Obstet Gynaecol 93:1121, 1986

Rasmussen NG, Hornnes PJ, Hegedüs L: Ultrasonographically determined thyroid size in pregnancy and postpartum: The goitrogenic effect of pregnancy. Am J Obstet Gynecol 160:1216, 1989

Raziel A, Rosenberg T, Schreyer P, Caspi E, Gilboa Y: Transient postpartum diabetes insipidus. Am J Obstet Gynecol 164:616, 1991

Reece EA, Coustan DR, Hayslett JP, Holford T, Coulehan J, O'Connor TZ, Hobbins JC: Diabetic nephropathy: Pregnancy performance and fetomaternal outcome. Am J Obstet Gynecol 159:56, 1988

Reece EA, Hobbins JC: Diabetic embryopathy: Pathogenesis, prenatal diagnosis, and prevention. Obstet Gynecol Surv 41:325, 1986

Rizzo T, Metzger BE, Burns WJ, Burns K: Correlations between antepartum maternal metabolism and intelligence of offspring. N Engl J Med 325:911, 1991

Rosenn B, Miodovnik M, Combs CA, Khoury J, Siddiqi TA: Pre-conception management of insulin-dependent diabetes: Improvement of pregnancy outcome. Obstet Gynecol 77:846, 1991

Rosenn B, Miodovnik M, Dignan SJP, Siddiqi TA, Khoury J, Mimouni F: Minor congenital malformations in infants of insulin-dependent diabetic women: Association with poor glycemic control. Obstet Gynecol 76:745, 1990

Rosen IB, Walfish PG: Pregnancy as a predisposing factor in thyroid neoplasia. Arch Surg 121:1287, 1986

Roti E, Emerson CH: Clinical Review 29: Postpartum thyroiditis. J Clin Endocrinol Metab 74:3, 1992

Salvesen DR, Brudenell MJ, Nicolaides KH: Fetal polycythemia and thrombocytopenia in pregnancies complicated by maternal diabetes mellitus. Am J Obstet Gynecol 166:1287, 1992

St. John Sutton MG, Sheps SG, Lie JT: Prevalence of clinically unsuspected pheochromocytoma. Review of a 50-year autopsy series. Mayo Clin Proc 56:354, 1981

Schenker JG, Granat M: Pheochromocytoma and pregnancy—An updated appraisal. Aust NZ J Obstet Gynaecol 22:1, 1982

Schneider JM, Curet LB, Olson RW, Shay G: Ambulatory care of the pregnant diabetic. Obstet Gynecol 56:144, 1980

Seaward PGR, Guidozzi F, Sonnendecker EWW: Addisonian crisis in pregnancy. Case report. Br J Obstet Gynaecol 96:1348, 1989

Selby JV, Fitzsimmons SC, Newman JM, Katz PP, Sepe S, Showstack J: The natural history and epidemiology of diabetic nephropathy: Implications for prevention and control. JAMA 263:1954, 1990

Sende P, Pantelakis N, Suzuki K, Bashore R: Plasma oxytocin level in pregnancy with diabetes insipidus. Clin Res 23:242A, 1975

Shangold MM, Dor N, Welt SI, Fleischman AR, Crenshaw MC Jr: Hyperparathyroidism and pregnancy: A review. Obstet Gynecol Surv 37:217, 1982

Sherif IH, Oyan WT, Bosairi S, Carrascal SM: Treatment of hyperthyroidism in pregnancy. Acta Obstet Gynecol Scand 70:461, 1991

Siddiqi T, Rosenn B, Mimouni F, Khoury J, Miodovnik M: Hypertension during pregnancy in insulin-dependent diabetic women. Obstet Gynecol 77:514, 1991

Stagnaro-Green A, Roman SH, Cobin RH, El-Harazy E, Alvarez-Marfany M, Davies TF: Detection of at-risk pregnancy by means of highly sensitive assays for thyroid autoantibodies. JAMA 264:1422, 1990

Stagnaro-Green A, Roman SH, Cobin RH, El-Harazy E, Wallenstein S, Davies TF: A prospective study of lymphocyte-initiated immunosuppression in normal pregnancy: Evidence of a T-cell etiology for postpartum thyroid dysfunction. J Clin Endocrinol Metab 74:645, 1992

Tachi J, Amino N, Tamaki H, Aozasa M, Iwatani Y, Miyai K: Long term follow-up and HLA association in patients with postpartum hypothyroidism. J Clin Endocrinol Metab 66:480, 1988

Tamaki H, Amino N, Takeoka K, Mitsuda N, Miyai K, Tanizawa O: Thyroxine requirement during pregnancy for replacement therapy of hypothyroidism. Obstet Gynecol 76:230, 1990

Thilly CH, Delange F, Lagasse R, Bourdoux P, Ramioul L, Berquist H, Ermans AM: Fetal hypothyroidism and maternal thyroid status in severe endemic goiter. J Clin Endocrinol Metab 47:354, 1978

Third International Workshop—Conference on Gestational Diabetes: November 8–10, 1990, Chicago, IL. Diabetes 40S2:1, 1991

Thompson DJ, Porter KB, Gunnells DJ, Wagner PC, Spinnato JA: Prophylactic insulin in the management of gestational diabetes. Obstet Gynecol 75:960, 1990

Turkalj I, Braun P, Krupp P: Surveillance of bromocriptine in pregnancy. JAMA 247:1589, 1982

Vanderpas JB, Rivera-Vanderpas MT, Bourdoux P, Luvivila K, Lagasse R, Perlmutter-Cremer N, Delange F, Lanoie L, Ermans AM, Thilly CH: Reversibility of severe hypothyroidism with supplementary iodine in patients with endemic cretinism. N Engl J Med 315:791, 1986

Vargas MT, Briones-Urbina R, Gladman D, Papsin FR, Walfish PG: Antithyroid microsomal autoantibodies and HLA-DR5 are associated with postpartum thyroid dysfunction: Evidence supporting an autoimmune pathogenesis. J Clin Endocrinol Metab 67:327, 1988

Veille J-C, Sivakoff M, Hanson R, Fanaroff AA: Interventricular septal thickness in fetuses of diabetic mothers. Obstet Gynecol 79:51, 1992

Walfish PG, Chan JYC: Postpartum hyperthyroidism. J Clin Endocrinol Metab 14:417, 1985

Watson WJ: Serial changes in the 50-g oral glucose test in pregnancy: Implications for screening. Obstet Gynecol 74:40, 1989

Wenstrom KD, Weiner CP, Williamson RA, Grant SS: Prenatal diagnosis of fetal hyperthyroidism using funipuncture. Obstet Gynecol 76:513, 1990

Whalley PJ: Hyperparathyroidism and pregnancy. Am J Obstet Gynecol 86:517, 1963

White P: Classification of obstetric diabetes. Am J Obstet Gynecol 130:228, 1978

Williams JW: The limitations and possibilities of prenatal care. JAMA 64:95, 1915

Yap AS, Clouston WM, Mortimer RH, Drake RF: Acromegaly first diagnosed in pregnancy: The role of bromocriptine therapy. Am J Obstet Gynecol 163:477, 1990

Zakarija M, McKenzie JM: Pregnancy-associated changes in the thyroid-stimulating antibody of Graves' disease and the relationship to neonatal hyperthyroidism. J Clin Endocrinol Metab 57:1036, 1983

CHAPTER 54
Connective-Tissue Disorders

Connective-tissue disorders, also referred to as collagen–vascular disorders, are a group of diseases principally characterized by connective-tissue abnormalities that are immunopathologically mediated as the consequence of a variety of autoantibodies. Another common name for this group of disorders is *immune-complex disease*, because many of these syndromes are thought to be mediated by deposition of immune complexes in specific organ or tissue sites, including the glomerulus and blood vessel walls. Some of these disorders—characterized by sterile inflammation, especially of the skin, joints, blood vessels, and kidney—are referred to as *rheumatic diseases*. In some cases, inherited noninflammatory disorders of collagen metabolism constitute the underlying pathogenic mechanisms, for example, Marfan and Ehlers–Danlos syndromes.

Although the pathogenesis for all of these disorders has not been elucidated, immunologically mediated tissue destruction of various organ systems is frequently the common denominator. Diseases in this category include systemic lupus erythematosus, rheumatoid arthritis, progressive systemic sclerosis (scleroderma), mixed connective-tissue disease, dermatomyositis, Sjögren syndrome, ankylosing spondylitis, Reiter and Behcet syndromes, and a multitude of vasculitis syndromes.

Because renal involvement is common with many of these syndromes, and because pregnancy is affected by glomerulopathic syndromes, a search for co-existing renal involvement is paramount to evaluation. Hypertension likewise is common, and exacerbation during pregnancy frequently forces early delivery. In some of these immune-mediated diseases, *antiphospholipid antibodies* are formed that can cause injury to the placenta or to the fetus. Conversely, they can arise de novo and do similar damage.

Immunological Aspects. The immune system basically protects cells, tissues, and organs perceived as *self* and attacks and destroys foreign or *non-self* antigenic material. The **major histocompatibility complex (MHC)** is a series of 40 to 50 genes located on the short arm of chromosome 6, and it is known as the **human leukocyte associated (HLA) complex.** These genetic loci code for distinct cell-surface glycoproteins, including transplantation antigens, and they are involved in self and non-self recognition. There are two classes: class I antigens include HLA-A, -B, and -C; class II antigens include HLA-DR, -DQ, and -DP. Through a variety of complex interactions, including T and B cell stimu-

lation and interaction with immunoglobulins and the complement system, non-self antigens (for example, bacterial toxins) are destroyed. The specific antibody produced is bound to the antigen, forming an *immune complex.* These complexes usually undergo phagocytosis, but may be deposited in tissues to cause inflammation and tissue damage. Immune complexes are thought to play a critical role in the pathophysiology of lupus erythematosus and many of the vasculitis syndromes.

Immune-mediated Disease and Pregnancy. Very few immune disorders are definitely proved to arise only during pregnancy. Maternal isoimmunization from fetal red cell or platelet antigens is the most common (see Chap. 44, p. 1004). Some theories of the cause of preeclampsia–eclampsia implicate an immunological basis (see Chap. 36, p. 767). Some causes of recurrent abortion also are attributed to immunological causes (see Chap. 31, p. 670).

There are some pregnancy-induced immunological alterations that potentially interface with connective-tissue disorders. Many of these are discussed in Chapter 8 (p. 224); they include: depression of cell-mediated immunity and some antibody responses, increased immunoglobulin-secreting cells, decreased inflammatory response, and increased levels of circulating immune complexes. Complement levels during pregnancy normally may be elevated, and there may be low-grade activation of the classical pathway. Serum levels of autoantibodies are not increased appreciably during pregnancy (El-Roeiy and associates, 1990). In general, it is thought that these changes have negligible effects on immune-mediated collagen–vascular disorders; however, it is an area of ongoing investigation.

Systemic Lupus Erythematosus

Lupus is a disease of unknown etiology in which tissues and cells are damaged by deposition of autoantibodies and immune complexes. Almost 90 percent of cases are in women, and its prevalence in women aged 15 to 65 is about 1 in 700 (Varner, 1991). Some autoantibodies produced in patients with lupus are shown in Table 54–1. A number of genetic, environmental, and sex hormonal factors result in abnormal hormonal and cellular immune responses and inadequate clearing of antibodies and immune complexes. Genetic influences are indicated by a higher concordance with monozygotic

TABLE 54–1. SOME AUTOANTIBODIES IN PATIENTS WITH SYSTEMIC LUPUS ERYTHEMATOSUS

Antibody	Incidence (%)	Clinical Associations
Antinuclear	95	Multiple antibodies; repeated negative test makes lupus unlikely
Anti-DNA	70	Associated with nephritis and clinical activity
Anti-Sm	30	Specific for lupus
Anti-RNP	40	Polymyositis, scleroderma, lupus, mixed connective-tissue disease
Anti-Ro (SSA)	30	Sjögren syndrome, cutaneous lupus, neonatal lupus, congenital heart block
Anti-La (SSB)	10	Always with anti-Ro; Sjögren syndrome
Anticardiolipin	50	Antiphospholipid antibody; increased thrombosis; spontaneous abortion; early preeclampsia; placental infarction, fetal death; prolonged partial thromboplastin time; false-positive syphilis serological tests
Antierythrocytic	60	Overt hemolysis uncommon
Antiplatelet	—	Thombocytopenia

Modified from Hahn (1991) with permission.

compared with dizygotic twins and a 10 percent frequency in patients with one affected family member. The relative risk of disease is increased threefold if HLA-DR2 or -DR3 genes are found. In general, estrogens enhance disease and testosterone reduces antibody response.

Clinical Findings. Lupus is notoriously variable in its presentation, course, and outcome. The revised criteria of the American Rheumatism Association for diagnosis of systemic lupus are shown in Table 54–2. If any 4 or more of these 11 criteria are present, serially or simultaneously, the diagnosis of lupus is made. Clinical manifestations may be confined initially to one organ system, with other systems becoming involved as the disease progresses, or it may be manifested initially by multisystem involvement (Table 54–3). The most common findings are arthritis, rash, pleuropericarditis, fever, photosensitivity, lymphadenopathy, and alopecia. Renal involvement is demonstrated in half of patients. In addition, Galve and colleagues (1988) demonstrated clinically important cardiac valvar lesions in 18 percent of 74 patients with lupus.

The overall 10-year survival for patients with lupus is about 70 percent (Hahn, 1991). Involvement of the brain, lungs, kidney, or heart worsen the prognosis. Leading causes of death are infections and renal failure.

Laboratory Findings. Identification of characteristic antibodies shown in Table 54–1 confirms the diagnosis of lupus. Determination of antinuclear antibodies (ANA) is the best screening test; however, a positive test is not specific for lupus. For example, low titers are found in some normal individuals, and other autoimmune diseases, acute viral infections, chronic inflammatory processes, and several drugs can cause a positive reaction. Almost all patients with lupus have a positive test. Thus, a positive ANA test supports the diagnosis of lupus but is not specific; whereas a negative ANA test makes the diagnosis unlikely but not impossible. Antibodies to double-stranded DNA (dsDNA) and to Sm (Smith) are relatively specific for lupus, whereas other antibodies shown in Table 54–1 are not.

Other laboratory findings include false-positive syphilis serology, prolonged partial thromboplastin time, and rheumatoid factors. Anemia is common, and there may be a positive direct Coombs test with hemolysis, leukopenia, and thrombocytopenia. Proteinuria and casts are found in the half of patients with glomerular lesions, and there may be renal insufficiency.

TABLE 54–2. CRITERIA OF AMERICAN RHEUMATISM ASSOCIATION FOR SYSTEMIC LUPUS ERYTHEMATOSUS[a]

Malar (butterfly) rash
Discoid rash
Photosensitivity
Oral ulcers (painless)
Arthritis (two or more joints)
Serositis (pleurisy, pericarditis)
Renal disorder (proteinuria, casts)
Neurological disorder (seizures, psychosis)
Hematological disorders (hemolysis, leukopenia, or thrombocytopenia)
Immunological disorder (positive LE preparation, anti-DNA or anti-Sm antibodies, false-positive syphilis serology)
Antinuclear antibody

[a] Diagnosis made if any four or more of these 11 criteria present, serially or simultaneously.
From Tan and associates (1982) with permission.

TABLE 54–3. CLINICAL MANIFESTATIONS OF SYSTEMIC LUPUS ERYTHEMATOSUS

Organ System	Clinical Manifestations	%
Systemic	Fatigue, malaise, fever, weight loss	95
Musculoskeletal	Arthralgias, myalgias, myopathy	95
Hematological	Anemia, hemolysis, leukopenia, thrombocytopenia, lupus anticoagulant	85
Cutaneous	Malar (butterfly) rash, discoid rash, photosensitivity, oral ulcers, alopecia, skin rashes	80
Neurological	Organic brain syndromes, psychosis, seizures	60
Cardiopulmonary	Pleuritis, pericarditis	60
Renal	Proteinuria, casts	50
Gastrointestinal	Anorexia, nausea, ascites, vasculitis	45
Thrombosis	Arterial and venous	15
Ocular	Conjunctivitis	15

Modified from Hahn (1991) with permission.

Treatment. Approximately 20 to 30 percent of patients have mild disease, which is not life-threatening but is disabling because of pain and fatigue. Their arthralgia and serositis are managed by nonsteroidal anti-inflammatory drugs, including aspirin. Life-threatening and severely disabling manifestations are managed with prednisone, 1 to 2 mg/kg per day. After the disease is controlled, glucocorticoid therapy is tapered to a daily dose of 10 to 15 mg given each morning.

The use of immunosuppressive agents such as azathioprine and cyclophosphamide is controversial. They are usually reserved for lupus nephritis or disease that is steroid resistant. Intravenous pulse dose of cyclophosphamide, 10 to 15 mg/kg given once every 4 weeks, is the most effective, but also the most toxic.

Lupus and Pregnancy. Nearly a half million individuals in the United States have lupus, and the great majority are women. Even so, only recently have there been reports describing sufficient numbers of women with lupus complicating pregnancy. Fine and co-workers (1981) analyzed their experiences with one or more pregnancies in 39 women with systemic lupus erythematosus to provide answers to the following questions:

1. ***Does pregnancy alter the natural history of systemic lupus erythematosus?*** They concluded that pregnancy was not accompanied by an increased prevalence of major systemic nonrenal manifestations of lupus unless immunosuppressive therapy was stopped because of pregnancy.
2. ***Are the effects of lupus on renal function exaggerated by pregnancy?*** They observed that for those women with minimal prepregnancy renal impairment, renal function remained good in the great majority, deteriorated but recovered postpartum in about 10 percent, and in another 10 percent deteriorated and remained impaired. It was difficult to distinguish clinically between preeclampsia and lupus nephritis as the cause of renal impairment. Induced abortions were not

accompanied by any discernible deleterious effect on renal function.
3. ***Should pharmacological treatment of systemic lupus be altered during pregnancy?*** Their experiences led them to recommend the use of glucocorticoids and azathioprine antepartum in doses no different from those used when not pregnant. Moreover, they concluded that there probably is merit in increasing the dosage during labor and for up to 2 months thereafter to minimize the risk of exacerbation.
4. ***How does systemic lupus affect the fetus and neonate?*** Stillbirths were frequent (24 percent), as were preterm births (33 percent) and fetal growth retardation (33 percent). Persistent proteinuria or reduced creatinine clearance were associated with a high prevalence of stillbirths and low-birthweight infants. When both proteinuria and appreciably reduced glomerular filtration coexisted, fetal wastage was very high. Talipes equinovarus was the only anomaly detected. Congenital heart block was not described.

Since this report, verification of most of these observations has been made by several groups (Table 54–4). The number of exacerbations is highly variable between studies, but these are not defined rigidly, even for nonpregnant patients. Thus, although it was commonly thought that lupus is exacerbated by pregnancy, most studies, especially those with controls, indicate that this is not the case (Varner, 1991).

Lockshin (1989) prospectively evaluated 80 pregnant women and observed that only 13 percent had lupus-specific disease exacerbation. Importantly, exclusion of prednisone-treated patients did not alter the conclusion that there was no evidence of pregnancy-aggravated disease. Mor-Yosef and associates (1984) summarized their results with 159 pregnancies and concluded that lupus usually was not exacerbated. Nearly 80 percent of their patients had no appreciable clinical changes.

TABLE 54–4. MATERNAL AND FETAL OUTCOMES IN PREGNANCIES COMPLICATED BY SYSTEMIC LUPUS ERYTHEMATOSUS

	Pregnancies	Exacerbations During Pregnancy (%)	Abortions[a] (%)	Stillborn	Neonatal Death	Growth Retarded	Preterm	Term
Fine and co-workers (1981)	52	Not increased	27	24	NS[b]	33	33	43
Gimovsky and colleagues (1984)	77	30	45	17	10	50	33	50
Mor-Yosef and associates (1984)	159	20	25	8	NS	NS	8	60
Mintz and co-workers (1986)	102	48	16	18	4	23	49	34
Nossent and Swaak (1990)	39	74	10	5	NS	NS	19	67
Nicklin (1991)	42	9	31	5	NS	9	24	36

(Perinatal Outcome (%): Stillborn, Neonatal Death, Growth Retarded, Preterm, Term)

[a] Includes induced and spontaneous abortions.
[b] NS = not stated.

Experiences from the Hopkins Lupus Pregnancy Center (Petri and colleagues, 1991) indicate a significantly increased incidence of flares during 40 pregnancies in 37 women. Mintz and co-workers (1986) reported data from a prospective study of 102 pregnancies in 75 women cared for from 1974 to 1983. They reported that while exacerbations were common during pregnancy (60 percent), these were no more likely than in a group of nonpregnant control women taking progestational contraceptives.

Burkett (1985) reviewed outcomes in 156 women with 242 pregnancies complicated by systemic lupus erythematosus. Nicklin (1991) similarly reviewed outcomes in 517 pregnancies in 294 women. They compared the high incidence of perinatal mortality, fetal growth retardation, and preterm delivery. Importantly, it was concluded that optimal pregnancy outcome was achieved when clinical conditions included prepregnancy remission for at least 6 months, along with good renal function estimated by serum creatinine of 1.5 mg/dL or less, creatinine clearance of 60 mL per minute or more, or proteinuria of less than 3 g per day.

Lupus Nephropathy and Pregnancy. Hayslett and Lynn (1980) analyzed pregnancy outcomes for a group of women with lupus nephropathy and concluded that women whose disease stays in remission usually have a good outcome. Packham and associates (1992) described their experiences with 64 pregnancies in 41 women with biopsy-proven lupus nephritis. They found similar outcomes in pregnancies before and after nephritis was diagnosed. Importantly, hypertension developed during almost half of pregnancies, and it frequently was early and severe. Likewise, proteinuria worsened in half of these women during pregnancy.

While most authorities recommend continuation of immunosuppressive therapy in women with nephritis, it is not clear at this time whether there is any advantage from increasing immunosuppressive dosage at delivery and during the puerperium. It has often been stated that this is the time that activation or exacerbation are most likely to develop, but evidence to support this is not striking. In the prospective study by Lockshin (1989), there was no evidence for postpartum exacerbation.

Effects on Fetus and Infant. As summarized in Table 54–4, most investigators report substantively increased rates of fetal growth retardation, preterm delivery, and perinatal mortality. Mor-Yosef and colleagues (1984) presented results from 159 pregnancies and reported 10 percent stillbirths and 10 percent preterm births. Gimovsky and associates (1984) and Mintz and co-workers (1986) confirmed a high incidence of growth-retarded, preterm, and stillborn infants, especially in women with active disease. Hanly and collaborators (1988) observed that placental size was smaller in lupus patients, and that pathological changes included infarction, hematomas,

immunoglobulin and complement deposition, and thickening of trophoblast basement membrane. In all of these studies, adverse outcomes were more likely if there was renal involvement and hypertension.

Because of these adverse effects, the fetus should be observed closely for adverse effects imposed by a hostile intrauterine environment. These would warrant prompt delivery unless perhaps the fetus is very preterm, in which case close monitoring is necessary until delivery.

Neonatal Lupus. Neonatal lupus erythematosus is caused by transplacental passage of IgG anti-SSA (Ro), anti-SSB (La), and probably other antibodies (Buyon and Winchester, 1990; Vetter and Rashkind, 1983). The syndrome is relatively uncommon. Lockshin and colleagues (1988) prospectively followed 91 infants born to women with lupus; four had definite neonatal lupus and four had possible disease.

Congenital heart block may develop as the consequence of diffuse myocarditis and fibrosis in the region between the atrioventricular node and bundle of His. Heart block may be tolerated or may lead to Stokes–Adams attacks or heart failure in the fetus or infant. Fetal ascites may not always be due to heart failure from bradycardia. Richards and associates (1990) described a fetus whose ascites cleared promptly with maternal corticosteroid therapy; however, heart block and bradycardia persisted. The neonate may require a pacemaker. Heart block also may develop in fetuses whose mothers appear normal but are destined subsequently to develop clinical lupus erythematosus or some other connective-tissue disease. **Cutaneous lupus, thrombocytopenia, and autoimmune hemolysis** are transient and clear within a few months (Lee and Weston, 1984).

McCune and colleagues (1987) described 24 children with congenital lupus: 12 had heart block, 10 cutaneous lesions, and two had both. Three died as neonates and 5 of 11 survivors had permanent pacemakers. Importantly, 3 of 12 subsequent liveborns in these women were affected similarly.

Singsen and colleagues (1985) recommend maternal and newborn screening of women at risk. Certainly, if SSA or SSB antibodies are detected in maternal blood, then careful ultrasound screening of the fetus should be conducted to detect any evidence of heart block so that plans can be made for delivery in a tertiary level center.

Management. Various laboratory procedures have been recommended to monitor systemic lupus activity during pregnancy. The sedimentation rate is uninterpretable because it is increased appreciably by pregnancy-induced hyperfibrinogenemia. Serial measurements of C_3, C_4, and CH_{50} components of complement have been recommended, and although falling or low levels more likely are associated with active disease, higher levels provide no guarantee against disease activation. In a retrospective study, Shibata and associates (1992) found that 5 of 6 women with lupus and fetal loss had low CH_{50} levels (less than 25 U/mL), while only 2 of 22 with a liveborn had these low levels. Varner and co-workers (1983), found no correlation between clinical manifestations of disease and C_3 and C_4 complement levels in nearly half of their pregnant patients. Our experiences have been similar.

Frequent hematological evaluation and assessment of renal and hepatic functions are essential to detect changes in disease activity during pregnancy and the puerperium. Hemolysis is characterized by a positive Coombs test, anemia, reticulocytosis, and unconjugated hyperbilirubinemia. Thrombocytopenia, leukopenia, or both, may develop. Increased serum transaminase activity reflects hepatic involvement, as does a rise in serum bilirubin. At times, azathioprine therapy will induce abnormalities in these tests of hepatic function. A urine specimen is screened at each visit to detect new-onset or worsening proteinuria. Overt proteinuria that persists is an ominous sign and is even more ominous if accompanied by other evidence for the nephrotic syndrome or an abnormal serum creatinine concentration.

In general, the prognosis becomes worse as the number of abnormal findings increase. Treatment is generally the same as for the nonpregnant woman, and if disease is severe, corticosteroid therapy is given. Azathioprine is used if there is steroid-resistant nephropathy, but cyclophosphamide is avoided unless life-threatening complications develop. The use of antimalarials to control disease activity during pregnancy is controversial. For short-term malarial therapy, chloroquine and hydroxychloroquine are used, but long-term therapy for lupus is less certain. Most authorities recommend that they be avoided (Gimovsky and Montoro, 1991).

Fetal growth is monitored closely and careful attention is given to development of hypertension. In women with anti-SSA or anti-SSB antibodies, a search for fetal cardiac dysfunction and arrhythmias is made using echocardiography. Other tests to monitor fetal well-being are done. Unless hypertension develops or there is evidence for fetal compromise or retarded growth, pregnancy is allowed to progress to term. Delivery decisions are made using obstetrical criteria. Peripartum corticosteroids in "stress doses" are given to women who are taking these drugs or who have recently done so.

Lupus Versus Preeclampsia–Eclampsia. Preeclampsia is common in all women with lupus, and superimposed preeclampsia is encountered even more often in those with lupus nephropathy. It may be difficult, if not impossible, to differentiate clinically lupus nephropathy from severe preeclampsia. Moreover, central nervous system involvement with systemic lupus may culminate in convulsions similar to those of eclampsia. Thrombocytopenia with or without hemolysis may further confuse the diagnosis. We have elected to manage such problem cases of systemic lupus as if they were the

consequences of preeclampsia–eclampsia, utilizing methods described in Chapter 36 (p. 792). At the same time, corticosteroid therapy is continued. It should be emphasized that the most common causes of death in these women when not pregnant are malignant hypertension with glomerulonephritis and neurological catastrophes such as seizures, strokes, and coma.

Some problems of differential diagnosis of preeclampsia–eclampsia from systemic lupus with vascular, renal, and central nervous system involvement during pregnancy and the puerperium are illustrated in the following woman cared for at Parkland Hospital:

A 21-year-old nullipara was observed throughout pregnancy. By term, her blood pressure had risen from its first trimester value of 100/60 to 130/80 mm Hg and intrapartum to 140/90. Edema was obvious, but proteinuria was not detected. She convulsed one hour after spontaneous delivery of a healthy infant who weighed 3985 g. Transiently, her blood pressure was elevated to 160/108 mm Hg and proteinuria appeared. The hematocrit, platelet count, and plasma creatinine were normal. She was treated with magnesium sulfate parenterally for 24 hours and had no more convulsions. One week later she was discharged normotensive and asymptomatic.

Two weeks after delivery, she experienced bizarre neurological changes, which included tremors and transient loss of vision and consciousness. The cranial computed tomographic scan was normal, but an electroencephalogram was abnormal. The antinuclear antibody titer was 1 : 640 and the serological test for syphilis was falsely positive. While hospitalized, she developed a malar (butterfly) rash. The diagnosis was systemic lupus erythematosus with central nervous system involvement. Did she have eclampsia 2 weeks before? We concluded that she did not, but rather that she had lupus.

Long-term Prognosis. If systemic lupus has been induced by a drug, the disease most likely will ameliorate when the drug is stopped. Otherwise, it is a lifelong disease. In general, women with systemic lupus and chronic vascular or renal disease should limit their family size because of the guarded maternal prognosis as well as increased adverse perinatal outcomes. Wallace and associates (1981) made the following observations on 609 cases of systemic lupus erythematosus: The 10-year survival was 87 percent for those without nephritis but 65 percent for those with nephritis. The most common causes of death were renal disease and sepsis.

Tubal sterilization may be advantageous. It is performed with greatest safety when the disease is reasonably quiescent. Oral contraceptives have not been recommended for women with systemic lupus because vascular disease is a relatively common component. Intrauterine devices should be prescribed with caution, especially if the woman is receiving immunosuppressive therapy.

Antiphospholipid Antibodies—Lupus Anticoagulant and Anticardiolipin Antibody. Over the years, a number of antibodies directed against negatively charged phospholipids have been described. Although these may be found in normal persons, they have been associated with thrombosis, thrombocytopenia, and adverse pregnancy outcomes. Antiphospholipid antibodies include those responsible for biological false-positive serological tests for syphilis, lupus anticoagulant (LAC), and anticardiolipin antibodies (ACA). Antiphospholipid and anticardiolipin antibodies are measured serologically using enzyme-linked immunosorbent assays (ELISA), whereas the lupus anticoagulant is characterized by a prolonged partial thromboplastin time (Harris, 1990b). The so called "anticoagulant" is a powerful thrombotic agent in vivo.

Following development of an assay for anticardiolipin antibody, it soon became apparent that a large number of patients with systemic lupus erythematosus have circulating antibodies directed against cardiolipin. As perhaps expected, there is considerable cross-reactivity. For example, Triplett and colleagues (1988) reported that about 70 percent of patients with lupus anticoagulant activity also have antiphospholipid antibody. Ninomiya and associates (1992) studied 349 lupus patients and found 27 percent to be positive for lupus anticoagulent and 35 percent to have anticardiolipin antibody. Half of each group were positive for both. Love and Santoro (1990) reviewed 29 series that included over 1000 patients with systemic lupus and reported an average frequency of 34 percent for lupus anticoagulant and 44 percent for anticardiolipin antibodies. Again, because both are antiphospholipid antibodies, there is overlap. In general, patients with lupus anticoagulant have higher levels of anticardiolipin antibodies and about a third of those with biological false-positive tests for syphilis have anticardiolipin antibodies (Branch, 1990). Conversely, only about 20 percent of patients with identifiable anticardiolipin have the lupus anticoagulant. Importantly, in patients with lupus, documentation of either anticardiolipin or lupus anticoagulant are risk factors for thrombosis, neurological disorders, or thrombocytopenia (Love and Santoro, 1990). Kutteh and Carr (1992) reviewed pregnancy outcomes in women attending the Parkland Hospital Lupus Clinic. Of those with anticardiolipin antibodies, 55 percent of pregnancies ended in early fetal loss, compared with only 20 percent of those with assays negative for these antibodies. Finally, Khamashta and colleagues (1990) reported that cardiac valvar disease is much more prevalent in lupus patients who have antiphospholipid antibodies.

Nonspecific antiphospholipid antibodies in low titers have been found in about 5 percent of all otherwise healthy nonpregnant populations screened (Harris, 1990b). Likewise, Lockwood and colleagues (1989) studied 737 normally pregnant women without a history of recurrent pregnancy loss and found that two (0.27 percent) had lupus anticoagulant and 16 (2.2 percent) had elevated concentrations of either IgM- or IgG-anticardiolipin antibodies. Bendon and associates (1990) screened 686 women whose mean gestation was 20 weeks. About 5 percent had either IgG- or IgM-anticardiolipin titers greater than three standard deviations from the nonpregnant mean. No correlation was found with antinuclear antibodies, lupus anticoagulant, or placental pathology. Harris and Spinnato (1991) studied 1449 consecutive pregnant women and found 1.8 percent positive for immunoglobulin G anticardiolipin and 4.3 percent for immunoglobulin M anticardiolipin. Most assays were low positive (see Diagnosis), and did not correlate with adverse outcome.

Diagnosis. Because standardization of laboratory methods is not yet uniform, there are conflicting views in interpretation of tests to diagnose these syndromes (Peaceman and associates, 1992). Efforts have been made to standardize the anticardiolipin antibody by using enzyme-linked immunosorbent assay. By agreement reached at the 1987 International Anti-Cardiolipin Workshop, values are reported in units and expressed as either *negative* or *low, medium,* or *high positive* (Harris and colleagues, 1987).

Tests for lupus anticoagulant are nonspecific coagulation tests, the endpoints of which are subject to the amount of phospholipid added to the assay. *The partial thromboplastin time* generally is prolonged because the anticoagulant interferes with conversion of prothrombin to thrombin in vitro by adhering to the phospholipid surface, thereby inhibiting attachment and assembly of other clotting factors. Tests considered more specific are the *tissue thromboplastin-inhibition test,* the dilute *Russell viper venom test,* and the *platelet neutralization procedure.* There currently is disagreement as to which of these is best for screening.

Effect on Pregnancy. Interest in these entities by obstetricians has resulted from the association of the lupus anticoagulant and anticardiolipin antibodies with decidual vasculopathy, placental infarction, fetal growth retardation, early-onset preeclampsia, and recurrent abortion and fetal death. These women, like those with lupus, also have a high incidence of venous and arterial thromboses, cerebral thrombosis, hemolytic anemia, thrombocytopenia, pulmonary hypertension, biologically false-positive tests for syphilis, and multiple abortions and fetal wastage (Derue and colleagues, 1985; Lockshin and associates, 1985). During 264 pregnancies in 68 women with lupus anticoagulant activity reviewed by Gant (1986), about one third had no symptoms, one third had a history of thrombotic episodes, and another third had systemic lupus. In addition, about one fourth each had a false-positive serological test for syphilis and a positive Coombs test.

Kochenour and colleagues (1987) described the clinical courses of three women who had lupus anticoagulant, anticardiolipin antibody, or both, who developed a postpartum syndrome of pleural effusion, pulmonary infiltrates, and fever. These women did not fulfill enough criteria for the diagnosis of lupus erythematosus, and the authors suggest that this is a specific pleuropulmonary and cardiac disease. Similarly, Kincaid-Smith and collaborators (1988) reported findings in renal biopsies in 12 pregnant women with renal failure and lupus anticoagulant. Four had serological evidence for lupus. They described fibrin thrombi in glomerular arterioles and described these as indistinguishable from findings in thrombotic microangulopathy.

Although there is no doubt that the lupus anticoagulant and anticardiolipin antibodies are associated with increased fetal wastage in some women, it is unclear as to the extent of these adverse sequelae in all women who have these antibodies. In most studies that describe recurrent abortions and fetal deaths, women were usually included because they had repeated adverse pregnancy outcomes. In the studies of pregnant women cited above, the incidence of antiphospholipid antibodies in general obstetrical populations is about 3 to 5 percent. Although these studies are too limited to draw conclusions concerning the impact of these antibodies on the incidence of bad outcomes, in the study by Lockwood and colleagues (1989), the two women with lupus anticoagulant had spontaneous abortions and 12 of 16 women with anticardiolipin antibodies had abortions, stillbirths, preterm delivery, or infants with fetal growth retardation.

The incidence of these antibodies may be increased in adverse obstetrical outcomes associated with the syndromes. Polzin and colleagues (1991) identified antiphospholipid antibodies in a fourth of 37 women with growth-retarded fetuses. None of the mothers had evidence for lupus anticoagulant. Branch and co-workers (1989) found a 16 percent incidence of antiphospholipid antibodies in 43 women with severe preeclampsia before 34 weeks' gestation. Six of these seven also had lupus anticoagulant. One of these women also had multiple cerebral infarctions (Fig. 54–1). Haddow and co-workers (1991) measured anticardiolipin antibodies in 309 pregnancies ending in fetal death and found no differences when they compared these with 618 viable pregnancies. Similarly, Infante-Rivard and associates (1991) did not find an increased incidence of lupus anticoagulants or IgG anticardiolipins in a case-control study of 331 women with spontaneous abortion or fetal death. Silver and colleagues (1992) described two infants with middle cerebral artery infarction born to mothers with anticardiolipin antibody. Although pregnant women with HIV infection commonly have elevated antibody, they seldom manifest the clinical syndrome.

Treatment. There is now evidence that many women who have suffered excessive reproductive losses associated with lupus anticoagulant will have improved outcomes if given treatment consisting of *low-dose aspirin* (about 75 mg), along with 20 to 80 mg of prednisone daily (Branch and associates, 1985; Lubbe and co-

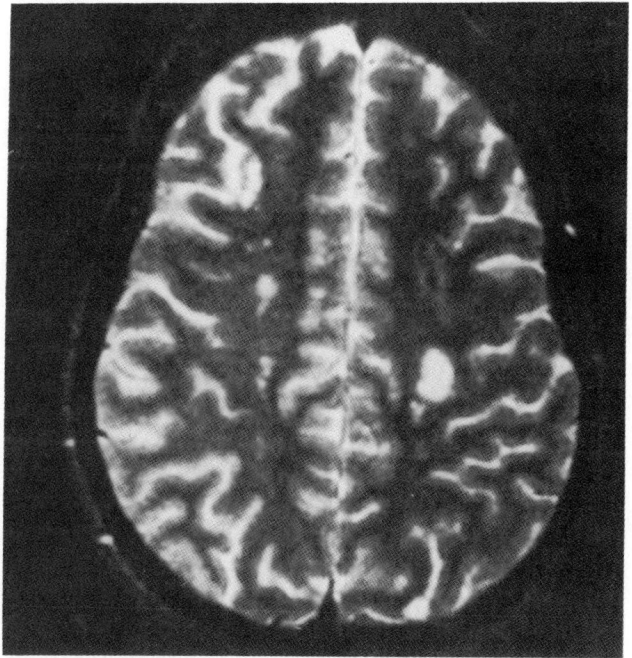

Fig. 54–1. A 23-year-old primigravida with falsely positive syphilis serology and severe preeclampsia and fetal growth retardation at 28 weeks. She had frequent episodes of transient monocular visual loss. Magnetic resonance of brain (T2 weighted image) disclosed multiple bright signals from both hemispheres, predominantly on the left, which were consistent with multiple infarctions. (From Branch and colleagues, 1989, with permission.)

workers, 1983). Gant (1986) reviewed treatment results and reported that the number of liveborn infants increased from 6 to 80 percent in women so treated. The effects of therapy are measured by reversal of clotting abnormalities (Fig. 54–2).

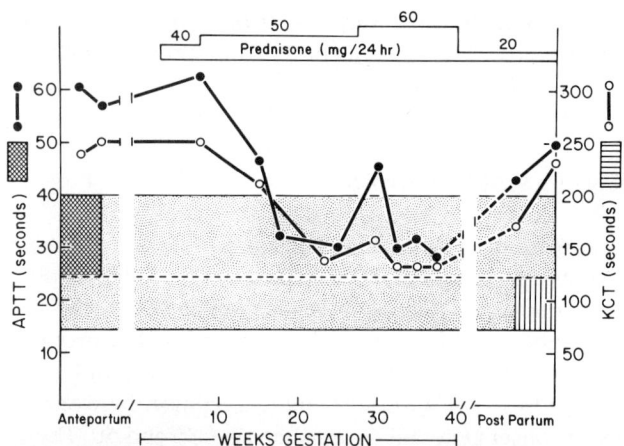

Fig. 54–2. Activated partial thromboplastin time (APTT) and kaolin clotting time (KCT) in a single patient before, during, and after pregnancy. Therapy during pregnancy consisted of aspirin, 75 mg daily, plus prednisone as illustrated. (Modified from Lubbe and associates, 1983, with permission.)

Rosove and associates (1990) gave heparin twice daily (mean daily dose, 25,000 units) to 14 women with anticardiolipin antibodies, lupus anticoagulant, or both. All had at least one prior pregnancy loss. Therapy was begun at 6 to 18 weeks and excluding one spontaneous abortion, 14 pregnancies resulted in liveborns. Katz and colleagues (1990) reported successful prolongation of pregnancy in a woman given high-dose immunoglobulin therapy. She developed severe preeclampsia at 24 weeks despite heparin and aspirin treatment beginning at 6 weeks. Immunoglobulin infusion caused anticardiolipin IgG levels to decrease, and those for IgM and IgA became undetectable. Preeclampsia worsened at 32 weeks and a healthy infant was delivered by cesarean section.

Despite improved outcomes, Branch and associates (1985) caution that fetal growth retardation and preeclampsia still are common. They also reported that low-dose aspirin and corticosteroid therapy are not universally successful. On the other hand, women with lupus and the lupus anticoagulant have had normal pregnancy outcomes without treatment (Stafford-Brady and colleagues, 1988). Similarly, women without lupus but with lupus anticoagulant and prior bad pregnancy outcomes also have had liveborn infants without treatment (Trudinger and associates, 1988). Lubbe and Liggins (1985) recommend that treatment be given only to those women with a history of fetal death. Lockshin and co-workers (1989) found that women with very high IgG antiphospholipid antibody titers (greater than 40 IgG phospholipid units), who also had a prior fetal death, had a dismal prognosis for subsequent pregnancy despite treatment. Specifically, 23 of 32 (70 percent) such women had a recurrent fetal death despite treatment with prednisone or aspirin or both. Cowchock and associates (1992), in a multicenter randomized trial, reported that low-dose aspirin plus low-dose heparin therapy was superior to low-dose aspirin combined with 40 mg prednisone daily to prevent recurrent fetal losses and "serious" maternal morbidity. Landy and colleagues (1992) reported that almost half of women given corticosteroids had complications from therapy, usually gestational diabetes.

Rheumatoid Arthritis

Rheumatoid arthritis is a chronic multisystem disease characterized by a variety of systemic manifestations. The noteworthy feature is inflammatory synovitis, usually involving the peripheral joints, and with a propensity for cartilage destruction, bony erosions, and joint deformities. The disease is more common in women, and its onset generally is between ages 35 and 50. There is a genetic predisposition and 30 percent of monozygous twins and 5 percent of dizygous twins are concordant (Lipsky, 1991). There is also an association with HLA-DR4. Hazes and colleagues (1990) reported a protective effect of pregnancy in development of rheumatoid arthritis.

Clinically, rheumatoid arthritis is a chronic polyarthritis. In addition to symptoms of synovitis, there is fatigue, anorexia, weakness, and vague musculoskeletal symptoms. The hands, wrists, knees, and feet are commonly involved. Pain, aggravated by movement, is accompanied by swelling and tenderness. The American Rheumatism Association (Arnett and colleagues, 1988) revised its 1958 criteria for diagnosis, which have a 90 percent specificity and sensitivity for the diagnosis. Extraarticular manifestations include rheumatoid nodules, vasculitis, pleuropulmonary symptoms, as well as others.

Management. Management is directed at pain relief, reduction of inflammation, and preservation of function. Treatment is important before cartilage loss is irreversible. Physical and occupational therapy and self-management instructions are essential. Aspirin or one of the nonsteroidal anti-inflammatory drugs are the cornerstone of therapy. Corticosteroids are avoided if possible, but low-dose therapy may be used with salicylates. A variety of disease-modifying drugs and immunosuppressive therapy are used for more severe disease. These include hydroxychloroquine, sulfasalazine, low-dose methotrexate, gold salts, and penicillamine (Harris, 1990a). Cyclosporine is reserved for the most severe cases. Orthopedic surgery for joint deformities, including replacement, is performed commonly.

Effects of Pregnancy. In 1938, Hench reported marked improvement in the inflammatory component of rheumatoid arthritis during pregnancy. The pattern of improvement was the same as in spontaneous remission and involved gradual amelioration of the signs and symptoms. Apparently because cortisol levels in plasma were considered to be markedly increased in pregnancy, Hench began to use cortisone to treat rheumatoid arthritis, and there was a favorable effect. Smith and West (1960) demonstrated subsequently that increased secretion of cortisol did not account for all of the remissions. Sex hormones supposedly interfere with a number of putative processes involved in arthritis pathogenesis, including immunoregulation and interactions with the cytokine system (DaSilva and Hall, 1992).

Unger and associates (1983) reported that two thirds of women with rheumatoid arthritis had diminished disease activity during pregnancy. In the group in which activity subsided, **pregnancy-associated α_2-glycoprotein** was considerably higher (mean 1250 mg/L) than in those in whom the disease remained the same or worsened (mean 470 mg/L). Pregnancy-associated glycoprotein is known to have immunosuppressive properties in vitro, and it is tempting to implicate the high level of this protein in the remission of rheumatoid arthritis in pregnancy, as Hench did for cortisol. Pope and associates (1983) reported that concentrations of immune complexes detected by the Clq-binding assay were decreased during pregnancy.

Neely and Persellin (1977) similarly identified amelioration of rheumatoid arthritis activity in 62 percent of 56 pregnancies; in the other 38 percent, there was either no change or the arthritis actually became worse. In four women, signs and symptoms of the disease first appeared during pregnancy. Thus, in some women the course occasionally may worsen during pregnancy, and sometimes the disease may first appear at that time. Silman and associates (1992) performed a case-controlled study with 88 women with rheumatoid arthritis and reported that pregnancy had a "protective effect" for disease onset, whereas there was a five- to six-fold increased likelihood of new disease onset in the first 3 months postpartum.

Østensen and Husby (1983) reported prospective observations in women with rheumatoid arthritis. They confirmed the remarkable amelioration of symptoms even during early pregnancy in women with rheumatoid arthritis as well as exacerbations within 12 weeks postpartum in 11 of 12 women. Conversely, these same investigators (Østensen and Husby, 1989) observed that a third of women with **ankylosing spondylitis** had unchanged disease activity throughout pregnancy and another third worsened. Pregnancy outcomes were relatively normal.

Østensen (1991) retrospectively reviewed outcomes of 76 pregnancies in 51 women with **juvenile rheumatoid arthritis.** Pregnancy had no effects on presentation of disease, but disease activity became quiescent or remained so during pregnancy. Postpartum flares were common, as discussed above for rheumatoid arthritis. Joint deformities were common in these women, and 15 of 20 cesarean deliveries were done for contracted pelves or joint prosthesis.

Perinatal Outcome. There are no obvious adverse effects of rheumatoid arthritis on pregnancy outcome, including preterm labor (Klipple and Cecere, 1989). Although Kaplan (1986) reported that women who go on to develop the disease have had a higher than expected incidence of spontaneous abortion, Nelson and colleagues (1992) noted that this is not the case.

Management. In most instances, these women can be reassured that successful pregnancy outcome is likely. Drugs most commonly used to treat rheumatoid arthritis in women not pregnant have been aspirin or nonsteroidal anti-inflammatory drugs in doses that, if used in pregnancy, might adversely affect the fetus and neonate. Concerns include impaired hemostasis, prolonged gestation, and premature closure of the ductus arteriosus (Briggs and colleagues, 1990). Nonetheless, these drugs usually have been the treatment of choice during pregnancy for symptomatic women. Prednisone and other corticosteroids are used as indicated. Gold compounds

have been used in pregnancy, and are in risk category C. Hydroxychloroquine is an antimalarial with which there is little pregnancy experience. It is a congener of chloroquine that is risk category C. Immunosuppressive therapy with azathioprine, cyclophosphamide, or methotrexate is not used routinely during pregnancy.

If cervical spine involvement exists, particular attention is warranted during pregnancy. Subluxation is common with such involvement, and pregnancy, at least theoretically, predisposes to this because of joint laxity discussed in Chapter 8 (p. 240). Intense involvement of certain joints may interfere with delivery; for example, severe hip deformities may preclude vaginal delivery.

Systemic Sclerosis (Scleroderma)

Systemic sclerosis is a multisystem disorder of unknown etiology characterized by fibrosis of skin, blood vessels, and visceral organs. The gastrointestinal tract, heart, lungs, and kidney are commonly involved. The **overlap syndrome** is when systemic sclerosis is found with features of other connective-tissue disorders. **Mixed connective-tissue disease** is a term used for the syndrome involving features of lupus, systemic sclerosis, polymyositis, rheumatoid arthritis, and high titers of anti-RNP antibodies (see Table 54–1).

The hallmark of the disease is overproduction of normal collagen. The result is fibrosis of skin and the gastrointestinal tract, especially the distal esophagus. Pulmonary interstitial fibrosis along with vascular changes may cause pulmonary hypertension. Antinuclear antibodies are found in 95 percent of patients, and immunoincompetence is common.

Common symptoms are Raynaud phenomenon (95 percent) and swelling of the distal extremities and face. Half of patients have symptoms from esophageal involvement, especially fullness and epigastric burning pain. Pulmonary involvement is common and causes dyspnea. Renal failure causes half of deaths due to systemic sclerosis. Mortality is high with renal or pulmonary involvement and 10-year survival is less than 50 percent.

There is no effective treatment. Therapy is symptomatic and directed at end-organ involvement. Corticosteroids are helpful for inflammatory myositis and hemolytic anemia.

Effects on Pregnancy. Systemic sclerosis is seen most commonly in women during the fourth decade, but its rarity prevents an accumulation of extensive data relative to its effect on pregnancy. Scleroderma formerly was considered to have a markedly deleterious effect upon pregnancy; however, Johnson and associates (1964) were more encouraging in their report of 36 pregnancies in 337 women in whom scleroderma developed before age 45. They concluded that pregnancy had little or no effect on the course of the disease, and that scleroderma had minimal effects on pregnancy. Conversely, from their review of 94 reported cases, Maymon and Fejgin (1989) found that a third had exacerbations of symptoms during pregnancy; 15 percent died of hypertension, renal failure, or cardiopulmonary complications; and there was a 20 percent fetal mortality rate. The majority of maternal deaths in this series were isolated case reports and do not reflect accurately the risks involved.

Steen and colleagues (1989) reported pregnancy outcomes in 69 women with scleroderma. Major complications included *renal crisis* in two women characterized by malignant hypertension and renal failure. One woman died at 25 weeks; the other was delivered preterm and died during hemodialysis 3 years later. The incidence of renal crisis was not considered different from that of nonpregnant women over the same period. Moreover, they did not find an increased incidence of preeclampsia or hypertension. Although the abortion rate was not increased, the risks for preterm delivery, fetal growth retardation, and perinatal mortality were increased, but not dramatically so. As some have reported for rheumatoid arthritis, a higher incidence of pre-diagnosis early pregnancy wastage was observed in these women in a case-controlled study (Silman and Black, 1988).

As perhaps expected, dysphagia and reflux esophagitis are aggravated by pregnancy. Treatment is described in Chapter 51 (p. 1147). Women with hypertension, renal or cardiac involvement, or pulmonary fibrosis do poorly. Women with renal insufficiency and malignant hypertension have an increased incidence of preeclampsia. A case of apparent eclampsia in a woman with scleroderma was reported to be fatal for both mother and fetus (Fear, 1968).

Vaginal delivery may be anticipated, unless the soft tissue changes wrought by scleroderma produce dystocia requiring abdominal delivery. Tracheal intubation for general anesthesia has special concerns because these women typically have limited ability to open their mouths (Black and Stevens, 1989). Because of esophageal dysfunction, aspiration also is more likely. For these reasons, epidural analgesia is preferable (Maymon and Fejgin, 1989).

Vasculitis Syndromes

Inflammation and damage to blood vessels may be primary or due to another disease. Most cases are presumed to be caused by immunopathogenic mechanisms, specifically, immune-complex deposition. These syndromes are difficult to classify because of overlap, but include classical polyarteritis nodosa, hypersensitivity vasculitis, Wegener granulomatosis, and giant-cell arteritis.

Polyarteritis Nodosa. Polyarteritis (periarteritis) nodosa is a rare disease with protean manifestations. The pathological lesion is necrotizing vasculitis of small- and medium-sized arteries. The classical variety is one of the progressive vasculitis syndromes characterized clinically by myalgia, neuropathy, gastrointestinal disorders, hypertension, and renal disease. A third of cases are associated with hepatitis B antigenemia. Even with corticosteroid and immunosuppressive treatment, almost half of patients die within a year of diagnosis.

Only a few documented cases of polyarteritis nodosa in association with pregnancy have been reported and the experience is too scant to draw any definitive conclusions other than that generally the combination is associated with an unfavorable maternal outcome. Certainly, if active arteritis is identified during pregnancy, mortality is high. Owen and Hauth (1989) reviewed the courses of 12 pregnant women. In seven women, polyarteritis first manifested during pregnancy, and it was rapidly fatal by 6 weeks postpartum. The diagnosis was not made until autopsy in six of the seven women. Five other women were in remission at conception. Four of these women continued pregnancy, resulting in one stillborn and three successful outcomes.

Wegener Granulomatosis. Wegener granulomatosis is necrotizing granulomatous vasculitis of the upper and lower respiratory tract along with glomeronephritis. It is uncommon and there have been only a few cases reported in association with pregnancy. Fields and colleagues (1991) reported a woman who became symptomatic at 17 weeks' gestation. She had renal failure and was treated successfully with cyclophosphamide, corticosteroids, and hemodialysis. A healthy infant was delivered by cesarean at 33 weeks. Palit and Clague (1990) reported a woman whose onset of disease was at 7 weeks. She had pulmonary hemorrhage, dyspnea, and mouth ulcers. Therapeutic abortion was done so that cyclophosphamide could be given, and she recovered.

Arteritis Syndromes. **Temporal arteritis** and **Takayasu arteritis** involve medium- and large-size arteries and both are uncommon. Takayasu arteritis, or so-called *pulseless disease*, is most prevalent in young women. It primarily affects the aorta and its main branches. Arteritis may respond to corticosteroid therapy. Surgical bypass sometimes is required to re-establish circulation. Severe renovascular hypertension, cardiac involvement, and pulmonary hypertension frequently preclude a good pregnancy outcome. Conversely, from their review of 14 cases, Nagey and colleagues (1983) reported good pregnancy outcomes. Other case reports and one series of four patients reported by Railton and Allen (1988) substantiate this optimism.

Most authors advise that blood pressure be taken in the lower extremity. Hemodynamic monitoring may be helpful if severe hypertension is identified (Winn and associates, 1988). Epidural analgesia has been advocated (Crofts and Wilson, 1991).

Dermatomyositis and Polymyositis

Dermatomyositis and polymyositis are uncommon acute, subacute, or chronic inflammatory diseases of unknown cause involving skin and muscle, in particular. Prevailing theories are that the syndromes are caused by either viral infections or autoimmune disorders. At least one third of cases are associated with one of the connective-tissue disorders, including rheumatoid arthritis, lupus, mixed connective-tissue disease, or scleroderma. The disease may manifest as a severe generalized myositis with a cutaneous eruption, fever, and a fatal outcome within a few days or weeks. It also may assume a chronic form, characterized by the gradual development of paresis with little, if any, cutaneous or systemic involvement. Laboratory manifestations include elevated muscle enzymes in serum, and an abnormal electromyogram. Confirmation is by biopsy. The disease usually responds to high-dose corticosteroid therapy, and cytotoxic drugs such as azathioprine, cyclophosphamide, and methotrexate are reserved for refractory cases.

About 15 percent of adults developing dermatomyositis have an associated malignant tumor. The time of appearance of the two diseases, however, may be separated by several years. Extirpation of the malignant lesion sometimes is followed by a permanent remission of the dermatomyositis. The most common sites of associated cancer are breast, lung, stomach, and ovary. The uterus and cervix also have been reported as primary sites.

There are only a few reports of dermatomyositis complicating pregnancy, thus it is difficult to draw any definite conclusions about the effect of one upon the other. England and associates (1986) described a woman with new-onset disease at 15 weeks' gestation. Her myositis responded to prednisone therapy, but immediately postpartum she developed severe hypertension. After discharge, she was noncompliant and died 6 weeks later. King and Chow (1985) reported five uneventful pregnancies in three women with dermatomyositis. In four of these, disease was inactive.

Gutierrez and colleagues (1984) reviewed outcomes in 10 pregnancies among seven women with active disease. They reported three abortions, three perinatal deaths, and five preterm deliveries. We have cared for one woman diagnosed and treated with prednisone before pregnancy. During and after the pregnancy, the woman actually improved, and the infant thrived.

Rosenzweig and colleagues (1989) reviewed 24 pregnancy outcomes in 18 women with primary polymyositis–dermatomyositis. In half, the diagnosis preceded pregnancy. Although they were in remission at conception, a fourth had an exacerbation in the second or third trimester. Excluding abortions, there were two perinatal deaths and two growth-retarded neonates.

In the other half of women in whom disease became manifest first during pregnancy, outcomes were less favorable. One woman died 6 weeks postpartum when she suffered a severe exacerbation. Excluding abortions, half of the eight pregnancies resulted in perinatal death. Two fetuses developed ascites, and two were growth-retarded.

Marfan Syndrome

Marfan syndrome is an autosomal dominant connective-tissue disorder that affects both sexes equally. There appears to be no racial or ethnic basis for the syndrome. There are many mild cases in which the intrinsic connective tissue lesion is subclinical with no effect on longevity. Although the specific defect is still controversial, there is a degeneration of the elastic lamina in the media of the aorta. The cardiovascular lesion is the most serious abnormality, involving most of the ascending aorta and predisposing to aortic dilatation or dissecting aneurysm. Early death in Marfan syndrome ultimately is caused by either valvar insufficiency and congestive heart failure or by rupture of a dissecting aneurysm. According to their review, Mor-Yosef and colleagues (1988) report an increased frequency of dissecting and ruptured aneurysms during pregnancy. These were more likely in the last trimester. The syndrome is discussed in detail in Chapter 48 (p. 1099).

Ehlers–Danlos Syndrome

Ehlers–Danlos syndrome is characterized by a variety of changes in connective tissue including hyperelasticity of the skin. In the more severe types of Ehlers–Danlos syndrome, there is a strong tendency for fatal rupture of any of several arteries, causing strokes or bleeding. Rupture of the colon or uterus has been described. There are at least 10 reported varieties, some autosomal dominant, some recessive, and some X-linked. There is overlap between these types, but the underlying molecular defect is unknown. Types I, II, and III are autosomally dominant and each accounts for about 30 percent of cases.

Women with Ehlers–Danlos syndrome have an increased frequency of preterm rupture of membranes, and preterm delivery is increased substantively. There is also increased antepartum and postpartum hemorrhage, and tissue fragility makes episiotomy repair and cesarean delivery difficult. Multiple musculoskeletal abnormalities may develop or worsen during pregnancy and back pain may be exacerbated (Klipple and Riordan, 1989). Case reports and literature reviews have been provided by Peaceman and Cruikshank (1987), Sakala and Harding (1991), Snyder and co-workers (1983), and Taylor and associates (1982).

References

Arnett FC, Edworthy SM, Bloch DA, McShane DJ, Fries JF, Cooper NS, Healy LA, Kaplan SR, Liang MH, Luthra HS: The American Rheumatism Association 1987 revised criteria for the classification of rheumatoid arthritis. Arthritis Rheum 31:315, 1988

Bendon RW, Hayden LE, Hurtubise PE, Getahun B, Siddiqi TA, Glueck HI, Luggen ME, Gartside PS: Prenatal screening for anticardiolipin antibody. Am J Perinatol 7:245, 1990

Black CM, Stevens WM: Scleroderma. Rheum Dis Clin North Am 15:193, 1989

Branch DW: Antiphospholipid antibodies and pregnancy. Semin Perinatol 14:139, 1990

Branch DW, Andres R, Digre KB, Rote NS, Scott JR: The association of antiphospholipid antibodies with severe preeclampsia. Obstet Gynecol 73:541, 1989

Branch DW, Scott JR, Kochenour NK, Hershgold E: Obstetric complications associated with lupus anticoagulant. N Engl J Med 313:1322, 1985

Briggs GG, Freeman RK, Yaffee SJ: Drugs in Pregnancy and Lactation, 3rd ed. Baltimore, Williams & Wilkins, 1990

Burkett G: Lupus nephropathy and pregnancy. Clin Obstet Gynecol 28:310, 1985

Buyon JP, Winchester R: Congenital complete heart block. Arthritis Rheum 33:609, 1990

Cowchock FS, Reece EA, Balaban D, Branch DW, Plouffe L: Repeated fetal losses associated with antiphospholipid antibodies: A collaborative randomized trial comparing prednisone with low-dose heparin treatment. Am J Obstet Gynecol 166:1318, 1992

Crofts SL, Wilson E: Epidural analgesia for labour in Takayasu's arteritis: Case report. Br J Obstet Gynaecol 98:408, 1991

DaSilva JA, Hall GM: The effects of gender and sex hormones on outcome in rheumatoid arthritis. Baillieres Clin Rheumatol 6:196, 1992

Derue GJ, Englert JH, Harris EN, Gharavi AE, Morgan SH, Hull RG: Fetal loss in systemic lupus: Association with anticardiolipin antibodies. J Obstet Gynaecol 5:207, 1985

El-Roeiy A, Myers SA, Gleicher N: The prevalence of autoantibodies and lupus anticoagulant in healthy pregnant women. Obstet Gynecol 75:390, 1990

England MJ, Perlmann T, Veriava Y: Dermatomyositis in Pregnancy: A case report. J Reprod Med 31:633, 1986

Fear RE: Eclampsia superimposed on scleroderma. Obstet Gynecol 31:69, 1968

Fields GL, Ossorio MA, Roy TM, Bunke CM: Wegener's granulomatosis complicated by pregnancy: A case report. J Reprod Med 36:463, 1991

Fine LG: UCLA Conference: Systemic lupus erythematosus in pregnancy. Ann Intern Med 94:667, 1981

Galve E, Candell-Riera J, Pigrau C, Permanyer-Miralda G, Garcia-Del-Castillo H, Soler-Soler J: Prevalence, morphologic types, and evolution of cardiac valvular disease in systemic lupus erythematosus. N Engl J Med 319:817, 1988

Gant NF: Lupus erythematosus, the lupus anticoagulant, and the anticardiolipin antibody. Williams Obstetrics, 17th ed (suppl 6). Norwalk, CT, Appleton & Lange, May/June 1986

Gimovsky ML, Montoro M: Systemic lupus erythematosus and other connective tissue diseases in pregnancy. Clin Obstet Gynecol 34:35, 1991

Gimovsky ML, Montoro M, Paul RH: Pregnancy outcome in women with systemic lupus erythematosus. Obstet Gynecol 63:686, 1984

Gutierrez G, Dagnino R, Mintz G: Polymyositis/dermatomyositis and pregnancy. Arthritis Rheum 27:291, 1984

Haddow JE, Rote NS, Dostal-Johnson D, Palomaki GE, Pulkkinen AJ, Knight GJ: Lack of an association between late fetal death and antiphospholipid antibody measurements in the second trimester. Am J Obstet Gynecol 165:1308, 1991

Hahn BH: Systemic lupus erythematosus. In Wilson JD, Braunwald E, Isselbacher KJ, Petersdorf RG, Martin JB, Fauci AS, Root RK (eds): Harrison's Principles of Internal Medicine, 12th ed. New York, McGraw-Hill, 1991, p 1432

Hanly JG, Gladman DD, Rose TH, Laskin CA, Urowitz MB: Lupus pregnancy: A prospective study of placental changes. Arthritis Rheum 31:358, 1988

Harris ED Jr: Rheumatoid arthritis. Pathophysiology and implications for therapy. N Engl J Med 322:1277, 1990a

Harris EN: A reassessment of the antiphospholipid syndrome. J Rheumatol 17:733, 1990b

Harris EN, Gharavi AE, Patel SP, Hughes GVR: Evaluation of the anti-cardiolipin antibody test: Report of an international workshop. Clin Exp Immunol 68:215, 1987

Harris EN, Spinnato JA: Should anticardiolipin tests be performed in otherwise healthy pregnant women? Am J Obstet Gynecol 165:1272, 1991

Hayslett JP, Lynn RI: Effect of pregnancy in patients with lupus nephropathy. Kidney Int 18:207, 1980

Hazes JMW, Dijkmans BAC, Vandenbroucke JP, De Vries RRP, Cats A: Pregnancy and the risk of developing rheumatoid arthritis. Arthritis Rheum 33:1770, 1990

Hench PG: Ameliorating effect of pregnancy on chronic atrophic (infectious rheumatoid) arthritis, fibrositis and intermittent hydrarthrosis. Proc Mayo Clin 13:161, 1938

Infante-Rivard C, David M, Gauthier R, Rivard GE: Lupus anticoagulants, anticardiolipin antibodies, and fetal loss: A case-control study. N Engl J Med 325:1063, 1991

Johnson TR, Banner EA, Winkelmann RK: Scleroderma and pregnancy. Obstet Gynecol 23:467, 1964

Johnstone FD, Kilpatrick DC, Burns SM: Anticardiolipin antibodies and pregnancy outcome in women with human immunodeficiency virus infection. Obstet Gynecol 80:92, 1992

Kaplan D: Fetal wastage in patients with rheumatoid arthritis. J Rheumatol 13:875, 1986

Katz VL, Thorp JM, Watson WJ, Fowler L, Heine RP: Human immunoglobulin therapy for preeclampsia associated with lupus anticoagulant and anticardiolipin antibody. Obstet Gynecol 76:986, 1990

Khamashta MA, Cervera R, Asherson RA, Font J, Gil A, Coltart DJ, Vázquez JJ, Paré C, Ingelmo M, Oliver J, Hughes GRV: Association of antibodies against phospholipids with heart valve disease in systemic lupus erythematosus. Lancet 335:1541, 1990

Kincaid-Smith P, Fairley KF, Kloss M: Lupus anticoagulant associated with renal thrombotic microangiopathy and pregnancy-related renal failure. Q J Med 258:795, 1988

King CR, Chow S: Dermatomyositis and pregnancy. Obstet Gynecol 66:589, 1985

Klipple GL, Cecere FA: Rheumatoid arthritis and pregnancy. Rheum Dis Clin North Am 15:213, 1989

Klipple GL, Riordan KK: Rare inflammatory and hereditary

connective tissue diseases. Rheum Dis Clin North Am 15:383, 1989

Kochenour NK, Branch W, Rote NS, Scott JR: A new postpartum syndrome associated with antiphospholipid antibodies. Obstet Gynecol 69:460, 1987

Kutteh WH, Carr BR: Recurrent pregnancy loss. In Carr BR, Blackwell RC (eds): Textbook of Reproductive Medicine. Norwalk, CT, Appleton & Lange, 1992

Landy HJ, Kessler C, Kelly WK, Weingold AB: Obstetric performance in patients with the lupus anticoagulant and/or anticardiolipin antibodies. Am J Perinatol 9:146, 1992

Lee LA, Weston WL: New findings in neonatal lupus syndrome. Am J Dis Child 138:233, 1984

Lipsky PE: Rheumatoid arthritis. In Wilson JD, Braunwald E, Isselbacher KJ, Petersdorf RG, Martin JB, Fauci AS, Root RK (eds): Harrison's Principles of Internal Medicine, 12th ed. New York, McGraw-Hill, 1991, p 1437

Lockshin MD: Pregnancy does not cause systemic lupus erythematosus to worsen. Arthritis Rheum 32:665, 1989

Lockshin MD, Bonfa E, Elkon K, Druzin ML: Neonatal lupus risk to newborns of mothers with systemic lupus erythematosus. Arthritis Rheum 31:697, 1988

Lockshin MD, Druzin ML, Goei S, Qamar T, Magid MS, Jovanovic L, Ferenc M: Antibody to cardiolipin as a predictor of fetal distress or death in pregnant patients with systemic lupus erythematosus. N Engl J Med 313:152, 1985

Lockshin MD, Druzin ML, Qamar T: Prednisone does not prevent recurrent fetal death in women with antiphospholipid antibody. Am J Obstet Gynecol 160:439, 1989

Lockwood CJ, Romero R, Feinberg RF, Clyne LP, Coster B, Hobbins JC: The prevalence and biologic significance of lupus anticoagulant and anticardiolipin antibodies in a general obstetric population. Am J Obstet Gynecol 161:369, 1989

Love PE, Santoro SA: Antiphospholipid antibodies: Anticardiolipin and the lupus anticoagulant in systemic lupus erythematosus (SLE) and in non-SLE disorders. Ann Intern Med 112:682, 1990

Lubbe WF, Buttler WS, Palmer SJ, Liggins GC: Fetal survival after prednisone suppression of maternal lupus-anticoagulant. Lancet 1:1361, 1983

Lubbe WF, Liggins GC: Lupus anticoagulant and pregnancy. Am J Obstet Gynecol 153:322, 1985

Maymon R, Fejgin M: Scleroderma in pregnancy. Obstet Gynecol Surv 44:530, 1989

McCune AB, Weston WL, Lee LA: Maternal and fetal outcome in neonatal lupus erythematosus. Ann Intern Med 106:520, 1987

Mintz G, Niz J, Gutiérrez G, Garcia-Alonso A, Karchmar S: Prospective study of pregnancy in systemic lupus erythematosus: Results of a multidisciplinary approach. J Rheumatol 13:732, 1986

Mor-Yosef S, Navot D, Rabinowitz R, Schenker JG: Collagen diseases in pregnancy. Obstet Gynecol Surv 39:67, 1984

Mor-Yosef S, Younis J, Granat M, Kedari A, Milgalter A, Schenker JG: Marfan's syndrome in pregnancy. Obstet Gynecol Surv 43:382, 1988

Nagey DA, Fortier KJ, Hayes BA, Linder J: Takayasu's arteritis in pregnancy: A case presentation demonstrating the absence of placental pathology. Am J Obstet Gynecol 147:463, 1983

Neely NT, Persellin RH: Activity of rheumatoid arthritis during pregnancy. Tex Med 73:59, 1977

Nelson JL, Voigt LF, Koepsell TD, Dugowson CE, Daling JR: Pregnancy outcome in women with rheumatoid arthritis before disease onset. J Rheumatol 19:18, 1992

Nicklin JL: Systemic lupus erythematosus and pregnancy at the Royal Women's Hospital, Brisbane 1979–1989. Aust NZ Obstet Gynecol 31:128, 1991

Ninomiya C, Taniguchi O, Kato T, Hirano T, Hashimoto H, Hirose S: Distribution and clinical significance of lupus anticoagulant and anticardiolipin antibody in 349 patients with systemic lupus. Intern Med 31:194, 1992

Nossent HC, Swaak TJG: Systemic lupus erythematosus. VI. Analysis of the interrelationship with pregnancy. J Rheumatol 17:771, 1990

Østensen M: Pregnancy in patients with a history of juvenile rheumatoid arthritis. Arthritis Rheum 34:881, 1991

Østensen M, Husby G: Ankylosing spondylitis and pregnancy. Rheum Dis Clin North Am 15:241, 1989

Østensen M, Husby G: A prospective clinical study of the effect of pregnancy on rheumatoid arthritis and ankylosing spondylitis. Arthritis Rheum 26:1155, 1983

Owen J, Hauth JC: Polyarteritis nodosa in pregnancy: A case report and brief literature review. Am J Obstet Gynecol 160:606, 1989

Packham DK, Lam SS, Nicholls K, Fairley KF, Kincaid-Smith PS: Lupus nephritis and pregnancy. Q J Med 83:315, 1992

Palit J, Clague RB: Wegener's granulomatosis presenting during first trimester of pregnancy. Br J Rheumatol 29:389, 1990

Peaceman AM, Cruikshank DP: Ehlers–Danlos syndrome and pregnancy: Association of type IV disease with maternal death. Obstet Gynecol 69:428, 1987

Peaceman AM, Silver RK, MacGregor SN, Socol ML: Interlaboratory variation in antiphospholipid antibody testing. Am J Obstet Gynecol 166:1780, 1992

Petri M, Howard D, Repke J: Frequency of lupus flare in pregnancy. The Hopkins Lupus Pregnancy Center experience. Arthritis Rheum 34:1538, 1991

Polzin WJ, Kopelman JN, Robinson RD, Read JA, Brady K: The association of antiphospholipid antibodies with pregnancies complicated by fetal growth restriction. Obstet Gynecol 78:1108, 1991

Pope RM, Yoshinoya S, Rutstein J, Persellin RH: Effect of pregnancy on immune complexes and rheumatoid factors in patients with rheumatoid arthritis. Am J Med 74:973, 1983

Railton A, Allen DG: Takayasu's arteritis in pregnancy. A report of 4 cases. S Afr Med J 73:123, 1988

Richards DS, Wagman AJ, Cabaniss ML: Ascites not due to congestive heart failure in a fetus with lupus-induced heart block. Obstet Gynecol 76:957, 1990

Rosenzweig BA, Rotmensch S, Binette SP, Phillippe M: Primary idiopathic polymyositis and dermatomyositis complicating pregnancy: Diagnosis and management. Obstet Gynecol Surv 44:162, 1989

Rosove MH, Tabsh K, Wasserstrum N, Howard P, Hahn B, Kalunian KC: Heparin therapy for pregnant women with lupus anticoagulant or anticardiolipin antibodies. Obstet Gynecol 75:630, 1990

Sakala EP, Harding MD: Ehlers–Danlos syndrome type III and pregnancy. J Reprod Med 36:622, 1991

Shibata S, Sasaki T, Hirabayashi Y, Seino J, Okamura K, Yoshinaga K, Morito N, Kasukawa R, Aotuka S, Yokohari R: Risk factors in the pregnancy of patients with systemic lupus erythematosus: Association of hypocomplementaemia with poor prognosis. Ann Rheum Dis 51:619, 1992

Silman A, Black CM: Increased incidence of spontaneous abortion and infertility in women with scleroderma before disease onset: A controlled study. Ann Rheum Dis 47:441, 1988

Silman A, Kay A, Brennan P: Timing of pregnancy in relation to the onset of rheumatoid arthritis. Arthritis Rheum 35:152, 1992

Singsen BH, Akhter JE, Weinstein MM, Sharp GC: Congenital complete heart block and SSA antibodies: Obstetric implications. Am J Obstet Gynecol 153; 495, 1985

Silver RK, MacGregor SN, Pasternak JF, Neely SE: Fetal stroke associated with elevated maternal anticardiolipin antibodies. Obstet Gynecol 80:497, 1992

Smith WD, West HF: Pregnancy and rheumatoid arthritis. Acta Rheumat Scand 6:189, 1960

Snyder RR, Gilstrap LC, Hauth JC: Ehlers–Danlos syndrome and pregnancy. Obstet Gynecol 61:649, 1983

Stafford-Brady FJ, Gladman DD, Urowitz MB: Successful pregnancy in systemic lupus erythematosus with an untreated lupus anticoagulant. Arch Intern Med 148:1647, 1988

Steen VD, Conte C, Day N, Ramsey-Goldman R, Medsger TA: Pregnancy in women with systemic sclerosis. Arthritis Rheum 32:151, 1989

Tan EM, Cohen AS, Fries JF, Masi AT, McShane DJ, Rothfield NF, Schaller JG, Talal N, Winchester RJ: The 1982 revised criteria for the classification of systemic lupus erythematosus. Arthritis Rheum 25:1271, 1982

Taylor DJ, Wilcox I, Russell JK: Ehlers–Danlos syndrome during pregnancy: A case report and review of the literature. Obstet Gynecol Surv 36:277, 1982

Triplett DA, Brandt JT, Musgrave KA, Orr CA: The relationship between lupus anticoagulants and antibodies to phospholipid. JAMA 259:550, 1988

Trudinger BJ, Stewart GJ, Cook CM, Connelly A, Exner T: Monitoring lupus anticoagulant-positive pregnancies with umbilical artery flow velocity waveforms. Obstet Gynecol 72:215, 1988

Unger A, Kay A, Griffin AJ, Panayi GS: Disease activity and pregnancy associated α_2-glycoprotein in rheumatoid arthritis. BMJ 286:750, 1983

Varner MW: Autoimmune disorders and pregnancy. Semin Perinatol 15:238, 1991

Varner MW, Meehan RT, Syrop CH, Strottman MP, Gopelrud CP: Pregnancy in patients with systemic lupus erythematosus. Am J Obstet Gynecol 145:1025, 1983

Vetter VL, Rashkind WJ: Congenital complete heart block and connective-tissue disorders. N Engl J Med 309:236, 1983

Wallace DJ, Podell T, Weiner J, Klinenberg JR, Forouzesh S, Dubois EL: Systemic lupus erythematosus—Survival patterns. JAMA 245:934, 1981

Winn HN, Setaro JF, Mazor M, Reece A, Black HR, Hobbins JC: Severe Takayasu's arteritis in pregnancy: The role of central hemodynamic monitoring. Am J Obstet Gynecol 159:1135, 1988

CHAPTER 55

Neurological and Psychiatric Disorders

NEUROLOGICAL DISORDERS

Neurological diseases may be encountered with some frequency in women of childbearing age and many of the disorders are physically and mentally disabling. These consequences are tragic, particularly when they occur in young women. Fortunately, most coincidental nervous system disorders are compatible with normal pregnancy outcome, and pregnancy seldom exacerbates underlying neurological disease. Exceptions to this generalization will be emphasized in the following discussion.

Diagnosis of Neurological Disease During Pregnancy. Neurological symptoms are complex and may involve cognitive as well as neuromuscular functions, therefore, they must often be distinguished from psychiatric disorders. With few exceptions, neurological diseases will not be appreciably affected by pregnancy. For example, as discussed in Chapter 8, even though in late pregnancy a woman may have mild parasthesias of the upper extremity due to accentuated cervical spine lordosis, this seldom mimics serious neurological disease.

Imaging of the Central Nervous System. Various imaging techniques have been developed during the past 20 years that have revolutionized the ability to visualize anatomical lesions responsible for neurological disease. Computed-tomography scanning and magnetic resonance imaging have opened new vistas for the diagnosis, classification, and management of many neurological and psychiatric disorders. In general, use of these diagnostic techniques should not be restricted merely because the woman is pregnant.

Cranial computed tomography with appropriate shielding is safe during pregnancy (see Chap 43, p. 985). In some diseases, it is used preferentially to magnetic resonance imaging, while in others, it is complimentary. Certainly, it is more widely available, and it is commonly used whenever rapid diagnosis is necessary to differentiate between medical and surgical management of an acute neurological catastrophe. In hemorrhagic lesions, tomography is likely superior to magnetic resonance imaging.

Magnetic resonance imaging (MRI) does not employ radiation and is thought to be devoid of fetal risks. It is helpful in diagnosing demyelinating diseases, screening for arteriovenous malformations, evaluation of congenital and developmental nervous system abnormalities, identifying posterior fossa lesions, and diagnos-

ing spinal cord diseases. A major disadvantage is the limited space available within the scanner, which makes it difficult to monitor critically ill patients. The claustrophobic conditions of the scanner may be difficult for some pregnant women to tolerate.

Cerebral vessel angiography with contrast injection, usually via femoral artery access, is a valuable adjunct to the diagnosis and treatment of some cerebrovascular diseases. If indicated, these techniques should not be withheld from the pregnant woman. Careful abdominal shielding may be used to limit x-ray exposure during fluoroscopy and film exposure.

Positron-emission tomography (PET) is based on a 3-dimensional reconstruction of brain sections using positron-emitting radionuclides. It is a relatively new technique which evaluates cerebral blood flow and oxygen and glucose metabolism. Unfortunately, the need for radioisotopes severely limits its use during pregnancy (see Chap. 43, p. 985).

Seizure Disorders

More than 2 million people in the United States have some form of epilepsy. Complex partial with secondary generalized seizures account for 60 percent of cases, generalized tonic-clonic seizures for 30 percent, and generalized absence (petit mal) for 5 percent (Shorvon, 1990). Seizures are caused by chronic, paroxysmal disorders of abnormal brain electrical activity. If accompanied by motor manifestations, they are termed convulsive seizures. These disorders may arise from neurological injury, a structural lesion, as a part of systemic illness, or they may be idiopathic.

Pathogenesis. Because a number of metabolic abnormalities and anatomical lesions can induce seizures, there is no pathognomonic lesion of epilepsy. The hallmark of the disease is the rhythmical and repetitive hypersynchronous neuronal discharge in a localized brain area. These electrical discharges are seen on electroencephalograms as spikes or waves. Seizures may be induced by (1) decreases in inhibitory mechanisms due to reductions in gamma-aminobutyric acid (GABA), (2) enhancement of excitatory synaptic mechanisms mediated by N-methyl-D-aspartate (NMDA), and (3) enhancement of neuronal burst firing. Antiepileptic drugs act on these mechanisms.

The diagnosis of idiopathic seizures is dependent

upon excluding known causes. Some identifiable causes of convulsive disorders in adolescents and young adults include trauma, alcohol and other drug-induced withdrawals, brain tumors, or arteriovenous malformations. A search for all of these, including biochemical abnormalities, is necessary when a new-onset seizure disorder is encountered in a pregnant woman. Lumbar puncture, skull x-rays, and arteriography have been largely replaced by evaluation either with computed tomography, magnetic resonance imaging, or sometimes both.

Epilepsy During Pregnancy. According to Nelson and Ellenberg (1982), the prevalence of epilepsy was 4.4 per 1000 in the 45,000 pregnant women included in the Collaborative Perinatal Project. The effect of pregnancy on the frequency of epileptic seizures has been argued for more than 100 years. Like many chronic diseases, in some women epilepsy appears to be worsened by pregnancy, in some it improves, but in the majority it appears to be unaffected. If seizures are well controlled before pregnancy, there is likely little risk of increased frequency during pregnancy. If seizures are poorly controlled before pregnancy, however, there is a likelihood of even further deterioration (Schmidt and associates, 1983).

In general, pregnant women with epilepsy have more overall complications as well as increased adverse perinatal outcomes. Bjerkedal and Bahana (1973) found a two- to three-fold increase in the incidence of pregnancy-induced hypertension, cesarean delivery, preterm delivery, low-birthweight infants, congenital malformations, and perinatal mortality in epileptic women. Nelson and Ellenberg (1982) reported similar findings from the Collaborative Perinatal Project, but they also found the incidence of cerebral palsy, seizures, and mental retardation to be significantly increased in the infants of epileptic mothers.

More recently, Wilhelm and colleagues (1990) compared outcomes in 98 pregnancies complicated by epilepsy with nonepileptic controls. In about one fourth of these women, epilepsy worsened; the important predictor of this was prepregnancy severity. They confirmed the data reported in the older studies cited above that the incidence of preeclampsia and preterm delivery was increased two- to three-fold compared with nonepileptic controls. The congenital malformation rate was 14 percent, compared with 3 percent in their general obstetrical population.

Management. The therapeutic goal for treatment of epilepsy during pregnancy is control of convulsions with the least amount of a drug likely to affect the fetus adversely. **Overwhelming evidence has accrued that use of several of the most effective antiepileptic drugs during pregnancy is accompanied by higher frequencies of fetal malformations.** Thus, monotherapy with the smallest effective dose is another goal.

Increased seizure activity during pregnancy has been attributed to impaired anticonvulsant absorption; however, this seems unlikely. Certainly, the commonly encountered nausea and vomiting of early pregnancy may at times preclude ingestion or availability of antiepileptic medications. Some women may reduce their medications dosage or abstain completely because of fear of adverse fetal effects. During labor, delivery, and the early puerperium, medication may be withheld deliberately or inadvertently, similarly increasing the likelihood of convulsions.

There is evidence that hepatic microsomal activity is induced during pregnancy, thus altering anticonvulsant metabolism. Clinical effects from this, however, are unclear. The effects of pregnancy on the metabolic clearance rate of some anticonvulsant drugs have been of interest for some years. For example, phenytoin is cleared more rapidly during pregnancy. Thus, with a constant dose, plasma levels are lower than when nonpregnant (Kochenour and co-workers, 1980; Lander and Eadie, 1991). Although it seems that this should increase the risk of seizures, this is offset during pregnancy by an increased amount of free or nonprotein-bound drug in plasma (Perucca and associates, 1981). **Thus, there is no evidence that anticonvulsant doses need to be increased empirically during pregnancy.**

The fall in anticonvulsant plasma levels that accompanies pregnancy has been interpreted by some as an indication for frequent measurements of plasma levels and an increase in dosage. This approach fails to recognize the enhanced therapeutic effect that results from decreased protein binding of the drug as pregnancy advances. Moreover, appropriate plasma levels throughout pregnancy, as yet, have not been established. Although Dalessio (1985) recommends that plasma levels be determined routinely, Lander and Eadie (1991) reported that seizure control was not improved by this practice. For the same reasons, we do not routinely measure these drug levels at Parkland Hospital. We prefer to measure serum levels of anticonvulsants in women who are not controlled using standard empirical doses or in women suspected of being noncompliant.

Effect of Anticonvulsants on Fetus-Infant. It is estimated that almost 12,000 children are born annually to women who take some type of anticonvulsant medication (Kelly, 1984). Although the precise pathophysiology of congenital malformations associated with seizure disorders has not been elucidated, it is well established that epileptic women, who chronically take anticonvulsant medications, have a two- to three-fold increased risk of malformed fetuses compared with nonepileptics (see Chap. 42, p. 965).

It remains unclear whether epilepsy per se causes the increased malformations or whether they are caused by anticonvulsant exposure or, more likely, the combination of a potentially teratogenic drug working in concert with a genetic predisposition. Characteristics of the anticonvulsant embryopathies are discussed in Chapter 42 (see p. 967). It has been postulated that the teratogenicity of various antiepileptic medications is mediated by toxic intermediary metabolites of the parent compound. The latter is related to a genetic defect in arene oxide detoxification that causes diminished *epoxide hydrolase enzyme* activity (Buehler and associates, 1990; Jones and co-workers, 1989; Strickler and colleagues, 1985).

Maternal phenytoin ingestion alone or with phenobarbital has been implicated in the neonatal deficiency of four vitamin K–dependent clotting factors (II, VII, IX, and X) (Mountain and co-workers, 1970). **Hemorrhagic disease of the newborn** described in this circumstance usually can be prevented by prompt parenteral administration of vitamin K to the newborn. It might be worthwhile, therefore, to give the mother vitamin K late in pregnancy or at least at the onset of labor to further minimize the risk of hemorrhage in the fetus and infant (see Chap. 44, p. 1017).

Other anticonvulsants are associated with an increased risk for fetal malformations. **Carbamazepine** is commonly prescribed and for many years it was believed to be the drug of choice for pregnant epileptics. However, Jones and co-workers (1989) reported findings strongly suggestive that carbamazepine is teratogenic and causes significant malformations. More recently, Rosa (1991) provided evidence from a Michigan Medicaid cohort that prenatal exposure to carbamazepine carries a 1 percent risk of spina bifida.

Phenobarbital is difficult to assess as a teratogen because it was once commonly used in conjunction with phenytoin. For these reasons, phenobarbital is a category D drug (Briggs and colleagues, 1990). **Trimethadione,** used principally for petit mal seizures, has been implicated in causing birth defects in excess of those associated with hydantoin, and this drug should be avoided in pregnancy (Briggs and colleagues, 1990). **Valproic acid** has been associated with a constellation of major and minor anomalies, but it is estimated to cause neural tube defects in 1 to 2 percent of exposed offspring (Centers for Disease Control, 1983). This risk apparently is greatest from 17 to 30 days postconception, and prenatal diagnosis is recommended for fetuses exposed during these times. This drug should not be given to pregnant women (see Chap. 42, p. 968).

Counseling. Consideration should be given to stopping anticonvulsant medication for the woman who wishes to conceive. The circumstances in which treatment may be stopped without likelihood of recurrence have been described by Delgado-Escueta and associates (1983). Generally, if the woman has not convulsed for a long time on medication and does not do so while off medication before conception, she is likely to have no prob-

lem during pregnancy. There is, however, a 25 to 40 percent chance of recurrence after stopping the medication even though a woman has been seizure-free for at least 2 years while taking medications (Pedley, 1988). Thus, precautions to protect her and others must be taken during the trial period off medication. **If she convulses, however, treatment during pregnancy is essential.** Pregnancy is not the best time to test medication withdrawal.

Several anticonvulsant drugs precipitate or aggravate folic acid deficiency, and megaloblastic anemia has been described. Folic acid administration has been claimed by some to increase the likelihood of convulsions; however, Hiilesmaa and associates (1983) found no such association. The benefits, if any, to be derived from folic acid supplementation in these circumstances are not apparent, and we do not prescribe supplemental folic acid.

At times, it may be difficult to differentiate between eclampsia and epilepsy in the hypertensive pregnant woman (see Chap. 36, p. 790). We have observed that parenteral magnesium sulfate most often promptly controls the convulsions of epilepsy as well as those of eclampsia.

Cerebrovascular Diseases

In the United States, cerebrovascular disease is the third leading cause of death after heart disease and cancer. Cerebrovascular disease refers to disorders of one or more blood vessels of the brain, and the majority of lesions that arise from these are from arterial diseases. The resultant pathological lesion is a **stroke,** which is an acute neurological injury arising from ischemia, embolization, occlusion, or a ruptured vessel (Kistler and colleagues, 1991). Other symptoms that may accompany stroke and cerebrovascular disease include cranial nerve pressure, vascular headache, or increased intracranial pressure with venous thrombosis.

Although distinctly uncommon in young women, disorders of cerebral circulation have continued to be a prominent cause of maternal deaths in the United States. Kaunitz and colleagues (1985) reported that cerebrovascular accidents caused 5 percent of 2067 nonabortion-related maternal deaths in the United States from 1974 to 1978. The Maternal Mortality Collaborative (Rochat and associates, 1988) reported that 10 percent of 507 direct maternal deaths from 1980 to 1985 were caused by strokes. Sachs and colleagues (1987) noted that whereas the incidence of intracranial hemorrhage as a cause of maternal death decreased three-fold over a 30-year period, it remained the third or fourth leading cause in Massachusetts.

The incidence of strokes in pregnant women varies depending on the population surveyed. For example, at Parkland Hospital, in a predominantly young and indigent population, the incidence of stroke in nearly 90,000 women was 1 in 6000 pregnancies (Simolke and co-workers, 1991). Three of these 15 women (20 percent) died as a result of their stroke, and six of the survivors (50 percent) had permanent neurological sequelae.

Ischemic Strokes

Cerebral Artery Thrombosis. The vast majority of strokes afflict older individuals and result from cerebral artery thrombosis caused by atherosclerosis. Arterial thrombosis during pregnancy is probably not more common than stroke from cerebral embolism or intracranial hemorrhage. In over 29,000 consecutive births at the Mayo Clinic, Wiebers and Whisnant (1985) identified only one case each of cerebral thrombosis and intracranial hemorrhage. In the almost 90,000 women reported from Parkland Hospital, Simolke and colleagues (1991) identified only two cases of cerebral artery thrombosis (Table 55–1). One of these women had other features of connective-tissue disease. Unexplained cerebral thrombosis and other thrombotic complications occur more frequently in women who have **antiphospholipid antibodies.** According to Branch (1990), up to one third of ischemic strokes in otherwise healthy patients under 50 years of age are caused by these antibodies (see Chap. 54, p. 1234).

Cerebral Venous Thrombosis. Lateral or superior **sagittal venous sinus thromboses** are rare in the absence of infection or trauma, but pregnancy, and especially the puerperium, are predisposing events. As discussed in Chapter 52 (p. 1194), venous thrombosis is more common in patients with protein C or S deficiency (Roos and colleagues, 1990). It is interesting that venous thrombosis is more common in undeveloped countries. For example, Srinivasan (1984) reported its incidence in Madurai, India, to be 1 in 250 deliveries. Such lesions are much less common in America and Europe. Specifically, Cross and colleagues (1968) reported the inci-

dence to be 1 in 20,000 pregnancies in Scotland, and Wiebers and Whisnant (1985) observed only one case among more than 29,000 deliveries at the Mayo Clinic. In the series from Parkland Hospital, two women with sagittal sinus thrombosis were identified for an incidence of 1 in 45,000 deliveries (Simolke and co-workers, 1991).

Venous thrombosis of the cerebral circulation is more common in the puerperium and frequently is heralded by seizures. Its management includes anticonvulsants to control seizures and antimicrobials if septic thrombophlebitis is suspected. Use of anticoagulants is controversial because bleeding may develop spontaneously. Prognosis is guarded. Coma and death may ensue rapidly, or, conversely, full recovery may follow.

Cerebral Embolism. Cerebral embolism most commonly involves the middle cerebral artery. This is the most frequently reported type of stroke during the latter half of pregnancy or early puerperium. The source of arterial occlusion may be unclear at first, but a diligent search will often identify the source of emboli to be associated with heart disease.

Management of embolic stroke consists of supportive measures and a consideration for anticoagulation once cerebral hemorrhage or infarction has been excluded. Because infarction follows cerebral embolization, it is sometimes confused with cerebral artery thrombosis. Many cases of cerebral embolism in young women never are found to have an underlying cause, and the risk of recurrence is speculative. On the other hand, if an underlying cause is identified, recurrence is more common unless treatment can be given. **Thus, it is important to pursue aggressively an etiology when these lesions are identified during pregnancy.** The most commonly found origin of emboli is the heart, and these may result from arrhythmias, especially atrial fibrillation associated with rheumatic valvar disease. They also may arise from a heart valve affected by old rheumatic disease or mitral valve prolapse. Finally, emboli from infective endocarditis must be considered (Cox and associates, 1988).

Hemorrhagic Strokes. Several lesions may cause serious intracranial hemorrhage. Hemorrhagic and ischemic strokes occur with about equal frequency during pregnancy (Table 55–1). **Intracerebral hemorrhage** into the substance of the brain associated with hypertension may complicate chronic essential hypertension with superimposed preeclampsia, or it may be associated with "pure" preeclampsia. Mercado and colleagues (1989) described a woman with postpartum intracerebral hemorrhage associated with hypertension and seizures caused by crack cocaine use. Lesions that cause **subarachnoid hemorrhage** over the surface of the brain are more likely to be associated with an otherwise normal pregnancy. These lesions are typically due to rup-

TABLE 55–1. TYPES OF STROKES DURING PREGNANCY OR PUERPERIUM IN 15 WOMEN CARED FOR AT PARKLAND HOSPITAL, 1984 TO 1990

Type of Stroke	Number
Ischemic strokes (9)	
Arterial thrombosis	2
Venous thrombosis	2
Arterial embolism	3
Vasculitis	1
Moyamoya disease	1
Hemorrhagic strokes (6)	
Hypertensive	3
Saccular aneurysm	1
Arteriovenous malformation	1
Unknown	1

From Simolke and associates (1991).

tured **saccular aneurysms** or bleeding **arteriovenous malformations;** they complicate about 1 in 15,000 pregnancies (Noronha, 1985).

Intracerebral Hemorrhage. Intracerebral hemorrhages are usually associated with hypertensive disorders, and three of the four women cared for at Parkland Hospital who suffered this type of stroke had pregnancy-induced hypertension (Fig. 55–1). Women especially likely to develop these serious neurovascular complications are usually older and have chronic underlying hypertension. Because of its location, this type of stroke frequently has a poor prognosis, and indeed, in these three women, one died and the other two suffered permanent neurological sequelae. These experiences underscore the importance of proper management for acute hypertension to prevent cerebrovascular pathology.

Subarachnoid Hemorrhage. Subarachnoid hemorrhage generally results from rupture of a **cerebral aneurysm** or bleeding from an **arteriovenous malformation.** The cardinal feature is sudden severe headache. According to Dias and associates (1990), bleeding from aneurysms is more common than arteriovenous malformations with a ratio of 3 : 1 during pregnancy. The reported incidence during pregnancy of approximately 1 in 10,000 does not differ from that in the general nonobstetrical population (Minielly and associates, 1979). Simolke and co-workers (1991) observed the incidence to be 1 in 45,000 pregnancies.

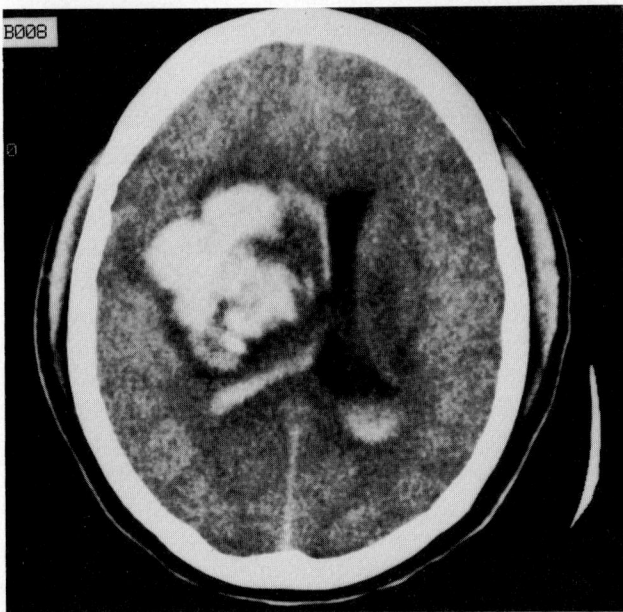

Fig. 55–1. Computed tomograph of massive, ultimately fatal right-sided intracerebral hemorrhage with associated contralateral hydrocephaly. The 23-year-old primigravid woman refused hospitalization for pregnancy-induced hypertension and she next was seen comatose with blood pressures as high as 260/160 mm Hg.

RUPTURED ANEURYSM. Bleeding from a ruptured aneurysm reportedly is more common during the second half of pregnancy, but about 20 percent bleed before midpregnancy (Dias and colleagues, 1990). There seems to be a relationship between pregnancy-associated hypertension and ruptured aneurysms. Henderson and Torbey (1988) described a case temporally related to crack cocaine smoking. Overall, the mortality rate of bleeding aneurysms during pregnancy is 35 percent (Dias and colleagues, 1990).

Prompt evaluation, usually including cerebral angiography, is important because rebleeding can be fatal and early neurosurgical intervention using clip ligation can prevent this. Giannotta and colleagues (1986) recommend that the workup be approached aggressively and as if these women were not pregnant. Treatment must be individualized. Whether to attempt repair of a potentially accessible vascular lesion during pregnancy is debatable. The advantages achieved by reducing the risk of a subsequent intracranial hemorrhage are obvious; however, the potential for adverse fetal effects from maternal hypotension and hypothermia during the surgical procedure is real. Because of maternal danger, it is our policy to favor repair, and if the woman is near term, cesarean delivery immediately followed by craniotomy has proven successful. Antifibrinolytic agents commonly are used in attempts to impede clot dissolution and in turn perhaps to reduce the risk of further hemorrhage. Because fibrinolytic activity already is reduced as the consequence of pregnancy per se, we have counseled against use of these agents in pregnancy or the immediate puerperium.

Following surgical repair, vaginal delivery is not prohibited. A major obstetrical problem concerns the management of delivery in women who survive intracranial hemorrhage, but in whom repair is not done. Some authorities, but certainly not all, favor cesarean delivery, and in cases in which the cerebral hemorrhage occurred shortly before or very early in pregnancy, some believe that therapeutic abortion is indicated. On the basis of a review of 142 cases of intracranial aneurysms that ruptured before or during pregnancy, Hunt and co-workers (1974) concluded that there is no contraindication to vaginal delivery. With an unrepaired aneurysm, Wiebers (1988) recommends cesarean delivery only if bleeding occurred in the third trimester.

ARTERIOVENOUS MALFORMATIONS. Vascular malformations causing subarachnoid hemorrhage are uncommon. According to Horton and co-workers (1990), the incidence of bleeding from cerebral arteriovenous malformations is not increased during pregnancy. Simolke and associates (1991) encountered only one case in nearly 90,000 deliveries cared for at our hospital (Fig. 55–2). Although it is commonly accepted that bleeding from these malformations occurs with similar frequency throughout gestation, Dias and colleagues (1990) reported an increased

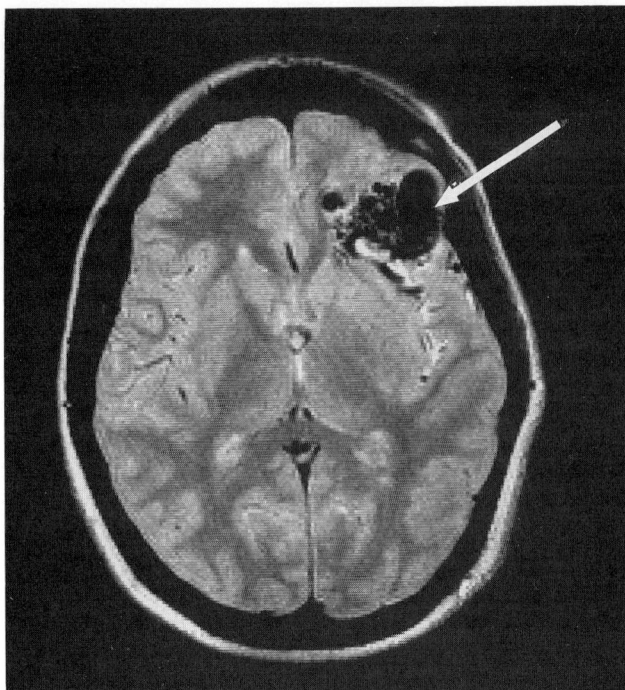

Fig. 55–2. Magnetic resonance image of a left-sided frontal lobe arteriovenous malformation. The lesion caused subarachnoid bleeding at 29 weeks in a 24-year-old primigravida who presented with severe headache, nausea, and vomiting. (From Simolke and colleagues, 1991, with permission.)

frequency with advancing gestational age. About 10 percent of initial bleeding episodes are fatal in nonpregnant patients (Itoyama and colleagues, 1989), but Dias and associates (1990) reported a mortality rate of 28 percent with similar bleeding events during pregnancy.

There is no general agreement in nonpregnant patients whether all of these lesions should be resected, even if they are accessible. Without surgical therapy, about 5 to 7 percent will bleed again within the first year, and perhaps 2 to 3 percent per year thereafter (Itoyama and associates, 1989). In pregnancy, management decisions to operate should be based on neurosurgical considerations. Because these lesions commonly rebleed, the conduct of labor and delivery following a bleeding episode during pregnancy from an inoperable lesion is more critical than for aneurysmal hemorrhage. Although Dias and colleagues (1990) found no evidence to support better maternal outcome with cesarean delivery, it seems best to avoid vaginal delivery if the malformation was not corrected surgically.

Migraine Headaches

The term **migraine** describes periodic, hemicranial, throbbing headaches that are often accompanied by nausea and vomiting. They usually begin in childhood, adolescence, or young adulthood and tend to diminish both in frequency of recurrence as well as severity with advancing years. In a recent national survey, Stewart and colleagues (1992) reported that 18 percent of women and 6 percent of men suffer from migraine headaches. Such headaches especially are common in young women, and frequently there is premenstrual provocation. The exact pathophysiology is uncertain, but there is general agreement that prodromal neurological symptoms are caused by cerebral artery vasoconstriction and decreased blood flow. Presumably, vasodilation follows and is responsible for the headache. Serotonin has been implicated in this mechanism (Lance, 1992).

Migraine or vascular headaches present in three clinical patterns. **Classical migraine** has prominent neurological prodromata such as visual scintillations, dazzling lines, photophobias, scotomatas, dizziness, and tinnitus. In **common migraine,** headache begins abruptly and it is frequently accompanied by nausea and vomiting. **Complicated migraine** is accompanied by neurological symptoms which may include parasthesias, paresis, and even temporary paralysis that resembles a stroke. Although full recovery usually occurs within minutes to hours, there may be permanent neurological residua.

Effects of Pregnancy. There is said to be dramatic improvement of migraine during pregnancy. Certainly, we seldom encounter severe migraines in pregnant women at Parkland Hospital. Uknis and Silberstein (1991) reviewed four studies in which nearly 800 pregnant women were surveyed. Almost 70 percent of women with prior migraines noted improvement during pregnancy. Perhaps paradoxically, in most of these studies, about 15 percent of migraine headaches first appeared during a pregnancy.

Management. Most migraine headaches respond to simple analgesics, such as aspirin or acetaminophen, especially if given early in the course of symptoms. Ergotamine preparations are successful in preventing headaches when taken during the prodrome. Almost 90 percent of classical migraines can be aborted by ergotamine. Because they cause vasoconstriction and have oxytocic properties, these drugs should be avoided if possible; however, their effects on the pregnant uterus are not nearly so profound as ergonovine. Once the headache has become intense, ergot is of little help. For severe headaches not responsive to aspirin or acetaminophen, codeine or meperidine is given along with promethazine for its antiemetic and sedative effects.

For women with frequent migraine attacks, prophylactic therapy is indicated. Propranolol, 20 to 40 mg three times daily, or atenolol, 50 to 100 mg daily, have been used with success. Calcium-channel blockers, nifedipine or verapamil (both category C), may be beneficial in preventing headaches in migraineurs. More recently, sumatriptan, a serotonin agonist, has been used successfully to treat migraine attacks (Sumatriptan International Study Group, 1991). Its use in pregnancy has not been evaluated.

Demyelinating and Degenerative Diseases

Demyelinating diseases comprise a group of neurological disorders that have in common focal or patchy destruction of central nervous system myelin sheaths accompanied by an inflammatory response. The degenerative diseases frequently are inherited, and they are characterized by gradually evolving and progressive neuronal death from unknown causes.

Multiple Sclerosis. This chronic demyelinating neurological disorder of unknown etiology usually begins in young adults. It may be immune mediated, and it is characterized clinically by recurrent attacks of focal or multifocal neurological dysfunction with random exacerbations and remissions. In many cases, the first attack is so mild that it goes unnoticed. Typically, early in the disease, attacks last 2 to 3 days, followed by complete recovery over several weeks. As these attacks become more frequent, recovery is not complete, and permanent deficits accrue. In a third of cases, multiple sclerosis pursues a progressive downhill course from its first manifestation.

Classical symptoms include impaired vision and over 40 percent of patients have *optic neuritis* during the course of disease. In fact, 75 percent of women who have isolated optic neuritis will go on to develop multiple sclerosis within 15 years. Other common symptoms are nystagmus, dysarthria, diminished vibratory sense, ataxia and intention tremor, limb weakness, spasticity, and bladder dysfunction. The diagnosis usually is made clinically and confirmed by magnetic resonance imaging. The characteristic multifocal white matter lesions are present in more than 90 percent of patients. The pathological hallmarks of these lesions are termed *plaques*, which represent discrete areas of demyelination.

There is no effective treatment. Corticosteroids may diminish the severity of acute flares, but they have no effect on permanent disability. Immunosuppressive therapy with azathioprine and cyclophosphamide has not been accepted by all as efficacious. Plasma exchange in combination with immunosuppressive therapy is under investigation.

Effect on Pregnancy. Multiple sclerosis rarely complicates pregnancy, and there is no evidence that pregnancy precipitates the disease in women who were destined to develop it. In most cases, pregnancy has no deleterious effect on the course of multiple sclerosis; however, about a third of women have an exacerbation during the first few months postpartum (Nelson and colleagues, 1988). Birk and co-workers (1990) summa-

rized six retrospective studies totaling nearly 900 pregnancies. Multiple sclerosis worsened during pregnancy in only 10 percent, but 30 percent had worsening in the puerperium. Conversely, Frith and McLeod (1988) cite data that pregnancy may ameliorate multiple sclerosis. They questioned 52 women and reported that during 85 pregnancies the relapse rate was significantly reduced during the first two trimesters. Although not decreased, relapses were not increased in the third trimester or up to 6 months postpartum.

If uncomplicated, multiple sclerosis has no adverse effects on pregnancy outcome. Women may become fatigued easier, and those with bladder dysfunction are prone to symptomatic urinary infection. Labor is unaffected, and the indications for cesarean delivery are obstetrical. Spinal analgesia anecdotally has been associated with exacerbations, but epidural analgesia is considered safe by some (Donaldson, 1989). Bader and colleagues (1988) performed epidural block for five women undergoing cesarean delivery and nine for labor analgesia. Although their observations suggested that 0.5 percent bupivacaine was associated with a higher relapse rate postpartum, they concluded that epidural analgesia was safe.

Perinatal outcome is not altered significantly, but the incidence of multiple sclerosis in the offspring is increased nearly 15-fold. Breast feeding is not associated with an increase in postpartum exacerbations (Nelson and colleagues, 1988).

Huntington Disease. Huntington disease is a degenerative disease of the cerebral cortex and basal ganglia. It is characterized by a combination of choreoathetotic movements and progressive dementia that usually begins in mid-adult life. The disease is more widely distributed than once thought, and there are an estimated 25,000 affected persons in the United States (Hayden and colleagues, 1987). Although it characteristically advances slowly over 15 to 20 years, the earlier the onset, the more severely progressive is the syndrome.

Huntington disease is inherited as an autosomal dominant trait, and the gene is localized to the terminal segment of the short arm of chromosome 4. With the description of several DNA probes, as well as the use of the polymerase chain reaction, prenatal diagnosis now is possible. Affected fetuses in some families can be predicted with great accuracy by linkage analysis (Skraastad and colleagues, 1991).

Myasthenia Gravis

Myasthenia gravis is an acquired immune-mediated neuromuscular disorder with a prevalence of about 1 in 10,000. The disease has a predilection for women of childbearing age and is more common in those with the HLA-B8 antigen. The disease is caused by autoimmune antibodies that are directed against acetylcholine receptors at the postsynaptic muscle membrane. This results in a significant decrease in such functional receptors. Thus, even though acetylcholine is released normally, it produces diminished endplate action potentials that do not always trigger muscle action potentials; this results in weakened muscle contractions.

Clinically, myasthenia is characterized by muscle weakness and fatigability. Cranial muscles are involved early and disparately, and diplopia and ptosis are common. Facial muscle weakness causes difficulty in smiling, chewing, and speech. In 85 percent of patients the weakness becomes generalized. The course of the disease is variable, but it tends to be marked by exacerbations and remissions, especially when it first becomes clinically apparent. Remissions seldom are complete or permanent. Systemic diseases or concurrent infections may precipitate myasthenic crises.

Myasthenia gravis is very manageable but not curable. Anticholinesterase medications impede degradation of acetylcholine and bring about improvement, but seldom normalcy of muscle function. **Pyridostigmine,** an analog of neostigmine, is the most commonly used preparation. Ironically, its side effects with overdosage are increased weakness, and this is sometimes difficult to differentiate from myasthenic symptoms.

Nearly all patients respond to immunosuppressive therapy with corticosteroids and azathioprine. Cyclosporine is effective and is given to patients who cannot tolerate azathioprine (Tindall and associates, 1987). Cyclophosphamide is used only for refractory cases. Clinical improvement has been reported following intravenously administered immunoglobulin, and this may be life-saving in some cases (Minnefor and Oleske, 1987).

About 10 percent of patients have a **thymoma** and this should be surgically removed. Even without a tumor, 85 percent of patients respond to thymectomy and about one third undergo drug-free remission.

Effects on Pregnancy. There is no predictable response to pregnancy in the woman with myasthenia gravis. Like many chronic diseases, it may undergo remission, exacerbate, or remain stable throughout pregnancy. According to their review, Fennell and Ringel (1987), as well as Plauché (1991) found that two thirds of women improve or are unchanged during pregnancy whereas the other third worsen. Although the disease has no adverse general effects on pregnancy outcome, Plauché (1991) reported nine maternal deaths among 322 pregnancies. Most of these were due to complications of myasthenia.

Management during pregnancy includes close observation with liberal bedrest and prompt treatment of infection. Most of our patients have responded well to **pyridostigmine** administered every 3 to 4 hours. Those in remission who become pregnant while taking corticosteroids or azathioprine should continue these medications. Acute myasthenia onset or its exacerbation—the so-called *myasthenic crisis*—demands prompt admission and supportive care. Plasmapheresis should be used for emergency situations (Fennell and Ringel, 1987). There is one report of thymectomy performed in a 17-week pregnant woman (Ip and colleagues, 1986).

Most women with myasthenia gravis tolerate labor without difficulty. Careful observation and prompt respiratory support is essential. Narcotics must be used with care and epidural or spinal analgesia are acceptable. Cesarean delivery is done for obstetrical indications. During the second stage of labor, some women may have impairment of voluntary expulsive efforts, and forceps delivery should be considered. Any drug with a curare-like effect must be used with extreme caution; for example, magnesium sulfate, muscle relaxants used with general anesthesia, and aminoglycoside antibiotics.

Neonatal Effects. Acetylcholine-receptor antibodies have been detected in most myasthenic patients, and these IgG antibodies are transferred readily from mother to fetus. Despite this, only about 15 percent of neonates develop symptoms. According to Donaldson and associates (1981), this is more likely if neonatal antibody levels are high. Transient symptomatic myasthenia gravis in the affected infant is typically demonstrated by a feeble cry, poor suckling, and respiratory distress which are corrected by parenteral neostigmine. Neonatal myasthenia also responds to small doses of edrophonium or pyridostigmine and most often completely subsides within 2 to 6 weeks. Without prompt recognition and treatment, including good nursing care, the affected neonate may succumb to respiratory insufficiency and aspiration due to muscular weakness. In most cases, the fetus appears to be protected while in utero by a factor, perhaps alphafetoprotein, that inhibits the interaction between the antibody and receptors (Noronha, 1985). Carr and colleagues (1991) reported a case in which serial plasmaphereses and prednisone were used to treat a woman who previously had delivered two infants with malformations presumably due to fetal myasthenia gravis.

Neuropathies

Peripheral neuropathy is a general term used to describe a disorder of peripheral nerve(s) due to a variety of possible causes. Its discovery should prompt a search for an etiology. Polyneuropathies are often associated with systemic diseases. For example, diabetes is the most common cause in women of childbearing ages. Drugs or environmental toxins also may cause a polyneuropathy, and there is an imposing list of genetically determined diseases. Mononeuropathies signify focal involvement of a single nerve trunk and imply a local causation such as trauma, compression, or entrapment.

Guillain-Barré Syndrome. This acute demyelinating polyneuropathy shows a similar worldwide incidence. In over two thirds of cases, it follows clinical or serological evidence for viral infections, especially cytomegalovirus and Epstein-Barr virus. Approximately 10 percent of cases develop within weeks following a surgical procedure. In 1977, there was an "epidemic" of Guillain-Barré syndrome following immunization against swine influenza. The disease is thought to be immune-mediated, but its pathogenesis is unclear. Current data support the concept of primary lymphocytic T-cell infiltration as an aberrant response to the precipitating infection (Ropper, 1992).

Clinical features include arreflexic paralysis with mild sensory disturbances. There also may be evidence for autonomic dysfunction, and the full syndrome takes 1 to 3 weeks to develop. Management is supportive, and these patients should be hospitalized because about 25 percent will need ventilatory assistance. Corticosteroids have not been effective. Plasmapheresis has been shown to be of benefit if begun within 1 to 2 weeks of symptoms, but if disease progression has plateaued, plasmapheresis is not helpful. Almost 85 percent of patients will have full recovery, but about 3 percent will die from complications of the acute condition.

Effect on Pregnancy. The incidence of Guillain-Barré syndrome likely is not affected by pregnancy. Hurley and colleagues (1991) described three pregnancies complicated by this syndrome and reviewed 31 others. About one third required ventilatory support, and overall maternal mortality was 13 percent. As in nonpregnant patients, after an insidious onset, paresis and paralysis most often continue to ascend, and respiratory insufficiency then becomes a common and serious problem. Bravo and associates (1982) successfully ventilated a mother for 5 weeks before delivery of a healthy infant who did not appear to be affected neurologically.

Pregnancy is not a contraindication to plasmapheresis. The Guillain-Barré Syndrome Study Group (1985) randomized nearly 250 affected nonpregnant patients to treatment with plasmapheresis. Benefits included a shorter duration of paralysis and a lessened severity. Hurley and associates (1991) described successful outcomes in three pregnant women with impending ventilatory failure in whom plasmapheresis was performed.

More recently, van der Meché and colleagues (1992) showed that high-dose intravenous immune globulin was as effective as plasma exchange for treatment of Guillain-Barré syndrome in nonpregnant patients. Indeed, Ropper (1992) postulates that globulin infusion will become the preferred treatment.

Bell Palsy. Cranial nerves are susceptible to disorders that rarely affect peripheral nerves. One of these, isolated facial nerve palsy, or Bell palsy, is relatively common. It is thought to be a viral-induced mononeuropathy. Its onset is usually abrupt with maximum weakness within 48 hours. In some cases, hyperacusis and loss of taste accompany varying degrees of facial muscle paralysis. Electromyography may be helpful in determining prognosis; if denervation extends beyond 10 days, healing will be delayed and likely incomplete.

Pregnancy and Bell Palsy. Pregnancy seems to be complicated by a disparate number of cases of Bell palsy. Prescott (1988) described that 12 percent of 461 female patients were pregnant. Falco and Eriksson (1989) report an incidence of 1 in 2500 births at Brigham and Women's Hospital. These cases typically develop in late gestation, and three fourths of the 55 cases reported by Prescott (1988) were in the third trimester.

Pregnancy does not alter the overall good prognosis for spontaneous recovery of Bell palsy, and nearly 90 percent of affected women will recover function within a few weeks to months. Treatment with short-term corticosteroids remains controversial, but the bulk of evidence suggests that these drugs do not hasten resolution (McGregor and associates, 1987; Prescott, 1988). Surgical decompression is not routinely recommended. Supportive care includes prevention of injury to the constantly exposed cornea, facial muscle massage, and reassurance that the woman will likely regain total neurological function.

Carpal Tunnel Syndrome. Hand symptoms, presumably caused by nerve compression, are common during pregnancy. The median nerve is especially vulnerable to compression within the carpal tunnel at the wrist. According to Voitk and colleagues (1983), as many as 25 percent of women complain of symptoms of median nerve compression. Conversely, McLennan and associates (1987) found that only 20 percent of women who reported hand symptoms had evidence for median nerve compression. In a carefully performed prospective investigation, Ekman-Ordeberg and colleagues (1987) verified carpal tunnel syndrome in 2.3 percent of almost 2400 pregnant women. Typically, a woman awakens with burning, numbness, or tingling in the thenar half of one or both hands. Symptoms are bilateral in 80 percent of cases. The fingers feel numb and useless.

Carpal tunnel syndrome is self-limited, and treatment is symptomatic. A splint applied to the very slightly flexed wrist and worn during sleep usually provides relief. Ekman-Ordeberg and colleagues (1987) reported that this relieved pain in 80 percent of 56 women. Only three required surgical decompression. The signs and symptoms most often regress after delivery, and in our experiences, surgical decompression and corticosteroid injections have not been necessary. If severe pain persists, however, these treatments should be considered.

The syndrome should be distinguished from **De Quervain tendinitis** caused by swelling of the conjoined tendons and sheaths near the distal radius. Schumacher and colleagues (1985) described six women with De Quervain tendinitis during pregnancy, and two also had carpel tunnel syndrome.

Spinal Cord Injury

Trauma, especially motor vehicle accidents, accounts for most spinal cord injuries. Typically, the cervical or thoracic spine is involved, and most patients are young adults. Lesions caused by trauma or tumor do not prevent conception, and pregnancy outcome usually is good. However, pregnancy will likely be complicated by urinary infections, anemia, pressure necrosis of skin, and aggravation of constipation. Hughes and colleagues (1991) described 17 such women, and all but one had a urinary infection during pregnancy. If the lesion is above T_{10}, cough reflex will be impaired, and pulmonary function should be determined before and carefully monitored throughout pregnancy.

Autonomic hyperreflexia is common with lesions above T_{5-6} because of splanchnic nerve overstimulation and lack of central inhibition. It is characterized by sudden sympathetic stimulation below the cord lesion causing a throbbing headache, facial flushing, and paroxysmal hypertension. A number of stimuli, including urethral, bladder, rectal, or cervical distention, caused by catheterization, rectal examination, or cervical dilatation, may precipitate dangerous hypertension which should be treated immediately (Young and associates, 1983).

Uterine contractions are not affected by cord lesions. Indeed, labor often is easy—even precipitous—and comparatively painless. If the lesion is below T_{12}, then contractions are felt normally. There is great concern that women with lesions above T_{12} may deliver at home unattended before they realize that labor has begun. Serial examinations with admission for advanced cervical dilation or effacement may prevent this, and the Committee on Obstetrics (1990) recommends weekly cervical examinations beginning at 28 weeks. These women also can be taught to palpate uterine contractions; alternatively, home tocodynamometry can be used. Hughes and associates (1991) recommend elective admission between 36 and 37 weeks.

Delivery is preferably vaginal. The Committee on Obstetrics (1990) recommends continuous cardiac rhythm monitoring along with intra-arterial pressure monitoring. Epidural or spinal analgesia is used to minimize autonomic hyperreflexia. In some cases, second-stage labor may be prolonged due to diminished expulsive efforts. Because trauma causing paraplegia also may cause pelvic deformity and, in turn, fetopelvic disproportion, cesarean delivery may be necessary. Greenspoon and Paul (1986), as well as Hughes and associates (1991) have provided concise reviews of care for these women.

Shunts for Maternal Hydrocephalus

About 20 cases of pregnancy have been described in women with ventriculoperitoneal shunts for hydrocephalus (Cusimano and colleagues, 1990; Houston and Clein, 1989). Pregnancy outcomes have usually been satisfactory. Although half of women with ventriculoperitoneal shunts have been reported to have shunt obstruction, typically late in pregnancy, this probably is reporting bias. A number of such women have been cared for at Parkland Hospital and in none has the shunt become obstructed. Symptoms of obstruction include headache, nausea and vomiting, and impaired consciousness. Computed tomography discloses acute hydrocephaly which can be relieved by tapping the shunt or pumping it several times daily. Complications are more common with ventriculoatrial shunts, at least in nonpregnant patients.

In women with shunts, vaginal delivery is preferred, and unless there is a meningomyelocele, epidural analgesia is permitted. Antimicrobial prophylaxis is indicated if the peritoneal cavity is entered for cesarean delivery or tubal sterilization.

Maternal Brain Death

A few instances of maternal brain death during pregnancy have been described in which life support systems and parenteral alimentation were utilized for extended periods of time while the fetus achieved maturity (Dillon and associates, 1982; Field and colleagues, 1988). In the case described by Bernstein and co-workers (1989), life support was begun at 15 weeks' gestation for a brain dead woman and continued until 32 weeks. The ethical, financial, and legal implications, both civil and criminal, that may arise from attempting—or not attempting—such care are profound!

Benign Intracranial Hypertension (Pseudotumor Cerebri)

Benign intracranial hypertension is characterized by headache, stiff neck, visual disturbances, and papilledema from increased intracranial pressure in an otherwise healthy individual. Its cause is thought to be overproduction or underabsorption of cerebrospinal fluid. It commonly is found in young women, especially those who are obese, or who recently have gained weight. It is probably not more prevalent during pregnancy as once believed (Ireland and associates, 1990). Criteria for diagnosis include elevated cerebrospinal fluid pressure, normal cerebrospinal fluid composition, and normal cranial computed tomography or magnetic resonance imaging. In some patients, spinal fluid protein concentration may be low. Interestingly, Bates and associates (1982) reported that men and nonpregnant women with this condition had significantly increased cerebrospinal fluid prolactin concentrations.

Usually, but not always, pseudotumor is self-limited; however, optic atrophy can cause blindness. Permanent visual impairment may develop in a significant number of patients. Treatment is aimed at prevention of visual defects by lowering the elevated pressure. Repetitive lumbar punctures to remove cerebrospinal fluid will lower pressure. If there is no ventriculomegaly, lumbar punctures are not associated with brainstem herniation. Drugs given to lower pressure include acetazolamide, furosemide, or dexamethasone. In rare cases, lumboperitoneal shunting of spinal fluid is necessary.

Effects of Pregnancy. There have been several reviews published about the effects of pregnancy on the course of benign intracranial hypertension (Digre and colleagues, 1984; Kassam and associates, 1983; Peterson and Kelly, 1985). The condition is usually detected by midpregnancy, is self-limited, and resolves postpartum. Headache is the presenting symptom in 95 percent of women, and almost 75 percent have blurred vision (Peterson and Kelly, 1985).

As discussed, it is arguable that the incidence of pseudotumor is increased in pregnancy. Katz and colleagues (1989) reported the incidence of pseudotumor cerebri complicating pregnancy to be about 1 in 1000. They described 11 such pregnancies and concluded that pregnancy increased the likelihood of symptoms in women who already had intracranial hypertension. They also reported a 30 percent recurrence rate.

Treatment of benign intracranial hypertension during pregnancy is identical to that for nonpregnant women. From their review of 54 pregnancies, Katz and associates (1989) did not find an increased incidence of adverse perinatal outcomes. Labor is permitted, the route of delivery is decided by obstetrical indications, and epidural analgesia is not contraindicated.

Chorea Gravidarum

Chorea gravidarum describes any chorea that occurs during pregnancy. Because cases in the past were linked to rheumatic fever, chorea now is a rare complication. Zegart and Schwarz (1968) identified only one case due to rheumatic fever in nearly 140,000 deliveries, and our experiences at Parkland Hospital are similar. In over half of these cases, the woman previously had suffered chorea which sooner or later spontaneously abated as it is likely to do during or after pregnancy. Recurrence in subsequent pregnancies occurs in perhaps 20 percent of patients. Pregnancy outcome probably is not affected. Chlorpromazine or haloperidol have been used to treat the disorder.

A more common cause of chorea is collagen-vascular disease, and up to 2 percent of patients with systemic lupus erythematosus exhibit chorea (Branch, 1990). Most of these patients have antiphospholipid antibodies (see Chap. 54, p. 1234).

PSYCHIATRIC DISORDERS

Pregnancy and the puerperium are at times sufficiently stressful to induce psychosis. Mental illness may represent remission or exacerbation of pre-existing psychiatric disorders, or it may be the onset of a new disorder.

Psychological Adjustment to Pregnancy. Pregnancy, despite often evoking overwhelming joy, is stressful for most women. In some women with ambivalent feelings about the pregnancy, stress may be appreciably increased. A woman's response to stress may be seen in a variety of subtle or not so subtle ways. For example, most women express concerns about whether their baby is "normal." For those whose fetus is at higher risk for a congenital malformation, stress is increased (Tunis and Golbus, 1991). As pregnancy progresses, the woman's somatic image becomes distorted, and she may have concerns about her physical attractiveness. Throughout pregnancy, and especially toward the end, plans should be made for child care and the lifestyle changes that will ensue after delivery. In a number of women, the fear of childbirth pain is particularly stressful.

Issues concerning mental health of the pregnant woman should not be overlooked. Screening for mental illness should be elicited during the first prenatal examination. This includes obtaining a history of any prior treatment of psychiatric disorders, including hospitalizations and outpatient care. Prior or current use of psychoactive medications should be documented and any use of alcohol and illicit drugs should be noted. Current symptoms that might indicate mental dysfunction should be investigated. According to Oates (1989), 15 to 20 percent of pregnant women will have mental health issues that need to be considered in their management.

Classification of Mental Disorders

In 1987, the American Psychiatric Association published its revised third edition of the Diagnostic and Statistical Manual (DSM-IIIR). This system, currently used in the United States, includes the diagnostic classification of mental disorders.

Major mood disorders include major depression, considered a unipolar disorder, and manic-depressive illness, considered a bipolar disorder. These may be primary or secondary. Primary disorders occur for the first time de novo, and both depressive and manic disorders are significantly influenced by genetic factors. Secondary mood disorders, especially depression, may develop in conjunction with other psychiatric illnesses (for example, schizophrenia and personality disorders), or they may be associated with medical illnesses. As many as two thirds of suicides in this country are associated with these major mood disorders.

Schizophrenic disorders are major forms of mental illness, and they are common with a lifetime prevalence rate of about 1 percent. The hallmarks of this psychosis include delusions, hallucinations, incoherence, and inappropriate affect. Four major types of schizophrenia are recognized: catatonic, disorganized, paranoid, and undifferentiated. Schizophrenia has a major genetic component, and there is 65 percent concordance with monozygotic twins. If one parent is schizophrenic, the empirical risk to their offspring is 5 to 10 percent. With appropriate treatment, the 5-year social recovery is 60 percent. For all patients, at 5 years, half are employed, 30 percent are mentally handicapped, and 10 percent require continued hospitalization.

Anxiety disorders refer to paroxysmal and persistent psychological feelings of dread, irritability, and ruminations that occur along with physiological changes such as sweating, dyspnea, insomnia, and trembling. Anxiety disorders are commonly encountered in everyday medical practices, and they are more easily recognized when subdivided into panic disorders, obsessive-compulsive disorders, posttraumatic stress disorders, and phobic disorders.

Personality disorders are a result of chronic misuse of certain coping mechanisms in an inappropriate, stereotyped, and maladaptive manner. The Diagnostic and Statistical Manual recognizes three *clusters* of personality disorders: (1) Paranoid, schizoid, and schizotypal personality disorders are characterized by oddness or eccentricity. (2) Histrionic, narcissistic, antisocial, and borderline disorders all are characterized by dramatic presentations along with self-centeredness and erratic behavior. (3) Avoidant, dependent, compulsive, and passive-aggressive personalities are characterized by underlying fear and anxiety. Genetic and environmental factors are important in the genesis of these disorders whose prevalence may be as high as 20 percent. Management is through psychotherapy; however, only about 20 percent of affected individuals recognize their problems and seek psychiatric help.

Effects of Pregnancy on Mental Illness

For nearly 150 years, the puerperium has been recognized as a time of great risk for mental illness (Brockington and colleagues, 1990). According to Gitlin and

Pasnau (1989), a severe and frequently psychotic episode follows delivery in 1 to 2 per 1000 births. The Diagnostic and Statistical Manual does not include puerperal psychoses as a separate listing. Still, a woman is 20 times more likely to require admission for a psychiatric illness in the month following delivery than she is in the previous two years. Platz and Kendell (1988) could not differentiate puerperal psychoses from those occurring at other times. Importantly, preexisting mental illness has a high recurrence rate in the puerperium. For women with an affective disorder, the risk of puerperal psychosis is 20 to 25 percent (Gitlin and Pasnau, 1989). Despite this predilection, suicide is uncommon during pregnancy and the year following delivery (Appleby, 1991).

It is difficult to distinguish biochemical factors as a primary cause of mental illness in the puerperium per se. This is true because the stress of childbirth in some women can precipitate mental illness. For example, women who give birth to twins are more likely to experience depression (Thorpe and associates, 1991). In their review, Tunis and Golbus (1991) noted increased anxiety in early and late pregnancy. Brockington and colleagues (1990) compared 88 women admitted to a psychiatric mother-and-baby unit with 80 randomly selected women who had completed an uncomplicated pregnancy. Surprisingly, although only 15 percent of women with mental illnesses had a provoking event during pregnancy, 36 percent of those who were healthy reported such events. These investigators, therefore, concluded that puerperal psychosis was not associated with environmental stress. Conversely, they found a strong association between prenatal depression and social stress.

Biochemical Changes. Wieck and associates (1991) reported that onset of affective psychoses was associated with increased sensitivity of dopamine receptors in the hypothalamus and other central nervous system sites. They postulated that these were triggered by falling estrogen levels that characterize the puerperium. Gitlin and Pasnau (1989) cited several studies in which attempts were made to establish a relationship between changes in hormone levels, tryptophan metabolism, and monoamine oxidase levels in platelets and postpartum mental changes.

Treatment During Pregnancy. A large number of psychotropic medications now are available for management of mental disorders. Some of these, their general use, and pregnancy-risk categories are shown in Table 55–2. They are discussed in greater detail in Chapter 42 (p. 968).

Antidepressants include tricylic compounds, monoamine oxidase inhibitors, tetracyclic compounds, and derivatives of other chemical classes such as fluoxetine. These drugs are commonly ingested for suicidal attempts,

TABLE 55–2. SOME COMMONLY USED PSYCHOTROPIC MEDICATIONS

Indication/Drug	Risk Category	Comments
Antidepressants		
Amitriptyline	D	Questionable teratogen
Imipramine	D	Questionable teratogen
Fluoxetine	B	Animal studies only
Antipsychotics		
Chlorpromazine	C	Not a proven teratogen
Clozapine	B	Animal studies only
Haloperidol	C	Limited data available
Anxiolytics		
Diazepam	D	Possibly teratogenic
Manic-Depressive Disorders		
Lithium	D	Fetal cardiovascular anomalies

Data from Briggs and colleagues (1990).

and their abuse follows that of alcohol-drug combinations and heroin as causes of drug-related deaths.

Antipsychotic medications sedate, tranquilize, and attenuate aggressive and impulsive behavior. They also cause disinterest and lack of initiative. They are primarily used for treatment of schizophrenia.

A large number of **anxiolytic medications** are available, and they are the drug of choice for generalized anxiety disorders. Benzodiazepines are prescribed most frequently, and diazepam is the prototype of their class. One characteristic is their very long elimination half-life, which for diazepam is 20 to 90 hours.

Use of these drugs results in a significant risk of withdrawal symptoms.

Lithium is the drug of choice for treating acute manic episodes and for the prevention of recurrent episodes of both mania and depression in bipolar disorders. Outside of pregnancy, it is considered very safe when used knowledgeably. When taken during early pregnancy, it has been associated with increased congenital malformations, especially cardiovascular, and it is classified as category D (Chap. 42, p. 969).

Electroconvulsive Therapy. Treatment of depression with electroshock during pregnancy has not been extensively evaluated. A review by Repke and Berger (1984) indicates that there is no fetal danger from such therapy. Griffiths and colleagues (1989) reported results obtained in a woman who underwent 11 such treatments from 23 to 31 weeks. They used thiamylal and succinylcholine anesthesia, intubation, and assisted ventilation during each treatment and observed that plasma levels of epinephrine, norepinephrine, and dopamine were elevated 2- to 3-fold within minutes of electroshock. Despite this, the fetal heart rate tracing and maternal heart rate, blood pressure and oxygen saturation remained normal. Varan and co-workers (1985) described a variable fetal heart rate deceleration characteristic of cord compression during electroconvulsive therapy. Sherer and associates (1991) described a woman who underwent seven weekly antepartum electroconvulsive treatments beginning at 30 weeks. Each treatment was followed by hypertension, uterine hypertonicity, and uterine bleeding (Fig. 55–3). Subsequently, placental abruption was shown to be the cause.

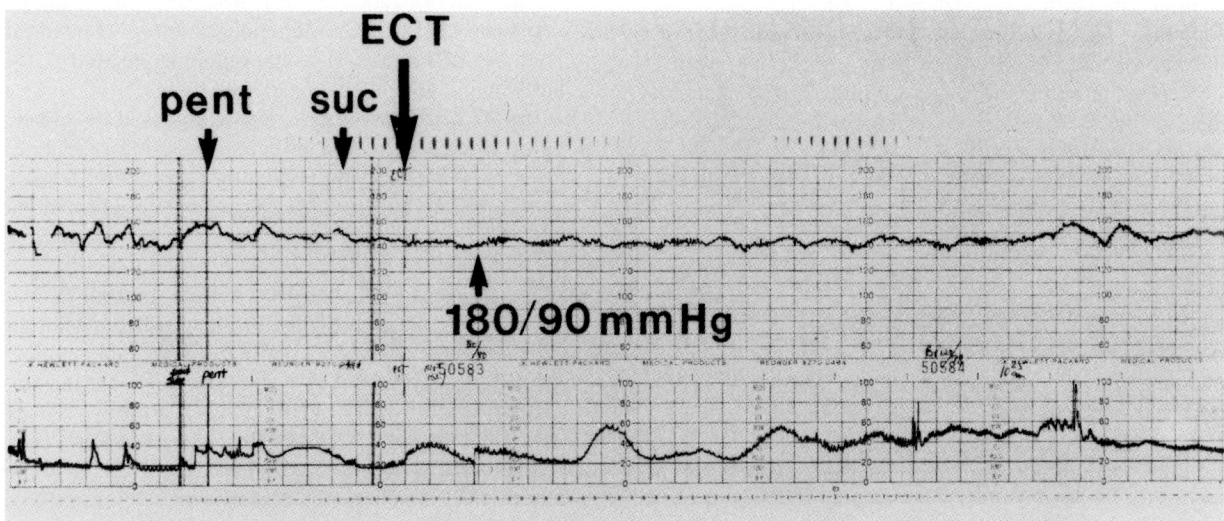

Fig. 55–3. Continuous fetal cardiotocography during electroconvulsive therapy at 34 weeks. Note regular uterine contractions and post-shock subsequent hypertonic-tetanic contractions. Medications before electroconvulsive therapy (ECT) and blood pressure after therapy are noted. (Pent = thiopental sodium; suc = succinylcholine; paper speed, 3 cm/min.) (From Sherer and colleagues, 1991, with permission.)

References

Appleby L: Suicide during pregnancy and in the first postnatal year. BMJ 302:137, 1991

Bader AM, Hunt CO, Datta S, Naulty JS, Ostheimer GW: Anesthesia for the obstetric patient with multiple sclerosis. J Clin Anesth 1:21, 1988

Bates GW, Whitworth NS, Parker JL, Johnson MP: Elevated cerebrospinal fluid prolactin concentration in women with pseudotumor cerebri. South Med J 75:807, 1982

Bernstein IM, Watson M, Simmons GM, Catalano PM, Davis G, Collins R: Maternal brain death and prolonged fetal survival. Obstet Gynecol 74:434, 1989

Birk K, Ford C, Smeltzer S, Ryan D, Miller R, Rudick RA: The clinical course of multiple sclerosis during pregnancy and the puerperium. Arch Neurol 47:738, 1990

Bjerkedal T, Bahana SL: The course and outcome of pregnancy in women with epilepsy. Acta Obstet Gynecol Scan 52:245, 1973

Branch DW: Antiphospholipid antibodies and pregnancy: Maternal implications. Semin Perinatol 14:139, 1990

Bravo RH, Katz M, Inturisi M, Cohen NH: Obstetric management of Landry-Guillain-Barré syndrome. Am J Obstet Gynecol 142:714, 1982

Briggs GG, Freeman RK, Yaffee SJ: Drugs in Pregnancy and Lactation, 3rd ed. Baltimore, Williams & Wilkins, 1990

Brockington IF, Martin C, Brown GW, Goldberg D, Margison F: Stress and puerperal psychosis. Br J Psych 157:331, 1990

Buehler BA, Delimont D, van Waes M, Finnell RH: Prenatal prediction of risk of the fetal hydantoin syndrome. N Engl J Med 322:1567, 1990

Carr SR, Gilchrist JM, Abuelo DN, Clark D: Treatment of antenatal myasthenia gravis. Obstet Gynecol 78:485, 1991

Centers for Disease Control: Valproate: A new cause of birth defects—report from Italy and follow-up from France. MMWR 32:439, 1983

Committee on Drugs, American Academy of Pediatrics: Psychotropic drugs in pregnancy and lactation. Pediatrics 69:241, 1982

Committee on Obstetrics: Maternal Fetal Medicine: ACOG Committee Opinion Number 83: Management of labor and delivery for patients with spinal cord injury. May, 1990

Cox SM, Hankins GDV, Leveno KJ, Cunningham FG: Bacterial endocarditis: A serious pregnancy complication. J Reprod Med 33:671, 1988

Cross JN, Castro PO, Jennett WB: Cerebral strokes associated with pregnancy and the puerperium. BMJ 3:214, 1968

Cusimano MD, Meffe FM, Gentili F, Sermer M: Ventriculoperitoneal shunt malfunction during pregnancy. Neurosurgery 27:969, 1990

Dalessio DJ: Seizure disorders and pregnancy. N Engl J Med 312:559, 1985

Delgado-Escueta AV, Treiman DM, Walsh GO: The treatable epilepsies. N Engl J Med 308:1508, 1983

Dias MS, Sekhar LN: Intracranial hemorrhage from aneurysms and arteriovenous malformations during pregnancy and the puerperium. Neurosurgery 27:855, 1990

Digre KB, Varner MW, Corbett JJ: Pseudotumor cerebri and pregnancy. Neurology 34:721, 1984

Dillon WP, Lee RV, Tronolone MJ, Buckwald S, Foote RJ: Life support and maternal death during pregnancy. JAMA 248:1089, 1982

Donaldson JO: Neurology of Pregnancy, 2nd ed. Philadelphia, Saunders, 1989

Donaldson JO: Stroke. Clin Obstet Gynecol 24:825, 1981

Donaldson JO, Penn AS, Lisak RP, Abramsky O, Brenner T, Schotland DL: Antiacetylcholine receptor antibody in neonatal myasthenia gravis. Am J Dis Child 135:222, 1981

Ekman-Ordeberg G, Sälgeback S, Ordeberg G: Carpal tunnel syndrome in pregnancy. A prospective study. Acta Obstet Gynecol Scand 66:233, 1987

Falco NA, Eriksson E: Idiopathic facial palsy in pregnancy and the puerperium. Surg Gynecol Obstet 169:337, 1989

Fennell DF, Ringel SP: Myasthenia gravis and pregnancy. Obstet Gynecol Surv 41:414, 1987

Field DR, Gates EA, Creasy RK, Jonsen AR, Laros RK Jr: Maternal brain death during pregnancy. JAMA 260:816, 1988

Frith JA, McLeod JG: Pregnancy and multiple sclerosis. J Neurol Neurosurg Psychiatry 51:495, 1988

Giannotta SL, Daniels J, Golde SH, Zelman V, Bayat A: Ruptured intracranial aneurysms during pregnancy. A report of four cases. J Reprod Med 31:139, 1986

Gitlin MJ, Pasnau RO: Psychiatric syndromes linked to reproductive function in women: A review of current knowledge. Am J Psychiatry 146:1413, 1989

Greenspoon JS, Paul RH: Paraplegia and quadriplegia: Special considerations during pregnancy and labor and delivery. Am J Obstet Gynecol 155:738, 1986

Griffiths EJ, Lorenz RP, Baxter S, Talon NS: Acute neurohumoral response to electroconvulsive therapy during pregnancy. A case report. J Reprod Med 34:907, 1989

Guillain-Barré Syndrome Study Group: Plasmapheresis and acute Guillain-Barré syndrome. Neurology 35:1096, 1985

Hayden MR, Kastelein JJP, Wilson RD, Hilbert C, Hewitt J, Langlois S, Fox S, Bloch M: First-trimester prenatal diagnosis for Huntington's disease with DNA probes. Lancet 1:1284, 1987

Henderson CE, Torbey M: Rupture of intracranial aneurysm associated with cocaine use during pregnancy. Am J Perinatol 5:142, 1988

Hiilesmaa VK, Teramo K, Granström M-L, Bardy AH: Serum folate concentration during pregnancy in women with epilepsy: Relation to antiepileptic drug concentrations, number of seizures, and fetal outcome. Br Med J 287:577, 1983

Horton JC, Chambers WA, Lyons SL, Adams RD, Kjellberg RN: Pregnancy and the risk of hemorrhage from cerebral arteriovenous malformations. Neurosurgery 27:867, 1990

Houston CS, Clein LJ: Ventriculoperitoneal shunt malfunction in a pregnant patient with meningomyelocele. CMAJ 141:701, 1989

Hughes SJ, Short DJ, Usherwood MMcD, Tebbutt H: Management of the pregnant women with spinal cord injuries. Br J Obstet Gynaecol 98:513, 1991

Hunt HB, Schrifin BS, Suzuki K: Ruptured berry aneurysms and pregnancy. Obstet Gynecol 43:827, 1974

Hurley TJ, Brunson AD, Archer RL, Lefler SF, Quirk JG: Landry Guillain-Barré Strohl syndrome in pregnancy: Report of three cases treated with plasmapheresis. Obstet Gynecol 78:482, 1991

Ireland B, Corbett JJ, Wallace RB: The search for causes of idiopathic intracranial hypertension. A preliminary case-control study. Arch Neurol 47:315, 1990

Ip MSM, So SY, Lam WK, Tang LCH, Mok CK: Thymectomy in

myasthenia gravis during pregnancy. Postgrad Med J 62:473, 1986

Itoyama Y, Uemura S, Ushio Y, Kuratsu J, Nonaka N: Natural course of unoperated intracranial arteriovenous malformation: Study of 50 cases. J Neurosurg 71:805, 1989

Jones KL, Lacro RV, Johnson KA, Adams J: Patterns of malformations in the children of women treated with carbamazepine during pregnancy. N Engl J Med 320:1661, 1989

Kassam SH, Hadi HA, Fadel HE, Sims W, Joy WM: Benign intracranial hypertension in pregnancy: Current diagnostic and therapeutic approach. Obstet Gynecol Surv 38:314 1983

Katz VL, Peterson R, Cefalo RC: Pseudotumor cerebri and pregnancy. Am J Perinatol 6:442, 1989

Kaunitz AM, Hughes JM, Grimes DA, Smith JC, Rochat RW, Kafrissen ME: Causes of maternal mortality in the United States. Obstet Gynecol 65:605, 1985

Kelly TE: Teratogenecity of anticonvulsant drugs, I. Review of the literature. Am J Med Genet 19:413, 1984

Kistler JP, Ropper AH, Martin JB: Cerebrovascular disease. In Wilson JD, Braunwald E, Isselbacher KJ, Petersdorf RG, Martin JB, Fauci AS, Root RK (eds): Harrison's Principles of Internal Medicine, 12th ed. New York, McGraw-Hill, 1991, p 1977

Kochenour NK, Emery MG, Sawchuk RJ: Phenytoin metabolism in pregnancy. Obstet Gynecol 56:577, 1980

Lance JW: Treatment of migraine. Lancet 339:1207, 1992

Lander CM, Eadie MJ: Plasma antiepileptic drug concentrations during pregnancy. Epilepsia 32:257, 1991

McGregor JA, Guberman A, Goodlin R: Idiopathic facial nerve paralysis (Bell's palsy) in late pregnancy and the early puerperium. Obstet Gynecol 69:435, 1987

McLennan HG, Oats JN, Walstab JE: Survey of hand symptoms in pregnancy. Med J Aust 147:542, 1987

Mercado A, Johnson G Jr, Calver D, Sokol RJ: Cocaine, pregnancy, and postpartum intracerebral hemorrhage. Obstet Gynecol 73:467, 1989

Minielly R, Yuzpe AA, Drake CG: Subarachnoid hemorrhage secondary to ruptured cerebral aneurysm in pregnancy. Obstet Gynecol 53:64, 1979

Minnefor AB, Oleske JM: Intravenous immune globulin: Efficacy and safety. Hosp Pract 22:171, 1987

Mountain KR, Hirsh J, Gallers AS: Neonatal coagulation defect due to anticonvulsant drug treatment in pregnancy. Lancet 1:265, 1970

Nelson KB, Ellenberg JH: Maternal seizure disorder, outcome of pregnancy, and neurologic abnormalities in the children. Neurology 32:1247, 1982

Nelson LM, Franklin GM, Jones MC, the Multiple Sclerosis Study Group: Risk of multiple sclerosis exacerbation during pregnancy and breast-feeding. JAMA 259:3441, 1988

Noronha A: Neurologic disorders during pregnancy and the puerperium. Clin Perinatol 12:695, 1985

Oates M: Management of major mental illness in pregnancy and the puerperium. Baillieres Clin Obstet Gynaecol 3:905, 1989

Pedley TA: Discontinuing antiepileptic drugs. N Engl J Med 318:982, 1988

Perucca E, Ruprah M, Richens A: Altered drug binding to serum proteins in pregnant women: Therapeutic relevance. J R Soc Med 74:422, 1981

Peterson CM, Kelly JV: Pseudotumor cerebri in pregnancy: Case reports and review of literature. Obstet Gynecol Surv 40:323, 1985

Platz C, Kendell RE: A matched-control follow-up and family study of "puerperal psychoses." Br J Psychiatry 153:90, 1988

Plauché WC: Myasthenia gravis in mothers and their newborns. Clin Obstet Gynecol 34:82, 1991

Prescott CAJ: Idiopathic facial nerve palsy. The effect of treatment with steroids. J Laryngol Otol 102:403, 1988

Repke JT, Berger NG: Electroconvulsive therapy in pregnancy. Obstet Gynecol 63:39S, 1984

Rochat RW, Koonin LM, Atrash HK, Jewett JJ and the Maternal Mortality Collaborative. Maternal mortality in the United States: Report from the Maternal Mortality Collaborative. Obstet Gynecol 72:91, 1988

Roos KL, Pascuzzi RM, Kuharik MA, Shapiro AD, Manco-Johnson M: Postpartum intracranial venous thrombosis associated with dysfunctional protein C and deficiency of protein S. Obstet Gynecol 76:492, 1990

Ropper AH: The Guillain-Barré syndrome. N Engl J Med 326:1130, 1992

Rosa FW: Spina bifida in infants of women treated with carbamazepine during pregnancy. N Engl J Med 324:674, 1991

Sachs BP, Brown DA, Driscoll SG, Schulman E, Acker D, Ransil BJ, Jewett JF: Maternal mortality in Massachusetts: Trends and prevention. N Engl J Med 316:667, 1987

Schmidt D, Canger R, Avanzini G, Battino D, Cusi C, Beck-Mannagetta G, Koch S, Rating D, Janz D: Change of seizure frequency in pregnant epileptic women. J Neurol Neurosurg Psychiatry 46:751, 1983

Schumacher HR Jr, Dorwart BB, Korzeniowski OM: Occurrence of De Quervain's tendinitis during pregnancy. Arch Intern Med 145:2083, 1985

Sherer DM, D'Amico ML, Warshal DP, Stern RA, Grunert HF, Abramowicz JS: Recurrent mild abruptio placenta occurring immediately after repeated electroconvulsive therapy in pregnancy. Am J Obstet Gynecol 165:652, 1991

Shorvon SD: Epidemiology, classification, natural history, and genetics of epilepsy. Lancet 336:93, 1990

Simolke GA, Cox SM, Cunningham FG: Cerebrovascular accidents complicating pregnancy and the puerperium. Obstet Gynecol 78:37, 1991

Skraastad MI, Verwest A, Bakker E, Vegter-van der Vlis M, van Leeuwend-Cornelisse I, Roos RAC, Pearson PL, van Ommen G-J B: Presymptomatic, prenatal, and exclusion testing for Huntington disease using seven closely linked DNA markers. Am J Med Genet 38:217, 1991

Srinivasan K: Ischemic cerebral vascular disease in the young. Two common causes in India. Stroke 15:733, 1984

Stewart WF, Lipton RB, Celentano DD, Reed ML: Prevalence of migraine headache in the United States: Relation to age, income, race and other sociodemographic factors. JAMA 267:64, 1992

Strickler SM, Dansky LV, Miller MA, Seni MH, Andermann E, Spielberg SP: Genetic predisposition to phenytoin-induced birth defects. Lancet 2:746, 1985

Sumatriptan International Study Group: Treatment of migraine attacks with sumatriptan. N Engl J Med 325:316, 1991

Thorpe K, Golding J, MacGillivray I, Greenwood R: Comparison of prevalence of depression in mothers of twins and mothers of singletons. BMJ 302:875, 1991

Tindall RS, Rollins JA, Phillips JT, Greenlee RG, Wells L, Belendiuk G: Preliminary results of a double-blind, randomized placebo-controlled trial of cyclosporine in myasthenia gravia. N Engl J Med 316:1987

Tunis SL, Golbus MS: Assessing mood states in pregnancy. Survey of the literature. Obstet Gynecol Surv 46:340, 1991

Uknis A, Silberstein SD: Migraine and Pregnancy. Headache 31:372, 1991

van der Meché FGA, Schmitz PIM, the Dutch Guillain-Barré Study Group: A randomized trial comparing intravenous immune globulin and plasma exchange in Guillain-Barré syndrome. N Eng J Med 326:1123, 1992

Varan LR, Gillieson MS, Skene DS, Sarwer-Foner GJ: ECT in an acutely psychotic pregnant woman with actively aggressive (homicidal) impulses. Can J Psychiatry 30:363, 1985

Voitk AJ, Mueller JC, Farlinger DE, Johnston RU: Carpel tunnel syndrome in pregnancy. Can Med Assoc J 129:277, 1983

Wiebers DO: Subarachnoid hemorrhage in pregnancy. Semin Neurol 8:226, 1988

Wiebers DO, Whisnant JP: The incidence of stroke among pregnant women in Rochester, Minn, 1955 through 1979. JAMA 253:3055, 1985

Wieck A, Kumar R, Hirst AD, Marks MN, Campbell IC, Checkley SA: Increased sensitivity of dopamine receptors and recurrence of affective psychosis after childbirth. BMJ 303:613, 1991

Wilhelm J, Morris D, Hotham N: Epilepsy and pregnancy—A review of 98 pregnancies. Aust NZ J Obstet Gynaecol 4:290, 1990

Young BK, Katz M, Klein SA: Pregnancy after spinal cord injury: Altered maternal and fetal response in labor. Obstet Gynecol 62:59, 1983

Zegart KN, Schwarz RH: Chorea gravidarum. Obstet Gynecol 32:24, 1968

CHAPTER 56
Dermatological Disorders

DISEASES OF THE SKIN

Most skin diseases are encountered with similar frequency in pregnant as in nonpregnant women. There are, however, a number of rather unique skin changes that are induced by the hormonal influences of pregnancy. For example, episodes of pruritus are common during pregnancy, and in many instances, itching is not accompanied by a skin eruption. The most common etiology of itching is intrahepatic cholestasis and bile salt retention, commonly known as pruritus gravidarum (Chap. 51, p. 1153). In addition, there is a group of pregnancy-specific dermatoses that usually are symptomatic and thus may be alarming. Importantly, some of these may be associated with adverse pregnancy outcomes.

Physiological Skin Changes in Pregnancy

A number of hormonal changes that are induced by normal pregnancy may have rather profound influences on the skin. As discussed in Chapters 6 and 8, fetoplacental production, stimulation, or alteration of metabolic clearance may increase the plasma availability of estrogens, progesterone, and a variety of androgens. Similarly, there are profound changes in the availability or concentrations of some adrenal steroids, including cortisol, aldosterone, and deoxycorticosterone. Presumably related to enlargement of the intermediate lobe of the pituitary gland, plasma levels of melanocyte-stimulating hormone (MSH) become remarkably elevated by the end of the second month of pregnancy. Finally, production of pro-opiomelanocortin has been demonstrated in placental extracts and this ultimately is a source of α- and β-melanocyte stimulating hormone.

Hyperpigmentation. According to Wong and Ellis (1984), some degree of skin darkening is observed in 90 percent of all pregnant women. Its exact cause is not known, but it is doubtful that elevated serum levels of melanocyte-stimulating hormone are responsible. Estrogens play a role in melanogenesis in mammals and may be the inciting factor. **Hyperpigmentation** is evident beginning early in pregnancy, and this is more marked in dark-skinned women. These effects, as perhaps expected, are more pronounced in naturally hyperpigmented areas such as the areolae, perineum, and umbilicus. Areas prone to friction, including the axillae

and inner thighs, may also become darkened. The linea alba becomes pigmented and is now called the **linea nigra.**

Pigmentation of the face, referred to as the mask of pregnancy, is also called **chloasma** or **melasma,** and is seen in at least half of pregnant women. Melasma is aggravated by sunlight or other ultraviolet light exposure; its severity may be altered by avoiding excessive exposure and using sunscreens. It is caused by melanin deposition into epidermal or dermal macrophages, and although the former usually regresses postpartum, dermal melanosis may persist up to 10 years in one third of women (Wong and Ellis, 1984). Oral contraceptives may aggravate melasma and should be avoided in susceptible women. If particularly disfiguring, topical application of 2 to 5 percent hydroxyquinone or 0.1 percent tretinoin ointment or cream may provide some improvement.

Benign or **melanocytic nevi** are found in some form in all persons. During pregnancy, these pigmented cutaneous tumors commonly enlarge and darken, and thus may be confused for a **malignant melanoma.** Although cutaneous nevi are shown histologically to have enlarged melanocytes and increased melanin deposition, there is no evidence that they undergo malignant transformation as a result of pregnancy (Winton and Lewis, 1982). According to the study by the World Health Organization Melanoma Program, the average malignant tumor is slightly but significantly thicker when discovered during pregnancy (MacKie and colleagues, 1991). These authors concluded that this represents either a delay in identification or pregnancy-induced melanoma stimulation. Malignant melanoma is discussed in detail in Chapter 57 (p. 1272).

Changes in Hair Growth. During pregnancy, presumably as a result of estrogen and perhaps androgen stimulation, there is an increased proportion of *anagen,* or growing hairs, to that of *telogen,* or resting hairs (Lynfield, 1960). Postpartum this ratio is reversed and shedding of hair becomes prominent. **Telogen effluvium** describes the rather abrupt hair loss that is seen beginning approximately 1 to 4 months postpartum. This process is sometimes characterized by alarming amounts of hair shedding usually associated with brushing or washing. Fortunately, the process is self-limited, and the woman may be reassured that normal hair growth is usually restored by 6 to 12 months.

Mild hirsutism is common during pregnancy, and

may be most noticeable on the face. Women who are predisposed genetically to coarse hair growth are affected most profoundly. More severe degrees of hirsutism are unusual, and if accompanied by other evidence for masculinization, should prompt consideration for another androgen source. We have seen pregnant women at Parkland Hospital who had virilization caused by adrenal tumors and luteomas (Chap. 8, p. 214).

Vascular Changes. Augmented cutaneous blood flow in pregnancy is associated with marked decreases in peripheral vascular resistance (Spetz, 1964). This is thought to serve to dissipate excess heat generated by increased metabolism. There are a number of presumably estrogen-induced changes in the small vessels that are encountered with some frequency. **Spider angiomas** are found in two thirds of white women and about 10 percent of African Americans during pregnancy (Wong and Ellis, 1984). Most of these vascular lesions regress postpartum. **Palmar erythema** is likewise more commonly noticed in whites (two thirds) than blacks (one third). **Capillary hemangiomas,** especially of the head and neck, are seen in about 5 percent of women during pregnancy.

One vascular condition that may be distressing is pregnancy **gingivitis,** which is caused by growth of the gum capillaries. This so-called **epulis of pregnancy** may become more severe as gestation progresses, but it may be controlled by proper dental hygiene and avoidance of trauma. Epulis should not be confused with **pyogenic granuloma** of pregnancy, which is also called **granuloma gravidarum.** These lesions are typical pyogenic granulomas, which are found in the oral cavity and often arise from the gingival papillae.

Dermatoses of Pregnancy

A number of dermatological conditions have been identified as being unique to pregnancy, or if not unique, encountered with a greater frequency during gestation. Except for **pruritus gravidarum,** which is probably a mild variant of intrahepatic cholestasis of pregnancy (see Chap. 51, p. 1153), most of these lesions are encountered uncommonly. Their gross appearances and clinical presentation sometimes may be confusing. Listed in Table 56–1 are some of the skin conditions that have been described.

Pruritic Urticarial Papules and Plaques of Pregnancy. Pruritic urticarial papules and plaques of pregnancy, also called PUPPP, is the most common pruritic dermatosis of pregnancy. It is characterized by an intensely pruritic cutaneous eruption that usually appears late during pregnancy (Table 56–1). The incidence has been reported to range from 0.25 to as high as 1 percent (Aronson and Halaska, 1991). Typically occurring late in pregnancy, erythematous urticarial papules and plaques

(Fig. 56–1) first develop on the abdomen, usually in the periumbilical area, and spread to the thighs and extremities (Alcalay and associates, 1987; Yancey and colleagues, 1984). Pruritus may be severe. In some women, the urticarial component predominates, while in others, the erythematous pattern is prominent. The erythematous patches are widespread. The face is usually spared, and seldom is there excoriation. **The disease is more common in nulliparas and seldom recurs in subsequent pregnancies.** It may resemble herpes gestationis, but there are no vesicles or bullae. Weiss and Hull (1992) describe a familial tendency and attribute the maternal response to a circulatory paternal factor.

On biopsy, immunofluorescent staining of dermis shows no immunoglobulin or complement deposition. Rather, there is a mild nonspecific lymphohistiocytic perivasculitis with an eosinophilic component. The absence of a linear band of C_3 in the basement membrane differentiates this dermatosis from herpes gestationis. Alcalay and associates (1988) found no differences between serum concentrations of β-chorionic gonadotropin, estradiol, and cortisol or urinary estriol excretion in 11 women with this dermatosis when compared with gestational-age-matched controls.

Treatment. Some women obtain relief from oral antihistamines and skin emollients, but most require topical corticosteroid creams or ointments for relief. Oral corticosteroids are given if these fail to relieve severe itching. The lesions invariably regress following delivery. Beltrani and Beltrani (1992) described a woman at 35 weeks whose pruritus was refractory to prednisone and whose symptoms were so severe that delivery by cesarean section was done. Pruritus resolved within hours and resolved totally in 2 days. There is no evidence that perinatal morbidity is increased (Yancey and associates, 1984).

Herpes Gestationis. Herpes gestationis, also called *pemphigoid gestationis,* is similar to bullous pemphigoid seen in elderly patients. Herpes gestationis is a serious but fortunately rare dermatological disease peculiar to pregnancy. According to Shornick (1987), the incidence is about 1 in 50,000 pregnancies. It has also been reported to accompany gestational trophoblastic disease. Unlike the name implies, it is not a viral-induced illness. This pruritic blistering skin eruption usually presents in multiparous women in late pregnancy, but may begin early in pregnancy or up to a week postpartum.

Herpes gestationis is characterized by an extremely pruritic widespread eruption with lesions that vary from erythematous and edematous papules to large, tense vesicles and bullae (Figs. 56–2 and 56–3). Common sites of involvement are the abdomen and the extremities. Exacerbations and remissions throughout pregnancy are common, and up to 80 percent of women suffer postpartum exacerbations (Shornick, 1987). In subsequent pregnancies the disease invariably recurs,

TABLE 56–1. DERMATOLOGICAL DISORDERS UNIQUE TO PREGNANCY

Disorder	Frequency	Clinical Characteristics	Histopathology	Perinatal Outcome	Treatment	Comments
Pruritus gravidarum	Common (1–2%)	Onset third trimester; intense pruritus; generalized; excoriations common	Noncharacteristic; excoriations common	Perinatal morbidity increased	Antipruritics, Cholestyramine	Possibly a mild form of cholestatic jaundice; recurs in subsequent pregnancy
Pruritic urticarial papules and plaques of pregnancy (PUPPP)	Common (0.25–1%)	Onset second or third trimester; intense pruritus; patchy or generalized; abdomen, thighs, arms, buttocks; erythematous papules, urticarial papules and plaques	Lymphocytic perivascular infiltrate; negative immunofluorescence	No adverse effects	Antipruritics, emollients, topical steroids, oral steroids if severe	Common in nulliparas; seldom recurs in subsequent pregnancy
Papular eruptions (prurigo gestationis and papular dermatitis)	(1:300–1:2400)	Onset second or third trimester; localized or generalized; 1–5 mm pruritic papules; excoriations common	Lymphocytic perivascular infiltrate; parakeratosis, acanthosis; negative immunofluorescence	Probably unaffected	Antipruritics, topical steroids, oral steroids if severe	Prurigo gestationis localized to forearms and trunk; papular dermatitis generalized; does not recur in subsequent pregnancy
Herpes gestationis	Rare (1:50,000)	Onset second or third trimester, sometimes 1–2 weeks postpartum; severe pruritus; abdomen, extremities, or generalized; urticarial papules and plaques, erythema, vesicles, and bullae	Edema; infiltrate of lymphocytes, histiocytes, and eosinophils; C$_3$ and IgG deposition at basement membrane	Possibly increased preterm birth; transient neonatal lesions (5–10%)	Antipruritics, topical steroids, oral steroids if severe	Also associated with gestational trophoblastic disease; exacerbations and remissions during pregnancy common; postpartum exacerbations very common; recurrence in subsequent pregnancies more severe
Impetigo herpetiformis	Rare	Onset third trimester; local, then generalized; erythema with marginal sterile pustules; mucous membranes involved; systemic symptoms	Microabscesses	Maternal sepsis common	Antibiotics, oral steroids	Possibly pustular psoriasis; persists for weeks to months postpartum; may recur with subsequent pregnancy

1261

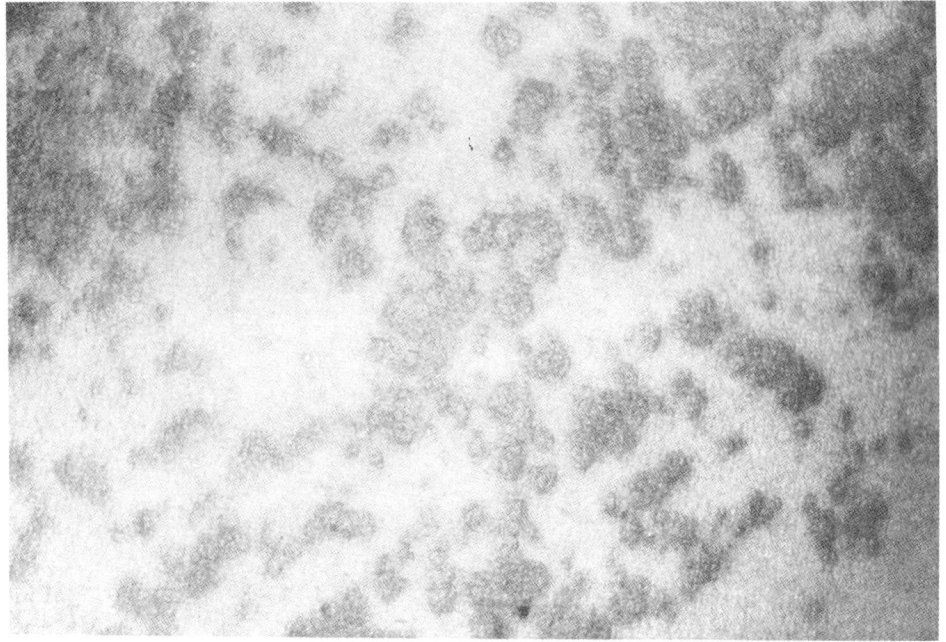

Fig. 56–1. Pruritic urticarial papules and plaques of pregnancy. Numerous edematous and erythematous papular lesions are present on the lower trunk. (From Yancey and colleagues, 1984, with permission.)

and it usually does so earlier and is more severe. Baxi and colleagues (1991) reported a woman in whom recurrence was documented in five pregnancies; however, each time the disease was less severe. Although morphological changes may develop in the small intestinal mucosa similar to those of adult celiac disease, they do not appear to cause significant malabsorption.

Katz and co-workers (1976) described a **herpes gestationis serum factor,** which is a thermostable immunoglobulin G protein. This serum factor reacts with amnionic tissue, and has been demonstrated to react with a 180-kd human epidermal antigen (Morrison and colleagues, 1988). Histologically, the classical finding in herpes gestationis is subepidermal edema with infiltrates of lymphocytes, histocytes, and eosinophils. Direct immunofluorescent techniques applied to a skin biopsy are of value for confirming the diagnosis, and C_3 complement and sometimes IgG, are deposited along the basement membrane zone.

Although the etiology of herpes gestationis is unknown, there is an inherited predisposition to its development. Specifically, there is a markedly increased incidence of HLA-DR3 and HLA-DR4 antigens in affected women. Although over half of women with herpes gestationis have these antigens, they are found in only 3 percent of unaffected women. According to Shornick (1987), these antigens are also associated with Graves disease, Hashimoto thyroiditis, Addison disease, type I diabetes, and systemic lupus erythematosus. Recently, Shornick and Black (1992b) reported that 11 percent of 75 women with herpes gestationis also had Graves disease.

Treatment. Pruritus may be quite severe. Some women obtain relief from topical steroids and antihistamines. If

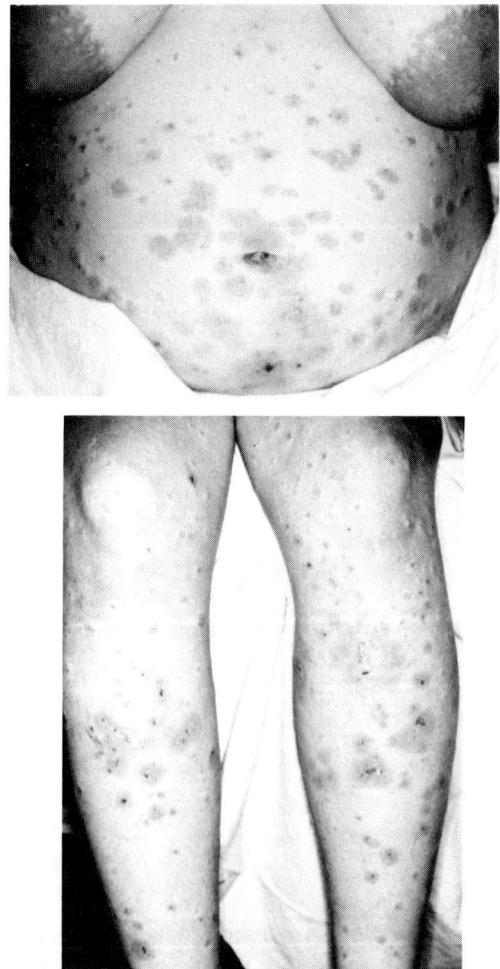

Fig. 56–2. Herpes gestationis at 30 weeks' gestation. Subsequently, remarkable relief from the intense pruritus, as well as considerable decrease in the intensity of the skin reaction, was provided by corticosteroid treatment.

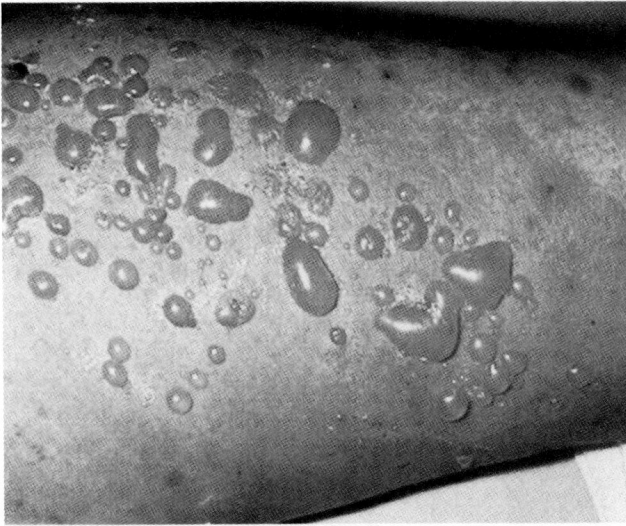

Fig. 56–3. Herpes gestationis with large, tense bullae on thigh. (From Holmes and Black, 1983, with permission.)

unsuccessful, orally administered prednisone in doses of 40 to 60 mg daily usually brings relief promptly and inhibits the formation of new lesions. The healed sites usually are not scarred but frequently are hyperpigmented.

Effect on Pregnancy. It is unclear if herpes gestationis causes adverse fetal outcomes. Lawley and colleagues (1978) reviewed the literature and reported a high incidence of preterm birth and stillborn infants. Holmes and Black (1984) reviewed 50 pregnancies, and Shornick and Black (1992a) reviewed 74; both reported an increased incidence of preterm delivery and small-for-gestational age infants, but not perinatal mortality.

Lesions similar to those of the mother have been reported to develop in up to 10 percent of neonates. These usually clear spontaneously within a few weeks (Shornick, 1987). C_3 complement deposited at the basement membrane of the newborn's skin and herpes gestationis factor in cord serum have been described by Katz and associates (1976).

Papular Eruptions of Pregnancy. According to Aronson and Halaska (1991) and Black (1989), papular eruptions of pregnancy include **prurigo gestationis** and **papular dermatitis,** which are variants of the same disease. The mild and more common variant, prurigo gestationis, is characterized by small, pruritic, rapidly excoriated lesions on the forearms and trunk. Lesions typically have their onset at 25 to 30 weeks, and vesicles or bullae do not develop (Black, 1989). Papular dermatitis, described by Spangler and colleagues in 1962, is a rare dermatitis of late pregnancy. It is characterized by a generalized pruritic eruption, the lesions of which consist of soft, red to violet to red-brown papules, some of which have a centrally hemorrhagic crust.

Pruritus is usually controlled with antihistamines and topical steroid creams. High-dose systemic steroid therapy is not requisite for good fetal outcome (Aronson and Halaska, 1991). In the earlier report by Spangler and associates (1962), perinatal mortality was reported to be increased. Aronson and colleagues (1984), however, found no adverse perinatal outcomes with 16 pregnancies complicated by papular eruptions.

Impetigo Herpetiformis. Impetigo herpetiformis is a rare pustular eruption that may be seen in late pregnancy. Some consider it to be a form of pustular psoriasis that occurs coincidental to pregnancy, while others consider it to be a distinct pregnancy dermatosis (Aronson and Halaska, 1991). Oumeish and associates (1982) have described a woman in whom this dermatosis recurred in nine successive pregnancies. In three pregnancies there was fetal hydrocephaly and there were two unexplained perinatal deaths. This woman also developed characteristic skin lesions when taking estrogen–progesterone oral contraceptives.

The hallmark lesions of impetigo herpetiformis are sterile pustules that form around the margin of erythematous patches (Fig. 56–4). The erythematous lesions characteristically begin at flexures and extend peripherally. Mucous membranes are usually involved. The characteristic histological lesion is a microabscess, and the spongelike epidermal cavity filled with neutrophils has been termed the **spongioform pustule of Kogoj.**

Pruritus is not severe, but constitutional symptoms are common. In addition to nausea, vomiting, diarrhea, and chills and fever, frequently there is hypoalbuminemia and hypocalcemia. Although the pustules are initially sterile, they may become secondarily infected after rupture, and sepsis is a serious concern. Treatment is given with systemic steroids along with antimicrobials to treat secondary infection and sepsis. The disease may persist for several weeks to months after delivery. Fetal morbidity and mortality is rated to the severity of maternal infection.

Preexisting Skin Disease and Pregnancy

A number of chronic dermatological disorders may complicate pregnancy. These may antedate pregnancy or manifest for the first time during pregnancy. Many of these, such as acne, psoriasis, and eczema, are like other chronic disorders, which usually have no predictable course during pregnancy. Thus, they may be unchanged, improve, or worsen as gestation progresses.

If **pemphigus** appears during pregnancy for the first time, it may be confused with herpes gestationis. Even with corticosteroid therapy, mortality is 10 percent secondary to sepsis caused by infection of denuded skin. It also may be associated with adverse pregnancy outcomes, and Ross and colleagues (1986) reviewed 29

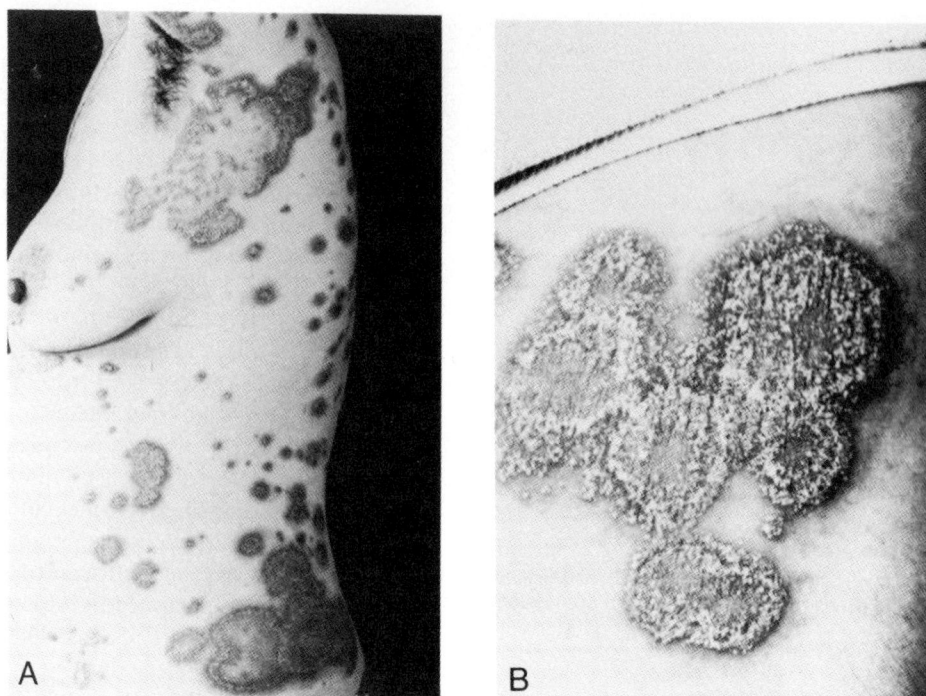

Fig. 56–4. Impetigo herpetiformis. **A.** Round polycyclic patches over sides of the trunk at the time of admission. **B.** Patches over the thigh, with fresh pustules in the periphery encircling crusted older lesions. (From Lotem and associates, 1989, with permission.)

cases and reported 4 stillborn infants. Lesions of **neurofibromatosis** may increase in size and number as a result of pregnancy. **Hansen disease** likely worsens during pregnancy, at least according to the review by Aronson and Halaska (1991). This is discussed in Chapter 58 (p. 1292).

Acne. Some women, but certainly not all, note that their acne improves during pregnancy. **The retinoic acid, isotretinoin (Accutane), is commonly prescribed for severe cystic acne, but unfortunately it has proven to be highly teratogenic.** Lammer and colleagues (1985) reported a 26-fold risk for craniofacial, cardiac, and central nervous system malformations in exposed fetuses (see Chap. 42, p. 971). Likewise, **etretinate,** a similar compound utilized for the treatment of psoriasis, has been classified as category X because of associated major anomalies. Moreover, this agent may be detected in the serum of women for as long as 2 years after cessation of therapy (DiGiovanna and associates, 1989). Conversely, topically applied **tretinoin** for acne treatment is not associated with fetal anomalies, and is a category C drug. **Benzoyl peroxide** is also in category C. Rothman and Pochi (1988) have reviewed oral and topical drugs used to treat acne during pregnancy.

Hidradenitis Suppurativa. This is a chronic, progressive inflammatory and suppurative disorder of skin and supporting structures characterized by apocrine gland plugging that leads to anhidrosis and bacterial infection. Subcutaneous extension causes scarring and sinus for-

mation. In most cases, skin involvement is in multiple apocrine gland sites, but it may be seen only in the axillae, groin, perineum, perirectal area, or under the breasts.

The disease is hormonally responsive and thus not seen until puberty. It has been said to be improved by pregnancy, but with postpartum exacerbations. In our experiences, it is not appreciably changed by pregnancy. Treatment is control of acute infections with either systemic antimicrobials or clindamycin ointment. Isotretinoin has been used in a limited fashion and with variable results in nonpregnant patients (Brown and associates, 1988), but as discussed above, it is a category X drug contraindicated during pregnancy. Definitive treatment is wide surgical excision, but this most often should be postponed during pregnancy.

References

Alcalay J, Ingber A, David M, Hazaz B, Sandbank M: Pruritic urticarial papules and plaques of pregnancy: A review of 21 cases. J Reprod Med 32:315, 1987

Alcalay J, Ingber A, Kafri B, Segal J, Kaufmann H, Hazaz B, Sandbank M: Hormonal evaluation and autoimmune background in pruritic urticarial papules and plaques of pregnancy. Am J Obstet Gynecol 158:417, 1988

Baxi LV, Kovilam OP, Collins MH, Walther RR: Recurrent herpes gestationis with postpartum flare: A case report. Am J Obstet Gynecol 164:778, 1991

Beltrani VP, Beltrani VS: Pruritic urticarial papules and plaques of pregnancy: A severe case requiring early delivery for relief of symptoms. J Am Acad Dermatol 26:2, 1992

Black MM: Prurigo of pregnancy, papular dermatitis of pregnancy, and pruritic folliculitis of pregnancy. Semin Dermatol 8:23, 1989

Brown CF, Gallup DG, Brown VM: Hidradenitis suppurativa of the anogenital region: Response to isotretinoin. Am J Obstet Gynecol 158:12, 1988

DiGiovanna JJ, Zech LA, Ruddel ME, Gantt G, Peck GL: Etretinate. Persistent serum levels after long-term therapy. Arch Dermatol 125:246, 1989

Holmes RC, Black MM: The fetal prognosis in pemphigoid gestationis (herpes gestationis). Br J Dermatol 110:67, 1984

Holmes RC, Black MM: Dermatosis of pregnancy. J Am Acad Dermatol 8:406, 1983

Katz SI, Hertz KC, Yaoita H: Immunopathology and characterization of the HG factor. J Clin Invest 57:1434, 1976

Lammer EJ, Chen DT, Hoar RM, Agnish ND, Benke PJ, Braun JT, Curry CJ, Fernhoff PM, Grix AW, Lott IT, Richard JM, Sun SC: Retinoic acid embryopathy. N Engl J Med 313:837, 1985

Lawley TJ, Stingl G, Katz SI: Fetal and maternal risk factors in herpes gestationis. Arch Dermatol 114:552, 1978

Lotem M, Katzenelson V, Rotem A, Hod M, Sandbank M: Impetigo herpetiformis: A variant of pustular psoriasis or a separate entity? J Am Acad Dermatol 20:338, 1989

Lynfield VL: Effect of pregnancy on the human hair cycle. J Invest Dermatol 35:323, 1960

MacKie RM, Bufalina R, Morabito A, Sutherland C, Cascinelli N: Lack of effect of pregnancy on outcome of melanoma. Lancet 337:653, 1991

Morrison LH, Labib RS, Zone JJ, Diaz LA, Anhault GJ: Herpes gestationis autoantibodies recognize a 180-kD human epidermal antigen. J Clin Invest 81:2023, 1988

Oumeish OY, Farraj SE, Bataineh AS: Some aspects of impetigo herpetiformis. Arch Dermatol 118:103, 1982

Ross MG, Kane B, Frieder R, Gurevitch A, Hayashi R: Pemphigus in pregnancy: A reevaluation of fetal risk. Am J Obstet Gynecol 155:30, 1986

Rothman KF, Pochi PE: Use of oral and topical agents for acne. J Am Acad Dermatol 19:431, 1988

Shornick JK, Black MM: Fetal risks in herpes gestationis. J Am Acad Dermatol 26:63, 1992a

Shornick JK, Black MM: Secondary autoimmune diseases in herpes gestationis (pemphigoid gestationis). J Am Acad Dermatol 26:563, 1992b

Shornick JK: Herpes gestationis. J Am Acad Dermatol 17:539, 1987

Spangler AS, Reddy W, Bardawil WA, Roby CC, Emerson K: Papular dermatitis of pregnancy: A new clinical entity. JAMA 181:577, 1962

Spetz S: Peripheral circulation during normal pregnancy. Acta Obstet Gynecol Scand 43:309, 1964

Weiss R, Hull P: Familial occurrence of pruritic urticarial papules and plaques of pregnancy. J Am Acad Dermatol 26:715, 1992

Winton GB, Lewis CW: Dermatoses of pregnancy. J Am Acad Dermatol 6:977, 1982

Wong RC, Ellis CN: Physiologic skin changes in pregnancy. J Am Acad Dermatol 10:929, 1984

Yancey KB, Hall RP, Lawley TJ: Pruritic urticarial papules and plaques of pregnancy: Clinical experience in 25 patients. J Am Acad Dermatol 10:473, 1984

CHAPTER 57
Neoplastic Diseases

Cancer during pregnancy is not rare. According to the Third National Cancer Survey (1975), about 13 percent of cancers in females develop during the childbearing years. From his review, Donegan (1983) estimated that 1 in 1000 women will be affected by cancer while pregnant. As shown in Table 57–1, the most frequent malignant tumors in women of childbearing age are those of the hemopoietic and lymphatic systems, thyroid, breast, cervix, ovary, colon, and malignant melanoma. Sachs and colleagues (1990) reviewed 886 maternal deaths in Massachusetts from 1954 to 1985, and reported that 5 percent were cancer-related. The most common cancers causing death in these pregnant women were those of the central nervous and hemopoietic systems.

The approach to the pregnant woman with cancer must be modified compared with that of a nonpregnant patient. Specific questions to be asked include: (1) Does pregnancy adversely influence maternal cancer? (2) What risk does cancer or its treatment pose to the fetus? (3) Should the pregnancy be terminated because it represents a significant obstacle for effective cancer therapy or because of the likelihood of grave danger to the fetus? (4) Should the pregnancy be allowed to continue under a very carefully defined regimen? (5) If the neoplasm exists before conception, is pregnancy contraindicated, and if so, what should be the advice for contraception? (6) Is pregnancy advisable following cancer treatment?

Principles of Cancer Therapy During Pregnancy

Surgery. Surgical intervention for suspected or proved malignant tumors may be indicated for diagnostic, staging, or therapeutic purposes. To generalize, extra-abdominal procedures are usually well tolerated by both mother and fetus, as are most intraperitoneal operations that do not interfere with the reproductive tract. If indicated, however, the ovaries may be removed safely after about 8 weeks' gestation because placental progesterone production is sufficient for pregnancy maintenance. Ovariectomy before this time may cause abortion which often can be prevented by progesterone administration (see Chap. 8, p. 213).

In the past, diagnostic and staging operations usually were deferred until the second trimester so as to minimize abortion risks. This probably is not necessary because documenting fetal life by ultrasound between 9 and 11 weeks indicates that 95 percent of fetuses will reach viability. Therapeutic surgery should be performed regardless of gestational age if the maternal well-being is imperiled.

Radiation Therapy. Depending on the dose, dose rate, field size, radiation energy, and gestational age, radiation can cause chromatin damage, which in turn may lead to cytogenetic anomalies or cell death (Beckman and Brent, 1986). As discussed in Chapter 43 (p. 981), the characteristic adverse effects of high-dose radiation are microcephaly and mental retardation. For example, children born to pregnant women exposed to atomic bomb explosions had a 2.4 percent incidence of mental retardation with 10 to 50 rad exposure, and this was increased to nearly 18 percent if exposure was 50 to 100 rad (Otake, 1984). The most critical time appeared to be between 8 to 15 weeks.

The National Council on Radiation Protection and Measurements (Brent, 1987) concluded that exposure of the embryo to less than 5 rad is associated with negligible risk for major malformations. It was further suggested that the threshold for radiation effects may be 15 to 20 rad. Although the most susceptible period appears to be during organogenesis, there is no gestational age that is considered safe for radiation exposure because late exposure can cause fetal growth retardation.

The necessity for therapeutic radiation raises issues such as abortion, teratogenesis, and fetal sequelae. Therapeutic radiation to the abdomen is contraindicated because of a high risk of fetal damage, unless of course abortion induction is one of its purposes. In some cases, for example, the head and neck, radiation therapy to supradiaphragmatic areas can be given relatively safely with abdominal shielding; however, in others, for example, the breasts, significant scatter doses can accrue to the fetus. Lippman and colleagues (1988) calculated fetal doses of up to 100 rad during radiotherapy for breast cancer if the uterus reached the xiphoid.

Chemotherapy

Effect on Pregnancy Outcome. Fetal hazards from chemotherapy exposure are encountered in women first diagnosed with cancer during pregnancy or in those who become pregnant while being given chemotherapy. Before chemotherapy, reproductive-age women are cautioned that pregnancy is inadvisable during treat-

TABLE 57–1. MOST FREQUENT MALIGNANCIES IN WOMEN IN CHILDBEARING AGE GROUPS

15 to 24 Years Old	25 to 34 Years Old	35 to 44 Years Old
Hodgkin Disease	Breast	Breast
Thyroid	Cervix	Cervix
Melanoma	Melanoma, Thyroid	Melanoma

From 1988 Annual Cancer Statistics Review, National Cancer Advisory Board.

ment. Some advise the woman to wait at least 12 months to conceive after chemotherapy completion. Early fetal wastage is possibly increased and, depending on the teratogenic potential of the drugs given, therapeutic abortion is considered. Most antineoplastic drugs should be considered potentially teratogenic, especially if given between 5 and 10 weeks' gestation and thus during organogenesis and the period of maximal susceptibility. Surprisingly, most antineoplastic drugs given after the first trimester are without obvious adverse sequelae, although long-term effects have not been evaluated thoroughly. As expected, most of the antineoplastic drugs shown in Table 57–2, are classified as category D.

Zemlickis and associates (1992a) reported four

TABLE 57–2. SOME DRUGS USED FOR TREATMENT OF NEOPLASMS

Class/Drug	Risk Category	Common Uses for Cancer Therapy
Alkylating agents		
Busulfan	D	Leukemias
Chlorambucil	D	Lymphomas, leukemias
Cyclophosphamide	D	Breast, ovary, lymphomas, leukemias
Melphalan	D	Ovary, leukemia, myeloma
Procarbazine	D	Lymphomas
Antimetabolites		
5-Fluorouracil	D	Breast, gastrointestinal
6-Mercaptopurine	D	Leukemias
Methotrexate	D	Trophoblastic disease, lymphomas, leukemias, breast
6-Thioguanine	D	Leukemias
Antibiotics		
Bleomycin	D	Cervix, lymphomas
Daunorubicin	D	Leukemias
Doxorubicin	D	Leukemias, lymphomas, breast
Other agents		
L-Asparaginase	C	Leukemia
Cisplatin	D	Ovary, cervix, sarcoma
Hydroxyurea	D	Leukemias
Prednisone	B	Lymphomas, leukemias, breast
Tamoxifen	D	Breast, uterus
Taxol	D	Breast, ovarian
Vinblastine	D	Breast, lymphomas, choriocarcinoma
Vincristine	D	Leukemias, lymphomas

spontaneous abortions and two of five fetuses with major malformations when chemotherapy was given to nine women during the first trimester. Eight women treated later in pregnancy had lower birthweight infants than controls, but no malformations. Doll and collaborators (1988) reviewed chemotherapy-induced teratogenesis. They found six instances (25 percent) of fetal malformations during 24 first-trimester exposures to combination chemotherapy compared with 24 of 139 (17 percent) exposed to single-agent therapy. Many of these women had been given folate antagonists and some were given concomitant radiation, and if these were excluded, the incidence of malformations with single-agent therapy was only 6 percent. In contrast, during the second and third trimesters there was no evidence for increased risk of teratogenesis, and of 131 cases there were only two (1.5 percent) fetal malformations. From their review, Koren and colleagues (1990) estimate the major malformation rate at 10 percent for first-trimester exposure.

Because the magnitude of secretion of chemotherapeutic agents in breast milk has not been established, breastfeeding is not recommended. There is concern for exposure of health-care workers to chemotherapeutic agents. Selevan and colleagues (1985) reported a twofold increased risk of fetal loss in nurses exposed during the first trimester, and they recommended caution during mixing and administering antineoplastic drugs. Late effects on offspring of women treated for cancer during pregnancy have been analyzed and Li and associates (1979) found only two childhood malignancies in a group of 146 women treated during 286 pregnancies. Similarly, Avilés and colleagues (1991) found no adverse sequelae in 43 children exposed to antineoplastic drugs in utero, and who were evaluated 3 to 19 years later.

Ovarian Function and Fertility After Cancer Therapy. There are concerns for long-term effects on ovarian function and fertility from radiation and chemotherapy for cancer. For example, treatment of advanced Hodgkin lymphoma with multiple-drug regimens results in azoospermia in many men (Waxman, 1985). In women there is depressed follicular maturation as well as ovarian fibrosis. Ovarian susceptibility depends on the woman's age and the drug dose given. Interestingly, the prepubertal ovary is more resistant to effects of chemotherapy.

Although some chemotherapy regimens induce amenorrhea, if fertility is not lost, or if it returns, there does not appear to be an increased incidence of abortion, fetal chromosomal damage, or fetal anomalies (Rustin and colleagues, 1984). Gershenson (1988) reviewed subsequent outcome in women successfully treated with chemotherapy for germ cell ovarian tumors, and although 68 percent had regular menses, the remainder had total or partial ablation of ovarian function. Affected women were significantly older at diagnosis.

Breast Carcinoma

Breast cancer is the most common malignancy of women of all age groups. Almost one of every 10 American women will eventually be afflicted. Thus, it is not surprising that breast cancer is encountered with some frequency during pregnancy. Its exact incidence is not known, but has been estimated to be about 1 in 3000 to 10,000 pregnancies (Donegan, 1983; Orr and Shingleton, 1983; Parente and associates, 1988).

Effects of Pregnancy on Breast Cancer. A large number of breast cancers have female sex hormone receptors and appear to be estrogen- or progesterone-dependent. Theoretically at least, they should be more aggressive because of the hyperestrogenemia and hyperprogesteronemia that characterize normal pregnancy. There is no proof of this, however, and two observations may serve to explain this. First, there is the widely held view that pregnancy is protective because the dominant estrogen is estriol that displaces the substantively more potent estradiol from tumor cell receptors. Second, Nugent and O'Connell (1985) reported that more than 70 percent of breast tumors in pregnant patients were estrogen-receptor negative. Paradoxically, this latter characteristic is seen in many of the more aggressive neoplasms in young women.

In reality, it appears that pregnancy does not exert much influence on the course of mammary cancer, thus therapeutic abortion does not improve its prognosis. In the extensive investigations of Westberg (1946), based on 224 cases of pregnant women and a control series of 3000 nonpregnant women with breast cancer, the difference in the survival rates scarcely was significant. Hochman and Schreiber (1953), and others since then, contended that the 5-year survival rate in breast cancer co-existing with pregnancy is primarily dependent on the stage of the disease at the time of diagnosis, and that interruption of pregnancy has no influence on the course. Thus, survival in pregnant women is comparable to the rates expected with similar disease stages in nonpregnant women (Zemlickis and associates, 1992b; King and colleagues, 1985; Nugent and O'Connell, 1985).

Although survival is stage-dependent, there may be serious delays in clinical assessment, diagnostic procedures, and treatment of pregnant women with breast tumors. Hormonally induced physiological breast changes tend to obscure breast masses, and this is particularly evident during lactation when there is lobular hyperplasia and galactostasis. This serves to at least partially explain the more advanced stages of cancer at diagnosis, which consequently have a worse prognosis. According to Jacob and Stringer (1990), 28 percent of pregnant women with breast cancer have stage I disease, 30 percent stage II, and 41 percent stages III and IV. As shown in Table 57–3, about three fourths of

TABLE 57–3. AXILLARY NODE INVOLVEMENT IN PREGNANCY-ASSOCIATED BREAST CANCER

Investigators	No.	Positive Nodes (%)
Holleb and Farrow (1962)	117	86 (74)
Rosemond (1963)	37	23 (62)
Haagensen (1971)	48	33 (69)
Ribeiro and Palmer (1977)	88	78 (89)
Clark and Reid (1978)	121	100 (83)
Donegan (1979)	24	17 (71)
Petrek and associates (1991)	56	34 (61)
Total	**491**	**371 (76)**

Modified from Lippman and colleagues (1988).

pregnant women had axillary node involvement. This is substantively higher than the 40 to 50 percent reported for nonpregnant women (Hoover, 1990).

King and colleagues (1985) described experiences with 63 pregnant women treated for breast carcinoma at the Mayo Clinic. They reported that 63 percent of these women had axillary nodal metastases compared with only 38 percent of similar-age nonpregnant women described by others. Ribeiro and colleagues (1986) also reported advanced stages of tumors diagnosed during pregnancy compared to nonpregnant women. Finally, Zemlickis and associates (1992b) reported their results with 118 pregnant women with breast cancer from the Princess Margaret Hospital in Toronto. These women had a 2.5-fold risk of metastatic disease compared with nonpregnant control women with breast cancer.

Diagnosis and Treatment. The diagnostic approach in the pregnant woman with a breast tumor is not different than for a nonpregnant woman. **Any suspicious breast mass found during pregnancy should prompt an aggressive plan to determine its cause, whether by mammography and fine-needle aspiration, or by open biopsy.** The risk of mammography is negligible for the fetus, if appropriate shielding is used. The dense breast tissue of pregnancy makes this test less reliable. Using fine-needle aspiration, it is possible to differentiate a cyst or galactocele from solid tumors. Excisional biopsy should be done if cytological results are negative but the mass persists. According to Barnavon and Wallack (1990) aspiration is 66 percent sensitive and 95 percent specific.

Once the diagnosis of breast malignancy is established, chest x-ray and limited metastatic search is performed. Whereas bone and liver scans probably are contraindicated, magnetic resonance imaging and ultrasonography are reasonable alternatives to assess for liver involvement.

Surgical treatment should not be delayed because of pregnancy. In the absence of metastatic disease, a modified radical mastectomy or a total mastectomy with axillary node staging can be performed (Donegan, 1983). Risks from these procedures are minimal, and the incidence of abortion is negligible following mastectomy. **Radiotherapy** is not recommended during pregnancy because abdominal scatter is considerable even with shielding (Hoover, 1990; Orr and Shingleton, 1983). Early in pregnancy the dose may be 10 to 20 rad, and when the uterus is near the xiphoid, fetal doses of 100 rad have been calculated (Lippman and associates, 1988). **Chemotherapy** was traditionally reserved for women with metastatic disease. Recent data indicate that women with node-positive cancer should be given adjuvant chemotherapy without delay, and many centers are advising such therapy even for node-negative patients (Hoover, 1990). It therefore seems advisable to give chemotherapy for node-positive disease if delivery is not anticipated soon.

Pregnancy Following Breast Cancer. About 10 percent of women treated for breast cancer subsequently become pregnant, and 70 percent of these do so within the first 5 years (Harvey, 1981; Hornstein and colleagues, 1982). There is little evidence to suggest that pregnancy after mastectomy for breast cancer adversely effects survival (Donegan, 1983; Harvey and associates, 1981; Sutton and colleagues, 1990). Similarly, there is no data to suggest that lactation adversely affects the course of breast cancer. Recommendations for future pregnancies in women successfully treated for breast malignancy are based on several factors, including consideration for recurrence. It seems reasonable to advise a delay of 2 to 3 years which is the most critical observation period for recurrence.

Lymphomas and Leukemias

Lymphomas

Hodgkin Disease. Hodgkin disease constitutes approximately 40 percent of malignant lymphomas. These tumors have a bimodal peak incidence, and the first peak is between 15 and 35 years of age. Hodgkin disease is the most common lymphoma encountered in childbearing-age women, and its concurrence with pregnancy is estimated to be about 1 in 6000. Our experiences indicate that the incidence is much lower than this. The most common finding is peripheral adenopathy, and neck nodes commonly are involved. Patients may be asymptomatic or they may present with fever, night sweats, malaise, weight loss, and pruritus. Diagnosis is established by histological examination of involved nodes.

The pregnant woman with Hodgkin disease presents special management considerations. A tenet of treatment is that careful staging is essential, and either local radiotherapy or systemic chemotherapy is indicated. The Ann Arbor staging system, shown in Table 57–4, was designed for Hodgkin lymphomas but is also used for other lym-

TABLE 57–4. ANN ARBOR STAGING SYSTEM FOR LYMPHOMAS

Stage	Findings
I	Involvement in single lymph node region or single extralymphatic site
II	Involvement of two or more lymph node regions on the same side of the diaphragm Includes localized involvement of extralymphatic site (stage II E)
III	Involvement of lymph node regions or extralymphatic sites on both sides of diaphragm
IV	Disseminated involvement of one or more extralymphatic organs, with or without lymph node involvement

Substage A = asymptomatic patient; substage B = patients with fever, sweats, or weight loss.

phomas. More recently, its revision termed the Cotswold classification, has been used (Urba and Longo, 1992). Pregnancy limits the widespread application of some radiographic studies of the chest, abdomen, and pelvis. Magnetic resonance imaging may prove a reasonable alternative to computed-tomographic scanning for evaluating thoracic and abdominal para-aortic lymph nodes. Staging laparotomy is done in nonpregnant patients routinely in many centers. Although this may be done in early pregnancy, it does not seem advisable in later pregnancy.

Treatment is individualized depending upon the suspected disease stage and pregnancy duration. Whereas radiotherapy is preferable for isolated cervical adenopathy, it is not recommended if the fields to be used will deliver significant radiation scatter to the fetus. Wong and colleagues (1990) estimated fetal exposure from 4400 rad delivered to the midline of the central supradiaphragmatic axis. Fetal dosage was calculated to 63, 88, and 220 rad in early, mid- and late pregnancy. Because of this, Ward and Weiss (1989) recommend dose and field modification. Nisce and colleagues (1986) temporarily modified their radiotherapeutic regime to deliver only 1500 to 2000 rad to supradiaphragmatic sites in seven women with a second- or third-trimester pregnancy. Despite this reduction to what were considered subcurative doses, fetal radiation exposure ranged from 2 to 50 rad and averaged about 20 rad. When evaluated at 6 to 11 years of age, all seven children were normal, but two mothers had died.

Chemotherapy probably is best avoided during early pregnancy, but it is a relatively safe option later. With obvious widespread disease, chemotherapy is given at diagnosis. Postponement of therapy until fetal maturity is achieved is considered reasonable by some if the diagnosis is made late in pregnancy and the mother is asymptomatic.

There are no convincing data that pregnancy adversely affects Hodgkin lymphoma; therefore, its interruption to improve the prognosis is unnecessary. Likewise, the disease does not cause increased pregnancy wastage. Holmes and Holmes (1978) analyzed 93 pregnancy outcomes when either the pregnant woman or the father had Hodgkin disease, and the great majority were satisfactory. Jacobs and associates (1981) reported their experiences from Stanford University and found that neither chemotherapy during the second and third trimesters, nor irradiation to the mediastinum and neck, appeared to adversely affect the fetus or neonate. **Pregnant women with Hodgkin disease are inordinately susceptible to infections and sepsis, and both radiotherapy or chemotherapy increases this susceptibility.**

FERTILITY AFTER TREATMENT. Horning and co-workers (1981) evaluated the reproductive potential of women after treatment for Hodgkin disease. They reported that 55 percent of women resumed normal menses after chemotherapy. No birth defects nor developmental abnormalities were evident in the 24 infants studied. The risk of second cancers, especially leukemia, is substantively increased in patients with Hodgkin disease. Tucker and colleagues (1988) reported this risk to be 18 percent within 15 years. When compared with radiotherapy given alone, Kaldor and associates (1990) reported that the risk for leukemia was increased almost nine-fold following chemotherapy.

Non-Hodgkin Lymphomas. Lymphomas that are not classified as Hodgkin disease recently have become the most common neoplasms among persons aged 20 to 40. Their incidence has risen sharply because of their relationship to the **acquired immunodeficiency syndrome.** Indeed, 5 to 10 percent of persons infected with human immunodeficiency virus will develop a lymphoma.

Currently the concurrence of non-Hodgkin lymphoma with pregnancy has been rare, although its incidence is expected to increase because of the rising incidence of human immunodeficiency virus infection. In a 50-year literature review, Ioachim (1985) found only 21 cases. Ward and Weiss (1989) found 75 cases complicating pregnancy in their review. Avilés and colleagues (1990) described their experiences with 16 pregnant women with these malignancies. Although one half were discovered in the first trimester, they began cytotoxic drug therapy and observed no fetal malformations. All but one offspring were healthy at 3 to 11 years. Eight of the 16 mothers who had remissions were alive 4 to 9 years later.

Extensive staging is required for non-Hodgkin lymphomas, and radiotherapy typically is used for stage I disease, whereas chemotherapy is recommended for most stage II and all stages III and IV tumors.

Leukemias. Except for acute lymphocytic leukemia, which is a childhood disorder, leukemias are more prev-

alent after age 40. Despite this, acute leukemias are among the most common malignant neoplasms of young women, but paradoxically, their incidence complicating pregnancy is cited to be 1 in 75,000 (McLain, 1974; Orr and Shingleton, 1983). This has also been our experience at Parkland Hospital and we have encountered only four women with leukemia in nearly 200,000 pregnancies. Caligiuri and Mayer (1989) compiled 350 reports of pregnancy complicated by leukemia. Of 72 newly diagnosed cases during pregnancy and reported since 1975, 44 had acute myelogenous leukemia, 20 acute lymphocytic leukemia, and eight had one of the chronic leukemias.

Effect on Pregnancy. In more recent times, there is an improved survival rate with these malignancies, and in three fourths of women who develop **acute leukemia** during pregnancy, remission usually can be induced with chemotherapy. Thus, maternal and fetal outcomes have improved substantively for leukemic patients in recent years (Catanzarite and Ferguson, 1984; Reynoso and colleagues, 1987). For example, McLain (1974) reported that the maternal mortality rate was 100 percent and perinatal mortality was 34 percent in 256 women with acute leukemia treated before 1970. According to Lewis and Laros (1986), maternal death during pregnancy due to acute leukemia has become negligible since 1970, although most of these unfortunate women die months to years following pregnancy. Survival also has improved for women with **chronic myelogenous** and **lymphocytic leukemias.**

Despite being improved, perinatal outcomes generally are poor for leukemic women. Reynoso and colleagues (1987) analyzed 58 reported cases of acute leukemia during pregnancy in a 10-year period. Nearly 75 percent of these were diagnosed during the second and third trimesters, half had acute myelogenous leukemia, and most cases were treated with chemotherapy with a reported remission rate of 75 percent. Only 40 percent of pregnancies in these women resulted in live-born infants. Similarly, Caligiuri and Mayer (1989) reported preterm delivery in about 50 percent of women diagnosed during pregnancy. The stillbirth rate also was increased.

Several cases of **congenital leukemia** in infants of nonleukemic mothers have been recorded, although no case of transmission of maternal leukemia to the fetus has been authenticated.

Management. In general, multiagent chemotherapy is given as soon as the diagnosis of leukemia is established, even if in the first trimester. Rare cases of spontaneous remission of acute leukemia after pregnancy have been reported (Antunez and colleagues, 1989), perhaps implicating a hormonal influence, but hormone receptors were not studied. Because there is no evidence that pregnancy has a deleterious effect on leukemia, termination is not recommended to improve the prognosis, but it is a consideration in early pregnancy to avoid teratogenesis from chemotherapy.

Significant complications in pregnancy that include infection and hemorrhage should be anticipated at the time of delivery in women with active disease. Manifestations include anemia, neutropenia, and thrombocytopenia. Vaginal delivery is preferable, and cesarean section is reserved for obstetrical indications.

Malignant Melanoma

Melanomas are relatively common in women of childbearing age. Their incidence in pregnancy is not known exactly, but the 2.8 per 1000 pregnancies cited by Smith (1969) is much higher than most experiences. Melanomas are most common in light-skinned Caucasians and over 90 percent originate in the skin from pigment-producing melanocytes, usually arising from a pre-existing nevus. Any suspicious behavior in a pigmented cutaneous lesion such as changes in contour, surface elevation, discoloration, itching, bleeding, or ulceration warrants a biopsy.

Melanomas are clinically staged: stage I has no palpable lymph nodes, stage II has palpable nodes, and in stage III there are distant metastases. Tumor thickness is the single most important predictor of survival in stage I patients. The Clark Classification is most widely used and includes five levels of involvement by depth into the epidermis, dermis, and subcutaneous fat.

Effect of Pregnancy. Earlier reports that pregnancy stimulates growth of malignant melanoma have not been

substantiated. As discussed in Chapters 8 (p. 215) and 56 (p. 1259), pregnancy is associated with increased melanocyte-stimulating hormones, and some melanomas contain sex steroid hormone receptors. Ellis (1991) has shown that pregnancy and estrogen-containing oral contraceptives probably increase dysplastic nevus changes, a forerunner to melanoma development. In his review of 11 studies, however, Holly (1986) concluded that there was no adverse effect on survival if melanoma was first diagnosed during pregnancy, or if pregnancy developed in a woman with previously recognized melanoma. Findings from the World Health Organization Melanoma Program (MacKie and colleagues, 1991) indicate that pregnant women in whom melanoma was diagnosed had significantly greater tumor thickness when compared with women diagnosed before or after pregnancy.

Primary surgical treatment for melanoma is determined by the stage of the disease and includes wide local resection and extensive lymph node dissection. Prophylactic chemotherapy or immunotherapy usually is avoided during pregnancy; however, chemotherapy for active disease is given if indicated by tumor stage, maternal prognosis, and gestational age. In most cases of metastatic melanoma, treatment is at best palliative.

Prognosis is determined by the stage of the lesion, and those with deep cutaneous invasion or regional node involvement have a much poorer prognosis. As discussed above, women who were pregnant when melanoma was diagnosed had thicker skin tumors. As shown in Figure 57–1, these women had a higher mortality rate when compared with women whose melanoma was diagnosed before or after pregnancy. However, survival is equivalent, stage-for-stage when pregnancy is compared

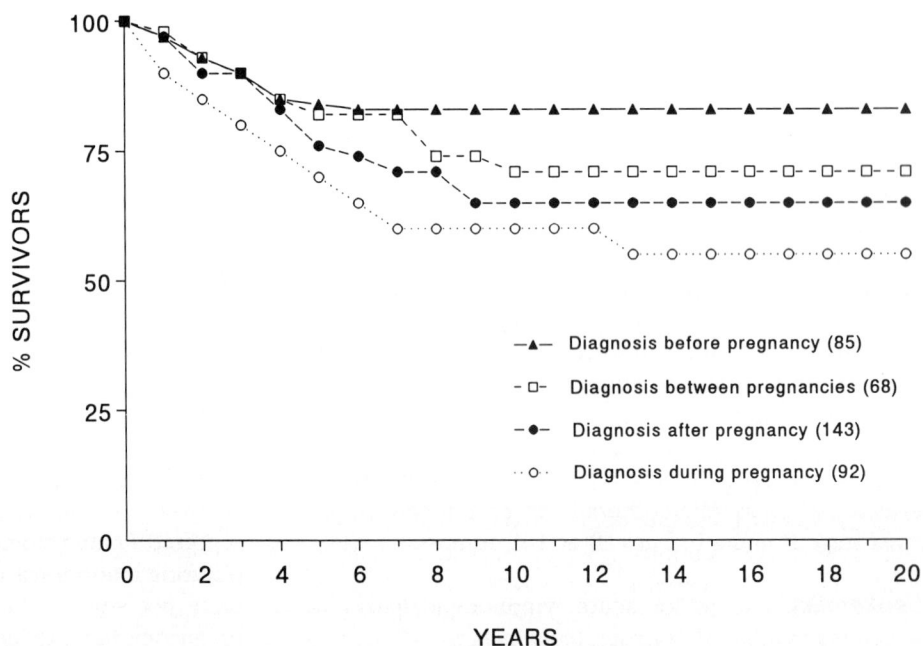

Fig. 57–1. Disease-free survival in 388 women with malignant melanoma. Decreased survival in women diagnosed during pregnancy is due to increased thickness of tumors. (Modified from MacKie and colleagues, 1991, with permission.)

—▲— Diagnosis before pregnancy (85)

–□– Diagnosis between pregnancies (68)

–●– Diagnosis after pregnancy (143)

···○··· Diagnosis during pregnancy (92)

% SURVIVORS

YEARS

with nonpregnancy. Slingluff and associates (1990) described their experiences with 100 pregnant women with melanoma. Mortality in the 6 to 8 year follow-up was similar (about 25 percent) to controls but lymph node metastases were increased. McManamny and colleagues (1989) had reported observations from 46 women who were either pregnant when melanoma was diagnosed or who became pregnant subsequent to treatment. They also found no adverse effects of pregnancy on survival. Because most recurrences manifest by 2 (60 percent) to 5 (90 percent) years, most recommend that future pregnancies be avoided for 3 to 5 years after treatment.

According to their review, Dildy and colleagues (1989) found that one third of reported cases of malignancies metastatic to the fetus or placenta have been malignant melanoma (see Chap. 35, p. 759). Although in some cases, the tumor undergoes regression in the neonate, many have succumbed to disease (Anderson and colleagues, 1989).

Genital Cancer

Cervical Neoplasia. Incidence data for cervical neoplasia complicating pregnancy varies widely and is based on collected series. Cervical dysplasia is quite common and Jolles (1989) cited an incidence in reproductive-age women of 25.7 per 1000. The incidence of carcinoma-in-situ was found to be 4.7 per 1000 women. According to Hacker and associates (1982), the average incidence of carcinoma-in-situ during pregnancy is about 1.3 per 1000 and for invasive carcinoma it is about 1 per 2200 pregnancies.

Intraepithelial Neoplasia. The effects of pregnancy and delivery on premalignant and malignant epithelial cervical lesions are not understood completely, and disagreements persist despite considerable interest displayed by numerous investigators (Hannigan, 1990). In the study by Kiguchi and co-workers (1981), pregnancy was not a potent stimulus for progression of dysplasia to invasive neoplasia. Progression from dysplasia to invasive carcinoma after delivery (0.4 percent) was almost half that for nonpregnant women (1 percent). Moreover, the regression rates of moderate and marked dysplasia within 6 months after delivery were higher than those for the general population.

According to Talebian and co-workers (1976), the incidence of abnormal cytology during pregnancy is about 3 percent, which is similar to that reported for nonpregnant women. Evaluation of an abnormal cytological smear is the same as for nonpregnant women with minor modifications. During pregnancy, colposcopic evaluation is easier to perform because the transformation zone is better exposed due to physiological eversion. Colposcopically directed biopsies are taken of any suspicious lesion. Biopsy sites may actively bleed because of hyperemia, and although this can be stopped easily with Monsel's solution, silver nitrate, or a vaginal pack, occasionally a suture is required. Multiple biopsies need not all be taken on one occasion. Instead, the squamocolumnar junction can be "mapped" and biopsies obtained over a period of time without hospitalization. Colposcopically directed biopsy during pregnancy is safe and reliable; its diagnostic accuracy is 99 percent and its complication rate is less than 1 percent (Hacker, 1982). In most cases, punch biopsies eliminate the need for conization.

During pregnancy, endocervical curettage is omitted to avoid risks of hemorrhage and membrane rupture. Cone biopsy usually is reserved to exclude invasive cancer, particularly if the biopsy shows microinvasion. If possible, conization is avoided because of an increased incidence of hemorrhage, abortion, and preterm labor (Table 57–5). Indeed, conization during pregnancy is less than satisfactory for at least three reasons: (1) The epithelium and underlying stroma within the cervical canal cannot be excised extensively because of the risk of membrane rupture. Of 376 conizations during pregnancy reviewed by Hacker and colleagues (1982), residual neoplasia was found in 43 percent of subsequent conization or hysterectomy specimens. (2) Blood loss during and after conization may be appreciable, and at times it is severe. Averette and colleagues (1970) reported that nearly 10 percent of 180 women required transfusion. (3) There is increased risk of abortion or preterm delivery during the current pregnancy and probably subsequent ones as well (Hannigan and associates, 1982; Larsson and co-workers, 1982).

If cytological changes of mild cervical intraepithelial

TABLE 57–5. BLEEDING COMPLICATIONS, ABORTIONS, AND PERINATAL MORTALITY (IN PERCENT) ASSOCIATED WITH CERVICAL CONIZATION DURING PREGNANCY

Study	Immediate Bleeding	Delayed Bleeding	Abortion	Perinatal Death Rate
Rogers and Williams (1967)	14	0	—	4
Daskal and Pitkin (1968)	5	5	17	6
Horowitz and associates (1969)	8	—	0	3
Averette and colleagues (1970)	7	4	27	5
Hannigan and co-workers (1982)	12	4	18	4
Average	9	4	18	5

Modified from Hannigan and colleagues (1982).

neoplasia (CIN I) are identified and subsequently confirmed, further follow-up during pregnancy may consist of colposcopic evaluation. In the absence of lesions detected by a satisfactory colposcopy, simply repeating the cervical smears later in pregnancy is usually adequate. Cytological changes that are suggestive of moderate or severe dysplasia (CIN II or CIN III) or invasive disease require colposcopically directed biopsies to identify the responsible lesion. Women with histologically confirmed intraepithelial neoplasia may be followed with cytology and colposcopically directed biopsies, allowed to deliver vaginally, and given definitive treatment after delivery. If cesarean hysterectomy is indicated for other reasons, it is kept in mind that it may be difficult to be certain that all the cervix has been removed.

Invasive Carcinoma of the Cervix. Pregnancy coexisting with invasive cervical carcinoma complicates both staging and treatment. Accurate identification of the extent of cancer is more difficult during pregnancy because induration of the base of the broad ligaments, which in nonpregnant women characterizes tumor spread beyond the cervix, may be less prominent during pregnancy. Thus, the extent of the tumor is more likely to be underestimated in the pregnant woman. Limited computed tomography of the pelvis is acceptable, but to avoid ionizing radiation, magnetic resonance imaging is a useful adjunct to ascertain extent of disease, including urinary tract involvement (Hannigan, 1990). Cystoscopy and sigmoidoscopy are performed to rule out mucosal involvement.

Although only a few institutions have had extensive experience with cervical carcinoma complicating pregnancy, some generalizations can be made. The survival rate for invasive carcinoma has not been profoundly different for pregnant and nonpregnant women within a given stage of disease, although studies have been retrospective and small. The mode of delivery has not been shown to affect maternal survival significantly, although experiences are limited because most women were delivered by hysterotomy or cesarean section (Hacker and colleagues, 1982). In general, when frankly invasive carcinoma is identified, most favor delivery by the abdominal route, if for no other reason than that the cervix would not lacerate during dilatation.

Management. Treatment of cervical cancer varies according to its stage and pregnancy duration. Treatment for microinvasive disease diagnosed by cone biopsy to exclude frankly invasive disease follows guidelines similar to those for intraepithelial disease. Thus, continuation of pregnancy and vaginal delivery is allowed, with therapy given postpartum.

Invasive cancer demands relatively prompt therapy. In general, during the first half of pregnancy, immediate treatment is advised, whereas during the latter half a reasonable option is to await not only fetal viabil-

ity, but fetal maturity (Greer and colleagues, 1989). Preferred treatment for selected patients with stage I and early stage IIA small diameter (less than 3 cm) invasive carcinoma is **radical hysterectomy plus pelvic lymphadenectomy.** Surgical treatment allows ovarian conservation and vaginal function, and minimizes exposure at an early age to the adverse effects of radiation on the intestinal and urinary tracts. Nisker and Shubat (1983) described 49 cases of stage IB cervical cancer complicating pregnancy, and reported a 29 percent severe complication rate from radiation therapy compared to only 7 percent in those treated by radical surgery. Surgical dissection during pregnancy actually may be facilitated by softening of uterine supportive structures. Before 20 weeks, hysterectomy usually is performed with the fetus in situ, however, in later pregnancy, hysterotomy may first be necessary. **Radiotherapy** is given for more extensive cancer. Early in pregnancy, external irradiation is given and if spontaneous abortion does not ensue, then curettage is performed. During the second trimester, spontaneous abortion may be delayed, and hysterotomy may be necessary in up to one fourth of cases. About a week following abortion, external radiation is begun, followed by intracavitary radium application. For pregnancy after 24 weeks, the risk of delay to allow fetal maturity is unknown, but consideration is given to allowing pulmonic maturity, and after this is verified, to follow by cesarean delivery (American College of Obstetricians and Gynecologists, 1989).

Prognosis. The overall prognosis for all stages of cervical cancer during pregnancy is probably similar to that for nonpregnant women. The results from several published reports are shown in Table 57–6. These aggregate results suggest no difference in survival when pregnant women are compared with nonpregnant women. In-

TABLE 57–6. FIVE-YEAR SURVIVAL RATES OF PREGNANT AND NONPREGNANT WOMEN TREATED FOR CERVICAL CANCER

Investigators	Pregnant No. (%)	Nonpregnant No. (%)
Creasman and associates (1970)		
Stage I	24 (85)	NS (80)
Stage II	18 (60)	NS (70)
Sablinska and colleagues (1977)		
Stage I	114 (72)	208 (76)
Stage II	116 (54)	270 (56)
Lee and co-workers (1981)		
Stage IA	3 (100)	30 (100)
Stage IB-surgery	17 (93)	156 (91)
Stage IB-radiation	4 (80)	32 (88)
Nisker and Shubat (1983)		
Stage IB	49 (70)	NS (87)

NS = not stated.
Modified from Lee and associates (1981).

cluded are 49 cases of stage IB cancer and reported by Nisker and Shubat (1983). These investigators found a 5-year survival of only 70 percent compared with 87 percent in nonpregnant women with similar stages, and although this difference was significant, the authors speculate that this might be due to understaging of the disease during pregnancy.

It is unknown if vaginal delivery through a cancerous cervix worsens the prognosis; however, most oncologists favor abdominal delivery based on theoretical considerations. Certainly, there are at least four case reports of recurrence in the episiotomy scar after vaginal delivery, such as that shown in Figure 57–2. Direct implantation of tumor cells is likely the mechanism of recurrence in these cases.

Ovarian Carcinoma. Malignant ovarian neoplasms are the fourth most common cause of death from cancer and the leading cause of death from genital tract cancers

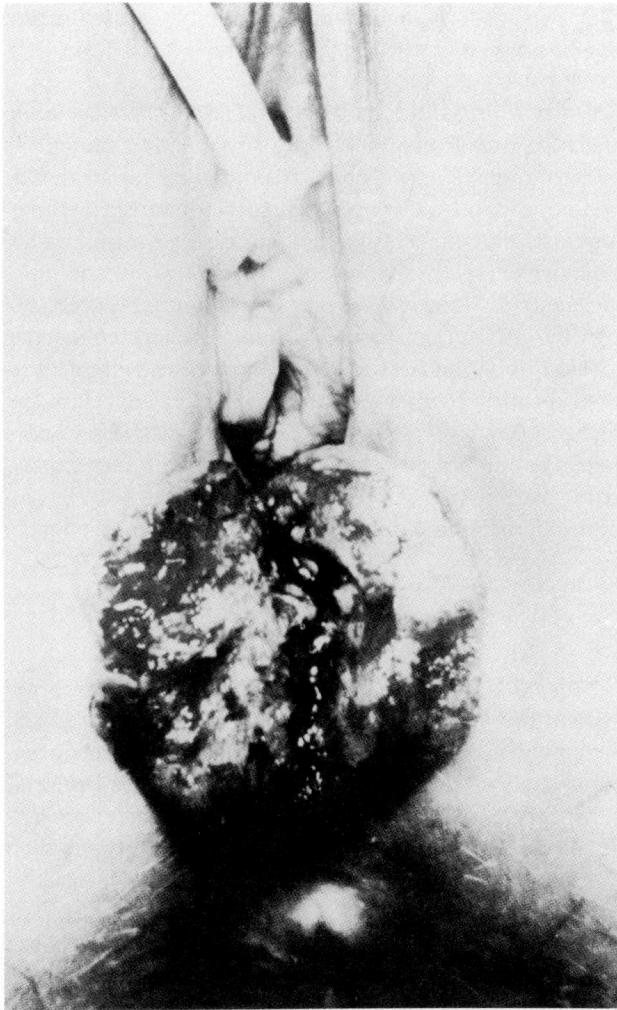

Fig. 57–2. Recurrent cancer in an episiotomy site 6 weeks after delivery in a woman with stage IB cervical carcinoma. (From Gordon and colleagues, 1989, with permission.)

in North American women. Their incidence during pregnancy is not accurately known, but it has been reported to average about 1 per 25,000 deliveries (Jacob and Stringer, 1990; Jolles, 1989). According to the American College of Obstetricians and Gynecologists (1990), about 1 of every 1000 pregnant women will undergo surgical exploration for an adnexal mass. During the 3-year period from 1989 through 1991, 24 pregnant women of nearly 45,000 delivered at Parkland Hospital had exploratory surgery for an adnexal mass. There were no malignant ovarian tumors. There were 18 benign tubal or ovarian cysts; of five ovarian neoplasms, there were four benign cystic teratomas, and one cystadenoma. The one malignancy was a sacral tumor. Because of the younger age of pregnant women, and because of the disparate number of corpus luteal cysts, the incidence of malignancy is lower. Indeed, according to several reviews, adnexal neoplasms diagnosed during pregnancy are malignant in only about 5 percent of cases compared with 15 to 20 percent in nonpregnant women (Hess and associates, 1988; Jacob and Stringer, 1990). Pregnancy apparently does not alter the prognosis of most ovarian malignancies, but complications such as torsion and rupture may increase the incidence of spontaneous abortion or preterm delivery.

Most women who have ovarian cancer are asymptomatic whether they are pregnant or not. At best, symptoms notoriously are vague and nonspecific, and flatulence, abdominal distention, and gastrointestinal discomfort may be attributed to pregnancy. Prior to widespread use of ultrasonic evaluation of pregnancy, most pelvic masses were detected by routine prenatal examination during the first trimester. Diagnosis during the second and third trimesters is more difficult because an adnexal tumor usually is obscured by the enlarging uterus. On the other hand, torsion may be more common as consequence of the enlarged uterus. In many centers, universal sonography is performed during pregnancy and the detection of adnexal masses has increased concomitantly. Certainly, sonography is indicated for women in whom there is a palpable adnexal mass, and it is helpful to differentiate functional cystic masses from solid or multiseptated masses. With the former, expectant management is acceptable, but the latter require surgery for diagnosis. Corpus luteum cysts usually, but not always, subside spontaneously by 14 weeks.

Management. If ovarian cancer is discovered at laparotomy, treatment is similar to that for the nonpregnant woman and this depends on the stage, histological type, and grade of the tumor. After frozen section verifies malignancy, complete surgical staging with careful inspection of all peritoneal and visceral surfaces is performed. **Malignant ovarian tumors confined apparently to one ovary require complete surgical staging, and this is recommended also in tumors of low malignant potential** (Yazigi and associates,

1988). Procedures include peritoneal washings for cytological examination, multiple biopsies of the diaphragmatic undersurface and pelvic and parietal peritoneum, wedge resection of the opposite ovary, partial omentectomy, and excisional biopsies of pelvic and aortic lymph nodes. Whereas in most advanced stages hysterectomy and bilateral adnexectomy is indicated, in certain circumstances it can be justified to remove the tumor and await fetal maturity. In some cases, chemotherapy is given while awaiting pulmonary maturation.

Prognosis. According to Jolles (1989), two thirds of ovarian cancers found during pregnancy are of the common epithelial types. The remainder are germ-cell tumors, and occasionally a stromal-cell tumor. There does not appear to be an adverse influence of pregnancy on these malignancies. About 70 cases of invasive **epithelial cell tumors** coexistent with pregnancy have been reported (Dgani and colleagues, 1989; Jubb, 1963; Van Dessel and co-workers, 1988). These are the most frequent ovarian malignancies in nonpregnant as well as pregnant women. Because of the relatively young age of the pregnant population, there is a higher proportion of less-advanced tumors. Thus, tumors with low-malignant potential and stage IA are seen more often compared with nonpregnant women.

Karlen and associates (1979) reviewed 27 cases of **dysgerminomas** during pregnancy and added one of their own. They found significant obstetrical complications in nearly half of the women and reported a 30 percent recurrence in apparent stage IA cases. Buller and colleagues (1992) described conservative surgical management to allow pregnancy progression in three women with dysgerminomas. They recommended follow-up with magnetic resonance imaging and tumor markers to monitor for recurrences. Young and associates (1984) reviewed 36 cases of **gonadal stromal tumors** which accounted for 4 percent of reported ovarian malignancies complicating pregnancy. All of these tumors were stage I and they had an excellent prognosis. An **endodermal sinus tumor** was diagnosed because of persistently elevated maternal serum alphafetoprotein levels (van der Zee and colleagues, 1991). The tumor had an overall bad prognosis in the 11 cases described thus far (Farahmand and associates, 1991).

Vulvar Cancer. Invasive **squamous cell carcinoma** of the vulva is primarily a disease of postmenopausal women, thus it is only rarely associated with pregnancy. Although Lutz and colleagues (1977) reported an incidence of one case in 8000 pregnancies, this seems excessive. For example, Moore and colleagues (1991) found only 12 cases in their review of English literature, and they added two cases of their own. **Vulvar intraepithelial neoplasia** is seen more often in young women; however, its potential for progression to invasive disease is unclear. Interestingly, the association with invasive disease and papillomavirus infection is not as closely linked as it is with cervical carcinoma (Crum and Burkett, 1989). Kuller and colleagues (1990) reviewed five cases of vulvar **sarcoma** discovered during pregnancy. In four of these, cure was obtained by a variety of therapies.

Any suspicious vulvar lesion should be biopsied. Treatment of invasive disease is individualized according to the clinical stage and depth of invasion, and it varies from wide local excision to radical vulvectomy with bilateral inguino-femoral lymphadenectomy. Surgical treatment is performed at any gestational age, except perhaps in later pregnancy in which it may be delayed until delivery. Vaginal delivery is not contraindicated if the vulvar incisions are well healed.

Uterine Leiomyomas

Benign uterine leiomyomas are common in older pregnant women, and especially in black women. Because they are seldom malignant, leiomyomas complicating pregnancy are considered in Chapter 22 (p. 533).

Leiomyomatosis Peritonealis Disseminata. Rarely at cesarean section or puerperal tubal ligation, numerous subperitoneal smooth muscle tumors are found that at first appear to be disseminated carcinomatosis. Leiomyomatosis peritonealis disseminata results from stimulation, probably by estrogen, of multicentric subcoelomic mesenchymal cells to become smooth muscle cells. According to the review by Minassian and colleagues (1986), about half of the 21 reported cases were discovered during pregnancy. Although surgical excision has been recommended, there is evidence that these tumors regress after pregnancy, and this has been our experience. Although rare, Rubin and associates (1986), reported a malignant variety of this neoplasm.

Cancer of the Gastrointestinal Tract

Colorectal Carcinoma. Colorectal carcinoma is the second most frequent malignancy in women of all age groups in the United States. It rarely complicates pregnancy because only 8 percent of cases are diagnosed before age 40. Although colon cancer has been reported in pregnant women from 19 to 48 years of age, less than 200 cases have been described (Nesbitt and associates, 1985).

The most common symptoms of colon cancer are abdominal pain, distention, nausea and vomiting, constipation, and rectal bleeding. The diagnosis may be delayed because these symptoms may be ascribed to the pregnancy. Gonsoulin and colleagues (1990) described a woman with colon carcinoma and hepatic metastases in whom maternal serum alphafetoprotein levels were elevated persistently after first being measured at 16 weeks' gestation. Certainly, if symptoms suggestive of colon disease persist, digital rectal examination and tests for occult blood and proctosigmoidoscopy are followed by colonoscopy if indicated. Seidman and colleagues (1992) described a woman in whom an intussuscepted colon cancer was diagnosed using magnetic resonance imaging.

From limited information available, it appears that the segmental distribution of the colon cancer lesions is the same as in nonpregnant women and 60 to 70 percent are palpable by rectal examination. Tumors above the peritoneal reflection are uncommon, and Tsukamoto and associates (1986) described only 20 cases in their review. Van Voorhis and Cruikshank (1989) recently reported two additional women with colon cancer who had persistent microcytic, hypochromic anemia from occult bleeding.

Management. Treatment of colon cancer follows the same general guidelines as for nonpregnant patients, and when there is no evidence for metastatic disease, surgery is performed. During the first half of the pregnancy, hysterectomy is not necessary in order to perform colon or rectal resection, and thus therapeutic abortion is not mandated. During later pregnancy, as well as in the presence of metastatic disease, delaying therapy to allow fetal maturation is considered. Vaginal delivery is usually permitted if obstetrical conditions are favorable, but rectal lesions below the pelvic brim may cause dystocia. Of course, hemorrhage, obstruction, or perforation may force surgical intervention (Donegan, 1983).

The prognosis for colon malignancies is similar to that for identical stages in nonpregnant patients, and there is no evidence that pregnancy influences the usual course of the disease. Carcinoembryonic antigen (CEA), a useful tumor marker for colon cancer, may be elevated during pregnancy and therefore is of little value.

Other Gastrointestinal Cancers. **Gastric cancer** is rarely associated with pregnancy, and most reported cases are from Japan. Hirabayashi and collaborators (1987) reviewed outcomes in 60 pregnant women with this malignancy seen over a 70-year period from 1916 to 1985. Delay in diagnosis during pregnancy was unfortunately common and the reported prognosis was consistently poor; 88 percent of women were dead within one year of diagnosis. As discussed in Chapter 51 (p. 1145), persistent upper gastrointestinal symptoms should be evaluated by endoscopy. Davis and Chen (1991) described a woman with gastric cancer who attributed her continued epigastric pain during pregnancy to pre-existing peptic ulcer disease.

At least 21 cases of **carcinoid tumors** complicating pregnancy have been reported. In his review, Durkin (1983) found that most cases were of gastrointestinal

origin, and some were incidentally diagnosed at cesarean section. **Pancreatic cancer** is very rare during pregnancy. Gamberdella (1984) found two previously reported cases and added a third. Bondeson and colleagues (1990) described an endocrine pancreatic malignancy in which the diagnosis was confused because of chorionic gonadotropin produced by an early pregnancy. Primary **hepatic cancer** during pregnancy is rare. Four cases were described by Purtilo and associates (1975) who found only one previously reported case.

Renal Tumors

Walker and Knight (1986) found 71 cases of primary renal neoplasms associated with pregnancy. Half were **renal cell carcinoma** and a palpable abdominal mass was the presenting finding in almost 90 percent of these women. Pain was the second most common presenting symptom (50 percent) and hematuria was found in half the cases. Only one fourth of those women had the classical triad of hematuria, pain, and a palpable mass. We have encountered only six pregnant women with this malignancy during the past 25 years at Parkland Hospital. These women either presented because of painless hematuria, or the tumor was found by abdominal palpation done routinely in conjunction with cesarean section. If suspected antepartum, the diagnosis can be confirmed by intravenous pyelography, ultrasonic-directed needle biopsy, magnetic resonance imaging, or limited computed tomography scanning as shown in Figure 57–3.

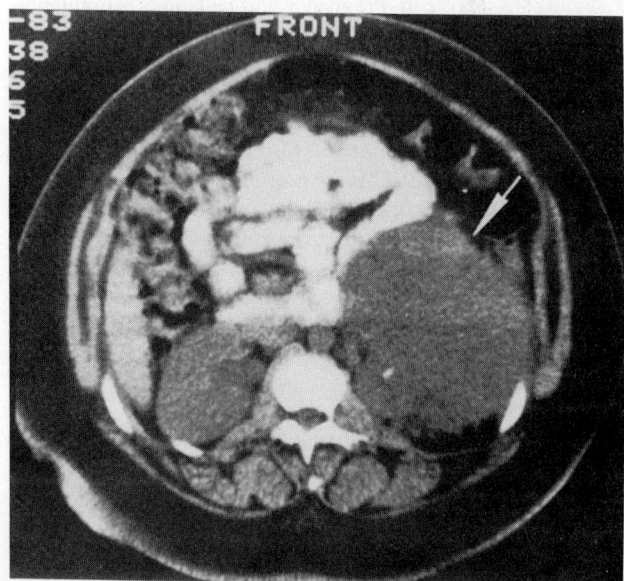

Fig. 57–3. Renal cell carcinoma. Computed axial tomography scan of the abdomen shows a solid mass arising from the left kidney (*arrow*). Right kidney is normal. (From Klein and colleagues, 1987.)

References

American College of Obstetricians and Gynecologists: Cancer of the ovary. Technical bulletin no. 141, May 1990

American College of Obstetricians and Gynecologists: Diagnosis and management of invasive cervical carcinomas. Technical bulletin no. 138, December 1989

Anderson JF, Kent S, Machin GA: Maternal malignant melanoma with placental metastasis: A case report with literature review. Pediatric Pathol 9:35, 1989

Antunez-de-Mayolo J, Ahn YS, Temple JD, Harrington WJ: Spontaneous remission of acute leukemia after the termination of pregnancy. Cancer 63:1621, 1989

Averette HE, Nasser N, Yankow SL, Little WA: Cervical conization in pregnancy. Am J Obstet Gynecol 106:543, 1970

Avilés A, Diaz-Maqueo JC, Talavera A, Guzmán R, Garcia EL: Growth and development of children of mothers treated with chemotherapy during pregnancy: Current status of 43 children. Am J Hematol 36:243, 1991

Avilés A, Diaz-Maqueo JC, Torras V, Garcia EL, Guzmán R: Non-Hodgkin lymphomas and pregnancy: Presentation of 16 cases. Gynecol Oncol 37:335, 1990

Barnavon Y, Wallack MK: Management of the pregnant patient with carcinoma of the breast. Surg Gynecol Obstet 171:347, 1990

Beckman DA, Brent RL: Mechanism of known environmental teratogens: Drugs and chemicals. Clin Perinatol 13:649, 1986

Bondeson AG, Bondeson L, Thompson NW: Early pregnancy masquerading as a marker for malignancy in a young woman with curable neoplasm of the pancreas. Br J Surg 77:108, 1990

Brent RL: Ionizing radiation. Contemp Ob/Gyn 30:20, 1987

Briggs GG, Freeman RK, Yaffee SJ: Drugs in Pregnancy and Lactation, 3rd ed. Baltimore, Williams & Wilkins, 1990

Buller RE, Darrow V, Manetta A, Porto M, DiSaia PJ: Conservative surgical management of dysgerminoma concomitant with pregnancy. Obstet Gynecol 78:887, 1992

Caligiuri MA, Mayer RJ: Pregnancy and leukemia. Semin Oncol 16:388, 1989

Catanzarite VA, Ferguson JE: Acute leukemia and pregnancy: A review of management and outcome, 1972–1982. Obstet Gynecol Surv 39:663, 1984

Clark RM, Reid J: Carcinoma of the breast in pregnancy and lactation. Int J Radiat Oncol Biol Phys 4:693, 1978

Creasman WT, Rutledge FN, Fletcher GH: Carcinoma of the cervix associated with pregnancy. Obstet Gynecol 36:495, 1970

Crum CP, Burkett BJ: Papillomavirus and vulvovaginal neoplasia. J Reprod Med 34:566, 1989

Daskal JL, Pitkin RM: Cone biopsy of the cervix during pregnancy. Obstet Gynecol 32:1, 1968

Davis JL, Chen MD: Gastric carcinoma presenting as an exacerbation of ulcers during pregnancy. A case report. J Repro Med 36:450, 1991

Dgani R, Shoham Z, Atar E, Zosmer A, Lancet M: Ovarian carcinoma during pregnancy: A study of 23 cases in Israel between the years 1960 and 1984. Gynecol Oncol 33:326, 1989

Dildy GA III, Moise KJ Jr, Carpenter RJ Jr, Klima T: Maternal malignancy metastatic to the products of conception: A review. Obstet Gynecol Surv 44:535, 1989

Doll DC, Ringenberg S, Yarbro JW: Management of cancer during pregnancy. Arch Intern Med 148:2058, 1988

Donegan WL: Cancer and pregnancy. CA 33:194, 1983

Donegan WL: Mammary carcinoma and pregnancy. Major Prob Clin Surg 5:448, 1979

Durkin JW: Carcinoid tumor and pregnancy. Am J Obstet Gynecol 145:757, 1983

Ellis DL: Pregnancy and sex steroid hormone effects on nevi of patients with the dysplastic nevus syndrome. J Am Acad Dermatol 25:467, 1991

Farahmand SM, Marchetti DL, Asirwatham JE, Dewey MR: Case report ovarian endodermal sinus tumor associated with pregnancy: Review of the literature. Gynecol Oncol 41:156, 1991

Gamberdella FR: Pancreatic carcinoma in pregnancy: A case report. Am J Obstet Gynecol 149:15, 1984

Gershenson DM: Menstrual and reproductive function after treatment with combination chemotherapy for malignant ovarian germ cell tumors. J Clin Oncol 6:270, 1988

Gonsoulin W, Mason B, Carpenter RJ Jr: Colon cancer in pregnancy with elevated maternal serum α-fetoprotein level at presentation. Am J Obstet Gynecol 163:1172, 1990

Gordon AN, Jensen R, Jones HW III: Squamous carcinoma of the cervix complicating pregnancy: Recurrence in episiotomy after vaginal delivery: Obstet Gynecol 73:850, 1989

Greer BE, Easterling TR, McLennan DA, Benedetti TJ, Cain JM, Figge DC, Tamimi HK, Jackson JC: Fetal and maternal considerations in the management of stage I-B cervical cancer during pregnancy. Gynecol Oncol 34:61, 1989

Haagensen CD: Diseases of the Breast, 2nd ed. Philadelphia, WB Saunders Co., 1971, p 660

Hacker NF, Berek JS, Lagasse LD, Charles EH, Savage EW, Moore JG: Carcinoma of the cervix associated with pregnancy. Obstet Gynecol 59:735, 1982

Hannigan EV: Cervical cancer in pregnancy. Clin Obstet Gynecol 33:837, 1990

Hannigan EV, Whitehouse HH, Atkinson WD, Becker SN: Cone biopsy during pregnancy. Obstet Gynecol 60:450, 1982

Harvey JC, Rosen PP, Ashikari R, Robbins GF, Kinne DW: The effect of pregnancy on the prognosis of carcinoma of the breast following radical mastectomy. Surg Gynecol Obstet 153:723, 1981

Hess LW, Peaceman A, O'Brien WF, Winkel CA, Cruikshank DP, Morrison JC: Adnexal mass occurring with intrauterine pregnancy: Report of fifty-four patients requiring laparotomy for definitive management. Am J Obstet Gynecol 158:1029, 1988

Hirabayashi M, Ueo H, Okudaira Y, Matsumata T, Hanawa S, Sugimachi K: Early gastric cancer and a concomitant pregnancy. Am Surg 53:730, 1987

Hochman A, Schreiber H: Pregnancy and cancer of the breast. Obstet Gynecol 2:268, 1953

Holleb AI, Farrow JH: The relation of carcinoma of the breast and pregnancy in 238 patients. Surg Gynecol Obstet 115:65, 1962

Holly EA: Melanoma and pregnancy. Recent Results. Cancer Res 102:118, 1986

Holmes GE, Holmes FF: Pregnancy outcomes of patients treated for Hodgkin's disease: A controlled study. Cancer 41:1317, 1978

Hoover HC Jr: Breast cancer during pregnancy and lactation. Surg Clin N Amer 70:1151, 1990

Horning SJ, Hoppe RT, Kaplan HS, Rosenberg SA: Female reproductive potential after treatment for Hodgkin's disease. N Engl J Med 304:1377, 1981

Hornstein E, Skornick Y, Rozin R: The management of breast carcinoma in pregnancy and lactation. J Surg Oncol 21:179, 1982

Horowitz A, Sabatelle R, Sall S: The risk of cone biopsy during pregnancy. J Reprod Med 3:9, 1969

Ioachim HL: Non-Hodgkin's lymphoma in pregnancy. Arch Pathol Lab Med 109:803, 1985

Jacob JH, Stringer CA: Diagnosis and management of cancer during pregnancy. Semin Perinatol 14:79, 1990

Jacobs C, Donaldson SS, Rosenberg SA, Kaplan HS: Management of the pregnant patient with Hodgkin's disease. Ann Intern Med 95:669, 1981

Jolles CJ: Gynecologic cancer associated with pregnancy. Semin Oncol 16:417, 1989

Jubb ED: Primary ovarian carcinoma in pregnancy. Am J Obstet Gynecol 85:345, 1963

Kaldor JM, Day NE, Clarke A, Van Leeuwen FE, Henry-Amar M, Fiorentino Mv, Bell J, Pedersen D, Band P, Assouline D, Koch M, Choi W, Prior P, Blair V, Langmark F, Kirn VP, Neal F, Peters D, Pfiffer R, Karjalainen S, Cuzick J, Sutcliffe SB, Somers R, Pellae-Cosset B, Pappagallo GL, Fraser P, Storm H, Stoval M: Leukemia following Hodgkin's disease: N Engl J Med 322:7, 1990

Karlen JR, Akbari A, Cook WA: Dysgerminoma associated with pregnancy. Obstet Gynecol 53:330, 1979

Kiguchi K, Bibbo M, Hasegawa T, Kurihara S, Tsutsui F, Wied G: Dysplasia during pregnancy: A cytologic follow-up study. J Reprod Med 26:66, 1981

King LA, Nevin PC, Williams PP, Carson LF: Treatment of advanced epithelial ovarian carcinoma in pregnancy with cisplatin-based chemotherapy. Gynecol Oncol 41:78, 1991

King RM, Welch JS, Martin JK, Coulam CB: Carcinoma of the breast associated with pregnancy. Surg Gynecol Obstet 160:228, 1985

Klein VR, Laifer S, Timoll EA, Repke JT: Renal cell carcinoma in pregnancy. Obstet Gynecol 69:531, 1987

Koren G, Weiner L, Lishner M, Zemlickis D, Finegen J: Cancer in pregnancy: Identification of unanswered questions on maternal and fetal risks. Obstet Gynecol Surv 45:509, 1990

Kuller JA, Zucker PK, Peng TCC: Vulvar leiomyosarcoma in pregnancy. Am J Obstet Gynecol 162:164, 1990

Larsson G, Grundsell H, Gullberg B, Svenneraud S: Outcome of pregnancy after conization. Acta Obstet Gynecol Scand 61:461, 1982

Lee RB, Neglia W, Park RC: Cervical carcinoma in pregnancy. Obstet Gynecol 58:584, 1981

Lewis BJ, Laros RK Jr: Leukemia and lymphoma. In Laros RK Jr (ed): Blood Disorders in Pregnancy. Philadelphia, Lea & Febiger, 1986, p 85

Li FP, Fine W, Jaffe N, Holmes GE, Holmes FF: Offspring of patients treated for cancer in childhood. J Natl Cancer Inst 62:1193, 1979

Lippman ME, Lichter AS, Danforth DN Jr: Diagnosis and management of breast cancer. Philadelphia, Saunders, 1988, p 415

Lutz MH, Underwood PB Jr, Rozier JC, Putney FW: Genital malignancy in pregnancy. Am J Obstet Gynecol 129:536, 1977

MacKie RM, Bufalino R, Morabito A, Sutherland C, Cacsinelli N: Lack of effect of pregnancy on outcome of melanoma. Lancet 337:653, 1991

McLain CR Jr: Leukemia in pregnancy. Clin Obstet Gynecol 17:185, 1974

McManamny DS, Moss ALH, Pocock PV, Briggs JC: Melanoma and pregnancy: A long-term follow-up. Br J Obstet Gynaecol 96:1419, 1989

Minassian SS, Frangipane W, Polin JI, Ellis M: Leiomyomatosis peritonealis disseminata: A case report and literature review. J Reprod Med 31:997, 1986

Moore DH, Fowler WC Jr, Currie JL, Walton LA: Squamous cell carcinoma of the vulva in pregnancy. Gynecol Oncol 41:74, 1991

Nesbitt JC, Moise KJ, Sawyers JL: Colorectal carcinoma in pregnancy. Arch Surg 120:636, 1985

Nisce LZ, Tome, MA, Shaoqin H, Lee BJ, Kutcher GJ: Management of coexisting Hodgkin's disease and pregnancy. Am J Clin Oncol 9:146, 1986

Nisker JA, Shubat M: Stage IB cervical carcinoma and pregnancy: Report of 49 cases. Am J Obstet Gynecol 145:203, 1983

Nugent P, O'Connell TX: Breast cancer and pregnancy. Arch Surg 120:1221, 1985

Orr JW Jr, Shingleton HM: Cancer in pregnancy. In Hickey RC (ed): Current Problems in Cancer. Chicago, Year Book, 1983, p 1

Otake M, Schull WJ: In utero exposure to A-bomb radiation and mental retardation: A reassessment. Br J Radiol 57:409, 1984

Parente JT, Amsel M, Lerner R, Chinea F: Breast cancer associated with pregnancy. Obstet Gynecol 71:861, 1988

Petrek JA, Dukoff R, Rogatko A: Prognosis of pregnancy-associated breast cancer. Cancer 67:869, 1991

Purtilo DT, Clark JV, Williams R: Primary hepatic malignancy in pregnant women. Am J Obstet Gynecol 121:41, 1975

Reynoso EE, Shepherd FA, Messner HA, Farquharson HA, Garvey MB, Baker MA: Acute leukemia during pregnancy: The Toronto leukemia study group experience with long-term follow-up of children exposed in utero to chemotherapeutic agents. J Clin Oncol 5:1098, 1987

Ribeiro G, Jones DA, Jones M: Carcinoma of the breast associated with pregnancy. Br J Surg 73:607, 1986

Ribeiro GG, Palmer MK: Breast carcinoma associated with pregnancy: A clinician's dilemma. BMJ 2:1524, 1977

Rogers RS III, Williams JH: The impact of the suspicious Papanicolaou smear on pregnancy: A study of nationwide attitudes and maternal and perinatal complications. Am J Obstet Gynecol 98:488, 1967

Rosemond GP: Carcinoma of the breast during pregnancy. Clin Obstet Gynecol 6:994, 1963

Rubin SC, Wheeler JE, Mikuta JJ: Malignant leiomyomatosis peritonealis disseminata. Obstet Gynecol 68:126, 1986

Rustin GJ, Booth M, Dent J, Salt S, Rustin F, Bagshawe KD: Pregnancy after chemotherapy for gestational trophoblastic tumours. BMJ 288:103, 1984

Sablinska R, Tarlowska L, Stelmachow J: Invasive carcinoma of the cervix associated with pregnancy: Correlation between patient age, advancement of cancer and gestation, and result of treatment. Gynecol Oncol 5:363, 1977

Sachs BP, Penzias AS, Brown DAJ, Driscoll SG, Jewett JF: Cancer-related maternal mortality in Massachusetts, 1954–1985. Gynecol Oncol 36:395, 1990

Seidman DS, Heyman Z, Ben-Ari GY, Mashiach S, Barkai G: Use of magnetic resonance imaging in pregnancy to diagnose intussusception induced by colonic cancer. Obstet Gynecol 79:822, 1992

Selevan SG, Lindbohm ML, Hornung RW, Hemminki K: A study of occupational exposure to antineoplastic drugs and fetal loss in nurses. N Engl J Med 313:1173, 1985

Slingluff CL, Reintgen DS, Vollmer RT, Seigler HF: Malignant melanoma arising during pregnancy. A study of 100 patients. Ann Surg 211:552, 1990

Smith RS, Randal P: Melanoma during pregnancy. Obstet Gynecol 34:825, 1969

Sutton R, Buzdar AU, Hortobagyi GN: Pregnancy and offspring after adjuvant chemotherapy in breast cancer patients. Cancer 65:847, 1990

Talebian F, Krumholz BA, Shayan A, Mann LI: Colposcopic evaluation of patients with abnormal cytologic smears during pregnancy. Obstet Gynecol 47:693, 1976

Third National Cancer Survey: Incidence data. Natl Cancer Inst Monogr 41:108, 1975

Tsukamoto N, Uchino H, Matsukuma K, Kamura T: Carcinoma of the colon presenting as bilateral ovarian tumors during pregnancy. Gynecol Oncol 24:385, 1986

Tucker MA, Coleman CN, Cox RS, Varghese A, Rosenberg SA: Risk of second cancers after treatment for Hodgkin's disease. N Engl J Med 318:76, 1988

Urba WJ, Longo DL: Hodgkin's disease. N Engl J Med 326:678, 1992

van der Zee AGJ, de Bruijin HWA, Bouma J, Aalders JG, Oosterhuis JW, de Vries EGE: Endodermal sinus tumor of the ovary during pregnancy: A case report. Am J Obstet Gynecol 164:504, 1991

Van Dessel T, Hameeteman TM, Wagenaar SS: Mucinous cystadenocarcinoma in pregnancy. Case report. Br J Obstet Gynaecol 95:527, 1988

Van Voorhis B, Cruikshank DP: Colon carcinoma complicating pregnancy. J Reprod Med 34:923, 1989

Walker JL, Knight EL: Renal cell carcinoma in pregnancy. Cancer 58:2343, 1986

Ward FT, Weiss RB: Lymphoma and pregnancy. Semin Oncol 16:397, 1989

Waxman J: Cancer, chemotherapy and fertility. BMJ 290:1096, 1985

Westberg SV: Prognosis of breast cancer for pregnant and nursing women. Acta Obstet Gynecol Scand (suppl 4) 25:1, 1946

White TT: Carcinoma of the breast associated with pregnancy. Northwest Med 57:477, 1958

Wong DJ, Strassner HT: Melanoma in pregnancy. Clin Obstet Gynecol 33:782, 1990

Yazigi R, Sandstad J, Munoz A: Primary staging in ovarian tumors of low malignant potential. Gynecol Oncol 31:402, 1988

Young RH, Dudley AG, Scully RE: Granulosa cell, Sertoli-Leydig cell, and unclassified sex cord-stromal tumors associated with pregnancy: A clinicopathological analysis of thirty-six cases. Gynecol Oncol 18:181, 1984

Zemlickis D, Lishner M, Degendorfer P, Panzarella T, Sutcliffe SB, Koren G: Fetal outcome after in utero exposure to cancer chemotherapy. Arch Intern Med 152:573, 1992a

Zemlickis D, Lishner M, Degendorfer P, Panzarella T, Burke B, Sutcliffe SB, Koren G: Maternal and fetal outcome after breast cancer in pregnancy. Am J Obstet Gynecol 166:781, 1992b

CHAPTER 58
Infections

The pregnant woman and her fetus are susceptible to many infections and infectious diseases. Some of these may be quite serious and life-threatening for the mother, whereas others may have a profound impact on fetal outcome by virtue of a high likelihood of teratogenesis. Considered now are some infections that pose unique problems created during a coexisting pregnancy.

Immunological Changes. There has been much speculation concerning possible effects of decreased immunological surveillance during pregnancy. These are principally engendered by maternal tolerance for the foreign-tissue antigens of the semiallogeneic fetal "graft."

Generally speaking, the pregnant woman is immunocompetent. As discussed in Chapter 8 (p. 224), although there are subtle changes in circulating immunoglobulin levels in pregnancy, these appear to be of no consequence. Polymorphonuclear leukocyte chemotaxis and adherence may be depressed beginning in midpregnancy. Assessment of cell-mediated immunity is difficult, but available evidence suggests that maternal lymphocytes are as fully competent as paternal and unrelated cells in producing a cytotoxic response (Stirrat, 1991).

Fetal and Newborn Immunology. The active immunological capacity of the fetus and neonate is compromised compared with that of older children and adults. According to Stirrat (1991), cell-mediated and humoral immunity begins to develop in the fetus by 9 to 15 weeks. Despite the ability to synthesize IgG, the primary fetal response to infection is IgM. Conversely, passive immunity is provided by the mother by IgG transferred actively across the placenta. By 16 weeks, transfer begins to increase rapidly, and by 26 weeks fetal concentrations are equivalent to those of the mother. At birth, the degree of passive immunity is much lower in preterm infants compared with older newborns.

Neonatal infection, especially in its early stages, may be difficult to diagnose because of failure to respond in a classical fashion. The signs of infection can be vague, and nonspecific. If infected in utero, there may be depression and acidosis at birth for no apparent reason. The infant may suck poorly, vomit, or develop abdominal distention. Respiratory insufficiency may develop, which is similar in many ways to idiopathic respiratory distress syndrome. The neonate may be lethargic or jittery. The response to sepsis may be hypothermia rather than hyperthermia, and the total leukocyte count and neutrophil counts may be depressed or not influenced by sepsis.

As shown in Table 58–1, bacteria, viruses, or parasites may gain access transplacentally, or they may cross the membranes even though intact. Fetal infections may develop early in pregnancy to produce obvious stigmata at birth. Conversely, organisms may colonize and infect the fetus during delivery; thus, preterm rupture of membranes, prolonged labor, and cervical examinations and manipulations may increase the risk of neonatal infection. Infection occurring less than 72 hours of age usually, but not always, is caused by bacteria acquired in utero or during delivery, whereas infections after that time most likely have been acquired after birth.

A major mechanism for inducing infection subsequent to birth is from those caring for the infant who may be colonized with the organism or may passively transfer it from another infected infant. The use of indwelling venous and arterial umbilical catheters demands scrupulous care to prevent infection. Ventilatory systems that involve moisture become contaminated quickly with bacteria and can be the source of life-threatening infection. **The very-low-birthweight infant who survives the first few days is at considerable risk of dying later from infection acquired in the intensive-care nursery.**

Any infant who appears ill should be suspected of having an infection. If infection is suspected at vaginal delivery, some recommend that cultures of a swabbing from the ear or of gastric aspirate may be taken, or amnionic fluid can be collected at cesarean section and promptly cultured. Because bacteria from the normal maternal flora almost always are found, the pragmatic use of such cultures is unproven. Subsequently, cultures of blood and cerebrospinal fluid of the infant may be essential for appropriate evaluation.

Bacteria most often responsible for sepsis in the newborn in the United States have varied during the past several decades. For example, in the 1930s and 1940s, group A β-hemolytic streptococci were involved principally. With the widespread use of penicillin, these infections were reduced remarkably, and next came the staphylococcus in the 1950s and coliforms and group B streptococcus in the 1970s.

TABLE 58–1. SOME CAUSES OF FETAL AND NEONATAL INFECTIONS

Intrauterine

Transplacental—rubella, cytomegalovirus, syphilis, toxoplasmosis, malaria, varicella-zoster, listeriosis, coxsackie, parvovirus, human immunodeficiency virus, other viruses

Ascending chorioamnionitis—bacteria associated with:
    Preterm rupture of membranes
    Preterm labor with intact membranes

Intrapartum

Maternal exposure—gonorrhea, herpesvirus, chlamydia, papillomavirus, group B streptococcus, hepatitis B, human immunodeficiency virus

External contamination—staphylococcus, coliforms, others

Neonatal

Human transmission—staphylococcus, viruses

Respiratory equipment and catheters—staphylococcus, coliforms

VIRAL INFECTIONS

Varicella-Zoster

Varicella-zoster virus is a DNA herpesvirus that remains latent in the dorsal root ganglia after primary infection. It may be reactivated years later to cause herpes zoster or shingles. Most adults have acquired chickenpox during childhood and are immune. The virus is highly contagious for nonimmune persons. Varicella infection in adults tends to be much more severe than in children. Although disputed, there is evidence that infection is especially severe during pregnancy. For example, Paryani and Arvin (1986) reported that 4 of 43, or about 10 percent of infected pregnant women, developed pneumonitis. Two of these women required ventilatory support and one died. Currently, treatment usually consists of oxygenation, assisted ventilation when necessary, and treatment with acyclovir given intravenously (Cox and colleagues, 1990). Although there are some reassurances that acyclovir is probably not teratogenic, its use is reserved for life-threatening infections (Andrews and colleagues, 1992).

Maternal herpes zoster infection is more common in older or immunocompromised patients. There is no evidence that zoster is more frequent or more severe in pregnant women. Eyal and associates (1983), in a review of 15 cases of zoster during pregnancy, concluded that there was little evidence that zoster caused congenital malformations.

Prevention. Administration of **varicella-zoster immunoglobulin (VZIG)** will either prevent or attenuate varicella infection in exposed susceptible individuals if given within 96 hours. The dose is 125 U/10 kg given intramuscularly. Immunoglobulin is recommended by the Centers for Disease Control (1984) for immuno-compromised susceptible adults who are exposed, but it is not recommended routinely for pregnant women. Because of the severity of varicella during pregnancy, however, some recommend immunoglobulin administration (McGregor and colleagues, 1987; Paryani and Arvin, 1986). Up to 80 to 90 percent of adults are immune from prior symptomatic or asymptomatic infection, thus antibody testing with enzyme-linked immunosorbent assay (ELISA) or fluorescent antibody to membrane antigen (FAMA) should be done, if possible, prior to immune globulin therapy. Demonstration of antibodies by complement fixation indicates relatively recent infection. A rising complement-fixation titer is evidence for current or very recent disease.

An experimental attenuated live-virus vaccine has been developed and, if successful, will probably be of value for susceptible nonpregnant women.

Fetal Effects. Maternal chickenpox during early pregnancy has been implicated to cause congenital malformations by transplacental infection (Stagno and Whitley, 1985). Isada and associates (1991) recovered viral DNA using chorionic villus sampling, but found no correlation with clinical disease in the fetus. Paryani and Arvin (1986) reported that 10 percent of maternal infections resulted in clinical evidence for fetal infection, and this risk was the same for all trimesters. Another 12 percent of fetuses exposed during the second or third trimester had immunological evidence for infection. Infection early in pregnancy resulted in severe congenital malformations including chorioretinitis, cerebral cortical atrophy, hydronephrosis, and cutaneous and bony leg defects (Fig. 58–1). Magliocco and colleagues (1992) described most of these findings in a term infant whose mother had chickenpox at 12 weeks' gestation. Conversely, Balducci and associates (1992) found no phys-

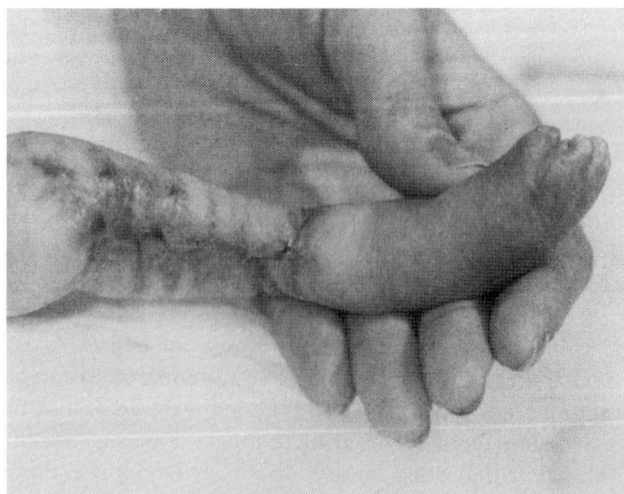

Fig. 58–1. Atrophy of the lower extremity with bony defects and scarring in a fetus infected during the first trimester by varicella. (From Paryani and Arvin, 1986, with permission.)

ical stigmata of congenital varicella syndrome in 36 infants whose mothers had classical chickenpox in the first trimester.

Fetal exposure later in pregnancy is associated with congenital varicella lesions, and zoster occasionally develops at several months of age. Fetal exposure to the virus just before or during delivery, and therefore before maternal antibody has been formed, poses a serious threat to the newborn. The incubation period for neonatal varicella infection is short, usually less than 2 weeks. In some instances, the infant will develop disseminated visceral and central nervous system disease which will likely be fatal. Varicella-zoster or zoster immunoglobulin (ZIG) should be administered to the neonate whenever the onset of maternal clinical disease was within 5 days before delivery or 2 days postpartum. Earlier observations established that perinatal mortality at other times was reduced drastically because passive maternal antibody was protective. Despite passive immunoglobulin therapy, Miller and colleagues (1989) reported that 15 percent of infants developed severe varicella infection.

Influenza

Influenza is caused by members of the *Orthomyxoviridae* family. Influenza A and B form one genus of these RNA viruses and are identified by nucleoprotein antigenic reactions. These are subclassified further by hemagglutinin (H) and neuraminidase (N) antigenic makeup. The viral strain then is characterized by its origin and the year isolated. For example, one component in the 1992–1993 trivalent vaccine was A/Texas/36/91 (H_1N_1), the 36th influenza A virus isolated from a patient in Texas in 1991 and having antigens of the H_1 hemagglutinin and N_1 neuraminidase subtypes.

Influenza A is more serious than influenza B and usually develops during winter epidemics. Infection usually is self-limited and not life-threatening for otherwise healthy adults. If pneumonia develops, the prognosis becomes serious (see Chap. 49, p. 1106). Although antibiotics are not effective against the influenza viruses, they are of value in the treatment of a secondary bacterial pneumonia. In the influenza pandemic of 1918, the pneumonic form of the infection was a grave complication of pregnancy. In a statistical study based on 1350 cases, Harris (1919) found a gross maternal mortality rate of 27 percent, which increased to 50 percent when pneumonia developed. The 1957 pandemic also affected pregnant women with particular frequency and ferocity. In August and September 1957, for instance, 50 percent of childbearing-age women who died of influenza in Minnesota were pregnant (Freeman and Barno, 1959). In the same year in that state, the leading cause of maternal death was influenza. In New York City, the incidence of influenza in pregnant women was 50 per-

cent higher than in nonpregnant controls and the mortality rate also was higher (Bass and Molloshok, 1960).

Prevention. Vaccination against influenza is recommended by the Centers for Disease Control (1992) for pregnant women who have chronic underlying medical disorders and health-care workers who are likely to be exposed to high-risk patients. The vaccine is considered safe for pregnant women, but unless there are high-risk conditions, it is recommended that vaccination be withheld until after the first trimester.

Amantadine is an antiviral agent with specific activity against influenza A viruses. Given prophylactically during epidemics, it is 70 to 90 percent effective in preventing influenza (Centers for Disease Control, 1992). If therapy is begun within 48 hours of onset of symptoms, amantadine reduces the duration of fever and systemic symptoms. It is reserved for nonimmunized women at high risk for influenza complications.

Fetal Effects. There is no firm evidence that influenza A virus causes congenital malformations (Korones, 1988; Larsen, 1982). Saxén and associates (1990) identified no association with increased first-trimester influenza in 248 mothers of anencephalic children. However, McGregor and colleagues (1984) have convincingly demonstrated that the virus can infect the fetus, at least late in pregnancy. Schizophrenia is more common in individuals born in late winter and early spring, and Barr and colleagues (1990) and O'Callaghan and co-workers (1991) have provided epidemiological evidence that midpregnancy fetal exposure in influenza A doubles this risk.

Mumps

This uncommon adult infectious disease is caused by an RNA paramyxovirus. Up to 80 to 90 percent of adults are seropositive. The virus primarily infects the salivary glands, but may involve the gonads, meninges, pancreas, and other organs. Treatment is symptomatic. Mumps during pregnancy is no more severe than in nonpregnant adults.

The live attenuated Jeryl–Lynn vaccine strain is recommended for children after one year of age. The vaccine is contraindicated in pregnant women (American College of Obstetricians and Gynecologists, 1991).

Fetal Effects. There is no firm evidence that mumps infection causes increased fetal wastage (Siegal and Fuerst, 1966). Fetal infection has been confirmed in a 10-week fetus (Kurtz and colleagues, 1982), and attenuated Jeryl–Lynn virus has been recovered from placental tissue of women given the live-attenuated vaccine 7 to 10 days before elective abortion (Yamauchi and co-workers, 1974). Manson and associates (1960) described 501 cases of mumps during pregnancy and reported that major fetal anomalies were not much different than in the general population. Siegel (1973) confirmed this in a cohort study. Congenital mumps is very rare.

Rubeola (Measles)

Most adults are immune to measles. Unfortunately, when measles becomes epidemic as it did during 1989, unvaccinated women may develop measles pneumonia with adverse maternal and perinatal outcomes (Stein and Greenspoon, 1991). In nonpregnant adults with measles, about 3 percent develop clinical pneumonia.

The virus does not appear to be teratogenic, but there is an increased frequency of abortion and low-birthweight infants with maternal measles (Christensen and co-workers, 1953; Siegel, 1973; Siegel and Fuerst, 1966). Moroi and colleagues (1991) reported that measles infection of the placenta caused death in a 25-week fetus who was not infected. If the woman develops measles shortly before birth, there is considerable risk of infection developing in the neonate and, in turn, some risk of death, especially in preterm infants. Passive immunization can be achieved by administering immune serum globulin, 5 mL given intramuscularly within 3 days of exposure. Vaccination should not be attempted during pregnancy; however, vaccination of susceptible women is recommended for routine postpartum care (American College of Obstetricians and Gynecologists, 1991).

Respiratory Viruses

The average adult has three to four acute viral respiratory illnesses each year. Probably three fourths of these infections are caused by more than 200 antigenetically distinct viruses. Illnesses caused by respiratory viruses cause the common cold, pharyngitis, laryngotracheobronchitis, bronchitis, and pneumonia. Virus that frequently cause these are common cold viruses, influenza viruses, adenoviruses, and respiratory syncytial viruses.

Rhinovirus, coronavirus, and adenovirus are major causes of the **common cold.** The first two are RNA viruses and usually produce a trivial, self-limited illness characterized by rhinorrhea, sneezing, and congestion. There are 100 distinct rhinovirus serotypes. The DNA-containing adenovirus is more likely to produce cough and lower respiratory tract involvement, including pneumonia.

It is thought that the pregnant woman may be slightly more susceptible to acute upper respiratory infections than the nonpregnant woman. This is difficult to prove. As discussed in Chapter 49 (p. 1105), pneumonia complicating pregnancy is often preceded by an acute upper respiratory viral infection.

It is worrisome that mothers suffering from common cold had a 4.5-fold increased risk of anencephaly when a 393-woman cohort of the Finnish Register of Congenital Malformations was analyzed (Kurppa and associates, 1991). These investigators further found that fever—a commonly quoted possible cause of anencephaly—was not found to be a factor.

Enterovirus Infections

Enteroviruses are a major subgroup of the RNA picornaviruses that include poliovirus, coxsackievirus, and echovirus. Even though they are trophic for intestinal epithelium, they can cause widespread infections that may include the central nervous system, skin, heart, and lungs. Occasionally, fulminant newborn disease is caused by enteroviral infections. Hepatitis A is an enterovirus 72 that is discussed in Chapter 51 (p. 1158).

Coxsackievirus. Coxsackie infections usually are clinically inapparent, but may cause aseptic meningitis, a polio-like illness, rashes, respiratory disease, or pleuritis, pericarditis, and myocarditis. The virus can be a serious complication of pregnancy because it can be fatal to the fetus-infant, although causing only minor symptoms in the mother.

In an earlier investigation, Brown and Karunas (1972) reported that congenital malformations were increased slightly in pregnant women who had serological evidence of some coxsackievirus, but not echovirus infections. According to Amstey and colleagues (1988), there is clinical evidence that the coxsackievirus seldom infects the fetus. Viremia in the fetus may cause hepatitis, myocarditis, and encephalomyelitis which can cause fetal death (Brady and Purdon, 1986). Finally, Garcia and associates (1991) reported that histological placentitis was common following maternal enteroviral infection. Thus, although fetal death is uncommon, it is possible that maternal coxsackievirus infection causes sublethal injuries of the embryo and fetus, thus producing congenital anomalies.

Poliovirus. Most polioviral infections are subclinical or mild. The virus is tropic for the central nervous system and symptomatic infections can cause paralytic disease—poliomyelitis. Inactivated subcutaneous polio vaccine is recommended for susceptible pregnant women who must travel to endemic areas or in other high-risk situations. Live oral polio vaccine has been used for mass vaccination during pregnancy without harmful fetal effects (Harjulehto and associates, 1989). With the widespread use of vaccination during childhood, polio has become rare in the United States. Siegel and Goldberg (1955), in a carefully controlled study in New York City, demonstrated that pregnant women not only were more susceptible to polio, but had a higher death rate. Although the perinatal loss was about 33 percent, rarely was the fetus infected. If maternal infection occurs late in pregnancy, the newborn may suffer fatal infection.

Parvovirus

Human B19 parvovirus causes **erythema infectiosum, or fifth disease.** This is a small, single-stranded DNA virus that replicates in rapidly proliferating cells, for example, erythroblast precursors. Viremia occurs during the prodrome, which is followed by clinical features including a bright red macular rash and erythroderma that affects the face giving a *slapped cheek* appearance. The rash, with accompanying arthralgias, may be due to immune-complex disease. In some women, the disease may be asymptomatic or without a rash. Confirmation of infection is by IgM specific antibody. About 50 percent of pregnant women are nonimmune, and there is no evidence that the mild infection is altered by pregnancy. The attack rate of susceptible adults in a school outbreak was 20 percent (Cartter and associates, 1991). In women with hemolytic anemia, for example, sickle cell disease, parvovirus infection may cause an aplastic crisis (see Chap. 52, p. 1179).

Maternal infection can be associated with adverse pregnancy outcomes, including abortion and fetal death. During an outbreak in Connecticut, the fetal loss rate was 5 percent in 39 infected women (Rodis and colleagues, 1990). In London, the Public Health Laboratory Service Working Party on Fifth Disease (1990) prospectively followed 190 women infected during pregnancy. The transplacental infection rate was 33 percent. Midpregnancy infection was associated with 12 percent fetal loss; overall the risk of fetal death was 9 percent.

There is no evidence that the virus is teratogenic, but fetal death usually is due to hydrops caused by anemia from erythroid aplasia.

Diagnosis is confirmed serologically by demonstrating parvovirus-specific IgM antibodies. For women with positive serology, ultrasonographic examination is indicated, and if there is hydrops, then fetal transfusion should be considered (Peters and Nicolaides, 1990; Rodis and colleagues, 1990; Sahakian and associates, 1991).

Rubella

Rubella, or German measles, a disease usually of minor import in the absence of pregnancy, has been directly responsible for inestimable pregnancy wastage, and even more importantly, for severe congenital malformations. The relation between maternal rubella and grave congenital malformations was first recognized by Gregg (1942), an Australian ophthalmologist.

Prevention. Although large epidemics of rubella have virtually disappeared in the United States because of immunization, the disease, with its horrific teratogenic potential, still prevails (Fig. 58–2). From 6 to 25 percent of women are susceptible, and the Centers for Disease Control (1991a) reported at least 26 outbreaks in 1990 and many of those infected were 20 years or older. As shown in the inset in Figure 58–2, the incidence of congenital rubella syndrome has increased since 1986. Lee and colleagues (1992) have shown that at least half of cases of congenital rubella were because of missed opportunities at vaccination.

To eradicate the disease completely, the following approach is recommended for immunizing the adult population, particularly women of childbearing age:

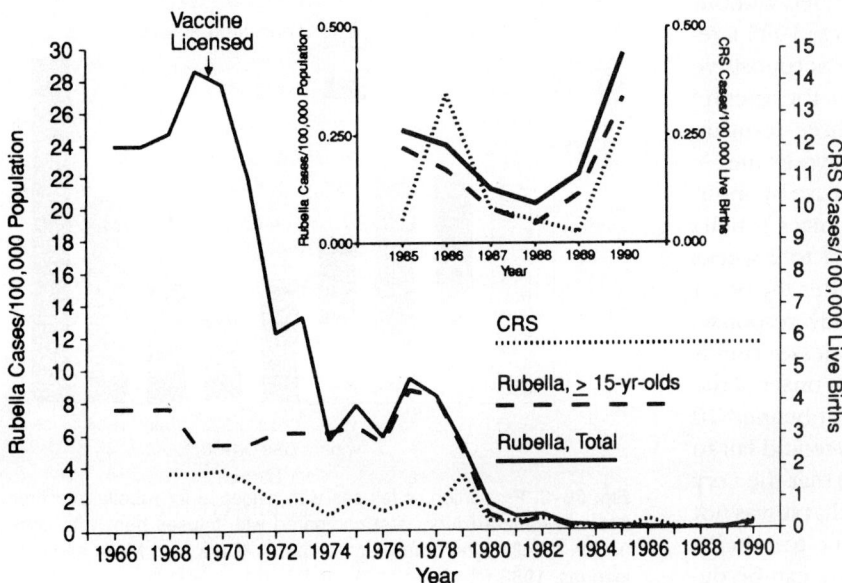

Fig. 58–2. Incidence rates of reported rubella and congenital rubella syndrome (CRS), United States, 1966 through 1990. (From Centers for Disease Control, 1991a).

1. Education of health-care providers and the general public on the dangers of rubella infection.
2. Vaccination of susceptible women as part of routine medical and gynecological care.
3. Vaccination of susceptible women visiting family planning clinics.
4. Identification and vaccination of unimmunized women immediately after childbirth or abortion.
5. Vaccination of nonpregnant susceptible women identified by premarital serology.
6. Vaccination of all susceptible hospital personnel who might be exposed to patients with rubella or who might have contact with pregnant women.

It is advised that rubella vaccination be avoided shortly before or during pregnancy because the vaccine is an attenuated live virus. The Centers for Disease Control (1990) have maintained a registry since 1971 to monitor the fetal effects of vaccination. Through 1989, 321 susceptible women who were immunized within 3 months of conception had been followed to term; fortunately, there is no evidence that the vaccine induces malformations.

Diagnosis. The diagnosis of rubella is often difficult. Not only are the clinical features of other illnesses quite similar, but about one fourth of rubella infections are subclinical despite viremia and infection of the embryo and fetus. Absence of rubella antibody indicates susceptibility. Antibody denotes an immune response to rubella viremia that may have been acquired anywhere from a few weeks to many years earlier. If maternal rubella antibody is demonstrated at the time of exposure to rubella or before, it is exceedingly unlikely that the fetus will be affected. Despite native or vaccine-induced immunity, subclinical rubella infections may develop during outbreaks. Although asymptomatic reinfection in early pregnancy has been described without fetal effects (Morgan-Capner and colleagues, 1985), fetal infection has been documented in five seropositive mothers (Best and associates, 1989). In two, therapeutic abortion was performed, and the other three term infants had all aspects of congenital rubella syndrome.

Viremia precedes clinically evident disease by about 1 week. The nonimmune person who acquires rubella viremia demonstrates peak antibody titers 1 to 2 weeks after the onset of the rash, or 2 to 3 weeks after the onset of viremia. The promptness of the antibody response, therefore, may complicate serodiagnosis unless serum is collected initially within a few days after the onset of the rash. If, for example, the first specimen was obtained 10 days after the rash, detection of antibodies would fail to differentiate between two possibilities: (1) that the very recent disease was actually rubella, or (2) that it was not rubella, but the person was already immune to rubella. Specific IgM antibody by radioimmunoassay can be de-

tected from early after onset of clinical disease. It peaks at 7 to 10 days, and persists for 4 weeks after appearance of the rash (American College of Obstetricians and Gynecologists, 1992b). In some cases, it may persist for a year. Importantly, rubella reinfection can give rise to transient low levels of IgM. There is no chemotherapeutic or antibiotic agent that will prevent viremia in nonimmune subjects exposed to rubella. The use of immunoglobulin is not recommended.

Congenital Rubella Syndrome. **With rubella, as with any fetal infection, the concept of an infected versus an affected infant must be understood.** Only about half of women with affected infants give a history of a rash during pregnancy. Rubella is a potent teratogen; Miller and colleagues (1982) have shown that 80 percent of women with rubella infection and a rash during the first 12 weeks have a fetus with congenital infection (Fig. 58–3). At 13 to 14 weeks this incidence was 54 percent, and it was 25 percent by the end of the second trimester. As the duration of pregnancy increases, fetal infections are less likely to cause congenital malformations. For example, rubella defects were seen in all infants with evidence of intrauterine infections before 11 weeks, but only in 35 percent of those infected at 13 to 16 weeks. Although no defects were found in 63 children infected after 16 weeks, they were followed only 2 years. The **extended rubella syndrome,** with progressive panencephalitis and type I diabetes, may not develop clinically until the second or third decade of life. Perhaps as many as one third of infants who are asymptomatic at birth may manifest such developmental injury (American College of Obstetricians and Gynecologists, 1988).

Thus, clinical manifestations of congenital rubella correlate with the timing of maternal infection and fetal

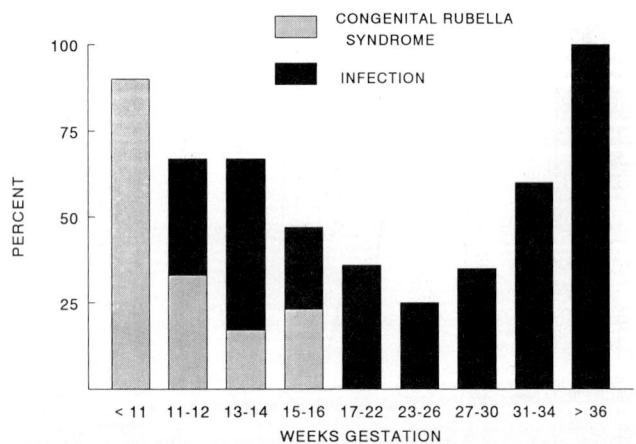

Fig. 58–3. Proportion of fetuses with evidence for rubella infection but no stigmata (*dark bars*) compared with fetuses born with congenital rubella syndrome (*hatched bars*). (Data from Miller and colleagues, 1982.)

organ development. Congenital rubella syndrome includes one or more of the following:

1. Eye lesions, including cataracts, glaucoma, microphthalmia, and various other abnormalities
2. Heart disease, including patent ductus arteriosus, septal defects, and pulmonary artery stenosis
3. Sensorineural deafness
4. Central nervous system defects, including meningoencephalitis
5. Retarded fetal growth
6. Thrombocytopenia and anemia
7. Hepatitis, hepatosplenomegaly, and jaundice
8. Chronic diffuse interstitial pneumonitis
9. Osseous changes
10. Chromosomal abnormalities

Infants born with congenital rubella may shed the virus for many months and thus be a threat to other infants, as well as to susceptible adults who come in contact with them.

Cytomegalovirus

Cytomegalovirus is a ubiquitous DNA herpesvirus that eventually infects most humans. It is the most common cause of perinatal infection and evidence for fetal infection is found in from 0.5 to 2 percent of all neonates. The virus is transmitted horizontally by droplet infection and contact with saliva and urine, vertically from mother to fetus-infant, and as a sexually transmitted disease. Day-care centers are a common source of acquisition of infection. Usually by 2 to 3 years of age, children acquire the infection from one another and then transmit it to their parents (Demmler, 1991; Pass, 1991).

Following primary infection, the virus becomes latent, and like other herpesvirus infections, there is periodic reactivation with viral shedding despite the presence of serum antibody. Humoral antibody is produced, but cell-mediated immunity appears to be the primary mechanism for recovery. Immunosuppressed states, whether naturally acquired or drug-induced, increase the propensity for serious cytomegalovirus infection. Presumably, decreased cell-mediated immune surveillance places the fetus-infant at high risk for sequelae of these infections.

Yow and Demmler (1992) have estimated the morbidity of perinatal cytomegalovirus infection since its public health importance was emphasized in 1971. In the ensuing 20 years, over 800,000 fetuses have been infected and 50,000 were born with symptomatic disease. Many have died, and most of the survivors have severe handicaps, including mental retardation, blindness, and deafness. Collectively, the annual cost for their care is nearly $2 billion. Another 120,000 infected children who were asymptomatic at birth have neurological impairments.

Maternal Infection. There is no evidence that pregnancy increases the risk or clinical severity of maternal cytomegalovirus infection. Most infections are asymptomatic, but about 15 percent of adults have a mononucleosis-like syndrome characterized by fever, pharyngitis, lymphadenopathy, and polyarthritis. As shown in Figure 58–4, the risk of seroconversion among susceptible women during pregnancy is from 1 to 4 percent. Immunity from previous infection can be demonstrated in up to 85 percent of pregnant women from lower socioeconomic backgrounds, whereas only half of women in higher income groups are seropositive. Primary infection, which is transmitted to the fetus in approximately 40 percent of cases, more often is associated with severe morbidity (Fowler and co-workers, 1992). Although transplacental infection is not universal, an infected fetus is more likely with maternal infection during the first half of pregnancy.

As with other herpesviruses, maternal immunity to cytomegalovirus does not prevent recurrence (reactivation), nor unfortunately does it prevent congenital infection. In fact, because most infections during pregnancy are recurrent, the majority of congenitally infected neonates are born to these women. Fortunately, congenital infections that result from recurrent infection are less often associated with clinically apparent sequelae than are those from primary infections.

Congenital Infection. Congenital cytomegalovirus infection, termed **cytomegalic inclusion disease,** causes a syndrome that includes low birthweight, microcephaly, intracranial calcifications, chorioretinitis, mental and motor retardation, sensorineural deficits, hepatosplenomegaly, jaundice, hemolytic anemia, and thrombocytopenic purpura. Perlman and Argyle (1992) reported that neurological involvement in preterm infants has more diverse clinical findings. They emphasized the need to consider cytomegaloviral infection in preterm infants with neurological findings, and suggest that such an encephalopathic process is progressive. Fortunately, of the estimated 40,000 infants born infected in the United States each year, only approximately 10 percent demonstrate this syndrome, which is more prevalent in neonates born to women with primary infection during the first half of pregnancy.

Fowler and colleagues (1992) recently reported long-term results from 197 newborns with congenital cytomegalovirus viremia followed at the University of Alabama. About 20 percent of infants in the primary-infection group had symptomatic infection at birth; none in the recurrent-infection group were symptomatic at birth. After a mean of 4.7 years, sequelae were identified in 25 percent of the primary-infection group and 8 percent of the recurrent-infection group. Overall,

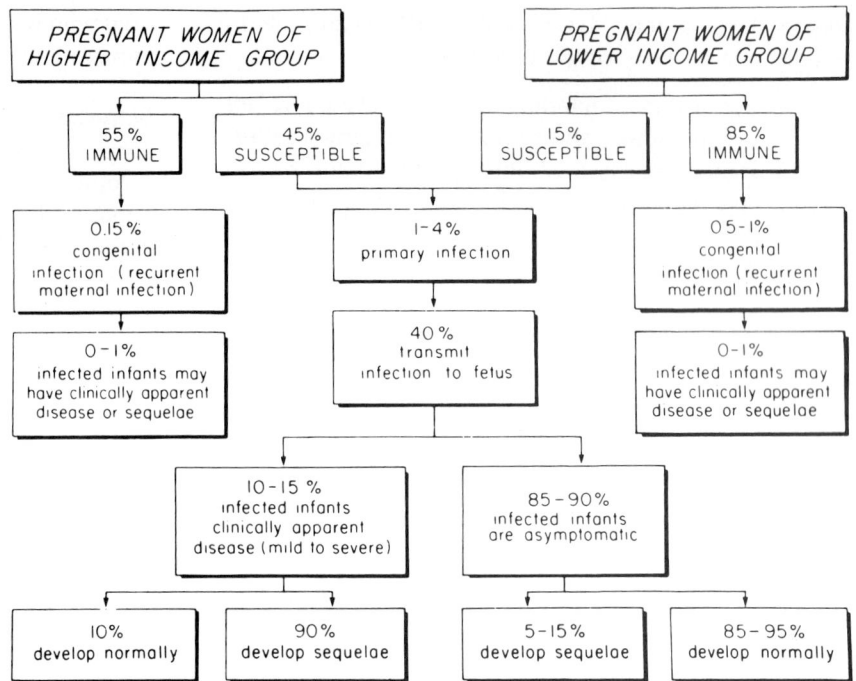

Fig. 58–4. Characteristics of cytomegalovirus infection in pregnancy. (From Stagno and Whitley, 1985, with permission.)

13 percent of primarily infected mothers had children whose intelligence quotient was less than 70 whereas none of the other children had mental impairment. Sensorineural hearing loss was found in 15 versus 5 percent of primary- and recurrent-infection groups, respectively.

Management. There is no effective therapy for maternal infection. Serological screening during pregnancy has limited value because (1) current knowledge does not allow accurate predictability of the sequelae of primary infection, (2) knowledge of immune status at conception serves no purpose because there is no vaccine, and (3) 1 to 2 percent of all infants excrete cytomegalovirus in the urine, and attempts to identify and isolate them are expensive and impractical (Demmler, 1991).

The predictive value of a positive maternal genitourinary culture or cervical cytology in assessing fetal risk for infection is likewise minimal. Asymptomatic cytomegalovirus excretion can be shown in up to 10 percent of pregnant women, and the majority have low-risk recurrent infections. **Primary infection** is diagnosed by four-fold increased IgG titers in paired acute and convalescent sera measured simultaneously, or preferentially by detecting IgM cytomegalovirus antibody in maternal serum. Recurrent infection usually is not accompanied by IgM antibody production. Unfortunately, neither of these methods is totally accurate to confirm maternal infection.

Counseling regarding fetal outcome must be individualized and it depends on the stage of gestation during which primary infection is documented. Even with a high infection rate with primary infection in the first half of pregnancy, the majority of infants develop normally.

Prenatal Diagnosis. In some cases, effects of fetal infection are detected by sonography (Fig. 58–5) or by computed tomography or magnetic resonance imaging (Koga and associates, 1990). Over 20 years ago, fetal cytomegalovirus infection was confirmed by amnionic fluid culture. As risks became better known for fetal

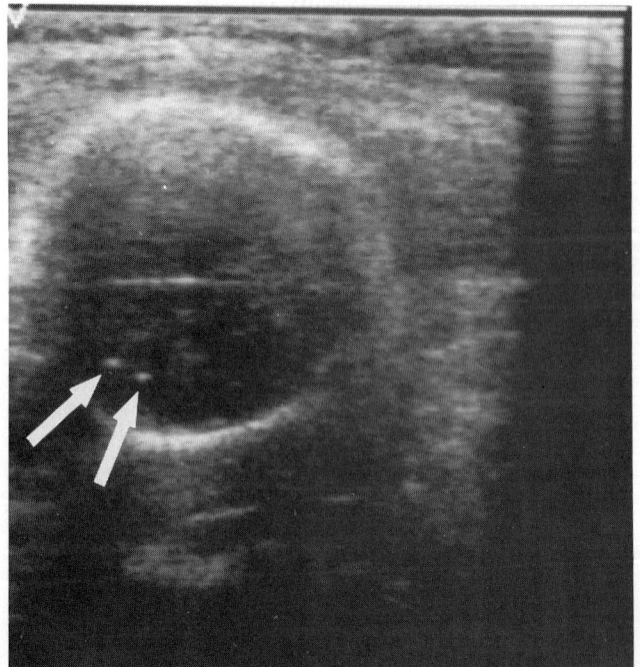

Fig. 58–5. Intracranial calcifications (*arrows*) seen by ultrasonography in a microcephalic fetus at about 30 weeks. (Courtesy of Dr. R. Santos.)

involvement, a number of investigators reported the efficacy of confirming suspected primary infections by amniocentesis for viral culture or by cordocentesis to detect IgM (Grose and Weiner, 1990).

Lynch and colleagues (1991) evaluated 12 fetuses by ultrasonography, amniocentesis, and cordocentesis and reported that viral isolation and elevated cord-blood total IgM were helpful to confirm infection. Importantly, noninfected fetuses were identified correctly. Hohlfeld and co-workers (1991) studied 15 Swiss women with primary infection and confirmed fetal infection in eight of these within 24 hours using the *shell vial assay* for viral antigen in amnionic fluid and fetal blood. In all cases, amniocentesis provided diagnostic results, but fetal blood analysis provided further information concerning fetal condition—anemia, thrombocytopenia, elevated hepatic enzymes, and total IgM.

Lamy and colleagues (1992) provided prospective data from a study done to evaluate fetal cytomegalovirus transmission in nearly 1800 Belgian women. At their initial prenatal visit, about half (861) were seronegative. They were tested serologically at each prenatal visit and 20 (2.3 percent) seroconverted before 22 weeks' gestation. Only seven allowed evaluation, and in five amnionic fluid cultures were positive for cytomegalovirus; abortions were performed and histopathological evaluation disclosed brain involvement in all five. The other two were uninfected.

BACTERIAL INFECTIONS

Group A Streptococcus

Infection caused by *Streptococcus pyogenes* is rarely encountered today. These infections are particularly virulent and the organism produces a number of toxins and enzymes. More recently, a resurgence in puerperal infections from group A streptococci has been observed (see Chap. 47, p. 1072). As discussed in Chapter 28 (p. 639), the organism produces a **toxic shock–like syndrome** that is highly fatal. We encountered 3 cases in 1992 and 2 caused maternal deaths. Prompt penicillin treatment, sometimes combined with surgical debridement, may be lifesaving. **Scarlet fever** is occasionally seen, and treatment is also given with penicillin. Rigid isolation is instituted and maintained in the pregnant woman. **Erysipelas** is an acute streptococcal skin infection and bacteremia is common. It is always a serious disease, but is particularly dangerous in pregnant women because of the potential hazard of puerperal infection.

Group B Streptococcus

Asymptomatic carriage of group B β-hemolytic streptococcus (*Streptococcus agalactiae*) is common in women, especially in the vagina and rectum. The Vaginal Infections and Prematurity Study Group (Regan and co-workers, 1991) reported that 15 to 20 percent of over 8000 pregnant women from five clinical centers had a lower genital-tract culture positive for group B streptococci done between 23 and 26 weeks. The organism has been implicated in several adverse pregnancy outcomes, including preterm labor, prematurely ruptured membranes, covert and overt chorioamnionitis, puerperal sepsis, as well as in fetal and neonatal infections. There also have been case reports of postpartum maternal osteomyelitis and mastitis caused by group B infection (Berkowitz and McCaffrey, 1990; Rench and Baker, 1989).

Epidemiology. Half of newborns of carrier women became colonized almost immediately at birth. Serious neonatal infections with group B streptococci are at least as prevalent as those from coliform organisms. During the 1970s, neonatal group B infections increased remarkably in frequency. In Victoria, Australia, group B infection caused one third of perinatal deaths due to infection (Fliegner and Garland, 1990).

It is clear that intrapartum fetal transmission from the colonized mother may lead to severe neonatal sepsis soon after birth. The overall attack rate of early-onset sepsis is about 1 to 2 per 1000 of all births. It is 10 per 1000 for babies born to colonized mothers, and approaches 40 per 1000 if there is preterm labor and delivery, prolonged membrane rupture, or intrapartum fever (American College of Obstetricians and Gynecologists, 1992a). Although preterm or low-birthweight infants are at highest risk, more than half of the cases of neonatal sepsis are in term neonates. Maternally transmitted antibodies protect most infants.

Neonatal Sepsis. With septicemia from group B streptococci that characterizes *early-onset disease*, signs of serious illness usually develop within 6 to 12 hours of birth. These include respiratory distress, apnea, and shock. At the outset, therefore, the illness must be differentiated from idiopathic respiratory distress syndrome (see Chap. 44, p. 991). The mortality rate with early-onset disease is about 25 percent, and preterm infants fare less well. Unfortunately, it is not uncommon for surviving infants to exhibit neurological sequelae apparently sustained during hypotension from the sepsis syndrome. *Late-onset* disease usually manifests as meningitis a week or more after birth. These cases are most often caused by serotype III organisms. Whereas the serotype with early-onset disease varies from infant to infant, it most often is concordant with organisms cultured from the maternal vagina. The mortality rate, although appreciable, is less for late-onset meningitis than for early-onset sepsis. Here again, neurological sequelae are common in survivors.

Screening. There is not comprehensive agreement concerning universal screening or treatment for maternal group B streptococcal carriage (Greenspoon and colleagues, 1991b). Targeted screening of "high risk" women was not found effective by the Vaginal Infections and Prematurity Study Group (Regan and co-workers, 1991). Whereas it is controversial whether these organisms cause preterm labor and prematurely ruptured membranes (Romero and colleagues, 1989), it is not disputed that they cause serious perinatal infections in pregnancies complicated by these events. A major problem with screening and attempts to eradicate the organism is a high recurrence rate. Despite this, because of a high colonization rate combined with a relatively low attack rate, screening was not considered to be cost-effective by the American College of Obstetricians and Gynecologists (1992a). Although the American Academy of Pediatrics (1992) favors antepartum screening, the American College of Obstetricians and Gynecologists (1993) has reaffirmed its recommendations cited below.

Because of these problems, efforts have been directed at rapid screening techniques and treatment schemes designed to prevent neonatal colonization, and thus sepsis. Culture remains most accurate, but its use is limited by the time required to obtain results. According to the Vaginal Infections and Prematurity Study Group (Carey and colleagues, 1990), Gram staining is neither sensitive nor specific. Enzyme-linked immunosorbent assays for streptococcal antigen have been evaluated by a number of investigators. Although under optimal circumstances this technology provides results within an hour, there are a large number of false-positive as well as false-negative results (Greenspoon and co-workers, 1991a; Towers and colleagues, 1990). According to Gentry and associates (1991), the test is highly sensitive to detect heavy colonization, but cultures are necessary to detect light growth.

Treatment and Prophylaxis. Steigman and associates (1978) reported an absence of early-onset group B streptococcal sepsis in 130,000 newborn infants given 50,000 units of aqueous penicillin G intramuscularly at birth as prophylaxis against gonococcal ophthalmia neonatorum. A prospective study of nearly 19,000 infants was then carried out by Siegal and co-workers (1980) at Parkland Hospital. About half of these infants were randomized to receive aqueous procaine penicillin G intramuscularly within 1 hour of birth as prophylaxis against ophthalmia neonatorum and also to evaluate its impact on group B infections. The incidence of streptococcal disease was significantly lowered in those given penicillin. It was worrisome, however, that the incidence of infection and mortality caused by penicillin-resistant nonstreptococcal organisms increased.

Pyati and co-workers (1983) subsequently reported that such penicillin prophylaxis was of little benefit in preventing early-onset group B disease in low-birthweight neonates. Many infants who did poorly were subsequently found to have positive cord blood cultures for streptococci. Thus, in these already infected fetuses, single-dose prophylaxis failed to treat adequately ongoing neonatal infection. These findings also served to emphasize the important association of group B streptococci with preterm delivery.

More recent emphasis has been on intrapartum treatment of mothers found to be colonized near the time of delivery. A number of regimens have been reviewed by Greenspoon and colleagues (1991b). Boyer and Gotoff (1986) randomized intrapartum and neonatal ampicillin treatment of colonized mothers. They observed decreased neonatal colonization (9 versus 51 percent) and early-onset sepsis (none versus 6 percent) in infants born to treated women. Garland and Fliegner (1991) from Melbourne, Australia, screened over 30,000 clinic patients at 32 weeks and treated asymptomatic carriers intrapartum with intravenous penicillin. Nearly 27,000 private patients admitted to their hospital were not screened. Although there were no group B infections in neonates of clinic patients, by contrast, there were 27 infections and eight deaths in the unscreened private control group.

Tuppurainen and Hallman (1989) reported similar results from a study in which almost 9000 women were screened on arrival to the delivery unit for heavy colonization using a rapid latex agglutination test. Importantly, of 412 women with a positive latex test, almost 40 percent delivered before results were available. The remaining almost 200 latex-positive women were randomized to receive intrapartum intravenous penicillin G, 5 million units every 6 hours. Whereas only one of 88 infants whose mothers were treated had early-onset group B sepsis, 10 of 111 of those not treated did so.

Morales and Lim (1987) showed that rapid streptococcal identification using coagglutination methods in women with preterm prematurely ruptured membranes, along with treatment given for those positive, reduced the incidence of chorioamnionitis and neonatal group B sepsis. Maxwell and Watson (1992) reported observations from 182 women with prematurely ruptured membranes between 26 and 33 weeks. Of these, about 20 percent subsequently were found to have cervical cultures positive for group B streptococcus. Intravenous ampicillin was given to all of these women upon admission and continued until cultures were reported negative at 72 hours. For the 34 with positive cultures, antibiotics were continued for 7 to 10 days. Neonatal sepsis was not increased in these.

Recommendations for Prophylaxis. At this time, universal screening is not recommended. According to the American College of Obstetricians and Gynecologists (1992a), if maternal group B colonization cannot be verified, then women with the following condition(s) would most likely benefit from intrapartum administration of ampicillin, penicillin G, or erythromycin: (1) preterm labor, (2) preterm prematurely ruptured membranes, (3) prolonged membrane rupture defined as greater than 18 hours, (4) sibling affected by symptomatic group B streptococcal infection, or (5) intrapartum maternal fever.

Prevention. Because some protection against serious neonatal infection is conferred by maternal antibody, it is logical that vaccination with capsular polysaccharide antigen may prove efficacious. From preliminary findings, Baker and colleagues (1988) reported that maternal immunization to type III antigen produces antibody in about 60 percent of women. This may provide passive neonatal immunity. Coleman and co-workers (1992) as well as the Institute of Medicine (1985) have cited vaccine development as attainable and as a priority.

Listeriosis

Listeria monocytogenes is an uncommon but probably underdiagnosed cause of neonatal sepsis. The organism is a Gram-positive aerobic motile bacillus that can be isolated from soil, water, and sewage. From 1 to 5 percent of adults have listeria in their feces. Foodborne transmission is important and outbreaks of listeriosis have been reported from manure-contaminated cabbage, pasteurized milk, and fresh Mexican-style cheese.

Listerial infections are more common in the very old or young, pregnant, or immunocompromised patients. Because cell-mediated immunity is important in defense, some have speculated that the pregnant woman is susceptible because this is decreased. The Listeriosis Study Group of the Centers for Disease Control (Gellin and colleagues, 1991), surveyed culture results from a population of 34 million persons in 1986 and estimated that there were 1700 cases of listeriosis. About one fourth were in pregnant women. Another review by them (Schuchat and associates, 1992) of over 18 million persons in 1988 through 1990 showed that about one third of reported culture-proven cases were in pregnant women. In an epidemic in Los Angeles County in 1985, caused by contaminated Mexican-style cheese, 65 percent of cases were in pregnant women or their fetusneonate.

Listeriosis during pregnancy may be asymptomatic or cause a febrile illness that is confused for influenza or pyelonephritis. The diagnosis usually is not apparent until the blood culture is reported as positive. Occult or clinical infection also may stimulate labor (Boucher and Yonekura, 1986). Maternal listeremia causes fetal infection that characteristically produces disseminated granulomatous lesions with microabscesses. Meconium passage is common with fetal infection.

The neonate is particularly susceptible to infection

and the mortality rate approaches 50 percent. In these cases, early-onset neonatal sepsis is common, whereas late-onset listeriosis manifests as meningitis after 3 to 4 weeks of age. In this regard, these infections are very similar to those caused by group B β-hemolytic streptococci. There is evidence that maternal antimicrobial treatment may be effective for fetal infection (Linnan and colleagues, 1988).

Treatment. Antimicrobial agents active against *L. monocytogenes* in vitro include penicillin G, ampicillin, erythromycin, sulfamethoxazole-trimethoprim, chloramphenicol, rifampin, tetracyclines, and aminoglycosides (Gellin and Broome, 1989). There are no clinical trials concerning efficacy, but a combination of ampicillin and gentamicin is usually recommended because of proven laboratory synergism. The efficacy of trimethoprim–sulfamethoxazole has been documented and it should be given to penicillin-allergic women. We recently encountered a 36-week pregnant woman who had a recurrently positive blood culture for *Listeria* a week after completing a 5-day course of intravenous erythromycin. She was asymptomatic, but intravenous ampicillin was given for another 10 days after which induction at term resulted in delivery of a normal infant.

Salmonella Infections

Salmonellosis. Salmonella infections continue to be a major cause of foodborne illness. The organisms are ubiquitous in warm-blooded animals and almost all of more than 2200 serovars cause human illness (Baird-Parker, 1990). Enteritis is contracted through contaminated food and symptoms include diarrhea, abdominal pain, fever, chills, nausea, and vomiting. Scialli and Rarick (1992) described a woman with enteritis and bacteremia from group C1 salmonella infection. Amnionic fluid cultures also were positive and infection caused fetal death at 15 weeks. Management is usually by intravenous fluid rehydration. Antimicrobials prolong the carrier state and are not given in uncomplicated infections.

Typhoid Fever. *Salmonella typhi* is spread by oral ingestion of contaminated food, water, or milk. In pregnant women, the disease is more likely to be encountered during epidemics (Duff and Engelsgjerd, 1983). According to their review, Dildy and associates (1990) reported that pregnancy complicated by typhoid fever in former years resulted in abortion or preterm labor in up to 80 percent of cases, with a fetal mortality rate of 60 percent and a maternal mortality rate of 25 percent. Subsequent experiences fortunately were much more favorable (Riggall and co-workers, 1974).

Chloramphenicol remains the treatment of choice, but ampicillin or trimethoprim-sulfamethoxazole may be given. Antityphoid vaccines appear to exert no harmful effects when administered to pregnant women. As discussed in Chapter 9 (p. 264), vaccine should be given in an epidemic or before travel to endemic areas (American College of Obstetricians and Gynecologists, 1991).

Shigellosis. Bacillary dysentery caused by *Shigella* species is a relatively common cause of inflammatory exudative diarrhea in adults. Bloody stools are common. Shigellosis is more common in children attending day-care centers. It is highly contagious with primary attack rates up to 75 percent and exposed family members may be infected in over 50 percent of cases (Guerrant and Bobak, 1991). Because of these factors, shigellosis is occasionally encountered in pregnant women. Clinical manifestations range from mild diarrhea to severe dysentery, abdominal cramping, tenesmus, fever, and systemic toxicity. Although shigellosis is self-limited, careful attention to treatment of dehydration is essential in severe cases. We have encountered women in whom secretory diarrhea exceeded 10 L per day! In severely ill women, the treatment of choice is trimethoprim–sulfamethoxazole, but ampicillin also may be given.

Hansen Disease. According to Maurus (1978), women with leprosy generally do well in pregnancy. Dapsone and clofazimine for treatment appear to be safe for use during pregnancy (Farb and associates, 1982). Rifampin therapy is also effective. Duncan (1980) reported an excessive incidence of low-birthweight infants born to women infected with *Mycobacterium leprae*, and this was not explained by treatment or maternal nutritional status. Fetal and placental infection must be rare because Duncan and associates (1984) were unable to demonstrate any morphological evidence of placental infection in 82 infected pregnant women. Neonatal infection apparently is acquired from skin-to-skin or droplet transmission.

Lyme Disease

Lyme disease is caused by the spirochete *Borrelia burgdorferi*. It is the most commonly reported vectorborne illness in the United States. Lyme borreliosis results from the bite of ticks of the genus *Ixodes*. Steere (1989) has reviewed the clinical course. Stage 1 is early local infection which causes a distinctive skin lesion, **erythema chronicum migrans,** which may be accompanied by a flu-like syndrome and regional adenopathy. If untreated, stage 2 disease, characterized by disseminated infection, may develop in days to weeks after inoculation. Multisystem involvement is common, but skin lesions, arthralgia and myalgia, carditis and meningitis predominate. If untreated after several weeks to months, stage 3 infection develops in perhaps half of patients. Native immunity is

acquired and the disease enters a chronic phase. Whereas some patients remain asymptomatic, others develop a variety of dermatological, rheumatic, or neurological manifestations.

Serological diagnosis has pitfalls and clinical diagnosis is important. Optimal treatment has not been established. In early infection, treatment with tetracycline is recommended for nonpregnant patients. Pregnant women are given erythromycin or amoxicillin. For later infection manifest by meningitis or carditis, high-dose intravenous penicillin G is recommended. Chronic arthritis is treated with amoxicillin and probenecid orally for 30 days, or with ceftriaxone or penicillin G intravenously for 14 days (Smith and co-workers, 1991).

Neonatal Infection. There is concern that infection may be teratogenic because other spirochetes, notably *Treponema pallidum* (see Chap. 59, p. 1299) cause congenital infection. Schlesinger and colleagues (1985) documented the persistence of spirochetes in fetal spleen, kidney, and bone marrow at 35 weeks in a woman who had Lyme disease during the first trimester. Similarly, Weber and associates (1988) demonstrated the organism in brain and liver of a term infant who died suddenly at 1 day of age. The mother had been treated and responded to oral penicillin for erythema migrans at 8 weeks. Markowitz and associates (1986) reviewed 19 cases complicating pregnancy, and reported that 25 percent had preterm labor, fetal death, or rash-like illness in the newborn. Smith and colleagues (1991) recently provided a review of Lyme disease complicating pregnancy.

PROTOZOAL INFECTIONS

Toxoplasmosis

Toxoplasmosis is a protozoal infection caused by *Toxoplasma gondii*. Infection is transmitted through encysted organisms by eating infected raw or undercooked meat and through contact with infected cat feces, or it can be acquired congenitally by transplacental transfer.

Effects on Pregnancy. Maternal immunity appears to protect against intrauterine parasite transmission; therefore, for congenital toxoplasmosis to develop, the mother must have acquired the infection during pregnancy. About one third of North American women acquire protective antibody before pregnancy, and this is higher in those keeping cats as pets.

Fatigue, muscle pains, and sometimes lymphadenopathy develop, but most often infection is subclinical. Infection in pregnancy may cause abortion or result in a liveborn with evidence of disease. The risk of fetal infection increases with duration of pregnancy, but overall it approaches 50 percent (McCabe and Remington,

1988). The virulence of fetal infection is greater the earlier that infection is acquired—fortunately, infection is less common earlier in pregnancy. Overall, less than 10 percent of newborns with congenital toxoplasmosis have signs of clinical illness at birth. Affected infants usually have evidence of generalized disease with low birthweight, hepatosplenomegaly, icterus, and anemia. Some infants primarily have neurological disease with convulsions, intracranial calcifications, and hydrocephaly or microcephaly. Both groups eventually develop chorioretinitis.

Screening. Until perhaps recently, serum screening for prenatal toxoplasmosis was not feasible because of technical difficulties in interpreting test results. Certainly, some women, usually those who own cats, will request serological testing. The American College of Obstetricians and Gynecologists (1988) recommends preconceptional serological screening. Recent knowledge gained from several European studies now may allow studies to evaluate systematic screening programs in the United States (McCabe and Remington, 1988).

If anti-toxoplasma IgG antibody is confirmed before pregnancy, then the woman is not at risk for a congenitally infected fetus. In most cases, however, serological testing is not done until the woman is pregnant. If antibody, usually determined by indirect fluorescence on enzyme-linked immunosorbent assay, is present in low titers, it probably represents previously acquired immunity. However, it could be IgM from recent infection, although IgM may persist for years and false-positive results may be due to rheumatoid factor (Fuccillo and associates, 1987). Unfortunately, differentiation between the two is difficult, and consultation from a state reference laboratory, the Centers for Disease Control, or the National Institutes of Health is advised.

The most accurate confirmation of active infection is a rise in IgG titer in two appropriately spaced but simultaneously tested serum samples. Very high titers—that is, greater than 1:512—more likely indicate recent or current illness. Sever and colleagues (1988) reported increased microcephaly, deafness, and mental retardation in women whose titers were 1:256 or higher.

A polymerase chain reaction (PCR) assay has been developed and initial reports indicate high specificity and sensitivity (Cazenave and colleagues, 1992). The technique permits prenatal diagnosis in one day by performing assay on amnionic fluid specimens.

Management. For the woman thought to have active disease, treatment is recommended by McCabe and Remington (1988). There is evidence that spiramycin, a macrolide antibiotic used widely in Europe, reduces the incidence of fetal infection, but it may not modify its severity. In a follow-up to preliminary work, Daffos and colleagues (1988) from Paris employed amnionic fluid and fetal blood sampling in 746 women with proven

infection up to 25 weeks. Maternal infection was diagnosed by toxoplasma-specific IgM antibody. All women with presumed infection were treated with spiramycin, 3 g daily throughout pregnancy. Only 6 percent of their fetuses were found to have infection, and 39 of these 42 were diagnosed by demonstrating IgM-specific antibody in serum obtained by umbilical vessel sampling. For these women, pyrimethamine and either sulfadoxine or sulfadiazine were added to the spiramycin regime. In the United States, spiramycin is available only through the Centers for Disease Control. Treatment may be given with pyrimethamine plus sulfadiazine; however, the efficacy of such management is not established.

Ghidini and colleagues (1991) from Milan reported no fetal abnormalities from congenital toxoplasmosis in 35 women treated after seroconversion was documented. Foulon and co-workers (1990b) from Brussels reported a 12 percent incidence of congenital toxoplasmosis in 50 women infected up to 20 weeks' gestation. They concluded that serological screening with invasive fetal diagnosis was safe and feasible. In another report, Foulon and associates (1990a) described a case in which prenatal diagnosis was confirmed by tissue culture of a chorionic villus biopsy.

Although these studies suggest that identification of women who seroconvert during early pregnancy, followed by cordocentesis and identification and treatment of infected fetuses (about 5 to 10 percent), as emphasized by Jeannel and associates (1990), the efficacy of spiramycin to prevent or modify fetal infection has not been evaluated in randomized placebo studies.

Malaria

There are four species of *Plasmodium* that cause human malaria: *vivax, ovale, malariae,* and *falciparum.* Organisms are transmitted by the bite of a female *Anopheles* mosquito. In 1992, the World Health Organization estimated that nearly 270 million persons worldwide are infected at any given time. Almost 40 percent of the world's population—2 billion people—are at risk of contracting the disease. Malaria has been effectively eradicated in Europe and most of North America except for parts of Mexico.

The disease is characterized by fever and flu-like symptoms including chills, headaches, myalgia, and malaise, which may occur at intervals. Symptoms are less severe in immune patients. Malaria may be associated with anemia and jaundice, and falciparum infections may cause kidney failure, coma, and death.

Effects on Pregnancy. The incidence of abortion and preterm labor is increased with malaria, although the likelihood of either relates to the severity of the disease and the promptness with which therapy is instituted. Infection tends to be more severe in primigravidas, probably related to a lower incidence of nonimmune patients. Increased fetal loss may be related to placental and fetal infection. The evidence for this is somewhat contradictory, however, because parasites rarely cross the placenta to infect the fetus. Covell (1950) studied this extensively in Africa and cited an incidence of neonatal malaria of 0.03 percent. According to Jones (1950), parasites have an affinity for decidual vessels and may involve the placenta extensively without affecting the fetus. Cot and colleagues (1992) showed that chloroquine chemoprophylaxis decreased placental infection in asymptomatic infected women to 4 percent compared with 19 percent of untreated controls; however, mean birthweight was not different.

There is a marked tendency toward recrudescence of the disease during pregnancy and the puerperium, and after surgical operations. Pregnancy enhances the severity of falciparum malaria, especially in nonimmune nulliparous women (Nathwani and colleagues, 1992).

Treatment. Commonly used antimalarial drugs are not contraindicated during pregnancy. Some of the newer antimalarial agents have antifolic acid activity, and may theoretically contribute to the development of megaloblastic anemia. In actual practice, this does not appear to be the case. In at least one study by Keuter and coworkers (1990), primigravidas were more likely to remain parasitemic after therapy for falciparum infection. For the woman with chloroquine-resistant falciparum infection, quinine is given orally. Because of the difficulty in obtaining quinine for parenteral administration, the Centers for Disease Control (1991b) currently recommends intravenous quinidine as the drug of choice to treat critically ill persons infected with falciparum malaria. Malin and associates (1990) report a successful outcome in a 26-week pregnant woman treated with intravenous quinine and exchange transfusion.

Prophylaxis. For travel to areas where chloroquine-resistant *P. falciparum* has not been reported, prophylaxis with chloroquine, 300 mg of base orally once a week, is initiated 1 to 2 weeks before the endemic area is entered and this is continued until 4 weeks after return to nonendemic areas (Centers for Disease Control, 1990). Travel to areas endemic for chloroquine-resistant *P. falciparum* should be avoided by pregnant women. Mefloquine or doxycycline are recommended for chemoprophylaxis in nonpregnant persons, but both are contraindicated in pregnancy, according to the Centers for Disease Control (1990).

Amebiasis

Most persons infected with *Entamoeba histolytica* are asymptomatic cyst-passers. Amoebic dysentery may take a fulminant course during pregnancy. Prognosis is worse if complicated by a hepatic abscess, which may be quite serious during pregnancy and rupture has been reported (Constantine and colleagues, 1987). Therapy is similar to that for the nonpregnant woman, and metronidazole is the drug of choice.

Mycotic Infections

In the past, disseminated *coccidiomycosis* during pregnancy commonly ended in maternal death. In more recent years, treatment with amphotericin B has been successfully employed in a number of cases. Disseminated infection during pregnancy is even less common with blastomycosis, cryptococcosis, or histoplasmosis, but their identification mandates prompt treatment with amphotericin B. Management of these infections is considered in Chapter 49 (p. 1108).

References

American Academy of Pediatrics Committee on Infectious Disease and Committee on Fetus and Newborn: Guidelines for prevention of group B streptococcal (GBS) infections by chemoprophylaxis. Pediatrics 90:7775, 1992

American College of Obstetricians and Gynecologists: Universal antepartum screening for maternal GBS not recommended. ACOG Newsletter 37:1, 1993

American College of Obstetricians and Gynecologists: Group B streptococcal infections in pregnancy. Technical bulletin no. 169, July 1992a

American College of Obstetricians and Gynecologists: Immunization during pregnancy. Technical bulletin no. 160, October 1991

American College of Obstetricians and Gynecologists: Perinatal viral and parasitic infections. Technical bulletin no. 114, March 1988

American College of Obstetricians and Gynecologists: Rubella and pregnancy. Technical bulletin no. 171, August 1992b

Amstey MS, Miller RK, Menegus MA, di Sant Ágnese PA: Enterovirus in pregnant women and the perfused placenta. Am J Obstet Gynecol 158:775, 1988

Andrews EB, Yankaskas BC, Cordero JF, Schoeffler K, Hampp S, and the Acyclovir in Pregnancy Registry Advisory Committee: Six years' experience. Obstet Gynecol 79:7, 1992

Baird-Parker AC: Foodborne illness: Foodborne salmonellosis. Lancet 336:1231, 1990

Baker CJ, Rench MA, Edwards MS, Carpenter RJ, Hays BM, Kasper DL: Immunization of pregnant women with a polysaccharide vaccine of group B streptococcus. N Engl J Med 319:1180, 1988

Balducci J, Rodis JF, Rosengren S, Vintzileos AM, Spivey G, Vosseller C: Pregnancy outcome following first-trimester varicella infection. Obstet Gynecol 79:5, 1992

Barr CE, Mednick SA, Munk-Jorgensen P: Exposure to influenza epidemics during gestation and adult schizophrenia. Arch Gen Psychiatry 47:869, 1990

Bass MH, Molloshok RE: In Guttmacher A, Rovinsky JJ (eds): Medical, Surgical, and Gynecological Complications of Pregnancy. Baltimore, Williams & Wilkins, 1960, p 526

Berkowitz K, McCaffrey R: Postpartum osteomyelitis caused by group B streptococcus. Am J Obstet Gynecol 163:1200, 1990

Best JM, Banatvala JE, Morgan-Capner P, Miller E: Fetal infection after maternal reinfection with rubella: Criteria for defining reinfection. BMJ 299:773, 1989

Boucher M, Yonekura ML: Perinatal listeriosis (early onset): Correlation of antenatal manifestations and neonatal outcome. Obstet Gynecol 68:593, 1986

Boyer KM, Gotoff SP: Prevention of early-onset neonatal Group B streptococcal disease with selective intrapartum chemoprophylaxis. N Engl J Med 314:1665, 1986

Brady WK, Purdon A Jr: Intrauterine fetal demise associated with enterovirus infection. South Med J 79:770, 1986

Brown GC, Karunas RS: Relationship of congenital anomalies and maternal infection with selected enteroviruses. Am J Epidemiol 95:207, 1972

Carey JC, Klebanoff MA, Regan JA, The Vaginal Infections and Prematurity Study Group: Evaluation of the gram stain as a screening tool for maternal carriage of group B beta-hemolytic streptococci. Obstet Gynecol 76:693, 1990

Cartter ML, Farley TA, Rosengren S, Quinn DL, Gillespie SM, Gary GW, Hadler JL: Occupational risk factors for infection with parvovirus B19 among pregnant women. J Infect Dis 163:292, 1991

Cazenave J, Forestier F, Bessiers M, Broussins B, Begueret J: Contribution of a new PCR assay to the prenatal diagnosis of congenital toxoplasmosis. Prenat Diag 12:119, 1992

Centers for Disease Control: Increase in rubella and congenital rubella. MMWR 40:93, 1991a

Centers for Disease Control: Prevention and control of influenza. Recommendations of the Immunization Practices Advisory Committee (ACIP). MMWR 41:1, 1992

Centers for Disease Control: Recommendations for the prevention of malaria among travelers. MMWR 39:1, 1990

Centers for Disease Control: Rubella prevention: Recommendations of the Immunization Practices Advisory Committee (ACIP). MMWR 39:1, 1990

Centers for Disease Control: Treatment of severe *Plasmodium falciparum* malaria with quinidine gluconate: Discontinuation of parenteral quinine from CDC drug service. MMWR 40:240, 1991b

Centers for Disease Control: Varicella-zoster immune globulin for the prevention of chickenpox. MMWR 33:84, 1984

Christensen PE, Schmidt H, Bang HO, Anderson V, Jordal B, Jensen O: An epidemic of measles in southern Greenland 1951. ACTA Med Scand 144:431, 1953

Coleman RT, Sherer DM, Maniscalco WM: Prevention of neonatal group B streptococcal infections: Advances in maternal vaccine development. Obstet Gynecol 80:301, 1992

Constantine G, Menon V, Luesley D: Amoebic peritonitis in pregnancy in the United Kingdom. Postgrad Med J 63:495, 1987

Cot M, Roisin A, Barro D, Yada JP, Verhave P, Carnevale P, Breart G: Effect of chloroquine chemoprophylaxis during pregnancy on birth weight: Results of a randomized trial. Am J Trop Med Hyg 46:21, 1992

Covell G: Congenital malaria. Trop Dis Bull 47:1174, 1950

Cox SM, Cunningham FG, Luby J: Management of varicella pneumonia complicating pregnancy. Am J Perinatol 7:300, 1990

Daffos F, Forestier F, Capella-Pavlovsky M, Thulliez P, Aufrant C, Valenti D, Cox W: Prenatal management of 746 pregnancies at risk for congenital toxoplasmosis. N Engl J Med 381:271, 1988

Demmler GJ: Summary of a workshop on surveillance for congenital cytomegalovirus disease. Rev Inf Dis 13:315, 1991

Dildy GA III, Martens MG, Faro S, Lee W: Typhoid fever in pregnancy: A case report. J Reprod Med 35:273, 1990

Duff P, Engelsgjerd B: Typhoid fever on an obstetrics–gynecology service. Am J Obstet Gynecol 145:113, 1983

Duncan ME: Babies of mothers with leprosy have small placentae, low birth weights and grow slowly. Br J Obstet Gynaecol 87:461, 1980

Duncan ME, Fox H, Harkness RA, Rees RJW: The placenta in leprosy. Placenta 5:189, 1984

Eyal A, Friedman M, Peretz BA, Paldi E: Pregnancy complicated by herpes zoster: A report of two cases and literature review. J Reprod Med 28:600, 1983

Farb H, West DP, Pedvis-Leftick A: Clofazimine in pregnancy complicated by leprosy. Obstet Gynecol 59:122, 1982

Fliegner JR, Garland SM: Perinatal mortality in Victoria, Australia: Role of group B streptococcus. Am J Obstet Gynecol 163:1609, 1990

Foulon W, Naessens A, de Catte L, Amy JJ: Detection of congenital toxoplasmosis by chorionic villus sampling and early amniocentesis. Am J Obstet Gynecol 163:1511, 1990a

Foulon W, Naessens A, Mahler T, de Waele M, de Catte L, de Meuter F: Prenatal diagnosis of congenital toxoplasmosis. Obstet Gynecol 76:769, 1990b

Fowler KB, Stagno S, Pass RF, Britt WJ, Boll TJ, Alford CA: The outcome of congenital cytomegalovirus infection in relation to maternal antibody status. N Engl J Med 326:663, 1992

Freeman DW, Barno A: Deaths from Asian influenza associated with pregnancy. Am J Obstet Gynecol 78:1172, 1959

Fuccillo DA, Madden DL, Tzan N, Sever JL: Difficulties associated with serological diagnosis of *Toxoplasma gondii* infections. Diagn Clin Immunol 5:8, 1987

Garcia AGP, Basso NG, Fonseca MEF, Zuardi JAT, Outanni HN: Enterovirus associated placental morphology: A light, virological, electron microscopic and immunohistologic study. Placenta 12:53, 1991

Garland SM, Fliegner JR: Group B streptococcus (GBS) and neonatal infections: The case for intrapartum chemoprophylaxis. Aust NZ J Obstet Gynaecol 31:2, 1991

Gellin BG, Broome CV: Listeriosis. JAMA 261:1313, 1989

Gellin BG, Broome CV, Bibb WF, Weaver RE, Gaventa S, Mascola L, Listeriosis Study Group: The epidemiology of listeriosis in the United States—1986. Am J Epidemiol 133:392, 1991

Gentry YM, Hillier SL, Eschenbach DA: Evaluation of a rapid enzyme immunoassay test for detection of group B *Streptococcus*. Obstet Gynecol 78:397, 1991

Ghidini A, Sirtori M, Spelta A, Vergani P: Results of a preventive program for congenital toxoplasmosis. J Reprod Med 36:268, 1991

Greenspoon JS, Fishman A, Wilcox JG, Greenspoon RT, Lewis W: Comparison of culture for group B streptococcus versus enzyme immunoassay and latex agglutination rapid tests: Results in 250 patients during labor. Obstet Gynecol 77:97, 1991a

Greenspoon JS, Wilcox JG, Kirschbaum TH: Group B streptococcus: The effectiveness of screening and chemoprophylaxis. Obstet Gynecol Surv 46:499, 1991b

Gregg NM: Congenital cataract following German measles in the mother. Trans Ophthalmol Soc Aust 3:35, 1942

Grose C, Weiner CP: Prenatal diagnosis of congenital cytomegalovirus infection: Two decades later. Am J Obstet Gynecol 163:447, 1990

Guerrant RL, Bobak DA: Bacterial and protozoal gastroenteritis. N Engl J Med 325:327, 1991

Harjulehto T, Aro T, Hovi T, Saxén L: Congenital malformations and oral poliovirus vaccination during pregnancy. Lancet 1:771, 1989

Harris JW: Influenza occurring in pregnant women. JAMA 72:978, 1919

Hohlfeld P, Vial Y, Maillard-Brignon C, Vaudaux B, Fawer CL: Cytomegalovirus fetal infection: Prenatal diagnosis. Obstet Gynecol 78:615, 1991

Institute of Medicine, Committee on Issues and Priorities for New Vaccine Development: Prospects for immunizing against streptococcal group B. In New Vaccine Development: Establishing priorities, Vol I. Diseases of Importance in the United States. Washington, DC, National Academy Press, 1985, p 424

Isada NB, Paar DP, Johnson MP, Evans MI, Holzgreve W, Quereshi F, Straus SE: In utero diagnosis of congenital varicella zoster virus infection by chorionic villus sampling and polymerase chain reaction. Am J Obstet Gynecol 165:6, 1991

Jeannel D, Costagliola D, Niel G, Hubert B, Danis M: What is known about the prevention of congenital toxoplasmosis? Lancet 336:359, 1990

Jones BS: Congenital malaria: 3 cases. BMJ 2:439, 1950

Keuter M, van Eijk A, Hoogstrate M, Raasveld M, van de Ree M, Ngwawe WA, Watkins WM, Were JBO, Brandling-Bennett AD: Comparison of chloroquine, pyrimethamine and sulfadoxine, and chlorproguanil and dapsone as treatment for falciparum malaria in pregnant and non-pregnant women, Kakamega district, Kenya. BMJ 301:466, 1990

Koga Y, Mizumoto M, Matsumoto Y, Hattori T, Tanaka S, Tanaka T, Fujimoto S: Prenatal diagnosis of fetal intracranial calcifications. Am J Obstet Gynecol 163:1543, 1990

Korones SB: Uncommon virus infections of the mother, fetus, and newborn: Influenza, mumps and measles. Clin Perinatol 15:259, 1988

Kurppa K, Holmberg PC, Kuosma E, Aro T, Saxén L: Anencephaly and maternal common cold. Teratology 44:51, 1991

Kurtz JB, Tomlinson AH, Pearson J: Mumps virus isolated from a fetus. BMJ 284:471, 1982

Lamy ME, Mulongo KN, Gadisseux JF, Lyon G, Gaudy V, Van Lierde M: Prenatal diagnosis of fetal cytomegalovirus infection. Am J Obstet Gynecol 166:91, 1992

Larsen JW Jr: Influenza and pregnancy. Clin Obstet Gynecol 25:599, 1982

Lee SH, Ewert DP, Frederick PD, Mascola L: Resurgence of congenital rubella syndrome in the 1990s. JAMA 267:2616, 1992

Linnan MJ, Mascola L, Lou XD, Goulet V, May S, Salminen C, Hird DW, Yonekura ML, Hayes P, Weaver R, Audurier A, Plikaytis BD, Fannin SL, Kleks A, Broome CV: Epidemic listeriosis associated with Mexican-style cheese. N Engl J Med 319:823, 1988

Lynch L, Daffos F, Emanuel D, Giovangrandi Y, Meisel R, Forestier F, Cathomas G, Berkowitz RL: Prenatal diagnosis of fetal cytomegalovirus. Am J Obstet Gynecol 165:714, 1991

Magliocco AM, Demetrick DJ, Sarnat HB, Hwang W: Varicella embryopathy. Arch Pathol Lab Med 116:181, 1992

Malin AS, Cass PL, Hudson, CN: Exchange transfusion for severe falciparum malaria in pregnancy. Br Med J 300:1240, 1990

Markowitz LE, Steere AC, Benach JL, Slade JD, Broome CV: Lyme disease during pregnancy. JAMA 255:3394, 1986

Maurus JN: Hansen's disease in pregnancy. Obstet Gynecol 52:22, 1978

Maxwell GL, Watson WJ: Preterm premature rupture of membranes: Results of expectant management in patients with cervical cultures positive for group B streptococcus or Neisseria gonorrhoeae. Am J Obstet Gynecol 166:945, 1992

McCabe R, Remington JS: Toxoplasmosis: The time has come. N Eng J Med 318:313, 1988

McGregor JA, Burns JC, Levin MJ, Burlington B, Meiklejohn G: Transplacental passage of influenza A/Bangkok (H_3N_2) mimicking amniotic fluid infection syndrome. Am J Obstet Gynecol 148:856, 1984

McGregor JA, Mark S, Crawford GP, Levin MJ: Varicella zoster antibody testing in the case of pregnant woman exposed to varicella. Am J Obstet Gynecol 157:218, 1987

Manson MM, Logan WPD, Loy RM: Rubella and other virus infections during pregnancy. London, Her Majesty's Stationery Office, 1960

Miller E, Cradock-Watson JE, Pollock TM: Consequences of confirmed maternal rubella at successive stages of pregnancy. Lancet 2:781, 1982

Miller E, Cradock-Watson JE, Ridehalgh MKS: Outcome in newborn babies given anti-varicella-zoster immunoglobulin after perinatal maternal infection with varicella-zoster virus. Lancet 2:371, 1989

Morales WJ, Lim D: Reduction of group B streptococcal maternal and neonatal infections in preterm pregnancies with premature rupture of membranes through a rapid identification test. Am J Obstet Gynecol 157:13, 1987

Morgan-Capner P, Hambling MH, Coleman TJ, Watkins RP, Stern H, Hodgson J, Dulake C, Boswell PA, Booth J, Best JM: Detection of rubella-specific IgM in subclinical rubella reinfection in pregnancy. Lancet 1:246, 1985

Moroi K, Saito S, Kurata T, Sata T, Yanagida M: Fetal death associated with measles virus infection of the placenta. Am J Obstet Gynecol 164:1107, 1991

Nathwani D, Currie PF, Douglas JG, Green ST, Smith NC: *Plasmodium falciparum* malaria in pregnancy: A review. Br J Obstet Gynaecol 99:118, 1992

O'Callaghan E, Sham P, Takei N, Glover G, Murray RM: Schizophrenia after prenatal exposure to 1957 A2 influenza epidemic. Lancet 337:1248, 1991

Paryani SG, Arvin AM: Intrauterine infection with varicella-zoster virus after maternal varicella. N Engl J Med 314:1542, 1986

Pass RF: Day-care centers and the spread of cytomegalovirus and parvovirus B19. Pediatr Ann 20:419, 1991

Perlman JM, Argyle C: Lethal cytomegalovirus infection in preterm infants: Clinical, radiological, and neuropathological findings. Ann Neurol 31:64, 1992

Peters MT, Nicolaides KH: Cordocentesis for the diagnosis and treatment of human fetal parvovirus infection. Obstet Gynecol 75:501, 1990

Public Health Laboratory Service Working Party on Fifth Disease: Prospective study of human parvovirus (B19) infection in pregnancy. BMJ 300:1166, 1990

Pyati SP, Pildes RS, Jacobs NM, Ramamurthy RS, Yeh TF, Raval DS, Lilien LD, Amma P, Metzger WI: Penicillin in infants weighing two kilograms or less with early-onset group B streptococcal disease. N Engl J Med 308:1383, 1983

Regan JA, Klebanoff MA, Nugent RP, The Vaginal Infections and Prematurity Study Group: The epidemiology of group B streptococcal colonization in pregnancy. Obstet Gynecol 77:604, 1991

Rench MA, Baker CJ: Group B streptococcal breast abscess in a mother and mastitis in her infant. Obstet Gynecol 73:875, 1989

Riggall F, Salkind G, Spellacy W: Typhoid fever complicating pregnancy. Obstet Gynecol 44:117, 1974

Rodis JF, Quinn DL, Gary GW Jr, Anderson LJ, Rosengren S, Cartter ML, Campbell WA, Vintzileos AM: Management and outcomes of pregnancies complicated by human B19 parvovirus infection: A prospective study. Am J Obstet Gynecol 163:1168, 1990

Romero R, Mazor M, Oyarzun E, Sitori M, Wu YK, Hobbins JC: Is there an association between colonization with group B streptococcus and prematurity? J Reprod Med 34:797, 1989

Sahakian V, Weiner CP, Naides SJ, Williamson RA, Scharosch LL: Intrauterine transfusion treatment of nonimmune hydrops fetalis secondary to human parvovirus B19 infection. Am J Obstet Gynecol 164:1090, 1991

Saxén L, Holmberg PC, Kurppa K, Kuosma E, Pyhälä R: Influenza epidemics and anencephaly. Am J Public Health 80:473, 1990

Scialli AR, Rarick TL: Salmonella sepsis and second-trimester pregnancy loss. Obstet Gynecol 79:820, 1992

Schlesinger PA, Duray PH, Burke BA, Steere AC, Stillman MT: Maternal-fetal transmission of lyme disease spirochet, *Borrelia burgdorferi*. Ann Intern Med 103:67, 1985

Schuchat A, Deaver KA, Wenger JD, Plikaytis BD, Mascola L, Pinner RW, Reingold AL, Broome CV, The Listeria Study Group: Role of foods in sporadic listeriosis, I. Case-control study of dietary risk factors. JAMA 267:2041, 1992

Sever JL, Ellenberg JH, Ley AC, Madden DL, Fuccillo DA, Tzan NR, Edmonds DM: Toxoplasmosis: Maternal and pediatric findings in 23,000 pregnancies. Pediatrics 82:181, 1988

Siegal JD, McCracken GH Jr, Threlkeld N, Milvenan B, Rosenfeld CR: Single-dose penicillin prophylaxis against neonatal group B streptococcal infections. N Engl J Med 303:769, 1980

Siegel M: Congenital malformations following chickenpox, measles, mumps, and hepatitis: Results of a cohort study. JAMA 226:1521, 1973

Siegel M, Fuerst HT: Low birth weight and maternal virus diseases: A prospective study of rubella, measles, mumps, chickenpox, and hepatitis. JAMA 197:88, 1966

Siegel M, Goldberg M: Incidence of poliomyelitis in pregnancy. N Engl J Med 253:841, 1955

Smith LG, Pearlman M, Smith LG, Faro S: Lyme Disease: A review with emphasis on the pregnant woman. Obstet Gynecol Surv 46:125, 1991

Stagno S, Whitley RJ: Herpesvirus infections of pregnancy. Part II. Herpes simplex virus and varicella—zoster virus infections. N Engl J Med 313:1327, 1985

Steere AC: Lyme Disease. N Engl J Med 321:586, 1989

Steigman AJ, Bottone EJ, Hanna BA: Control of perinatal group B streptococcal sepsis: Efficacy of single injection of aqueous penicillin at birth. Mt Sinai J Med 45:685, 1978

Stein SJ, Greenspoon JS: Rubeola during pregnancy. Obstet Gynecol 78:925, 1991

Stirrat G: The immune system. In Hytten F, Chamberlain G (eds): Clinical Physiology in Obstetrics. Blackwell, London, 1991, p 101

Towers CV, Garite TJ, Friedman WW, Pircon RA, Nageotte MP: Comparison of a rapid enzyme-linked immunosorbent assay test and the gram stain for detection of group B streptococcus in high-risk antepartum patients. Am J Obstet Gynecol 163:965, 1990

Tuppurainen N, Hallman M: Prevention of neonatal group B streptococcal disease: Intrapartum detection and chemoprophylaxis of heavily colonized parturients. Obstet Gynecol 73:583, 1989

Weber K, Bratzke H-J, Neubert U, Wilske B, Duray PH: *Borrelia burgdorferi* in a newborn despite oral penicillin for Lyme borreliosis during pregnancy. Pediatr Infect Dis J 7:286, 1988

Yamauchi T, Wilson C, St Geme JW: Transmission of live, attenuated mumps virus to the human placenta. N Engl J Med 290:710, 1974

Yow MD, Demmler GJ: Congenital cytomegalovirus disease—20 years is long enough. N Engl J Med 326:703, 1992

CHAPTER 59
Sexually Transmitted Diseases

There are more than 20 infectious diseases that may be transmitted by sexual contact, and pregnancy confers immunity to none of them. Equally as important to maternal health and well-being is the potential impact that some of these diseases may have on the developing fetus. Women at highest risk for most of these diseases are sexually active, single adolescents who are often unaware of signs of sexually transmitted diseases in their sexual partners. Because many woman cannot be identified to be at increased risk for some infections, some clinicians choose to screen all prenatal patients for many of these infections. Consequently, as a part of routine prenatal testing, common sexually transmitted diseases that are often sought include syphilis, gonorrhea, chlamydia, hepatitis B virus, human papillomavirus, and in a growing number of settings, human immunodeficiency virus.

When all sexually transmitted diseases are considered together, they represent one of the most common medical complications of pregnancy, especially in indigent, urban populations plagued by drug abuse and prostitution. For example, in the prenatal clinics of Parkland Hospital, chlamydial infection is found in 12 percent of women, gonorrhea in 2 to 3 percent, syphilis in 2 to 3 percent, genital herpes in about 1 percent, and human immunodeficiency infection in 0.3 percent (Wendel and Cunningham, 1991). It can readily be seen that screening, identification, education, and treatment should be important components of prenatal care for women at increased risk for these common infections. In many of the following treatment protocols for sexually transmitted diseases, we attempt to adhere to the intensive, but frequently modified, treatment schedules provided periodically by the Centers for Disease Control. These usually are published for distribution in the *Morbidity and Mortality Weekly Report (MMWR)*.

Syphilis

There have recently been marked increases in the incidence of syphilis in pregnant women in many areas of the United States. This is not surprising because the rates of syphilis in reproductive-age women are the highest that have been observed since the 1940s (Centers for Disease Control, 1992a). Ricci and associates (1989) and Minkoff and colleagues (1990b) reported associations with maternal syphilis and drug abuse, particularly crack cocaine, and lack of prenatal care. An-

tepartum syphilis can profoundly effect pregnancy outcome by causing preterm labor, fetal death, and neonatal infection by transplacental or perinatal infection (Wendel, 1988). Fortunately, of the many congenital infections, syphilis is not only the most readily prevented, but it also is one of the most susceptible to therapy.

Clinical Manifestations. Primary syphilis follows an incubation period of 10 to 90 days, but usually less than 6 weeks. During pregnancy, the primary genital lesion, or sometimes multiple lesions, may be of such small size or be so located as to go unnoticed. For example, a **cervical chancre** is more common in pregnant women, probably because of inoculation of the friable cervix. In some instances, however, the lesion may be somewhat larger than usual, presumably because of increased genital vascularity. The primary lesion or chancre persists from 2 to 6 weeks and then heals spontaneously, but the chancre is often accompanied by the development of nontender, enlarged inguinal lymph nodes.

Approximately 6 to 8 weeks after healing of the chancre, secondary syphilis usually appears in the form of a highly variable skin rash. About 15 percent of women still have a chancre. The lesions of secondary syphilis may be mild and go unnoticed in 25 percent of patients. In some, lesions are limited to the genitalia, where they appear usually as elevated areas, or **condylomata lata,** which occasionally cause vulvar ulcerations (Fig. 59–1). In many women there is no history of a local sore or rash. At times the first suggestion of the disease is the delivery of an infant who either may be stillborn or liveborn but severely afflicted with congenital syphilis.

Fetal and Neonatal Infection. In the past, syphilis accounted for nearly a third of stillborns and, indeed, delivery of a macerated fetus was considered diagnostic of infection with *Treponema pallidum.* Today, syphilis has a smaller but persistent role in the genesis of fetal deaths, and as emphasized by the Centers for Disease Control (1989a), the number of cases of congenital infection has paralleled the 240 percent increase in adult syphilis from 1986 through 1988. Half of these mothers had inadequate prenatal care, and thus infection was not diagnosed. **Half of congenitally infected infants were born to women who received prenatal care but in whom serological screening was not done, and thus maternal syphilis was not treated.** Dorf-

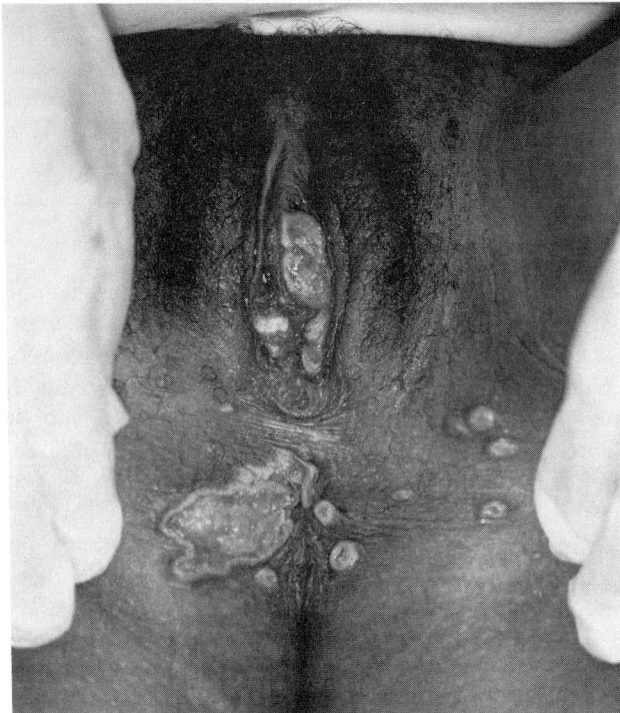

Fig. 59–1. Genital condylomata lata of secondary syphilis. (From Wendel and Cunningham, 1991.)

man and Glaser (1990) and Sanchez and colleagues (1991) described several cases of congenital syphilis that were missed because recent maternal infection had not allowed an antibody response by the time of delivery.

PATHOLOGY. Syphilis is a chronic infection, and the spirochete causes lesions in the internal organs that include interstitial changes in the lungs (*pneumonia alba of Virchow*), liver (*hypertrophic cirrhosis*), spleen, and pancreas. Any stage of syphilis during pregnancy can result in an infected and affected fetus. More recent infections are more likely to be associated with fetal morbidity. Syphilitic infection also causes *osteochondritis* in the long bones, which is most readily recognizable radiographically at the lower ends of the femur, tibia, and radius.

Under the influence of syphilitic infection, the placenta becomes large and pale. Microscopically, villi appear to have lost their characteristic arborescent appearance and to have become thicker and club shaped. There is a marked decrease in the number of blood vessels, which in advanced cases almost entirely disappear as a result of endarteritis and proliferation of the stromal cells. Perhaps related to this, Lucas and colleagues (1991) demonstrated increased vascular resistance in uterine and umbilical arteries of infected pregnancies. Spirochetes are sparsely scattered throughout the placenta even when they are present in large numbers in fetal organs. They may be demonstrated by examination under the darkfield microscope of scrapings from the intima of the vessels of the fresh cord.

Serological Diagnosis. A suitable serological screening test such as the *Venereal Disease Research Laboratory (VDRL) slide test* or the *rapid plasma reagin (RPR) test* is performed at the first prenatal visit. Testing is required by law. Fortunately, serological tests for syphilis almost always will be positive by 4 to 6 weeks after contracting the disease. Because such reagin tests lack specificity, a treponemal test such as the *fluorescent treponemal antibody absorption test (FTA-ABS)* or the *microhemagglutination assay for antibodies to Treponema pallidum (MHA-TP)* is used to confirm a positive result. Especially for women at high risk for syphilis, a second nontreponemal test should be done during the third trimester. The Centers for Disease Control (1988) recommends that all pregnant women have repeat serological screening at delivery. Cord blood screening is an insensitive test to detect early congenital syphilis.

Fetal Diagnosis. Wendel and colleagues (1989) have shown that motile spirochetes can be seen in amnionic fluid obtained transabdominally in women with syphilis and fetal death. These same workers later reported that the polymerase chain reaction was 100 percent specific for detection of *Treponema pallidum* in amnionic fluid and neonatal serum and spinal fluid. Figure 59–2 shows an infant with congenital lues who has a large abdomen owing mostly to marked hepatosplenomegaly. His placenta weighed almost as much as the infant!

Treatment. Penicillin remains the treatment of choice; however, treatment of syphilis during pregnancy has not been evaluated rigorously. Such therapy is dual; it is given to eradicate maternal infection as well as to prevent congenital syphilis. The principal difficulty in defining successful treatment has been because fetal syphilis could not be confirmed. Although the prenatal diagnosis of severe fetal syphilis can be made by funipuncture, its clinical utility is not yet clear (Wendel and associates, 1991).

It has been observed retrospectively that benzathine penicillin G cures early maternal infection and prevents neonatal syphilis in 98 percent of cases (Zenker and Rolfs, 1990). As shown in Table 59–1, the current Centers for Disease Control guidelines for treatment of syphilis in pregnancy include the same dosage schedule of long-acting benzathine penicillin G as for nonpregnant adults. Skin testing is encouraged to confirm the risk of an IgE-mediated allergic reaction to penicillin. If skin tests are reactive, penicillin desensitization as described by Wendel and associates (1985) is recommended and is followed by benzathine penicillin G treatment.

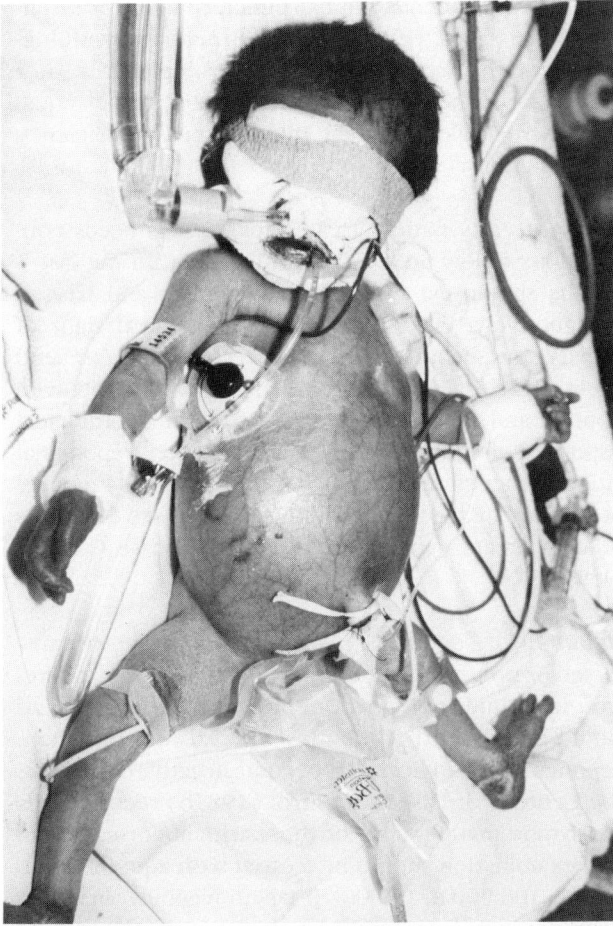

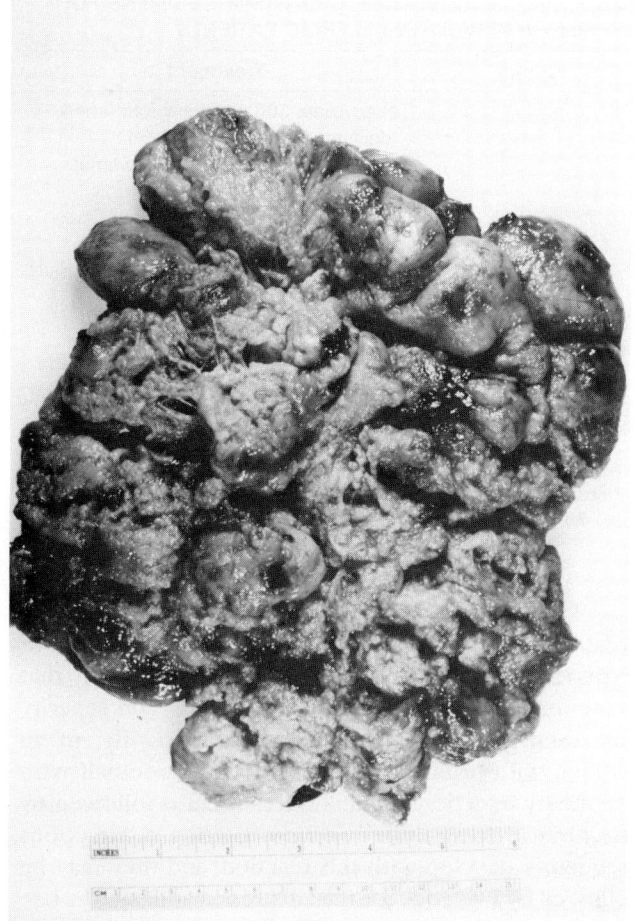

A   **B**

Fig. 59–2. Congenital syphilis. **A.** A 29-week infant gravely ill with congenital lues. Note the enlarged abdomen caused by marked hepatosplenomegaly plus ascites. **B.** The large syphilitic placenta of the same infant. The placenta weighed 1200 g, almost the birthweight of the infant. (Photographs courtesy of Dr. G. Wendel.)

Alternative therapy during pregnancy with one of the non-penicillin regimens shown in Table 59–2 is discouraged by the Centers for Disease Control because of reported treatment failures in preventing congenital syphilis, especially with erythromycin (Wendel, 1988; Zenker and Rolfs, 1990). The recommended alternative is to desensitize these women to penicillin after which benzathine penicillin G is used. If this is not practical, then we agree with Fiumara (1984) that tetracycline should be given. Treatment of early syphilis with newer cephalosporins, particularly ceftriaxone, looks promising (Hook and co-workers, 1988), but there is not enough information about their transplacental pharmacokinetics to currently recommend their use in pregnancy.

There is concern that despite recommended treatment during pregnancy, almost 20 percent of newborns have obvious clinical stigmata of congenital syphilis (Centers for Disease Control, 1988). Half of these method failures were identified in mothers not given

TABLE 59–1. RECOMMENDED TREATMENT FOR PREGNANT WOMEN WITH SYPHILIS

Category	Treatment
Early syphilis[a]	Benzathine penicillin G, 2.4 million units intramuscularly as a single injection
Syphilis of more than 1 year's duration[b]	Benzathine penicillin G, 2.4 million units intramuscularly weekly for 3 doses
Neurosyphilis	Aqueous crystalline penicillin G, 2–4 million units intravenously every 4 hrs for 10–14 days, followed by benzathine penicillin G, 2.4 million units intramuscularly weekly for 3 doses
	or
	Aqueous procaine penicillin G, 2.4 million units intramuscularly daily, plus probenecid 500 mg orally four times daily, both for 10–14 days, followed by benzathine penicillin G, 2.4 million units intramuscularly weekly for three doses

[a] Primary, secondary, and latent syphilis of less than 1 year's duration.
[b] Latent syphilis of unknown or more than 1 year's duration; cardiovascular or late benign syphilis.
From the Centers for Disease Control (1988a and 1989b).

TABLE 59–2. ALTERNATIVE TREATMENT REGIMENS FOR SYPHILIS IN PENICILLIN-ALLERGIC PATIENTS

Category	Treatment
Early syphilis	Tetracycline, 500 mg orally four times daily for 2 weeks[a]
	Doxycycline, 100 mg orally two times daily for 2 weeks[a]
	Erythromycin, 500 mg orally four times daily for 2 weeks
	Ceftriaxone, 250 mg intramuscularly daily for 10 days[b]
Syphilis of more than 1 year's duration	Tetracycline, 500 mg orally four times daily for 4 weeks[a]
	Doxycycline, 100 mg orally two times daily for 4 weeks[a]
Neurosyphilis	Non-penicillin treatment not recommended

[a] Tetracycline therapy is generally avoided during pregnancy.
[b] Probably effective; limited clinical experience.
From the Centers for Disease Control (1989b).

treatment until the third trimester. This also has been our experience at Parkland Hospital, and it seems likely that these fetal infections are of such duration and severity that there is irreversible damage. Importantly, in all women with primary syphilis and about one half with secondary infection, penicillin treatment is followed by the *Jarisch-Herxheimer reaction*. Uterine contractions frequently develop with this reaction, and they may be followed by evidence for fetal distress manifested as late fetal heart rate decelerations (Klein and colleagues, 1990). Lucas and co-workers (1991) used Doppler velocimetry studies and demonstrated associated acute vascular-resistance changes. Finally, obvious fetal involvement, characterized by ultrasonic evidence for ascites, is associated with almost universally bad fetal outcome, despite therapy. Hill and Maloney (1991) and Satin and colleagues (1992) have described fetuses with hepatosplenomegaly, gastrointestinal tract obstruction, and placentomegaly. Barton and co-workers (1992) found that delivery and neonatal treatment may be the best option for hydropic fetuses with congenital syphilis.

Prior to syphilotherapy, all women should be offered counseling and testing for antibody to human immunodeficiency virus because of the frequent association of these two infections and implications for therapy.

Lumbar Puncture. Whether to perform a lumbar puncture for cerebrospinal fluid analysis remains controversial (Wiesel and colleagues, 1985). Many asymptomatic patients have spinal fluid abnormalities with primary, secondary, and early latent syphilis, but most do not develop neurosyphilis after treatment with one of the currently recommended regimens (Lukehart and co-workers, 1988). Ideally, individuals with latent syphilis of greater than 1 years' duration should have spinal fluid analysis, but Hart (1986) recommends that management be individualized. The Centers for Disease Control

(1989b) recommends lumbar puncture in latent syphilis of more than 1 years' duration if there are neurological symptoms, treatment failures, serological test titer of 1 : 32 or higher, if non-penicillin therapy is planned, or if there is concomitant human immunodeficiency viral infection.

Follow-up. Any patient treated for syphilis needs conscientious follow-up. Sexual contacts within the last 3 months should be evaluated for syphilis and treated presumptively, even if seronegative. Clinical signs of primary or secondary syphilis resolve over several weeks. Maternal quantitative serologies are followed monthly and again at delivery to confirm a serological response to treatment. The quantitative non-treponemal antibody titer should decline four-fold by 3 to 4 months for primary or secondary syphilis, and by 6 to 8 months for early latent syphilis (Centers for Disease Control, 1989b).

Treatment of Congenital Syphilis. Every infant with suspected or proven congenital syphilis should have a cerebrospinal fluid examination prior to treatment, and should be followed at monthly intervals until the nontreponemal serological tests become negative or serofast. The Centers for Disease Control (1989b) recommends that symptomatic infants or those with abnormal spinal fluid examination should be treated with aqueous penicillin G, 100,000 to 150,000 U/kg intravenously in two to three divided doses each day for at least 10 days, or aqueous procaine penicillin G, 50,000 U/kg intramuscularly each day for a minimum of 10 days.

Asymptomatic seropositive infants with a normal spinal fluid examination can be treated with a single dose of benzathine penicillin G, 50,000 U/kg intramuscularly.

Infants born of mothers treated with erythromycin for syphilis during pregnancy should be retreated as though they have congenital syphilis.

Gonorrhea

The prevalence of gonorrhea during pregnancy varies from 0.5 to 7 percent and reflects the risk status of the population (Wendel and Cunningham, 1991). Risk factors include being single, adolescence, poverty, drug abuse, prostitution, other sexually transmitted diseases, and lack of prenatal care. Gonococcal infection is also a marker for concomitant chlamydial infection in about 40 percent of infected pregnant woman (Christmas and associates, 1989).

In most pregnant women, gonococcal infection is limited to the lower genital tract, including the cervix, urethra, and periurethral and vestibular glands. Acute salpingitis is rare but develops if cervical infection ascends before obliteration of the uterine cavity through fusion of the chorion and decidua at 12 weeks. Reactivated or persistent preexisting infection can cause a tubo-ovarian abscess, but this is rare. The diagnosis of acute salpingitis during pregnancy is made by excluding appendicitis, septic abortion, adnexal torsion, and ectopic pregnancy.

There is some evidence that pregnancy alters the clinical presentation of gonorrhea. For example, some clinicians have reported increased rates of oropharyngeal and anal infections in pregnancy (Corman and associates, 1974; Holmes and colleagues, 1971). The increased incidence of non-cervical infection may be from altered sexual practices because of pregnancy, cultural customs, or both. It is also interesting that pregnant women account for a disproportionate amount (7 to 40 percent) of disseminated gonococcal infection in women (Al-Suleiman and co-workers, 1983; Holmes and colleagues, 1971). These observations may reflect heightened medical attention during pregnancy or they may be due to increased gonococcal dissemination from engorged pelvic vasculature.

Effect on Pregnancy. Gonococcal infection may have deleterious effects on pregnancy outcome in any trimester. There is an association between untreated gonococcal cervicitis and septic spontaneous abortion or infection after induced abortion (Burkman and associates, 1976). Preterm delivery, prematurely ruptured membranes, chorioamnionitis, and postpartum infection are more common in women with *Neisseria gonorrhoeae* detected at delivery (Alger and associates, 1988; Edwards and co-workers, 1978). Elliott and associates (1990) found that the attributable risk for preterm birth was 14 percent. *N. gonorrhoeae* carriage marks women at increased risk for adverse pregnancy outcome, and treatment reduces that risk (Stoll and colleagues, 1982). Maxwell and Watson (1992) reported that expectant management of the culture-positive woman was reasonable even with prematurely ruptured membranes as long as antimicrobial treatment was given promptly.

Because of these factors, a screening cervical culture is recommended by most authorities at the first prenatal visit or prior to an induced abortion. In high-risk populations, the Centers for Disease Control (1989b) recommends that a repeat culture be obtained after 28 weeks' gestation.

Treatment. In many areas, antimicrobial-resistant *N. gonorrhoeae*, particularly penicillinase-producing strains, have rendered some β-lactam drugs ineffective for therapy (Centers for Disease Control, 1990b). For these reasons, Moran and Zenilman (1990) recommend that the treatment of gonorrhea in pregnant women be guided by gonococcal culture and susceptibility testing. As shown in Table 59–3, ceftriaxone is recommended for gonococcal infection at any anatomical site. In regions

TABLE 59–3. TREATMENT FOR GONOCOCCAL INFECTIONS DURING PREGNANCY

Ceftriaxone, 250 mg intramuscularly
or
Amoxicillin, 3 g orally after 1 g probenecid orally
or
Spectinomycin, 2 g intramuscularly

For possible concomitant chlamydial infection, one of the above is given with erythromycin base, 500 mg, or stearate, 500 mg, or ethylsuccinate, 800 mg orally four times daily for 7 days

From the Centers for Disease Control (1989b).

with a low prevalence of β-lactam resistance, oral amoxicillin with probenecid is reasonable and inexpensive therapy. Spectinomycin is recommended for women allergic to penicillin. Cavanee and associates (1993) reported that treatment with ceftriaxone, spectinomycin, or amoxicillin with probenecid produced similar cure rates in 252 pregnant women with asymptomatic endocervical gonorrhea. One fourth of these women had concomitant rectal infection.

Screening for syphilis and *Chlamydia trachomatis* should precede treatment, if possible. If chlamydial testing is unavailable, presumptive therapy is given as shown in Table 59–3. Treatment for sexual contacts and maternal test-of-cure cultures help to insure efficacy of therapy. Because gonococcal reinfection is common, repeat screening in late pregnancy should be considered for women treated earlier during pregnancy.

Disseminated Gonococcal Infections. There are several acceptable treatment schedules for *arthritis* and *dermatitis* including aqueous crystalline penicillin G intravenously at the outset, and either ampicillin or amoxicillin, 500 mg by mouth four times daily to complete 7 days of therapy. Tetracycline is recommended in case of penicillin allergy, unless the woman is pregnant. Then erythromycin can be used as described above.

For gonococcal *endocarditis* and *meningitis*, long-term high-dose penicillin is given intravenously. Endocarditis rarely complicates pregnancy, but it may be fatal (Bataskov and colleagues, 1991).

Infants of Mothers with Gonorrhea. Ceftriaxone, 50 mg/kg but not to exceed 125 mg, is given intravenously or intramuscularly in a single injection. The drug should be used with caution in infants with hyperbilirubinemia, especially low-birthweight infants.

All infants are given prophylaxis against eye infection (see Chap. 17, p. 451). Infants who develop gonococcal ophthalmia should be evaluated for disseminated infection. Gonococcal ophthalmia may be treated with intravenously or intramuscularly administered ceftriaxone, 25 to 50 mg/kg daily for 7 days. Isolation is recommended until treated for 24 hours. Local care of the eyes by an expert is also important. Topical antibiotic preparations are not appropriate. Both parents also should be treated for gonorrhea.

Chlamydial Infections

Chlamydia trachomatis is an obligate intracellular bacterium that has several serotypes, including those that cause *lymphogranuloma venereum.* The most commonly encountered strains are those that attach only to columnar or transitional cell epithelium and cause cervical, but not vulvar, infection. The replication rate for chlamydiae is long compared with other bacteria, and chlamydial infections are characterized by their low-grade indolence, often associated with a paucity of clinical findings.

Maternal Infections. According to the Centers for Disease Control (1985), genital infection with *Chlamydia trachomatis* is the most common sexually transmitted bacterial disease in women. Cultures from the cervix are positive in up to one fourth of pregnant women, and its incidence depends on the demographic make-up of the population (Table 59–4). The prevalence of symptomatic and asymptomatic genital infections in private obstetrical patients is under 2 percent, but it is up to 24 percent in some groups of young, inner-city women attending public clinics (McGregor and French, 1991; Ryan and colleagues, 1990; Rettig, 1988; Wendel and Cunningham, 1991).

Symptomatic Infection. Chlamydial infection may be associated with several clinical syndromes that include **urethritis, mucopurulent cervicitis,** and **acute salpingitis** (Table 59–4). Despite this, most pregnant women have subclinical or asymptomatic infection. The predictive ability of mucopurulent cervicitis to indicate *C. trachomatis* in pregnant women is uncertain (Brunham and co-workers, 1984; Moscicki and colleagues, 1987).

TABLE 59–4. CHLAMYDIAL INFECTIONS

Women at High Risk	Symptomatic Syndromes
Less than 20 years of age	**Maternal**
Unmarried	Mucopurulent cervicitis
Lower socioeconomic status	Nongonococcal urethritis
Inner-city population	Proctitis
Multiple sexual partners	Acute salpingitis
Other sexually transmitted diseases	Conjunctivitis
	Neonatal
	Conjunctivitis
	Pneumonia

From the Centers for Disease Control (1985).

Asymptomatic Infection and Pregnancy Outcome. There is no doubt that perinatal transmission is associated with neonatal **conjunctivitis** and **pneumonia** (Hammerschlag and colleagues, 1989; Schachter and co-workers, 1986a). Vertical transmission occurs in at least half of infants delivered vaginally to infected women (McGregor and French, 1991). There is evidence that eye prophylaxis for gonococcal infection with silver nitrate, erythromycin, or tetracycline will prevent many cases of chlamydial conjunctivitis (see Chap. 17, p. 451).

Although many investigators have examined the effects of asymptomatic chlamydial infection on pregnancy outcome, its role remains controversial (Gibbs and associates, 1992). Some authorities have found that untreated maternal cervical chlamydial infection increases the risk for preterm delivery, prematurely ruptured membranes, and perinatal mortality (Alger, 1988; Gravett, 1986; Martin, 1982; and Martius, 1988; and their many colleagues). Conversely, other investigators have found that only women with recent chlamydial infection, confirmed by anti-chlamydial IgM antibody testing, are at risk for these adverse outcomes (Berman and co-workers, 1987; Sweet and associates, 1987). Moreover, although Cohen (1990) and Ryan (1990) and their colleagues reported a reduction in these adverse events in women treated with erythromycin, preliminary data from the Vaginal Infections and Prematurity Study Group showed no improvement in pregnancy outcome with treatment (Martin, 1990). This latter study was a large, multicenter, randomized, placebo-controlled, blinded investigation carried out under the auspices of the National Institutes of Health.

There is evidence that recent-onset chlamydial infection may have a worse prognosis. Sweet and colleagues (1987) prospectively studied 270 pregnant women with untreated cervical chlamydial infection and compared their pregnancy outcomes with chlamydia-negative controls. There were no differences in the incidences of preterm labor, prematurely ruptured membranes, chorioamnionitis, neonatal sepsis, or postpartum uterine infections. However, they found that women with evidence for recent infection characterized by IgM antibody to *C. trachomatis* were more likely to have preterm labor or prematurely ruptured membranes. Berman and colleagues (1987) also reported this association in 1152 Navajo women whose cervical carriage rate for chlamydia was 22 percent.

Chlamydial infection is not associated with an increased risk of chorioamnionitis (Gibbs and Schachter, 1987) nor metritis and pelvic cellulitis after cesarean section (Blanco and colleagues, 1985). However, delayed postpartum uterine infection with *C. trachomatis* has been described by Hoyme and associates (1986). The syndrome, which develops 2 to 3 weeks postpartum, is distinct from early metritis. It causes vaginal bleeding or discharge, low-grade fever, lower abdominal pain, and uterine tenderness.

Neonatal Infections

Conjunctivitis. Ophthalmic chlamydial infections are one of the most common causes of preventable blindness in undeveloped countries. Inclusion conjunctivitis develops in as many as one third of neonates born to mothers with cervical infection. Symptomatic conjunctivitis tends to appear later than disease caused by *N. gonorrhoeae,* and the two must be differentiated using culture or Gram and Giemsa staining because treatment is not the same.

Pneumonitis. Approximately 10 percent of infants born through an infected cervix develop chlamydial pneumonitis within 1 to 3 months (McGregor and French, 1991). Clinically, bilateral pulmonary infiltrates and chronic cough are often associated with poor weight gain. As in their incubation, these infections resolve slowly, even with treatment.

Screening. The role for routine screening cultures for *C. trachomatis* during pregnancy remains unclear. Laga (1988) and Hammerschlag (1989) and their co-workers reported that newborn eye prophylaxis with silver nitrate solution or erythromycin or tetracycline ointment, given to prevent neonatal gonococcal and chlamydial ophthalmic infection, are associated with chlamydial conjunctivitis in up to 20 percent of exposed infants. The annual cost of sequelae of neonatal chlamydial infection in the United States was estimated by Washington and associates (1987) to be almost $53 million.

According to Schachter (1989), the direct fluorescent antibody test and the enzyme immunoassay test have a sensitivity of 85 percent and a specificity of 98 percent. Currently, universal *C. trachomatis* prenatal screening is not considered cost-effective for direct antigen testing unless the prevalence of infection exceeds 6 percent; for cultures, the prevalence must be about 15 percent (Nettleman and Bell, 1991). Newer DNA probes and polymerase chain reaction may make detection cheaper and quicker. Currently, the Centers for Disease Control (1989b) recommends *C. trachomatis* diagnostic testing, if possible, at the first prenatal visit for all pregnant women, and again in the third trimester for those at high risk (Table 59–4). Conversely, the American College of Obstetricians and Gynecologists (1992a) recommends targeted screening of high-risk populations.

Treatment. The currently recommended regimen and its alternatives for treatment of chlamydial infection in pregnant women are shown in Table 59–5. Erythromycin taken orally for at least 7 days will eradicate maternal infection in over 90 percent of pregnant women (Crombleholme, 1990; McNeeley, 1989; Schachter, 1986b; and their associates). For women who cannot tolerate erythromycin because of gastrointestinal side effects, the dosage is reduced by one half and the dura-

TABLE 59–5. TREATMENT OF *CHLAMYDIA TRACHOMATIS* DURING PREGNANCY

Regimens	Dosage
Recommended	Erythromycin base, 500 mg orally, four times daily for 7 days[a]
Alternatives	Erythromycin ethylsuccinate, 800 mg orally, four times daily for 7 days[a]
	Amoxicillin, 500 mg orally, three times daily for 7 days[b]

[a] If intolerance develops, the dosage may be reduced by 50 percent and the duration of administration doubled.
[b] Limited data available in pregnancy.
From the Centers for Disease Control (1989b).

tion of therapy doubled. McNeeley and colleagues (1989) reported that erythromycin base, 1 g daily given orally for only 7 days was equally efficacious. Crombleholme and co-workers (1990) found that amoxicillin, 1.5 g daily for 7 days is as effective as erythromycin base, and with significantly fewer side effects and thus better compliance. There are no data concerning the new oral macrolide antibiotic, azithromycin, for use in pregnancy. It has been classified as category B and in nonpregnant adults it has proven effective for chlamydial infections given as a single 1-g dose (Johnson, 1991).

Erythromycin estolate, tetracyclines, and quinolones should not be used during pregnancy. Sex partners within the prior 30 days should be examined and treated for chlamydial infection.

Lymphogranuloma Venereum. The LGV serovars of *C. trachomatis* cause lymphogranuloma venereum. The primary genital infection is transient and seldom recognized. Inguinal adenitis may follow and at times lead to suppuration. It may be confused with chancroid. Ultimately, the lymphatics of the lower genital tract and perirectal tissues may be involved with sclerosis and fibrosis, which can cause vulvar elephantiasis and especially severe rectal stricture. Fistula formation involving the rectum, perineum, and vulva also may be quite troublesome.

In the absence of pregnancy, doxycycline, 100 mg orally twice daily for 21 days is recommended (Centers for Disease Control, 1989b). Otherwise, erythromycin or sulfisoxazole, 500 mg four times daily is given for 21 days. Some of these infections that we have encountered at Parkland Hospital have been long-standing, and there was little response to multiple antimicrobial regimens that in one case included erythromycin, sulfamethoxazole, tetracycline, and chloramphenicol.

Herpes Simplex Virus Infections

Management of pregnancy complicated by maternal genital infection with herpesvirus remains a frustrating

TABLE 59–6. CLINICAL MANIFESTATIONS OF GENITAL HERPES SIMPLEX VIRUS (HSV) INFECTIONS

Infection	History of Herpes	Anti-HSV Antibody	Clinical Severity	Systemic Symptoms	Duration of Lesions
First episode					
Primary	Absent	Absent	Severe	Present	2–3 weeks
Non-primary	Orolabial (variable)	Present	Moderate	Attenuated	2–3 weeks
Recurrent					
Symptomatic	Present	Present	Mild	Absent	< 1–2 weeks
Asymptomatic	Present	Present	Inapparent	Absent	< 1 week

From Wendel and Cunningham (1991).

exercise for the obstetrician. There are currently no available rapid diagnostic tests that document reliably contemporary infection. Moreover, there are minimal data to estimate risks for the neonate exposed to recurrent maternal infection.

Virology. Two types of herpes simplex virus (HSV) have been distinguished based on immunological as well as clinical differences. Type 1 is responsible for most nongenital herpetic infections, but infrequently involves the genital tract. Type 2 virus is recovered almost exclusively from the genital tract and is transmitted in the great majority of instances by sexual contact (National Institutes of Health, 1985). The incidence of antibodies specific for type 2 herpes increases with age and varies considerably with the population studied, for example, it approaches 100 percent among prostitutes. In the absence of antibody, exposure to a sexual partner with active herpetic lesions will in the majority of instances result in clinical disease.

Clinical Infection. Clinical syndromes vary depending on whether there has been previous infection, and even prior orolabial infection with type 1 virus may modify an initial type 2 genital infection (Table 59–6). The prevalence of asymptomatic infection is widely underestimated, and in a national seroepidemiological survey from 1976 to 1980, 20 percent of women had antibody to type 2 virus (Johnson and colleagues, 1989). The risks for type 2 antibody were greatest among black and previously married women.

First-episode Infection. Primary infection with herpesvirus is frequently symptomatic. Some first-episodes are mild or asymptomatic, probably due to some immunity from cross-reacting antibody from childhood-acquired type 1 infection. The typical incubation period of 3 to 6 days is followed by a papular eruption with itching or tingling which then becomes painful and vesicular with multiple vulvar and perineal lesions that may coalesce (Fig. 59–3). Inguinal adenopathy may be severe. Transient systemic influenza-like symptoms are common and are presumably caused by viremia. Occasionally, hepatitis, encephalitis, or pneumonia may develop. Frieden

and colleagues (1990) reviewed experiences with herpes encephalitis complicating pregnancy. Of six reported cases, only two women lived, including their patient.

The vulvar and perineal vesicles are traumatized easily, eventually ulcerate, but usually do not become secondarily infected. Vulvar lesions are likely to be extremely painful and may cause considerable debility. Urinary retention may develop because of the pain induced by micturition or because of sacral nerve involvement. In 2 to 4 weeks, all signs and symptoms of

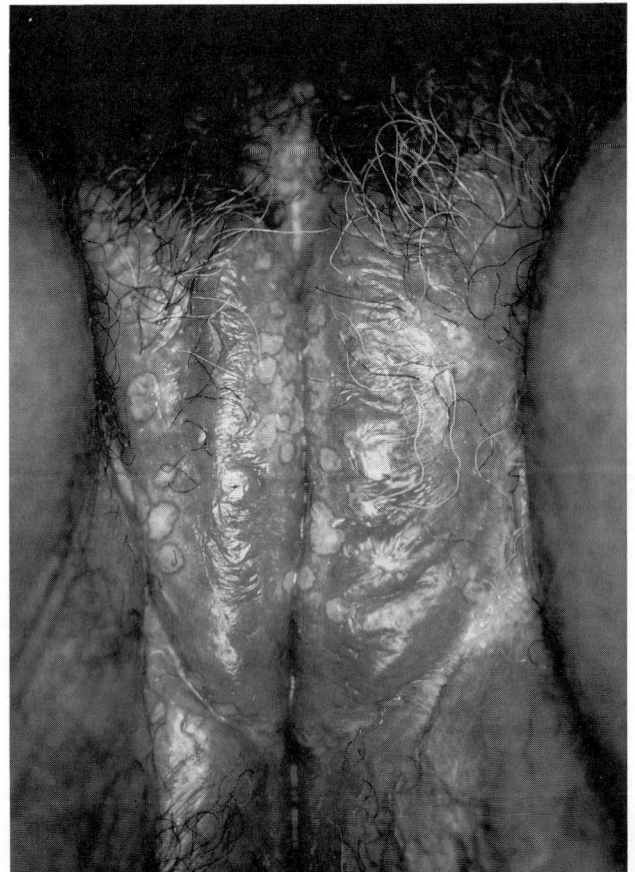

Fig. 59–3. First-episode primary genital herpes simplex virus infection. (From Wendel and Cunningham, 1991.)

infection disappear, but later recurrences are common because of viral reactivation within the nerve ganglia. Cervical involvement is common and may be inapparent clinically.

Recurrent Infections. During the latency period in which viral particles reside in nerve ganglia, reactivation is common and mediated through variable but poorly understood stimuli. Reactivation is termed recurrent infection and results in herpesvirus shedding (Table 59–6). These lesions generally are fewer in number, less tender, and shed virus for shorter periods (2 to 5 days) than those of primary infection, and typically they recur at the same sites. Although commonly involved in primary disease, cervical involvement is less frequent with recurrent infections (Brown and colleagues, 1985; Yeager and Arvin, 1984).

Diagnosis of Herpesvirus Infection. Recovery of virus by *tissue culture* is most optimal for confirmation of clinically apparent infection and asymptomatic recurrences. The sensitivity of culture is nearly 95 percent before the lesions undergo crusting as long as specimens are obtained and handled properly. There are virtually no false-positives. With symptomatic recurrences, more than half of the cultures will be positive after 48 hours, but it may take longer to demonstrate cytopathic effects with asymptomatic recurrences because of a smaller inoculum.

Cytological examination after alcohol fixation and Papanicolaou staining is used commonly as a rapid means of diagnosis of clinical recurrences, and smears taken from scrapings of the base of lesions may show large multinucleated cells and eosinophilic viral inclusion bodies. This method is limited by its specificity for cervical infection and sensitivity for genital ulcer disease. For example, common cytomegalovirus cervical infection (see Chap. 58, p. 1287) is difficult to distinguish from herpesvirus by Pap smear. *Enzyme-linked immunosorbent assay* (ELISA) techniques have been evaluated for rapid diagnosis of direct smears and are promising (Baker and colleagues, 1989); currently, however, there is little experience with these tests during pregnancy. Likewise, Hardy and associates (1990) have reported preliminary salutary results with *polymerase chain reaction* to identify viral sequences.

ANTIBODIES. Several assay systems are available commercially and in research settings to detect anti-HSV antibody. About one third of private patients test positive for type-specific antibodies to HSV-2 glycoprotein G (Gibbs and Mead, 1992; Johnson and associates, 1989). Kulhanjian and colleagues (1992) have proposed that serological screening of couples during pregnancy for HSV-2 antibodies would stimulate the need for sexual precautions if discordancy were found, that is, a seronegative woman with a positive partner. Unfortunately, as emphasized by Gibbs and Mead (1992), there currently is no reliable commercially available assay to differentiate HSV-1 from HSV-2 antibody.

Treatment. There is really no effective treatment. *Acyclovir* used topically perhaps modifies the symptomatology. Oral or parenteral preparations attenuate clinical infection as well as the duration of viral shedding, but have not been used extensively during pregnancy and are not routinely recommended. For intense discomfort, analgesics and topical anesthetics may provide some relief, and severe urinary retention is treated with an indwelling bladder catheter. The safety of acyclovir given during pregnancy has not been established. However, in a recent report from the acyclovir registry of 168 liveborns who had been exposed to acyclovir during the first trimester, there were only nine with congenital malformations (Andrews and colleagues, 1992). Treatment is not recommended for the pregnant woman with normal immune function who has uncomplicated primary genital herpes infection, because treatment has not been shown to decrease the risk of abortion or preterm labor. With disseminated herpes infection that is potentially life-threatening, parenteral acyclovir is justified (Brown and Baker, 1989).

Many women with *human immunodeficiency viral infection* also have genital herpes, and treatment failures with recommended doses of acyclovir have been reported. Higher dosages of acyclovir may be beneficial for immunoincompetent women with immunodeficiency virus infection and severe recurrent genital herpes (Stone and Whittington, 1990).

Acyclovir is of little benefit in recurrent genital herpes in adults. It has not been evaluated as suppressive therapy given during pregnancy to prevent recurrences near term. Suppressive therapy given orally reduces the signs and symptoms of recurrent infection, but does not completely eliminate asymptomatic viral shedding and may be associated with potential fetal nephrotoxicity (Stone and Whittington, 1990; Straus and co-workers, 1989). Frenkel and colleagues (1991) have shown that 200 or 400 mg given three times daily is well-tolerated in late pregnancy; it concentrates in amnionic fluid, but does not accumulate or cause adverse effects in the newborn.

Clinical Course During Pregnancy. The clinical course in pregnancy is well known for recurrent infections in young women with recently acquired genital herpes infection. Approximately 80 percent will have an average of two to four **symptomatic** recurrences during pregnancy (Brown, 1985; Harger, 1989; Vontver, 1982; and their colleagues). Concomitant cervical shedding is identified in about 15 percent of women with clinically evident vulvar recurrences.

Brown (1985) and Arvin (1986) and their coworkers found that about 10 percent of the recurrences in pregnancy will be **asymptomatic,** and these more frequently are from the perineum than the cervix. The incidence of positive cultures at any time during pregnancy or at delivery for nonpregnant women who had herpes is only 1 to 2 percent. Although clinical recurrences appear to be slightly more common in late pregnancy, asymptomatic cervical shedding of herpesvirus is unaffected by the duration of pregnancy. Additionally, "remote recurrences," that is, those on the buttocks, back, thigh, and anus have low rates of concomitant cervical virus shedding, and this allows consideration for vaginal delivery (Harger and colleagues, 1989; Wittek and co-workers, 1984).

Neonatal Disease. Infection is transmitted only rarely across the placenta or intact membranes. The fetus almost always becomes infected by virus shed from the cervix or lower genital tract. The virus then either invades the uterus following membrane rupture or contacts the fetus at delivery. The incidence of neonatal herpesvirus infection has increased, and Sullivan-Bolyai and associates (1983) reported an increase in King County, Washington, from 2.6 per 100,000 livebirths in 1969 to 12 per 100,000 in 1981.

Newborn infection takes on one of three forms: (1) disseminated, with involvement of major viscera (Fig. 59–4), (2) localized, with involvement confined to the central nervous system, eyes, skin or mucosa, or (3) asymptomatic. Nearly half of infected neonates are preterm and their risk of infection correlates with whether there is primary or recurrent maternal infection. Nahmias and colleagues (1971) reported a 50 percent risk

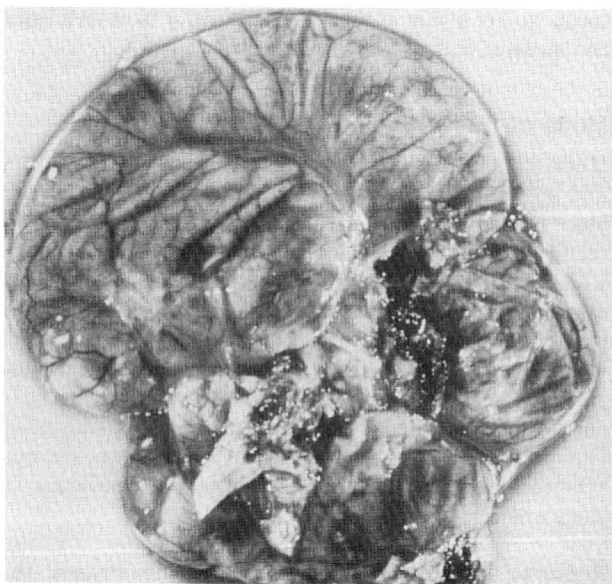

Fig. 59–4. Cross-section showing necrotic brain tissue in a newborn infant who died from disseminated herpesvirus infection.

of neonatal infection with primary maternal infection, but only 4 to 5 percent with recurrent infection. Prober and associates (1987) reported that none of 34 neonates exposed to recurrent viral shedding at delivery became infected. This is thought to be due to a smaller viral inoculum with recurrent infection and also to transplacentally acquired antibody, which decreases the incidence and severity of neonatal disease (Prober and colleagues, 1987; Yeager and Arvin, 1984).

Localized infection is usually associated with a good outcome. Even with treatment with acyclovir or vidarabine, disseminated neonatal infection is associated with a mortality rate of at least 60 percent (Whitley and colleagues, 1991a, 1991b). Importantly, serious ophthalmic and central nervous system damage has been identified in at least half of survivors. Because treatment of the neonate has been disappointing, considerable emphasis is placed on prevention of contact between fetus and virus during delivery.

Whereas the episodic nature of asymptomatic viral shedding is well appreciated, its predictability is of particular concern in pregnant women who have recurrent genital infections. The reported prevalence rates for isolation of genital tract herpesvirus vary considerably depending on the population studied, but equally important is whether women were included (or excluded) because of prior symptomatic infection. Prober and colleagues (1988) obtained specimens for culture from mothers and infants at the time of nearly 7000 deliveries without regard to the maternal history of genital herpes. Only 14 (0.2 percent) were positive for herpesvirus, and 12 of these women had recurrent infections. In a similar study, Brown and associates (1991) cultured nearly 16,000 women in early labor. Only 56 (0.35 percent) were positive, and one third of these had serological evidence for a recently acquired but subclinical first infection. Although one third of these infants developed neonatal infection, only one of 34 did in women with recurrent infection.

Effect on Pregnancy Outcome. Adverse pregnancy outcomes are most likely when the initial outbreak of genital herpes is during pregnancy. These risks are greatest when there is first-episode primary infection and no cross-reacting antibody to type 1 herpesvirus (Table 59–6). First-episode nonprimary infections are associated with milder symptoms and clinical findings that resolve quicker when compared with primary genital type 2 infection. Concomitant cervical infection is frequent with first-episode primary genital herpes and the viral inoculum tends to be high. After a primary infection during pregnancy, asymptomatic recurrences are more common than clinically detected recurrent infections (Brown and colleagues, 1985, 1987). Concomitant perineal and cervical recurrences are more common after either type of first-episode infection in pregnancy.

First-episode infection in early pregnancy is probably not associated with an increased rate of spontaneous abortion. Fagnant and Monif (1989) reviewed the literature and described 15 cases of congenital herpetic infection acquired during early pregnancy. Brown and colleagues (1989) found that late pregnancy primary infection results in an increased incidence of preterm labor.

Antepartum Management. Because of the severity of neonatal infection, cesarean delivery has been used widely in instances when genital herpetic lesions are suspected or a recent culture has been positive for virus. Although the unproven threat of asymptomatic viral shedding by women previously diagnosed as having genital herpes is not sufficient grounds for cesarean section, it is certainly prudent to choose cesarean delivery if there is *reasonable* chance that virus is being shed.

The premise that all neonatal infections can be avoided by carefully screening the obstetrical population is incorrect. A history consistent with a recurrent maternal genital infection is elicited in only one fourth of mothers of infected infants (Yeager and Arvin, 1984). Many of the remaining women have peripartum primary infection, undiagnosed recurrent infection, or a sexual partner with recurrent genital infection. Another source of neonatal infection is from oral lesions in the mother, family members, or even health personnel.

Several points should be emphasized with respect to women with a history of recurrent genital infection. The presence, absence, or frequency of recurrences does not predict asymptomatic shedding at delivery. Such shedding appears to be an entirely random event of short duration, usually less than 7 days (Wittek and associates, 1984). Indeed, according to some, there is more than a 95 percent chance of a negative culture 7 days after an episode of asymptomatic shedding during pregnancy.

In the past, there were many proposed protocols advocating the use of weekly genital cultures to detect asymptomatic shedding. Although 1 to 5 percent of randomly selected women have been shown to shed virus asymptomatically near term, cultures taken during labor rarely are positive (Hankins and colleagues, 1984). The Centers for Disease Control estimated that $1.8 million would be spent yearly in the United States to prevent each case of neonatal infection in women with recurrent herpes infections (Binkin and associates, 1984). Moreover, only 11 neonatal deaths and 3.7 cases of severe mental retardation would be averted, but 3 to 4 women would die from complications of cesarean sections performed because of positive viral cultures. Finally, it is estimated that only one fourth of women shedding virus at the time of delivery would be identified.

Arvin and colleagues (1986) provided data that serial genital cultures for herpesvirus are not predictive of the risk for neonatal infection. They studied 414 pregnant women with a history of recurrent genital herpes infections and found that in none of these women did antepartum cultures predict the 1.4 percent with positive cultures at delivery. Accordingly, the American College of Obstetricians and Gynecologists (1988), the Infectious Disease Society for Obstetrics and Gynecology (Gibbs and colleagues, 1988), as well as the Canadian Paediatric Society (1992), now recommend the following approach: (1) Cultures are taken to confirm the diagnosis when a pregnant woman has lesions suggestive of herpesvirus infection. If there are no visible lesions at the onset of labor, then vaginal delivery is acceptable. (2) Weekly surveillance cultures of women with a history of herpesvirus infection but without lesions are not necessary and vaginal delivery is acceptable. (3) Amniocentesis in an attempt to confirm fetal infection is not recommended. Thus, cesarean delivery is performed if primary or recurrent lesions are visualized near the time of labor or when the membranes are ruptured or if there are prodromal symptoms of a recurrence.

Ruptured Membranes. With ruptured membranes, the "4-hour rule" has commonly been applied: if genital herpes is diagnosed or strongly suspected, and the membranes have been ruptured less than 4 to 6 hours, cesarean delivery is performed; otherwise, vaginal delivery is allowed. With recurrent perineal or vulvar lesions, this plan is not always justified because only about 20 to 40 percent of these women have concomitant cervical (and thus membrane-contiguous) infection. In the absence of previous examination or instrumentation, there is no evidence that these external lesions cause ascending membrane and fetal infection. We disregard the duration of membrane rupture in formulating a plan of delivery for women with perineal lesions, and unless there are other contradictory factors, for example, gross immaturity, we deliver these women by cesarean section.

Care of the Neonate. An exposed infant of a mother known or suspected of having genital herpes should be isolated and cultures taken for herpes. Additionally, liver function and spinal fluid should be examined serially along with close infant observation for up to 2 weeks. It is considered unnecessary to separate baby and mother when the mother has herpetic lesions. Instead, she may be instructed to wash her hands carefully and avoid any contact between her lesions, her hands, and the baby. Breast feeding has been allowed under these conditions; however, this has been implicated in at least one case of disseminated neonatal infection. Some have recommended that parents and personnel with oral herpetic lesions be isolated from newborn infants, although according to the American College of Obstetricians and Gynecologists (1988), this is not necessary.

Acquired Immunodeficiency Syndrome (AIDS)

Acquired immunodeficiency syndrome was first described in 1981 when a cluster of patients was found to have defective cellular immunity and *Pneumocystis carinii* pneumonia. By 1992, the World Health Organization projected that 40 million persons would be infected worldwide by the year 2000. A report by the Harvard University Global AIDS Policy Coalition predicts the number to be 110 million.

The etiological agents of the immunodeficiency syndrome are **human immunodeficiency viruses,** HIV-1 and HIV-2, which are RNA retroviruses capable of inducing severe immunological dysfunction in T-4 helper lymphocytes. Most cases worldwide in 1992 are caused by HIV-1 infection and HIV-2 infection is endemic in West Africa (O'Brien and colleagues, 1992). Retroviruses have genomes that encode *reverse transcriptase,* which allows DNA to be transcribed from RNA. Thus, the virus can make DNA copies of its own genome in host cells. Transmission is similar to hepatitis B virus, and sexual intercourse, especially among male homosexuals, is the major mode of transmission. It also is transmitted by blood or blood-contaminated products, and infected mothers may infect their infants.

The Centers for Disease Control (1992b) estimates the prevalence of asymptomatic infection in the United States by late 1991 at 1 to 1.5 million persons. More than 200,000 cases of AIDS had been reported in the United States, and more than half have died. Among adult cases in the United States, 60 percent are in homosexual or bisexual men who do not use intravenous drugs, 20 percent are among heterosexual men and women who use intravenous drugs, 7 percent among homosexual or bisexual men who use intravenous drugs, and 1 percent are in hemophiliacs. About 10 percent of infected individuals are women, and more than half of those are related to use of intravenous drugs or heterosexual relationships with intravenous drug users.

Pathogenesis. The common denominator of AIDS is profound immunosuppression, principally of cell-mediated immunity, which gives rise to a variety of opportunistic infections and neoplasms. Thymus-derived lymphocytes—*T-lymphocytes*—defined phenotypically by the CD4 surface antigen, are the principal targets. The CD4 site serves as a receptor for the virus, which then is internalized and uses reverse transcriptase to transcribe its genomic RNA and DNA. Thus, viral DNA is integrated into the cellular DNA for the life of the cell, which is shortened by infection. After infection, over time the number of T cells drops insidiously and progressively, resulting eventually in profound immunosuppression. Monocyte-macrophages may also be infected, and microglial brain cell infection may cause neuropsychiatric abnormalities. HIV-infected persons also have increased incidence of neoplasms, notably Kaposi sarcoma, B-cell and non-Hodgkins lymphomas, and some carcinomas.

Clinical Manifestations. The exact incubation period from infection to clinical disease is unknown; however, it usually is 2 to 3 months. Figure 59–5 shows a schematic model of the natural history of HIV-1 infection. The stimuli that cause further progression from asymptomatic viremia to the immunodeficiency syndrome are presently unclear, but the mean time is estimated to be about 10 years; approximately 75 percent of patients with serological evidence for infection will develop some symptoms within 7 years (Fauci and Lane, 1991). Some have less severe manifestations characterized by immune dysfunction and generalized lymphadenopathy (CDC Group III). When infection is associated with symptoms of malaise, fatigue, weight loss, and fever, then AIDS is diagnosed. These may be further complicated by Kaposi sarcoma and multiple opportunistic infections, including oral thrush, herpes simplex, tuberculosis, cytomegalovirus, pneumocystis, toxoplasmosis, and others. Neurological disease is common, and about half of patients have central nervous system symptoms. The mortality rate of AIDS is extremely high, and 60 to 80 percent who develop the syndrome die within 2 years.

Serological Testing. **Enzyme-linked immunosorbent assays (ELISA)** are used to determine the presence of antibodies to HIV. Currently used tests have sensitivities and specificities of 99 percent when repeatedly positive. The Centers for Disease Control recommends that all positive tests be followed by additional testing of the same serum sample using a **Western blot test** that identifies antibodies to specific viral proteins. Although highly specific, this technique is less sensitive than immunoassay because more antibody is required for a positive result, and thus the Western blot test may

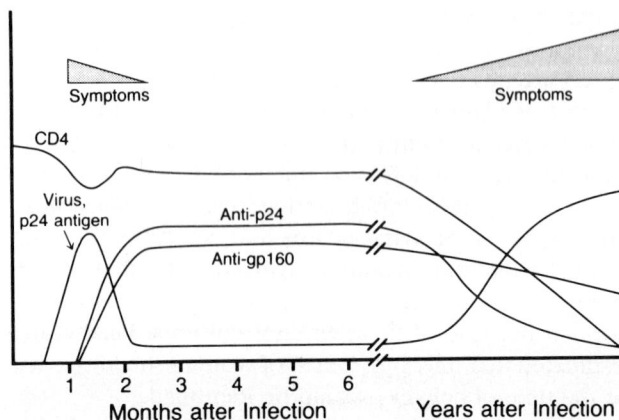

Fig. 59–5. Schematic model of the natural history of HIV-1 infection. (From Clark and colleagues, 1991, with permission.)

have false-negative results. Identification of the p24 core antigen indicates virus and not antibody. This test has many false-negative results in healthy patients. Some laboratories are capable of culturing live virus from infected cells. Work is in progress to develop a test based on the **polymerase chain reaction** which amplifies viral genes.

Screening. There is disagreement as to who should be screened, and more importantly, how positive results should be managed. Certainly it is reasonable to test all blood products, and the American Red Cross found immunodeficiency virus antibody in 0.22 percent of the first 100,000 units screened (American Medical Association, 1985). Thus, if there are nearly 40,000 positive tests from 20 million blood units processed annually, even assuming false-positive test results of 95 percent, only a relatively small number of units are discarded. Of greater concern are the donors with incubating virus who test seronegative. Ward and colleagues (1988) estimate that 1 of 40,000 units from donors screened as negative will be infective. In June, 1992, the Food and Drug Administration also mandated testing of all blood donors for HIV-2.

Opinions currently vary as to the advisability of routine prenatal HIV screening. The Institute of Medicine (1991) recommends universal but voluntary screening. The American College of Obstetricians and Gynecologists (1992b) recommends that screening be offered to all women, and encourages it if they are at risk. Table 59–7 gives risk factors for pregnant women or their sexual partner(s).

Maternal and Fetus-Infant Infection. There is insufficient experience to ascertain the risk of fetal infection from pregnant women with asymptomatic HIV infection, or those with clinical immunodeficiency syndromes. Of the more than 200,000 cases of AIDS reported through late 1991, over 3000 were in children (Centers for Disease Control, 1992b). Many of these were less than one year of age and nearly three fourths were born to mothers from groups with known risk

TABLE 59–7. RISK FACTORS FOR WOMEN OR THEIR SEXUAL PARTNER(S) FOR ACQUIRING HUMAN IMMUNODEFICIENCY VIRUS INFECTION

Illicit drug abuse—especially intravenous drug use
Current or previous multiple sexual partners; trading sex for drugs
Transfusion with blood products before adequate screening in 1985
Bisexual activity
Origin in HIV-endemic areas
Symptoms of HIV-related illnesses
History of or current sexually transmitted disease

From the American College of Obstetricians and Gynecologists (1992b), with permission.

factors associated with increased prevalence of HIV infection such as those listed in Table 59–7.

To determine maternal seroprevalence, Gwinn and colleagues (1991) tested nearly 2 million newborns for HIV-positivity from 38 states born in 1988 and 1989. Nationwide, they estimated that 1.5 women per 1000 were infected; for New York City it was 5.8 per 1000, and for the District of Columbia it was 5.5 per 1000. Inner-city populations are even higher, for example, Landesman and co-workers (1987) found a 2 percent seroprevalence rate for 602 cord blood specimens collected at Kings County Hospital in Brooklyn. Lindsay and associates (1991) showed that inner-city prenatal patients in Atlanta were more likely seropositive if they had not registered for prenatal care. Importantly, although in all of these studies women were from an inner-city minority population, only about one half were considered high risk by factors outlined in Table 59–7. Serosurveys like these underpin recommendations that serological testing and counseling be offered to all pregnant women.

The rate of perinatal transmission of HIV is uncertain, and studies are hampered by passive maternal antibody that persists for up to 18 months. An average of several studies is about 30 percent (American College of Obstetrics and Gynecologists, 1992a), but the European Collaborative Study (1991, 1992) found persistent seropositivity in only 14 percent of 721 children at 18 months. Risk factors included maternal p24 antigenemia and a CD4 count less than 700/μL. Vertical transmission was almost four times more common with delivery before 34 weeks. Perinatal transmission is either by transplacental infection or is contracted at birth (Ehrnst and colleagues, 1991). The viral antigen and nucleic acid has been identified in fetal and placental tissue in early pregnancies terminated by elective abortion (Lewis and co-workers, 1990). There is no doubt that postnatal HIV-1 mother-to-infant transmission occurs (Van de Perre and associates, 1991). Many women who are delivered of infants who subsequently develop AIDS have been asymptomatic during pregnancy. Gloeb and colleagues (1988) reported that 35 percent of 50 seropositive women had preterm labor and delivery. Conversely, Minkoff and co-workers (1990a) found minimal obstetrical impact in seropositive women. According to the American College of Obstetricians and Gynecologists (1992b), there is no evidence that preterm birth, low-birthweight, or other pregnancy complications are increased in asymptomatic seropositive women.

The possibility exists that during pregnancy clinical illness is more likely to develop, presumably because of suppressed cell-mediated immunity. Biggar and associates (1989) showed accelerated loss of CD4 cells during pregnancy, implying an increased risk of symptomatic infection. In the report by Scott and colleagues (1985), of 16 asymptomatic infected mothers, one third had developed AIDS and another half AIDS-related complex within 30 months of delivery. Similarly, Minkoff and co-workers (1987) observed that almost half of women had one of these syndromes by 24 months following delivery. Progression of asymptomatic infection to clinical immunodeficiency syndromes is usually at a much slower rate in nonpregnant homosexuals and drug abusers. However, there have been no large controlled studies on the natural history of disease progression or CD4 lymphocyte depletion in women. Those who transmit the virus perinatally may be at unique risk for disease progression. At least until fetal and maternal risks can be defined better, it is reasonable to advise that pregnancy be avoided in seropositive women.

Prevention of Transmission. For the pregnant woman with symptomatic infection, or who is seropositive but asymptomatic, the same precautions should be followed as for nonpregnant individuals with these findings. Precautions for antepartum, peripartum, and pediatric care of infected mothers and infants are similar to those for hepatitis B, with avoidance of exposure to blood and body fluids. **Unfortunately, if heightened awareness of these precautions is reserved for women known to be seropositive, a large number of women with incubating infection or who are asymptomatic but undiagnosed will pose a larger threat to medical personnel.**

Because transplacental viral transfer is thought to be the major mode of vertical transmission, at the present time there is no reason to think that cesarean delivery will decrease the chance of peripartum transmission (American College of Obstetricians and Gynecologists, 1992b). Preliminary data from the European Collaborative Study (1992), however, indicate perhaps some protective effect of delivery by cesarean section, that is, there is evidence for peripartum transmission. Similarly, the risks of transmission attributable to fetal scalp monitoring, episiotomy, or operative vaginal delivery currently are uncertain. Using viral culture or polymerase chain reaction, Krivine and co-workers (1992) provided further evidence that infection occurs near delivery. The effects of maternal antiviral therapy on the fetus are conjectural at this time. Fortunato and associates (1989) found active transfer of zidovudine in the perfused cotyledon system.

The Centers for Disease Control (1987) emphasizes that because medical history and examination cannot identify reliably all patients infected with immunodeficiency virus or other bloodborne pathogens, blood and body-fluid precautions should be used consistently in all patients. These precautions are: (1) All health-care workers who participate in invasive procedures, including surgical procedures or obstetrical deliveries, must use appropriate barrier precautions to prevent skin and mucous-membrane contact with blood and other body fluids of all patients. Gloves, surgical masks, and protective eyewear (goggles) must be worn for all invasive procedures

that commonly result in the generation of droplets, splashing of blood or other body fluids, or the generation of bone chips. Fluid-resistant gowns or aprons that provide an effective barrier should be worn during invasive procedures that are likely to result in the splashing of blood or other body fluids. Those who perform or assist in vaginal or cesarean deliveries should wear gloves and gowns when handling the placenta or the infant until blood and amnionic fluid have been removed from the infant's skin, and should wear gloves during care of the cord. Mouth-suction devices for clearing the airway should be avoided. (2) If a glove is torn or there is a needlestick or other injury, the glove should be removed and a new glove used as promptly as patient safety permits. The needle or instrument involved in the incident also should be removed from the sterile field.

For health-care workers exposed significantly to contaminated fluids, for example, a needle-stick injury, counseling regarding zidovudine prophylaxis should be given (Centers for Disease Control, 1990a).

Management. In many of the earliest treatment studies, pregnant women were excluded. To ascertain the delicate balance between maternal health and fetal safety, the National Institute of Health has declared a high priority to perform clinical trials to treat pregnant women and decrease mother-to-fetus transmission (Stratton and colleagues, 1992).

Counseling is mandatory for the HIV-positive woman early in pregnancy, if possible. If she chooses to continue pregnancy, ongoing counseling for psychological support is important. Testing for other sexually transmitted diseases, as well as tuberculosis, is done. Vaccination is given for hepatitis B, influenza, and perhaps pneumococcal infection.

The American College of Obstetricians and Gynecologists (1992b) recommends CD4 cell count determinations during each trimester. If those are less than $500/\mu L$, consideration is given to zidovudine therapy. The benefits of zidovudine therapy for women with CD4 counts between 200 and $500/\mu L$ is unclear at this time (Sperling and colleagues, 1992a). However, if this count is below $200/\mu L$, antiviral therapy along with primary prophylaxis for *P. carinii* pneumonia is recommended with either sulfamethoxazole–trimethoprim or aerosolized pentamidine. Preliminary data from the AIDS Clinical Trials Group indicate that zidovudine is well tolerated in pregnancy, and there were no associated teratogenic effects when the drug was given in early pregnancy (Sperling and colleagues, 1992b). Pneumocystis pneumonia is treated with oral or intravenous sulfamethoxazole–trimethoprim or pentamidine (see Chap. 49, p. 1108). Other symptomatic opportunistic infections include toxoplasmosis, herpesvirus infections, and candidiasis.

In nonpregnant patients, zidovudine has been shown to slow the progression of AIDS in HIV-positive patients whose CD4 counts have dropped to below 500/μL. Sperling and associates (1992a) reviewed current management and treatment options for HIV-infected women.

Human Papillomavirus

Several types of human papillomaviruses (HPV) cause mucocutaneous warts. **Condylomata acuminata** are also called genital warts and usually are caused by types 6 and 11. The virus also can cause **laryngeal papillomatosis** in children, and evidence is consistent that types 6 and 11 in some cases may be transmitted by aspiration of infected material at delivery. Viral types 16, 18, 31, 33, and 35 have been implicated in the cause of **cervical intraepithelial neoplasia** and possibly invasive cancer, as well as other female genital cancers (see Chap. 57, p. 1273). Preliminary data from Taiwan indicate that the virus may be transmitted transplacentally (Tseng and colleagues, 1992).

Condylomata Acuminata. For unknown reasons, genital warts frequently increase in number and size during pregnancy, sometimes filling the vagina or covering the perineum making it difficult to perform vaginal delivery or episiotomy (Fig. 59–6). Even in women without grossly visible lesions, Snyder and co-workers (1990) but not Goldaber and associates (in press), found an association with papillomavirus infection and episiotomy breakdown. Certainly, the mucorrhea throughout pregnancy offers ideal moist conditions for their growth. Accelerated viral replication with advancing pregnancy has been hypothesized to explain the growth of perineal lesions, progression of some to cervical neoplasm, and increased detection of viral DNA from the cervix in some studies of pregnant women (Gary and colleagues, 1985; Rando and co-workers, 1989). Not all investigators have found such an association with pregnancy (Kemp and associates, 1992). Because papillomavirus infection can be subclinical and multifocal, most women with vulvar lesions also have cervical infection, and vice versa (Spitzer and colleagues, 1989). Vulvar lesions often improve rapidly or disappear postpartum, possibly related to loss of either vascularity, excessive moisture, or the alleged immunosuppression of pregnancy.

Treatment. Treatment may be very unsatisfactory, but it is usual for these lesions to clear rapidly following delivery. During pregnancy, washing of the external genitalia, plus cleansing of the vagina by gentle douching (see Chap. 9, p. 263), followed by thorough drying of the external genitalia, performed at least once daily, may inhibit proliferation of the warts as well as minimize discomfort.

Because lesions commonly regress after delivery, it is not always necessary to try to eradicate them during

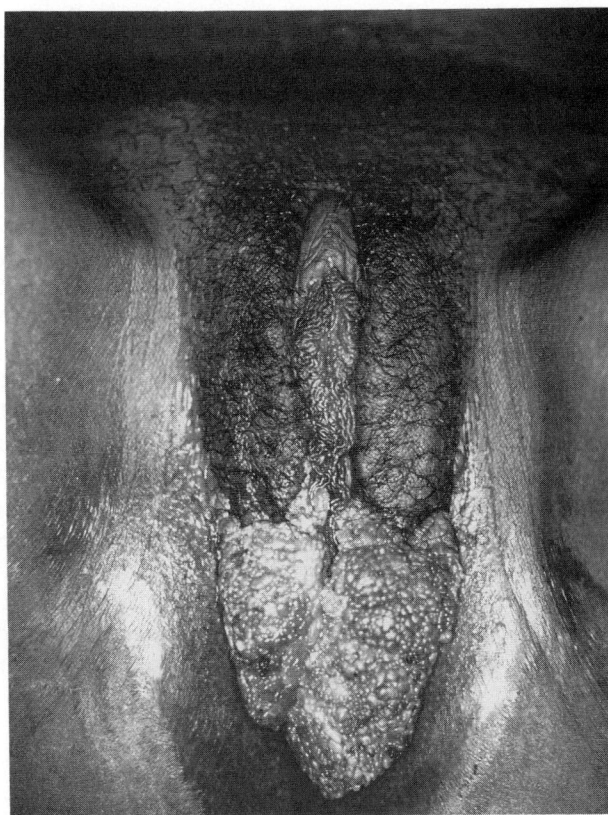

Fig. 59–6. Extensive vulvar condylomata acuminata in a woman near term. (From Wendel and Cunningham, 1991.)

pregnancy. If they produce discomfort, then they are treated. Therapy is directed toward minimizing toxicity to the mother and fetus and debulking the genital warts in the late second or third trimester so that recurrence is less likely prior to delivery. **Trichloroacetic acid,** 50 or 80 percent, both in 70 percent ethanol, applied topically three times weekly or once a week, respectively, is the least expensive mode of therapy (Ferenczy, 1989). Cryotherapy and laser ablation of visible lesions are preferred modes of therapy in pregnancy (Bergman and colleagues, 1984; Ferenczy, 1984). Schwartz and associates (1988) reported good results in 31 of 32 women treated with combination laser and 85 percent trichloracetic acid therapy. Unfortunately, others have reported failures in about one third of women treated in the first and early second trimester. **Podophyllin resin, 5-fluorouracil cream,** and **interferon** therapy should not be used in pregnancy due to concerns about maternal and fetal toxicity.

Occasionally, condylomata acuminata attain enormous size as shown in Figure 59–6, and these may even necessitate cesarean section. If the woman is seen several weeks before delivery, the large lesions sometimes can be removed by excision, electrocautery, cryosurgery, or laser ablation. Matsunaga and colleagues (1987) reported successful results in 51 women with rather extensive cervical or labial lesions. Enthusiasm has been expressed for use of the carbon-dioxide laser during pregnancy to remove large lesions under anesthesia (Ferenczy, 1984).

Neonatal Infection. An indeterminate, but probably small number of infants and children born to women with genital papillomavirus lesions will become infected and develop **laryngeal papillomatosis.** In one study, over 44,000 children were followed for 7 years and there were no cases of laryngeal papillomatosis identified (Shah and colleagues, 1986). These papillomas are usually found on the true vocal cords and HPV-6 or 11 were identified in 92 percent of 57 cases (Abramson and colleagues, 1987). They are persistent, recurrent, and disfiguring. The question has been posed that cesarean section might avoid infection of the fetus-infant, but this is not recommended currently (Ferenczy, 1989; Hallden and Majmudar, 1986). In at least one case, elective repeat cesarean section was done at term; however, the child developed extensive respiratory papillomatosis at 7 months (Shah and associates, 1986).

Chancroid

Hemophilus ducreyi can cause painful non-indurated genital ulcers, or soft chancre, at times accompanied by painful inguinal lymphadenopathy. Chancroid is common in some developing countries. Although it had become rare in the United States, in 1987 its incidence was increased 10-fold over the previous 10 years and drug use and sex-for-drugs were shown to be important risk factors for infection (Schmid and co-workers, 1987). Diagnosis should be confirmed by culture obtained from the ulcers or in aspirates from the enlarged nodes. Recommended treatment is erythromycin, 500 mg orally four times daily for 7 days or ceftriaxone, 250 mg in a single intramuscular dose (Centers for Disease Control, 1989b). Trimethoprim 160 mg–sulfamethoxazole 800 mg orally twice a day for 7 days is an alternative regimen.

Trichomonas Infections

Trichomonas vaginalis was identified in 13 percent of nearly 14,000 women cultured at midpregnancy by the Vaginal Infections and Prematurity Study Group (Cotch and colleagues, 1991). Symptomatic infection is much less common and vaginitis is characterized by symptoms of a yellow discharge, abnormal odor, and vulvar pruritus. On examination, these women usually have a purulent vaginal discharge, vulvovaginal erythema, and *colpitis macularis* or "strawberry cervix."

Trichomonads are demonstrated readily in a wet mount of vaginal secretions as flagellated, ovoid, motile organisms that are somewhat larger than leukocytes.

The sensitivity of this technique depends on the concentration of organisms, the degree of dilution, and the experience of the examiner, but is generally considered to be 65 to 80 percent. Trichomonads are identified most accurately by culture using Diamond medium; however, direct immunofluorescent monoclonal antibody staining is a sensitive and specific alternative (Krieger and co-workers, 1988).

According to their review, Gibbs and colleagues (1992) concluded that the association of preterm delivery with antepartum colonization with *T. vaginalis* is controversial. Minkoff and associates (1984) found that trichomonas infestation was associated with an increased incidence of prematurely ruptured membranes near term, but not preterm prematurely ruptured membranes, nor preterm labor and delivery. The Vaginal Infections and Prematurity Study Group (Martin, 1990) used multivariate analysis and reported significant associations between trichomoniasis and preterm prematurely ruptured membranes, preterm delivery, and low-birthweight infants. Further prospective investigation is warranted before adopting widespread screening and treatment to eradicate this organism in hope of decreasing its possible deleterious effects on pregnancy outcome.

Treatment. Metronidazole, the only trichomonacidal drug available in the United States, is quite effective in eradicating *T. vaginalis.* Oral administration is the preferred route of administration. Lossick (1990) reviewed extensively the clinical experiences with metronidazole and found that 250 mg given 3 times daily for 7 days, and 2 g as a single dose, had median cure rates of 92 and 96 percent, respectively. The drug uniformly is successful in most treatment regimens; an exception is a single 1-g dose (Lossick, 1990). Unfortunately, there are few data regarding efficacy of any regimen in pregnancy.

Men apparently have transient infection with *T. vaginalis.* Although the need for concomitant treatment is uncertain, most investigators have found higher relapse rates in women whose partners were not treated. Lossick (1990) recommends that steady sex partners be treated, and the Centers for Disease Control (1989b) recommends that all partners be treated.

Fetal Effects of Therapy. Metronidazole crosses the placenta and enters the fetal circulation. The drug is carcinogenic in rodents and mutagenic in bacteria, and thus there is concern for teratogenicity if metronidazole is taken during early pregnancy. The bulk of data, discussed in Chapter 42 (p. 964), suggests that the drug is safe, even when given early in pregnancy. Nevertheless, the Centers for Disease Control (1989b) recommends treatment only if there are severe symptoms after the first trimester. Lossick (1990) cautions against the use of metronidazole at any stage in pregnancy, and recommends vaginally applied clotrimazole as palliative therapy.

Other Sexually Transmitted Diseases

There are many more infections and infestations that can be acquired as the consequence of sexual intercourse. Among others, these include hepatitis B and C (see Chap. 51, p. 1157), *candida vulvovaginitis* (see Chap. 9, p. 268), *scabies,* and *pediculosis pubis.* Sexual partners at risk of fecal–oral transmission may acquire any of a number of enteric infections.

References

Abramson AL, Steinberg BM, Winkler B: Laryngeal papillomatosis: Clinical histopathologic and molecular studies. Laryngoscope 87:678, 1987

Alger LS, Lovchik JC, Hebel JR, Blackmon LR, Crenshaw MC: The association of *Chlamydia trachomatis, Neisseria gonorrhoeae*, and group B streptococci with preterm rupture of the membranes and pregnancy outcome. Am J Obstet Gynecol 159:397, 1988

Al-Suleiman SA, Grimes EM, Jonas HS: Disseminated gonococcal infections. Obstet Gynecol 61:48, 1983

American College of Obstetricians and Gynecologists: Guidelines for Perinatal Care, 3rd ed. Washington DC, 1992a

American College of Obstetricians and Gynecologists: Human immunodeficiency virus infections. Technical bulletin no. 169, June 1992b

American College of Obstetricians and Gynecologists: Perinatal herpes simplex virus infections. Technical bulletin no. 122, November 1988

American Medical Association Council on Scientific Affairs: Status report on the acquired immunodeficiency syndrome: Human T-cell lymphotrophic virus III testing. JAMA 254:1342, 1985

Andrews EB, Yankaskas BC, Cardero JF, Schaeffer X, Hampp S, Acyclovir in Pregnancy Registry Advisory Committee: Acyclovir in pregnancy registry: Six years' experience. Obstet Gynecol 76:7, 1992

Arvin AM, Hensleigh PA, Prober CG, Au DS, Yasukawa LL, Wittek AE, Palumbo PE, Paryani SG, Yeager AS: Failure of antepartum maternal cultures to predict the infant's risk of exposure to herpes simplex virus at delivery. N Engl J Med 315:796, 1986

Baker DA, Gonik B, Milch PO, Berkowitz A, Lipson S, Verma U: Clinical evaluation of a new herpes simplex virus ELISA: A rapid diagnostic test for herpes simplex virus. Obstet Gynecol 73:322, 1989

Barton JR, Thorpe EM Jr, Shaver DC, Hager WD, Sibai BM: Nonimmune hydrops fetalis associated with maternal infection with syphilis. Am J Obstet Gynecol 167:56, 1992

Bataskov KL, Hariharan S, Horowitz MD, Neibart RM, Cox MM: Gonococcal endocarditis complicating pregnancy: A case report and literature review. Obstet Gynecol 78:494, 1991

Bergman A, Bhatia NN, Broen EM: Cryotherapy for treatment of genital condyloma during pregnancy. J Reprod Med 29:432, 1984

Berman SM, Harrison HR, Boyce WT, Haffner WJJ, Lewis M, Arthur JB: Low birth weight, prematurity, and postpartum endometritis. JAMA 257:1189, 1987

Biggar RJ, Pahwa S, Minkoff H, Mendes H, Willoughby A, Landesman S, Goedert JJ: Immunosuppression in pregnant women infected with human immunodeficiency virus. Am J Obstet Gynecol 161:1239, 1989

Binkin NJ, Koplan JP, Cates W: Preventing neonatal herpes: The value of weekly viral cultures in pregnant women with recurrent genital herpes. JAMA 251:2816, 1984

Blanco JD, Diaz KC, Lipscomb KA, Bruun D, Gibbs RS: *Chlamydia trachomatis* isolation in patients with endometritis after cesarean section. Am J Obstet Gynecol 152:278, 1985

Brown ZA, Baker DA: Acyclovir therapy during pregnancy. Obstet Gynecol 73:526, 1989

Brown ZA, Benedetti J, Ashley R, Burchett S, Selke S, Berry S, Vontver LA, Corey L: Neonatal herpes simplex virus infection in relation to asymptomatic maternal infection at the time of labor. N Engl J Med 324:1247, 1991

Brown ZA, Vontver LA, Benedetti J, Critchlow CW, Hickok DE, Sells CJ, Berry S, Corey L: Genital herpes in pregnancy: Risk factors associated with recurrences and asymptomatic shedding. Am J Obstet Gynecol 153:24, 1985

Brown ZA, Vontver LA, Benedetti J, Critchlow CW, Sells CJ, Berry S, Corey L: Effects on infants of a first episode of genital herpes during pregnancy. N Engl J Med 317:1246, 1987

Brunham RC, Paavonen J, Stevens CE, Kiviat N, Kuo C-C, Critchlow CW, Holmes KK: Mucopurulent cervicitis—the ignored counterpart in women of urethritis in men. N Engl J Med 311:1, 1984

Burkman RT, Tonascia JA, Atienza MF, King TM: Untreated endocervical gonorrhea and endometritis following elective abortion. Am J Obstet Gynecol 126:648, 1976

Canadian Paediatric Society, Infectious Diseases and Immunization Committee: Toward the rational management of herpes infection in pregnant women and their newborn infants. Can Med Assoc J 146:1557, 1992

Cavenee MR, Farris JR, Spalding TR, Barnes DL, Castaneda YS, Wendel GD: Treatment of gonorrhea in pregnancy. Obstet Gynecol 83:33, 1993

Centers for Disease Control: *Chlamydia trachomatis* infections. Policy guidelines for prevention and control. MMWR 34:53, 1985

Centers for Disease Control: Congenital syphilis—New York City, 1986–1988. MMWR 38:826, 1989a

Centers for Disease Control: Guidelines for the prevention and control of congenital syphilis. MMWR 37:1, 1988

Centers for Disease Control: Plasmid-mediated antimicrobial resistance in *Neisseria gonorrhoeae*—United States, 1988 and 1989. MMWR 39:284, 1990b

Centers for Disease Control: Public health service statement on management of occupational exposure to human immunodeficiency virus, including considerations regarding zidovudine postexposure use. MMWR 39:1, 1990a

Centers for Disease Control: Recommendations for prevention of HIV transmission in health-care settings. MMWR 36:1s, 1987

Centers for Disease Control: Regional and temporal trends in the surveillance of syphilis, United States, 1986–1990. MMWR 40:29, 1992a

Centers for Disease Control: The second 100,000 cases of acquired immunodeficiency syndrome—United States, June 1981–December 1991. MMWR 41:28, 1992b

Centers for Disease Control: 1989 sexually transmitted diseases treatment guidelines. MMWR 38:1, 1989b

Christmas JT, Wendel GD, Bawdon RE, Farris R, Cartwright G, Little BB: Concomitant infection with *Neisseria gonorrhoeae* and *Chlamydia trachomatis* in pregnancy. Obstet Gynecol 74:295, 1989

Clark SJ, Saag MS, Decker WD, Campbell-Hill S, Roberson JL, Veldkamp PJ, Kappes JC, Hahn BH, Shaw GM: High titers of cytopathic virus in plasma of patients with symptomatic primary HIV-1 infection. N Engl J Med 324:954, 1991

Cohen I, Veille J-C, Calkins BM: Improved pregnancy outcome following successful treatment of chlamydial infection. JAMA 263:3160, 1990

Corman LC, Levison ME, Knight R, Carrington ER, Kaye D: The high frequency of pharyngeal gonococcal infection in a prenatal clinic population. JAMA 230:568, 1974

Cotch MF, Pastorek JG II, Nugent RP, Yerg DE, Martin DH, Eschenbach EA, for the Vaginal Infections and Prematurity Study Group: Demographic and behavioral predictors of *Trichomonas vaginalis* infection among pregnant women. Obstet Gynecol 78:1087, 1991

Crombleholme WR, Schachter J, Grossman M, Landers DV, Sweet RL: Amoxicillin therapy for *Chlamydia trachomatis* in pregnancy. Obstet Gynecol 75:752, 1990

Dorfman DH, Glaser JH: Congenital syphilis presenting in infants after the newborn period. N Engl J Med 323:1299, 1990

Edwards L, Barrada MI, Hamann AA, Hakanson EY: Gonorrhea in pregnancy. Am J Obstet Gynecol 132:637, 1978

Ehrnst A, Lindgren S, Dictor M, Johansson B, Sönnerborg, Czajkowski J, Sundin G, Bohlin AB: HIV in pregnant women and their offspring: Evidence for late transmission. Lancet 338:203, 1991

Elliott B, Brunham RC, Laga M, Piot P, Ndinya-Achola JO, Maitha G, Cheang M, Plummer FA: Maternal gonococcal infection as a preventable risk factor for low birth weight. J Infect Dis 161:531, 1990

European Collaborative Study: Risk factors for mother-to-child transmission of HIV-1. Lancet 339:1007, 1992

Fagnant RJ, Monif GRG: How rare is congenital herpes simplex? A literature review. J Reprod Med 34:417, 1989

Fauci AS, Lane HC: The acquired immunodeficiency syndrome (AIDS). In Wilson JD, Braunwald E, Isselbacher KJ, Petersdorf RG, Martin JB, Fauci AS, Root RK (eds): Harrison's Principles of Internal Medicine, 12th ed. New York, McGraw-Hill, 1991, p 1402

Ferenczy A: HPV-associated lesions in pregnancy and their clinical complications. Clin Obstet Gynecol 32:191, 1989

Ferenczy A: Treating genital condyloma during pregnancy with the carbon dioxide laser. Am J Obstet Gynecol 148:9, 1984

Fiumara NJ: Letters to the editor. Sex Transm Dis 11:49, 1984

Fortunato SJ, Bawdon RE, Swan KF, Sobhi S: Transfer of azidothymidine (AZT) across the in vitro perfused human placenta. Abstract presented at the 36th annual meeting of the Society for Gynecological Investigation, San Diego, March 1989

Frenkel LM, Brown ZA, Bryson YJ, Corey L, Unadkat JD, Hensleigh PA, Arvin AM, Prober CG, Connor JR: Pharmacokinetics of acyclovir in the term human pregnancy and neonate. Am J Obstet Gynecol 164:569, 1991

Frieden FJ, Ordorica SA, Goodgold AL, Hoskins IA, Silverman F,

Young BK: Successful pregnancy with isolated herpes simplex virus encephalitis: Case report and review of the literature. Obstet Gynecol 75:511, 1990

Gary R, Jones R: Relationship between cervical condylomata, pregnancy and subclinical papillomavirus infection. J Reprod Med 30:393, 1985

Gibbs RS, Amstey MS, Sweet RL, Mead PB, Sever JL: Management of genital herpes infection in pregnancy. Obstet Gynecol 71:779, 1988

Gibbs RS, Mead PB: Preventing neonatal herpes—current strategies. N Engl J Med 326:946 1992

Gibbs RS, Romero R, Hillier SL, Eschenbach DA, Sweet RL: A review of premature birth and subclinical infection. Am J Obstet Gynecol 166:1515, 1992

Gibbs RS, Schachter J: Chlamydial serology in patients with intra-amniotic infection and controls. Sex Transm Dis 14:213, 1987

Gloeb DJ, O'Sullivan MJ, Efantis J: Human immunodeficiency virus infection in women. Am J Obstet Gynecol 159:756, 1988

Goldaber KG, Wendel PJ, McIntire DD, Wendel GD Jr: Postpartum perineal morbidity after fourth degree perineal repair. Am J Obstet Gynecol (in press)

Gravett MG, Nelson HP, DeRouen T, Critchlow C, Eschenbach DA, Holmes KK: Independent associations of bacterial vaginosis and *Chlamydia trachomatis* infection with adverse pregnancy outcome. JAMA 256:1899, 1986

Gwinn M, Pappaioanou M, George JR, Hannon WH, Wasser SC, Redus MA, Hoff R, Grady GF, Willoughby A, Novello AC, Petersen LR, Dondero TJ, Curran JW: Prevalence of HIV infection in childbearing women in the United States: Surveillance using newborn blood samples. JAMA 265:1704, 1991

Hallden C, Majmudar B: The relationship between juvenile laryngeal papillomatosis and maternal *Condylomata acuminata*. J Reprod Med 31:804, 1986

Hammerschlag MR, Cummings C, Roblin PM, Williams TH, Delke I: Efficacy of neonatal ocular prophylaxis for the prevention of chlamydial and gonococcal conjunctivitis. N Engl J Med 320:769, 1989

Hankins GVD, Cunningham FG, Luby JP, Butler SL, Stroud J, Roark M: Asymptomatic genital excretion of herpes simplex virus during early labor. Am J Obstet Gynecol 150:100, 1984

Hardy DA, Arvin AM, Yasukawa LL, Bronzan RN, Lewinsohn DM, Hensleigh PA, Prober CG: Use of polymerase chain reaction for successful identification of asymptomatic genital infection with herpes simplex virus in pregnant women at delivery. J Infect Dis 162:1031, 1990

Harger JH, Amortegui AJ, Meyer MP, Pazin GJ: Characteristics of recurrent genital herpes simplex infections in pregnant women. Obstet Gynecol 73:367, 1989

Hart G: Syphilis tests in diagnostic and therapeutic decision making. Ann Intern Med 104:368, 1986

Hill LM, Maloney JB: An unusual constellation of sonographic findings associated with congenital syphilis. Obstet Gynecol 78:895, 1991

Holmes KK, Counts GW, Beaty HN: Disseminated gonococcal infection. Ann Int Med 74:979, 1971

Holmes KK, Lukhart SA: Syphilis. In Wilson JD, Braunwald E, Isselbacher KJ, Petersdorf RG, Martin JB, Fauci AS, Root RK (eds): Harrison's Principles of Internal Medicine, 12th ed. New York, McGraw-Hill, 1991, p 1402

Hook EW, Roddy RE, Hansfield HH: Ceftriaxone therapy for incubating and early syphilis. J Infect Dis 158:881, 1988

Hoyme UB, Kiviat N, Eschenbach DA: The microbiology and treatment of late postpartum endometritis. Obstet Gynecol 68:226, 1986

Institute of Medicine, Committee on Prenatal and Newborn Screening for HIV Infection: HIV screening of pregnant women and newborns. Washington, DC, National Academy Press, 1991

Johnson RB: The role of azalide antibiotics in the treatment of chlamydia. Am J Obstet Gynecol 164:1794, 1991

Johnson RE, Nahmias AJ, Magder LS, Lee FK, Brooks CA, Snowden CB: A seroepidemiologic surgery of the prevalence of herpes simplex virus type 2 infection in the United States. N Engl J Med 321:7, 1989

Kemp EA, Hakenewerth AM, Laurent SL, Gravitt PE, Stoerker J: Human papillomavirus prevalence in pregnancy. Obstet Gynecol 79:649, 1992

Klein VR, Cox SM, Mitchell MD, Wendel GD: The Jarisch-Herxheimer reaction complicating syphilotherapy in pregnancy. Obstet Gynecol 75:375, 1990

Krieger JN, Tam MR, Stevens CE, Nielsen IO, Hale J, Kiviat NB, Holmes KK: Diagnosis of trichomoniasis. JAMA 259:1223, 1988

Krivine A, Firtion G, Cao L, Francoual C, Henrion R, Lebon P: HIV replication during the first weeks of life. Lancet 339:1187, 1992

Kulhanjian JA, Soroush V, Au DS, Bronzan RN, Yasukawa LL, Weylman LE, Arvin AM, Prober CG: Identification of women at unsuspected risk of primary infection with herpes simplex virus type 2 during pregnancy. N Engl J Med 326:916, 1992

Laga M, Plummer FA, Piot P, Datta P, Namaara W, Ndinya-Achola JO, Nzanze H, Maitha G, Ronald AR, Pamba HO, Brunham RC: Prophylaxis of gonococcal and chlamydial ophthalmia neonatorum: A comparison of silver nitrate and tetracycline. N Engl J Med 318:653, 1988

Landesman S, Minkoff H, Holman S, McCalla S, Sijin O: Serosurgery of human immunodeficiency virus infection in parturients: Applications for human immunodeficiency virus testing programs of pregnant women. JAMA 258:2701, 1987

Lewis SH, Reynolds-Kohler C, Fox HE, Nelson JA: HIV-1 in trophoblastic and villous Hofbauer cells, and haematological precursors in eight-week fetuses. Lancet 335:565, 1990

Lindsay MK, Feng TI, Peterson HB, Slade BA, Willis S, Klein L: Routine human immunodeficiency virus infection screening in unregistered and registered inner-city parturients. Obstet Gynecol 77:599, 1991

Lossick JG: Treatment of sexually transmitted vaginosis/vaginitis. Rev Infect Dis 12:S665, 1990

Lucas MJ, Theriot SK, Wendel GD: Doppler systolic–diastolic ratios in pregnancies complicated by syphilis. Obstet Gynecol 77:217, 1991

Lukehart SA, Hook EW, Baker-Zander SA, Collier AC, Critchlow CW, Hansfield HH: Invasion of the central nervous system by *Treponema pallidum*: Implications of diagnosis and treatment. Ann Inter Med 109:855, 1988

Martin DH, Koutsky L, Eschenbach DA, Daling JR, Alexander ER, Benedetti JK, Holmes KK: Prematurity and perinatal mortality in pregnancies complicated by maternal *Chlamydia trachomatis* infections. JAMA 247:1585, 1982

Martin DH, Vaginal Infections and Prematurity Study Group: Erythromycin treatment of *Chlamydia trachomatis* infections during pregnancy. Abstract 683, presented at 30th Interscience Conference on Antimicrobial Agents and Chemotherapy. Atlanta, October 1990

Martius J, Krohn MA, Hillier SL, Stamm WE, Holmes KK, Eschenbach DA: Relationships of vaginal *Lactobacillus* species, cervical *Chlamydia trachomatis*, and bacterial vaginosis to preterm birth. Obstet Gynecol 71:89, 1988

Matsunaga J, Bergman A, Bhatia NN: Genital condylomata acuminata in pregnancy: Effectiveness, safety and pregnancy outcome following cryotherapy. Br J Obstet Gynaecol 94:168, 1987

Maxwell GL, Watson WJ: Preterm premature rupture of membranes: Results of expectant management in patients with cervical cultures positive for group B streptococcus or *Neisseria gonorrhoeae*. Am J Obstet Gynecol 166:945, 1992

McGregor JA, French JI: *Chlamydia trachomatis* infection during pregnancy. Am J Obstet Gynecol 164:1782, 1991

McNeely GS, Ryan GM, Baselski V: Treatment of chlamydial infections of the cervix during pregnancy. Sex Transm Dis 16:60, 1989

Minkoff H, Grunebaum AN, Schwarz RH, Feldman J, Cummings M, Crombleholme W, Clark L, Pringle G, McCormack WM: Risk factor for prematurity and premature rupture of membranes: A prospective study of the vaginal flora in pregnancy. Am J Obstet Gynecol 150:965, 1984

Minkoff HL, Henderson C, Mendez H, Gail MH, Holman S, Willoughby A, Goedett JJ, Rubinstein A, Stratton P, Walsh JH, Landesman SH: Pregnancy outcomes among mothers infected with human immunodeficiency virus and uninfected control subjects. Am J Obstet Gynecol 163:1598, 1990a

Minkoff HL, McCalla S, Delke I, Stevens R, Salwen M, Feldman J: The relationship of cocaine use to syphilis and human immunodeficiency virus infections among inner city parturient women. Am J Obstet Gynecol 163:521, 1990b

Minkoff H, Nanda D, Menez R, Fikrig S: Pregnancies resulting in infants with acquired immunodeficiency syndrome or AIDS-related complex: Follow-up of mothers, children, and subsequently born siblings. Obstet Gynecol 69:288, 1987

Moran JS, Zenilman JM: Therapy for gonococcal infections: Options in 1989. Rev Infect Dis 12:S633, 1990

Moscicki B, Shafer MA, Millstein SG, Irvin CE, Schachter J: The use and limitations of endocervical Gram stains and mucopurulent cervicitis as predictors for *Chlamydia trachomatis* in female adolescents. Am J Obstet Gynecol 157:65, 1987

Nahmias AJ, Josey WE, Naib ZM, Freeman MG, Fernandez RJ, Wheeler JH: Perinatal risk associated with maternal genital herpes simplex virus infection. Am J Obstet Gynecol 110:825, 1971

National Institutes of Health Conference: Herpes simplex virus infection: Biology, treatment and prevention. Ann Intern Med 103:404, 1985

Nettleman MD, Bell TA: Cost-effectiveness of prenatal testing for *Chlamydia trachomatis*. Am J Obstet Gynecol 164:1289, 1991

O'Brien TR, George JR, Holmberg SD: Human immunodeficiency virus type 2 infection in the United States. Epidemiology, diagnosis, and public health implications. JAMA 267:2775, 1992

Prober CG, Hensleigh PA, Boucher FD, Yasukawa LL, Au DS, Arvin AM: Use of routine viral cultures at delivery to identify neonates exposed to herpes simplex virus. N Engl J Med 318:887, 1988

Prober CG, Sullender WM, Yasukawa LL, Au DS, Yeager AS, Arvin AM: Low risk of herpes simplex virus infections in neonates exposed to the virus at the time of vaginal delivery to mothers with recurrent genital herpes simplex virus infections. N Engl J Med 316:240, 1987

Rando RF, Lindheim S, Hasty L, Sedlacek TV, Woodland M, Eder C: Increased frequency of detection of human papillomavirus deoxyribonucleic acid in exfoliated cervical cells during pregnancy. Am J Obstet Gynecol 161:50, 1989

Rettig PJ: Perinatal infections with *Chlamydia trachomatis*. Clin Perinatol 15:321, 1988

Ricci JM, Fojaco RM, O'Sullivan MJ: Congenital syphilis: The University of Miami/Jackson Memorial Medical Center experience, 1986–1988. Obstet Gynecol 74:687, 1989

Ryan GM, Abdella TN, McNeeley SG, Baselski V, Drummond DE: *Chlamydia trachomatis* infection in pregnancy and effect of treatment on outcome. Am J Obstet Gynecol 162:34, 1990

Sanchez PJ, Wendel GD, Norgard MV: Congenital syphilis associated with negative results of maternal serologic tests at delivery. Am J Dis Child 145:967, 1991

Satin AJ, Twickler DM, Wendel GD Jr: Congenital syphilis associated with dilation of fetal small bowel: A case report. J Ultrasound Med 11:49, 1992

Schachter J: Why we need a program for the control of chlamydia trachomatis. N Engl J Med 320:803, 1989

Schachter J, Grossman M, Sweet RL, Holt J, Jordan C, Bishop E: Prospective study of perinatal transmission of *Chlamydia trachomatis*. JAMA 255:3374, 1986a

Schachter J, Sweet RL, Grossman M, Landers D, Robbie M, Bishop E: Experience with the routine use of erythromycin for chlamydial infections in pregnancy. N Engl J Med 314:276, 1986b

Schmid GP, Sanders LL, Blount JH, Alexander ER: Chancroid in the United States: Reestablishment of an old disease. JAMA 258:3265, 1987

Schwartz DB, Greenberg MD, Daoud Y, Reid R: Genital condylomas in pregnancy: Use of trichloroacetic acid and laser therapy. Am J Obstet Gynecol 158:1407, 1988

Scott GB, Fischi MA, Klimas N, Fletcher MF, Dickinson GM, Levine RS, Parks WP: Mothers of infants with the acquired immunodeficiency syndrome: Evidence for both symptomatic and asymptomatic carriers. JAMA 253:363, 1985

Shah K, Kashima H, Polk BF, Shah F, Abbey H, Abramson A: Rarity of cesarean delivery in cases of juvenile-onset respiratory papillomatosis. Obstet Gynecol 68:795, 1986

Snyder RR, Hammond TL, Hankins GDV: Human papillomavirus associated with poor healing of episiotomy repairs. Obstet Gynecol 76:664, 1990

Sperling RS, Stratton P, Members of the Obstetric–Gynecologic Working Group of the AIDS Clinical Trials Group of the National Institute of Allergy and Infectious Diseases: Treatment options for human immunodeficiency virus–infected pregnant women. Obstet Gynecol 79:443, 1992a

Sperling RS, Stratton P, O'Sullivan MJ, Boyer P, Watts DH,

Lambert JS, Hammill H, Livingston EG, Gloeb DJ, Minkoff H, Fox HE: A survey of zidovudine use in pregnant women with human immunodeficiency virus infection. N Engl J Med 326:857, 1992b

Spitzer M, Krumholz BA, Seltzer VL: The multicentric nature of disease related to human papillomavirus infection of the female lower genital tract. Obstet Gynecol 73:303, 1989

Stoll BJ, Kanto WP, Glass RI, Pushkin J: Treated maternal gonorrhea without adverse effect on outcome of pregnancy. South Med J 75:1236, 1982

Stone KM, Whittington WL: Treatment of genital herpes. Rev Infect Dis 12:S610, 1990

Stratton P, Mofenson LM, Willoughby AD: Human immunodeficiency virus infection in pregnant women under care at AIDS Clinical Trials Centers in the United States. Obstet Gynecol 79:364, 1992

Straus SE, Seidlin M, Takiff HE, Rooney JF, Felser JM, Smith HA, Roane P, Johnson F, Hallahan C, Ostrove JM, Nusinoff-Lehrman S: Effect of oral acyclovir treatment on symptomatic and asymptomatic virus shedding in recurrent genital herpes. Sex Transm Dis 16:107, 1989

Sullivan-Bolyai J, Hull HF, Wilson C, Corey L: Neonatal herpes simplex virus infection in King County, Washington. JAMA 250:3059, 1983

Sweet RL, Landers CV, Walker C, Schachter J: *Chlamydia trachomatis* infection and pregnancy outcome. Am J Obstet Gynecol 156:824, 1987

Tseng CJ, Lin CY, Wang RL, Chen LJ, Chang YL, Hsieh TT, Pao CC: Possible transplacental transmission of human papillomaviruses. Am J Obstet Gynecol 166:35, 1992

Van de Perre P, Simonon A, Msellati P, Hitimana D-G, Vaira D, Bazubagira A, Van Goethem C, Stevens A-M, Karita E, Sondag-Thull D, Dabis F, Lepage P: Postnatal transmission of human immunodeficiency virus type 1 from mother to infant. N Engl J Med 325:593, 1991

Vontver LA, Hickok DE, Brown Z, Reid L, Corey L: Recurrent genital herpes simplex virus infection in pregnancy: Infant outcome and frequency of asymptomatic recurrences. Am J Obstet Gynecol 143:75, 1982

Ward JW, Holmbert DS, Allen JR, Cohn DL, Critchley SE, Kleinman SH, Lenes BA, Ravenholt O, Davis JR, Quinn MG, Jaffee HW: Transmission of human immunodeficiency virus (HIV) by blood transfusions screened as negative for HIV antibody. N Engl J Med 318:473, 1988

Washington AE, Johnson RE, Sanders LL: *Chlamydia trachomatis* infections in the United States: What are they costing us? JAMA 257:2070, 1987

Wendel GD: Gestational and congenital syphilis. Clin Perinatol 15:287, 1988

Wendel GD, Cunningham FG: Sexually transmitted diseases in pregnancy. Williams Obstetrics, 18th ed (suppl 13). Norwalk, CT, Appleton & Lange, August/September 1991

Wendel GD, Maberry MC, Christmas JT, Goldberg MS, Norgard MV: Examination of amniotic fluid in diagnosing congenital syphilis with fetal death. Obstet Gynecol 74:967, 1989

Wendel GD, Sanchez PJ, Peters MT, Harstad TW, Potter LL, Norgard MV: Identification of *Treponema pallidum* in amniotic fluid and fetal blood from pregnancies complicated by congenital syphilis. Obstet Gynecol 78:890, 1991

Wendel GD, Stark RJ, Jamison RR, Molina RD, Sullivan TJ: Penicillin allergy and desensitization in serious infections during pregnancy. N Engl J Med 312:1229, 1985

Whitley R, Arvin A, Prober C, Burchett S, Corey L, Powell D, Plotkin S, Starr S, Alford C, Connor J, Jacobs R, Nahmias A, Soong SJ, National Institute of Allergy and Infectious Diseases Collaborative Antiviral Study Group: A controlled trial comparing vidarabine with acyclovir in neonatal herpes simplex virus infection. N Engl J Med 324:444, 1991a

Whitley R, Arvin A, Prober C, Corey L, Burchett S, Plotkin S, Starr S, Jacobs R, Powell D, Nahmias A, Sumaya C, Edwards K, Alford C, Caddell G, Soong SJ, National Institute of Allergy and Infectious Diseases Collaborative Antiviral Study Group: Predictors of morbidity and mortality in neonates with herpes simplex virus infections. N Engl J Med 324:450, 1991b

Wiesel J, Rose DN, Silver AL, Sacks HS, Bernstein RH: Lumbar puncture in asymptomatic late syphilis: An analysis of the benefits and risks. Arch Inter Med 145:465, 1985

Wittek AE, Yeager AS, Au DS, Hensleigh PA: Asymptomatic shedding of herpes simplex virus from the cervix and lesion site during pregnancy: Correlation of antepartum shedding with shedding at delivery. Am J Dis Child 138:439, 1984

Yeager AS, Arvin AM: Reasons for the absence of a history of recurrent genital infections in mothers of neonates infected with herpes simplex virus. Pediatrics 73:188, 1984

Zenker PN, Rolfs RT: Treatment of syphilis, 1989. Rev Infect Dis 12:S590, 1990

■ XIV ■
Family Planning

■

CHAPTER 60
Medical Contraception

The practice of obstetrics in the United States has been influenced by forces from outside the medical community more than any other specialty to date. In no other branch of medicine are social, religious, and political forces more obvious than in family planning. While clearly the majority of fertile American women would prefer to avoid pregnancy in any one given year, they and their physicians are confronted continuously by these forces. Thus, in spite of countless lawsuits alleging that contraception causes fetal malformations, and a variety of new formulations, the physician must continue to counsel and prescribe in an area in which confusion is common, change seems continual, and scientific evidence often is conflicting or even ignored by legal and judicial communities.

Who Needs Contraception?

The sexually active couple, both of whom are fertile but do not desire pregnancy, needs to use effective contraception. **When no contraception is used by presumably fertile sex partners, about 90 percent of women will conceive within 1 year.** Young women who do not want to be pregnant are best advised to use contraception whenever they become sexually active, no matter how young. At least some girls, and perhaps the majority, ovulate before their first menstrual period.

Contraceptive advice for the woman nearing menopause is a more difficult question because it is impossible to predict when fertility has ended. Results of one study of women ages 40 to 50 support the view that ovulation is related more closely to regularity of menstruation than to age (Metcalf, 1979). *When menstruation remained regular, there was evidence of ovulation in almost every cycle.* A recent history of oligomenorrhea or of increasing cycle length was associated with a diminished frequency but not the complete absence of ovulation. Even the presence of hot flushes, amenorrhea, and elevated levels of follicle-stimulating hormone do not absolutely guarantee against subsequent ovulation (Metcalf and Donald, 1979). Primordial follicles with apparently normal oocytes have been observed in ovaries removed from women over 50 years of age.

Even so, pregnancies are rare in women over 50, and extremely rare after age 52 (Francis, 1970). Therefore, older women probably are best advised as follows: regular menstrual periods imply recurrent ovulation irrespective of age; however, pregnancy is rare after age 50. A woman younger than this who has not menstruated for 2 years is very unlikely to ovulate spontaneously and to conceive, although there are reported instances in which conception occurred more than 2 years after the onset of documented hypergonadotropic, hypoestrogenic amenorrhea (Szlachter and co-workers, 1979).

Commonly Employed Contraceptive Techniques

Methods of contraception of variable effectiveness currently employed include (1) oral steroidal contraceptives, (2) injected or implanted steroidal contraceptives, (3) intrauterine devices, (4) physical, chemical, or physicochemical barrier techniques, (5) withdrawal, (6) sexual abstinence around the time of ovulation, (7) breast feeding, and (8) permanent sterilization.

The results of a 1989 national survey of contraceptive use by women of reproductive age are presented in Figure 60–1. Estimates of the failure rate *during the first year of use* with each of these techniques are presented in Table 60–1. It is emphasized that failures from patient misuse of the method are included. Effective education, as well as motivation, undoubtedly would have appreciably reduced the cited failure rates. The results of the

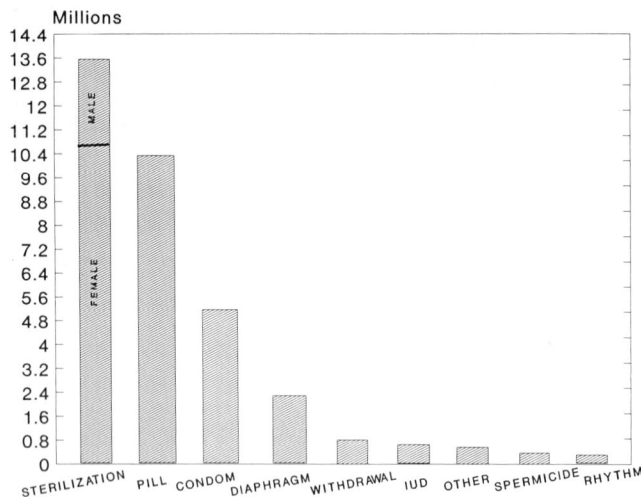

Fig. 60-1. Contraceptive methods used in 1989 by women aged 15 to 44. (Data adapted from Mosher and Pratt, 1990, with permission.)

Oxford Family Planning Association contraceptive study provide strong support for this view (Vessey and coworkers, 1982). Their failure rates for more than 17,000 women who had been observed for an average of about 9 years are among the lowest reported. Failure rates for various contraceptive techniques per 100 woman-years of use were as follows: estrogen plus progestin oral contraceptives, 0.16 to 0.32; intrauterine devices, 0.4 to 2.4; diaphragm, 1.9; and condom, 3.6. Mature women who continued to use one technique for a long time typically experienced a very low failure rate.

Elective abortion is not a contraceptive technique. It serves, at times, as a less than ideal remedy for contraceptive failure or neglect. The medical and surgical techniques for inducing abortion are discussed extensively in Chapter 31. The synthetic 19-norsteroid competitive progesterone antagonist, RU 486, has been reported to be an effective orally administered abortifacient either alone or in combination with a prostaglandin if administered within 6 weeks of the last menstrual period (Cameron and colleagues, 1988; Couzinet and associates, 1986; Grimes and associates, 1988). The compound competes with progesterone at the endometrial receptor level. Das and Catt (1987) also demonstrated in vitro receptor blockade on syncytiotrophoblast where RU 486 impaired production of chorionic gonadotropin, placental lactogen, and progesterone. Nieman and colleagues (1987) reported that a single oral dose of RU 486 during the midluteal phase will reliably induce menses. Menstruation began within 72 hours after RU 486 administration and was not prevented by augmented progesterone production induced by the concomitant administration of chorionic gonadotropin. The potential usefulness of RU 486 as a once-a-month oral contraceptive is obvious, provided that long-term safety and appropriate dosage and timing can be estab-

lished. Even then, the abortifacient action of the drug will preclude its being accepted by some women. The agent ultimately may provide an alternative to surgical techniques currently employed.

Epostane, a 3β-hydroxysteroid dehydrogenase inhibitor, produced early pregnancy termination in 84 percent of women given the drug orally (Crooij and colleagues, 1988). Epostane prevents conversion of pregnenolone to progesterone.

HORMONAL CONTRACEPTIVES

Hormonal contraceptives are available in a variety of oral, injectable, and implantable forms. Generally, oral contraceptives are a combination of estrogen and progestins or a progestin only (the so-called "mini pill"). The injectable or implantable hormonal contraceptives usually are progestins alone.

When introduced in 1960, hormonal contraceptives represented a dramatic departure from previous traditional methods; they also created a unique therapeutic dilemma. As stated in the 1986 report of an advisory committee to the Food and Drug Administration, "Never will so many people have taken such potent drugs voluntarily over such a protracted period for an objective other than for the control of disease." Indeed, in 1988, 10.7 million women in the United States used one of the variety of oral contraceptives available for fertility control (Mosher and Pratt, 1990).

Estrogen Plus Progestin Contraceptives

The oral contraceptives employed most often consist of a combination of an estrogen and a progestational agent taken daily for 3 weeks and omitted for 1 week, during which time withdrawal uterine bleeding normally occurs.

Mechanisms of Action. The contraceptive actions of the estrogen–progestin steroidal medication are multiple, but the most important effect is to prevent ovulation by suppression of hypothalamic releasing factors. This suppresses pituitary secretion of follicle-stimulating and luteinizing hormones (Fig. 60–2). To understand hormonal contraception, it is essential to know the endocrine and nonendocrine actions of only one estrogen and five progestins.

Estrogen alone in sufficient dose will inhibit ovulation by suppressing pituitary gonadotropins. Implantation also is likely inhibited by altering normal endometrial maturation. Although estrogen accelerates ovum transport, progestins cause slowing; thus, their possible role in altered tubal and uterine motility is unclear.

Progestins produce thick, scanty, cellular cervical mucus that impairs sperm transport. Also, sperm capac-

TABLE 60–1. LOWEST EXPECTED, TYPICAL, AND LOWEST REPORTED RATES FOR ORAL, INJECTABLE, AND IMPLANTABLE CONTRACEPTIVE METHODS AND CONTINUATION RATES FOR WOMEN IN THE UNITED STATES

Method	Women Pregnant in First Year of Use (%)			Women Continuing Use at 1 Year[a] (%)	
	Lowest Expected[b]	*Typical*[c]	*Lowest Reported*[d]	*Excluding Pregnancy*	*Including Pregnancy*
Chance[e]	85	85	43.1	—	—
Medical					
Oral contraceptives	—	3	—	75	73
Combined	0.1	—	0	—	—
Progestin-only	0.5	—	1.1	—	—
Injectable progestin[f]	—	—	—	70	70
DMPA	0.3	0.3	0	—	—
NET	0.4	0.4	0	—	—
Implants	—	—	—	90	90
Norplant	0.04	0.04	0	—	—
Norplant-2	0.03	0.03	0	—	—
Mechanical					
Intrauterine device	—	3	—	75	73
Progestasert	2.0	—	1.9	—	—
Copper T 380A	0.8	—	0.5	—	—
Spermicides[g]	3	21	0	55	43
Periodic abstinence	—	20	—	84	67
Calendar	9	—	14.4[h]	—	—
Ovulation Method[i]	3	—	10.5[h]	—	—
Symptothermal	2	—	12.6	—	—
Postovulation	1	—	2.0[h]	—	—
Cap[j]	6	18	8.0	77	63
Diaphragm[j]	6	18	2.1	69	57
Condom[k]	2	12	4.2	73	64
Sponge					
Parous women	9	28	27.7	73	53
Nulliparous women	6	18	13.9	73	60
Sterilization					
Female	0.2	0.4	0	—	—
Male	0.1	0.15	0	—	—

[a] Among couples attempting to avoid pregnancy, the percentage who continue to use a method for one year.
[b] Among couples who initiate use of a method (not necessarily for the first time) and who use it *perfectly* (both consistently and correctly); the authors' best guess of the percentage expected to experience an accidental pregnancy during the first year if they do not stop use for any other reason.
[c] Among *typical* couples who initiate use of a method (not necessarily for the first time), the percentage who experience an accidental pregnancy during the first year if they do not stop use for any other reason.
[d] In the literature on contraceptive failure, the *lowest reported* percentage who experienced an accidental pregnancy during the first year following initiation of use (not necessarily for the first time) if they did not stop use for any other reason (see note i).
[e] The lowest expected and typical percents are based on data from populations where contraception is not used and from women who cease using contraception in order to become pregnant. These represent the best guess of the percent who would conceive among women now relying on reversible methods of contraception if they abandoned contraception altogether. The lowest reported percent is based on women in the U.S. who use no contraception even though they do not wish to become pregnant. This group is selected for low fecundity or low coital frequency, and some fraction may use an unreported variant of periodic abstinence.
[f] DMPA = Depo-medoxyprogesterone acetate; NET = Norethindrone.
[g] Foams and vaginal suppositories.
[h] Too low, because rate is based on more than one year of exposure.
[i] Cervical mucus (ovulation) method supplemented by calendar in the pre-ovulatory and basal body temperature in the post-ovulatory phases.
[j] With spermicidal cream or jelly.
[k] Without spermicides.
Modified from Trussell and colleagues (1990), with permission.

itation is likely inhibited. Similar to estrogens, progestins produce an endometrium that is unfavorable to blastocyst implantation. Finally, progestins also can inhibit ovulation by suppressing gonadotropins.

The net or combined effect of estrogen and progestin with respect to contraception is extremely effective ovulation suppression, sperm penetration blockage by cervical mucus, and unfavorable endometrium for implantation if the first two mechanisms fail. As the consequence of these actions, estrogen plus progestin combined oral contraceptives, *if taken daily for 3 weeks out of every 4,* provide virtually absolute protection against conception. An important exception, however, is the period of about a week immediately following initiation of an oral contraceptive. Indeed, ovulation actually may be triggered by starting oral contraceptives in a woman with a maturing follicle who is soon to ovulate spontaneously.

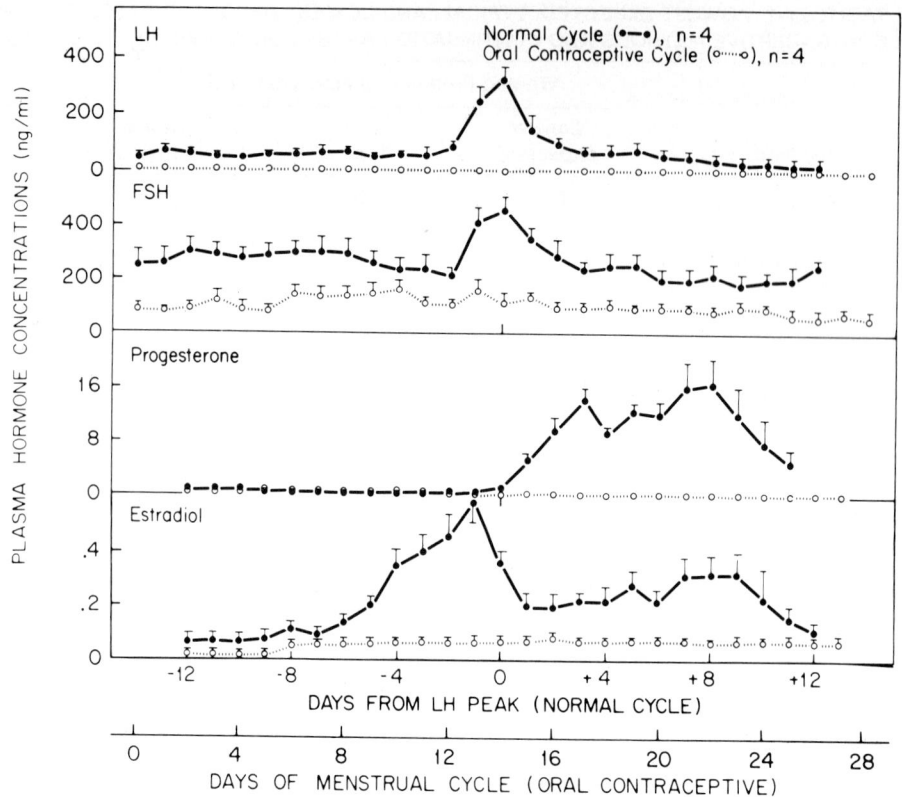

Fig. 60-2. Plasma levels of luteinizing hormone (LH), follicle-stimulating hormone (FSH), progesterone, and 17-β estradiol in four ovulatory women and in four women who were ingesting one tablet daily of an oral contraceptive that contained 80 μg of mestranol and 1 mg of norethindrone. Note the suppression of all four hormones in the women taking the oral contraceptives. (From Carr and colleagues, 1979, with permission.)

Pharmacology

Estrogens. In the United States, the only estrogens available are *ethinyl estradiol* or its 3-methyl ether, *mestranol*. To be bioactive, the methyl group at carbon 3 of mestranol must be removed by hepatic conversion into ethinyl estradiol. The exact conversion factor for potency of mestranol to ethinyl estradiol is not known, but it probably is 1.2 to 1.5 on a microgram basis (Heinen, 1974). The vast majority of all prescriptions for combined oral contraceptives in the United States are for 50 μg doses or less of estrogen, and *all of these contain only ethinyl estradiol.*

Progestins. Only 19-nortestosterone derivatives are currently used for progestins because derivatives of 17α-acetoxyprogesterone in high doses produce breast tumors in female beagles. Of the four compounds currently available in the United States (Fig. 60–3), only norgestrel has two isomers. Levonorgestrel is the bioactive isomer and *Nordette* contains 0.15 mg of this compound. *Lo/Ovral* contains 0.3 mg of dl-norgestrel (a combination of dextro and levo forms), of which only half is in the active levo form.

Three new potent progestins—*desogestrel, norgestimate,* and *gestodene*—currently are undergoing extensive study in both the United States and Europe for possible use in oral contraceptives (Fig. 60–3). Preliminary reports suggest that low doses may be associated with minimal metabolic changes but excellent cycle control (Runnebaum and Rabe, 1987). It is anticipated that these new progestins may soon be approved for commercial sale in both fixed dose and phasic pills.

All progestins were initially chosen because of their progestational potencies, and they were ranked in that manner based on that by Greenblatt (1967) who used a delay-of-menses assay on human estrogen-primed endometrium (Table 60–2). Swyer (1982) and Dorflinger (1985) since have added newer scales of progestational potency (Table 60–2). The potency is different for each compound when they are compared for estrogenic (Table 60–3), anti-estrogenic (Table 60–4), and androgenic effects (Table 60–5). All of these actions for each compound must be considered when prescribing appropriate oral contraception for a specific patient. For example, if a low androgenic effect were desired for a woman because of acne, a good choice of combination pill would be one containing 35 μg of ethinyl estradiol and 0.4 to 0.5 mg of norethindrone. An even better choice might be the newly approved *Ortho-Cyclen,* which contains 0.25 mg of norgestimate and 35 μg of ethinyl estradiol. *Norgestimate has less androgenic effect than any other currently available progestin.* In combination with this estrogen dose, it reduces free testosterone and increases sex-binding globulin and high density lipoprotein (HDL). Finally, norgestimate does not adversely affect coagulation values (Hatcher and associates, 1990).

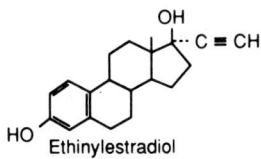

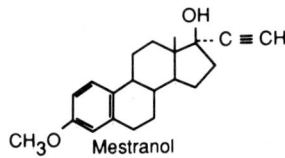

A. Estrogens

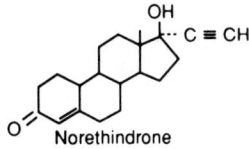

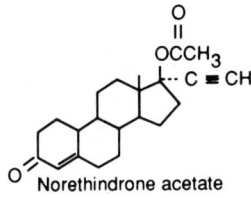

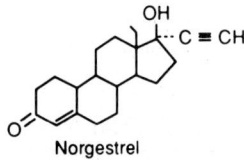

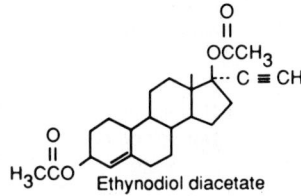

B. Progestins available in United States

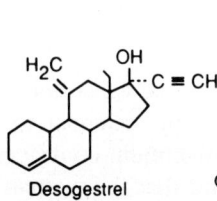

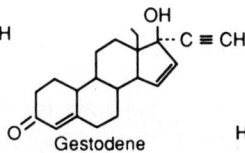

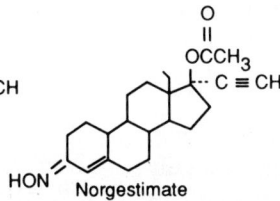

C. Progestins soon to be available in United States

Fig. 60–3. Structural formulas of contraceptive steroids currently in use. (Norgestimate was approved for use in late 1992.)

It is apparent that these progestins have variable estrogenic, androgenic, and progestational effects. Not surprisingly, they also have profound effects on plasma lipids, lipoproteins, clotting factors, vessel disease, diabetes, and a variety of nonendocrine effects (see Adverse and Beneficial Effects).

Dosage and Administration. Since oral contraceptives have come into use, the amounts of estrogen and progestin contained in each tablet have been reduced considerably. Effective contraception can be achieved with doses of the steroids that are quite small compared to those originally used. This is important, because most adverse effects are dose-related. The lowest acceptable dose is governed by the medication's ability to prevent unacceptable breakthrough bleeding (Edelman and associates, 1983). Daily estrogen content usually is 30 to 35 μg of ethinyl estradiol. Oral contraceptive tablets that

TABLE 60–2. RELATIVE PROGESTATIONAL POTENCY OF PROGESTINS IN CURRENTLY AVAILABLE ORAL CONTRACEPTIVES

Progestin Dose (mg)	Trade Name[a]	Progestin Relative Potency		
		Greenblatt (1967)	Swyer (1982)	Dorflinger (1985)
Norethindrone 0.4	Ovcon-35	0.4	0.4	0.4
Norethindrone 0.5	Brevicon Modicon	0.5	0.5	0.5
Norethindrone 1.0	Norinyl 1/35 Ortho 1/35	1.0	1.0	1.0
Norethindrone 1.0 Acetate	Loestrin 1/20	2.0	0.5	1.0
L-Norgestrel 0.15	Nordette Levien	9.0	0.45	3.0
Norgestrel 0.30	Lo/Ovral	9.0	0.9	3.0
Ethynodiol Diacetate 1.0	Demulen 1/35	15.0	0.5	1.0

[a] All drugs contain 35 μg or less of ethinyl estradiol.

TABLE 60–3. RELATIVE ESTROGENIC EFFECT OF PROGESTINS IN CURRENTLY AVAILABLE ORAL CONTRACEPTIVES

Progestin	Dose (mg)	Trade Name[a]	Estrogenic Relative Potency
Norgestrel	0.3	Lo/Ovral	0
Norethindrone	1.0	Norinyl and Ortho 1/35	1.0
Norethindrone acetate	1.0	Loestrin 1/20	1.5
Ethynodiol diacetate	1.0	Demulen 1/35	3.4

[a] All drugs contain 35 μg or less of ethinyl estradiol.
Adapted from Hatcher and associates (1990); Jones and Edgren (1973).

contain as little as 20 μg of ethinyl estradiol per tablet are available commercially, but no tablet sold in the United States contains more than 50 μg (FDA, 1988). The amount of progestin varies in two ways: (1) among older, now well-evaluated formulations, progestin dose remains constant throughout the cycle, and (2) in some newer preparations, the progestin dosage varies throughout the cycle.

To prevent ovulation induction, as well as to help recognize preexisting early pregnancy, it is generally recommended that women begin oral contraceptives within the first 7 days of the menstrual cycle. Many women, however, start their use after delivery or abortion, before return of spontaneous menses. If their use is initiated at any time other than during or immediately after a normal menstrual cycle, or within 3 weeks of delivery, another means of birth control should be used throughout the first week to avoid the risk of pregnancy due to induced ovulation (p. 1323).

To obtain maximum protection and promote regular use of oral contraceptives, most suppliers offer dispensers that provide 21 sequentially and individually wrapped, color-coded tablets containing hormones, followed by seven inert tablets of another color (Fig. 60–4).

TABLE 60–4. RELATIVE ANTI-ESTROGENIC EFFECT OF PROGESTINS IN CURRENTLY AVAILABLE ORAL CONTRACEPTIVES

Progestin	Dose (mg)	Trade Name[a]	Anti-estrogenic Relative Potency
Ethynodiol diacetate	1.0	Demulen 1/35	1.0
Norethindrone	1.0	Norinyl and Ortho 1/35	2.5
Norgestrel	0.3	Lo/Ovral	15.0[b]
Norethindrone acetate	1.0	Loestrin 1/20	25.0

[a] All drugs contain 35 μg or less of ethinyl estradiol.
[b] Estimate based on Norgestrel 0.5 = 18.5 relative anti-estrogenic potency.
Adapted from Dickey (1991); Hatcher and associates (1990).

TABLE 60–5. RELATIVE ANDROGENIC EFFECT OF PROGESTINS IN CURRENTLY AVAILABLE ORAL CONTRACEPTIVES

Progestin	Dose (mg)	Trade Name[a]	Androgenic Relative Potency
Norethindrone	0.4	Ovacon-35	0.14
Norethindrone	0.5	Brevicon/Modicon	0.17
Ethynodiol diacetate	1.0	Demulen 1/35	0.21
Norethindrone	0.5–0.75–1.0	Ortho-Novum 7/7/7	0.26
L-Norgestrel	0.05–0.075–0.12	Triphasil/ TriLevlen	0.29
Norethindrone	1.0	Norinyl and Ortho 1/35	0.34
L-Norgestrel	0.15	Nordette/Levlen	0.47
Norgestrel	0.30	Lo/Ovral	0.47
Norethindrone acetate	1.0	Loestrin 1/20	0.52

[a] All drugs contain 35 μg or less of ethinyl estradiol.
Adapted from Dickey (1991); Hatcher and associates (1990).

Many of these have the day of the week imprinted next to each tablet or with a variable calendar that may be affixed. It is important for maximum contraceptive efficiency and for peace of mind that the woman adopt an effective scheme for assuring daily (or nightly) self-administration. One technique is to keep her pill supply

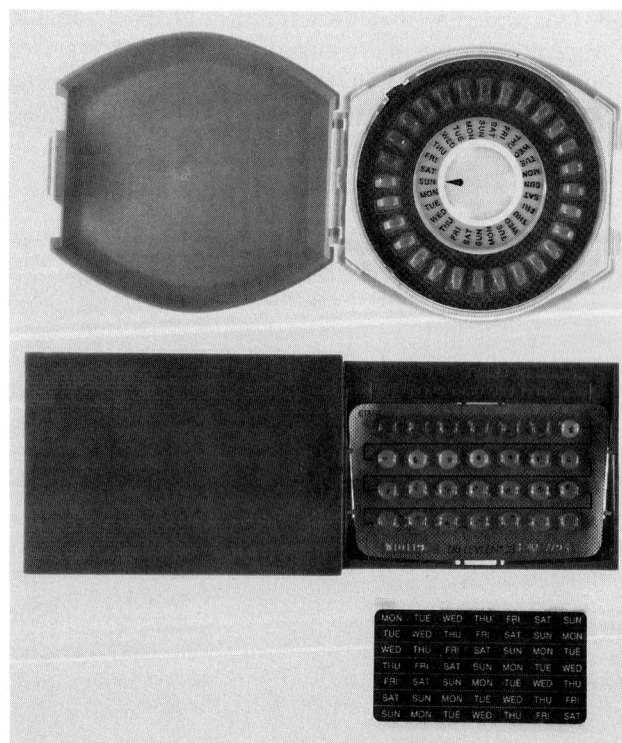

Fig. 60–4. Oral contraceptive tablets in a container.

and toothbrush close to each other and to swallow a pill at tooth brushing time either in the morning or evening. If one dose is missed, nothing serious will happen; it may be desirable to double the next dose to minimize break-through bleeding and to "stay on schedule." If several doses are missed, another form of effective contraception (a barrier technique) should be used. The pill can be started after withdrawal bleeding. Without bleeding, the possibility of pregnancy must be considered and excluded prior to resumption of oral contraceptive use.

Phasic Pills. These preparations were developed in an effort to reduce the amount of total progestin ingested per cycle without sacrificing contraceptive efficacy or cycle control. The reduction in progestin dose is achieved by beginning the contraceptive cycle with a low dose of progestin and increasing this later in the cycle. For example, a combined pill containing 35 μg of ethinyl estradiol plus 1.0 mg of norethindrone (*Ortho 1+35; Norinyl 1+35*) supplies 21 mg of progestin per cycle versus a similar triphasic combination (*Ortho 7-7-7*), which supplies 15.75 mg of norethindrone per cycle (Table 60–5). Another non-phasic formulation (*Ovacon-35*), however, supplies only 8.4 mg of norethindrone per cycle. Thus, if compliance is a problem, a simpler formulation with fewer different colored pills—some triphasic pills used four different colored pills—might be advisable; however, compliance has been good even in teen-aged women (Woods and associates, 1992). The lower dose of the less androgenic compound would also result in a lesser risk of adverse metabolic effects.

Triphasic formulations are highly effective in preventing pregnancy (Ellis, 1987; Toews and colleagues, 1987). The theoretical advantage is a reduction in metabolic changes that are attributable to the progestin, and thereby a reduction in those adverse effects from such metabolic changes. Unfortunately, beneficial effects of oral progestins may also be reduced. The triphasic oral contraceptives initially marketed in 1984 in the United States have achieved great popularity, and they now account for a large portion of new oral contraceptive prescriptions. Estrogen dose may be kept constant, or it may be increased temporarily later in the cycle, but in all preparations, it is kept to approximately 30 to 40 μg of ethinyl estradiol.

Despite the cited advantages, both theoretical and actual, there are distinct disadvantages to triphasic formulations. These include: (1) confusion due to multi colored pills, (2) breakthrough bleeding (spotting) which almost is doubled compared with non-phasic pills (Hatcher and colleagues, 1990), (3) loss of flexibility due to difficulty in "doubling up" if a pill is missed and different manufacturers recommending different "start up" times, for example, *Tri-norinyl* and *Ortho 7-7-7* must be started on a Sunday while *Triphasil* may be started on day 1 of menses.

Drug Interactions. Oral contraceptives are not known to interfere with the action of other drugs, but phenytoin and rifampin are believed to increase break-through bleeding and reduce contraceptive effectiveness of pills containing less than 50 μg ethinyl estradiol (Back and associates, 1980; Hatcher and colleagues, 1990). The mechanism is not entirely clear, but some antibiotics such as rifampin, ampicillin, and sulfonamides alter gut bacterial flora that possibly metabolizes oral contraceptives or alters their absorption. Certainly, any agent such as phenytoin or sulfonamides that stimulate hepatic enzymes might be expected to accelerate the enzymatic degradation of these synthetic hormones. Other agents, for example, barbiturates, are known to induce hepatic hydroxylation enzymes. Thus, if oral contraceptives are to be given in combination with barbiturates, phenytoin, or rifampin, then the minimal estrogen dose should be 50 μg of ethinyl estradiol. A barrier technique with vaginal spermicide likely should be used also.

Safety of Oral Contraceptives. At the outset, concern was raised for the safety of users of oral contraceptives. Fortunately, no major consequences have occurred, and in general, use of oral contraceptives, when appropriately monitored as outlined below, has proven to be safe for most women. The possibility of adverse effects from oral contraceptives has received so much attention for so long that the major adverse effect among their users may be the anxiety that has been created by almost incessant publicity. Unfortunately, physicians as well as the public are frequently confused by the many and often conflicting reports.

Beneficial Effects. The combined estrogen plus progestin pill taken 3 out of every 4 weeks is the most effective reversible form of contraception available. Failure rates of 0.32 per 100 woman-years or lower have been documented (Vessey and co-workers, 1982). Other reported beneficial effects include reduced menstrual blood loss and less iron-deficiency anemia; less dysmenorrhea, functional ovarian cysts, and salpingitis; fewer premenstrual complaints; less endometrial and ovarian cancer; reduction in various benign breast diseases and possibly breast cancer; and less rheumatoid arthritis (Andersch and Hahn, 1981; Centers for Disease Control, 1983a, 1983b, 1983c; Holt and colleagues, 1992; Mishell, 1982; Ory, 1982). Ory (1982) estimated that oral contraceptives significantly reduce hospitalizations for a variety of diseases (Table 60–6).

Possible Adverse Effects

Metabolic Effects. Oral contraceptives have a wide range of metabolic effects that are often combined and overlapping. For purposes of simplicity, these are presented separately.

TABLE 60–6. ESTIMATED RATE AND NUMBER OF HOSPITALIZATIONS PER SPECIFIC DISEASE EACH YEAR IN THE UNITED STATES

Disease	Rate per 100,000 Oral Contraceptive Users	Number of Hospitalizations Prevented[a]
Benign breast disease	235	20,000
Ovarian retention cysts	35	3000
Iron-deficiency anemia[b]	320	27,200
Pelvic inflammatory disease		
Total episodes[b]	600	51,000
Hospitalizations	156	13,300
Ectopic pregnancy	117	9900
Rheumatoid arthritis[b]	32	2700
Endometrial cancer[c]	5	2000
Ovarian cancer[c]	4	1700

[a] Except where noted, figures in this column refer to hospitalizations prevented based on 8.5 million oral contraceptive users.
[b] Episodes prevented regardless of whether hospitalizations occurred.
[c] Based on estimated 39 million women who never used oral contraceptives.
Modified from Ory (1982), with permission.

CHANGES SIMILAR TO PREGNANCY. Metabolic changes, often qualitatively similar to those of pregnancy, have been identified in women taking oral contraceptives. For example, plasma thyroxine and thyroid binding proteins are elevated, whereas triiodothyronine resin uptake is lowered. Plasma cortisol concentration increases with a nearly comparable increase in transcortin. It is extremely important, therefore, that evaluation of these laboratory tests and others be considered vis-a-vis the woman who takes oral contraceptives.

LIPOPROTEINS AND LIPIDS. The estrogen in a combined pill appears to decrease the serum concentration of low-density lipoprotein (LDL) cholesterol and to increase high-density lipoprotein (HDL) cholesterol, but some progestins cause the reverse (Stadel, 1981). The importance of such changes in the genesis of *arterial vascular disease* such as myocardial infarction or stroke in users of oral contraceptives is not clear but is cause for concern (Knopp, 1988; Meade, 1988; Mishell, 1988). Almost certainly, the adverse changes noted in HDL–LDL ratios are the consequences of the 19-nortestosterone progestins, and these changes are likely related to the specific progestin and its dose (Kauppinen-Mäkelin and colleagues, 1992). Importantly, progestins can change the relative amounts of total HDL, HDL_2, and HDL_3 (Tikkanen and associates, 1981, 1982). It is believed that the HDL_2 fraction provides cardiovascular protection (Miller and co-workers, 1982). Therefore, the estrogen and progestin effects on the specific HDL_2 fraction are of special importance because oral contraceptives may alter a woman's cardiovascular risks even though total HDL cholesterol values are unchanged. Briggs (1982) reported no change in total HDL with *Triphasil* (levo-

norgestrel) use, but Hatcher and colleagues (1990) found that it decreased HDL_2 and increased HDL_3. Apparently, norethindrone-containing oral contraceptives do not alter HDL_2 fractions (Hatcher and associates, 1990; Krauss and colleagues, 1983). More recently, however, Patsch and co-workers (1989) reported that two triphasic formulations containing norethindrone and one containing levonorgestrel all had similar effects on total HDL, HDL_2, and LDL.

The definitive study is yet to be conducted, and may never be. Certainly, no final recommendation can be made with respect to levonorgestrel-containing compounds. A prudent choice, if lipoproteins are a concern, would be to use a low dose of norethindrone, or possibly a norgestimate containing oral contraceptive which were recently approved for use.

CARBOHYDRATES. Contraceptive steroids may intensify pre-existing *diabetes* or may prove sufficiently diabetogenic to induce clinically apparent disease in susceptible women. The risk of the latter appears low because in the great majority of women the effect on carbohydrate metabolism is slight. Phillips and Duffy (1973), for example, identified serum glucose levels 1 hour after oral administration of 75 g of glucose to average 11 mg/dL more in users of oral contraceptives than in nonusers. As with pregnancy, diabetogenic effects are most often reversible when oral contraceptives are terminated (Wingrave and associates, 1979).

Estrogen–progestin oral contraceptive use in women who had *gestational diabetes* has been discouraged by some. Initially, concern centered around the possible acceleration of the appearance of permanent diabetes. Kalkhoff (1980) suggested that whereas the incidence of diabetes among normal women taking estrogen–progestin oral contraceptives is almost identical to that in a general population of women, the incidence of diabetes among women with previous gestational diabetes taking oral contraceptives is increased 10-fold. Because the number of women with previous gestational diabetes studied while taking oral contraceptives is very small, and the proportion of gestational diabetics who are expected to become diabetic later in life is very large, the ability of oral contraceptives to hasten the onset of permanent disease in gestational diabetics is still an important unanswered question.

More recently, concern about oral contraceptive use in women with previous gestational diabetes has centered around possible associations between mild hyperglycemia or hyperinsulinemia and an increased risk for cardiovascular disease. In this context, a report by Skouby and associates (1985) is encouraging. These investigators described a small group of women with previous gestational diabetes who were using a triphasic oral contraceptive pill (levonorgestrel). They reported that glucose, insulin, and glucagon response, as well as serum cholesterol, high-density lipoproteins, and low-density lipoproteins were unchanged compared with pretreatment values. Not all reports have been as optimistic. Wynn and Godsland (1986) reported in a long-term study of women taking 30 μg of ethinyl estradiol and 0.15 mg of levonorgestrel (*Nordette*) that there was a progressive deterioration of glucose tolerance. There was less effect when the progestin used was 1 mg of norethindrone. Thus, norgestrel appears to have the greatest antagonizing effect on insulin and glucose metabolism, and this effect becomes more pronounced over time (Hatcher and colleagues, 1990; Spellacy and associates, 1981, 1982; Wynn and Godsland, 1986).

Argument persists as to whether women with *overt* diabetes should use oral contraceptives. Our policy is as follows: **No women with systemic chronic disease should be given an oral contraceptive except in circumstances where it can be verified that the merits from its use clearly outweigh any risks.**

PROTEINS. The estrogens used in oral contraceptives are known to induce an increase in hepatic production of a variety of *globulins*. Increased production of *angiotensinogen* appears to be dose related. Because angiotensinogen is converted by renin to angiotensin I, this has been suspected to be associated with the development of so-called "pill hypertension" (see p. 1331). *Fibrinogen*, and likely Factors II, VII, IX, X, XII, and XIII, are increased in direct proportion to the amount of estrogen in the formulation (Meade, 1982). The relationship of these increased clotting factors to venous and arterial thrombosis are discussed on page 1330; but the incidence of both forms of thrombosis appear to be directly estrogen dose related (Mann, 1982).

LIVER DISEASE. *Cholestasis* and *cholestatic jaundice* are uncommon complications in users of oral contraceptives; the signs and symptoms clear when the medication is stopped. A somewhat increased risk of surgically identified gallstones and *gallbladder disease* was reported for users of higher-dose oral contraceptives, but not for women using the 50 μg or smaller estrogen doses (Strom and colleagues, 1986). It appears that oral contraceptives may accelerate the development of gallbladder disease in women who are susceptible, but there is no overall increased long-term risk (Kay, 1984; Royal College of General Practitioners, 1982). There is no reason to withhold oral contraceptives from women recovered from viral hepatitis.

Neoplasia. Hormonal contraception as a definite cause of cancer appears to be unlikely in view of the intense scrutiny that has been applied to all aspects of this form of contraception. There is, of course, a possibility that such an association may develop because most of the women who began taking oral contraceptives in the early 1960s are not yet elderly. Nonetheless, thus far no convincing evidence has been published to support such an association (Cancer and Steroid Hormone Study, 1986, 1987a, 1987b; Prentice and Thomas, 1987; Schlessman, 1988). In fact, a protective effect against ovarian and endometrial cancer was shown. There are, however, conflicting reports concerning the risks of premalignant and malignant changes of the liver, pituitary, cervix, and breast. Therefore, each of these areas is considered separately.

HEPATIC HYPERPLASIA AND CANCER. Use of estrogen plus progestin contraceptives has been linked circumstantially with the development of *hepatic focal nodular hyperplasia* and actual tumor formation that most often, but not always, is benign. This association has been observed in women using high-dose estrogen containing formulations (usually mestranol) for prolonged periods. In fact, Neuberger and associates (1986) reported an association between prolonged oral contraceptive use and *hepatocellular carcinoma* in women under age 50. In contrast, conclusions derived from a multicenter World Health Organization study (1989) support the view that there is no increased risk of hepatic cancer associated with oral contraceptive use even in countries with an increased prevalence of liver cancer.

Benign hepatic nodules have increased vascularity with extensive proliferation of large and small thin-walled blood vessels. The lesions on rupture can be complicated by bleeding, hemoperitoneum, and shock, which proved fatal in 8 of 24 cases cited by Antoniades and colleagues (1975). The liver may become enlarged to palpation, and imaging studies disclose a space-occupying lesion(s). If identified before rupture, resection of the lesion, along with stopping the oral contraceptives, has been recommended. Some liver lesions appear to have disappeared after discontinuing oral contraceptives. Increased growth and vascularity during pregnancy or the puerperium, leading to rupture, and death, have been described (Kent and co-workers, 1978).

PITUITARY ADENOMAS. Although it has been suggested that oral contraceptives might increase the risk of pituitary *prolactinomas*, the Pituitary Adenoma Study Group (1983) provided contrary evidence. The awareness in recent years that these neoplasms may cause menstrual irregularities, along with imaging technology to visualize them, has resulted in the diagnosis even before steroidal contraceptives are given.

CERVIX. There is a correlation between the risk of preinvasive cervical cancer and oral contraceptive use, and the risk of invasive cancer increases after 5 years of use (Beral and colleagues, 1988; Schlesselman and co-workers, 1988; Vessey and associates, 1983b). It is unclear if these associations are casually related. For example, oral contraceptive users do not have the benefit of barrier or spermicidal protection from the human papillomavirus, and they more frequently are screened cytologically for cervical cancer (Butterworth and associates, 1992). Thus, the observed association may be casually and not causally related. Regardless, cervical cytologic screening should occur no less often than yearly.

BREAST CANCER. It is not clear at this time whether oral contraceptives contribute to the development of *breast cancer.* Several studies have failed to clarify this issue. In the largest study to date, no increased risk for breast cancer among oral contraceptive users was demonstrated (Cancer and Steroid Hormone Study, 1986). Moreover, the risk did not vary according to preparation or duration of use. Whereas a New Zealand study (Paul and colleagues, 1986) confirmed these findings, a Swedish study (Meirik and associates, 1986) contained evidence of a slightly increased risk of breast cancer among women who used oral contraceptives for 12 or more years. If there is an increased risk of breast malignancy from use of estrogen plus progestin oral contraceptives, the risk must be small (Kay and Hannerford, 1988; Pike and associates, 1983; Prentice and Thomas, 1987; Reuter and associates, 1992; Schlesselman and co-workers, 1988; Vessey and colleagues, 1983a).

Long-term studies for evaluation of the newer low-dose oral contraceptives have not been performed. Finally, the 1 in 9 attack rate of breast cancer would make it difficult for a small increased incidence to be detected. The Food and Drug Administration (1984) has not changed its recommendations regarding oral contraceptive prescribing and the risks for breast cancer.

Nutrition. Aberrations in the levels of several *nutrients* have been described for women who use oral contraceptives. These typically are similar to changes induced by normal pregnancy. Lower plasma levels in users compared with nonusers have been described by some investigators, but not all, for ascorbic acid, folic acid, vitamin B_{12}, niacin, riboflavin, and zinc.

PYRIDOXINE DEFICIENCY. Biochemical changes compatible with, but not necessarily proof of, vitamin B_6 (pyridoxine) deficiency have been documented with oral contraceptive use, but do not differ from those of normal pregnancy (Wynn, 1975). Estrogens induce the rate-limiting liver enzyme, *tryptophan oxygenase*, which enhances tryptophan metabolism in a way that suggests pyridoxine deficiency (Wynn, 1975) (also see Depression, p. 1332). To abolish these, as much as 20 to 30 mg of pyridoxine, or 10 times the usual intake, must be ingested! Because altered tryptophan metabolism persists in contraceptive users even when other indices of vitamin B_6 nutrition are normal, Leklem and co-workers (1975) believe that oral contraceptives specifically af-

fect tryptophan metabolism by some other means. The similarity of changes in tryptophan and pyridoxine metabolism to those of normal pregnancy strongly implies that estrogen–progestin contraceptives do not induce clinically significant pathological changes.

DECREASED IRON-DEFICIENCY ANEMIA AND DYSMENORRHEA. Combined estrogen–progestin oral contraceptives conserve *iron* by reducing menstrual blood loss. Nilsson and Sölvell (1967) compared hemoglobin shed by apparently normal women during spontaneous menses with that following estrogen–progestin contraceptives, and they found that contraceptives reduced by half the amount of hemoglobin shed. It is apparent that women who typically lose more than the average amount of blood with their periods may benefit from oral contraceptives. Moreover, women with *dysmenorrhea* from endometriosis or from idiopathic causes are likely to enjoy appreciable relief from pain while using combined oral contraceptives. At times, while using the combined medication, blood loss is so scant that the woman believes that she is pregnant, especially if she has missed one or more tablets. She may then stop taking the medication and soon thereafter conceive. Increasing the estrogen dose particularly for the first 7 days of a cycle usually will alleviate amenorrhea.

Cardiovascular Effects

VENOUS THROMBOSIS AND EMBOLISM. The risk of *deep vein thrombosis* and *pulmonary embolism* has been estimated to be increased by 3 to 11 times in women who used oral contraceptives (Realini and Goldzieher, 1985; Stadel, 1981). Moreover, contraceptive use during the month before an operative procedure appears to increase significantly the risk of postoperative thromboembolism. These risks clearly are dose related (Mann, 1982). In 1988, American manufacturers stopped production of preparations containing more than 50 μg of estrogen.

The mechanism by which estrogen–progestin contraceptives enhance the risk of venous thrombosis and thromboembolism is unclear. Development of distinctive vascular intimal and medial lesions with associated occlusive thrombi has been described (Irey and co-workers, 1970). Moreover, platelet aggregation may be accelerated, and both plasma antithrombin III activity and endothelial plasminogen activator are likely to be reduced somewhat while using estrogen plus progestin oral contraceptives (Stadel, 1981).

The enhanced risk of thromboembolism appears to decrease rapidly once the contraceptive is stopped. Women who develop thromboembolism while taking estrogen-containing contraceptives, however, also appear to be at increased risk of thromboembolism during pregnancy and the early puerperium (Badaracco and Vessey, 1974; Vessey, 1974).

ARTERIAL THROMBOSIS. This form of thrombosis has also been attributed to use of estrogen plus progestin contraceptives, but it does not appear to be related to atherosclerotic lesions. Instead, thrombotic lesions appear to be more frequent. The relative risk of stroke is increased four-fold in users compared with nonusers and appears to be confined largely to women age 35 or older (Stadel, 1981). Smoking is a strong co-factor.

HYPERTENSION. An association between oral contraceptives and hypertension became apparent in the late 1960s, when several reports appeared of the occasional woman who, while using an estrogen-progestin contraceptive, became overtly hypertensive. Usually, but not always, blood pressure returned to normal when the medication was stopped. Oral contraceptives, presumably in response to estrogen, were shown to increase plasma angiotensinogen (renin substrate) to levels near those found in normal pregnancy. Although the great majority of women using oral contraceptives demonstrate these changes, most do not become hypertensive. Progestin appears to contribute to the hypertension. Weir (1982) observed that women who developed hypertension while taking estrogen–progestin oral contraceptives and who become normotensive after stopping the contraceptive, redeveloped hypertension when oral contraception was reinstituted, even if the contraceptive employed contained no estrogen. Fisch and Frank (1977) evaluated blood pressures of a large number of women taking oral contraceptives and identified the mean systolic and diastolic blood pressures to be only 5 to 6 and 1 to 2 mm Hg higher, respectively, than in the age-adjusted control group. Not surprisingly, the risk of hypertension attributable to oral contraceptives increases with age (Stadel, 1981).

Unfortunately, normotensive women who are destined to become hypertensive in response to oral contraceptives usually cannot be identified in advance. The development of hypertension during pregnancy does not preclude subsequent use of oral contraceptives. Pritchard and Pritchard (1977) evaluated the pressor response to oral contraceptives in young black women who had developed overt pregnancy-induced hypertension but postpartum had diastolic blood pressures of 90 mm Hg or less when oral contraceptives were started. The contraceptive provided 50 μg of mestranol and 1 mg of norethindrone daily. Over an average of 1 year, only 6 percent demonstrated a rise in diastolic pressure above 90 mm Hg, a frequency not remarkably different from that observed in initially normotensive young nulligravid black women who used the same kind of oral contraceptive. Moreover, Fisch and Frank (1977) found no significant association between hypertension from use of oral contraceptives and previous hypertension during pregnancy.

We do not administer oral contraceptives to hypertensive women in our family planning clinics. Moreover, blood pressure is measured when contraceptive refills are provided 3 months after starting the medication, and every 9 to 12 months thereafter. Smoking is discouraged. Whenever hypertension is detected, the oral contraceptive is stopped and another form of contraception is substituted.

MYOCARDIAL INFARCTION. All data related to myocardial infarction and oral contraceptives prior to the use of 50 μg or less ethinyl estradiol and lower dose progestins, and studies in which smokers were not excluded, in essence, are obsolete. Specifically, smoking has been shown to be an independent risk factor for myocardial infarction, which is enhanced synergistically by oral contraceptives (Craft and Hannaford, 1989). The critical points with respect to smoking and oral contraceptives appears to be at greater than 15 cigarettes per day for current and past smokers and age greater than 35 (Craft and Hannaford, 1989).

The cause of increased risk with smoking and oral contraceptives is not entirely known, but it is likely related in a major way to an increased concentration of platelet-activating factor (PAF) resulting from cigarette smoke (Miyaura and associates, 1992). Both cigarette smoke and estrogen result in a decreased plasma concentration of platelet-activating factor acetylhydrolase (PAF-AH), the enzyme that destroys platelet activating factor (Miyaura and associates, 1991, 1992). The combined effects result in decreased destruction of platelet activating factor; this in turn results in an increased plasma level of platelet-activating factor and increased platelet aggregation. This supports the observations of Mileikowsky and associates (1988) who reported that platelet aggregation was increased only in oral contraceptive users who smoked. These authors also observed decreased plasma levels of prostacyclin only in the women who smoked. This resulted in an increased thromboxane to prostacyclin ratio in smokers, adding further to platelet aggregation and vasoconstriction.

The relationship of estrogen and cigarette smoke on platelet activating factor and an increased incidence of myocardial infarction is compatible with the observed lesions seen with these infarcts. Specifically, they appear to be the result of thrombosis rather than atherosclerosis. Stampfer and associates (1988) and Rosenberg and colleagues (1990) found no increased risk of myocardial infarction in women who had taken oral contraceptives in the past. Thus, pill-induced atherosclerosis does not appear to be a factor in the etiology of smoking and oral contraceptive related myocardial infarction. **Currently used low-dose oral contraceptives are not associated with an increased risk of myocardial infarction in nonsmokers** (Craft and Hannaford, 1989; Porter and co-workers, 1985; Rosenberg and colleagues, 1990). The American College of Obstetricians and Gynecologists (1985) cited no contraindication for oral contraceptives in nonsmoking women past age 35. Finally, the Food and Drug Administration revised their labeling of oral contraceptives to remove restrictions for nonsmoking women past age 40 (Contraception Report, 1992).

MIGRAINE HEADACHES. The frequency and intensity of attacks of *migraine headaches* may be enhanced appreciably by estrogen plus progestin contraceptives. We prefer to avoid these contraceptives in a woman with migraines, not only because they are likely to be unacceptable to her, but also because some migraine symptoms and signs are indistinguishable from mild or impending stroke.

Effects on Reproduction

"POSTPILL" AMENORRHEA. When estrogen–progestin contraception is discontinued, ovulation usually, but not always, resumes promptly. Similar to the postpartum period, within 3 months after discontinuance, at least 90 percent of women who previously ovulated regularly will have done so again, but Bracken and associates (1990) noted there was a reduced conception rate for at least six cycles after stopping oral contraceptives. This was even longer in older women. *Post-pill amenorrhea* poses no long-term threat to fertility (Hull and associates, 1981; Linn and colleagues, 1982). In the rare instance in which *anovulation* persists and is not caused by unrecognized early pregnancy or pituitary adenoma or by premature menopause, ovulation usually can be induced successfully.

CONGENITAL DEFECTS. Whether recent oral contraceptive use before pregnancy or continued use during early unrecognized pregnancy might adversely affect the fetus has been the source of much concern. Linn and co-workers (1983) did not find an increased risk for major fetal malformations among users of oral contraceptives, diaphragms, or foam barrier techniques. Even so, the woman who thinks that she may be pregnant should be advised to stop the oral contraceptive *(but use another contraceptive technique!)* until it can be established whether or not she is pregnant.

In earlier studies, fetal limb-reduction deformities were reported in pregnancies conceived while taking, or soon after taking, combination oral contraceptives (Janevich and co-workers, 1974; Nora and Nora, 1975). Rothman and Louik (1978) and Savolainen and associates (1981), however, found little difference for major malformations between infants whose mothers recently had used oral contraceptives and those who had not. Lammer and Cordero (1986) found no association between any major malformation and oral contraceptive exposure in early pregnancy (see Chap. 42, p. 972).

LACTATION. Use of combined oral contraceptive hormones by nursing mothers reduces the amount of *breast milk;* however, only very small quantities of the hormones are excreted in milk. Because progestin-only oral contraceptives have little effect on lactation and provide excellent contraception, they should be used for the lactating woman (see p. 1334).

Other Effects. Cervical mucorrhea is fairly common in response to the estrogen component, and the mucus at times may be irritating to the vagina and vulva. *Vaginitis* or *vulvovaginitis,* especially that caused by *Candida,* also may develop. Antibiotic therapy in pill users increases the frequency of such infections.

Hyperpigmentation of the face and forehead (*chloasma*) is more likely in women who demonstrated such a change during pregnancy. Almost all women using combination contraceptives have increased pigmentation of their breast areola and vulva. *Acne* may improve or, at times, be aggravated, often dependent on the progestin used. Combined contraceptives suppress gonadotropins and thus diminish ovarian androstenedione secretion with resultant testosterone production. If a low androgenic progestin such as norethindrone or norgestimate is used in the combination pill, overall androgen effect is reduced and acne will likely decrease.

Uterine *myomas* most likely are not increased in size by oral contraceptives (Parazzini and colleagues, 1992).

Weight gain has been a troublesome complaint from women who use oral contraceptives, although an increase in weight is far from a uniform phenomenon. Some of the weight may be caused by fluid retention, but it is likely to be a consequence of increased dietary intake.

Oral contraceptives often ameliorate primary *dysmenorrhea* and dysmenorrhea associated with endometriosis (Robinson and colleagues, 1992). Their use may even reduce the risk of a woman developing severe endometriosis.

Low-dose estrogen formulations are not associated with *depression,* but oral contraceptives containing 50 μg or more of estrogen were associated directly with depression in a dose-dependent manner (Kay, 1984). The mechanism for this is unclear but might involve a decrease in brain serotonin. This may be the consequence of tryptophan, the serotonin precursor, being inactivated by estrogen stimulated hepatic enzymes.

Risk of Death. The risk of death from oral contraceptives is very low if the woman is under 35, has no systemic illness, and does not smoke. Porter and associates (1987) reported their experiences with nearly 55,000 woman-years of oral contraceptive use in the Group Health Cooperative of Puget Sound, and attributed only one death to their use. The risk of dying as the consequence of using an oral contraceptive certainly is less than that of pregnancy, even though the risk with the latter is quite low (Harlap and associates, 1991).

Similar results have been reported from England. Vessey and colleagues (1989) in a 20-year follow-up study of over 17,000 women reported that the overall risk of death in women taking oral contraceptives was 0.9 compared with women of similar age using barrier methods for contraception. Deaths due to cancer and their relative risk were breast, 0.9; cervix, 3.3; and ovary, 0.4. The death risk from cardiovascular disease was 1.5—most cardiovascular deaths occurred in smokers!

Postpartum Use. Women who do not nurse their children, and especially those who have undergone abortions, may ovulate before 6 to 7 weeks after pregnancy ends (Chap. 18, p. 470). There is an advantage, therefore, to starting oral contraceptives before the traditional "6-weeks postpartum check." On the other hand, increased risks of adverse effects, especially venous thromboembolism, might be anticipated from use of estrogen–progestin contraceptives earlier in the puerperium. The use of 50 μg or smaller estrogen doses has reduced this risk greatly, and thus far, in our now extensive experience in which oral contraceptives have been started during the third week postpartum, there has been no evidence of increased morbidity.

Cost. Unfortunately, the cost of oral contraceptives has increased remarkably. Their price does not likely reflect the cost of the ingredients. In 1987, fixed dose estrogen–progestin contraceptives containing norethindrone and either 35 μg or 50 μg of estrogen were first marketed as *generic products* in this country. Because United States regulations allow a 25 percent variance in bioavailability, poor cycle control might follow their use in women as they change from one generic manufacturer to another.

Contraindications for Combined Oral Contraceptives.

Contraindications for these agents can be conveniently separated into absolute and relative. If there is an absolute contraindication, combined oral contraceptive pills likely should never be used for **contraceptive purposes**. With a relative contraindication, the woman and her physician should have excellent reasons that outweigh the risks before using these pills. Some of these are listed in Table 60–7.

Progestational Agents Alone

Oral Progestins Alone. So-called *mini-pills*, which are shown in Table 60–8, consist solely of 0.5 mg or less of a progestin used daily. They have not achieved widespread popularity because of a much higher incidence

TABLE 60–7. SOME CONTRAINDICATIONS TO USE OF ORAL CONTRACEPTIVES

Absolute
Thrombophlebitis or thromboembolic disorders
Prior thrombophlebitis or thromboembolic disorders
Cerebrovascular or coronary artery disease
Known or suspected breast carcinoma
Known or suspected endometrial carcinoma
Known or suspected estrogen-dependent neoplasia
Undiagnosed abnormal genital bleeding
Hepatic adenoma, carcinoma, or benign liver tumors
Known or suspected pregnancy
Markedly impaired liver function
Liver tumor that developed during previous use of oral contraceptive or other estrogen-containing products

Relative
Migraine or vascular headaches
Cardiac or renal dysfunction
Gestational diabetes or prediabetes
Hypertension
Depression
Varicose veins
Age > 35 for a smoker
Sickle cell (SS) or sickle C (SC) disease
Cholestatic jaundice during pregnancy
Hepatitis or mononucleosis during past year
Asthma
First-order family history of fatal or nonfatal nonrheumatic cardiovascular disease or diabetes before age 50
Use of drugs known to interact with oral contraceptives
Ulcerative colitis

Modified from Dickey (1991).

of irregular bleeding and a higher pregnancy rate. As with all forms of progestin-only contraception, when failure results in pregnancy, there is an increased risk that it is ectopic (see Chap. 32, p. 691). These agents, when used alone, impair fertility without always inhibiting ovulation. This likely results from inducing cervical mucus that impedes sperm penetration and from altering endometrial maturation sufficiently to thwart successful blastocyst implantation. Contraceptive effectiveness is greatest if there is ovulation suppression that paradoxically results in an increased incidence of abnormal uterine bleeding. Therefore, if menses are not dis-

TABLE 60–8. COMPOSITION OF PROGESTIN-ONLY ORAL CONTRACEPTIVES

Progestin	Dose (μg)	Brand Names
Norethindrone	350	Micronor, Nor-QD, Noriday
Norethindrone	75	Micro-Novum
Norgestrel	75	Ovrette, Neogest
Levonorgestrel	30	Microlut, Microval, Noregeston
Ethynodial diacetate	500	Femulen

Modified from Hatcher and associates (1990).

turbed, or only minimally disturbed, ovulation is likely not suppressed, and the pregnancy risk is greater. Actual pregnancy rates with progestin-only pills range from 1.1 to 9.6 pregnancies per 100 women in the first year of use (Trussel and Kost, 1987). Guillebaud (1985) reported a lower rate of 0.9 pregnancies per 100 married women with a decreasing rate observed with advancing age (25 to 29 years, 3.1; 30 to 34 years, 2.0; 35 to 39 years, 1.0; 40 or older, 0.3 pregnancies per 100 married women).

Benefits. Benefits are similar to the combined oral contraceptives (see p. 1327). In addition, these formulations have not been shown to increase the risk of cardiovascular disease or malignancy (Guillebaud, 1985). They are less likely to increase blood pressure or cause headaches (Vessey and colleagues, 1985). They have minimal effects on carbohydrate metabolism and allegedly cause less depression, dysmenorrhea, and premenstrual symptoms. When used by lactating women, these agents are virtually 100 percent effective, and they have less effect on milk production (Bertrabet and colleagues, 1987; Guillebaud, 1985; Shikary and associates, 1987). Smokers who cannot use combined oral contraceptives after age 35 can use these agents. These pills are a good choice for older smokers because, as noted above, the failure rate decreases with advancing age. Finally, the formulations can be used in women with altered glucose tolerance and, with caution and frequent blood pressure monitoring, in women who had hypertension or headaches while taking combination contraceptives.

A newer and increasingly popular indication for pills that contain only norgestrel or levonorgestrel is to use these for 4 to 6 months in women considering implantable contraception (*Norplant*), or in women with certain medical disorders, such as hypertension or diabetes. If no adverse effects are noted using 30 μg levonorgestrel doses (see p. 1335), the implantable contraception system **possibly** can be utilized.

Disadvantages. The major disadvantages are contraceptive failure and an increased incidence of ectopic pregnancy when contraception fails (Chap. 32, p. 691). Irregular uterine bleeding is a distinct disadvantage and can consist of amenorrhea, spotting, breakthrough bleeding, and prolonged periods of amenorrhea or menorrhagia. Ovarian functional cysts occur with a greater frequency in women using these agents. Another disadvantage is that to be effective they must be taken at the same or nearly the same time daily (Gillebaud, 1985).

Contraindications. Progestin-only pills are contraindicated in women, especially older women, with unexplained uterine bleeding. A history of a previous ectopic pregnancy or previous functional ovarian cysts also should be considered as relative contraindications.

Injectable Progestin Contraceptives. The advantages of injected progestins include a contraceptive effectiveness comparable to combined oral contraceptives (World Health Organization, 1983), long-lasting action with injections required only 4 to 6 times a year, and minimal impairment of lactation. Medroxyprogesterone acetate (*Depo-Provera*) and norethindrone ethanthate (*Norgest*) have been used effectively in more than 90 countries for many years. *Depo-Provera* only recently has been approved for contraceptive use in the United States. Their mechanisms of action appear to be multiple and include ovulation inhibition, increased cervical mucus viscosity, and production of an endometrium unfavorable for ovum implantation.

Disadvantages of these compounds include prolonged amenorrhea, uterine bleeding during and after its use, and prolonged anovulation after discontinuation. Return of fertility is delayed but not prevented. Hypertension and thromboembolism are not contraindications, because there is no estrogen component. Triglycerides and HDL-cholesterol are both reduced in long-term users, but LDL-cholesterol is not increased (Deslypere and associates, 1985). These agents modify glucose metabolism only slightly in long-term users. Finally, the risks of breast, cervix, and hepatic malignancy do not appear to be increased, and the risk of ovarian and endometrial cancers is decreased in women using this contraception (Liskin and Blackburn, 1987).

Medroxyprogesterone acetate is injected deeply into the upper outer quadrant of the buttock without massage to insure the drug is released slowly. The usual dose is 150 mg every 90 days (World Health Organization, 1983). Within days, this results in plasma levels of approximately 1.5 to 3 ng/mL which gradually decline to 0.2 ng/mL at 6 months and become undetectable by 7 to 9 months (Ortiz and colleagues, 1977).

Norethindrone ethanthate is injected in a similar manner in a dose of 200 mg, but it must be reinjected every 60 days (World Health Organization, 1983). Within a week of injection, plasma levels of norethindrone plateau at 10 to 17 ng/mL and remain at these values for about three to four weeks. After this time, the levels fall to approximately 4 ng/mL for 30 to 60 days (Goebelsmann and colleagues, 1979).

The advantages, disadvantages, and contraindications for injectable progestins are the same as those for oral progestins.

Progestin Implants (Norplant System). The *Norplant System* provides levonorgestrel in six silastic containers that are implanted subdermally. Each is 34 mm long, 2.4 mm in diameter, and contains 36 mg of levonorgestrel. The combined 216-mg dose results in an almost immediate plasma release of about 80 μg per day for the first 6 to 8 weeks. By 2 to 6 months after insertion, the release rate is about 30 to 35 μg per day, gradually decreasing to 25 μg per day by 60 months when it should be removed (Hatcher and colleagues, 1990). A newer system, which utilizes only two levonorgestrel-containing rods (Norplant-2), is being evaluated (Population Council, 1986). In this system, levonorgestrel is dispersed homogeneously within a rod of silastic rather than being placed in a silastic tube.

Contraceptive Effectiveness. During 18,530 woman-months of use, 19 pregnancies were reported in women using levonorgestrel implants, 11 of which occurred in years 6 to 8 (Diaz and colleagues, 1987). Data from the Population Council (Sivin, 1988), based on more than 12,000 woman-years of experience, indicates a failure rate in the first year of 0.04 per 100 woman-years. The rate was 0.2 in the second year, and rates of 0.9, 0.5, and 1.1 were reported in the third, fourth, and fifth years. Thus, this form of contraception is one of the most effective available. Importantly, after termination of use, normal fertility is promptly restored (Sivin and colleagues, 1992).

Mode of Action. Ovulation is not always inhibited. Up to one third of cycles may be ovulatory based upon serum progesterone determinations of 3 ng/mL (Brache and associates, 1990). This estimate is likely overestimated by a factor of two, based upon normal progesterone values during ovulatory cycles (see Chap. 2, p. 45). Even so, with progestin-induced changes in cervical mucus and endometrium, the contraceptive effect is extremely effective. Finally, despite early reports that contraceptive effectiveness was dependent on and inversely proportional to body weight in excess of 70 kg, the development of a newer delivery system utilizing a thinner silastic tube has partially eliminated this concern.

Advantages and Disadvantages. These are almost identical to oral progestins (p. 1334) except for their effect on carbohydrate metabolism. Konje and associates (1992) reported that after six months use glucose and insulin values were altered even in non-diabetic women. They cautioned that these changes were not significant in normal women, but they were concerns in potential diabetics. Because of minor surgery involved, there are problems associated with local infection. If the capsules are not inserted as directed, removal is more difficult.

CONTRAINDICATIONS. Contraindications are the same as those for oral progestins (see p. 1335). Importantly, as emphasized by the American Medical Association Board of Trustees (1992), these agents are not to be used by governmental agencies to coerce women into using contraception in return for receipt of benefits.

Vaginal Progestin Rings. Vaginal time-release rings containing levonorgestrel or progesterone are undergo-

ing clinical trials (Liskin and Blackburn, 1987). These devices have the obvious advantage of easy insertion and removal, advantages not available with injectable or implantable progestins. They are not currently approved for use in the United States.

POSTCOITAL CONTRACEPTION

Estrogens and Progestins. Stilbestrol administered after intercourse to prevent unwanted pregnancy has come to be known as the *morning-after pill.* Kuchara (1971) reported no pregnancies in 1000 women who had inadequate contraceptive protection at the time of intercourse but within 3 days began to take stilbestrol, 25 mg twice daily for the next 5 days.

Pregnancy prevention has also been reported with a variety of other hormonal regimens (Table 60–9) and with copper-containing intrauterine devices. Best results are obtained if the steroidal agents are administered within 72 hours of sexual intercourse. The ethinyl estradiol regimens usually consist of 2.5 mg morning and evening for 5 days. The conjugated estrogen technique consists of 15 mg morning and evening for 5 days. These high-dose regimens (including stilbestrol) are extremely effective with failure rates varying between 0.6 and 1.6 percent (Table 60–9). No controls were included in the summarized results presented in Table 60–9. Nonetheless, if 7 of 100 women who have coitus at midcycle actually conceive as estimated by Dixon and associates (1980), then these high-dose treatment regimens are likely very effective.

TABLE 60–9. POSTCOITAL CONTRACEPTION: OBSERVED PREGNANCY RATES

Drug and Dosage	No. of Patients[a]	No. of Pregnancies	Pregnancy Rate (%)	Follow Up (%)
Ethinyl estradiol 2–5 mg/day × 5 days	2336	13	0.6	100
Ethinyl estradiol 5 mg/day × 5 days	832	6	0.7	87
Diethylstilbestrol 25–50 mg/day × 5 days	545	4	0.7	100
Conjugated estrogens 30 mg/day × 5 days	430	7	1.6	94
Ethinyl estradiol 200 μg +Norgestrel 2mg/day × 1 day	3553	63	1.8	83
Danazol 800 mg/day	668	17	2.5	100
Danazol 1200 mg/day	330	3	0.9	100

[a] Treated within 72 hours of exposure. No controls were included in any of the studies.
Adapted from Fasoli and associates (1989).

Nausea and Vomiting. Nausea and vomiting may be severe with estrogen regimens, especially with stilbestrol and ethinyl estradiol. We routinely prescribe an oral antiemetic such as phenergan one hour before breakfast and the evening meal. Rectal suppositories may also be used. The high-dose estrogen then is taken after the meal. Because of these problems, Yuzpe and Lancee (1977) proposed a lower estrogen dose combined with a progestin. They administered two *Ovral* tablets (100 μg ethinyl estradiol and 0.5 mg norgestrel) morning and evening. This is less effective (1.8 versus 0.7 percent) compared with higher-dose estrogen therapy, but compliance is improved. This preparation was not approved for this use and is no longer available in the United States (FDA, 1988).

Danazol. Rowlands and colleagues (1983) used danazol as a postcoital contraceptive in 400 mg morning and evening doses for 5 days. Initial failure rates were 6 percent, no better than expected without therapy. If the total experience with danazol is considered, however, the failure rate with 800 mg per day is 2.5 percent, and that can be reduced to 1.9 percent by increasing the dose to 1200 mg per day (Table 60–9). Compliance is improved with danazol, but cost is prohibitive. Because of the short duration of use, androgenic side effects are not prominent.

Copper-containing Intrauterine Devices. Fasoli and co-workers (1989) reviewed postcoital contraception and summarized results from nine studies. They included results from 879 women who accepted some type of copper-containing intrauterine device as their sole means of postcoital contraception. Only one pregnancy was reported, and it aborted spontaneously.

Intrauterine postcoital contraception should likely not be utilized in nulligravid women. It should also probably not be used for women with multiple sexual partners or those with a history of pelvic inflammatory disease because of the increased risk for ectopic pregnancy if the method fails (see Chap. 32, p. 691).

RU 486 and Epostane. These agents are discussed in Chapter 31 (p. 685). They are not available in the United States for the provision of abortion. Both agents logically should be ideal agents to use for postcoital contraception. They would be expected to block progesterone production (epostane) or action (RU 486), and thus prevent implantation. This would produce a so-called *menstrual induction.* Glasier and colleagues (1991, 1992) confirmed the effectiveness of mifepristone (RU 486) as an effective postcoital contraceptive. A single 600 mg oral dose of RU 486 prevented any pregnancies in 402 women at risk of pregnancy compared with four pregnancies in 398 women who twice received 100 μg of ethinyl estradiol and 1 mg of norgestrel 12 hours apart.

As of early 1992, neither drug is available for use in the United States. Grimes and Cook (1992) have made a convincing argument that mifepristone for postcoital contraception will lower the induced abortion rate.

Failure of Postcoital Contraception. The use of any postcoital contraceptive method is associated with failures. This can likely be reduced by employing a barrier technique until the next menses to prevent fertilization after use of the postcoital method. It must be remembered that estrogen administration prior to ovulation may induce ovulation. Finally, if menses are delayed for more than 3 weeks past their expected onset, pregnancy is likely. Serum chorionic gonadotropin should be measured to diagnose pregnancy as early as possible. This will allow the woman time to make a choice concerning her pregnancy.

Lactation

Breast feeding is important to infant health and to childspacing. For mothers who are nursing their infants, ovulation during the first 10 weeks after delivery is very unlikely according to Pérez (1981). Nursing is not a very reliable method of family planning, however, for women whose infants are on a 3- to 4-hour, daytime-only feeding schedule and are receiving other food (see Chap. 18, p. 471). **Waiting for first menses involves a risk of pregnancy because ovulation may antedate menstruation.** Certainly, after the first menses, contraception is essential unless the woman desires another pregnancy. Estrogen-progestin contraceptives are thought by some to reduce both the rate and the duration of milk production. The benefits from prevention of pregnancy by the use of combined oral contraceptives would appear to outweigh the risks in selected patients, but progestin-only oral contraceptives appear to be the best choice (see p. 1334).

Intrauterine devices have been recommended for the lactating, but potentially ovulating, sexually active woman (see Chap. 61, p. 1341). An increased rate of uterine perforation has been identified in lactating women with an intrauterine device, perhaps as the consequence of vigorous myometrial contractions and involution brought about by the release of oxytocin in response to suckling (Heartwell and Schlesselman, 1983). The risk is not so great however, that intrauterine devices should not be used.

References

American College of Obstetricians and Gynecologists: Contraception for women in their later reproductive years. ACOG Committee Opinion No. 41, December 1985

American Medical Association Board of Trustees: Requirements or incentives by government for the use of long-acting contraceptives. JAMA 267:1818, 1992

Andersch B, Hahn L: Premenstrual complaints, II. Influence of oral contraceptives. Acta Obstet Gynecol Scand 60:579, 1981

Antoniades K, Campbell WN, Hecksher RH, Kessler WB, McCarthy GE Jr: Liver cell adenoma and oral contraceptives. JAMA 234:628, 1975

Back DJ, Breckenridge AM, Crawford FE, Hall JM, MacIver M, Orme ML, Rowe PH, Smith E, Watts MJ: The effects of rifampicin on the pharmacokinetics of ethinyl estradiol in women. Contraception 21:135, 1980

Badaracco MA, Vessey MP: Recurrence of venous thromboembolic disease and use of oral contraceptives. BMJ 1:215, 1974

Beral V, Hannaford PC, Kay C: Oral contraceptive use and malignancies of the genital tract. Lancet 2:1331, 1988

Betrabet SS, Shikary ZK, Toddywalla VS, Toddywalla SP, Patel D, Saxena BN: ICMR Task Force Study on hormonal contraception. Transfer of norethindrone (NET) and levonorgestrel (LNG) from a single tablet into the infant's circulation through the mother's milk. Contraception 35:517, 1987.

Brache V, Alvarez-Sanchez F, Faundes A, Tejada AS, Cochon L: Ovarian endocrine function through 5 years of continuous treatment with Norplant® subdermal contraceptive implants. Contraception 41:169, 1990

Bracken MB, Hillenbrand KG, Holford TR: Contraception delay after oral contraceptive use: The effect of estrogen dose. Fertil Steril 53:21, 1990

Briggs NH: Implications and assessments of metabolic effects of oral contraceptives. In New Considerations In Oral Contraception. New York, BMI Publications, 1982, p 131

Butterworth CE Jr, Hatch KD, Macaluso M, Cole P, Sauberlich HE, Soong SJ, Borst M, Baker V: Folate deficiency and cervical dysplasia. JAMA 267:528, 1992

Cameron IT, Baird DT: Early pregnancy termination: A comparison between vacuum aspiration and medical abortion using prostaglandin (16, 16 dimethyl-trans-Δ-PGE$_1$ methyl ester) or the antiprogesterone RU 486. Br J Obstet Gynaecol 95:271, 1988

Cancer and Steroid Hormone Study of the Centers for Disease Control and the National Institute of Child Health and Development: Combination oral contraceptive use and the risk of endometrial cancer. JAMA 257:796, 1987a

Cancer and Steroid Hormone Study of the Centers for Disease Control and the National Institute of Child Health and Development: The reduction in risk of ovarian cancer associated with oral-contraceptive use. N Engl J Med 316:650, 1987b

Cancer and Steroid Hormone Study of the Centers for Disease Control and the National Institute of Child Health and Development: Oral-contraceptive use and the risk of breast cancer. N Engl J Med 315:405, 1986

Carr BR, Parker CR Jr, Madden JD, MacDonald PC, Porter JC: Plasma levels of adrenocorticotropin and cortisol in women receiving oral contraceptive steroid treatment. J Clin Endocrinol Metab 49:346, 1979

Centers for Disease Control: Oral contraceptive use and the risk of breast cancer. JAMA 249:1591, 1983a

Centers for Disease Control: Oral contraceptive use and the risk of ovarian cancer. JAMA 249:1596, 1983b

Centers for Disease Control: Oral contraceptive use and the risk of endometrial cancer. JAMA 249:1600, 1983c

Contraception Report 3:4, May, 1992

Couzinet B, Le Strat N, Ulmann A, Baulieu EE, Schaison G: Termination of early pregnancy by the progesterone antagonist RU 486 (mifepristone). N Engl J Med 315:1555, 1986

Craft P, Hannaford PC: Risk factors for acute myocardial infarction in women: Evidence from the Royal College of General Practitioners' Oral Contraceptive Study. BMJ 298:165, 1989

Crooij MJ, De Nooyer CCA, Rao BR, Berends GT, Gooren LJG, Janssens J: Termination of early pregnancy by the 3β-hydroxysteroid dehydrogenase inhibitor epostane. N Engl J Med 319:813, 1988

Das C, Catt KJ: Antifertility actions of the progesterone antagonist RU 486 include direct inhibition of placental hormone secretion. Lancet 2:599, 1987

Diaz S, Pavez M, Miranda P, Johansson ED, Croxatto HB: Long-term followup of women treated with Norplant implants. Contraception 35:551, 1987

Dickey RP: Managing Contraceptive Pill Patients, 6th ed. Durant, Oklahoma, Creative Informatics, Inc., 1991, pp 207, 208

Deslypere JP, Thiery M, Vermenulen A: Effect of long-term hormonal contraception on plasma lipids. Contraception 31:633, 1985

Dixon GW, Schlesselman JJ, Ory HW, Blye RP: Ethinyl estradiol and conjugated estrogens as postcoital contraceptives. JAMA 244:1336, 1980

Dorflinger LJ: Relative potency of progestins used in oral contraceptives. Contraception 31:357, 1985

Edelman DA, Kothenbeutel R, Levinski MJ, Kelly SE: Comparative trials of low-dose combined oral contraceptives. J Reprod Med 28:195, 1983

Ellis JW: Multiphasic oral contraceptives: Efficacy and metabolic impact. J Reprod Med 32:38, 1987

Fasoli M, Parazzini F, Cecchetti G, La Vecchia C: Post-coital contraception: An overview of published studies. Contraception 39:459, 1989

FDA: Drug Bulletin 14:2, 1984

FDA: Drug Bulletin 16:2, 1986

FDA: Drug Bulletin 18:19, 1988

Fisch IR, Frank J: Oral contraceptives and blood pressure. JAMA 237:2499, 1977

Francis WJA: Reproduction at menarche and menopause in women. J Reprod Fertil (suppl) 12:89, 1970

Glasier A, Thong KJ, Dewar M, Mackie M, Baird DT: Postcoital contraception with mifepristone. Lancet 337:1414, 1991

Glasier A, Thong KJ, Dewar M, Mackie M, Baird DT: Mifepristone (RU 486) compared with high-dose estrogen and progestagen for emergency postcoital contraception. N Engl J Med 327:1041, 1992

Goebelsmann U, Stanczyk FZ, Brenner PF, Goebelsmann AE, Gentzschein EK, Mishell DR Jr: Serum norethindrone (NET) concentrations following intramusculalr NET enanthate injection. Effect upon serum LH, FSH, estradiol and progesterone. Contraception 19:283, 1979

Greenblatt RB: Progestational agents in clinical practice. Med Science 18:37, 1967

Grimes DA, Cook RJ: Mifepristone (RU 486)—an abortifacient to prevent abortion? N Engl J Med 327:1088, 1988

Grimes DA, Mishell DR Jr, Soupe D, Lacarra M: Early abortion with a single dose of the antiprogestin RU-486. Am J Obstet Gynecol 158:1307, 1988

Guillebaud J: Contraception: Your Questions Answered. New York, Pitman, 1985

Harlap S, Kost K, Forrest JD: Preventing pregnancy, protecting health: A new look at birth control choices in the United States. New York and Washington, DC. The Alan Guttmacher Institute, 1991

Hatcher RA, Stewart F, Trussel J, Kowal P, Guest F, Stewart GK, Cates W: Contraceptive Technology, 15th ed. New York, Irvington, 1990, pp 256, 259, 261, 264, 266

Heartwell SF, Schlesselman S: Risk of uterine perforation among users of intrauterine devices. Obstet Gynecol 61:31, 1983

Heinen G: The discriminating use of combination and sequential preparations in hormonal inhibition of ovulation. Contraception 4:393, 1974

Holt VL, Daling JR, McKnight B, Moore D, Stergachis A, Weiss NS: Functional ovarian cysts in relation to the use of monophasic and triphasic oral contraceptives. Obstet Gynecol 79:529, 1992

Hull MGR, Savage PE, Bromham DR, Jackson JAM: Normal fertility in women with post-pill amenorrhea. Lancet 1:1329, 1981

Irey NS, Nanion WC, Taylor HB: Vascular lesions in women taking oral contraceptives. Arch Pathol 89:1, 1970

Janevich DT, Piper JM, Glebatis DM: Oral contraceptives and congenital limb reduction defects. N Engl J Med 291:697, 1974

Jones RC, Edgren RA: The effects of various steroids on the vaginal histology in the rat. Fertil Steril 24:284, 1973

Kalkhoff RK: Relative sensitivity of postpartum gestational diabetic women to oral contraceptive agents and other metabolic stress. Diabetes Care 3:421, 1980

Kauppinen-Mäkelin R, Kuusi T, Ylikorkala O, Tikkanen MJ: Contraceptives containing desogestrel or levonorgestrel have different effects on serum lipoproteins and post-heparin plasma lipase activities. Clin Endocrinol 36:203, 1992

Kay CR: The Royal College of General Practitioners' Oral Contraception Study: Some recent observations. Clin Obstet Gynaecol 11:759, 1984

Kay CR, Hannaford PC: Breast cancer and the pill—A further report from the Royal College of General Practitioners' Oral Contraceptive Study. Br J Cancer 58:676, 1988

Kent DR, Nissen ED, Nissen SE, Ziehm DJ: Effect of pregnancy on liver tumor associated with oral contraceptives. Obstet Gynecol 51:148, 1978

Knopp RH: Cardiovascular effects of endogenous and exogenous sex hormones over a woman's lifetime. Am J Obstet Gynecol 158:1630, 1988

Konje JC, Otolorin EO, Ladipo OA: The effect of continuous subdermal levonorgestrel (Norplant) on carbohydrate metabolism. Am J Obstet Gynecol 166:15, 1992

Krauss RM, Roy S, Mishell DR Jr, Casagrande J, Pike MC: Effects of two low-dose oral contraceptives on serum lipids and lipoproteins: Differential changes in high-density lipoprotein subclasses. Am J Obstet Gynecol 145:446, 1983

Kuchara LK: Postcoital contraception with diethylstilbestrol. JAMA 218:562, 1971

Lammer EJ, Cordero JF: Exogenous sex hormone exposure and the risk for major malformations. JAMA 255:3128, 1986

Leklem JE, Brown RR, Rose DP, Linkswiler HM: Vitamin B$_6$ requirements of women using oral contraceptives. Am J Clin Nutr 28:535, 1975

Linn S, Schoenbaum SC, Monson RR, Rosner B, Ryan KJ: Delay in conception for former "pill" users. JAMA 247:629, 1982

Linn S, Schoenbaum SC, Monson RR, Rosner B, Stubblefield PG, Ryan KJ: Lack of association between contraceptive usage and congenital malformations in offspring. Am J Obstet Gynecol 147:923, 1983

Liskin L, Blackburn R: Hormonal contraception: New long-acting methods. Popul Rep [K]3: 1987

Mann JI: Progestogens in cardiovascular disease: An introduction to the epidemiologic data. Am J Obstet Gynecol 142:752, 1982

Meade TW: Risks and mechanisms of cardiovascular events in users of oral contraceptives. Am J Obstet Gynecol 158:1646, 1988

Meade TW: Oral contraceptives, clotting factors and thrombosis. Am J Obstet Gynecol 142:758, 1982

Meirik O, Lund E, Adami H, Bergstrom R, Christoffersen T, Bergsö P: Oral contraceptive use and breast cancer in young women: A joint national case-control study in Sweden and Norway. Lancet 1:650, 1986

Metcalf MG: Incidence of ovulatory cycles in women approaching the menopause. J Biosoc Sci 11:39, 1979

Metcalf MG, Donald RA: Fluctuating ovarian function in a perimenopausal woman. Aust NZ Med J 89:45, 1979

Mileikowsky GN, Nadler JL, Huey F, Francis R, Roy S: Evidence that smoking alters prostacyclin formation and platelet aggregation in women who use oral contraceptives. Am J Obstet Gynecol 159:1547, 1988

Miller NE, Hammett F, Saltissi S, Rao S, van Zeller H, Coltart J, Lewis B: Relation of angiographically defined coronary artery disease to plasma lipoprotein subfractions and apolipoproteins. BMJ 282:1741, 1982

Mishell DR Jr: Noncontraceptive health benefits of oral contraceptives. Am J Obstet Gynecol 142:809, 1982

Mishell DR Jr: Use of oral contraceptives in women of older reproductive age. Am J Obstet Gynecol 158:1652, 1988

Miyaura S, Eguchi H, Johnston JM: Effect of a cigarette smoke extract on the metabolism of the proinflammatory autocoid, platelet-activating factor. Circ Res 70:341, 1992

Miyaura S, Maki N, Byrd W, Johnston JM: The hormonal regulation of platelet-activating factor acetylhydrolase activity in plasma. Lipids 26:1015, 1991

Mosher WD, Pratt WF: Contraceptive use in the United States, 1973–1988. Patient Educ Conns 16:163, 1990

Neuberger J, Forman D, Doll R, Williams R: Oral contraceptives and hepatocellular carcinoma. BMJ 292:1355, 1986

Nieman LK, Choate TM, Chrousos GP, Healy DL, Morin M, Renquist D, Merriam GR, Spitz IM, Bardin CW, Baulieu EE, Loriaux DL: The progesterone antagonist RU 486: A potential new contraceptive agent. N Engl J Med 316:187, 1987

Nilsson L, Sölvell L: Clinical studies on oral contraceptives. Acta Obstet Gynecol Scand (suppl) 8:46, 1967

Nora AH, Nora JJ: A syndrome of multiple congenital anomalies associated with teratogenic exposure. Arch Environ Health 30:17, 1975

Ortiz A, Hirol M, Stanczyk FZ, Goebelsmann U, Mishell DR: Serum medroxyprogesterone acetate (MPA) concentrations and ovarian function following intramuscular injection of depo-MPA. J Clin Endocrinol Metab 44:32, 1977

Ory HW: The noncontraceptive health benefits from oral contraceptive use. Fam Plann Perspect 14:182, 1982

Parazzini F, Negri E, La Vecchia C, Fedele L, Rabaiotti M,

Luchini L: Oral contraceptive use and risk of uterine fibroids. Obstet Gynecol 79:430, 1992

Patsch W, Brown SA, Gatto AM Jr, Young RL: The effects of triphasic oral contraceptives on plasma lipids and lipoproteins. Am J Obstet Gynecol 161:1396, 1989

Paul C, Skegg DCG, Spears GFS, Kaldor JM: Oral contraceptives and breast cancer: A national study. BMJ 293:723, 1986

Pérez A: Natural family planning: Postpartum period. Int J Fertil 26:219, 1981

Phillips N, Duffy T: One-hour glucose tolerance in relation to the use of oral contraceptive drugs. Am J Obstet Gynecol 116:91, 1973

Pike MC, Henderson BE, Krailo MD, Duke A, Roy S: Breast cancer in young women and use of oral contraceptives: Possible modifying effect of formulation and age at use. Lancet 2:926, 1983

Pituitary Adenoma Study Group: Pituitary adenomas and oral contraceptives: A multi-center case controlled study. Fertil Steril 39:753, 1983

Population Council. Norplant fact sheet. Norplant Worldwide 5:2, August 1986

Porter JB, Jick H, Walker AM: Mortality among oral contraceptive users. Obstet Gynecol 70:29, 1987

Porter JB, Hunter JR, Jick H, Stergachis A: Oral contraceptives and nonfatal vascular disease. Obstet Gynecol 66:1, 1985

Prentice RL, Thomas DB: On the epidemiology of oral contraceptives and disease. Adv Cancer Res 49:285, 1987

Pritchard JA, Pritchard SA: Blood pressure response to estrogen–progestin oral contraceptive after pregnancy-induced hypertension. Am J Obstet Gynecol 129:733, 1977

Realini JP, Goldzieher JW: Oral contraceptives and cardiovascular disease: A critique of the epidemiologic studies. Am J Obstet Gynecol 152:729, 1985

Reuter KL, Baker SP, Krolikowski FJ: Risk factors for breast cancer in women undering mammography. AJR 158:273, 1992

Robinson JC, Plichta S, Weisman CS, Nathanson CA, Ensminger M: Dysmenorrhea and use of oral contraceptives in adolescent women attending a family planning clinic. Am J Obstet Gynecol 166:578, 1992

Rosenberg L, Palmer JR, Lesk SM, Shapiro S: Oral contraceptives use and the risk of myocardial infarction. Am J Epidemiol 131:1009, 1990

Rothman KJ, Louik C: Oral contraceptives and birth defects. N Engl J Med 299:522, 1978

Rowlands S, Guillebaud J, Bounds W, Booth M: Side effects of danazol compared with an ethinylestradiol/norgestrel combination when used for postcoital contraception. Contraception 27:39, 1983

Royal College of General Practitioners' Oral Contraceptive Study: Oral contraceptives and gallbladder disease. Lancet 2:957, 1982

Runnebaum B, Rabe T: New progestogens in oral contraceptives. Am J Obstet Gynecol 157:1059, 1987

Savolainen E, Saksela E, Saxen L: Teratogenic hazards of oral contraceptives analyzed in a national malformation register. Am J Obstet Gynecol 140:521, 1981

Schlesselman JJ, Stadel BV, Murray P, Lai S: Breast cancer in relation to early use of oral contraceptives: No evidence of latent effect. JAMA 259:1828, 1988

Shikary ZK, Betrabet SS, Patel ZM, Patel S, Joshi JV, Toddywala VS, Toddywala SP, Patel DM, Jhaveri K, Saxena BN: ICMR Task Force Study on hormonal contraception. Transfer of levonorgestrel (LNG) administered through different drug delivery systems from the maternal circulation via breast milk. Contraception 35:477, 1987

Sivin I: International experience with norplant and norplant-2 contraceptives. Stud Fam Plann 19:81, 1988

Sivin I, Stern J, Diaz S, Pavéz M, Alvarez F, Brache V, Mishell DR Jr, Lacarra M, McCarthy T, Holma P, Darney P, Klaisle C, Olsson SE, Odlind V: Rates and outcomes of planned pregnancy after use of Norplant capsules, Norplant II rods, or levonorgestrel-releasing or copper TCu 380 Ag intrauterine contraceptive devices. Am J Obstet Gynecol 166:1208, 1992

Skouby SO, Kühl C, Mølsted-Pedersen L, Petersen K, Christensen MS: Triphasic oral contraception: Metabolic effects in normal women and those with previous gestational diabetes. Am J Obstet Gynecol 153:495, 1985

Spellacy WN, Buhi WC, Birk SA: Prospective studies of carbohydrate metabolism in "normal" women using norgestrel for 18 months. Fertil Steril 35:167, 1981

Spellacy WN, Buhi WC, Birk SA, Vann Arnarn JB: Carbohydrate metabolism studies in women using Brevicon, a low-estrogen type of oral contraceptive for one year. Am J Obstet Gynecol 142:105, 1982

Stadel BV: Oral contraceptives and cardiovascular disease. N Engl J Med 305:612, 672, 1981

Stampfer MJ, Willett WC, Colditz GA, Speizer FE, Hennekens CH: A prospective study of past use of oral contraceptive agents and risk of cardiovascular diseases. N Engl J Med 319:1313, 1988

Strom BL, Tamragouri RN, Morse ML, Lazar EL, West SL, Stolley PD, Jones JK: Oral contraceptives and other risk factors for gallbladder diseases. Clin Pharmacol Ther 39:335, 1986

Swyer GI: Potency of progestogens in oral contraceptives—further delay of menses data. Contraception 26:23, 1982

Szlachter BN, Nachtigall LE, Epstein J, Young BK, Weiss G: Premature menopause: A reversible entity? Obstet Gynecol 54:396, 1979

Tikkanen MJ, Nikkilä EA, Kuusi T, Sipinen S: Reduction of plasma high density lipoprotein$_2$ cholesterol and increase of post heparin plasma hepatic lipase activity during progestin treatment. Clin Chem Acta 115:63, 1981

Tikkanen MJ, Nikkilä EA, Kuusi T, Sipinen SU: High density lipoprotein$_2$ and hepatic lipase: Reciprocal changes produced by estrogen and norgestrel. J Clin Endocrinol Metab 54:1113, 1982

Toews M, Boone S, Watson M, Whillans J: A multicenter phase IV study of Ortho 7/7/7 tablets in previous users of oral contraceptives. Curr Ther Res 41:509, 1987

Trussell J, Hatcher R, Cates W, Stewart F, Kost K: Contraceptive failure in the United States: An update. Stud Fam Plann 21, 1990

Trussel J, Kost K: Contraceptive failure in the United States: A critical review of the literature. Stud Fam Plann 18:237, 1987

Vessey MP: Thromboembolism, cancer, and oral contraceptives. Clin Obstet Gynecol 17:65, 1974

Vessey MP, Baron J, Doll R, McPherson K, Yeates D: Oral contraceptives and breast cancer: Final report of an epidemiological study. Br J Cancer 47:455, 1983a

Vessey MP, Lawless M, Yeates D: Efficacy of different contraceptive methods. Lancet 1:841, 1982

Vessey MP, Lawless M, Yeates D, McPherson K: Progestin-only oral contraception: Findings in a large prospective study with special reference to effectiveness. Br J Fam Plann 10:117, 1985

Vessey MP, McPherson K, Lawless M, Yeates D: Neoplasia of the cervix uteri and contraception: A possible adverse effect of the pill. Lancet 2:930, 1983b

Vessey MP, Villard-Mackintosh L, McPherson K, Yeates D: Mortality among oral contraceptive users: 20 year follow up of women in a cohort study. BMJ 299:1487, 1989

Weir RJ: Effect on blood pressure of changing from high to low dose steroid preparations in women with oral contraceptive induced hypertension. Scott Med J 27:212, 1982

Williams NB: Contraceptive Technology 1986–1987. New York, Irvington, 1986, p 183

Wingrave AJ, Kay CR, Vessey MP: Oral contraceptives and diabetes mellitus. BMJ 1:23, 1979

Woods ER, Grace E, Havens KK, Merola JL, Emans SJ: Contraceptive compliance with a levonorgestrel triphasic and a norethindrone monophasic oral contraceptive in adolescent patients. Am J Obstet Gynecol 166:901, 1992

World Health Organization: Combined oral contraceptives and liver cancer. Int J Cancer 43:254, 1989

World Health Organization, Special Programme of Research, Development and Research Training in Human Reproduction, Task Force on Long-acting Systemic Agents for the Regulation of Fertility: Multinational comparative clinical evaluation of two long-acting injectable contraceptive steroids: Norethindrone enanthate and medroxyprogesterone acetate—final report. Contraception 28:1, 1983

Wynn V: Vitamins and oral contraceptive use. Lancet 1:561, 1975

Wynn V, Godsland I: Effects of oral contraceptives on carbohydrate metabolism. J Reprod Med (suppl 9) 31:892, 1986

Yuzpe AA, Lancee WJ: Ethinylestradiol and dl-norgestrel as a postcoital contraceptive. Fertil Steril 28:932, 1977

CHAPTER 61

Mechanical Methods of Contraception

Intrauterine Contraceptive Devices

Since early in this century, attempts have been made—sporadically at the outset but becoming very intense by 1960—to design an intrauterine device that would prevent pregnancy without causing adverse effects. One intriguing but unconfirmed story describes the insertion of small stones into camels' uteri to prevent pregnancy during long caravans.

At one time in the United States, approximately 7 percent of sexually active women used an intrauterine device for contraception. Two devices currently approved are shown in Figure 61–1. The pregnancy rates in larger studies generally vary from 0.5 to 5 per 100 woman-years (Population Reports, 1982a).

By 1986, the two most popular intrauterine devices used by American women had been withdrawn voluntarily from the market by their manufacturers. The announced reason for the withdrawal of the Lippes loop and Cu 7 was the financial burden of defense in liability cases. Nearly 2 million women were suddenly left with doubts as to their ability to continue use of this effective, generally safe contraceptive method, which was approved by the Food and Drug Administration. At that time, about half of the women in the United States wearing intrauterine devices were acceptable candidates for oral contraceptive therapy. Some of the remaining women continued to use the inert plastic devices, which could be left in place indefinitely. Many women, however, had to choose between alternative, albeit less effective, contraceptive measures and permanent sterilization. Fortunately, the Progestasert (Fig. 61–1) continued to be marketed in the United States in limited quantities but at a very high cost to the consumer. Although developed much earlier by the nonprofit Population Council, the copper T model 380A (Fig. 61–1) did not become commercially available in the United States until 1988. It too is very expensive.

Theoretical Advantages. Ideally, an intrauterine device would be inserted once, and would provide complete protection against pregnancy. It would neither be expelled spontaneously nor have to be removed for adverse effects; and after removal to allow a planned pregnancy, it would have induced no changes to prevent normal pregnancy. To date, these objectives have not been fully achieved by any device.

Types of Intrauterine Devices. In general, devices are of two varieties: (1) chemically inert and composed of a nonabsorbable material, most often polyethylene, impregnated with barium sulfate for radiopacity; and (2) chemically active in which there is more or less continuous elution from the device of copper or a progestational agent.

Of the chemically inert devices, the *Lippes loop* had been quite popular before it was withdrawn from the market in 1985. Even so, many American women continue to wear these devices that were inserted before that time.

Progestasert. The Progestasert is a T-shaped ethylene vinyl acetate co-polymer with a vertical stem containing 38 mg of progesterone and barium sulfate in a silicone base. The progesterone source supplies approximately 65 μg/day into the uterine cavity. This does not alter plasma progesterone values. The device is 36 mm long and 32 mm wide, and has a single dark blue to black string attached to the base of the stem (Fig. 61–1). For insertion, the withdrawal technique must be used (see p. 1346).

A device similar to the Progestasert, but containing levonorgestrel, is currently being tested in Europe. Its major advantage appears to be the need to replace it only once every 5 years, compared with yearly for the Progestasert.

Copper T 380A. The Copper T 380A is also T shaped, but it is composed of polyethylene and barium sulfate. The stem is wound with 314 mm^2 of fine copper wire, and the arms each have 33 mm^2 copper bracelets, thus totalling 380 mm^2 of copper. Two strings extend from the base of the stem (Fig. 61–1). Originally, the strings were blue, but they now are an off-white color. The "A" designation is to identify this model as having an enlarged bulbous stem base. This allegedly reduces the incidence of cervical and lower uterine perforations by the distal tip. **It is important to note that this device should not be "loaded" into its inserter tube more than 5 minutes before it is inserted.**

Mechanisms of Action. The mechanisms by which these devices effect contraception have not been defined precisely. Interference with successful implantation of the fertilized ovum, which at one time was believed to be the mode of action, may be its least

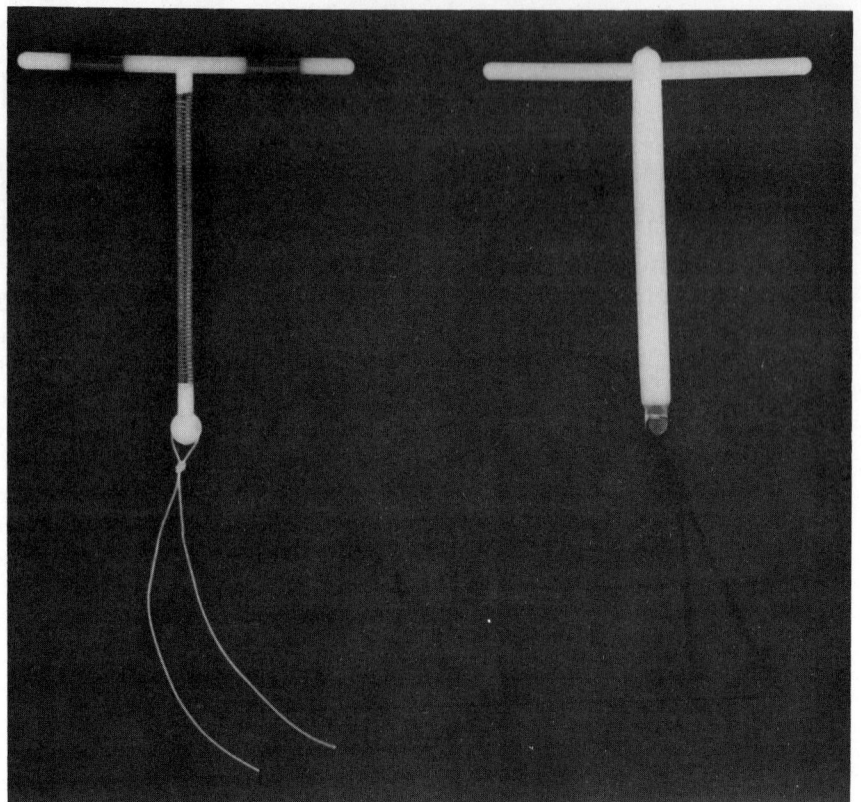

Fig. 61–1. Intrauterine contraceptive devices available in 1993. At left is a Copper T 380A (Courtesy of GynoPharma, Somerville, New Jersey) and to the right is a Progestasert (Courtesy of ALZA Corp., Palo Alto, CA).

important action. Specifically, an intense local inflammatory response is induced, especially by copper-containing devices, that in turn leads to lysosomal activation and other inflammatory actions that are spermicidal (Alverez and associates, 1988; Moyer and Mishell, 1971; Ortiz and Croxatto, 1987; Population Reports, 1982a). In the unlikely event fertilization does occur, the same inflammatory actions are directed against the blastocyst. The report by Lippes and co-workers (1978) that insertion of a Copper T or Cu7 device up to 7 days after coitus effectively prevented pregnancy strongly supports the concept that copper-bearing devices also can compromise the blastocyst (see Chap. 60, p. 1335). Providing support for such a mechanism are the observations of Buhler and Papiernik (1983), who described two successive pregnancies in each of four women who had been fitted with intrauterine devices but who chronically were taking anti-inflammatory drugs. For the chemically inert devices, contraceptive effectiveness generally increases with increased size and extent of contact with endometrium.

Certain metals, especially copper, greatly enhance the contraceptive action of inert devices, likely by inducing a more intense local intrauterine inflammatory response. For example, one small T-shaped polyethylene device allowed a pregnancy rate of about 18 per 100 woman-years until the addition of fine copper ribbon with a surface area of 200 mm^2. The pregnancy rate then dropped to about 2 per 100 woman-years. A local,

rather than systemic, action from copper must be of major importance, because metallic copper placed in one uterine horn of a rabbit prevents blastocyst implantation there, but not in the adjacent horn (Zipper and co-workers, 1971).

An additional mechanism includes possibly accelerated tubal motility likely induced by the intrauterine inflammatory response. Also, the endometrium is an extremely hostile site for implantation even if fertilization and successful tubal transport have occurred. Finally, the endometrium is atrophic in long-time Progestasert users.

Effectiveness. Intrauterine devices have one-year and long-term continuation rates second only to implantable contraceptives (Table 60–1). One-year continuation rates are equal to oral contraceptives. This almost certainly is due to their effectiveness and a once-only approach to contraception.

The effectiveness of the devices is similar to overall effectiveness of oral contraceptives. Even so, as shown in Table 60–1, the typical first-year failure rate with a Progestasert is almost four times greater than with the Copper T 380A (1.9 versus 0.5 percent). The Copper T 380A is one of the most effective contraceptive means available. Importantly, the unintended pregnancy rate decreases progressively after the first year of use (Vessey and associates, 1983). This must in part be due to true method failures and not user failures.

Adverse Effects. Numerous complications have been described with use of various intrauterine devices. For the most part, however, common side effects have not been serious, while the serious side effects have not been common. Moreover, with progressive use and advancing user age, unintended pregnancy, expulsion, and bleeding complications decrease in frequency. Finally, with discontinuation, fertility is not impaired (Sivin and colleagues, 1992).

Uterine Perforation and Abortion. The earliest adverse effects are those associated with insertion. They include clinically apparent or silent *uterine perforation,* either while sounding the uterus or during insertion of the device, and *abortion of an unsuspected pregnancy.* The frequency of these complications depends upon operator skill and the precautions taken to avoid interrupting a pregnancy. Although devices may migrate spontaneously into and through the uterine wall, most perforations occur, or at least begin, at the time of insertion.

Uterine Cramping and Bleeding. Uterine *cramping* and some *bleeding* are likely to develop soon after insertion and they persist for variable periods. Cramping at the time of insertion can be minimized by administering a nonsteroidal anti-inflammatory agent approximately 1 hour prior. The occasional increase in cramping with menses also can be controlled in a similar manner. These prostaglandin synthase inhibitors should not be used at other times throughout the cycle because they decrease the contraceptive effectiveness of the devices likely through their anti-inflammatory actions (Buhler and Papiernik, 1983).

Menorrhagia. Blood loss with menstruation is commonly increased by a factor of about two, and may be so great as to cause iron-deficiency anemia. Therefore, it is wise to check the hemoglobin or hematocrit, and possibly the plasma ferritin level, annually in women with intrauterine devices as well as any time they complain of heavy menstruation. This is a troubling side effect, and approximately 15 percent of women using intrauterine devices have them removed for this problem (Hatcher and co-workers, 1990).

The Progestasert, because of its localized progesterone action, is associated with a low incidence of menorrhagia and anemia. For example, normal menstruation results in blood loss of about 35 mL. Mean blood loss with most copper-containing devices is approximately 50 to 60 mL per cycle, but can be more (Guillebaud and colleagues, 1979). Mean blood loss with the Progestasert is about 25 mL per cycle.

Infection. As an aid for ascertaining appropriate placement in the uterine cavity, most devices have an attached synthetic filament. This so-called tail protrudes through the external os and is cut off so that approximately 2 cm is visible through the cervix. There has been concern from the outset that the tail might act as a wick to promote invasion of the uterine cavity by pathogenic bacteria. Purrier and co-workers (1979) identified potentially pathogenic bacteria colonizing mucus that coated the tails of more than half of devices.

Pelvic infections, including septic abortion, have developed with a variety of intrauterine devices. *Tuboovarian abscesses,* which may be unilateral, have been described by Dawood and Birnbaum (1975), Taylor and associates (1973, 1975), and several others. With suspected infection, the device should be removed, and the woman treated with effective antibiotics. She must be observed closely because there have been deaths from sepsis associated with the use of these devices. Even so, such mortality is probably lower than that attributed to estrogen plus progestin oral contraceptives or to pregnancy. Nonetheless, because of the risk of salpingitis, pelvic peritonitis, and pelvic abscess, and as a consequence, sterility, use of an intrauterine device is usually discouraged for women under the age of 25 or those of low parity. Vessey and associates (1983) provided data that reinforce their earlier observations that after removing the devices from parous women, they have no prolonged impairment of fertility. They concluded that pelvic infection sufficient to impair fertility must be very uncommon, at least in parous users of such devices.

Subsequently, Daling (1985) and Cramer (1985) and their associates provided data consistent with the view that intrauterine devices are associated with increased infertility due to tubal factors. These effects were negligible with copper-bearing devices, but more apparent in nulliparous women, especially if they had multiple sexual partners and used the now discontinued Dalkon shield. Interestingly, Lee and Rubin (1988) reported that married women and those with only one sexual partner had no higher risk of developing pelvic inflammatory disease than controls **after** the first 4 months of use.

Immediately following insertion of an intrauterine device, bacteria can be recovered from the uterine cavity for several days, but at appreciably lower rates after the first 24 hours (Mishell and colleagues, 1966). More recent data are consistent with a small increased risk of pelvic inflammatory disease for only up to the first 20 days following insertion (Farley and associates, 1992). Thus, the major risk of infection is due to the insertion process and does not increase with long-term use. In fact, long-term use of copper and hormonal-containing devices results in pelvic inflammatory disease rates comparable with oral contraceptive users. After 45 to 60 days, the uterine cavity is sterile. Thus, any infection after this time should be considered to be sexually transmitted and appropriately treated (Lee and associates, 1983; Mishell and colleagues, 1966). The newer copper and progestin-releasing devices also may reduce the incidence of pelvic inflammatory disease in women using these devices (Editorial, 1992).

Actinomyces-like structures identified in Papanicolaou smears and the prolonged use of an intrauterine device have been linked. The clinical importance of this finding is not clear, but it is worrisome. In most studies, an increased prevalence of *Actinomyces israelii* or actinomyces-like organisms was apparent only after several years of use. Furthermore, the organisms were found much less frequently when a copper-bearing device was used, rather than an inert one, possibly because the former was changed more frequently. Of importance, the percentage of women reporting gynecological symptoms did not differ significantly between users with and without actinomyces-like organisms seen on smear (Petitti and associates, 1983). Keebler and coworkers (1983) identified actinomyces in 12.6 percent of device users. Once the smear became positive for actinomyces bodies, all subsequent smears remained positive until the device was removed. Most agree that, if signs or symptoms of infection develop in women who harbor actinomyces bodies, the device should be removed and antibiotic therapy instituted. Recent evidence is suggestive that *Eubacterium nodatum* may be confused with *Actinomyces israelii* on Papanicolaou smears (Hill, 1992). The bacterium can cause pelvic infection and, if identified, the intrauterine device should probably be removed even in asymptomatic women. In the absence of signs or symptoms of pelvic infection, however, there is considerable disagreement as to whether uniform removal of the device or simply close observation is the correct approach. We remove the device, treat with antibiotics, provide an alternative method of contraception, and replace the device at a later time if requested.

Pregnancy with a Device In Utero. As emphasized in Chapter 9, it is important to identify all pregnant women who might be harboring a device, whether it be intrauterine or extrauterine. A device within the pregnant uterus is risky for the woman and her fetus. A device residing beyond the uterus may be dangerous for the woman. Appropriate steps should be taken at delivery to identify and assure removal of the device.

When pregnancy is recognized and the tail of the device is visible through the cervix, it should be removed. This will help reduce subsequent complications such as late abortion, sepsis, and preterm birth. Tatum and co-workers (1976) observed the abortion rate to be 54 percent with the device left in situ, compared with 25 percent if promptly removed. Moreover, with the device remaining in situ, the frequency of low birthweight, chiefly from preterm delivery, was 20 percent, compared with about 5 percent if the device was removed early. Vessey and associates (1979a) confirmed these observations. If the tail is not visible, no attempt to

locate and remove the device should be made because this may result in abortion. There have been anecdotal reports of successful sonographically assisted removal of devices without visible strings; however, we have had no experience with such attempts.

The likelihood of second-trimester abortion is approximately 50 percent if an intrauterine device remains in a pregnant uterus; moreover, the abortion also is more likely to be septic (Lewit, 1970; Vessey and associates, 1974a). Sepsis is at times fulminant and often fatal. Because of these risks, a woman with a device in utero should be offered the option of a pregnancy termination (American College of Obstetricians and Gynecologists, 1992). Women pregnant with a device in utero who demonstrate any evidence of uterine infection must have intensive antibiotic therapy and prompt uterine evacuation of pregnancy products and the device. The following case illustrates the dangers of a device coexisting with a pregnancy:

> A woman conceived with a Lippes loop in place, and attempts to visualize the strings and remove it were unsuccessful. She elected to continue the pregnancy, and did well until 20 weeks, when she was admitted to a community hospital because of chills and fever. The membranes were intact, the cervix was closed, there were no contractions, and no pelvic or uterine tenderness was elicited. Blood cultures were obtained and broad-spectrum antimicrobials begun. She felt better initially, but in 24 hours she had another chill accompanied by a temperature of 40° C. The initial blood cultures were sterile; however, others done at this time were subsequently positive for *Escherichia coli*. Also at this time, she began to develop clinical and x-ray evidence for permeability pulmonary edema caused by injury from endotoxin (see Chap. 47, p. 1069). Labor began spontaneously, and the 20-week fetus was delivered shortly thereafter. The loop was laying on the fetal chest and not embedded in the placenta.
>
> The pulmonary injury improved slowly over the next few days, but despite continued intravenous antimicrobial therapy, consumptive coagulopathy developed 7 days later. This was presumed to be due to continued sepsis. Computed tomography (Fig. 61–2) disclosed evidence of uterine necrosis, and at laparotomy, the uterus and both adnexae were found to be necrotic. There was also septic ovarian vein thrombophlebitis. Hysterectomy and bilateral adnexectomy were performed. After an extremely complicated and prolonged postoperative course, which included renal failure that required hemodialysis, she ultimately survived.

An increased incidence of fetal malformations has not been noted with pregnancies complicated by the presence of any intrauterine device.

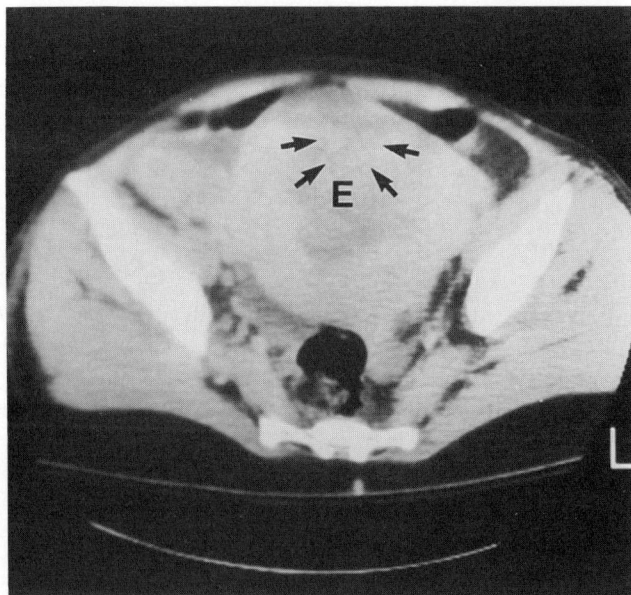

Fig. 61–2. Computed tomography showing uterine necrosis from an intrauterine device-related infection at 20 weeks' gestation. Arrows surround areas of hypodensity indicating necrosis. (E = endometrial cavity.) (Courtesy of Drs. K. Waldrep and L. Swygert.)

Ectopic Pregnancies. Although most intrauterine pregnancies are prevented, the device provides less protection against extrauterine nidation. There has been concern that use of an intrauterine device inordinately increases the risk of ectopic pregnancy, but Vessey and co-workers (1979b) found that the risk remained rather constant with duration of use at 1.2 per 1000 woman-years. With a contraceptive failure, however, the risk for an ectopic pregnancy increases significantly and may be increased even more in women using Progestaserts (see Chap. 32, p. 691). Because the device does not prevent extrauterine pregnancy reliably, women already at high risk for an ectopic pregnancy—those with previous salpingitis, ectopic pregnancy, or tubal surgery—are poor candidates for an intrauterine device.

Contraindications. As described in Chapter 60 (p. 1333), contraindications may be separated into absolute and relative contraindications. If a woman has an absolute contraindication, the device should not be used. In the case of a relative contraindication, another contraceptive method should be used because, unlike oral contraceptives, intrauterine devices provide no additional benefits other than contraception. If a device is used in a woman with a relative contraindication, carefully documented informed consent should be obtained.

Absolute Contraindications

1. Active, recent, or recurrent pelvic infections
2. Pregnancy, known or suspected
3. Undiagnosed, irregular, or abnormal uterine bleeding
4. Cervical or uterine malignancy

Relative Contraindications

1. Nulliparous
2. At risk for sexually transmitted diseases—that is, multiple sexual partners, diabetic, immunosuppressive therapy, purulent cervicitis
3. Exposure or risk of exposure to human immunodeficiency virus
4. History of ectopic pregnancy
5. History of fallopian tube reconstructive surgery
6. Impaired coagulation
7. Impaired physical or mental ability to check for device string
8. Wilson disease
9. Valvar heart disease
10. Endometriosis
11. Uterine leiomyoma

Procedures for Insertion. The Food and Drug Administration requires that before an intrauterine device is inserted, the women must be given a brochure detailing the side effects and apparent risks from its use. Most devices have a special inserter, usually a sterile graduated plastic tube into which the device is withdrawn just before insertion (Fig. 61–3). Timing of insertion influences the ease of placement as well as the pregnancy and expulsion rates. Insertion near the end of normal menstruation, when the cervix is usually softer and the canal somewhat more dilated, may facilitate insertion and at the same time exclude early pregnancy. Insertion, however, need not be limited to this time. For the woman who is sure she is not pregnant and does not want to be pregnant, insertion may be carried out anytime during the ovulation cycle. Even though she engaged in coitus during the previous week, she is unlikely to conceive if a Copper T device is used (Lippes and associates, 1978). (See also Chap. 60, p. 1336.)

Insertion at the time of delivery or very soon thereafter is followed by an unsatisfactorily high expulsion rate. The recommendation has been made, therefore, to withhold insertion for at least 8 weeks to reduce expulsion as well as to minimize the risk of perforation. We have observed, however, that earlier insertion has not led to perforation or expulsion rates significantly higher than for insertion remote from pregnancy. In the absence of infection, the device may be inserted immediately after early abortion.

A satisfactory technique for insertion and plan for follow-up are outlined below:

1. Obtain a careful gynecological history. Contraindications to the use of an intrauterine device include untreated gonorrhea even though asymp-

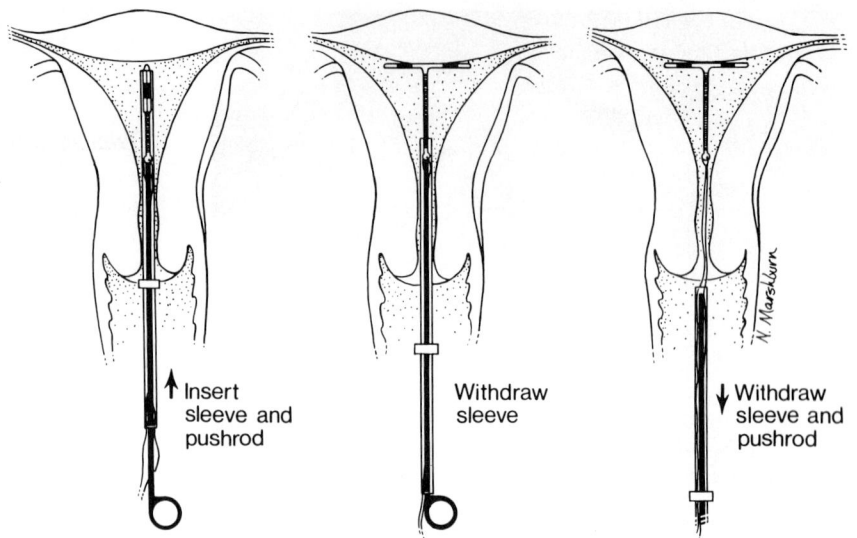

↑ Insert
sleeve and
pushrod

Withdraw
sleeve

↓ Withdraw
sleeve and
pushrod

Fig. 61–3. Insertion of Copper T 380A using the withdrawal technique. (Redrawn from Porter and associates, 1983, with permission.)

tomatic, recent pelvic infection or history of recurrent pelvic infections, severe dysmenorrhea, cervical stenosis, uterine cavity abnormalities, menorrhagia, anemia, and coagulation abnormalities. The woman who has had a previous ectopic pregnancy should be counseled against the use of a device because she already is at considerable risk of another ectopic pregnancy, and an intrauterine device does not prevent ectopic pregnancy efficiently.

2. Describe the various problems associated with use of an intrauterine device and obtain informed consent.

3. Perform a thorough pelvic examination especially to identify the position and size of the uterus and adnexa. If abnormalities are found, an intrauterine device is often contraindicated.

4. Visualize the cervix and grasp it with a tenaculum. Use sterile instruments and a sterile intrauterine device. Wipe the cervix and the vaginal walls with an antiseptic solution. The uterus should be sounded to identify the direction and depth of the uterine cavity. Before identifying the depth of the uterine cavity with a sound, the cervical canal and uterine cavity are first straightened by applying gentle traction on the tenaculum. The movable flange on the barrel of the inserter should be adjusted to the depth to which the device should be inserted. The inserter, with the device contained within its most distal portion, is then gently inserted to the uterine fundus. After rotating the inserter so that the device is positioned high in the transverse plane of the uterus, the inserter is removed while the device is held in the fundus by the plastic rod within the inserter. **Thus, the device is not pushed out of the tube, but rather it is held**

in place by the rod while the inserter tube is withdrawn (Fig. 61–3).

5. Cut the marker tail 2 cm from the external os, remove the tenaculum, observe for bleeding from the tenaculum puncture sites, and if there is no bleeding, remove the speculum.

6. Provide analgesia with aspirin or codeine to allay cramps. Advise the woman to report promptly any apparent adverse effects.

Expulsion. Loss of the device from the uterus is most common during the first month of use. The woman should be instructed to palpate the strings protruding from the cervix by either sitting on the edge of a chair or squatting down and then advancing the middle finger into the vagina until the cervix is reached. The woman should be checked in 1 month, usually after menses, for appropriate placement by identifying the tail protruding appropriately from the cervix. Barrier contraception may be desirable during this time, especially if a device has been expelled previously.

Locating a Lost Device. When the tail of a device cannot be visualized, the device may have been expelled, or it may have perforated the uterus. In either event, pregnancy is likely. Conversely, the tail simply may be in the uterine cavity along with a normally positioned device. Often, gentle probing of the uterine cavity with a Randall stone clamp or a rod with a terminal hook will retrieve the string. The simple assumption that the device has been expelled, and thus another should be inserted can be carried to extremes. For example, we observed a woman in whom two Dalkon shields and one Lippes loop were found adherent to the placenta at delivery! Almost certainly, each tail was drawn into the uterine cavity by the rapidly growing pregnant uterus. Fortunately, the pregnancy was otherwise uncomplicated.

When the tail is not visible and the device is not felt by gentle probing of the uterine cavity, sonography is done to ascertain if the device is within the uterine cavity. If these findings are negative or inconclusive, then a plain x-ray of the abdomen and pelvis is taken with a sound inserted into the uterine cavity. Instillation of radiocontrast for hysterography may be done, and hysteroscopy is yet another alternative. Obviously none of these maneuvers except sonography should be performed during early pregnancy.

An open device of inert material, such as the Lippes loop, located outside the uterus may or may not do harm. Perforations of large and small bowel and bowel fistulas, with attendant morbidity, have been reported remote from the time of insertion. Closed devices are no longer used because they can cause *bowel obstruction.* An extrauterine copper-bearing device induces an intense local inflammatory reaction and adherence to the inflamed structure. Although chemically inert devices have been removed easily from the peritoneal cavity by laparoscopy or through a posterior colpotomy, copper-bearing devices are likely to be too firmly adherent for removal by these techniques.

A device may penetrate the uterine wall in varying degrees. At times part of the device may extend into the peritoneal cavity while the remainder is firmly fixed in the myometrium. In one case, at the time of repeat cesarean delivery, part of a Lippes loop that was inserted 3 years before was found protruding from the fundus posteriorly. Omentum was firmly adherent to the uterus around the protruding loop. Devices also can penetrate into the cervix and actually protrude into the vagina. This is more common with the Cu 7 and earlier Copper T devices without the bulb on the stem tip. Although successful nidation may occur with the device in the fundus of the uterus, a more likely cause for pregnancy with a device in situ is displacement of the device into the uterine isthmus and cervix.

Replacement. Chemically inert devices may be left in the uterus indefinitely. In some cases, the polyethylene compound becomes encrusted with calcium salts, and endometrial erosion causes bleeding that prompts replacement. Copper-bearing devices have to be replaced periodically. The new copper-bearing device, Copper T 380 A is approved in the United States for 8 years of continuous use. The progesterone-bearing intrauterine device, Progestasert, should be replaced annually.

Local Barrier Methods

For many years, condoms, vaginal spermicidal agents, and vaginal diaphragms have been used for contraception with variable success (Table 60–1). More recently, a female condom has been approved for use in the United States.

Condoms

Male Condom. In the United States, the condom represents the only reversible, effective, "male method" of contraception. Condoms do provide effective contraception, and their failure rate with experienced and strongly motivated couples has been as low as 3 or 4 per 100 couple-years of exposure (Vessey and co-workers, 1982). Generally, and during the first year of use especially, the failure rate is much higher (Table 60–1). Trussel and colleagues (1990) also noted that women above the age of 30 had fewer unintended pregnancies than those under 25. Perhaps the recent availability in the United States of condoms with spermicidal lubricants will lower the failure rate.

When used properly, condoms provide considerable but not absolute protection against a broad range of sexually transmitted diseases, including gonorrhea, syphilis, herpes, chlamydia, and trichomoniasis. They also possibly prevent and ameliorate premalignant changes in the cervix (Population Reports, 1982b). Feldblum and Fortney (1988) reviewed the few published studies and concluded that there is some evidence that use of condoms provides protection, although not absolute, from infection with the *human immunodeficiency virus* (see Chap. 59, p. 1310). The Centers for Disease Control recommends their use for patients at risk for infection with the virus, and this includes women with multiple sex partners. Consequently, the use of condoms has escalated, exponentially in the past few years, but not necessarily for contraception. It is estimated that 40 million couples in the world use condoms for birth control, and in Japan, 50 percent of married couples use this method of contraception.

> Historically, the original condoms were made of intestine and other material, but with the introduction of rubber, the condom became much more effective, less expensive, and more widely available. The origin of the word "condom" is unknown. It has been stated, probably incorrectly, that this refers to Dr. Condom, a physician who provided King Charles II with a means of preventing more illegitimate offspring. Casanova (1725–1798) is said to have mentioned condoms several times in his exhaustive memoirs.
>
> Often the earliest father–son discussion of sex and reproduction was stimulated by the presence of condom-dispensing machines in the men's room of service stations. It is of interest that condoms were available widely at a time when attempts to make other family planning techniques available were discouraged lest they promote sexual promiscuity or offend someone's religious beliefs. The condoms, or "prophylactics," in the gasoline stations, were allegedly provided only to prevent sexually transmitted diseases—a use that now certainly has become popular.

Female Condom (*Vaginal Pouch*). The Food and Drug Administration refers to female condoms as vaginal pouches. Before approval for marketing, a vaginal pouch must be proven to prevent pregnancy and sexually transmitted diseases, including human immunodeficiency virus (Contraceptive Technology Update, 1991). Three devices will be available; all appear to provide effective contraception and, at least, some protection from sexually transmitted diseases.

BIKINI CONDOM. The condom resembles a G-string panty and is composed of 0.12 mm latex, which is about twice as thick as a typical male condom. The actual condom, which contains a water-based lubricant, is rolled up within the panty crotch, and is unrolled upon penile penetration. The device is said to have a 0.5 percent breakage rate compared with an average male condom of 1 to 2 percent, and it can be used 5 to 10 times.

WOMEN'S CHOICE CONDOM. This device is similar to a male condom, but wider and thicker by about 30 percent. Its open end has a 2-inch flexible ring that hangs from the vaginal opening. The upper internal end of the condom consists of a thickened latex dome similar to a diaphragm. It contains a silicone lubricant both inside and outside, and it is inserted with a tampon-like applicator.

REALITY CONDOM. This is a polyurethane sheath with one flexible polyurethane ring at each end. The open ring remains outside the vagina, and the closed internal ring is fitted under the symphysis like a diaphragm (Fig. 61–4). In vitro tests have shown it to be impermeable to human immunodeficiency virus, cytomegalovirus, and hepatitis-B virus. It has a 0.6 percent breakage rate. The slippage and displacement rate is about 3 percent compared with an 8 percent rate for male condoms. Overall, acceptability has been about 60 percent for women and 80 percent for men. This condom was approved by the FDA Advisory Panel in December, 1992.

Intravaginal Spermicidal Contraceptives. These contraceptive agents are marketed variously as creams, jellies, suppositories, film, and foam in aerosol containers as well as sponges (Fig. 61–5). They are used widely in this country, especially by women who find oral contraceptives or an intrauterine device unacceptable. They are useful especially for women who need temporary protection, for example, during the first week after starting oral contraceptives or while nursing.

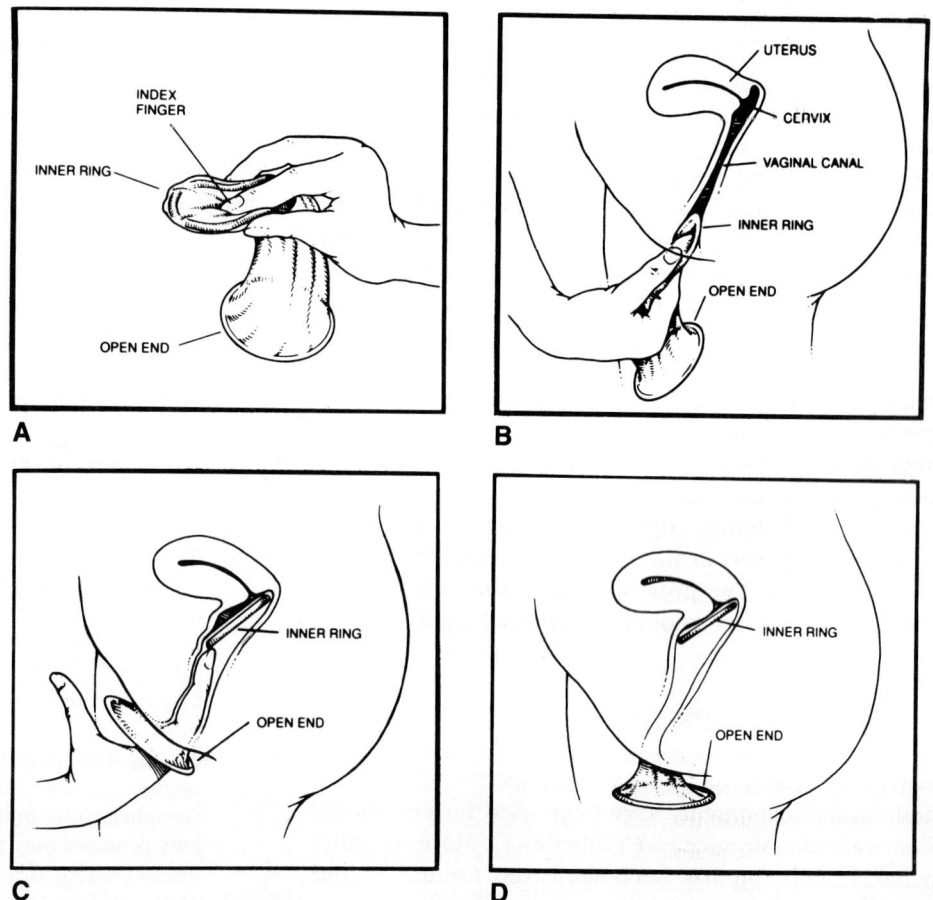

Fig. 61–4. "Reality" female condom insertion and positioning. **A.** Inner ring is squeezed for insertion. **B.** Sheath is inserted similarly to a diaphragm. **C.** Inner ring is pushed up as far as it can go with index finger. **D.** Vaginal pouch is in place. (Figure from Wisconsin Pharmacal Company, Jackson, Wisconsin, and Contraception Report, 1992, with permission.)

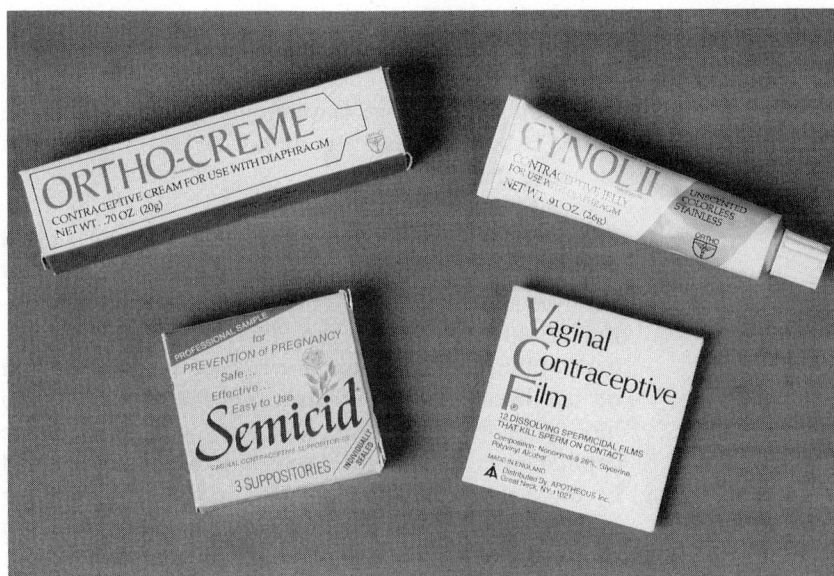

Fig. 61–5. Vaginal contraceptive agents: cream, jelly, suppository, and film.

Most agents can be purchased without a prescription. Typically, they work by providing a physical barrier to sperm penetration as well as a chemical spermicidal action. The active spermicidal ingredient is nonoxynol-9. **To be highly effective, the spermicides must be deposited high in the vagina in contact with the cervix shortly before intercourse.** Their duration of maximal spermicidal effectiveness is usually no more than 1 hour. Thereafter they must be reinserted before repeat intercourse. Douching should be avoided for at least 6 hours after intercourse.

High pregnancy rates are primarily attributable to inconsistent use rather than to method failure—that is, they are user failures. If inserted regularly and correctly, foam preparations probably result in no more than 5 to 12 pregnancies per 100 woman-years of use (Population Reports, 1984; Trussel and associates, 1990; Vessey and colleagues, 1982). Moreover, the spermicides in current use appear to provide at least partial protection against some sexually transmitted diseases, including gonorrhea and probably papillomavirus and human immunodeficiency virus (Feldblum and Fortney, 1988).

Malformations. Although an earlier preliminary study suggested that the use of vaginal spermicides might be associated with an increased frequency of malformations, in well-designed studies by Mills and co-workers (1982) and Shapiro and associates (1982), no association was identified between malformations and maternal spermicide exposure before or after the last menstrual period. In 1986, the Food and Drug Administration concluded that evidence *does not* support an association between spermicide use and congenital malformations.

In spite of the scientific evidence to the contrary, a court decision (*Wells v. Ortho Pharmaceutical*) was rendered in favor of the plaintiff in a suit alleging that congenital malformations were caused by maternal spermicide exposure. The decision was upheld by an appellate court. Subsequently, Louik and colleagues (1987) reported results from their case-controlled surveillance system, in which they examined specifically for possible effects of periconceptual use of spermicides on specific fetal malformations. They found no association with spermicide use and Down syndrome, hypospadias, limb-reduction defects, neoplasms, or neural tube defects. Warburton and associates (1987) reported no increased risk of trisomies with spermicide use. Finally, Strobino and colleagues (1988) did not identify increased congenital malformations in a cohort study.

Diaphragm Plus Spermicidal Agent. The vaginal diaphragm, consisting of circular rubber dome of various diameters supported by a circumferentially placed metal spring, is very effective when used in combination with a spermicidal jelly or cream. The spermicidal agent is applied to the superior surface both along the rim and centrally. The device is then placed in the vagina so that the cervix, vaginal fornices, and anterior vaginal wall are partitioned effectively from the remainder of the vagina and the penis. At the same time, the centrally placed spermicidal agent is held against the cervix by the diaphragm. When appropriately positioned, the rim is lodged superiorly deep in the posterior vaginal fornix, and inferiorly the rim lies in close proximity to the inner surface of the symphysis immediately below the urethra (Fig. 61–6). If the diaphragm is too small, it will not remain in place. If too large, it will be uncomfortable when it is forced into position. A cystocele or uterine prolapse is very likely to result in instability and therefore expulsion. Because the variables of size and spring flexibility must be specified, the diaphragm is available only by prescription.

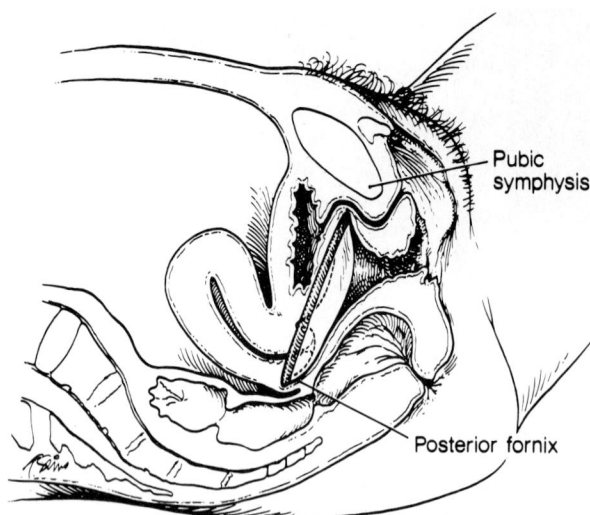

Fig. 61–6. A diaphragm in place creates a physical barrier between the vagina and cervix and importantly provides for intimate contact between the contraceptive jelly or cream and the cervix.

The diaphragm and spermicidal agent can be inserted hours before intercourse, but if more than 2 hours elapse, additional spermicide should be placed in the upper vagina for maximum protection and be reapplied before each coital episode. The diaphragm should not be removed for at least 6 hours after intercourse. Because toxic-shock syndrome has been described following its use (Alcid and associates, 1982), it may be worthwhile to remove the diaphragm at the end of 6 hours, or at least the next morning, to minimize this very uncommon event.

The diaphragm requires a high level of motivation for proper use that, when expended, is accompanied by a low pregnancy rate. Vessey and colleagues (1982) reported a pregnancy rate of only 1.9 to 2.4 per 100 woman-years for established diaphragm users. The unintended pregnancy rate is lower in women past 35 than in those under 30 (Vessey and colleagues, 1982). Finally, contraceptive sponge and diaphragm use results in a decreased incidence in sexually transmitted diseases compared with condom use and tubal sterilization (Rosenberg and colleagues, 1992).

Sponge and Cervical Cap

Contraceptive Sponge. Contraceptive sponges placed in the upper vagina continue to undergo extensive evaluation. One polyurethane sponge soaked with a spermicide has been approved by the Food and Drug Administration and is marketed under the trade name *Today.* It has been claimed to be about as effective as other vaginal methods, but McIntyre and Higgins (1986) reported higher contraceptive failure rates, especially in parous women, compared with diaphragm use. Edelman

and North (1987), however, did not note a parity difference in failure rates in their expanded studies.

The risk of toxic shock syndrome is small, but it is increased if the sponge is used during menses. Because of this risk, the sponge should not be left in the vagina for more than 24 hours.

Cervical Cap. After falling into disuse in the United States for several decades, the Prentif cavity-rim *cervical cap* was approved for use (Food and Drug Administration, 1988). The flexible, cup-like device, made of natural rubber, is fitted around the base of the cervix. It can be self-inserted and allowed to remain in place for no more than 48 hours. It should be used with a spermicide applied once at insertion. According to trials conducted by the National Institutes of Health, the cap is comparable in effectiveness to the diaphragm, and at least two thirds of the failures were user related (see Table 60–1). Unfortunately, the cost is high, and the fitting is critical for the device to be successful.

Periodic (Rhythmic) Abstinence

Ideally, sexual abstinence during and around the time of ovulation should prevent pregnancy; unfortunately, this is not always the case. For example, pregnancy rates with various methods of periodic abstinence (rhythm methods, "natural" family planning) have been placed at from 5 to 40 per 100 woman-years (Population Reports, 1981). Four methods of contraceptive periodic abstinence currently are being practiced and were reviewed in detail by Klaus (1982).

Calendar Rhythm Method. Ovulation most often occurs about 14 days before the onset of the next menstrual period, but unfortunately, not necessarily 14 days after the onset of the last menstrual period. Therefore, the *calendar rhythm method* is not reliable. In 1982, the International Planned Parenthood Federation concluded that "couples electing to use periodic abstinence should, however, be clearly informed that the method is not considered an effective method of family planning."

The human ovum probably is susceptible to successful fertilization only for about 12 to no more than 24 hours after ovulation. Motile sperm have been identified in cervical mucus as many as 7 days after coitus or artificial insemination and in oviducts of women undergoing laparotomy as long as 85 hours after coitus (Ahlgren, 1975). It is unlikely, however, that sperm retain the capability for successful fertilization for this long a period.

Temperature Rhythm Method. This method relies on *slight* changes in morning basal body temperature that usually occur just before ovulation. The temperature rhythm method is much more likely to be successful if, during each menstrual cycle, intercourse is avoided until well after the ovulatory temperature rise. For this method to be most effective, the woman must abstain from intercourse from the first day of menses through the third day after the increase in basal body temperature. For obvious reasons, this is not a popular method of contraception.

Cervical Mucus Rhythm Method. The *cervical mucus rhythm,* or so-called *Billings method,* depends upon awareness of vaginal "dryness" and "wetness" as the consequence of changes in the amount and kind of cervical mucus formed at different times in the menstrual cycle. Abstinence is required from the beginning of menses until 4 days after slippery mucus is identified. This method has not achieved popularity. A small, hand-held device that detects small variations in electrolyte concentrations in vaginal or oral secretions is also claimed to be capable of predicting ovulation 5 to 7 days in advance, however, Roumen and Dieben (1988) found it to be of no use in predicting the day of ovulation.

Sympto-thermal Method. This method combines the use of changes in cervical mucus (onset of fertile period), changes in basal body temperature (end of fertile period), and calculations to estimate the time of ovulation. This is a more complex system to learn and apply, and it does not improve reliability appreciably (Table 60–1).

For the interested reader, the December 1991, Supplement to the American Journal of Obstetrics and Gynecology was devoted to the subject of natural family planning. Twenty-seven separate papers were included on this subject, as well as a final discussion and recommendations (Queenan and associates, 1991).

REFERENCES

Ahlgren M: Sperm transport to and survival in the human fallopian tube. Gynecol Invest 6:206, 1975

Alcid DV, Kothari N, Quinn EP, Geismar L, Glowinsky LZ: Toxic-shock syndrome associated with diaphragm use for only nine hours. Lancet 1:1363, 1982

Alvarez F, Brache V, Fernandez E, Guerrero B, Builoff E, Hess R, Salvatierra AM, Zacharias S: New insights on the mode of action of intrauterine contraceptive devices in women. Fertil Steril 49:768, 1988

American College of Obstetricians and Gynecologists: The intrauterine device. Technical bulletin no. 164, February 1992

Buhler M, Papiernik E: Successive pregnancies in women fitted with intrauterine devices who take anti-inflammatory drugs. Lancet 1:483, 1983

Contracep Rep 3:13, 1992

Cramer DW, Schiff I, Schoenbaum SC, Gibson M, Belisle S, Albrecht A, Stillman RJ, Berger MJ, Wilson E, Stadel BV, Seibel M: Tubal infertility and the intrauterine device. N Engl J Med 312:941, 1985

Daling JR, Weiss NS, Metch BJ, Chow WH, Soderstrom RM, Moore DE, Spadoni LR, Stadel BV: Primary tubal infertility in relation to the use of an intrauterine device. N Engl J Med 312:937, 1985

Dawood MY, Birnbaum SJ: Unilateral tubo-ovarian abscess and intrauterine contraceptive device. Obstet Gynecol 46:429, 1975

Edelman DA, North BB: Updated pregnancy rates for the Today contraceptive sponge. Am J Obstet Gynecol 157:1164, 1987

Editorial: Does infection occur with modern intrauterine devices? Lancet 339:783, 1992

Farley TMM, Rosenberg MJ, Rowe PJ, Chen J-H, Meirik O: Intrauterine devices and pelvic inflammatory disease: An international perspective. Lancet 339:785, 1992

Feldblum PJ, Fortney JA: Condoms, spermicides and the transmission of human immunodeficiency virus: A review of the literature. Am J Public Health 78:52, 1988

Female condoms scheduled to reach US market this year. Contracep Technol Update 12:117, 1991.

Food and Drug Administration: *Drug Bulletin* 18:18, 1988

Food and Drug Administration: *Drug Bulletin* 16:21, 1986

Guillebaud J, Barnett MD, Gordon YB: Plasma ferritin levels as an index of iron deficiency in women using intrauterine devices. Br J Obstet Gynaecol 86:51, 1979

Hatcher RA, Stewart F, Trussel J, Kowal P, Guest F, Stewart GK, Cates W: Contraceptive Technology. 15th ed. New York, Irvington, 1990, p 370

Hill GB: Eubacterium nodatum mimics actinomyces in intrauterine device-associated infections and other settings within the female genital tract. Obstet Gynecol 79:534, 1992

International Planned Parenthood Federation, International Medical Advisory Panel: Statement on periodic abstinence for family planning. IPPF Med Bull 18:2, 1982

Keebler C, Chatwani A, Schwartz R: Actinomyces infection associated with intrauterine contraceptive devices. Am J Obstet Gynecol 145:596, 1983

Klaus H: Natural family planning: A review. Obstet Gynecol Surv 37:128, 1982

Lee NC, Rubin GL: The intrauterine device and pelvic inflammatory disease revisited: New results from the woman's health study. Obstet Gynecol 72:1, 1988

Lee NC, Rubin GL, Ory HW, Burknan RT: Type of intrauterine device and the risk of pelvic inflammatory disease. Obstet Gynecol 62:1, 1983

Lewit S: Outcome of pregnancy with an intrauterine device. Contraception 2:47, 1970

Lippes J, Tatum HJ, Maulid D, Zielezny M: A continuation of the study of postcoital IUDs. Paper presented at the annual meeting of the Association of Planned Parenthood Physicians, San Diego, October 25, 1978

Louik C, Mitchell AA, Werler MM, Hanson JW, Shapiro S: Maternal exposure to spermicides in relation to certain birth defects. N Engl J Med 317:474, 1987

McIntyre SL, Higgins JE: Parity and use-effectiveness with the contraceptive sponge. Am J Obstet Gynecol 155:796, 1986

Mills JL, Harley EE, Reed GF, Berendes HW: Are spermicides teratogenic? JAMA 248:2148, 1982

Mishell DR Jr, Bell JH, Good RG, Moyer DL: The intrauterine device: A bacteriologic study of the endometrial cavity. Am J Obstet Gynecol 96:119, 1966

Moyer DL, Mishell DR Jr: Reactions of human endometrium to the intrauterine foreign body, II. Long-term effects on the endometrial histology and cytology. Am J Obstet Gynecol 111:66, 1971

Ortiz ME, Croxatto HB: The mode of action of IUDs. Contraception 36:37, 1987

Petitti DB, Yamamoto D, Morgenstern N: Factors associated with actinomyces-like organisms on Papanicolaou smear in users of intrauterine contraceptive devices. Am J Obstet Gynecol 145:339, 1983

Population Reports: Barrier Method—New developments in vaginal contraception. Series H, no. 7, January-February 1984, p 157

Population Reports: IUDs: An appropriate contraception for many women. Series B, no. 4, July 1982a, p 101

Population Reports: Update on condoms—Products, protection, promotion. Series H, no. 6, September-October 1982b, p 121

Population Reports: Periodic abstinence: How well do new approaches work? Series L, no. 3, September 1981, p 33

Porter CW, Waife RS, Holtrap HR: The health provider's guide to contraception, international ed. Watertown, MA, Pathfinder Fund, 1983

Purrier BGA, Sparks RA, Watt PJ, Elstein M: In vitro study of the possible role of the intrauterine contraceptive device tail in ascending infection of the genital tract. Br J Obstet Gynaecol 86:374, 1979

Queenan JT, Jennings VH, Spieler JM, von Hertzen H, eds: Natural family planning: Current knowledge and new strategies for the 1990s. Am J Obstet Gynecol 165(suppl):1977, 1991

Rosenberg MJ, Davidson AJ, Chen J-H, Judson FN, Douglas JM: Barrier contraceptives and sexually transmitted diseases in women: A comparison of female-dependent methods and condoms. Am J Pub Health 82:669, 1992

Roumen FJME, Dieben TOM: Ovulation prediction by monitoring salivary electrical resistance with the Cue fertility monitor. Obstet Gynecol 71:49, 1988

Shapiro S, Slone D, Heinonin OP, Kaufman DW, Rosenberg L, Mitchell AA, Helmrich SP: Birth defects and vaginal spermicides. JAMA 247:2381, 1982

Sivin I, Stern J, Diaz S, Pavéz M, Alvarez F, Brache V, Mishell DR Jr, Lacarra M, McCarthy T, Holma P, Darney P, Klaisle C, Olsson S-E, Odlind V: Rates and outcomes of planned pregnancy after use of Norplant capsules, Norplant II rods, or levonorgestrel-releasing or copper TCu-380Ag intrauterine contraceptive devices. Am J Obstet Gynecol 166:1208, 1992

Strobino B, Kline J, Warburton D: Spermicide use and pregnancy outcome. Am J Public Health 78:260, 1988

Tatum HJ, Schmidt FH, Jain AK: Management and outcome of pregnancies associated with Copper-T intrauterine contraceptive device. Am J Obstet Gynecol 126:869, 1976

Taylor ES, McMillan JH, Greer BE, Droegemueller W, Thompson HE: The intrauterine device and tubo-ovarian abscess. Am J Obstet Gynecol 123:338, 1975

Taylor WW, Martin FG, Pritchard SA, Pritchard JA: Complications from Majzlin spring intrauterine device. Obstet Gynecol 14:404, 1973

Trussel R, Hatcher R, Cates W, Stewart F, Kost K: Contraceptive failure in the United States: An update. Studies Fam Plan 21:51, 1990

Vessey MP, Johnson B, Doll R, Peto R: Outcome of pregnancy in women using intrauterine devices. Lancet 1:495, 1974

Vessey MP, Lawless M, McPherson K, Yeates D: Fertility after stopping use of intrauterine contraceptive device. BMJ 286:106, 1983

Vessey M, Lawless M, Yeates D: Efficacy of different contraceptive methods. Lancet 1:841, 1982

Vessey MP, Meisler L, Flavel R, Yeates D: Outcome of pregnancy in women using different methods of contraception. Br J Obstet Gynaecol 86:548, 1979a

Vessey MP, Yeates D, Flavel R: Risk of ectopic pregnancy and duration of use of an intrauterine device. Lancet 2:501, 1979b

Warburton D, Neugut RH, Lustenberger A, Nicholas AG, Kline J: Lack of association between spermicide use and trisomy. N Engl J Med 317:478, 1987

Wisconsin Pharmacal Corporation. REALITY, the female condom (press release). January 1992

Zipper JA, Tatum JH, Medel M, Pastene L, Rivera M: Contraception through the use of intrauterine metals, I. Copper as an adjunct to the T device. Am J Obstet Gynecol 109:771, 1971

CHAPTER 62
Surgical Contraception

Prevalence. Surgical sterilization of one or both sexual partners is the most popular form of contraception among couples of reproductive age (Fig. 60–1). According to the Association for Voluntary Sterilization (1989), there were 976,000 sterilization procedures performed in the United States in 1987; 66 percent were performed in women.

Until recently, sterilization of women as a family planning technique was frowned upon by important segments of society, including some churches, medical groups, and a variety of political bodies. For example, until 1969, the American College of Obstetricians and Gynecologists recommended that a woman 30 years of age should have four living children before qualifying for sterilization. Even now, multiple restrictions imposed by the federal government serve to discourage voluntary sterilization among financially underprivileged women by threatening to sever federal funding to the organizations that provide the service. These restrictive and sometimes archaic federal practices will likely appear as ridiculous to future generations as do the men (certainly not women) who devised and promulgated them. For example, the American College of Obstetricians and Gynecologists (1988) currently has a much more enlightened view of surgical sterilization compared with legislative and executive governmental branches.

Female Sterilization

Over 5 million women underwent tubal sterilization in the United States during the 1970s. Mortality rates of approximately 3 per 100,000 for all tubal sterilizations have been reported, and this compares favorably when compared with maternal mortality rates of approximately 14 per 100,000 live births (Hatcher and colleagues, 1990). Medically speaking, the operation can be performed at any time, and many are done at cesarean delivery. For women who deliver vaginally, the early puerperium is a particularly convenient time. Because the fundus is near the umbilicus and the oviducts are accessible directly beneath the abdominal wall for several days after delivery, the operation is technically simple and hospitalization need not be prolonged.

Sterilization immediately following vaginal delivery has some disadvantages. Because the mother is usually multiparous, she was more likely delivered without receiving anesthesia appropriate for entering the peritoneal cavity. The likelihood of postpartum hemorrhage in multiparous women subsides remarkably after the first 12 puerperal hours. Importantly, the status of the newborn can be determined much more precisely several hours after birth.

It was previously recommended that puerperal sterilization by partial resection of the oviducts be accomplished during the first 72 puerperal hours to minimize infection from ascending bacterial invasion of the fallopian tubes. This is no longer believed to be valid because no correlation has been seen between time interval and postoperative morbidity. At Parkland Hospital, puerperal tubal ligation is performed in the obstetrical surgical suite the morning after delivery to minimize hospital stay.

Puerperal Tubal Sterilization. The first tubal sterilization reported in the United States more than 100 years ago consisted of ligating the oviducts with a strong silk ligature about 1 inch from their uterine attachment following the woman's second cesarean delivery (Lungren, 1881). Literally, the woman had her tubes tied. Subsequently, it became apparent that an unacceptably high failure rate followed ligation without tubal resection. A variety of techniques are now employed to disrupt tubal patency; several are considered below.

Irving Procedure. The Irving procedure is least likely to fail. Briefly, the procedure, as illustrated in Figure 62–1A, involves severing the oviduct and separating it from the mesosalpinx sufficiently to create a medial segment of tube. The distal stump of the proximal segment of tube is buried within a tunnel in the myometrium posteriorly, and the proximal end of the distal tubal segment is buried within the mesosalpinx. The procedure requires considerably more exposure than do most other techniques, and the likelihood of hemorrhage is greater.

Pomeroy Procedure. Of all abdominal techniques that divide the tube, the simplest, reasonably effective method is the Pomeroy procedure (Fig. 62–1B). It generally has been considered important that plain catgut be used to ligate the knuckle of tube, because the rationale of this procedure is based on prompt absorption of the ligature and subsequent separation of the severed tubal ends, which most often become sealed over by fibrosis.

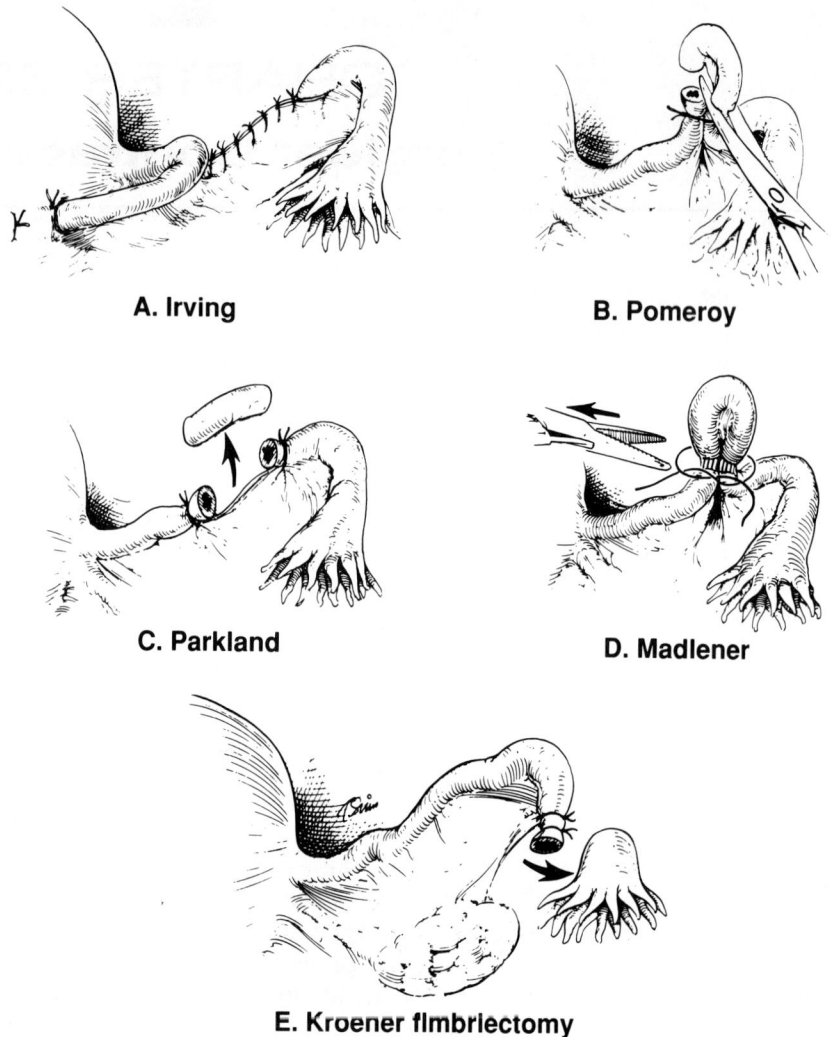

A. Irving

B. Pomeroy

C. Parkland

D. Madlener

E. Kroener fimbriectomy

Fig. 62–1. Various techniques for tubal sterilization. **A.** Irving procedure: the medial cut end of the oviduct is buried in the myometrium posteriorly and the distal cut end is buried in the mesosalpinx. **B.** Pomeroy procedure: a loop of oviduct is ligated and the knuckle of tube above the ligature is excised. **C.** Parkland procedure: a midsegment of tube is separated from the mesosalpinx at an avascular site and the separated tubal segment is ligated proximally and distally and then excised. **D.** Madlener procedure: a knuckle of oviduct is crushed and then ligated without resection. **E.** Kroener procedure: the tube is ligated across the ampulla, and the distal portion of the ampulla, including all of the fimbriae, is resected.

Parkland Procedure. The procedure developed at Parkland Hospital in the 1960s was designed to avoid the initial intimate approximation of the cut ends of the oviduct that is inherent with the Pomeroy procedure (Fig. 62–1C). A small infraumbilical abdominal wall incision is made, and a small Richardson retractor inserted. The oviduct is identified positively by grasping the midportion in a Babcock clamp and confirming by direct identification of distal fimbriae. This prevents confusing the round ligament with the midportion of the oviduct. **Whenever the oviduct is inadvertently dropped, it is mandatory to repeat completely the identification procedure just described!**

An avascular site (Fig. 62–2A) in the mesosalpinx adjacent to the oviduct is then perforated with a small hemostat and the jaws are opened to separate the oviduct from the adjacent mesosalpinx for about 2.5 cm. The freed oviduct is ligated proximally and distally with 0 chromic suture, and the intervening segment of about 2 cm is excised with sharp scissors (Fig. 62–2B). After inspection for hemostasis, the oviduct segments are replaced and the procedure is repeated on the other side.

Both resected segments of oviduct are labeled and submitted for histological confirmation. Excluding the rare instance in which the operator failed to resect the fallopian tube, the failure rate has been approximately 1 in 400 procedures.

Madlener Procedure. The Madlener procedure is similar to the Pomeroy operation except that a knuckle of tube is crushed and ligated with nonabsorbable suture but not resected (Fig. 62–1D). This procedure is mentioned only to discourage its use. Our experience with this procedure resulted in a failure rate of about 7 percent.

Fimbriectomy. Removal of all of the distal tube to effect sterilization was recommended by Kroener (1969) and others. Kroener doubly ligated the oviduct with silk suture and then excised the fimbriated end (Fig. 62–1E). Although he reported no failures, others have, and in some instances, the rate has been unacceptable. Taylor (1972), for example, observed six pregnancies among about 200 women subjected to fimbriectomy.

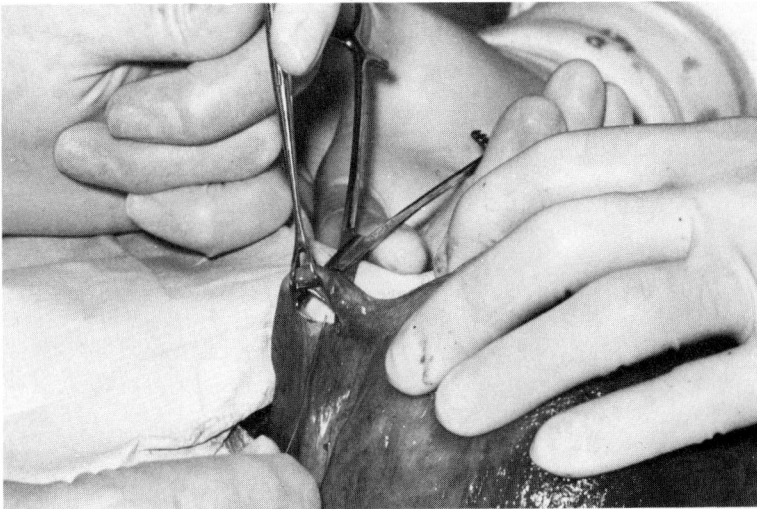

A

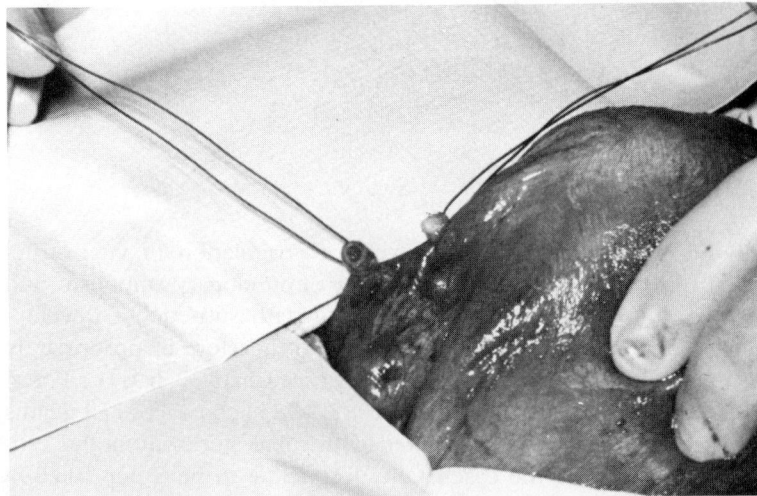

B

Fig. 62–2. Sterilization at cesarean delivery. **A.** An avascular site in the mesosalpinx adjacent to the midportion of the oviduct has been identified, and a small hemostat inserted through the avascular site. The jaws of the clamp have been opened to separate mesosalpinx from tube for about 2.5 cm. A ligature is being inserted. **B.** The segment of oviduct separated from mesosalpinx has been ligated and resected.

When the oviducts subsequently were examined, a small amount of fimbrial tissue usually had been left. Metz (1977) identified seven failures among 388 women who underwent this procedure. Catgut suture had been used, and the resected surface had been lightly electrocoagulated. In the cases that failed, tuboperitoneal fistulas lined with tubal epithelium were found in the remaining ampullary portion of tube.

Postoperative Care. After puerperal sterilization, analgesia should be provided for abdominal soreness, which at times is aggravated in multiparous women by "afterbirth pains." Meperidine, 50 to 75 mg intramuscularly, given intermittently as needed during the first 24 hours, provides excellent analgesia. Within 8 hours, most women can ambulate, eat a regular diet, and care for and nurse their babies. Hospital discharge usually is possible on the day after the procedure.

Nonpuerperal Tubal Sterilization. The techniques, including modifications that have been recommended to accomplish sterilization through tubal occlusion, are almost bewildering in number. Basically, they consist of (1) ligation and resection at laparotomy as described above for puerperal sterilization, (2) the permanent application of a variety of rings or clips to the fallopian tubes, usually through a laparoscope or culpotomy incision, and (3) electrocoagulation of a segment of the oviducts, again usually through a laparoscope.

Laparotomy. Sterilization can be a much more formidable procedure once the uterus has involuted completely and returned to the true pelvis. Much of the difficulty in obtaining exposure is removed if the uterus and adnexa are pushed out of the true pelvis to beneath the abdominal wall above the symphysis using a manipulator previously inserted into the uterus with the handle protruding from the vagina. Utilizing this technique, "minilaparotomies" can be performed through a 3-cm incision made suprapubically and tubal sterilization can be effected (Fig. 62–3).

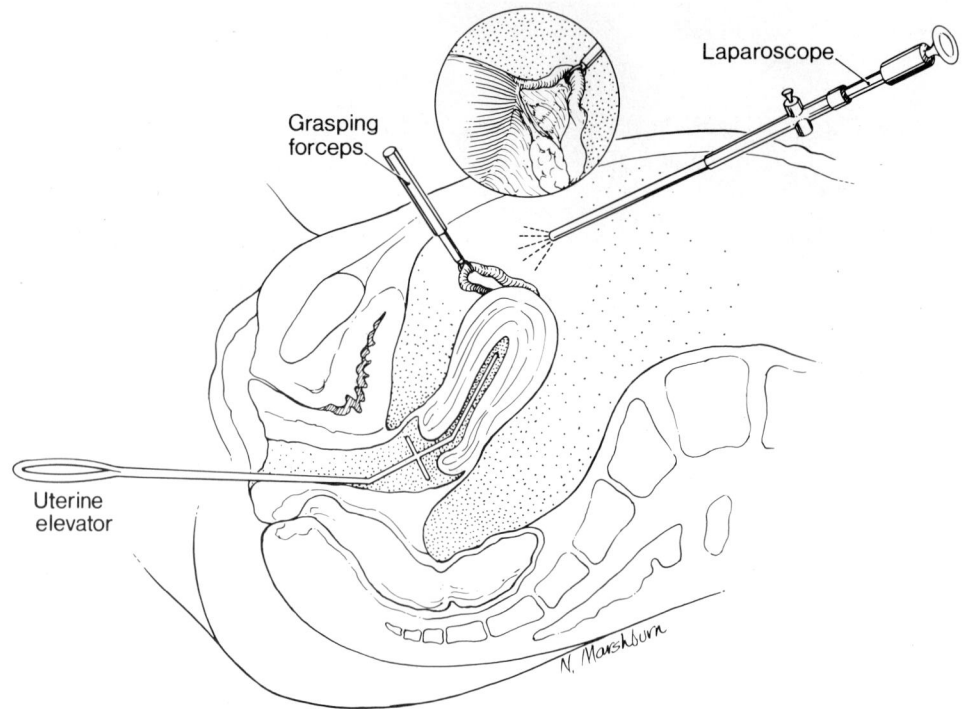

Fig. 62–3. Tubal sterilization using laparoscopic technique. Note pneumoperitoneum to ensure adequate visualization and exposure for surgery, and the laparoscopically directed instrument grasping one fallopian tube prior to cauterization or application of a clip or ring. A uterine elevator is used to move the uterine fundus toward the anterior abdominal wall.

Colpotomy. Vaginal tubal sterilization can usually be performed for women delivered vaginally once the uterus has involuted and pregnancy-induced hyperemia has subsided. The peritoneal cavity is entered through the posterior vaginal fornix (colpotomy, culdotomy), the oviducts are grasped and drawn into view, and then either a Pomeroy type resection or a fimbriectomy is performed. As expected, because the operation is performed through the vagina, this approach has a higher infection rate.

Laparoscopy. Enthusiasm was generated for interval as well as post-abortal sterilizations using *laparoscopy* by an article in *Life* magazine on July 28, 1972 that referred to the technique as "Band-Aid" surgery (Fig. 62–3). Commonly, the woman is cared for in an ambulatory surgical setting. Anesthesia, usually general with endotracheal intubation, is induced, and after producing pneumoperitoneum with carbon dioxide, the sterilization procedure is accomplished. Most often the woman can be discharged several hours later. The actual disruption of tubal continuity has been accomplished using loops, clips, and electrocauterization with and without transection of the tube. Because electrocauterization destroys a large segment of tube, surgical reversal is often not possible. Therefore, many recommend that women under 25, or those of low parity, should not have an electrocautery procedure performed.

Hazards from Tubal Sterilization.

The principal hazards associated with tubal sterilization are anesthetic complications, inadvertent coagulation of vital structures, the rare occurrence of pulmonary embolism, and failure to produce sterility with subsequent development of an unrecognized and therefore inappropriately treated ectopic pregnancy (see Chap. 32, p. 691). Peterson and co-workers (1982, 1983) considered all deaths temporally associated with tubal sterilization and estimated the case-fatality frequency to be 8 per 100,000 procedures. When only deaths directly attributable to the procedure were considered, this rate was 4 per 100,000. The leading cause of death, general anesthesia without tracheal intubation, almost certainly could have been avoided in most cases by use of a tracheal tube or another form of anesthesia.

Results of a multicenter, multinational randomized study of minilaparotomy with tubal ligation plus a midsegment resection procedure compared with laparoscopy and tubal electrocoagulation have been provided by the World Health Organization Task Force on Female Sterilization (1982). Significant complications were identified in 1.5 percent of the former and 0.9 percent of the latter. They concluded, however, that minilaparotomy is the preferred approach for such a service when provided away from a major institution.

DeStefano and co-workers (1983) identified intraoperative or postoperative complications in 1.7 percent of a large number of women who underwent nonpuerperal laparoscopic tubal electrocoagulation for sterilization. Factors identified to increase morbidity were previous abdominal or pelvic surgery, a history of previous pelvic infection, obesity, diabetes, and general anesthesia rather than local analgesia. These same factors undoubtedly would increase the risk of morbidity with minilaparotomy.

Tubal Sterilization Failures. No method of tubal sterilization is without failure, and subsequent pregnancy, both uterine as well as ectopic, may result from failure of the method itself or from improper performance of the procedure.

Causes of Tubal Sterilization Failure. Soderstrom (1985) reviewed in detail causes of failures in 47 women referred because of failed sterilization procedures and concluded the following: (1) Resection method failures most often followed spontaneous reanastomosis or fistula formation. Fimbriectomy particularly was vulnerable to reanastomosis because the fimbria was not always removed. (2) Mechanical devices failed when the device was defective or placed improperly. (3) Tissue damage was evident but incomplete with failures following bipolar electrocoagulation, whereas failures following unipolar electrocoagulation were caused by fistula formation. He further concluded that most sterilization failures are not preventable.

Puerperal Tubal Sterilization Failure. For reasons that are hard to identify, an increased failure rate for sterilization at the time of cesarean delivery has been reported by some. With the technique for tubal sterilization used at Parkland Hospital and described above (Figs. 62–1C and 62–2), no difference has been identified (Husbands and co-workers, 1970).

Ectopic Pregnancy. If a tubal sterilization fails, the resulting pregnancy likely will be ectopic (see Chap. 32, p. 692). Approximately 50 percent of pregnancies after electrocoagulation are ectopic compared with 10 percent following failure of a ring, clip, or tubal resection method (Hatcher and colleagues, 1990). These must be compared with an ectopic pregnancy rate in nonsterilized women of about 1 percent. **Any symptoms of pregnancy in a woman after tubal sterilization must be investigated and an ectopic pregnancy excluded.**

"Post–Tubal Ligation Syndrome." The possibility has been raised of a "post–tubal ligation syndrome," variably characterized by pelvic discomfort, ovarian cyst formation, and especially menorrhagia. That tubal ligation induces any of these changes remains to be established. Kasonde and Bonnar (1976) actually measured menstrual blood loss before and for 6 to 12 months after tubal sterilization. They found that the operation made no significant difference in menstrual blood loss. They also reported that women who presented with menorrhagia soon after sterilization usually had the problem beforehand, or they had been using oral contraceptives, which reduced blood loss. After sterilization and discon-

tinuing the oral contraceptives, they reverted to their normal spontaneous heavier periods. DeStefano and co-workers (1983) followed nearly 2500 women for 2 years after tubal sterilization and reported that, except for menstrual pain, there was no increase in the prevalence of adverse menstrual function among women who had undergone unipolar electrocoagulation. In fact, 50 percent or more of women with adverse menstrual function before sterilization had an improvement over the 2 years following the sterilization procedure. DeStefano and colleagues (1985) amplified their earlier work by including a control group of women whose partners had undergone vasectomy. They reported that abnormal menstrual bleeding seldom developed unless it was reported before sterilization. Shy and colleagues (1992) reported similar results. Interestingly, women with menstrual irregularities before sterilization were less likely than controls to revert spontaneously to normal cyclic menses later. Vessey and associates (1983) compared the frequency of gynecological and psychological disorders among women who had undergone tubal sterilization with those in women whose husbands had undergone vasectomy, and found little difference between the two groups.

Some women who had undergone tubal sterilization were reported by Hargrove and Abraham (1981) to have high serum estradiol and low serum progesterone levels compared with controls. Ladehoff and co-workers (1980), however, identified no change in ovarian endocrine function following tubal sterilization. Other investigators have failed to identify luteal phase dysfunction after tubal sterilization, except possibly after techniques that can cause obstruction of the utero-ovarian artery (Alvarez-Sanchez and colleagues, 1981; Corson and co-workers, 1981; Donnez and associates, 1981).

Although complete transection of the oviduct is mandatory, it is desirable at the same time to preserve blood supply through the adjacent mesosalpinx to minimize the possibility of "postligation" abnormalities attributed by some to tubal sterilization. The Parkland technique (Fig. 62–1C) should not compromise ovarian blood supply. Interestingly, El-Minawi and associates (1983), by means of venography, commonly identified uterovaginal and ovarian varicosities after the Pomeroy and some other procedures but not following the Parkland technique.

Restoration of Fertility. Despite the recent enthusiasm for performing "microsurgery" on oviducts previously divided surgically, no woman should undergo tubal sterilization believing that her fertility can be restored by such means. Sterilization reversal is costly, difficult, and uncertain. Restoration of tubal continuity and function is technically feasible, but success rates vary with the extent of tubal destruction or removal at the time of sterilization (Hatcher and colleagues, 1990). The overall success rate probably is no more than 50 percent. If any doubt exists in the mind of the woman, sterilization should not be done.

Hysterectomy. For the woman who desires no more children, hysterectomy has many theoretical advantages. The only known potential of the uterus, other than child bearing, is to harbor disease. In the absence of uterine or other pelvic disease, however, hysterectomy for sterilization at the time of cesarean delivery, early in the puerperium, or even remote from pregnancy is difficult to justify (Barclay and associates, 1976; Laros and Work, 1975). Mortality rates for hysterectomy vary from 5 to 25 per 100,000 in women ages 35 to 44 (Wingo and colleagues, 1985). With cesarean hysterectomy, blood loss nearly always is greater than with cesarean plus tubal sterilization, leading to much more frequent use of transfusions and their sequelae. Urinary tract injury also is appreciably more common.

Hysteroscopy. Sterilization utilizing hysteroscopy to visualize the tubal ostia and somehow obliterate them is a worthy goal and has received considerable attention. To date, the failure rate and other problems limit the clinical utility of this approach (Zatuchni and colleagues, 1983).

Male Sterilization

Male sterilization, or vasectomy, has emerged as a popular form of family planning. It is estimated that annually more than 300,000 men undergo vasectomy in the United States. Through a small incision in the scrotum, the lumen of the vas deferens is disrupted to block the passage of sperm from the testes (Fig. 62–4). The pro-

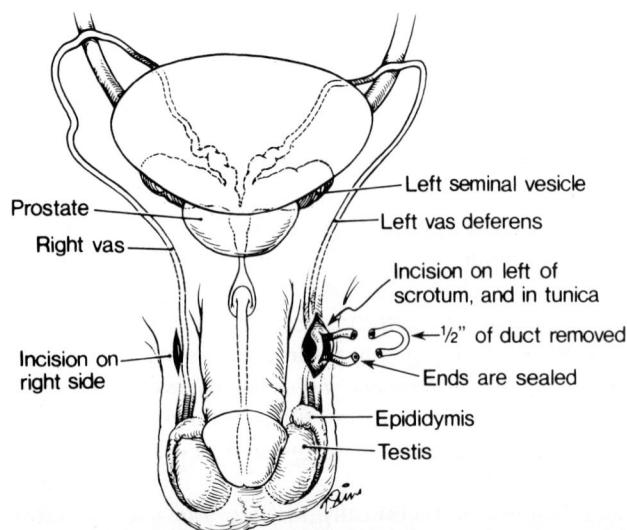

Prostate
Right vas
Left seminal vesicle
Left vas deferens
Incision on left of scrotum, and in tunica
½" of duct removed
Incision on right side
Ends are sealed
Epididymis
Testis

Fig. 62–4. Male reproductive system showing the site of vasectomy.

cedure is usually performed using local analgesia within 20 minutes on an outpatient basis. The procedure has less morbidity and is less expensive than female sterilization, but at least one mortality has been reported (Viddeleer and Lycklama À Nijeholt, 1992). The cost of vasectomy has been estimated to be only about one fifth that of tubal sterilization. In Dallas in 1993, the cost of vasectomy was $500 compared with $2700 for outpatient tubal ligation (Ms. Kathy Mitchell, personal communication).

A disadvantage of vasectomy is that sterility is not immediate. Complete expulsion of sperm stored in the reproductive tract beyond the interrupted vas deferens may take a week to several months. The time appears to depend in part on the frequency of ejaculation. Semen should be checked until two consecutive sperm counts are zero. During this period, another form of contraception must be used. The failure rate for vasectomy is estimated to be about 1 in 100 (Population Reports, 1975).

Restoration of fertility after a successful vasectomy does not always succeed. A review of several reports suggests that odds for success are about 50 percent, with somewhat higher rates following microsurgical reanastomosis. As with women, the risks of regret after sterilization appear to relate primarily to immaturity at the time of sterilization (Howard, 1982). Three factors that appear to be important in restoration of fertility after previous vasectomy are (1) the application of meticulous microsurgical techniques for reanastomosis, (2) the length of time after vasectomy, because chronic obstruction of the vas and possibly the development of sperm antibodies reduce progressively the capacity for spermatogenesis, and (3) the presence or absence of sperm granulomas.

Long-term semen storage collected before vasectomy remains an experimental procedure. The cost of storing frozen semen is high, the availability of facilities is limited, and the results remain uncertain (Beck, 1978).

Sperm antibodies can be identified rather often after vasectomy. Concern was raised over the possibility that the immune response might cause harmful systemic changes. Moreover, in some preliminary studies on previously vasectomized monkeys, atherosclerosis appeared to be increased. Carefully made observations on a very large number of men who had undergone vasectomy several years before have not identified an increase in cardiovascular disease, circulating immune complexes, or damage to blood vessels of the retina (Giovannucci and colleagues, 1992; Linnet and coworkers, 1982; Petitti, 1982; Walker and associates, 1981; Goldacre and colleagues, 1983). There also is no evidence of an increased incidence of testicular or prostatic cancer following vasectomy (Giovannucci and colleagues, 1992; Noticeboard, 1991).

Open-ended Vasectomy. A new variant of the classical vasectomy has been reported. The modification is to leave the testicular end of the vas deferens open and fulgurate approximately 1.5 cm of the abdominal end of the tube. The method is alleged to (1) decrease the frequency of congestive epididymitis without increasing the incidence of sperm granulomas, and (2) increase the success rate of subsequent reversal procedures (Errey and Edwards, 1986; Moss, 1985).

References

Alvarez-Sanchez F, Segal SJ, Brache V, Adejuwon CA, Leon P, Faundes A: Pituitary-ovarian function after tubal ligation. Fertil Steril 36:606, 1981

American College of Obstetricians and Gynecologists: Sterilization. Technical Bulletin no. 113, February 1988

Association for Voluntary Surgical Contraception News 27:1, 1989

Barclay DL, Hawks BL, Frueh DM, Power JD, Struble RH: Elective cesarean hysterectomy: A five year comparison with cesarean section. Am J Obstet Gynecol 124:900, 1976

Beck WW Jr: Artificial insemination and preservation of semen. Urol Clin N Am 5:593, 1978

Corson SL, Levinson CJ, Batzer FR, Otis C: Hormonal levels following sterilization and hysterectomy. J Reprod Med 26:363, 1981

DeStefano F, Greenspan JR, Dicker RC, Peterson HB, Strauss LT, Rubin GL: Complications of interval laparoscopic tubal sterilization. Obstet Gynecol 61:153, 1983

DeStefano F, Perlman JA, Peterson HB, Diamond EL: Long-term risk of menstrual disturbances after tubal sterilization. Am J Obstet Gynecol 152:835, 1985

Donnez J, Wauters M, Thomas K: Luteal function after tubal sterilization. Obstet Gynecol 57:65, 1981

El-Minawi MF, Masor N, Reda MS: Pelvic venous changes after tubal sterilization. J Reprod Med 28:641, 1983

Errey BB, Edwards IS: Open-ended vasectomy: An assessment. Fertil Steril 45:843, 1986

Giovannucci E, Tosteson TD, Speizer FE, Vessey MP, Colditz GA: A long-term study of mortality in men who have undergone vasectomy. N Engl J Med 326:1392, 1992

Goldacre JM, Holford TR, Vessey MP: Cardiovascular disease and vasectomy. N Engl J Med 308:805, 1983

Hargrove JT, Abraham GE: Endocrine profile of patients with post-tubal ligation syndrome. J Reprod Med 26:359, 1981

Hatcher RA, Stewart F, Trussel J, Kowal P, Guest F, Stewart GK, Cates W: Contraceptive Technology, 15th ed. New York, Irvington, 1990, pp 391, 403, 416

Howard G: Who asks for vasectomy reversal and why? BMJ 285:490, 1982

Husbands, ME Jr, Pritchard JA, Pritchard SA: Failure of tubal sterilization accompanying cesarean section. Am J Obstet Gynecol 107:966, 1970

Kasonde JM, Bonnar J: Effect of sterilization on menstrual blood loss. Br J Obstet Gynaecol 83:572, 1976

Kroener WF Jr: Surgical sterilization by fimbriectomy. Am J Obstet Gynecol 104:247, 1969

Ladehoff P, Lindholm P, Qvist K, Sorenson T: Gonadotropins and estrogens before and after laparoscopic sterilization. Acta Obstet Gynecol Scand 93 (suppl):77, 1980

Laros RK Jr, Work BA Jr: Female sterilization, III. Vaginal hysterectomy. Am J Obstet Gynecol 122:693, 1975

Linnet L, Moller NPH, Bernth-Perersen P, Ehlers N, Brandslund I, Svehag SE: No increase in arteriosclerotic retinopathy or activity in tests for circulating immune complexes 5 years after vasectomy. Fertil Steril 37:798, 1982

Lungren SS: A case of cesarean twice. Am J Obstet Dis Women Child 14:78, 1881

Metz KGP: Failures following fimbriectomy. Fertil Steril 28:66, 1977

Moss WM: Vasectomy failure after use of an open-ended technique. Fertil Steril 43:667, 1985

Noticeboard: Vasectomy and cancer. Lancet 338:1586, 1991

Peterson HB, DeStefano F, Greenspan JR, Ory HW: Mortality risk associated with tubal sterilization in United States hospitals. Am J Obstet Gynecol 143:125, 1982

Peterson HB, DeStefano F, Rubin GL, Greenspan JR, Lee NC, Ory HW: Deaths attributed to tubal sterilization in the United States, 1977 to 1981. Am J Obstet Gynecol 146:131, 1983

Petitti DB: Atherosclerotic disease in men 10 or more years after vasectomy. Presented at the annual meeting of the Association of Planned Parenthood Professionals, Baltimore, November 19, 1982

Population Reports: Vasectomy—What are the problems? Series D, No. 1, January 1975, p 41

Shy KK, Stergachis A, Grothaus LG, Wagner EH, Hecht J, Anderson G: Tubal sterilization and risk of subsequent hospital admission for menstrual disorders. Am J Obstet Gynecol 166:1698, 1992

Soderstrom RM: Sterilization failures and their causes. Am J Obstet Gynecol 152:395, 1985

Taylor TS: Editorial comment. Obstet Gynecol Surv 27:168, 1972

Vessey MP, Huggins G, Lawless M, Yeates D: Tubal sterilization: Findings in a large prospective study. Br J Obstet Gynaecol 90:203, 1983

Viddeleer AC, Lycklama À Nijeholt GAB: Lethal Fournier's gangrene following vasectomy. J Urol 147:1613, 1992

Walker AM, Hunter JR, Watkins RN, Jick H, Danford A, Alhadeff L, Rothman KF: Vasectomy and non-fatal myocardial infarction. Lancet 1:13, 1981

Wingo PA, Huezo CM, Rubin GL, Ory HW, Peterson HB: The mortality risk associated with hysterectomy. Am J Obstet Gynecol 152:803, 1985

World Health Organization Task Force on Female Sterilization: Minilaparotomy or laparoscopy for sterilization: A multicenter, multinational randomized study. Am J Obstet Gynecol 143:645, 1982

Zatuchni GI, Shelton JD, Goldsmith A, Sciarra JJ (eds): Female transcervical sterilization. In PARFR Series on Fertility Regulation. Philadelphia, Harper & Row, 1983

■ Index ■

Page numbers followed by t and f indicate tables and figures, respectively.

Juan I Posada
San Joaquin
General Hospital
1-23-1995